Access the BNF y...

The *British National Formulary* (BNF) and *BNF for Childre...* ... ... online via MedicinesComplete, ensuring healthcare professionals always have the latest prescribing advice.

You can be alerted to all the latest updates by signing up to the BNF eNewsletter at www.bnf.org/newsletter.

ONLINE

 MedicinesComplete

BNF on MedicinesComplete
Access BNF and *BNF for Children* on MedicinesComplete and receive the very latest drug information through monthly online updates.

 FormularyComplete

FormularyComplete Create, edit and manage your own local formulary content built upon the trusted prescribing advice of the BNF and *BNF for Children*.

BNF on Evidence Search
Search the BNF and *BNF for Children* alongside other authoritative clinical and non-clinical evidence and best practice at http://evidence.nhs.uk from NICE.

MOBILE

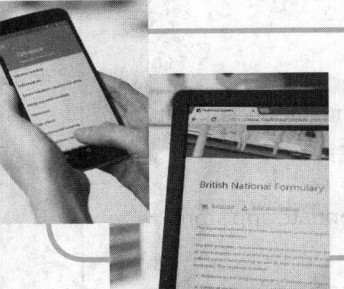

BNF app – Stay up to date anywhere with the BNF app available for iOS, Android and Blackberry.

BNF eBook – Available as an ePDF via a range of suppliers. See www.pharmpress.com/bnf.

BNF on MedicinesComplete – Now mobile responsive.

PRINT

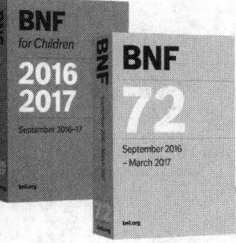

BNF subscription – if you prefer to access BNF in print, take advantage of our subscription option. We will send you the new BNF as soon as the book is published. One or two year packages (including or excluding BNFC) are available. Discounted pricing is also available on bulk sales.

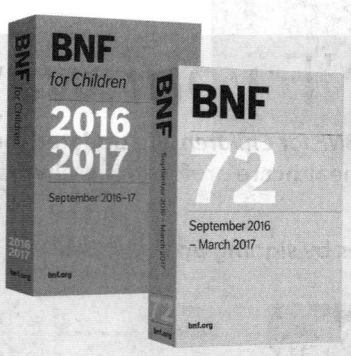
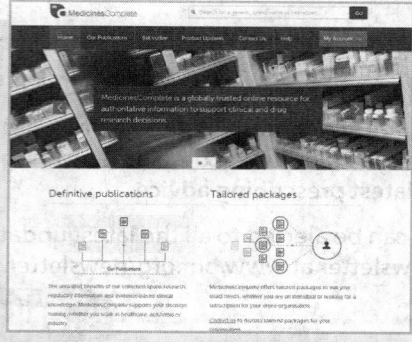

Eligible health professionals will now receive one print copy a year – the September issue – to supplement online access. If you are entitled to an NHS copy please refer to page ii for full details on distribution, call 01268 495 609 or email **bnf@binleys.com**.

How to purchase

Purchase direct from Pharmaceutical Press by visiting **www.pharmpress.com/bnf**

For enquiries about the BNF or BNFC in print, contact **direct@macmillan.co.uk**
Tel: **+44 (0) 1256 302 699**

For enquiries concerning MedicinesComplete, FormularyComplete, or bulk orders of the print edition, contact **pharmpress@rpharms.com**
Tel: **+44 (0) 20 7572 2266**

Download mobile apps by visiting your appropriate app store. Available for iOS, Android and Blackberry

For pricing information please visit the website at **www.pharmpress.com/bnf**

For international sales contact your local sales agent. Contact details at **www.pharmpress.com/agents**

Stay up to date – sign up to the BNF eNewsletter at **www.bnf.org/newsletter**

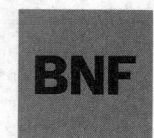
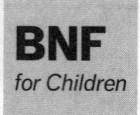

BNF
72

September 2016
– March 2017

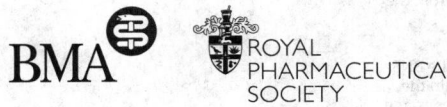

BMA

ROYAL
PHARMACEUTICAL
SOCIETY

Published jointly by
BMJ Group
Tavistock Square, London, WC1H 9JP, UK

and

Pharmaceutical Press
Pharmaceutical Press is the publishing division of the Royal Pharmaceutical Society.
66-68 East Smithfield, London E1W 1AW, UK

Copyright © BMJ Group and the Royal Pharmaceutical Society of Great Britain 2016.

ISBN: 978 0 85711 273 6

ISBN: 978 0 85711 303 0 (NHS edition)

ISBN: 978 0 85711 305 4 (ePDF)

Printed by GGP Media GmbH, Pößneck, Germany

Typeset by Data Standards Ltd, UK

Text designed by Peter Burgess

A catalogue record for this book is available from the British Library.

Requesting copies of BNF publications
Paper copies may be obtained through any bookseller or direct from:

Pharmaceutical Press
c/o Macmillan Distribution (MDL)
Brunel Rd
Houndmills
Basingstoke
Hampshire
RG21 6XS
Tel: +44 (0) 1256 302 699
Fax: +44 (0) 1256 812 521
direct@macmillan.co.uk

For all bulk orders of more than 20 copies:
Tel: +44 (0) 207 572 2266
pharmpress@rpharms.com

The BNF is available online through MedicinesComplete and as mobile apps; a PDA version is also available. In addition, BNF content can be integrated into a local formulary by using BNF on FormularyComplete; see www.bnf.org for details.

The BNF is also available on www.evidence.nhs.uk and eligible users can download smartphone apps from the relevant app stores.

Distribution of printed BNFs
In **England**, NICE purchases print editions of the BNF (September editions only) for distribution within the NHS. For details of who is eligible to receive a copy and further contact details, please refer to the NICE website: www.nice.org.uk/mpc/BritishNationalFormulary.jsp. If you are entitled to an NHS copy of BNF, please call (0) 1268 495 609 or email: bnf@binleys.com.

In **Scotland**, email: nss.psd-bnf@nhs.net

In **Wales**, contact NHS Wales Shared Services Partnership—Contractor Services:
Tel: 01792 607420

In **Northern Ireland**, email: ni.bnf@hscni.net

About BNF content
The BNF is designed as a digest for rapid reference and it may not always include all the information necessary for prescribing and dispensing. Also, less detail is given on areas such as obstetrics, malignant disease, and anaesthesia since it is expected that those undertaking treatment will have specialist knowledge and access to specialist literature. *BNF for Children* should be consulted for detailed information on the use of medicines in children. The BNF should be interpreted in the light of professional knowledge and supplemented as necessary by specialised publications and by reference to the product literature. Information is also available from Medicines Information Services.

Please refer to digital versions of BNF for the most up-to-date content. BNF is published in print but interim updates are issued and published in the digital versions of BNF. The publishers work to ensure that the information is as accurate and up-to-date as possible at the date of publication, but knowledge and best practice in this field change regularly. BNF's accuracy and currency cannot be guaranteed and neither the publishers nor the authors accept any responsibility for errors or omissions. While considerable efforts have been made to check the material in this publication, it should be treated as a guide only. Prescribers, pharmacists and other healthcare professionals are advised to check www.bnf.org for information about key updates and corrections.

Pharmaid
Numerous requests have been received from developing countries for BNFs. The Pharmaid scheme of the Commonwealth Pharmacists Association will dispatch old BNFs to certain Commonwealth countries. For more information on this scheme see www.commonwealthpharmacy.org/about/projects/pharmaid/. If you would like to donate your copy email: admin@commonwealthpharmacy.org

Preface

The BNF is a joint publication of the British Medical Association and the Royal Pharmaceutical Society. It is published under the authority of a Joint Formulary Committee which comprises representatives of the two professional bodies, the UK Health Departments, the Medicines and Healthcare products Regulatory Agency, and a national guideline producer. The Dental Advisory Group oversees the preparation of advice on the drug management of dental and oral conditions; the Group includes representatives of the British Dental Association and a representative from the UK Health Departments. The Nurse Prescribers' Advisory Group advises on the content relevant to nurses and includes representatives from different parts of the nursing community and from the UK Health Departments.

The BNF aims to provide prescribers, pharmacists, and other healthcare professionals with sound up-to-date information about the use of medicines.

The BNF includes key information on the selection, prescribing, dispensing and administration of medicines. Medicines generally prescribed in the UK are covered and those considered less suitable for prescribing are clearly identified. Little or no information is included on medicines promoted for purchase by the public.

Information on drugs is drawn from the manufacturers' product literature, medical and pharmaceutical literature, UK health departments, regulatory authorities, and professional bodies. Advice is constructed from clinical literature and reflects, as far as possible, an evaluation of the evidence from diverse sources. The BNF also takes account of authoritative national guidelines and emerging safety concerns. In addition, the editorial team receives advice on all therapeutic areas from expert clinicians; this ensures that the BNF's recommendations are relevant to practice.

The BNF is designed as a digest for rapid reference and it may not always include all the information necessary for prescribing and dispensing. Also, less detail is given on areas such as obstetrics, malignant disease, and anaesthesia since it is expected that those undertaking treatment will have specialist knowledge and access to specialist literature. *BNF for Children* should be consulted for detailed information on the use of medicines in children. The BNF should be interpreted in the light of professional knowledge and supplemented as necessary by specialised publications and by reference to the product literature. Information is also available from medicines information services, see Medicines Information Services (see inside front cover).

It is **important** to use the most recent BNF information for making clinical decisions. The print edition of the BNF is updated in March and September each year. Monthly updates are provided online via Medicines Complete and the NHS Evidence portal. The more important changes are listed under Changes; changes listed online are cumulative (from one print edition to the next), and can be printed off each month to show the main changes since the last print edition as an aide memoire for those using print copies.

The BNF Publications website (www.bnf.org) includes additional information of relevance to healthcare professionals. Other digital formats of the BNF—including versions for mobile devices and integration into local formularies—are also available.

BNF Publications welcomes comments from healthcare professionals. Comments and constructive criticism should be sent to:

British National Formulary,
Royal Pharmaceutical Society,
66–68 East Smithfield
London
E1W 1AW
editor@bnf.org

The contact email for manufacturers or pharmaceutical companies wishing to contact BNF Publications is manufacturerinfo@bnf.org

Contents

Acknowledgements

The Joint Formulary Committee is grateful to individuals and organisations that have provided advice and information to the BNF.

The principal contributors for this update were:

K.W. Ah-See, M.N. Badminton, A.K. Bahl, P.R.J. Barnes, D. Bilton, S.L. Bloom, M.F. Bultitude, I.F. Burgess, D.J. Burn, C.E. Dearden, D.W. Denning, P.N. Durrington, D.A.C. Elliman, P. Emery, M.D. Feher, B.G. Gazzard, A.M. Geretti, N.J.L. Gittoes, P.J. Goadsby, M. Gupta, T.L. Hawkins, B.G. Higgins, S.P. Higgins, S.H.D. Jackson, A. Jones, D.M. Keeling, J.R. Kirwan, P.G. Kopelman, T.H. Lee, A. Lekkas, D.N.J. Lockwood, A.M. Lovering, M.G. Lucas, L. Luzzatto, P.D. Mason, D.A. McArthur, K.E.L. McColl, L.M. Melvin, E. Miller, R.M. Mirakian, P. Morrison, S.M.S. Nasser, C. Nelson-Piercy, J.M. Neuberger, D.J. Nutt, L.P. Ormerod, R. Patel, W.J. Penny, A.B. Provan, M.M. Ramsay, A.S.C. Rice, D.J. Rowbotham, J.W. Sander, J.A.T. Sandoe, M. Schacter, S.E. Slater, J. Soar, S.C.E. Sporton, M.D. Stewart, S. Thomas, J.P. Thompson, A.D. Weeks, A. Wilcock, A.P.R. Wilson, M.M. Yaqoob.

Expert advice on the management of oral and dental conditions was kindly provided by M. Addy, P. Coulthard, A. Crighton, M.A.O. Lewis, J.G. Meechan, N.D. Robb, C. Scully, R.A. Seymour, R. Welbury, and J.M. Zakrzewska. S. Kaur provided valuable advice on dental prescribing policy.

Members of the British Association of Dermatologists' Therapy & Guidelines Subcommittee, D.A. Buckley, N. Chiang, M. Cork, K. Gibbon, R.Y.P. Hunasehally, G.A. Johnston, T.A. Leslie, E.C. Mallon, P.M. McHenry, J. Natkunarajah, C. Saunders, S. Ungureanu, S. Wakelin, F.S. Worsnop, A.G. Brain (Secretariat), and M.F. Mohd Mustapa (Secretariat) have provided valuable advice.

Members of the Advisory Committee on Malaria Prevention, R.H. Behrens, D. Bell, P.L. Chiodini, V. Field, F. Genasi, L. Goodyer, A. Green, J. Jones, G. Kassianos, D.G. Lalloo, D. Patel, H. Patel, M. Powell, D.V. Shingadia, N.O. Subair, C.J.M. Whitty, M. Blaze (Secretariat), and V. Smith (Secretariat) have provided valuable advice.

The UK Ophthalmic Pharmacy Group have also provided valuable advice.

The MHRA have provided valuable assistance.

Correspondents in the pharmaceutical industry have provided information on new products and commented on products in the BNF.

Numerous doctors, pharmacists, nurses, and others have sent comments and suggestions.

BNF interactions are provided by C.L. Preston, S.L. Jones, H.K. Sandhu, and S. Sutton.

The BNF has valuable access to the Martindale data banks by courtesy of A. Brayfield and staff.

Valuable technical assistance provided by J. Macdonald, H. Benson, R. Calle, J. Cater, D. Granger, N. Judd, M. Mebrate, K. Parsons, B. Stephenson, J. Stott and I. White.

S. Frau, P.D. Lee, J. Martin, L. Mistry, S. Sacranie, and A. Sparshatt provided considerable assistance during the production of this update of the BNF.

BNF Staff

BNF DIRECTOR
Karen Baxter
BSc, MSc, MRPharmS

HEAD OF CONTENT
Kate Towers
BPharm (AU), GCClinPharm

CONTENT MANAGERS
Kristina Fowlie
MPharm, CertPharmPract, MRPharmS
Heenaben Patel
MPharm, DipClinPharm, MRPharmS

QUALITY AND PROCESS MANAGER
Angela M.G. McFarlane
BSc, DipClinPharm

CLINICAL WRITERS
Naimah Callachand
MPharm

Thomas F. Corbett
BScPharm (IRL), MPharm (IRL)

Joyce Donnelly
MPharm, MRPharmS
Belén Granell Villén
BSc, DipClinPharm
Basma Hossin
MPharm, PhD
Maeve A.M. Lynn
MPharm, CertClinPharm
Claire McSherry
BPharm (NZ), PGCertClinPharm (NZ)
Kere Odumah
MPharm
Paridhi K. Prashar
MPharm, MRPharmS
Dominique Shakir
MPharm, MRPharmS, IP, PGDip
Jacob M. Warner
BPharm (AU)
Sharyn Young
BPharm (NZ), PGDipClinPharm (NZ)

CLINICAL ASSISTANTS
Elizabeth King

EDITORIAL ASSISTANTS
Jaya Venkitachalam
BSc, MRes

SENIOR BNF ADMINISTRATOR
Heidi Homar
BA

MANAGING DIRECTOR, PHARMACEUTICAL PRESS
Alina Lourie
B.Ed, MSc

SENIOR MEDICAL ADVISER
Derek G. Waller
BSc, MB, BS, DM, FRCP

Nurse Prescribers' Advisory Group 2015-2016

How BNF Publications are constructed

Overview

The BNF is an independent professional publication that addresses the day-to-day prescribing information needs of healthcare professionals. Use of this resource throughout the health service helps to ensure that medicines are used safely, effectively, and appropriately.

Hundreds of changes are made between print editions, and are published monthly in a number of digital formats. The most clinically significant updates are listed under Changes p. xix.

The BNF is unique in bringing together authoritative, independent guidance on best practice with clinically validated drug information. Validation of information follows a standardised process, reviewing emerging evidence, best-practice guidelines, and advice from a network of clinical experts. Where the evidence base is weak, further validation is undertaken through a process of peer review. The process and its governance are outlined in greater detail in the sections that follow.

Joint Formulary Committee

The Joint Formulary Committee (JFC) is responsible for the content of the BNF. The JFC includes pharmacy, medical, nursing and lay representatives; there are also representatives from the Medicines and Healthcare products Regulatory Agency (MHRA), the UK Health Departments, and a national guideline producer. The JFC decides on matters of policy and reviews amendments to the BNF in the light of new evidence and expert advice.

Dental Advisory Group

The Dental Advisory Group oversees the preparation of advice on the drug management of dental and oral conditions; the group includes representatives from the British Dental Association and a representative from the UK Health Departments.

Nurse Prescribers' Advisory Group

The Nurse Prescribers' Advisory Group oversees the list of drugs approved for inclusion in the Nurse Prescribers' Formulary; the group includes representatives from a range of nursing disciplines and stakeholder organisations.

Expert advisers

The BNF uses about 60 expert clinical advisers (including doctors, pharmacists, nurses, and dentists) throughout the UK to help with clinical content. The role of these expert advisers is to review existing text and to comment on amendments drafted by the clinical writers. These clinical experts help to ensure that the BNF remains reliable by:

- commenting on the relevance of the text in the context of best clinical practice in the UK;
- checking draft amendments for appropriate interpretation of any new evidence;
- providing expert opinion in areas of controversy or when reliable evidence is lacking;
- providing independent advice on drug interactions, prescribing in hepatic impairment, renal impairment, pregnancy, breast-feeding, children, the elderly, palliative care, and the emergency treatment of poisoning.

In addition to consulting with regular advisers, the BNF calls on other clinical specialists for specific developments when particular expertise is required.

The BNF works closely with a number of expert bodies that produce clinical guidelines. Drafts or pre-publication copies of guidelines are often received for comment and assimilation into the BNF.

Editorial team

BNF clinical writers have all worked as pharmacists or possess a pharmacy degree and a further, relevant post-graduate qualification, and have a sound understanding of how drugs are used in clinical practice. As a team, the clinical writers are responsible for editing, maintaining, and updating BNF content. They follow a systematic prioritisation process in response to updates to the evidence base in order to ensure the most clinically important topics are reviewed as quickly as possible. In parallel the team of clinical writers undertakes a process of rolling revalidation, aiming to review all of the content in the BNF over a 3- to 4-year period.

Amendments to the text are drafted when the clinical writers are satisfied that any new information is reliable and relevant. A set of standard criteria define when content is referred to expert advisers, the Joint Formulary Committee or other advisory groups, or submitted for peer review.

Clinical writers prepare the text for publication and undertake a number of validation checks on the knowledge at various stages of the production process.

Sources of BNF information

The BNF uses a variety of sources for its information; the main ones are shown below.

Summaries of product characteristics

The BNF reviews summaries of product characteristics (SPCs) of all new products as well as revised SPCs for existing products. The SPCs are the principal source of product information and are carefully processed. Such processing involves:

- verifying the approved names of all relevant ingredients including 'non-active' ingredients (the BNF is committed to using approved names and descriptions as laid down by the Human Medicine Regulations 2012);
- comparing the indications, cautions, contra-indications, and side-effects with similar existing drugs. Where these are different from the expected pattern, justification is sought for their inclusion or exclusion;
- seeking independent data on the use of drugs in pregnancy and breast-feeding;
- incorporating the information into the BNF using established criteria for the presentation and inclusion of the data;
- checking interpretation of the information by a second clinical writer before submitting to a content manager; changes relating to doses receive a further check;
- identifying potential clinical problems or omissions and seeking further information from manufacturers or from expert advisers;
- constructing, with the help of expert advisers, a comment on the role of the drug in the context of similar drugs.

Much of this processing is applicable to the following sources as well.

Literature

Clinical writers monitor core medical and pharmaceutical journals. Research papers and reviews relating to drug therapy are carefully processed. When a difference between the advice in the BNF and the paper is noted, the new information is assessed for reliability (using tools based on SIGN methodology) and relevance to UK clinical practice. If necessary, new text is drafted and discussed with expert advisers and the Joint Formulary Committee. The BNF enjoys a close working relationship with a number of national information providers.

In addition to the routine process, which is used to identify 'triggers' for changing the content, systematic literature searches are used to identify the best quality evidence available to inform an update. Clinical writers receive training in critical appraisal, literature evaluation, and search strategies.

Consensus guidelines

The advice in the BNF is checked against consensus guidelines produced by expert bodies. The quality of the guidelines is assessed using adapted versions of the AGREE II tool. A number of bodies make drafts or pre-publication copies of the guidelines available to the BNF; it is therefore possible to ensure that a consistent message is disseminated. The BNF routinely processes guidelines from the National Institute for Health and Care Excellence (NICE), the Scottish Medicines Consortium (SMC), and the Scottish Intercollegiate Guidelines Network (SIGN).

Reference sources

Textbooks and reference sources are used to provide background information for the review of existing text or for the construction of new text. The BNF team works closely with the editorial team that produces *Martindale: The Complete Drug Reference*. The BNF has access to *Martindale* information resources and each team keeps the other informed of significant developments and shifts in the trends of drug usage.

Peer review

Although every effort is made to identify the most robust data available, inevitably there are areas where the evidence base is weak or contradictory. While the BNF has the valuable support of expert advisers and the Joint Formulary Committee, the recommendations made may be subject to a further level of scrutiny through peer review to ensure they reflect best practice.

Content for peer review is posted on bnf.org and interested parties are notified via a number of channels, including the BNF e-newsletter.

Statutory information

The BNF routinely processes relevant information from various Government bodies including Statutory Instruments and regulations affecting the Prescriptions only Medicines Order. Official compendia such as the British Pharmacopoeia and its addenda are processed routinely to ensure that the BNF complies with the relevant sections of the Human Medicines Regulations 2012.

The BNF maintains close links with the Home Office (in relation to controlled drug regulations) and the Medicines and Healthcare products Regulatory Agency (including the British Pharmacopoeia Commission). Safety warnings issued by the Commission on Human Medicines (CHM) and guidelines on drug are issued by the UK health departments are processed as a matter of routine.

Relevant professional statements issued by the Royal Pharmaceutical Society are included in the BNF as are guidelines from bodies such as the Royal College of General Practitioners.

Medicines and devices

NHS Prescription Services (from the NHS Business Services Authority) provides non-clinical, categorical information (including prices) on the medicines and devices included in the BNF.

Comments from readers

Readers of the BNF are invited to send in comments. Numerous letters and emails are received by the BNF team. Such feedback helps to ensure that the BNF provides practical and clinically relevant information. Many changes in the presentation and scope of the BNF have resulted from comments sent in by users.

Comments from industry

Close scrutiny of BNF by the manufacturers provides an additional check and allows them an opportunity to raise issues about BNF's presentation of the role of various drugs; this is yet another check on the balance of BNF's advice. All comments are looked at with care and, where necessary, additional information and expert advice are sought.

Market research

Market research is conducted at regular intervals to gather feedback on specific areas of development.

Assessing the evidence

From January 2016, recommendations made in BNF publications have been evidence graded to reflect the strength of the recommendation. The addition of evidence grading is to support clinical decision making based on the best available evidence.

The BNF aims to revalidate all content over a rolling 3- to 4-year period and evidence grading will be applied to recommendations as content goes through the revalidation process. Therefore, initially, only a small number of recommendations will have been graded.

Grading system

The BNF has adopted a five level grading system from A to E, based on the former SIGN grading system. This grade is displayed next to the recommendation within the text.

Evidence used to make a recommendation is assessed for validity using standardised methodology tools based on AGREE II and assigned a level of evidence. The recommendation is then given a grade that is extrapolated from the level of evidence, and an assessment of the body of evidence and its applicability.

Evidence assigned a level 1- or 2- score has an unacceptable level of bias or confounding and is not used to form recommendations.

Levels of evidence

- **Level 1++**
  High quality meta-analyses, systematic reviews of randomised controlled trials (RCTs), or RCTs with a very low risk of bias.

- **Level 1+**
  Well-conducted meta-analyses, systematic reviews, or RCTs with a low risk of bias.

- **Level 1-**
  Meta-analyses, systematic reviews, or RCTs with a high risk of bias.

- **Level 2++**
  High quality systematic reviews of case control or cohort studies; or high quality case control or cohort studies with a very low risk of confounding or bias and a high probability that the relationship is causal.

- **Level 2+**
  Well-conducted case control or cohort studies with a low risk of confounding or bias and a moderate probability that the relationship is causal.

- **Level 2-**
  Case control or cohort studies with a high risk of confounding or bias and a significant risk that the relationship is not causal.

- **Level 3**
  Non-analytic studies, e.g. case reports, case series.

- **Level 4**
  Expert advice or clinical experience from respected authorities.

Grades of recommendation

- **Grade A: High strength**
  NICE-accredited guidelines; or guidelines that pass AGREE II assessment; or at least one meta-analysis, systematic review, or RCT rated as 1++, and directly applicable to the target population; or a body of evidence consisting principally of studies rated as 1+, directly applicable to the target population, and demonstrating overall consistency of results.

- **Grade B: Moderate strength**
  A body of evidence including studies rated as 2++, directly applicable to the target population, and demonstrating overall consistency of results; or extrapolated evidence from studies rated as 1++ or 1+.

- **Grade C: Low strength**
  A body of evidence including studies rated as 2+, directly applicable to the target population and demonstrating overall consistency of results; or extrapolated evidence from studies rated as 2++.

- **Grade D: Very low strength**
  Evidence level 3; or extrapolated evidence from studies rated as 2+; or tertiary reference source created by a transparent, defined methodology, where the basis for recommendation is clear.

- **Grade E: Practice point**
  Evidence level 4.

How to use BNF Publications in print

How to use the BNF

This edition of the BNF continues to display the fundamental change to the structure of the content that was first shown in BNF 70. The changes were made to bring consistency and clarity to BNF content, and to the way that the content is arranged within print and digital products, increasing the ease with which information can be found.

For reference, the most notable changes to the structure of the content include:

- Drug monographs – where possible, all information that relates to a single drug is contained within its drug monograph, moving information previously contained in the prescribing notes. Drug monographs have also changed structurally: additional sections have been added, ensuring greater regularity around where information is located within the publication.
- Drug class monographs – where substantial amounts of information are common to all drugs within a drug class (e.g. macrolides p. 486), a drug class monograph has been created to contain the common information.
- Medicinal forms – categorical information about marketed medicines, such as price and pack size, continues to be sourced directly from the Dictionary of Medicines and Devices provided by the NHS Business Services Authority. However, clinical information curated by the BNF team has been clearly separated from the categorical pricing and pack size information and is included in the relevant section of the drug monograph.
- Section numbering – the BNF section numbering has been removed. This section numbering tied the content to a rigid structure and enforced the retention of defunct classifications, such as mercurial diuretics, and hindered the relocation of drugs where therapeutic use had altered. It also caused constraints between the BNF and BNF *for Children*, where drugs had different therapeutic uses in children.
- Appendix 4 – the content has been moved to individual drug monographs. The introductory notes have been replaced with a new guidance section, Guidance on intravenous infusions p. 15.

Introduction

In order to achieve the safe, effective, and appropriate use of medicines, healthcare professionals must be able to use the BNF effectively, and keep up to date with significant changes in the BNF that are relevant to their clinical practice. This *How to Use the BNF* is key in reinforcing the details of the new structure of the BNF to all healthcare professionals involved with prescribing, monitoring, supplying, and administering medicines, as well as supporting the learning of students training to join these professions.

Structure of the BNF

This BNF edition continues to broadly follows the high-level structure of earlier editions of the BNF (i.e. those published before BNF 70):

Front matter, comprising information on how to use the BNF, the significant content changes in each edition, and guidance on various prescribing matters (e.g. prescription writing, the use of intravenous drugs, particular considerations for special patient populations).

Chapters, containing drug monographs describing the uses, doses, safety issues and other considerations involved in the use of drugs; drug class monographs; and treatment summaries, covering guidance on the selection of drugs. Monographs and treatment summaries are divided into chapters based on specific aspects of medical care, such as Chapter 5, Infections, or Chapter 16, Emergency treatment

of poisoning; or drug use related to a particular system of the body, such as Chapter 2, Cardiovascular.

Within each chapter, content is organised alphabetically by therapeutic use (e.g. Airways disease, obstructive), with the treatment summaries first, (e.g. asthma), followed by the monographs of the drugs used to manage the conditions discussed in the treatment summary. Within each therapeutic use, the drugs are organised alphabetically by classification (e.g. Antimuscarinics, Beta$_2$-agonist bronchodilators) and then alphabetically within each classification (e.g. Aclidinium bromide, Glycopyrronium bromide, Ipratropium bromide).

Appendices, covering interactions, borderline substances, cautionary and advisory labels, and woundcare.

Back matter, covering the lists of medicines approved by the NHS for Dental and Nurse Practitioner prescribing, proprietary and specials manufacturers' contact details, and the index. Yellow cards are also included, to facilitate the reporting of adverse events, as well as quick reference guides for life support and key drug doses in medical emergencies, for ease of access.

Navigating the BNF

The contents page provides the high-level layout of information within the BNF; and in addition, each chapter begins with a small contents section, describing the therapeutic uses covered within that chapter. Once in a chapter, location is guided by the side of the page showing the chapter number (the *thumbnail*), alongside the chapter title. The top of the page includes the therapeutic use (the *running head*) alongside the page number.

Once on a page, visual cues aid navigation: treatment summary information is in black type, with therapeutic use titles similarly styled in black, whereas the use of colour indicates drug-related information, including drug classification titles, drug class monographs, and drug monographs.

Although navigation is possible by browsing, primarily access to the information is via the index, which covers the titles of drug class monographs, drug monographs, and treatment summaries. The index also includes the names of branded medicines and other topics of relevance, such as abbreviations, guidance sections, tables, and images.

Content types

Treatment summaries

Treatment summaries are of three main types;

- an overview of delivering a drug to a particular body system (e.g. Skin conditions, management p. 1063)
- a comparison between a group or groups of drugs (e.g. beta-adrenoceptor blockers (systemic) p. 133)
- an overview of the drug management or prophylaxis of common conditions intended to facilitate rapid appraisal of options (e.g. Hypertension p. 127, or Malaria, prophylaxis p. 552).

In order to select safe and effective medicines for individual patients, information in the treatment summaries must be used in conjunction with other prescribing details about the drugs and knowledge of the patient's medical and drug history.

Monographs

Overview

In earlier editions (i.e. before BNF 70), a systemically administered drug with indications for use in different body systems was split across the chapters relating to those body systems. So, for example, codeine phosphate p. 413 was found in chapter 1, for its antimotility effects and chapter 4 for its analgesic effects. However, the monograph in chapter

1 contained only the dose and some selected safety precautions.

Now, all of the information for the systemic use of a drug is contained within one monograph, so codeine phosphate p. 413 is now included in chapter 4. This carries the advantage of providing all of the information in one place, so the user does not need to flick back and forth across several pages to find all of the relevant information for that drug. Cross references are included in chapter 1, where the management of diarrhoea is discussed, to the drug monograph to assist navigation.

Where drugs have systemic and local uses, for example, chloramphenicol, and the considerations around drug use are markedly different according to the route of administration, the monograph is split, as with earlier editions, into the relevant chapters.

This means that the majority of drugs are still placed in the same chapters and sections as earlier editions, and although there may be some variation in order, all of the relevant information will be easier to locate.

One of the most significant changes to the monograph structure is the increased granularity, with a move from around 9 sections to over 20 sections; sections are only included when relevant information has been identified. The following information describes these sections and their uses in more detail.

Nomenclature

Monograph titles follow the convention of recommended international non-proprietary names (rINNs), or, in the absence of a rINN, British Approved Names. Relevant synonyms are included below the title and, in some instances a brief description of the drug action is included. Over future editions these drug action statements will be rolled out for all drugs.

In some monographs, immediately below the nomenclature or drug action, there are a number of cross references or flags used to signpost the user to any additional information they need to consider about a drug. This is most common for drugs formulated in combinations, where users will be signposted to the monographs for the individual ingredients (e.g. senna with ispaghula husk p. 55) or for drugs that are related to a drug class monograph (see Drug class monographs, below).

Indication and dose

User feedback has highlighted that one of the main uses of the BNF is identifying indications and doses of drugs. Therefore, indication and dose information has been promoted to the top of the monograph and highlighted by a coloured panel to aid quick reference.

The indication and dose section is more highly structured than in earlier editions, giving greater clarity around which doses should be used for which indications and by which route. In addition, if the dose varies with a specific preparation or formulation, that dosing information has been moved out of the preparations section and in to the indication and dose panel, under a heading of the preparation name.

Doses are either expressed in terms of a definite frequency (e.g. 1 g 4 times daily) or in the total daily dose format (e.g. 6 g daily in 3 divided doses); the total daily dose should be divided into individual doses (in the second example, the patient should receive 2 g 3 times daily).

Doses for specific patient groups (e.g. the elderly) may be included if they are different to the standard dose. Doses for children can be identified by the relevant age range and may vary according to their age or body-weight.

In earlier editions of the BNF, age ranges and weight ranges overlapped. For clarity and to aid selection of the correct dose, wherever possible these age and weight ranges now do not overlap. When interpreting age ranges it is important to understand that a patient is considered to be 64 up until the point of their 65th birthday, meaning that an age range of adult 18 to 64 is applicable to a patient from the day of their 18th birthday until the day before their 65th birthday. All age ranges should be interpreted in this way. Similarly, when interpreting weight ranges, it should be understood that a weight of up to 30 kg is applicable to a patient up to, but not including, the point that they tip the scales at 30 kg and a weight range of 35 to 59 kg is applicable to a patient as soon as they tip the scales at 35 kg right up until, but not including, the point that they tip the scales at 60 kg. All weight ranges should be interpreted in this way.

In all circumstances, it is important to consider the patient in question and their physical condition, and select the dose most appropriate for the individual.

Other information relevant to Indication and dose

The dose panel also contains, where known, an indication of **pharmacokinetic considerations** that may affect the choice of dose, and **dose equivalence** information, which may aid the selection of dose when switching between drugs or preparations.

The BNF includes **unlicensed use** of medicines when the clinical need cannot be met by licensed medicines; such use should be supported by appropriate evidence and experience. When the BNF recommends an unlicensed medicine or the 'off-label' use of a licensed medicine, this is shown below the indication and dose panel in the unlicensed use section.

Minimising harm and drug safety

The drug chosen to treat a particular condition should minimise the patient's susceptibility to adverse effects and, where co-morbidities exist, have minimal detrimental effects on the patient's other diseases. To achieve this, the *Contra-indications*, *Cautions* and *Side-effects* of the relevant drug should be reviewed.

The information under Cautions can be used to assess the risks of using a drug in a patient who has co-morbidities that are also included in the Cautions for that drug—if a safer alternative cannot be found, the drug may be prescribed while monitoring the patient for adverse-effects or deterioration in the co-morbidity. Contra-indications are far more restrictive than Cautions and mean that the drug should be avoided in a patient with a condition that is contra-indicated.

The impact that potential side-effects may have on a patient's quality of life should also be assessed. For instance, in a patient who has difficulty sleeping, it may be preferable to avoid a drug that frequently causes insomnia.

Clinically relevant *Side-effects* for drugs are included in the monographs or class monographs. Side-effects are listed in order of frequency, where known, and arranged alphabetically. The frequency of side-effects follows the regulatory standard:

- Very common — occurs more frequently than 1 in 10 administrations of a drug
- Common — occurs between 1 in 10 and 1 in 100 administrations of a drug
- Uncommon — between 1 in 100 and 1 in 1,000 administrations of a drug
- Rare — between 1 in 1,000 and 1 in 10,000 administrations of a drug
- Very rare — occurs less than 1 in 10,000 administrations of a drug
- Frequency not known

An exhaustive list of side-effects is not included, particularly for drugs that are used by specialists (e.g. cytotoxic drugs and drugs used in anaesthesia). The BNF also omits effects that are likely to have little clinical consequence (e.g. transient increase in liver enzymes).

Recognising that hypersensitivity reactions can occur with virtually all medicines, this effect is generally not listed, unless the drug carries an increased risk of such reactions, when the information is included under *Allergy and cross sensitivity*.

Typical layout of a monograph and associated medicinal forms

❶ Class Monographs and drug monographs
In most cases, all information that relates to an individual drug is contained in its drug monograph and there is no symbol. Class monographs have been created where substantial amounts of information are common to all drugs within a drug class, these are indicated by a flag symbol in a circle:

Drug monographs with a corresponding class monograph are indicated by a tab with a flag symbol:

The page number of the corresponding class monograph is indicated within the tab. For further information, see How to use BNF Publications

❷ Drug classifications
Used to inform users of the class of a drug and to assist in finding other drugs of the same class. May be based on pharmacological class (e.g. opioids) but can also be associated with the use of the drug (e.g. cough suppressants)

❸ Review date
The date of last review of the content

❹ Specific preparation name
If the dose varies with a specific preparation or formulation it appears under a heading of the preparation name

❺ Evidence grading
Evidence grading to reflect the strengths of recommendations will be applied as content goes through the revalidation process. A five level evidence grading system based on the former SIGN grading system has been adopted. The grades Ⓐ Ⓑ Ⓒ Ⓓ Ⓔ are displayed next to the recommendations within the text, and are preceded by the symbol: EvGr

For further information, see How BNF Publications are constructed

---

Class monograph ❶

CLASSIFICATION ❷
F 1234

Drug monograph ❶
❸ 1.6.2016

(Synonym) another name by which a drug may be known
- **DRUG ACTION** how a drug exerts its effect in the body

- **INDICATIONS AND DOSE**
Indications are the clinical reasons a drug is used. The dose of a drug will often depend on the indications
Indication
▸ ROUTE
▸ Age groups: [Child/Adult/Elderly]
  Dose and frequency of administration (max. dose)
SPECIFIC PREPARATION NAME ❹
Indication
▸ ROUTE
▸ Age groups: [Child/Adult/Elderly]
  Dose and frequency of administration (max. dose)
DOSE EQUIVALENCE AND CONVERSION information around the bioequivalence between formulations of the same drug, or equivalent doses of drugs that are members of the same class
PHARMACOKINETICS how the body affects a drug (absorption, distribution, metabolism, and excretion)
POTENCY a measure of drug activity expressed in terms of the concentration required to produce an effect of given intensity
DOSES AT EXTREMES OF BODY-WEIGHT dosing information for patients who are overweight or underweight

- **UNLICENSED USE** describes the use of medicines outside the terms of their UK licence (off-label use), or use of medicines that have no licence for use in the UK

> **IMPORTANT SAFETY INFORMATION**
> Information produced and disseminated by drug regulators often highlights serious risks associated with the use of a drug, and may include advice that is mandatory

- **CONTRA-INDICATIONS** circumstances when a drug should be avoided
- **CAUTIONS** details of precautions required
- **INTERACTIONS** when one drug changes the effects of another drug; the mechanisms underlying drug interactions are explained in Appendix 1
- **SIDE-EFFECTS** listed in order of frequency, where known, and arranged alphabetically
- **ALLERGY AND CROSS-SENSITIVITY** for drugs that carry an increased risk of hypersensitivity reactions
- **CONCEPTION AND CONTRACEPTION** potential for a drug to have harmful effects on an unborn child when prescribing for a woman of childbearing age or for a man trying to father a child; information on the effect of drugs on the efficacy of latex condoms or diaphragms
- **PREGNANCY** advice on the use of a drug during pregnancy
- **BREAST FEEDING** EvGr advice on the use of a drug during breast feeding Ⓐ ❺

- HEPATIC IMPAIRMENT advice on the use of a drug in hepatic impairment
- RENAL IMPAIRMENT advice on the use of a drug in renal impairment
- PRE-TREATMENT SCREENING covers one off tests required to assess the suitability of a patient for a particular drug
- MONITORING REQUIREMENTS specifies any special monitoring requirements, including information on monitoring the plasma concentration of drugs with a narrow therapeutic index
- EFFECTS ON LABORATORY TESTS for drugs that can interfere with the accuracy of seemingly unrelated laboratory tests
- TREATMENT CESSATION specifies whether further monitoring or precautions are advised when the drug is withdrawn
- DIRECTIONS FOR ADMINISTRATION practical information on the preparation of intravenous drug infusions; general advice relevant to other routes of administration
- PRESCRIBING AND DISPENSING INFORMATION practical information around how a drug can be prescribed and dispensed including details of when brand prescribing is necessary
- HANDLING AND STORAGE includes information on drugs that can cause adverse effects to those who handle them before they are taken by, or administered to, a patient; advice on storage conditions
- PARENT AND CARER ADVICE for drugs with a special need for counselling
- PROFESSION SPECIFIC INFORMATION provides details of the restrictions certain professions such as dental practitioners or nurse prescribers need to be aware of when prescribing on the NHS
- NATIONAL FUNDING/ACCESS DECISIONS details of NICE Technology Appraisals and SMC advice
- LESS SUITABLE FOR PRESCRIBING preparations that are considered by the Joint Formulary Committee to be less suitable for prescribing
- EXCEPTION TO LEGAL CATEGORY advice and information on drugs which may be sold without a prescription under specific conditions

---

- MEDICINAL FORMS

Form
CAUTIONARY AND ADVISORY LABELS if applicable
EXCIPIENTS clinically important but not comprehensive [consult manufacturer information for full details]
ELECTROLYTES if clinically significant quantities occur
▶ Preparation name (Manufacturer/Non-proprietary)
  Drug name and strength pack sizes [PoM] ⑥ Prices

Combinations available this indicates a combination preparation is available and a cross reference page number is provided to locate this preparation

⑥ Legal categories

[PoM] This symbol has been placed against those preparations that are available only on a prescription issued by an appropriate practitioner. For more detailed information see *Medicines, Ethics and Practice*, London, Pharmaceutical Press (always consult latest edition)

[CD1] [CD2] [CD3] [CD4-1] [CD4-2] These symbols indicate that the preparations are subject to the prescription requirements of the Misuse of Drugs Act

For regulations governing prescriptions for such preparations, see Controlled Drugs and Drug Dependence

Not all monographs include all possible sections; sections are only included when relevant information has been identified

The *Important safety advice* section in the BNF, delineated by a coloured outline box, highlights important safety concerns, often those raised by regulatory authorities or guideline producers. Safety warnings issued by the Commission on Human Medicines (CHM) or Medicines and Healthcare products Regulatory Agency (MHRA) are found here.

Drug selection should aim to minimise drug interactions. If it is necessary to prescribe a potentially serious combination of drugs, patients should be monitored appropriately. The mechanisms underlying drug interactions are explained in Appendix 1, followed by details of drug interactions.

Use of drugs in specific patient populations

Drug selection should aim to minimise the potential for drug accumulation, adverse drug reactions, and exacerbation of pre-existing hepatic or renal disease. If it is necessary to prescribe drugs whose effect is altered by hepatic or renal disease, appropriate drug dose adjustments should be made, and patients should be monitored adequately. The general principles for prescribing are outlined under Prescribing in hepatic impairment p. 18, and Prescribing in renal impairment p. 18. Information about drugs that should be avoided or used with caution in hepatic disease or renal impairment can be found in drug monographs under *Hepatic impairment* and *Renal impairment* (e.g. fluconazole p. 540).

Similarly, drug selection should aim to minimise harm to the fetus, nursing infant, and mother. The infant should be monitored for potential side-effects of drugs used by the *mother during pregnancy or breast-feeding*. The general principles for prescribing are outlined under Prescribing in pregnancy p. 20 and Prescribing in breast-feeding p. 20. The Treatment Summaries provide guidance on the drug treatment of common conditions that can occur during pregnancy and breast-feeding (e.g. Asthma p. 219). Information about the use of specific drugs during pregnancy and breast-feeding can be found in their drug monographs under *Pregnancy*, and *Breast-feeding* (e.g. fluconazole p. 540).

A section, *Conception and contraception*, containing information around considerations for females of childbearing potential or men who might father a child (e.g. isotretinoin p. 1114) has been included.

Administration and monitoring

When selecting the most appropriate drug, it may be necessary to screen the patient for certain genetic markers or metabolic states. This information is included within a section called *Pre-treatment screening* (e.g. abacavir p. 587). This section covers one-off tests required to assess the suitability of a patient for a particular drug.

Once the drug has been selected, it needs to be given in the most appropriate manner. A *Directions for administration* section contains the information about intravenous administration previously located in Appendix 4. This provides practical information on the preparation of intravenous drug infusions, including compatibility of drugs with standard intravenous infusion fluids, method of dilution or reconstitution, and administration rates. In addition, general advice relevant to other routes of administration is provided within this section (e.g. fentanyl p. 416).

After selecting and administering the most appropriate drug by the most appropriate route, patients should be monitored to ensure they are achieving the expected benefits from drug treatment without any unwanted side-effects. The *Monitoring* section specifies any special monitoring requirements, including information on monitoring the plasma concentration of drugs with a narrow therapeutic index (e.g. theophylline p. 250). Monitoring may, in certain cases, be affected by the impact of a drug on laboratory tests (e.g. hydroxocobalamin p. 887), and this information is included in *Effects on laboratory tests*.

In some cases, when a drug is withdrawn, further monitoring or precautions may be advised (e.g. clonidine hydrochloride p. 131): these are covered under *Treatment cessation*.

Choice and supply

The prescriber and the patient should agree on the health outcomes that the patient desires and on the strategy for achieving them (see *Taking Medicines to Best Effect*). Taking the time to explain to the patient (and carers) the rationale and the potential adverse effects of treatment may improve adherence. For some medicines there is a special need for counselling (e.g. appropriate posture during administration of doxycycline p. 513); this is shown in *Patient and carer advice*.

Other information contained in the latter half of the monograph also helps prescribers and those dispensing medicines choose medicinal forms (by indicating information such as flavour or when branded products may not be interchangeable (e.g. diltiazem hydrochloride p. 143), assess the suitability of a drug for prescribing, understand the NHS funding status for a drug (e.g. sildenafil p. 736), or assess when a patient may be able to purchase a drug without prescription (e.g. loperamide hydrochloride p. 59).

Medicinal forms

In the BNF, preparations follow immediately after the monograph for the drug that is their main ingredient.

In earlier editions, when a particular preparation had safety information, dose advice or other clinical information specific to the product, it was contained within the preparations section. This information has been moved to the relevant section in the main body of the monograph under a heading of the name of the specific medicinal form (e.g. peppermint oil p. 42).

The medicinal forms (formerly preparations) section provides information on the type of formulation (e.g. tablet), the amount of active drug in a solid dosage form, and the concentration of active drug in a liquid dosage form. The legal status is shown for prescription-only medicines and controlled drugs, as well as pharmacy medicines and medicines on the general sales list. Practitioners are reminded, by a statement under the heading of "Medicinal Forms" that not all products containing a specific drug ingredient may be similarly licensed. To be clear on the precise licensing status of specific medicinal forms, practitioners should check the product literature for the particular product being prescribed or dispensed.

Details of all medicinal forms available on the dm+d for each drug in BNF Publications appears online on MedicinesComplete. In print editions, due to space constraints, only certain branded products are included in detail. Where medicinal forms are listed they should not be inferred as equivalent to the other brands listed under the same form heading. For example, all the products listed under a heading of "Modified release capsule" will be available as modified release capsules, however, the brands listed under that form heading may have different release profiles, the available strengths may vary and/or the products may have different licensing information. As with earlier editions of the BNF, practitioners must ensure that the particular product being prescribed or dispensed is appropriate.

As medicinal forms are derived from dm+d data, some drugs may appear under names derived from that data; this may vary slightly from those in previous BNF versions, e.g. sodium acid phosphate, is now sodium dihydrogen phosphate anhydrous.

Patients should be prescribed a preparation that complements their daily routine, and that provides the right dose of drug for the right indication and route of administration. When dispensing liquid preparations, a sugar-free preparation should always be used in preference to one containing sugar. Patients receiving medicines containing cariogenic sugars should be advised of appropriate dental hygiene measures to prevent caries.

In earlier editions, the BNF only included excipients and electrolyte information for proprietary medicines. This information is now covered at the level of the dose form (e.g. tablet). It is not possible to keep abreast of all of the generic products available on the UK market, and so this information serves as a reminder to the healthcare professional that, if the presence of a particular excipient is of concern, they should check the product literature for the particular product being prescribed or dispensed.

Cautionary and advisory labels that pharmacists are recommended to add when dispensing are included in the medicinal forms section. Details of these labels can be found in Appendix 3, Guidance for cautionary and advisory labels p. 1365. As these labels have now been applied at the level of the dose form, a full list of medicinal products with their relevant labels would be extensive. This list has therefore been removed, but the information is retained within the monograph.

In the case of compound preparations, the prescribing information for all constituents should be taken into account.

Prices in the BNF
Basic NHS **net prices** are given in the BNF to provide an indication of relative cost. Where there is a choice of suitable preparations for a particular disease or condition the relative cost may be used in making a selection. Cost-effective prescribing must, however, take into account other factors (such as dose frequency and duration of treatment) that affect the total cost. The use of more expensive drugs is justified if it will result in better treatment of the patient, or a reduction of the length of an illness, or the time spent in hospital.

Prices are regularly updated using the Drug Tariff and proprietary price information published by the NHS dictionary of medicines and devices (dm+d, www.dmd.nhs.uk). The weekly updated dm+d data (including prices) can be accessed using the dm+d browser of the NHS Business Services Authority (https://apps.nhsbsa.nhs.uk/DMDBrowser/DMDBrowser.do). Prices have been calculated from the net cost used in pricing NHS prescriptions and generally reflect whole dispensing packs. Prices for extemporaneously prepared preparations are not provided in the BNF as prices vary between different manufacturers. In Appendix 4, prices stated are per dressing or bandage.

BNF prices are not suitable for quoting to patients seeking private prescriptions or contemplating over-the-counter purchases because they do not take into account VAT, professional fees, and other overheads.

A fuller explanation of costs to the NHS may be obtained from the Drug Tariff. Separate drug tariffs are applicable to England and Wales (www.ppa.org.uk/ppa/edt_intro.htm), Scotland (www.isdscotland.org/Health-Topics/Prescribing-and-Medicines/Scottish-Drug-Tariff/), and Northern Ireland (www.hscbusiness.hscni.net/services/2034.htm); prices in the different tariffs may vary.

Drug class monographs
In earlier editions of the BNF, information relating to a class of drugs sharing the same properties (e.g. tetracyclines p. 513), was contained within the prescribing notes. In the updated structure, drug class monographs have been created to contain the common information; this ensures such information is easier to find, and has a more regularised structure.

For consistency and ease of use, the class monograph follows the same structure as a drug monograph. Class monographs are indicated by the presence of a flag ⊖ (e.g. beta-adrenoceptor blockers (systemic) p. 133). If a drug monograph has a corresponding class monograph, that needs to be considered in tandem, in order to understand the full information about a drug, the monograph is also indicated by a flag ⟦1234⟧ (e.g. metoprolol tartrate p. 140). Within this flag, the page number of the drug class

monograph is provided (e.g. 1234), to help navigate the user to this information. This is particularly useful where occasionally, due to differences in therapeutic use, the drug monograph may not directly follow the drug class monograph (e.g. sotalol hydrochloride p. 97).

Evidence grading
The BNF has adopted a five level evidence grading system (see How BNF Publications are constructed p. ix). Recommendations that are evidence graded can be identified by a symbol appearing immediately before the recommendation. The evidence grade is displayed at the end of the recommendation.

Other content
Nutrition
Appendix 2, Borderline substances p. 1334, includes tables of ACBS-approved enteral feeds and nutritional supplements based on their energy and protein content. There are separate tables for specialised formulae for specific clinical conditions. Classified sections on foods for special diets and nutritional supplements for metabolic diseases are also included.

Wound dressings
A table on wound dressings in Appendix 4, Wound management products and elasticated garments p. 1368, allows an appropriate dressing to be selected based on the appearance and condition of the wound. Further information about the dressing can be found by following the cross-reference to the relevant classified section in the Appendix.

Advanced wound contact dressings have been classified in order of increasing absorbency.

Other useful information
Finding significant changes in the BNF
- *Changes*, provides a list of significant changes, dose changes, classification changes, new names, and new preparations that have been incorporated into the BNF, as well as a list of preparations that have been discontinued and removed from the BNF. Changes listed online are cumulative (from one print edition to the next), and can be printed off each month to show the main changes since the last print edition as an aide memoire for those using print copies. So many changes are made for each update of the BNF, that not all of them can be accommodated in the Changes section. We encourage healthcare professionals to regularly review the prescribing information on drugs that they encounter frequently;
- *Changes to the Dental Practitioners' Formulary*, are located at the end of the Dental List;
- *E-newsletter*, the BNF & BNFC e-newsletter service is available free of charge. It alerts healthcare professionals to details of significant changes in the clinical content of these publications and to the way that this information is delivered. Newsletters also review clinical case studies, provide tips on using these publications effectively, and highlight forthcoming changes to the publications. To sign up for e-newsletters go to www.bnf.org.
- An e-learning programme developed in collaboration with the Centre for Pharmacy Postgraduate Education (CPPE), enables pharmacists to identify and assess how significant changes in the BNF affect their clinical practice. The module can be found at www.cppe.ac.uk.

Using other sources for medicines information
The BNF is designed as a digest for rapid reference. Less detail is given on areas such as obstetrics, malignant disease, and anaesthesia since it is expected that those undertaking treatment will have specialist knowledge and access to specialist literature. *BNF for Children* should be consulted for detailed information on the use of medicines in children. The BNF should be interpreted in the light of professional knowledge and supplemented as necessary by specialised

publications and by reference to the product literature.
Information is also available from medicines information
services.

Changes

Monthly updates are provided online via MedicinesComplete and the NHS Evidence portal. The changes listed below are cumulative (from one print edition to the next).

Significant changes

Significant changes that will appear in the print edition of BNF 72 (September 2016–March 2017):

- Abiraterone acetate p. 831 for treating metastatic hormone-relapsed prostate cancer before chemotherapy is indicated [NICE guidance].
- Adalimumab p. 957, etanercept p. 961, infliximab p. 964, certolizumab pegol p. 959, golimumab p. 962, tocilizumab p. 954 and abatacept p. 956 for rheumatoid arthritis not previously treated with DMARDs or after conventional DMARDs only have failed [NICE guidance].
- Apremilast p. 966 for treating moderate to severe plaque psoriasis [NICE guidance] and for treating active psoriatic arthritis [NICE guidance].
- Asthma: updated guidance on management of chronic asthma and acute asthma.
- Bisphosphonates: risk of osteonecrosis of the external auditory canal [MHRA/CHM advice].
- Bortezomib p. 868 for previously untreated mantle cell lymphoma [NICE guidance].
- Breast cancer: update guidance on management.
- Daclatasvir p. 568 for treating chronic hepatitis C [NICE guidance].
- Diverticular disease and diverticulitis: updated guidance on management.
- Drug allergy (suspected or confirmed): new guidance.
- Edoxaban p. 113 for treating and preventing deep-vein thrombosis and pulmonary embolism [NICE guidance] and for preventing stroke and systemic embolism in non-valvular atrial fibrillation [NICE guidance].
- Enzalutamide p. 832 for treating metastatic hormone-relapsed prostate cancer before chemotherapy is indicated [NICE guidance].
- Erlotinib p. 852 and gefitinib p. 854 for treating non-small cell lung cancer that has progressed after prior chemotherapy [NICE guidance].
- Ezetimibe p. 181 for treating primary heterozygous-familial and non-familial hypercholesterolaemia [NICE guidance].
- Idelalisib p. 856 for treating chronic lymphocytic leukaemia [NICE guidance].
- Irritable bowel syndrome: updated guidance on management.
- Levonorgestrel p. 729 releasing intra-uterine device: brand name prescribing [MHRA/CHM advice].
- Live attenuated vaccines [MHRA/CHM advice].
- Mirabegron p. 707: measures to minimise risk of severe hypertension and associated cerebrovascular and cardiac events.
- Mycophenolate mofetil p. 765: new pregnancy-prevention advice for women and men.
- Nicorandil p. 194: risk of ulcer complications.
- Nintedanib p. 867 for previously treated locally advanced, metastatic, or locally recurrent non-small cell lung cancer [NICE guidance] and for treating idiopathic pulmonary fibrosis [NICE guidance].
- Obesity: updated guidance on management.
- Olaparib p. 869 for maintenance treatment of relapsed, platinum-sensitive, BRCA mutation-positive ovarian, fallopian tube, and peritoneal cancer after response to second-line or subsequent platinum-based chemotherapy [NICE guidance].
- Ombitasvir with paritaprevir and ritonavir p. 569 (*Viekirax*®) with or without dasabuvir p. 575, for treatment of chronic hepatitis C [NICE guidance].
- Paclitaxel p. 817 as albumin-bound nanoparticles in combination with gemcitabine for previously untreated metastatic pancreatic cancer [NICE guidance].
- Pembrolizumab p. 780 for treating advanced melanoma after disease progression with ipilimumab p. 778 [NICE Guidance] and for advanced melanoma not previously treated with ipilimumab [NICE guidance].
- Prostate cancer: updated guidance on management.
- Ramucirumab p. 782 for treating advanced gastric cancer or gastro-oesophageal junction adenocarcinoma previously treated with chemotherapy [NICE guidance].
- Ruxolitinib p. 862 for treating disease-related splenomegaly or symptoms in adults with myelofibrosis [NICE guidance].
- Secukinumab p. 954 (*Cosentyx*®) for the treatment of plaque psoriasis [NICE guidance].
- Sodium valproate p. 298 and risk of abnormal pregnancy outcomes [updated MHRA/CHM advice].
- Sofosbuvir with ledipasvir p. 572 for the treatment of chronic hepatitis C [NICE guidance].
- TNF-alpha inhibitors for ankylosing spondylitis and non-radiographic axial spondyloarthritis [NICE guidance].
- Tolvaptan p. 605 (*Jinarc*®) for the treatment of autosomal dominant polycystic kidney disease [NICE guidance].
- Topotecan p. 818, pegylated liposomal doxorubicin hydrochloride p. 798, paclitaxel p. 817, trabectedin p. 812 and gemcitabine p. 805 for treating recurrent ovarian cancer [NICE guidance].
- Trastuzumab emtansine p. 786 for treating HER2-positive unresectable locally advanced or metastatic breast cancer [NICE guidance].
- Valproic acid p. 323 and risk of abnormal pregnancy outcomes [updated MHRA/CHM advice].
- Valsartan with sacubitril p. 176 (Sacubitril valsartan) for treating symptomatic chronic heart failure with reduced ejection fraction [NICE guidance].
- Vedolizumab p. 40 for treating moderately to severely active Crohn's disease [NICE guidance].
- Vortioxetine p. 349 for treating major depressive episodes [NICE guidance].

Dose changes

Changes in dose statements that will appear in the print edition of BNF 72 (September 2016–March 2017):

- Ceftriaxone p. 480
- Hydroxyzine hydrochloride p. 262
- Nicorandil p. 194
- Nystatin p. 1062
- Prucalopride p. 52 [licensed for use in men].
- Thalidomide p. 845 [reduced dose in patients aged 76 years and over]
- Ulipristal acetate p. 727 [uterine fibroids]

Classification changes

Classification changes that will appear in the print edition of BNF 72 (September 2016–March 2017):

New names

Name changes that will appear in the print edition of BNF 72 (September 2016–March 2017):

Deleted preparations

Preparations discontinued in the print edition of BNF 72 (September 2016–March 2017):
- *Preotact*® injection [parathyroid hormone].
- *TriNovum*® tablets [ethinylestradiol with norethisterone p. 725].

New preparations

New preparations that will appear in the print edition of BNF 72 (September 2016–March 2017):
- *Akynzeo*® capsules [palonosetron with netupitant p. 399].

- *Bramox*® tablets [midodrine hydrochloride p. 172].
- *Brintellix*® [vortioxetine p. 349].
- *Cholib*® [simvastatin with fenofibrate p. 189].
- *Cosentyx*® injection [secukinumab p. 954].
- *Cyramza*® [ramucirumab p. 782].
- *Entresto*® tablets [valsartan with sacubitril p. 176].
- *Eperzan*® [albiglutide p. 629].
- *Exviera*® tablets [dasabuvir p. 575].
- *Harvoni*® tablets [sofosbuvir with ledipasvir p. 572].
- *Intuniv*® tablets [guanfacine p. 321].
- *Keytruda*® [pembrolizumab p. 780].
- *Lixiana*® tablets [edoxaban p. 113].
- *Lynparza*® capsules [olaparib p. 869].
- *Ofev*® capsules [nintedanib p. 867].
- *Orphacol*® capsules [cholic acid p. 79].
- *Spiolto Respimat*® inhalation solution [tiotropium with olodaterol p. 229].
- *Synjardy*® tablets [empagliflozin with metformin p. 636].
- *Taptiqom*® eyedrops [tafluprost with timolol p. 1031].
- *Trulicity*® injection [dulaglutide p. 629].
- *Ultibro Breezhaler*® [glycopyrronium with indacaterol p. 228].
- *Vargatef*® capsules [nintedanib p. 867].
- *Viekirax*® tablets [ombitasvir with paritaprevir and ritonavir p. 569].

Guidance on prescribing

General guidance

Medicines should be prescribed only when they are necessary, and in all cases the benefit of administering the medicine should be considered in relation to the risk involved. This is particularly important during pregnancy, when the risk to both mother and fetus must be considered. It is important to discuss treatment options carefully with the patient to ensure that the patient is content to take the medicine as prescribed. In particular, the patient should be helped to distinguish the adverse effects of prescribed drugs from the effects of the medical disorder. When the beneficial effects of the medicine are likely to be delayed, the patient should be advised of this.

Taking medicines to best effect

Difficulties in adherence to drug treatment occur regardless of age. Factors contributing to poor compliance with prescribed medicines include:

- prescription not collected or not dispensed;
- purpose of medicine not clear;
- perceived lack of efficacy;
- real or perceived adverse effects;
- patients' perception of the risk and severity of side-effects may differ from that of the prescriber;
- instructions for administration not clear;
- physical difficulty in taking medicines (e.g. swallowing the medicine, handling small tablets, or opening medicine containers);
- unattractive formulation (e.g. unpleasant taste);
- complicated regimen.

The prescriber and the patient should agree on the health outcomes that the patient desires and on the strategy for achieving them ('concordance'). The prescriber should be sensitive to religious, cultural, and personal beliefs that can affect a patient's acceptance of medicines.

Taking the time to explain to the patient (and relatives) the rationale and the potential adverse effects of treatment may improve adherence. Reinforcement and elaboration of the physician's instructions by the pharmacist and other members of the healthcare team also helps. Advising the patient of the possibility of alternative treatments may encourage the patient to seek advice rather than merely abandon unacceptable treatment.

Simplifying the drug regimen may help; the need for frequent administration may reduce adherence, although there appears to be little difference in adherence between once-daily and twice-daily administration. Combination products reduce the number of drugs taken but at the expense of the ability to titrate individual doses.

Biosimilar medicines

A biosimilar medicine is a new biological product that is similar to a medicine that has already been authorised to be marketed (the biological reference medicine) in the European Union. The active substance of a biosimilar medicine is similar, but not identical, to the biological reference medicine. Biological products are different from standard chemical products in terms of their complexity and although theoretically there should be no important differences between the biosimilar and the biological reference medicine in terms of safety or efficacy, when prescribing biological products, it is good practice to use the brand name. This will ensure that substitution of a biosimilar medicine does not occur when the medicine is dispensed. Biosimilar medicines have black triangle status at the time of initial marketing. It is important to report suspected adverse

reactions to biosimilar medicines using the Yellow Card Scheme. For biosimilar medicines, adverse reaction reports should clearly state the brand name and the batch number of the suspected medicine.

The following biological medicines are available as biosimilar preparations and should therefore always be prescribed by brand name:

- Epoetin alfa p. 874
- Etanercept p. 961
- Filgrastim p. 890
- Follitropin alfa p. 673
- Infliximab p. 964
- Insulin glargine p. 643
- Somatropin p. 676

Complementary and alternative medicine

An increasing amount of information on complementary and alternative medicine is becoming available. The scope of the BNF is restricted to the discussion of conventional medicines but reference is made to complementary treatments if they affect conventional therapy (e.g. interactions with St John's wort). Further information on herbal medicines is available at www.mhra.gov.uk.

Abbreviation of titles

In general, titles of drugs and preparations should be written in full. Unofficial abbreviations should not be used as they may be misinterpreted.

Non-proprietary titles

Where non-proprietary ('generic') titles are given, they should be used in prescribing. This will enable any suitable product to be dispensed, thereby saving delay to the patient and sometimes expense to the health service. The only exception is where there is a demonstrable difference in clinical effect between each manufacturer's version of the formulation, making it important that the patient should always receive the same brand; in such cases, the brand name or the manufacturer should be stated. Non-proprietary titles should not be invented for the purposes of prescribing generically since this can lead to confusion, particularly in the case of compound and modified-release preparations. Titles used as headings for monographs may be used freely in the United Kingdom but in other countries may be subject to restriction.

Many of the non-proprietary titles used in this book are titles of monographs in the European Pharmacopoeia, British Pharmacopoeia, or British Pharmaceutical Codex 1973. In such cases the preparations must comply with the standard (if any) in the appropriate publication, as required by the Human Medicines Regulations 2012.

Proprietary titles

Names followed by the symbol® are or have been used as proprietary names in the United Kingdom. These names may in general be applied only to products supplied by the owners of the trade marks.

Marketing authorisation and BNF advice

In general the *doses, indications, cautions, contra-indications,* and *side-effects* in the BNF reflect those in the manufacturers' data sheets or Summaries of Product Characteristics (SPCs) which, in turn, reflect those in the corresponding marketing authorisations (formerly known as Product Licences). The BNF does not generally include proprietary medicines that are not supported by a valid Summary of Product Characteristics or when the marketing

Guidance on prescribing

authorisation holder has not been able to supply essential information. When a preparation is available from more than one manufacturer, the BNF reflects advice that is the most clinically relevant regardless of any variation in the marketing authorisations. Unlicensed products can be obtained from 'special-order' manufacturers or specialist importing companies.

Where an unlicensed drug is included in the BNF, this is indicated in square brackets after the entry. When the BNF suggests a use (or route) that is outside the licensed indication of a product ('off-label' use), this too is indicated. Unlicensed use of medicines becomes necessary if the clinical need cannot be met by licensed medicines; such use should be supported by appropriate evidence and experience.

The doses stated in the BNF are intended for general guidance and represent, unless otherwise stated, the usual range of doses that are generally regarded as being suitable for adults.

Prescribing unlicensed medicines

Prescribing medicines outside the recommendations of their marketing authorisation alters (and probably increases) the prescriber's professional responsibility and potential liability. The prescriber should be able to justify and feel competent in using such medicines, and also inform the patient or the patient's carer that the prescribed medicine is unlicensed.

Oral syringes

An **oral syringe** is supplied when oral liquid medicines are prescribed in doses other than multiples of 5 mL. The oral syringe is marked in 0.5 mL divisions from 1 to 5 mL to measure doses of less than 5 mL (other sizes of oral syringe may also be available). It is provided with an adaptor and an instruction leaflet. The 5–*mL spoon* is used for doses of 5 mL (or multiples thereof).

Important To avoid inadvertent intravenous administration of oral liquid medicines, only an appropriate oral or enteral syringe should be used to measure an oral liquid medicine (if a medicine spoon or graduated measure cannot be used); these syringes should not be compatible with intravenous or other parenteral devices. Oral and enteral syringes should be clearly labelled 'Oral' or 'Enteral' in a large font size; it is the healthcare practitioner's responsibility to label the syringe with this information if the manufacturer has not done so.

Excipients

Branded oral liquid preparations that do not contain *fructose, glucose,* or *sucrose* are described as 'sugar-free' in the BNF. Preparations containing hydrogenated glucose syrup, mannitol, maltitol, sorbitol, or xylitol are also marked 'sugar-free' since there is evidence that they do not cause dental caries. Patients receiving medicines containing cariogenic sugars should be advised of appropriate dental hygiene measures to prevent caries. Sugar-free preparations should be used whenever possible.

Where information on the presence of *aspartame, gluten, sulfites, tartrazine, arachis (peanut) oil* or *sesame oil* is available, this is indicated in the BNF against the relevant preparation.

Information is provided on selected excipients in skin preparations, in vaccines, and on *selected preservatives* and *excipients* in eye drops and injections.

The presence of *benzyl alcohol* and *polyoxyl castor oil* (polyethoxylated castor oil) in injections is indicated in the BNF. Benzyl alcohol has been associated with a fatal toxic syndrome in preterm neonates, and therefore, parenteral preparations containing the preservative should not be used in neonates. Polyoxyl castor oils, used as vehicles in intravenous injections, have been associated with severe anaphylactoid reactions.

The presence of *propylene glycol* in oral or parenteral medicines is indicated in the BNF; it can cause adverse effects if its elimination is impaired, e.g. in renal failure, in neonates and young children, and in slow metabolisers of the substance. It may interact with disulfiram p. 451 and metronidazole p. 492.

The *lactose* content in most medicines is too small to cause problems in most lactose-intolerant patients. However in severe lactose intolerance, the lactose content should be determined before prescribing. The amount of lactose varies according to manufacturer, product, formulation, and strength.

Important In the absence of information on excipients in the BNF and in the product literature (available at www.medicines.org.uk/emc), contact the manufacturer (see Index of Proprietary Manufacturers) if it is essential to check details.

Extemporaneous preparation

A product should be dispensed extemporaneously only when no product with a marketing authorisation is available. The BP direction that a preparation must be *freshly prepared* indicates that it must be made not more than 24 hours before it is issued for use. The direction that a preparation should be *recently prepared* indicates that deterioration is likely if the preparation is stored for longer than about 4 weeks at 15–25° C.

The term **water** used without qualification means either potable water freshly drawn direct from the public supply and suitable for drinking or freshly boiled and cooled purified water. The latter should be used if the public supply is from a local storage tank or if the potable water is unsuitable for a particular preparation (Water for injections).

Drugs and driving

Prescribers and other healthcare professionals should advise patients if treatment is likely to affect their ability to perform skilled tasks (e.g. driving). This applies especially to drugs with sedative effects; patients should be warned that these effects are increased by alcohol. General information about a patient's fitness to drive is available from the Driver and Vehicle Licensing Agency at www.dvla.gov.uk.

A new offence of driving, attempting to drive, or being in charge of a vehicle, with certain specified controlled drugs in excess of specified limits, came into force on 2nd March 2015. This offence is an addition to the existing rules on drug impaired driving and fitness to drive, and applies to two groups of drugs—commonly abused drugs, including amfetamines, cannabis, cocaine, and ketamine p. 1179, and drugs used mainly for medical reasons, such as opioids and benzodiazepines. Anyone found to have any of the drugs (including related drugs, for example, apomorphine hydrochloride p. 382) above specified limits in their blood will be guilty of an offence, whether their driving was impaired or not. This also includes prescribed drugs which metabolise to those included in the offence, for example, selegiline hydrochloride p. 391. However, the legislation provides a statutory "medical defence" for patients taking drugs for medical reasons in accordance with instructions, *if their driving was not impaired*—it continues to be an offence to drive if actually impaired. Patients should therefore be advised to continue taking their medicines as prescribed, and when driving, to carry suitable evidence that the drug was prescribed, or sold, to treat a medical or dental problem, and that it was taken according to the instructions given by the prescriber, or information provided with the medicine (e.g. a repeat prescription form or the medicine's patient information leaflet). Further information is available from the Department for Transport at www.gov.uk/government/collections/drug-driving.

Patents

In the BNF, certain drugs have been included notwithstanding the existence of actual or potential patent rights. In so far as such substances are protected by Letters Patent, their inclusion in this Formulary neither conveys, nor implies, licence to manufacture.

Health and safety

When handling chemical or biological materials particular attention should be given to the possibility of allergy, fire, explosion, radiation, or poisoning. Substances such as corticosteroids, some antimicrobials, phenothiazines, and many cytotoxics, are irritant or very potent and should be handled with caution. Contact with the skin and inhalation of dust should be avoided.

Safety in the home

Patients must be warned to keep all medicines out of the reach of children. All solid dose and all oral and external liquid preparations must be dispensed in a reclosable *child-resistant container* unless:

- the medicine is in an original pack or patient pack such as to make this inadvisable;
- the patient will have difficulty in opening a child-resistant container;
- a specific request is made that the product shall not be dispensed in a child-resistant container;
- no suitable child-resistant container exists for a particular liquid preparation.

All patients should be advised to dispose of *unwanted medicines* by returning them to a supplier for destruction.

Labelling of prescribed medicines

There is a legal requirement for the following to appear on the label of any prescribed medicine:

- name of the patient;
- name and address of the supplying pharmacy;
- date of dispensing;
- name of the medicine;
- directions for use of the medicine;
- precautions relating to the use of the medicine.

The Royal Pharmaceutical Society recommends that the following also appears on the label:

- the words 'Keep out of the sight and reach of children';
- where applicable, the words 'Use this medicine only on your skin'.

A pharmacist can exercise professional skill and judgement to amend or include more appropriate wording for the name of the medicine, the directions for use, or the precautions relating to the use of the medicine.

Non-proprietary names of compound preparations

Non-proprietary names of **compound preparations** which appear in the BNF are those that have been compiled by the British Pharmacopoeia Commission or another recognised body; whenever possible they reflect the names of the active ingredients.

Prescribers should avoid creating their own compound names for the purposes of generic prescribing; such names do not have an approved definition and can be misinterpreted.

Special care should be taken to avoid errors when prescribing compound preparations; in particular the hyphen in the prefix 'co-' should be retained.

Special care should also be taken to avoid creating generic names for **modified-release** preparations where the use of these names could lead to confusion between formulations with different lengths of action.

EEA and Swiss prescriptions

Pharmacists can dispense prescriptions issued by doctors and dentists from the European Economic Area (EEA) or Switzerland (except prescriptions for controlled drugs in Schedules 1, 2, or 3, or for drugs without a UK marketing authorisation). Prescriptions should be written in ink or otherwise so as to be indelible, should be dated, should state the name of the patient, should state the address of the prescriber, should contain particulars indicating whether the prescriber is a doctor or dentist, and should be signed by the prescriber.

Security and validity of prescriptions

The Councils of the British Medical Association and the Royal Pharmaceutical Society have issued a joint statement on the security and validity of prescriptions.
In particular, prescription forms should:

- not be left unattended at reception desks;
- not be left in a car where they may be visible; and
- when not in use, be kept in a locked drawer within the surgery and at home.

Where there is any doubt about the authenticity of a prescription, the pharmacist should contact the prescriber. If this is done by telephone, the number should be obtained from the directory rather than relying on the information on the prescription form, which may be false.

Patient group direction (PGD)

In most cases, the most appropriate clinical care will be provided on an individual basis by a prescriber to a specific individual patient. However, a Patient Group Direction for supply and administration of medicines by other healthcare professionals can be used where it would benefit patient care without compromising safety.

A Patient Group Direction is a written direction relating to the supply and administration (or administration only) of a licensed prescription-only medicine (including some Controlled Drugs in specific circumstances) by certain classes of healthcare professionals; the Direction is signed by a doctor (or dentist) and by a pharmacist. Further information on Patient Group Directions is available in Health Service Circular HSC 2000/026 (England), HDL (2001) 7 (Scotland), and WHC (2000) 116 (Wales); see also the Human Medicines Regulations 2012.

NICE and Scottish Medicines Consortium

Advice issued by the National Institute for Health and Care Excellence (NICE) is included in the BNF when relevant. The BNF also includes advice issued by the Scottish Medicines Consortium (SMC) when a medicine is restricted or not recommended for use within NHS Scotland. If advice within a NICE Single Technology Appraisal differs from SMC advice, the Scottish Executive expects NHS Boards within NHS Scotland to comply with the SMC advice. Details of the advice together with updates can be obtained from www.nice.org.uk and from www.scottishmedicines.org.uk.

Prescription writing

Shared care

In its guidelines on responsibility for prescribing (circular EL (91) 127) between hospitals and general practitioners, the Department of Health has advised that legal responsibility for prescribing lies with the doctor who signs the prescription.

Requirements

Prescriptions should be written legibly in ink or otherwise so as to be indelible (it is permissible to issue carbon copies of NHS prescriptions as long as they are signed in ink), should be dated, should state the name and address of the patient, the address of the prescriber, an indication of the type of prescriber, and should be signed in ink by the prescriber (computer-generated facsimile signatures do not meet the legal requirement). The age and the date of birth of the patient should preferably be stated, and it is a legal requirement in the case of prescription-only medicines to state the age for children under 12 years. These recommendations are acceptable for **prescription-only medicines**. Prescriptions for controlled drugs have additional legal requirements.

Wherever appropriate the prescriber should state the current weight of the child to enable the dose prescribed to be checked. Consideration should also be given to including the dose per unit mass e.g. mg/kg or the dose per m^2 body-surface area e.g. mg/m^2 where this would reduce error. The following should be noted:

- The strength or quantity to be contained in capsules, lozenges, tablets etc. should be stated by the prescriber. In particular, strength of liquid preparations should be clearly stated (e.g. 125 mg/5 mL).
- The unnecessary use of decimal points should be avoided, e.g. 3 mg, not 3.0 mg. Quantities of 1 gram or more should be written as 1 g etc. Quantities less than 1 gram should be written in milligrams, e.g. 500 mg, not 0.5 g. Quantities less than 1 mg should be written in micrograms, e.g. 100 micrograms, not 0.1 mg. When decimals are unavoidable a zero should be written in front of the decimal point where there is no other figure, e.g. 0.5 mL, not .5 mL. Use of the decimal point is acceptable to express a range, e.g. 0.5 to 1 g.
- 'Micrograms' and 'nanograms' should **not** be abbreviated. Similarly 'units' should **not** be abbreviated.
- The term 'millilitre' (ml or mL) is used in medicine and pharmacy, and cubic centimetre, c.c., or cm^3 should not be used. (The use of capital 'L' in mL is a printing convention throughout the BNF; both 'mL' and 'ml' are recognised SI abbreviations).
- Dose and dose frequency should be stated; in the case of preparations to be taken 'as required' a **minimum dose interval** should be specified. Care should be taken to ensure children receive the correct dose of the active drug. Therefore, the dose should normally be stated in terms of the mass of the active drug (e.g. '125 mg 3 times daily'); terms such as '5 mL' or '1 tablet' should be avoided except for compound preparations. When doses other than multiples of 5 mL are prescribed for *oral liquid preparations* the dose-volume will be provided by means of an **oral syringe**, (except for preparations intended to be measured with a pipette). Suitable quantities:
  - Elixirs, Linctuses, and Paediatric Mixtures (5-mL dose), 50, 100, or 150 mL
  - Adult Mixtures (10 mL dose), 200 or 300 mL
  - Ear Drops, Eye drops, and Nasal Drops, 10 mL (or the manufacturer's pack)
  - Eye Lotions, Gargles, and Mouthwashes, 200 mL
- The names of drugs and preparations should be written clearly and **not** abbreviated, using approved titles **only**;

avoid creating generic titles for modified-release preparations).

- The quantity to be supplied may be stated by indicating the number of days of treatment required in the box provided on NHS forms. In most cases the exact amount will be supplied. This does not apply to items directed to be used as required—if the dose and frequency are not given then the quantity to be supplied needs to be stated. When several items are ordered on one form the box can be marked with the number of days of treatment provided the quantity is added for any item for which the amount cannot be calculated.
- Although directions should preferably be in **English without abbreviation**, it is recognised that some Latin abbreviations are used.

Sample prescription

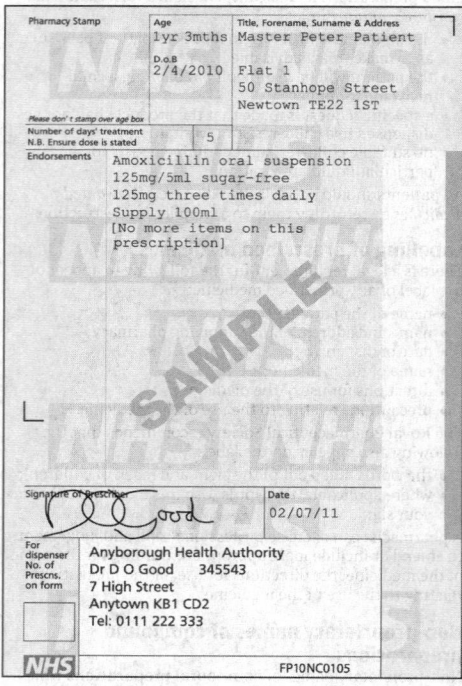

Prescribing by dentists

Until new prescribing arrangements are in place for NHS prescriptions, dentists should use form FP10D (GP14 in Scotland, WP10D in Wales) to prescribe only those items listed in the Dental Practitioners' Formulary. The Human Medicines Regulations 2012 does not set any limitations upon the number and variety of substances which the dentist may administer to patients in the surgery or may order by private prescription—provided the relevant legal requirements are observed the dentist may use or order whatever is required for the clinical situation. There is no statutory requirement for the dentist to communicate with a patient's medical practitioner when prescribing for dental use. There are, however, occasions when this would be in the patient's interest and such communication is to be encouraged. For legal requirements relating to prescriptions of Controlled Drugs, see Controlled drugs and drug dependence p. 7.

Computer-issued prescriptions

For computer-issued prescriptions the following advice, based on the recommendations of the Joint GP Information Technology Committee, should also be noted:

1   The computer must print out the date, the patient's surname, one forename, other initials, and address, and may also print out the patient's title and date of birth. The age of children under 12 years and of adults over 60 years must be printed in the box available; the age of children under 5 years should be printed in years and months. A facility may also exist to print out the age of patients between 12 and 60 years.

2   The doctor's name must be printed at the bottom of the prescription form; this will be the name of the doctor responsible for the prescription (who will normally sign it). The doctor's surgery address, reference number, and Primary Care Trust (PCT, Health Board in Scotland, Local Health Board in Wales) are also necessary. In addition, the surgery telephone number should be printed.

3   When prescriptions are to be signed by general practitioner registrars, assistants, locums, or deputising doctors, the name of the doctor printed at the bottom of the form must still be that of the responsible principal.

4   Names of medicines must come from a dictionary held in the computer memory, to provide a check on the spelling and to ensure that the name is written in full. The computer can be programmed to recognise both the non-proprietary and the proprietary name of a particular drug and to print out the preferred choice, but must not print out both names. For medicines not in the dictionary, separate checks are required—the user must be warned that no check was possible and the entire prescription must be entered in the lexicon.

5   The dictionary may contain information on the usual doses, formulations, and pack sizes to produce standard predetermined prescriptions for common preparations, and to provide a check on the validity of an individual prescription on entry.

6   The prescription must be printed in English without abbreviation; information may be entered or stored in abbreviated form. The dose must be in numbers, the frequency in words, and the quantity in numbers in brackets, thus: 40 mg four times daily (112). It must also be possible to prescribe by indicating the length of treatment required.

7   The BNF recommendations should be followed as listed above.

8   Checks may be incorporated to ensure that all the information required for dispensing a particular drug has been filled in. For instructions such as 'as directed' and 'when required', the maximum daily dose should normally be specified.

9   Numbers and codes used in the system for organising and retrieving data must never appear on the form.

10 Supplementary warnings or advice should be written in full, should not interfere with the clarity of the prescription itself, and should be in line with any warnings or advice in the BNF; numerical codes should not be used.

11 A mechanism (such as printing a series of nonspecific characters) should be incorporated to cancel out unused space, or wording such as 'no more items on this prescription' may be added after the last item. Otherwise the doctor should delete the space manually.

12 To avoid forgery the computer may print on the form the number of items to be dispensed (somewhere separate from the box for the pharmacist). The number of items per form need be limited only by the ability of the printer to produce clear and well-demarcated instructions with sufficient space for each item and a spacer line before each fresh item.

13 Handwritten alterations should only be made in exceptional circumstances—it is preferable to print out a new prescription. Any alterations must be made in the doctor's own handwriting and countersigned; computer records should be updated to fully reflect any alteration. Prescriptions for drugs used for contraceptive purposes (but which are not promoted as contraceptives) may need to be marked in handwriting with the symbol ♀, (or endorsed in another way to indicate that the item is prescribed for contraceptive purposes).

14 Prescriptions for controlled drugs can be printed from the computer, but the prescriber's signature must be handwritten (See Controlled Drugs and Drug Dependence; the prescriber may use a date stamp).

15 The strip of paper on the side of the FP10SS (GP10SS in Scotland, WP10SS in Wales) may be used for various purposes but care should be taken to avoid including confidential information. It may be advisable for the patient's name to appear at the top, but this should be preceded by 'confidential'.

16 In rural dispensing practices prescription requests (or details of medicines dispensed) will normally be entered in one surgery. The prescriptions (or dispensed medicines) may then need to be delivered to another surgery or location; if possible the computer should hold up to 10 alternatives.

17 Prescription forms that are reprinted or issued as a duplicate should be labelled clearly as such.

Emergency supply of medicines

Emergency supply requested by member of the public

Pharmacists are sometimes called upon by members of the public to make an emergency supply of medicines. The Human Medicines Regulations 2012 allows exemptions from the Prescription Only requirements for emergency supply to be made by a person lawfully conducting a retail pharmacy business provided:

a) that the pharmacist has interviewed the person requesting the prescription-only medicine and is satisfied:

   i) that there is immediate need for the prescription-only medicine and that it is impracticable in the circumstances to obtain a prescription without undue delay;

   ii) that treatment with the prescription-only medicine has on a previous occasion been prescribed for the person requesting it;

   iii) as to the dose that it would be appropriate for the person to take;

b) that no greater quantity shall be supplied than will provide 5 days' treatment of phenobarbital p. 304, *phenobarbital sodium*, or Controlled Drugs in Schedules 4 or 5 (doctors or dentists from the European Economic Area and Switzerland, or their patients, cannot request an emergency supply of Controlled Drugs in Schedules 1, 2, or 3, or drugs that do not have a UK marketing authorisation) or 30 days' treatment for other prescription-only medicines, except when the prescription-only medicine is:

   i) insulin, an ointment or cream, or a preparation for the relief of asthma in an aerosol dispenser when the smallest pack can be supplied;

   ii) an oral contraceptive when a full cycle may be supplied;

   iii) an antibiotic in liquid form for oral administration when the smallest quantity that will provide a full course of treatment can be supplied;

c) that an entry shall be made by the pharmacist in the prescription book stating:

   i) the date of supply;

   ii) the name, quantity and, where appropriate, the pharmaceutical form and strength;

   iii) the name and address of the patient;

   iv) the nature of the emergency;

d) that the container or package must be labelled to show:

   i) the date of supply;

   ii) the name, quantity and, where appropriate, the pharmaceutical form and strength;

   iii) the name of the patient;

   iv) the name and address of the pharmacy;

   v) the words 'Emergency supply';

   vi) the words 'Keep out of the reach of children' (or similar warning);

e) that the prescription-only medicine is not a substance specifically excluded from the emergency supply provision, and does not contain a Controlled Drug specified in Schedules 1, 2, or 3 to the Misuse of Drugs Regulations 2001 except for phenobarbital p. 304 or *phenobarbital sodium* for the treatment of epilepsy: for details see *Medicines, Ethics and Practice,* London, Pharmaceutical Press (always consult latest edition). Doctors or dentists from the European Economic Area and Switzerland, or their patients, cannot request an emergency supply of Controlled Drugs in Schedules 1, 2, or 3, or drugs that do not have a UK marketing authorisation.

Emergency supply requested by prescriber

Emergency supply of a prescription-only medicine may also be made at the request of a doctor, a dentist, a supplementary prescriber, a community practitioner nurse prescriber, a nurse, pharmacist, or optometrist independent prescriber, or a doctor or dentist from the European Economic Area or Switzerland, provided:

a) that the pharmacist is satisfied that the prescriber by reason of some emergency is unable to furnish a prescription immediately;

b) that the prescriber has undertaken to furnish a prescription within 72 hours;

c) that the medicine is supplied in accordance with the directions of the prescriber requesting it;

d) that the medicine is not a Controlled Drug specified in Schedules 1, 2, or 3 to the Misuse of Drugs Regulations 2001 except for phenobarbital p. 304 or *phenobarbital sodium* for the treatment of epilepsy: for details see *Medicines, Ethics and Practice,* London, Pharmaceutical Press (always consult latest edition); (Doctors or dentists from the European Economic Area and Switzerland, or their patients, cannot request an emergency supply of Controlled Drugs in Schedules 1, 2, or 3, or drugs that do not have a UK marketing authorisation).

e) that an entry shall be made in the prescription book stating:

   i) the date of supply;

   ii) the name, quantity and, where appropriate, the pharmaceutical form and strength;

   iii) the name and address of the practitioner requesting the emergency supply;

   iv) the name and address of the patient;

   v) the date on the prescription;

   vi) when the prescription is received the entry should be amended to include the date on which it is received.

Royal Pharmaceutical Society's guidelines

1. The pharmacist should consider the medical consequences of not supplying a medicine in an emergency.

2. If the pharmacist is unable to make an emergency supply of a medicine the pharmacist should advise the patient how to obtain essential medical care.

For conditions that apply to supplies made at the request of a patient see Medicines, Ethics and Practice, London Pharmaceutical Press, (always consult latest edition).

Controlled drugs and drug dependence

Regulations and classification

The Misuse of Drugs Act, 1971 prohibits certain activities in relation to 'Controlled Drugs', in particular their manufacture, supply, and possession. The penalties applicable to offences involving the different drugs are graded broadly according to the *harmfulness attributable to a drug when it is misused* and for this purpose the drugs are defined in the following three classes:

- **Class A** includes: alfentanil p. 1177, cocaine, diamorphine hydrochloride (heroin) p. 415, dipipanone hydrochloride, lysergide (LSD), methadone hydrochloride p. 456, methylenedioxymethamfetamine (MDMA, 'ecstasy'), morphine, opium, pethidine hydrochloride p. 426, phencyclidine, remifentanil p. 1178, and class B substances when prepared for injection.
- **Class B** includes: oral amfetamines, barbiturates, cannabis, cannabis resin, codeine phosphate p. 413, ethylmorphine, glutethimide, ketamine p. 1179, nabilone p. 394, pentazocine p. 426 phenmetrazine, and pholcodine p. 271.
- **Class C** includes: certain drugs related to the amfetamines such as benzfetamine and chlorphentermine, buprenorphine p. 409, mazindol, meprobamate p. 316 pemoline, pipradrol, most benzodiazepines, tramadol hydrochloride p. 427, zaleplon p. 445, zolpidem tartrate p. 446, zopiclone p. 446, androgenic and anabolic steroids, clenbuterol, chorionic gonadotrophin (HCG), non-human chorionic gonadotrophin, somatotropin, somatrem, and somatropin p. 676.

The Misuse of Drugs Regulations 2001 (and subsequent amendments) define the classes of person who are authorised to supply and possess controlled drugs while acting in their professional capacities and lay down the conditions under which these activities may be carried out. In the regulations drugs are divided into five schedules each specifying the requirements governing such activities as import, export, production, supply, possession, prescribing, and record keeping which apply to them.

- **Schedule 1** includes drugs such as lysergide which is not used medicinally. Possession and supply are prohibited except in accordance with Home Office authority.
- **Schedule 2** includes drugs such as diamorphine hydrochloride (heroin) p. 415, morphine p. 421, nabilone p. 394, remifentanil p. 1178, pethidine hydrochloride p. 426, secobarbital, glutethimide, the amfetamines, sodium oxybate and cocaine and are subject to the full controlled drug requirements relating to prescriptions, safe custody (except for secobarbital), the need to keep registers, etc. (unless exempted in Schedule 5).
- **Schedule 3** includes the barbiturates (except secobarbital, now Schedule 2), buprenorphine p. 409, mazindol, meprobamate p. 316, midazolam p. 310, pentazocine p. 426, phentermine, temazepam p. 443, and tramadol hydrochloride p. 427. They are subject to the special prescription requirements. Safe custody requirements do apply, except for any 5,5 disubstituted barbituric acid (e.g. phenobarbital), mazindol, meprobamate p. 316, midazolam p. 310, pentazocine p. 426, phentermine, tramadol hydrochloride p. 427, or any stereoisomeric form or salts of the above. Records in registers do not need to be kept (although there are requirements for the retention of invoices for 2 years).
- **Schedule 4** includes in Part I benzodiazepines (except temazepam p. 443 and midazolam p. 310, which are in Schedule 3), zaleplon p. 445, zolpidem tartrate p. 446, and zopiclone p. 446 which are subject to minimal control. Part II includes androgenic and anabolic

steroids, clenbuterol, chorionic gonadotrophin (HCG), non-human chorionic gonadotrophin, somatotropin, somatrem, and somatropin p. 676. Controlled drug prescription requirements do not apply and Schedule 4 Controlled Drugs are not subject to safe custody requirements.
- **Schedule 5** includes those preparations which, because of their strength, are exempt from virtually all Controlled Drug requirements other than retention of invoices for two years.

Prescriptions

Preparations in Schedules 1, 2, 3, and 4 of the Misuse of Drugs Regulations 2001 (and subsequent amendments) are identified throughout the BNF and *BNF for children* using the following symbols:

CD1	for preparations in Schedule 1
CD2	for preparations in Schedule 2
CD3	for preparations in Schedule 3
CD4-1	for preparations in Schedule 4 (Part I)
CD4-2	for preparations in Schedule 4 (Part II)

The principal legal requirements relating to medical prescriptions are listed below (see also Department of Health Guidance).

Prescription requirements Prescriptions for Controlled Drugs that are subject to prescription requirements (all preparations in Schedules 2 and 3) must be indelible and must be *signed* by the prescriber, be *dated*, and specify the prescriber's *address*. A machine-written prescription is acceptable, but the prescriber's signature must be handwritten. Advanced electronic signatures can be accepted for Schedule 2 and 3 Controlled Drugs where the Electronic Prescribing Service (EPS) is used. All prescriptions for Controlled Drugs that are subject to the prescription requirements must always state:

- the name and address of the patient;
- in the case of a preparation, the form, (the dosage form e.g. tablets must be included on a Controlled Drugs prescription irrespective of whether it is implicit in the proprietary name e.g. *MST Continus* or whether only one form is available), and where appropriate the strength of the preparation (when more than one strength of a preparation exists the strength required must be specified);
- for liquids, the total volume in millilitres (in both words and figures) of the preparation to be supplied; for dosage units, the number (in both words and figures) of dosage units to be supplied; in any other case, the total quantity (in both words and figures) of the Controlled Drug to be supplied;
- the dose (the instruction 'one as directed' constitutes a dose but 'as directed' does not);
- the words 'for dental treatment only' if issued by a dentist.

A pharmacist is **not** allowed to dispense a Controlled Drug unless all the information required by law is given on the prescription. In the case of a prescription for a Controlled Drug in Schedule 2 or 3, a pharmacist can amend the prescription if it specifies the total quantity only in words or in figures or if it contains minor typographical errors, provided that such amendments are indelible and clearly attributable to the pharmacist (implementation date for *N. Ireland* not confirmed). Failure to comply with the regulations concerning the writing of prescriptions will result in inconvenience to patients and carers and delay in

Controlled drugs and drug dependence

supplying the necessary medicine. A prescription for a Controlled Drug in Schedules 2, 3, or 4 is valid for 28 days from the date stated thereon (the prescriber may forward-date the prescription; the start date may also be specified in the body of the prescription).

Instalments and 'repeats'

A prescription may order a Controlled Drug to be dispensed by instalments; the amount of instalments and the intervals to be observed must be specified. A total of 14 days' treatment by instalment of any drug listed in Schedule 2 of the Misuse of Drugs Regulations, buprenorphine p. 409, and diazepam p. 313 may be prescribed in England. In *England*, forms FP10(MDA) (blue) and FP10H(MDA) (blue) should be used. In *Scotland*, forms GP10 (peach), HBP (blue), or HBPA (pink) should be used. In *Wales* a total of 14 days' treatment by instalment of any drug listed in Schedules 2–5 of the Misuse of Drugs Regulations may be prescribed. In *Wales*, form WP10(MDA) or form WP10HP(AD) should be used. Instalment prescriptions must be dispensed in accordance with the directions in the prescription. However, the Home Office has approved specific wording which may be included in an instalment prescription to cover certain situations; for example, if a pharmacy is closed on the day when an instalment is due. For details, see *Medicines, Ethics and Practice*, London, Pharmaceutical Press (always consult latest edition) or see *Drug Misuse and Dependence: UK Guidelines on Clinical Management* (2007), available at www.nta.nhs.uk/uploads/clinical_guidelines_2007.pdf.

Prescriptions ordering 'repeats' on the same form are **not** permitted for Controlled Drugs in Schedules 2 or 3.

Private prescriptions

Private prescriptions for Controlled Drugs in Schedules 2 and 3 must be written on specially designated forms provided by Primary Care Trusts in England, Health Boards in Scotland, Local Health Boards in Wales, or the Northern Ireland Central Services Agency; in addition, prescriptions must specify the *prescriber's identification number*. Prescriptions to be supplied by a pharmacist in hospital are exempt from the requirements for private prescriptions.

Department of Health guidance

Guidance (June 2006) issued by the Department of Health in England on prescribing and dispensing of Controlled Drugs requires:

- in general, prescriptions for Controlled Drugs in Schedules 2, 3, and 4 to be limited to a supply of up to 30 days' treatment; exceptionally, to cover a justifiable clinical need and after consideration of any risk, a prescription can be issued for a longer period, but the reasons for the decision should be recorded on the patient's notes;
- the patient's identifier to be shown on NHS and private prescriptions for Controlled Drugs in Schedules 2 and 3.

Further information is available at www.gov.uk/dh.

See sample prescription:

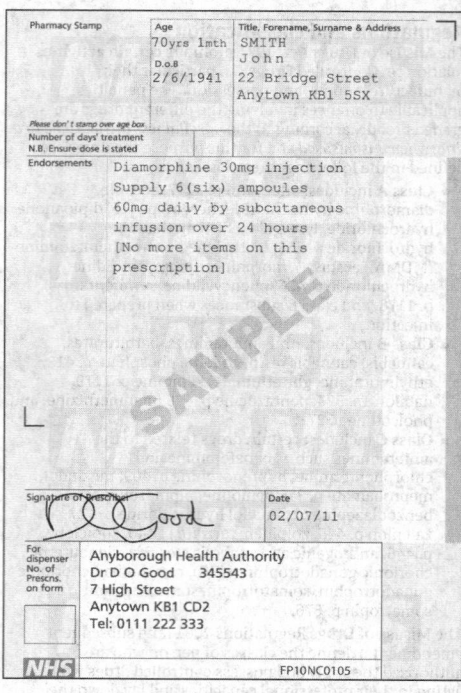

Dependence and misuse

The most serious drugs of addiction are **cocaine**, **diamorphine hydrochloride p. 415** (heroin), **morphine p. 421**, and the **synthetic opioids**. For arrangements for prescribing of diamorphine, dipipanone, or cocaine for addicts, see Prescribing of diamorphine (heroin), dipipanone, and cocaine for addicts.

Despite marked reduction in the prescribing of **amfetamines**, there is concern that abuse of illicit amfetamine and related compounds is widespread. **Benzodiazepines** are commonly misused. However, the misuse of **barbiturates** is now uncommon, in line with declining medicinal use and consequent availability. **Cannabis** (Indian hemp) has no approved medicinal use and cannot be prescribed by doctors. Its use is illegal but widespread. Cannabis is a mild hallucinogen seldom accompanied by a desire to increase the dose; withdrawal symptoms are unusual. However, cannabis extract is licensed as a medicinal product. **Lysergide** (lysergic acid diethylamide, LSD) is a much more potent hallucinogen; its use can lead to severe psychotic states which can be life-threatening.

There are concerns over increases in the availability and misuse of other drugs with variously combined hallucinogenic, anaesthetic, or sedative properties. These include ketamine p. 1179 and gamma-hydroxybutyrate (sodium oxybate, GHB).

Supervised consumption

Individuals prescribed opioid substitution therapy can take their daily dose under the supervision of a doctor, nurse, or pharmacist during the dose stabilisation phase (usually the first 3 months of treatment), after a relapse or period of instability, or if there is a significant increase in the dose of methadone. Supervised consumption should continue (in accordance with local protocols) until the prescriber is confident that the patient is compliant with their treatment.

Prescribing drugs likely to cause dependence or misuse

The prescriber has three main responsibilities:

- To avoid creating dependence by introducing drugs to patients without sufficient reason. In this context, the proper use of the morphine-like drugs is well understood. The dangers of other Controlled Drugs are less clear because recognition of dependence is not easy and its effects, and those of withdrawal, are less obvious.
- To see that the patient does not gradually increase the dose of a drug, given for good medical reasons, to the point where dependence becomes more likely. This tendency is seen especially with hypnotics and anxiolytics. The prescriber should keep a close eye on the amount prescribed to prevent patients from accumulating stocks. A minimal amount should be prescribed in the first instance, or when seeing a new patient for the first time.
- To avoid being used as an unwitting source of supply for addicts and being vigilant to methods for obtaining medicines. Methods include visiting more than one doctor, fabricating stories, and forging prescriptions.

Patients under temporary care should be given only small supplies of drugs unless they present an unequivocal letter from their own doctor. Doctors should also remember that their own patients may be attempting to collect prescriptions from other prescribers, especially in hospitals. It is sensible to reduce dosages steadily or to issue weekly or even daily prescriptions for small amounts if it is apparent that dependence is occurring.

The stealing and misuse of prescription forms could be minimised by the following precautions:

- do not leave unattended if called away from the consulting room or at reception desks; do not leave in a car where they may be visible; when not in use, keep in a locked drawer within the surgery and at home;
- draw a diagonal line across the blank part of the form under the prescription;
- write the quantity in words and figures when prescribing drugs prone to abuse; this is obligatory for controlled drugs;
- alterations are best avoided but if any are made they should be clear and unambiguous; add initials against altered items;
- if prescriptions are left for collection they should be left in a safe place in a sealed envelope.

Travelling abroad

Prescribed drugs listed in Schedule 4 Part II (CD Anab) and Schedule 5 of the Misuse of Drugs Regulations 2001 are not subject to export or import licensing. However, patients intending to travel abroad for more than 3 months carrying any amount of drugs listed in Schedules 2, 3, or 4 Part I (CD Benz) will require a personal export/import licence. Further details can be obtained at www.gov.uk/guidance/controlled-drugs-licences-fees-and-returns or from the Home Office by contacting licensing_enquiry.aadu@homeoffice.gsi.gov.uk. In cases of emergency, telephone (020) 7035 6330. Applications must be supported by a covering letter from the prescriber and should give details of:

- the patient's name and address;
- the quantities of drugs to be carried;
- the strength and form in which the drugs will be dispensed;
- the country or countries of destination;
- the dates of travel to and from the United Kingdom.

Applications for licences should be sent to the Home Office, Drugs Licensing & Compliance Unit, Fry Building, 2 Marsham Street, London, SW1P 4DF.
Alternatively, completed application forms can be emailed to dlcucommsofficer@homeoffice.gsi.gov.uk with a copy of the covering letter from the prescriber as a pdf. A minimum of two weeks should be allowed for processing the application. Patients travelling for less than 3 months do not require a personal export/import licence for carrying Controlled Drugs, but are advised to carry a letter from the prescribing doctor. Those travelling for more than 3 months are advised to make arrangements to have their medication prescribed by a practitioner in the country they are visiting.
Doctors who want to take Controlled Drugs abroad while accompanying patients may similarly be issued with licences. Licences are not normally issued to doctors who want to take Controlled Drugs abroad solely in case a family emergency should arise.
Personal export/import licences do not have any legal status outside the UK and are issued only to comply with the Misuse of Drugs Act and to facilitate passage through UK Customs and Excise control. For clearance in the country to be visited it is necessary to approach that country's consulate in the UK.

Notification of patients receiving structured drug treatment for substance dependence

In **England**, doctors should report cases where they are providing structured drug treatment for substance dependence to their local National Drug Treatment Monitoring System (NDTMS) Team. General information about NDTMS can be found at www.nta.nhs.uk/ndtms.aspx. Enquiries about NDTMS, and how to submit data, should initially be directed to
EvidenceApplicationTeam@phe.gov.uk

In **Scotland**, doctors should report cases to the Substance Misuse Programme (SMP).

Tel: (0131) 275 6348

In **Northern Ireland**, the Misuse of Drugs (Notification of and Supply to Addicts) (Northern Ireland) Regulations 1973 require doctors to send particulars of persons whom they consider to be addicted to certain controlled drugs to the Chief Medical Officer of the Department of Health and Social Services. The Northern Ireland contacts are:
Medical contact:

Dr Ian McMaster, C3 Castle Buildings, Belfast, BT4 3FQ
Tel: (028) 9052 2421, Fax: (028) 9052 0718
ian.mcmaster@dhsspsni.gov.uk

Administrative contact:

Public Health Information & Research Branch, Annex 2, Castle Building, Belfast, BT4 3SQ
Tel: (028) 9052 2520

Public Health Information & Research Branch also maintains the Northern Ireland Drug Misuse Database (NIDMD) which collects detailed information on those presenting for treatment, on drugs misused and injecting behaviour; participation is not a statutory requirement.
In **Wales**, doctors should report cases where they are providing structured drug treatment for substance dependence on the Welsh National Database for Substance Misuse; enquiries should be directed to: substance.misuse-queries@wales.nhs.uk.

Prescribing of diamorphine (heroin), dipipanone, and cocaine for addicts

The Misuse of Drugs (Supply to Addicts) Regulations 1997 require that only medical practitioners who hold a special licence issued by the Home Secretary may prescribe, administer, or supply diamorphine hydrochloride p. 415, dipipanone (*Diconal*®), or cocaine in the treatment of drug addiction; other practitioners must refer any addict who requires these drugs to a treatment centre. Whenever possible the addict will be introduced by a member of staff from the treatment centre to a pharmacist whose agreement has been obtained and whose pharmacy is conveniently sited for the patient. Prescriptions for weekly supplies will be sent to the pharmacy by post and will be dispensed on a daily basis as indicated by the doctor. If any alterations of the arrangements are requested by the addict, the portion of the prescription affected must be represcribed and not merely altered.

General practitioners and other doctors do not require a special licence for prescribing diamorphine hydrochloride p. 415, dipipanone, and cocaine for patients (including addicts) for *relieving pain* from organic disease or injury.

Adverse reactions to drugs

Yellow card scheme

Any drug may produce unwanted or unexpected adverse reactions. Rapid detection and recording of adverse drug reactions is of vital importance so that unrecognised hazards are identified promptly and appropriate regulatory action is taken to ensure that medicines are used safely. Healthcare professionals and coroners are urged to report suspected adverse drug reactions directly to the Medicines and Healthcare products Regulatory Agency (MHRA) through the Yellow Card Scheme using the electronic form at www.mhra.gov.uk/yellowcard. Alternatively, prepaid Yellow Cards for reporting are available from the address below and are also bound in the inside back cover of the BNF.

Send Yellow Cards to:

FREEPOST YELLOW CARD
(No other address details required).
Tel: 0800 731 6789

Suspected adverse drug reactions to any therapeutic agent should be reported, including drugs (self-medication as well as those prescribed), blood products, vaccines, radiographic contrast media, complementary and herbal products. For biosimilar medicines and vaccines, adverse reaction reports should clearly state the brand name and the batch number of the suspected medicine or vaccine.

Suspected adverse drug reactions should be reported through the Yellow Card Scheme at www.mhra.gov.uk/yellowcard. Yellow Cards can be used for reporting suspected adverse drug reactions to medicines, vaccines, herbal or complementary products, whether self-medicated or prescribed. This includes suspected adverse drug reactions associated with misuse, overdose, medication errors or from use of unlicensed and off-label medicines. Yellow Cards can also be used to report medical device incidents, defective medicines, and suspected fake medicines.

Spontaneous reporting is particularly valuable for recognising possible new hazards rapidly. An adverse reaction should be reported even if it is not certain that the drug has caused it, or if the reaction is well recognised, or if other drugs have been given at the same time. Reports of overdoses (deliberate or accidental) can complicate the assessment of adverse drug reactions, but provide important information on the potential toxicity of drugs.

A freephone service is available to all parts of the UK for advice and information on suspected adverse drug reactions; contact the National Yellow Card Information Service at the MHRA on 0800 731 6789. Outside office hours a telephone-answering machine will take messages.

The following Yellow Card Centres can be contacted for further information:

Yellow Card Centre Northwest
2nd Floor, 70 Pembroke Place, Liverpool, L69 3GF
Tel: (0151) 794 8122

Yellow Card Centre Wales
Cardiff University, Department of Pharmacology, Therapeutics and Toxicology, Heath Park, Cardiff, CF14 4XN
Tel: (029) 2074 4181

Yellow Card Centre Northern & Yorkshire
Regional Drug and Therapeutics Centre, 16/17 Framlington Place, Newcastle upon Tyne, NE2 4AB
Tel: (0191) 213 7855

Yellow Card Centre West Midlands
City Hospital, Dudley Road, Birmingham, B18 7QH
Tel: (0121) 507 5672

Yellow Card Centre Scotland
CARDS, Royal Infirmary of Edinburgh, 51 Little France Crescent, Old Dalkeith Road, Edinburgh, EH16 4SA
Tel: (0131) 242 2919
YCCScotland@luht.scot.nhs.uk

The MHRA's database facilitates the monitoring of adverse drug reactions. More detailed information on reporting and a list of products currently under additional monitoring can be found on the MHRA website: www.mhra.gov.uk.

MHRA Drug Safety Update

Drug Safety Update is a monthly newsletter from the MHRA and the Commission on Human Medicines (CHM); it is available at www.mhra.gov.uk/drugsafetyupdate.

Self-reporting

Patients and their carers can also report suspected adverse drug reactions to the MHRA. Reports can be submitted directly to the MHRA through the Yellow Card Scheme using the electronic form at www.mhra.gov.uk/yellowcard, by telephone on 0808 100 3352, or by downloading the Yellow Card form from www.mhra.gov.uk. Alternatively, patient Yellow Cards are available from pharmacies and GP surgeries. Information for patients about the Yellow Card Scheme is available in other languages at www.mhra.gov.uk/yellowcard.

Prescription-event monitoring

In addition to the MHRA's Yellow Card Scheme, an independent scheme monitors the safety of new medicines using a different approach. The Drug Safety Research Unit identifies patients who have been prescribed selected new medicines and collects data on clinical events in these patients. The data are submitted on a voluntary basis by general practitioners on green forms. More information about the scheme and the Unit's educational material is available from www.dsru.org.

Newer drugs and vaccines

Only limited information is available from clinical trials on the safety of new medicines. Further understanding about the safety of medicines depends on the availability of information from routine clinical practice.

The black triangle symbol identifies newly licensed medicines that require additional monitoring by the European Medicines Agency. Such medicines include new active substances, biosimilar medicines, and medicines that the European Medicines Agency consider require additional monitoring. The black triangle symbol also appears in the Patient Information Leaflets for relevant medicines, with a brief explanation of what it means. Products usually retain a black triangle for 5 years, but this can be extended if required.

Spontaneous reporting is particularly valuable for recognising possible new hazards rapidly. For medicines showing the black triangle symbol, the MHRA asks that **all** suspected reactions (including those considered not to be serious) are reported through the Yellow Card Scheme. An adverse reaction should be reported even if it is not certain that the drug has caused it, or if the reaction is well recognised, or if other drugs have been given at the same time.

Established drugs and vaccines

Healthcare professionals and coroners are asked to report all suspected reactions to established drugs (including over-the-counter, herbal, and unlicensed medicines and medicines used off-label) and vaccines that are **serious, medically significant, or result in harm.** Serious reactions include those that are fatal, life-threatening, disabling, incapacitating, or which result in or prolong hospitalisation, or a congenital abnormality; they should be reported even if the effect is well recognised. Examples include anaphylaxis, blood disorders, endocrine disturbances, effects on fertility, haemorrhage from any site, renal impairment, jaundice, ophthalmic disorders, severe CNS effects, severe skin reactions, reactions in pregnant women, and any drug interactions. Reports of serious adverse reactions are required to enable comparison with other drugs of a similar class. Reports of overdoses (deliberate or accidental) can complicate the assessment of adverse drug reactions, but provide important information on the potential toxicity of drugs.

For established drugs there is no need to report well-known, relatively minor side-effects, such as dry mouth with tricyclic antidepressants or constipation with opioids.

Medication errors

Adverse drug reactions where harm occurs as a result of a medication error are reportable as a Yellow Card or through the local risk management systems into the National Reporting and Learning System (NRLS). If reported to the NRLS, these will be shared with the MHRA. If the NRLS is not available and harm occurs, report using a Yellow Card.

Adverse reactions to medical devices

Suspected adverse reactions to medical devices including dental or surgical materials, intra-uterine devices, and contact lens fluids should be reported. Information on reporting these can be found at: www.mhra.gov.uk.

Side-effects in the BNF

The BNF includes clinically relevant side-effects for most drugs; an exhaustive list is not included for drugs that are used by specialists (e.g. cytotoxic drugs and drugs used in anaesthesia). Where causality has not been established, side-effects in the manufacturers' literature may be omitted from the BNF.

Recognising that hypersensitivity reactions can occur with virtually all medicines, this effect is not generally listed, unless the drug carries an increased risk of such reactions. The BNF also omits effects that are likely to have little clinical consequence (e.g. transient increase in liver enzymes).

Side-effects are generally listed in order of frequency and arranged broadly by body systems. Occasionally a rare side-effect might be listed first if it is considered to be particularly important because of its seriousness. In the product literature the frequency of side-effects is generally described as follows:

Description of the frequency of side-effects	
Very common	greater than 1 in 10
Common	1 in 100 to 1 in 10
Uncommon [formerly 'less commonly' in BNF publications]	1 in 1000 to 1 in 100
Rare	1 in 10 000 to 1 in 1000
Very rare	less than 1 in 10 000

Special problems

Delayed drug effects Some reactions (e.g. cancers, chloroquine retinopathy, and retroperitoneal fibrosis) may become manifest months or years after exposure. Any suspicion of such an association should be reported directly to the MHRA through the Yellow Card Scheme.

The elderly Particular vigilance is required to identify adverse reactions in the elderly.

Congenital abnormalities When an infant is born with a congenital abnormality or there is a malformed aborted fetus doctors are asked to consider whether this might be an adverse reaction to a drug and to report all drugs (including self-medication) taken during pregnancy.

Children Particular vigilance is required to identify and report adverse reactions in children, including those resulting from the unlicensed use of medicines; **all** suspected reactions should be reported directly to the MHRA through the Yellow Card Scheme (see also Adverse Drug Reactions in Children).

Prevention of adverse reactions

Adverse reactions may be prevented as follows:

- never use any drug unless there is a good indication. If the patient is pregnant do not use a drug unless the need for it is imperative;
- allergy and idiosyncrasy are important causes of adverse drug reactions. Ask if the patient had previous reactions to the drug or formulation;
- ask if the patient is already taking other drugs including self-medication drugs, health supplements, complementary and alternative therapies; interactions may occur;
- age and hepatic or renal disease may alter the metabolism or excretion of drugs, so that much smaller doses may be needed. Genetic factors may also be responsible for variations in metabolism, and therefore for the adverse effect of the drug; notably of isoniazid p. 532 and the tricyclic antidepressants;
- prescribe as few drugs as possible and give very clear instructions to the elderly or any patient likely to misunderstand complicated instructions;
- whenever possible use a familiar drug; with a new drug, be particularly alert for adverse reactions or unexpected events;
- consider if excipients (e.g. colouring agents) may be contributing to the adverse reaction. If the reaction is minor, a trial of an alternative formulation of the same drug may be considered before abandoning the drug;
- warn the patient if serious adverse reactions are liable to occur.

Drug allergy (suspected or confirmed)

Suspected drug allergy is any reaction caused by a drug with clinical features compatible with an immunological mechanism. All drugs have the potential to cause adverse drug reactions, but not all of these are allergic in nature. A reaction is more likely to be caused by drug allergy if:

- The reaction occurred while the patient was being treated with the drug, or
- The drug is known to cause this pattern of reaction, or
- The patient has had a similar reaction to the same drug or drug-class previously.

A suspected reaction is less likely to be caused by a drug allergy if there is a possible non-drug cause or if there are only gastro-intestinal symptoms present.

The following signs, allergic patterns and timing of onset can be used to help decide whether to suspect drug allergy:

Immediate, rapidly-evolving reactions (onset usually less than 1 hour after drug exposure)

- Anaphylaxis, with erythema, urticaria or angioedema, and hypotension and/or bronchospasm. See also Antihistamines, allergen immunotherapy and allergic emergencies p. 253
- Urticaria or angioedema without systemic features
- Exacerbation of asthma e.g. with non-steroidal anti-inflammatory drugs (NSAIDs)

*Non-immediate reactions, **without** systemic involvement* (onset usually 6–10 days after first drug exposure or 3 days after second exposure)

- Cutaneous reactions, e.g. widespread red macules and/or papules, or, fixed drug eruption (localised inflamed skin)

*Non-immediate reactions, **with** systemic involvement* (onset may be variable, usually 3 days to 6 weeks after first drug exposure, depending on features, or 3 days after second exposure)

- Cutaneous reactions with systemic features, e.g. drug reaction with eosinophilia and systemic signs (DRESS) or drug hypersensitivity syndrome (DHS), characterised by widespread red macules, papules or erythroderma, fever, lymphadenopathy, liver dysfunction or eosinophilia
- Toxic epidermal necrolysis or Stevens–Johnson syndrome
- Acute generalised exanthematous pustulosis (AGEP)

EvGr Suspected drug allergy information should be clearly and accurately documented in clinical notes and prescriptions, and shared among all healthcare professionals. Patients should be given information about which drugs and drug-classes to avoid and encouraged to share their drug allergy status. ◇

EvGr If a drug allergy is suspected, consider stopping the suspected drug and advising the patient or carer to avoid this drug in future. Symptoms of the acute reaction should be treated, in hospital if severe. Patients presenting with a suspected anaphylactic reaction, or a severe or non-immediate cutaneous reaction, should be referred to a specialist drug allergy service. Patients presenting with a suspected drug allergic reaction or anaphylaxis to NSAIDs, and local and general anaesthetics may also need to be referred to a specialist drug allergy service, e.g. in cases of anaphylactoid reactions or to determine future treatment options. Patients presenting with a suspected drug allergic reaction or anaphylaxis associated with beta-lactam antibiotics should be referred to a specialist drug allergy service if their disease or condition can only be treated by a beta-lactam antibiotic or they are likely to need beta-lactam antibiotics frequently in the future (e.g. immunodeficient patients). ◇ For further information see Drug allergy: diagnosis and management. NICE Clinical Guideline 183 (September 2014) www.nice.org.uk/guidance/cg183.

Oral side-effects of drugs

Drug-induced disorders of the mouth may be due to a local action on the mouth or to a systemic effect manifested by oral changes. In the latter case urgent referral to the patient's medical practitioner may be necessary.

Oral mucosa Medicaments left in contact with or applied directly to the oral mucosa can lead to inflammation or ulceration; the possibility of allergy should also be borne in mind.

Aspirin tablets p. 109 allowed to dissolve in the sulcus for the treatment of toothache can lead to a white patch followed by ulceration.

Flavouring agents, particularly **essential oils**, may sensitise the skin, but mucosal swelling is not usually prominent.

The oral mucosa is particularly vulnerable to ulceration in patients treated with cytotoxic drugs, e.g. methotrexate p. 807. Other drugs capable of causing oral ulceration include **ACE inhibitors, gold, nicorandil p. 194, NSAIDs, pancreatin p. 85, penicillamine p. 952, proguanil hydrochloride p. 562,** and **protease inhibitors**.

Erythema multiforme or Stevens-Johnson syndrome may follow the use of a wide range of drugs including **antibacterials, antiretrovirals, sulfonamide derivatives,** and **anticonvulsants**; the oral mucosa may be extensively ulcerated, with characteristic target lesions on the skin. Oral lesions of toxic epidermal necrolysis have been reported with a similar range of drugs.

Lichenoid eruptions are associated with **ACE inhibitors, NSAIDs,** methyldopa p. 131, chloroquine p. 560, **oral antidiabetics, thiazide diuretics,** and **gold**.

Candidiasis can complicate treatment with **antibacterials** and **immunosuppressants** and is an occasional side-effect of **corticosteroid inhalers**.

Teeth and jaw *Brown staining* of the teeth frequently follows the use of chlorhexidine mouthwash, spray or gel p. 1053, but can readily be removed by polishing. **Iron** salts in liquid form can stain the enamel black. Superficial staining has been reported rarely with co-amoxiclav suspension p. 501. *Intrinsic staining* of the teeth is most commonly caused by **tetracyclines**. They will affect the teeth if given at any time from about the fourth month *in utero* until the age of twelve years; they are contra-indicated during pregnancy, in breast-feeding women, and in children under 12 years. All tetracyclines can cause permanent, unsightly staining in children, the colour varying from yellow to grey.

Excessive ingestion of **fluoride** leads to *dental fluorosis* with mottling of the enamel and areas of hypoplasia or pitting; fluoride supplements occasionally cause mild mottling (white patches) if the dose is too large for the child's age (taking into account the fluoride content of the local drinking water and of toothpaste).

The risk of *osteonecrosis of the jaw* is substantially greater for patients receiving intravenous bisphosphonates in the treatment of cancer than for patients receiving oral bisphosphonates for osteoporosis or Paget's disease. All patients receiving bisphosphonates should have a dental check-up (and any necessary remedial work should be performed) before bisphosphonate treatment, or as soon as possible after starting treatment. Patients with cancer receiving bevacizumab p. 774 or sunitinib p. 863 may also be at risk of osteonecrosis of the jaw.

Periodontium *Gingival overgrowth* (gingival hyperplasia) is a side-effect of phenytoin p. 294 and sometimes of ciclosporin p. 758 or of nifedipine p. 148 (and some other calcium-channel blockers).

Thrombocytopenia may be drug related and may cause bleeding at the gingival margins, which may be spontaneous or may follow mild trauma (such as toothbrushing).

Salivary glands The most common effect that drugs have on the salivary glands is to *reduce flow* (xerostomia). Patients with a persistently dry mouth may have poor oral hygiene; they are at an increased risk of dental caries and oral infections (particularly candidiasis). Many drugs have been implicated in xerostomia, particularly **antimuscarinics** (anticholinergics), **antidepressants** (including tricyclic antidepressants, and selective serotonin re-uptake inhibitors), **alpha-blockers, antihistamines, antipsychotics, baclofen p. 973, bupropion hydrochloride p. 453, clonidine hydrochloride p. 131, $5HT_1$ agonists, opioids,** and tizanidine p. 974. Excessive use of **diuretics** can also result in xerostomia.

Some drugs (e.g. clozapine p. 363, neostigmine p. 971) can *increase saliva production* but this is rarely a problem unless the patient has associated difficulty in swallowing.

Pain in the salivary glands has been reported with some **antihypertensives** (e.g. clonidine hydrochloride p. 131, methyldopa p. 131) and with **vinca alkaloids**.

Swelling of the salivary glands can occur with **iodides, antithyroid drugs, phenothiazines,** and **sulfonamides**.

Taste There can be *decreased* taste acuity or *alteration* in taste sensation. Many drugs are implicated, including amiodarone hydrochloride p. 94, **calcitonin, ACE inhibitors**, carbimazole p. 698, clarithromycin p. 487, **gold,** griseofulvin p. 545, **lithium salts,** metformin hydrochloride p. 624, metronidazole p. 492, penicillamine p. 952, phenindione p. 126, propafenone hydrochloride p. 93, **protease inhibitors,** terbinafine p. 1079, and zopiclone p. 446.

Defective medicines

During the manufacture or distribution of a medicine an error or accident may occur whereby the finished product does not conform to its specification. While such a defect may impair the therapeutic effect of the product and could adversely affect the health of a patient, it should **not** be confused with an Adverse Drug Reaction where the product conforms to its specification.

The Defective Medicines Report Centre assists with the investigation of problems arising from licensed medicinal products thought to be defective and co-ordinates any necessary protective action. Reports on suspect defective medicinal products should include the brand or the non-proprietary name, the name of the manufacturer or supplier, the strength and dosage form of the product, the product licence number, the batch number or numbers of the product, the nature of the defect, and an account of any action already taken in consequence. The Centre can be contacted at:

The Defective Medicines Report Centre
Medicines and Healthcare products Regulatory Agency,
151 Buckingham Palace Road, London, SW1W 9SZ
Tel: (020) 3080 6574
dmrc@mhra.gsi.gov.uk

Guidance on intravenous infusions

Intravenous additives policies

A local policy on the addition of drugs to intravenous fluids should be drawn up by a multi-disciplinary team in each Strategic Health Authority (or equivalent) and issued as a document to the members of staff concerned.

Centralised additive services are provided in a number of hospital pharmacy departments and should be used in preference to making additions on wards.

The information that follows should be read in conjunction with local policy documents.

Guidelines

- Drugs should only be added to infusion containers when constant plasma concentrations are needed or when the administration of a more concentrated solution would be harmful.
- In general, only one drug should be added to any infusion container and the components should be compatible. Ready-prepared solutions should be used whenever possible. Drugs should not normally be added to blood products, mannitol, or sodium bicarbonate. Only specially formulated additives should be used with fat emulsions or amino-acid solutions.
- Solutions should be thoroughly mixed by shaking and checked for absence of particulate matter before use.
- Strict asepsis should be maintained throughout and in general the giving set should not be used for more than 24 hours (for drug admixtures).
- The infusion container should be labelled with the patient's name, the name and quantity of additives, and the date and time of addition (and the new expiry date or time). Such additional labelling should not interfere with information on the manufacturer's label that is still valid. When possible, containers should be retained for a period after use in case they are needed for investigation.
- It is good practice to examine intravenous infusions from time to time while they are running. If cloudiness, crystallisation, change of colour, or any other sign of interaction or contamination is observed the infusion should be discontinued.

Problems

Microbial contamination The accidental entry and subsequent growth of micro-organisms converts the infusion fluid pathway into a potential vehicle for infection with micro-organisms, particularly species of *Candida*, *Enterobacter*, and *Klebsiella*. Ready-prepared infusions containing the additional drugs, or infusions prepared by an additive service (when available) should therefore be used in preference to making extemporaneous additions to infusion containers on wards etc. However, when this is necessary strict aseptic procedure should be followed.

Incompatibility Physical and chemical incompatibilities may occur with loss of potency, increase in toxicity, or other adverse effect. The solutions may become opalescent or precipitation may occur, but in many instances there is no visual indication of incompatibility. Interaction may take place at any point in the infusion fluid pathway, and the potential for incompatibility is increased when more than one substance is added to the infusion fluid.

Common incompatibilities Precipitation reactions are numerous and varied and may occur as a result of pH, concentration changes, 'salting-out' effects, complexation or other chemical changes. Precipitation or other particle formation must be avoided since, apart from lack of control of dosage on administration, it may initiate or exacerbate adverse effects. This is particularly important in the case of

drugs which have been implicated in either thrombophlebitis (e.g. diazepam) or in skin sloughing or necrosis caused by extravasation (e.g. sodium bicarbonate and certain cytotoxic drugs). It is also especially important to effect solution of colloidal drugs and to prevent their subsequent precipitation in order to avoid a pyrogenic reaction (e.g. amphotericin).

It is considered undesirable to mix beta-lactam antibiotics, such as semi-synthetic penicillins and cephalosporins, with proteinaceous materials on the grounds that immunogenic and allergenic conjugates could be formed.

A number of preparations undergo significant loss of potency when added singly or in combination to large volume infusions. Examples include ampicillin in infusions that contain glucose or lactates. The breakdown products of dacarbazine have been implicated in adverse effects.

Blood Because of the large number of incompatibilities, drugs should not normally be added to blood and blood products for infusion purposes. Examples of incompatibility with blood include hypertonic mannitol solutions (irreversible crenation of red cells), dextrans (rouleaux formation and interference with cross-matching), glucose (clumping of red cells), and oxytocin (inactivated).

If the giving set is not changed after the administration of blood, but used for other infusion fluids, a fibrin clot may form which, apart from blocking the set, increases the likelihood of microbial growth.

Intravenous fat emulsions These may break down with coalescence of fat globules and separation of phases when additions such as antibacterials or electrolytes are made, thus increasing the possibility of embolism. Only specially formulated products such as *Vitlipid N®* may be added to appropriate intravenous fat emulsions.

Other infusions Infusions that frequently give rise to incompatibility include amino acids, mannitol, and sodium bicarbonate.

Bactericides Bactericides such as chlorocresol 0.1% or phenylmercuric nitrate 0.001% are present in some injection solutions. The total volume of such solutions added to a container for infusion on one occasion should not exceed 15 mL.

Method

Ready-prepared infusions should be used whenever available. **Potassium chloride** is usually available in concentrations of 20, 27, and 40 mmol/litre in sodium chloride intravenous infusion (0.9%), glucose intravenous infusion (5%) or sodium chloride and glucose intravenous infusion. **Lidocaine hydrochloride** is usually available in concentrations of 0.1 or 0.2% in glucose intravenous infusion (5%).

When addition is required to be made extemporaneously, any product reconstitution instructions such as those relating to concentration, vehicle, mixing, and handling precautions should be strictly followed using an aseptic technique throughout. Once the product has been reconstituted, addition to the infusion fluid should be made immediately in order to minimise microbial contamination and, with certain products, to prevent degradation or other formulation change which may occur; e.g. reconstituted ampicillin injection degrades rapidly on standing, and also may form polymers which could cause sensitivity reactions. It is also important in certain instances that an infusion fluid of specific pH be used (e.g. **furosemide** injection requires dilution in infusions of pH greater than 5.5).

When drug additions are made it is important to mix thoroughly; additions should not be made to an infusion container that has been connected to a giving set, as mixing is hampered. If the solutions are not thoroughly mixed a concentrated layer of the additive may form owing to differences in density. **Potassium chloride** is particularly prone to this 'layering' effect when added without adequate mixing to infusions packed in non-rigid infusion containers; if such a mixture is administered it may have a serious effect on the heart.

A time limit between addition and completion of administration must be imposed for certain admixtures to guarantee satisfactory drug potency and compatibility. For admixtures in which degradation occurs without the formation of toxic substances, an acceptable limit is the time taken for 10% decomposition of the drug. When toxic substances are produced stricter limits may be imposed. Because of the risk of microbial contamination a maximum time limit of 24 hours may be appropriate for additions made elsewhere than in hospital pharmacies offering central additive service.

Certain injections must be protected from light during continuous infusion to minimise oxidation, e.g. dacarbazine and sodium nitroprusside.

Dilution with a small volume of an appropriate vehicle and administration using a motorised infusion pump is advocated for preparations such as unfractionated heparin where strict control over administration is required. In this case the appropriate dose may be dissolved in a convenient volume (e.g. 24–48 mL) of sodium chloride intravenous infusion (0.9%).

Information provided in the *BNF*

The *BNF* gives information about preparations given by three methods:

- continuous infusion;
- intermittent infusion;
- addition via the drip tubing.

Drugs for **continuous infusion** must be diluted in a large volume infusion. Penicillins and cephalosporins are not usually given by continuous infusion because of stability problems and because adequate plasma and tissue concentrations are best obtained by intermittent infusion. Where it is necessary to administer them by continuous infusion, detailed literature should be consulted.

Drugs that are both compatible and clinically suitable may be given by **intermittent infusion** in a relatively small volume of infusion over a short period of time, e.g. 100 mL in 30 minutes. The method is used if the product is incompatible or unstable over the period necessary for continuous infusion; the limited stability of ampicillin or amoxicillin in large volume glucose or lactate infusions may be overcome in this way.

Intermittent infusion is also used if adequate plasma and tissue concentrations are not produced by continuous infusion as in the case of drugs such as dacarbazine, gentamicin, and ticarcillin.

An in-line burette may be used for intermittent infusion techniques in order to achieve strict control over the time and rate of administration, especially for infants and children and in intensive care units. Intermittent infusion may also make use of the 'piggy-back' technique provided that no additions are made to the primary infusion. In this method the drug is added to a small secondary container connected to a Y-type injection site on the primary infusion giving set; the secondary solution is usually infused within 30 minutes.

Addition *via* the drip tubing is indicated for a number of cytotoxic drugs in order to minimise extravasation. The preparation is added aseptically via the rubber septum of the injection site of a fast-running infusion. In general, drug preparations intended for a bolus effect should be given directly into a separate vein where possible. Failing this, administration may be made via the drip tubing provided that the preparation is compatible with the infusion fluid when given in this manner.

Drugs given by intravenous infusion The BNF includes information on addition to *Glucose intravenous infusion* 5 and 10%, and *Sodium chloride intravenous infusion* 0.9%. Compatibility with glucose 5% and with sodium chloride 0.9% indicates compatibility with *Sodium chloride and glucose intravenous infusion*. Infusion of a large volume of hypotonic solution should be avoided therefore care should be taken if water for injections is used. The information relates to the proprietary preparations indicated; for other preparations suitability should be checked with the manufacturer.

Prescribing in children

Overview
For detailed advice on medicines used for children, consult *BNF for Children*.

Children, and particularly neonates, differ from adults in their response to drugs. Special care is needed in the neonatal period (first 28 days of life) and doses should always be calculated with care. At this age, the risk of toxicity is increased by reduced drug clearance and differing target organ sensitivity.

Whenever possible, intramuscular injections should be **avoided** in children because they are painful.

Where possible, medicines for children should be prescribed within the terms of the marketing authorisation (product licence). However, many children may require medicines not specifically licensed for paediatric use.

Although medicines cannot be promoted outside the limits of the licence, the Human Medicines Regulations 2012 does not prohibit the use of unlicensed medicines. It is recognised that the informed use of unlicensed medicines or of licensed medicines for unlicensed applications ('off-label' use) is often necessary in paediatric practice.

Adverse drug reactions in children
Suspected adverse drug reactions in children and young adults under 18 years should be reported through the Yellow Card Scheme. Yellow cards can be used for reporting suspected adverse drug reactions to medicines, vaccines, herbal or complementary products, whether self-medicated or prescribed. This includes suspected adverse drug reactions associated with misuse, overdose, medication errors or from use of unlicensed and off-label medicines. Yellow Cards can also be used to report medical device incidents, defective medicines, and suspected fake medicines.

Report all suspected adverse drug reactions that are:

- **serious, medically significant or result in harm.** Serious events are fatal, life-threatening, a congenital abnormality, disabling or incapacitating, or resulting in hospitalisation;
- associated with **newer drugs and vaccines;** the most up to date list of black triangle medicines is available at: www.mhra.gov.uk/blacktriangle

If in doubt whether to report a suspected adverse drug reaction, please complete a Yellow Card.

The identification and reporting of adverse reactions to drugs in children and neonates is particularly important because:

- the action of the drug and its pharmacokinetics in children (especially in the very young) may be different from that in adults;
- drugs may not have been extensively tested in children;
- many drugs are not specifically licensed for use in children and are used either 'off-label' or as unlicensed products;
- drugs may affect the way a child grows and develops or may cause delayed adverse reactions which do not occur in adults;
- suitable formulations may not be available to allow precise dosing in children or they may contain excipients that should be used with caution in children;
- the nature and course of illnesses and adverse drug reactions may differ between adults and children.

Even if reported through the British Paediatric Surveillance Unit's Orange Card Scheme, any identified suspected adverse drug reactions should also be submitted to the Yellow Card Scheme.

Adverse drug reactions where harm occurs as a result of a medication error are reportable as a Yellow Card or through the local risk management systems into the National Reporting and Learning System (NRLS). If reported to the NRLS, these will be shared with the MHRA. If the NRLS is not available and harm occurs, report using a Yellow Card.

Prescription writing
Prescriptions should be written according to the guidelines in Prescription Writing. Inclusion of age is a legal requirement in the case of prescription-only medicines for children under 12 years of age, but it is preferable to state the age for **all** prescriptions for children.

It is particularly important to state the strengths of capsules or tablets. Although liquid preparations are particularly suitable for children, they may contain sugar which encourages dental decay. Sugar-free medicines are preferred for long-term treatment.

Many children are able to swallow tablets or capsules and may prefer a solid dose form; involving the child and parents in choosing the formulation is helpful.

When a prescription for a liquid oral preparation is written and the dose ordered is smaller than 5 mL an **oral syringe** will be supplied. Parents should be advised not to add any medicines to the infant's feed, since the drug may interact with the milk or other liquid in it; moreover the ingested dosage may be reduced if the child does not drink all the contents.

Parents must be warned to keep **all** medicines out of reach of children.

Rare paediatric conditions
Information on substances such as *biotin* and *sodium benzoate* used in rare metabolic conditions is included in *BNF for Children*; further information can be obtained from:

Alder Hey Children's Hospital
Drug Information Centre, Liverpool, L12 2AP
Tel: (0151) 252 5381

Great Ormond Street Hospital for Children
Pharmacy, Great Ormond St, London, WC1N 3JH
Tel: (020) 7405 9200

Dosage in children
Children's doses in the BNF are stated in the individual drug entries.

Doses are generally based on body-weight (in kilograms) or specific age ranges. In the BNF and BNF for *Children*, the term neonate is used to describe a newborn infant aged 0–28 days. The terms child or children are used generically to describe the entire range from infant to adolescent (1 month–17 years). An age range is specified when the dose information applies to a narrower age range than a child from 1 month–17 years.

Dose calculation
Many children's doses are standardised by **weight** (and therefore require multiplying by the body-weight in kilograms to determine the child's dose); occasionally, the doses have been standardised by **body surface area** (in m²). These methods should be used rather than attempting to calculate a child's dose on the basis of doses used in adults. For most drugs the adult maximum dose should not be exceeded. For example if the dose is stated as 8 mg/kg (max. 300 mg), a child weighing 10 kg should receive 80 mg but a child weighing 40 kg should receive 300 mg (rather than 320 mg).

Young children may require a higher dose per kilogram than adults because of their higher metabolic rates. Other problems need to be considered. For example, calculation by body-weight in the overweight child may result in much higher doses being administered than necessary; in such

Prescribing in hepatic impairment

cases, dose should be calculated from an ideal weight, related to height and age.

Body surface area (BSA) estimates are sometimes preferable to body-weight for calculation of paediatric doses since many physiological phenomena correlate better with body surface area. Body surface area can be estimated from weight. For more information, refer to *BNF for Children*. Where the dose for children is not stated, prescribers should consult *BNF for Children* or seek advice from a medicines information centre.

Dose frequency
Antibacterials are generally given at regular intervals throughout the day. Some flexibility should be allowed in children to avoid waking them during the night. For example, the night-time dose may be given at the child's bedtime.

Where new or potentially toxic drugs are used, the manufacturers' recommended doses should be carefully followed.

Prescribing in hepatic impairment

Overview
Liver disease may alter the response to drugs in several ways as indicated below, and drug prescribing should be kept to a minimum in all patients with severe liver disease. The main problems occur in patients with jaundice, ascites, or evidence of encephalopathy.

Impaired drug metabolism
Metabolism by the liver is the main route of elimination for many drugs, but hepatic reserve is large and liver disease has to be severe before important changes in drug metabolism occur. Routine liver-function tests are a poor guide to the capacity of the liver to metabolise drugs, and in the individual patient it is not possible to predict the extent to which the metabolism of a particular drug may be impaired. A few drugs, e.g. rifampicin p. 527 and fusidic acid p. 519, are excreted in the bile unchanged and can accumulate in patients with intrahepatic or extrahepatic obstructive jaundice.

Hypoproteinaemia
The hypoalbuminaemia in severe liver disease is associated with reduced protein binding and increased toxicity of some highly protein-bound drugs such as phenytoin p. 294 and prednisolone p. 614.

Reduced clotting
Reduced hepatic synthesis of blood-clotting factors, indicated by a prolonged prothrombin time, increases the

sensitivity to oral anticoagulants such as warfarin sodium p. 126 and phenindione p. 126.

Hepatic encephalopathy
In severe liver disease many drugs can further impair cerebral function and may precipitate hepatic encephalopathy. These include all sedative drugs, opioid analgesics, those diuretics that produce hypokalaemia, and drugs that cause constipation.

Fluid overload
Oedema and ascites in chronic liver disease can be exacerbated by drugs that give rise to fluid retention e.g. NSAIDs and corticosteroids.

Hepatotoxic drugs
Hepatotoxicity is either dose-related or unpredictable (idiosyncratic). Drugs that cause dose-related toxicity may do so at lower doses in the presence of hepatic impairment than in individuals with normal liver function, and some drugs that produce reactions of the idiosyncratic kind do so more frequently in patients with liver disease. These drugs should be avoided or used very carefully in patients with liver disease.

Where care is needed when prescribing in hepatic impairment, this is indicated under the relevant drug in the BNF.

Prescribing in renal impairment

Issues encountered in renal impairment
The use of drugs in patients with reduced renal function can give rise to problems for several reasons:

- reduced renal excretion of a drug or its metabolites may cause toxicity;
- sensitivity to some drugs is increased even if elimination is unimpaired;
- many side-effects are tolerated poorly by patients with renal impairment;
- some drugs are not effective when renal function is reduced.

Many of these problems can be avoided by reducing the dose or by using alternative drugs.

Principles of dose adjustment in renal impairment
The level of renal function below which the dose of a drug must be reduced depends on the proportion of the drug eliminated by renal excretion and its toxicity.

For many drugs with only minor or no dose-related side-effects very precise modification of the dose regimen is unnecessary and a simple scheme for dose reduction is sufficient.

For more toxic drugs with a small safety margin or patients at extremes of weight, dose regimens based on creatinine clearance should be used. When both efficacy and toxicity are closely related to plasma-drug concentration, recommended regimens should be regarded only as a guide to initial treatment; subsequent doses must be adjusted according to clinical response and plasma-drug concentration.

Renal function declines with age; many elderly patients have renal impairment but, because of reduced muscle mass, this may not be indicated by a raised serum creatinine. It is wise to assume at least mild impairment of renal function when prescribing for the elderly.

The total daily maintenance dose of a drug can be reduced either by reducing the size of the individual doses or by increasing the interval between doses. For some drugs, although the size of the maintenance dose is reduced it is important to give a loading dose if an immediate effect is required. This is because it takes about five times the half-life of the drug to achieve steady-state plasma concentrations. Because the plasma half-life of drugs excreted by the kidney is prolonged in renal impairment it can take many doses for the reduced dosage to achieve a therapeutic plasma concentration. The loading dose should usually be the same size as the initial dose for a patient with normal renal function.

Nephrotoxic drugs should, if possible, be avoided in patients with renal disease because the consequences of nephrotoxicity are likely to be more serious when renal reserve is already reduced.

Dose recommendations are based on the severity of renal impairment.

Renal function is measured either in terms of estimated **glomerular filtration rate** (eGFR) calculated from a formula derived from the Modification of Diet in Renal Disease study ('MDRD formula' that uses serum creatinine, age, sex, and race (for Afro-Caribbean patients)) or it can be expressed as **creatinine clearance** (best derived from a 24-hour urine collection but often calculated from the Cockcroft and Gault formula (CG).

Cockcroft and Gault Formula

$$\text{Estimated Creatinine Clearance in mL/minute} = \frac{(140 - \text{Age}) \times \text{Weight} \times \text{Constant}}{\text{Serum creatinine}}$$

Age in years
Weight in kilograms; use ideal body-weight
Serum creatinine in micromol/litre
Constant = 1.23 for men; 1.04 for women

The serum-creatinine concentration is sometimes used instead as a measure of renal function but it is only a **rough guide** to drug dosing.

Important Renal function in adults is increasingly being reported on the basis of estimated glomerular filtration rate (eGFR) normalised to a body surface area of $1.73\,m^2$ and derived from the Modification of Diet in Renal Disease (MDRD) formula. However, published information on the effects of renal impairment on drug elimination is usually stated in terms of creatinine clearance as a surrogate for glomerular filtration rate (GFR).

The information on dosage adjustment in the BNF is expressed in terms of eGFR, rather than creatinine clearance, for most drugs (exceptions include toxic drugs and patients at extremes of weight). Although the two measures of renal function are not interchangeable, in practice, for most drugs and for most patients (over 18 years) of average build and height, eGFR (MDRD 'formula') can be used to determine dosage adjustments in place of creatinine clearance. An individual's absolute glomerular filtration rate can be calculated from the eGFR as follows: $\text{GFR}_{\text{Absolute}} = \text{eGFR} \times$ (individual's body surface area/1.73)

Toxic drugs For potentially toxic drugs with a small safety margin, creatinine clearance (calculated from the Cockcroft and Gault formula) should be used to adjust drug dosages in addition to plasma-drug concentration and clinical response.

Patients at extremes of weight In patients at both extremes of weight (BMI of less than $18.5\,kg/m^2$ or greater than $30\,kg/m^2$) the absolute glomerular filtration rate or creatinine clearance (calculated from the Cockcroft and Gault formula) should be used to adjust drug dosages. In the BNF, values for eGFR, creatinine clearance (for toxic drugs), or another measure of renal function are included where possible. However, where such values are not available, the BNF reflects the terms used in the published information.

Degrees of renal impairment defined using estimated glomerular filtration rate (eGFR)

Chronic kidney disease in adults: UK guidelines for identification, management and referral (March 2006) define renal function as follows:	
Degree of impairment	eGFR mL/minute/$1.73\,m^2$
Normal - Stage 1	More than 90 (with other evidence of kidney damage)
Mild - Stage 2	60–89 (with other evidence of kidney damage)
Moderate[1]- Stage 3	30–59
Severe - Stage 4	15–29
Established renal failure - Stage 5	Less than 15

1. NICE clinical guideline 73 (September 2008)—Chronic kidney disease: Stage 3A eGFR 45-59, Stage 3B eGFR 30-44

Drug prescribing should be kept to the minimum in all patients with severe renal disease.

If even mild renal impairment is considered likely on clinical grounds, renal function should be checked before prescribing **any** drug which requires dose modification. Where care is needed when prescribing in renal impairment, this is indicated under the relevant drug in the BNF.

Dialysis

For prescribing in patients on continuous ambulatory peritoneal dialysis (CAPD) or haemodialysis, consult specialist literature.

Prescribing in pregnancy

Overview

Drugs can have harmful effects on the embryo or fetus at any time during pregnancy. It is important to bear this in mind when prescribing for a woman of *childbearing age* or for men *trying* to *father* a child.

During the *first trimester* drugs can produce congenital malformations (teratogenesis), and the period of greatest risk is from the third to the eleventh week of pregnancy. During the *second* and *third trimesters* drugs can affect the growth or functional development of the fetus, or they can have toxic effects on fetal tissues.

Drugs given shortly before term or during labour can have adverse effects on labour or on the neonate after delivery.

Not all the damaging effects of intra-uterine exposure to drugs are obvious at birth, some may only manifest later in life. Such late-onset effects include malignancy, e.g. adenocarcinoma of the vagina after puberty in females exposed to diethylstilbestrol in the womb, and adverse effects on intellectual, social, and functional development. The BNF and *BNF for Children* identifies drugs which:

- may have harmful effects in pregnancy and indicates the trimester of risk
- are not known to be harmful in pregnancy

The information is based on human data, but information from *animal* studies has been included for some drugs when its omission might be misleading. Maternal drug doses may require adjustment during pregnancy due to changes in maternal physiology but this is beyond the scope of the *BNF* and *BNF for Children*.

Where care is needed when prescribing in pregnancy, this is indicated under the relevant drug in the BNF and *BNF for Children*.

Important

Drugs should be prescribed in pregnancy only if the expected benefit to the mother is thought to be greater than the risk to the fetus, and all drugs should be avoided if possible during the first trimester. Drugs which have been extensively used in pregnancy and appear to be usually safe should be prescribed in preference to new or untried drugs; and the smallest effective dose should be used. Few drugs have been shown conclusively to be teratogenic in humans, but no drug is safe beyond all doubt in early pregnancy. Screening procedures are available when there is a known risk of certain defects.

Absence of information does not imply safety. It should be noted that the BNF and *BNF for Children* provide independent advice and may not always agree with the product literature.

Information on drugs and pregnancy is also available from the UK Teratology Information Service. www.uktis.org. Tel: 0344 892 0909 (09.00–17:00 Monday to Friday; urgent enquiries only outside these hours).

Prescribing in breast-feeding

Overview

Breast-feeding is beneficial; the immunological and nutritional value of breast milk to the infant is greater than that of formula feeds.

Although there is concern that drugs taken by the mother might affect the infant, there is very little information on this. In the absence of evidence of an effect, the potential for harm to the infant can be inferred from:

- the amount of drug or active metabolite of the drug delivered to the infant (dependent on the pharmacokinetic characteristics of the drug in the mother);
- the efficiency of absorption, distribution, and elimination of the drug by the infant (infant pharmacokinetics);
- the nature of the effect of the drug on the infant (pharmacodynamic properties of the drug in the infant).

The amount of drug transferred in breast milk is rarely sufficient to produce a discernible effect on the infant. This applies particularly to drugs that are poorly absorbed and need to be given parenterally. However, there is a theoretical possibility that a small amount of drug present in breast milk can induce a hypersensitivity reaction.

A clinical effect can occur in the infant if a pharmacologically significant quantity of the drug is present in milk. For some drugs (e.g. fluvastatin p. 187), the ratio between the concentration in milk and that in maternal plasma may be high enough to expose the infant to adverse effects. Some infants, such as those born prematurely or who have jaundice, are at a slightly higher risk of toxicity.

Some drugs inhibit the infant's sucking reflex (e.g. phenobarbital p. 304) while others can affect lactation (e.g. bromocriptine p. 383).

The BNF identifies drugs:

- that should be used with caution or are contra-indicated in breast-feeding;
- that can be given to the mother during breastfeeding because they are present in milk in amounts which are too small to be harmful to the infant;
- that might be present in milk in significant amount but are not known to be harmful.

Where care is needed when prescribing in breast-feeding, this is indicated under the relevant drug in the BNF.

Important

For many drugs insufficient evidence is available to provide guidance and it is advisable to administer only essential drugs to a mother during breast-feeding. Because of the inadequacy of information on drugs in breast-feeding, absence of information does not imply safety.

Prescribing in palliative care

Overview

Palliative care is an approach that improves the quality of life of patients and their families facing life-threatening illness, through the prevention and relief of suffering by means of early identification and impeccable assessment and treatment of pain and other problems, physical, psychosocial, and spiritual. Careful assessment of symptoms and needs of the patient should be undertaken by a multidisciplinary team.

Specialist palliative care is available in most areas as day hospice care, home-care teams (often known as Macmillan teams), in-patient hospice care, and hospital teams. Many acute hospitals and teaching centres now have consultative, hospital-based teams.

Hospice care of terminally ill patients has shown the importance of symptom control and psychosocial support of the patient and family. Families should be included in the care of the patient if they wish.

Many patients wish to remain at home with their families. Although some families may at first be afraid of caring for the patient at home, support can be provided by community nursing services, social services, voluntary agencies and hospices together with the general practitioner. The family may be reassured by the knowledge that the patient will be admitted to a hospital or hospice if the family cannot cope.

Drug treatment The number of drugs should be as few as possible, for even the taking of medicine may be an effort. Oral medication is usually satisfactory unless there is severe nausea and vomiting, dysphagia, weakness, or coma, when parenteral medication may be necessary.

Pain

Pain management in palliative care is focused on achieving control of pain by administering the right drug in the right dose at the right time. Analgesics can be divided into three broad classes: non-opioid (paracetamol p. 406, NSAID), opioid (e.g. codeine phosphate p. 413 'weak', morphine p. 421 'strong') and adjuvant (e.g. antidepressants, antiepileptics). Drugs from the different classes are used alone or in combination according to the type of pain and response to treatment. Analgesics are more effective in preventing pain than in the relief of established pain; it is important that they are given regularly.

Paracetamol or a **NSAID** given regularly will often be sufficient to manage mild pain. If non-opioid analgesics alone are not sufficient, then an opioid analgesic alone or in combination with a non-opioid analgesic at an adequate dosage, may be helpful in the control of moderate pain. Codeine phosphate or tramadol hydrochloride p. 427 can be considered for moderate pain. If these preparations do not control the pain then morphine is the most useful opioid analgesic. Alternatives to morphine, including transdermal buprenorphine p. 409, transdermal fentanyl p. 416, hydromorphone hydrochloride p. 420, methadone hydrochloride p. 456, or oxycodone hydrochloride p. 424, should be initiated by those with experience in palliative care. Initiation of an opioid analgesic should not be delayed by concern over a theoretical likelihood of psychological dependence (addiction).

Bone metastases In addition to the above approach, radiotherapy, **bisphosphonates**, and radioactive isotopes of strontium ranelate p. 661 (*Metastron*® available from GE Healthcare) may be useful for pain due to bone metastases.

Neuropathic pain Patients with **neuropathic pain** may benefit from a trial of a tricyclic antidepressant. An antiepileptic may be added or substituted if pain persists; gabapentin p. 287 and pregabalin p. 295 are licensed for neuropathic pain. Ketamine p. 1179 is sometimes used under specialist supervision for neuropathic pain that responds poorly to opioid analgesics. Pain due to nerve compression may be reduced by a corticosteroid such as dexamethasone p. 610, which reduces oedema around the tumour, thus reducing compression. Nerve blocks or regional anaesthesia techniques (including the use of epidural and intrathecal catheters) can be considered when pain is localised to a specific area.

Pain management with opioids

Oral route Treatment with morphine p. 421 is given by mouth as immediate-release or modified-release preparations. During the titration phase the initial dose is based on the previous medication used, the severity of the pain, and other factors such as presence of renal impairment, increasing age, or frailty. The dose is given either as an immediate-release preparation 4-hourly or as a modified-release preparation 12-hourly, in addition to rescue doses. If pain occurs between regular doses of morphine ('breakthrough pain'), an additional dose ('rescue dose') of immediate-release morphine should be given. An additional dose should also be given 30 minutes before an activity that causes pain, such as wound dressing. The standard dose of a strong opioid for breakthrough pain is usually one-tenth to one-sixth of the regular 24-hour dose, repeated every 2–4 hours as required (up to hourly may be needed if pain is severe or in the last days of life). Review pain management if rescue analgesic is required frequently (twice daily or more). Each patient should be assessed on an individual basis. Formulations of fentanyl p. 416 that are administered nasally, buccally or sublingually are also licensed for breakthrough pain.

When adjusting the dose of morphine, the number of rescue doses required and the response to them should be taken into account; increments of morphine should not exceed one-third to one-half of the total daily dose every 24 hours. Thereafter, the dose should be adjusted with careful assessment of the pain, and the use of adjuvant analgesics should also be considered. Upward titration of the dose of morphine stops when either the pain is relieved or unacceptable adverse effects occur, after which it is necessary to consider alternative measures.

Morphine immediate-release 30mg 4-hourly (or modified-release 100 mg 12-hourly) is usually adequate for most patients; some patients require morphine immediate-release up to 200mg 4-hourly (or modified-release 600 mg 12-hourly), occasionally more is needed.

Once their pain is controlled, patients started on 4-hourly immediate-release morphine can be transferred to the same total 24-hour dose of morphine given as the modified-release preparation for 12-hourly or 24-hourly administration. The first dose of the modified-release preparation is given with, or within 4 hours of, the last dose of the immediate-release preparation. For preparations suitable for 12-hourly or 24-hourly administration see modified-release preparations under morphine p. 421. Increments should be made to the dose, not to the frequency of administration. The patient must be monitored closely for efficacy and side-effects, particularly constipation, and nausea and vomiting. A suitable laxative should be prescribed routinely.

Oxycodone hydrochloride p. 424 can be used in patients who require an opioid but cannot tolerate morphine. If the patient is already receiving an opioid, oxycodone hydrochloride should be started at a dose equivalent to the current analgesic (see below). Oxycodone hydrochloride immediate-release preparations can be given for breakthrough pain.

Prescribing in palliative care (side margin)

Equivalent doses of opioid analgesics

This table is only an **approximate** guide (doses may not correspond with those given in clinical practice); patients should be carefully monitored after any change in medication and dose titration may be required.

Analgesic/Route	Dose
Codeine: PO	100 mg
Diamorphine: IM, IV, SC	3 mg
Dihydrocodeine: PO	100 mg
Hydromorphone: PO	2 mg
Morphine: PO	10 mg
Morphine: IM, IV, SC	5 mg
Oxycodone: PO	6.6 mg
Tramadol: PO	100 mg

PO = by mouth; IM = intramuscular; IV = intravenous; SC = subcutaneous

Parenteral route The equivalent parenteral dose of morphine p. 421 (subcutaneous, intramuscular, or intravenous) is about half of the oral dose. If the patient becomes unable to swallow, generally morphine is administered as a continuous subcutaneous infusion (for details, see Continuous Subcutaneous Infusions below). Diamorphine hydrochloride p. 415 is sometimes preferred, because being more soluble, it can be given in a smaller volume. The equivalent subcutaneous dose of diamorphine hydrochloride is about one-third of the oral dose of morphine.

If the patient can resume taking medicines by mouth, then oral morphine may be substituted for subcutaneous infusion of morphine or diamorphine hydrochloride, see table above of approximate equivalent doses of morphine and diamorphine hydrochloride. The infusion is discontinued when the first oral dose of morphine is given.

Rectal route Morphine p. 421 is also available for rectal administration as suppositories; alternatively oxycodone hydrochloride p. 424 suppositories can be obtained on special order.

Transdermal route Transdermal preparations of fentanyl p. 416 and buprenorphine p. 409 are available, they are not suitable for acute pain or in patients whose analgesic requirements are changing rapidly because the long time to steady state prevents rapid titration of the dose. Prescribers should ensure that they are familiar with the correct use of transdermal preparations, see under buprenorphine p. 409 and fentanyl p. 416 (inappropriate use has caused fatalities). Immediate-release morphine p. 421 can be given for breakthrough pain.

The following 24-hour oral doses of morphine are considered to be *approximately* equivalent to the buprenorphine and fentanyl patches shown, however when switching due to possible opioid-induced hyperalgesia, reduce the calculated equivalent dose of the new opioid by one-quarter to one-half.

Buprenorphine patches are *approximately* equivalent to the following 24-hour doses of oral morphine

morphine salt 12 mg daily	≡ *BuTrans*® '5' patch: 7-day patches
morphine salt 24 mg daily	≡ *BuTrans*® '10' patch: 7-day patches
morphine salt 48 mg daily	≡ *BuTrans*® '20' patch: 7-day patches
morphine salt 84 mg daily	≡ *Transtec*® '35' patch: 4-day patches
morphine salt 126 mg daily	≡ *Transtec*® '52.5' patch: 4-day patches
morphine salt 168 mg daily	≡ *Transtec*® '70' patch: 4-day patches

Conversion ratios vary and these figures are a guide only. Morphine equivalences for transdermal opioid preparations have been approximated to allow comparison with available preparations of oral morphine.

72-hour Fentanyl patches are *approximately* equivalent to the following 24-hour doses of oral morphine

morphine salt 30 mg daily	≡ fentanyl '12' patch
morphine salt 60 mg daily	≡ fentanyl '25' patch
morphine salt 120 mg daily	≡ fentanyl '50' patch
morphine salt 180 mg daily	≡ fentanyl '75' patch
morphine salt 240 mg daily	≡ fentanyl '100' patch

Fentanyl equivalences in this table are for patients on well-tolerated opioid therapy for long periods; for patients who are opioid naive or who have been stable on oral morphine or other immediate release opioid for only several weeks, see Transdermal Route. Conversion ratios vary and these figures are a guide only. Morphine equivalences for transdermal opioid preparations have been approximated to allow comparison with available preparations of oral morphine.

Symptom control

Several recommendations in this section involve unlicensed indications or routes.

Anorexia Anorexia may be helped by prednisolone p. 614 or dexamethasone p. 610.

Bowel colic and excessive respiratory secretions Bowel colic and excessive respiratory secretions may be reduced by a subcutaneous injection of hyoscine hydrobromide p. 401, hyoscine butylbromide p. 77, or glycopyrronium bromide p. 227. These antimuscarinics are generally given every 4 hours when required, but hourly use is occasionally necessary, particularly in excessive respiratory secretions. If symptoms persist, they can be given regularly via a continuous infusion device. Care is required to avoid the discomfort of dry mouth.

Capillary bleeding Capillary bleeding can be treated with tranexamic acid p. 99 by mouth; treatment is usually discontinued one week after the bleeding has stopped, or, if necessary, it can be continued at a reduced dose. Alternatively, gauze soaked in tranexamic acid 100 mg/mL or adrenaline/epinephrine solution 1 mg/mL (1 in 1000) p. 205 can be applied to the affected area.

Vitamin K may be useful for the treatment and prevention of bleeding associated with prolonged clotting in liver disease. In severe chronic cholestasis, absorption of vitamin K may be impaired; either parenteral or water-soluble oral vitamin K (see phytomenadione p. 945 and menadiol sodium phosphate p. 945) should be considered.

Constipation Constipation is a common cause of distress and is almost invariable after administration of an opioid analgesic. It should be prevented if possible by the regular administration of laxatives; a faecal softener with a peristaltic stimulant (e.g. co-danthramer p. 53) or lactulose solution p. 49 with a senna preparation p. 55 should be used. Methylnaltrexone bromide p. 56 is licensed for the treatment of opioid-induced constipation.

Convulsions Patients with cerebral tumours or uraemia may be susceptible to convulsions. Prophylactic treatment with phenytoin p. 294 or carbamazepine p. 283 should be considered. When oral medication is no longer possible, diazepam p. 313 given rectally, or phenobarbital p. 304 by injection is continued as prophylaxis. For the use of midazolam p. 310 by subcutaneous infusion using a continuous infusion device see below.

Dry mouth Dry mouth may be relieved by good mouth care and measures such as chewing sugar-free gum, sucking ice or pineapple chunks, or the use of artificial saliva, dry mouth associated with candidiasis can be treated by oral preparations of nystatin p. 1062 or miconazole p. 1061, alternatively, fluconazole p. 540 can be given by mouth. Dry mouth may be caused by certain medications including opioids, antimuscarinic drugs (e.g. hyoscine), antidepressants and some antiemetics; if possible, an alternative preparation should be considered.

Dysphagia A corticosteroid such as dexamethasone p. 610 may help, temporarily, if there is an obstruction due to tumour. See also *Dry mouth*, above.

Dyspnoea Breathlessness at rest may be relieved by regular oral morphine p. 421 in carefully titrated doses. Diazepam p. 313 may be helpful for dyspnoea associated with anxiety. A corticosteroid, such as dexamethasone p. 610, may also be helpful if there is bronchospasm or partial obstruction.

Fungating tumours Fungating tumours can be treated by regular dressing and antibacterial drugs; systemic treatment with metronidazole p. 492 is often required to reduce malodour but topical metronidazole p. 1074 is also used.

Gastro-intestinal pain The pain of bowel colic may be reduced by loperamide hydrochloride p. 59. Hyoscine hydrobromide p. 401 may also be helpful, given sublingually as *Kwells* ® tablets. Subcutaneous injections of hyoscine butylbromide p. 77, hyoscine hydrobromide, and glycopyrronium bromide p. 1170 can also be used to treat bowel colic.

Gastric distension pain due to pressure on the stomach may be helped by a preparation incorporating an antacid with an antiflatulent and a prokinetic such as domperidone p. 394 before meals.

Hiccup Hiccup due to gastric distension may be helped by a preparation incorporating an antacid with an antiflatulent. If this fails, metoclopramide hydrochloride p. 395 by mouth or by subcutaneous or intramuscular injection can be added; if this also fails, baclofen p. 973, or nifedipine p. 148, or chlorpromazine hydrochloride p. 353 can be tried.

Insomnia Patients with advanced cancer may not sleep because of discomfort, cramps, night sweats, joint stiffness, or fear. There should be appropriate treatment of these problems before hypnotics are used. Benzodiazepines, such as temazepam p. 443, may be useful.

Intractable cough Intractable cough may be relieved by moist inhalations or by regular administration of oral morphine p. 421. Methadone hydrochloride linctus p. 456 should be avoided because it has a long duration of action and tends to accumulate.

Muscle spasm The pain of muscle spasm can be helped by a muscle relaxant such as diazepam p. 313 or baclofen p. 973.

Nausea and vomiting Nausea and vomiting are common in patients with advanced cancer. Ideally, the cause should be determined before treatment with an antiemetic is started. A prokinetic antiemetic may be a preferred choice for first-line therapy.

Nausea and vomiting may occur with opioid therapy particularly in the initial stages but can be prevented by giving an antiemetic such as haloperidol p. 354 or metoclopramide hydrochloride p. 395. An antiemetic is usually necessary only for the first 4 or 5 days and therefore combined preparations containing an opioid with an antiemetic are not recommended because they lead to unnecessary antiemetic therapy (and associated side-effects when used long-term).

Metoclopramide hydrochloride has a prokinetic action and is used by mouth for nausea and vomiting associated with gastritis, gastric stasis, and functional bowel obstruction. Drugs with antimuscarinic effects antagonise prokinetic drugs and, if possible, should not be used concurrently. Haloperidol is used by mouth for most metabolic causes of vomiting (e.g. hypercalcaemia, renal failure).

Cyclizine p. 393 is given by mouth. It is used for nausea and vomiting due to mechanical bowel obstruction, raised intracranial pressure, and motion sickness.

Levomepromazine p. 403 is used as an antiemetic; it is given by mouth or by subcutaneous injection at bedtime. For the dose by subcutaneous infusion see below. Dexamethasone p. 610 by mouth can be used as an adjunct.

Antiemetic therapy should be reviewed every 24 hours; it may be necessary to substitute the antiemetic or to add another one.

For the administration of antiemetics by subcutaneous infusion using a continuous infusion device, see below. For the treatment of nausea and vomiting associated with cancer chemotherapy see Cytotoxic drugs p. 787.

Pruritus Pruritus, even when associated with obstructive jaundice, often responds to simple measures such as application of emollients. In the case of obstructive jaundice, further measures include administration of colestyramine p. 180).

Raised intracranial pressure Headache due to raised intracranial pressure often responds to a high dose of a corticosteroid, such as dexamethasone p. 610 and should be given before 6 p.m. to reduce the risk of insomnia.

Restlessness and confusion Restlessness and confusion may require treatment with an antipsychotic, e.g. haloperidol p. 354 or levomepromazine p. 403, by mouth or by subcutaneous injection, both repeated every 2 hours if required. The dose and frequency is adjusted according to the level of patient distress and the response. A regular maintenance dose should also be considered, given twice daily either by mouth or by subcutaneous injection; alternatively use a continuous infusion device. Levomepromazine is licensed to treat pain in palliative care—this use is reserved for distressed patients with severe pain unresponsive to other measures (seek specialist advice).

Continuous subcutaneous infusions

Although drugs can usually be administered *by mouth* to control the symptoms of advanced cancer, the parenteral route may sometimes be necessary. Repeated administration of *intramuscular injections* can be difficult in a cachectic patient. This has led to the use of portable continuous infusion devices, such as syringe drivers, to give a *continuous subcutaneous infusion*, which can provide good control of symptoms with little discomfort or inconvenience to the patient.

Indications for the **parenteral route** are:

- the patient is unable to take medicines by mouth owing to *nausea and vomiting, dysphagia, severe weakness*, or *coma*
- there is *malignant bowel obstruction* in patients for whom further surgery is inappropriate (avoiding the need for an intravenous infusion or for insertion of a nasogastric tube)
- occasionally when the patient *does not wish* to take regular medication by mouth.

Syringe driver rate settings Staff using syringe drivers should be **adequately trained** and different rate settings should be **clearly identified** and **differentiated**; incorrect use of syringe drivers is a common cause of medication errors.

Bowel colic and excessive respiratory secretions Hyoscine hydrobromide p. 401 effectively reduces respiratory secretions and bowel colic and is sedative (but occasionally causes paradoxical agitation).
Hyoscine butylbromide p. 77 is used for bowel colic and for excessive respiratory secretions, and is less sedative than hyoscine hydrobromide.
Glycopyrronium bromide p. 1170 may also be used to treat bowel colic or excessive respiratory secretions.

Confusion and restlessness Haloperidol p. 354 has little sedative effect.
Levomepromazine p. 403 has a sedative effect.
Midazolam p. 310 is a sedative and an antiepileptic that may be used in addition to an antipsychotic drug in a very restless patient. Midazolam is also used for myoclonus.

Convulsions If a patient has previously been receiving an antiepileptic drug *or* has a primary or secondary cerebral tumour *or* is at risk of convulsion (e.g. owing to uraemia) antiepileptic medication should not be stopped. Midazolam p. 310 is the benzodiazepine antiepileptic of choice for *continuous subcutaneous infusion*.

Nausea and vomiting Haloperidol p. 354 and levomepromazine p. 403 can both be given as a *subcutaneous infusion* but sedation can limit the dose of levomepromazine. Cyclizine is particularly likely to precipitate if mixed with diamorphine or other drugs (see under Mixing and Compatibility, below)
Metoclopramide hydrochloride p. 395 can cause skin reactions.
Octreotide p. 835, which stimulates water and electrolyte absorption and inhibits water secretion in the small bowel, can be used by subcutaneous infusion to reduce intestinal secretions and to reduce vomiting due to bowel obstruction.

Pain control Diamorphine hydrochloride p. 415 is the preferred opioid since its high solubility permits a large dose to be given in a small volume (see under Mixing and Compatibility, below). The table shows approximate equivalent doses of morphine and diamorphine hydrochloride.

Mixing and compatibility The general principle that injections should be given into separate sites (and should not be mixed) does not apply to the use of syringe drivers in palliative care. Provided that there is evidence of compatibility, selected injections can be mixed in syringe drivers. Not all types of medication can be used in a subcutaneous infusion. In particular, chlorpromazine hydrochloride p. 353, prochlorperazine p. 357, and diazepam p. 313 are **contra-indicated** as they cause skin reactions at the injection site; to a lesser extent cyclizine p. 393 and levomepromazine p. 403 also sometimes cause local irritation.
In theory injections dissolved in water for injections are more likely to be associated with pain (possibly owing to

their hypotonicity). The use of physiological saline (sodium chloride 0.9% p. 901) however increases the likelihood of precipitation when more than one drug is used; moreover subcutaneous infusion rates are so slow (0.1– 0.3 mL/hour) that pain is not usually a problem when water is used as a diluent.

Compatibility with diamorphine Diamorphine can be given by *subcutaneous infusion* in a strength of up to 250 mg/mL; up to a strength of 40 mg/mL either *water for injections* or *physiological saline* (sodium chloride 0.9%) is a suitable diluent—above that strength only *water for injections* is used (to avoid precipitation).
The following can be mixed with *diamorphine*:

- **Cyclizine**, may precipitate at concentrations above 10 mg/mL *or* in the presence of sodium chloride 0.9% *or* as the concentration of diamorphine relative to cyclizine increases; mixtures of diamorphine and cyclizine are also likely to precipitate after 24 hours.
- **Dexamethasone**, special care is needed to avoid precipitation of dexamethasone when preparing it.
- **Haloperidol**, mixtures of haloperidol and diamorphine are likely to precipitate after 24 hours if haloperidol concentration is above 2 mg/mL.
- **Hyoscine butylbromide**
- **Hyoscine hydrobromide**
- **Levomepromazine**
- **Metoclopramide**, under some conditions infusions containing metoclopramide become discoloured; such solutions should be discarded.
- **Midazolam**

Subcutaneous infusion solution should be monitored regularly both to check for precipitation (and discolouration) and to ensure that the infusion is running at the correct rate.

Problems encountered with syringe drivers The following are problems that may be encountered with syringe drivers and the action that should be taken:

- if the subcutaneous infusion runs *too quickly* check the rate setting and the calculation;
- if the subcutaneous infusion runs *too slowly* check the start button, the battery, the syringe driver, the cannula, and make sure that the injection site is not inflamed;
- if there is an *injection site reaction* make sure that the site does not need to be changed—firmness or swelling at the site of injection is not in itself an indication for change, but pain or obvious inflammation is.

Equivalent doses of morphine sulfate and diamorphine hydrochloride given over 24 hours

These equivalences are *approximate only* and should be adjusted according to response

ORAL MORPHINE	PARENTERAL MORPHINE	PARENTERAL DIAMORPHINE
Oral morphine sulfate **over 24 hours**	Subcutaneous infusion of morphine sulfate **over 24 hours**	Subcutaneous infusion of diamorphine hydrochloride **over 24 hours**
30 mg	15 mg	10 mg
60 mg	30 mg	20 mg
90 mg	45 mg	30 mg
120 mg	60 mg	40 mg
180 mg	90 mg	60 mg
240 mg	120 mg	80 mg
360 mg	180 mg	120 mg
480 mg	240 mg	160 mg
600 mg	300 mg	200 mg
780 mg	390 mg	260 mg
960 mg	480 mg	320 mg
1200 mg	600 mg	400 mg

If breakthrough pain occurs give a subcutaneous (preferable) or intramuscular injection equivalent to one-tenth to one-sixth of the total 24-hour subcutaneous infusion dose. It is kinder to give an intermittent bolus injection *subcutaneously*—absorption is smoother so that the risk of adverse effects at peak absorption is avoided (an even better method is to use a subcutaneous butterfly needle). To minimise the risk of infection no individual subcutaneous infusion solution should be used for longer than 24 hours.

Prescribing in the elderly

Overview

Old people, especially the very old, require special care and consideration from prescribers. *Medicines for Older People*, a component document of the National Service Framework for Older People (Department of Health. National Service Framework for Older People. London: Department of Health, March 2001), describes how to maximise the benefits of medicines and how to avoid excessive, inappropriate, or inadequate consumption of medicines by older people.

Appropriate prescribing

Elderly patients often receive multiple drugs for their multiple diseases. This greatly increases the risk of drug interactions as well as adverse reactions, and may affect compliance. The balance of benefit and harm of some medicines may be altered in the elderly. Therefore, elderly patients' medicines should be reviewed regularly and medicines which are not of benefit should be stopped. Non-pharmacological measures may be more appropriate for symptoms such as headache, sleeplessness, and light-headedness when associated with social stress as in widowhood, loneliness, and family dispersal.

In some cases prophylactic drugs are inappropriate if they are likely to complicate existing treatment or introduce unnecessary side-effects, especially in elderly patients with poor prognosis or with poor overall health. However, elderly patients should not be denied medicines which may help them, such as anticoagulants or antiplatelet drugs for atrial fibrillation, antihypertensives, statins, and drugs for osteoporosis.

Form of medicine

Frail elderly patients may have difficulty swallowing tablets; if left in the mouth, ulceration may develop. They should always be encouraged to take their tablets or capsules with enough fluid, and whilst in an upright position to avoid the possibility of oesophageal ulceration. It can be helpful to discuss with the patient the possibility of taking the drug as a liquid if available.

Manifestations of ageing

In the very old, manifestations of normal ageing may be mistaken for disease and lead to inappropriate prescribing. In addition, age-related muscle weakness and difficulty in maintaining balance should not be confused with neurological disease. Disorders such as light-headedness not associated with postural or postprandial hypotension are unlikely to be helped by drugs.

Sensitivity

The nervous system of elderly patients is more sensitive to many commonly used drugs, such as opioid analgesics, benzodiazepines, antipsychotics, and antiparkinsonian drugs, all of which must be used with caution. Similarly, other organs may also be more susceptible to the effects of drugs such as anti-hypertensives and NSAIDs.

Pharmacokinetics

Pharmacokinetic changes can markedly increase the tissue concentration of a drug in the elderly, especially in debilitated patients.

The most important effect of age is reduced renal clearance. Many aged patients thus *excrete drugs slowly*, and are *highly susceptible to nephrotoxic drugs*. Acute illness can lead to rapid reduction in renal clearance, especially if accompanied by dehydration. Hence, a patient stabilised on a drug with a narrow margin between the therapeutic and the toxic dose (e.g. digoxin p. 98) can rapidly develop adverse effects in the aftermath of a myocardial infarction or a respiratory-tract infection. The hepatic metabolism of lipid soluble drugs is reduced in elderly patients because there is a reduction in liver volume. This is important for drugs with a narrow therapeutic window.

Adverse reactions

Adverse reactions often present in the elderly in a vague and non-specific fashion. *Confusion* is often the presenting symptom (caused by almost any of the commonly used drugs). Other common manifestations are *constipation* (with antimuscarinics and many tranquillisers) and postural *hypotension* and *falls* (with diuretics and many psychotropics).

Hypnotics

Many hypnotics with long half-lives have serious hangover effects, including drowsiness, unsteady gait, slurred speech, and confusion. Hypnotics with short half-lives should be used but they too can present problems. Short courses of hypnotics are occasionally useful for helping a patient through an acute illness or some other crisis but every effort must be made to avoid dependence. Benzodiazepines impair balance, which can result in falls.

Diuretics

Diuretics are overprescribed in old age and should **not** be used on a long-term basis to treat simple gravitational oedema which will usually respond to increased movement, raising the legs, and support stockings. A few days of diuretic treatment may speed the clearing of the oedema but it should rarely need continued drug therapy.

NSAIDs

Bleeding associated with aspirin and other NSAIDs is more common in the elderly who are more likely to have a fatal or serious outcome. NSAIDs are also a special hazard in patients with cardiac disease or renal impairment which may again place older patients at particular risk.

Owing to the *increased susceptibility of the elderly* to the *side-effects of NSAIDs* the following recommendations are made:

- for *osteoarthritis, soft-tissue lesions*, and *back pain*, first try measures such as weight reduction (if obese), warmth, exercise, and use of a walking stick;
- for *osteoarthritis, soft-tissue lesions, back pain*, and *pain in rheumatoid arthritis*, paracetamol p. 406 should be used first and can often provide adequate pain relief;
- alternatively, a low-dose NSAID (e.g. ibuprofen p. 987 up to 1.2 g daily) may be given;
- for pain relief when either drug is inadequate, paracetamol in a full dose plus a low-dose NSAID may be given;
- if necessary, the NSAID dose can be increased or an opioid analgesic given with paracetamol;
- do not give two NSAIDs at the same time.

Prophylaxis of NSAID-induced peptic ulcers may be required if continued NSAID treatment is necessary see, *NSAID-associated ulcers* under Peptic ulceration p. 64.

Other drugs

Other drugs which commonly cause adverse reactions are *antiparkinsonian drugs, antihypertensives, psychotropics*, and digoxin p. 98. The usual maintenance dose of digoxin in very old patients is 125 micrograms daily (62.5 micrograms in those with renal disease); lower doses are often inadequate but toxicity is common in those given 250 micrograms daily. Drug-induced blood disorders are much more common in the elderly. Therefore drugs with a tendency to cause bone marrow depression (e.g. co-trimoxazole p. 511, mianserin hydrochloride p. 339) should be avoided unless there is no acceptable alternative.

The elderly generally require a lower maintenance dose of warfarin sodium p. 126 than younger adults; once again, the outcome of bleeding tends to be more serious.

Guidelines

Always consider whether a drug is indicated at all.

Limit range It is a sensible policy to prescribe from a limited range of drugs and to be thoroughly familiar with their effects in the elderly.

Reduce dose Dosage should generally be substantially lower than for younger patients and it is common to start with about 50% of the adult dose. Some drugs (e.g. long-acting antidiabetic drugs such as glibenclamide p. 637) should be avoided altogether.

Review regularly Review repeat prescriptions regularly. In many patients it may be possible to stop some drugs, provided that clinical progress is monitored. It may be necessary to reduce the dose of some drugs as renal function declines.

Simplify regimens Elderly patients benefit from simple treatment regimens. Only drugs with a clear indication should be prescribed and whenever possible given once or twice daily. In particular, regimens which call for a confusing array of dosage intervals should be avoided.

Explain clearly Write full instructions on every prescription (*including* repeat prescriptions) so that containers can be properly labelled with full directions. Avoid imprecisions like 'as directed'. Child-resistant containers may be unsuitable.

Repeats and disposal Instruct patients what to do when drugs run out, and also how to dispose of any that are no longer necessary. Try to prescribe matching quantities. If these guidelines are followed most elderly people will cope adequately with their own medicines. If not then it is essential to enrol the help of a third party, usually a relative or a friend.

Drugs and sport

Anti-doping

UK Anti-Doping, the national body responsible for the UK's anti-doping policy, advises that athletes are personally responsible should a prohibited substance be detected in their body. An advice card listing examples of permitted and prohibited substances is available from:

UK Anti-doping
Oceanic House
1a Cockspur Street
London
SW1Y 5BG
Tel: (020) 7766 7350
information@ukad.org.uk
www.ukad.org.uk

General Medical Council's advice

Doctors who prescribe or collude in the provision of drugs or treatment with the intention of improperly enhancing an individual's performance in sport contravene the GMC's guidance, and such actions would usually raise a question of a doctor's continued registration. This does not preclude the provision of any care or treatment where the doctor's intention is to protect or improve the patient's health.

Prescribing in dental practice

General guidance

Advice on the drug management of dental and oral conditions has been integrated into the main text. For ease of access, guidance on such conditions is usually identified by means of a relevant heading (e.g. Dental and Orofacial Pain) in the appropriate sections of the BNF.

The following is a list of topics of particular relevance to dentists.

> Prescribing by dentists, see Prescription writing p. 4
> Oral side-effects of drugs, see Adverse reactions to drugs p. 11
> Medical emergencies in dental practice, see below
> Medical problems in dental practice, see p. 30

Drug management of dental and oral conditions
Dental and orofacial pain, see Analgesics p. 404

> Neuropathic pain p. 438
> Non-opioid analgesics and compound analgesic preparations, see Analgesics p. 403
> Opioid analgesics, see Analgesics p. 403
> Non-steroidal anti-inflammatory drugs p. 975

Oral infections

> Bacterial infections, see Antibacterials, principles of therapy p. 459
>
>> Phenoxymethylpenicillin p. 497
>> Broad-spectrum penicillins (amoxicillin p. 498 and ampicillin p. 499)
>> Cephalosporins (cefalexin p. 476 and cefradine p. 477)
>> Tetracyclines p. 513
>> Macrolides (clarithromycin p. 487, erythromycin p. 488 and azithromycin p. 486)
>> Clindamycin p. 485
>> Metronidazole p. 492
>> Fusidic acid p. 519
>
> Fungal infections
>
>> Local treatment, see Oropharyngeal fungal infections p. 1060
>> Systemic treatment, see Antifungals, systemic use p. 536
>
> Viral infections
>
>> Herpetic gingivostomatitis, local treatment, see Oropharyngeal viral infections p. 1062
>> Herpetic gingivostomatitis, systemic treatment, see Oropharyngeal viral infections p. 1062 and Herpesvirus infections p. 575
>> Herpes labialis p. 1072

Anaesthetics, anxiolytics and hypnotics

> Sedation, anaesthesia, and resuscitation in dental practice p. 1164
> Hypnotics, see Hypnotics and anxiolytics p. 439
> Sedation for dental procedures, see Hypnotics and anxiolytics p. 439
> Local anaesthesia p. 1181

Minerals

> Fluorides p. 1055

Oral ulceration and inflammation p. 1056
Mouthwashes, gargles and dentifrices, see Mouthwashes and other preparations for oropharyngeal use p. 1053
Dry mouth, see Treatment of dry mouth p. 1051
Aromatic inhalations, see Aromatic inhalations, cough preparations and systemic nasal decongestants p. 270
Nasal decongestants, see Aromatic inhalations, cough preparations and systemic nasal decongestants p. 270

Dental Practitioners' Formulary p. 1394

Medical emergencies in dental practice

This section provides guidelines on the management of the more common medical emergencies which may arise in dental practice. Dentists and their staff should be familiar with standard resuscitation procedures, but in all circumstances it is advisable to summon medical assistance as soon as possible. See also **algorithm** of the procedure for Cardiopulmonary resuscitation inside back cover.

The drugs referred to in this section include:

> Adrenaline/epinephrine Injection, adrenaline 1 in 1000, (adrenaline 1 mg/mL as acid tartrate), 1 mL amps p. 205
> Aspirin Dispersible Tablets 300 mg p. 109
> Glucagon Injection, glucagon (as hydrochloride), 1- unit vial (with solvent) p. 652
> Glucose (for administration by mouth) p. 903
> Glyceryl trinitrate Spray p. 201
> Midazolam Oromucosal Solution p. 310, midazolam 5 mg/mL p. 310
> Oxygen
> Salbutamol Aerosol Inhalation, salbutamol 100 micrograms/metered inhalation p. 233

Adrenal insufficiency

Adrenal insufficiency may follow prolonged therapy with corticosteroids and can persist for years after stopping. A patient with adrenal insufficiency may become hypotensive under the stress of a dental visit (important: see individual monographs for details of corticosteroid cover before dental surgical procedures under general anaesthesia).

Management

- Lay the patient flat
- Give **oxygen**
- Transfer patient urgently to hospital

Anaphylaxis

A severe allergic reaction may follow oral or parenteral administration of a drug. Anaphylactic reactions in dentistry may follow the administration of a drug or contact with substances such as latex in surgical gloves. In general, the more rapid the onset of the reaction the more profound it tends to be. Symptoms may develop within minutes and rapid treatment is essential.

Anaphylactic reactions may also be associated with *additives* and *excipients* in foods and medicines. Refined arachis (peanut) oil, which may be present in some medicinal products, is unlikely to cause an allergic reaction— nevertheless it is wise to check the full formula of preparations which may contain allergens (including those for topical application, particularly if they are intended for use in the mouth or for application to the nasal mucosa).

Symptoms and signs

- Paraesthesia, flushing, and swelling of face
- Generalised itching, especially of hands and feet
- Bronchospasm and laryngospasm (with wheezing and difficulty in breathing)
- Rapid weak pulse together with fall in blood pressure and pallor; finally cardiac arrest

Management

First-line treatment includes securing the airway, restoration of blood pressure (laying the patient flat and raising the feet, or in the recovery position if unconscious or nauseous and at risk of vomiting), and administration of adrenaline/epinephrine injection p. 205. This is given **intramuscularly** in a dose of 500 micrograms (0.5 mL adrenaline injection 1 in 1000); a dose of 300 micrograms (0.3 mL adrenaline injection 1 in 1000) may be appropriate for immediate self-administration. The dose is repeated if necessary at 5-minute intervals according to blood pressure, pulse, and respiratory function. **Oxygen** administration is also of primary importance. Arrangements should be made to transfer the patient to hospital urgently.

Asthma

Patients with asthma may have an attack while at the dental surgery. Most attacks will respond to 2 puffs of the patient's short-acting beta$_2$ agonist inhaler such as salbutamol 100 micrograms/puff p. 233; further puffs are required if the patient does not respond rapidly. If the patient is unable to use the inhaler effectively, further puffs should be given through a large-volume spacer device (or, if not available, through a plastic or paper cup with a hole in the bottom for the inhaler mouthpiece). If the response remains unsatisfactory, or if further deterioration occurs, then the patient should be transferred urgently to hospital. Whilst awaiting transfer, **oxygen** should be given with salbutamol 5 mg or terbutaline sulfate 10 mg p. 235 by nebuliser; if a nebuliser is unavailable, then 2–10 puffs of salbutamol 100 micrograms/metered inhalation should be given (preferably by a large-volume spacer), and repeated every 10–20 minutes if necessary. If asthma is part of a more generalised anaphylactic reaction, an intramuscular injection of adrenaline/epinephrine p. 205 (as detailed under Anaphylaxis) should be given.

Patients with severe chronic asthma or whose asthma has deteriorated previously during a dental procedure may require an increase in their prophylactic medication before a dental procedure. This should be discussed with the patient's medical practitioner and may include increasing the dose of inhaled or oral corticosteroid.

Cardiac emergencies

If there is a history of *angina* the patient will probably carry glyceryl trinitrate spray or tablets p. 201 (or isosorbide dinitrate tablets p. 202) and should be allowed to use them. Hospital admission is not necessary if symptoms are mild and resolve rapidly with the patient's own medication. See also Coronary Artery Disease below.

Arrhythmias may lead to a sudden reduction in cardiac output with loss of consciousness. Medical assistance should be summoned. For advice on pacemaker interference, see also Pacemakers below.

The pain of *myocardial infarction* is similar to that of angina but generally more severe and more prolonged. For general advice see also Coronary Artery Disease below.

Symptoms and signs of myocardial infarction:

- Progressive onset of severe, crushing pain across front of chest; pain may radiate towards the shoulder and down arm, or into neck and jaw
- Skin becomes pale and clammy
- Nausea and vomiting are common
- Pulse may be weak and blood pressure may fall
- Breathlessness

Initial management of myocardial infarction:

Call immediately for medical assistance and an ambulance, as appropriate.

Allow the patient to rest in the position that feels most comfortable; in the presence of breathlessness this is likely to be sitting position, whereas the syncopal patient should be laid flat; often an intermediate position (dictated by the patient) will be most appropriate. **Oxygen** may be administered.

Sublingual glyceryl trinitrate p. 201 may relieve pain. Intramuscular injection of drugs should be avoided because absorption may be too slow (particularly when cardiac output is reduced) and pain relief is inadequate. Intramuscular injection also increases the risk of local bleeding into the muscle if the patient is given a thrombolytic drug.

Reassure the patient as much as possible to relieve further anxiety. If available, aspirin p. 109 in a single dose of 300 mg should be given. A note (to say that aspirin has been given) should be sent with the patient to the hospital. For further details on the initial management of myocardial infarction, see Management of ST-Segment Elevation Myocardial Infarction.

If the patient collapses and loses consciousness attempt standard resuscitation measures. See also **algorithm** of the procedure for Cardiopulmonary resuscitation inside back cover.

Epileptic seizures

Patients with epilepsy must continue with their normal dosage of anticonvulsant drugs when attending for dental treatment. It is not uncommon for epileptic patients not to volunteer the information that they are epileptic but there should be little difficulty in recognising a tonic-clonic (grand mal) seizure.

Symptoms and signs

- There may be a brief warning (but variable)
- Sudden loss of consciousness, the patient becomes rigid, falls, may give a cry, and becomes cyanotic (tonic phase)
- After 30 seconds, there are jerking movements of the limbs; the tongue may be bitten (clonic phase)
- There may be frothing from mouth and urinary incontinence
- The seizure typically lasts a few minutes; the patient may then become flaccid but remain unconscious. After a variable time the patient regains consciousness but may remain confused for a while

Management

During a convulsion try to ensure that the patient is not at risk from injury but make no attempt to put anything in the mouth or between the teeth (in mistaken belief that this will protect the tongue). Give **oxygen** to support respiration if necessary.

Do not attempt to restrain convulsive movements.

After convulsive movements have subsided place the patient in the coma (recovery) position and check the airway.

After the convulsion the patient may be confused ('post-ictal confusion') and may need reassurance and sympathy. The patient should not be sent home until fully recovered. Seek medical attention or transfer the patient to hospital if it was the first episode of epilepsy, or if the convulsion was atypical, prolonged (or repeated), or if injury occurred. Medication should only be given if convulsive seizures are prolonged (convulsive movements lasting 5 minutes or longer) or repeated rapidly.

Midazolam oromucosal solution p. 310 can be given by the buccal route in adults as a single dose of 10 mg [unlicensed]. For further details on the management of status epilepticus, including details of paediatric doses of midazolam, see Drugs used in status epilepticus (Epilepsy p. 279).

Focal seizures similarly need very little active management (in an automatism only a minimum amount of restraint should be applied to prevent injury). Again, the patient should be observed until post-ictal confusion has completely resolved.

Hypoglycaemia

Insulin-treated diabetic patients attending for dental treatment under local anaesthesia should inject insulin and eat meals as normal. If food is omitted the blood glucose will fall to an abnormally low level (hypoglycaemia). Patients can often recognise the symptoms themselves and this state responds to sugar in water or a few lumps of sugar. Children may not have such prominent changes but may appear unduly lethargic.

Symptoms and signs

- Shaking and trembling
- Sweating
- 'Pins and needles' in lips and tongue
- Hunger
- Palpitation
- Headache (occasionally)
- Double vision
- Difficulty in concentration
- Slurring of speech
- Confusion
- Change of behaviour; truculence
- Convulsions
- Unconsciousness

Management

Initially glucose 10–20 g is given by mouth either in liquid form or as granulated sugar or sugar lumps. Approximately 10 g of glucose is available from non-diet versions of *Lucozade® Energy Original* 55 mL, *Coca- Cola®* 100 mL, *Ribena® Blackcurrant* 19 mL (to be diluted), 2 teaspoons sugar, and also from 3 sugar lumps. (Proprietary products of quick-acting carbohydrate (e.g. GlucoGel®, Dextrogel®, GSF-Syrup®, Rapilose® gel) are available on prescription for the patient to keep to hand in case of hypoglycaemia.) If necessary this may be repeated in 10–15 minutes.

If glucose cannot be given by mouth, if it is ineffective, or if the hypoglycaemia causes unconsciousness, **glucagon** 1 mg (1 unit) should be given by intramuscular (or subcutaneous) injection; a child under 8 years or of body-weight under 25 kg should be given 500 micrograms. Once the patient regains consciousness oral glucose should be administered as above. If glucagon is ineffective or contra-indicated, the patient should be transferred urgently to hospital. The patient must also be admitted to hospital if hypoglycaemia is caused by an oral antidiabetic drug.

Syncope

Insufficient blood supply to the brain results in loss of consciousness. The commonest cause is a vasovagal attack or simple faint (syncope) due to emotional stress.

Symptoms and signs

- Patient feels faint
- Low blood pressure
- Pallor and sweating
- Yawning and slow pulse
- Nausea and vomiting
- Dilated pupils
- Muscular twitching

Management

- Lay the patient as flat as is reasonably comfortable and, in the absence of associated breathlessness, raise the legs to improve cerebral circulation
- Loosen any tight clothing around the neck
- Once consciousness is regained, give sugar in water or a cup of sweet tea

Other possible causes Postural hypotension can be a consequence of rising abruptly or of standing upright for too long; antihypertensive drugs predispose to this. When rising, susceptible patients should take their time. Management is as for a vasovagal attack.

Under stressful circumstances, some patients hyperventilate. This gives rise to feelings of faintness but does not usually result in syncope. In most cases reassurance is all that is necessary; rebreathing from cupped hands or a bag may be helpful but calls for careful supervision.

Adrenal insufficiency or arrhythmias are other possible causes of syncope.

Medical problems in dental practice

Individuals presenting at the dental surgery may also suffer from an unrelated medical condition; this may require modification to the management of their dental condition. If the patient has systemic disease or is taking other medication, the matter may need to be discussed with the patient's general practitioner or hospital consultant.

Allergy

Patients should be asked about any history of allergy; those with a history of atopic allergy (asthma, eczema, hay fever, etc.) are at special risk. Those with a history of a severe allergy or of anaphylactic reactions are at high risk—it is essential to confirm that they are not allergic to any medication, or to any dental materials or equipment (including latex gloves). See also Anaphylaxis above.

Arrhythmias

Patients, especially those who suffer from heart failure or who have sustained a myocardial infarction, may have irregular cardiac rhythm. Atrial fibrillation is a common arrhythmia even in patients with normal hearts and is of little concern except that dentists should be aware that such patients may be receiving anticoagulant therapy. The patient's medical practitioner should be asked whether any special precautions are necessary. Premedication (e.g. with temazepam p. 443) may be useful in some instances for very anxious patients.

See also Cardiac emergencies above, and Dental Anaesthesia (Local anaesthesia p. 1181).

Cardiac prostheses

For an account of the risk of infective endocarditis in patients with prosthetic heart valves, see Infective Endocarditis below. For advice on patients receiving anticoagulants, see Thromboembolic disease below.

Coronary artery disease

Patients are vulnerable for at least 4 weeks following a myocardial infarction or following any sudden increase in the symptoms of angina. It would be advisable to check with the patient's medical practitioner before commencing treatment. See also Cardiac Emergencies above.

Treatment with low-dose aspirin (75 mg daily), clopidogrel p. 110, or dipyridamole p. 111 should not be stopped routinely nor should the dose be altered before dental procedures.

A Working Party of the British Society for Antimicrobial Chemotherapy has not recommended antibiotic prophylaxis for patients following coronary artery bypass surgery.

Cyanotic heart disease

Patients with cyanotic heart disease are at risk in the dental chair, particularly if they have pulmonary hypertension. In such patients a syncopal reaction increases the shunt away from the lungs, causing more hypoxia which worsens the syncopal reaction—a vicious circle that may prove fatal. The advice of the cardiologist should be sought on any patient with congenital cyanotic heart disease. Treatment in hospital is more appropriate for some patients with this condition.

Hypertension

Patients with hypertension are likely to be receiving antihypertensive drugs. Their blood pressure may fall dangerously low under general anaesthesia, see also under Dental Anaesthesia (Local anaesthesia p. 1181).

Immunosuppression and indwelling intraperitoneal catheters

Advice of a Working Party of the British Society for Antimicrobial Chemotherapy is that patients who are immunosuppressed (including transplant patients) and patients with indwelling intraperitoneal catheters do not require antibiotic prophylaxis for dental treatment provided there is no other indication for prophylaxis.

The Working Party has commented that there is little evidence that dental treatment is followed by infection in immunosuppressed and immunodeficient patients nor is there evidence that dental treatment is followed by infection in patients with indwelling intraperitoneal catheters.

Infective endocarditis

While almost any dental procedure can cause bacteraemia, there is no clear association with the development of infective endocarditis. Routine daily activities such as tooth brushing also produce a bacteraemia and may present a greater risk of infective endocarditis than a single dental procedure.

Antibacterial prophylaxis and chlorhexidine mouthwash p. 1053 are **not** recommended for the prevention of endocarditis in patients undergoing dental procedures. Such prophylaxis may expose patients to the adverse effects of antimicrobials when the evidence of benefit has not been proven.

Reduction of oral bacteraemia

Patients at risk of endocarditis including those with valve replacement, acquired valvular heart disease with stenosis or regurgitation, structural congenital heart disease (including surgically corrected or palliated structural conditions, but excluding isolated atrial septal defect, fully repaired ventricular septal defect, fully repaired patent ductus arteriosus, and closure devices considered to be endothelialised), hypertrophic cardiomyopathy, or a previous episode of infective endocarditis, should be advised to maintain the highest possible standards of oral hygiene in order to reduce the:

- need for dental extractions or other surgery;
- chances of severe bacteraemia if dental surgery is needed;
- possibility of 'spontaneous' bacteraemia.

Postoperative care

Patients at risk of endocarditis including those with valve replacement, acquired valvular heart disease with stenosis or regurgitation, structural congenital heart disease (including surgically corrected or palliated structural conditions, but excluding isolated atrial septal defect, fully repaired ventricular septal defect, fully repaired patent ductus arteriosus, and closure devices considered to be endothelialised), hypertrophic cardiomyopathy, or a previous episode of infective endocarditis, should be warned to report to the doctor or dentist any unexplained illness that develops after dental treatment.

Any infection in patients at risk of endocarditis should be investigated promptly and treated appropriately to reduce the risk of endocarditis.

Patients on anticoagulant therapy

For general advice on dental surgery in patients receiving oral anticoagulant therapy see Thromboembolic Disease below.

Joint prostheses

Advice of a Working Party of the British Society for Antimicrobial Chemotherapy is that patients with prosthetic joint implants (including total hip replacements) do not require antibiotic prophylaxis for dental treatment. The Working Party considers that it is unacceptable to expose patients to the adverse effects of antibiotics when there is no evidence that such prophylaxis is of any benefit, but that those who develop any intercurrent infection require prompt treatment with antibiotics to which the infecting organisms are sensitive.

The Working Party has commented that joint infections have rarely been shown to follow dental procedures and are even more rarely caused by oral streptococci.

Pacemakers

Pacemakers prevent asystole or severe bradycardia. Some ultrasonic scalers, electronic apex locators, electro-analgesic devices, and electrocautery devices interfere with the normal function of pacemakers (including shielded pacemakers) and should not be used. The manufacturer's literature should be consulted whenever possible. If severe bradycardia occurs in a patient fitted with a pacemaker, electrical equipment should be switched off and the patient placed supine with the legs elevated. If the patient loses consciousness and the pulse remains slow or is absent, cardiopulmonary resuscitation may be needed. Call immediately for medical assistance and an ambulance, as appropriate.

A Working Party of the British Society for Antimicrobial Chemotherapy does not recommend antibacterial prophylaxis for patients with pacemakers.

Thromboembolic disease

Patients receiving a **heparin** or an oral anticoagulant such as warfarin sodium p. 126, acenocoumarol p. 126 (nicoumalone), phenindione p. 126, apixaban p. 112, dabigatran etexilate p. 123 or rivaroxaban p. 115 may be liable to excessive bleeding after extraction of teeth or other dental surgery. Often dental surgery can be delayed until the anticoagulant therapy has been completed.

For a patient requiring long-term therapy with warfarin sodium p. 126, the patient's medical practitioner should be consulted and the International Normalised Ratio (INR) should be assessed 72 hours before the dental procedure. This allows sufficient time for dose modification if necessary. In those with an unstable INR (including those who require weekly monitoring of their INR, or those who have had some INR measurements greater than 4.0 in the last 2 months), the INR should be assessed within 24 hours of the dental procedure. Patients requiring minor dental procedures (including extractions) who have an INR below 4.0 may continue warfarin sodium without dose adjustment. There is no need to check the INR for a patient requiring a non-invasive dental procedure.

If it is necessary to remove several teeth, a single extraction should be done first; if this goes well further teeth may be extracted at subsequent visits (two or three at a time). Measures should be taken to minimise bleeding during and after the procedure. This includes the use of sutures and a haemostatic such as oxidised cellulose, collagen sponge or resorbable gelatin sponge. Scaling and root planing should initially be restricted to a limited area to assess the potential for bleeding.

For a patient on long-term warfarin sodium, the advice of the clinician responsible for the patient's anticoagulation should be sought if:

- the INR is unstable, or if the INR is greater than 4.0;
- the patient has thrombocytopenia, haemophilia, or other disorders of haemostasis, or suffers from liver impairment, alcoholism, or renal failure;
- the patient is receiving antiplatelet drugs, cytotoxic drugs or radiotherapy.

Intramuscular injections are *contra-indicated* in patients taking anticoagulants with an INR above the therapeutic range, and in those with any disorder of haemostasis. In patients taking anticoagulants who have a stable INR within the therapeutic range, intramuscular injections should be avoided if possible; if an intramuscular injection is

Prescribing in dental practice

necessary, the patient should be informed of the increased
risk of localised bleeding and monitored carefully.

A local anaesthetic containing a vasoconstrictor should be
given by infiltration, or by intraligamentary or mental nerve
injection if possible. If regional nerve blocks cannot be
avoided the local anaesthetic should be given cautiously
using an aspirating syringe.

Drugs which have potentially serious interactions with
anticoagulants include aspirin and other NSAIDs,
carbamazepine, imidazole and triazole antifungals
(including miconazole), erythromycin, clarithromycin, and
metronidazole; for details of these and other interactions
with anticoagulants, see Appendix 1 (dabigatran etexilate,
heparins, phenindione, rivaroxaban, and coumarins).

Although studies have failed to demonstrate an interaction,
common experience in anticoagulant clinics is that the INR
can be altered following a course of an oral broad-spectrum
antibiotic, such as ampicillin or amoxicillin.

Information on the treatment of patients who take
anticoagulants is available at www.npsa.nhs.uk/patientsafety/
alerts-and-directives/alerts/anticoagulant.

Liver disease

Liver disease may alter the response to drugs and drug
prescribing should be kept to a minimum in patients with
severe liver disease. Problems are likely mainly in patients
with *jaundice, ascites,* or evidence of *encephalopathy*.

For guidance on prescribing for patients with hepatic
impairment, see Prescribing in hepatic impairment p. 18.
Where care is needed when prescribing in hepatic
impairment, this is indicated under the relevant drug in the
BNF.

Renal impairment

The use of drugs in patients with reduced renal function can
give rise to many problems. Many of these problems can be
avoided by reducing the dose or by using alternative drugs.
Special care is required in renal transplantation and
immunosuppressed patients; if necessary such patients
should be referred to specialists.

For guidance on prescribing in patients with renal
impairment, see Prescribing in renal impairment p. 18.
Where care is needed when prescribing in renal impairment,
this is indicated under the relevant drug in the BNF.

Pregnancy

Drugs taken during pregnancy can be harmful to the fetus
and should be prescribed only if the expected benefit to the
mother is thought to be greater than the risk to the fetus; all
drugs should be avoided if possible during the first trimester.
For guidance on prescribing in pregnancy, see Prescribing in
pregnancy p. 20. Where care is needed when prescribing in
pregnancy, this is indicated under the relevant drug in the
BNF.

Breast-feeding

Some drugs taken by the mother whilst breast-feeding can be
transferred to the breast milk, and may affect the infant.
For guidance on prescribing in breast-feeding, see
Prescribing in breast-feeding p. 20. Where care is needed
when prescribing in breast-feeding, this is indicated under
the relevant drug in the BNF.

Chapter 1
Gastro-intestinal system

CONTENTS

1   Chronic bowel disorders

Chronic bowel disorders

Overview

Once tumours are ruled out individual symptoms of chronic bowel disorders need specific treatment including dietary manipulation as well as drug treatment and the maintenance of a liberal fluid intake.

Clostridium difficile infection

Clostridium difficile infection is caused by colonisation of the colon with *Clostridium difficile* and production of toxin. It often follows antibiotic therapy and is usually of acute onset, but may become chronic. It is a particular hazard of ampicillin p. 499, amoxicillin p. 498, co-amoxiclav p. 501, second- and third-generation cephalosporins, clindamycin p. 485, and quinolones, but few antibiotics are free of this side-effect. Treatment options include metronidazole p. 492, vancomycin p. 484, and fidaxomicin p. 518.

Malabsorption syndromes

Individual conditions need specific management and also general nutritional consideration. Coeliac disease (gluten enteropathy) usually needs a gluten-free diet and pancreatic insufficiency needs pancreatin supplements.

For further information on foods for special diets (ACBS), see Borderline substances.

1.1   Diverticular disease and diverticulitis

Diverticular disease and diverticulitis   24.2.2016

Description of condition

Diverticular disease is a condition where diverticula (sac-like protrusions of mucosa through the muscular colonic wall) cause intermittent lower abdominal pain in the absence of inflammation or infection. The prevalence of diverticula increases with age, with the majority of patients older than 50 years.

Diverticulitis occurs when the diverticula become inflamed and infected, causing marked lower abdominal pain usually accompanied by fever and general malaise, and occasionally, with large rectal bleeds. Complicated diverticulitis includes episodes associated with an abscess, free perforation, fistula, obstruction, or stricture.

To ensure that an accurate diagnosis of diverticular disease and diverticulitis is made, consider and exclude all other causes of lower abdominal pain prior to treatment.

Aims of treatment

The aim of treatment is to relieve symptoms of diverticular disease, cure episodes of diverticulitis, and reduce the risk of recurrences and complications.

Drug treatment

[EvGr] A high-fibre diet is recommended for the treatment of symptomatic diverticular disease, although evidence supporting this is inconsistent and of low quality. Bulk-forming drugs have also been used, but evidence of their effectiveness is lacking. [A]

[EvGr] Treatment of uncomplicated diverticulitis includes a low residue diet and bowel rest. Antibacterials are recommended only when the patient presents with signs of infection or is immunocompromised, as there is no evidence to support routine administration. [A]

[EvGr] Patients with complicated diverticulitis or with severe presentation, require hospital admission, treatment with intravenous antibacterials (covering Gram-negative organisms and anaerobes), and bowel rest. [A]

[EvGr] There is insufficient evidence to justify the role of fibre, rifaximin p. 522, antispasmodics, mesalazine p. 35, and probiotics in the prevention or treatment of diverticulitis. [A]

[EvGr] Elective surgery to provide symptomatic relief or prevent recurrence, should be considered for patients following recovery from an episode of complicated diverticulitis. This includes episodes associated with free perforation, abscess, fistula, obstruction, or stricture. Urgent sigmoid colectomy is required for patients with diffuse peritonitis or for those in whom non-operative management of acute diverticulitis fails. [A]

Gastro-intestinal system

1.2 Inflammatory bowel disease

Inflammatory bowel disease

Management of acute ulcerative colitis and Crohn's disease

Chronic inflammatory bowel diseases include *ulcerative colitis* and *Crohn's disease*. Effective management requires drug therapy, attention to nutrition, and in severe or chronic active disease, surgery.

Aminosalicylates (balsalazide sodium p. 35, mesalazine p. 35, olsalazine sodium p. 38, and sulfasalazine p. 38), **corticosteroids** (hydrocortisone p. 612, beclometasone dipropionate p. 39, budesonide p. 39, and prednisolone p. 614), and **drugs that affect the immune response** are used in the treatment of inflammatory bowel disease.

Treatment of acute ulcerative colitis and Crohn's disease

Acute mild to moderate disease affecting the rectum (proctitis) or the recto-sigmoid is treated initially with local application of an aminosalicylate; alternatively, a local corticosteroid can be used but it is less effective. A combination of a local aminosalicylate and a local corticosteroid can be used for proctitis that does not respond to a local aminosalicylate alone. Foam preparations and suppositories are especially useful when patients have difficulty retaining liquid enemas.

Diffuse inflammatory bowel disease or disease that does not respond to local therapy requires oral treatment. Mild disease affecting the proximal colon can be treated with an oral aminosalicylate alone; a combination of a local and an oral aminosalicylate can be used in proctitis or distal colitis. Refractory or moderate inflammatory bowel disease usually requires adjunctive use of an oral corticosteroid such as prednisolone for 4–8 weeks. Modified-release budesonide is licensed for Crohn's disease affecting the ileum and the ascending colon; it causes fewer systemic side-effects than oral prednisolone but may be less effective. Beclometasone dipropionate by mouth is licensed as an adjunct to mesalazine for mild to moderate ulcerative colitis, but it is not known whether it is as effective as other corticosteroids.

Severe inflammatory bowel disease or disease that is not responding to an oral corticosteroid requires hospital admission and treatment with an intravenous corticosteroid (such as hydrocortisone or methylprednisolone p. 613); other therapy may include intravenous fluid and electrolyte replacement, and possibly parenteral nutrition. Specialist supervision is required for patients who fail to respond adequately to these measures. Patients with severe ulcerative colitis that has not responded to intravenous corticosteroids, may benefit from a short course of intravenous ciclosporin p. 758 [unlicensed indication]. Patients with unresponsive or chronically active Crohn's disease may benefit from azathioprine p. 757, mercaptopurine p. 806 [unlicensed indication], or once-weekly methotrexate p. 807 [unlicensed indication]; these drugs have a slower onset of action.

Infliximab p. 964 is licensed for the management of severe active Crohn's disease and severe ulcerative colitis in patients whose condition has not responded adequately to treatment with a corticosteroid and a conventional drug that affects the immune response, or who are intolerant of them.

Adalimumab p. 957 is licensed for the treatment of severe active Crohn's disease and severe ulcerative colitis in patients whose condition has not responded adequately to treatment with a corticosteroid and a conventional drug that affects the immune response, or who are intolerant of them. For inducing remission, adalimumab can be used in combination with a corticosteroid, but it may be given alone if a corticosteroid is inappropriate or is not tolerated.

Adalimumab may also be used for Crohn's disease in patients who have relapsed while taking infliximab or who cannot tolerate infliximab because of hypersensitivity reactions.

Golimumab p. 962 is licensed for the treatment of severe ulcerative colitis in patients whose condition has not responded adequately to conventional therapy, or who are intolerant of it.

Vedolizumab p. 40 is licensed for the treatment of moderate to severe active Crohn's disease and ulcerative colitis in patients who have had an inadequate response with, lost response to, or are intolerant to either conventional therapy or a tumour necrosis factor alpha inhibitor.

Maintenance of remission of acute ulcerative colitis and Crohn's disease

Smoking cessation reduces the risk of relapse in Crohn's disease and should be encouraged. **Aminosalicylates** are efficacious in the maintenance of remission of ulcerative colitis, but there is no evidence of efficacy in the maintenance of remission of Crohn's disease. Corticosteroids are **not** suitable for maintenance treatment because of their side-effects. In resistant or frequently relapsing cases either azathioprine or mercaptopurine [unlicensed indication], given under close supervision may be helpful. Methotrexate is tried in Crohn's disease if azathioprine or mercaptopurine cannot be used [unlicensed indication]. Maintenance therapy with infliximab should be considered for patients with Crohn's disease or ulcerative colitis who respond to the initial induction course of infliximab; fixed-interval dosing is superior to intermittent dosing. Adalimumab is licensed for maintenance therapy in Crohn's disease and ulcerative colitis. Golimumab is licensed for maintenance therapy in ulcerative colitis.

Fistulating Crohn's disease

Treatment may not be necessary for simple, asymptomatic perianal fistulas. Metronidazole p. 492 or ciprofloxacin p. 506 can improve symptoms of fistulating Crohn's disease but complete healing occurs rarely [unlicensed indication]. Metronidazole is usually given for 1 month but no longer than 3 months because of concerns about peripheral neuropathy. Ciprofloxacin by mouth is given twice daily. Other antibacterials should be given if specifically indicated (e.g. sepsis associated with fistulas and perianal disease) and for managing bacterial overgrowth in the small bowel. Fistulas may also require surgical exploration and local drainage.

Either azathioprine or mercaptopurine is used as a second-line treatment for fistulating Crohn's disease and continued for maintenance [unlicensed indication]. Infliximab is used for fistulating Crohn's disease refractory to conventional treatments; fixed-interval dosing is superior to intermittent dosing. Maintenance therapy with infliximab should be considered for patients who respond to the initial induction course of infliximab. Adalimumab can be used if there is intolerance to infliximab [unlicensed indication].

Adjunctive treatment of inflammatory bowel disease

Due attention should be paid to diet; high-fibre or low-residue diets should be used as appropriate.

Antimotility drugs such as codeine phosphate p. 413 and loperamide hydrochloride p. 59, and antispasmodic drugs may precipitate paralytic ileus and megacolon in active ulcerative colitis; treatment of the inflammation is more logical. An osmotic laxative, such as a macrogol, may be required in proctitis. Diarrhoea resulting from the loss of bile-salt absorption (e.g. in terminal ileal disease or bowel resection) may improve with colestyramine p. 180, which binds bile salts.

Drugs used in chronic bowel disorders

Aminosalicylates

Sulfasalazine is a combination of 5-aminosalicylic acid ('5-ASA') and sulfapyridine; sulfapyridine acts only as a carrier to the colonic site of action but still causes side-effects. In the newer aminosalicylates, mesalazine (5-aminosalicylic acid), balsalazide sodium (a pro-drug of 5-aminosalicylic acid) and olsalazine sodium (a dimer of 5-aminosalicylic acid which cleaves in the lower bowel), the sulfonamide-related side-effects of sulfasalazine are avoided, but 5-aminosalicylic acid alone can still cause side-effects including blood disorders and lupus-like syndrome also seen with sulfasalazine p. 38.

Drugs affecting the immune response

Azathioprine p. 757, ciclosporin p. 758, mercaptopurine p. 806, and methotrexate p. 807 have a role in the treatment of inflammatory bowel disease.

Folic acid p. 886 should be given to reduce the possibility of methotrexate toxicity [unlicensed indication]. Folic acid is usually given once weekly on a different day to the methotrexate; alternative regimens may be used in some settings.

Cytokine modulators

Infliximab p. 964, adalimumab p. 957, and golimumab p. 962 are monoclonal antibodies which inhibit the pro-inflammatory cytokine, tumour necrosis factor alpha. They should be used under specialist supervision. Adequate resuscitation facilities must be available when infliximab is used.

AMINOSALICYLATES

Aminosalicylates ⊖

- **SIDE-EFFECTS**
- ▸ **Rare** Acute pancreatitis · agranulocytosis · alopecia · aplastic anaemia · arthralgia · blood disorders · eosinophilia · fibrosing alveolitis · hepatitis · interstitial nephritis · leucopenia · lung disorders · lupus erythematosus-like syndrome · methaemoglobinaemia · myalgia · myocarditis · nephrotic syndrome · neutropenia · pericarditis · peripheral neuropathy · renal dysfunction · skin reactions · Stevens-Johnson syndrome · thrombocytopenia
- ▸ **Frequency not known** Abdominal pain · diarrhoea · exacerbation of symptoms of colitis · headache · hypersensitivity reactions · nausea · rash · urticaria · vomiting

  SIDE-EFFECTS, FURTHER INFORMATION
- ▸ **Blood Disorders** A blood count should be performed and the drug stopped immediately if there is suspicion of a blood dyscrasia.
- **ALLERGY AND CROSS-SENSITIVITY** Contra-indicated in salicylate hypersensitivity.
- **RENAL IMPAIRMENT**
  Monitoring
  Renal function should be monitored more frequently in renal impairment.
- **MONITORING REQUIREMENTS** Renal function should be monitored before starting an oral aminosalicylate, at 3 months of treatment, and then annually during treatment.
- **PATIENT AND CARER ADVICE**
  Blood disorders Patients receiving aminosalicylates, and their carers, should be advised to report any unexplained bleeding, bruising, purpura, sore throat, fever or malaise that occurs during treatment.

⚑ above
Balsalazide sodium

- **INDICATIONS AND DOSE**

Treatment of mild to moderate ulcerative colitis, acute attack
- ▸ BY MOUTH
- ▸ Adult: 2.25 g 3 times a day until remission occurs or for up to maximum of 12 weeks

Maintenance of remission of ulcerative colitis
- ▸ BY MOUTH
- ▸ Adult: 1.5 g twice daily (max. per dose 3 g), adjusted according to response; maximum 6 g per day

- **CAUTIONS** History of asthma
- **SIDE-EFFECTS** Cholelithiasis
- **PREGNANCY** Manufacturer advises avoid.
- **BREAST FEEDING** Diarrhoea may develop in the infant. Monitor breast-fed infants for diarrhoea.
- **HEPATIC IMPAIRMENT** Avoid in severe impairment.
- **RENAL IMPAIRMENT** Manufacturer advises avoid in moderate to severe impairment.

- **MEDICINAL FORMS**
There can be variation in the licensing of different medicines containing the same drug.
Capsule
CAUTIONARY AND ADVISORY LABELS 21, 25
- ▸ Colazide (Almirall Ltd)
  Balsalazide disodium 750 mg Colazide 750mg capsules | 130 capsule [PoM] £30.42 DT price = £30.42

⚑ above
Mesalazine

- **INDICATIONS AND DOSE**

ASACOL® MR 400MG TABLETS

Treatment of mild to moderate ulcerative colitis, acute attack
- ▸ BY MOUTH
- ▸ Child 12-17 years: 800 mg 3 times a day
- ▸ Adult: 2.4 g daily in divided doses

Maintenance of remission of ulcerative colitis and Crohn's ileo-colitis
- ▸ BY MOUTH
- ▸ Child 12-17 years: 400-800 mg 2-3 times a day
- ▸ Adult: 1.2-2.4 g daily in divided doses

ASACOL® MR 800MG TABLETS

Treatment of mild to moderate ulcerative colitis, acute attack
- ▸ BY MOUTH
- ▸ Adult: 2.4-4.8 g daily in divided doses

Maintenance of remission of ulcerative colitis
- ▸ BY MOUTH
- ▸ Adult: Up to 2.4 g once daily, alternatively up to 2.4 g daily in divided doses

Maintenance of remission of Crohn's ileo-colitis
- ▸ BY MOUTH
- ▸ Adult: Up to 2.4 g daily in divided doses continued →

ASACOL® FOAM ENEMA

Treatment of acute attack of mild to moderate ulcerative colitis affecting the rectosigmoid region
▸ BY RECTUM
▸ Adult: 1 g daily for 4–6 weeks, to be administered into the rectum

Treatment of acute attack of mild to moderate ulcerative colitis, affecting the descending colon
▸ BY RECTUM
▸ Adult: 2 g once daily for 4–6 weeks, to be administered into the rectum

ASACOL® SUPPOSITORIES

Treatment of acute attack of mild to moderate ulcerative colitis and maintenance of remission
▸ BY RECTUM
▸ Adult: 0.75–1.5 g daily in divided doses, last dose to be administered at bedtime

IPOCOL®

Treatment of mild to moderate ulcerative colitis, acute attack
▸ BY MOUTH
▸ Adult: 2.4 g daily in divided doses

Maintenance of remission of ulcerative colitis
▸ BY MOUTH
▸ Adult: 1.2–2.4 g daily in divided doses

MEZAVANT® XL

Treatment of mild to moderate ulcerative colitis, acute attack
▸ BY MOUTH
▸ Adult: 2.4 g once daily, increased if necessary to 4.8 g once daily, review treatment at 8 weeks

Maintenance of remission of ulcerative colitis
▸ BY MOUTH
▸ Adult: 2.4 g once daily

OCTASA®

Treatment of mild to moderate ulcerative colitis, acute attack
▸ BY MOUTH
▸ Adult: 2.4–4.8 g once daily, alternatively 2.4–4.8 g daily in divided doses, dose over 2.4 g daily in divided doses only

Maintenance of remission of ulcerative colitis and Crohn's ileo-colitis
▸ BY MOUTH
▸ Adult: 1.2–2.4 g once daily, alternatively daily in divided doses

PENTASA® GRANULES

Treatment of mild to moderate ulcerative colitis, acute attack
▸ BY MOUTH
▸ Child 5–17 years (body-weight up to 40 kg): 10–20 mg/kg 3 times a day
▸ Child 5–17 years (body-weight 40 kg and above): 1–2 g twice daily, total daily dose may alternatively be given in 3–4 divided doses
▸ Adult: Up to 4 g once daily, alternatively up to 4 g daily in 2–4 divided doses

Maintenance of remission of ulcerative colitis
▸ BY MOUTH
▸ Child 5–17 years (body-weight up to 40 kg): 7.5–15 mg/kg twice daily, total daily dose may alternatively be given in 3 divided doses
▸ Child 5–17 years (body-weight 40 kg and above): 2 g once daily
▸ Adult: 2 g once daily

PENTASA® RETENTION ENEMA

Treatment of acute attack of mild to moderate ulcerative colitis or maintenance of remission
▸ BY RECTUM
▸ Adult: 1 g once daily, dose to be administered at bedtime

Treatment of acute attack of mild to moderate ulcerative colitis affecting the rectosigmoid region
▸ BY RECTUM
▸ Child 12–17 years: 1 g once daily, dose to be administered at bedtime

PENTASA® SUPPOSITORIES

Treatment of acute attack, ulcerative proctitis
▸ BY RECTUM
▸ Child 15–17 years: 1 g daily for 2–4 weeks
▸ Adult: 1 g daily for 2–4 weeks

Maintenance, ulcerative proctitis
▸ BY RECTUM
▸ Child 15–17 years: 1 g daily
▸ Adult: 1 g daily

PENTASA® TABLETS

Treatment of mild to moderate ulcerative colitis, acute attack
▸ BY MOUTH
▸ Adult: Up to 4 g once daily, alternatively up to 4 g daily in 2–3 divided doses

Maintenance of remission of ulcerative colitis
▸ BY MOUTH
▸ Adult: 2 g once daily

SALOFALK® ENEMA

Treatment of acute attack of mild to moderate ulcerative colitis or maintenance of remission
▸ BY RECTUM
▸ Adult: 2 g once daily, dose to be administered at bedtime

SALOFALK® GRANULES

Treatment of mild to moderate ulcerative colitis, acute attack
▸ BY MOUTH
▸ Child 5–17 years (body-weight up to 40 kg): 30–50 mg/kg once daily, dose preferably given in the morning, alternatively 10–20 mg/kg 3 times a day
▸ Child 5–17 years (body-weight 40 kg and above): 1.5–3 g once daily, dose preferably given in the morning, alternatively 0.5–1 g 3 times a day
▸ Adult: 1.5–3 g once daily, dose preferably taken in the morning, alternatively 0.5–1 g 3 times a day

Maintenance of remission of ulcerative colitis
▸ BY MOUTH
▸ Child 5–17 years (body-weight up to 40 kg): 7.5–15 mg/kg twice daily, total daily dose may alternatively be given in 3 divided doses
▸ Child 5–17 years (body-weight 40 kg and above): 500 mg 3 times a day
▸ Adult: 500 mg 3 times a day

SALOFALK® RECTAL FOAM

Treatment of mild ulcerative colitis affecting sigmoid colon and rectum
▸ BY RECTUM
▸ Child 12–17 years: 2 g once daily, dose to be administered into the rectum at bedtime, alternatively 2 g daily in 2 divided doses
▸ Adult: 2 g once daily, dose to be administered into the rectum at bedtime, alternatively 2 g daily in 2 divided doses

SALOFALK® SUPPOSITORIES

Treatment of acute attack of mild to moderate ulcerative colitis affecting the rectum, sigmoid colon and descending colon

▸ BY RECTUM

▸ Adult: 0.5–1 g 2–3 times a day, adjusted according to response, dose to be given using 500 mg suppositories

Treatment of acute attack of mild to moderate ulcerative colitis affecting the rectum

▸ BY RECTUM

▸ Adult: 1 g daily, preferably at bedtime, dose to be given using 1 g suppositories

SALOFALK® TABLETS

Treatment of mild to moderate ulcerative colitis, acute attack

▸ BY MOUTH

▸ Child 5–17 years (body-weight up to 40 kg): 10–20 mg/kg 3 times a day

▸ Child 5–17 years (body-weight 40 kg and above): 0.5–1 g 3 times a day

▸ Adult: 0.5–1 g 3 times a day

Maintenance of remission of ulcerative colitis

▸ BY MOUTH

▸ Child 5–17 years (body-weight up to 40 kg): 7.5–15 mg/kg twice daily, total daily dose may alternatively be given in 3 divided doses

▸ Child 5–17 years (body-weight 40 kg and above): 500 mg 3 times a day

▸ Adult: 500 mg 3 times a day

DOSE EQUIVALENCE AND CONVERSION
There is no evidence to show that any one oral preparation of mesalazine is more effective than another; however, the delivery characteristics of oral mesalazine preparations may vary.

● UNLICENSED USE
▸ With oral use in children *Asacol*® (all preparations) not licensed for use in children under 18 years. *Pentasa*® granules and *Salofalk*® tablets and granules not licensed for use in children under 6 years.
▸ With rectal use in children *Pentasa*® suppositories not licensed for use in children under 15 years. *Pentasa*® enema not licensed for use in children. *Salofalk*® rectal foam no dose recommendations for children (age range not specified by manufacturer).

● CONTRA-INDICATIONS Blood clotting abnormalities (in children)

● CAUTIONS Elderly (in adults) · pulmonary disease

● INTERACTIONS The manufacturers of some mesalazine gastro-resistant and modified-release medicines (*Asacol*® MR tablets, *Ipocol*®, *Salofalk*® granules) suggest that preparations that lower stool pH (e.g. lactulose) may prevent the release of mesalazine.

● SIDE-EFFECTS
▸ **Rare** Dizziness
▸ **Very rare** Oligospermia (reversible)

● PREGNANCY Negligible quantities cross placenta.

● BREAST FEEDING Diarrhoea reported in breast-fed infants, but negligible amounts of mesalazine detected in breast milk.
Monitor breast-fed infant for diarrhoea.

● HEPATIC IMPAIRMENT Avoid in severe impairment.

● RENAL IMPAIRMENT
▸ In adults Use with caution. Avoid if eGFR less than 20 mL/minute/1.73 m^2.
▸ In children Use with caution. Avoid if estimated glomerular filtration rate less than 20 mL/minute/1.73 m^2.

● DIRECTIONS FOR ADMINISTRATION
PENTASA® TABLETS Tablets may be halved, quartered, or dispersed in water, but should not be chewed.
SALOFALK® GRANULES Granules should be placed on tongue and washed down with water without chewing.
PENTASA® GRANULES Granules should be placed on tongue and washed down with water or orange juice without chewing.
▸ In children Contents of one sachet should be weighed and divided immediately before use; discard any remaining granules.

● PRESCRIBING AND DISPENSING INFORMATION There is no evidence to show that any one oral preparation of mesalazine is more effective than another; however, the delivery characteristics of oral mesalazine preparations may vary.
Flavours of granule formulations of *Salofalk*® may include vanilla.

● PATIENT AND CARER ADVICE
If it is necessary to switch a patient to a different brand of mesalazine, the patient should be advised to report any changes in symptoms.
Some products may require special administration advice; patients and carers should be informed.
Medicines for Children leaflet: Mesalazine (oral) for inflammatory bowel disease www.medicinesforchildren.org.uk/mesalazine-oral-for-inflammatory-bowel-disease
Medicines for Children leaflet: Mesalazine foam enema for inflammatory bowel disease www.medicinesforchildren.org.uk/mesalazine-foam-enema-for-inflammatory-bowel-disease
Medicines for Children leaflet: Mesalazine liquid enema for inflammatory bowel disease www.medicinesforchildren.org.uk/mesalazine-liquid-enema-for-inflammatory-bowel-disease
Medicines for Children leaflet: Mesalazine suppositories for inflammatory bowel disease www.medicinesforchildren.org.uk/mesalazine-suppositories-for-inflammatory-bowel-disease

● MEDICINAL FORMS
There can be variation in the licensing of different medicines containing the same drug.
Modified-release tablet
CAUTIONARY AND ADVISORY LABELS 21 (does not apply to Pentasa® tablets), 25 (does not apply to Pentasa® tablets)
▸ Mezavant XL (Shire Pharmaceuticals Ltd)
Mesalazine 1.2 gram Mezavant XL 1200mg tablets | 60 tablet [PoM] £42.95 DT price = £42.95
▸ Pentasa (Ferring Pharmaceuticals Ltd)
Mesalazine 500 mg Pentasa 500mg modified-release tablets | 100 tablet [PoM] £30.74 DT price = £30.74
Mesalazine 1 gram Pentasa 1g modified-release tablets | 60 tablet [PoM] £36.89 DT price = £36.89
Gastro-resistant tablet
CAUTIONARY AND ADVISORY LABELS 5 (does not apply to Octasa®), 25
▸ Asacol MR (Allergan Ltd)
Mesalazine 400 mg Asacol 400mg MR gastro-resistant tablets | 84 tablet [PoM] £27.45 DT price = £27.45 | 168 tablet [PoM] £54.90
Mesalazine 800 mg Asacol 800mg MR gastro-resistant tablets | 84 tablet [PoM] £54.90 DT price = £54.90
▸ Ipocol (Sandoz Ltd)
Mesalazine 400 mg Ipocol 400mg gastro-resistant tablets | 120 tablet [PoM] £17.68
▸ Octasa MR (Tillotts Pharma Ltd)
Mesalazine 400 mg Octasa 400mg MR gastro-resistant tablets | 90 tablet [PoM] £19.50 DT price = £19.50 | 120 tablet [PoM] £26.00
Mesalazine 800 mg Octasa 800mg MR gastro-resistant tablets | 90 tablet [PoM] £47.50 DT price = £47.50 | 180 tablet [PoM] £95.00 DT price = £95.00
▸ Salofalk (Dr. Falk Pharma UK Ltd)
Mesalazine 250 mg Salofalk 250mg gastro-resistant tablets | 100 tablet [PoM] £16.19
Mesalazine 500 mg Salofalk 500mg gastro-resistant tablets | 100 tablet [PoM] £32.38

Modified-release granules

CAUTIONARY AND ADVISORY LABELS 25 (does not apply to Pentasa® granules)

EXCIPIENTS: May contain Aspartame

▸ Pentasa (Ferring Pharmaceuticals Ltd)

Mesalazine 1 gram Pentasa 1g modified-release granules sachets sugar-free | 50 sachet [PoM] £30.74 DT price = £30.74

Mesalazine 2 gram Pentasa 2g modified-release granules sachets sugar-free | 60 sachet [PoM] £73.78 DT price = £73.78

Mesalazine 4 gram Pentasa 4g modified-release granules sachets sugar-free | 30 sachet [PoM] £73.78

▸ Salofalk (Dr. Falk Pharma UK Ltd)

Mesalazine 500 mg Salofalk 500mg gastro-resistant modified-release granules sachets sugar-free | 100 sachet [PoM] £28.74

Mesalazine 1 gram Salofalk 1g gastro-resistant modified-release granules sachets sugar-free | 50 sachet [PoM] £28.74 DT price = £28.74

Mesalazine 1.5 gram Salofalk 1.5g gastro-resistant modified-release granules sachets sugar-free | 60 sachet [PoM] £48.85 DT price = £48.85

Mesalazine 3 gram Salofalk 3g gastro-resistant modified-release granules sachets sugar-free | 60 sachet [PoM] £97.70 DT price = £97.70

Foam

EXCIPIENTS: May contain Cetostearyl alcohol (including cetyl and stearyl alcohol), disodium edetate, hydroxybenzoates (parabens), polysorbates, propylene glycol, sodium metabisulfite

▸ Asacol (Allergan Ltd)

Mesalazine 1 gram per 1 application Asacol 1g/application foam enema | 14 dose [PoM] £26.72

▸ Salofalk (Dr. Falk Pharma UK Ltd)

Mesalazine 1 gram per 1 application Salofalk 1g/application foam enema | 14 dose [PoM] £30.17

Suppository

▸ Asacol (Allergan Ltd)

Mesalazine 250 mg Asacol 250mg suppositories | 20 suppository [PoM] £4.82 DT price = £4.82

Mesalazine 500 mg Asacol 500mg suppositories | 10 suppository [PoM] £4.82 DT price = £4.82

▸ Pentasa (Ferring Pharmaceuticals Ltd)

Mesalazine 1 gram Pentasa 1g suppositories | 28 suppository [PoM] £40.01 DT price = £40.01

▸ Salofalk (Dr. Falk Pharma UK Ltd)

Mesalazine 500 mg Salofalk 500mg suppositories | 30 suppository [PoM] £14.81

Mesalazine 1 gram Salofalk 1g suppositories | 30 suppository [PoM] £29.62

Enema

▸ Pentasa (Ferring Pharmaceuticals Ltd)

Mesalazine 10 mg per 1 ml Pentasa Mesalazine 1g/100ml enema | 7 enema [PoM] £17.73 DT price = £17.73

▸ Salofalk (Dr. Falk Pharma UK Ltd)

Mesalazine 33.9 mg per 1 ml Salofalk 2g/59ml enema | 7 enema [PoM] £29.92

◤ 35

| Olsalazine sodium

● **INDICATIONS AND DOSE**

Treatment of acute attack of mild ulcerative colitis

▸ BY MOUTH

▸ Adult: 1 g daily in divided doses, doses to be taken after meals, then increased if necessary up to 3 g daily in divided doses (max. per dose 1 g), dose to be increased over 1 week

Maintenance of remission of mild ulcerative colitis

▸ BY MOUTH

▸ Adult: Maintenance 500 mg twice daily, dose to be taken after food

● SIDE-EFFECTS

▸ **Common or very common** Watery diarrhoea

▸ **Frequency not known** Blurred vision · palpitation · photosensitivity · pyrexia · tachycardia

● PREGNANCY Manufacturer advises avoid unless potential benefit outweighs risk.

● BREAST FEEDING

Monitoring

Monitor breast-fed infants for diarrhoea.

● RENAL IMPAIRMENT Use with caution; manufacturer advises avoid in significant impairment.

● DIRECTIONS FOR ADMINISTRATION Capsules can be opened and contents sprinkled on food.

● MEDICINAL FORMS

There can be variation in the licensing of different medicines containing the same drug. Forms available from special-order manufacturers include: oral suspension, oral solution

Tablet

CAUTIONARY AND ADVISORY LABELS 21

▸ Olsalazine sodium (Non-proprietary)

Olsalazine sodium 500 mg Olsalazine 500mg tablets | 60 tablet [PoM] £85.00–£161.00 DT price = £161.00

Capsule

CAUTIONARY AND ADVISORY LABELS 21

▸ Olsalazine sodium (Non-proprietary)

Olsalazine sodium 250 mg Olsalazine 250mg capsules | 112 capsule [PoM] £75.00–£144.00 DT price = £144.00

◤ 35

| Sulfasalazine

(Sulphasalazine)

● **INDICATIONS AND DOSE**

Treatment of acute attack of mild to moderate and severe ulcerative colitis | Active Crohn's disease

▸ BY MOUTH

▸ Adult: 1–2 g 4 times a day until remission occurs, corticosteroids may also be given, if necessary

▸ BY RECTUM

▸ Adult: 0.5–1 g twice daily, administered alone or in conjunction with oral therapy, morning and night after a bowel movement

Maintenance of remission of mild to moderate and severe ulcerative colitis

▸ BY MOUTH

▸ Adult: 500 mg 4 times a day

▸ BY RECTUM

▸ Adult: 0.5–1 g twice daily, administered alone or in conjunction with oral therapy, morning and night after a bowel movement

Active rheumatoid arthritis (administered on expert advice)

▸ BY MOUTH

▸ Adult: Initially 500 mg daily, increased in steps of 500 mg every 1 week, increased to 2–3 g daily in divided doses, enteric coated tablets to be administered

● CAUTIONS Acute porphyrias p. 918 · G6PD deficiency · history of allergy · history of asthma · maintain adequate fluid intake · risk of haematological toxicity · risk of hepatic toxicity · slow acetylator status

● INTERACTIONS → Appendix 1 (aminosalicylates).

● SIDE-EFFECTS

▸ **Common or very common** Blood disorders · cough · dizziness · fever · Heinz body anaemia · insomnia · megaloblastic anaemia · proteinuria · pruritus · stomatitis · taste disturbances · tinnitus

▸ **Uncommon** Alopecia · convulsions · depression · dyspnoea · vasculitis

▸ **Frequency not known** Anaphylaxis · aseptic meningitis · ataxia · crystalluria · disturbances of smell · epidermal necrolysis · exfoliative dermatitis · gastro-intestinal intolerance · hallucinations · hypersensitivity reactions · leucopenia (especially in patients with rheumatoid arthritis) · loss of appetite · neutropenia (especially in patients with rheumatoid arthritis) · oligospermia ·

parotitis · photosensitivity · rashes · serum sickness · some
soft contact lenses may be stained · thrombocytopenia
(especially in patients with rheumatoid arthritis) · yellow-
orange discoloration of other body fluids · yellow-orange
discoloration of skin · yellow-orange discoloration of urine

SIDE-EFFECTS, FURTHER INFORMATION
▸ Gastro-intestinal side effects　Upper gastro-intestinal side-
effects common over 4 g daily.
▸ Blood disorders　Haematological abnormalities occur usually
in the first 3 to 6 months of treatment and are reversible
on cessation of treatment.
● PREGNANCY　Theoretical risk of neonatal haemolysis in
third trimester; adequate folate supplements should be
given to mother.
● BREAST FEEDING　Small amounts in milk (1 report of
bloody diarrhoea); theoretical risk of neonatal haemolysis
especially in G6PD-deficient infants.
● HEPATIC IMPAIRMENT　Use with caution.
● RENAL IMPAIRMENT　Risk of toxicity, including crystalluria,
in moderate impairment—ensure high fluid intake. Avoid
in severe impairment.
● MONITORING REQUIREMENTS
▸ Blood disorders　Close monitoring of full blood counts
(including differential white cell count and platelet count)
is necessary initially, and at monthly intervals during the
first 3 months.
▸ Renal function　Although the manufacturer recommends
renal function tests in rheumatic diseases, evidence of
practical value is unsatisfactory.
▸ Liver function　Liver function tests should be performed at
monthly intervals for first 3 months.
● PATIENT AND CARER ADVICE
Contact lenses　Some soft contact lenses may be stained.

● MEDICINAL FORMS
There can be variation in the licensing of different medicines
containing the same drug. Forms available from special-order
manufacturers include: oral suspension

Tablet
CAUTIONARY AND ADVISORY LABELS　14
▸ Sulfasalazine (Non-proprietary)
　Sulfasalazine 500 mg　Sulfasalazine 500mg tablets |
　112 tablet PoM £18.00 DT price = £6.13
▸ Salazopyrin (Pfizer Ltd)
　Sulfasalazine 500 mg　Salazopyrin 500mg tablets | 112 tablet PoM
　£6.97 DT price = £6.13

Gastro-resistant tablet
CAUTIONARY AND ADVISORY LABELS　5, 14, 25
▸ Sulfasalazine (Non-proprietary)
　Sulfasalazine 500 mg　Sulfasalazine 500mg gastro-resistant tablets
　| 100 tablet PoM no price available | 112 tablet PoM £27.00 DT
　price = £8.63
▸ Salazopyrin EN (Pfizer Ltd)
　Sulfasalazine 500 mg　Salazopyrin EN-Tabs 500mg |
　112 tablet PoM £8.43 DT price = £8.63
▸ Sulazine EC (Genesis Pharmaceuticals Ltd, Teva UK Ltd)
　Sulfasalazine 500 mg　Sulazine EC 500mg tablets | 112 tablet PoM
　£8.00 DT price = £8.63

Oral suspension
CAUTIONARY AND ADVISORY LABELS　14
EXCIPIENTS: May contain Alcohol
▸ Sulfasalazine (Non-proprietary)
　Sulfasalazine 50 mg per 1 ml　Sulfasalazine 250mg/5ml oral
　suspension sugar free sugar-free | 500 ml PoM £44.09 DT price =
　£43.42

Suppository
CAUTIONARY AND ADVISORY LABELS　14
▸ Salazopyrin (Pfizer Ltd)
　Sulfasalazine 500 mg　Salazopyrin 500mg suppositories |
　10 suppository PoM £3.30

CORTICOSTEROIDS

Beclometasone dipropionate
(Beclomethasone dipropionate)

● INDICATIONS AND DOSE
**Adjunct to aminosalicylates in acute mild to moderate
ulcerative colitis**
▸ BY MOUTH
▸ Adult:　5 mg daily maximum duration of treatment of
4 weeks, dose to be taken in the morning

● SIDE-EFFECTS　Constipation · drowsiness
● HEPATIC IMPAIRMENT　Manufacturer advises avoid in
severe impairment—no information available.

● MEDICINAL FORMS
There can be variation in the licensing of different medicines
containing the same drug.
Modified-release tablet
CAUTIONARY AND ADVISORY LABELS　25
▸ Clipper (Chiesi Ltd)
　Beclometasone dipropionate 5 mg　Clipper 5mg gastro-resistant
　modified-release tablets | 30 tablet PoM £56.56

Budesonide

● INDICATIONS AND DOSE
BUDENOFALK® CAPSULES
**Mild to moderate Crohn's disease affecting the ileum or
ascending colon | Chronic diarrhoea due to collagenous
colitis**
▸ BY MOUTH
▸ Adult:　3 mg 3 times a day for up to 8 weeks, reduce dose
for the last 2 weeks of treatment
Autoimmune hepatitis, induction of remission
▸ BY MOUTH
▸ Adult:　3 mg 3 times a day
Autoimmune hepatitis, maintenance
▸ BY MOUTH
▸ Adult:　3 mg twice daily
BUDENOFALK® GRANULES
**Mild to moderate Crohn's disease affecting the ileum or
ascending colon | Collagenous colitis**
▸ BY MOUTH
▸ Adult:　9 mg daily for up to 8 weeks, to be taken in the
morning, dose to be reduced for the last two weeks of
treatment
BUDENOFALK® RECTAL FOAM
Ulcerative colitis affecting sigmoid colon and rectum
▸ BY RECTUM
▸ Adult:　1 metered application once daily for up to
8 weeks
DOSE EQUIVALENCE AND CONVERSION
For *Budenofalk*® rectal foam: 1 metered application is
equivalent to budesonide 2 mg.
ENTOCORT® CAPSULES
**Mild to moderate Crohn's disease affecting the ileum or
ascending colon**
▸ BY MOUTH
▸ Adult:　9 mg once daily for up to 8 weeks; reduce dose
for the last 2–4 weeks of treatment, to be taken in the
morning　　　　　　　　　　　　continued →

1

Gastro-intestinal system

ENTOCORT® ENEMA

Ulcerative colitis involving rectal and recto-sigmoid disease

▸ BY RECTUM
▸ Adult: 1 enema daily for 4 weeks, to be administered at bedtime

- CAUTIONS
▸ With systemic use Autoimmune hepatitis
- HEPATIC IMPAIRMENT
▸ With systemic use When used in autoimmune hepatitis liver function tests should be monitored every 2 weeks for 1 month, then at least every 3 months.
- DIRECTIONS FOR ADMINISTRATION Granules should be placed on tongue and washed down with water without chewing.
- PRESCRIBING AND DISPENSING INFORMATION Flavours of granule formulations may include lemon.
  ENTOCORT® CAPSULES Dispense modified-release capsules in original container (contains desiccant).
- PATIENT AND CARER ADVICE Patients or carers should be given advice on how to administer budesonide granules.
- NATIONAL FUNDING/ACCESS DECISIONS
  BUDENOFALK® CAPSULES
  Scottish Medicines Consortium (SMC) Decisions
▸ With oral use The *Scottish Medicines Consortium* has advised (April 2015) that *Budenofalk*® gastro-resistant capsules are accepted for restricted use within NHS Scotland for the treatment of autoimmune hepatitis in non-cirrhotic patients who are intolerant of conventional oral corticosteroids (prednisolone) with severe corticosteroid-related side effects (actual or anticipated) such as psychosis, poorly controlled diabetes or osteoporosis.

- MEDICINAL FORMS
  There can be variation in the licensing of different medicines containing the same drug.
  Modified-release capsule
  CAUTIONARY AND ADVISORY LABELS 5, 10, 25
  ▸ Entocort CR (Tillotts Pharma Ltd)
  Budesonide 3 mg Entocort CR 3mg capsules | 100 capsule [PoM]
  £99.00 DT price = £99.00
  Gastro-resistant capsule
  CAUTIONARY AND ADVISORY LABELS 5, 10, 22, 25
  ▸ Budenofalk (Dr. Falk Pharma UK Ltd)
  Budesonide 3 mg Budenofalk 3mg gastro-resistant capsules | 100 capsule [PoM] £75.05 DT price = £75.05
  Gastro-resistant granules
  CAUTIONARY AND ADVISORY LABELS 5, 10, 22, 25
  ▸ Budenofalk (Dr. Falk Pharma UK Ltd)
  Budesonide 9 mg Budenofalk 9mg gastro-resistant granules sachets | 60 sachet [PoM] £135.00
  Foam
  EXCIPIENTS: May contain Cetostearyl alcohol (including cetyl and stearyl alcohol), disodium edetate, propylene glycol, sorbic acid
  ▸ Budenofalk (Dr. Falk Pharma UK Ltd)
  Budesonide 2 mg per 1 actuation Budenofalk 2mg foam enema | 14 dose [PoM] £57.11
  Enema
  ▸ Entocort (Tillotts Pharma Ltd)
  Budesonide 20 microgram per 1 ml Entocort 2mg/100ml enema | 7 enema [PoM] £39.60

IMMUNOSUPPRESSANTS > MONOCLONAL ANTIBODIES, ANTI-LYMPHOCYTE

Vedolizumab

4.4.2016

- DRUG ACTION Vedolizumab is a monoclonal antibody that binds specifically to the $\alpha_4\beta_7$ integrin, which is expressed on gut homing T helper lymphocytes and causes a reduction in gastrointestinal inflammation.

- INDICATIONS AND DOSE
  Moderate to severe active ulcerative colitis in patients who have had an inadequate response with, lost response to, or are intolerant to either conventional therapy or a tumour necrosis factor alpha inhibitor (under expert supervision)
  ▸ BY INTRAVENOUS INFUSION
  ▸ Adult: Initially 300 mg, then 300 mg after 2 weeks, followed by 300 mg after 4 weeks, followed by 300 mg every 8 weeks, dose to be given over 30 minutes, if treatment is interrupted or response decreases, dosing frequency may be increased—consult product literature; review treatment if no response within 10 weeks of initial dose
  Moderate to severe active Crohn's disease in patients who have had an inadequate response with, lost response to, or are intolerant to either conventional therapy or a tumour necrosis factor alpha inhibitor (under expert supervision)
  ▸ BY INTRAVENOUS INFUSION
  ▸ Adult: Initially 300 mg, then 300 mg after 2 weeks, followed by 300 mg after 4 weeks, followed by 300 mg every 8 weeks, dose to be given over 30 minutes, if no response is observed, an additional dose of 300 mg may be given 10 weeks after initial dose; if treatment is interrupted or response decreases, dosing frequency may be increased—consult product literature; review treatment if no response within 14 weeks of initial dose

- CONTRA-INDICATIONS Severe active infection
- CAUTIONS Controlled chronic severe infection · history of recurring severe infection · previous treatment with natalizumab (wait at least 12 weeks between natalizumab use and initiation of vedolizumab unless potential benefit outweighs risk) · previous treatment with rituximab
  CAUTIONS, FURTHER INFORMATION
  ▸ Risk of infection Patients must be screened for tuberculosis before starting treatment; if latent tuberculosis is diagnosed, appropriate treatment must be initiated prior to vedolizumab treatment; if tuberculosis is diagnosed during treatment, discontinue vedolizumab until infection is resolved.
  Patients should be brought up to date with current immunisation schedule before initiating treatment.
- INTERACTIONS → Appendix 1 (vedolizumab).
- SIDE-EFFECTS
  ▸ **Common or very common** Acne · arthralgia · back pain · constipation · cough · dyspepsia · eczema · erythema · flatulence · gastroenteritis · headache · hypertension · infection (increased susceptibility to viral, fungal and bacterial infections) · malaise · muscle spasms · muscular weakness · nasal congestion · nasopharyngitis · nausea · night sweats · oropharyngeal pain · paraesthesia · pharyngitis · pruritus · pyrexia · rash · sinusitis
  ▸ **Uncommon** Folliculitis · infusion-related reactions
  ▸ **Frequency not known** Dizziness
  SIDE-EFFECTS, FURTHER INFORMATION
  ▸ Infusion-related reactions Infusion-related and hypersensitivity reactions have been reported. Patients should be observed continuously during each infusion for signs and symptoms of acute hypersensitivity reactions;

they should also be observed for 2 hours after the initial two infusions, and for 1 hour after subsequent infusions. Discontinue treatment if a severe infusion-related or other severe reaction occurs and initiate appropriate treatment (e.g. adrenaline and antihistamines); if a mild to moderate infusion-related reaction occurs, interrupt infusion or reduce infusion rate and initiate appropriate treatment (if reaction subsides the infusion may be continued)— consider pretreatment with an antihistamine, hydrocortisone, and/or paracetamol prior to subsequent infusions in patients who experience mild to moderate infusion-related reactions.

● CONCEPTION AND CONTRACEPTION Manufacturer advises effective contraception required during and for at least 18 weeks after treatment.

● PREGNANCY Manufacturer advises use only if potential benefit outweighs risk.

● BREAST FEEDING Manufacturer advises avoid—present in milk in *animal* studies.

● MONITORING REQUIREMENTS
▸ Manufacturer advises monitor closely for infection before, during and after treatment—potential increased risk of opportunistic infection.
▸ Manufacturer advises monitor for new onset or worsening neurological signs and symptoms (withhold treatment if progressive multifocal leukoencephalopathy (PML) is suspected).

● DIRECTIONS FOR ADMINISTRATION For *intravenous infusion* (*Entyvio* ®), give intermittently *in* Sodium chloride 0.9%; allow vial to reach room temperature then reconstitute with 4.8 mL of water for injection (using a syringe with a 21–25 gauge needle); gently swirl vial for at least 15 seconds, do not shake vigorously or invert; allow to stand for up to 20 minutes (gently swirl vial if needed), leave for an additional 10 minutes if not dissolved; gently invert vial three times, withdraw 5 mL of reconstituted solution (using a syringe with a 21–25 gauge needle), and add to 250 mL of infusion fluid; gently mix and give over 30 minutes.

● PATIENT AND CARER ADVICE Patients should be provided with a patient alert card.

● NATIONAL FUNDING/ACCESS DECISIONS
NICE technology appraisals (TAs)
▸ **Vedolizumab for treating moderately to severely active Crohn's disease after prior therapy (August 2015)** NICE TA352
Vedolizumab is recommended as an option for the treatment of moderate to severe active Crohn's disease in adults if:
● a tumour necrosis factor-alpha inhibitor has failed (that is, the disease has responded inadequately or has lost response to treatment) **or**
● a tumour necrosis factor-alpha inhibitor cannot be tolerated or is contra-indicated,
● **and** the manufacturer provides vedolizumab with the discount agreed in the patient access scheme.
Vedolizumab should be given as a planned course of treatment until treatment fails, or surgery is needed, or until 12 months after starting treatment, whichever is the shorter. Treatment should be continued only if there is clear evidence of a response. Patients who continue treatment should be reassessed at least every 12 months to determine whether ongoing treatment is still clinically appropriate.
    Patients currently receiving vedolizumab whose disease does not meet the above criteria should be able to continue treatment until they and their clinician consider it appropriate to stop.
www.nice.org.uk/TA352
Scottish Medicines Consortium (SMC) Decisions
The *Scottish Medicines Consortium* has advised (July 2015) that vedolizumab (*Entyvio* ®) is accepted for restricted use

within NHS Scotland for the treatment of adult patients with moderately to severely active Crohn's disease who have had an inadequate response with, lost response to, or were intolerant to a TNFα antagonist; it is also accepted for use in NHS Scotland for the treatment of adult patients with moderately to severely active ulcerative colitis who have had an inadequate response with, lost response to, or were intolerant to either conventional therapy or a TNFα antagonist.

● MEDICINAL FORMS
There can be variation in the licensing of different medicines containing the same drug.
Powder for solution for infusion
▸ Entyvio (Takeda UK Ltd) ▼
    Vedolizumab 300 mg Entyvio 300mg powder for concentrate for solution for infusion vials | 1 vial [PoM] £2,050.00

1.3   Irritable bowel syndrome

Irritable bowel syndrome   24.2.2016

Description of condition
Irritable bowel syndrome (IBS) is a common, chronic, relapsing, and often life-long condition, mainly affecting people aged between 20 and 30 years. It is more common in women. Symptoms include abdominal pain or discomfort, disordered defaecation (either diarrhoea, or constipation with straining, urgency, and incomplete evacuation), passage of mucus, and bloating. Symptoms are usually relieved by defaecation. Obtaining an accurate clinical diagnosis of IBS prior to treatment is crucial.

Aims of treatment
The treatment of IBS is focused on symptom control, in order to improve quality of life.

Non-drug treatment
EvGr Diet and lifestyle changes are important for effective self-management of IBS. Patients should be encouraged to increase physical activity, and advised to eat regularly, without missing meals or leaving long gaps between meals. Dietary advice should also include, limiting fresh fruit consumption to no more than 3 portions per day. The fibre intake of patients with IBS should be reviewed. If an increase in dietary fibre is required, soluble fibre such as ispaghula husk p. 47, or foods high in soluble fibre such as oats, are recommended. Intake of insoluble fibre (e.g. bran) and 'resistant starch' should be reduced or discouraged as they may exacerbate symptoms. Fluid intake (mostly water) should be increased to at least 8 cups each day and the intake of caffeine, alcohol and fizzy drinks reduced. The artificial sweetener sorbitol should be avoided in patients with diarrhoea. Where probiotics are being used, continue for at least 4 weeks while monitoring the effect. Ⓐ

EvGr If a patient's symptoms persist following lifestyle and dietary advice, single food avoidance and exclusion diets may be an option under the supervision of a dietitian or medical specialist. Ⓐ

Drug treatment

[EvGr] The choice of drug treatment depends on the nature and severity of the symptoms. Many drug treatment options for IBS are available over-the-counter. ⚠

[EvGr] Antispasmodic drugs (such as alverine citrate p. 78, mebeverine hydrochloride p. 78 and peppermint oil below) can be taken in addition to dietary and lifestyle changes. A laxative (excluding lactulose p. 49 as it may cause bloating) can be used to treat constipation. Patients who have not responded to laxatives from the different classes and who have had constipation for at least 12 months, can be treated with linaclotide below. Loperamide hydrochloride p. 59 is the first-line choice of anti-motility drug for relief of diarrhoea. Patients with IBS should be advised how on to adjust their dose of laxative or anti-motility drug according to stool consistency, with the aim of achieving a soft, well-formed stool. ⚠ See Constipation p. 46, for information on other drugs used for chronic constipation.

[EvGr] A low-dose tricyclic antidepressant, such as amitriptyline hydrochloride p. 341 [unlicensed indication], can be used for abdominal pain or discomfort as a second-line option in patients who have not responded to antispasmodics, anti-motility drugs, or laxatives. A selective serotonin reuptake inhibitor may be considered in those who do not respond to a tricyclic antidepressant [unlicensed indication]. ⚠

[EvGr] Psychological intervention can be offered to patients who have no relief of IBS symptoms after 12 months of drug treatment. ⚠

Useful Resources

Irritable bowel syndrome in adults: diagnosis and management. Clinical guideline 61. February 2015
www.nice.org.uk/guidance/cg61

ANTISPASMODICS

Mebeverine with ispaghula husk   4.2.2016

The properties listed below are those particular to the combination only. For the properties of the components please consider, mebeverine hydrochloride p. 78, ispaghula husk p. 47.

- ● INDICATIONS AND DOSE
Irritable bowel syndrome
  ▶ BY MOUTH
  ▶ Child 12–17 years: 1 sachet twice daily, in water, morning and evening, 30 minutes before food and 1 sachet daily if required, taken 30 minutes before midday meal
  ▶ Adult: 1 sachet twice daily, in water, morning and evening, 30 minutes before food and 1 sachet daily if required, taken 30 minutes before midday meal

- ● DIRECTIONS FOR ADMINISTRATION Contents of one sachet should be stirred into a glass (approx. 150 mL) of cold water and drunk immediately.

- ● PATIENT AND CARER ADVICE Patients or carers should be given advice on how to administer ispaghula husk with mebeverine granules.

- ● MEDICINAL FORMS
There can be variation in the licensing of different medicines containing the same drug.
Effervescent granules
CAUTIONARY AND ADVISORY LABELS 13, 22
EXCIPIENTS: May contain Aspartame
ELECTROLYTES: May contain Potassium
  ▶ Fybogel Mebeverine (Reckitt Benckiser Healthcare (UK) Ltd)
  Mebeverine hydrochloride 135 mg, Ispaghula husk
  3.5 gram Fybogel Mebeverine effervescent granules sachets orange sugar-free | 10 sachet [P] £4.22 DT price = £4.22

Peppermint oil

- ● INDICATIONS AND DOSE
COLPERMIN®
Relief of abdominal colic and distension, particularly in irritable bowel syndrome
  ▶ BY MOUTH
  ▶ Child 15–17 years: 1–2 capsules 3 times a day for up to 3 months if necessary, capsule to be swallowed whole with water
  ▶ Adult: 1–2 capsules 3 times a day for up to 3 months if necessary, capsule to be swallowed whole with water
MINTEC®
Relief of abdominal colic and distension, particularly in irritable bowel syndrome
  ▶ BY MOUTH
  ▶ Adult: 1–2 capsules 3 times a day for up to 2–3 months if necessary, dose to be taken before meals, swallowed whole with water

- ● CAUTIONS Sensitivity to menthol
- ● SIDE-EFFECTS
  ▶ Rare Allergic reactions · ataxia · bradycardia · headache · muscle tremor · rash
  ▶ Frequency not known Heartburn · perianal irritation
- ● PREGNANCY Not known to be harmful.
- ● BREAST FEEDING Significant levels of menthol in breast milk unlikely.
- ● DIRECTIONS FOR ADMINISTRATION Capsules should not be broken or chewed because peppermint oil may irritate mouth or oesophagus.

- ● MEDICINAL FORMS
There can be variation in the licensing of different medicines containing the same drug.
Modified-release capsule
CAUTIONARY AND ADVISORY LABELS 5, 22, 25
EXCIPIENTS: May contain Arachis (peanut) oil
  ▶ Colpermin (McNeil Products Ltd)
  Peppermint oil 200 microlitre Colpermin gastro-resistant modified-release capsule | 20 capsule [GSL] £3.33 | 100 capsule [GSL] £12.18 DT price = £12.18
Gastro-resistant capsule
CAUTIONARY AND ADVISORY LABELS 5, 22, 25
  ▶ Mintec (Almirall Ltd)
  Peppermint oil 200 microlitre Mintec 0.2ml gastro-resistant capsules | 84 capsule [GSL] £7.04 DT price = £7.04

LAXATIVES > GUANYLATE CYCLASE-C RECEPTOR AGONISTS

Linaclotide   24.2.2016

- ● INDICATIONS AND DOSE
Moderate to severe irritable bowel syndrome with constipation
  ▶ BY MOUTH
  ▶ Adult: 290 micrograms once daily, dose to be taken at least 30 minutes before meals, review treatment if no response after 4 weeks

- ● CONTRA-INDICATIONS Gastro-intestinal obstruction · inflammatory bowel disease
- ● CAUTIONS Predisposition to fluid and electrolyte disturbances
- ● SIDE-EFFECTS
  ▶ Common or very common Abdominal distension · abdominal pain · diarrhoea · dizziness · flatulence
  ▶ Uncommon Decreased appetite · dehydration · faecal incontinence · hypokalaemia · orthostatic hypotension

SIDE-EFFECTS, FURTHER INFORMATION
▸ Diarrhoea Manufacturer advises if diarrhoea severe or prolonged, consider suspending treatment.

● PREGNANCY Manufacturer advises avoid.

● BREAST FEEDING Unlikely to be present in milk in significant amounts, but manufacturer advises avoid.

● PRESCRIBING AND DISPENSING INFORMATION Dispense capsules in original container (contains desiccant); discard any capsules remaining 18 weeks after opening.

● NATIONAL FUNDING/ACCESS DECISIONS
Scottish Medicines Consortium (SMC) Decisions
The *Scottish Medicines Consortium* has advised (May 2013) that linaclotide (*Constella*®) is accepted for restricted use within NHS Scotland for moderate to severe irritable bowel syndrome in patients whose condition has not responded adequately to all other treatments, or who are intolerant of them.

● MEDICINAL FORMS
There can be variation in the licensing of different medicines containing the same drug.
Capsule
CAUTIONARY AND ADVISORY LABELS 22
▸ Linaclotide (Non-proprietary) ▼
  Linaclotide 290 microgram Linaclotide 290microgram capsules |
  28 capsule [PoM] no price available
▸ Constella (Allergan Ltd) ▼
  Linaclotide 290 microgram Constella 290microgram capsules |
  28 capsule [PoM] £37.56

2   Constipation and bowel cleansing

2.1   Bowel cleansing

Drugs used for Bowel cleansing not listed below
Bisacodyl, p. 53 · Docusate sodium, p. 57 · Magnesium sulfate, p. 911

LAXATIVES > OSMOTIC LAXATIVES

Citric acid with magnesium carbonate
(Formulated as a bowel cleansing preparation)

● INDICATIONS AND DOSE
Bowel evacuation for surgery, colonoscopy or radiological examination
▸ BY MOUTH
▸ Child 5–9 years: One-third of a sachet to be given at 8 a.m. the day before the procedure and, one-third of a sachet to be given between 2 and 4 p.m. the day before the procedure
▸ Child 10–17 years: 0.5–1 sachet, given at 8 a.m. the day before the procedure and 0.5–1 sachet, given between 2 and 4 p.m. the day before the procedure
▸ Adult: 1 sachet, given 8 a.m. the day before the procedure and 1 sachet, given between 2 and 4 p.m. the day before the procedure, use half the dose in frail elderly patients

● CONTRA-INDICATIONS Acute severe colitis · gastric retention · gastro-intestinal obstruction · gastro-intestinal perforation · toxic megacolon

● CAUTIONS Children · colitis (avoid if acute severe colitis) · debilitated · elderly (in adults) · hypovolaemia (should be corrected before administration of bowel cleansing preparations) · impaired gag reflex or possibility of regurgitation or aspiration · patients with fluid and electrolyte disturbances

CAUTIONS, FURTHER INFORMATION
Adequate hydration should be maintained during treatment.

● INTERACTIONS Other oral drugs should not be taken one hour before or after administration of bowel cleansing preparations because absorption may be impaired.
▸ In adults Consider withholding ACE inhibitors, angiotensin-II receptor antagonists, and NSAIDs on the day that bowel cleansing preparations are given and for up to 72 hours after the procedure. Also consider withholding diuretics on the day that bowel cleansing preparations are given.

● SIDE-EFFECTS
▸ **Common or very common** Abdominal distention · abdominal pain · nausea · vomiting
▸ **Uncommon** Dehydration · dizziness · electrolyte disturbances · headache

SIDE-EFFECTS, FURTHER INFORMATION
▸ Abdominal pain Abdominal pain is usually transient and can be reduced by taking preparation more slowly.

● PREGNANCY Use with caution.

● BREAST FEEDING Use with caution.

● HEPATIC IMPAIRMENT Avoid in hepatic coma if risk of renal failure.

● RENAL IMPAIRMENT
▸ In adults Avoid if eGFR less than 30 mL/minute/1.73 m^2—risk of hypermagnesaemia.
▸ In children Avoid if estimated glomerular filtration rate less than 30 mL/minute/1.73 m^2—risk of hypermagnesaemia.

● MONITORING REQUIREMENTS Renal function should be measured before starting treatment in patients at risk of fluid and electrolyte disturbances.

● DIRECTIONS FOR ADMINISTRATION One sachet should be reconstituted with 200 mL of hot water; the solution should be allowed to cool for approx. 30 minutes before drinking.

● PRESCRIBING AND DISPENSING INFORMATION Reconstitution of one sachet containing 11.57 g magnesium carbonate and 17.79 g anhydrous citric acid produces a solution containing magnesium citrate with 118 mmol Mg^{2+}.
  Flavours of oral powders may include lemon and lime.

● PATIENT AND CARER ADVICE Low residue or fluid only diet (e.g. water, fruit squash, clear soup, black tea or coffee) recommended before procedure (according to prescriber's advice) and copious intake of clear fluids recommended until procedure. Patient or carers should be given advice on how to administer oral powder.

● MEDICINAL FORMS
There can be variation in the licensing of different medicines containing the same drug.
Effervescent powder
CAUTIONARY AND ADVISORY LABELS 13, 10
ELECTROLYTES: May contain Magnesium
▸ Citramag (Sanochemia Diagnostics UK Ltd)
  Magnesium carbonate heavy 11.57 gram, Citric acid anhydrous 17.79 gram Citramag effervescent powder sachets sugar-free |
  10 sachet [P] £18.92

Macrogol 3350 with anhydrous sodium sulfate, ascorbic acid, potassium chloride, sodium ascorbate and sodium chloride

(Polyethylene glycols)

● INDICATIONS AND DOSE

MOVIPREP®

Bowel evacuation for surgery, colonoscopy or radiological examination

▶ BY MOUTH

▶ Adult: 1 litre daily for 2 doses: first dose of reconstituted solution taken on the evening before procedure and the second dose on the morning of procedure, alternatively 2 litres daily for 1 dose; reconstituted solution to be taken on the evening before the procedure, treatment should be completed at least 1 hour before colonoscopy

● CONTRA-INDICATIONS Acute severe colitis · G6PD deficiency · gastric retention · gastro-intestinal obstruction · gastro-intestinal perforation · toxic megacolon

● CAUTIONS Colitis (avoid if acute severe colitis) · debilitated patients · elderly · fluid and electrolyte disturbances · heart failure · hypovolaemia (should be corrected before administration of bowel cleansing preparations) · impaired gag reflex or possibility of regurgitation or aspiration

● INTERACTIONS Consider withholding ACE inhibitors, angiotensin-II receptor antagonists, and NSAIDs on the day that bowel cleansing preparations are given and for up to 72 hours after the procedure. Also consider withholding diuretics on the day that bowel cleansing preparations are given.

● SIDE-EFFECTS

▶ **Common or very common** Abdominal distention · abdominal pain · nausea · vomiting

▶ **Uncommon** Dehydration · dizziness · electrolyte disturbances · headache

▶ **Frequency not known** Anal discomfort · fatigue · sleep disturbances

SIDE-EFFECTS, FURTHER INFORMATION

▶ Abdominal pain Abdominal pain is usually transient and can be reduced by taking preparation more slowly.

● PREGNANCY Manufacturers advise use only if essential— no information available.

● BREAST FEEDING Manufacturers advise use only if essential—no information available.

● RENAL IMPAIRMENT Caution if eGFR less than 30 mL/minute/1.73 m².

● MONITORING REQUIREMENTS Renal function should be measured before starting treatment in patients at risk of fluid and electrolyte disturbances.

● DIRECTIONS FOR ADMINISTRATION

MOVIPREP® One pair of sachets (A and B) should be reconstituted in 1 litre of water and taken over 1–2 hours. 1 litre of other clear fluid should also be taken during treatment.

● PRESCRIBING AND DISPENSING INFORMATION Flavours of oral powder formulations may include lemon or orange.

MOVIPREP® 1 pair of sachets (A+B) when reconstituted with 1 litre of water provides Na⁺ 181.6 mmol (Na⁺ 56.2 mmol absorbable), K⁺ 14.2 mmol, Cl⁻ 59.8 mmol.

● PATIENT AND CARER ADVICE Patient information leaflet. Solid food should not be taken during treatment until procedure completed.
Treatment can be stopped if bowel motions become watery and clear.

● MEDICINAL FORMS
There can be variation in the licensing of different medicines containing the same drug.
Form unstated
CAUTIONARY AND ADVISORY LABELS 10, 13
EXCIPIENTS: May contain Aspartame
ELECTROLYTES: May contain Chloride, potassium, sodium
▶ Moviprep (Norgine Pharmaceuticals Ltd)
  Moviprep oral powder sachets sugar-free | 4 sachet [P] £9.87

Macrogol 3350 with anhydrous sodium sulfate, potassium chloride, sodium bicarbonate and sodium chloride

(Formulated as a bowel cleansing preparation)

● INDICATIONS AND DOSE

Bowel cleansing before radiological examination, colonoscopy, or surgery

▶ INITIALLY BY MOUTH

▶ Adult: Initially 2 litres daily for 2 doses: first dose of reconstituted solution taken on the evening before procedure and the second dose on the morning of procedure, alternatively (by mouth) initially 250 mL every 10–15 minutes, reconstituted solution to be administered, alternatively (by nasogastric tube) initially 20–30 mL/minute, starting on the day before procedure until 4 litres have been consumed

● CONTRA-INDICATIONS Acute severe colitis · gastric retention · gastro-intestinal obstruction · gastro-intestinal perforation · toxic megacolon

● CAUTIONS Colitis (avoid if acute severe colitis) · debilitated patients · elderly · fluid and electrolyte disturbances · heart failure · hypovolaemia (should be corrected before administration of bowel cleansing preparations) · impaired gag reflex or possibility of regurgitation or aspiration

● INTERACTIONS Consider withholding ACE inhibitors, angiotensin-II receptor antagonists, and NSAIDs on the day that bowel cleansing preparations are given and for up to 72 hours after the procedure. Also consider withholding diuretics on the day that bowel cleansing preparations are given.

● SIDE-EFFECTS

▶ **Common or very common** Abdominal distention · abdominal pain · nausea · vomiting

▶ **Uncommon** Anal discomfort · dehydration · dizziness · electrolyte disturbances · fatigue · headache · sleep disturbances

SIDE-EFFECTS, FURTHER INFORMATION

▶ Abdominal pain Abdominal pain is usually transient and can be reduced by taking preparation more slowly.

● PREGNANCY Manufacturers advise use only if essential— no information available.

● BREAST FEEDING Manufacturers advise use only if essential—no information available.

● MONITORING REQUIREMENTS Renal function should be measured before starting treatment in patients at risk of fluid and electrolyte disturbances.

● DIRECTIONS FOR ADMINISTRATION 1 sachet should be reconstituted with 1 litre of water. Flavouring such as clear fruit cordials may be added if required. After reconstitution the solution should be kept in a refrigerator and discarded if unused after 24 hours.

● PRESCRIBING AND DISPENSING INFORMATION Each *Klean-Prep*® sachet provides Na⁺ 125 mmol, K⁺ 10 mmol, Cl⁻ 35 mmol and HCO³⁻ 20mmol when reconstituted with 1 litre of water.

● PATIENT AND CARER ADVICE Solid food should not be taken for 2 hours before starting treatment. Adequate hydration should be maintained during treatment. Treatment can be stopped if bowel motions become watery and clear.

● MEDICINAL FORMS
There can be variation in the licensing of different medicines containing the same drug.
Powder
CAUTIONARY AND ADVISORY LABELS 10, 13
EXCIPIENTS: May contain Aspartame
ELECTROLYTES: May contain Bicarbonate, chloride, potassium, sodium
▸ Klean-Prep (Norgine Pharmaceuticals Ltd)
    Potassium chloride 742.5 mg, Sodium chloride 1.465 gram, Sodium bicarbonate 1.685 gram, Sodium sulfate anhydrous 5.685 gram, Polyethylene glycol 3350 59 gram Klean-Prep oral powder 69g sachets sugar-free | 4 sachet P £9.98

LAXATIVES ⟩ STIMULANT LAXATIVES

Magnesium citrate with sodium picosulfate
(Formulated as a bowel cleansing preparation)

● INDICATIONS AND DOSE
CITRAFLEET® SACHETS
Bowel evacuation on day before radiological examination, endoscopy, or surgery
▸ BY MOUTH
▸ Adult: 1 sachet taken before 8 a.m, then 1 sachet after 6–8 hours
PHARMACOKINETICS
For *Citrafleet*® sachets: Acts within 3 hours of first dose.

PICOLAX® SACHETS
Bowel evacuation on day before radiological procedure, endoscopy, or surgery
▸ BY MOUTH
▸ Child 1 year: 0.25 sachet taken before 8 a.m, then 0.25 sachet after 6–8 hours
▸ Child 2-3 years: 0.5 sachet taken before 8 a.m, then 0.5 sachet after 6–8 hours
▸ Child 4-8 years: 1 sachet taken before 8 a.m, then 0.5 sachet after 6–8 hours
▸ Child 9-17 years: 1 sachet taken before 8 a.m, then 1 sachet after 6–8 hours
▸ Adult: 1 sachet taken before 8 a.m, then 1 sachet after 6–8 hours
PHARMACOKINETICS
For *Picolax*® sachets: Acts within 3 hours of first dose.

● CONTRA-INDICATIONS Acute severe colitis · ascites · congestive cardiac failure · gastric retention · gastro-intestinal obstruction · gastro-intestinal perforation · gastro-intestinal ulceration · toxic megacolon
● CAUTIONS Cardiac disease (avoid in congestive cardiac failure) · children · colitis (avoid if acute severe colitis) · debilitated patients · elderly (in adults) · fluid and electrolyte disturbances · hypovolaemia (should be corrected before administration) · impaired gag reflex or possibility of regurgitation or aspiration · recent gastro-intestinal surgery
● SIDE-EFFECTS
▸ **Common or very common** Abdominal distention · abdominal pain (usually transient—reduced by taking more slowly) · nausea · vomiting
▸ **Uncommon** Dehydration · dizziness · electrolyte disturbances · headache
▸ **Frequency not known** Anal discomfort · fatigue · rash · sleep disturbances

● PREGNANCY Caution.
● BREAST FEEDING Caution.
● HEPATIC IMPAIRMENT Avoid in hepatic coma if risk of renal failure.
● RENAL IMPAIRMENT
▸ In adults Avoid if eGFR less than 30 mL/minute/1.73 m^2—risk of hypermagnesaemia.
▸ In children Avoid if estimated glomerular filtration rate less than 30 mL/minute/1.73 m^2—risk of hypermagnesaemia.
● DIRECTIONS FOR ADMINISTRATION One sachet of sodium picosulfate with magnesium citrate powder should be reconstituted with 150 mL (approx. half a glass) of cold water; patients should be warned that heat is generated during reconstitution and that the solution should be allowed to cool before drinking.
PICOLAX® SACHETS One sachet should be reconstituted with 150 mL (approx. half a glass) of cold water.
CITRAFLEET® SACHETS One sachet should be reconstituted with 150 mL (approx. half a glass) of cold water.
● PRESCRIBING AND DISPENSING INFORMATION Flavours of oral powder formulations may include lemon.
PICOLAX® SACHETS One reconstituted sachet contains K$^+$ 5 mmol and Mg^{2+} 87 mmol.
CITRAFLEET® SACHETS One reconstituted sachet contains K$^+$ 5 mmol and Mg^{2+} 86 mmol.
● PATIENT AND CARER ADVICE Low residue diet recommended on the day before procedure and copious intake of water or other clear fluids recommended during treatment. Patients or carers should be given advice on how to administer sodium picosulfate with magnesium citrate oral powder.
PICOLAX® SACHETS Low residue diet recommended on the day before procedure and copious intake of water or other clear fluids recommended during treatment.
   Patients and carers should be given advice on how to administer oral powder; they should be warned that heat is generated during reconstitution and that the solution should be allowed to cool before drinking.
CITRAFLEET® SACHETS Low residue diet recommended on the day before procedure and copious intake of water or other clear fluids recommended during treatment.
   Patients and carers should be given advice on how to administer oral powder; they should be warned that heat is generated during reconstitution and that the solution should be allowed to cool before drinking.

● MEDICINAL FORMS
There can be variation in the licensing of different medicines containing the same drug.
Powder
CAUTIONARY AND ADVISORY LABELS 10, 13
ELECTROLYTES: May contain Magnesium, potassium
▸ CitraFleet (Casen Recordati S.L.)
    Sodium picosulfate 10 mg, Magnesium oxide light 3.5 gram, Citric acid anhydrous 10.97 gram CitraFleet oral powder 15.08g sachets sugar-free | 2 sachet P £3.25
▸ Picolax (Ferring Pharmaceuticals Ltd)
    Sodium picosulfate 10 mg, Magnesium oxide 3.5 gram, Citric acid anhydrous 12 gram Picolax oral powder 16.1g sachets sugar-free | 2 sachet P £3.39

2.2 Constipation

Constipation

Overview

Before prescribing laxatives it is important to be sure that the patient *is* constipated and that the constipation is *not* secondary to an underlying undiagnosed complaint.

It is also important for those who complain of constipation to understand that bowel habit can vary considerably in frequency without doing harm. Some people tend to consider themselves constipated if they do not have a bowel movement each day. A useful definition of constipation is the passage of hard stools less frequently than the patient's own normal pattern and this can be explained to the patient.

Misconceptions about bowel habits have led to excessive laxative use. Abuse may lead to hypokalaemia.

Thus, laxatives should generally be **avoided** except where straining will exacerbate a condition (such as angina) or increase the risk of rectal bleeding as in haemorrhoids. Laxatives are also of value in *drug-induced constipation*, for the expulsion of *parasites* after anthelmintic treatment, and to clear the alimentary tract *before surgery and radiological procedures*. Prolonged treatment of constipation is sometimes necessary.

Laxatives also have a role in the treatment of irritable bowel syndrome.

Also see the prevention of opioid-induced constipation in palliative care.

The laxatives that follow have been divided into 5 main groups. This simple classification disguises the fact that some laxatives have a complex action.

Bulk-forming laxatives

Bulk-forming laxatives are of value if the diet is deficient in fibre. Bulk-forming laxatives are of particular value in those with small hard stools, but should not be required unless fibre cannot be increased in the diet. A balanced diet, including adequate fluid intake and fibre is of value in preventing constipation.

Bulk-forming laxatives can be used in the management of patients with *colostomy, ileostomy, haemorrhoids, anal fissure, chronic diarrhoea associated with diverticular disease, irritable bowel syndrome*, and as adjuncts in *ulcerative colitis*. Adequate fluid intake must be maintained to avoid intestinal obstruction. Unprocessed wheat bran, taken with food or fruit juice, is a most effective bulk-forming preparation. Finely ground bran, though more palatable, has poorer water-retaining properties, but can be taken as bran bread or biscuits in appropriately increased quantities. Oat bran is also used.

Methylcellulose p. 48, ispaghula husk p. 47, and sterculia p. 48 are useful in patients who cannot tolerate bran. Methylcellulose also acts as a faecal softener.

Stimulant laxatives

Stimulant laxatives include bisacodyl p. 53, sodium picosulfate p. 55, and members of the **anthraquinone** group, senna p. 55, co-danthramer p. 53 and co-danthrusate p. 54. The indications for co-danthramer and co-danthrusate are limited by its potential carcinogenicity (based on rodent carcinogenicity studies) and evidence of genotoxicity. Powerful stimulants such as **cascara** (an anthraquinone) and **castor oil** are obsolete. Docusate sodium p. 57 probably acts both as a stimulant and as a softening agent.

Stimulant laxatives increase intestinal motility and often cause abdominal cramp; they should be avoided in intestinal obstruction. Excessive use of stimulant laxatives can cause diarrhoea and related effects such as hypokalaemia;

however, prolonged use may be justifiable in some circumstances.

Glycerol suppositories p. 54 act as a lubricant and as a rectal stimulant by virtue of the mildly irritant action of glycerol.

Unstandardised preparations of cascara, frangula, rhubarb, and senna should be **avoided** as their laxative action is unpredictable. Aloes, colocynth, and jalap should be **avoided** as they have a drastic purgative action.

The **parasympathomimetics** bethanechol chloride p. 712, neostigmine p. 971, and pyridostigmine bromide p. 972 enhance parasympathetic activity in the gut and increase intestinal motility. They are rarely used for their gastro-intestinal effects. Organic obstruction of the gut must first be excluded and they should not be used shortly after bowel anastomosis.

Other stimulant laxatives

Unstandardised preparations of cascara, frangula, rhubarb, and senna should be **avoided** as their laxative action is unpredictable. Aloes, colocynth, and jalap should be **avoided** as they have a drastic purgative action.

Faecal softeners

Liquid paraffin p. 57, the traditional lubricant, has disadvantages. Bulk laxatives and non-ionic surfactant 'wetting' agents e.g. docusate sodium also have softening properties. Such drugs are useful for oral administration in the management of haemorrhoids and anal fissure; glycerol is useful for rectal use.

Enemas containing arachis oil p. 56 (ground-nut oil, peanut oil) lubricate and soften impacted faeces and promote a bowel movement.

Osmotic laxatives

Osmotic laxatives increase the amount of water in the large bowel, either by drawing fluid from the body into the bowel or by retaining the fluid they were administered with.

Lactulose p. 49 is a semi-synthetic disaccharide which is not absorbed from the gastro-intestinal tract. It produces an osmotic diarrhoea of low faecal pH, and discourages the proliferation of ammonia-producing organisms. It is therefore useful in the treatment of *hepatic encephalopathy*.

Macrogols are inert polymers of ethylene glycol which sequester fluid in the bowel; giving fluid with macrogols may reduce the dehydrating effect sometimes seen with osmotic laxatives.

Saline purgatives such as magnesium hydroxide p. 51 are commonly abused but are satisfactory for occasional use; adequate fluid intake should be maintained. Magnesium salts, such as magnesium sulfate p. 911 are useful where rapid bowel evacuation is required. **Sodium salts** should be avoided as they may give rise to sodium and water retention in susceptible individuals. **Phosphate enemas** are useful in bowel clearance before radiology, endoscopy, and surgery.

Other drugs used in constipation

Linaclotide p. 42 is a guanylate cyclase-C receptor agonist that is licensed for the treatment of moderate to severe irritable bowel syndrome associated with constipation. It increases intestinal fluid secretion and transit, and decreases visceral pain. It is metabolised within the gastro-intestinal tract and is virtually undetectable in the plasma after therapeutic doses.

Lubiprostone p. 49 is a chloride-channel activator that is licensed for the treatment of chronic idiopathic constipation in adults whose condition has not responded adequately to lifestyle changes (including dietary changes).

Prucalopride p. 52 is a selective serotonin 5HT4-receptor agonist with prokinetic properties. It is licensed for the treatment of chronic constipation in women, when other laxatives have failed to provide an adequate response.

Bowel cleansing preparations

Bowel cleansing preparations are used before colonic surgery, colonoscopy, or radiological examination to ensure the bowel is free of solid contents. They are not treatments for constipation.

Pregnancy

If dietary and lifestyle changes fail to control constipation in pregnancy, moderate doses of poorly absorbed laxatives may be used. A bulk-forming laxative should be tried first. An osmotic laxative, such as lactulose, can also be used. Bisacodyl or senna may be suitable, if a stimulant effect is necessary.

Constipation in children

Laxatives should be prescribed by a healthcare professional experienced in the management of constipation in children. Delays of greater than 3 days between stools may increase the likelihood of pain on passing hard stools leading to anal fissure, anal spasm and eventually to a learned response to avoid defaecation.

In *infants*, increased intake of fluids, particularly fruit juice containing sorbitol (e.g. prune, pear, or apple), may be sufficient to soften the stool. In infants under 1 year of age with mild constipation, lactulose p. 49 can be used to soften the stool; either an oral preparation containing macrogols or, rarely, glycerol suppositories p. 54 can be used to clear faecal impaction. The infant should be referred to a hospital paediatric specialist if these measures fail.

The diet of *children over 1 year of age* should be reviewed to ensure that it includes an adequate intake of fibre and fluid. An osmotic laxative containing macrogols can also be used, particularly in children with chronic constipation; lactulose is an alternative in children who cannot tolerate a macrogol. If there is an inadequate response to the osmotic laxative, a **stimulant laxative** can be added.

Treatment of faecal impaction may initially increase symptoms of soiling and abdominal pain. In children over 1 year of age with faecal impaction, an oral preparation containing macrogols is used to clear faecal mass and to establish and maintain soft well-formed stools. If disimpaction does not occur after 2 weeks, a **stimulant laxative** can be added. If the impacted mass is not expelled following treatment with macrogols and a stimulant laxative, a sodium citrate enema can be administered. Although rectal administration of laxatives may be effective, this route is frequently distressing for the child and may lead to persistence of withholding. A **phosphate enema** may be administered under specialist supervision if disimpaction does not occur after a sodium citrate enema; a **bowel cleansing preparation** is an alternative. Manual evacuation under anaesthetic may be necessary if disimpaction does not occur after oral and rectal treatment, or if the child is afraid.

Long-term regular use of laxatives is essential to maintain well-formed stools and prevent recurrence of faecal impaction; intermittent use may provoke relapses. In children with chronic constipation, laxatives should be continued for several weeks after a regular pattern of bowel movements or toilet training is established. The dose of laxatives should then be tapered gradually, over a period of months, according to response. Some children may require laxative therapy for several years.

Chronic constipation

For children with chronic constipation, it may be necessary to exceed the licensed doses of some laxatives. Parents and carers of children should be advised to adjust the dose of laxative in order to establish a regular pattern of bowel movements in which stools are soft, well-formed, and passed without discomfort. Laxatives should be administered at a time that produces an effect that is likely to fit in with the child's toilet routine.

> **Drugs used for Constipation not listed below** Sodium citrate, p. 713

LAXATIVES > BULK-FORMING LAXATIVES

Ispaghula husk   24.2.2016

- ● DRUG ACTION Bulk-forming laxatives relieve constipation by increasing faecal mass which stimulates peristalsis.

- ● INDICATIONS AND DOSE

Constipation

▶ BY MOUTH
  ▸ Child 1 month–5 years: 2.5–5 mL twice daily, dose to be taken only when prescribed by a doctor, as half or whole level spoonful in water, preferably after meals, morning and evening
  ▸ Child 6–11 years: 2.5–5 mL twice daily, dose to be given as a half or whole level spoonful in water, preferably after meals, morning and evening
  ▸ Child 12–17 years: 1 sachet twice daily, dose to be given in water preferably after meals, morning and evening
  ▸ Adult: 1 sachet twice daily, dose to be given in water preferably taken after food, morning and evening

DOSE EQUIVALENCE AND CONVERSION
1 sachet equivalent to 2 level 5 ml spoonful.

- ● CONTRA-INDICATIONS Colonic atony · faecal impaction · intestinal obstruction · reduced gut motility

- ● CAUTIONS Adequate fluid intake should be maintained to avoid intestinal obstruction

- ● SIDE-EFFECTS Abdominal distension · flatulence · gastro-intestinal impaction · gastro-intestinal obstruction · hypersensitivity

- ● DIRECTIONS FOR ADMINISTRATION Dose to be taken with at least 150 mL liquid.

- ● PRESCRIBING AND DISPENSING INFORMATION Flavours of soluble granules formulations may include plain, lemon, or orange.

- ● HANDLING AND STORAGE Ispaghula husk contains potent allergens. Individuals exposed to the product (including those handling the product) can develop hypersensitivity reactions such as rhinitis, conjunctivitis, bronchospasm and in some cases, anaphylaxis.

- ● PATIENT AND CARER ADVICE Manufacturer advises that preparations that swell in contact with liquid should always be carefully swallowed with water and should not be taken immediately before going to bed. Patients and their carers should be advised that the full effect may take some days to develop and should be given advice on how to administer ispaghula husk.

- ● MEDICINAL FORMS
There can be variation in the licensing of different medicines containing the same drug.

Granules
CAUTIONARY AND ADVISORY LABELS 13
EXCIPIENTS: May contain Aspartame
▸ Ispaghula husk (Non-proprietary)
  Ispaghula husk 3.5 gram Ispaghula husk 3.5g granules sachets gluten free | 30 sachet GSL £2.48

Effervescent granules
CAUTIONARY AND ADVISORY LABELS 13
EXCIPIENTS: May contain Aspartame
▸ Ispaghula husk (Non-proprietary)
  Ispaghula husk 3.5 gram Ispaghula husk 3.5g effervescent granules sachets gluten free sugar free sugar-free | 30 sachet P no price available DT price = £2.48
▸ Fybogel (Reckitt Benckiser Healthcare (UK) Ltd)
  Ispaghula husk 3.5 gram Fybogel 3.5g effervescent granules sachets plain SF sugar-free | 30 sachet DT price = £2.48
  Fybogel Orange 3.5g effervescent granules sachets SF sugar-free | 30 sachet GSL £2.48 DT price = £2.48

Fybogel Lemon 3.5g effervescent granules sachets SF sugar-free | 30 sachet GSL £2.48 DT price = £2.48
▸ Fybogel Hi-Fibre (Reckitt Benckiser Healthcare (UK) Ltd)
Ispaghula husk 3.5 gram Fybogel Hi-Fibre Orange 3.5g effervescent granules sachets sugar-free | 10 sachet GSL £2.26 sugar-free | 30 sachet GSL £4.85 DT price = £2.48
Fybogel Hi-Fibre Lemon 3.5g effervescent granules sachets sugar-free | 10 sachet GSL £2.26
▸ Ispagel (Bristol Laboratories Ltd)
Ispaghula husk 3.5 gram Ispagel Orange 3.5g effervescent granules sachets sugar-free | 10 sachet GSL £1.65 sugar-free | 30 sachet GSL £2.25 DT price = £2.48

Combinations available: *Senna with ispaghula husk*, p. 55

Methylcellulose

● **DRUG ACTION** Bulk-forming laxatives relieve constipation by increasing faecal mass which stimulates peristalsis.

● **INDICATIONS AND DOSE**

Constipation | Diarrhoea
▸ **BY MOUTH USING TABLETS**
▸ Adult: 3–6 tablets twice daily

● **CONTRA-INDICATIONS** Colonic atony · difficulty in swallowing · faecal impaction · infective bowel disease · intestinal obstruction

● **CAUTIONS** Adequate fluid intake should be maintained to avoid intestinal obstruction
CAUTIONS, FURTHER INFORMATION
It may be necessary to supervise elderly or debilitated patients or those with intestinal narrowing or decreased motility to ensure adequate fluid intake.

● **SIDE-EFFECTS** Abdominal distension (especially during the first few days of treatment) · flatulence (especially during the first few days of treatment) · gastro-intestinal impaction · gastro-intestinal obstruction · hypersensitivity

● **DIRECTIONS FOR ADMINISTRATION** In constipation the dose should be taken with at least 300 mL liquid. In diarrhoea, ileostomy, and colostomy control, avoid liquid intake for 30 minutes before and after dose.

● **PATIENT AND CARER ADVICE** Patients and their carers should be advised that the full effect may take some days to develop. Preparations that swell in contact with liquid should always be carefully swallowed with water and should not be taken immediately before going to bed.

● **MEDICINAL FORMS**
There can be variation in the licensing of different medicines containing the same drug.
Tablet
▸ Celevac (AMCo)
Methylcellulose "450" 500 mg Celevac 500mg tablets | 112 tablet GSL £4.64 DT price = £4.64

Sterculia

19.2.2016

● **DRUG ACTION** Sterculia is a bulk-forming laxative. It relieves constipation by increasing faecal mass which stimulates peristalsis.

● **INDICATIONS AND DOSE**

Constipation
▸ **BY MOUTH**
▸ Child 6–11 years: 0.5–1 sachet 1–2 times a day, alternatively, half to one heaped 5-mL spoonful once or twice a day; washed down without chewing with plenty of liquid after meals
▸ Child 12–17 years: 1–2 sachets 1–2 times a day, alternatively, one to two heaped 5-mL spoonfuls once or twice a day; washed down without chewing with plenty of liquid after meals

▸ Adult: 1–2 sachets 1–2 times a day, alternatively, one to two heaped 5-mL spoonfuls once or twice a day; washed down without chewing with plenty of liquid after meals

● **CONTRA-INDICATIONS** Colonic atony · difficulty in swallowing · faecal impaction · intestinal obstruction

● **CAUTIONS** Adequate fluid intake should be maintained to avoid intestinal obstruction
CAUTIONS, FURTHER INFORMATION
▸ In adults It may be necessary to supervise elderly or debilitated patients or those with intestinal narrowing or decreased motility to ensure adequate fluid intake.

● **SIDE-EFFECTS** Abdominal distension (especially during the first few days of treatment) · flatulence (especially during the first few days of treatment) · gastro-intestinal impaction · gastro-intestinal obstruction · hypersensitivity

● **DIRECTIONS FOR ADMINISTRATION** May be mixed with soft food (e.g. yoghurt) before swallowing, followed by plenty of liquid.

● **PATIENT AND CARER ADVICE** Patients and their carers should be advised that the full effect may take some days to develop. Preparations that swell in contact with liquid should always be carefully swallowed with water and should not be taken immediately before going to bed.

● **MEDICINAL FORMS**
There can be variation in the licensing of different medicines containing the same drug.
Granules
CAUTIONARY AND ADVISORY LABELS 25, 27
▸ Normacol (Norgine Pharmaceuticals Ltd)
Sterculia 620 mg per 1 gram Normacol granules 7g sachets | 60 sachet GSL £6.35 DT price = £5.77
Normacol granules | 500 gram GSL £7.54 DT price = £6.85

Sterculia with frangula

The properties listed below are those particular to the combination only. For the properties of the components please consider, sterculia above.

● **INDICATIONS AND DOSE**

After haemorrhoidectomy
▸ **BY MOUTH**
▸ Adult: 1–2 sachets 1–2 times a day, alternatively, 1–2 heaped 5 mL spoonfuls once or twice a day; washed down without chewing with plenty of liquid after meals

Constipation
▸ **BY MOUTH**
▸ Adult: 1–2 sachets 1–2 times a day, alternatively, 1–2 heaped 5 mL spoonfuls once or twice a day; washed down without chewing with plenty of liquid after meals

● **PREGNANCY** Manufacturer advises avoid.

● **BREAST FEEDING** Manufacturer advises avoid.

● **PATIENT AND CARER ADVICE** Patients and their carers should be advised that the full effect may take some days to develop. Preparations that swell in contact with liquid should always be carefully swallowed with water and should not be taken immediately before going to bed.

● **MEDICINAL FORMS**
There can be variation in the licensing of different medicines containing the same drug.
Granules
▸ Normacol Plus (Norgine Pharmaceuticals Ltd)
Frangula 80 mg per 1 gram, Sterculia 620 mg per 1 gram Normacol Plus granules 7g sachets | 60 sachet GSL £6.78 DT price = £6.16
Normacol Plus granules | 500 gram GSL £8.05 DT price = £7.32

LAXATIVES > CHLORIDE-CHANNEL AGONISTS

Lubiprostone   23.3.2016

- **DRUG ACTION** Lubiprostone is a chloride-channel activator that acts locally in the gut to increase intestinal fluid secretion and intestinal motility, resulting in a laxative effect.

- **INDICATIONS AND DOSE**
Chronic idiopathic constipation when response to lifestyle changes (including diet) inadequate
  ▶ BY MOUTH
    ▸ Adult: 24 micrograms twice daily for 2–4 weeks, discontinue if no response after initial 2 weeks

- **CONTRA-INDICATIONS** Gastro-intestinal obstruction
- **SIDE-EFFECTS**
▶ **Common or very common** Abdominal discomfort · abdominal distension · abdominal pain · diarrhoea · dizziness · dyspepsia · dyspnoea · flatulence · headache · hot flush · hyperhidrosis · nausea · oedema · palpitation
▶ **Uncommon** Chest pain · muscle spasm · syncope · vomiting
▶ **Frequency not known** Influenza-like symptoms · rash · tachycardia

- **PREGNANCY** Manufacturer advises avoid—toxicity in *animal* studies.
- **BREAST FEEDING** Unknown if excreted in milk. EvGr If benefits of use outweigh the risk, monitor infant for side effects (e.g. diarrhoea). E
- **HEPATIC IMPAIRMENT** In moderate to severe impairment initially 24 micrograms once daily; if tolerated, and if necessary, increased to 24 micrograms twice daily.
- **PRESCRIBING AND DISPENSING INFORMATION** Dispense capsules in original container; discard any capsules remaining 4 weeks after opening.
- **NATIONAL FUNDING/ACCESS DECISIONS**
NICE technology appraisals (TAs)
▶ Lubiprostone for treating chronic idiopathic constipation (July 2014) NICE TA318
Lubiprostone is recommended as an option for treating chronic idiopathic constipation for adults in whom treatment with at least 2 laxatives from different classes, at the highest tolerated recommended doses for at least 6 months, has failed to provide adequate relief and for whom invasive treatment for constipation is being considered. If treatment with lubiprostone is not effective after 2 weeks, the patient should be re-examined and the benefit of continuing treatment reconsidered.
   Lubiprostone should only be prescribed by a clinician with experience of treating chronic idiopathic constipation, after careful review of the patient's previous courses of laxative treatments.
www.nice.org.uk/TA318
Scottish Medicines Consortium (SMC) Decisions
The *Scottish Medicines Consortium* has advised (July 2014) that lubiprostone (*Amitiza*)® is **not** recommended for use within NHS Scotland.

- **MEDICINAL FORMS**
There can be variation in the licensing of different medicines containing the same drug.
Capsule
CAUTIONARY AND ADVISORY LABELS 21
  ▸ Amitiza (Sucampo Pharma Europe Ltd) ▼
    Lubiprostone 24 microgram Amitiza 24microgram capsules | 28 capsule PoM £29.68 | 56 capsule PoM £53.48

LAXATIVES > OSMOTIC LAXATIVES

Lactulose

- **INDICATIONS AND DOSE**
Constipation
  ▶ BY MOUTH
    ▸ Child 1–11 months: 2.5 mL twice daily, adjusted according to response
    ▸ Child 1–4 years: 2.5–10 mL twice daily, adjusted according to response
    ▸ Child 5–17 years: 5–20 mL twice daily, adjusted according to response
    ▸ Adult: Initially 15 mL twice daily, adjusted according to response
Hepatic encephalopathy (portal systemic encephalopathy)
  ▶ BY MOUTH
    ▸ Adult: Adjusted according to response to 30–50 mL 3 times a day, subsequently adjusted to produce 2–3 soft stools per day
PHARMACOKINETICS
Lactulose may take up to 48 hours to act.

- **UNLICENSED USE** Lactulose doses in the BNF may differ from those in product literature.
- **CONTRA-INDICATIONS** Galactosaemia · intestinal obstruction
- **CAUTIONS** Lactose intolerance
- **INTERACTIONS** → Appendix 1 (lactulose).
- **SIDE-EFFECTS**
▶ **Common or very common** Abdominal discomfort · cramps · flatulence · nausea · vomiting
  SIDE-EFFECTS, FURTHER INFORMATION
  ▸ Nausea Nausea can be reduced by administration with water, fruit juice or meals.
- **PREGNANCY** Not known to be harmful.
- **PATIENT AND CARER ADVICE**
Medicines for Children leaflet: Lactulose for constipation www.medicinesforchildren.org.uk/lactulose-for-constipation

- **MEDICINAL FORMS**
There can be variation in the licensing of different medicines containing the same drug.
Oral solution
  ▸ Lactulose (Non-proprietary)
    Lactulose 666.667 mg per 1 ml Lactulose 10g/15ml oral solution 15ml sachets sugar free sugar-free | 10 sachet P £2.50 DT price = £2.50
    Lactulose 680 mg per 1 ml Lactulose 3.1-3.7g/5ml oral solution | 300 ml P £2.73 | 500 ml P £4.55 DT price = £2.50
  ▸ Duphalac (BGP Products Ltd)
    Lactulose 680 mg per 1 ml Duphalac 3.35g/5ml syrup | 200 ml P £1.92
  ▸ Lactugal (Intrapharm Laboratories Ltd)
    Lactulose 680 mg per 1 ml Lactugal 3.1-3.7g/5ml oral solution | 500 ml P £4.56 DT price = £2.50 | 2000 ml P £16.42

Macrogol 3350 with potassium chloride, sodium bicarbonate and sodium chloride

- **INDICATIONS AND DOSE**
Chronic constipation (dose for non-proprietary 'full-strength' sachets)
  ▶ BY MOUTH
    ▸ Child 12–17 years: 1–3 sachets daily in divided doses usually for up to 2 weeks; maintenance 1–2 sachets daily

continued →

▸ Adult: 1–3 sachets daily in divided doses usually for up to 2 weeks; maintenance 1–2 sachets daily

Faecal impaction (dose for non-proprietary 'full-strength' sachets)

▸ BY MOUTH

▸ Child 12-17 years: 4 sachets on first day, then increased in steps of 2 sachets daily, total daily dose to be drunk within a 6 hour period, after disimpaction, switch to maintenance laxative therapy if required; maximum 8 sachets per day

▸ Adult: 4 sachets on first day, then increased in steps of 2 sachets daily, total daily dose to be drunk within a 6 hour period, after disimpaction, switch to maintenance laxative therapy if required; maximum 8 sachets per day

MOVICOL-HALF®

Chronic constipation

▸ BY MOUTH

▸ Child 12-17 years: 2–6 sachets daily in divided doses usually for up to 2 weeks; maintenance 2–4 sachets daily

▸ Adult: 2–6 sachets daily in divided doses usually for up to 2 weeks; maintenance 2–4 sachets daily

Faecal impaction

▸ BY MOUTH

▸ Child 12-17 years: Initially 8 sachets daily on first day, then increased in steps of 4 sachets daily, total daily dose to be drunk within 6 hours, after disimpaction, switch to maintenance laxative therapy; maximum 16 sachets per day

▸ Adult: Initially 8 sachets daily on first day, then increased in steps of 4 sachets daily, total daily dose to be drunk within 6 hours, after disimpaction, switch to maintenance laxative therapy; maximum 16 sachets per day

MOVICOL-PAEDIATRIC®

Chronic constipation | Prevention of faecal impaction

▸ BY MOUTH

▸ Child 2-5 years: 1 sachet daily, adjust dose to produce regular soft stools; maximum 4 sachets per day

▸ Child 6-11 years: 2 sachets daily, adjust dose to produce regular soft stools; maximum 4 sachets per day

Faecal impaction

▸ BY MOUTH

▸ Child 5-11 years: Initially 4 sachets daily on first day, then increased in steps of 2 sachets daily, total daily dose to be taken over a 12-hour period, after disimpaction, switch to maintenance laxative therapy; maximum 12 sachets per day

MOVICOL® LIQUID

Chronic constipation

▸ BY MOUTH

▸ Child 12-17 years: 25 mL 1–3 times a day usually for up to 2 weeks; maintenance 25 mL 1–2 times a day

▸ Adult: 25 mL 1–3 times a day usually for up to 2 weeks; maintenance 25 mL 1–2 times a day

MOVICOL® ORAL POWDER

Chronic constipation

▸ BY MOUTH

▸ Child 12-17 years: 1–3 sachets daily in divided doses usually for up to 2 weeks; maintenance 1–2 sachets daily

▸ Adult: 1–3 sachets daily in divided doses usually for up to 2 weeks; maintenance 1–2 sachets daily

Faecal impaction

▸ BY MOUTH

▸ Child 12-17 years: Initially 4 sachets daily on first day, then increased in steps of 2 sachets daily, total daily dose to be drunk within a 6 hour period, after

disimpaction, switch to maintenance laxative therapy if required; maximum 8 sachets per day

▸ Adult: Initially 4 sachets daily on first day, then increased in steps of 2 sachets daily, total daily dose to be drunk within a 6 hour period, after disimpaction, switch to maintenance laxative therapy if required; maximum 8 sachets per day

● UNLICENSED USE MOVICOL-PAEDIATRIC® *Movicol® Paediatric* not licensed for use in faecal impaction in children under 5 years, or for chronic constipation in children under 2 years.

● CONTRA-INDICATIONS Crohn's disease · intestinal obstruction · intestinal perforation · paralytic ileus · severe inflammatory conditions of the intestinal tract · toxic megacolon · ulcerative colitis

MOVICOL-PAEDIATRIC® Cardiovascular impairment · renal impairment

● CAUTIONS Cardiovascular impairment (should not take more than 2 'full-strength' sachets or 4 'half-strength' sachets in any one hour) · discontinue if symptoms of fluid and electrolyte disturbance

MOVICOL-PAEDIATRIC® Impaired consciousness (with high doses) · impaired gag reflex (with high doses) · reflux oesophagitis (with high doses)

● INTERACTIONS → Appendix 1 (macrogols).

● SIDE-EFFECTS Abdominal distention · addominal pain · flatulence · nausea

● PREGNANCY Limited data, but manufacturer advises that it can be used.

● BREAST FEEDING Manufacturer advises that it can be used.

● RENAL IMPAIRMENT MOVICOL-PAEDIATRIC® Contra-indicated in renal impairment.

● DIRECTIONS FOR ADMINISTRATION Contents of each 'full strength' sachet of oral powder to be dissolved in half a glass (approx. 125 mL) of water; after reconstitution the solution should be kept in a refrigerator and discarded if unused after 6 hours.

MOVICOL® LIQUID 25 mL of oral concentrate to be diluted with half a glass (approx. 100 mL) of water. After dilution the solution should be discarded if unused after 24 hours.

MOVICOL-PAEDIATRIC® Contents of each sachet to be dissolved in quarter of a glass (approx. 60–65 mL) of water; after reconstitution the solution should be kept in a refrigerator and discarded if unused after 24 hours.

MOVICOL® ORAL POWDER Contents of each sachet to be dissolved in half a glass (approx. 125 mL) of water; after reconstitution the solution should be kept in a refrigerator and discarded if unused after 6 hours.

MOVICOL-HALF® Contents of each sachet to be dissolved in quarter of a glass (approx. 60–65 mL) of water; after reconstitution the solution should be kept in a refrigerator and discarded if unused after 6 hours.

● PRESCRIBING AND DISPENSING INFORMATION Flavours of oral liquid formulations may include orange.

Flavours of oral powder formulations may include chocolate, lime and lemon, or plain.

MOVICOL® LIQUID 25 mL of oral concentrate when diluted with 100 mL water provides K^+ 5.4 mmol/litre.

MOVICOL® ORAL POWDER Amount of potassium chloride varies according to flavour of *Movicol®* as follows: plain-flavour (sugar-free) = 50.2 mg/sachet; lime and lemon flavour = 46.6 mg/sachet; chocolate flavour = 31.7 mg/sachet. 1 sachet when reconstituted with 125 mL water provides K^+ 5.4 mmol/litre.

● PATIENT AND CARER ADVICE Medicines for Children leaflet: Movicol for constipation www.medicinesforchildren.org.uk/movicol-for-constipation

Patients or carers should be counselled on how to take the oral powder and oral solution.

MOVICOL® LIQUID Patients or carers should be counselled on how to take *Movicol*® oral solution.

MOVICOL® ORAL POWDER Patients or carers should be counselled on how to take *Movicol*® oral powder.

MOVICOL-HALF® Patients or carers should be given advice on how to administer *Movicol-Half*® oral powder.

● MEDICINAL FORMS
There can be variation in the licensing of different medicines containing the same drug.

Oral solution
CAUTIONARY AND ADVISORY LABELS 13
ELECTROLYTES: May contain Bicarbonate, chloride, potassium, sodium
▶ Macrogol 3350 with potassium chloride, sodium bicarbonate and sodium chloride (Non-proprietary)

Bicarbonate 17 mmol per 1 litre, Chloride 53 mmol per 1 litre, Macrogol '3350' 13.125 gram, Potassium 5.4 mmol per 1 litre, Sodium 65 mmol per 1 litre Macrogol compound oral liquid NPF sugar free sugar-free | 500 ml Ⓟ no price available
▶ Movicol (Norgine Pharmaceuticals Ltd)

Bicarbonate 17 mmol per 1 litre, Chloride 53 mmol per 1 litre, Macrogol '3350' 13.125 gram, Potassium 5.4 mmol per 1 litre, Sodium 65 mmol per 1 litre Movicol Liquid sugar-free | 500 ml Ⓟ £5.15

Powder
CAUTIONARY AND ADVISORY LABELS 13
ELECTROLYTES: May contain Bicarbonate, chloride, potassium, sodium
▶ Macrogol 3350 with potassium chloride, sodium bicarbonate and sodium chloride (Non-proprietary)

Bicarbonate 17 mmol per 1 litre, Chloride 53 mmol per 1 litre, Macrogol '3350' 13.125 gram, Potassium 5.4 mmol per 1 litre, Sodium 65 mmol per 1 litre Macrogol compound oral powder sachets sugar free sugar-free | 20 sachet Ⓟ £4.45 sugar-free | 30 sachet Ⓟ £6.68 DT price = £4.27

Bicarbonate 17 mmol per 1 litre, Chloride 53 mmol per 1 litre, Macrogol '3350' 6.563 gram, Potassium 5.4 mmol per 1 litre, Sodium 65 mmol per 1 litre Macrogol compound half-strength oral powder sachets NPF sugar free sugar-free | 20 sachet ⓅoM no price available sugar-free | 30 sachet ⓅoM no price available
▶ CosmoCol (Stirling Anglian Pharmaceuticals Ltd)

Bicarbonate 17 mmol per 1 litre, Chloride 53 mmol per 1 litre, Macrogol '3350' 13.125 gram, Potassium 5.4 mmol per 1 litre, Sodium 65 mmol per 1 litre CosmoCol Orange Lemon and Lime oral powder sachets sugar-free | 20 sachet Ⓟ £2.75 sugar-free | 30 sachet Ⓟ £3.95 DT price = £4.27
CosmoCol Plain oral powder sachets sugar-free | 30 sachet Ⓟ £3.95 DT price = £4.27
CosmoCol Orange Flavour oral powder sachets sugar-free | 20 sachet Ⓟ £2.75 sugar-free | 30 sachet Ⓟ £3.95 DT price = £4.27
CosmoCol Lemon and Lime Flavour oral powder sachets sugar-free | 20 sachet Ⓟ £3.56 sugar-free | 30 sachet Ⓟ £5.34 DT price = £4.27
Bicarbonate 17 mmol per 1 litre, Chloride 53 mmol per 1 litre, Macrogol '3350' 6.563 gram, Potassium 5.4 mmol per 1 litre, Sodium 65 mmol per 1 litre CosmoCol Half oral powder 6.9g sachets sugar-free | 30 sachet Ⓟ £2.99
CosmoCol Paediatric oral powder 6.9g sachets sugar-free | 30 sachet ⓅoM £2.99
▶ Laxido (Galen Ltd)

Bicarbonate 17 mmol per 1 litre, Chloride 53 mmol per 1 litre, Macrogol '3350' 13.125 gram, Potassium 5.4 mmol per 1 litre, Sodium 65 mmol per 1 litre Laxido Orange oral powder sachets sugar-free | 20 sachet Ⓟ £2.85 sugar-free | 30 sachet Ⓟ £4.27 DT price = £4.27

Bicarbonate 17 mmol per 1 litre, Chloride 53 mmol per 1 litre, Macrogol '3350' 6.563 gram, Potassium 5.4 mmol per 1 litre, Sodium 65 mmol per 1 litre Laxido Paediatric Plain oral powder 6.9g sachets sugar-free | 30 sachet ⓅoM £2.99
▶ Macilax (Teva UK Ltd)

Bicarbonate 17 mmol per 1 litre, Chloride 53 mmol per 1 litre, Macrogol '3350' 13.125 gram, Potassium 5.4 mmol per 1 litre, Sodium 65 mmol per 1 litre Macilax oral powder 13.8g sachets sugar-free | 20 sachet Ⓟ £3.20 sugar-free | 30 sachet Ⓟ £4.81 DT price = £4.27 sugar-free | 50 sachet Ⓟ £8.01

Bicarbonate 17 mmol per 1 litre, Chloride 53 mmol per 1 litre, Macrogol '3350' 6.563 gram, Potassium 5.4 mmol per 1 litre,

Sodium 65 mmol per 1 litre Macilax Paediatric oral powder 6.9g sachets sugar-free | 30 sachet Ⓟ £3.15
▶ Molaxole (Meda Pharmaceuticals Ltd)

Bicarbonate 17 mmol per 1 litre, Chloride 53 mmol per 1 litre, Macrogol '3350' 13.125 gram, Potassium 5.4 mmol per 1 litre, Sodium 65 mmol per 1 litre Molaxole oral powder sachets sugar-free | 20 sachet Ⓟ £3.78 sugar-free | 30 sachet Ⓟ £5.68 DT price = £4.27
▶ Movicol (Norgine Pharmaceuticals Ltd)

Bicarbonate 17 mmol per 1 litre, Chloride 53 mmol per 1 litre, Macrogol '3350' 13.125 gram, Potassium 5.4 mmol per 1 litre, Sodium 65 mmol per 1 litre Movicol Plain oral powder 13.7g sachets sugar-free | 30 sachet Ⓟ £7.72 DT price = £4.27 sugar-free | 50 sachet Ⓟ £12.85
Movicol Chocolate oral powder 13.9g sachets sugar-free | 30 sachet Ⓟ £7.72 DT price = £4.27
Movicol oral powder 13.8g sachets lemon & lime sugar-free | 20 sachet Ⓟ £5.15 sugar-free | 30 sachet Ⓟ £7.72 DT price = £4.27 sugar-free | 50 sachet Ⓟ £12.85
Bicarbonate 17 mmol per 1 litre, Chloride 53 mmol per 1 litre, Macrogol '3350' 6.563 gram, Potassium 5.4 mmol per 1 litre, Sodium 65 mmol per 1 litre Movicol-Half oral powder 6.9g sachets sugar-free | 20 sachet Ⓟ £3.37 sugar-free | 30 sachet Ⓟ £5.06
Movicol Paediatric Plain oral powder 6.9g sachets sugar-free | 30 sachet ⓅoM £4.38
Movicol Paediatric Chocolate oral powder 6.9g sachets sugar-free | 30 sachet ⓅoM £4.38

Magnesium hydroxide

● INDICATIONS AND DOSE

Constipation
▶ BY MOUTH
▶ Adult: 30−45 mL as required, dose to be given mixed with water at bedtime

● CONTRA-INDICATIONS Acute gastro-intestinal conditions
● CAUTIONS Debilitated patients · elderly
● INTERACTIONS → Appendix 1 (antacids).
● SIDE-EFFECTS Colic
● HEPATIC IMPAIRMENT Avoid in hepatic coma if risk of renal failure.
● RENAL IMPAIRMENT Avoid or reduce dose. Increased risk of toxicity in renal impairment.
● PRESCRIBING AND DISPENSING INFORMATION When prepared extemporaneously, the BP states Magnesium Hydroxide Mixture, BP consists of an aqueous suspension containing about 8% hydrated magnesium oxide.

● MEDICINAL FORMS
There can be variation in the licensing of different medicines containing the same drug.
Oral suspension
▶ Magnesium hydroxide (Non-proprietary)

Magnesium hydroxide 83 mg per 1 ml Phillips' Milk of Magnesia 415mg/5ml oral suspension sugar-free | 200 ml Ⓖⓢⓛ £3.22 DT price = £3.22

Combinations available: *Liquid paraffin with magnesium hydroxide*, p. 57

Sodium acid phosphate with sodium phosphate

● INDICATIONS AND DOSE

Constipation (using Phosphates Enema BP Formula B) | Bowel evacuation before abdominal radiological procedures, endoscopy, and surgery (using Phosphates Enema BP Formula B)
▶ BY RECTUM
▶ Child 3−6 years: 45−65 mL once daily
▶ Child 7-11 years: 65−100 mL once daily

continued →

- Child 12–17 years: 100–128 mL once daily
- Adult: 128 mL daily

FLEET® READY-TO-USE ENEMA

Constipation | Bowel evacuation before abdominal radiological procedures | Bowel evacuation before endoscopy | Bowel evacuation before surgery
▶ BY RECTUM
▶ Adult: 118 mL

FLEET®PHOSPHO-SODA

Bowel evacuation before colonic surgery | Bowel evacuation before colonoscopy | Bowel evacuation before radiological examination
▶ BY MOUTH
▶ Adult: 45 mL twice daily, each dose must be diluted with half a glass (120 mL) of cold water, followed by one full glass (240 mL) of cold water, timing of doses is dependent on the time of the procedure, for morning procedure, the first dose should be taken at 7 a.m. and second at 7 p.m. on day before the procedure.; for afternoon procedure, first dose should be taken at 7 p.m. on day before and second dose at 7 a.m. on day of the procedure

PHARMACOKINETICS
For *Fleet® Phospho-soda*: Onset of action is within half to 6 hours of first dose.

● CONTRA-INDICATIONS
▶ With oral use Acute severe colitis (in adults) · ascites (in adults) · congestive cardiac failure (in adults) · gastric retention (in adults) · gastro-intestinal obstruction · gastro-intestinal perforation (in adults) · toxic megacolon (in adults)
▶ With rectal use Conditions associated with increased colonic absorption · gastro-intestinal obstruction · inflammatory bowel disease

● CAUTIONS
▶ With oral use Cardiac disease (avoid in congestive cardiac failure) (in adults) · colitis (avoid if acute severe colitis) (in adults) · elderly and debilitated patients (in adults) · fluid and electrolyte disturbances (in adults) · hypovolaemia (should be corrected before administration) (in adults) · impaired gag reflex or possibility of regurgitation or aspiration (in adults)
▶ With rectal use Ascites · congestive heart failure · elderly and debilitated patients (in adults) · electrolyte disturbances · uncontrolled hypertension

● INTERACTIONS
▶ With oral use in adults Other oral drugs should not be taken one hour before or after administration of bowel cleansing preparations because absorption may be impaired. Consider withholding ACE inhibitors, angiotensin-II receptor antagonists, and NSAIDs on the day that bowel cleansing preparations are given and for up to 72 hours after the procedure. Also consider withholding diuretics on the day that bowel cleansing preparations are given.

● SIDE-EFFECTS
▶ **Common or very common**
▶ With oral use Abdominal distension (in adults) · abdominal pain (usually transient—reduced by taking more slowly) (in adults) · nausea (in adults) · vomiting (in adults)
▶ **Uncommon**
▶ With oral use Dehydration (in adults) · dizziness (in adults) · headache (in adults)
▶ **Frequency not known**
▶ With oral use Arrhythmias (in adults) · asthenia (in adults) · chest pain (in adults) · electrolyte disturbances · renal failure (in adults)
▶ With rectal use Electrolyte disturbances · local irritation

● PREGNANCY
▶ With oral use in adults Caution.

● BREAST FEEDING
▶ With oral use in adults Caution.

● HEPATIC IMPAIRMENT Use with caution in cirrhosis.

● RENAL IMPAIRMENT
▶ With oral use in adults Avoid if eGFR less than 60 mL/minute/1.73 m^2.
▶ With rectal use Use with caution.

● MONITORING REQUIREMENTS
▶ With oral use in adults Renal function should be measured before starting treatment in patients at risk of fluid and electrolyte disturbances.

● DIRECTIONS FOR ADMINISTRATION
FLEET®PHOSPHO-SODA Copious intake of water or other clear fluids (e.g. clear soup, strained fruit juice without pulp, black tea or coffee) recommended until midnight before morning procedure and until 8 a.m. before afternoon procedure. At least one glass (approx 240 mL) of water or other clear fluid should also be taken immediately before each dose.

● PRESCRIBING AND DISPENSING INFORMATION When prepared extemporaneously, the BP states Phosphates Enema BP Formula B consists of sodium dihydrogen phosphate dihydrate 12.8 g, disodium phosphate dodecahydrate 10.24 g, purified water, freshly boiled and cooled, to 128 mL.

● PATIENT AND CARER ADVICE
FLEET®PHOSPHO-SODA Intake of solid food should be stopped for at least 6 hours before starting treatment and until procedure completed.
Patients or carers should be advised that adequate hydration should be maintained during treatment.
Patients or carers should be given advice on administration of *Fleet Phospho-soda®* oral solution.

● MEDICINAL FORMS
There can be variation in the licensing of different medicines containing the same drug.
Oral solution
CAUTIONARY AND ADVISORY LABELS 10
ELECTROLYTES: May contain Phosphate, sodium
▶ Fleet Phospho-soda (Casen Recordati S.L.)
Disodium hydrogen phosphate dodecahydrate 240 mg per 1 ml, Sodium dihydrogen phosphate dihydrate 542 mg per 1 ml Fleet Phospho-soda oral solution sugar-free | 90 ml Ⓟ £4.79
Enema
▶ Sodium acid phosphate with sodium phosphate (Non-proprietary)
Disodium hydrogen phosphate dodecahydrate 80 mg per 1 ml, Sodium dihydrogen phosphate dihydrate 100 mg per 1 ml Phosphates enema (Formula B) 128ml long tube | 1 enema Ⓟ £27.93 DT price = £27.93
Phosphates enema (Formula B) 128ml standard tube | 1 enema Ⓟ £3.98 DT price = £3.98
▶ Fleet Ready-to-use (Casen Recordati S.L.)
Disodium hydrogen phosphate dodecahydrate 80 mg per 1 ml, Sodium dihydrogen phosphate dihydrate 181 mg per 1 ml Fleet Ready-to-use 133ml enema | 1 enema Ⓟ £0.68

LAXATIVES ⟩ SELECTIVE 5-HT$_4$ RECEPTOR AGONISTS

Prucalopride
24.2.2016

● DRUG ACTION A selective serotonin 5HT$_4$-receptor agonist with prokinetic properties.

● INDICATIONS AND DOSE
Chronic constipation when other laxatives fail to provide an adequate response
▶ BY MOUTH
▶ Adult: 2 mg once daily, review treatment if no response after 4 weeks

▸ **Elderly:** Initially 1 mg once daily, increased if necessary to 2 mg once daily, review treatment if no response after 4 weeks

● CONTRA-INDICATIONS Crohn's disease · intestinal obstruction · intestinal perforation · toxic megacolon · ulcerative colitis

● CAUTIONS History of arrhythmias · history of ischaemic heart disease

● SIDE-EFFECTS

▸ **Common or very common** Abdominal pain · decreased appetite · diarrhoea · dizziness · dyspepsia · fatigue · flatulence · headache · nausea · polyuria · rectal bleeding · vomiting

▸ **Uncommon** Fever · malaise · palpitation · tremor

SIDE-EFFECTS, FURTHER INFORMATION

Manufacturer advises that side-effects generally occur at the start of treatment and are usually transient.

● CONCEPTION AND CONTRACEPTION Manufacturer recommends effective contraception during treatment.

● PREGNANCY Manufacturer advises avoid—limited data available.

● BREAST FEEDING Manufacturer advises avoid—present in milk.

● HEPATIC IMPAIRMENT In severe impairment, manufacturer advises reduced dose of 1 mg once daily; increased if necessary to 2 mg once daily.

● RENAL IMPAIRMENT Manufacturer recommends a reduced dose of 1 mg daily if eGFR less than 30 mL/minute/1.73 m^2.

● PATIENT AND CARER ADVICE

Driving and skilled tasks

Manufacturer advises that dizziness and fatigue may initially affect ability to drive or operate machinery.

● NATIONAL FUNDING/ACCESS DECISIONS

NICE technology appraisals (TAs)

▸ **Prucalopride for the treatment of chronic constipation in women (December 2010)** NICE TA211

Prucalopride is recommended as an option for the treatment of chronic constipation in women for whom treatment with at least 2 laxatives from different classes, at the highest tolerated recommended doses for at least 6 months, has failed to provide adequate relief and invasive treatment for constipation is being considered. If treatment with prucalopride is not effective after 4 weeks, the patient should be re-examined and the benefit of continuing treatment reconsidered.

Prucalopride should only be prescribed by a clinician with experience of treating chronic constipation, after careful review of the patient's previous courses of laxative treatments.

www.nice.org.uk/TA211

Scottish Medicines Consortium (SMC) Decisions

The *Scottish Medicines Consortium* has advised (June 2011) that prucalopride (*Resolor®*) is not recommended for use within NHS Scotland for the symptomatic treatment of chronic constipation of women in whom laxatives fail to provide adequate relief.

● MEDICINAL FORMS

There can be variation in the licensing of different medicines containing the same drug.

Tablet

▸ Resolor (Shire Pharmaceuticals Ltd)

Prucalopride (as Prucalopride succinate) **1 mg** Resolor 1mg tablets | 28 tablet [PoM] £38.69 DT price = £38.69

Prucalopride (as Prucalopride succinate) **2 mg** Resolor 2mg tablets | 28 tablet [PoM] £59.52 DT price = £59.52

LAXATIVES ⟩ STIMULANT LAXATIVES

Bisacodyl

● INDICATIONS AND DOSE

Constipation

▸ BY MOUTH

▸ Child 4-17 years: 5–20 mg once daily, adjusted according to response, dose to be taken at night

▸ Adult: 5–10 mg once dailyIncreased if necessary up to 20 mg once daily, dose to be taken at night

▸ BY RECTUM

▸ Child 2-17 years: 5–10 mg once daily, adjusted according to response

▸ Adult: 10 mg once daily, dose to be taken in the morning

Bowel clearance before radiological procedures and surgery

▸ INITIALLY BY MOUTH

▸ Adult: 10 mg twice daily, does to be taken in the morning and evening on the day before procedure and (by rectum) 10 mg, to be administered 1–2 hours before procedure the following day

PHARMACOKINETICS

Tablets act in 10–12 hours; suppositories act in 20–60 minutes.

● CONTRA-INDICATIONS Acute abdominal conditions (in children) · acute inflammatory bowel disease · acute surgical abdominal conditions (in adults) · intestinal obstruction · severe dehydration

● CAUTIONS Excessive use of stimulant laxatives can cause diarrhoea and related effects such as hypokalaemia · risk of electrolyte imbalance with prolonged use (in children)

● SIDE-EFFECTS

GENERAL SIDE-EFFECTS

Abdominal cramp · colitis · nausea · vomiting

SPECIFIC SIDE-EFFECTS

▸ With rectal use Local irritation

● PREGNANCY May be suitable for constipation in pregnancy, if a stimulant effect is necessary.

● MEDICINAL FORMS

There can be variation in the licensing of different medicines containing the same drug. Forms available from special-order manufacturers include: oral suspension, suppository, enema

Gastro-resistant tablet

CAUTIONARY AND ADVISORY LABELS 5, 25

▸ Bisacodyl (Non-proprietary)

Bisacodyl **5 mg** Bisacodyl 5mg gastro-resistant tablets | 60 tablet [P] £3.25 DT price = £1.85 | 100 tablet [P] £5.40 | 500 tablet [P] £25.73 | 1000 tablet [P] £51.45

Suppository

▸ Bisacodyl (Non-proprietary)

Bisacodyl **10 mg** Bisacodyl 10mg suppositories | 12 suppository [P] £3.53 DT price = £3.53

Enema

▸ Bisacodyl (Non-proprietary)

Bisacodyl **333.333 microgram per 1 ml** Fleet Bisacodyl 10mg/30ml enema | 1 enema [PoM] no price available

---

Co-danthramer

● INDICATIONS AND DOSE

Constipation in terminally ill patients (standard strength capsules)

▸ BY MOUTH USING CAPSULES

▸ Child 6-11 years: 1 capsule once daily, dose should be taken at night continued →

- Child 12–17 years: 1–2 capsules once daily, dose should be taken at night
- Adult: 1–2 capsules once daily, dose should be taken at night

Constipation in terminally ill patients (strong capsules)
- BY MOUTH USING CAPSULES
- Child 12–17 years: 1–2 capsules once daily, dose should be given at night
- Adult: 1–2 capsules once daily, dose should be given at night

Constipation in terminally ill patients (standard strength suspension)
- BY MOUTH USING ORAL SUSPENSION
- Child 2–11 years: 2.5–5 mL once daily, dose should be taken at night
- Child 12–17 years: 5–10 mL once daily, dose should be taken at night
- Adult: 5–10 mL once daily, dose should be taken at night

Constipation in terminally ill patients (strong suspension)
- BY MOUTH USING ORAL SUSPENSION
- Child 12–17 years: 5 mL once daily, dose should be taken at night
- Adult: 5 mL once daily, dose should be taken at night

DOSE EQUIVALENCE AND CONVERSION
Co-danthramer (standard strength) capsules contain dantron 25 mg with poloxamer '188' 200 mg per capsule.
Co-danthramer (standard strength) oral suspension contains dantron 25 mg with poloxamer '188' 200 mg per 5 mL.
Co-danthramer **strong** capsules contain dantron 37.5 mg with poloxamer '188' 500 mg.
Co-danthramer **strong** oral suspension contains dantron 75 mg with poloxamer '188' 1 g per 5 mL.
Co-danthramer suspension 5 mL = one co-danthramer capsule, **but** strong co-danthramer suspension 5 mL = two strong co-danthramer capsules.

- CONTRA-INDICATIONS Acute abdominal conditions (in children) · acute inflammatory bowel disease · acute surgical abdominal conditions (in adults) · intestinal obstruction · severe dehydration
- CAUTIONS Excessive use of stimulant laxatives can cause diarrhoea and related effects such as hypokalaemia · may cause local irritation · *rodent* studies indicate potential carcinogenic risk
  CAUTIONS, FURTHER INFORMATION
- Local irritation Avoid prolonged contact with skin (as in incontinent patients or infants wearing nappies—risk of irritation and excoriation).
- SIDE-EFFECTS Abdominal cramp · urine may be coloured red
- PREGNANCY Manufacturers advise avoid—limited information available.
- BREAST FEEDING Manufacturers advise avoid—no information available.
- MEDICINAL FORMS
  There can be variation in the licensing of different medicines containing the same drug.
  Oral suspension
  CAUTIONARY AND ADVISORY LABELS 14 (urine red)
  - Co-danthramer (Non-proprietary)
    Dantron 5 mg per 1 ml, Poloxamer 188 40 mg per 1 ml Co-danthramer 25mg/200mg/5ml oral suspension sugar free sugar-free | 300 ml [PoM] £146.39 DT price = £146.27
    Dantron 15 mg per 1 ml, Poloxamer 188 200 mg per 1 ml Co-danthramer 75mg/1000mg/5ml oral suspension sugar free sugar-free | 300 ml [PoM] £293.63 DT price = £293.39

Co-danthrusate
20.4.2016

- INDICATIONS AND DOSE
Constipation in terminally ill patients
- BY MOUTH USING CAPSULES
- Child 6–11 years: 1 capsule once daily, to be taken at night
- Child 12–17 years: 1–3 capsules once daily, to be taken at night
- Adult: 1–3 capsules once daily, to be taken at night
- BY MOUTH USING ORAL SUSPENSION
- Child 6–11 years: 5 mL once daily, to be taken at night
- Child 12–17 years: 5–15 mL once daily, to be taken at night
- Adult: 5–15 mL once daily, to be taken at night

DOSE EQUIVALENCE AND CONVERSION
Co-danthrusate suspension contains dantron 50 mg and docusate 60 mg per 5 mL.
Co-danthrusate capsules contain dantron 50 mg and docusate 60 mg per capsule.

- CONTRA-INDICATIONS Acute abdominal conditions (in children) · acute inflammatory bowel disease · acute surgical abdominal conditions (in adults) · intestinal obstruction · severe dehydration
- CAUTIONS Excessive use of stimulant laxatives can cause diarrhoea and related effects such as hypokalaemia · may cause local irritation · *rodent* studies indicate potential carcinogenic risk
  CAUTIONS, FURTHER INFORMATION
- Local irritation Avoid prolonged contact with skin (as in incontinent patients or infants wearing nappies—risk of irritation and excoriation).
- SIDE-EFFECTS Abdominal cramp · urine may be coloured red
- PREGNANCY Manufacturers advise avoid—limited information available.
- BREAST FEEDING Manufacturers advise avoid—no information available.
- MEDICINAL FORMS
  There can be variation in the licensing of different medicines containing the same drug.
  Capsule
  CAUTIONARY AND ADVISORY LABELS 14 (urine red)
  - Co-danthrusate (Non-proprietary)
    Dantron 50 mg, Docusate sodium 60 mg Co-danthrusate 50mg/60mg capsules | 63 capsule [PoM] £52.50 DT price = £52.50
  Oral suspension
  CAUTIONARY AND ADVISORY LABELS 14 (urine red)
  - Co-danthrusate (Non-proprietary)
    Dantron 10 mg per 1 ml, Docusate sodium 12 mg per 1 ml Co-danthrusate 50mg/60mg/5ml oral suspension sugar free sugar-free | 200 ml [PoM] £89.92

Glycerol
(Glycerin)

- INDICATIONS AND DOSE
Constipation
- BY RECTUM
- Child 1–11 months: 1 g as required
- Child 1–11 years: 2 g as required
- Child 12–17 years: 4 g as required
- Adult: 4 g as required

- DIRECTIONS FOR ADMINISTRATION Moisten suppositories with water before insertion.
- PRESCRIBING AND DISPENSING INFORMATION When prepared extemporaneously, the BP states Glycerol

Suppositories, BP consists of gelatin 140 mg, glycerol 700 mg, purified water to 1 g.

- **PATIENT AND CARER ADVICE**
Medicines for Children leaflet: Glycerin (glycerol) suppositories for constipation www.medicinesforchildren.org.uk/glycerin-glycerol-suppositories-for-constipation

- **MEDICINAL FORMS**
There can be variation in the licensing of different medicines containing the same drug. Forms available from special-order manufacturers include: suppository

Suppository
- Glycerol (Non-proprietary)
   Gelatin 140 mg per 1 gram, Glycerol 700 mg per 1 gram Glycerol 2g suppositories | 12 suppository GSL £1.73 DT price = £1.67 | Glycerol 1g suppositories | 12 suppository GSL £1.69 DT price = £1.04 | Glycerol 4g suppositories | 12 suppository GSL £1.54 DT price = £1.39

Senna
13.6.2016

- **DRUG ACTION** Senna is a stimulant laxative. After metabolism of sennosides in the gut the anthrone component stimulates peristalsis thereby increasing the motility of the large intestine.

- **INDICATIONS AND DOSE**

Constipation
- BY MOUTH USING TABLETS
- Child 6-17 years: 7.5–30 mg once daily, adjusted according to response
- Adult: 7.5–15 mg daily (max. per dose 30 mg daily), dose usually taken at bedtime; initial dose should be low then gradually increased, higher doses may be prescribed under medical supervision
- BY MOUTH USING SYRUP
- Child 1 month-3 years: 3.75–15 mg once daily, adjusted according to response
- Child 4-17 years: 3.75–30 mg once daily, adjusted according to response
- Adult: 7.5–15 mg once daily (max. per dose 30 mg daily), dose usually taken at bedtime, higher doses may be prescribed under medical supervision

PHARMACOKINETICS
Onset of action 8–12 hours.

- **UNLICENSED USE** *Tablets* not licensed for use in children under 6 years. *Syrup* not licensed for use in children under 2 years.
   Doses in BNF adhere to national guidelines and may differ from those in product literature.

- **CONTRA-INDICATIONS** Intestinal obstruction · undiagnosed abdominal pain

- **SIDE-EFFECTS** Abdominal spasm · discoloration of urine · pruritus

   SIDE-EFFECTS, FURTHER INFORMATION
   Prolonged or excessive use of stimulant laxatives can cause diarrhoea and related effects such as hypokalaemia.

- **PREGNANCY** EvGr Specialist sources indicate suitable for use in pregnancy. ◇

- **BREAST FEEDING** EvGr Specialist sources indicate suitable for use in breast-feeding in infants over 1 month. ◇

- **PATIENT AND CARER ADVICE**
Medicines for Children leaflet: Senna for constipation www.medicinesforchildren.org.uk/senna-for-constipation

- **NATIONAL FUNDING/ACCESS DECISIONS**
NHS restrictions *Senokot*® tablets

- **EXCEPTIONS TO LEGAL CATEGORY** Senna is on sale to the public for use in children over 12 years; doses on packs may vary from those in BNF Publications.

- **MEDICINAL FORMS**
There can be variation in the licensing of different medicines containing the same drug.
Tablet
- Senna (Non-proprietary)
   Sennoside B (as Sennosides) 7.5 mg
   Senna 7.5mg tablets | 20 tablet P £0.99 | 20 tablet GSL £0.99 | 60 tablet P £3.47 DT price = £3.01 | 60 tablet GSL £1.70 DT price = £3.01 | 100 tablet GSL £2.10 | 100 tablet P £2.10 | 1000 tablet GSL no price available

Oral solution
- Senokot (Forum Health Products Ltd, Reckitt Benckiser Healthcare (UK) Ltd)
   Sennoside B (as Sennosides) 1.5 mg per 1 ml Senokot 7.5mg/5ml Syrup Pharmacy sugar free sugar-free | 500 ml P £3.99 DT price = £3.99 | Senokot 7.5mg/5ml syrup sugar free sugar-free | 150 ml GSL £3.49

Senna with ispaghula husk
24.2.2016

The properties listed below are those particular to the combination only. For the properties of the components please consider, senna above, ispaghula husk p. 47.

- **INDICATIONS AND DOSE**

Constipation
- BY MOUTH
- Child 12-17 years: 5–10 g once daily, to be taken at night, 5 g equivalent to one level spoonful of granules
- Adult: 5–10 g once daily, to be taken at night, 5 g equivalent to one level spoonful of granules

- **SIDE-EFFECTS** Urine coloured yellow or red-brown

- **PREGNANCY** Manufacturer advises avoid during first trimester. To be used only intermittently and only if dietary and lifestyle changes fail.

- **DIRECTIONS FOR ADMINISTRATION** Take at night with at least 150 mL liquid..

- **MEDICINAL FORMS**
There can be variation in the licensing of different medicines containing the same drug.
Granules
CAUTIONARY AND ADVISORY LABELS 25
EXCIPIENTS: May contain Sucrose
- Manevac (Meda Pharmaceuticals Ltd)
   Senna fruit 124 mg per 1 gram, Ispaghula 542 mg per 1 gram Manevac granules | 400 gram P £9.25 DT price = £9.25

Sodium picosulfate
6.5.2016

(Sodium picosulphate)

- **DRUG ACTION** Sodium picosulfate is a stimulant laxative. After metabolism in the colon it stimulates the mucosa thereby increasing the motility of the large intestine.

- **INDICATIONS AND DOSE**

Constipation
- BY MOUTH
- Child 1 month-3 years: 2.5–10 mg once daily, adjusted according to response
- Child 4-17 years: 2.5–20 mg once daily, adjusted according to response
- Adult: 5–10 mg once daily, dose to be taken at bedtime

PHARMACOKINETICS
Onset of action 6–12 hours.

- **UNLICENSED USE** Sodium picosulfate doses in BNF Publications adhere to national guidelines and may differ from those in product literature.

- **CONTRA-INDICATIONS** Intestinal obstruction · undiagnosed abdominal pain

- SIDE-EFFECTS
- ▶ **Common or very common** Abdominal cramp
- ▶ **Uncommon** Dizziness · nausea · vomiting
- ▶ **Frequency not known** Angioedema · pruritus · rash · syncope

SIDE-EFFECTS, FURTHER INFORMATION
Prolonged or excessive use can cause diarrhoea and related effects such as hypokalaemia.
- PREGNANCY Manufacturer states evidence limited but not known to be harmful.
- BREAST FEEDING [EvGr] Specialist sources indicate suitable for use in breast-feeding in infants over 1 month—not known to be present in milk. ⓓ
- PATIENT AND CARER ADVICE
Medicines for Children leaflet: Sodium picosulfate for constipation www.medicinesforchildren.org.uk/sodium-picosulfate-for-constipation

- MEDICINAL FORMS
There can be variation in the licensing of different medicines containing the same drug.

Oral solution
EXCIPIENTS: May contain Alcohol
- ▶ Sodium picosulfate (Non-proprietary)
Sodium picosulfate 1 mg per 1 ml
Sodium picosulfate 5mg/5ml oral solution sugar free sugar-free | 100 ml [P] £2.37 sugar-free | 300 ml [P] £7.10 DT price = £7.10
- ▶ Dulco-Lax (sodium picosulfate) (Boehringer Ingelheim Self-Medication Division)
Sodium picosulfate 1 mg per 1 ml Dulcolax Pico 5mg/5ml liquid sugar-free | 100 ml [P] £1.85 sugar-free | 300 ml [P] £4.40 DT price = £7.10

OPIOID RECEPTOR ANTAGONISTS

Methylnaltrexone bromide

12.4.2016

- DRUG ACTION Methylnaltrexone bromide is a peripherally acting opioid-receptor antagonist. It therefore blocks the gastro-intestinal (constipating) effects of opioids without altering their central analgesic effects.

- INDICATIONS AND DOSE

Opioid-induced constipation in patients with chronic pain (except palliative care patients with advanced illness)
- ▶ BY SUBCUTANEOUS INJECTION
- ▶ Adult: 12 mg once daily if required, to be given as 4–7 doses weekly

Adjunct to other laxatives in opioid-induced constipation in advanced illness (palliative care patients)
- ▶ BY SUBCUTANEOUS INJECTION
- ▶ Adult (body-weight up to 38 kg): 150 micrograms/kg once daily on alternate days for maximum duration of treatment 4 months, two consecutive doses may be given 24 hours apart if no response to treatment on the preceding day
- ▶ Adult (body-weight 38–61 kg): 8 mg once daily on alternate days for maximum duration of treatment 4 months, two consecutive doses may be given 24 hours apart if no response to treatment on the preceding day
- ▶ Adult (body-weight 62–114 kg): 12 mg once daily on alternate days for maximum duration of treatment 4 months, two consecutive doses may be given 24 hours apart if no response to treatment on the preceding day
- ▶ Adult (body-weight 115 kg and above): 150 micrograms/kg once daily on alternate days for maximum duration of treatment 4 months, two consecutive doses may be given 24 hours apart if no response to treatment on the preceding day

PHARMACOKINETICS
May act within 30–60 minutes.

- CONTRA-INDICATIONS Acute surgical abdominal conditions · gastro-intestinal obstruction
- CAUTIONS Diverticular disease (when active) · faecal impaction · gastro-intestinal tract lesions (known or suspected) · patients with colostomy · patients with peritoneal catheter
- SIDE-EFFECTS
- ▶ **Common or very common** Abdominal pain · diarrhoea · dizziness · flatulence · injection site reactions · nausea · opioid withdrawal symptoms (usually mild to moderate) · vomiting
- ▶ **Frequency not known** Gastro-intestinal perforation
Overdose
Symptoms of overdosage include orthostatic hypotension.
- PREGNANCY Manufacturer advises use unless essential—toxicity at high doses in *animal* studies.
- BREAST FEEDING Manufacturer advises use only if potential benefit outweighs risk—present in milk in *animal* studies.
- HEPATIC IMPAIRMENT Manufacturer advises avoid in severe impairment—no information available.
- RENAL IMPAIRMENT If eGFR less than 30 mL/minute/1.73 m^2, reduce dose as follows: body-weight under 62 kg, 75 micrograms/kg on alternate days; body-weight 62–114 kg, 8 mg on alternate days; body-weight over 114 kg, 75 micrograms/kg on alternate days.
- DIRECTIONS FOR ADMINISTRATION Rotate injection site.
- HANDLING AND STORAGE Protect from light.

- MEDICINAL FORMS
There can be variation in the licensing of different medicines containing the same drug.
Solution for injection
- ▶ Relistor (Swedish Orphan Biovitrum Ltd)
Methylnaltrexone bromide 20 mg per 1 ml Relistor 12mg/0.6ml solution for injection vials | 1 vial [PoM] £21.05 | 7 vial [PoM] £147.35

SOFTENING DRUGS

Arachis oil

- INDICATIONS AND DOSE

To soften impacted faeces
- ▶ BY RECTUM
- ▶ Adult: 130 mL as required

- CAUTIONS Hypersensitivity to soya · intestinal obstruction
- ALLERGY AND CROSS-SENSITIVITY Contra-indicated if history of hypersensitivity to arachis oil or peanuts.
- DIRECTIONS FOR ADMINISTRATION Warm enema in warm water before use.

- MEDICINAL FORMS
There can be variation in the licensing of different medicines containing the same drug.
Enema
- ▶ Arachis oil (Non-proprietary)
Arachis oil 1 ml per 1 ml Arachis oil 130ml enema | 1 enema [P] £37.50 DT price = £37.50

Docusate sodium

(Dioctyl sodium sulphosuccinate)

- **INDICATIONS AND DOSE**

Chronic constipation
- ▶ BY MOUTH
- ▶ Child 6 months-1 year: 12.5 mg 3 times a day, adjusted according to response, use paediatric oral solution
- ▶ Child 2–11 years: 12.5–25 mg 3 times a day, adjusted according to response, use paediatric oral solution
- ▶ Child 12-17 years: Up to 500 mg daily in divided doses, adjusted according to response
- ▶ Adult: Up to 500 mg daily in divided doses, adjusted according to response
- ▶ BY RECTUM
- ▶ Adult: 120 mg for 1 dose

Adjunct in abdominal radiological procedures
- ▶ BY MOUTH
- ▶ Adult: 400 mg, to be administered with barium meal
- ▶ BY RECTUM
- ▶ Adult: 120 mg for 1 dose

PHARMACOKINETICS
- ▶ With oral use or rectal use Oral preparations act within 1–2 days; response to rectal administration usually occurs within 20 minutes.

- UNLICENSED USE *Adult oral solution and capsules* not licensed for use in children under 12 years.
- CONTRA-INDICATIONS Avoid in intestinal obstruction
- CAUTIONS Do not give with liquid paraffin · excessive use of stimulant laxatives can cause diarrhoea and related effects such as hypokalaemia · rectal preparations not indicated if haemorrhoids or anal fissure
- SIDE-EFFECTS Abdominal cramp · diarrhoea (excessive use) · hypokalaemia · rash
- PREGNANCY Not known to be harmful—manufacturer advises caution.
- BREAST FEEDING
- ▶ With oral use Present in milk following oral administration— manufacturer advises caution.
- ▶ With rectal use Rectal administration not known to be harmful.
- DIRECTIONS FOR ADMINISTRATION
- ▶ With oral use in children For administration *by mouth*, solution may be mixed with milk or squash.
- MEDICINAL FORMS
There can be variation in the licensing of different medicines containing the same drug.

Capsule
- ▶ Dioctyl (UCB Pharma Ltd)
 Docusate sodium 100 mg Dioctyl 100mg capsules | 30 capsule P £2.09 DT price = £2.09 | 100 capsule P £6.98

Oral solution
- ▶ Docusol (Typharm Ltd)
 Docusate sodium 2.5 mg per 1 ml Docusol Paediatric 12.5mg/5ml oral solution sugar-free | 300 ml P £5.29 DT price = £5.29
 Docusate sodium 10 mg per 1 ml Docusol Adult 50mg/5ml oral solution sugar-free | 300 ml P £5.49 DT price = £5.49

Enema
- ▶ Norgalax (Essential Pharma Ltd)
 Docusate sodium 12 mg per 1 gram Norgalax 120mg/10g enema | 6 enema P £28.00

Liquid paraffin

- **INDICATIONS AND DOSE**

Constipation
- ▶ BY MOUTH
- ▶ Adult: 10–30 mL daily if required, to be administered at night

- CAUTIONS Avoid prolonged use
- SIDE-EFFECTS Anal irritation after prolonged use · anal seepage of paraffin after prolonged use · granulomatous reactions caused by absorption of small quantities of liquid paraffin (especially from the emulsion) · interference with the absorption of fat-soluble vitamins · lipoid pneumonia
- PRESCRIBING AND DISPENSING INFORMATION When prepared extemporaneously, the BP states Liquid Paraffin Oral Emulsion, BP consists of liquid paraffin 5 mL, vanillin 5 mg, chloroform 0.025 mL, benzoic acid solution 0.2 mL, methylcellulose-20 200 mg, saccharin sodium 500 micrograms, water to 10 mL.
- PATIENT AND CARER ADVICE Oral emulsion should not be taken immediately before going to bed.
- LESS SUITABLE FOR PRESCRIBING Liquid Paraffin Oral Emulsion BP is less suitable for prescribing.
- MEDICINAL FORMS
There can be variation in the licensing of different medicines containing the same drug.
Form unstated
- ▶ Liquid paraffin (Non-proprietary)
 Liquid paraffin light 1 ml per 1 ml Liquid paraffin light liquid | 500 ml GSL £3.97 DT price = £3.97 | 2000 ml GSL £11.48

Liquid paraffin with magnesium hydroxide

The properties listed below are those particular to the combination only. For the properties of the components please consider, liquid paraffin above, magnesium hydroxide p. 51.

- **INDICATIONS AND DOSE**

Constipation
- ▶ BY MOUTH
- ▶ Adult: 5–20 mL as required

- PRESCRIBING AND DISPENSING INFORMATION Liquid paraffin and magnesium hydroxide preparations are on sale to the public.
 When prepared extemporaneously, the BP states Liquid Paraffin and Magnesium Hydroxide Oral Emulsion, BP consists of 25% liquid paraffin in aqueous suspension containing 6% hydrated magnesium oxide.
- LESS SUITABLE FOR PRESCRIBING Liquid paraffin with magnesium hydroxide is less suitable for prescribing.
- MEDICINAL FORMS
There can be variation in the licensing of different medicines containing the same drug.
No licensed medicines listed.

3   Diarrhoea

Acute diarrhoea

Management of acute diarrhoea

The priority in acute diarrhoea, as in gastro-enteritis, is the prevention or reversal of fluid and electrolyte depletion. This is particularly important in infants and in frail and elderly patients. **Oral rehydration preparations** are used in the prevention or reversal of fluid and electrolyte depletion. Severe depletion of fluid and electrolytes requires immediate admission to hospital and urgent replacement.

Antimotility drugs

Antimotility drugs relieve symptoms of acute diarrhoea by binding to opioid receptors in the gastrointestinal tract and thereby prolonging the duration of intestinal transit. They are used in the management of uncomplicated acute diarrhoea in adults, however, are **not** recommended for acute diarrhoea in young children; fluid and electrolyte replacement are of primary importance in severe cases of acute diarrhoea and may also be necessary in cases of dehydration.

Loperamide hydrochloride p. 59 is used due to its action on opioid receptors in the gastrointestinal tract and because it does not readily cross the blood-brain barrier.Loperamide hydrochloride can also be used for faecal incontinence [unlicensed indication] after the underlying cause of incontinence has been addressed.

Antimotility drugs have a role in Inflammatory bowel disease p. 34 and in Stoma care p. 87.

Antispasmodics

Antispasmodics are occasionally of value in treating abdominal cramp associated with diarrhoea but they should **not** be used for primary treatment. Antispasmodics and antiemetics should be **avoided** in young children with gastro-enteritis because they are rarely effective and have troublesome side-effects.

Antibacterial drugs

Antibacterial drugs are generally unnecessary in simple gastro-enteritis because the complaint usually resolves quickly without them, and infective diarrhoeas in the UK often have a viral cause. Systemic bacterial infection does, however, need appropriate systemic treatment.Ciprofloxacin p. 506 is occasionally used for prophylaxis against travellers' diarrhoea, but routine use is **not** recommended. Lactobacillus preparations have not been shown to be effective.

Adsorbents and bulk-forming drugs

Adsorbents such as kaolin p. 60 are **not** recommended for *acute diarrhoeas*. Bulk-forming drugs, such as ispaghula husk p. 47, methylcellulose p. 48, and sterculia p. 48 are useful in controlling diarrhoea associated with diverticular disease.

Colestyramine p. 180 binds unabsorbed bile salts and provides symptomatic relief of diarrhoea following ileal disease or resection.

Enkephalinase inhibitors

Racecadotril p. 60 is a pro-drug of thiorphan. Thiorphan is an enkephalinase inhibitor that inhibits the breakdown of endogenous opioids, thereby reducing intestinal secretions. Racecadotril is licensed, as an adjunct to rehydration, for the symptomatic treatment of uncomplicated acute diarrhoea; it should only be used in children over 3 months of age when usual supportive measures, including oral rehydration, are insufficient to control the condition. Racecadotril does not affect the duration of intestinal transit.

Drugs used for Diarrhoea not listed below Codeine phosphate, p. 413

ANTIDIARRHOEALS ›
ANTIPROPULSIVES

☞ 408

Co-phenotrope

● **INDICATIONS AND DOSE**

Adjunct to rehydration in acute diarrhoea
▸ BY MOUTH
▸ Child 4–8 years: 1 tablet 3 times a day
▸ Child 9–11 years: 1 tablet 4 times a day
▸ Child 12–15 years: 2 tablets 3 times a day
▸ Child 16–17 years: Initially 4 tablets, followed by 2 tablets every 6 hours until diarrhoea controlled
▸ Adult: Initially 4 tablets, followed by 2 tablets every 6 hours until diarrhoea controlled

Control of faecal consistency after colostomy or ileostomy
▸ BY MOUTH
▸ Child 4–8 years: 1 tablet 3 times a day
▸ Child 9–11 years: 1 tablet 4 times a day
▸ Child 12–15 years: 2 tablets 3 times a day
▸ Child 16–17 years: Initially 4 tablets, then 2 tablets 4 times a day
▸ Adult: Initially 4 tablets, then 2 tablets 4 times a day

● UNLICENSED USE Not licensed for use in children under 4 years.

● CONTRA-INDICATIONS Gastro-intestinal obstruction · intestinal atony · myasthenia gravis (but some antimuscarinics may be used to decrease muscarinic side-effects of anticholinesterases) · paralytic ileus · prostatic enlargement (in adults) · pyloric stenosis · severe ulcerative colitis · significant bladder outflow obstruction · toxic megacolon · urinary retention

● CAUTIONS Presence of subclinical doses of atropine may give rise to atropine side-effects in susceptible individuals or in overdosage · young children are particularly susceptible to **overdosage**; symptoms may be delayed and observation is needed for at least 48 hours after ingestion

● INTERACTIONS → Appendix 1 (antimuscarinics, opioid analgesics).

● SIDE-EFFECTS
▸ **Very rare** Angle-closure glaucoma
▸ **Frequency not known** Abdominal pain · anorexia · confusion (particularly in the elderly) (in adults) · constipation · dilation of the pupils with loss of accomodation · dry mouth · dryness of the skin · fever · flushing · giddiness · nausea · photophobia · reduced bronchial secretions · transient bradycardia (followed by tachycardia, palpitation and arrhythmias) · urinary retention · urinary urgency · vomiting

● PREGNANCY Manufacturer advises caution.

● BREAST FEEDING May be present in milk.

● HEPATIC IMPAIRMENT Avoid in jaundice.

● DIRECTIONS FOR ADMINISTRATION For administration *by mouth* tablets may be crushed.

● PRESCRIBING AND DISPENSING INFORMATION A mixture of diphenoxylate hydrochloride and atropine sulfate in the mass proportions 100 parts to 1 part respectively.

- EXCEPTIONS TO LEGAL CATEGORY Co-phenotrope 2.5/0.025 can be sold to the public for adults and children over 16 years (provided packs do not contain more than 20 tablets) as an adjunct to rehydration in acute diarrhoea (max. daily dose 10 tablets).

- MEDICINAL FORMS
There can be variation in the licensing of different medicines containing the same drug.
Tablet
  ‣ Co-phenotrope (Non-proprietary)
    Atropine sulfate 25 microgram, Diphenoxylate hydrochloride 2.5 mg Lomotil 2.5mg/25microgram tablets | 100 tablet PoM no price available Schedule 5 (CD Inv)

⚑ 408

Kaolin with morphine

- INDICATIONS AND DOSE
Acute diarrhoea
▶ BY MOUTH
  ‣ Adult: 10 mL every 6 hours, dose to be given in water

- CONTRA-INDICATIONS Acute abdomen · delayed gastric emptying · heart failure secondary to chronic lung disease · phaeochromocytoma

- CAUTIONS Cardiac arrhythmias · pancreatitis · severe cor pulmonale

- SIDE-EFFECTS Abdominal pain · agitation · amenorrhoea · anorexia · asthenia · bronchospasm · delirium · disorientation · dyspepsia · exacerbation of pancreatitis · excitation · hypertension · hypothermia · inhibition of cough reflex · malaise · muscle fasciculation · myoclonus · nystagmus · paraesthesia · paralytic ileus · raised intracranial pressure · restlessness · rhabdomyolysis · seizures · syncope · taste disturbance

- BREAST FEEDING Therapeutic doses unlikely to affect infant.

- RENAL IMPAIRMENT Avoid use or reduce dose; opioid effects increased and prolonged and increased cerebral sensitivity occurs.

- PRESCRIBING AND DISPENSING INFORMATION When prepared extemporaneously, the BP states Kaolin and Morphine Mixture, BP consists of light kaolin or light kaolin (natural) 20%, sodium bicarbonate 5%, and chloroform and morphine tincture 4% in a suitable vehicle. Contains anhydrous morphine 550–800 micrograms/10 mL.

- LESS SUITABLE FOR PRESCRIBING Kaolin and Morphine Mixture, BP (Kaolin and Morphine Oral Suspension) is less suitable for prescribing.

- MEDICINAL FORMS
There can be variation in the licensing of different medicines containing the same drug.
Oral suspension
  ‣ Kaolin with morphine (Non-proprietary)
    Chloroform 5 ml per 1 litre, Morphine hydrochloride 91.6 microgram per 1 ml, Sodium bicarbonate 50 mg per 1 ml, Kaolin light 200 mg per 1 ml Kaolin and Morphine mixture | 200 ml P £1.50 DT price = £1.50 Schedule 5 (CD Inv)

Loperamide hydrochloride

- INDICATIONS AND DOSE
Symptomatic treatment of acute diarrhoea
▶ BY MOUTH
  ‣ Child 4-7 years: 1 mg 3–4 times a day for up to 3 days only
  ‣ Child 8-11 years: 2 mg 4 times a day for up to 5 days

  ‣ Child 12-17 years: Initially 4 mg, followed by 2 mg for up to 5 days, dose to be taken after each loose stool; usual dose 6–8 mg daily; maximum 16 mg per day
  ‣ Adult: Initially 4 mg, followed by 2 mg for up to 5 days, dose to be taken after each loose stool; usual dose 6–8 mg daily; maximum 16 mg per day

Chronic diarrhoea
▶ BY MOUTH
  ‣ Adult: Initially 4–8 mg daily in divided doses, adjusted according to response; maintenance up to 16 mg daily in 2 divided doses

Faecal incontinence
▶ BY MOUTH
  ‣ Adult: Initially 500 micrograms daily, adjusted according to response, maximum daily dose to be given in divided doses; maximum 16 mg per day

Pain of bowel colic in palliative care
▶ BY MOUTH
  ‣ Adult: 2–4 mg 4 times a day

- UNLICENSED USE
▶ In children Not licensed for use in children for chronic diarrhoea. *Capsules* not licensed for use in children under 8 years. *Syrup* not licensed for use in children under 4 years.
▶ In adults Use for faecal incontinence is an unlicensed indication.

- CONTRA-INDICATIONS Active ulcerative colitis · antibiotic-associated colitis · conditions where abdominal distension develops · conditions where inhibition of peristalsis should be avoided

- CAUTIONS Not recommended for children under 12 years

- INTERACTIONS → Appendix 1 (loperamide).

- SIDE-EFFECTS
▶ **Common or very common** Dizziness · flatulence · headache · nausea
▶ **Uncommon** Abdominal pain · drowsiness · dry mouth · dyspepsia · rash · vomiting
▶ **Rare** Fatigue · hypertonia · paralytic ileus · Stevens-Johnson syndrome · toxic epidermal necrolysis · urinary retention

- PREGNANCY Manufacturers advise avoid—no information available.

- BREAST FEEDING Amount probably too small to be harmful.

- HEPATIC IMPAIRMENT Risk of accumulation—manufacturer advises caution.

- PATIENT AND CARER ADVICE
Medicines for Children leaflet: Loperamide for diarrhoea www.medicinesforchildren.org.uk/loperamide-for-diarrhoea

- EXCEPTIONS TO LEGAL CATEGORY Loperamide can be sold to the public, for use in adults and children over 12 years, provided it is licensed and labelled for the treatment of acute diarrhoea.
▶ In adults Loperamide can be sold to the public, provided it is licensed and labelled for the treatment of acute diarrhoea associated with irritable bowel syndrome (after initial diagnosis by a doctor) in adults over 18 years of age.

- MEDICINAL FORMS
There can be variation in the licensing of different medicines containing the same drug. Forms available from special-order manufacturers include: oral suspension, oral solution
Tablet
  ‣ Loperamide hydrochloride (Non-proprietary)
    Loperamide hydrochloride 2 mg Loperamide 2mg tablets | 30 tablet PoM £2.25 DT price = £2.15
  ‣ Norimode (Tillomed Laboratories Ltd)
    Loperamide hydrochloride 2 mg Norimode 2mg tablets | 30 tablet PoM £2.15 DT price = £2.15

▸ Normaloe (Tillomed Laboratories Ltd)
Loperamide hydrochloride 2 mg Normaloe 2mg tablets |
12 tablet P £1.70

Orodispersible tablet
▸ Imodium (McNeil Products Ltd)
Loperamide hydrochloride 2 mg Imodium Instants 2mg
orodispersible tablets sugar-free | 6 tablet GSL £2.45 sugar-free |
12 tablet GSL £3.76
Imodium Instant Melts 2mg orodispersible tablets sugar-free |
12 tablet P £3.75 sugar-free | 18 tablet P £5.02 DT price = £5.02

Capsule
▸ Loperamide hydrochloride (Non-proprietary)
Loperamide hydrochloride 2 mg Loperamide 2mg capsules |
6 capsule GSL no price available | 12 capsule P £1.94 |
30 capsule PoM £2.99 DT price = £1.39
▸ Imodium (McNeil Products Ltd)
Loperamide hydrochloride 2 mg Imodium LiquiCaps 2mg Soft
capsules | 6 capsule GSL £2.45
Imodium 2mg Soft capsules | 12 capsule P £3.79
Imodium IBS Relief 2mg capsules | 12 capsule P £3.79
Imodium Classic 2mg capsules | 12 capsule P £3.31 |
18 capsule P £4.13
Imodium Original 2mg capsules | 6 capsule GSL £1.88

Oral solution
▸ Imodium (Janssen-Cilag Ltd)
Loperamide hydrochloride 200 microgram per 1 ml Imodium
1mg/5ml oral solution sugar-free | 100 ml PoM £1.17 DT price =
£1.17

Loperamide with simeticone

The properties listed below are those particular to the
combination only. For the properties of the components
please consider, loperamide hydrochloride p. 59, simeticone
p. 64.

● INDICATIONS AND DOSE
Acute diarrhoea with abdominal colic
▸ BY MOUTH
▸ Child 12-17 years: Initially 1 tablet, then 1 tablet, after
each loose stool, for up to 2 days; maximum 4 tablets
per day
▸ Adult: Initially 2 tablets, then 1 tablet, after each loose
stool, for up to 2 days; maximum 4 tablets per day

● MEDICINAL FORMS
There can be variation in the licensing of different medicines
containing the same drug.
Tablet
▸ Imodium Plus (McNeil Products Ltd)
**Loperamide hydrochloride 2 mg, Dimeticone (as Simeticone)
125 mg** Imodium Plus Comfort tablets | 6 tablet GSL £2.51
Imodium Plus caplets | 12 tablet P £3.66

**ANTIDIARRHOEALS ❭ ENKEPHALINASE
INHIBITORS**

Racecadotril
11.2.2016

● INDICATIONS AND DOSE
**Adjunct to rehydration, for the symptomatic treatment of
uncomplicated acute diarrhoea**
▸ BY MOUTH USING CAPSULES
▸ Adult: Initially 100 mg, then 100 mg 3 times a day until
diarrhoea stops; maximum duration of treatment
7 days, dose to be taken preferably before food
▸ BY MOUTH USING GRANULES
▸ Child 3 months-17 years (body-weight up to 9 kg): 10 mg
3 times a day until diarrhoea stops; maximum duration
of treatment 7 days
▸ Child 3 months-17 years (body-weight 9-12 kg): 20 mg
3 times a day until diarrhoea stops; maximum duration
of treatment 7 days

▸ Child 3 months-17 years (body-weight 13-27 kg): 30 mg
3 times a day until diarrhoea stops; maximum duration
of treatment 7 days
▸ Child 3 months-17 years (body-weight 28 kg and
above): 60 mg 3 times a day until diarrhoea stops;
maximum duration of treatment 7 days

● CONTRA-INDICATIONS Antibiotic-associated diarrhoea
● SIDE-EFFECTS
▸ **Common or very common** Headache (in adults)
▸ **Uncommon** Erythema · rash
▸ **Frequency not known** Angioedema · pruritus · urticaria
SIDE-EFFECTS, FURTHER INFORMATION
▸ Skin reactions Severe skin reactions have been reported—
discontinue treatment immediately.
● PREGNANCY Manufacturer advises avoid—no information
available.
● BREAST FEEDING Manufacturer advises avoid—no
information available.
● HEPATIC IMPAIRMENT
▸ In adults Manufacturer advises caution.
▸ In children Manufacturer advises avoid.
● RENAL IMPAIRMENT
▸ In adults Manufacturer advises caution.
▸ In children Manufacturer advises avoid.
● DIRECTIONS FOR ADMINISTRATION Granules may be added
to food or mixed with water or bottle feeds and then taken
immediately.
● PATIENT AND CARER ADVICE Patients and carers should be
given advice on how to administer racecadotril granules.
● NATIONAL FUNDING/ACCESS DECISIONS
Scottish Medicines Consortium (SMC) Decisions
The *Scottish Medicines Consortium*, has advised (July 2014)
that racecadotril (*Hidrasec*®) is **not** recommended for use
within NHS Scotland for the treatment of acute diarrhoea
in children because there is insufficient evidence that it
improves the recovery rate.

● MEDICINAL FORMS
There can be variation in the licensing of different medicines
containing the same drug.
Granules
EXCIPIENTS: May contain Sucrose
▸ Hidrasec (Lincoln Medical Ltd)
Racecadotril 10 mg Hidrasec Infants 10mg granules sachets |
20 sachet PoM £8.42
Racecadotril 30 mg Hidrasec Children 30mg granules sachets |
20 sachet PoM £8.42

ANTIDIARRHOEALS ❭ INTESTINAL ADSORBENTS

Kaolin

● INDICATIONS AND DOSE
Diarrhoea (not recommended for acute diarrhoea)
▸ BY MOUTH
▸ Adult: 10-20 mL every 4 hours

● INTERACTIONS → Appendix 1 (kaolin).
● PRESCRIBING AND DISPENSING INFORMATION Flavours of
oral liquid formulations may include peppermint.
When prepared extemporaneously, the BP states Kaolin
Mixture, BP consists of light kaolin or light kaolin (natural)
20%, light magnesium carbonate 5%, sodium bicarbonate
5% in a suitable vehicle with a peppermint flavour.
● LESS SUITABLE FOR PRESCRIBING Kaolin Mixture BP is less
suitable for prescribing.
● MEDICINAL FORMS
There can be variation in the licensing of different medicines
containing the same drug.
No licensed medicines listed.

4   Disorders of gastric acid and ulceration

4.1   Dyspepsia

Dyspepsia

Overview

Dyspepsia covers upper abdominal pain, fullness, early satiety, bloating, and nausea. It can occur with gastric and duodenal ulceration and, gastric cancer, but most commonly it is of uncertain origin.

Urgent endoscopic investigation is required if dyspepsia is accompanied by 'alarm features' (e.g. bleeding, dysphagia, recurrent vomiting, or weight loss). Urgent investigation should also be considered for patients over 55 years with unexplained, recent-onset dyspepsia that has not responded to treatment.

Patients with dyspepsia should be advised about lifestyle changes (avoidance of excess alcohol and of aggravating foods such as fats); other measures include weight reduction, smoking cessation, and raising the head of the bed. Some medications may cause dyspepsia—these should be stopped, if possible.

Antacids may provide some symptomatic relief, however if symptoms persist in *uninvestigated dyspepsia*, treatment involves a **proton pump inhibitor** for up to 4 weeks. A proton pump inhibitor can be used intermittently to control symptoms long term. Patients with uninvestigated dyspepsia, who do not respond to an initial trial with a proton pump inhibitor, should be tested for *Helicobacter pylori* and given eradication therapy if *H. pylori* is present. Alternatively, particularly in populations where *H. pylori* infection is more likely, the 'test and treat' strategy for *H. pylori* can be used before a trial with a proton pump inhibitor.

If *H. pylori* is present in patients with *functional (investigated, non-ulcer) dyspepsia*, eradication therapy should be provided. If symptoms persist, treatment with either a **proton pump inhibitor** or a **histamine H₂-receptor antagonist** can be given for 4 weeks. These antisecretory drugs can be used intermittently to control symptoms long term. However, most patients with functional dyspepsia do not benefit symptomatically from *H. pylori* eradication therapy or antisecretory drugs.

ANTACIDS

Antacids

Overview

Antacids (usually containing aluminium or magnesium compounds) can often relieve symptoms in *ulcer dyspepsia* and in *non-erosive gastro-oesophageal reflux* ; they are also sometimes used in functional (non-ulcer) dyspepsia but the evidence of benefit is uncertain. Antacids are best given when symptoms occur or are expected, usually between meals and at bedtime, although additional doses may be required. Conventional doses of liquid magnesium–aluminium antacids promote ulcer healing, but less well than antisecretory drugs; proof of a relationship between healing and neutralising capacity is lacking. Liquid preparations are more effective than tablet preparations.

Aluminium- and **magnesium-containing** antacids (e.g. aluminium hydroxide p. 913, magnesium carbonate p. 63, co-magaldrox p. 62 and magnesium trisilicate p. 63), being relatively insoluble in water, are long-acting if retained in the stomach. They are suitable for most antacid purposes. Magnesium-containing antacids tend to be laxative whereas aluminium-containing antacids may be constipating; antacids containing both magnesium and aluminium may reduce these colonic side-effects. Aluminium accumulation does not appear to be a risk if renal function is normal.

The acid-neutralising capacity of preparations that contain more than one antacid may be the same as simpler preparations. Complexes such as **hydrotalcite** confer no special advantage.

Sodium bicarbonate should no longer be prescribed alone for the relief of dyspepsia but it is present as an ingredient in many indigestion remedies. However, it retains a place in the management of urinary-tract disorders and acidosis.

Bismuth-containing antacids (unless chelates) are not recommended because absorbed bismuth can be neurotoxic, causing encephalopathy; they tend to be constipating. **Calcium-containing** antacids can induce rebound acid secretion: with modest doses the clinical significance is doubtful, but prolonged high doses also cause hypercalcaemia and alkalosis, and can precipitate the milk-alkali syndrome.

Simeticone

Simeticone (activated dimeticone) p. 64 is added to an antacid as an antifoaming agent to relieve flatulence. These preparations may be useful for the relief of hiccup in palliative care.

Alginates

Alginates taken in combination with an antacid increases the viscosity of stomach contents and can protect the oesophageal mucosa from acid reflux. Some alginate-containing preparations form a viscous gel ('raft') that floats on the surface of the stomach contents, thereby reducing symptoms of reflux.

The amount of additional ingredient or antacid in individual preparations varies widely, as does their sodium content, so that preparations may not be freely interchangeable.

ANTACIDS > ALGINATE

Alginic acid

> ● **INDICATIONS AND DOSE**
>
> GAVISCON INFANT® POWDER SACHETS
>
> **Management of gastro-oesophageal reflux disease**
> ▶ BY MOUTH
> ▶ Child 1–23 months (body-weight up to 4.5 kg): 1 dose as required, to be mixed with feeds (or water, for breast-fed infants); maximum 6 doses per day
> ▶ Child 1–23 months (body-weight 4.5 kg and above): 2 doses as required, to be mixed with feeds (or water, for breast-fed infants); maximum 12 doses per day

● CONTRA-INDICATIONS Intestinal obstruction · preterm neonates · where excessive water loss likely (e.g. fever, diarrhoea, vomiting, high room temperature)

● INTERACTIONS → Appendix 1 (antacids).
Not to be used with other preparations containing thickening agents.
Antacids should preferably not be taken at the same time as other drugs since they may impair absorption.
Antacids may damage enteric coatings designed to prevent dissolution in the stomach.

● HEPATIC IMPAIRMENT In patients with fluid retention, avoid antacids containing large amounts of sodium. Avoid antacids containing magnesium salts in hepatic coma if there is a risk of renal failure.

● RENAL IMPAIRMENT In patients with fluid retention, avoid antacids containing large amounts of sodium.

Gastro-intestinal system

1

- PRESCRIBING AND DISPENSING INFORMATION Each half of the dual-sachet is identified as 'one dose'.

  To avoid errors prescribe with directions in terms of 'dose'.

- MEDICINAL FORMS
  There can be variation in the licensing of different medicines containing the same drug.

  Powder
  ELECTROLYTES: May contain Sodium
  ▸ Gaviscon Infant (Forum Health Products Ltd)
  Magnesium alginate 87.5 mg, Sodium alginate 225 mg Gaviscon Infant oral powder sachets sugar-free | 15 dual dose sachet GSL £4.39

Sodium alginate with potassium bicarbonate

The properties listed below are those particular to the combination only. For the properties of the components please consider, alginic acid p. 61.

- INDICATIONS AND DOSE
  Management of mild symptoms of dyspepsia and gastro-oesophageal reflux disease
  ▸ BY MOUTH USING CHEWABLE TABLETS
  ▸ Child 6–11 years (under medical advice only): 1 tablet, to be chewed after meals and at bedtime
  ▸ Child 12–17 years: 1–2 tablets, to be chewed after meals and at bedtime
  ▸ Adult: 1–2 tablets, to be chewed after meals and at bedtime
  ▸ BY MOUTH USING ORAL SUSPENSION
  ▸ Child 2–11 years (under medical advice only): 2.5–5 mL, to be taken after meals and at bedtime
  ▸ Child 12–17 years: 5–10 mL, to be taken after meals and at bedtime
  ▸ Adult: 5–10 mL, to be taken after meals and at bedtime

- PRESCRIBING AND DISPENSING INFORMATION Flavours of oral liquid formulations may include aniseed or peppermint.

- MEDICINAL FORMS
  There can be variation in the licensing of different medicines containing the same drug.

  Chewable tablet
  EXCIPIENTS: May contain Aspartame
  ELECTROLYTES: May contain Potassium, sodium
  ▸ Sodium alginate with potassium bicarbonate (Non-proprietary)
  Potassium bicarbonate 100 mg, Sodium alginate 500 mg Sodium alginate 500mg / Potassium bicarbonate 100mg chewable tablets sugar free sugar-free | 60 tablet GSL no price available DT price = £3.07
  ▸ Brands may include Gaviscon Advance

  Oral suspension
  ELECTROLYTES: May contain Potassium, sodium
  ▸ Gaviscon Advance (Reckitt Benckiser Healthcare (UK) Ltd)
  Potassium bicarbonate 20 mg per 1 ml, Sodium alginate 100 mg per 1 ml Gaviscon Advance oral suspension aniseed sugar-free | 150 ml P £3.23 sugar-free | 300 ml P £5.82
  Gaviscon Advance oral suspension peppermint sugar-free | 300 ml P £5.82

Co-magaldrox

The properties listed below are those particular to the combination only. For the properties of the components please consider, aluminium hydroxide p. 913, magnesium hydroxide p. 51.

- INDICATIONS AND DOSE
  MAALOX®
  Dyspepsia
  ▸ BY MOUTH
  ▸ Child 14–17 years: 10–20 mL, to be taken 20–60 minutes after meals, and at bedtime or when required
  ▸ Adult: 10–20 mL, to be taken 20–60 minutes after meals, and at bedtime or when required
  MUCOGEL®
  Dyspepsia
  ▸ BY MOUTH
  ▸ Child 12–17 years: 10–20 mL 3 times a day, to be taken 20–60 minutes after meals, and at bedtime, or when required
  ▸ Adult: 10–20 mL 3 times a day, to be taken 20–60 minutes after meals, and at bedtime, or when required

- PRESCRIBING AND DISPENSING INFORMATION Co-magaldrox is a mixture of aluminium hydroxide and magnesium hydroxide; the proportions are expressed in the form x/y where x and y are the strengths in milligrams per unit dose of magnesium hydroxide and aluminium hydroxide respectively.
  MUCOGEL® Mucogel® suspension is low in sodium.
  MAALOX® Maalox® suspension is low in sodium.

- MEDICINAL FORMS
  There can be variation in the licensing of different medicines containing the same drug.

  Oral suspension
  ▸ Maalox (Sanofi)
  Magnesium hydroxide 39 mg per 1 ml, Aluminium hydroxide gel dried 44 mg per 1 ml Maalox oral suspension sugar-free | 500 ml GSL £3.35
  ▸ Mucogel (Chemidex Pharma Ltd)
  Magnesium hydroxide 39 mg per 1 ml, Aluminium hydroxide gel dried 44 mg per 1 ml Mucogel oral suspension sugar-free | 500 ml GSL £2.99

Co-simalcite

- INDICATIONS AND DOSE
  Dyspepsia
  ▸ BY MOUTH
  ▸ Child 8–11 years: 5 mL 4 times a day as required, to be taken between meals and at bedtime
  ▸ Child 12–17 years: 10 mL 4 times a day as required, to be taken between meals and at bedtime
  ▸ Adult: 10 mL 4 times a day as required, to be taken between meals and at bedtime

- CONTRA-INDICATIONS Hypophosphataemia · infants · neonates
  CONTRA-INDICATIONS, FURTHER INFORMATION
  ▸ Aluminium-containing antacids Aluminium-containing antacids should not be used in neonates and infants because accumulation may lead to increased plasma-aluminium concentrations.

- INTERACTIONS → Appendix 1 (antacids).
  Antacids should preferably not be taken at the same time as other drugs since they may impair absorption.
  Antacids may damage enteric coatings designed to prevent dissolution in the stomach.
- SIDE-EFFECTS
  SIDE-EFFECTS, FURTHER INFORMATION
- Constipation and diarrhoea Magnesium-containing antacids tend to be laxative whereas aluminium-containing antacids may be constipating; antacids containing both magnesium and aluminium may reduce these colonic side-effects.
- HEPATIC IMPAIRMENT Avoid; can cause constipation which can precipitate coma. Avoid in hepatic coma; risk of renal failure.
- RENAL IMPAIRMENT Antacids containing magnesium salts should be avoided or used at a reduced dose because there is an increased risk of toxicity.
- In adults There is a risk of accumulation and aluminium toxicity with antacids containing aluminium salts. Absorption of aluminium from aluminium salts is increased by citrates, which are contained in many effervescent preparations (such as effervescent analgesics).
- In children Aluminium-containing antacids should not be used in children with renal impairment, because accumulation may lead to increased plasma-aluminium concentrations.
- PRESCRIBING AND DISPENSING INFORMATION *Altacite Plus* ® is low in Na⁺.

- MEDICINAL FORMS
  There can be variation in the licensing of different medicines containing the same drug.

  Oral suspension
  - Altacite Plus (Peckforton Pharmaceuticals Ltd)
    Simeticone 25 mg per 1 ml, Hydrotalcite 100 mg per 1 ml Altacite Plus oral suspension sugar-free | 100 ml P £4.00 sugar-free | 500 ml P £5.20 DT price = £5.20

Simeticone with aluminium hydroxide and magnesium hydroxide

The properties listed below are those particular to the combination only. For the properties of the components please consider, simeticone p. 64, aluminium hydroxide p. 913.

- INDICATIONS AND DOSE

  Dyspepsia
  - BY MOUTH
  - Child 12–17 years: 5–10 mL 4 times a day, to be taken after meals and at bedtime, or when required
  - Adult: 5–10 mL 4 times a day, to be taken after meals and at bedtime, or when required

- MEDICINAL FORMS
  There can be variation in the licensing of different medicines containing the same drug.

  Oral suspension
  - Maalox Plus (Sanofi)
    Simeticone 5 mg per 1 ml, Magnesium hydroxide 39 mg per 1 ml, Aluminium hydroxide gel dried 44 mg per 1 ml Maalox Plus oral suspension sugar-free | 500 ml GSL £3.90

ANTACIDS > MAGNESIUM

Magnesium carbonate

- INDICATIONS AND DOSE

  Dyspepsia
  - BY MOUTH USING ORAL SUSPENSION
  - Adult: 10 mL 3 times a day, dose to be taken in water

- CONTRA-INDICATIONS Hypophosphataemia
- INTERACTIONS → Appendix 1 (antacids).
  Antacids should preferably not be taken at the same time as other drugs since they may impair absorption.
  Antacids may damage enteric coatings designed to prevent dissolution in the stomach.
- SIDE-EFFECTS Belching due to liberated carbon dioxide · diarrhoea
- HEPATIC IMPAIRMENT In patients with fluid retention, avoid antacids containing large amounts of sodium. Avoid antacids containing magnesium salts in hepatic coma if there is a risk of renal failure.
- RENAL IMPAIRMENT Avoid or use at a reduced dose; increased risk of toxicity. Magnesium carbonate mixture has a high sodium content; avoid in patients with fluid retention.
- PRESCRIBING AND DISPENSING INFORMATION When prepared extemporaneously, the BP states Aromatic Magnesium Carbonate Mixture, BP consists of light magnesium carbonate 3%, sodium bicarbonate 5%, in a suitable vehicle containing aromatic cardamom tincture.

- MEDICINAL FORMS
  There can be variation in the licensing of different medicines containing the same drug.
  No licensed medicines listed.

Magnesium trisilicate

- INDICATIONS AND DOSE

  Dyspepsia
  - BY MOUTH USING CHEWABLE TABLETS
  - Adult: 1–2 tablets as required

- CONTRA-INDICATIONS Hypophosphataemia
- INTERACTIONS → Appendix 1 (antacids).
  Antacids should preferably not be taken at the same time as other drugs since they may impair absorption.
  Antacids may damage enteric coatings designed to prevent dissolution in the stomach.
- SIDE-EFFECTS Belching due to liberated carbon dioxide · diarrhoea · silica-based renal stones (with long-term treatment)
- HEPATIC IMPAIRMENT Avoid in hepatic coma; risk of renal failure.
- RENAL IMPAIRMENT Avoid or used at a reduced dose (increased risk of toxicity).

- MEDICINAL FORMS
  There can be variation in the licensing of different medicines containing the same drug.
  No licensed medicines listed.

Gastro-intestinal system

1

Magnesium trisilicate with magnesium carbonate and sodium bicarbonate

The properties listed below are those particular to the combination only. For the properties of the components please consider, magnesium trisilicate p. 63, magnesium carbonate p. 63, sodium bicarbonate p. 898.

● **INDICATIONS AND DOSE**

Dyspepsia
▶ BY MOUTH
▶ Child 5–11 years: 5–10 mL 3 times a day, alternatively as required, dose to be made up with water
▶ Child 12–17 years: 10–20 mL 3 times a day, alternatively as required, dose to be made up with water
▶ Adult: 10–20 mL 3 times a day, alternatively as required, dose to be made up with water

● **CONTRA-INDICATIONS** Hypophosphataemia · Severe renal failure
● **CAUTIONS** Heart failure · hypermagnesaemia · hypertension · metabolic alkalosis · respiratory alkalosis
● **INTERACTIONS** → Appendix 1 (antacids).
Antacids should preferably not be taken at the same time as other drugs since they may impair absorption. Antacids may damage enteric coatings designed to prevent dissolution in the stomach.
● **SIDE-EFFECTS** Belching due to liberated carbon dioxide · diarrhoea
● **HEPATIC IMPAIRMENT** In patients with fluid retention avoid antacids containing large amounts of sodium. Avoid antacids containing magnesium salts in hepatic coma if there is a risk of renal failure.
● **RENAL IMPAIRMENT** Magnesium trisilicate and magnesium carbonate mixtures have high sodium content; avoid in patients with fluid retention.
● **PRESCRIBING AND DISPENSING INFORMATION** When prepared extemporaneously, the BP states Magnesium Trisilicate Mixture, BP consists of 5% each of magnesium trisilicate, light magnesium carbonate, and sodium bicarbonate in a suitable vehicle with a peppermint flavour.
● **MEDICINAL FORMS**
There can be variation in the licensing of different medicines containing the same drug.
Oral suspension
▶ Magnesium trisilicate with magnesium carbonate and sodium bicarbonate (Non-proprietary)
  Magnesium carbonate light 50 mg per 1 ml, Magnesium trisilicate 50 mg per 1 ml, Sodium bicarbonate 50 mg per 1 ml Magnesium trisilicate oral suspension | 200 ml GSL £1.50 DT price = £1.50

ANTIFOAMING DRUGS

Simeticone

(Activated dimeticone)

● **DRUG ACTION** Simeticone (activated dimeticone) is an antifoaming agent.

● **INDICATIONS AND DOSE**

DENTINOX®

Colic | Wind pains
▶ BY MOUTH
▶ Child 1 month–1 year: 2.5 mL, to be taken with or after each feed; may be added to bottle feed; maximum 6 doses per day

INFACOL®

Colic | Wind pains
▶ BY MOUTH
▶ Child 1 month–1 year: 0.5–1 mL, to be taken before feeds

● **PRESCRIBING AND DISPENSING INFORMATION**
DENTINOX® The brand name *Dentinox®* is also used for other preparations including teething gel.
● **PATIENT AND CARER ADVICE**
INFACOL® Patients or carers should be given advice on use of the *Infacol®* dropper.
● **LESS SUITABLE FOR PRESCRIBING**
INFACOL® *Infacol®* is less suitable for prescribing (evidence of benefit in infantile colic uncertain).
DENTINOX® *Dentinox®* colic drops are less suitable for prescribing (evidence of benefit in infantile colic uncertain).
● **MEDICINAL FORMS**
There can be variation in the licensing of different medicines containing the same drug.
Oral suspension
▶ Infacol (Forest Laboratories UK Ltd)
  Simeticone 40 mg per 1 ml Infacol 40mg/ml oral suspension sugar-free | 50 ml GSL £2.71 DT price = £2.71
Oral drops
▶ Dentinox Infant (Dendron Ltd)
  Simeticone 8.4 mg per 1 ml Dentinox Infant colic drops | 100 ml GSL £1.73

Combinations available: *Simeticone with aluminium hydroxide and magnesium hydroxide,* p. 63

4.2 Gastric and duodenal ulceration

Peptic ulceration

Overview

Peptic ulceration commonly involves the stomach, duodenum, and lower oesophagus; after gastric surgery it involves the gastro-enterostomy stoma. Healing can be promoted by general measures, stopping smoking and taking antacids and by antisecretory drug treatment, but relapse is common when treatment ceases. Nearly all duodenal ulcers and most gastric ulcers not associated with NSAIDs are caused by *Helicobacter pylori*.

Helicobacter pylori infection

Eradication of *Helicobacter pylori* reduces recurrence of gastric and duodenal ulcers and the risk of rebleeding. It also causes regression of most localised gastric mucosa associated lymphoid-tissue (MALT) lymphomas. The presence of *H. pylori* should be confirmed before starting eradication treatment. Acid inhibition combined with antibacterial treatment is highly effective in the eradication of *H. pylori*; reinfection is rare. Antibiotic associated colitis is an uncommon risk.

For initial treatment, a one-week triple-therapy regimen that comprises a proton pump inhibitor, clarithromycin p. 487, and *either* amoxicillin p. 498 *or* metronidazole p. 492 can be used. However, if a patient has been treated with metronidazole for other infections, a regimen containing a proton pump inhibitor, amoxicillin and clarithromycin is preferred for initial therapy. If a patient has been treated with a macrolide for other infections, a regimen containing a proton pump inhibitor, amoxicillin and metronidazole is preferred for initial therapy. These regimens eradicate *H. pylori* in about 85% of cases. There is usually no need to

Recommended regimens for *Helicobacter pylori* eradication

Acid suppressant	Antibacterial			Price for 7-day course
	Amoxicillin	Clarithromycin	Metronidazole	
Esomeprazole 20 mg twice daily	1 g twice daily	500 mg twice daily	–	£6.63
		250 mg twice daily	400 mg twice daily	£4.30
Lansoprazole 30 mg twice daily	1 g twice daily	500 mg twice daily	–	£5.52
	1 g twice daily	–	400 mg twice daily	£3.70
	–	250 mg twice daily	400 mg twice daily	£3.19
Omeprazole 20 mg twice daily	1 g twice daily	500 mg twice daily	–	£5.36
	500 mg 3 times a day	–	400 mg 3 times a day	£3.40
	–	250 mg twice daily	400 mg twice daily	£3.03
Pantoprazole 40 mg twice daily	1 g twice daily	500 mg twice daily	–	£5.48
	–	250 mg twice daily	400 mg twice daily	£3.15
Rabeprazole sodium 20 mg twice daily	1 g twice daily	500 mg twice daily	–	£6.04
	–	250 mg twice daily	400 mg twice daily	£3.71

continue antisecretory treatment (with a proton pump inhibitor or H$_2$-receptor antagonist), however, if the ulcer is large, or complicated by haemorrhage or perforation, then antisecretory treatment is continued for a further 3 weeks. Treatment failure usually indicates antibacterial resistance or poor compliance. Resistance to amoxicillin is rare. However, resistance to clarithromycin and metronidazole is common and can develop during treatment.

Two-week triple-therapy regimens offer the possibility of higher eradication rates compared to one-week regimens, but adverse effects are common and poor compliance is likely to offset any possible gain.

Two-week dual-therapy regimens using a proton pump inhibitor and a single antibacterial are licensed, but produce low rates of *H. pylori* eradication and are **not** recommended.

Tinidazole p. 493 is also used occasionally for *H. pylori* eradication as an alternative to metronidazole; tinidazole should be combined with antisecretory drugs and other antibacterials.

Routine retesting, to confirm eradication, is not necessary unless the patient has gastric MALT lymphoma or complicated *H. pylori* associated peptic ulcer.

A two-week regimen comprising a proton pump inhibitor *plus* tripotassium dicitratobismuthate p. 66, *plus* tetracycline p. 515, *plus* metronidazole can be used for eradication failure. Alternatively, the patient can be referred for endoscopy and treatment based on the results of culture and sensitivity testing.

See under *NSAID-associated ulcers* for the role of *H. pylori* eradication therapy in patients starting or taking a NSAID. Also see Dyspepsia p. 61 for *H. pylori* eradication in patients with dyspepsia.

Test for *Helicobacter pylori*

^{13}C-Urea breath test kits are available for the diagnosis of gastro-duodenal infection with *Helicobacter pylori*. The test involves collection of breath samples before and after ingestion of an oral solution of ^{13}C-urea; the samples are sent for analysis by an appropriate laboratory. The test should not be performed within 4 weeks of treatment with an antibacterial or within 2 weeks of treatment with an antisecretory drug. A specific ^{13}C-urea breath test kit for children is available (*Helicobacter Test INFAI for children of the age* 3–11 ®). However, the appropriateness of testing for *H. pylori* infection in children has not been established.

NSAID-associated ulcers

Gastro-intestinal bleeding and ulceration can occur with NSAID use. The risk of serious upper gastro-intestinal side-effects varies between individual NSAIDs. Whenever possible, the NSAID should be **withdrawn** if an ulcer occurs.

Patients at high risk of developing gastro-intestinal complications with a NSAID include those aged over 65 years, those with a history of peptic ulcer disease or

serious gastro-intestinal complication, those taking other medicines that increase the risk of gastro-intestinal side-effects, or those with serious co-morbidity (e.g. cardiovascular disease, diabetes, renal or hepatic impairment). In those at risk of ulceration, a proton pump inhibitor can be considered for protection against gastric and duodenal ulcers associated with non-selective NSAIDs; a H$_2$-receptor antagonist such as ranitidine p. 68 given at twice the usual dose or misoprostol p. 70 are alternatives. Colic and diarrhoea may limit the dose of misoprostol. Its use is most appropriate for the frail or very elderly from whom NSAIDs cannot be withdrawn. A combination of a cyclo-oxygenase-2 selective inhibitor with a proton pump inhibitor may be more appropriate for those with a history of upper gastro-intestinal bleeding or 3 or more risk factors for gastro-intestinal ulceration, but see NSAIDs and Cardiovascular Events.

NSAID use and *H. pylori* infection are independent risk factors for gastro-intestinal bleeding and ulceration. In patients already taking a NSAID, eradication of *H. pylori* is unlikely to reduce the risk of NSAID-induced bleeding or ulceration. However, in patients with dyspepsia or a history of gastric or duodenal ulcer, who are *H. pylori* positive, and who are about to start long-term treatment with a non-selective NSAID, eradication of *H. pylori* may reduce the overall risk of ulceration.

In a patient who has developed an ulcer, if the *NSAID can be discontinued*, a proton pump inhibitor usually produces the most rapid healing; alternatively, the ulcer can be treated with a H$_2$-receptor antagonist or misoprostol. On healing, patients should be tested for *H. pylori* and given eradication therapy if *H. pylori* is present (see also Test for *Helicobacter pylori*).

If *treatment with a non-selective NSAID needs to continue*, the following options are suitable:

- Treat ulcer with a proton pump inhibitor and on healing continue the proton pump inhibitor (dose not normally reduced because asymptomatic ulcer recurrence may occur);
- Treat ulcer with a proton pump inhibitor and on healing switch to misoprostol for maintenance therapy (colic and diarrhoea may limit the dose of misoprostol);
- Treat ulcer with a proton pump inhibitor and switch non-selective NSAID to a cyclo-oxygenase-2 selective inhibitor, but see NSAIDs and Cardiovascular Events; on healing, continuation of the proton pump inhibitor in patients with a history of upper gastro-intestinal bleeding may provide further protection against recurrence.

If *treatment with a cyclo-oxygenase-2 selective inhibitor needs to continue,* treat ulcer with a proton pump inhibitor; on healing continuation of the proton pump inhibitor in patients with a history of upper gastro-intestinal bleeding may provide further protection against recurrence.

GASTROPROTECTIVE COMPLEXES AND CHELATORS

Chelates and complexes

Overview

Tripotassium dicitratobismuthate below is a bismuth chelate effective in healing gastric and duodenal ulcers. See under Peptic ulceration p. 64 for the role of tripotassium dicitratobismuthate in a *Helicobacter pylori* eradication regimen for those who have not responded to first-line regimens.

The bismuth content of tripotassium dicitratobismuthate is low but absorption has been reported; encephalopathy (described with older high-dose bismuth preparations) has not been reported.

Sucralfate below may act by protecting the mucosa from acid-pepsin attack in gastric and duodenal ulcers. It is a complex of aluminium hydroxide and sulfated sucrose but has minimal antacid properties.

Sucralfate

● INDICATIONS AND DOSE

Benign gastric ulceration | Benign duodenal ulceration
▸ BY MOUTH
▸ Child 15-17 years: 2 g twice daily, dose to be taken on rising and at bedtime, alternatively 1 g 4 times a day for 4–6 weeks, or in resistant cases up to 12 weeks, dose to be taken 1 hour before meals and at bedtime; maximum 8 g per day
▸ Adult: 2 g twice daily, dose to be taken on rising and at bedtime, alternatively 1 g 4 times a day for 4–6 weeks, or in resistant cases up to 12 weeks, dose to be taken 1 hour before meals and at bedtime; maximum 8 g per day

Chronic gastritis
▸ BY MOUTH
▸ Adult: 2 g twice daily, dose to be taken on rising and at bedtime, alternatively 1 g 4 times a day for 4–6 weeks or in resistant cases up to 12 weeks, dose to be taken 1 hour before meals and at bedtime; maximum 8 g per day

Prophylaxis of stress ulceration in child under intensive care
▸ BY MOUTH
▸ Child 15-17 years: 1 g 6 times a day; maximum 8 g per day

Prophylaxis of stress ulceration
▸ BY MOUTH
▸ Adult: 1 g 6 times a day; maximum 8 g per day

● UNLICENSED USE
▸ In children Not licensed for use in children under 15 years. Tablets not licensed for prophylaxis of stress ulceration.

● CAUTIONS Patients under intensive care (**Important:** reports of bezoar formation)

CAUTIONS, FURTHER INFORMATION
▸ Bezoar formation Following reports of bezoar formation associated with sucralfate, caution is advised in seriously ill patients, especially those receiving concomitant enteral feeds or those with predisposing conditions such as delayed gastric emptying.

● INTERACTIONS → Appendix 1 (sucralfate).

● SIDE-EFFECTS
▸ **Common or very common** Constipation
▸ **Uncommon** Back pain · bezoar formation · diarrhoea · dizziness · drowsiness · dry mouth · eadache · flatulence · gastric discomfort · indigestion · nausea · rash

● PREGNANCY No evidence of harm; absorption from gastrointestinal tract negligible.

● BREAST FEEDING Amount probably too small to be harmful.

● RENAL IMPAIRMENT Use with caution; aluminium is absorbed and may accumulate.

● DIRECTIONS FOR ADMINISTRATION Administration of sucralfate and enteral feeds should be separated by 1 hour and for administration by *mouth*, sucralfate should be given 1 hour before meals. *Oral suspension* blocks fine-bore feeding tubes. Crushed *tablets* may be dispersed in water.

● PRESCRIBING AND DISPENSING INFORMATION Flavours of oral liquid formulations may include aniseed and caramel.

● MEDICINAL FORMS
There can be variation in the licensing of different medicines containing the same drug. Forms available from special-order manufacturers include: tablet, oral suspension
Tablet
CAUTIONARY AND ADVISORY LABELS 5
▸ Sucralfate (Non-proprietary)
Sucralfate 1 gram Sulcrate 1g tablets | 100 tablet no price available

Tripotassium dicitratobismuthate

● INDICATIONS AND DOSE

Eradication failure of *Helicobacter pylori* infection (in combination with omeprazole, tetracycline and metronidazole)
▸ BY MOUTH
▸ Adult: 120 mg 4 times a day for 2 weeks

Benign gastric and duodenal ulceration
▸ BY MOUTH
▸ Adult: 240 mg twice daily, alternatively 120 mg 4 times a day both dosage regimens taken for 28 days followed by a further 28 days if necessary, maintenance dose not indicated but course may be repeated after interval of 1 month

● INTERACTIONS → Appendix 1 (tripotassium dicitratobismuthate).

● SIDE-EFFECTS
▸ **Common or very common** May blacken faeces · may darken tongue
▸ **Uncommon** Constipation · diarrhoea · nausea · pruritus · rash · vomiting

● PREGNANCY Manufacturer advises avoid on theoretical grounds.

● BREAST FEEDING No information available.

● RENAL IMPAIRMENT Avoid in severe impairment.

● DIRECTIONS FOR ADMINISTRATION To be swallowed with half a glass of water. Twice-daily dosage to be taken 30 minutes before breakfast and main evening meal. Four-times-daily dosage to be taken as follows: one dose 30 minutes before breakfast, midday meal and main evening meal, and one dose 2 hours after main evening meal.

● PATIENT AND CARER ADVICE Milk should not be drunk by itself during treatment but small quantities may be taken in tea or coffee or on cereal. Antacids, fruit, or fruit juice should not be taken half an hour before or after a dose. Patients and carers should be aware that the patient may develop darkened tongue and blackened faeces.

● MEDICINAL FORMS
There can be variation in the licensing of different medicines containing the same drug.
No licensed medicines listed.

H$_2$-RECEPTOR ANTAGONISTS

H$_2$-receptor antagonists

Overview

Histamine H$_2$-receptor antagonists heal *gastric and duodenal ulcers* by reducing gastric acid output as a result of histamine H$_2$-receptor blockade; they are also used to relieve symptoms of *gastro-oesophageal reflux disease*. H$_2$-receptor antagonists should not normally be used for *Zollinger-Ellison syndrome* because proton pump inhibitors are more effective.

Maintenance treatment with low doses for the prevention of peptic ulcer disease has largely been replaced in *Helicobacter pylori* positive patients by eradication regimens.

In adults, H$_2$-receptor antagonists are used for the treatment of *functional dyspepsia* and may be used for the treatment of *uninvestigated dyspepsia* without alarm features.

H$_2$-receptor antagonist therapy can promote healing of NSAID-associated ulcers (particularly duodenal).

Treatment with a H$_2$-receptor antagonist has not been shown to be beneficial in haematemesis and melaena, but prophylactic use reduces the frequency of bleeding from *gastroduodenal erosions in hepatic coma*, and possibly in other conditions requiring intensive care. H$_2$- receptor antagonists also reduce the risk of *acid aspiration* in obstetric patients at delivery (Mendelson's syndrome).

H$_2$-receptor antagonists

- CAUTIONS Signs and symptoms of gastric cancer (in adults)

  CAUTIONS, FURTHER INFORMATION
  - Gastric cancer
  - In adults H$_2$-receptor antagonists might mask symptoms of gastric cancer; particular care is required in patients presenting with 'alarm features' in such cases gastric malignancy should be ruled out before treatment.

- SIDE-EFFECTS
  - **Common or very common** Diarrhoea · dizziness · headache
  - **Uncommon** Erythema multiforme · rash · toxic epidermal necrolysis
  - **Rare** Arthralgia · blood disorders · bradycardia · cholestatic jaundice · confusion · depression · hallucinations · hepatitis · leucopenia · myalgia · pancytopenia · psychiatric reactions · thrombocytopenia
  - **Frequency not known** Gynaecomastia · impotence

  SIDE-EFFECTS, FURTHER INFORMATION
  - Psychiatric reactions Psychiatric reactions, including confusion, depression, and hallucinations occur particularly in the elderly or the very ill.

▶ above

Cimetidine

- INDICATIONS AND DOSE

  Benign duodenal ulceration
  ▶ BY MOUTH
  - Adult: 400 mg twice daily for at least 4 weeks, to be taken with breakfast and at night, alternatively 800 mg once daily for at least 4 weeks, to be taken at night; increased if necessary up to 400 mg 4 times a day; maintenance 400 mg once daily, to be taken at night, alternatively maintenance 400 mg twice daily, to be taken in the morning and at night

  Benign gastric ulceration
  ▶ BY MOUTH
  - Adult: 400 mg twice daily for 6 weeks, to be taken with breakfast and at night, alternatively 800 mg daily for 6 weeks, to be taken at night; increased if necessary up to 400 mg 4 times a day; maintenance 400 mg once daily, to be taken at night, alternatively maintenance 400 mg twice daily, to be taken in the morning and at night

  NSAID-associated ulceration
  ▶ BY MOUTH
  - Adult: 400 mg twice daily for 8 weeks, to be taken with breakfast and at night, alternatively 800 mg daily for 8 weeks, to be taken at night; increased if necessary up to 400 mg 4 times a day; maintenance 400 mg twice daily, to be taken in the morning and at night

  Reflux oesophagitis
  ▶ BY MOUTH
  - Adult: 400 mg 4 times a day for 4–8 weeks

  Prophylaxis of stress ulceration
  ▶ BY MOUTH
  - Adult: 200–400 mg every 4–6 hours

  Gastric acid reduction in obstetrics
  ▶ BY MOUTH
  - Adult: Initially 400 mg, to be administered at start of labour, then increased if necessary up to 400 mg every 4 hours, do not use syrup in prophylaxis of acid aspiration; maximum 2.4 g per day

  Gastric acid reduction during surgical procedures
  ▶ BY MOUTH
  - Adult: 400 mg, to be given 90–120 minutes before induction of general anaesthesia

  Short-bowel syndrome
  ▶ BY MOUTH
  - Adult: 400 mg twice daily, adjusted according to response, to be taken with breakfast and at bedtime

  To reduce degradation of pancreatic enzyme supplements
  ▶ BY MOUTH
  - Adult: 0.8–1.6 g daily in 4 divided doses, dose to be taken 1–1½ hours before meals

- INTERACTIONS → Appendix 1 (histamine H$_2$-antagonists).

- SIDE-EFFECTS
  - **Common or very common** Malaise
  - **Uncommon** Tachycardia
  - **Rare** Interstitial nephritis
  - **Very rare** Alopecia · galactorrhoea · pancreatitis · vasculitis

- PREGNANCY Manufacturer advises avoid unless essential.

- BREAST FEEDING Significant amount present in milk—not known to be harmful but manufacturer advises avoid.

- HEPATIC IMPAIRMENT Reduce dose. Increased risk of confusion.

- RENAL IMPAIRMENT Reduce dose to 200 mg 4 times daily if eGFR 30–50 mL/minute/1.73 m^2. Reduce dose to 200 mg 3 times daily if eGFR 15–30 mL/minute/1.73 m^2. Reduce dose to 200 mg twice daily if eGFR less than 15 mL/minute/1.73 m^2. Occasional risk of confusion.

- EXCEPTIONS TO LEGAL CATEGORY Cimetidine can be sold to the public for adults and children over 16 years (provided packs do not contain more than 2 weeks' supply) for the short-term symptomatic relief of heartburn, dyspepsia, and hyperacidity (max. single dose 200 mg, max. daily dose 800 mg), and for the prophylactic management of nocturnal heartburn (single night-time dose 100 mg).

- MEDICINAL FORMS
  There can be variation in the licensing of different medicines containing the same drug. Forms available from special-order manufacturers include: oral suspension

  Tablet
  ▶ Cimetidine (Non-proprietary)
    Cimetidine 200 mg Cimetidine 200mg tablets | 60 tablet PoM no price available DT price = £40.00

Cimetidine 400 mg Cimetidine 400mg tablets | 60 tablet PoM
£5.69 DT price = £8.76
Cimetidine 800 mg Cimetidine 800mg tablets | 30 tablet PoM
£9.09 DT price = £9.09
▸ Tagamet (Chemidex Pharma Ltd)
Cimetidine 200 mg Tagamet 200mg tablets | 120 tablet PoM
£19.58
Cimetidine 400 mg Tagamet 400mg tablets | 60 tablet PoM
£22.62 DT price = £8.76
Cimetidine 800 mg Tagamet 800mg tablets | 30 tablet PoM
£22.62 DT price = £9.09

Oral solution
EXCIPIENTS: May contain Propylene glycol
▸ Cimetidine (Non-proprietary)
Cimetidine 40 mg per 1 ml Cimetidine 200mg/5ml oral solution
sugar free sugar-free | 300 ml PoM £14.24–£14.25 DT price = £14.25
▸ Tagamet (Essential Pharma Ltd)
Cimetidine 40 mg per 1 ml Tagamet 200mg/5ml syrup |
600 ml PoM £28.49 DT price = £28.49

Famotidine
F 67

● INDICATIONS AND DOSE

Treatment of benign gastric and duodenal ulceration
▸ BY MOUTH
▸ Adult: 40 mg once daily for 4–8 weeks, dose to be taken
at night

Maintenance treatment of duodenal ulceration
▸ BY MOUTH
▸ Adult: 20 mg once daily, dose to be taken at night

Reflux oesophagitis
▸ BY MOUTH
▸ Adult: 20–40 mg twice daily for 6–12 weeks;
maintenance 20 mg twice daily

● INTERACTIONS → Appendix 1 (histamine H_2-antagonists).
● SIDE-EFFECTS
▸ **Common or very common** Constipation
▸ **Uncommon** Fatigue · vomiting · anorexia · dry mouth ·
flatulence · nausea · taste disorders
▸ **Very rare** Chest tightness · interstitial pneumonia ·
paraesthesia · seizures
● PREGNANCY Manufacturer advises avoid unless potential
benefit outweighs risk.
● BREAST FEEDING Present in milk—not known to be
harmful but manufacturer advises avoid.
● RENAL IMPAIRMENT Use normal dose every 36–48 hours or
use half normal dose if eGFR less than
50 mL/minute/1.73 m². Seizures reported very rarely.
● EXCEPTIONS TO LEGAL CATEGORY Famotidine can be sold
to the public for adults and children over 16 years
(provided packs do not contain more than 2 weeks' supply)
for the short-term symptomatic relief of heartburn,
dyspepsia, and hyperacidity, and for the prevention of
these symptoms when associated with consumption of
food or drink including when they cause sleep disturbance
(max. single dose 10 mg, max. daily dose 20 mg).

● MEDICINAL FORMS
There can be variation in the licensing of different medicines
containing the same drug.
Tablet
▸ Famotidine (Non-proprietary)
Famotidine 20 mg Famotidine 20mg tablets | 28 tablet PoM
£22.00 DT price = £21.26
Famotidine 40 mg Famotidine 40mg tablets | 28 tablet PoM
£39.00 DT price = £38.95

Nizatidine
F 67

● INDICATIONS AND DOSE

Benign gastric, duodenal or NSAID-associated ulceration
▸ BY MOUTH
▸ Adult: 300 mg once daily for 4–8 weeks, dose to be
taken in the evening, alternatively 150 mg twice daily
for 4–8 weeks; maintenance 150 mg once daily, dose to
be taken at night

Gastro-oesophageal reflux disease
▸ BY MOUTH
▸ Adult: 150–300 mg twice daily for up to 12 weeks

● INTERACTIONS → Appendix 1 (histamine H_2-antagonists).
● SIDE-EFFECTS
▸ **Common or very common** Sweating
▸ **Rare** Fever · hyperuricaemia · nausea · vasculitis
● PREGNANCY Manufacturer advises avoid unless essential.
● BREAST FEEDING Amount too small to be harmful.
● HEPATIC IMPAIRMENT Manufacturer advises caution.
● RENAL IMPAIRMENT Use half normal dose if eGFR
20–50 mL/minute/1.73 m². Use one-quarter normal dose if
eGFR less than 20 mL/minute/1.73 m².
● EXCEPTIONS TO LEGAL CATEGORY Nizatidine can be sold to
the public for the prevention and treatment of symptoms
of food-related heartburn and meal-induced indigestion in
adults and children over 16 years; max. single dose 75 mg,
max. daily dose 150 mg for max. 14 days.

● MEDICINAL FORMS
There can be variation in the licensing of different medicines
containing the same drug. Forms available from special-order
manufacturers include: oral suspension, oral solution
Capsule
▸ Nizatidine (Non-proprietary)
Nizatidine 150 mg Nizatidine 150mg capsules | 30 capsule PoM
£12.20 DT price = £4.03
Nizatidine 300 mg Nizatidine 300mg capsules | 30 capsule PoM
£15.43 DT price = £15.43

Ranitidine
F 67

● INDICATIONS AND DOSE

Benign gastric ulceration | Duodenal ulceration
▸ BY MOUTH
▸ Child 1-5 months: 1 mg/kg 3 times a day (max. per dose
3 mg/kg 3 times a day)
▸ Child 6 months-2 years: 2–4 mg/kg twice daily
▸ Child 3-11 years: 2–4 mg/kg twice daily (max. per dose
150 mg)
▸ Child 12-17 years: 150 mg twice daily, alternatively
300 mg once daily, dose to be taken at night
▸ Adult: 150 mg twice daily for 4–8 weeks, alternatively
300 mg once daily for 4–8 weeks, dose to be taken at
night

Chronic episodic dyspepsia
▸ BY MOUTH
▸ Adult: 150 mg twice daily for 6 weeks, alternatively
300 mg once daily for 6 weeks, dose to be taken at night

NSAID-associated gastric ulceration
▸ BY MOUTH
▸ Adult: 150 mg twice daily for up to 8 weeks,
alternatively 300 mg once daily for up to 8 weeks, dose
to be taken at night

NSAID-associated duodenal ulcer
▸ BY MOUTH
▸ Adult: 300 mg twice daily for 4 weeks, to achieve a
higher healing rate

**Prophylaxis of NSAID-associated gastric ulcer |
Prophylaxis of NSAID-associated duodenal ulcer**
▸ BY MOUTH
▸ Adult: 300 mg twice daily

Gastro-oesophageal reflux disease
▸ BY MOUTH
▸ Adult: 150 mg twice daily for up to 8 weeks or if
necessary 12 weeks, alternatively 300 mg once daily for
up to 8 weeks or if necessary 12 weeks, dose to be taken
at night

Moderate to severe gastro-oesophageal reflux disease
▸ BY MOUTH
▸ Adult: 600 mg daily in 2–4 divided doses for up to
12 weeks

**Long-term treatment of healed gastro-oesophageal reflux
disease**
▸ BY MOUTH
▸ Adult: 150 mg twice daily

**Gastric acid reduction (prophylaxis of acid aspiration) in
obstetrics**
▸ BY MOUTH
▸ Adult: 150 mg, dose to be given at onset of labour, then
150 mg every 6 hours

**Gastric acid reduction (prophylaxis of acid aspiration) in
surgical procedures**
▸ INITIALLY BY INTRAMUSCULAR INJECTION, OR BY SLOW
INTRAVENOUS INJECTION
▸ Adult: 50 mg, to be given 45–60 minutes before
induction of anaesthesia, intravenous injection diluted
to 20 mL and given over at least 2 minutes,
alternatively (by mouth) 150 mg, to be given 2 hours
before induction of anaesthesia and also when possible
on the preceding evening

Prophylaxis of stress ulceration
▸ INITIALLY BY SLOW INTRAVENOUS INJECTION
▸ Adult: 50 mg every 8 hours, dose to be diluted to 20 mL
and given over at least 2 minutes, then (by mouth)
150 mg twice daily, may be given when oral feeding
commences

**Reflux oesophagitis and other conditions where gastric
acid reduction is beneficial**
▸ BY MOUTH
▸ Child 1–5 months: 1 mg/kg 3 times a day (max. per dose
3 mg/kg 3 times a day)
▸ Child 6 months–2 years: 2–4 mg/kg twice daily
▸ Child 3–11 years: 2–4 mg/kg twice daily (max. per dose
150 mg); increased to up to 5 mg/kg twice daily (max.
per dose 300 mg), dose increase for severe gastro-
oesophageal disease
▸ Child 12–17 years: 150 mg twice daily, alternatively
300 mg once daily, dose to be taken at night, then
increased if necessary to 300 mg twice daily for up to
12 weeks in moderate to severe gastro-oesophageal
reflux disease, alternatively increased if necessary to
150 mg 4 times a day for up to 12 weeks in moderate to
severe gastro-oesophageal reflux disease

**Conditions where reduction of gastric acidity is beneficial
and oral route not available**
▸ BY INTRAMUSCULAR INJECTION
▸ Adult: 50 mg every 6–8 hours
▸ BY SLOW INTRAVENOUS INJECTION
▸ Adult: 50 mg, dose to be diluted to 20 mL and given
over at least 2 minutes; may be repeated every
6–8 hours

● UNLICENSED USE
▸ In children *Oral* preparations not licensed for use in
children under 3 years.
▸ In adults Doses given for prophylaxis of NSAID-associated
gastric or duodenal ulcer, and prophylaxis of stress
ulceration, are not licensed.

● INTERACTIONS → Appendix 1 (histamine H_2-antagonists).

● SIDE-EFFECTS
▸ Uncommon Blurred vision
▸ Frequency not known Alopecia · interstitial nephritis ·
involuntary movement disorders · pancreatitis

● PREGNANCY Manufacturer advises avoid unless essential,
but not known to be harmful.

● BREAST FEEDING Significant amount present in milk, but
not known to be harmful.

● RENAL IMPAIRMENT
▸ In adults Use half normal dose if eGFR less than
50 mL/minute/1.73 m^2.
▸ In children Use half normal dose if estimated glomerular
filtration rate less than 50 mL/minute/1.73 m^2.

● DIRECTIONS FOR ADMINISTRATION For *intravenous infusion*
(*Zantac*®), give intermittently in Glucose 5% or Sodium
Chloride 0.9%.

● PATIENT AND CARER ADVICE
In fat malabsorption syndrome, give oral doses 1–2 hours
before food to enhance effects of pancreatic enzyme
replacement.
Medicines for Children leaflet: Ranitidine for acid reflux www.
medicinesforchildren.org.uk/ranitidine-for-acid-reflux

● EXCEPTIONS TO LEGAL CATEGORY Ranitidine can be sold to
the public for adults and children over 16 years (provided
packs do not contain more than 2 weeks' supply) for the
short-term symptomatic relief of heartburn, dyspepsia,
and hyperacidity, and for the prevention of these
symptoms when associated with consumption of food or
drink (max. single dose 75 mg, max. daily dose 300 mg).

● MEDICINAL FORMS
There can be variation in the licensing of different medicines
containing the same drug. Forms available from special-order
manufacturers include: oral suspension, oral solution, infusion

Tablet
▸ Ranitidine (Non-proprietary)
Ranitidine (as Ranitidine hydrochloride) 75 mg price available
Ranitidine (as Ranitidine hydrochloride) 150 mg Ranitidine
150mg tablets | 60 tablet [P] no price available DT price = £1.15 |
60 tablet [PoM] £2.50 DT price = £1.15
Ranitidine (as Ranitidine hydrochloride) 300 mg Ranitidine
300mg tablets | 30 tablet [P] no price available DT price = £1.17 |
30 tablet [PoM] £1.61 DT price = £1.17
▸ Ranitil (Tillomed Laboratories Ltd)
Ranitidine (as Ranitidine hydrochloride) 150 mg Ranitil 150mg
tablets | 60 tablet [PoM] £18.13 DT price = £1.15
Ranitidine (as Ranitidine hydrochloride) 300 mg Ranitil 300mg
tablets | 30 tablet [PoM] £17.64 DT price = £1.17
▸ Zantac (Omega Pharma Ltd, GlaxoSmithKline UK Ltd)
Ranitidine (as Ranitidine hydrochloride) 150 mg Zantac 150mg
tablets | 60 tablet [PoM] £1.30 DT price = £1.15
Ranitidine (as Ranitidine hydrochloride) 300 mg Zantac 300mg
tablets | 30 tablet [PoM] £1.30 DT price = £1.17

Effervescent tablet
CAUTIONARY AND ADVISORY LABELS 13
ELECTROLYTES: May contain Sodium
▸ Ranitidine (Non-proprietary)
Ranitidine (as Ranitidine hydrochloride) 150 mg Ranitidine
150mg effervescent tablets | 60 tablet [PoM] £35.00 DT price = £34.76
Ranitidine (as Ranitidine hydrochloride) 300 mg Ranitidine
300mg effervescent tablets | 30 tablet [PoM] £35.00 DT price = £34.76

Oral solution
EXCIPIENTS: May contain Alcohol
▸ Ranitidine (Non-proprietary)
**Ranitidine (as Ranitidine hydrochloride) 15 mg per
1 ml** Ranitidine 75mg/5ml oral solution sugar free sugar-free |
100 ml [PoM] £2.10-£2.88 sugar-free | 300 ml [PoM] £21.55 DT price
= £6.45
▸ Zantac (GlaxoSmithKline UK Ltd)
Ranitidine (as Ranitidine hydrochloride) 15 mg per 1 ml Zantac
150mg/10ml syrup sugar-free | 300 ml [PoM] £20.76 DT price = £6.45

Solution for injection

▸ Ranitidine (Non-proprietary)

Ranitidine (as Ranitidine hydrochloride) 25 mg per 1 ml Ranitidine 50mg/2ml solution for injection ampoules | 5 ampoule [PoM] £2.69–£5.00

▸ Zantac (GlaxoSmithKline UK Ltd)

Ranitidine (as Ranitidine hydrochloride) 25 mg per 1 ml Zantac 50mg/2ml solution for injection ampoules | 5 ampoule [PoM] £2.82

PROSTAGLANDIN ANALOGUES AND PROSTAMIDES > PROSTAGLANDINS, GASTROPROTECTIVE

Misoprostol

● DRUG ACTION Misoprostol is a synthetic prostaglandin analogue that has antisecretory and protective properties, promoting healing of gastric and duodenal ulcers. It also acts as a potent uterine stimulant.

● INDICATIONS AND DOSE

Benign gastric ulceration | Benign duodenal ulceration | NSAID-associated ulceration

▸ BY MOUTH

▹ Adult: 800 micrograms daily in 2–4 divided doses continued for at least 4 weeks or may be continued for up to 8 weeks if required, dose to be taken with breakfast (or main meals) and at bedtime

Prophylaxis of NSAID-induced gastric ulcer | Prophylaxis of duodenal ulcer

▸ BY MOUTH

▹ Adult: 200 micrograms 4 times a day, reduced if not tolerated to 200 micrograms 2–3 times a day, use lower dose is less effective

● CAUTIONS Conditions where hypotension might precipitate severe complications (e.g. cerebrovascular disease, cardiovascular disease) · inflammatory bowel disease

● INTERACTIONS → Appendix 1 (misoprostol)

● SIDE-EFFECTS

▸ **Common or very common** Diarrhoea

▸ **Frequency not known** Abdominal pain · abnormal vaginal bleeding · dizziness · dyspepsia · flatulence · intermenstrual bleeding · menorrhagia · nausea · postmenopausal bleeding · rashes · vomiting

SIDE-EFFECTS, FURTHER INFORMATION

▸ Diarrhoea May occasionally be severe and require withdrawal, reduced by giving single doses not exceeding 200 micrograms and by avoiding magnesium-containing antacids.

● CONCEPTION AND CONTRACEPTION Manufacturer advises that misoprostol should not be used in women of childbearing age unless pregnancy has been excluded. In such patients it is advised that misoprostol should only be used if the patient takes *effective contraceptive measures* and has been advised of the *risks of taking misoprostol if pregnant.*

● PREGNANCY Avoid—potent uterine stimulant (has been used to induce abortion). Teratogenic risk in first trimester.

● BREAST FEEDING Present in milk, but amount probably too small to be harmful.

● MEDICINAL FORMS

There can be variation in the licensing of different medicines containing the same drug.

Tablet

CAUTIONARY AND ADVISORY LABELS 21

▸ Misoprostol (Non-proprietary)

Misoprostol 100 microgram Apo-Misoprostol 100microgram tablets | 100 tablet [PoM] no price available

▸ Cytotec (Pfizer Ltd)

Misoprostol 200 microgram Cytotec 200microgram tablets | 56 tablet [PoM] no price available | 60 tablet [PoM] £10.03 DT price = £10.03

PROTON PUMP INHIBITORS

Proton pump inhibitors

Overview

Proton pump inhibitors are effective short-term treatments for *gastric* and *duodenal ulcers*; they are also used in combination with antibacterials for the eradication of *Helicobacter pylori* (see specific regimens). Following endoscopic treatment of severe peptic ulcer bleeding, an intravenous, high-dose proton pump inhibitor reduces the risk of rebleeding and the need for surgery. Proton pump inhibitors can be used for the treatment of *dyspepsia* and *gastro-oesophageal reflux disease.*

Proton pump inhibitors are also used for the prevention and treatment of NSAID-associated ulcers. In patients who need to continue NSAID treatment after an ulcer has healed, the dose of proton pump inhibitor should normally not be reduced because asymptomatic ulcer deterioration may occur.

A proton pump inhibitor can be used to reduce the degradation of pancreatic enzyme supplements in patients with cystic fibrosis. They can also be used to control excessive secretion of gastric acid in *Zollinger–Ellison syndrome*; high doses are often required.

Proton pump inhibitors

● DRUG ACTION Proton pump inhibitors inhibit gastric acid secretion by blocking the hydrogen-potassium adenosine triphosphatase enzyme system (the 'proton pump') of the gastric parietal cell.

> IMPORTANT SAFETY INFORMATION
>
> MHRA ADVICE: PROTON PUMP INHIBITORS (PPIS): VERY LOW RISK OF SUBACUTE CUTANEOUS LUPUS ERYTHEMATOSUS (SEPTEMBER 2015)
>
> Very infrequent cases of subacute cutaneous lupus erythematosus (SCLE) have been reported in patients taking PPIs. Drug-induced SCLE can occur weeks, months or even years after exposure to the drug.
>
> If a patient treated with a PPI develops lesions—especially in sun-exposed areas of the skin—and it is accompanied by arthralgia:
>
> ● advise them to avoid exposing the skin to sunlight;
> ● consider SCLE as a possible diagnosis;
> ● consider discontinuing PPI treatment unless it is imperative for a serious acid-related condition; a patient who develops SCLE with a particular PPI may be at risk of the same reaction with another;
> ● in most cases, symptoms resolve on PPI withdrawal; topical or systemic steroids might be necessary for treatment of SCLE only if there are no signs of remission after a few weeks or months.

● CAUTIONS Can increase the risk of fractures (particularly when used at high doses for over a year in the elderly) (in adults) · may increase the risk of gastro-intestinal infections (including *Clostridium difficile* infection) · may mask the symptoms of gastric cancer (in adults) · patients at risk of osteoporosis

CAUTIONS, FURTHER INFORMATION

▸ Risk of osteoporosis Patients at risk of osteoporosis should maintain an adequate intake of calcium and vitamin D, and if necessary, receive other preventative therapy.

▸ Gastric cancer
▸ In adults Particular care is required in those presenting
with 'alarm features', in such cases gastric malignancy
should be ruled out before treatment.

● SIDE-EFFECTS
▸ **Common or very common** Abdominal pain · constipation ·
diarrhoea · flatulence · gastro-intestinal disturbances ·
headache · nausea · vomiting
▸ **Uncommon** Arthralgia · dizziness · dry mouth · fatigue ·
myalgia · paraesthesia · peripheral oedema · pruritus · rash ·
sleep disturbances
▸ **Rare** Alopecia · anaphylaxis · blood disorders ·
bronchospasm · confusion · depression · fever ·
gynaecomastia · hallucinations · hepatitis · hypersensitivity
reactions · hypomagnesaemia (usually after 1 year of
treatment, but sometimes after 3 months of treatment) ·
hyponatraemia · interstitial nephritis · jaundice ·
leucocytosis · leucopenia · pancytopenia · photosensitivity
· Stevens-Johnson syndrome · stomatitis · sweating · taste
disturbance · thrombocytopenia · toxic epidermal
necrolysis · visual disturbances
SIDE-EFFECTS, FURTHER INFORMATION
Rebound acid hypersecretion and protracted dyspepsia
may occur after stopping prolonged treatment with a
proton pump inhibitor.

● MONITORING REQUIREMENTS Measurement of serum-
magnesium concentrations should be considered before
and during prolonged treatment with a proton pump
inhibitor, especially when used with other drugs that cause
hypomagnesaemia or with digoxin.

● PRESCRIBING AND DISPENSING INFORMATION A proton
pump inhibitor should be prescribed for appropriate
indications at the lowest effective dose for the shortest
period; the need for long-term treatment should be
reviewed periodically.

F 70

Esomeprazole

● INDICATIONS AND DOSE
NSAID-associated gastric ulcer
▸ BY MOUTH
▸ Adult: 20 mg once daily for 4–8 weeks
▸ BY INTRAVENOUS INJECTION, OR BY INTRAVENOUS INFUSION
▸ Adult: 20 mg daily continue until oral administration
possible, injection to be given over at least 3 minutes
**Prophylaxis of NSAID-associated gastric ulcer in patients
with an increased risk of gastroduodenal complications
who require continued NSAID treatment**
▸ BY MOUTH
▸ Adult: 20 mg daily
Prophylaxis of NSAID-associated gastric or duodenal ulcer
▸ BY INTRAVENOUS INJECTION, OR BY INTRAVENOUS INFUSION
▸ Adult: 20 mg daily continue until oral administration
possible, injection to be given over at least 3 minutes
**Gastro-oesophageal reflux disease (in the presence of
erosive reflux oesophagitis)**
▸ BY MOUTH
▸ Child 1-11 years (body-weight 10-19 kg): 10 mg once daily
for 8 weeks
▸ Child 1-11 years (body-weight 20 kg and above): 10–20 mg
once daily for 8 weeks
▸ Child 12-17 years: Initially 40 mg once daily for 4 weeks,
continued for further 4 weeks if not fully healed or
symptoms persist; maintenance 20 mg daily
▸ Adult: Initially 40 mg once daily for 4 weeks, continued
for further 4 weeks if not fully healed or symptoms
persist; maintenance 20 mg daily

▸ BY INTRAVENOUS INJECTION, OR BY INTRAVENOUS INFUSION
▸ Adult: 40 mg daily continue until oral administration
possible, injection to be given over at least 3 minutes
**Symptomatic treatment of gastro-oesophageal reflux
disease (in the absence of oesophagitis)**
▸ BY MOUTH
▸ Child 1-11 years (body-weight 10 kg and above): 10 mg
once daily for up to 8 weeks
▸ Child 12-17 years: 20 mg once daily for up to 4 weeks
▸ Adult: 20 mg once daily for up to 4 weeks, then 20 mg
daily if required
▸ BY INTRAVENOUS INJECTION, OR BY INTRAVENOUS INFUSION
▸ Adult: 20 mg once daily continue until oral
administration is possible, injection to be given over at
least 3 minutes
Zollinger–Ellison syndrome
▸ BY MOUTH
▸ Adult: Initially 40 mg twice daily, adjusted according to
response; usual dose 80–160 mg daily, daily doses
above 80 mg should be given in 2 divided doses
**Severe peptic ulcer bleeding (following endoscopic
treatment)**
▸ INITIALLY BY INTRAVENOUS INFUSION
▸ Adult: Initially 80 mg, to be given over 30 minutes,
then (by continuous intravenous infusion) 8 mg/hour
for 72 hours, then (by mouth) 40 mg once daily for
4 weeks
***Helicobacter pylori* eradication in combination with
clarithromycin and amoxicillin or metronidazole**
▸ BY MOUTH
▸ Adult: 20 mg twice daily

● UNLICENSED USE Tablets and capsules not licensed for use
in children 1–11 years.
● INTERACTIONS → Appendix 1 (proton pump inhibitors).
● PREGNANCY Manufacturer advises caution—no
information available.
● BREAST FEEDING Manufacturer advises avoid—no
information available.
● HEPATIC IMPAIRMENT
▸ In adults In severe hepatic impairment max. 20 mg daily.
Severe peptic ulcer bleeding in severe hepatic impairment,
initial intravenous infusion of 80 mg, then by continuous
intravenous infusion, 4 mg/hour for 72 hours.
▸ In children 1–11 years max. 10 mg daily in severe
impairment. 12–17 years max. 20 mg daily in severe
impairment.
● RENAL IMPAIRMENT Manufacturer advises caution in
severe renal insufficiency.
● DIRECTIONS FOR ADMINISTRATION
▸ With intravenous use in adults For *intravenous infusion*
(*Nexium* ®), give continuously *or* intermittently in Sodium
Chloride 0.9%; reconstitute 40–80 mg with up to 100 ml
infusion fluid; for intermittent infusion, give requisite
dose over 10–30 minutes; stable for 12 hours in Sodium
Chloride 0.9%.
▸ With oral use Do not chew or crush capsules; swallow whole
or mix capsule contents in water and drink within
30 minutes. Do not crush or chew tablets; swallow whole
or disperse in water and drink within 30 minutes. Disperse
the contents of each sachet of gastro-resistant granules in
approx. 15 mL water. Stir and leave to thicken for a few
minutes; stir again before administration and use within
30 minutes; rinse container with 15 mL water to obtain full
dose. For administration through a gastric tube, consult
product literature.
● PATIENT AND CARER ADVICE
▸ With oral use Counselling on administration of gastro-
resistant capsules, tablets, and granules advised.

- MEDICINAL FORMS
  There can be variation in the licensing of different medicines containing the same drug. Forms available from special-order manufacturers include: oral suspension

Gastro-resistant tablet

▸ Esomeprazole (Non-proprietary)
Esomeprazole (as Esomeprazole magnesium trihydrate)
20 mg Esomeprazole 20mg gastro-resistant tablets | 28 tablet [PoM] £18.50 DT price = £3.31
Esomeprazole (as Esomeprazole magnesium trihydrate)
40 mg Esomeprazole 40mg gastro-resistant tablets | 28 tablet · [PoM] £25.19 DT price = £4.18
▸ Nexium (AstraZeneca UK Ltd, Pfizer Consumer Healthcare Ltd)
Esomeprazole (as Esomeprazole magnesium trihydrate)
20 mg Nexium 20mg gastro-resistant tablets | 28 tablet [PoM] £18.50 DT price = £3.31
Esomeprazole (as Esomeprazole magnesium trihydrate)
40 mg Nexium 40mg gastro-resistant tablets | 28 tablet [PoM] £25.19 DT price = £4.18

Gastro-resistant capsule

▸ Esomeprazole (Non-proprietary)
Esomeprazole (as Esomeprazole magnesium dihydrate)
20 mg Esomeprazole 20mg gastro-resistant capsules | 28 capsule [PoM] £12.95 DT price = £3.40
Esomeprazole (as Esomeprazole magnesium dihydrate)
40 mg Esomeprazole 40mg gastro-resistant capsules | 28 capsule [PoM] £17.63 DT price = £3.96
▸ Emozul (Consilient Health Ltd)
Esomeprazole (as Esomeprazole magnesium dihydrate)
20 mg Emozul 20mg gastro-resistant capsules | 28 capsule [PoM] £3.40 DT price = £3.40
Esomeprazole (as Esomeprazole magnesium dihydrate)
40 mg Emozul 40mg gastro-resistant capsules | 28 capsule [PoM] £3.96 DT price = £3.96

Gastro-resistant granules

CAUTIONARY AND ADVISORY LABELS 25
▸ Nexium (AstraZeneca UK Ltd)
Esomeprazole (as Esomeprazole magnesium trihydrate)
10 mg Nexium 10mg gastro-resistant granules sachets | 28 sachet [PoM] £25.19 DT price = £25.19

Powder for solution for injection

▸ Esomeprazole (Non-proprietary)
Esomeprazole (as Esomeprazole sodium) 40 mg Esomeprazole 40mg powder for solution for injection vials | 1 vial [PoM] £3.07–£3.13 (Hospital only)
▸ Nexium (AstraZeneca UK Ltd)
Esomeprazole (as Esomeprazole sodium) 40 mg Nexium I.V 40mg powder for solution for injection vials | 1 vial [PoM] £4.25 (Hospital only)

F 70

Lansoprazole

- INDICATIONS AND DOSE

***Helicobacter pylori* eradication in combination with amoxicillin and clarithromycin; or in combination with amoxicillin and metronidazole; or in combination with clarithromycin and metronidazole**

▸ BY MOUTH
▸ Adult: 30 mg twice daily

Benign gastric ulcer

▸ BY MOUTH
▸ Adult: 30 mg once daily for 8 weeks, dose to be taken in the morning

Duodenal ulcer

▸ BY MOUTH
▸ Adult: 30 mg once daily for 4 weeks, dose to be taken in the morning; maintenance 15 mg once daily

NSAID-associated duodenal ulcer | NSAID-associated gastric ulcer

▸ BY MOUTH
▸ Adult: 30 mg once daily for 4 weeks, continued for further 4 weeks if not fully healed

Prophylaxis of NSAID-associated duodenal ulcer | Prophylaxis of NSAID-associated gastric ulcer

▸ BY MOUTH
▸ Adult: 15–30 mg once daily

Zollinger–Ellison syndrome (and other hypersecretory conditions)

▸ BY MOUTH
▸ Adult: Initially 60 mg once daily, adjusted according to response, daily doses of 120 mg or more given in two divided doses

Gastro-oesophageal reflux disease

▸ BY MOUTH
▸ Adult: 30 mg once daily for 4 weeks, continued for further 4 weeks if not fully healed; maintenance 15–30 mg once daily, doses to be taken in the morning

Acid-related dyspepsia

▸ BY MOUTH
▸ Adult: 15–30 mg once daily for 2-4 weeks, doses to be taken in the morning

- UNLICENSED USE Lansoprazole doses in BNF may differ from those in product literature.
- INTERACTIONS → Appendix 1 (proton pump inhibitors).
- SIDE-EFFECTS
▸ Very rare Colitis · raised serum cholesterol · raised triglycerides
▸ Frequency not known Anorexia · glossitis · impotence · pancreatitis · petechiae · purpura · restlessness · tremor
- PREGNANCY Manufacturer advises avoid.
- BREAST FEEDING Avoid—present in milk in *animal* studies.
- HEPATIC IMPAIRMENT Use half normal dose in moderate to severe liver disease.
- DIRECTIONS FOR ADMINISTRATION Orodispersible tablets should be placed on the tongue, allowed to disperse and swallowed, or may be swallowed whole with a glass of water. Alternatively, tablets can be dispersed in a small amount of water and administered by an oral syringe or nasogastric tube.
- PATIENT AND CARER ADVICE Counselling on administration of orodispersible tablet advised.
- PROFESSION SPECIFIC INFORMATION

Dental practitioners' formulary

▸ With oral use Lansoprazole capsules may be prescribed.

- MEDICINAL FORMS
  There can be variation in the licensing of different medicines containing the same drug. Forms available from special-order manufacturers include: oral suspension, oral solution, powder

Orodispersible tablet

CAUTIONARY AND ADVISORY LABELS 5, 22
EXCIPIENTS: May contain Aspartame
▸ Lansoprazole (Non-proprietary)
Lansoprazole 15 mg Lansoprazole 15mg orodispersible tablets | 28 tablet [PoM] £3.99 DT price = £2.42
Lansoprazole 30 mg Lansoprazole 30mg orodispersible tablets | 28 tablet [PoM] £6.99 DT price = £4.18
▸ Zoton FasTab (Pfizer Ltd)
Lansoprazole 15 mg Zoton FasTab 15mg | 28 tablet [PoM] £2.99 DT price = £2.42
Lansoprazole 30 mg Zoton FasTab 30mg | 28 tablet [PoM] £5.50 DT price = £4.18

Gastro-resistant capsule

CAUTIONARY AND ADVISORY LABELS 5, 22, 25
▸ Lansoprazole (Non-proprietary)
Lansoprazole 15 mg Lansoprazole 15mg gastro-resistant capsules | 28 capsule [PoM] £12.92 DT price = £0.97
Lansoprazole 30 mg Lansoprazole 30mg gastro-resistant capsules | 28 capsule [PoM] £23.63 DT price = £1.37

► 70

Omeprazole

● INDICATIONS AND DOSE

Helicobacter pylori **eradication in combination with amoxicillin and clarithromycin; or in combination with amoxicillin and metronidazole; or in combination with clarithromycin and metronidazole**
▸ BY MOUTH
▸ Adult: 20 mg twice daily

Eradication failure of *Helicobacter pylori* infection in combination with tripotassium dicitratobismuthate, tetracycline and metronidazole
▸ BY MOUTH
▸ Adult: 20 mg twice daily

Benign gastric ulceration
▸ BY MOUTH
▸ Adult: 20 mg once daily for 8 weeks, increased if necessary to 40 mg once daily, in severe or recurrent cases

Duodenal ulceration
▸ BY MOUTH
▸ Adult: 20 mg once daily for 4 weeks, increased if necessary to 40 mg once daily, in severe or recurrent cases

Prevention of relapse in gastric ulcer
▸ BY MOUTH
▸ Adult: 20 mg once daily, increased if necessary to 40 mg once daily

Prevention of relapse in duodenal ulcer
▸ BY MOUTH
▸ Adult: 20 mg once daily, dose may range between 10–40 mg daily

NSAID-associated duodenal ulcer | NSAID-associated gastric ulcer | NSAID-associated gastroduodenal erosions
▸ BY MOUTH
▸ Adult: 20 mg once daily for 4 weeks, continued for a further 4 weeks if not fully healed

Prophylaxis in patients with a history of NSAID-associated duodenal ulcer who require continued NSAID treatment | Prophylaxis in patients with a history of NSAID-associated gastric ulcer who require continued NSAID treatment | Prophylaxis in patients with a history of NSAID-associated gastroduodenal lesions who require continued NSAID treatment | Prophylaxis in patients with a history of NSAID-associated dyspeptic symptoms who require continued NSAID treatment
▸ BY MOUTH
▸ Adult: 20 mg once daily

Zollinger–Ellison syndrome
▸ BY MOUTH
▸ Adult: Initially 60 mg once daily; usual dose 20–120 mg daily, total daily doses greater than 80 mg should be given in 2 divided doses
▸ BY INTRAVENOUS INJECTION, OR BY INTRAVENOUS INFUSION
▸ Adult: Initially 60 mg once daily, adjusted according to response, total daily doses greater than 60 mg should be given in 2 divided doses, injection to be given over 5 minutes, infusion to be given over 20–30 minutes

Gastro-oesophageal reflux disease
▸ BY MOUTH
▸ Adult: 20 mg once daily for 4 weeks, continued for a further 4–8 weeks if not fully healed; maintenance 20 mg once daily

Gastro-oesophageal reflux disease refractory to other treatment
▸ BY MOUTH
▸ Adult: 40 mg once daily for 8 weeks; maintenance 20 mg once daily

Acid reflux disease (long-term management)
▸ BY MOUTH
▸ Adult: 10 mg once daily, increased to 20 mg once daily, dose only increased if symptoms return

Acid-related dyspepsia
▸ BY MOUTH
▸ Adult: 10–20 mg once daily for 2–4 weeks according to response

Treatment and prevention of benign gastric ulcers | Treatment and prevention of duodenal ulcers | Treatment and prevention of NSAID-associated ulcers | Treatment and prevention of gastro-oesophageal reflux disease
▸ BY INTRAVENOUS INJECTION, OR BY INTRAVENOUS INFUSION
▸ Adult: 40 mg once daily until oral administration possible, injection to be given over 5 minutes, infusion to be given over 20–30 minutes

Major peptic ulcer bleeding (following endoscopic treatment)
▸ INITIALLY BY INTRAVENOUS INFUSION
▸ Adult: Initially 80 mg, to be given over 40–60 minutes, then (by continuous intravenous infusion) 8 mg/hour for 72 hours, subsequent dose then changed to oral therapy

● UNLICENSED USE Treatment of major peptic ulcer bleeding (following endoscopic treatment) is an unlicensed indication.

● INTERACTIONS → Appendix 1 (proton pump inhibitors).

● SIDE-EFFECTS Agitation · impotence

● PREGNANCY Not known to be harmful.

● BREAST FEEDING Present in milk but not known to be harmful.

● HEPATIC IMPAIRMENT Not more than 20 mg daily should be needed.

● DIRECTIONS FOR ADMINISTRATION For administration by *mouth*, swallow whole, or disperse *Losec MUPS®* tablets in water, *or* mix capsule contents or *Losec MUPS®* tablets with fruit juice or yoghurt. Preparations consisting of an e/c tablet within a capsule should **not** be opened.
▸ With intravenous use For *intravenous infusion* (*Losec®*), give intermittently or continuously in Glucose 5% or Sodium chloride 0.9%; reconstitute each 40 mg vial with infusion fluid and dilute to 100 mL; for intermittent infusion give 40 mg over 20–30 minutes; stable for 3 hours in glucose 5% or 12 hours in sodium chloride 0.9%.

● PATIENT AND CARER ADVICE
▸ With oral use Counselling on administration advised.

● PROFESSION SPECIFIC INFORMATION
Dental practitioners' formulary
Gastro-resistant omeprazole capsules may be prescribed.

● EXCEPTIONS TO LEGAL CATEGORY
▸ With oral use Omeprazole 10 mg tablets can be sold to the public for the short-term relief of reflux-like symptoms (e.g. heartburn) in adults over 18 years, max. daily dose 20 mg for max. 4 weeks, and a pack size of 28 tablets.

● MEDICINAL FORMS
There can be variation in the licensing of different medicines containing the same drug. Forms available from special-order manufacturers include: oral suspension, oral solution

Gastro-resistant tablet
CAUTIONARY AND ADVISORY LABELS 25
▸ Omeprazole (Non-proprietary)
 Omeprazole 10 mg Omeprazole 10mg gastro-resistant tablets | 28 tablet [PoM] £18.91 DT price = £7.90
 Omeprazole (as Omeprazole magnesium) 10 mg Omeprazole 10mg dispersible gastro-resistant tablets | 28 tablet [PoM] £8.94 DT price = £7.75
 Omeprazole 20 mg Omeprazole 20mg gastro-resistant tablets | 28 tablet [PoM] £28.56 DT price = £5.87

Omeprazole (as Omeprazole magnesium) 20 mg Omeprazole 20mg dispersible gastro-resistant tablets | 28 tablet [PoM] £12.53 DT price = £11.60

Omeprazole 40 mg Omeprazole 40mg gastro-resistant tablets | 7 tablet [PoM] £15.00 DT price = £4.97

Omeprazole (as Omeprazole magnesium) 40 mg Omeprazole 40mg dispersible gastro-resistant tablets | 7 tablet [PoM] £6.78 DT price = £5.80

▸ Losec (AstraZeneca UK Ltd)

Omeprazole (as Omeprazole magnesium) 10 mg Losec MUPS 10mg gastro-resistant tablets | 28 tablet [PoM] £7.75 DT price = £7.75

Omeprazole (as Omeprazole magnesium) 20 mg Losec MUPS 20mg gastro-resistant tablets | 28 tablet [PoM] £11.60 DT price = £11.60

Omeprazole (as Omeprazole magnesium) 40 mg Losec MUPS 40mg gastro-resistant tablets | 7 tablet [PoM] £5.80 DT price = £5.80

▸ Mezzopram (Sandoz Ltd)

Omeprazole (as Omeprazole magnesium) 10 mg Mezzopram 10mg gastro-resistant tablets | 28 tablet [PoM] £6.58 DT price = £7.75

Omeprazole (as Omeprazole magnesium) 20 mg Mezzopram 20mg gastro-resistant tablets | 28 tablet [PoM] £9.86 DT price = £11.60

Omeprazole (as Omeprazole magnesium) 40 mg Mezzopram 40mg gastro-resistant tablets | 7 tablet [PoM] £4.93 DT price = £5.80

Gastro-resistant capsule

▸ Omeprazole (Non-proprietary)

Omeprazole 10 mg Omeprazole 10mg gastro-resistant capsules | 28 capsule [PoM] £9.30 DT price = £0.92

Omeprazole 20 mg Omeprazole 20mg gastro-resistant capsules | 28 capsule [PoM] £13.50 DT price = £0.92

Omeprazole 40 mg Omeprazole 40mg gastro-resistant capsules | 7 capsule [PoM] £6.58 DT price = £0.78 | 28 capsule [PoM] £21.65

▸ Losec (AstraZeneca UK Ltd)

Omeprazole 10 mg Losec 10mg gastro-resistant capsules | 28 capsule [PoM] £9.30 DT price = £0.92

Omeprazole 20 mg Losec 20mg gastro-resistant capsules | 28 capsule [PoM] £13.92 DT price = £0.92

Omeprazole 40 mg Losec 40mg gastro-resistant capsules | 7 capsule [PoM] £6.96 DT price = £0.78

▸ Mepradec (Discovery Pharmaceuticals)

Omeprazole 10 mg Mepradec 10mg gastro-resistant capsules | 28 capsule [PoM] £0.92 DT price = £0.92

Omeprazole 20 mg Mepradec 20mg gastro-resistant capsules | 28 capsule [PoM] £0.92 DT price = £0.92

Powder for solution for infusion

▸ Omeprazole (Non-proprietary)

Omeprazole (as Omeprazole sodium) 40 mg Omeprazole 40mg powder for solution for infusion vials | 5 vial [PoM] £32.45 (Hospital only) | 5 vial [PoM] £16.54

▸70

Pantoprazole

● **INDICATIONS AND DOSE**

***Helicobacter pylori* eradication in combination with amoxicillin and clarithromycin; or in combination with clarithromycin and metronidazole**

▸ BY MOUTH

▸ Adult: 40 mg twice daily

Benign gastric ulcer

▸ BY MOUTH

▸ Adult: 40 mg daily for 8 weeks; increased if necessary up to 80 mg daily, dose increased in severe cases

Gastric ulcer

▸ BY INTRAVENOUS INJECTION, OR BY INTRAVENOUS INFUSION

▸ Adult: 40 mg daily until oral administration can be resumed, injection to be given over at least 2 minutes

Duodenal ulcer

▸ BY MOUTH

▸ Adult: 40 mg daily for 4 weeks; increased if necessary up to 80 mg daily, dose increased in severe cases

▸ BY INTRAVENOUS INJECTION, OR BY INTRAVENOUS INFUSION

▸ Adult: 40 mg daily until oral administration can be resumed, injection to be given over at least 2 minutes

Prophylaxis of NSAID-associated gastric ulcer in patients with an increased risk of gastroduodenal complications who require continued NSAID treatment | Prophylaxis of NSAID-associated duodenal ulcer in patients with an increased risk of gastroduodenal complications who require continued NSAID treatment

▸ BY MOUTH

▸ Adult: 20 mg daily

Gastro-oesophageal reflux disease

▸ BY MOUTH

▸ Adult: 20–80 mg daily for 4 weeks, continued for further 4 weeks if not fully healed, dose to be taken in the morning; maintenance 20 mg daily and increased to 40 mg daily, increased only if symptoms return

▸ BY INTRAVENOUS INJECTION, OR BY INTRAVENOUS INFUSION

▸ Adult: 40 mg daily until oral administration can be resumed, injection to be given over at least 2 minutes

Zollinger–Ellison syndrome (and other hypersecretory conditions)

▸ BY MOUTH

▸ Adult: Initially 80 mg daily (max. per dose 80 mg), adjusted according to response

▸ Elderly: 40 mg daily

▸ BY INTRAVENOUS INJECTION, OR BY INTRAVENOUS INFUSION

▸ Adult: Initially 80 mg, alternatively 160 mg in 2 divided doses, if rapid acid control required, then 80 mg once daily (max. per dose 80 mg), adjusted according to response

● INTERACTIONS → Appendix 1 (proton pump inhibitors).

● SIDE-EFFECTS Hyperlipidaemia · weight changes

● PREGNANCY Manufacturer advises avoid unless potential benefit outweighs risk—fetotoxic in *animals*.

● BREAST FEEDING Manufacturer advises avoid unless potential benefit outweighs risk—small amount present in milk.

● HEPATIC IMPAIRMENT Max. 20 mg daily in severe impairment and cirrhosis. Monitor liver function in hepatic impairment (discontinue if deterioration).

● RENAL IMPAIRMENT Max. oral dose 40 mg daily.

● DIRECTIONS FOR ADMINISTRATION For *intravenous infusion* (*Protium*®), give intermittently in Glucose 5% or Sodium chloride 0.9%; reconstitute 40 mg with 10 mL sodium chloride 0.9% and dilute with 100 mL of infusion fluid; give 40 mg over 15 minutes.

● EXCEPTIONS TO LEGAL CATEGORY Pantoprazole 20 mg tablets can be sold to the public for the short-term treatment of reflux symptoms (e.g. heartburn) in adults over 18 years, max. daily dose 20 mg for max. 4 weeks.

● MEDICINAL FORMS
There can be variation in the licensing of different medicines containing the same drug. Forms available from special-order manufacturers include: oral suspension

Gastro-resistant tablet

CAUTIONARY AND ADVISORY LABELS 25

▸ Pantoprazole (Non-proprietary)

Pantoprazole (as Pantoprazole sodium sesquihydrate) 20 mg Pantoprazole 20mg gastro-resistant tablets | 28 tablet [PoM] £11.83 DT price = £0.96

Pantoprazole (as Pantoprazole sodium sesquihydrate) 40 mg Pantoprazole 40mg gastro-resistant tablets | 28 tablet [PoM] £20.57 DT price = £1.15

Powder for solution for injection

▸ Pantoprazole (Non-proprietary)

Pantoprazole (as Pantoprazole sodium sesquihydrate) 40 mg Pantoprazole 40mg powder for solution for injection vials | 1 vial [PoM] £5.00 | 5 vial [PoM] £22.50-£23.25

▸ Protium (Nycomed UK Ltd)

Pantoprazole (as Pantoprazole sodium sesquihydrate) 40 mg Protium I.V. 40mg powder for solution for injection vials | 5 vial [PoM] £25.53

Rabeprazole sodium 70

- **INDICATIONS AND DOSE**

Benign gastric ulcer
▶ BY MOUTH
▶ Adult: 20 mg daily for 8 weeks, dose to be taken in the morning

Duodenal ulcer
▶ BY MOUTH
▶ Adult: 20 mg daily for 4 weeks, dose to be taken in the morning

Gastro-oesophageal reflux disease
▶ BY MOUTH
▶ Adult: 20 mg once daily for 4-8 weeks; maintenance 10-20 mg daily

Gastro-oesophageal reflux disease (symptomatic treatment in the absence of oesophagitis)
▶ BY MOUTH
▶ Adult: 10 mg daily for up to 4 weeks, then 10 mg daily if required

Zollinger–Ellison syndrome
▶ BY MOUTH
▶ Adult: Initially 60 mg once daily, adjusted according to response, doses above 100 mg daily given in 2 divided doses; maximum 120 mg per day

***Helicobacter pylori* eradication in combination with amoxicillin or metronidazole and clarithromycin**
▶ BY MOUTH
▶ Adult: 20 mg twice daily

- INTERACTIONS → Appendix 1 (proton pump inhibitors).

- SIDE-EFFECTS
▶ **Common or very common** Cough · influenza like syndrome · rhinitis
▶ **Uncommon** Chest pain · nervousness
▶ **Rare** Anorexia · weight gain

- PREGNANCY Manufacturer advises avoid—no information available.

- BREAST FEEDING Manufacturer advises avoid—no information available.

- HEPATIC IMPAIRMENT Manufacturer advises caution in severe hepatic dysfunction.

- MEDICINAL FORMS
There can be variation in the licensing of different medicines containing the same drug.

Gastro-resistant tablet
CAUTIONARY AND ADVISORY LABELS 25
▶ Rabeprazole sodium (Non-proprietary)
Rabeprazole sodium 10 mg Rabeprazole 10mg gastro-resistant tablets | 28 tablet [PoM] £11.56 DT price = £1.65
Rabeprazole sodium 20 mg Rabeprazole 20mg gastro-resistant tablets | 28 tablet [PoM] £19.55 DT price = £1.87
▶ Pariet (Eisai Ltd)
Rabeprazole sodium 10 mg Pariet 10mg gastro-resistant tablets | 28 tablet [PoM] £5.78 DT price = £1.65
Rabeprazole sodium 20 mg Pariet 20mg gastro-resistant tablets | 28 tablet [PoM] £11.34 DT price = £1.87

4.3 Gastro-oesophageal reflux disease

Gastro-oesophageal reflux disease

Management

Gastro-oesophageal reflux disease (including non-erosive gastro-oesophageal reflux and erosive oesophagitis) is associated with heartburn, acid regurgitation, and

sometimes, difficulty in swallowing (dysphagia); oesophageal inflammation (oesophagitis), ulceration, and stricture formation may occur and there is an association with asthma.

The management of gastro-oesophageal reflux disease includes drug treatment, lifestyle changes and, in some cases, surgery. Initial treatment is guided by the severity of symptoms and treatment is then adjusted according to response. The extent of healing depends on the severity of the disease, the treatment chosen, and the duration of therapy.

Patients with gastro-oesophageal reflux disease should be advised about lifestyle changes (avoidance of excess alcohol and of aggravating foods such as fats); other measures include weight reduction, smoking cessation, and raising the head of the bed.

For *mild symptoms* of gastro-oesophageal reflux disease, initial management may include the use of **antacids** and **alginates**. Alginate-containing antacids can form a 'raft' that floats on the surface of the stomach contents to reduce reflux and protect the oesophageal mucosa. **Histamine H_2-receptor antagonists** may relieve symptoms and permit reduction in antacid consumption. However, **proton pump inhibitors** provide more effective relief of symptoms than H2-receptor antagonists. When symptoms abate, treatment is titrated down to a level which maintains remission (e.g. by giving treatment intermittently).

For *severe symptoms* of gastro-oesophageal reflux disease or for patients with a proven or severe pathology (e.g. *oesophagitis, oesophageal ulceration, oesophagopharyngeal reflux, Barrett's oesophagus*), initial management involves the use of a **proton pump inhibitor**; patients need to be reassessed if symptoms persist despite treatment for 4–6 weeks with a proton pump inhibitor. When symptoms abate, treatment is titrated down to a level which maintains remission (e.g. by reducing the dose of the proton pump inhibitor or by giving it intermittently, or by substituting treatment with a histamine H_2-receptor antagonist). However, for endoscopically confirmed *erosive, ulcerative,* or *stricturing* disease, or *Barrett's oesophagus*, treatment with a proton pump inhibitor usually needs to be maintained at the minimum effective dose.

Pregnancy
If dietary and lifestyle changes fail to control gastro-oesophageal reflux disease in pregnancy, an antacid or an alginate can be used. If this is ineffective, ranitidine p. 68 can be tried. Omeprazole p. 73 is reserved for women with severe or complicated reflux disease.

Gastro-oesophageal reflux disease in children

Gastro-oesophageal reflux disease is common in infancy but most symptoms resolve without treatment between 12 and 18 months of age. In infants, mild or moderate reflux without complications can be managed initially by changing the frequency and volume of feed; a feed thickener or thickened formula feed can be used (with advice of a dietitian). If necessary, a suitable alginate-containing preparation can be used instead of thickened feeds. For older children, life-style changes similar to those for adults may be helpful followed if necessary by treatment with an alginate-containing preparation.

Children who do not respond to these measures or who have problems such as respiratory disorders or suspected oesophagitis need to be referred to hospital; an H_2-receptor antagonist may be needed to reduce acid secretion. If the oesophagitis is resistant to H_2-receptor blockade, the proton pump inhibitor omeprazole can be tried.

> **Drugs used for Gastro-oesophageal reflux disease not listed below** Cimetidine, p. 67 · Esomeprazole, p. 71 · Famotidine, p. 68 · Lansoprazole, p. 72 · Nizatidine, p. 68 · Pantoprazole, p. 74 · Rabeprazole sodium, above

Gastro-intestinal system

1

ANTACIDS > ALGINATE

Sodium alginate with calcium carbonate and sodium bicarbonate

The properties listed below are those particular to the combination only. For the properties of the components please consider, alginic acid p. 61, sodium bicarbonate p. 898, calcium carbonate p. 906.

- ● INDICATIONS AND DOSE
  Mild symptoms of gastro-oesophageal reflux disease
  ▸ BY MOUTH
  ▸ Child 6–11 years: 5–10 mL, to be taken after meals and at bedtime
  ▸ Child 12–17 years: 10–20 mL, to be taken after meals and at bedtime
  ▸ Adult: 10–20 mL, to be taken after meals and at bedtime

- ● PRESCRIBING AND DISPENSING INFORMATION Flavours of oral liquid formulations may include aniseed or peppermint.
- ● PATIENT AND CARER ADVICE
  Medicines for Children leaflet: Gaviscon for gastro-oesophageal reflux disease www.medicinesforchildren.org.uk/gaviscon-gastro-oesophageal-reflux-disease

- ● MEDICINAL FORMS
  There can be variation in the licensing of different medicines containing the same drug.
  Oral suspension
  ELECTROLYTES: May contain Sodium
  ▸ Sodium alginate with calcium carbonate and sodium bicarbonate (Non-proprietary)
  Calcium carbonate 16 mg per 1 ml, Sodium bicarbonate 26.7 mg per 1 ml, Sodium alginate 50 mg per 1 ml Alginate raft-forming oral suspension sugar free peppermint sugar-free | 500 ml GSL no price available DT price = £1.95
  Alginate raft-forming oral suspension sugar free aniseed sugar-free | 500 ml GSL no price available DT price = £1.95
  ▸ Brands may include Acidex, Entrocalm Heartburn and Indigestion Relief, Gaviscon, Gaviscon Cool, Gaviscon Liquid Relief, Peptac

4.4 *Helicobacter pylori* diagnosis

DIAGNOSTIC AGENTS

Urea (13C)

- ● INDICATIONS AND DOSE
  Diagnosis of gastro-duodenal *Helicobacter pylori* infection
  ▸ BY MOUTH
  ▸ Adult: (consult product literature)

- ● MEDICINAL FORMS
  There can be variation in the licensing of different medicines containing the same drug.
  Tablet
  ▸ Diabact UBT (Seahorse Laboratories Ltd)
  Urea [13-C] 50 mg diabact UBT 50mg tablets | 1 tablet PoM £21.25 | 10 tablet PoM no price available (Hospital only)
  Soluble tablet
  ▸ Pylobactell (Torbet Laboratories Ltd)
  Urea [13-C] 100 mg Pylobactell breath test kit | 1 kit PoM £20.75
  Powder
  ▸ Helicobacter Test INFAI (INFAI UK Ltd)
  Urea [13-C] 75 mg Helicobacter Test INFAI breath test kit sugar-free | 1 kit PoM £21.70

5 Food allergy

Food allergy

Management

Allergy with classical symptoms of vomiting, colic and diarrhoea caused by specific foods such as cow's milk or shellfish should be managed by strict avoidance. The condition should be distinguished from symptoms of occasional food intolerance in those with irritable bowel syndrome. Sodium cromoglicate p. 247 may be helpful as an adjunct to dietary avoidance.

> **Other drugs used for Food allergy** Chlorphenamine maleate, p. 260

6 Gastro-intestinal smooth muscle spasm

Antispasmodics

Antimuscarinics

The intestinal smooth muscle relaxant properties of antimuscarinic and other antispasmodic drugs may be useful in *irritable bowel syndrome*.

Antimuscarinics (formerly termed 'anticholinergics') reduce intestinal motility. They can be used for the management of *irritable bowel syndrome*.

Antimuscarinics that are used for gastro-intestinal smooth muscle spasm include the tertiary amines atropine sulfate p. 1169 and dicycloverine hydrochloride p. 77 and the quaternary ammonium compounds propantheline bromide p. 78 and hyoscine butylbromide p. 77. The quaternary ammonium compounds are less lipid soluble than atropine sulfate and are less likely to cross the blood–brain barrier; they are also less well absorbed from the gastro-intestinal tract.

Dicycloverine hydrochloride has a much less marked antimuscarinic action than atropine sulfate and may also have some direct action on smooth muscle. Hyoscine butylbromide is advocated as a gastro-intestinal antispasmodic, but it is poorly absorbed; the injection is useful in endoscopy and radiology. Atropine sulfate and the belladonna alkaloids are outmoded treatments, any clinical virtues being outweighed by atropinic side-effects.

Other indications for antimuscarinic drugs include arrhythmias, asthma and airways disease, motion sickness, parkinsonism, urinary incontinence, mydriasis and cycloplegia, premedication, and as an antidote to organophosphorus poisoning.

Other antispasmodics

Alverine citrate p. 78, mebeverine hydrochloride p. 78, and peppermint oil p. 42 are believed to be direct relaxants of intestinal smooth muscle and may relieve pain in *irritable bowel syndrome*. They have no serious adverse effects but, like all antispasmodics, should be avoided in paralytic ileus.

ANTIMUSCARINICS ☞ 703

Dicycloverine hydrochloride

(Dicyclomine hydrochloride)

● **INDICATIONS AND DOSE**

Symptomatic relief of gastro-intestinal disorders characterised by smooth muscle spasm

▸ BY MOUTH
▸ Child 6-23 months: 5–10 mg 3–4 times a day, dose to be taken 15 minutes before feeds
▸ Child 2-11 years: 10 mg 3 times a day
▸ Child 12-17 years: 10–20 mg 3 times a day
▸ Adult: 10–20 mg 3 times a day

● CONTRA-INDICATIONS Child under 6 months

● PREGNANCY Not known to be harmful; manufacturer advises use only if essential.

● BREAST FEEDING Avoid—present in milk; apnoea reported in infant.

● EXCEPTIONS TO LEGAL CATEGORY Dicycloverine hydrochloride can be sold to the public provided that max. single dose is 10 mg and max. daily dose is 60 mg.

● MEDICINAL FORMS
There can be variation in the licensing of different medicines containing the same drug.

Tablet
▸ Dicycloverine hydrochloride (Non-proprietary)
Dicycloverine hydrochloride 10 mg Dicycloverine 10mg tablets | 100 tablet [PoM] £190.80 DT price = £159.30
Dicycloverine hydrochloride 20 mg Dicycloverine 20mg tablets | 84 tablet [PoM] £203.42 DT price = £169.86

Oral solution
▸ Dicycloverine hydrochloride (Non-proprietary)
Dicycloverine hydrochloride 2 mg per 1 ml Dicycloverine 10mg/5ml oral solution | 100 ml [PoM] no price available | 120 ml [PoM] £189.49 DT price = £158.25 | 300 ml [PoM] no price available

Dicycloverine hydrochloride with aluminium hydroxide, magnesium oxide and simeticone

The properties listed below are those particular to the combination only. For the properties of the components please consider, dicycloverine hydrochloride above, aluminium hydroxide p. 913, simeticone p. 64.

● **INDICATIONS AND DOSE**

Symptomatic relief of gastro-intestinal disorders characterised by smooth muscle spasm

▸ BY MOUTH
▸ Child 12-17 years: 10–20 mL every 4 hours as required
▸ Adult: 10–20 mL every 4 hours as required

● MEDICINAL FORMS
There can be variation in the licensing of different medicines containing the same drug.

Oral suspension
▸ Kolanticon (Peckforton Pharmaceuticals Ltd)
Dicycloverine hydrochloride 500 microgram per 1 ml, Simeticone 4 mg per 1 ml, Magnesium oxide light 20 mg per 1 ml, Aluminium hydroxide dried 40 mg per 1 ml Kolanticon gel sugar-free | 200 ml [P] £4.00 sugar-free | 500 ml [P] £6.00

☞ 703

Hyoscine butylbromide

● **INDICATIONS AND DOSE**

Symptomatic relief of gastro-intestinal or genito-urinary disorders characterised by smooth muscle spasm

▸ BY MOUTH
▸ Child 6-11 years: 10 mg 3 times a day
▸ Child 12-17 years: 20 mg 4 times a day
▸ Adult: 20 mg 4 times a day

Irritable bowel syndrome

▸ BY MOUTH
▸ Adult: 10 mg 3 times a day; increased if necessary up to 20 mg 4 times a day

Acute spasm | Spasm in diagnostic procedures

▸ INITIALLY BY INTRAMUSCULAR INJECTION, OR BY SLOW INTRAVENOUS INJECTION
▸ Adult: 20 mg, then (by intramuscular injection or by slow intravenous injection) 20 mg after 30 minutes if required, dose may be repeated more frequently in endoscopy; maximum 100 mg per day

Excessive respiratory secretions in palliative care

▸ BY MOUTH
▸ Child 1 month-1 year: 300–500 micrograms/kg 3–4 times a day (max. per dose 5 mg)
▸ Child 2-4 years: 5 mg 3–4 times a day
▸ Child 5-11 years: 10 mg 3–4 times a day
▸ Child 12-17 years: 10–20 mg 3–4 times a day
▸ BY INTRAMUSCULAR INJECTION, OR BY INTRAVENOUS INJECTION
▸ Child 1 month-4 years: 300–500 micrograms/kg 3–4 times a day (max. per dose 5 mg)
▸ Child 5-11 years: 5–10 mg 3–4 times a day
▸ Child 12-17 years: 10–20 mg 3–4 times a day
▸ BY SUBCUTANEOUS INJECTION
▸ Adult: 20 mg every 4 hours if required, adjusted according to response to up to 20 mg every 1 hour
▸ BY SUBCUTANEOUS INFUSION
▸ Adult: 20–120 mg/24 hours

Bowel colic (in palliative care)

▸ BY MOUTH
▸ Child 1 month-1 year: 300–500 micrograms/kg 3–4 times a day (max. per dose 5 mg)
▸ Child 2-4 years: 5 mg 3–4 times a day
▸ Child 5-11 years: 10 mg 3–4 times a day
▸ Child 12-17 years: 10–20 mg 3–4 times a day
▸ BY INTRAMUSCULAR INJECTION, OR BY INTRAVENOUS INJECTION
▸ Child 1 month-4 years: 300–500 micrograms/kg 3–4 times a day (max. per dose 5 mg)
▸ Child 5-11 years: 5–10 mg 3–4 times a day
▸ Child 12-17 years: 10–20 mg 3–4 times a day
▸ BY SUBCUTANEOUS INJECTION
▸ Adult: 20 mg every 4 hours if required, adjusted according to response to up to 20 mg every 1 hour
▸ BY SUBCUTANEOUS INFUSION
▸ Adult: 60–300 mg/24 hours

PHARMACOKINETICS
Administration by mouth is associated with poor absorption.

● UNLICENSED USE
▸ In children *Tablets* not licensed for use in children under 6 years. *Injection* not licensed for use in children (age range not specified by manufacturer).

● PREGNANCY Manufacturer advises avoid.

● BREAST FEEDING Amount too small to be harmful.

Gastro-intestinal system

1

- DIRECTIONS FOR ADMINISTRATION
  ‣ With oral use in children For administration by *mouth*, injection solution may be used; content of ampoule may be stored in a refrigerator for up to 24 hours after opening.
  ‣ With intravenous use in children For *intravenous injection*, may be diluted with Glucose 5% or Sodium Chloride 0.9%; give over at least 1 minute.
- EXCEPTIONS TO LEGAL CATEGORY Hyoscine butylbromide tablets can be sold to the public for medically confirmed irritable bowel syndrome, provided single dose does not exceed 20 mg, daily dose does not exceed 80 mg, and pack does not contain a total of more than 240 mg.

- MEDICINAL FORMS
  There can be variation in the licensing of different medicines containing the same drug. Forms available from special-order manufacturers include: oral suspension, oral solution
  Tablet
  ‣ Buscopan (Boehringer Ingelheim Ltd)
    Hyoscine butylbromide 10 mg Buscopan 10mg tablets | 56 tablet [PoM] £3.00 DT price = £3.00
  Solution for injection
  ‣ Buscopan (Boehringer Ingelheim Ltd)
    Hyoscine butylbromide 20 mg per 1 ml Buscopan 20mg/1ml solution for injection ampoules | 10 ampoule [PoM] £2.92 DT price = £2.92

▶ 703

Propantheline bromide

- INDICATIONS AND DOSE
  Symptomatic relief of gastro-intestinal disorders characterised by smooth muscle spasm
  ‣ BY MOUTH
  ‣ Child 12-17 years: 15 mg 3 times a day, dose to be taken at least one hour before food and 30 mg, dose to be taken at night; maximum 120 mg per day
  ‣ Adult: 15 mg 3 times a day, dose to be taken at least one hour before food and 30 mg, dose to be taken at night; maximum 120 mg per day

  Adult enuresis
  ‣ BY MOUTH
  ‣ Adult: Initially 15 mg 3 times a day, dose to be taken at least one hour before food and 30 mg, dose to be taken at bedtime, subsequently adjusted according to response; maximum 120 mg per day

- UNLICENSED USE
  ‣ In children *Tablets* not licensed for use in children under 12 years.
- SIDE-EFFECTS Facial flushing
- PREGNANCY Manufacturer advises avoid unless essential—no information available.
- BREAST FEEDING May suppress lactation.
- HEPATIC IMPAIRMENT Manufacturer advises caution.
- RENAL IMPAIRMENT Manufacturer advises caution.

- MEDICINAL FORMS
  There can be variation in the licensing of different medicines containing the same drug. Forms available from special-order manufacturers include: oral suspension, oral solution
  Tablet
  CAUTIONARY AND ADVISORY LABELS 23
  ‣ Propantheline bromide (Non-proprietary)
    Propantheline bromide 15 mg Propantheline bromide 15mg tablets | 100 tablet [PoM] no price available
  ‣ Pro-Banthine (ProStrakan Ltd)
    Propantheline bromide 15 mg Pro-Banthine 15mg tablets | 112 tablet [PoM] £20.74 DT price = £20.74

ANTISPASMODICS

Alverine citrate

24.2.2016

- INDICATIONS AND DOSE
  Symptomatic relief of gastro-intestinal disorders characterised by smooth muscle spasm | Dysmenorrhoea
  ‣ BY MOUTH
  ‣ Child 12-17 years: 60–120 mg 1–3 times a day
  ‣ Adult: 60–120 mg 1–3 times a day

- CONTRA-INDICATIONS Intestinal obstruction · paralytic ileus
- SIDE-EFFECTS Dizziness · dyspnoea · headache · hepatitis · jaundice (resolves with cessation) · nausea · pruritus · wheezing
- PREGNANCY Manufacturer advises avoid—limited information available
- BREAST FEEDING Manufacturer advises avoid—limited information available.
- PATIENT AND CARER ADVICE
  Driving and skilled tasks
  Dizziness may affect performance of skilled tasks (e.g. driving).

- MEDICINAL FORMS
  There can be variation in the licensing of different medicines containing the same drug.
  Capsule
  ‣ Alverine citrate (Non-proprietary)
    Alverine citrate 60 mg Alverine 60mg capsules | 100 capsule [P] £19.49 DT price = £19.48
    Alverine citrate 120 mg Alverine 120mg capsules | 60 capsule [P] £23.30 DT price = £23.11
  ‣ Audmonal (Auden McKenzie (Pharma Division) Ltd)
    Alverine citrate 60 mg Audmonal 60mg capsules | 100 capsule [P] £14.80 DT price = £19.48
    Alverine citrate 120 mg Audmonal Forte 120mg capsules | 60 capsule [P] £17.75 DT price = £23.11
  ‣ Spasmonal (Meda Pharmaceuticals Ltd)
    Alverine citrate 60 mg Spasmonal 60mg capsules | 100 capsule [P] £16.45 DT price = £19.48
    Alverine citrate 120 mg Spasmonal Forte 120mg capsules | 60 capsule [P] £19.42 DT price = £23.11

Mebeverine hydrochloride

- INDICATIONS AND DOSE
  Adjunct in gastro-intestinal disorders characterised by smooth muscle spasm
  ‣ BY MOUTH USING IMMEDIATE-RELEASE MEDICINES
  ‣ Child 10-17 years: 135–150 mg 3 times a day, dose preferably taken 20 minutes before meals
  ‣ Adult: 135–150 mg 3 times a day, dose preferably taken 20 minutes before meals
  Irritable bowel syndrome
  ‣ BY MOUTH USING MODIFIED-RELEASE MEDICINES
  ‣ Child 12-17 years: 200 mg twice daily
  ‣ Adult: 200 mg twice daily

- UNLICENSED USE
  ‣ In children *Tablets and liquid* not licensed for use in children under 10 years. *Granules* not licensed for use in children under 12 years. *Modified-release capsules* not licensed for use in children under 18 years.
- CONTRA-INDICATIONS Paralytic ileus
- SIDE-EFFECTS Allergic reactions · angioedema · rash · urticaria
- PREGNANCY Not known to be harmful—manufacturers advise avoid.

- BREAST FEEDING Manufacturers advise avoid—no information available.
- PATIENT AND CARER ADVICE
  Medicines for Children leaflet: Mebeverine for intestinal spasm www.medicinesforchildren.org.uk/mebeverine-for-intestinal-spasms

  Patients or carers should be given advice on the timing of administration of mebeverine hydrochloride tablets and oral suspension.
- EXCEPTIONS TO LEGAL CATEGORY
  ▸ In adults Mebeverine hydrochloride can be sold to the public for symptomatic relief of irritable bowel syndrome provided that max. single dose is 135 mg and max. daily dose is 405 mg; for uses other than symptomatic relief of irritable bowel syndrome provided that max. single dose is 100 mg and max. daily dose is 300 mg.
- MEDICINAL FORMS
  There can be variation in the licensing of different medicines containing the same drug.

  Tablet
  ▸ Mebeverine hydrochloride (Non-proprietary)
    Mebeverine hydrochloride 135 mg Mebeverine 135mg tablets | 15 tablet PoM £4.50 | 100 tablet PoM £20.00 DT price = £7.59
  ▸ Colofac (BGP Products Ltd)
    Mebeverine hydrochloride 135 mg Colofac 135mg tablets | 100 tablet PoM £9.02 DT price = £7.59

  Modified-release capsule
  CAUTIONARY AND ADVISORY LABELS 25
  ▸ Colofac MR (BGP Products Ltd)
    Mebeverine hydrochloride 200 mg Colofac MR 200mg capsules | 60 capsule PoM £6.92 DT price = £6.92

  Oral suspension
  ▸ Mebeverine hydrochloride (Non-proprietary)
    Mebeverine hydrochloride (as Mebeverine pamoate) 10 mg per 1 ml Mebeverine 50mg/5ml oral suspension sugar free sugar-free | 300 ml PoM £163.43 DT price = £163.43

7 Liver disorders and related conditions

7.1 Biliary disorders

Biliary disorders

Drugs affecting biliary composition and flow

The use of laparoscopic cholecystectomy and of endoscopic biliary techniques has limited the place of the bile acid ursodeoxycholic acid p. 80 in gallstone disease. Ursodeoxycholic acid is suitable for patients with unimpaired gall bladder function, small or medium-sized radiolucent stones, and whose mild symptoms are not amenable to other treatment. Long-term prophylaxis may be needed after complete dissolution of the gallstones has been confirmed because they may recur in up to 25% of patients within one year of stopping treatment.

Ursodeoxycholic acid is also used in primary biliary cirrhosis; liver tests improve in most patients but the effect on overall survival is uncertain.

Cholic acid below may be used to improve the flow of bile in those with inborn errors of primary bile acid synthesis.

A **terpene** mixture (*Rowachol*®) raises biliary cholesterol solubility. It is not considered to be a useful adjunct.

Bile acid sequestrants

Colestyramine p. 180 is an anion-exchange resin that is not absorbed from the gastro-intestinal tract. It relieves diarrhoea and pruritus by forming an insoluble complex with bile acids in the intestine.

Pancreatin

Supplements of pancreatin are given by mouth to compensate for reduced or absent exocrine secretion in cystic fibrosis, and following pancreatectomy, gastrectomy, or chronic pancreatitis. Pancreatin may also be necessary if a tumour (e.g. pancreatic cancer) obstructs outflow from the pancreas.

Pancreatin preparations			
Preparation	Protease units	Amylase units	Lipase units
Creon® 10 000 capsule, e/c granules	600	8000	10 000
Creon® Micro e/c granules (per 100 mg)	200	3600	5000
Pancrex® granules (per gram)	300	4000	5000
Pancrex V® capsule, powder	430	9000	8000
Pancrex V '125'® capsule, powder	160	3300	2950
Pancrex V® e/c tablet	110	1700	1900
Pancrex V® Forte e/c tablet	330	5000	5600
Pancrex V® powder (per gram)	1400	30 000	25 000

Higher-strength pancreatin preparations			
Preparation	Protease units	Amylase units	Lipase units
Creon® 25 000 capsule, e/c pellets	1000	18 000	25 000
Creon® 40 000 capsule, e/c granules	1600	25 000	40 000
Nutrizym 22® capsule, e/c minitablets	1100	19 800	22 000
Pancrease HL® capsule, e/c minitablets	1250	22 500	25 000

BILE ACIDS

Cholic acid
21.3.2016

- DRUG ACTION Cholic acid is the predominant primary bile acid in humans, which can be used to provide a source of bile acid in patients with inborn deficiencies in bile acid synthesis.

- INDICATIONS AND DOSE
  Inborn errors of primary bile acid synthesis (initiated by a specialist)
  ▸ BY MOUTH
  ▸ Adult: Usual dose 5–15 mg/kg daily; increased in steps of 50 mg daily in divided doses if required, dose to be given with food at the same time each day; Usual maximum 500 mg/24 hours

- INTERACTIONS → Appendix 1 (bile acids).

- SIDE-EFFECTS Diarrhoea · gallstones (long term use) · pruritus
  SIDE-EFFECTS, FURTHER INFORMATION
  Patients presenting with pruritus and/or persistent diarrhoea should be investigated for potential overdose by a serum and/or urine bile acid assay.

- PREGNANCY Limited data available—not known to be harmful, manufacturer advises continue treatment.
  Manufacturer advises monitor patient parameters more frequently in pregnancy.

- BREAST FEEDING Present in milk but not known to be harmful.

- HEPATIC IMPAIRMENT Manufacturer advises monitor closely.

- **MONITORING REQUIREMENTS** Manufacturer advises monitor serum and/or urine bile-acid concentrations every 3 months for the first year, then every 6 months for three years, then annually; monitor liver function tests at the same or greater frequency.
- **DIRECTIONS FOR ADMINISTRATION** Manufacturer advises capsules may be opened and the content added to infant formula, juice, fruit compote, or yoghurt for administration.
- **PATIENT AND CARER ADVICE** Counselling advised on administration.

- **MEDICINAL FORMS**
  There can be variation in the licensing of different medicines containing the same drug.
  Capsule
  CAUTIONARY AND ADVISORY LABELS 25
  ▸ Kolbam (Lucane Pharma Ltd) ▼
    Cholic acid 50 mg Kolbam 50mg capsules | 90 capsule [PoM] £3,240.00
    Cholic acid 250 mg Kolbam 250mg capsules | 90 capsule [PoM] £11,340.00
  ▸ Orphacol (Laboratoires CTRS) ▼
    Cholic acid 50 mg Orphacol 50mg capsules | 30 capsule [PoM] £1,860.00 | 60 capsule [PoM] £3,720.00
    Cholic acid 250 mg Orphacol 250mg capsules | 30 capsule [PoM] £6,630.00

Ursodeoxycholic acid

- **INDICATIONS AND DOSE**
  Dissolution of gallstones
  ▸ BY MOUTH
  ▸ Adult: 8–12 mg/kg once daily, dose to be taken at bedtime, alternatively 8–12 mg/kg daily in 2 divided doses for up to 2 years; treatment is continued for 3–4 months after stones dissolve

  Primary biliary cirrhosis
  ▸ BY MOUTH
  ▸ Adult: 12–16 mg/kg daily in 3 divided doses for 3 months, then 12–16 mg/kg once daily, dose to be taken at bedtime

- **CONTRA-INDICATIONS** Acute inflammation of the gall bladder · frequent episodes of biliary colic · inflammatory diseases and other conditions of the colon, liver or small intestine which interfere with enterohepatic circulation of bile salts · non-functioning gall bladder · radio-opaque stones
- **CAUTIONS** Liver disease
- **INTERACTIONS** → Appendix 1 (bile acids).
- **SIDE-EFFECTS**
  ▸ **Common or very common** Diarrhoea
  ▸ **Very rare** Abdominal pain · gallstone calcification · urticaria
  ▸ **Frequency not known** Nausea · pruritus · vomiting
- **PREGNANCY** No evidence of harm but manufacturer advises avoid.
- **BREAST FEEDING** Not known to be harmful but manufacturer advises avoid.
- **HEPATIC IMPAIRMENT** Avoid in chronic liver disease (but used in primary biliary cirrhosis).
- **MONITORING REQUIREMENTS** In primary biliary cirrhosis, monitor liver function every 4 weeks for 3 months, then every 3 months.
- **PATIENT AND CARER ADVICE** Patients should be given dietary advice (including avoidance of excessive cholesterol and calories).

- **MEDICINAL FORMS**
  There can be variation in the licensing of different medicines containing the same drug. Forms available from special-order manufacturers include: oral suspension, oral solution
  Tablet
  CAUTIONARY AND ADVISORY LABELS 21
  ▸ Ursodeoxycholic acid (Non-proprietary)
    Ursodeoxycholic acid 150 mg Ursodeoxycholic acid 150mg tablets | 60 tablet [PoM] £19.02 DT price = £19.02
    Ursodeoxycholic acid 300 mg Ursodeoxycholic acid 300mg tablets | 60 tablet [PoM] £47.63 DT price = £47.63
  ▸ Destolit (Norgine Pharmaceuticals Ltd)
    Ursodeoxycholic acid 150 mg Destolit 150mg tablets | 60 tablet [PoM] £18.39 DT price = £19.02
  ▸ Ursofalk (Dr. Falk Pharma UK Ltd)
    Ursodeoxycholic acid 500 mg Ursofalk 500mg tablets | 100 tablet [PoM] £80.00
  Capsule
  CAUTIONARY AND ADVISORY LABELS 21
  ▸ Ursodeoxycholic acid (Non-proprietary)
    Ursodeoxycholic acid 250 mg Ursodeoxycholic acid 250mg capsules | 60 capsule [PoM] £25.93 DT price = £25.29
  ▸ Ursofalk (Dr. Falk Pharma UK Ltd)
    Ursodeoxycholic acid 250 mg Ursofalk 250mg capsules | 60 capsule [PoM] £30.17 DT price = £25.29 | 100 capsule [PoM] £31.88
  Oral suspension
  CAUTIONARY AND ADVISORY LABELS 21
  ▸ Ursofalk (Dr. Falk Pharma UK Ltd)
    Ursodeoxycholic acid 50 mg per 1 ml Ursofalk 250mg/5ml oral suspension sugar-free | 250 ml [PoM] £26.98 DT price = £26.98

TERPENES

Borneol with camphene, cineole, menthol, menthone and pinene

- **INDICATIONS AND DOSE**
  Biliary disorders
  ▸ BY MOUTH
  ▸ Adult: 1–2 capsules 3 times a day, to be taken before food

- **LESS SUITABLE FOR PRESCRIBING** *Rowachol®* is less suitable for prescribing.

- **MEDICINAL FORMS**
  There can be variation in the licensing of different medicines containing the same drug.
  Gastro-resistant capsule
  CAUTIONARY AND ADVISORY LABELS 22
  ▸ Rowachol (Meadow Laboratories Ltd)
    Cineole 2 mg, Borneol 5 mg, Camphene 5 mg, Menthone 6 mg, Pinene 17 mg, Menthol 32 mg Rowachol gastro-resistant capsules | 50 capsule [PoM] £7.35

7.2 Oesophageal varices

Drugs used for Oesophageal varices not listed below
Vasopressin, p. 605

PITUITARY AND HYPOTHALAMIC HORMONES AND ANALOGUES > VASOPRESSIN AND ANALOGUES

Terlipressin acetate

● **INDICATIONS AND DOSE**

GLYPRESSIN® INJECTION

Bleeding from oesophageal varices
▸ BY INTRAVENOUS INJECTION
▸ Adult (body-weight up to 50 kg): Initially 2 mg every 4 hours until bleeding controlled, then reduced to 1 mg every 4 hours if required, maximum duration 48 hours
▸ Adult (body-weight 50 kg and above): Initially 2 mg every 4 hours until bleeding controlled, reduced if not tolerated to 1 mg every 4 hours, maximum duration 48 hours

VARIQUEL® INJECTION

Bleeding from oesophageal varices
▸ BY INTRAVENOUS INJECTION
▸ Adult (body-weight up to 50 kg): Initially 1 mg, then 1 mg every 4–6 hours for up to 72 hours, to be administered over 1 minute
▸ Adult (body-weight 50–69 kg): Initially 1.5 mg, then 1 mg every 4–6 hours for up to 72 hours, to be administered over 1 minute
▸ Adult (body-weight 70 kg and above): Initially 2 mg, then 1 mg every 4–6 hours for up to 72 hours, to be administered over 1 minute

● CAUTIONS Arrhythmia · elderly · electrolyte and fluid disturbances · heart disease · history of QT-interval prolongation · respiratory disease · septic shock · uncontrolled hypertension · vascular disease

● INTERACTIONS Caution with concomitant use of drugs that prolong the QT-interval.

● SIDE-EFFECTS
▸ **Common or very common** Abdominal cramps · arrhythmia · bradycardia · diarrhoea · headache · hypertension · hypotension · pallor · peripheral ischaemia
▸ **Uncommon** Angina · bronchospasm · convulsions · hot flushes · hyponatraemia · intestinal ischaemia · myocardial infarction · nausea · pulmonary oedema · respiratory failure · tachycardia · vomiting
▸ **Rare** Dyspnoea
▸ **Very rare** Hyperglycaemia · stroke
▸ **Frequency not known** Heart failure · skin necrosis

● PREGNANCY Avoid unless benefits outweigh risk—uterine contractions and increased intra-uterine pressure in early pregnancy, and decreased uterine blood flow reported.

● BREAST FEEDING Avoid unless benefits outweigh risk—no information available.

● RENAL IMPAIRMENT Use with caution in chronic renal failure.

● MEDICINAL FORMS
There can be variation in the licensing of different medicines containing the same drug.
Solution for injection
▸ Glypressin (Ferring Pharmaceuticals Ltd)
Terlipressin acetate 120 microgram per 1 ml Glypressin 1mg/8.5ml solution for injection ampoules | 5 ampoule [PoM] no price available

▸ Variquel (Sinclair IS Pharma Plc)
Terlipressin acetate 200 microgram per 1 ml Variquel 1mg/5ml solution for injection vials | 5 vial [PoM] £89.98 (Hospital only)
Powder and solvent for solution for injection
▸ Glypressin (Ferring Pharmaceuticals Ltd)
Terlipressin acetate 1 mg Glypressin 1mg powder and solvent for solution for injection vials | 5 vial [PoM] £92.33
▸ Variquel (Sinclair IS Pharma Plc)
Terlipressin acetate 1 mg Variquel 1mg powder and solvent for solution for injection vials | 5 vial [PoM] £89.48

8 Obesity

Obesity   1.6.2016

Description of condition

Obesity is directly linked to many health problems including cardiovascular disease, type 2 diabetes, fatty liver disease, gallstones, and gastro-oesophageal reflux disease. It is also linked to psychological and psychiatric morbidities.

In adults, obesity is generally classified as a body mass index (BMI) of $\geq 30\,kg/m^2$, though BMI should be interpreted with caution as it is not a direct measure of adiposity, particularly in patients who are very muscular or have muscle weakness or atrophy.

Waist circumference should also be considered as it may provide an indication of total body fat and a risk of obesity-related health problems. Men with a waist circumference ≥ 94 cm (≥ 90 cm for Asian men), and women with a waist circumference of ≥ 80 cm are at increased risk of obesity-related health problems. A waist circumference of ≥ 102 cm in men and ≥ 88 cm in women indicates a very high risk of obesity-related health problems.

Aims of treatment

Management should be aimed at modest, sustainable weight loss and maintenance of a healthy weight, to reduce the risk factors associated with obesity.

Overview

[EvGr] Obesity should be managed in an appropriate setting by staff who have been trained in the management of obesity. Patients should be monitored for changes in weight, as well as changes in blood pressure and blood lipids, and for other associated conditions. ⟨A⟩

[EvGr] An initial assessment should consider potential underlying causes (e.g. hypothyroidism) and a review of the appropriateness of current medications which are known to cause weight gain, e.g. atypical antipsychotics, beta-adrenoceptor blocking drugs, insulin (when used in the treatment of type 2 diabetes), lithium carbonate, lithium citrate, sodium valproate, sulphonylureas, thiazolidinediones, and tricyclic antidepressants. ⟨A⟩

Lifestyle changes

[EvGr] Patients should be encouraged to engage in a sustainable weight management programme which includes strategies to change behaviour, increase physical activity, and improve diet and eating behaviour. ⟨A⟩

Drug treatment

[EvGr] Drug treatment should **never** be used as the sole element of treatment and should be used as part of an overall weight management plan. An anti-obesity drug should be considered only for those with a BMI of $\geq 30\,kg/m^2$, in whom diet, exercise and behaviour changes fail to achieve a realistic reduction in weight. In the presence of associated risk factors, it may be appropriate to prescribe an anti-obesity drug to individuals with a BMI of $\geq 28\,kg/m^2$. A vitamin and mineral supplement may also be considered if there is concern about inadequate micronutrient intake, particularly for vulnerable groups such as in the elderly and younger patients. ⟨A⟩

EvGr The effect of management should be monitored on a regular basis with reinforcement of supporting lifestyle advice. Rates of weight loss may be slower in patients with type 2 diabetes, so less strict goals than in those without diabetes may be appropriate. Ⓐ

EvGr Orlistat below, is the only drug currently available in the UK that is recommended specifically for the management of obesity; it acts by reducing the absorption of dietary fat. Ⓐ

EvGr Orlistat is licensed for use as an adjunct in the management of obesity in patients with a BMI of $\geq 30 \text{ kg/m}^2$, or, in individuals with a BMI of $\geq 28 \text{ kg/m}^2$ in the presence of other risk factors. Treatment with orlistat may also be used to maintain weight loss rather than to continue to lose weight. Discontinuation of treatment with orlistat should be considered after 12 weeks if weight loss has not exceeded 5% since the start of treatment. Ⓐ

Drugs which produce a feeling of satiety (such as methylcellulose p. 48 and sterculia p. 48 [unlicensed indications]) have been used in an attempt to control appetite, but there is little evidence for their efficacy. Various centrally acting appetite suppressants, including stimulants and serotonergic drugs (such as dexfenfluramine, fenfluramine, sibutramine, and rimonabant), have been used in the management of obesity but have been withdrawn or are no longer recommended due to serious safety concerns or their addictive potential.

Surgery

EvGr Bariatric surgery may be considered for patients who have a BMI of $\geq 40 \text{ kg/m}^2$ (Obesity III, morbid obesity), or between 35–39.9 kg/m² (Obesity II) and a significant disease (such as type 2 diabetes or high blood pressure) which could be improved with weight loss, and if all appropriate non-surgical measures has been tried but clinically beneficial weight loss has not been achieved or maintained. Ⓐ

Useful Resources

Obesity: identification, assessment and management. Clinical Guideline 189. National Institute for Health and Care Excellence. November 2014.
www.nice.org.uk/guidance/cg189

PERIPHERALLY ACTING ANTIOBESITY DRUGS >
LIPASE INHIBITORS

❙ Orlistat

● DRUG ACTION Orlistat, a lipase inhibitor, reduces the absorption of dietary fat.

● **INDICATIONS AND DOSE**

Adjunct in obesity (in conjunction with a mildly hypocaloric diet in individuals with a body mass index (BMI) of 30 kg/m² or more or in individuals with a BMI of 28 kg/m² or more in the presence of other risk factors such as type 2 diabetes, hypertension, or hypercholesterolaemia)

▸ BY MOUTH

▸ Adult: 120 mg up to 3 times a day, dose to be taken immediately before, during, or up to 1 hour after each main meal, continue treatment beyond 12 weeks only if weight loss since start of treatment exceeds 5% (target for initial weight loss may be lower in patients with type 2 diabetes), if a meal is missed or contains no fat, the dose of orlistat should be omitted

● CONTRA-INDICATIONS Cholestasis · chronic malabsorption syndrome

● CAUTIONS Chronic kidney disease · may impair absorption of fat-soluble vitamins · volume depletion

CAUTIONS, FURTHER INFORMATION
Vitamin supplementation (especially of vitamin D) may be considered if there is concern about deficiency of fat-soluble vitamins.

● INTERACTIONS → Appendix 1 (orlistat).

▸ **Multivitamins** If a multivitamin supplement is required, it should be taken at least 2 hours after orlistat dose or at bedtime.

● SIDE-EFFECTS

▸ **Common or very common** Abdominal distension (gastro-intestinal effects minimised by reduced fat intake) · abdominal pain (gastro-intestinal effects minimised by reduced fat intake) · anxiety · faecal incontinence · faecal urgency · flatulence · gingival disorders · headache · hypoglycaemia · liquid stools · malaise · menstrual disturbances · oily leakage from rectum · oily stools · respiratory infections · tooth disorders · urinary tract infection

▸ **Frequency not known** Bullous eruptions · cholelithiasis · diverticulitis · hepatitis · hypothyroidism · oxalate nephropathy · rectal bleeding

● PREGNANCY Use with caution.

● BREAST FEEDING Avoid—no information available.

● MEDICINAL FORMS
There can be variation in the licensing of different medicines containing the same drug.

Capsule
▸ Orlistat (Non-proprietary)
  Orlistat 120 mg Orlistat 120mg capsules | 84 capsule PoM £30.05
  DT price = £20.07
▸ Alli (GlaxoSmithKline Consumer Healthcare)
  Orlistat 60 mg Alli 60mg capsules | 42 capsule Ⓟ £19.20 | 84 capsule Ⓟ £29.10 | 120 capsule Ⓟ £36.32
▸ Beacita (Actavis UK Ltd)
  Orlistat 120 mg Beacita 120mg capsules | 84 capsule PoM £31.63
  DT price = £20.07
▸ Xenical (Roche Products Ltd)
  Orlistat 120 mg Xenical 120mg capsules | 84 capsule PoM £31.63
  DT price = £20.07

9　Rectal and anal disorders

Rectal and anal disorders

Overview

Anal and perianal pruritus, soreness, and excoriation are best treated by application of bland ointments and suppositories. These conditions occur commonly in patients suffering from haemorrhoids, fistulas, and proctitis. Cleansing with attention to any minor faecal soiling, adjustment of the diet to avoid hard stools, the use of bulk-forming materials such as bran and a high residue diet are helpful. In proctitis these measures may supplement treatment with corticosteroids or sulfasalazine p. 38.

When necessary, topical preparations containing **local anaesthetics** or **corticosteroids** are used, provided perianal thrush has been excluded. Perianal thrush is treated with a topical antifungal preparation.

Soothing haemorrhoidal preparations

Soothing preparations containing mild astringents such as bismuth subgallate, zinc oxide, and hamamelis may give symptomatic relief in haemorrhoids. Many proprietary preparations also contain lubricants, vasoconstrictors, or mild antiseptics.

Local anaesthetics are used to relieve pain associated with *haemorrhoids* and *pruritus ani* but good evidence is lacking. Lidocaine hydrochloride ointment p. 1187 is used before emptying the bowel to relieve pain associated with *anal fissure*. Alternative local anaesthetics include tetracaine

p. 1023, cinchocaine (dibucaine), and pramocaine (pramoxine), but they are more irritant. Local anaesthetic ointments can be absorbed through the rectal mucosa therefore excessive application should be **avoided**, particularly in infants and children. Preparations containing local anaesthetics should be used for short periods only (no longer than a few days) since they may cause sensitisation of the anal skin.

Compound haemorrhoidal preparations with corticosteroids
Corticosteroids are often combined with local anaesthetics and soothing agents in preparations for haemorrhoids. They are suitable for occasional short-term use after exclusion of infections, such as herpes simplex; prolonged use can cause atrophy of the anal skin.

Rectal sclerosants
Oily phenol injection is used to inject haemorrhoids particularly when unprolapsed.

Anal fissures

The management of *anal fissures* requires stool softening by increasing dietary fibre in the form of bran or by using a bulk-forming laxative. Short-term use of local anaesthetic preparations may help. If these measures are inadequate, the patient should be referred for specialist treatment in hospital. The use of a topical nitrate (e.g. glyceryl trinitrate 0.4% ointment p. 201) may be considered. Before considering surgery, topical diltiazem hydrochloride 2% may be used twice daily [unlicensed indication] in patients with chronic anal fissures unresponsive to topical nitrates.

Rectal and anal disorders in children

Haemorrhoids in children are rare. Treatment is usually symptomatic and the use of a locally applied cream is appropriate for short periods; however, local anaesthetics can cause stinging initially and this may aggravate the child's fear of defaecation.

9.1 Haemorrhoids

CORTICOSTEROIDS

Benzyl benzoate with bismuth oxide, bismuth subgallate, hydrocortisone acetate, peru balsam and zinc oxide

● INDICATIONS AND DOSE

Haemorrhoids | Pruritus ani
▸ BY RECTUM USING OINTMENT
▸ Adult: Apply twice daily for no longer than 7 days, to be applied morning and night, an additional dose should be applied after a bowel movement
▸ BY RECTUM USING SUPPOSITORIES
▸ Adult: 1 suppository twice daily for no longer than 7 days, to be inserted night and morning, additional dose after a bowel movement

● CAUTIONS Local anaesthetic component can be absorbed through the rectal mucosa (avoid excessive application) · local anaesthetic component may cause sensitisation (use for short periods only—no longer than a few days)

● PRESCRIBING AND DISPENSING INFORMATION A proprietary brand *Anusol Plus HC*® (ointment and suppositories) is on sale to the public.

● MEDICINAL FORMS
There can be variation in the licensing of different medicines containing the same drug.

Suppository
▸ Benzyl benzoate with bismuth oxide, bismuth subgallate, hydrocortisone acetate, peru balsam and zinc oxide (Non-proprietary)
  Hydrocortisone acetate 10 mg, Bismuth oxide 24 mg, Benzyl benzoate 33 mg, Peru Balsam 49 mg, Bismuth subgallate 59 mg, Zinc oxide 296 mg Anusol Soothing Relief suppositories | 12 suppository GSL £3.34
▸ Anusol-Hc (McNeil Products Ltd)
  Hydrocortisone acetate 10 mg, Bismuth oxide 24 mg, Benzyl benzoate 33 mg, Peru Balsam 49 mg, Bismuth subgallate 59 mg, Zinc oxide 296 mg Anusol HC suppositories | 12 suppository PoM £1.74
  Anusol Plus HC suppositories | 12 suppository P £3.03

Ointment
▸ Benzyl benzoate with bismuth oxide, bismuth subgallate, hydrocortisone acetate, peru balsam and zinc oxide (Non-proprietary)
  Hydrocortisone acetate 2.5 mg per 1 gram, Bismuth oxide 8.75 mg per 1 gram, Benzyl benzoate 12.5 mg per 1 gram, Peru Balsam 18.75 mg per 1 gram, Bismuth subgallate 22.5 mg per 1 gram, Zinc oxide 107.5 mg per 1 gram Anusol Soothing Relief ointment | 15 gram GSL £3.34
▸ Anusol-Hc (McNeil Products Ltd)
  Hydrocortisone acetate 2.5 mg per 1 gram, Bismuth oxide 8.75 mg per 1 gram, Benzyl benzoate 12.5 mg per 1 gram, Peru Balsam 18.75 mg per 1 gram, Bismuth subgallate 22.5 mg per 1 gram, Zinc oxide 107.5 mg per 1 gram Anusol Plus HC ointment | 15 gram P £3.03
  Anusol HC ointment | 30 gram PoM £2.49

Benzyl benzoate with bismuth oxide, hydrocortisone acetate, peru balsam, pramocaine hydrochloride and zinc oxide

● INDICATIONS AND DOSE

Haemorrhoids | Pruritus ani
▸ BY RECTUM
▸ Adult: Apply twice daily for no longer than 7 days, to be applied morning and night and after a bowel movement

● CAUTIONS Local anaesthetic component can be absorbed through the rectal mucosa (avoid excessive application) · local anaesthetic component may cause sensitisation (use for short periods only—no longer than a few days)

● MEDICINAL FORMS
There can be variation in the licensing of different medicines containing the same drug.

Cream
▸ Anugesic-Hc (Pfizer Ltd)
  Hydrocortisone acetate 5 mg per 1 gram, Bismuth oxide 8.75 mg per 1 gram, Pramocaine hydrochloride 10 mg per 1 gram, Benzyl benzoate 12 mg per 1 gram, Peru Balsam 18.5 mg per 1 gram, Zinc oxide 123.5 mg per 1 gram Anugesic-HC cream | 30 gram PoM £3.71

Cinchocaine hydrochloride with fluocortolone caproate and fluocortolone pivalate

● **INDICATIONS AND DOSE**

Haemorrhoids | Pruritus ani
▸ BY RECTUM USING OINTMENT
▸ Adult: Apply twice daily for 5–7 days, apply 3–4 times a day if required, on the first day of treatment, then apply once daily for a few days after symptoms have cleared
▸ BY RECTUM USING SUPPOSITORIES
▸ Adult: Initially 1 suppository daily for 5–7 days, to be inserted after a bowel movement, then 1 suppository once daily on alternate days for 1 week

Haemorrhoids (severe cases) | Pruritus ani (severe cases)
▸ BY RECTUM USING SUPPOSITORIES
▸ Adult: Initially 1 suppository 2–3 times a day for 5–7 days, then 1 suppository once daily on alternate days for 1 week

● **CAUTIONS** Local anaesthetic component can be absorbed through the rectal mucosa (avoid excessive application) · local anaesthetic component may cause sensitisation (use for short periods only—no longer than a few days)

● **MEDICINAL FORMS**
There can be variation in the licensing of different medicines containing the same drug.
Suppository
▸ Ultraproct (Meadow Laboratories Ltd)
  Fluocortolone pivalate 610 microgram, Fluocortolone caproate 630 microgram, Cinchocaine hydrochloride 1 mg Ultraproct suppositories | 12 suppository PoM £4.06
Ointment
▸ Ultraproct (Meadow Laboratories Ltd)
  Fluocortolone pivalate 920 microgram per 1 gram, Fluocortolone caproate 950 microgram per 1 gram, Cinchocaine hydrochloride 5 mg per 1 gram Ultraproct ointment | 30 gram PoM £8.27

Cinchocaine with hydrocortisone

● **INDICATIONS AND DOSE**

PROCTOSEDYL® OINTMENT

Haemorrhoids | Pruritus ani
▸ TO THE SKIN, OR BY RECTUM
▸ Child: Apply twice daily, to be administered morning and night and after a bowel movement. Apply externally or by rectum. Do not use for longer than 7 days
▸ Adult: Apply twice daily, to be administered morning and night and after a bowel movement. Apply externally or by rectum. Do not use for longer than 7 days

PROCTOSEDYL® SUPPOSITORIES

Haemorrhoids | Pruritus ani
▸ BY RECTUM
▸ Child 12–17 years: 1 suppository, insert suppository night and morning and after a bowel movement. Do not use for longer than 7 days
▸ Adult: 1 suppository, insert suppository night and morning and after a bowel movement. Do not use for longer than 7 days

UNIROID-HC® OINTMENT

Haemorrhoids | Pruritus ani
▸ TO THE SKIN, OR BY RECTUM
▸ Child 12–17 years: Apply twice daily, and apply after a bowel movement, apply externally or by rectum, do not use for longer than 7 days
▸ Adult: Apply twice daily, and apply after a bowel movement, apply externally or by rectum, do not use for longer than 7 days

UNIROID-HC® SUPPOSITORIES

Haemorrhoids | Pruritus ani
▸ BY RECTUM
▸ Child 12–17 years: 1 suppository, insert twice daily and after a bowel movement. Do not use for longer than 7 days
▸ Adult: 1 suppository, insert twice daily and after a bowel movement. Do not use for longer than 7 days

● **CAUTIONS** Local anaesthetic component can be absorbed through the rectal mucosa (avoid excessive application, particularly in children and infants) · local anaesthetic component may cause sensitisation (use for short periods only—no longer than a few days)

● **MEDICINAL FORMS**
There can be variation in the licensing of different medicines containing the same drug.
Suppository
▸ Proctosedyl (Sanofi)
  Cinchocaine hydrochloride 5 mg, Hydrocortisone 5 mg Proctosedyl suppositories | 12 suppository PoM £5.08
▸ Uniroid HC (Chemidex Pharma Ltd)
  Cinchocaine hydrochloride 5 mg, Hydrocortisone 5 mg Uniroid HC suppositories | 12 suppository PoM £1.91
Ointment
▸ Proctosedyl (Sanofi)
  Cinchocaine hydrochloride 5 mg per 1 gram, Hydrocortisone 5 mg per 1 gram Proctosedyl ointment | 30 gram PoM £10.34
▸ Uniroid HC (Chemidex Pharma Ltd)
  Cinchocaine hydrochloride 5 mg per 1 gram, Hydrocortisone 5 mg per 1 gram Uniroid HC ointment | 30 gram PoM £4.23

Cinchocaine with prednisolone

● **INDICATIONS AND DOSE**

Haemorrhoids | Pruritus ani
▸ BY RECTUM USING OINTMENT
▸ Adult: Apply twice daily for 5–7 days, apply 3–4 times a day on the first day if necessary, then apply once daily for a few days after symptoms have cleared
▸ BY RECTUM USING SUPPOSITORIES
▸ Adult: 1 suppository daily for 5–7 days, to be inserted after a bowel movement

Haemorrhoids (severe cases) | Pruritus ani (severe cases)
▸ BY RECTUM USING SUPPOSITORIES
▸ Adult: Initially 1 suppository 2–3 times a day, then 1 suppository daily for a total of 5–7 days, to be inserted after a bowel movement

● **CAUTIONS** Local anaesthetic component can be absorbed through the rectal mucosa (avoid excessive application) · local anaesthetic component may cause sensitisation (use for short periods only—no longer than a few days)

● **MEDICINAL FORMS**
There can be variation in the licensing of different medicines containing the same drug.
Suppository
▸ Scheriproct (Bayer Plc)
  Cinchocaine hydrochloride 1 mg, Prednisolone hexanoate 1.3 mg Scheriproct suppositories | 12 suppository PoM £1.38 DT price = £1.38
Ointment
▸ Scheriproct (Bayer Plc)
  Prednisolone hexanoate 1.9 mg per 1 gram, Cinchocaine hydrochloride 5 mg per 1 gram Scheriproct ointment | 30 gram PoM £2.94 DT price = £2.94

Hydrocortisone with lidocaine

● **INDICATIONS AND DOSE**

Haemorrhoids | Pruritus ani
▸ BY RECTUM USING AEROSOL SPRAY
▸ Adult: 1 spray up to 3 times a day for no longer than 7 days without medical advice, spray once over the affected area
▸ BY RECTUM USING OINTMENT
▸ Adult: Apply several times daily, for short term use only

● CAUTIONS Local anaesthetic component can be absorbed through the rectal mucosa (avoid excessive application) · local anaesthetic component may cause sensitisation (use for short periods only—no longer than a few days)

● MEDICINAL FORMS
There can be variation in the licensing of different medicines containing the same drug.

Ointment
▸ Hydrocortisone with lidocaine (Non-proprietary)
  Hydrocortisone acetate 2.75 mg per 1 gram, Lidocaine 50 mg per 1 gram Lidocaine 5% / Hydrocortisone acetate 0.275% ointment | 20 gram [PoM] no price available DT price = £4.19
▸ Xyloproct (AstraZeneca UK Ltd)
  Hydrocortisone acetate 2.75 mg per 1 gram, Lidocaine 50 mg per 1 gram Xyloproct 5%/0.275% ointment | 20 gram [PoM] £4.19 DT price = £4.19

Spray
▸ Germoloids HC (Bayer Plc)
  Hydrocortisone 2 mg per 1 gram, Lidocaine hydrochloride 10 mg per 1 gram Germoloids HC spray | 30 ml [GSL] £5.20
▸ Perinal (Dermal Laboratories Ltd)
  Hydrocortisone 2 mg per 1 gram, Lidocaine hydrochloride 10 mg per 1 gram Perinal spray | 30 ml [P] £6.11

Hydrocortisone with pramocaine

● **INDICATIONS AND DOSE**

Haemorrhoids | Proctitis
▸ BY RECTUM
▸ Adult: 1 applicatorful 2–3 times a day and 1 applicatorful, after a bowel movement, do not use for longer than 7 days; maximum 4 applicatorfuls per day

● CAUTIONS Local anaesthetic component can be absorbed through the rectal mucosa (avoid excessive application) · local anaesthetic component may cause sensitisation (use for short periods only—no longer than a few days)

● MEDICINAL FORMS
There can be variation in the licensing of different medicines containing the same drug.

Foam
▸ Proctofoam HC (Meda Pharmaceuticals Ltd)
  Hydrocortisone acetate 10 mg per 1 gram, Pramocaine hydrochloride 10 mg per 1 gram Proctofoam HC foam enema | 40 dose [PoM] £6.07 DT price = £6.07

SCLEROSANTS

Phenol

● **INDICATIONS AND DOSE**

Haemorrhoids (particularly when unprolapsed)
▸ BY SUBMUCOSAL INJECTION
▸ Adult: 2–3 mL, dose (using phenol 5%) to be injected into the submucosal layer at the base of the pile; several injections may be given at different sites, max. total injected 10 mL at any one time

● SIDE-EFFECTS Irritation · tissue necrosis

● PRESCRIBING AND DISPENSING INFORMATION When prepared extemporaneously, the BP states Oily Phenol Injection, BP consists of phenol 5% in a suitable fixed oil.

● MEDICINAL FORMS
There can be variation in the licensing of different medicines containing the same drug. Forms available from special-order manufacturers include: solution for injection

Solution for injection
▸ Phenol (Non-proprietary)
  Phenol 50 mg per 1 ml Oily phenol 5% solution for injection 5ml ampoules | 10 ampoule [PoM] £50.31-£55.34
  Oily phenol 5% solution for injection 2ml ampoules | 10 ampoule [PoM] £38.03

10 Reduced exocrine secretions

PANCREATIC ENZYMES

Pancreatin

● DRUG ACTION Supplements of pancreatin are given to compensate for reduced or absent exocrine secretion. They assist the digestion of starch, fat, and protein.

● **INDICATIONS AND DOSE**

CREON® 10000

Pancreatic insufficiency
▸ BY MOUTH
▸ Child: Initially 1–2 capsules, dose to be taken with each meal either taken whole or contents mixed with acidic fluid or soft food (then swallowed immediately without chewing)
▸ Adult: Initially 1–2 capsules, dose to be taken with each meal either taken whole or contents mixed with acidic fluid or soft food (then swallowed immediately without chewing)

CREON® 25000

Pancreatic insufficiency
▸ BY MOUTH
▸ Child 2-17 years: Initially 1–2 capsules, dose to be taken with each meal either taken whole or contents mixed with acidic fluid or soft food (then swallowed immediately without chewing)
▸ Adult: Initially 1–2 capsules, dose to be taken with each meal either taken whole or contents mixed with acidic fluid or soft food (then swallowed immediately without chewing)

CREON® 40000

Pancreatic insufficiency
▸ BY MOUTH
▸ Child 2-17 years: Initially 1–2 capsules, dose to be taken with each meal either taken whole or contents mixed with acidic fluid or soft food (then swallowed immediately without chewing)
▸ Adult: Initially 1–2 capsules, dose to be taken with each meal either taken whole or contents mixed with acidic fluid or soft food (then swallowed immediately without chewing)   continued →

Gastro-intestinal system

1

CREON® MICRO

Pancreatic insufficiency

▶ BY MOUTH

▶ Child: Initially 100 mg, to be taken before each feed or meal; granules can be mixed with a small amount of milk or soft food and administered immediately (manufacturer recommends mixing with acidic liquid or pureed fruit before administration), granules should not be chewed before swallowing

▶ Adult: Initially 100 mg, to be taken before each feed or meal; granules can be mixed with a small amount of milk or soft food and administered immediately (manufacturer recommends mixing with acidic liquid or pureed fruit before administration), granules should not be chewed before swallowing

DOSE EQUIVALENCE AND CONVERSION
For *Creon® Micro*: 100 mg granules = one measured scoopful (scoop supplied with product).

NUTRIZYM 22® GASTRO-RESISTANT CAPSULES

Pancreatic insufficiency

▶ BY MOUTH

▶ Adult: Initially 1–2 capsules, dose to be taken with meals and 1 capsule as required, dose to be taken with snacks, doses should be swallowed whole or contents taken with water or mixed with soft food (then swallowed immediately without chewing)

PANCREASE HL®

Pancreatic insufficiency

▶ BY MOUTH

▶ Child 15–17 years: Initially 1–2 capsules, dose to be taken during each meal and 1 capsule, to be taken with snacks, all doses either taken whole or contents mixed with slightly acidic liquid or soft food (then swallowed immediately without chewing)

▶ Adult: Initially 1–2 capsules, dose to be taken during each meal and 1 capsule, to be taken with snacks, all doses either taken whole or contents mixed with slightly acidic liquid or soft food (then swallowed immediately without chewing)

PANCREX®

Pancreatic insufficiency

▶ BY MOUTH

▶ Child 2–17 years: 5–10 g, to be taken just before meals, washed down or mixed with milk or water

▶ Adult: 5–10 g, to be taken just before meals, washed down or mixed with milk or water

PANCREX® V

Pancreatic insufficiency

▶ BY MOUTH

▶ Child 1–11 months: 1–2 capsules, contents of capsule to be mixed with feeds

▶ Child 1–17 years: 2–6 capsules, dose to be taken with each meal either swallowed whole or sprinkled on food

▶ Adult: 2–6 capsules, dose to be taken with each meal either swallowed whole or sprinkled on food

PANCREX® V POWDER

Pancreatic insufficiency

▶ BY MOUTH

▶ Child: 0.5–2 g, to be taken before or with meals, washed down or mixed with milk or water

▶ Adult: 0.5–2 g, to be taken before or with meals, washed down or mixed with milk or water

PANCREX® V TABLETS

Pancreatic insufficiency

▶ BY MOUTH

▶ Child 2–17 years: 5–15 tablets, to be taken before meals

▶ Adult: 5–15 tablets, to be taken before meals

PANCREX® V TABLETS FORTE

Pancreatic insufficiency

▶ BY MOUTH

▶ Child 2–17 years: 6–10 tablets, to be taken before meals

▶ Adult: 6–10 tablets, to be taken before meals

● CONTRA-INDICATIONS
PANCREASE HL® Should not be used in children aged 15 years or less with cystic fibrosis

● CAUTIONS Can irritate the perioral skin and buccal mucosa if retained in the mouth · excessive doses can cause perianal irritation

● INTERACTIONS → Appendix 1 (pancreatin).

● SIDE-EFFECTS Abdominal discomfort · hyperuricaemia (associated with very high doses) · hyperuricosuria (associated with very high doses) · mucosal irritation · nausea · skin irritation · vomiting

● PREGNANCY Not known to be harmful.

● DIRECTIONS FOR ADMINISTRATION Enteric-coated preparations deliver a higher enzyme concentration in the duodenum (provided the capsule contents are swallowed whole without chewing). Since pancreatin is inactivated by heat, excessive heat should be avoided if preparations are mixed with liquids or food; the resulting mixtures should not be kept for more than one hour. Gastro-resistant granules should be mixed with milk, slightly acidic soft food or liquid such as apple juice, and then swallowed immediately without chewing. Any left-over food or liquid containing pancreatin should be discarded. Capsules containing enteric-coated granules can be opened and the granules administered in the same way. Pancreatin is inactivated by gastric acid therefore pancreatin preparations are best taken with food (or immediately before or after food).

▶ In adults Gastric acid secretion may be reduced by giving cimetidine or ranitidine an hour beforehand. Concurrent use of antacids also reduces gastric acidity.

▶ In children In children with cystic fibrosis with persistent fat malabsorption despite optimal use of enzyme replacement, an H_2-receptor antagonist or a proton pump inhibitor may improve fat digestion and absorption.

● PRESCRIBING AND DISPENSING INFORMATION
Preparations may contain pork pancreatin—consult product literature.

● HANDLING AND STORAGE Hypersensitivity reactions occur occasionally and may affect those handling the powder.

● PATIENT AND CARER ADVICE
Medicines for Children leaflet: Pancreatin for pancreatic insufficiency www.medicinesforchildren.org.uk/pancreatin-for-pancreatic-insufficiency

Patients or carers should be given advice on administration.

It is important to ensure adequate hydration at all times in patients receiving higher-strength pancreatin preparations.

● MEDICINAL FORMS
There can be variation in the licensing of different medicines containing the same drug.

Gastro-resistant tablet
CAUTIONARY AND ADVISORY LABELS 5, 25

▶ Pancrex (Essential Pharmaceuticals Ltd)
Protease 110 unit, Amylase 1700 unit, Lipase 1900 unit Pancrex V gastro-resistant tablets | 300 tablet ℗ £38.79
Protease 330 unit, Amylase 5000 unit, Lipase 5600 unit Pancrex V Forte gastro-resistant tablets | 300 tablet ℗ £48.11

Capsule

▶ Pancrex (Essential Pharmaceuticals Ltd)
Protease 160 unit, Lipase 2950 unit, Amylase 3300 unit Pancrex V 125mg capsule | 300 capsule ℗ £42.07
Protease 430 unit, Lipase 8000 unit, Amylase 9000 unit Pancrex V capsules | 300 capsule ℗ £53.20

Gastro-resistant capsule

▸ Creon (BGP Products Ltd)
  Protease 600 unit, Amylase 8000 unit, Lipase 10000 unit Creon 10000 gastro-resistant capsules | 100 capsule Ⓟ £12.93
  Protease 1000 unit, Amylase 18000 unit, Lipase 25000 unit Creon 25000 gastro-resistant capsules | 100 capsule PoM £28.25
  Protease 1600 unit, Amylase 25000 unit, Lipase 40000 unit Creon 40000 gastro-resistant capsules | 100 capsule PoM £41.80

▸ Nutrizym (Merck Serono Ltd)
  Protease 1100 unit, Amylase 19800 unit, Lipase 22000 unit Nutrizym 22 gastro-resistant capsules | 100 capsule PoM £33.33

▸ Pancrease (Janssen-Cilag Ltd)
  Protease 1250 unit, Amylase 22500 unit, Lipase 25000 unit Pancrease HL gastro-resistant capsules | 100 capsule PoM £40.38

Gastro-resistant granules

CAUTIONARY AND ADVISORY LABELS 25

▸ Creon (BGP Products Ltd)
  Protease 200 unit, Amylase 3600 unit, Lipase 5000 unit Creon Micro Pancreatin 60.12mg gastro-resistant granules | 20 gram Ⓟ £31.50

▸ Pancrex (Essential Pharmaceuticals Ltd)
  Protease 300 unit, Amylase 4000 unit, Lipase 5000 unit Pancrex gastro-resistant granules | 300 gram Ⓟ £57.00

Powder

▸ Pancrex (Essential Pharmaceuticals Ltd)
  Protease 1400 unit, Lipase 25000 unit, Amylase 30000 unit Pancrex V oral powder sugar-free | 300 gram Ⓟ £58.88

11 Stoma care

Stoma care

24.2.2016

Description of condition

A stoma is an artificial opening on the abdomen to divert flow of faeces or urine into an external pouch located outside of the body. This procedure may be temporary or permanent. Colostomy and ileostomy are the most common forms of stoma but a gastrostomy, jejunostomy, duodenostomy or caecostomy may also be performed. Understanding the type and extent of surgical intervention in each patient is crucial in managing the patient's pharmaceutical needs correctly.

Overview

Prescribing for patients with stoma calls for special care due to modifications in drug delivery, resulting in a higher risk of sub-optimal absorption. The following is a brief account of some of the main points to be borne in mind.

Enteric-coated and modified-release medicines are **unsuitable**, particularly in patients with an ileostomy, as there may not be sufficient release of active ingredient. Soluble tablets, liquids, capsules or uncoated tablets are more suitable due to their quicker dissolution. When a solid-dose form such as a capsule or a tablet is given, the contents of the ostomy bag should be checked for any remnants.

Preparations containing sorbitol as an excipient should be avoided, due to its laxative side effects.

Analgesics

Opioid analgesics may cause troublesome constipation in colostomy patients. When a non-opioid analgesic is required, paracetamol is usually suitable. Anti-inflammatory analgesics may cause gastric irritation and bleeding; faecal output should be monitored for traces of blood.

Antacids

The tendency to diarrhoea from magnesium salts or constipation from aluminium or calcium salts may be increased in patients with stoma.

Antisecretory drugs

The gastric acid secretion often increases stoma output. Proton pump inhibitors and somatostatin analogues (octreotide p. 835 and lanreotide p. 834) are often used to reduce this risk.

Antidiarrhoeal drugs

Loperamide hydrochloride p. 59 and codeine phosphate p. 413 reduce intestinal motility and decrease water and sodium output from an ileostomy. Loperamide hydrochloride circulates through the enterohepatic circulation, which is disrupted in patients with a short bowel; high doses of loperamide hydrochloride may be required. Codeine phosphate can be added if response with loperamide hydrochloride alone is inadequate.

Digoxin

Patients with a stoma are particularly susceptible to hypokalaemia if taking digoxin p. 98, due to fluid and sodium depletion. Potassium supplements or a potassium-sparing diuretic may be advisable with monitoring for early signs of toxicity.

Diuretics

Diuretics should be used with caution in patients with an ileostomy or with urostomy as they may become excessively dehydrated and potassium depletion may easily occur. It is usually advisable to use a potassium-sparing diuretic.

Iron preparations

Iron preparations may cause loose stools and sore skin in these patients. If this is troublesome and if iron is definitely indicated, an intramuscular iron preparation should be used. Modified-release preparations should be avoided for the reasons given above.

Laxatives

Laxatives should not be used in patients with an ileostomy where possible as they may cause rapid and severe loss of water and electrolytes.

Colostomy patients may suffer from constipation and whenever possible should be treated by increasing fluid intake or dietary fibre. Bulk-forming drugs can be tried. If they are insufficient, as small a dose as possible of a stimulant laxative such as senna p. 55 can be used with caution.

Potassium supplements

Liquid formulations are preferred to modified-release formulations. The daily dose should be split to avoid osmotic diarrhoea.

Care of stoma

Patients and their carers are usually given advice about the use of cleansing agents, protective creams, lotions, deodorants, or sealants whilst in hospital, either by the surgeon or by stoma care nurses. Voluntary organisations offer help and support to patients with stoma.

Chapter 2
Cardiovascular system

CONTENTS

1 Arrhythmias

Arrhythmias

Overview

Management of an arrhythmia requires precise diagnosis of the type of arrhythmia, and electrocardiography is essential; underlying causes such as heart failure require appropriate treatment.

Ectopic beats

If ectopic beats are spontaneous and the patient has a normal heart, treatment is rarely required and reassurance to the patient will often suffice. If they are particularly troublesome, beta-blockers are sometimes effective and may be safer than other suppressant drugs.

Atrial fibrillation

Treatment of patients with atrial fibrillation aims to reduce symptoms and prevent complications, especially stroke. All patients with atrial fibrillation should be assessed for their risk of stroke and thromboembolism. Atrial fibrillation can be managed by either controlling the ventricular rate ('rate control') or by attempting to restore and maintain sinus rhythm ('rhythm control'). At any stage if treatment fails to control symptoms, or, if symptoms reoccur after cardioversion and specialised management is required, referral should be made within 4 weeks. If drug treatment fails to control the symptoms of atrial fibrillation or is unsuitable, ablation strategies can be considered. Review anticoagulation, stroke, and bleeding risk at least annually in all patients with atrial fibrillation.

Acute presentation

All patients with life-threatening haemodynamic instability caused by new-onset atrial fibrillation should undergo emergency electrical cardioversion without delaying to achieve anticoagulation. In patients presenting acutely but without life-threatening haemodynamic instability, rate or rhythm control can be offered if the onset of arrhythmia is less than 48 hours; rate control is preferred if onset is more than 48 hours or uncertain. Consideration of pharmacological or electrical cardioversion should be based on clinical circumstances. If pharmacological cardioversion

has been agreed, intravenous amiodarone hydrochloride p. 94, or alternatively flecainide acetate p. 92, can be used (amiodarone hydrochloride is preferred if there is structural heart disease). If urgent rate control is required, a beta-blocker or verapamil hydrochloride p. 150 can be given intravenously.

Cardioversion

Sinus rhythm can be restored by electrical cardioversion, or pharmacological cardioversion with an oral or intravenous antiarrhythmic drug e.g. flecainide acetate or amiodarone hydrochloride. If atrial fibrillation has been present for more than 48 hours, electrical cardioversion is preferred and should not be attempted until the patient has been fully anticoagulated for at least 3 weeks; if this is not possible, parenteral anticoagulation should be commenced, and a left atrial thrombus ruled out immediately before cardioversion; oral anticoagulation should be given after cardioversion and continued for at least 4 weeks; prior to cardioversion, offer rate control as appropriate.

Drug treatment

Rate control is the preferred first-line drug treatment strategy for atrial fibrillation except in patients with new-onset atrial fibrillation, heart failure secondary to atrial fibrillation, atrial flutter suitable for an ablation strategy, atrial fibrillation with a reversible cause, or if rhythm control is more suitable based on clinical judgement. Ventricular rate can be controlled with a standard beta-blocker (not sotalol hydrochloride p. 97) or a rate-limiting calcium channel blocker such as diltiazem hydrochloride p. 143 [unlicensed indication], or verapamil hydrochloride as monotherapy. Choice of drug should be based on individual symptoms, heart rate, comorbidities, and patient preference. Digoxin p. 98 is usually only effective for controlling the ventricular rate at rest, and should therefore only be used as monotherapy in predominantly sedentary patients with non-paroxysmal atrial fibrillation. When a single drug fails to adequately control the ventricular rate, a combination of two drugs including a beta-blocker, digoxin, or diltiazem hydrochloride can be used. If symptoms are not controlled with a combination of two drugs, a rhythm-control strategy should be considered. If ventricular function is diminished, the combination of a beta-blocker (that is licensed for use in heart failure) and digoxin is preferred. Digoxin is also used when atrial fibrillation is accompanied by congestive heart failure.

If drug treatment is required to maintain sinus rhythm ('rhythm control') post-cardioversion, a standard beta-blocker is used. If a standard beta-blocker is not appropriate or is ineffective, consider an oral anti-arrhythmic drug such as sotalol hydrochloride, flecainide acetate, propafenone hydrochloride p. 93, or amiodarone hydrochloride; dronedarone p. 95 may be considered in paroxysmal or persistent atrial fibrillation (see NICE guidance). If necessary, amiodarone hydrochloride can be started 4 weeks before and continuing for up to 12 months after electrical cardioversion to increase success of the procedure, and to maintain sinus rhythm. Flecainide acetate or propafenone hydrochloride should not be given when there is known ischaemic or structural heart disease. Consider amiodarone hydrochloride in patients with left ventricular impairment or heart failure.

Paroxysmal atrial fibrillation

In symptomatic paroxysmal atrial fibrillation, ventricular rhythm is controlled with a standard beta-blocker. Alternatively, if symptoms persist or a standard beta-blocker is not appropriate, an oral anti-arrhythmic drug such as dronedarone (see NICE guidance), sotalol hydrochloride, flecainide acetate, propafenone hydrochloride, or amiodarone hydrochloride can be given (see also Paroxysmal supraventricular tachycardia and Supraventricular arrhythmias). In selected patients with infrequent episodes of symptomatic paroxysmal atrial fibrillation, sinus rhythm can be restored using the 'pill-in-the-pocket' approach; this involves the patient taking oral flecainide acetate or propafenone hydrochloride to self-treat an episode of atrial fibrillation when it occurs.

Stroke prevention

All patients with atrial fibrillation should be assessed for their risk of stroke and the need for thromboprophylaxis; this needs to be balanced with the patient's risk of bleeding; a NICE guideline (NICE clinical guideline 180 (June 2014). Atrial fibrillation: The management of atrial fibrillation) recommends using the CHA_2DS_2-VASc assessment tool for stroke risk and the HAS-BLED tool for bleeding risk prior to and during anticoagulation. Risk factors for stroke taken into account by CHA_2DS_2-VASc include prior ischaemic stroke, transient ischaemic attacks, or thromboembolic events, heart failure, left ventricular systolic dysfunction, vascular disease, diabetes, hypertension, females, and patients over 65 years. Patients with a very low risk of stroke (CHA_2DS_2-VASc score of 0 for men or 1 for women) do not require an antithrombotic for stroke prevention. Parenteral anticoagulation should be offered to patients with new-onset atrial fibrillation who are receiving subtherapeutic or no anticoagulation therapy until assessment is made, and appropriate anticoagulation is started. Oral anticoagulation should be offered to patients with confirmed diagnosis of atrial fibrillation in whom sinus rhythm has not been successfully restored within 48 hours of onset, patients who have had, or are at high risk of recurrence of atrial fibrillation such as those with structural heart disease, prolonged history of atrial fibrillation (more than 12 months), a history of failed attempts at cardioversion, and patients whom the risk of stroke outweighs the risk of bleeding. Anticoagulation treatment should not be withheld solely because of the risk of falls, and choice of treatment should be based on clinical features and patient preferences. Oral anticoagulation may be with a vitamin K antagonist (e.g warfarin sodium p. 126, or in non-valvular atrial fibrillation with apixaban p. 112, dabigatran etexilate p. 123, or rivaroxaban p. 115. Anticoagulants are also indicated during cardioversion procedures. Aspirin p. 109 is less effective than warfarin sodium at preventing emboli; the modest benefit is offset by the risk of bleeding, and aspirin should not be offered as monotherapy solely for stroke prevention in atrial fibrillation. If anticoagulant treatment is contra-indicated or

not tolerated, left atrial appendage occlusion can be considered.

Atrial flutter

Like atrial fibrillation, treatment options for atrial flutter involve either controlling the ventricular rate or attempting to restore and maintain sinus rhythm. However, atrial flutter generally responds less well to drug treatment than atrial fibrillation.

Control of the ventricular rate is usually an interim measure pending restoration of sinus rhythm. Ventricular rate can be controlled by administration of a beta-blocker, diltiazem hydrochloride p. 143 [unlicensed indication], or verapamil hydrochloride p. 150; an intravenous beta-blocker or verapamil hydrochloride is preferred for rapid control. Digoxin p. 98 can be added if rate control remains inadequate, and may be particularly useful in those with heart failure.

Conversion to sinus rhythm can be achieved by electrical cardioversion (by cardiac pacing or direct current), pharmacological cardioversion, or catheter ablation. If the duration of atrial flutter is unknown, or it has lasted for over 48 hours, cardioversion should not be attempted until the patient has been fully anticoagulated for at least 3 weeks; if this is not possible, parenteral anticoagulation should be commenced and a left atrial thrombus ruled out immediately before cardioversion; oral anticoagulation should be given after cardioversion and continued for at least 4 weeks.

Direct current cardioversion is usually the treatment of choice when rapid conversion to sinus rhythm is necessary (e.g. when atrial flutter is associated with haemodynamic compromise); catheter ablation is preferred for the treatment of recurrent atrial flutter. There is a limited role for anti-arrhythmic drugs as their use is not always successful. Flecainide acetate p. 92 or propafenone hydrochloride p. 93 can slow atrial flutter, resulting in 1:1 conduction to the ventricles, and should therefore be prescribed in conjunction with a ventricular rate controlling drug such as a beta-blocker, diltiazem hydrochloride [unlicensed indication], or verapamil hydrochloride. Amiodarone hydrochloride p. 94 can be used when other drug treatments are contra-indicated or ineffective.

All patients should be assessed for their risk of stroke and the need for thromboprophylaxis; the choice of anticoagulant is based on the same criteria as for atrial fibrillation.

Paroxysmal supraventricular tachycardia

This will often terminate spontaneously or with reflex vagal stimulation such as a Valsalva manoeuvre, immersing the face in ice-cold water, or carotid sinus massage; such manoeuvres should be performed with ECG monitoring.

If the effects of reflex vagal stimulation are transient or ineffective, or if the arrhythmia is causing severe symptoms, intravenous adenosine p. 96 should be given. If adenosine is ineffective or contra-indicated, intravenous verapamil hydrochloride is an alternative, but it should be avoided in patients recently treated with beta-blockers.

Failure to terminate paroxysmal supraventricular tachycardia with reflex vagal stimulation or drug treatment may suggest an arrhythmia of atrial origin, such as focal atrial tachycardia or atrial flutter.

Treatment with direct current cardioversion is needed in haemodynamically unstable patients or when the above measures have failed to restore sinus rhythm (and an alternative diagnosis has not been found).

Recurrent episodes of paroxysmal supraventricular tachycardia can be treated by catheter ablation, or prevented with drugs such as diltiazem hydrochloride, verapamil hydrochloride, beta-blockers including sotalol hydrochloride p. 97, flecainide acetate or propafenone hydrochloride.

Arrhythmias after myocardial infarction

In patients with a paroxysmal tachycardia or rapid irregularity of the pulse it is best not to administer an anti-arrhythmic until an ECG record has been obtained. Bradycardia, particularly if complicated by hypotension, should be treated with an intravenous dose of atropine sulfate p. 1169 the dose may be repeated if necessary. If there is a risk of asystole, or if the patient is unstable and has failed to respond to atropine sulfate, adrenaline/epinephrine p. 205 should be given by intravenous infusion, and the dose adjusted according to response.

For further advice, refer to the most recent recommendations of the Resuscitation Council (UK) available at www.resus.org.uk.

Ventricular tachycardia

Pulseless ventricular tachycardia or ventricular fibrillation should be treated with immediate defibrillation (see Cardiopulmonary resuscitation).

Patients with unstable sustained ventricular tachycardia, who continue to deteriorate with signs of hypotension or reduced cardiac output, should receive direct current cardioversion to restore sinus rhythm. If this fails, intravenous amiodarone hydrochloride should be administered and direct current cardioversion repeated.

Patients with sustained ventricular tachycardia who are haemodynamically stable can be treated with intravenous anti-arrhythmic drugs. Amiodarone hydrochloride is the preferred drug. Flecainide acetate, propafenone hydrochloride, and, although less effective, lidocaine hydrochloride p. 92 have all been used. If sinus rhythm is not restored, direct current cardioversion or pacing should be considered. Catheter ablation is an alternative if cessation of the arrhythmia is not urgent. Non-sustained ventricular tachycardia can be treated with a beta-blocker.

All patients presenting with ventricular tachycardia should be referred to a specialist. Following restoration of sinus rhythm, patients who remain at high risk of cardiac arrest will require maintenance therapy. Most patients will be treated with an implantable cardioverter defibrillator. Beta-blockers or sotalol hydrochloride (in place of a standard beta-blocker), or amiodarone hydrochloride (in combination with a standard beta-blocker), can be used in addition to the device in some patients; alternatively, they can be used alone when use of an implantable cardioverter defibrillator is not appropriate.

Torsade de pointes

Torsade de pointes is a form of ventricular tachycardia associated with a long QT syndrome (usually drug-induced, but other factors including hypokalaemia, severe bradycardia, and genetic predisposition are also implicated). Episodes are usually self-limiting, but are frequently recurrent and can cause impairment or loss of consciousness. If not controlled, the arrhythmia can progress to ventricular fibrillation and sometimes death. Intravenous infusion of magnesium sulfate p. 911 is usually effective. A beta-blocker (but not sotalol hydrochloride) and atrial (or ventricular) pacing can be considered. Anti-arrhythmics can further prolong the QT interval, thus worsening the condition.

Drugs for arrhythmias

Anti-arrhythmic drugs can be classified clinically into those that act on supraventricular arrhythmias (e.g. verapamil hydrochloride), those that act on both supraventricular and ventricular arrhythmias (e.g. amiodarone hydrochloride), and those that act on ventricular arrhythmias (e.g. lidocaine hydrochloride).

Anti-arrhythmic drugs can also be classified according to their effects on the electrical behaviour of myocardial cells during activity (the Vaughan Williams classification) although this classification is of less clinical significance:

- Class I: membrane stabilising drugs (e.g. lidocaine, flecainide)
- Class II: beta-blockers
- Class III: amiodarone; sotalol (also Class II)
- Class IV: calcium-channel blockers (includes verapamil but not dihydropyridines)

The negative inotropic effects of anti-arrhythmic drugs tend to be additive. Therefore special care should be taken if two or more are used, especially if myocardial function is impaired. Most drugs that are effective in countering arrhythmias can also provoke them in some circumstances; moreover, hypokalaemia enhances the arrhythmogenic (pro-arrhythmic) effect of many drugs.

Supraventricular arrhythmias

Adenosine p. 96 is usually the treatment of choice for terminating paroxysmal supraventricular tachycardia. As it has a very short duration of action (half-life only about 8 to 10 seconds, but prolonged in those taking dipyridamole p. 111), most side-effects are short lived. Unlike verapamil hydrochloride p. 150, adenosine can be used after a beta-blocker. Verapamil hydrochloride may be preferable to adenosine in asthma.

Oral administration of a **cardiac glycoside** (such as digoxin p. 98) slows the ventricular response in cases of atrial fibrillation and atrial flutter. However, intravenous infusion of digoxin is rarely effective for rapid control of ventricular rate. Cardiac glycosides are contra-indicated in supraventricular arrhythmias associated with accessory conducting pathways (e.g. Wolff- Parkinson-White syndrome).

Verapamil hydrochloride is usually effective for supraventricular tachycardias. An initial intravenous dose (**important:** serious beta-blocker interaction hazard) may be followed by oral treatment; hypotension may occur with large doses. It should not be used for tachyarrhythmias where the QRS complex is wide (i.e. broad complex) unless a supraventricular origin has been established beyond reasonable doubt. It is also contra-indicated in atrial fibrillation or atrial flutter associated with accessory conducting pathways (e.g. Wolff-Parkinson-White syndrome). It should not be used in children with arrhythmias without specialist advice; some supraventricular arrhythmias in childhood can be accelerated by verapamil hydrochloride with dangerous consequences.

Intravenous administration of a **beta-blocker** such as esmolol hydrochloride p. 140 or propranolol hydrochloride p. 136, can achieve rapid control of the ventricular rate.

Drugs for both supraventricular and ventricular arrhythmias include amiodarone hydrochloride p. 94, **beta-blockers**, disopyramide p. 91, flecainide acetate p. 92, **procainamide** (available from 'special-order' manufacturers or specialist importing companies) and propafenone hydrochloride p. 93.

Supraventricular and ventricular arrhythmias

Amiodarone hydrochloride is used in the treatment of arrhythmias, particularly when other drugs are ineffective or contra-indicated. It can be used for paroxysmal supraventricular, nodal and ventricular tachycardias, atrial fibrillation and flutter, and ventricular fibrillation. It can also be used for tachyarrhythmias associated with Wolff-Parkinson- White syndrome. It should be initiated only under hospital or specialist supervision. Amiodarone hydrochloride may be given by intravenous infusion as well as by mouth, and has the advantage of causing little or no myocardial depression. Unlike oral amiodarone hydrochloride, intravenous amiodarone hydrochloride acts relatively rapidly.

Intravenous injection of amiodarone hydrochloride can be used in cardiopulmonary resuscitation for ventricular fibrillation or pulseless tachycardia unresponsive to other interventions.

Amiodarone hydrochloride has a very long half-life (extending to several weeks) and only needs to be given once daily (but high doses can cause nausea unless divided). Many weeks or months may be required to achieve steady-state plasma-amiodarone concentration; this is particularly important when drug interactions are likely.

Beta-blockers act as anti-arrhythmic drugs principally by attenuating the effects of the sympathetic system on automaticity and conductivity within the heart. Sotalol hydrochloride p. 97 has a role in the management of ventricular arrhythmias.

Disopyramide can be given by intravenous injection to control arrhythmias after myocardial infarction (including those not responding to lidocaine hydrochloride p. 92), but it impairs cardiac contractility. Oral administration of disopyramide is useful, but it has an antimuscarinic effect which limits its use in patients susceptible to angle-closure glaucoma or with prostatic hyperplasia.

Flecainide acetate belongs to the same general class as lidocaine hydrochloride and may be of value for serious symptomatic ventricular arrhythmias. It may also be indicated for junctional re-entry tachycardias and for paroxysmal atrial fibrillation. However, it can precipitate serious arrhythmias in a small minority of patients (including those with otherwise normal hearts).

Propafenone hydrochloride is used for the prophylaxis and treatment of ventricular arrhythmias and also for some supraventricular arrhythmias. It has complex mechanisms of action, including weak beta-blocking activity (therefore caution is needed in obstructive airways disease—contra-indicated if severe).

Drugs for supraventricular arrhythmias include adenosine, **cardiac glycosides**, and verapamil hydrochloride. Drugs for ventricular arrhythmias include lidocaine hydrochloride.

Mexiletine and procainamide are both available from 'special-order' manufacturers or specialist importing companies. Mexiletine can be used for life-threatening ventricular arrhythmias; procainamide is given by intravenous injection to control ventricular arrhythmias.

Ventricular arrhythmias

Intravenous lidocaine hydrochloride can be used for the treatment of ventricular tachycardia in haemodynamically stable patients, and ventricular fibrillation and pulseless ventricular tachycardia in cardiac arrest refractory to defibrillation, however it is no longer the anti-arrhythmic drug of first choice.

Drugs for both supraventricular and ventricular arrhythmias include amiodarone hydrochloride, **beta-blockers**, disopyramide, flecainide acetate, **procainamide** (available from 'special- order' manufacturers or specialist importing companies), and propafenone hydrochloride.

Mexiletine is available from 'special-order' manufacturers or specialist importing companies for treatment of life-threatening ventricular arrhythmias.

> **Drugs used for Arrhythmias not listed below** Acebutolol, p. 138 · Atenolol p. 138 · Metoprolol tartrate, p. 140 · Nadolol, p. 135 · Oxprenolol hydrochloride, p. 136

ANTIARRHYTHMICS 〉 CLASS IA

Disopyramide

● **INDICATIONS AND DOSE**

Prevention and treatment of ventricular and supraventricular arrhythmias, including after myocardial infarction | Maintenance of sinus rhythm after cardioversion

▸ BY MOUTH USING IMMEDIATE-RELEASE MEDICINES
▸ Adult: 300–800 mg daily in divided doses
▸ BY MOUTH USING MODIFIED-RELEASE MEDICINES
▸ Adult: 250–375 mg every 12 hours

● CONTRA-INDICATIONS Bundle-branch block associated with first-degree AV block · second- and third-degree AV block or bifascicular block (unless pacemaker fitted) · severe heart failure (unless secondary to arrhythmia) · severe sinus node dysfunction

● CAUTIONS Atrial flutter or atrial tachycardia with partial block · avoid in Acute porphyrias p. 918 · elderly · heart failure (avoid if severe) · myasthenia gravis · prostatic enlargement · structural heart disease · susceptibility to angle-closure glaucoma

● INTERACTIONS → Appendix 1 (disopyramide).

● SIDE-EFFECTS Angle-closure glaucoma · antimuscarinic effects · AV block · blurred vision · cholestatic jaundice · dry mouth · gastro-intestinal irritation · hypoglycaemia · hypotension · myocardial depression · psychosis · urinary retention · ventricular tachycardia, ventricular fibrillation or torsade de pointes (usually associated with prolongation of QRS complex or QT interval)

● PREGNANCY Manufacturer advises use only if potential benefit outweighs risk; may induce labour if used in third trimester.

● BREAST FEEDING Present in milk—use only if essential. Monitor infant for antimuscarinic effects.

● HEPATIC IMPAIRMENT Half-life prolonged—may need dose reduction. Avoid modified-release preparation.

● RENAL IMPAIRMENT Reduce dose by increasing dose interval; adjust according to response. Avoid modified-release preparation.

● MONITORING REQUIREMENTS
▸ Monitor for hypotension, hypoglycaemia, ventricular tachycardia, ventricular fibrillation or torsade de pointes (discontinue if occur).
▸ Monitor serum potassium.

● MEDICINAL FORMS
There can be variation in the licensing of different medicines containing the same drug. Forms available from special-order manufacturers include: capsule, oral suspension, oral solution

Modified-release tablet
CAUTIONARY AND ADVISORY LABELS 25
▸ Rythmodan Retard (Sanofi)
  Disopyramide (as Disopyramide phosphate) 250 mg Rythmodan Retard 250mg tablets | 60 tablet [PoM] £32.08 DT price = £32.08

Capsule
▸ Disopyramide (Non-proprietary)
  Disopyramide 100 mg Disopyramide 100mg capsules | 84 capsule [PoM] £25.00 DT price = £22.09
  Disopyramide 150 mg Disopyramide 150mg capsules | 84 capsule [PoM] £33.40 DT price = £27.58
▸ Rythmodan (Sanofi)
  Disopyramide 100 mg Rythmodan 100mg capsules | 84 capsule [PoM] £14.14 DT price = £22.09

Cardiovascular system

2

ANTIARRHYTHMICS > CLASS IB

Lidocaine hydrochloride

(Lignocaine hydrochloride)

- **INDICATIONS AND DOSE**

Cardiopulmonary resuscitation (as an alternative if amiodarone is not available)
▸ BY INTRAVENOUS INJECTION
▸ Adult: 1 mg/kg, do not exceed 3 mg/kg over the first hour

Ventricular arrhythmias, especially after myocardial infarction in patients without gross circulatory impairment
▸ INITIALLY BY INTRAVENOUS INJECTION
▸ Adult: 100 mg, to be given as a bolus dose over a few minutes, followed immediately by (by intravenous infusion) 4 mg/minute for 30 minutes, then (by intravenous infusion) 2 mg/minute for 2 hours, then (by intravenous infusion) 1 mg/minute, reduce concentration further if infusion continued beyond 24 hours (ECG monitoring and specialist advice for infusion), following intravenous injection lidocaine has a short duration of action (lasting for 15–20 minutes). If an intravenous infusion is not immediately available the initial intravenous injection of 100 mg can be repeated if necessary once or twice at intervals of not less than 10 minutes

Ventricular arrhythmias, especially after myocardial infarction in lighter patients or those whose circulation is severely impaired
▸ INITIALLY BY INTRAVENOUS INJECTION
▸ Adult: Initially 50 mg, to be given as a bolus dose over a few minutes, followed immediately by (by intravenous infusion) 4 mg/minute for 30 minutes, then (by intravenous infusion) 2 mg/minute for 2 hours, then (by intravenous infusion) 1 mg/minute, reduce concentration further if infusion continued beyond 24 hours (ECG monitoring and specialist advice for infusion), following intravenous injection lidocaine has a short duration of action (lasting for 15–20 minutes). If an intravenous infusion is not immediately available the initial intravenous injection of 50 mg can be repeated if necessary once or twice at intervals of not less than 10 minutes

- **CONTRA-INDICATIONS** All grades of atrioventricular block · severe myocardial depression · sino-atrial disorders
- **CAUTIONS** Acute porphyria (consider infusion with glucose for its anti-porphyrinogenic effects) · congestive cardiac failure (consider lower dose) · post cardiac surgery (consider lower dose)
- **INTERACTIONS** → Appendix 1 (lidocaine)
- **SIDE-EFFECTS**
▸ **Common or very common** Bradycardia (may lead to cardiac arrest) · confusion · convulsions · dizziness (particularly if injection too rapid) · drowsiness (particularly if injection too rapid) · hypotension (may lead to cardiac arrest) · paraesthesia (particularly if injection too rapid) · respiratory depression
▸ **Rare** Anaphylaxis
- **PREGNANCY** Crosses the placenta but not known to be harmful in *animal* studies—use if benefit outweighs risk.
- **BREAST FEEDING** Present in milk but amount too small to be harmful.
- **HEPATIC IMPAIRMENT** Caution—increased risk of side-effects.

- **RENAL IMPAIRMENT** Possible accumulation of lidocaine and active metabolite; caution in severe impairment.
- **MONITORING REQUIREMENTS**
▸ Monitor ECG and have resuscitation facilities available.

- **MEDICINAL FORMS**
There can be variation in the licensing of different medicines containing the same drug.
Solution for injection
▸ Lidocaine hydrochloride (Non-proprietary)
Lidocaine hydrochloride 5 mg per 1 ml Lidocaine 50mg/10ml (0.5%) solution for injection ampoules | 10 ampoule [PoM] £7.00
Lidocaine hydrochloride 10 mg per 1 ml Lidocaine 100mg/10ml (1%) solution for injection Mini-Plasco ampoules | 20 ampoule [PoM] £10.89
Lidocaine 100mg/10ml (1%) solution for injection ampoules | 10 ampoule [PoM] £4.50 DT price = £4.01
Lidocaine 100mg/10ml (1%) solution for injection Sure-Amp ampoules | 20 ampoule [PoM] £8.80
Lidocaine 200mg/20ml (1%) solution for injection vials | 10 vial [PoM] £18.00–£19.00
Lidocaine 200mg/20ml (1%) solution for injection ampoules | 10 ampoule [PoM] £7.00–£8.75 DT price = £8.75
Lidocaine 50mg/5ml (1%) solution for injection ampoules | 10 ampoule [PoM] £2.35–£3.10 DT price = £2.36
Lidocaine 20mg/2ml (1%) solution for injection ampoules | 10 ampoule [PoM] £3.50 DT price = £1.98
Lidocaine 50mg/5ml (1%) solution for injection Sure-Amp ampoules | 20 ampoule [PoM] £6.00
Lidocaine hydrochloride 20 mg per 1 ml Lidocaine 100mg/5ml (2%) solution for injection ampoules | 10 ampoule [PoM] £2.40–£3.80 DT price = £2.41
Lidocaine 400mg/20ml (2%) solution for injection vials | 10 vial [PoM] £18.50–£19.50
Lidocaine 200mg/10ml (2%) solution for injection Mini-Plasco ampoules | 20 ampoule [PoM] £14.52
Lidocaine 40mg/2ml (2%) solution for injection ampoules | 10 ampoule [PoM] £4.00 DT price = £2.11
Lidocaine 100mg/5ml (2%) solution for injection Sure-Amp ampoules | 20 ampoule [PoM] £6.00
Lidocaine 400mg/20ml (2%) solution for injection ampoules | 10 ampoule [PoM] £8.00–£9.00 DT price = £9.00

ANTIARRHYTHMICS > CLASS IC

Flecainide acetate

- **INDICATIONS AND DOSE**

AV nodal reciprocating tachycardia, arrhythmias associated with accessory conducting pathways (e.g. Wolff-Parkinson-White syndrome), disabling symptoms of paroxysmal atrial fibrillation in patients without left ventricular dysfunction (arrhythmias of recent onset will respond more readily) (specialist supervision in hospital) | Ventricular tachyarrhythmias resistant to other treatment (specialist supervision in hospital)
▸ INITIALLY BY SLOW INTRAVENOUS INJECTION
▸ Adult: Initially 2 mg/kg (max. per dose 150 mg), to be given over 10–30 minutes with ECG monitoring, followed by (by intravenous infusion) 1.5 mg/kg/hour if required for 1 hour, then (by intravenous infusion) reduced to 100–250 micrograms/kg/hour for up to 24 hours, maximum cumulative dose of 600 mg in first 24 hours, then transfer to oral treatment

Supraventricular arrhythmias
▸ BY MOUTH USING IMMEDIATE-RELEASE MEDICINES
▸ Adult: Initially 50 mg twice daily, increased if necessary up to 300 mg daily
▸ BY MOUTH USING MODIFIED-RELEASE MEDICINES
▸ Adult: 200 mg daily

Ventricular arrhythmias (initiated under direction of hospital consultant)
▶ BY MOUTH USING IMMEDIATE-RELEASE MEDICINES
▸ Adult: Initially 100 mg twice daily for 3–5 days, maximum 400 mg daily reserved for rapid control or in heavily built patients; for maintenance, reduce to the lowest dose that controls the arrhythmia

DOSE EQUIVALENCE AND CONVERSION
Patients stabilised on 200 mg daily immediate-release flecainide may be transferred to modified-release medicines.

● UNLICENSED USE Capsules, tablets and injection: licensed for AV nodal reciprocating tachycardia, arrhythmias associated with accessory conducting pathways (e.g. Wolff-Parkinson-White syndrome), disabling symptoms of paroxysmal atrial fibrillation in patients without left ventricular dysfunction (arrhythmias of recent onset will respond more readily). Immediate-release tablets only: licensed for symptomatic sustained ventricular tachycardia, disabling symptoms of premature ventricular contractions and/or non-sustained ventricular tachycardia in patients resistant to or intolerant of other therapy. Injection only: licensed for ventricular tachyarrhythmias resistant to other treatment.

● CONTRA-INDICATIONS Abnormal left ventricular function · atrial conduction defects (unless pacing rescue available) · bundle branch block (unless pacing rescue available) · control of arrhythmias in acute situations (for modified-release forms only) · distal block (unless pacing rescue available) · haemodynamically significant valvular heart disease · heart failure · history of myocardial infarction and either asymptomatic ventricular ectopics or asymptomatic non-sustained ventricular tachycardia · long-standing atrial fibrillation where conversion to sinus rhythm not attempted · second-degree or greater AV block (unless pacing rescue available) · sinus node dysfunction (unless pacing rescue available)

● CAUTIONS Atrial fibrillation following heart surgery · elderly (accumulation may occur) · patients with pacemakers (especially those who may be pacemaker dependent because stimulation threshold may rise appreciably)

● INTERACTIONS → Appendix 1 (flecainide).

● SIDE-EFFECTS
▸ **Common or very common** Asthenia · dizziness · dyspnoea · fatigue · fever · oedema · pro-arrhythmic effects · visual disturbances
▸ **Rare** Amnesia · confusion · convulsions · depression · dyskinesia · hallucinations · peripheral neuropathy · pneumonitis
▸ **Frequency not known** Anaemia · anorexia · anxiety · ataxia · corneal deposits · drowsiness · flushing · gastrointestinal disturbances · headache · hepatic dysfunction · hypersensitivity reactions · increased antinuclear antibodies · increased sweating · insomnia · leucopenia · paraesthesia · photosensitivity · rash · syncope · thrombocytopenia · tinnitus · tremor · urticaria · vertigo

● PREGNANCY Used in pregnancy to treat maternal and fetal arrhythmias in specialist centres; toxicity reported in *animal* studies; infant hyperbilirubinaemia also reported.

● BREAST FEEDING Significant amount present in milk but not known to be harmful.

● HEPATIC IMPAIRMENT Avoid or reduce dose in severe impairment.

● RENAL IMPAIRMENT Reduce initial oral dose to max. 100 mg daily or reduce intravenous dose by 50%, if eGFR less than 35 mL/minute/1.73 m^2.

● MONITORING REQUIREMENTS
▸ With intravenous use ECG monitoring and resuscitation facilities must be available.

● DIRECTIONS FOR ADMINISTRATION For *intravenous infusion* (*Tambocor®*), give continuously or intermittently in Glucose 5% or Sodium Chloride 0.9%. Minimum volume in infusion fluids containing chlorides 500 mL.

● MEDICINAL FORMS
There can be variation in the licensing of different medicines containing the same drug. Forms available from special-order manufacturers include: oral suspension, oral solution
Tablet
▸ Flecainide acetate (Non-proprietary)
  Flecainide acetate 50 mg Flecainide 50mg tablets | 60 tablet [PoM] £19.50 DT price = £3.02
  Flecainide acetate 100 mg Flecainide 100mg tablets | 60 tablet [PoM] £29.00 DT price = £3.89
▸ Tambocor (Meda Pharmaceuticals Ltd)
  Flecainide acetate 50 mg Tambocor 50mg tablets | 60 tablet [PoM] £11.57 DT price = £3.02
  Flecainide acetate 100 mg Tambocor 100mg tablets | 60 tablet [PoM] £16.53 DT price = £3.89
Modified-release capsule
CAUTIONARY AND ADVISORY LABELS 25
▸ Tambocor XL (Meda Pharmaceuticals Ltd)
  Flecainide acetate 200 mg Tambocor XL 200mg capsules | 30 capsule [PoM] £14.77
Solution for injection
▸ Tambocor (Meda Pharmaceuticals Ltd)
  Flecainide acetate 10 mg per 1 ml Tambocor 150mg/15ml solution for injection ampoules | 5 ampoule [PoM] £21.99

Propafenone hydrochloride

● INDICATIONS AND DOSE

Ventricular arrhythmias (specialist supervision in hospital) | Paroxysmal supraventricular tachyarrhythmias which include paroxysmal atrial flutter or fibrillation and paroxysmal re-entrant tachycardias involving the AV node or accessory pathway, where standard therapy ineffective or contra-indicated (specialist supervision in hospital)
▶ BY MOUTH
▸ Adult: Initially 150 mg 3 times a day, dose to be taken after food, monitor ECG and blood pressure, if QRS interval prolonged by more than 20%, reduce dose or discontinue until ECG returns to normal limits; increased if necessary to 300 mg twice daily (max. per dose 300 mg 3 times a day), dose to be increased at intervals of at least 3 days, reduce total daily dose for patients under 70 kg
▸ Elderly: Initially 150 mg 3 times a day, dose to be taken after food, monitor ECG and blood pressure, if QRS interval prolonged by more than 20%, reduce dose or discontinue until ECG returns to normal limits; increased if necessary to 300 mg twice daily (max. per dose 300 mg 3 times a day), dose to be increased at intervals of at least 5 days, reduce total daily dose for patients under 70 kg

● CONTRA-INDICATIONS Atrial conduction defects (unless adequately paced) · Brugada syndrome · bundle branch block (unless adequately paced) · cardiogenic shock (except arrhythmia induced) · distal block (unless adequately paced) · electrolyte disturbances · marked hypotension · myasthenia gravis · myocardial infarction within last 3 months · second degree or greater AV block (unless adequately paced) · severe bradycardia · severe obstructive pulmonary disease (due to weak beta-blocking activity) · sinus node dysfunction (unless adequately paced) · uncontrolled congestive heart failure with left ventricular ejection fraction less than 35%

- CAUTIONS Elderly · great caution in mild to moderate obstructive airways disease owing to beta-blocking activity · heart failure · pacemaker patients · potential for conversion of paroxysmal atrial fibrillation to atrial flutter with 2:1 or 1:1 conduction block
- INTERACTIONS → Appendix 1 (propafenone).
- SIDE-EFFECTS
  - **Common or very common** Bradycardia · abdominal pain · anxiety · atrioventricular block · blurred vision · chest pain · constipation · diarrhoea · dizziness · dry mouth · dyspnoea · headache · intraventricular blocks · malaise · nausea · palpitation · sino-atrial block · sleep disorders · tachycardia · taste disturbance · vomiting
  - **Uncommon** Abdominal distension · anorexia · ataxia · erectile dysfunction · flatulence · hypotension · paraesthesia · pro-arrhythmic effects · rash · syncope · thrombocytopenia · vertigo
  - **Frequency not known** Agranulocytosis · cholestasis · confusion · convulsions · extrapyramidal symptoms · granulocytopenia · hepatitis · jaundice · leucopenia · lupus erythematosus-like syndrome · reduced sperm count (reversible on withdrawal) · restlessness
- PREGNANCY Use only if potential benefit outweighs risk.
- BREAST FEEDING Use with caution—present in milk.
- PATIENT AND CARER ADVICE
  Driving and skilled tasks
  May affect performance of skilled tasks e.g. driving.

- MEDICINAL FORMS
  There can be variation in the licensing of different medicines containing the same drug. Forms available from special-order manufacturers include: oral suspension, oral solution
  Tablet
  CAUTIONARY AND ADVISORY LABELS 21, 25
  - Propafenone hydrochloride (Non-proprietary)
    Propafenone hydrochloride 150 mg Propafenone 150mg tablets | 90 tablet PoM £7.37 DT price = £7.37
    Propafenone hydrochloride 300 mg Propafenone 300mg tablets | 60 tablet PoM no price available DT price = £9.34
  - Arythmol (BGP Products Ltd)
    Propafenone hydrochloride 150 mg Arythmol 150mg tablets | 90 tablet PoM £7.37 DT price = £7.37
    Propafenone hydrochloride 300 mg Arythmol 300mg tablets | 60 tablet PoM £9.34 DT price = £9.34

ANTIARRHYTHMICS > CLASS III

Amiodarone hydrochloride

- INDICATIONS AND DOSE
  Treatment of arrhythmias, particularly when other drugs are ineffective or contra-indicated (including paroxysmal supraventricular, nodal and ventricular tachycardias, atrial fibrillation and flutter, ventricular fibrillation, and tachyarrhythmias associated with Wolff-Parkinson-White syndrome) (initiated in hospital or under specialist supervision)
  - BY MOUTH
  - Adult: 200 mg 3 times a day for 1 week, then reduced to 200 mg twice daily for a further week, followed by maintenance dose, usually 200 mg daily or the minimum dose required to control arrhythmia
  - BY INTRAVENOUS INFUSION
  - Adult: Initially 5 mg/kg, to be given over 20–120 minutes with ECG monitoring, subsequent infusions given if necessary according to response; maximum 1.2 g per day

Ventricular fibrillation or pulseless ventricular tachycardia refractory to defibrillation (for cardiopulmonary resuscitation)
- INITIALLY BY INTRAVENOUS INJECTION
- Adult: Initially 300 mg, dose to be considered after administration of adrenaline, dose should be given from a pre-filled syringe or diluted in 20 mL Glucose 5%, then (by intravenous injection) 150 mg if required, followed by (by intravenous infusion) 900 mg/24 hours

> IMPORTANT SAFETY INFORMATION
> MHRA/CHM ADVICE: SOFOSBUVIR WITH DACLATASVIR; SOFOSBUVIR AND LEDIPASVIR (MAY 2015); SIMEPREVIR WITH SOFOSBUVIR (AUGUST 2015): RISK OF SEVERE BRADYCARDIA AND HEART BLOCK WHEN TAKEN WITH AMIODARONE
> Avoid concomitant use unless other antiarrhythmics cannot be given.

- CONTRA-INDICATIONS
  GENERAL CONTRA-INDICATIONS
  Avoid in severe conduction disturbances (unless pacemaker fitted) · avoid in sinus node disease (unless pacemaker fitted) · iodine sensitivity · sino-atrial heart block (except in cardiac arrest) · sinus bradycardia (except in cardiac arrest) · thyroid dysfunction
  SPECIFIC CONTRA-INDICATIONS
  - With intravenous use Avoid bolus injection in cardiomyopathy · avoid bolus injection in congestive heart failure · avoid in circulatory collapse · avoid in severe arterial hypotension · avoid in severe respiratory failure
- CAUTIONS
  GENERAL CAUTIONS
  Acute porphyrias p. 918 · conduction disturbances (in excessive dosage) · elderly · heart failure · hypokalaemia · severe bradycardia (in excessive dosage)
  SPECIFIC CAUTIONS
  - With intravenous use Moderate and transient fall in blood pressure (circulatory collapse precipitated by rapid administration or overdosage) · severe hepatocellular toxicity
- INTERACTIONS → Appendix 1 (amiodarone).
  Amiodarone has a long half-life; there is a potential for drug interactions to occur for several weeks (or even months) after treatment with it has been stopped. Use extreme caution or avoid concomitant use of drugs that prolong QT interval.
- SIDE-EFFECTS
  GENERAL SIDE-EFFECTS
  - **Common or very common** Bradycardia · hyperthyroidism · hypothyroidism · jaundice · nausea · persistent slate grey skin discoloration · phototoxicity · pulmonary toxicity (including pneumonitis and fibrosis) · raised serum transaminases (may require dose reduction or withdrawal if accompanied by acute liver disorders) · reversible corneal microdeposits (sometimes with night glare) · sleep disorders · taste disturbances · tremor · vomiting
  - **Uncommon** Conduction disturbances · onset or worsening of arrhythmia · peripheral myopathy (usually reversible on withdrawal) · peripheral neuropathy (usually reversible on withdrawal)
  - **Very rare** Alopecia · aplastic anaemia · ataxia · benign intracranial hypertension · bronchospasm (in patients with severe respiratory failure) · chronic liver disease · cirrhosis · epididymo-orchitis · exfoliative dermatitis · haemolytic anaemia · headache · hypersensitivity · impaired vision due to optic neuritis or optic neuropathy (including blindness) · impotence · rash · sinus arrest · thrombocytopenia · vasculitis · vertigo
  - **Frequency not known** Hot flushes · hypotension · respiratory distress syndrome · sweating

SPECIFIC SIDE-EFFECTS

► **Common or very common**
► With intravenous use Injection-site reactions
► **Very rare**
► With intravenous use Anaphylaxis on rapid injection

SIDE-EFFECTS, FURTHER INFORMATION

► Corneal microdeposits Most patients taking amiodarone develop corneal microdeposits (reversible on withdrawal of treatment); these rarely interfere with vision, but drivers may be dazzled by headlights at night. However, if vision is impaired or if optic neuritis or optic neuropathy occur, amiodarone must be stopped to prevent blindness and expert advice sought.

► Thyroid function Amiodarone contains iodine and can cause disorders of thyroid function; both hypothyroidism and hyperthyroidism can occur. Thyrotoxicosis may be very refractory, and amiodarone should usually be withdrawn at least temporarily to help achieve control; treatment with carbimazole may be required. Hypothyroidism can be treated with replacement therapy without withdrawing amiodarone if it is essential; careful supervision is required.

► Hepatotoxicity Amiodarone is also associated with hepatotoxicity and treatment should be discontinued if severe liver function abnormalities or clinical signs of liver disease develop.

► Pulmonary toxicity Pneumonitis should always be suspected if new or progressive shortness of breath or cough develops in a patient taking amiodarone.

► Peripheral neuropathy Fresh neurological symptoms should raise the possibility of peripheral neuropathy.

● PREGNANCY Possible risk of neonatal goitre; use only if no alternative.

● BREAST FEEDING Avoid; present in milk in significant amounts; theoretical risk of neonatal hypothyroidism from release of iodine.

● MONITORING REQUIREMENTS

► Thyroid function tests should be performed before treatment and then every 6 months. Clinical assessment of thyroid function alone is unreliable. Thyroxine (T4) may be raised in the absence of hyperthyroidism; therefore tri-iodothyronine (T3), T4, and thyroid-stimulating hormone (thyrotrophin, TSH) should all be measured. A raised T3 and T4 with a very low or undetectable TSH concentration suggests the development of thyrotoxicosis.

► Liver function tests required before treatment and then every 6 months.

► Serum potassium concentration should be measured before treatment.

► Chest x-ray required before treatment.

► With intravenous use ECG monitoring and resuscitation facilities must be available. Monitor liver transaminases closely.

  If concomitant use of amiodarone with sofosbuvir and daclatasvir, simeprevir and sofosbuvir, or sofosbuvir and ledipasvir cannot be avoided because other anti-arrhythmics are not tolerated or contra-indicated, patients should be closely monitored, particularly during the first weeks of treatment. Patients at high risk of bradycardia should be monitored continuously for 48 hours in an appropriate clinical setting after starting concomitant treatment. Patients who have stopped amiodarone within the last few months and need to start sofosbuvir and daclatasvir, simeprevir and sofosbuvir, or sofosbuvir and ledipasvir should be monitored.

● DIRECTIONS FOR ADMINISTRATION

► With intravenous use For *intravenous infusion* (*Cordarone X®*), give continuously or intermittently in Glucose 5%. Suggested initial infusion volume 250 mL given over 20–120 minutes; for repeat infusions up to 1.2 g in max. 500 mL; should not be diluted to less than

600 micrograms/mL. See cardio-pulmonary resuscitation for details of infusion in extreme emergency. Incompatible with Sodium Chloride infusion fluids; avoid equipment containing the plasticizer di-2-ethylhexphthalate (DEHP).

► With oral use For administration *by mouth*, tablets may be crushed and dispersed in water; injection solution should **not** be given orally (irritant).

● PATIENT AND CARER ADVICE Because of the possibility of phototoxic reactions, patients should be advised to shield the skin from light during treatment and for several months after discontinuing amiodarone; a wide-spectrum sunscreen to protect against both long-wave ultraviolet and visible light should be used.

  If taking amiodarone with concomitant sofosbuvir and daclatasvir, simeprevir and sofosbuvir, or sofosbuvir and ledipasvir, patients and their carers should be told how to recognise signs and symptoms of bradycardia and heart block and advised to seek immediate medical attention if symptoms such as shortness of breath, light-headedness, palpitations, fainting, unusual tiredness or chest pain develop.

● MEDICINAL FORMS
There can be variation in the licensing of different medicines containing the same drug. Forms available from special-order manufacturers include: oral suspension, oral solution

Tablet
CAUTIONARY AND ADVISORY LABELS 11
► Amiodarone hydrochloride (Non-proprietary)
  Amiodarone hydrochloride 100 mg Amiodarone 100mg tablets | 28 tablet PoM £4.25 DT price = £0.96
  Amiodarone hydrochloride 200 mg Amiodarone 200mg tablets | 28 tablet PoM £7.80 DT price = £1.45
► Cordarone X (Sanofi)
  Amiodarone hydrochloride 100 mg Cordarone X 100 tablets | 28 tablet PoM £4.28 DT price = £0.96
  Amiodarone hydrochloride 200 mg Cordarone X 200 tablets | 28 tablet PoM £6.99 DT price = £1.45

Solution for injection
EXCIPIENTS: May contain Benzyl alcohol
► Amiodarone hydrochloride (Non-proprietary)
  Amiodarone hydrochloride 30 mg per 1 ml Amiodarone 300mg/10ml solution for injection pre-filled syringes | 1 pre-filled disposable injection PoM £13.80
  Amiodarone hydrochloride 50 mg per 1 ml Amiodarone 150mg/3ml concentrate for solution for injection ampoules | 10 ampoule PoM £15.00
► Cordarone X (Sanofi)
  Amiodarone hydrochloride 50 mg per 1 ml Cordarone X 150mg/3ml solution for injection ampoules | 6 ampoule PoM £9.60

Dronedarone

● DRUG ACTION Dronedarone is a multi-channel blocking anti-arrhythmic drug.

● INDICATIONS AND DOSE

Maintenance of sinus rhythm after cardioversion in clinically stable patients with paroxysmal or persistent atrial fibrillation, when alternative treatments are unsuitable (initiated under specialist supervision)
► BY MOUTH
► Adult: 400 mg twice daily

● CONTRA-INDICATIONS Atrial conduction defects · bradycardia · complete bundle branch block · distal block · existing or previous heart failure or left ventricular systolic dysfunction · haemodynamically unstable patients · liver toxicity associated with previous amiodarone use · lung toxicity associated with previous amiodarone use · permanent atrial fibrillation · prolonged QT interval · second- or third- degree AV block · sick sinus syndrome (unless pacemaker fitted) · sinus node dysfunction

Cardiovascular system

2

- CAUTIONS Coronary artery disease · correct hypokalaemia and hypomagnesaemia before starting and during treatment
- INTERACTIONS → Appendix 1 (dronedarone).
- SIDE-EFFECTS
▸ **Common or very common** Bradycardia · gastro-intestinal disturbances · heart failure · malaise · pruritus · QT-interval prolongation · raised serum creatinine · rash
▸ **Uncommon** Dermatitis · eczema · erythema · interstitial lung disease (investigate if symptoms such as dyspnoea or dry cough develop and discontinue treatment if confirmed) · photosensitivity · pneumonitis (investigate if symptoms such as dyspnoea or dry cough develop and discontinue treatment if confirmed) · pulmonary fibrosis (investigate if symptoms such as dyspnoea or dry cough develop and discontinue treatment if confirmed) · taste disturbance
▸ **Rare** Liver injury (including life-threatening acute liver failure)

SIDE-EFFECTS, FURTHER INFORMATION
▸ Liver injury Liver injury, including life-threatening acute liver failure reported rarely; discontinue treatment if 2 consecutive alanine aminotransferase concentrations exceed 3 times upper limit of normal.
▸ Heart failure New onset or worsening heart failure reported. If heart failure or left ventricular systolic dysfunction develops, discontinue treatment.
- PREGNANCY Manufacturer advises avoid—toxicity in *animal* studies.
- BREAST FEEDING Manufacturer advises avoid—present in milk in *animal* studies.
- HEPATIC IMPAIRMENT Avoid in severe impairment.
- RENAL IMPAIRMENT Avoid if eGFR less than 30 mL/minute/1.73 m^2.
- MONITORING REQUIREMENTS
▸ Ongoing monitoring should occur under specialist supervision.
▸ Monitor for heart failure.
▸ Perform ECG at least every 6 months—consider discontinuation if atrial fibrillation reoccurs.
▸ Measure serum creatinine before treatment and 7 days after initiation—if raised, measure again after a further 7 days and consider discontinuation if creatinine continues to rise.
▸ Monitor liver function before treatment, 1 week and 1 month after initiation of treatment, then monthly for 6 months, then every 3 months for 6 months and periodically thereafter.
- PATIENT AND CARER ADVICE
Heart failure Patients or their carers should be told how to recognise signs of heart failure and advised to seek prompt medical attention if symptoms such as weight gain, dependent oedema, or dyspnoea develop or worsen.
Hepatic disorders Patients or their carers should be told how to recognise signs of liver disorder and advised to seek prompt medical attention if symptoms such as abdominal pain, anorexia, nausea, vomiting, fever, malaise, itching, dark urine, or jaundice develop.
- NATIONAL FUNDING/ACCESS DECISIONS

NICE technology appraisals (TAs)
▸ **Dronedarone for the treatment of non-permanent atrial fibrillation** (December 2012) NICE TA197
Dronedarone is an option for the maintenance of sinus rhythm after successful cardioversion in paroxysmal or persistent atrial fibrillation which is not controlled by first-line therapy (usually including beta-blockers), **and** after alternative options have been considered in patients:
  - who have at least 1 of the following cardiovascular risk factors: hypertension requiring drugs of at least 2 different classes, diabetes mellitus, previous transient ischaemic attack, stroke or systemic embolism, left atrial

diameter of 50 mm or greater, or age 70 years or older **and**
  - who do not have left ventricular systolic dysfunction nor a history of, or current, heart failure
Patients who do not meet the above criteria who are currently receiving dronedarone should have the option to continue treatment until they and their clinicians consider it appropriate to stop.
www.nice.org.uk/TA197

- MEDICINAL FORMS
There can be variation in the licensing of different medicines containing the same drug.
Tablet
CAUTIONARY AND ADVISORY LABELS 21
▸ Dronedarone (Non-proprietary)
Dronedarone (as Dronedarone hydrochloride)
400 mg Dronedarone 400mg tablets | 60 tablet [PoM] no price available
▸ Multaq (Sanofi)
Dronedarone (as Dronedarone hydrochloride) 400 mg Multaq 400mg tablets | 20 tablet [PoM] £22.50 DT price = £22.50 | 60 tablet [PoM] £67.50

ANTIARRHYTHMICS ⟩ OTHER

Adenosine

- INDICATIONS AND DOSE

Rapid reversion to sinus rhythm of paroxysmal supraventricular tachycardias, including those associated with accessory conducting pathways (e.g. Wolff-Parkinson-White syndrome) | Used to aid in diagnosis of broad or narrow complex supraventricular tachycardias
▸ BY RAPID INTRAVENOUS INJECTION
▸ Adult: Initially 6 mg, administer into central or large peripheral vein and give over 2 seconds, cardiac monitoring required, followed by 12 mg after 1–2 minutes if required, then 12 mg after 1–2 minutes if required, increments should not be given if high level AV block develops at any particular dose

Rapid reversion to sinus rhythm of paroxysmal supraventricular tachycardias, including those associated with accessory conducting pathways (e.g. Wolff-Parkinson-White syndrome) in patients with a heart transplant | Aid to diagnosis of broad or narrow complex supraventricular tachycardias in patients with a heart transplant
▸ BY RAPID INTRAVENOUS INJECTION
▸ Adult: Initially 3 mg, administer into a central or large peripheral vein and give over 2 seconds, followed by 6 mg after 1–2 minutes if required, then 12 mg after 1–2 minutes if required, patients with a heart transplant are very sensitive to the effects of adenosine

Used in conjunction with radionuclide myocardial perfusion imaging in patients who cannot exercise adequately or for whom exercise is inappropriate
▸ BY INTRAVENOUS INFUSION
▸ Adult: (consult product literature)

DOSE ADJUSTMENTS DUE TO INTERACTIONS
If essential to give with dipyridamole reduce adenosine dose to a quarter of the usual dose.

- UNLICENSED USE Adenosine doses in the BNF may differ from those in the product literature.
- CONTRA-INDICATIONS Asthma · chronic obstructive lung disease · decompensated heart failure · long QT syndrome · second- or third-degree AV block and sick sinus syndrome (unless pacemaker fitted) · severe hypotension
- CAUTIONS Atrial fibrillation with accessory pathway (conduction down anomalous pathway may increase) ·

atrial flutter with accessory pathway (conduction down anomalous pathway may increase) · autonomic dysfunction · bundle branch block · first-degree AV block · heart transplant · left main coronary artery stenosis · left to right shunt · pericardial effusion · pericarditis · QT-interval prolongation · recent myocardial infarction · severe heart failure · stenotic carotid artery disease with cerebrovascular insufficiency · stenotic valvular heart disease · uncorrected hypovolaemia

- INTERACTIONS → Appendix 1 (adenosine); also possibility of interaction with drugs tending to impair myocardial conduction.

- SIDE-EFFECTS
▸ **Common or very common** Angina (discontinue) · apprehension · arrhythmia (discontinue if asystole or severe bradycardia occur) · AV block · dizziness · dyspnoea · flushing · headache · nausea · sinus pause
▸ **Uncommon** Blurred vision · hyperventilation · metallic taste · palpitation · sweating · weakness
▸ **Very rare** Bronchospasm · injection-site reactions · transient worsening of intracranial hypertension
▸ **Frequency not known** Cardiac arrest · convulsions · hypotension (discontinue if severe) · respiratory failure (discontinue) · syncope · vomiting

- PREGNANCY Large doses may produce fetal toxicity; manufacturer advises use only if potential benefit outweighs risk.

- BREAST FEEDING No information available—unlikely to be present in milk owing to short half-life.

- MONITORING REQUIREMENTS Monitor ECG and have resuscitation facilities available.

- DIRECTIONS FOR ADMINISTRATION For *rapid intravenous injection* give over 2 seconds into central or large peripheral vein followed by rapid Sodium Chloride 0.9% flush; injection solution may be diluted with Sodium Chloride 0.9% if required.

- MEDICINAL FORMS
There can be variation in the licensing of different medicines containing the same drug. Forms available from special-order manufacturers include: solution for injection, infusion, solution for infusion

Solution for injection
ELECTROLYTES: May contain Sodium
▸ Adenosine (Non-proprietary)
   Adenosine 3 mg per 1 ml Adenosine 6mg/2ml solution for injection vials | 6 vial [PoM] £26.70–£29.24 (Hospital only)
▸ Adenocor (Sanofi)
   Adenosine 3 mg per 1 ml Adenocor 6mg/2ml solution for injection vials | 6 vial [PoM] £29.94 (Hospital only)

Solution for infusion
ELECTROLYTES: May contain Sodium
▸ Adenosine (Non-proprietary)
   Adenosine 3 mg per 1 ml Adenosine 30mg/10ml solution for infusion vials | 6 vial [PoM] £70.00–£85.57 (Hospital only)
▸ Adenoscan (Sanofi)
   Adenosine 3 mg per 1 ml Adenoscan 30mg/10ml solution for infusion vials | 6 vial [PoM] £85.57

BETA-ADRENOCEPTOR BLOCKERS ⟩
NON-SELECTIVE

F 133

Sotalol hydrochloride

- INDICATIONS AND DOSE

Symptomatic non-sustained ventricular tachyarrhythmias | Prophylaxis of paroxysmal atrial tachycardia or fibrillation, paroxysmal AV re-entrant tachycardias (both nodal and involving accessory pathways), and paroxysmal supraventricular tachycardia after cardiac surgery | Maintenance of sinus rhythm following cardioversion of atrial fibrillation or flutter
▸ BY MOUTH
▸ Adult: Initially 80 mg daily in 1–2 divided doses, then increased to 160–320 mg daily in 2 divided doses, dose to be increased gradually at intervals of 2–3 days

Life-threatening arrhythmias including ventricular tachyarrhythmias
▸ BY MOUTH
▸ Adult: Initially 80 mg daily in 1–2 divided doses, then increased to 160–320 mg daily in 2 divided doses, dose to be increased gradually at intervals of 2–3 days, higher doses of 480–640 mg daily may be required for life-threatening ventricular arrhythmias (under specialist supervision)

IMPORTANT SAFETY INFORMATION
Sotalol may prolong the QT interval, and it occasionally causes life threatening ventricular arrhythmias (**important**: particular care is required to avoid hypokalaemia in patients taking sotalol—electrolyte disturbances, particularly hypokalaemia and hypomagnesaemia should be corrected before sotalol started and during use).

- CONTRA-INDICATIONS Long QT syndrome (congenital or acquired) · torsade de pointes
- CAUTIONS Diarrhoea (severe or prolonged)
- INTERACTIONS Extreme caution or avoid concomitant use of drugs that prolong QT interval.
- SIDE-EFFECTS Arrhythmogenic (pro-arrhythmic) effect (torsade de pointes—increased risk in females)
- BREAST FEEDING Water soluble beta-blockers such as sotalol are present in breast milk in greater amounts than other beta blockers.
- RENAL IMPAIRMENT Use half normal dose if eGFR 30–60 mL/minute/1.73 m^2; use one-quarter normal dose if eGFR 10–30 mL/minute/1.73 m^2. Avoid if eGFR less than 10 mL/minute/1.73 m^2.
- MONITORING REQUIREMENTS Measurement of corrected QT interval, and monitoring of ECG and electrolytes required; correct hypokalaemia, hypomagnesaemia, or other electrolyte disturbances.

- MEDICINAL FORMS
There can be variation in the licensing of different medicines containing the same drug. Forms available from special-order manufacturers include: oral suspension, oral solution

Tablet
CAUTIONARY AND ADVISORY LABELS 8
▸ Sotalol hydrochloride (Non-proprietary)
   Sotalol hydrochloride 40 mg Sotalol 40mg tablets | 28 tablet [PoM] £3.00 DT price = £1.09
   Sotalol hydrochloride 80 mg Sotalol 80mg tablets | 28 tablet [PoM] £3.75 DT price = £1.30 | 56 tablet [PoM] no price available
   Sotalol hydrochloride 160 mg Sotalol 160mg tablets | 28 tablet [PoM] £6.25 DT price = £5.93

▸ Beta-Cardone (Focus Pharmaceuticals Ltd)
Sotalol hydrochloride 200 mg Beta-Cardone 200mg tablets |
28 tablet [PoM] £2.40 DT price = £2.40
▸ Sotacor (Bristol-Myers Squibb Pharmaceuticals Ltd)
Sotalol hydrochloride 80 mg Sotacor 80mg tablets |
30 tablet [PoM] £3.28

CARDIAC GLYCOSIDES

Cardiac glycosides

Digoxin-specific antibody

Serious cases of digoxin toxicity should be discussed with the
National Poisons Information Service (see further
information, under Emergency treatment of poisoning
p. 1194). Digoxin-specific antibody p. 1203 fragments are
indicated for the treatment of known or strongly suspected
life-threatening digoxin toxicity associated with ventricular
arrhythmias or bradyarrhythmias unresponsive to atropine
sulfate p. 1169 and when measures beyond the withdrawal of
digoxin below and correction of any electrolyte
abnormalities are considered necessary.

Digoxin

Digoxin is most useful for controlling ventricular response in
persistent and permanent atrial fibrillation and atrial flutter.
Digoxin also has a role in heart failure.

For management of atrial fibrillation the maintenance
dose of digoxin can usually be determined by the ventricular
rate at rest, which should not usually be allowed to fall
persistently below 60 beats per minute.

Digoxin is now rarely used for rapid control of heart rate
(see management of supraventricular arrhythmias). Even
with intravenous administration, response may take many
hours; persistence of tachycardia is therefore not an
indication for exceeding the recommended dose. The
intramuscular route is **not** recommended.

In patients with heart failure who are in sinus rhythm a
loading dose is not required, and a satisfactory plasma-
digoxin concentration can be achieved over a period of about
a week.

Digoxin has a long half-life and maintenance doses need
to be given only once daily (although higher doses may be
divided to avoid nausea); renal function is the most
important determinant of digoxin dosage.

Unwanted effects depend both on the concentration of
digoxin in the plasma and on the sensitivity of the
conducting system or of the myocardium, which is often
increased in heart disease. It can sometimes be difficult to
distinguish between toxic effects and clinical deterioration
because symptoms of both are similar. The plasma
concentration alone cannot indicate toxicity reliably, but the
likelihood of toxicity increases progressively through the
range 1.5 to 3 micrograms/litre for digoxin. Digoxin should
be used with special care in the elderly, who may be
particularly susceptible to digitalis toxicity.

Regular monitoring of plasma-digoxin concentration
during maintenance treatment is not necessary unless
problems are suspected. Hypokalaemia predisposes the
patient to digitalis toxicity; it is managed by giving a
potassium-sparing diuretic or, if necessary, potassium
supplementation.

If toxicity occurs, digoxin should be withdrawn; serious
manifestations require urgent specialist management.
Digoxin-specific antibody fragments are available for
reversal of life-threatening overdosage.

Digoxin

● DRUG ACTION Digoxin is a cardiac glycoside that increases
the force of myocardial contraction and reduces
conductivity within the atrioventricular (AV) node.

● INDICATIONS AND DOSE

Rapid digitalisation, for atrial fibrillation or flutter
▸ BY MOUTH
▸ Adult: 0.75–1.5 mg in divided doses, dose to be given
over 24 hours, reduce dose in the elderly

Maintenance, for atrial fibrillation or flutter
▸ BY MOUTH
▸ Adult: Maintenance 125–250 micrograms daily, dose
according to renal function and initial loading dose,
reduce dose in the elderly

Heart failure (for patients in sinus rhythm)
▸ BY MOUTH
▸ Adult: 62.5–125 micrograms once daily, reduce dose in
the elderly

Emergency loading dose, for atrial fibrillation or flutter
▸ INITIALLY BY INTRAVENOUS INFUSION
▸ Adult: Loading dose 0.75–1 mg, to be given over at
least 2 hours, then (by mouth) maintenance, loading
dose is rarely necessary, maintenance dose to be
started on the day following the loading dose, reduce
dose in the elderly

DOSE EQUIVALENCE AND CONVERSION
Dose may need to be reduced if digoxin (or another
cardiac glycoside) has been given in the preceding
2 weeks.
When switching from intravenous to oral route may need
to increase dose by 20–33% to maintain the same
plasma-digoxin concentration.

● UNLICENSED USE Digoxin doses in the BNF may differ
from those in product literature.

● CONTRA-INDICATIONS Constrictive pericarditis (unless to
control atrial fibrillation or improve systolic dysfunction—
but use with caution) · hypertrophic cardiomyopathy
(unless concomitant atrial fibrillation and heart failure—
but use with caution) · intermittent complete heart block ·
myocarditis · second degree AV block · supraventricular
arrhythmias associated with accessory conducting
pathways e.g. Wolff-Parkinson-White syndrome (although
can be used in infancy) · ventricular tachycardia or
fibrillation

● CAUTIONS Hypercalcaemia (risk of digitalis toxicity) ·
hypokalaemia (risk of digitalis toxicity) ·
hypomagnesaemia (risk of digitalis toxicity) · hypoxia (risk
of digitalis toxicity) · recent myocardial infarction · severe
respiratory disease · sick sinus syndrome · thyroid disease

● INTERACTIONS → Appendix 1 (cardiac glycosides).

● SIDE-EFFECTS
▸ **Common or very common** Arrhythmias · blurred vision ·
conduction disturbances · diarrhoea · dizziness ·
eosinophilia · nausea · rash · vomiting · yellow vision
▸ **Uncommon** Depression
▸ **Very rare** Anorexia · apathy · confusion · fatigue ·
gynaecomastia on long-term use · headache · intestinal
ischaemia and necrosis · psychosis · thrombocytopenia ·
weakness

Overdose
If toxicity occurs, digoxin should be withdrawn; serious
manifestations require urgent specialist management.

● PREGNANCY May need dosage adjustment.

● BREAST FEEDING Amount too small to be harmful.

● RENAL IMPAIRMENT Reduce dose. Monitor plasma-digoxin
concentration in renal impairment.

- **MONITORING REQUIREMENTS**
- ► For plasma-digoxin concentration assay, blood should be taken at least 6 hours after a dose.
- ► Monitor serum electrolytes and renal function. Toxicity increased by electrolyte disturbances.
- **DIRECTIONS FOR ADMINISTRATION**
- ► With intravenous use Avoid rapid intravenous administration (risk of hypertension and reduced coronary flow). For *intravenous infusion (Lanoxin®)*, give intermittently in Glucose 5% or Sodium chloride 0.9%; dilute to a concentration of not more than 62.5 micrograms/mL. To be given over at least 2 hours.
- ► With oral use For *oral* administration, oral solution must **not** be diluted.
- **PATIENT AND CARER ADVICE** Patient counselling is advised for digoxin elixir (use pipette).

- **MEDICINAL FORMS**
  There can be variation in the licensing of different medicines containing the same drug. Forms available from special-order manufacturers include: oral suspension, oral solution, solution for injection

  Tablet
  - ► Digoxin (Non-proprietary)
    Digoxin 62.5 microgram Digoxin 62.5microgram tablets | 28 tablet [PoM] £9.99 DT price = £2.87 | 500 tablet [PoM] no price available
    Digoxin 125 microgram Digoxin 125microgram tablets | 28 tablet [PoM] £5.02 DT price = £3.02
    Digoxin 250 microgram Digoxin 250microgram tablets | 28 tablet [PoM] £5.09 DT price = £2.85 | 500 tablet [PoM] no price available
  - ► Lanoxin (Aspen Pharma Trading Ltd)
    Digoxin 62.5 microgram Lanoxin PG 62.5microgram tablets | 500 tablet [PoM] £8.09
    Digoxin 125 microgram Lanoxin 125 tablets | 500 tablet [PoM] £8.09
    Digoxin 250 microgram Lanoxin 250microgram tablets | 500 tablet [PoM] £8.09

  Oral solution
  - ► Lanoxin (Aspen Pharma Trading Ltd)
    Digoxin 50 microgram per 1 ml Lanoxin PG 50micrograms/ml elixir | 60 ml [PoM] £5.35 DT price = £5.35

  Solution for injection
  EXCIPIENTS: May contain Alcohol, propylene glycol
  - ► Digoxin (Non-proprietary)
    Digoxin 100 microgram per 1 ml Lanoxin Injection Pediatric 100micrograms/1ml solution for injection ampoules | 10 ampoule [PoM] no price available

  Solution for infusion
  - ► Digoxin (Non-proprietary)
    Digoxin 250 microgram per 1 ml Digoxin 500micrograms/2ml solution for infusion ampoules | 10 ampoule [PoM] £7.00
  - ► Lanoxin (Aspen Pharma Trading Ltd)
    Digoxin 250 microgram per 1 ml Lanoxin 500micrograms/2ml solution for infusion ampoules | 5 ampoule [PoM] £3.30

2   Bleeding disorders

Antifibrinolytic drugs and haemostatics

Overview

Fibrin dissolution can be impaired by the administration of tranexamic acid below, which inhibits fibrinolysis. It can be used to prevent bleeding or to treat bleeding associated with excessive fibrinolysis (e.g. in surgery, dental extraction, obstetric disorders, and traumatic hyphaema) and in the management of menorrhagia. Tranexamic acid may also be used in hereditary angioedema, epistaxis, and in thrombolytic overdose.

Desmopressin p. 603 is used in the management of mild to moderate haemophilia and von Willebrand's disease. It is also used for fibrinolytic response testing.

Etamsylate p. 100 reduces capillary bleeding in the presence of a normal number of platelets; it does not act by fibrin stabilisation, but probably by correcting abnormal adhesion. Etamsylate is less effective than other treatments in the management of heavy menstrual bleeding and its use is no longer recommended.

ANTIHAEMORRHAGICS > ANTIFIBRINOLYTICS

Tranexamic acid

- **INDICATIONS AND DOSE**

  Local fibrinolysis
  - ► BY MOUTH
  - ► Adult: 1–1.5 g 2–3 times a day, alternatively 15–25 mg/kg 2–3 times a day
  - ► INITIALLY BY SLOW INTRAVENOUS INJECTION
  - ► Adult: 0.5–1 g 2–3 times a day, to be administered at a rate not exceeding 100 mg/minute, dose may be followed by continuous infusion; (by continuous intravenous infusion) 25–50 mg/kg, dose to be given over 24 hours

  Menorrhagia
  - ► BY MOUTH
  - ► Adult: 1 g 3 times a day for up to 4 days, to be initiated when menstruation has started; maximum 4 g per day

  Hereditary angioedema
  - ► BY MOUTH
  - ► Adult: 1–1.5 g 2–3 times a day, for short-term prophylaxis of hereditary angioedema, tranexamic acid is started several days before planned procedures which may trigger an acute attack of hereditary angioedema (e.g. dental work) and continued for 2–5 days afterwards

  Epistaxis
  - ► BY MOUTH
  - ► Adult: 1 g 3 times a day for 7 days

  General fibrinolysis
  - ► BY SLOW INTRAVENOUS INJECTION
  - ► Adult: 1 g every 6–8 hours, alternatively 15 mg/kg every 6–8 hours, dose to be given at a rate not exceeding 100 mg/minute

- **UNLICENSED USE** Use of tranexamic acid by continuous intravenous infusion for treatment of local fibrinolysis is an unlicensed route of administration.
- **CONTRA-INDICATIONS** Fibrinolytic conditions following disseminated intravascular coagulation (unless predominant activation of fibrinolytic system with severe bleeding) · history of convulsions · thromboembolic disease
- **CAUTIONS** Irregular menstrual bleeding (establish cause before initiating therapy) · massive haematuria (avoid if risk of ureteric obstruction) · patients receiving oral contraceptives (increased risk of thrombosis)
  CAUTIONS, FURTHER INFORMATION
  - ► Menorrhagia Before initiating treatment for menorrhagia, exclude structural or histological causes or fibroids causing distortion of uterine cavity.
- **SIDE-EFFECTS**
  - ► **Common or very common** Diarrhoea (reduce dose) · nausea · vomiting
  - ► **Uncommon** Dermatitis
  - ► **Rare** Impairment of colour vision (discontinue) · thromboembolic events · visual disturbances (discontinue)
  - ► **Frequency not known** Convulsions (usually with high doses) · hypotension (on rapid intravenous injection) · malaise (on rapid intravenous injection)

- PREGNANCY No evidence of teratogenicity in *animal* studies; manufacturer advises use only if potential benefit outweighs risk—crosses the placenta.
- BREAST FEEDING Small amount present in milk—antifibrinolytic effect in infant unlikely.
- RENAL IMPAIRMENT Reduce dose—consult product literature for details.
- MONITORING REQUIREMENTS Regular liver function tests in long-term treatment of hereditary angioedema.
- DIRECTIONS FOR ADMINISTRATION For *intravenous infusion* (*Cyklokapron®*), give continuously in Glucose 5% or Sodium chloride 0.9%.
- MEDICINAL FORMS There can be variation in the licensing of different medicines containing the same drug. Forms available from special-order manufacturers include: oral suspension, oral solution

Tablet
▸ Tranexamic acid (Non-proprietary)
Tranexamic acid 500 mg Tranexamic acid 500mg tablets | 60 tablet PoM £18.87 DT price = £4.42
▸ Cyklokapron (Meda Pharmaceuticals Ltd)
Tranexamic acid 500 mg Cyklokapron 500mg tablets | 60 tablet PoM £14.30 DT price = £4.42

Solution for injection
▸ Tranexamic acid (Non-proprietary)
Tranexamic acid 100 mg per 1 ml Tranexamic acid 500mg/5ml solution for injection ampoules | 5 ampoule PoM £7.50 (Hospital only) | 10 ampoule PoM £15.47 (Hospital only)
▸ Cyklokapron (Pfizer Ltd)
Tranexamic acid 100 mg per 1 ml Cyklokapron 500mg/5ml solution for injection ampoules | 10 ampoule PoM £15.47

ANTIHAEMORRHAGICS > HAEMOSTATICS

Etamsylate

(Ethamsylate)

- INDICATIONS AND DOSE
Short-term blood loss in menorrhagia
▸ BY MOUTH
▸ Adult: 500 mg 4 times a day during menstruation

- CONTRA-INDICATIONS Acute porphyrias p. 918
- CAUTIONS Exclude structural or histological causes of menorrhagia, or fibroids causing distortion of the uterine cavity, before initiating treatment
- SIDE-EFFECTS Diarrhoea · fever (discontinue treatment) · headache · nausea · rashes · vomiting
- BREAST FEEDING Present in milk—manufacturer advises avoid.
- LESS SUITABLE FOR PRESCRIBING Less suitable for prescribing.
- MEDICINAL FORMS There can be variation in the licensing of different medicines containing the same drug. Forms available from special-order manufacturers include: oral solution

2.1 Coagulation factor deficiencies

BLOOD AND RELATED PRODUCTS > COAGULATION PROTEINS

Dried prothrombin complex

(Human prothrombin complex)

- INDICATIONS AND DOSE
Treatment and peri-operative prophylaxis of haemorrhage in patients with congenital deficiency of factors II, VII, IX, or X if purified specific coagulation factors not available | Treatment and peri-operative prophylaxis of haemorrhage in patients with acquired deficiency of factors II, VII, IX, or X (e.g. during warfarin treatment)
▸ BY INTRAVENOUS INFUSION
▸ Adult: (consult haematologist)

Major bleeding in patients on warfarin following phytomenadione (initiated under specialist supervision)
▸ BY INTRAVENOUS INFUSION
▸ Adult: 25–50 units/kg

- CONTRA-INDICATIONS Angina · history of heparin induced thrombocytopenia · recent myocardial infarction (except in life-threatening haemorrhage following overdosage of oral anticoagulants, and before induction of fibrinolytic therapy)
- CAUTIONS Disseminated intravascular coagulation · history of myocardial infarction or coronary heart disease · postoperative use · risk of thrombosis
- SIDE-EFFECTS
▸ Rare Headache
▸ Very rare Anaphylaxis · antibody formation · hypersensitivity reactions · pyrexia
▸ Frequency not known Disseminated intravascular coagulation · nephrotic syndrome · thrombotic events
- HEPATIC IMPAIRMENT Monitor closely in hepatic impairment (risk of thromboembolic complications).
- PRESCRIBING AND DISPENSING INFORMATION Dried prothrombin complex is prepared from human plasma by a suitable fractionation technique, and contains factor IX, together with variable amounts of factors II, VII, and X.
  Available from CSL Behring (*Beriplix® P/N*), Octapharma (*Octaplex®*).
- MEDICINAL FORMS There can be variation in the licensing of different medicines containing the same drug. No licensed medicines identified.

Factor IX fraction, dried

- INDICATIONS AND DOSE
Treatment and prophylaxis of haemorrhage in congenital factor IX deficiency (haemophilia B)
▸ BY INTRAVENOUS INJECTION, OR BY CONTINUOUS INTRAVENOUS INFUSION
▸ Adult: (consult haematologist)

- CONTRA-INDICATIONS Disseminated intravascular coagulation
- CAUTIONS Risk of thrombosis—principally with former low purity products
- SIDE-EFFECTS Allergic reactions · chills · dizziness · fever · gastro-intestinal disturbances · headache

- **PRESCRIBING AND DISPENSING INFORMATION** Dried factor IX fraction is prepared from human plasma by a suitable fractionation technique; it may also contain clotting factors II, VII, and X.

- **MEDICINAL FORMS**
There can be variation in the licensing of different medicines containing the same drug.

Powder and solvent for solution for injection

▸ AlphaNine (Grifols UK Ltd)

Factor IX high purity 1000 unit AlphaNine 1,000unit powder and solvent for solution for injection vials | 1 vial PoM £390.00
Factor IX high purity 1500 unit AlphaNine 1,500unit powder and solvent for solution for injection vials | 1 vial PoM no price available

▸ Haemonine (Biotest (UK) Ltd)

Factor IX high purity 500 unit Haemonine 500unit powder and solvent for solution for injection vials | 1 vial PoM £255.00 (Hospital only)
Factor IX high purity 1000 unit Haemonine 1,000unit powder and solvent for solution for injection vials | 1 vial PoM £510.00 (Hospital only)

▸ Mononine (CSL Behring UK Ltd)

Factor IX high purity 1000 unit Mononine 1,000unit powder and solvent for solution for injection vials | 1 vial PoM £478.43

▸ Replenine-VF (Bio Products Laboratory Ltd)

Factor IX high purity 500 unit Replenine-VF 500unit powder and solvent for solution for injection vials | 1 vial PoM £180.00 | 10 vial PoM no price available
Factor IX high purity 1000 unit Replenine-VF 1,000unit powder and solvent for solution for injection vials | 1 vial PoM £360.00 | 10 vial PoM no price available

Powder and solvent for solution for infusion

▸ BeneFIX (Pfizer Ltd)

Nonacog alfa 250 unit BeneFIX 250unit powder and solvent for solution for infusion vials | 1 vial PoM £151.80 (Hospital only)
Nonacog alfa 500 unit BeneFIX 500unit powder and solvent for solution for infusion vials | 1 vial PoM £303.60 (Hospital only)
Nonacog alfa 1000 unit BeneFIX 1,000unit powder and solvent for solution for infusion vials | 1 vial PoM £607.20 (Hospital only)
Nonacog alfa 2000 unit BeneFIX 2,000unit powder and solvent for solution for infusion vials | 1 vial PoM £1,214.40 (Hospital only)
Nonacog alfa 3000 unit BeneFIX 3,000unit powder and solvent for solution for infusion vials | 1 vial PoM £1,821.60 (Hospital only)

Factor VIIa (recombinant)

(Eptacog alfa (activated))

- **INDICATIONS AND DOSE**

Treatment and prophylaxis of haemorrhage in patients with haemophilia A or B with inhibitors to factors VIII or IX, acquired haemophilia, factor VII deficiency, or Glanzmann's thrombasthenia

▸ BY INTRAVENOUS INJECTION
▸ Adult: (consult haematologist)

- **CAUTIONS** Disseminated intravascular coagulation · risk of thrombosis

- **SIDE-EFFECTS**
▸ **Uncommon** Deep vein thrombosis · fever · pulmonary embolism · rash · venous thromboembolic events
▸ **Rare** Angina · arterial thrombotic events · cerebrovascular accident · coagulation disorders · headache · myocardial infarction · nausea
▸ **Frequency not known** Anaphylaxis · angioedema · flushing

- **MEDICINAL FORMS**
There can be variation in the licensing of different medicines containing the same drug.

Powder and solvent for solution for injection

▸ NovoSeven (Novo Nordisk Ltd)

Eptacog alfa activated 50000 unit NovoSeven 1mg (50,000units) powder and solvent for solution for injection pre-filled syringes | 1 pre-filled disposable injection PoM £525.20 (Hospital only)
NovoSeven 1mg (50,000units) powder and solvent for solution for injection vials | 1 vial PoM £525.20 (Hospital only)

Eptacog alfa activated 100000 unit NovoSeven 2mg (100,000units) powder and solvent for solution for injection vials | 1 vial PoM £1,050.40 (Hospital only)
NovoSeven 2mg (100,000units) powder and solvent for solution for injection pre-filled syringes | 1 pre-filled disposable injection PoM £1,050.40 (Hospital only)

Eptacog alfa activated 250000 unit NovoSeven 5mg (250,000units) powder and solvent for solution for injection pre-filled syringes | 1 pre-filled disposable injection PoM £2,626.00 (Hospital only)
NovoSeven 5mg (250,000units) powder and solvent for solution for injection vials | 1 vial PoM £2,626.00 (Hospital only)

Eptacog alfa activated 400000 unit NovoSeven 8mg (400,000units) powder and solvent for solution for injection vials | 1 vial PoM £4,201.60 (Hospital only)
NovoSeven 8mg (400,000units) powder and solvent for solution for injection pre-filled syringes | 1 pre-filled disposable injection £4,201.60 (Hospital only)

Factor VIII fraction, dried

(Human coagulation factor VIII, dried)

- **INDICATIONS AND DOSE**

Treatment and prophylaxis of haemorrhage in congenital factor VIII deficiency (haemophilia A), acquired factor VIII deficiency | Von Willebrand's disease

▸ BY INTRAVENOUS INJECTION, OR BY INTRAVENOUS INFUSION, OR BY CONTINUOUS INTRAVENOUS INFUSION
▸ Adult: (consult haematologist)

- **CAUTIONS** Intravascular haemolysis after large or frequently repeated doses in patients with blood groups A, B, or AB—less likely with high potency concentrates

- **SIDE-EFFECTS** Anaphylaxis · angioedema · antibody formation · blurred vision · chills · coughing · dizziness · drowsiness · dyspnoea · fever · flushing · gastro-intestinal disturbances · headache · hypersensitivity reactions · hypotension · palpitation · paraesthesia · taste disturbances · urticaria

- **MONITORING REQUIREMENTS** Monitor for development of factor VIII inhibitors.

- **PRESCRIBING AND DISPENSING INFORMATION** Dried factor VIII fraction is prepared from human plasma by a suitable fractionation technique; it may also contain varying amounts of von Willebrand factor. *Optivate®, Fanhdi®,* and *Octanate®* are not indicated for use in von Willebrand's disease.

  Recombinant human coagulation factor VIII including octocog alfa, moroctocog alfa, and simoctocog alfa are not indicated for use in von Willebrand's disease.

- **MEDICINAL FORMS**
There can be variation in the licensing of different medicines containing the same drug.

Powder and solvent for solution for injection

▸ Advate (Baxalta UK Ltd)

Octocog alfa 250 unit Advate 250unit powder and solvent for solution for injection vials | 1 vial PoM no price available
Octocog alfa 500 unit Advate 500unit powder and solvent for solution for injection vials | 1 vial PoM no price available
Octocog alfa 1000 unit Advate 1,000unit powder and solvent for solution for injection vials | 1 vial PoM no price available
Octocog alfa 2000 unit Advate 2,000unit powder and solvent for solution for injection vials | 1 vial PoM no price available

▸ Elocta (Swedish Orphan Biovitrum Ltd) ▼

Efmoroctocog alfa 250 unit Elocta 250unit powder and solvent for solution for injection vials | 1 vial PoM no price available (Hospital only)
Efmoroctocog alfa 500 unit Elocta 500unit powder and solvent for solution for injection vials | 1 vial PoM no price available (Hospital only)
Efmoroctocog alfa 1000 unit Elocta 1,000unit powder and solvent for solution for injection vials | 1 vial PoM no price available (Hospital only)

Efmoroctocog alfa 1500 unit Elocta 1,500unit powder and solvent for solution for injection vials | 1 vial [PoM] no price available (Hospital only)

Efmoroctocog alfa 2000 unit Elocta 2,000unit powder and solvent for solution for injection vials | 1 vial [PoM] no price available (Hospital only)

Efmoroctocog alfa 3000 unit Elocta 3,000unit powder and solvent for solution for injection vials | 1 vial [PoM] no price available (Hospital only)

▸ Fanhdi (Grifols UK Ltd)

Factor VIII high purity 500 unit Fanhdi 500unit powder and solvent for solution for injection vials | 1 vial [PoM] £165.00 (Hospital only)

Factor VIII high purity 1000 unit Fanhdi 1,000unit powder and solvent for solution for injection vials | 1 vial [PoM] £330.00 (Hospital only)

Factor VIII high purity 1500 unit Fanhdi 1,500unit powder and solvent for solution for injection vials | 1 vial [PoM] £495.00

▸ Haemoctin (Biotest (UK) Ltd)

Factor VIII high purity 250 unit Haemoctin 250unit powder and solvent for solution for injection vials | 1 vial [PoM] £127.50 (Hospital only)

Factor VIII high purity 500 unit Haemoctin 500unit powder and solvent for solution for injection vials | 1 vial [PoM] £255.00 (Hospital only)

Factor VIII high purity 1000 unit Haemoctin 1,000unit powder and solvent for solution for injection vials | 1 vial [PoM] £510.00 (Hospital only)

▸ Helixate NexGen (CSL Behring UK Ltd)

Octocog alfa 250 unit Helixate NexGen 250unit powder and solvent for solution for injection vials | 1 vial [PoM] £118.57

Octocog alfa 500 unit Helixate NexGen 500unit powder and solvent for solution for injection vials | 1 vial [PoM] £237.15

Octocog alfa 1000 unit Helixate NexGen 1,000unit powder and solvent for solution for injection vials | 1 vial [PoM] £474.30

Octocog alfa 2000 unit Helixate NexGen 2,000unit powder and solvent for solution for injection vials | 1 vial [PoM] £948.60

▸ Kogenate (Bayer Plc)

Octocog alfa 250 unit Kogenate Bayer 250unit powder and solvent for solution for injection vials | 1 vial [PoM] £157.50

Octocog alfa 500 unit Kogenate Bayer 500unit powder and solvent for solution for injection vials | 1 vial [PoM] £315.00

Octocog alfa 1000 unit Kogenate Bayer 1,000unit powder and solvent for solution for injection vials | 1 vial [PoM] £630.00

Octocog alfa 2000 unit Kogenate Bayer 2,000unit powder and solvent for solution for injection vials | 1 vial [PoM] £1,260.00

▸ Nuwiq (Octapharma Ltd) ▾

Simoctocog alfa 250 unit Nuwiq 250unit powder and solvent for solution for injection vials | 1 vial [PoM] £190.00 (Hospital only)

Simoctocog alfa 500 unit Nuwiq 500unit powder and solvent for solution for injection vials | 1 vial [PoM] £380.00 (Hospital only)

Simoctocog alfa 1000 unit Nuwiq 1,000unit powder and solvent for solution for injection vials | 1 vial [PoM] £760.00 (Hospital only)

Simoctocog alfa 2000 unit Nuwiq 2,000unit powder and solvent for solution for injection vials | 1 vial [PoM] £1,520.00 (Hospital only)

Powder and solvent for solution for infusion

▸ Advate (Baxalta UK Ltd)

Octocog alfa 1500 unit Advate 1,500unit powder and solvent for solution for infusion vials | 1 vial [PoM] no price available

Octocog alfa 3000 unit Advate 3,000unit powder and solvent for solution for infusion vials | 1 vial [PoM] no price available

▸ Kogenate (Bayer Plc)

Octocog alfa 3000 unit Kogenate Bayer 3,000unit powder and solvent for solution for injection vials | 1 vial [PoM] £1,890.00

Factor XIII fraction, dried

(Human fibrin-stabilising factor, dried)

● **INDICATIONS AND DOSE**

Congenital factor XIII deficiency

▸ BY INTRAVENOUS INJECTION, OR BY INTRAVENOUS INFUSION
▸ Adult: (consult haematologist)

● SIDE-EFFECTS
▸ **Rare** Allergic reactions · fever

● MEDICINAL FORMS
There can be variation in the licensing of different medicines containing the same drug.

Powder and solvent for solution for injection

▸ Fibrogammin P (CSL Behring UK Ltd)

Factor XIII 250 unit Fibrogammin 250unit powder and solvent for solution for injection vials | 1 vial [PoM] £90.59

Factor XIII 1250 unit Fibrogammin 1,250unit powder and solvent for solution for injection vials | 1 vial [PoM] £452.95

Fibrinogen, dried

(Human fibrinogen)

● **INDICATIONS AND DOSE**

Treatment of haemorrhage in congenital hypofibrinogenaemia or afibrinogenaemia

▸ BY INTRAVENOUS INJECTION, OR BY INTRAVENOUS INFUSION
▸ Adult: (consult haematologist)

● CAUTIONS Risk of thrombosis

● SIDE-EFFECTS
▸ **Rare** Allergic reactions · fever
▸ **Very rare** Myocardial infarction · pulmonary embolism · thromboembolic events

● PREGNANCY Manufacturer advises not known to be harmful—no information available.

● BREAST FEEDING Manufacturer advises avoid—no information available.

● PRESCRIBING AND DISPENSING INFORMATION Fibrinogen is prepared from human plasma.

● MEDICINAL FORMS
There can be variation in the licensing of different medicines containing the same drug.

Powder for solution for infusion

▸ Riastap (CSL Behring UK Ltd)

Fibrinogen 1 gram Riastap 1g powder for solution for infusion vials | 1 vial [PoM] £340.00

Protein C concentrate

● **INDICATIONS AND DOSE**

Congenital protein C deficiency

▸ BY INTRAVENOUS INJECTION
▸ Adult: (consult haematologist)

● CAUTIONS Hypersensitivity to heparins

● SIDE-EFFECTS
▸ **Very rare** Bleeding · dizziness · fever · hypersensitivity reactions

● PRESCRIBING AND DISPENSING INFORMATION Protein C is prepared from human plasma.

● MEDICINAL FORMS
There can be variation in the licensing of different medicines containing the same drug.

Powder and solvent for solution for injection

▸ Ceprotin (Baxalta UK Ltd)

Protein C 500 unit Ceprotin 500unit powder and solvent for solution for injection vials | 1 vial [PoM] no price available

Protein C 1000 unit Ceprotin 1000unit powder and solvent for solution for injection vials | 1 vial [PoM] no price available

BLOOD AND RELATED PRODUCTS ›
HAEMOSTATIC PRODUCTS

Factor VIII inhibitor bypassing fraction

- ● **INDICATIONS AND DOSE**

Treatment and prophylaxis of haemorrhage in patients with congenital factor VIII deficiency (haemophilia A) and factor VIII inhibitors | Treatment of haemorrhage in non-haemophiliac patients with acquired factor VIII inhibitors
  ▸ BY INTRAVENOUS INFUSION, OR BY INTRAVENOUS INJECTION
  ▸ Adult: (consult haematologist)

- ● CONTRA-INDICATIONS Disseminated intravascular coagulation
- ● SIDE-EFFECTS Anaphylaxis · disseminated intravascular coagulation · flushing · hypersensitivity · hypotension · myocardial infarction · paraesthesia · pyrexia · rash · thrombosis · urticaria
- ● PRESCRIBING AND DISPENSING INFORMATION
Preparations with factor VIII inhibitor bypassing activity are prepared from human plasma.

- ● MEDICINAL FORMS
There can be variation in the licensing of different medicines containing the same drug.
Powder and solvent for solution for injection
  ▸ FEIBA Imuno (Baxalta UK Ltd)
  Factor VIII inhibitor bypassing fraction 500 unit FEIBA 500unit powder and solvent for solution for injection vials | 1 vial [PoM] no price available
Powder and solvent for solution for infusion
  ▸ FEIBA Imuno (Baxalta UK Ltd)
  Factor VIII inhibitor bypassing fraction 1000 unit FEIBA 1,000unit powder and solvent for solution for infusion vials | 1 vial [PoM] no price available

BLOOD AND RELATED PRODUCTS › PLASMA PRODUCTS

Fresh frozen plasma

- ● **INDICATIONS AND DOSE**

Replacement of coagulation factors or other plasma proteins where their concentration or functional activity is critically reduced
  ▸ BY INTRAVENOUS INFUSION
  ▸ Adult: (consult haematologist)
Major bleeding in patients on warfarin following phytomenadione (if dried prothrombin complex is unavailable)
  ▸ Adult: 15 mL/kilogram

- ● CONTRA-INDICATIONS Avoid use as a volume expander · IgA deficiency with confirmed antibodies to IgA
- ● CAUTIONS Cardiac decompensation · need for compatibility · pulmonary oedema · severe protein S deficiency (avoid products with low protein S activity e.g. OctaplasLG®)
- ● SIDE-EFFECTS
  ▸ **Common or very common** Nausea · pruritus · rash
  ▸ **Uncommon** Oedema · vomiting
  ▸ **Rare** Agitation · allergic reactions · bronchospasm · cardiorespiratory collapse · chills · fever · tachycardia
  ▸ **Very rare** Arrhythmia · hypertension · thromboembolism
- ● PRESCRIBING AND DISPENSING INFORMATION Fresh frozen plasma is prepared from the supernatant liquid obtained by centrifugation of one donation of whole blood.

A preparation of solvent/detergent treated human plasma (frozen) from pooled donors is available from Octapharma (*OctaplasLG®*).

- ● MEDICINAL FORMS
There can be variation in the licensing of different medicines containing the same drug.
No licensed medicines identified.

2.2 Subarachnoid haemorrhage

CALCIUM-CHANNEL BLOCKERS
➤ 142

Nimodipine

- ● DRUG ACTION Nimodipine is a dihydropyridine calcium-channel blocker.

- ● **INDICATIONS AND DOSE**

Prevention of ischaemic neurological defects following aneurysmal subarachnoid haemorrhage
  ▸ BY MOUTH
  ▸ Adult: 60 mg every 4 hours, to be started within 4 days of aneurysmal subarachnoid haemorrhage and continued for 21 days

Treatment of ischaemic neurological defects following aneurysmal subarachnoid haemorrhage
  ▸ BY INTRAVENOUS INFUSION
  ▸ Adult (body-weight up to 70 kg): Initially up to 0.5 mg/hour, increased after 2 hours if no severe fall in blood pressure; increased to 2 mg/hour and continue for at least 5 days (max. 14 days); if surgical intervention during treatment, continue for at least 5 days after surgery; max. total duration of nimodipine use 21 days, to be given via central catheter
  ▸ Adult (body-weight 70 kg and above): Initially 1 mg/hour, increased after 2 hours if no severe fall in blood pressure; increased to 2 mg/hour and continue for at least 5 days (max. 14 days); if surgical intervention during treatment, continue for at least 5 days after surgery; max. total duration of nimodipine use 21 days, to be given via central catheter

Treatment of ischaemic neurological defects following aneurysmal subarachnoid haemorrhage in patients with unstable blood pressure
  ▸ BY INTRAVENOUS INFUSION
  ▸ Adult: Initially up to 0.5 mg/hour, increased after 2 hours if no severe fall in blood pressure; increased to 2 mg/hour and continue for at least 5 days (max. 14 days); if surgical intervention during treatment, continue for at least 5 days after surgery; max. total duration of nimodipine use 21 days, to be given via central catheter

- ● CONTRA-INDICATIONS Acute porphyrias p. 918 · unstable angina · within 1 month of myocardial infarction
- ● CAUTIONS Cerebral oedema · hypotension · severely raised intracranial pressure
- ● INTERACTIONS → Appendix 1 (calcium-channel blockers, alcohol (infusion only)).
Avoid concomitant administration with other calcium-channel blockers, beta-blocker and nephrotoxic drugs.
- ● SIDE-EFFECTS Flushing · gastro-intestinal disorders · headache · hypotension · ileus · nausea · sweating and feeling of warmth · thrombocytopenia · variation in heart-rate
- ● PREGNANCY Manufacturer advises use only if potential benefit outweighs risk.
- ● BREAST FEEDING Manufacturer advises avoid—present in milk.

2

Cardiovascular system

● HEPATIC IMPAIRMENT

Monitoring
Elimination reduced in cirrhosis—monitor blood pressure.

● RENAL IMPAIRMENT

Monitoring
▶ With intravenous use Manufacturer advises monitor renal function closely in renal impairment.

▶ DIRECTIONS FOR ADMINISTRATION Avoid concomitant administration of nimodipine infusion and tablets.

▶ With oral use For administration *by mouth*, tablets may be crushed or halved but are light sensitive—administer immediately.

▶ With intravenous use For *intravenous infusion*, give *via* drip tubing in Glucose 5% or Sodium chloride 0.9%. Not to be added to infusion container; administer via an infusion pump through a Y-piece into a central catheter; incompatible with polyvinyl chloride giving sets or containers; protect infusion from light.

▶ With intravenous use Polyethylene, polypropylene, or glass apparatus should be used. PVC should be avoided.

● MEDICINAL FORMS
There can be variation in the licensing of different medicines containing the same drug. Forms available from special-order manufacturers include: oral suspension

Tablet
▶ Nimotop (Bayer Plc)
Nimodipine 30 mg Nimotop 30mg tablets | 100 tablet [PoM] £40.00

Solution for infusion
▶ Nimotop (Bayer Plc)
Nimodipine 200 microgram per 1 ml Nimotop 0.02% solution for infusion 50ml vials | 5 vial [PoM] £68.00 (Hospital only)

3   Blood clots
3.1   Blocked catheters and lines

> **Drugs used for Blocked catheters and lines not listed below** Heparin (unfractionated), p. 120 · Urokinase, p. 124

ANTITHROMBOTIC DRUGS > PROSTAGLANDINS, CARDIOVASCULAR

Epoprostenol

(Prostacyclin)

● DRUG ACTION Epoprostenol is a prostaglandin and a potent vasodilator. It is also a powerful inhibitor of platelet aggregation.

● INDICATIONS AND DOSE

Inhibition of platelet aggregation during renal dialysis when heparins are unsuitable or contra-indicated | **Treatment of primary pulmonary hypertension resistant to other treatments, usually with oral anti-coagulation (initiated by a specialist)**

▶ BY CONTINUOUS INTRAVENOUS INFUSION
▶ Adult: (consult product literature)

PHARMACOKINETICS
Short half-life of approximately 3 minutes, therefore it must be administered by continuous intravenous infusion.

● CONTRA-INDICATIONS Severe left ventricular dysfunction

● CAUTIONS Avoid abrupt withdrawal when used for primary pulmonary hypertension (risk of rebound pulmonary hypertension) · extreme caution in coronary artery disease · haemorrhagic diathesis · pulmonary veno-occlusive disease · reconstituted solution highly alkaline—avoid

extravasation (irritant to tissues) · risk of pulmonary oedema (dose titration for pulmonary hypertension should be in hospital)

● INTERACTIONS Caution with concomitant use of drugs that increase risk of bleeding.

● SIDE-EFFECTS

▶ **Common or very common** Abdominal pain · anxiety · arthralgia · bleeding · bradycardia · chest pain · diarrhoea · flushing · headache · hypotension · jaw pain · nausea · rash · sepsis · tachycardia · thrombocytopenia · vomiting

▶ **Uncommon** Dry mouth · sweating

▶ **Very rare** Agitation · hyperthyroidism · malaise · pallor

▶ **Frequency not known** Hyperglycaemia · pulmonary oedema (avoid chronic use if occurs during dose titration)

● PREGNANCY Use if potential benefit outweighs risk.

● BREAST FEEDING Manufacturer advises avoid—no information available.

● MONITORING REQUIREMENTS Anticoagulant monitoring required when given with anticoagulants.

● TREATMENT CESSATION Avoid abrupt withdrawal when used for primary pulmonary hypertension (risk of rebound pulmonary hypertension).

● DIRECTIONS FOR ADMINISTRATION For *intravenous infusion* (*Flolan*®), give continuously in Sodium chloride 0.9%; reconstitute using the filter and solvent (glycine buffer diluent) provided to make a concentrate; may be diluted further (consult product literature); for *pulmonary hypertension* dilute further with glycine buffer diluent only and administer via a central venous catheter (can give via peripheral vein until central venous access established); for *renal dialysis* may be diluted further with sodium chloride 0.9%; protect infusion from light. For *intravenous infusion* (*Veletri*®), give continuously in Sodium chloride 0.9%; reconstitute each vial with 5 mL sodium chloride 0.9% then dilute to required concentration with sodium chloride 0.9% (consult product literature); administer through an in-line 0.22 micron filter; for *pulmonary hypertension*, administer via a central venous catheter (can give via peripheral vein until central venous access established); protect infusion from direct sunlight.

● MEDICINAL FORMS
There can be variation in the licensing of different medicines containing the same drug.

Powder for solution for infusion
▶ Veletri (Actelion Pharmaceuticals UK Ltd)
Epoprostenol (as Epoprostenol sodium) 500 microgram Veletri 500microgram powder for solution for infusion vials | 1 vial [PoM] £24.44
Epoprostenol (as Epoprostenol sodium) 1.5 mg Veletri 1.5mg powder for solution for infusion vials | 1 vial [PoM] £49.24

Powder and solvent for solution for infusion
▶ Epoprostenol (Non-proprietary)
Epoprostenol (as Epoprostenol sodium)
500 microgram Epoprostenol 500microgram powder and solvent for solution for infusion vials | 1 vial [PoM] £22.22
Epoprostenol (as Epoprostenol sodium) 1.5 mg Epoprostenol 1.5mg powder and solvent for solution for infusion vials | 1 vial [PoM] £49.24

▶ Flolan (GlaxoSmithKline UK Ltd)
Epoprostenol (as Epoprostenol sodium) 500 microgram Flolan 500microgram powder and solvent for solution for infusion vials | 1 vial [PoM] £22.22
Epoprostenol (as Epoprostenol sodium) 1.5 mg Flolan 1.5mg powder and solvent for solution for infusion vials | 1 vial [PoM] £44.76

3.2   Thromboembolism

Venous thromboembolism

Overview

Venous thromboembolism includes deep-vein thrombosis and pulmonary embolism, and occurs as a result of thrombus formation in a vein.

Prophylaxis of venous thromboembolism

All patients admitted to hospital should undergo a risk assessment for venous thromboembolism on admission. Patients considered to be at high risk include those anticipated to have a substantial reduction in mobility, those with obesity, malignant disease, history of venous thromboembolism, thrombophilic disorder, or patients over 60 years. Patients with risk factors for bleeding (e.g. acute stroke, thrombocytopenia, acquired or untreated inherited bleeding disorders) should only receive pharmacological prophylaxis when the risk of bleeding does not outweigh the risk of venous thromboembolism. NICE clinical guideline 92 (January 2010) provides a full list of risk factors, and gives recommendations for prophylaxis. A venous thromboembolism risk assessment checklist is also available from the Department of Health (www.gov.uk/dh).

Patients scheduled for surgery should be offered mechanical prophylaxis (e.g. anti-embolism stockings) on admission if appropriate; prophylaxis should continue until the patient is sufficiently mobile. Choice of mechanical prophylaxis will depend on factors such as the type of surgery, suitability for the patient, and their condition.

Patients undergoing general or orthopaedic surgery, who are considered to be at high risk of venous thromboembolism, should be offered pharmacological prophylaxis. Choice of prophylaxis will depend on the type of surgery, suitability for the patient, and local policy. A low molecular weight heparin is suitable in all types of general and orthopaedic surgery; heparin (unfractionated) p. 120 is preferred for patients in renal failure. Fondaparinux sodium p. 114 is an option for patients undergoing hip or knee replacement surgery, hip fracture surgery, gastro-intestinal, bariatric, or day surgery procedures. The oral anticoagulants apixaban p. 112, dabigatran etexilate p. 123, and rivaroxaban p. 115 are indicated for thromboprophylaxis following hip or knee replacement surgery.

Pharmacological prophylaxis in general surgery should usually continue for 5–7 days, or until sufficient mobility has been re-established. Pharmacological prophylaxis should be extended to 28 days after major cancer surgery in the abdomen or pelvis. Hip or knee replacement surgery, and hip fracture surgery, require an extended duration of pharmacological prophylaxis, depending on the preparation used (consult product literature).

General medical patients who are considered to be at high risk of venous thromboembolism should be offered pharmacological prophylaxis on admission. Choice of prophylaxis will depend on the medical condition, suitability for the patient, and local policy. Patients should receive either a low molecular weight heparin, heparin (unfractionated) (if patient in renal failure), or fondaparinux sodium. Prophylaxis should continue until the patient is no longer considered to be at significant risk of venous thromboembolism. Mechanical prophylaxis (e.g. anti-embolism stockings) can be offered to medical patients in whom pharmacological prophylaxis is contra-indicated, and continued until the patient is sufficiently mobile.

Edoxaban p. 113, an inhibitor of factor Xa, is given orally for the treatment and prophylaxis of venous thromboembolism, although, it should not be used as an alternative to unfractionated heparin in pulmonary embolism in patients with haemodynamic instability, or who may receive thrombolysis or pulmonary embolectomy. Duration of therapy should be determined by balancing the benefit of treatment with the bleeding risk; shorter duration of treatment (at least 3 months) should be based on transient risk factors i.e. recent surgery, trauma, immobilisation, and longer durations should be based on permanent risk factors or idiopathic deep-vein thrombosis or pulmonary embolism. Edoxaban is also licensed for the prophylaxis of stroke and systemic embolism in patients with non-valvular atrial fibrillation and at least one other risk factor.

Treatment of venous thromboembolism

For the initial treatment of deep-vein thrombosis and pulmonary embolism a low molecular weight heparin is used; alternatively, heparin (unfractionated) is given as an intravenous loading dose, followed by continuous intravenous infusion (using an infusion pump) or (for deep-vein thrombosis only) by intermittent subcutaneous injection. Intermittent intravenous injection of heparin (unfractionated) is no longer recommended. An oral anticoagulant (usually warfarin sodium p. 126) is started at the same time as unfractionated or low molecular weight heparin (the heparin needs to be continued for at least 5 days and until the INR is ≥2 for at least 24 hours). Laboratory monitoring for heparin (unfractionated), preferably on a daily basis, is essential; determination of the activated partial thromboplastin time (APTT) is the most widely used measure (for heparin (unfractionated). A low molecular weight heparin or, in some circumstances, heparin (unfractionated) is also used in regimens for the management of myocardial infarction and unstable angina.

Management of venous thromboembolism in pregnancy

Heparins are used for the management of venous thromboembolism in pregnancy because they do not cross the placenta. Low molecular weight heparins are preferred because they have a lower risk of osteoporosis and of heparin-induced thrombocytopenia. Low molecular weight heparins are eliminated more rapidly in pregnancy, requiring alteration of the dosage regimen for drugs such as dalteparin sodium p. 118, enoxaparin sodium p. 119, and tinzaparin sodium p. 121. Treatment should be stopped at the onset of labour and advice sought from a specialist on continuing therapy after birth.

Extracorporeal circuits

Heparin (unfractionated) is also used in the maintenance of extracorporeal circuits in cardiopulmonary bypass and haemodialysis.

Haemorrhage

If haemorrhage occurs it is usually sufficient to withdraw unfractionated or low molecular weight heparin, but if rapid reversal of the effects of the heparin is required, protamine sulfate p. 1203 is a specific antidote (but only partially reverses the effects of low molecular weight heparins).

Management of stroke

Overview

Stroke is associated with a significant risk of morbidity and mortality. Patients presenting with acute symptoms should be immediately transferred to hospital for accurate diagnosis of stroke type, and urgent initiation of appropriate treatment; patients should be managed by a specialist multidisciplinary stroke team.

The following notes give an overview of the initial and long-term management of transient ischaemic attack, ischaemic stroke, and intracerebral haemorrhage.

Transient ischaemic attack

Patients suspected of having a transient ischaemic attack should immediately receive aspirin p. 109 (patients with aspirin hypersensitivity, or those intolerant of aspirin despite the addition of a proton pump inhibitor, should receive clopidogrel p. 110 [unlicensed use] as an alternative). Following a confirmed diagnosis, patients should receive treatment for secondary prevention (see Long-term Management, under Ischaemic Stroke).

Ischaemic stroke

Initial management

Alteplase p. 199 is recommended in the treatment of acute ischaemic stroke if it can be administered within 4.5 hours of symptom onset; it should be given by medical staff experienced in the administration of thrombolytics and the treatment of acute stroke, preferably within a specialist stroke centre. Treatment with aspirin should be initiated 24 hours after thrombolysis (or as soon as possible within 48 hours of symptom onset in patientsnot receiving thrombolysis); patients with aspirin hypersensitivity, or those intolerant of aspirin despite the addition of a proton pump inhibitor, should receive clopidogrel [unlicensed use] as an alternative.

Anticoagulants are not recommended as an alternative to antiplatelet drugs in acute ischaemic stroke in patients who are in sinus rhythm. However, parenteral anticoagulants may be indicated in patients who are symptomatic of, or at high risk of developing, deep vein thrombosis or pulmonary embolism; warfarin sodium p. 126 should not be commenced in the acute phase of ischaemic stroke.

Anticoagulants should be considered after cardio-embolic ischaemic stroke in patients with atrial fibrillation, however patients presenting with atrial fibrillation following a disabling ischaemic stroke should receive aspirin before being considered for anticoagulant treatment. Patients already receiving anticoagulation for a prosthetic heart valve who experience a disabling ischaemic stroke and are at significant risk of haemorrhagic transformation, should have their anticoagulant treatment stopped for 7 days and substituted with aspirin.

Treatment of hypertension in the acute phase of ischaemic stroke can result in reduced cerebral perfusion, and should therefore only be instituted in the event of a hypertensive emergency, or in those patients considered for thrombolysis.

Long-term management

Patients should receive long-term treatment following a transient ischaemic attack or an ischaemic stroke to reduce the risk of further cardiovascular events.

Following a *transient ischaemic attack*, long-term treatment with modified-release dipyridamole in combination with aspirin is recommended. If patients are intolerant of aspirin, or it is contra-indicated, then modified-release dipyridamole p. 111 alone is recommended; if patients are intolerant of dipyridamole, or it is contra-indicated, then aspirin alone is recommended. Patients who are intolerant of both aspirin and dipyridamole should receive clopidogrel alone [unlicensed use].

Following an *ischaemic stroke* (not associated with atrial fibrillation), clopidogrel is recommended as long-term treatment. If clopidogrel is contra-indicated or not tolerated, patients should receive modified-release dipyridamole in combination with aspirin; if both aspirin and clopidogrel are contra-indicated or not tolerated, then modified-release dipyridamole alone is recommended; if both dipyridamole and clopidogrel are contra-indicated or not tolerated, then aspirin alone is recommended.

Patients with stroke associated with atrial fibrillation should be reviewed for long-term treatment with warfarin sodium or an alternative anticoagulant (see Initial Management under Ischaemic Stroke).

Anticoagulants are not routinely recommended in the long-term prevention of recurrent stroke, except in patients with atrial fibrillation.

A statin should be initiated 48 hours after stroke symptom onset, irrespective of the patient's serum-cholesterol concentration.

Following the acute phase of ischaemic stroke, blood pressure should be measured and treatment initiated to achieve a target blood pressure of <130/80 mmHg. Beta-blockers should not be used in the management of hypertension following a stroke, unless they are indicated for a co-existing condition.

All patients should be advised to make lifestyle modifications that include beneficial changes to diet, exercise, weight, alcohol intake, and smoking.

Intracerebral haemorrhage

Initial Management

Surgical intervention may be required following intracerebral haemorrhage to remove the haematoma and relieve intracranial pressure. Patients taking anticoagulants should have this treatment stopped and reversed; anticoagulant therapy has, however, been used in patients with intracerebral haemorrhage who are symptomatic of deep vein thrombosis or pulmonary embolism; placement of a caval filter is an alternative in this situation.

Long-term management

Aspirin therapy should only be given to patients at a high risk of a cardiac ischaemic event. Anticoagulant therapy is not recommended following an intracerebral haemorrhage, even in those with atrial fibrillation, unless the patient is at very high risk of an ischaemic stroke or cardiac ischaemic events; advice from a specialist should be sought in this situation. Blood pressure should be measured and treatment initiated where appropriate, taking care to avoid hypoperfusion. Statins should be avoided following intracerebral haemorrhage, however they can be used with caution when the risk of a vascular event outweighs the risk of further haemorrhage.

Oral anticoagulants

Overview

The main use of anticoagulants is to prevent thrombus formation or extension of an existing thrombus in the slower-moving venous side of the circulation, where the thrombus consists of a fibrin web enmeshed with platelets and red cells.

Anticoagulants are of less use in preventing thrombus formation in arteries, for in faster-flowing vessels thrombi are composed mainly of platelets with little fibrin.

Coumarins and phenindione

The oral anticoagulants warfarin sodium p. 126, acenocoumarol p. 126 and phenindione p. 126, antagonise the effects of vitamin K, and take at least 48 to 72 hours for the anticoagulant effect to develop fully; warfarin sodium is the drug of choice. If an immediate effect is required, unfractionated or low molecular weight heparin must be given concomitantly.

These oral anticoagulants should not be used in cerebral artery thrombosis or peripheral artery occlusion as first-line therapy; aspirin p. 109 is more appropriate for reduction of risk in transient ischaemic attacks. Unfractionated or a low molecular weight heparin (see under Parenteral anticoagulants p. 108) is usually preferred for the prophylaxis of venous thromboembolism in patients undergoing surgery; alternatively, warfarin sodium can be continued in selected patients currently taking long-term warfarin sodium and who are at high risk of thromboembolism (seek expert advice).

Dose
The base-line prothrombin time should be determined but the initial dose should not be delayed whilst awaiting the result.

Target INR
The following indications and target INRs for adults for warfarin take into account recommendations of the British Society for Haematology guidelines on oral anticoagulation with warfarin—fourth edition. *Br J Haematol* 2011; **154**: 311–324:

An INR which is within 0.5 units of the target value is generally satisfactory; larger deviations require dosage adjustment. Target values (rather than ranges) are now recommended.

INR 2.5 for:

- treatment of deep-vein thrombosis or pulmonary embolism (including those associated with antiphospholipid syndrome or for recurrence in patients no longer receiving warfarin sodium)
- atrial fibrillation
- cardioversion—target INR should be achieved at least 3 weeks before cardioversion and anticoagulation should continue for at least 4 weeks after the procedure (higher target values, such as an INR of 3, can be used for up to 4 weeks before the procedure to avoid cancellations due to low INR)
- dilated cardiomyopathy
- mitral stenosis or regurgitation in patients with either atrial fibrillation, a history of systemic embolism, a left atrial thrombus, or an enlarged left atrium
- bioprosthetic heart valves in the mitral position (treat for 3 months), or in patients with a history of systemic embolism (treat for at least 3 months), or with a left atrial thrombus at surgery (treat until clot resolves), or with other risk factors (e.g. atrial fibrillation or a low ventricular ejection fraction)
- acute arterial embolism requiring embolectomy (consider long-term treatment)
- myocardial infarction

INR 3.5 for:

- recurrent deep-vein thrombosis or pulmonary embolism in patients currently receiving anticoagulation and with an INR above 2;

Mechanical prosthetic heart valves:

- the recommended target INR depends on the type and location of the valve, and patient-related risk factors
- consider increasing the INR target or adding an antiplatelet drug, if an embolic event occurs whilst anticoagulated at the target INR.

Duration
The risks of thromboembolism recurrence and anticoagulant-related bleeding should be considered when deciding the duration of anticoagulation.

The following durations of warfarin sodium for the treatment of deep-vein thrombosis and pulmonary embolism reflect the recommendations of the British Society for Haematology (Guidelines on Oral Anticoagulation with Warfarin—fourth edition. *Br J Haematol* 2011; **154**: 311–324):

- 6 weeks for isolated calf-vein deep-vein thrombosis
- 3 months for venous thromboembolism provoked by surgery or other transient risk factor (e.g. combined oral contraceptive use, pregnancy, plaster cast)
- *at least* 3 months for unprovoked proximal deep-vein thrombosis or pulmonary embolism; long-term anticoagulation may be required.

Haemorrhage
The main adverse effect of all oral anticoagulants is haemorrhage. Checking the INR and omitting doses when appropriate is essential; if the anticoagulant is stopped but not reversed, the INR should be measured 2–3 days later to ensure that it is falling. The cause of an elevated INR should be investigated. The following recommendations (which take into account the recommendations of the British Society for Haematology Guidelines on Oral Anticoagulation with Warfarin—fourth edition. *Br J Haematol* 2011; **154**: 311–324) are based on the result of the INR and whether there is major or minor bleeding; the recommendations apply to adults taking warfarin:

- Major bleeding—stop warfarin sodium; give phytomenadione p. 945 (vitamin K₁) by slow intravenous injection; give dried prothrombin complex p. 100 (factors II, VII, IX, and X); if dried prothrombin complex unavailable, fresh frozen plasma can be given but is less effective; recombinant factor VIIa is not recommended for emergency anticoagulation reversal
- INR >8.0, minor bleeding—stop warfarin sodium; give phytomenadione (vitamin K₁) by slow intravenous injection; repeat dose of phytomenadione if INR still too high after 24 hours; restart warfarin sodium when INR <5.0
- INR >8.0, no bleeding—stop warfarin sodium; give phytomenadione (vitamin K₁) by mouth using the intravenous preparation orally [unlicensed use]; repeat dose of phytomenadione if INR still too high after 24 hours; restart warfarin when INR <5.0
- INR 5.0–8.0, minor bleeding—stop warfarin sodium; give phytomenadione (vitamin K₁) by slow intravenous injection; restart warfarin sodium when INR <5.0
- INR 5.0–8.0, no bleeding—withhold 1 or 2 doses of warfarin sodium and reduce subsequent maintenance dose
- Unexpected bleeding at therapeutic levels—always investigate possibility of underlying cause e.g. unsuspected renal or gastro-intestinal tract pathology

Peri-operative anticoagulation
Warfarin sodium should usually be stopped 5 days before elective surgery; phytomenadione (vitamin K₁) by mouth (using the intravenous preparation orally [unlicensed use]) should be given the day before surgery if the INR is ≥1.5. If haemostasis is adequate, warfarin sodium can be resumed at the normal maintenance dose on the evening of surgery or the next day.

Patients stopping warfarin sodium prior to surgery who are considered to be at high risk of thromboembolism (e.g. those with a venous thromboembolic event within the last 3 months, atrial fibrillation with previous stroke or transient ischaemic attack, or mitral mechanical heart valve) may require interim therapy ('bridging') with a low molecular weight heparin (using treatment dose). The low molecular weight heparin should be stopped at least 24 hours before surgery; if the surgery carries a high risk of bleeding, the low molecular weight heparin should not be restarted until at least 48 hours after surgery.

Patients on warfarin sodium p. 126 who require emergency surgery that can be delayed for 6–12 hours can be given intravenous phytomenadione p. 945 (vitamin K₁) to reverse the anticoagulant effect. If surgery cannot be delayed, dried prothrombin complex p. 100 can be given in addition to intravenous phytomenadione (vitamin K₁) and the INR checked before surgery.

Combined anticoagulant and antiplatelet therapy
Existing antiplatelet therapy following an acute coronary syndrome or percutaneous coronary intervention should be continued for the necessary duration according to the indication being treated. The addition of warfarin sodium, when indicated (e.g. for venous thromboembolism or atrial fibrillation) should be considered following an assessment of

the patient's risk of bleeding and discussion with a cardiologist. The duration of treatment with dual therapy (e.g. aspirin p. 109 and warfarin sodium) or triple therapy (e.g. aspirin with clopidogrel p. 110 and warfarin sodium) should be kept to a minimum where possible. The risk of bleeding with aspirin and warfarin sodium dual therapy is lower than with clopidogrel and warfarin sodium dual therapy Depending on the indications being treated and the patient's risk of thromboembolism, it may be possible to withhold antiplatelet therapy until warfarin sodium therapy is complete, or *vice versa* (on specialist advice) in order to reduce the length of time on dual or triple therapy.

Parenteral anticoagulants

Overview

The main use of anticoagulants is to prevent thrombus formation or extension of an existing thrombus in the slower-moving venous side of the circulation, where the thrombus consists of a fibrin web enmeshed with platelets and red cells.

Anticoagulants are of less use in preventing thrombus formation in arteries, for in faster-flowing vessels thrombi are composed mainly of platelets with little fibrin.

Heparin

Heparin initiates anticoagulation rapidly but has a short duration of action. It is often referred to as **'standard'** or heparin (unfractionated) p. 120 to distinguish it from the **low molecular weight heparins**, which have a longer duration of action. Although a low molecular weight heparin is generally preferred for routine use, heparin (unfractionated) can be used in those at high risk of bleeding because its effect can be terminated rapidly by stopping the infusion.

Low molecular weight heparins

Low molecular weight heparins (dalteparin sodium p. 118, enoxaparin sodium p. 119, and tinzaparin sodium p. 121) are usually preferred over heparin (unfractionated) in the *prevention* of Venous thromboembolism p. 105 because they are as effective and they have a lower risk of heparin-induced thrombocytopenia. The standard prophylactic regimen does not require anticoagulant monitoring. The duration of action of low molecular weight heparins is longer than that of heparin (unfractionated) and *once-daily subcutaneous* administration is possible for some indications, making them convenient to use.

Low molecular weight heparins are generally preferred over heparin (unfractionated) in the *treatment* of deep vein thrombosis and pulmonary embolism, and are also used in the treatment of myocardial infarction, unstable coronary artery disease (see under Acute coronary syndromes p. 195) and for the prevention of clotting in extracorporeal circuits.

Dalteparin sodium and tinzaparin sodium (only 20 000 unit/mL syringe) are also licensed for the extended treatment and prophylaxis of venous thromboembolism in patients with solid tumours; treatment is recommended for a duration of 6 months. Treatment should be initiated by healthcare professionals experienced in the treatment of venous thromboembolism.

Heparinoids

Danaparoid sodium p. 117 is a heparinoid used for prophylaxis of deep-vein thrombosis in patients undergoing general or orthopaedic surgery. Providing there is no evidence of cross-reactivity, it also has a role in patients who develop heparin-induced thrombocytopenia.

Argatroban

An oral anticoagulant can be given with argatroban monohydrate p. 121, but it should only be started once thrombocytopenia has substantially resolved.

Hirudins

Bivalirudin, a hirudin analogue, is a thrombin inhibitor which is licensed for unstable angina or non-ST-segment elevation myocardial infarction in patients planned for urgent or early intervention, and as an anticoagulant for patients undergoing percutaneous coronary intervention (including patients with ST-segment elevation myocardial infarction undergoing primary percutaneous coronary intervention—see also Management of ST-segment elevation myocardial infarction (STEMI) in Acute coronary syndromes p. 195).

Heparin flushes

The use of heparin flushes should be kept to a minimum. For maintaining patency of peripheral venous catheters, sodium chloride injection 0.9% is as effective as heparin flushes. The role of heparin flushes in maintaining patency of arterial and central venous catheters is unclear.

Epoprostenol

Epoprostenol (prostacyclin) can be given to inhibit platelet aggregation during renal dialysis when heparins are unsuitable or contra-indicated. It is also licensed for the treatment of primary pulmonary hypertension resistant to other treatment, usually with oral anticoagulation; it should be initiated by specialists in pulmonary hypertension. Epoprostenol is a potent vasodilator. It has a short half-life of approximately 3 minutes and therefore it must be administered by continuous intravenous infusion.

Fondaparinux

Fondaparinux sodium is a synthetic pentasaccharide that inhibits activated factor X.

> **Drugs used for Thromboembolism not listed below**
> Streptokinase, p. 199

ANTITHROMBOTIC DRUGS > ANTIPLATELET DRUGS

Antiplatelet drugs

Overview

Antiplatelet drugs decrease platelet aggregation and inhibit thrombus formation in the arterial circulation, because in faster-flowing vessels, thrombi are composed mainly of platelets with little fibrin.

Use of aspirin p. 109 in primary prevention of cardiovascular events, in patients with or without diabetes, is of unproven benefit. Long-term use of aspirin is of benefit in established cardiovascular disease (secondary prevention); unduly high blood pressure must be controlled before aspirin is given. If the patient is at a high risk of gastro-intestinal bleeding, a proton pump inhibitor can be added.

Aspirin is given following coronary bypass surgery. It is also used in atrial fibrillation, for intermittent claudication, for stable angina and acute coronary syndromes, for use following placement of coronary stents and for use in stroke.

Clopidogrel p. 110 is licensed for the prevention of atherothrombotic events in patients with a history of symptomatic ischaemic disease. Clopidogrel, in combination with low-dose aspirin, is also licensed for acute coronary syndrome without ST-segment elevation; in these circumstances the combination is given for up to 12 months (most benefit occurs during the first 3 months; there is no evidence of benefit beyond 12 months). Clopidogrel, in combination with low-dose aspirin, is also licensed for acute myocardial infarction with ST-segment elevation; the combination is licensed for at least 4 weeks, but the optimum treatment duration has not been established. In patients undergoing percutaneous coronary intervention, clopidogrel is used as an adjunct with aspirin. Patients who are not already taking clopidogrel should receive a loading dose prior to procedure.

Clopidogrel is also licensed, in combination with low-dose aspirin, for the prevention of atherothrombotic and thromboembolic events in patients with atrial fibrillation (and at least one risk factor for a vascular event), and for whom warfarin sodium p. 126 is unsuitable.

Use of clopidogrel with aspirin increases the risk of bleeding. Clopidogrel monotherapy may be an alternative when aspirin is contra-indicated, for example in those with aspirin hypersensitivity, or when aspirin is not tolerated despite the addition of a proton pump inhibitor (see also NICE guidance).

Clopidogrel also has uses in stroke.

Dipyridamole p. 111 is used by mouth as an adjunct to oral anticoagulation for prophylaxis of thromboembolism associated with prosthetic heart valves. Modified-release preparations are licensed for secondary prevention of ischaemic stroke and transient ischaemic attacks.

Prasugrel p. 197, in combination with aspirin, is licensed for the prevention of atherothrombotic events in patients with acute coronary syndrome undergoing percutaneous coronary intervention; the combination is usually given for up to 12 months.

Ticagrelor p. 197, in combination with aspirin, is licensed for the prevention of atherothrombotic events in patients with acute coronary syndrome; the combination is usually given for up to 12 months.

Cangrelor p. 191, in combination with aspirin, is licensed for the reduction of thrombotic cardiovascular events in patients with coronary artery disease undergoing percutaneous coronary intervention (PCI) who have not received treatment with oral clopidogrel, prasugrel or ticagrelor prior to the procedure and in whom oral therapy with these drugs is not suitable. Cangrelor is to be used under expert supervision only.

Antiplatelet drugs and coronary stents

Patients selected for percutaneous coronary intervention, with the placement of a coronary stent, will require dual antiplatelet therapy with aspirin and either cangrelor, clopidogrel, prasugrel, or ticagrelor. Aspirin therapy should continue indefinitely. Clopidogrel is recommended for 1 month following elective percutaneous coronary intervention with placement of a bare-metal stent, and for 12 months if percutaneous coronary intervention with placement of a bare-metal stent was for an acute coronary syndrome; clopidogrel should be given for 12 months following placement of a drug-eluting stent. Clopidogrel should not be discontinued prematurely in patients with a drug-eluting stent—there is an increased risk of stent thrombosis as a result of the eluted drug slowing the re-endothelialisation process. Patients considered to be at high risk of developing late stent thrombosis with a drug-eluting stent may require a longer duration of treatment with clopidogrel. Prasugrel or ticagrelor are alternatives to clopidogrel in certain patients undergoing percutaneous coronary intervention.

Glycoprotein IIb/IIIa inhibitors

Glycoprotein IIb/IIIa inhibitors prevent platelet aggregation by blocking the binding of fibrinogen to receptors on platelets. Abciximab p. 192 is a monoclonal antibody which binds to glycoprotein IIb/IIIa receptors and to other related sites; it is licensed as an adjunct to heparin (unfractionated) p. 120 and aspirin for the prevention of ischaemic complications in high-risk patients undergoing percutaneous transluminal coronary intervention. Abciximab should be used once only (to avoid additional risk of thrombocytopenia). Eptifibatide p. 192 (in combination with heparin (unfractionated) and aspirin) and tirofiban p. 193 (in combination with heparin (unfractionated), aspirin, and clopidogrel) also inhibit glycoprotein IIb/IIIa receptors; they are licensed for use to prevent early myocardial infarction in patients with unstable angina or non-ST-segment-elevation myocardial infarction. Tirofiban is also licensed for use in combination with heparin (unfractionated), aspirin, and clopidogrel, for the reduction of major cardiovascular events in patients with ST-segment elevation myocardial infarction intended for primary percutaneous coronary intervention. Abciximab, eptifibatide and tirofiban should be used by specialists only.

Epoprostenol p. 104 is also used to inhibit platelet aggregation during renal dialysis when heparins are unsuitable or contra-indicated.

Aspirin

(Acetylsalicylic Acid)

● **INDICATIONS AND DOSE**

Cardiovascular disease (secondary prevention)
▶ BY MOUTH
▸ Adult: 75 mg daily

Management of unstable angina and non-ST-segment elevation myocardial infarction (NSTEMI) | Management of ST-segment elevation myocardial infarction (STEMI)
▶ BY MOUTH
▸ Adult: 300 mg, chewed or dispersed in water

Suspected transient ischaemic attack
▶ BY MOUTH
▸ Adult: 300 mg once daily until diagnosis established

Transient ischaemic attack (long-term treatment in combination with dipyridamole) | Ischaemic stroke not associated with atrial fibrillation (in combination with dipyridamole if clopidogrel contra-indicated or not tolerated) | Ischaemic stroke not associated with atrial fibrillation (used alone if clopidogrel and dipyridamole contra-indicated or not tolerated)
▶ BY MOUTH
▸ Adult: 75 mg once daily

Acute ischaemic stroke
▶ BY MOUTH
▸ Adult: 300 mg once daily for 14 days, to be initiated 24 hours after thrombolysis or as soon as possible within 48 hours of symptom onset in patients not receiving thrombolysis

Atrial fibrillation following a disabling ischaemic stroke (before being considered for anticoagulant treatment)
▶ BY MOUTH
▸ Adult: 300 mg once daily for 14 days

Following disabling ischaemic stroke in patients receiving anticoagulation for a prosthetic heart valve and who are at significant risk of haemorrhagic transformation
▶ BY MOUTH
▸ Adult: 300 mg once daily, anticoagulant treatment stopped for 7 days and to be substituted with aspirin

Following coronary by-pass surgery
▶ BY MOUTH
▸ Adult: 75–300 mg daily

Mild to moderate pain | Pyrexia
▶ BY MOUTH
▸ Adult: 300–900 mg every 4–6 hours as required; maximum 4 g per day continued →

2

Cardiovascular system

▸ BY RECTUM
▸ Adult: 450–900 mg every 4 hours; maximum 3.6 g per day

● CONTRA-INDICATIONS Active peptic ulceration · bleeding disorders (antiplatelet dose) · children under 16 years (risk of Reye's syndrome) · haemophilia · previous peptic ulceration (analgesic dose) · severe cardiac failure (analgesic dose)

CONTRA-INDICATIONS, FURTHER INFORMATION
▸ Reye's syndrome Owing to an association with Reye's syndrome, aspirin-containing preparations should not be given to children under 16 years, unless specifically indicated, e.g. for Kawasaki disease.

● CAUTIONS Allergic disease · anaemia · asthma · dehydration · elderly · G6PD deficiency · preferably avoid during fever or viral infection in children (risk of Reye's syndrome) · previous peptic ulceration (but manufacturers may advise avoidance of low-dose aspirin in history of peptic ulceration) · thyrotoxicosis · uncontrolled hypertension

● INTERACTIONS → Appendix 1 (aspirin).
Caution with concomitant use of drugs that increase risk of bleeding.

● SIDE-EFFECTS Blood disorders (with analgesic doses) · bronchospasm · confusion (with analgesic doses) · gastro-intestinal haemorrhage (occasionally major) · gastro-intestinal irritation (with slight asymptomatic blood loss at higher doses) · haemorrhage including subconjunctival haemorrhage (reported with antiplatelet doses) · increased bleeding time · skin reactions in hypersensitive patients · tinnitus (with analgesic doses)

Overdose
The main features of salicylate poisoning are hyperventilation, tinnitus, deafness, vasodilatation, and sweating. Coma is uncommon but indicates very severe poisoning.
   For specific details on the management of poisoning, see *Aspirin*, under Emergency treatment of poisoning p. 1194.

● ALLERGY AND CROSS-SENSITIVITY Aspirin is **contra-indicated** in history of hypersensitivity to aspirin or any other NSAID—which includes those in whom attacks of asthma, angioedema, urticaria, or rhinitis have been precipitated by aspirin or any other NSAID.

● PREGNANCY Use antiplatelet doses with caution during third trimester; impaired platelet function and risk of haemorrhage; delayed onset and increased duration of labour with increased blood loss; avoid analgesic doses if possible in last few weeks (low doses probably not harmful); high doses may be related to intra-uterine growth restriction, teratogenic effects, closure of fetal ductus arteriosus in utero and possibly persistent pulmonary hypertension of newborn; kernicterus may occur in jaundiced neonates.

● BREAST FEEDING Avoid—possible risk of Reye's syndrome; regular use of high doses could impair platelet function and produce hypoprothrombinaemia in infant if neonatal vitamin K stores low.

● HEPATIC IMPAIRMENT Avoid in severe impairment—increased risk of gastro-intestinal bleeding.

● RENAL IMPAIRMENT Use with caution; avoid in severe impairment; sodium and water retention; deterioration in renal function; increased risk of gastro-intestinal bleeding.

● PRESCRIBING AND DISPENSING INFORMATION BP directs that when no strength is stated the 300 mg strength should be dispensed, and that when soluble aspirin tablets are prescribed, dispersible aspirin tablets shall be dispensed.

● PROFESSION SPECIFIC INFORMATION
Dental practitioners' formulary
Aspirin Dispersible Tablets 300 mg may be prescribed.

● EXCEPTIONS TO LEGAL CATEGORY Can be sold to the public provided packs contain no more than 32 capsules or tablets; pharmacists can sell multiple packs up to a total quantity of 100 capsules or tablets in justifiable circumstances.

● MEDICINAL FORMS
There can be variation in the licensing of different medicines containing the same drug. Forms available from special-order manufacturers include: capsule, oral suspension, oral solution

Tablet
CAUTIONARY AND ADVISORY LABELS 21, 32
▸ Aspirin (Non-proprietary)
Aspirin 75 mg Aspirin 75mg tablets | 28 tablet PoM £1.13 DT price = £0.98
Aspirin 300 mg Aspirin 300mg tablets | 16 tablet GSL no price available | 32 tablet P £3.35 DT price = £3.35 | 32 tablet GSL £3.35 DT price = £3.35 | 100 tablet PoM £10.47

Dispersible tablet
CAUTIONARY AND ADVISORY LABELS 13, 21, 32
▸ Aspirin (Non-proprietary)
Aspirin 75 mg Aspirin 75mg dispersible tablets | 28 tablet GSL £1.04 DT price = £0.68 | 28 tablet P £0.75 DT price = £0.68 | 100 tablet P £0.64 DT price = £2.43 | 100 tablet GSL £1.27 DT price = £2.43 | 1000 tablet PoM £31.28
Aspirin 300 mg Aspirin 300mg dispersible tablets | 32 tablet PoM no price available DT price = £1.09 | 32 tablet P £1.12 DT price = £1.09 | 100 tablet PoM £4.28 DT price = £3.41 | 1000 tablet PoM £37.80

Gastro-resistant tablet
CAUTIONARY AND ADVISORY LABELS 5, 25, 32
▸ Aspirin (Non-proprietary)
Aspirin 75 mg Aspirin 75mg gastro-resistant tablets | 28 tablet GSL £0.80 DT price = £0.73 | 28 tablet P £0.80–£0.93 DT price = £0.73 | 56 tablet PoM no price available | 56 tablet P £1.93 | 56 tablet GSL £1.60
Aspirin 300 mg Aspirin 300mg gastro-resistant tablets | 100 tablet PoM £20.34 DT price = £20.34
▸ Micropirin (Dexcel-Pharma Ltd)
Aspirin 75 mg Micropirin 75mg gastro-resistant tablets | 28 tablet P £1.45 DT price = £0.73 | 56 tablet P £2.87
▸ Nu-Seals (Alliance Pharmaceuticals Ltd)
Aspirin 75 mg Nu-Seals 75 gastro-resistant tablets | 56 tablet P £3.12

Clopidogrel

● INDICATIONS AND DOSE

Prevention of atherothrombotic events in percutaneous coronary intervention (adjunct with aspirin) in patients not already on clopidogrel
▸ BY MOUTH
▸ Adult: Loading dose 300 mg, to be taken prior to the procedure, alternatively loading dose 600 mg, higher dose may produce a greater and more rapid inhibition of platelet aggregation

Transient ischaemic attack for patients with aspirin hypersensitivity, or those intolerant of aspirin despite the addition of a proton pump inhibitor | Acute ischaemic stroke for patients with aspirin hypersensitivity, or those intolerant of aspirin despite the addition of a proton pump inhibitor
▸ BY MOUTH
▸ Adult: 75 mg once daily

Prevention of atherothrombotic events in peripheral arterial disease or within 35 days of myocardial infarction, or within 6 months of ischaemic stroke
▸ BY MOUTH
▸ Adult: 75 mg once daily

Prevention of artherothrombotic events in acute coronary syndrome without ST-segment elevation (given with aspirin)
▶ BY MOUTH
▸ Adult: Initially 300 mg, then 75 mg daily for up to 12 months

Prevention of artherothrombotic events in acute myocardial infarction with ST-segment elevation (given with aspirin)
▶ BY MOUTH
▸ Adult 18-75 years: Initially 300 mg, then 75 mg for at least 4 weeks
▸ Adult 76 years and over: 75 mg daily for at least 4 weeks

Prevention of atherothrombotic and thromboembolic events in patients with atrial fibrillation and at least one risk factor for a vascular event (with aspirin) and for whom warfarin is unsuitable
▶ BY MOUTH
▸ Adult: 75 mg once daily

● UNLICENSED USE 600 mg loading dose prior to percutaneous coronary intervention is an unlicensed dose. Use in transient ischaemic attack or acute ischaemic stroke, in patients with aspirin hypersensitivity or intolerant of aspirin, is unlicensed.

● CONTRA-INDICATIONS Active bleeding

● CAUTIONS Discontinue 7 days before elective surgery if antiplatelet effect not desirable · patients at risk of increased bleeding from trauma, surgery, or other pathological conditions

● INTERACTIONS → Appendix 1 (clopidogrel).
Caution with concomitant use of drugs that increase risk of bleeding.

● SIDE-EFFECTS
▶ Common or very common Abdominal pain · bleeding disorders (including gastro-intestinal and intracranial) · diarrhoea · dyspepsia
▶ Uncommon Constipation · decreased platelets · dizziness · duodenal ulcers · eosinophilia · flatulence · gastric ulcer · gastritis · headache · leucopenia · nausea · paraesthesia · pruritus · rash · vomiting
▶ Rare Vertigo
▶ Very rare Acquired haemophilia · acute liver failure · agranulocytosis · arthralgia · blood disorders · bronchospasm · colitis · confusion · eosinophilic pneumonia · fever · glomerulonephritis · hallucinations · hepatitis · hypersensitivity-like reactions · interstitial pneumonitis · lichen planus · pancreatitis · pancytopenia · severe thrombocytopenia · Stevens-Johnson syndrome · stomatitis · taste disturbance · thrombocytopenic purpura · toxic epidermal necrolysis · vasculitis

● ALLERGY AND CROSS-SENSITIVITY Caution with history of hypersensitivity reactions to thienopyridines (e.g. prasugrel).

● PREGNANCY Manufacturer advises avoid—no information available.

● BREAST FEEDING Manufacturer advises avoid.

● HEPATIC IMPAIRMENT Manufacturer advises caution (risk of bleeding). Avoid in severe impairment.

● RENAL IMPAIRMENT Manufacturer advises caution.

● NATIONAL FUNDING/ACCESS DECISIONS

NICE technology appraisals (TAs)
▶ Clopidogrel and modified-release dipyridamole in the prevention of occlusive vascular events (December 2010)
NICE TA210
The guidance applies to patients who have had an occlusive vascular event, or who have established peripheral arterial disease. The guidance does not apply to patients who have had, or are at risk of, stroke associated with atrial fibrillation, or who need prophylaxis for

occlusive events following coronary revascularisation or carotid artery procedures.
Clopidogrel monotherapy is recommended as an option to prevent occlusive vascular events in patients who have had:
● an ischaemic stroke, or who have peripheral arterial disease or multivascular disease, **or**
● a myocardial infarction, only if aspirin is contra-indicated or not tolerated.
www.nice.org.uk/TA210

Scottish Medicines Consortium (SMC) Decisions
The *Scottish Medicines Consortium* has advised (February 2004) that clopidogrel be accepted for restricted use for the treatment of confirmed acute coronary syndrome (without ST-segment elevation), in combination with aspirin. Clopidogrel should be initiated in hospital inpatients **only**.
The *Scottish Medicines Consortium* has also advised (July 2007) that clopidogrel be accepted for restricted use for patients with ST-segment elevation acute myocardial infarction in combination with aspirin; treatment with clopidogrel is restricted to 4 weeks only.

● MEDICINAL FORMS
There can be variation in the licensing of different medicines containing the same drug. Forms available from special-order manufacturers include: oral suspension, oral solution
Tablet
▶ Clopidogrel (Non-proprietary)
Clopidogrel 75 mg Clopidogrel 75mg tablets | 28 tablet [PoM] £30.53 DT price = £1.48 | 30 tablet [PoM] £38.00
▶ Grepid (Beacon Pharmaceuticals Ltd)
Clopidogrel 75 mg Grepid 75mg tablets | 30 tablet [PoM] £32.28
▶ Plavix (Sanofi)
Clopidogrel 75 mg Plavix 75mg tablets | 30 tablet [PoM] £35.64
Clopidogrel (as Clopidogrel hydrogen sulfate) 300 mg Plavix 300mg tablets | 30 tablet [PoM] £142.54 DT price = £142.54

Dipyridamole

● INDICATIONS AND DOSE

Secondary prevention of ischaemic stroke (not associated with atrial fibrillation) and transient ischaemic attacks (used alone or with aspirin) | Adjunct to oral anticoagulation for prophylaxis of thromboembolism associated with prosthetic heart valves
▶ BY MOUTH USING MODIFIED-RELEASE MEDICINES
▸ Adult: 200 mg twice daily, to be taken preferably with food

Adjunct to oral anticoagulation for prophylaxis of thromboembolism associated with prosthetic heart valves
▶ BY MOUTH USING IMMEDIATE-RELEASE MEDICINES
▸ Adult: 300–600 mg daily in 3–4 divided doses

Myocardial imaging—diagnostic use only
▶ BY INTRAVENOUS INJECTION
▸ Adult: (consult product literature)

● CAUTIONS Aortic stenosis · coagulation disorders · heart failure · hypotension · left ventricular outflow obstruction · may exacerbate migraine · myasthenia gravis (risk of exacerbation) · rapidly worsening angina · recent myocardial infarction

● INTERACTIONS → Appendix 1 (dipyridamole).
Caution with concomitant use of drugs that increase risk of bleeding.

● SIDE-EFFECTS Angioedema · dizziness · gastro-intestinal effects · hot flushes · hypersensitivity reactions · hypotension · increased bleeding after surgery · increased bleeding during surgery · myalgia · rash · severe bronchospasm · tachycardia · throbbing headache · thrombocytopenia · urticaria · worsening symptoms of coronary heart disease

- PREGNANCY Not known to be harmful.
- BREAST FEEDING Manufacturers advise use only if essential—small amount present in milk.
- PRESCRIBING AND DISPENSING INFORMATION Modified-release capsules should be dispensed in original container (pack contains a desiccant) and any capsules remaining should be discarded 6 weeks after opening.
- NATIONAL FUNDING/ACCESS DECISIONS

NICE technology appraisals (TAs)
- Clopidogrel and modified-release dipyridamole in the prevention of occlusive vascular events (December 2010) NICE TA210

The guidance applies to patients who have had an occlusive vascular event, or who have established peripheral arterial disease. The guidance does not apply to patients who have had, or are at risk of, stroke associated with atrial fibrillation, or who need prophylaxis for occlusive events following coronary revascularisation or carotid artery procedures.

Modified-release dipyridamole, in combination with aspirin, is recommended as an option to prevent occlusive vascular events in patients who have had:
- a transient ischaemic attack, **or**
- an ischaemic stroke, only if clopidogrel is contra-indicated or not tolerated.

Modified-release dipyridamole monotherapy is recommended as an option to prevent occlusive vascular events in patients who have had:
- an ischaemic stroke, only if aspirin and clopidogrel are contra-indicated or not tolerated, **or**
- a transient ischaemic attack, only if aspirin is contra-indicated or not tolerated.

www.nice.org.uk/TA210

- MEDICINAL FORMS

There can be variation in the licensing of different medicines containing the same drug. Forms available from special-order manufacturers include: oral suspension, oral solution

Tablet
CAUTIONARY AND ADVISORY LABELS 22
- Dipyridamole (Non-proprietary)
  Dipyridamole 25 mg Dipyridamole 25mg tablets | 84 tablet [PoM] £9.40 DT price = £9.40
  Dipyridamole 100 mg Dipyridamole 100mg tablets | 84 tablet [PoM] £12.50 DT price = £4.48
- Persantin (Boehringer Ingelheim Ltd)
  Dipyridamole 100 mg Persantin 100mg tablets | 84 tablet [PoM] £6.30 DT price = £4.48

Modified-release capsule
CAUTIONARY AND ADVISORY LABELS 21, 25
- Dipyridamole (Non-proprietary)
  Dipyridamole 200 mg Dipyridamole 200mg modified-release capsules | 60 capsule [PoM] £10.06 DT price = £10.06
- Attia (Dr Reddy's Laboratories (UK) Ltd)
  Dipyridamole 200 mg Attia 200mg modified-release capsules | 60 capsule [PoM] £9.56 DT price = £10.06
- Ofcram PR (Focus Pharmaceuticals Ltd)
  Dipyridamole 200 mg Ofcram PR 200mg capsules | 60 capsule [PoM] £10.06 DT price = £10.06
- Persantin Retard (Consilient Health Ltd, Boehringer Ingelheim Ltd)
  Dipyridamole 200 mg Persantin Retard 200mg capsules | 60 capsule [PoM] £8.55–£10.06 DT price = £10.06

Oral suspension
- Dipyridamole (Non-proprietary)
  Dipyridamole 10 mg per 1 ml Dipyridamole 50mg/5ml oral suspension sugar free sugar-free | 150 ml [PoM] £41.06 DT price = £41.06
  Dipyridamole 40 mg per 1 ml Dipyridamole 200mg/5ml oral suspension sugar free sugar-free | 150 ml [PoM] £109.35–£131.22 DT price = £120.29

Solution for injection
- Persantin (Boehringer Ingelheim Ltd)
  Dipyridamole 5 mg per 1 ml Persantin 10mg/2ml solution for injection ampoules | 5 ampoule [PoM] £0.82

Dipyridamole with aspirin

The properties listed below are those particular to the combination only. For the properties of the components please consider, dipyridamole p. 111, aspirin p. 109.

- INDICATIONS AND DOSE

Secondary prevention of ischaemic stroke and transient ischaemic attacks
- BY MOUTH USING MODIFIED-RELEASE MEDICINES
- Adult: 25/200 mg twice daily

- PRESCRIBING AND DISPENSING INFORMATION Dispense in original container (pack contains a desiccant) and discard any capsules remaining 6 weeks after opening.

- MEDICINAL FORMS
There can be variation in the licensing of different medicines containing the same drug.
Modified-release capsule
CAUTIONARY AND ADVISORY LABELS 21, 25, 32
- Dipyridamole with aspirin (Non-proprietary)
  Aspirin 25 mg, Dipyridamole 200 mg Dipyridamole 200mg modified-release / Aspirin 25mg capsules | 100 capsule [PoM] no price available
- Asasantin Retard (Boehringer Ingelheim Ltd)
  Aspirin 25 mg, Dipyridamole 200 mg Asasantin Retard capsules | 60 capsule [PoM] £9.84 DT price = £9.84
- Molita (Dr Reddy's Laboratories (UK) Ltd)
  Aspirin 25 mg, Dipyridamole 200 mg Molita 200mg/25mg modified-release capsules | 100 capsule [PoM] £9.35

ANTITHROMBOTIC DRUGS > FACTOR XA INHIBITORS

Apixaban

- DRUG ACTION Apixaban is a direct inhibitor of activated factor X (factor Xa).

- INDICATIONS AND DOSE

Prophylaxis of venous thromboembolism following knee replacement surgery
- BY MOUTH
- Adult: 2.5 mg twice daily for 10–14 days, to be started 12–24 hours after surgery

Prophylaxis of venous thromboembolism following hip replacement surgery
- BY MOUTH
- Adult: 2.5 mg twice daily for 32–38 days, to be started 12–24 hours after surgery

Treatment of deep-vein thrombosis | Treatment of pulmonary embolism
- BY MOUTH
- Adult: Initially 10 mg twice daily for 7 days, then maintenance 5 mg twice daily

Prophylaxis of recurrent deep-vein thrombosis | Prophylaxis of recurrent pulmonary embolism
- BY MOUTH
- Adult: 2.5 mg twice daily, following completion of 6 months anticoagulant treatment

Prophylaxis of stroke and systemic embolism in non-valvular atrial fibrillation and at least one risk factor such as previous stroke or transient ischaemic attack, symptomatic heart failure, diabetes mellitus, hypertension, or age ≥ 75 years
- BY MOUTH
- Adult 18-79 years: 5 mg twice daily
- Adult 80 years and over (body-weight up to 61 kg): 2.5 mg twice daily
- Adult 80 years and over (body-weight 61 kg and above): 5 mg twice daily

DOSE EQUIVALENCE AND CONVERSION
For information on changing from, or to, other anticoagulants, consult product literature.

- **CONTRA-INDICATIONS** Active bleeding · malignant neoplasms · oesophageal varices · recent brain surgery · recent gastro-intestinal ulcer · recent intracranial haemorrhage · recent ophthalmic surgery · recent spine surgery · significant risk of major bleeding · vascular aneurysm

- **CAUTIONS** Anaesthesia with postoperative indwelling epidural catheter (risk of paralysis—monitor neurological signs and wait 20–30 hours after apixaban dose before removing catheter and do not give next dose until at least 5 hours after catheter removal) · prosthetic heart valve (efficacy not established) · risk of bleeding

- **INTERACTIONS** → Appendix 1 (apixaban). Caution in concomitant use of drugs that increase risk of bleeding.

- **SIDE-EFFECTS**
- **Common or very common** Anaemia · bruising · haemorrhage · nausea
- **Uncommon** Hypotension · rash · thrombocytopenia

- **PREGNANCY** Manufacturer advises avoid—no information available.

- **BREAST FEEDING** Manufacturer advises avoid—present in milk in *animal* studies.

- **HEPATIC IMPAIRMENT** Avoid in severe impairment and in hepatic disease associated with coagulopathy.

- **RENAL IMPAIRMENT**
- When used for prophylaxis of stroke and systemic embolism in atrial fibrillation Reduce dose to 2.5 mg twice daily if creatinine clearance 15–29 mL/minute, or if serum-creatinine ≥133 micromol/litre and age ≥80 years or body-weight ≤60 kg.
- When used for prophylaxis of venous thromboembolism following knee or hip replacement surgery, prophylaxis of recurrent deep-vein thrombosis or pulmonary embolism, and treatment of deep-vein thrombosis or pulmonary embolism Use with caution if creatinine clearance 15–29 mL/minute.

  Manufacturer advises avoid if creatinine clearance less than 15 mL/minute—no information available.

- **MONITORING REQUIREMENTS**
- Patients should be monitored for signs of bleeding or anaemia; treatment should be stopped if severe bleeding occurs.
- No routine anticoagulant monitoring required (INR tests are unreliable).

- **PRESCRIBING AND DISPENSING INFORMATION** Duration of treatment should be determined by balancing the benefit of treatment with the bleeding risk; shorter duration of treatment (at least 3 months) should be based on transient risk factors i.e recent surgery, trauma, immobilisation.

  Apixaban should not be used as an alternative to unfractionated heparin in pulmonary embolism in patients with haemodynamic instability, or who may receive thrombolysis or pulmonary embolectomy.

- **NATIONAL FUNDING/ACCESS DECISIONS**
  NICE technology appraisals (TAs)
- Apixaban for the prevention of venous thromboembolism after total hip or knee replacement in adults (January 2012) NICE TA245
  Apixaban is an option for the prevention of venous thromboembolism in adults after elective hip or knee replacement surgery.
  www.nice.org.uk/TA245
- Apixaban for the prevention of stroke and systemic embolism in non-valvular atrial fibrillation (February 2013) NICE TA275
  Apixaban is an option for the prevention of stroke and systemic embolism in non-valvular atrial fibrillation in

accordance with its licensed indication; with one or more of the following risk factors:
- previous stroke or transient ischaemic attack
- symptomatic heart failure
- age ≥75 years
- diabetes mellitus
- hypertension
The risks and benefits of apixaban compared to warfarin, dabigatran etexilate, and rivaroxaban should be discussed with the patient.
www.nice.org.uk/TA275

- Apixaban for the treatment and secondary prevention of deep vein thrombosis and/or pulmonary embolism (June 2015) NICE TA341
  Apixaban is an option for the treatment and prevention of recurrent deep vein thrombosis and pulmonary embolism in adults.
  www.nice.org.uk/TA341

- **MEDICINAL FORMS**
  There can be variation in the licensing of different medicines containing the same drug.
  Tablet
  - Eliquis (Bristol-Myers Squibb Pharmaceuticals Ltd)
    Apixaban 2.5 mg Eliquis 2.5mg tablets | 10 tablet [PoM] £9.50 | 20 tablet [PoM] £19.00 | 60 tablet [PoM] £57.00 DT price = £57.00
    Apixaban 5 mg Eliquis 5mg tablets | 28 tablet [PoM] £26.60 | 56 tablet [PoM] £53.20 DT price = £53.20

Edoxaban
25.4.2016

- **DRUG ACTION** Edoxaban is a direct and reversible inhibitor of activated factor X (factor Xa), which prevents conversion of prothrombin to thrombin and prolongs clotting time, thereby reducing the risk of thrombus formation.

- **INDICATIONS AND DOSE**

  Prophylaxis of stroke and systemic embolism in non-valvular atrial fibrillation, in patients with at least one risk factor (such as congestive heart failure, hypertension, aged 75 years and over, diabetes mellitus, previous stroke or transient ischaemic attack)
  - BY MOUTH
  - Adult (body-weight up to 61 kg): 30 mg once daily
  - Adult (body-weight 61 kg and above): 60 mg once daily

  Treatment of deep-vein thrombosis | Prophylaxis of recurrent deep-vein thrombosis | Treatment of pulmonary embolism | Prophylaxis of recurrent pulmonary embolism
  - BY MOUTH
  - Adult (body-weight up to 61 kg): 30 mg once daily, duration of treatment adjusted according to risk factors—consult product literature, treatment should follow initial use of parenteral anticoagulant for at least 5 days
  - Adult (body-weight 61 kg and above): 60 mg once daily, duration of treatment adjusted according to risk factors—consult product literature), treatment should follow initial use of parenteral anticoagulant for at least 5 days

  DOSE ADJUSTMENTS DUE TO INTERACTIONS
  Maximum dose of 30 mg once daily with concomitant ciclosporin, dronedarone, erythromycin, or ketoconazole.

  DOSE EQUIVALENCE AND CONVERSION
  For information on changing from, or to, other anticoagulants, consult product literature.

- **CONTRA-INDICATIONS** Active bleeding · arteriovenous malformations · current or recent gastro-intestinal ulceration · hepatic disease (associated with coagulopathy and clinically relevant bleeding risk) · known or suspected oesophageal varices · major intraspinal or intracerebral vascular abnormalities · presence of malignant neoplasms at high risk of bleeding · recent brain or spinal injury · recent brain, spinal or ophthalmic surgery · recent intracranial haemorrhage · uncontrolled severe hypertension · vascular aneurysms

  CONTRA-INDICATIONS, FURTHER INFORMATION
  ▸ **Risk for major bleeding** Edoxaban treatment is contra-indicated in patients with significant risk factors for major bleeding, these include those listed above.
- **CAUTIONS** Moderate to severe mitral stenosis (safety and efficacy not established) · prosthetic heart valve (safety and efficacy not established) · risk of bleeding · surgery
  CAUTIONS, FURTHER INFORMATION
  ▸ **Surgery** Manufacturer recommends to discontinue treatment at least 24 hours before a surgical procedure; the risk of bleeding should be weighed against the urgency of the intervention—consult product literature.
- **INTERACTIONS** → Appendix 1 (edoxaban). Caution with concomitant use of drugs that increase risk of bleeding.
- **SIDE-EFFECTS**
  ▸ **Common or very common** Anaemia · epistaxis · haemorrhage · nausea · pruritus · rash
  ▸ **Uncommon** Urticaria
  ▸ **Rare** Allergic oedema
  SIDE-EFFECTS, FURTHER INFORMATION
  ▸ **Management of bleeding** Should a bleeding complication arise in a patient receiving edoxaban, the manufacturer recommends to delay the next dose or treatment should be discontinued as appropriate.
- **PREGNANCY** Manufacturer advises avoid—toxicity in *animal* studies.
- **BREAST FEEDING** Manufacturer advises avoid—present in milk in *animal* studies.
- **HEPATIC IMPAIRMENT** Manufacturer advises avoid in severe impairment; use with caution in mild to moderate impairment.
- **RENAL IMPAIRMENT** Manufacturer advises reduce dose to 30 mg once daily in moderate to severe impairment; avoid in end-stage renal disease or in patients undergoing dialysis.
- **MONITORING REQUIREMENTS**
  ▸ Manufacturer advises monitor renal function before treatment and when clinically indicated during treatment; monitor hepatic function before treatment and repeat periodically if treatment duration longer than 1 year.
  ▸ Manufacturer advises monitor for signs of mucosal bleeding and anaemia in patients at increased risk; treatment should be stopped if severe bleeding occurs.
  ▸ No routine anticoagulant monitoring required (INR tests are unreliable).
- **PATIENT AND CARER ADVICE** Patients should be provided with an alert card and advised to keep it with them at all times.
- **NATIONAL FUNDING/ACCESS DECISIONS**
  NICE technology appraisals (TAs)
  ▸ Edoxaban for treating and preventing deep vein thrombosis and pulmonary embolism (August 2015) NICE TA354
  Edoxaban (*Lixiana*®) is recommended as an option for treating and preventing recurrent deep vein thrombosis and pulmonary embolism.
  www.nice.org.uk/guidance/ta354
  ▸ Edoxaban for preventing stroke and systemic embolism in non-valvular atrial fibrillation (September 2015) NICE TA355
  Edoxaban (*Lixiana*®) is an option for the prevention of stroke and systemic embolism in non-valvular atrial fibrillation, with one or more of the following risk factors:

- previous stroke or transient ischaemic attack
- congestive heart failure
- age ≥75 years
- diabetes mellitus
- hypertension

The risks and benefits of edoxaban treatment compared to warfarin, apixaban, dabigatran etexilate, and rivaroxaban should be discussed with the patient.
www.nice.org.uk/TA355

- **MEDICINAL FORMS**
  There can be variation in the licensing of different medicines containing the same drug.
  Tablet
  ▸ Lixiana (Daiichi Sankyo UK Ltd) ▼
  Edoxaban (as Edoxaban tosilate) 15 mg Lixiana 15mg tablets | 10 tablet [PoM] £18.50
  Edoxaban (as Edoxaban tosilate) 30 mg Lixiana 30mg tablets | 28 tablet [PoM] £51.80
  Edoxaban (as Edoxaban tosilate) 60 mg Lixiana 60mg tablets | 28 tablet [PoM] £51.80

Fondaparinux sodium

- **DRUG ACTION** Fondaparinux sodium is a synthetic pentasaccharide that inhibits activated factor X.

- **INDICATIONS AND DOSE**
  Prophylaxis of venous thromboembolism in patients after undergoing major orthopaedic surgery of the hip or leg, or abdominal surgery
  ▸ BY SUBCUTANEOUS INJECTION
  ▸ Adult: Initially 2.5 mg, dose to be given 6 hours after surgery, then 2.5 mg once daily
  Prophylaxis of venous thromboembolism in medical patients immobilised because of acute illness
  ▸ BY SUBCUTANEOUS INJECTION
  ▸ Adult: 2.5 mg once daily
  Treatment of superficial-vein thrombosis
  ▸ BY SUBCUTANEOUS INJECTION
  ▸ Adult (body-weight 50 kg and above): 2.5 mg once daily for at least 30 days (max. 45 days if high risk of thromboembolic complications), treatment should be stopped 24 hours before surgery and restarted at least 6 hours post operatively
  Treatment of unstable angina and non-ST-segment elevation myocardial infarction
  ▸ BY SUBCUTANEOUS INJECTION
  ▸ Adult: 2.5 mg once daily for up to 8 days (or until hospital discharge if sooner), treatment should be stopped 24 hours before coronary artery bypass graft surgery (where possible) and restarted 48 hours post operatively
  Treatment of ST-segment elevation myocardial infarction
  ▸ INITIALLY BY INTRAVENOUS INJECTION, OR BY INTRAVENOUS INFUSION
  ▸ Adult: Initially 2.5 mg daily for the first day, then (by subcutaneous injection) 2.5 mg once daily for up to 8 days (or until hospital discharge if sooner), treatment should be stopped 24 hours before coronary artery bypass graft surgery (where possible) and restarted 48 hours post operatively
  Treatment of deep-vein thrombosis and pulmonary embolism
  ▸ BY SUBCUTANEOUS INJECTION
  ▸ Adult (body-weight up to 50 kg): 5 mg every 24 hours, an oral anticoagulant (usually warfarin) is started at the same time as fondaparinux (fondaparinux should be continued for at least 5 days and until INR ≥ 2 for at least 24 hours)

▸ Adult (body-weight 50-100 kg): 7.5 mg every 24 hours, an oral anticoagulant (usually warfarin) is started at the same time as fondaparinux (fondaparinux should be continued for at least 5 days and until INR $\geq$ 2 for at least 24 hours)

▸ Adult (body-weight 101 kg and above): 10 mg every 24 hours, an oral anticoagulant (usually warfarin) is started at the same time as fondaparinux (fondaparinux should be continued for at least 5 days and until INR $\geq$ 2 for at least 24 hours)

● **CONTRA-INDICATIONS** Active bleeding · bacterial endocarditis

● **CAUTIONS** Active gastro-intestinal ulcer disease · bleeding disorders · brain surgery · elderly patients · low body-weight · ophthalmic surgery · recent intracranial haemorrhage · risk of catheter thrombus during percutaneous coronary intervention · spinal or epidural anaesthesia (risk of spinal haematoma—avoid if using treatment doses) · spinal surgery

● **INTERACTIONS** → Appendix 1 (fondaparinux). Caution with concomitant use of drugs that increase risk of bleeding.

● **SIDE-EFFECTS**

▸ **Common or very common** Anaemia · bleeding · purpura

▸ **Uncommon** Chest pain · dyspnoea · gastro-intestinal disturbances · hepatic impairment · oedema · pruritus · rash · thrombocythaemia · thrombocytopenia

▸ **Rare** Anxiety · confusion · cough · dizziness · drowsiness · flushing · headache · hyperbilirubinaemia · hypokalaemia · hypotension · injection-site reactions · vertigo

▸ **Frequency not known** Atrial fibrillation · pyrexia · tachycardia

● **PREGNANCY** Manufacturer advises avoid unless potential benefit outweighs possible risk—no information available.

● **BREAST FEEDING** Present in milk in *animal* studies—manufacturer advises avoid.

● **HEPATIC IMPAIRMENT** Caution in severe impairment (increased risk of bleeding).

● **RENAL IMPAIRMENT**

▸ When used for prophylaxis of venous thromboembolism and treatment of superficial-vein thrombosis Reduce dose to 1.5 mg daily if eGFR 20–50 mL/minute/1.73 m^2. Increased risk of bleeding in renal impairment.

▸ When used for treatment of acute coronary syndromes or prophylaxis of venous thromboembolism and treatment of superficial-vein thrombosis Avoid if eGFR less than 20 mL/minute/1.73 m^2.

▸ When used for treatment of venous thromboembolism Use with caution if eGFR 30–50 mL/minute/1.73 m^2, avoid if eGFR less than 30 mL/minute/1.73 m^2.

● **DIRECTIONS FOR ADMINISTRATION** For *intravenous infusion* (*Arixtra*®), give intermittently in Sodium chloride 0.9%. For ST-segment elevation myocardial infarction, add requisite dose to 25-50 mL infusion fluid and give over 1-2 minutes.

● **MEDICINAL FORMS**
There can be variation in the licensing of different medicines containing the same drug.
Solution for injection
▸ Fondaparinux sodium (Non-proprietary)
Fondaparinux sodium 5 mg per 1 ml Fondaparinux sodium 2.5mg/0.5ml solution for injection pre-filled syringes | 10 pre-filled disposable injection PoM £59.65
Fondaparinux sodium 12.5 mg per 1 ml Fondaparinux sodium 5mg/0.4ml solution for injection pre-filled syringes | 10 pre-filled disposable injection PoM £110.70
Fondaparinux sodium 10mg/0.8ml solution for injection pre-filled syringes | 10 pre-filled disposable injection PoM £110.70
Fondaparinux sodium 7.5mg/0.6ml solution for injection pre-filled syringes | 10 pre-filled disposable injection PoM £110.70

▸ Arixtra (Aspen Pharma Trading Ltd)
Fondaparinux sodium 5 mg per 1 ml Arixtra 2.5mg/0.5ml solution for injection pre-filled syringes | 10 pre-filled disposable injection PoM £62.79
Arixtra 1.5mg/0.3ml solution for injection pre-filled syringes | 10 pre-filled disposable injection PoM £62.79 (Hospital only)
Fondaparinux sodium 12.5 mg per 1 ml Arixtra 7.5mg/0.6ml solution for injection pre-filled syringes | 10 pre-filled disposable injection PoM £116.53
Arixtra 5mg/0.4ml solution for injection pre-filled syringes | 10 pre-filled disposable injection PoM £116.53
Arixtra 10mg/0.8ml solution for injection pre-filled syringes | 10 pre-filled disposable injection PoM £116.53

Rivaroxaban

● **DRUG ACTION** Rivaroxaban is a direct inhibitor of activated factor X (factor Xa).

● **INDICATIONS AND DOSE**
Prophylaxis of venous thromboembolism following knee replacement surgery
▸ BY MOUTH
▸ Adult: 10 mg once daily for 2 weeks, to be started 6–10 hours after surgery

Prophylaxis of venous thromboembolism following hip replacement surgery
▸ BY MOUTH
▸ Adult: 10 mg once daily for 5 weeks, to be started 6–10 hours after surgery

Initial treatment of deep-vein thrombosis | Initial treatment of pulmonary embolism
▸ BY MOUTH
▸ Adult: Initially 15 mg twice daily for 21 days, to be taken with food

Continued treatment of deep-vein thrombosis (following initial treatment) | Continued treatment of pulmonary embolism (following initial treatment) | Prophylaxis of recurrent deep-vein thrombosis | Prophylaxis of recurrent pulmonary embolism
▸ BY MOUTH
▸ Adult: 20 mg once daily, to be taken with food

Prophylaxis of stroke and systemic embolism in patients with non-valvular atrial fibrillation and with at least one of the following risk factors: congestive heart failure, hypertension, previous stroke or transient ischaemic attack, age $\geq$ 75 years, or diabetes mellitus
▸ BY MOUTH
▸ Adult: 20 mg once daily, to be taken with food

Prophylaxis of atherothrombotic events following an acute coronary syndrome with elevated cardiac biomarkers (in combination with aspirin alone or aspirin and clopidogrel)
▸ BY MOUTH
▸ Adult: 2.5 mg twice daily usual duration 12 months

DOSE EQUIVALENCE AND CONVERSION
For information on changing from, or to, other anticoagulants—consult product literature.

● **CONTRA-INDICATIONS** Active bleeding · in *acute coronary syndrome*—previous stroke · in *acute coronary syndrome*—transient ischaemic attack · malignant neoplasms · oesophageal varices · recent brain surgery · recent gastro-intestinal ulcer · recent intracranial haemorrhage · recent ophthalmic surgery · recent spine surgery · significant risk of major bleeding · vascular aneurysm

● **CAUTIONS** Anaesthesia with postoperative indwelling epidural catheter (risk of paralysis—monitor neurological signs and wait at least 18 hours after rivaroxaban dose before removing catheter and do not give next dose until at least 6 hours after catheter removal) · bronchiectasis · prosthetic heart valve (efficacy not established) · risk of bleeding · rivaroxaban should not be used as an alternative to unfractionated heparin in pulmonary embolism in patients with haemodynamic instability, or who may receive thrombolysis or pulmonary embolectomy · severe hypertension · vascular retinopathy

● INTERACTIONS → Appendix 1 (rivaroxaban). Caution in concomitant use of drugs that increase risk of bleeding.

● SIDE-EFFECTS

▸ **Common or very common** Abdominal pain · constipation · diarrhoea · dizziness · dyspepsia · haemorrhage · headache · hypotension · nausea · pain in extremities · pruritus · rash · renal impairment · vomiting

▸ **Uncommon** Angioedema · dry mouth · malaise · syncope · tachycardia · thrombocythaemia

▸ **Rare** Jaundice · oedema

● PREGNANCY Manufacturer advises avoid—toxicity in *animal* studies.

● BREAST FEEDING Manufacturer advises avoid—present in milk in *animal* studies.

● HEPATIC IMPAIRMENT Avoid in liver disease with coagulopathy.

● RENAL IMPAIRMENT

▸ When used for treatment of deep-vein thrombosis or pulmonary embolism and prophylaxis of recurrent deep-vein thrombosis and pulmonary embolism Initially 15 mg twice daily for 21 days, then 20 mg once daily (but consider reducing to 15 mg once daily if risk of bleeding outweighs risk of recurrent deep-vein thrombosis or pulmonary embolism) if creatinine clearance 15–49 mL/minute.

▸ When used for prophylaxis of stroke and systemic embolism in atrial fibrillation Reduce dose to 15 mg once daily if creatinine clearance 15–49 mL/minute.

▸ When used for prophylaxis of venous thromboembolism following knee or hip replacement surgery and prophylaxis of atherothrombotic events in acute coronary syndrome Use with caution if creatinine clearance 15–29 mL/minute.

Use with caution if concomitant use of drugs that increase plasma-rivaroxaban concentration (consult product literature).

Avoid if creatinine clearance less than 15 mL/minute; manufacturer recommends Cockroft and Gault formula to calculate creatinine clearance.

● MONITORING REQUIREMENTS

▸ Patients should be monitored for signs of bleeding or anaemia; treatment should be stopped if severe bleeding occurs.

▸ No routine anticoagulant monitoring required (INR tests are unreliable).

● DIRECTIONS FOR ADMINISTRATION Tablets may be crushed and mixed with water or apple puree just before administration.

● PRESCRIBING AND DISPENSING INFORMATION Low-dose rivaroxaban, in combination with aspirin alone *or* aspirin and clopidogrel, is licensed for the prevention of atherothrombotic events following an acute coronary syndrome with elevated cardiac biomarkers. Treatment should be started as soon as possible after the patient has been stabilised following the acute coronary event, at the earliest 24 hours after admission to hospital, and at the time when parenteral anticoagulation therapy would normally be discontinued; the usual duration of treatment is 12 months.

● NATIONAL FUNDING/ACCESS DECISIONS

NICE technology appraisals (TAs)

▸ **Rivaroxaban for the prevention of venous thromboembolism after total hip or total knee replacement in adults (April 2009)** NICE TA170

Rivaroxaban is an option for the prophylaxis of venous thromboembolism in adults after total hip replacement or total knee replacement surgery.
www.nice.org.uk/TA170

▸ **Rivaroxaban for the prevention of stroke and systemic embolism in atrial fibrillation (May 2012)** NICE TA256

Rivaroxaban is an option for the prevention of stroke and systemic embolism (in accordance with its licensed indication) in patients with non-valvular atrial fibrillation and with at least one of the following risk factors:

● previous stroke or transient ischaemic attack
● congestive heart failure
● age ≥75 years
● diabetes mellitus
● hypertension

The risks and benefits of rivaroxaban compared with warfarin should be discussed with the patient.
www.nice.org.uk/TA256

▸ **Rivaroxaban for the treatment of deep-vein thrombosis and prevention of recurrent venous thrombosis and pulmonary embolism (July 2012)** NICE TA261

Rivaroxaban is an option for the treatment of deep-vein thrombosis and prevention of recurrent deep-vein thrombosis and pulmonary embolism in adults after diagnosis of acute deep-vein thrombosis.
www.nice.org.uk/TA261

▸ **Rivaroxaban for treating pulmonary embolism and preventing recurrent venous thromboembolism (June 2013)** NICE TA287

Rivaroxaban is an option for treating pulmonary embolism and preventing recurrent deep-vein thrombosis and pulmonary embolism in adults.
www.nice.org.uk/TA287

▸ **Rivaroxaban for preventing adverse outcomes after acute management of acute coronary syndrome (March 2015)** NICE TA335

Rivaroxaban is an option within its marketing authorisation, in combination with aspirin plus clopidogrel or aspirin alone, for preventing atherothrombotic events in patients who have had an acute coronary syndrome with elevated cardiac biomarkers.

The patient's risk of bleeding should be carefully assessed before treatment is initiated and the risks and benefits of rivaroxaban in combination with aspirin plus clopidogrel or with aspirin alone, compared with aspirin plus clopidogrel or aspirin alone should be discussed with the patient.

A decision on continuation of treatment should be taken no later than 12 months after starting treatment.
www.nice.org.uk/TA335

Scottish Medicines Consortium (SMC) Decisions

The *Scottish Medicines Consortium* has advised (January 2012) that rivaroxaban (*Xarelto*®) is accepted for restricted use within NHS Scotland for the prevention of stroke and systemic embolism in accordance with the licensed indication; use is restricted to patients with poor INR control despite compliance with coumarin anticoagulant therapy, or to patients who are allergic to, or unable to tolerate, a coumarin anticoagulant.

● MEDICINAL FORMS
There can be variation in the licensing of different medicines containing the same drug.

Tablet

▸ Xarelto (Bayer Plc) ▼

Rivaroxaban 2.5 mg Xarelto 2.5mg tablets | 56 tablet PoM £50.40 DT price = £50.40

Rivaroxaban 10 mg Xarelto 10mg tablets | 10 tablet PoM £18.00 | 30 tablet PoM £54.00 DT price = £54.00 | 100 tablet PoM £180.00

Rivaroxaban 15 mg Xarelto 15mg tablets | 14 tablet PoM £25.20 | 28 tablet PoM £50.40 DT price = £50.40 | 42 tablet PoM £75.60 | 100 tablet PoM £180.00

Rivaroxaban 20 mg Xarelto 20mg tablets | 28 tablet PoM £50.40 DT price = £50.40 | 100 tablet PoM £180.00

ANTITHROMBOTIC DRUGS > HEPARINOIDS

Danaparoid sodium

- **INDICATIONS AND DOSE**

Prevention of deep-vein thrombosis in general or orthopaedic surgery
▶ BY SUBCUTANEOUS INJECTION
▶ Adult: 750 units twice daily for 7–10 days, initiate treatment before operation, with last pre-operative dose 1–4 hours before surgery

Thromboembolic disease in patients with history of heparin-induced thrombocytopenia
▶ INITIALLY BY INTRAVENOUS INJECTION
▶ Adult (body-weight up to 55 kg): Initially 1250 units, then (by continuous intravenous infusion) 400 units/hour for 2 hours, then (by continuous intravenous infusion) 300 units/hour for 2 hours, then (by continuous intravenous infusion) 200 units/hour for 5 days
▶ Adult (body-weight 55–89 kg): Initially 2500 units, then (by continuous intravenous infusion) 400 units/hour for 2 hours, then (by continuous intravenous infusion) 300 units/hour for 2 hours, then (by continuous intravenous infusion) 200 units/hour for 5 days
▶ Adult (body-weight 90 kg and above): Initially 3750 units, then (by continuous intravenous infusion) 400 units/hour for 2 hours, then (by continuous intravenous infusion) 300 units/hour for 2 hours, then (by continuous intravenous infusion) 200 units/hour for 5 days

- **CONTRA-INDICATIONS** Active peptic ulcer (unless this is the reason for operation) · acute bacterial endocarditis · diabetic retinopathy · epidural anaesthesia (with treatment doses) · haemophilia and other haemorrhagic disorders · recent cerebral haemorrhage · severe hypertension · spinal anaesthesia (with treatment doses) · thrombocytopenia (unless patient has heparin-induced thrombocytopenia)
- **CAUTIONS** Antibodies to heparins (risk of antibody-induced thrombocytopenia) · body-weight over 90 kg · recent bleeding · risk of bleeding
- **INTERACTIONS** → Appendix 1 (danaparoid). Caution with concomitant use of drugs that increase risk of bleeding.
- **SIDE-EFFECTS** Bleeding · hypersensitivity reactions · rash
- **PREGNANCY** Manufacturer advises avoid—limited information available but not known to be harmful.
- **BREAST FEEDING** Amount probably too small to be harmful but manufacturer advises avoid.
- **HEPATIC IMPAIRMENT** Caution in moderate impairment (increased risk of bleeding). Avoid in severe impairment unless patient has heparin-induced thrombocytopenia and no alternative available.
- **RENAL IMPAIRMENT** Use with caution in moderate impairment. Avoid in severe impairment unless patient has heparin-induced thrombocytopenia and no alternative available. Increased risk of bleeding in renal impairment, monitor anti-Factor Xa activity.
- **MONITORING REQUIREMENTS** Monitor anti factor Xa activity in patients with body-weight over 90 kg.
- **DIRECTIONS FOR ADMINISTRATION** For *intravenous infusion* (*Orgaran*®), give continuously in Glucose 5% or Sodium chloride 0.9%.

- **MEDICINAL FORMS**
There can be variation in the licensing of different medicines containing the same drug.
Solution for injection
▶ Orgaran (Aspen Pharma Trading Ltd)
Danaparoid sodium 1250 unit per 1 ml Orgaran 750units/0.6ml solution for injection ampoules | 10 ampoule PoM £266.73

ANTITHROMBOTIC DRUGS > HEPARINS

Heparins

- **CONTRA-INDICATIONS** Acute bacterial endocarditis · after major trauma · epidural anaesthesia with treatment doses · haemophilia · other haemorrhagic disorders · peptic ulcer · recent cerebral haemorrhage · recent surgery to eye · recent surgery to nervous system · severe hypertension · spinal anaesthesia with treatment doses · thrombocytopenia (including history of heparin-induced thrombocytopenia)
- **CAUTIONS** Elderly
- **INTERACTIONS** → Appendix 1 (heparins). Caution with concomitant use of drugs that increase risk of bleeding.
- **SIDE-EFFECTS**
▶ **Rare** Alopecia (on prolonged use) · anaphylaxis · angioedema · hyperkalaemia · hypersensitivity reactions · injection-site reactions · osteoporosis (risk lower with low molecular weight heparins) · priapism · rebound hyperlipidaemia (following unfractionated heparin withdrawal) · skin necrosis · urticaria
▶ **Frequency not known** Haemorrhage · thrombocytopenia
SIDE-EFFECTS, FURTHER INFORMATION
▶ **Haemorrhage** If haemorrhage occurs it is usually sufficient to withdraw unfractionated or low molecular weight heparin, but if rapid reversal of the effects of the heparin is required, protamine sulfate is a specific antidote (but only partially reverses the effects of low molecular weight heparins).
▶ Heparin-induced thrombocytopenia Clinically important heparin-induced thrombocytopenia is immune-mediated and does not usually develop until after 5–10 days; it can be complicated by thrombosis.
Signs of heparin-induced thrombocytopenia include a 30% reduction of platelet count, thrombosis, or skin allergy. If heparin-induced thrombocytopenia is strongly suspected or confirmed, the heparin should be **stopped** and an alternative anticoagulant, such as danaparoid, should be given. Ensure platelet counts return to normal range in those who require warfarin.
▶ Hyperkalaemia Inhibition of aldosterone secretion by unfractionated or low molecular weight heparin can result in hyperkalaemia; patients with diabetes mellitus, chronic renal failure, acidosis, raised plasma potassium or those taking potassium-sparing drugs seem to be more susceptible. The risk appears to increase with duration of therapy.
- **ALLERGY AND CROSS-SENSITIVITY** Hypersensitivity to unfractionated or low molecular weight heparin.
- **MONITORING REQUIREMENTS**
▶ Heparin-induced thrombocytopenia Platelet counts should be measured just before treatment with unfractionated or low molecular weight heparin, and regular monitoring of platelet counts may be required if given for longer than 4 days. See the British Society for Haematology's Guidelines on the diagnosis and management of heparin-induced thrombocytopenia: second edition. *Br J Haematol* 2012; **159**: 528–540.
▶ Hyperkalaemia Plasma-potassium concentration should be measured in patients at risk of hyperkalaemia before starting the heparin and monitored regularly thereafter, particularly if treatment is to be continued for longer than 7 days.

Cardiovascular system

2

Dalteparin sodium

F 117

● INDICATIONS AND DOSE

FRAGMIN®

Treatment of deep-vein thrombosis, with oral anticoagulant treatment | Treatment of pulmonary embolism, with oral anticoagulant treatment
▸ BY SUBCUTANEOUS INJECTION
▸ Adult: 200 units/kg daily (max. per dose 18 000 units) until adequate oral anticoagulation established

Treatment of deep-vein thrombosis, with oral anticoagulant treatment (in patients at increased risk of haemorrhage) | Treatment of pulmonary embolism, with oral anticoagulant treatment (in patients at increase risk of haemorrhage)
▸ BY SUBCUTANEOUS INJECTION
▸ Adult: 100 units/kg twice daily until adequate oral anticoagulation established

Unstable coronary artery disease
▸ BY SUBCUTANEOUS INJECTION
▸ Adult: 120 units/kg every 12 hours (max. per dose 10 000 units twice daily) for 5–8 days

Prevention of clotting in extracorporeal circuits
▸ TO THE DEVICE AS A FLUSH
▸ Adult: (consult product literature)

FRAGMIN® GRADUATED SYRINGES

Unstable coronary artery disease (including non-ST-segment-elevation myocardial infarction)
▸ BY SUBCUTANEOUS INJECTION
▸ Adult: 120 units/kg every 12 hours (max. per dose 10 000 units twice daily) for up to 8 days

Patients with unstable coronary artery disease (including non-ST-segment-elevation myocardial infarction) awaiting angiography or revascularisation and having already had 8 days treatment with dalteparin
▸ BY SUBCUTANEOUS INJECTION
▸ Adult (body-weight up to 70 kg and male): 5000 units every 12 hours until the day of the procedure (max. 45 days).
▸ Adult (body-weight up to 80 kg and female): 5000 units every 12 hours until the day of the procedure (max. 45 days).
▸ Adult (body-weight 70 kg and above and male): 7500 units every 12 hours until the day of the procedure (max. 45 days).
▸ Adult (body-weight 80 kg and above and female): 7500 units every 12 hours until the day of the procedure (max. 45 days).

FRAGMIN® SINGLE-DOSE SYRINGES

Prophylaxis of deep-vein thrombosis in surgical patients—moderate risk
▸ BY SUBCUTANEOUS INJECTION
▸ Adult: Initially 2500 units for 1 dose, dose to be given 1–2 hours before surgery, then 2500 units every 24 hours

Prophylaxis of deep-vein thrombosis in surgical patients—high risk
▸ BY SUBCUTANEOUS INJECTION
▸ Adult: Initially 2500 units for 1 dose, dose to be administered 1–2 hours before surgery, followed by 2500 units after 8–12 hours, then 5000 units every 24 hours, alternatively initially 5000 units for 1 dose, dose to be given on the evening before surgery, followed by 5000 units after 24 hours, then 5000 units every 24 hours

Prophylaxis of deep-vein thrombosis in medical patients
▸ BY SUBCUTANEOUS INJECTION
▸ Adult: 5000 units every 24 hours

Treatment of deep-vein thrombosis, with oral anticoagulant treatment | Treatment of pulmonary embolism, with oral anticoagulant treatment
▸ BY SUBCUTANEOUS INJECTION
▸ Adult (body-weight up to 46 kg): 7500 units once daily until adequate oral anticoagulation established
▸ Adult (body-weight 46–56 kg): 10 000 units once daily until adequate oral anticoagulation established
▸ Adult (body-weight 57–68 kg): 12 500 units once daily until adequate oral anticoagulation established
▸ Adult (body-weight 69–82 kg): 15 000 units once daily until adequate oral anticoagulation established
▸ Adult (body-weight 83 kg and above): 18 000 units once daily until adequate oral anticoagulation established

Extended treatment and prophylaxis of venous thromboembolism in patients with solid tumours
▸ BY SUBCUTANEOUS INJECTION
▸ Adult (body-weight 40–45 kg): 7500 units once daily for 30 days, then 7500 units once daily for a further 5 months, interrupt treatment or reduce dose in chemotherapy-induced thrombocytopenia—consult product literature
▸ Adult (body-weight 46–56 kg): 10 000 units once daily for 30 days, then 7500 units once daily for a further 5 months, interrupt treatment or reduce dose in chemotherapy-induced thrombocytopenia—consult product literature
▸ Adult (body-weight 57–68 kg): 12 500 units once daily for 30 days, then 10 000 units once daily for a further 5 months, interrupt treatment or reduce dose in chemotherapy-induced thrombocytopenia—consult product literature
▸ Adult (body-weight 69–82 kg): 15 000 units once daily for 30 days, then 12 500 units once daily for a further 5 months, interrupt treatment or reduce dose in chemotherapy-induced thrombocytopenia—consult product literature
▸ Adult (body-weight 83–98 kg): 18 000 units once daily for 30 days, then 15 000 units once daily for a further 5 months, interrupt treatment or reduce dose in chemotherapy-induced thrombocytopenia—consult product literature
▸ Adult (body-weight 99 kg and above): 18 000 units once daily for 30 days, then 18 000 units once daily for a further 5 months, interrupt treatment or reduce dose in chemotherapy-induced thrombocytopenia—consult product literature

Treatment of venous thromboembolism in pregnancy
▸ BY SUBCUTANEOUS INJECTION
▸ Adult (body-weight up to 50 kg): 5000 units twice daily, use body-weight in early pregnancy to calculate the dose
▸ Adult (body-weight 50–69 kg): 6000 units twice daily, use body-weight in early pregnancy to calculate the dose
▸ Adult (body-weight 70–89 kg): 8000 units twice daily, use body-weight in early pregnancy to calculate the dose
▸ Adult (body-weight 90 kg and above): 10 000 units twice daily, use body-weight in early pregnancy to calculate the dose

● UNLICENSED USE Not licensed for treatment of venous thromboembolism in pregnancy.

● PREGNANCY Not known to be harmful, low molecular weight heparins do not cross the placenta. Multidose vial contains benzyl alcohol—manufacturer advises avoid.

● BREAST FEEDING Due to the relatively high molecular weight and inactivation in the gastro-intestinal tract, passage into breast-milk and absorption by the nursing infant are likely to be negligible, however manufacturers advise avoid.

- HEPATIC IMPAIRMENT Dose reduction may be required in severe impairment—risk of bleeding may be increased.
- RENAL IMPAIRMENT Risk of bleeding may be increased—dose reduction may be required. Use of unfractionated heparin may be preferable.
- MONITORING REQUIREMENTS
- For monitoring during treatment of deep-vein thrombosis and of pulmonary embolism, blood should be taken 3–4 hours after a dose (recommended plasma concentration of anti-Factor Xa 0.5–1 unit/mL); monitoring not required for once-daily treatment regimen and not generally necessary for twice-daily regimen.
- Routine monitoring of anti-Factor Xa activity is not usually required during treatment with dalteparin, but may be necessary in patients at increased risk of bleeding (e.g. in renal impairment and those who are underweight or overweight).
- NATIONAL FUNDING/ACCESS DECISIONS

Scottish Medicines Consortium (SMC) Decisions
The *Scottish Medicines Consortium* has advised (February 2011) that dalteparin (*Fragmin*®) is accepted for restricted use within NHS Scotland as extended treatment of symptomatic venous thromboembolism and prevention of its recurrence in patients with solid tumours.

- MEDICINAL FORMS
There can be variation in the licensing of different medicines containing the same drug.

Solution for injection
EXCIPIENTS: May contain Benzyl alcohol
- Fragmin (Pfizer Ltd)
  Dalteparin sodium 2500 unit per 1 ml Fragmin 10,000units/4ml solution for injection ampoules | 10 ampoule PoM £51.22
  Dalteparin sodium 10000 unit per 1 ml Fragmin 10,000units/1ml solution for injection pre-filled syringes | 5 pre-filled disposable injection PoM £28.23
  Fragmin 10,000units/1ml solution for injection ampoules | 10 ampoule PoM £51.22
  Dalteparin sodium 12500 unit per 1 ml Fragmin 2,500units/0.2ml solution for injection pre-filled syringes | 10 pre-filled disposable injection PoM £18.58
  Dalteparin sodium 25000 unit per 1 ml Fragmin 18,000units/0.72ml solution for injection pre-filled syringes | 5 pre-filled disposable injection PoM £50.82
  Fragmin 15,000units/0.6ml solution for injection pre-filled syringes | 5 pre-filled disposable injection PoM £42.34
  Fragmin 5,000units/0.2ml solution for injection pre-filled syringes | 10 pre-filled disposable injection PoM £28.23
  Fragmin 12,500units/0.5ml solution for injection pre-filled syringes | 5 pre-filled disposable injection PoM £35.29
  Fragmin 7,500units/0.3ml solution for injection pre-filled syringes | 10 pre-filled disposable injection PoM £42.34
  Fragmin 100,000units/4ml solution for injection vials | 1 vial PoM £48.66
  Fragmin 10,000units/0.4ml solution for injection pre-filled syringes | 5 pre-filled disposable injection PoM £28.23

117

Enoxaparin sodium

- INDICATIONS AND DOSE

Treatment of venous thromboembolism in pregnancy
- BY SUBCUTANEOUS INJECTION
- Adult (body-weight up to 50 kg): 40 mg twice daily, dose based on early pregnancy body-weight
- Adult (body-weight 50–69 kg): 60 mg twice daily, dose based on early pregnancy body-weight
- Adult (body-weight 70–89 kg): 80 mg twice daily, dose based on early pregnancy body-weight
- Adult (body-weight 90 kg and above): 100 mg twice daily, dose based on early pregnancy body-weight

Prophylaxis of deep-vein thrombosis, especially in surgical patients—moderate risk
- BY SUBCUTANEOUS INJECTION
- Adult: 20 mg for 1 dose, dose to be given approximately 2 hours before surgery, then 20 mg every 24 hours

Prophylaxis of deep-vein thrombosis, especially surgical patients—high risk (e.g. orthopaedic surgery)
- BY SUBCUTANEOUS INJECTION
- Adult: 40 mg for 1 dose, dose to be given 12 hours before surgery, then 40 mg every 24 hours

Prophylaxis of deep-vein thrombosis in medical patients
- BY SUBCUTANEOUS INJECTION
- Adult: 40 mg every 24 hours

Treatment of deep-vein thrombosis | Treatment of pulmonary embolism
- BY SUBCUTANEOUS INJECTION
- Adult: 1.5 mg/kg every 24 hours until adequate oral anticoagulation established

Treatment of acute ST-segment elevation myocardial infarction (patients not undergoing percutaneous coronary intervention)
- INITIALLY BY INTRAVENOUS INJECTION
- Adult 18–74 years: Initially 30 mg, followed by (by subcutaneous injection) 1 mg/kg for 1 dose, then (by subcutaneous injection) 1 mg/kg every 12 hours (max. per dose 100 mg) for up to 8 days, maximum dose applies for the first two subcutaneous doses only
- BY SUBCUTANEOUS INJECTION
- Adult 75 years and over: 750 micrograms/kg every 12 hours (max. per dose 75 mg), maximum dose applies for the first two doses only

Treatment of acute ST-segment elevation myocardial infarction (patients undergoing percutaneous coronary intervention)
- INITIALLY BY INTRAVENOUS INJECTION
- Adult 18–74 years: Initially 30 mg, followed by (by subcutaneous injection) 1 mg/kg for 1 dose, then (by subcutaneous injection) 1 mg/kg every 12 hours (max. per dose 100 mg) for up to 8 days, maximum dose applies for the first two subcutaneous doses only, then (by intravenous injection) 300 micrograms/kg for 1 dose, dose to be given at the time of procedure if the last subcutaneous dose was given more than 8 hours previously
- INITIALLY BY SUBCUTANEOUS INJECTION
- Adult 75 years and over: 750 micrograms/kg every 12 hours (max. per dose 75 mg), maximum dose applies for the first two doses only, then (by intravenous injection) 300 micrograms/kg for 1 dose, dose to be given at the time of procedure if the last subcutaneous dose was given more than 8 hours previously

Unstable angina | Non-ST-segment-elevation myocardial infarction
- BY SUBCUTANEOUS INJECTION
- Adult: 1 mg/kg every 12 hours usually for 2–8 days (minimum 2 days)

Prevention of clotting in extracorporeal circuits
- TO THE DEVICE AS A FLUSH
- Adult: (consult product literature)

DOSE EQUIVALENCE AND CONVERSION
1 mg equivalent to 100 units.

- UNLICENSED USE Not licensed for treatment of venous thromboembolism in pregnancy.
- CAUTIONS Low body-weight (increased risk of bleeding)
- PREGNANCY Not known to be harmful, low molecular weight heparins do not cross the placenta. Multidose vial contains benzyl alcohol—avoid.
- BREAST FEEDING Due to the relatively high molecular weight of enoxaparin and inactivation in the gastro-

intestinal tract, passage into breast-milk and absorption by the nursing infant are likely to be negligible; however manufacturers advise avoid.

● HEPATIC IMPAIRMENT Manufacturer advises caution—no information available.

● RENAL IMPAIRMENT Risk of bleeding increased; reduce dose if eGFR less than 30 mL/minute/1.73 m² —consult product literature for details. Use of unfractionated heparin may be preferable.

● MONITORING REQUIREMENTS Routine monitoring of anti-Factor Xa activity is not usually required during treatment with enoxaparin, but may be necessary in patients at increased risk of bleeding (e.g. in renal impairment and those who are underweight or overweight).

● DIRECTIONS FOR ADMINISTRATION When administered in conjunction with a thrombolytic, enoxaparin should be given between 15 minutes before and 30 minutes after the start of thrombolytic therapy.

● MEDICINAL FORMS
There can be variation in the licensing of different medicines containing the same drug.
Solution for injection
EXCIPIENTS: May contain Benzyl alcohol
▸ Clexane (Sanofi)
Enoxaparin sodium 100 mg per 1 ml Clexane 60mg/0.6ml solution for injection pre-filled syringes | 10 pre-filled disposable injection [PoM] £39.26 DT price = £39.26
Clexane 300mg/3ml solution for injection multidose vials | 1 vial [PoM] £21.33
Clexane 80mg/0.8ml solution for injection pre-filled syringes | 10 pre-filled disposable injection [PoM] £55.13 DT price = £55.13
Clexane 40mg/0.4ml solution for injection pre-filled syringes | 10 pre-filled disposable injection [PoM] £30.27 DT price = £30.27
Clexane 100mg/1ml solution for injection pre-filled syringes | 10 pre-filled disposable injection [PoM] £72.30 DT price = £72.30
Clexane 20mg/0.2ml solution for injection pre-filled syringes | 10 pre-filled disposable injection [PoM] £20.86 DT price = £20.86
Enoxaparin sodium 150 mg per 1 ml Clexane Forte 120mg/0.8ml solution for injection pre-filled syringes | 10 pre-filled disposable injection [PoM] £87.93 DT price = £87.93
Clexane Forte 150mg/1ml solution for injection pre-filled syringes | 10 pre-filled disposable injection [PoM] £99.91 DT price = £99.91

⚑ 117

Heparin (unfractionated)

● INDICATIONS AND DOSE

Treatment of mild to moderate pulmonary embolism | Treatment of unstable angina | Treatment of acute peripheral arterial occlusion
▸ INITIALLY BY INTRAVENOUS INJECTION
▸ Adult: Loading dose 5000 units, alternatively (by intravenous injection) loading dose 75 units/kg, followed by (by continuous intravenous infusion) 18 units/kg/hour, laboratory monitoring essential— preferably on a daily basis, and dose adjusted accordingly

Treatment of severe pulmonary embolism
▸ INITIALLY BY INTRAVENOUS INJECTION
▸ Adult: Loading dose 10 000 units, followed by (by continuous intravenous infusion) 18 units/kg/hour, laboratory monitoring essential—preferably on a daily basis, and dose adjusted accordingly

Treatment of deep-vein thrombosis
▸ INITIALLY BY INTRAVENOUS INJECTION
▸ Adult: Loading dose 5000 units, alternatively (by intravenous injection) loading dose 75 units/kg, followed by (by continuous intravenous infusion) 18 units/kg/hour, alternatively (by subcutaneous injection) 15 000 units every 12 hours, laboratory monitoring essential—preferably on a daily basis, and dose adjusted accordingly

Thromboprophylaxis in medical patients
▸ BY SUBCUTANEOUS INJECTION
▸ Adult: 5000 units every 8–12 hours

Thrombophylaxis in surgical patients
▸ BY SUBCUTANEOUS INJECTION
▸ Adult: 5000 units for 1 dose, to be taken 2 hours before surgery, then 5000 units every 8–12 hours

Thromboprophylaxis during pregnancy
▸ BY SUBCUTANEOUS INJECTION
▸ Adult: 5000–10 000 units every 12 hours, to be administered with monitoring, **Important**: prevention of prosthetic heart-valve thrombosis in pregnancy calls for **specialist management**

Haemodialysis
▸ INITIALLY BY INTRAVENOUS INJECTION
▸ Adult: Initially 1000–5000 units, followed by (by continuous intravenous infusion) 250–1000 units/hour

Prevention of clotting in extracorporeal circuits
▸ TO THE DEVICE AS A FLUSH
▸ Adult: (consult product literature)

To maintain patency of catheters, cannulas, other indwelling intravenous infusion devices
▸ TO THE DEVICE AS A FLUSH
▸ Adult: 10–200 units, to be flushed through every 4–8 hours, not for therapeutic use

● PREGNANCY Does not cross the placenta; maternal osteoporosis reported after prolonged use; multidose vials may contain benzyl alcohol—some manufacturers advise avoid.

● BREAST FEEDING Not excreted into milk due to high molecular weight.

● HEPATIC IMPAIRMENT Risk of bleeding increased—reduce dose or avoid in severe impairment (including oesophageal varices).

● RENAL IMPAIRMENT Risk of bleeding increased in severe impairment—dose may need to be reduced.

● DIRECTIONS FOR ADMINISTRATION For *intravenous infusion*, give continuously in Glucose 5% or Sodium chloride 0.9%; administration with a motorised pump is advisable.

● PRESCRIBING AND DISPENSING INFORMATION Doses listed take into account the guidelines of the British Society for Haematology.

● MEDICINAL FORMS
There can be variation in the licensing of different medicines containing the same drug. Forms available from special-order manufacturers include: solution for injection, solution for infusion
Solution for injection
EXCIPIENTS: May contain Benzyl alcohol
▸ Heparin (unfractionated) (Non-proprietary)
Heparin sodium 1000 unit per 1 ml Heparin sodium 1,000units/1ml solution for injection ampoules | 10 ampoule [PoM] £14.85
Heparin sodium 5,000units/5ml solution for injection vials | 10 vial [PoM] £16.50–£37.41
Heparin sodium 20,000units/20ml solution for injection ampoules | 10 ampoule [PoM] £70.80–£70.88
Heparin sodium 5,000units/5ml solution for injection ampoules | 10 ampoule [PoM] £37.45–£37.47
Heparin sodium 10,000units/10ml solution for injection ampoules | 10 ampoule [PoM] £64.50–£64.59
Heparin sodium 5000 unit per 1 ml Heparin sodium 5,000units/1ml solution for injection ampoules | 10 ampoule [PoM] £29.04
Heparin sodium 25,000units/5ml solution for injection vials | 10 vial [PoM] £45.00–£84.60
Heparin sodium 25,000units/5ml solution for injection ampoules | 10 ampoule [PoM] £75.78
Heparin calcium 25000 unit per 1 ml Heparin calcium 5,000units/0.2ml solution for injection ampoules | 10 ampoule [PoM] £44.70

Heparin sodium 25000 unit per 1 ml Heparin sodium 25,000units/1ml solution for injection ampoules | 10 ampoule PoM £76.95

Heparin sodium 5,000units/0.2ml solution for injection ampoules | 10 ampoule PoM £37.35

Infusion

▸ Heparin (unfractionated) (Non-proprietary)

Heparin sodium 2 unit per 1 ml Heparin sodium 1,000units/500ml infusion Viaflex bags | 1 bag PoM no price available

Heparin sodium 2,000units/1,000ml infusion Viaflex bags | 1 bag PoM no price available

Heparin sodium 5 unit per 1 ml Heparin sodium 5,000units/1litre infusion Viaflex bags | 1 bag PoM no price available

Intravenous flush

EXCIPIENTS: May contain Benzyl alcohol

▸ Heparin (unfractionated) (Non-proprietary)

Heparin sodium 10 unit per 1 ml Heparin sodium 50units/5ml patency solution ampoules | 10 ampoule PoM £14.96

Heparin sodium 50units/5ml I.V. flush solution ampoules | 10 ampoule PoM £14.96

Heparin sodium 100 unit per 1 ml Heparin sodium 200units/2ml I.V. flush solution ampoules | 10 ampoule PoM £15.68

Heparin sodium 200units/2ml patency solution ampoules | 10 ampoule PoM £15.68

F 117

Tinzaparin sodium

● **INDICATIONS AND DOSE**

INNOHEP® 10,000 UNITS/ML

Prophylaxis of deep-vein thrombosis (general surgery)

▸ BY SUBCUTANEOUS INJECTION

▸ **Adult:** 3500 units for 1 dose, dose to be given 2 hours before surgery, then 3500 units every 24 hours

Prophylaxis of deep-vein thrombosis (orthopaedic surgery)

▸ BY SUBCUTANEOUS INJECTION

▸ **Adult:** Initially 50 units/kg for 1 dose, dose to be given 2 hours before surgery, then 50 units/kg every 24 hours, alternatively initially 4500 units for 1 dose, dose to be given 12 hours before surgery, then 4500 units every 24 hours

Prevention of clotting in extracorporeal circuits

▸ TO THE DEVICE AS A FLUSH

▸ **Adult:** (consult product literature)

INNOHEP® 20,000 UNITS/ML

Extended treatment of venous thromboembolism in patients with solid tumours | Prophylaxis of venous thromboembolism in patients with solid tumours

▸ BY SUBCUTANEOUS INJECTION

▸ **Adult:** 175 units/kg once daily for up to 6 months

Treatment of deep-vein thrombosis | Treatment of pulmonary embolism

▸ BY SUBCUTANEOUS INJECTION

▸ **Adult:** 175 units/kg once daily until adequate oral anticoagulation established, treatment regimens do not require anticoagulation monitoring

Treatment of venous thromboembolism in pregnancy

▸ BY SUBCUTANEOUS INJECTION

▸ **Adult:** 175 units/kg once daily, dose based on early pregnancy body-weight, treatment regimens do not require anticoagulation monitoring

● UNLICENSED USE Not licensed for the treatment of venous thromboembolism in pregnancy.

● SIDE-EFFECTS

▸ Uncommon Headache

● PREGNANCY Not known to be harmful, low molecular weight heparins do not cross the placenta. Vials contain benzyl alcohol—manufacturer advises avoid.

● BREAST FEEDING Due to the relatively high molecular weight of tinzaparin and inactivation in the gastro-

intestinal tract, passage into breast-milk and absorption by the nursing infant are likely to be negligible; however manufacturer advise avoid.

● RENAL IMPAIRMENT Manufacturer advises caution if eGFR less than 30 mL/minute/1.73 m². Risk of bleeding may be increased. Unfractionated heparin may be preferable. In renal impairment monitoring of anti-Factor Xa may be required if eGFR less than 30 mL/minute/1.73 m².

● MONITORING REQUIREMENTS Routine monitoring of anti-Factor Xa activity is not usually required during treatment with tinzaparin, but may be necessary in patients at increased risk of bleeding (e.g. in renal impairment and those who are underweight or overweight).

● MEDICINAL FORMS There can be variation in the licensing of different medicines containing the same drug.

Solution for injection

EXCIPIENTS: May contain Benzyl alcohol, sulfites

▸ Innohep (LEO Pharma)

Tinzaparin sodium 10000 unit per 1 ml Innohep 20,000units/2ml solution for injection vials | 10 vial PoM £105.66

Tinzaparin sodium 20000 unit per 1 ml Innohep 18,000units/0.9ml solution for injection pre-filled syringes | 6 pre-filled disposable injection PoM £64.25 | 10 pre-filled disposable injection PoM £107.08

Innohep 8,000units/0.4ml solution for injection pre-filled syringes | 6 pre-filled disposable injection PoM £28.56 | 10 pre-filled disposable injection PoM £47.60

Innohep 40,000units/2ml solution for injection vials | 1 vial PoM £34.20

Innohep 16,000units/0.8ml solution for injection pre-filled syringes | 6 pre-filled disposable injection PoM £57.12 | 10 pre-filled disposable injection PoM £95.20

Innohep 12,000units/0.6ml solution for injection pre-filled syringes | 6 pre-filled disposable injection PoM £42.84 | 10 pre-filled disposable injection PoM £71.40

Innohep 14,000units/0.7ml solution for injection pre-filled syringes | 6 pre-filled disposable injection PoM £49.98 | 10 pre-filled disposable injection PoM £83.30

Innohep 10,000units/0.5ml solution for injection pre-filled syringes | 6 pre-filled disposable injection PoM £35.70 | 10 pre-filled disposable injection PoM £59.50

ANTITHROMBOTIC DRUGS 〉 THOMBIN INHIBITORS, DIRECT

Argatroban monohydrate

● **INDICATIONS AND DOSE**

Anticoagulation in patients with heparin-induced thrombocytopenia type II who require parenteral antithrombotic treatment

▸ INITIALLY BY CONTINUOUS INTRAVENOUS INFUSION

▸ **Adult:** Initially 2 micrograms/kg/minute, dose to be adjusted according to activated partial thromboplastin time, (by intravenous infusion) increased to up to 10 micrograms/kg/minute maximum duration of treatment 14 days

Anticoagulation in patients with heparin-induced thrombocytopenia type II who require parenteral antithrombotic treatment (for dose in cardiac surgery, percutaneous coronary intervention, or critically ill patients)

▸ BY CONTINUOUS INTRAVENOUS INFUSION

▸ **Adult:** (consult product literature)

Anticoagulation in patients with heparin-induced thrombocytopenia type II who require parenteral antithrombotic treatment (when initiating concomitant warfarin treatment)

▸ BY CONTINUOUS INTRAVENOUS INFUSION

▸ **Adult:** Reduced to 2 micrograms/kg/minute, dose should be temporarily reduced and INR measured after 4–6 hours; warfarin should be initiated at continued →

2

Cardiovascular system

intended maintenance dose (do not give loading dose of warfarin); consult product literature for further details

- CAUTIONS Bleeding disorders · diabetic retinopathy · gastro-intestinal ulceration · immediately after lumbar puncture · major surgery (especially of brain, spinal cord, or eye) · risk of bleeding · severe hypertension · spinal anaesthesia
- INTERACTIONS → Appendix 1 (argatroban). Caution with concomitant use of drugs that increase risk of bleeding.
- SIDE-EFFECTS
  - Common or very common Haemorrhage · nausea · purpura
  - Uncommon Alopecia · constipation · deafness · diarrhoea · dizziness · fever · gastritis · headache · hepatic failure · hepatomegaly · hiccups · hyperbilirubinaemia · hypertension · hypoglycaemia · hyponatraemia · hypotension · malaise · muscle weakness · myalgia · rash · renal impairment · sweating · syncope · tachycardia · visual disturbance · vomiting
- PREGNANCY Manufacturer advises avoid unless essential—limited information available.
- BREAST FEEDING Avoid—no information available.
- HEPATIC IMPAIRMENT Reduce initial dose to 500 nanograms/kg/minute in moderate impairment. Avoid in severe impairment *or* in patients with hepatic impairment undergoing percutaneous coronary intervention.
- MONITORING REQUIREMENTS Determine activated partial thromboplastin time 2 hours after start of treatment, then 2 or 4 hours after infusion rate altered (consult product literature), and at least once daily thereafter.
- DIRECTIONS FOR ADMINISTRATION For *intravenous infusion* (*Exembol®*) give continuously in Glucose 5% or Sodium chloride 0.9%. Dilute each 2.5-mL vial with 250 mL infusion fluid.

- MEDICINAL FORMS
There can be variation in the licensing of different medicines containing the same drug.
Solution for infusion
EXCIPIENTS: May contain Ethanol
  - Exembol (Mitsubishi Tanabe Pharma Europe Ltd)
  Argatroban monohydrate 100 mg per 1 ml Exembol 250mg/2.5ml concentrate for solution for infusion vials | 1 vial [PoM] no price available

Bivalirudin

- DRUG ACTION Bivalirudin, a hirudin analogue, is a thrombin inhibitor.

- INDICATIONS AND DOSE
Unstable angina or non-ST-segment elevation myocardial infarction in patients planned for urgent or early intervention (in addition to aspirin and clopidogrel)
  - INITIALLY BY INTRAVENOUS INJECTION
  - Adult: Initially 100 micrograms/kg, then (by intravenous infusion) 250 micrograms/kg/hour (for up to 72 hours in medically managed patients)
Unstable angina or non-ST-segment elevation myocardial infarction (in addition to aspirin and clopidogrel) in patients proceeding to percutaneous coronary intervention or coronary artery bypass surgery without cardiopulmonary bypass
  - INITIALLY BY INTRAVENOUS INJECTION
  - Adult: Initially 100 micrograms/kg for 1 dose, then (by intravenous injection) 500 micrograms/kg for 1 dose, then (by intravenous infusion) 1.75 mg/kg/hour for duration of procedure; (by intravenous infusion) reduced to 250 micrograms/kg/hour for 4–12 hours as

necessary following percutaneous coronary intervention, for patients proceeding to coronary artery bypass surgery with cardiopulmonary bypass, discontinue intravenous infusion 1 hour before procedure and treat with unfractionated heparin

Anticoagulation in patients undergoing percutaneous coronary intervention including patients with ST-segment elevation myocardial infarction undergoing primary percutaneous coronary intervention (in addition to aspirin and clopidogrel)
  - INITIALLY BY INTRAVENOUS INJECTION
  - Adult: Initially 750 micrograms/kg, followed immediately by (by intravenous infusion) 1.75 mg/kg/hour during procedure and for up to 4 hours after procedure, then (by intravenous infusion) reduced to 250 micrograms/kg/hour for a further 4–12 hours if necessary

- CONTRA-INDICATIONS Active bleeding · bleeding disorders · severe hypertension · subacute bacterial endocarditis
- CAUTIONS Brachytherapy procedures · previous exposure to lepirudin (theoretical risk from lepirudin antibodies)
- INTERACTIONS → Appendix 1 (bivalirudin). Caution with concomitant use of drugs that increase risk of bleeding.
- SIDE-EFFECTS
  - Common or very common Bleeding (discontinue) · ecchymosis
  - Uncommon Allergic reactions · anaemia · headache · hypotension · isolated reports of anaphylaxis · nausea · thrombocytopenia
  - Rare Back pain · bradycardia · dyspnoea · tachycardia · thrombosis · vomiting
- PREGNANCY Manufacturer advises avoid unless potential benefit outweighs risk—no information available.
- BREAST FEEDING Manufacturer advises caution—no information available.
- RENAL IMPAIRMENT
  - When used for percutaneous coronary intervention Reduce rate of infusion to 1.4 mg/kg/hour if eGFR 30–60 mL/minute/1.73 m^2 and monitor blood clotting parameters. Avoid if eGFR less than 30 mL/minute/1.73 m^2.
- DIRECTIONS FOR ADMINISTRATION For *intravenous infusion* (*Angiox®*), give continuously in Glucose 5% or Sodium chloride 0.9%. Reconstitute each 250-mg vial with 5 mL water for injections then withdraw 5 mL and dilute to 50 mL with infusion fluid.
- NATIONAL FUNDING/ACCESS DECISIONS
NICE technology appraisals (TAs)
  - Bivalirudin for the treatment of ST-segment elevation myocardial infarction (July 2011) NICE TA230
Bivalirudin in combination with aspirin and clopidogrel is recommended for the treatment of adults with ST-segment elevation myocardial infarction undergoing primary percutaneous coronary intervention.
www.nice.org.uk/TA230
Scottish Medicines Consortium (SMC) Decisions
The *Scottish Medicines Consortium* has advised (November 2008) that bivalirudin (*Angiox®*) is accepted for restricted use within NHS Scotland for patients with acute coronary syndromes planned for urgent or early intervention who would have been considered for treatment with unfractionated heparin in combination with a glycoprotein IIb/IIIa inhibitor; it should not be used as an alternative to heparin alone.
The *Scottish Medicines Consortium* has advised (August 2010) that bivalirudin (*Angiox®*) is accepted for restricted use within NHS Scotland as an anticoagulant in patients undergoing percutaneous coronary intervention who

would have been considered for treatment with unfractionated heparin in combination with a glycoprotein IIb/IIIa inhibitor; it should not be used as an alternative to heparin alone.

● MEDICINAL FORMS
There can be variation in the licensing of different medicines containing the same drug.

Powder for solution for injection
▸ Angiox (The Medicines Company UK Ltd)
  Bivalirudin 250 mg Angiox 250mg powder for solution for injection vials | 10 vial [PoM] no price available

Dabigatran etexilate

● DRUG ACTION Dabigatran etexilate is a direct thrombin inhibitor with a rapid onset of action.

● INDICATIONS AND DOSE

Prophylaxis of venous thromboembolism following total knee replacement surgery
▸ BY MOUTH
  ▸ Adult 18-74 years: 110 mg, to be taken 1–4 hours after surgery, followed by 220 mg once daily for 9 days, to be taken 12–24 hours after initial dose
  ▸ Adult 75 years and over: 75 mg, to be taken 1–4 hours after surgery, followed by 150 mg once daily for 9 days, to be taken 12–24 hours after initial dose

Prophylaxis of venous thromboembolism following total knee replacement surgery in patients receiving concomitant treatment with amiodarone or verapamil
▸ BY MOUTH
  ▸ Adult 18-74 years: 110 mg, to be taken 1–4 hours after surgery, followed by 150 mg once daily for 9 days, to be taken 12–24 hours after initial dose
  ▸ Adult 75 years and over: 75 mg, to be taken 1–4 hours after surgery, followed by 150 mg once daily for 9 days, to be taken 12–24 hours after initial dose

Prophylaxis of venous thromboembolism following total hip replacement surgery
▸ BY MOUTH
  ▸ Adult 18-74 years: 110 mg, to be taken 1–4 hours after surgery, followed by 220 mg once daily for 27–34 days, to be taken 12–24 hours after initial dose
  ▸ Adult 75 years and over: 75 mg, to be taken 1–4 hours after surgery, followed by 150 mg once daily for 27–34 days, to be taken 12–24 hours after initial dose

Prophylaxis of venous thromboembolism following total hip replacement surgery in patients receiving concomitant treatment with amiodarone or verapamil
▸ BY MOUTH
  ▸ Adult 18-74 years: 110 mg, to be taken 1–4 hours after surgery, followed by 150 mg daily for 27–34 days, to be taken 12–24 hours after initial dose
  ▸ Adult 75 years and over: 75 mg, to be taken 1–4 hours after surgery, followed by 150 mg once daily for 27–34 days, to be taken 12–24 hours after initial dose

Treatment of deep-vein thrombosis | Treatment of pulmonary embolism | Prophylaxis of recurrent deep-vein thrombosis | Prophylaxis of recurrent pulmonary embolism
▸ BY MOUTH
  ▸ Adult 18-74 years: 150 mg twice daily, following at least 5 days treatment with a parenteral anticoagulant
  ▸ Adult 75-79 years: 110–150 mg twice daily, following at least 5 days treatment with a parenteral anticoagulant
  ▸ Adult 80 years and over: 110 mg twice daily, following at least 5 days treatment with a parenteral anticoagulant

Treatment of deep-vein thrombosis in patients with moderate renal impairment | Treatment of deep-vein thrombosis in patients at increased risk of bleeding | Treatment of pulmonary embolism in patients with moderate renal impairment | Treatment of pulmonary embolism in patients at increased risk of bleeding | Prophylaxis of recurrent deep-vein thrombosis in patients with moderate renal impairment | Prophylaxis of recurrent deep-vein thrombosis in patients at increased risk of bleeding | Prophylaxis of recurrent pulmonary embolism in patients with moderate renal impairment | Prophylaxis of recurrent pulmonary embolism in patients at increased risk of bleeding
▸ BY MOUTH
  ▸ Adult: 110–150 mg twice daily, following at least 5 days treatment with a parenteral anticoagulant

Treatment of deep-vein thrombosis in patients receiving concomitant treatment with verapamil | Treatment of pulmonary embolism in patients receiving concomitant treatment with verapamil | Prophylaxis of recurrent deep-vein thrombosis in patients receiving concomitant treatment with verapamil | Prophylaxis of recurrent pulmonary embolism in patients receiving concomitant treatment with verapamil
▸ BY MOUTH
  ▸ Adult: 110 mg twice daily, following at least 5 days treatment with a parenteral anticoagulant

Prophylaxis of stroke and systemic embolism in non-valvular atrial fibrillation and with one or more risk factors such as previous stroke or transient ischaemic attack, symptomatic heart failure, age ≥ 75 years, diabetes mellitus, or hypertension
▸ BY MOUTH
  ▸ Adult 18-74 years: 150 mg twice daily
  ▸ Adult 75-79 years: 110–150 mg twice daily
  ▸ Adult 80 years and over: 110 mg twice daily

Prophylaxis of stroke and systemic embolism in non-valvular atrial fibrillation and with one or more risk factors such as previous stroke or transient ischaemic attack, symptomatic heart failure, age ≥ 75 years, diabetes mellitus, or hypertension in patients receiving concomitant treatment with verapamil
▸ BY MOUTH
  ▸ Adult: 110 mg twice daily

Prophylaxis of stroke and systemic embolism in non-valvular atrial fibrillation and with one or more risk factors such as previous stroke or transient ischaemic attack, symptomatic heart failure, age ≥ 75 years, diabetes mellitus, or hypertension, in patients at increased risk of bleeding | Prophylaxis of stroke and systemic embolism in non-valvular atrial fibrillation and with one or more risk factors such as previous stroke or transient ischaemic attack, symptomatic heart failure, age ≥ 75 years, diabetes mellitus, or hypertension, in patients with moderate renal impairment
▸ BY MOUTH
  ▸ Adult: 110–150 mg twice daily

DOSE EQUIVALENCE AND CONVERSION
For information on changing from, or to, other anticoagulants, consult product literature.

● CONTRA-INDICATIONS Active bleeding · do not use as anticoagulant for prosthetic heart valve · malignant neoplasms · oesophageal varices · recent brain surgery · recent gastro-intestinal ulcer · recent intracranial haemorrhage · recent ophthalmic surgery · recent spine surgery · significant risk of major bleeding · vascular aneurysm

- CAUTIONS Anaesthesia with postoperative indwelling epidural catheter (risk of paralysis—give initial dose at least 2 hours after catheter removal and monitor neurological signs) · bacterial endocarditis · bleeding disorders · body-weight less than 50 kg · elderly · gastritis · gastro-oesophageal reflux · oesophagitis · recent biopsy · recent major trauma · thrombocytopenia

- INTERACTIONS → Appendix 1 (dabigatran).
Caution in concomitant use of drugs that increase risk of bleeding.

- SIDE-EFFECTS
- **Common or very common** Abdominal pain · anaemia · diarrhoea · dyspepsia · haemorrhage · nausea
- **Uncommon** Dysphagia · gastro-intestinal ulcer · gastro-oesophageal reflux · hepatobiliary disorders · oesophagitis · thrombocytopenia · vomiting

- PREGNANCY Manufacturer advises avoid unless essential—toxicity in *animal* studies.

- BREAST FEEDING Manufacturer advises avoid—no information available.

- HEPATIC IMPAIRMENT Avoid in severe liver disease, especially if prothrombin time already prolonged.

- RENAL IMPAIRMENT
- When used for prophylaxis of venous thromboembolism following knee or hip replacement surgery Reduce initial dose to 75 mg and subsequent doses to 150 mg once daily if creatinine clearance 30–50 mL/minute; reduce dose to 75 mg once daily if creatinine clearance 30–50 mL/minute and patient receiving concomitant treatment with verapamil.
- When used for treatment of deep-vein thrombosis and pulmonary embolism, prophylaxis of recurrent deep-vein thrombosis and pulmonary embolism, prophylaxis of stroke and systemic embolism in non-valvular atrial fibrillation Consider reduced dose of 110 mg twice daily if creatinine clearance 30–50 mL/minute, based on individual assessment of thromboembolic risk and risk of bleeding.

Avoid if creatinine clearance less than 30 mL/minute.

In renal impairment monitor renal function at least annually (manufacturer recommends Cockroft and Gault formula to calculate creatinine clearance).

- MONITORING REQUIREMENTS
- Patients should be monitored for signs of bleeding or anaemia; treatment should be stopped if severe bleeding occurs.
- No routine anticoagulant monitoring required (INR tests are unreliable).
- Assess renal function (manufacturer recommends Cockroft and Gault formula to calculate creatinine clearance) before treatment in all patients and at least annually in elderly.

- DIRECTIONS FOR ADMINISTRATION When given concomitantly with amiodarone or verapamil, doses should be taken at the same time.

- PRESCRIBING AND DISPENSING INFORMATION Dabigatran etexilate, is given orally for prophylaxis of venous thromboembolism in adults after total hip replacement or total knee replacement surgery; it is also licensed for the treatment of deep-vein thrombosis and pulmonary embolism, and prophylaxis of recurrent deep-vein thrombosis and pulmonary embolism in adults. Duration of treatment should be determined by balancing the benefit of treatment with the bleeding risk; shorter duration of treatment (at least 3 months) should be based on transient risk factors i.e recent surgery, trauma, immobilisation, and longer duration of treatment should be based on permanent risk factors, or idiopathic deep-vein thrombosis or pulmonary embolism.

- NATIONAL FUNDING/ACCESS DECISIONS
NICE technology appraisals (TAs)
- Dabigatran etexilate for the prevention of venous thromboembolism after hip or knee replacement surgery in adults (September 2008) NICE TA157
Dabigatran etexilate is an option for the prophylaxis of venous thromboembolism in adults after total hip replacement or total knee replacement surgery.
www.nice.org.uk/TA157

- Dabigatran etexilate for the prevention of stroke and systemic embolism in atrial fibrillation (March 2012) NICE TA249
Dabigatran etexilate is an option for the prevention of stroke and systemic embolism in patients with non-valvular atrial fibrillation and with one or more of the following risk factors:
  - previous stroke, transient ischaemic attack, or systemic embolism
  - left ventricular ejection fraction <40%
  - symptomatic heart failure
  - age ≥75 years
  - age ≥65 years in patients with diabetes mellitus, coronary artery disease, or hypertension
The risks and benefits of dabigatran compared to warfarin should be discussed with the patient.
www.nice.org.uk/TA249

- Dabigatran etexilate for the treatment and secondary prevention of deep vein thrombosis and /or pulmonary embolism (December 2014) NICE TA327
Dabigatran etexilate is recommended, within its marketing authorisation, as an option for treating and for preventing recurrent deep vein thrombosis and pulmonary embolism in adults.
www.nice.org.uk/TA327

- MEDICINAL FORMS
There can be variation in the licensing of different medicines containing the same drug.
Capsule
CAUTIONARY AND ADVISORY LABELS 25
- Pradaxa (Boehringer Ingelheim Ltd)
Dabigatran etexilate (as Dabigatran etexilate mesilate)
75 mg Pradaxa 75mg capsules | 10 capsule PoM £8.50 | 60 capsule PoM £51.00 DT price = £51.00
Dabigatran etexilate (as Dabigatran etexilate mesilate)
110 mg Pradaxa 110mg capsules | 10 capsule PoM £8.50 | 60 capsule PoM £51.00 DT price = £51.00
Dabigatran etexilate (as Dabigatran etexilate mesilate)
150 mg Pradaxa 150mg capsules | 60 capsule PoM £51.00 DT price = £51.00

ANTITHROMBOTIC DRUGS > TISSUE PLASMINOGEN ACTIVATORS

Urokinase

- INDICATIONS AND DOSE
Deep-vein thrombosis (thromboembolic occlusive vascular disease)
- BY INTRAVENOUS INFUSION
- Adult: Initially 4400 units/kg, to be given over 10–20 minutes, followed by 100 000 units/hour for 2–3 days

Pulmonary embolism (thromboembolic occlusive vascular disease)
- BY INTRAVENOUS INFUSION
- Adult: Initially 4400 units/kg, to be given over 10–20 minutes, followed by 4400 units/kg/hour for 12 hours

Occlusive peripheral arterial disease (thromboembolic occlusive vascular disease)
- BY INTRA-ARTERIAL INFUSION
- Adult: (consult product literature)

Occluded central venous catheters (blocked by fibrin clots)

▶ BY INTRAVENOUS INJECTION

▸ Adult: Inject directly into occluded catheter, to be dissolved in sodium chloride 0.9% to a concentration of 5000 units/mL; use a volume sufficient to fill the catheter lumen; leave for 20–60 minutes then aspirate the lysate; repeat if necessary

Occluded arteriovenous haemodialysis shunts (blocked by fibrin clots)

▶ BY INTRAVENOUS INFUSION, OR BY INTRA-ARTERIAL INFUSION

▸ Adult: (consult product literature)

SYNER-KINASE®

Deep-vein thrombosis (thromboembolic occlusive vascular disease)

▶ BY INTRAVENOUS INFUSION

▸ Adult: Initially 4400 units/kg, to be given over 10 minutes, dose to be made up in 15 mL sodium chloride 0.9%, followed by 4400 units/kg/hour for 12–24 hours

Pulmonary embolism (thromboembolic occlusive vascular disease)

▶ INITIALLY BY INTRAVENOUS INFUSION

▸ Adult: Initially 4400 units/kg, to be given over 10 minutes, dose to be made up in 15 mL sodium chloride 0.9%, followed by (by intravenous infusion) 4400 micrograms/kg/hour for 12 hours, alternatively (by intra-arterial injection) initially 15 000 units/kg, to be injected into pulmonary artery, subsequent doses adjusted according to response; maximum 3 doses per day

Occlusive peripheral arterial disease

▶ BY INTRA-ARTERIAL INFUSION

▸ Adult: (consult product literature)

Occluded intravenous catheters and cannulas (blocked by fibrin clots)

▶ BY INTRA-ARTERIAL INJECTION, OR BY INTRAVENOUS INJECTION

▸ Adult: 5000–25 000 units, to be injected directly into catheter or cannula, dose dissolved in suitable volume of sodium chloride 0.9% to fill the catheter or cannula lumen; leave for 20–60 minutes then aspirate the lysate; repeat if necessary

● BREAST FEEDING Manufacturer advises avoid—no information available.

● HEPATIC IMPAIRMENT Dose reduction may be required.

● RENAL IMPAIRMENT Dose reduction may be required.

● DIRECTIONS FOR ADMINISTRATION For *intravenous infusion* (*Syner-KINASE*®), give continuously or intermittently in Sodium chloride 0.9%.

● MEDICINAL FORMS
There can be variation in the licensing of different medicines containing the same drug.

Powder for solution for injection

▸ Urokinase (Non-proprietary)
Urokinase 10000 unit Urokinase 10,000unit powder for solution for injection vials | 1 vial [PoM] £33.79
Urokinase 50000 unit Urokinase 50,000unit powder for solution for injection vials | 1 vial [PoM] £69.70
Urokinase 100000 unit Urokinase 100,000unit powder for solution for injection vials | 1 vial [PoM] £106.17
Urokinase 250000 unit Urokinase 250,000unit powder for solution for injection vials | 1 vial [PoM] £185.65
Urokinase 500000 unit Urokinase 500,000unit powder for solution for injection vials | 1 vial [PoM] £365.00
▸ Syner-KINASE (Syner-Med (Pharmaceutical Products) Ltd)
Urokinase 10000 unit Syner-KINASE 10,000unit powder for solution for injection vials | 1 vial [PoM] £35.95
Urokinase 25000 unit Syner-KINASE 25,000unit powder for solution for injection vials | 1 vial [PoM] £45.95

Urokinase 100000 unit Syner-KINASE 100,000unit powder for solution for injection vials | 1 vial [PoM] £112.95
Urokinase 250000 unit Syner-KINASE 250,000unit powder for solution for injection vials | 1 vial [PoM] no price available
Urokinase 500000 unit Syner-KINASE 500,000unit powder for solution for injection vials | 1 vial [PoM] no price available

ANTITHROMBOTIC DRUGS > VITAMIN K ANTAGONISTS

Vitamin K antagonists

● CONTRA-INDICATIONS Avoid use within 48 hours postpartum · haemorrhagic stroke · significant bleeding

● CAUTIONS Bacterial endocarditis (use only if warfarin otherwise indicated) · conditions in which risk of bleeding is increased · history of gastrointestinal bleeding · peptic ulcer · postpartum (delay warfarin until risk of haemorrhage is low—usually 5–7 days after delivery) · recent ischaemic stroke · recent surgery · uncontrolled hypertension

● INTERACTIONS → Appendix 1 (coumarins, phenindione). Major changes in diet (especially involving salads and vegetables) and in alcohol consumption may affect warfarin control.
Caution if concomitant use of drugs that increase risk of bleeding. Avoid cranberry juice.

● SIDE-EFFECTS Alopecia · diarrhoea · haemorrhage · hepatic dysfunction · jaundice · nausea · pancreatitis · purpura · pyrexia · rash · skin necrosis (increased risk in patients with protein C or protein S deficiency) · vomiting · 'purple toes'

● CONCEPTION AND CONTRACEPTION Women of child-bearing age should be warned of the danger of teratogenicity.

● PREGNANCY Should not be given in the first trimester of pregnancy. Warfarin, acenocoumarol, and phenindione cross the placenta with risk of congenital malformations, and placental, fetal, or neonatal haemorrhage, especially during the last few weeks of pregnancy and at delivery. Therefore, if at all possible, they should be avoided in pregnancy, especially in the first and third trimesters (difficult decisions may have to be made, particularly in women with prosthetic heart valves, atrial fibrillation, or with a history of recurrent venous thrombosis or pulmonary embolism). Stopping these drugs before the sixth week of gestation may largely avoid the risk of fetal abnormality.

● MONITORING REQUIREMENTS
▶ The base-line prothrombin time should be determined but the initial dose should not be delayed whilst awaiting the result.
▶ It is essential that the INR be determined daily or on alternate days in early days of treatment, *then* at longer intervals (depending on response), *then* up to every 12 weeks.
▶ Change in patient's clinical condition, particularly associated with liver disease, intercurrent illness, or drug administration, necessitates more frequent testing.

● PATIENT AND CARER ADVICE Anticoagulant treatment booklets should be issued to all patients or their carers; these booklets include advice for patients on anticoagulant treatment, an alert card to be carried by the patient at all times, and a section for recording of INR results and dosage information. In **England**, **Wales**, and **Northern Ireland**, they are available for purchase from:
Gorse Street, Chadderton
Oldham
OL9 9QH
Tel: 0845 610 1112

GP practices can obtain supplies through their Local Area Team stores. NHS Trusts can order supplies from www.nhsforms.co.uk or by emailing nhsforms@mmm.com.

In **Scotland**, treatment booklets and starter information packs can be obtained by emailing stockorders.dppas@theapsgroup.com or by fax on (0131) 6299 967

Electronic copies of the booklets and further advice are also available at www.npsa.nhs.uk/nrls/alerts-and-directives/alerts/anticoagulant.

☞ 125

Acenocoumarol

(Nicoumalone)

● INDICATIONS AND DOSE

Prophylaxis of embolisation in rheumatic heart disease and atrial fibrillation | Prophylaxis after insertion of prosthetic heart valve | Prophylaxis and treatment of venous thrombosis and pulmonary embolism | Transient ischaemic attacks

▸ BY MOUTH

▸ Adult: Initially 2–4 mg once daily for 2 days, alternatively initially 6 mg on day 1, then 4 mg on day 2; maintenance 1–8 mg daily, adjusted according to response, dose to be taken at the same time each day, lower doses may be required in patients over 65 years, liver disease, severe heart failure with hepatic congestion, and malnutrition

● CAUTIONS Patients over 65 years

● SIDE-EFFECTS
▸ Rare Anorexia
▸ Very rare Vasculitis

● BREAST FEEDING Risk of haemorrhage; increased by vitamin k deficiency—manufacturer recommends prophylactic vitamin K for the infant (consult product literature).

● HEPATIC IMPAIRMENT Use with caution in mild to moderate impairment. Avoid in severe impairment, especially if prothrombin time is already prolonged.

● RENAL IMPAIRMENT Caution in mild to moderate impairment. Avoid in severe impairment.

● PATIENT AND CARER ADVICE Anticoagulant card to be provided.

● MEDICINAL FORMS
There can be variation in the licensing of different medicines containing the same drug.

Tablet
CAUTIONARY AND ADVISORY LABELS 10
▸ Acenocoumarol (Non-proprietary)
Acenocoumarol 1 mg Acenocoumarol 1mg tablets | 100 tablet [PoM] no price available DT price = £4.62
▸ Sinthrome (Merus Labs Luxco S.a R.L.)
Acenocoumarol 1 mg Sinthrome 1mg tablets | 100 tablet [PoM] £4.62 DT price = £4.62

☞ 125

Phenindione

● INDICATIONS AND DOSE

Prophylaxis of embolisation in rheumatic heart disease and atrial fibrillation | Prophylaxis after insertion of prosthetic heart valve | Prophylaxis and treatment of venous thrombosis and pulmonary embolism

▸ BY MOUTH

▸ Adult: Initially 200 mg on day 1, then 100 mg on day 2, then, adjusted according to response; maintenance 50–150 mg daily

● SIDE-EFFECTS Agranulocytosis · eosinophilia · exanthema · exfoliative dermatitis · fever · hypersensitivity reactions ·

leucopenia · micro-adenopathy · renal damage · urine coloured pink or orange

● BREAST FEEDING Avoid. Risk of haemorrhage; increased by vitamin K deficiency.

● HEPATIC IMPAIRMENT Avoid in severe impairment, especially if prothrombin time is already prolonged.

● RENAL IMPAIRMENT Caution in mild to moderate impairment. Avoid in severe impairment.

● PATIENT AND CARER ADVICE Anticoagulant card to be provided.

Patient counselling is advised for phenindione tablets (may turn urine pink or orange).

● MEDICINAL FORMS
There can be variation in the licensing of different medicines containing the same drug.

Tablet
CAUTIONARY AND ADVISORY LABELS 10, 14
▸ Phenindione (Non-proprietary)
Phenindione 10 mg Phenindione 10mg tablets | 28 tablet [PoM] £519.98 DT price = £519.98
Phenindione 25 mg Phenindione 25mg tablets | 28 tablet [PoM] £519.98 DT price = £519.98
Phenindione 50 mg Phenindione 50mg tablets | 28 tablet [PoM] £51.84

☞ 125

Warfarin sodium

● INDICATIONS AND DOSE

Prophylaxis of embolisation in rheumatic heart disease and atrial fibrillation | Prophylaxis after insertion of prosthetic heart valve | Prophylaxis and treatment of venous thrombosis and pulmonary embolism | Transient ischaemic attacks

▸ BY MOUTH

▸ Adult: Initially 5–10 mg, to be taken on day 1; subsequent doses dependent on the prothrombin time, reported as INR (international normalised ratio), a lower induction dose can be given over 3–4 weeks in patients who do not require rapid anticoagulation, elderly patients to be given a lower induction dose; maintenance 3–9 mg daily, to be taken at the same time each day

● PREGNANCY Babies of mothers taking warfarin at the time of delivery need to be offered immediate prophylaxis with intramuscular phytomenadione (vitamin K_1).

● BREAST FEEDING Not present in milk in significant amounts and appears safe. Risk of haemorrhage which is increased by vitamin K deficiency.

● HEPATIC IMPAIRMENT Avoid in severe impairment, especially if prothrombin time is already prolonged.

● RENAL IMPAIRMENT Use with caution in mild to moderate impairment. In severe renal impairment, monitor INR more frequently.

● PATIENT AND CARER ADVICE Anticoagulant card to be provided.

● MEDICINAL FORMS
There can be variation in the licensing of different medicines containing the same drug. Forms available from special-order manufacturers include: capsule, oral suspension, oral solution

Tablet
CAUTIONARY AND ADVISORY LABELS 10
▸ Warfarin sodium (Non-proprietary)
Warfarin sodium 500 microgram Warfarin 500microgram tablets | 28 tablet [PoM] £1.92 DT price = £1.54
Warfarin sodium 1 mg Warfarin 1mg tablets | 28 tablet [PoM] £1.16 DT price = £0.76 | 500 tablet [PoM] £14.82
Warfarin sodium 3 mg Warfarin 3mg tablets | 28 tablet [PoM] £1.20 DT price = £0.79 | 500 tablet [PoM] £15.71

Warfarin sodium 4 mg Coumadin 4mg tablets | 100 tablet [PoM] no price available
Warfarin sodium 5 mg Warfarin 5mg tablets | 28 tablet [PoM] £1.29 DT price = £0.82 | 500 tablet [PoM] no price available
▶ Marevan (AMCo)
Warfarin sodium 1 mg Marevan 1mg tablets | 28 tablet [PoM] £0.31 DT price = £0.76
Warfarin sodium 3 mg Marevan 3mg tablets | 28 tablet [PoM] £0.35 DT price = £0.79
Warfarin sodium 5 mg Marevan 5mg tablets | 28 tablet [PoM] £0.47 DT price = £0.82

Oral suspension
CAUTIONARY AND ADVISORY LABELS 10
▶ Warfarin sodium (Non-proprietary)
Warfarin sodium 1 mg per 1 ml Warfarin 1mg/ml oral suspension sugar free sugar-free | 150 ml [PoM] £108.00 DT price = £108.00

4 Blood pressure conditions
4.1 Hypertension

Hypertension

Overview

Lowering raised blood pressure decreases the risk of stroke, coronary events, heart failure, and renal impairment. Advice on antihypertensive therapy in this section takes into account the recommendations of NICE clinical guidance 127 (August 2011), Hypertension—Clinical management of primary hypertension in adults.

Possible causes of hypertension (e.g. renal disease, endocrine causes), contributory factors, risk factors, and the presence of any complications of hypertension, such as left ventricular hypertrophy, should be established. Patients should be given advice on lifestyle changes to reduce blood pressure or cardiovascular risk; these include smoking cessation, weight reduction, reduction of excessive intake of alcohol and caffeine, reduction of dietary salt, reduction of total and saturated fat, increasing exercise, and increasing fruit and vegetable intake.

Thresholds and targets for treatment

Patients presenting with a blood pressure of 140/90 mmHg or higher when measured in a clinic setting, should be offered ambulatory blood pressure monitoring (or home blood pressure monitoring if ambulatory blood pressure monitoring is unsuitable) to confirm the diagnosis and stage of hypertension.

Stage 1 hypertension:
* Clinic blood pressure 140/90 mmHg or higher, *and* ambulatory daytime average or home blood pressure average 135/85 mmHg or higher
* Treat patients under 80 years who have stage 1 hypertension and target-organ damage (e.g. left ventricular hypertrophy, chronic kidney disease, hypertensive retinopathy), cardiovascular disease, renal disease, diabetes, or a 10 year cardiovascular risk ≥20%; in the absence of these conditions, advise lifestyle changes and review annually. For patients under 40 years with stage 1 hypertension but **no** overt target-organ damage, cardiovascular disease, renal disease, or diabetes, consider seeking specialist advice for evaluation of secondary causes of hypertension

Stage 2 hypertension:
* Clinic blood pressure 160/100 mmHg or higher, *and* ambulatory daytime average or home blood pressure average 150/95 mmHg or higher
* Treat all patients who have stage 2 hypertension, regardless of age

Severe hypertension:
* Clinic systolic blood pressure ≥180 mmHg or clinic diastolic blood pressure ≥110 mmHg; treat promptly—see Hypertensive Crises, below.

A target clinic blood pressure below 140/90 mmHg is suggested for patients under 80 years; a target ambulatory or home blood pressure average (during the patient's waking hours) of below 135/85 mmHg is suggested for patients under 80 years; see also Hypertension in the Elderly, below. A target clinic blood pressure below 130/80 mmHg should be considered for those with established atherosclerotic cardiovascular disease, or diabetes in the presence of kidney, eye, or cerebrovascular disease. In some individuals it may not be possible to reduce blood pressure below the suggested targets despite the use of appropriate therapy.

Drug treatment of hypertension

A single antihypertensive drug is often inadequate in the management of hypertension, and additional antihypertensive drugs are usually added in a step-wise manner until control is achieved. Unless it is necessary to lower the blood pressure urgently (see Hypertensive Crises), an interval of at least 4 weeks should be allowed to determine response; clinicians should ensure antihypertensive drugs are titrated to the optimum or maximum tolerated dose at each step of treatment. Response to drug treatment may be affected by age and ethnicity.

Patients under 55 years:
Step 1
* **ACE inhibitor**; if not tolerated, offer an **angiotensin-II receptor antagonist**. If both ACE inhibitors and angiotensin-II receptor antagonists are contra-indicated or not tolerated, consider a **beta-blocker**; beta-blockers, especially when combined with a thiazide diuretic, should be avoided for the routine treatment of uncomplicated hypertension in patients with diabetes or at high risk of developing diabetes

Step 2
* ACE inhibitor or angiotensin-II receptor antagonist in combination with a **calcium-channel blocker**. If a calcium-channel blocker is not tolerated or if there is evidence of, or a high risk of, heart failure, give a **thiazide-related diuretic** (e.g. chlortalidone or indapamide). If a beta-blocker was given at Step 1, add a calcium channel blocker in preference to a thiazide-related diuretic (see Step 1)

Step 3
* ACE inhibitor or angiotensin-II receptor antagonist in combination with a calcium-channel blocker *and* a thiazide-related diuretic

Step 4 (resistant hypertension)
* Consider seeking specialist advice
* Add low-dose **spironolactone** [unlicensed indication], *or* use high-dose thiazide related diuretic if plasma-potassium concentration above 4.5 mmol/litre
* Monitor renal function and electrolytes
* If additional diuretic therapy is contra-indicated, ineffective, or not tolerated, consider an **alpha-blocker** *or* a beta-blocker

Patients over 55 years, and patients of any age who are of African or Caribbean family origin:
Step 1
* Calcium-channel blocker; if not tolerated or if there is evidence of, or a high risk of, heart failure, give a thiazide-related diuretic (e.g. chlortalidone or indapamide)

Step 2
* Calcium-channel blocker *or* thiazide-related diuretic in combination with an ACE inhibitor or angiotensin-II receptor antagonist (an angiotensin-II receptor antagonist

in combination with a calcium-channel blocker is preferred in patients of African or Caribbean family origin)

Steps 3 and 4

- Treat as for patients under 55 years

Other measures to reduce cardiovascular risk

Aspirin p. 109 reduces the risk of cardiovascular events and myocardial infarction. Unduly high blood pressure must be controlled before aspirin is given. Unless contra-indicated, aspirin is recommended for all patients with established cardiovascular disease. Use of aspirin in primary prevention, in those with or without diabetes, is of unproven benefit. For the role of aspirin in the prevention of stroke in patients with atrial fibrillation, see Arrhythmias p. 88.

Statins are also of benefit in cardiovascular disease or in those who are at high risk of developing cardiovascular disease.

Hypertension in the elderly

Benefit from antihypertensive therapy is evident up to at least 80 years of age, but it is probably inappropriate to apply a strict age limit when deciding on drug therapy. Patients who reach 80 years of age while taking antihypertensive drugs should continue treatment, provided that it continues to be of benefit and does not cause significant side-effects. If patients are aged over 80 years when diagnosed with stage 1 hypertension, the decision to treat should be based on the presence of other comorbidities; patients with stage 2 hypertension should be treated as for patients over 55 years. A target clinic blood pressure below 150/90 mmHg is suggested for patients over 80 years; the suggested target ambulatory or home blood pressure average (during the patient's waking hours) is below 145/85 mmHg.

Isolated systolic hypertension

Isolated systolic hypertension (systolic pressure ≥160 mmHg, diastolic pressure < 90 mmHg) is common in patients over 60 years, and is associated with an increased cardiovascular disease risk; it should be treated as for patients with both a raised systolic and diastolic blood pressure. Patients with severe postural hypotension should be referred to a specialist.

Hypertension in diabetes

For patients with diabetes, a target clinic blood pressure below 140/80 mmHg is suggested (below 130/80 mmHg is advised if kidney, eye, or cerebrovascular disease are also present). However, in some individuals, it may not be possible to achieve this level of control despite appropriate therapy. Most patients require a combination of antihypertensive drugs.

Hypertension is common in type 2 diabetes, and antihypertensive treatment prevents macrovascular and microvascular complications. In type 1 diabetes, hypertension usually indicates the presence of diabetic nephropathy. An ACE inhibitor (or an angiotensin-II receptor antagonist) may have a specific role in the management of diabetic nephropathy; in patients with type 2 diabetes, an ACE inhibitor (or an angiotensin-II receptor antagonist) can delay progression of microalbuminuria to nephropathy.

Hypertension in renal disease

A target clinic blood pressure below 140/90 mmHg is suggested (below 130/80 mmHg is advised in patients with chronic kidney disease and diabetes, or if proteinuria exceeds 1 g in 24 hours). An ACE inhibitor (or an angiotensin-II receptor antagonist) should be considered for patients with proteinuria; however, ACE inhibitors should be used with caution in renal impairment. Thiazide diuretics may be ineffective and high doses of loop diuretics may be required.

Hypertension in pregnancy

Hypertensive complications in pregnancy can be hazardous for both the mother and the fetus, and are associated with a significant risk of morbidity and mortality; complications can occur in pregnant women with pre-existing chronic hypertension, or in those who develop hypertension in the latter half of pregnancy.

Labetalol hydrochloride p. 135 is widely used for treating hypertension in pregnancy. Methyldopa p. 131 is considered safe for use in pregnancy. Modified-release preparations of nifedipine p. 148 [unlicensed] are also used.

The following advice takes into account the recommendations of NICE Clinical Guideline 107 (August 2010), Hypertension in Pregnancy.

Pregnant women with chronic hypertension who are already receiving antihypertensive treatment should have their drug therapy reviewed. In uncomplicated chronic hypertension, a target blood pressure of <150/100 mmHg is recommended; women with target-organ damage as a result of chronic hypertension, and in women with chronic hypertension who have given birth, a target blood pressure of <140/90 mmHg is advised. Long-term antihypertensive treatment should be reviewed 2 weeks following the birth. Women managed with methyldopa during pregnancy should discontinue treatment and restart their original antihypertensive medication within 2 days of the birth.

Pregnant women are at high risk of developing pre-eclampsia if they have chronic kidney disease, diabetes mellitus, autoimmune disease, chronic hypertension, or if they have had hypertension during a previous pregnancy; these women are advised to take aspirin p. 109 once daily [unlicensed indication] from week 12 of pregnancy until the baby is born. Women with more than one moderate risk factor (first pregnancy, aged ≥40 years, pregnancy interval >10 years, BMI ≥ 35 kg/m^2 at first visit, multiple pregnancy, or family history of pre-eclampsia) for developing pre-eclampsia are also advised to take aspirin once daily [unlicensed indication] from week 12 of pregnancy until the baby is born.

Women with pre-eclampsia or gestational hypertension who present with a blood pressure over 150/100 mmHg, should receive initial treatment with oral labetalol hydrochloride to achieve a target blood pressure of <150 mmHg systolic, and diastolic 80–100 mmHg. If labetalol hydrochloride is unsuitable, methyldopa or modified-release nifedipine may be considered. Women with gestational hypertension or pre-eclampsia who have been managed with methyldopa during pregnancy should discontinue treatment within 2 days of the birth. Women with a blood pressure of ≥160/110 mmHg who require critical care during pregnancy or after birth should receive immediate treatment with either oral or intravenous labetalol hydrochloride, intravenous hydralazine hydrochloride p. 166, or oral modified-release nifedipine to achieve a target blood pressure of <150 mmHg systolic, and diastolic 80–100 mmHg.

Also see use of magnesium sulfate p. 911 in pre-eclampsia and eclampsia.

Hypertensive crises

If blood pressure is reduced too quickly in the management of hypertensive crises, there is a risk of reduced organ perfusion leading to cerebral infarction, blindness, deterioration in renal function, and myocardial ischaemia.

A *hypertensive emergency* is defined as severe hypertension with acute damage to the target organs (e.g. signs of papilloedema or retinal haemorrhage, or the presence of clinical conditions such as acute coronary syndromes, acute aortic dissection, acute pulmonary oedema, hypertensive encephalopathy, acute cerebral infarction, intracerebral or subarachnoid haemorrhage, eclampsia, or rapidly progressing renal failure); prompt treatment with intravenous antihypertensive therapy is generally required. Over the first few minutes or within 2 hours, blood pressure should be reduced by 20–25%. When intravenous therapy is indicated, treatment options include sodium nitroprusside p. 168 [unlicensed], nicardipine hydrochloride p. 147, labetalol hydrochloride, glyceryl trinitrate p. 201, phentolamine mesilate p. 167, hydralazine hydrochloride, or esmolol hydrochloride p. 140; choice of drug is dependent on concomitant conditions and clinical status of the patient.

Severe hypertension (blood pressure ≥ 180/110 mmHg) without acute target-organ damage is defined as a *hypertensive urgency*; blood pressure should be reduced gradually over 24–48 hours with oral antihypertensive therapy, such as labetalol hydrochloride, or the calcium-channel blockers amlodipine p. 142 or felodipine p. 145. Use of sublingual nifedipine is not recommended.

Also see advice on short-term management of hypertensive episodes in phaeochromocytoma.

Phaeochromocytoma

Long-term management of phaeochromocytoma involves surgery. However, surgery should not take place until there is adequate blockade of both alpha- and beta-adrenoceptors; the optimal choice of drug therapy remains unclear. Alpha-blockers are used in the short-term management of hypertensive episodes in phaeochromocytoma. Once alpha blockade is established, tachycardia can be controlled by the cautious addition of a beta-blocker; a cardioselective beta-blocker is preferred.

Phenoxybenzamine hydrochloride p. 167, a powerful alpha-blocker, is effective in the management of phaeochromocytoma but it has many side-effects. Phentolamine mesilate is a short-acting alpha-blocker used mainly during surgery of phaeochromocytoma; its use for the diagnosis of phaeochromocytoma has been superseded by measurement of catecholamines in blood and urine.

Metirosine (available from 'special-order' manufacturers or specialist importing companies) inhibits the enzyme tyrosine hydroxylase, and hence the synthesis of catecholamines. It is rarely used in the pre-operative management of phaeochromocytoma, and long term in patients unsuitable for surgery; an alpha-adrenoceptor blocking drug may also be required. Metirosine should **not** be used to treat essential hypertension.

Antihypertensive drugs

Vasodilator antihypertensive drugs

Vasodilators have a potent hypotensive effect, especially when used in combination with a beta-blocker and a thiazide. **Important:** see Hypertension (hypertensive crises) for a warning on the hazards of a very rapid fall in blood pressure.

Hydralazine hydrochloride p. 166 is given by mouth as an adjunct to other antihypertensives for the treatment of resistant hypertension but is rarely used; when used alone it causes tachycardia and fluid retention.

Sodium nitroprusside p. 168 [unlicensed] is given by intravenous infusion to control severe hypertensive emergencies when parenteral treatment is necessary.

Minoxidil p. 167 should be reserved for the treatment of severe hypertension resistant to other drugs. Vasodilatation is accompanied by increased cardiac output and tachycardia and the patients develop fluid retention. For this reason the addition of a beta-blocker and a diuretic (usually furosemide p. 210, in high dosage) are mandatory. Hypertrichosis is troublesome and renders this drug unsuitable for females.

Prazosin p. 709, doxazosin p. 708, and terazosin p. 711 have alpha-blocking and vasodilator properties.

Ambrisentan p. 169, bosentan p. 169, iloprost p. 168, macitentan p. 170, sildenafil p. 736, and tadalafil p. 737 are

licensed for the treatment of pulmonary arterial hypertension and should be used under specialist supervision. Epoprostenol p. 104 can be used in patients with primary pulmonary hypertension resistant to other treatments. Bosentan is also licensed to reduce the number of new digital ulcers in patients with systemic sclerosis and ongoing digital ulcer disease. Riociguat p. 170 is licensed for the treatment of pulmonary arterial hypertension and chronic thromboembolic pulmonary hypertension; it should be used under specialist supervision.

Sitaxentan has been withdrawn from the market because the benefit of treatment does not outweigh the risk of severe hepatotoxicity.

Centrally acting antihypertensive drugs

Methyldopa p. 131 is a centrally acting antihypertensive; it may be used for the management of hypertension in pregnancy.

Clonidine hydrochloride p. 131 has the disadvantage that sudden withdrawal of treatment may cause severe rebound hypertension.

Moxonidine p. 132, a centrally acting drug, is licensed for mild to moderate essential hypertension. It may have a role when thiazides, calcium-channel blockers, ACE inhibitors, and beta-blockers are not appropriate or have failed to control blood pressure.

Adrenergic neurone blocking drugs

Adrenergic neurone blocking drugs prevent the release of noradrenaline from postganglionic adrenergic neurones. These drugs do not control supine blood pressure and may cause postural hypotension. For this reason they have largely fallen from use, but may be necessary with other therapy in resistant hypertension.

Guanethidine monosulfate p. 168, which also depletes the nerve endings of noradrenaline, is licensed for rapid control of blood pressure, however alternative treatments are preferred.

Alpha-adrenoceptor blocking drugs

Prazosin has post-synaptic alpha-blocking and vasodilator properties and rarely causes tachycardia. It may, however, reduce blood pressure rapidly after the first dose and should be introduced with caution. Doxazosin, indoramin p. 709, and terazosin have properties similar to those of prazosin.

Alpha-blockers can be used with other antihypertensive drugs in the treatment of resistant hypertension.

Prostatic hyperplasia

Alfuzosin hydrochloride p. 707, doxazosin, indoramin, prazosin, tamsulosin hydrochloride p. 710, and terazosin are indicated for benign prostatic hyperplasia.

Drugs affecting the renin-angiotensin system

Angiotensin-converting enzyme inhibitors

Angiotensin-converting enzyme inhibitors (ACE inhibitors) inhibit the conversion of angiotensin I to angiotensin II. They have many uses and are generally well tolerated. The main indications of ACE inhibitors are shown below.

Heart failure

ACE inhibitors are used in all grades of heart failure, usually combined with a beta-blocker. Potassium supplements and potassium-sparing diuretics should be discontinued before introducing an ACE inhibitor because of the risk of hyperkalaemia. However, a low dose of spironolactone p. 175 may be beneficial in severe heart failure and can be used with an ACE inhibitor provided serum potassium is monitored carefully. Profound first-dose hypotension may occur when

ACE inhibitors are introduced to patients with heart failure who are already taking a high dose of a loop diuretic (e.g. furosemide 80 mg daily or more). Temporary withdrawal of the loop diuretic reduces the risk, but may cause severe rebound pulmonary oedema. Therefore, for patients on high doses of loop diuretics, the ACE inhibitor may need to be initiated under specialist supervision. An ACE inhibitor can be initiated in the community in patients who are receiving a low dose of a diuretic or who are not otherwise at risk of serious hypotension; nevertheless, care is required and a very low dose of the ACE inhibitor is given initially.

Hypertension
An ACE inhibitor may be the most appropriate initial drug for hypertension in younger Caucasian patients; Afro-Caribbean patients, those aged over 55 years, and those with primary aldosteronism respond less well. ACE inhibitors are particularly indicated for hypertension in patients with type 1 diabetes with nephropathy. They may reduce blood pressure very rapidly in some patients particularly in those receiving diuretic therapy.

Diabetic nephropathy
ACE inhibitors have a role in the management of diabetic nephropathy.

Prophylaxis of cardiovascular events
ACE inhibitors are used in the early and long-term management of patients who have had a myocardial infarction. ACE inhibitors may also have a role in preventing cardiovascular events.

Initiation under specialist supervision
ACE inhibitors should be initiated under specialist supervision and with careful clinical monitoring in those with severe heart failure or in those:

- receiving multiple or high-dose diuretic therapy (e.g. more than 80 mg of furosemide daily or its equivalent);
- receiving concomitant angiotensin-II receptor antagonist or aliskiren;
- with hypovolaemia;
- with hyponatraemia (plasma-sodium concentration below 130 mmol/litre);
- with hypotension (systolic blood pressure below 90 mmHg);
- with unstable heart failure;
- receiving high-dose vasodilator therapy;
- known renovascular disease.

Renal effects
Renal function and electrolytes should be checked before starting ACE inhibitors (or increasing the dose) and monitored during treatment (more frequently if features mentioned below present); hyperkalaemia and other side-effects of ACE inhibitors are more common in those with impaired renal function and the dose may need to be reduced. Although ACE inhibitors now have a specialised role in some forms of renal disease, including chronic kidney disease, they also occasionally cause impairment of renal function which may progress and become severe in other circumstances (at particular risk are the elderly). A specialist should be involved if renal function is significantly reduced as a result of treatment with an ACE inhibitor.

Concomitant treatment with NSAIDs increases the risk of renal damage, and potassium-sparing diuretics (or potassium-containing salt substitutes) increase the risk of hyperkalaemia.

In patients with severe bilateral renal artery stenosis (or severe stenosis of the artery supplying a single functioning kidney), ACE inhibitors reduce or abolish glomerular filtration and are likely to cause severe and progressive renal failure. They are therefore not recommended in patients known to have these forms of critical renovascular disease.

ACE inhibitor treatment is unlikely to have an adverse effect on overall renal function in patients with severe unilateral renal artery stenosis and a normal contralateral kidney, but glomerular filtration is likely to be reduced (or even abolished) in the affected kidney and the long-term consequences are unknown.

ACE inhibitors are therefore best avoided in patients with known or suspected renovascular disease, unless the blood pressure cannot be controlled by other drugs. If ACE inhibitors are used, they should be initiated only under specialist supervision and renal function should be monitored regularly.

ACE inhibitors should also be used with particular caution in patients who may have undiagnosed and clinically silent renovascular disease. This includes patients with peripheral vascular disease or those with severe generalised atherosclerosis.

ACE inhibitors in combination with other drugs
See also, *Concomitant use of drugs affecting the renin-angiotensin system*, below.

Concomitant diuretics
ACE inhibitors can cause a very rapid fall in blood pressure in volume-depleted patients; treatment should therefore be initiated with very low doses. If the dose of diuretic is greater than 80 mg furosemide or equivalent, the ACE inhibitor should be initiated under close supervision and in some patients the diuretic dose may need to be reduced or the diuretic discontinued at least 24 hours beforehand (may not be possible in heart failure—risk of pulmonary oedema). If high-dose diuretic therapy cannot be stopped, close observation is recommended after administration of the first dose of ACE inhibitor, for at least 2 hours or until the blood pressure has stabilised.

Combination products
Products incorporating an ACE inhibitor with a thiazide diuretic or a calcium-channel blocker are available for the management of hypertension. Use of these combination products should be reserved for patients whose blood pressure has not responded adequately to a single antihypertensive drug and who have been stabilised on the individual components of the combination in the same proportions.

Angiotensin-II receptor antagonists

Azilsartan medoxomil p. 160, candesartan cilexetil p. 161, eprosartan p. 161, irbesartan p. 161, losartan potassium p. 162, olmesartan medoxomil p. 163, telmisartan p. 164, and valsartan p. 164 are angiotensin-II receptor antagonists with many properties similar to those of the ACE inhibitors. However, unlike ACE inhibitors, they do not inhibit the breakdown of bradykinin and other kinins, and thus are less likely to cause the persistent dry cough which can complicate ACE inhibitor therapy. They are therefore a useful alternative for patients who have to discontinue an ACE inhibitor because of persistent cough.

An angiotensin-II receptor antagonist may be used as an alternative to an ACE inhibitor in the management of heart failure or diabetic nephropathy. Candesartan cilexetil and valsartan are also licensed as adjuncts to ACE inhibitors under specialist supervision, in the management of heart failure when other treatments are unsuitable.

Renal effects
Angiotensin-II receptor antagonists should be used with caution in renal artery stenosis (see also Renal effects under Angiotensin-converting enzyme inhibitors, above).

Renin inhibitor
Aliskiren is a renin inhibitor that is licensed for the treatment of hypertension.

Concomitant use of drugs affecting the renin-angiotensin system

Combination therapy with two drugs affecting the renin-angiotensin system (ACE inhibitors, angiotensin-II receptor antagonists, and aliskiren p. 165 is not recommended due to an increased risk of hyperkalaemia, hypotension, and renal impairment, compared to use of a single drug. Patients with diabetic nephropathy are particularly susceptible to developing hyperkalaemia and should not be given an ACE inhibitor with an angiotensin-II receptor antagonist. There is some evidence that the benefits of combination use of an ACE inhibitor with candesartan or valsartan may outweigh the risks in selected patients with heart failure for whom other treatments are unsuitable, however, the concomitant use of this combination, together with an aldosterone antagonist or a potassium-sparing diuretic is not recommended.

For patients currently taking combination therapy, the need for continued combined therapy should be reviewed. If combination therapy is considered essential, it should be carried out under specialist supervision, with close monitoring of blood pressure, renal function, and electrolytes (particularly potassium); monitoring should be considered at the start of treatment, then monthly, and also after any change in dose or during intercurrent illness.

> **Drugs used for Hypertension not listed below** Co-triamterzide, p. 214 · Metolazone, p. 214 · Torasemide, p. 211 · Triamterene with chlortalidone, p. 213 · Xipamide, p. 214

ANTIHYPERTENSIVES, CENTRALLY ACTING

| Clonidine hydrochloride

- **INDICATIONS AND DOSE**

Hypertension
▶ BY MOUTH
▸ Adult: Initially 50–100 micrograms 3 times a day, increase dose every second or third day, usual maximum dose 1.2 mg daily

Prevention of recurrent migraine | Prevention of vascular headache
▶ BY MOUTH
▸ Adult: Initially 50 micrograms twice daily for 2 weeks, then increased if necessary to 75 micrograms twice daily

- **UNLICENSED USE** Clonidine may also be used for Tourette syndrome and sedation—unlicensed indications.
- **CONTRA-INDICATIONS** Severe bradyarrhythmia secondary to second- or third-degree AV block or sick sinus syndrome
- **CAUTIONS** Cerebrovascular disease · constipation · heart failure · history of depression · mild to moderate bradyarrhythmia · polyneuropathy · Raynaud's syndrome or other occlusive peripheral vascular disease
- **INTERACTIONS** → Appendix 1 (clonidine).
- **SIDE-EFFECTS**
▶ **Common or very common** Constipation · depression · dizziness · drowsiness · dry mouth · headache · malaise · nausea · postural hypotension · salivary gland pain · sexual dysfunction · sleep disturbances · vomiting
▶ **Uncommon** Bradycardia · delusion · hallucination · paraesthesia · pruritus · rash · Raynaud's syndrome · urticaria
▶ **Rare** Alopecia · AV block · colonic pseudo-obstruction · decreased lacrimation · gynaecomastia · nasal dryness
▶ **Frequency not known** Bradyarrhythmia · confusion · fluid retention · hepatitis · impaired visual accommodation

- **PREGNANCY** May lower fetal heart rate. Avoid oral use unless potential benefit outweighs risk. Avoid using injection.
- **BREAST FEEDING** Avoid—present in milk.
- **RENAL IMPAIRMENT** Use with caution in severe impairment—reduce initial dose and increase gradually.
- **TREATMENT CESSATION** In hypertension, must be withdrawn gradually to avoid severe rebound hypertension.
- **PATIENT AND CARER ADVICE**
Driving and skilled tasks
Drowsiness may affect performance of skilled tasks (e.g. driving); effects of alcohol may be enhanced.
- **LESS SUITABLE FOR PRESCRIBING** Clonidine is less suitable for prescribing.

- **MEDICINAL FORMS**
There can be variation in the licensing of different medicines containing the same drug. Forms available from special-order manufacturers include: oral suspension, oral solution
Tablet
CAUTIONARY AND ADVISORY LABELS 3, 8
▸ Clonidine hydrochloride (Non-proprietary)
  Clonidine hydrochloride 25 microgram Clonidine 25microgram tablets | 112 tablet [PoM] £12.79 DT price = £6.15
▸ Catapres (Boehringer Ingelheim Ltd)
  Clonidine hydrochloride 100 microgram Catapres 100microgram tablets | 100 tablet [PoM] £8.04 DT price = £8.04
▸ Dixarit (Boehringer Ingelheim Ltd)
  Clonidine hydrochloride 25 microgram Dixarit 25microgram tablets | 112 tablet [PoM] £6.99 DT price = £6.15

| Methyldopa

- **INDICATIONS AND DOSE**

Hypertension
▶ BY MOUTH
▸ Adult: Initially 250 mg 2–3 times a day, dose should be increased gradually at intervals of at least 2 days; maximum 3 g per day
▸ Elderly: Initially 125 mg twice daily, dose should be increased gradually; maximum 2 g per day

- **CONTRA-INDICATIONS** Acute porphyria · depression · phaeochromocytoma
- **CAUTIONS** History of depression
- **INTERACTIONS** → Appendix 1 (methyldopa).
- **SIDE-EFFECTS** Amenorrhoea · arthralgia · asthenia · Bell's palsy · bone-marrow depression · bradycardia · decreased libido · depression · dizziness · drug fever · dry mouth · eosinophilia · exacerbation of angina · failure of ejaculation · gastro-intestinal disturbances · gynaecomastia · haemolytic anaemia · headache · hepatitis · hyperprolactinaemia · hypersensitivity reactions · impaired mental acuity · impotence · jaundice · leucopenia · lupus erythematosus-like syndrome · mild psychosis · myalgia · myocarditis · nasal congestion · nightmares · oedema · pancreatitis · paraesthesia · parkinsonism · pericarditis · postural hypotension · rashes · sedation · sialadenitis · stomatitis · thrombocytopenia · toxic epidermal necrolysis
SIDE-EFFECTS, FURTHER INFORMATION
Side-effects are minimised if the daily dose is kept below 1 g.
- **PREGNANCY** Not known to be harmful.
- **BREAST FEEDING** Amount too small to be harmful.
- **HEPATIC IMPAIRMENT** Manufacturer advises caution in history of liver disease. Avoid in active liver disease.
- **RENAL IMPAIRMENT** Start with small dose. Increased sensitivity to hypotensive and sedative effect.

- MONITORING REQUIREMENTS Monitor blood counts and liver-function before treatment and at intervals during first 6–12 weeks or if unexplained fever occurs.
- EFFECT ON LABORATORY TESTS Interference with laboratory tests. Positive direct Coombs' test in up to 20% of patients (may affect blood cross-matching).
- PATIENT AND CARER ADVICE
  Driving and skilled tasks
  Drowsiness may affect performance of skilled tasks (e.g. driving); effects of alcohol may be enhanced.
- MEDICINAL FORMS
  There can be variation in the licensing of different medicines containing the same drug. Forms available from special-order manufacturers include: oral suspension, oral solution
  Tablet
  CAUTIONARY AND ADVISORY LABELS 3, 8
  ▸ Methyldopa (Non-proprietary)
    Methyldopa anhydrous 125 mg Methyldopa 125mg tablets | 56 tablet [PoM] £121.70 DT price = £112.95
    Methyldopa anhydrous 250 mg Methyldopa 250mg tablets | 56 tablet [PoM] £11.53 DT price = £5.35
    Methyldopa anhydrous 500 mg Methyldopa 500mg tablets | 56 tablet [PoM] £18.05 DT price = £9.58
  ▸ Aldomet (Aspen Pharma Trading Ltd)
    Methyldopa anhydrous 250 mg Aldomet 250mg tablets | 60 tablet [PoM] £6.15
    Methyldopa anhydrous 500 mg Aldomet 500mg tablets | 30 tablet [PoM] £4.55

Moxonidine

- INDICATIONS AND DOSE
  Mild to moderate essential hypertension
  ▸ BY MOUTH
  ▸ Adult: 200 micrograms once daily for 3 weeks, dose to be taken in the morning, then increased if necessary to 400 micrograms daily in 1–2 divided doses (max. per dose 400 micrograms), maximum daily dose to be given in 2 divided doses; maximum 600 micrograms per day

- CONTRA-INDICATIONS Bradycardia · conduction disorders · second- or third-degree AV block · severe heart failure · sick sinus syndrome · sino-atrial block
- CAUTIONS First-degree AV block · moderate heart failure · severe coronary artery disease · unstable angina
- INTERACTIONS → Appendix 1 (moxonidine).
- SIDE-EFFECTS
  ▸ Common or very common Back pain · diarrhoea · dizziness · dry mouth · dyspepsia · insomnia · nausea · pruritus · rash · somnolence · vomiting
  ▸ Uncommon Angioedema · bradycardia · neck pain · nervousness · oedema · tinnitus
- PREGNANCY Manufacturer advises avoid—no information available.
- BREAST FEEDING Present in milk—manufacturer advises avoid.
- RENAL IMPAIRMENT Max. single dose 200 micrograms and max. daily dose 400 micrograms if eGFR 30–60 mL/minute/1.73 m². Avoid if eGFR less than 30 mL/minute/1.73 m².
- TREATMENT CESSATION Avoid abrupt withdrawal (if concomitant treatment with beta-blocker has to be stopped, discontinue beta-blocker first, then moxonidine after a few days).

- MEDICINAL FORMS
  There can be variation in the licensing of different medicines containing the same drug.
  Tablet
  CAUTIONARY AND ADVISORY LABELS 3
  ▸ Moxonidine (Non-proprietary)
    Moxonidine 200 microgram Moxonidine 200microgram tablets | 28 tablet [PoM] £10.40 DT price = £1.47
    Moxonidine 300 microgram Moxonidine 300microgram tablets | 28 tablet [PoM] £12.30 DT price = £1.59
    Moxonidine 400 microgram Moxonidine 400microgram tablets | 28 tablet [PoM] £14.24 DT price = £1.68
  ▸ Physiotens (BGP Products Ltd)
    Moxonidine 200 microgram Physiotens 200microgram tablets | 28 tablet [PoM] £9.72 DT price = £1.47
    Moxonidine 300 microgram Physiotens 300microgram tablets | 28 tablet [PoM] £11.49 DT price = £1.59
    Moxonidine 400 microgram Physiotens 400microgram tablets | 28 tablet [PoM] £13.26 DT price = £1.68

BETA-ADRENOCEPTOR BLOCKERS

Beta-adrenoceptor blocking drugs

Overview

Beta-adrenoceptor blocking drugs (beta-blockers) block the beta-adrenoceptors in the heart, peripheral vasculature, bronchi, pancreas, and liver.

Many beta-blockers are now available and in general they are all equally effective. There are, however, differences between them, which may affect choice in treating particular diseases or individual patients.

Intrinsic sympathomimetic activity (ISA, partial agonist activity) represents the capacity of beta-blockers to stimulate as well as to block adrenergic receptors. Oxprenolol hydrochloride p. 136, pindolol p. 136, acebutolol p. 138, and celiprolol hydrochloride p. 139 have intrinsic sympathomimetic activity; they tend to cause less bradycardia than the other beta-blockers and may also cause less coldness of the extremities.

Some beta-blockers are lipid soluble and some are water soluble. Atenolol p. 138, celiprolol hydrochloride, nadolol p. 135, and sotalol hydrochloride p. 97 are the most water-soluble; they are less likely to enter the brain, and may therefore cause less sleep disturbance and nightmares. Water-soluble beta-blockers are excreted by the kidneys and dosage reduction is often necessary in renal impairment.

Beta-blockers with a relatively short duration of action have to be given two or three times daily. Many of these are, however, available in modified-release formulations so that administration once daily is adequate for hypertension. For angina twice-daily treatment may sometimes be needed even with a modified-release formulation. Some beta-blockers, such as atenolol, bisoprolol fumarate p. 139, celiprolol hydrochloride, and nadolol, have an intrinsically longer duration of action and need to be given only once daily.

Beta-blockers slow the heart and can depress the myocardium; they are contra-indicated in patients with second- or third-degree heart block. Beta-blockers should also be avoided in patients with worsening unstable heart failure; care is required when initiating a beta-blocker in those with stable heart failure.

Labetalol hydrochloride p. 135, celiprolol hydrochloride, carvedilol p. 134, and nebivolol p. 141 are beta-blockers that have, in addition, an arteriolar vasodilating action, by diverse mechanisms, and thus lower peripheral resistance. There is no evidence that these drugs have important advantages over other beta-blockers in the treatment of hypertension.

Beta-blockers can precipitate bronchospasm and should therefore usually be avoided in patients with a history of asthma. When there is no suitable alternative, it may be necessary for a patient with well-controlled asthma, or chronic obstructive pulmonary disease (without significant reversible airways obstruction), to receive treatment with a beta-blocker for a co-existing condition (e.g. heart failure or following myocardial infarction). In this situation, a cardioselective beta-blocker should be selected and initiated at a low dose by a specialist; the patient should be closely monitored for adverse effects. Atenolol, bisoprolol fumarate, metoprolol tartrate p. 140, nebivolol, and (to a lesser extent) acebutolol, have less effect on the beta$_2$ (bronchial) receptors and are, therefore, relatively *cardioselective*, but they are not *cardiospecific*. They have a lesser effect on airways resistance but are not free of this side-effect.

Beta-blockers are also associated with fatigue, coldness of the extremities (may be less common with those with ISA), and sleep disturbances with nightmares (may be less common with the water-soluble beta-blockers).

Beta-blockers can affect carbohydrate metabolism, causing hypoglycaemia or hyperglycaemia in patients with or without diabetes; they can also interfere with metabolic and autonomic responses to hypoglycaemia, thereby masking symptoms such as tachycardia. However, beta-blockers are not contra-indicated in diabetes, although the cardioselective beta-blockers may be preferred. Beta-blockers should be avoided altogether in those with frequent episodes of hypoglycaemia. Beta-blockers, especially when combined with a thiazide diuretic, should be avoided for the routine treatment of uncomplicated hypertension in patients with diabetes or in those at high risk of developing diabetes.

Hypertension
The mode of action of beta-blockers in hypertension is not understood, but they reduce cardiac output, alter baroceptor reflex sensitivity, and block peripheral adrenoceptors. Some beta-blockers depress plasma renin secretion. It is possible that a central effect may also partly explain their mode of action.

Beta-blockers are effective for reducing blood pressure but other antihypertensives are usually more effective for reducing the incidence of stroke, myocardial infarction, and cardiovascular mortality, especially in the elderly. Other antihypertensives are therefore preferred for routine initial treatment of uncomplicated hypertension.

In general, the dose of a beta-blocker does not have to be high.

Beta-blockers can be used to control the pulse rate in patients with *phaeochromocytoma*. However, they should never be used alone as beta-blockade without concurrent alpha-blockade may lead to a hypertensive crisis. For this reason phenoxybenzamine hydrochloride p. 167 should always be used together with the beta-blocker.

Angina
By reducing cardiac work beta-blockers improve exercise tolerance and relieve symptoms in patients with *angina* (see management of stable angina and acute coronary syndromes for further details). As with hypertension there is no good evidence of the superiority of any one drug, although occasionally a patient will respond better to one beta-blocker than to another. There is some evidence that sudden withdrawal may cause an exacerbation of angina and therefore gradual reduction of dose is preferable when beta-blockers are to be stopped. There is a risk of precipitating heart failure when beta-blockers and verapamil are used together in established ischaemic heart disease.

Myocardial infarction
For specific comments see management of ST-segment elevation myocardial infarction and non-ST-segment elevation myocardial infarction.

Several studies have shown that some beta-blockers can reduce the recurrence rate of *myocardial infarction*. However, uncontrolled heart failure, hypotension, bradyarrhythmias,

and obstructive airways disease render beta-blockers unsuitable in some patients following a myocardial infarction. Atenolol and metoprolol tartrate may reduce early mortality after intravenous and subsequent oral administration in the acute phase, while acebutolol, metoprolol tartrate, propranolol hydrochloride p. 136, and timolol maleate p. 137 have protective value when started in the early convalescent phase. The evidence relating to other beta-blockers is less convincing; some have not been tested in trials of secondary prevention.

Arrhythmias
Beta-blockers act as *anti-arrhythmic drugs* principally by attenuating the effects of the sympathetic system on automaticity and conductivity within the heart. They can be used in conjunction with digoxin to control the ventricular response in atrial fibrillation, especially in patients with thyrotoxicosis. Beta-blockers are also useful in the management of supraventricular tachycardias, and are used to control those following myocardial infarction.

Esmolol hydrochloride p. 140 is a relatively cardioselective beta-blocker with a very short duration of action, used intravenously for the short-term treatment of supraventricular arrhythmias, sinus tachycardia, or hypertension, particularly in the peri-operative period. It may also be used in other situations, such as acute myocardial infarction, when sustained beta-blockade might be hazardous.

Sotalol hydrochloride p. 97, a non-cardioselective beta-blocker with additional class III anti-arrhythmic activity, is used for prophylaxis in paroxysmal supraventricular arrhythmias. It also suppresses ventricular ectopic beats and non-sustained ventricular tachycardia. It has been shown to be more effective than lidocaine in the termination of spontaneous sustained ventricular tachycardia due to coronary disease or cardiomyopathy. However, it may induce torsade de pointes in susceptible patients.

Heart failure
Beta-blockers may produce benefit in heart failure by blocking sympathetic activity. Bisoprolol fumarate p. 139 and carvedilol p. 134 reduce mortality in any grade of stable heart failure; nebivolol p. 141 is licensed for stable mild to moderate heart failure in patients over 70 years. Treatment should be initiated by those experienced in the management of heart failure.

Thyrotoxicosis
Beta-blockers are used in pre-operative preparation for thyroidectomy. Administration of propranolol hydrochloride p. 136 can reverse clinical symptoms of *thyrotoxicosis* within 4 days. Routine tests of increased thyroid function remain unaltered. The thyroid gland is rendered less vascular thus making surgery easier.

Other uses
Beta-blockers have been used to alleviate some symptoms of *anxiety*; probably patients with palpitation, tremor, and tachycardia respond best. Beta-blockers are also used in the *prophylaxis of migraine*. Betaxolol p. 1025, carteolol hydrochloride p. 1025, levobunolol hydrochloride p. 1025, and timolol maleate p. 1025 are used topically in *glaucoma*.

Beta-adrenoceptor blockers (systemic)

- CONTRA-INDICATIONS Asthma · cardiogenic shock · hypotension · marked bradycardia · metabolic acidosis · phaeochromocytoma (apart from specific use with alpha-blockers) · Prinzmetal's angina · second-degree AV block · severe peripheral arterial disease · sick sinus syndrome · third-degree AV block · uncontrolled heart failure

CONTRA-INDICATIONS, FURTHER INFORMATION
▸ Bronchospasm Beta-blockers, including those considered to be cardioselective, should usually be avoided in patients with a history of asthma, bronchospasm or a history of obstructive airways disease. However, when there is no alternative, a cardioselective beta-blocker can be given to these patients with caution and under specialist supervision. In such cases the risk of inducing bronchospasm should be appreciated and appropriate precautions taken.

● CAUTIONS Diabetes · first-degree AV block · history of obstructive airways disease (introduce cautiously) · myasthenia gravis · portal hypertension (risk of deterioration in liver function) · psoriasis · symptoms of hypoglycaemia may be masked · symptoms of thyrotoxicosis may be masked

● INTERACTIONS → Appendix 1 (beta-blockers).
▸ Verapamil and beta-blockers Verapamil injection should not be given to patients recently treated with beta-blockers because of the risk of hypotension and asystole. The suggestion that when verapamil injection has been given first, an interval of 30 minutes before giving a beta-blocker is sufficient has not been confirmed.
It may also be hazardous to give verapamil and a beta-blocker together by mouth (should only be contemplated if myocardial function well preserved).
There is a risk of precipitating heart failure when beta-blockers and verapamil are used together in established ischaemic heart disease.

● SIDE-EFFECTS
▸ Rare Dry eyes (reversible on withdrawal) · rashes (reversible on withdrawal)
▸ Frequency not known Alopecia · bradycardia · bronchospasm · coldness of the extremities · conduction disorders · dizziness · dyspnoea · exacerbation of intermittent claudication · exacerbation of psoriasis · exacerbation of Raynaud's phenomenon · fatigue · gastro-intestinal disturbances · headache · heart failure · hyperglycaemia (in patients with or without diabetes) · hypoglycaemia (in patients with or without diabetes) · hypotension · paraesthesia · peripheral vasoconstriction · psychoses · purpura · sexual dysfunction · sleep disturbances (with nightmares) · symptoms of hypoglycaemia masked · thrombocytopenia · vertigo · visual disturbances

SIDE-EFFECTS, FURTHER INFORMATION
▸ Bradycardia With administration by intravenous injection, excessive bradycardia can occur and may be countered with **intravenous injection** of atropine sulfate.

Overdose
Therapeutic overdosages with beta-blockers may cause lightheadedness, dizziness, and possibly syncope as a result of bradycardia and hypotension; heart failure may be precipitated or exacerbated. For details on the management of poisoning, see Beta-blockers, under Emergency treatment of poisoning p. 1194.

● ALLERGY AND CROSS-SENSITIVITY Caution is advised in patients with a history of hypersensitivity—may increase sensitivity to allergens and result in more serious hypersensitivity response. Furthermore beta-adrenoceptor blockers may reduce response to adrenaline (epinephrine).

● PREGNANCY Beta-blockers may cause intra-uterine growth restriction, neonatal hypoglycaemia, and bradycardia; the risk is greater in severe hypertension.

● BREAST FEEDING With systemic use in the mother, infants should be monitored as there is a risk of possible toxicity due to beta-blockade. However, the amount of most beta-blockers present in milk is too small to affect infants.

● MONITORING REQUIREMENTS Monitor lung function (in patients with a history of obstructive airway disease).

● TREATMENT CESSATION Avoid abrupt withdrawal especially in ischaemic heart disease. Sudden cessation of a beta-blocker can cause a rebound worsening of myocardial ischaemia and therefore gradual reduction of dose is preferable when beta-blockers are to be stopped.

BETA-ADRENOCEPTOR BLOCKERS ›
ALPHA- AND BETA-ADRENOCEPTOR BLOCKERS

F 133

Carvedilol

● INDICATIONS AND DOSE
Hypertension
▸ BY MOUTH
▸ Adult: Initially 12.5 mg once daily for 2 days, then increased to 25 mg once daily; increased if necessary up to 50 mg daily, dose to be increased at intervals of at least 2 weeks and can be given as a single dose or in divided doses
▸ Elderly: Initially 12.5 mg daily, initial dose may provide satisfactory control

Angina
▸ BY MOUTH
▸ Adult: Initially 12.5 mg twice daily for 2 days, then increased to 25 mg twice daily

Adjunct to diuretics, digoxin, or ACE inhibitors in symptomatic chronic heart failure
▸ BY MOUTH
▸ Adult: Initially 3.125 mg twice daily, dose to be taken with food, then increased to 6.25 mg twice daily, then increased to 12.5 mg twice daily, then increased to 25 mg twice daily, dose should be increased at intervals of at least 2 weeks up to the highest tolerated dose, max. 25 mg twice daily in patients with severe heart failure or body-weight less than 85 kg; max. 50 mg twice daily in patients over 85 kg

● CONTRA-INDICATIONS Acute or decompensated heart failure requiring intravenous inotropes

● SIDE-EFFECTS Allergic skin reactions · angina · AV block · changes in liver enzymes · depressed mood · disturbances of micturition · influenza-like symptoms · leucopenia · nasal stuffiness · postural hypotension · thrombocytopenia · wheezing

● PREGNANCY Information on the safety of carvedilol during pregnancy is lacking. If carvedilol is used close to delivery, infants should be monitored for signs of alpha-blockade (as well as beta-blockade).

● BREAST FEEDING Infants should be monitored as there is a risk of possible toxicity due to alpha-blockade (in addition to beta-blockade).

● HEPATIC IMPAIRMENT Avoid in hepatic impairment.

● MONITORING REQUIREMENTS Monitor renal function during dose titration in patients with heart failure who also have renal impairment, low blood pressure, ischaemic heart disease, or diffuse vascular disease.

● MEDICINAL FORMS
There can be variation in the licensing of different medicines containing the same drug. Forms available from special-order manufacturers include: oral suspension
Tablet
CAUTIONARY AND ADVISORY LABELS 8
▸ Carvedilol (Non-proprietary)
Carvedilol 3.125 mg Carvedilol 3.125mg tablets | 28 tablet PoM
£8.00 DT price = £0.89
Carvedilol 6.25 mg Carvedilol 6.25mg tablets | 28 tablet PoM
£8.99 DT price = £0.98
Carvedilol 12.5 mg Carvedilol 12.5mg tablets | 28 tablet PoM £9.99
DT price = £0.99
Carvedilol 25 mg Carvedilol 25mg tablets | 28 tablet PoM £12.50
DT price = £1.15

F 133

Labetalol hydrochloride

- **INDICATIONS AND DOSE**

Controlled hypotension in anaesthesia
▸ BY INTRAVENOUS INFUSION, OR BY INTRAVENOUS INJECTION
▸ Adult: (consult product literature or local protocols)

Hypertension of pregnancy
▸ BY INTRAVENOUS INFUSION
▸ Adult: Initially 20 mg/hour, then increased if necessary to 40 mg/hour after 30 minutes, then increased if necessary to 80 mg/hour after 30 minutes, then increased if necessary to 160 mg/hour after 30 minutes, adjusted according to response; Usual maximum 160 mg/hour
▸ BY MOUTH
▸ Adult: Use dose for hypertension

Hypertension following myocardial infarction
▸ BY INTRAVENOUS INFUSION
▸ Adult: 15 mg/hour, then increased to up to 120 mg/hour, dose to be increased gradually

Hypertensive emergencies
▸ BY INTRAVENOUS INJECTION
▸ Adult: 50 mg, to be given over at least 1 minute, then 50 mg every 5 minutes if required until a satisfactory response occurs; maximum 200 mg per course
▸ BY INTRAVENOUS INFUSION
▸ Adult: Initially 2 mg/minute until a satisfactory response is achieved, then discontinue; usual dose 50–200 mg

Hypertension
▸ BY MOUTH
▸ Adult: Initially 100 mg twice daily, dose to be increased at intervals of 14 days; usual dose 200 mg twice daily, increased if necessary up to 800 mg daily in 2 divided doses, to be taken with food, higher doses to be given in 3–4 divided doses; maximum 2.4 g per day
▸ Elderly: Initially 50 mg twice daily, dose to be increased at intervals of 14 days; usual dose 200 mg twice daily, increased if necessary up to 800 mg daily in 2 divided doses, to be taken with food, higher doses to be given in 3–4 divided doses; maximum 2.4 g per day
▸ BY INTRAVENOUS INJECTION
▸ Adult: 50 mg, dose to be given over at least 1 minute, then 50 mg after 5 minutes if required; maximum 200 mg per course
▸ BY INTRAVENOUS INFUSION
▸ Adult: Initially 2 mg/minute until a satisfactory response is achieved, then discontinue; usual dose 50–200 mg

- **CAUTIONS** Liver damage
- **SIDE-EFFECTS**
▸ **Rare** Lichenoid rash
▸ **Frequency not known** Difficulty in micturition · epigastric pain · liver damage · nausea · postural hypotension · vomiting · weakness
- **PREGNANCY** The use of labetalol in maternal hypertension is not known to be harmful, except possibly in the first trimester. If labetalol is used close to delivery, infants should be monitored for signs of alpha-blockade (as well as beta blockade).
- **BREAST FEEDING** Infants should be monitored as there is a risk of possible toxicity due to alpha-blockade (in addition to beta-blockade).
- **HEPATIC IMPAIRMENT** Avoid—severe hepatocellular injury reported.
- **RENAL IMPAIRMENT** Dose reduction may be required.

- **MONITORING REQUIREMENTS**
▸ **Liver damage** Severe hepatocellular damage reported after both short-term and long-term treatment. Appropriate laboratory testing needed at first symptom of liver dysfunction and if laboratory evidence of damage (or if jaundice) labetalol should be stopped and not restarted.
- **EFFECT ON LABORATORY TESTS** Interferes with laboratory tests for catecholamines.
- **DIRECTIONS FOR ADMINISTRATION** For *intravenous infusion*, give intermittently in Glucose 5% *or* Sodium chloride and glucose. Dilute to a concentration of 1 mg/mL; suggested volume 200 mL; adjust rate with in-line burette. Avoid upright position during and for 3 hours after intravenous administration.

- **MEDICINAL FORMS**
There can be variation in the licensing of different medicines containing the same drug. Forms available from special-order manufacturers include: oral suspension, oral solution

Tablet
CAUTIONARY AND ADVISORY LABELS 8, 21
▸ Labetalol hydrochloride (Non-proprietary)
 Labetalol hydrochloride 100 mg Labetalol 100mg tablets | 56 tablet [PoM] £7.21 DT price = £5.81
 Labetalol hydrochloride 200 mg Labetalol 200mg tablets | 56 tablet [PoM] £9.97 DT price = £8.83
 Labetalol hydrochloride 400 mg Labetalol 400mg tablets | 56 tablet [PoM] £23.14 DT price = £23.14
▸ Trandate (Focus Pharmaceuticals Ltd)
 Labetalol hydrochloride 50 mg Trandate 50mg tablets | 56 tablet [PoM] £3.79 DT price = £3.79
 Labetalol hydrochloride 100 mg Trandate 100mg tablets | 56 tablet [PoM] £4.64 DT price = £5.81 | 250 tablet [PoM] £15.62
 Labetalol hydrochloride 200 mg Trandate 200mg tablets | 56 tablet [PoM] £7.41 DT price = £8.83 | 250 tablet [PoM] £24.76
 Labetalol hydrochloride 400 mg Trandate 400mg tablets | 56 tablet [PoM] £10.15 DT price = £23.14

Solution for injection
▸ Labetalol hydrochloride (Non-proprietary)
 Labetalol hydrochloride 5 mg per 1 ml Labetalol 100mg/20ml solution for injection ampoules | 5 ampoule [PoM] £44.44-£53.33

BETA-ADRENOCEPTOR BLOCKERS ›
NON-SELECTIVE

F 133

Nadolol

- **INDICATIONS AND DOSE**

Hypertension
▸ BY MOUTH
▸ Adult: Initially 80 mg once daily, then increased in steps of up to 80 mg every 1 week if required, doses higher than the maximum are rarely necessary; maximum 240 mg per day

Angina
▸ BY MOUTH
▸ Adult: Initially 40 mg once daily, then increased if necessary up to 160 mg daily, doses should be increased at weekly intervals, maximum dose rarely is used; maximum 240 mg per day

Arrhythmias
▸ BY MOUTH
▸ Adult: Initially 40 mg once daily, then increased if necessary up to 160 mg once daily, doses should be increased at weekly intervals; reduced to 40 mg daily if bradycardia occurs

Migraine prophylaxis
▸ BY MOUTH
▸ Adult: Initially 40 mg once daily, then increased in steps of 40 mg every 1 week, adjusted according to response; maintenance 80–160 mg once daily

continued →

Cardiovascular system
2

2

Cardiovascular system

Thyrotoxicosis (adjunct)
▶ BY MOUTH
▹ Adult: 80–160 mg once daily

● BREAST FEEDING Water soluble beta-blockers such as nadolol are present in breast milk in greater amounts than other beta blockers.
● HEPATIC IMPAIRMENT Manufacturer advises caution.
● RENAL IMPAIRMENT Increase dosage interval if eGFR less than 50 mL/minute/1.73 m^2.

● MEDICINAL FORMS
There can be variation in the licensing of different medicines containing the same drug. Forms available from special-order manufacturers include: tablet, oral suspension, oral solution
Tablet
CAUTIONARY AND ADVISORY LABELS 8
▹ Corgard (Sanofi)
Nadolol 80 mg Corgard 80mg tablets | 28 tablet [PoM] £5.00 DT price = £5.00

[F] 133

Oxprenolol hydrochloride

● INDICATIONS AND DOSE
Hypertension | Angina
▶ BY MOUTH USING IMMEDIATE-RELEASE MEDICINES
▹ Adult: 80–160 mg daily in 2–3 divided doses, then increased if necessary up to 320 mg daily
▶ BY MOUTH USING MODIFIED-RELEASE MEDICINES
▹ Adult: Initially 160 mg once daily, then increased if necessary up to 320 mg daily
Arrhythmias
▶ BY MOUTH USING IMMEDIATE-RELEASE MEDICINES
▹ Adult: 40–240 mg daily in 2–3 divided doses; maximum 240 mg per day
Anxiety symptoms (short-term use)
▶ BY MOUTH USING IMMEDIATE-RELEASE MEDICINES
▹ Adult: 40–80 mg daily in 1–2 divided doses

● HEPATIC IMPAIRMENT Reduce dose.

● MEDICINAL FORMS
There can be variation in the licensing of different medicines containing the same drug. Forms available from special-order manufacturers include: oral solution
Tablet
CAUTIONARY AND ADVISORY LABELS 8
▹ Oxprenolol hydrochloride (Non-proprietary)
Oxprenolol hydrochloride 20 mg Oxprenolol 20mg tablets | 56 tablet [PoM] £5.37 DT price = £5.37
Oxprenolol hydrochloride 40 mg Oxprenolol 40mg tablets | 56 tablet [PoM] £7.22 DT price = £7.22
Oxprenolol hydrochloride 80 mg Oxprenolol 80mg tablets | 56 tablet [PoM] £11.70
Modified-release tablet
CAUTIONARY AND ADVISORY LABELS 8, 25
▹ Oxprenolol hydrochloride (Non-proprietary)
Oxprenolol hydrochloride 160 mg Oxprenolol 160mg modified-release tablets | 28 tablet [PoM] no price available
▹ Slow-Trasicor (AMCo)
Oxprenolol hydrochloride 160 mg Slow-Trasicor 160mg tablets | 28 tablet [PoM] £7.96

[F] 133

Pindolol

● INDICATIONS AND DOSE
Hypertension
▶ BY MOUTH
▹ Adult: Initially 5 mg 2–3 times a day, alternatively 15 mg once daily, doses to be increased as required at weekly intervals; maintenance 15–30 mg daily; maximum 45 mg per day

Angina
▶ BY MOUTH
▹ Adult: 2.5–5 mg up to 3 times a day

● RENAL IMPAIRMENT May adversely affect renal function in severe impairment—manufacturer advises avoid.

● MEDICINAL FORMS
There can be variation in the licensing of different medicines containing the same drug.
Tablet
CAUTIONARY AND ADVISORY LABELS 8
▹ Pindolol (Non-proprietary)
Pindolol 5 mg Pindolol 5mg tablets | 100 tablet [PoM] £15.00 DT price = £8.22
▹ Visken (AMCo)
Pindolol 5 mg Visken 5mg tablets | 56 tablet [PoM] £5.85
Pindolol 15 mg Visken 15mg tablets | 28 tablet [PoM] £10.55

Pindolol with clopamide

The properties listed below are those particular to the combination only. For the properties of the components please consider, pindolol above.

● INDICATIONS AND DOSE
Hypertension
▶ BY MOUTH
▹ Adult: Initially 1 tablet daily for 2–3 weeks, increased if necessary to 2 tablets once daily, dose to be taken in the morning; maximum 3 tablets per day

● MEDICINAL FORMS
There can be variation in the licensing of different medicines containing the same drug.
Tablet
CAUTIONARY AND ADVISORY LABELS 8
▹ Viskaldix (AMCo)
Clopamide 5 mg, Pindolol 10 mg Viskaldix tablets | 28 tablet [PoM] £6.70 DT price = £6.70

[F] 133

Propranolol hydrochloride

● INDICATIONS AND DOSE
Thyrotoxicosis (adjunct)
▶ BY MOUTH
▹ Adult: 10–40 mg 3–4 times a day
Thyrotoxic crisis
▶ BY INTRAVENOUS INJECTION
▹ Adult: 1 mg, to be given over 1 minute, dose may be repeated if necessary at intervals of 2 minutes, maximum total dose is 5 mg in anaesthesia; maximum 10 mg per course
Hypertension
▶ BY MOUTH
▹ Adult: Initially 80 mg twice daily, dose should be increased at weekly intervals as required; maintenance 160–320 mg daily
Prophylaxis of variceal bleeding in portal hypertension
▶ BY MOUTH
▹ Adult: Initially 40 mg twice daily, then increased to 80 mg twice daily (max. per dose 160 mg twice daily), dose to be adjusted according to heart rate
Phaeochromocytoma (only with an alpha-blocker) in preparation for surgery
▶ BY MOUTH
▹ Adult: 60 mg daily for 3 days before surgery

Phaeochromocytoma (only with an alpha-blocker) in patients unsuitable for surgery
▶ BY MOUTH
▶ Adult: 30 mg daily

Angina
▶ BY MOUTH
▶ Adult: Initially 40 mg 2–3 times a day; maintenance 120–240 mg daily

Hypertrophic cardiomyopathy | Anxiety tachycardia
▶ BY MOUTH
▶ Adult: 10–40 mg 3–4 times a day

Anxiety with symptoms such as palpitation, sweating and tremor
▶ BY MOUTH
▶ Adult: 40 mg once daily, then increased if necessary to 40 mg 3 times a day

Prophylaxis after myocardial infarction
▶ BY MOUTH
▶ Adult: Initially 40 mg 4 times a day for 2–3 days, then 80 mg twice daily, start treatment 5 to 21 days after infarction

Essential tremor
▶ BY MOUTH
▶ Adult: Initially 40 mg 2–3 times a day; maintenance 80–160 mg daily

Migraine prophylaxis
▶ BY MOUTH
▶ Adult: 80–240 mg daily in divided doses

Arrhythmias
▶ BY MOUTH
▶ Adult: 10–40 mg 3–4 times a day
▶ BY INTRAVENOUS INJECTION
▶ Adult: 1 mg, to be given over 1 minute, dose may be repeated if necessary at intervals of 2 minutes, maximum 10 mg per course (5 mg in anaesthesia)

● SIDE-EFFECTS
▶ **Rare** Dry eyes (reversible on withdrawal)

● HEPATIC IMPAIRMENT Reduce oral dose.

● RENAL IMPAIRMENT Manufacturer advises caution; dose reduction may be required.

● PRESCRIBING AND DISPENSING INFORMATION Modified-release preparations can be used for once daily administration.

● MEDICINAL FORMS
There can be variation in the licensing of different medicines containing the same drug. Forms available from special-order manufacturers include: oral suspension, oral solution

Tablet
CAUTIONARY AND ADVISORY LABELS 8
▶ Propranolol hydrochloride (Non-proprietary)
Propranolol hydrochloride 10 mg Propranolol 10mg tablets | 28 tablet [PoM] £1.47 DT price = £0.85
Propranolol hydrochloride 40 mg Propranolol 40mg tablets | 28 tablet [PoM] £1.85 DT price = £0.89
Propranolol hydrochloride 80 mg Propranolol 80mg tablets | 28 tablet [PoM] no price available | 56 tablet [PoM] £9.33 DT price = £1.93
Propranolol hydrochloride 160 mg Propranolol 160mg tablets | 56 tablet [PoM] £6.23 DT price = £5.65

Modified-release capsule
CAUTIONARY AND ADVISORY LABELS 8, 25
▶ Propranolol hydrochloride (Non-proprietary)
Propranolol hydrochloride 80 mg Propranolol 80mg modified-release capsules | 28 capsule [PoM] £6.98 DT price = £4.95
Propranolol hydrochloride 160 mg Propranolol 160mg modified-release capsules | 28 capsule [PoM] £4.88 DT price = £5.13
▶ Bedranol SR (Almus Pharmaceuticals Ltd, Sandoz Ltd)
Propranolol hydrochloride 80 mg Bedranol SR 80mg capsules | 28 capsule [PoM] £4.16 DT price = £4.95
Propranolol hydrochloride 160 mg Bedranol SR 160mg capsules | 28 capsule [PoM] £5.09 DT price = £5.13

▶ Beta-Prograne (Actavis UK Ltd, Tillomed Laboratories Ltd, Teva UK Ltd)
Propranolol hydrochloride 160 mg Beta-Prograne 160mg modified-release capsules | 28 capsule [PoM] £6.11 DT price = £5.13
▶ Half Beta-Prograne (Tillomed Laboratories Ltd, Teva UK Ltd, Actavis UK Ltd)
Propranolol hydrochloride 80 mg Half Beta-Prograne 80mg modified-release capsules | 28 capsule [PoM] £4.95 DT price = £4.95

Oral solution
CAUTIONARY AND ADVISORY LABELS 8
▶ Propranolol hydrochloride (Non-proprietary)
Propranolol hydrochloride 1 mg per 1 ml Propranolol 5mg/5ml oral solution sugar free sugar-free | 150 ml [PoM] £15.50 DT price = £12.50
Propranolol hydrochloride 2 mg per 1 ml Propranolol 10mg/5ml oral solution sugar free sugar-free | 150 ml [PoM] £20.45 DT price = £16.45
Propranolol hydrochloride 8 mg per 1 ml Propranolol 40mg/5ml oral solution sugar free sugar-free | 150 ml [PoM] £31.50 DT price = £31.50
Propranolol hydrochloride 10 mg per 1 ml Propranolol 50mg/5ml oral solution sugar free sugar-free | 150 ml [PoM] £24.98 DT price = £19.98
▶ Syprol (Rosemont Pharmaceuticals Ltd)
Propranolol hydrochloride 1 mg per 1 ml Syprol 5mg/5ml oral solution sugar-free | 150 ml [PoM] £12.50 DT price = £12.50
Propranolol hydrochloride 2 mg per 1 ml Syprol 10mg/5ml oral solution sugar-free | 150 ml [PoM] £16.45 DT price = £16.45
Propranolol hydrochloride 8 mg per 1 ml Syprol 40mg/5ml oral solution sugar-free | 150 ml [PoM] £31.50 DT price = £31.50
Propranolol hydrochloride 10 mg per 1 ml Syprol 50mg/5ml oral solution sugar-free | 150 ml [PoM] £19.98 DT price = £19.98

☞ 133

Timolol maleate

● INDICATIONS AND DOSE

Hypertension
▶ BY MOUTH
▶ Adult: Initially 10 mg daily in 1–2 divided doses, then increased if necessary up to 60 mg daily, doses to be increased gradually. Doses above 30 mg daily given in divided doses, usual maintenance 10–30 mg daily; maximum 60 mg per day

Angina
▶ BY MOUTH
▶ Adult: Initially 5 mg twice daily, then increased in steps of 10 mg daily (max. per dose 30 mg twice daily), to be increased every 3–4 days

Prophylaxis after myocardial infarction
▶ BY MOUTH
▶ Adult: Initially 5 mg twice daily for 2 days, then increased if tolerated to 10 mg twice daily

Migraine prophylaxis
▶ BY MOUTH
▶ Adult: 10–20 mg daily in 1–2 divided doses

● BREAST FEEDING Manufacturer advises avoidance.

● HEPATIC IMPAIRMENT Dose reduction may be necessary.

● RENAL IMPAIRMENT Manufacturer advises caution—dose reduction may be required.

● MEDICINAL FORMS
There can be variation in the licensing of different medicines containing the same drug.

Tablet
CAUTIONARY AND ADVISORY LABELS 8
▶ Timolol maleate (Non-proprietary)
Timolol maleate 10 mg Timolol 10mg tablets | 30 tablet [PoM] £16.24–£19.49 DT price = £19.12

Timolol with amiloride and hydrochlorothiazide

The properties listed below are those particular to the combination only. For the properties of the components please consider, timolol maleate p. 137, amiloride hydrochloride p. 212, hydrochlorothiazide p. 153.

- **INDICATIONS AND DOSE**

Hypertension
▶ BY MOUTH
▶ Adult: 1–2 tablets daily

- **MEDICINAL FORMS**
There can be variation in the licensing of different medicines containing the same drug.
Tablet
CAUTIONARY AND ADVISORY LABELS 8
▶ Timolol with amiloride and hydrochlorothiazide (Non-proprietary)
Amiloride hydrochloride 2.5 mg, Timolol maleate 10 mg, Hydrochlorothiazide 25 mg Timolol 10mg / Amiloride 2.5mg / Hydrochlorothiazide 25mg tablets | 28 tablet [PoM] £29.87

Timolol with bendroflumethiazide

The properties listed below are those particular to the combination only. For the properties of the components please consider, timolol maleate p. 137, bendroflumethiazide p. 152.

- **INDICATIONS AND DOSE**

Hypertension
▶ BY MOUTH
▶ Adult: 1–2 tablets daily; maximum 4 tablets per day

- **MEDICINAL FORMS**
There can be variation in the licensing of different medicines containing the same drug.
Tablet
CAUTIONARY AND ADVISORY LABELS 8
▶ Timolol with bendroflumethiazide (Non-proprietary)
Bendroflumethiazide 2.5 mg, Timolol maleate 10 mg Timolol 10mg / Bendroflumethiazide 2.5mg tablets | 30 tablet [PoM] £11.08-£26.60 DT price = £18.84

BETA-ADRENOCEPTOR BLOCKERS >
SELECTIVE

F 133

Acebutolol

- **INDICATIONS AND DOSE**

Hypertension
▶ BY MOUTH
▶ Adult: Initially 400 mg daily for 2 weeks, alternatively initially 200 mg twice daily for 2 weeks, then increased if necessary to 400 mg twice daily; maximum 1.2 g per day

Angina
▶ BY MOUTH
▶ Adult: Initially 400 mg daily, alternatively initially 200 mg twice daily; maximum 1.2 g per day

Arrhythmias
▶ BY MOUTH
▶ Adult: 0.4–1.2 g daily in 2–3 divided doses

Severe angina
▶ BY MOUTH
▶ Adult: Initially 300 mg 3 times a day; maximum 1.2 g per day

- **BREAST FEEDING** Acebutolol and water soluble beta-blockers are present in breast milk in greater amounts than other beta-blockers.

- **RENAL IMPAIRMENT** Halve dose if eGFR 25–50 mL/minute/1.73 m^2; use quarter dose if eGFR less than 25 mL/minute/1.73 m^2; do not administer more than once daily.

- **MEDICINAL FORMS**
There can be variation in the licensing of different medicines containing the same drug.
Tablet
CAUTIONARY AND ADVISORY LABELS 8
▶ Acebutolol (Non-proprietary)
Acebutolol (as Acebutolol hydrochloride) 400 mg Acebutolol 400mg tablets | 28 tablet [PoM] £18.62 DT price = £18.62
▶ Sectral (Sanofi)
Acebutolol (as Acebutolol hydrochloride) 400 mg Sectral 400mg tablets | 28 tablet [PoM] £18.62 DT price = £18.62
Capsule
CAUTIONARY AND ADVISORY LABELS 8
▶ Acebutolol (Non-proprietary)
Acebutolol (as Acebutolol hydrochloride) 100 mg Acebutolol 100mg capsules | 84 capsule [PoM] £14.97 DT price = £14.97
Acebutolol (as Acebutolol hydrochloride) 200 mg Acebutolol 200mg capsules | 56 capsule [PoM] £19.18 DT price = £19.18
▶ Sectral (Sanofi)
Acebutolol (as Acebutolol hydrochloride) 100 mg Sectral 100mg capsules | 84 capsule [PoM] £14.97 DT price = £14.97
Acebutolol (as Acebutolol hydrochloride) 200 mg Sectral 200mg capsules | 56 capsule [PoM] £19.18 DT price = £19.18

F 133

Atenolol

- **INDICATIONS AND DOSE**

Hypertension
▶ BY MOUTH
▶ Adult: 25–50 mg daily, higher doses are rarely necessary

Angina
▶ BY MOUTH
▶ Adult: 100 mg daily in 1–2 divided doses

Arrhythmias
▶ BY MOUTH
▶ Adult: 50–100 mg daily
▶ BY INTRAVENOUS INJECTION
▶ Adult: 2.5 mg every 5 minutes (max. per dose 10 mg), repeated if necessary, given at a rate of 1 mg/minute
▶ BY INTRAVENOUS INFUSION
▶ Adult: 150 micrograms/kg every 12 hours if required, to be given over 20 minutes

Migraine prophylaxis
▶ BY MOUTH
▶ Adult: 50–200 mg daily in divided doses

Early intervention within 12 hours of myocardial infarction
▶ INITIALLY BY INTRAVENOUS INJECTION
▶ Adult: Initially 5 mg, to be given over 5 minutes, followed by (by mouth) 50 mg after 15 minutes, then (by mouth) 50 mg after 12 hours, then (by mouth) 100 mg daily

- **UNLICENSED USE** Use of atenolol for migraine prophylaxis is an unlicensed indication.

- **BREAST FEEDING** Water soluble beta-blockers such as atenolol are present in breast milk in greater amounts than other beta blockers.

- **RENAL IMPAIRMENT**
▶ With oral use Max. 50 mg daily if eGFR 15–35 mL/minute/1.73 m^2; max. 25 mg daily or 50 mg on alternate days if eGFR less than 15 mL/minute/1.73 m^2.
▶ With intravenous use Max. 10 mg on alternate days if eGFR 15–35 mL/minute/1.73 m^2; max. 10 mg every 4 days if eGFR less than 15 mL/minute/1.73 m^2.

- DIRECTIONS FOR ADMINISTRATION For *intravenous infusion* (*Tenormin*®), give intermittently in Glucose 5% or Sodium chloride 0.9%. Suggested infusion time 20 minutes.

- MEDICINAL FORMS
There can be variation in the licensing of different medicines containing the same drug. Forms available from special-order manufacturers include: oral suspension, oral solution

Tablet
CAUTIONARY AND ADVISORY LABELS 8
  ▸ Atenolol (Non-proprietary)
    Atenolol 25 mg Atenolol 25mg tablets | 28 tablet [PoM] £1.39 DT price = £0.70
    Atenolol 50 mg Atenolol 50mg tablets | 28 tablet [PoM] £1.44 DT price = £0.77
    Atenolol 100 mg Atenolol 100mg tablets | 28 tablet [PoM] £1.74 DT price = £0.73
  ▸ Tenormin (AstraZeneca UK Ltd)
    Atenolol 50 mg Tenormin LS 50mg tablets | 28 tablet [PoM] £5.11 DT price = £0.77
    Atenolol 100 mg Tenormin 100mg tablets | 28 tablet [PoM] £6.49 DT price = £0.73

Oral solution
  ▸ Atenolol (Non-proprietary)
    Atenolol 5 mg per 1 ml Atenolol 25mg/5ml oral solution sugar free sugar-free | 300 ml [PoM] £6.72 DT price = £5.59

Solution for injection
  ▸ Tenormin (AstraZeneca UK Ltd)
    Atenolol 500 microgram per 1 ml Tenormin 5mg/10ml solution for injection ampoules | 10 ampoule [PoM] £34.45 (Hospital only)

Atenolol with nifedipine

The properties listed below are those particular to the combination only. For the properties of the components please consider, atenolol p. 138, nifedipine p. 148.

- INDICATIONS AND DOSE

Hypertension
  ▸ BY MOUTH
  ▸ Adult: 1 capsule daily, increased if necessary to 1 capsule twice daily
  ▸ Elderly: 1 capsule daily

Angina
  ▸ BY MOUTH
  ▸ Adult: 1 capsule twice daily

- PRESCRIBING AND DISPENSING INFORMATION Only indicated when calcium-channel blocker or beta-blocker alone proves inadequate.

- MEDICINAL FORMS
There can be variation in the licensing of different medicines containing the same drug.
Modified-release capsule
CAUTIONARY AND ADVISORY LABELS 8, 25
  ▸ Tenif (AstraZeneca UK Ltd)
    Nifedipine 20 mg, Atenolol 50 mg Tenif 50mg/20mg modified-release capsules | 28 capsule [PoM] £12.76 DT price = £12.76

₣ 133

Bisoprolol fumarate

- INDICATIONS AND DOSE

Hypertension | Angina
  ▸ BY MOUTH
  ▸ Adult: 5–10 mg once daily; maximum 20 mg per day

Adjunct in heart failure
  ▸ BY MOUTH
  ▸ Adult: Initially 1.25 mg once daily for 1 week, dose to be taken in the morning, then increased if tolerated to 2.5 mg once daily for 1 week, then increased if tolerated to 3.75 mg once daily for 1 week, then increased if tolerated to 5 mg once daily for 4 weeks,

then increased if tolerated to 7.5 mg once daily for 4 weeks, then increased if tolerated to 10 mg once daily; maximum 10 mg per day

- CONTRA-INDICATIONS Acute or decompensated heart failure requiring intravenous inotropes · sino–atrial block
- CAUTIONS Ensure heart failure not worsening before increasing dose
- SIDE-EFFECTS
  ▸ **Uncommon** Cramp · depression · muscle weakness
  ▸ **Rare** Hearing impairment · hypertriglyceridaemia · syncope
  ▸ **Very rare** Conjunctivitis
- HEPATIC IMPAIRMENT Max. 10 mg daily in severe impairment.
- RENAL IMPAIRMENT Reduce dose if eGFR less than 20 mL/minute/1.73 m^2 (max. 10 mg daily).

- MEDICINAL FORMS
There can be variation in the licensing of different medicines containing the same drug. Forms available from special-order manufacturers include: oral suspension, oral solution

Tablet
CAUTIONARY AND ADVISORY LABELS 8
  ▸ Bisoprolol fumarate (Non-proprietary)
    Bisoprolol fumarate 1.25 mg Bisoprolol 1.25mg tablets | 28 tablet [PoM] £13.00 DT price = £0.87
    Bisoprolol fumarate 2.5 mg Bisoprolol 2.5mg tablets | 28 tablet [PoM] £14.00 DT price = £0.83
    Bisoprolol fumarate 3.75 mg Bisoprolol 3.75mg tablets | 28 tablet [PoM] £6.50 DT price = £1.13
    Bisoprolol fumarate 5 mg Bisoprolol 5mg tablets | 28 tablet [PoM] £5.89 DT price = £0.76
    Bisoprolol fumarate 7.5 mg Bisoprolol 7.5mg tablets | 28 tablet [PoM] £7.50 DT price = £4.32
    Bisoprolol fumarate 10 mg Bisoprolol 10mg tablets | 28 tablet [PoM] £5.89 DT price = £0.79
  ▸ Cardicor (Merck Serono Ltd)
    Bisoprolol fumarate 1.25 mg Cardicor 1.25mg tablets | 28 tablet [PoM] £2.35 DT price = £0.87
    Bisoprolol fumarate 2.5 mg Cardicor 2.5mg tablets | 28 tablet [PoM] £2.35 DT price = £0.83
    Bisoprolol fumarate 3.75 mg Cardicor 3.75mg tablets | 28 tablet [PoM] £4.90 DT price = £1.13
    Bisoprolol fumarate 5 mg Cardicor 5mg tablets | 28 tablet [PoM] £5.90 DT price = £0.76
    Bisoprolol fumarate 7.5 mg Cardicor 7.5mg tablets | 28 tablet [PoM] £5.90 DT price = £4.32
    Bisoprolol fumarate 10 mg Cardicor 10mg tablets | 28 tablet [PoM] £5.90 DT price = £0.79
  ▸ Congescor (Tillomed Laboratories Ltd)
    Bisoprolol fumarate 1.25 mg Congescor 1.25mg tablets | 28 tablet [PoM] £5.90 DT price = £0.87
    Bisoprolol fumarate 2.5 mg Congescor 2.5mg tablets | 28 tablet [PoM] £3.90 DT price = £0.83

₣ 133

Celiprolol hydrochloride

- INDICATIONS AND DOSE

Mild to moderate hypertension
  ▸ BY MOUTH
  ▸ Adult: 200 mg once daily, dose to be taken in the morning, then increased if necessary to 400 mg once daily

- SIDE-EFFECTS
  ▸ **Rare** Depression · pneumonitis
  ▸ **Frequency not known** Hot flushes
- BREAST FEEDING Manufacturers advise avoidance.
- HEPATIC IMPAIRMENT Consider dose reduction.
- RENAL IMPAIRMENT Reduce dose by half if eGFR 15–40 mL/minute/1.73 m^2. Avoid if eGFR less than 15 mL/minute/1.73 m^2.

● MEDICINAL FORMS
There can be variation in the licensing of different medicines containing the same drug. Forms available from special-order manufacturers include: oral suspension

Tablet
CAUTIONARY AND ADVISORY LABELS 8, 22
▸ Celiprolol hydrochloride (Non-proprietary)
Celiprolol hydrochloride 200 mg Celiprolol 200mg tablets | 28 tablet [PoM] £25.50 DT price = £20.63
Celiprolol hydrochloride 400 mg Celiprolol 400mg tablets | 28 tablet [PoM] £49.50 DT price = £29.12
▸ Celectol (Zentiva)
Celiprolol hydrochloride 200 mg Celectol 200mg tablets | 28 tablet [PoM] £19.83 DT price = £20.63
Celiprolol hydrochloride 400 mg Celectol 400mg tablets | 28 tablet [PoM] £39.65 DT price = £29.12

⟁ 133,151

Co-tenidone

● INDICATIONS AND DOSE

Hypertension
▸ BY MOUTH
▸ Adult: 50/12.5 mg daily, alternatively increased if necessary to 100/25 mg daily, doses higher than 50 mg atenolol rarely necessary

DOSE EQUIVALENCE AND CONVERSION
A mixture of atenolol and chlortalidone in mass proportions corresponding to 4 parts of atenolol and 1 part chlortalidone.

● SIDE-EFFECTS Allergic interstitial nephritis · jaundice
● PREGNANCY Avoid. Diuretics not used to treat hypertension in pregnancy.
● BREAST FEEDING Atenolol present in milk in greater amounts than some other beta-blockers. Possible toxicity due to beta-blockade—monitor infant. Large doses of chlortalidone may suppress lactation.
● RENAL IMPAIRMENT Avoid if eGFR less than 30 mL/minute/1.73 m^2—consider alternative treatment.

● MEDICINAL FORMS
There can be variation in the licensing of different medicines containing the same drug. Forms available from special-order manufacturers include: oral suspension, oral solution

Tablet
CAUTIONARY AND ADVISORY LABELS 8
▸ Co-tenidone (Non-proprietary)
Chlortalidone 12.5 mg, Atenolol 50 mg Co-tenidone 50mg/12.5mg tablets | 28 tablet [PoM] £4.85 DT price = £1.88
Chlortalidone 25 mg, Atenolol 100 mg Co-tenidone 100mg/25mg tablets | 28 tablet [PoM] £4.85 DT price = £1.86
▸ Tenoret (AstraZeneca UK Ltd)
Chlortalidone 12.5 mg, Atenolol 50 mg Tenoret 50mg/12.5mg tablets | 28 tablet [PoM] £5.18 DT price = £1.88
▸ Tenoretic (AstraZeneca UK Ltd)
Chlortalidone 25 mg, Atenolol 100 mg Tenoretic 100mg/25mg tablets | 28 tablet [PoM] £5.18 DT price = £1.88

⟁ 133

Esmolol hydrochloride

● INDICATIONS AND DOSE

Short-term treatment of supraventricular arrhythmias (including atrial fibrillation, atrial flutter, sinus tachycardia) | Tachycardia and hypertension in peri-operative period
▸ BY INTRAVENOUS INFUSION
▸ Adult: 50–200 micrograms/kg/minute, consult product literature for details of dose titration and doses during peri-operative period

● SIDE-EFFECTS Thrombophlebitis · venous irritation
● BREAST FEEDING Manufacturer advises avoidance.
● RENAL IMPAIRMENT Manufacturer advises caution.

● MEDICINAL FORMS
There can be variation in the licensing of different medicines containing the same drug.

Solution for injection
▸ Brevibloc (Baxter Healthcare Ltd)
Esmolol hydrochloride 10 mg per 1 ml Brevibloc Premixed 100mg/10ml solution for injection vials | 5 vial [PoM] no price available

Solution for infusion
▸ Brevibloc (Baxter Healthcare Ltd)
Esmolol hydrochloride 10 mg per 1 ml Brevibloc Premixed 2.5g/250ml infusion bags | 1 bag [PoM] £89.69

⟁ 133

Metoprolol tartrate

● INDICATIONS AND DOSE

Hypertension
▸ BY MOUTH USING IMMEDIATE-RELEASE MEDICINES
▸ Adult: Initially 100 mg daily, increased if necessary to 200 mg daily in 1–2 divided doses, high doses are rarely required; maximum 400 mg per day
▸ BY MOUTH USING MODIFIED-RELEASE MEDICINES
▸ Adult: 200 mg once daily

Angina
▸ BY MOUTH USING IMMEDIATE-RELEASE MEDICINES
▸ Adult: 50–100 mg 2–3 times a day
▸ BY MOUTH USING MODIFIED-RELEASE MEDICINES
▸ Adult: 200–400 mg daily

Arrhythmias
▸ BY MOUTH USING IMMEDIATE-RELEASE MEDICINES
▸ Adult: Usual dose 50 mg 2–3 times a day, then increased if necessary up to 300 mg daily in divided doses
▸ BY INTRAVENOUS INJECTION
▸ Adult: Up to 5 mg, dose to be given at a rate of 1–2 mg/minute, then up to 5 mg after 5 minutes if required, total dose of 10–15 mg

Migraine prophylaxis
▸ BY MOUTH USING IMMEDIATE-RELEASE MEDICINES
▸ Adult: 100–200 mg daily in divided doses
▸ BY MOUTH USING MODIFIED-RELEASE MEDICINES
▸ Adult: 200 mg daily

Hyperthyroidism (adjunct)
▸ BY MOUTH USING IMMEDIATE-RELEASE MEDICINES
▸ Adult: 50 mg 4 times a day

In surgery
▸ BY SLOW INTRAVENOUS INJECTION
▸ Adult: Initially 2–4 mg, given at induction or to control arrhythmias developing during anaesthesia, then 2 mg, repeated if necessary; maximum 10 mg per course

Early intervention within 12 hours of infarction
▸ INITIALLY BY INTRAVENOUS INJECTION
▸ Adult: Initially 5 mg every 2 minutes, to a max. of 15 mg, followed by (by mouth) 50 mg every 6 hours for 48 hours, to be taken 15 minutes after intravenous injection; (by mouth) maintenance 200 mg daily in divided doses

● HEPATIC IMPAIRMENT Reduce dose in severe impairment.

- MEDICINAL FORMS
There can be variation in the licensing of different medicines containing the same drug. Forms available from special-order manufacturers include: capsule, oral suspension, oral solution

Tablet
CAUTIONARY AND ADVISORY LABELS 8
▸ Metoprolol tartrate (Non-proprietary)
Metoprolol tartrate 50 mg Metoprolol 50mg tablets |
28 tablet [PoM] £3.00 DT price = £1.31 | 56 tablet [PoM] £3.52
Metoprolol tartrate 100 mg Metoprolol 100mg tablets |
28 tablet [PoM] £3.00 DT price = £1.50 | 56 tablet [PoM] £4.64
▸ Lopresor (Recordati Pharmaceuticals Ltd)
Metoprolol tartrate 50 mg Lopresor 50mg tablets | 56 tablet [PoM]
£2.57
Metoprolol tartrate 100 mg Lopresor 100mg tablets |
56 tablet [PoM] £6.68

Modified-release tablet
CAUTIONARY AND ADVISORY LABELS 8, 25
▸ Lopresor SR (Recordati Pharmaceuticals Ltd)
Metoprolol tartrate 200 mg Lopresor SR 200mg tablets |
28 tablet [PoM] £9.80

Solution for injection
▸ Betaloc (AstraZeneca UK Ltd)
Metoprolol tartrate 1 mg per 1 ml Betaloc I.V. 5mg/5ml solution for
injection ampoules | 5 ampoule [PoM] £5.02 (Hospital only)

◤ 133

Nebivolol

- INDICATIONS AND DOSE

Essential hypertension
▸ BY MOUTH
▸ Adult: 5 mg daily
▸ Elderly: Initially 2.5 mg daily, then increased if
necessary to 5 mg daily

Hypertension in patient with renal impairment
▸ BY MOUTH
▸ Adult: Initially 2.5 mg once daily, then increased if
necessary to 5 mg once daily

Adjunct in stable mild to moderate heart failure
▸ BY MOUTH
▸ Adult 70 years and over: Initially 1.25 mg once daily for
1–2 weeks, then increased if tolerated to 2.5 mg once
daily for 1–2 weeks, then increased if tolerated to 5 mg
once daily for 1–2 weeks, then increased if tolerated to
10 mg once daily

- CONTRA-INDICATIONS Acute or decompensated heart
failure requiring intravenous inotropes
- SIDE-EFFECTS Depression · oedema
- BREAST FEEDING Manufacturers advise avoidance.
- HEPATIC IMPAIRMENT No information available—
manufacturer advises avoid.
- RENAL IMPAIRMENT Manufacturer advises avoid in heart
failure if serum creatinine greater than 250 micromol/litre.

- MEDICINAL FORMS
There can be variation in the licensing of different medicines
containing the same drug.

Tablet
CAUTIONARY AND ADVISORY LABELS 8
▸ Nebivolol (Non-proprietary)
Nebivolol (as Nebivolol hydrochloride) 2.5 mg Nebivolol 2.5mg
tablets | 28 tablet [PoM] £69.84 DT price = £41.67
Nebivolol (as Nebivolol hydrochloride) 5 mg Nebivolol 5mg tablets
| 28 tablet [PoM] £22.00 DT price = £1.36
Nebivolol (as Nebivolol hydrochloride) 10 mg Nebivolol 10mg
tablets | 28 tablet [PoM] £3.96 DT price = £3.96
▸ Nebilet (A. Menarini Farmaceutica Internazionale SRL)
Nebivolol (as Nebivolol hydrochloride) 5 mg Nebilet 5mg tablets |
28 tablet [PoM] £9.23 DT price = £1.36

CALCIUM-CHANNEL BLOCKERS

Calcium-channel blockers

Overview

Calcium-channel blockers differ in their predilection for the various possible sites of action and, therefore, their therapeutic effects are disparate, with much greater variation than those of beta-blockers. There are important differences between verapamil hydrochloride p. 150, diltiazem hydrochloride p. 143, and the dihydropyridine calcium-channel blockers (amlodipine p. 142, felodipine p. 145, lacidipine p. 146, lercanidipine hydrochloride p. 146, nicardipine hydrochloride p. 147, nifedipine p. 148, and nimodipine p. 103). Verapamil hydrochloride and diltiazem hydrochloride should usually be **avoided** in heart failure because they may further depress cardiac function and cause clinically significant deterioration.

Verapamil hydrochloride is used for the treatment of angina, hypertension, and arrhythmias. It is a highly negatively inotropic calcium channel-blocker and it reduces cardiac output, slows the heart rate, and may impair atrioventricular conduction. It may precipitate heart failure, exacerbate conduction disorders, and cause hypotension at high doses and should **not** be used with beta-blockers. Constipation is the most common side-effect.

Nifedipine relaxes vascular smooth muscle and dilates coronary and peripheral arteries. It has more influence on vessels and less on the myocardium than does verapamil hydrochloride, and unlike verapamil hydrochloride has no anti-arrhythmic activity. It rarely precipitates heart failure because any negative inotropic effect is offset by a reduction in left ventricular work.

Nicardipine hydrochloride has similar effects to those of nifedipine and may produce less reduction of myocardial contractility. Amlodipine and felodipine also resemble nifedipine and nicardipine hydrochloride in their effects and do not reduce myocardial contractility and they do not produce clinical deterioration in heart failure. They have a longer duration of action and can be given once daily. Nifedipine, nicardipine hydrochloride, amlodipine, and felodipine are used for the treatment of angina or hypertension. All are valuable in forms of angina associated with coronary vasospasm. Side-effects associated with vasodilatation such as flushing and headache (which become less obtrusive after a few days), and ankle swelling (which may respond only partially to diuretics) are common.

Intravenous nicardipine hydrochloride is licensed for the treatment of acute life-threatening hypertension, for example in the event of malignant arterial hypertension or hypertensive encephalopathy; aortic dissection, when a short-acting beta-blocker is not suitable, or in combination with a beta-blocker when beta-blockade alone is not effective; severe pre-eclampsia, when other intravenous anti-hypertensives are not recommended or are contra-indicated; and for treatment of postoperative hypertension..

Isradipine p. 146, lacidipine and lercanidipine hydrochloride have similar effects to those of nifedipine and nicardipine hydrochloride; they are indicated for hypertension only.

Nimodipine is related to nifedipine but the smooth muscle relaxant effect preferentially acts on cerebral arteries. Its use is confined to prevention and treatment of vascular spasm following aneurysmal subarachnoid haemorrhage.

Diltiazem hydrochloride is effective in most forms of angina; the longer-acting formulation is also used for hypertension. It may be used in patients for whom beta-blockers are contra-indicated or ineffective. It has a less negative inotropic effect than verapamil hydrochloride and significant myocardial depression occurs rarely. Nevertheless because of the risk of bradycardia it should be used with caution in association with beta-blockers.

2

Unstable angina

Calcium-channel blockers do not reduce the risk of myocardial infarction in unstable angina. The use of diltiazem hydrochloride or verapamil hydrochloride should be reserved for patients resistant to treatment with beta-blockers.

Calcium-channel blockers

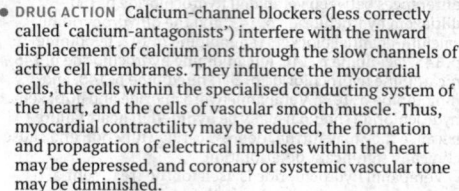

- DRUG ACTION Calcium-channel blockers (less correctly called 'calcium-antagonists') interfere with the inward displacement of calcium ions through the slow channels of active cell membranes. They influence the myocardial cells, the cells within the specialised conducting system of the heart, and the cells of vascular smooth muscle. Thus, myocardial contractility may be reduced, the formation and propagation of electrical impulses within the heart may be depressed, and coronary or systemic vascular tone may be diminished.

- SIDE-EFFECTS

Overdose
Features of calcium-channel blocker poisoning include nausea, vomiting, dizziness, agitation, confusion, and coma in severe poisoning. Metabolic acidosis and hyperglycaemia may occur.

For details on the management of poisoning, see Calcium-channel blockers, under Emergency treatment of poisoning p. 1194.

- TREATMENT CESSATION There is some evidence that sudden withdrawal of calcium-channel blockers may be associated with an exacerbation of myocardial ischaemia.

↗ above

Amlodipine

- DRUG ACTION Amlodipine is a dihydropyridine calcium-channel blocker.

- **INDICATIONS AND DOSE**

Prophylaxis of angina
▸ BY MOUTH
▸ Adult: Initially 5 mg once daily; maximum 10 mg per day

Hypertension
▸ BY MOUTH
▸ Adult: Initially 5 mg once daily; maximum 10 mg per day

DOSE EQUIVALENCE AND CONVERSION
Tablets from various suppliers may contain different salts (e.g. amlodipine besilate, amlodipine maleate, and amlodipine mesilate) but the strength is expressed in terms of amlodipine (base); tablets containing different salts are considered interchangeable.

- CONTRA-INDICATIONS Cardiogenic shock · significant aortic stenosis · unstable angina
- INTERACTIONS → Appendix 1 (calcium-channel blockers).
- SIDE-EFFECTS
▸ **Common or very common** Abdominal pain · dizziness · fatigue · flushing · headache · nausea · oedema · palpitation · sleep disturbances
▸ **Uncommon** Alopecia · arthralgia · asthenia · back pain · chest pain · dry mouth · dyspnoea · gastro-intestinal disturbances · gynaecomastia · hypotension · impotence · mood changes · muscle cramps · myalgia · paraesthesia · pruritus · purpura · rashes · rhinitis · skin discolouration · sweating · syncope · taste disturbances · tinnitus · tremor · urinary disturbances · visual disturbances · weight changes
▸ **Very rare** Angioedema · arrhythmias · cholestasis · coughing · gastritis · gingival hyperplasia · hepatitis ·

hyperglycaemia · jaundice · myocardial infarction · pancreatitis · peripheral neuropathy · tachycardia · thrombocytopenia · urticaria · vasculitis
▸ **Frequency not known** Erythema multiforme

Overdose
In overdose, the dihydropyridine calcium-channel blockers cause severe hypotension secondary to profound peripheral vasodilatation.

- PREGNANCY No information available—manufacturer advises avoid, but risk to fetus should be balanced against risk of uncontrolled maternal hypertension.

- BREAST FEEDING Manufacturer advises avoid—no information available.

- HEPATIC IMPAIRMENT May need dose reduction—half-life prolonged.

- DIRECTIONS FOR ADMINISTRATION Tablets may be dispersed in water.

- MEDICINAL FORMS
There can be variation in the licensing of different medicines containing the same drug. Forms available from special-order manufacturers include: oral suspension, oral solution

Tablet
▸ Amlodipine (Non-proprietary)
 Amlodipine 5 mg Amlodipine 5mg tablets | 28 tablet [PoM] £9.42 DT price = £0.72
 Amlodipine 10 mg Amlodipine 10mg tablets | 28 tablet [PoM] £14.07 DT price = £0.77
▸ Amlostin (Discovery Pharmaceuticals)
 Amlodipine 5 mg Amlostin 5mg tablets | 28 tablet [PoM] £0.73 DT price = £0.72
 Amlodipine 10 mg Amlostin 10mg tablets | 28 tablet [PoM] £0.77 DT price = £0.77
▸ Istin (Pfizer Ltd)
 Amlodipine 5 mg Istin 5mg tablets | 28 tablet [PoM] £11.08 DT price = £0.72
 Amlodipine 10 mg Istin 10mg tablets | 28 tablet [PoM] £16.55 DT price = £0.77

Oral solution
▸ Amlodipine (Non-proprietary)
 Amlodipine 1 mg per 1 ml Amlodipine 5mg/5ml oral solution sugar free sugar-free | 150 ml [PoM] £77.82 DT price = £76.65
 Amlodipine 2 mg per 1 ml Amlodipine 10mg/5ml oral solution sugar free sugar-free | 150 ml [PoM] £118.89 DT price = £117.11

Combinations available: *Olmesartan with amlodipine*, p. 163 · *Olmesartan with amlodipine and hydrochlorothiazide*, p. 163

Amlodipine with valsartan

The properties listed below are those particular to the combination only. For the properties of the components please consider, amlodipine above, valsartan p. 164.

- **INDICATIONS AND DOSE**

Hypertension in patients stabilised on the individual components in the same proportions
▸ BY MOUTH
▸ Adult: (consult product literature)

- MEDICINAL FORMS
There can be variation in the licensing of different medicines containing the same drug.

Tablet
▸ Exforge (Novartis Pharmaceuticals UK Ltd)
 Amlodipine (as Amlodipine besilate) 5 mg, Valsartan 80 mg Exforge 5mg/80mg tablets | 28 tablet [PoM] £20.11 DT price = £20.11
 Amlodipine (as Amlodipine besilate) 10 mg, Valsartan 160 mg Exforge 10mg/160mg tablets | 28 tablet [PoM] £26.51 DT price = £26.51
 Amlodipine (as Amlodipine besilate) 5 mg, Valsartan 160 mg Exforge 5mg/160mg tablets | 28 tablet [PoM] £26.51 DT price = £26.51

Diltiazem hydrochloride

► 142

● INDICATIONS AND DOSE

Prophylaxis and treatment of angina
► BY MOUTH
► Adult: Initially 60 mg 3 times a day, adjusted according to response; maximum 360 mg per day
► Elderly: Initially 60 mg twice daily, adjusted according to response; maximum 360 mg per day

ADIZEM-SR® CAPSULES

Mild to moderate hypertension
► BY MOUTH
► Adult: 120 mg twice daily, dose form not appropriate for initial dose titration

Angina
► BY MOUTH
► Adult: Initially 90 mg twice daily; increased if necessary to 180 mg twice daily, dose form not appropriate for initial dose titration in the elderly

ADIZEM-SR® TABLETS

Mild to moderate hypertension
► BY MOUTH
► Adult: 120 mg twice daily, dose form not appropriate for initial dose titration

Angina
► BY MOUTH
► Adult: Initially 90 mg twice daily; increased if necessary to 180 mg twice daily, dose form not appropriate for initial dose titration in the elderly

ADIZEM-XL®

Angina | Mild to moderate hypertension
► BY MOUTH
► Adult: Initially 240 mg once daily, increased if necessary to 300 mg once daily
► Elderly: Initially 120 mg once daily, increased if necessary up to 300 mg once daily

ANGITIL® SR

Angina | Mild to moderate hypertension
► BY MOUTH
► Adult: Initially 90 mg twice daily; increased if necessary to 120–180 mg twice daily

ANGITIL® XL

Angina | Mild to moderate hypertension
► BY MOUTH
► Adult: Initially 240 mg once daily; increased if necessary to 300 mg once daily, dose form not appropriate for initial dose titration in the elderly

DILCARDIA® SR

Angina | Mild to moderate hypertension
► BY MOUTH
► Adult: Initially 90 mg twice daily; increased if necessary to 180 mg twice daily
► Elderly: Initially 60 mg twice daily; increased if necessary to 90 mg twice daily

DILZEM® SR

Angina | Mild to moderate hypertension
► BY MOUTH
► Adult: Initially 90 mg twice daily; increased if necessary up to 180 mg twice daily
► Elderly: Initially 60 mg twice daily; increased if necessary up to 180 mg twice daily

DILZEM® XL

Angina | Mild to moderate hypertension
► BY MOUTH
► Adult: Initially 180 mg once daily; increased if necessary to 360 mg once daily

► Elderly: Initially 120 mg once daily; increased if necessary to 360 mg once daily

SLOZEM®

Angina | Mild to moderate hypertension
► BY MOUTH
► Adult: Initially 240 mg once daily; increased if necessary to 360 mg once daily
► Elderly: Initially 120 mg once daily; increased if necessary to 360 mg once daily

TILDIEM RETARD®

Mild to moderate hypertension
► BY MOUTH
► Adult: Initially 90–120 mg twice daily; increased if necessary to 360 mg daily in divided doses
► Elderly: Initially 120 mg once daily; increased if necessary to 120 mg twice daily

Angina
► BY MOUTH
► Adult: Initially 90–120 mg twice daily; increased if necessary to 480 mg daily in divided doses
► Elderly: Up to 120 mg twice daily, dose form not appropriate for initial dose titration

TILDIEM® LA

Angina | Mild to moderate hypertension
► BY MOUTH
► Adult: Initially 200 mg once daily, to be taken with or before food, increased if necessary to 300–400 mg once daily; maximum 500 mg per day
► Elderly: Initially 200 mg once daily, increased if necessary to 300 mg once daily

VIAZEM® XL

Angina | Mild to moderate hypertension
► BY MOUTH
► Adult: Initially 180 mg once daily, adjusted according to response to 240 mg once daily; maximum 360 mg per day
► Elderly: Initially 120 mg once daily, adjusted according to response

ZEMTARD®

Angina
► BY MOUTH
► Adult: 180–300 mg once daily, increased if necessary to 480 mg once daily
► Elderly: Initially 120 mg once daily, increased if necessary to 480 mg once daily

Mild to moderate hypertension
► BY MOUTH
► Adult: 180–300 mg once daily, increased if necessary to 360 mg once daily
► Elderly: Initially 120 mg once daily, increased if necessary to 360 mg once daily

● CONTRA-INDICATIONS Acute porphyrias p. 918 · left ventricular failure with pulmonary congestion · second- or third-degree AV block (unless pacemaker fitted) · severe bradycardia · sick sinus syndrome
● CAUTIONS Bradycardia (avoid if severe) · first degree AV block · heart failure · prolonged PR interval · significantly impaired left ventricular function
● INTERACTIONS → Appendix 1 (calcium-channel blockers).
● SIDE-EFFECTS
► Common or very common Asthenia · AV block · bradycardia · dizziness · gastro-intestinal disturbances · headache · hot flushes · hypotension · malaise · oedema (notably of ankles) · palpitation · sino-atrial block
► Rare Erythema multiforme · exfoliative dermatitis · photosensitivity · rashes
► Frequency not known Depression · extrapyramidal symptoms · gum hyperplasia · gynaecomastia · hepatitis

Overdose

In overdose, diltiazem has a profound cardiac depressant effect causing hypotension and arrhythmias, including complete heart block and asystole.

- PREGNANCY Avoid.
- BREAST FEEDING Significant amount present in milk—no evidence of harm but avoid unless no safer alternative.
- HEPATIC IMPAIRMENT Reduce dose.

ADIZEM-XL® Dose for angina and mild to moderate hypertension—initially 120 mg once daily.

ANGITIL® XL Dose form not appropriate for initial dose titration.

DILCARDIA® SR Dose for angina and mild to moderate hypertension—initially 60 mg twice a day; maximum 90 mg twice a day.

DILZEM® XL Dose for angina and mild to moderate hypertension—initially 120 mg once daily.

SLOZEM® Dose for angina and mild to moderate hypertension—initially 120 mg once daily.

TILDIEM® LA Dose for angina and mild to moderate hypertension—initially 200 mg daily; increased if necessary to 300 mg daily.

TILDIEM RETARD® Dose for mild to moderate hypertension—initially 120 mg once a day; increased if necessary to 120 mg twice a day.

For treatment of angina, dose form not appropriate for initial titration; up to 120 mg twice a day may be required.

VIAZEM® XL Dose for angina and mild to moderate hypertension—initially 120 mg once daily, adjusted according to response.

ZEMTARD® Dose for angina and mild to moderate hypertension—initially 120 mg once daily.

- RENAL IMPAIRMENT Start with smaller dose.

ADIZEM-XL® Dose for angina and mild to moderate hypertension—initially 120 mg once daily.

ANGITIL® XL Dose form not appropriate for initial dose titration.

DILCARDIA® SR Dose for angina and mild to moderate hypertension—initially 60 mg twice a day; maximum 90 mg twice a day.

DILZEM® XL Dose for angina and mild to moderate hypertension—initially 120 mg once daily.

SLOZEM® Dose for angina and mild to moderate hypertension—initially 120 mg once daily.

TILDIEM® LA Dose for angina and mild to moderate hypertension—initially 200 mg daily; increased if necessary to 300 mg daily.

TILDIEM RETARD® Dose for mild to moderate hypertension—initially 120 mg once a day; increased if necessary to 120 mg twice a day.

For treatment of angina, dose form not appropriate for initial titration; up to 120 mg twice a day may be required.

VIAZEM® XL Dose for angina and mild to moderate hypertension—initially 120 mg once daily, adjusted according to response.

ZEMTARD® Dose for angina and mild to moderate hypertension—initially 120 mg once daily.

- PRESCRIBING AND DISPENSING INFORMATION The standard formulations containing 60 mg diltiazem hydrochloride are licensed as generics and there is no requirement for brand name dispensing. Although their means of formulation has called for the strict designation 'modified-release', their duration of action corresponds to that of tablets requiring administration more frequently.

Different versions of modified-release preparations containing more than 60 mg diltiazem hydrochloride may not have the same clinical effect. To avoid confusion between these different formulations of diltiazem, prescribers should specify the brand to be dispensed.

- PATIENT AND CARER ADVICE

TILDIEM RETARD® Tablet membrane may pass through gastro-intestinal tract unchanged, but being porous has no effect on efficacy.

- MEDICINAL FORMS

There can be variation in the licensing of different medicines containing the same drug. Forms available from special-order manufacturers include: oral suspension, oral solution

Modified-release tablet

CAUTIONARY AND ADVISORY LABELS 25

▸ Diltiazem hydrochloride (Non-proprietary)

Diltiazem hydrochloride 60 mg Diltiazem 60mg modified-release tablets | 84 tablet [PoM] £41.87 DT price = £41.50 | 100 tablet [PoM] £49.40

Diltiazem hydrochloride 90 mg Diltiazem 90mg modified-release tablets | 56 tablet [PoM] no price available

Diltiazem hydrochloride 120 mg Diltiazem 120mg modified-release tablets | 56 tablet [PoM] no price available

▸ Tildiem (Sanofi)

Diltiazem hydrochloride 60 mg Tildiem 60mg modified-release tablets | 90 tablet [PoM] £7.96

▸ Tildiem Retard (Sanofi)

Diltiazem hydrochloride 90 mg Tildiem Retard 90mg tablets | 56 tablet [PoM] £7.27

Diltiazem hydrochloride 120 mg Tildiem Retard 120mg tablets | 56 tablet [PoM] £7.15

Modified-release capsule

CAUTIONARY AND ADVISORY LABELS 25

▸ Diltiazem hydrochloride (Non-proprietary)

Diltiazem hydrochloride 60 mg Diltiazem 60mg modified-release capsules | 56 capsule [PoM] £6.04 DT price = £6.04

Diltiazem hydrochloride 90 mg Diltiazem 90mg modified-release capsules | 56 capsule [PoM] £8.50 DT price = £8.50

Diltiazem hydrochloride 120 mg Diltiazem 120mg modified-release capsules | 28 capsule [PoM] £48.40 | 56 capsule [PoM] £8.40

Diltiazem hydrochloride 180 mg Diltiazem 180mg modified-release capsules | 28 capsule [PoM] £54.20 | 56 capsule [PoM] no price available

Diltiazem hydrochloride 240 mg Diltiazem 240mg modified-release capsules | 28 capsule [PoM] no price available DT price = £11.52

Diltiazem hydrochloride 300 mg Diltiazem 300mg modified-release capsules | 28 capsule [PoM] no price available DT price = £9.01

Diltiazem hydrochloride 360 mg Diltiazem 360mg modified-release capsules | 28 capsule [PoM] no price available

▸ Adizem-SR (Napp Pharmaceuticals Ltd)

Diltiazem hydrochloride 90 mg Adizem-SR 90mg capsules | 56 capsule [PoM] £8.50 DT price = £8.50

Diltiazem hydrochloride 120 mg Adizem-SR 120mg capsules | 56 capsule [PoM] £9.45

Diltiazem hydrochloride 180 mg Adizem-SR 180mg capsules | 56 capsule [PoM] £14.15

▸ Adizem-XL (Napp Pharmaceuticals Ltd)

Diltiazem hydrochloride 120 mg Adizem-XL 120mg capsules | 28 capsule [PoM] £9.14

Diltiazem hydrochloride 180 mg Adizem-XL 180mg capsules | 28 capsule [PoM] £10.37

Diltiazem hydrochloride 200 mg Adizem-XL 200mg capsules | 28 capsule [PoM] £6.30 DT price = £6.29

Diltiazem hydrochloride 240 mg Adizem-XL 240mg capsules | 28 capsule [PoM] £11.52 DT price = £11.52

Diltiazem hydrochloride 300 mg Adizem-XL 300mg capsules | 28 capsule [PoM] £9.14 DT price = £9.01

▸ Angitil SR (Chiesi Ltd)

Diltiazem hydrochloride 90 mg Angitil SR 90 capsules | 56 capsule [PoM] £7.03 DT price = £8.50

Diltiazem hydrochloride 120 mg Angitil SR 120 capsules | 56 capsule [PoM] £6.91

Diltiazem hydrochloride 180 mg Angitil SR 180 capsules | 56 capsule [PoM] £13.27

▸ Angitil XL (Chiesi Ltd)

Diltiazem hydrochloride 240 mg Angitil XL 240 capsules | 28 capsule [PoM] £7.94 DT price = £11.52

Diltiazem hydrochloride 300 mg Angitil XL 300 capsules | 28 capsule [PoM] £6.98 DT price = £9.01

- Dilcardia SR (Mylan Ltd)
  Diltiazem hydrochloride 60 mg Dilcardia SR 60mg capsules | 56 capsule PoM £6.03 DT price = £6.04
  Diltiazem hydrochloride 90 mg Dilcardia SR 90mg capsules | 56 capsule PoM £9.61 DT price = £8.50
  Diltiazem hydrochloride 120 mg Dilcardia SR 120mg capsules | 56 capsule PoM £10.69
- Dilzem SR (Teva UK Ltd)
  Diltiazem hydrochloride 60 mg Dilzem SR 60 capsules | 56 capsule PoM £6.04 DT price = £6.04
  Diltiazem hydrochloride 90 mg Dilzem SR 90 capsules | 56 capsule PoM £11.29 DT price = £8.50
  Diltiazem hydrochloride 120 mg Dilzem SR 120 capsules | 56 capsule PoM £12.89
- Dilzem XL (Teva UK Ltd)
  Diltiazem hydrochloride 120 mg Dilzem XL 120 capsules | 28 capsule PoM £7.78
  Diltiazem hydrochloride 180 mg Dilzem XL 180 capsules | 28 capsule PoM £11.55
  Diltiazem hydrochloride 240 mg Dilzem XL 240 capsules | 28 capsule PoM £11.03 DT price = £11.52
- Slozem (Merck Serono Ltd)
  Diltiazem hydrochloride 120 mg Slozem 120mg capsules | 28 capsule PoM £7.00
  Diltiazem hydrochloride 180 mg Slozem 180mg capsules | 28 capsule PoM £7.80
  Diltiazem hydrochloride 240 mg Slozem 240mg capsules | 28 capsule PoM £8.20 DT price = £11.52
  Diltiazem hydrochloride 300 mg Slozem 300mg capsules | 28 capsule PoM £8.50 DT price = £9.01
- Tildiem LA (Sanofi)
  Diltiazem hydrochloride 200 mg Tildiem LA 200 capsules | 28 capsule PoM £6.29 DT price = £6.29
  Diltiazem hydrochloride 300 mg Tildiem LA 300 capsules | 28 capsule PoM £9.01 DT price = £9.01
- Viazem XL (Thornton & Ross Ltd)
  Diltiazem hydrochloride 120 mg Viazem XL 120mg capsules | 28 capsule PoM £6.60
  Diltiazem hydrochloride 180 mg Viazem XL 180mg capsules | 28 capsule PoM £7.36
  Diltiazem hydrochloride 240 mg Viazem XL 240mg capsules | 28 capsule PoM £7.74 DT price = £11.52
  Diltiazem hydrochloride 300 mg Viazem XL 300mg capsules | 28 capsule PoM £8.03 DT price = £9.01
  Diltiazem hydrochloride 360 mg Viazem XL 360mg capsules | 28 capsule PoM £13.85
- Zemtard XL (Galen Ltd)
  Diltiazem hydrochloride 120 mg Zemtard 120 XL capsules | 28 capsule PoM £5.19
  Diltiazem hydrochloride 180 mg Zemtard 180 XL capsules | 28 capsule PoM £5.27
  Diltiazem hydrochloride 240 mg Zemtard 240 XL capsules | 28 capsule PoM £5.36 DT price = £11.52
  Diltiazem hydrochloride 300 mg Zemtard 300 XL capsules | 28 capsule PoM £5.70 DT price = £9.01

F 142

Felodipine

- **DRUG ACTION** Felodipine is a dihydropyridine calcium-channel blocker.

- **INDICATIONS AND DOSE**

Prophylaxis of angina

▶ BY MOUTH
- Adult: Initially 5 mg once daily; increased if necessary to 10 mg once daily, to be taken in the morning
- Elderly: Initially 2.5 mg once daily; increased if necessary to 10 mg once daily, to be taken in the morning

Hypertension

▶ BY MOUTH
- Adult: Initially 5 mg once daily; usual maintenance 5–10 mg once daily, to be taken in the morning, doses above 20 mg daily rarely needed
- Elderly: Initially 2.5 mg daily; usual maintenance 5–10 mg once daily, to be taken in the morning, doses above 20 mg daily rarely needed

- **CONTRA-INDICATIONS** Cardiac outflow obstruction · significant cardiac valvular obstruction (e.g. aortic stenosis) · uncontrolled heart failure · unstable angina · within 1 month of myocardial infarction
- **CAUTIONS** Predisposition to tachycardia · severe left ventricular dysfunction · withdraw if cardiogenic shock develops · withdraw if existing pain worsens shortly after initiating treatment · withdraw if ischaemic pain occurs shortly after initiating treatment
- **INTERACTIONS** → Appendix 1 (calcium-channel blockers).
- **SIDE-EFFECTS**
  - **Common or very common** Flushing · headache · peripheral oedema
  - **Uncommon** Abdominal pain · dizziness · malaise · nausea · palpitation · paraesthesia · pruritus · rash · tachycardia
  - **Rare** Arthralgia · impotence · myalgia · syncope · vomiting
  - **Very rare** Gum hyperplasia · leucocytoclastic vasculitis · photosensitivity · urinary frequency
- **PREGNANCY** Avoid; toxicity in *animal* studies; may inhibit labour.
- **BREAST FEEDING** Present in milk but amount probably too small to be harmful.
- **HEPATIC IMPAIRMENT** Dose reduction may be required.

- **MEDICINAL FORMS**
There can be variation in the licensing of different medicines containing the same drug. Forms available from special-order manufacturers include: oral solution

Modified-release tablet

CAUTIONARY AND ADVISORY LABELS 25

- Felodipine (Non-proprietary)
  Felodipine 2.5 mg Felodipine 2.5mg modified-release tablets | 28 tablet PoM no price available DT price = £6.31
  Felodipine 5 mg Felodipine 5mg modified-release tablets | 28 tablet PoM £4.21 DT price = £4.21
  Felodipine 10 mg Felodipine 10mg modified-release tablets | 28 tablet PoM £5.66 DT price = £5.66
- Cardioplen XL (Chiesi Ltd)
  Felodipine 2.5 mg Cardioplen XL 2.5mg tablets | 28 tablet PoM £5.68 DT price = £6.31
  Felodipine 5 mg Cardioplen XL 5mg tablets | 28 tablet PoM £3.87 DT price = £4.21
  Felodipine 10 mg Cardioplen XL 10mg tablets | 28 tablet PoM £4.81 DT price = £5.66
- Felendil XL (Teva UK Ltd)
  Felodipine 2.5 mg Folpik XL 2.5mg tablets | 28 tablet PoM £6.31 DT price = £6.31
  Felodipine 5 mg Folpik XL 5mg tablets | 28 tablet PoM £4.21 DT price = £4.21
  Felodipine 10 mg Folpik XL 10mg tablets | 28 tablet PoM £7.21 DT price = £5.66
- Felogen XL (Mylan Ltd)
  Felodipine 5 mg Felogen XL 5mg tablets | 28 tablet PoM £4.21 DT price = £4.21
  Felodipine 10 mg Felogen XL 10mg tablets | 28 tablet PoM £5.66 DT price = £5.66
- Felotens XL (Genus Pharmaceuticals Ltd)
  Felodipine 2.5 mg Felotens XL 2.5mg tablets | 28 tablet PoM £5.68 DT price = £6.31
  Felodipine 5 mg Felotens XL 5mg tablets | 28 tablet PoM £3.79 DT price = £4.21
  Felodipine 10 mg Felotens XL 10mg tablets | 28 tablet PoM £5.10 DT price = £5.66
- Neofel XL (Kent Pharmaceuticals Ltd, Actavis UK Ltd, Almus Pharmaceuticals Ltd)
  Felodipine 2.5 mg Neofel XL 2.5mg tablets | 28 tablet PoM £6.31 DT price = £6.31
  Felodipine 5 mg Neofel XL 5mg tablets | 28 tablet PoM £4.21 DT price = £4.21
  Felodipine 10 mg Neofel XL 10mg tablets | 28 tablet PoM £5.66 DT price = £5.66
- Parmid XL (Sandoz Ltd)
  Felodipine 2.5 mg Parmid XL 2.5mg tablets | 28 tablet PoM £5.36 DT price = £6.31

2

Cardiovascular system

▸ Pinefeld XL (Tillomed Laboratories Ltd)
Felodipine 10 mg Pinefeld XL 10mg tablets | 28 tablet [PoM] £11.98 DT price = £5.66
▸ Plendil (AstraZeneca UK Ltd)
Felodipine 2.5 mg Plendil 2.5mg modified-release tablets | 28 tablet [PoM] £6.31 DT price = £6.31
Felodipine 5 mg Plendil 5mg modified-release tablets | 28 tablet [PoM] £4.21 DT price = £4.21
Felodipine 10 mg Plendil 10mg modified-release tablets | 28 tablet [PoM] £5.66 DT price = £5.66
▸ Vascalpha (Almus Pharmaceuticals Ltd, Actavis UK Ltd)
Felodipine 5 mg Vascalpha 5mg modified-release tablets | 28 tablet [PoM] £7.16–£7.29 DT price = £4.21
Felodipine 10 mg Vascalpha 10mg modified-release tablets | 28 tablet [PoM] £9.63–£9.81 DT price = £5.66

Combinations available: *Ramipril with felodipine*, p. 159

F 142

Isradipine

● **INDICATIONS AND DOSE**

Hypertension
▸ BY MOUTH
▸ **Adult:** 2.5 mg twice daily for 3–4 weeks, then increased if necessary to 5 mg twice daily, dose increased exceptionally up to 10 mg twice daily
▸ **Elderly:** 1.25 mg twice daily, increased if necessary after 3–4 weeks according to response; maintenance 2.5–5 mg once daily may be sufficient

● CONTRA-INDICATIONS Acute porphyrias p. 918 · cardiogenic shock · during or within 1 month of myocardial infarction · unstable angina
● CAUTIONS Chronic heart failure · poor cardiac reserve · severe aortic stenosis · sick sinus syndrome (if pacemaker not fitted)
● INTERACTIONS → Appendix 1 (calcium-channel blockers).
● SIDE-EFFECTS
▸ **Common or very common** Abdominal discomfort · dizziness · dyspnoea · fatigue · flushing · headache · palpitation · peripheral oedema · polyuria · rash · tachycardia
▸ **Uncommon** Hypotension · weight gain
▸ **Very rare** Anaemia · anorexia · anxiety · arrhythmia · arthralgia · blood disorders · bradycardia · cough · depression · drowsiness · erectile dysfunction · gum hyperplasia · heart failure · hypersensitivity reactions · leucopenia · nausea · paraesthesia · thrombocytopenia · visual disturbance · vomiting
▸ **Frequency not known** Gynaecomastia · hepatitis
Overdose
In overdose, the dihydropyridine calcium-channel blockers cause severe hypotension secondary to profound peripheral vasodilatation.
● PREGNANCY May inhibit labour. Risk to fetus should be balanced against risk of uncontrolled maternal hypertension.
● BREAST FEEDING Manufacturer advises avoid—present in milk in *animal* studies.
● HEPATIC IMPAIRMENT 1.25 mg twice daily, increased if necessary after 3–4 weeks according to response; maintenance dose of 2.5 mg or 5 mg once daily may be sufficient.
● RENAL IMPAIRMENT Use with caution.
● MEDICINAL FORMS
There can be variation in the licensing of different medicines containing the same drug.
Tablet
▸ Isradipine (Non-proprietary)
Isradipine 2.5 mg Isradipine 2.5mg tablets | 56 tablet [PoM] £187.50 DT price = £184.56

F 142

Lacidipine

● DRUG ACTION Lacidipine is a dihydropyridine calcium-channel blocker.

● **INDICATIONS AND DOSE**

Hypertension
▸ BY MOUTH
▸ **Adult:** Initially 2 mg daily; increased if necessary to 4 mg daily, then increased if necessary to 6 mg daily, dose increases should occur at intervals of 3–4 weeks, to be taken preferably in the morning

● CONTRA-INDICATIONS Acute porphyrias p. 918 · aortic stenosis · avoid within 1 month of myocardial infarction · cardiogenic shock · unstable angina
● CAUTIONS Cardiac conduction abnormalities · poor cardiac reserve
● INTERACTIONS → Appendix 1 (calcium-channel blockers).
● SIDE-EFFECTS
▸ **Common or very common** Dizziness · flushing · headache · oedema · palpitation
▸ **Rare** Aggravation of angina · asthenia · erythema · gastro-intestinal disturbances · gum hyperplasia · mood disturbances · muscle cramps · polyuria · pruritus · skin rash
Overdose
In overdose, the dihydropyridine calcium-channel blockers cause severe hypotension secondary to profound peripheral vasodilatation.
● PREGNANCY Manufacturer advises avoid; may inhibit labour.
● BREAST FEEDING Manufacturer advises avoid—no information available.
● HEPATIC IMPAIRMENT Antihypertensive effect possibly increased.

● MEDICINAL FORMS
There can be variation in the licensing of different medicines containing the same drug.
Tablet
▸ Lacidipine (Non-proprietary)
Lacidipine 2 mg Lacidipine 2mg tablets | 28 tablet [PoM] £6.85 DT price = £2.55
Lacidipine 4 mg Lacidipine 4mg tablets | 28 tablet [PoM] £6.85 DT price = £2.61
▸ Molap (Rivopharm (UK) Ltd)
Lacidipine 4 mg Molap 4mg tablets | 28 tablet [PoM] £3.66 DT price = £2.61
▸ Motens (GlaxoSmithKline UK Ltd)
Lacidipine 2 mg Motens 2mg tablets | 28 tablet [PoM] £2.95 DT price = £2.55
Lacidipine 4 mg Motens 4mg tablets | 28 tablet [PoM] £3.10 DT price = £2.61

F 142

Lercanidipine hydrochloride

● DRUG ACTION Lercanidipine is a dihydropyridine calcium-channel blocker.

● **INDICATIONS AND DOSE**

Mild to moderate hypertension
▸ BY MOUTH
▸ **Adult:** Initially 10 mg once daily; increased if necessary to 20 mg daily, dose can be adjusted after 2 weeks

● CONTRA-INDICATIONS Acute porphyrias p. 918 · aortic stenosis · uncontrolled heart failure · unstable angina · within 1 month of myocardial infarction
● CAUTIONS Left ventricular dysfunction · sick sinus syndrome (if pacemaker not fitted)

- INTERACTIONS → Appendix 1 (calcium-channel blockers).
- SIDE-EFFECTS
► **Uncommon** Dizziness · flushing · headache · palpitation · peripheral oedema · tachycardia
► **Rare** Angina · asthenia · drowsiness · gastro-intestinal disturbances · myalgia · polyuria · rash
► **Very rare** Gingival hyperplasia · hypotension · myocardial infarction

Overdose
In overdose, the dihydropyridine calcium-channel blockers cause severe hypotension secondary to profound peripheral vasodilatation.

- PREGNANCY Manufacturer advises avoid—no information available.
- BREAST FEEDING Manufacturer advises avoid.
- HEPATIC IMPAIRMENT Avoid in severe disease.
- RENAL IMPAIRMENT Avoid if eGFR less than 30 mL/minute/1.73 m^2.

- MEDICINAL FORMS
There can be variation in the licensing of different medicines containing the same drug.

Tablet
CAUTIONARY AND ADVISORY LABELS 22
► Lercanidipine hydrochloride (Non-proprietary)
   Lercanidipine hydrochloride 10 mg Lercanidipine 10mg tablets | 28 tablet (PoM) £12.99 DT price = £5.74
   Lercanidipine hydrochloride 20 mg Lercanidipine 20mg tablets | 28 tablet (PoM) £15.99 DT price = £6.66
► Zanidip (Recordati Pharmaceuticals Ltd)
   Lercanidipine hydrochloride 10 mg Zanidip 10mg tablets | 28 tablet (PoM) £5.70 DT price = £5.74
   Lercanidipine hydrochloride 20 mg Zanidip 20mg tablets | 28 tablet (PoM) £10.82 DT price = £6.66

☞ 142

Nicardipine hydrochloride

- DRUG ACTION Nicardipine is a dihydropyridine calcium-channel blocker.

- INDICATIONS AND DOSE

Prophylaxis of angina
► BY MOUTH USING IMMEDIATE-RELEASE MEDICINES
► Adult: Initially 20 mg 3 times a day, then increased to 30 mg 3 times a day, dose increased after at least 3 days; usual dose 60–120 mg daily

Mild to moderate hypertension
► BY MOUTH USING IMMEDIATE-RELEASE MEDICINES
► Adult: Initially 20 mg 3 times a day, then increased to 30 mg 3 times a day, dose increased after at least 3 days; usual dose 60–120 mg daily
► BY MOUTH USING MODIFIED-RELEASE MEDICINES
► Adult: Initially 30 mg twice daily; increased if necessary up to 45 mg twice daily. usual dose 30–60 mg twice daily

Life-threatening hypertension (specialist use only) | Post-operative hypertension (specialist use only)
► BY CONTINUOUS INTRAVENOUS INFUSION
► Adult: Initially 3–5 mg/hour for 15 minutes, increased in steps of 0.5–1 mg every 15 minutes, adjusted according to response, maximum rate 15 mg/hour, reduce dose gradually when target blood pressure achieved; maintenance 2–4 mg/hour
► Elderly: Initially 1–5 mg/hour, then adjusted in steps of 500 micrograms/hour after 30 minutes, adjusted according to response, maximum rate 15 mg/hour

Life-threatening hypertension in patients with hepatic or renal impairment (specialist use only) | Postoperative hypertension in patients with hepatic or renal impairment (specialist use only)
► BY CONTINUOUS INTRAVENOUS INFUSION
► Adult: Initially 1–5 mg/hour, then adjusted in steps of 500 micrograms/hour after 30 minutes, adjusted according to response, maximum rate 15 mg/hour

Acute life-threatening hypertension in pregnancy (specialist use only)
► BY CONTINUOUS INTRAVENOUS INFUSION
► Adult: Initially 1–5 mg/hour, then adjusted in steps of 500 micrograms/hour after 30 minutes, adjusted according to response, usual maximum rate 4 mg/hour in treatment of pre-eclampsia (maximum rate 15 mg/hour)

- CONTRA-INDICATIONS
GENERAL CONTRA-INDICATIONS
Acute porphyrias p. 918 · cardiogenic shock · significant or advanced aortic stenosis · unstable or acute attacks of angina

SPECIFIC CONTRA-INDICATIONS
► With intravenous use Avoid within 8 days of myocardial infarction · compensatory hypertension
► With oral use Avoid within 1 month of myocardial infarction

- CAUTIONS Congestive heart failure · elderly · elevated intracranial pressure · portal hypertension · pulmonary oedema · significantly impaired left ventricular function · stroke · withdraw if ischaemic pain occurs or existing pain worsens within 30 minutes of initiating treatment or increasing dose

- INTERACTIONS → Appendix 1 (calcium-channel blockers).
- SIDE-EFFECTS Atrioventricular block · depression · dizziness · drowsiness · dyspnoea · flushing · frequency of micturition · gastro-intestinal disturbances · gingival hyperplasia · headache · hypotension · impotence · insomnia · nausea · palpitations · paraesthesia · paralytic ileus · peripheral oedema · pruritus · pulmonary oedema · rashes · tachycardia · thrombocytopenia · tinnitus · vomiting

SIDE-EFFECTS, FURTHER INFORMATION
► Hypotension and reflex tachycardia Systemic hypotension and reflex tachycardia with rapid reduction of blood pressure may occur—during intravenous use consider stopping infusion or decreasing dose by half.

Overdose
In overdose, the dihydropyridine calcium-channel blockers cause severe hypotension secondary to profound peripheral vasodilatation.

- PREGNANCY May inhibit labour. Not to be used in multiple pregnancy (twins or more) unless there is no other acceptable alternative. Toxicity in *animal* studies. Risk of severe maternal hypotension and fatal foetal hypoxia— avoid excessive decrease in blood pressure. For treatment of acute life-threatening hypertension only.
- BREAST FEEDING Manufacturer advises avoid—present in breast milk.
- HEPATIC IMPAIRMENT
► With oral use Use with caution—consider using lowest initial dose and extending dosing interval according to individual response.
► With intravenous use Use with caution—use lower initial dose.
- RENAL IMPAIRMENT
► With oral use Consider using lowest initial dose and extending dosing interval according to individual response.
► With intravenous use Use with caution—use lower initial dose.

2

Cardiovascular system

- MONITORING REQUIREMENTS Monitor blood pressure and heart rate at least every 5 minutes during intravenous infusion, and then until stable, and continue monitoring for at least 12 hours after end of infusion.
- DIRECTIONS FOR ADMINISTRATION Intravenous nicardipine should only be administered under the supervision of a specialist and in a hospital or intensive care setting in which patients can be closely monitored.

  For *intravenous infusion* give continuously *in* Glucose 5%; dilute dose in infusion fluid to a final concentration of 100–200 micrograms/mL (undiluted solution *via* central venous line only) and give *via* volumetric infusion pump or syringe driver; protect from light; to minimise peripheral venous irritation, change site of infusion every 12 hours; risk of adsorption on to plastic of infusion set in the presence of saline solutions; incompatible with bicarbonate or alkaline solutions—consult product literature.

- MEDICINAL FORMS
  There can be variation in the licensing of different medicines containing the same drug. Forms available from special-order manufacturers include: oral suspension, oral solution

Capsule
- Nicardipine hydrochloride (Non-proprietary)
  Nicardipine hydrochloride 20 mg Nicardipine 20mg capsules | 56 capsule PoM £8.38 DT price = £6.00
  Nicardipine hydrochloride 30 mg Nicardipine 30mg capsules | 56 capsule PoM £9.73 DT price = £6.37
- Cardene (Astellas Pharma Ltd)
  Nicardipine hydrochloride 20 mg Cardene 20mg capsules | 56 capsule PoM £6.00 DT price = £6.00
  Nicardipine hydrochloride 30 mg Cardene 30mg capsules | 56 capsule PoM £6.96 DT price = £6.37

Modified-release capsule
CAUTIONARY AND ADVISORY LABELS 25
- Cardene SR (Astellas Pharma Ltd)
  Nicardipine hydrochloride 30 mg Cardene SR 30mg capsules | 56 capsule PoM £7.15 DT price = £7.15
  Nicardipine hydrochloride 45 mg Cardene SR 45mg capsules | 56 capsule PoM £10.40 DT price = £10.40

Solution for infusion
- Nicardipine hydrochloride (Non-proprietary)
  Nicardipine hydrochloride 1 mg per 1 ml Nicardipine 10mg/10ml solution for injection ampoules | 5 ampoule PoM £50.00
  Nicardipine hydrochloride 2.5 mg per 1 ml Cardene I.V. 25mg/10ml solution for infusion ampoules | 10 ampoule PoM no price available

▸ 142

Nifedipine

- DRUG ACTION Nifedipine is a dihydropyridine calcium-channel blocker.

- INDICATIONS AND DOSE

Raynaud's syndrome
▸ BY MOUTH USING IMMEDIATE-RELEASE MEDICINES
- Adult: Initially 5 mg 3 times a day, then adjusted according to response to 20 mg 3 times a day

Angina prophylaxis (not recommended)
▸ BY MOUTH USING IMMEDIATE-RELEASE MEDICINES
- Adult: Initially 5 mg 3 times a day, then adjusted according to response to 20 mg 3 times a day

Postponement of premature labour
▸ BY MOUTH USING IMMEDIATE-RELEASE MEDICINES
- Adult: Initially 20 mg, followed by 10–20 mg 3–4 times a day, adjusted according to uterine activity

Hiccup in palliative care
▸ BY MOUTH
- Adult: 10 mg 3 times a day

ADALAT RETARD®

Hypertension | Angina prophylaxis
▸ BY MOUTH
- Adult: 10 mg twice daily, adjusted according to response to 40 mg twice daily

ADALAT®

Angina prophylaxis (not recommended) | Raynaud's phenomenon
▸ BY MOUTH USING IMMEDIATE-RELEASE MEDICINES
- Adult: Initially 5 mg 3 times a day, then adjusted according to response to 20 mg 3 times a day

DOSE EQUIVALENCE AND CONVERSION
For *Adalat*®: Adalat liquid gel capsules contain 5 mg nifedipine in 0.17 mL and 10 mg nifedipine in 0.34 mL.

ADALAT® LA

Hypertension
▸ BY MOUTH
- Adult: 20–30 mg once daily, increased if necessary up to 90 mg once daily

Angina prophylaxis
▸ BY MOUTH
- Adult: 30 mg once daily, increased if necessary up to 90 mg once daily

ADIPINE® MR

Hypertension | Angina prophylaxis
▸ BY MOUTH
- Adult: 10 mg twice daily, adjusted according to response to 40 mg twice daily

ADIPINE® XL

Hypertension | Angina prophylaxis
▸ BY MOUTH
- Adult: 30 mg daily, increased if necessary up to 90 mg daily

CORACTEN® SR

Hypertension | Angina prophylaxis
▸ BY MOUTH
- Adult: Initially 10 mg twice daily, increased if necessary up to 40 mg twice daily

CORACTEN® XL

Hypertension | Angina prophylaxis
▸ BY MOUTH
- Adult: Initially 30 mg daily, increased if necessary up to 90 mg daily

FORTIPINE® LA 40

Hypertension | Angina prophylaxis
▸ BY MOUTH
- Adult: Initially 40 mg once daily, increased if necessary to 80 mg daily in 1–2 divided doses

NIFEDIPRESS® MR

Hypertension | Angina prophylaxis
▸ BY MOUTH
- Adult: 10 mg twice daily, adjusted according to response to 40 mg twice daily

TENSIPINE® MR

Hypertension | Angina prophylaxis
▸ BY MOUTH
- Adult: Initially 10 mg twice daily, adjusted according to response to 40 mg twice daily

VALNI® XL

Severe hypertension | Prophylaxis of angina
▸ BY MOUTH
- Adult: 30 mg once daily, increased if necessary up to 90 mg once daily

- UNLICENSED USE Not licensed for use in postponing premature labour.

- CONTRA-INDICATIONS Acute attacks of angina · cardiogenic shock · significant aortic stenosis · unstable angina · within 1 month of myocardial infarction
- CAUTIONS Diabetes mellitus · elderly · heart failure · poor cardiac reserve · severe hypotension · short-acting formulations are not recommended for angina or long-term management of hypertension; their use may be associated with large variations in blood pressure and reflex tachycardia · significantly impaired left ventricular function (heart failure deterioration observed) · withdraw if ischaemic pain occurs or existing pain worsens shortly after initiating treatment

ADALAT® LA Crohn's disease · decreased lumen diameter of the gastro-intestinal tract · history of gastro-intestinal obstruction · history of oesophageal obstruction · inflammatory bowel disease

CAUTIONS, FURTHER INFORMATION
Dose form not appropriate for use where there is a history of oesophageal or gastro-intestinal obstruction, decreased lumen diameter of the gastro-intestinal tract, or inflammatory bowel disease (including Crohn's disease).

VALNI® XL Decreased lumen diameter of gastro-intestinal tract · history of gastro-intestinal obstruction · history of oesophageal obstruction · ileostomy after proctocolectomy · inflammatory bowel disease

CAUTIONS, FURTHER INFORMATION
Dose form not appropriate for use where there is a history of oesophageal or gastro-intestinal obstruction, decreased lumen diameter of the gastro-intestinal tract, inflammatory bowel disease, or ileostomy after proctocolectomy.

- INTERACTIONS → Appendix 1 (calcium-channel blockers).
- SIDE-EFFECTS
  ▸ **Common or very common** Asthenia · dizziness · gastro-intestinal disturbance · headache · hypotension · lethargy · oedema · palpitation · vasodilatation
  ▸ **Uncommon** Angioedema · anxiety · chills · dyspnoea · dysuria · epistaxis · erectile dysfunction · hypersensitivity reactions · jaundice · joint swelling · migraine · myalgia · nasal congestion · nocturia · paraesthesia · polyuria · pruritus · rash · sleep disturbance · sweating · syncope · tachycardia · tremor · urticaria · vertigo · visual disturbance
  ▸ **Rare** Anorexia · gum hyperplasia · hyperglycaemia · male infertility · mood disturbances · photosensitivity reactions · purpura
  ▸ **Frequency not known** Agranulocytosis · anaphylaxis · bezoar formation (with some modified-release preparations) · dysphagia · gynaecomastia · intestinal obstruction · intestinal ulcer

Overdose
In overdose, the dihydropyridine calcium-channel blockers cause severe hypotension secondary to profound peripheral vasodilatation.

- PREGNANCY May inhibit labour; manufacturer advises avoid before week 20, but risk to fetus should be balanced against risk of uncontrolled maternal hypertension. Use only if other treatment options are not indicated or have failed.
- BREAST FEEDING Amount too small to be harmful but manufacturers advise avoid.
- HEPATIC IMPAIRMENT Dose reduction may be required in severe liver disease.
  Some modified-release formulations may not be suitable for dose titration in hepatic disease—consult product literature.
  ADALAT® LA Dose form not appropriate.
  VALNI® XL Dose form not appropriate.

- DIRECTIONS FOR ADMINISTRATION
  FORTIPINE® LA 40 Take with or just after food, or a meal.
- PRESCRIBING AND DISPENSING INFORMATION Different versions of modified-release preparations may not have the same clinical effect. To avoid confusion between these different formulations of nifedipine, prescribers should specify the brand to be dispensed.
- PATIENT AND CARER ADVICE
  ADALAT® LA Tablet membrane may pass through gastro-intestinal tract unchanged, but being porous has no effect on efficacy.

- MEDICINAL FORMS
  There can be variation in the licensing of different medicines containing the same drug. Forms available from special-order manufacturers include: oral suspension, oral drops

Modified-release tablet
CAUTIONARY AND ADVISORY LABELS 25
▸ Adalat LA (Bayer Plc)
  Nifedipine 20 mg Adalat LA 20 tablets | 28 tablet [PoM] £5.27
  Nifedipine 30 mg Adalat LA 30 tablets | 28 tablet [PoM] £6.85 DT price = £6.85
  Nifedipine 60 mg Adalat LA 60 tablets | 28 tablet [PoM] £9.03 DT price = £9.03
▸ Adalat retard (Bayer Plc)
  Nifedipine 10 mg Adalat retard 10mg tablets | 56 tablet [PoM] £7.34 DT price = £7.34
  Nifedipine 20 mg Adalat retard 20mg tablets | 56 tablet [PoM] £8.81
▸ Adipine MR (Chiesi Ltd)
  Nifedipine 10 mg Adipine MR 10 tablets | 56 tablet [PoM] £3.73 DT price = £7.34
  Nifedipine 20 mg Adipine MR 20 tablets | 56 tablet [PoM] £5.21
▸ Adipine XL (Chiesi Ltd)
  Nifedipine 30 mg Adipine XL 30mg tablets | 28 tablet [PoM] £4.70 DT price = £6.85
  Nifedipine 60 mg Adipine XL 60mg tablets | 28 tablet [PoM] £7.10 DT price = £9.03
▸ Fortipine LA (AMCo)
  Nifedipine 40 mg Fortipine LA 40 tablets | 30 tablet [PoM] £14.40 DT price = £14.40
  Nifedipine 60 mg Neozipine XL 60mg tablets | 28 tablet [PoM] £9.03 DT price = £9.03
▸ Nifedipress MR (Dexcel-Pharma Ltd)
  Nifedipine 10 mg Nifedipress MR 10 tablets | 56 tablet [PoM] £9.32 DT price = £7.34
  Nifedipine 20 mg Nifedipress MR 20 tablets | 56 tablet [PoM] £10.06
▸ Tensipine MR (Genus Pharmaceuticals Ltd)
  Nifedipine 10 mg Tensipine MR 10 tablets | 56 tablet [PoM] £3.65 DT price = £7.34
  Nifedipine 20 mg Tensipine MR 20 tablets | 56 tablet [PoM] £4.67
▸ Valni XL (Zentiva)
  Nifedipine 30 mg Valni XL 30mg tablets | 28 tablet [PoM] £9.14 DT price = £6.85
  Nifedipine 60 mg Valni XL 60mg tablets | 28 tablet [PoM] £21.85 DT price = £9.03

Capsule
▸ Nifedipine (Non-proprietary)
  Nifedipine 5 mg Nifedipine 5mg capsules | 84 capsule [PoM] £19.99 DT price = £16.21
  Nifedipine 10 mg Nifedipine 10mg capsules | 84 capsule [PoM] £21.00 DT price = £11.36
▸ Adalat (Bayer Plc)
  Nifedipine 5 mg Adalat 5mg capsules | 90 capsule [PoM] £5.73
  Nifedipine 10 mg Adalat 10mg capsules | 90 capsule [PoM] £7.30

Modified-release capsule
CAUTIONARY AND ADVISORY LABELS 25
▸ Coracten SR (UCB Pharma Ltd)
  Nifedipine 10 mg Coracten SR 10mg capsules | 60 capsule [PoM] £3.90 DT price = £3.90
  Nifedipine 20 mg Coracten SR 20mg capsules | 60 capsule [PoM] £5.41 DT price = £5.41
▸ Coracten XL (UCB Pharma Ltd)
  Nifedipine 30 mg Coracten XL 30mg capsules | 28 capsule [PoM] £4.89 DT price = £4.89
  Nifedipine 60 mg Coracten XL 60mg capsules | 28 capsule [PoM] £7.34 DT price = £7.34

Oral drops

▸ Nifedipine (Non-proprietary)
Nifedipine 20 mg per 1 ml Nifedipin-ratiopharm 20mg/ml oral drops
| 30 ml [PoM] no price available | 100 ml [PoM] no price available

Combinations available: *Atenolol with nifedipine*, p. 139

⚑ 142

Verapamil hydrochloride

● INDICATIONS AND DOSE

Treatment of supraventricular arrhythmias
▸ BY MOUTH USING IMMEDIATE-RELEASE MEDICINES
▸ Adult: 40–120 mg 3 times a day
▸ BY SLOW INTRAVENOUS INJECTION
▸ Adult: 5–10 mg, to be given over 2 minutes, preferably with ECG monitoring
▸ Elderly: 5–10 mg, to be given over 3 minutes, preferably with ECG monitoring

Paroxysmal tachyarrhythmias
▸ BY SLOW INTRAVENOUS INJECTION
▸ Adult: Initially 5–10 mg, followed by 5 mg after 5–10 minutes if required, to be given over 2 minutes, preferably with ECG monitoring
▸ Elderly: Initially 5–10 mg, followed by 5 mg after 5–10 minutes if required, to be given over 3 minutes, preferably with ECG monitoring

Angina
▸ BY MOUTH USING IMMEDIATE-RELEASE MEDICINES
▸ Adult: 80–120 mg 3 times a day

Hypertension
▸ BY MOUTH USING IMMEDIATE-RELEASE MEDICINES
▸ Adult: 240–480 mg daily in 2–3 divided doses

Prophylaxis of cluster headache (initiated under specialist supervision)
▸ BY MOUTH USING IMMEDIATE-RELEASE MEDICINES
▸ Adult: 240–960 mg daily in 3–4 divided doses

HALF SECURON® SR

Hypertension (in patients new to verapamil)
▸ BY MOUTH
▸ Adult: Initially 120 mg daily, increased if necessary up to 480 mg daily, doses above 240 mg daily as 2 divided doses

Hypertension
▸ BY MOUTH
▸ Adult: 240 mg daily, increased if necessary up to 480 mg daily, doses above 240 mg daily as 2 divided doses

Angina
▸ BY MOUTH
▸ Adult: 240 mg twice daily, may sometimes be reduced to once daily

Prophylaxis after myocardial infarction where beta-blockers not appropriate
▸ BY MOUTH
▸ Adult: 360 mg daily in divided doses, started at least 1 week after infarction, given as either 240 mg in the morning and 120 mg in the evening *or* 120 mg 3 times daily

SECURON® SR

Hypertension (in patients new to verapamil)
▸ BY MOUTH
▸ Adult: Initially 120 mg daily, increased if necessary up to 480 mg daily, doses above 240 mg daily as 2 divided doses

Hypertension
▸ BY MOUTH
▸ Adult: 240 mg daily, increased if necessary up to 480 mg daily, doses above 240 mg daily as 2 divided doses

Angina
▸ BY MOUTH
▸ Adult: 240 mg twice daily, may sometimes be reduced to once daily

Prophylaxis after myocardial infarction where beta-blockers not appropriate
▸ BY MOUTH
▸ Adult: 360 mg daily in divided doses, started at least 1 week after infarction, given as either 240 mg in the morning and 120 mg in the evening *or* 120 mg 3 times daily

UNIVER®

Hypertension (in patients new to verapamil)
▸ BY MOUTH
▸ Adult: Initially 120 mg daily; maximum 480 mg per day

Hypertension
▸ BY MOUTH
▸ Adult: 240 mg daily; maximum 480 mg per day

Angina
▸ BY MOUTH
▸ Adult: 360 mg daily; maximum 480 mg per day

VERAPRESS® MR

Hypertension
▸ BY MOUTH
▸ Adult: 240 mg daily, increased if necessary to 240 mg twice daily

Angina
▸ BY MOUTH
▸ Adult: 240 mg twice daily, may sometimes be reduced to once daily

VERTAB® SR 240

Mild to moderate hypertension
▸ BY MOUTH
▸ Adult: 240 mg daily, increased if necessary to 240 mg twice daily

Angina
▸ BY MOUTH
▸ Adult: 240 mg twice daily, may sometimes be reduced to once daily

● UNLICENSED USE
▸ With oral use Prophylaxis of cluster headaches is an unlicensed indication.

● CONTRA-INDICATIONS Acute porphyrias p. 918 · atrial flutter or fibrillation associated with accessory conducting pathways (e.g. Wolff-Parkinson-White-syndrome) · bradycardia · cardiogenic shock · history of heart failure (even if controlled by therapy) · history of significantly impaired left ventricular function (even if controlled by therapy) · hypotension · second- and third-degree AV block · sick sinus syndrome · sino-atrial block

● CAUTIONS Acute phase of myocardial infarction (avoid if bradycardia, hypotension, left ventricular failure) · first-degree AV block

● INTERACTIONS → Appendix 1 (calcium-channel blockers).
▸ Verapamil and beta-blockers Verapamil injection should not be given to patients recently treated with beta-blockers because of the risk of hypotension and asystole. The suggestion that when verapamil injection has been given first, an interval of 30 minutes before giving a beta-blocker is sufficient has not been confirmed. It may also be hazardous to give verapamil and a beta-blocker together by mouth (should only be contemplated if myocardial function well preserved).

● SIDE-EFFECTS
▸ Common or very common Constipation
▸ Uncommon Ankle oedema · dizziness · fatigue · flushing · headache · nausea · vomiting

Cardiovascular system

- **Rare** Allergic reactions · angioedema · arthralgia · asystole · bradycardia · erythema · erythromelalgia · gingival hyperplasia after long-term treatment · gynaecomastia after long-term treatment · heart block · heart failure · hypotension · increased prolactin concentration · myalgia · paraesthesia · pruritus · Stevens-Johnson syndrome · urticaria

  SIDE-EFFECTS, FURTHER INFORMATION
- Intravenous administration or high doses Hypotension, heart failure, bradycardia, heart block, and asystole are side-effects associated with intravenous administration or high doses.

  Overdose
  In overdose, verapamil has a profound cardiac depressant effect causing hypotension and arrhythmias, including complete heart block and asystole.

- PREGNANCY May reduce uterine blood flow with fetal hypoxia. Manufacturer advises avoid in first trimester unless absolutely necessary. May inhibit labour.

- BREAST FEEDING Amount too small to be harmful.

- HEPATIC IMPAIRMENT Oral dose may need to be reduced.

- MEDICINAL FORMS
  There can be variation in the licensing of different medicines containing the same drug. Forms available from special-order manufacturers include: oral suspension, oral solution
  Tablet
  ▸ Verapamil hydrochloride (Non-proprietary)
  Verapamil hydrochloride 40 mg Verapamil 40mg tablets | 84 tablet [PoM] £2.07 DT price = £1.65
  Verapamil hydrochloride 80 mg Verapamil 80mg tablets | 84 tablet [PoM] £2.33 DT price = £1.90
  Verapamil hydrochloride 120 mg Verapamil 120mg tablets | 28 tablet [PoM] £2.01 DT price = £1.47
  Verapamil hydrochloride 160 mg Verapamil 160mg tablets | 56 tablet [PoM] £33.84 DT price = £28.20

  Modified-release tablet
  CAUTIONARY AND ADVISORY LABELS 25
  ▸ Half Securon (BGP Products Ltd)
  Verapamil hydrochloride 120 mg Half Securon SR 120mg tablets | 28 tablet [PoM] £7.71 DT price = £7.71
  ▸ Securon SR (BGP Products Ltd)
  Verapamil hydrochloride 240 mg Securon SR 240mg tablets | 28 tablet [PoM] £5.55 DT price = £5.55
  ▸ Verapress MR (Dexcel-Pharma Ltd)
  Verapamil hydrochloride 240 mg Verapress MR 240mg tablets | 28 tablet [PoM] £9.90 DT price = £5.55
  ▸ Vertab SR (Chiesi Ltd)
  Verapamil hydrochloride 240 mg Vertab SR 240 tablets | 28 tablet [PoM] £5.45 DT price = £5.55

  Modified-release capsule
  CAUTIONARY AND ADVISORY LABELS 25
  EXCIPIENTS: May contain Propylene glycol
  ▸ Univer (Teva UK Ltd)
  Verapamil hydrochloride 120 mg Univer 120mg modified-release capsules | 28 capsule [PoM] £4.86 DT price = £4.86
  Verapamil hydrochloride 180 mg Univer 180mg modified-release capsules | 56 capsule [PoM] £11.38 DT price = £11.38
  Verapamil hydrochloride 240 mg Univer 240mg modified-release capsules | 28 capsule [PoM] £7.67 DT price = £7.67

  Oral solution
  ▸ Verapamil hydrochloride (Non-proprietary)
  Verapamil hydrochloride 8 mg per 1 ml Verapamil 40mg/5ml oral solution sugar free sugar-free | 150 ml [PoM] £39.00 DT price = £36.90
  ▸ Zolvera (Rosemont Pharmaceuticals Ltd)
  Verapamil hydrochloride 8 mg per 1 ml Zolvera 40mg/5ml oral solution sugar-free | 150 ml [PoM] £36.90 DT price = £36.90

  Solution for injection
  ▸ Securon (BGP Products Ltd)
  Verapamil hydrochloride 2.5 mg per 1 ml Securon IV 5mg/2ml solution for injection ampoules | 5 ampoule [PoM] £5.41

DIURETICS › POTASSIUM-SPARING DIURETICS › OTHER

Amiloride with cyclopenthiazide

The properties listed below are those particular to the combination only. For the properties of the components please consider, amiloride hydrochloride p. 212, cyclopenthiazide p. 214.

- INDICATIONS AND DOSE
  Hypertension
  ▸ BY MOUTH
  ▸ **Adult:** 1–2 tablets daily, dose to be taken in the morning

- MEDICINAL FORMS
  There can be variation in the licensing of different medicines containing the same drug.
  Tablet
  EXCIPIENTS: May contain Gluten
  ▸ Navispare (AMCo)
  Cyclopenthiazide 250 microgram, Amiloride hydrochloride 2.5 mg Navispare 2.5mg/250microgram tablets | 28 tablet [PoM] £3.24 DT price = £3.24

DIURETICS › THIAZIDES AND RELATED DIURETICS

Thiazides and related diuretics

- CONTRA-INDICATIONS Addison's disease · hypercalcaemia · hyponatraemia · refractory hypokalaemia · symptomatic hyperuricaemia

- CAUTIONS Diabetes · gout · hyperaldosteronism · malnourishment · nephrotic syndrome · systemic lupus erythematosus

  CAUTIONS, FURTHER INFORMATION
  ▸ Potassium loss Hypokalaemia can occur with both thiazide and loop diuretics. The risk of hypokalaemia depends on the duration of action as well as the potency and is thus greater with thiazides than with an equipotent dose of a loop diuretic.
  Hypokalaemia is dangerous in severe cardiovascular disease and in patients also being treated with cardiac glycosides. Often the use of potassium-sparing diuretics avoids the need to take potassium supplements.
  Potassium supplements or potassium-sparing diuretics are seldom necessary when thiazides are used in the routine treatment of hypertension.
  In hepatic failure, hypokalaemia caused by diuretics can precipitate encephalopathy, particularly in alcoholic cirrhosis.
  ▸ Elderly Lower initial doses of diuretics should be used in the elderly because they are particularly susceptible to the side-effects. The dose should then be adjusted according to renal function. Diuretics should not be used continuously on a long-term basis to treat simple gravitational oedema (which will usually respond to increased movement, raising the legs, and support stockings).
  ▸ Existing conditions Thiazides and related diuretics can exacerbate diabetes, gout, and systemic lupus erythematosus.

- INTERACTIONS → Appendix 1 (diuretics).

- SIDE-EFFECTS
  ▸ **Common or very common** Altered plasma-lipid concentrations · gout · hypercalcaemia · hyperglycaemia · hyperuricaemia · hypochloraemic alkalosis · hypokalaemia · hypomagnesaemia · hyponatraemia · metabolic and electrolyte disturbances · mild gastrointestinal disturbances · postural hypotension

2

Cardiovascular system

• **Uncommon** Agranulocytosis · blood disorders · impotence · leucopenia · thrombocytopenia
• **Frequency not known** Cardiac arrhythmias · dizziness · headache · hypersensitivity reactions · intrahepatic cholestasis · pancreatitis · paraesthesia · photosensitivity · pneumonitis · pulmonary oedema · severe skin reactions · visual disturbances
• PREGNANCY Thiazides and related diuretics should not be used to treat gestational hypertension. They may cause neonatal thrombocytopenia, bone marrow suppression, jaundice, electrolyte disturbances, and hypoglycaemia; placental perfusion may also be reduced. Stimulation of labour, uterine inertia, and meconium staining have also been reported.
• HEPATIC IMPAIRMENT Caution in mild to moderate impairment. Avoid in severe liver disease. Hypokalaemia may precipitate coma in hepatic impairment, although hypokalaemia can be prevented by using a potassium-sparing diuretic. There is an increased risk of hypomagnesaemia in alcoholic cirrhosis.
• RENAL IMPAIRMENT Thiazides and related diuretics are ineffective if eGFR is less than 30 mL/minute/1.73 m^2 and should be avoided. Metolazone remains effective if eGFR is less than 30 mL/minute/1.73 m^2 but is associated with a risk of excessive diuresis. Electrolytes should be monitored in renal impairment.
• MONITORING REQUIREMENTS Electrolytes should be monitored, particularly with high doses and long-term use.

Bendroflumethiazide ☞ 151

(Bendrofluazide)

• **INDICATIONS AND DOSE**

Oedema
▸ BY MOUTH
 ▸ Adult: Initially 5–10 mg once daily or on alternate days, dose to be taken in the morning, then maintenance 5–10 mg 1–3 times a week

Hypertension
▸ BY MOUTH
 ▸ Adult: 2.5 mg daily, dose to be taken in the morning, higher doses are rarely necessary

• BREAST FEEDING The amount present in milk is too small to be harmful. Large doses may suppress lactation.

• MEDICINAL FORMS
There can be variation in the licensing of different medicines containing the same drug. Forms available from special-order manufacturers include: oral suspension, oral solution

Tablet
 ▸ Bendroflumethiazide (Non-proprietary)
 Bendroflumethiazide 2.5 mg Bendroflumethiazide 2.5mg tablets | 28 tablet [PoM] £3.68 DT price = £0.67 | 500 tablet [PoM] £65.71
 Bendroflumethiazide 5 mg Bendroflumethiazide 5mg tablets | 28 tablet [PoM] £7.36 DT price = £0.97 | 500 tablet [PoM] £73.60
 ▸ Aprinox (AMCo)
 Bendroflumethiazide 2.5 mg Aprinox 2.5mg tablets | 500 tablet [PoM] £27.31
 ▸ Neo-Naclex (AMCo)
 Bendroflumethiazide 2.5 mg Neo-Naclex 2.5mg tablets | 28 tablet [PoM] £0.33 DT price = £0.67

Combinations available: *Timolol with bendroflumethiazide,* p. 138

Co-amilozide ☞ 151

• **INDICATIONS AND DOSE**

Hypertension
▸ BY MOUTH
 ▸ Adult: Initially 2.5/25 mg daily, increased if necessary up to 5/50 mg daily

Congestive heart failure
▸ BY MOUTH
 ▸ Adult: Initially 2.5/25 mg daily; increased if necessary up to 10/100 mg daily, reduce dose for maintenance if possible

Oedema and ascites in cirrhosis of the liver
▸ BY MOUTH
 ▸ Adult: Initially 5/50 mg daily; increased if necessary up to 10/100 mg daily, reduce dose for maintenance if possible

DOSE EQUIVALENCE AND CONVERSION
A mixture of amiloride hydrochloride and hydrochlorothiazide in the mass proportions of 1 part amiloride hydrochloride to 10 parts hydrochlorothiazide.

• CONTRA-INDICATIONS Anuria · hyperkalaemia
• CAUTIONS Diabetes mellitus · elderly
• SIDE-EFFECTS Abdominal pain · agitation · alopecia · angina · anorexia · arrhythmias · arthralgia · confusion · constipation · cough · diarrhoea · dizziness · dry mouth · dyspepsia · dyspnoea · encephalopathy · fever · flatulence · flushing · gastro-intestinal bleeding · headache · hyperkalaemia · insomnia · jaundice · malaise · muscle cramp · nasal congestion · nausea · palpitation · paraesthesia · postural hypotension · pruritus · raised intra-ocular pressure · rash · respiratory distress · restlessness · sexual dysfunction · sweating · thirst · tinnitus · tremor · urinary disturbances · visual disturbance · vomiting · weakness
• BREAST FEEDING Avoid—no information regarding amiloride component available. Amount of hydrochlorothiazide in milk probably too small to be harmful. Large doses of hydrochlorothiazide may suppress lactation.
• RENAL IMPAIRMENT Manufacturers advise avoid in severe impairment. Monitor plasma-potassium concentration (high risk of hyperkalaemia in renal impairment).
• MONITORING REQUIREMENTS Monitor electrolytes.

• MEDICINAL FORMS
There can be variation in the licensing of different medicines containing the same drug. Forms available from special-order manufacturers include: oral solution

Tablet
 ▸ Co-amilozide (Non-proprietary)
 Amiloride hydrochloride 2.5 mg, Hydrochlorothiazide 25 mg Co-amilozide 2.5mg/25mg tablets | 28 tablet [PoM] £7.95 DT price = £6.05
 Amiloride hydrochloride 5 mg, Hydrochlorothiazide 50 mg Co-amilozide 5mg/50mg tablets | 28 tablet [PoM] £1.16 DT price = £1.05
 ▸ Moduret (Merck Sharp & Dohme Ltd)
 Amiloride hydrochloride 2.5 mg, Hydrochlorothiazide 25 mg Moduret 25 tablets | 28 tablet [PoM] £0.86 DT price = £6.05
 ▸ Moduretic (Merck Sharp & Dohme Ltd)
 Amiloride hydrochloride 5 mg, Hydrochlorothiazide 50 mg Moduretic 5mg/50mg tablets | 28 tablet [PoM] £1.29 DT price = £1.05

Hydrochlorothiazide

F 151

- **INDICATIONS AND DOSE**

Indications listed in combination monographs (available in the UK only in combination with other drugs)
- ▶ BY MOUTH
- ▶ Adult: Doses listed in combination monographs

- **MEDICINAL FORMS**
There can be variation in the licensing of different medicines containing the same drug. Forms available from special-order manufacturers include: tablet, oral suspension, oral solution

Combinations available: Co-zidocapt, p. 154 ·
Enalapril with hydrochlorothiazide, p. 155 ·
Irbesartan with hydrochlorothiazide, p. 162 ·
Lisinopril with hydrochlorothiazide, p. 156 ·
Losartan with hydrochlorothiazide, p. 163 ·
Olmesartan with amlodipine and hydrochlorothiazide, p. 163 ·
Olmesartan with hydrochlorothiazide, p. 164 ·
Quinapril with hydrochlorothiazide, p. 158 ·
Telmisartan with hydrochlorothiazide, p. 164 ·
Timolol with amiloride and hydrochlorothiazide, p. 138 ·
Valsartan with hydrochlorothiazide, p. 165

Indapamide

F 151

- **INDICATIONS AND DOSE**

Essential hypertension
- ▶ BY MOUTH USING IMMEDIATE-RELEASE MEDICINES
- ▶ Adult: 2.5 mg daily, dose to be taken in the morning
- ▶ BY MOUTH USING MODIFIED-RELEASE MEDICINES
- ▶ Adult: 1.5 mg daily, dose to be taken preferably in the morning

- **CAUTIONS** Acute porphyrias p. 918
- **SIDE-EFFECTS** Diuresis (with doses above 2.5 mg daily) · palpitation
- **ALLERGY AND CROSS-SENSITIVITY** Contra-indicated if history of hypersensitivity to sulfonamides.
- **BREAST FEEDING** Present in milk—manufacturer advises avoid.

- **MEDICINAL FORMS**
There can be variation in the licensing of different medicines containing the same drug. Forms available from special-order manufacturers include: oral suspension

Tablet
- ▶ Indapamide (Non-proprietary)
  Indapamide hemihydrate 2.5 mg Indapamide 2.5mg tablets | 28 tablet PoM £40.99 DT price = £1.30 | 30 tablet PoM £27.99 | 56 tablet PoM £52.00
- ▶ Natrilix (Servier Laboratories Ltd)
  Indapamide hemihydrate 2.5 mg Natrilix 2.5mg tablets | 30 tablet PoM £3.40 | 60 tablet PoM £6.80

Modified-release tablet
CAUTIONARY AND ADVISORY LABELS 25
- ▶ Indapamide (Non-proprietary)
  Indapamide 1.5 mg Indapamide 1.5mg modified-release tablets | 30 tablet PoM £8.00 DT price = £3.40
- ▶ Cardide SR (Teva UK Ltd)
  Indapamide 1.5 mg Cardide SR 1.5mg tablets | 30 tablet PoM £4.32 DT price = £3.40
- ▶ Indipam XL (Actavis UK Ltd)
  Indapamide 1.5 mg Indipam XL 1.5mg tablets | 30 tablet PoM £4.32 DT price = £3.40
- ▶ Natrilix SR (Servier Laboratories Ltd)
  Indapamide 1.5 mg Natrilix SR 1.5mg tablets | 30 tablet PoM £3.40 DT price = £3.40
- ▶ Rawel XL (Consilient Health Ltd)
  Indapamide 1.5 mg Rawel XL 1.5mg tablets | 30 tablet PoM £2.89 DT price = £3.40

- ▶ Tensaid XL (Mylan Ltd)
  Indapamide 1.5 mg Tensaid XL 1.5mg tablets | 30 tablet PoM £3.40 DT price = £3.40

Combinations available: Perindopril arginine with indapamide, p. 157

DRUGS ACTING ON THE RENIN-ANGIOTENSIN SYSTEM > ACE INHIBITORS

Angiotensin-converting enzyme inhibitors

- **CONTRA-INDICATIONS** The combination of an ACE inhibitor with aliskiren is contra-indicated in patients with an eGFR less than 60 mL/minute/1.73 m^2 · the combination of an ACE inhibitor with aliskiren is contra-indicated in patients with diabetes mellitus
- **CAUTIONS** Afro-Caribbean patients (may respond less well to ACE inhibitors) · concomitant diuretics · first dose hypotension (especially in patients taking high doses of diuretics, on a low-sodium diet, on dialysis, dehydrated, or with heart failure) · peripheral vascular disease or generalised atherosclerosis (risk of clinically silent renovascular disease) · primary aldosteronism (patients may respond less well to ACE inhibitors) · the risk of agranulocytosis is possibly increased in collagen vascular disease (blood counts recommended) · use with care (or avoid) in those with a history of idiopathic or hereditary angioedema · use with care in patients with hypertrophic cardiomyopathy · use with care in patients with severe or symptomatic aortic stenosis (risk of hypotension)
CAUTIONS, FURTHER INFORMATION
- ▶ Anaphylactoid reactions To prevent anaphylactoid reactions, ACE inhibitors should be avoided during dialysis with high-flux polyacrylonitrile membranes and during low-density lipoprotein apheresis with dextran sulfate; they should also be withheld before desensitisation with wasp or bee venom.
- **INTERACTIONS** → Appendix 1 (ACE inhibitors).
- **SIDE-EFFECTS** Pruritus · abdominal pain · altered liver function tests · angioedema (onset may be delayed; higher incidence reported in Afro-Caribbean patients) · arthralgia · blood disorders · bronchospasm · cholestatic jaundice · constipation · diarrhoea · dizziness · dyspepsia · eosinophilia · fatigue · fever · fulminant hepatic necrosis · haemolytic anaemia · headache · hepatic failure · hepatitis · hyperkalaemia · hypoglycaemia · leucocytosis · leucopenia · malaise · myalgia · nausea · neutropenia · pancreatitis · paraesthesia · persistent dry cough · photosensitivity · positive antinuclear antibody · profound hypotension · raised erythrocyte sedimentation rate · rash · renal impairment · rhinitis · serositis · sinusitis · sore throat · taste disturbance · thrombocytopenia · urticaria · vasculitis · vomiting
SIDE-EFFECTS, FURTHER INFORMATION
- ▶ Hepatic effects In light of reports of cholestatic jaundice, hepatitis, fulminant hepatic necrosis, and hepatic failure, ACE inhibitors should be discontinued if marked elevation of hepatic enzymes or jaundice occur.
- **ALLERGY AND CROSS-SENSITIVITY** ACE inhibitors are contra-indicated in patients with hypersensitivity to ACE inhibitors (including angioedema).
- **PREGNANCY** ACE inhibitors should be avoided in pregnancy unless essential. They may adversely affect fetal and neonatal blood pressure control and renal function; skull defects and oligohydramnios have also been reported.
- **BREAST FEEDING** Information on the use of ACE inhibitors in breast-feeding is limited.

2

Cardiovascular system

- RENAL IMPAIRMENT Use with caution, starting with low dose, and adjust according to response. Hyperkalaemia and other side-effects of ACE inhibitors are more common in those with impaired renal function and the dose may need to be reduced.
- MONITORING REQUIREMENTS Renal function and electrolytes should be checked before starting ACE inhibitors (or increasing the dose) and monitored during treatment (more frequently if side effects mentioned are present).
- DIRECTIONS FOR ADMINISTRATION For hypertension the first dose should preferably be given at bedtime.

⌐ 153

Captopril

- INDICATIONS AND DOSE

Hypertension
▸ BY MOUTH
  ▸ Adult: Initially 12.5–25 mg twice daily, then increased if necessary up to 150 mg daily in 2 divided doses, doses to be increased at intervals of at least 2 weeks, once-daily dosing may be appropriate if other concomitant antihypertensive drugs taken
  ▸ Elderly: Initially 6.25 mg twice daily, then increased if necessary up to 150 mg daily in 2 divided doses, doses to be increased at intervals of at least 2 weeks, once-daily dosing may be appropriate if other concomitant antihypertensive drugs taken

Essential hypertension if used in volume depletion, cardiac decompensation, or renovascular hypertension
▸ BY MOUTH
  ▸ Adult: Initially 6.25–12.5 mg for 1 dose (under close medical supervision), then 6.25–12.5 mg twice daily; increased if necessary up to 100 mg daily in 1–2 divided doses, doses to be increased at intervals of at least 2 weeks, once-daily dosing may be appropriate if other concomitant antihypertensive drugs taken

Heart failure
▸ BY MOUTH
  ▸ Adult (under close medical supervision): Initially 6.25–12.5 mg 2–3 times a day, then increased if tolerated to up to 150 mg daily in divided doses, dose to be increased gradually at intervals of at least 2 weeks

Short-term treatment within 24 hours of onset of myocardial infarction in clinically stable patients
▸ BY MOUTH
  ▸ Adult: Initially 6.25 mg, then increased to 12.5 mg after 2 hours, followed by 25 mg after 12 hours; increased if tolerated to 50 mg twice daily for 4 weeks

Prophylaxis of symptomatic heart failure after myocardial infarction in clinically stable patients with asymptomatic left ventricular dysfunction (starting 3–16 days after infarction) (under close medical supervision)
▸ BY MOUTH
  ▸ Adult: Initially 6.25 mg daily, then increased to 12.5 mg 3 times a day for 2 days, then increased if tolerated to 25 mg 3 times a day, then increased if tolerated to 75–150 mg daily in 2–3 divided doses, doses exceeding 75 mg per day to be increased gradually

Diabetic nephropathy in type 1 diabetes mellitus
▸ BY MOUTH
  ▸ Adult: 75–100 mg daily in divided doses

- SIDE-EFFECTS
▸ **Common or very common** Alopecia · dry mouth · dyspnoea · sleep disorder
▸ **Uncommon** Angina · arrhythmia · flushing · pallor · palpitation · Raynaud's syndrome · tachycardia
▸ **Rare** Anorexia · stomatitis

▸ **Very rare** Allergic alveolitis · blurred vision · cardiac arrest · cardiogenic shock · cerebrovascular events · confusion · depression · eosinophilic pneumonia · glossitis · gynaecomastia · hyponatraemia · impotence · peptic ulcer · photosensitivity · Stevens-Johnson syndrome · syncope

- BREAST FEEDING Avoid in first few weeks after delivery, particularly in preterm infants—risk of profound neonatal hypotension; can be used in mothers breast-feeding older infants if essential but monitor infant's blood pressure.
- RENAL IMPAIRMENT Reduce dose; max. initial dose 50 mg if eGFR above 40 mL/minute/1.73 m^2; max. initial dose 25 mg daily (do not exceed 100 mg daily) if eGFR 20–40 mL/minute/1.73 m^2; max. initial dose 12.5 mg daily (do not exceed 75 mg daily) if eGFR 10–20 mL/minute/1.73 m^2; max. initial dose 6.25 mg daily (do not exceed 37.5 mg daily) if eGFR less than 10 mL/minute/1.73 m^2.

- MEDICINAL FORMS
There can be variation in the licensing of different medicines containing the same drug. Forms available from special-order manufacturers include: tablet, capsule, oral suspension, oral solution

Tablet
▸ Captopril (Non-proprietary)
  Captopril 12.5 mg Captopril 12.5mg tablets | 56 tablet [PoM] £2.80 DT price = £2.44 | 100 tablet [PoM] £5.00
  Captopril 25 mg Captopril 25mg tablets | 56 tablet [PoM] £4.52 DT price = £3.32 | 100 tablet [PoM] £8.07
  Captopril 50 mg Captopril 50mg tablets | 56 tablet [PoM] £5.83 DT price = £2.47 | 100 tablet [PoM] £10.41
▸ Capoten (Bristol-Myers Squibb Pharmaceuticals Ltd)
  Captopril 25 mg Capoten 25mg tablets | 28 tablet [PoM] £5.26
▸ Ecopace (AMCo)
  Captopril 12.5 mg Ecopace 12.5mg tablets | 56 tablet [PoM] £0.48 DT price = £2.44
  Captopril 25 mg Ecopace 25mg tablets | 56 tablet [PoM] £0.60 DT price = £3.32
  Captopril 50 mg Ecopace 50mg tablets | 56 tablet [PoM] £0.72 DT price = £2.47

Oral solution
ELECTROLYTES: May contain Sodium
▸ Noyada (Martindale Pharmaceuticals Ltd)
  Captopril 1 mg per 1 ml Noyada 5mg/5ml oral solution sugar-free | 100 ml [PoM] £98.21 DT price = £98.21
  Captopril 5 mg per 1 ml Noyada 25mg/5ml oral solution sugar-free | 100 ml [PoM] £108.94 DT price = £108.94

Co-zidocapt

The properties listed below are those particular to the combination only. For the properties of the components please consider, captopril above, hydrochlorothiazide p. 153.

- INDICATIONS AND DOSE

Mild to moderate hypertension in patients stabilised on the individual components in the same proportions
▸ BY MOUTH
  ▸ Adult: (consult product literature)

- MEDICINAL FORMS
There can be variation in the licensing of different medicines containing the same drug.
Tablet
▸ Co-zidocapt (Non-proprietary)
  Hydrochlorothiazide 12.5 mg, Captopril 25 mg Co-zidocapt 12.5mg/25mg tablets | 28 tablet [PoM] £11.00
  Hydrochlorothiazide 25 mg, Captopril 50 mg Co-zidocapt 25mg/50mg tablets | 28 tablet [PoM] £14.00
▸ Capozide (Bristol-Myers Squibb Pharmaceuticals Ltd)
  Hydrochlorothiazide 25 mg, Captopril 50 mg Capozide 25mg/50mg tablets | 30 tablet [PoM] £7.52

Enalapril maleate ☞ 153

● **INDICATIONS AND DOSE**

Hypertension
▸ BY MOUTH
▸ Adult: Initially 5 mg once daily, lower initial doses may be required when used in addition to diuretic or in renal impairment; maintenance 20 mg once daily; maximum 40 mg per day

Heart failure
▸ BY MOUTH
▸ Adult (under close medical supervision): Initially 2.5 mg once daily, increased if tolerated to 10–20 mg twice daily, dose to be increased gradually over 2–4 weeks

Prevention of symptomatic heart failure in patients with asymptomatic left ventricular dysfunction
▸ BY MOUTH
▸ Adult (under close medical supervision): Initially 2.5 mg once daily, increased if tolerated to 10–20 mg twice daily, dose to be increased gradually over 2–4 weeks

● SIDE-EFFECTS
▸ **Common or very common** Asthenia · blurred vision · depression · dyspnoea
▸ **Uncommon** Alopecia · anorexia · arrhythmias · confusion · drowsiness · dry mouth · flushing · hyponatraemia · ileus · impotence · insomnia · muscle cramps · nervousness · palpitation · peptic ulcer · sweating · tinnitus · vertigo
▸ **Rare** Abnormal dreams · allergic alveolitis · exfoliative dermatitis · glossitis · gynaecomastia · pemphigus · pulmonary infiltrates · Raynaud's syndrome · Stevens-Johnson syndrome · stomatitis · toxic epidermal necrolysis
▸ **Very rare** Gastro-intestinal angioedema

● BREAST FEEDING Avoid in first few weeks after delivery, particularly in preterm infants—risk of profound neonatal hypotension; can be used in mothers breast-feeding older infants if essential but monitor infant's blood pressure.

● HEPATIC IMPAIRMENT Enalapril is a prodrug and requires close monitoring in patients with hepatic impairment.

● RENAL IMPAIRMENT Max. initial dose 2.5 mg daily if eGFR less than 30 mL/minute/1.73 m^2.

● DIRECTIONS FOR ADMINISTRATION Tablets may be crushed and suspended in water immediately before use.

● MEDICINAL FORMS
There can be variation in the licensing of different medicines containing the same drug. Forms available from special-order manufacturers include: oral suspension, oral solution
Tablet
▸ Enalapril maleate (Non-proprietary)
Enalapril maleate 2.5 mg Enalapril 2.5mg tablets | 28 tablet PoM £3.60 DT price = £2.38
Enalapril maleate 5 mg Enalapril 5mg tablets | 28 tablet PoM £4.13 DT price = £0.87
Enalapril maleate 10 mg Enalapril 10mg tablets | 28 tablet PoM £5.64 DT price = £0.89
Enalapril maleate 20 mg Enalapril 20mg tablets | 28 tablet PoM £6.63 DT price = £1.42
▸ Innovace (Merck Sharp & Dohme Ltd)
Enalapril maleate 2.5 mg Innovace 2.5mg tablets | 28 tablet PoM £5.35 DT price = £2.38
Enalapril maleate 5 mg Innovace 5mg tablets | 28 tablet PoM £7.51 DT price = £0.87
Enalapril maleate 10 mg Innovace 10mg tablets | 28 tablet PoM £10.53 DT price = £0.89
Enalapril maleate 20 mg Innovace 20mg tablets | 28 tablet PoM £12.51 DT price = £1.42

Enalapril with hydrochlorothiazide

The properties listed below are those particular to the combination only. For the properties of the components please consider, enalapril maleate above, hydrochlorothiazide p. 153.

● **INDICATIONS AND DOSE**

Mild to moderate hypertension in patients stabilised on the individual components in the same proportions
▸ BY MOUTH
▸ Adult: (consult product literature)

● MEDICINAL FORMS
There can be variation in the licensing of different medicines containing the same drug.
Tablet
▸ Enalapril with hydrochlorothiazide (Non-proprietary)
Hydrochlorothiazide 12.5 mg, Enalapril maleate 20 mg Enalapril 20mg / Hydrochlorothiazide 12.5mg tablets | 28 tablet PoM £20.00 DT price = £19.98
▸ Innozide (Merck Sharp & Dohme Ltd)
Hydrochlorothiazide 12.5 mg, Enalapril maleate 20 mg Innozide 20mg/12.5mg tablets | 28 tablet PoM £13.90 DT price = £19.98

☞ 153

Fosinopril sodium

● **INDICATIONS AND DOSE**

Hypertension
▸ BY MOUTH
▸ Adult: Initially 10 mg daily for 4 weeks, then increased if necessary up to 40 mg daily, doses over 40 mg not shown to increase efficacy

Congestive heart failure (adjunct) (under close medical supervision)
▸ BY MOUTH
▸ Adult: Initially 10 mg once daily, then increased if tolerated to 40 mg once daily, doses to be increased gradually

● SIDE-EFFECTS Chest pain · musculoskeletal pain
● BREAST FEEDING Not recommended; alternative treatment options, with better established safety information during breast-feeding, are available.
● HEPATIC IMPAIRMENT

Monitoring
Fosinopril is a prodrug and requires close monitoring in patients with hepatic impairment.

● MEDICINAL FORMS
There can be variation in the licensing of different medicines containing the same drug. Forms available from special-order manufacturers include: oral suspension, oral solution
Tablet
▸ Fosinopril sodium (Non-proprietary)
Fosinopril sodium 10 mg Fosinopril 10mg tablets | 28 tablet PoM £28.50 DT price = £10.70
Fosinopril sodium 20 mg Fosinopril 20mg tablets | 28 tablet PoM £38.98 DT price = £12.51

☞ 153

Imidapril hydrochloride

● **INDICATIONS AND DOSE**

Essential hypertension
▸ BY MOUTH
▸ Adult: Initially 5 mg daily, increased if necessary to 10 mg daily, dose to be taken before food, doses to be increased at intervals of at least 3 weeks; maximum 20 mg per day

continued →

2

Cardiovascular system

▸ Elderly: Initially 2.5 mg daily, increased if necessary to 10 mg daily, dose to be taken before food, doses to be increased at intervals of at least 3 weeks

Essential hypertension in patients with heart failure, angina or cerebrovascular disease, or in renal or hepatic impairment
▸ BY MOUTH
▸ Adult: Initially 2.5 mg daily, increased if necessary to 10 mg daily, dose to be taken before food, dose to be increased at intervals of at least 3 weeks; maximum 20 mg per day

● SIDE-EFFECTS Blurred vision · bronchitis · confusion · depression · dry mouth · dyspnoea · glossitis · ileus · impotence · sleep disturbances · tinnitus

● BREAST FEEDING Not recommended; alternative treatment options, with better established safety information during breast-feeding, are available.

● HEPATIC IMPAIRMENT
Monitoring
Imidapril is a prodrug and requires close monitoring in patients with hepatic impairment.

● RENAL IMPAIRMENT Initial dose 2.5 mg daily if eGFR 30–80 mL/minute/1.73 m^2. Avoid if eGFR less than 30 mL/minute/1.73 m^2.

● MEDICINAL FORMS
There can be variation in the licensing of different medicines containing the same drug.
Tablet
▸ Tanatril (Mitsubishi Tanabe Pharma Europe Ltd)
  Imidapril hydrochloride 5 mg Tanatril 5mg tablets | 28 tablet [PoM] £6.40 DT price = £6.40
  Imidapril hydrochloride 10 mg Tanatril 10mg tablets | 28 tablet [PoM] £7.22 DT price = £7.22
  Imidapril hydrochloride 20 mg Tanatril 20mg tablets | 28 tablet [PoM] £8.67 DT price = £8.67

F 153

Lisinopril

● INDICATIONS AND DOSE
Hypertension
▸ BY MOUTH
▸ Adult: Initially 10 mg once daily; usual maintenance 20 mg once daily; maximum 80 mg per day

Hypertension, when used in addition to diuretic, in cardiac decompensation or in volume depletion
▸ BY MOUTH
▸ Adult: Initially 2.5–5 mg once daily; usual maintenance 20 mg once daily; maximum 80 mg per day

Short-term treatment following myocardial infarction in haemodynamically stable patients—systolic blood pressure over 120 mmHg
▸ BY MOUTH
▸ Adult: Initially 5 mg, taken within 24 hours of myocardial infarction, followed by 5 mg, to be taken 24 hours after initial dose, then 10 mg, to be taken 24 hours after second dose, then 10 mg once daily for 6 weeks (or continued if heart failure), temporarily reduce maintenance dose to 5 mg and if necessary 2.5 mg daily if systolic blood pressure 100 mmHg or less during treatment; withdraw if prolonged hypotension occurs during treatment (systolic blood pressure less than 90 mmHg for more than 1 hour)

Short-term treatment following myocardial infarction in haemodynamically stable patients—systolic blood pressure 100–120 mmHg
▸ BY MOUTH
▸ Adult: Initially 2.5 mg once daily, maintenance 5 mg once daily, increase to maintenance dose only after at

least 3 days of the initial dose, should not be started after myocardial infarction if systolic blood pressure less than 100 mmHg, temporarily reduce maintenance dose to 2.5 mg daily if systolic blood pressure 100 mmHg or less during treatment; withdraw if prolonged hypotension occurs (systolic blood pressure less than 90 mmHg for more than 1 hour)

Renal complications of diabetes mellitus
▸ BY MOUTH
▸ Adult: Initially 2.5–5 mg once daily, adjusted according to response; usual dose 10–20 mg once daily

Heart failure (adjunct) (under close medical supervision)
▸ BY MOUTH
▸ Adult: Initially 2.5 mg once daily; increased in steps of up to 10 mg at least every 2 weeks; maximum 35 mg per day

● SIDE-EFFECTS
▸ **Uncommon** Raynaud's syndrome · vertigo · asthenia · cerebrovascular accident · confusion · impotence · mood changes · myocardial infarction · palpitation · sleep disturbances · tachycardia
▸ **Rare** Alopecia · dry mouth · gynaecomastia · psoriasis
▸ **Very rare** Allergic alveolitis · pemphigus · profuse sweating · pulmonary infiltrates · Stevens-Johnson syndrome · toxic epidermal necrolysis

● BREAST FEEDING Not recommended; alternative treatment options, with better established safety information during breast-feeding, are available.

● RENAL IMPAIRMENT Max. initial doses 5–10 mg daily if eGFR 30–80 mL/minute/1.73 m^2 (max. 40 mg daily); 2.5–5 mg daily if eGFR 10–30 mL/minute/1.73 m^2 (max. 40 mg daily); 2.5 mg daily if eGFR less than 10 mL/minute/1.73 m^2.

● MEDICINAL FORMS
There can be variation in the licensing of different medicines containing the same drug. Forms available from special-order manufacturers include: oral suspension, oral solution
Tablet
▸ Lisinopril (Non-proprietary)
  Lisinopril 2.5 mg Lisinopril 2.5mg tablets | 28 tablet [PoM] £1.51 DT price = £0.72
  Lisinopril 5 mg Lisinopril 5mg tablets | 28 tablet [PoM] £7.80 DT price = £0.74
  Lisinopril 10 mg Lisinopril 10mg tablets | 28 tablet [PoM] £9.60 DT price = £0.76
  Lisinopril 20 mg Lisinopril 20mg tablets | 28 tablet [PoM] £10.90 DT price = £0.85
▸ Zestril (AstraZeneca UK Ltd)
  Lisinopril 5 mg Zestril 5mg tablets | 28 tablet [PoM] £4.71 DT price = £0.74
  Lisinopril 10 mg Zestril 10mg tablets | 28 tablet [PoM] £7.38 DT price = £0.76
  Lisinopril 20 mg Zestril 20mg tablets | 28 tablet [PoM] £6.51 DT price = £0.85
Oral solution
▸ Lisinopril (Non-proprietary)
  Lisinopril 1 mg per 1 ml Lisinopril 5mg/5ml oral solution sugar free sugar-free | 150 ml [PoM] £154.11 DT price = £154.11

Lisinopril with hydrochlorothiazide

The properties listed below are those particular to the combination only. For the properties of the components please consider, lisinopril above, hydrochlorothiazide p. 153.

● INDICATIONS AND DOSE
Mild to moderate hypertension in patients stabilised on the individual components in the same proportions
▸ BY MOUTH
▸ Adult: (consult product literature)

● MEDICINAL FORMS
There can be variation in the licensing of different medicines containing the same drug.

Tablet

▸ Lisinopril with hydrochlorothiazide (Non-proprietary)
  Lisinopril 10 mg, Hydrochlorothiazide 12.5 mg Lisinopril 10mg / Hydrochlorothiazide 12.5mg tablets | 28 tablet [PoM] £12.99 DT price = £4.99
  Hydrochlorothiazide 12.5 mg, Lisinopril 20 mg Lisinopril 20mg / Hydrochlorothiazide 12.5mg tablets | 28 tablet [PoM] £14.65 DT price = £6.94

▸ Carace Plus (Merck Sharp & Dohme Ltd)
  Hydrochlorothiazide 12.5 mg, Lisinopril 20 mg Carace 20 Plus tablets | 28 tablet [PoM] £11.43 DT price = £6.94

▸ Zestoretic 10 (AstraZeneca UK Ltd)
  Lisinopril 10 mg, Hydrochlorothiazide 12.5 mg Zestoretic 10 tablets | 28 tablet [PoM] £6.81 DT price = £4.99

▸ Zestoretic 20 (AstraZeneca UK Ltd)
  Hydrochlorothiazide 12.5 mg, Lisinopril 20 mg Zestoretic 20 tablets | 28 tablet [PoM] £11.52 DT price = £6.94

⌐ 153

Moexipril hydrochloride

● INDICATIONS AND DOSE

Essential hypertension (monotherapy)
▸ BY MOUTH
▸ Adult: Initially 7.5 mg once daily, adjusted according to response; maintenance 7.5–15 mg once daily; maximum 30 mg per day
▸ Elderly: Initially 3.75 mg once daily, adjusted according to response; maintenance 7.5–15 mg once daily; maximum 30 mg per day

Essential hypertension when used in addition with nifedipine or other antihypertensive drug
▸ BY MOUTH
▸ Adult: Initially 3.75 mg once daily, adjusted according to response; maintenance 7.5–15 mg once daily; maximum 30 mg per day

● CAUTIONS Significant mitral valve stenosis

● SIDE-EFFECTS
▸ Very rare Numbness
▸ Frequency not known Alopecia · angina · appetite · arrhythmias · blurred vision · cerebrovascular accident · confusion · depression · drowsiness · dry mouth · dyspnoea · flushing · hyperuricaemia · impotence · myocardial infarction · palpitation · pemphigus · sleep disturbance · Stevens-Johnson syndrome · sweating · syncope · tachycardia · tinnitus · toxic epidermal necrolysis · weight changes

● BREAST FEEDING Not recommended; alternative treatment options, with better established safety information during breast-feeding, are available.

● HEPATIC IMPAIRMENT Initial dose 3.75 mg once daily. Moexipril is a prodrug and requires close monitoring in patients with hepatic impairment.

● RENAL IMPAIRMENT If eGFR less than 40 mL/minute/1.73 m^2, initial dose 3.75 mg once daily titrated to max. 15 mg once daily.

● MEDICINAL FORMS
There can be variation in the licensing of different medicines containing the same drug.
No licensed medicines listed.

⌐ 153

Perindopril arginine

● INDICATIONS AND DOSE

Hypertension
▸ BY MOUTH
▸ Adult: Initially 5 mg once daily for 1 month, dose to be taken in the morning, then, adjusted according to response; maximum 10 mg per day
▸ Elderly: Initially 2.5 mg once daily for 1 month, dose to be taken in the morning, then, adjusted according to response; maximum 10 mg per day

Hypertension, if used in addition to diuretic, or in cardiac decompensation or volume depletion
▸ BY MOUTH
▸ Adult: Initially 2.5 mg once daily for 1 month, dose to be taken in the morning, then, adjusted according to response; maximum 10 mg per day

Symptomatic heart failure (adjunct) (under close medical supervision)
▸ BY MOUTH
▸ Adult: Initially 2.5 mg once daily for 2 weeks, then increased if tolerated to 5 mg once daily, dose to be taken in the morning

Prophylaxis of cardiac events following myocardial infarction or revascularisation in stable coronary artery disease
▸ BY MOUTH
▸ Adult: Initially 5 mg once daily for 2 weeks, then increased if tolerated to 10 mg once daily, dose to be taken in the morning
▸ Elderly: Initially 2.5 mg once daily for 1 week, then increased if tolerated to 5 mg once daily for 1 week, then increased if tolerated to 10 mg once daily to be taken in the morning

● SIDE-EFFECTS Asthenia · mood disturbances · sleep disturbances

● HEPATIC IMPAIRMENT

Monitoring
Perindopril is a prodrug and requires close monitoring in patients with hepatic impairment.

● RENAL IMPAIRMENT Max. initial dose 2.5 mg once daily if eGFR 30–60 mL/minute/1.73 m^2; 2.5 mg once daily on alternate days if eGFR 15–30 mL/minute/1.73 m^2.

● MEDICINAL FORMS
There can be variation in the licensing of different medicines containing the same drug.

Tablet
CAUTIONARY AND ADVISORY LABELS 22
▸ Coversyl Arginine (Servier Laboratories Ltd)
  Perindopril arginine 2.5 mg Coversyl Arginine 2.5mg tablets | 30 tablet [PoM] £4.43 DT price = £4.43
  Perindopril arginine 5 mg Coversyl Arginine 5mg tablets | 30 tablet [PoM] £6.28 DT price = £6.28
  Perindopril arginine 10 mg Coversyl Arginine 10mg tablets | 30 tablet [PoM] £10.65 DT price = £10.65

Perindopril arginine with indapamide

The properties listed below are those particular to the combination only. For the properties of the components please consider, perindopril arginine above, indapamide p. 153.

● INDICATIONS AND DOSE

Hypertension not adequately controlled by perindopril alone
▸ BY MOUTH
▸ Adult: (consult product literature)

- MEDICINAL FORMS
There can be variation in the licensing of different medicines containing the same drug.

Tablet
CAUTIONARY AND ADVISORY LABELS 22
- Coversyl Arginine Plus (Servier Laboratories Ltd)
  Indapamide 1.25 mg, Perindopril arginine 5 mg Coversyl Arginine Plus 5mg/1.25mg tablets | 30 tablet [PoM] £9.51 DT price = £9.51

F 153

Perindopril erbumine

- INDICATIONS AND DOSE

Hypertension
- BY MOUTH
- Adult: Initially 4 mg once daily for 1 month, dose to be taken in the morning, then, adjusted according to response; maximum 8 mg per day
- BY MOUTH
- Elderly: Initially 2 mg once daily for 1 month, dose to be taken in the morning, then, adjusted according to response; maximum 8 mg per day

Hypertension, if used in addition to diuretic, or in cardiac decompensation or volume depletion
- BY MOUTH
- Adult: Initially 2 mg once daily for 1 month, dose to be taken in the morning, then, adjusted according to response; maximum 8 mg per day

Heart failure (adjunct) (under close medical supervision)
- BY MOUTH
- Adult: Initially 2 mg once daily for at least 2 weeks, dose to be taken in the morning, then increased if tolerated to 4 mg once daily

Prophylaxis of cardiac events following myocardial infarction or revascularisation in stable coronary artery disease
- BY MOUTH
- Adult: Initially 4 mg once daily for 2 weeks, dose to be taken in the morning, then increased if tolerated to 8 mg once daily
- Elderly: Initially 2 mg once daily for 1 week, then increased if tolerated to 4 mg once daily for 1 week, then increased if tolerated to 8 mg once daily

- SIDE-EFFECTS Asthenia · mood disturbances · sleep disturbances
- BREAST FEEDING Not recommended; alternative treatment options, with better established safety information during breast-feeding, are available.
- HEPATIC IMPAIRMENT
Monitoring
Perindopril is a prodrug and requires close monitoring in patients with hepatic impairment.
- RENAL IMPAIRMENT Max. initial dose 2 mg once daily if eGFR 30–60 mL/minute/1.73 m^2; 2 mg once daily on alternate days if eGFR 15–30 mL/minute/1.73 m^2.

- MEDICINAL FORMS
There can be variation in the licensing of different medicines containing the same drug. Forms available from special-order manufacturers include: oral suspension, oral solution

Tablet
CAUTIONARY AND ADVISORY LABELS 22
- Perindopril erbumine (Non-proprietary)
  Perindopril erbumine 2 mg Perindopril erbumine 2mg tablets | 30 tablet [PoM] £4.41 DT price = £1.00 | 56 tablet [PoM] £3.34 | 60 tablet [PoM] £13.90
  Perindopril erbumine 4 mg Perindopril erbumine 4mg tablets | 30 tablet [PoM] £4.50 DT price = £1.16 | 56 tablet [PoM] £3.38 | 60 tablet [PoM] £27.80
  Perindopril erbumine 8 mg Perindopril erbumine 8mg tablets | 30 tablet [PoM] £5.95 DT price = £1.14 | 56 tablet [PoM] £3.88 | 60 tablet [PoM] £40.00

F 153

Quinapril

- INDICATIONS AND DOSE

Essential hypertension
- BY MOUTH
- Adult: Initially 10 mg once daily; maintenance 20–40 mg daily in up to 2 divided doses; maximum 80 mg per day
- Elderly: Initially 2.5 mg once daily; maintenance 20–40 mg daily in up to 2 divided doses; maximum 80 mg per day

Essential hypertension if used in addition to diuretic
- BY MOUTH
- Adult: Initially 2.5 mg once daily; maintenance 20–40 mg daily in up to 2 divided doses; maximum 80 mg per day

Heart failure (adjunct) (under close medical supervision)
- BY MOUTH
- Adult: Initially 2.5 mg daily, increased if tolerated to 10–20 mg daily in 1–2 divided doses, doses to be increased gradually; maximum 40 mg per day

- SIDE-EFFECTS Impotence · asthenia · back pain · blurred vision · chest pain · depression · flatulence · insomnia · nervousness · oedema
- BREAST FEEDING Avoid in the first few weeks after delivery, particularly in preterm infants, due to the risk of profound neonatal hypotension; if essential, may be used in mothers breast-feeding older infants—the infant's blood pressure should be monitored.
- HEPATIC IMPAIRMENT
Monitoring
Quinapril is a prodrug and requires close monitoring in patients with hepatic impairment.
- RENAL IMPAIRMENT Max. initial dose 2.5 mg once daily if eGFR less than 40 mL/minute/1.73 m^2.

- MEDICINAL FORMS
There can be variation in the licensing of different medicines containing the same drug.
Tablet
- Quinapril (Non-proprietary)
  Quinapril (as Quinapril hydrochloride) 5 mg Quinapril 5mg tablets | 28 tablet [PoM] £8.59 DT price = £8.57
  Quinapril (as Quinapril hydrochloride) 10 mg Quinapril 10mg tablets | 28 tablet [PoM] £8.59 DT price = £8.57
  Quinapril (as Quinapril hydrochloride) 20 mg Quinapril 20mg tablets | 28 tablet [PoM] £3.05 DT price = £1.47
  Quinapril (as Quinapril hydrochloride) 40 mg Quinapril 40mg tablets | 28 tablet [PoM] £3.51 DT price = £1.95
- Accupro (Pfizer Ltd)
  Quinapril (as Quinapril hydrochloride) 5 mg Accupro 5mg tablets | 28 tablet [PoM] £8.60 DT price = £8.57
  Quinapril (as Quinapril hydrochloride) 10 mg Accupro 10mg tablets | 28 tablet [PoM] £8.60 DT price = £8.57
  Quinapril (as Quinapril hydrochloride) 20 mg Accupro 20mg tablets | 28 tablet [PoM] £10.79 DT price = £1.47
  Quinapril (as Quinapril hydrochloride) 40 mg Accupro 40mg tablets | 28 tablet [PoM] £9.75 DT price = £1.95

Quinapril with hydrochlorothiazide

The properties listed below are those particular to the combination only. For the properties of the components please consider, quinapril above, hydrochlorothiazide p. 153.

- INDICATIONS AND DOSE

Hypertension in patients stabilised on the individual components in the same proportions
- BY MOUTH
- Adult: (consult product literature)

Cardiovascular system

- MEDICINAL FORMS
There can be variation in the licensing of different medicines containing the same drug.

Tablet

▸ Quinapril with hydrochlorothiazide (Non-proprietary)
  **Quinapril (as Quinapril hydrochloride) 10 mg,
  Hydrochlorothiazide 12.5 mg** Quinapril 10mg / Hydrochlorothiazide 12.5mg tablets | 28 tablet PoM £11.75 DT price = £11.75

▸ Accuretic (Pfizer Ltd)
  **Quinapril (as Quinapril hydrochloride) 10 mg,
  Hydrochlorothiazide 12.5 mg** Accuretic 12.5mg/10mg tablets | 28 tablet PoM £11.75 DT price = £11.75

🕮 153

Ramipril

- INDICATIONS AND DOSE

Hypertension
▸ BY MOUTH
▸ Adult: Initially 1.25–2.5 mg once daily, increased if necessary up to 10 mg once daily, dose to be increased at intervals of 2–4 weeks

Symptomatic heart failure (adjunct) (under close medical supervision)
▸ BY MOUTH
▸ Adult: Initially 1.25 mg once daily, increased if tolerated to 10 mg daily, preferably taken in 2 divided doses, increase dose gradually at intervals of 1–2 weeks

Prophylaxis after myocardial infarction in patients with clinical evidence of heart failure (started at least 48 hours after infarction)
▸ BY MOUTH
▸ Adult: Initially 2.5 mg twice daily for 3 days, then increased to 5 mg twice daily

Prophylaxis after myocardial infarction in patients with clinical evidence of heart failure (started at least 48 hours after infarction) when initial dose not tolerated
▸ BY MOUTH
▸ Adult: 1.25 mg twice daily for 2 days, then increased to 2.5 mg twice daily, then increased to 5 mg twice daily, withdraw treatment if dose cannot be increased to 2.5 mg twice daily

Prevention of cardiovascular events in patients with atherosclerotic cardiovascular disease or with diabetes mellitus and at least one additional risk factor for cardiovascular disease
▸ BY MOUTH
▸ Adult: Initially 2.5 mg once daily for 1–2 weeks, then increased to 5 mg once daily for a further 2–3 weeks, then increased to 10 mg once daily

Nephropathy (consult product literature)
▸ BY MOUTH
▸ Adult: Initially 1.25 mg once daily for 2 weeks, then increased to 2.5 mg once daily for a further 2 weeks, then increased if tolerated to 5 mg once daily

- SIDE-EFFECTS
▸ **Common or very common** Bronchitis · dyspnoea · muscle cramps · stomatitis · syncope
▸ **Uncommon** Angina · anxiety · arrhythmias · chest pain · decreased libido · depression · dry mouth · flushing · impotence · loss of appetite · myocardial infarction · nervousness · palpitations · peripheral oedema · sweating · tachycardia · visual disturbances
▸ **Rare** Confusion · conjunctivitis · impaired hearing · onycholysis · tinnitus · tremor
▸ **Frequency not known** Alopecia · cerebrovascular accident · erythema multiforme · gynaecomastia · hyponatraemia · pemphigoid exanthema · precipitation or exacerbation of Raynaud's syndrome · skin reactions · sleep disturbance · Stevens-Johnson syndrome · toxic epidermal necrolysis

- BREAST FEEDING Not recommended; alternative treatment options, with better established safety information during breast-feeding, are available.
- HEPATIC IMPAIRMENT Max. daily dose 2.5 mg. Ramipril is a prodrug and requires close monitoring in patients with hepatic impairment.
- RENAL IMPAIRMENT Max. daily dose 5 mg if eGFR 30–60 mL/minute/1.73 m^2; max. initial dose 1.25 mg once daily (do not exceed 5 mg daily) if eGFR less than 30 mL/minute/1.73 m^2.

- MEDICINAL FORMS
There can be variation in the licensing of different medicines containing the same drug. Forms available from special-order manufacturers include: oral suspension, oral solution

Tablet
▸ Ramipril (Non-proprietary)
  Ramipril 1.25 mg Ramipril 1.25mg tablets | 28 tablet PoM £5.25 DT price = £0.91
  Ramipril 2.5 mg Ramipril 2.5mg tablets | 28 tablet PoM £7.49 DT price = £0.91
  Ramipril 5 mg Ramipril 5mg tablets | 28 tablet PoM £10.40 DT price = £0.94
  Ramipril 10 mg Ramipril 10mg tablets | 28 tablet PoM £14.20 DT price = £1.04
▸ Tritace (Sanofi)
  Ramipril 1.25 mg Tritace 1.25mg tablets | 28 tablet PoM £5.09 DT price = £0.91
  Ramipril 2.5 mg Tritace 2.5mg tablets | 7 tablet PoM no price available | 28 tablet PoM £7.22 DT price = £0.91
  Ramipril 5 mg Tritace 5mg tablets | 21 tablet PoM no price available | 28 tablet PoM £10.05 DT price = £0.94
  Ramipril 10 mg Tritace 10mg tablets | 7 tablet PoM no price available | 28 tablet PoM £13.68 DT price = £1.04

Capsule
▸ Ramipril (Non-proprietary)
  Ramipril 1.25 mg Ramipril 1.25mg capsules | 28 capsule PoM £1.80 DT price = £0.87
  Ramipril 2.5 mg Ramipril 2.5mg capsules | 28 capsule PoM £1.90 DT price = £0.89
  Ramipril 5 mg Ramipril 5mg capsules | 28 capsule PoM £2.05 DT price = £0.97
  Ramipril 10 mg Ramipril 10mg capsules | 28 capsule PoM £2.20 DT price = £1.03

Oral solution
▸ Ramipril (Non-proprietary)
  Ramipril 500 microgram per 1 ml Ramipril 2.5mg/5ml oral solution sugar free sugar-free | 150 ml PoM £96.00 DT price = £96.00

Ramipril with felodipine

The properties listed below are those particular to the combination only. For the properties of the components please consider, ramipril above, felodipine p. 145.

- INDICATIONS AND DOSE

Hypertension in patients stabilised on the individual components in the same proportions
▸ BY MOUTH
▸ Adult: (consult product literature)

- MEDICINAL FORMS
There can be variation in the licensing of different medicines containing the same drug.

Modified-release tablet
CAUTIONARY AND ADVISORY LABELS 25
▸ Triapin (Sanofi)
  Felodipine 2.5 mg, Ramipril 2.5 mg Triapin 2.5mg/2.5mg modified-release tablets | 28 tablet PoM £24.55
  Felodipine 5 mg, Ramipril 5 mg Triapin 5mg/5mg modified-release tablets | 28 tablet PoM £16.13 DT price = £16.13

☞ 153

Trandolapril

● INDICATIONS AND DOSE

Mild to moderate hypertension
▶ BY MOUTH
▸ Adult: Initially 500 micrograms once daily; increased to 1–2 mg once daily, dose to be increased at intervals of 2–4 weeks; maximum 4 mg per day

Prophylaxis after myocardial infarction in patients with left ventricular dysfunction (starting as early as 3 days after infarction)
▶ BY MOUTH
▸ Adult: Initially 500 micrograms once daily, then increased to up to 4 mg once daily, doses to be increased gradually

● SIDE-EFFECTS Alopecia · angina · arrhythmias · asthenia · bronchitis · cerebral haemorrhage · dry mouth · dyspnoea · hot flushes · ileus · myocardial infarction · nervousness · palpitation · psoriasis-like efflorescence · skin reactions · sleep disturbances · Stevens-Johnson syndrome · sweating · syncope · tachycardia · toxic epidermal necrolysis · transient ischaemic attacks

SIDE-EFFECTS, FURTHER INFORMATION
▸ Symptomatic hypotension If symptomatic hypotension develops during titration, do not increase dose further; if possible, reduce dose of any adjunctive treatment and if this is not effective or feasible, reduce dose of trandolapril.

● BREAST FEEDING Not recommended; alternative treatment options, with better established safety information during breast-feeding, are available.

● HEPATIC IMPAIRMENT
Monitoring
Trandolapril is a prodrug and requires close monitoring in patients with hepatic impairment.

● RENAL IMPAIRMENT Max. 2 mg daily if eGFR less than $10 \, mL/minute/1.73 \, m^2$.

● MEDICINAL FORMS
There can be variation in the licensing of different medicines containing the same drug. Forms available from special-order manufacturers include: oral suspension
Capsule
▸ Trandolapril (Non-proprietary)
Trandolapril 500 microgram Trandolapril 500microgram capsules | 14 capsule [PoM] £1.66 DT price = £1.66
Trandolapril 1 mg Trandolapril 1mg capsules | 28 capsule [PoM] £19.99 DT price = £19.99
Trandolapril 2 mg Trandolapril 2mg capsules | 28 capsule [PoM] £5.49 DT price = £4.95
Trandolapril 4 mg Trandolapril 4mg capsules | 28 capsule [PoM] £13.25 DT price = £13.24

DRUGS ACTING ON THE RENIN-ANGIOTENSIN SYSTEM › ANGIOTENSIN II RECEPTOR ANTAGONISTS

Angiotensin II receptor antagonists

● CONTRA-INDICATIONS The combination of an angiotensin-II receptor antagonist with aliskiren is contra-indicated in patients with an eGFR less than 60 mL/minute/1.73 m² · the combination of an angiotensin-II receptor antagonist with aliskiren is contra-indictated in patients with diabetes mellitus

● CAUTIONS Afro-Caribbean patients—particularly those with left ventricular hypertrophy (may not benefit from an angiotensin-II receptor antagonist) · aortic or mitral valve stenosis · elderly (lower initial doses may be appropriate) ·

hypertrophic cardiomyopathy · patients with a history of angioedema · patients with primary aldosteronism (may not benefit from an angiotensin-II receptor antagonist) · renal artery stenosis

● INTERACTIONS → Appendix 1 (angiotensin-II receptor antagonists).

● SIDE-EFFECTS Hyperkalaemia · angioedema (may be delayed onset) · symptomatic hypotension including dizziness (particularly in patients with intravascular volume depletion, e.g. those taking high-dose diuretics)

● PREGNANCY Angiotensin-II receptor antagonists should be avoided in pregnancy unless essential. They may adversely affect fetal and neonatal blood pressure control and renal function; neonatal skull defects and oligohydramnios have also been reported.

● BREAST FEEDING Information on the use of angiotensin-II receptor antagonists in breast-feeding is limited. They are not recommended in breast-feeding and alternative treatment options, with better established safety information during breast-feeding, are available.

● RENAL IMPAIRMENT Use with caution, starting with low dose, and adjust according to response.

● MONITORING REQUIREMENTS Monitor plasma-potassium concentration, particularly in the elderly and in patients with renal impairment.

☞ above

Azilsartan medoxomil

● INDICATIONS AND DOSE

Hypertension
▶ BY MOUTH
▸ Adult 18–74 years: Initially 40 mg once daily, increased if necessary to 80 mg once daily
▸ Adult 75 years and over: Initially 20–40 mg once daily, increased if necessary to 80 mg once daily

Hypertension with intravascular volume depletion
▶ BY MOUTH
▸ Adult: Initially 20–40 mg daily, increased if necessary to 80 mg daily

● CAUTIONS Heart failure

● SIDE-EFFECTS
▶ **Common or very common** Diarrhoea · raised creatine kinase
▶ **Uncommon** Hyperuricaemia · peripheral oedema · raised creatinine · malaise

● HEPATIC IMPAIRMENT Manufacturer advises to consider initial dose of 20 mg in mild to moderate impairment (limited information available). Manufacturer advises avoid in severe impairment (no information available). Manufacturer advises monitor closely in mild to moderate hepatic impairment (limited information available).

● RENAL IMPAIRMENT Manufacturer advises caution in severe impairment—no information available.

● MEDICINAL FORMS
There can be variation in the licensing of different medicines containing the same drug.
Tablet
▸ Edarbi (Takeda UK Ltd) ▼
Azilsartan medoxomil 20 mg Edarbi 20mg tablets | 28 tablet [PoM] £16.80 DT price = £16.80
Azilsartan medoxomil 40 mg Edarbi 40mg tablets | 28 tablet [PoM] £16.80 DT price = £16.80
Azilsartan medoxomil 80 mg Edarbi 80mg tablets | 28 tablet [PoM] £19.95 DT price = £19.95

2

Cardiovascular system

Candesartan cilexetil
F 160

● **INDICATIONS AND DOSE**

Hypertension
▶ BY MOUTH
▸ Adult: Initially 8 mg once daily, increased if necessary up to 32 mg once daily, doses to be increased at intervals of 4 weeks; usual dose 8 mg once daily

Hypertension with intravascular volume depletion
▶ BY MOUTH
▸ Adult: Initially 4 mg once daily, increased if necessary up to 32 mg daily, doses to be increased at intervals of 4 weeks; usual dose 8 mg once daily

Heart failure with impaired left ventricular systolic function when ACE inhibitors are not tolerated | Heart failure with impaired left ventricular systolic function in conjunction with an ACE inhibitor (under expert supervision)
▶ BY MOUTH
▸ Adult: Initially 4 mg once daily, increased at intervals of at least 2 weeks to 'target' dose of 32 mg once daily or to maximum tolerated dose

● **CONTRA-INDICATIONS** Cholestasis
● **SIDE-EFFECTS**
▶ **Common or very common** Headache · vertigo
▶ **Very rare** Arthralgia · back pain · blood disorders · cough · hepatitis · hyponatraemia · myalgia · nausea · pruritus · rash · urticaria

● **HEPATIC IMPAIRMENT** Initially 4 mg once daily in mild or moderate impairment. Avoid in severe hepatic impairment.

● **RENAL IMPAIRMENT** Initially 4 mg daily. Use with caution if eGFR less than 15 mL/minute/1.73 m^2—limited experience.

● **MEDICINAL FORMS**
There can be variation in the licensing of different medicines containing the same drug. Forms available from special-order manufacturers include: oral suspension, oral solution
Tablet
▸ Candesartan cilexetil (Non-proprietary)
 Candesartan cilexetil 2 mg Candesartan 2mg tablets | 7 tablet [PoM] £3.40 DT price = £1.02
 Candesartan cilexetil 4 mg Candesartan 4mg tablets | 7 tablet [PoM] £3.88 DT price = £0.68 | 28 tablet [PoM] £9.78
 Candesartan cilexetil 8 mg Candesartan 8mg tablets | 28 tablet [PoM] £9.89 DT price = £1.05
 Candesartan cilexetil 16 mg Candesartan 16mg tablets | 28 tablet [PoM] £12.72 DT price = £1.26
 Candesartan cilexetil 32 mg Candesartan 32mg tablets | 28 tablet [PoM] £16.13 DT price = £1.79
▸ Amias (Takeda UK Ltd)
 Candesartan cilexetil 2 mg Amias 2mg tablets | 7 tablet [PoM] £3.58 DT price = £1.02
 Candesartan cilexetil 4 mg Amias 4mg tablets | 7 tablet [PoM] £3.88 DT price = £0.68 | 28 tablet [PoM] £9.78
 Candesartan cilexetil 8 mg Amias 8mg tablets | 28 tablet [PoM] £9.89 DT price = £1.05
 Candesartan cilexetil 16 mg Amias 16mg tablets | 28 tablet [PoM] £12.72 DT price = £1.26
 Candesartan cilexetil 32 mg Amias 32mg tablets | 28 tablet [PoM] £16.13 DT price = £1.79

Eprosartan
F 160

● **INDICATIONS AND DOSE**

Hypertension
▶ BY MOUTH
▸ Adult: 600 mg once daily

● **SIDE-EFFECTS**
▶ **Common or very common** Headache · nausea · rhinitis · diarrhoea · malaise · vomiting

● **HEPATIC IMPAIRMENT** Caution in mild or moderate liver disease. Avoid in severe impairment.

● **RENAL IMPAIRMENT** Caution if eGFR less than 30 mL/minute/1.73 m^2.

● **MEDICINAL FORMS**
There can be variation in the licensing of different medicines containing the same drug. Forms available from special-order manufacturers include: oral suspension, oral solution
Tablet
CAUTIONARY AND ADVISORY LABELS 21
▸ Eprosartan (Non-proprietary)
 Eprosartan (as Eprosartan mesilate) 300 mg Eprosartan 300mg tablets | 28 tablet [PoM] £7.31 DT price = £7.06
 Eprosartan (as Eprosartan mesilate) 400 mg Eprosartan 400mg tablets | 56 tablet [PoM] £25.85 DT price = £20.78
 Eprosartan (as Eprosartan mesilate) 600 mg Eprosartan 600mg tablets | 28 tablet [PoM] £14.31 DT price = £13.82
▸ Teveten (BGP Products Ltd)
 Eprosartan (as Eprosartan mesilate) 300 mg Teveten 300mg tablets | 28 tablet [PoM] £7.31 DT price = £7.06
 Eprosartan (as Eprosartan mesilate) 600 mg Teveten 600mg tablets | 28 tablet [PoM] £14.31 DT price = £13.82

Irbesartan
F 160

● **INDICATIONS AND DOSE**

Hypertension
▶ BY MOUTH
▸ Adult 18–74 years: Initially 150 mg once daily, increased if necessary to 300 mg once daily
▸ Adult 75 years and over: Initially 75–150 mg once daily, increased if necessary to 300 mg once daily

Hypertension in patients receiving haemodialysis
▶ BY MOUTH
▸ Adult: Initially 75–150 mg once daily, increased if necessary to 300 mg once daily

Renal disease in hypertensive type 2 diabetes mellitus
▶ BY MOUTH
▸ Adult 18–74 years: Initially 150 mg once daily, increased if tolerated to 300 mg once daily
▸ Adult 75 years and over: Initially 75–150 mg once daily, increased if tolerated to 300 mg once daily

Renal disease in hypertensive type 2 diabetes mellitus in patients receiving haemodialysis
▶ BY MOUTH
▸ Adult: Initially 75–150 mg once daily, increased if tolerated to 300 mg once daily

● **SIDE-EFFECTS**
▶ **Common or very common** Fatigue · musculoskeletal pain · nausea · vomiting
▶ **Uncommon** Chest pain · cough · diarrhoea · dyspepsia · flushing · sexual dysfunction · tachycardia
▶ **Rare** Rash · urticaria
▶ **Very rare** Arthralgia · cutaneous vasculitis · headache · hepatitis · myalgia · renal dysfunction · taste disturbance · tinnitus

● **MEDICINAL FORMS**
There can be variation in the licensing of different medicines containing the same drug. Forms available from special-order manufacturers include: oral suspension
Tablet
▸ Irbesartan (Non-proprietary)
 Irbesartan 75 mg Irbesartan 75mg tablets | 28 tablet [PoM] £9.21 DT price = £1.02
 Irbesartan 150 mg Irbesartan 150mg tablets | 28 tablet [PoM] £11.25 DT price = £1.30

2

Cardiovascular system

Irbesartan 300 mg Irbesartan 300mg tablets | 28 tablet [PoM]
£15.13 DT price = £1.81
▸ Aprovel (Sanofi)
Irbesartan 75 mg Aprovel 75mg tablets | 28 tablet [PoM] £9.69 DT
price = £1.02
Irbesartan 150 mg Aprovel 150mg tablets | 28 tablet [PoM] £11.84
DT price = £1.30
Irbesartan 300 mg Aprovel 300mg tablets | 28 tablet [PoM] £15.93
DT price = £1.81
▸ Ifirmasta (Consilient Health Ltd)
Irbesartan 75 mg Ifirmasta 75mg tablets | 28 tablet [PoM] £8.23 DT
price = £1.02
Irbesartan 150 mg Ifirmasta 150mg tablets | 28 tablet [PoM] £10.06
DT price = £1.30
Irbesartan 300 mg Ifirmasta 300mg tablets | 28 tablet [PoM]
£13.54 DT price = £1.81
▸ Sabervel (Aspire Pharma Ltd)
Irbesartan 75 mg Sabervel 75mg tablets | 28 tablet [PoM] £9.69 DT
price = £1.02
Irbesartan 150 mg Sabervel 150mg tablets | 28 tablet [PoM] £11.84
DT price = £1.30
Irbesartan 300 mg Sabervel 300mg tablets | 28 tablet [PoM]
£15.93 DT price = £1.81

Irbesartan with hydrochlorothiazide

The properties listed below are those particular to the
combination only. For the properties of the components
please consider, irbesartan p. 161, hydrochlorothiazide
p. 153.

● **INDICATIONS AND DOSE**

**Hypertension not adequately controlled with irbesartan
alone**
▸ BY MOUTH
▸ Adult: (consult product literature)

● **MEDICINAL FORMS**
There can be variation in the licensing of different medicines
containing the same drug.
Tablet
▸ Irbesartan with hydrochlorothiazide (Non-proprietary)
Hydrochlorothiazide 12.5 mg, Irbesartan 150 mg Irbesartan
150mg / Hydrochlorothiazide 12.5mg tablets | 28 tablet [PoM] £10.06
DT price = £5.42
Hydrochlorothiazide 25 mg, Irbesartan 300 mg Irbesartan 300mg
/ Hydrochlorothiazide 25mg tablets | 28 tablet [PoM] £13.54 DT price
= £6.46
Hydrochlorothiazide 12.5 mg, Irbesartan 300 mg Irbesartan
300mg / Hydrochlorothiazide 12.5mg tablets | 28 tablet [PoM] £13.54
DT price = £1.68
▸ CoAprovel (Sanofi)
Hydrochlorothiazide 12.5 mg, Irbesartan 150 mg CoAprovel
150mg/12.5mg tablets | 28 tablet [PoM] £11.84 DT price = £5.42
Hydrochlorothiazide 25 mg, Irbesartan 300 mg CoAprovel
300mg/25mg tablets | 28 tablet [PoM] £15.93 DT price = £6.46
Hydrochlorothiazide 12.5 mg, Irbesartan 300 mg CoAprovel
300mg/12.5mg tablets | 28 tablet [PoM] £15.93 DT price = £1.68

F 160

Losartan potassium

● **INDICATIONS AND DOSE**

Diabetic nephropathy in type 2 diabetes mellitus
▸ BY MOUTH
▸ Adult 18-75 years: Initially 50 mg once daily for several
weeks, then increased if necessary to 100 mg once daily
▸ Adult 76 years and over: Initially 25 mg once daily for
several weeks, then increased if necessary to 100 mg
once daily

**Chronic heart failure when ACE inhibitors are unsuitable
or contra-indicated**
▸ BY MOUTH
▸ Adult: Initially 12.5 mg once daily, increased if
tolerated to up to 150 mg once daily, doses to be
increased at weekly intervals

**Hypertension (including reduction of stroke risk in
hypertension with left ventricular hypertrophy)**
▸ BY MOUTH
▸ Adult 18-75 years: Initially 50 mg once daily for several
weeks, then increased if necessary to 100 mg once daily
▸ Adult 76 years and over: Initially 25 mg once daily for
several weeks, then increased if necessary to 100 mg
once daily

Hypertension with intravascular volume depletion
▸ BY MOUTH
▸ Adult 18-75 years: Initially 25 mg once daily for several
weeks, then increased if necessary up to 100 mg once
daily

● CAUTIONS Severe heart failure
● SIDE-EFFECTS
▸ **Common or very common** Vertigo
▸ **Uncommon** Angina · dyspnoea · gastro-intestinal
disturbances · headache · malaise · oedema · palpitation ·
pruritus · rash · sleep disorders · urticaria
▸ **Rare** Atrial fibrillation · cerebrovascular accident ·
hepatitis · paraesthesia · syncope
▸ **Frequency not known** Anaemia · anaphylaxis · arthralgia ·
cough · depression · erectile dysfunction · Henoch-
Schönlein purpura · hyponatraemia · myalgia · pancreatitis
· photosensitivity · renal impairment · rhabdomyolysis ·
thrombocytopenia · tinnitus · vasculitis
● HEPATIC IMPAIRMENT Consider dose reduction in mild to
moderate impairment. Manufacturer advises avoid in
severe impairment—no information available.
● PRESCRIBING AND DISPENSING INFORMATION Flavours of
oral liquid formulations may include berry-citrus.

● **MEDICINAL FORMS**
There can be variation in the licensing of different medicines
containing the same drug. Forms available from special-order
manufacturers include: oral suspension, oral solution
Tablet
▸ Losartan potassium (Non-proprietary)
Losartan potassium 12.5 mg Losartan 12.5mg tablets |
28 tablet [PoM] £30.00 DT price = £5.15
Losartan potassium 25 mg Losartan 25mg tablets | 28 tablet [PoM]
£16.18 DT price = £0.82
Losartan potassium 50 mg Losartan 50mg tablets | 28 tablet [PoM]
£12.80 DT price = £0.89
Losartan potassium 100 mg Losartan 100mg tablets |
28 tablet [PoM] £16.18 DT price = £1.05
▸ Cozaar (Merck Sharp & Dohme Ltd)
Losartan potassium 12.5 mg Cozaar 12.5mg tablets |
28 tablet [PoM] £8.09 DT price = £5.15
Losartan potassium 25 mg Cozaar 25mg tablets | 28 tablet [PoM]
£16.18 DT price = £0.82
Losartan potassium 50 mg Cozaar 50mg tablets | 28 tablet [PoM]
£12.80 DT price = £0.89
Losartan potassium 100 mg Cozaar 100mg tablets |
28 tablet [PoM] £16.18 DT price = £1.05
Oral suspension
▸ Cozaar (Merck Sharp & Dohme Ltd)
Losartan potassium 2.5 mg per 1 ml Cozaar 2.5mg/ml oral
suspension sugar-free | 200 ml [PoM] £53.68

Losartan with hydrochlorothiazide

The properties listed below are those particular to the combination only. For the properties of the components please consider, losartan potassium p. 162, hydrochlorothiazide p. 153.

● INDICATIONS AND DOSE

Hypertension not adequately controlled with losartan alone
▶ BY MOUTH
▸ Adult: (consult product literature)

● MEDICINAL FORMS
There can be variation in the licensing of different medicines containing the same drug.
Tablet
▸ Losartan with hydrochlorothiazide (Non-proprietary)
Hydrochlorothiazide 12.5 mg, Losartan potassium 50 mg Losartan 50mg / Hydrochlorothiazide 12.5mg tablets | 28 tablet [PoM] £13.75 DT price = £1.40
Hydrochlorothiazide 25 mg, Losartan potassium 100 mg Losartan 100mg / Hydrochlorothiazide 25mg tablets | 28 tablet [PoM] £16.18 DT price = £1.51
Hydrochlorothiazide 12.5 mg, Losartan potassium 100 mg Losartan 100mg / Hydrochlorothiazide 12.5mg tablets | 28 tablet [PoM] £16.18 DT price = £10.51
▸ Cozaar-Comp (Merck Sharp & Dohme Ltd)
Hydrochlorothiazide 12.5 mg, Losartan potassium 50 mg Cozaar-Comp 50mg/12.5mg tablets | 28 tablet [PoM] £12.80 DT price = £1.40
Hydrochlorothiazide 25 mg, Losartan potassium 100 mg Cozaar-Comp 100mg/25mg tablets | 28 tablet [PoM] £16.18 DT price = £1.51
Hydrochlorothiazide 12.5 mg, Losartan potassium 100 mg Cozaar-Comp 100mg/12.5mg tablets | 28 tablet [PoM] £16.18 DT price = £10.51

160

Olmesartan medoxomil

● INDICATIONS AND DOSE

Hypertension
▶ BY MOUTH
▸ Adult: Initially 10 mg daily, increased if necessary to 20 mg daily; maximum 40 mg per day

● CONTRA-INDICATIONS Biliary obstruction
● SIDE-EFFECTS
▶ **Common or very common** Arthritis · chest pain · cough · fatigue · gastro-intestinal disturbances · haematuria · hypertriglyceridaemia · hyperuricaemia · influenza-like symptoms · musculoskeletal pain · peripheral oedema · pharyngitis · rhinitis · urinary-tract infection
▶ **Uncommon** Angina · rash · vertigo
▶ **Very rare** Headache · myalgia · pruritus · thrombocytopenia · urticaria
● HEPATIC IMPAIRMENT Dose should not exceed 20 mg daily in moderate impairment. Manufacturer advises avoid in severe impairment—no information available.
● RENAL IMPAIRMENT Max. 20 mg daily if eGFR 20–60 mL/minute/1.73 m^2. Avoid if eGFR less than 20 mL/minute/1.73 m^2.

● MEDICINAL FORMS
There can be variation in the licensing of different medicines containing the same drug. Forms available from special-order manufacturers include: oral suspension, oral solution
Tablet
▸ Olmetec (Daiichi Sankyo UK Ltd)
Olmesartan medoxomil 10 mg Olmetec 10mg tablets | 28 tablet [PoM] £10.95 DT price = £10.95
Olmesartan medoxomil 20 mg Olmetec 20mg tablets | 28 tablet [PoM] £12.95 DT price = £12.95
Olmesartan medoxomil 40 mg Olmetec 40mg tablets | 28 tablet [PoM] £17.50 DT price = £17.50

Olmesartan with amlodipine

The properties listed below are those particular to the combination only. For the properties of the components please consider, olmesartan medoxomil above, amlodipine p. 142.

● INDICATIONS AND DOSE

Hypertension in patients stabilised on the individual components in the same proportions
▶ BY MOUTH
▸ Adult: (consult product literature)

● MEDICINAL FORMS
There can be variation in the licensing of different medicines containing the same drug.
Tablet
▸ Sevikar (Daiichi Sankyo UK Ltd)
Amlodipine (as Amlodipine besilate) 5 mg, Olmesartan medoxomil 20 mg Sevikar 20mg/5mg tablets | 28 tablet [PoM] £16.95
Amlodipine (as Amlodipine besilate) 10 mg, Olmesartan medoxomil 40 mg Sevikar 40mg/10mg tablets | 28 tablet [PoM] £16.95
Amlodipine (as Amlodipine besilate) 5 mg, Olmesartan medoxomil 40 mg Sevikar 40mg/5mg tablets | 28 tablet [PoM] £16.95

Olmesartan with amlodipine and hydrochlorothiazide

The properties listed below are those particular to the combination only. For the properties of the components please consider, olmesartan medoxomil above, amlodipine p. 142, hydrochlorothiazide p. 153.

● INDICATIONS AND DOSE

Hypertension in patients stabilised on the individual components in the same proportions, or for hypertension not adequately controlled with olmesartan and amlodipine
▶ BY MOUTH
▸ Adult: (consult product literature)

● MEDICINAL FORMS
There can be variation in the licensing of different medicines containing the same drug.
Tablet
▸ Sevikar HCT (Daiichi Sankyo UK Ltd)
Amlodipine besilate 5 mg, Hydrochlorothiazide 12.5 mg, Olmesartan medoxomil 20 mg Sevikar HCT 20mg/5mg/12.5mg tablets | 28 tablet [PoM] £16.95
Amlodipine besilate 5 mg, Hydrochlorothiazide 25 mg, Olmesartan medoxomil 40 mg Sevikar HCT 40mg/5mg/25mg tablets | 28 tablet [PoM] £16.95
Amlodipine besilate 10 mg, Hydrochlorothiazide 25 mg, Olmesartan medoxomil 40 mg Sevikar HCT 40mg/10mg/25mg tablets | 28 tablet [PoM] £16.95
Amlodipine besilate 5 mg, Hydrochlorothiazide 12.5 mg, Olmesartan medoxomil 40 mg Sevikar HCT 40mg/5mg/12.5mg tablets | 28 tablet [PoM] £16.95
Amlodipine besilate 10 mg, Hydrochlorothiazide 12.5 mg, Olmesartan medoxomil 40 mg Sevikar HCT 40mg/10mg/12.5mg tablets | 28 tablet [PoM] £16.95

Olmesartan with hydrochlorothiazide

The properties listed below are those particular to the combination only. For the properties of the components please consider, olmesartan medoxomil p. 163, hydrochlorothiazide p. 153.

● **INDICATIONS AND DOSE**

Hypertension not adequately controlled with olmesartan alone
▶ BY MOUTH
▶ Adult: (consult product literature)

● **MEDICINAL FORMS**
There can be variation in the licensing of different medicines containing the same drug.
Tablet
▶ Olmetec Plus (Daiichi Sankyo UK Ltd)
Hydrochlorothiazide 12.5 mg, Olmesartan medoxomil 20 mg Olmetec Plus 20mg/12.5mg tablets | 28 tablet [PoM] £12.95 DT price = £12.95
Olmesartan medoxomil 20 mg, Hydrochlorothiazide 25 mg Olmetec Plus 20mg/25mg tablets | 28 tablet [PoM] £12.95 DT price = £12.95
Hydrochlorothiazide 12.5 mg, Olmesartan medoxomil 40 mg Olmetec Plus 40mg/12.5mg tablets | 28 tablet [PoM] £17.50 DT price = £17.50

F 160

Telmisartan

● **INDICATIONS AND DOSE**

Hypertension
▶ BY MOUTH
▶ Adult: Initially 20–40 mg once daily for at least 4 weeks, increased if necessary up to 80 mg once daily

Prevention of cardiovascular events in patients with established atherosclerotic cardiovascular disease, or type 2 diabetes mellitus with target-organ damage
▶ BY MOUTH
▶ Adult: 80 mg once daily

● **SIDE-EFFECTS**
▶ **Common or very common** Arthralgia · back pain · chest pain · eczema · gastro-intestinal disturbances · influenza-like symptoms · leg cramps · myalgia · pharyngitis · sinusitis · urinary-tract infection
▶ **Uncommon** Abnormal vision · anxiety · dry mouth · flatulence · increased sweating · tendinitis-like symptoms · vertigo
▶ **Rare** Blood disorders · bradycardia · depression · dyspnoea · eosinophilia · increase in uric acid · insomnia · pruritus · rash · tachycardia
▶ **Frequency not known** Asthenia · syncope

● **HEPATIC IMPAIRMENT** 20–40 mg once daily in mild or moderate impairment. Avoid in severe impairment or biliary obstruction.

● **RENAL IMPAIRMENT** Manufacturer advises initial dose of 20 mg once daily in severe impairment.

● **MEDICINAL FORMS**
There can be variation in the licensing of different medicines containing the same drug.
Tablet
▶ Telmisartan (Non-proprietary)
Telmisartan 20 mg Telmisartan 20mg tablets | 28 tablet [PoM] £10.55 DT price = £1.07
Telmisartan 40 mg Telmisartan 40mg tablets | 28 tablet [PoM] £12.93 DT price = £1.09
Telmisartan 80 mg Telmisartan 80mg tablets | 28 tablet [PoM] £1.56–£16.15 DT price = £1.41
▶ Micardis (Boehringer Ingelheim Ltd)
Telmisartan 20 mg Micardis 20mg tablets | 28 tablet [PoM] £11.10 DT price = £1.07

Telmisartan 40 mg Micardis 40mg tablets | 28 tablet [PoM] £13.61 DT price = £1.09
Telmisartan 80 mg Micardis 80mg tablets | 28 tablet [PoM] £17.00 DT price = £1.41
▶ Tolura (Consilient Health Ltd)
Telmisartan 20 mg Tolura 20mg tablets | 28 tablet [PoM] £11.10 DT price = £1.07
Telmisartan 40 mg Tolura 40mg tablets | 28 tablet [PoM] £13.61 DT price = £1.09
Telmisartan 80 mg Tolura 80mg tablets | 28 tablet [PoM] £17.00 DT price = £1.41

Telmisartan with hydrochlorothiazide

The properties listed below are those particular to the combination only. For the properties of the components please consider, telmisartan above, hydrochlorothiazide p. 153.

● **INDICATIONS AND DOSE**

Hypertension not adequately controlled by telmisartan alone
▶ BY MOUTH
▶ Adult: (consult product literature)

● **MEDICINAL FORMS**
There can be variation in the licensing of different medicines containing the same drug.
Tablet
▶ Telmisartan with hydrochlorothiazide (Non-proprietary)
Hydrochlorothiazide 12.5 mg, Telmisartan 40 mg Telmisartan 40mg / Hydrochlorothiazide 12.5mg tablets | 28 tablet [PoM] £13.61 DT price = £13.61
Hydrochlorothiazide 25 mg, Telmisartan 80 mg Telmisartan 80mg / Hydrochlorothiazide 25mg tablets | 28 tablet [PoM] £16.15–£17.00 DT price = £17.00
Hydrochlorothiazide 12.5 mg, Telmisartan 80 mg Telmisartan 80mg / Hydrochlorothiazide 12.5mg tablets | 28 tablet [PoM] £16.15–£17.00 DT price = £17.00
▶ Actelsar HCT (Actavis UK Ltd)
Hydrochlorothiazide 12.5 mg, Telmisartan 40 mg Actelsar HCT 40mg/12.5mg tablets | 28 tablet [PoM] £13.61 DT price = £13.61
Hydrochlorothiazide 25 mg, Telmisartan 80 mg Actelsar HCT 80mg/25mg tablets | 28 tablet [PoM] £17.00 DT price = £17.00
Hydrochlorothiazide 12.5 mg, Telmisartan 80 mg Actelsar HCT 80mg/12.5mg tablets | 28 tablet [PoM] £17.00 DT price = £17.00
▶ MicardisPlus (Boehringer Ingelheim Ltd)
Hydrochlorothiazide 12.5 mg, Telmisartan 40 mg MicardisPlus 40mg/12.5mg tablets | 28 tablet [PoM] £13.61 DT price = £13.61
Hydrochlorothiazide 25 mg, Telmisartan 80 mg MicardisPlus 80mg/25mg tablets | 28 tablet [PoM] £17.00 DT price = £17.00
Hydrochlorothiazide 12.5 mg, Telmisartan 80 mg MicardisPlus 80mg/12.5mg tablets | 28 tablet [PoM] £17.00 DT price = £17.00
▶ Tolucombi (Consilient Health Ltd)
Hydrochlorothiazide 12.5 mg, Telmisartan 40 mg Tolucombi 40mg/12.5mg tablets | 28 tablet [PoM] £13.61 DT price = £13.61
Hydrochlorothiazide 25 mg, Telmisartan 80 mg Tolucombi 80mg/25mg tablets | 28 tablet [PoM] £17.00 DT price = £17.00
Hydrochlorothiazide 12.5 mg, Telmisartan 80 mg Tolucombi 80mg/12.5mg tablets | 28 tablet [PoM] £17.00 DT price = £17.00

F 160

Valsartan

● **INDICATIONS AND DOSE**

Hypertension
▶ BY MOUTH
▶ Adult: Initially 80 mg once daily, increased if necessary up to 320 mg daily, doses to be increased at intervals of 4 weeks

Hypertension with intravascular volume depletion
▶ BY MOUTH
▶ Adult: Initially 40 mg once daily, increased if necessary up to 320 mg daily, doses to be increased at intervals of 4 weeks

Heart failure when ACE inhibitors cannot be used, or in conjunction with an ACE inhibitor when a beta-blocker cannot be used | Heart failure, in conjunction with an ACE inhibitor when a beta-blocker cannot be used (under expert supervision)
▶ BY MOUTH
▸ Adult: Initially 40 mg twice daily, increased to up to 160 mg twice daily, doses to be increased at intervals of at least 2 weeks

Myocardial infarction with left ventricular failure or left ventricular systolic dysfunction (adjunct)
▶ BY MOUTH
▸ Adult: Initially 20 mg twice daily, increased if necessary up to 160 mg twice daily, doses to be increased over several weeks if tolerated

● CONTRA-INDICATIONS Biliary cirrhosis · cholestasis
● SIDE-EFFECTS
▶ **Common or very common** Renal impairment
▶ **Uncommon** Acute renal failure · cough · fatigue · gastro-intestinal disturbance · headache · syncope
▶ **Frequency not known** Hypersensitivity reactions · myalgia · neutropenia · pruritus · rash · serum sickness · thrombocytopenia · vasculitis

● HEPATIC IMPAIRMENT Max. dose 80 mg daily in mild to moderate impairment. Avoid in severe hepatic impairment.

● RENAL IMPAIRMENT Use with caution if eGFR less than 10 mL/minute/1.73 m^2—no information available.

● MEDICINAL FORMS
There can be variation in the licensing of different medicines containing the same drug. Forms available from special-order manufacturers include: oral suspension, oral solution

Tablet
▸ Valsartan (Non-proprietary)
Valsartan 40 mg Valsartan 40mg tablets | 7 tablet PoM £3.49 DT price = £2.66 | 28 tablet PoM no price available
Valsartan 80 mg Valsartan 80mg tablets | 28 tablet PoM £13.69 DT price = £13.69
Valsartan 160 mg Valsartan 160mg tablets | 28 tablet PoM £14.69 DT price = £14.69
Valsartan 320 mg Valsartan 320mg tablets | 28 tablet PoM £20.23 DT price = £14.32

Capsule
▸ Valsartan (Non-proprietary)
Valsartan 40 mg Valsartan 40mg capsules | 28 capsule PoM £13.97 DT price = £1.00
Valsartan 80 mg Valsartan 80mg capsules | 28 capsule PoM £13.97 DT price = £1.06
Valsartan 160 mg Valsartan 160mg capsules | 28 capsule PoM £18.41 DT price = £1.48

Oral solution
▸ Diovan (Novartis Pharmaceuticals UK Ltd)
Valsartan 3 mg per 1 ml Diovan 3mg/1ml oral solution | 160 ml PoM £7.20

Combinations available: *Amlodipine with valsartan*, p. 142

Valsartan with hydrochlorothiazide

The properties listed below are those particular to the combination only. For the properties of the components please consider, valsartan p. 164, hydrochlorothiazide p. 153.

● INDICATIONS AND DOSE
Hypertension not adequately controlled by valsartan alone
▶ BY MOUTH
▸ Adult: (consult product literature)

● MEDICINAL FORMS
There can be variation in the licensing of different medicines containing the same drug.
Tablet
▸ Valsartan with hydrochlorothiazide (Non-proprietary)
Hydrochlorothiazide 12.5 mg, Valsartan 80 mg Valsartan 80mg / Hydrochlorothiazide 12.5mg tablets | 28 tablet PoM £13.97 DT price = £8.27
Hydrochlorothiazide 25 mg, Valsartan 160 mg Valsartan 160mg / Hydrochlorothiazide 25mg tablets | 28 tablet PoM £18.41 DT price = £10.77
Hydrochlorothiazide 12.5 mg, Valsartan 160 mg Valsartan 160mg / Hydrochlorothiazide 12.5mg tablets | 28 tablet PoM £18.41 DT price = £1.98
▸ Co-Diovan (Novartis Pharmaceuticals UK Ltd)
Hydrochlorothiazide 12.5 mg, Valsartan 80 mg Co-Diovan 80mg/12.5mg tablets | 28 tablet PoM £16.76 DT price = £8.27
Hydrochlorothiazide 25 mg, Valsartan 160 mg Co-Diovan 160mg/25mg tablets | 28 tablet PoM £22.09 DT price = £10.77
Hydrochlorothiazide 12.5 mg, Valsartan 160 mg Co-Diovan 160mg/12.5mg tablets | 28 tablet PoM £22.09 DT price = £1.98

DRUGS ACTING ON THE RENIN-ANGIOTENSIN SYSTEM 〉 RENIN INHIBITORS

Aliskiren

● DRUG ACTION Renin inhibitors inhibit renin directly; renin converts angiotensinogen to angiotensin I.

● INDICATIONS AND DOSE
Essential hypertension either alone or in combination with other antihypertensives
▶ BY MOUTH
▸ Adult: 150 mg once daily, increased if necessary to 300 mg once daily

● CONTRA-INDICATIONS Concomitant treatment with an ACE inhibitor or an angiotensin-II receptor antagonist in patients with an eGFR less than 60 mL/minute/1.73 m^2 · concomitant treatment with an ACE inhibitor or an angiotensin-II receptor antagonist in patients with diabetes mellitus · hereditary angioedema · idiopathic angioedema

● CAUTIONS Combination treatment with an ACE inhibitor · combination treatment with an angiotensin-II receptor antagonist · concomitant use of diuretics (first doses may cause hypotension—initiate with care) · history of angioedema · moderate to severe congestive heart failure · patients at risk of renal impairment · salt depletion (first doses may cause hypotension—initiate with care) · volume depletion (first doses may cause hypotension—initiate with care)

CAUTIONS, FURTHER INFORMATION
● Concomitant use of drugs affecting the renin-angiotensin system Combination therapy with two drugs affecting the renin-angiotensin system (ACE inhibitors, angiotensin-II receptor antagonists, and aliskiren) is not recommended due to an increased risk of hyperkalaemia, hypotension, and renal impairment, compared to use of a single drug. Patients with diabetic nephropathy are particularly susceptible to developing hyperkalaemia and should not be given an ACE inhibitor with an angiotensin-II receptor antagonist. There is some evidence that the benefits of combination use of an ACE inhibitor with candesartan or valsartan may outweigh the risks in selected patients with heart failure for whom other treatments are unsuitable, however, the concomitant use of this combination, together with an aldosterone antagonist or a potassium-sparing diuretic is not recommended. For patients currently taking combination therapy, the need for continued combined therapy should be reviewed. If combination therapy is considered essential, it should be carried out under specialist supervision, with close monitoring of blood pressure, renal function, and

Cardiovascular system

2

Cardiovascular system

electrolytes (particularly potassium); monitoring should be considered at the start of treatment, then monthly, and also after any change in dose or during intercurrent illness.

● INTERACTIONS → Appendix 1 (aliskiren).

● SIDE-EFFECTS

▶ **Common or very common** Arthralgia · dizziness · hyperkalaemia · diarrhoea

▶ **Uncommon** Acute renal failure (reversible on discontinuation of treatment) · hypotension · palpitation · peripheral oedema · cough · pruritus · rash · Stevens-Johnson syndrome · toxic epidermal necrolysis · urticaria

▶ **Rare** Anaemia · angioedema · erythema

▶ **Frequency not known** Liver disorders · nausea · vertigo · vomiting

SIDE-EFFECTS, FURTHER INFORMATION
If diarrhoea severe or persistent discontinue treatment.

● PREGNANCY Manufacturer advises avoid—no information available; other drugs acting on the renin-angiotensin system have been associated with fetal malformations and neonatal death.

● BREAST FEEDING Present in milk in *animal* studies—manufacturer advises avoid.

● RENAL IMPAIRMENT Avoid if eGFR is less than 30 mL/minute/1.73 m^2— no information available. Use with caution in renal artery stenosis—no information available. Monitor plasma-potassium concentration in renal impairment.

● MONITORING REQUIREMENTS Monitor patients with a history of angioedema closely during treatment.

● NATIONAL FUNDING/ACCESS DECISIONS
Scottish Medicines Consortium (SMC) Decisions
The *Scottish Medicines Consortium* has advised (January 2010) that aliskiren (*Rasilez* ®) is **not** recommended for use within NHS Scotland.

● MEDICINAL FORMS
There can be variation in the licensing of different medicines containing the same drug.
Tablet
CAUTIONARY AND ADVISORY LABELS 21
▶ Rasilez (Novartis Pharmaceuticals UK Ltd)
Aliskiren (as Aliskiren hemifumarate) 150 mg Rasilez 150mg tablets | 28 tablet [PoM] £28.51 DT price = £28.51
Aliskiren (as Aliskiren hemifumarate) 300 mg Rasilez 300mg tablets | 28 tablet [PoM] £34.27 DT price = £34.27

VASODILATORS 〉 VASODILATOR ANTIHYPERTENSIVES

Hydralazine hydrochloride

● INDICATIONS AND DOSE
Moderate to severe hypertension (adjunct)
▶ BY MOUTH
▶ Adult: Initially 25 mg twice daily, increased if necessary up to 50 mg twice daily
Heart failure (with long acting nitrate) (initiated in hospital or under specialist supervision)
▶ BY MOUTH
▶ Adult: Initially 25 mg 3–4 times a day, subsequent doses to be increased every 2 days if necessary; usual maintenance 50–75 mg 4 times a day
Hypertensive emergencies (including during pregnancy) | Hypertension with renal complications
▶ BY INTRAVENOUS INFUSION
▶ Adult: Initially 200–300 micrograms/minute; usual maintenance 50–150 micrograms/minute
▶ BY SLOW INTRAVENOUS INJECTION
▶ Adult: 5–10 mg, to be diluted with 10 mL sodium chloride 0.9%; dose may be repeated after 20–30 minutes

● CONTRA-INDICATIONS Acute porphyrias p. 918 · cor pulmonale · dissecting aortic aneurysm · high output heart failure · idiopathic systemic lupus erythematosus · myocardial insufficiency due to mechanical obstruction · severe tachycardia

● CAUTIONS Cerebrovascular disease · coronary artery disease (may provoke angina, avoid after myocardial infarction until stabilised) · occasionally blood pressure reduction too rapid even with low parenteral doses

● INTERACTIONS → Appendix 1 (hydralazine).

● SIDE-EFFECTS

▶ **Rare** Rashes

▶ **Frequency not known** Abnormal liver function · agitation · anorexia · anxiety · arthralgia · blood disorders · dizziness · dyspnoea · fever · fluid retention · flushing · gastro-intestinal disturbances · haematuria · haemolytic anaemia · headache · hypotension · increased lacrimation · jaundice · leucopenia · myalgia · nasal congestion · palpitation · paraesthesia · peripheral neuritis · polyneuritis · proteinuria · raised plasma creatinine · systemic lupus erythematosus-like syndrome after long-term therapy with over 100 mg daily (or less in women and in slow acetylator individuals) · tachycardia · thrombocytopenia

SIDE-EFFECTS, FURTHER INFORMATION
The incidence of side-effects is lower if the dose is kept below 100 mg daily, but systemic lupus erythematosus should be suspected if there is unexplained weight loss, arthritis, or any other unexplained ill health.

● PREGNANCY Neonatal thrombocytopenia reported, but risk should be balanced against risk of uncontrolled maternal hypertension. Manufacturer advises avoid before third trimester.

● BREAST FEEDING Present in milk but not known to be harmful.
Monitor infant in breast-feeding.

● HEPATIC IMPAIRMENT Reduce dose.

● RENAL IMPAIRMENT Reduce dose if eGFR less than 30 mL/minute/1.73 m^2.

● MONITORING REQUIREMENTS Manufacturer advises test for antinuclear factor and for proteinuria every 6 months and check acetylator status before increasing dose above 100 mg daily, but evidence of clinical value unsatisfactory.

● DIRECTIONS FOR ADMINISTRATION For *intravenous infusion* (*Apresoline* ®) give continuously in Sodium chloride 0.9%. Suggested infusion volume 500 mL.

● MEDICINAL FORMS
There can be variation in the licensing of different medicines containing the same drug. Forms available from special-order manufacturers include: oral suspension, oral solution
Tablet
EXCIPIENTS: May contain Gluten, propylene glycol
▶ Hydralazine hydrochloride (Non-proprietary)
Hydralazine hydrochloride 10 mg Apo-Hydralazine 10mg tablets | 100 tablet [PoM] no price available
Hydralazine hydrochloride 25 mg Hydralazine 25mg tablets | 56 tablet [PoM] £8.56 DT price = £7.71 | 84 tablet [PoM] £14.00
Hydralazine hydrochloride 50 mg Hydralazine 50mg tablets | 56 tablet [PoM] £15.74 DT price = £13.15
▶ Apresoline (AMCo)
Hydralazine hydrochloride 25 mg Apresoline 25mg tablets | 84 tablet [PoM] £3.38
Powder for solution for injection
▶ Hydralazine hydrochloride (Non-proprietary)
Hydralazine hydrochloride 20 mg Hydralazine 20mg powder for concentrate for solution for injection ampoules | 5 ampoule [PoM] £64.50
▶ Apresoline (AMCo)
Hydralazine hydrochloride 20 mg Apresoline 20mg powder for solution for injection ampoules | 5 ampoule [PoM] £11.09

Minoxidil

- **INDICATIONS AND DOSE**

Severe hypertension, in addition to a diuretic and a beta-blocker

▶ BY MOUTH
- Adult: Initially 5 mg daily in 1–2 divided doses, then increased in steps of 5–10 mg, increased at intervals of at least 3 days, seldom necessary to exceed 50 mg daily; maximum 100 mg per day
- Elderly: Initially 2.5 mg daily in 1–2 divided doses, then increased in steps of 5–10 mg, increased at intervals of at least 3 days, seldom necessary to exceed 50 mg daily; maximum 100 mg per day

- **CONTRA-INDICATIONS** Phaeochromocytoma
- **CAUTIONS** Acute porphyrias p. 918 · after myocardial infarction (until stabilised) · angina
- **INTERACTIONS** → Appendix 1 (vasodilator antihypertensives).
- **SIDE-EFFECTS** Breast tenderness · gastro-intestinal disturbances · hypertrichosis · peripheral oedema · rashes · reversible rise in creatinine and blood urea nitrogen · sodium retention · tachycardia · water retention · weight gain
- **PREGNANCY** Avoid—possible toxicity including reduced placental perfusion. Neonatal hirsutism reported.
- **BREAST FEEDING** Present in milk but not known to be harmful.
- **RENAL IMPAIRMENT** Use with caution in significant impairment.

- **MEDICINAL FORMS**
There can be variation in the licensing of different medicines containing the same drug.

Tablet
- Loniten (Pfizer Ltd)
Minoxidil 2.5 mg Loniten 2.5mg tablets | 60 tablet [PoM] £8.88 DT price = £8.88
Minoxidil 5 mg Loniten 5mg tablets | 60 tablet [PoM] £15.83 DT price = £15.83
Minoxidil 10 mg Loniten 10mg tablets | 60 tablet [PoM] £30.68 DT price = £30.68

4.1a Hypertension associated with phaeochromocytoma

Drugs used for Hypertension associated with phaeochromocytoma not listed below Propranolol hydrochloride, p. 136

VASODILATORS > PERIPHERAL VASODILATORS

Phenoxybenzamine hydrochloride

- **INDICATIONS AND DOSE**

Hypertension in phaeochromocytoma

▶ BY MOUTH
- Adult: Initially 10 mg daily, increased in steps of 10 mg daily until hypertension controlled or treatment not tolerated; maintenance 1–2 mg/kg daily in 2 divided doses

- **CONTRA-INDICATIONS** During recovery period after myocardial infarction (usually 3–4 weeks) · history of cerebrovascular accident
- **CAUTIONS** Avoid contact with skin (risk of contact sensitisation) · avoid in Acute porphyrias p. 918 · carcinogenic in *animals* · cerebrovascular disease ·

congestive heart failure · elderly · severe ischaemic heart disease
- **SIDE-EFFECTS**
▶ **Rare** Gastro-intestinal disturbances
▶ **Frequency not known** Inhibition of ejaculation · lassitude · miosis · nasal congestion · postural hypotension (with dizziness and marked compensatory tachycardia)
- **PREGNANCY** Hypotension may occur in newborn.
- **BREAST FEEDING** May be present in milk.
- **RENAL IMPAIRMENT** Use with caution.
- **HANDLING AND STORAGE** Owing to risk of contact sensitisation healthcare professionals should avoid contamination of hands.

- **MEDICINAL FORMS**
There can be variation in the licensing of different medicines containing the same drug. Forms available from special-order manufacturers include: oral suspension, oral solution

Capsule
- Phenoxybenzamine hydrochloride (Non-proprietary)
Phenoxybenzamine hydrochloride 10 mg Phenoxybenzamine 10mg capsules | 30 capsule [PoM] £97.38 DT price = £97.38

Phentolamine mesilate

- **INDICATIONS AND DOSE**

Hypertensive episodes due to phaeochromocytoma e.g. during surgery

▶ BY INTRAVENOUS INJECTION
- Adult: 2–5 mg, repeated if necessary

Diagnosis of phaeochromocytoma

▶ BY INTRAVENOUS INJECTION, OR BY INTRAMUSCULAR INJECTION
- Adult: (consult product literature)

- **CONTRA-INDICATIONS** Angina · coronary insufficiency · evidence of coronary artery disease · history of myocardial infarction · hypotension
- **CAUTIONS** Elderly · gastritis · peptic ulcer
- **INTERACTIONS** → Appendix 1 (alpha-blockers).
- **SIDE-EFFECTS** Acute or prolonged hypotension · angina · arrhythmias · chest pain · diarrhoea · dizziness · flushing · nasal congestion · nausea · postural hypotension · tachycardia · vomiting
- **PREGNANCY** Use with caution—may cause marked decrease in maternal blood pressure with resulting fetal anoxia.
- **BREAST FEEDING** Manufacturer advises avoid—no information available.
- **RENAL IMPAIRMENT** Manufacturer advises caution—no information available.
- **MONITORING REQUIREMENTS** Monitor blood pressure and heart rate.

- **MEDICINAL FORMS**
There can be variation in the licensing of different medicines containing the same drug.
No licensed medicines listed.

Cardiovascular system

2

4.1b Hypertensive crises

ANTIADRENERGIC AGENTS, PERIPHERALLY ACTING

Guanethidine monosulfate

- **INDICATIONS AND DOSE**

Hypertensive crisis (but no longer recommended)
▸ BY INTRAMUSCULAR INJECTION
▸ Adult: 10–20 mg, dose may be repeated after 3 hours if necessary

- CONTRA-INDICATIONS Heart failure · phaeochromocytoma
- CAUTIONS Asthma · cerebral arteriosclerosis · coronary arteriosclerosis · history of peptic ulceration
- INTERACTIONS → Appendix 1 (adrenergic neurone blockers).
- SIDE-EFFECTS Diarrhoea · drowsiness · failure of ejaculation · fluid retention · headache · nasal congestion · postural hypotension
- PREGNANCY Postural hypotension and reduced uteroplacental perfusion. Should not be used to treat hypertension in pregnancy.
- RENAL IMPAIRMENT Reduce dose if eGFR 40–65 mL/minute/1.73 m². Avoid if eGFR less than 40 mL/minute/1.73 m².
- LESS SUITABLE FOR PRESCRIBING Guanethidine monosulfate is less suitable for prescribing.

- MEDICINAL FORMS
There can be variation in the licensing of different medicines containing the same drug.
Solution for injection
▸ Guanethidine monosulfate (Non-proprietary)
  Guanethidine monosulfate 10 mg per 1 ml Guanethidine 10mg/1ml solution for injection ampoules | 5 ampoule PoM £224.15

VASODILATORS › VASODILATOR ANTIHYPERTENSIVES

Sodium nitroprusside

- **INDICATIONS AND DOSE**

Hypertensive emergencies
▸ BY INTRAVENOUS INFUSION
▸ Adult: Initially 0.5–1.5 micrograms/kg/minute, adjusted in steps of 500 nanograms/kg/minute every 5 minutes, usual dose 0.5–8 micrograms/kg/minute, use lower doses if already receiving other antihypertensives, stop if response unsatisfactory with max. dose in 10 minutes, lower initial dose of 300 nanograms/kg/minute has been used

Maintenance of blood pressure at 30–40% lower than pretreatment diastolic blood pressure
▸ BY INTRAVENOUS INFUSION
▸ Adult: 20–400 micrograms/minute, use lower doses for patients being treated with other antihypertensives

Controlled hypotension in anaesthesia during surgery
▸ BY INTRAVENOUS INFUSION
▸ Adult: Up to 1.5 micrograms/kg/minute

Acute or chronic heart failure
▸ BY INTRAVENOUS INFUSION
▸ Adult: Initially 10–15 micrograms/minute, increased every 5–10 minutes as necessary; usual dose 10–200 micrograms/minute normally for max. 3 days

- UNLICENSED USE Not licensed for use in the UK.

- CONTRA-INDICATIONS Compensatory hypertension · Leber's optic atrophy · severe vitamin B₁₂ deficiency
- CAUTIONS Elderly · hyponatraemia · hypothermia · hypothyroidism · impaired cerebral circulation · ischaemic heart disease
- INTERACTIONS → Appendix 1 (sodium nitroprusside).
- SIDE-EFFECTS Abdominal pain · acute transient phlebitis · anxiety · dizziness · headache · nausea · palpitation · perspiration · reduced platelet count · retching · retrosternal discomfort

SIDE-EFFECTS, FURTHER INFORMATION
▸ Side-effects associated with over rapid reduction in blood pressure: Headache, dizziness, nausea, retching, abdominal pain, perspiration, palpitation, anxiety, retrosternal discomfort—reduce infusion rate if any of these side-effects occur.

Overdose
Side-effects caused by excessive plasma concentration of the cyanide metabolite include tachycardia, sweating, hyperventilation, arrhythmias, marked metabolic acidosis (discontinue and give antidote, see cyanide in Emergency treatment of poisoning p. 1194).

- PREGNANCY Avoid prolonged use—potential for accumulation of cyanide in fetus.
- BREAST FEEDING No information available. Caution advised due to thiocyanate metabolite.
- HEPATIC IMPAIRMENT Use with caution. Avoid in hepatic failure—cyanide or thiocyanate metabolites may accumulate.
- RENAL IMPAIRMENT Avoid prolonged use—cyanide or thiocyanate metabolites may accumulate.
- MONITORING REQUIREMENTS Monitor blood pressure (including intra-arterial blood pressure) and blood-cyanide concentration, and if treatment exceeds 3 days, also blood thiocyanate concentration.
- TREATMENT CESSATION Avoid sudden withdrawal—terminate infusion over 15–30 minutes.
- DIRECTIONS FOR ADMINISTRATION For *continuous intravenous infusion* in Glucose 5%, infuse *via* infusion device to allow precise control. For further details, consult product literature. Protect infusion from light.

- MEDICINAL FORMS
There can be variation in the licensing of different medicines containing the same drug.
Powder and solvent for solution for infusion
▸ Sodium nitroprusside (Non-proprietary)
  Sodium nitroprusside dihydrate 50 mg Sodium nitroprusside 50mg powder and solvent for solution for infusion vials | 1 vial PoM no price available

4.1c Pulmonary hypertension

ANTITHROMBOTIC DRUGS › PROSTAGLANDINS, CARDIOVASCULAR

Iloprost

- **INDICATIONS AND DOSE**

Idiopathic or familial pulmonary arterial hypertension (initiated under specialist supervision)
▸ BY INHALATION OF NEBULISED SOLUTION
▸ Adult: Initially 2.5 micrograms for 1 dose, increased to 5 micrograms for 1 dose, increased if tolerated to 5 micrograms 6–9 times a day, adjusted according to response; reduced if not tolerated to 2.5 micrograms 6–9 times a day, reduce to lower maintenance dose if high dose not tolerated

- CONTRA-INDICATIONS Conditions which increase risk of haemorrhage · congenital or acquired valvular defects of the myocardium · decompensated cardiac failure (unless under close medical supervision) · pulmonary veno-occlusive disease · severe arrhythmias · unstable angina · within 3 months of cerebrovascular events · within 6 months of myocardial infarction
- CAUTIONS Acute pulmonary infection · chronic obstructive pulmonary disease · hypotension (do not initiate if systolic blood pressure below 85 mmHg) · severe asthma · unstable pulmonary hypertension with advanced right heart failure
- INTERACTIONS → Appendix 1 (iloprost).
- SIDE-EFFECTS
- ▶ **Common or very common** Chest pain · cough · diarrhoea · dyspnoea · haemorrhage · headache · hypotension · jaw pain · nausea · oral irritation · rash · throat pain · vomiting
- ▶ **Frequency not known** Bronchospasm · taste disturbance · thrombocytopenia · wheezing
- PREGNANCY Use if potential benefit outweighs risk.
- BREAST FEEDING Manufacturer advises avoid—no information available.
- HEPATIC IMPAIRMENT Initially 2.5 micrograms at intervals of 3–4 hours (max. 6 times daily), adjusted according to response (consult product literature). Elimination reduced.
- DIRECTIONS FOR ADMINISTRATION For *inhaled treatment*, to minimise accidental exposure use only with nebulisers listed in *Ventavis* ® product literature in a well ventilated room.
- PRESCRIBING AND DISPENSING INFORMATION Delivery characteristics of nebuliser devices may vary—only switch devices under medical supervision.
- NATIONAL FUNDING/ACCESS DECISIONS
Scottish Medicines Consortium (SMC) Decisions
The *Scottish Medicines Consortium* has advised (November 2005) that iloprost (*Ventavis* ®) is accepted for restricted use within NHS Scotland in patients in whom bosentan is ineffective or not tolerated, and should only be prescribed by specialists in the Scottish Pulmonary Vascular Unit.

- MEDICINAL FORMS
There can be variation in the licensing of different medicines containing the same drug.
Nebuliser liquid
 ▶ Ventavis (Bayer Plc)
   Iloprost (as Iloprost trometamol) 10 microgram per 1 ml Ventavis 10micrograms/ml nebuliser solution 1ml ampoules | 30 ampoule [PoM] £400.19 | 168 ampoule [PoM] £2,241.08

ENDOTHELIN RECEPTOR ANTAGONISTS

Ambrisentan

- INDICATIONS AND DOSE
Pulmonary arterial hypertension (initiated under specialist supervision)
 ▶ BY MOUTH
 ▶ Adult: 5 mg once daily, increased if necessary to 10 mg once daily
DOSE ADJUSTMENTS DUE TO INTERACTIONS
Max. 5 mg daily with concomitant ciclosporin.

- CONTRA-INDICATIONS Idiopathic pulmonary fibrosis
- CAUTIONS Not to be initiated in significant anaemia
- INTERACTIONS → Appendix 1 (ambrisentan).
- SIDE-EFFECTS
- ▶ **Common or very common** Abdominal pain · anaemia · chest pain · constipation · diarrhoea · dizziness · dyspnoea · epistaxis · flushing · headache · heart failure · hypotension ·

malaise · nausea · palpitation · peripheral oedema · upper respiratory-tract disorders · vomiting
- ▶ **Uncommon** Autoimmune hepatitis · hepatic injury · syncope
- CONCEPTION AND CONTRACEPTION Exclude pregnancy before treatment and ensure effective contraception during treatment. Monthly pregnancy tests advised.
- PREGNANCY Avoid (teratogenic in *animal studies*).
- BREAST FEEDING Manufacturer advises avoid—no information available.
- HEPATIC IMPAIRMENT Avoid in severe impairment.
- RENAL IMPAIRMENT Use with caution if eGFR less than 30 mL/minute/1.73 m^2.
- MONITORING REQUIREMENTS
- ▶ Monitor haemoglobin concentration or haematocrit after 1 month and 3 months of starting treatment, and periodically thereafter (reduce dose or discontinue treatment if significant decrease in haemoglobin concentration or haematocrit observed).
- ▶ Monitor liver function before treatment, and monthly thereafter—discontinue if liver enzymes raised significantly or if symptoms of liver impairment develop.
- NATIONAL FUNDING/ACCESS DECISIONS
Scottish Medicines Consortium (SMC) Decisions
The *Scottish Medicines Consortium* has advised (October 2008) that ambrisentan (*Volibris* ®) should be prescribed only by specialists in the Scottish Pulmonary Vascular Unit or other similar specialists.

- MEDICINAL FORMS
There can be variation in the licensing of different medicines containing the same drug.
Tablet
 ▶ Volibris (GlaxoSmithKline UK Ltd)
   Ambrisentan 5 mg Volibris 5mg tablets | 30 tablet [PoM] £1,618.08
   Ambrisentan 10 mg Volibris 10mg tablets | 30 tablet [PoM] £1,618.08

Bosentan

- INDICATIONS AND DOSE
Pulmonary arterial hypertension (initiated under specialist supervision)
 ▶ BY MOUTH
 ▶ Adult: Initially 62.5 mg twice daily for 4 weeks, then increased to 125 mg twice daily (max. per dose 250 mg); maximum 500 mg per day
Systemic sclerosis with ongoing digital ulcer disease (to reduce number of new digital ulcers)
 ▶ BY MOUTH
 ▶ Adult: Initially 62.5 mg twice daily for 4 weeks, then increased to 125 mg twice daily

- CONTRA-INDICATIONS Acute porphyrias p. 918
- CAUTIONS Not to be initiated if systemic systolic blood pressure is below 85 mmHg
- INTERACTIONS → Appendix 1 (bosentan).
- SIDE-EFFECTS
- ▶ **Common or very common** Anaemia · diarrhoea · flushing · gastro-oesophageal reflux · headache · hypotension · oedema · palpitation · syncope
- ▶ **Uncommon** Leucopenia · neutropenia · thrombocytopenia
- ▶ **Rare** Liver cirrhosis · liver failure
- CONCEPTION AND CONTRACEPTION Effective contraception required during administration (hormonal contraception not considered effective). Monthly pregnancy tests advised.
- PREGNANCY Avoid (teratogenic in *animal* studies).

2

Cardiovascular system

- BREAST FEEDING Manufacturer advises avoid—no information available.
- HEPATIC IMPAIRMENT Avoid in moderate and severe impairment.
- MONITORING REQUIREMENTS
▶ Monitor haemoglobin before and during treatment (monthly for first 4 months, then 3-monthly).
▶ Monitor liver function before treatment, at monthly intervals during treatment, and 2 weeks after dose increase (reduce dose or suspend treatment if liver enzymes raised significantly)—discontinue if symptoms of liver impairment.
- TREATMENT CESSATION Avoid abrupt withdrawal—withdraw treatment gradually.

- MEDICINAL FORMS
There can be variation in the licensing of different medicines containing the same drug.
Tablet
▶ Tracleer (Actelion Pharmaceuticals UK Ltd)
Bosentan (as Bosentan monohydrate) 62.5 mg Tracleer 62.5mg tablets | 56 tablet PoM £1,510.21
Bosentan (as Bosentan monohydrate) 125 mg Tracleer 125mg tablets | 56 tablet PoM £1,510.21

Macitentan

- INDICATIONS AND DOSE
Pulmonary arterial hypertension (initiated under specialist supervision)
▶ BY MOUTH
▶ Adult: 10 mg daily

- CONTRA-INDICATIONS Severe anaemia
- CAUTIONS Patients over 75 years · pulmonary veno-occlusive disease
- INTERACTIONS → Appendix 1 (macitentan).
- SIDE-EFFECTS
▶ **Common or very common** Anaemia · bronchitis · headache · hypotension · upper respiratory-tract disorders · urinary-tract infection
▶ **Frequency not known** Leucopenia · thrombocytopenia
- CONCEPTION AND CONTRACEPTION Manufacturer advices exclude pregnancy before treatment and ensure effective contraception during and for one month after stopping treatment. Monthly pregnancy tests advised.
- PREGNANCY Toxicity in *animal* studies.
- BREAST FEEDING Manufacturer advises avoid—present in milk in *animal* studies.
- HEPATIC IMPAIRMENT Do not initiate if serum transaminases exceed 3 times upper limit of normal. Avoid in moderate and severe impairment.
- RENAL IMPAIRMENT Manufacturer advises caution in severe impairment and avoid in patients undergoing dialysis (no information available). In renal impairment consider monitoring blood pressure (risk of hypotension).
- MONITORING REQUIREMENTS
▶ Monitor liver function before treatment, then monthly thereafter (discontinue if unexplained persistent raised serum transaminases or signs of hepatic injury—can restart on advice on hepatologist if liver function tests return to normal and no hepatic injury).
▶ Monitor haemoglobin concentration before treatment and then as indicated.
- PATIENT AND CARER ADVICE Patient card should be provided.
  Patients should be told how to recognise signs of liver disorder and advised to seek immediate medical attention if symptoms such as dark urine, nausea, vomiting, fatigue, abdominal pain, or pruritus develop.

- NATIONAL FUNDING/ACCESS DECISIONS
Scottish Medicines Consortium (SMC) Decisions
The *Scottish Medicines Consortium* has advised (March 2014) that macitentan (*Opsumit®*) should be initiated and prescribed only by specialists in the Scottish Pulmonary Vascular Unit or other similar specialists.

- MEDICINAL FORMS
There can be variation in the licensing of different medicines containing the same drug.
Tablet
▶ Opsumit (Actelion Pharmaceuticals UK Ltd) ▼
Macitentan 10 mg Opsumit 10mg tablets | 30 tablet PoM £2,306.00

GUANYLATE CYCLASE STIMULATORS

Riociguat

- INDICATIONS AND DOSE
Chronic thromboembolic pulmonary hypertension that is recurrent or persistent following surgery, or is inoperable (initiated under specialist supervision) | Monotherapy or in combination with an endothelin receptor antagonist for idiopathic or hereditary pulmonary arterial hypertension, or pulmonary arterial hypertension associated with connective tissue disease (initiated under specialist supervision)
▶ BY MOUTH
▶ Adult: Initially 1 mg 3 times a day for 2 weeks, increased in steps of 0.5 mg 3 times a day, dose to be increased every 2 weeks, increased to up to 2.5 mg 3 times a day (max. per dose 2.5 mg 3 times a day), increase up to maximum dose only if systolic blood pressure ≥ 95 mmHg and no signs of hypotension, if treatment interrupted for 3 or more days, restart at 1 mg three times daily for 2 weeks and titrate as before, during titration, reduce dose by 0.5 mg three times daily if systolic blood pressure falls below 95 mmHg and patient shows signs of hypotension

- CONTRA-INDICATIONS History of serious haemoptysis · previous bronchial artery embolisation · pulmonary veno-occlusive disease
- CAUTIONS Autonomic dysfunction · elderly (risk of hypotension) · hypotension (do not initiate if systolic blood pressure below 95 mmHg) · hypovolaemia · severe left ventricular outflow obstruction
CAUTIONS, FURTHER INFORMATION
▶ Smoking Smoking cessation advised (response possibly reduced); dose adjustment may be necessary if smoking started or stopped during treatment.
- INTERACTIONS → Appendix 1 (riociguat).
- SIDE-EFFECTS
▶ **Common or very common** Anaemia · constipation · diarrhoea · dizziness · dyspepsia · dysphagia · epistaxis · gastritis · gastro-oesophageal reflux · haemoptysis · headache · hypotension · nasal congestion · nausea · palpitation · peripheral oedema · vomiting
▶ **Uncommon** Pulmonary haemorrhage
- CONCEPTION AND CONTRACEPTION Effective contraception required during treatment. Monthly pregnancy tests advised.
- PREGNANCY Avoid—toxicity in *animal* studies.
- BREAST FEEDING Manufacturer advises avoid—present in milk in *animal* studies.
- HEPATIC IMPAIRMENT Titrate dose cautiously in moderate impairment. Manufacturer advises avoid in severe impairment—no information available.

- RENAL IMPAIRMENT Titrate dose cautiously—risk of hypotension. Manufacturer advises avoid if eGFR less than 30 mL/minute/1.73 m^2—limited information available.
- DIRECTIONS FOR ADMINISTRATION Tablets may be crushed and mixed with water or soft foods and swallowed immediately.
- PATIENT AND CARER ADVICE Smoking cessation advised (response possibly reduced). Patients should inform prescriber if smoking started or stopped during treatment; dose adjustment may be necessary.
- NATIONAL FUNDING/ACCESS DECISIONS

Scottish Medicines Consortium (SMC) Decisions
The *Scottish Medicines Consortium* has advised (November 2014) that riociguat (*Adempas*®) is accepted for restricted use within NHS Scotland for the treatment of chronic thromboembolic pulmonary hypertension in patients for whom a phosphodiesterase type-5 inhibitor is inappropriate, not tolerated, or ineffective, and should only be prescribed by specialists in the Scottish Pulmonary Vascular Unit.

- MEDICINAL FORMS
There can be variation in the licensing of different medicines containing the same drug.

Tablet
▸ Adempas (Merck Sharp & Dohme Ltd) ▼
  Riociguat 500 microgram Adempas 0.5mg tablets | 42 tablet PoM £997.36
  Riociguat 1 mg Adempas 1mg tablets | 42 tablet PoM £997.36
  Riociguat 1.5 mg Adempas 1.5mg tablets | 42 tablet PoM £997.36
  Riociguat 2 mg Adempas 2mg tablets | 42 tablet PoM £997.36 | 84 tablet PoM £1,994.72
  Riociguat 2.5 mg Adempas 2.5mg tablets | 84 tablet PoM £1,994.72

4.2   Hypotension and shock

Sympathomimetics

Inotropic sympathomimetics

Shock
Shock is a medical emergency associated with a high mortality. The underlying causes of shock such as haemorrhage, sepsis, or myocardial insufficiency should be corrected. The profound hypotension of shock must be treated promptly to prevent tissue hypoxia and organ failure. Volume replacement is essential to correct the hypovolaemia associated with haemorrhage and sepsis but may be detrimental in cardiogenic shock. Depending on haemodynamic status, cardiac output may be improved by the use of sympathomimetic inotropes such as adrenaline/epinephrine p. 205, dobutamine p. 204 or dopamine hydrochloride below. In septic shock, when fluid replacement and inotropic support fail to maintain blood pressure, the vasoconstrictor noradrenaline/norepinephrine p. 173 may be considered. In cardiogenic shock peripheral resistance is frequently high and to raise it further may worsen myocardial performance and exacerbate tissue ischaemia.

The use of sympathomimetic inotropes and vasoconstrictors should preferably be confined to the intensive care setting and undertaken with invasive haemodynamic monitoring.

See also advice on the management of anaphylactic shock in Antihistamines, allergen immunotherapy and allergic emergencies p. 253.

Vasoconstrictor sympathomimetics

Vasoconstrictor sympathomimetics raise blood pressure transiently by acting on alpha-adrenergic receptors to constrict peripheral vessels. They are sometimes used as an emergency method of elevating blood pressure where other measures have failed.

The danger of vasoconstrictors is that although they raise blood pressure they also reduce perfusion of vital organs such as the kidney.

Spinal and epidural anaesthesia may result in sympathetic block with resultant hypotension. Management may include intravenous fluids (which are usually given prophylactically), oxygen, elevation of the legs, and injection of a pressor drug such as ephedrine hydrochloride p. 248. As well as constricting peripheral vessels ephedrine hydrochloride also accelerates the heart rate (by acting on beta receptors). Use is made of this dual action of ephedrine hydrochloride to manage associated bradycardia (although intravenous injection of atropine sulfate p. 1169 may also be required if bradycardia persists).

SYMPATHOMIMETICS > INOTROPIC

Dopamine hydrochloride

- DRUG ACTION Dopamine is a cardiac stimulant which acts on beta$_1$ receptors in cardiac muscle, and increases contractility with little effect on rate.

- INDICATIONS AND DOSE

Cardiogenic shock in infarction or cardiac surgery
▸ BY INTRAVENOUS INFUSION
▸ Adult: Initially 2–5 micrograms/kg/minute

- CONTRA-INDICATIONS Phaeochromocytoma · tachyarrhythmia
- CAUTIONS Correct hypovolaemia · hyperthyroidism · low dose in shock due to acute myocardial infarction
- INTERACTIONS → Appendix 1 (sympathomimetics).
- SIDE-EFFECTS
▸ **Common or very common** Chest pain · dyspnoea · headache · hypotension · nausea · palpitation · tachycardia · vasoconstriction · vomiting
▸ **Uncommon** Bradycardia · gangrene · hypertension · mydriasis
▸ **Rare** Fatal ventricular arrhythmias
- PREGNANCY No evidence of harm in *animal* studies—manufacturer advises use only if potential benefit outweighs risk.
- BREAST FEEDING May suppress lactation—not known to be harmful.
- DIRECTIONS FOR ADMINISTRATION Dopamine concentrate for intravenous infusion to be diluted before use.
  For *intravenous infusion* give continuously in Glucose 5% or Sodium chloride 0.9%. Dilute to max. concentration of 3.2 mg/mL; incompatible with bicarbonate.

- MEDICINAL FORMS
There can be variation in the licensing of different medicines containing the same drug. Forms available from special-order manufacturers include: solution for infusion

Solution for infusion
▸ Dopamine hydrochloride (Non-proprietary)
  Dopamine hydrochloride 40 mg per 1 ml Dopamine 200mg/5ml solution for infusion ampoules | 5 ampoule PoM £19.42-£20.00 | 10 ampoule PoM £9.04
  Dopamine 200mg/5ml concentrate for solution for infusion ampoules | 10 ampoule PoM no price available
  Dopamine hydrochloride 160 mg per 1 ml Dopamine 800mg/5ml solution for infusion ampoules | 10 ampoule PoM £34.00

2

Cardiovascular system

SYMPATHOMIMETICS ⟩ VASOCONSTRICTOR

Metaraminol

● **INDICATIONS AND DOSE**

Acute hypotension
▶ BY INTRAVENOUS INFUSION
▸ Adult: 15–100 mg, adjusted according to response

Emergency treatment of acute hypotension
▶ INITIALLY BY INTRAVENOUS INJECTION
▸ Adult: Initially 0.5–5 mg, then (by intravenous infusion) 15–100 mg, adjusted according to response

● CONTRA-INDICATIONS Hypertension

● CAUTIONS Cirrhosis · coronary vascular thrombosis · diabetes mellitus · elderly · extravasation at injection site may cause necrosis · following myocardial infarction · hypercapnia · hyperthyroidism · hypoxia · mesenteric vascular thrombosis · peripheral vascular thrombosis · Prinzmetal's variant angina · uncorrected hypovolaemia

CAUTIONS, FURTHER INFORMATION
▸ Hypertensive response Metaraminol has a longer duration of action than noradrenaline, and an excessive vasopressor response may cause a prolonged rise in blood pressure.

● INTERACTIONS → Appendix 1 (sympathomimetics).

● SIDE-EFFECTS Angle-closure glaucoma · anorexia · anxiety · arrhythmias · bradycardia · confusion · dyspnoea · fatal ventricular arrhythmia reported in Laennec's cirrhosis · headache · hypertension · hypoxia · insomnia · nausea · palpitation · peripheral ischaemia · psychosis · tachycardia · tremor · urinary retention · vomiting · weakness

● PREGNANCY May reduce placental perfusion—manufacturer advises use only if potential benefit outweighs risk.

● BREAST FEEDING Manufacturer advises caution—no information available.

● MONITORING REQUIREMENTS Monitor blood pressure and rate of flow frequently.

● DIRECTIONS FOR ADMINISTRATION For *intravenous infusion* (*Aramine*®), give continuously or via drip tubing in Glucose 5% or Sodium chloride 0.9%. Suggested volume 500 mL.

● MEDICINAL FORMS
There can be variation in the licensing of different medicines containing the same drug. Forms available from special-order manufacturers include: solution for injection
Solution for injection
▸ Metaraminol (Non-proprietary)
Metaraminol (as Metaraminol tartrate) 10 mg per 1 ml Metaraminol 10mg/1ml solution for injection ampoules | 10 ampoule PoM £31.97

Midodrine hydrochloride   1.4.2016

● DRUG ACTION Midodrine hydrochloride is a pro-drug of desglymidodrine. Desglymidodrine is a sympathomimetic agent, which acts on peripheral alpha-adrenergic receptors to increase arterial resistance, resulting in an increase in blood pressure.

● **INDICATIONS AND DOSE**

Severe orthostatic hypotension due to autonomic dysfunction when corrective factors have been ruled out and other forms of treatment are inadequate
▶ BY MOUTH
▸ Adult: Initially 2.5 mg 3 times a day, increased if necessary up to 10 mg 3 times a day, dose to be increased at weekly intervals, according to blood

pressure measurements; usual maintenance 10 mg 3 times a day, avoid administration at night; the last daily dose should be taken at least 4 hours before bedtime

● CONTRA-INDICATIONS Aortic aneurysm · blood vessel spasm · bradycardia · cardiac conduction disturbances · cerebrovascular occlusion · congestive heart failure · hypertension · hyperthyroidism · myocardial infarction · narrow-angle glaucoma · pheochromocytoma · proliferative diabetic retinopathy · serious obliterative blood vessel disease · serious prostate disorder · urinary retention

● CAUTIONS Atherosclerotic cardiovascular disease (especially with symptoms of intestinal angina or claudication of the legs) · autonomic dysfunction · elderly (manufacturer recommends cautious dose titration) · prostate disorders

● INTERACTIONS → Appendix 1 (sympathomimetics).

● SIDE-EFFECTS
▶ **Common or very common** Chills · dyspepsia · flushing · headache · nausea · paraesthesia · piloerection · pruritus · rash · stomatitis · supine hypertension (dose dependent) · urinary disorders
▶ **Uncommon** Excitability · irritability · reflex bradycardia · restlessness · sleep disorders
▶ **Rare** Hepatic dysfunction · palpitations · tachycardia
▶ **Frequency not known** Abdominal pain · anxiety · confusion · diarrhoea · vomiting

SIDE-EFFECTS, FURTHER INFORMATION
▸ Supine hypertension Manufacturer advises that treatment must be stopped if supine hypertension is not controlled by reducing the dose.

● CONCEPTION AND CONTRACEPTION Manufacturer recommends effective contraception during treatment in women of childbearing potential.

● PREGNANCY Manufacturer advises avoid—toxicity in *animal* studies.

● BREAST FEEDING Manufacturer advises avoid—no information available.

● RENAL IMPAIRMENT Manufacturer advises avoid in severe or acute impairment.

● MONITORING REQUIREMENTS
▸ Manufacturer advises measure hepatic and renal function before treatment and at regular intervals during treatment.
▸ Manufacturer advises regular monitoring of supine and standing blood pressure due to the risk of hypertension in the supine position.

● PATIENT AND CARER ADVICE Manufacturer advises that patients report symptoms of supine hypertension (such as chest pain, palpitations, shortness of breath, headache and blurred vision) immediately. The risk of supine hypertension at night can be reduced by raising the head of the bed.

● MEDICINAL FORMS
There can be variation in the licensing of different medicines containing the same drug.
Tablet
▸ Midodrine hydrochloride (Non-proprietary)
Midodrine hydrochloride 2.5 mg Gutron 2.5mg tablets | 50 tablet PoM no price available
Midodrine hydrochloride 5 mg Gutron 5mg tablets | 50 tablet PoM no price available
▸ Bramox (Brancaster Pharma Ltd)
Midodrine hydrochloride 2.5 mg Bramox 2.5mg tablets | 100 tablet PoM £55.05 DT price = £55.05
Midodrine hydrochloride 5 mg Bramox 5mg tablets | 100 tablet PoM £75.05 DT price = £75.05

Noradrenaline/norepinephrine

- **INDICATIONS AND DOSE**

Acute hypotension
▶ BY INTRAVENOUS INFUSION
▸ Adult: Initially 0.16–0.33 mL/minute, adjusted according to response, to be given via central venous catheter, of a solution containing noradrenaline 40 micrograms(base)/mL

DOSE EQUIVALENCE AND CONVERSION
1 mg of noradrenaline base is equivalent to 2 mg of noradrenaline acid tartrate. **Doses expressed as the base.**

- **CONTRA-INDICATIONS** Hypertension
- **CAUTIONS** Coronary vascular thrombosis · diabetes mellitus · elderly · extravasation at injection site may cause necrosis · following myocardial infarction · hypercapnia · hyperthyroidism · hypoxia · mesenteric vascular thrombosis · peripheral vascular thrombosis · Prinzmetal's variant angina · uncorrected hypovolaemia
- **INTERACTIONS** → Appendix 1 (sympathomimetics).
- **SIDE-EFFECTS** Angle-closure glaucoma · anorexia · anxiety · arrhythmias · bradycardia · confusion · dyspnoea · headache · hypertension · hypoxia · insomnia · nausea · palpitation · peripheral ischaemia · psychosis · tachycardia · tremor · urinary retention · vomiting · weakness
- **PREGNANCY** Avoid—may reduce placental perfusion.
- **MONITORING REQUIREMENTS** Monitor blood pressure and rate of flow frequently.
- **DIRECTIONS FOR ADMINISTRATION** For treatment of acute hypotension in adults, use a solution containing noradrenaline 40 micrograms (base)/mL. For *intravenous infusion*, give continuously in Glucose 5% or Sodium Chloride and glucose via a controlled infusion device. For administration via syringe pump, dilute 2 mg (2 mL of solution) noradrenaline base with 48 mL infusion fluid. For administration via drip counter dilute 20 mg (20 mL of solution) noradrenaline base with 480 mL infusion fluid; give through a central venous catheter; incompatible with alkalis.
- **PRESCRIBING AND DISPENSING INFORMATION** For a period of time, preparations on the UK market may be described as either noradrenaline base or noradrenaline acid tartrate; doses in the BNF are expressed as the base.

- **MEDICINAL FORMS**
There can be variation in the licensing of different medicines containing the same drug. Forms available from special-order manufacturers include: infusion, solution for infusion

Solution for infusion
▶ Noradrenaline/norepinephrine (Non-proprietary)
  Noradrenaline (as Noradrenaline acid tartrate) 1 mg per 1 ml Noradrenaline (Norepinephrine) 4mg/4ml concentrate for solution for infusion ampoules | 10 ampoule PoM £44.00
  Noradrenaline (base) 8mg/8ml concentrate for solution for infusion ampoules | 10 ampoule PoM £116.00
  Noradrenaline (base) 2mg/2ml solution for infusion ampoules | 5 ampoule PoM £12.00 (Hospital only)
  Noradrenaline (base) 4mg/4ml solution for infusion ampoules | 5 ampoule PoM £22.00 (Hospital only)
  Noradrenaline (base) 4mg/4ml concentrate for solution for infusion ampoules | 10 ampoule PoM £58.00
  Noradrenaline (Norepinephrine) 2mg/2ml concentrate for solution for Infusion ampoules | 5 ampoule PoM £11.00

Phenylephrine hydrochloride

- **INDICATIONS AND DOSE**

Acute hypotension
▶ BY SUBCUTANEOUS INJECTION, OR BY INTRAMUSCULAR INJECTION
▸ Adult: Initially 2–5 mg, followed by 1–10 mg, after at least 15 minutes if required
▶ BY SLOW INTRAVENOUS INJECTION
▸ Adult: 100–500 micrograms, repeated as necessary after at least 15 minutes
▶ BY INTRAVENOUS INFUSION
▸ Adult: Initially up to 180 micrograms/minute, reduced to 30–60 micrograms/minute, adjusted according to response

- **CONTRA-INDICATIONS** Hypertension · severe hyperthyroidism
- **CAUTIONS** Coronary disease · coronary vascular thrombosis · diabetes · elderly · extravasation at injection site may cause necrosis · following myocardial infarction · hypercapnia · hyperthyroidism · hypoxia · mesenteric vascular thrombosis · peripheral vascular thrombosis · Prinzmetal's variant angina · susceptibility to angle-closure glaucoma · uncorrected hypovolaemia

  CAUTIONS, FURTHER INFORMATION
▸ Hypertensive response Phenylephrine has a longer duration of action than noradrenaline (norepinephrine), and an excessive vasopressor response may cause a prolonged rise in blood pressure.
- **INTERACTIONS** → Appendix 1 (sympathomimetics). Phenylephrine may interact with systemically administered monoamine-oxidase inhibitors.
- **SIDE-EFFECTS** Angle-closure glaucoma · anorexia · anxiety · arrhythmias · bradycardia (also reflex bradycardia) · confusion · dyspnoea · headache · hypertension · hypoxia · insomnia · nausea · palpitation · peripheral ischaemia · psychosis · tachycardia · tremor · urinary retention · vomiting · weakness
- **PREGNANCY** Avoid if possible; malformations reported following use in first trimester; fetal hypoxia and bradycardia reported in late pregnancy and labour.
- **MONITORING REQUIREMENTS** Contra-indicated in hypertension—monitor blood pressure and rate of flow frequently.
- **DIRECTIONS FOR ADMINISTRATION** For *intravenous infusion* give intermittently in Glucose 5% or Sodium chloride 0.9%. Dilute 10 mg in 500 mL infusion fluid.

- **MEDICINAL FORMS**
There can be variation in the licensing of different medicines containing the same drug. Forms available from special-order manufacturers include: solution for injection

Solution for injection
▶ Phenylephrine hydrochloride (Non-proprietary)
  Phenylephrine (as Phenylephrine hydrochloride) 50 microgram per 1 ml Phenylephrine 500micrograms/10ml solution for injection pre-filled syringes | 1 pre-filled disposable injection PoM £15.00 | 10 pre-filled disposable injection PoM £150.00
  Phenylephrine hydrochloride 100 microgram per 1 ml Phenylephrine 1mg/10ml solution for injection ampoules | 10 ampoule PoM £40.00
  Phenylephrine hydrochloride 10 mg per 1 ml Phenylephrine 10mg/1ml solution for injection ampoules | 10 ampoule PoM £99.12

2

Cardiovascular system

5 Heart failure

Heart failure

Drug treatment

Drug treatment of **heart failure** associated with a reduced left ventricular ejection fraction (left ventricular systolic dysfunction) is covered below; optimal management of heart failure with a preserved left ventricular ejection fraction has not been established.

The treatment of chronic heart failure aims to relieve symptoms, improve exercise tolerance, reduce the incidence of acute exacerbations, and reduce mortality. An **ACE inhibitor**, titrated to a 'target dose' (or the maximum tolerated dose if lower), together with a **beta-blocker**, form the basis of treatment for all patients with heart failure due to left ventricular systolic dysfunction.

An ACE inhibitor is generally advised for patients with asymptomatic left ventricular systolic dysfunction or symptomatic heart failure. An **angiotensin-II receptor antagonist** may be a useful alternative for patients who, because of side-effects such as cough, cannot tolerate ACE inhibitors; a relatively high dose of the angiotensin-II receptor antagonist may be required to produce benefit. Candesartan cilexetil p. 161 or valsartan p. 164 may be given under specialist supervision as adjuncts to an ACE inhibitor in the treatment of heart failure when other treatments are unsuitable; the concomitant use of this combination, together with an aldosterone antagonist or a potassium-sparing diuretic is not recommended. The combination of valsartan with sacubitril p. 176, an angiotensin-II receptor antagonist with a neprilysin inhibitor, may be a suitable alternative for those patients already stabilised on an ACE inhibitor or angiotensin-II receptor antagonist.

The beta-blockers bisoprolol fumarate p. 139 and carvedilol p. 134 are of value in any grade of stable heart failure due to left ventricular systolic dysfunction; nebivolol p. 141 is licensed for stable mild to moderate heart failure in patients over 70 years. Beta-blocker treatment should be started by those experienced in the management of heart failure, at a very low dose and titrated very slowly over a period of weeks or months. Symptoms may deteriorate initially, calling for adjustment of concomitant therapy.

The aldosterone antagonist spironolactone p. 175 can be added to an ACE inhibitor and a beta-blocker in patients who continue to remain symptomatic (particularly in those with moderate to severe heart failure); low doses of spironolactone reduce symptoms and mortality in these patients. If spironolactone cannot be used, eplerenone below may be considered for the management of heart failure after an acute myocardial infarction with evidence of left ventricular systolic dysfunction, or for chronic mild heart failure with left ventricular systolic dysfunction. Close monitoring of serum creatinine, eGFR, and potassium is necessary, particularly following any change in treatment or any change in the patient's clinical condition.

Patients who cannot tolerate an ACE inhibitor or an angiotensin-II receptor antagonist, or in whom they are contra-indicated, may be given isosorbide dinitrate p. 202 with hydralazine hydrochloride p. 166 but this combination may be poorly tolerated. The combination of isosorbide dinitrate and hydralazine hydrochloride may be considered in addition to standard therapy with an ACE inhibitor and a beta-blocker in patients who remain symptomatic (particularly in patients of African or Caribbean origin who have moderate to severe heart failure).

Digoxin p. 98 improves symptoms of heart failure and exercise tolerance and reduces hospitalisation due to acute exacerbations but it does not reduce mortality. Digoxin is reserved for patients with worsening or severe heart failure

due to left ventricular systolic dysfunction who remain symptomatic despite treatment with an ACE inhibitor and a beta-blocker in combination with either an aldosterone antagonist, candesartan cilexetil, or isosorbide dinitrate with hydralazine hydrochloride.

Patients with fluid overload should also receive either a loop or a thiazide diuretic (with salt or fluid restriction where appropriate). A **thiazide diuretic** may be of benefit in patients with mild heart failure and good renal function; however, thiazide diuretics are ineffective in patients with poor renal function (eGFR less than 30 mL/minute/1.73 m^2) and a **loop diuretic** is preferred. If diuresis with a single diuretic is insufficient, a combination of a loop diuretic and a thiazide diuretic may be tried; addition of metolazone p. 214 may also be considered but the resulting diuresis may be profound and care is needed to avoid potentially dangerous electrolyte disturbances.

> **Drugs used for Heart failure not listed below**
>
> Bendroflumethiazide, p. 152 · Captopril, p. 154 · Chlortalidone, p. 213 · Co-amilozide, p. 152 · Cyclopenthiazide, p. 214 · Enalapril maleate, p. 155 · Fosinopril sodium, p. 155 · Glyceryl trinitrate, p. 201 · Isosorbide mononitrate, p. 203 · Ivabradine, p. 194 · Lisinopril, p. 156 · Losartan potassium, p. 162 · Metoprolol tartrate, p. 140 · Perindopril arginine, p. 157 · Perindopril erbumine, p. 158 · Prazosin, p. 709 · Quinapril, p. 158 · Ramipril, p. 159 · Sodium nitroprusside, p. 168

DIURETICS 〉 POTASSIUM-SPARING DIURETICS 〉 ALDOSTERONE ANTAGONISTS

Co-flumactone

The properties listed below are those particular to the combination only. For the properties of the components please consider, spironolactone p. 175.

● **INDICATIONS AND DOSE**

Congestive heart failure
▸ BY MOUTH
▸ Adult: Initially 100/100 mg daily; maintenance 25/25–200/200 mg daily, maintenance dose not recommended because spironolactone generally given in lower dose

● **LESS SUITABLE FOR PRESCRIBING** Co-flumactone tablets are less suitable for prescribing.

● **MEDICINAL FORMS**
There can be variation in the licensing of different medicines containing the same drug.
Tablet
▸ Aldactide (Pfizer Ltd)
  Hydroflumethiazide 25 mg, Spironolactone 25 mg Aldactide 25 tablets | 100 tablet PoM £20.23 DT price = £20.23
  Hydroflumethiazide 50 mg, Spironolactone 50 mg Aldactide 50 tablets | 28 tablet PoM £10.70 | 100 tablet PoM £38.23 DT price = £38.23

Eplerenone

● **INDICATIONS AND DOSE**

Adjunct in stable patients with left ventricular ejection fraction ≤40% with evidence of heart failure, following myocardial infarction (start therapy within 3–14 days of event) | Adjunct in chronic mild heart failure with left ventricular ejection fraction ≤30%
▸ BY MOUTH
▸ Adult: Initially 25 mg daily, then increased to 50 mg daily, increased within 4 weeks of initial treatment

● **CONTRA-INDICATIONS** Hyperkalaemia

- CAUTIONS Elderly
- INTERACTIONS → Appendix 1 (diuretics).
  Concomitant use of potassium-sparing diuretics or potassium supplements is contra-indicated.
- SIDE-EFFECTS
  ▸ **Common or very common** Azotaemia · constipation · cough · diarrhoea · dizziness · hyperkalaemia · hypotension · muscle spasm · musculoskeletal pain · nausea · pruritus · rash · renal impairment · syncope
  ▸ **Uncommon** Arterial thrombosis · atrial fibrillation · back pain · cholecystitis · dehydration · dyslipidaemia · eosinophilia · epidermal growth factor receptor decreased · flatulence · gynaecomastia · headache · hyperglycaemia · hypoaesthesia · hyponatraemia · hypothyroidism · insomnia · malaise · pharyngitis · postural hypotension · pyelonephritis · sweating · tachycardia · vomiting
  ▸ **Frequency not known** Angioedema
- PREGNANCY Manufacturer advises caution—no information available.
- BREAST FEEDING Manufacturer advises use only if potential benefit outweighs risk.
- HEPATIC IMPAIRMENT Avoid in severe impairment.
- RENAL IMPAIRMENT Initially 25 mg on alternate days if eGFR 30–60 mL/minute/1.73 m², adjust dose according to serum-potassium concentration—consult product literature. Avoid if eGFR less than 30 mL/minute/1.73 m². Increased risk of hyperkalaemia in renal impairment—close monitoring required.
- MONITORING REQUIREMENTS Monitor plasma-potassium concentration before treatment, during initiation, and when dose changed.

- MEDICINAL FORMS
  There can be variation in the licensing of different medicines containing the same drug.
  Tablet
  ▸ Eplerenone (Non-proprietary)
    Eplerenone 25 mg Eplerenone 25mg tablets | 28 tablet PoM £42.72 DT price = £12.33
    Eplerenone 50 mg Eplerenone 50mg tablets | 28 tablet PoM £42.72 DT price = £12.60
  ▸ Inspra (Pfizer Ltd)
    Eplerenone 25 mg Inspra 25mg tablets | 28 tablet PoM £42.72 DT price = £12.33
    Eplerenone 50 mg Inspra 50mg tablets | 28 tablet PoM £42.72 DT price = £12.60

Spironolactone

- INDICATIONS AND DOSE
  Oedema | Ascites in cirrhosis of the liver
  ▸ BY MOUTH
  ▸ Adult: 100–400 mg daily, adjusted according to response
  Malignant ascites
  ▸ BY MOUTH
  ▸ Adult: Initially 100–200 mg daily, then increased if necessary to 400 mg daily, maintenance dose adjusted according to response
  Nephrotic syndrome
  ▸ BY MOUTH
  ▸ Adult: 100–200 mg daily
  Oedema in congestive heart failure
  ▸ BY MOUTH
  ▸ Adult: Initially 100 mg daily, alternatively initially 25–200 mg daily, dose may be taken as a single dose or divided doses, maintenance dose adjusted according to response

Moderate to severe heart failure (adjunct)
  ▸ BY MOUTH
  ▸ Adult: Initially 25 mg once daily, then adjusted according to response to 50 mg once daily
Resistant hypertension (adjunct)
  ▸ BY MOUTH
  ▸ Adult: 25 mg once daily
Primary hyperaldosteronism in patients awaiting surgery
  ▸ BY MOUTH
  ▸ Adult: 100–400 mg daily, may be used for long-term maintenance if surgery inappropriate, use lowest effective dose

- UNLICENSED USE Resistant hypertension (adjunct) unlicensed indication.
- CONTRA-INDICATIONS Addison's disease · anuria · hyperkalaemia
- CAUTIONS Acute porphyrias p. 918 · elderly · potential metabolic products carcinogenic in *rodents*
- INTERACTIONS → Appendix 1 (diuretics).
  Potassium supplements must **not** be given with potassium-sparing diuretics.
  Administration of a potassium-sparing diuretic to a patient receiving an ACE inhibitor or an angiotensin-II receptor antagonist can also cause severe hyperkalaemia.
- SIDE-EFFECTS Acute renal failure · agranulocytosis · alopecia · benign breast tumour · breast pain · changes in libido · confusion · dizziness · drowsiness · electrolyte disturbances · gastro-intestinal disturbances · gynaecomastia · hepatotoxicity · hyperkalaemia (discontinue) · hypertrichosis · hyperuricaemia · hyponatraemia · leg cramps · leucopenia · malaise · menstrual disturbances · rash · Stevens-Johnson syndrome · thrombocytopenia
- PREGNANCY Use only if potential benefit outweighs risk—feminisation of male fetus in *animal* studies.
- BREAST FEEDING Metabolites present in milk, but amount probably too small to be harmful.
- RENAL IMPAIRMENT Avoid in acute renal insufficiency or severe impairment. Monitor plasma-potassium concentration (high risk of hyperkalaemia in renal impairment).
- MONITORING REQUIREMENTS Monitor electrolytes—discontinue if hyperkalaemia occurs (in *severe heart failure* monitor potassium and creatinine 1 week after initiation and after any dose increase, monthly for first 3 months, then every 3 months for 1 year, and then every 6 months).

- MEDICINAL FORMS
  There can be variation in the licensing of different medicines containing the same drug. Forms available from special-order manufacturers include: oral suspension, oral solution
  Tablet
  CAUTIONARY AND ADVISORY LABELS 21
  ▸ Spironolactone (Non-proprietary)
    Spironolactone 25 mg Spironolactone 25mg tablets | 28 tablet PoM £1.95 DT price = £1.23
    Spironolactone 50 mg Spironolactone 50mg tablets | 28 tablet PoM £6.00 DT price = £1.74
    Spironolactone 100 mg Spironolactone 100mg tablets | 28 tablet PoM £6.24 DT price = £2.04 | 30 tablet PoM no price available
  ▸ Aldactone (Pfizer Ltd)
    Spironolactone 25 mg Aldactone 25mg tablets | 100 tablet PoM £8.89
    Spironolactone 50 mg Aldactone 50mg tablets | 100 tablet PoM £17.78
    Spironolactone 100 mg Aldactone 100mg tablets | 28 tablet PoM £9.96 DT price = £2.04 | 100 tablet PoM £35.56

2 Cardiovascular system

DRUGS ACTING ON THE RENIN-ANGIOTENSIN SYSTEM > ANGIOTENSIN II RECEPTOR ANTAGONISTS

Valsartan with sacubitril

17.6.2016

The properties listed below are those particular to the combination only. For the properties of the components please consider, valsartan p. 164.

- DRUG ACTION Sacubitril (a prodrug) inhibits the breakdown of natriuretic peptides resulting in varied effects including increased diuresis, natriuresis, and vasodilation.

- INDICATIONS AND DOSE

Symptomatic chronic heart failure with reduced ejection fraction (in patients not currently taking an ACE inhibitor or angiotensin II receptor antagonist, or stabilised on low doses of either of these agents)
- BY MOUTH
- Adult: Initially 26/24 mg twice daily for 3–4 weeks, increased if tolerated to 51/49 mg twice daily for 3–4 weeks, then increased if tolerated to 103/97 mg twice daily

Symptomatic chronic heart failure with reduced ejection fraction (in patients currently stabilised on an ACE inhibitor or angiotensin II receptor antagonist)
- BY MOUTH
- Adult: Initially 51/49 mg twice daily for 2–4 weeks, increased if tolerated to 103/97 mg twice daily, consider a starting dose of 26/24 mg if systolic blood pressure less than 110 mmHg

DOSE EQUIVALENCE AND CONVERSION
Entresto® tablets contain valsartan and sacubitril; the proportions are expressed in the form x/y where x and y are the strength in milligrams of valsartan and sacubitril respectively. Valsartan, in this formulation, is more bioavailable than other tablet formulations—26 mg, 51 mg, and 103 mg valsartan is equivalent to 40 mg, 80 mg and 160 mg, respectively. Furthermore, note that the 26/24 mg, 51/49 mg and 103/97 mg strengths are sometimes referred to as a total of both drug strengths, that is, 50 mg, 100 mg and 200 mg, respectively.

- CONTRA-INDICATIONS Concomitant use of ACE inhibitor (separate administration by 36 hours) · systolic blood pressure less than 100 mmHg
- INTERACTIONS → Appendix 1 (angiotensin-II receptor antagonists, sacubitril)
- SIDE-EFFECTS
- Common or very common Anaemia · diarrhoea · gastritis · hypoglycaemia · hypokalaemia · nausea · vertigo
- PREGNANCY Manufacturer advises avoid—toxicity with sacubitril in *animal* studies.
- BREAST FEEDING Manufacturer advises avoid—present in milk in *animal* studies.
- HEPATIC IMPAIRMENT Manufacturer advises starting dose of 26/24 mg twice daily in moderate impairment. Contra-indicated in severe impairment.
- RENAL IMPAIRMENT Manufacturer recommends a starting dose of 26/24 mg twice daily if eGFR less than 30 mL/minute/1.73m². Also consider this starting dose if eGFR 30 to 60 mL/minute/1.73m².
- NATIONAL FUNDING/ACCESS DECISIONS

NICE technology appraisals (TAs)
- Sacubitril valsartan for treating symptomatic chronic heart failure with reduced ejection fraction (April 2016) NICE TA388 Sacubitril valsartan is recommended as an option for treating symptomatic chronic heart failure with reduced ejection fraction, only in adults:

- with New York Heart Association class II to IV symptoms **and**
- a left ventricular ejection fraction of 35% or less **and**
- who are already taking a stable dose of an ACE inhibitor or angiotensin II receptor antagonist.
www.nice.org.uk/ta388

- MEDICINAL FORMS There can be variation in the licensing of different medicines containing the same drug.
Tablet
- Entresto (Novartis Pharmaceuticals UK Ltd) ▼
  Sacubitril 24 mg, Valsartan 26 mg Entresto 24mg/26mg tablets | 28 tablet [PoM] £45.78
  Sacubitril 49 mg, Valsartan 51 mg Entresto 49mg/51mg tablets | 28 tablet [PoM] £45.78 | 56 tablet [PoM] £91.56
  Sacubitril 97 mg, Valsartan 103 mg Entresto 97mg/103mg tablets | 56 tablet [PoM] £91.56

PHOSPHODIESTERASE TYPE-3 INHIBITORS

Enoximone

- DRUG ACTION Enoximone is a phosphodiesterase type-3 inhibitor that exerts most effect on the myocardium; it has positive inotropic properties and vasodilator activity.

- INDICATIONS AND DOSE

Congestive heart failure where cardiac output reduced and filling pressures increased
- BY SLOW INTRAVENOUS INJECTION
- Adult: Initially 0.5–1 mg/kg, rate not exceeding 12.5 mg/minute, then 500 micrograms/kg every 30 minutes until satisfactory response or total of 3 mg/kg given; maintenance, initial dose of up to 3 mg/kg may be repeated every 3–6 hours as required
- BY INTRAVENOUS INFUSION
- Adult: Initially 90 micrograms/kg/minute, dose to be given over 10–30 minutes, followed by 5–20 micrograms/kg/minute, dose to be given as either a continuous or intermittent infusion; maximum 24 mg/kg per day

- CAUTIONS Heart failure associated with hypertrophic cardiomyopathy, stenotic or obstructive valvular disease or other outlet obstruction
- INTERACTIONS → Appendix 1 (phosphodiesterase type-3 inhibitors).
- SIDE-EFFECTS Chills · diarrhoea · ectopic beats · fever · headache · hypotension · insomnia · nausea · oliguria · supraventricular arrhythmias (more likely in patients with pre-existing arrhythmias) · upper and lower limb pain · urinary retention · ventricular tachycardia (more likely in patients with pre-existing arrhythmias) · vomiting
- PREGNANCY Manufacturer advises use only if potential benefit outweighs risk.
- BREAST FEEDING Manufacturer advises caution—no information available.
- HEPATIC IMPAIRMENT Dose reduction may be required.
- RENAL IMPAIRMENT Consider dose reduction.
- MONITORING REQUIREMENTS Monitor blood pressure, heart rate, ECG, central venous pressure, fluid and electrolyte status, renal function, platelet count and hepatic enzymes.
- DIRECTIONS FOR ADMINISTRATION Incompatible with glucose solutions. Use only plastic containers or syringes; crystal formation if glass used. Avoid extravasation.
  For *intravenous infusion* (Perfan®), give continuously or intermittently in Sodium chloride 0.9% or Water for injections; dilute to a concentration of 2.5 mg/mL.
- PRESCRIBING AND DISPENSING INFORMATION Sustained haemodynamic benefit has been observed after

administration of phosphodiesterase type-3 inhibitors, but there is no evidence of any beneficial effect on survival.

● MEDICINAL FORMS
There can be variation in the licensing of different medicines containing the same drug.
Solution for injection
EXCIPIENTS: May contain Alcohol, propylene glycol
▸ Perfan (Myogen GmbH)
  Enoximone 5 mg per 1 ml Perfan 100mg/20ml solution for injection
  ampoules | 10 ampoule [PoM] no price available (Hospital only)

Milrinone

● DRUG ACTION Milrinone is a phosphodiesterase type-3 inhibitor that exerts most effect on the myocardium; it has positive inotropic properties and vasodilator activity.

● INDICATIONS AND DOSE

Short-term treatment of severe congestive heart failure unresponsive to conventional maintenance therapy (not immediately after myocardial infarction) | Acute heart failure, including low output states following heart surgery
▸ INITIALLY BY INTRAVENOUS INJECTION
▸ Adult: Initially 50 micrograms/kg, given over 10 minutes, followed by (by intravenous infusion) 375–750 nanograms/kg/minute usually given following surgery for up to 12 hours or in congestive heart failure for 48-72 hours; maximum 1.13 mg/kg per day

● CONTRA-INDICATIONS Severe hypovolaemia

● CAUTIONS Correct hypokalaemia · heart failure associated with hypertrophic cardiomyopathy, stenotic or obstructive valvular disease or other outlet obstruction

● INTERACTIONS → Appendix 1 (phosphodiesterase type-3 inhibitors).

● SIDE-EFFECTS
▸ **Common or very common** Ectopic beats · headache · hypotension · supraventricular arrhythmias (more likely in patients with pre-existing arrhythmias) · ventricular tachycardia
▸ **Uncommon** Chest pain · hypokalaemia · thrombocytopenia · tremor · ventricular fibrillation
▸ **Very rare** Anaphylaxis · bronchospasm · rash

● PREGNANCY Manufacturer advises use only if potential benefit outweighs risk.

● BREAST FEEDING Manufacturer advises avoid—no information available.

● RENAL IMPAIRMENT Reduce dose and monitor response if eGFR less than 50 mL/minute/1.73 m^2—consult product literature for details.

● MONITORING REQUIREMENTS Monitor blood pressure, heart rate, ECG, central venous pressure, fluid and electrolyte status, renal function, platelet count and hepatic enzymes.

● DIRECTIONS FOR ADMINISTRATION Avoid extravasation. For *intravenous injection*, may be given either undiluted or diluted before use. For *intravenous infusion* (Primacor®) give continuously in Glucose 5% or Sodium chloride 0.9%; dilute to a suggested concentration of 200 micrograms/mL.

● PRESCRIBING AND DISPENSING INFORMATION Sustained haemodynamic benefit has been observed after administration of phosphodiesterase type-3 inhibitors, but there is no evidence of any beneficial effect on survival.

● MEDICINAL FORMS
There can be variation in the licensing of different medicines containing the same drug. Forms available from special-order manufacturers include: solution for infusion
Solution for injection
▸ Primacor (Sanofi)
  Milrinone 1 mg per 1 ml Primacor 10mg/10ml solution for injection
  ampoules | 10 ampoule [PoM] £199.06

SYMPATHOMIMETICS ⟩ INOTROPIC

Dopexamine hydrochloride

● DRUG ACTION Dopexamine acts on beta$_2$ receptors in cardiac muscle to produce a positive inotropic effect; and on peripheral dopamine receptors to increase renal perfusion; it is reported not to induce vasoconstriction.

● INDICATIONS AND DOSE

Inotropic support and vasodilator in exacerbations of chronic heart failure and in heart failure associated with cardiac surgery
▸ BY INTRAVENOUS INFUSION
▸ Adult: 0.5 microgram/kg/minute, to be administered into central or large peripheral vein, then increased if necessary to 1 microgram/kg/minute, increased if necessary up to 6 micrograms/kg/minute, in increments of 0.5–1 microgram/kg/minute at intervals of not less than 15 minutes

● CONTRA-INDICATIONS Aortic stenosis · hypertrophic cardiomyopathy · left ventricular outlet obstruction · phaeochromocytoma · thrombocytopenia

● CAUTIONS Correct hypovolaemia before starting and during treatment · hyperglycaemia · hyperthyroidism · hypokalaemia · myocardial infarction · recent angina

● INTERACTIONS → Appendix 1 (sympathomimetics).

● SIDE-EFFECTS
▸ **Common or very common** Angina · arrhythmias · bradycardia · dyspnoea · headache · myocardial infarction · nausea · reversible thrombocytopenia · sweating · tachycardia · tremor · vomiting

● PREGNANCY No information available—manufacturer advises avoid.

● MONITORING REQUIREMENTS Monitor blood pressure, pulse, plasma potassium, and blood glucose.

● TREATMENT CESSATION Avoid abrupt withdrawal.

● DIRECTIONS FOR ADMINISTRATION Concentrate for intravenous infusion to be diluted before use. For *continuous intravenous infusion*, dilute to a concentration of 400 or 800 micrograms/mL with Glucose 5% or Sodium Chloride 0.9%; max. concentration via large peripheral vein 1 mg/mL, concentrations up to 4 mg/mL may be infused via central vein; give via infusion pump or other device which provides accurate control of rate; contact with metal in infusion apparatus should be minimised; incompatible with bicarbonate.

● MEDICINAL FORMS
There can be variation in the licensing of different medicines containing the same drug.
Solution for infusion
▸ Dopacard (Teva UK Ltd)
  Dopexamine hydrochloride 10 mg per 1 ml Dopacard 50mg/5ml
  concentrate for solution for infusion ampoules | 10 ampoule [PoM]
  £252.00 (Hospital only)

6   Hyperlipidaemia

Lipid-regulating drugs

Primary and secondary prevention of cardiovascular disease

Preventative measures should be taken in individuals with a high risk of developing cardiovascular disease (primary prevention) and to prevent recurrence of events in those with established cardiovascular disease (secondary prevention).

Primary prevention

Individuals at high risk of developing cardiovascular disease include those who have diabetes mellitus, chronic kidney disease (eGFR < 60 mL/minute/1.73 m^2) and/or albuminuria, and those with familial hypercholesterolaemia. The risk also increases with age; those aged 85 years and over are at particularly high risk, especially if they smoke or have hypertension. Preventative measures are also required for other individuals who are considered to be at high risk of developing atherosclerotic cardiovascular disease based on risk estimated using risk calculators (see Risk calculators); those with a 10-year risk of cardiovascular disease of 10% or more stand to benefit most from drug treatment. Patients with a 10-year cardiovascular risk of less than 10% may benefit from an assessment of their lifetime risk (using the JBS3 tool—see Risk calculators for more detail), discussion on the impact of lifestyle interventions and, if necessary, drug therapy.

Risk calculators

Risk assessment calculators are recommended by both NICE (clinical guideline 181 (July 2014). Lipid Modification—Cardiovascular risk assessment and the modification of blood lipids for the primary and secondary prevention of cardiovascular disease) and JBS3 (Joint British Societies' consensus recommendations for the prevention of cardiovascular disease 2014). They should not be used in patients at high cardiovascular risk. Both calculators are unsuitable for assessing risk in those aged 85 years and over, and NICE advises against using a risk assessment tool in those with type 1 diabetes mellitus.

The QRISK®2 risk calculator www.qrisk.org/ is recommended by NICE clinical guideline 181, and the JBS3 risk calculator www.jbs3risk.com/pages/risk_calculator.htm is endorsed by JBS3. Both tools assess cardiovascular risk—coronary heart disease (angina and myocardial infarction), stroke, and transient ischaemic attack, on the basis of lipid profile, systolic blood pressure, gender, age, ethnicity, smoking status, BMI, chronic kidney disease, diabetes mellitus, atrial fibrillation, treated hypertension, rheumatoid arthritis, or a family history of premature cardiovascular disease. Risk assessment tools underestimate risk in patients with additional risk due to existing conditions or medication, such as:

- serious mental disorder
- autoimmune disorders such as systemic lupus erythematosus and other systemic inflammatory disorders
- antiretroviral treatment
- medication causing dyslipidaemia as a side-effect e.g. antipsychotics, corticosteroids, or immunosuppressants
- triglyceride concentration > 4.5 mmol/litre

Cardiovascular disease risk is also underestimated in those who are already taking antihypertensive or lipid-regulating drugs, and in those who have recently stopped smoking. Severe obesity (BMI > 40 kg/m^2) also increases cardiovascular risk; the need for further treatment of risk

factors in patients below the cardiovascular risk threshold for treatment should be based on clinical judgement.

Preventative measures for primary prevention

All patients at high risk of cardiovascular disease should be advised to make lifestyle modifications that include beneficial changes to diet, exercise, weight management, alcohol consumption, and smoking cessation.

Offer a statin as first-line drug treatment if lifestyle modifications are inappropriate or ineffective (see also Statins for the prevention of cardiovascular disease). Lipid-regulating drug treatment must be combined with advice on diet and lifestyle measures, and where appropriate, treatment of comorbidities and secondary causes of dyslipidaemia.

Secondary prevention

Statins should be offered to all patients, including the elderly, with cardiovascular disease such as those with coronary heart disease (including history of angina or acute myocardial infarction), occlusive arterial disease (including peripheral vascular disease, non-haemorrhagic stroke, or transient ischaemic attacks).

Preventative measures for secondary prevention

Patients should be advised to make lifestyle modifications that include beneficial changes to diet, exercise, weight management, alcohol consumption, and smoking cessation, however, initiation of lipid-regulating drug treatment should not be delayed to manage modifiable risk factors, and must be combined with advice on diet and lifestyle measures, and where appropriate, treatment of co-morbidities and secondary causes of dyslipidaemia.

Statins for the prevention of cardiovascular disease

A statin reduces the risk of cardiovascular disease events, and is the drug of first choice for primary and secondary prevention of cardiovascular disease. Before starting treatment with statins, secondary causes of dyslipidaemia should be addressed; these include uncontrolled diabetes mellitus, hepatic disease, nephrotic syndrome, and excessive alcohol consumption. Patients with hypothyroidism should receive adequate thyroid replacement therapy (before assessing the requirement for lipid-regulating treatment if for primary prevention) because correcting hypothyroidism itself may resolve the lipid abnormality. Untreated hypothyroidism increases the risk of myositis with lipid-regulating drugs.

For the purpose of reducing cardiovascular risk, NICE Clinical Guideline 181 (NICE clinical guideline 181 (July 2014). Lipid Modification—Cardiovascular risk assessment and the modification of blood lipids for the primary and secondary prevention of cardiovascular disease) defines statins by the percentage reduction in LDL-cholesterol they achieve:

For *primary prevention*, NICE Clinical Guideline 181 recommends that atorvastatin p. 186 a high-intensity statin (when prescribed at a dose of at least 20 mg/day), should be offered to those with a 10-year risk of cardiovascular disease of 10% or more; patients aged 85 years and over may benefit from atorvastatin to reduce the risk of non-fatal myocardial infarction. For *secondary prevention*, atorvastatin is also recommended. Patients taking a low- or medium-intensity statin should discuss the benefits and risks of switching to a high intensity statin at their next medication review.

A statin should be considered for *all* adults with type 1 diabetes mellitus, particularly those aged 40 years and over, or who have had diabetes for more than 10 years, or who have established nephropathy, or other risk factors for cardiovascular disease. JBS3 recommendations (Joint British Societies' consensus recommendations for the prevention of cardiovascular disease (JBS3) 2014) in diabetes mellitus differ in certain respects from NICE Clinical Guideline 181 (NICE clinical guideline 181 (July 2014). Lipid Modification—Cardiovascular risk assessment and the modification of blood lipids for the primary and secondary prevention of cardiovascular disease)—see JBS3 recommendations for further details. In type 2 diabetes, assess level of risk using the risk calculator and treat for primary prevention if necessary.

Total cholesterol, HDL-cholesterol, and non-HDL cholesterol concentrations should be checked 3 months after starting treatment with a high intensity statin. NICE Clinical Guideline 181 recommends aiming for a reduction in non-HDL cholesterol concentration greater than 40%; JBS3 recommends a target non-HDL cholesterol concentration below 2.5 mol/litre. If these are not achieved, ensure lifestyle modifications are optimised and consider increasing the dose of the statin if started on less than atorvastatin 80 mg and the patient is judged to be at higher risk because of comorbidities, risk score or, using clinical judgement.

Specialist advice should be sought about treatment options for patients at high risk of cardiovascular disease or those with existing cardiovascular disease, who are intolerant of three different statins.

Fibrates should not be routinely used for primary or secondary prevention. Nicotinic acid p. 184, **bile acid sequestrants**, and **omega-3 fatty acid compounds** are not recommended for primary or secondary prevention.

Hypercholesterolaemia, hypertriglyceridaemia, and familial hypercholesterolaemia

A statin is also the drug of first choice for treating hypercholesterolaemia and moderate hypertriglyceridaemia. Severe hyperlipidaemia not adequately controlled with a maximal dose of a statin may require the use of an additional lipid-regulating drug such as ezetimibe p. 181; such treatment should generally be supervised by a specialist.

A number of conditions, some familial, are characterised by very high LDL-cholesterol concentration, high triglyceride concentration, or both. Fenofibrate p. 183 may be added to statin therapy if triglycerides remain high even after the LDL-cholesterol concentration has been reduced adequately; nicotinic acidmay also be used to further lower triglyceride or LDL-cholesterol concentration.

Combination of a statin with a fibrate or with nicotinic acid carries an increased risk of side-effects (including rhabdomyolysis) and should be under specialist supervision; monitoring of liver function and creatine kinase should also be considered. The concomitant administration of gemfibrozil with a statin increases the risk of rhabdomyolysis considerably—this combination should **not** be used.

A statin is recommended for all patients with familial hypercholesterolaemia. A 'high-intensity' statin (as defined in NICE Clinical Guideline 71, August 2008. Identification and management of familial hypercholesterolaemia) e.g. rosuvastatin p. 188 (initiated by a specialist) or atorvastatin p. 186 should be considered in order to achieve the recommended reduction in LDL-cholesterol concentration of greater than 50% from baseline; a 'high-intensity' statin is one that produces a greater LDL-cholesterol reduction than simvastatin 40 mg. Patients with heterozygous familial hypercholesterolaemia who have contra-indications to, or are intolerant of, statins should receive ezetimibe. The combination of a statin and ezetimibe can be considered if a statin alone fails to provide adequate control (or if intolerance limits dose titration), and when a switch to an alternative statin is being considered. Patients for whom statins and ezetimibe are inappropriate, should be referred to a specialist for the consideration of treatment with a bile acid sequestrant, nicotinic acid, or a fibrate.

The prescribing of drug therapy in homozygous familial hypercholesterolaemia should be undertaken in a specialist centre.

Reduction in low-density lipoprotein cholesterol

Therapy intensity	Drug	Daily dose (reduction in LDL cholesterol)
High-intensity	Atorvastatin	20mg (43%)
		40mg (49%)
		80mg (55%)
	Rosuvastatin	10mg (43%)
		20mg (48%)
		40mg (53%)
	Simvastatin	80mg (42%)
Medium-intensity	Atorvastatin	10mg (37%)
	Fluvastatin	80mg (33%)
	Rosuvastatin	5mg (38%)
	Simvastatin	20mg (32%)
		40mg (37%)
Low-intensity	Fluvastatin	20mg (21%)
		40mg (27%)
	Pravastatin	10mg (20%)
		20mg (24%)
		40mg (29%)
	Simvastatin	10mg (27%)

Advice from the MHRA: there is an increased risk of myopathy associated with high-dose (80 mg) simvastatin. The 80 mg dose should be considered only in patients with severe hypercholesterolaemia and high risk of cardiovascular complications who have not achieved their treatment goals on lower doses, when the benefits are expected to outweigh the potential risks.

Statins

Statins are more effective than other lipid-regulating drugs at lowering LDL-cholesterol concentration but they are less effective than the fibrates in reducing triglyceride concentration. However, statins reduce cardiovascular disease events and total mortality irrespective of the initial cholesterol concentration.

Bile acid sequestrants

Bile acid sequestrants effectively reduce LDL-cholesterol but can aggravate hypertriglyceridaemia. Treatment with bile acid sequestrants may be appropriate under specialist supervision if statins and ezetimibe are inappropriate, and when LDL-cholesterol is severely raised, for example in familial hypercholesterolaemia.

Fibrates

Fibrates are mainly used in those whose serum-triglyceride concentration is greater than 10 mol/litre or in those who cannot tolerate a statin (specialist use).

Lomitapide

Lomitapide p. 189 is licensed as an adjunct to dietary measures and other lipid-regulating drugs for the treatment of homozygous familial hypercholesterolaemia.

Nicotinic acid group

The value of nicotinic acid is limited by its side-effects, especially vasodilatation.

Nicotinic acid is used by specialists in combination with a statin if the statin alone cannot adequately control dyslipidaemia (raised LDL-cholesterol, triglyceridaemia, and low HDL-cholesterol).

Acipimox p. 184 seems to have fewer side-effects than nicotinic acid but may be less effective in its lipid-regulating capabilities.

Omega-3 fatty acid compounds

There is no evidence that omega-3 fatty acid compounds reduce the risk of cardiovascular disease.

> **Drugs used for Hyperlipidaemia not listed below** Inositol nicotinate, p. 216

LIPID MODIFYING DRUGS > BILE ACID
SEQUESTRANTS

Bile acid sequestrants

- DRUG ACTION Bile acid sequestrants act by binding bile acids, preventing their reabsorption; this promotes hepatic conversion of cholesterol into bile acids; the resultant increased LDL-receptor activity of liver cells increases the clearance of LDL-cholesterol from the plasma.
- CAUTIONS Interference with the absorption of fat-soluble vitamins (supplements of vitamins A, D, K, and folic acid may be required when treatment is prolonged).
- SIDE-EFFECTS Constipation · diarrhoea · gastro-intestinal discomfort · hypertriglyceridaemia (aggravation) · hypoprothrombinaemia associated with vitamin K deficiency · increased risk of bleeding · nausea · vomiting
- PREGNANCY Bile acid sequestrants should be used with caution as although the drugs are not absorbed, they may cause fat-soluble vitamin deficiency on prolonged use.
- BREAST FEEDING Bile acid sequestrants should be used with caution as although the drugs are not absorbed, they may cause fat-soluble vitamin deficiency on prolonged use.

⌐ above

Colesevelam hydrochloride

- INDICATIONS AND DOSE

Primary hypercholesterolaemia as an adjunct to dietary measures (monotherapy)
▸ BY MOUTH
▸ Adult: 3.75 g daily in 1–2 divided doses; maximum 4.375 g per day

Primary hypercholesterolaemia as an adjunct to dietary measures, in combination with a statin | Primary and familial hypercholesterolaemia, in combination with ezetimibe, either with or without a statin
▸ BY MOUTH
▸ Adult: 2.5–3.75 g daily in 1–2 divided doses, may be taken at the same time as the statin and ezetimibe

- CONTRA-INDICATIONS Biliary obstruction · bowel obstruction
- CAUTIONS Gastro-intestinal motility disorders · inflammatory bowel disease · major gastro-intestinal surgery
- INTERACTIONS → Appendix 1 (colesevelam).
- SIDE-EFFECTS Headache · myalgia
- HEPATIC IMPAIRMENT Manufacturer advises caution.
- MONITORING REQUIREMENTS Patients receiving ciclosporin should have their blood-ciclosporin concentration monitored before, during, and after treatment with colesevelam.
- DIRECTIONS FOR ADMINISTRATION Other drugs should be taken at least 4 hours before or after colesevelam to reduce possible interference with absorption.
- PATIENT AND CARER ADVICE Patient counselling on administration is advised for colesevelam hydrochloride tablets (avoid other drugs at same time).

- MEDICINAL FORMS
There can be variation in the licensing of different medicines containing the same drug.
Tablet
CAUTIONARY AND ADVISORY LABELS 21
▸ Cholestagel (Sanofi)
Colesevelam hydrochloride 625 mg Cholestagel 625mg tablets | 180 tablet [PoM] £96.10 DT price = £96.10

⌐ above

Colestipol hydrochloride

- INDICATIONS AND DOSE

Hyperlipidaemias, particularly type IIa, in patients who have not responded adequately to diet and other appropriate measures
▸ BY MOUTH
▸ Adult: Initially 5 g 1–2 times a day, increased in steps of 5 g every 1 month if required, total daily dose may be given in 1–2 divided doses; maximum 30 g per day

- INTERACTIONS → Appendix 1 (colestipol).
- DIRECTIONS FOR ADMINISTRATION The contents of each sachet should be mixed with at least 100 mL of water or other suitable liquid such as fruit juice or skimmed milk; alternatively it can be mixed with thin soups, cereals, yoghurt, or pulpy fruits ensuring at least 100 mL of liquid is provided.
  Other drugs should be taken at least 1 hour before or 4–6 hours after colestipol to reduce possible interference with absorption.
- PATIENT AND CARER ADVICE Patient counselling on administration is advised for colestipol hydrochloride granules (avoid other drugs at same time).

- MEDICINAL FORMS
There can be variation in the licensing of different medicines containing the same drug.
Tablet
▸ Colestipol hydrochloride (Non-proprietary)
Colestipol hydrochloride 1 gram Colestid 1g tablets | 120 tablet [PoM] no price available
Granules
CAUTIONARY AND ADVISORY LABELS 13
▸ Colestid (Pfizer Ltd)
Colestipol hydrochloride 5 gram Colestid 5g granules sachets plain sugar-free | 30 sachet [PoM] £15.05
Colestid Orange 5g granules sachets sugar-free | 30 sachet [PoM] £15.05

⌐ above

Colestyramine

(Cholestyramine)

- INDICATIONS AND DOSE

Hyperlipidaemias, particularly type IIa, in patients who have not responded adequately to diet and other appropriate measures | Primary prevention of coronary heart disease in men aged 35–59 years with primary hypercholesterolaemia who have not responded to diet and other appropriate measures
▸ BY MOUTH
▸ Adult: Initially 4 g daily, increased in steps of 4 g every 1 week; increased to 12–24 g daily in 1–4 divided doses, adjusted according to response; maximum 36 g per day

Pruritus associated with partial biliary obstruction and primary biliary cirrhosis
▸ BY MOUTH
▸ Adult: 4–8 g once daily

Diarrhoea associated with Crohn's disease, ileal resection, vagotomy, diabetic vagal neuropathy, and radiation
▸ BY MOUTH
▸ Adult: Initially 4 g daily, increased in steps of 4 g every 1 week; increased to 12–24 g daily in 1–4 divided doses, adjusted according to response, if no response within 3 days an alternative therapy should be initiated; maximum 36 g per day

Accelerated elimination of teriflunomide
▸ BY MOUTH
▸ Adult: 8 g 3 times a day for 11 days; reduced to 4 g 3 times a day, dose should only be reduced if not tolerated

Accelerated elimination of leflunomide (washout procedure)
▸ BY MOUTH
▸ Adult: 8 g 3 times a day for 11 days

● CONTRA-INDICATIONS Complete biliary obstruction (not likely to be effective)
● INTERACTIONS → Appendix 1 (colestyramine).
● SIDE-EFFECTS
▸ **Rare** Intestinal obstruction
▸ **Frequency not known** Hyperchloraemic acidosis (on prolonged use)
● DIRECTIONS FOR ADMINISTRATION The contents of each sachet should be mixed with at least 150 mL of water or other suitable liquid such as fruit juice, skimmed milk, thin soups, and pulpy fruits with a high moisture content.
    Other drugs should be taken at least 1 hour before or 4–6 hours after colestyramine to reduce possible interference with absorption.
● PATIENT AND CARER ADVICE Patient counselling on administration is advised for colestyramine powder (avoid other drugs at same time).

● MEDICINAL FORMS
There can be variation in the licensing of different medicines containing the same drug. Forms available from special-order manufacturers include: oral suspension, oral solution

Powder
CAUTIONARY AND ADVISORY LABELS 13
EXCIPIENTS: May contain Aspartame, sucrose
▸ Colestyramine (Non-proprietary)
    Colestyramine anhydrous 4 gram Colestyramine 4g oral powder sachets | 50 sachet PoM no price available
    Colestyramine 4g oral powder sachets sugar free sugar-free | 50 sachet PoM £30.00–£32.78 DT price = £31.85
▸ Questran (Bristol-Myers Squibb Pharmaceuticals Ltd)
    Colestyramine anhydrous 4 gram Questran 4g oral powder sachets | 50 sachet PoM £10.76
▸ Questran Light (Bristol-Myers Squibb Pharmaceuticals Ltd)
    Colestyramine anhydrous 4 gram Questran Light 4g oral powder sachets sugar-free | 50 sachet PoM £16.15 DT price = £31.85

LIPID MODIFYING DRUGS > CHOLESTEROL ABSORPTION INHIBITORS

Ezetimibe   19.5.2016

● DRUG ACTION Ezetimibe inhibits the intestinal absorption of cholesterol.
    If used alone, it has a modest effect on lowering LDL-cholesterol, with little effect on other lipoproteins.

● INDICATIONS AND DOSE

Adjunct to dietary measures and statin treatment in primary hypercholesterolaemia | Adjunct to dietary measures and statin in homozygous familial hypercholesterolaemia | Primary hypercholesterolaemia (if statin inappropriate or not tolerated) | Adjunct to dietary measures in homozygous sitosterolaemia
▸ BY MOUTH
▸ Adult: 10 mg daily

● INTERACTIONS → Appendix 1 (ezetimibe).
There is an increased risk of rhabdomyolysis if ezetimibe is used in combination with a statin.
● SIDE-EFFECTS
▸ **Common or very common** Fatigue · gastro-intestinal disturbances · headache · myalgia
▸ **Rare** Anaphylaxis · angioedema · arthralgia · hepatitis · hypersensitivity reactions · rash
▸ **Very rare** Cholecystitis · cholelithiasis · myopathy · pancreatitis · raised creatine kinase · rhabdomyolysis · thrombocytopenia
● PREGNANCY Manufacturer advises use only if potential benefit outweighs risk—no information available.
● BREAST FEEDING Manufacturer advises avoid—present in milk in *animal* studies.
● HEPATIC IMPAIRMENT Avoid in moderate and severe impairment—may accumulate.
● NATIONAL FUNDING/ACCESS DECISIONS

NICE technology appraisals (TAs)
▸ **Ezetimibe for treating primary heterozygous-familial and non-familial hypercholesterolaemia (February 2016)** NICE TA385 This guidance should be used with NICE's guidelines on cardiovascular disease: risk assessment and reduction, including lipid modification and familial hypercholesterolaemia: identification and management (see Lipid-regulating drugs p. 178).
    Ezetimibe, alone, is recommended as an option for the treatment of primary (heterozygous-familial or non-familial) hypercholesterolaemia in adult patients in whom initial statin therapy is contra-indicated, or who are intolerant of initial statin therapy.
    Ezetimibe, in combination with initial statin therapy, is also recommended as an option for the treatment of primary (heterozygous-familial or non-familial) hypercholesterolaemia in adult patients when:
    ● serum total or low-density lipoprotein (LDL) cholesterol concentration is not appropriately controlled either after appropriate dose titration of initial statin therapy or because dose titration is limited by intolerance to the initial statin therapy **and**
    ● a change from initial statin therapy to an alternative statin is being considered.
When prescribing ezetimibe in combination with statin, ezetimibe should be prescribed on the basis of lowest acquisition cost.
www.nice.org.uk/TA385

Cardiovascular system

2

● MEDICINAL FORMS
There can be variation in the licensing of different medicines containing the same drug.

Tablet
▸ Ezetrol (Merck Sharp & Dohme Ltd)
Ezetimibe 10 mg Ezetrol 10mg tablets | 28 tablet [PoM] £26.31 DT price = £26.31

Combinations available: *Simvastatin with ezetimibe*, p. 189

LIPID MODIFYING DRUGS > FIBRATES

Bezafibrate

● DRUG ACTION Fibrates act by decreasing serum triglycerides; they have variable effect on LDL-cholestrol.

● INDICATIONS AND DOSE

Adjunct to diet and other appropriate measures in mixed hyperlipidaemia if statin contra-indicated or not tolerated | Adjunct to diet and other appropriate measures in severe hypertriglyceridaemia
▸ BY MOUTH USING IMMEDIATE-RELEASE MEDICINES
▹ Adult: 200 mg 3 times a day
▸ BY MOUTH USING MODIFIED-RELEASE MEDICINES
▹ Adult: 400 mg once daily, modified-release dose form is not appropriate in patients with renal impairment

● CONTRA-INDICATIONS Gall bladder disease · hypoalbuminaemia · nephrotic syndrome · photosensitivity to fibrates

● CAUTIONS Correct hypothyroidism before initiating treatment

● INTERACTIONS → Appendix 1 (fibrates).
Combination of a fibrate with a statin increases the risk of muscle effects (especially rhabdomyolysis) and should be used with caution.

● SIDE-EFFECTS
▸ **Common or very common** Abdominal distension · anorexia · diarrhoea · nausea
▸ **Uncommon** Alopecia · cholestasis · dizziness · erectile dysfunction · headache · myotoxicity (with myasthenia, myalgia, or very rarely rhabdomyolysis)—special risk in renal impairment · photosensitivity reactions · pruritus · rash · renal failure · urticaria
▸ **Rare** Pancreatitis · peripheral neuropathy
▸ **Very rare** Anaemia · gallstones · increased platelet count · interstitial lung disease · leucopenia · pancytopenia · Stevens-Johnson syndrome · thrombocytopenic purpura · toxic epidermal necrolysis

● PREGNANCY Manufacturers advise avoid—no information available.

● BREAST FEEDING Manufacturer advises avoid—no information available.

● HEPATIC IMPAIRMENT Avoid in severe liver disease.

● RENAL IMPAIRMENT Reduce dose to 400 mg daily if eGFR 40–60 mL/minute/1.73 m^2. Reduce dose to 200 mg every 1–2 days if eGFR 15–40 mL/minute/1.73 m^2.
Myotoxicity Special care needed in patients with renal disease, as progressive increases in serum creatinine concentration or failure to follow dosage guidelines may result in myotoxicity (rhabdomyolysis); discontinue if myotoxicity suspected or creatine kinase concentration increases significantly.
   Avoid *immediate-release* preparations if eGFR less than 15 mL/minute/1.73 m^2.
   Avoid *modified-release* preparations if eGFR less than 60 mL/minute/1.73 m^2.

● MONITORING REQUIREMENTS Consider monitoring of liver function and creatine kinase when fibrates used in combination with a statin.

● PRESCRIBING AND DISPENSING INFORMATION Fibrates are mainly used in those whose serum-triglyceride concentration is greater than 10 mmol/litre or in those who cannot tolerate a statin (specialist use).

● MEDICINAL FORMS
There can be variation in the licensing of different medicines containing the same drug. Forms available from special-order manufacturers include: oral suspension

Tablet
CAUTIONARY AND ADVISORY LABELS 21
▸ Bezafibrate (Non-proprietary)
Bezafibrate 200 mg Bezafibrate 200mg tablets | 100 tablet [PoM] £8.50 DT price = £4.51
▸ Bezalip (Actavis UK Ltd)
Bezafibrate 200 mg Bezalip 200mg tablets | 100 tablet [PoM] £8.63 DT price = £4.51

Modified-release tablet
CAUTIONARY AND ADVISORY LABELS 21, 25
▸ Bezafibrate (Non-proprietary)
Bezafibrate 400 mg Bezafibrate 400mg modified-release tablets | 28 tablet [PoM] no price available | 30 tablet [PoM] £7.63 DT price = £7.63
▸ Bezalip Mono (Actavis UK Ltd)
Bezafibrate 400 mg Bezalip Mono 400mg modified-release tablets | 30 tablet [PoM] £7.63 DT price = £7.63
▸ Fibrazate XL (Sandoz Ltd)
Bezafibrate 400 mg Fibrazate XL 400mg tablets | 30 tablet [PoM] £6.87 DT price = £7.63

Ciprofibrate

● DRUG ACTION Fibrates act by decreasing serum triglycerides; they have variable effect on LDL-cholestrol.

● INDICATIONS AND DOSE

Adjunct to diet and other appropriate measures in mixed hyperlipidaemia if statin contra-indicated or not tolerated | Adjunct to diet and other appropriate measures in severe hypertriglyceridaemia
▸ BY MOUTH
▹ Adult: 100 mg daily

● CONTRA-INDICATIONS Gall bladder disease · hypoalbuminaemia · nephrotic syndrome · photosensitivity to fibrates

● CAUTIONS Correct hypothyroidism before initiating treatment

● INTERACTIONS → Appendix 1 (fibrates)
Combination of a fibrate with a statin increases the risk of muscle effects (especially rhabdomyolysis) and should be used with caution.

● SIDE-EFFECTS
▸ **Common or very common** Abdominal distension · anorexia · diarrhoea · nausea
▸ **Uncommon** Alopecia · cholestasis · dizziness · erectile dysfunction · headache · myotoxicity (with myasthenia, myalgia, or very rarely rhabdomyolysis)—special risk in renal impairment · photosensitivity reactions · pruritus · rash · renal failure · urticaria
▸ **Rare** Pancreatitis · peripheral neuropathy
▸ **Very rare** Anaemia · gallstones · increased platelet count · interstitial lung disease · leucopenia · pancytopenia · Stevens-Johnson syndrome · thrombocytopenic purpura · toxic epidermal necrolysis
▸ **Frequency not known** Pneumonitis · pulmonary fibrosis

● PREGNANCY Manufacturers advise avoid—toxicity in *animal* studies.

● BREAST FEEDING Manufacturer advises avoid—present in milk in *animal* studies.

● HEPATIC IMPAIRMENT Use with caution in mild to moderate impairment. Avoid in severe impairment.

- RENAL IMPAIRMENT Reduce dose to 100 mg on alternate days in moderate impairment. Avoid in severe impairment. Myotoxicity Special care needed in patients with renal disease, as progressive increases in serum creatinine concentration or failure to follow dosage guidelines may result in myotoxicity (rhabdomyolysis); discontinue if myotoxicity suspected or creatine kinase concentration increases significantly.
- MONITORING REQUIREMENTS
‣ Liver function tests recommended every 3 months for first year (discontinue treatment if significantly raised).
‣ Consider monitoring liver function and creatine kinase when fibrates used in combination with a statin.
- PRESCRIBING AND DISPENSING INFORMATION Fibrates are mainly used in those whose serum-triglyceride concentration is greater than 10 mmol/litre or in those who cannot tolerate a statin (specialist use).

- MEDICINAL FORMS
There can be variation in the licensing of different medicines containing the same drug.
Tablet
‣ Ciprofibrate (Non-proprietary)
  Ciprofibrate 100 mg Ciprofibrate 100mg tablets | 28 tablet PoM
  £134.21 DT price = £112.06

Fenofibrate

- DRUG ACTION Fibrates act by decreasing serum triglycerides; they have variable effect on LDL-cholestrol.

- INDICATIONS AND DOSE
Adjunct to diet and other appropriate measures in mixed hyperlipidaemia if statin contra-indicated or not tolerated | Adjunct to diet and other appropriate measures in severe hypertriglyceridaemia | Adjunct to statin in mixed hyperlipidaemia if triglycerides and HDL-cholesterol inadequately controlled in patients at high cardiovascular risk
‣ BY MOUTH USING CAPSULES
‣ Adult: Initially 200 mg daily, then increased if necessary to 267 mg daily, maximum 200 mg daily with concomitant statin, 200 mg capsules not appropriate for use in renal impairment, 267 mg capsules not appropriate for initial dose titration, or in renal impairment
‣ BY MOUTH USING TABLETS
‣ Adult: 160 mg daily, tablets not appropriate in renal impairment

- CONTRA-INDICATIONS Gall bladder disease · pancreatitis (unless due to severe hypertriglyceridaemia) · photosensitivity to ketoprofen
- CAUTIONS Correct hypothyroidism before initiating treatment
- INTERACTIONS → Appendix 1 (fibrates).
Combination of a fibrate with a statin increases the risk of muscle effects (especially rhabdomyolysis) and should be used with caution.
- SIDE-EFFECTS
‣ **Common or very common** Abdominal distension · anorexia · diarrhoea · nausea
‣ **Uncommon** Alopecia · cholestasis · dizziness · erectile dysfunction · headache · myotoxicity (with myasthenia, myalgia, or very rarely rhabdomyolysis)—special risk in renal impairment · pancreatitis · photosensitivity reactions · pruritus · pulmonary embolism · rash · renal failure · urticaria
‣ **Rare** Hepatitis · peripheral neuropathy
‣ **Very rare** Anaemia · gallstones · increased platelet count · interstitial lung disease · leucopenia · pancytopenia ·

Stevens-Johnson syndrome · thrombocytopenic purpura · toxic epidermal necrolysis
‣ **Frequency not known** Interstitial pneumopathies
- PREGNANCY Avoid—embryotoxicity in *animal* studies.
- BREAST FEEDING Manufacturers advise avoid—no information available.
- HEPATIC IMPAIRMENT Avoid.
- RENAL IMPAIRMENT Reduce dose to 134 mg daily if eGFR less than 60 mL/minute/1.73 m². Reduce dose to 67 mg daily if eGFR less than 20 mL/minute/1.73 m². Avoid if eGFR less than 15 mL/minute/1.73 m².
Myotoxicity Special care needed in patients with renal disease, as progressive increases in serum creatinine concentration or failure to follow dosage guidelines may result in myotoxicity (rhabdomyolysis); discontinue if myotoxicity suspected or creatine kinase concentration increases significantly.
- MONITORING REQUIREMENTS
‣ Liver function tests recommended every 3 months for first year (discontinue treatment if significantly raised).
‣ Consider monitoring liver function and creatine kinase when fibrates used in combination with a statin.
- PRESCRIBING AND DISPENSING INFORMATION Fibrates are mainly used in those whose serum-triglyceride concentration is greater than 10 mmol/litre or in those who cannot tolerate a statin (specialist use).

- MEDICINAL FORMS
There can be variation in the licensing of different medicines containing the same drug.
Tablet
CAUTIONARY AND ADVISORY LABELS 21
‣ Fenofibrate (Non-proprietary)
  Fenofibrate micronised 160 mg Fenofibrate micronised 160mg tablets | 28 tablet PoM £6.69 DT price = £6.69
‣ Supralip (BGP Products Ltd)
  Fenofibrate micronised 160 mg Supralip 160mg tablets | 28 tablet PoM £6.69 DT price = £6.69
Capsule
CAUTIONARY AND ADVISORY LABELS 21
‣ Fenofibrate (Non-proprietary)
  Fenofibrate micronised 67 mg Fenofibrate micronised 67mg capsules | 90 capsule PoM £23.30 DT price = £22.37
  Fenofibrate micronised 200 mg Fenofibrate micronised 200mg capsules | 28 capsule PoM £21.75 DT price = £7.38
  Fenofibrate micronised 267 mg Fenofibrate micronised 267mg capsules | 28 capsule PoM £21.75 DT price = £4.33
‣ Lipantil Micro (BGP Products Ltd)
  Fenofibrate micronised 67 mg Lipantil Micro 67 capsules | 90 capsule PoM £23.30 DT price = £22.37
  Fenofibrate micronised 200 mg Lipantil Micro 200 capsules | 28 capsule PoM £14.23 DT price = £7.38
  Fenofibrate micronised 267 mg Lipantil Micro 267 capsules | 28 capsule PoM £21.75 DT price = £4.33

Combinations available: *Simvastatin with fenofibrate*, p. 189

Gemfibrozil

- **DRUG ACTION** Fibrates act by decreasing serum triglycerides; they have variable effect on LDL-cholesterol.

- **INDICATIONS AND DOSE**

Adjunct to diet and other appropriate measures in mixed hyperlipidaemia if statin contra-indicated or not tolerated | Adjunct to diet and other appropriate measures in primary hypercholesterolaemia if statin contra-indicated or not tolerated | Adjunct to diet and other appropriate measures in severe hypertriglyceridaemia | Adjunct to diet and other appropriate measures in primary prevention of cardiovascular disease in men with hyperlipidaemias if statin contra-indicated or not tolerated

  ▸ BY MOUTH
  ▸ Adult: 1.2 g daily in 2 divided doses, maintenance 0.9–1.2 g daily

- **CONTRA-INDICATIONS** History of gall-bladder or biliary tract disease including gallstones · photosensitivity to fibrates

- **CAUTIONS** Correct hypothyroidism before initiating treatment · elderly

- **INTERACTIONS** → Appendix 1 (fibrates).
The combination of gemfibrozil and a statin should preferably be avoided; high risk of muscle effects (especially rhabdomyolysis).

- **SIDE-EFFECTS**
  ▸ **Common or very common** Abdominal pain · constipation · diarrhoea · dyspepsia · eczema · fatigue · flatulence · headache · nausea · rash · vertigo · vomiting
  ▸ **Uncommon** Atrial fibrillation
  ▸ **Rare** Hepatitis · paraesthesia · alopecia · anaemia · angioedema · appendicitis · blurred vision · bone-marrow suppression · cholestatic jaundice · depression · disturbances in hepatic function · dizziness · drowsiness · eosinophilia · exfoliative dermatitis · leucopenia · myalgia · myasthenia · myopathy · myositis accompanied by increase in creatine kinase (discontinue if raised significantly) · pancreatitis · photosensitivity · pruritus · sexual dysfunction · thrombocytopenia · urticaria

- **PREGNANCY** Manufacturers advise avoid unless essential— toxicity in *animal* studies.

- **BREAST FEEDING** Manufacturer advises avoid—no information available.

- **HEPATIC IMPAIRMENT** Avoid.

- **RENAL IMPAIRMENT** Initially 900 mg daily if eGFR 30–80 mL/minute/1.73 m^2. Avoid if eGFR less than 30 mL/minute/1.73 m^2.
  Myotoxicity Special care needed in patients with renal disease, as progressive increases in serum creatinine concentration or failure to follow dosage guidelines may result in myotoxicity (rhabdomyolysis); discontinue if myotoxicity suspected or creatine kinase concentration increases significantly.

- **MONITORING REQUIREMENTS**
  ▸ Monitor blood counts for first year.
  ▸ Monitor liver-function (discontinue treatment if abnormalities persist).
  ▸ Consider monitoring creatine kinase if used in combination with a statin.

- **PRESCRIBING AND DISPENSING INFORMATION** Fibrates are mainly used in those whose serum-triglyceride concentration is greater than 10 mmol/litre or in those who cannot tolerate a statin (specialist use).

- **MEDICINAL FORMS**
There can be variation in the licensing of different medicines containing the same drug.
Tablet
CAUTIONARY AND ADVISORY LABELS 22
  ▸ Gemfibrozil (Non-proprietary)
  Gemfibrozil 600 mg Gemfibrozil 600mg tablets | 30 tablet [PoM] £15.00 | 56 tablet [PoM] £34.99 DT price = £34.97
  ▸ Lopid (Pfizer Ltd)
  Gemfibrozil 600 mg Lopid 600mg tablets | 56 tablet [PoM] £35.57 DT price = £34.97
Capsule
CAUTIONARY AND ADVISORY LABELS 22
  ▸ Lopid (Pfizer Ltd)
  Gemfibrozil 300 mg Lopid 300mg capsules | 100 capsule [PoM] £31.76 DT price = £31.76

LIPID MODIFYING DRUGS > NICOTINIC ACID DERIVATIVES

Acipimox

- **INDICATIONS AND DOSE**

Adjunct or alternative treatment in hyperlipidaemias of types IIb and IV in patients who have not responded adequately to other lipid-regulating drugs such as a statin or fibrate, and lifestyle changes (including diet, exercise, and weight reduction)
  ▸ BY MOUTH
  ▸ Adult: 250 mg 2–3 times a day

- **CONTRA-INDICATIONS** Peptic ulcer

- **SIDE-EFFECTS**
  ▸ **Common or very common** Abdominal pain · dyspepsia · flushing · headache · malaise · urticaria
  ▸ **Uncommon** Anaphylactoid reaction · arthralgia · bronchospasm · erythema · myalgia · myositis · nausea · pruritus · rash
  ▸ **Frequency not known** Diarrhoea · dry eyes · vasodilatation

- **PREGNANCY** Manufacturer advises avoid—no information available.

- **BREAST FEEDING** Manufacturer advises avoid—no information available.

- **RENAL IMPAIRMENT** Reduce dose to 250 mg 1–2 times daily if eGFR 30–60 mL/minute/1.73 m^2. Avoid if eGFR less than 30 mL/minute/1.73 m^2.

- **MONITORING REQUIREMENTS** Monitor hepatic and renal function.

- **MEDICINAL FORMS**
There can be variation in the licensing of different medicines containing the same drug.
Capsule
CAUTIONARY AND ADVISORY LABELS 21
  ▸ Olbetam (Pfizer Ltd)
  Acipimox 250 mg Olbetam 250mg capsules | 90 capsule [PoM] £46.33 DT price = £46.33

Nicotinic acid

- **DRUG ACTION** In doses of 1.5 to 3 g daily, it lowers both cholesterol and triglyceride concentrations by inhibiting synthesis; it also increases HDL-cholesterol.

- **INDICATIONS AND DOSE**

Adjunct to statin in dyslipidaemia or used alone if statin not tolerated
  ▸ BY MOUTH
  ▸ Adult: (consult product literature)

- **CONTRA-INDICATIONS** Active peptic ulcer disease · arterial bleeding

- CAUTIONS Acute myocardial infarction · diabetes mellitus · gout · history of peptic ulceration · unstable angina
- INTERACTIONS → Appendix 1 (nicotinic acid).
- SIDE-EFFECTS
‣ **Common or very common** Abdominal pain · diarrhoea · dyspepsia · flushing · nausea · pruritus · rash · vomiting
‣ **Uncommon** Dizziness · headache · hypophosphataemia · increase in uric acid · palpitation · peripheral oedema · prolonged prothrombin time · reduced platelet count · shortness of breath · tachycardia
‣ **Rare** Hypotension · insomnia · myalgia · myasthenia · myopathy · reduced glucose tolerance · rhinitis · syncope
‣ **Very rare** Anorexia · rhabdomyolysis · visual disturbance
‣ **Frequency not known** Jaundice

SIDE-EFFECTS, FURTHER INFORMATION
‣ Prostaglandin-mediated symptoms Prostaglandin-mediated symptoms (such as flushing) can be reduced by low initial doses taken with meals or, if patient taking aspirin, aspirin dose should be taken 30 minutes before nicotinic acid.

- PREGNANCY No information available—manufacturer advises avoid unless potential benefit outweighs risk.
- BREAST FEEDING Present in milk—avoid.
- HEPATIC IMPAIRMENT Avoid in severe impairment. Discontinue if severe abnormalities in liver function tests. Manufacturer advises monitor liver function in mild to moderate hepatic impairment.
- RENAL IMPAIRMENT Manufacturer advises use with caution—no information available.

- MEDICINAL FORMS
There can be variation in the licensing of different medicines containing the same drug. Forms available from special-order manufacturers include: tablet, modified-release tablet, capsule

Capsule
‣ Nicotinic acid (Non-proprietary)
  Nicotinic acid 500 mg Solgar Niacin 500mg capsules | 100 capsule no price available

LIPID MODIFYING DRUGS > STATINS

Statins

- DRUG ACTION Statins competitively inhibit 3-hydroxy-3-methylglutaryl coenzyme A (HMG CoA) reductase, an enzyme involved in cholesterol synthesis, especially in the liver.
- CAUTIONS Elderly · high alcohol intake · history of liver disease · hypothyroidism · patients at increased risk of muscle toxicity, including myopathy or rhabdomyolysis (e.g. those with a personal or family history of muscular disorders, previous history of muscular toxicity and a high alcohol intake)

CAUTIONS, FURTHER INFORMATION
‣ Muscle effects Muscle toxicity can occur with all statins, however the likelihood increases with higher doses and in certain patients (see below). Statins should be used with caution in patients at increased risk of muscle toxicity, including those with a personal or family history of muscular disorders, previous history of muscular toxicity, a high alcohol intake, renal impairment or hypothyroidism.
  In patients at increased risk of muscle effects, a statin should not usually be started if the baseline creatine kinase concentration is more than 5 times the upper limit of normal (some patients may present with an extremely elevated baseline creatine kinase concentration, for example because of a physical occupation or rigorous exercise—specialist advice should be sought regarding consideration of statin therapy in these patients).
‣ Hypothyroidism Hypothyroidism should be managed adequately before starting treatment with a statin.

- INTERACTIONS → Appendix 1 (statins).
There is an increased incidence of myopathy if a statin is given with a fibrate (the combination of a statin and gemfibrozil should preferably be avoided), with lipid-lowering doses of nicotinic acid, with fusidic acid (risk of rhabdomyolysis—the combination of a statin and fusidic acid should be avoided; temporarily discontinue statin and restart 7 days after last fusidic acid dose), or with drugs that increase the plasma-statin concentration, such as macrolide antibiotics, imidazole and triazole antifungals, and ciclosporin; close monitoring of liver function and, if muscular symptoms occur, of creatine kinase is necessary.

- SIDE-EFFECTS
‣ **Rare** Hepatitis · jaundice
‣ **Very rare** Hepatic failure. · interstitial lung disease · lupus erythematosus-like reactions · pancreatitis
‣ **Frequency not known** Alopecia · altered liver function tests · amnesia · arthralgia · asthenia · depression · dizziness · fatigue · gastro-intestinal disturbances · headache · hyperglycaemia · hypersensitivity reactions · may be associated with the development of diabetes mellitus (particularly in those already at risk of the condition) · myalgia · myopathy · myositis · paraesthesia · peripheral neuropathy · pruritus · rash · rhabdomyolysis · sexual dysfunction · sleep disturbance · thrombocytopenia · urticaria · visual disturbance

SIDE-EFFECTS, FURTHER INFORMATION
‣ Muscle effects The risk of myopathy, myositis, and rhabdomyolysis associated with statin use is rare. Although myalgia has been reported commonly in patients receiving statins, muscle toxicity truly attributable to statin use is rare. Muscle toxicity can occur with all statins, however the likelihood increases with higher doses.
  If muscular symptoms or raised creatine kinase occur during treatment, other possible causes (e.g. rigorous physical activity, hypothyroidism, infection, recent trauma, and drug or alcohol addiction) should be excluded before statin therapy is implicated, particularly if statin treatment has previously been tolerated for more than 3 months. When a statin is suspected to be the cause of myopathy, and creatine kinase concentration is markedly elevated (more than 5 times upper limit of normal), or if muscular symptoms are severe, treatment should be discontinued. If symptoms resolve and creatine kinase concentrations return to normal, the statin should be reintroduced at a lower dose and the patient monitored closely; an alternative statin should be prescribed if unacceptable side-effects are experienced with a particular statin. Statins should not be discontinued in the event of small, asymptomatic elevations of creatine kinase. Routine monitoring of creatine kinase is unnecessary in asymptomatic patients.
  Statins should not be discontinued if there is an increase in the blood-glucose concentration or HbA$_{1C}$ as the benefits continue to outweigh the risks.
‣ Interstitial lung disease If patients develop symptoms such as dyspnoea, cough, and weight loss, they should seek medical attention.

- CONCEPTION AND CONTRACEPTION Adequate contraception is required during treatment and for 1 month afterwards.
- PREGNANCY Statins should be avoided in pregnancy (discontinue 3 months before attempting to conceive) as congenital anomalies have been reported and the decreased synthesis of cholesterol possibly affects fetal development.
- HEPATIC IMPAIRMENT Statins should be used with caution in those with a history of liver disease. Avoid in active liver disease or when there are unexplained persistent elevations in serum transaminases.

- MONITORING REQUIREMENTS
▶ Before starting treatment with statins, at least one full lipid profile (non-fasting) should be measured, including total cholesterol, HDL-cholesterol, non-HDL-cholesterol (calculated as total cholesterol minus HDL-cholesterol), and triglyceride concentrations, thyroid-stimulating hormone, and renal function should also be assessed.
▶ Liver function There is little information available on a rational approach to liver-function monitoring; however, NICE suggests that liver enzymes should be measured before treatment, and repeated within 3 months and at 12 months of starting treatment, unless indicated at other times by signs or symptoms suggestive of hepatotoxicity (NICE clinical guideline 181 (July 2014). Lipid Modification—Cardiovascular risk assessment and the modification of blood lipids for the primary and secondary prevention of cardiovascular disease).

  Those with serum transaminases that are raised, but less than 3 times the upper limit of the reference range, should **not** be routinely excluded from statin therapy. Those with serum transaminases of more than 3 times the upper limit of the reference range should discontinue statin therapy.
▶ Creatine kinase Before initiation of statin treatment, creatine kinase concentration should be measured in patients who have had persistent, generalised, unexplained muscle pain (whether associated or not with previous lipid-regulating drugs); if the concentration is more than 5 times the upper limit of normal, a repeat measurement should be taken after 7 days. If the repeat concentration remains above 5 times the upper limit, statin treatment should not be started; if concentrations are still raised but less than 5 times the upper limit, the statin should be started at a lower dose.
▶ Diabetes Patients at high risk of diabetes mellitus should have fasting blood-glucose concentration or HbA$_{1C}$ checked before starting statin treatment, and then repeated after 3 months.
- PATIENT AND CARER ADVICE Advise patients to report promptly unexplained muscle pain, tenderness, or weakness.

🖙 185

Atorvastatin

- INDICATIONS AND DOSE
Primary hypercholesterolaemia in patients who have not responded adequately to diet and other appropriate measures | Combined (mixed) hyperlipidaemia in patients who have not responded adequately to diet and other appropriate measures
▶ BY MOUTH
▶ Adult: Usual dose 10 mg once daily; increased if necessary up to 80 mg once daily, dose to be increased at intervals of at least 4 weeks

Heterozygous familial hypercholesterolaemia in patients who have not responded adequately to diet and other appropriate measures | Homozygous familial hypercholestrolaemia in patients who have not responded adequately to diet and other appropriate measures
▶ BY MOUTH
▶ Adult: Initially 10 mg once daily, then increased to 40 mg once daily, dose to be increased at intervals of at least 4 weeks; maximum 80 mg per day

Primary prevention of cardiovascular events in patients at high risk of a first cardiovascular event
▶ BY MOUTH
▶ Adult: 20 mg once daily, dose can be increased if necessary

Secondary prevention of cardiovascular events
▶ BY MOUTH
▶ Adult: 80 mg once daily
DOSE ADJUSTMENTS DUE TO INTERACTIONS
Reduced dose required (max. 10 mg daily) with concomitant ciclosporin, or tipranavir combined with ritonavir—seek specialist advice.
Maximum dose of 40 mg daily when combined with anion-exchange resin for heterozygous familial hypercholesterolaemia.

- UNLICENSED USE Not licensed for use in secondary prevention of cardiovascular events.
  Starting dose of 20 mg once daily is not licensed for the primary prevention of cardiovascular events.
- CAUTIONS Haemorrhagic stroke
- SIDE-EFFECTS
▶ **Common or very common** Back pain · epistaxis · hyperglycaemia · nasopharyngitis · pharyngeolaryngeal pain
▶ **Uncommon** Anorexia · blurred vision · chest pain · hypoglycaemia · malaise · neck pain · peripheral oedema · pyrexia · tinnitus · weight gain
▶ **Rare** Cholestasis · Stevens-Johnson syndrome · toxic epidermal necrolysis
▶ **Very rare** Gynaecomastia · hearing loss
- BREAST FEEDING Manufacturer advises avoid—no information available.
- RENAL IMPAIRMENT In chronic kidney disease, for primary and secondary prevention of cardiovascular events [unlicensed starting dose in *primary* prevention; unlicensed in *secondary* prevention], initially 20 mg once daily, increased if necessary (on specialist advice if eGFR < 30 mL/minute/1.73 m^2); max. 80 mg once daily.
- PATIENT AND CARER ADVICE Patient counselling is advised for atorvastatin tablets (muscle effects).

- MEDICINAL FORMS
There can be variation in the licensing of different medicines containing the same drug. Forms available from special-order manufacturers include: oral suspension, oral solution
Tablet
▶ Atorvastatin (Non-proprietary)
  Atorvastatin (as Atorvastatin calcium trihydrate)
  10 mg Atorvastatin 10mg tablets | 28 tablet [PoM] £13.00 DT price = £0.95 | 90 tablet [PoM] £41.78
  Atorvastatin (as Atorvastatin calcium trihydrate)
  20 mg Atorvastatin 20mg tablets | 28 tablet [PoM] £24.64 DT price = £1.12 | 90 tablet [PoM] £79.20
  Atorvastatin (as Atorvastatin calcium trihydrate)
  30 mg Atorvastatin 30mg tablets | 28 tablet [PoM] £24.50 DT price = £24.50
  Atorvastatin (as Atorvastatin calcium trihydrate)
  40 mg Atorvastatin 40mg tablets | 28 tablet [PoM] £24.64 DT price = £1.28 | 90 tablet [PoM] £79.20
  Atorvastatin (as Atorvastatin calcium trihydrate)
  60 mg Atorvastatin 60mg tablets | 28 tablet [PoM] £28.00 DT price = £28.00
  Atorvastatin (as Atorvastatin calcium trihydrate)
  80 mg Atorvastatin 80mg tablets | 28 tablet [PoM] £28.21 DT price = £2.18 | 90 tablet [PoM] £90.67
▶ Lipitor (Pfizer Ltd)
  Atorvastatin (as Atorvastatin calcium trihydrate) 10 mg Lipitor 10mg tablets | 28 tablet [PoM] £13.00 DT price = £0.95
  Atorvastatin (as Atorvastatin calcium trihydrate) 20 mg Lipitor 20mg tablets | 28 tablet [PoM] £24.64 DT price = £1.12
  Atorvastatin (as Atorvastatin calcium trihydrate) 40 mg Lipitor 40mg tablets | 28 tablet [PoM] £24.64 DT price = £1.28
  Atorvastatin (as Atorvastatin calcium trihydrate) 80 mg Lipitor 80mg tablets | 28 tablet [PoM] £28.21 DT price = £2.18

Chewable tablet

CAUTIONARY AND ADVISORY LABELS 24

‣ Lipitor (Pfizer Ltd)

Atorvastatin (as Atorvastatin calcium trihydrate) 10 mg Lipitor 10mg chewable tablets sugar-free | 30 tablet [PoM] £13.80 DT price = £13.80

Atorvastatin (as Atorvastatin calcium trihydrate) 20 mg Lipitor 20mg chewable tablets sugar-free | 30 tablet [PoM] £26.40 DT price = £26.40

F 185

Fluvastatin

● INDICATIONS AND DOSE

Adjunct to diet in primary hypercholesterolaemia or combined (mixed) hyperlipidaemia (types IIa and IIb)

▸ BY MOUTH USING IMMEDIATE-RELEASE MEDICINES

‣ Adult: Initially 20–40 mg daily, dose to be taken in the evening, increased if necessary up to 80 mg daily in 2 divided doses, dose to be adjusted at intervals of at least 4 weeks

▸ BY MOUTH USING MODIFIED-RELEASE MEDICINES

‣ Adult: 80 mg daily, dose form is not appropriate for initial dose titration

Prevention of coronary events after percutaneous coronary intervention

▸ BY MOUTH USING IMMEDIATE-RELEASE MEDICINES

‣ Adult: 80 mg daily

▸ BY MOUTH USING MODIFIED-RELEASE MEDICINES

‣ Adult: 80 mg daily, dose form is not appropriate for initial dose titration

● SIDE-EFFECTS

▸ Very rare Vasculitis

● BREAST FEEDING Manufacturer advises avoid—no information available.

● RENAL IMPAIRMENT Manufacturer advises doses above 40 mg daily should be initiated with caution if eGFR less than 30 mL/minute/1.73 m^2.

● PATIENT AND CARER ADVICE Patient counselling is advised for fluvastatin tablets/capsules (muscle effects).

● NATIONAL FUNDING/ACCESS DECISIONS

Scottish Medicines Consortium (SMC) Decisions

The *Scottish Medicines Consortium* has advised (February 2004) that fluvastatin is accepted for restricted use for the secondary prevention of coronary events after percutaneous coronary angioplasty; if the patient has previously been receiving another statin, then there is no need to change the statin.

● MEDICINAL FORMS

There can be variation in the licensing of different medicines containing the same drug.

Modified-release tablet

CAUTIONARY AND ADVISORY LABELS 25

‣ Fluvastatin (Non-proprietary)

Fluvastatin (as Fluvastatin sodium) 80 mg Fluvastatin 80mg modified-release tablets | 28 tablet [PoM] no price available DT price = £19.20

‣ Dorisin XL (Aspire Pharma Ltd)

Fluvastatin (as Fluvastatin sodium) 80 mg Dorisin XL 80mg tablets | 28 tablet [PoM] £19.20 DT price = £19.20

‣ Lescol XL (Novartis Pharmaceuticals UK Ltd)

Fluvastatin (as Fluvastatin sodium) 80 mg Lescol XL 80mg tablets | 28 tablet [PoM] £19.20 DT price = £19.20

‣ Luvinsta XL (Actavis UK Ltd)

Fluvastatin (as Fluvastatin sodium) 80 mg Luvinsta XL 80mg tablets | 28 tablet [PoM] £19.20 DT price = £19.20

‣ Nandovar XL (Sandoz Ltd)

Fluvastatin (as Fluvastatin sodium) 80 mg Nandovar XL 80mg tablets | 28 tablet [PoM] £16.32 DT price = £19.20

‣ Pinmactil (Mylan Ltd)

Fluvastatin (as Fluvastatin sodium) 80 mg Pinmactil 80mg modified-release tablets | 28 tablet [PoM] £19.20 DT price = £19.20

Capsule

▸ Fluvastatin (Non-proprietary)

Fluvastatin (as Fluvastatin sodium) 20 mg Fluvastatin 20mg capsules | 28 capsule [PoM] £6.96 DT price = £2.16

Fluvastatin (as Fluvastatin sodium) 40 mg Fluvastatin 40mg capsules | 28 capsule [PoM] £7.42 DT price = £2.38

‣ Lescol (Novartis Pharmaceuticals UK Ltd)

Fluvastatin (as Fluvastatin sodium) 20 mg Lescol 20mg capsules | 28 capsule [PoM] £15.26 DT price = £2.16

Fluvastatin (as Fluvastatin sodium) 40 mg Lescol 40mg capsules | 28 capsule [PoM] £15.26 DT price = £2.38

F 185

Pravastatin sodium

● INDICATIONS AND DOSE

Adjunct to diet for primary hypercholesterolaemia or combined (mixed) hyperlipidaemias in patients who have not responded adequately to dietary control

▸ BY MOUTH

‣ Adult: 10–40 mg daily, dose to be taken at night, dose to be adjusted at intervals of at least 4 weeks

Prevention of cardiovascular events in patients with previous myocardial infarction or unstable angina | Adjunct to diet to prevent cardiovascular events in patients with hypercholesterolaemia

▸ BY MOUTH

‣ Adult: 40 mg daily, dose to be taken at night

Reduction of hyperlipidaemia in patients receiving immunosuppressive therapy following solid-organ transplantation

▸ BY MOUTH

‣ Adult: Initially 20 mg daily, then increased if necessary up to 40 mg daily, dose to be taken at night, close medical supervision is required if dose is increased to maximum dose

● SIDE-EFFECTS

▸ Uncommon Abnormal urination · dysuria · nocturia · urinary frequency

▸ Very rare Fulminant hepatic necrosis

● BREAST FEEDING Manufacturer advises avoid—small amount of drug present in breast milk.

● RENAL IMPAIRMENT Manufacturer advises initial dose of 10 mg once daily in moderate to severe impairment.

● PATIENT AND CARER ADVICE Patient counselling is advised for pravastatin tablets (muscle effects).

● MEDICINAL FORMS

There can be variation in the licensing of different medicines containing the same drug. Forms available from special-order manufacturers include: oral suspension, oral solution

Tablet

▸ Pravastatin sodium (Non-proprietary)

Pravastatin sodium 10 mg Pravastatin 10mg tablets | 28 tablet [PoM] £16.10 DT price = £0.91

Pravastatin sodium 20 mg Pravastatin 20mg tablets | 28 tablet [PoM] £29.60 DT price = £1.08

Pravastatin sodium 40 mg Pravastatin 40mg tablets | 28 tablet [PoM] £29.60 DT price = £1.37

2

Cardiovascular system

Rosuvastatin

⌐ 185

● **INDICATIONS AND DOSE**

Primary hypercholesterolaemia (type IIa including heterozygous familial hypercholesterolaemia), mixed dyslipidaemia (type IIb), or homozygous familial hypercholesterolaemia in patients who have not responded adequately to diet and other appropriate measures

▸ BY MOUTH

▸ Adult 18–69 years: Initially 5–10 mg once daily, then increased if necessary to 20 mg once daily, dose to be increased at intervals of at least 4 weeks

▸ Adult (patients of Asian origin): Initially 5 mg once daily, then increased if necessary up to 20 mg once daily, dose to be increased at intervals of at least 4 weeks.

▸ Adult 70 years and over: Initially 5 mg once daily, then increased if necessary up to 20 mg once daily, dose to be increased at intervals of at least 4 weeks

Primary hypercholesterolaemia (type IIa including heterozygous familial hypercholesterolaemia), mixed dyslipidaemia (type IIb), or homozygous familial hypercholesterolaemia in patients who have not responded adequately to diet and other appropriate measures and who have risk factors for myopathy or rhabdomyolysis

▸ BY MOUTH

▸ Adult: Initially 5 mg once daily, then increased if necessary up to 20 mg once daily, dose to be increased at intervals of at least 4 weeks

Severe primary hypercholesterolaemia (type IIa including heterozygous familial hypercholesterolaemia), mixed dyslipidaemia (type IIb), or homozygous familial hypercholesterolaemia in patients who have not responded adequately to diet and other appropriate measures, in patients with high cardiovascular risk (under expert supervision)

▸ BY MOUTH

▸ Adult: Initially 5–10 mg once daily, increased if necessary to 20 mg once daily, then increased if necessary to 40 mg once daily, dose to be increased at intervals of at least 4 weeks

Prevention of cardiovascular events in patients at high risk of a first cardiovascular event

▸ BY MOUTH

▸ Adult 18–69 years: 20 mg once daily

▸ Adult (patients of Asian origin): Initially 5 mg once daily, then increased if necessary up to 20 mg once daily.

▸ Adult 70 years and over: Initially 5 mg once daily, then increased if necessary up to 20 mg once daily

Prevention of cardiovascular events in patients at high risk of a first cardiovascular event and with risk factors for myopathy or rhabdomyolysis

▸ BY MOUTH

▸ Adult: Initially 5 mg once daily, then increased if necessary up to 20 mg once daily

DOSE ADJUSTMENTS DUE TO INTERACTIONS
Initially 5 mg once daily with concomitant fibrate increased if necessary to max. 20 mg daily. For dose adjustments with concomitant atazanavir, clopidogrel, darunavir, dronedarone, eltrombopag, ezetimibe, itraconazole, lopinavir, or tipranavir, consult product literature. Maximum dose 5 mg with concomitant ombitasvir, paritaprevir, and ritonavir given with dasabuvir, but maximum 10 mg daily with concomitant ombitasvir, paritaprevir, and ritonavir given without dasabuvir.

● CAUTIONS Patients of Asian origin

● **SIDE-EFFECTS**

▸ **Common or very common** Proteinuria

▸ **Very rare** Gynaecomastia · haematuria

▸ **Frequency not known** Oedema · Stevens-Johnson syndrome

● BREAST FEEDING Manufacturer advises avoid—no information available.

● RENAL IMPAIRMENT Initially 5 mg once daily (do not exceed 20 mg daily) if eGFR 30–60 mL/minute/1.73 m^2. Avoid if eGFR less than 30 mL/minute/1.73 m^2.

● PATIENT AND CARER ADVICE Patient counselling is advised for rosuvastatin tablets (muscle effects).

● **MEDICINAL FORMS**
There can be variation in the licensing of different medicines containing the same drug. Forms available from special-order manufacturers include: oral suspension

Tablet

▸ Crestor (AstraZeneca UK Ltd)

Rosuvastatin (as Rosuvastatin calcium) 5 mg Crestor 5mg tablets | 28 tablet PoM £18.03 DT price = £18.03

Rosuvastatin (as Rosuvastatin calcium) 10 mg Crestor 10mg tablets | 28 tablet PoM £18.03 DT price = £18.03

Rosuvastatin (as Rosuvastatin calcium) 20 mg Crestor 20mg tablets | 28 tablet PoM £26.02 DT price = £26.02

Rosuvastatin (as Rosuvastatin calcium) 40 mg Crestor 40mg tablets | 28 tablet PoM £29.69 DT price = £29.69

Simvastatin

⌐ 185

● **INDICATIONS AND DOSE**

Primary hypercholesterolaemia, or combined (mixed) hyperlipidaemia in patients who have not responded adequately to diet and other appropriate measures

▸ BY MOUTH

▸ Adult: 10–20 mg once daily, then increased if necessary up to 80 mg once daily, adjusted at intervals of at least 4 weeks, dose to be taken at night; 80 mg dose only for those with severe hypercholesterolaemia and at high risk of cardiovascular complications

Homozygous familial hypercholesterolaemia in patients who have not responded adequately to diet and other appropriate measures

▸ BY MOUTH

▸ Adult: Initially 40 mg once daily, then increased if necessary up to 80 mg once daily, adjusted at intervals of at least 4 weeks, dose to be taken at night; 80 mg dose only for those with severe hypercholesterolaemia and at high risk of cardiovascular complications

Prevention of cardiovascular events in patients with atherosclerotic cardiovascular disease or diabetes mellitus

▸ BY MOUTH

▸ Adult: Initially 20–40 mg once daily, increased if necessary up to 80 mg once daily, adjusted at intervals of at least 4 weeks, dose to be taken at night; 80 mg dose only for those with severe hypercholesterolaemia and at high risk of cardiovascular complications

DOSE ADJUSTMENTS DUE TO INTERACTIONS
Max. 10 mg daily with concomitant bezafibrate or ciprofibrate.
Max. 20 mg daily with concomitant amiodarone, verapamil, diltiazem, amlodipine, or ranolazine.
Max. 40 mg daily with concomitant lomitapide.

● **SIDE-EFFECTS**

▸ **Rare** Anaemia

▸ **Frequency not known** Tendinopathy

● BREAST FEEDING Manufacturer advises avoid—no information available.

● RENAL IMPAIRMENT Doses above 10 mg daily should be used with caution if eGFR less than 30 mL/minute/1.73 m^2.

- PATIENT AND CARER ADVICE Patient counselling is advised for simvastatin tablets/oral suspension (muscle effects).
- EXCEPTIONS TO LEGAL CATEGORY Simvastatin 10 mg tablets can be sold to the public to reduce risk of first coronary event in individuals at moderate risk of coronary heart disease (approx. 10–15 % risk of major event in 10 years), max. daily dose 10 mg and pack size of 28 tablets; treatment should form part of a programme to reduce risk of coronary heart disease.

- MEDICINAL FORMS
There can be variation in the licensing of different medicines containing the same drug. Forms available from special-order manufacturers include: oral suspension, oral solution

Tablet
- Simvastatin (Non-proprietary)
  Simvastatin 10 mg Simvastatin 10mg tablets | 28 tablet PoM £18.00 DT price = £0.67
  Simvastatin 20 mg Simvastatin 20mg tablets | 28 tablet PoM £29.60 DT price = £0.77
  Simvastatin 40 mg Simvastatin 40mg tablets | 28 tablet PoM £29.60 DT price = £0.86
  Simvastatin 80 mg Simvastatin 80mg tablets | 28 tablet PoM £29.61 DT price = £1.71
- Simvador (Discovery Pharmaceuticals)
  Simvastatin 10 mg Simvador 10mg tablets | 28 tablet PoM £0.67 DT price = £0.67
  Simvastatin 20 mg Simvador 20mg tablets | 28 tablet PoM £0.77 DT price = £0.77
  Simvastatin 40 mg Simvador 40mg tablets | 28 tablet PoM £0.86 DT price = £0.86
  Simvastatin 80 mg Simvador 80mg tablets | 28 tablet PoM £1.71 DT price = £1.71
- Zocor (Merck Sharp & Dohme Ltd)
  Simvastatin 10 mg Zocor 10mg tablets | 28 tablet PoM £18.03 DT price = £0.67
  Simvastatin 20 mg Zocor 20mg tablets | 28 tablet PoM £29.69 DT price = £0.77
  Simvastatin 40 mg Zocor 40mg tablets | 28 tablet PoM £29.69 DT price = £0.86
  Simvastatin 80 mg Zocor 80mg tablets | 28 tablet PoM £29.69 DT price = £1.71

Oral suspension
EXCIPIENTS: May contain Propylene glycol
- Simvastatin (Non-proprietary)
  Simvastatin 4 mg per 1 ml Simvastatin 20mg/5ml oral suspension sugar free sugar-free | 150 ml PoM £119.40 DT price = £119.40
  Simvastatin 8 mg per 1 ml Simvastatin 40mg/5ml oral suspension sugar free sugar-free | 150 ml PoM £182.40 DT price = £182.40

Simvastatin with ezetimibe

The properties listed below are those particular to the combination only. For the properties of the components please consider, simvastatin p. 188, ezetimibe p. 181.

- INDICATIONS AND DOSE

Homozygous familial hypercholesterolaemia, primary hypercholesterolaemia, and mixed hyperlipidaemia in patients over 10 years stabilised on the individual components in the same proportions, or for patients not adequately controlled by statin alone
- BY MOUTH
- Adult: (consult product literature)

- MEDICINAL FORMS
There can be variation in the licensing of different medicines containing the same drug.

Tablet
- Inegy (Merck Sharp & Dohme Ltd)
  Ezetimibe 10 mg, Simvastatin 20 mg Inegy 10mg/20mg tablets | 28 tablet PoM £33.42 DT price = £33.42
  Ezetimibe 10 mg, Simvastatin 40 mg Inegy 10mg/40mg tablets | 28 tablet PoM £38.98 DT price = £38.98
  Ezetimibe 10 mg, Simvastatin 80 mg Inegy 10mg/80mg tablets | 28 tablet PoM £41.21 DT price = £41.21

Simvastatin with fenofibrate

19.4.2016

The properties listed below are those particular to the combination only. For the properties of the components please consider, simvastatin p. 188, fenofibrate p. 183.

- INDICATIONS AND DOSE

Adjunct to diet and exercise in mixed dyslipidaemia, when LDL-cholesterol levels are adequately controlled with the corresponding dose of simvastatin monotherapy (in patients at high cardiovascular risk)
- BY MOUTH
- Adult: 20/145 mg once daily, alternatively 40/145 mg once daily, dose should be based on previous simvastatin monotherapy dose

- CAUTIONS History of pulmonary embolism
- SIDE-EFFECTS
- Common or very common Gastroenteritis
- Uncommon Dermatitis · eczema
- RENAL IMPAIRMENT Manufacturer advises avoid if eGFR less than 60 mL/minute/1.73 m^2; use with caution if eGFR 60–89 mL/minute/1.73 m^2.

- MEDICINAL FORMS
There can be variation in the licensing of different medicines containing the same drug.

Tablet
CAUTIONARY AND ADVISORY LABELS 25
EXCIPIENTS: May contain Butylated hydroxyanisole, lecithin
- Cholib (BGP Products Ltd)
  Simvastatin 20 mg, Fenofibrate 145 mg Cholib 145mg/20mg tablets | 30 tablet PoM £7.71
  Simvastatin 40 mg, Fenofibrate 145 mg Cholib 145mg/40mg tablets | 30 tablet PoM £8.33

LIPID MODIFYING DRUGS 〉 OTHER

Lomitapide

- DRUG ACTION Lomitapide, an inhibitor of microsomal triglyceride transfer protein (MTP), reduces lipoprotein secretion and circulating concentrations of lipoprotein-borne lipids such as cholesterol and triglycerides.

- INDICATIONS AND DOSE

Adjunct to dietary measures and other lipid-regulating drugs with or without low-density lipoprotein apheresis in homozygous familial hypercholesterolaemia (under expert supervision)
- BY MOUTH
- Adult: Initially 5 mg daily for 2 weeks, dose to be taken at least 2 hours after evening meal, then increased if necessary to 10 mg daily, for at least 4 weeks, then increased to 20 mg daily for at least 4 weeks, then increased in steps of 20 mg daily, adjusted at intervals of at least 4 weeks; maximum 60 mg per day

- CONTRA-INDICATIONS Significant or chronic bowel disease
- CAUTIONS Concomitant use of hepatotoxic drugs · lomitapide can interfere with the absorption of fat-soluble nutrients and supplementation of vitamin E and fatty acids is required · patients over 65 years
- INTERACTIONS → Appendix 1 (lomitapide).
- SIDE-EFFECTS
- Common or very common Bloating · abdominal pain · appetite changes · constipation · diarrhoea · dizziness · dyspepsia · ecchymosis · eructation · erythematous rash · flatulence · gastro-oesophageal reflux disease · gastroenteritis · haemorrhoids · headache · hepatic steatosis · hepatomegaly · hypokalaemia · leucopenia · malaise · migraine · muscle spasms · nausea · neutropenia ·

2

Cardiovascular system

raised serum transaminases · tenesmus · vomiting · weight loss
- **Uncommon** Abnormal gait · anaemia · arthralgia · chest pain · drowsiness · dry mouth · dry skin · eye swelling · gastro-intestinal haemorrhage · haematemesis · haematuria · hyperbilirubinaemia · joint swelling · myalgia · pain in extremities · paraesthesia · proteinuria · pyrexia · sweating · vertigo

SIDE-EFFECTS, FURTHER INFORMATION
- **Raised transaminases** Reduce dose if serum transaminases raised during treatment (consult product literature).

● CONCEPTION AND CONTRACEPTION Manufacturer advises exclude pregnancy before treatment and ensure effective contraception used.

● PREGNANCY Avoid—teratogenicity and embryotoxicity in *animal* studies.

● BREAST FEEDING Manufacturer advises avoid—no information available.

● HEPATIC IMPAIRMENT Reduce dose if serum transaminases raised during treatment (consult product literature). Max. 40 mg daily in mild impairment. Avoid in moderate to severe impairment, or if unexplained persistent abnormal liver function tests.

● RENAL IMPAIRMENT Max. 40 mg daily in end-stage renal disease.

● MONITORING REQUIREMENTS
- Monitor liver function tests before treatment, then at least monthly and before each dose increase for first year, then at least every 3 months and before each dose increase thereafter.
- Screen for hepatic steatosis and fibrosis before treatment, then annually thereafter.

● MEDICINAL FORMS
There can be variation in the licensing of different medicines containing the same drug.

Capsule
- Lojuxta (Aegerion Pharmaceuticals Ltd) ▼
  Lomitapide 5 mg Lojuxta 5mg capsules | 28 capsule [PoM] £17,765.00
  Lomitapide 10 mg Lojuxta 10mg capsules | 28 capsule [PoM] £17,765.00
  Lomitapide 20 mg Lojuxta 20mg capsules | 28 capsule [PoM] £17,765.00

Omega-3-acid ethyl esters

● INDICATIONS AND DOSE
Adjunct to diet and statin in type IIb or III hypertriglyceridaemia | Adjunct to diet in type IV hypertriglyceridaemia
- BY MOUTH
- Adult: Initially 2 capsules daily, dose to be taken with food, increased if necessary to 4 capsules daily

Adjunct in secondary prevention in those who have had a myocardial infarction in the preceding 3 months
- BY MOUTH
- Adult: 1 capsule daily, dose to be taken with food

● CAUTIONS Anticoagulant treatment (bleeding time increased) · haemorrhagic disorders

● SIDE-EFFECTS
- **Common or very common** Dyspepsia · nausea
- **Uncommon** Abdominal pain · dizziness · gastritis · taste disturbances
- **Rare** Acne · headache · hepatic disorders · hyperglycaemia · rash
- **Very rare** Gastro-intestinal haemorrhage · hypotension · increased white cell count · nasal dryness · urticaria

● PREGNANCY Manufacturers advise use only if potential benefit outweighs risk—no information available.

● BREAST FEEDING Manufacturers advise avoid—no information available.

● HEPATIC IMPAIRMENT Monitor liver function in hepatic impairment.

● NATIONAL FUNDING/ACCESS DECISIONS
Scottish Medicines Consortium (SMC) Decisions
The *Scottish Medicines Consortium* has advised (November 2002) that omega-3-acid ethyl esters are **not** recommended for use within NHS Scotland for the treatment of hypertriglyceridaemia.

● MEDICINAL FORMS
There can be variation in the licensing of different medicines containing the same drug.

Capsule
CAUTIONARY AND ADVISORY LABELS 21
- Omega-3-acid ethyl esters (Non-proprietary)
  Docosahexaenoic acid 380 mg, Eicosapentaenoic acid 460 mg Eicosapentaenoic acid 460mg / Docosahexaenoic acid 380mg capsules | 28 capsule [PoM] no price available DT price = £14.24 | 28 capsule £14.24 DT price = £14.24 | 100 capsule [PoM] £50.86
- Dualtis (BGP Products Ltd)
  Docosahexaenoic acid 380 mg, Eicosapentaenoic acid 460 mg Dualtis 1000mg capsules | 28 capsule [P] £11.37 DT price = £14.24
- Nebbaro (Zentiva)
  Docosahexaenoic acid 380 mg, Eicosapentaenoic acid 460 mg Nebbaro 1000mg capsules | 28 capsule [P] £8.48 DT price = £14.24
- Omacor (BGP Products Ltd)
  Docosahexaenoic acid 380 mg, Eicosapentaenoic acid 460 mg Omacor capsules | 28 capsule [P] £14.24 DT price = £14.24 | 100 capsule [P] £50.84
- Omega 3 (Glenmark Generics (Europe) Ltd, Alissa Healthcare Research Ltd)
  Docosahexaenoic acid 380 mg, Eicosapentaenoic acid 460 mg Omega 3-acid-ethyl esters 1000mg capsules | 28 capsule [PoM] £6.00 DT price = £14.24 | 100 capsule [PoM] £21.00 Omega 3 1000mg capsules | 28 capsule no price available DT price = £14.24
- Prestylon (Teva UK Ltd)
  Docosahexaenoic acid 380 mg, Eicosapentaenoic acid 460 mg Prestylon 1g capsules | 28 capsule [PoM] £10.68 DT price = £14.24 | 100 capsule [PoM] £38.13
- Teromeg (AMCo)
  Docosahexaenoic acid 380 mg, Eicosapentaenoic acid 460 mg Teromeg 1000mg capsules | 28 capsule [PoM] £11.39 DT price = £14.24 | 100 capsule [PoM] £40.67

7 Myocardial ischaemia

Stable angina

Overview
It is important to distinguish stable angina from unstable angina. *Stable angina* usually results from atherosclerotic plaques in the coronary arteries that restrict blood flow and oxygen supply to the heart; it is often precipitated by exertion and relieved by rest. Treatment involves management of acute anginal pain, and long term management to prevent angina attacks and to reduce the risk of cardiovascular events.

Management
Acute attacks of stable angina should be managed with sublingual glyceryl trinitrate p. 201 which can be taken immediately before performing activities that are known to bring on an attack. If attacks occur more than twice a week, regular drug therapy is required and should be introduced in a step-wise manner according to response.

Patients with stable angina should be given a **beta-blocker** or a **calcium-channel blocker**. In those with left-ventricular dysfunction, beta-blocker treatment should be started at a very low dose and titrated very slowly over a period of weeks or months. If a beta-blocker or a calcium-channel blocker alone fails to control symptoms adequately, a combination of a beta-blocker and a dihydropyridine calcium-channel blocker (e.g. amlodipine p. 142, felodipine p. 145, modified-release nifedipine p. 148) should be used; if this combination is not appropriate due to intolerance of, or contra-indication to, either beta-blockers or calcium-channel blockers, addition of a long-acting **nitrate**, ivabradine p. 194, nicorandil p. 194, or ranolazine p. 193 can be considered.

For those patients in whom both beta-blockers and calcium-channel blockers are not tolerated or are contra-indicated, monotherapy with a long-acting nitrate, ivabradine, nicorandil, or ranolazine should be considered.

Response to treatment should be assessed every 2–4 weeks after initiating or changing drug therapy; the drug should be titrated (according to symptom control) to the maximum tolerated dose. Consider referring the patient to a specialist if a combination of two drugs fails to control symptoms. Addition of a third antianginal drug should only be considered if symptom control is not achieved with two drugs and the patient is either due to undergo a revascularisation procedure, or a revascularisation procedure is considered inappropriate. See the use of antiplatelet drugs in patients undergoing coronary stenting.

For long-term prevention of cardiovascular events, see Prevention of cardiovascular events.

Antianginal drugs

Nitrates, calcium-channel blockers, and potassium channel activators (use in adults only) have a vasodilating and, consequently, blood pressure lowering effect. Vasodilators can act in heart failure by arteriolar dilatation which reduces both peripheral vascular resistance and left ventricular pressure during systole resulting in improved cardiac output. They can also cause venous dilatation which results in dilatation of capacitance vessels, increase of venous pooling, and diminution of venous return to the heart (decreasing left ventricular end-diastolic pressure).

Nicorandil, a potassium-channel activator with a nitrate component, has both arterial and venous vasodilating properties and is licensed for the prevention and long-term treatment of angina. Nicorandil has similar efficacy to other antianginal drugs in controlling symptoms; it may produce additional symptomatic benefit in combination with other antianginal drugs [unlicensed indication].

Ivabradine lowers the heart rate by its action on the sinus node. It is licensed for the treatment of angina in patients who are in normal sinus rhythm in combination with a beta-blocker, or when beta-blockers are contra-indicated or not tolerated. Ivabradine, in combination with standard therapy including a beta-blocker (unless contra-indicated or not tolerated), is also licensed for mild to severe stable chronic heart failure in patients who are in sinus rhythm.

Ranolazine is licensed as adjunctive therapy in patients who are inadequately controlled or intolerant of first-line antianginal drugs.

Drugs used for Myocardial ischaemia not listed below
Acebutolol, p. 138 · Aspirin, p. 109 · Atenolol, p. 138 · Bisoprolol fumarate, p. 139 · Bivalirudin, p. 122 · Carvedilol, p. 134 · Diltiazem hydrochloride, p. 143 · Fondaparinux sodium, p. 114 · Metoprolol tartrate, p. 140 · Nadolol, p. 135 · Nicardipine hydrochloride, p. 147 · Oxprenolol hydrochloride, p. 136 · Pindolol, p. 136 · Propranolol hydrochloride, p. 136 · Timolol maleate, p. 137 · Verapamil hydrochloride, p. 150

ANTITHROMBOTIC DRUGS > ANTIPLATELET DRUGS

Cangrelor
16.2.2016

- **DRUG ACTION** Cangrelor is a direct P2Y$_{12}$ platelet receptor antagonist that blocks adenosine diphosphate induced platelet activation and aggregation.

- **INDICATIONS AND DOSE**

In combination with aspirin for the reduction of thrombotic cardiovascular events in patients with coronary artery disease undergoing percutaneous coronary intervention (PCI) who have not received an oral P2Y$_{12}$ inhibitor (e.g. clopidogrel, prasugrel, ticagrelor) prior to the PCI procedure and in whom oral therapy with a P2Y$_{12}$ inhibitor is not suitable (under expert supervision)
  - ▸ INITIALLY BY INTRAVENOUS INJECTION
  - ▸ Adult: Initially 30 micrograms/kg, to be given as a bolus dose, followed immediately by (by intravenous infusion) 4 micrograms/kg/minute, start treatment before percutaneous coronary intervention and continue infusion for at least 2 hours or for the duration of intervention if longer; maximum duration of infusion 4 hours

- **CONTRA-INDICATIONS** Active bleeding · history of stroke · history of transient ischaemic attack · patients at increased risk of bleeding (e.g. impaired haemostasis, irreversible coagulation disorders, major surgery or trauma, uncontrolled severe hypertension)

- **CAUTIONS** Disease states associated with increased bleeding risk

- **INTERACTIONS** Caution with concomitant use of drugs that increase risk of bleeding

- **SIDE-EFFECTS**
  - ▸ **Common or very common** Dyspnoea · ecchymosis · haematoma · haemorrhage (including gastro-intestinal and intracranial)
  - ▸ **Uncommon** Acute renal failure · cardiac tamponade · epistaxis · haemoptysis · rash · retroperitoneal haemorrhage (fatalities reported) · urticaria
  - ▸ **Rare** Anaemia · bruising · thrombocytopenia
  - ▸ **Very rare** Menorrhagia

- **PREGNANCY** Manufacturer advises avoid—toxicity in animal studies.

- **BREAST FEEDING** Manufacturer advises potential risk to infant —no information available.

- **RENAL IMPAIRMENT** Manufacturer advises caution in severe renal impairment—increased risk of bleeding.

- **DIRECTIONS FOR ADMINISTRATION** For intravenous bolus injection and intravenous infusion, reconstitute each 50 mg vial with 5 mL of water for injection and gently swirl, do not shake vigorously. Withdraw 5 mL of reconstituted solution, add to 250 mL of either Sodium Chloride 0.9% or Glucose 5% and mix thoroughly. The bolus injection and infusion should be administered from the infusion solution.

- MEDICINAL FORMS
There can be variation in the licensing of different medicines containing the same drug.
Powder for solution for injection
  - ▸ Kengrexal (The Medicines Company UK Ltd) ▼
  Cangrelor (as Cangrelor tetrasodium) 50 mg Kengrexal 50mg powder for concentrate for solution for injection / infusion vials | 10 vial [PoM] £2,500.00 (Hospital only)

Cardiovascular system

2

ANTITHROMBOTIC DRUGS > GLYCOPROTEIN IIB/IIIA INHIBITORS

Abciximab

● INDICATIONS AND DOSE

Prevention of ischaemic cardiac complications in patients undergoing percutaneous coronary intervention (specialist use only)
▸ INITIALLY BY INTRAVENOUS INJECTION
▸ Adult: Initially 250 micrograms/kg, to be given over 1 minute, then (by intravenous infusion) 125 nanograms/kg/minute (max. per dose 10 micrograms/minute), to be started 10–60 minutes before percutaneous coronary intervention and continue for 12 hours

Short-term prevention of myocardial infarction in patients with unstable angina not responding to conventional treatment and who are scheduled for percutaneous coronary intervention (specialist use only)
▸ INITIALLY BY INTRAVENOUS INJECTION
▸ Adult: Initially 250 micrograms/kg, to be given over 1 minute, then (by intravenous infusion) 125 nanograms/kg/minute (max. per dose 10 micrograms/minute), to be started up to 24 hours before possible percutaneous coronary intervention and continue infusion for 12 hours after intervention

● CONTRA-INDICATIONS Active internal bleeding · arteriovenous malformation or aneurysm · haemorrhagic diathesis · hypertensive retinopathy · intracranial neoplasm · intracranial or intraspinal surgery or trauma within last 2 months · major surgery within last 2 months · severe hypertension · stroke within last 2 years · thrombocytopenia · vasculitis

● CAUTIONS Discontinue if uncontrollable serious bleeding occurs or emergency cardiac surgery needed (consult product literature for details of procedures to minimise bleeding) · elderly

● INTERACTIONS Caution with concomitant use of drugs that increase risk of bleeding.

● SIDE-EFFECTS
▸ **Common or very common** Back pain · bleeding manifestations · bradycardia · chest pain · fever · headache · hypotension · nausea · puncture site pain · thrombocytopenia · vomiting
▸ **Rare** Adult respiratory distress · cardiac tamponade · hypersensitivity reactions

● PREGNANCY Manufacturer advises use only if potential benefit outweighs risk—no information available.

● BREAST FEEDING Manufacturer advises avoid—no information available.

● HEPATIC IMPAIRMENT Avoid in severe liver disease—increased risk of bleeding.

● RENAL IMPAIRMENT Caution in severe impairment—increased risk of bleeding.

● MONITORING REQUIREMENTS
▸ Measure baseline prothrombin time, activated clotting time, activated partial thromboplastin time, platelet count, haemoglobin and haematocrit.
▸ Monitor haemoglobin and haematocrit 12 hours and 24 hours after start of treatment and platelet count 2–4 hours and 24 hours after start of treatment.

● DIRECTIONS FOR ADMINISTRATION For *intravenous infusion* (*ReoPro*®), give continuously in Glucose 5% or Sodium Chloride 0.9%. Dilute requisite dose in infusion fluid and give via infusion pump; filter upon dilution through a non-pyrogenic low proteinbinding 0.2, 0.22, or 5 micron filter or upon administration through an in-line non-progenic low protein-binding 0.2 or 0.22 micron filter.

● MEDICINAL FORMS
There can be variation in the licensing of different medicines containing the same drug.
Solution for injection
▸ ReoPro (Eli Lilly and Company Ltd)
Abciximab 2 mg per 1 ml ReoPro 10mg/5ml solution for injection vials | 1 vial [PoM] £250.24

Eptifibatide

● INDICATIONS AND DOSE

In combination with aspirin and unfractionated heparin for the prevention of early myocardial infarction in patients with unstable angina or non-ST-segment-elevation myocardial infarction and with last episode of chest pain within 24 hours (specialist use only)
▸ INITIALLY BY INTRAVENOUS INJECTION
▸ Adult: Initially 180 micrograms/kg, then (by intravenous infusion) 2 micrograms/kg/minute for up to 72 hours (up to 96 hours if percutaneous coronary intervention during treatment)

● CONTRA-INDICATIONS Abnormal bleeding within 30 days · aneurysm · arteriovenous malformation · haemorrhagic diathesis · history of haemorrhagic stroke · increased INR · increased prothrombin time · intracranial disease · major surgery or severe trauma within 6 weeks · neoplasm · severe hypertension · stroke within last 30 days · thrombocytopenia

● CAUTIONS Discontinue if emergency cardiac surgery necessary · discontinue if intra-aortic balloon pump necessary · discontinue if thrombolytic therapy necessary · risk of bleeding—discontinue immediately if uncontrolled serious bleeding

● INTERACTIONS Caution with concomitant drugs that increase risk of bleeding—discontinue immediately if uncontrolled serious bleeding.

● SIDE-EFFECTS
▸ **Common or very common** Bleeding manifestations
▸ **Very rare** Anaphylaxis · rash

● PREGNANCY Manufacturer advises use only if potential benefit outweighs risk—no information available.

● BREAST FEEDING Manufacturer advises avoid—no information available.

● HEPATIC IMPAIRMENT Avoid in severe liver disease—increased risk of bleeding.

● RENAL IMPAIRMENT Reduce infusion to 1 microgram/kg/minute if eGFR 30–50 mL/minute/1.73 m^2. Avoid if eGFR less than 30 mL/minute/1.73 m^2.

● MONITORING REQUIREMENTS
▸ Measure baseline prothrombin time, activated partial thromboplastin time, platelet count, haemoglobin, haematocrit and serum creatinine.
▸ Monitor haemoglobin, haematocrit and platelets within 6 hours after start of treatment, then at least once daily.

● MEDICINAL FORMS
There can be variation in the licensing of different medicines containing the same drug.
Solution for injection
▸ Integrilin (GlaxoSmithKline UK Ltd)
Eptifibatide 2 mg per 1 ml Integrilin 20mg/10ml solution for injection vials | 1 vial [PoM] £13.61 (Hospital only)
Solution for infusion
▸ Integrilin (GlaxoSmithKline UK Ltd)
Eptifibatide 750 microgram per 1 ml Integrilin 75mg/100ml solution for infusion vials | 1 vial [PoM] £42.79 (Hospital only)

Tirofiban

- **INDICATIONS AND DOSE**

In combination with unfractionated heparin, aspirin, and clopidogrel for prevention of early myocardial infarction in patients with unstable angina or non-ST-segment-elevation myocardial infarction (NSTEMI) and with last episode of chest pain within 12 hours (with angiography planned for 4–48 hours after diagnosis) (initiated under specialist supervision)
  - ▸ BY INTRAVENOUS INFUSION
  - ▸ Adult: Initially 400 nanograms/kg/minute for 30 minutes, then 100 nanograms/kg/minute for at least 48 hours (continue during and for 12–24 hours after percutaneous coronary intervention), maximum duration of treatment 108 hours

In combination with unfractionated heparin, aspirin, and clopidogrel for prevention of early myocardial infarction in patients with unstable angina or non-ST-segment-elevation myocardial infarction (NSTEMI) and with last episode of chest pain within 12 hours (with angiography within 4 hours of diagnosis) (initiated under specialist supervision)
  - ▸ INITIALLY BY INTRAVENOUS INJECTION
  - ▸ Adult: 25 micrograms/kg, to be given over 3 minutes at start of percutaneous coronary intervention, then (by intravenous infusion) 150 nanograms/kg/minute for 12–24 hours, maximum duration of treatment 48 hours

In combination with unfractionated heparin, aspirin, and clopidogrel for reduction of major cardiovascular events in patients with ST-segment elevation myocardial infarction (STEMI) intended for primary percutaneous coronary intervention (PCI) (initiated under specialist supervision)
  - ▸ INITIALLY BY INTRAVENOUS INJECTION
  - ▸ Adult: 25 micrograms/kg, to be given over 3 minutes at start of percutaneous coronary intervention, then (by intravenous infusion) 150 nanograms/kg/minute for 12–24 hours, maximum duration of treatment 48 hours

- CONTRA-INDICATIONS Abnormal bleeding within 30 days · history of aneurysm · history of arteriovenous malformation · history of haemorrhagic stroke · history of intracranial disease · history of neoplasm · increased INR · increased prothrombin time · severe hypertension · stroke within 30 days · thrombocytopenia

- CAUTIONS Active peptic ulcer (within 3 months) · acute pericarditis · anaemia · aortic dissection · cardiogenic shock · discontinue if intra-aortic balloon pump necessary · discontinue if thrombolytic therapy necessary · discontinue immediately if serious or uncontrollable bleeding occurs · discontiue if emergency cardiac surgery necessary · elderly · faecal occult blood · haematuria · haemorrhagic retinopathy · low body-weight · major surgery within 3 months (avoid if within 6 weeks) · organ biopsy or lithotripsy within last 2 weeks · puncture of non-compressible vessel within 24 hours · risk of bleeding (within 3 months) · severe heart failure · severe trauma within 3 months (avoid if within 6 weeks) · traumatic or protracted cardiopulmonary resuscitation within last 2 weeks · uncontrolled severe hypertension · vasculitis

- INTERACTIONS → Appendix 1 (tirofiban). Concomitant drugs that increase risk of bleeding (including within 48 hours of thrombolytic administration).

- SIDE-EFFECTS Bleeding manifestations · fever · headache · nausea · reversible thrombocytopenia

- PREGNANCY Manufacturer advises use only if potential benefit outweighs risk—no information available.

- BREAST FEEDING Manufacturer advises avoid—no information available.

- HEPATIC IMPAIRMENT Caution in mild to moderate liver disease. Avoid in severe liver disease—increased risk of bleeding.

- RENAL IMPAIRMENT Use half normal dose if eGFR less than 30 mL/minute/1.73 m². Increased risk of bleeding. Monitor carefully if eGFR less than 60 mL/minute/1.73 m².

- MONITORING REQUIREMENTS Monitor platelet count, haemoglobin and haematocrit before treatment, 2–6 hours after start of treatment and then at least once daily.

- DIRECTIONS FOR ADMINISTRATION For *intravenous infusion* (*Aggrastat*®), give continuously in Glucose 5% or Sodium chloride 0.9%. Withdraw 50 mL infusion fluid from 250 mL bag and replace with 50 mL tirofiban concentrate (250 micrograms/mL) to give a final concentration of 50 micrograms/mL.

- MEDICINAL FORMS There can be variation in the licensing of different medicines containing the same drug.

Infusion
ELECTROLYTES: May contain Sodium
  - ▸ Aggrastat (Correvio GmbH)
    Tirofiban (as Tirofiban hydrochloride) 50 microgram per 1 ml Aggrastat 12.5mg/250ml infusion bags | 1 bag [PoM] no price available (Hospital only)

Solution for infusion
ELECTROLYTES: May contain Sodium
  - ▸ Aggrastat (Correvio GmbH)
    Tirofiban (as Tirofiban hydrochloride) 250 microgram per 1 ml Aggrastat 12.5mg/50ml concentrate for solution for infusion vials | 1 vial [PoM] no price available (Hospital only)

PIPERAZINE DERIVATIVES

Ranolazine

- **INDICATIONS AND DOSE**

As adjunctive therapy in the treatment of stable angina in patients inadequately controlled or intolerant of first-line antianginal therapies
  - ▸ BY MOUTH
  - ▸ Adult: Initially 375 mg twice daily for 2–4 weeks, then increased to 500 mg twice daily, then adjusted according to response to 750 mg twice daily; reduced if not tolerated to 375–500 mg twice daily

- CAUTIONS Body-weight less than 60 kg · elderly · moderate to severe congestive heart failure · QT interval prolongation

- INTERACTIONS → Appendix 1 (ranolazine).

- SIDE-EFFECTS
  - ▸ **Common or very common** Asthenia · constipation · dizziness · headache · nausea · vomiting
  - ▸ **Uncommon** Abdominal pain · anorexia · anxiety · chromaturia · confusion · cough · dehydration · drowsiness · dry mouth · dyspepsia · dysponea · dysuria · epistaxis · flatulence · haematuria · hallucination · hot flush · hypoaesthesia · hypotension · insomnia · joint swelling · lethargy · muscle cramp · pain in extremities · peripheral oedema · prolonged QT interval · pruritus · sweating · syncope · tinnitus · tremor · visual disturbance · weight loss
  - ▸ **Rare** Allergic dermatitis · amnesia · angioedema · cold extremities · erectile dysfunction · erosive duodenitis · impaired hearing · loss of consciousness · pancreatitis · parosmia · rash · renal failure · throat tightness · urticaria

- PREGNANCY Manufacturer advises avoid unless essential—no information available.

- BREAST FEEDING Manufacturer advises avoid—no information available.

- HEPATIC IMPAIRMENT Use with caution in mild impairment; avoid in moderate and severe impairment.

- RENAL IMPAIRMENT Use with caution if eGFR 30–80 mL/minute/1.73 m^2; avoid if eGFR less than 30 mL/minute/1.73 m^2.
- PATIENT AND CARER ADVICE Patient alert card to be provided.
- NATIONAL FUNDING/ACCESS DECISIONS
  Scottish Medicines Consortium (SMC) Decisions
  The *Scottish Medicines Consortium* has advised (October 2012) that ranolazine (*Ranexa*®) is **not** recommended for use within NHS Scotland.

- MEDICINAL FORMS
  There can be variation in the licensing of different medicines containing the same drug.
  Modified-release tablet
  CAUTIONARY AND ADVISORY LABELS 25
  ▶ Ranexa (A. Menarini Farmaceutica Internazionale SRL)
  Ranolazine 375 mg Ranexa 375mg modified-release tablets | 60 tablet PoM £48.98 DT price = £48.98
  Ranolazine 500 mg Ranexa 500mg modified-release tablets | 60 tablet PoM £48.98 DT price = £48.98
  Ranolazine 750 mg Ranexa 750mg modified-release tablets | 60 tablet PoM £48.98 DT price = £48.98

SELECTIVE SINUS NODE I$_F$ INHIBITORS

Ivabradine

- **INDICATIONS AND DOSE**
  Treatment of angina in patients in normal sinus rhythm
  ▶ BY MOUTH
  ▶ Adult: Initially 5 mg twice daily for 3–4 weeks, then increased if necessary to 7.5 mg twice daily; reduced if not tolerated to 2.5–5 mg twice daily, heart rate at rest should not be allowed to fall below 50 beats per minute
  ▶ Elderly: Initially 2.5 mg twice daily, heart rate at rest should not be allowed to fall below 50 beats per minute

  Mild to severe chronic heart failure
  ▶ BY MOUTH
  ▶ Adult: Initially 5 mg twice daily for 2 weeks, then increased if necessary to 7.5 mg twice daily; reduced if not tolerated to 2.5 mg twice daily, heart rate at rest should not be allowed to fall below 50 beats per minute

- CONTRA-INDICATIONS Acute myocardial infarction · cardiogenic shock · congenital QT syndrome · do not initiate for angina if heart rate below 70 beats per minute · do not initiate for chronic heart failure if heart rate below 75 beats per minute · immediately after cerebrovascular accident · patients dependent on pacemaker · second- and third-degree heart block · severe hypotension · sick-sinus syndrome · sino-atrial block · unstable angina · unstable or acute heart failure
- CAUTIONS Atrial fibrillation or other arrhythmias (treatment ineffective) · elderly · in angina, consider stopping if there is no or limited symptom improvement after 3 months · intraventricular conduction defects · mild to moderate hypotension (avoid if severe) · retinitis pigmentosa
- INTERACTIONS → Appendix 1 (ivabradine).
- SIDE-EFFECTS
  ▶ **Common or very common** Atrial fibrillation · blurred vision · bradycardia · dizziness · first-degree heart block · headache · phosphenes · ventricular extrasystoles · visual disturbances
  ▶ **Uncommon** Angioedema · constipation · diarrhoea · dyspnoea · eosinophilia · hyperuricaemia · muscle cramps · nausea · palpitations · raised plasma-creatinine concentration · rash · supraventricular extrasystoles · vertigo
  ▶ **Very rare** Second and third-degree heart block · sick sinus syndrome

- PREGNANCY Manufacturer advises avoid—*toxicity* in animal studies.
- BREAST FEEDING Present in milk in *animal* studies—manufacturer advises avoid.
- HEPATIC IMPAIRMENT Manufacturer advises caution in moderate impairment. Avoid in severe impairment.
- RENAL IMPAIRMENT Manufacturer advises use with caution if eGFR less than 15 mL/minute/1.73 m^2—no information available.
- MONITORING REQUIREMENTS
  ▶ Monitor regularly for atrial fibrillation (consider benefits and risks of continued treatment if atrial fibrillation occurs).
  ▶ Monitor for bradycardia, especially after any dose increase, and discontinue if resting heart rate persistently below 50 beats per minute or continued symptoms of bradycardia despite dose reduction.
- NATIONAL FUNDING/ACCESS DECISIONS
  NICE technology appraisals (TAs)
  ▶ **Ivabradine for the treatment of chronic heart failure (November 2012)** NICE TA267
  Ivabradine, in combination with standard therapy including a beta-blocker (unless contra-indicated or not tolerated), an ACE inhibitor, and an aldosterone antagonist, is an option for treating mild to severe stable chronic heart failure in patients who:
  - have a left ventricular ejection fraction of ≤ 35%, *and*
  - are in sinus rhythm with a heart rate of ≥75 beats per minute
  Ivabradine should be initiated only by a heart failure specialist after 4 weeks of stable optimal standard therapy; monitoring and dose titration should be carried out by a heart failure specialist, or a GP with special interest in heart failure, or by a heart failure specialist nurse.
  www.nice.org.uk/TA267
  Scottish Medicines Consortium (SMC) Decisions
  The *Scottish Medicines Consortium* has advised (September 2012) that ivabradine (*Procoralan*®) is accepted for restricted use within NHS Scotland in accordance with its licensed indication for heart failure only if resting heart rate remains ≥75 beats per minute despite optimal standard therapy.

- MEDICINAL FORMS
  There can be variation in the licensing of different medicines containing the same drug.
  Tablet
  ▶ Procoralan (Servier Laboratories Ltd) ▼
  Ivabradine (as Ivabradine hydrochloride) 5 mg Procoralan 5mg tablets | 56 tablet PoM £40.17 DT price = £40.17
  Ivabradine (as Ivabradine hydrochloride) 7.5 mg Procoralan 7.5mg tablets | 56 tablet PoM £40.17 DT price = £40.17

VASODILATORS › POTASSIUM-CHANNEL OPENERS

Nicorandil

24.2.2016

- **INDICATIONS AND DOSE**
  Prophylaxis and treatment of stable angina (second-line)
  ▶ BY MOUTH
  ▶ Adult: Initially 5–10 mg twice daily, then increased if tolerated to 40 mg twice daily; usual dose 10–20 mg twice daily, use lower initial dose regimen if patient susceptible to headache

- CONTRA-INDICATIONS Acute pulmonary oedema · cardiogenic shock · hypovolaemia · left ventricular failure with low filling pressures · severe hypotension
- CAUTIONS Acute myocardial infarction with acute left ventricular failure and low filling pressures · diverticular

disease (risk of fistula formation or bowel perforation) ·
G6PD deficiency · heart failure (class III–IV) ·
hyperkalaemia · low systolic blood pressure

● INTERACTIONS → Appendix 1 (nicorandil).

● SIDE-EFFECTS
▶ **Common or very common** Cutaneous vasodilation with
flushing · dizziness · headache (especially on initiation,
usually transitory) · increase in heart rate (at high doses) ·
nausea · rectal bleeding · vomiting · weakness
▶ **Uncommon** Angioedema · hypotension · myalgia · oral
ulceration
▶ **Rare** Abdominal pain · anal ulceration · cholestasis ·
gastrointestinal ulceration · hepatitis · jaundice · pruritus ·
rash · skin ulceration
▶ **Very rare** Eye ulceration
▶ **Frequency not known** Gastrointestinal haemorrhage
    SIDE-EFFECTS, FURTHER INFORMATION
▶ Nicorandil-induced ulceration Nicorandil can cause serious
skin, mucosal, and eye ulceration; including
gastrointestinal ulcers, which may progress to perforation,
haemorrhage, fistula or abscess. Stop treatment if
ulceration occurs and consider an alternative.

● PREGNANCY Manufacturer advises use only if potential
benefit outweighs risk—no information available.

● BREAST FEEDING No information available—manufacturer
advises avoid.

● PATIENT AND CARER ADVICE
Driving and skilled tasks
Patients should be warned not to drive or operate
machinery until it is established that their performance is
unimpaired.

● MEDICINAL FORMS
There can be variation in the licensing of different medicines
containing the same drug.
Tablet
  ▶ Nicorandil (Non-proprietary)
    Nicorandil 10 mg Nicorandil 10mg tablets | 60 tablet [PoM] £7.71 DT
    price = £2.52
    Nicorandil 20 mg Nicorandil 20mg tablets | 60 tablet [PoM] £14.64
    DT price = £4.82
  ▶ Ikorel (Zentiva)
    Nicorandil 10 mg Ikorel 10mg tablets | 60 tablet [PoM] £7.71 DT
    price = £2.52
    Nicorandil 20 mg Ikorel 20mg tablets | 60 tablet [PoM] £14.64 DT
    price = £4.82

7.1   Acute coronary syndromes

Acute coronary syndromes

Overview
Acute coronary syndromes encompass a spectrum of
conditions which include unstable angina, and myocardial
infarction with or without ST-segment elevation. Patients
with different acute coronary syndromes may present
similarly; definitive diagnosis is made on the basis of clinical
presentation, ECG changes, and measurement of
biochemical cardiac markers.

Unstable angina and non-ST-segment elevation myocardial infarction (NSTEMI)
These are related acute coronary syndromes that fall
between the classifications of stable angina and ST-segment
elevation myocardial infarction (STEMI). They usually occur
as a result of atheromatous plaque rupture, and are often
characterised by stable angina that suddenly worsens,
recurring or prolonged angina at rest, or new onset of severe
angina. Patients with unstable angina have no evidence of

myocardial necrosis, whereas in NSTEMI, myocardial
necrosis (less significant than with STEMI) will be evident.
There is a risk of progression to STEMI or sudden death,
particularly in patients who experience pain at rest.

Management of unstable angina and non-ST-segment elevation myocardial infarction (NSTEMI)
These conditions are managed similarly; the aims of
management are to provide supportive care and pain relief
during the acute attack and to prevent further cardiac events
and death. For advice on the management of patients with
acute ST-segment elevation myocardial infarction (STEMI),
see below.

Initial management
Oxygen should be administered if there is evidence of
hypoxia, pulmonary oedema, or continuing myocardial
ischaemia; hyperoxia should be avoided and particular care
is required in patients with chronic obstructive airways
disease.

Nitrates are used to relieve ischaemic pain. If sublingual
glyceryl trinitrate p. 201 is not effective, intravenous or
buccal glyceryl trinitrate or intravenous isosorbide dinitrate
p. 202 is given. If pain continues, diamorphine hydrochloride
p. 415 or morphine p. 421 can be given by slow intravenous
injection; an antiemetic such as metoclopramide
hydrochloride p. 395 should also be given.

Aspirin p. 109 (chewed or dispersed in water) is given for
its antiplatelet effect. If aspirin is given before arrival at
hospital, a note saying that it has been given should be sent
with the patient. Clopidogrel p. 110 should also be given.
Prasugrel p. 197 is an alternative to clopidogrel in certain
patients undergoing percutaneous coronary intervention
(see NICE guidance). Ticagrelor p. 197 is also an alternative
to clopidogrel (see NICE guidance). Patients should also
receive either heparin (unfractionated) p. 120, a **low
molecular weight heparin**, or fondaparinux sodium p. 114.

Patients without contra-indications should receive **beta-blockers** which should be continued indefinitely. In patients
without left ventricular dysfunction and in whom beta-blockers are inappropriate, diltiazem hydrochloride p. 143 or
verapamil hydrochloride p. 150 can be given.

The glycoprotein IIb/IIIa inhibitors eptifibatide p. 192 (in
combination with heparin (unfractionated) and aspirin) and
tirofiban p. 193 (in combination with heparin
(unfractionated), aspirin, and clopidogrel) can be used for
unstable angina or for NSTEMI in patients at a high risk of
either myocardial infarction or death.

In intermediate- and high-risk patients, abciximab p. 192
or eptifibatide (in combination with heparin (unfractionated)
and aspirin), or tirofiban (in combination with heparin
(unfractionated), aspirin, and clopidogrel) can also be used
in patients undergoing percutaneous coronary intervention,
to reduce the immediate risk of vascular occlusion. In
intermediate- and high-risk patients in whom early
intervention is planned, bivalirudin p. 122 can be considered
as an alternative to the combination of a glyocprotein
IIb/IIIa inhibitor plus a heparin.

Revascularisation procedures are often appropriate for
patients with unstable angina or NSTEMI; the use of
antiplatelet drugs in patients undergoing coronary stenting.

Long-term management
The need for long-term angina treatment or for coronary
angiography should be assessed. Most patients will require
standard angina treatment to prevent recurrence of
symptoms.

ST-segment elevation myocardial infarction (STEMI)
This is an acute coronary syndrome where atheromatous
plaque rupture leads to thrombosis and myocardial
ischaemia, with irreversible necrosis of the heart muscle,
often leading to long-term complications. STEMI can also
occasionally occur as a result of coronary spasm or

embolism, arteritis, spontaneous thrombosis, or sudden severe elevation in blood pressure.

Management of ST-segment elevation myocardial infarction (STEMI)

These notes give an overview of the initial and long-term management of myocardial infarction with ST segment elevation (STEMI). For advice on the management of non-ST-segment elevation myocardial infarction (NSTEMI) and unstable angina, see above. The aims of management of STEMI are to provide supportive care and pain relief, to promote reperfusion and to reduce mortality. Oxygen, nitrates, and diamorphine hydrochloride or morphine can provide initial support and pain relief; aspirin and percutaneous coronary intervention or thrombolytics promote reperfusion; anticoagulants help to reduce re-occlusion and systemic embolisation; long-term use of aspirin, beta-blockers, ACE inhibitors, and statins help to reduce mortality further.

Local guidelines for the management of myocardial infarction should be followed where they exist.

Initial management

Oxygen should be administered if there is evidence of hypoxia, pulmonary oedema, or continuing myocardial ischaemia; hyperoxia should be avoided and particular care is required in patients with chronic obstructive airways disease.

The pain (and anxiety) of myocardial infarction is managed with slow intravenous injection of diamorphine hydrochloride or morphine; an antiemetic such as metoclopramide hydrochloride (or, if left ventricular function is not compromised, cyclizine p. 393) by intravenous injection should also be given.

Aspirin (chewed or dispersed in water) is given for its antiplatelet effect. If aspirin is given before arrival at hospital, a note saying that it has been given should be sent with the patient. Clopidogrel, should also be given. Prasugrel, is an alternative to clopidogrel in certain patients undergoing percutaneous coronary intervention (see NICE guidance). Ticagrelor, is also an alternative to clopidogrel (see NICE guidance).

Patency of the occluded artery can be restored by percutaneous coronary intervention or by giving a **thrombolytic drug**, unless contra-indicated. Percutaneous coronary intervention is the preferred method; a **glycoprotein IIb/IIIa inhibitor** can be used to reduce the risk of immediate vascular occlusion in intermediate- and high-risk patients. Patients undergoing percutaneous coronary intervention should also receive either heparin (unfractionated) or a low molecular weight heparin (e.g. enoxaparin sodium p. 119); bivalirudin is an alternative to the combination of a glycoprotein IIb/IIIa inhibitor plus a heparin (see also NICE guidance). In patients who cannot be offered percutaneous coronary intervention within 90 minutes of diagnosis, a thrombolytic drug should be administered along with either heparin (unfractionated) (for maximum 2 days), a low molecular weight heparin (e.g. enoxaparin sodium), or fondaparinux sodium. See use of antiplatelet drugs in patients undergoing coronary stenting in Antiplatelet drugs p. 108.

Patients who do not receive reperfusion therapy (with percutaneous coronary intervention or a thrombolytic) should be treated with either fondaparinux sodium, enoxaparin sodium, or heparin (unfractionated). Prescribers should consult product literature and local protocols (where they exist) for details of anticoagulant dose and duration.

Nitrates are used to relieve ischaemic pain. If sublingual glyceryl trinitrate p. 201 is not effective, intravenous glyceryl trinitrate or isosorbide dinitrate p. 202 is given.

Early administration of some **beta-blockers** has been shown to be of benefit and should be given to patients without contra-indications.

ACE inhibitors, and angiotensin-II receptor antagonists if an ACE inhibitor cannot be used, are also of benefit to patients who have no contra-indications; in hypertensive and normotensive patients treatment with an ACE inhibitor, or an angiotensin-II receptor antagonist, can be started within 24 hours of the myocardial infarction and continued for at least 5–6 weeks (see below for long-term treatment).

All patients should be closely monitored for hyperglycaemia; those with diabetes or raised blood-glucose concentration should receive insulin p. 644.

Long-term management

Long-term management following STEMI involves the use of several drugs which should ideally be started before the patient is discharged from hospital.

Aspirin p. 109 should be given to all patients, unless contra-indicated. The addition of clopidogrel p. 110 has been shown to reduce morbidity and mortality. Prasugrel p. 197 or ticagrelor p. 197 are alternatives to clopidogrel in certain patients. For those intolerant of clopidogrel, and who are at low risk of bleeding, the combination of warfarin sodium p. 126 and aspirin should be considered. In those intolerant of both aspirin and clopidogrel, warfarin sodium alone can be used. Warfarin sodium should be continued for those who are already being treated for another indication, such as atrial fibrillation, with the addition of aspirin if there is a low risk of bleeding. The combination of aspirin with clopidogrel or warfarin sodium increases the risk of bleeding. Low-dose rivaroxaban p. 115, in combination with aspirin alone *or* aspirin and clopidogrel, is licensed for the prevention of atherothrombotic events following STEMI—see Prevention of cardiovascular events. For details of antiplatelet drug duration following coronary stenting—see also Antiplatelet drugs and coronary stents in Antiplatelet drugs p. 108.

Beta-blockers should be given to all patients in whom they are not contra-indicated. Acebutolol p. 138, metoprolol tartrate p. 140, propranolol hydrochloride p. 136 and timolol maleate p. 137 are suitable; for patients with left ventricular dysfunction, carvedilol p. 134, bisoprolol fumarate p. 139, or long-acting metoprolol tartrate may be appropriate

Diltiazem hydrochloride p. 143 [unlicensed] or verapamil hydrochloride p. 150 can be considered if a beta-blocker cannot be used; however, they are contra-indicated in those with left ventricular dysfunction. Other calcium-channel blockers have no place in routine long-term management after a myocardial infarction.

An **ACE inhibitor** should be considered for all patients, especially those with evidence of left ventricular dysfunction. If an ACE inhibitor cannot be used, an angiotensin-II receptor antagonist may be used for patients with heart failure. A relatively high dose of either the ACE inhibitor or angiotensin-II receptor antagonist may be required to produce benefit.

Nitrates are used for patients with angina.

Eplerenone p. 174 is licensed for use following a myocardial infarction in those with left ventricular dysfunction and evidence of heart failure.

See also the role of **statins** in preventing recurrent cardiovascular events in Lipid-regulating drugs p. 178.

Prevention of cardiovascular events

Patients with stable angina, unstable angina, or NSTEMI should be given advice and treatments to reduce their cardiovascular risk. The importance of life-style changes, especially stopping smoking, should be emphasised. Aspirin should be given indefinitely. Antihypertensive treatment should be initiated if appropriate, and a **statin** should also be given.

In patients with stable angina, addition of an **ACE inhibitor** should be considered for patients with diabetes (and should be continued if indicated for a co-morbidity).

In patients with unstable angina or NSTEMI, clopidogrel is given, in combination with aspirin, for up to 12 months—

most benefit occurs during the first 3 months. Prasugrel or ticagrelor are alternatives to clopidogrel in certain patients. An ACE inhibitor should also be given.

Low-dose rivaroxaban, in combination with aspirin alone *or* aspirin and clopidogrel, is licensed for the prevention of atherothrombotic events following an acute coronary syndrome with elevated cardiac biomarkers.

> **Drugs used for Acute coronary syndromes not listed below** Captopril, p. 154 · Dalteparin sodium, p. 118 · Lisinopril, p. 156 · Perindopril arginine, p. 157 · Perindopril erbumine, p. 158 · Ramipril, p. 159 · Trandolapril, p. 160 · Valsartan, p. 164

ANTITHROMBOTIC DRUGS > ANTIPLATELET DRUGS

Prasugrel

● **INDICATIONS AND DOSE**

In combination with aspirin for the prevention of atherothrombotic events in patients with acute coronary syndrome undergoing percutaneous coronary intervention

▸ BY MOUTH

▸ Adult 18–74 years (body-weight up to 60 kg): Initially 60 mg for 1 dose, then 5 mg once daily usually for up to 12 months

▸ Adult 18–74 years (body-weight 60 kg and above): Initially 60 mg for 1 dose, then 10 mg once daily usually for up to 12 months

▸ Adult 75 years and over: Initially 60 mg for 1 dose, then 5 mg once daily usually for up to 12 months

Patients undergoing coronary angiography within 48 hours of admission for unstable angina or NSTEMI

▸ BY MOUTH

▸ Adult: Loading dose 60 mg, not to be administered until the time of percutaneous coronary intervention in order to minimise the risk of bleeding, maintenance dose of 10 mg or 5 mg daily should then be selected as appropriate based on age and weight

Alternative to clopidogrel in certain patients undergoing percutaneous coronary intervention

▸ BY MOUTH

▸ Adult: 60 mg, as a single dose

● **CONTRA-INDICATIONS** Active bleeding · history of stroke or transient ischaemic attack

● **CAUTIONS** Body-weight less than 60 kg · discontinue at least 7 days before elective surgery if antiplatelet effect not desirable · elderly · patients at increased risk of bleeding (e.g. from recent trauma, surgery, gastro-intestinal bleeding, or active peptic ulcer disease)

● **INTERACTIONS** → Appendix 1 (prasugrel). Caution with concomitant use of drugs that increase risk of bleeding.

● **SIDE-EFFECTS**

▸ **Common or very common** Anaemia · gastro-intestinal haemorrhage · haematoma · haematuria · haemorrhage · intracranial haemorrhage · rash

▸ **Uncommon** Angioedema · hypersensitivity reactions

▸ **Rare** Thrombocytopenia

▸ **Frequency not known** Thrombotic thrombocytopenic purpura

● **ALLERGY AND CROSS-SENSITIVITY** Caution in patients with history of hypersensitivity reactions to thienopyridines (e.g. clopidogrel).

● **PREGNANCY** Manufacturer advises use only if potential benefit outweighs risk.

● **BREAST FEEDING** Manufacturer advises avoid—no information available.

● **HEPATIC IMPAIRMENT** Use with caution in moderate impairment—increased risk of bleeding. Avoid in severe impairment.

● **RENAL IMPAIRMENT** Use with caution—increased risk of bleeding.

● **NATIONAL FUNDING/ACCESS DECISIONS**

NICE technology appraisals (TAs)

▸ **Prasugrel with percutaneous coronary intervention for treating acute coronary syndromes (July 2014)** NICE TA317 Prasugrel 10 mg in combination with aspirin is recommended as an option, within its marketing authorisation, for preventing atherothrombotic events in adults with acute coronary syndrome (unstable angina (UA), non-ST segment elevation myocardial infarction (NSTEMI) or ST segment elevation myocardial infarction (STEMI)) having primary or delayed percutaneous coronary intervention.
www.nice.org.uk/TA317

Scottish Medicines Consortium (SMC) Decisions
The *Scottish Medicines Consortium* has advised (August 2009) that prasugrel (*Efient®*), in combination with aspirin, be accepted for restricted use within NHS Scotland for the prevention of atherothrombotic events in patients with acute coronary syndrome undergoing percutaneous coronary intervention who are eligible to receive the 10 mg dose of prasugrel.

● **MEDICINAL FORMS**
There can be variation in the licensing of different medicines containing the same drug.

Tablet

▸ Efient (Eli Lilly and Company Ltd)
  Prasugrel (as Prasugrel hydrochloride) 5 mg Efient 5mg tablets | 28 tablet [PoM] £47.56 DT price = £47.56
  Prasugrel (as Prasugrel hydrochloride) 10 mg Efient 10mg tablets | 28 tablet [PoM] £47.56 DT price = £47.56

Ticagrelor

● **INDICATIONS AND DOSE**

In combination with aspirin for the prevention of atherothrombotic events in patients with acute coronary syndrome

▸ BY MOUTH

▸ Adult: Initially 180 mg for 1 dose, then 90 mg twice daily usually for up to 12 months

Alternative to clopidogrel in patients undergoing percutaneous coronary intervention

▸ BY MOUTH

▸ Adult: 180 mg, as a single dose

● **CONTRA-INDICATIONS** Active bleeding · history of intracranial haemorrhage

● **CAUTIONS** Asthma · bradycardia (unless pacemaker fitted) · chronic obstructive pulmonary disease · discontinue 7 days before elective surgery if antiplatelet effect not desirable · history of hyperuricaemia · patients at increased risk of bleeding (e.g. from recent trauma, surgery, gastro-intestinal bleeding, or coagulation disorders) · second- or third-degree AV block (unless pacemaker fitted) · sick sinus syndrome (unless pacemaker fitted)

● **INTERACTIONS** Caution with concomitant use of drugs that increase risk of bleeding.

● **SIDE-EFFECTS**

▸ **Common or very common** Bruising · dyspnoea · haemorrhage

▸ **Uncommon** Abdominal pain · diarrhoea · dizziness · dyspepsia · gastritis · headache · nausea · pruritus · rash · vomiting

2

Cardiovascular system

▶ **Rare** Confusion · constipation · hyperuricaemia · paraesthesia · raised serum creatinine · vertigo

● PREGNANCY Manufacturer advises avoid—toxicity in *animal* studies.

● BREAST FEEDING Manufacturer advises avoid—present in milk in *animal* studies.

● HEPATIC IMPAIRMENT Avoid in moderate or severe impairment—no information available.

● MONITORING REQUIREMENTS Monitor renal function 1 month after initiation.

● NATIONAL FUNDING/ACCESS DECISIONS

NICE technology appraisals (TAs)

▶ **Ticagrelor for the treatment of acute coronary syndromes (October 2011)** NICE TA236

Ticagrelor, in combination with low-dose aspirin, is recommended for up to 12 months as a treatment option in adults with acute coronary syndromes, that is, people:

● with ST-segment elevation myocardial infarction—defined as ST elevation or new left bundle branch block on electrocardiogram—that cardiologists intend to treat with primary percutaneous coronary intervention, **or**

● with non-ST-segment elevation myocardial infarction (NSTEMI), **or**

● admitted to hospital with unstable angina—defined as ST or T wave changes on electrocardiogram suggestive of ischaemia plus one of the characteristics defined below. Before ticagrelor is continued beyond the initial treatment, the diagnosis of unstable angina should first be confirmed, ideally by a cardiologist. Characteristics to be used in defining treatment with ticagrelor for unstable angina are:

● age 60 years or older;

● previous myocardial infarction or previous coronary artery bypass grafting;

● coronary artery disease with stenosis of 50% or more in at least two vessels;

● previous ischaemic stroke;

● previous transient ischaemic attack, carotid stenosis of at least 50%, or cerebral revascularisation;

● diabetes mellitus;

● peripheral arterial disease, **or**

● chronic renal dysfunction (creatinine clearance less than 60 mL/minute/1.73 m^2).

www.nice.org.uk/TA236

● MEDICINAL FORMS

There can be variation in the licensing of different medicines containing the same drug.

Tablet

▶ Brilique (AstraZeneca UK Ltd)

Ticagrelor 60 mg Brilique 60mg tablets | 56 tablet [PoM] £54.60
Ticagrelor 90 mg Brilique 90mg tablets | 56 tablet [PoM] £54.60 DT price = £54.60

ANTITHROMBOTIC DRUGS ›TISSUE PLASMINOGEN ACTIVATORS

Fibrinolytic drugs

Overview

The value of thrombolytic drugs for the treatment of *myocardial infarction* has been established. Streptokinase p. 199 and alteplase p. 199 have been shown to reduce mortality. Reteplase p. 199 and tenecteplase p. 200 are also licensed for acute myocardial infarction. Thrombolytic drugs are indicated for any patient with acute myocardial infarction for whom the benefit is likely to outweigh the risk of treatment. Trials have shown that the benefit is greatest in those with ECG changes that include ST segment elevation (especially in those with anterior infarction) and in patients with bundle branch block. Patients should not be denied

thrombolytic treatment on account of age alone because mortality in the elderly is high and the reduction in mortality is the same as in younger patients. Alteplase should be given within 6–12 hours of symptom onset, reteplase and streptokinase within 12 hours of symptom onset, but ideally all should be given within 1 hour; use after 12 hours requires specialist advice. Tenecteplase should be given as early as possible and usually within 6 hours of symptom onset.

Alteplase, streptokinase and urokinase p. 124 can be used for other thromboembolic disorders such as deep-vein thrombosis and pulmonary embolism. Alteplase is also used for acute ischaemic stroke.

Urokinase is also licensed to restore the patency of occluded intravenous catheters and cannulas blocked with fibrin clots.

Fibrinolytics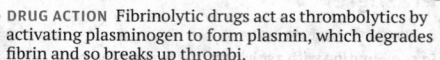

● DRUG ACTION Fibrinolytic drugs act as thrombolytics by activating plasminogen to form plasmin, which degrades fibrin and so breaks up thrombi.

● CONTRA-INDICATIONS Active pulmonary disease with cavitation · acute pancreatitis · aneurysm · aortic dissection · bacterial endocarditis · bleeding diatheses · coagulation defects · coma · heavy vaginal bleeding · history of cerebrovascular disease (especially recent events or with any residual disability) · oesophageal varices · pericarditis · recent haemorrhage · recent surgery (including dental extraction) · recent symptoms of possible peptic ulceration · recent trauma · severe hypertension

● CAUTIONS Conditions in which thrombolysis might give rise to embolic complications such as enlarged left atrium with atrial fibrillation (risk of dissolution of clot and subsequent embolisation) · elderly · external chest compression · hypertension · risk of bleeding (including that from venepuncture or invasive procedures)

● INTERACTIONS Caution with recent or concomitant use of drugs that increase the risk of bleeding.

● SIDE-EFFECTS Allergic reactions · anaphylaxis · angina (when used in myocardial infarction) · back pain · bleeding · bleeding (usually limited to the site of injection, but can occur from other sites) · cerebral oedema (caused by reperfusion) · convulsions · fever · flushing · hypotension · intracerebral haemorrhage · nausea · pulmonary oedema (caused by reperfusion) · rash · recurrent ischaemia (when used in myocardial infarction) · reperfusion arrhythmias (when used in myocardial infarction) · uveitis · vomiting

SIDE-EFFECTS, FURTHER INFORMATION

▶ **Bleeding** Serious bleeding calls for discontinuation of the thrombolytic and may require administration of coagulation factors and antifibrinolytic drugs (e.g. tranexamic acid). Rarely further embolism may occur (either due to clots that break away from the original thrombus or to cholesterol crystal emboli).

▶ **Hypotension** Hypotension can usually be controlled by elevating the patient's legs, or by reducing the rate of infusion or stopping it temporarily.

● PREGNANCY Thrombolytic drugs can possibly lead to premature separation of the placenta in the first 18 weeks of pregnancy. There is also a risk of maternal haemorrhage throughout pregnancy and post-partum, and also a theoretical risk of fetal haemorrhage throughout pregnancy.

● HEPATIC IMPAIRMENT Avoid in severe hepatic impairment as there is an increased risk of bleeding.

Alteplase

☞198

(rt-PA; Tissue-type plasminogen activator)

● INDICATIONS AND DOSE

Acute myocardial infarction, accelerated regimen
▸ INITIALLY BY INTRAVENOUS INJECTION
▸ Adult (body-weight up to 65 kg): Initially 15 mg, to be initiated within 6 hours of symptom onset, followed by (by intravenous infusion) 0.75 mg/kg, to be given over 30 minutes, then (by intravenous infusion) 0.5 mg/kg, to be given over 60 minutes, maximum total dose of 100 mg administered over 90 minutes
▸ Adult (body-weight 65 kg and above): Initially 15 mg, to be initiated within 6 hours of symptom onset, followed by (by intravenous infusion) 50 mg, to be given over 30 minutes, then (by intravenous infusion) 35 mg, to be given over 60 minutes, maximum total dose of 100 mg administered over 90 minutes

Acute myocardial infarction
▸ INITIALLY BY INTRAVENOUS INJECTION
▸ Adult: Initially 10 mg, to be initiated within 6–12 hours of symptom onset, followed by (by intravenous infusion) 50 mg, to be given over 60 minutes, then (by intravenous infusion) 10 mg for 4 infusions, each 10 mg infusion dose to be given over 30 minutes, total dose of 100 mg over 3 hours; maximum 1.5 mg/kg in patients less than 65 kg

Pulmonary embolism
▸ INITIALLY BY INTRAVENOUS INJECTION
▸ Adult: Initially 10 mg, to be given over 1–2 minutes, followed by (by intravenous infusion) 90 mg, to be given over 2 hours, maximum 1.5 mg/kg in patients less than 65 kg

Acute ischaemic stroke (under specialist neurology physician only)
▸ BY INTRAVENOUS INFUSION
▸ Adult 18–79 years: Initially 900 micrograms/kg (max. per dose 90 mg), treatment **must** begin within 4.5 hours of symptom onset, to be given over 60 minutes, the initial 10% of dose is to be administered by intravenous injection and the remainder by intravenous infusion

ACTILYSE CATHFLO®

Thrombolytic treatment of occluded central venous access devices (including those used for haemodialysis)
▸ BY INTRAVENOUS INJECTION
▸ Adult: (consult product literature)

● CONTRA-INDICATIONS
▸ When used for acute ischaemic stroke Convulsion accompanying stroke · history of stroke in patients with diabetes · hyperglycaemia · hypoglycaemia · severe stroke · stroke in last 3 months
● INTERACTIONS Contra-indicated if concomitant treatment with oral anticoagulants.
● SIDE-EFFECTS Risk of cerebral bleeding increased in acute stroke
● ALLERGY AND CROSS-SENSITIVITY Contra-indicated if history of hypersensitivity to gentamicin (residue from manufacturing process).
● MONITORING REQUIREMENTS
▸ When used for acute ischaemic stroke Monitor for intracranial haemorrhage, and monitor blood pressure (antihypertensive recommended if systolic above 180 mmHg or diastolic above 105 mmHg).
● DIRECTIONS FOR ADMINISTRATION For *intravenous infusion* (*Actilyse*®), give intermittently or continuously in Sodium chloride 0.9%; dissolve in water for injections to a concentration of 1 mg/mL or 2 mg/mL and infuse

intravenously; alternatively dilute the solution further in the infusion fluid to a concentration of not less than 200 micrograms/mL; not to be infused in glucose solution.
● NATIONAL FUNDING/ACCESS DECISIONS
NICE technology appraisals (TAs)
▸ Alteplase for the treatment of acute ischaemic stroke (September 2012) NICE TA264
Alteplase is recommended for the treatment of acute ischaemic stroke in adults in accordance with its licensed indication if:
● treatment is started as early as possible within 4.5 hours of onset of stroke symptoms, *and*
● intracranial haemorrhage has been excluded by appropriate imaging techniques.
www.nice.org.uk/TA264

● MEDICINAL FORMS
There can be variation in the licensing of different medicines containing the same drug. Forms available from special-order manufacturers include: solution for injection
Powder and solvent for solution for injection
▸ Actilyse (Boehringer Ingelheim Ltd)
Alteplase 10 mg Actilyse 10mg powder and solvent for solution for injection vials | 1 vial PoM £144.00
Alteplase 20 mg Actilyse 20mg powder and solvent for solution for injection vials | 1 vial PoM £216.00
▸ Actilyse Cathflo (Boehringer Ingelheim Ltd)
Alteplase 2 mg Actilyse Cathflo 2mg powder and solvent for solution for injection vials | 5 vial PoM £225.00 (Hospital only)
Powder and solvent for solution for infusion
▸ Actilyse (Boehringer Ingelheim Ltd)
Alteplase 50 mg Actilyse 50mg powder and solvent for solution for infusion vials | 1 vial PoM £360.00

Reteplase

☞198

● INDICATIONS AND DOSE
Acute myocardial infarction
▸ BY INTRAVENOUS INJECTION
▸ Adult: 10 units, initiated within 12 hours of onset of symptoms, dose to be given over not more than 2 minutes, followed by 10 units after 30 minutes

● BREAST FEEDING Manufacturer advises avoid breastfeeding for 24 hours after dose (express and discard milk during this time).

● MEDICINAL FORMS
There can be variation in the licensing of different medicines containing the same drug.
No licensed medicines listed.

Streptokinase

☞198

● INDICATIONS AND DOSE
Acute myocardial infarction
▸ BY INTRAVENOUS INFUSION
▸ Adult: 1 500 000 units, to be initiated within 12 hours of symptom onset, dose to be given over 60 minutes

Deep-vein thrombosis | Pulmonary embolism | Acute arterial thromboembolism | Central retinal venous or arterial thrombosis
▸ BY INTRAVENOUS INFUSION
▸ Adult: 250 000 units, dose to be given over 30 minutes, then 100 000 units every 1 hour for up to 12–72 hours, duration is adjusted according to condition with monitoring of clotting parameters (consult product literature)

● SIDE-EFFECTS
▸ **Rare** Guillain-Barré syndrome

- **ALLERGY AND CROSS-SENSITIVITY** Contra-indicated if previous allergic reaction to either streptokinase or anistreplase (no longer available). Prolonged persistence of antibodies to streptokinase and anistreplase (no longer available) can reduce the effectiveness of subsequent treatment; therefore, streptokinase should not be used again beyond 4 days of first administration of either streptokinase or anistreplase.

- **DIRECTIONS FOR ADMINISTRATION** For *intravenous infusion* (*Streptase*®), give continuously or intermittently; reconstitute with sodium chloride 0.9%, then dilute further with Glucose 5% or Sodium Chloride 0.9% after reconstitution.

- **MEDICINAL FORMS**
There can be variation in the licensing of different medicines containing the same drug.
Powder for solution for infusion
  ▸ Streptokinase (Non-proprietary)
    Streptokinase 1.5 mega u Biofactor Streptokinase 1.5million unit powder for solution for infusion vials | 1 vial [PoM] £83.44
    Streptokinase 250000 unit Biofactor Streptokinase 250,000unit powder for solution for infusion vials | 1 vial [PoM] £15.91
    Streptokinase 750000 unit Biofactor Streptokinase 750,000unit powder for solution for infusion vials | 1 vial [PoM] £41.72

🏃 198

Tenecteplase

- **INDICATIONS AND DOSE**
Acute myocardial infarction
  ▸ BY INTRAVENOUS INJECTION
  ▸ Adult: 30–50 mg (max. per dose 50 mg), dose to be given over 10 seconds and Initiated within 6 hours of symptom onset, dose varies according to body weight—consult product literature

- **BREAST FEEDING** Manufacturer advises avoid breast-feeding for 24 hours after dose (express and discard milk during this time).

- **MEDICINAL FORMS**
There can be variation in the licensing of different medicines containing the same drug.
Powder and solvent for solution for injection
  ▸ Metalyse (Boehringer Ingelheim Ltd)
    Tenecteplase 8000 unit Metalyse 8,000unit powder and solvent for solution for injection vials | 1 vial [PoM] £502.25
    Tenecteplase 10000 unit Metalyse 10,000unit powder and solvent for solution for injection vials | 1 vial [PoM] £502.25

NITRATES

Nitrates

Overview

Nitrates have a useful role in *angina*. Although they are potent coronary vasodilators, their principal benefit follows from a reduction in venous return which reduces left ventricular work. Unwanted effects such as flushing, headache, and postural hypotension may limit therapy, especially when angina is severe or when patients are unusually sensitive to the effects of nitrates.

Sublingual glyceryl trinitrate p. 201 is one of the most effective drugs for providing rapid symptomatic relief of angina, but its effect lasts only for 20 to 30 minutes; the 300-microgram tablet is often appropriate when glyceryl trinitrate is first used. The *aerosol* spray provides an alternative method of rapid relief of symptoms for those who find difficulty in dissolving sublingual preparations. Duration of action may be prolonged by *transdermal* preparations (but tolerance may develop).

Isosorbide dinitrate p. 202 is active *sublingually* and is a more stable preparation for those who only require nitrates infrequently. It is also effective by mouth for prophylaxis; although the effect is slower in onset, it may persist for several hours. Duration of action of up to 12 hours is claimed for *modified-release* preparations. The activity of isosorbide dinitrate may depend on the production of active metabolites, the most important of which is isosorbide mononitrate p. 203. Isosorbide mononitrate itself is also licensed for angina prophylaxis; modified-release formulations (for once daily administration) are available.

Glyceryl trinitrate or isosorbide dinitrate may be tried by *intravenous injection* when the sublingual form is ineffective in patients with chest pain due to myocardial infarction or severe ischaemia. Intravenous injections are also useful in the treatment of congestive heart failure.

Nitrates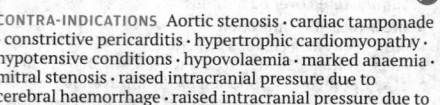

- **CONTRA-INDICATIONS** Aortic stenosis · cardiac tamponade · constrictive pericarditis · hypertrophic cardiomyopathy · hypotensive conditions · hypovolaemia · marked anaemia · mitral stenosis · raised intracranial pressure due to cerebral haemorrhage · raised intracranial pressure due to head trauma · toxic pulmonary oedema

- **CAUTIONS** Heart failure due to obstruction · hypothermia · hypothyroidism · hypoxaemia · malnutrition · metal-containing transdermal systems should be removed before magnetic resonance imaging procedures, cardioversion, or diathermy · recent history of myocardial infarction · susceptibility to angle-closure glaucoma · tolerance · ventilation and perfusion abnormalities

  CAUTIONS, FURTHER INFORMATION
  ▸ Tolerance Many patients on long-acting or transdermal nitrates rapidly develop tolerance (with reduced therapeutic effects). Reduction of blood-nitrate concentrations to low levels for 4 to 12 hours each day usually maintains effectiveness in such patients. If tolerance is suspected during the use of transdermal patches they should be left off for 8–12 hours (usually overnight) in each 24 hours; in the case of modified-release tablets of isosorbide dinitrate (and conventional formulations of isosorbide mononitrate), the second of the two daily doses should be given after about 8 hours rather than after 12 hours. Conventional formulations of isosorbide mononitrate should not usually be given more than twice daily unless small doses are used; modified-release formulations of isosorbide mononitrate should only be given once daily, and used in this way do not produce tolerance.

- **INTERACTIONS** → Appendix 1 (nitrates).

- **SIDE-EFFECTS**
  GENERAL SIDE-EFFECTS
  ▸ **Common or very common** Dizziness · postural hypotension · tachycardia · throbbing headache
  ▸ **Uncommon** Flushing · heartburn · nausea · rash · syncope · temporary hypoxaemia · vomiting
  ▸ **Very rare** Angle-closure glaucoma
  ▸ **Frequency not known** Paradoxical bradycardia
  SPECIFIC SIDE-EFFECTS
  ▸ **Uncommon**
  ▸ With transdermal use Application site reactions with transdermal patches
  ▸ **Frequency not known**
  ▸ With intravenous use Abdominal pain · apprehension · diaphoresis · muscle twitching · palpitation · prolonged administration has been associated with methaemoglobinaemia · restlessness · retrosternal discomfort · severe hypotension

SIDE-EFFECTS, FURTHER INFORMATION

▸ With intravenous use Specific side-effects following injection (particularly if given too rapidly) include severe hypotension, diaphoresis, apprehension, restlessness, muscle twitching, retrosternal discomfort, palpitation, abdominal pain; prolonged administration has been associated with methaemoglobinaemia.

● ALLERGY AND CROSS-SENSITIVITY Contra-indicated in nitrate hypersensitivity.

● BREAST FEEDING No information available—manufacturers advise use only if potential benefit outweighs risk.

● HEPATIC IMPAIRMENT Caution in severe impairment.

● RENAL IMPAIRMENT Manufacturers advise use with caution in severe impairment.

● MONITORING REQUIREMENTS Monitor blood pressure and heart rate during intravenous infusion.

● TREATMENT CESSATION Avoid abrupt withdrawal.

⮜ 200

Glyceryl trinitrate

● INDICATIONS AND DOSE

Prophylaxis and treatment of angina
▸ BY SUBLINGUAL ADMINISTRATION USING SUBLINGUAL TABLETS
▸ Adult: 0.3–1 mg, dose may be repeated as required

Control of hypertension and myocardial ischaemia during and after cardiac surgery | Induction of controlled hypotension during surgery | Congestive heart failure | Unstable angina
▸ BY INTRAVENOUS INFUSION
▸ Adult: 10–200 micrograms/minute (max. per dose 400 micrograms/minute), adjusted according to response, consult product literature for recommended starting doses specific to indication

Treatment or prophylaxis of angina
▸ BY SUBLINGUAL ADMINISTRATION USING AEROSOL SPRAY
▸ Adult: 1–2 sprays, dose be administered under tongue and then close mouth

Anal fissure
▸ BY RECTUM USING OINTMENT
▸ Adult: Apply 2.5 centimetres every 12 hours until pain stops. Max. duration of use 8 weeks, apply to anal canal, 2.5 cm of ointment contains 1.5 mg of glyceryl trinitrate

DEPONIT®

Prophylaxis of angina
▸ BY TRANSDERMAL APPLICATION
▸ Adult: One '5' or one '10' patch to be applied to lateral chest wall, upper arm, thigh, abdomen, or shoulder; increase to two '10' patches every 24 hours if necessary, to be replaced every 24 hours, siting replacement patch on different area

MINITRAN®

Prophylaxis of angina
▸ BY TRANSDERMAL APPLICATION
▸ Adult: One '5' patch to be applied to chest or upper arm; replace every 24 hours, siting replacement patch on different area, dose to be adjusted according to response

Maintenance of venous patency ('5' patch only)
▸ BY TRANSDERMAL APPLICATION
▸ Adult: (consult product literature)

NITRO-DUR®

Prophylaxis of angina
▸ BY TRANSDERMAL APPLICATION
▸ Adult: One '0.2mg/h' patch to be applied to chest or outer upper arm and replaced every 24 hours, siting

replacement patch on different area, dose adjusted according to response; maximum 15 mg per day

PERCUTOL®

Prophylaxis of angina
▸ TO THE SKIN
▸ Adult: Usual dose 1–2 inches every 3–4 hours as required, to be measured on to *Applirule*® and applied (usually to chest, arm, or thigh) without rubbing in and secured with surgical tape, approx. 800 micrograms/hour absorbed from 1 inch of ointment.

Prophylaxis of angina (to determine dose)
▸ TO THE SKIN
▸ Adult: ½ inch to be administered on first day then increased by ½ inch/day until headache occurs, then reduced by ½ inch, to be measured on to *Applirule*® and applied (usually to chest, arm, or thigh) without rubbing in and secured with surgical tape, approx. 800 micrograms/hour absorbed from 1 inch of ointment.

TRANSIDERM-NITRO®

Prophylaxis of angina
▸ BY TRANSDERMAL APPLICATION
▸ Adult: One '5' or one '10' patch to be applied to lateral chest wall and replaced every 24 hours, siting replacement patch on different area, max. two '10' patches daily

Prophylaxis of phlebitis and extravasation ('5' patch only)
▸ BY TRANSDERMAL APPLICATION
▸ Adult: (consult product literature)

● SIDE-EFFECTS
▸ With rectal use Burning · diarrhoea · itching · rectal bleeding

● PREGNANCY Not known to be harmful.

● DIRECTIONS FOR ADMINISTRATION
▸ With intravenous use For *intravenous infusion* (*Nitrocine*®, *Nitronal*®), give continuously in Glucose 5% or Sodium Chloride 0.9%. For *Nitrocine*®, suggested infusion concentration 100 micrograms/mL; incompatible with polyvinyl chloride infusion containers such as *Viaflex*® or *Steriflex*®; use glass or polyethylene containers or give via a syringe pump.
▸ With intravenous use Glass or polyethylene apparatus is preferable; loss of potency will occur if PVC is used. Glyceryl trinitrate 1 mg/ml to be diluted before use or given undiluted with syringe pump. Glyceryl trinitrate 5 mg/ml to be diluted before use.

● PRESCRIBING AND DISPENSING INFORMATION
▸ With sublingual use Glyceryl trinitrate tablets should be supplied in glass containers of not more than 100 tablets, closed with a foil-lined cap, and containing no cotton wool wadding; they should be discarded after 8 weeks in use.

● PATIENT AND CARER ADVICE Rectal ointment should be discarded 8 weeks after first opening.
PERCUTOL® Patients or carers should be given advice on how to administer glyceryl trinitrate ointment.

● NATIONAL FUNDING/ACCESS DECISIONS
Scottish Medicines Consortium (SMC) Decisions
The *Scottish Medicines Consortium* has advised (January 2008) that glyceryl trinitrate 0.4% ointment (*Rectogesic*®) is **not** recommended for use within NHS Scotland for the relief of pain associated with chronic anal fissure.

● MEDICINAL FORMS

There can be variation in the licensing of different medicines containing the same drug. Forms available from special-order manufacturers include: ointment

Sublingual tablet

CAUTIONARY AND ADVISORY LABELS 16

▸ Glyceryl trinitrate (Non-proprietary)

Glyceryl trinitrate 300 microgram GTN 300microgram sublingual tablets | 100 tablet Ⓟ £2.30 DT price = £2.30
Glyceryl trinitrate 300microgram sublingual tablets | 100 tablet Ⓟ no price available DT price = £2.30

Glyceryl trinitrate 500 microgram Glyceryl trinitrate 500microgram sublingual tablets | 100 tablet Ⓟ £14.31 DT price = £9.53

Glyceryl trinitrate 600 microgram Glyceryl trinitrate 600microgram sublingual tablets | 100 tablet Ⓟ no price available

Sublingual spray

CAUTIONARY AND ADVISORY LABELS 15

▸ Glyceryl trinitrate (Non-proprietary)

Glyceryl trinitrate 400 microgram per 1 dose Glyceryl trinitrate 400micrograms/dose pump sublingual spray | 180 dose Ⓟ £3.10 DT price = £3.10 | 200 dose Ⓟ £6.50 DT price = £3.44
Glyceryl trinitrate 400micrograms/dose aerosol sublingual spray | 180 dose Ⓟ £3.20 DT price = £3.00 | 200 dose Ⓟ £6.50 DT price = £3.50

▸ Coro-Nitro (J M Loveridge Ltd)

Glyceryl trinitrate 400 microgram per 1 dose Coro-Nitro 400micrograms/dose pump sublingual spray | 200 dose Ⓖⓢⓛ £3.44 DT price = £3.44

▸ Glytrin (Aspire Pharma Ltd)

Glyceryl trinitrate 400 microgram per 1 dose Glytrin 400micrograms/dose aerosol sublingual spray | 200 dose Ⓟ £3.44 DT price = £3.50

▸ Nitrolingual (Merck Serono Ltd)

Glyceryl trinitrate 400 microgram per 1 dose Nitrolingual 400micrograms/dose pump sublingual spray | 75 dose Ⓟ no price available (Hospital only) | 180 dose Ⓟ £3.10 DT price = £3.10 | 200 dose Ⓟ £3.44 DT price = £3.44

▸ Nitromin (Teva UK Ltd)

Glyceryl trinitrate 400 microgram per 1 dose Nitromin 400micrograms/dose pump sublingual spray | 180 dose Ⓟ £2.63 DT price = £3.10 | 200 dose Ⓟ £2.71 DT price = £3.44

Solution for infusion

EXCIPIENTS: May contain Ethanol, propylene glycol

▸ Glyceryl trinitrate (Non-proprietary)

Glyceryl trinitrate 1 mg per 1 ml Glyceryl trinitrate 50mg/50ml solution for infusion vials | 1 vial ⓅⓞⓂ £15.90 | 25 vial ⓅⓞⓂ no price available

Glyceryl trinitrate 5 mg per 1 ml Glyceryl trinitrate 50mg/10ml solution for infusion ampoules | 5 ampoule ⓅⓞⓂ £64.90
Glyceryl trinitrate 25mg/5ml solution for infusion ampoules | 5 ampoule ⓅⓞⓂ £32.45

▸ Nitrocine (UCB Pharma Ltd)

Glyceryl trinitrate 1 mg per 1 ml Nitrocine 10mg/10ml solution for infusion ampoules | 10 ampoule ⓅⓞⓂ £58.75 (Hospital only)

▸ Nitronal (Merck Serono Ltd)

Glyceryl trinitrate 1 mg per 1 ml Nitronal 5mg/5ml solution for infusion ampoules | 10 ampoule ⓅⓞⓂ £18.04
Nitronal 50mg/50ml solution for infusion vials | 1 vial ⓅⓞⓂ £14.76

Transdermal patch

▸ Deponit (UCB Pharma Ltd)

Glyceryl trinitrate 5 mg per 24 hour Deponit 5 transdermal patches | 28 patch Ⓟ £12.77

Glyceryl trinitrate 10 mg per 24 hour Deponit 10 transdermal patches | 28 patch Ⓟ £14.06

▸ Minitran (Meda Pharmaceuticals Ltd)

Glyceryl trinitrate 5 mg per 24 hour Minitran 5 transdermal patches | 30 patch Ⓟ £11.62

Glyceryl trinitrate 10 mg per 24 hour Minitran 10 transdermal patches | 30 patch Ⓟ £12.87

Glyceryl trinitrate 15 mg per 24 hour Minitran 15 transdermal patches | 30 patch Ⓟ £14.19

▸ Nitro-Dur (Merck Sharp & Dohme Ltd)

Glyceryl trinitrate 5 mg per 24 hour Nitro-Dur 0.2mg/hour transdermal patches | 28 patch Ⓟ £10.59

Glyceryl trinitrate 10 mg per 24 hour Nitro-Dur 0.4mg/hour transdermal patches | 28 patch Ⓟ £11.72

Glyceryl trinitrate 15 mg per 24 hour Nitro-Dur 0.6mg/hour transdermal patches | 28 patch Ⓟ £12.90

▸ Transiderm-Nitro (Novartis Pharmaceuticals UK Ltd)

Glyceryl trinitrate 5 mg per 24 hour Transiderm-Nitro 5 transdermal patches | 28 patch Ⓟ £20.46

Glyceryl trinitrate 10 mg per 24 hour Transiderm-Nitro 10 transdermal patches | 28 patch Ⓟ £22.49

Ointment

EXCIPIENTS: May contain Wool fat and related substances including lanolin

▸ Percutol (Aspire Pharma Ltd)

Glyceryl trinitrate 20 mg per 1 gram Percutol 2% ointment | 60 gram Ⓟ £79.00 DT price = £79.00

Rectal ointment

EXCIPIENTS: May contain Propylene glycol, wool fat and related substances including lanolin

▸ Rectogesic (ProStrakan Ltd)

Glyceryl trinitrate 4 mg per 1 gram Rectogesic 0.4% rectal ointment | 30 gram ⓅⓞⓂ £39.30 DT price = £39.30

Ⓕ 200

Isosorbide dinitrate

● INDICATIONS AND DOSE

Prophylaxis and treatment of angina

▸ BY MOUTH USING IMMEDIATE-RELEASE MEDICINES
▸ Adult: 30–120 mg daily in divided doses
▸ BY INTRAVENOUS INFUSION
▸ Adult: 2–10 mg/hour, increased if necessary up to 20 mg/hour
▸ BY SUBLINGUAL ADMINISTRATION USING AEROSOL SPRAY
▸ Adult: 1–3 sprays, to be administered under tongue whilst holding breath, allow a 30 second interval between each dose

Left ventricular failure

▸ BY MOUTH USING IMMEDIATE-RELEASE MEDICINES
▸ Adult: 40–160 mg daily in divided doses, increased if necessary up to 240 mg daily in divided doses
▸ BY INTRAVENOUS INFUSION
▸ Adult: Initially 2–10 mg/hour, increased if necessary up to 20 mg/hour

Prophylaxis of angina

▸ BY MOUTH USING MODIFIED-RELEASE MEDICINES
▸ Adult: 40 mg daily in 1–2 divided doses, increased if necessary to 60–80 mg daily in 2–3 divided doses

● PREGNANCY May cross placenta—manufacturers advise avoid unless potential benefit outweighs risk.

● DIRECTIONS FOR ADMINISTRATION For intravenous infusion (Isoket 0.05%®, Isoket 0.1%®), give continuously in Glucose 5% or Sodium chloride 0.9%. Adsorbed to some extent by polyvinyl chloride infusion containers; preferably use glass or polyethylene containers or give via a syringe pump; Isoket 0.05%® can alternatively be administered undiluted using a syringe pump with a glass or rigid plastic syringe. Glass or polyethylene infusion apparatus is preferable; loss of potency if PVC used.

● MEDICINAL FORMS

There can be variation in the licensing of different medicines containing the same drug. Forms available from special-order manufacturers include: oral suspension, oral solution

Tablet

▸ Isosorbide dinitrate (Non-proprietary)

Isosorbide dinitrate 10 mg Isosorbide dinitrate 10mg tablets | 56 tablet Ⓟ £13.41 DT price = £13.41

Isosorbide dinitrate 20 mg Isosorbide dinitrate 20mg tablets | 56 tablet ⓅⓞⓂ no price available DT price = £14.38 | 56 tablet Ⓟ £14.38 DT price = £14.38

Modified-release tablet

CAUTIONARY AND ADVISORY LABELS 25

▸ Isosorbide dinitrate (Non-proprietary)

Isosorbide dinitrate 20 mg Isosorbide dinitrate 20mg modified-release tablets | 56 tablet Ⓟ no price available DT price = £2.58

Isosorbide dinitrate 40 mg Isosorbide dinitrate 40mg modified-release tablets | 56 tablet Ⓟ no price available DT price = £6.36

▸ Isoket Retard (UCB Pharma Ltd)
Isosorbide dinitrate 20 mg Isoket Retard 20 tablets | 56 tablet P
£2.58 DT price = £2.58
Isosorbide dinitrate 40 mg Isoket Retard 40 tablets | 56 tablet P
£6.36 DT price = £6.36
Solution for injection
▸ Isosorbide dinitrate (Non-proprietary)
Isosorbide dinitrate 1 mg per 1 ml Isosorbide dinitrate 10mg/10ml
concentrate for solution for injection ampoules | 10 ampoule PoM
£21.80
▸ Isoket (UCB Pharma Ltd)
Isosorbide dinitrate 1 mg per 1 ml Isoket 0.1% solution for injection
10ml ampoules | 10 ampoule PoM £26.93 (Hospital only)
Solution for infusion
▸ Isosorbide dinitrate (Non-proprietary)
Isosorbide dinitrate 500 microgram per 1 ml Isosorbide dinitrate
25mg/50ml solution for infusion vials | 10 vial PoM £50.40
Isosorbide dinitrate 1 mg per 1 ml Isosorbide dinitrate 50mg/50ml
concentrate for solution for infusion vials | 10 vial PoM £66.50

◀ 200

Isosorbide mononitrate

● **INDICATIONS AND DOSE**

Prophylaxis of angina | Adjunct in congestive heart failure
▸ BY MOUTH USING IMMEDIATE-RELEASE MEDICINES
▸ Adult: Initially 20 mg 2–3 times a day, alternatively
initially 40 mg twice daily, increased if necessary up to
120 mg daily in divided doses

**Prophylaxis of angina (for patients who have not
previously had a nitrate) | Adjunct in congestive heart
failure (for patients who have not previously had a
nitrate)**
▸ BY MOUTH USING IMMEDIATE-RELEASE MEDICINES
▸ Adult: Initially 10 mg twice daily, increased if necessary
up to 120 mg daily in divided doses

CHEMYDUR® 60XL

Prophylaxis of angina
▸ BY MOUTH
▸ Adult: Initially 0.5 tablet daily for 2–4 days, to
minimise possibility of headache, then 1 tablet daily,
increased if necessary to 2 tablets daily, dose to be
taken in the morning

ELANTAN® LA

Prophylaxis of angina
▸ BY MOUTH
▸ Adult: 25–50 mg once daily, then increased if necessary
to 50–100 mg once daily, dose to be taken in the
morning, the lowest effective dose should be used

IMDUR®

Prophylaxis of angina
▸ BY MOUTH
▸ Adult: Initially 0.5 tablet once daily, to minimise the
occurrence of headache, then 1 tablet once daily, then
increased if necessary to 2 tablets once daily, dose to be
taken in the morning

ISIB® 60XL

Prophylaxis of angina
▸ BY MOUTH
▸ Adult: Initially 0.5 tablet once daily for 2–4 days, to
minimise the occurrence of headache, then 1 tablet
once daily, increased if necessary to 2 tablets once
daily, dose to be taken in the morning

ISMO RETARD®

Prophylaxis of angina
▸ BY MOUTH
▸ Adult: 1 tablet once daily, dose to be taken in the
morning

ISODUR®

Prophylaxis of angina
▸ BY MOUTH
▸ Adult: 25–50 mg once daily, then increased if necessary
to 50–100 mg once daily, dose to be taken in the
morning

ISOTARD®

Prophylaxis of angina
▸ BY MOUTH
▸ Adult: 25–60 mg once daily, if headaches occur with
60 mg tablet, half a 60 mg tablet may be given for
2–4 days, then increased if necessary to 50–120 mg
once daily, dose to be taken in the morning

MODISAL® XL

Prophylaxis of angina
▸ BY MOUTH
▸ Adult: Initially 0.5 tablet once daily for 2–4 days, to
minimise the occurrence of headache, then 1 tablet
once daily, increased if necessary to 2 tablets once
daily, dose to be taken in the morning

MONOMAX® SR

Prophylaxis of angina
▸ BY MOUTH
▸ Adult: 40–60 mg daily, increased if necessary to 120 mg
daily, dose to be taken in the morning

MONOMAX® XL

Prophylaxis of angina
▸ BY MOUTH
▸ Adult: Initially 0.5 tablet once daily for 2–4 days, to
minimise occurrence of headache, then 1 tablet once
daily, increased if necessary to 2 tablets once daily,
dose to be taken in the morning

MONOMIL® XL

Prophylaxis of angina
▸ BY MOUTH
▸ Adult: Initially 0.5 tablet daily for 2–4 days, to
minimise possibility of headache, then 1 tablet daily,
increased if necessary to 2 tablets once daily, to be
taken in the morning

MONOSORB® XL60

Prophylaxis of angina
▸ BY MOUTH
▸ Adult: Initially 0.5 tablet once daily for the first
2–4 days, to minimise the occurrence of headache,
then 1 tablet once daily, increased if necessary to
2 tablets once daily, dose to be taken in the morning

ZEMON®

Prophylaxis of angina
▸ BY MOUTH
▸ Adult: Initially 30 mg once daily for 2–4 days, to
minimise the occurrence of headache, then 40–60 mg
once daily, increased if necessary to 80–120 mg once
daily, dose to be taken in the morning

● PREGNANCY Manufacturers advise avoid unless potential
benefit outweighs risk.

● MEDICINAL FORMS
There can be variation in the licensing of different medicines
containing the same drug. Forms available from special-order
manufacturers include: oral suspension, oral solution

Tablet
CAUTIONARY AND ADVISORY LABELS 25
▸ Isosorbide mononitrate (Non-proprietary)
Isosorbide mononitrate 10 mg Isosorbide mononitrate 10mg
tablets | 56 tablet P £48.25 DT price = £1.58
Isosorbide mononitrate 20 mg Isosorbide mononitrate 20mg
tablets | 56 tablet P £62.25 DT price = £1.24 | 56 tablet PoM no
price available DT price = £1.24

Isosorbide mononitrate 40 mg Isosorbide mononitrate 40mg tablets | 56 tablet (P) £36.75 DT price = £1.83 | 56 tablet [PoM] no price available DT price = £1.83
▸ Ismo (Intrapharm Laboratories Ltd)
Isosorbide mononitrate 10 mg Ismo 10 tablets | 60 tablet (P) £3.31
Isosorbide mononitrate 20 mg Ismo 20 tablets | 60 tablet (P) £4.85

Modified-release tablet
CAUTIONARY AND ADVISORY LABELS 25
▸ Chemydur 60XL (AMCo)
Isosorbide mononitrate 60 mg Chemydur 60XL tablets | 28 tablet [PoM] £3.49 DT price = £10.50
▸ Imdur (AstraZeneca UK Ltd)
Isosorbide mononitrate 60 mg Imdur 60mg modified-release tablets | 28 tablet (P) £10.50 DT price = £10.50
▸ Isib XL (Sinclair IS Pharma Plc)
Isosorbide mononitrate 60 mg Isib 60XL tablets | 28 tablet (P) £8.15 DT price = £10.50
▸ Ismo Retard (Intrapharm Laboratories Ltd)
Isosorbide mononitrate 40 mg Ismo Retard 40mg tablets | 30 tablet (P) £10.71
▸ Isotard XL (ProStrakan Ltd)
Isosorbide mononitrate 25 mg Isotard 25XL tablets | 28 tablet (P) £6.75 DT price = £6.75
Isosorbide mononitrate 40 mg Isotard 40XL tablets | 28 tablet (P) £6.75
Isosorbide mononitrate 50 mg Isotard 50XL tablets | 28 tablet (P) £6.75 DT price = £6.75
Isosorbide mononitrate 60 mg Isotard 60XL tablets | 28 tablet (P) £5.75 DT price = £10.50
▸ Modisal XL (Ennogen Pharma Ltd)
Isosorbide mononitrate 40 mg Modisal XL 40mg tablets | 28 tablet [PoM] £50.64
▸ Monomax XL (Chiesi Ltd)
Isosorbide mononitrate 60 mg Monomax XL 60mg tablets | 28 tablet (P) £5.25 DT price = £10.50
▸ Monomil XL (Teva UK Ltd)
Isosorbide mononitrate 60 mg Monomil XL 60mg tablets | 28 tablet [PoM] £3.49 DT price = £10.50
▸ Monosorb XL (Kent Pharmaceuticals Ltd, Almus Pharmaceuticals Ltd, Dexcel-Pharma Ltd)
Isosorbide mononitrate 60 mg Monosorb XL 60 tablets | 28 tablet (P) £15.35–£16.66 DT price = £10.50
▸ Zemon XL (Kent Pharmaceuticals Ltd)
Isosorbide mononitrate 40 mg Zemon 40 XL tablets | 28 tablet [PoM] £14.25

Modified-release capsule
CAUTIONARY AND ADVISORY LABELS 25
▸ Elantan LA (UCB Pharma Ltd)
Isosorbide mononitrate 25 mg Elantan LA25 capsules | 28 capsule (P) £3.40 DT price = £3.40
Isosorbide mononitrate 50 mg Elantan LA50 capsules | 28 capsule (P) £3.69 DT price = £3.69
▸ Isodur XL (Galen Ltd)
Isosorbide mononitrate 25 mg Isodur 25XL capsules | 28 capsule (P) £4.63 DT price = £3.40
Isosorbide mononitrate 50 mg Isodur 50XL capsules | 28 capsule (P) £6.45 DT price = £3.69
▸ Monomax SR (Chiesi Ltd)
Isosorbide mononitrate 40 mg Monomax SR 40 capsules | 28 capsule (P) £6.52 DT price = £6.52
Isosorbide mononitrate 60 mg Monomax SR 60 capsules | 28 capsule (P) £8.86 DT price = £8.86

SYMPATHOMIMETICS ⟩ INOTROPIC

Dobutamine

- **DRUG ACTION** Dobutamine is a cardiac stimulant which acts on beta$_1$ receptors in cardiac muscle, and increases contractility with little effect on rate.

● INDICATIONS AND DOSE

Inotropic support in infarction, cardiac surgery, cardiomyopathies, septic shock, cardiogenic shock, and during positive end expiratory pressure ventilation
▸ BY INTRAVENOUS INFUSION
▸ Adult: Usual dose 2.5–10 micrograms/kg/minute, adjusted according to response, alternatively 0.5–40 micrograms/kg/minute

Cardiac stress testing
▸ BY INTRAVENOUS INFUSION
▸ Adult: (consult product literature)

- **CONTRA-INDICATIONS** Phaeochromocytoma
- **CAUTIONS** Acute heart failure · acute myocardial infarction · arrhythmias · correct hypercapnia before starting and during treatment · correct hypovolaemia before starting and during treatment · correct hypoxia before starting and during treatment · correct metabolic acidosis before starting and during treatment · diabetes mellitus · elderly · extravasation may cause tissue necrosis · extreme caution or avoid in marked obstruction of cardiac ejection (such as idiopathic hypertrophic subaortic stenosis) · hyperthyroidism · ischaemic heart disease · occlusive vascular disease · severe hypotension · susceptibility to angle-closure glaucoma · tachycardia · tolerance may develop with continuous infusions longer than 72 hours
- **INTERACTIONS** → Appendix 1 (sympathomimetics).
- **SIDE-EFFECTS**
▸ **Rare** Psychosis
▸ **Very rare** Angle-closure glaucoma · AV block · bradycardia · cardiac arrest · coronary artery spasm · hypokalaemia · myocardial infarction · petechial bleeding
▸ **Frequency not known** Anxiety · arrhythmias · bronchospasm · cerebral haemorrhage · chest pain · dyspnoea · eosinophilia · fever · headache · hypertension (marked increase in systolic blood pressure indicates overdose) · hypotension · increased urinary urgency · myoclonic spasm · nausea · palpitation · paraesthesia · phlebitis · pruritus of scalp · pulmonary oedema · rash · reduced platelet aggregation (on prolonged use) · tachycardia · tremor · vomiting
- **PREGNANCY** No evidence of harm in *animal* studies—manufacturers advise use only if potential benefit outweighs risk.
- **BREAST FEEDING** Manufacturers advise avoid—no information available.
- **MONITORING REQUIREMENTS** Monitor serum-potassium concentration.
- **DIRECTIONS FOR ADMINISTRATION** Dobutamine injection should be diluted before use or given undiluted with syringe pump. Dobutamine concentrate for intravenous infusion should be diluted before use.
  For *intravenous infusion*, give continuously in Glucose 5% or Sodium chloride 0.9%. Dilute to a concentration of 0.5–1 mg/mL and give via an infusion pump; give higher concentration (max. 5 mg/mL) through central venous catheter; incompatible with bicarbonate and other strong alkaline solutions.

- MEDICINAL FORMS
There can be variation in the licensing of different medicines containing the same drug.
Solution for infusion
EXCIPIENTS: May contain Sulfites
- Dobutamine (Non-proprietary)
Dobutamine (as Dobutamine hydrochloride) 5 mg per 1 ml Dobutamine 250mg/50ml solution for infusion vials | 1 vial PoM £7.50
Dobutamine (as Dobutamine hydrochloride) 12.5 mg per 1 ml Dobutamine 250mg/20ml concentrate for solution for infusion ampoules | 5 ampoule PoM £26.00–£26.25

7.1a Cardiac arrest

Cardiopulmonary resuscitation

Overview

The algorithm for cardiopulmonary resuscitation (Life support algorithm (image) p. inside back cover) reflects the most recent recommendations of the Resuscitation Council (UK). These guidelines are available at www.resus.org.uk.

Cardiac arrest can be associated with ventricular fibrillation, pulseless ventricular tachycardia, asystole, and pulseless electrical activity (electromechanical dissociation). Adrenaline/epinephrine below 1 in 10000 (100 micrograms/mL) is recommended by intravenous injection repeated every 3–5 minutes if necessary. Administration through a central line results in a faster response than peripheral administration, however placement of a central line must not interfere with chest compressions; drugs administered peripherally must be followed by a flush of at least 20 mL Sodium Chloride 0.9% injection to aid entry into the central circulation. Intravenous injection of amiodarone hydrochloride p. 94 should be considered after adrenaline/epinephrine to treat ventricular fibrillation or pulseless ventricular tachycardia in cardiac arrest refractory to defibrillation. An additional dose of amiodarone hydrochloride can be given if necessary, followed by an intravenous infusion of amiodarone hydrochloride. Lidocaine hydrochloride p. 92, is an alternative if amiodarone hydrochloride is not available. Atropine sulfate p. 1169 is no longer recommended in the treatment of asystole or pulseless electrical activity.

During cardiopulmonary arrest if intravenous access cannot be obtained, the intraosseous route can be used instead. Drug administration via the endotracheal route is no longer recommended.

For the management of acute anaphylaxis, see allergic emergencies under Antihistamines, allergen immunotherapy and allergic emergencies p. 253.

SYMPATHOMIMETICS > VASOCONSTRICTOR

Adrenaline/epinephrine

- DRUG ACTION Acts on both alpha and beta receptors and increases both heart rate and contractility (beta$_1$ effects); it can cause peripheral vasodilation (a beta$_2$ effect) or vasoconstriction (an alpha effect).

- INDICATIONS AND DOSE
Cardiopulmonary resuscitation
▸ BY INTRAVENOUS INJECTION
- Adult: 1 mg every 3–5 minutes as required, a 1 in 10000 (100 micrograms/mL) solution is recommended

Acute hypotension
▸ BY CONTINUOUS INTRAVENOUS INFUSION
- Child: Initially 100 nanograms/kg/minute, adjusted according to response, higher doses up to 1.5 micrograms/kg/minute have been used in acute hypotension

Emergency treatment of acute anaphylaxis (under expert supervision) | Angioedema (if laryngeal oedema is present) (under expert supervision)
▸ BY INTRAMUSCULAR INJECTION
- Child 1 month–5 years: 150 micrograms, doses may be repeated several times if necessary at 5 minute intervals according to blood pressure, pulse, and respiratory function, suitable syringe to be used for measuring small volume; injected preferably into the anterolateral aspect of the middle third of the thigh
- Child 6–11 years: 300 micrograms, doses may be repeated several times if necessary at 5 minute intervals according to blood pressure, pulse, and respiratory function, to be injected preferably into the anterolateral aspect of the middle third of the thigh
- Child 12–17 years: 500 micrograms, to be injected preferably into the anterolateral aspect of the middle third of the thigh, doses may be repeated several times if necessary at 5 minute intervals according to blood pressure, pulse, and respiratory function, 300 micrograms (0.3 mL) to be administered if child small or prepubertal
- Adult: 500 micrograms, to be injected preferably into the anterolateral aspect of the middle third of the thigh, doses may be repeated several times if necessary at 5 minute intervals according to blood pressure, pulse, and respiratory function

Acute anaphylaxis when there is doubt as to the adequacy of the circulation (specialist use only) | Angioedema (if laryngeal oedema is present) (specialist use only)
▸ BY SLOW INTRAVENOUS INJECTION
- Adult: 50 micrograms, using 0.5 mL of the dilute 1 in 10 000 adrenaline injection, dose to be repeated according to response, if multiple doses required, adrenaline should be given as a slow intravenous infusion stopping when a response has been obtained

Control of bradycardia in patients with arrhythmias after myocardial infarction, if there is a risk of asystole, or if the patient is unstable and has failed to respond to atropine
▸ BY INTRAVENOUS INFUSION
- Adult: 2–10 micrograms/minute, adjusted according to response

EMERADE® 150 MICROGRAMS
Acute anaphylaxis (for self-administration)
▸ BY INTRAMUSCULAR INJECTION
- Child (body-weight up to 15 kg): 150 micrograms, then 150 micrograms after 5–15 minutes as required
- Child (body-weight 15–30 kg): 150 micrograms, then 150 micrograms after 5–15 minutes as required, on the basis of a dose of 10 micrograms/kg, 300 micrograms may be more appropriate for some children

EMERADE® 300 MICROGRAMS
Acute anaphylaxis (for self-administration)
▸ BY INTRAMUSCULAR INJECTION
- Child (body-weight 30 kg and above): 300 micrograms, then 300 micrograms after 5–15 minutes as required
- Adult (body-weight 30 kg and above): 300 micrograms, then 300 micrograms after 5–15 minutes as required

continued →

EMERADE® 500 MICROGRAMS

Acute anaphylaxis (for self-administration for patients at risk of severe anaphylaxis)
▸ BY INTRAMUSCULAR INJECTION
▸ Child 12–17 years: 500 micrograms, then 500 micrograms after 5–15 minutes as required
▸ Adult: 500 micrograms, then 500 micrograms after 5–15 minutes as required

EPIPEN® AUTO-INJECTOR 0.3MG

Acute anaphylaxis (for self-administration)
▸ BY INTRAMUSCULAR INJECTION
▸ Child (body-weight 30 kg and above): 300 micrograms, then 300 micrograms after 5–15 minutes as required
▸ Adult (body-weight 30 kg and above): 300 micrograms, then 300 micrograms after 5–15 minutes as required

EPIPEN® JR AUTO-INJECTOR 0.15MG

Acute anaphylaxis (for self-administration)
▸ BY INTRAMUSCULAR INJECTION
▸ Child (body-weight up to 15 kg): 150 micrograms, then 150 micrograms after 5–15 minutes as required
▸ Child (body-weight 15-30 kg): 150 micrograms, then 150 micrograms after 5–15 minutes as required, on the basis of a dose of 10 micrograms/kg, 300 micrograms may be more appropriate for some children

JEXT® 150 MICROGRAMS

Acute anaphylaxis (for self-administration)
▸ BY INTRAMUSCULAR INJECTION
▸ Child (body-weight up to 15 kg): 150 micrograms, then 150 micrograms after 5–15 minutes as required
▸ Child (body-weight 15-30 kg): 150 micrograms, then 150 micrograms after 5–15 minutes as required, on the basis of a dose of 10 micrograms/kg, 300 micrograms may be more appropriate for some children

JEXT® 300 MICROGRAMS

Acute anaphylaxis (for self-administration)
▸ BY INTRAMUSCULAR INJECTION
▸ Child (body-weight 30 kg and above): 300 micrograms, then 300 micrograms after 5–15 minutes as required
▸ Adult (body-weight 30 kg and above): 300 micrograms, then 300 micrograms after 5–15 minutes as required

● UNLICENSED USE
▸ With intramuscular use for acute anaphylaxis in children Auto-injectors delivering 150-microgram dose of adrenaline may not be licensed for use in children with body-weight under 15 kg.
▸ With intravenous use for acute hypotension in children Adrenaline 1 in 1000 (1 mg/mL) solution is not licensed for intravenous administration.

IMPORTANT SAFETY INFORMATION
SAFE PRACTICE
Intravenous route should be used with **extreme care** by specialists only.

● CAUTIONS Arteriosclerosis (in adults) · arrhythmias · cerebrovascular disease · cor pulmonale · diabetes mellitus · elderly (in adults) · hypercalcaemia · hyperreflexia · hypertension · hyperthyroidism · hypokalaemia · ischaemic heart disease · obstructive cardiomyopathy · occlusive vascular disease · organic brain damage · phaeochromocytoma · prostate disorders · psychoneurosis · severe angina · susceptibility to angle-closure glaucoma
CAUTIONS, FURTHER INFORMATION
Cautions listed are only for non-life-threatening situations.
● INTERACTIONS → Appendix 1 (sympathomimetics)
Severe anaphylaxis in patients taking beta-blockers may not respond to adrenaline—consider bronchodilator therapy. Furthermore, adrenaline can cause severe

hypertension and bradycardia in those taking non-cardioselective beta-blockers.

● SIDE-EFFECTS Angina · angle-closure glaucoma · anorexia · anxiety · arrhythmias · cold extremities · confusion · difficulty in micturition · dizziness · dry mouth · dyspnoea · headache · hyperglycaemia · hypersalivation · hypertension (risk of cerebral haemorrhage) · hypokalaemia · insomnia · metabolic acidosis · mydriasis · myocardial infarction · nausea · pallor · palpitation · psychosis · pulmonary oedema (on excessive dosage or extreme sensitivity) · restlessness · sweating · tachycardia · tissue necrosis at injection site · tissue necrosis of bowel · tissue necrosis of extremities · tissue necrosis of kidneys · tissue necrosis of liver · tremor · urinary retention · vomiting · weakness
● PREGNANCY May reduce placental perfusion and cause tachycardia, cardiac irregularities, and extrasystoles in fetus. Can delay second stage of labour. Manufacturers advise use only if benefit outweighs risk.
● BREAST FEEDING Present in milk but unlikely to be harmful as poor oral bioavailability.
● RENAL IMPAIRMENT Manufacturers advise use with caution in severe impairment.
● MONITORING REQUIREMENTS Monitor blood pressure and ECG.
● DIRECTIONS FOR ADMINISTRATION
Acute hypotension
▸ With intravenous use in children For *continuous intravenous infusion*, dilute with Glucose 5% or Sodium Chloride 0.9% and give through a central venous catheter. Incompatible with bicarbonate and alkaline solutions. *Neonatal intensive care*, dilute 3 mg/kg body-weight to a final volume of 50 mL with infusion fluid; an intravenous infusion rate of 0.1 mL/hour provides a dose of 100 nanograms/kg/minute; infuse through a central venous catheter. Incompatible with bicarbonate and alkaline solutions. These infusions are usually made up with adrenaline 1 in 1000 (1 mg/mL) solution.
Cardiopulmonary resuscitation
▸ With intravenous use in adults Administration through a central line results in a faster response than peripheral administration, however placement of a central line must not interfere with chest compressions; drugs administered peripherally must be followed by a flush of at least 20 mL Sodium Chloride 0.9% injection to aid entry into the central circulation.
● PRESCRIBING AND DISPENSING INFORMATION It is important, in acute anaphylaxis where intramuscular injection might still succeed, time should not be wasted seeking intravenous access.
     Great vigilance is needed to ensure that the *correct strength* of adrenaline injection is used; anaphylactic shock kits need to make a *very clear distinction* between the 1 in 10 000 strength and the 1 in 1000 strength.
     Patients with severe allergy should be instructed in the self-administration of adrenaline by intramuscular injection.
     Packs for self-administration need to be **clearly labelled with instructions** on how to administer adrenaline (intramuscularly, preferably at the midpoint of the outer thigh, through light clothing if necessary) so that in the case of rapid collapse someone else is able to give it. It is important to ensure individuals at risk and their carers understand that:
● two injection devices should be carried at all times to treat symptoms until medical assistance is available; if, after the first injection, the individual does not start to feel better, the second injection should be given 5 to 15 minutes after the first;
● an ambulance should be called after every administration, even if symptoms improve;

- the individual should lie down with their legs raised (unless they have breathing difficulties, in which case they should sit up) and should not be left alone.

Adrenaline for administration by intramuscular injection is available in 'auto-injectors' (e.g. *Emerade*®, *EpiPen*®, or *Jext*®), pre-assembled syringes fitted with a needle suitable for very rapid administration (if necessary by a bystander or a healthcare provider if it is the only preparation available); injection technique is device specific.

To ensure patients receive the auto-injector device that they have been trained to use, prescribers should specify the brand to be dispensed.

- **PATIENT AND CARER ADVICE** Individuals at considerable risk of anaphylaxis need to carry (or have available) adrenaline at all times and the patient, or their carers, need to be *instructed in advance* when and how to inject it.

JEXT® 300 MICROGRAMS 1.1 mL of the solution remains in the auto-injector device after use.

JEXT® 150 MICROGRAMS 1.25 mL of the solution remains in the auto-injector device after use.

EPIPEN® JR AUTO-INJECTOR 0.15MG 1.7 mL of the solution remains in the auto-injector device after use.

EMERADE® 300 MICROGRAMS 0.2 mL of the solution remains in the auto-injector device after use.

EPIPEN® AUTO-INJECTOR 0.3MG 1.7 mL of the solution remains in the auto-injector device after use.

EMERADE® 500 MICROGRAMS No solution remains in the auto-injector device after use.

EMERADE® 150 MICROGRAMS 0.35 mL of the solution remains in the auto-injector device after use.

Medicines for Children leaflet: Adrenaline auto-injector for anaphylaxis www.medicinesforchildren.org.uk/adrenaline-for-anaphylaxis

- **EXCEPTIONS TO LEGAL CATEGORY** POM restriction does not apply to the intramuscular administration of up to 1 mg of adrenaline injection 1 in 1000 (1 mg/mL) for the emergency treatment of anaphylaxis.

- **MEDICINAL FORMS** There can be variation in the licensing of different medicines containing the same drug. Forms available from special-order manufacturers include: solution for injection

Solution for injection
EXCIPIENTS: May contain Sulfites

▸ Adrenaline/epinephrine (Non-proprietary)
Adrenaline 100 microgram per 1 ml Adrenaline (base) 100micrograms/1ml (1 in 10,000) dilute solution for injection ampoules | 10 ampoule [PoM] £60.09
Adrenaline (base) 1mg/10ml (1 in 10,000) dilute solution for injection pre-filled syringes | 1 pre-filled disposable injection [PoM] £6.87
Adrenaline (base) 1mg/10ml (1 in 10,000) dilute solution for injection Minijet pre-filled syringes | 1 pre-filled disposable injection [PoM] £6.99
Adrenaline (as Adrenaline acid tartrate) 100 microgram per 1 ml Adrenaline (base) 1mg/10ml (1 in 10,000) dilute solution for injection ampoules | 1 ampoule [PoM] £43.53 | 10 ampoule [PoM] £69.65
Adrenaline (base) 500micrograms/5ml (1 in 10,000) dilute solution for injection ampoules | 10 ampoule [PoM] £64.02
Adrenaline 1 mg per 1 ml Adrenaline (base) for anaphylaxis 1mg/1ml (1 in 1,000) solution for injection pre-filled syringes | 1 pre-filled disposable injection [PoM] £10.40
Adrenaline (base) 1mg/1ml (1 in 1,000) solution for injection Minijet pre-filled syringes 21 gauge | 1 pre-filled disposable injection [PoM] £15.00
Adrenaline (base) 1mg/1ml (1 in 1,000) solution for injection pre-filled syringes | 1 pre-filled disposable injection [PoM] £10.40–£30.00
Adrenaline (base) 1mg/1ml (1 in 1,000) solution for injection Minijet pre-filled syringes 25 gauge | 1 pre-filled disposable injection [PoM] £13.90
Adrenaline (as Adrenaline acid tartrate) 1 mg per 1 ml Adrenaline (base) 5mg/5ml (1 in 1,000) solution for injection ampoules | 10 ampoule [PoM] £73.66

Adrenaline (base) 500micrograms/0.5ml (1 in 1,000) solution for injection ampoules | 10 ampoule [PoM] £58.08–£58.41 DT price = £58.25
Adrenaline (base) 1mg/1ml (1 in 1,000) solution for injection ampoules | 10 ampoule [PoM] £5.82 DT price = £5.81

▸ Emerade (Imed Systems Ltd)
Adrenaline 1 mg per 1 ml Emerade 300micrograms/0.3ml (1 in 1,000) solution for injection auto-injectors | 1 pre-filled disposable injection [PoM] £26.94 DT price = £26.45
Adrenaline (as Adrenaline acid tartrate) 1 mg per 1 ml Emerade 150micrograms/0.15ml (1 in 1,000) solution for injection auto-injectors | 1 pre-filled disposable injection [PoM] £26.94
Emerade 500micrograms/0.5ml (1 in 1,000) solution for injection auto-injectors | 1 pre-filled disposable injection [PoM] £28.74

▸ EpiPen (Meda Pharmaceuticals Ltd)
Adrenaline 500 microgram per 1 ml EpiPen Jr. 150micrograms/0.3ml (1 in 2,000) solution for injection auto-injectors | 1 pre-filled disposable injection [PoM] £26.45 | 2 pre-filled disposable injection [PoM] £52.90
Adrenaline 1 mg per 1 ml EpiPen 300micrograms/0.3ml (1 in 1,000) solution for injection auto-injectors | 1 pre-filled disposable injection [PoM] £26.45 DT price = £26.45 | 2 pre-filled disposable injection [PoM] £52.90

▸ Jext (ALK-Abello Ltd)
Adrenaline 1 mg per 1 ml Jext 300micrograms/0.3ml (1 in 1,000) solution for injection auto-injectors | 1 pre-filled disposable injection [PoM] £23.99 DT price = £26.45
Adrenaline (as Adrenaline acid tartrate) 1 mg per 1 ml Jext 150micrograms/0.15ml (1 in 1,000) solution for injection auto-injectors | 1 pre-filled disposable injection [PoM] £23.99

8   Oedema

Diuretics

Overview

Thiazides are used to relieve oedema due to chronic heart failure and, in lower doses, to reduce blood pressure.

Loop diuretics are used in pulmonary oedema due to left ventricular failure and in patients with chronic heart failure.

Combination diuretic therapy may be effective in patients with oedema resistant to treatment with one diuretic. Vigorous diuresis, particularly with loop diuretics, may induce acute hypotension; rapid reduction of plasma volume should be avoided.

Thiazides and related diuretics

Thiazides and related compounds are moderately potent diuretics; they inhibit sodium reabsorption at the beginning of the distal convoluted tubule. They act within 1 to 2 hours of oral administration and most have a duration of action of 12 to 24 hours; they are usually administered early in the day so that the diuresis does not interfere with sleep.

In the management of *hypertension* a low dose of a thiazide produces a maximal or near-maximal blood pressure lowering effect, with very little biochemical disturbance. Higher doses cause more marked changes in plasma potassium, sodium, uric acid, glucose, and lipids, with little advantage in blood pressure control. Chlortalidone p. 213 and indapamide p. 153 are the preferred diuretics in the management of hypertension. Thiazides also have a role in chronic heart failure.

Bendroflumethiazide p. 152 can be used for mild or moderate heart failure; it is licensed for the treatment of hypertension but is no longer considered the first-line diuretic for this indication, although patients with stable and controlled blood pressure currently taking bendroflumethiazide can continue treatment.

Chlortalidone, a thiazide-related compound, has a longer duration of action than the thiazides and may be given on alternate days to control oedema. It is also useful if acute retention is liable to be precipitated by a more rapid diuresis or if patients dislike the altered pattern of micturition caused by other diuretics. Chlortalidone can also be used under close supervision for the treatment of ascites due to cirrhosis in stable patients.

Xipamide p. 214 and indapamideare chemically related to chlortalidone. Indapamide is claimed to lower blood pressure with less metabolic disturbance, particularly less aggravation of diabetes mellitus.

Metolazone p. 214 is particularly effective when combined with a loop diuretic (even in renal failure); profound diuresis can occur and the patient should therefore be monitored carefully.

The thiazide diuretics benzthiazide, clopamide, cyclopenthiazide p. 214, hydrochlorothiazide, and hydroflumethiazide do not offer any significant advantage over other thiazides and related diuretics.

Loop diuretics

Loop diuretics are used in pulmonary oedema due to left ventricular failure; intravenous administration produces relief of breathlessness and reduces pre-load sooner than would be expected from the time of onset of diuresis. Loop diuretics are also used in patients with chronic heart failure. Diuretic-resistant oedema (except lymphoedema and oedema due to peripheral venous stasis or calcium-channel blockers) can be treated with a loop diuretic combined with a thiazide or related diuretic (e.g. bendroflumethiazide or metolazone).

If necessary, a loop diuretic can be added to antihypertensive treatment to achieve better control of blood pressure in those with resistant hypertension, or in patients with impaired renal function or heart failure.

Loop diuretics can exacerbate diabetes (but hyperglycaemia is less likely than with thiazides) and gout. If there is an enlarged prostate, urinary retention can occur, although this is less likely if small doses and less potent diuretics are used initially.

Furosemide p. 210 and bumetanide p. 209 are similar in activity; both act within 1 hour of oral administration and diuresis is complete within 6 hours so that, if necessary, they can be given twice in one day without interfering with sleep. Following intravenous administration furosemide has a peak effect within 30 minutes. The diuresis associated with these drugs is dose related.

Torasemide p. 211 has properties similar to those of furosemideand bumetanide, and is indicated for oedema and for hypertension.

Potassium-sparing diuretics and aldosterone antagonists

Amiloride hydrochloride p. 212 and triamterene p. 213 on their own are weak diuretics. They cause retention of potassium and are therefore given with thiazide or loop diuretics as a more effective alternative to potassium supplements. See compound preparations with thiazides or loop diuretics.

Potassium supplements must **not** be given with potassium- sparing diuretics. Administration of a potassium sparing diuretic to a patient receiving an ACE inhibitor or an angiotensin-II receptor antagonist can also cause severe hyperkalaemia.

Aldosterone antagonists

Spironolactone p. 175 potentiates thiazide or loop diuretics by antagonising aldosterone; it is a potassium-sparing diuretic. Spironolactone is of value in the treatment of oedema and ascites caused by cirrhosis of the liver; furosemide can be used as an adjunct. Low doses of spironolactone are beneficial in moderate to severe heart failure and when used in resistant hypertension [unlicensed indication].

Spironolactone is also used in primary hyperaldosteronism (Conn's syndrome). It is given before surgery or if surgery is

not appropriate, in the lowest effective dose for maintenance.

Eplerenone p. 174 is licensed for use as an adjunct in left ventricular dysfunction with evidence of heart failure after a myocardial infarction; it is also licensed as an adjunct in chronic mild heart failure with left ventricular systolic dysfunction.

Potassium supplements must **not** be given with aldosterone antagonists

Potassium-sparing diuretics with other diuretics

Although it is preferable to prescribe thiazides and potassium-sparing diuretics separately, the use of fixed combinations may be justified if compliance is a problem. Potassium-sparing diuretics are not usually necessary in the routine treatment of hypertension, unless hypokalaemia develops.

Other diuretics

Mannitol p. 211 is an osmotic diuretic that can be used to treat cerebral oedema and raised intra-ocular pressure.

Mercurial diuretics are effective but are now almost never used because of their nephrotoxicity.

The carbonic anhydrase inhibitor acetazolamide p. 1026 is a weak diuretic and is little used for its diuretic effect. It is used for prophylaxis against mountain sickness [unlicensed indication] but is not a substitute for acclimatisation.

Acetazolamide and eye drops of dorzolamide p. 1027 and brinzolamide p. 1027 inhibit the formation of aqueous humour and are used in glaucoma.

Diuretics with potassium

Many patients on diuretics do not need potassium supplements. For many of those who do, the amount of potassium in combined preparations may not be enough, and for this reason their use is to be discouraged.

Diuretics with potassium and potassium-sparing diuretics should **not** usually be given together. Diuretics and potassium supplements should be prescribed separately for children.

> **Drugs used for Oedema not listed below** Diamorphine hydrochloride, p. 415

DIURETICS > LOOP DIURETICS

Loop diuretics

- **DRUG ACTION** Loop diuretics inhibit reabsorption from the ascending limb of the loop of Henlé in the renal tubule and are powerful diuretics.

- **CONTRA-INDICATIONS** Anuria · comatose and precomatose states associated with liver cirrhosis · renal failure due to nephrotoxic or hepatotoxic drugs · severe hypokalaemia · severe hyponatraemia

- **CAUTIONS** Can exacerbate diabetes (but hyperglycaemia less likely than with thiazides) · can excacerbate gout · hypotension should be corrected before initiation of treatment · hypovolaemia should be corrected before initiation of treatment · urinary retention can occur in prostatic hyperplasia

  CAUTIONS, FURTHER INFORMATION
  ▸ Elderly Lower initial doses of diuretics should be used in the elderly because they are particularly susceptible to the side-effects. The dose should then be adjusted according to renal function. Diuretics should not be used continuously on a long-term basis to treat simple gravitational oedema (which will usually respond to increased movement, raising the legs, and support stockings).

▸ **Potassium loss** Hypokalaemia can occur with both thiazide and loop diuretics. The risk of hypokalaemia depends on the duration of action as well as the potency and is thus greater with thiazides than with an equipotent dose of a loop diuretic.

Hypokalaemia is dangerous in severe cardiovascular disease and in patients also being treated with cardiac glycosides. Often the use of potassium-sparing diuretics avoids the need to take potassium supplements.

In hepatic failure, hypokalaemia caused by diuretics can precipitate encephalopathy, particularly in alcoholic cirrhosis.

▸ **Urinary retention** If there is an enlarged prostate, urinary retention can occur, although this is less likely if small doses and less potent diuretics are used initially; an adequate urinary output should be established before initiating treatment.

● INTERACTIONS → Appendix 1 (diuretics).

● SIDE-EFFECTS

▸ **Very rare** Hyperuricaemia

▸ **Frequency not known** Acute urinary retention · blood disorders · bone-marrow depression · deafness (usually with high doses and rapid intravenous administration, and in renal impairment) · electrolyte disturbances · hepatic encephalopathy · hyperglycaemia (less common than with thiazides) · hypersensitivity reactions · hypocalcaemia · hypochloraemia · hypokalaemia · hypomagnesaemia · hyponatraemia · leucopenia · metabolic alkalosis · mild gastro-intestinal disturbances · pancreatitis · photosensitivity · postural hypotension · pruritus · rash · temporary increase in serum-cholesterol and triglyceride concentration · thrombocytopenia · tinnitus (usually with high doses and rapid intravenous administration, and in renal impairment) · visual disturbances

● HEPATIC IMPAIRMENT Hypokalaemia induced by loop diuretics may precipitate hepatic encephalopathy and coma—potassium-sparing diuretics can be used to prevent this. Diuretics can increase the risk of hypomagnesaemia in alcoholic cirrhosis, leading to arrhythmias.

● RENAL IMPAIRMENT High doses of loop diuretics may occasionally be needed in renal impairment. High doses or rapid intravenous administration can cause tinnitus and deafness.

● MONITORING REQUIREMENTS Monitor electrolytes during treatment.

▸ 208

Bumetanide

● INDICATIONS AND DOSE

Oedema

▸ BY MOUTH

▸ **Adult:** 1 mg, dose to be taken in the morning, then 1 mg after 6–8 hours if required

▸ **Elderly:** 500 micrograms daily, this lower dose may be sufficient in elderly patients

Oedema, severe cases

▸ BY MOUTH

▸ **Adult:** Initially 5 mg daily, increased in steps of 5 mg every 12–24 hours, adjusted according to response

● SIDE-EFFECTS Breast pain · gynaecomastia · musculoskeletal pain (associated with high doses in renal failure)

● PREGNANCY Bumetanide should not be used to treat gestational hypertension because of the maternal hypovolaemia associated with this condition.

● BREAST FEEDING No information available. May inhibit lactation.

● MEDICINAL FORMS
There can be variation in the licensing of different medicines containing the same drug. Forms available from special-order manufacturers include: oral suspension

Tablet

▸ Bumetanide (Non-proprietary)

Bumetanide 1 mg Bumetanide 1mg tablets | 28 tablet PoM £3.00 DT price = £1.18

Bumetanide 5 mg Bumetanide 5mg tablets | 28 tablet PoM £7.00 DT price = £6.98

Oral solution

▸ Bumetanide (Non-proprietary)

Bumetanide 200 microgram per 1 ml Bumetanide 1mg/5ml oral solution sugar free sugar-free | 150 ml PoM £168.00 DT price = £168.00

Combinations available: *Amiloride with bumetanide,* p. 213

Co-amilofruse

● INDICATIONS AND DOSE

Oedema

▸ BY MOUTH

▸ **Adult:** 2.5/20–10/80 mg daily, dose to be taken in the morning

DOSE EQUIVALENCE AND CONVERSION
A mixture of amiloride hydrochloride and furosemide (frusemide) in the mass proportions of 1 part amiloride hydrochloride to 8 parts furosemide (frusemide).

● CONTRA-INDICATIONS Addison's disease · anuria · comatose or precomatose states associated with liver cirrhosis · dehydration · hyperkalaemia · hypovolaemia · renal failure · severe hypokalaemia · severe hyponatraemia

● CAUTIONS Correct hypovolaemia before using in oliguria · diabetes mellitus · elderly · gout · hepatorenal syndrome · hypoproteinaemia · hypotension · impaired micturition · prostatic enlargement

● INTERACTIONS → Appendix 1 (diuretics).

● SIDE-EFFECTS Agranulocytosis · anaphylaxis · aplastic anaemia · blood disorders · bone marrow depression (withdraw treatment) · confusion · deafness (usually in renal impairment or in hypoproteinaemia) · dry mouth · eosinophilia · exfoliative dermatitis · gastro-intestinal disturbances · gout · haemolytic anaemia · hepatic encephalopathy · hyperglycaemia · hypersensitivity reactions · hyperuricaemia · hypocalcaemia · hypokalaemia (due to furosemide—may be followed by hyperkalaemia due to amiloride) · hypomagnesaemia · hyponatraemia · hypotension · intrahepatic cholestasis · leucopenia · metabolic alkalosis or acidosis · pancreatitis · paraesthesia · photosensitivity · purpura · rashes · Stevens-Johnson syndrome · temporary increase in serum cholesterol and triglyceride concentrations · thrombocytopenia · tinnitus · toxic epidermal necrolysis

● PREGNANCY Not used to treat hypertension in pregnancy.

● BREAST FEEDING Manufacturers advise avoid—no information regarding amiloride component available. Amount of furosemide in milk too small to be harmful. Furosemide may inhibit lactation.

● HEPATIC IMPAIRMENT Increased risk of hypomagnesaemia in alcoholic cirrhosis.

● RENAL IMPAIRMENT Risk of hyperkalaemia in renal impairment but may need higher doses. Avoid if eGFR less than 30 mL/minute/1.73 m^2. Monitor plasma-potassium concentration.

● MONITORING REQUIREMENTS Monitor electrolytes.

2

Cardiovascular system

- MEDICINAL FORMS

There can be variation in the licensing of different medicines containing the same drug. Forms available from special-order manufacturers include: oral suspension, oral solution

Tablet

▸ Co-amilofruse (Non-proprietary)

Amiloride hydrochloride 2.5 mg, Furosemide 20 mg Co-amilofruse 2.5mg/20mg tablets | 28 tablet [PoM] £10.95 DT price = £2.10 | 56 tablet [PoM] £4.66

Amiloride hydrochloride 5 mg, Furosemide 40 mg Co-amilofruse 5mg/40mg tablets | 28 tablet [PoM] £13.95 DT price = £2.03 | 56 tablet [PoM] £4.48

Amiloride hydrochloride 10 mg, Furosemide 80 mg Co-amilofruse 10mg/80mg tablets | 28 tablet [PoM] £19.95 DT price = £15.52

▸ Frumil (Sanofi)

Amiloride hydrochloride 2.5 mg, Furosemide 20 mg Frumil LS 20mg/2.5mg tablets | 28 tablet [PoM] £4.32 DT price = £2.10 | 56 tablet [PoM] £8.49

Amiloride hydrochloride 5 mg, Furosemide 40 mg Frumil 40mg/5mg tablets | 28 tablet [PoM] £5.29 DT price = £2.03 | 56 tablet [PoM] £10.35

F 208

Furosemide

(Frusemide)

- INDICATIONS AND DOSE

Oedema

▸ BY MOUTH

▸ Adult: Initially 40 mg daily, dose to be taken in the morning, then maintenance 20–40 mg daily

▸ INITIALLY BY INTRAMUSCULAR INJECTION, OR BY SLOW INTRAVENOUS INJECTION, OR BY INTRAVENOUS INFUSION

▸ Adult: Initially 20–50 mg, then (by intramuscular injection or by intravenous injection or by intravenous infusion) increased in steps of 20 mg every 2 hours if required, doses greater than 50 mg given by intravenous infusion only; maximum 1.5 g per day

Resistant oedema

▸ BY MOUTH

▸ Adult: 80–120 mg daily

▸ INITIALLY BY INTRAMUSCULAR INJECTION, OR BY SLOW INTRAVENOUS INJECTION, OR BY INTRAVENOUS INFUSION

▸ Adult: Initially 20–50 mg, then (by intramuscular injection or by intravenous injection or by intravenous infusion) increased in steps of 20 mg every 2 hours if required, doses greater than 50 mg given by intravenous infusion only; maximum 1.5 g per day

Resistant hypertension

▸ BY MOUTH

▸ Adult: 40–80 mg daily

▸ INITIALLY BY INTRAMUSCULAR INJECTION, OR BY SLOW INTRAVENOUS INJECTION, OR BY INTRAVENOUS INFUSION

▸ Adult: Initially 20–50 mg, then (by intramuscular injection or by intravenous injection or by intravenous infusion) increased in steps of 20 mg every 2 hours if required, doses greater than 50 mg given by intravenous infusion only; maximum 1.5 g per day

- CAUTIONS Hepatorenal syndrome · hypoproteinaemia may reduce diuretic effect and increase risk of side-effects

- SIDE-EFFECTS Gout · intrahepatic cholestasis

- PREGNANCY Furosemide should not be used to treat gestational hypertension because of the maternal hypovolaemia associated with this condition.

- BREAST FEEDING Amount too small to be harmful. May inhibit lactation.

- DIRECTIONS FOR ADMINISTRATION Intravenous administration rate should not usually exceed 4 mg/minute however single doses of up to 80 mg may be administered more rapidly; a lower rate of infusion may be necessary in renal impairment. For *intravenous infusion*

(*Lasix®*), give continuously in Sodium chloride 0.9%; infusion pH must be above 5.5; glucose solutions are unsuitable.

- MEDICINAL FORMS

There can be variation in the licensing of different medicines containing the same drug. Forms available from special-order manufacturers include: oral suspension, oral solution

Tablet

▸ Furosemide (Non-proprietary)

Furosemide 20 mg Furosemide 20mg tablets | 28 tablet [PoM] £1.02 DT price = £0.73

Furosemide 40 mg Furosemide 40mg tablets | 28 tablet [PoM] £1.03 DT price = £0.70 | 1000 tablet [PoM] £35.00

Furosemide 500 mg Furosemide 500mg tablets | 28 tablet [PoM] £70.00 DT price = £37.09

▸ Diuresal (Ennogen Pharma Ltd)

Furosemide 500 mg Diuresal 500mg tablets | 28 tablet [PoM] £44.80 DT price = £37.09

Oral solution

EXCIPIENTS: May contain Alcohol

▸ Furosemide (Non-proprietary)

Furosemide 4 mg per 1 ml Furosemide 20mg/5ml oral solution sugar free sugar-free | 150 ml [PoM] £14.49 DT price = £14.49

Furosemide 8 mg per 1 ml Furosemide 40mg/5ml oral solution sugar free sugar-free | 150 ml [PoM] £18.69 DT price = £18.69

Furosemide 10 mg per 1 ml Furosemide 50mg/5ml oral solution sugar free sugar-free | 150 ml [PoM] £20.21 DT price = £20.21

▸ Frusol (Rosemont Pharmaceuticals Ltd)

Furosemide 4 mg per 1 ml Frusol 20mg/5ml oral solution sugar-free | 150 ml [PoM] £12.07 DT price = £14.49

Furosemide 8 mg per 1 ml Frusol 40mg/5ml oral solution sugar-free | 150 ml [PoM] £15.58 DT price = £18.69

Furosemide 10 mg per 1 ml Frusol 50mg/5ml oral solution sugar-free | 150 ml [PoM] £16.84 DT price = £20.21

Solution for injection

▸ Furosemide (Non-proprietary)

Furosemide 10 mg per 1 ml Furosemide 250mg/25ml solution for injection ampoules | 10 ampoule [PoM] £25.00–£40.00

Furosemide 50mg/5ml solution for injection ampoules | 10 ampoule [PoM] £4.50–£7.60

Furosemide 20mg/2ml solution for injection ampoules | 10 ampoule [PoM] £4.50

▸ Lasix (Sanofi)

Furosemide 10 mg per 1 ml Lasix 20mg/2ml solution for injection ampoules | 5 ampoule [PoM] £3.74

Combinations available: *Spironolactone with furosemide,* p. 212

Furosemide with potassium chloride

The properties listed below are those particular to the combination only. For the properties of the components please consider, furosemide above, potassium chloride p. 917.

- INDICATIONS AND DOSE

Oedema

▸ BY MOUTH

▸ Adult: (consult product literature)

- DIRECTIONS FOR ADMINISTRATION Furosemide with modified-release potassium chloride tablets should be swallowed whole with plenty of fluid during meals while sitting or standing.

- PATIENT AND CARER ADVICE Patients or carers should be given advice on how to administer furosemide with potassium chloride tablets.

- LESS SUITABLE FOR PRESCRIBING Furosemide with potassium chloride tablets are less suitable for prescribing.

- MEDICINAL FORMS
There can be variation in the licensing of different medicines containing the same drug.
Modified-release tablet
CAUTIONARY AND ADVISORY LABELS 25, 27
  ▸ Diumide-K Continus (Teofarma)
    Furosemide 40 mg, Potassium chloride 600 mg Diumide-K Continus tablets | 30 tablet PoM £3.00

Furosemide with triamterene

The properties listed below are those particular to the combination only. For the properties of the components please consider, furosemide p. 210, triamterene p. 213.

- INDICATIONS AND DOSE
Oedema
  ▸ BY MOUTH
  ▸ Adult: 0.5–2 tablets daily, dose to be taken in the morning

- CONTRA-INDICATIONS Anuria · comatose or precomatose states associated with liver cirrhosis · dehydration · hyperkalaemia · hypovolaemia · renal failure · severe hypokalaemia · severe hyponatraemia

- CAUTIONS Diabetes mellitus · elderly · gout · hepatorenal syndrome · hypotension · impaired micturition · may cause blue fluorescence of urine · prostatic enlargement

- INTERACTIONS → Appendix 1 (diuretics).

- SIDE-EFFECTS
  ▸ **Rare** Agranulocytosis · anaphylaxis · aplastic anaemia · blood disorders · bone marrow depression (withdraw treatment) · deafness (usually in renal impairment or in hypoproteinaemia) · eosinophilia · exfoliative dermatitis · haemolytic anaemia · hypersensitivity reactions · intrahepatic cholestasis · leucopenia · pancreatitis · paraesthesia · photosensitivity · purpura · rash · thrombocytopenia · tinnitus (usually in renal impairment or in hypoproteinaemia)
  ▸ **Frequency not known** Dry mouth · electrolyte disturbances · gastro-intestinal disturbances · gout · hyperglycaemia (less common than with thiazides) · hyperkalaemia · hyperuricaemia · hypocalcaemia · hypokalaemia · hypomagnesaemia · hyponatraemia · hypotension · metabolic alkalosis · temporary increase in plasma cholesterol and triglyceride concentration · triamterene found in kidney stones

- BREAST FEEDING Triamterene present in milk—manufacturer advises avoid. Furosemide may inhibit lactation.

- HEPATIC IMPAIRMENT Increased risk of hypomagnesaemia in alcoholic cirrhosis. Hypokalaemia may precipitate coma.

- RENAL IMPAIRMENT May need high doses. Avoid in severe impairment. Monitor plasma-potassium concentration in renal impairment (high risk of hyperkalaemia).

- MONITORING REQUIREMENTS Monitor electrolytes.

- PATIENT AND CARER ADVICE Urine may look slightly blue in some lights.

- MEDICINAL FORMS
There can be variation in the licensing of different medicines containing the same drug.
Tablet
CAUTIONARY AND ADVISORY LABELS 14
  ▸ Frusene (Orion Pharma (UK) Ltd)
    Furosemide 40 mg, Triamterene 50 mg Frusene 50mg/40mg tablets | 56 tablet PoM £4.34 DT price = £4.34

⬛ 208

Torasemide

- INDICATIONS AND DOSE
Oedema
  ▸ BY MOUTH
  ▸ Adult: 5 mg once daily, to be taken preferably in the morning, then increased if necessary to 20 mg once daily; maximum 40 mg per day
Hypertension
  ▸ BY MOUTH
  ▸ Adult: 2.5 mg daily, then increased if necessary to 5 mg once daily

- SIDE-EFFECTS
  ▸ **Rare** Limb paraesthesia
  ▸ **Frequency not known** Dry mouth

- PREGNANCY Manufacturer advises avoid—toxicity in *animal* studies.

- BREAST FEEDING Manufacturer advises avoid—no information available.

- MEDICINAL FORMS
There can be variation in the licensing of different medicines containing the same drug.
Tablet
  ▸ Torasemide (Non-proprietary)
    Torasemide 5 mg Torasemide 5mg tablets | 28 tablet PoM £14.50 DT price = £5.53
    Torasemide 10 mg Torasemide 10mg tablets | 28 tablet PoM £18.75 DT price = £8.14
  ▸ Torem (Meda Pharmaceuticals Ltd)
    Torasemide 2.5 mg Torem 2.5mg tablets | 28 tablet PoM £3.78 DT price = £3.78
    Torasemide 5 mg Torem 5mg tablets | 28 tablet PoM £5.53 DT price = £5.53
    Torasemide 10 mg Torem 10mg tablets | 28 tablet PoM £8.14 DT price = £8.14

DIURETICS > OSMOTIC DIURETICS

Mannitol

- INDICATIONS AND DOSE
Cerebral oedema
  ▸ BY INTRAVENOUS INFUSION
  ▸ Adult: 0.25–2 g/kg, repeated if necessary, to be administered over 30-60 minutes, dose may be repeated 1–2 times after 4–8 hours
Raised intra-ocular pressure
  ▸ BY INTRAVENOUS INFUSION
  ▸ Adult: 0.25–2 g/kg, repeated if necessary, to be administered over 30–60 minutes, dose may be repeated 1–2 times after 4–8 hours

- CONTRA-INDICATIONS Anuria · intracranial bleeding (except during craniotomy) · severe cardiac failure · severe dehydration · severe pulmonary oedema

- CAUTIONS Extravasation causes inflammation and thrombophlebitis

- INTERACTIONS → Appendix 1 (mannitol).

- SIDE-EFFECTS
  ▸ **Uncommon** Electrolyte imbalance · fluid imbalance · hypotension · thrombophlebitis
  ▸ **Rare** Anaphylaxis · arrhythmia · blurred vision · chest pain · chills · convulsions · cramp · dehydration · dizziness · dry mouth · fever · focal osmotic nephrosis · headache · hypersensitivity reactions · hypertension · nausea · oedema · pulmonary oedema · raised intracranial pressure · rhinitis · skin necrosis · thirst · urinary retention · urticaria · vomiting
  ▸ **Very rare** Acute renal failure · congestive heart failure

- PREGNANCY Manufacturer advises avoid unless essential— no information available.
- BREAST FEEDING Manufacturer advises avoid unless essential—no information available.
- RENAL IMPAIRMENT Use with caution in severe impairment.
- PRE-TREATMENT SCREENING Assess cardiac function before treatment.
- MONITORING REQUIREMENTS Monitor fluid and electrolyte balance, serum osmolality, and cardiac, pulmonary and renal function.
- DIRECTIONS FOR ADMINISTRATION For mannitol 20%, an in-line filter is recommended (15-micron filters have been used).

- MEDICINAL FORMS
There can be variation in the licensing of different medicines containing the same drug. Forms available from special-order manufacturers include: infusion, solution for infusion
Infusion
  ▸ Mannitol (Non-proprietary)
    Mannitol 100 mg per 1 ml Mannitol 50g/500ml (10%) infusion Viaflo bags | 1 bag [PoM] no price available | 20 bag [PoM] no price available
    Mannitol 50g/500ml (10%) infusion Viaflex bags | 1 bag [PoM] no price available | 20 bag [PoM] no price available
    Polyfusor K mannitol 10% infusion 500ml bottles | 1 bottle [PoM] £4.46 | 12 bottle [PoM] no price available
    Mannitol 150 mg per 1 ml Mannitol 75g/500ml (15%) infusion Viaflo bags | 20 bag [PoM] no price available
    Mannitol 200 mg per 1 ml Mannitol 100g/500ml (20%) infusion Viaflex bags | 1 bag [PoM] no price available | 20 bag [PoM] no price available
    Polyfusor M mannitol 20% infusion 500ml bottles | 1 bottle [PoM] £5.86 | 12 bottle [PoM] no price available
    Mannitol 50g/250ml (20%) infusion Viaflex bags | 1 bag [PoM] no price available | 30 bag [PoM] no price available
    Mannitol 100g/500ml (20%) infusion Viaflo bags | 1 bag [PoM] no price available | 20 bag [PoM] no price available

DIURETICS > POTASSIUM-SPARING DIURETICS > ALDOSTERONE ANTAGONISTS

Spironolactone with furosemide
The properties listed below are those particular to the combination only. For the properties of the components please consider, spironolactone p. 175, furosemide p. 210.

- INDICATIONS AND DOSE
Resistant oedema
  ▸ BY MOUTH
  ▸ Adult: 20/50–80/200 mg daily

- MEDICINAL FORMS
There can be variation in the licensing of different medicines containing the same drug.
Capsule
  ▸ Lasilactone (Sanofi)
    Furosemide 20 mg, Spironolactone 50 mg Lasilactone 20mg/50mg capsules | 28 capsule [PoM] £7.97

DIURETICS > POTASSIUM-SPARING DIURETICS > OTHER

Amiloride hydrochloride

- INDICATIONS AND DOSE
Oedema (monotherapy)
  ▸ BY MOUTH
  ▸ Adult: Initially 10 mg daily, alternatively initially 5 mg twice daily, adjusted according to response; maximum 20 mg per day

Potassium conservation when used as an adjunct to thiazide or loop diuretics for hypertension or congestive heart failure
  ▸ BY MOUTH
  ▸ Adult: Initially 5–10 mg daily

Potassium conservation when used as an adjunct to thiazide or loop diuretics for hepatic cirrhosis with ascites
  ▸ BY MOUTH
  ▸ Adult: Initially 5 mg daily

- CONTRA-INDICATIONS Addison's disease · anuria · hyperkalaemia
- CAUTIONS Diabetes mellitus · elderly
- INTERACTIONS → Appendix 1 (diuretics).
- SIDE-EFFECTS Abdominal pain · agitation · alopecia · angina · anorexia · arrhythmias · arthralgia · confusion · constipation · cough · diarrhoea · dizziness · dry mouth · dyspepsia · dyspnoea · encephalopathy · flatulence · gastro-intestinal bleeding · headache · hyperkalaemia · insomnia · jaundice · malaise · muscle cramp · nasal congestion · nausea · palpitation · paraesthesia · postural hypotension · pruritus · raised intra-ocular pressure · rash · sexual dysfunction · thirst · tinnitus · tremor · urinary disturbances · visual disturbance · vomiting · weakness
- PREGNANCY Not to be used to treat gestational hypertension.
- BREAST FEEDING Manufacturer advises avoid—no information available.
- RENAL IMPAIRMENT Manufacturers advise avoid in severe impairment. Monitor plasma-potassium concentration (high risk of hyperkalaemia in renal impairment).
- MONITORING REQUIREMENTS Monitor electrolytes.

- MEDICINAL FORMS
There can be variation in the licensing of different medicines containing the same drug. Forms available from special-order manufacturers include: oral suspension, oral solution
Tablet
  ▸ Amiloride hydrochloride (Non-proprietary)
    Amiloride hydrochloride 5 mg Amiloride 5mg tablets | 28 tablet [PoM] £6.72 DT price = £4.31
Oral solution
EXCIPIENTS: May contain Propylene glycol
  ▸ Amiloride hydrochloride (Non-proprietary)
    Amiloride hydrochloride 1 mg per 1 ml Amiloride 5mg/5ml oral solution sugar free sugar-free | 150 ml [PoM] no price available DT price = £37.35
  ▸ Amilamont (Rosemont Pharmaceuticals Ltd)
    Amiloride hydrochloride 1 mg per 1 ml Amilamont 5mg/5ml oral solution sugar free sugar-free | 150 ml [PoM] £37.35 DT price = £37.35

Amiloride with bumetanide

The properties listed below are those particular to the combination only. For the properties of the components please consider, amiloride hydrochloride p. 212, bumetanide p. 209.

● **INDICATIONS AND DOSE**

Oedema
▶ BY MOUTH
▶ Adult: 1–2 tablets daily

● MEDICINAL FORMS
There can be variation in the licensing of different medicines containing the same drug.
Tablet
▶ Amiloride with bumetanide (Non-proprietary)
  Bumetanide 1 mg, Amiloride hydrochloride 5 mg Amiloride 5mg / Bumetanide 1mg tablets | 28 tablet [PoM] £29.60 DT price = £29.60

Triamterene

● **INDICATIONS AND DOSE**

Oedema | Potassium conservation with thiazide and loop diuretics
▶ BY MOUTH
▶ Adult: Initially 150–250 mg daily for 1 week, then reduced to 150–250 mg daily on alternate days, dose to be taken in divided doses after breakfast and lunch; lower initial dose when given with other diuretics

● CONTRA-INDICATIONS Addison's disease · anuria · hyperkalaemia
● CAUTIONS Diabetes mellitus · elderly · gout · may cause blue fluorescence of urine
● INTERACTIONS → Appendix 1 (triamterene).
● SIDE-EFFECTS
▶ **Common or very common** Diarrhoea · hyperkalaemia · nausea · vomiting
▶ **Uncommon** Dry mouth · headache · hyperuricaemia · rash
▶ **Rare** Megaloblastic anaemia · pancytopenia · photosensitivity · serum-sickness
▶ **Very rare** Renal failure (reversible on discontinuation) · triamterene found in kidney stones
▶ **Frequency not known** Jaundice · malaise · slight decrease in blood pressure
● PREGNANCY Not used to treat gestational hypertension. Avoid unless essential.
● BREAST FEEDING Present in milk—manufacturer advises avoid.
● HEPATIC IMPAIRMENT Use with caution. Avoid in progressive impairment.
● RENAL IMPAIRMENT Avoid in progressive impairment. Monitor plasma-potassium concentration (high risk of hyperkalaemia in renal impairment).
● MONITORING REQUIREMENTS Monitor electrolytes.
● PATIENT AND CARER ADVICE Urine may look slightly blue in some lights.

● MEDICINAL FORMS
There can be variation in the licensing of different medicines containing the same drug.
Capsule
CAUTIONARY AND ADVISORY LABELS 14, 21
▶ Triamterene (Non-proprietary)
  Triamterene 50 mg Triamterene 50mg capsules | 30 capsule [PoM] £41.90 DT price = £41.90

Combinations available: *Co-triamterzide,* p. 214 · *Furosemide with triamterene,* p. 211

Triamterene with chlortalidone

The properties listed below are those particular to the combination only. For the properties of the components please consider, triamterene above, chlortalidone below.

● **INDICATIONS AND DOSE**

Hypertension | Oedema
▶ BY MOUTH
▶ Adult: 50/50–100/100 mg once daily, dose to be taken in the morning
DOSE EQUIVALENCE AND CONVERSION
Dose expressed as x/y mg of triamterene/chlortalidone.

● MEDICINAL FORMS
There can be variation in the licensing of different medicines containing the same drug.
Tablet
CAUTIONARY AND ADVISORY LABELS 14, 21
▶ Kalspare (DHP Healthcare Ltd)
  Chlortalidone 50 mg, Triamterene 50 mg Kalspare tablets | 28 tablet [PoM] £9.90

DIURETICS > THIAZIDES AND RELATED DIURETICS
⚑ 151

Chlortalidone

(Chlorthalidone)

● **INDICATIONS AND DOSE**

Ascites due to cirrhosis in stable patients (under close supervision) | Oedema due to nephrotic syndrome
▶ BY MOUTH
▶ Adult: Up to 50 mg daily
Hypertension
▶ BY MOUTH
▶ Adult: 25 mg daily, dose to be taken in the morning, then increased if necessary to 50 mg daily
Mild to moderate chronic heart failure
▶ BY MOUTH
▶ Adult: 25–50 mg daily, dose to be taken in the morning, then increased if necessary to 100–200 mg daily, reduce to lowest effective dose for maintenance
Nephrogenic diabetes insipidus | Partial pituitary diabetes insipidus
▶ BY MOUTH
▶ Adult: Initially 100 mg twice daily, then reduced to 50 mg daily

● SIDE-EFFECTS
▶ **Rare** Allergic interstitial nephritis · jaundice
● BREAST FEEDING The amount present in milk is too small to be harmful. Large doses may suppress lactation.

● MEDICINAL FORMS
There can be variation in the licensing of different medicines containing the same drug. Forms available from special-order manufacturers include: oral suspension
Tablet
▶ Chlortalidone (Non-proprietary)
  Chlortalidone 25 mg Chlortalidone 25mg tablets | 100 tablet [PoM] no price available
  Chlortalidone 50 mg Chlortalidone 50mg tablets | 30 tablet [PoM] £88.00 DT price = £88.00

Combinations available: *Triamterene with chlortalidone,* above

Co-triamterzide

The properties listed below are those particular to the combination only. For the properties of the components please consider, triamterene p. 213, hydrochlorothiazide p. 153.

● **INDICATIONS AND DOSE**

Hypertension

▶ BY MOUTH
▹ Adult: 50/25 mg daily, increased if necessary up to 200/100 mg daily, dose to be taken after breakfast

Oedema

▶ BY MOUTH
▹ Adult: 50/25 mg twice daily, to be taken after breakfast and after midday meal, increased if necessary to 150/75 mg daily, to be taken as 100/50 mg after breakfast and 50/25 mg after midday meal; maintenance 50/25 mg daily, alternatively maintenance 100/50 mg once daily on alternate days; maximum 200/100 mg per day

DOSE EQUIVALENCE AND CONVERSION
Dose expressed as x/y mg of triamterene/hydrochlorothiazide.

● **PATIENT AND CARER ADVICE** Urine may look slightly blue in some lights.

● **MEDICINAL FORMS**
There can be variation in the licensing of different medicines containing the same drug.
Tablet
CAUTIONARY AND ADVISORY LABELS 14, 21
▹ Dyazide (AMCo)
Hydrochlorothiazide 25 mg, Triamterene 50 mg Dyazide 50mg/25mg tablets | 30 tablet [PoM] £0.95 DT price = £0.95

F 151

Cyclopenthiazide

● **INDICATIONS AND DOSE**

Heart failure

▶ BY MOUTH
▹ Adult: 250–500 micrograms daily, take in the morning, then increased if necessary to 1 mg daily, reduce to lowest effective dose for maintenance

Hypertension

▶ BY MOUTH
▹ Adult: Initially 250 micrograms daily, take in the morning, then increased if necessary to 500 micrograms daily

Oedema

▶ BY MOUTH
▹ Adult: Up to 500 micrograms daily for a short period

● **SIDE-EFFECTS**
▶ Rare Depression

● **BREAST FEEDING** The amount present in milk is too small to be harmful. Large doses may suppress lactation.

● **MEDICINAL FORMS**
There can be variation in the licensing of different medicines containing the same drug.
Tablet
EXCIPIENTS: May contain Gluten
▹ Navidrex (AMCo)
Cyclopenthiazide 500 microgram Navidrex 500microgram tablets | 28 tablet [PoM] £1.27

F 151

Metolazone

● **INDICATIONS AND DOSE**

Oedema

▶ BY MOUTH
▹ Adult: 5–10 mg daily, dose to be taken in the morning; increased if necessary to 20 mg daily, dose increased in resistant oedema; maximum 80 mg per day

Hypertension

▶ BY MOUTH
▹ Adult: Initially 5 mg daily, dose to be taken in the morning; maintenance 5 mg once daily on alternate days

● CAUTIONS Acute porphyrias p. 918

● SIDE-EFFECTS Chest pain · chills

● BREAST FEEDING The amount present in milk is too small to be harmful. Large doses may suppress lactation.

● DIRECTIONS FOR ADMINISTRATION Tablets may be crushed and mixed with water immediately before use.

● MEDICINAL FORMS
There can be variation in the licensing of different medicines containing the same drug. Forms available from special-order manufacturers include: tablet, oral suspension, oral solution
Tablet
▹ Metolazone (Non-proprietary)
Metolazone 2.5 mg Zaroxolyn 2.5mg tablets | 100 tablet [PoM] no price available
Metolazone 5 mg Zaroxolyn 5mg tablets | 50 tablet [PoM] no price available

F 151

Xipamide

● **INDICATIONS AND DOSE**

Oedema

▶ BY MOUTH
▹ Adult: Initially 40 mg daily, dose to be taken in the morning, increased if necessary to 80 mg daily, higher dose to be used in resistant cases; maintenance 20 mg daily, dose to be taken in the morning

Hypertension

▶ BY MOUTH
▹ Adult: 20 mg daily, dose to be taken in the morning

● CAUTIONS Acute porphyrias p. 918

● BREAST FEEDING No information available.

● MEDICINAL FORMS
There can be variation in the licensing of different medicines containing the same drug.
Tablet
▹ Diurexan (Meda Pharmaceuticals Ltd)
Xipamide 20 mg Diurexan 20mg tablets | 140 tablet [PoM] £19.46 DT price = £19.46

9　Vascular disease

Peripheral vascular disease

Classification and management

Peripheral vascular disease can be either occlusive (e.g. *intermittent claudication*) in which occlusion of the peripheral arteries is caused by atherosclerosis, or vasospastic (e.g. *Raynaud's syndrome*). Peripheral arterial occlusive disease is associated with an increased risk of cardiovascular events; this risk is reduced by measures such as smoking cessation, effective control of blood pressure, regulating blood lipids, optimising glycaemic control in diabetes, taking aspirin p. 109 in a dose of 75 mg daily, and possibly weight reduction in obesity. Exercise training can improve symptoms of intermittent claudication; revascularisation procedures may be appropriate.

Naftidrofuryl oxalate p. 216 can alleviate symptoms of intermittent claudication and improve pain-free walking distance in moderate disease. Patients taking naftidrofuryl oxalate should be assessed for improvement after 3–6 months.

Cilostazol below is licensed for use in intermittent claudication to improve walking distance in patients without peripheral tissue necrosis who do not have pain at rest; use is restricted to second-line treatment where lifestyle modifications and other appropriate interventions have failed to improve symptoms. Cilostazol should be initiated by those experienced in the management of intermittent claudication. Patients receiving cilostazol should be assessed for improvement after 3 months; consider discontinuation of treatment if there is no clinically relevant improvement in walking distance.

Inositol nicotinate p. 216 and pentoxifylline p. 217 are not established as being effective for the treatment of intermittent claudication.

Management of *Raynaud's syndrome* includes avoidance of exposure to cold and stopping smoking. More severe symptoms may require vasodilator treatment, which is most often successful in primary Raynaud's syndrome. Nifedipine p. 148 is useful for reducing the frequency and severity of vasospastic attacks. Alternatively, naftidrofuryl oxalate may produce symptomatic improvement; inositol nicotinate (a nicotinic acid derivative) may also be considered. Pentoxifylline, prazosin p. 709, and moxisylyte p. 216 are not established as being effective for the treatment of Raynaud's syndrome.

Vasodilator therapy is not established as being effective for *chilblains*.

ANTITHROMBOTIC DRUGS > ANTIPLATELET DRUGS

Cilostazol

- **INDICATIONS AND DOSE**

Intermittent claudication in patients without rest pain and no peripheral tissue necrosis

- ▸ BY MOUTH
- ▸ Adult: 100 mg twice daily, to be taken 30 minutes before food, cilostazol should be initiated by those experienced in the management of intermittent claudication, patients receiving cilostazol should be assessed for improvement after 3 months; consider discontinuation of treatment if there is no clinically relevant improvement in walking distance

DOSE ADJUSTMENTS DUE TO INTERACTIONS
Reduce dose to 50 mg twice daily with concomitant use of potent inhibitors of cytochrome P450 enzymes CYP3A4 (e.g. clarithromycin, itraconazole, ketoconazole, protease inhibitors) or CYP2C19, or with erythromycin or omeprazole.

- **CONTRA-INDICATIONS** Active peptic ulcer · congestive heart failure · coronary intervention in previous 6 months · haemorrhagic stroke in previous 6 months · history of severe tachyarrhythmia · myocardial infarction in previous 6 months · poorly controlled hypertension · predisposition to bleeding · proliferative diabetic retinopathy · prolongation of QT interval · severe atrial flutter · unstable angina
- **CAUTIONS** Atrial fibrillation · atrial or ventricular ectopy · diabetes mellitus (higher risk of intraocular bleeding) ·

mild to moderate atrial flutter · stable coronary disease · surgery

- **INTERACTIONS** → Appendix 1 (cilostazol).
Caution with concomitant use of drugs that increase risk of bleeding.
Contra-indicated with concomitant use of 2 or more antiplatelets or anticoagulants.
- **SIDE-EFFECTS**
- ▸ **Common or very common** Abdominal pain · angina · anorexia · arrhythmia · diarrhoea · dizziness · dyspepsia · ecchymosis · flatulence · headache · malaise · nausea · oedema · palpitation · pharyngitis · pruritus · rash · rhinitis · tachycardia · vomiting
- ▸ **Uncommon** Abnormal dreams · anaemia · anxiety · congestive heart failure · cough · diabetes mellitus · dyspnoea · gastritis · haemorrhage · hyperglycaemia · insomnia · myalgia · myocardial infarction · pneumonia · postural hypotension
- ▸ **Rare** Bleeding disorders · increased urinary frequency · renal impairment · thrombocythaemia
- ▸ **Frequency not known** Agranulocytosis · aplastic anemia · conjunctivitis · hepatitis · hot flushes · hypertension · leucopenia · pancytopenia · pyrexia · Stevens-Johnson syndrome · thrombocytopenia · tinnitus · toxic epidermal necrolysis

SIDE-EFFECTS, FURTHER INFORMATION
- ▸ Blood Disorders A blood count should be performed and the drug stopped immediately if there is suspicion of a blood dyscrasia.
- **PREGNANCY** Avoid—toxicity in *animal* studies.
- **BREAST FEEDING** Present in milk in *animal* studies—manufacturer advises avoid.
- **HEPATIC IMPAIRMENT** Avoid in moderate or severe liver disease.
- **RENAL IMPAIRMENT** Avoid if eGFR less than 25 mL/minute/1.73 m².
- **PATIENT AND CARER ADVICE**
Blood disorders Patients should be advised to report any unexplained bleeding, bruising, sore throat, or fever.
- **NATIONAL FUNDING/ACCESS DECISIONS**

NICE technology appraisals (TAs)
- ▸ Cilostazol, naftidrofuryl oxalate, pentoxifylline and inositol nicotinate for the treatment of intermittent claudication in people with peripheral arterial disease (May 2011) NICE TA223 Cilostazol is not recommended for the treatment of intermittent claudication in patients with peripheral arterial disease; patients currently receiving this treatment should have the option to continue until they and their clinician consider it appropriate to stop.
www.nice.org.uk/TA223

Scottish Medicines Consortium (SMC) Decisions
The *Scottish Medicines Consortium* has advised (October 2005) that cilostazol is not recommended for the treatment of intermittent claudication within NHS Scotland.

- **MEDICINAL FORMS**
There can be variation in the licensing of different medicines containing the same drug.

Tablet
- ▸ Cilostazol (Non-proprietary) ▼
Cilostazol 50 mg Cilostazol 50mg tablets | 56 tablet PoM £40.05 DT price = £40.05
Cilostazol 100 mg Cilostazol 100mg tablets | 56 tablet PoM £31.70 DT price = £4.02
- ▸ Pletal (Otsuka Pharmaceuticals (U.K.) Ltd) ▼
Cilostazol 50 mg Pletal 50mg tablets | 56 tablet PoM £35.31 DT price = £40.05
Cilostazol 100 mg Pletal 100mg tablets | 56 tablet PoM £33.37 DT price = £4.02

LIPID MODIFYING DRUGS > NICOTINIC ACID DERIVATIVES

Inositol nicotinate

- **INDICATIONS AND DOSE**

Peripheral vascular disease
- ▸ BY MOUTH
- ▸ Adult: 3 g daily in 2–3 divided doses; maximum 4 g per day

- **CONTRA-INDICATIONS** Acute phase of a cerebrovascular accident · recent myocardial infarction
- **CAUTIONS** Cerebrovascular insufficiency · unstable angina
- **SIDE-EFFECTS** Dizziness · flushing · headache · hypotension · nausea · oedema · paraesthesia · rash · syncope · vomiting
- **PREGNANCY** No information available—manufacturer advises avoid unless potential benefit outweighs risk.
- **NATIONAL FUNDING/ACCESS DECISIONS**

  NICE technology appraisals (TAs)
  - ▸ Cilostazol, naftidrofuryl oxalate, pentoxifylline and inositol nicotinate for the treatment of intermittent claudication in people with peripheral arterial disease (May 2011) NICE TA223 Inositol nicotinate is not recommended for the treatment of intermittent claudication in patients with peripheral arterial disease; patients currently receiving treatment should have the option to continue until they and their clinician consider it appropriate to stop.
    www.nice.org.uk/TA223

- **LESS SUITABLE FOR PRESCRIBING** Less suitable for prescribing.

- **MEDICINAL FORMS**
  There can be variation in the licensing of different medicines containing the same drug. Forms available from special-order manufacturers include: oral suspension
  Tablet
  - ▸ Hexopal (Genus Pharmaceuticals Ltd)
    Inositol nicotinate 500 mg Hexopal 500mg tablets | 100 tablet Ⓟ £26.15 DT price = £30.76
    Inositol nicotinate 750 mg Hexopal Forte 750mg tablets | 112 tablet Ⓟ £43.37 DT price = £51.03
  Capsule
  - ▸ Inositol nicotinate (Non-proprietary)
    Inositol nicotinate 500 mg Solgar No-Flush Niacin 500mg capsules | 50 capsule no price available

VASODILATORS > FLAVONOIDS

Oxerutins

- **INDICATIONS AND DOSE**

Relief of symptoms of oedema associated with chronic venous insufficiency
- ▸ BY MOUTH
- ▸ Adult: 500 mg twice daily

- **SIDE-EFFECTS** Flushing · headache · mild gastro-intestinal disturbances · rash
- **LESS SUITABLE FOR PRESCRIBING** Oxerutins (rutosides) are not vasodilators and are not generally regarded as effective preparations as capillary sealants or for the treatment of cramps; they are less suitable for prescribing.

- **MEDICINAL FORMS**
  There can be variation in the licensing of different medicines containing the same drug.
  Capsule
  - ▸ Paroven (Novartis Consumer Health UK Ltd)
    Oxerutins 250 mg Paroven 250mg capsules | 120 capsule Ⓟ £16.81 DT price = £16.81

VASODILATORS > PERIPHERAL VASODILATORS

Moxisylyte

(Thymoxamine)

- **INDICATIONS AND DOSE**

Primary Raynaud's syndrome (short-term treatment)
- ▸ BY MOUTH
- ▸ Adult: Initially 40 mg 4 times a day, increased if necessary to 80 mg 4 times a day, increase dose if poor initial response, discontinue after 2 weeks if no response

- **CONTRA-INDICATIONS** Active liver disease
- **CAUTIONS** Diabetes mellitus
- **SIDE-EFFECTS** Cholestatic jaundice · diarrhoea · dizziness · flushing · headache · hepatic reactions · hepatitis · nausea
- **PREGNANCY** Manufacturer advises avoid.
- **LESS SUITABLE FOR PRESCRIBING** Less suitable for prescribing.

- **MEDICINAL FORMS**
  There can be variation in the licensing of different medicines containing the same drug.
  Tablet
  CAUTIONARY AND ADVISORY LABELS 21
  - ▸ Opilon (ProStrakan Ltd)
    Moxisylyte (as Moxisylyte hydrochloride) 40 mg Opilon 40mg tablets | 112 tablet Ⓟ₀ₘ £90.22 DT price = £90.22

Naftidrofuryl oxalate

- **INDICATIONS AND DOSE**

Peripheral vascular disease
- ▸ BY MOUTH
- ▸ Adult: 100–200 mg 3 times a day, patients taking naftidrofuryl should be assessed for improvement after 3–6 months

Cerebral vascular disease
- ▸ BY MOUTH
- ▸ Adult: 100 mg 3 times a day, patients taking naftidrofuryl should be assessed for improvement after 3–6 months

- **SIDE-EFFECTS** Epigastric pain · hepatic failure · hepatitis · nausea · rash
- **NATIONAL FUNDING/ACCESS DECISIONS**

  NICE technology appraisals (TAs)
  - ▸ Cilostazol, naftidrofuryl oxalate, pentoxifylline and inositol nicotinate for the treatment of intermittent claudication in people with peripheral arterial disease (May 2011) NICE TA223 Naftidrofuryl oxalate is an option for the treatment of intermittent claudication in patients with peripheral arterial disease in whom vasodilator therapy is considered appropriate.
    www.nice.org.uk/TA223

- **MEDICINAL FORMS**
  There can be variation in the licensing of different medicines containing the same drug. Forms available from special-order manufacturers include: oral solution
  Capsule
  CAUTIONARY AND ADVISORY LABELS 25, 27
  - ▸ Naftidrofuryl oxalate (Non-proprietary)
    Naftidrofuryl oxalate 100 mg Naftidrofuryl 100mg capsules | 84 capsule Ⓟₒₘ £25.00 DT price = £5.27
  - ▸ Praxilene (Merck Serono Ltd)
    Naftidrofuryl oxalate 100 mg Praxilene 100mg capsules | 84 capsule Ⓟₒₘ £8.10 DT price = £5.27

Pentoxifylline

(Oxpentifylline)

- **INDICATIONS AND DOSE**

Peripheral vascular disease | Venous leg ulcer (adjunct)
- ▶ BY MOUTH
  - ▶ Adult: 400 mg 2–3 times a day

- UNLICENSED USE Use of pentoxifylline as adjunct therapy for venous leg ulcers is an unlicensed indication.
- CONTRA-INDICATIONS Acute myocardial infarction · cerebral haemorrhage · extensive retinal haemorrhage · severe cardiac arrhythmias
- CAUTIONS Avoid in Acute porphyrias p. 918 · coronary artery disease · hypotension
- INTERACTIONS → Appendix 1 (pentoxifylline).
- SIDE-EFFECTS
- ▶ **Rare** Angina · hypotension
- ▶ **Very rare** Bleeding
- ▶ **Frequency not known** Agitation · diarrhoea · dizziness · flushing · headache · intra-hepatic cholestasis · nausea · sleep disturbances · tachycardia · thrombocytopenia · vomiting
- PREGNANCY Manufacturer advises avoid—no information available.
- BREAST FEEDING Present in milk—manufacturer advises use only if potential benefit outweighs risk.
- HEPATIC IMPAIRMENT Manufacturer advises reduce dose in severe impairment.
- RENAL IMPAIRMENT Reduce dose by 30–50% if eGFR less than 30 mL/minute/1.73 m^2.
- NATIONAL FUNDING/ACCESS DECISIONS

NICE technology appraisals (TAs)
- ▶ Cilostazol, naftidrofuryl oxalate, pentoxifylline and inositol nicotinate for the treatment of intermittent claudication in people with peripheral arterial disease (May 2011) NICE TA223 Pentoxifylline is not recommended for the treatment of intermittent claudication in patients with peripheral arterial disease; patients currently receiving this treatment should have the option to continue until they and their clinician consider it appropriate to stop.
www.nice.org.uk/TA223
- LESS SUITABLE FOR PRESCRIBING Less suitable for prescribing.

- MEDICINAL FORMS
There can be variation in the licensing of different medicines containing the same drug. Forms available from special-order manufacturers include: oral solution
Modified-release tablet
CAUTIONARY AND ADVISORY LABELS 21, 25
- ▶ Trental (Sanofi)
  Pentoxifylline 400 mg Trental 400 modified-release tablets | 90 tablet [PoM] £19.39 DT price = £19.39

9.1 Vein malformations

SCLEROSANTS

Sodium tetradecyl sulfate

- **INDICATIONS AND DOSE**

Sclerotherapy of reticular veins and spider veins in legs and varicose veins
- ▶ BY INTRAVENOUS INJECTION
  - ▶ Adult: Test dose recommended before each treatment (consult product literature)

- CONTRA-INDICATIONS Acute infection · asthma · blood disorders · deep vein thrombosis · high risk of thromboembolism · hyperthyroidism · inability to walk · neoplasm · occlusive arterial disease · phlebitis · pulmonary embolism · recent acute superficial thrombophlebitis · recent surgery · respiratory disease · significant valvular incompetence in deep veins · skin disease · symptomatic patent foramen ovale (if administered as foam) · uncontrolled diabetes mellitus · varicose veins caused by tumours (unless tumour removed)
- CAUTIONS Arterial disease · asymptomatic patent foramen ovale (use smaller volumes and avoid Valsalva manoeuvre immediately after administration) · extravasation may cause necrosis of tissues · history of migraine (use smaller volumes) · resuscitation facilities must be available · venous insufficiency with lymphoedema (pain and inflammation may worsen)
- SIDE-EFFECTS
- ▶ **Common or very common** Local burning · local pain · phlebitis · skin discoloration · superficial thrombophlebitis · telangiectatic matting
- ▶ **Uncommon** Deep vein thrombosis · scotoma
- ▶ **Rare** Chest pain · cough · headache · migraine · paraesthesia · shortness of breath · vasovagal reactions
- ▶ **Very rare** Anaphylaxis · circulatory collapse · diarrhoea · dry mouth · fever · hot flushes · hypersensitivity reactions · nausea · necrosis of skin and tissues · palpitation · pulmonary embolism · sloughing of skin and tissues · stroke · swollen tongue · transient ischaemic attack · vasculitis · vomiting · weakness
- PREGNANCY Avoid unless benefits outweigh risks—no information available.
- BREAST FEEDING Use with caution—no information available.

- MEDICINAL FORMS
There can be variation in the licensing of different medicines containing the same drug.
Solution for injection
EXCIPIENTS: May contain Benzyl alcohol
- ▶ Fibro-Vein (STD Pharmaceutical Products Ltd)
  Sodium tetradecyl sulfate 2 mg per 1 ml Fibrovein 0.2% solution for injection 5ml vials | 10 vial [PoM] £70.00
  Sodium tetradecyl sulfate 5 mg per 1 ml Fibrovein 0.5% solution for injection 2ml ampoules | 5 ampoule [PoM] £18.00
  Sodium tetradecyl sulfate 10 mg per 1 ml Fibrovein 1% solution for injection 2ml ampoules | 5 ampoule [PoM] £21.50
  Sodium tetradecyl sulfate 30 mg per 1 ml Fibrovein 3% solution for injection 2ml ampoules | 5 ampoule [PoM] £32.00
  Fibrovein 3% solution for injection 5ml vials | 10 vial [PoM] £158.50

Chapter 3
Respiratory system

CONTENTS

Respiratory system, drug delivery

Inhalation

This route delivers the drug directly to the airways; the dose required is smaller than when given by mouth and side-effects are reduced.

Inhaler devices

These include *pressurised metered-dose inhalers*, *breath-actuated inhalers*, and *dry powder inhalers*. Many patients can be taught to use a pressurised metered-dose inhaler effectively but some patients, particularly the elderly and children, find them difficult to use. *Spacer devices* can help such patients because they remove the need to co-ordinate actuation with inhalation. Dry powder inhalers may be useful in adults and children over 5 years who are unwilling or unable to use a pressurised metered-dose inhaler. Alternatively, breath-actuated inhalers are suitable for adults and older children provided they can use the device effectively.

Pressurised metered-dose inhalers are an effective and convenient method of drug administration in mild to moderate asthma.

On changing from a pressurised metered-dose inhaler to a dry powder inhaler, patients may notice a lack of sensation in the mouth and throat previously associated with each actuation. Coughing may also occur.

The patient should be instructed carefully on the use of the inhaler and it is important to check that the inhaler continues to be used correctly because inadequate inhalation technique may be mistaken for a lack of response to the drug.

Spacer devices

Spacer devices remove the need for coordination between actuation of a pressurised metered-dose inhaler and inhalation. The spacer device reduces the velocity of the aerosol and subsequent impaction on the oropharynx and allows more time for evaporation of the propellant so that a larger proportion of the particles can be inhaled and deposited in the lungs. Spacer devices are particularly useful for patients with poor inhalation technique, for children, for patients requiring high doses of inhaled corticosteroids, for nocturnal asthma, and for patients prone to candidiasis with inhaled corticosteroids. The size of the spacer is important, the larger spacers with a one-way valve (*Volumatic*®) being most effective. It is important to prescribe a spacer device that is compatible with the metered-dose inhaler, see devices below. Spacer devices should not be regarded as interchangeable; patients should be advised not to switch between spacer devices.

Use and care of spacer devices

Patients should inhale from the spacer device as soon as possible after actuation because the drug aerosol is very short-lived; single-dose actuation is recommended. Tidal breathing is as effective as single breaths. The device should be cleaned once a month by washing in mild detergent and then allowed to dry in air without rinsing; the mouthpiece should be wiped clean of detergent before use. Some manufacturers recommend more frequent cleaning, but this should be avoided since any electrostatic charge may affect drug delivery. Spacer devices should be replaced every 6–12 months.

Nebulisers

Solutions for nebulisation are available for use in severe acute asthma. They are administered over 5–10 minutes from a nebuliser usually driven by oxygen in hospital.

Patients with a severe attack of asthma should preferably have oxygen during nebulisation since beta$_2$ agonists can increase arterial hypoxaemia.

A nebuliser converts a solution of a drug into an aerosol for inhalation. It is used to deliver higher doses of drug to the airways than is usual with standard inhalers. The main indications for use of a nebuliser are to deliver:

- a beta$_2$ agonist or ipratropium bromide p. 228 to a patient with an *acute exacerbation* of asthma or of chronic obstructive pulmonary disease;
- a beta$_2$ agonist, corticosteroid, or ipratropium bromide on a *regular basis* to a patient with severe asthma or reversible airways obstruction when the patient is unable to use other inhalational devices;
- an antibiotic (such as colistimethate sodium p. 504) or a mucolytic to a patient with cystic fibrosis;
- Budesonide p. 240 or adrenaline/epinephrine p. 205 to a child with severe croup;
- Pentamidine isetionate p. 547 for the prophylaxis and treatment of pneumocystis pneumonia.

The use of nebulisers in chronic persistent asthma and chronic obstructive pulmonary disease should be considered only:

- after a review of the diagnosis;
- after review of therapy (see also Chronic Obstructive Pulmonary Disease) and the patient's ability to use hand-held devices;
- after increased doses of inhaled therapy from hand-held inhalers (with a spacer if necessary) have been tried for 2 weeks;
- if the patient remains breathless, despite correctly using optimal therapy.

Before prescribing a nebuliser, a home trial should preferably be undertaken to monitor response for up to 2 weeks on standard treatment and up to 2 weeks on nebulised treatment. If prescribed, patients must:

- have clear instructions from a doctor, specialist nurse, physiotherapist, or pharmacist on the use of the nebuliser (including maintenance and cleaning) and on peak-flow monitoring;
- be instructed not to treat acute attacks at home without also seeking help;
- have regular follow up by a doctor, specialist nurse or physiotherapist after about 1 month and annually thereafter.

The proportion of a nebuliser solution that reaches the lungs depends on the type of nebuliser and although it can be as high as 30%, it is more frequently close to 10% and sometimes below 10%. The remaining solution is left in the nebuliser as residual volume or is deposited in the mouthpiece and tubing. The extent to which the nebulised solution is deposited in the airways or alveoli depends on the droplet size, pattern of breath inhalation, and condition of the lung. Droplets with a mass median diameter of 1–5 microns are deposited in the airways and are therefore appropriate for asthma, whereas a particle size of 1–2 microns is needed for alveolar deposition of pentamidine isetionate to combat pneumocystis infection. The type of nebuliser is therefore chosen according to the deposition required and according to the viscosity of the solution.

Jet nebulisers
Jet nebulisers are more widely used than ultrasonic nebulisers. Most jet nebulisers require an optimum gas flow rate of 6–8 litres/minute and in hospital can be driven by piped air or oxygen; in acute asthma the nebuliser should be driven by oxygen. Domiciliary oxygen cylinders do not provide an adequate flow rate therefore an electrical compressor is required for domiciliary use.

For patients at risk of hypercapnia, such as those with chronic obstructive pulmonary disease, oxygen can be dangerous and the nebuliser should be driven by air. If oxygen is required, it should be given simultaneously by nasal cannula.

Tubing
The Department of Health has reminded users of the need to use the correct grade of tubing when connecting a nebuliser to a medical gas supply or compressor.

Ultrasonic nebulisers
Ultrasonic nebulisers produce an aerosol by ultrasonic vibration of the drug solution and therefore do not require a gas flow; they are not suitable for the nebulisation of some drugs, such as dornase alfa p. 269 and nebulised suspensions.

Nebuliser diluent
Nebulisation may be carried out using an undiluted nebuliser solution or it may require dilution beforehand. The usual diluent is sterile sodium chloride 0.9% (physiological saline).

In England and Wales nebulisers and compressors are not available on the NHS (but they are free of VAT); some nebulisers (but not compressors) are available on form GP10A in Scotland (for details consult Scottish Drug Tariff).

Oral

The oral route is used when administration by inhalation is not possible. Systemic side-effects occur more frequently when a drug is given orally rather than by inhalation. Drugs given by mouth for the treatment of asthma include beta$_2$ agonists, corticosteroids, theophylline p. 250, and leukotriene receptor antagonists.

Parenteral

Drugs such as beta$_2$ agonists, corticosteroids, and aminophylline p. 249 can be given by injection in acute severe asthma when administration by nebulisation is inadequate or inappropriate. If the patient is being treated in the community, urgent transfer to hospital should be arranged.

Peak flow meters

When used in addition to symptom-based monitoring, peak flow monitoring has not been proven to improve asthma control in either adults or children, however measurement of peak flow may be of benefit in adult patients who are 'poor perceivers' and hence slow to detect deterioration in their asthma, and for those with more severe asthma.

When peak flow meters are used, patients must be given clear guidelines as to the action they should take if their peak flow falls below a certain level. Patients can be encouraged to adjust some of their own treatment (within specified limits) according to changes in peak flow rate.

Peak flow charts should be issued to patients where appropriate, and are available to purchase from:

3M Security Print and Systems Limited. Gorse Street, Chadderton, Oldham, OL9 9QH. Tel: 0845 610 1112

GP practices can obtain supplies through their Area Team stores.

NHS Hospitals can order supplies from www.nhsforms.co.uk or by emailing nhsforms@mmm.com.

In Scotland, peak flow charts can be obtained by emailing stockorders.dppas@apsgroup.co.uk.

NICE technology appraisals (TAs)
Inhaler devices for children under 5 years with chronic asthma (August 2000) NICE TA10
A child's needs and likelihood of good compliance should govern the choice of inhaler and spacer device; only then should cost be considered.

- corticosteroid and bronchodilator therapy should be delivered by pressurised metered-dose inhaler and spacer device, with a facemask if necessary;
- if this is not effective, and depending on the child's condition, nebulised therapy may be considered and, in children over 3 years, a dry powder inhaler may also be considered.

www.nice.org.uk/TA10

Inhaler devices for children 5–15 years with chronic asthma (March 2002) NICE TA38
A child's needs, ability to develop and maintain effective technique, and likelihood of good compliance should govern the choice of inhaler and spacer device; only then should cost be considered.

- corticosteroid therapy should be routinely delivered by a pressurised metered-dose inhaler and spacer device;
- for other inhaled drugs, particularly bronchodilators, a wider range of devices should be considered;
- children and their carers should be trained in the use of the chosen device; suitability of the device should be reviewed at least annually. Inhaler technique and compliance should be monitored.

www.nice.org.uk/TA38

1   Airways disease, obstructive

Asthma   31.3.2016

Description of condition

Asthma is a common chronic inflammatory condition of the airways characterised by bronchoconstriction. The most frequent symptoms are cough, wheezing, chest tightness, and shortness of breath. The bronchoconstriction is usually reversible (either spontaneously or with the aid of

3

Respiratory system

medication) leading to intermittent symptoms, but in some patients with chronic asthma the inflammation may result in irreversible airway obstruction. Occasionally, asthma symptoms can get gradually or suddenly worse provoking an acute asthma attack that, if severe, may require hospitalisation.

Aims of treatment

In clinical practice, patients may choose to balance the aims of asthma management against the potential side-effects or inconvenience of taking medication necessary to achieve perfect control. Complete control of asthma is defined as no daytime symptoms, no night-time awakening due to asthma, no asthma attacks, no need for rescue medication, no limitations on activity including exercise, and normal lung function (in practical terms FEV_1 and/or peak flow > 80% predicted or best).

Lifestyle changes

[EvGr] Weight loss in overweight patients may lead to an improvement in asthma symptoms. Parents with asthma should be advised about the danger to themselves and to their children with asthma, of smoking, and be offered appropriate support to stop smoking. Breathing exercise programmes (including physiotherapist-taught methods) can be offered as an adjuvant to drug treatment in order to improve quality of life and reduce symptoms. (A)

Management of chronic asthma

[EvGr] A stepwise approach aims to stop symptoms quickly and to improve peak flow. Start at the step most appropriate to initial severity of asthma. The aim is to achieve early control and to maintain it by *stepping up* treatment as necessary and *stepping down* treatment when control is good. Before initiating a new drug consider whether diagnosis is correct, check compliance and inhaler technique, and eliminate trigger factors for acute attacks. (A)

Adult and child over 5 years
Step 1—Mild intermittent asthma

- [EvGr] Start inhaled short-acting beta₂ agonist (such as salbutamol p. 233 or terbutaline sulfate p. 235) as required (A)

[EvGr] Patients using more than one short-acting bronchodilator inhaler a month should have their asthma urgently assessed and action taken to improve poorly controlled asthma. Inhaled ipratropium bromide p. 228, (or, if over 12 years, short-acting beta₂ agonist tablets and syrup, or theophylline p. 250) also act as short-acting bronchodilators but inhaled short-acting beta₂ agonists are preferred. (A)

[EvGr] Move to **step 2** if the patient presents with any one of the following features; is using an inhaled beta₂ agonist three times a week or more, being symptomatic three times a week or more, experiencing night-time symptoms at least once a week, or has had an asthma attack in the last 2 years. (A)

Step 2—Regular preventer therapy

- [EvGr] Consider adding regular inhaled standard-dose corticosteroid (alternatives to inhaled corticosteroid are leukotriene receptor antagonists, theophylline, inhaled sodium cromoglicate p. 247, or inhaled nedocromil sodium p. 247, but are less effective) (A)

[EvGr] Start the inhaled corticosteroid at a dose appropriate to severity of disease and adjust to the lowest effective dose at which control of asthma is maintained. Inhaled corticosteroids (except ciclesonide p. 242) should be initially taken twice daily, however, the same total daily dose can be considered once a day if good control is established. (A)

Note, inhaled standard-dose corticosteroid
Adult and child over 12 years: 200–800 micrograms/day beclometasone dipropionate p. 238 or equivalent

Child 5–12 years: 200–400 micrograms/day beclometasone dipropionate or equivalent

[EvGr] Beclometasone dipropionate and budesonide p. 240 are approximately equivalent in clinical practice although there may be variations with different drug delivery devices. Fluticasone p. 242 and mometasone furoate p. 244 provide equal clinical activity to beclometasone dipropionate and budesonide at half the dosage. (A)

[EvGr] In children, administration of high doses of inhaled corticosteroids may be associated with systemic side-effects, including growth failure, reduced bone mineral density, and adrenal suppression, see individual drug monographs for monitoring information. (A)

[EvGr] If asthma is not adequately controlled, move to **step 3**. (A)

Step 3—Initial add-on therapy

- [EvGr] Consider adding a regular inhaled long-acting beta₂ agonist (LABA) such as formoterol fumarate p. 231 or salmeterol p. 232 (or, in adults only, indacaterol p. 232 or olodaterol p. 232) to be used in conjunction with an inhaled corticosteroid (see also CHM advice for formoterol fumarate and salmeterol) (A)

[EvGr] If the patient is gaining some benefit from addition of a LABA but control is *inadequate* then continue the LABA and increase dose of inhaled corticosteroid to top end of inhaled standard-dose corticosteroid range. If there is *no response* to the LABA, discontinue and increase dose of inhaled corticosteroid. If control is still inadequate, start a trial of either a leukotriene receptor antagonist (montelukast p. 245, or zafirlukast p. 246 if over 12 years) or modified-release theophylline. (A)

Step 4—Persistent poor control
Consider the following options:

- [EvGr] Increase dose of inhaled corticosteroid (a spacer should be used), *or* (A)
- [EvGr] Add a leukotriene receptor antagonist, modified-release theophylline, or modified-release oral beta₂ agonist (caution in patients already taking a LABA) (A)

  Note, increased inhaled corticosteroid dose
  Adult and child over 12 years: up to 2000 micrograms/day beclometasone dipropionate or equivalent
  Child 5–12 years: up to 800 micrograms/day beclometasone dipropionate or equivalent

[EvGr] Before proceeding to **step 5**, refer patients with inadequately controlled asthma to specialist care. (A)

Step 5—Continuous or frequent use of oral corticosteroids

- [EvGr] Add a regular oral corticosteroid (prednisolone p. 614, as single daily dose) at lowest dose to provide adequate control; continue high-dose inhaled corticosteroid (in exceptional cases, this may exceed licensed doses) (A)

Child under 5 years
Step 1—Mild intermittent asthma

- [EvGr] Inhaled short-acting beta₂ agonist (such as salbutamol or terbutaline sulfate) as required (A)

[EvGr] Children identified to be using more than one short-acting bronchodilator inhaler a month should have their asthma urgently assessed and action taken to improve poorly controlled asthma. (A)

[EvGr] Move to **step 2** if the child presents with any one of the following features; is using an inhaled beta₂ agonist three times a week or more, being symptomatic three times a week or more, experiencing night-time symptoms at least once a week. (A)

Step 2—Regular preventer therapy

- [EvGr] Consider adding regular standard-dose inhaled corticosteroid (A)

- [EvGr] If the child is unable to take an inhaled corticosteroid, a leukotriene receptor antagonist (such as montelukast) is an effective first-line preventer (A)

[EvGr] Start inhaled corticosteroid at a dose appropriate to severity of disease and adjust to the lowest effective dose at which control of asthma is maintained. (A)

Note, inhaled standard-dose corticosteroid
Child under 5 years: 200–400 micrograms/day beclometasone dipropionate or equivalent

[EvGr] Beclometasone dipropionate and budesonide are approximately equivalent in clinical practice although there may be variations with different drug delivery devices. Fluticasone p. 242 provides equal activity to beclometasone dipropionate p. 238 and budesonide p. 240 at half the dosage. (A)

[EvGr] Administration of high doses of inhaled corticosteroids in children may be associated with systemic side-effects, including growth failure, reduced bone mineral density and adrenal suppression. (A)

[EvGr] If asthma is not adequately controlled, move to **step 3**. (A)

Step 3—Initial add-on therapy

- [EvGr] In children 2–5 years, add a leukotriene receptor antagonist if not added during step 2. If a leukotriene receptor antagonist was added at step 2, reconsider addition of standard-dose inhaled corticosteroid (A)
- [EvGr] In children under 2 years, consider proceeding to **step 4** (A)

Step 4—Persistent poor control

- [EvGr] Refer child to respiratory paediatrician (A)

Stepping down

[EvGr] Once asthma is controlled, it is recommended to step down therapy and continue to regularly review the patient. When deciding which drug to step down first and at what rate, the severity of asthma, the side-effects of treatment, duration on current dose, the beneficial effect achieved, and the patient's preference, should be considered. (A)

[EvGr] Patient should be maintained at the lowest possible dose of inhaled corticosteroid. Reductions should be considered every three months, decreasing the dose by approximately 25–50% each time. Reduce the dose slowly as patients deteriorate at different rates. (A)

Management of acute asthma

Adults
The nature of treatment required for the management of acute asthma depends on the level of severity, described as follows:

Moderate acute asthma

- Increasing symptoms
- Peak flow > 50-75% best or predicted
- No features of acute severe asthma

Severe acute asthma
Any one of the following:

- Peak flow 33-50% best or predicted
- Respiratory rate ≥ 25/min
- Heart rate ≥ 110/min
- Inability to complete sentences in one breath

Life-threatening acute asthma
Any one of the following, in a patient with severe asthma:

- Peak flow < 33% best or predicted
- Arterial oxygen saturation (SpO$_2$) < 92%
- Partial arterial pressure of oxygen (PaO$_2$) < 8 kPa
- Normal partial arterial pressure of carbon dioxide (PaCO$_2$) (4.6–6.0 kPa)
- Silent chest
- Cyanosis
- Poor respiratory effort
- Arrhythmia
- Exhaustion
- Altered conscious level
- Hypotension

Near-fatal acute asthma

- Raised PaCO$_2$, requiring mechanical ventilation with raised inflation pressures, or both

[EvGr] Patients with moderate asthma should be treated at home or in primary care according to response to treatment, while patients with severe or life-threatening acute asthma should start treatment as soon as possible and be admitted to hospital immediately following initial assessment. (A)

[EvGr] Supplementary oxygen should be given to all hypoxaemic patients with acute severe asthma to maintain a SpO$_2$ level between 94–98%. (A)

[EvGr] First-line treatment for acute asthma is a high-dose inhaled short-acting beta$_2$ agonist (salbutamol p. 233 or terbutaline sulfate p. 235) given as soon as possible. A pressurised metered dose inhaler with spacer device is preferred in patients with non-life-threatening acute asthma. Whereas, in patients with life-threatening acute asthma, a beta$_2$ agonist administered by an oxygen-driven nebuliser is recommended. If the response to an initial dose of short-acting beta$_2$ agonist is poor, consider continuous nebulisation with an appropriate nebuliser. Intravenous beta$_2$ agonists are reserved for those patients in whom inhaled therapy cannot be used reliably. (A)

[EvGr] In all cases of acute asthma, patients should be prescribed an adequate dose of oral prednisolone p. 614 once daily for at least 5 days or until recovery. Parenteral hydrocortisone p. 612 or intramuscular methylprednisolone p. 613 are alternatives in patients who are unable to take oral prednisolone. (A)

[EvGr] Nebulised ipratropium bromide p. 228 may be combined with a nebulised beta$_2$ agonist in patients with acute severe or life-threatening asthma or in those with a poor initial response to beta$_2$ agonist therapy to provide greater bronchodilation. (A)

[EvGr] There is some evidence that magnesium sulfate p. 911 has bronchodilator effects. A single intravenous dose of magnesium sulfate may be considered in patients with severe acute asthma (peak flow < 50% best or predicted) who have not had a good initial response to inhaled bronchodilator therapy [unlicensed use]. In an acute asthma attack, intravenous aminophylline p. 249 is not likely to produce any additional bronchodilation compared to standard therapy with inhaled bronchodilators and corticosteroids. However, in some patients with near-fatal or life-threatening acute asthma with a poor response to initial therapy, intravenous aminophylline may provide some benefit. Magnesium sulfate by intravenous infusion or aminophylline should only be used after consultation with, or on the recommendation of, senior medical staff. (A)

Child over 2 years
The nature of treatment required for the management of acute asthma depends on the level of severity, described as follows:

Moderate acute asthma

- Able to talk in sentences
- Arterial oxygen saturation (SpO$_2$) ≥ 92%
- Peak flow ≥ 50% best or predicted
- Heart rate ≤ 140/minute in children aged 2–5 years; heart rate ≤ 125/minute in children over 5 years
- Respiratory rate ≤ 40/minute in children aged 2–5 years; respiratory rate ≤ 30/minute in children over 5 years

Severe acute asthma

- Can't complete sentences in one breath or too breathless to talk or feed
- SpO$_2$ < 92%
- Peak flow 33–50% best or predicted
- Heart rate > 140/minute in children aged 2–5 years; heart

rate > 125/minute in children aged over 5 years
- Respiratory rate > 40/minute in children aged 2–5 years; respiratory rate > 30/minute in children aged over 5 years

Life-threatening acute asthma

Any one of the following in a child with severe asthma:
- SpO_2 < 92%
- Peak flow < 33% best or predicted
- Silent chest
- Cyanosis
- Poor respiratory effort
- Hypotension
- Exhaustion
- Confusion

[EvGr] Following initial assessment, supplementary high flow oxygen should be given to all children with life-threatening acute asthma or SpO_2 < 94% to achieve normal saturations of 94–98%. (A)

[EvGr] First-line treatment for acute asthma is an inhaled short-acting beta₂ agonist (salbutamol or terbutaline sulfate) given as soon as possible, ideally via a metered dose inhaler and spacer device in mild to moderate acute asthma. Children with severe or life-threatening acute asthma should be transferred to hospital urgently. (A)

[EvGr] In all cases of acute asthma, children should be prescribed an adequate once daily dose of oral prednisolone. Treatment for up to 3 days is usually sufficient, but the length of course should be tailored to the number of days necessary to bring about recovery. Intravenous hydrocortisone should be reserved for severely affected children who are unable to retain oral medication. (A)

[EvGr] Nebulised ipratropium bromide can be combined with beta₂ agonist treatment for children with severe or life-threatening acute asthma or in those with a poor initial response to beta₂ agonist therapy to provide greater bronchodilation. Consider adding magnesium sulfate p. 911 to nebulised salbutamol p. 233 and ipratropium bromide p. 228 in the first hour in children with a short duration of acute severe asthma symptoms presenting with an oxygen saturation less than 92%. (A)

[EvGr] Children with continuing severe asthma despite frequent nebulised beta₂ agonists and ipratropium bromide plus oral corticosteroids, and those with life-threatening features, need urgent review by a specialist with a view to transfer to a high dependency unit or paediatric intensive care unit (PICU) to receive second-line intravenous therapies. (A)

[EvGr] In a severe asthma attack where the child has not responded to initial inhaled therapy, early addition of a single bolus dose of intravenous salbutamol may be an option. Continuous intravenous infusion of salbutamol, administered under specialist supervision with continuous ECG and electrolyte monitoring, should be considered in children with unreliable inhalation or severe refractory asthma. Aminophylline p. 249 may be considered in children with severe or life-threatening acute asthma unresponsive to maximal doses of bronchodilators and corticosteroids. Aminophylline is not recommended in children with mild to moderate acute asthma. Intravenous magnesium sulfate has been used for acute asthma [unlicensed use] although its place in management is not yet established. (A)

Child under 2 years

[EvGr] Inhaled short-acting beta₂ agonists are the initial treatment of choice for acute asthma in children under 2 years. For mild to moderate acute asthma attacks, a metered-dose inhaler with a spacer and mask is the optimal drug delivery device. In a hospital setting, consider oral prednisolone daily for up to 3 days, early in the management of severe asthma attacks. For more severe symptoms, inhaled ipratropium bromide in combination with an inhaled beta₂ agonist is also an option. (A)

Follow up in all cases

[EvGr] Episodes of acute asthma may be a failure of preventative therapy, review is required to prevent further episodes. A careful history should be taken to establish the reason for the asthma attack. Inhaler technique should be checked and regular treatment should be reviewed. Patients should be given a written asthma action plan aimed at preventing relapse, optimising treatment, and preventing delay in seeking assistance in future attacks. It is essential that the patient's GP practice is informed within 24 hours of discharge from the emergency department or hospital following an asthma attack. Patients who have had a near-fatal asthma attack should be kept under specialist supervision indefinitely. A respiratory specialist should follow up all patients admitted with a severe asthma attack for at least one year after the admission. (A)

Exercise-induced asthma

[EvGr] For most patients, exercise-induced asthma is an illustration of poorly controlled asthma and regular treatment including inhaled corticosteroids should therefore be reviewed. If exercise is a specific problem in patients already taking inhaled corticosteroids who are otherwise well controlled, consider adding either a leukotriene receptor antagonist, a long-acting beta₂ agonist, an oral beta₂ agonist, sodium cromoglicate p. 247 or nedocromil sodium p. 247, or theophylline p. 250. An inhaled short-acting beta₂ agonists used immediately before exercise is the drug of choice. (A)

Pregnancy and breast-feeding

[EvGr] Women with asthma should be closely monitored during pregnancy. It is particularly important that asthma should be well controlled during pregnancy; when this is achieved asthma has no important effects on pregnancy, labour, or on the fetus. Women planning to become pregnant should be counselled about the importance of taking their asthma medication regularly to maintain good control. Drugs for asthma should preferably be administered by inhalation to minimise exposure of the fetus. Short-acting beta₂ agonists, long-acting beta₂ agonists, oral and inhaled corticosteroids, sodium cromoglicate, nedocromil sodium, and oral and intravenous theophyllines can be used as normal during pregnancy. There is limited information on use of leukotriene receptor antagonists during pregnancy, however they may be used if potential benefit outweighs risk. Drugs for asthma, including corticosteroid tablets, can be used as normal and in-line with manufacturers' recommendations in breast-feeding. (A)

[EvGr] Severe acute attacks of asthma can have an adverse effect on pregnancy and should be treated promptly in hospital with conventional therapy, including nebulisation of a beta₂ agonist and oral or parenteral administration of a corticosteroid; prednisolone p. 614 is the preferred corticosteroid for oral administration since very little of the drug reaches the fetus. Oxygen should be given immediately to maintain arterial oxygen saturation of 94–98% and prevent maternal and fetal hypoxia. (A)

Useful Resources

British guideline on the management of asthma. British Thoracic Society and Scottish Intercollegiate Guidelines Network. Quick Reference Guide 141. October 2014.
sign.ac.uk/pdf/QRG141.pdf

British guideline on the management of asthma. British Thoracic Society and Scottish Intercollegiate Guidelines Network. Full guidance - A national clinical guideline 141. October 2014.
sign.ac.uk/pdf/SIGN141.pdf

Bronchodilators

Adrenoceptor agonists (sympathomimetics)

Selective beta$_2$ agonists produce bronchodilation. A short-acting beta$_2$ agonist is used for immediate relief of asthma symptoms while some long-acting beta$_2$ agonists are added to an inhaled corticosteroid in patients requiring prophylactic treatment.

The selective beta$_2$ agonists (selective beta$_2$-adrenoceptor agonists, selective beta$_2$ stimulants) such as salbutamol p. 233 or terbutaline sulfate p. 235 are the safest and most effective short-acting beta$_2$ agonists for asthma. Less selective beta$_2$ agonists such as ephedrine hydrochloride p. 248 is less suitable and less safe for use as a bronchodilator than the selective beta$_2$ agonists, because it is more likely to cause arrhythmias and other side-effects; it should be avoided whenever possible.

Adrenaline/epinephrine p. 205 (which has both alpha-and beta-adrenoceptor agonist properties) is used in the emergency management of acute allergic and anaphylactic reactions, in angioedema, in cardiopulmonary resuscitation, and in the management of severe croup.

Short-acting beta$_2$ agonists

Mild to moderate symptoms of asthma respond rapidly to the inhalation of a selective short-acting beta$_2$ agonist such as salbutamol or terbutaline sulfate. If beta$_2$ agonist inhalation is needed more often than twice a week, or if night-time symptoms occur at least once a week, or if the patient has suffered an exacerbation in the last 2 years, then prophylactic treatment should be considered using a stepped approach.

A short-acting beta$_2$ agonist inhaled immediately before exertion reduces *exercise-induced asthma*; however, frequent exercise-induced asthma probably reflects poor overall control and calls for reassessment of asthma treatment.

Long-acting beta$_2$ agonists

Formoterol fumarate p. 231 (eformoterol) and salmeterol p. 232 are longer-acting beta$_2$ agonists which are administered by inhalation. They should be used for asthma only in patients who regularly use an inhaled corticosteroid. They have a role in the long-term management of chronic asthma and can be useful in nocturnal asthma.

Salmeterol should not be used for the relief of an asthma attack; it has a slower onset of action than salbutamol or terbutaline sulfate. Formoterol fumarate is licensed for short-term symptom relief and for the prevention of exercise-induced bronchospasm; its speed of onset of action is similar to that of salbutamol.

Combination inhalers that contain a long-acting beta$_2$ agonist and a corticosteroid ensure that long-acting beta$_2$ agonists are not used without concomitant corticosteroids, but reduce the flexibility to adjust the dose of each component.

Indacaterol p. 232 and olodaterol p. 232 are long-acting beta$_2$ agonists licensed for chronic obstructive pulmonary disease in adults; they are not indicated for the relief of acute bronchospasm.

Vilanterol is a long-acting beta$_2$ agonist available only in a combination inhaler with fluticasone furoate *or* with umeclidinium p. 229.

Oral

Oral preparations of beta$_2$ agonists may be used by patients who cannot manage the inhaled route. They are sometimes used for children and the elderly, but inhaled beta$_2$ agonists are more effective and have fewer side-effects. The longer-acting oral preparations, including bambuterol hydrochloride p. 230, may be of value in nocturnal asthma but they have a limited role and inhaled long-acting beta$_2$ agonists are usually preferred.

Parenteral

Salbutamol or terbutaline sulfate can be given intravenously for severe or life-threatening acute asthma; patients should be carefully monitored and the dose adjusted according to response and heart rate. The regular use of beta$_2$ agonists by the subcutaneous route is not recommended since the evidence of benefit is uncertain and it may be difficult to withdraw such treatment once started. In adults, beta$_2$ agonists may also be given by intramuscular injection.

Children

Selective beta$_2$ agonists are useful even in children under the age of 18 months. They are most effective by the inhaled route; a pressurised metered-dose inhaler should be used with a spacer device in children under 5 years. A beta$_2$ agonist may also be given by mouth but administration by inhalation is preferred; a long-acting inhaled beta$_2$ agonist may be used where appropriate. In severe attacks nebulisation using a selective beta$_2$ agonist or ipratropium bromide p. 228 is advisable.

Antimuscarinic bronchodilators

Ipratropium bromide can provide short-term relief in chronic asthma, but short-acting beta$_2$ agonists act more quickly and are preferred. Ipratropium bromide by nebulisation can be added to other standard treatment in life-threatening asthma or if acute asthma fails to improve with standard therapy.

The aerosol inhalation of ipratropium bromide can be used for short-term relief in mild chronic obstructive pulmonary disease in patients who are not using a long-acting inhaled antimuscarinic drug. Its maximal effect occurs 30–60 minutes after use; its duration of action is 3 to 6 hours and bronchodilation can usually be maintained with treatment 3 times a day.

Aclidinium bromide p. 227, glycopyrronium bromide p. 227, tiotropium p. 229, and umeclidinium are licensed for the maintenance treatment of adults with chronic obstructive pulmonary disease. They are not suitable for the relief of acute bronchospasm. Tiotropium (via *Respimat*® device) is also licensed as an adjunct to inhaled corticosteroids and long-acting beta$_2$ agonists for the maintenance treatment of patients with asthma who have suffered one or more severe exacerbations in the last year.

Theophylline

Theophylline p. 250 is a xanthine used as a bronchodilator in *asthma* and stable *chronic obstructive pulmonary disease*; it is not generally effective in exacerbations of chronic obstructive pulmonary disease. Theophylline may have an additive effect when used in conjunction with small doses of beta$_2$ agonists; the combination may increase the risk of side-effects, including hypokalaemia.

Theophylline is given by injection as aminophylline p. 249, a mixture of theophylline with ethylenediamine, which is 20 times more soluble than theophylline alone. Aminophylline injection is needed rarely for severe acute asthma.

Compound bronchodilator preparations

In general, patients are best treated with single-ingredient preparations, such as a selective beta$_2$ agonist or ipratropium bromide, so that the dose of each drug can be adjusted. This flexibility is lost with compound bronchodilator preparations. However, a combination product may be appropriate for patients stabilised on individual components in the same proportion.

Chronic obstructive pulmonary disease

Management

Smoking cessation reduces the progressive decline in lung function in chronic obstructive pulmonary disease (COPD, chronic bronchitis, or emphysema). Infection can complicate chronic obstructive pulmonary disease and may be prevented by vaccination (pneumococcal polysaccharide conjugate vaccine (adsorbed) p. 1152 and influenza vaccine p. 1157).

A trial of a high-dose inhaled corticosteroid *or* an oral corticosteroid is recommended for patients with moderate or severe airflow obstruction if the diagnosis is in doubt.

Symptoms of chronic obstructive pulmonary disease may be alleviated by an inhaled **short-acting beta$_2$ agonist** or a **short-acting antimuscarinic bronchodilator** used as required.

When the airways obstruction is more severe, regular inhaled therapy should be used. It is important to check compliance and inhaler technique before initiating a new drug.

If the Forced Expiratory Volume in 1 second (FEV$_1$), is 50% of predicted or more, *either* a long-acting antimuscarinic bronchodilator *or* a long-acting beta$_2$ agonist should be used. Short-acting antimuscarinic bronchodilators should be discontinued when a long-acting antimuscarinic bronchodilator is started. A long-acting beta$_2$ agonist with a corticosteroid in a combination inhaler can be used for patients who remain symptomatic despite regular treatment with a long-acting beta$_2$ agonist.

If FEV$_1$ is less than 50% of predicted, *either* a long-acting antimuscarinic bronchodilator *or* a long-acting beta$_2$ agonist with a corticosteroid in a combination inhaler should be used.

In any patient who remains breathless or continues to have exacerbations, triple therapy with a long-acting beta$_2$ agonist and a corticosteroid in a combination inhaler *plus* a long-acting antimuscarinic bronchodilator should be used.

If an inhaled corticosteroid is not appropriate, a long-acting antimuscarinic bronchodilator can be used with a long-acting beta$_2$ agonist, (see Use of inhaled therapies in chronic obstructive pulmonary disease algorithm, below).

If symptoms persist or if the patient is unable to use an inhaler, oral modified-release aminophylline p. 249 or theophylline p. 250 can be used.

Indacaterol p. 232 is a long-acting beta$_2$ agonist licensed for the maintenance treatment of chronic obstructive pulmonary disease.

In patients with severe chronic obstructive pulmonary disease associated with chronic bronchitis and a history of frequent exacerbations, roflumilast p. 248 is licensed as an adjunct to existing bronchodilator treatment.

A **mucolytic** drug may be considered for a patient with a chronic productive cough.

Long-term **oxygen** therapy prolongs survival in patients with severe chronic obstructive pulmonary disease and hypoxaemia.

During an exacerbation of chronic obstructive pulmonary disease, bronchodilator therapy can be administered through a nebuliser if necessary and oxygen given if appropriate. Aminophylline can be given intravenously if response to nebulised bronchodilators is poor. A short course of **oral corticosteroid**, such as prednisolone for 7–14 days, should be given if increased breathlessness interferes with daily activities. **Antibacterial** treatment is required if sputum becomes more purulent than usual, or if there are other signs of infection.

Patients who have had an episode of hypercapnic respiratory failure should be given a 24% or 28% Venturi mask and an *oxygen alert card* endorsed with the oxygen saturations required during previous exacerbations. Patients and their carers should be instructed to show the card to emergency healthcare providers in the event of an exacerbation.

Oxygen alert card based on British Thoracic Society guideline for emergency oxygen use in adult patients (October 2008)

> **Oxygen alert card**
>
> Name: _____
>
> I am at risk of type II respiratory failure with a raised CO$_2$ level.
>
> Please use my _____% Venturi mask to achieve an oxygen saturation of _____% to _____% during exacerbations.
>
> Use compressed air to drive nebulisers (with nasal oxygen at 2 litres/minute). If compressed air not available, limit oxygen-driven nebulisers to 6 minutes.

Oxygen alert card is available at www.brit-thoracic.org.uk.

Croup

Management

Mild croup is largely self-limiting, but treatment with a single dose of a corticosteroid (e.g. dexamethasone p. 610) by mouth may be of benefit.

More severe croup (or mild croup that might cause complications) calls for hospital admission; a single dose of a corticosteroid (e.g. dexamethasone or prednisolone p. 614 by mouth) should be administered before transfer to hospital. In hospital, dexamethasone (by mouth or by injection) or budesonide p. 240 (by nebulisation) will often reduce symptoms; the dose may need to be repeated after 12 hours if necessary.

For severe croup not effectively controlled with corticosteroid treatment, nebulised adrenaline/epinephrine solution 1 in 1000 (1 mg/mL) p. 205 should be given with close clinical monitoring; the effects of nebulised adrenaline/epinephrine last 2–3 hours and the child needs to be monitored carefully for recurrence of the obstruction.

Oxygen

Overview

Oxygen should be regarded as a drug. It is prescribed for hypoxaemic patients to increase alveolar oxygen tension and decrease the work of breathing. The concentration of oxygen required depends on the condition being treated; the administration of an inappropriate concentration of oxygen can have serious or even fatal consequences.

Oxygen is probably the most common drug used in medical emergencies. It should be prescribed initially to achieve a normal or near–normal oxygen saturation; in most acutely ill patients with a normal or low arterial carbon dioxide (P_aCO_2), oxygen saturation should be 94–98% oxygen saturation. However, in some clinical situations such as cardiac arrest and carbon monoxide poisoning it is more appropriate to aim for the highest possible oxygen saturation until the patient is stable. A lower target of 88–92% oxygen saturation is indicated for patients at risk of hypercapnic respiratory failure.

Use of inhaled therapies in chronic obstructive pulmonary disease

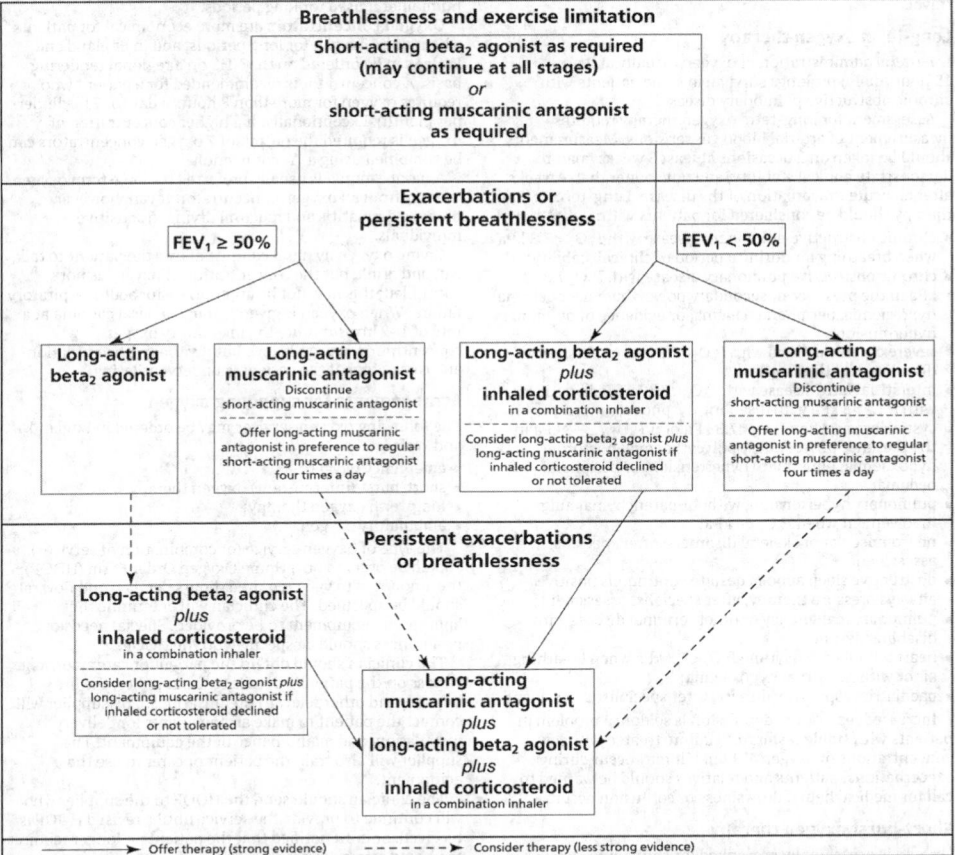

Advice on the use of inhaled therapies in chronic obstructive pulmonary disease is based on the recommendations of the National Institute for Health and Care Excellence (2010). Management of chronic obstructive pulmonary disease in adults in primary and secondary care. London: NICE. Available from www.nice.org.uk/CG101 Reproduced with permission

High concentration oxygen therapy is safe in uncomplicated cases of conditions such as pneumonia, pulmonary thromboembolism, pulmonary fibrosis, shock, severe trauma, sepsis, or anaphylaxis. In such conditions low arterial oxygen (P_aO_2) is usually associated with low or normal arterial carbon dioxide (P_aCO_2), and therefore there is little risk of hypoventilation and carbon dioxide retention.

In acute severe asthma, the arterial carbon dioxide (P_aCO_2) is usually subnormal but as asthma deteriorates it may rise steeply (particularly in children). These patients usually require high concentrations of oxygen and if the arterial carbon dioxide (P_aCO_2) remains high despite other treatment, intermittent positive-pressure ventilation needs to be considered urgently.

Low concentration oxygen therapy (controlled oxygen therapy) is reserved for patients at risk of hypercapnic respiratory failure, which is more likely in those with:

- chronic obstructive pulmonary disease;
- advanced cystic fibrosis;
- severe non-cystic fibrosis bronchiectasis;
- severe kyphoscoliosis or severe ankylosing spondylitis;
- severe lung scarring caused by tuberculosis;

- musculoskeletal disorders with respiratory weakness, especially if on home ventilation;
- an overdose of opioids, benzodiazepines, or other drugs causing respiratory depression.

Until blood gases can be measured, initial oxygen should be given using a controlled concentration of 28% or less, titrated towards a target oxygen saturation of 88–92%. The aim is to provide the patient with enough oxygen to achieve an acceptable arterial oxygen tension without worsening carbon dioxide retention and respiratory acidosis. Patients may carry an *oxygen alert card*.

Domiciliary oxygen
Oxygen should only be prescribed for use in the home after careful evaluation in hospital by respiratory experts. Patients should be advised of the risks of continuing to smoke when receiving oxygen therapy, including the risk of fire. Smoking cessation therapy should be recommended before home oxygen prescription.

Air travel
Some patients with arterial hypoxaemia require supplementary oxygen for air travel. The patient's

requirement should be discussed with the airline before travel.

Long-term oxygen therapy

Long-term administration of oxygen (usually at least 15 hours daily) prolongs survival in some patients with chronic obstructive pulmonary disease.

Assessment for long-term oxygen therapy requires measurement of arterial blood gas tensions. Measurements should be taken on 2 occasions at least 3 weeks apart to demonstrate clinical stability, and not sooner than 4 weeks after an acute exacerbation of the disease. Long-term oxygen therapy should be considered for patients with:

- chronic obstructive pulmonary disease with P_aO_2 <7.3 kPa when breathing air during a period of clinical stability;
- chronic obstructive pulmonary disease with P_aO_2 7.3–8 kPa in the presence of secondary polycythaemia, nocturnal hypoxaemia, peripheral oedema, or evidence of pulmonary hypertension;
- severe chronic asthma with P_aO_2 <7.3 kPa or persistent disabling breathlessness;
- interstitial lung disease with P_aO_2 <8 kPa and in patients with P_aO_2 >8 kPa with disabling dyspnoea;
- cystic fibrosis when P_aO_2 <7.3 kPa or if P_aO_2 7.3–8 kPa in the presence of secondary polycythaemia, nocturnal hypoxaemia, pulmonary hypertension, or peripheral oedema;
- pulmonary hypertension, without parenchymal lung involvement when P_aO_2 <8 kPa;
- neuromuscular or skeletal disorders, after specialist assessment;
- obstructive sleep apnoea despite continuous positive airways pressure assessment, after specialist assessment;
- pulmonary malignancy or other terminal disease with disabling dyspnoea;
- heart failure with daytime P_aO_2 <7.3 kPa when breathing air or with nocturnal hypoxaemia;
- paediatric respiratory disease, after specialist assessment.

Increased respiratory depression is seldom a problem in patients with stable respiratory failure treated with low concentrations of oxygen although it may occur during exacerbations; patients and relatives should be warned to call for medical help if drowsiness or confusion occur.

Short-burst oxygen therapy

Oxygen is occasionally prescribed for short-burst (intermittent) use for episodes of breathlessness not relieved by other treatment in patients with severe chronic obstructive pulmonary disease, interstitial lung disease, heart failure, and in palliative care. It is important, however, that the patient does not rely on oxygen instead of obtaining medical help or taking more specific treatment. Short-burst oxygen therapy can be used to improve exercise capacity and recovery; it should only be continued if there is proven improvement in breathlessness or exercise tolerance.

Ambulatory oxygen therapy

Ambulatory oxygen is prescribed for patients on long-term oxygen therapy who need to be away from home on a regular basis. Patients who are not on long-term oxygen therapy can be considered for ambulatory oxygen therapy if there is evidence of exercise-induced oxygen desaturation and of improvement in blood oxygen saturation and exercise capacity with oxygen. Ambulatory oxygen therapy is not recommended for patients with heart failure or those who smoke.

Oxygen therapy equipment

Under the NHS oxygen may be supplied as **oxygen cylinders**. Oxygen flow can be adjusted as the cylinders are equipped with an oxygen flow meter with 'medium' (2 litres/minute) and 'high' (4 litres/minute) settings. Oxygen

delivered from a cylinder should be passed through a humidifier if used for long periods.

Oxygen concentrators are more economical for patients who require oxygen for long periods, and in England and Wales can be ordered on the NHS on a regional tendering basis. A concentrator is recommended for a patient who requires oxygen for more than 8 hours a day (or 21 cylinders per month). Exceptionally, if a higher concentration of oxygen is required the output of 2 oxygen concentrators can be combined using a 'Y' connection.

A nasal cannula is usually preferred for long-term oxygen therapy from an oxygen concentrator. It can, however, produce dermatitis and mucosal drying in sensitive individuals.

Giving oxygen by nasal cannula allows the patient to talk, eat, and drink, but the concentration of oxygen is not controlled; this may not be appropriate for acute respiratory failure. When oxygen is given through a nasal cannula at a rate of 1–2 litres/minute the inspiratory oxygen concentration is usually low, but it varies with ventilation and can be high if the patient is underventilating.

Arrangements for supplying oxygen

The following oxygen services may be ordered in England and Wales:

- emergency oxygen;
- short-burst (intermittent) oxygen therapy;
- long-term oxygen therapy;
- ambulatory oxygen.

The type of oxygen service (or combination of services) should be ordered on a Home Oxygen Order Form (HOOF); the amount of oxygen required (hours per day) and flow rate should be specified. The clinician will determine the appropriate equipment to be provided. Special needs or preferences should be specified on the HOOF.

The clinician should obtain the patient or carers consent, to pass on the patient's details to the supplier, the fire brigade, and other relevant organisations. The supplier will contact the patient to make arrangements for delivery, installation, and maintenance of the equipment. The supplier will also train the patient or carer to use the equipment.

The clinician should send the HOOF to the supplier who will continue to provide the service until a revised HOOF is received, or until notified that the patient no longer requires the home oxygen service.

- East of England, North East: BOC Medical: Tel: 0800 136 603 Fax: 0800 169 9989
- South West: Air Liquide: Tel: 0808 202 2229 Fax: 0191 497 4340
- London, East Midlands, North West: Air Liquide: Tel: 0500 823 773 Fax: 0800 781 4610
- Yorkshire and Humberside, West Midlands, Wales: Air Products: Tel: 0800 373 580 Fax: 0800 214 709
- South East Coast, South Central: Dolby Vivisol: Tel: 08443 814 402 Fax: 0800 781 4610

In **Scotland** refer the patient for assessment by a respiratory consultant. If the need for a concentrator is confirmed the consultant will arrange for the provision of a concentrator through the Common Services Agency. Prescribers should complete a Scottish Home Oxygen Order Form (SHOOF) and email it to Health Facilities Scotland. Health Facilities Scotland will then liaise with their contractor to arrange the supply of oxygen. Further information can be obtained at: www.dolbyvivisol.com/our-services/healthcare-professionals/home-oxygen-services-sco.aspx.

In **Northern Ireland** oxygen concentrators and cylinders should be prescribed on form HS21; oxygen concentrators are supplied by a local contractor. Prescriptions for oxygen cylinders and accessories can be dispensed by pharmacists contracted to provide domiciliary oxygen services.

ANTIMUSCARINICS

Antimuscarinics (inhaled)   9.2.2016

- CAUTIONS Bladder outflow obstruction · paradoxical bronchospasm · prostatic hyperplasia · susceptibility to angle-closure glaucoma
- INTERACTIONS → Appendix 1 (antimuscarinics). However, note that interactions do not *generally* apply to antimuscarinics used by inhalation.
- SIDE-EFFECTS
- ▶ **Common or very common** Constipation · cough · diarrhoea · dry mouth · gastro-intestinal motility disorder · headache · sinusitis
- ▶ **Uncommon** Angle-closure glaucoma · atrial fibrillation · blurred vision · dizziness · gastro-oesophageal reflux disease (in adults) · mydriasis · nasopharyngitis · nausea · palpitation · paradoxical bronchospasm · pharyngitis · rash · tachycardia · throat irritation · urinary retention
- ▶ **Rare** Dental caries

☞ above

Aclidinium bromide   19.2.2016

- INDICATIONS AND DOSE

Maintenance treatment of chronic obstructive pulmonary disease
- ▶ BY INHALATION OF POWDER
- ▶ Adult: 375 micrograms twice daily

DOSE EQUIVALENCE AND CONVERSION
Each 375 microgram inhalation of aclidinium bromide delivers 322 micrograms of aclidinium.

- CAUTIONS Arrhythmia (when newly diagnosed within last 3 months) · heart failure (hospitalisation with moderate or severe heart failure within last 12 months) · myocardial infarction within last 6 months · unstable angina
- SIDE-EFFECTS
- ▶ **Uncommon** Dysphonia · stomatitis
- PREGNANCY Manufacturer advises use only if potential benefit outweighs risk.
- BREAST FEEDING Manufacturer advises only use if potential benefits outweigh risks.
- PATIENT AND CARER ADVICE Patients or carers should be given advice on appropriate inhaler technique.

- MEDICINAL FORMS
There can be variation in the licensing of different medicines containing the same drug.
Inhalation powder
- ▶ Aclidinium bromide (Non-proprietary) ▼
  Aclidinium bromide 375 microgram per 1 dose Aclidinium bromide 375micrograms/dose dry powder inhaler | 60 dose PoM no price available DT price = £28.60
- ▶ Eklira (AstraZeneca UK Ltd) ▼
  Aclidinium bromide 375 microgram per 1 dose Eklira 322micrograms/dose Genuair | 60 dose PoM £28.60 DT price = £28.60

Aclidinium bromide with formoterol   19.2.2016

The properties listed below are those particular to the combination only. For the properties of the components please consider, aclidinium bromide above, formoterol fumarate p. 231.

- INDICATIONS AND DOSE

Maintenance treatment of chronic obstructive pulmonary disease
- ▶ BY INHALATION OF POWDER
- ▶ Adult: 1 inhalation twice daily

- CAUTIONS Convulsive disorders · phaeochromocytoma
- PATIENT AND CARER ADVICE Patients or carers should be given advice on appropriate inhaler technique.

- MEDICINAL FORMS
There can be variation in the licensing of different medicines containing the same drug.
Inhalation powder
- ▶ Aclidinium bromide with formoterol (Non-proprietary) ▼
  Formoterol fumarate dihydrate 11.8 microgram per 1 dose, Aclidinium bromide 396 microgram per 1 dose Aclidinium bromide 396micrograms/dose / Formoterol 11.8micrograms/dose dry powder inhaler | 60 dose PoM no price available
- ▶ Duaklir (AstraZeneca UK Ltd) ▼
  Formoterol fumarate dihydrate 11.8 microgram per 1 dose, Aclidinium bromide 396 microgram per 1 dose Duaklir 340micrograms/dose / 12micrograms/dose Genuair | 60 dose PoM £32.50

☞ above

Glycopyrronium bromide

(Glycopyrrolate)

- INDICATIONS AND DOSE

Maintenance treatment of chronic obstructive pulmonary disease
- ▶ BY INHALATION OF POWDER
- ▶ Adult: 50 micrograms once daily

DOSE EQUIVALENCE AND CONVERSION
For inhalation of powder, each 50 microgram capsule of glycopyrronium delivers 44 micrograms of glycopyrronium.

- CAUTIONS Arrhythmia (excluding chronic stable atrial fibrillation) · history of myocardial infarction · history of QT-interval prolongation · left ventricular failure · unstable ischaemic heart disease
- SIDE-EFFECTS
- ▶ **Common or very common** Insomnia
- ▶ **Uncommon** Epistaxis · hyperglycaemia · hypoaesthesia · malaise · rhinitis
- PREGNANCY Manufacturer advises use only if potential benefit outweighs risk.
- BREAST FEEDING Manufacturer advises use only if potential benefit outweighs risk.
- RENAL IMPAIRMENT Use with caution if eGFR less than 30 mL/minute/1.73 m^2.
- PATIENT AND CARER ADVICE Patients or carers should be given advice on how to administer glycopyrronium for inhalation.

- MEDICINAL FORMS
There can be variation in the licensing of different medicines containing the same drug.
Inhalation powder
- ▶ Glycopyrronium bromide (Non-proprietary) ▼
  Glycopyrronium bromide 55 microgram Glycopyrronium bromide 55microgram inhalation powder capsules with device | 6 capsule PoM no price available | 30 capsule PoM no price available
- ▶ Seebri Breezhaler (Novartis Pharmaceuticals UK Ltd) ▼
  Glycopyrronium bromide 55 microgram Seebri Breezhaler 44microgram inhalation powder capsules with device | 6 capsule PoM no price available (Hospital only) | 30 capsule PoM £27.50

3

Respiratory system

3

Respiratory system

Glycopyrronium with indacaterol 17.2.2016

The properties listed below are those particular to the combination only. For the properties of the components please consider, glycopyrronium bromide p. 227, indacaterol p. 232.

● **INDICATIONS AND DOSE**

Maintenance treatment of chronic obstructive pulmonary disease
▸ BY INHALATION OF POWDER
▸ Adult: 1 inhalation daily

● CAUTIONS Convulsive disorders
● PATIENT AND CARER ADVICE Patients or carers should be given advice on appropriate inhaler technique and reminded that the capsules are not for oral administration.

● MEDICINAL FORMS
There can be variation in the licensing of different medicines containing the same drug.
Inhalation powder
▸ Ultibro Breezhaler (Novartis Pharmaceuticals UK Ltd) ▼
Glycopyrronium bromide 54 microgram per 1 dose, Indacaterol (as Indacaterol maleate) 85 microgram per 1 dose Ultibro Breezhaler 85microgram/43microgram inhalation powder capsules with device | 12 capsule [PoM] £13.00 | 30 capsule [PoM] £32.50

 227

Ipratropium bromide 24.2.2016

● **INDICATIONS AND DOSE**

Reversible airways obstruction
▸ BY INHALATION OF AEROSOL
▸ Child 1 month–5 years: 20 micrograms 3 times a day
▸ Child 6–11 years: 20–40 micrograms 3 times a day
▸ Child 12–17 years: 20–40 micrograms 3–4 times a day
Reversible airways obstruction, particularly in chronic obstructive pulmonary disease
▸ BY INHALATION OF AEROSOL
▸ Adult: 20–40 micrograms 3–4 times a day
▸ BY INHALATION OF NEBULISED SOLUTION
▸ Adult: 250–500 micrograms 3–4 times a day
Acute bronchospasm
▸ BY INHALATION OF NEBULISED SOLUTION
▸ Child 1 month–5 years: 125–250 micrograms as required; maximum 1 mg per day
▸ Child 6–11 years: 250 micrograms as required; maximum 1 mg per day
▸ Child 12–17 years: 500 micrograms as required, doses higher than max. can be given under medical supervision; maximum 2 mg per day
▸ Adult: 500 micrograms as required, doses higher than max. can be given under medical supervision; maximum 2 mg per day
Severe or life-threatening acute asthma
▸ BY INHALATION OF NEBULISED SOLUTION
▸ Child 1 month–11 years: 250 micrograms every 20–30 minutes for the first 2 hours, then 250 micrograms every 4–6 hours as required
▸ Child 12–17 years: 500 micrograms every 4–6 hours as required
▸ Adult: 500 micrograms every 4–6 hours as required
PHARMACOKINETICS
The maximal effect of inhaled ipratropium occurs 30–60 minutes after use; its duration of action is 3 to 6 hours and bronchodilation can usually be maintained with treatment 3 times a day.

● UNLICENSED USE [EvGr] The dose of ipratropium for severe or life-threatening acute asthma is unlicensed. Ⓐ
● CAUTIONS Cystic fibrosis

● CAUTIONS, FURTHER INFORMATION
▸ Glaucoma *Acute angle-closure glaucoma* has been reported with nebulised ipratropium, particularly when given with nebulised salbutamol (and possibly other beta₂ agonists); care needed to protect the patient's eyes from nebulised drug or from drug powder.

● SIDE-EFFECTS
▸ **Uncommon** Laryngospasm · pharyngeal oedema · stomatitis · vomiting
▸ **Rare** Ocular accommodation disorder
● PREGNANCY Manufacturer advises only use if potential benefit outweighs the risk.
● BREAST FEEDING No information available—manufacturer advises only use if potential benefit outweighs risk.
● DIRECTIONS FOR ADMINISTRATION If dilution of ipratropium bromide nebuliser solution is necessary use only sterile sodium chloride 0.9%.
● PATIENT AND CARER ADVICE Patients or carers should be given advice on appropriate inhaler technique.

● MEDICINAL FORMS
There can be variation in the licensing of different medicines containing the same drug.
Pressurised inhalation
▸ Ipratropium bromide (Non-proprietary)
Ipratropium bromide 20 microgram per 1 dose Ipratropium bromide 20micrograms/dose inhaler CFC free | 200 dose [PoM] £5.00 DT price = £5.56
▸ Atrovent (Boehringer Ingelheim Ltd)
Ipratropium bromide 20 microgram per 1 dose Atrovent 20micrograms/dose inhaler CFC free | 200 dose [PoM] £5.56 DT price = £5.56
Nebuliser liquid
▸ Ipratropium bromide (Non-proprietary)
Ipratropium bromide 250 microgram per 1 ml Ipratropium bromide 500micrograms/2ml nebuliser liquid unit dose vials | 20 unit dose [PoM] £8.93 DT price = £2.95
Ipratropium bromide 250micrograms/1ml nebuliser liquid unit dose vials | 20 unit dose [PoM] £4.52 DT price = £4.44
Ipratropium 250micrograms/1ml nebuliser liquid Steri-Neb unit dose vials | 20 unit dose [PoM] £14.99 DT price = £4.44
Ipratropium 500micrograms/2ml nebuliser liquid Steri-Neb unit dose vials | 20 unit dose [PoM] £15.99 DT price = £2.95
▸ Atrovent UDV (Boehringer Ingelheim Ltd)
Ipratropium bromide 250 microgram per 1 ml Atrovent 500micrograms/2ml nebuliser liquid UDVs | 20 unit dose [PoM] £4.87 DT price = £2.95 | 60 unit dose [PoM] £14.59
Atrovent 250micrograms/1ml nebuliser liquid UDVs | 20 unit dose [PoM] £4.14 DT price = £4.44 | 60 unit dose [PoM] £12.44
▸ Respontin (GlaxoSmithKline UK Ltd)
Ipratropium bromide 250 microgram per 1 ml Respontin 250micrograms/1ml Nebules | 20 unit dose [PoM] £4.78 DT price = £4.44
Respontin 500micrograms/2ml Nebules | 20 unit dose [PoM] £5.60 DT price = £2.95

Ipratropium with salbutamol 17.2.2016

The properties listed below are those particular to the combination only. For the properties of the components please consider, ipratropium bromide above, salbutamol p. 233.

● **INDICATIONS AND DOSE**

Bronchospasm in chronic obstructive pulmonary disease
▸ BY INHALATION OF NEBULISED SOLUTION
▸ Adult: 0.5/2.5 mg 3–4 times a day

● PRESCRIBING AND DISPENSING INFORMATION A mixture of ipratropium bromide and salbutamol (as sulphate); the proportions are expressed in the form x/y where x and y are the strengths in milligrams of ipratropium and salbutamol respectively.

- MEDICINAL FORMS

There can be variation in the licensing of different medicines containing the same drug.

Nebuliser liquid

▸ Ipratropium with salbutamol (Non-proprietary)

Ipratropium bromide 200 microgram per 1 ml, Salbutamol (as Salbutamol sulfate) 1 mg per 1 ml Salbutamol 2.5mg/2.5ml / Ipratropium bromide 500micrograms/2.5ml nebuliser liquid unit dose vials | 60 unit dose [PoM] no price available

▸ Combivent (Boehringer Ingelheim Ltd)

Ipratropium bromide 200 microgram per 1 ml, Salbutamol (as Salbutamol sulfate) 1 mg per 1 ml Combivent nebuliser liquid 2.5ml UDVs | 60 unit dose [PoM] £24.10

▸ Ipramol (Teva UK Ltd)

Ipratropium bromide 200 microgram per 1 ml, Salbutamol (as Salbutamol sulfate) 1 mg per 1 ml Ipramol nebuliser solution 2.5ml Steri-Neb unit dose vials | 60 unit dose [PoM] £23.83

F 227

Tiotropium
24.2.2016

- INDICATIONS AND DOSE

Maintenance treatment of chronic obstructive pulmonary disease

▸ BY INHALATION OF POWDER

▸ Adult: 18 micrograms once daily

SPIRIVA RESPIMAT®

Maintenance treatment of chronic obstructive pulmonary disease | Adjunct to inhaled corticosteroids and long-acting beta$_2$ agonists for the maintenance treatment of patients with asthma who have suffered one or more severe exacerbations in the last year

▸ BY INHALATION OF AEROSOL

▸ Adult: 5 micrograms once daily

- CAUTIONS Arrhythmia (unstable, life-threatening or requiring intervention in the previous 12 months) · heart failure (hospitalisation for moderate to severe heart failure in the previous 12 months) · myocardial infarction in the previous 6 months

- SIDE-EFFECTS

▸ **Common or very common** Epistaxis · oropharyngeal candidiasis · taste disturbance

▸ **Uncommon** Dysphonia

▸ **Rare** Gingivitis · glossitis · insomnia · stomatitis

▸ **Frequency not known** Dehydration · joint swelling

- PREGNANCY Manufacturer advises avoid—limited data available.

- BREAST FEEDING Manufacturer advises avoid—no information available.

- RENAL IMPAIRMENT Plasma-tiotropium concentration raised. Manufacturer advises use only if potential benefit outweighs risk if eGFR less than 50 mL/minute/1.73 m².

- PRESCRIBING AND DISPENSING INFORMATION

SPIRIVA RESPIMAT® Use *Spiriva Respimat*® only when patient unable to use *Spiriva Handihaler*® device.

- PATIENT AND CARER ADVICE Patients or carers should be given advice on appropriate inhaler technique and reminded that the powder inhalation capsules are not for oral administration.

- NATIONAL FUNDING/ACCESS DECISIONS

SPIRIVA RESPIMAT®

Scottish Medicines Consortium (SMC) Decisions

The *Scottish Medicines Consortium* has advised (November 2007) that *Spiriva Respimat*® is restricted for use in chronic obstructive pulmonary disease in patients who have poor manual dexterity and difficulty using the *Handihaler*® device.

- MEDICINAL FORMS

There can be variation in the licensing of different medicines containing the same drug.

Pressurised inhalation

▸ Spiriva Respimat (Boehringer Ingelheim Ltd)

Tiotropium (as Tiotropium bromide) 2.5 microgram per 1 dose Spiriva Respimat 2.5micrograms/dose solution for inhalation cartridge with device | 60 dose [PoM] £23.00 DT price = £33.50

Inhalation powder

▸ Spiriva (Boehringer Ingelheim Ltd)

Tiotropium (as Tiotropium bromide) 18 microgram Spiriva 18microgram inhalation powder capsules | 30 capsule [PoM] £33.50 DT price = £33.50 | 60 capsule [PoM] £67.00

Spiriva 18microgram inhalation powder capsules with HandiHaler | 30 capsule [PoM] £34.87 DT price = £34.87

Tiotropium with olodaterol
15.2.2016

The properties listed below are those particular to the combination only. For the properties of the components please consider, tiotropium above, olodaterol p. 232.

- INDICATIONS AND DOSE

Maintenance treatment of chronic obstructive pulmonary disease

▸ BY INHALATION OF AEROSOL

▸ Adult: 2 puffs once daily

- SIDE-EFFECTS

▸ **Rare** Laryngitis

▸ **Frequency not known** Skin ulcer

- PATIENT AND CARER ADVICE Patient or carers should be given advice on appropriate inhaler technique.

- MEDICINAL FORMS

There can be variation in the licensing of different medicines containing the same drug.

Pressurised inhalation

▸ Spiolto Respimat (Boehringer Ingelheim Ltd)

Olodaterol (as Olodaterol hydrochloride) 2.5 microgram per 1 dose, Tiotropium (as Tiotropium bromide) 2.5 microgram per 1 dose Spiolto Respimat 2.5micrograms/dose / 2.5micrograms/dose solution for inhalation cartridge with device | 60 dose [PoM] £32.50 DT price = £32.50

F 227

Umeclidinium
19.2.2016

- INDICATIONS AND DOSE

Maintenance treatment of chronic obstructive pulmonary disease

▸ BY INHALATION OF POWDER

▸ Adult: 55 micrograms once daily

DOSE EQUIVALENCE AND CONVERSION

Each 65 microgram inhalation of umeclidinium bromide delivers 55 micrograms of umeclidinium.

- CAUTIONS Cardiac disorders (particularly cardiac rhythm disorders)

- PREGNANCY Manufacturer advises use only if potential benefit outweighs risk.

- BREAST FEEDING Manufacturer advises avoid—no information available.

- HEPATIC IMPAIRMENT Manufacturer advises to use with caution in severe impairment—no information available.

- PATIENT AND CARER ADVICE Patient or carers should be given advice on appropriate inhaler technique.

Respiratory system

3

- MEDICINAL FORMS
There can be variation in the licensing of different medicines containing the same drug.
Inhalation powder
‣ Incruse Ellipta (GlaxoSmithKline UK Ltd) ▼
Umeclidinium bromide 65 microgram per 1 dose Incruse Ellipta 55micrograms/dose dry powder inhaler | 30 dose PoM £27.50 DT price = £27.50

Umeclidinium with vilanterol
19.2.2016

The properties listed below are those particular to the combination only. For the properties of the components please consider, umeclidinium p. 229.

- INDICATIONS AND DOSE
Maintenance treatment of chronic obstructive pulmonary disease
‣ BY INHALATION OF POWDER
‣ Adult: 1 inhalation once daily

- CONTRA-INDICATIONS Severe pre-eclampsia
- CAUTIONS Arrhythmias · cardiovascular disease · diabetes (risk of hyperglycaemia and ketoacidosis) · hypertension · hyperthyroidism · hypokalaemia · susceptibility to QT-interval prolongation
CAUTIONS, FURTHER INFORMATION
‣ Hypokalaemia Potentially serious hypokalaemia may result in severe asthma, because this effect may be potentiated by concomitant treatment with theophylline and its derivatives, corticosteroids, diuretics, and by hypoxia.
- INTERACTIONS → Appendix 1 (antimuscarinics, sympathomimetics beta₂).
- SIDE-EFFECTS Angioedema · arrhythmias · behavioural disturbances · collapse · fine tremor (particularly in the hands) · hyperglycaemia · hypersensitivity reactions · hypokalaemia (with high doses) · hypotension · ketoacidosis · muscle cramps · myocardial ischaemia · nervous tension · peripheral vasodilation · sleep disturbances · urticaria
- MONITORING REQUIREMENTS
‣ In severe asthma, plasma-potassium concentration should be monitored (risk of hypokalaemia).
‣ In patients with diabetes, monitor blood glucose (risk of hyperglycaemia and ketoacidosis, especially when beta₂ agonist given intravenously).
- PATIENT AND CARER ADVICE Patient or carers should be given advice on appropriate inhaler technique.

- MEDICINAL FORMS
There can be variation in the licensing of different medicines containing the same drug.
Inhalation powder
‣ Umeclidinium with vilanterol (Non-proprietary) ▼
Vilanterol (as Vilanterol trifenatate) 22 microgram per 1 dose, Umeclidinium bromide 65 microgram per 1 dose Umeclidinium bromide 65micrograms/dose / Vilanterol 22micrograms/dose dry powder inhaler | 30 dose PoM no price available
‣ Anoro Ellipta (GlaxoSmithKline UK Ltd) ▼
Vilanterol (as Vilanterol trifenatate) 22 microgram per 1 dose, Umeclidinium bromide 65 microgram per 1 dose Anoro Ellipta 55micrograms/dose / 22micrograms/dose dry powder inhaler | 30 dose PoM £32.50

BETA₂-ADRENOCEPTOR AGONISTS, SELECTIVE

Beta₂-adrenoceptor agonists, selective
12.2.2016

- CONTRA-INDICATIONS Severe pre-eclampsia
- CAUTIONS Arrhythmias · cardiovascular disease · diabetes (risk of hyperglycaemia and ketoacidosis, especially with intravenous use) · high doses of beta₂ agonists can be dangerous in some children (in children) · hypertension · hyperthyroidism · hypokalaemia · susceptibility to QT-interval prolongation
CAUTIONS, FURTHER INFORMATION
‣ Hypokalaemia Potentially serious hypokalaemia may result from beta₂ agonist therapy. Particular caution is required in severe asthma, because this effect may be potentiated by concomitant treatment with theophylline and its derivatives, corticosteroids, diuretics, and by hypoxia.
- INTERACTIONS → Appendix 1 (sympathomimetics, beta₂). Hypokalaemia may be potentiated by concomitant treatment with theophylline and its derivatives, corticosteroids, and diuretics.
- SIDE-EFFECTS Angioedema · arrhythmias · behavioural disturbances · collapse · fine tremor (particularly in the hands) · headache · hyperglycaemia (especially when given intravenously) · hypersensitivity reactions · hypokalaemia (with high doses) · hypotension · ketoacidosis (especially when given intravenously) · muscle cramps · myocardial ischaemia · nervous tension · palpitation · paradoxical bronchospasm (occasionally severe) · peripheral vasodilation · rash · sleep disturbances · tachycardia · urticaria
- PREGNANCY Women planning to become pregnant should be counselled about the importance of taking their asthma medication regularly to maintain good control.
- MONITORING REQUIREMENTS
‣ In severe asthma, plasma-potassium concentration should be monitored (risk of hypokalaemia).
‣ In patients with diabetes, monitor blood glucose (risk of hyperglycaemia and ketoacidosis, especially when beta₂ agonist given intravenously).
- PATIENT AND CARER ADVICE
‣ When used by inhalation The **dose**, the frequency, and the maximum number of inhalations in 24 hours of the beta₂ agonist should be **stated explicitly** to the patient or their carer. The patient or their carer should be advised to seek medical advice when the prescribed dose of beta₂ agonist fails to provide the usual degree of symptomatic relief because this usually indicates a worsening of the asthma and the patient may require a prophylactic drug. Patients or their carers should be advised to follow manufacturers' instructions on the care and cleansing of inhaler devices.

BETA₂-ADRENOCEPTOR AGONISTS, SELECTIVE > LONG-ACTING
 above

Bambuterol hydrochloride
- DRUG ACTION Bambuterol is a pro-drug of terbutaline.

- INDICATIONS AND DOSE
Asthma (patients who have previously tolerated beta₂-agonists) | Other conditions associated with reversible airways obstruction (patients who have previously tolerated beta₂-agonists)
‣ BY MOUTH
‣ Adult: 20 mg once daily, dose to be taken at bedtime

Asthma (patients who have not previously tolerated beta$_2$-agonists) | Other conditions associated with reversible airways obstruction (patients who have not previously tolerated beta$_2$-agonists)
▶ BY MOUTH
▸ Adult: Initially 10 mg once daily for 1–2 weeks, then increased if necessary to 20 mg once daily, dose to be taken at bedtime

● PREGNANCY Manufacturer advises avoid—no information available.
● BREAST FEEDING Manufacturer advises avoid—no information available.
● HEPATIC IMPAIRMENT Avoid in severe impairment.
● RENAL IMPAIRMENT Reduce initial dose by half if eGFR less than 50 mL/minute/1.73 m^2.

● MEDICINAL FORMS
There can be variation in the licensing of different medicines containing the same drug.
Tablet
▸ Bambec (AstraZeneca UK Ltd)
  Bambuterol hydrochloride 10 mg Bambec 10mg tablets |
  28 tablet [PoM] £14.46 DT price = £14.46
  Bambuterol hydrochloride 20 mg Bambec 20mg tablets |
  28 tablet [PoM] £15.77 DT price = £15.77

☞ 230

Formoterol fumarate

(Eformoterol fumarate)

● INDICATIONS AND DOSE
Reversible airways obstruction in patients requiring long-term regular bronchodilator therapy | Nocturnal asthma in patients requiring long-term regular bronchodilator therapy | Prophylaxis of exercise-induced bronchospasm in patients requiring long-term regular bronchodilator therapy | Chronic asthma in patients who regularly use an inhaled corticosteroid
▶ BY INHALATION OF POWDER
▸ Child 6-11 years: 12 micrograms twice daily, a daily dose of 24 micrograms of formoterol should be sufficient for the majority of children, particularly for younger age-groups; higher doses should be used rarely, and only when control is not maintained on the lower dose
▸ Child 12-17 years: 12 micrograms twice daily, dose may be increased in more severe airway obstruction; increased to 24 micrograms twice daily, a daily dose of 24 micrograms of formoterol should be sufficient for the majority of children, particularly for younger age-groups; higher doses should be used rarely, and only when control is not maintained on the lower dose
▸ Adult: 12 micrograms twice daily, dose may be increased in more severe airway obstruction; increased to 24 micrograms twice daily
▶ BY INHALATION OF AEROSOL
▸ Child 12-17 years: 12 micrograms twice daily, dose may be increased in more severe airway obstruction; increased to 24 micrograms twice daily, a daily dose of 24 micrograms of formoterol should be sufficient for the majority of children, particularly for younger age-groups; higher doses should be used rarely, and only when control is not maintained on the lower dose
▸ Adult: 12 micrograms twice daily, dose may be increased in more severe airway obstruction; increased to 24 micrograms twice daily

Chronic obstructive pulmonary disease
▶ BY INHALATION OF POWDER
▸ Adult: 12 micrograms twice daily

▶ BY INHALATION OF AEROSOL
▸ Adult: 12 micrograms twice daily (max. per dose 24 micrograms), for symptom relief additional doses may be taken to maximum daily dose; maximum 48 micrograms per day
OXIS®
Chronic asthma
▶ BY INHALATION OF POWDER
▸ Child 6-17 years: 6–12 micrograms 1–2 times a day (max. per dose 12 micrograms), occasionally doses up to the maximum daily may be needed, reassess treatment if additional doses required on more than 2 days a week; maximum 48 micrograms per day
▸ Adult: 6–12 micrograms 1–2 times a day, increased if necessary up to 24 micrograms twice daily (max. per dose 36 micrograms), occasionally doses up to the maximum daily may be needed, reassess treatment if additional doses required on more than 2 days a week; maximum 72 micrograms per day
Relief of bronchospasm
▶ BY INHALATION OF POWDER
▸ Child 6-17 years: 6–12 micrograms
▸ Adult: 6–12 micrograms
Prophylaxis of exercise-induced bronchospasm
▶ BY INHALATION OF POWDER
▸ Child 6-17 years: 6–12 micrograms, dose to be taken before exercise
▸ Adult: 12 micrograms, dose to be taken before exercise
Chronic obstructive pulmonary disease
▶ BY INHALATION OF POWDER
▸ Adult: 12 micrograms 1–2 times a day (max. per dose 24 micrograms), for symptom relief additional doses up to maximum daily dose can be taken; maximum 48 micrograms per day
PHARMACOKINETICS
At recommended inhaled doses, the duration of action of formoterol is about 12 hours.

IMPORTANT SAFETY INFORMATION
CHM ADVICE
To ensure safe use, the CHM has advised that for the management of chronic asthma, long-acting beta$_2$ agonist (formoterol) should:
● be added only if regular use of standard-dose inhaled corticosteroids has failed to control asthma adequately;
● not be initiated in patients with rapidly deteriorating asthma;
● be introduced at a low dose and the effect properly monitored before considering dose increase;
● be discontinued in the absence of benefit;
● not be used for the relief of exercise-induced asthma symptoms unless regular inhaled corticosteroids are also used;
● be reviewed as clinically appropriate: stepping down therapy should be considered when good long-term asthma control has been achieved.

● SIDE-EFFECTS
▶ Very rare QT-interval prolongation
▶ **Frequency not known** Dizziness · nausea · pruritus · taste disturbances
● PREGNANCY Inhaled drugs for asthma can be taken as normal during pregnancy.
● BREAST FEEDING Inhaled drugs for asthma can be taken as normal during breast-feeding.
● PATIENT AND CARER ADVICE Advise patients not to exceed prescribed dose, and to follow manufacturer's directions; if a previously effective dose of inhaled formoterol fails to provide adequate relief, a doctor's advice should be

obtained as soon as possible. Patients should be advised to report any deterioration in symptoms following initiation of treatment with a long-acting beta₂ agonist. Patient or carer should be given advice on how to administer formoterol fumarate inhalers.

● MEDICINAL FORMS
There can be variation in the licensing of different medicines containing the same drug.
Pressurised inhalation
▸ Atimos Modulite (Chiesi Ltd)
Formoterol fumarate dihydrate 12 microgram per 1 dose Atimos Modulite 12micrograms/dose inhaler | 100 dose PoM £30.06 DT price = £30.06
Inhalation powder
▸ Easyhaler (formoterol) (Orion Pharma (UK) Ltd)
Formoterol fumarate dihydrate 12 microgram per 1 dose Formoterol Easyhaler 12micrograms/dose dry powder inhaler | 120 dose PoM £23.75 DT price = £23.75
▸ Foradil (Novartis Pharmaceuticals UK Ltd)
Formoterol fumarate dihydrate 12 microgram Foradil 12microgram inhalation powder capsules with device | 60 capsule PoM £28.06 DT price = £28.06
▸ Oxis Turbohaler (AstraZeneca UK Ltd)
Formoterol fumarate dihydrate 6 microgram per 1 dose Oxis 6 Turbohaler | 60 dose PoM £24.80 DT price = £24.80
Formoterol fumarate dihydrate 12 microgram per 1 dose Oxis 12 Turbohaler | 60 dose PoM £24.80 DT price = £24.80

Combinations available: *Aclidinium bromide with formoterol*, p. 227 · *Beclometasone with formoterol*, p. 239 · *Budesonide with formoterol*, p. 241 · *Fluticasone with formoterol*, p. 242

F 230

Indacaterol

● INDICATIONS AND DOSE
Maintenance treatment of chronic obstructive pulmonary disease
▸ BY INHALATION OF POWDER
▸ Adult: 150 micrograms once daily, then increased to 300 micrograms once daily

● CAUTIONS Convulsive disorders
● SIDE-EFFECTS
▸ Common or very common Cough · dizziness · nasopharyngitis · oropharyngeal pain · peripheral oedema · rhinorrhoea · sinusitis
▸ Uncommon Atrial fibrillation · chest pain · paraesthesia · pruritus
● PREGNANCY Manufacturer advises use only if potential benefit outweighs risk.
● BREAST FEEDING Manufacturer advises avoid—present in milk in *animal* studies.
● HEPATIC IMPAIRMENT Use with caution in severe impairment—no information available.
● PATIENT AND CARER ADVICE Patients or carers should be given advice on how to administer indacaterol inhalation powder.

● MEDICINAL FORMS
There can be variation in the licensing of different medicines containing the same drug.
Inhalation powder
▸ Onbrez Breezhaler (Novartis Pharmaceuticals UK Ltd)
Indacaterol (as Indacaterol maleate) 150 microgram Onbrez Breezhaler 150microgram inhalation powder capsules with device | 30 capsule PoM £32.19 DT price = £32.19
Indacaterol (as Indacaterol maleate) 300 microgram Onbrez Breezhaler 300microgram inhalation powder capsules with device | 30 capsule PoM £32.19 DT price = £32.19

Combinations available: *Glycopyrronium with indacaterol*, p. 228

F 230

Olodaterol

● INDICATIONS AND DOSE
Maintenance treatment of chronic obstructive pulmonary disease
▸ BY INHALATION
▸ Adult: 5 micrograms once daily
DOSE EQUIVALENCE AND CONVERSION
2 puffs is equivalent to 5 micrograms.

● CAUTIONS Aneurysm · convulsive disorders
● SIDE-EFFECTS
▸ Uncommon Dizziness · nasopharyngitis
▸ Rare Arthralgia · hypertension
● PREGNANCY Manufacturer advises avoid—no information available.
● BREAST FEEDING Manufacturer advises avoid— present in milk in *animal* studies.
● HEPATIC IMPAIRMENT Use with caution in severe hepatic impairment—no information available.
● PATIENT AND CARER ADVICE Patients or carers should be given advice on how to administer olodaterol solution for inhalation.

● MEDICINAL FORMS
There can be variation in the licensing of different medicines containing the same drug.
Pressurised inhalation
▸ Striverdi Respimat (Boehringer Ingelheim Ltd) ▼
Olodaterol (as Olodaterol hydrochloride) 2.5 microgram per 1 dose Striverdi Respimat 2.5micrograms/dose solution for inhalation cartridge with device | 60 dose PoM £26.35 DT price = £26.35

Combinations available: *Tiotropium with olodaterol*, p. 229

F 230

Salmeterol

● INDICATIONS AND DOSE
Reversible airways obstruction in patients requiring long-term regular bronchodilator therapy | Nocturnal asthma in patients requiring long-term regular bronchodilator therapy | Prevention of exercise-induced bronchospasm in patients requiring long-term regular bronchodilator therapy | Chronic asthma only in patients who regularly use an inhaled corticosteroid (not for immediate relief of acute asthma)
▸ BY INHALATION OF AEROSOL, OR BY INHALATION OF POWDER
▸ Child 5–11 years: 50 micrograms twice daily
▸ Child 12–17 years: 50 micrograms twice daily, dose may be increased in more severe airway obstruction; increased to 100 micrograms twice daily
▸ Adult: 50 micrograms twice daily, dose may be increased in more severe airway obstruction; increased to 100 micrograms twice daily
Chronic obstructive pulmonary disease
▸ BY INHALATION OF AEROSOL, OR BY INHALATION OF POWDER
▸ Adult: 50 micrograms twice daily
PHARMACOKINETICS
At recommended inhaled doses, the duration of action of salmeterol is about 12 hours.

● UNLICENSED USE *Neovent* ® not licensed for use in children under 12 years.

Respiratory system

3

CHM ADVICE

To ensure safe use, the CHM has advised that for the management of chronic asthma, long-acting beta$_2$ agonist (salmeterol) should:

- be added only if regular use of standard-dose inhaled corticosteroids has failed to control asthma adequately;
- not be initiated in patients with rapidly deteriorating asthma;
- be introduced at a low dose and the effect properly monitored before considering dose increase;
- be discontinued in the absence of benefit;
- not be used for the relief of exercise-induced asthma symptoms unless regular inhaled corticosteroids are also used;
- be reviewed as clinically appropriate: stepping down therapy should be considered when good long-term asthma control has been achieved.

- **SIDE-EFFECTS** Arthralgia · dizziness · nausea
- **PREGNANCY** Inhaled drugs for asthma can be taken as normal during pregnancy.
- **BREAST FEEDING** Inhaled drugs for asthma can be taken as normal during breast-feeding.
- **PATIENT AND CARER ADVICE**
  Advise patients that salmeterol should **not** be used for relief of acute attacks, not to exceed prescribed dose, and to follow manufacturer's directions; if a previously effective dose of inhaled salmeterol fails to provide adequate relief, a doctor's advice should be obtained as soon as possible.

  Patients should be advised to report any deterioration in symptoms following initiation of treatment with a long-acting beta$_2$ agonist.

  Medicines for Children leaflet: Salmeterol inhaler for asthma prevention (prophylaxis) www.medicinesforchildren.org.uk/salmeterol-inhaler-for-asthma-prevention

- **MEDICINAL FORMS**
  There can be variation in the licensing of different medicines containing the same drug.

  Pressurised inhalation
  - Salmeterol (Non-proprietary)
    Salmeterol (as Salmeterol xinafoate) 25 microgram per 1 dose Salmeterol 25micrograms/dose inhaler CFC free | 120 dose [PoM] £29.26 DT price = £29.26
  - Neovent (Kent Pharmaceuticals Ltd)
    Salmeterol (as Salmeterol xinafoate) 25 microgram per 1 dose Neovent 25micrograms/dose inhaler CFC free | 120 dose [PoM] £29.26 DT price = £29.26
  - Serevent Evohaler (GlaxoSmithKline UK Ltd)
    Salmeterol (as Salmeterol xinafoate) 25 microgram per 1 dose Serevent 25micrograms/dose Evohaler | 120 dose [PoM] £29.26 DT price = £29.26
  - Vertine (Teva UK Ltd)
    Salmeterol (as Salmeterol xinafoate) 25 microgram per 1 dose Vertine 25micrograms/dose inhaler CFC free | 120 dose [PoM] £23.40 DT price = £29.26

  Inhalation powder
  - Serevent Accuhaler (GlaxoSmithKline UK Ltd)
    Salmeterol (as Salmeterol xinafoate) 50 microgram per 1 dose Serevent 50micrograms/dose Accuhaler | 60 dose [PoM] £29.26 DT price = £29.26

  Combinations available: *Fluticasone with salmeterol*, p. 243

BETA$_2$-ADRENOCEPTOR AGONISTS, SELECTIVE ⟩ SHORT-ACTING

☞ 230

Salbutamol

(Albuterol)

- **INDICATIONS AND DOSE**

Asthma | Other conditions associated with reversible airways obstruction
- ▸ BY MOUTH USING IMMEDIATE-RELEASE MEDICINES
- ▸ Adult: 4 mg 3–4 times a day, maximum single dose 8 mg (but unlikely to provide much extra benefit or to be tolerated), inhalation route preferred over oral route, use elderly dose for sensitive patients
- ▸ Elderly: Initially 2 mg 3–4 times a day, maximum single dose 8 mg (but unlikely to provide much extra benefit or to be tolerated), inhalation route preferred over oral route
- ▸ BY SUBCUTANEOUS INJECTION, OR BY INTRAMUSCULAR INJECTION
- ▸ Adult: 500 micrograms every 4 hours if required
- ▸ BY SLOW INTRAVENOUS INJECTION
- ▸ Adult: 250 micrograms, repeated if necessary, injection to be diluted to a concentration of 50 micrograms/mL, reserve intravenous beta$_2$ agonists for those in whom inhaled therapy cannot be used reliably
- ▸ BY INTRAVENOUS INFUSION
- ▸ Adult: Initially 5 micrograms/minute, adjusted according to response and heart rate, usual dose 3–20 micrograms/minute, higher doses may be required, reserve intravenous beta$_2$ agonists for those in whom inhaled therapy cannot be used reliably
- ▸ BY INHALATION OF AEROSOL
- ▸ Adult: 100–200 micrograms, up to 4 times a day for persistent symptoms
- ▸ BY INHALATION OF NEBULISED SOLUTION
- ▸ Adult: 2.5–5 mg, repeated up to 4 times daily or more frequently in severe cases

Prophylaxis of allergen- or exercise-induced bronchospasm
- ▸ BY INHALATION OF AEROSOL
- ▸ Adult: 200 micrograms

Acute asthma
- ▸ BY INTRAVENOUS INJECTION
- ▸ Child 1–23 months: 5 micrograms/kg for 1 dose, dose to be administered over 5 minutes, reserve intravenous beta$_2$ agonists for those in whom inhaled therapy cannot be used reliably or there is no current effect
- ▸ Child 2–17 years: 15 micrograms/kg (max. per dose 250 micrograms) for 1 dose, dose to be administered over 5 minutes, reserve intravenous beta$_2$ agonists for those in whom inhaled therapy cannot be used reliably or there is no current effect

Moderate, severe, or life-threatening acute asthma
- ▸ BY INHALATION OF NEBULISED SOLUTION
- ▸ Child 1 month–4 years: 2.5 mg, repeat every 20–30 minutes or when required, give via oxygen-driven nebuliser if available
- ▸ Child 5–11 years: 2.5–5 mg, repeat every 20–30 minutes or when required, give via oxygen-driven nebuliser if available
- ▸ Child 12–17 years: 5 mg, repeat every 20–30 minutes or when required, give via oxygen-driven nebuliser if available
- ▸ Adult: 5 mg, repeat every 20–30 minutes or when required, give via oxygen-driven nebuliser if available

continued →

Moderate and severe acute asthma
▶ BY INHALATION OF AEROSOL
▶ Child: 2–10 puffs, each puff is to be inhaled separately, repeat every 10–20 minutes or when required, give via large volume spacer (and a close-fitting face mask in children under 3 years), each puff is equivalent to 100 micrograms
▶ Adult: 2–10 puffs, each puff is to be inhaled separately, repeat every 10–20 minutes or when required, give via large volume spacer, each puff is equivalent to 100 micrograms

Exacerbation of reversible airways obstruction (including nocturnal asthma) | Prophylaxis of allergen- or exercise-induced bronchospasm
▶ BY INHALATION OF AEROSOL
▶ Child: 100–200 micrograms, up to 4 times a day for persistent symptoms
▶ BY MOUTH
▶ Child 1 month–1 year: 100 micrograms/kg 3–4 times a day (max. per dose 2 mg), inhalation route preferred over oral route
▶ Child 2–5 years: 1–2 mg 3–4 times a day, inhalation route preferred over oral route
▶ Child 6–11 years: 2 mg 3–4 times a day, inhalation route preferred over oral route
▶ Child 12–17 years: 2–4 mg 3–4 times a day, inhalation route preferred over oral route

Chronic asthma
▶ BY MOUTH USING MODIFIED-RELEASE MEDICINES
▶ Child 3–11 years: 4 mg twice daily
▶ Child 12–17 years: 8 mg twice daily
▶ Adult: 8 mg twice daily

Uncomplicated premature labour (between 22 and 37 weeks of gestation) (specialist supervision in hospital)
▶ BY INTRAVENOUS INFUSION
▶ Adult: Initially 10 micrograms/minute, rate increased gradually according to response at 10-minute intervals until contractions diminish then increase rate slowly until contractions cease (maximum rate 45 micrograms/minute), maintain rate for 1 hour after contractions have stopped, then gradually reduce by 50% every 6 hours, maximum duration 48 hours

ASMASAL CLICKHALER®

Acute bronchospasm
▶ BY INHALATION OF POWDER
▶ Adult: 1–2 puffs, up to 4 times daily for persistent symptoms

Prophylaxis of allergen- or exercise-induced bronchospasm
▶ BY INHALATION OF POWDER
▶ Adult: 1–2 puffs

EASYHALER® SALBUTAMOL

Acute bronchospasm
▶ BY INHALATION OF POWDER
▶ Adult: Initially 100–200 micrograms, increased if necessary to 400 micrograms; maximum 800 micrograms per day

Prophylaxis of allergen- or exercise-induced bronchospasm
▶ BY INHALATION OF POWDER
▶ Adult: 200 micrograms

PULVINAL® SALBUTAMOL

Acute bronchospasm
▶ BY INHALATION OF POWDER
▶ Child 5–17 years: Initially 200 micrograms, up to 800 micrograms daily for persistent symptoms
▶ Adult: Initially 200 micrograms, up to 800 micrograms daily for persistent symptoms

Prophylaxis of allergen- or exercise-induced bronchospasm
▶ BY INHALATION OF POWDER
▶ Child 5–17 years: 200 micrograms
▶ Adult: 200 micrograms

SALBULIN NOVOLIZER®

Acute bronchospasm
▶ BY INHALATION OF POWDER
▶ Adult: Initially 100–200 micrograms, up to 800 micrograms daily for persistent symptoms

Prophylaxis of allergen- or exercise-induced bronchospasm
▶ BY INHALATION OF POWDER
▶ Adult: 200 micrograms

VENTOLIN ACCUHALER®

Acute bronchospasm
▶ BY INHALATION OF POWDER
▶ Adult: Initially 200 micrograms, up to 4 times daily for persistent symptoms

Prophylaxis of allergen- or exercise-induced bronchospasm
▶ BY INHALATION OF POWDER
▶ Adult: 200 micrograms

PHARMACOKINETICS
At recommended inhaled doses, the duration of action of salbutamol is about 3 to 5 hours.

● UNLICENSED USE Syrup and tablets not licensed for use in children under 2 years. Modified-release tablets not licensed for use in children under 3 years. Injection not licensed for use in children under 12 years.
● CONTRA-INDICATIONS
▶ When used for uncomplicated premature labour under specialist supervision Abruptio placenta · antepartum haemorrhage · cord compression · eclampsia · history of cardiac disease · intra-uterine fetal death · intra-uterine infection · placenta praevia · pulmonary hypertension · severe pre-eclampsia · significant risk factors for myocardial ischaemia · threatened miscarriage
● CAUTIONS
▶ With intravenous use Mild to moderate pre-eclampsia (when used for uncomplicated premature labour) · suspected cardiovascular disease (should be assessed by a cardiologist before initiating therapy for uncomplicated premature labour)
● SIDE-EFFECTS
GENERAL SIDE-EFFECTS
Lactic acidosis (with high doses) · nausea
SPECIFIC SIDE-EFFECTS
▶ When used for uncomplicated premature labour Bronchospasm · muscle tension · pulmonary oedema · vomiting
● BREAST FEEDING Inhaled drugs for asthma can be taken as normal during breast-feeding.
● MONITORING REQUIREMENTS In uncomplicated premature labour it is important to monitor blood pressure, pulse rate (should not exceed 120 beats per minute), ECG (discontinue treatment if signs of myocardial ischaemia develop), blood glucose and lactate concentrations, and the patient's fluid and electrolyte status (avoid over-hydration—discontinue drug immediately and initiate diuretic therapy if pulmonary oedema occurs).
● DIRECTIONS FOR ADMINISTRATION
▶ With intravenous use in children Dilute to a concentration of 50 micrograms/mL with Glucose 5%, Sodium Chloride 0.9%, or Water for injections.
▶ When used by inhalation For nebulisation, dilute nebuliser solution with a suitable volume of sterile Sodium Chloride 0.9% solution according to nebuliser type and duration of administration; salbutamol and ipratropium bromide

solutions are compatible and can be mixed for nebulisation.

▸ With intravenous use in adults For *bronchodilation* by *continuous intravenous infusion*, dilute to a concentration of 200 micrograms/mL with glucose 5% or sodium chloride 0.9%. For *premature labour* by *continuous intravenous infusion*, dilute with glucose 5% to a concentration of 200 micrograms/mL for use in a syringe pump *or* for other infusion methods (preferably *via* controlled infusion device), dilute to a concentration of 20 micrograms/mL; close attention to patient's fluid and electrolyte status essential.

● **PATIENT AND CARER ADVICE**
Medicines for Children leaflet: Salbutamol inhaler for asthma and wheeze www.medicinesforchildren.org.uk/salbutamol-inhaler-for-asthma-and-wheeze

▸ When used by inhalation *For inhalation by aerosol or dry powder*, advise patients and carers not to exceed prescribed dose and to follow manufacturer's directions; if a previously effective dose of inhaled salbutamol fails to provide at least 3 hours relief, a doctor's advice should be obtained as soon as possible. *For inhalation by nebuliser*, the dose given by nebuliser is substantially higher than that given by inhaler. Patients should therefore be warned that it is dangerous to exceed the prescribed dose and they should seek medical advice if they fail to respond to the usual dose of the respirator solution.

● **MEDICINAL FORMS**
There can be variation in the licensing of different medicines containing the same drug.

Tablet
▸ Salbutamol (Non-proprietary)
Salbutamol (as Salbutamol sulfate) 2 mg Salbutamol 2mg tablets | 28 tablet [PoM] £113.09 DT price = £104.95
Salbutamol (as Salbutamol sulfate) 4 mg Salbutamol 4mg tablets | 28 tablet [PoM] £115.76 DT price = £107.43

Oral solution
▸ Salbutamol (Non-proprietary)
Salbutamol (as Salbutamol sulfate) 400 microgram per 1 ml Salbutamol 2mg/5ml oral solution sugar free sugar-free | 150 ml [PoM] no price available DT price = £0.72
▸ Ventolin (GlaxoSmithKline UK Ltd)
Salbutamol (as Salbutamol sulfate) 400 microgram per 1 ml Ventolin 2mg/5ml syrup sugar-free | 150 ml [PoM] £0.72 DT price = £0.72

Solution for injection
▸ Ventolin (GlaxoSmithKline UK Ltd)
Salbutamol (as Salbutamol sulfate) 500 microgram per 1 ml Ventolin 500micrograms/1ml solution for injection ampoules | 5 ampoule [PoM] £1.91

Solution for infusion
▸ Ventolin (GlaxoSmithKline UK Ltd)
Salbutamol (as Salbutamol sulfate) 1 mg per 1 ml Ventolin 5mg/5ml solution for infusion ampoules | 10 ampoule [PoM] £24.81

Pressurised inhalation
▸ Salbutamol (Non-proprietary)
Salbutamol (as Salbutamol sulfate) 100 microgram per 1 dose Salbutamol 100micrograms/dose inhaler CFC free | 200 dose [PoM] £1.50 DT price = £1.50
▸ AirSalb (Sandoz Ltd)
Salbutamol (as Salbutamol sulfate) 100 microgram per 1 dose AirSalb 100micrograms/dose inhaler CFC free | 200 dose [PoM] £1.50 DT price = £1.50
▸ Airomir (Teva UK Ltd)
Salbutamol (as Salbutamol sulfate) 100 microgram per 1 dose Airomir 100micrograms/dose inhaler | 200 dose [PoM] £1.97 DT price = £1.50
▸ Airomir Autohaler (Teva UK Ltd)
Salbutamol (as Salbutamol sulfate) 100 microgram per 1 dose Airomir 100micrograms/dose Autohaler | 200 dose [PoM] £6.02 DT price = £6.30
▸ Asmavent (Kent Pharmaceuticals Ltd)
Salbutamol (as Salbutamol sulfate) 100 microgram per 1 dose Asmavent 100micrograms/dose inhaler CFC free | 200 dose [PoM] £1.50 DT price = £1.50

▸ Salamol (Teva UK Ltd)
Salbutamol (as Salbutamol sulfate) 100 microgram per 1 dose Salamol 100micrograms/dose inhaler CFC free | 200 dose [PoM] £1.46 DT price = £1.50
▸ Salamol Easi-Breathe (Teva UK Ltd)
Salbutamol (as Salbutamol sulfate) 100 microgram per 1 dose Salbutamol 100micrograms/dose Easi-Breathe inhaler | 200 dose [PoM] £6.30 DT price = £6.30
▸ Ventolin Evohaler (GlaxoSmithKline UK Ltd)
Salbutamol (as Salbutamol sulfate) 100 microgram per 1 dose Ventolin 100micrograms/dose Evohaler | 200 dose [PoM] £1.50 DT price = £1.50

Inhalation powder
▸ Easyhaler (salbutamol) (Orion Pharma (UK) Ltd)
Salbutamol 100 microgram per 1 dose Easyhaler Salbutamol sulfate 100micrograms/dose dry powder inhaler | 200 dose [PoM] £3.31 DT price = £3.31
Salbutamol 200 microgram per 1 dose Easyhaler Salbutamol sulfate 200micrograms/dose dry powder inhaler | 200 dose [PoM] £6.63 DT price = £6.63
▸ Salbulin Novolizer (Meda Pharmaceuticals Ltd)
Salbutamol (as Salbutamol sulfate) 100 microgram per 1 dose Salbulin Novolizer 100micrograms/dose inhalation powder | 200 dose [PoM] £4.95
Salbulin Novolizer 100micrograms/dose inhalation powder refill | 200 dose [PoM] £2.75
▸ Ventolin Accuhaler (GlaxoSmithKline UK Ltd)
Salbutamol 200 microgram per 1 dose Ventolin 200micrograms/dose Accuhaler | 60 dose [PoM] £3.00 DT price = £3.00

Nebuliser liquid
▸ Salbutamol (Non-proprietary)
Salbutamol (as Salbutamol sulfate) 1 mg per 1 ml Salbutamol 2.5mg/2.5ml nebuliser liquid unit dose vials | 20 unit dose [PoM] £7.00 DT price = £1.91
Salbutamol (as Salbutamol sulfate) 2 mg per 1 ml Salbutamol 5mg/2.5ml nebuliser liquid unit dose vials | 20 unit dose [PoM] £7.35 DT price = £3.82
▸ Salamol Steri-Neb (Teva UK Ltd)
Salbutamol (as Salbutamol sulfate) 1 mg per 1 ml Salamol 2.5mg/2.5ml nebuliser liquid Steri-Neb unit dose vials | 20 unit dose [PoM] £1.91 DT price = £1.91
Salbutamol (as Salbutamol sulfate) 2 mg per 1 ml Salamol 5mg/2.5ml nebuliser liquid Steri-Neb unit dose vials | 20 unit dose [PoM] £3.82 DT price = £3.82
▸ Ventolin (GlaxoSmithKline UK Ltd)
Salbutamol (as Salbutamol sulfate) 5 mg per 1 ml Ventolin 5mg/ml respirator solution | 20 ml [PoM] £2.18 DT price = £2.18
▸ Ventolin Nebules (GlaxoSmithKline UK Ltd)
Salbutamol (as Salbutamol sulfate) 1 mg per 1 ml Ventolin 2.5mg Nebules | 20 unit dose [PoM] £1.65 DT price = £1.91
Salbutamol (as Salbutamol sulfate) 2 mg per 1 ml Ventolin 5mg Nebules | 20 unit dose [PoM] £2.78 DT price = £3.82

Combinations available: *Ipratropium with salbutamol*, p. 228

◀ 230

Terbutaline sulfate

● **INDICATIONS AND DOSE**

Asthma | Other conditions associated with reversible airways obstruction
▸ BY MOUTH
▸ Adult: Initially 2.5 mg 3 times a day for 1–2 weeks, then increased to up to 5 mg 3 times a day, use by inhalation preferred over by mouth
▸ BY SUBCUTANEOUS INJECTION, OR BY SLOW INTRAVENOUS INJECTION
▸ Adult: 250–500 micrograms up to 4 times a day, reserve intravenous beta₂ agonists for those in whom inhaled therapy cannot be used reliably or there is no current effect
▸ BY CONTINUOUS INTRAVENOUS INFUSION
▸ Adult: 90–300 micrograms/hour for 8-10 hours, to be administered as a solution containing 3–5 micrograms/mL, high doses require close monitoring, reserve intravenous beta₂ continued →

Respiratory system

3

3

Respiratory system

agonists for those in whom inhaled therapy cannot be used reliably or there is no current effect

▶ BY INHALATION OF POWDER

▸ Adult: 500 micrograms up to 4 times a day, for persistent symptoms

▶ BY INHALATION OF NEBULISED SOLUTION

▸ Adult: 5–10 mg 2–4 times a day, additional doses may be necessary in severe acute asthma

Acute asthma

▶ BY SUBCUTANEOUS INJECTION, OR BY SLOW INTRAVENOUS INJECTION

▸ Child 2-14 years: 10 micrograms/kg up to 4 times a day (max. per dose 300 micrograms), reserve intravenous beta₂ agonists for those in whom inhaled therapy cannot be used reliably or there is no current effect

▸ Child 15-17 years: 250–500 micrograms up to 4 times a day, reserve intravenous beta₂ agonists for those in whom inhaled therapy cannot be used reliably or there is no current effect

▶ BY CONTINUOUS INTRAVENOUS INFUSION

▸ Child: Loading dose 2–4 micrograms/kg, then 1–10 micrograms/kg/hour, dose to be adjusted according to response and heart rate, close monitoring is required for doses above 10 micrograms/kg/hour, reserve intravenous beta₂ agonists for those in whom inhaled therapy cannot be used reliably or there is no current effect

Moderate, severe, or life-threatening acute asthma

▶ BY INHALATION OF NEBULISED SOLUTION

▸ Child 1 month-4 years: 5 mg, repeat every 20–30 minutes or when required, give via oxygen-driven nebuliser if available

▸ Child 5-11 years: 5–10 mg, repeat every 20–30 minutes or when required, give via oxygen-driven nebuliser if available

▸ Child 12-17 years: 10 mg, repeat every 20–30 minutes or when required, give via oxygen-driven nebuliser if available

▸ Adult: 10 mg, repeat every 20–30 minutes or when required, give via oxygen-driven nebuliser if available

Exacerbation of reversible airways obstruction (including nocturnal asthma) | Prevention of exercise-induced bronchospasm

▶ BY INHALATION OF POWDER

▸ Child 5-17 years: 500 micrograms up to 4 times a day, for occasional use only

▶ BY MOUTH

▸ Child 1 month-6 years: 75 micrograms/kg 3 times a day (max. per dose 2.5 mg), administration by mouth is not recommended

▸ Child 7-14 years: 2.5 mg 2–3 times a day, administration by mouth is not recommended

▸ Child 15-17 years: Initially 2.5 mg 3 times a day, then increased if necessary to 5 mg 3 times a day, administration by mouth is not recommended

Uncomplicated premature labour (between 22 and 37 weeks of gestation) (specialist supervision in hospital)

▶ BY INTRAVENOUS INFUSION

▸ Adult: Initially 5 micrograms/minute for 20 minutes, then increased in steps of 2.5 micrograms/minute every 20 minutes until contractions have ceased (more than 10 micrograms/minute should **seldom** be given— 20 micrograms/minute should **not** be exceeded), continue for 1 hour, then reduced in steps of 2.5 micrograms/minute every 20 minutes to lowest dose that maintains suppression (maximum total duration 48 hours)

PHARMACOKINETICS

At recommended inhaled doses, the duration of action of terbutaline is about 3 to 5 hours.

● UNLICENSED USE Injection not licensed for use in children under 2 years.

● CONTRA-INDICATIONS

▸ When used for uncomplicated premature labour Abruptio placenta · antepartum haemorrhage · cord compression · eclampsia · history of cardiac disease · intra-uterine fetal death · intra-uterine infection · placenta praevia · pulmonary hypertension · severe pre-eclampsia · significant risk factors for myocardial ischaemia · threatened miscarriage

● CAUTIONS Mild to moderate pre-eclampsia (when used for uncomplicated premature labour) · suspected cardiovascular disease (should be assessed by a cardiologist before initiating therapy for uncomplicated premature labour)

● SIDE-EFFECTS

GENERAL SIDE-EFFECTS
Nausea

SPECIFIC SIDE-EFFECTS

▸ When used for uncomplicated premature labour Muscle tension · pulmonary oedema · vomiting

● PREGNANCY Inhaled drugs for asthma can be taken as normal during pregnancy.

● BREAST FEEDING Inhaled drugs for asthma can be taken as normal during breast-feeding.

● MONITORING REQUIREMENTS In uncomplicated premature labour it is important to monitor blood pressure, pulse rate (should not exceed 120 beats per minute), ECG (discontinue treatment if signs of myocardial ischaemia develop), blood glucose and lactate concentrations, and the patient's fluid and electrolyte status (avoid over-hydration—discontinue drug immediately and initiate diuretic therapy if pulmonary oedema occurs).

● DIRECTIONS FOR ADMINISTRATION

▸ With intravenous use in children For *continuous intravenous infusion*, dilute to a concentration of 5 micrograms/mL with Glucose 5% or Sodium Chloride 0.9%; if fluid-restricted, dilute to a concentration of 100 micrograms/mL.

▸ When used by inhalation For *nebulisation*, dilute nebuliser solution with sterile Sodium Chloride 0.9% solution according to nebuliser type and duration of administration; terbutaline and ipratropium bromide solutions are compatible and may be mixed for nebulisation.

▸ With intravenous use in adults For *bronchodilation* by *continuous intravenous infusion*, dilute 1.5–2.5 mg with 500 mL glucose 5% or sodium chloride 0.9% and give over 8–10 hours. For *premature labour* by *continuous intravenous infusion*, dilute in glucose 5% and give *via* controlled infusion device preferably a syringe pump; if syringe pump available dilute to a concentration of 100 micrograms/mL; if syringe pump not available dilute to a concentration of 10 micrograms/mL; close attention to patient's fluid and electrolyte status essential.

● PATIENT AND CARER ADVICE

▸ When used by inhalation For *inhalation by dry powder*, advise patients and carers not to exceed prescribed dose and to follow manufacturer's directions; if a previously effective dose of inhaled terbutaline fails to provide at least 3 hours relief, a doctor's advice should be obtained as soon as possible. For *inhalation by nebuliser*, the dose given by nebuliser is substantially higher than that given by inhaler. Patients should therefore be warned that it is dangerous to exceed the prescribed dose and they should seek medical advice if they fail to respond to the usual dose of the respirator solution.

● MEDICINAL FORMS
There can be variation in the licensing of different medicines containing the same drug. Forms available from special-order manufacturers include: solution for injection

Tablet
▸ Bricanyl (AstraZeneca UK Ltd)
  Terbutaline sulfate 5 mg Bricanyl 5mg tablets | 100 tablet [PoM] £4.91 DT price = £4.91

Oral solution
▸ Bricanyl (AstraZeneca UK Ltd)
  Terbutaline sulfate 300 microgram per 1 ml Bricanyl 1.5mg/5ml syrup sugar-free | 100 ml [PoM] £2.80 DT price = £2.80

Solution for injection
▸ Bricanyl (AstraZeneca UK Ltd)
  Terbutaline sulfate 500 microgram per 1 ml Bricanyl 2.5mg/5ml solution for injection ampoules | 10 ampoule [PoM] £16.74
  Bricanyl 500micrograms/1ml solution for injection ampoules | 5 ampoule [PoM] £2.16

Inhalation powder
▸ Bricanyl Turbohaler (AstraZeneca UK Ltd)
  Terbutaline sulfate 500 microgram per 1 dose Bricanyl 500micrograms/dose Turbohaler | 100 dose [PoM] £6.92 DT price = £6.92

Nebuliser liquid
▸ Terbutaline sulfate (Non-proprietary)
  Terbutaline sulfate 2.5 mg per 1 ml Terbutaline 5mg/2ml nebuliser liquid unit dose vials | 20 unit dose [PoM] £4.04 DT price = £4.04
▸ Bricanyl Respules (AstraZeneca UK Ltd)
  Terbutaline sulfate 2.5 mg per 1 ml Bricanyl 5mg/2ml Respules | 20 unit dose [PoM] £5.82 DT price = £4.04

CORTICOSTEROIDS

Airways disease, use of corticosteroids

Asthma

Inhaled corticosteroids

An inhaled corticosteroid used for 3–4 weeks may help to distinguish asthma from chronic obstructive pulmonary disease; clear improvement over 3–4 weeks suggests asthma.

Corticosteroids are effective in *asthma*; they reduce airway inflammation (and hence reduce oedema and secretion of mucus into the airway).

An inhaled corticosteroid is used regularly for prophylaxis of asthma when patients require a beta$_2$ agonist more than twice a week, or if symptoms disturb sleep at least once a week, or if the patient has suffered an exacerbation in the last 2 years requiring a systemic corticosteroid. *Regular use of* inhaled corticosteroids reduces the risk of exacerbation of asthma.

Current and previous smoking reduces the effectiveness of inhaled corticosteroids and higher doses may be necessary.

Corticosteroid inhalers must be used regularly for maximum benefit; alleviation of symptoms usually occurs 3 to 7 days after initiation. Beclometasone dipropionate p. 238, budesonide p. 240, fluticasone p. 242, and mometasone furoate p. 244 appear to be equally effective. Preparations that combine a corticosteroid with a long-acting beta$_2$ agonist may be helpful for patients stabilised on the individual components in the same proportion.

In adults using an inhaled corticosteroid and a long-acting beta$_2$ agonist for the prophylaxis of asthma, but who are poorly controlled, *Symbicort* ® or *DuoResp Spiromax* ® (both containing budesonide with formoterol p. 241) can be used as relievers (instead of a short-acting beta$_2$ agonist), in addition to their regular use for the prophylaxis of asthma. *Symbicort* ® can also be used in this way in adults using an inhaled corticosteroid with a dose greater than beclometasone dipropionate 400 micrograms daily, but who are poorly controlled (standard doses of other inhaled corticosteroids can be used). When starting this treatment, the total regular daily dose of inhaled corticosteroid should

not be reduced. Patients must be carefully instructed on the appropriate dose and management of exacerbations before initiating this therapy. Patients using budesonide with formoterol as a reliever once a day or more should have their treatment reviewed regularly. The use of *Symbicort* ® for both reliever and maintenance therapy is also used by some specialists in children 12–18 years [unlicensed]. *Fostair* ® can also be used in adults as a reliever (instead of a short-acting beta$_2$ agonist) in addition to its regular use for the prophylaxis of asthma. It may be particularly useful for patients with poorly controlled asthma requiring reliever therapy, or for those who have had previous exacerbations of asthma which needed medical intervention. Patients requiring frequent daily use of *Fostair* ® as a reliever should have their maintenance treatment reviewed. This approach has not been investigated with combination inhalers containing other corticosteroids and long-acting beta$_2$ agonists.

High doses of inhaled corticosteroid can be prescribed for patients who respond only partially to standard doses with a long-acting beta$_2$ agonist or another long-acting bronchodilator. High doses should be continued only if there is clear benefit over the lower dose. The recommended maximum dose of an inhaled corticosteroid should not generally be exceeded. However, if a higher dose is required, then it should be initiated and supervised by a specialist. The use of high doses of inhaled corticosteroid can minimise the requirement for an oral corticosteroid.

Oral corticosteroids

Systemic corticosteroid therapy may be necessary during episodes of stress, such as severe infection, or if the asthma is worsening, when higher doses are needed and access of inhaled drug to small airways may be reduced; patients may need a reserve supply of corticosteroid tablets.

In chronic asthma, when the response to other drugs has been inadequate, longer term administration of an oral corticosteroid may be necessary; in such cases high doses of an inhaled corticosteroid should be continued to minimise oral corticosteroid requirements. Patients taking long-term oral corticosteroids for asthma can often be transferred to an inhaled corticosteroid but the transfer must be slow, with gradual reduction in the dose of the oral corticosteroid, and at a time when the asthma is well controlled.

An acute attack of asthma should be treated with a short course of an oral corticosteroid starting with a high dose. Patients whose asthma has deteriorated rapidly usually respond quickly to corticosteroids. The dose can usually be stopped abruptly; tapering is not needed provided that the patient receives an inhaled corticosteroid in an adequate dose (apart from those on maintenance oral corticosteroid treatment or where oral corticosteroids are required for 3 or more weeks). In patients who have needed several courses of oral corticosteroids and in whom the possibility of a period on maintenance corticosteroids is being considered, it may be useful to taper the corticosteroid dose gradually to identify a threshold dose for asthma control. This should only be done after other standard options for controlling asthma have been tried.

An oral corticosteroid should normally be taken as a single dose in the morning to reduce the disturbance to circadian cortisol secretion. Dosage should always be titrated to the lowest dose that controls symptoms. Regular peak-flow measurements help to optimise the dose.

Parenteral corticosteroids

Hydrocortisone injection p. 612 has a role in the emergency treatment of acute severe asthma.

Chronic obstructive pulmonary disease

Inhaled corticosteroids

In *chronic obstructive pulmonary disease* inhaled corticosteroid therapy may reduce exacerbations when given in combination with an inhaled long-acting beta$_2$ agonist.

Respiratory system

3

Oral corticosteroids

During an acute exacerbation of chronic obstructive pulmonary disease, prednisolone p. 614 should be given; treatment can be stopped abruptly. Prolonged treatment with oral prednisolone is of no benefit and maintenance treatment is not normally recommended.

Corticosteroids (inhaled)

● INTERACTIONS → Appendix 1 (corticosteroids). Interactions do not generally apply to corticosteroids used for inhalation unless specified.

● SIDE-EFFECTS

▶ **Very rare** Paradoxical bronchospasm

▶ **Frequency not known** Adrenal crisis (with prolonged high doses) · adrenal suppression (with prolonged high doses) · aggression (particularly in children) · anxiety · behavioural changes (particularly in children) · bruising · candidiasis of the mouth · candidiasis of the throat · cataracts · coma (with prolonged high doses) · Cushing's syndrome (with moon face, striae and acne) · depression · dysphonia · glaucoma (with prolonged high doses) · hoarseness · hyperactivity (particularly in children) · hyperglycaemia (usually only with high doses) · irritability (particularly in children) · lower respiratory tract infections in older patients with chronic obstructive pulmonary disease (with high doses) · pneumonia in older patients with chronic obstructive pulmonary disease (with high doses) · reduced growth velocity (in children) · reduced mineral bone density (with long-term treatment of high doses) · side-effects applicable to systemic corticosteroids may also apply if absorption occurs following inhaled use · sleep disturbances · throat irritation

SIDE-EFFECTS, FURTHER INFORMATION

▶ Candidiasis The risk of oral candidiasis can be reduced by using a spacer device with the corticosteroid inhaler; rinsing the mouth with water after inhalation of a dose may also be helpful. An anti-fungal oral suspension or oral gel can be used to treat oral candidiasis without discontinuing corticosteroid therapy.

▶ Paradoxical bronchospasm The potential for paradoxical bronchospasm (calling for discontinuation and alternative therapy) should be borne in mind—mild bronchospasm may be prevented by inhalation of a short-acting beta$_2$ agonist beforehand (or by transfer from an aerosol inhalation to a dry powder inhalation).

● PREGNANCY Inhaled drugs for asthma can be taken as normal during pregnancy.

● BREAST FEEDING Inhaled corticosteroids for asthma can be taken as normal during breast-feeding.

● MONITORING REQUIREMENTS

▶ In children The height and weight of children receiving prolonged treatment with inhaled corticosteroids should be monitored annually; if growth is slowed, referral to a paediatrician should be considered.

● NATIONAL FUNDING/ACCESS DECISIONS

NICE technology appraisals (TAs)

▶ Inhaled corticosteroids for the treatment of chronic asthma in children under 12 years (November 2007) NICE TA131

▶ In children For children under 12 years with chronic asthma in whom treatment with an inhaled corticosteroid is considered appropriate, the least costly product that is suitable for an individual child (taking into consideration NICE TAs 38 and 10), within its marketing authorisation, is recommended. For children under 12 years with chronic asthma in whom treatment with an inhaled corticosteroid and a long-acting beta$_2$ agonist is considered appropriate, the following apply:

● the use of a combination inhaler within its marketing authorisation is recommended as an option;

● the decision to use a combination inhaler or two agents in separate inhalers should be made on an individual basis, taking into consideration therapeutic need and the likelihood of treatment adherence;

● if a combination inhaler is chosen, then the least costly inhaler that is suitable for the individual child is recommended.

www.nice.org.uk/TA131

▶ Inhaled corticosteroids for the treatment of chronic asthma in adults and children over 12 years (March 2008) NICE TA138

For adults and children over 12 years with chronic asthma in whom treatment with an inhaled corticosteroid is considered appropriate, the least costly product that is suitable for an individual (taking into consideration NICE TAs 38 and 10), within its marketing authorisation is recommended.

For adults and children over 12 years with chronic asthma in whom treatment with an inhaled corticosteroid and a long-acting beta$_2$ agonist is considered appropriate, the following apply:

● the use of a combination inhaler within its marketing authorisation is recommended as an option;

● the decision to use a combination inhaler or two agents in separate inhalers should be made on an individual basis, taking into consideration therapeutic need, and the likelihood of treatment adherence;

● if a combination inhaler is chosen, then the least costly inhaler that is suitable for the individual is recommended.

www.nice.org.uk/TA138

◀ above

Beclometasone dipropionate

(Beclomethasone dipropionate)

● INDICATIONS AND DOSE

Prophylaxis of asthma

▶ BY INHALATION OF POWDER

▶ Child 5-11 years: 100–200 micrograms twice daily, dose to be adjusted as necessary

▶ Child 12-17 years: 200–400 micrograms twice daily; increased if necessary up to 800 micrograms twice daily, dose to be adjusted as necessary

▶ Adult: 200–400 micrograms twice daily; increased if necessary up to 800 micrograms twice daily, dose to be adjusted as necessary

ASMABEC CLICKHALER®

Prophylaxis of asthma

▶ BY INHALATION OF POWDER

▶ Child 6-11 years: 100–200 micrograms twice daily, dose to be adjusted as necessary

▶ Child 12-17 years: 100–400 micrograms twice daily (max. per dose 1 mg twice daily), dose to be adjusted as necessary

▶ Adult: 100–400 micrograms twice daily (max. per dose 1 mg twice daily), dose to be adjusted as necessary

CLENIL MODULITE®

Prophylaxis of asthma

▶ BY INHALATION OF AEROSOL

▶ Child 2-11 years: 100–200 micrograms twice daily

▶ Child 12-17 years: 200–400 micrograms twice daily, adjusted according to response; increased if necessary up to 1 mg twice daily

▶ Adult: 200–400 micrograms twice daily, adjusted according to response; increased if necessary up to 1 mg twice daily

QVAR® PREPARATIONS

Prophylaxis of asthma

▶ BY INHALATION OF AEROSOL
▶ Child 12-17 years: 50–200 micrograms twice daily; increased if necessary up to 400 micrograms twice daily
▶ Adult: 50–200 micrograms twice daily; increased if necessary up to 400 micrograms twice daily

POTENCY

Qvar® has extra-fine particles, is more potent than traditional beclometasone dipropionate CFC-containing inhalers and is approximately twice as potent as *Clenil Modulite®*.

DOSE EQUIVALENCE AND CONVERSION

Dose adjustments may be required for some inhaler devices, see under individual preparations.

● UNLICENSED USE *Easyhaler® Beclometasone Dipropionate* is not licensed for use in children under 18 years. *Clenil Modulite®* -200 and -250 are not licensed for use in children under 12 years. *Qvar®* is not licensed for use in children under 12 years.

IMPORTANT SAFETY INFORMATION

MHRA/CHM ADVICE (JULY 2008)

Beclometasone dipropionate CFC-free pressurised metered-dose inhalers (*Qvar®* and *Clenil Modulite®*) are **not** interchangeable and should be prescribed by brand name; *Qvar®* has extra-fine particles, is more potent than traditional beclometasone dipropionate CFC-containing inhalers, and is approximately twice as potent as *Clenil Modulite®*.

● PRESCRIBING AND DISPENSING INFORMATION The MHRA has advised (July 2008) that beclometasone dipropionate CFC-free inhalers should be prescribed by brand name.

CLENIL MODULITE® *Clenil Modulite®* is not interchangeable with other CFC-free beclometasone dipropionate inhalers.

QVAR® PREPARATIONS When switching a patient with well-controlled asthma from another corticosteroid inhaler, initially a 100-microgram metered dose of *Qvar®* should be prescribed for 200–250 micrograms of beclometasone dipropionate or budesonide and for 100 micrograms of fluticasone propionate. When switching a patient with poorly controlled asthma from another corticosteroid inhaler, initially a 100-microgram metered dose of *Qvar®* should be prescribed for 100 micrograms of beclometasone dipropionate, budesonide, or fluticasone propionate; the dose of *Qvar®* should be adjusted according to response.

● PATIENT AND CARER ADVICE Steroid card should be issued with high doses of inhaled beclometasone dipropionate. Medicines for Children leaflet: Beclometasone for asthma prevention (prophylaxis) www.medicinesforchildren.org.uk/beclometasone-inhaler-asthma-prevention-prophylaxis-0

● PROFESSION SPECIFIC INFORMATION

Dental practitioners' formulary

Clenil Modulite® 50 micrograms/metered inhalation may be prescribed.

● MEDICINAL FORMS
There can be variation in the licensing of different medicines containing the same drug.

Pressurised inhalation

CAUTIONARY AND ADVISORY LABELS 8, 10
▶ Beclometasone dipropionate (Non-proprietary)
Beclometasone dipropionate 50 microgram per 1 dose Beclometasone 50micrograms/dose inhaler CFC free | 200 dose [PoM] no price available
Beclometasone dipropionate 100 microgram per 1 dose Beclometasone 100micrograms/dose inhaler CFC free | 200 dose [PoM] £54.20

Beclometasone dipropionate 200 microgram per 1 dose Beclometasone 200micrograms/dose inhaler CFC free | 200 dose [PoM] no price available
▶ Clenil Modulite (Chiesi Ltd)
Beclometasone dipropionate 50 microgram per 1 dose Clenil Modulite 50micrograms/dose inhaler | 200 dose [PoM] £3.70
Beclometasone dipropionate 100 microgram per 1 dose Clenil Modulite 100micrograms/dose inhaler | 200 dose [PoM] £7.42
Beclometasone dipropionate 200 microgram per 1 dose Clenil Modulite 200micrograms/dose inhaler | 200 dose [PoM] £16.17
Beclometasone dipropionate 250 microgram per 1 dose Clenil Modulite 250micrograms/dose inhaler | 200 dose [PoM] £16.29
▶ Qvar (Teva UK Ltd)
Beclometasone dipropionate 50 microgram per 1 dose Qvar 50 inhaler | 200 dose [PoM] £7.87
Beclometasone dipropionate 100 microgram per 1 dose Qvar 100 inhaler | 200 dose [PoM] £17.21
▶ Qvar Autohaler (Teva UK Ltd)
Beclometasone dipropionate 50 microgram per 1 dose Qvar 50 Autohaler | 200 dose [PoM] £7.87 DT price = £7.87
Beclometasone dipropionate 100 microgram per 1 dose Qvar 100 Autohaler | 200 dose [PoM] £17.21 DT price = £17.21
▶ Qvar Easi-Breathe (Teva UK Ltd)
Beclometasone dipropionate 50 microgram per 1 dose Qvar 50micrograms/dose Easi-Breathe inhaler | 200 dose [PoM] £7.74 DT price = £7.87
Beclometasone dipropionate 100 microgram per 1 dose Qvar 100micrograms/dose Easi-Breathe inhaler | 200 dose [PoM] £16.95 DT price = £17.21

Inhalation powder

CAUTIONARY AND ADVISORY LABELS 8, 10
▶ Asmabec Clickhaler (Focus Pharmaceuticals Ltd)
Beclometasone dipropionate 100 microgram per 1 dose Asmabec 100 Clickhaler | 200 dose [PoM] £9.81
▶ Easyhaler (beclometasone) (Orion Pharma (UK) Ltd)
Beclometasone dipropionate 200 microgram per 1 dose Easyhaler Beclometasone 200micrograms/dose dry powder inhaler | 200 dose [PoM] £14.93

▌Beclometasone with formoterol

The properties listed below are those particular to the combination only. For the properties of the components please consider, beclometasone dipropionate p. 238, formoterol fumarate p. 231.

● INDICATIONS AND DOSE

Asthma maintenance therapy

▶ BY INHALATION OF AEROSOL, OR BY INHALATION OF POWDER
▶ Adult: 100/6–200/12 micrograms twice daily; maximum 400/24 micrograms per day

Asthma, maintenance and reliever therapy

▶ BY INHALATION OF AEROSOL
▶ Adult: Maintenance 100/6 micrograms twice daily; 100/6 micrograms as required for relief of symptoms; maximum 800/48 micrograms per day

Chronic obstructive pulmonary disease with forced expiratory volume in 1 second < 50% of predicted

▶ BY INHALATION OF AEROSOL
▶ Adult: 200/12 micrograms twice daily

DOSE EQUIVALENCE AND CONVERSION

For inhalation of aerosol, when switching patients from other beclometasone dipropionate and formoterol fumarate inhalers, *Fostair®* 100/6 can be prescribed for patients already using beclometasone dipropionate 250 micrograms in another CFC-free inhaler; the dose of *Fostair®* should be adjusted according to response. For inhalation of powder, when switching patients from other beclometasone dipropionate formulations with non-extrafine particle size distribution, the dose should be adjusted according to response. continued →

3

Respiratory system

1 puff is equivalent to 100 micrograms beclometasone dipropionate and 6 micrograms formoterol fumarate.

> **IMPORTANT SAFETY INFORMATION**
> MHRA/CHM ADVICE (JULY 2008)
> *Fostair*® contains extra-fine particles of beclometasone dipropionate and is more potent than traditional beclometasone dipropionate CFC-free inhalers. The dose of beclometasone dipropionate in *Fostair*® should be lower than non-extra-fine formulations of beclometasone dipropionate and will need to be adjusted to the individual needs of the patient.

- PATIENT AND CARER ADVICE With high doses, a steroid card should be supplied.
  Patients or carers should be given advice on how to administer beclometasone with formoterol aerosol for inhalation.

- MEDICINAL FORMS
  There can be variation in the licensing of different medicines containing the same drug.
  Pressurised inhalation
  CAUTIONARY AND ADVISORY LABELS 8, 10
  ▸ Fostair (Chiesi Ltd)
  Formoterol fumarate dihydrate 6 microgram, Beclometasone dipropionate 200 microgram Fostair 200micrograms/dose / 6micrograms/dose inhaler | 120 dose [PoM] £29.32
  Formoterol fumarate dihydrate 6 microgram per 1 dose, Beclometasone dipropionate 100 microgram per 1 dose Fostair 100micrograms/dose / 6micrograms/dose inhaler | 120 dose [PoM] £29.32 DT price = £29.32
  Inhalation powder
  CAUTIONARY AND ADVISORY LABELS 8, 10
  ▸ Fostair NEXThaler (Chiesi Ltd)
  Formoterol fumarate dihydrate 6 microgram per 1 dose, Beclometasone dipropionate 100 microgram per 1 dose Fostair NEXThaler 100micrograms/dose / 6micrograms/dose dry powder inhaler | 120 dose [PoM] £29.32
  Formoterol fumarate dihydrate 6 microgram per 1 dose, Beclometasone dipropionate 200 microgram per 1 dose Fostair NEXThaler 200micrograms/dose / 6micrograms/dose dry powder inhaler | 120 dose [PoM] £29.32

◀ 238

Budesonide

- INDICATIONS AND DOSE
  Prophylaxis of mild to moderate asthma (in patients stabilised on twice daily dose)
  ▶ BY INHALATION OF POWDER
  ▸ Child 6-11 years: 200–400 micrograms once daily, dose to be given in the evening
  ▸ Child 12-17 years: 200–400 micrograms once daily (max. per dose 800 micrograms), dose to be given in the evening
  ▸ Adult: 200–400 micrograms once daily (max. per dose 800 micrograms), dose to be given in the evening
  Prophylaxis of asthma
  ▶ BY INHALATION OF POWDER
  ▸ Child 6-11 years: 100–400 micrograms twice daily, dose to be adjusted as necessary
  ▸ Child 12-17 years: 100–800 micrograms twice daily, dose to be adjusted as necessary
  ▸ Adult: 100–800 micrograms twice daily, dose to be adjusted as necessary
  ▶ BY INHALATION OF NEBULISED SUSPENSION
  ▸ Child 6 months-11 years: 125–500 micrograms twice daily, adjusted according to response; maximum 2 mg per day
  ▸ Child 12-17 years: Initially 0.25–1 mg twice daily, adjusted according to response, doses higher than

recommended max. may be used in severe disease; maximum 2 mg per day
▸ Adult: Initially 0.25–1 mg twice daily, adjusted according to response, doses higher than recommended max. may be used in severe disease; maximum 2 mg per day

BUDELIN NOVOLIZER®
Prophylaxis of asthma
▶ BY INHALATION OF POWDER
▸ Adult: 200–800 micrograms twice daily, dose is adjusted as necessary
Alternative in mild to moderate asthma, for patients previously stabilised on a twice daily dose
▶ BY INHALATION OF POWDER
▸ Adult: 200–400 micrograms once daily (max. per dose 800 micrograms), to be taken in the evening

PULMICORT® RESPULES
Prophylaxis of asthma
▶ BY INHALATION OF NEBULISED SUSPENSION
▸ Child 3 months-11 years: Initially 0.5–1 mg twice daily, reduced to 250–500 micrograms twice daily
▸ Child 12-17 years: Initially 1–2 mg twice daily, reduced to 0.5–1 mg twice daily
▸ Adult: Initially 1–2 mg twice daily, reduced to 0.5–1 mg twice daily

PULMICORT® TURBOHALER
Prophylaxis of asthma
▶ BY INHALATION OF POWDER
▸ Adult: 100–800 micrograms twice daily, dose to be adjusted as necessary
Alternative in mild to moderate asthma, for patients previously stabilised on a twice daily dose
▶ BY INHALATION OF POWDER
▸ Adult: 200–400 micrograms once daily (max. per dose 800 micrograms), to be taken in the evening
POTENCY
Dose adjustments may be required for some inhaler devices, see under individual preparations.

- UNLICENSED USE *Pulmicort*® nebuliser solution not licensed for use in children under 3 months.
- DIRECTIONS FOR ADMINISTRATION Budesonide nebuliser suspension is not suitable for use in ultrasonic nebulisers.
- PATIENT AND CARER ADVICE With high doses, a steroid card should be supplied. Patients or carers should be given advice on how to administer budesonide dry powder inhaler and nebuliser suspension.
  Medicines for Children leaflet: Budesonide inhaler for asthma prevention (prophylaxis) www.medicinesforchildren.org.uk/budesonide-inhaler-asthma-prevention-prophylaxis
  BUDELIN NOVOLIZER® Patients or carers should be given advice on adminstration of *Budelin NovolizerA*®.

- MEDICINAL FORMS
  There can be variation in the licensing of different medicines containing the same drug.
  Inhalation powder
  CAUTIONARY AND ADVISORY LABELS 8, 10
  ▸ Budelin Novolizer (Meda Pharmaceuticals Ltd)
  Budesonide 200 microgram per 1 dose Budelin Novolizer 200micrograms/dose inhalation powder | 100 dose [PoM] £14.86
  Budelin Novolizer 200micrograms/dose inhalation powder refill | 100 dose [PoM] £9.59
  ▸ Easyhaler (budesonide) (Orion Pharma (UK) Ltd)
  Budesonide 100 microgram per 1 dose Easyhaler Budesonide 100micrograms/dose dry powder inhaler | 200 dose [PoM] £8.86 DT price = £11.84
  Budesonide 200 microgram per 1 dose Easyhaler Budesonide 200micrograms/dose dry powder inhaler | 200 dose [PoM] £17.71
  Budesonide 400 microgram per 1 dose Easyhaler Budesonide 400micrograms/dose dry powder inhaler | 100 dose [PoM] £17.71

▸ Pulmicort Turbohaler (AstraZeneca UK Ltd)
Budesonide 100 microgram per 1 dose Pulmicort 100 Turbohaler | 200 dose PoM £11.84 DT price = £11.84
Budesonide 200 microgram per 1 dose Pulmicort 200 Turbohaler | 100 dose PoM £11.84 DT price = £11.84
Budesonide 400 microgram per 1 dose Pulmicort 400 Turbohaler | 50 dose PoM £13.86 DT price = £13.86

Nebuliser liquid
CAUTIONARY AND ADVISORY LABELS 8, 10
▸ Budesonide (Non-proprietary)
Budesonide 250 microgram per 1 ml Budesonide 500micrograms/2ml nebuliser liquid unit dose vials | 20 unit dose PoM £63.00 DT price = £24.70
Budesonide 500 microgram per 1 ml Budesonide 1mg/2ml nebuliser liquid unit dose vials | 20 unit dose PoM £42.41 DT price = £34.62
▸ Pulmicort Respules (AstraZeneca UK Ltd)
Budesonide 250 microgram per 1 ml Pulmicort 0.5mg Respules | 20 unit dose PoM £26.42 DT price = £24.70
Budesonide 500 microgram per 1 ml Pulmicort 1mg Respules | 20 unit dose PoM £40.00 DT price = £34.62

Budesonide with formoterol

The properties listed below are those particular to the combination only. For the properties of the components please consider, budesonide p. 240, formoterol fumarate p. 231.

● INDICATIONS AND DOSE

DUORESP SPIROMAX® 160MICROGRAMS/4.5MICROGRAMS

Asthma maintenance therapy
▸ BY INHALATION OF POWDER
▸ Adult: 1–2 inhalations twice daily, increased if necessary up to 4 inhalations twice daily

Asthma, maintenance and reliever therapy
▸ BY INHALATION OF POWDER
▸ Adult: 2 inhalations daily in 1–2 divided doses, increased if necessary to 2 inhalations twice daily. 1 inhalation (max. per dose 6 inhalations) as required, for relief of symptoms, a total daily dose of up to 12 inhalations can be used for a limited time but medical assessment is recommended if more than 8 inhalations daily are needed

Chronic obstructive pulmonary disease with forced expiratory volume in 1 second < 50% of predicted
▸ BY INHALATION OF POWDER
▸ Adult: 2 inhalations twice daily

DUORESP SPIROMAX® 320MICROGRAMS/9MICROGRAMS

Asthma, maintenance therapy
▸ BY INHALATION OF POWDER
▸ Adult: 1 inhalation twice dailyIncreased if necessary up to 2 inhalations twice daily

Chronic obstructive pulmonary disease with forced expiratory volume in 1 second < 50% of predicted
▸ BY INHALATION OF POWDER
▸ Adult: 1 inhalation twice daily

SYMBICORT 100/6 TURBOHALER®

Asthma, maintenance therapy
▸ BY INHALATION OF POWDER
▸ Child 6-17 years: Initially 1–2 puffs twice daily; reduced to 1 puff daily, dose reduced only if control is maintained
▸ Adult: Initially 1–2 puffs twice daily, increased if necessary up to 4 puffs twice daily; reduced to 1 puff daily, dose reduced only if control is maintained

Asthma, maintenance and reliever therapy
▸ BY INHALATION OF POWDER
▸ Adult: Maintenance 2 puffs daily in 1–2 divided doses; 1 puff as required for relief of symptoms, increased if necessary up to 6 puffs as required, max. 8 puffs per

day; up to 12 puffs daily can be used for a limited time but medical assessment should be considered

SYMBICORT 200/6 TURBOHALER®

Asthma, maintenance therapy
▸ BY INHALATION OF POWDER
▸ Child 12-17 years: Initially 1–2 puffs twice daily; reduced to 1 puff daily, dose reduced only if control is maintained
▸ Adult: Initially 1–2 puffs twice daily, increased if necessary up to 4 puffs twice daily; reduced to 1 puff daily, dose reduced only if control is maintained

Asthma, maintenance and reliever therapy
▸ BY INHALATION OF POWDER
▸ Adult: Maintenance 2 puffs daily in 1–2 divided doses, increased if necessary to 2 puffs twice daily; 1 puff as required for relief of symptoms, increased if necessary up to 6 puffs as required, max. 8 puffs per day; up to 12 puffs daily can be used for a limited time but medical assessment should be considered

Chronic obstructive pulmonary disease with forced expiratory volume in 1 second < 50% of predicted
▸ BY INHALATION OF POWDER
▸ Adult: 2 puffs twice daily

SYMBICORT 400/12 TURBOHALER®

Asthma, maintenance therapy
▸ BY INHALATION OF POWDER
▸ Child 12-17 years: Initially 1 puff twice daily; reduced to 1 puff daily, dose reduced only if control is maintained
▸ Adult: Initially 1 puff twice daily, increased if necessary up to 2 puffs twice daily; reduced to 1 puff daily, dose reduced only if control is maintained

Chronic obstructive pulmonary disease with forced expiratory volume in 1 second <50% of predicted
▸ BY INHALATION OF POWDER
▸ Adult: 1 puff twice daily

● PATIENT AND CARER ADVICE With high doses, a steroid card should be supplied.
Patients counselling is advised for budesonide with formoterol dry powder inhalation (administration).

● MEDICINAL FORMS
There can be variation in the licensing of different medicines containing the same drug.
Inhalation powder
CAUTIONARY AND ADVISORY LABELS 8, 10 (high doses)
▸ DuoResp Spiromax (Teva UK Ltd)
Formoterol fumarate dihydrate 6 microgram per 1 dose, Budesonide 200 microgram per 1 dose DuoResp Spiromax 160micrograms/dose / 4.5micrograms/dose dry powder inhaler | 120 dose PoM £29.97 DT price = £38.00
Formoterol fumarate dihydrate 12 microgram per 1 dose, Budesonide 400 microgram per 1 dose DuoResp Spiromax 320micrograms/dose / 9micrograms/dose dry powder inhaler | 60 dose PoM £29.97 DT price = £38.00
▸ Symbicort Turbohaler (AstraZeneca UK Ltd)
Formoterol fumarate dihydrate 6 microgram per 1 dose, Budesonide 100 microgram per 1 dose Symbicort 100/6 Turbohaler | 120 dose PoM £33.00 DT price = £33.00
Formoterol fumarate dihydrate 6 microgram per 1 dose, Budesonide 200 microgram per 1 dose Symbicort 200/6 Turbohaler | 120 dose PoM £38.00 DT price = £38.00
Formoterol fumarate dihydrate 12 microgram per 1 dose, Budesonide 400 microgram per 1 dose Symbicort 400/12 Turbohaler | 60 dose PoM £38.00 DT price = £38.00

Respiratory system

3

Ciclesonide

📖 238

- **INDICATIONS AND DOSE**

Prophylaxis of asthma
- ▶ BY INHALATION OF AEROSOL
- ▶ Child 12-17 years: 160 micrograms once daily; reduced to 80 micrograms daily, if control maintained
- ▶ Adult: Initially 160 micrograms once daily; reduced to 80 micrograms once daily, if control maintained; increased if necessary up to 320 micrograms twice daily, in severe asthma

- **UNLICENSED USE**
- ▶ In adults High dose recommended in severe asthma is unlicensed.
- **SIDE-EFFECTS** Nausea · taste disturbance
- **PATIENT AND CARER ADVICE** Patients or carers should be given advice on how to administer ciclesonide aerosol inhaler.

- **MEDICINAL FORMS**
There can be variation in the licensing of different medicines containing the same drug.
Pressurised inhalation
CAUTIONARY AND ADVISORY LABELS 8
- ▶ Alvesco (Takeda UK Ltd)
  Ciclesonide 80 microgram per 1 dose Alvesco 80 inhaler | 120 dose [PoM] £32.83 DT price = £32.83
  Ciclesonide 160 microgram per 1 dose Alvesco 160 inhaler | 60 dose [PoM] £19.31 DT price = £19.31 | 120 dose [PoM] £38.62 DT price = £38.62

Fluticasone

📖 238

4.1.2016

- **INDICATIONS AND DOSE**

Prophylaxis of asthma
- ▶ BY INHALATION OF POWDER
- ▶ Child 5-15 years: Initially 50–100 micrograms twice daily (max. per dose 200 micrograms twice daily), dose to be adjusted as necessary
- ▶ Child 16-17 years: Initially 100–500 micrograms twice daily (max. per dose 1 mg twice daily), dose may be increased according to severity of asthma. Doses above 500 micrograms twice daily initiated by a specialist
- ▶ Adult: Initially 100–500 micrograms twice daily (max. per dose 1 mg twice daily), dose may be increased according to severity of asthma. Doses above 500 micrograms twice daily initiated by a specialist
- ▶ BY INHALATION OF AEROSOL
- ▶ Child 4-15 years: Initially 50–100 micrograms twice daily (max. per dose 200 micrograms twice daily), dose to be adjusted as necessary
- ▶ Child 16-17 years: Initially 100–500 micrograms twice daily (max. per dose 1 mg twice daily), dose may be increased according to severity of asthma. Doses above 500 micrograms twice daily initiated by a specialist
- ▶ Adult: Initially 100–500 micrograms twice daily (max. per dose 1 mg twice daily), dose may be increased according to severity of asthma. Doses above 500 micrograms twice daily initiated by a specialist
- ▶ BY INHALATION OF NEBULISED SUSPENSION
- ▶ Child 4-15 years: 1 mg twice daily
- ▶ Child 16-17 years: 0.5–2 mg twice daily
- ▶ Adult: 0.5–2 mg twice daily

- **SIDE-EFFECTS** Arthralgia · dyspepsia
- **DIRECTIONS FOR ADMINISTRATION** Fluticasone nebuliser liquid may be diluted with sterile sodium chloride 0.9%. It is not suitable for use in ultrasonic nebulisers.

- **PATIENT AND CARER ADVICE** With high doses, a steroid card should be supplied.
  Patients or carers should be given advice on how to administer all fluticasone inhalations preparations. Medicines for Children leaflet: Fluticasone inhaler for asthma prevention (prophylaxis) www.medicinesforchildren.org.uk/fluticasone-inhaler-for-asthma-prevention

- **MEDICINAL FORMS**
There can be variation in the licensing of different medicines containing the same drug.
Pressurised inhalation
CAUTIONARY AND ADVISORY LABELS 8, 10
- ▶ Flixotide Evohaler (GlaxoSmithKline UK Ltd)
  Fluticasone propionate 50 microgram per 1 dose Flixotide 50micrograms/dose Evohaler | 120 dose [PoM] £5.44 DT price = £5.44
  Fluticasone propionate 125 microgram per 1 dose Flixotide 125micrograms/dose Evohaler | 120 dose [PoM] £21.26 DT price = £21.26
  Fluticasone propionate 250 microgram per 1 dose Flixotide 250micrograms/dose Evohaler | 120 dose [PoM] £36.14 DT price = £36.14

Inhalation powder
CAUTIONARY AND ADVISORY LABELS 8, 10
- ▶ Flixotide Accuhaler (GlaxoSmithKline UK Ltd)
  Fluticasone propionate 50 microgram per 1 dose Flixotide 50micrograms/dose Accuhaler | 60 dose [PoM] £6.38 DT price = £6.38
  Fluticasone propionate 100 microgram per 1 dose Flixotide 100micrograms/dose Accuhaler | 60 dose [PoM] £8.93 DT price = £8.93
  Fluticasone propionate 250 microgram per 1 dose Flixotide 250micrograms/dose Accuhaler | 60 dose [PoM] £21.26 DT price = £21.26
  Fluticasone propionate 500 microgram per 1 dose Flixotide 500micrograms/dose Accuhaler | 60 dose [PoM] £36.14 DT price = £36.14

Nebuliser liquid
CAUTIONARY AND ADVISORY LABELS 8, 10
- ▶ Flixotide Nebule (GlaxoSmithKline UK Ltd)
  Fluticasone propionate 250 microgram per 1 ml Flixotide 0.5mg/2ml Nebules | 10 unit dose [PoM] £9.34
  Fluticasone propionate 1 mg per 1 ml Flixotide 2mg/2ml Nebules | 10 unit dose [PoM] £37.35

Fluticasone with formoterol

The properties listed below are those particular to the combination only. For the properties of the components please consider, fluticasone above, formoterol fumarate p. 231.

- **INDICATIONS AND DOSE**

FLUTIFORM® 50

Prophylaxis of asthma
- ▶ BY INHALATION OF AEROSOL
- ▶ Child 12-17 years: 2 puffs twice daily
- ▶ Adult: 2 puffs twice daily

FLUTIFORM® 125

Prophylaxis of asthma
- ▶ BY INHALATION OF AEROSOL
- ▶ Child 12-17 years: 2 puffs twice daily
- ▶ Adult: 2 puffs twice daily

FLUTIFORM® 250

Prophylaxis of asthma
- ▶ BY INHALATION OF AEROSOL
- ▶ Adult: 2 puffs twice daily

- **PATIENT AND CARER ADVICE** With high doses, a steroid card should be provided. Patients or carers should be given advice on how to administer fluticasone with formoterol aerosol inhalation.

• MEDICINAL FORMS
There can be variation in the licensing of different medicines containing the same drug.

Pressurised inhalation
CAUTIONARY AND ADVISORY LABELS 8, 10 (high doses)
▶ Flutiform (Napp Pharmaceuticals Ltd)
Formoterol fumarate dihydrate 5 microgram per 1 dose, Fluticasone propionate 50 microgram per 1 dose Flutiform 50micrograms/dose / 5micrograms/dose inhaler | 120 dose [PoM] £14.40 DT price = £14.40
Formoterol fumarate dihydrate 5 microgram per 1 dose, Fluticasone propionate 125 microgram per 1 dose Flutiform 125micrograms/dose / 5micrograms/dose inhaler | 120 dose [PoM] £28.00 DT price = £28.00
Formoterol fumarate dihydrate 10 microgram per 1 dose, Fluticasone propionate 250 microgram per 1 dose Flutiform 250micrograms/dose / 10micrograms/dose inhaler | 120 dose [PoM] £45.56 DT price = £45.56

Fluticasone with salmeterol

The properties listed below are those particular to the combination only. For the properties of the components please consider, fluticasone p. 242, salmeterol p. 232.

• INDICATIONS AND DOSE

SERETIDE 100 ACCUHALER®

Prophylaxis of asthma
▶ BY INHALATION OF POWDER
▶ Child 5-17 years: 1 inhalation twice daily, reduced to 1 inhalation daily, use reduced dose only if control maintained
▶ Adult: 1 inhalation twice daily, reduced to 1 inhalation daily, use reduced dose only if control maintained

SERETIDE 250 ACCUHALER®

Prophylaxis of asthma
▶ BY INHALATION OF POWDER
▶ Child 12-17 years: 1 inhalation twice daily
▶ Adult: 1 inhalation twice daily

SERETIDE 500 ACCUHALER®

Prophylaxis of asthma
▶ BY INHALATION OF POWDER
▶ Child 12-17 years: 1 inhalation twice daily
▶ Adult: 1 inhalation twice daily

Chronic obstructive pulmonary disease with forced expiratory volume in 1 second <60% of predicted
▶ BY INHALATION OF POWDER
▶ Adult: 1 inhalation twice daily

SERETIDE 50 EVOHALER®

Prophylaxis of asthma
▶ BY INHALATION OF AEROSOL
▶ Child 5-17 years: 2 puffs twice daily, reduced to 2 puffs once daily, use reduced dose only if control maintained
▶ Adult: 2 puffs twice daily, reduced to 2 puffs once daily, use reduced dose only if control maintained

SERETIDE 125 EVOHALER®

Prophylaxis of asthma
▶ BY INHALATION OF AEROSOL
▶ Child 12-17 years: 2 puffs twice daily
▶ Adult: 2 puffs twice daily

SERETIDE 250 EVOHALER®

Prophylaxis of asthma
▶ BY INHALATION OF AEROSOL
▶ Child 12-17 years: 2 puffs twice daily
▶ Adult: 2 puffs twice daily

• PATIENT AND CARER ADVICE With preparations containing greater than 100 micrograms fluticasone, a steroid card should be provided.
Patients or carers should be given advice on how to administer fluticasone with salmeterol dry powder inhalation and aerosol inhalation.

• NATIONAL FUNDING/ACCESS DECISIONS

Scottish Medicines Consortium (SMC) Decisions
The *Scottish Medicines Consortium* has advised (December 2008) that *Seretide 500 Accuhaler*® is **not** recommended for use within NHS Scotland for chronic obstructive pulmonary disease in patients with a forced expiratory volume in 1 second (FEV₁) less than 60% and greater than 50% of the predicted normal value, with significant symptoms despite regular bronchodilator therapy, and a history of repeated exacerbations.

• MEDICINAL FORMS
There can be variation in the licensing of different medicines containing the same drug.

Pressurised inhalation
CAUTIONARY AND ADVISORY LABELS 8, 10 (excluding Seretide 50 Evohaler®)
▶ Seretide Evohaler (GlaxoSmithKline UK Ltd)
Salmeterol (as Salmeterol xinafoate) 25 microgram per 1 dose, Fluticasone propionate 50 microgram per 1 dose Seretide 50 Evohaler | 120 dose [PoM] £18.00 DT price = £18.00
Salmeterol (as Salmeterol xinafoate) 25 microgram per 1 dose, Fluticasone propionate 125 microgram per 1 dose Seretide 125 Evohaler | 120 dose [PoM] £35.00 DT price = £35.00
Salmeterol (as Salmeterol xinafoate) 25 microgram per 1 dose, Fluticasone propionate 250 microgram per 1 dose Seretide 250 Evohaler | 120 dose [PoM] £59.48 DT price = £59.48

Inhalation powder
CAUTIONARY AND ADVISORY LABELS 8, 10 (excluding Seretide 100 Accuhaler®)
▶ Seretide Accuhaler (GlaxoSmithKline UK Ltd)
Salmeterol (as Salmeterol xinafoate) 50 microgram per 1 dose, Fluticasone propionate 100 microgram per 1 dose Seretide 100 Accuhaler | 60 dose [PoM] £18.00 DT price = £18.00
Salmeterol (as Salmeterol xinafoate) 50 microgram per 1 dose, Fluticasone propionate 250 microgram per 1 dose Seretide 250 Accuhaler | 60 dose [PoM] £35.00 DT price = £35.00
Salmeterol (as Salmeterol xinafoate) 50 microgram per 1 dose, Fluticasone propionate 500 microgram per 1 dose Seretide 500 Accuhaler | 60 dose [PoM] £40.92 DT price = £40.92

Fluticasone with vilanterol

The properties listed below are those particular to the combination only. For the properties of the components please consider, fluticasone p. 242.

• INDICATIONS AND DOSE

RELVAR ELLIPTA® 184 MICROGRAMS/22 MICROGRAMS

Prophylaxis of asthma
▶ BY INHALATION OF POWDER
▶ Child 12-17 years: 1 inhalation once daily
▶ Adult: 1 inhalation once daily

RELVAR ELLIPTA® 92 MICROGRAMS/22 MICROGRAMS

Prophylaxis of asthma
▶ BY INHALATION OF POWDER
▶ Child 12-17 years: 1 inhalation once daily
▶ Adult: 1 inhalation once daily

Chronic obstructive pulmonary disease with forced expiratory volume in 1 second < 70% of predicted
▶ BY INHALATION OF POWDER
▶ Adult: 1 inhalation once daily   continued →

DOSE EQUIVALENCE AND CONVERSION
RELVAR ELLIPTA® 184 MICROGRAMS/22 MICROGRAMS
1 inhalation (delivered dose) of fluticasone *furoate*
184 micrograms once daily is approximately equivalent to
fluticasone *propionate* 500 micrograms twice daily.
RELVAR ELLIPTA® 92 MICROGRAMS/22 MICROGRAMS
1 inhalation (delivered dose) of fluticasone *furoate*
92 micrograms once daily is approximately equivalent to
fluticasone *propionate* 250 micrograms twice daily.

- SIDE-EFFECTS Abdominal pain · back pain
- PREGNANCY Manufacturer advises use only if potential
  benefit outweighs risk.
- BREAST FEEDING Manufacturer advises avoid—no
  information available.
- HEPATIC IMPAIRMENT Max. dose fluticasone furoate
  92 micrograms, vilanterol 22 micrograms.
  RELVAR ELLIPTA®
  184 MICROGRAMS/22 MICROGRAMS Avoid in moderate to
  severe impairment.
- PATIENT AND CARER ADVICE A steroid card should be
  provided.
    Patients or carers should be given advice on how to
  administer fluticasone with vilanterol powder for
  inhalation.
- NATIONAL FUNDING/ACCESS DECISIONS
  Scottish Medicines Consortium (SMC) Decisions
  The *Scottish Medicines Consortium* has advised (March
  2014) that fluticasone furoate/vilanterol (*Relvar Ellipta* ®) is
  accepted for restricted use within NHS Scotland in patients
  with severe chronic obstructive pulmonary disease with a
  forced expiratory volume in 1 second (FEV$_1$) less than 50%
  of the predicted normal value.

- MEDICINAL FORMS
  There can be variation in the licensing of different medicines
  containing the same drug.
  Inhalation powder
  CAUTIONARY AND ADVISORY LABELS 8, 10
  ▸ Relvar Ellipta (GlaxoSmithKline UK Ltd) ▼
    **Vilanterol 22 microgram per 1 dose, Fluticasone furoate
    92 microgram per 1 dose** Relvar Ellipta 92micrograms/dose /
    22micrograms/dose dry powder inhaler | 30 dose [PoM] £22.00
    **Vilanterol 22 microgram per 1 dose, Fluticasone furoate
    184 microgram per 1 dose** Relvar Ellipta 184micrograms/dose /
    22micrograms/dose dry powder inhaler | 30 dose [PoM] £29.50

⟟ 238

Mometasone furoate

- INDICATIONS AND DOSE
Prophylaxis of asthma
▸ BY INHALATION OF POWDER
▸ Child 12–17 years: Initially 400 micrograms daily in
  1–2 divided doses, single dose to be inhaled in the
  evening, reduced to 200 micrograms once daily, if
  control maintained
▸ Adult: Initially 400 micrograms daily in 1–2 divided
  doses, single dose to be inhaled in the evening, reduced
  to 200 micrograms once daily, if control maintained
Prophylaxis of severe asthma
▸ BY INHALATION OF POWDER
▸ Child 12–17 years: Increased if necessary up to
  400 micrograms twice daily
▸ Adult: Increased if necessary up to 400 micrograms
  twice daily

- SIDE-EFFECTS
▸ **Common or very common** Headache
▸ **Uncommon** Dyspepsia · palpitation · weight gain

- PATIENT AND CARER ADVICE Patients or carers should be
  given advice on how to administer mometasone by inhaler.
  With high doses, a steroid card should be supplied.
  Medicines for Children leaflet: Mometasone furoate inhaler for
  asthma prevention (prophylaxis) www.medicinesforchildren.org.
  uk/mometasone-furoate-inhaler-for-asthma-prevention-
  prophylaxis
- NATIONAL FUNDING/ACCESS DECISIONS
  Scottish Medicines Consortium (SMC) Decisions
  The *Scottish Medicines Consortium* has advised (November
  2003) that *Asmanex* ® is restricted for use following failure
  of first-line inhaled corticosteroids.

- MEDICINAL FORMS
  There can be variation in the licensing of different medicines
  containing the same drug.
  Inhalation powder
  CAUTIONARY AND ADVISORY LABELS 8, 10
  ▸ Asmanex Twisthaler (Merck Sharp & Dohme Ltd)
    Mometasone furoate 200 microgram per 1 dose Asmanex
    200micrograms/dose Twisthaler | 30 dose [PoM] £15.70 DT price =
    £15.70 | 60 dose [PoM] £23.54 DT price = £23.54
    Mometasone furoate 400 microgram per 1 dose Asmanex
    400micrograms/dose Twisthaler | 30 dose [PoM] £21.78 DT price =
    £21.78 | 60 dose [PoM] £36.05 DT price = £36.05

DRUGS FOR RESPIRATORY DISEASES ›
MONOCLONAL ANTIBODIES

Omalizumab

- INDICATIONS AND DOSE
Prophylaxis of severe persistent allergic asthma
▸ BY SUBCUTANEOUS INJECTION
▸ Adult: Dose according to immunoglobulin E
  concentration and body-weight (consult product
  literature)
**Add-on therapy for chronic spontaneous urticaria in
patients who have had an inadequate response to H$_1$
antihistamine treatment**
▸ BY SUBCUTANEOUS INJECTION
▸ Adult: 300 mg every 4 weeks

- CAUTIONS Autoimmune disease · susceptibility to
  helmintic infection—discontinue if infection does not
  respond to anthelmintic
- SIDE-EFFECTS
▸ **Common or very common** Abdominal pain · arthralgia ·
  headache · injection-site reactions · pyrexia · sinusitis ·
  upper respiratory tract infection
▸ **Uncommon** Bronchospasm · cough · diarrhoea · dizziness ·
  drowsiness · dyspepsia · flushing · influenza-like illness ·
  malaise · nausea · paraesthesia · pharyngitis ·
  photosensitivity · postural hypotension · pruritus · rash ·
  syncope · urticaria · weight gain
▸ **Rare** Angioedema · antibody formation · laryngoedema ·
  parasitic infection
▸ **Frequency not known** Alopecia · arterial thromboembolic
  events · Churg-Strauss syndrome · joint swelling · myalgia ·
  serum sickness (including fever and lymphadenopathy) ·
  thrombocytopenia

SIDE-EFFECTS, FURTHER INFORMATION
▸ Churg-Strauss syndrome Churg-Strauss syndrome has
  occurred rarely in patients given omalizumab; the reaction
  is usually associated with the reduction of oral
  corticosteroid therapy. Churg-Strauss syndrome can
  present as eosinophilia, vasculitic rash, cardiac
  complications, worsening pulmonary symptoms, or
  peripheral neuropathy.
▸ Hypersensitivity reactions Hypersensitivity reactions can also
  occur immediately following treatment with omalizumab
  or sometimes more than 24 hours after the first injection.

- PREGNANCY Manufacturer advises avoid unless essential—crosses the placenta.
- BREAST FEEDING Manufacturer advises avoid—present in milk in *animal* studies.
- HEPATIC IMPAIRMENT Manufacturer advises caution—no information available.
- RENAL IMPAIRMENT Manufacturer advises caution—no information available.
- NATIONAL FUNDING/ACCESS DECISIONS

NICE technology appraisals (TAs)

▸ Omalizumab for severe persistent allergic asthma (April 2013) NICE TA278

Omalizumab is recommended as an option for treating severe persistent confirmed allergic IgE-mediated asthma as an add-on to optimised standard therapy in patients aged 6 years and over:
- who need continuous or frequent treatment with oral corticosteroids (defined as 4 or more courses in the previous year), **and**
- only if the manufacturer makes omalizumab available with the discount agreed in the patient access scheme.

Optimised standard therapy is defined as a full trial of and, if tolerated, documented compliance with inhaled high-dose corticosteroids, long-acting beta$_2$ agonists, leukotriene receptor antagonists, theophyllines, oral corticosteroids, and smoking cessation if clinically appropriate.

Patients currently receiving omalizumab whose disease does not meet the criteria should be able to continue treatment until they and their clinician consider it appropriate to stop.
www.nice.org.uk/TA278

▸ Omalizumab for previously treated chronic spontaneous urticaria (June 2015) NICE TA339

Omalizumab is an option as add-on therapy for the treatment of severe chronic spontaneous urticaria in patients 12 years and over, only if:
- the severity of the condition is assessed objectively, for example, using a weekly urticaria activity score of 28 or more,
- the patient's condition has not responded to standard treatment with H$_1$-antihistamines and leukotriene receptor antagonists,
- omalizumab is stopped at or before the fourth dose if the condition has not responded,
- omalizumab is stopped at the end of a course of treatment (6 doses) if the condition has responded and is restarted only if the condition relapses,
- omalizumab is administered under the management of a secondary care specialist in dermatology, immunology or allergy,
- the manufacturer provides omalizumab with the discount agreed in the patient access scheme.

Patients currently receiving omalizumab whose disease does not meet the above criteria should have the option to continue treatment until they and their clinician consider it appropriate to stop.
www.nice.org.uk/TA339

Scottish Medicines Consortium (SMC) Decisions

The *Scottish Medicines Consortium* has advised (December 2014) that omalizumab (*Xolair*®) is accepted for restricted use within NHS Scotland for the treatment of chronic spontaneous urticaria in patients aged 12 years and over, who have had an inadequate response to combination therapy with H$_1$-antihistamines, leukotriene receptor antagonists and H$_2$-antihistamines, used according to current treatment guidelines.

- MEDICINAL FORMS
There can be variation in the licensing of different medicines containing the same drug.
Solution for injection
▸ Xolair (Novartis Pharmaceuticals UK Ltd)
Omalizumab 150 mg per 1 ml Xolair 150mg/1ml solution for injection pre-filled syringes | 1 pre-filled disposable injection [PoM] £256.15
Xolair 75mg/0.5ml solution for injection pre-filled syringes | 1 pre-filled disposable injection [PoM] £128.07

LEUKOTRIENE RECEPTOR ANTAGONISTS

Leukotriene receptor antagonists

The leukotriene receptor antagonists, montelukast below and zafirlukast p. 246, block the effects of cysteinyl leukotrienes in the airways. They are effective in asthma when used alone or with an inhaled corticosteroid.

Montelukast has not been shown to be more effective than a standard dose of inhaled corticosteroid, but the two drugs appear to have an additive effect. The leukotriene receptor antagonists may be of benefit in exercise-induced asthma and in those with concomitant rhinitis, but they are less effective in those with severe asthma who are also receiving high doses of other drugs.

Montelukast

- INDICATIONS AND DOSE

Prophylaxis of asthma
▸ BY MOUTH
▸ Child 6 months–5 years: 4 mg once daily, dose to be taken in the evening
▸ Child 6–14 years: 5 mg once daily, dose to be taken in the evening
▸ Child 15–17 years: 10 mg once daily, dose to be taken in the evening
▸ Adult: 10 mg once daily, dose to be taken in the evening

Symptomatic relief of seasonal allergic rhinitis in patients with asthma.
▸ BY MOUTH
▸ Child 15–17 years: 10 mg once daily, dose to be taken in the evening
▸ Adult: 10 mg once daily, dose to be taken in the evening

- INTERACTIONS → Appendix 1 (leukotriene receptor antagonists).

- SIDE-EFFECTS
▸ **Common or very common** Abdominal pain · headache · hyperkinesia (in young children) · thirst
▸ **Uncommon** Abnormal dreams · aggressive behaviour · agitation · anxiety · arthralgia · bruising · depression · dizziness · drowsiness · dry mouth · dyspepsia · epistaxis · hostility · hypoaesthesia · irritability · malaise · muscle cramps · myalgia · oedema · paraesthesia · psychomotor hyperactivity · restlessness · seizures · sleep disturbances · sleep-walking
▸ **Rare** Disturbance in attention · increased bleeding tendency · memory impairment · palpitation · tremor
▸ **Very rare** Churg-Strauss syndrome · disorientation · erythema multiforme · erythema nodosum · hallucinations · hepatic disorders · hepatic eosinophilic infiltration · suicidal behaviour · suicidal thoughts

SIDE-EFFECTS, FURTHER INFORMATION
Churg-Strauss syndrome has occurred very rarely in association with the use of montelukast; in many of the reported cases the reaction followed the reduction or withdrawal of oral corticosteroid therapy. Prescribers

3

Respiratory system

should be alert to the development of eosinophilia, vasculitic rash, worsening pulmonary symptoms, cardiac complications, or peripheral neuropathy.

- **PREGNANCY** Manufacturer advises avoid unless essential. There is limited evidence for the safe use of montelukast during pregnancy; however, it can be taken as normal in women who have shown a significant improvement in asthma not achievable with other drugs before becoming pregnant.
- **BREAST FEEDING** Manufacturer advises avoid unless essential.
- **DIRECTIONS FOR ADMINISTRATION** Granules may be swallowed or mixed with cold, soft food (not liquid) and taken immediately.
- **PRESCRIBING AND DISPENSING INFORMATION** Flavours of chewable tablet formulations may include cherry.
- **PATIENT AND CARER ADVICE** Patients or carers should be given advice on how to administer montelukast granules. Medicines for Children leaflet: Montelukast for asthma www.medicinesforchildren.org.uk/montelukast-for-asthma
- **NATIONAL FUNDING/ACCESS DECISIONS**
SINGULAIR® GRANULES

Scottish Medicines Consortium (SMC) Decisions
The *Scottish Medicines Consortium* has advised (June 2007) that *Singulair*® granules are restricted for use as an alternative to low-dose inhaled corticosteroids for children 2–14 years with mild persistent asthma who have not recently had serious asthma attacks that required oral corticosteroid use and who are not capable of using inhaled corticosteroids; *Singulair*® granules should be initiated by a specialist in paediatric asthma.

SINGULAIR® CHEWABLE TABLETS

Scottish Medicines Consortium (SMC) Decisions
The *Scottish Medicines Consortium* has advised (June 2007) that *Singulair*® chewable tablets are restricted for use as an alternative to low-dose inhaled corticosteroids for children 2–14 years with mild persistent asthma who have not recently had serious asthma attacks that required oral corticosteroid use and who are not capable of using inhaled corticosteroids; *Singulair*® chewable tablets should be initiated by a specialist in paediatric asthma.

- **MEDICINAL FORMS**
There can be variation in the licensing of different medicines containing the same drug.
Tablet
  - Montelukast (Non-proprietary)
  Montelukast (as Montelukast sodium) 10 mg Montelukast 10mg tablets | 28 tablet PoM £26.97 DT price = £1.54
  - Singulair (Merck Sharp & Dohme Ltd)
  Montelukast (as Montelukast sodium) 10 mg Singulair 10mg tablets | 28 tablet PoM £26.97 DT price = £1.54
Chewable tablet
CAUTIONARY AND ADVISORY LABELS 23, 24
EXCIPIENTS: May contain Aspartame
  - Montelukast (Non-proprietary)
  Montelukast (as Montelukast sodium) 4 mg Montelukast 4mg chewable tablets sugar free sugar-free | 28 tablet PoM £25.69 DT price = £1.35
  Montelukast (as Montelukast sodium) 5 mg Montelukast 5mg chewable tablets sugar free sugar-free | 28 tablet PoM £25.69 DT price = £1.58
  - Singulair (Merck Sharp & Dohme Ltd)
  Montelukast (as Montelukast sodium) 4 mg Singulair Paediatric 4mg chewable tablets sugar-free | 28 tablet PoM £25.69 DT price = £1.35
  Montelukast (as Montelukast sodium) 5 mg Singulair Paediatric 5mg chewable tablets sugar-free | 28 tablet PoM £25.69 DT price = £1.58

Granules
  - Montelukast (Non-proprietary)
  Montelukast (as Montelukast sodium) 4 mg Montelukast 4mg granules sachets sugar free sugar-free | 28 sachet PoM £24.41 DT price = £4.05
  - Singulair (Merck Sharp & Dohme Ltd)
  Montelukast (as Montelukast sodium) 4 mg Singulair Paediatric 4mg granules sachets sugar-free | 28 sachet PoM £25.69 DT price = £4.05

Zafirlukast

- **INDICATIONS AND DOSE**
Prophylaxis of asthma
  - BY MOUTH
  - Child 12–17 years: 20 mg twice daily
  - Adult: 20 mg twice daily

- **CAUTIONS** Elderly
- **INTERACTIONS** → Appendix 1 (leukotriene receptor antagonists).
- **SIDE-EFFECTS**
  - **Common or very common** Gastro-intestinal disturbances · headache · respiratory infections
  - **Uncommon** Insomnia · malaise
  - **Rare** Angioedema · arthralgia · bleeding disorders · hepatitis · hyperbilirubinaemia · hypersensitivity reactions · myalgia · skin reactions · thrombocytopenia
  - **Very rare** Agranulocytosis · Churg-Strauss syndrome

  SIDE-EFFECTS, FURTHER INFORMATION
  - Hepatic disorder Patients or their carers should be told how to recognise development of liver disorder and advised to seek medical attention if symptoms or signs such as persistent nausea, vomiting, malaise, or jaundice develop.

  Churg-Strauss syndrome has occurred very rarely in association with the use of zafirlukast; in many of the reported cases the reaction followed the reduction or withdrawal of oral corticosteroid therapy. Prescribers should be alert to the development of eosinophilia, vasculitic rash, worsening pulmonary symptoms, cardiac complications, or peripheral neuropathy.

- **PREGNANCY** Manufacturer advises use only if potential benefit outweighs risk. There is limited evidence for the safe use of zafirlukast during pregnancy; however, it can be taken as normal in women who have shown a significant improvement in asthma not achievable with other drugs before becoming pregnant.
- **BREAST FEEDING** Present in milk—manufacturer advises avoid.
- **HEPATIC IMPAIRMENT** Manufacturer advises avoid.
- **RENAL IMPAIRMENT**
  - In adults Manufacturer advises caution in moderate to severe impairment.
  - In children Manufacturer advises caution.

- **PATIENT AND CARER ADVICE**
Medicines for Children leaflet: Zafirlukast for asthma prevention (prophylaxis) www.medicinesforchildren.org.uk/zafirlukast-for-asthma-prevention

- **MEDICINAL FORMS**
There can be variation in the licensing of different medicines containing the same drug.
Tablet
CAUTIONARY AND ADVISORY LABELS 23
  - Accolate (AstraZeneca UK Ltd)
  Zafirlukast 20 mg Accolate 20mg tablets | 56 tablet PoM £17.75 DT price = £17.75

MAST-CELL STABILISERS

Cromoglicate and related therapy

Overview

The mode of action of sodium cromoglicate below and nedocromil sodium below is not completely understood. They may be of value in asthma with an allergic basis, but, in practice, it is difficult to predict who will benefit; they could probably be given for 4 to 6 weeks to assess response. Dose frequency is adjusted according to response but is usually 3 to 4 times a day initially; this may subsequently be reduced.

In general, *prophylaxis* with sodium cromoglicate is less effective than prophylaxis with corticosteroid inhalations. There is evidence of efficacy of nedocromil sodium in children aged 5–12 years. Sodium cromoglicate and nedocromil sodium are of no value in the treatment of acute attacks of asthma.

Sodium cromoglicate can prevent exercise-induced asthma. However, exercise-induced asthma may reflect poor overall control and the patient should be reassessed.

Sodium cromoglicate and nedocromil sodium may also have a role in allergic conjunctivitis; sodium cromoglicate is used also in allergic rhinitis and allergy-related diarrhoea.

Nedocromil sodium

● INDICATIONS AND DOSE

Prophylaxis of asthma

▸ BY INHALATION OF AEROSOL

▸ Child 5-17 years: Initially 4 mg 4 times a day, when control achieved may be possible to reduce to twice daily

▸ Adult: Initially 4 mg 4 times a day, when control achieved may be possible to reduce to twice daily

DOSE EQUIVALENCE AND CONVERSION
2 puffs = 4 mg.

● UNLICENSED USE

▸ When used by inhalation in children Not licensed for use in children under 6 years.

● SIDE-EFFECTS

▸ **Common or very common** Abdominal pain · dyspepsia · nausea · pharyngitis · vomiting

▸ **Rare** Taste disturbances

▸ **Frequency not known** Bronchospasm · cough · headache · paradoxical bronchospasm · throat irritation

SIDE-EFFECTS, FURTHER INFORMATION

▸ Paradoxical bronchospasm If paradoxical bronchospasm occurs, a short-acting beta$_2$ agonist such as salbutamol or terbutaline should be used to control symptoms; treatment with nedocromil should be discontinued.

● PREGNANCY Inhaled drugs can be taken as normal during pregnancy.

● BREAST FEEDING Inhaled drugs can be taken as normal during breast-feeding.

● TREATMENT CESSATION Withdrawal should be done gradually over a period of one week—symptoms of asthma may recur.

● PRESCRIBING AND DISPENSING INFORMATION Flavours of inhalers may include mint.

● PATIENT AND CARER ADVICE Regular use is necessary. Patient counselling is advised for Nedocromil aerosol for inhalation (administration).

● MEDICINAL FORMS
There can be variation in the licensing of different medicines containing the same drug.
Pressurised inhalation
CAUTIONARY AND ADVISORY LABELS 8
▸ Tilade (Sanofi)
   Nedocromil sodium 2 mg per 1 dose Tilade 2mg/dose inhaler CFC free | 112 dose PoM £39.94

Sodium cromoglicate

(Sodium cromoglycate)

● INDICATIONS AND DOSE

Prophylaxis of asthma

▸ BY INHALATION OF AEROSOL

▸ Child 5-17 years: Initially 10 mg 4 times a day, additional dose may also be taken before exercise, increased if necessary to 10 mg 6–8 times a day; maintenance 5 mg 4 times a day, 5 mg is equivalent to 1 puff

▸ Adult: Initially 10 mg 4 times a day, additional dose may also be taken before exercise, increased if necessary to 10 mg 6–8 times a day; maintenance 5 mg 4 times a day, 5 mg is equivalent to 1 puff

Food allergy (in conjunction with dietary restriction)

▸ BY MOUTH

▸ Child 2-13 years: Initially 100 mg 4 times a day for 2–3 weeks, then increased if necessary up to 40 mg/kg daily, then reduced according to response, to be taken before meals

▸ Child 14-17 years: Initially 200 mg 4 times a day for 2–3 weeks, then increased if necessary up to 40 mg/kg daily, then reduced according to response, to be taken before meals

▸ Adult: Initially 200 mg 4 times a day for 2–3 weeks, then increased if necessary up to 40 mg/kg daily, then reduced according to response, to be taken before meals

● CAUTIONS

▸ When used by inhalation Discontinue if eosinophilic pneumonia occurs

● SIDE-EFFECTS

▸ When used by inhalation Bronchospasm · cough · eosinophilic pneumonia · headache · paradoxical bronchospasm · rhinitis · throat irritation

▸ With oral use Joint pain · occasional nausea · rashes

SIDE-EFFECTS, FURTHER INFORMATION

▸ Paradoxical bronchospasm

▸ When used by inhalation If paradoxical bronchospasm occurs, a short-acting beta$_2$ agonist such as salbutamol or terbutaline should be used to control symptoms; treatment with sodium cromoglicate should be discontinued.

● PREGNANCY Not known to be harmful. Inhaled drugs can be taken as normal during pregnancy.

● BREAST FEEDING Unlikely to be present in milk. Inhaled drugs can be taken as normal during breast-feeding.

● TREATMENT CESSATION

▸ When used by inhalation Withdrawal of sodium cromoglicate should be done gradually over a period of one week— symptoms of asthma may recur.

● DIRECTIONS FOR ADMINISTRATION

▸ With oral use Capsules may be swallowed whole or the contents dissolved in hot water and diluted with cold water before taking.

● PATIENT AND CARER ADVICE

▸ With oral use Patient counselling is advised for sodium

Respiratory system

3

3

Respiratory system

cromoglicate capsules (administration).
▸ When used by inhalation Patient counselling is advised for sodium cromoglicate pressurised inhalation (administration).

● MEDICINAL FORMS
There can be variation in the licensing of different medicines containing the same drug. Forms available from special-order manufacturers include: oral solution, nebuliser liquid

Capsule
CAUTIONARY AND ADVISORY LABELS 22
▸ Nalcrom (Sanofi)
  Sodium cromoglicate 100 mg Nalcrom 100mg capsules | 100 capsule [PoM] £41.14 DT price = £41.14

Pressurised inhalation
CAUTIONARY AND ADVISORY LABELS 8
▸ Intal (Sanofi)
  Sodium cromoglicate 5 mg per 1 dose Intal 5mg/dose inhaler CFC free | 112 dose [PoM] £18.33

PHOSPHODIESTERASE TYPE-4 INHIBITORS

Roflumilast

● DRUG ACTION Roflumilast is a phosphodiesterase type-4 inhibitor with anti-inflammatory properties.

● INDICATIONS AND DOSE

Adjunct to bronchodilators for the maintenance treatment of patients with severe chronic obstructive pulmonary disease associated with chronic bronchitis and a history of frequent exacerbations
▸ BY MOUTH
▸ Adult: 500 micrograms once daily

● CONTRA-INDICATIONS Cancer (except basal cell carcinoma) · concomitant treatment with immunosuppressive drugs (except short-term systemic corticosteroids) · history of depression associated with suicidal ideation or behaviour · moderate to severe cardiac failure · severe acute infectious disease · severe immunological disease

● CAUTIONS History of psychiatric illness (discontinue if new or worsening psychiatric symptoms occur) · latent infection (such as tuberculosis, viral hepatitis, herpes infection)

● INTERACTIONS Caution with concomitant use of drugs likely to cause psychiatric events (discontinue if new or worsening psychiatric symptoms occur).
Appendix 1 (roflumilast).

● SIDE-EFFECTS
▸ **Common or very common** Abdominal pain · decreased appetite · diarrhoea · headache · insomnia · nausea · weight loss
▸ **Uncommon** Anxiety · back pain · dizziness · dyspepsia · gastritis · gastro-oesophageal reflux · malaise · muscle spasm · myalgia · palpitation · rash · tremor · vertigo · vomiting
▸ **Rare** Constipation · depression · gynaecomastia · haematochezia · nervousness · raised creatine kinase · respiratory tract infections · suicidal behaviour · suicidal ideation · taste disturbances · urticaria

● CONCEPTION AND CONTRACEPTION Women of child-bearing age should use effective contraception.

● PREGNANCY Manufacturer advises avoid—toxicity in *animal* studies.

● BREAST FEEDING Manufacturer advises avoid—present in milk in *animal* studies.

● HEPATIC IMPAIRMENT Caution in mild impairment. Avoid in moderate to severe impairment.

● MONITORING REQUIREMENTS Monitor body-weight.

● PATIENT AND CARER ADVICE Patients should be given a patient card before starting treatment and advised to record body-weight at regular intervals.

● NATIONAL FUNDING/ACCESS DECISIONS

NICE technology appraisals (TAs)
▸ Roflumilast for the management of severe chronic obstructive pulmonary disease (January 2012) NICE TA244
Roflumilast is recommended only in the context of research as part of a clinical trial for adults with severe chronic obstructive pulmonary disease associated with chronic bronchitis with a history of frequent exacerbations as an add-on to bronchodilator treatment. Patients receiving roflumilast should have the option to continue treatment until they and their clinicians consider it appropriate to stop.
www.nice.org.uk/TA244

● MEDICINAL FORMS
There can be variation in the licensing of different medicines containing the same drug.

Tablet
▸ Daxas (Takeda UK Ltd) ▼
  Roflumilast 500 microgram Daxas 500microgram tablets | 30 tablet [PoM] £37.71 DT price = £37.71

SYMPATHOMIMETICS › VASOCONSTRICTOR

Ephedrine hydrochloride

● INDICATIONS AND DOSE

Reversal of hypotension from spinal or epidural anaesthesia
▸ BY SLOW INTRAVENOUS INJECTION
▸ Adult: 3–6 mg every 3–4 minutes (max. per dose 9 mg), adjusted according to response, injection solution to contain ephedrine hydrochloride 3 mg/ml; maximum 30 mg per course

Reversible airways obstruction
▸ BY MOUTH
▸ Adult: 15–60 mg 3 times a day

Neuropathic oedema
▸ BY MOUTH
▸ Adult: 30–60 mg 3 times a day

● UNLICENSED USE
▸ With oral use Not licensed for neuropathic oedema.

● CAUTIONS
GENERAL CAUTIONS
Diabetes mellitus · elderly · hypertension · hyperthyroidism · ischaemic heart disease · prostatic hypertrophy (risk of acute urinary retention)
SPECIFIC CAUTIONS
▸ With intravenous use Susceptibility to angle-closure glaucoma

● INTERACTIONS → Appendix 1 (sympathomimetics).

● SIDE-EFFECTS
▸ **Common or very common**
▸ With intravenous use Anginal pain · anorexia · anxiety · arrhythmias · changes in blood-glucose concentration · confusion · difficulty in micturition · dizziness · dyspnoea · flushing · headache · hypersalivation · insomnia · nausea · psychoses · restlessness · sweating · tachycardia · tremor · urine retention · vasoconstriction with hypertension · vasodilation with hypotension · vomiting
▸ With oral use Anxiety · arrhythmias · insomnia · restlessness · tachycardia · tremor
▸ **Very rare**
▸ With intravenous use Angle-closure glaucoma
▸ **Frequency not known**
▸ With intravenous use Bradycardia
▸ With oral use Cold extremities · dry mouth
▸ With systemic use Increased lacrimation (can have adverse effects on contact lens wear)

- **PREGNANCY**
- ▸ With oral use Manufacturer advises avoid.
- ▸ With intravenous use Increased fetal heart rate reported with parenteral ephedrine.
- **BREAST FEEDING** Present in milk; manufacturer advises avoid—irritability and disturbed sleep reported.
- **RENAL IMPAIRMENT**
- ▸ With intravenous use or oral use Use with caution.
- **LESS SUITABLE FOR PRESCRIBING**
- ▸ With oral use Ephedrine tablets are less suitable and less safe for use as a bronchodilator than the selective beta₂ agonists.
- **EXCEPTIONS TO LEGAL CATEGORY** For exceptions relating to ephedrine tablets see *Medicines, Ethics and Practice*, London, Pharmaceutical Press (always consult latest edition).

- **MEDICINAL FORMS**
  There can be variation in the licensing of different medicines containing the same drug. Forms available from special-order manufacturers include: oral suspension, oral solution, solution for injection

  Tablet
  - ▸ Ephedrine hydrochloride (Non-proprietary)
    Ephedrine hydrochloride 15 mg Ephedrine hydrochloride 15mg tablets | 28 tablet PoM £22.83 DT price = £20.73
    Ephedrine hydrochloride 30 mg Ephedrine hydrochloride 30mg tablets | 28 tablet PoM £32.58 DT price = £32.26

  Solution for injection
  - ▸ Ephedrine hydrochloride (Non-proprietary)
    Ephedrine hydrochloride 3 mg per 1 ml Ephedrine 30mg/10ml solution for injection ampoules | 10 ampoule PoM £73.21
    Ephedrine 30mg/10ml solution for injection pre-filled syringes | 1 pre-filled disposable injection PoM £7.59-£9.50 | 12 pre-filled disposable injection PoM £114.00
    Ephedrine hydrochloride 30 mg per 1 ml Ephedrine 30mg/1ml solution for injection ampoules | 10 ampoule PoM £4.31-£4.74

XANTHINES

Aminophylline

- **INDICATIONS AND DOSE**

Severe acute asthma in patients not previously treated with theophylline
- ▸ BY SLOW INTRAVENOUS INJECTION
- ▸ Child: 5 mg/kg (max. per dose 500 mg), to be followed by intravenous infusion
- ▸ Adult: 250–500 mg (max. per dose 5 mg/kg), to be followed by intravenous infusion

Severe acute asthma
- ▸ BY INTRAVENOUS INFUSION
- ▸ Child 1 month-11 years: 1 mg/kg/hour, adjusted according to plasma-theophylline concentration
- ▸ Child 12-17 years: 500–700 micrograms/kg/hour, adjusted according to plasma-theophylline concentration
- ▸ Adult: 500–700 micrograms/kg/hour, adjusted according to plasma-theophylline concentration
- ▸ Elderly: 300 micrograms/kg/hour, adjusted according to plasma-theophylline concentration

Severe acute exacerbation of chronic obstructive pulmonary disease in patients not previously treated with theophylline
- ▸ BY SLOW INTRAVENOUS INJECTION
- ▸ Adult: 250–500 mg (max. per dose 5 mg/kg), to be followed by intravenous infusion

Severe acute exacerbation of chronic obstructive pulmonary disease
- ▸ BY INTRAVENOUS INFUSION
- ▸ Adult: 500–700 micrograms/kg/hour, adjusted according to plasma-theophylline concentration

- ▸ Elderly: 300 micrograms/kg/hour, adjusted according to plasma-theophylline concentration

Chronic asthma
- ▸ BY MOUTH USING MODIFIED-RELEASE MEDICINES
- ▸ Child (body-weight 40 kg and above): Initially 225 mg twice daily for 1 week, then increased if necessary to 450 mg twice daily, adjusted according to plasma-theophylline concentration

Reversible airway obstruction
- ▸ BY MOUTH USING MODIFIED-RELEASE MEDICINES
- ▸ Adult (body-weight 40 kg and above): Initially 225 mg twice daily for 1 week, then increased if necessary to 450 mg twice daily, adjusted according to plasma-theophylline concentration

PHYLLOCONTIN CONTINUS® FORTE

Reversible airways obstruction
- ▸ BY MOUTH USING MODIFIED-RELEASE MEDICINES
- ▸ Adult: Initially 350 mg twice daily for 1 week, then increased if necessary to 700 mg twice daily, increase dose according to plasma-theophylline concentration

DOSE ADJUSTMENTS DUE TO INTERACTIONS
Dose adjustment may be necessary if smoking started or stopped during treatment.

DOSES AT EXTREMES OF BODY-WEIGHT
To avoid excessive dosage in obese patients, dose should be calculated on the basis of ideal weight for height.

PHARMACOKINETICS
Aminophylline is a stable mixture or combination of theophylline and ethylenediamine; the ethylenediamine confers greater solubility in water.
Theophylline is metabolised in the liver. The plasma-theophylline concentration is increased in heart failure, hepatic impairment, and in viral infections. The plasma-theophylline concentration is decreased in smokers, and by alcohol consumption. Differences in the half-life of aminophylline are important because the toxic dose is close to the therapeutic dose.

- **UNLICENSED USE** Aminophylline injection not licensed for use in children under 6 months.
- **CAUTIONS** Arrhythmias following rapid intravenous injection · cardiac arrhythmias or other cardiac disease · elderly (increased plasma-theophylline concentration) (in adults) · epilepsy · fever · hypertension · hyperthyroidism · peptic ulcer · risk of hypokalaemia
- **INTERACTIONS** → Appendix 1 (aminophylline).
- **SIDE-EFFECTS** Arrhythmias (especially if given rapidly by intravenous injection) · CNS stimulation · convulsions (especially if given rapidly by intravenous injection) · diarrhoea · gastric irritation · headache · hypotension (especially if given rapidly by intravenous injection) · insomnia · nausea · palpitation · tachycardia · vomiting

  SIDE-EFFECTS, FURTHER INFORMATION
- ▸ Hypokalaemia Potentially serious hypokalaemia may result from beta₂ agonist therapy. Particular caution is required in severe asthma, because this effect may be potentiated by concomitant treatment with theophylline and its derivatives, corticosteroids, and diuretics, and by hypoxia. Plasma-potassium concentration should therefore be monitored in severe asthma.

  Overdose
  Theophylline and related drugs are often prescribed as modified-release formulations and toxicity can therefore be delayed. They cause vomiting (which may be severe and intractable), agitation, restlessness, dilated pupils, sinus tachycardia, and hyperglycaemia. More serious effects are haematemesis, convulsions, and supraventricular and ventricular arrhythmias. Severe hypokalaemia may develop rapidly.
  For specific details on the management of poisoning, see

Theophylline, under Emergency treatment of poisoning p. 1199.

- ● ALLERGY AND CROSS-SENSITIVITY Allergy to ethylenediamine can cause urticaria, erythema, and exfoliative dermatitis.
- ● PREGNANCY Neonatal irritability and apnoea have been reported. Theophylline can be taken as normal during pregnancy as it is particularly important that asthma should be well controlled during pregnancy.
- ● BREAST FEEDING Present in milk—irritability in infant reported; modified-release preparations preferable. Theophylline can be taken as normal during breast-feeding.
- ● HEPATIC IMPAIRMENT Reduce dose.
- ● MONITORING REQUIREMENTS
- ▸ Aminophylline is monitored therapeutically in terms of plasma-theophylline concentrations.
- ▸ Measurement of plasma-theophylline concentration may be helpful and is **essential** if a loading dose of intravenous aminophylline is to be given to patients who are already taking theophylline, because serious side-effects such as convulsions and arrhythmias can occasionally precede other symptoms of toxicity.
- ▸ In most individuals, a plasma-theophylline concentration of 10–20 mg/litre (55–110 micromol/litre) is required for satisfactory bronchodilation, although a lower plasma-theophylline concentration of 5–15 mg/litre may be effective. Adverse effects can occur within the range 10–20 mg/litre and both the frequency and severity increase at concentrations above 20 mg/litre.
- ▸ If aminophylline is given intravenously, a blood sample should be taken 4–6 hours after starting treatment.
- ▸ With oral use Plasma-theophylline concentration is measured 5 days after starting oral treatment and at least 3 days after any dose adjustment. A blood sample should usually be taken 4–6 hours after an oral dose of a modified-release preparation (sampling times may vary—consult local guidelines).
- ● DIRECTIONS FOR ADMINISTRATION
- ▸ With intravenous use For *intravenous injection*, give **very slowly** over at least 20 minutes (with close monitoring).
- ▸ With intravenous use in adults For *intravenous infusion*, give continuously in Glucose 5% *or* Sodium Chloride 0.9%.
- ▸ With intravenous use in children For *intravenous infusion*, dilute to a concentration of 1 mg/mL with Glucose 5% *or* Sodium Chloride 0.9%.
- ▸ With intramuscular use Aminophylline is too irritant for intramuscular use.
- ● PRESCRIBING AND DISPENSING INFORMATION
  Patients taking oral theophylline or aminophylline should not normally receive a loading dose of intravenous aminophylline.
   Consider intravenous aminophylline for treatment of severe and life-threatening acute asthma only after consultation with senior medical staff.
  Modified release The rate of absorption from modified-release preparations can vary between brands. If a prescription for a modified-release oral aminophylline preparation does not specify a brand name, the pharmacist should contact the prescriber and agree the brand to be dispensed. Additionally, it is essential that a patient discharged from hospital should be maintained on the brand on which that patient was stabilised as an in-patient.
  PHYLLOCONTIN CONTINUS® FORTE *Phyllocontin Continus*® Forte tablets are for smokers and other patients where theophylline half-life is shorter.

- ● MEDICINAL FORMS
  There can be variation in the licensing of different medicines containing the same drug. Forms available from special-order manufacturers include: solution for infusion
  Modified-release tablet
  CAUTIONARY AND ADVISORY LABELS 25
  ▸ Aminophylline (Non-proprietary)
    Aminophylline hydrate 225 mg Aminophylline hydrate 225mg modified-release tablets | 56 tablet Ⓟ no price available DT price = £2.40
  ▸ Phyllocontin Continus (Napp Pharmaceuticals Ltd)
    Aminophylline hydrate 225 mg Phyllocontin Continus 225mg tablets | 56 tablet Ⓟ £2.40 DT price = £2.40
    Aminophylline hydrate 350 mg Phyllocontin Forte Continus 350mg tablets | 56 tablet Ⓟ £4.22 DT price = £4.22
  Solution for injection
  ▸ Aminophylline (Non-proprietary)
    Aminophylline 25 mg per 1 ml Aminophylline 250mg/10ml solution for injection ampoules | 10 ampoule PoM £6.50 DT price = £6.50

Theophylline

- ● INDICATIONS AND DOSE

NUELIN SA® 175MG TABLETS

Reversible airways obstruction | Severe acute asthma | Chronic asthma
- ▸ BY MOUTH USING MODIFIED-RELEASE MEDICINES
- ▸ Adult: 175–350 mg every 12 hours
Chronic asthma
- ▸ BY MOUTH USING MODIFIED-RELEASE MEDICINES
- ▸ Child 6–11 years: 175 mg every 12 hours
- ▸ Child 12–17 years: 175–350 mg every 12 hours

NUELIN SA® 250 TABLETS

Reversible airways obstruction | Severe acute asthma | Chronic asthma
- ▸ BY MOUTH USING MODIFIED-RELEASE MEDICINES
- ▸ Adult: 250–500 mg every 12 hours
Chronic asthma
- ▸ BY MOUTH USING MODIFIED-RELEASE MEDICINES
- ▸ Child 6–11 years: 125–250 mg every 12 hours
- ▸ Child 12–17 years: 250–500 mg every 12 hours

SLO-PHYLLIN®

Chronic asthma
- ▸ BY MOUTH USING MODIFIED-RELEASE MEDICINES
- ▸ Child 2–5 years: 60–120 mg every 12 hours
- ▸ Child 6–11 years: 125–250 mg every 12 hours
- ▸ Child 12–17 years: 250–500 mg every 12 hours
Reversible airways obstruction | Severe acute asthma | Chronic asthma
- ▸ BY MOUTH USING MODIFIED-RELEASE MEDICINES
- ▸ Adult: 250–500 mg every 12 hours

UNIPHYLLIN CONTINUS®

Chronic asthma
- ▸ BY MOUTH USING MODIFIED-RELEASE MEDICINES
- ▸ Child 2–11 years: 9 mg/kg every 12 hours (max. per dose 200 mg), dose may be increased in some children with chronic asthma; increased to 10–16 mg/kg every 12 hours (max. per dose 400 mg), may be appropriate to give larger evening or morning dose to achieve optimum therapeutic effect when symptoms most severe; in patients whose night or daytime symptoms persist despite other therapy, who are not currently receiving theophylline, total daily requirement may be added as single evening or morning dose
- ▸ Child 12–17 years: 200 mg every 12 hours, adjusted according to response to 400 mg every 12 hours, may be appropriate to give larger evening or morning dose to achieve optimum therapeutic effect when symptoms most severe; in patients whose night or daytime

symptoms persist despite other therapy, who are not currently receiving theophylline, total daily requirement may be added as single evening or morning dose

Reversible airways obstruction | Severe acute asthma | Chronic asthma
▸ BY MOUTH USING MODIFIED-RELEASE MEDICINES
▸ Adult: 200 mg every 12 hours, adjusted according to response to 400 mg every 12 hours, may be appropriate to give larger evening or morning dose to achieve optimum therapeutic effect when symptoms most severe; in patients whose night or daytime symptoms persist despite other therapy, who are not currently receiving theophylline, total daily requirement may be added as single evening or morning dose

DOSE ADJUSTMENTS DUE TO INTERACTIONS
Dose adjustment may be necessary if smoking started or stopped during treatment.

PHARMACOKINETICS
Theophylline is metabolised in the liver. The plasma-theophylline concentration is increased in heart failure, hepatic impairment, and in viral infections. The plasma-theophylline concentration is decreased in smokers, and by alcohol consumption. Differences in the half-life of theophylline are important because the toxic dose is close to the therapeutic dose.

● UNLICENSED USE
SLO-PHYLLIN® *Slo-phyllin*® capsules not licensed for use in children under 2 years.
● CAUTIONS Cardiac arrhythmias or other cardiac disease · elderly (increased plasma-theophylline concentration) · epilepsy · fever · hypertension · hyperthyroidism · peptic ulcer · risk of hypokalaemia
● INTERACTIONS → Appendix 1 (theophylline).
● SIDE-EFFECTS Arrhythmias · CNS stimulation · convulsions · diarrhoea · gastric irritation · headache · insomnia · nausea · palpitation · tachycardia · vomiting
SIDE-EFFECTS, FURTHER INFORMATION
▸ Hypokalaemia Potentially serious hypokalaemia may result from beta$_2$ agonist therapy. Particular caution is required in severe asthma, because this effect may be potentiated by concomitant treatment with theophylline and its derivatives, corticosteroids, and diuretics, and by hypoxia. Plasma-potassium concentration should therefore be monitored in severe asthma.

Overdose
Theophylline in overdose can cause vomiting (which may be severe and intractable), agitation, restlessness, dilated pupils, sinus tachycardia, and hyperglycaemia. More serious effects are haematemesis, convulsions, and supraventricular and ventricular arrhythmias. Severe hypokalaemia may develop rapidly.
    For details on the management of poisoning, see Theophylline, under Emergency treatment of poisoning p. 1199.
● PREGNANCY Neonatal irritability and apnoea have been reported. Theophylline can be taken as normal during pregnancy as it is particularly important that asthma should be well controlled during pregnancy.
● BREAST FEEDING Present in milk—irritability in infant reported; modified-release preparations preferable. Theophylline can be taken as normal during breast-feeding.
● HEPATIC IMPAIRMENT Reduce dose.
● MONITORING REQUIREMENTS
▸ In most individuals, a plasma-theophylline concentration of 10–20 mg/litre (55–110 micromol/litre) is required for satisfactory bronchodilation, although a lower plasma-theophylline concentration of 5–15 mg/litre may be

effective. Adverse effects can occur within the range 10–20 mg/litre and both the frequency and severity increase at concentrations above 20 mg/litre.
▸ Plasma-theophylline concentration is measured 5 days after starting oral treatment and at least 3 days after any dose adjustment. A blood sample should usually be taken 4–6 hours after an oral dose of a modified-release preparation (sampling times may vary—consult local guidelines).
● DIRECTIONS FOR ADMINISTRATION
SLO-PHYLLIN®
▸ In adults Swallow whole with fluid or swallow enclosed granules with soft food (e.g. yoghurt).
▸ In children Contents of the capsule (enteric-coated granules) may be sprinkled on to a spoonful of soft food (e.g. yoghurt) and swallowed without chewing.
● PRESCRIBING AND DISPENSING INFORMATION The rate of absorption from modified-release preparations can vary between brands. If a prescription for a modified-release oral theophylline preparation does not specify a brand name, the pharmacist should contact the prescriber and agree the brand to be dispensed. Additionally, it is essential that a patient discharged from hospital should be maintained on the brand on which that patient was stabilised as an in-patient.
● PATIENT AND CARER ADVICE
SLO-PHYLLIN® Patient or carer should be given advice on how to administer theophylline modified release capsules.

● MEDICINAL FORMS
There can be variation in the licensing of different medicines containing the same drug.
Modified-release tablet
CAUTIONARY AND ADVISORY LABELS 21, 25
▸ Nuelin SA (Meda Pharmaceuticals Ltd)
Theophylline 175 mg Nuelin SA 175mg tablets | 60 tablet ℙ £6.38 DT price = £6.38
Theophylline 250 mg Nuelin SA 250 tablets | 60 tablet ℙ £8.92 DT price = £8.92
▸ Uniphyllin Continus (Napp Pharmaceuticals Ltd)
Theophylline 200 mg Uniphyllin Continus 200mg tablets | 56 tablet ℙ £2.96
Theophylline 300 mg Uniphyllin Continus 300mg tablets | 56 tablet ℙ £4.77
Theophylline 400 mg Uniphyllin Continus 400mg tablets | 56 tablet ℙ £5.65 DT price = £5.65
Modified-release capsule
CAUTIONARY AND ADVISORY LABELS 25
▸ Slo-Phyllin (Merck Serono Ltd)
Theophylline 60 mg Slo-Phyllin 60mg capsules | 56 capsule ℙ £2.76 DT price = £2.76
Theophylline 125 mg Slo-Phyllin 125mg capsules | 56 capsule ℙ £3.48 DT price = £3.48
Theophylline 250 mg Slo-Phyllin 250mg capsules | 56 capsule ℙ £4.34 DT price = £4.34

Nebuliser solutions
● HYPERTONIC SODIUM CHLORIDE SOLUTIONS

● INDICATIONS AND DOSE
MUCOCLEAR® 3%
Mobilise lower respiratory tract secretions in mucous consolidation (e.g. cystic fibrosis) | Mild to moderate acute viral bronchiolitis in infants
▸ BY INHALATION OF NEBULISED SOLUTION
▸ Adult: 4 mL 2–4 times a day, temporary irritation, such as coughing, hoarseness, or reversible bronchoconstriction may occur; an inhaled bronchodilator can be used before treatment with hypertonic sodium chloride to reduce the risk of these adverse effects

MucoClear 3% inhalation solution 4ml ampoules (Pari Medical Ltd) **Sodium chloride 30 mg per 1 ml** | 20 ampoule · NHS indicative price = £12.98 · Drug Tariff (Part IXa) | 60 ampoule · NHS indicative price = £27.00 · Drug Tariff (Part IXa)

● INDICATIONS AND DOSE
MUCOCLEAR® 6%

Mobilise lower respiratory tract secretions in mucous consolidation (e.g. cystic fibrosis)
▸ BY INHALATION OF NEBULISED SOLUTION
▸ Adult: 4 mL twice daily, temporary irritation, such as coughing, hoarseness, or reversible bronchoconstriction may occur; an inhaled bronchodilator can be used before treatment with hypertonic sodium chloride to reduce the risk of these adverse effects

MucoClear 6% inhalation solution 4ml ampoules (Pari Medical Ltd) **Sodium chloride 60 mg per 1 ml** | 20 ampoule · NHS indicative price = £12.98 · Drug Tariff (Part IXa) | 60 ampoule · NHS indicative price = £27.00 · Drug Tariff (Part IXa)

● INDICATIONS AND DOSE
NEBUSAL®

Mobilise lower respiratory tract secretions in mucous consolidation (e.g. cystic fibrosis)
▸ BY INHALATION OF NEBULISED SOLUTION
▸ Adult: 4 mL up to twice daily, temporary irritation, such as coughing, hoarseness, or reversible bronchoconstriction may occur; an inhaled bronchodilator can be used before treatment with hypertonic sodium chloride to reduce the risk of these adverse effects

Nebusal 7% inhalation solution 4ml vials (Forest Laboratories UK Ltd) **Sodium chloride 70 mg per 1 ml** | 60 vial · NHS indicative price = £27.00 · Drug Tariff (Part IXa)

Peak flow meters

● LOW RANGE PEAK FLOW METERS
MEDI® LOW RANGE
Range 40–420 litres/minute.
Compliant to standard EN ISO 23747:2007 except for scale range.

Medi peak flow meter low range (Medicareplus International Ltd) | 1 device · NHS indicative price = £6.50 · Drug Tariff (Part IXa) price = £6.50
MINI-WRIGHT® LOW RANGE
Range 30–400 litres/minute.
Compliant to standard EN ISO 23747:2007 except for scale range.

Mini-wright peak flow meter low range (Clement Clarke International Ltd) | 1 device · NHS indicative price = £6.50 · Drug Tariff (Part IXa) price = £7.14
POCKETPEAK® LOW RANGE
Range 50–400 litres/minute.
Compliant to standard EN ISO 23747:2007 except for scale range.

nSpire Pocket Peak peak flow meter low range (nSpire Health Ltd) | 1 device · NHS indicative price = £6.53 · Drug Tariff (Part IXa) price = £6.50

● STANDARD RANGE PEAK FLOW METERS
AIRZONE®
Range 60–720 litres/minute.
Conforms to standard EN ISO 23747:2007.

AirZone peak flow meter standard range (Clement Clarke International Ltd) | 1 device · NHS indicative price = £4.69 · Drug Tariff (Part IXa) price = £4.50

MEDI® STANDARD RANGE
Range 60–800 litres/minute.
Conforms to standard EN ISO 23747:2007.

Medi peak flow meter standard range (Medicareplus International Ltd) | 1 device · NHS indicative price = £4.50 · Drug Tariff (Part IXa) price = £4.50
MICROPEAK®
Range 60–900 litres/minute.
Conforms to standard EN ISO 23747:2007.

MicroPeak peak flow meter standard range (Micro Medical Ltd) | 1 device · NHS indicative price = £6.50 · Drug Tariff (Part IXa) price = £4.50
MINI-WRIGHT® STANDARD RANGE
Range 60–800 litres/minute.
Conforms to standard EN ISO 23747:2007.

Mini-Wright peak flow meter standard range (Clement Clarke International Ltd) | 1 device · NHS indicative price = £7.08 · Drug Tariff (Part IXa) price = £4.50
PIKO-1®
Range 15–999 litres/minute.
Conforms to standard EN ISO 23747:2007.

nSpire PiKo-1 peak flow meter standard range (nSpire Health Ltd) | 1 device · NHS indicative price = £9.50 · Drug Tariff (Part IXa) price = £4.50
PINNACLE®
Range 60–900 litres/minute.
Conforms to standard EN ISO 23747:2007.

Fyne Dynamics Pinnacle peak flow meter standard range (Fyne Dynamics Ltd) | 1 device · NHS indicative price = £6.50 · Drug Tariff (Part IXa) price = £4.50
POCKETPEAK® STANDARD RANGE
Range 60–800 litres/minute.
Conforms to standard EN ISO 23747:2007.

nSpire Pocket Peak peak flow meter standard range (nSpire Health Ltd) | 1 device · NHS indicative price = £6.53 · Drug Tariff (Part IXa) price = £4.50
VITALOGRAPH®
Range 50–800 litres/minute.
Conforms to standard EN ISO 23747:2007.

Vitalograph peak flow meter standard range (Vitalograph Ltd) | 1 device · NHS indicative price = £4.83 · Drug Tariff (Part IXa) price = £4.50

Spacers

● SPACERS
A2A SPACER®
For use with all pressurised (aerosol) inhalers.

A2A Spacer (Clement Clarke International Ltd) | 1 device · NHS indicative price = £4.15 · Drug Tariff (Part IXa)

A2A Spacer with medium mask (Clement Clarke International Ltd) | 1 device · NHS indicative price = £6.68 · Drug Tariff (Part IXa)

A2A Spacer with small mask (Clement Clarke International Ltd) | 1 device · NHS indicative price = £6.68 · Drug Tariff (Part IXa)
ABLE SPACER®
Small-volume device. For use with all pressurised (aerosol) inhalers.

Able Spacer (Clement Clarke International Ltd) | 1 device · NHS indicative price = £4.39 · Drug Tariff (Part IXa)

Able Spacer with medium mask (Clement Clarke International Ltd) | 1 device · NHS indicative price = £7.16 · Drug Tariff (Part IXa)

Able Spacer with small mask (Clement Clarke International Ltd) | 1 device · NHS indicative price = £7.16 · Drug Tariff (Part IXa)
AEROCHAMBER PLUS®
Medium-volume device. For use with all pressurised (aerosol) inhalers.

AeroChamber Plus (GlaxoSmithKline UK Ltd) | 1 device · NHS indicative price = £4.81 · Drug Tariff (Part IXa)

AeroChamber Plus with adult mask (GlaxoSmithKline UK Ltd) | 1 device · NHS indicative price = £8.02 · Drug Tariff (Part IXa)

AeroChamber Plus with child mask (GlaxoSmithKline UK Ltd) |
1 device · NHS indicative price = £8.02 · Drug Tariff (Part IXa)

AeroChamber Plus with infant mask (GlaxoSmithKline UK Ltd) |
1 device · NHS indicative price = £8.02 · Drug Tariff (Part IXa)

BABYHALER®

For paediatric use with *Flixotide*®, and *Ventolin*® inhalers.

● PRESCRIBING AND DISPENSING INFORMATION
Not available for NHS prescription.

Babyhaler (Allen & Hanburys Ltd) | 1 device · No NHS indicative price
available · Drug Tariff (Part IXa)

HALERAID®

Device to place over pressurised (aerosol) inhalers to aid
when strength in hands is impaired (e.g. in arthritis). For
use with *Flixotide*®, *Seretide*®, *Serevent*®, and *Ventolin*®
inhalers.

● PRESCRIBING AND DISPENSING INFORMATION
Not available for NHS prescription.

Haleraid-120 (Allen & Hanburys Ltd) | 1 device · No NHS indicative
price available · Drug Tariff (Part IXa)

Haleraid-200 (Allen & Hanburys Ltd) | 1 device · No NHS indicative
price available · Drug Tariff (Part IXa)

OPTICHAMBER®

For use with all pressurised (aerosol) inhalers.

OptiChamber (Respironics (UK) Ltd) | 1 device · NHS indicative price =
£4.28 · Drug Tariff (Part IXa)

OPTICHAMBER® DIAMOND

For use with all pressurised (aerosol) inhalers.

OptiChamber Diamond (Respironics (UK) Ltd) | 1 device · NHS
indicative price = £4.49 · Drug Tariff (Part IXa)

OptiChamber Diamond with large LiteTouch mask 5 years-
adult (Respironics (UK) Ltd) | 1 device · NHS indicative price = £7.49 ·
Drug Tariff (Part IXa)

OptiChamber Diamond with medium LiteTouch mask 1-5 years
(Respironics (UK) Ltd) | 1 device · NHS indicative price = £7.49 · Drug
Tariff (Part IXa)

OptiChamber Diamond with small LiteTouch mask 0-
18 months (Respironics (UK) Ltd) | 1 device · NHS indicative price =
£7.49 · Drug Tariff (Part IXa)

POCKET CHAMBER®

Small volume device. For use with all pressurised (aerosol)
inhalers.

Pocket Chamber (nSpire Health Ltd) | 1 device · NHS indicative price
= £4.18 · Drug Tariff (Part IXa)

Pocket Chamber with adult mask (nSpire Health Ltd) | 1 device ·
NHS indicative price = £9.75 · Drug Tariff (Part IXa)

Pocket Chamber with child mask (nSpire Health Ltd) | 1 device ·
NHS indicative price = £9.75 · Drug Tariff (Part IXa)

Pocket Chamber with infant mask (nSpire Health Ltd) | 1 device ·
NHS indicative price = £9.75 · Drug Tariff (Part IXa)

Pocket Chamber with teenager mask (nSpire Health Ltd) |
1 device · NHS indicative price = £9.75 · Drug Tariff (Part IXa)

SPACE CHAMBER PLUS®

For use with all pressurised (aerosol) inhalers.

Space Chamber Plus (Medical Developments International Ltd) |
1 device · NHS indicative price = £4.26 · Drug Tariff (Part IXa)

Space Chamber Plus with large mask (Medical Developments
International Ltd) | 1 device · NHS indicative price = £6.98 · Drug Tariff
(Part IXa)

Space Chamber Plus with medium mask (Medical Developments
International Ltd) | 1 device · NHS indicative price = £6.98 · Drug Tariff
(Part IXa)

Space Chamber Plus with small mask (Medical Developments
International Ltd) | 1 device · NHS indicative price = £6.98 · Drug Tariff
(Part IXa)

VOLUMATIC®

Large-volume device. For use with *Clenil Modulite*®,
Flixotide®, *Seretide*®, *Serevent*®, and *Ventolin*® inhalers.

Volumatic (GlaxoSmithKline UK Ltd) | 1 device · NHS indicative price =
£3.81 · Drug Tariff (Part IXa)

Volumatic with paediatric mask (GlaxoSmithKline UK Ltd) |
1 device · NHS indicative price = £6.70 · Drug Tariff (Part IXa)

VORTEX®

Medium-volume device. For use with all pressurised
(aerosol) inhalers.

Vortex Spacer (Pari Medical Ltd) | 1 device · NHS indicative price =
£6.28 · Drug Tariff (Part IXa)

Vortex with child mask 0-2 years (Pari Medical Ltd) | 1 device ·
NHS indicative price = £7.99 · Drug Tariff (Part IXa)

Vortex with child mask 2 years+ (Pari Medical Ltd) | 1 device · NHS
indicative price = £7.99 · Drug Tariff (Part IXa)

2 Allergic conditions

Antihistamines, allergen immunotherapy and allergic emergencies

Antihistamines

All antihistamines are of potential value in the treatment of
nasal allergies, particularly seasonal allergic rhinitis
(hayfever), and they may be of some value in vasomotor
rhinitis. They reduce rhinorrhoea and sneezing but are
usually less effective for nasal congestion. Antihistamines
are used topically in the eye, in the nose, and on the skin.

Oral antihistamines are also of some value in preventing
urticaria and are used to treat urticarial rashes, pruritus, and
insect bites and stings; they are also used in drug allergies.
Injections of chlorphenamine maleate p. 260 or
promethazine hydrochloride p. 264 are used as an adjunct to
adrenaline/epinephrine p. 205 in the emergency treatment
of anaphylaxis and angioedema. Antihistamines (including
cinnarizine p. 400, cyclizine p. 393, and promethazine
teoclate p. 400) may also have a role in nausea and vomiting.
Buclizine is included as an anti-emetic in a preparation for
migraine. Antihistamines may also have a role in occasional
insomnia.

All older antihistamines cause sedation but alimemazine
tartrate p. 259 and **promethazine** may be more sedating
whereas chlorphenamine maleate and cyclizine may be less
so. This sedating activity is sometimes used to manage the
pruritus associated with some allergies. There is little
evidence that any one of the older, 'sedating' antihistamines
is superior to another and patients vary widely in their
response.

Non-sedating antihistamines such as acrivastine p. 255,
bilastine p. 255, cetirizine hydrochloride p. 256,
desloratadine p. 256 (an active metabolite of loratadine
p. 258), fexofenadine hydrochloride p. 257 (an active
metabolite of terfenadine), levocetirizine hydrochloride
p. 257 (an isomer of cetirizine hydrochloride), loratadine,
and mizolastine p. 259 cause less sedation and psychomotor
impairment than the older antihistamines because they
penetrate the blood brain barrier only to a slight extent.

Allergen immunotherapy

Immunotherapy using allergen vaccines containing house
dust mite, animal dander (cat or dog), or extracts of grass
and tree pollen can reduce symptoms of asthma and allergic
rhinoconjunctivitis. A vaccine containing extracts of wasp
and bee venom is used to reduce the risk of severe
anaphylaxis and systemic reactions in individuals with
hypersensitivity to wasp and bee stings. An oral preparation
of grass pollen extract (*Grazax*®) is also licensed for disease-
modifying treatment of grass pollen-induced rhinitis and
conjunctivitis. Those requiring immunotherapy must be
referred to a hospital specialist for accurate diagnosis,
assessment, and treatment.

Omalizumab p. 244 is a monoclonal antibody that binds to
immunoglobulin E (IgE). It is used as additional therapy in

individuals with proven IgE-mediated sensitivity to inhaled allergens, whose severe persistent allergic asthma cannot be controlled adequately with high dose inhaled corticosteroid together with a long-acting beta₂ agonist. Omalizumab should be initiated by physicians in specialist centres experienced in the treatment of severe persistent asthma. Omalizumab is also indicated as add-on therapy for the treatment of chronic spontaneous urticaria in patients who have had an inadequate response to H₁ antihistamine treatment.

Allergic emergencies

Anaphylaxis

Anaphylaxis is a severe, life-threatening, generalised or systemic hypersensitivity reaction. It is characterised by the rapid onset of respiratory and/or circulatory problems and is usually associated with skin and mucosal changes; prompt treatment is required. Patients with pre-existing asthma, especially poorly controlled asthma, are at particular risk of life-threatening reactions. Insect stings are a recognised risk (in particular wasp and bee stings). Latex and certain foods, including eggs, fish, cow's milk protein, peanuts, sesame, shellfish, soy, and tree nuts may also precipitate anaphylaxis. Medicinal products particularly associated with anaphylaxis include blood products, vaccines, hyposensitising (allergen) preparations, antibacterials, aspirin and other NSAIDs, and neuromuscular blocking drugs. In the case of drugs, anaphylaxis is more likely after parenteral administration; resuscitation facilities must always be available for injections associated with special risk. Anaphylactic reactions may also be associated with *additives and excipients* in foods and medicines. Refined arachis (peanut) oil, which may be present in some medicinal products, is unlikely to cause an allergic reaction— nevertheless it is wise to check the full formula of preparations which may contain allergens.

Treatment of anaphylaxis

Adrenaline/epinephrine provides physiological reversal of the immediate symptoms associated with hypersensitivity reactions such as *anaphylaxis* and *angioedema*.

First-line treatment includes:

- securing the airway, restoration of blood pressure (laying the patient flat and raising the legs, or in the recovery position if unconscious or nauseous and at risk of vomiting);
- administering adrenaline/epinephrine (by **intramuscular** injection in a dose of 500 micrograms (a dose of 300 micrograms may be appropriate for *immediate self-administration*); the dose should be repeated if necessary at 5-minute intervals according to blood pressure, pulse, and respiratory function. Patients receiving beta-blockers require special consideration;
- administering high-flow **oxygen** and **intravenous fluids** is also of primary importance;
- administering an antihistamine, such as chlorphenamine maleate, by slow intravenous injection or intramuscular injection is a useful adjunctive treatment, given after adrenaline.
- Administering an intravenous corticosteroid such as hydrocortisone p. 612 (preferably as sodium succinate) is of secondary value in the initial management of anaphylaxis because the onset of action is delayed for several hours, but should be given to prevent further deterioration in severely affected patients.

Continuing respiratory deterioration requires further treatment with **bronchodilators** including inhaled or intravenous salbutamol p. 233, inhaled ipratropium bromide p. 228, intravenous aminophylline p. 249, or intravenous magnesium sulfate p. 911 [unlicensed indication] (as for acute severe asthma); in addition to oxygen, assisted respiration and possibly emergency tracheotomy may be necessary.

When a patient is so ill that there is doubt about the adequacy of the circulation, the initial injection of adrenaline/epinephrine may need to be given as a *dilute solution by the intravenous route*.

Cardiopulmonary arrest may follow an anaphylactic reaction; resuscitation should be started immediately.

On discharge, patients should be considered for further treatment with an oral antihistamine and an oral corticosteroid for up to 3 days to reduce the risk of further reaction. Patients should be instructed to return to hospital if symptoms recur and to contact their general practitioner for follow-up.

Patients who are suspected of having had an anaphylactic reaction should be referred to a specialist for specific allergy diagnosis. Avoidance of the allergen is the principal treatment; if appropriate, an adrenaline/epinephrine auto-injector should be given for self-administration or a replacement supplied.

Intramuscular adrenaline (epinephrine)

The *intramuscular route* is the *first choice route* for the administration of adrenaline/epinephrine in the management of anaphylaxis. Adrenaline/epinephrine is best given as an intramuscular injection into the anterolateral aspect of the middle third of the thigh; it has a rapid onset of action after intramuscular administration and in the shocked patient its absorption from the intramuscular site is faster and more reliable than from the subcutaneous site.

Patients with severe allergy should be instructed in the self-administration of adrenaline/epinephrine p. 205 by intramuscular injection.

Prompt injection of adrenaline/epinephrine is of paramount importance. The adrenaline/epinephrine doses recommended for the emergency treatment of anaphylaxis by appropriately trained healthcare professionals are based on the revised recommendations of the Working Group of the Resuscitation Council (UK).

Dose of intramuscular injection of adrenaline (epinephrine) for the emergency treatment of anaphylaxis by healthcare professionals

Age	Dose	Volume of adrenaline
▸ Child 1 month–5 years	150 micrograms	0.15 mL 1 in 1000 (1 mg/mL) adrenaline[1]
▸ Child 6–11 years	300 micrograms	0.3 mL 1 in 1000 (1 mg/mL) adrenaline
▸ Child 12–17 years	500 micrograms	0.5 mL 1 in 1000 (1 mg/mL) adrenaline[2]
▸ Adult	500 micrograms	0.5 mL 1 in 1000 (1 mg/mL) adrenaline

These doses may be repeated several times if necessary at 5-minute intervals according to blood pressure, pulse and respiratory function.

1. Use suitable syringe for measuring small volume
2. 300 micrograms (0.3 mL) if child is small or prepubertal

Intravenous adrenaline (epinephrine)

Intravenous adrenaline/epinephrine should be given only by those experienced in its use, in a setting where patients can be carefully monitored.

When the patient is severely ill and there is real doubt about the adequacy of the circulation and absorption after intramuscular injection, adrenaline/epinephrine can be given by **slow** *intravenous injection* repeated according to response; if multiple doses are required, adrenaline/epinephrine should be given as a **slow** intravenous infusion *stopping when a response has been obtained*.

It is important that, where intramuscular injection might still succeed, time should not be wasted seeking intravenous access.

The intravenous route is also used for *cardiac resuscitation*.

Angioedema

Angioedema is dangerous if *laryngeal oedema* is present. In this circumstance adrenaline/epinephrine injection and **oxygen** should be given as described under **Anaphylaxis**; antihistamines and corticosteroids should also be given. Tracheal intubation may be necessary.

Hereditary angioedema

The treatment of hereditary angioedema should be under specialist supervision. Unlike allergic angioedema, adrenaline/epinephrine, corticosteroids, and antihistamines should not be used for the treatment of acute attacks, including attacks involving laryngeal oedema, as they are ineffective and may delay appropriate treatment—intubation may be necessary. The administration of C1-esterase inhibitor p. 267, an endogenous complement blocker derived from human plasma, (in fresh frozen plasma or in partially purified form) can terminate acute attacks of *hereditary angioedema*; it can also be used for short-term prophylaxis before dental, medical or surgical procedures. Conestat alfa p. 267 and icatibant p. 268 are licensed for the treatment of acute attacks of hereditary angioedema in adults with C1-esterase inhibitor deficiency.

Tranexamic acid p. 99 and danazol p. 670 [unlicensed indication] are used for short-term and long-term prophylaxis of hereditary angioedema. Short-term prophylaxis with tranexamic acid or danazol is started several days before planned procedures (e.g. dental work) and continued for 2–5 days afterwards. Danazol should be avoided in children because of its androgenic effects.

ANTIHISTAMINES > NON-SEDATING

Acrivastine

● **INDICATIONS AND DOSE**

Symptomatic relief of allergy such as hayfever, chronic idiopathic urticaria
▸ BY MOUTH
▸ Child 12-17 years: 8 mg 3 times a day
▸ Adult: 8 mg 3 times a day

● CONTRA-INDICATIONS Avoid in Acute porphyrias p. 918 (some antihistamines are thought to be safe) · elderly

● CAUTIONS Epilepsy

● INTERACTIONS → Appendix 1 (antihistamines).
Sedative antihistamine interactions apply to a lesser extent to the non-sedating antihistamines.

● SIDE-EFFECTS
▸ **Uncommon** Antimuscarinic effects · gastro-intestinal disturbances · headache · psychomotor impairment
▸ **Rare** Anaphylaxis · angioedema · angle-closure glaucoma (in adults) · arrhythmias · blood disorders · bronchospasm · confusion · convulsions · depression · dizziness · extrapyramidal effects · hypersensitivity reactions · hypotension · liver dysfunction · palpitation · photosensitivity reactions · rashes · sleep disturbances · tremor
▸ **Frequency not known** Blurred vision · drowsiness · dry mouth · urinary retention

SIDE-EFFECTS, FURTHER INFORMATION
Non-sedating antihistamines such as acrivastine cause less sedation and psychomotor impairment than the older antihistamines because they penetrate the blood brain barrier only to a slight extent.

If drowsiness occurs, it may diminish after a few days of treatment.

Children and the elderly are more susceptible to side-effects.

● ALLERGY AND CROSS-SENSITIVITY Contra-indicated if history of hypersensitivity to triprolidine.

● PREGNANCY Most manufacturers of antihistamines advise avoiding their use during pregnancy; however, there is no evidence of teratogenicity.

● BREAST FEEDING Most antihistamines are present in breast milk in varying amounts; although not known to be harmful, most manufacturers advise avoiding their use in mothers who are breast-feeding.

● RENAL IMPAIRMENT Avoid in severe impairment.

● PATIENT AND CARER ADVICE
Driving and skilled tasks
▸ In adults Although drowsiness is rare, nevertheless patients should be advised that it can occur and may affect performance of skilled tasks (e.g. driving); excess alcohol should be avoided.
▸ In children Although drowsiness is rare, nevertheless children and their carers should be advised that it can occur and may affect performance of skilled tasks (e.g. cycling or driving); alcohol should be avoided.

● MEDICINAL FORMS
There can be variation in the licensing of different medicines containing the same drug.
Capsule
▸ Benadryl Allergy Relief (McNeil Products Ltd)
Acrivastine 8 mg Benadryl Allergy Relief 8mg capsules | 24 capsule Ⓟ £4.95

Bilastine

● **INDICATIONS AND DOSE**

Symptomatic relief of allergic rhinoconjunctivitis and urticaria
▸ BY MOUTH
▸ Child 12-17 years: 20 mg once daily
▸ Adult: 20 mg once daily

● CONTRA-INDICATIONS Avoid in Acute porphyrias p. 918 (some antihistamines are thought to be safe)

● CAUTIONS Epilepsy

● INTERACTIONS → Appendix 1 (antihistamines).
Sedative antihistamine interactions apply to a lesser extent to the non-sedating antihistamines.

● SIDE-EFFECTS
▸ **Common or very common** Headache · malaise
▸ **Uncommon** Abdominal pain · anxiety · diarrhoea · dizziness · dyspnoea · gastritis · increased appetite · insomnia · oral herpes · prolongation of the QT interval · pyrexia · thirst · tinnitus · vertigo · weight gain

SIDE-EFFECTS, FURTHER INFORMATION
Children and the elderly are more susceptible to side-effects.

Non-sedating antihistamines such as bilastine cause less sedation and psychomotor impairment than the older antihistamines because they penetrate the blood brain barrier only to a slight extent.

● PREGNANCY Avoid—limited information available. Most manufacturers of antihistamines advise avoiding their use during pregnancy; however, there is no evidence of teratogenicity.

● BREAST FEEDING Avoid—no information available. Most antihistamines are present in breast milk in varying amounts; although not known to be harmful, most manufacturers advise avoiding their use in mothers who are breast-feeding.

● DIRECTIONS FOR ADMINISTRATION Take tablet 1 hour before or 2 hours after food or fruit juice.

3

Respiratory system

• PATIENT AND CARER ADVICE
Patients or carers should be given advice on how to administer bilastine tablets.

Driving and skilled tasks
Although drowsiness is rare, nevertheless patients should be advised that it can occur and may affect performance of skilled tasks (e.g. cycling or driving); alcohol should be avoided.

• MEDICINAL FORMS
There can be variation in the licensing of different medicines containing the same drug.
No licensed medicines listed.

Cetirizine hydrochloride

• INDICATIONS AND DOSE

Symptomatic relief of allergy such as hay fever, chronic idiopathic urticaria, atopic dermatitis
▶ BY MOUTH
▸ Child 2–5 years: 2.5 mg twice daily
▸ Child 6–11 years: 5 mg twice daily
▸ Child 12–17 years: 10 mg once daily
▸ Adult: 10 mg once daily

• UNLICENSED USE
▸ In children Not licensed for use in children under 2 years.

• CONTRA-INDICATIONS Avoid in Acute porphyrias p. 918 (some antihistamines are thought to be safe)

• CAUTIONS Epilepsy

• INTERACTIONS → Appendix 1 (antihistamines). Sedative antihistamine interactions apply to a lesser extent to the non-sedating antihistamines.

• SIDE-EFFECTS
▶ **Uncommon** Antimuscarinic effects · blurred vision · dry mouth · gastro-intestinal disturbances · headache · psychomotor impairment · urinary retention
▶ **Rare** Anaphylaxis · angioedema · angle-closure glaucoma (in adults) · arrhythmias · blood disorders · bronchospasm · confusion · convulsions · depression · dizziness · extrapyramidal effects · hypersensitivity reactions · hypotension · liver dysfunction · palpitation · photosensitivity reactions · rashes · sleep disturbances · tremor
▶ **Frequency not known** Drowsiness

SIDE-EFFECTS, FURTHER INFORMATION
Non-sedating antihistamines such as cetirizine cause less sedation and psychomotor impairment than the older antihistamines because they penetrate the blood brain barrier only to a slight extent.
  If drowsiness occurs, it may diminish after a few days of treatment.
  Children and the elderly are more susceptible to side-effects.

• PREGNANCY Most manufacturers of antihistamines advise avoiding their use during pregnancy; however, there is no evidence of teratogenicity.

• BREAST FEEDING Most antihistamines are present in breast milk in varying amounts; although not known to be harmful, most manufacturers advise avoiding their use in mothers who are breast-feeding.

• RENAL IMPAIRMENT
▸ In adults Use half normal dose if eGFR 30–50 mL/minute/1.73 m^2. Use half normal dose and reduce dose frequency to alternate days if eGFR 10–30 mL/minute/1.73 m^2. Avoid if eGFR less than 10 mL/minute/1.73 m^2.
▸ In children Use half normal dose if estimated glomerular filtration rate 30–50 mL/minute/1.73 m^2. Use half normal dose and reduce dose frequency to alternate days if

estimated glomerular filtration rate 10–30 mL/minute/1.73 m^2. Avoid if estimated glomerular filtration rate less than 10 mL/minute/1.73 m^2.

• PATIENT AND CARER ADVICE
Medicines for Children leaflet: Cetirizine hydrochloride for hay fever www.medicinesforchildren.org.uk/cetirizine-hay-fever-0

Driving and skilled tasks
Although drowsiness is rare, nevertheless patients should be advised that it can occur and may affect performance of skilled tasks (e.g. cycling or driving); alcohol should be avoided.

• PROFESSION SPECIFIC INFORMATION

Dental practitioners' formulary
Cetirizine Tablets 10 mg may be prescribed.
  Cetirizine Oral Solution 5 mg/5 mL may be prescribed.

• MEDICINAL FORMS
There can be variation in the licensing of different medicines containing the same drug.

Tablet
▸ Cetirizine hydrochloride (Non-proprietary)
  Cetirizine hydrochloride 10 mg Cetirizine 10mg tablets | 7 tablet P £1.40 | 14 tablet GSL no price available | 30 tablet PoM £1.26 DT price = £0.81 | 30 tablet P £8.29 DT price = £0.81
▸ Pollenshield (Actavis UK Ltd)
  Cetirizine hydrochloride 10 mg Pollenshield Hayfever 10mg tablets | 30 tablet P £2.17 DT price = £0.81
▸ Zirtek (UCB Pharma Ltd)
  Cetirizine hydrochloride 10 mg Zirtek Allergy 10mg tablets | 21 tablet P £5.33 | 30 tablet P £8.12 DT price = £0.81

Oral solution
EXCIPIENTS: May contain Propylene glycol
▸ Cetirizine hydrochloride (Non-proprietary)
  Cetirizine hydrochloride 1 mg per 1 ml Cetirizine 1mg/ml oral solution sugar free sugar-free | 200 ml P no price available DT price = £1.58 sugar-free | 200 ml PoM £3.50 DT price = 1.58
▸ Benadryl Allergy (McNeil Products Ltd)
  Cetirizine hydrochloride 1 mg per 1 ml Benadryl Allergy Children's 1mg/ml oral solution sugar-free | 100 ml P £3.21
  Benadryl Allergy 1mg/ml oral solution sugar-free | 100 ml P £3.15
▸ Zirtek (UCB Pharma Ltd)
  Cetirizine hydrochloride 1 mg per 1 ml Zirtek Allergy 1mg/ml oral solution sugar-free | 150 ml P £3.70 sugar-free | 200 ml P £9.77 DT price = £1.58

Desloratadine

• INDICATIONS AND DOSE

Symptomatic relief of allergy such as allergic rhinitis, urticaria, chronic idiopathic urticaria
▶ BY MOUTH
▸ Child 1–5 years: 1.25 mg once daily
▸ Child 6–11 years: 2.5 mg once daily
▸ Child 12–17 years: 5 mg once daily
▸ Adult: 5 mg once daily

PHARMACOKINETICS
Desloratadine is a metabolite of loratadine.

• CAUTIONS Acute porphyrias p. 918 · epilepsy

• INTERACTIONS → Appendix 1 (antihistamines). Sedative antihistamine interactions apply to a lesser extent to the non-sedating antihistamines.

• SIDE-EFFECTS
▶ **Uncommon** Antimuscarinic effects · blurred vision · dry mouth · gastro-intestinal disturbances · headache · psychomotor impairment · urinary retention
▶ **Rare** Anaphylaxis · angioedema · angle-closure glaucoma (in adults) · arrhythmias · blood disorders · bronchospasm · confusion · convulsions · depression · dizziness · extrapyramidal effects · hypersensitivity reactions · hypotension · liver dysfunction · myalgia · palpitation ·

photosensitivity reactions · rashes · sleep disturbances · tremor
▸ **Very rare** Hallucinations
▸ **Frequency not known** Drowsiness

SIDE-EFFECTS, FURTHER INFORMATION
Non-sedating antihistamines such as desloratadine cause less sedation and psychomotor impairment than the older antihistamines because they penetrate the blood brain barrier only to a slight extent.

If drowsiness occurs, it may diminish after a few days of treatment.

Children and the elderly are more susceptible to side-effects.

● ALLERGY AND CROSS-SENSITIVITY Contra-indicated if history of hypersensitivity to loratadine.
● PREGNANCY Most manufacturers of antihistamines advise avoiding their use during pregnancy; however, there is no evidence of teratogenicity.
● BREAST FEEDING Most antihistamines are present in breast milk in varying amounts; although not known to be harmful, most manufacturers advise avoiding their use in mothers who are breast-feeding.
● RENAL IMPAIRMENT Use with caution in severe impairment.
● PRESCRIBING AND DISPENSING INFORMATION Flavours of oral liquid formulations may include bubblegum.
● PATIENT AND CARER ADVICE
Driving and skilled tasks
Although drowsiness is rare, nevertheless patients should be advised that it can occur and may affect performance of skilled tasks (e.g. cycling or driving); excess alcohol should be avoided.

● MEDICINAL FORMS
There can be variation in the licensing of different medicines containing the same drug.
Tablet
▸ Desloratadine (Non-proprietary)
  Desloratadine 5 mg Desloratadine 5mg tablets | 30 tablet PoM £6.77 DT price = £1.23
▸ Neoclarityn (Merck Sharp & Dohme Ltd)
  Desloratadine 5 mg Neoclarityn 5mg tablets | 30 tablet PoM £6.77 DT price = £1.23
Oral solution
EXCIPIENTS: May contain Propylene glycol, sorbitol
▸ Desloratadine (Non-proprietary)
  Desloratadine 500 microgram per 1 ml Desloratadine 2.5mg/5ml oral solution sugar free sugar-free | 100 ml PoM no price available sugar-free | 150 ml PoM £8.00–£10.15 DT price = £10.15
▸ Neoclarityn (Merck Sharp & Dohme Ltd)
  Desloratadine 500 microgram per 1 ml Neoclarityn 2.5mg/5ml oral solution sugar-free | 100 ml PoM £6.77 sugar-free | 150 ml PoM £10.15 DT price = £10.15

Fexofenadine hydrochloride

● INDICATIONS AND DOSE
Symptomatic relief of seasonal allergic rhinitis
▸ BY MOUTH
▸ Child 6–11 years: 30 mg twice daily
▸ Child 12–17 years: 120 mg once daily
▸ Adult: 120 mg once daily
Symptomatic relief of chronic idiopathic urticaria
▸ BY MOUTH
▸ Child 12–17 years: 180 mg once daily
▸ Adult: 180 mg once daily
PHARMACOKINETICS
Fexofenadine is a metabolite of terfenadine.

● CAUTIONS Epilepsy

● INTERACTIONS → Appendix 1 (antihistamines). Sedative antihistamine interactions apply to a lesser extent to the non-sedating antihistamines.
● SIDE-EFFECTS
▸ **Uncommon** Antimuscarinic effects · blurred vision · dry mouth · gastro-intestinal disturbances · headache · psychomotor impairment · urinary retention
▸ **Rare** Anaphylaxis · angioedema · angle-closure glaucoma (in adults) · arrhythmias · blood disorders · bronchospasm · confusion · convulsions · depression · dizziness · extrapyramidal effects · hypersensitivity reactions · hypotension · liver dysfunction · palpitation · photosensitivity reactions · rashes · sleep disturbances · tremor
▸ **Frequency not known** Drowsiness
SIDE-EFFECTS, FURTHER INFORMATION
Non-sedating antihistamines such as fexofenadine cause less sedation and psychomotor impairment than the older antihistamines because they penetrate the blood brain barrier only to a slight extent.

If drowsiness occurs, it may diminish after a few days of treatment.

Children and the elderly are more susceptible to side-effects.

● PREGNANCY Most manufacturers of antihistamines advise avoiding their use during pregnancy; however, there is no evidence of teratogenicity.
● BREAST FEEDING Most antihistamines are present in breast milk in varying amounts; although not known to be harmful, most manufacturers advise avoiding their use in mothers who are breast-feeding.
● PATIENT AND CARER ADVICE
Driving and skilled tasks
Although drowsiness is rare, nevertheless patients should be advised that it can occur and may affect performance of skilled tasks (e.g. cycling or driving); alcohol should be avoided.

● MEDICINAL FORMS
There can be variation in the licensing of different medicines containing the same drug. Forms available from special-order manufacturers include: oral suspension, oral solution
Tablet
CAUTIONARY AND ADVISORY LABELS 5
▸ Fexofenadine hydrochloride (Non-proprietary)
  Fexofenadine hydrochloride 120 mg Fexofenadine 120mg tablets | 30 tablet PoM £7.15 DT price = £2.28
  Fexofenadine hydrochloride 180 mg Fexofenadine 180mg tablets | 30 tablet PoM £9.65 DT price = £3.24
▸ Telfast (Sanofi)
  Fexofenadine hydrochloride 30 mg Telfast 30mg tablets | 60 tablet PoM £5.46 DT price = £5.46
  Fexofenadine hydrochloride 120 mg Telfast 120mg tablets | 30 tablet PoM £5.99 DT price = £2.28
  Fexofenadine hydrochloride 180 mg Telfast 180mg tablets | 30 tablet PoM £7.58 DT price = £3.24

Levocetirizine hydrochloride

● INDICATIONS AND DOSE
Symptomatic relief of allergy such as hay fever, urticaria
▸ BY MOUTH
▸ Child 6–17 years: 5 mg once daily
▸ Adult: 5 mg once daily
PHARMACOKINETICS
Levocetirizine is an isomer of cetirizine.

● UNLICENSED USE Tablets not licensed for use in children under 6 years.
● CONTRA-INDICATIONS Avoid in Acute porphyrias p. 918 (some antihistamines are thought to be safe)

- CAUTIONS Epilepsy
- INTERACTIONS → Appendix 1 (antihistamines). Sedative antihistamine interactions apply to a lesser extent to the non-sedating antihistamines.
- SIDE-EFFECTS
▸ **Uncommon** Antimuscarinic effects · blurred vision · dry mouth · gastro-intestinal disturbances · headache · psychomotor impairment · urinary retention
▸ **Rare** Anaphylaxis · angioedema · angle-closure glaucoma (in adults) · arrhythmias · blood disorders · bronchospasm · confusion · convulsions · depression · dizziness · extrapyramidal effects · hypersensitivity reactions · hypotension · liver dysfunction · palpitation · photosensitivity reactions · rashes · sleep disturbances · tremor
▸ **Very rare** Weight gain
▸ **Frequency not known** Drowsiness
SIDE-EFFECTS, FURTHER INFORMATION
Non-sedating antihistamines such as levocetirizine cause less sedation and psychomotor impairment than the older antihistamines because they penetrate the blood brain barrier only to a slight extent.
  If drowsiness occurs, it may diminish after a few days of treatment.
  Children and the elderly are more susceptible to side-effects.

- PREGNANCY Most manufacturers of antihistamines advise avoiding their use during pregnancy; however, there is no evidence of teratogenicity.

- BREAST FEEDING Most antihistamines are present in breast milk in varying amounts; although not known to be harmful, most manufacturers advise avoiding their use in mothers who are breast-feeding.

- RENAL IMPAIRMENT
▸ In adults 5 mg on alternate days if eGFR 30–50 mL/minute/1.73 m². 5 mg every 3 days if eGFR 10–30 mL/minute/1.73 m². Avoid if eGFR less than 10 mL/minute/1.73 m².
▸ In children Reduce dose frequency to alternate days if estimated glomerular filtration rate 30–50 mL/minute/1.73 m². Reduce dose frequency to every 3 days if estimated glomerular filtration rate 10–30 mL/minute/1.73 m². Avoid if estimated glomerular filtration rate less than 10 mL/minute/1.73 m².

- PATIENT AND CARER ADVICE
Driving and skilled tasks
Although drowsiness is rare, nevertheless patients should be advised that it can occur and may affect performance of skilled tasks (e.g. cycling or driving); alcohol should be avoided.

- MEDICINAL FORMS
There can be variation in the licensing of different medicines containing the same drug.
Tablet
▸ Levocetirizine hydrochloride (Non-proprietary)
  Levocetirizine dihydrochloride 5 mg Levocetirizine 5mg tablets | 30 tablet PoM £4.39 DT price = £4.28
▸ Xyzal (UCB Pharma Ltd)
  Levocetirizine dihydrochloride 5 mg Xyzal 5mg tablets | 30 tablet PoM £4.39 DT price = £4.28
Oral solution
▸ Xyzal (UCB Pharma Ltd)
  Levocetirizine dihydrochloride 500 microgram per 1 ml Xyzal 0.5mg/ml oral solution sugar-free | 200 ml PoM £6.00 DT price = £6.00

Loratadine

- INDICATIONS AND DOSE
Symptomatic relief of allergy such as hay fever, chronic idiopathic urticaria
▸ BY MOUTH
▸ Child 2–11 years (body-weight up to 31 kg): 5 mg once daily
▸ Child 2–11 years (body-weight 31 kg and above): 10 mg once daily
▸ Child 12–17 years: 10 mg once daily
▸ Adult: 10 mg once daily

- CAUTIONS Acute porphyrias p. 918 · epilepsy
- INTERACTIONS → Appendix 1 (antihistamines). Sedative antihistamine interactions apply to a lesser extent to the non-sedating antihistamines. Interactions do not generally apply to antihistamines used for topical action (including inhalation).
- SIDE-EFFECTS
▸ **Uncommon** Antimuscarinic effects · blurred vision · dry mouth · gastro-intestinal disturbances · Headache · psychomotor impairment · urinary retention
▸ **Rare** Anaphylaxis · angioedema · angle-closure glaucoma (in adults) · arrhythmias · blood disorders · bronchospasm · confusion · convulsions · depression · dizziness · extrapyramidal effects · hypersensitivity reactions · hypotension · liver dysfunction · palpitation · photosensitivity reactions · rashes · sleep disturbances · tremor
▸ **Frequency not known** Drowsiness
SIDE-EFFECTS, FURTHER INFORMATION
Non-sedating antihistamines such as loratadine cause less sedation and psychomotor impairment than the older antihistamines because they penetrate the blood brain barrier only to a slight extent.
  If drowsiness occurs, it may diminish after a few days of treatment.
  Children and the elderly are more susceptible to side-effects.

- PREGNANCY Most manufacturers of antihistamines advise avoiding their use during pregnancy; however, there is no evidence of teratogenicity.

- BREAST FEEDING Most antihistamines are present in breast milk in varying amounts; although not known to be harmful, most manufacturers advise avoiding their use in mothers who are breast-feeding.

- HEPATIC IMPAIRMENT Reduce dose frequency to alternate days in severe impairment.

- PATIENT AND CARER ADVICE
Driving and skilled tasks
Although drowsiness is rare, nevertheless patients and their carers should be advised that it can occur and may affect performance of skilled tasks (e.g. cycling or driving); alcohol should be avoided.

- PROFESSION SPECIFIC INFORMATION
Dental practitioners' formulary
Loratadine 10 mg tablets may be prescribed.
  Loratadine syrup 5 mg/5 mL may be prescribed.

- MEDICINAL FORMS
There can be variation in the licensing of different medicines containing the same drug.
Tablet
▸ Loratadine (Non-proprietary)
  Loratadine 10 mg Loratadine 10mg tablets | 14 tablet GSL no price available | 30 tablet P £8.20 DT price = £0.86
▸ Clarityn (Loratadine) (Bayer Plc)
  Loratadine 10 mg Clarityn Allergy 10mg tablets | 60 tablet P £8.85

Oral solution

EXCIPIENTS: May contain Propylene glycol
▸ Loratadine (Non-proprietary)
 Loratadine 1 mg per 1 ml Loratadine 5mg/5ml oral solution |
 100 ml P £4.85 DT price = £1.80 | 100 ml PoM £2.63 DT price =
 £1.80 | 120 ml P £2.40-£2.47 | 120 ml PoM £2.40
▸ Clarityn (Loratadine) (Bayer Plc)
 Loratadine 1 mg per 1 ml Clarityn Allergy 5mg/5ml syrup |
 70 ml GSL £2.43

Oral lyophilisate

▸ Clarityn (Loratadine) (Bayer Plc)
 Loratadine 10 mg Clarityn Rapide Allergy 10mg tablets sugar-free |
 10 tablet GSL £3.24

Mizolastine

● INDICATIONS AND DOSE

Symptomatic relief of allergy such as hay fever, urticaria
▸ BY MOUTH
 ▸ Child 12-17 years: 10 mg once daily
 ▸ Adult: 10 mg once daily

● CONTRA-INDICATIONS Avoid in Acute porphyrias p. 918
 (some antihistamines are thought to be safe) · cardiac
 disease · hypokalaemia · susceptibility to QT-interval
 prolongation
● CAUTIONS Epilepsy
● INTERACTIONS → Appendix 1 (antihistamines).
 Sedative antihistamine interactions apply to a lesser
 extent to the non-sedating antihistamines.
● SIDE-EFFECTS
▸ **Common or very common** Anxiety · asthenia · weight gain
▸ **Uncommon** Antimuscarinic effects · arthralgia · blurred
 vision · dry mouth · gastro-intestinal disturbances ·
 headache · myalgia · psychomotor impairment · urinary
 retention
▸ **Rare** Anaphylaxis · angioedema · angle-closure glaucoma
 (in adults) · arrhythmias · blood disorders · bronchospasm ·
 confusion · convulsions · depression · dizziness ·
 extrapyramidal effects · hypersensitivity reactions ·
 hypotension · liver dysfunction · palpitation ·
 photosensitivity reactions · rashes · sleep disturbances ·
 tremor
▸ **Frequency not known** Drowsiness
 SIDE-EFFECTS, FURTHER INFORMATION
 Non-sedating antihistamines such as mizolastine cause
 less sedation and psychomotor impairment than the older
 antihistamines because they penetrate the blood brain
 barrier only to a slight extent.
  If drowsiness occurs, it may diminish after a few days of
 treatment.
  Children and the elderly are more susceptible to side-
 effects.
● PREGNANCY Most manufacturers of antihistamines advise
 avoiding their use during pregnancy; however, there is no
 evidence of teratogenicity.
● BREAST FEEDING Most antihistamines are present in
 breast milk in varying amounts; although not known to be
 harmful, most manufacturers advise avoiding their use in
 mothers who are breast-feeding.
● HEPATIC IMPAIRMENT Manufacturer advises avoid in
 significant impairment.
● PATIENT AND CARER ADVICE
 Driving and skilled tasks
 Although drowsiness is rare, nevertheless patients and
 their carers should be advised that it can occur and may
 affect performance of skilled tasks (e.g. cycling or driving);
 alcohol should be avoided.

● MEDICINAL FORMS
 There can be variation in the licensing of different medicines
 containing the same drug.
 Modified-release tablet
 CAUTIONARY AND ADVISORY LABELS 25
 ▸ Mizollen (Sanofi)
  Mizolastine 10 mg Mizollen 10mg modified-release tablets |
  30 tablet PoM £6.92 DT price = £6.92

ANTIHISTAMINES > SEDATING

Alimemazine tartrate
(Trimeprazine tartrate)

● INDICATIONS AND DOSE

Urticaria | Pruritus
▸ BY MOUTH
 ▸ Child 2-4 years: 2.5 mg 3–4 times a day
 ▸ Child 5-11 years: 5 mg 3–4 times a day
 ▸ Child 12-17 years: 10 mg 2–3 times a day, in severe cases
  up to maximum daily dose has been used; maximum
  100 mg per day
 ▸ Adult: 10 mg 2–3 times a day, in severe cases up to
  maximum daily dose has been used; maximum 100 mg
  per day
 ▸ Elderly: 10 mg 1–2 times a day

● UNLICENSED USE Not licensed for use in children under
 2 years.
● CONTRA-INDICATIONS Children under 2 years except on
 specialist advice (safety of such use has not been
 established) · epilepsy · hepatic dysfunction · history of
 narrow angle glaucoma · hypothyroidism · many
 antihistamines should be avoided in Acute porphyrias
 p. 918 but alimemazine is thought to be safe · myasthenia
 gravis · Parkinson's disease · phaeochromocytoma ·
 prostatic hypertrophy (in adults) · renal dysfunction
● CAUTIONS Cardiovascular diseases (due to tachycardia-
 inducing and hypotensive effects of phenothiazines) ·
 elderly (in adults) · exposure to sunlight should be avoided
 during treatment with high doses · pyloroduodenal
 obstruction · urinary retention · volume depleted patients
 who are more susceptible to orthostatic hypotension
● INTERACTIONS → Appendix 1 (antihistamines).
● SIDE-EFFECTS
▸ **Rare** Anaphylaxis · angioedema · bronchospasm ·
 hypersensitivity reactions
▸ **Frequency not known** Acute dystonia · agitation ·
 agranulocytosis · akathisia · akinesia · angle-closure
 glaucoma · anti-muscarinic effects · arrhythmias (may be
 predisposed by hypokalaemia and cardiac disease) · blurred
 vision · contact sensitisation · convulsions · drowsiness ·
 dry mouth · dyskinesia · gastro-intestinal disturbances ·
 headache · hyperprolactinaemia · hypotension · insomnia ·
 jaundice · leukopenia (on prolonged high dose) · nasal
 stuffiness · neuroleptic malignant syndrome · ocular
 changes · pallor (in children) · paradoxical excitement ·
 parkinsonism · photosensitivity · postural hypotension (in
 elderly) (in adults) · postural hypotension (in volume
 depletion) · rashes · respiratory depression · rigidity ·
 tardive dyskinesia (usually after prolonged high doses) ·
 tremor · urinary retention
 SIDE-EFFECTS, FURTHER INFORMATION
 Patients on high dosage may develop photosensitivity and
 should avoid exposure to direct sunlight.
  Children and the elderly are more susceptible to side-
 effects.
  Drowsiness is a significant side-effect with most of the
 older antihistamines although paradoxical stimulation
 may occur rarely, especially with high doses or in children
 and the elderly. Drowsiness may diminish after a few days

3

Respiratory system

3

Respiratory system

of treatment and is considerably less of a problem with the newer antihistamines.

- PREGNANCY Most manufacturers of antihistamines advise avoiding their use during pregnancy; however, there is no evidence of teratogenicity. Use in the latter part of the third trimester may cause adverse effects in neonates such as irritability, paradoxical excitability, and tremor.
- BREAST FEEDING Most antihistamines are present in breast milk in varying amounts; although not known to be harmful, most manufacturers advise avoiding their use in mothers who are breast-feeding.
- HEPATIC IMPAIRMENT Avoid in severe liver disease— increased risk of coma.
- RENAL IMPAIRMENT Avoid.
- PATIENT AND CARER ADVICE

Driving and skilled tasks
Drowsiness may affect performance of skilled tasks (e.g. driving); sedating effects enhanced by alcohol.

- MEDICINAL FORMS
There can be variation in the licensing of different medicines containing the same drug. Forms available from special-order manufacturers include: oral solution

Tablet
CAUTIONARY AND ADVISORY LABELS 2
▸ Alimemazine tartrate (Non-proprietary)
   Alimemazine tartrate 10 mg Alimemazine 10mg tablets | 25 tablet [PoM] no price available | 28 tablet [PoM] £67.81 DT price = £62.16

Oral solution
CAUTIONARY AND ADVISORY LABELS 2
▸ Alimemazine tartrate (Non-proprietary)
   Alimemazine tartrate 1.5 mg per 1 ml Alimemazine 7.5mg/5ml oral solution | 100 ml [PoM] £124.74 DT price = £114.35
   Alimemazine tartrate 6 mg per 1 ml Alimemazine 30mg/5ml oral solution | 100 ml [PoM] £180.00 DT price = £176.65

Chlorphenamine maleate

(Chlorpheniramine maleate)

- INDICATIONS AND DOSE

Symptomatic relief of allergy such as hay fever, urticaria, food allergy, drug reactions | Relief of itch associated with chickenpox
▸ BY MOUTH
▸ Child 1–23 months: 1 mg twice daily
▸ Child 2–5 years: 1 mg every 4–6 hours; maximum 6 mg per day
▸ Child 6–11 years: 2 mg every 4–6 hours; maximum 12 mg per day
▸ Child 12–17 years: 4 mg every 4–6 hours; maximum 24 mg per day
▸ Adult: 4 mg every 4–6 hours; maximum 24 mg per day
▸ Elderly: 4 mg every 4–6 hours; maximum 12 mg per day
▸ BY INTRAMUSCULAR INJECTION, OR BY INTRAVENOUS INJECTION
▸ Child 1–5 months: 250 micrograms/kg (max. per dose 2.5 mg), repeated if necessary; maximum 4 doses per day
▸ Child 6 months–5 years: 2.5 mg, repeated if necessary; maximum 4 doses per day
▸ Child 6–11 years: 5 mg, repeated if necessary; maximum 4 doses per day
▸ Child 12–17 years: 10 mg, repeated if necessary; maximum 4 doses per day
▸ Adult: 10 mg, repeated if necessary; maximum 4 doses per day

Emergency treatment of anaphylactic reactions
▸ BY INTRAMUSCULAR INJECTION, OR BY INTRAVENOUS INJECTION
▸ Child 1–5 months: 250 micrograms/kg (max. per dose 2.5 mg), repeated if necessary; maximum 4 doses per day
▸ Child 6 months–5 years: 2.5 mg, repeated if necessary; maximum 4 doses per day
▸ Child 6–11 years: 5 mg, repeated if necessary; maximum 4 doses per day
▸ Child 12–17 years: 10 mg, repeated if necessary; maximum 4 doses per day
▸ Adult: 10 mg, repeated if necessary; maximum 4 doses per day

- UNLICENSED USE
▸ In children *Injection* not licensed for use in neonates. *Tablets* not licensed for use in children under 6 years. *Syrup* not licensed for use in children under 1 year.

> **IMPORTANT SAFETY INFORMATION**
> MHRA/CHM ADVICE (MARCH 2008 AND FEBRUARY 2009) OVER-THE-COUNTER COUGH AND COLD MEDICINES FOR CHILDREN
> Children under 6 years should not be given over-the-counter cough and cold medicines containing chlorphenamine.

- CONTRA-INDICATIONS Many antihistamines should be avoided in Acute porphyrias p. 918 but chlorphenamine is thought to be safe · neonate (due to significant antimuscarinic activity)
- CAUTIONS Epilepsy · prostatic hypertrophy (in adults) · pyloroduodenal obstruction · susceptibility to angle-closure glaucoma · urinary retention
- INTERACTIONS → Appendix 1 (antihistamines).
- SIDE-EFFECTS
GENERAL SIDE-EFFECTS
▸ **Common or very common** Blurred vision · dry mouth · gastro-intestinal disturbances · headache · psychomotor impairment · urinary retention
▸ **Rare** Anaphylaxis · angioedema · angle-closure glaucoma (in adults) · arrhythmias · bronchospasm · confusion · convulsions · depression · dizziness · extrapyramidal effects · hypersensitivity reactions · hypotension · liver dysfunction · palpitation · photosensitivity reactions · sleep disturbances · tremor
▸ **Frequency not known** Antimuscarinic effects · blood disorders · exfoliative dermatitis · rashes · tinnitus
SPECIFIC SIDE-EFFECTS
▸ With intramuscular or intravenous use CNS stimulation · irritant effects · transient hypotension
SIDE-EFFECTS, FURTHER INFORMATION
Children and the elderly are more susceptible to side-effects.
   Drowsiness is a significant side-effect with most of the older antihistamines although paradoxical stimulation may occur rarely, especially with high doses or in children and the elderly. Drowsiness may diminish after a few days of treatment and is considerably less of a problem with the newer antihistamines.

- PREGNANCY Most manufacturers of antihistamines advise avoiding their use during pregnancy; however, there is no evidence of teratogenicity. Use in the latter part of the third trimester may cause adverse effects in neonates such as irritability, paradoxical excitability, and tremor.
- BREAST FEEDING Most antihistamines are present in breast milk in varying amounts; although not known to be harmful, most manufacturers advise avoiding their use in mothers who are breast-feeding.
- HEPATIC IMPAIRMENT Avoid in severe liver disease— increased risk of coma.

- **DIRECTIONS FOR ADMINISTRATION** For *intravenous injection*, give over 1 minute; if small dose required, dilute with Sodium Chloride 0.9%.
- **PATIENT AND CARER ADVICE**

  Driving and skilled tasks

  Drowsiness may affect performance of skilled tasks (e.g. cycling or driving); sedating effects enhanced by alcohol.

  Medicines for Children leaflet: Chlorphenamine maleate for allergy symptoms www.medicinesforchildren.org.uk/chlorphenamine-maleate-allergy-symptoms-0
- **PROFESSION SPECIFIC INFORMATION**

  Dental practitioners' formulary

  Chlorphenamine tablets may be prescribed.
  Chlorphenamine oral solution may be prescribed.
- **EXCEPTIONS TO LEGAL CATEGORY**
  ‣ With intramuscular use or intravenous use Prescription only medicine restriction does not apply to chlorphenamine injection where administration is for saving life in emergency.

- **MEDICINAL FORMS**

  There can be variation in the licensing of different medicines containing the same drug. Forms available from special-order manufacturers include: oral solution

  Tablet

  CAUTIONARY AND ADVISORY LABELS 2
  ‣ Chlorphenamine maleate (Non-proprietary)

  Chlorphenamine maleate 4 mg Chlorphenamine 4mg tablets | 28 tablet P £1.08 DT price = £0.75 | 30 tablet P no price available
  ‣ Hayleve (Genesis Pharmaceuticals Ltd)

  Chlorphenamine maleate 4 mg Hayleve 4mg tablets | 28 tablet P £0.84 DT price = £0.75
  ‣ Piriton (GlaxoSmithKline Consumer Healthcare)

  Chlorphenamine maleate 4 mg Piriton 4mg tablets | 500 tablet P £4.06

  Piriton Allergy 4mg tablets | 30 tablet P £2.06 | 60 tablet P £3.73
  ‣ Pollenase (chlorphenamine) (E M Pharma)

  Chlorphenamine maleate 4 mg Pollenase Antihistamine 4mg tablets | 30 tablet P £1.20

  Oral solution

  CAUTIONARY AND ADVISORY LABELS 2
  ‣ Chlorphenamine maleate (Non-proprietary)

  Chlorphenamine maleate 400 microgram per 1 ml Chlorphenamine 2mg/5ml oral solution sugar free sugar-free | 150 ml P £2.62 DT price = £2.62
  ‣ Allerief (Orbis Consumer Products Ltd)

  Chlorphenamine maleate 400 microgram per 1 ml Allerief 2mg/5ml oral solution sugar-free | 150 ml P £2.22 DT price = £2.62
  ‣ Piriton (GlaxoSmithKline Consumer Healthcare)

  Chlorphenamine maleate 400 microgram per 1 ml Piriton 2mg/5ml syrup | 150 ml P £2.62 DT price = £2.62

  Solution for injection
  ‣ Chlorphenamine maleate (Non-proprietary)

  Chlorphenamine maleate 10 mg per 1 ml Chlorphenamine 10mg/1ml solution for injection ampoules | 5 ampoule PoM £22.48-£22.50 DT price = £22.50

Clemastine

- **INDICATIONS AND DOSE**

  Symptomatic relief of allergy such as hay fever, urticaria
  ‣ BY MOUTH
  ‣ Adult: 1 mg twice daily, increased if necessary up to 6 mg daily

- **CONTRA-INDICATIONS** Avoid in Acute porphyrias p. 918 (some antihistamines are thought to be safe)
- **CAUTIONS** Epilepsy · prostatic hypertrophy · pyloroduodenal obstruction · susceptibility to angle-closure glaucoma · urinary retention
- **INTERACTIONS** → Appendix 1 (antihistamines).

- **SIDE-EFFECTS**
  ‣ **Rare** Anaphylaxis · angioedema · angle-closure glaucoma · arrhythmias · blood disorders · bronchospasm · confusion · convulsions · depression · dizziness · extrapyramidal effects · hypersensitivity reactions · hypotension · liver dysfunction · palpitation · photosensitivity reactions · rashes · sleep disturbances · tremor
  ‣ **Frequency not known** Antimuscarinic effects · blurred vision · drowsiness · dry mouth · gastro-intestinal disturbances · headache · psychomotor impairment · urinary retention

  SIDE-EFFECTS, FURTHER INFORMATION

  Elderly patients are more susceptible to side-effects.
  Drowsiness is a significant side-effect with most of the older antihistamines although paradoxical stimulation may occur rarely, especially with high doses or in the elderly. Drowsiness may diminish after a few days of treatment and is considerably less of a problem with the newer antihistamines.
- **PREGNANCY** Most manufacturers of antihistamines advise avoiding their use during pregnancy; however, there is no evidence of teratogenicity. Use in the latter part of the third trimester may cause adverse effects in neonates such as irritability, paradoxical excitability, and tremor.
- **BREAST FEEDING** Most antihistamines are present in breast milk in varying amounts; although not known to be harmful, most manufacturers advise avoiding their use in mothers who are breast-feeding.
- **HEPATIC IMPAIRMENT** Avoid in severe liver disease—increased risk of coma.
- **PATIENT AND CARER ADVICE**

  Driving and skilled tasks

  Drowsiness may affect performance of skilled tasks (e.g. driving); sedating effects enhanced by alcohol.

- **MEDICINAL FORMS**

  There can be variation in the licensing of different medicines containing the same drug.

  Tablet

  CAUTIONARY AND ADVISORY LABELS 2
  ‣ Tavegil (Novartis Consumer Health UK Ltd)

  Clemastine (as Clemastine hydrogen fumarate) 1 mg Tavegil 1mg tablets | 60 tablet P £5.00 DT price = £5.00

Cyproheptadine hydrochloride

- **INDICATIONS AND DOSE**

  Symptomatic relief of allergy such as hay fever, urticaria | Pruritus
  ‣ BY MOUTH
  ‣ Adult: 4 mg 3 times a day, usual dose 4–20 mg daily; maximum 32 mg per day

- **CONTRA-INDICATIONS** Avoid in Acute porphyrias p. 918 (some antihistamines are thought to be safe)
- **CAUTIONS** Epilepsy · prostatic hypertrophy · pyloroduodenal obstruction · susceptibility to angle-closure glaucoma · urinary retention
- **INTERACTIONS** → Appendix 1 (antihistamines).
- **SIDE-EFFECTS**
  ‣ **Rare** Anaphylaxis · angioedema · angle-closure glaucoma · arrhythmias · blood disorders · bronchospasm · confusion · convulsions · depression · dizziness · extrapyramidal effects · hypersensitivity reactions · hypotension · liver dysfunction · palpitation · photosensitivity reactions · rashes · sleep disturbances · tremor
  ‣ **Frequency not known** Antimuscarinic effects · blurred vision · drowsiness · dry mouth · gastro-intestinal disturbances · headache · psychomotor impairment · urinary retention

SIDE-EFFECTS, FURTHER INFORMATION
Elderly patients are more susceptible to side-effects.

Drowsiness is a significant side-effect with most of the older antihistamines although paradoxical stimulation may occur rarely, especially with high doses or in the elderly. Drowsiness may diminish after a few days of treatment and is considerably less of a problem with the newer antihistamines.

- PREGNANCY Most manufacturers of antihistamines advise avoiding their use during pregnancy; however, there is no evidence of teratogenicity. Use in the latter part of the third trimester may cause adverse effects in neonates such as irritability, paradoxical excitability, and tremor.

- BREAST FEEDING Most antihistamines are present in breast milk in varying amounts; although not known to be harmful, most manufacturers advise avoiding their use in mothers who are breast-feeding.

- HEPATIC IMPAIRMENT Avoid in severe liver disease—increased risk of coma.

- PATIENT AND CARER ADVICE
Driving and skilled tasks
Drowsiness may affect performance of skilled tasks (e.g. driving); sedating effects enhanced by alcohol.

- MEDICINAL FORMS
There can be variation in the licensing of different medicines containing the same drug. Forms available from special-order manufacturers include: oral suspension, oral solution
Tablet
CAUTIONARY AND ADVISORY LABELS 2
▸ Periactin (Auden McKenzie (Pharma Division) Ltd)
Cyproheptadine hydrochloride 4 mg Periactin 4mg tablets |
30 tablet Ⓟ £5.99 DT price = £5.99

Hydroxyzine hydrochloride

22.2.2016

- DRUG ACTION Hydroxyzine is a sedating antihistamine which exerts its actions by antagonising the effects of histamine.

- **INDICATIONS AND DOSE**
Pruritus
▸ BY MOUTH
▸ **Child 6 months-5 years:** 5–15 mg daily in divided doses, dose adjusted according to weight; maximum 2 mg/kg per day
▸ **Child 6-17 years (body-weight up to 40 kg):** Initially 15–25 mg daily in divided doses, dose increased as necessary, adjusted according to weight; maximum 2 mg/kg per day
▸ **Child 6-17 years (body-weight 40 kg and above):** Initially 15–25 mg daily in divided doses, increased if necessary to 50–100 mg daily in divided doses, dose adjusted according to weight
▸ **Adult:** Initially 25 mg daily, dose to be taken at night; increased if necessary to 25 mg 3–4 times a day
▸ **Elderly:** Initially 25 mg daily, dose to be taken at night; increased if necessary to 25 mg twice daily

- UNLICENSED USE *Ucerax* ® preparations not licensed for use in children under 1 year.

| IMPORTANT SAFETY INFORMATION |
MHRA/CHM ADVICE: RISK OF QT-INTERVAL PROLONGATION AND TORSADE DE POINTES (APRIL 2015)
▸ **In adults**
Following concerns of heart rhythm abnormalities, the safety and efficacy of hydroxyzine has been reviewed by the European Medicines Agency. The review concludes that hydroxyzine is associated with a small risk of QT-interval prolongation and torsade de pointes; these events are most likely to occur in patients who have risk

factors for QT prolongation, e.g. concomitant use of drugs that prolong the QT-interval, cardiovascular disease, family history of sudden cardiac death, significant electrolyte imbalance (low plasma-potassium or plasma-magnesium concentrations), or significant bradycardia. To minimise the risk of such adverse effects, the following dose restrictions have been made and new cautions and contra-indications added:
- Hydroxyzine is contra-indicated in patients with prolonged QT-interval or who have risk factors for QT-interval prolongation;
- Avoid use in the elderly due to increased susceptibility to the side-effects of hydroxyzine;
- Consider the risks of QT-interval prolongation and torsade de pointes before prescribing to patients taking drugs that lower heart rate or plasma-potassium concentration;
- In adults, the maximum daily dose is 100 mg;
- In the elderly, the maximum daily dose is 50 mg (if use of hydroxyzine cannot be avoided);
- The lowest effective dose for the shortest period of time should be prescribed.

MHRA/CHM ADVICE: RISK OF QT-INTERVAL PROLONGATION AND TORSADE DE POINTES (APRIL 2015)
▸ **In children**
Following concerns of heart rhythm abnormalities, the safety and efficacy of hydroxyzine has been reviewed by the European Medicines Agency. The review concludes that hydroxyzine is associated with a small risk of QT-interval prolongation and torsade de pointes; these events are most likely to occur in patients who have risk factors for QT prolongation, e.g. concomitant use of drugs that prolong the QT-interval, cardiovascular disease, family history of sudden cardiac death, significant electrolyte imbalance (low plasma-potassium or plasma-magnesium concentrations), or significant bradycardia. To minimise the risk of such adverse effects, the following dose restrictions have been made and new cautions and contra-indications added:
- Hydroxyzine is contra-indicated in patients with prolonged QT-interval or who have risk factors for QT-interval prolongation;
- Consider the risks of QT-interval prolongation and torsade de pointes before prescribing to patients taking drugs that lower heart rate or plasma-potassium concentration;
- In children with body-weight up to 40 kg, the maximum daily dose is 2 mg/kg;
- The lowest effective dose for the shortest period of time should be prescribed.

- CONTRA-INDICATIONS Acquired or congenital QT interval prolongation · avoid in Acute porphyrias p. 918 (some antihistamines are thought to be safe) · predisposition to QT interval prolongation
CONTRA-INDICATIONS, FURTHER INFORMATION
▸ QT interval prolongation Risk factors for QT interval prolongation include significant electrolyte imbalance, bradycardia, cardiovascular disease, and family history of sudden cardiac death.

- CAUTIONS Bladder outflow obstruction · breathing problems · cardiovascular disease · children · decreased gastrointestinal motility · dementia · elderly · epilepsy · hypertension · hyperthyroidism · myasthenia gravis · prostatic hypertrophy (in adults) · pyloroduodenal obstruction · stenosing peptic ulcer · susceptibility to angle-closure glaucoma · urinary retention
CAUTIONS, FURTHER INFORMATION
▸ In adults Elderly patients are particularly susceptible to side-effects; manufacturers advise avoid or reduce dose.
▸ Children Children have an increased susceptibility to side-effects, particularly CNS effects.

● INTERACTIONS → Appendix 1 (antihistamines).

● SIDE-EFFECTS
▶ **Common or very common** Dry mouth · fatigue · headache
▶ **Uncommon** Constipation · dizziness · insomnia · nausea
▶ **Rare** Blood disorders · bronchospasm · liver dysfunction · rashes
▶ **Frequency not known** Agitation · alopecia · anorexia · anxiety · blurred vision · coma · confusion · convulsions (with high doses) · depression · diarrhoea · drowsiness · dyskinesia (after stopping use) · extrapyramidal effects · flushing · hallucinations · hypotension · impotence · labrynthitis · menstrual disturbances · myalgia · palpitation · priapsim · psychomotor impairment · sleep disturbances · tachycardia · tinnitus · tremor (with high doses) · urinary retention · ventricular arrhythmias · vertigo · vomiting

SIDE-EFFECTS, FURTHER INFORMATION
Drowsiness is a significant side-effect with most of the older antihistamines although paradoxical stimulation may occur rarely, especially with high doses or in the elderly. Drowsiness may diminish after a few days of treatment and is considerably less of a problem with the newer antihistamines.

● ALLERGY AND CROSS-SENSITIVITY Manufacturer advises hydroxyzine should be avoided in patients with previous hypersensitivity to cetirizine or other piperazine derivatives, and aminophylline.

● PREGNANCY Manufacturers advise avoid—toxicity in *animal* studies with higher doses. Use in the latter part of the third trimester may cause irritability, paradoxical excitability, and tremor in the neonate.

● BREAST FEEDING Manufacturer advises avoid—expected to be present in milk but effect unknown.

● HEPATIC IMPAIRMENT Manufacturer advises reduce daily dose by one-third. Manufacturer advises avoid in severe liver disease—increased risk of coma.

● RENAL IMPAIRMENT Manufacturers advise reduce daily dose by half in moderate to severe renal impairment.

● EFFECT ON LABORATORY TESTS May interfere with methacholine test—manufacturer advises stop treatment 96 hours prior to test. May interfere with skin testing for allergy—manufacturer advises stop treatment one week prior to test.

● PATIENT AND CARER ADVICE
Driving and skilled tasks
Drowsiness may affect performance of skilled tasks (e.g. cycling or driving); sedating effects enhanced by alcohol.

● MEDICINAL FORMS
There can be variation in the licensing of different medicines containing the same drug. Forms available from special-order manufacturers include: oral suspension, oral solution
Tablet
CAUTIONARY AND ADVISORY LABELS 2
▸ Atarax (Alliance Pharmaceuticals Ltd)
  Hydroxyzine hydrochloride 10 mg Atarax 10mg tablets |
  84 tablet [PoM] £1.20 DT price = £1.20
  Hydroxyzine hydrochloride 25 mg Atarax 25mg tablets |
  28 tablet [PoM] £0.62 DT price = £0.62

Ketotifen

● INDICATIONS AND DOSE
Allergic rhinitis
▶ BY MOUTH
▸ Child 3-17 years: 1 mg twice daily
▸ Adult: 1 mg twice daily, increased if necessary to 2 mg twice daily, to be taken with food

Allergic rhinitis in readily sedated patients
▶ BY MOUTH
▸ Adult: Initially 0.5–1 mg once daily, dose to be taken at night

● CONTRA-INDICATIONS Avoid in Acute porphyrias p. 918 (some antihistamines are thought to be safe)

● CAUTIONS Epilepsy · prostatic hypertrophy (in adults) · pyloroduodenal obstruction · susceptibility to angle-closure glaucoma · urinary retention

● INTERACTIONS → Appendix 1 (antihistamines). Sedative antihistamine interactions apply to a lesser extent to the non-sedating antihistamines.

● SIDE-EFFECTS
▶ **Common or very common** Excitation (in adults) · irritability · nervousness
▶ **Uncommon** Cystitis
▶ **Rare** Weight gain
▶ **Very rare** Stevens-Johnson syndrome
▶ **Frequency not known** Anaphylaxis · angioedema · angle-closure glaucoma (in adults) · antimuscarinic effects · arrhythmias · blood disorders · blurred vision · bronchospasm · confusion · convulsions · depression · dizziness · dry mouth · extrapyramidal effects · gastro-intestinal disturbances · headache · hypersensitivity reactions · hypotension · liver dysfunction · palpitation · photosensitivity reactions · psychomotor impairment · rashes · sleep disturbances · tremor · urinary retention

SIDE-EFFECTS, FURTHER INFORMATION
Elderly are more suceptible to side effects.
Drowsiness is a significant side-effect with most of the older antihistamines although paradoxical stimulation may occur rarely, especially with high doses or in children and the elderly. Drowsiness may diminish after a few days of treatment and is considerably less of a problem with the newer antihistamines.

● PREGNANCY Most manufacturers of antihistamines advise avoiding their use during pregnancy; however, there is no evidence of teratogenicity. Use in the latter part of the third trimester may cause adverse effects in neonates such as irritability, paradoxical excitability, and tremor.

● BREAST FEEDING Most antihistamines are present in breast milk in varying amounts; although not known to be harmful, most manufacturers advise avoiding their use in mothers who are breast-feeding.

● HEPATIC IMPAIRMENT Avoid in severe liver disease—increased risk of coma.

● PATIENT AND CARER ADVICE
Driving and skilled tasks
Drowsiness may affect performance of skilled tasks (e.g. driving or cycling); sedating effects enhanced by alcohol.

● MEDICINAL FORMS
There can be variation in the licensing of different medicines containing the same drug.
Tablet
CAUTIONARY AND ADVISORY LABELS 2, 21
▸ Zaditen (CD Pharma AB)
  Ketotifen (as Ketotifen fumarate) 1 mg Zaditen 1mg tablets |
  60 tablet [PoM] £7.53
Oral solution
CAUTIONARY AND ADVISORY LABELS 2, 21
▸ Zaditen (CD Pharma AB)
  Ketotifen (as Ketotifen fumarate) 200 microgram per 1 ml Zaditen 1mg/5ml elixir sugar-free | 300 ml [PoM] £8.91 DT price = £8.91

Promethazine hydrochloride

● **INDICATIONS AND DOSE**

Symptomatic relief of allergy such as hay fever and urticaria | Insomnia associated with urticaria and pruritus
▶ BY MOUTH
▸ Child 2–4 years: 5 mg twice daily, alternatively 5–15 mg once daily, dose to be taken at night
▸ Child 5–9 years: 5–10 mg twice daily, alternatively 10–25 mg once daily, dose to be taken at night
▸ Child 10–17 years: 10–20 mg 2–3 times a day, alternatively 25 mg once daily, dose to be taken at night, increased if necessary to 25 mg twice daily
▸ Adult: 10–20 mg 2–3 times a day
▶ BY DEEP INTRAMUSCULAR INJECTION
▸ Adult: 25–50 mg (max. per dose 100 mg)

Emergency treatment of anaphylactic reactions
▶ BY SLOW INTRAVENOUS INJECTION
▸ Adult: 25–50 mg, to be administered as a solution containing 2.5 mg/mL in water for injections; maximum 100 mg per course

Sedation (short-term use)
▶ BY MOUTH
▸ Child 2–4 years: 15–20 mg
▸ Child 5–9 years: 20–25 mg
▸ Child 10–17 years: 25–50 mg
▸ Adult: 25–50 mg
▶ BY DEEP INTRAMUSCULAR INJECTION
▸ Adult: 25–50 mg

Nausea | Vomiting | Vertigo | Labyrinthine disorders | Motion sickness
▶ BY MOUTH
▸ Child 2–4 years: 5 mg, to be taken at bedtime on night before travel, repeat following morning if necessary
▸ Child 5–9 years: 10 mg, to be taken at bedtime on night before travel, repeat following morning if necessary
▸ Child 10–17 years: 20–25 mg, to be taken at bedtime on night before travel, repeat following morning if necessary
▸ Adult: 20–25 mg, to be taken at bedtime on night before travel, repeat following morning if necessary

● UNLICENSED USE Not licensed for use for sedation in children under 2 years.

> **IMPORTANT SAFETY INFORMATION**
> MHRA/CHM ADVICE (MARCH 2008 AND FEBRUARY 2009) OVER-THE-COUNTER COUGH AND COLD MEDICINES FOR CHILDREN
> Children under 6 years should not be given over-the-counter cough and cold medicines containing promethazine.

● CONTRA-INDICATIONS Many antihistamines should be avoided in Acute porphyrias p. 918 but promethazine is thought to be safe · should not be given to children under 2 years, except on specialist advice, because the safety of such use has not been established

● CAUTIONS
GENERAL CAUTIONS
Epilepsy · prostatic hypertrophy (in adults) · pyloroduodenal obstruction · severe coronary artery disease · susceptibility to angle-closure glaucoma · urinary retention
SPECIFIC CAUTIONS
▶ With intravenous use Avoid extravasation with intravenous injection

● INTERACTIONS → Appendix 1 (antihistamines).

● **SIDE-EFFECTS**
GENERAL SIDE-EFFECTS
▶ **Rare** Anaphylaxis · angioedema · angle-closure glaucoma · arrhythmias · blood disorders · bronchospasm · confusion · convulsions · depression · dizziness · extrapyramidal effects · hypersensitivity reactions · hypotension · liver dysfunction · palpitation · photosensitivity reactions · rashes · sleep disturbances · tremor
▶ **Frequency not known** Antimuscarinic effects · blurred vision · drowsiness · dry mouth · gastro-intestinal disturbances · headache · psychomotor impairment · restlessness · urinary retention
SPECIFIC SIDE-EFFECTS
▶ With intramuscular use Injection pain (in adults)
SIDE-EFFECTS, FURTHER INFORMATION
Children and the elderly are more susceptible to side-effects.
  Drowsiness is a significant side-effect with most of the older antihistamines although paradoxical stimulation may occur rarely, especially with high doses or in children and the elderly. Drowsiness may diminish after a few days of treatment and is considerably less of a problem with the newer antihistamines.

● PREGNANCY Most manufacturers of antihistamines advise avoiding their use during pregnancy; however, there is no evidence of teratogenicity. Use in the latter part of the third trimester may cause adverse effects in neonates such as irritability, paradoxical excitability, and tremor.

● BREAST FEEDING Most antihistamines are present in breast milk in varying amounts; although not known to be harmful, most manufacturers advise avoiding their use in mothers who are breast-feeding.

● HEPATIC IMPAIRMENT Avoid in severe liver disease—increased risk of coma.

● RENAL IMPAIRMENT Use with caution.

● PATIENT AND CARER ADVICE
Driving and skilled tasks
Drowsiness may affect the performance of skilled tasks (e.g. cycling or driving); sedating effects enhanced by alcohol.

● PROFESSION SPECIFIC INFORMATION
Dental practitioners' formulary
Promethazine Hydrochloride Tablets 10 mg or 25 mg may be prescribed.
  Promethazine Hydrochloride Oral Solution (elixir) 5 mg/5 mL may be prescribed.

● LESS SUITABLE FOR PRESCRIBING Promethazine is less suitable for prescribing for sedation.

● EXCEPTIONS TO LEGAL CATEGORY Prescription only medicine restriction does not apply to promethazine hydrochloride injection where administration is for saving life in emergency.

● MEDICINAL FORMS
There can be variation in the licensing of different medicines containing the same drug. Forms available from special-order manufacturers include: oral suspension, oral solution
Tablet
CAUTIONARY AND ADVISORY LABELS 2
▸ Promethazine hydrochloride (Non-proprietary)
  Promethazine hydrochloride 10 mg Promethazine hydrochloride 10mg tablets | 56 tablet PoM £3.30 DT price = £2.96
▸ Phenergan (Sanofi)
  Promethazine hydrochloride 10 mg Phenergan 10mg tablets | 56 tablet P £2.96 DT price = £2.96
  Promethazine hydrochloride 25 mg Phenergan 25mg tablets | 56 tablet P £4.65 DT price = £4.65

Oral solution

CAUTIONARY AND ADVISORY LABELS 2

EXCIPIENTS: May contain Sulfites

ELECTROLYTES: May contain Sodium

▸ Phenergan (Sanofi)

Promethazine hydrochloride 1 mg per 1 ml Phenergan 5mg/5ml elixir sugar-free | 100 ml [P] £2.85 DT price = £2.85

Solution for injection

EXCIPIENTS: May contain Sulfites

▸ Phenergan (Sanofi)

Promethazine hydrochloride 25 mg per 1 ml Phenergan 25mg/1ml solution for injection ampoules | 10 ampoule [PoM] £6.74

VACCINES > ALLERGEN-TYPE VACCINES

Bee venom extract

- **INDICATIONS AND DOSE**

Hypersensitivity to bee venom

▸ BY SUBCUTANEOUS INJECTION

▸ Adult: (consult product literature)

IMPORTANT SAFETY INFORMATION

DESENSITISING VACCINES

In view of concerns about the safety of desensitising vaccines, it is recommended that they are used by specialists and only for the following indications:

- seasonal allergic hay fever (caused by pollen) that has not responded to anti-allergic drugs;
- hypersensitivity to wasp and bee venoms.

Desensitising vaccines should generally be avoided or used with particular care in patients with asthma.

- CONTRA-INDICATIONS Consult product literature
- CAUTIONS Consult product literature
- INTERACTIONS → Appendix 1 (bee venom extracts). Contra-indicated in patients taking beta-blockers (adrenaline may be ineffective in case of a hypersensitivity reaction).
- SIDE-EFFECTS

SIDE-EFFECTS, FURTHER INFORMATION

Consult product literature.

▸ Hypersensitivity reactions Hypersensitivity reactions to immunotherapy (especially to wasp and bee venom extracts) can be life-threatening; bronchospasm usually develops within 1 hour and anaphylaxis within 30 minutes of injection. Therefore, cardiopulmonary resuscitation must be immediately available and patients need to be monitored for at least 1 hour after injection. If symptoms or signs of hypersensitivity develop (e.g. rash, urticaria, bronchospasm, faintness), **even when mild**, the patient should be observed until these have **resolved completely**.

- PREGNANCY Avoid.
- PRESCRIBING AND DISPENSING INFORMATION Each set of allergen extracts usually contains vials for the administration of graded amounts of allergen to patients undergoing hyposensitisation. Maintenance sets containing vials at the highest strength are also available. Product literature must be consulted for details of allergens, vial strengths, and administration.
- NATIONAL FUNDING/ACCESS DECISIONS

NICE technology appraisals (TAs)

▸ *Pharmalgen®* for bee and wasp venom allergy (February 2012) NICE TA246

Pharmalgen® is an option for the treatment of IgE-mediated bee and wasp venom allergy in those who have had:

- a severe systemic reaction to bee or wasp venom;
- a moderate systemic reaction to bee or wasp venom and

who have a raised baseline serum-tryptase concentration, a high risk of future stings, or anxiety about future stings.

Treatment with *Pharmalgen®* should be initiated and monitored in a specialist centre experienced in venom immunotherapy.

www.nice.org.uk/TA246

- MEDICINAL FORMS

There can be variation in the licensing of different medicines containing the same drug.

Powder and solvent for solution for injection

▸ Bee Venom (ALK-Abello Ltd)

Bee venom 1.2 microgram Pharmalgen Bee Venom 1.2microgram powder and solvent for solution for injection vials | 1 vial [PoM] no price available

Bee venom 12 microgram Pharmalgen Bee Venom 12microgram powder and solvent for solution for injection vials | 1 vial [PoM] no price available

Bee venom 120 microgram Pharmalgen Bee Venom maintenance set 120microgram powder and solvent for solution for injection vials | 1 vial [PoM] no price available | 4 vial [PoM] £150.00

Bee venom 120 nanogram Pharmalgen Bee Venom 120nanogram powder and solvent for solution for injection vials | 1 vial [PoM] no price available

Grass pollen extract

- **INDICATIONS AND DOSE**

Treatment of seasonal allergic hay fever due to grass pollen in patients who have failed to respond to anti-allergy drugs

▸ BY SUBCUTANEOUS INJECTION

▸ Adult: (consult product literature)

Treatment of seasonal allergic hay fever due to grass pollen in patients who have failed to respond to anti-allergy drugs (initiated under specialist supervision)

▸ BY MOUTH

▸ Adult: 1 tablet daily, treatment to be started at least 4 months before start of pollen season and continue for up to 3 years

---

IMPORTANT SAFETY INFORMATION

DESENSITISING VACCINES

In view of concerns about the safety of desensitising vaccines, it is recommended that they are used by specialists and only for the following indications:

- seasonal allergic hay fever (caused by pollen) that has not responded to anti-allergic drugs;
- hypersensitivity to wasp and bee venoms.

Desensitising vaccines should generally be avoided or used with particular care in patients with asthma.

- CONTRA-INDICATIONS Consult product literature
- CAUTIONS Consult product literature
- INTERACTIONS Desensitising vaccines should be avoided in patients taking beta-blockers (adrenaline may be ineffective in case of a hypersensitivity reaction), or ACE inhibitors (risk of severe anaphylactoid reactions).
- SIDE-EFFECTS

SIDE-EFFECTS, FURTHER INFORMATION

Consult product literature.

▸ Hypersensitivity reactions Hypersensitivity reactions to immunotherapy can be life-threatening; bronchospasm usually develops within 1 hour and anaphylaxis within 30 minutes of injection. Therefore, cardiopulmonary resuscitation must be immediately available and patients need to be monitored for at least 1 hour after injection. If symptoms or signs of hypersensitivity develop (e.g. rash, urticaria, bronchospasm, faintness), **even when mild**, the patient should be observed until these have **resolved completely**.

- PREGNANCY Should be avoided in pregnant women—consult product literature.
- MONITORING REQUIREMENTS The first dose of grass pollen extract should be (*Grazax*®) should be taken under medical supervision and the patient should be monitored for 20–30 minutes.
- DIRECTIONS FOR ADMINISTRATION Oral lyophilisates should be placed under the tongue and allowed to disperse. Advise patient not to swallow for 1 minute, or eat or drink for 5 minutes after taking the tablet. The first should be taken under medical supervision and the patient should be monitored for 20–30 minutes.
- PRESCRIBING AND DISPENSING INFORMATION Each set of allergen extracts usually contains vials for the administration of graded amounts of allergen to patients undergoing hyposensitisation. Maintenance sets containing vials at the highest strength are also available. Product literature must be consulted for details of allergens, vial strengths, and administration.
- PATIENT AND CARER ADVICE
  - With oral use Patients or carers should be given advice on how to administer oral lyophilisates.
- MEDICINAL FORMS
  There can be variation in the licensing of different medicines containing the same drug.
  Oral lyophilisate
  ▸ Grazax (ALK-Abello Ltd)
  Phleum pratense 75000 SQ-T Grazax 75,000 SQ-T oral lyophilisates sugar-free | 30 tablet PoM £80.12
  Suspension for Injection
  ▸ Pollinex Grasses + Rye (Allergy Therapeutics (UK) Ltd)
  Pollinex Grasses + Rye suspension for injection treatment and extension course vials | 4 vial PoM £450.00

Tree pollen extract

- INDICATIONS AND DOSE
  Treatment of seasonal allergic hay fever due to tree pollen in patients who have failed to respond to anti-allergy drugs
  ▸ BY SUBCUTANEOUS INJECTION
  ▸ Adult: (consult product literature)

> IMPORTANT SAFETY INFORMATION
> DESENSITISING VACCINES
> In view of concerns about the safety of desensitising vaccines, it is recommended that they are used by specialists and only for the following indications:
> - seasonal allergic hay fever (caused by pollen) that has not responded to anti-allergic drugs;
> - hypersensitivity to wasp and bee venoms.
> Desensitising vaccines should generally be avoided or used with particular care in patients with asthma.

- CONTRA-INDICATIONS Consult product literature
- CAUTIONS Consult product literature
- INTERACTIONS Desensitising vaccines should be avoided in patients taking beta-blockers (adrenaline may be ineffective in case of a hypersensitivity reaction), or ACE inhibitors (risk of severe anaphylactoid reactions).
- SIDE-EFFECTS
  SIDE-EFFECTS, FURTHER INFORMATION
  Consult product literature.
  ▸ Hypersensitivity reactions Hypersensitivity reactions to immunotherapy (especially to wasp and bee venom extracts) can be life-threatening; bronchospasm usually develops within 1 hour and anaphylaxis within 30 minutes of injection. Therefore, cardiopulmonary resuscitation must be immediately available and patients need to be

monitored for at least 1 hour after injection. If symptoms or signs of hypersensitivity develop (e.g. rash, urticaria, bronchospasm, faintness, **even when mild**, the patient should be observed until these have **resolved completely**.

- PREGNANCY Should be avoided in pregnant women—consult product literature.
- PRESCRIBING AND DISPENSING INFORMATION Each set of allergen extracts usually contains vials for the administration of graded amounts of allergen to patients undergoing hyposensitisation. Maintenance sets containing vials at the highest strength are also available. Product literature must be consulted for details of allergens, vial strengths, and administration.
- MEDICINAL FORMS
  There can be variation in the licensing of different medicines containing the same drug.
  Suspension for injection
  ▸ Pollinex Trees (Allergy Therapeutics (UK) Ltd)
  Pollinex Trees No 3 suspension for injection 1ml vials | 1 vial PoM no price available
  Pollinex Trees No 2 suspension for injection 1ml vials | 1 vial PoM no price available
  Pollinex Trees No 1 suspension for injection 1ml vials | 1 vial PoM no price available
  ▸ Pollinex Trees (Allergy Therapeutics (UK) Ltd)
  Pollinex Trees suspension for injection treatment and extension course vials | 4 vial PoM £450.00

Wasp venom extract

- INDICATIONS AND DOSE
  Hypersensitivity to wasp venom
  ▸ BY SUBCUTANEOUS INJECTION
  ▸ Adult: (consult product literature)

> IMPORTANT SAFETY INFORMATION
> DESENSITISING VACCINES
> In view of concerns about the safety of desensitising vaccines, it is recommended that they are used by specialists and only for the following indications:
> - seasonal allergic hay fever (caused by pollen) that has not responded to anti-allergic drugs;
> - hypersensitivity to wasp and bee venoms.
> Desensitising vaccines should generally be avoided or used with particular care in patients with asthma.

- CONTRA-INDICATIONS Consult product literature
- CAUTIONS Consult product literature
- INTERACTIONS → Appendix 1 (wasp venom extracts). Contra-indicated in patients taking beta-blockers (adrenaline may be ineffective in case of a hypersensitivity reaction).
- SIDE-EFFECTS
  SIDE-EFFECTS, FURTHER INFORMATION
  Consult product literature.
  ▸ Hypersensitivity reactions Hypersensitivity reactions to immunotherapy (especially to wasp and bee venom extracts) can be life-threatening; bronchospasm usually develops within 1 hour and anaphylaxis within 30 minutes of injection. Therefore, cardiopulmonary resuscitation must be immediately available and patients need to be monitored for at least 1 hour after injection. If symptoms or signs of hypersensitivity develop (e.g. rash, urticaria, bronchospasm, faintness, **even when mild**, the patient should be observed until these have **resolved completely**.
- PREGNANCY Avoid.
- PRESCRIBING AND DISPENSING INFORMATION Each set of allergen extracts usually contains vials for the administration of graded amounts of allergen to patients undergoing hyposensitisation. Maintenance sets

containing vials at the highest strength are also available. Product literature must be consulted for details of allergens, vial strengths, and administration.

● NATIONAL FUNDING/ACCESS DECISIONS

NICE technology appraisals (TAs)

▸ *Pharmalgen*® for bee and wasp venom allergy (February 2012) NICE TA246

Pharmalgen® is an option for the treatment of IgE-mediated bee and wasp venom allergy in those who have had:

● a severe systemic reaction to bee or wasp venom;
● a moderate systemic reaction to bee or wasp venom and who have a raised baseline serum-tryptase concentration, a high risk of future stings, or anxiety about future stings.

Treatment with *Pharmalgen*® should be initiated and monitored in a specialist centre experienced in venom immunotherapy.

www.nice.org.uk/TA246

● MEDICINAL FORMS

There can be variation in the licensing of different medicines containing the same drug.

Powder and solvent for solution for injection

▸ Wasp Venom (ALK-Abello Ltd)

Wasp venom 1.2 microgram Pharmalgen Wasp Venom 1.2microgram powder and solvent for solution for injection vials | 1 vial `PoM` no price available

Wasp venom 12 microgram Pharmalgen Wasp Venom 12microgram powder and solvent for solution for injection vials | 1 vial `PoM` no price available

Wasp venom 120 nanogram Pharmalgen Wasp Venom 120nanogram powder and solvent for solution for injection vials | 1 vial `PoM` no price available

Wasp venom 120 microgram Pharmalgen Wasp Venom maintenance set 120microgram vaccine powder and solvent for solution for injection vials | 1 vial `PoM` no price available | 4 vial `PoM` £150.00

2.1 Angioedema

Drugs used for Angioedema not listed below
Adrenaline/epinephrine p. 205

DRUGS USED IN HEREDITARY ANGIOEDEMA ›
COMPLEMENT REGULATORY PROTEINS

C1-esterase inhibitor

● INDICATIONS AND DOSE

BERINERT®

Acute attacks of hereditary angioedema (under expert supervision)

▸ BY SLOW INTRAVENOUS INJECTION, OR BY INTRAVENOUS INFUSION

▸ Adult: 20 units/kg

Short-term prophylaxis of hereditary angioedema before dental, medical, or surgical procedures (under expert supervision)

▸ BY SLOW INTRAVENOUS INJECTION, OR BY INTRAVENOUS INFUSION

▸ Adult: 1000 units for 1 dose, to be administered less than 6 hours before procedure

CINRYZE®

Acute attacks of hereditary angioedema (under expert supervision)

▸ BY SLOW INTRAVENOUS INJECTION

▸ Adult: 1000 units, repeated if necessary for 1 dose, dose may be repeated if necessary

Short-term prophylaxis of hereditary angioedema before dental, medical, or surgical procedures (under expert supervision)

▸ BY SLOW INTRAVENOUS INJECTION

▸ Adult: 1000 units for 1 dose, to be administered up to 24 hours before procedure

Long-term prophylaxis of severe, recurrent attacks of hereditary angioedema where acute treatment is inadequate, or when oral prophylaxis is inadequate or not tolerated (under expert supervision)

▸ BY SLOW INTRAVENOUS INJECTION

▸ Adult: 1000 units every 3–4 days, interval between doses to be adjusted according to response

● CAUTIONS Vaccination against hepatitis A and hepatitis B may be required

● SIDE-EFFECTS Fever · headache · thrombosis (with high doses)

● PREGNANCY Manufacturer advises avoid unless essential.

● PRESCRIBING AND DISPENSING INFORMATION C1-esterase inhibitor is prepared from human plasma.

● MEDICINAL FORMS

There can be variation in the licensing of different medicines containing the same drug.

Powder and solvent for solution for injection
ELECTROLYTES: May contain Sodium

▸ Berinert P (CSL Behring UK Ltd)

C1-esterase inhibitor 500 unit Berinert 500unit powder and solvent for solution for injection vials | 1 vial `PoM` £467.50

C1-esterase inhibitor 1500 unit Berinert 1,500unit powder and solvent for solution for injection vials | 1 vial `PoM` £1,402.50

▸ Cinryze (Shire Pharmaceuticals Ltd) ▼

C1-esterase inhibitor 500 unit Cinryze 500unit powder and solvent for solution for injection vials | 2 vial `PoM` £1,336.00

Conestat alfa

● INDICATIONS AND DOSE

Acute attacks of hereditary angioedema in patients with C1-esterase inhibitor deficiency

▸ BY SLOW INTRAVENOUS INJECTION

▸ Adult (body-weight up to 84 kg): 50 units/kg for 1 dose, to be administered over 5 minutes, dose may be repeated if necessary; maximum 2 doses per day

▸ Adult (body-weight 84 kg and above): 4200 units for 1 dose, to be administered over 5 minutes, dose may be repeated if necessary; maximum 2 doses per day

● CONTRA-INDICATIONS Rabbit allergy

● SIDE-EFFECTS

▸ Common or very common Headache

▸ Uncommon Abdominal discomfort · diarrhoea · nausea · paraesthesia · throat irritation · urticaria · vertigo

● PREGNANCY Use only if potential benefit outweighs risk—toxicity in *animal* studies.

● BREAST FEEDING Use only if potential benefit outweighs risk—no information available.

● PRE-TREATMENT SCREENING Test for immunoglobulin E (IgE) antibodies against rabbit allergens before starting treatment.

● MONITORING REQUIREMENTS Repeat immunoglobulin E (IgE) antibody testing annually or after 10 treatments—consult product literature.

Respiratory system

3

- MEDICINAL FORMS
There can be variation in the licensing of different medicines containing the same drug.
Powder for solution for injection
▸ Ruconest (Swedish Orphan Biovitrum Ltd)
   Conestat alfa 2100 unit Ruconest 2,100unit powder for solution for injection vials | 1 vial PoM £750.00

DRUGS USED IN HEREDITARY ANGIOEDEMA ›
SELECTIVE BRADYKININ B₂ ANTAGONISTS

Icatibant

- INDICATIONS AND DOSE
Acute attacks of hereditary angioedema in patients with C1-esterase inhibitor deficiency
▸ BY SUBCUTANEOUS INJECTION
▸ Adult: 30 mg for 1 dose, then 30 mg after 6 hours if required, then 30 mg after 6 hours if required; maximum 3 doses per day

- CAUTIONS Ischaemic heart disease · stroke
- SIDE-EFFECTS Dizziness · erythema · headache · injection-site reactions · nausea · pruritus · pyrexia · rash
- PREGNANCY Manufacturer advises use only if potential benefit outweighs risk—toxicity in *animal* studies.
- BREAST FEEDING Manufacturer advises avoid for 12 hours after administration.

- MEDICINAL FORMS
There can be variation in the licensing of different medicines containing the same drug.
Solution for injection
▸ Firazyr (Shire Pharmaceuticals Ltd)
   Icatibant (as Icatibant acetate) 10 mg per 1 ml Firazyr 30mg/3ml solution for injection pre-filled syringes | 1 pre-filled disposable injection PoM £1,395.00

3 Conditions affecting sputum viscosity

Mucolytics for cystic fibrosis

Overview

Mucolytics are prescribed to facilitate expectoration by reducing sputum viscosity. In some patients with chronic obstructive pulmonary disease and a chronic productive cough, mucolytics can reduce exacerbations; mucolytic therapy should be stopped if there is no benefit after a 4-week trial. Steam inhalation with postural drainage is effective in bronchiectasis and in some cases of chronic bronchitis.

Dornase alfa p. 269 is used to reduce sputum viscosity in patients with cystic fibrosis.

Nebulised hypertonic sodium chloride (3–7%) is used to mobilise lower respiratory tract secretions in mucus consolidation (e.g cystic fibrosis). Nebulised hypertonic sodium chloride solution (3%) is used for mild to moderate acute viral bronchiolitis in infants.

Mannitol p. 269, administered by inhalation, improves mucus clearance and is licensed for the treatment of cystic fibrosis as an add-on therapy to standard care.

MUCOLYTICS

Carbocisteine

- INDICATIONS AND DOSE
Reduction of sputum viscosity
▸ BY MOUTH
▸ Adult: Initially 2.25 g daily in divided doses, then reduced to 1.5 g daily in divided doses, as condition improves

- CONTRA-INDICATIONS Active peptic ulceration
- CAUTIONS History of peptic ulceration (may disrupt the gastric mucosal barrier)
- SIDE-EFFECTS
▸ **Rare** Gastro-intestinal bleeding
▸ **Frequency not known** Erythema multiforme · Stevens-Johnson syndrome
- PREGNANCY Manufacturer advises avoid in first trimester.
- BREAST FEEDING No information available.
- PRESCRIBING AND DISPENSING INFORMATION Flavours of oral liquid formulations may include cherry, raspberry, cinnamon, or rum.

- MEDICINAL FORMS
There can be variation in the licensing of different medicines containing the same drug.
Capsule
▸ Carbocisteine (Non-proprietary)
   Carbocisteine 375 mg Carbocisteine 375mg capsules | 120 capsule PoM £18.98 DT price = £11.50
▸ Mucodyne (Sanofi)
   Carbocisteine 375 mg Mucodyne 375mg capsules | 120 capsule PoM £18.98 DT price = £11.50
Oral solution
▸ Carbocisteine (Non-proprietary)
   Carbocisteine 75 mg per 1 ml Carbocisteine 750mg/10ml oral solution 10ml sachets sugar free sugar-free | 15 sachet PoM £3.85 DT price = £3.85
▸ Mucodyne (Sanofi)
   Carbocisteine 50 mg per 1 ml Mucodyne 250mg/5ml syrup | 300 ml PoM £8.39 DT price = £8.39

Erdosteine

- INDICATIONS AND DOSE
Symptomatic treatment of acute exacerbations of chronic bronchitis
▸ BY MOUTH
▸ Adult: 300 mg twice daily for up to 10 days

- CAUTIONS History of peptic ulceration (may disrupt the gastric mucosal barrier)
- SIDE-EFFECTS
▸ **Very rare** Abdominal pain · diarrhoea · headache · nausea · rash · taste disturbance · urticaria · vomiting
- PREGNANCY Manufacturer advises avoid—no information available.
- BREAST FEEDING Manufacturer advises avoid—no information available.
- HEPATIC IMPAIRMENT Manufacturer advises max. 300 mg daily in mild to moderate impairment. Avoid in severe impairment.
- RENAL IMPAIRMENT Avoid if eGFR less than 25 mL/minute/1.73 m² —no information available.
- NATIONAL FUNDING/ACCESS DECISIONS
Scottish Medicines Consortium (SMC) Decisions
The *The Scottish Medicines Consortium* (October 2007) has advised that erdosteine (*Erdotin*®) is not recommended for the symptomatic treatment of acute exacerbations of chronic bronchitis.

- MEDICINAL FORMS
There can be variation in the licensing of different medicines containing the same drug.
Capsule
▶ Erdotin (Galen Ltd)
Erdosteine 300 mg Erdotin 300mg capsules | 20 capsule [PoM] £4.25 DT price = £4.25

3.1 Cystic fibrosis

MUCOLYTICS

Dornase alfa

(Phosphorylated glycosylated recombinant human deoxyribonuclease 1 (rhDNase))

- DRUG ACTION Dornase alfa is a genetically engineered version of a naturally occurring human enzyme which cleaves extracellular deoxyribonucleic acid (DNA).

- INDICATIONS AND DOSE
Management of cystic fibrosis patients with a forced vital capacity (FVC) of greater than 40% of predicted to improve pulmonary function
▶ BY INHALATION OF NEBULISED SOLUTION
▶ Adult: 2500 units once daily, administered by jet nebuliser, patients over 21 years may benefit from twice daily dosage
DOSE EQUIVALENCE AND CONVERSION
Dornase alfa 1000 units is equivalent to 1 mg

- SIDE-EFFECTS
▶ Rare Chest pain · conjunctivitis · dyspepsia · dysphonia · dyspnoea · laryngitis · pharyngitis · pyrexia · rash · rhinitis · urticaria
- PREGNANCY No evidence of teratogenicity; manufacturer advises use only if potential benefit outweighs risk.
- BREAST FEEDING Amount probably too small to be harmful—manufacturer advises caution.
- DIRECTIONS FOR ADMINISTRATION Dornase alfa is administered by inhalation using a jet nebuliser, usually once daily at least 1 hour before physiotherapy; however, alternate-day therapy may be as effective as daily treatment.
For use undiluted with jet nebulisers only; ultrasonic nebulisers are unsuitable.

- MEDICINAL FORMS
There can be variation in the licensing of different medicines containing the same drug.
Nebuliser liquid
▶ Pulmozyme (Roche Products Ltd)
Dornase alfa 1 mg per 1 ml Pulmozyme 2.5mg nebuliser liquid 2.5ml ampoules | 30 ampoule [PoM] £496.43 DT price = £496.43

Ivacaftor

- INDICATIONS AND DOSE
Treatment of cystic fibrosis in patients who have a G551D mutation in the cystic fibrosis transmembrane conductance regulator (CFTR) gene (under expert supervision)
▶ BY MOUTH
▶ Adult: 150 mg every 12 hours
DOSE ADJUSTMENTS DUE TO INTERACTIONS
Reduce dose to 150 mg twice a week with concomitant use of itraconazole, ketoconazole, posaconazole, voriconazole, telithromycin, and clarithromycin.
Reduce dose to 150 mg once daily with concomitant use of fluconazole and erythromycin.

- CONTRA-INDICATIONS Organ transplantation (no information available)
- INTERACTIONS → Appendix 1 (ivacaftor). Avoid grapefruit and Seville oranges.
- SIDE-EFFECTS
▶ Common or very common Abdominal pain · diarrhoea · dizziness · ear discomfort · headache · nasal congestion · nasopharyngitis · oropharyngeal pain · pharyngeal oedema · rash · rhinitis · tinnitus · upper respiratory-tract infection
▶ Uncommon Gynaecomastia · vestibular disorder
- PREGNANCY Manufacturer advises use only if potential benefit outweighs risk—no information available.
- BREAST FEEDING Manufacturer advises use only if potential benefit outweighs risk—no information available.
- HEPATIC IMPAIRMENT Max. 150 mg once daily in moderate impairment; in severe impairment, manufacturer recommends use only if potential benefit outweighs risk—starting dose 150 mg on alternate days, dosing interval adjusted according to clinical response and tolerability.
- RENAL IMPAIRMENT Caution in severe impairment.
- PRE-TREATMENT SCREENING If the patient's genotype is unknown, a validated genotyping method should be performed to confirm the presence of the G551D mutation in at least one allele of the CFTR gene before starting treatment.
- MONITORING REQUIREMENTS Test liver function before treatment, every 3 months during the first year of treatment, then annually thereafter.
- DIRECTIONS FOR ADMINISTRATION Tablets should be taken with fat-containing food.
- PRESCRIBING AND DISPENSING INFORMATION Ivacaftor should be prescribed by a physician experienced in the treatment of cystic fibrosis.
- PATIENT AND CARER ADVICE Patients or carers should be given advice on how to administer ivacaftor tablets.

- MEDICINAL FORMS
There can be variation in the licensing of different medicines containing the same drug.
Tablet
CAUTIONARY AND ADVISORY LABELS 25
▶ Kalydeco (Vertex Pharmaceuticals (UK) Ltd) ▼
Ivacaftor 150 mg Kalydeco 150mg tablets | 56 tablet [PoM] £14,000.00
Granules
▶ Kalydeco (Vertex Pharmaceuticals (UK) Ltd) ▼
Ivacaftor 50 mg Kalydeco 50mg granules sachets sugar-free | 56 sachet [PoM] £14,000.00
Ivacaftor 75 mg Kalydeco 75mg granules sachets sugar-free | 56 sachet [PoM] £14,000.00

Mannitol

- INDICATIONS AND DOSE
Treatment of cystic fibrosis as an add-on therapy to standard care
▶ BY INHALATION OF POWDER
▶ Adult: Maintenance 400 mg twice daily, an initiation dose assessment must be carried out under medical supervision, for details of the initiation dose regimen, consult product literature

- CONTRA-INDICATIONS Bronchial hyperresponsiveness to inhaled mannitol · impaired lung function (forced expiratory volume in 1 second < 30% of predicted) · non-CF bronchiectasis
- CAUTIONS Asthma · haemoptysis
- INTERACTIONS → Appendix 1 (mannitol).

- SIDE-EFFECTS
  - ► **Common or very common** Cough · haemoptysis · headache · pharyngolaryngeal pain · throat irritation · vomiting · wheezing
  - ► **Uncommon** Acne · arthralgia · bronchospasm · dizziness · dysphonia · dyspnoea · ear pain · eructation · flatulence · gastro-oesophageal reflux disease · glossodynia · hyperventilation · influenza-like illness · malaise · nausea · oral candidiasis · pharyngitis · pruritus · pyrexia · rash · rhinorrhoea · stomatitis · transient insomnia
- PREGNANCY Manufacturer advises avoid.
- BREAST FEEDING Manufacturer advises avoid.
- PRE-TREATMENT SCREENING Patients must be assessed for bronchial hyperresponsiveness to inhaled mannitol before starting the therapeutic dose regimen; an initiation dose assessment must be carried out under medical supervision—for details of the initiation dose regimen, consult product literature.
- DIRECTIONS FOR ADMINISTRATION The dose should be administered 5–15 minutes after a bronchodilator and before physiotherapy; the second daily dose should be taken 2–3 hours before bedtime.
- PATIENT AND CARER ADVICE Patients or carers should be given advice on how to administer mannitol inhalation powder.
- NATIONAL FUNDING/ACCESS DECISIONS

  NICE technology appraisals (TAs)
  - ► **Mannitol dry powder for inhalation for treating cystic fibrosis** (November 2012) NICE TA266

  Mannitol dry powder for inhalation is recommended as an option for treating cystic fibrosis in adults:
  - who cannot use dornase alfa (rhDNase) because of ineligibility, intolerance or inadequate response to dornase alfa (rhDNase), **and**
  - whose lung function is rapidly declining (forced expiratory volume in 1 second decline greater than 2% annually), **and**
  - for whom other osmotic agents are not considered appropriate.

  www.nice.org.uk/TA266

  Scottish Medicines Consortium (SMC) Decisions
  The *Scottish Medicines Consortium*, has advised (November 2013) that mannitol (*Bronchitol®*) is accepted for restricted use within NHS Scotland for the treatment of cystic fibrosis in adults aged 18 years and over as an add-on therapy to best standard of care. Mannitol is restricted to patients who are not currently using dornase alfa due to lack of response, intolerance, or ineligibility and have rapidly declining lung function and in whom other osmotic agents are considered unsuitable.

- MEDICINAL FORMS
  There can be variation in the licensing of different medicines containing the same drug.

  Inhalation powder
  - ► Mannitol (Non-proprietary)

    Mannitol 5 mg Osmohale 5mg inhalation powder capsules | 1 capsule PoM no price available

    Mannitol 10 mg Osmohale 10mg inhalation powder capsules | 1 capsule PoM no price available

    Mannitol 20 mg Osmohale 20mg inhalation powder capsules | 1 capsule PoM no price available

    Mannitol 40 mg Osmohale 40mg inhalation powder capsules | 15 capsule PoM no price available
  - ► Bronchitol (Chiesi Ltd)

    Mannitol 40 mg Bronchitol 40mg inhalation powder capsules with two devices | 280 capsule PoM £231.66

    Bronchitol 40mg inhalation powder capsules with device | 10 capsule PoM no price available

4 Cough and congestion

Aromatic inhalations, cough preparations and systemic nasal decongestants

Aromatic inhalations in adults

Inhalations containing volatile substances such as eucalyptus oil are traditionally used and although the vapour may contain little of the additive it encourages deliberate inspiration of warm moist air which is often comforting in bronchitis; boiling water should not be used owing to the risk of scalding. Inhalations are also used for the relief of nasal obstruction in acute rhinitis or sinusitis. Eucalyptus with menthol p. 272 inhalation is used to relieve sinusitis affecting the maxillary antrum.

Cough preparations in adults

Cough suppressants

Cough may be a symptom of an underlying disorder, such as asthma, gastro-oesophageal reflux disease, or rhinitis, which should be addressed before prescribing cough suppressants. Cough may be a side-effect of another drug, such as an ACE inhibitor, or it can be associated with smoking or environmental pollutants. Cough can also have a significant habit component. When there is no identifiable cause, cough suppressants may be useful, for example if sleep is disturbed. They may cause sputum retention and this may be harmful in patients with chronic bronchitis and bronchiectasis.

Codeine phosphate p. 413 may be effective but it is constipating and can cause dependence; **dextromethorphan** and pholcodine p. 271 have fewer side-effects.

Sedating antihistamines are used as the cough suppressant component of many compound cough preparations on sale to the public; all tend to cause drowsiness which may reflect their main mode of action.

Palliative care

Diamorphine hydrochloride p. 415 and methadone hydrochloride p. 456 have been used to control distressing cough in terminal lung cancer although morphine p. 421 is now preferred. In other circumstances they are contra-indicated because they induce sputum retention and ventilatory failure as well as causing opioid dependence. Methadone hydrochloride linctus should be avoided because it has a long duration of action and tends to accumulate.

Demulcent and expectorant cough preparations

Demulcent cough preparations contain soothing substances such as syrup or glycerol and some patients believe that such preparations relieve a dry irritating cough. Preparations such as **simple linctus** have the advantage of being harmless and inexpensive; **paediatric simple linctus** is particularly useful in children.

Expectorants are claimed to promote expulsion of bronchial secretions, but there is no evidence that any drug can specifically facilitate expectoration.

Compound preparations are on sale to the public for the treatment of cough and colds but should not be used in children under 6 years; the rationale for some is dubious. Care should be taken to give the correct dose and to not use more than one preparation at a time.

Systemic nasal decongestants

Nasal decongestants for administration by mouth may not be as effective as preparations for local application but they do not give rise to rebound nasal congestion on withdrawal. Pseudoephedrine hydrochloride p. 1045 is available over the counter; it has few sympathomimetic effects.

Aromatic inhalations in children

The use of strong aromatic decongestants (applied as rubs or to pillows) is not advised for infants under the age of 3 months. Carers of young infants in whom nasal obstruction with mucus is a problem can readily be taught appropriate techniques of suction aspiration but sodium chloride 0.9% p. 901 given as nasal drops is preferred; administration before feeds may ease feeding difficulties caused by nasal congestion.

Cough preparations in children

The use of over-the-counter cough suppressants containing codeine phosphate should be avoided in children under 12 years and in children of any age known to be CYP2D6 ultra-rapid metabolisers. Cough suppressants containing similar opioid analgesics such as dextromethorphan and pholcodine are not generally recommended in children and should be avoided in children under 6 years.

MHRA/CHM advice (March 2008 and February 2009)

Children under 6 years should not be given over-the-counter cough and cold medicines containing the following ingredients:

- brompheniramine, chlorphenamine maleate p. 260, diphenhydramine, doxylamine, promethazine, or triprolidine (antihistamines);
- dextromethorphan or pholcodine (cough suppressants);
- guaifenesin or ipecacuanha (expectorants);
- phenylephrine hydrochloride p. 173, pseudoephedrine hydrochloride, ephedrine hydrochloride p. 248, oxymetazoline, or xylometazoline hydrochloride p. 1046 (decongestants).

Over-the-counter cough and cold medicines can be considered for children aged 6–12 years after basic principles of best care have been tried, but treatment should be restricted to five days or less. Children should not be given more than 1 cough or cold preparation at a time because different brands may contain the same active ingredient; care should be taken to give the correct dose.

COUGH AND COLD PREPARATIONS > COUGH SUPPRESSANTS

Pholcodine

- **INDICATIONS AND DOSE**

Dry cough

▸ BY MOUTH USING LINCTUS

- ▸ Child 6-11 years: 2–5 mg 3–4 times a day
- ▸ Child 12-17 years: 5–10 mg 3–4 times a day
- ▸ Adult: 5–10 mg 3–4 times a day

IMPORTANT SAFETY INFORMATION

MHRA/CHM ADVICE (MARCH 2008 AND FEBRUARY 2009) OVER-THE-COUNTER COUGH AND COLD MEDICINES FOR CHILDREN

Children under 6 years should not be given over-the-counter cough and cold medicines containing pholcodine (cough suppressant).

Over-the-counter cough and cold medicines can be considered for children aged 6–12 years after basic principles of best care have been tried, but treatment should be restricted to 5 days or less. Children should not be given more than 1 cough or cold preparation at a time because different brands may contain the same active ingredient; care should be taken to give the correct dose.

- CONTRA-INDICATIONS Bronchiectasis · bronchiolitis (in children) · chronic bronchitis · chronic obstructive pulmonary disease (in adults) · patients at risk of respiratory failure

- CAUTIONS Asthma · chronic cough · persistent cough · productive cough
- INTERACTIONS → Appendix 1 (pholcodine).
- SIDE-EFFECTS Confusion · constipation · dizziness · drowsiness · excitation · nausea · rash · sputum retention · vomiting
- PREGNANCY Manufacturer advises avoid unless potential benefit outweighs risk.
- BREAST FEEDING Manufacturer advises avoid unless potential benefit outweighs risk—no information available.
- HEPATIC IMPAIRMENT Avoid in hepatic impairment.
- RENAL IMPAIRMENT Use with caution in renal impairment. Avoid in severe renal impairment.
- PRESCRIBING AND DISPENSING INFORMATION Pholcodine is not generally recommended for children.

  Flavours of oral liquid formulations may include orange.

  When prepared extemporaneously, the BP states Pholcodine Linctus, BP consists of pholcodine 5 mg/5 mL in a suitable flavoured vehicle, containing citric acid monohydrate 1% and Pholcodine Linctus, Strong, BP consists of pholcodine 10 mg/5 mL in a suitable flavoured vehicle, containing citric acid monohydrate 2%

- MEDICINAL FORMS
There can be variation in the licensing of different medicines containing the same drug.

Oral solution

▸ Pholcodine (Non-proprietary)

   Pholcodine 1 mg per 1 ml Pholcodine 5mg/5ml linctus | 200 ml P
   £1.29 DT price = £1.29 Schedule 5 (CD Inv)
   Pholcodine 5mg/5ml linctus sugar free | 200 ml P £1.31 DT price =
   £1.31 Schedule 5 (CD Inv) sugar-free | 2000 ml P £13.10 Schedule 5
   (CD Inv)

   Pholcodine 2 mg per 1 ml Pholcodine 10mg/5ml linctus strong sugar
   free | 2000 ml P £10.88 DT price = £9.88 Schedule 5 (CD Inv)
   Pholcodine 10mg/5ml linctus strong | 200 ml P £1.61 Schedule 5
   (CD Inv)

▸ Galenphol (Thornton & Ross Ltd)

   Pholcodine 400 microgram per 1 ml Galenphol Paediatric 2mg/5ml
   linctus sugar-free | 2000 ml P £4.50 DT price = £4.50 Schedule 5 (CD
   Inv)

   Pholcodine 1 mg per 1 ml Galenphol 5mg/5ml linctus sugar-free |
   2000 ml P £8.50 Schedule 5 (CD Inv)

   Pholcodine 2 mg per 1 ml Galenphol Strong 10mg/5ml linctus sugar-
   free | 2000 ml P £9.88 DT price = £9.88 Schedule 5 (CD Inv)

▸ Pavacol-D (Alliance Pharmaceuticals Ltd)

   Pholcodine 1 mg per 1 ml Pavacol-D 5mg/5ml mixture sugar-free |
   150 ml P £1.69 Schedule 5 (CD Inv) sugar-free | 300 ml P
   £2.55 Schedule 5 (CD Inv)

COUGH AND COLD PREPARATIONS > OTHER

Citric acid

(Formulated as Simple Linctus)

- **INDICATIONS AND DOSE**

Cough

▸ BY MOUTH

- ▸ Adult: 5 mL 3–4 times a day, this dose is for Simple Linctus, BP (2.5%)

- PRESCRIBING AND DISPENSING INFORMATION Flavours of oral liquid formulations may include anise.

  When prepared extemporaneously, the BP states Simple Linctus, BP consists of citric acid monohydrate 2.5%, in a suitable vehicle with an anise flavour.

3

Respiratory system

- **MEDICINAL FORMS**
  There can be variation in the licensing of different medicines containing the same drug.
  Oral solution
  ‣ Citric acid (Non-proprietary)
    Citric acid monohydrate 25 mg per 1 ml Simple linctus sugar free sugar-free | 200 ml GSL £1.21 DT price = £0.89 sugar-free | 2000 ml GSL £8.40

MENTHOL AND DERIVATIVES

Eucalyptus with menthol

- **INDICATIONS AND DOSE**
  Aromatic inhalation for relief of nasal congestion
  ‣ BY INHALATION
  ‣ Adult: Add one teaspoonful to a pint of hot, **not** boiling, water and inhale the vapour

- **PRESCRIBING AND DISPENSING INFORMATION** When prepared extemporaneously, the BP states Menthol and Eucalyptus Inhalation, BP 1980 consists of racementhol or levomenthol 2 g, eucalyptus oil 10 mL, light magnesium carbonate 7 g, water to 100 mL.

- **PROFESSION SPECIFIC INFORMATION**
  Dental practitioners' formulary
  Menthol and Eucalyptus Inhalation BP, 1980 may be prescribed.

- **MEDICINAL FORMS**
  There can be variation in the licensing of different medicines containing the same drug.
  Inhalation vapour
  ‣ Eucalyptus with menthol (Non-proprietary)
    Eucalyptus oil 100 microlitre per 1 ml, Menthol 20 mg per 1 ml, Magnesium carbonate light 70 mg per 1 ml Menthol and Eucalyptus inhalation | 100 ml GSL £1.34–£1.36 DT price = £1.35

RESINS

Benzoin tincture

(Friars' Balsam)

- **INDICATIONS AND DOSE**
  Aromatic inhalation for relief of nasal congestion
  ‣ BY INHALATION
  ‣ Child: Add 5 mL to a pint of hot, **not** boiling, water and inhale the vapour; repeat after 4 hours if necessary
  ‣ Adult: Add 5 mL to a pint of hot, **not** boiling, water and inhale the vapour; repeat after 4 hours if necessary

- **SIDE-EFFECTS** Allergic contact dermatitis
- **PRESCRIBING AND DISPENSING INFORMATION** Not recommended (applied as a rub or to pillows) for infants under 3 months.
  When prepared extemporaneously, the BP states Benzoin Tincture, Compound, BP consists of balsamic acids approx. 4.5%.

- **MEDICINAL FORMS**
  There can be variation in the licensing of different medicines containing the same drug.
  Liquid
  CAUTIONARY AND ADVISORY LABELS 15
  ‣ Benzoin tincture (Non-proprietary)
    Balsamic acids 16.5 mg per 1 ml Benzoin tincture | 500 ml GSL £12.62–£22.78 DT price = £12.62

5 Idiopathic pulmonary fibrosis

Drugs used for Idiopathic pulmonary fibrosis not listed below Nintedanib, p. 867

ANTIFIBROTICS

Pirfenidone

- **DRUG ACTION** The exact mechanism of action of pirfenidone is not yet understood, but it is believed to slow down the progression of idiopathic pulmonary fibrosis by exerting both antifibrotic and anti-inflammatory properties.

- **INDICATIONS AND DOSE**
  Treatment of mild to moderate idiopathic pulmonary fibrosis (initiated under specialist supervision)
  ‣ BY MOUTH
  ‣ Adult: Initially 267 mg 3 times a day for 7 days, then increased to 534 mg 3 times a day for 7 days, then increased to 801 mg 3 times a day
  DOSE ADJUSTMENTS DUE TO INTERACTIONS
  Caution with concomitant use with ciprofloxacin—reduce dose of pirfenidone to 534 mg three times daily with high-dose ciprofloxacin (750 mg twice daily).
  Caution with concomitant use of drugs known to cause photosensitivity—if photosensitivity reaction or rash occurs, dose adjustment or treatment interruption may be required (consult product literature).

- **CONTRA-INDICATIONS** Cigarette smoking
- **CAUTIONS**
  CAUTIONS, FURTHER INFORMATION
  ‣ Photosensitivity Avoid exposure to direct sunlight—if photosensitivity reaction or rash occurs, dose adjustment or treatment interruption may be required (consult product literature).
  ‣ Treatment interruption If treatment is interrupted for 14 consecutive days or more, the initial 2 week titration regimen should be repeated; if treatment is interrupted for less than 14 consecutive days, the dose can be resumed at the previous daily dose without titration.
- **INTERACTIONS** → Appendix 1 (pirfenidone).
- **SIDE-EFFECTS**
  ‣ **Common or very common** Abdominal discomfort · anorexia · arthralgia · constipation · diarrhoea · dizziness · dry skin · dysgeusia · dyspepsia · erythema · flatulence · gastritis · gastro-oesophageal reflux disease · headache · hot flush · insomnia · malaise · myalgia · nausea · non-cardiac chest pain · photosensitivity reaction · pruritus · raised hepatic enzymes · rash · somnolence · upper respiratory tract infection · urinary tract infection · vomiting · weight loss
  ‣ **Rare** Raised bilirubin in combination with raised hepatic transaminases
  SIDE-EFFECTS, FURTHER INFORMATION
  Gastrointestinal side-effects may require dose reduction or treatment interruption—consult product literature.
- **PREGNANCY** Manufacturer advises avoid—no information available.
- **BREAST FEEDING** Manufacturer advises avoid—no information available.
- **HEPATIC IMPAIRMENT** Use with caution in mild to moderate hepatic impairment, particularly if concomitant use of CYP1A2 inhibitors. Avoid use in severe hepatic impairment.

- **RENAL IMPAIRMENT** Avoid use if eGFR less than 30 mL/minute/1.73 m^2.
- **MONITORING REQUIREMENTS**
  - Monitor for weight loss.
  - Test liver function before treatment, then at monthly intervals for the next 6 months, and then every 3 months thereafter; review if abnormal liver function tests—dose reduction, treatment interruption or discontinuation may be required (consult product literature).
- **PATIENT AND CARER ADVICE**
  Driving and skilled tasks
  Dizziness or malaise may affect performance of skilled tasks (e.g. driving).
- **NATIONAL FUNDING/ACCESS DECISIONS**
  NICE technology appraisals (TAs)
  - Pirfenidone for treating idiopathic pulmonary fibrosis (April 2013) NICE TA282
  Pirfenidone is recommended as an option for treating idiopathic pulmonary fibrosis only if:
  - the patient has a forced vital capacity (FVC) between 50% and 80% predicted, **and**
  - the manufacturer provides pirfenidone with the discount agreed in the patient access scheme.Treatment should be discontinued if there is evidence of disease progression, defined as a decline in predicted FVC of 10% or more within any 12 month period.

  Patients currently receiving pirfenidone that is not recommended according to the above criteria should have the option to continue treatment until they and their clinician consider it appropriate to stop.
  www.nice.org.uk/TA282

  Scottish Medicines Consortium (SMC) Decisions
  The *Scottish Medicines Consortium* has advised (August 2013) that pirfenidone is accepted for restricted use within NHS Scotland for the treatment of mild to moderate idiopathic pulmonary fibrosis. Pirfenidone is restricted for use in patients with a predicted forced vital capacity less than or equal to 80%, and only whilst pirfenidone is available at the price agreed in the patient access scheme.

- **MEDICINAL FORMS**
  There can be variation in the licensing of different medicines containing the same drug.
  Capsule
  CAUTIONARY AND ADVISORY LABELS 21, 25
  - Esbriet (Roche Products Ltd) ▼
    Pirfenidone 267 mg Esbriet 267mg capsules | 63 capsule [PoM] £501.92 | 252 capsule [PoM] £2,007.70 | 270 capsule [PoM] £2,151.10

6   Respiratory depression, respiratory distress syndrome and apnoea

Respiratory stimulants

Overview

Respiratory stimulants (analeptic drugs) have a limited place in the treatment of ventilatory failure in patients with chronic obstructive pulmonary disease. They are effective only when given by intravenous injection or infusion and have a short duration of action. Their use has largely been replaced by ventilatory support including nasal intermittent positive pressure ventilation. However, occasionally when ventilatory support is contra-indicated and in patients with hypercapnic respiratory failure who are becoming drowsy or comatose, respiratory stimulants in the short term may arouse patients sufficiently to co-operate and clear their secretions.

Respiratory stimulants can also be harmful in respiratory failure since they stimulate non-respiratory as well as respiratory muscles. They should only be given under **expert supervision** in hospital and must be combined with active physiotherapy. There is at present no oral respiratory stimulant available for long-term use in chronic respiratory failure.

RESPIRATORY STIMULANTS

Doxapram hydrochloride

- **INDICATIONS AND DOSE**
  Postoperative respiratory depression
  - INITIALLY BY INTRAVENOUS INJECTION
  - **Adult:** Initially 1–1.5 mg/kg, to be administered over at least 30 seconds, repeated if necessary after intervals of one hour, alternatively (by intravenous infusion) 2–3 mg/minute, adjusted according to response
  Acute respiratory failure
  - BY INTRAVENOUS INFUSION
  - **Adult:** 1.5–4 mg/minute, adjusted according to response, to be given concurrently with oxygen and whenever possible monitor with frequent measurement of blood gas tensions

- **CONTRA-INDICATIONS** Cerebral oedema · cerebrovascular accident · coronary artery disease · epilepsy and other convulsive disorders · hyperthyroidism · physical obstruction of respiratory tract · severe hypertension · status asthmaticus
- **CAUTIONS** Give with beta$_2$ agonist in bronchoconstriction · give with oxygen in severe irreversible airways obstruction or severely decreased lung compliance (because of increased work load of breathing) · hypertension · impaired cardiac reserve · phaeochromocytoma
- **INTERACTIONS** → Appendix 1 (doxapram).
- **SIDE-EFFECTS** Arrhythmias · bradycardia · bronchospasm · chest pain · confusion · convulsions · cough · dizziness · dyspnoea · extrasystoles · flushing · hallucination · headache · hyperactivity · hypertension · incontinence · laryngospasm · muscle spasms · nausea · perineal warmth · pyrexia · tachycardia · urinary retention · vomiting
- **PREGNANCY** No evidence of harm, but manufacturer advises avoid unless benefit outweighs risk.
- **HEPATIC IMPAIRMENT** Use with caution.
- **MONITORING REQUIREMENTS** Frequent arterial blood gas and pH measurements are necessary during treatment to ensure correct dosage.

- **MEDICINAL FORMS**
  There can be variation in the licensing of different medicines containing the same drug.
  Solution for injection
  - Doxapram hydrochloride (Non-proprietary)
    Doxapram hydrochloride 20 mg per 1 ml Doxapram 100mg/5ml solution for injection ampoules | 5 ampoule [PoM] £110.00
  Infusion
  - Doxapram hydrochloride (Non-proprietary)
    Doxapram hydrochloride 2 mg per 1 ml Doxapram 1g/500ml infusion bags | 1 bag [PoM] no price available

Chapter 4
Nervous system

CONTENTS

1 Dementia

Dementia

Management

Acetylcholinesterase inhibiting drugs are used in the treatment of Alzheimer's disease, specifically for mild to moderate disease. Rivastigmine p. 276 is also licensed for mild to moderate dementia associated with Parkinson's disease. The evidence to support the use of these drugs relates to their cognitive enhancement.

Treatment with drugs for dementia should be initiated and supervised only by a specialist experienced in the management of dementia.

Benefit is assessed by repeating the cognitive assessment at around 3 months. Such assessment cannot demonstrate how the disease may have progressed in the absence of treatment but it can give a good guide to response. Up to half the patients given these drugs will show a slower rate of cognitive decline. Drugs for dementia should be discontinued in those thought not to be responding. Many specialists repeat the cognitive assessment 4 to 6 weeks after discontinuation to assess deterioration; if significant deterioration occurs during this short period, consideration should be given to restarting therapy.

Drugs used for Dementia not listed below Risperidone, p. 368

ANTICHOLINESTERASES > CENTRALLY ACTING

Donepezil hydrochloride

● DRUG ACTION Donepezil is a reversible inhibitor of acetylcholinesterase.

● INDICATIONS AND DOSE

Mild to moderate dementia in Alzheimer's disease
► BY MOUTH
▸ Adult: Initially 5 mg once daily for one month, then increased if necessary up to 10 mg daily, doses to be given at bedtime

● CAUTIONS Asthma · chronic obstructive pulmonary disease · sick sinus syndrome · supraventricular conduction abnormalities · susceptibility to peptic ulcers

● INTERACTIONS → Appendix 1 (parasympathomimetics). Caution with concomitant antipsychotic treatment—increased risk of neuroleptic malignant syndrome.

● SIDE-EFFECTS
▸ **Common or very common** Abnormal dreams · aggression · agitation · anorexia · diarrhoea · dizziness · fatigue · hallucinations · headache · insomnia · muscle cramps · nausea · pruritus · rash · syncope · urinary incontinence · vomiting
▸ **Uncommon** Bradycardia · duodenal ulcers · gastric ulcers · gastro-intestinal haemorrhage · seizures
▸ **Rare** AV block · extrapyramidal symptoms · hepatitis · potential for bladder outflow obstruction · sino-atrial block
▸ **Very rare** Neuroleptic malignant syndrome
SIDE-EFFECTS, FURTHER INFORMATION
Acetylcholinesterase inhibitors can cause unwanted dose-related cholinergic effects and should be started at a low dose and the dose increased according to response and tolerability.

● HEPATIC IMPAIRMENT Caution in mild to moderate impairment. No information available for severe impairment.

● DIRECTIONS FOR ADMINISTRATION Donepezil orodispersible tablet should be placed on the tongue, allowed to disperse, and swallowed.

- **PATIENT AND CARER ADVICE** Patient or carers should be given advise on how to administer donepezil hydrochloride orodispersible tablets.

- **NATIONAL FUNDING/ACCESS DECISIONS**

NICE technology appraisals (TAs)

▶ Donepezil, galantamine, rivastigmine, and memantine for the treatment of Alzheimer's disease (March 2011) NICE TA217
Donepezil can be used for the treatment of mild to moderate Alzheimer's disease. Treatment should only be prescribed under the following conditions:
- Alzheimer's disease must be diagnosed and treatment initiated by a specialist; treatment can be continued by general practitioners under a shared-care protocol;
- the carer's view of the condition should be sought before and during treatment;
- treatment should continue only if it is considered to have a worthwhile effect on cognitive, global, functional, or behavioural symptoms.

Healthcare professionals should not rely solely on assessment scales to determine the severity of Alzheimer's disease when the patient has learning or other disabilities, or other communication difficulties.
www.nice.org.uk/TA217

- **MEDICINAL FORMS**
There can be variation in the licensing of different medicines containing the same drug. Forms available from special-order manufacturers include: oral suspension

Tablet
▶ Donepezil hydrochloride (Non-proprietary)
Donepezil hydrochloride 5 mg Donepezil 5mg tablets |
28 tablet [PoM] £59.85 DT price = £1.13
Donepezil hydrochloride 10 mg Donepezil 10mg tablets |
28 tablet [PoM] £83.89 DT price = £1.45
▶ Aricept (Eisai Ltd)
Donepezil hydrochloride 5 mg Aricept 5mg tablets |
28 tablet [PoM] £59.85 DT price = £1.13
Donepezil hydrochloride 10 mg Aricept 10mg tablets |
28 tablet [PoM] £83.89 DT price = £1.45

Orodispersible tablet
▶ Donepezil hydrochloride (Non-proprietary)
Donepezil hydrochloride 5 mg Donepezil 5mg orodispersible tablets
| 28 tablet [PoM] £59.85
Donepezil 5mg orodispersible tablets sugar free sugar-free |
28 tablet [PoM] £6.05–£7.99 DT price = £6.68
Donepezil hydrochloride 10 mg Donepezil 10mg orodispersible
tablets sugar free sugar-free | 28 tablet [PoM] £8.39–£8.99 DT price =
£8.57
Donepezil 10mg orodispersible tablets | 28 tablet [PoM] £83.89
▶ Aricept Evess (Eisai Ltd)
Donepezil hydrochloride 5 mg Aricept Evess 5mg orodispersible
tablets sugar-free | 28 tablet [PoM] £59.85 DT price = £6.68
Donepezil hydrochloride 10 mg Aricept Evess 10mg orodispersible
tablets sugar-free | 28 tablet [PoM] £83.89 DT price = £8.57

Oral solution
▶ Donepezil hydrochloride (Non-proprietary)
Donepezil hydrochloride 1 mg per 1 ml Donepezil 1mg/ml oral
solution sugar free sugar-free | 150 ml [PoM] £48.00 DT price = £47.91

Galantamine
3.3.2016

- **DRUG ACTION** Galantamine is a reversible inhibitor of acetylcholinesterase and it also has nicotinic receptor agonist properties.

- **INDICATIONS AND DOSE**

Mild to moderately severe dementia in Alzheimer's disease
▶ BY MOUTH USING IMMEDIATE-RELEASE MEDICINES
▶ Adult: Initially 4 mg twice daily for 4 weeks, increased to 8 mg twice daily for at least 4 weeks; maintenance 8–12 mg twice daily

▶ BY MOUTH USING MODIFIED-RELEASE CAPSULES
▶ Adult: Initially 8 mg once daily for 4 weeks, increased to 16 mg once daily for at least 4 weeks; maintenance 16–24 mg daily

- **CAUTIONS** Avoid in gastro-intestinal obstruction · avoid in urinary outflow obstruction · avoid whilst recovering from bladder surgery · avoid whilst recovering from gastro-intestinal surgery · cardiac disease · chronic obstructive pulmonary disease · congestive heart failure · electrolyte disturbances · history of seizures · history of severe asthma · pulmonary infection · sick sinus syndrome · supraventricular conduction abnormalities · susceptibility to peptic ulcers · unstable angina

- **INTERACTIONS** → Appendix 1 (parasympathomimetics).

- **SIDE-EFFECTS**
▶ **Common or very common** Abdominal pain · bradycardia · decreased appetite · depression · diarrhoea · dizziness · dyspepsia · fatigue · hallucination · headache · hypertension · malaise · muscle spasm · nausea · syncope · tremor · vomiting · weight loss
▶ **Uncommon** Arrhythmias · blurred vision · dehydration · first-degree AV block · flushing · hypersomnia · hypotension · muscular weakness · palpitation · paraesthesia · retching · seizures · sweating · taste disturbance · tinnitus
▶ **Rare** Acute generalized exanthematous pustulosis · erythema multiforme · exacerbation of Parkinson's disease · hepatitis · Stevens-Johnson syndrome

SIDE-EFFECTS, FURTHER INFORMATION
Acetylcholinesterase inhibitors can cause unwanted dose-related cholinergic effects and should be started at a low dose and the dose increased according to response and tolerability.
▶ Serious skin reactions Serious skin reactions (including Stevens-Johnson syndrome and acute generalized exanthematous pustulosis) have been reported—manufacturer advises discontinue at the first appearance of skin rash.

- **PREGNANCY** Use with caution—toxicity in *animal* studies.

- **BREAST FEEDING** Avoid—no information available.

- **HEPATIC IMPAIRMENT** For *immediate-release* preparations in moderate impairment, initially 4 mg once daily (preferably in the morning) for at least 7 days, then 4 mg twice daily for at least 4 weeks; max. 8 mg twice daily; avoid in severe impairment. For *modified-release* preparations in moderate impairment, initially 8 mg on alternate days (preferably in the morning) for 7 days, then 8 mg once daily for 4 weeks; max. 16 mg daily; avoid in severe impairment.

- **RENAL IMPAIRMENT** Avoid if eGFR less than 9 mL/minute/1.73 m^2.

- **PATIENT AND CARER ADVICE** Manufacturer recommends that patients are warned of the signs of serious skin reactions; they should be advised to stop taking galantamine immediately and seek medical advice if symptoms occur.

- **NATIONAL FUNDING/ACCESS DECISIONS**

NICE technology appraisals (TAs)
▶ Donepezil, galantamine, rivastigmine, and memantine for the treatment of Alzheimer's disease (March 2011) NICE TA217
Galantamine can be used for the treatment of mild to moderate Alzheimer's disease. Treatment should only be prescribed under the following conditions:
- Alzheimer's disease must be diagnosed and treatment initiated by a specialist; treatment can be continued by general practitioners under a shared-care protocol;
- the carer's view of the condition should be sought before and during treatment;

4

Nervous system

- treatment should continue only if it is considered to have a worthwhile effect on cognitive, global, functional, or behavioural symptoms.

Healthcare professionals should not rely solely on assessment scales to determine the severity of Alzheimer's disease when the patient has learning or other disabilities, or other communication difficulties.

www.nice.org.uk/TA217

- MEDICINAL FORMS
There can be variation in the licensing of different medicines containing the same drug. Forms available from special-order manufacturers include: tablet

Tablet

CAUTIONARY AND ADVISORY LABELS 3, 21

▸ Galantamine (Non-proprietary)

Galantamine (as Galantamine hydrobromide) 8 mg Galantamine 8mg tablets | 56 tablet (PoM) £59.25–£64.90 DT price = £61.13

Galantamine (as Galantamine hydrobromide) 12 mg Galantamine 12mg tablets | 56 tablet (PoM) £71.25–£79.80 DT price = £74.10

▸ Reminyl (Shire Pharmaceuticals Ltd)

Galantamine (as Galantamine hydrobromide) 8 mg Reminyl 8mg tablets | 56 tablet (PoM) £68.32 DT price = £61.13

Galantamine (as Galantamine hydrobromide) 12 mg Reminyl 12mg tablets | 56 tablet (PoM) £84.00 DT price = £74.10

Modified-release capsule

CAUTIONARY AND ADVISORY LABELS 3, 21, 25

▸ Acumor XL (Mylan Ltd)

Galantamine (as Galantamine hydrobromide) 8 mg Acumor XL 8mg capsules | 28 capsule (PoM) £49.26 DT price = £51.88

Galantamine (as Galantamine hydrobromide) 16 mg Acumor XL 16mg capsules | 28 capsule (PoM) £61.65 DT price = £64.90

Galantamine (as Galantamine hydrobromide) 24 mg Acumor XL 24mg capsules | 28 capsule (PoM) £75.81 DT price = £79.80

▸ Consion XL (Dr Reddy's Laboratories (UK) Ltd)

Galantamine (as Galantamine hydrobromide) 8 mg Consion XL 8mg capsules | 28 capsule (PoM) £25.94 DT price = £51.88

Galantamine (as Galantamine hydrobromide) 16 mg Consion XL 16mg capsules | 28 capsule (PoM) £32.45 DT price = £64.90

Galantamine (as Galantamine hydrobromide) 24 mg Consion XL 24mg capsules | 28 capsule (PoM) £39.90 DT price = £79.80

▸ Elmino (Zentiva)

Galantamine (as Galantamine hydrobromide) 8 mg Elmino XL 8mg capsules | 28 capsule (PoM) £51.88 DT price = £51.88

Galantamine (as Galantamine hydrobromide) 16 mg Elmino XL 16mg capsules | 28 capsule (PoM) £64.90 DT price = £64.90

Galantamine (as Galantamine hydrobromide) 24 mg Elmino XL 24mg capsules | 28 capsule (PoM) £79.80 DT price = £79.80

▸ Galantex XL (Creo Pharma Ltd)

Galantamine (as Galantamine hydrobromide) 8 mg Galantex XL 8mg capsules | 28 capsule (PoM) £25.42 DT price = £51.88

Galantamine (as Galantamine hydrobromide) 16 mg Galantex XL 16mg capsules | 28 capsule (PoM) £31.80 DT price = £64.90

Galantamine (as Galantamine hydrobromide) 24 mg Galantex XL 24mg capsules | 28 capsule (PoM) £39.10 DT price = £79.80

▸ Galsya XL (Consilient Health Ltd)

Galantamine (as Galantamine hydrobromide) 8 mg Galsya XL 8mg capsules | 28 capsule (PoM) £44.09 DT price = £51.88

Galantamine (as Galantamine hydrobromide) 16 mg Galsya XL 16mg capsules | 28 capsule (PoM) £55.16 DT price = £64.90

Galantamine (as Galantamine hydrobromide) 24 mg Galsya XL 24mg capsules | 28 capsule (PoM) £67.83 DT price = £79.80

▸ Gatalin XL (Aspire Pharma Ltd)

Galantamine (as Galantamine hydrobromide) 8 mg Gatalin XL 8mg capsules | 28 capsule (PoM) £25.94 DT price = £51.88

Galantamine (as Galantamine hydrobromide) 16 mg Gatalin XL 16mg capsules | 28 capsule (PoM) £32.45 DT price = £64.90

Galantamine (as Galantamine hydrobromide) 24 mg Gatalin XL 24mg capsules | 28 capsule (PoM) £39.90 DT price = £79.80

▸ Gazylan XL (Teva UK Ltd)

Galantamine (as Galantamine hydrobromide) 8 mg Gazylan XL 8mg capsules | 28 capsule (PoM) £25.41 DT price = £51.88

Galantamine (as Galantamine hydrobromide) 16 mg Gazylan XL 16mg capsules | 28 capsule (PoM) £31.79 DT price = £64.90

Galantamine (as Galantamine hydrobromide) 24 mg Gazylan XL 24mg capsules | 28 capsule (PoM) £39.09 DT price = £79.80

▸ Lotprosin XL (Actavis UK Ltd)

Galantamine (as Galantamine hydrobromide) 8 mg Lotprosin XL 8mg capsules | 28 capsule (PoM) £51.88 DT price = £51.88

Galantamine (as Galantamine hydrobromide) 16 mg Lotprosin XL 16mg capsules | 28 capsule (PoM) £64.90 DT price = £64.90

Galantamine (as Galantamine hydrobromide) 24 mg Lotprosin XL 24mg capsules | 28 capsule (PoM) £79.80 DT price = £79.80

▸ Luventa XL (Fontus Health Ltd)

Galantamine (as Galantamine hydrobromide) 8 mg Luventa XL 8mg capsules | 28 capsule (PoM) £25.42 DT price = £51.88

Galantamine (as Galantamine hydrobromide) 16 mg Luventa XL 16mg capsules | 28 capsule (PoM) £31.80 DT price = £64.90

Galantamine (as Galantamine hydrobromide) 24 mg Luventa XL 24mg capsules | 28 capsule (PoM) £39.10 DT price = £79.80

▸ Reminyl XL (Shire Pharmaceuticals Ltd)

Galantamine (as Galantamine hydrobromide) 8 mg Reminyl XL 8mg capsules | 28 capsule (PoM) £51.88 DT price = £51.88

Galantamine (as Galantamine hydrobromide) 16 mg Reminyl XL 16mg capsules | 28 capsule (PoM) £64.90 DT price = £64.90

Galantamine (as Galantamine hydrobromide) 24 mg Reminyl XL 24mg capsules | 28 capsule (PoM) £79.80 DT price = £79.80

Oral solution

CAUTIONARY AND ADVISORY LABELS 3, 21

▸ Galantamine (Non-proprietary)

Galantamine (as Galantamine hydrobromide) 4 mg per 1 ml Galantamine 20mg/5ml oral solution sugar free sugar-free | 100 ml (PoM) £437.00

▸ Reminyl (Shire Pharmaceuticals Ltd)

Galantamine (as Galantamine hydrobromide) 4 mg per 1 ml Reminyl 4mg/ml oral solution sugar-free | 100 ml (PoM) £120.00

Rivastigmine

- DRUG ACTION Rivastigmine is a reversible non-competitive inhibitor of acetylcholinesterases.

- INDICATIONS AND DOSE

Mild to moderate dementia in Alzheimer's disease

▸ BY MOUTH

▸ Adult: Initially 1.5 mg twice daily, increased in steps of 1.5 mg twice daily, dose to be increased at intervals of at least 2 weeks according to response and tolerance; usual dose 3–6 mg twice daily (max. per dose 6 mg twice daily), if treatment interrupted for more than several days, retitrate from 1.5 mg twice daily

▸ BY TRANSDERMAL APPLICATION USING PATCHES

▸ Adult: Apply 4.6 mg/24 hours daily for at least 4 weeks, increased if tolerated to 9.5 mg/24 hours daily for a further 6 months, then increased if necessary to 13.3 mg/24 hours daily, increase to 13.3 mg/24 hours patch if well tolerated and cognitive deterioration or functional decline demonstrated; use caution in patients with body-weight less than 50 kg, if treatment interrupted for more than 3 days, retitrate from 4.6 mg/24 hours patch

Mild to moderate dementia in Parkinson's disease

▸ BY MOUTH

▸ Adult: Initially 1.5 mg twice daily, increased in steps of 1.5 mg twice daily, dose to be increased at intervals of at least 2 weeks according to response and tolerance; usual dose 3–6 mg twice daily (max. per dose 6 mg twice daily), if treatment interrupted for more than several days, retitrate from 1.5 mg twice daily

DOSE EQUIVALENCE AND CONVERSION

When switching from oral to transdermal therapy, patients taking 3–6 mg by mouth daily should initially switch to 4.6 mg/24 hours patch, then titrate as above. Patients taking 9 mg by mouth daily should switch to 9.5 mg/24 hours patch if oral dose stable and well tolerated; if oral dose not stable or well tolerated. patients should switch to 4.6 mg/24 hours patch, then titrate as above. Patients taking 12 mg by mouth daily should switch to 9.5 mg/24 hours patch. The first patch should be applied on the day following the last oral dose

- CAUTIONS Bladder outflow obstruction · conduction abnormalities · duodenal ulcers · gastric ulcers · history of asthma · history of chronic obstructive pulmonary disease · history of seizures · risk of fatal overdose with patch administration errors · sick sinus syndrome · susceptibility to ulcers
- INTERACTIONS → Appendix 1 (parasympathomimetics).
- SIDE-EFFECTS
  ▸ **Common or very common** Abdominal pain · agitation · anorexia · anxiety · bradycardia · confusion · diarrhoea · dizziness · drowsiness · dyspepsia · extrapyramidal symptoms · headache · increased salivation · insomnia · malaise · nausea · sweating · tremor · urinary incontinence · vomiting · weight loss · worsening of Parkinson's disease
  ▸ **Uncommon** Atrial fibrillation · AV block · depression · syncope
  ▸ **Rare** Angina · duodenal ulceration · gastric ulceration · rash · seizures
  ▸ **Very rare** Gastro-intestinal haemorrhage · hallucinations · hypertension · pancreatitis · tachycardia
  ▸ **Frequency not known** Aggression · dehydration · hepatitis · restlessness · sick sinus syndrome · skin hypersensitivity reactions

  SIDE-EFFECTS, FURTHER INFORMATION
  Transdermal administration less likely to cause gastro-intestinal disturbance.
  Treatment should be interrupted if gastro-intestinal side-effects occur and withheld until their resolution—retitrate dose if necessary.
  Acetylcholinesterase inhibitors can cause unwanted dose-related cholinergic effects and should be started at a low dose and the dose increased according to response and tolerability.

- HEPATIC IMPAIRMENT Titrate according to individual tolerability in mild to moderate impairment. Use with caution in severe impairment—no information available.
- RENAL IMPAIRMENT Titrate according to individual tolerability.
- MONITORING REQUIREMENTS Monitor body-weight.
- DIRECTIONS FOR ADMINISTRATION
  ▸ With transdermal use Apply patches to clean, dry, non-hairy, non-irritated skin on back, upper arm, or chest, removing after 24 hours and siting a replacement patch on a different area (avoid using the same area for 14 days).
- PATIENT AND CARER ADVICE
  EXELON® PATCHES Advise patients and carers of patch administration instructions, particularly to remove the previous day's patch before applying the new patch—consult product literature.
- NATIONAL FUNDING/ACCESS DECISIONS

  NICE technology appraisals (TAs)
  ▸ **Donepezil, galantamine, rivastigmine, and memantine for the treatment of Alzheimer's disease (March 2011)** NICE TA217
  Rivastigmine can be used for the treatment of mild to moderate Alzheimer's disease. Treatment should only be prescribed under the following conditions:
  - Alzheimer's disease must be diagnosed and treatment initiated by a specialist; treatment can be continued by general practitioners under a shared-care protocol;
  - the carer's view of the condition should be sought before and during treatment;
  - treatment should continue only if it is considered to have a worthwhile effect on cognitive, global, functional, or behavioural symptoms.
  Healthcare professionals should not rely solely on assessment scales to determine the severity of Alzheimer's disease when the patient has learning or other disabilities, or other communication difficulties.
  www.nice.org.uk/TA217

EXELON® PATCHES

Scottish Medicines Consortium (SMC) Decisions
The *Scottish Medicines Consortium* has advised (October 2007) that *Exelon*® patches should be restricted for use in patients with moderately severe Alzheimer's disease under the conditions of the NICE guidance (September 2007) and when a transdermal patch is an appropriate choice of formulation.

- MEDICINAL FORMS
  There can be variation in the licensing of different medicines containing the same drug.

Capsule
CAUTIONARY AND ADVISORY LABELS 21, 25
▸ Rivastigmine (Non-proprietary)
  Rivastigmine (as Rivastigmine hydrogen tartrate)
  1.5 mg Rivastigmine 1.5mg capsules | 28 capsule [PoM] £33.25 DT price = £2.17 | 56 capsule [PoM] £66.51
  Rivastigmine (as Rivastigmine hydrogen tartrate)
  3 mg Rivastigmine 3mg capsules | 28 capsule [PoM] £33.25 DT price = £2.57 | 56 capsule [PoM] £66.51
  Rivastigmine (as Rivastigmine hydrogen tartrate)
  4.5 mg Rivastigmine 4.5mg capsules | 28 capsule [PoM] £33.25 DT price = £14.69 | 56 capsule [PoM] £66.51
  Rivastigmine (as Rivastigmine hydrogen tartrate)
  6 mg Rivastigmine 6mg capsules | 28 capsule [PoM] £33.25 DT price = £15.98 | 56 capsule [PoM] £66.51
▸ Exelon (Novartis Pharmaceuticals UK Ltd)
  Rivastigmine (as Rivastigmine hydrogen tartrate) 1.5 mg Exelon 1.5mg capsules | 28 capsule [PoM] £33.25 DT price = £2.17 | 56 capsule [PoM] £66.51
  Rivastigmine (as Rivastigmine hydrogen tartrate) 3 mg Exelon 3mg capsules | 28 capsule [PoM] £33.25 DT price = £2.57 | 56 capsule [PoM] £66.51
  Rivastigmine (as Rivastigmine hydrogen tartrate) 4.5 mg Exelon 4.5mg capsules | 28 capsule [PoM] £33.25 DT price = £14.69 | 56 capsule [PoM] £66.51
  Rivastigmine (as Rivastigmine hydrogen tartrate) 6 mg Exelon 6mg capsules | 28 capsule [PoM] £33.25 DT price = £15.98 | 56 capsule [PoM] £66.51
▸ Kerstipon (Aspire Pharma Ltd)
  Rivastigmine (as Rivastigmine hydrogen tartrate)
  1.5 mg Kerstipon 1.5mg capsules | 28 capsule [PoM] £33.25 DT price = £2.17
  Rivastigmine (as Rivastigmine hydrogen tartrate) 3 mg Kerstipon 3mg capsules | 28 capsule [PoM] £33.25 DT price = £2.57
  Rivastigmine (as Rivastigmine hydrogen tartrate)
  4.5 mg Kerstipon 4.5mg capsules | 28 capsule [PoM] £33.25 DT price = £14.69
  Rivastigmine (as Rivastigmine hydrogen tartrate) 6 mg Kerstipon 6mg capsules | 28 capsule [PoM] £33.25 DT price = £15.98
▸ Nimvastid (Consilient Health Ltd)
  Rivastigmine (as Rivastigmine hydrogen tartrate)
  1.5 mg Nimvastid 1.5mg capsules | 28 capsule [PoM] £28.26 DT price = £2.17
  Rivastigmine (as Rivastigmine hydrogen tartrate) 3 mg Nimvastid 3mg capsules | 28 capsule [PoM] £28.26 DT price = £2.57
  Rivastigmine (as Rivastigmine hydrogen tartrate)
  4.5 mg Nimvastid 4.5mg capsules | 28 capsule [PoM] £28.26 DT price = £14.69
  Rivastigmine (as Rivastigmine hydrogen tartrate)
  6 mg Nimvastid 6mg capsules | 28 capsule [PoM] £28.26 DT price = £15.98

Oral solution
CAUTIONARY AND ADVISORY LABELS 21
▸ Rivastigmine (Non-proprietary)
  Rivastigmine (as Rivastigmine hydrogen tartrate) 2 mg per 1 ml Rivastigmine 2mg/ml oral solution | 120 ml [PoM] £81.75-£94.18
  Rivastigmine 2mg/ml oral solution sugar free sugar-free | 120 ml [PoM] £96.82 DT price = £96.82
▸ Exelon (Novartis Pharmaceuticals UK Ltd)
  Rivastigmine (as Rivastigmine hydrogen tartrate) 2 mg per 1 ml Exelon 2mg/ml oral solution sugar-free | 120 ml [PoM] £99.14 DT price = £96.82

Transdermal patch

▸ Rivastigmine (Non-proprietary)

Rivastigmine 4.6 mg per 24 hour Rivastigmine 4.6mg/24hours transdermal patches | 30 patch [PoM] £77.97 DT price = £77.97
Rivastigmine 9.5 mg per 24 hour Rivastigmine 9.5mg/24hours transdermal patches | 30 patch [PoM] £15.48 DT price = £14.80
Rivastigmine 13.3 mg per 24 hour Rivastigmine 13.3mg/24hours transdermal patches | 30 patch [PoM] £77.97 DT price = £77.97

▸ Alzest (Dr Reddy's Laboratories (UK) Ltd)

Rivastigmine 4.6 mg per 24 hour Alzest 4.6mg/24hours transdermal patches | 30 patch [PoM] £35.10 DT price = £77.97
Rivastigmine 9.5 mg per 24 hour Alzest 9.5mg/24hours transdermal patches | 30 patch [PoM] £15.47 DT price = £14.80

▸ Eluden (Mylan Ltd)

Rivastigmine 4.6 mg per 24 hour Eluden 4.6mg/24hours transdermal patches | 30 patch [PoM] £74.07 DT price = £77.97
Rivastigmine 9.5 mg per 24 hour Eluden 9.5mg/24hours transdermal patches | 30 patch [PoM] £74.07 DT price = £14.80

▸ Exelon (Novartis Pharmaceuticals UK Ltd)

Rivastigmine 4.6 mg per 24 hour Exelon 4.6mg/24hours transdermal patches | 30 patch [PoM] £77.97 DT price = £77.97
Rivastigmine 9.5 mg per 24 hour Exelon 9.5mg/24hours transdermal patches | 30 patch [PoM] £77.97 DT price = £14.80
Rivastigmine 13.3 mg per 24 hour Exelon 13.3mg/24hours transdermal patches | 30 patch [PoM] £77.97 DT price = £77.97

▸ Prometax (Novartis Pharmaceuticals UK Ltd)

Rivastigmine 4.6 mg per 24 hour Prometax 4.6mg/24hours transdermal patches | 30 patch [PoM] £77.97 DT price = £77.97
Rivastigmine 9.5 mg per 24 hour Prometax 9.5mg/24hours transdermal patches | 30 patch [PoM] £77.97 DT price = £14.80

▸ Rivatev (Teva UK Ltd)

Rivastigmine 4.6 mg per 24 hour Erastig 4.6mg/24hours transdermal patches | 30 patch [PoM] £74.07 DT price = £77.97
Rivastigmine 9.5 mg per 24 hour Erastig 9.5mg/24hours transdermal patches | 30 patch [PoM] £74.07 DT price = £14.80
Rivastigmine 13.3 mg per 24 hour Erastig 13.3mg/24hours transdermal patches | 30 patch [PoM] £73.90 DT price = £77.97

▸ Voleze (Focus Pharmaceuticals Ltd)

Rivastigmine 4.6 mg per 24 hour Voleze 4.6mg/24hours transdermal patches | 30 patch [PoM] £77.97 DT price = £77.97
Rivastigmine 9.5 mg per 24 hour Voleze 9.5mg/24hours transdermal patches | 30 patch [PoM] £77.97 DT price = £14.80
Rivastigmine 13.3 mg per 24 hour Voleze 13.3mg/24hours transdermal patches | 30 patch [PoM] £77.97 DT price = £77.97

DOPAMINERGIC DRUGS > NMDA RECEPTOR ANTAGONISTS

Memantine hydrochloride

● **DRUG ACTION** Memantine is a glutamate receptor antagonist.

● **INDICATIONS AND DOSE**

Moderate to severe dementia in Alzheimer's disease
▸ BY MOUTH
▸ Adult: Initially 5 mg once daily, increased in steps of 5 mg every 1 week; maximum 20 mg per day

● **CAUTIONS** History of convulsions

● **INTERACTIONS** → Appendix 1 (memantine).

● **SIDE-EFFECTS**
▸ **Common or very common** Constipation · dizziness · drowsiness · dyspnoea · headache · hypertension
▸ **Uncommon** Abnormal gait · confusion · fatigue · hallucinations · heart failure · thrombosis · vomiting
▸ **Very rare** Seizures
▸ **Frequency not known** Depression · pancreatitis · psychosis · suicidal ideation

● **HEPATIC IMPAIRMENT** Avoid in severe impairment—no information available.

● **RENAL IMPAIRMENT** Reduce dose to 10 mg daily if eGFR 30–49 mL/minute/1.73 m^2, if well tolerated after at least 7 days dose can be increased in steps to 20 mg daily; reduce dose to 10 mg daily if eGFR

5–29 mL/minute/1.73 m^2. Avoid if eGFR less than 5 mL/minute/1.73 m^2.

● **DIRECTIONS FOR ADMINISTRATION** Oral solution should be dosed onto a spoon or into a glass of water.

● **NATIONAL FUNDING/ACCESS DECISIONS**

NICE technology appraisals (TAs)
▸ **Donepezil, galantamine, rivastigmine, and memantine for the treatment of Alzheimer's disease (March 2011)** NICE TA217
Memantine can be used for moderate Alzheimer's disease in patients who are unable to take acetylcholinesterase inhibitors, and for patients with severe disease; combination treatment with memantine and an acetylcholinesterase inhibitor is not recommended. Treatment should only be prescribed under the following conditions:
● Alzheimer's disease must be diagnosed and treatment initiated by a specialist; treatment can be continued by general practitioners under a shared-care protocol;
● the carer's view of the condition should be sought before and during treatment;
● treatment should continue only if it is considered to have a worthwhile effect on cognitive, global, functional, or behavioural symptoms.
Healthcare professionals should not rely solely on assessment scales to determine the severity of Alzheimer's disease when the patient has learning or other disabilities, or other communication difficulties.
www.nice.org.uk/TA217

● **MEDICINAL FORMS**
There can be variation in the licensing of different medicines containing the same drug.

Tablet
▸ Memantine hydrochloride (Non-proprietary)

Memantine hydrochloride 10 mg Memantine 10mg tablets | 28 tablet [PoM] £69.01 DT price = £1.20 | 56 tablet [PoM] £69.01 | 112 tablet [PoM] £12.08
Memantine hydrochloride 20 mg Memantine 20mg tablets | 28 tablet [PoM] £69.01 DT price = £1.52

▸ Ebixa (Lundbeck Ltd)

Memantine hydrochloride 5 mg Ebixa 5mg tablets | 7 tablet [PoM] no price available
Memantine hydrochloride 10 mg Ebixa 10mg tablets | 7 tablet [PoM] no price available | 28 tablet [PoM] £34.50 DT price = £1.20 | 56 tablet [PoM] £69.01
Memantine hydrochloride 15 mg Ebixa 15mg tablets | 7 tablet [PoM] no price available
Memantine hydrochloride 20 mg Ebixa 20mg tablets | 7 tablet [PoM] no price available | 28 tablet [PoM] £69.01 DT price = £1.52

▸ Maruxa (Consilient Health Ltd)

Memantine hydrochloride 10 mg Maruxa 10mg tablets | 28 tablet [PoM] £29.32 DT price = £1.20
Memantine hydrochloride 20 mg Maruxa 20mg tablets | 28 tablet [PoM] £58.65 DT price = £1.52

▸ Nemdatine (Actavis UK Ltd)

Memantine hydrochloride 5 mg Nemdatine 5mg tablets | 7 tablet [PoM] no price available
Memantine hydrochloride 10 mg Nemdatine 10mg tablets | 7 tablet [PoM] no price available | 28 tablet [PoM] £34.50 DT price = £1.20 | 56 tablet [PoM] £69.01
Memantine hydrochloride 15 mg Nemdatine 15mg tablets | 7 tablet [PoM] no price available
Memantine hydrochloride 20 mg Nemdatine 20mg tablets | 7 tablet [PoM] no price available | 28 tablet [PoM] £69.01 DT price = £1.52

▸ Ebixa (Lundbeck Ltd)

Ebixa tablets treatment initiation pack | 28 tablet [PoM] £43.13

▸ Nemdatine (Actavis UK Ltd)

Nemdatine tablets treatment initiation pack | 28 tablet [PoM] £43.12

Orodispersible tablet
▸ Valios (Dr Reddy's Laboratories (UK) Ltd)

Memantine hydrochloride 10 mg Valios 10mg orodispersible tablets sugar free sugar-free | 28 tablet [PoM] £32.78
Memantine hydrochloride 20 mg Valios 20mg orodispersible tablets sugar free sugar-free | 28 tablet [PoM] £65.56

Oral solution

▸ Memantine hydrochloride (Non-proprietary)

Memantine hydrochloride 10 mg per 1 ml Memantine 10mg/ml oral solution sugar free sugar-free | 50 ml [PoM] £61.61 DT price = £57.67 sugar-free | 100 ml [PoM] £123.23

▸ Ebixa (Lundbeck Ltd)

Memantine hydrochloride 10 mg per 1 ml Ebixa 5mg/0.5ml pump actuation oral solution sugar-free | 50 ml [PoM] £61.61 DT price = £57.67 sugar-free | 100 ml [PoM] £123.23

2 Epilepsy and other seizure disorders

Epilepsy

Control of the epilepsies

The object of treatment is to prevent the occurrence of seizures by maintaining an effective dose of one or more antiepileptic drugs. Careful adjustment of doses is necessary, starting with low doses and increasing gradually until seizures are controlled or there are significant adverse effects.

When choosing an antiepileptic drug, the presenting epilepsy syndrome should first be considered. If the syndrome is not clear, the seizure type should determine the choice of treatment. Concomitant medication, co-morbidity, age, and sex should also be taken into account.

The dosage frequency is often determined by the plasma-drug half-life, and should be kept as low as possible to encourage adherence with the prescribed regimen. Most antiepileptics, when used in the usual dosage, can be given twice daily. Lamotrigine p. 289, perampanel p. 293, phenobarbital p. 294, and phenytoin p. 304, which have long half-lives, can be given once daily at bedtime. However, with large doses, some antiepileptics may need to be given more frequently to avoid adverse effects associated with high peak plasma-drug concentration.

Management

When monotherapy with a first-line antiepileptic drug has failed, monotherapy with a second drug should be tried; the diagnosis should be checked before starting an alternative drug if the first drug showed lack of efficacy. The change from one antiepileptic drug to another should be cautious, slowly withdrawing the first drug only when the new regimen has been established. Combination therapy with two or more antiepileptic drugs may be necessary, but the concurrent use of antiepileptic drugs increases the risk of adverse effects and drug interactions. If combination therapy does not bring about worthwhile benefits, revert to the regimen (monotherapy or combination therapy) that provided the best balance between tolerability and efficacy. A single antiepileptic drug should be prescribed wherever possible.

MHRA/CHM advice: Antiepileptic drugs: new advice on switching between different manufacturers' products for a particular drug (November 2013)

The CHM has reviewed spontaneous adverse reactions received by the MHRA and publications that reported potential harm arising from switching of antiepileptic drugs in patients previously stabilised on a branded product to a generic. The CHM concluded that reports of loss of seizure control and/or worsening of side-effects around the time of switching between products could be explained as chance associations, but that a causal role of switching could not be ruled out in all cases. The following guidance has been issued to help minimise risk:

• Different antiepileptic drugs vary considerably in their characteristics, which influences the risk of whether switching between different manufacturers' products of a

particular drug may cause adverse effects or loss of seizure control;

• Antiepileptic drugs have been divided into three risk-based categories to help healthcare professionals decide whether it is necessary to maintain continuity of supply of a specific manufacturer's product. These categories are listed below;

• If it is felt desirable for a patient to be maintained on a specific manufacturer's product this should be prescribed either by specifying a brand name, or by using the generic drug name and name of the manufacturer (otherwise known as the Marketing Authorisation Holder);

• This advice relates only to antiepileptic drug use for treatment of epilepsy; it does not apply to their use in other indications (e.g. mood stabilisation, neuropathic pain);

• Please report on a Yellow Card any suspected adverse reactions to antiepileptic drugs;

• Dispensing pharmacists should ensure the continuity of supply of a particular product when the prescription specifies it. If the prescribed product is unavailable, it may be necessary to dispense a product from a different manufacturer to maintain continuity of treatment of that antiepileptic drug. Such cases should be discussed and agreed with both the prescriber and patient (or carer);

• Usual dispensing practice can be followed when a specific product is not stated.

Category 1
Phenytoin, carbamazepine p. 283, phenobarbital, primidone p. 305. For these drugs, doctors are advised to ensure that their patient is maintained on a specific manufacturer's product.

Category 2
Valproate, lamotrigine, perampanel, retigabine p. 297, rufinamide p. 297, clobazam p. 306, clonazepam p. 307, oxcarbazepine p. 292, eslicarbazepine acetate p. 285, zonisamide p. 303, topiramate p. 301. For these drugs, the need for continued supply of a particular manufacturer's product should be based on clinical judgement and consultation with the patient and/or carer taking into account factors such as seizure frequency and treatment history.

Category 3
Levetiracetam p. 291, lacosamide p. 288, tiagabine p. 301, gabapentin p. 287,pregabalin p. 295, ethosuximide p. 285, vigabatrin p. 302. For these drugs, it is usually unnecessary to ensure that patients are maintained on a specific manufacturer's product unless there are specific concerns such as patient anxiety, and risk of confusion or dosing errors Interactions.

Antiepileptic hypersensitivity syndrome

Antiepileptic hypersensitivity syndrome is a rare but potentially fatal syndrome associated with some antiepileptic drugs (**carbamazepine, lacosamide, lamotrigine, oxcarbazepine, phenobarbital, phenytoin, primidone,** and **rufinamide**); rarely cross-sensitivity occurs between some of these antiepileptic drugs. Some other antiepileptics (**eslicarbazepine, stiripentol,** and **zonisamide**) have a theoretical risk. The symptoms usually start between 1 and 8 weeks of exposure; fever, rash, and lymphadenopathy are most commonly seen. Other systemic signs include liver dysfunction, haematological, renal, and pulmonary abnormalities, vasculitis, and multi-organ failure. If signs or symptoms of hypersensitivity syndrome occur, the drug should be withdrawn immediately, and the patient must not be re-exposed, and expert advice should be sought.

Interactions

Interactions between antiepileptics are complex and may increase toxicity without a corresponding increase in

4

Nervous system

antiepileptic effect. Interactions are usually caused by hepatic enzyme induction or inhibition; displacement from protein binding sites is not usually a problem. These interactions are highly variable and unpredictable.

Withdrawal

Antiepileptic drugs should be withdrawn under specialist supervision. Avoid abrupt withdrawal, particularly of barbiturates and benzodiazepines, because this can precipitate severe rebound seizures. Reduction in dosage should be gradual and, in the case of barbiturates, withdrawal of the drug may take months.

The decision to withdraw antiepileptic drugs from a seizure-free patient, and its timing, is often difficult and depends on individual circumstances. Even in patients who have been seizure-free for several years, there is a significant risk of seizure recurrence on drug withdrawal. In patients receiving several antiepileptic drugs, only one drug should be withdrawn at a time.

Driving

Patients with epilepsy may drive a motor vehicle (but not a large goods or passenger carrying vehicle) provided that they have been seizure-free for one year or, if subject to attacks only while asleep, have established a 3-year period of asleep attacks without awake attacks. Those affected by drowsiness should not drive or operate machinery.

Guidance issued by the Drivers Medical Unit of the Driver and Vehicle Licensing Agency (DVLA) recommends that patients should be advised not to drive during medication changes or withdrawal of antiepileptic drugs, and for 6 months afterwards.

Patients who have had a first or single epileptic seizure must not drive for 6 months (5 years in the case of large goods or passenger carrying vehicles) after the event; driving may then be resumed, provided the patient has been assessed by a specialist as fit to drive because no abnormality was detected on investigation.

Pregnancy

Women of child-bearing potential should discuss with a specialist the impact of both epilepsy, and its treatment, on the outcome of pregnancy.

There is an increased risk of teratogenicity associated with the use of antiepileptic drugs (especially if used during the first trimester and particularly if the patient takes two or more antiepileptic drugs). Valproate is associated with the highest risk of major and minor congenital malformations (in particular neural tube defects), and long-term developmental disorders. There is also an increased risk of teratogenicity with phenytoin, primidone, phenobarbital, lamotrigine, and carbamazepine. Topiramate carries an increased risk of cleft palate if taken in the first trimester of pregnancy. There is not enough evidence to establish the risk of teratogenicity with other antiepileptic drugs.

Prescribers should also consider carefully the choice of antiepileptic therapy in pre-pubescent girls who may later become pregnant. Women of child-bearing potential who take antiepileptic drugs should be given advice about the need for an effective contraception method to avoid unplanned pregnancy. Some antiepileptic drugs can reduce the efficacy of hormonal contraceptives, and the efficacy of some antiepileptics may be affected by hormonal contraceptives.

Women who want to become pregnant should be referred to a specialist for advice in advance of conception. For some women, the severity of seizure or the seizure type may not pose a serious threat, and drug withdrawal may be considered; therapy may be resumed after the first trimester. If treatment with antiepileptic drugs must continue throughout pregnancy, then monotherapy is preferable at the lowest effective dose.

Once an unplanned pregnancy is discovered it is usually too late for changes to be made to the treatment regimen; the risk of harm to the mother and fetus from convulsive seizures outweighs the risk of continued therapy. The likelihood of a woman who is taking antiepileptic drugs having a baby with no malformations is at least 90%, and it is important that women do not stop taking essential treatment because of concern over harm to the fetus. To reduce the risk of neural tube defects, folate supplementation is advised before conception and throughout the first trimester. In the case of sodium valproate p. 298 and valproic acid p. 323 an urgent consultation is required to reconsider the benefits and risks of valproate therapy.

The concentration of antiepileptic drugs in the plasma can change during pregnancy. Doses of phenytoin, carbamazepine, and lamotrigine should be adjusted on the basis of plasma-drug concentration monitoring; the dose of other antiepileptic drugs should be monitored carefully during pregnancy and after birth, and adjustments made on a clinical basis. Plasma-drug concentration monitoring during pregnancy is also useful to check compliance. Additionally, in patients taking topiramate or levetiracetam, it is recommended that fetal growth should be monitored. Women who have seizures in the second half of pregnancy should be assessed for eclampsia before any change is made to antiepileptic treatment. Status epilepticus should be treated according to the standard protocol.

Routine injection of vitamin K at birth minimises the risk of neonatal haemorrhage associated with antiepileptics. Withdrawal effects in the newborn may occur with some antiepileptic drugs, in particular benzodiazepines and phenobarbital.

Epilepsy and Pregnancy Register

All pregnant women with epilepsy, whether taking medication or not, should be encouraged to notify the UK Epilepsy and Pregnancy Register (Tel: 0800 389 1248).

Breast-feeding

Women taking antiepileptic monotherapy should generally be encouraged to breast-feed; if a woman is on combination therapy or if there are other risk factors, such as premature birth, specialist advice should be sought.

All infants should be monitored for sedation, feeding difficulties, adequate weight gain, and developmental milestones. Infants should also be monitored for adverse effects associated with the antiepileptic drug particularly with newer antiepileptics, if the antiepileptic is readily transferred into breast-milk causing high infant serum-drug concentrations (e.g. ethosuximide, lamotrigine, primidone, and zonisamide), or if slower metabolism in the infant causes drugs to accumulate (e.g. phenobarbital and lamotrigine). Serum-drug concentration monitoring should be undertaken in breast-fed infants if suspected adverse reactions develop; if toxicity develops it may be necessary to introduce formula feeds to limit the infant's drug exposure, or to wean the infant off breast-milk altogether.

Primidone, phenobarbital, and the benzodiazepines are associated with an established risk of drowsiness in breast-fed babies and caution is required.

Withdrawal effects may occur in infants if a mother suddenly stops breast-feeding, particularly if she is taking phenobarbital, primidone, or lamotrigine.

Focal seizures with or without secondary generalisation

Carbamazepine p. 283 and lamotrigine p. 289 are first-line options for treating newly diagnosed focal seizures; oxcarbazepine p. 292, sodium valproate and levetiracetam p. 291 may be used if carbamazepine or lamotrigine are unsuitable or not tolerated. If monotherapy is unsuccessful with two of these first-line antiepileptic drugs, adjunctive treatment may be considered. Options for adjunctive treatment include carbamazepine, clobazam p. 306, gabapentin p. 287, lamotrigine, levetiracetam, oxcarbazepine, sodium valproate, or topiramate p. 301. If adjunctive treatment is ineffective or not tolerated, a tertiary epilepsy specialist should be consulted who may consider eslicarbazepine acetate p. 285, lacosamide p. 288, phenobarbital p. 304, phenytoin p. 294, pregabalin p. 295, tiagabine p. 301, vigabatrin p. 302 and zonisamide p. 303.

Generalised seizures

Tonic-clonic seizures

Sodium valproate is the first-line treatment for newly diagnosed generalised tonic-clonic seizures (except in female patients who are premenopausal, see *Valproate* below). Lamotrigine is the alternative choice if sodium valproate is not suitable, but may exacerbate myoclonic seizures. In those with established epilepsy with generalised tonic-clonic seizures only, lamotrigine or sodium valproate may be prescribed as the first-line treatment.

Carbamazepine and oxcarbazepine may also be considered in newly diagnosed and established tonic-clonic seizures, but may exacerbate myoclonic and absence seizures. Clobazam, lamotrigine, levetiracetam, sodium valproate or topiramate may be used as adjunctive treatment if monotherapy is ineffective or not tolerated.

Absence seizures

Ethosuximide p. 285, or sodium valproate (except in female patients who are premenopausal, see *Valproate* below), are the drugs of choice in absence seizures and syndromes; lamotrigine p. 289 is a suitable alternative when ethosuximide p. 285 and sodium valproate p. 298 are unsuitable, ineffective or not tolerated. Sodium valproate should be used as the first choice if there is a high risk of generalised tonic-clonic seizures. A combination of any two of these drugs may be used if monotherapy is ineffective. Clobazam p. 306, clonazepam p. 307, levetiracetam p. 291, topiramate p. 301 or zonisamide p. 303 may be considered by a tertiary epilepsy specialist if adjunctive treatment fails. Carbamazepine p. 283, gabapentin p. 287, oxcarbazepine p. 292, phenytoin p. 294, pregabalin p. 295, tiagabine p. 301 and vigabatrin p. 302 are not recommended in absence seizures or syndromes.

Myoclonic seizures

Myoclonic seizures (myoclonic jerks) occur in a variety of syndromes, and response to treatment varies considerably. Sodium valproate is the drug of choice in newly diagnosed myoclonic seizures (except in female patients who are premenopausal, see *Valproate* below); topiramate and levetiracetam are alternative options if sodium valproate is unsuitable but consideration should be given to the less favourable side-effect profile of topiramate. A combination of two of these drugs may be used if monotherapy is ineffective or not tolerated. If adjunctive treatment fails, a tertiary epilepsy specialist should be consulted and may consider clobazam, clonazepam, zonisamide or piracetam p. 371. Carbamazepine, gabapentin, oxcarbazepine, phenytoin, pregabalin, tiagabine and vigabatrin are not recommended for the treatment of myoclonic seizures.

Sodium valproate and levetiracetam are effective in treating the generalised tonic-clonic seizures that coexist with myoclonic seizures in idiopathic generalised epilepsy.

Atonic and tonic seizures

Atonic and tonic seizures are usually seen in childhood, in specific epilepsy syndromes, or associated with cerebral damage or mental retardation. They may respond poorly to the traditional drugs. Sodium valproate is the drug of choice (except in female patients who are premenopausal, see *Valproate* below); lamotrigine can be added as adjunctive treatment. If adjunctive treatment is ineffective or not tolerated, a tertiary epilepsy specialist should be consulted, and may consider rufinamide p. 297 or topiramate. Carbamazepine, gabapentin, oxcarbazepine, pregabalin,

tiagabine or vigabatrin are not recommended in atonic and tonic seizures.

Epilepsy syndromes

Some drugs are licensed for use in particular epilepsy syndromes, such as lamotrigine and rufinamide in Lennox-Gastaut syndrome. The epilepsy syndromes are specific types of epilepsy that are characterised according to a number of features including seizure type, age of onset, and EEG characteristics.

Antiepileptic drugs

Carbamazepine and related antiepileptics

Carbamazepine is a drug of choice for simple and complex focal seizures and is a first-line treatment option for generalised tonic-clonic seizures. It can be used as adjunctive treatment for focal seizures when monotherapy has been ineffective. It is essential to initiate carbamazepine therapy at a low dose and build this up slowly.

Carbamazepine may exacerbate tonic, atonic, myoclonic and absence seizures and is therefore not recommended if these seizures are present.

Oxcarbazepine is licensed as monotherapy or adjunctive therapy for the treatment of focal seizures with or without secondary generalised tonic-clonic seizures. It can also be considered for the treatment of primary generalised tonic-clonic seizures [unlicensed]. Oxcarbazepine is not recommended in tonic, atonic, absence or myoclonic seizures due to the risk of seizure exacerbation.

Eslicarbazepine acetate p. 285 is licensed for adjunctive treatment in adults with focal seizures with or without secondary generalisation.

Ethosuximide

Ethosuximide is a first-line treatment option for absence seizures. It may also be prescribed as adjunctive treatment for absence seizures when monotherapy is ineffective. Ethosuximide is also licensed for myoclonic seizures.

Gabapentin and pregabalin

Gabapentin and pregabalin are used for the treatment of focal seizures with or without secondary generalisation. They are not recommended if tonic, atonic, absence or myoclonic seizures are present. Both are also licensed for the treatment of neuropathic pain. Pregabalin is licensed for the treatment of generalised anxiety disorder. Gabapentin is an effective treatment for migraine prophylaxis [unlicensed].

Lamotrigine

Lamotrigine is an antiepileptic drug recommended as a first-line treatment for focal seizures and primary and secondary generalised tonic-clonic seizures. It is also licensed for typical absence seizures in children (but efficacy may not be maintained in all children) and is an unlicensed treatment option in adults if first-line treatments have been unsuccessful. Lamotrigine can also be used as adjunctive treatment in atonic or tonic seizures if first-line treatment has failed [unlicensed]. Myoclonic seizures may be exacerbated by lamotrigine and it can cause serious rashes especially in children; dose recommendations should be adhered to closely.

Lamotrigine is used either as sole treatment or as an adjunct to treatment with other antiepileptic drugs. Valproate increases plasma-lamotrigine concentration, whereas the enzyme-inducing antiepileptics reduce it; care is therefore required in choosing the appropriate initial dose and subsequent titration. When the potential for interaction is not known, treatment should be initiated with lower doses, such as those used with valproate.

Levetiracetam

Levetiracetam is used for monotherapy and adjunctive treatment of focal seizures with or without secondary generalisation, and for adjunctive treatment of myoclonic seizures in patients with juvenile myoclonic epilepsy and primary generalised tonic-clonic seizures. Levetiracetam may be prescribed alone and in combination for the treatment of myoclonic seizures, and under specialist supervision for absence seizures [both unlicensed].

Phenobarbital and primidone

Phenobarbital p. 304 is effective for tonic-clonic and focal seizures but may be sedative in adults. It may be tried for atypical absence, atonic, and tonic seizures. Rebound seizures may be a problem on withdrawal.

Primidone p. 305 is largely converted to phenobarbital and this is probably responsible for its antiepileptic action. A low initial dose of primidone is essential.

Phenytoin

Phenytoin is licensed for tonic-clonic and focal seizures but may exacerbate absence or myoclonic seizures and should be avoided if these seizures are present. It has a narrow therapeutic index and the relationship between dose and plasma-drug concentration is non-linear; small dosage increases in some patients may produce large increases in plasma concentration with acute toxic side-effects. Similarly, a few missed doses or a small change in drug absorption may result in a marked change in plasma-drug concentration. Monitoring of plasma-drug concentration improves dosage adjustment.

When only parenteral administration is possible, fosphenytoin sodium p. 286, a pro-drug of phenytoin, may be convenient to give. Unlike phenytoin (which should only be given intravenously), fosphenytoin sodium may also be given by intramuscular injection.

Rufinamide

Rufinamide is licensed for the adjunctive treatment of seizures in Lennox-Gastaut syndrome. It may be considered by a tertiary specialist for the treatment of refractory tonic or atonic seizures [unlicensed].

Topiramate

Topiramate can be given alone or as adjunctive treatment in generalised tonic-clonic seizures or focal seizures with or without secondary generalisation. It can be used as adjunctive treatment for seizures associated with Lennox-Gastaut syndrome and for absence, tonic and atonic seizures under specialist supervision [unlicensed]. It can also be considered as an option in myoclonic seizures [unlicensed]. Topiramate p. 301 is also licensed for prophylaxis of migraine.

Valproate

Sodium valproate p. 298 is effective in controlling tonic-clonic seizures, particularly in primary generalised epilepsy. It is a drug of choice in primary generalised tonic-clonic seizures, focal seizures, generalised absences and myoclonic seizures, and can be tried in atypical absence seizures. It is recommended as a first-line option in atonic and tonic seizures. Sodium valproate has widespread metabolic effects and monitoring of liver function tests and full blood count is essential. Valproate should not be used in female children, in females of childbearing potential, and pregnant females, unless alternative treatments are ineffective or not tolerated, because of its high teratogenic potential; the benefits and risks of valproate therapy should be carefully reconsidered at regular treatment reviews, see *Important safety information* in the sodium valproate and valproic acid p. 323 drug monographs.

Valproic acid (as semisodium valproate) is licensed for acute mania associated with bipolar disorder.

Zonisamide

Zonisamide p. 303 can be used alone for the treatment of focal seizures with or without secondary generalisation in adults with newly diagnosed epilepsy, and as adjunctive treatment for refractory focal seizures with or without secondary generalisation in adults and children aged 6 years and above. It can also be used under the supervision of a specialist for refractory absence and myoclonic seizures [unlicensed indications].

Benzodiazepines

Clobazam p. 306 may be used as adjunctive therapy in the treatment of generalised tonic-clonic and refractory focal seizures. It may be prescribed under the care of a specialist for refractory absence and myoclonic seizures. Clonazepam p. 307 may be prescribed by a specialist for refractory absence and myoclonic seizures, but its sedative side-effects may be prominent.

Other drugs

Acetazolamide p. 1026, a carbonic anhydrase inhibitor, has a specific role in treating epilepsy associated with menstruation. Piracetam p. 371 is used as adjunctive treatment for cortical myoclonus.

Status epilepticus

Convulsive status epilepticus

Immediate measures to manage status epilepticus include positioning the patient to avoid injury, supporting respiration including the provision of oxygen, maintaining blood pressure, and the correction of any hypoglycaemia. Parenteral thiamine p. 938 should be considered if alcohol abuse is suspected; pyridoxine hydrochloride p. 937 should be given if the status epilepticus is caused by pyridoxine hydrochloride deficiency.

Seizures lasting longer than 5 minutes should be treated urgently with intravenous lorazepam p. 308 (repeated once after 10 minutes if seizures recur or fail to respond). Intravenous diazepam p. 313 is effective but it carries a high risk of thrombophlebitis (reduced by using an emulsion formulation). Absorption of diazepam from intramuscular injection or from suppositories is too slow for treatment of status epilepticus. Patients should be monitored for respiratory depression and hypotension.

Where facilities for resuscitation are not immediately available, diazepam can be administered as a rectal solution or midazolam oromucosal solution p. 310 can be given into the buccal cavity.

Important

If, after initial treatment with benzodiazepines, seizures recur or fail to respond 25 minutes after onset, phenytoin sodium, fosphenytoin sodium p. 286, or phenobarbital sodium should be used; contact intensive care unit if seizures continue. If these measures fail to control seizures 45 minutes after onset, anaesthesia with thiopental sodium p. 308, midazolam, or a non-barbiturate anaesthetic such as propofol p. 1165 [unlicensed indication], should be instituted with full intensive care support.

Phenytoin sodium can be given by slow intravenous injection, followed by the maintenance dosage if appropriate.

Alternatively, fosphenytoin sodium (a pro-drug of phenytoin), can be given more rapidly and when given intravenously causes fewer injection-site reactions than phenytoin sodium. Although it can also be given intramuscularly, absorption is too slow by this route for treatment of status epilepticus. Doses of fosphenytoin sodium should be expressed in terms of phenytoin sodium.

Non-convulsive status epilepticus

The urgency to treat non-convulsive status epilepticus depends on the severity of the patient's condition. If there is incomplete loss of awareness, usual oral antiepileptic therapy should be continued or restarted. Patients who fail to respond to oral antiepileptic therapy or have complete lack of awareness can be treated in the same way as for convulsive status epilepticus, although anaesthesia is rarely needed.

Febrile convulsions

Brief febrile convulsions need no specific treatment; antipyretic medication (e.g. paracetamol p. 406), is commonly used to reduce fever and prevent further convulsions but evidence to support this practice is lacking. *Prolonged febrile convulsions* (those lasting 5 minutes or longer), or *recurrent febrile convulsions* without recovery must be treated actively (as for convulsive status epilepticus). Long-term anticonvulsant prophylaxis for febrile convulsions is rarely indicated.

> **Drugs used for Epilepsy and other seizure disorders not listed below** Magnesium sulfate, p. 911

ANTIEPILEPTICS

Carbamazepine

● **INDICATIONS AND DOSE**

Focal and secondary generalised tonic-clonic seizures | Primary generalised tonic-clonic seizures
▸ BY MOUTH USING IMMEDIATE-RELEASE MEDICINES
▸ Adult: Initially 100–200 mg 1–2 times a day, increased in steps of 100–200 mg every 2 weeks; usual dose 0.8–1.2 g daily in divided doses; increased if necessary up to 1.6–2 g daily in divided doses
▸ Elderly: Reduce initial dose
▸ BY RECTUM
▸ Adult: Up to 1 g daily in 4 divided doses for up to 7 days, for short-term use when oral therapy temporarily not possible
DOSE EQUIVALENCE AND CONVERSION
Suppositories of 125 mg may be considered to be approximately equivalent in therapeutic effect to tablets of 100 mg but final adjustment should always depend on clinical response (plasma concentration monitoring recommended).

Trigeminal neuralgia
▸ BY MOUTH USING IMMEDIATE-RELEASE MEDICINES
▸ Adult: Initially 100 mg 1–2 times a day, some patients may require higher initial dose, increase gradually according to response; usual dose 200 mg 3–4 times a day, increased if necessary up to 1.6 g daily

Prophylaxis of bipolar disorder unresponsive to lithium
▸ BY MOUTH USING IMMEDIATE-RELEASE MEDICINES
▸ Adult: Initially 400 mg daily in divided doses, increased until symptoms controlled; usual dose 400–600 mg daily; maximum 1.6 g per day

Adjunct in acute alcohol withdrawal
▸ BY MOUTH USING IMMEDIATE-RELEASE MEDICINES
▸ Adult: Initially 800 mg daily in divided doses, then reduced to 200 mg daily for usual treatment duration of 7–10 days, dose to be reduced gradually over 5 days

Diabetic neuropathy
▸ BY MOUTH USING IMMEDIATE-RELEASE MEDICINES
▸ Adult: Initially 100 mg 1–2 times a day, increased gradually according to response; usual dose 200 mg 3–4 times a day, increased if necessary up to 1.6 g daily

Focal and generalised tonic-clonic seizures
▸ BY MOUTH USING IMMEDIATE-RELEASE MEDICINES
▸ Child 1 month–11 years: Initially 5 mg/kg once daily, dose to be taken at night, alternatively initially 2.5 mg/kg twice daily, then increased in steps of 2.5–5 mg/kg every 3–7 days as required; maintenance 5 mg/kg 2–3 times a day, increased if necessary up to 20 mg/kg daily
▸ Child 12-17 years: Initially 100–200 mg 1–2 times a day, then increased to 200–400 mg 2–3 times a day,

increased if necessary up to 1.8 g daily, dose should be increased slowly

CARBAGEN® SR

Focal and secondary generalised tonic-clonic seizures | Primary generalised tonic-clonic seizures
▸ BY MOUTH
▸ Adult: Initially 100–400 mg daily in 1–2 divided doses, increased in steps of 100–200 mg every 2 weeks, dose should be increased slowly; usual dose 0.8–1.2 g daily in 1–2 divided doses, increased if necessary up to 1.6–2 g daily in 1–2 divided doses
▸ Elderly: Reduce initial dose

Trigeminal neuralgia
▸ BY MOUTH
▸ Adult: Initially 100–200 mg daily in 1–2 divided doses, some patients may require higher initial dose, increase gradually according to response; usual dose 600–800 mg daily in 1–2 divided doses, increased if necessary up to 1.6 g daily in 1–2 divided doses

Prophylaxis of bipolar disorder unresponsive to lithium
▸ BY MOUTH
▸ Adult: Initially 400 mg daily in 1–2 divided doses, increased until symptoms controlled; usual dose 400–600 mg daily in 1–2 divided doses; maximum 1.6 g per day

Focal and generalised tonic-clonic seizures | Prophylaxis of bipolar disorder
▸ BY MOUTH
▸ Child 5-11 years: Initially 5 mg/kg daily in 1–2 divided doses, then increased in steps of 2.5–5 mg/kg every 3–7 days as required, dose should be increased slowly; maintenance 10–15 mg/kg daily in 1–2 divided doses, increased if necessary up to 20 mg/kg daily in 1–2 divided doses
▸ Child 12-17 years: Initially 100–400 mg daily in 1–2 divided doses, then increased to 400–1200 mg daily in 1–2 divided doses, increased if necessary up to 1.8 g daily in 1–2 divided doses, dose should be increased slowly

TEGRETOL® PROLONGED RELEASE

Focal and secondary generalised tonic-clonic seizures | Primary generalised tonic-clonic seizures
▸ BY MOUTH
▸ Adult: Initially 100–400 mg daily in 2 divided doses, increased in steps of 100–200 mg every 2 weeks, dose should be increased slowly; usual dose 0.8–1.2 g daily in 2 divided doses, increased if necessary up to 1.6–2 g daily in 2 divided doses
▸ Elderly: Reduce initial dose

Focal and generalised tonic-clonic seizures | Prophylaxis of bipolar disorder
▸ BY MOUTH
▸ Child 5-11 years: Initially 5 mg/kg daily in 2 divided doses, then increased in steps of 2.5–5 mg/kg every 3–7 days as required; maintenance 10–15 mg/kg daily in 2 divided doses, increased if necessary up to 20 mg/kg daily in 2 divided doses
▸ Child 12-17 years: Initially 100–400 mg daily in 2 divided doses, dose should be increased slowly; maintenance 400–1200 mg daily in 2 divided doses, increased if necessary up to 1.8 g daily in 2 divided doses

Trigeminal neuralgia
▸ BY MOUTH
▸ Adult: Initially 100–200 mg daily in 2 divided doses, some patients may require higher initial dose. After initial dose, increase according to response; usual dose 600–800 mg daily in 2 divided doses, increased if necessary up to 1.6 g daily in 2 divided doses, dose should be increased slowly continued →

Prophylaxis of bipolar disorder unresponsive to lithium
▶ BY MOUTH
▶ Adult: Initially 400 mg daily in 2 divided doses, increased until symptoms controlled; usual dose 400–600 mg daily in 2 divided doses; maximum 1.6 g per day

● UNLICENSED USE Use in the treatment of alcohol withdrawal is an unlicensed indication. Use in diabetic neuropathy is an unlicensed indication.
● CONTRA-INDICATIONS Acute porphyrias p. 918 · AV conduction abnormalities (unless paced) · history of bone-marrow depression
● CAUTIONS Cardiac disease · history of haematological reactions to other drugs · may exacerbate absence and myoclonic seizures · skin reactions · susceptibility to angle-closure glaucoma
CAUTIONS, FURTHER INFORMATION
Consider vitamin D supplementation in patients who are immobilised for long periods or who have inadequate sun exposure or dietary intake of calcium.
▶ Blood, hepatic, or skin disorders Carbamazepine should be withdrawn immediately in cases of aggravated liver dysfunction or acute liver disease. Leucopenia that is severe, progressive, or associated with clinical symptoms requires withdrawal (if necessary under cover of a suitable alternative).
● INTERACTIONS → Appendix 1 (carbamazepine).
● SIDE-EFFECTS
▶ **Common or very common** Allergic skin reactions · aplastic anaemia · ataxia · blood disorders · blurring of vision · dermatitis · dizziness · drowsiness · dry mouth · eosinophilia · fatigue · haemolytic anaemia · headache · hyponatraemia (leading in rare cases to water intoxication) · leucopenia · nausea · oedema · thrombocytopenia · unsteadiness · urticaria · vomiting
▶ **Uncommon** Constipation · diarrhoea · involuntary movements (including nystagmus) · visual disturbances
▶ **Rare** Abdominal pain · aggression · agitation · anorexia · cardiac conduction disorders · confusion · delayed multi-organ hypersensitivity disorder · depression · dysarthria · hallucinations · hepatitis · hypertension · hypotension · jaundice · lymph node enlargement · muscle weakness · paraesthesia · peripheral neuropathy · restlessness · systemic lupus erythematosus · vanishing bile duct syndrome
▶ **Very rare** Arthralgia · muscle spasm · acne · alopecia · alterations in skin pigmentation · angle-closure glaucoma · aseptic meningitis · AV block with syncope · circulatory collapse · conjunctivitis · dyspnoea · exacerbation of coronary artery disease · galactorrhoea · gynaecomastia · hearing disorders · hepatic failure · hirsutism · hypercholesterolaemia · impaired male fertility · interstitial nephritis · muscle pain · neuroleptic malignant syndrome · osteomalacia · osteoporosis · pancreatitis · photosensitivity · pneumonia · pneumonitis · psychosis · pulmonary hypersensitivity · purpura · renal failure · sexual dysfunction · Stevens-Johnson syndrome · stomatitis · sweating · taste disturbance · thromboembolism · thrombophlebitis · toxic epidermal necrolysis · urinary frequency · urinary retention
▶ **Frequency not known** Suicidal ideation
SIDE-EFFECTS, FURTHER INFORMATION
Some side-effects (such as headache, ataxia, drowsiness, nausea, vomiting, blurring of vision, dizziness, unsteadiness, and allergic skin reactions) are dose-related, and may be dose-limiting. These side-effects are more common at the start of treatment and in the elderly. Patients should be offered a modified-release preparation to reduce the risk of side-effects; altering the timing of medication may also be beneficial.

Overdose
For details on the management of poisoning, see Active elimination techniques, under Emergency treatment of poisoning p. 1194.
● ALLERGY AND CROSS-SENSITIVITY Antiepileptic hypersensitivity syndrome associated with carbamazepine. See under Epilepsy p. 279 for more information. Caution—cross-sensitivity reported with oxcarbazepine and with phenytoin.
● PREGNANCY
Monitoring
Doses should be adjusted on the basis of plasma-drug concentration monitoring.
● BREAST FEEDING Amount probably too small to be harmful.
  Monitor infant for possible adverse reactions.
● HEPATIC IMPAIRMENT Metabolism impaired in advanced liver disease.
● RENAL IMPAIRMENT Use with caution.
● PRE-TREATMENT SCREENING Test for HLA-B*1502 allele in individuals of Han Chinese or Thai origin (avoid unless no alternative—risk of Stevens-Johnson syndrome in presence of HLA-B*1502 allele).
● MONITORING REQUIREMENTS
▶ Plasma concentration for optimum response 4–12 mg/litre (20–50 micromol/litre) measured after 1–2 weeks.
▶ Manufacturer recommends blood counts and hepatic and renal function tests (but evidence of practical value uncertain).
● TREATMENT CESSATION When stopping treatment with carbamazepine for bipolar disorder, reduce the dose gradually over a period of at least 4 weeks.
● DIRECTIONS FOR ADMINISTRATION
TEGRETOL® PROLONGED RELEASE *Tegretol® Prolonged Release* tablets can be halved but should not be chewed.
● PRESCRIBING AND DISPENSING INFORMATION
Switching between formulations Different formulations of oral preparations may vary in bioavailability. Patients being treated for epilepsy should be maintained on a specific manufacturer's product.
● PATIENT AND CARER ADVICE
Medicines for Children leaflet: Carbamazepine (oral) for preventing seizures www.medicinesforchildren.org.uk/carbamazepine-oral-preventing-seizures-0
Blood, hepatic, or skin disorders Patients or their carers should be told how to recognise signs of blood, liver, or skin disorders, and advised to seek immediate medical attention if symptoms such as fever, rash, mouth ulcers, bruising, or bleeding develop.
● PROFESSION SPECIFIC INFORMATION
Dental practitioners' formulary
Carbamazepine Tablets may be prescribed.

● MEDICINAL FORMS
There can be variation in the licensing of different medicines containing the same drug. Forms available from special-order manufacturers include: oral suspension, oral solution
Tablet
CAUTIONARY AND ADVISORY LABELS 3, 8
▶ Carbamazepine (Non-proprietary)
Carbamazepine 100 mg Carbamazepine 100mg tablets | 28 tablet PoM £6.75 | 84 tablet PoM no price available DT price = £2.07
Carbamazepine 200 mg Carbamazepine 200mg tablets | 28 tablet PoM £5.83 DT price = £5.26 | 84 tablet PoM no price available
Carbamazepine 400 mg Carbamazepine 400mg tablets | 28 tablet PoM no price available | 56 tablet PoM £6.15 DT price = £5.02

▸ Carbagen (Mylan Ltd)
Carbamazepine 100 mg Carbagen 100mg tablets | 28 tablet [PoM]
£5.74 | 56 tablet [PoM] no price available (Hospital only) |
84 tablet [PoM] no price available DT price = £2.07 (Hospital only)
Carbamazepine 200 mg Carbagen 200mg tablets | 28 tablet [PoM]
£4.99 DT price = £5.26 | 56 tablet [PoM] no price available (Hospital
only) | 84 tablet [PoM] no price available (Hospital only)
Carbamazepine 400 mg Carbagen 400mg tablets | 28 tablet [PoM]
£4.27 | 56 tablet [PoM] no price available DT price = £5.02 (Hospital
only)
▸ Tegretol (Novartis Pharmaceuticals UK Ltd)
Carbamazepine 100 mg Tegretol 100mg tablets | 84 tablet [PoM]
£2.07 DT price = £2.07
Carbamazepine 200 mg Tegretol 200mg tablets | 84 tablet [PoM]
£3.83
Carbamazepine 400 mg Tegretol 400mg tablets | 56 tablet [PoM]
£5.02 DT price = £5.02

Modified-release tablet
CAUTIONARY AND ADVISORY LABELS 3, 8, 25
▸ Carbagen SR (Mylan Ltd)
Carbamazepine 200 mg Carbagen SR 200mg tablets |
56 tablet [PoM] £4.16 DT price = £5.20
Carbamazepine 400 mg Carbagen SR 400mg tablets |
56 tablet [PoM] £8.20 DT price = £10.24
▸ Tegretol Retard (Novartis Pharmaceuticals UK Ltd)
Carbamazepine 200 mg Tegretol Prolonged Release 200mg tablets
| 56 tablet [PoM] £5.20 DT price = £5.20
Carbamazepine 400 mg Tegretol Prolonged Release 400mg tablets
| 56 tablet [PoM] £10.24 DT price = £10.24

Oral suspension
CAUTIONARY AND ADVISORY LABELS 3, 8
▸ Carbamazepine (Non-proprietary)
Carbamazepine 20 mg per 1 ml Carbamazepine 100mg/5ml oral
suspension sugar free sugar-free | 300 ml [PoM] £7.13 DT price =
£6.12
▸ Tegretol (Novartis Pharmaceuticals UK Ltd)
Carbamazepine 20 mg per 1 ml Tegretol 100mg/5ml liquid sugar-
free | 300 ml [PoM] £6.12 DT price = £6.12

Suppository
CAUTIONARY AND ADVISORY LABELS 3, 8
▸ Tegretol (Novartis Pharmaceuticals UK Ltd)
Carbamazepine 125 mg Tegretol 125mg suppositories |
5 suppository [PoM] £8.03
Carbamazepine 250 mg Tegretol 250mg suppositories |
5 suppository [PoM] £10.71

Eslicarbazepine acetate

● INDICATIONS AND DOSE

**Adjunctive treatment in adults with focal seizures with or
without secondary generalisation**
▸ BY MOUTH
▸ Adult: Initially 400 mg once daily for 1–2 weeks, then
  increased to 800 mg once daily (max. per dose 1.2 g)

● CONTRA-INDICATIONS Second- or third-degree AV block
● CAUTIONS Elderly · hyponatraemia · PR-interval
prolongation
● INTERACTIONS → Appendix 1 (eslicarbazepine).
Caution—avoid concomitant administration of drugs that
prolong PR interval.
● SIDE-EFFECTS
▸ **Common or very common** Dizziness · drowsiness · fatigue ·
gastro-intestinal disturbances · headache · impaired
coordination · rash · tremor · visual disturbances
▸ **Uncommon** Agitation · alopecia · anaemia · appetite
changes · bradycardia · chest pain · chills · confusion ·
convulsions · dehydration · dry mouth · dysaesthesia ·
dysarthria · dystonia · electrolyte imbalance · epistaxis ·
gingival hyperplasia · hyperactivity · hypertension ·
hyponatraemia · hypotension · hypothyroidism · impaired
memory · insomnia · liver disorders · malaise ·
menstruation changes · mood changes · movement
disorders · myalgia · nail disorder · nocturia · nystagmus ·
palpitation · parosmia · peripheral neuropathy · peripheral

oedema · psychosis · stomatitis · sweating · taste
disturbance · tinnitus · urinary tract infection · weight
changes
▸ **Very rare** Leucopenia · pancreatitis · thrombocytopenia
▸ **Frequency not known** PR-interval prolongation · suicidal
ideation
● ALLERGY AND CROSS-SENSITIVITY Antiepileptic
hypersensitivity syndrome theoretically associated with
eslicarbazepine. See under Epilepsy p. 279 for more
information.
● PREGNANCY
Monitoring
The dose should be monitored carefully during pregnancy
and after birth, and adjustments made on a clinical basis.
● HEPATIC IMPAIRMENT Avoid in severe impairment—no
information available.
● RENAL IMPAIRMENT Reduce initial dose to 400 mg every
other day for 2 weeks then 400 mg once daily if eGFR
30–60 mL/minute/1.73 m^2, adjusted according to response.
Avoid if eGFR less than 30 mL/minute/1.73 m^2.
● PRE-TREATMENT SCREENING Test for HLA-B*1502 allele in
individuals of Han Chinese or Thai origin (avoid unless no
alternative— risk of Stevens-Johnson syndrome in
presence of HLA-B*1502 allele).
● MONITORING REQUIREMENTS Monitor plasma-sodium
concentration in patients at risk of hyponatraemia and
discontinue treatment if hyponatraemia occurs.
● PRESCRIBING AND DISPENSING INFORMATION
Switching between formulations Care should be taken when
switching between oral formulations. The need for
continued supply of a particular manufacturer's product
should be based on clinical judgement and consultation
with the patient or their carer, taking into account factors
such as seizure frequency and treatment history.
● NATIONAL FUNDING/ACCESS DECISIONS
Scottish Medicines Consortium (SMC) Decisions
The *Scottish Medicines Consortium* has advised (October
2010) that eslicarbazepine (*Zebinix* ®) is accepted for
restricted use within NHS Scotland as adjunctive therapy
in adults with focal seizures with or without secondary
generalisation. It is restricted for use in refractory
epilepsy.
● MEDICINAL FORMS
There can be variation in the licensing of different medicines
containing the same drug.
Tablet
CAUTIONARY AND ADVISORY LABELS 8
▸ Zebinix (Eisai Ltd)
Eslicarbazepine acetate 800 mg Zebinix 800mg tablets |
30 tablet [PoM] £136.00

Ethosuximide

● INDICATIONS AND DOSE

**Absence seizures | Atypical absence seizures (adjunct) |
Myoclonic seizures**
▸ BY MOUTH
▸ Child 1 month-5 years: Initially 5 mg/kg twice daily
  (max. per dose 125 mg), dose to be increased every
  5–7 days; maintenance 10–20 mg/kg twice daily (max.
  per dose 500 mg), total daily dose may rarely be given
  in 3 divided doses
▸ Child 6-17 years: Initially 250 mg twice daily, then
  increased in steps of 250 mg every 5–7 days; usual dose
  500–750 mg twice daily, increased if necessary up to
  1 g twice daily
▸ Adult: Initially 500 mg daily in 2 divided doses, then
  increased in steps of 250 mg every 5–7 days; continued →

Nervous system

4

usual dose 1–1.5 g daily in 2 divided doses, increased if necessary up to 2 g daily

- CAUTIONS Avoid in Acute porphyrias p. 918
- INTERACTIONS → Appendix 1 (ethosuximide).
- SIDE-EFFECTS
- **Common or very common** Anorexia · abdominal pain · diarrhoea · gastro-intestinal disturbances · nausea · vomiting · weight loss
- **Uncommon** Aggression · ataxia · dizziness · drowsiness · euphoria · fatigue · headache · hiccup · impaired concentration · irritability
- **Rare** Depression · dyskinesia · gingival hypertrophy · increased libido · myopia · photophobia · psychosis · rash · sleep disturbances · tongue swelling · vaginal bleeding
- **Frequency not known** Agranulocytosis · aplastic anaemia · blood disorders · hyperactivity · increase in seizure frequency · leucopenia · pancytopenia · Stevens-Johnson syndrome · suicidal ideation · systemic lupus erythematosus

SIDE-EFFECTS, FURTHER INFORMATION
- Blood disorders Blood counts required if features of infection.

- PREGNANCY
Monitoring
The dose should be monitored carefully during pregnancy and after birth, and adjustments made on a clinical basis.
- BREAST FEEDING Present in milk. Hyperexcitability and sedation reported.
- HEPATIC IMPAIRMENT Use with caution.
- RENAL IMPAIRMENT Use with caution.
- PATIENT AND CARER ADVICE
Medicines for Children leaflet: Ethosuximide for preventing seizures www.medicinesforchildren.org.uk/ethosuximide-for-preventing-seizures
Blood disorders Patients or their carers should be told how to recognise signs of blood disorders, and advised to seek immediate medical attention if symptoms such as fever, mouth ulcers, bruising, or bleeding develop.

- MEDICINAL FORMS
There can be variation in the licensing of different medicines containing the same drug.
Capsule
CAUTIONARY AND ADVISORY LABELS 8
- Ethosuximide (Non-proprietary)
Ethosuximide 250 mg Ethosuximide 250mg capsules | 56 capsule [PoM] £73.20 DT price = £73.20
Oral solution
CAUTIONARY AND ADVISORY LABELS 8
- Emeside (Essential Pharma Ltd)
Ethosuximide 50 mg per 1 ml Emeside 250mg/5ml syrup | 200 ml [PoM] £6.60 DT price = £4.22
- Zarontin (Pfizer Ltd)
Ethosuximide 50 mg per 1 ml Zarontin 250mg/5ml syrup | 200 ml [PoM] £4.22 DT price = £4.22

Fosphenytoin sodium

- DRUG ACTION Fosphenytoin is a pro-drug of phenytoin.

- INDICATIONS AND DOSE
Status epilepticus
▸ BY INTRAVENOUS INFUSION
- Adult: Initially 20 mg(PE)/kg, dose to be administered at a rate of 100–150 mg(PE)/minute, then 4–5 mg (PE)/kg daily in 1–2 divided doses, dose to be administered at a rate of 50–100 mg(PE)/minute, dose to be adjusted according to response and trough plasma-phenytoin concentration

- Elderly: Consider 10–25% reduction in dose or infusion rate

Prophylaxis or treatment of seizures associated with neurosurgery or head injury
▸ BY INTRAMUSCULAR INJECTION, OR BY INTRAVENOUS INFUSION
- Adult: Initially 10–15 mg(PE)/kg, intravenous infusion to be administered at a rate of 50–100 mg(PE)/minute, then 4–5 mg(PE)/kg daily in 1–2 divided doses, intravenous infusion to be administered at a rate of 50–100 mg(PE)/minute, dose to be adjusted according to response and trough plasma-phenytoin concentration
- Elderly: Consider 10–25% reduction in dose or infusion rate

Temporary substitution for oral phenytoin
▸ BY INTRAMUSCULAR INJECTION, OR BY INTRAVENOUS INFUSION
- Adult: Same dose and same dosing frequency as oral phenytoin therapy, intravenous infusion to be administered at a rate of 50–100 mg(PE)/minute
- Elderly: Consider 10–25% reduction in dose or infusion rate

DOSE EQUIVALENCE AND CONVERSION
Doses are expressed as phenytoin sodium equivalent (PE); fosphenytoin sodium 1.5 mg ≡ phenytoin sodium 1 mg.

- UNLICENSED USE Fosphenytoin sodium doses in BNF may differ from those in product literature.
- CONTRA-INDICATIONS Acute porphyrias p. 918 · second-degree heart block · sino-atrial block · sinus bradycardia · Stokes-Adams syndrome · third-degree heart block
- CAUTIONS Heart failure · hypotension · injection solutions alkaline (irritant to tissues) · respiratory depression · resuscitation facilities must be available
- INTERACTIONS → Appendix 1 (fosphenytoin).
- SIDE-EFFECTS
- **Common or very common** Alterations in respiratory function · arrhythmias · asthenia · cardiovascular collapse · cardiovascular depression (particularly if injection too rapid) · chills · CNS depression (particularly if injection too rapid) · dry mouth · dysarthria · ecchymosis · euphoria · hypotension · incoordination · pruritus · respiratory arrest · taste disturbance · tinnitus · vasodilatation · visual disturbances
- **Uncommon** Decreased reflexes · hypoacusis · hypoaesthesia · increased reflexes · muscle spasm · muscle weakness · pain · stupor
- **Frequency not known** Confusion · extrapyramidal disorder · hyperglycaemia · purple glove syndrome · tonic seizures · twitching

SIDE-EFFECTS, FURTHER INFORMATION
- Cardiovascular reactions Intravenous infusion of fosphenytoin has been associated with severe cardiovascular reactions including asystole, ventricular fibrillation, and cardiac arrest. Hypotension, bradycardia, and heart block have also been reported. The following are recommended:
  - monitor heart rate, blood pressure, and respiratory function for duration of infusion;
  - observe patient for at least 30 minutes after infusion;
  - if hypotension occurs, reduce infusion rate or discontinue;
  - reduce dose or infusion rate in elderly, and in renal or hepatic impairment.
- ALLERGY AND CROSS-SENSITIVITY Cross-sensitivity reported with carbamazepine.
- PREGNANCY Changes in plasma-protein binding make interpretation of plasma-phenytoin concentrations difficult—monitor unbound fraction. The dose should be

monitored carefully during pregnancy and after birth, and adjustments made on a clinical basis.

- **BREAST FEEDING** Small amounts present in milk, but not known to be harmful.
- **HEPATIC IMPAIRMENT** Consider 10–25% reduction in dose or infusion rate (except initial dose for status epilepticus).
- **RENAL IMPAIRMENT** Consider 10–25% reduction in dose or infusion rate (except initial dose for status epilepticus).
- **PRE-TREATMENT SCREENING** HLA-B* 1502 allele in individuals of Han Chinese or Thai origin—avoid unless essential (increased risk of Stevens-Johnson syndrome).
- **MONITORING REQUIREMENTS**
  - Manufacturer recommends blood counts (but evidence of practical value uncertain).
  - With intravenous use Monitor heart rate, blood pressure, ECG, and respiratory function for during infusion.
- **DIRECTIONS FOR ADMINISTRATION** For *intermittent intravenous infusion (Pro-Epanutin®)*, give *in* Glucose 5% *or* Sodium chloride 0.9%; dilute to a concentration of 1.5–25 mg (phenytoin sodium equivalent (PE))/mL.
- **PRESCRIBING AND DISPENSING INFORMATION** Prescriptions for fosphenytoin sodium should state the dose in terms of phenytoin sodium equivalent (PE); fosphenytoin sodium 1.5 mg ≡ phenytoin sodium 1 mg.

- **MEDICINAL FORMS**
  There can be variation in the licensing of different medicines containing the same drug.

  Solution for injection
  ELECTROLYTES: May contain Phosphate
  - Pro-Epanutin (Pfizer Ltd)
    Fosphenytoin sodium 75 mg per 1 ml Pro-Epanutin 750mg/10ml concentrate for solution for injection vials | 10 vial [PoM] £400.00 (Hospital only)

Gabapentin

- **INDICATIONS AND DOSE**

Adjunctive treatment of focal seizures with or without secondary generalisation
- BY MOUTH
  - Child 6–11 years: 10 mg/kg once daily (max. per dose 300 mg) on day 1, then 10 mg/kg twice daily (max. per dose 300 mg) on day 2, then 10 mg/kg 3 times a day (max. per dose 300 mg) on day 3; usual dose 25–35 mg/kg daily in 3 divided doses, some children may not tolerate daily increments; longer intervals (up to weekly) may be more appropriate, daily dose maximum to be given in 3 divided doses; maximum 70 mg/kg per day
  - Child 12–17 years: Initially 300 mg once daily on day 1, then 300 mg twice daily on day 2, then 300 mg 3 times a day on day 3, alternatively initially 300 mg 3 times a day on day 1, then increased in steps of 300 mg every 2–3 days in 3 divided doses, adjusted according to response; usual dose 0.9–3.6 g daily in 3 divided doses (max. per dose 1.6 g 3 times a day), some children may not tolerate daily increments; longer intervals (up to weekly) may be more appropriate
  - Adult: Initially 300 mg once daily on day 1, then 300 mg twice daily on day 2, then 300 mg 3 times a day on day 3, alternatively initially 300 mg 3 times a day on day 1, then increased in steps of 300 mg every 2–3 days in 3 divided doses, adjusted according to response; usual dose 0.9–3.6 g daily in 3 divided doses (max. per dose 1.6 g 3 times a day)

Monotherapy for focal seizures with or without secondary generalisation
- BY MOUTH
  - Child 12-17 years: Initially 300 mg once daily on day 1, then 300 mg twice daily on day 2, then 300 mg 3 times a day on day 3, alternatively initially 300 mg 3 times a day on day 1, then increased in steps of 300 mg every 2–3 days in 3 divided doses, adjusted according to response; usual dose 0.9–3.6 g daily in 3 divided doses (max. per dose 1.6 g 3 times a day), some children may not tolerate daily increments; longer intervals (up to weekly) may be more appropriate
  - Adult: Initially 300 mg once daily on day 1, then 300 mg twice daily on day 2, then 300 mg 3 times a day on day 3, alternatively initially 300 mg 3 times a day on day 1, then increased in steps of 300 mg every 2–3 days in 3 divided doses, adjusted according to response; usual dose 0.9–3.6 g daily in 3 divided doses (max. per dose 1.6 g 3 times a day)

Peripheral neuropathic pain
- BY MOUTH
  - Adult: Initially 300 mg once daily on day 1, then 300 mg twice daily on day 2, then 300 mg 3 times a day on day 3, alternatively initially 300 mg 3 times a day on day 1, then increased in steps of 300 mg every 2–3 days in 3 divided doses, adjusted according to response; maximum 3.6 g per day

Migraine prophylaxis
- BY MOUTH
  - Adult: Initially 300 mg daily, then increased to up to 2.4 g daily in divided doses, adjusted according to response

- **UNLICENSED USE**
  - In children Not licensed for use in children under 6 years. Not licensed at doses over 50 mg/kg daily in children under 12 years.
  - In adults Not licensed for migraine prophylaxis.

> **IMPORTANT SAFETY INFORMATION**
> The levels of propylene glycol, acesulfame K and saccharin sodium may exceed the recommended WHO daily intake limits if high doses of gabapentin oral solution (Rosemont brand) are given to adolescents or adults with low body-weight (39–50 kg)—consult product literature.

- **CAUTIONS** Diabetes mellitus · elderly (in adults) · high doses of oral solution in adolescents and adults with low body-weight · history of psychotic illness · mixed seizures (including absences)
- **INTERACTIONS** → Appendix 1 (gabapentin).
- **SIDE-EFFECTS**
  - **Common or very common** Abdominal pain · abnormal reflexes · abnormal thoughts · acne · amnesia · anorexia · anxiety · arthralgia · ataxia · confusion · constipation · convulsions · cough · depression · diarrhoea · dizziness · drowsiness · dry mouth · dry throat · dyspepsia · dyspnoea · emotional lability · fever · flatulence · flu syndrome · gingivitis · headache · hostility · hypertension · impotence · increased appetite · insomnia · leucopenia · malaise · movement disorders · myalgia · nausea · nervousness · nystagmus · oedema · paraesthesia · pharyngitis (in adults) · pruritus · rash · rhinitis · speech disorder · tremor · twitching · vasodilatation · vertigo · visual disturbances · vomiting · weight gain
  - **Uncommon** Palpitations
  - **Frequency not known** Acute renal failure · alopecia · blood glucose fluctuations in patients with diabetes · breast hypertrophy · gynaecomastia · hallucinations · hepatitis · hypersensitivity syndrome · incontinence · pancreatitis ·

Stevens-Johnson syndrome · suicidal ideation · thrombocytopenia · tinnitus

- PREGNANCY

Monitoring
The dose should be monitored carefully during pregnancy and after birth, and adjustments made on a clinical basis.
- BREAST FEEDING Present in milk—manufacturer advises use only if potential benefit outweighs risk.
- RENAL IMPAIRMENT
  - In adults Reduce dose to 0.6–1.8 g daily in 3 divided doses if eGFR 50–80 mL/minute/1.73 m². Reduce dose to 300–900 mg daily in 3 divided doses if eGFR 30–50 mL/minute/1.73 m². Reduce dose to 300 mg on alternate days (up to max. 600 mg daily) in 3 divided doses if eGFR 15–30 mL/minute/1.73 m². Reduce dose to 300 mg on alternate days (up to max. 300 mg daily) in 3 divided doses if eGFR less than 15 mL/minute/1.73 m²—consult product literature.
  - In children Reduce dose if estimated glomerular filtration rate less than 80 mL/minute/1.73 m²; consult product literature.
- EFFECT ON LABORATORY TESTS False positive readings with some urinary protein tests.
- DIRECTIONS FOR ADMINISTRATION Capsules can be opened but the bitter taste is difficult to mask.
- PATIENT AND CARER ADVICE
  Medicines for Children leaflet: Gabapentin for preventing seizures www.medicinesforchildren.org.uk/gabapentin-for-preventing-seizures

- MEDICINAL FORMS
  There can be variation in the licensing of different medicines containing the same drug. Forms available from special-order manufacturers include: oral suspension, oral solution

Tablet
CAUTIONARY AND ADVISORY LABELS 3, 5, 8
- Gabapentin (Non-proprietary)
  Gabapentin 600 mg Gabapentin 600mg tablets | 100 tablet [PoM] £106.00 DT price = £7.62
  Gabapentin 800 mg Gabapentin 800mg tablets | 100 tablet [PoM] £98.13 DT price = £25.93
- Neurontin (Pfizer Ltd)
  Gabapentin 600 mg Neurontin 600mg tablets | 100 tablet [PoM] £84.80 DT price = £7.62
  Gabapentin 800 mg Neurontin 800mg tablets | 100 tablet [PoM] £98.13 DT price = £25.93

Capsule
CAUTIONARY AND ADVISORY LABELS 3, 5, 8
- Gabapentin (Non-proprietary)
  Gabapentin 100 mg Gabapentin 100mg capsules | 100 capsule [PoM] £22.00 DT price = £2.12
  Gabapentin 300 mg Gabapentin 300mg capsules | 100 capsule [PoM] £42.40 DT price = £3.47
  Gabapentin 400 mg Gabapentin 400mg capsules | 100 capsule [PoM] £49.06 DT price = £3.62
- Neurontin (Pfizer Ltd)
  Gabapentin 100 mg Neurontin 100mg capsules | 100 capsule [PoM] £18.29 DT price = £2.12
  Gabapentin 300 mg Neurontin 300mg capsules | 100 capsule [PoM] £42.40 DT price = £3.47
  Gabapentin 400 mg Neurontin 400mg capsules | 100 capsule [PoM] £49.06 DT price = £3.62

Oral solution
CAUTIONARY AND ADVISORY LABELS 3, 5, 8
EXCIPIENTS: May contain Propylene glycol
ELECTROLYTES: May contain Potassium, sodium
- Gabapentin (Non-proprietary)
  Gabapentin 50 mg per 1 ml Neurontin 250mg/5ml oral solution | 470 ml no price available
  Gabapentin 50mg/ml oral solution sugar free sugar-free | 150 ml [PoM] £69.00 DT price = £69.00

Lacosamide

- INDICATIONS AND DOSE

Adjunctive treatment of focal seizures with or without secondary generalisation
▸ BY MOUTH, OR BY INTRAVENOUS INFUSION
▸ Child 16-17 years: Initially 50 mg twice daily, infusion to be administered over 15–60 minutes (for up to 5 days), then increased, if tolerated, in steps of 50 mg twice daily, adjusted according to response, dose to be increased in weekly intervals; maintenance 100 mg twice daily (max. per dose 200 mg twice daily)
▸ Adult: Initially 50 mg twice daily, infusion to be administered over 15–60 minutes (for up to 5 days), then increased, if tolerated, in steps of 50 mg twice daily, adjusted according to response, dose to be increased in weekly intervals; maintenance 100 mg twice daily (max. per dose 200 mg twice daily)

Adjunctive treatment of focal seizures with or without secondary generalisation (alternative loading dose regimen when it is necessary to rapidly attain therapeutic plasma concentrations) (under close medical supervision)
▸ BY MOUTH, OR BY INTRAVENOUS INFUSION
▸ Child 16-17 years: Loading dose 200 mg, infusion to be administered over 15–60 minutes (for up to 5 days), followed by maintenance 100 mg twice daily, to be given 12 hours after initial dose, then increased, if tolerated, in steps of 50 mg twice daily (max. per dose 200 mg twice daily), adjusted according to response, dose to be increased in weekly intervals
▸ Adult: Loading dose 200 mg, infusion to be administered over 15–60 minutes (for up to 5 days), followed by maintenance 100 mg twice daily, to be given 12 hours after initial dose, then increased, if tolerated, in steps of 50 mg twice daily (max. per dose 200 mg twice daily), adjusted according to response, dose to be increased in weekly intervals

- CONTRA-INDICATIONS Second- or third-degree AV block
- CAUTIONS Conduction problems · elderly (in adults) · risk of PR-interval prolongation · severe cardiac disease
- INTERACTIONS → Appendix 1 (lacosamide). Caution with concomitant use of drugs that prolong PR interval.
- SIDE-EFFECTS
  ▸ Common or very common Abnormal gait · blurred vision · cognitive disorder · constipation · depression · dizziness · drowsiness · fatigue · flatulence · headache · impaired coordination · nausea · nystagmus · pruritus · tremor · vomiting
  ▸ Rare Multi-organ hypersensitivity reaction
  ▸ Frequency not known Aggression · agitation · agranulocytosis · atrial fibrillation · atrial flutter · AV block · bradycardia · confusion · dry mouth · dysarthria · dyspepsia · euphoria · hypoesthesia · irritability · muscle spasm · PR-interval prolongation · psychosis · rash · suicidal ideation · tinnitus
- ALLERGY AND CROSS-SENSITIVITY Antiepileptic hypersensitivity syndrome associated with lacosamide. See under Epilepsy p. 279 for more information.
- PREGNANCY

Monitoring
The dose should be monitored carefully during pregnancy and after birth, and adjustments made on a clinical basis.
- BREAST FEEDING Manufacturer advises avoid—present in milk in *animal* studies.
- HEPATIC IMPAIRMENT Titrate with caution in mild to moderate impairment if co-existing renal impairment. Caution in severe impairment—no information available.

- **RENAL IMPAIRMENT** Loading dose regimen can be considered in mild to moderate impairment—titrate above 200 mg with caution. Titrate with caution in severe impairment, max. 250 mg daily.
- In adults Consult product literature for loading dose if eGFR less than 30 mL/minute/1.73 m².
- In children Consult product literature for loading dose if estimated glomerular filtration rate is less than 30 mL/minute/1.73 m².
- **DIRECTIONS FOR ADMINISTRATION**
- With intravenous use in children For *intravenous infusion*, give undiluted or dilute with Glucose 5% *or* Sodium Chloride 0.9%.
- With intravenous use in adults For *intravenous infusion* (*Vimpat®*), give intermittently in Glucose 5% *or* Sodium Chloride 0.9%. May be administered undiluted.
- **PRESCRIBING AND DISPENSING INFORMATION** Flavours of syrup may include strawberry.
- **PATIENT AND CARER ADVICE**
Medicines for Children leaflet: Lacosamide for preventing seizures www.medicinesforchildren.org.uk/lacosamide-for-preventing-seizures
- **NATIONAL FUNDING/ACCESS DECISIONS**
Scottish Medicines Consortium (SMC) Decisions
The *Scottish Medicines Consortium* has advised (January 2009) that lacosamide (*Vimpat®*) is accepted for restricted use within NHS Scotland as adjunctive treatment for focal seizures with or without secondary generalisation in patients from 16 years. It is restricted for specialist use in refractory epilepsy.

- **MEDICINAL FORMS**
There can be variation in the licensing of different medicines containing the same drug.
Tablet
CAUTIONARY AND ADVISORY LABELS 8
- Vimpat (UCB Pharma Ltd)
Lacosamide 50 mg Vimpat 50mg tablets | 14 tablet [PoM] £10.81 DT price = £10.81
Lacosamide 100 mg Vimpat 100mg tablets | 14 tablet [PoM] £21.62 | 56 tablet [PoM] £86.50 DT price = £86.50
Lacosamide 150 mg Vimpat 150mg tablets | 14 tablet [PoM] £32.44 | 56 tablet [PoM] £129.74 DT price = £129.74
Lacosamide 200 mg Vimpat 200mg tablets | 56 tablet [PoM] £144.16 DT price = £144.16
Oral solution
CAUTIONARY AND ADVISORY LABELS 8
EXCIPIENTS: May contain Aspartame, propylene glycol
ELECTROLYTES: May contain Sodium
- Vimpat (UCB Pharma Ltd)
Lacosamide 10 mg per 1 ml Vimpat 10mg/ml syrup sugar-free | 200 ml [PoM] £25.74 DT price = £25.74
Solution for infusion
ELECTROLYTES: May contain Sodium
- Vimpat (UCB Pharma Ltd)
Lacosamide 10 mg per 1 ml Vimpat 200mg/20ml solution for infusion vials | 1 vial [PoM] £29.70

Lamotrigine

- **INDICATIONS AND DOSE**

Monotherapy of focal seizures | Monotherapy of primary and secondary generalised tonic-clonic seizures | Monotherapy of seizures associated with Lennox-Gastaut syndrome
- BY MOUTH
- Child 12-17 years: Initially 25 mg once daily for 14 days, then increased to 50 mg once daily for further 14 days, then increased in steps of up to 100 mg every 7–14 days; maintenance 100–200 mg daily in 1–2 divided doses; increased if necessary up to 500 mg

daily, dose titration should be repeated if restarting after interval of more than 5 days
- Adult: Initially 25 mg once daily for 14 days, then increased to 50 mg once daily for 14 days, then increased in steps of up to 100 mg every 7–14 days; maintenance 100–200 mg daily in 1–2 divided doses; increased if necessary up to 500 mg daily, dose titration should be repeated if restarting after interval of more than 5 days

Adjunctive therapy of focal seizures with valproate | Adjunctive therapy of primary and secondary generalised tonic-clonic seizures with valproate | Adjunctive therapy of seizures associated with Lennox-Gastaut syndrome with valproate
- BY MOUTH
- Child 2-11 years (body-weight up to 13 kg): Initially 2 mg once daily on alternate days for first 14 days, then 300 micrograms/kg once daily for further 14 days, then increased in steps of up to 300 micrograms/kg every 7–14 days; maintenance 1–5 mg/kg daily in 1–2 divided doses, dose titration should be repeated if restarting after interval of more than 5 days; maximum 200 mg per day
- Child 2-11 years (body-weight 13 kg and above): Initially 150 micrograms/kg once daily for 14 days, then 300 micrograms/kg once daily for further 14 days, then increased in steps of up to 300 micrograms/kg every 7–14 days; maintenance 1–5 mg/kg daily in 1–2 divided doses, dose titration should be repeated if restarting after interval of more than 5 days; maximum 200 mg per day
- Child 12-17 years: Initially 25 mg once daily on alternate days for 14 days, then 25 mg once daily for further 14 days, then increased in steps of up to 50 mg every 7–14 days; maintenance 100–200 mg daily in 1–2 divided doses, dose titration should be repeated if restarting after interval of more than 5 days
- Adult: Initially 25 mg once daily on alternate days for 14 days, then 25 mg once daily for further 14 days, then increased in steps of up to 50 mg every 7–14 days; maintenance 100–200 mg daily in 1–2 divided doses, dose titration should be repeated if restarting after interval of more than 5 days

Adjunctive therapy of focal seizures (with enzyme inducing drugs) without valproate | Adjunctive therapy of primary and secondary generalised tonic-clonic seizures (with enzyme inducing drugs) without valproate | Adjunctive therapy of seizures associated with Lennox-Gastaut syndromes (with enzyme inducing drugs) without valproate
- BY MOUTH
- Child 2-11 years: Initially 300 micrograms/kg twice daily for 14 days, then 600 micrograms/kg twice daily for further 14 days, then increased in steps of up to 1.2 mg/kg every 7–14 days; maintenance 5–15 mg/kg daily in 1–2 divided doses, dose titration should be repeated if restarting after interval of more than 5 days; maximum 400 mg per day
- Child 12-17 years: Initially 50 mg once daily for 14 days, then 50 mg twice daily for further 14 days, then increased in steps of up to 100 mg every 7–14 days; maintenance 200–400 mg daily in 2 divided doses, increased if necessary up to 700 mg daily, dose titration should be repeated if restarting after interval of more than 5 days
- Adult: Initially 50 mg once daily for 14 days, then 50 mg twice daily for further 14 days, then increased in steps of up to 100 mg every 7–14 days; maintenance 200–400 mg daily in 2 divided doses, increased if necessary up to 700 mg daily, dose titration should be repeated if restarting after interval of more than 5 days continued →

Adjunctive therapy of focal seizures (without enzyme inducing drugs) without valproate | Adjunctive therapy of primary and secondary generalised tonic-clonic seizures (without enzyme inducing drugs) without valproate | Adjunctive therapy of seizures associated with Lennox-Gastaut syndromes (without enzyme inducing drugs) without valproate

▶ BY MOUTH
▶ Child 2-11 years: Initially 300 micrograms/kg daily in 1–2 divided doses for 14 days, then 600 micrograms/kg daily in 1–2 divided doses for further 14 days, then increased in steps of up to 600 micrograms/kg every 7–14 days; maintenance 1–10 mg/kg daily in 1–2 divided doses, dose titration should be repeated if restarting after interval of more than 5 days; maximum 200 mg per day
▶ Child 12-17 years: Initially 25 mg once daily for 14 days, then increased to 50 mg once daily for further 14 days, then increased in steps of up to 100 mg every 7–14 days; maintenance 100–200 mg daily in 1–2 divided doses, dose titration should be repeated if restarting after interval of more than 5 days
▶ Adult: Initially 25 mg once daily for 14 days, then increased to 50 mg once daily for further 14 days, then increased in steps of up to 100 mg every 7–14 days; maintenance 100–200 mg daily in 1–2 divided doses, dose titration should be repeated if restarting after interval of more than 5 days

Monotherapy or adjunctive therapy of bipolar disorder (without enzyme inducing drugs) without valproate

▶ BY MOUTH
▶ Adult: Initially 25 mg once daily for 14 days, then 50 mg daily in 1–2 divided doses for further 14 days, then 100 mg daily in 1–2 divided doses for further 7 days; maintenance 200 mg daily in 1–2 divided doses, patients stabilised on lamotrigine for bipolar disorder may require dose adjustments if other drugs are added to or withdrawn from their treatment regimens—consult product literature, dose titration should be repeated if restarting after interval of more than 5 days; maximum 400 mg per day

Adjunctive therapy of bipolar disorder with valproate

▶ BY MOUTH
▶ Adult: Initially 25 mg once daily on alternate days for 14 days, then 25 mg once daily for further 14 days, then 50 mg daily in 1–2 divided doses for further 7 days; maintenance 100 mg daily in 1–2 divided doses, patients stabilised on lamotrigine for bipolar disorder may require dose adjustments if other drugs are added to or withdrawn from their treatment regimens—consult product literature, dose titration should be repeated if restarting after interval of more than 5 days; maximum 200 mg per day

Adjunctive therapy of bipolar disorder (with enzyme inducing drugs) without valproate

▶ BY MOUTH
▶ Adult: Initially 50 mg once daily for 14 days, then 50 mg twice daily for further 14 days, then increased to 100 mg twice daily for further 7 days, then increased to 150 mg twice daily for further 7 days; maintenance 200 mg twice daily, patients stabilised on lamotrigine for bipolar disorder may require dose adjustments if other drugs are added to or withdrawn from their treatment regimens—consult product literature, dose

titration should be repeated if restarting after interval of more than 5 days

---

IMPORTANT SAFETY INFORMATION
SAFE PRACTICE
Do not confuse the different combinations or indications.

● CAUTIONS Myoclonic seizures (may be exacerbated) · Parkinson's disease (may be exacerbated) (in adults)
● INTERACTIONS → Appendix 1 (lamotrigine).
● SIDE-EFFECTS
▶ **Common or very common** Blurred vision · aggression · agitation · arthralgia · ataxia · back pain · diarrhoea · diplopia · dizziness · drowsiness · dry mouth · headache · insomnia · nausea · nystagmus · rash · tremor · vomiting
▶ **Rare** Conjunctivitis
▶ **Very rare** Anaemia · blood disorders · confusion · exacerbation of Parkinson's disease (in adults) · hallucination · hepatic failure · hypersensitivity syndrome · increase in seizure frequency · leucopenia · lupus erythematosus-like reactions · movement disorders · pancytopenia · thrombocytopenia · unsteadiness
▶ **Frequency not known** Aseptic meningitis · suicidal ideation
SIDE-EFFECTS, FURTHER INFORMATION
▶ Skin reactions Serious skin reactions including Stevens-Johnson syndrome and toxic epidermal necrolysis have developed (especially in children); most rashes occur in the first 8 weeks. Rash is sometimes associated with hypersensitivity syndrome and is more common in patients with history of allergy or rash from other antiepileptic drugs. Consider withdrawal if rash or signs of hypersensitivity syndrome develop. Factors associated with increased risk of serious skin reactions include concomitant use of valproate, initial lamotrigine dosing higher than recommended, and more rapid dose escalation than recommended.
● ALLERGY AND CROSS-SENSITIVITY Antiepileptic hypersensitivity syndrome associated with lamotrigine. See under Epilepsy p. 279 for more information.
● PREGNANCY
Monitoring
Doses should be adjusted on the basis of plasma-drug concentration monitoring.
● BREAST FEEDING Present in milk, but limited data suggest no harmful effect on infant.
● HEPATIC IMPAIRMENT Halve dose in moderate impairment. Quarter dose in severe impairment.
● RENAL IMPAIRMENT Consider reducing maintenance dose in significant impairment. Caution in renal failure; metabolite may accumulate.
● TREATMENT CESSATION Avoid abrupt withdrawal (taper off over 2 weeks or longer) unless serious skin reaction occurs.
● PRESCRIBING AND DISPENSING INFORMATION Patients being treated for epilepsy may need to be maintained on a specific manufacturer's branded or generic lamotrigine product.
Switching between formulations Care should be taken when switching between oral formulations in the treatment of epilepsy. The need for continued supply of a particular manufacturer's product should be based on clinical judgement and consultation with the patient or their carer, taking into account factors such as seizure frequency and treatment history.
● PATIENT AND CARER ADVICE
Medicines for Children leaflet: Lamotrigine for preventing seizures www.medicinesforchildren.org.uk/lamotrigine-for-preventing-seizures

Skin reactions Warn patients and carers to see their doctor immediately if rash or signs or symptoms of hypersensitivity syndrome develop.

Blood disorders Patients and their carers should be alert for symptoms and signs suggestive of bone-marrow failure, such as anaemia, bruising, or infection. Aplastic anaemia, bone-marrow depression, and pancytopenia have been associated rarely with lamotrigine.

● MEDICINAL FORMS

There can be variation in the licensing of different medicines containing the same drug. Forms available from special-order manufacturers include: oral suspension, oral solution

Tablet

CAUTIONARY AND ADVISORY LABELS 8

▸ Lamotrigine (Non-proprietary)

Lamotrigine 25 mg Lamotrigine 25mg tablets | 56 tablet [PoM] £20.41 DT price = £1.41

Lamotrigine 50 mg Lamotrigine 50mg tablets | 56 tablet [PoM] £9.00 DT price = £1.39

Lamotrigine 100 mg Lamotrigine 100mg tablets | 56 tablet [PoM] £5.87 DT price = £1.65

Lamotrigine 200 mg Lamotrigine 200mg tablets | 56 tablet [PoM] £12.00 DT price = £2.99

▸ Lamictal (GlaxoSmithKline UK Ltd)

Lamotrigine 25 mg Lamictal 25mg tablets | 56 tablet [PoM] £23.53 DT price = £1.41

Lamotrigine 50 mg Lamictal 50mg tablets | 56 tablet [PoM] £40.02 DT price = £1.39

Lamotrigine 100 mg Lamictal 100mg tablets | 56 tablet [PoM] £69.04 DT price = £1.65

Lamotrigine 200 mg Lamictal 200mg tablets | 56 tablet [PoM] £117.35 DT price = £2.99

Dispersible tablet

CAUTIONARY AND ADVISORY LABELS 8, 13

▸ Lamotrigine (Non-proprietary)

Lamotrigine 5 mg Lamotrigine 5mg dispersible tablets sugar free sugar-free | 28 tablet [PoM] £15.00 DT price = £2.42

Lamotrigine 25 mg Lamotrigine 25mg dispersible tablets sugar free sugar-free | 56 tablet [PoM] £20.41 DT price = £2.37

Lamotrigine 100 mg Lamotrigine 100mg dispersible tablets sugar free sugar-free | 56 tablet [PoM] £6.98 DT price = £2.15

▸ Lamictal (GlaxoSmithKline UK Ltd)

Lamotrigine 2 mg Lamictal 2mg dispersible tablets sugar-free | 30 tablet [PoM] £12.54 DT price = £12.54

Lamotrigine 5 mg Lamictal 5mg dispersible tablets sugar-free | 28 tablet [PoM] £9.38 DT price = £2.42

Lamotrigine 25 mg Lamictal 25mg dispersible tablets sugar-free | 56 tablet [PoM] £23.53 DT price = £2.37

Lamotrigine 100 mg Lamictal 100mg dispersible tablets sugar-free | 56 tablet [PoM] £69.04 DT price = £2.15

Levetiracetam

● INDICATIONS AND DOSE

Monotherapy of focal seizures with or without secondary generalisation

▸ BY MOUTH, OR BY INTRAVENOUS INFUSION

▸ Child 16-17 years: Initially 250 mg once daily for 1 week, then increased to 250 mg twice daily, then increased in steps of 250 mg twice daily (max. per dose 1.5 g twice daily), adjusted according to response, dose to be increased every 2 weeks

▸ Adult: Initially 250 mg once daily for 1–2 weeks, then increased to 250 mg twice daily, then increased in steps of 250 mg twice daily (max. per dose 1.5 g twice daily), adjusted according to response, dose to be increased every 2 weeks

Adjunctive therapy of focal seizures with or without secondary generalisation

▸ BY MOUTH

▸ Child 1-5 months: Initially 7 mg/kg once daily, then increased in steps of up to 7 mg/kg twice daily (max. per dose 21 mg/kg twice daily), dose to be increased every 2 weeks

▸ Child 6 months-17 years (body-weight up to 50 kg): Initially 10 mg/kg once daily, then increased in steps of up to 10 mg/kg twice daily (max. per dose 30 mg/kg twice daily), dose to be increased every 2 weeks

▸ Child 12-17 years (body-weight 50 kg and above): Initially 250 mg twice daily, then increased in steps of 500 mg twice daily (max. per dose 1.5 g twice daily), dose to be increased every 2–4 weeks

▸ Adult: Initially 250 mg twice daily, then increased in steps of 500 mg twice daily (max. per dose 1.5 g twice daily), dose to be increased every 2–4 weeks

▸ BY INTRAVENOUS INFUSION

▸ Child 4-17 years (body-weight up to 50 kg): Initially 10 mg/kg once daily, then increased in steps of up to 10 mg/kg twice daily (max. per dose 30 mg/kg twice daily), dose to be increased every 2 weeks

▸ Child 12-17 years (body-weight 50 kg and above): Initially 250 mg twice daily, then increased in steps of 500 mg twice daily (max. per dose 1.5 g twice daily), dose to be increased every 2 weeks

▸ Adult: Initially 250 mg twice daily, then increased in steps of 500 mg twice daily (max. per dose 1.5 g twice daily), dose to be increased every 2–4 weeks

Adjunctive therapy of myoclonic seizures and tonic-clonic seizures

▸ BY MOUTH, OR BY INTRAVENOUS INFUSION

▸ Child 12-17 years (body-weight up to 50 kg): Initially 10 mg/kg once daily, then increased in steps of up to 10 mg/kg twice daily (max. per dose 30 mg/kg twice daily), dose to be increased every 2 weeks

▸ Child 12-17 years (body-weight 50 kg and above): Initially 250 mg twice daily, then increased in steps of 500 mg twice daily (max. per dose 1.5 g twice daily), dose to be increased every 2 weeks

▸ Adult: Initially 250 mg twice daily, then increased in steps of 500 mg twice daily (max. per dose 1.5 g twice daily), dose to be increased every 2–4 weeks

● UNLICENSED USE

▸ In adults Levetiracetam doses in BNF may differ from those in product literature.

▸ With oral use in children *Granules* not licensed for use in children under 6 years, for initial treatment in children with body-weight less than 25 kg, or for the administration of doses below 250 mg.

● INTERACTIONS → Appendix 1 (levetiracetam).

● SIDE-EFFECTS

▸ **Common or very common** Abdominal pain · aggression · anorexia · anxiety · ataxia · convulsion · cough · depression · diarrhoea · dizziness · drowsiness · dyspepsia · headache · insomnia · irritability · malaise · nasopharyngitis · nausea · rash · tremor · vertigo · vomiting

▸ **Uncommon** Agitation · alopecia · amnesia · blurred vision · confusion · diplopia · eczema · impaired attention · leucopenia · myalgia · paraesthesia · pruritus · psychosis · suicidal ideation · thrombocytopenia · weight changes

▸ **Rare** Agranulocytosis · choreoathetosis · drug reaction with eosinophilia and systemic symptoms (DRESS) · dyskinesia · erythema multiforme · hepatic failure · hyponatraemia · neutropenia · pancreatitis · pancytopenia · Stevens-Johnson syndrome · toxic epidermal necrolysis

▸ **Frequency not known** Completed suicide · pancytopenia

● PREGNANCY

Monitoring

The dose should be monitored carefully during pregnancy and after birth, and adjustments made on a clinical basis.

It is recommended that the fetal growth should be monitored.

● BREAST FEEDING Present in milk—manufacturer advises avoid.

● HEPATIC IMPAIRMENT
▸ In adults Halve dose in severe hepatic impairment if eGFR less than 60 mL/minute/1.73 m².
▸ In children Halve dose in severe hepatic impairment if estimated glomerular filtration rate less than 60 mL/minute/1.73 m².

● RENAL IMPAIRMENT
▸ In children Reduce dose if estimated glomerular filtration rate less than 80 mL/minute/1.73 m² (consult product literature).
▸ In adults Maximum 2 g daily if eGFR 50–80 mL/minute/1.73 m². Maximum 1.5 g daily if eGFR 30–50 mL/minute/1.73 m². Maximum 1 g daily if eGFR less than 30 mL/minute/1.73 m².

● DIRECTIONS FOR ADMINISTRATION
▸ With intravenous use For *intravenous infusion* (*Keppra*®), dilute requisite dose with at least 100 mL Glucose 5% or Sodium Chloride 0.9%; give over 15 minutes.
▸ With oral use For administration of *oral solution*, requisite dose may be diluted in a glass of water.

● PRESCRIBING AND DISPENSING INFORMATION If switching between oral therapy and intravenous therapy (for those temporarily unable to take oral medication), the intravenous dose should be the same as the established oral dose.

● PATIENT AND CARER ADVICE
Medicines for Children leaflet: Levetiracetam for preventing seizures www.medicinesforchildren.org.uk/levetiracetam-for-preventing-seizures

● MEDICINAL FORMS
There can be variation in the licensing of different medicines containing the same drug. Forms available from special-order manufacturers include: oral suspension, oral solution

Tablet
CAUTIONARY AND ADVISORY LABELS 8
▸ Levetiracetam (Non-proprietary)
Levetiracetam 250 mg Levetiracetam 250mg tablets | 60 tablet PoM £28.01 DT price = £2.60
Levetiracetam 500 mg Levetiracetam 500mg tablets | 60 tablet PoM £49.32 DT price = £3.75
Levetiracetam 750 mg Levetiracetam 750mg tablets | 60 tablet PoM £84.02 DT price = £5.26
Levetiracetam 1 gram Levetiracetam 1g tablets | 60 tablet PoM £95.34 DT price = £6.96
▸ Keppra (UCB Pharma Ltd)
Levetiracetam 250 mg Keppra 250mg tablets | 60 tablet PoM £28.01 DT price = £2.60
Levetiracetam 500 mg Keppra 500mg tablets | 60 tablet PoM £49.32 DT price = £3.75
Levetiracetam 750 mg Keppra 750mg tablets | 60 tablet PoM £84.02 DT price = £5.26
Levetiracetam 1 gram Keppra 1g tablets | 60 tablet PoM £95.34 DT price = £6.96
▸ Matever (Aspire Pharma Ltd)
Levetiracetam 250 mg Matever 250mg tablets | 60 tablet PoM £28.01 DT price = £2.60
Levetiracetam 500 mg Matever 500mg tablets | 60 tablet PoM £49.32 DT price = £3.75
Levetiracetam 750 mg Matever 750mg tablets | 60 tablet PoM £84.02 DT price = £5.26
Levetiracetam 1 gram Matever 1g tablets | 60 tablet PoM £95.34 DT price = £6.96

Granules
CAUTIONARY AND ADVISORY LABELS 8
▸ Desitrend (Desitin Pharma Ltd)
Levetiracetam 250 mg Desitrend 250mg granules sachets sugar-free | 60 sachet PoM £22.41
Levetiracetam 500 mg Desitrend 500mg granules sachets sugar-free | 60 sachet PoM £39.46
Levetiracetam 1 gram Desitrend 1000mg granules sachets sugar-free | 60 sachet PoM £76.27

Oral solution
CAUTIONARY AND ADVISORY LABELS 8
▸ Levetiracetam (Non-proprietary)
Levetiracetam 100 mg per 1 ml Levetiracetam 100mg/ml oral solution sugar free sugar-free | 150 ml PoM £27.00-£33.48 sugar-free | 300 ml PoM £66.95 DT price = £6.88
▸ Desitrend (Desitin Pharma Ltd)
Levetiracetam 100 mg per 1 ml Desitrend 100mg/ml oral solution sugar-free | 300 ml PoM £15.90 DT price = £6.88
▸ Keppra (UCB Pharma Ltd)
Levetiracetam 100 mg per 1 ml Keppra 100mg/ml oral solution sugar-free | 150 ml PoM £33.48 sugar-free | 300 ml PoM £66.95 DT price = £6.88

Solution for infusion
ELECTROLYTES: May contain Sodium
▸ Levetiracetam (Non-proprietary)
Levetiracetam 100 mg per 1 ml Levetiracetam 500mg/5ml concentrate for solution for infusion vials | 1 vial PoM £127.31 | 10 vial PoM £114.57-£127.31
Levetiracetam 500mg/5ml solution for infusion vials | 10 vial £127.31
▸ Desitrend (Desitin Pharma Ltd)
Levetiracetam 100 mg per 1 ml Desitrend 500mg/5ml concentrate for solution for infusion ampoules | 10 ampoule PoM £127.31
▸ Keppra (UCB Pharma Ltd)
Levetiracetam 100 mg per 1 ml Keppra 500mg/5ml concentrate for solution for infusion vials | 10 vial PoM £127.31
▸ Matever (Aspire Pharma Ltd)
Levetiracetam 100 mg per 1 ml Matever 500mg/5ml concentrate for solution for infusion vials | 10 vial PoM £127.31

Oxcarbazepine

● INDICATIONS AND DOSE
Monotherapy for the treatment of focal seizures with or without secondary generalised tonic-clonic seizures
▸ BY MOUTH
▸ Child 6-17 years: Initially 4–5 mg/kg twice daily (max. per dose 300 mg), then increased in steps of up to 5 mg/kg twice daily, adjusted according to response, dose to be adjusted at weekly intervals; maximum 46 mg/kg per day
▸ Adult: Initially 300 mg twice daily, then increased in steps of up to 600 mg daily, adjusted according to response, dose to be adjusted at weekly intervals; usual dose 0.6–2.4 g daily in divided doses

Adjunctive therapy for the treatment of focal seizures with or without secondary generalised tonic-clonic seizures
▸ BY MOUTH
▸ Child 6-17 years: Initially 4–5 mg/kg twice daily (max. per dose 300 mg), then increased in steps of up to 5 mg/kg twice daily, adjusted according to response, dose to be adjusted at weekly intervals; maintenance 15 mg/kg twice daily; maximum 46 mg/kg per day
▸ Adult: Initially 300 mg twice daily, then increased in steps of up to 600 mg daily, adjusted according to response, dose to be adjusted at weekly intervals; usual dose 0.6–2.4 g daily in divided doses

Treatment of primary generalised tonic-clonic seizures
▸ BY MOUTH
▸ Adult: Initially 300 mg twice daily, then increased in steps of up to 600 mg daily, adjusted according to response, dose to be increased at weekly intervals; usual dose 0.6–2.4 g daily in divided doses

DOSE ADJUSTMENTS DUE TO INTERACTIONS
In adjunctive therapy, the dose of concomitant antiepileptics may need to be reduced when using high doses of oxcarbazepine.

● UNLICENSED USE
▸ In adults Not licensed for the treatment of primary generalised tonic-clonic seizures.

- CAUTIONS Avoid in Acute porphyrias p. 918 · cardiac conduction disorders · heart failure · hyponatraemia
- INTERACTIONS → Appendix 1 (oxcarbazepine).
- SIDE-EFFECTS
  - **Common or very common** Abdominal pain · acne · agitation · alopecia · amnesia · asthenia · ataxia · confusion · constipation · depression · diarrhoea · diplopia · dizziness · drowsiness · headache · hyponatraemia · impaired concentration · nausea · nystagmus · rash · tremor · visual disorders · vomiting
  - **Uncommon** Leucopenia · urticaria
  - **Very rare** Arrhythmias · atrioventricular block · hepatitis · multi-organ hypersensitivity disorders · pancreatitis · Stevens-Johnson syndrome · systemic lupus erythematosus · thrombocytopenia · toxic epidermal necrolysis
  - **Frequency not known** Aplastic anaemia · bone marrow depression · hypertension · hypothyroidism · neutropenia · osteoporotic bone disorders · pancytopenia · suicidal ideation
- ALLERGY AND CROSS-SENSITIVITY Caution in patients with hypersensitivity to carbamazepine. Antiepileptic hypersensitivity syndrome associated with oxcarbazepine. See under Epilepsy p. 279 for more information.
- PREGNANCY
  Monitoring
  The dose should be monitored carefully during pregnancy and after birth, and adjustments made on a clinical basis.
- BREAST FEEDING Amount probably too small to be harmful but manufacturer advises avoid.
- HEPATIC IMPAIRMENT Caution in severe impairment—no information available.
- RENAL IMPAIRMENT
  - In adults Halve initial dose if eGFR less than 30 mL/minute/1.73 m^2; increase according to response at intervals of at least 1 week.
  - In children Halve initial dose if estimated glomerular filtration rate less than 30 mL/minute/1.73 m^2, increase according to response at intervals of at least 1 week.
  - PRE-TREATMENT SCREENING Test for HLA-B*1502 allele in individuals of Han Chinese or Thai origin (avoid unless no alternative—risk of Stevens-Johnson syndrome in presence of HLA-B*1502 allele).
- MONITORING REQUIREMENTS
  - Monitor plasma-sodium concentration in patients at risk of hyponatraemia.
  - Monitor body-weight in patients with heart failure.
- PRESCRIBING AND DISPENSING INFORMATION Patients may need to be maintained on a specific manufacturer's branded or generic oxcarbazepine product.
  Switching between formulations Care should be taken when switching between oral formulations. The need for continued supply of a particular manufacturer's product should be based on clinical judgement and consultation with the patient or their carer, taking into account factors such as seizure frequency and treatment history.
- PATIENT AND CARER ADVICE
  Medicines for Children: Oxcarbazepine for preventing seizures www.medicinesforchildren.org.uk/oxcarbazepine-for-preventing-seizures
  Blood, hepatic, or skin disorders Patients or their carers should be told how to recognise signs of blood, liver, or skin disorders, and advised to seek immediate medical attention if symptoms such as lethargy, confusion, muscular twitching, fever, rash, blistering, mouth ulcers, bruising, or bleeding develop.

- MEDICINAL FORMS
  There can be variation in the licensing of different medicines containing the same drug. Forms available from special-order manufacturers include: oral suspension
  Tablet
  CAUTIONARY AND ADVISORY LABELS 3, 8
  - Oxcarbazepine (Non-proprietary)
    Oxcarbazepine 150 mg Oxcarbazepine 150mg tablets | 50 tablet [PoM] £11.14 DT price = £8.60
    Oxcarbazepine 300 mg Oxcarbazepine 300mg tablets | 50 tablet [PoM] £22.61 DT price = £6.09
    Oxcarbazepine 600 mg Oxcarbazepine 600mg tablets | 50 tablet [PoM] £45.19 DT price = £38.96
  - Trileptal (Novartis Pharmaceuticals UK Ltd)
    Oxcarbazepine 150 mg Trileptal 150mg tablets | 50 tablet [PoM] £12.24 DT price = £8.60
    Oxcarbazepine 300 mg Trileptal 300mg tablets | 50 tablet [PoM] £24.48 DT price = £6.09
    Oxcarbazepine 600 mg Trileptal 600mg tablets | 50 tablet [PoM] £48.96 DT price = £38.96
  Oral suspension
  CAUTIONARY AND ADVISORY LABELS 3, 8
  EXCIPIENTS: May contain Propylene glycol
  - Trileptal (Novartis Pharmaceuticals UK Ltd)
    Oxcarbazepine 60 mg per 1 ml Trileptal 60mg/ml oral suspension sugar-free | 250 ml [PoM] £48.96

Perampanel

- INDICATIONS AND DOSE
  Adjunctive treatment of focal seizures with or without secondary generalised seizures
  - BY MOUTH
  - Child 12-17 years: Initially 2 mg once daily, dose to be taken before bedtime, then increased, if tolerated, in steps of 2 mg at intervals of at least every 2 weeks, adjusted according to response; maintenance 4–8 mg once daily; maximum 12 mg per day
  - Adult: Initially 2 mg once daily, dose to be taken before bedtime, then increased, if tolerated, in steps of 2 mg at intervals of at least every 2 weeks, adjusted according to response; maintenance 4–8 mg once daily; maximum 12 mg per day
  DOSE ADJUSTMENTS DUE TO INTERACTIONS
  Titrate at intervals of at least 1 week with concomitant carbamazepine, fosphenytoin, oxcarbazepine, or phenytoin.
- INTERACTIONS → Appendix 1 (perampanel).
- SIDE-EFFECTS Aggression · anxiety · ataxia · back pain · blurred vision · changes in appetite · confusion · diplopia · dizziness · drowsiness · dysarthria · gait disturbance · irritability · malaise · nausea · suicidal behaviour · suicidal ideation · vertigo · weight increase
- PREGNANCY Manufacturer advises avoid.
  The dose should be monitored carefully during pregnancy and after birth, and adjustments made on a clinical basis.
- BREAST FEEDING Avoid—present in milk in *animal* studies.
- HEPATIC IMPAIRMENT Increase at intervals of at least 2 weeks, up to max. 8 mg daily in mild or moderate impairment. Avoid in severe impairment.
- RENAL IMPAIRMENT Avoid in moderate or severe impairment.
- PRESCRIBING AND DISPENSING INFORMATION
  Switching between formulations Care should be taken when switching between oral formulations. The need for continued supply of a particular manufacturer's product should be based on clinical judgement and consultation with the patient or their carer, taking into account factors such as seizure frequency and treatment history.
  Patients may need to be maintained on a specific manufacturer's branded or generic perampanel product.

● MEDICINAL FORMS
There can be variation in the licensing of different medicines containing the same drug.

Tablet
CAUTIONARY AND ADVISORY LABELS 3, 8, 25
▶ Fycompa (Eisai Ltd) ▼
Perampanel 2 mg Fycompa 2mg tablets | 7 tablet [PoM] £35.00 | 28 tablet [PoM] £140.00
Perampanel 4 mg Fycompa 4mg tablets | 28 tablet [PoM] £140.00
Perampanel 6 mg Fycompa 6mg tablets | 28 tablet [PoM] £140.00
Perampanel 8 mg Fycompa 8mg tablets | 28 tablet [PoM] £140.00
Perampanel 10 mg Fycompa 10mg tablets | 28 tablet [PoM] £140.00
Perampanel 12 mg Fycompa 12mg tablets | 28 tablet [PoM] £140.00

Phenytoin

● INDICATIONS AND DOSE
Tonic-clonic seizures | Focal seizures | Prevention and treatment of seizures during or following neurosurgery or severe head injury
▶ BY MOUTH
▶ Child 1 month–11 years: Initially 1.5–2.5 mg/kg twice daily, then adjusted according to response to 2.5–5 mg/kg twice daily (max. per dose 7.5 mg/kg twice daily), dose also adjusted according to plasma-phenytoin concentration; maximum 300 mg per day
▶ Child 12–17 years: Initially 75–150 mg twice daily, then adjusted according to response to 150–200 mg twice daily (max. per dose 300 mg twice daily), dose also adjusted according to plasma-phenytoin concentration
▶ Adult: Initially 3–4 mg/kg daily, alternatively 150–300 mg once daily, alternatively 150–300 mg daily in 2 divided doses, alternatively maintenance 200–500 mg daily, to be taken preferably with or after food, dose to be increased gradually as necessary (with plasma-phenytoin concentration monitoring), exceptionally, higher doses may be used

Status epilepticus | Acute symptomatic seizures associated with head trauma or neurosurgery
▶ INITIALLY BY SLOW INTRAVENOUS INJECTION, OR BY INTRAVENOUS INFUSION
▶ Child 1 month–11 years: Loading dose 20 mg/kg, then (by slow intravenous injection or by intravenous infusion) 2.5–5 mg/kg twice daily, to be given with blood pressure and ECG monitoring
▶ Child 12–17 years: Loading dose 20 mg/kg, then (by intravenous infusion or by slow intravenous injection) up to 100 mg 3–4 times a day, to be given with blood pressure and ECG monitoring
▶ Adult: Loading dose 20 mg/kg (max. per dose 2 g), to be given at a rate not exceeding 1 mg/kg/minute (max. 50 mg per minute), to be given with blood pressure and ECG monitoring, then (by intravenous infusion or by slow intravenous injection or by mouth) maintenance 100 mg every 6–8 hours adjusted according to plasma-concentration monitoring, to be given with blood pressure and ECG monitoring

DOSE EQUIVALENCE AND CONVERSION
Preparations containing phenytoin sodium are **not** bioequivalent to those containing phenytoin base (such as *Epanutin Infatabs*® and *Epanutin*® suspension); 100 mg of phenytoin sodium is approximately equivalent in therapeutic effect to 92 mg phenytoin base. The dose is the same for all phenytoin products when initiating therapy. However, if switching between these products the difference in phenytoin content may be clinically significant. Care is needed when making changes between formulations and plasma-phenytoin concentration monitoring is recommended.

● UNLICENSED USE
▶ With oral use in children Licensed for use in children (age range not specified by manufacturer).
▶ With intravenous use Phenytoin doses in BNF publications may differ from those in product literature.

● CONTRA-INDICATIONS
GENERAL CONTRA-INDICATIONS
Acute porphyrias p. 918
SPECIFIC CONTRA-INDICATIONS
▶ With intravenous use Second- and third-degree heart block · sino-atrial block · sinus bradycardia · Stokes-Adams syndrome

● CAUTIONS
GENERAL CAUTIONS
Enteral feeding (interrupt feeding for 2 hours before and after dose; more frequent monitoring may be necessary)
SPECIFIC CAUTIONS
▶ With intravenous use Heart failure · hypotension · injection solutions alkaline (irritant to tissues) · respiratory depression · resuscitation facilities must be available
CAUTIONS, FURTHER INFORMATION
Consider vitamin D supplementation in patients who are immobilised for long periods or who have inadequate sun exposure or dietary intake of calcium.
    Intramuscular phenytoin should not be used (absorption is slow and erratic).

● INTERACTIONS → Appendix 1 (phenytoin).

● SIDE-EFFECTS
GENERAL SIDE-EFFECTS
▶ **Common or very common** Acne · anorexia · coarsening of facial appearance · constipation · dizziness · drowsiness · gingival hypertrophy and tenderness (maintain good oral hygiene) · headache · hirsutism · insomnia · nausea · paraesthesia · rash · transient nervousness · tremor · vomiting
▶ **Rare** Leucopenia · aplastic anaemia · blood disorders · dyskinesia · hepatotoxicity · lupus erythematosus · lymphadenopathy · megaloblastic anaemia · osteomalacia · peripheral neuropathy · polyarteritis nodosa · Stevens-Johnson syndrome · thrombocytopenia · toxic epidermal necrolysis
▶ **Frequency not known** Hypersensitivity syndrome · interstitial nephritis · pneumonitis · polyarthropathy · suicidal ideation
SPECIFIC SIDE-EFFECTS
▶ **Common or very common**
▶ With intravenous use Alterations in respiratory function · arrhythmias · cardiovascular collapse · cardiovascular depression (particularly if injection too rapid) · CNS depression (particularly if injection too rapid) · hypotension · respiratory arrest
▶ **Frequency not known**
▶ With intravenous use Purple glove syndrome · tonic seizures
SIDE-EFFECTS, FURTHER INFORMATION
▶ Hepatotoxicity Discontinue immediately and do not re-administer.
▶ Rash Discontinue; if mild re-introduce cautiously but discontinue immediately if recurrence.
▶ Use in adolescents Phenytoin may cause coarsening of the facial appearance, acne, hirsutism, and gingival hyperplasia and so may be particularly undesirable in adolescent patients.
▶ Bradycardia and hypotension
▶ With intravenous use Reduce rate of administration if bradycardia or hypotension occurs.

Overdose
Symptoms of phenytoin toxicity include nystagmus, diplopia, slurred speech, ataxia, confusion, and hyperglycaemia.

- ALLERGY AND CROSS-SENSITIVITY Cross-sensitivity reported with carbamazepine. Antiepileptic hypersensitivity syndrome associated with phenytoin. See under Epilepsy p. 279 for more information.
- PREGNANCY Changes in plasma-protein binding make interpretation of plasma-phenytoin concentrations difficult—monitor unbound fraction. Doses should be adjusted on the basis of plasma-drug concentration monitoring.
- BREAST FEEDING Small amounts present in milk, but not known to be harmful.
- HEPATIC IMPAIRMENT Reduce dose to avoid toxicity.
- PRE-TREATMENT SCREENING HLAB* 1502 allele in individuals of Han Chinese or Thai origin—avoid unless essential (increased risk of Stevens- Johnson syndrome).
- MONITORING REQUIREMENTS
  - In adults The usual total plasma-phenytoin concentration for optimum response is 10–20 mg/litre (or 40–80 micromol/litre). In pregnancy, the elderly, and certain disease states where protein binding may be reduced, careful interpretation of total plasma-phenytoin concentration is necessary; it may be more appropriate to measure free plasma-phenytoin concentration.
  - In children Therapeutic plasma-phenytoin concentrations reduced in first 3 months of life because of reduced protein binding. Trough plasma concentration for optimum response: neonate–3 months, 6–15 mg/litre (25–60 micromol/litre); child 3 months–18 years, 10–20 mg/litre (40–80 micromol/litre).
  - Manufacturer recommends blood counts (but evidence of practical value uncertain).
  - With intravenous use Monitor ECG and blood pressure.
- DIRECTIONS FOR ADMINISTRATION
  - With intravenous use in children Before and after administration flush intravenous line with Sodium Chloride 0.9%. For *intravenous injection*, give into a large vein at rate not exceeding 1 mg/kg/minute (max. 50 mg/minute). For *intravenous infusion*, dilute to a concentration not exceeding 10 mg/mL with Sodium Chloride 0.9% and give into a large vein through an in-line filter (0.22–0.50 micron) at a rate not exceeding 1 mg/kg/minute (max. 50 mg/minute); complete administration within 1 hour of preparation.
  - With intravenous use in adults For *intravenous infusion* (*Epanutin*®), give intermittently in Sodium chloride 0.9%. Flush intravenous line with Sodium chloride 0.9% before and after infusion; dilute in 50–100 mL infusion fluid (final concentration not to exceed 10 mg/mL) and give into a large vein through an in-line filter (0.22–0.50 micron) at a rate not exceeding 1 mg/kg/minute (max. 50 mg/minute); complete administration within 1 hour of preparation. To avoid local venous irritation each injection or infusion should be preceded and followed by an injection of sterile physiological saline through the same needle or catheter.
- PRESCRIBING AND DISPENSING INFORMATION Switching between formulations Different formulations of oral preparations may vary in bioavailability. Patients being treated for epilepsy should be maintained on a specific manufacturer's product.
- PATIENT AND CARER ADVICE Medicines for Children leaflet: Phenytoin for preventing seizures www.medicinesforchildren.org.uk/phenytoin-for-preventing-seizures
  Blood or skin disorders Patients or their carers should be told how to recognise signs of blood or skin disorders, and advised to seek immediate medical attention if symptoms such as fever, rash, mouth ulcers, bruising, or bleeding develop. Leucopenia that is severe, progressive, or associated with clinical symptoms requires withdrawal (if necessary under cover of a suitable alternative).

- MEDICINAL FORMS There can be variation in the licensing of different medicines containing the same drug. Forms available from special-order manufacturers include: oral suspension, oral solution

Tablet
CAUTIONARY AND ADVISORY LABELS 8
  - Phenytoin (Non-proprietary)
    Phenytoin sodium 100 mg Phenytoin sodium 100mg tablets | 28 tablet PoM £117.00 DT price = £26.75 | 100 tablet PoM no price available

Chewable tablet
CAUTIONARY AND ADVISORY LABELS 8, 24
  - Epanutin (Phenytoin) (Pfizer Ltd)
    Phenytoin 50 mg Epanutin Infatabs 50mg chewable tablets | 200 tablet PoM £13.18

Capsule
CAUTIONARY AND ADVISORY LABELS 8
  - Phenytoin (Non-proprietary)
    Phenytoin sodium 25 mg Phenytoin sodium 25mg capsules | 28 capsule PoM £15.74 DT price = £15.74
    Phenytoin sodium 50 mg Phenytoin sodium 50mg capsules | 28 capsule PoM £15.98 DT price = £15.98
    Phenytoin sodium 100 mg Phenytoin sodium 100mg capsules | 84 capsule PoM £68.76 DT price = £54.00
    Phenytoin sodium 300 mg Phenytoin sodium 300mg capsules | 28 capsule PoM £57.38 DT price = £57.38

Oral suspension
CAUTIONARY AND ADVISORY LABELS 8
  - Epanutin (Phenytoin) (Pfizer Ltd)
    Phenytoin 6 mg per 1 ml Epanutin 30mg/5ml oral suspension | 500 ml PoM £4.27 DT price = £4.27

Solution for injection
EXCIPIENTS: May contain Alcohol, propylene glycol
ELECTROLYTES: May contain Sodium
  - Phenytoin (Non-proprietary)
    Phenytoin sodium 50 mg per 1 ml Phenytoin sodium 250mg/5ml solution for injection ampoules | 5 ampoule PoM £15.50–£24.40 | 10 ampoule PoM no price available
  - Epanutin (Phenytoin sodium) (Pfizer Ltd)
    Phenytoin sodium 50 mg per 1 ml Epanutin Ready-Mixed Parenteral 250mg/5ml solution for injection ampoules | 10 ampoule PoM £48.79

Pregabalin

- INDICATIONS AND DOSE

Peripheral and central neuropathic pain
  - BY MOUTH
  - Adult: Initially 150 mg daily in 2–3 divided doses, then increased if necessary to 300 mg daily in 2–3 divided doses, dose to be increased after 3–7 days, then increased if necessary up to 600 mg daily in 2–3 divided doses, dose to be increased after 7 days

Adjunctive therapy for focal seizures with or without secondary generalisation
  - BY MOUTH
  - Adult: Initially 25 mg twice daily, then increased in steps of 50 mg daily, dose to be increased at 7 day intervals, increased to 300 mg daily in 2–3 divided doses for 7 days, then increased if necessary up to 600 mg daily in 2–3 divided doses

Generalised anxiety disorder
  - BY MOUTH
  - Adult: Initially 150 mg daily in 2–3 divided doses, then increased in steps of 150 mg daily if required, dose to be increased at 7 day intervals, increased if necessary up to 600 mg daily in 2–3 divided doses

- UNLICENSED USE Pregabalin doses in BNF may differ from those in product literature.
- CAUTIONS Conditions that may precipitate encephalopathy · severe congestive heart failure
- INTERACTIONS → Appendix 1 (pregabalin).

4

Nervous system

- SIDE-EFFECTS
- ► **Common or very common** Appetite changes · blurred vision · confusion · constipation · diplopia · disturbances in muscle control and movement · dizziness · drowsiness · dry mouth · euphoria · flatulence · impaired attention · impaired memory · insomnia · irritability · malaise · oedema · paraesthesia · sexual dysfunction · speech disorder · visual disturbances · visual field defects · vomiting · weight gain
- ► **Uncommon** Abdominal distension · abnormal dreams · agitation · arthralgia · chills · cognitive impairment · depersonalisation · depression · dry eye · dyspnoea · dysuria · first-degree AV block · flushing · gastro-oesophageal reflux disease · hallucinations · hyperacusis · hypersalivation · hypertension · hypoglycaemia · hypotension · hypotension · lacrimation · myalgia · nasal dryness · nasopharyngitis · panic attacks · rash · stupor · sweating · syncope · tachycardia · taste disturbance · thirst · thrombocytopenia · urinary incontinence
- ► **Rare** Arrhythmia · ascites · bradycardia · breast discharge · breast hypertrophy · breast pain · cold extremities · cough · dysphagia · epistaxis · hyperglycaemia · hypokalaemia · leucopenia · menstrual disturbances · neutropenia · oliguria · pancreatitis · parosmia · renal failure · rhabdomyolysis · rhinitis · urticaria · weight loss
- ► **Frequency not known** Aggression · congestive heart failure · convulsions · diarrhoea · encephalopathy · headache · keratitis · nausea · pruritus · QT-interval prolongation · Stevens-Johnson syndrome · suicidal ideation · urinary retention
- RENAL IMPAIRMENT Initially 75 mg daily and maximum 300 mg daily if eGFR 30–60 mL/minute/1.73 m^2. Initially 25–50 mg daily and maximum 150 mg daily in 1–2 divided doses if eGFR 15–30 mL/minute/1.73 m^2. Initially 25 mg once daily and maximum 75 mg once daily if eGFR less than 15 mL/minute/1.73 m^2.
- TREATMENT CESSATION Avoid abrupt withdrawal (taper over at least 1 week).
- PRESCRIBING AND DISPENSING INFORMATION Flavours of oral liquid formulations may include strawberry.
- NATIONAL FUNDING/ACCESS DECISIONS

Scottish Medicines Consortium (SMC) Decisions

The *Scottish Medicines Consortium* has advised (July 2007) that pregabalin (*Lyrica* ®) is not recommended for the treatment of central neuropathic pain.

The *Scottish Medicines Consortium* has advised (April 2009) that pregabalin (*Lyrica* ®) is accepted for restricted use within NHS Scotland for the treatment of peripheral neuropathic pain in adults who have not achieved adequate pain relief with, or have not tolerated, first- or second-line treatments; discontinue treatment if sufficient benefit is not achieved within 8 weeks of reaching the maximum tolerated dose.

- MEDICINAL FORMS
There can be variation in the licensing of different medicines containing the same drug. Forms available from special-order manufacturers include: oral suspension, oral solution

Capsule

CAUTIONARY AND ADVISORY LABELS 3, 8
- ► Pregabalin (Non-proprietary)
  Pregabalin 25 mg Pregabalin 25mg capsules | 56 capsule [PoM] £64.40 DT price = £64.40 | 84 capsule [PoM] £96.60
  Pregabalin 50 mg Pregabalin 50mg capsules | 56 capsule [PoM] no price available | 84 capsule [PoM] £96.60 DT price = £96.60
  Pregabalin 75 mg Pregabalin 75mg capsules | 56 capsule [PoM] £64.40 DT price = £64.40
  Pregabalin 100 mg Pregabalin 100mg capsules | 84 capsule [PoM] £96.60 DT price = £96.60
  Pregabalin 150 mg Pregabalin 150mg capsules | 56 capsule [PoM] £64.40 DT price = £64.40
  Pregabalin 200 mg Pregabalin 200mg capsules | 84 capsule [PoM] £96.60 DT price = £96.60

Pregabalin 225 mg Pregabalin 225mg capsules | 56 capsule [PoM] £64.40 DT price = £64.40
Pregabalin 300 mg Pregabalin 300mg capsules | 56 capsule [PoM] £64.40 DT price = £64.40
- ► Alzain (Dr Reddy's Laboratories (UK) Ltd)
  Pregabalin 25 mg Alzain 25mg capsules | 56 capsule [PoM] £45.08 DT price = £64.40
  Pregabalin 50 mg Alzain 50mg capsules | 56 capsule [PoM] £45.08 | 84 capsule [PoM] £67.62 DT price = £96.60
  Pregabalin 75 mg Alzain 75mg capsules | 56 capsule [PoM] £45.08 DT price = £64.40
  Pregabalin 100 mg Alzain 100mg capsules | 84 capsule [PoM] £67.62 DT price = £96.60
  Pregabalin 150 mg Alzain 150mg capsules | 56 capsule [PoM] £45.08 DT price = £64.40
  Pregabalin 200 mg Alzain 200mg capsules | 84 capsule [PoM] £67.62 DT price = £96.60
  Pregabalin 225 mg Alzain 225mg capsules | 56 capsule [PoM] £45.08 DT price = £64.40
  Pregabalin 300 mg Alzain 300mg capsules | 56 capsule [PoM] £45.08 DT price = £64.40
- ► Lecaent (Actavis UK Ltd)
  Pregabalin 25 mg Lecaent 25mg capsules | 56 capsule [PoM] £64.39 DT price = £64.40 | 84 capsule [PoM] £96.59
  Pregabalin 50 mg Lecaent 50mg capsules | 84 capsule [PoM] £96.59 DT price = £96.60
  Pregabalin 75 mg Lecaent 75mg capsules | 56 capsule [PoM] £64.39 DT price = £64.40
  Pregabalin 100 mg Lecaent 100mg capsules | 84 capsule [PoM] £96.59 DT price = £96.60
  Pregabalin 150 mg Lecaent 150mg capsules | 56 capsule [PoM] £64.39 DT price = £64.40
  Pregabalin 200 mg Lecaent 200mg capsules | 84 capsule [PoM] £96.59 DT price = £96.60
  Pregabalin 225 mg Lecaent 225mg capsules | 56 capsule [PoM] £64.39 DT price = £64.40
  Pregabalin 300 mg Lecaent 300mg capsules | 56 capsule [PoM] £64.39 DT price = £64.40
- ► Lyrica (Pfizer Ltd)
  Pregabalin 25 mg Lyrica 25mg capsules | 56 capsule [PoM] £64.40 DT price = £64.40 | 84 capsule [PoM] £96.60
  Pregabalin 50 mg Lyrica 50mg capsules | 84 capsule [PoM] £96.60 DT price = £96.60
  Pregabalin 75 mg Lyrica 75mg capsules | 56 capsule [PoM] £64.40 DT price = £64.40
  Pregabalin 100 mg Lyrica 100mg capsules | 84 capsule [PoM] £96.60 DT price = £96.60
  Pregabalin 150 mg Lyrica 150mg capsules | 56 capsule [PoM] £64.40 DT price = £64.40
  Pregabalin 200 mg Lyrica 200mg capsules | 84 capsule [PoM] £96.60 DT price = £96.60
  Pregabalin 225 mg Lyrica 225mg capsules | 56 capsule [PoM] £64.40 DT price = £64.40
  Pregabalin 300 mg Lyrica 300mg capsules | 56 capsule [PoM] £64.40 DT price = £64.40
- ► Rewisca (Consilient Health Ltd)
  Pregabalin 25 mg Rewisca 25mg capsules | 56 capsule [PoM] £45.40 DT price = £64.40
  Pregabalin 50 mg Rewisca 50mg capsules | 84 capsule [PoM] £68.10 DT price = £96.60
  Pregabalin 75 mg Rewisca 75mg capsules | 56 capsule [PoM] £45.40 DT price = £64.40
  Pregabalin 100 mg Rewisca 100mg capsules | 84 capsule [PoM] £68.10 DT price = £96.60
  Pregabalin 150 mg Rewisca 150mg capsules | 56 capsule [PoM] £45.40 DT price = £64.40
  Pregabalin 200 mg Rewisca 200mg capsules | 84 capsule [PoM] £68.10 DT price = £96.60
  Pregabalin 225 mg Rewisca 225mg capsules | 56 capsule [PoM] £45.40 DT price = £64.40
  Pregabalin 300 mg Rewisca 300mg capsules | 56 capsule [PoM] £45.40 DT price = £64.40

Oral solution

CAUTIONARY AND ADVISORY LABELS 3, 8
- ► Pregabalin (Non-proprietary)
  Pregabalin 20 mg per 1 ml Pregabalin 20mg/ml oral solution sugar-free sugar-free | 473 ml [PoM] £94.51
- ► Lyrica (Pfizer Ltd)
  Pregabalin 20 mg per 1 ml Lyrica 20mg/ml oral solution sugar-free | 473 ml [PoM] £99.48

Retigabine

● INDICATIONS AND DOSE

Adjunctive treatment of drug-resistant focal seizures with or without secondary generalisation when other appropriate drug combinations have proved inadequate or have not been tolerated

▶ BY MOUTH
▶ Adult: Initially up to 300 mg daily in 3 divided doses, then increased in steps of up to 150 mg every 1 week, adjusted according to response; maintenance 0.6–1.2 g daily
▶ Elderly: Initially 150 mg daily in 3 divided doses, then increased in steps of up to 150 mg every 1 week, adjusted according to response; maximum 900 mg per day

● CAUTIONS Known QT-interval prolongation · risk of urinary retention

CAUTIONS, FURTHER INFORMATION
▶ QT-interval prolongation Patients with known QT-interval prolongation, or with the following risk factors for QT interval prolongation, should be carefully monitored while taking retigabine: cardiac failure, ventricular hypertrophy, electrolyte abnormalities, or concomitant treatment with drugs that can prolong QT interval.

● INTERACTIONS → Appendix 1 (retigabine).

● SIDE-EFFECTS
▶ **Common or very common** Amnesia · anxiety · blurred vision · confusion · constipation · diplopia · discoloration of lips · discoloration of nails · discoloration of ocular tissue · discoloration of skin · dizziness · drowsiness · dry mouth · dysuria · haematuria · impaired attention · impaired coordination · impaired speech · increased appetite · malaise · myoclonus · nausea · paraesthesia · peripheral oedema · psychosis · tremor · vertigo · visual impairment · weight gain
▶ **Uncommon** Dyspepsia · dysphagia · hypokinesia · nephrolithiasis · rash · suicidal ideation · sweating · urinary retention

● PREGNANCY
Monitoring
The dose should be monitored carefully during pregnancy and after birth, and adjustments made on a clinical basis.

● HEPATIC IMPAIRMENT Reduce dose by 50% in moderate to severe impairment; increase by 50 mg every week according to response up to maximum 600 mg daily (450 mg in elderly).

● RENAL IMPAIRMENT Reduce dose by 50% if eGFR less than 50 mL/minute/1.73 m^2; increase by 50 mg every week according to response up to maximum 600 mg daily (450 mg in elderly).

● MONITORING REQUIREMENTS
▶ Ophthalmological monitoring A comprehensive ophthalmological examination (including visual acuity test, slit-lamp examination, and dilated fundoscopy) should be performed at initiation of treatment and at least every 6 months thereafter during treatment. Changes in vision or retinal pigment should lead to re-assessment of the benefits and risks of continuing treatment—discontinue unless no other treatment options are available. Monitoring should be increased if treatment is continued.
▶ Monitor for discoloration of ocular tissue and visual impairment.
▶ Monitor for blue-grey discoloration of nails, lips and skin—continue treatment only if potential benefit outweighs risk.

● PRESCRIBING AND DISPENSING INFORMATION
Switching between formulations Care should be taken when switching between oral formulations. The need for continued supply of a particular manufacturer's product should be based on clinical judgement and consultation with the patient or their carer, taking into account factors such as seizure frequency and treatment history.

Patients may need to be maintained on a specific manufacturer's branded or generic retigabine product.

● NATIONAL FUNDING/ACCESS DECISIONS
NICE technology appraisals (TAs)
▶ Retigabine for the adjunctive treatment of partial onset seizures in epilepsy (July 2011) NICE TA232
Retigabine is recommended as an option for the adjunctive treatment of partial onset seizures with or without secondary generalisation in adults aged 18 years and older with epilepsy, only when previous treatment with carbamazepine, clobazam, gabapentin, lamotrigine, levetiracetam, oxcarbazepine, sodium valproate, and topiramate has not provided an adequate response, or has not been tolerated.
www.nice.org.uk/TA232

Scottish Medicines Consortium (SMC) Decisions
The *Scottish Medicines Consortium* has advised (June 2011) that retigabine (*Trobalt*®®) is accepted for restricted use within NHS Scotland as adjunctive therapy in adults with focal seizures with or without secondary generalisation. It is restricted for use in refractory epilepsy.

● MEDICINAL FORMS
There can be variation in the licensing of different medicines containing the same drug.
Tablet
CAUTIONARY AND ADVISORY LABELS 8, 14, 25
▶ Trobalt (GlaxoSmithKline UK Ltd)
Retigabine 50 mg Trobalt 50mg tablets | 21 tablet [PoM] £4.87 | 84 tablet [PoM] £19.46
Retigabine 100 mg Trobalt 100mg tablets | 21 tablet [PoM] £9.73 | 42 tablet [PoM] no price available | 84 tablet [PoM] £38.93
Retigabine 200 mg Trobalt 200mg tablets | 84 tablet [PoM] £77.86
Retigabine 300 mg Trobalt 300mg tablets | 84 tablet [PoM] £116.78
Retigabine 400 mg Trobalt 400mg tablets | 84 tablet [PoM] £127.68
▶ Trobalt (GlaxoSmithKline UK Ltd)
Trobalt tablets starter pack | 63 tablet [PoM] £24.33

Rufinamide

● INDICATIONS AND DOSE

Adjunctive treatment of seizures in Lennox-Gastaut syndrome

▶ BY MOUTH
▶ Child 4-17 years (body-weight up to 30 kg): Initially 100 mg twice daily, then increased in steps of 100 mg twice daily (max. per dose 500 mg twice daily), adjusted according to response, dose to be increased at intervals of not less than 2 days
▶ Child 4-17 years (body-weight 30-49 kg): Initially 200 mg twice daily, then increased in steps of 200 mg twice daily (max. per dose 900 mg twice daily), adjusted according to response, dose to be increased at intervals of not less than 2 days
▶ Child 4-17 years (body-weight 50-69 kg): Initially 200 mg twice daily, then increased in steps of 200 mg twice daily (max. per dose 1.2 g twice daily), adjusted according to response, dose to be increased at intervals of not less than 2 days
▶ Child 4-17 years (body-weight 70 kg and above): Initially 200 mg twice daily, then increased in steps of 200 mg twice daily (max. per dose 1.6 g twice daily), adjusted according to response, dose to be increased at intervals of not less than 2 days

continued →

4

Nervous system

▸ Adult (body-weight 30–49 kg): Initially 200 mg twice daily, then increased in steps of 200 mg twice daily (max. per dose 900 mg twice daily), adjusted according to response, dose to be increased at intervals of not less than 2 days
▸ Adult (body-weight 50–69 kg): Initially 200 mg twice daily, then increased in steps of 200 mg twice daily (max. per dose 1.2 g twice daily), adjusted according to response, dose to be increased at intervals of not less than 2 days
▸ Adult (body-weight 70 kg and above): Initially 200 mg twice daily, then increased in steps of 200 mg twice daily (max. per dose 1.6 g twice daily), adjusted according to response, dose to be increased at intervals of not less than 2 days

Adjunctive treatment of seizures in Lennox-Gastaut syndrome with valproate
▸ BY MOUTH
▸ Child 4–17 years (body-weight up to 30 kg): Initially 100 mg twice daily, then increased in steps of 100 mg twice daily (max. per dose 300 mg twice daily), adjusted according to response, dose to be increased at intervals of not less than 2 days

● INTERACTIONS → Appendix 1 (rufinamide).
● SIDE-EFFECTS Abdominal pain · acne · anorexia · anxiety · back pain · blurred vision · constipation · diarrhoea · diplopia · dizziness · drowsiness · dyspepsia · epistaxis · fatigue · gait disturbances · headache · hyperactivity · hypersensitivity syndrome · impaired coordination · increase in seizure frequency · influenza-like symptoms · insomnia · nausea · nystagmus · oligomenorrhoea · rash · rhinitis · tremor · vomiting · weight loss
● ALLERGY AND CROSS-SENSITIVITY Antiepileptic hypersensitivity syndrome associated with rufinamide. See under Epilepsy p. 279 for more information.
● PREGNANCY
Monitoring
The dose should be monitored carefully during pregnancy and after birth, and adjustments made on a clinical basis.
● BREAST FEEDING Manufacturer advises avoid—no information available.
● HEPATIC IMPAIRMENT Caution and careful dose titration in mild to moderate impairment. Avoid in severe impairment.
● DIRECTIONS FOR ADMINISTRATION Tablets may be crushed and given in half a glass of water.
● PRESCRIBING AND DISPENSING INFORMATION
Switching between formulations Care should be taken when switching between oral formulations. The need for continued supply of a particular manufacturer's product should be based on clinical judgement and consultation with the patient or their carer, taking into account factors such as seizure frequency and treatment history.
Patients may need to be maintained on a specific manufacturer's branded or generic rufinamide product.
● PATIENT AND CARER ADVICE
Counselling on antiepileptic hypersensitivity syndrome is advised.
Medicines for Children leaflet: Rufinamide for preventing seizures www.medicinesforchildren.org.uk/rufinamide-for-preventing-seizures
● NATIONAL FUNDING/ACCESS DECISIONS
Scottish Medicines Consortium (SMC) Decisions
The *Scottish Medicines Consortium* has advised (October 2008) that rufinamide (*Inovelon* ®) is accepted for restricted use within NHS Scotland as adjunctive therapy in the treatment of seizures associated with Lennox-Gastaut syndrome in patients 4 years and above. It is restricted for

use when alternative traditional antiepileptic drugs are unsatisfactory.

● MEDICINAL FORMS
There can be variation in the licensing of different medicines containing the same drug.
Tablet
CAUTIONARY AND ADVISORY LABELS 8, 21
▸ Inovelon (Eisai Ltd)
   Rufinamide 100 mg Inovelon 100mg tablets | 10 tablet [PoM] £5.15
   Rufinamide 200 mg Inovelon 200mg tablets | 60 tablet [PoM] £61.77
   Rufinamide 400 mg Inovelon 400mg tablets | 60 tablet [PoM] £102.96
Oral suspension
CAUTIONARY AND ADVISORY LABELS 8, 21
EXCIPIENTS: May contain Propylene glycol
▸ Inovelon (Eisai Ltd)
   Rufinamide 40 mg per 1 ml Inovelon 40mg/ml oral suspension sugar-free | 460 ml [PoM] £94.71

Sodium valproate
9.6.2016

● INDICATIONS AND DOSE
All forms of epilepsy
▸ BY MOUTH USING IMMEDIATE-RELEASE MEDICINES
▸ Child 1 month–11 years: Initially 10–15 mg/kg daily in 1–2 divided doses (max. per dose 600 mg); maintenance 25–30 mg/kg daily in 2 divided doses, doses up to 60 mg/kg daily in 2 divided doses may be used in infantile spasms; monitor clinical chemistry and haematological parameters if dose exceeds 40 mg/kg daily
▸ Child 12–17 years: Initially 600 mg daily in 1–2 divided doses, increased in steps of 150–300 mg every 3 days; maintenance 1–2 g daily in 2 divided doses; maximum 2.5 g per day
▸ Adult: Initially 600 mg daily in 1–2 divided doses, then increased in steps of 150–300 mg every 3 days; maintenance 1–2 g daily, alternatively maintenance 20–30 mg/kg daily; maximum 2.5 g per day
Initiation of valproate treatment
▸ INITIALLY BY INTRAVENOUS INJECTION
▸ Adult: Initially 10 mg/kg, (usually 400–800 mg), followed by (by intravenous infusion or by intravenous injection) up to 2.5 g daily in 2–4 divided doses, alternatively (by continuous intravenous infusion) up to 2.5 g daily; (by intravenous injection or by intravenous infusion or by continuous intravenous infusion) usual dose 1–2 g daily, alternatively (by intravenous injection or by intravenous infusion or by continuous intravenous infusion) usual dose 20–30 mg/kg daily, intravenous injection to be administered over 3–5 minutes
Continuation of valproate treatment
▸ BY INTRAVENOUS INJECTION, OR BY INTRAVENOUS INFUSION, OR BY CONTINUOUS INTRAVENOUS INFUSION
▸ Adult: If switching from oral therapy to intravenous therapy give the same dose as current oral daily dose, give over 3–5 minutes by intravenous injection *or* in 2–4 divided doses by intravenous infusion
Migraine prophylaxis
▸ BY MOUTH USING IMMEDIATE-RELEASE MEDICINES
▸ Adult: Initially 200 mg twice daily, then increased if necessary to 1.2–1.5 g daily in divided doses
EPILIM CHRONOSPHERE®
All forms of epilepsy
▸ BY MOUTH
▸ Adult: Total daily dose to be given in 1–2 divided doses (consult product literature)

EPILIM CHRONO®

All forms of epilepsy

▸ BY MOUTH

▸ Adult: Total daily dose to be given in 1–2 divided doses (consult product literature)

EPISENTA® CAPSULES

All forms of epilepsy

▸ BY MOUTH

▸ Adult: Total daily dose to be given in 1–2 divided doses (consult product literature)

Mania

▸ BY MOUTH

▸ Adult: Initially 750 mg daily in 1–2 divided doses, adjusted according to response, usual dose 1–2 g daily in 1–2 divided doses, doses greater than 45 mg/kg daily require careful monitoring

EPISENTA® GRANULES

All forms of epilepsy

▸ BY MOUTH

▸ Adult: Total daily dose to be given in 1–2 divided doses (consult product literature)

Mania

▸ BY MOUTH

▸ Adult: Initially 750 mg daily in 1–2 divided doses, adjusted according to response, usual dose 1–2 g daily in 1–2 divided doses, doses greater than 45 mg/kg daily require careful monitoring

EPIVAL®

All forms of epilepsy

▸ BY MOUTH

▸ Adult: Total daily dose to be given in 1–2 divided doses (consult product literature)

● UNLICENSED USE Not licensed for migraine prophylaxis.

> **IMPORTANT SAFETY INFORMATION**
>
> MHRA/CHM ADVICE: VALPROATE AND RISK OF ABNORMAL PREGNANCY OUTCOMES
>
> Infants exposed to valproate in utero are at a high risk of serious developmental disorders (up to 30–40% risk) and congenital malformations (approx. 11% risk). Valproate should not be used in female children, females of childbearing potential or during pregnancy unless alternative treatments are ineffective or not tolerated.

● CONTRA-INDICATIONS Acute porphyrias p. 918 · known or suspected mitochondrial disorders (higher rate of acute liver failure and liver-related deaths) · personal or family history of severe hepatic dysfunction

● CAUTIONS Systemic lupus erythematosus

CAUTIONS, FURTHER INFORMATION

Consider vitamin D supplementation in patients that are immobilised for long periods or who have inadequate sun exposure or dietary intake of calcium.

▸ Liver toxicity Liver dysfunction (including fatal hepatic failure) has occurred in association with valproate (especially in children under 3 years and in those with metabolic or degenerative disorders, organic brain disease or severe seizure disorders associated with mental retardation) usually in first 6 months and usually involving multiple antiepileptic therapy. Raised liver enzymes during valproate treatment are usually transient but patients should be reassessed clinically and liver function (including prothrombin time) monitored until return to normal—discontinue if abnormally prolonged prothrombin time (particularly in association with other relevant abnormalities).

● INTERACTIONS → Appendix 1 (sodium valproate).

● SIDE-EFFECTS

▸ **Common or very common** Aggression · anaemia · confusion · convulsion · deafness · diarrhoea · extrapyramidal disorders · gastric irritation · haemorrhage · headache · hyponatraemia · memory impairment · menstrual disturbance · nausea · nystagmus · somnolence · stupor · thrombocytopenia · transient hair loss (regrowth may be curly) · tremor · weight gain

▸ **Uncommon** Angioedema · ataxia · coma · encephalopathy · increased alertness · lethargy · leucopenia · pancytopenia · paraesthesia · peripheral oedema · rash · reduced bone mineral density · syndrome of inappropriate secretion of antidiuretic hormone · vasculitis

▸ **Rare** Behavioural disturbance · blood disorders · bone marrow failure · dementia (in adults) · drowsiness · drug rash with eosinophilia and systemic symptoms (DRESS) syndrome · enuresis · Fanconi's syndrome · hallucinations · hearing loss · hyperactivity · hyperammonaemia · hypothyroidism · learning disorders · male infertility · myelodysplastic syndrome · polycystic ovaries · Stevens-Johnson syndrome · systemic lupus erythematosus · toxic epidermal necrolysis

▸ **Very rare** Acne · gynaecomastia · hepatic dysfunction · hirsutism · increase in bleeding time · pancreatitis

▸ **Frequency not known** Hypersensitivity reactions · suicidal ideation

SIDE-EFFECTS, FURTHER INFORMATION

▸ Hepatic dysfunction Withdraw treatment immediately if persistent vomiting and abdominal pain, anorexia, jaundice, oedema, malaise, drowsiness, or loss of seizure control.

▸ Pancreatitis Discontinue treatment if symtoms of pancreatitis develop.

● CONCEPTION AND CONTRACEPTION Valproate is associated with teratogenic risks and should not be used in females of child-bearing potential unless there is no safer alternative—this should be fully considered and discussed before prescribing for females of child-bearing age. Exclude pregnancy before treatment—effective contraception advised in females of child-bearing potential. In females planning to become pregnant, all efforts should be made to switch to appropriate alternative treatment prior to conception.

● PREGNANCY Valproate is associated with the highest risk of major and minor congenital malformations (in particular neural tube defects), and long-term neurodevelopmental effects. Valproate should not be used during pregnancy unless there is no safer alternative and only after a careful discussion of the risks. If valproate is to be used during pregnancy, the lowest effective dose should be prescribed in divided doses or as modified-release tablets to avoid peaks in plasma-valproate concentrations; doses greater than 1 g daily are associated with an increased risk of teratogenicity. Neonatal bleeding (related to hypofibrinaemia) reported. Neonatal hepatotoxicity also reported.

  Specialist prenatal monitoring should be instigated when valproate has been taken in pregnancy.

  The dose should be monitored carefully during pregnancy and after birth, and adjustments made on a clinical basis.

● BREAST FEEDING Present in milk—risk of haematological disorders in breast-fed newborns and infants.

● HEPATIC IMPAIRMENT Avoid if possible—hepatotoxicity and hepatic failure may occasionally occur (usually in first 6 months). Avoid in active liver disease.

● RENAL IMPAIRMENT Reduce dose.

● MONITORING REQUIREMENTS

▸ Plasma-valproate concentrations are not a useful index of efficacy, therefore routine monitoring is unhelpful.

▸ Monitor liver function before therapy and during first

4

Nervous system

6 months especially in patients most at risk.
▸ Measure full blood count and ensure no undue potential for bleeding before starting and before surgery.
● EFFECT ON LABORATORY TESTS False-positive urine tests for ketones.
● TREATMENT CESSATION [EvGr] Avoid abrupt withdrawal; if treatment with valproate is stopped, reduce the dose gradually over at least 4 weeks. Ⓐ
● DIRECTIONS FOR ADMINISTRATION For *intravenous infusion* (*Epilim*®, *Episenta*®), give continuously or intermittently in Glucose 5% or Sodium Chloride 0.9%. Reconstitute *Epilim*® with solvent provided then dilute with infusion fluid.

EPIVAL® Tablets may be halved but not crushed or chewed.

EPISENTA® CAPSULES Contents of capsule may be mixed with soft food or drink that is cold or at room temperature and swallowed immediately without chewing.

EPILIM® SYRUP May be diluted, preferably in Syrup BP; use within 14 days.

EPISENTA® GRANULES Granules may be mixed with soft food or drink that is cold or at room temperature and swallowed immediately without chewing.

EPILIM CHRONOSPHERE® Granules may be mixed with soft food or drink that is cold or at room temperature, and swallowed immediately without chewing.

● PRESCRIBING AND DISPENSING INFORMATION
Switching between formulations Care should be taken when switching between oral formulations in the treatment of epilepsy. The need for continued supply of a particular manufacturer's product should be based on clinical judgement and consultation with the patient or their carer, taking into account factors such as seizure frequency and treatment history.

Patients being treated for epilepsy may need to be maintained on a specific manufacturer's branded or generic oral sodium valproate product.

EPILIM CHRONOSPHERE® Prescribe dose to the nearest whole 50-mg sachet.
● PATIENT AND CARER ADVICE
Risk of abnormal pregnancy outcomes A patient guide and card should be provided to all female patients.
Medicines for Children leaflet: Sodium valproate for preventing seizures www.medicinesforchildren.org.uk/sodium-valproate-for-preventing-seizures
Blood or hepatic disorders Patients or their carers should be told how to recognise signs and symptoms of blood or liver disorders and advised to seek immediate medical attention if symptoms develop.
Pancreatitis Patients or their carers should be told how to recognise signs and symptoms of pancreatitis and advised to seek immediate medical attention if symptoms such as abdominal pain, nausea, or vomiting develop.
MHRA advice: Valproate and risk of abnormal pregnancy outcomes
Female patients and their carers should be counselled on the risk of valproate treatment during pregnancy. Ensure female patients are provided with relevant resources, to support their understanding of the risks. In particular the prescriber must ensure the patient understands:
● the risks associated with valproate during pregnancy;
● the need to use effective contraception;
● the need for regular review of treatment;
● the need to rapidly consult if she is planning a pregnancy or becomes pregnant

EPISENTA® CAPSULES Patients and carers should be counselled on the administration of capsules.

EPISENTA® GRANULES Patients and carers should be counselled on the administration of granules.

EPILIM CHRONOSPHERE® Patients and carers should be counselled on the administration of granules.

● MEDICINAL FORMS
There can be variation in the licensing of different medicines containing the same drug. Forms available from special-order manufacturers include: oral suspension, oral solution, suppository

Tablet
CAUTIONARY AND ADVISORY LABELS 8, 10, 21
▸ Epilim (Sanofi) ▼
Sodium valproate 100 mg Epilim 100mg crushable tablets | 100 tablet [PoM] £5.60 DT price = £5.60

Modified-release tablet
CAUTIONARY AND ADVISORY LABELS 8, 10, 21, 25
▸ Epilim Chrono (Sanofi) ▼
Sodium valproate 200 mg Epilim Chrono 200 tablets | 100 tablet [PoM] £11.65 DT price = £11.65
Sodium valproate 300 mg Epilim Chrono 300 tablets | 100 tablet [PoM] £17.47 DT price = £17.47
Sodium valproate 500 mg Epilim Chrono 500 tablets | 100 tablet [PoM] £29.10
▸ Epival CR (Chanelle Medical UK Ltd) ▼
Sodium valproate 300 mg Epival CR 300mg tablets | 100 tablet [PoM] £12.13 DT price = £17.47
Sodium valproate 500 mg Epival CR 500mg tablets | 100 tablet [PoM] £20.21

Gastro-resistant tablet
CAUTIONARY AND ADVISORY LABELS 5, 8, 10, 25
▸ Sodium valproate (Non-proprietary) ▼
Sodium valproate 200 mg Sodium valproate 200mg gastro-resistant tablets | 100 tablet [PoM] £7.70 DT price = £4.16
Sodium valproate 500 mg Sodium valproate 500mg gastro-resistant tablets | 100 tablet [PoM] £21.99 DT price = £7.98
▸ Epilim (Sanofi) ▼
Sodium valproate 200 mg Epilim 200 gastro-resistant tablets | 100 tablet [PoM] £7.70 DT price = £4.16
Sodium valproate 500 mg Epilim 500 gastro-resistant tablets | 100 tablet [PoM] £19.25 DT price = £7.98

Modified-release capsule
CAUTIONARY AND ADVISORY LABELS 8, 10, 21, 25
▸ Episenta (Desitin Pharma Ltd) ▼
Sodium valproate 150 mg Episenta 150mg modified-release capsules | 100 capsule [PoM] £7.00
Sodium valproate 300 mg Episenta 300mg modified-release capsules | 100 capsule [PoM] £13.00

Modified-release granules
CAUTIONARY AND ADVISORY LABELS 8, 10, 21, 25
▸ Epilim Chronosphere MR (Sanofi) ▼
Sodium valproate 50 mg Epilim Chronosphere MR 50mg granules sachets sugar-free | 30 sachet [PoM] £30.00
Sodium valproate 100 mg Epilim Chronosphere MR 100mg granules sachets sugar-free | 30 sachet [PoM] £30.00 DT price = £30.00
Sodium valproate 250 mg Epilim Chronosphere MR 250mg granules sachets sugar-free | 30 sachet [PoM] £30.00 DT price = £30.00
Sodium valproate 500 mg Epilim Chronosphere MR 500mg granules sachets sugar-free | 30 sachet [PoM] £30.00 DT price = £30.00
Sodium valproate 750 mg Epilim Chronosphere MR 750mg granules sachets sugar-free | 30 sachet [PoM] £30.00 DT price = £30.00
Sodium valproate 1 gram Epilim Chronosphere MR 1000mg granules sachets sugar-free | 30 sachet [PoM] £30.00 DT price = £30.00
▸ Episenta (Desitin Pharma Ltd) ▼
Sodium valproate 500 mg Episenta 500mg modified-release granules sachets sugar-free | 100 sachet [PoM] £21.00 DT price = £21.00
Sodium valproate 1 gram Episenta 1000mg modified-release granules sachets sugar-free | 100 sachet [PoM] £41.00 DT price = £41.00

Oral solution
CAUTIONARY AND ADVISORY LABELS 8, 10, 21
▸ Sodium valproate (Non-proprietary) ▼
Sodium valproate 40 mg per 1 ml Sodium valproate 200mg/5ml oral solution sugar free sugar-free | 300 ml [PoM] £4.77–£7.78 DT price = £4.30
▸ Epilim (Sanofi) ▼
Sodium valproate 40 mg per 1 ml Epilim 200mg/5ml liquid sugar-free | 300 ml [PoM] £7.78 DT price = £4.30
Epilim 200mg/5ml syrup | 300 ml [PoM] £9.33 DT price = £9.33

Solution for injection

▸ Sodium valproate (Non-proprietary) ▼
Sodium valproate 100 mg per 1 ml Sodium valproate 400mg/4ml solution for injection ampoules | 5 ampoule [PoM] £57.90

▸ Episenta (Desitin Pharma Ltd) ▼
Sodium valproate 100 mg per 1 ml Episenta 300mg/3ml solution for injection ampoules | 5 ampoule [PoM] £35.00

Powder and solvent for solution for injection

▸ Sodium valproate (Non-proprietary) ▼
Sodium valproate 400 mg Sodium valproate 400mg powder and solvent for solution for injection vials | 4 vial [PoM] £49.00

▸ Epilim (Sanofi) ▼
Sodium valproate 400 mg Epilim Intravenous 400mg powder and solvent for solution for injection vials | 1 vial [PoM] £13.32

Tiagabine

● **INDICATIONS AND DOSE**

Adjunctive treatment for focal seizures with or without secondary generalisation that are not satisfactorily controlled by other antiepileptics (with enzyme-inducing drugs)

▸ BY MOUTH

▸ Child 12-17 years: Initially 5–10 mg daily in 1–2 divided doses, then increased in steps of 5–10 mg/24 hours every 1 week; maintenance 30–45 mg daily in 2–3 divided doses

▸ Adult: Initially 5–10 mg daily in 1–2 divided doses, then increased in steps of 5–10 mg/24 hours every 1 week; maintenance 30–45 mg daily in 2–3 divided doses

Adjunctive treatment for focal seizures with or without secondary generalisation that are not satisfactorily controlled by other antiepileptics (without enzyme-inducing drugs)

▸ BY MOUTH

▸ Child 12-17 years: Initially 5–10 mg daily in 1–2 divided doses, then increased in steps of 5–10 mg/24 hours every 1 week; maintenance 15–30 mg daily in 2–3 divided doses

▸ Adult: Initially 5–10 mg daily in 1–2 divided doses, then increased in steps of 5–10 mg/24 hours every 1 week; maintenance 15–30 mg daily in 2–3 divided doses

● CAUTIONS Avoid in Acute porphyrias p. 918
  CAUTIONS, FURTHER INFORMATION
  Tiagabine should be avoided in absence, myoclonic, tonic and atonic seizures due to risk of seizure exacerbation.

● INTERACTIONS → Appendix 1 (tiagabine).

● SIDE-EFFECTS

▸ **Common or very common** Diarrhoea · dizziness · emotional lability · impaired concentration · nervousness · speech impairment · tiredness · tremor

▸ **Rare** Bruising · confusion · depression · drowsiness · non-convulsive status epilepticus · psychosis · suicidal ideation · visual disturbances

▸ **Frequency not known** Leucopenia

● PREGNANCY
  Monitoring
  The dose should be monitored carefully during pregnancy and after birth, and adjustments made on a clinical basis.

● HEPATIC IMPAIRMENT In mild to moderate impairment reduce dose, prolong the dose interval, or both. Avoid in severe impairment.

● PATIENT AND CARER ADVICE
  Medicines for Children leaflet: Tiagabine for preventing seizures www.medicinesforchildren.org.uk/tiagabine-for-preventing-seizures
  Driving and skilled tasks
  May impair performance of skilled tasks (e.g. driving).

● MEDICINAL FORMS
There can be variation in the licensing of different medicines containing the same drug. Forms available from special-order manufacturers include: oral suspension

Tablet
CAUTIONARY AND ADVISORY LABELS 21

▸ Gabitril (Teva UK Ltd)
Tiagabine (as Tiagabine hydrochloride monohydrate) 5 mg Gabitril 5mg tablets | 100 tablet [PoM] £52.04
Tiagabine (as Tiagabine hydrochloride monohydrate) 10 mg Gabitril 10mg tablets | 100 tablet [PoM] £104.09
Tiagabine (as Tiagabine hydrochloride monohydrate) 15 mg Gabitril 15mg tablets | 100 tablet [PoM] £156.13

Topiramate

● **INDICATIONS AND DOSE**

Monotherapy of generalised tonic-clonic seizures or focal seizures with or without secondary generalisation

▸ BY MOUTH

▸ Child 6-17 years: Initially 0.5–1 mg/kg once daily (max. per dose 25 mg) for 1 week, dose to be taken at night, then increased in steps of 250–500 micrograms/kg twice daily, dose to be increased by a maximum of 25 mg twice daily at intervals of 1–2 weeks; usual dose 50 mg twice daily (max. per dose 7.5 mg/kg twice daily), if child cannot tolerate titration regimens recommended above then smaller steps or longer interval between steps may be used; maximum 500 mg per day

▸ Adult: Initially 25 mg once daily for 1 week, dose to be taken at night, then increased in steps of 25–50 mg every 1–2 weeks, dose to be taken in 2 divided doses; usual dose 100–200 mg daily in 2 divided doses, adjusted according to response, doses of 1 g daily have been used in refractory epilepsy; maximum 500 mg per day

Adjunctive treatment of generalised tonic-clonic seizures or focal seizures with or without secondary generalisation | Adjunctive treatment for seizures associated with Lennox-Gastaut syndrome

▸ BY MOUTH

▸ Child 2-17 years: Initially 1–3 mg/kg once daily (max. per dose 25 mg) for 1 week, dose to be taken at night, then increased in steps of 0.5–1.5 mg/kg twice daily, dose to be increased by a maximum of 25 mg twice daily at intervals of 1–2 weeks; usual dose 2.5–4.5 mg/kg twice daily (max. per dose 7.5 mg/kg twice daily), if child cannot tolerate recommended titration regimen then smaller steps or longer interval between steps may be used; maximum 400 mg per day

▸ Adult: Initially 25–50 mg once daily for 1 week, dose to be taken at night, then increased in steps of 25–50 mg every 1–2 weeks, dose to be taken in 2 divided doses; usual dose 200–400 mg daily in 2 divided doses; maximum 400 mg per day

Migraine prophylaxis

▸ BY MOUTH

▸ Adult: Initially 25 mg once daily for 1 week, dose to be taken at night, then increased in steps of 25 mg every 1 week; usual dose 50–100 mg daily in 2 divided doses; maximum 200 mg per day

● CAUTIONS Avoid in Acute porphyrias p. 918 · risk of metabolic acidosis · risk of nephrolithiasis—ensure adequate hydration (especially in strenuous activity or warm environment)

● INTERACTIONS → Appendix 1 (topiramate).

● SIDE-EFFECTS

▸ **Common or very common** Abdominal pain · aggression · agitation · alopecia · anaemia · anxiety · appetite changes ·

Nervous system

4

arthralgia · cognitive impairment · confusion · constipation · depression · diarrhoea · dizziness · drowsiness · dry mouth · dyspepsia · dyspnoea · epistaxis · gastritis · impaired attention · impaired coordination · irritability · malaise · mood changes · movement disorders · muscle spasm · muscular weakness · myalgia · nausea · nephrolithiasis · nystagmus · paraesthesia · pruritus · rash · seizures · sleep disturbance · speech disorder · taste disturbance · tinnitus · tremor · urinary disorders · visual disturbances · vomiting

▶ **Uncommon** Abdominal distension · altered sense of smell · blepharospasm · blood disorders · bradycardia · dry eye · flatulence · flushing · gingival bleeding · glossodynia · haematuria · halitosis · hearing loss · hypokalaemia · hypotension · increased lacrimation · influenza-like symptoms · leucopenia · metabolic acidosis · mydriasis · neutropenia · palpitation · pancreatitis · panic attack · peripheral neuropathy · photophobia · postural hypotension · psychosis · reduced sweating · salivation · sexual dysfunction · skin discoloration · suicidal ideation · thirst · thrombocytopenia · urinary calculus

▶ **Rare** Abnormal skin odour · calcinosis · hepatic failure · hepatitis · periorbital oedema · Raynaud's syndrome · Stevens-Johnson syndrome · unilateral blindness

▶ **Very rare** Angle-closure glaucoma

▶ **Frequency not known** Encephalopathy · hyperammonaemia · maculopathy · toxic epidermal necrolysis

▶ SIDE-EFFECTS, FURTHER INFORMATION

▶ **Acute myopia with secondary angle-closure glaucoma** Topiramate has been associated with acute myopia with secondary angle-closure glaucoma, typically occurring within 1 month of starting treatment. Choroidal effusions resulting in anterior displacement of the lens and iris have also been reported. If raised intra-ocular pressure occurs:
- seek specialist ophthalmological advice;
- use appropriate measures to reduce intra-ocular pressure;
- stop topiramate as rapidly as feasible

● PREGNANCY Increased risk of cleft palate if taken in the first trimester of pregnancy.

The dose should be monitored carefully during pregnancy and after birth, and adjustments made on a clinical basis.

It is recommended that the fetal growth should be monitored.

● BREAST FEEDING Manufacturer advises avoid—present in milk.

● HEPATIC IMPAIRMENT Use with caution in moderate to severe impairment—clearance may be reduced.

● RENAL IMPAIRMENT

▶ In adults Half usual starting and maintenance dose if eGFR less than 70 mL/minute/1.73 m^2—reduced clearance and longer time to steady-state plasma concentration.

▶ In children Half usual starting and maintenance dose if estimated glomerular filtration less than 70 mL/minute/1.73 m^2—reduced clearance and longer time to steady-state plasma concentration. Use with caution.

● DIRECTIONS FOR ADMINISTRATION

TOPAMAX® CAPSULES Swallow whole or sprinkle contents of capsule on soft food and swallow immediately without chewing.

● PRESCRIBING AND DISPENSING INFORMATION

Switching between formulations Care should be taken when switching between oral formulations in the treatment of epilepsy. The need for continued supply of a particular manufacturer's product should be based on clinical judgement and consultation with the patient or their carer, taking into account factors such as seizure frequency and treatment history.

Patients being treated for epilepsy may need to be maintained on a specific manufacturer's branded or generic topiramate product.

● PATIENT AND CARER ADVICE

Medicines for Children leaflet: Topiramate for preventing seizures www.medicinesforchildren.org.uk/topiramate-for-preventing-seizures

TOPAMAX® CAPSULES Patients or carers should be given advice on how to administer Topamax® capsules.

● MEDICINAL FORMS

There can be variation in the licensing of different medicines containing the same drug. Forms available from special-order manufacturers include: oral suspension, oral solution

Tablet

CAUTIONARY AND ADVISORY LABELS 3, 8

▶ Topiramate (Non-proprietary)

Topiramate 25 mg Topiramate 25mg tablets | 60 tablet PoM £7.62 DT price = £1.64

Topiramate 50 mg Topiramate 50mg tablets | 60 tablet PoM £12.83 DT price = £2.05

Topiramate 100 mg Topiramate 100mg tablets | 60 tablet PoM £57.60 DT price = £2.63

Topiramate 200 mg Topiramate 200mg tablets | 60 tablet PoM £111.50 DT price = £14.03

▶ Topamax (Janssen-Cilag Ltd)

Topiramate 25 mg Topamax 25mg tablets | 60 tablet PoM £19.29 DT price = £1.64

Topiramate 50 mg Topamax 50mg tablets | 60 tablet PoM £31.69 DT price = £2.05

Topiramate 100 mg Topamax 100mg tablets | 60 tablet PoM £56.76 DT price = £2.63

Topiramate 200 mg Topamax 200mg tablets | 60 tablet PoM £110.23 DT price = £14.03

Capsule

CAUTIONARY AND ADVISORY LABELS 3, 8

▶ Topiramate (Non-proprietary)

Topiramate 15 mg Topiramate 15mg capsules | 60 capsule PoM £28.11 DT price = £23.73

Topiramate 25 mg Topiramate 25mg capsules | 60 capsule PoM £25.95 DT price = £14.74

Topiramate 50 mg Topiramate 50mg capsules | 60 capsule PoM £62.81 DT price = £52.19

▶ Topamax (Janssen-Cilag Ltd)

Topiramate 15 mg Topamax 15mg sprinkle capsules | 60 capsule PoM £14.79 DT price = £23.73

Topiramate 25 mg Topamax 25mg sprinkle capsules | 60 capsule PoM £22.18 DT price = £14.74

Topiramate 50 mg Topamax 50mg sprinkle capsules | 60 capsule PoM £36.45 DT price = £52.19

Vigabatrin

● INDICATIONS AND DOSE

Adjunctive treatment of focal seizures with or without secondary generalisation not satisfactorily controlled with other antiepileptics (under expert supervision)

▶ BY MOUTH

▶ Child 1-23 months: Initially 15–20 mg/kg twice daily (max. per dose 250 mg), to be increased over 2–3 weeks to usual maintenance dose, usual maintenance 30–40 mg/kg twice daily (max. per dose 75 mg/kg)

▶ Child 2-11 years: Initially 15–20 mg/kg twice daily (max. per dose 250 mg), to be increased over 2–3 weeks to usual maintenance dose, usual maintenance 30–40 mg/kg twice daily (max. per dose 1.5 g)

▶ Child 12-17 years: Initially 250 mg twice daily, to be increased over 2–3 weeks to usual maintenance dose, usual maintenance 1–1.5 g twice daily

▶ Adult: Initially 1 g once daily, alternatively initially 1 g daily in 2 divided doses, then increased in steps of 500 mg every 1 week, adjusted according to response; usual dose 2–3 g daily; maximum 3 g per day

▸ BY RECTUM
▸ **Child 1-23 months:** Initially 15–20 mg/kg twice daily (max. per dose 250 mg), to be increased over 2–3 weeks to usual maintenance dose, usual maintenance 30–40 mg/kg twice daily (max. per dose 75 mg/kg)
▸ **Child 2-11 years:** Initially 15–20 mg/kg twice daily (max. per dose 250 mg), to be increased over 2–3 weeks to usual maintenance dose, usual maintenance 30–40 mg/kg twice daily (max. per dose 1.5 g)
▸ **Child 12-17 years:** Initially 250 mg twice daily, to be increased over 2–3 weeks to usual maintenance dose, usual maintenance 1–1.5 g twice daily

● UNLICENSED USE Granules not licensed for rectal use. Tablets not licensed to be crushed and dispersed in liquid. Vigabatrin doses in BNF publications may differ from those in product literature.

● CONTRA-INDICATIONS Visual field defects

● CAUTIONS Elderly (in adults) · history of behavioural problems · history of depression · history of psychosis
CAUTIONS, FURTHER INFORMATION
Vigabatrin may worsen absence, myoclonic, tonic and atonic seizures.
▸ Visual field defects Vigabatrin is associated with visual field defects. The onset of symptoms varies from 1 month to several years after starting. In most cases, visual field defects have persisted despite discontinuation, and further deterioration after discontinuation cannot be excluded. Product literature advises visual field testing before treatment and at 6-month intervals. Patients and their carers should be warned to report any new visual symptoms that develop and those with symptoms should be referred for an urgent ophthalmological opinion. Gradual withdrawal of vigabatrin should be considered.

● INTERACTIONS → Appendix 1 (vigabatrin).

● SIDE-EFFECTS
▸ **Common or very common** Abdominal pain · aggression · agitation · blurred vision · depression · diplopia · dizziness · drowsiness · excitation (in children) · fatigue · headache · impaired concentration · impaired memory · irritability · nausea · nervousness · nystagmus · oedema · paraesthesia · paranoia · speech disorder · tremor · visual field defects · vomiting · weight gain
▸ **Uncommon** Ataxia · mania · occasional increase in seizure frequency (especially if myoclonic) · psychosis · rash
▸ **Rare** Peripheral retinal neuropathy · retinal disorders · suicidal ideation
▸ **Very rare** Hepatitis · optic atrophy · optic neuritis
▸ **Frequency not known** Movement disorders in infantile spasms
SIDE-EFFECTS, FURTHER INFORMATION
Encephalopathic symptoms including marked sedation, stupor, and confusion with non-specific slow wave EEG can occur *rarely*—reduce dose or withdraw.
▸ Visual field defects About one-third of patients treated with vigabatrin have suffered visual field defects; counselling and **careful monitoring** for this side-effect are required.

● PREGNANCY
Monitoring
The dose should be monitored carefully during pregnancy and after birth, and adjustments made on a clinical basis.

● BREAST FEEDING Present in milk—manufacturer advises avoid.

● RENAL IMPAIRMENT
▸ In adults Consider reduced dose or increased dose interval if eGFR less than 60 mL/minute/1.73 m^2.
▸ In children Consider reduced dose or increased dose interval if estimated glomerular filtration rate less than 60 mL/minute/1.73 m^2.

● MONITORING REQUIREMENTS Closely monitor neurological function.

● DIRECTIONS FOR ADMINISTRATION
▸ With oral use The contents of a sachet should be dissolved in water or a soft drink immediately before taking. Tablets may be crushed and dispersed in liquid.
▸ With rectal use Dissolve contents of sachet in small amount of water and administer rectally [unlicensed use].

● PATIENT AND CARER ADVICE
Patients and their carers should be warned to report any new visual symptoms that develop.
Medicines for Children leaflet: Vigabatrin for preventing seizures www.medicinesforchildren.org.uk/vigabatrin-for-preventing-seizures

● MEDICINAL FORMS
There can be variation in the licensing of different medicines containing the same drug. Forms available from special-order manufacturers include: oral solution
Tablet
CAUTIONARY AND ADVISORY LABELS 3, 8
▸ Sabril (Sanofi)
Vigabatrin **500 mg** Sabril 500mg tablets | 100 tablet [PoM] £44.41 DT price = £44.41
Powder
CAUTIONARY AND ADVISORY LABELS 3, 8, 13
▸ Sabril (Sanofi)
Vigabatrin **500 mg** Sabril 500mg oral powder sachets sugar-free | 50 sachet [PoM] £24.60 DT price = £24.60

Zonisamide

● INDICATIONS AND DOSE

Monotherapy for treatment of focal seizures with or without secondary generalisation in adults with newly diagnosed epilepsy
▸ BY MOUTH
▸ **Adult:** Initially 100 mg once daily for 2 weeks, then increased in steps of 100 mg every 2 weeks, usual maintenance dose 300 mg once daily; maximum 500 mg per day

Adjunctive treatment for refractory focal seizures with or without secondary generalisation
▸ BY MOUTH
▸ **Child 6-17 years (body-weight 20-54 kg):** Initially 1 mg/kg once daily for 7 days, then increased in steps of 1 mg/kg every 7 days, usual maintenance 6–8 mg/kg once daily (max. per dose 500 mg once daily), dose to be increased at 2-week intervals in patients who are **not** receiving concomitant carbamazepine, phenytoin, phenobarbital or other potent inducers of cytochrome P450 enzyme CYP3A4
▸ **Child 6-17 years (body-weight 55 kg and above):** Initially 1 mg/kg once daily for 7 days, then increased in steps of 1 mg/kg every 7 days, usual maintenance 300–500 mg once daily, dose to be increased at 2-week intervals in patients who are **not** receiving concomitant carbamazepine, phenytoin, phenobarbital or other potent inducers of cytochrome P450 enzyme CYP3A4
▸ **Adult:** Initially 50 mg daily in 2 divided doses for 7 days, then increased to 100 mg daily in 2 divided doses, then increased in steps of 100 mg every 7 days, usual maintenance 300–500 mg daily in 1–2 divided doses, dose to be increased at 2-week intervals in patients who are **not** receiving concomitant carbamazepine, phenytoin, phenobarbital or other potent inducers of cytochrome P450 enzyme CYP3A4

● CAUTIONS Elderly (in adults) · low body-weight or poor appetite—monitor weight throughout treatment (fatal cases of weight loss reported in children) · metabolic acidosis—monitor serum bicarbonate concentration in children and those with other risk factors (consider dose reduction or discontinuation if metabolic acidosis develops) · risk factors for renal stone formation (particularly predisposition to nephrolithiasis).

CAUTIONS, FURTHER INFORMATION
Avoid overheating and ensure adequate hydration especially in children, during strenuous activity or if in warm environment (fatal cases of heat stroke reported in children).

● INTERACTIONS → Appendix 1 (zonisamide).
▸ In adults Caution with concomitant use of drugs that increase risk of hyperthermia, metabolic acidosis, or nephrolithiasis.
▸ In children Caution with concomitant use of drugs that increase risk of nephrolithiasis. Contra-indicated with use of drugs that increase risk of hyperthermia or metabolic acidosis.

● SIDE-EFFECTS
▸ **Common or very common** Abdominal pain · agitation · alopecia · anorexia · ataxia · confusion · constipation · depression · diarrhoea · diplopia · dizziness · drowsiness · ecchymosis · fatigue · impaired attention · impaired memory · insomnia · irritability · nausea · nystagmus · paraesthesia · peripheral oedema · pruritus · psychosis · pyrexia · rash (consider withdrawal) · speech disorder · tremor · weight loss
▸ **Uncommon** Aggression · cholecystitis · cholelithiasis · dyspepsia · hypokalaemia · pneumonia · seizures · suicidal ideation · urinary calculus · urinary tract infection · vomiting
▸ **Very rare** Amnesia · aspiration · blood disorders · coma · dyspnoea · hallucinations · heat stroke · hepatitis · hydronephrosis · impaired sweating · metabolic acidosis · myasthenic syndrome · neuroleptic malignant syndrome · pancreatitis · renal failure · renal tubular acidosis · rhabdomyolysis · Stevens-Johnson syndrome · toxic epidermal necrolysis

● ALLERGY AND CROSS-SENSITIVITY Contra-indicated in sulfonamide hypersensitivity.
    Antiepileptic hypersensitivity syndrome theoretically associated with zonisamide. See under Epilepsy p. 279 for more information.

● CONCEPTION AND CONTRACEPTION Manufacturer advises women of childbearing potential should use adequate contraception during treatment and for 4 weeks after last dose.

● PREGNANCY
Monitoring
The dose should be monitored carefully during pregnancy and after birth, and adjustments made on a clinical basis.

● BREAST FEEDING Manufacturer advises avoid for 4 weeks after last dose.

● HEPATIC IMPAIRMENT Initially increase dose at 2-week intervals if mild or moderate impairment. Avoid in severe impairment.

● RENAL IMPAIRMENT Initially increase dose at 2-week intervals; discontinue if renal function deteriorates.

● TREATMENT CESSATION Avoid abrupt withdrawal (consult product literature for recommended withdrawal regimens in children).

● PRESCRIBING AND DISPENSING INFORMATION
Switching between formulations Care should be taken when switching between oral formulations. The need for continued supply of a particular manufacturer's product should be based on clinical judgement and consultation with the patient or carer, taking into account factors such as seizure frequency and treatment history.
    Patients may need to be maintained on a specific manufacturer's branded or generic zonisamide product.

● PATIENT AND CARER ADVICE
Children and their carers should be made aware of how to prevent and recognise overheating and dehydration. Medicines for Children leaflet: Zonisamide for preventing seizures www.medicinesforchildren.org.uk/zonisamide-for-preventing-seizures

● NATIONAL FUNDING/ACCESS DECISIONS
Scottish Medicines Consortium (SMC) Decisions
The *Scottish Medicines Consortium* has advised (February 2014) that zonisamide (*Zonegran*®) is accepted for restricted use within NHS Scotland as adjunctive treatment of focal seizures, with or without secondary generalisation, in adolescents and children aged 6 years and above. It is restricted to use on advice from specialists in paediatric neurology or epilepsy.

● MEDICINAL FORMS
There can be variation in the licensing of different medicines containing the same drug. Forms available from special-order manufacturers include: oral suspension, oral solution

Capsule
CAUTIONARY AND ADVISORY LABELS 3, 8, 10
▸ Zonisamide (Non-proprietary)
Zonisamide 25 mg Zonisamide 25mg capsules | 14 capsule [PoM]
£8.38–£9.26 DT price = £8.82
Zonisamide 50 mg Zonisamide 50mg capsule | 56 capsule [PoM]
£47.04 DT price = £47.04
Zonisamide 50mg capsules | 56 capsule [PoM] £44.69–£49.40 DT price
= £47.04
Zonisamide 100 mg Zonisamide 100mg capsules | 56 capsule [PoM]
£59.58–£65.85 DT price = £62.72
Zonisamide 100mg capsule | 56 capsule [PoM] £62.72 DT price =
£62.72
▸ Zonegran (Eisai Ltd)
Zonisamide 25 mg Zonegran 25mg capsules | 14 capsule [PoM]
£8.82 DT price = £8.82
Zonisamide 50 mg Zonegran 50mg capsules | 56 capsule [PoM]
£47.04 DT price = £47.04
Zonisamide 100 mg Zonegran 100mg capsules | 56 capsule [PoM]
£62.72 DT price = £62.72

ANTIEPILEPTICS > BARBITURATES

Phenobarbital
(Phenobarbitone)

● INDICATIONS AND DOSE
All forms of epilepsy except typical absence seizures
▸ BY MOUTH
▸ Child 1 month-11 years: Initially 1–1.5 mg/kg twice daily, then increased in steps of 2 mg/kg daily as required; maintenance 2.5–4 mg/kg 1–2 times a day
▸ Child 12–17 years: 60–180 mg once daily
▸ Adult: 60–180 mg once daily, dose to be taken at night
Status epilepticus
▸ BY INTRAVENOUS INJECTION
▸ Adult: 10 mg/kg (max. per dose 1 g), dose to be administered at a rate not more than 100 mg/minute, injection to be diluted 1 in 10 with water for injections
▸ BY SLOW INTRAVENOUS INJECTION
▸ Child 1 month-11 years: Initially 20 mg/kg, dose to be administered at a rate no faster than 1 mg/kg/minute, then 2.5–5 mg/kg 1–2 times a day
▸ Child 12–17 years: Initially 20 mg/kg (max. per dose 1 g), dose to be administered at a rate no faster than 1 mg/kg/minute, then 300 mg twice daily

DOSE EQUIVALENCE AND CONVERSION
For therapeutic purposes phenobarbital and phenobarbital sodium may be considered equivalent in effect.

● CAUTIONS Avoid in Acute porphyrias p. 918 · children · debilitated · elderly (in adults) · history of alcohol abuse ·

history of drug abuse · respiratory depression (avoid if severe)

CAUTIONS, FURTHER INFORMATION

Consider vitamin D supplementation in patients who are immobilised for long periods or who have inadequate sun exposure or dietary intake of calcium.

● INTERACTIONS → Appendix 1 (phenobarbital).

● SIDE-EFFECTS

▸ **Common or very common** Agranulocytosis · allergic skin reactions · ataxia · behavioural disturbances · cholestasis · depression · drowsiness · hallucinations · hepatitis · hyperactivity particularly in the elderly and in children · hypotension · impaired cognition · impaired memory · irritability · lethargy · megaloblastic anaemia (may be treated with folic acid) · nystagmus · osteomalacia · paradoxical excitement (in adults) · respiratory depression · thrombocytopenia

▸ **Very rare** Antiepileptic Hypersensitivity Syndrome · Stevens-Johnson syndrome · suicidal ideation · toxic epidermal necrolysis

▸ **Frequency not known** Hyperkinesia (in children)

Overdose

For details on the management of poisoning, see Active elimination techniques, under Emergency treatment of poisoning p. 1194.

● ALLERGY AND CROSS-SENSITIVITY Antiepileptic hypersensitivity syndrome associated with phenobarbital. See under Epilepsy p. 279 for more information.

● PREGNANCY

Monitoring

The dose should be monitored carefully during pregnancy and after birth, and adjustments made on a clinical basis.

● BREAST FEEDING Avoid if possible; drowsiness may occur.

● HEPATIC IMPAIRMENT May precipitate coma. Avoid in severe impairment.

● RENAL IMPAIRMENT Use with caution.

● MONITORING REQUIREMENTS

▸ Plasma-phenobarbital concentration for optimum response is 15–40 mg/litre (60–180 micromol/litre); however, monitoring the plasma-drug concentration is less useful than with other drugs because tolerance occurs.

● TREATMENT CESSATION Avoid abrupt withdrawal (dependence with prolonged use).

● DIRECTIONS FOR ADMINISTRATION

▸ With oral use For administration by *mouth*, tablets may be crushed.

▸ With intravenous use in adults Solution for injection must be diluted before intravenous administration.

▸ With intravenous use in children For *intravenous injection*, dilute to a concentration of 20 mg/mL with Water for Injections; give over 20 minutes (no faster than 1 mg/kg/minute).

● PRESCRIBING AND DISPENSING INFORMATION

Some hospitals supply **alcohol-free** formulations of varying phenobarbital strengths.

Switching between formulations Different formulations of oral preparations may vary in bioavailability. Patients should be maintained on a specific manufacturer's product.

● PATIENT AND CARER ADVICE

Medicines for Children leaflet: Phenobarbital for preventing seizures www.medicinesforchildren.org.uk/phenobarbital-for-preventing-seizures

● MEDICINAL FORMS

There can be variation in the licensing of different medicines containing the same drug. Forms available from special-order manufacturers include: tablet, capsule, oral suspension, oral solution

Tablet

CAUTIONARY AND ADVISORY LABELS 2, 8

▸ Phenobarbital (Non-proprietary)

Phenobarbital 15 mg Phenobarbital 15mg tablets | 28 tablet PoM £24.95 DT price = £22.14 CD3

Phenobarbital 30 mg Phenobarbital 30mg tablets | 28 tablet PoM £5.99 DT price = £0.79 CD3

Phenobarbital 60 mg Phenobarbital 60mg tablets | 28 tablet PoM £7.99 DT price = £6.07 CD3

Oral solution

CAUTIONARY AND ADVISORY LABELS 2, 8

▸ Phenobarbital (Non-proprietary)

Phenobarbital 3 mg per 1 ml Phenobarbital 15mg/5ml elixir | 500 ml PoM £83.00 DT price = £83.00 CD3

Solution for injection

EXCIPIENTS: May contain Propylene glycol

▸ Phenobarbital (Non-proprietary)

Phenobarbital sodium 15 mg per 1 ml Phenobarbital 15mg/1ml solution for injection ampoules | 10 ampoule PoM £19.68 CD3

Phenobarbital sodium 30 mg per 1 ml Phenobarbital 30mg/1ml solution for injection ampoules | 10 ampoule PoM £69.88–£76.87 CD3

Phenobarbital sodium 60 mg per 1 ml Phenobarbital 60mg/1ml solution for injection ampoules | 10 ampoule PoM £81.73 CD3

Phenobarbital sodium 200 mg per 1 ml Phenobarbital 200mg/1ml solution for injection ampoules | 10 ampoule PoM £60.57–£66.63 CD3

Primidone

● INDICATIONS AND DOSE

All forms of epilepsy except typical absence seizures

▸ BY MOUTH

▸ Child 1 month-1 year: Initially 125 mg daily, dose to be taken at bedtime, then increased in steps of 125 mg every 3 days, adjusted according to response; maintenance 125–250 mg twice daily

▸ Child 2-4 years: Initially 125 mg once daily, dose to be taken at bedtime, then increased in steps of 125 mg every 3 days, adjusted according to response; maintenance 250–375 mg twice daily

▸ Child 5-8 years: Initially 125 mg once daily, dose to be taken at bedtime, then increased in steps of 125 mg every 3 days, adjusted according to response; maintenance 375–500 mg twice daily

▸ Child 9-17 years: Initially 125 mg once daily, dose to be taken at bedtime, then increased in steps of 125 mg every 3 days, increased to 250 mg twice daily, then increased in steps of 250 mg every 3 days (max. per dose 750 mg twice daily), adjusted according to response

▸ Adult: Initially 125 mg once daily, dose to be taken at bedtime, then increased in steps of 125 mg every 3 days, increased to 500 mg daily in 2 divided doses, then increased in steps of 250 mg every 3 days, adjusted according to response; maintenance 0.75–1.5 g daily in 2 divided doses

Essential tremor

▸ BY MOUTH

▸ Adult: Initially 50 mg daily, then adjusted according to response to up to 750 mg daily, dose to be increased over 2–3 weeks

● CAUTIONS Avoid in acute porphyria · children · debilitated · elderly (in adults) · history of alcohol abuse · history of drug abuse · respiratory depression (avoid if severe)

4

Nervous system

Nervous system

4

CAUTIONS, FURTHER INFORMATION
Consider vitamin D supplementation in patients who are immobilised for long periods or who have inadequate sun exposure or dietary intake of calcium.

● INTERACTIONS → Appendix 1 (primidone).

● SIDE-EFFECTS
▸ **Common or very common** Agranulocytosis · allergic skin reactions · ataxia · behavioural disturbances · cholestasis · depression · drowsiness · hallucinations · hepatitis · hyperactivity (in children) · hyperactivity particularly in the elderly (in adults) · hypotension · impaired cognition · impaired memory · irritability · lethargy · megaloblastic anaemia (may be treated with folic acid) · nausea · nystagmus · osteomalacia · paradoxical excitement (in adults) · respiratory depression · thrombocytopenia · visual disturbances
▸ **Uncommon** Dizziness · headache · vomiting
▸ **Rare** Arthralgia · lupus erythematosus · psychosis
▸ **Very rare** Antiepileptic Hypersensitivity Syndrome · Stevens-Johnson syndrome · suicidal ideation · toxic epidermal necrolysis
▸ **Frequency not known** Dupuytren's contracture
● ALLERGY AND CROSS-SENSITIVITY Antiepileptic hypersensitivity syndrome associated with primidone. See under Epilepsy p. 279 for more information.
● PREGNANCY
Monitoring
The dose should be monitored carefully during pregnancy and after birth, and adjustments made on a clinical basis.
● HEPATIC IMPAIRMENT Reduce dose. May precipitate coma.
● RENAL IMPAIRMENT Use with caution.
● MONITORING REQUIREMENTS
▸ Monitor plasma concentrations of derived phenobarbital; plasma concentration for optimum response is 15–40 mg/litre (60–180 micromol/litre).
● TREATMENT CESSATION Avoid abrupt withdrawal (dependence with prolonged use).
● PRESCRIBING AND DISPENSING INFORMATION
Switching between formulations Different formulations of oral preparations may vary in bioavailability. Patients being treated for epilepsy should be maintained on a specific manufacturer's product.

● MEDICINAL FORMS
There can be variation in the licensing of different medicines containing the same drug. Forms available from special-order manufacturers include: capsule, oral suspension
Tablet
CAUTIONARY AND ADVISORY LABELS 2, 8
▸ Primidone (Non-proprietary)
Primidone 50 mg Primidone 50mg tablets | 100 tablet [PoM] £95.65–£112.37 DT price = £104.54
Primidone 250 mg Primidone 250mg tablets | 90 tablet [PoM] no price available | 100 tablet [PoM] £99.65–£121.94 DT price = £112.59
Oral suspension
▸ Primidone (Non-proprietary)
Primidone 25 mg per 1 ml Liskantin Saft 125mg/5ml oral suspension | 250 ml [PoM] no price available

HYPNOTICS, SEDATIVES AND ANXIOLYTICS > BENZODIAZEPINES

◤ 312

Clobazam

● INDICATIONS AND DOSE
Adjunct in epilepsy
▸ BY MOUTH
▸ Child 6-17 years: Initially 5 mg daily, dose to be increased if necessary at intervals of 5 days, maintenance 0.3–1 mg/kg daily, daily doses of up to

30 mg may be given as a single dose at bedtime, higher doses should be divided; maximum 60 mg per day
▸ Adult: 20–30 mg daily, then increased if necessary up to 60 mg daily

Anxiety (short-term use)
▸ BY MOUTH
▸ Adult: 20–30 mg daily in divided doses, alternatively 20–30 mg once daily, dose to be taken at bedtime; increased if necessary up to 60 mg daily in divided doses, dose only increased in severe anxiety (in hospital patients), for debilitated patients, use elderly dose
▸ Elderly: 10–20 mg daily

● UNLICENSED USE Not licensed for use in children under 6 years.
● CONTRA-INDICATIONS Chronic psychosis (in adults) · hyperkinesis · not for use alone to treat anxiety associated with depression (in adults) · obsessional states · phobic states · respiratory depression
● CAUTIONS Muscle weakness · organic brain changes · personality disorder (within the fearful group—dependent, avoidant, obsessive-compulsive) may increase risk of dependence
CAUTIONS, FURTHER INFORMATION
The effectiveness of clobazam may decrease significantly after weeks or months of continuous therapy.
● SIDE-EFFECTS
▸ **Common or very common** Amnesia · ataxia (especially in the elderly) · confusion (especially in the elderly) · dependence · drowsiness the next day · lightheadedness the next day · muscle weakness · paradoxical increase in aggression
▸ **Uncommon** Changes in libido (in adults) · dizziness · dysarthria · gastro-intestinal disturbances · gynaecomastia · headache (in adults) · hypotension (in adults) · incontinence · salivation changes · slurred speech (in adults) · tremor · urinary retention (in adults) · vertigo (in adults) · visual disturbances
▸ **Rare** Apnoea · blood disorders · changes in libido (in children) · headache (in children) · hypotension (in children) · jaundice · respiratory depression · skin reactions · urinary retention (in children) · vertigo (in children)
▸ **Frequency not known** Delusions (in children) · excitement (in children) · hallucinations (in children) · irritability (in children) · psychosis (in children) · restlessness (in children)
● BREAST FEEDING Benzodiazepines are present in milk, and should be avoided if possible during breast-feeding.
 All infants should be monitored for sedation, feeding difficulties, adequate weight gain, and developmental milestones.
● HEPATIC IMPAIRMENT Start with smaller initial doses or reduce dose. Can precipitate coma. Avoid in severe impairment.
● RENAL IMPAIRMENT Start with small doses in severe impairment.
● MONITORING REQUIREMENTS
▸ In children Routine measurement of plasma concentrations of antiepileptic drugs is not usually justified, because the target concentration ranges are arbitrary and often vary between individuals. However, plasma drug concentrations may be measured in children with worsening seizures, status epilepticus, suspected noncompliance, or suspected toxicity. Similarly, haematological and biochemical monitoring should not be undertaken unless clinically indicated.
● PRESCRIBING AND DISPENSING INFORMATION
Switching between formulations Care should be taken when switching between oral formulations in the treatment of

epilepsy. The need for continued supply of a particular manufacturer's product should be based on clinical judgement and consultation with the patient or their carer, taking into account factors such as seizure frequency and treatment history.

Patients being treated for epilepsy may need to be maintained on a specific manufacturer's branded or generic clobazam product.

● PATIENT AND CARER ADVICE
Medicines for Children leaflet: Clobazam for preventing seizures www.medicinesforchildren.org.uk/clobazam-preventing-seizures-0

● NATIONAL FUNDING/ACCESS DECISIONS
NHS restrictions Clobazam is not prescribable under the NHS except for epilepsy and endorsed 'SLS'.

● MEDICINAL FORMS
There can be variation in the licensing of different medicines containing the same drug. Forms available from special-order manufacturers include: capsule, oral suspension

Tablet
CAUTIONARY AND ADVISORY LABELS 2, 19, 8
▸ Clobazam (Non-proprietary)
  Clobazam 10 mg Clobazam 10mg tablets | 30 tablet [PoM] £3.59 DT price = £3.29 [CD4-1]
▸ Frisium (Sanofi)
  Clobazam 10 mg Frisium 10mg tablets | 30 tablet [PoM] £2.51 DT price = £3.29 [CD4-1]

Oral suspension
CAUTIONARY AND ADVISORY LABELS 2, 19, 8
▸ Clobazam (Non-proprietary)
  Clobazam 1 mg per 1 ml Clobazam 5mg/5ml oral suspension sugar free sugar-free | 150 ml [PoM] £90.00 DT price = £90.00 [CD4-1] sugar-free | 250 ml [PoM] £150.00 [CD4-1]
  Clobazam 2 mg per 1 ml Clobazam 10mg/5ml oral suspension sugar free sugar-free | 150 ml [PoM] £95.00–£97.50 DT price = £95.00 [CD4-1] sugar-free | 250 ml [PoM] £162.50 [CD4-1]
▸ Perizam (Rosemont Pharmaceuticals Ltd)
  Clobazam 1 mg per 1 ml Perizam 1mg/ml oral suspension sugar-free | 150 ml [PoM] £90.00 DT price = £90.00 [CD4-1]
  Clobazam 2 mg per 1 ml Perizam 2mg/ml oral suspension sugar-free | 150 ml [PoM] £95.00 DT price = £95.00 [CD4-1]
▸ Tapclob (Martindale Pharmaceuticals Ltd)
  Clobazam 1 mg per 1 ml Tapclob 5mg/5ml oral suspension sugar-free | 150 ml [PoM] £90.00 DT price = £90.00 [CD4-1] sugar-free | 250 ml [PoM] £150.00 [CD4-1]
  Clobazam 2 mg per 1 ml Tapclob 10mg/5ml oral suspension sugar-free | 150 ml [PoM] £95.00 DT price = £95.00 [CD4-1] sugar-free | 250 ml [PoM] £158.34 [CD4-1]

▶ 312

Clonazepam

● INDICATIONS AND DOSE
All forms of epilepsy
▸ BY MOUTH
▸ **Child 1-11 months:** Initially 250 micrograms once daily for 4 nights, dose to be increased over 2–4 weeks, usual dose 0.5–1 mg daily, dose to be taken at night; may be given in 3 divided doses if necessary
▸ **Child 1-4 years:** Initially 250 micrograms once daily for 4 nights, dose to be increased over 2–4 weeks, usual dose 1–3 mg daily, dose to be taken at night; may be given in 3 divided doses if necessary
▸ **Child 5-11 years:** Initially 500 micrograms once daily for 4 nights, dose to be increased over 2–4 weeks, usual dose 3–6 mg daily, dose to be taken at night; may be given in 3 divided doses if necessary
▸ **Child 12-17 years:** Initially 1 mg once daily for 4 nights, dose to be increased over 2–4 weeks, usual dose 4–8 mg daily, dose usually taken at night; may be given in 3–4 divided doses if necessary

All forms of epilepsy | Myoclonus
▸ BY MOUTH
▸ **Adult:** Initially 1 mg once daily for 4 nights, dose to be increased over 2–4 weeks, usual dose 4–8 mg daily, adjusted according to response, dose usually taken at night; may be given in 3–4 divided doses if necessary
▸ **Elderly:** Initially 500 micrograms once daily for 4 nights, dose to be increased over 2–4 weeks, usual dose 4–8 mg daily, adjusted according to response, dose usually taken at night; may be given in 3–4 divided doses if necessary

Panic disorders (with or without agoraphobia) resistant to antidepressant therapy
▸ BY MOUTH
▸ **Adult:** 1–2 mg daily

● UNLICENSED USE Clonazepam doses in BNF may differ from those in product literature. Use for panic disorders (with or without agoraphobia) resistant to antidepressant therapy is an unlicensed indication.

● CONTRA-INDICATIONS Coma · current alcohol abuse · current drug abuse · respiratory depression

● CAUTIONS Acute porphyrias p. 918 · airways obstruction · brain damage · cerebellar ataxia · depression · spinal ataxia · suicidal ideation
CAUTIONS, FURTHER INFORMATION
The effectiveness of clonazepam may decrease significantly after weeks or months of continuous therapy.

● SIDE-EFFECTS
▸ **Common or very common** Amnesia · bronchial hypersecretion in infants and small children · co-ordination disturbances · confusion · dependence · dizziness · drowsiness · fatigue · muscle hypotonia · nystagmus · poor concentration · restlessness · salivary hypersecretion in infants and small children · withdrawal symptoms (in children)
▸ **Rare** Aggression · anxiety · blood disorders · dysarthria · gastro-intestinal symptoms · headache · paradoxical effects · pruritus · respiratory depression · reversible hair loss · sexual dysfunction · skin pigmentation changes · suicidal ideation (in adults) · urinary incontinence · urticaria · visual disturbances on long-term treatment
▸ **Very rare** Increase in seizure frequency

● BREAST FEEDING Present in milk, and should be avoided if possible during breast-feeding.
  All infants should be monitored for sedation, feeding difficulties, adequate weight gain, and developmental milestones.

● HEPATIC IMPAIRMENT Start with smaller initial doses or reduce dose. Can precipitate coma. Avoid in severe impairment.

● RENAL IMPAIRMENT Start with small doses in severe impairment.

● MONITORING REQUIREMENTS
▸ In children Routine measurement of plasma concentrations of antiepileptic drugs is not usually justified, because the target concentration ranges are arbitrary and often vary between individuals. However, plasma drug concentrations may be measured in children with worsening seizures, status epilepticus, suspected noncompliance, or suspected toxicity. Similarly, haematological and biochemical monitoring should not be undertaken unless clinically indicated.

● PRESCRIBING AND DISPENSING INFORMATION
Switching between formulations Care should be taken when switching between oral formulations in the treatment of epilepsy. The need for continued supply of a particular manufacturer's product should be based on clinical judgement and consultation with the patient or their carer, taking into account factors such as seizure frequency and treatment history.

Patients being treated for epilepsy may need to be maintained on a specific manufacturer's branded or generic oral clonazepam product.

● PATIENT AND CARER ADVICE
Medicines for Children leaflet: Clonazepam for preventing seizures www.medicinesforchildren.org.uk/clonazepam-preventing-seizures-0

● MEDICINAL FORMS
There can be variation in the licensing of different medicines containing the same drug. Forms available from special-order manufacturers include: orodispersible tablet, oral suspension, oral solution, oral drops

Tablet
CAUTIONARY AND ADVISORY LABELS 2, 8
▸ Clonazepam (Non-proprietary)
Clonazepam 500 microgram Clonazepam 500microgram tablets | 100 tablet PoM £30.11 DT price = £24.95 CD4-1
Clonazepam 2 mg Clonazepam 2mg tablets | 100 tablet PoM £33.41 DT price = £27.69 CD4-1

Oral solution
CAUTIONARY AND ADVISORY LABELS 2, 8
EXCIPIENTS: May contain Ethanol
▸ Clonazepam (Non-proprietary)
Clonazepam 100 microgram per 1 ml Clonazepam 500micrograms/5ml oral solution sugar free sugar-free | 150 ml PoM £83.40 DT price = £69.50 CD4-1
Clonazepam 400 microgram per 1 ml Clonazepam 2mg/5ml oral solution sugar free sugar-free | 150 ml PoM £108.36 DT price = £108.36 CD4-1

Oral drops
▸ Clonazepam (Non-proprietary)
Clonazepam 2.5 mg per 1 ml Rivotril 2.5mg/1ml drops sugar-free | 10 ml PoM no price available CD4-1

Oral lyophilisate
▸ Clonazepam (Non-proprietary)
Clonazepam 500 microgram Klonopin 0.5mg oral lyophilisates sugar-free | 60 tablet PoM no price available CD4-1

2.1 Status epilepticus

Drugs used for status epilepticus not listed below
Fosphenytoin sodium p. 286 · Phenobarbital p. 304 · Phenytoin p. 294

ANTIEPILEPTICS 〉 BARBITURATES

Thiopental sodium

(Thiopentone sodium)

● INDICATIONS AND DOSE
Status epilepticus (only if other measures fail)
▸ BY SLOW INTRAVENOUS INJECTION
▸ Adult: 75–125 mg for 1 dose, to be administered as a 2.5% (25 mg/mL) solution
Induction of anaesthesia
▸ BY SLOW INTRAVENOUS INJECTION
▸ Adult: Initially 100–150 mg, to be administered over 10–15 seconds usually as a 2.5% (25 mg/mL) solution, followed by 100–150 mg after 0.5–1 minute if required, dose to be given in fit and premedicated adults; debilitated patients or adults over 65 years may require a lower dose or increased administration time, alternatively initially up to 4 mg/kg (max. per dose 500 mg)
Anaesthesia of short duration
▸ BY SLOW INTRAVENOUS INJECTION
▸ Adult: Initially 100–150 mg, to be administered over 10–15 seconds usually as a 2.5% (25 mg/mL) solution, followed by 100–150 mg after 0.5–1 minute if required,

dose to be given in fit and premedicated adults; debilitated patients or adults over 65 years may require a lower dose or increased administration time, alternatively initially up to 4 mg/kg (max. per dose 500 mg)
Reduction of raised intracranial pressure if ventilation controlled
▸ BY SLOW INTRAVENOUS INJECTION
▸ Adult: 1.5–3 mg/kg, repeated if necessary

IMPORTANT SAFETY INFORMATION
Thiopental sodium should only be administered by, or under the direct supervision of, personnel experienced in its use, with adequate training in anaesthesia and airway management, and when resuscitation equipment is available.

● CONTRA-INDICATIONS Acute porphyrias p. 918 · myotonic dystrophy
● CAUTIONS Acute circulatory failure (shock) · avoid intra-arterial injection · cardiovascular disease · elderly · fixed cardiac output · hypovolaemia · reconstituted solution is highly alkaline (extravasation causes tissue necrosis and severe pain)
● INTERACTIONS → Appendix 1 (anaesthetics, general).
● SIDE-EFFECTS Arrhythmias · cough · headache · hypersensitivity reactions · hypotension · laryngeal spasm · myocardial depression · rash · sneezing
● PREGNANCY May depress neonatal respiration when used during delivery.
● BREAST FEEDING Breast-feeding can be resumed as soon as mother has recovered sufficiently from anaesthesia.
● HEPATIC IMPAIRMENT Use with caution—reduce dose.
● RENAL IMPAIRMENT Caution in severe impairment.
● PATIENT AND CARER ADVICE
Driving and skilled tasks
Patients given sedatives and analgesics during minor outpatient procedures should be very carefully warned about the risk of driving or undertaking skilled tasks afterwards. For a short general anaesthetic the risk extends to **at least 24 hours** after administration. Responsible persons should be available to take patients home. The dangers of taking **alcohol** should also be emphasised.

● MEDICINAL FORMS
There can be variation in the licensing of different medicines containing the same drug. Forms available from special-order manufacturers include: solution for injection
Powder for solution for injection
▸ Thiopental sodium (Non-proprietary)
Thiopental sodium 500 mg Thiopental 500mg powder for solution for injection vials | 25 vial PoM £172.50

HYPNOTICS, SEDATIVES AND ANXIOLYTICS 〉 BENZODIAZEPINES

▶ 312

Lorazepam

● INDICATIONS AND DOSE
Short-term use in anxiety
▸ BY MOUTH
▸ Adult: 1–4 mg daily in divided doses, for debilitated patients, use elderly dose
▸ Elderly: 0.5–2 mg daily in divided doses
Short-term use in insomnia associated with anxiety
▸ BY MOUTH
▸ Adult: 1–2 mg daily, to be taken at bedtime

Acute panic attacks

▶ BY INTRAMUSCULAR INJECTION, OR BY SLOW INTRAVENOUS INJECTION
▶ Adult: 25–30 micrograms/kg every 6 hours if required; usual dose 1.5–2.5 mg every 6 hours if required, intravenous injection to be administered into a large vein, only use intramuscular route when oral and intravenous routes not possible

Conscious sedation for procedures

▶ BY MOUTH
▶ Adult: 2–3 mg, to be taken the night before operation; 2–4 mg, to be taken 1–2 hours before operation
▶ BY SLOW INTRAVENOUS INJECTION
▶ Adult: 50 micrograms/kg, to be administered 30–45 minutes before operation
▶ BY INTRAMUSCULAR INJECTION
▶ Adult: 50 micrograms/kg, to be administered 60–90 minutes before operation

Premedication

▶ BY MOUTH
▶ Adult: 2–3 mg, to be taken the night before operation; 2–4 mg, to be taken 1–2 hours before operation
▶ BY SLOW INTRAVENOUS INJECTION
▶ Adult: 50 micrograms/kg, to be administered 30–45 minutes before operation
▶ BY INTRAMUSCULAR INJECTION
▶ Adult: 50 micrograms/kg, to be administered 60–90 minutes before operation

Status epilepticus | Febrile convulsions | Convulsions caused by poisoning

▶ BY SLOW INTRAVENOUS INJECTION
▶ Child 1 month–11 years: 100 micrograms/kg (max. per dose 4 mg) for 1 dose, then 100 micrograms/kg after 10 minutes (max. per dose 4 mg) if required for 1 dose, to be administered into a large vein
▶ Child 12–17 years: 4 mg for 1 dose, then 4 mg after 10 minutes if required for 1 dose, to be administered into a large vein
▶ Adult: 4 mg for 1 dose, then 4 mg after 10 minutes if required for 1 dose, to be administered into a large vein

● UNLICENSED USE
▶ In children Not licensed for use in febrile convulsions. Not licensed for use in convulsions caused by poisoning.

> IMPORTANT SAFETY INFORMATION
> ANAESTHESIA
> Benzodiazepines should only be administered for anaesthesia by, or under the direct supervision of, personnel experienced in their use, with adequate training in anaesthesia and airway management.

● CONTRA-INDICATIONS Avoid injections containing benzyl alcohol in neonates · chronic psychosis (in adults) · CNS depression · compromised airway · hyperkinesis · not for use alone to treat depression (or anxiety associated with depression) (in adults) · obsessional states · phobic states · respiratory depression
● CAUTIONS Personality disorder (within the fearful group—dependent, avoidant, obsessive-compulsive) may increase risk of dependence · muscle weakness · organic brain changes · parenteral administration
CAUTIONS, FURTHER INFORMATION
▶ Paradoxical effects A paradoxical increase in hostility and aggression may be reported by patients taking benzodiazepines. The effects range from talkativeness and excitement to aggressive and antisocial acts. Adjustment of the dose (up or down) sometimes attenuates the impulses. Increased anxiety and perceptual disorders are other paradoxical effects.

▶ Special precautions for parenteral administration
▶ With intramuscular use or intravenous use When given parenterally, facilities for managing respiratory depression with mechanical ventilation must be available. Close observation required until full recovery from sedation.
● SIDE-EFFECTS
▶ **Common or very common** Amnesia · ataxia (in children) · ataxia (especially in the elderly) (in adults) · confusion (in children) · confusion (especially in the elderly) (in adults) · dependence · drowsiness the next day · lightheadedness the next day · muscle weakness · paradoxical increase in aggression
▶ **Uncommon** Changes in libido (in adults) · dizziness · dysarthria · gastro-intestinal disturbances · gynaecomastia · headache (in adults) · hypotension (in adults) · incontinence · salivation changes · slurred speech (in adults) · tremor · urinary retention (in adults) · vertigo (in adults) · visual disturbances
▶ **Rare** Apnoea · blood disorders · changes in libido (in children) · headache (in children) · hypotension (in children) · jaundice · respiratory depression · skin reactions · urinary retention (in children) · vertigo (in children)
▶ **Frequency not known** Delusions (in children) · excitement (in children) · hallucinations (in children) · irritability (in children) · marked respiratory depression, particularly with high dose and intravenous use (facilities for its treatment are essential) · pain (on intravenous injection) · psychosis (in children) · restlessness (in children) · thrombophlebitis (on intravenous injection)
● BREAST FEEDING Benzodiazepines are present in milk, and should be avoided if possible during breast-feeding.
● HEPATIC IMPAIRMENT Start with smaller initial doses or reduce dose. Can precipitate coma. Avoid in severe impairment.
▶ In adults If treatment is necessary, benzodiazepines with shorter half-lives are safer.
● RENAL IMPAIRMENT Start with small doses in severe impairment.
● DIRECTIONS FOR ADMINISTRATION
▶ With intravenous use in children For *intravenous injection*, dilute with an equal volume of Sodium Chloride 0.9% (for neonates, dilute injection solution to a concentration of 100 micrograms/mL). Give over 3–5 minutes; max. rate 50 micrograms/kg over 3 minutes.
▶ With intramuscular use in adults For intramuscular injection, solution for injection should be diluted with an equal volume of water for injections or sodium chloride 0.9% (but only use when oral and intravenous routes not possible).
▶ With intravenous use in adults For slow intravenous injection, solution for injection should be diluted with an equal volume of water for injections or sodium chloride 0.9%.
● PATIENT AND CARER ADVICE
Driving and skilled tasks
May impair judgement and increase reaction time, and so affect ability to drive or operate machinery; they increase the effects of alcohol. Moreover the hangover effects of a night dose may impair driving on the following day.
   Patients given sedatives and analgesics during minor outpatient procedures should be very carefully warned about the risks of undertaking skilled tasks (e.g. driving) afterwards. For intravenous benzodiazepines the risk extends to **at least 24 hours** after administration. Responsible persons should be available to take patients home afterwards. The dangers of taking **alcohol** should be emphasised.

● MEDICINAL FORMS
There can be variation in the licensing of different medicines
containing the same drug. Forms available from special-order
manufacturers include: oral suspension, oral solution, solution
for injection

Tablet
CAUTIONARY AND ADVISORY LABELS 2, 19
▸ Lorazepam (Non-proprietary)
Lorazepam 1 mg Lorazepam 1mg tablets | 28 tablet PoM £12.21
DT price = £2.02 CD4-1 | 30 tablet PoM no price available CD4-1
Lorazepam 2.5 mg Lorazepam 2.5mg tablets | 28 tablet PoM
£12.50 DT price = £2.90 CD4-1 | 30 tablet PoM no price
available CD4-1

Solution for injection
EXCIPIENTS: May contain Benzyl alcohol, propylene glycol
▸ Ativan (Pfizer Ltd)
Lorazepam 4 mg per 1 ml Ativan 4mg/1ml solution for injection
ampoules | 10 ampoule PoM £3.54 CD4-1

⬛ 312

Midazolam

● INDICATIONS AND DOSE

Status epilepticus | Febrile convulsions
▸ BY BUCCAL ADMINISTRATION
▸ Child 1-2 months: 300 micrograms/kg (max. per dose
2.5 mg), then 300 micrograms/kg after 10 minutes
(max. per dose 2.5 mg) if required
▸ Child 3-11 months: 2.5 mg, then 2.5 mg after 10 minutes
if required
▸ Child 1-4 years: 5 mg, then 5 mg after 10 minutes if
required
▸ Child 5-9 years: 7.5 mg, then 7.5 mg after 10 minutes if
required
▸ Child 10-17 years: 10 mg, then 10 mg after 10 minutes if
required
▸ Adult: 10 mg, then 10 mg after 10 minutes if required

Conscious sedation for procedures
▸ BY SLOW INTRAVENOUS INJECTION
▸ Adult: Initially 2–2.5 mg, to be administered
5–10 minutes before procedure at a rate of
approximately 2 mg/minute, increased in steps of 1 mg
if required, usual total dose is 3.5–5 mg; maximum
7.5 mg per course
▸ Elderly: Initially 0.5–1 mg, to be administered
5–10 minutes before procedure at a rate of
approximately 2 mg/minute, increased in steps of
0.5–1 mg if required; maximum 3.5 mg per course

Sedative in combined anaesthesia
▸ INITIALLY BY INTRAVENOUS INJECTION
▸ Adult: 30–100 micrograms/kg, repeated if necessary,
alternatively (by continuous intravenous infusion)
30–100 micrograms/kg/hour
▸ Elderly: Lower doses needed

Premedication
▸ BY DEEP INTRAMUSCULAR INJECTION
▸ Adult: 70–100 micrograms/kg, to be administered
20–60 minutes before induction, for debilitated
patients, use elderly dose
▸ Elderly: 25–50 micrograms/kg, to be administered
20–60 minutes before induction
▸ BY INTRAVENOUS INJECTION
▸ Adult: 1–2 mg, repeated if necessary, to be
administered 5–30 minutes before procedure, for
debilitated patients, use elderly dose
▸ Elderly: 0.5 mg, repeated if necessary, initial dose to be
administered 5–30 minutes before procedure, repeat
dose slowly as required

Induction of anaesthesia (but rarely used)
▸ BY SLOW INTRAVENOUS INJECTION
▸ Adult: 150–200 micrograms/kg daily in divided doses
(max. per dose 5 mg), dose to be given at intervals of

2 minutes, maximum total dose 600 micrograms/kg, for
debilitated patients, use elderly dose
▸ Elderly: 50–150 micrograms/kg daily in divided doses
(max. per dose 5 mg), dose to be given at intervals of
2 minutes, maximum total dose 600 micrograms/kg

Sedation of patient receiving intensive care
▸ INITIALLY BY SLOW INTRAVENOUS INJECTION
▸ Adult: Initially 30–300 micrograms/kg, dose to be given
in steps of 1–2.5 mg every 2 minutes, then (by slow
intravenous injection or by continuous intravenous
infusion) 30–200 micrograms/kg/hour, reduce dose (or
reduce or omit initial dose) in hypovolaemia,
vasoconstriction, or hypothermia, lower doses may be
adequate if opioid analgesic also used

**Confusion and restlessness in palliative care (adjunct to
antipsychotic)**
▸ BY SUBCUTANEOUS INFUSION
▸ Adult: Initially 10–20 mg/24 hours, adjusted according
to response; usual dose 20–60 mg/24 hours

Convulsions in palliative care
▸ BY CONTINUOUS SUBCUTANEOUS INFUSION
▸ Adult: Initially 20–40 mg/24 hours

● UNLICENSED USE Oromucosal solution not licensed for use
in children under 3 months. Oromucosal solution not
licensed for use in adults over 18 years. Unlicensed
oromucosal formulations are also available and may have
different doses—refer to product literature.

> IMPORTANT SAFETY INFORMATION
> ANAESTHESIA
> Benzodiazepines should only be administered for
> anaesthesia by, or under the direct supervision of,
> personnel experienced in their use, with adequate
> training in anaesthesia and airway management.
>
> PRESCRIBING OF MIDAZOLAM IN PALLIATIVE CARE
> The use of high-strength midazolam (5 mg/mL in 2 mL
> and 10 mL ampoules, or 2 mg/mL in 5 mL ampoules)
> should be considered in palliative care and other
> situations where a higher strength may be more
> appropriate to administer the prescribed dose, and
> where the risk of overdosage has been assessed. It is
> advised that flumazenil is available when midazolam is
> used, to reverse the effects if necessary.

● CONTRA-INDICATIONS CNS depression · compromised
airway · severe respiratory depression
● CAUTIONS Cardiac disease · children (particularly if
cardiovascular impairment) · concentration of midazolam
in children under 15 kg not to exceed 1 mg/mL · debilitated
patients (reduce dose) (in children) · hypothermia ·
hypovolaemia (risk of severe hypotension) · neonates · risk
of airways obstruction and hypoventilation in children
under 6 months (monitor respiratory rate and oxygen
saturation) · vasoconstriction
CAUTIONS, FURTHER INFORMATION
▸ Recovery when used for sedation Midazolam has a fast onset
of action, recovery is faster than for other benzodiazepines
such as diazepam, but may be significantly longer in the
elderly, in patients with a low cardiac output, or after
repeated dosing.
● SIDE-EFFECTS Amnesia · anaphylaxis · ataxia · blood
disorders · bronchospasm · cardiac arrest · changes in libido
(in adults) · confusion · convulsions (more common in
neonates) · depression of consciousness · dizziness ·
drowsiness · dry mouth · dysarthria · euphoria · fatigue (in
children) · gastro-intestinal disturbances · hallucinations ·
headache · heart rate changes · hiccups · hypotension ·
incontinence · increased appetite · injection-site reactions
· involuntary movements · jaundice · laryngospasm ·
muscle weakness · paradoxical aggression (especially in

children and elderly) · paradoxical excitement (especially in children and elderly) · respiratory arrest (particularly with high doses or on rapid injection) · respiratory depression (may be severe with sedative and peri-operative use—facilities for its treatment are essential) · respiratory depression (particularly with high doses or on rapid injection) · restlessness (with sedative and peri-operative use) (in children) · salivation changes · severe disinhibition (with sedative and peri-operative use) (in children) · skin reactions · thrombosis · urinary retention · vertigo · visual disturbances

SIDE-EFFECTS, FURTHER INFORMATION

▸ **Sedation** Midazolam is associated with profound sedation when high doses are given or when it is used with certain other drugs.

Overdose

There have been reports of overdosage when high strength midazolam has been used for conscious sedation. The use of high-strength midazolam (5 mg/mL in 2 mL and 10 mL ampoules, or 2 mg/mL in 5 mL ampoules) should be restricted to general anaesthesia, intensive care, palliative care, or other situations where the risk has been assessed. It is advised that flumazenil is available when midazolam is used, to reverse the effects if necessary.

● BREAST FEEDING Small amount present in milk—avoid breast-feeding for 24 hours after administration (although amount probably too small to be harmful after single doses).

● HEPATIC IMPAIRMENT Use with caution particularly in sedative doses; can precipitate coma. For status epilepticus and febrile convulsions: use with caution in mild to moderate impairment; avoid in severe impairment.

● RENAL IMPAIRMENT Use with caution in chronic renal failure.

● DIRECTIONS FOR ADMINISTRATION For *intravenous infusion* (*Hypnovel*®), give continuously *in* Glucose 5% *or* Sodium chloride 0.9%.

● PATIENT AND CARER ADVICE
Patients or carers should be given advice on how to administer midazolam oromucosal solution.

Patients given sedatives and analgesics during minor outpatient procedures should be very carefully warned about the risks of undertaking skilled tasks (e.g. driving) afterwards. For intravenous benzodiazepines the risk extends to **at least 24 hours** after administration. Responsible persons should be available to take patients home afterwards. The dangers of taking **alcohol** should be emphasised.
Medicines for Children leaflet: Midazolam for stopping seizures www.medicinesforchildren.org.uk/midazolam-for-stopping-seizures

● MEDICINAL FORMS
There can be variation in the licensing of different medicines containing the same drug. Forms available from special-order manufacturers include: oromucosal solution, solution for injection, infusion, solution for infusion

Tablet
▸ Midazolam (Non-proprietary)
Midazolam maleate 7.5 mg Dormicum 7.5mg tablets | 30 tablet PoM no price available CD3
Midazolam maleate 15 mg Dormicum 15mg tablets | 30 tablet PoM no price available CD3

Oral solution
▸ Midazolam (Non-proprietary)
Midazolam (as Midazolam hydrochloride) 2 mg per 1 ml Midazolam 2mg/ml oral solution sugar free sugar-free | 118 ml PoM no price available CD3

Oromucosal solution
CAUTIONARY AND ADVISORY LABELS 2
▸ Buccolam (Shire Pharmaceuticals Ltd)
Midazolam (as Midazolam hydrochloride) 5 mg per 1 ml Buccolam 7.5mg/1.5ml oromucosal solution pre-filled oral

syringes | 4 unit dose PoM £89.00 CD3 sugar-free | 4 unit dose PoM £89.00 DT price = £89.00 CD3
Buccolam 10mg/2ml oromucosal solution pre-filled oral syringes | 4 unit dose PoM £91.50 CD3 sugar-free | 4 unit dose PoM £91.50 DT price = £91.50 CD3
Buccolam 5mg/1ml oromucosal solution pre-filled oral syringes sugar-free | 4 unit dose PoM £85.50 DT price = £85.50 CD3 | 4 unit dose PoM £85.50 CD3
Buccolam 2.5mg/0.5ml oromucosal solution pre-filled oral syringes | 4 unit dose PoM £82.00 CD3 sugar-free | 4 unit dose PoM £82.00 DT price = £82.00 CD3

Solution for injection
▸ Midazolam (Non-proprietary)
Midazolam (as Midazolam hydrochloride) 1 mg per 1 ml Midazolam 5mg/5ml solution for injection ampoules | 10 ampoule PoM £6.00 CD3
Midazolam 2mg/2ml solution for injection ampoules | 10 ampoule PoM £5.00 CD3
Midazolam (as Midazolam hydrochloride) 2 mg per 1 ml Midazolam 10mg/5ml solution for injection ampoules | 10 ampoule PoM £9.80 CD3 | 10 ampoule PoM no price available (Hospital only) CD3
Midazolam (as Midazolam hydrochloride) 5 mg per 1 ml Midazolam 50mg/10ml solution for injection ampoules | 10 ampoule PoM £78.00 CD3
Midazolam 10mg/2ml solution for injection ampoules | 10 ampoule PoM £7.97 DT price = £6.90 CD3
▸ Hypnovel (Roche Products Ltd)
Midazolam (as Midazolam hydrochloride) 5 mg per 1 ml Hypnovel 10mg/2ml solution for injection ampoules | 10 ampoule PoM £7.11 DT price = £6.90 CD3

Solution for infusion
▸ Midazolam (Non-proprietary)
Midazolam (as Midazolam hydrochloride) 1 mg per 1 ml Midazolam 50mg/50ml solution for infusion vials | 1 vial PoM £9.56–£11.00 CD3
Midazolam (as Midazolam hydrochloride) 2 mg per 1 ml Midazolam 100mg/50ml solution for infusion vials | 1 vial PoM £9.05–£12.50 CD3

3   Mental health disorders

3.1   Anxiety

Drugs used for Anxiety not listed below Duloxetine, p. 336 · Escitalopram, p. 334 · Lorazepam, p. 308 · Moclobemide, p. 331 · Oxprenolol hydrochloride, p. 136 · Paroxetine, p. 335 · Pericyazine, p. 355 · Perphenazine, p. 356 · Pregabalin, p. 295 · Trazodone hydrochloride, p. 338 · Trifluoperazine, p. 358 · Venlafaxine, p. 337

ANTIDEPRESSANTS ⟩ SEROTONIN RECEPTOR AGONISTS

Buspirone hydrochloride

● INDICATIONS AND DOSE

Anxiety (short-term use)
▸ BY MOUTH
▸ Adult: 5 mg 2–3 times a day, increased if necessary up to 45 mg daily, dose to be increased at intervals of 2–3 days; usual dose 15–30 mg daily in divided doses

● CONTRA-INDICATIONS Acute porphyrias p. 918 · epilepsy

● CAUTIONS Does not alleviate symptoms of benzodiazepine withdrawal

CAUTIONS, FURTHER INFORMATION
A patient taking a benzodiazepine still needs to have the benzodiazepine withdrawn gradually; it is advisable to do this before starting buspirone.

● INTERACTIONS → Appendix 1 (anxiolytics and hypnotics).

Nervous system

4

- SIDE-EFFECTS
  - ▶ **Common or very common** Dizziness · excitement · headache · nausea · nervousness
  - ▶ **Rare** Chest pain · confusion · drowsiness · dry mouth · fatigue · palpitation · seizures · sweating · tachycardia
- PREGNANCY Avoid.
- BREAST FEEDING Avoid.
- HEPATIC IMPAIRMENT Reduce dose in mild to moderate disease. Avoid in severe disease.
- RENAL IMPAIRMENT Reduce dose. Avoid if eGFR less than 20 mL/minute/1.73 m².
- PATIENT AND CARER ADVICE

  Driving and skilled tasks
  May affect performance of skilled tasks (e.g. driving); effects of alcohol may be enhanced.

- MEDICINAL FORMS
  There can be variation in the licensing of different medicines containing the same drug. Forms available from special-order manufacturers include: oral suspension, oral solution

  Tablet
  - ▶ Buspirone hydrochloride (Non-proprietary)
    Buspirone hydrochloride 5 mg Buspirone 5mg tablets | 30 tablet (PoM) £13.30 DT price = £4.03
    Buspirone hydrochloride 10 mg Buspirone 10mg tablets | 30 tablet (PoM) £15.62 DT price = £4.92

HYPNOTICS, SEDATIVES AND ANXIOLYTICS ›
BENZODIAZEPINES

Benzodiazepines

- CONTRA-INDICATIONS Acute pulmonary insufficiency · marked neuromuscular respiratory weakness · sleep apnoea syndrome · unstable myasthenia gravis
- CAUTIONS Avoid prolonged use (and abrupt withdrawal thereafter) · debilitated patients (reduce dose) (in adults) · elderly (reduce dose) (in adults) · history of alcohol dependence or abuse · history of drug dependence or abuse · myasthenia gravis · respiratory disease
  CAUTIONS, FURTHER INFORMATION
  - ▶ **Paradoxical effects** A paradoxical increase in hostility and aggression may be reported by patients taking benzodiazepines. The effects range from talkativeness and excitement to aggressive and antisocial acts. Adjustment of the dose (up or down) sometimes attenuates the impulses. Increased anxiety and perceptual disorders are other paradoxical effects.
- INTERACTIONS → Appendix 1 (anxiolytics and hypnotics).
- SIDE-EFFECTS

  Overdose
  Benzodiazepines taken alone cause drowsiness, ataxia, dysarthria, nystagmus, and occasionally respiratory depression, and coma. For details on the management of poisoning, see Benzodiazepines, under Emergency treatment of poisoning p. 1194.

- PREGNANCY Risk of neonatal withdrawal symptoms when used during pregnancy. Avoid regular use and use only if there is a clear indication such as seizure control. High doses administered during late pregnancy or labour may cause neonatal hypothermia, hypotonia, and respiratory depression.
- RENAL IMPAIRMENT Increased cerebral sensitivity to benzodiazepines.
- PATIENT AND CARER ADVICE

  Driving and skilled tasks
  Drowsiness may persist the next day and affect performance of skilled tasks (e.g. driving); effects of alcohol enhanced.

For information on 2015 legislation regarding driving whilst taking certain controlled drugs, including benzodiazepines, see *Drugs and driving* under Guidance on prescribing p. 1.

⌐ above

Alprazolam

- INDICATIONS AND DOSE

  Short-term use in anxiety
  - ▶ BY MOUTH
  - ▶ **Adult:** 250–500 micrograms 3 times a day, increased if necessary up to 3 mg daily, for debilitated patients, use elderly dose
  - ▶ **Elderly:** 250 micrograms 2–3 times a day, increased if necessary up to 3 mg daily

- CONTRA-INDICATIONS Chronic psychosis · hyperkinesis · not for use alone to treat depression (or anxiety associated with depression) · obsessional states · phobic states · respiratory depression
- CAUTIONS Muscle weakness · organic brain changes · personality disorder (within the fearful group—dependent, avoidant, obsessive-compulsive) may increase risk of dependence
- SIDE-EFFECTS
  - ▶ **Common or very common** Amnesia · ataxia (especially in the elderly) · confusion (especially in the elderly) · dependence · drowsiness the next day · lightheadedness the next day · muscle weakness · paradoxical increase in aggression
  - ▶ **Uncommon** Changes in libido · dizziness · dysarthria · gastro-intestinal disturbances · gynaecomastia · headache · hypotension · incontinence · salivation changes · slurred speech · tremor · urinary retention · vertigo · visual disturbances
  - ▶ **Rare** Apnoea · blood disorders · jaundice · respiratory depression · skin reactions
- BREAST FEEDING Benzodiazepines are present in milk, and should be avoided if possible during breast-feeding.
- HEPATIC IMPAIRMENT Start with smaller initial doses or reduce dose. Can precipitate coma. If treatment is necessary, benzodiazepines with shorter half-lives (such as temazepam or oxazepam) are safer.
  Avoid in severe impairment.
- RENAL IMPAIRMENT Start with small doses in severe impairment.
- PATIENT AND CARER ADVICE

  Driving and skilled tasks
  May impair judgement and increase reaction time, and so affect ability to drive or operate machinery; they increase the effects of alcohol. Moreover the hangover effects of a night dose may impair driving on the following day.

- NATIONAL FUNDING/ACCESS DECISIONS
  NHS restrictions Alprazolam tablets are not prescribable under the NHS.

- MEDICINAL FORMS
  There can be variation in the licensing of different medicines containing the same drug.

  Tablet
  CAUTIONARY AND ADVISORY LABELS 2
  - ▶ Xanax (Pfizer Ltd)
    Alprazolam 250 microgram Xanax 250microgram tablets | 60 tablet (PoM) £3.18 (CD4-1)
    Alprazolam 500 microgram Xanax 500microgram tablets | 60 tablet (PoM) £6.09 (CD4-1)

☞ 312

Chlordiazepoxide hydrochloride

● INDICATIONS AND DOSE

Short-term use in anxiety
▸ BY MOUTH
▸ Adult: 10 mg 3 times a day, increased if necessary to 60–100 mg daily in divided doses, for debilitated patients, use elderly dose
▸ Elderly: 5 mg 3 times a day, increased if necessary to 30–50 mg daily in divided doses

Treatment of alcohol withdrawal in moderate dependence
▸ BY MOUTH
▸ Adult: 10–30 mg 4 times a day, dose to be gradually reduced over 5–7 days, consult local protocols for titration regimens

Treatment of alcohol withdrawal in severe dependence
▸ BY MOUTH
▸ Adult: 10–50 mg 4 times a day and 10–40 mg as required for the first 2 days, dose to be gradually reduced over 7–10 days, consult local protocols for titration regimens; maximum 250 mg per day

● CONTRA-INDICATIONS Chronic psychosis · hyperkinesis · not for use alone to treat depression (or anxiety associated with depression) · obsessional states · phobic states · respiratory depression

● CAUTIONS Muscle weakness · organic brain changes · personality disorder (within the fearful group—dependent, avoidant, obsessive-compulsive) may increase risk of dependence

● SIDE-EFFECTS
▸ **Common or very common** Amnesia · ataxia (especially in the elderly) · confusion (especially in the elderly) · dependence · drowsiness the next day · lightheadedness the next day · muscle weakness · paradoxical increase in aggression
▸ **Uncommon** Changes in libido · dizziness · dysarthria · gastro-intestinal disturbances · gynaecomastia · headache · hypotension · incontinence · salivation changes · slurred speech · tremor · urinary retention · vertigo · visual disturbances
▸ **Rare** Apnoea · blood disorders · jaundice · respiratory depression · skin reactions

● BREAST FEEDING Benzodiazepines are present in milk, and should be avoided if possible during breast-feeding.

● HEPATIC IMPAIRMENT Start with smaller initial doses or reduce dose. Can precipitate coma. If treatment is necessary, benzodiazepines with shorter half-lives (such as temazepam or oxazepam) are safer.
    Avoid in severe impairment.

● RENAL IMPAIRMENT Start with small doses in severe impairment.

● PATIENT AND CARER ADVICE
Driving and skilled tasks
May impair judgement and increase reaction time, and so affect ability to drive or operate machinery; chlordiazepoxide increases the effects of alcohol. Moreover the hangover effects of a night dose may impair driving on the following day.

● NATIONAL FUNDING/ACCESS DECISIONS
NHS restrictions Librium® is not prescribable under the NHS.

● MEDICINAL FORMS
There can be variation in the licensing of different medicines containing the same drug. Forms available from special-order manufacturers include: oral suspension, oral solution

Tablet
CAUTIONARY AND ADVISORY LABELS 2
▸ Chlordiazepoxide hydrochloride (Non-proprietary)
    Chlordiazepoxide (as Chlordiazepoxide hydrochloride)
    10 mg Chlordiazepoxide 10mg tablets | 100 tablet PoM £49.50 DT price = £49.50 CD4-1 | 500 tablet PoM no price available CD4-1

Capsule
CAUTIONARY AND ADVISORY LABELS 2
▸ Chlordiazepoxide hydrochloride (Non-proprietary)
    Chlordiazepoxide hydrochloride 5 mg Chlordiazepoxide 5mg capsules | 28 capsule PoM £3.50 CD4-1 | 100 capsule PoM £11.50 DT price = £11.50 CD4-1
    Chlordiazepoxide hydrochloride 10 mg Chlordiazepoxide 10mg capsules | 28 capsule PoM £5.00 CD4-1 | 100 capsule PoM £17.80 DT price = £17.80 CD4-1
▸ Librium (Meda Pharmaceuticals Ltd)
    Chlordiazepoxide hydrochloride 5 mg Librium 5mg capsules | 100 capsule PoM £5.38 DT price = £11.50 CD4-1
    Chlordiazepoxide hydrochloride 10 mg Librium 10mg capsules | 100 capsule PoM £7.46 DT price = £17.80 CD4-1

☞ 312

Diazepam

● INDICATIONS AND DOSE

Muscle spasm of varied aetiology
▸ BY MOUTH
▸ Adult: 2–15 mg daily in divided doses, then increased if necessary to 60 mg daily, adjusted according to response, dose only increased in spastic conditions

Acute muscle spasm
▸ BY INTRAMUSCULAR INJECTION, OR BY SLOW INTRAVENOUS INJECTION
▸ Adult: 10 mg, then 10 mg after 4 hours if required, intravenous injection to be administered into a large vein at a rate of no more than 5 mg/minute

Tetanus
▸ BY INTRAVENOUS INJECTION
▸ Child: 100–300 micrograms/kg every 1–4 hours
▸ Adult: 100–300 micrograms/kg every 1–4 hours
▸ BY INTRAVENOUS INFUSION, OR BY NASODUODENAL TUBE
▸ Child: 3–10 mg/kg, adjusted according to response, to be given over 24 hours
▸ Adult: 3–10 mg/kg, adjusted according to response, to be given over 24 hours

Muscle spasm in cerebral spasticity or in postoperative skeletal muscle spasm
▸ BY MOUTH
▸ Child 1-11 months: Initially 250 micrograms/kg twice daily
▸ Child 1-4 years: Initially 2.5 mg twice daily
▸ Child 5-11 years: Initially 5 mg twice daily
▸ Child 12-17 years: Initially 10 mg twice daily; maximum 40 mg per day

Anxiety
▸ BY MOUTH
▸ Adult: 2 mg 3 times a day, then increased if necessary to 15–30 mg daily in divided doses, for debilitated patients, use elderly dose
▸ Elderly: 1 mg 3 times a day, then increased if necessary to 7.5–15 mg daily in divided doses

Insomnia associated with anxiety
▸ BY MOUTH
▸ Adult: 5–15 mg daily, to be taken at bedtime

continued →

4

Nervous system

Severe acute anxiety | Control of acute panic attacks | Acute alcohol withdrawal
▸ BY INTRAMUSCULAR INJECTION, OR BY SLOW INTRAVENOUS INJECTION
▸ Adult: 10 mg, then 10 mg after at least 4 hours if required, intravenous injection to be administered into a large vein, at a rate of not more than 5 mg/minute

Acute drug-induced dystonic reactions
▸ BY INTRAVENOUS INJECTION
▸ Adult: 5–10 mg, then 5–10 mg after at least 10 minutes as required, to be administered into a large vein, at a rate of not more than 5 mg/minute

Acute anxiety and agitation
▸ BY RECTUM
▸ Adult: 500 micrograms/kg, then 500 micrograms/kg after 12 hours as required
▸ Elderly: 250 micrograms/kg, then 250 micrograms/kg after 12 hours as required

Premedication
▸ BY MOUTH
▸ Adult: 5–10 mg, to be given 1–2 hours before procedure, for debilitated patients, use elderly dose
▸ Elderly: 2.5–5 mg, to be given 1–2 hours before procedure
▸ BY INTRAVENOUS INJECTION
▸ Adult: 100–200 micrograms/kg, to be administered into a large vein at a rate of not more than 5 mg/minute, immediately before procedure

Sedation in dental procedures carried out in hospital
▸ BY MOUTH
▸ Adult: Up to 20 mg, to be given 1–2 hours before procedure

Conscious sedation for procedures, and in conjunction with local anaesthesia
▸ BY MOUTH
▸ Adult: 5–10 mg, to be given 1–2 hours before procedure, for debilitated patients, use elderly dose
▸ Elderly: 2.5–5 mg, to be given 1–2 hours before procedure

Sedative cover for minor surgical and medical procedures
▸ BY INTRAVENOUS INJECTION
▸ Adult: 10–20 mg, to be administered into a large vein over 2–4 minutes, immediately before procedure

Status epilepticus | Febrile convulsions | Convulsions due to poisoning
▸ BY INTRAVENOUS INJECTION
▸ Child 1 month–11 years: 300–400 micrograms/kg (max. per dose 10 mg), then 300–400 micrograms/kg after 10 minutes if required, to be given over 3–5 minutes
▸ Child 12–17 years: 10 mg, then 10 mg after 10 minutes if required, to be given over 3–5 minutes
▸ Adult: 10 mg, then 10 mg after 10 minutes if required, administered at a rate of 1 mL (5 mg) per minute
▸ BY RECTUM
▸ Child 1 month–1 year: 5 mg, then 5 mg after 10 minutes if required
▸ Child 2–11 years: 5–10 mg, then 5–10 mg after 10 minutes if required
▸ Child 12–17 years: 10–20 mg, then 10–20 mg after 10 minutes if required
▸ Adult: 10–20 mg, then 10–20 mg after 10–15 minutes if required
▸ Elderly: 10 mg, then 10 mg after 10–15 minutes if required

Life-threatening acute drug-induced dystonic reactions
▸ BY INTRAVENOUS INJECTION
▸ Child 1 month–11 years: 100 micrograms/kg, repeated if necessary, to be given over 3–5 minutes
▸ Child 12–17 years: 5–10 mg, repeated if necessary, to be given over 3–5 minutes

Dyspnoea associated with anxiety in palliative care
▸ BY MOUTH
▸ Adult: 5–10 mg daily
Pain of muscle spasm in palliative care
▸ BY MOUTH
▸ Adult: 5–10 mg daily

● UNLICENSED USE
▸ With rectal use in children *Diazepam Desitin*®, *Diazepam Rectubes*®, and *Stesolid Rectal Tubes*® not licensed for use in children under 1 year.

> IMPORTANT SAFETY INFORMATION
> ANAESTHESIA
> Benzodiazepines should only be administered for anaesthesia by, or under the direct supervision of, personnel experienced in their use, with adequate training in anaesthesia and airway management.

● CONTRA-INDICATIONS Avoid injections containing benzyl alcohol in neonates · chronic psychosis (in adults) · CNS depression · compromised airway · hyperkinesis · not for use alone to treat depression (or anxiety associated with depression) (in adults) · obsessional states · phobic states · respiratory depression
● CAUTIONS
GENERAL CAUTIONS
Muscle weakness · organic brain changes · parenteral administration (close observation required until full recovery from sedation) · personality disorder (within the fearful group—dependent, avoidant, obsessive-compulsive) may increase risk of dependence
SPECIFIC CAUTIONS
▸ With intravenous use High risk of venous thrombophlebitis with intravenous use (reduced by using an emulsion formulation)
CAUTIONS, FURTHER INFORMATION
▸ Special precautions for intravenous injection
▸ With intravenous use When given intravenously facilities for reversing respiratory depression with mechanical ventilation must be immediately available.
● SIDE-EFFECTS
GENERAL SIDE-EFFECTS
▸ **Common or very common** Amnesia · ataxia (in children) · ataxia (especially in the elderly) (in adults) · confusion (in children) · confusion (especially in the elderly) (in adults) · dependence · drowsiness the next day · lightheadedness the next day · muscle weakness · paradoxical increase in aggression
▸ **Uncommon** Changes in libido (in adults) · dizziness · dysarthria · gastro-intestinal disturbances · gynaecomastia · headache (in adults) · hypotension (in adults) · incontinence · salivation changes · slurred speech (in adults) · tremor · urinary retention (in adults) · vertigo (in adults) · visual disturbances
▸ **Rare** Apnoea · blood disorders · changes in libido (in children) · headache (in children) · hypotension (in children) · jaundice · respiratory depression · skin reactions · urinary retention (in children) · vertigo (in children)
▸ **Frequency not known** Delusions (in children) · excitement (in children) · hallucinations (in children) · hypotonia (when used for muscle spasm) · irritability (in children) · marked respiratory depression, particularly with high dose (facilities for its treatment are essential) · psychosis (in children) · restlessness (in children)
SPECIFIC SIDE-EFFECTS
▸ With intravenous use Pain · thrombophlebitis · venous thrombosis (in adults)
● PREGNANCY Women who have seizures in the second half of pregnancy should be assessed for eclampsia before any

change is made to antiepileptic treatment. Status epilepticus should be treated according to the standard protocol.

Epilepsy and Pregnancy Register All pregnant women with epilepsy, whether taking medication or not, should be encouraged to notify the UK Epilepsy and Pregnancy Register (Tel: 0800 389 1248).

● BREAST FEEDING Present in milk, and should be avoided if possible during breast-feeding.

● HEPATIC IMPAIRMENT Start with smaller initial doses or reduce dose. Can precipitate coma. If treatment is necessary, benzodiazepines with shorter half lives are safer, such as temazepam or oxazepam.
  Avoid in severe impairment.

● RENAL IMPAIRMENT Start with small doses in severe impairment.

● DIRECTIONS FOR ADMINISTRATION
▸ With intravenous use in children For *continuous intravenous infusion* of diazepam emulsion, dilute to a concentration of max. 400 micrograms/mL with Glucose 5% or 10%; max. 6 hours between addition and completion of infusion. For *continuous intravenous infusion* of diazepam solution, dilute to a concentration of max. 50 micrograms/mL with Glucose 5% or Sodium Chloride 0.9%.
▸ With intravenous use Diazepam is adsorbed by plastics of infusion bags and giving sets. Emulsion formulation preferred for intravenous injection.
▸ With intravenous use in adults For *intravenous infusion* (solution) (*Diazepam*, Wockhardt), give continuously *in* Glucose 5% or Sodium chloride 0.9%. Dilute to a concentration of not more than 10 mg in 200 mL. For *intravenous infusion* (emulsion) (*Diazemuls*®), give continuously *in* Glucose 5% or 10%. May be diluted to a max. concentration of 200 mg in 500 mL; max. 6 hours between addition and completion of administration. May be given *via* drip tubing *in* Glucose 5% or 10% or Sodium chloride 0.9%.
▸ With intramuscular use or intravenous use in adults Solution for injection should not be diluted, except for intravenous infusion.
▸ With intramuscular use in adults Only use intramuscular route when oral and intravenous routes not possible.

● PATIENT AND CARER ADVICE
  Driving and skilled tasks
  May impair judgement and increase reaction time, and so affect ability to drive or perform skilled tasks; they increase the effects of alcohol. Moreover the hangover effects of a night dose may impair performance on the following day.
  Patients given sedatives and analgesics during minor outpatient procedures should be very carefully warned about the risks of undertaking skilled tasks (e.g. driving) afterwards. For intravenous benzodiazepines the risk extends to **at least 24 hours** after administration. Responsible persons should be available to take patients home afterwards. The dangers of taking **alcohol** should be emphasised.
  Medicines for Children leaflet: Diazepam (rectal) for stopping seizures www.medicinesforchildren.org.uk/diazepam-rectal-stopping-seizures-0
  Medicines for Children leaflet: Diazepam for muscle spasm www.medicinesforchildren.org.uk/diazepam-for-muscle-spasm

● PROFESSION SPECIFIC INFORMATION
  Dental practitioners' formulary
  Diazepam Tablets may be prescribed.
  Diazepam Oral Solution 2 mg/5 mL may be prescribed.

● MEDICINAL FORMS
  There can be variation in the licensing of different medicines containing the same drug. Forms available from special-order manufacturers include: oral suspension, oral solution, suppository

Tablet
CAUTIONARY AND ADVISORY LABELS 2, 19
▸ Diazepam (Non-proprietary)
  Diazepam 2 mg Diazepam 2mg tablets | 28 tablet [PoM] £3.80 DT price = £0.76 [CD4-1] | 1000 tablet [PoM] £135.71 [CD4-1]
  Diazepam 5 mg Diazepam 5mg tablets | 28 tablet [PoM] £6.80 DT price = £0.79 [CD4-1] | 1000 tablet [PoM] £242.85 [CD4-1]
  Diazepam 10 mg Diazepam 10mg tablets | 28 tablet [PoM] £9.80 DT price = £0.91 [CD4-1] | 500 tablet [PoM] £175.00 [CD4-1]

Oral suspension
▸ Diazepam (Non-proprietary)
  Diazepam 400 microgram per 1 ml Diazepam 2mg/5ml oral suspension | 100 ml [PoM] £31.75 [CD4-1]
  Diazepam 1 mg per 1 ml Diazepam 5mg/5ml oral suspension | 100 ml [PoM] £55.00 [CD4-1]

Oral solution
CAUTIONARY AND ADVISORY LABELS 2, 19
▸ Diazepam (Non-proprietary)
  Diazepam 400 microgram per 1 ml Diazepam 2mg/5ml oral solution sugar free sugar-free | 100 ml [PoM] £40.49 DT price = £31.75 [CD4-1]

Solution for injection
EXCIPIENTS: May contain Benzyl alcohol, ethanol, propylene glycol
▸ Diazepam (Non-proprietary)
  Diazepam 5 mg per 1 ml Diazepam 10mg/2ml solution for injection ampoules | 10 ampoule [PoM] £4.00–£5.50 DT price = £5.50 [CD4-1]

Emulsion for injection
▸ Diazemuls (Actavis UK Ltd)
  Diazepam 5 mg per 1 ml Diazemuls 10mg/2ml emulsion for injection ampoules | 10 ampoule [PoM] £9.05 [CD4-1]

Enema
CAUTIONARY AND ADVISORY LABELS 2, 19
▸ Diazepam (Non-proprietary)
  Diazepam 2 mg per 1 ml Diazepam 5mg RecTubes | 5 tube [PoM] £5.85 DT price = £5.85 [CD4-1]
  Diazepam 2.5mg/1.25ml rectal solution tube | 5 tube [PoM] no price available [CD4-1]
  Diazepam 2.5mg RecTubes | 5 tube [PoM] £5.65 [CD4-1]
  Diazepam 5mg/2.5ml rectal solution tube | 5 tube [PoM] £6.30 DT price = £5.85 [CD4-1]
  Diazepam 4 mg per 1 ml Diazepam 10mg RecTubes | 5 tube [PoM] £7.35 DT price = £7.35 [CD4-1]
  Diazepam 10mg/2.5ml rectal solution tube | 5 tube [PoM] £8.00 DT price = £7.35 [CD4-1]
▸ Stesolid (Actavis UK Ltd)
  Diazepam 2 mg per 1 ml Stesolid 5mg rectal tube | 5 tube [PoM] £6.89 DT price = £5.85 [CD4-1]
  Diazepam 4 mg per 1 ml Stesolid 10mg rectal tube | 5 tube [PoM] £8.78 DT price = £7.35 [CD4-1]

◤ 312

Oxazepam

● INDICATIONS AND DOSE
  Anxiety (short-term use)
  ▸ BY MOUTH
  ▸ **Adult:** 15–30 mg 3–4 times a day, for debilitated patients, use elderly dose
  ▸ **Elderly:** 10–20 mg 3–4 times a day
  Insomnia associated with anxiety
  ▸ BY MOUTH
  ▸ **Adult:** 15–25 mg once daily (max. per dose 50 mg), dose to be taken at bedtime

● CONTRA-INDICATIONS Chronic psychosis · hyperkinesis · not for use alone to treat depression (or anxiety associated with depression) · obsessional states · phobic states · respiratory depression

● CAUTIONS Muscle weakness · organic brain changes · personality disorder (within the fearful group—dependent, avoidant, obsessive-compulsive) may increase risk of dependence

4

Nervous system

Nervous system

4

CAUTIONS, FURTHER INFORMATION
▶ Paradoxical effects A paradoxical increase in hostility and aggression may be reported by patients taking benzodiazepines. The effects range from talkativeness and excitement to aggressive and antisocial acts. Adjustment of the dose (up or down) sometimes attenuates the impulses. Increased anxiety and perceptual disorders are other paradoxical effects.

● SIDE-EFFECTS
▶ **Common or very common** Amnesia · ataxia (especially in the elderly) · confusion (especially in the elderly) · dependence · drowsiness the next day · lightheadedness the next day · muscle weakness · paradoxical increase in aggression
▶ **Uncommon** Changes in libido · dizziness · dysarthria · gastro-intestinal disturbances · gynaecomastia · headache · hypotension · incontinence · salivation changes · slurred speech · tremor · urinary retention · vertigo · visual disturbances
▶ **Rare** Apnoea · blood disorders · jaundice · respiratory depression · skin reactions

● BREAST FEEDING Benzodiazepines are present in milk, and should be avoided if possible during breast-feeding.

● HEPATIC IMPAIRMENT Start with smaller initial doses or reduce dose. Can precipitate coma. If treatment is necessary, benzodiazepines with shorter half-lives are safer.
    Avoid in severe impairment.

● RENAL IMPAIRMENT Start with small doses in severe impairment.

● PATIENT AND CARER ADVICE
Driving and skilled tasks
May impair judgement and increase reaction time, and so affect ability to drive or operate machinery; they increase the effects of alcohol. Moreover the hangover effects of a night dose may impair driving on the following day.

● MEDICINAL FORMS
There can be variation in the licensing of different medicines containing the same drug. Forms available from special-order manufacturers include: oral suspension

Tablet
CAUTIONARY AND ADVISORY LABELS 2
▶ Oxazepam (Non-proprietary)
    Oxazepam 10 mg Oxazepam 10mg tablets | 28 tablet [PoM] £1.32 DT price = £1.20 [CD4-1]
    Oxazepam 15 mg Oxazepam 15mg tablets | 28 tablet [PoM] £1.43 DT price = £1.23 [CD4-1]

HYPNOTICS, SEDATIVES AND ANXIOLYTICS ›
NON-BENZODIAZEPINE HYPNOTICS AND SEDATIVES

Meprobamate

● INDICATIONS AND DOSE
Short-term use in anxiety—not recommended
▶ BY MOUTH
▶ Adult: 400 mg 3–4 times a day
▶ Elderly: Up to 200 mg 3–4 times a day

IMPORTANT SAFETY INFORMATION
The European Medicines Agency has recommended (January 2012) the suspension of all marketing authorisations for meprobamate because the risks, particularly of serious CNS side-effects, outweigh the benefits.

● CONTRA-INDICATIONS Acute porphyrias p. 918 · acute pulmonary insufficiency · respiratory depression

● CAUTIONS Abrupt withdrawal (may precipitate convulsions) · avoid prolonged use · debilitated · elderly · epilepsy (may induce seizures) · history of alcohol abuse · history of drug abuse · marked personality disorder · muscle weakness · respiratory disease

● INTERACTIONS → Appendix 1 (anxiolytics and hypnotics).

● SIDE-EFFECTS
▶ **Common or very common** Amnesia · ataxia (especially in the elderly) · confusion (especially in the elderly) · dependence · drowsiness the next day · lightheadedness the next day · muscle weakness · paradoxical increase in aggression
▶ **Uncommon** Changes in libido · dizziness · dysarthria · gastro-intestinal disturbances · gynaecomastia · headache · hypotension · incontinence · salivation changes · slurred speech · tremor · urinary retention · vertigo · visual disturbances
▶ **Rare** Agranulocytosis · apnoea · blood disorders · jaundice · rashes · respiratory depression · skin reactions
▶ **Frequency not known** CNS effects · paradoxical excitement · paraesthesia · weakness

● PREGNANCY Avoid if possible.

● BREAST FEEDING Avoid. Concentration in milk may exceed maternal plasma concentrations fourfold and may cause drowsiness in infant.

● HEPATIC IMPAIRMENT Can precipitate coma.

● RENAL IMPAIRMENT Start with small doses in severe impairment. Increased cerebral sensitivity.

● PATIENT AND CARER ADVICE
Driving and skilled tasks
Drowsiness may affect performance of skilled tasks (e.g. driving); effects of alcohol enhanced.

● LESS SUITABLE FOR PRESCRIBING Meprobamate is less suitable for prescribing.

● MEDICINAL FORMS
There can be variation in the licensing of different medicines containing the same drug. Forms available from special-order manufacturers include: oral suspension, oral solution

Tablet
CAUTIONARY AND ADVISORY LABELS 2
▶ Meprobamate (Non-proprietary)
    Meprobamate 400 mg Meprobamate 400mg tablets | 84 tablet [PoM] £197.65 DT price = £197.64 [CD3]

3.2 Attention deficit hyperactivity disorder

Attention deficit hyperactivity disorder

Management
Central nervous system stimulants include the **amfetamines** (dexamfetamine sulfate p. 319 and lisdexamfetamine mesilate p. 320) **and related drugs** (e.g. methylphenidate hydrochloride p. 318). They have very few indications and in particular, should **not** be used to treat depression, obesity, senility, debility, or for relief of fatigue.

    CNS stimulants should be prescribed for children with severe and persistent symptoms of attention deficit hyperactivity disorder (ADHD), when the diagnosis has been confirmed by a specialist; children with moderate symptoms of ADHD can be treated with CNS stimulants when psychological interventions have been unsuccessful or are unavailable. Prescribing of CNS stimulants may be continued by general practitioners, under a shared-care arrangement. Treatment of ADHD often needs to be continued into adolescence, and may need to be continued into adulthood.

Drug treatment of ADHD should be part of a comprehensive treatment programme. The choice of medication should take into consideration co-morbid conditions (such as tic disorders, Tourette syndrome, and epilepsy), the adverse effect profile, potential for drug misuse, tolerance and dependance; and preferences of the patient and carers. Methylphenidate hydrochloride and atomoxetine below are used for the management of ADHD; dexamfetamine sulfate and lisdexamfetamine mesilate are an alternative in children who do not respond to these drugs. Guanfacine p. 321, a non-stimulant alpha$_2$-adrenoceptor agonist, can be used in children for whom stimulants are not suitable, not tolerated, or ineffective. Therapeutic response to guanfacine should be evaluated every 3 months for the first year and then at least yearly, when prescribed for extended periods.

The need to continue drug treatment for ADHD should be reviewed at least annually. This may involve suspending treatment.

CNS STIMULANTS ⟩ CENTRALLY ACTING SYMPATHOMIMETICS

Atomoxetine

● **INDICATIONS AND DOSE**

Attention deficit hyperactivity disorder (initiated by a specialist)
▸ BY MOUTH
▸ Child 6-17 years (body-weight up to 70 kg): Initially 500 micrograms/kg daily for 7 days, dose is increased according to response; maintenance 1.2 mg/kg daily, total daily dose may be given either as a single dose in the morning or in 2 divided doses with last dose no later than early evening, high daily doses to be given under the direction of a specialist; maximum 1.8 mg/kg per day; maximum 120 mg per day
▸ Child 6-17 years (body-weight 70 kg and above): Initially 40 mg daily for 7 days, dose is increased according to response; maintenance 80 mg daily, total daily dose may be given either as a single dose in the morning or in 2 divided doses with last dose no later than early evening, high daily doses to be given under the direction of a specialist; maximum 120 mg per day
▸ Adult (body-weight up to 70 kg): Initially 500 micrograms/kg daily for 7 days, dose is increased according to response; maintenance 1.2 mg/kg daily, total daily dose may be given either as a single dose in the morning or in 2 divided doses with last dose no later than early evening, high daily doses to be given under the direction of a specialist; maximum 1.8 mg/kg per day; maximum 120 mg per day
▸ Adult (body-weight 70 kg and above): Initially 40 mg daily for 7 days, dose is increased according to response; maintenance 80-100 mg daily, total daily dose may be given either as a single dose in the morning or in 2 divided doses with last dose no later than early evening, high daily doses to be given under the direction of a specialist; maximum 120 mg per day

● **UNLICENSED USE**
▸ In children Doses above 100 mg daily not licensed.
▸ In adults Dose maximum of 120 mg not licensed.
   Atomoxetine doses in BNF may differ from those in product literature.

● **CONTRA-INDICATIONS** Phaeochromocytoma · severe cardiovascular disease · severe cerebrovascular disease

● **CAUTIONS** QT-interval prolongation · aggressive behaviour · cardiovascular disease · cerebrovascular disease · emotional lability · history of seizures · hostility · hypertension · mania · psychosis · structural cardiac abnormalities · susceptibility to angle-closure glaucoma · tachycardia

● **INTERACTIONS** → Appendix 1 (atomoxetine).
   Avoid concomitant use of drugs that prolong QT interval.

● **SIDE-EFFECTS**
▸ **Common or very common** Abdominal pain · anorexia · anxiety · chills · constipation · depression · dermatitis · dizziness · drowsiness · dry mouth · dyspepsia · flatulence · flushing · headache · increased blood pressure · irritability · lethargy · malaise · mydriasis · nausea · palpitation · paraesthesia · prostatitis · rash · sexual dysfunction · sleep disturbances · sweating · tachycardia · taste disturbances · tremor · urinary dysfunction · vomiting
▸ **Uncommon** Aggression · cold extremities · emotional lability · hostility · hypoaesthesia · menstrual disturbances · muscle spasms · pruritus · psychosis · QT-interval prolongation · suicidal ideation · syncope · tics
▸ **Rare** Raynaud's phenomenon · seizures
▸ **Very rare** Angle-closure glaucoma · hepatic disorders

● **PREGNANCY** Manufacturer advises avoid unless potential benefit outweighs risk.

● **BREAST FEEDING** Avoid-present in milk in *animal* studies.

● **HEPATIC IMPAIRMENT** Halve dose in moderate impairment. Quarter dose in severe impairment.

● **MONITORING REQUIREMENTS**
▸ Monitor for appearance or worsening of anxiety, depression or tics.
▸ Pulse, blood pressure, psychiatric symptoms, appetite, weight and height should be recorded at initiation of therapy, following each dose adjustment, and at least every 6 months thereafter.

● **PATIENT AND CARER ADVICE**
Medicines for Children leaflet: Atomoxetine for attention deficit hyperactivity disorder (ADHD) www.medicinesforchildren.org.uk/atomoxetine-attention-deficit-hyperactivity-disorder-adhd
Suicidal ideation Following reports of suicidal thoughts and behaviour, patients and their carers should be informed about the risk and told to report clinical worsening, suicidal thoughts or behaviour, irritability, agitation, or depression.
Hepatic impairment Following rare reports of hepatic disorders, patients and carers should be advised of the risk and be told how to recognise symptoms; prompt medical attention should be sought in case of abdominal pain, unexplained nausea, malaise, darkening of the urine, or jaundice.

● **NATIONAL FUNDING/ACCESS DECISIONS**

NICE technology appraisals (TAs)
▸ **Methylphenidate, atomoxetine and dexamfetamine for attention deficit hyperactivity disorder (ADHD) (March 2006)**
NICE TA98
Atomoxetine is recommended, within its licensed indications, as an option for the management of ADHD in children and adolescents.
www.nice.org.uk/TA98

● **MEDICINAL FORMS**
There can be variation in the licensing of different medicines containing the same drug. Forms available from special-order manufacturers include: oral suspension, oral solution
Capsule
CAUTIONARY AND ADVISORY LABELS 3
▸ Strattera (Eli Lilly and Company Ltd)
   Atomoxetine (as Atomoxetine hydrochloride) 10 mg Strattera
   10mg capsules | 7 capsules PoM £13.28 | 28 capsule PoM £53.09
   DT price = £53.09
   Atomoxetine (as Atomoxetine hydrochloride) 18 mg Strattera
   18mg capsules | 7 capsules PoM £13.28 | 28 capsule PoM £53.09
   DT price = £53.09
   Atomoxetine (as Atomoxetine hydrochloride) 25 mg Strattera
   25mg capsules | 7 capsule PoM £13.28 | 28 capsule PoM £53.09
   DT price = £53.09
   Atomoxetine (as Atomoxetine hydrochloride) 40 mg Strattera
   40mg capsules | 7 capsule PoM £13.28 | 28 capsule PoM £53.09
   DT price = £53.09

4

Nervous system

Nervous system

4

Atomoxetine (as Atomoxetine hydrochloride) **60 mg** Strattera
60mg capsules | 28 capsule [PoM] £53.09 DT price = £53.09
Atomoxetine (as Atomoxetine hydrochloride) **80 mg** Strattera
80mg capsules | 28 capsule [PoM] £70.79 DT price = £70.79
Atomoxetine (as Atomoxetine hydrochloride) **100 mg** Strattera
100mg capsules | 28 capsule [PoM] £70.79 DT price = £70.79

Oral solution
CAUTIONARY AND ADVISORY LABELS 3
▸ Strattera (Eli Lilly and Company Ltd)
Atomoxetine (as Atomoxetine hydrochloride) **4 mg per
1 ml** Strattera 4mg/1ml oral solution sugar-free | 300 ml [PoM]
£85.00 DT price = £85.00

Methylphenidate hydrochloride

● INDICATIONS AND DOSE
**Attention deficit hyperactivity disorder (initiated under
specialist supervision)**
▸ BY MOUTH USING IMMEDIATE-RELEASE MEDICINES
▸ Child 6-17 years: Initially 5 mg 1–2 times a day,
increased in steps of 5–10 mg daily if required, at
weekly intervals, increased if necessary up to 60 mg
daily in 2–3 divided doses, increased if necessary up to
2.1 mg/kg daily in 2–3 divided doses, the licensed
maximum dose is 60 mg daily in 2–3 doses, higher dose
(up to a maximum of 90 mg daily) under the direction
of a specialist, discontinue if no response after
1 month, if effect wears off in evening (with rebound
hyperactivity) a dose at bedtime may be appropriate
(establish need with trial bedtime dose). Treatment
may be started using a modified-release preparation
▸ Adult: Initially 5 mg 2–3 times a day, dose is increased
if necessary at weekly intervals according to response,
increased if necessary up to 100 mg daily in 2–3 divided
doses, if effect wears off in evening (with rebound
hyperactivity) a dose at bedtime may be appropriate
(establish need with trial bedtime dose). Treatment
may be started using a modified-release preparation

Narcolepsy
▸ BY MOUTH USING IMMEDIATE-RELEASE MEDICINES
▸ Adult: 10–60 mg daily in divided doses; usual dose
20–30 mg daily in divided doses, dose to be taken
before meals

CONCERTA® XL
Attention deficit hyperactivity disorder
▸ BY MOUTH
▸ Child 6-17 years: Initially 18 mg once daily, dose to be
taken in the morning, increased in steps of 18 mg every
1 week, adjusted according to response; increased if
necessary up to 2.1 mg/kg daily, licensed max. dose is
54 mg once daily, to be increased to higher dose only
under direction of specialist; discontinue if no
response after 1 month; maximum 108 mg per day
▸ Adult: Initially 18 mg once daily, dose to be taken in
the morning; adjusted at weekly intervals according to
response; maximum 108 mg per day

DOSE EQUIVALENCE AND CONVERSION
Total daily dose of 15 mg of standard-release formulation
is considered equivalent to Concerta® XL 18 mg once
daily.

EQUASYM® XL
Attention deficit hyperactivity disorder
▸ BY MOUTH
▸ Child 6-17 years: Initially 10 mg once daily, dose to be
taken in the morning before breakfast; increased
gradually at weekly intervals if necessary; increased if
necessary up to 2.1 mg/kg daily, licensed max. dose is
60 mg daily, to be increased to higher dose only under
direction of specialist; discontinue if no response after
1 month; maximum 90 mg per day

▸ Adult: Initially 10 mg once daily, dose to be taken in
the morning before breakfast; increased gradually at
weekly intervals if necessary; maximum 100 mg per day

MEDIKINET® XL
Attention deficit hyperactivity disorder
▸ BY MOUTH
▸ Child 6-17 years: Initially 10 mg once daily, dose to be
taken in the morning with breakfast; adjusted at
weekly intervals according to response; increased if
necessary up to 2.1 mg/kg daily, licensed max. dose is
60 mg daily, to be increased to higher dose only under
direction of specialist; discontinue if no response after
1 month; maximum 90 mg per day
▸ Adult: Initially 10 mg once daily, dose to be taken in
the morning with breakfast; adjusted at weekly
intervals according to response; maximum 100 mg per
day

● UNLICENSED USE Doses over 60 mg daily not licensed;
doses of Concerta XL over 54 mg daily not licensed.
▸ In children Not licensed for use in children under 6 years.
▸ In adults Not licensed for use in narcolepsy. Not licensed
for use in adults for attention deficit hyperactivity
disorder.

● CONTRA-INDICATIONS Anorexia nervosa · arrhythmias ·
cardiomyopathy, · cardiovascular disease · cerebrovascular
disorders · heart failure · hyperthyroidism ·
phaeochromocytoma · psychosis · severe depression ·
severe hypertension · structural cardiac abnormalities ·
suicidal ideation · uncontrolled bipolar disorder · vasculitis

● CAUTIONS Agitation · alcohol dependence · anxiety · drug
dependence · epilepsy (discontinue if increased seizure
frequency) · family history of Tourette syndrome ·
susceptibility to angle-closure glaucoma · tics
CONCERTA® XL Dysphagia (dose form not appropriate) ·
restricted gastro-intestinal lumen (dose form not
appropriate)

● INTERACTIONS → Appendix 1 (sympathomimetics).

● SIDE-EFFECTS
▸ **Common or very common** Abdominal pain · aggression ·
alopecia · anorexia · arrhythmias · arthralgia · asthenia ·
changes in blood pressure · cough · depression · diarrhoea ·
dizziness · drowsiness · dry mouth · dyspepsia · fever ·
growth restriction · headache · insomnia · irritability ·
movement disorders · nasopharyngitis · nausea ·
nervousness · palpitation · pruritus · rash · reduced weight
gain · tachycardia · tics · vomiting
▸ **Uncommon** Abnormal dreams · confusion · constipation ·
dyspnoea · epistaxis · haematuria · muscle cramps · suicidal
ideation · urinary frequency
▸ **Rare** Angina · sweating · visual disturbances;
▸ **Very rare** Angle-closure glaucoma · blood disorders ·
cerebral arteritis · dependence · erythema multiforme ·
exfoliative dermatitis · hepatic dysfunction · leucopenia ·
myocardial infarction · neuroleptic malignant syndrome ·
psychosis · seizures · thrombocytopenia · tolerance ·
Tourette syndrome
▸ **Frequency not known** Bradycardia · convulsions ·
supraventricular tachycardia

● PREGNANCY Limited experience—avoid unless potential
benefit outweighs risk.

● BREAST FEEDING Limited information available—avoid.

● MONITORING REQUIREMENTS
▸ Monitor for psychiatric disorders.
▸ Pulse, blood pressure, psychiatric symptoms, appetite,
weight and height should be recorded at initiation of
therapy, following each dose adjustment, and at least
every 6 months thereafter.

● TREATMENT CESSATION Avoid abrupt withdrawal.

- DIRECTIONS FOR ADMINISTRATION

MEDIKINET® XL Contents of capsule can be sprinkled on a tablespoon of apple sauce or yoghurt (then swallowed immediately without chewing).

EQUASYM® XL Contents of capsule can be sprinkled on a tablespoon of apple sauce then swallowed immediately without chewing).

- PRESCRIBING AND DISPENSING INFORMATION Different versions of modified-release preparations may not have the same clinical effect. To avoid confusion between these different formulations of methylphenidate, prescribers should specify the brand to be dispensed.

CONCERTA® XL Consists of an immediate-release component (22% of the dose) and a modified-release component (78% of the dose).

MEDIKINET® XL Consists of an immediate-release component (50% of the dose) and a modified-release component (50% of the dose).

EQUASYM® XL Consists of an immediate-release component (30% of the dose) and a modified-release component (70% of the dose).

- PATIENT AND CARER ADVICE

Driving and skilled tasks

Drugs and Driving Prescribers and other healthcare professionals should advise patients if treatment is likely to affect their ability to perform skilled tasks (e.g. driving). This applies especially to drugs with sedative effects; patients should be warned that these effects are increased by alcohol. General information about a patient's fitness to drive is available from the Driver and Vehicle Licensing Agency at www.dvla.gov.uk.

2015 legislation regarding driving whilst taking certain drugs, may also apply to methylphenidate, see *Drugs and driving* under Guidance on prescribing p. 1.

CONCERTA® XL Tablet membrane may pass through gastro-intestinal tract unchanged.

- NATIONAL FUNDING/ACCESS DECISIONS

NICE technology appraisals (TAs)

▸ **Methylphenidate, atomoxetine and dexamfetamine for attention deficit hyperactivity disorder (ADHD) (March 2006)** NICE TA98

Methylphenidate is recommended, within its licensed indications, as an option for the management of ADHD in children and adolescents.

www.nice.org.uk/TA98

- MEDICINAL FORMS

There can be variation in the licensing of different medicines containing the same drug. Forms available from special-order manufacturers include: oral suspension, oral solution

Tablet

▸ Methylphenidate hydrochloride (Non-proprietary)
Methylphenidate hydrochloride 5 mg Methylphenidate 5mg tablets | 30 tablet [PoM] £3.44 DT price = £3.03 [CD2]
Methylphenidate hydrochloride 10 mg Methylphenidate 10mg tablets | 30 tablet [PoM] £7.17 DT price = £5.49 [CD2]
Methylphenidate hydrochloride 20 mg Methylphenidate 20mg tablets | 30 tablet [PoM] £11.12 DT price = £10.92 [CD2]
▸ Medikinet (Flynn Pharma Ltd)
Methylphenidate hydrochloride 5 mg Medikinet 5mg tablets | 30 tablet [PoM] £3.03 DT price = £3.03 [CD2]
Methylphenidate hydrochloride 10 mg Medikinet 10mg tablets | 30 tablet [PoM] £5.49 DT price = £5.49 [CD2]
Methylphenidate hydrochloride 20 mg Medikinet 20mg tablets | 30 tablet [PoM] £10.92 DT price = £10.92 [CD2]
▸ Ritalin (Novartis Pharmaceuticals UK Ltd)
Methylphenidate hydrochloride 10 mg Ritalin 10mg tablets | 30 tablet [PoM] £6.68 DT price = £5.49 [CD2]
▸ Tranquilyn (Genesis Pharmaceuticals Ltd)
Methylphenidate hydrochloride 5 mg Tranquilyn 5mg tablets | 30 tablet [PoM] £3.03 DT price = £3.03 [CD2]
Methylphenidate hydrochloride 10 mg Tranquilyn 10mg tablets | 30 tablet [PoM] £5.49 DT price = £5.49 [CD2]

Methylphenidate hydrochloride 20 mg Tranquilyn 20mg tablets | 30 tablet [PoM] £10.92 DT price = £10.92 [CD2]

Modified-release tablet

CAUTIONARY AND ADVISORY LABELS 25
▸ Concerta XL (Janssen-Cilag Ltd)
Methylphenidate hydrochloride 18 mg Concerta XL 18mg tablets | 30 tablet [PoM] £31.19 DT price = £31.19 [CD2]
Methylphenidate hydrochloride 27 mg Concerta XL 27mg tablets | 30 tablet [PoM] £36.81 DT price = £36.81 [CD2]
Methylphenidate hydrochloride 36 mg Concerta XL 36mg tablets | 30 tablet [PoM] £42.45 DT price = £42.45 [CD2]
Methylphenidate hydrochloride 54 mg Concerta XL 54mg tablets | 30 tablet [PoM] £73.62 DT price = £60.48 [CD2]

Modified-release capsule

CAUTIONARY AND ADVISORY LABELS 25
▸ Equasym XL (Shire Pharmaceuticals Ltd)
Methylphenidate hydrochloride 10 mg Equasym XL 10mg capsules | 30 capsule [PoM] £25.00 DT price = £25.00 [CD2]
Methylphenidate hydrochloride 20 mg Equasym XL 20mg capsules | 30 capsule [PoM] £30.00 DT price = £30.00 [CD2]
Methylphenidate hydrochloride 30 mg Equasym XL 30mg capsules | 30 capsule [PoM] £35.00 DT price = £35.00 [CD2]
▸ Medikinet XL (Flynn Pharma Ltd)
Methylphenidate hydrochloride 5 mg Medikinet XL 5mg capsules | 30 capsule [PoM] £24.04 [CD2]
Methylphenidate hydrochloride 10 mg Medikinet XL 10mg capsules | 30 capsule [PoM] £24.04 DT price = £25.00 [CD2]
Methylphenidate hydrochloride 20 mg Medikinet XL 20mg capsules | 30 capsule [PoM] £28.86 DT price = £30.00 [CD2]
Methylphenidate hydrochloride 30 mg Medikinet XL 30mg capsules | 30 capsule [PoM] £33.66 DT price = £35.00 [CD2]
Methylphenidate hydrochloride 40 mg Medikinet XL 40mg capsules | 30 capsule [PoM] £57.72 DT price = £57.72 [CD2]
Methylphenidate hydrochloride 50 mg Medikinet XL 50mg capsules | 30 capsule [PoM] £62.52 [CD2]
Methylphenidate hydrochloride 60 mg Medikinet XL 60mg capsules | 30 capsule [PoM] £67.32 [CD2]

CNS STIMULANTS > CENTRALLY ACTING SYMPATHOMIMETICS > AMFETAMINES

Dexamfetamine sulfate

(Dexamphetamine sulfate)

- INDICATIONS AND DOSE

Narcolepsy

▸ BY MOUTH
▸ **Adult:** Initially 10 mg daily in divided doses, increased in steps of 10 mg every 1 week, maintenance dose to be given in 2–4 divided doses; maximum 60 mg per day
▸ **Elderly:** Initially 5 mg daily in divided doses, increased in steps of 5 mg every 1 week, maintenance dose to be given in 2–4 divided doses; maximum 60 mg per day

Refractory attention deficit hyperactivity disorder (initiated under specialist supervision)

▸ BY MOUTH
▸ **Child 6–17 years:** Initially 2.5 mg 2–3 times a day, increased in steps of 5 mg once weekly if required, increased if necessary up to 1 mg/kg daily, maintenance dose to be given in 2–4 divided doses, up to 20 mg daily (40 mg daily has been required in some children)
▸ **Adult:** Initially 5 mg twice daily, dose is increased at weekly intervals according to response, maintenance dose to be given in 2–4 divided doses; maximum 60 mg per day

- UNLICENSED USE

▸ **In adults** Not licensed for use in adults for refractory attention deficit hyperactivity disorder.

- CONTRA-INDICATIONS Advanced arteriosclerosis (in adults) · agitated states · cardiovascular disease · history of alcohol abuse · history of drug abuse · hyperexcitability · hyperthyroidism · moderate hypertension · severe hypertension · structural cardiac abnormalities

Nervous system

4

- CAUTIONS Anorexia · bipolar disorder · history of epilepsy (discontinue if seizures occur) · mild hypertension · psychosis · susceptibility to angle-closure glaucoma · tics · Tourette syndrome

  CAUTIONS, FURTHER INFORMATION
- Tics and Tourette syndrome Discontinue use if tics occur.
- Growth restriction in children Monitor height and weight as growth restriction may occur during prolonged therapy (drug-free periods may allow catch-up in growth but withdraw slowly to avoid inducing depression or renewed hyperactivity).
- INTERACTIONS → Appendix 1 (sympathomimetics).
- SIDE-EFFECTS
- **Common or very common** Abdominal cramps · acidosis · aggression · alopecia · anhedonia · anorexia · anxiety · ataxia · cardiomyopathy · cardiovascular collapse · cerebral vasculitis · chest pain · confusion · depression · diarrhoea · dizziness · dry mouth · dysphoria · euphoria · growth restriction in children · headache · hyperactivity · hyperpyrexia (in children) · hyperreflexia · hypertension · hypotension · impaired concentration · irritability · ischaemic colitis · malaise · mydriasis · myocardial infarction · nausea · nervousness · neuroleptic malignant syndrome · obsessive-compulsive behaviour · palpitations · panic attack · paranoia · psychosis · pyrexia (in adults) · rash · renal impairment · restlessness · rhabdomyolysis · seizures · sexual dysfunction · sleep disturbances · stroke · sweating · tachycardia · taste disturbance · Tourette syndrome (in predisposed individuals) · tremor · urticaria · visual disturbances · weight loss
- **Very rare** Angle-closure glaucoma
- **Frequency not known** Choreoathetoid movements (in predisposed individuals) · dyskinesia (in predisposed individuals) · increased appetite · tics (in predisposed individuals)

  Overdose
  Amfetamines cause wakefulness, excessive activity, paranoia, hallucinations, and hypertension followed by exhaustion, convulsions, hyperthermia, and coma. See Stimulants under Emergency treatment of poisoning p. 1194.
- PREGNANCY Avoid (retrospective evidence of uncertain significance suggesting possible embryotoxicity).
- BREAST FEEDING Significant amount in milk—avoid.
- RENAL IMPAIRMENT Use with caution.
- MONITORING REQUIREMENTS
- Monitor growth in children.
- Monitor for aggressive behaviour or hostility during initial treatment.
- Pulse, blood pressure, psychiatric symptoms, appetite, weight and height should be recorded at initiation of therapy, following each dose adjustment, and at least every 6 months thereafter.
- TREATMENT CESSATION Avoid abrupt withdrawal.
- DIRECTIONS FOR ADMINISTRATION
- With oral use in children Tablets can be halved.
- PRESCRIBING AND DISPENSING INFORMATION Data on safety and efficacy of long-term use not complete.
- PATIENT AND CARER ADVICE
  Driving and skilled tasks
  Drugs and Driving Prescribers and other healthcare professionals should advise patients if treatment is likely to affect their ability to perform skilled tasks (e.g. driving). This applies especially to drugs with sedative effects; patients should be warned that these effects are increased by alcohol. General information about a patient's fitness to drive is available from the Driver and Vehicle Licensing Agency at www.dvla.gov.uk.
  For information on 2015 legislation regarding driving whilst taking certain controlled drugs, including

amfetamines, see *Drugs and driving* under Guidance on prescribing p. 1.
- NATIONAL FUNDING/ACCESS DECISIONS
  NICE technology appraisals (TAs)
- Methylphenidate, atomoxetine and dexamfetamine for attention deficit hyperactivity disorder (ADHD) (March 2006) NICE TA98
  Dexamfetamine is recommended, within its licensed indications, as an option for the management of ADHD in children and adolescents.
  www.nice.org.uk/TA98
- MEDICINAL FORMS
  There can be variation in the licensing of different medicines containing the same drug. Forms available from special-order manufacturers include: oral suspension, oral solution

  Tablet
- Dexamfetamine sulfate (Non-proprietary)
  Dexamfetamine sulfate 5 mg Dexamfetamine 5mg tablets | 28 tablet [PoM] £24.75 DT price = £24.75 [CD2]
- Amfexa (Flynn Pharma Ltd)
  Dexamfetamine sulfate 5 mg Amfexa 5mg tablets | 30 tablet [PoM] £19.89 [CD2]

  Oral solution
- Dexamfetamine sulfate (Non-proprietary)
  Dexamfetamine sulfate 1 mg per 1 ml Dexamfetamine 5mg/5ml oral solution sugar free sugar-free | 150 ml [PoM] £29.44-£34.35 [CD2] sugar-free | 500 ml [PoM] £114.49 DT price = £114.49 [CD2]

Lisdexamfetamine mesilate

- DRUG ACTION Lisdexamfetamine is a prodrug of dexamfetamine.

- INDICATIONS AND DOSE
  Attention deficit hyperactivity disorder refractory to methylphenidate (initiated by a specialist)
- BY MOUTH
- Child 6–17 years: Initially 30 mg once daily, increased in steps of 20 mg every 1 week if required, dose to be taken in the morning, discontinue if response insufficient after 1 month; maximum 70 mg per day
- Adult: Initially 30 mg once daily, increased in steps of 20 mg every 1 week if required, dose to be taken in the morning, discontinue if response insufficient after 1 month; maximum 70 mg per day

- UNLICENSED USE
- In adults Not licensed for use in adults for attention deficit hyperactivity disorder.
- CONTRA-INDICATIONS Advanced arteriosclerosis · agitated states · hyperexcitability · hyperthyroidism · moderate hypertension · severe hypertension · symptomatic cardiovascular disease
- CAUTIONS Anorexia · bipolar disorder · history of alcohol abuse · history of cardiac abnormalities · history of cardiovascular disease · history of drug abuse · may lower seizure threshold (discontinue if seizures occur) · psychosis · susceptibility to angle-closure glaucoma · tics · Tourette syndrome

  CAUTIONS, FURTHER INFORMATION
- Tics and Tourette syndrome Discontinue use if tics occur.
- Growth restriction in children Monitor height and weight as growth restriction may occur during prolonged therapy (drug-free periods may allow catch-up in growth but withdraw slowly to avoid inducing depression or renewed hyperactivity).
- INTERACTIONS → Appendix 1 (sympathomimetics).
- SIDE-EFFECTS
- **Common or very common** Abdominal cramps · aggression · decreased appetite · diarrhoea · dizziness · drowsiness · dry mouth · dyspnoea · growth restriction in children ·

headache · labile mood · malaise · mydriasis · nausea · pyrexia · sleep disturbances · tics · vomiting · weight loss
▸ **Uncommon** Anorexia · anxiety · depression · dermatillomania · dysphoria · hallucination · hypertension · logorrhoea · mania · palpitation · paranoia · rash · restlessness · sexual dysfunction · sweating · tachycardia · tremor · visual disturbances
▸ **Very rare** Angle-closure glaucoma
▸ **Frequency not known** Cardiomyopathy · choreoathetoid movements (in predisposed individuals) · dyskinesia (in predisposed individuals) · euphoria · seizures · Tourette syndrome (in predisposed individuals)

Overdose
Amfetamines cause wakefulness, excessive activity, paranoia, hallucinations, and hypertension followed by exhaustion, convulsions, hyperthermia, and coma. See Stimulants under Emergency treatment of poisoning p. 1194.

● PREGNANCY Manufacturer advises use only if potential benefit outweighs risk.

● BREAST FEEDING Manufacturer advises avoid—present in human milk.

● RENAL IMPAIRMENT Max. dose 50 mg daily in severe impairment.

● MONITORING REQUIREMENTS
▸ Monitor for aggressive behaviour or hostility during initial treatment.
▸ Monitor growth in children.
▸ Pulse, blood pressure, psychiatric symptoms, appetite, weight and height should be recorded at initiation of therapy, following each dose adjustment, and at least every 6 months thereafter.

● TREATMENT CESSATION Avoid abrupt withdrawal.

● DIRECTIONS FOR ADMINISTRATION Swallow whole or mix contents of capsule in yoghurt or a glass of water or orange juice; contents should be dispersed completely and consumed immediately.

● PATIENT AND CARER ADVICE
Patients and carers should be counselled on the administration of capsules.

Driving and skilled tasks
Drugs and Driving Prescribers and other healthcare professionals should advise patients if treatment is likely to affect their ability to perform skilled tasks (e.g. driving). This applies especially to drugs with sedative effects; patients should be warned that these effects are increased by alcohol. General information about a patient's fitness to drive is available from the Driver and Vehicle Licensing Agency at www.dvla.gov.uk.
For information on 2015 legislation regarding driving whilst taking certain controlled drugs, including amfetamines, see *Drugs and driving* under Guidance on prescribing p. 1.

● MEDICINAL FORMS
There can be variation in the licensing of different medicines containing the same drug.

Capsule
CAUTIONARY AND ADVISORY LABELS 3, 25
▸ Elvanse (Shire Pharmaceuticals Ltd) ▼
Lisdexamfetamine dimesylate 20 mg Elvanse 20mg capsules | 28 capsule PoM £54.62 CD2
Lisdexamfetamine dimesylate 30 mg Elvanse Adult 30mg capsules | 28 capsule PoM £58.24 DT price = £58.24 CD2
Elvanse 30mg capsules | 28 capsule PoM £58.24 DT price = £58.24 CD2
Lisdexamfetamine dimesylate 40 mg Elvanse 40mg capsules | 28 capsule PoM £62.82 CD2
Lisdexamfetamine dimesylate 50 mg Elvanse Adult 50mg capsules | 28 capsule PoM £68.60 DT price = £68.60 CD2
Elvanse 50mg capsules | 28 capsule PoM £68.60 DT price = £68.60 CD2

Lisdexamfetamine dimesylate 60 mg Elvanse 60mg capsules | 28 capsule PoM £75.18 CD2
Lisdexamfetamine dimesylate 70 mg Elvanse 70mg capsules | 28 capsule PoM £83.16 DT price = £83.16 CD2
Elvanse Adult 70mg capsules | 28 capsule PoM £83.16 DT price = £83.16 CD2

SYMPATHOMIMETICS ⟩ ALPHA₂-ADRENOCEPTOR AGONISTS

Guanfacine
26.5.2016

● INDICATIONS AND DOSE
Attention deficit hyperactivity disorder in children for whom stimulants are not suitable, not tolerated or ineffective (initiated under specialist supervision)
▸ BY MOUTH
▸ Child 6-12 years (body-weight 25 kg and above): Initially 1 mg once daily; adjusted in steps of 1 mg every week if necessary and if tolerated; maintenance 0.05–0.12 mg/kg once daily (max. per dose 4 mg), for optimal weight-adjusted dose titrations, consult product literature
▸ Child 13-17 years (body-weight 34-41.4 kg): Initially 1 mg once daily; adjusted in steps of 1 mg every week if necessary and if tolerated; maintenance 0.05–0.12 mg/kg once daily (max. per dose 4 mg), for optimal weight-adjusted dose titrations, consult product literature
▸ Child 13-17 years (body-weight 41.5-49.4 kg): Initially 1 mg once daily; adjusted in steps of 1 mg every week if necessary and if tolerated; maintenance 0.05–0.12 mg/kg once daily (max. per dose 5 mg), for optimal weight-adjusted dose titrations, consult product literature
▸ Child 13-17 years (body-weight 49.5-58.4 kg): Initially 1 mg once daily; adjusted in steps of 1 mg every week if necessary and if tolerated; maintenance 0.05–0.12 mg/kg once daily (max. per dose 6 mg), for optimal weight-adjusted dose titrations, consult product literature
▸ Child 13-17 years (body-weight 58.5 kg and above): Initially 1 mg once daily; adjusted in steps of 1 mg every week if necessary and if tolerated; maintenance 0.05–0.12 mg/kg once daily (max. per dose 7 mg), for optimal weight-adjusted dose titrations, consult product literature

● CAUTIONS Bradycardia (risk of torsade de pointes) · heart block (risk of torsade de pointes) · history of cardiovascular disease · history of QT-interval prolongation · hypokalaemia (risk of torsade de pointes)

● INTERACTIONS → Appendix 1 (guanfacine).
Caution with concomitant use of drugs that prolong QT-interval.

● SIDE-EFFECTS
▸ **Common or very common** Abdominal pain · anxiety · bradycardia · constipation · decreased appetite · depression · diarrhoea · dizziness · dry mouth · enuresis · headache · hypotension · irritability · malaise · mood lability · nausea · rash · sleep disturbance · somnolence · vomiting · weight increase
▸ **Uncommon** Agitation · chest pain · convulsion · dyspepsia · first-degree AV block · hallucination · pallor · pollakiuria · pruritus · sinus arrhythmia · syncope · tachycardia
▸ **Rare** Hypertension
▸ **Frequency not known** Suicidal ideation
SIDE-EFFECTS, FURTHER INFORMATION
▸ Somnolence and sedation Somnolence and sedation may occur, predominantly during the first 2-3 weeks of treatment and with dose increases; manufacturer advises

4

Nervous system

to consider dose reduction or discontinuation of treatment if symptoms are clinically significant or persistent.

Overdose

Features may include hypotension, initial hypertension, bradycardia, lethargy, and respiratory depression. Manufacturer advises that patients who develop lethargy should be observed for development of more serious toxicity for up to 24 hours.

● CONCEPTION AND CONTRACEPTION Manufacturer recommends effective contraception in females of childbearing potential.

● PREGNANCY Manufacturer advises avoid—toxicity in *animal* studies.

● BREAST FEEDING Manufacturer advises avoid—present in milk in *animal* studies.

● HEPATIC IMPAIRMENT Manufacturer advises consider dose reduction.

● RENAL IMPAIRMENT Manufacturer advises consider dose reduction in severe impairment and end-stage renal disease.

● MONITORING REQUIREMENTS
  ▸ Manufacturer advises to conduct a baseline evaluation to identify patients at risk of somnolence, sedation, hypotension, bradycardia, QT-prolongation, and arrhythmia; this should include assessment of cardiovascular status. Monitor for signs of these adverse effects weekly during dose titration and then every 3 months during the first year of treatment, and every 6 months thereafter. Monitor BMI prior to treatment and then every 3 months for the first year of treatment, and every 6 months thereafter. More frequent monitoring is advised following dose adjustments.
  ▸ Monitor blood pressure and pulse during dose downward titration and following discontinuation of treatment.

● TREATMENT CESSATION Manufacturer advises avoid abrupt withdrawal; consider dose tapering to minimise potential withdrawal effects.

● DIRECTIONS FOR ADMINISTRATION Manufacturer advises avoid administration with high fat meals (may increase absorption).

● PATIENT AND CARER ADVICE Patients or carers should be counselled on administration of guanfacine modified-release tablets.

Missed doses

Manufacturer advises that patients and carers should inform their prescriber if more than one dose is missed; consider dose re-titration.

Driving and skilled tasks

Manufacturer advises patients and carers should be counselled about the effects on driving and performance of skilled tasks—increased risk of dizziness and syncope.

● MEDICINAL FORMS
There can be variation in the licensing of different medicines containing the same drug.

Modified-release tablet

CAUTIONARY AND ADVISORY LABELS 25, 2
  ▸ Intuniv (Shire Pharmaceuticals Ltd) ▼
  Guanfacine (as Guanfacine hydrochloride) 1 mg Intuniv 1mg modified-release tablets | 28 tablet [PoM] £56.00
  Guanfacine (as Guanfacine hydrochloride) 2 mg Intuniv 2mg modified-release tablets | 28 tablet [PoM] £58.52
  Guanfacine (as Guanfacine hydrochloride) 3 mg Intuniv 3mg modified-release tablets | 28 tablet [PoM] £65.52
  Guanfacine (as Guanfacine hydrochloride) 4 mg Intuniv 4mg modified-release tablets | 28 tablet [PoM] £76.16

3.3 Bipolar disorder and mania

Drugs for mania and hypomania

Antimanic drugs are used to control acute attacks and to prevent recurrence of episodes of mania or hypomania. Long-term treatment of bipolar disorder should continue for at least two years from the last manic episode and up to five years if the patient has risk factors for relapse.

An antidepressant drug may also be required for the treatment of co-existing depression, but should be avoided in patients with rapid-cycling bipolar disorder, a recent history of hypomania, or with rapid mood fluctuations.

Benzodiazepines

Use of benzodiazepines (such as lorazepam p. 308) may be helpful in the initial stages of treatment for behavioural disturbance or agitation; they should not be used for long periods because of the risk of dependence.

Antipsychotic drugs

Antipsychotic drugs (normally olanzapine p. 365, quetiapine p. 367, or risperidone p. 368) are useful in acute episodes of mania and hypomania; if the response to antipsychotic drugs is inadequate, lithium or valproate may be added. An antipsychotic drug may be used concomitantly with lithium or valproate in the initial treatment of severe acute mania.

Olanzapine can be used for the long-term management of bipolar disorder in patients whose manic episode responded to olanzapine therapy. It can be given either as monotherapy, or in combination with lithium or valproate if the patient has frequent relapses or continuing functional impairment.

Asenapine p. 324, a second-generation antipsychotic, is licensed for the treatment of moderate to severe manic episodes associated with bipolar disorder.

When discontinuing antipsychotics, the dose should be reduced gradually over at least 4 weeks if the patient is continuing with other antimanic drugs; if the patient is not continuing with other antimanic drugs or if there is a history of manic relapse, a withdrawal period of up to 3 months should be considered.

Carbamazepine

Carbamazepine p. 283 may be used under specialist supervision for the prophylaxis of bipolar disorder (manic-depressive disorder) in patients unresponsive to a combination of other prophylactic drugs; it is used in patients with rapid-cycling manic-depressive illness (4 or more affective episodes per year). The dose of carbamazepine should not normally be increased if an acute episode of mania occurs.

Valproate

Valproate (valproic acid p. 323 (as the semisodium salt) and sodium valproate p. 298) is used for the treatment of manic episodes associated with bipolar disorder. It must be started and supervised by a specialist experienced in managing bipolar disorder. Valproate (valproic acid and sodium valproate) is also used for the prophylaxis of bipolar disorder. Valproic acid and sodium valproate should not be used in female children, in females of childbearing potential and pregnant females, unless alternative treatments are ineffective or not tolerated, because of its high teratogenic potential; the benefit and risk of valproate therapy should be carefully reconsidered at regular treatment reviews. In patients with frequent relapse or continuing functional impairment, consider switching therapy to lithium or olanzapine, or adding lithium or olanzapine to valproate. If a patient taking valproate experiences an acute episode of mania that is not ameliorated by increasing the valproate dose, consider concomitant therapy with olanzapine, quetiapine, or risperidone.

Lithium

Lithium salts are used in the prophylaxis and treatment of mania, hypomania and depression in bipolar disorder (manic-depressive disorder), and in the prophylaxis and treatment of recurrent unipolar depression. Lithium is also used as concomitant therapy with antidepressant medication in patients who have had an incomplete response to treatment for acute bipolar depression and to augment other antidepressants in patients with treatment-resistant depression [unlicensed indication]. It is also licensed for the treatment of aggressive or self-harming behaviour.

The decision to give prophylactic lithium requires specialist advice, and must be based on careful consideration of the likelihood of recurrence in the individual patient, and the benefit of treatment weighed against the risks. The full prophylactic effect of lithium may not occur for six to twelve months after the initiation of therapy. Olanzapine or valproate (given alone or as adjunctive therapy with lithium) are alternative prophylactic treatments in patients who experience frequent relapses or continued functional impairment.

> **Drugs used for Bipolar disorder and mania not listed below** Aripiprazole, p. 362 · Chlorpromazine hydrochloride, p. 353 · Haloperidol, p. 354 · Lamotrigine, p. 289 · Paliperidone, p. 366 · Perphenazine, p. 356 · Prochlorperazine, p. 357 · Zuclopenthixol acetate, p. 359

ANTIEPILEPTICS

Valproic acid   9.6.2016

- **INDICATIONS AND DOSE**

Treatment of manic episodes associated with bipolar disorder

▸ BY MOUTH
  ▸ Adult: Initially 750 mg daily in 2–3 divided doses, then increased to 1–2 g daily, adjusted according to response, doses greater than 45 mg/kg daily require careful monitoring

Migraine prophylaxis

▸ BY MOUTH
  ▸ Adult: Initially 250 mg twice daily, then increased if necessary to 1 g daily in divided doses

DOSE EQUIVALENCE AND CONVERSION
Semisodium valproate comprises equimolar amounts of sodium valproate and valproic acid.

CONVULEX®

Epilepsy

▸ BY MOUTH
  ▸ Adult: Initially 600 mg daily in 2–4 divided doses, increased in steps of 150–300 mg every 3 days; usual maintenance 1–2 g daily in 2–4 divided doses, max. 2.5 g daily in 2–4 divided doses

DOSE EQUIVALENCE AND CONVERSION
Convulex® has a 1:1 dose relationship with products containing sodium valproate, but nevertheless care is needed if switching or making changes.

- **UNLICENSED USE** Not licensed for migraine prophylaxis.

> **IMPORTANT SAFETY INFORMATION**
> MHRA/CHM ADVICE: VALPROATE AND RISK OF ABNORMAL PREGNANCY OUTCOMES
> Infants exposed to valproate in utero are at a high risk of serious developmental disorders (up to 30–40% risk) and congenital malformations (approx. 11% risk). Valproate should not be used in female children, females of

childbearing potential or during pregnancy unless alternative treatments are ineffective or not tolerated.

- CONTRA-INDICATIONS Acute porphyrias p. 918 · known or suspected mitochondrial disorders (higher rate of acute liver failure and liver-related deaths) · personal or family history of severe hepatic dysfunction
- CAUTIONS Systemic lupus erythematosus
  CAUTIONS, FURTHER INFORMATION
  Consider vitamin D supplementation in patients that are immobilised for long periods or who have inadequate sun exposure or dietary intake of calcium.
  ▸ Liver toxicity Liver dysfunction (including fatal hepatic failure) has occurred in association with valproate (especially in children under 3 years and in those with metabolic or degenerative disorders, organic brain disease or severe seizure disorders associated with mental retardation) usually in first 6 months and usually involving multiple antiepileptic therapy. Raised liver enzymes during valproate treatment are usually transient but patients should be reassessed clinically and liver function (including prothrombin time) monitored until return to normal—discontinue if abnormally prolonged prothrombin time (particularly in association with other relevant abnormalities).
- INTERACTIONS → Appendix 1 (valproic acid).
- SIDE-EFFECTS
  ▸ **Common or very common** Diarrhoea · gastric irritation · hyperammonaemia · nausea · thrombocytopenia · transient hair loss (regrowth may be curly) · weight gain
  ▸ **Uncommon** Aggression · ataxia · behavioural disturbances · hyperactivity · increased alertness · tremor · vasculitis
  ▸ **Rare** Anaemia · blood disorders · confusion · drowsiness · hallucinations · hearing loss · hepatic dysfunction · lethargy · leucopenia · pancytopenia · rash · stupor
  ▸ **Very rare** Acne · coma · dementia · encephalopathy · enuresis · extrapyramidal symptoms · Fanconi's syndrome · gynaecomastia · hirsutism · hyponatraemia · increase in bleeding time · pancreatitis · peripheral oedema · reduced bone mineral density · Stevens-Johnson syndrome · suicidal ideation · toxic epidermal necrolysis
  ▸ **Frequency not known** Drug rash with eosinophilia and systemic symptoms (DRESS) syndrome · hypersensitivity reactions · male infertility · menstrual disturbances · syndrome of inappropriate secretion of antidiuretic hormone
  SIDE-EFFECTS, FURTHER INFORMATION
  ▸ Hepatic dysfunction Withdraw treatment immediately if persistent vomiting and abdominal pain, anorexia, jaundice, oedema, malaise, drowsiness, or loss of seizure control.
  ▸ Pancreatitis Discontinue treatment if symptoms of pancreatitis develop.
- CONCEPTION AND CONTRACEPTION Valproate is associated with teratogenic risks and should not be used in females of child-bearing potential unless there is no safer alternative—this should be fully considered and discussed before prescribing for females of child-bearing age. Effective contraception advised in females of child-bearing potential. In females planning to become pregnant, all efforts should be made to switch to appropriate alternative treatment prior to conception.
- PREGNANCY Valproate is associated with the highest risk of major and minor congenital malformations (in particular neural tube defects), and long-term neurodevelopmental effects. Valproate should not be used during pregnancy unless there is no safer alternative and only after a careful discussion of the risks. If valproate is to be used during pregnancy, the lowest effective dose should be prescribed in divided doses to avoid peaks in plasma-valproate concentrations; doses greater than 1 g daily are

associated with an increased risk of teratogenicity. Neonatal bleeding (related to hypofibrinaemia). Neonatal hepatotoxicity also reported.

Specialist prenatal monitoring should be instigated when valproate has been taken in pregnancy.

The dose should be monitored carefully during pregnancy and after birth, and adjustments made on a clinical basis.

- BREAST FEEDING Present in milk—risk of haematological disorders in breast-fed newborns and infants.
- HEPATIC IMPAIRMENT Avoid if possible—hepatotoxicity and hepatic failure may occasionally occur (usually in first 6 months). Avoid in active liver disease.
- RENAL IMPAIRMENT Reduce dose.
- MONITORING REQUIREMENTS
  ‣ Monitor closely if dose greater than 45 mg/kg daily.
  ‣ Monitor liver function before therapy and during first 6 months especially in patients most at risk.
  ‣ Measure full blood count and ensure no undue potential for bleeding before starting and before surgery.
- EFFECT ON LABORATORY TESTS False-positive urine tests for ketones.
- TREATMENT CESSATION (EvGr) Avoid abrupt withdrawal; if treatment with valproate is stopped, reduce the dose gradually over at least 4 weeks. ⟨A⟩
- PRESCRIBING AND DISPENSING INFORMATION
CONVULEX® Patients being treated for epilepsy may need to be maintained on a specific manufacturer's branded or generic oral valproic acid product.
- PATIENT AND CARER ADVICE
Risk of abnormal pregnancy outcomes A patient guide and card should be provided to all female patients.
Blood or hepatic disorders Patients or their carers should be told how to recognise signs and symptoms of blood or liver disorders and advised to seek immediate medical attention if symptoms develop.
Pancreatitis Patients or their carers should be told how to recognise signs and symptoms of pancreatitis and advised to seek immediate medical attention if symptoms such as abdominal pain, nausea, or vomiting develop.
MHRA advice: Valproate and risk of abnormal pregnancy outcomes
Female patients and their carers should be counselled on the risk of valproate treatment during pregnancy. Ensure female patients are provided with relevant resources, to support their understanding of the risks. In particular the prescriber must ensure the patient understands:
- the risks associated with valproate during pregnancy;
- the need to use effective contraception;
- the need for regular review of treatment;
- the need to rapidly consult if she is planning a pregnancy or becomes pregnant

- MEDICINAL FORMS
There can be variation in the licensing of different medicines containing the same drug. Forms available from special-order manufacturers include: oral suspension, oral solution

Gastro-resistant tablet
CAUTIONARY AND ADVISORY LABELS 10, 21, 25
‣ Depakote (Sanofi) ▼
Valproic acid (as Valproate semisodium) 250 mg Depakote 250mg gastro-resistant tablets | 90 tablet (PoM) £17.08 DT price = £17.08
Valproic acid (as Valproate semisodium) 500 mg Depakote 500mg gastro-resistant tablets | 90 tablet (PoM) £34.11 DT price = £34.11
Gastro-resistant capsule
CAUTIONARY AND ADVISORY LABELS 8, 21, 25, 10
‣ Valproic acid (Non-proprietary)
Valproic acid (as Valproate semisodium) 125 mg Depakote 125mg sprinkle gastro-resistant capsules | 100 capsule (PoM) no price available

‣ Convulex (Pfizer Ltd) ▼
Valproic acid 150 mg Convulex 150mg gastro-resistant capsules | 100 capsule (PoM) £3.68
Valproic acid 300 mg Convulex 300mg gastro-resistant capsules | 100 capsule (PoM) £7.35
Valproic acid 500 mg Convulex 500mg gastro-resistant capsules | 100 capsule (PoM) £12.25

ANTIPSYCHOTICS 〉 SECOND-GENERATION

⌕ 352

Asenapine

- INDICATIONS AND DOSE
Monotherapy for the treatment of moderate to severe manic episodes associated with bipolar disorder
  ‣ BY MOUTH
  ‣ Adult: Initially 10 mg twice daily, reduced to 5 mg twice daily, adjusted according to response
Combination therapy for the treatment of moderate to severe manic episodes associated with bipolar disorder
  ‣ BY MOUTH
  ‣ Adult: Initially 5 mg twice daily, increased if necessary to 10 mg twice daily, adjusted according to response

- CAUTIONS Dementia with Lewy Bodies
- SIDE-EFFECTS Anxiety · dysphagia · glossodynia · hypersalivation · rhabdomyolysis · speech disturbance · taste disturbance · tongue swelling · transient oral hypoaesthesia · transient paraesthesia
- PREGNANCY Use only if potential benefit outweighs risk—toxicity in *animal* studies.
- BREAST FEEDING Avoid—no information available.
- HEPATIC IMPAIRMENT Use with caution in moderate impairment. Avoid in severe impairment.
- RENAL IMPAIRMENT Use with caution if eGFR less than 15 mL/minute/1.73 m^2—no information available.
- PATIENT AND CARER ADVICE Patient or carer should be given advice on how to administer asenapine sublingual tablet.

- MEDICINAL FORMS
There can be variation in the licensing of different medicines containing the same drug.
Sublingual tablet
CAUTIONARY AND ADVISORY LABELS 2, 26
‣ Sycrest (Lundbeck Ltd)
Asenapine (as Asenapine maleate) 5 mg Sycrest 5mg sublingual tablets sugar-free | 60 tablet (PoM) £102.60 DT price = £102.60
Asenapine (as Asenapine maleate) 10 mg Sycrest 10mg sublingual tablets sugar-free | 60 tablet (PoM) £102.60 DT price = £102.60

ANTIPSYCHOTICS 〉 LITHIUM SALTS

Lithium salts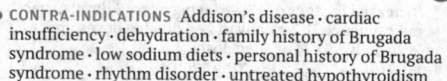

- CONTRA-INDICATIONS Addison's disease · cardiac insufficiency · dehydration · family history of Brugada syndrome · low sodium diets · personal history of Brugada syndrome · rhythm disorder · untreated hypothyroidism
- CAUTIONS Avoid abrupt withdrawal · cardiac disease · concurrent ECT (may lower seizure threshold) · diuretic treatment (risk of toxicity) · elderly (reduce dose) · epilepsy (may lower seizure threshold) · myasthenia gravis · psoriasis (risk of exacerbation) · QT interval prolongation · review dose as necessary in diarrhoea · review dose as necessary in intercurrent infection (especially if sweating profusely) · review dose as necessary in vomiting · surgery
CAUTIONS, FURTHER INFORMATION
‣ Long-term use Long-term use of lithium has been associated with thyroid disorders and mild cognitive and memory impairment. Long-term treatment should therefore be undertaken only with careful assessment of

risk and benefit, and with monitoring of thyroid function every 6 months (more often if there is evidence of deterioration).

The need for continued therapy should be assessed regularly and patients should be maintained on lithium after 3–5 years only if benefit persists.

- INTERACTIONS → Appendix 1 (lithium).
Caution with concomitant use of drugs and any therapy that may lower seizure threshold.
Caution with concomitant use of drugs that prolong the QT interval.
Lithium toxicity is made worse by sodium depletion, therefore concurrent use of diuretics (particularly thiazides) is hazardous and should be avoided.
- SIDE-EFFECTS
▸ **Very rare** Nystagmus
▸ **Frequency not known** Acneiform eruptions · alopecia · anorexia · arrhythmia · arthralgia · AV block · benign intracranial hypertension · bradycardia · cardiomyopathy · cognitive impairment · dry mouth · dysgeusia · ECG changes · electrolyte imbalance · encephalopathy · euthyroid goitre · extrapyramidal side-effects · fine tremor · gastritis · gastro-intestinal disturbances · hallucinations · hyperparathyroidism · hypersalivation · hyperthyroidism · hypothyroidism · kidney changes · leucocytosis · malaise · memory loss · myalgia · myasthenia gravis · nephrogenic diabetes insipidus · nephrotic syndrome · oedema · other skin disorders · parathyroid adenoma · peripheral neuropathy · polydipsia · psoriasis exacerbation · QT interval prolongation · Raynaud's phenomena · renal impairment · sexual dysfunction · sinus node dysfunction · speech disorder · thyroid changes · vertigo · weight changes

Overdose
Signs of intoxication require withdrawal of treatment and include increasing gastro-intestinal disturbances (vomiting, diarrhoea), visual disturbances, polyuria, muscle weakness, fine tremor increasing to coarse tremor, CNS disturbances (confusion and drowsiness increasing to lack of coordination, restlessness, stupor); abnormal reflexes, myoclonus, incontinence, hypernatraemia. With severe overdosage seizures, cardiac arrhythmias (including sino-atrial block, bradycardia and first-degree heart block), blood pressure changes, circulatory failure, renal failure, coma and sudden death reported.

For details on the management of poisoning, see Lithium, under Emergency treatment of poisoning p. 1194.

- CONCEPTION AND CONTRACEPTION Manufacturer advises effective contraception during treatment for women of child bearing potential.
- PREGNANCY Dose requirements increased during the second and third trimesters (but on delivery return abruptly to normal). Avoid if possible, particularly in the first trimester (risk of teratogenicity, including cardiac abnormalities).
Close monitoring of serum-lithium concentration advised in pregnancy (risk of toxicity in neonate).
- BREAST FEEDING Present in milk and risk of toxicity in infant—avoid.
- RENAL IMPAIRMENT Caution in mild to moderate impairment. Avoid in severe impairment. In renal impairment monitor serum-lithium concentration closely and adjust dose accordingly.
- MONITORING REQUIREMENTS
▸ Serum concentrations Lithium salts have a narrow therapeutic/toxic ratio and should therefore not be prescribed unless facilities for monitoring serum-lithium concentrations are available.
▸ Samples should be taken 12 hours after the dose to achieve a serum-lithium concentration of 0.4–1 mmol/litre (lower end of the range for maintenance therapy and elderly patients).

▸ A target serum-lithium concentration of 0.8–1 mmol/litre is recommended for acute episodes of mania, and for patients who have previously relapsed or have sub-syndromal symptoms. It is important to determine the optimum range for each individual patient.
▸ Routine serum-lithium monitoring should be performed weekly after initiation and after each dose change until concentrations are stable, then every 3 months thereafter. Additional serum-lithium measurements should be made if a patient develops significant intercurrent disease or if there is a significant change in a patient's sodium or fluid intake.
▸ Renal function should be monitored at baseline and every 6 months thereafter (more often if there is evidence of deterioration or if the patient has other risk factors, such as starting ACE inhibitors, NSAIDs, or diuretics).
▸ Assess cardiac and thyroid function before initiating, and thereafter every 6 months on stabilised regimens.
- TREATMENT CESSATION While there is no clear evidence of withdrawal or rebound psychosis, abrupt discontinuation of lithium increases the risk of relapse. If lithium is to be discontinued, the dose should be reduced gradually over a period of at least 4 weeks (preferably over a period of up to 3 months). Patients and their carers should be warned of the risk of relapse if lithium is discontinued abruptly. If lithium is stopped or is to be discontinued abruptly, consider changing therapy to an atypical antipsychotic or valproate.
- PATIENT AND CARER ADVICE
Patients should be advised to report signs and symptoms of lithium toxicity, hypothyroidism, renal dysfunction (including polyuria and polydipsia), and benign intracranial hypertension (persistent headache and visual disturbance).
Maintain adequate fluid intake and avoid dietary changes which reduce or increase sodium intake.
Driving and skilled tasks May impair performance of skilled tasks (e.g. driving, operating machinery).
Lithium treatment packs A lithium treatment pack should be given to patients on initiation of treatment with lithium. The pack consists of a patient information booklet, lithium alert card, and a record book for tracking serum-lithium concentration. Packs may be purchased from
3M
0845 610 1112
nhsforms@mmm.uk.com

F 324

Lithium carbonate

- INDICATIONS AND DOSE

Treatment and prophylaxis of mania | Treatment and prophylaxis of bipolar disorder | Treatment and prophylaxis of recurrent depression | Treatment and prophylaxis of aggressive or self-harming behaviour
▸ BY MOUTH
▸ Adult: Dose adjusted to achieve a serum-lithium concentration of 0.4–1 mmol/litre 12 hours after a dose on days 4–7 of treatment, then every week until dosage has remained constant for 4 weeks and every 3 months thereafter, doses are initially divided throughout the day, but once daily administration is preferred when serum-lithium concentration stabilised continued →

4

Nervous system

CAMCOLIT® IMMEDIATE-RELEASE TABLET

Treatment of mania | Treatment of bipolar disorder | Treatment of recurrent depression | Treatment of aggressive or self-harming behaviour
▸ BY MOUTH
▸ Adult: Initially 1–1.5 g daily, dose adjusted to achieve a serum-lithium concentration of 0.4–1 mmol/litre 12 hours after a dose on days 4–7 of treatment, then every week until dosage has remained constant for 4 weeks and every 3 months thereafter, doses are initially divided throughout the day, but once daily administration is preferred when serum-lithium concentration stabilised
▸ Elderly: Reduce initial dose, dose adjusted to achieve a serum-lithium concentration of 0.4–1 mmol/litre 12 hours after a dose on days 4–7 of treatment, then every week until dosage has remained constant for 4 weeks and every 3 months thereafter, doses are initially divided throughout the day, but once daily administration is preferred when serum-lithium concentration stabilised

Prophylaxis of mania | Prophylaxis of bipolar disorder | Prophylaxis of recurrent depression | Prophylaxis of aggressive or self-harming behaviour
▸ BY MOUTH
▸ Adult: Initially 300–400 mg daily, dose adjusted to achieve a serum-lithium concentration of 0.4–1 mmol/litre 12 hours after a dose on days 4–7 of treatment, then every week until dosage has remained constant for 4 weeks and every 3 months thereafter, doses are initially divided throughout the day, but once daily administration is preferred when serum-lithium concentration stabilised

CAMCOLIT® MODIFIED-RELEASE TABLET

Treatment of mania | Treatment of bipolar disorder | Treatment of recurrent depression | Treatment of aggressive or self-harming behaviour
▸ BY MOUTH
▸ Adult: Initially 1–1.5 g daily, dose adjusted to achieve a serum-lithium concentration of 0.4–1 mmol/litre 12 hours after a dose on days 4–7 of treatment, then every week until dosage has remained constant for 4 weeks and every 3 months thereafter, doses are initially divided throughout the day, but once daily administration is preferred when serum-lithium concentration stabilised
▸ Elderly: Reduce initial dose, dose adjusted to achieve a serum-lithium concentration of 0.4–1 mmol/litre 12 hours after a dose on days 4–7 of treatment, then every week until dosage has remained constant for 4 weeks and every 3 months thereafter, doses are initially divided throughout the day, but once daily administration is preferred when serum-lithium concentration stabilised

Prophylaxis of mania | Prophylaxis of bipolar disorder | Prophylaxis of recurrent depression | Prophylaxis of aggressive or self-harming behaviour
▸ BY MOUTH
▸ Adult: Initially 300–400 mg daily, dose adjusted to achieve a serum-lithium concentration of 0.4–1 mmol/litre 12 hours after a dose on days 4–7 of treatment, then every week until dosage has remained constant for 4 weeks and every 3 months thereafter, doses are initially divided throughout the day, but once daily administration is preferred when serum-lithium concentration stabilised

LISKONUM®

Treatment of mania | Treatment of bipolar disorder | Treatment of recurrent depression | Treatment of aggressive or self-harming behaviour
▸ BY MOUTH
▸ Adult: Initially 450–675 mg twice daily, dose adjusted to achieve a serum-lithium concentration of 0.4–1 mmol/litre 12 hours after a dose on days 4–7 of treatment, then every week until dosage has remained constant for 4 weeks and every 3 months thereafter, doses are initially divided throughout the day, but once daily administration is preferred when serum-lithium concentration stabilised
▸ Elderly: Initially 225 mg twice daily, dose adjusted to achieve a serum-lithium concentration of 0.4–1 mmol/litre 12 hours after a dose on days 4–7 of treatment, then every week until dosage has remained constant for 4 weeks and every 3 months thereafter, doses are initially divided throughout the day, but once daily administration is preferred when serum-lithium concentration stabilised

Prophylaxis of mania | Prophylaxis of bipolar disorder | Prophylaxis of recurrent depression | Prophylaxis of aggressive or self-harming behaviour
▸ BY MOUTH
▸ Adult: Initially 450 mg twice daily, dose adjusted to achieve a serum-lithium concentration of 0.4–1 mmol/litre 12 hours after a dose on days 4–7 of treatment, then every week until dosage has remained constant for 4 weeks and every 3 months thereafter, doses are initially divided throughout the day, but once daily administration is preferred when serum-lithium concentration stabilised
▸ Elderly: Initially 225 mg twice daily, dose adjusted to achieve a serum-lithium concentration of 0.4–1 mmol/litre 12 hours after a dose on days 4–7 of treatment, then every week until dosage has remained constant for 4 weeks and every 3 months thereafter, doses are initially divided throughout the day, but once daily administration is preferred when serum-lithium concentration stabilised

PRIADEL® TABLETS

Treatment and prophylaxis of mania | Treatment and prophylaxis of bipolar disorder | Treatment and prophylaxis of recurrent depression | Treatment and prophylaxis of aggressive or self-harming behaviour
▸ BY MOUTH
▸ Adult (body-weight up to 50 kg): Initially 200–400 mg daily, dose adjusted to achieve a serum-lithium concentration of 0.4–1 mmol/litre 12 hours after a dose on days 4–7 of treatment, then every week until dosage has remained constant for 4 weeks and every 3 months thereafter, doses are initially divided throughout the day, but once daily administration is preferred when serum-lithium concentration stabilised
▸ Adult (body-weight 50 kg and above): Initially 0.4–1.2 g once daily, alternatively initially 0.4–1.2 g daily in 2 divided doses, dose adjusted to achieve a serum-lithium concentration of 0.4–1 mmol/litre 12 hours after a dose on days 4–7 of treatment, then every week until dosage has remained constant for 4 weeks and every 3 months thereafter, doses are initially divided throughout the day, but once daily administration is preferred when serum-lithium concentration stabilised
▸ Elderly: Initially 200–400 mg daily, dose adjusted to achieve a serum-lithium concentration of 0.4–1 mmol/litre 12 hours after a dose on days 4–7 of treatment, then every week until dosage has remained constant for 4 weeks and every 3 months thereafter, doses are initially divided throughout the day, but once

daily administration is preferred when serum-lithium concentration stabilised

DOSE EQUIVALENCE AND CONVERSION

Preparations vary widely in bioavailability; changing the preparation requires the same precautions as initiation of treatment.

● **MEDICINAL FORMS**

There can be variation in the licensing of different medicines containing the same drug. Forms available from special-order manufacturers include: oral suspension

Tablet

CAUTIONARY AND ADVISORY LABELS 10

▸ Lithium carbonate (Non-proprietary)

Lithium carbonate 250 mg Lithium carbonate 250mg tablets | 100 tablet [PoM] £48.18 DT price = £48.18

Modified-release tablet

CAUTIONARY AND ADVISORY LABELS 10, 25

▸ Lithium carbonate (Non-proprietary)

Lithium carbonate 400 mg Lithium carbonate 400mg modified-release tablets | 100 tablet [PoM] no price available DT price = £4.02

▸ Camcolit (Essential Pharma Ltd)

Lithium carbonate 400 mg Camcolit 400 modified-release tablets | 100 tablet [PoM] £48.18 DT price = £4.02

▸ Liskonum (GlaxoSmithKline UK Ltd)

Lithium carbonate 450 mg Liskonum 450mg modified-release tablets | 60 tablet [PoM] £2.88 DT price = £2.88

▸ Priadel (lithium carbonate) (Sanofi)

Lithium carbonate 200 mg Priadel 200mg modified-release tablets | 100 tablet [PoM] £2.76 DT price = £2.76

Lithium carbonate 400 mg Priadel 400mg modified-release tablets | 100 tablet [PoM] £4.02 DT price = £4.02

📖 324

Lithium citrate

● **INDICATIONS AND DOSE**

Treatment and prophylaxis of mania | Treatment and prophylaxis of bipolar disorder | Treatment and prophylaxis of recurrent depression | Treatment and prophylaxis of aggressive or self-harming behaviour

▸ BY MOUTH

▸ Adult: Dose adjusted to achieve a serum-lithium concentration of 0.4–1 mmol/litre 12 hours after a dose on days 4–7 of treatment, then every week until dosage has remained constant for 4 weeks and every 3 months thereafter; doses are initially divided throughout the day, but once daily administration is preferred when serum-lithium concentration stabilised

DOSE EQUIVALENCE AND CONVERSION

Preparations vary widely in bioavailability; changing the preparation requires the same precautions as initiation of treatment.

LI-LIQUID®

Treatment and prophylaxis of mania | Treatment and prophylaxis of bipolar disorder | Treatment and prophylaxis of recurrent depression | Treatment and prophylaxis of aggressive or self-harming behaviour

▸ BY MOUTH

▸ Adult (body-weight up to 50 kg): Initially 509 mg twice daily, dose adjusted to achieve a serum-lithium concentration of 0.4–1 mmol/litre 12 hours after a dose on days 4–7 of treatment, then every week until dosage has remained constant for 4 weeks and every 3 months thereafter, doses are initially divided throughout the day, but once daily administration is preferred when serum-lithium concentration stabilised

▸ Adult (body-weight 50 kg and above): Initially 1.018–3.054 g daily in 2 divided doses, dose adjusted to achieve a serum-lithium concentration of 0.4–1 mmol/litre 12 hours after a dose on days 4–7 of treatment, then every week until dosage has remained

constant for 4 weeks and every 3 months thereafter, doses are initially divided throughout the day, but once daily administration is preferred when serum-lithium concentration stabilised

▸ Elderly: Initially 509 mg twice daily, dose adjusted to achieve a serum-lithium concentration of 0.4–1 mmol/litre 12 hours after a dose on days 4–7 of treatment, then every week until dosage has remained constant for 4 weeks and every 3 months thereafter, doses are initially divided throughout the day, but once daily administration is preferred when serum-lithium concentration stabilised

DOSE EQUIVALENCE AND CONVERSION

For *Li-Liquid®*: Lithium citrate tetrahydrate 509 mg is equivalent to lithium carbonate 200 mg.

Preparations vary widely in bioavailability; changing the preparation requires the same precautions as initiation of treatment.

PRIADEL® LIQUID

Treatment and prophylaxis of mania | Treatment and prophylaxis of bipolar disorder | Treatment and prophylaxis of recurrent depression | Treatment and prophylaxis of aggressive or self-harming behaviour

▸ BY MOUTH

▸ Adult (body-weight up to 50 kg): Initially 520 mg twice daily, dose adjusted to achieve a serum-lithium concentration of 0.4–1 mmol/litre 12 hours after a dose on days 4–7 of treatment, then every week until dosage has remained constant for 4 weeks and every 3 months thereafter, doses are initially divided throughout the day, but once daily administration is preferred when serum-lithium concentration stabilised

▸ Adult (body-weight 50 kg and above): Initially 1.04–3.12 g daily in 2 divided doses, dose adjusted to achieve a serum-lithium concentration of 0.4–1 mmol/litre 12 hours after a dose on days 4–7 of treatment, then every week until dosage has remained constant for 4 weeks and every 3 months thereafter, doses are initially divided throughout the day, but once daily administration is preferred when serum-lithium concentration stabilised

▸ Elderly: Initially 520 mg twice daily, dose adjusted to achieve a serum-lithium concentration of 0.4–1 mmol/litre 12 hours after a dose on days 4–7 of treatment, then every week until dosage has remained constant for 4 weeks and every 3 months thereafter, doses are initially divided throughout the day, but once daily administration is preferred when serum-lithium concentration stabilised

DOSE EQUIVALENCE AND CONVERSION

For *Priadel®* liquid: Lithium citrate tetrahydrate 520 mg is equivalent to lithium carbonate 204 mg.

Preparations vary widely in bioavailability; changing the preparation requires the same precautions as initiation of treatment.

● **MEDICINAL FORMS**

There can be variation in the licensing of different medicines containing the same drug.

Oral solution

CAUTIONARY AND ADVISORY LABELS 10

▸ Lithium citrate (Non-proprietary)

Lithium citrate 101.8 mg per 1 ml Lithium citrate 509mg/5ml oral solution | 150 ml [PoM] no price available

Lithium citrate 104 mg per 1 ml Lithium citrate 520mg/5ml oral solution sugar free sugar-free | 150 ml [PoM] no price available

Lithium citrate 203.6 mg per 1 ml Lithium citrate 1.018g/5ml oral solution | 150 ml [PoM] no price available

▸ Li-Liquid (Rosemont Pharmaceuticals Ltd)

Lithium citrate 101.8 mg per 1 ml Li-Liquid 509mg/5ml oral solution | 150 ml [PoM] £5.79

4

Nervous system

Lithium citrate 203.6 mg per 1 ml Li-Liquid 1.018g/5ml oral
solution | 150 ml PoM £11.58
▸ Priadel (lithium citrate) (Sanofi)
Lithium citrate 104 mg per 1 ml Priadel 520mg/5ml liquid sugar-
free | 150 ml PoM £6.73

3.4 Depression

Antidepressant drugs

Overview

Antidepressant drugs are effective for treating moderate to
severe depression associated with psychomotor and
physiological changes such as loss of appetite and sleep
disturbance; improvement in sleep is usually the first benefit
of therapy. Ideally, patients with moderate to severe
depression should be treated with psychological therapy in
addition to drug therapy. Antidepressant drugs are also
effective for dysthymia (lower grade chronic depression
(typically of at least 2 years duration)).

Antidepressant drugs should not be used routinely in mild
depression, and psychological therapy should be considered
initially; however, a trial of antidepressant therapy may be
considered in cases refractory to psychological treatments or
in those associated with psychosocial or medical problems.
Drug treatment of mild depression may also be considered in
patients with a history of moderate or severe depression.

Choice

The major classes of antidepressant drugs include the
tricyclic and related antidepressants, the selective serotonin
re-uptake inhibitors (SSRIs), and the monoamine oxidase
inhibitors (MAOIs). A number of antidepressant drugs
cannot be accommodated easily into this classification.

There is little to choose between the different classes of
antidepressant drugs in terms of efficacy, so choice should be
based on the individual patient's requirements, including
the presence of concomitant disease, existing therapy,
suicide risk, and previous response to antidepressant
therapy. Since there may be an interval of 2 weeks before the
antidepressant action takes place, electroconvulsive
treatment may be required in severe depression when delay
is hazardous or intolerable. During the first few weeks of
treatment, there is an increased potential for agitation,
anxiety, and suicidal ideation.

SSRIs are better tolerated and are safer in overdose than
other classes of antidepressants and should be considered
first-line for treating depression. In patients with unstable
angina or who have had a recent myocardial infarction,
sertraline p. 336 has been shown to be safe.

Tricyclic antidepressants have similar efficacy to SSRIs but
are more likely to be discontinued because of side-effects;
toxicity in overdosage is also a problem. SSRIs are less
sedating and have fewer antimuscarinic and cardiotoxic
effects than tricyclic antidepressants.

MAOIs have dangerous interactions with some foods and
drugs, and should be reserved for use by specialists.

Although anxiety is often present in depressive illness
(and may be the presenting symptom), the use of an
antipsychotic or an anxiolytic may mask the true diagnosis.
Anxiolytics or antipsychotic drugs should therefore be used
with caution in depression but they are useful adjuncts in
agitated patients. Augmenting antidepressants with
antipsychotics under specialist supervision may also be
necessary in patients who have depression with psychotic
symptoms.

St John's wort (*Hypericum perforatum*) is a popular herbal
remedy on sale to the public for treating mild depression. It
should not be prescribed or recommended for depression
because St John's wort can induce drug metabolising
enzymes and a number of important interactions with

conventional drugs, including conventional antidepressants,
have been identified. Furthermore, the amount of active
ingredient varies between different preparations of St John's
wort and switching from one to another can change the
degree of enzyme induction. If a patient stops taking St
John's wort, the concentration of interacting drugs may
increase, leading to toxicity.

Management

Patients should be reviewed every 1–2 weeks at the start of
antidepressant treatment. Treatment should be continued
for at least 4 weeks (6 weeks in the elderly) before
considering whether to switch antidepressant due to lack of
efficacy. In cases of partial response, continue for a further
2–4 weeks (elderly patients may take longer to respond).

Following remission, antidepressant treatment should be
continued at the same dose for at least 6 months (about
12 months in the elderly), or for at least 12 months in
patients receiving treatment for generalised anxiety disorder
(as the likelihood of relapse is high). Patients with a history
of recurrent depression should receive maintenance
treatment for at least 2 years.

Hyponatraemia and antidepressant therapy

Hyponatraemia (usually in the elderly and possibly due to
inappropriate secretion of antidiuretic hormone) has been
associated with all types of antidepressants; however, it has
been reported more frequently with SSRIs than with other
antidepressants. Hyponatraemia should be considered in all
patients who develop drowsiness, confusion, or convulsions
while taking an antidepressant.

Suicidal behaviour and antidepressant therapy

The use of antidepressants has been linked with suicidal
thoughts and behaviour; children, young adults, and
patients with a history of suicidal behaviour are particularly
at risk. Where necessary patients should be monitored for
suicidal behaviour, self-harm, or hostility, particularly at the
beginning of treatment or if the dose is changed.

Serotonin syndrome

Serotonin syndrome or serotonin toxicity is a relatively
uncommon adverse drug reaction caused by excessive
central and peripheral serotonergic activity. Onset of
symptoms, which range from mild to lifethreatening, can
occur within hours or days following the initiation, dose
escalation, or overdose of a serotonergic drug, the addition
of a new serotonergic drug, or the replacement of one
serotonergic drug by another without allowing a long
enough washout period in-between, particularly when the
first drug is an irreversible MAOI or a drug with a long half-
life. Severe toxicity, which is a medical emergency, usually
occurs with a combination of serotonergic drugs, one of
which is generally an MAOI.

The characteristic symptoms of serotonin syndrome fall
into 3 main areas, although features from each group may
not be seen in all patients—neuromuscular hyperactivity
(such as tremor, hyperreflexia, clonus, myoclonus, rigidity),
autonomic dysfunction (tachycardia, blood pressure
changes, hyperthermia, diaphoresis, shivering, diarrhoea),
and altered mental state (agitation, confusion, mania).

Treatment consists of withdrawal of the serotonergic
medication and supportive care; specialist advice should be
sought.

Failure to respond

Failure to respond to initial treatment with an SSRI may
require an increase in the dose, or switching to a different
SSRI or mirtazapine p. 340. Other second-line choices
include lofepramine p. 346, moclobemide p. 331, and
reboxetine p. 332. Other tricyclic antidepressants and
venlafaxine p. 337 should be considered for more severe
forms of depression; irreversible MAOIs should only be
prescribed by specialists. Failure to respond to a second
antidepressant may require the addition of another

antidepressant of a different class, or use of an augmenting agent (such as lithium, aripiprazole p. 362 [unlicensed], olanzapine p. 365 [unlicensed], quetiapine p. 367, or risperidone p. 368 [unlicensed]), but such adjunctive treatment should be initiated only by doctors with special experience of these combinations. Electroconvulsive therapy may be initiated in severe refractory depression.

Anxiety disorders and obsessive-compulsive disorder

Management of acute anxiety generally involves the use of a benzodiazepine or buspirone hydrochloride p. 311. For chronic anxiety (of longer than 4 weeks' duration) it may be appropriate to use an antidepressant. Combined therapy with a benzodiazepine may be required until the antidepressant takes effect. Patients with *generalised anxiety disorder*, a form of chronic anxiety, should be offered psychological treatment before initiating an antidepressant. If drug treatment is needed, an SSRI such as escitalopram p. 334, paroxetine p. 335, or sertraline p. 336 [unlicensed], can be used. Duloxetine p. 336 and venlafaxine p. 337 (serotonin and noradrenaline reuptake inhibitors) are also recommended for the treatment of generalised anxiety disorder; if the patient cannot tolerate SSRIs or serotonin and noradrenaline reuptake inhibitors (or if treatment has failed to control symptoms), pregabalin p. 295 can be considered.

Panic disorder, obsessive-compulsive disorder, post-traumatic stress disorder, and phobic states such as *social anxiety disorder* are treated with SSRIs. Clomipramine hydrochloride p. 342 or imipramine hydrochloride p. 345 can be used second-line in panic disorder [unlicensed]; clomipramine hydrochloride can also be used second-line for obsessive-compulsive disorder. Moclobemide p. 331 is licensed for the treatment of social anxiety disorder.

Tricyclic and related antidepressant drugs

Choice

Tricyclic and related antidepressants block the re-uptake of both serotonin and noradrenaline, although to different extents. For example, clomipramine hydrochloride is more selective for serotonergic transmission, and imipramine hydrochloride is more selective for noradrenergic transmission. Tricyclic and related antidepressant drugs can be roughly divided into those with additional sedative properties and those that are less sedating. Agitated and anxious patients tend to respond best to the sedative compounds, whereas withdrawn and apathetic patients will often obtain most benefit from the less sedating ones. Those with **sedative** properties include amitriptyline hydrochloride p. 341, clomipramine hydrochloride, dosulepin hydrochloride p. 343, doxepin p. 344, mianserin hydrochloride p. 339, trazodone hydrochloride p. 338, and trimipramine p. 348. Those with **less sedative** properties include imipramine hydrochloride, lofepramine p. 346, and nortriptyline p. 347.

Tricyclic and related antidepressants also have varying degrees of antimuscarinic side-effects and cardiotoxicity in overdosage, which may be important in individual patients. Lofepramine has a lower incidence of side-effects and is less dangerous in overdosage but is infrequently associated with hepatic toxicity. Imipramine hydrochloride is also well established, but has more marked antimuscarinic side-effects than other tricyclic and related antidepressants. Amitriptyline hydrochloride and dosulepin hydrochloride are effective but they are particularly dangerous in overdosage and are not recommended for the treatment of depression; dosulepin hydrochloride should be initiated by a specialist.

Dosage

About 10 to 20% of patients fail to respond to tricyclic and related antidepressant drugs and inadequate dosage may account for some of these failures. It is important to use doses that are sufficiently high for effective treatment but

not so high as to cause toxic effects. Low doses should be used for initial treatment in the **elderly**. In most patients the long half-life of tricyclic antidepressant drugs allows **once-daily** administration, usually at night; the use of modified-release preparations is therefore unnecessary.

Some tricyclic antidepressants are used in the management of *panic* and other *anxiety disorders*. Some tricyclic antidepressants may also have a role in some forms of *neuralgia* and in *nocturnal enuresis* in children.

Children and adolescents

Studies have shown that tricyclic antidepressants are not effective for treating depression in children.

Monoamine-oxidase inhibitors

Monoamine-oxidase inhibitors are used much less frequently than tricyclic and related antidepressants, or SSRIs and related antidepressants because of the dangers of dietary and drug interactions and the fact that it is easier to prescribe MAOIs when tricyclic antidepressants have been unsuccessful than vice versa.

Tranylcypromine p. 331 has a greater stimulant action than phenelzine p. 331 or isocarboxazid p. 331 and is more likely to cause a hypertensive crisis. Isocarboxazid and phenelzine are more likely to cause hepatotoxicity than tranylcypromine.

Moclobemide should be reserved as a second line treatment.

Phobic patients and depressed patients with atypical, hypochondriacal, or hysterical features are said to respond best to MAOIs. However, MAOIs should be tried in any patients who are refractory to treatment with other antidepressants as there is occasionally a dramatic response. Response to treatment may be delayed for 3 weeks or more and may take an additional 1 or 2 weeks to become maximal.

Other antidepressant drugs

The thioxanthene flupentixol (Fluanxol ®) p. 354 has antidepressant properties when given by mouth in low doses. Flupentixol is also used for the treatment of psychoses.

Vortioxetine p. 349, an antidepressant thought to directly modulate serotonergic receptor activity and inhibit the re-uptake of serotonin, is recommended in patients whose condition has responded inadequately to 2 antidepressants within the current episode.

> **Drugs used for Depression not listed below** Lithium carbonate, p. 325 · Lithium citrate, p. 327

ANTIDEPRESSANTS > MELATONIN RECEPTOR AGONISTS

Agomelatine

- **DRUG ACTION** A melatonin receptor agonist and a selective serotonin-receptor antagonist; it does not affect the uptake of serotonin, noradrenaline, or dopamine.

● INDICATIONS AND DOSE

Major depression

▸ BY MOUTH
▹ Adult: 25 mg daily, dose to be taken at bedtime, dose to be increased if necessary after 2 weeks, increased if necessary to 50 mg daily, dose to be taken at bedtime

DOSE ADJUSTMENTS DUE TO INTERACTIONS
Caution—dose adjustment may be necessary if smoking started or stopped during treatment.

- **CONTRA-INDICATIONS** Dementia · patients over 75 years of age

4 Nervous system

- CAUTIONS Bipolar disorder · diabetes · excessive alcohol consumption · hypomania · mania · non-alcoholic fatty liver disease · obesity
- INTERACTIONS → Appendix 1 (agomelatine). Caution with concomitant use of drugs associated with hepatic injury.
- SIDE-EFFECTS
- ▶ **Common or very common** Abdominal pain · agitation · anxiety · back pain · constipation · diarrhoea · dizziness · drowsiness · fatigue · headache · increased serum transaminases · nausea · sleep disturbances · sweating · vomiting
- ▶ **Uncommon** Blurred vision · eczema · paraesthesia · restless legs syndrome · tinnitus
- ▶ **Rare** Hepatic failure · hepatic injury · hepatitis · rash · weight changes
- ▶ **Frequency not known** Pruritus · suicidal behaviour
SIDE-EFFECTS, FURTHER INFORMATION
- ▶ Suicidal behaviour The use of antidepressants has been linked with suicidal thoughts and behaviour; children, young adults, and patients with a history of suicidal behaviour are particularly at risk. Where necessary patients should be monitored for suicidal behaviour, self-harm, or hostility, particularly at the beginning of treatment or if the dose is changed.
- PREGNANCY Manufacturer advises avoid.
- BREAST FEEDING Avoid—present in milk in *animal* studies.
- HEPATIC IMPAIRMENT Avoid. Do not start if serum transaminases exceed 3 times the upper limit of reference range.
- RENAL IMPAIRMENT Caution in moderate to severe impairment.
- MONITORING REQUIREMENTS Test liver function before treatment and after 3, 6, 12 and 24 weeks of treatment, and then regularly thereafter when clinically indicated (restart monitoring schedule if dose increased); discontinue if serum transaminases exceed 3 times the upper limit of reference range or symptoms of liver disorder.
- PATIENT AND CARER ADVICE Patients should be given a booklet with more information on the risk of hepatic side-effects.
Hepatotoxicity Patients should be told how to recognise signs of liver disorder, and advised to seek immediate medical attention if symptoms such as dark urine, light coloured stools, jaundice, bruising, fatigue, abdominal pain, or pruritus develop.

- MEDICINAL FORMS
There can be variation in the licensing of different medicines containing the same drug.
Tablet
- ▶ Valdoxan (Servier Laboratories Ltd)
Agomelatine 25 mg Valdoxan 25mg tablets | 28 tablet [PoM] £30.00 DT price = £30.00

ANTIDEPRESSANTS › MONOAMINE-OXIDASE INHIBITORS

Monoamine-oxidase inhibitors

- DRUG ACTION MAOIs inhibit monoamine oxidase, thereby causing an accumulation of amine neurotransmitters.
- CONTRA-INDICATIONS Cerebrovascular disease · not indicated in manic phase · phaeochromocytoma
- CAUTIONS Acute porphyria · avoid in agitated patients · blood disorders · cardiovascular disease · concurrent electroconvulsive therapy · diabetes mellitus · elderly (great caution) · epilepsy · severe hypertensive reactions to certain drugs and foods · surgery

- INTERACTIONS → Appendix 1 (MAOIs). The metabolism of some amine drugs such as *indirect-acting sympathomimetics* (present in many cough and decongestant preparations) is inhibited and their pressor action may be potentiated; the pressor effect of tyramine (in some foods, such as mature cheese, pickled herring, broad bean pods, and *Bovril*®, *Oxo*®, *Marmite*® or any similar meat or yeast extract or fermented soya bean extract) may also be dangerously potentiated. These interactions may cause a dangerous rise in blood pressure. An early warning symptom may be a throbbing headache. The danger of interaction persists for up to 2 weeks after treatment with MAOIs is discontinued.
Some psychiatrists use selected tricyclics in conjunction with MAOIs but this is hazardous, indeed potentially lethal, except in experienced hands and there is no evidence that the combination is more effective than when either constituent is used alone.
- SIDE-EFFECTS
- ▶ **Common or very common** Dizziness · postural hypotension (especially in elderly)
- ▶ **Uncommon** Agitation · arrhythmias · blurred vision · confusion · constipation · convulsions · difficulty in micturition · drowsiness · dry mouth · elevated liver enzymes · euphoria · fatigue · gastro-intestinal disturbances · hallucinations · headache · hyperreflexia · insomnia · leucopenia · myoclonic movement · nervousness · nystagmus · oedema · psychotic episodes with hypomanic behaviour · purpura · rashes · sexual disturbances · suicidal behaviour · sweating · tremors · weakness · weight gain with inappropriate appetite
- ▶ **Rare** Fatal progressive hepatocellular necrosis
- ▶ **Frequency not known** Jaundice · hyponatraemia · paraesthesia · peripheral neuritis · peripheral neuropathy (may be due to pyridoxine deficiency)
SIDE-EFFECTS, FURTHER INFORMATION
- ▶ Risk of postural hypotension and hypertensive responses Discontinue use if palpitations or frequent headaches occur.
- PREGNANCY Increased risk of neonatal malformations—manufacturer advises avoid unless there are compelling reasons.
- HEPATIC IMPAIRMENT MAOIs may cause idiosyncratic hepatotoxicity if used in patients with hepatic impairment.
- MONITORING REQUIREMENTS Monitor blood pressure (risk of postural hypotension and hypertensive responses).
- TREATMENT CESSATION
Withdrawal If possible avoid abrupt withdrawal.
    MAOIs are associated with withdrawal symptoms on cessation of therapy. Symptoms include agitation, irritability, ataxia, movement disorders, insomnia, drowsiness, vivid dreams, cognitive impairment, and slowed speech. Withdrawal symptoms occasionally experienced when discontinuing MAOIs include hallucinations and paranoid delusions. If possible MAOIs should be withdrawn slowly.
    Withdrawal effects may occur within 5 days of stopping treatment with antidepressant drugs; they are usually mild and self-limiting, but in some cases may be severe. The risk of withdrawal symptoms is increased if the antidepressant is stopped suddenly after regular administration for 8 weeks or more. The dose should preferably be reduced gradually over about 4 weeks, or longer if withdrawal symptoms emerge (6 months in patients who have been on long-term maintenance treatment).
- PATIENT AND CARER ADVICE
Patients should be advised to eat only fresh foods and avoid food that is suspected of being stale or 'going off'. This is especially important with meat, fish, poultry or offal; game should be avoided. The danger of interaction

persists for up to 2 weeks after treatment with MAOIs is discontinued.

Patients should also be advised to avoid alcoholic drinks or de-alcoholised (low alcohol) drinks.

Driving and skilled tasks
Drowsiness may affect performance of skilled tasks (e.g. driving).

ANTIDEPRESSANTS > MONOAMINE-OXIDASE A AND B INHIBITORS, IRREVERSIBLE

F 330

Isocarboxazid

● INDICATIONS AND DOSE
Depressive illness
▸ BY MOUTH
▸ Adult: Initially 30 mg daily until improvement occurs, initial dose may be given in single or divided doses, dose may be increased if necessary after 4 weeks, increased to 60 mg daily for 4–6 weeks, dose to be increased under close supervision only, then reduced to 10–20 mg daily, usual maintenance dose, but up to 40 mg daily may be required
▸ Elderly: 5–10 mg daily

● BREAST FEEDING Avoid.
● HEPATIC IMPAIRMENT Avoid in hepatic impairment.
● RENAL IMPAIRMENT Use with caution.
● LESS SUITABLE FOR PRESCRIBING Less suitable for prescribing.

● MEDICINAL FORMS
There can be variation in the licensing of different medicines containing the same drug. Forms available from special-order manufacturers include: oral suspension
Tablet
CAUTIONARY AND ADVISORY LABELS 3, 10
▸ Isocarboxazid (Non-proprietary)
Isocarboxazid 10 mg Isocarboxazid 10mg tablets | 56 tablet P͟o͟M͟
£179.95 DT price = £179.95

F 330

Phenelzine

● INDICATIONS AND DOSE
Depressive illness
▸ BY MOUTH
▸ Adult: Initially 15 mg 3 times a day, response is usually seen within first week; dose may be increased if necessary after 2 weeks if response is not evident, increased if necessary to 15 mg 4 times a day, doses up to 30 mg three times a day may be used in hospital patients; response may not become apparent for up to 4 weeks; once satisfactory response has been achieved, reduce dose gradually to lowest suitable maintenance dose (15 mg on alternate days may be adequate)

● BREAST FEEDING Avoid—no information available.
● HEPATIC IMPAIRMENT Avoid in hepatic impairment or if abnormal liver function tests.
● LESS SUITABLE FOR PRESCRIBING Less suitable for prescribing.

● MEDICINAL FORMS
There can be variation in the licensing of different medicines containing the same drug.
Tablet
CAUTIONARY AND ADVISORY LABELS 3, 10
▸ Nardil (ProStrakan Ltd)
Phenelzine (as Phenelzine sulfate) 15 mg Nardil 15mg tablets | 100 tablet P͟o͟M͟ £22.50 DT price = £22.50

F 330

Tranylcypromine

● INDICATIONS AND DOSE
Depressive illness
▸ BY MOUTH
▸ Adult: Initially 10 mg twice daily, dose to be taken at a time no later than 3 p.m, dose may be increased if necessary after 1 week, increased if necessary to 10 mg daily, dose to be taken in the morning and 20 mg daily, dose to be taken in the afternoon, doses above 30 mg daily, under close supervision only; maintenance 10 mg daily

● CONTRA-INDICATIONS Congestive heart failure · history of hepatic disease · hyperthyroidism
● INTERACTIONS The combination of tranylcypromine with clomipramine is particularly **dangerous**.
● SIDE-EFFECTS
▸ **Common or very common** Insomnia
▸ **Uncommon** Hypernatraemia · lupus erythematous-like syndrome · speech disturbances
▸ **Very rare** Angle-closure glaucoma · hypertensive crises with throbbing headache · liver damage (less frequent than with phenelzine)
▸ **Frequency not known** Blood dyscrasias
SIDE-EFFECTS, FURTHER INFORMATION
▸ Hypertensive crisis Hypertensive crisis and throbbing headache requiring discontinuation of treatment is more frequent than with other MAOIs.
● BREAST FEEDING Present in milk in *animal* studies.
● HEPATIC IMPAIRMENT Avoid if history of hepatic disease or if abnormal liver function tests.
● LESS SUITABLE FOR PRESCRIBING Less suitable for prescribing.

● MEDICINAL FORMS
There can be variation in the licensing of different medicines containing the same drug.
Tablet
CAUTIONARY AND ADVISORY LABELS 3, 10
▸ Tranylcypromine (Non-proprietary)
Tranylcypromine (as Tranylcypromine sulfate) 10 mg Tranylcypromine 10mg tablets | 28 tablet P͟o͟M͟ £243.98 DT price = £239.48

ANTIDEPRESSANTS > MONOAMINE-OXIDASE A INHIBITORS, REVERSIBLE

Moclobemide

● DRUG ACTION Moclobemide is reported to act by reversible inhibition of monoamine oxidase type A (it is therefore termed a RIMA).

● INDICATIONS AND DOSE
Depressive illness
▸ BY MOUTH
▸ Adult: Initially 300 mg daily in divided doses, adjusted according to response; usual dose 150–600 mg daily, dose to be taken after food

continued →

Nervous system

4

Social anxiety disorder
▶ BY MOUTH
▶ Adult: Initially 300 mg daily for 3 days, then increased to 600 mg daily in 2 divided doses continued for 8–12 weeks to assess efficacy

● CONTRA-INDICATIONS Acute confusional states · phaeochromocytoma
● CAUTIONS Avoid in agitated or excited patients (or give with sedative for up to 2–3 weeks) · may provoke manic episodes in bipolar disorders · thyrotoxicosis
● INTERACTIONS → Appendix 1 (moclobemide). The risk of drug interactions is claimed to be less than with the traditional (irreversible) MAOIs, but patients still need to avoid sympathomimetics such as ephedrine and pseudoephedrine. In addition, moclobemide should not be given with another antidepressant. Owing to its short duration of action no treatment-free period is required after it has been stopped but it should not be started until at least a week after a tricyclic or related antidepressant or an SSRI or related antidepressant has been stopped (at least 5 weeks in the case of fluoxetine), or for at least a week after an MAOI has been stopped.
● SIDE-EFFECTS
▶ Rare Galactorrhoea · hyponatraemia · raised liver enzymes
▶ Frequency not known Agitation · confusional states · dizziness · dry mouth · gastrointestinal disorders · headache · oedema · paraesthesia · restlessness · skin reactions · sleep disturbances · visual disturbances
● PREGNANCY Safety in pregnancy has not been established—manufacturer advises avoid unless there are compelling reasons.
● BREAST FEEDING Amount too small to be harmful, but patient information leaflet advises avoid.
● HEPATIC IMPAIRMENT Reduce dose in severe hepatic disease.
● TREATMENT CESSATION Withdrawal effects may occur within 5 days of stopping treatment with antidepressant drugs; they are usually mild and self-limiting, but in some cases may be severe. The risk of withdrawal symptoms is increased if the antidepressant is stopped suddenly after regular administration for 8 weeks or more. The dose should preferably be reduced gradually over about 4 weeks, or longer if withdrawal symptoms emerge (6 months in patients who have been on long-term maintenance treatment).
● PATIENT AND CARER ADVICE Moclobemide is claimed to cause less potentiation of the pressor effect of tyramine than the traditional (irreversible) MAOIs, but patients should avoid consuming large amounts of tyramine-rich food (such as mature cheese, yeast extracts and fermented soya bean products).

● MEDICINAL FORMS
There can be variation in the licensing of different medicines containing the same drug. Forms available from special-order manufacturers include: oral suspension
Tablet
CAUTIONARY AND ADVISORY LABELS 10, 21
▶ Moclobemide (Non-proprietary)
Moclobemide 150 mg Moclobemide 150mg tablets | 30 tablet PoM £22.12 DT price = £22.02
Moclobemide 300 mg Moclobemide 300mg tablets | 30 tablet PoM £15.00 DT price = £13.99
▶ Manerix (Meda Pharmaceuticals Ltd)
Moclobemide 150 mg Manerix 150mg tablets | 30 tablet PoM £9.33 DT price = £22.02
Moclobemide 300 mg Manerix 300mg tablets | 30 tablet PoM £13.99 DT price = £13.99

ANTIDEPRESSANTS > NORADRENALINE REUPTAKE INHIBITORS

Reboxetine

● DRUG ACTION Reboxetine is a selective inhibitor of noradrenaline re-uptake.

● INDICATIONS AND DOSE
Major depression
▶ BY MOUTH
▶ Adult: 4 mg twice daily for 3–4 weeks, then increased if necessary to 10 mg daily in divided doses; maximum 12 mg per day

● CAUTIONS Bipolar disorder · history of cardiovascular disease · history of epilepsy · prostatic hypertrophy · susceptibility to angle-closure glaucoma · urinary retention
● INTERACTIONS → Appendix 1 (reboxetine).
● SIDE-EFFECTS
▶ Common or very common Anorexia · chills · constipation · dizziness · dry mouth · headache · impaired visual accommodation · impotence · insomnia · lowering of plasma-potassium concentration on prolonged administration in the elderly · nausea · palpitation · postural hypotension · sweating · tachycardia · urinary retention · vasodilation
▶ Very rare Angle-closure glaucoma
▶ Frequency not known Aggression · agitation · anxiety · cold extremities · hallucinations · hypertension · hyponatraemia · irritability · paraesthesia · rash · Raynaud's syndrome · suicidal behaviour · testicular pain · vomiting
● PREGNANCY Use only if potential benefit outweighs risk—limited information available.
● BREAST FEEDING Small amount present in milk—use only if potential benefit outweighs risk.
● HEPATIC IMPAIRMENT Initial dose 2 mg twice daily, increased according to tolerance.
● RENAL IMPAIRMENT Initial dose 2 mg twice daily, increased according to tolerance.
● TREATMENT CESSATION Caution— avoid abrupt withdrawal.
● PATIENT AND CARER ADVICE
Driving and skilled tasks
Counselling advised.

● MEDICINAL FORMS
There can be variation in the licensing of different medicines containing the same drug.
Tablet
▶ Edronax (Pfizer Ltd)
Reboxetine (as Reboxetine mesilate) 4 mg Edronax 4mg tablets | 60 tablet PoM £18.91 DT price = £18.91

ANTIDEPRESSANTS > SELECTIVE SEROTONIN RE-UPTAKE INHIBITORS

Selective serotonin re-uptake inhibitors

● DRUG ACTION Selectively inhibit the re-uptake of serotonin (5-hydroxytryptamine, 5-HT).
● CONTRA-INDICATIONS Poorly controlled epilepsy · SSRIs should not be used if the patient enters a manic phase.
● CAUTIONS Cardiac disease · concurrent electroconvulsive therapy · diabetes mellitus · epilepsy (discontinue if convulsions develop) · history of bleeding disorders (especially gastro-intestinal bleeding) · history of mania · susceptibility to angle-closure glaucoma

- INTERACTIONS → Appendix 1 (antidepressants, SSRI). Caution with other drugs that increase the risk of bleeding.
- SIDE-EFFECTS
  ► **Common or very common** Abdominal pain (dose-related) · constipation (dose-related) · diarrhoea (dose-related) · dyspepsia (dose-related) · gastro-intestinal effects (dose-related) · nausea (dose-related) · vomiting (dose-related)
  ► **Uncommon** Serotonin syndrome
  ► **Very rare** Angle-closure glaucoma
  ► **Frequency not known** Anaphylaxis · angioedema · anorexia with weight loss · anxiety · arthralgia · asthenia · bleeding disorders · convulsions · dizziness · drowsiness · dry mouth · dyskinesias · ecchymoses · galactorrhoea · hallucinations · headache · hypersensitivity reactions · hypomania · hyponatraemia · increased appetite · insomnia · mania · movement disorders · myalgia · nervousness · photosensitivity · purpura · rash · sexual dysfunction · suicidal behaviour · sweating · tremor · urinary retention · urticaria · visual disturbances · weight gain

  SIDE-EFFECTS, FURTHER INFORMATION
  ► Hypersensitivity reactions If hypersensitivity reactions (including rash) occur, consider discontinuation—may be sign of impending serious systemic reaction, possibly associated with vasculitis.

  Overdose
  Symptoms of poisoning by selective serotonin re-uptake inhibitors include nausea, vomiting, agitation, tremor, nystagmus, drowsiness, and sinus tachycardia; convulsions may occur. Rarely, severe poisoning results in the serotonin syndrome, with marked neuropsychiatric effects, neuromuscular hyperactivity, and autonomic instability; hyperthermia, rhabdomyolysis, renal failure, and coagulopathies may develop.

  For details on the management of poisoning, see Selective serotonin re-uptake inhibitors, under Emergency treatment of poisoning p. 1194.
- PREGNANCY Manufacturers advise against during pregnancy unless the potential benefit outweighs the risk. There is a small increased risk of congenital heart defects when taken during early pregnancy. If used during the third trimester there is a risk of neonatal withdrawal symptoms, and persistent pulmonary hypertension in the newborn has been reported.
- TREATMENT CESSATION Gastro-intestinal disturbances, headache, anxiety, dizziness, paraesthesia, electric shock sensation in the head, neck, and spine, tinnitus, sleep disturbances, fatigue, influenza-like symptoms, and sweating are the most common features of abrupt withdrawal of an SSRI or marked reduction of the dose; palpitation and visual disturbances can occur less commonly. The dose should be tapered over at least a few weeks to avoid these effects. For some patients, it may be necessary to withdraw treatment over a longer period; consider obtaining specialist advice if symptoms persist.

  Withdrawal effects may occur within 5 days of stopping treatment with antidepressant drugs; they are usually mild and self-limiting, but in some cases may be severe. The risk of withdrawal symptoms is increased if the antidepressant is stopped suddenly after regular administration for 8 weeks or more. The dose should preferably be reduced gradually over about 4 weeks, or longer if withdrawal symptoms emerge (6 months in patients who have been on long-term maintenance treatment).
- PATIENT AND CARER ADVICE
  Driving and skilled tasks
  May also impair performance of skilled tasks (e.g. driving, operating machinery).

F 332

Citalopram

- INDICATIONS AND DOSE
  Depressive illness
  ► BY MOUTH USING TABLETS
  ► Adult: 20 mg once daily, increased in steps of 20 mg daily if required, dose to be increased at intervals of 3–4 weeks; maximum 40 mg per day
  ► Elderly: 10–20 mg once daily; maximum 20 mg per day
  ► BY MOUTH USING ORAL DROPS
  ► Adult: 16 mg once daily, increased in steps of 16 mg daily if required, dose to be increased at intervals of 3–4 weeks; maximum 32 mg per day
  ► Elderly: 8–16 mg daily; maximum 16 mg per day

  Panic disorder
  ► BY MOUTH USING TABLETS
  ► Adult: Initially 10 mg daily, increased in steps of 10 mg daily if required, dose to be increased gradually; usual dose 20–30 mg daily; maximum 40 mg per day
  ► Elderly: Initially 10 mg daily, increased in steps of 10 mg daily if required, dose to be increased gradually; maximum 20 mg per day
  ► BY MOUTH USING ORAL DROPS
  ► Adult: Initially 8 mg once daily, increased in steps of 8 mg if required, dose to be increased gradually; usual dose 16–24 mg daily; maximum 32 mg per day
  ► Elderly: Initially 8 mg once daily, increased in steps of 8 mg if required, dose to be increased gradually; maximum 16 mg per day

  DOSE EQUIVALENCE AND CONVERSION
  4 oral drops (8 mg) is equivalent in therapeutic effect to 10 mg tablet.

- CONTRA-INDICATIONS QT-interval prolongation
- CAUTIONS Susceptibility to QT-interval prolongation
- INTERACTIONS Avoid concomitant administration of drugs that prolong QT interval.
- SIDE-EFFECTS Taste disturbance · abnormal dreams · aggression · amnesia · bradycardia · confusion · coughing · euphoria · haemorrhage · hepatitis · hypokalaemia · impaired concentration · increased salivation · malaise · micturition disorders · migraine · mydriasis · oedema · palpitation · paradoxical increased anxiety during initial treatment of panic disorder (reduce dose) · paraesthesia · polyuria · postural hypotension · pruritus · QT-interval prolongation · rhinitis · tachycardia · tinnitus · yawning
- BREAST FEEDING Present in milk—use with caution.
- HEPATIC IMPAIRMENT Use doses at lower end of range; for *tablets* up to maximum 20 mg; for *oral solution* up to maximum 16 mg.
- RENAL IMPAIRMENT No information available for eGFR less than 20 mL/minute/1.73 m^2.
- DIRECTIONS FOR ADMINISTRATION *Cipramil*® oral drops should be mixed with water, orange juice, or apple juice before taking.
- PATIENT AND CARER ADVICE
  Counselling on administration of oral drops is advised.
  Driving and skilled tasks
  Patients should be advised of the effects of citalopram on driving and skilled tasks.

- MEDICINAL FORMS
  There can be variation in the licensing of different medicines containing the same drug.
  Tablet
  ► Citalopram (Non-proprietary)
  Citalopram (as Citalopram hydrobromide) 10 mg Citalopram 10mg tablets | 28 tablet PoM £8.90 DT price = £0.77
  Citalopram (as Citalopram hydrobromide) 20 mg Citalopram 20mg tablets | 28 tablet PoM £15.99 DT price = £0.82

4

Nervous system

4

Nervous system

Citalopram (as Citalopram hydrobromide) 40 mg Citalopram 40mg tablets | 28 tablet [PoM] £27.00 DT price = £0.96
▸ Cipramil (Lundbeck Ltd)
Citalopram (as Citalopram hydrobromide) 20 mg Cipramil 20mg tablets | 28 tablet [PoM] £8.95 DT price = £0.82

Oral drops
EXCIPIENTS: May contain Alcohol
▸ Citalopram (Non-proprietary)
Citalopram (as Citalopram hydrochloride) 40 mg per
1 ml Citalopram 40mg/ml oral drops sugar free sugar-free |
15 ml [PoM] £20.16 DT price = £5.17
▸ Cipramil (Lundbeck Ltd)
Citalopram (as Citalopram hydrochloride) 40 mg per
1 ml Cipramil 40mg/ml drops sugar-free | 15 ml [PoM] £10.08 DT price = £5.17

⬛ 332

Escitalopram

● DRUG ACTION Escitalopram is the active enantiomer of citalopram.

● INDICATIONS AND DOSE

Depressive illness | Generalised anxiety disorder | Obsessive-compulsive disorder
▸ BY MOUTH
▸ Adult: 10 mg once daily; increased if necessary up to 20 mg daily
▸ Elderly: Initially 5 mg once daily; maximum 10 mg per day

Panic disorder
▸ BY MOUTH
▸ Adult: Initially 5 mg once daily for 7 days, then increased to 10 mg daily; maximum 20 mg per day
▸ Elderly: Initially 2.5 mg once daily; maximum 10 mg per day

Social anxiety disorder
▸ BY MOUTH
▸ Adult: Initially 10 mg once daily for 2–4 weeks, dose to be adjusted after 2-4 weeks of treatment; usual dose 5–20 mg daily

● CONTRA-INDICATIONS QT-interval prolongation
● CAUTIONS Susceptibility to QT-interval prolongation
● INTERACTIONS Avoid concomitant administration of drugs that prolong QT interval.
● SIDE-EFFECTS
▸ **Common or very common** Abnormal dreams · fatigue · paraesthesia · pyrexia · restlessness · sinusitis · yawning
▸ **Uncommon** Alopecia · bruxism · confusion · epistaxis · menstrual disturbances · mydriasis · oedema · pruritus · syncope · tachycardia · taste disturbance · tinnitus
▸ **Rare** Aggression · bradycardia · depersonalisation
▸ **Frequency not known** Hepatitis · paradoxical increased anxiety during initial treatment of panic disorder (reduce dose) · postural hypotension · QT interval prolongation · thrombocytopenia
● BREAST FEEDING Present in breast milk; avoid.
● HEPATIC IMPAIRMENT Initial dose 5 mg daily for 2 weeks, thereafter increased to max. 10 mg daily according to response; particular caution in severe impairment.
● RENAL IMPAIRMENT Caution if eGFR less than 30 mL/minute/1.73m².
● DIRECTIONS FOR ADMINISTRATION Oral drops can be mixed with water, orange juice, or apple juice before taking.
● PATIENT AND CARER ADVICE
Counselling on administration of oral drops advised.
Driving and skilled tasks
Patients should be counselled about the effects on driving.

● MEDICINAL FORMS
There can be variation in the licensing of different medicines containing the same drug.
Tablet
▸ Escitalopram (Non-proprietary)
Escitalopram (as Escitalopram oxalate) 5 mg Escitalopram 5mg tablets | 28 tablet [PoM] £8.52 DT price = £0.99
Escitalopram (as Escitalopram oxalate) 10 mg Escitalopram 10mg tablets | 28 tablet [PoM] £14.55 DT price = £1.17
Escitalopram (as Escitalopram oxalate) 20 mg Escitalopram 20mg tablets | 28 tablet [PoM] £23.94 DT price = £1.48
▸ Cipralex (Lundbeck Ltd)
Escitalopram (as Escitalopram oxalate) 5 mg Cipralex 5mg tablets | 28 tablet [PoM] £8.97 DT price = £0.99
Escitalopram (as Escitalopram oxalate) 10 mg Cipralex 10mg tablets | 28 tablet [PoM] £14.91 DT price = £1.17
Escitalopram (as Escitalopram oxalate) 20 mg Cipralex 20mg tablets | 28 tablet [PoM] £25.20 DT price = £1.48
Oral drops
▸ Escitalopram (Non-proprietary)
Escitalopram (as Escitalopram oxalate) 20 mg per
1 ml Escitalopram 20mg/ml oral drops sugar free sugar-free |
15 ml [PoM] no price available
▸ Cipralex (Lundbeck Ltd)
Escitalopram (as Escitalopram oxalate) 20 mg per 1 ml Cipralex 20mg/ml oral drops sugar-free | 15 ml [PoM] £20.16

⬛ 332

Fluoxetine

● INDICATIONS AND DOSE

Major depression
▸ BY MOUTH
▸ Adult: Initially 20 mg daily, dose is increased after 3–4 weeks if necessary, and at appropriate intervals thereafter, daily dose may be administered as a single or divided dose; maximum 60 mg per day
▸ Elderly: Initially 20 mg daily, dose is increased after 3–4 weeks if necessary, and at appropriate intervals thereafter, daily dose may be administered as a single or divided dose, usual maximum dose is 40 mg daily but doses up to 60 mg daily can be used

Bulimia nervosa
▸ BY MOUTH
▸ Adult: 60 mg daily, daily dose may be administered as a single or divided dose
▸ Elderly: Up to 40 mg daily, daily dose may be administered as a single or divided dose, usual maximum dose is 40 mg daily but doses up to 60 mg daily can be used

Obsessive-compulsive disorder
▸ BY MOUTH
▸ Adult: 20 mg daily, increased if necessary up to 60 mg daily, daily dose may be administered as a single or divided dose, dose to be increased gradually, review treatment if inadequate response after 10 weeks; maximum 60 mg per day
▸ Elderly: 20 mg daily, increased if necessary up to 40 mg daily, daily dose may be administered as a single or divided dose, dose to be increased gradually, review treatment if inadequate response after 10 weeks, usual maximum dose is 40 mg daily but doses up to 60 mg daily can be used

PHARMACOKINETICS
Consider the long half-life of fluoxetine when adjusting dosage (or in overdosage).

● SIDE-EFFECTS Alopecia · changes in blood sugar · chills · confusion · diarrhoea · dysphagia · dyspnoea · euphoria · flushing · haemorrhage · hepatitis · hypotension · impaired concentration · malaise · neuroleptic malignant syndrome-like event · palpitation · pharyngitis · priapism · pulmonary fibrosis · pulmonary inflammation · sleep disturbances ·

taste disturbance · toxic epidermal necrolysis · urinary frequency · vasodilatation · yawning

- BREAST FEEDING Present in milk—avoid.
- HEPATIC IMPAIRMENT Reduce dose or increase dose interval.
- DIRECTIONS FOR ADMINISTRATION Dispersible tablets can be dispersed in water for administration or swallowed whole with plenty of water.
- PATIENT AND CARER ADVICE
Patients and carers should be counselled on the administration of dispersible tablets.

Driving and skilled tasks
Patients should be counselled about the effects on driving and skilled tasks.

- MEDICINAL FORMS
There can be variation in the licensing of different medicines containing the same drug. Forms available from special-order manufacturers include: tablet, oral suspension, oral solution

Dispersible tablet
CAUTIONARY AND ADVISORY LABELS 10
- Olena (AMCo)
Fluoxetine (as Fluoxetine hydrochloride) 20 mg Olena 20mg dispersible tablets sugar-free | 28 tablet PoM £3.44 DT price = £3.44

Capsule
- Fluoxetine (Non-proprietary)
Fluoxetine (as Fluoxetine hydrochloride) 10 mg Fluoxetine 10mg capsules | 30 capsule PoM £55.00
Fluoxetine (as Fluoxetine hydrochloride) 20 mg Fluoxetine 20mg capsules | 30 capsule PoM £20.00 DT price = £0.92
Fluoxetine (as Fluoxetine hydrochloride) 60 mg Fluoxetine 60mg capsules | 30 capsule PoM £144.00 DT price = £11.26
- Oxactin (Discovery Pharmaceuticals)
Fluoxetine (as Fluoxetine hydrochloride) 20 mg Oxactin 20mg capsules | 30 capsule PoM £0.91 DT price = £0.92
- Prozac (Eli Lilly and Company Ltd)
Fluoxetine (as Fluoxetine hydrochloride) 20 mg Prozac 20mg capsules | 30 capsule PoM £1.50 DT price = £0.92

Oral solution
- Fluoxetine (Non-proprietary)
Fluoxetine (as Fluoxetine hydrochloride) 4 mg per 1 ml Fluoxetine 20mg/5ml oral solution | 70 ml PoM £12.75 DT price = £2.86
Fluoxetine 20mg/5ml oral solution sugar free sugar-free | 70 ml PoM £5.56
- Prozac (Eli Lilly and Company Ltd)
Fluoxetine (as Fluoxetine hydrochloride) 4 mg per 1 ml Prozac 20mg/5ml liquid | 70 ml PoM £11.12 DT price = £2.86
- Prozep (Chemidex Pharma Ltd)
Fluoxetine (as Fluoxetine hydrochloride) 4 mg per 1 ml Prozep 20mg/5ml oral solution sugar-free | 70 ml PoM £12.95

F 332

Fluvoxamine maleate

- INDICATIONS AND DOSE

Depressive illness
- BY MOUTH
- Adult: Initially 50–100 mg daily, dose to be taken in the evening, dose to be increased gradually, increased if necessary up to 300 mg daily, doses over 150 mg daily are given in divided doses; maintenance 100 mg daily

Obsessive-compulsive disorder
- BY MOUTH
- Adult: Initially 50 mg daily, dose to be taken in the evening, dose is increased gradually if necessary after several weeks, increased if necessary up to 300 mg daily; maintenance 100–300 mg daily, doses over 150 mg daily are given in divided doses, if no improvement in obsessive-compulsive disorder within 10 weeks, treatment should be reconsidered

- SIDE-EFFECTS
- **Common or very common** Malaise · palpitation · tachycardia
- **Uncommon** Ataxia · confusion · postural hypotension

- **Rare** Abnormal liver function, usually symptomatic (discontinue treatment)
- **Frequency not known** Neuroleptic malignant syndrome-like event · paraesthesia · taste disturbance
- BREAST FEEDING Present in milk—avoid.
- HEPATIC IMPAIRMENT Start with low dose.
- RENAL IMPAIRMENT Start with low dose.
- PATIENT AND CARER ADVICE

Driving and skilled tasks
Patients should be counselled about the effects on driving and skilled tasks.

- MEDICINAL FORMS
There can be variation in the licensing of different medicines containing the same drug. Forms available from special-order manufacturers include: oral suspension

Tablet
- Fluvoxamine maleate (Non-proprietary)
Fluvoxamine maleate 50 mg Fluvoxamine 50mg tablets | 60 tablet PoM £29.99 DT price = £25.57
Fluvoxamine maleate 100 mg Fluvoxamine 100mg tablets | 30 tablet PoM £29.99 DT price = £25.57
- Faverin (BGP Products Ltd)
Fluvoxamine maleate 50 mg Faverin 50mg tablets | 60 tablet PoM £17.10 DT price = £25.57
Fluvoxamine maleate 100 mg Faverin 100mg tablets | 30 tablet PoM £17.10 DT price = £25.57

F 332

Paroxetine

- INDICATIONS AND DOSE

Major depression | Social anxiety disorder | Post-traumatic stress disorder | Generalised anxiety disorder
- BY MOUTH
- Adult: 20 mg daily, dose to be taken in the morning, no evidence of greater efficacy at higher doses; maximum 50 mg per day
- Elderly: 20 mg daily, dose to be taken in the morning, no evidence of greater efficacy at higher doses; maximum 40 mg per day

Obsessive-compulsive disorder
- BY MOUTH
- Adult: Initially 20 mg daily, dose to be taken in the morning, increased in steps of 10 mg, dose to be increased gradually, increased to 40 mg daily, no evidence of greater efficacy at higher doses; maximum 60 mg per day
- Elderly: Initially 20 mg daily, dose to be taken in the morning, increased in steps of 10 mg, dose to be increased gradually; maximum 40 mg per day

Panic disorder
- BY MOUTH
- Adult: Initially 10 mg daily, dose to be taken in the morning, increased in steps of 10 mg, dose to be increased gradually, increased to 40 mg daily, no evidence of greater efficacy at higher doses; maximum 60 mg per day
- Elderly: Initially 10 mg daily, dose to be taken in the morning, increased in steps of 10 mg, dose to be increased gradually; maximum 40 mg per day

- CAUTIONS Achlorhydria · high gastric pH
CAUTIONS, FURTHER INFORMATION
- Achlorhydria or high gastric pH Causes reduced absorption of the oral suspension.
- SIDE-EFFECTS
- **Common or very common** Abnormal dreams · raised cholesterol · yawning
- **Uncommon** Arrhythmias · confusion · urinary incontinence
- **Rare** Depersonalisation · neuroleptic malignant syndrome-like event · panic attacks · paradoxical increased

anxiety during initial treatment of panic disorder (reduce dose) · restless legs syndrome
- ▶ **Very rare** Acute glaucoma · hepatic disorders · hepatitis · peripheral oedema · priapism
- ▶ **Frequency not known** Extrapyramidal reactions · orofacial dystonias · tinnitus · withdrawal reactions
- ● PREGNANCY Increased risk of congenital malformations, especially if used in the first trimester.
- ● BREAST FEEDING Present in milk but amount too small to be harmful.
- ● HEPATIC IMPAIRMENT Reduce dose.
- ● RENAL IMPAIRMENT Reduce dose if eGFR less than 30 mL/minute/1.73 m².
- ● TREATMENT CESSATION Associated with a higher risk of withdrawal reactions.
- ● PATIENT AND CARER ADVICE

Driving and skilled tasks
Patients should be counselled about the effect on driving.

- ● MEDICINAL FORMS
There can be variation in the licensing of different medicines containing the same drug. Forms available from special-order manufacturers include: oral suspension, oral solution

Tablet
CAUTIONARY AND ADVISORY LABELS 21
- ▶ Paroxetine (Non-proprietary)
  Paroxetine (as Paroxetine hydrochloride) 10 mg Paroxetine 10mg tablets | 28 tablet [PoM] £18.65 DT price = £16.82
  Paroxetine (as Paroxetine hydrochloride) 20 mg Paroxetine 20mg tablets | 30 tablet [PoM] £3.00 DT price = £1.85
  Paroxetine (as Paroxetine hydrochloride) 30 mg Paroxetine 30mg tablets | 30 tablet [PoM] £4.04 DT price = £1.64
- ▶ Seroxat (GlaxoSmithKline UK Ltd)
  Paroxetine (as Paroxetine hydrochloride) 10 mg Seroxat 10mg tablets | 28 tablet [PoM] £14.21 DT price = £16.82
  Paroxetine (as Paroxetine hydrochloride) 20 mg Seroxat 20mg tablets | 30 tablet [PoM] £15.23 DT price = £1.85
  Paroxetine (as Paroxetine hydrochloride) 30 mg Seroxat 30mg tablets | 30 tablet [PoM] £26.74 DT price = £1.64

Oral suspension
CAUTIONARY AND ADVISORY LABELS 5, 21
- ▶ Seroxat (GlaxoSmithKline UK Ltd)
  Paroxetine (as Paroxetine hydrochloride) 2 mg per 1 ml Seroxat 20mg/10ml liquid sugar-free | 150 ml [PoM] £9.12 DT price = £9.12

🔗 332

Sertraline

- ● INDICATIONS AND DOSE

Depressive illness
- ▶ BY MOUTH
  - ▶ Adult: Initially 50 mg daily, then increased in steps of 50 mg at intervals of at least 1 week if required; maintenance 50 mg daily; maximum 200 mg per day

Obsessive-compulsive disorder
- ▶ BY MOUTH
  - ▶ Adult: Initially 50 mg daily, then increased in steps of 50 mg at intervals of at least 1 week if required; maximum 200 mg per day

Panic disorder | Post-traumatic stress disorder | Social anxiety disorder
- ▶ BY MOUTH
  - ▶ Adult: Initially 25 mg daily for 1 week, then increased to 50 mg daily, then increased in steps of 50 mg at intervals of at least 1 week if required, increase only if response is partial and if drug is tolerated; maximum 200 mg per day

- ● SIDE-EFFECTS Aggression · amnesia · bronchospasm · hepatitis · hypercholesterolaemia · hyperprolactinaemia · hypertension · hypoglycaemia · hypothyroidism · jaundice · leucopenia · liver failure · menstrual irregularities · palpitation · pancreatitis · paraesthesia · postural

hypotension · stomatitis · tachycardia · tinnitus · urinary incontinence
- ● BREAST FEEDING Not known to be harmful but consider discontinuing breast-feeding.
- ● HEPATIC IMPAIRMENT Reduce dose or increase dose interval in mild or moderate impairment. Avoid in severe impairment.
- ● RENAL IMPAIRMENT Use with caution.
- ● PATIENT AND CARER ADVICE

Driving and skilled tasks
Patients should be counselled on the effects on driving and skilled tasks.

- ● MEDICINAL FORMS
There can be variation in the licensing of different medicines containing the same drug. Forms available from special-order manufacturers include: oral suspension

Tablet
- ▶ Sertraline (Non-proprietary)
  Sertraline (as Sertraline hydrochloride) 50 mg Sertraline 50mg tablets | 28 tablet [PoM] £19.25 DT price = £1.28
  Sertraline (as Sertraline hydrochloride) 100 mg Sertraline 100mg tablets | 28 tablet [PoM] £29.09 DT price = £1.39
- ▶ Lustral (Pfizer Ltd)
  Sertraline (as Sertraline hydrochloride) 50 mg Lustral 50mg tablets | 28 tablet [PoM] £17.82 DT price = £1.28
  Sertraline (as Sertraline hydrochloride) 100 mg Lustral 100mg tablets | 28 tablet [PoM] £29.16 DT price = £1.39

ANTIDEPRESSANTS > SEROTONIN AND NORADRENALINE RE-UPTAKE INHIBITORS

Duloxetine

- ● DRUG ACTION Inhibits the re-uptake of serotonin and noradrenaline.

- ● INDICATIONS AND DOSE

Major depressive disorder
- ▶ BY MOUTH
  - ▶ Adult: 60 mg once daily

Generalised anxiety disorder
- ▶ BY MOUTH
  - ▶ Adult: Initially 30 mg once daily, increased if necessary to 60 mg once daily; maximum 120 mg per day

Diabetic neuropathy
- ▶ BY MOUTH
  - ▶ Adult: 60 mg once daily, discontinue if inadequate response after 2 months; review treatment at least every 3 months, maximum dose to be given in divided doses; maximum 120 mg per day

Moderate to severe stress urinary incontinence
- ▶ BY MOUTH
  - ▶ Adult (female): 40 mg twice daily, patient should be assessed for benefit and tolerability after 2–4 weeks, alternatively initially 20 mg twice daily for 2 weeks, this can minimise side effects, then increased to 40 mg twice daily, the patient should be assessed for benefit and tolerability after 2–4 weeks.

- ● CAUTIONS Bleeding disorders · cardiac disease · elderly · history of mania · history of seizures · hypertension (avoid if uncontrolled) · raised intra-ocular pressure · susceptibility to angle-closure glaucoma
- ● INTERACTIONS → Appendix 1 (duloxetine). Caution with concomitant use of drugs that increase risk of bleeding.
- ● SIDE-EFFECTS
- ▶ **Common or very common** Abdominal pain · abnormal dreams · anorexia · anxiety · constipation · decreased appetite · diarrhoea · dizziness · drowsiness · dry mouth · dyspepsia · fatigue · flatulence · headache · hot flush ·

insomnia · nausea · nervousness · palpitation · paraesthesia · pruritus · sexual dysfunction · sweating · tremor · visual disturbances · vomiting · weakness · weight changes
▶ **Uncommon** Bruxism · cold extremities · dysphagia · gastritis · halitosis · hepatitis · hypertension · hypothyroidism · impaired attention · impaired temperature regulation · movement disorders · muscle twitching · musculoskeletal pain · photosensitivity · postural hypotension · raised cholesterol · stomatitis · syncope · tachycardia · taste disturbance · thirst · urinary disorders · vertigo
▶ **Rare** Mania
▶ **Very rare** Angle-closure glaucoma
▶ **Frequency not known** Anaphylaxis · angioedema · chest pain · hallucinations · hypersensitivity reactions · hyponatraemia · rash · seizures · Stevens-Johnson syndrome · suicidal behaviour · supraventricular arrhythmia · urticaria
● PREGNANCY Toxicity in *animal* studies—avoid in patients with stress urinary incontinence; in other conditions use only if potential benefit outweighs risk. Risk of neonatal withdrawal symptoms if used near term.
● BREAST FEEDING Present in milk—manufacturer advises avoid.
● HEPATIC IMPAIRMENT Manufacturer advises avoid.
● RENAL IMPAIRMENT Avoid if eGFR less than 30 mL/minute/1.73 m^2.
● TREATMENT CESSATION Nausea, vomiting, headache, anxiety, dizziness, paraesthesia, sleep disturbances, and tremor are the most common features of abrupt withdrawal or marked reduction of the dose; dose should be reduced over at least 1–2 weeks.
● NATIONAL FUNDING/ACCESS DECISIONS

CYMBALTA®

Scottish Medicines Consortium (SMC) Decisions
▶ With oral use for Diabetic neuropathy The *Scottish Medicines Consortium* has advised (September 2006) that duloxetine (*Cymbalta* ®) should be restricted for use by specialists when other treatments for diabetic peripheral neuropathic pain are unsuitable or inadequate.

● MEDICINAL FORMS
There can be variation in the licensing of different medicines containing the same drug.

Gastro-resistant capsule
CAUTIONARY AND ADVISORY LABELS 2
▶ Duloxetine (Non-proprietary)
  Duloxetine (as Duloxetine hydrochloride) 20 mg Duloxetine 20mg gastro-resistant capsules | 28 capsule [PoM] £18.48 DT price = £8.90
  Duloxetine (as Duloxetine hydrochloride) 30 mg Duloxetine 30mg gastro-resistant capsules | 28 capsule [PoM] £22.40 DT price = £8.47
  Duloxetine (as Duloxetine hydrochloride) 40 mg Duloxetine 40mg gastro-resistant capsules | 56 capsule [PoM] £36.96 DT price = £16.74
  Duloxetine (as Duloxetine hydrochloride) 60 mg Duloxetine 60mg gastro-resistant capsules | 28 capsule [PoM] £27.72 DT price = £9.43
▶ Cymbalta (Eli Lilly and Company Ltd)
  Duloxetine (as Duloxetine hydrochloride) 30 mg Cymbalta 30mg gastro-resistant capsules | 28 capsule [PoM] £22.40 DT price = £8.47
  Duloxetine (as Duloxetine hydrochloride) 60 mg Cymbalta 60mg gastro-resistant capsules | 28 capsule [PoM] £27.72 DT price = £9.43
▶ Duciltia (CEB Pharma Ltd)
  Duloxetine (as Duloxetine hydrochloride) 30 mg Duciltia 30mg gastro-resistant capsules | 28 capsule [PoM] £22.40 DT price = £8.47
  Duloxetine (as Duloxetine hydrochloride) 60 mg Duciltia 60mg gastro-resistant capsules | 28 capsule [PoM] £27.72 DT price = £9.43
▶ Yentreve (Eli Lilly and Company Ltd)
  Duloxetine (as Duloxetine hydrochloride) 20 mg Yentreve 20mg gastro-resistant capsules | 28 capsule [PoM] £18.48 DT price = £8.90
  Duloxetine (as Duloxetine hydrochloride) 40 mg Yentreve 40mg gastro-resistant capsules | 56 capsule [PoM] £36.96 DT price = £16.74

Venlafaxine

● DRUG ACTION A serotonin and noradrenaline re-uptake inhibitor.

● INDICATIONS AND DOSE
Major depression
▶ BY MOUTH USING IMMEDIATE-RELEASE MEDICINES
▶ Adult: Initially 75 mg daily in 2 divided doses, then increased if necessary up to 375 mg daily, dose to be increased if necessary at intervals of at least 2 weeks, faster dose titration may be necessary in some patients; maximum 375 mg per day
▶ BY MOUTH USING MODIFIED-RELEASE MEDICINES
▶ Adult: Initially 75 mg once daily, increased if necessary up to 375 mg once daily, dose to be increased if necessary at intervals of at least 2 weeks, faster dose titration may be necessary in some patients; maximum 375 mg per day

Generalised anxiety disorder
▶ BY MOUTH USING MODIFIED-RELEASE MEDICINES
▶ Adult: 75 mg once daily, increased if necessary up to 225 mg once daily, dose to be increased at intervals of at least 2 weeks; maximum 225 mg per day

Social anxiety disorder
▶ BY MOUTH USING MODIFIED-RELEASE MEDICINES
▶ Adult: 75 mg once daily, there is no evidence of greater efficacy at higher doses, increased if necessary up to 225 mg once daily, dose to be increased if necessary at intervals of at least 2 weeks; maximum 225 mg per day

● CONTRA-INDICATIONS Conditions associated with high risk of cardiac arrhythmia · uncontrolled hypertension
● CAUTIONS Diabetes · heart disease (monitor blood pressure) · history of bleeding disorders · history of epilepsy · history or family history of mania · susceptibility to angle-closure glaucoma
● INTERACTIONS → Appendix 1 (venlafaxine). Concomitant use of drugs that increase risk of bleeding.
● SIDE-EFFECTS
▶ **Common or very common** Abnormal dreams · anorexia · anxiety · anxiety (on withdrawal) · asthenia · changes in serum cholesterol · chills · confusion · constipation · difficulty with micturition · dizziness · dizziness (on withdrawal) · drowsiness · dry mouth · gastro-intestinal disturbances (on withdrawal) · headache · headache (on withdrawal) · hypertension · hypertonia · insomnia · menstrual disturbances · mydriasis · nausea · nervousness · palpitation · paraesthesia (on withdrawal) · sensory disturbances · sexual dysfunction · sleep disturbances (on withdrawal) · sweating · sweating (on withdrawal) · tremor · tremor (on withdrawal) · vasodilatation · visual disturbances · vomiting · weight changes · yawning
▶ **Uncommon** Agitation · alopecia · angioedema · apathy · arrhythmias · bleeding disorders · bruxism · diarrhoea · ecchymosis · gastro-intestinal haemorrhage · hallucinations · incoordination · myoclonus · photosensitivity · postural hypotension · rash · taste disturbance · tinnitus · urinary retention
▶ **Rare** Akathisia · extrapyramidal symptoms · hypomania · mania · seizures · urinary incontinence
▶ **Very rare** Angle-closure glaucoma
▶ **Frequency not known** Aggression · blood dyscrasias · delirium · hepatitis · hyperprolactinaemia · hypotension · neuroleptic malignant syndrome · pancreatitis · pruritus · QT interval prolongation · rhabdomyolysis · Stevens-Johnson syndrome · suicidal behaviour · syndrome of inappropriate anti-diuretic hormone secretion · urticaria · vertigo

4

Nervous System

- PREGNANCY Avoid unless potential benefit outweighs risk—toxicity in *animal* studies. Risk of withdrawal effects in neonate.
- BREAST FEEDING Present in milk—avoid.
- HEPATIC IMPAIRMENT Consider reducing dose by 50% in mild or moderate impairment; use with caution and reduce dose by at least 50% in severe impairment.
- RENAL IMPAIRMENT Use half normal dose (immediate-release tablets may be given once daily) if eGFR less than 30 mL/minute/1.73 m². Use with caution.
- TREATMENT CESSATION Associated with a higher risk of withdrawal effects compared with other antidepressants.
  Gastro-intestinal disturbances, headache, anxiety, dizziness, paraesthesia, tremor, sleep disturbances, and sweating are most common features of withdrawal if treatment stopped abruptly or if dose reduced markedly; dose should be reduced over several weeks.
- PATIENT AND CARER ADVICE
  Driving and skilled tasks
  May affect performance of skilled tasks (e.g. driving).

- MEDICINAL FORMS
  There can be variation in the licensing of different medicines containing the same drug. Forms available from special-order manufacturers include: oral suspension, oral solution

Tablet
CAUTIONARY AND ADVISORY LABELS 3
▸ Venlafaxine (Non-proprietary)
  Venlafaxine (as Venlafaxine hydrochloride) 37.5 mg Venlafaxine 37.5mg tablets | 56 tablet PoM £4.90 DT price = £2.33
  Venlafaxine (as Venlafaxine hydrochloride) 75 mg Venlafaxine 75mg tablets | 56 tablet PoM £30.00 DT price = £2.21
▸ ViePax (Dexcel-Pharma Ltd)
  Venlafaxine (as Venlafaxine hydrochloride) 37.5 mg ViePax 37.5mg tablets | 56 tablet PoM £21.07 DT price = £2.33
  Venlafaxine (as Venlafaxine hydrochloride) 75 mg ViePax 75mg tablets | 56 tablet PoM £35.13 DT price = £2.21

Modified-release tablet
CAUTIONARY AND ADVISORY LABELS 3, 21, 25
▸ Sunveniz XL (Sun Pharmaceuticals UK Ltd)
  Venlafaxine (as Venlafaxine hydrochloride) 75 mg Sunveniz XL 75mg tablets | 30 tablet PoM £11.14 DT price = £11.20
  Venlafaxine (as Venlafaxine hydrochloride) 150 mg Sunveniz XL 150mg tablets | 30 tablet PoM £18.64 DT price = £18.70
▸ Venladex XL (Dexcel-Pharma Ltd)
  Venlafaxine (as Venlafaxine hydrochloride) 75 mg Venladex XL 75mg tablets | 28 tablet PoM £11.20
  Venlafaxine (as Venlafaxine hydrochloride) 150 mg Venladex XL 150mg tablets | 28 tablet PoM £18.70
▸ Venlalic XL (DB Ashbourne Ltd)
  Venlafaxine (as Venlafaxine hydrochloride) 37.5 mg Venlalic XL 37.5mg tablets | 30 tablet PoM £6.60 DT price = £6.60
  Venlafaxine (as Venlafaxine hydrochloride) 75 mg Venlalic XL 75mg tablets | 30 tablet PoM £11.20 DT price = £11.20
  Venlafaxine (as Venlafaxine hydrochloride) 150 mg Venlalic XL 150mg tablets | 30 tablet PoM £18.70 DT price = £18.70
  Venlafaxine (as Venlafaxine hydrochloride) 225 mg Venlalic XL 225mg tablets | 30 tablet PoM £33.60 DT price = £33.60
▸ ViePax XL (Dexcel-Pharma Ltd)
  Venlafaxine (as Venlafaxine hydrochloride) 75 mg ViePax XL 75mg tablets | 28 tablet PoM £10.44
  Venlafaxine (as Venlafaxine hydrochloride) 150 mg ViePax XL 150mg tablets | 28 tablet PoM £17.44

Modified-release capsule
CAUTIONARY AND ADVISORY LABELS 3, 21, 25
▸ Venlafaxine (Non-proprietary)
  Venlafaxine (as Venlafaxine hydrochloride) 75 mg Venlafaxine 75mg modified-release capsules | 28 capsule PoM £22.50 DT price = £22.08
  Venlafaxine (as Venlafaxine hydrochloride) 150 mg Venlafaxine 150mg modified-release capsules | 28 capsule PoM no price available DT price = £36.81
▸ Alventa XL (Consilient Health Ltd)
  Venlafaxine (as Venlafaxine hydrochloride) 75 mg Alventa XL 75mg capsules | 28 capsule PoM £19.12 DT price = £22.08

Venlafaxine (as Venlafaxine hydrochloride) 150 mg Alventa XL 150mg capsules | 28 capsule PoM £31.88 DT price = £36.81
▸ Amphero XL (Mylan Ltd)
  Venlafaxine (as Venlafaxine hydrochloride) 75 mg Amphero XL 75mg capsules | 28 capsule PoM £15.46 DT price = £22.08
  Venlafaxine (as Venlafaxine hydrochloride) 150 mg Amphero XL 150mg capsules | 28 capsule PoM £25.77 DT price = £36.81
▸ Depefex XL (Chiesi Ltd)
  Venlafaxine (as Venlafaxine hydrochloride) 75 mg Depefex XL 75mg capsules | 28 capsule PoM £10.40 DT price = £22.08
  Venlafaxine (as Venlafaxine hydrochloride) 150 mg Depefex XL 150mg capsules | 28 capsule PoM £17.40 DT price = £36.81
▸ Efexor XL (Pfizer Ltd)
  Venlafaxine (as Venlafaxine hydrochloride) 75 mg Efexor XL 75mg capsules | 28 capsule PoM £22.08 DT price = £22.08
  Venlafaxine (as Venlafaxine hydrochloride) 150 mg Efexor XL 150mg capsules | 28 capsule PoM £36.81 DT price = £36.81
  Venlafaxine (as Venlafaxine hydrochloride) 225 mg Efexor XL 225mg capsules | 28 capsule PoM £47.11
▸ Politid XL (Actavis UK Ltd)
  Venlafaxine (as Venlafaxine hydrochloride) 75 mg Politid XL 75mg capsules | 28 capsule PoM £23.41 DT price = £22.08
  Venlafaxine (as Venlafaxine hydrochloride) 150 mg Politid XL 150mg capsules | 28 capsule PoM £39.03 DT price = £36.81
▸ Rodomel XL (Teva UK Ltd)
  Venlafaxine (as Venlafaxine hydrochloride) 75 mg Rodomel XL 75mg capsules | 28 capsule PoM £17.91 DT price = £22.08
  Venlafaxine (as Venlafaxine hydrochloride) 150 mg Rodomel XL 150mg capsules | 28 capsule PoM £29.85 DT price = £36.81
▸ Tonpular XL (Wockhardt UK Ltd)
  Venlafaxine (as Venlafaxine hydrochloride) 75 mg Tonpular XL 75mg capsules | 28 capsule PoM £7.00 DT price = £22.08
  Venlafaxine (as Venlafaxine hydrochloride) 150 mg Tonpular XL 150mg capsules | 28 capsule PoM £12.00 DT price = £36.81
▸ Venaxx XL (AMCo)
  Venlafaxine (as Venlafaxine hydrochloride) 75 mg Venaxx XL 75mg capsules | 28 capsule PoM £10.40 DT price = £22.08
  Venlafaxine (as Venlafaxine hydrochloride) 150 mg Venaxx XL 150mg capsules | 28 capsule PoM £17.40 DT price = £36.81
▸ Venlablue XL (Bluefish Pharmaceuticals AB)
  Venlafaxine (as Venlafaxine hydrochloride) 37.5 mg Venlablue XL 37.5mg capsules | 28 capsule PoM £5.25
  Venlafaxine (as Venlafaxine hydrochloride) 75 mg Venlablue XL 75mg capsules | 28 capsule PoM £6.95 DT price = £22.08
  Venlafaxine (as Venlafaxine hydrochloride) 150 mg Venlablue XL 150mg capsules | 28 capsule PoM £9.95 DT price = £36.81
▸ Venlaneo XL (Kent Pharmaceuticals Ltd)
  Venlafaxine (as Venlafaxine hydrochloride) 75 mg Venlaneo XL 75mg capsules | 28 capsule PoM £22.08 DT price = £22.08
  Venlafaxine (as Venlafaxine hydrochloride) 150 mg Venlaneo XL 150mg capsules | 28 capsule PoM £36.81 DT price = £36.81
▸ Vensir XL (Morningside Healthcare Ltd)
  Venlafaxine (as Venlafaxine hydrochloride) 75 mg Vensir XL 75mg capsules | 28 capsule PoM £2.60 DT price = £22.08
  Venlafaxine (as Venlafaxine hydrochloride) 150 mg Vensir XL 150mg capsules | 28 capsule PoM £3.90 DT price = £36.81
▸ Vexarin XL (Mylan Ltd)
  Venlafaxine (as Venlafaxine hydrochloride) 150 mg Vexarin XL 150mg capsules | 28 capsule PoM £18.70 DT price = £36.81

ANTIDEPRESSANTS > SEROTONIN UPTAKE INHIBITORS

Trazodone hydrochloride

- INDICATIONS AND DOSE

Depressive illness (particularly where sedation is required)
▸ BY MOUTH
▸ Adult: Initially 150 mg daily in divided doses, dose to be taken after food, alternatively initially 150 mg once daily, dose to be taken at bedtime, increased if necessary to 300 mg daily; increased if necessary to 600 mg daily in divided doses, higher dose for use in hospital patients only
▸ Elderly: Initially 100 mg daily in divided doses, dose to be taken after food, alternatively initially 100 mg once

daily, dose to be taken at bedtime, increased if
necessary to 300 mg daily; increased if necessary to
600 mg daily in divided doses, higher dose for use in
hospital patients only

Anxiety
▶ BY MOUTH
▸ Adult: 75 mg daily, increased if necessary to 300 mg
daily

● CONTRA-INDICATIONS Acute porphyrias p. 918 ·
arrhythmias · during the manic phase of bipolar disorder ·
heart block · immediate recovery period after myocardial
infarction

● CAUTIONS Cardiovascular disease · chronic constipation ·
diabetes · epilepsy · history of bipolar disorder · history of
psychosis · hyperthyroidism (risk of arrhythmias) ·
increased intra-ocular pressure · patients with a significant
risk of suicide · phaeochromocytoma (risk of arrhythmias) ·
prostatic hypertrophy · susceptibility to angle-closure
glaucoma · urinary retention
CAUTIONS, FURTHER INFORMATION
Treatment should be stopped if the patient enters a manic
phase.
  Elderly patients are particularly susceptible to many of
the side-effects of tricyclic antidepressants; low initial
doses should be used, with close monitoring, particularly
for psychiatric and cardiac side-effects.

● INTERACTIONS Antidepressants, tricyclic (related).

● SIDE-EFFECTS
▸ **Rare** Extrapyramidal symptoms · paralytic ileus
▸ **Very rare** Precipitation of angle-closure glaucoma
▸ **Frequency not known** Changes in blood sugar · dry mouth ·
postural hypotension · agitation · alopecia · anorexia ·
anxiety · arrhythmia · arthralgia · blurred vision · breast
enlargement · chills (on withdrawal) · confusion ·
constipation · convulsions · delusions · dizziness ·
drowsiness · dysarthria · dyspepsia · dyspnoea · ECG
changes · galactorrhoea · gynaecomastia · haematological
reactions · hallucinations · headache (on withdrawal) ·
heart block · hepatic reactions · hypersalivation ·
hypertension · hypomania · hyponatraemia · increased
appetite · influenza-like symptoms (on withdrawal) ·
insomnia (on withdrawal) · irritability · mania · movement
disorders (on withdrawal) · myalgia · myalgia (on
withdrawal) · nausea · nausea (on withdrawal) · palpitation
· paraesthesia · photosensitivity · priapism (discontinue
immediately) · pruritus · rash · sexual dysfunction · sleep
disturbances · sudden death of patients with cardiac
disease · sweating · sweating (on withdrawal) · tachycardia ·
taste disturbance · tinnitus · tremor · urinary retention ·
urticaria · vivid dreams (on withdrawal) · vomiting · weight
gain · weight loss
SIDE-EFFECTS, FURTHER INFORMATION
The patient should be encouraged to persist with
treatment as some tolerance to these side-effects seems to
develop. They are reduced if low doses are given initially
and then gradually increased, but this must be balanced
against the need to obtain a full therapeutic effect as soon
as possible.

Overdose
The tricyclic-related antidepressant drugs may be
associated with a lower risk of cardiotoxicity in
overdosage.
  Tricyclic and related antidepressants cause dry mouth,
coma of varying degree, hypotension, hypothermia,
hyperreflexia, extensor plantar responses, convulsions,
respiratory failure, cardiac conduction defects, and
arrhythmias. Dilated pupils and urinary retention also
occur. For details on the management of poisoning see
Tricyclic and related antidepressants under Emergency
treatment of poisoning p. 1194.

● PREGNANCY Avoid during first trimester—limited
information available. Monitor infant for signs of
withdrawal if used until delivery.

● BREAST FEEDING The amount secreted into breast milk is
too small to be harmful.

● HEPATIC IMPAIRMENT Sedative effects are increased in
hepatic impairment. Avoid in severe liver disease.

● RENAL IMPAIRMENT Use with caution in severe
impairment.

● TREATMENT CESSATION Withdrawal effects may occur
within 5 days of stopping treatment with antidepressant
drugs; they are usually mild and self-limiting, but in some
cases may be severe. The risk of withdrawal symptoms is
increased if the antidepressant is stopped suddenly after
regular administration for 8 weeks or more. The dose
should preferably be reduced gradually over about 4 weeks,
or longer if withdrawal symptoms emerge (6 months in
patients who have been on long-term maintenance
treatment). If possible tricyclic and related antidepressants
should be withdrawn slowly.

● PRESCRIBING AND DISPENSING INFORMATION Limited
quantities of tricyclic antidepressants should be prescribed
at any one time because their cardiovascular and
epileptogenic effects are dangerous in overdosage.

● PATIENT AND CARER ADVICE
Driving and skilled tasks
Drowsiness may affect the performance of skilled tasks
(e.g. driving).
  Effects of alcohol enhanced.

● MEDICINAL FORMS
There can be variation in the licensing of different medicines
containing the same drug. Forms available from special-order
manufacturers include: oral suspension, oral solution

Tablet
CAUTIONARY AND ADVISORY LABELS 2, 21
▸ Trazodone hydrochloride (Non-proprietary)
  Trazodone hydrochloride 150 mg Trazodone 150mg tablets |
  28 tablet [PoM] £51.00 DT price = £24.13
▸ Molipaxin (Zentiva)
  Trazodone hydrochloride 150 mg Molipaxin 150mg tablets |
  28 tablet [PoM] £16.08 DT price = £24.13

Capsule
CAUTIONARY AND ADVISORY LABELS 2, 21
▸ Trazodone hydrochloride (Non-proprietary)
  Trazodone hydrochloride 50 mg Trazodone 50mg capsules |
  84 capsule [PoM] £52.50 DT price = £21.19
  Trazodone hydrochloride 100 mg Trazodone 100mg capsules |
  56 capsule [PoM] £61.50 DT price = £25.95
▸ Molipaxin (Zentiva)
  Trazodone hydrochloride 50 mg Molipaxin 50mg capsules |
  84 capsule [PoM] £23.92 DT price = £21.19
  Trazodone hydrochloride 100 mg Molipaxin 100mg capsules |
  56 capsule [PoM] £28.14 DT price = £25.95

Oral solution
CAUTIONARY AND ADVISORY LABELS 2, 21
▸ Trazodone hydrochloride (Non-proprietary)
  Trazodone hydrochloride 10 mg per 1 ml Trazodone 50mg/5ml
  oral solution sugar free sugar-free | 120 ml [PoM] £195.03 DT price =
  £138.20

ANTIDEPRESSANTS > TETRACYCLIC
ANTIDEPRESSANTS

Mianserin hydrochloride

● INDICATIONS AND DOSE
**Depressive illness (particularly where sedation is
required)**
▶ BY MOUTH
▸ Adult: Initially 30–40 mg daily in divided doses,
alternatively initially 30–40 mg once daily, continued →

4

Nervous system

dose to be taken at bedtime, increase dose gradually as necessary; usual dose 30–90 mg

▸ Elderly: Initially 30 mg daily in divided doses, alternatively initially 30 mg once daily, dose to be taken at bedtime, increase dose gradually as necessary; usual dose 30–90 mg

● CONTRA-INDICATIONS Acute porphyrias p. 918 · arrhythmias · during the manic phase of bipolar disorder · heart block · immediate recovery period after myocardial infarction

● CAUTIONS Cardiovascular disease · chronic constipation · diabetes · epilepsy · history of bipolar disorder · history of psychosis · hyperthyroidism (risk of arrhythmias) · increased intra-ocular pressure · patients with a significant risk of suicide · phaeochromocytoma (risk of arrhythmias) · prostatic hypertrophy · susceptibility to angle-closure glaucoma · urinary retention

CAUTIONS, FURTHER INFORMATION
Treatment should be stopped if the patient enters a manic phase.

Elderly patients are particularly susceptible to many of the side-effects of tricyclic antidepressants; low initial doses should be used, with close monitoring, particularly for psychiatric and cardiac side-effects.

● INTERACTIONS Antidepressants, tricyclic (related).

● SIDE-EFFECTS

▸ Common or very common Agitation · anxiety · arrhythmia · blurred vision · confusion · dizziness · dry mouth · ECG changes · heart block · irritability · paraesthesia · postural hypotension · sleep disturbances · sudden death of patients with cardiac disease · tachycardia

▸ Rare Dysarthria · extrapyramidal symptoms · paralytic ileus · tremor · urinary retention

▸ Very rare Constipation · neuroleptic malignant syndrome · precipitation of angle-closure glaucoma

▸ Frequency not known Alopecia · anorexia · arthralgia · arthritis · blood dyscrasias · breast enlargement · changes in blood sugar · chills (on withdrawal) · convulsions · delusions · galactorrhoea · gynaecomastia · haematological reactions · hallucinations · headache (on withdrawal) · hepatic reactions · hypomania · hyponatraemia · increased appetite · influenza-like symptoms (on withdrawal) · Insomnia (on withdrawal) · jaundice · mania · movement disorders (on withdrawal) · myalgia (on withdrawal) · nausea · nausea (on withdrawal) · oedema · photosensitivity · pruritus · rash · sexual dysfunction · suicidal behaviour · sweating · sweating (on withdrawal) · taste disturbance · tinnitus · urticaria · vivid dreams (on withdrawal) · vomiting · weight gain · weight loss

SIDE-EFFECTS, FURTHER INFORMATION
The patient should be encouraged to persist with treatment as some tolerance to these side-effects seems to develop. They are reduced if low doses are given initially and then gradually increased, but this must be balanced against the need to obtain a full therapeutic effect as soon as possible.

Overdose
The tricyclic-related antidepressant drugs may be associated with a lower risk of cardiotoxicity in overdosage.

Tricyclic and related antidepressants cause dry mouth, coma of varying degree, hypotension, hypothermia, hyperreflexia, extensor plantar responses, convulsions, respiratory failure, cardiac conduction defects, and arrhythmias. Dilated pupils and urinary retention also occur. For details on the management of poisoning see Tricyclic and related antidepressants under Emergency treatment of poisoning p. 1194.

● PREGNANCY Avoid.

● BREAST FEEDING The amount secreted into breast milk is too small to be harmful.

● HEPATIC IMPAIRMENT Sedative effects are increased in hepatic impairment. Avoid in severe liver disease.

● RENAL IMPAIRMENT Caution in renal impairment.

● MONITORING REQUIREMENTS A full **blood count** is recommended every 4 weeks during the first 3 months of treatment; clinical monitoring should continue subsequently and treatment should be stopped and a full blood count obtained if *fever, sore throat, stomatitis,* or other signs of infection develop.

● TREATMENT CESSATION Withdrawal effects may occur within 5 days of stopping treatment with antidepressant drugs; they are usually mild and self-limiting, but in some cases may be severe. The risk of withdrawal symptoms is increased if the antidepressant is stopped suddenly after regular administration for 8 weeks or more. The dose should preferably be reduced gradually over about 4 weeks, or longer if withdrawal symptoms emerge (6 months in patients who have been on long-term maintenance treatment). If possible tricyclic and related antidepressants should be withdrawn slowly.

● PRESCRIBING AND DISPENSING INFORMATION Limited quantities of tricyclic antidepressants should be prescribed at any one time because their cardiovascular and epileptogenic effects are dangerous in overdosage.

● PATIENT AND CARER ADVICE
Driving and skilled tasks
Drowsiness may affect the performance of skilled tasks (e.g. driving).
Effects of alcohol enhanced.

● MEDICINAL FORMS
There can be variation in the licensing of different medicines containing the same drug. Forms available from special-order manufacturers include: oral suspension, oral solution
Tablet
CAUTIONARY AND ADVISORY LABELS 2, 25
▸ Mianserin hydrochloride (Non-proprietary)
Mianserin hydrochloride 10 mg Mianserin 10mg tablets | 28 tablet [PoM] £8.25 DT price = £8.25
Mianserin hydrochloride 30 mg Mianserin 30mg tablets | 28 tablet [PoM] £18.34 DT price = £18.34

Mirtazapine

● DRUG ACTION Mirtazapine is a presynaptic alpha$_2$-adrenoreceptor antagonist which increases central noradrenergic and serotonergic neurotransmission.

● INDICATIONS AND DOSE
Major depression
▸ BY MOUTH
▸ Adult: Initially 15–30 mg daily for 2–4 weeks, dose to be taken at bedtime, then adjusted according to response to up to 45 mg once daily, alternatively up to 45 mg daily in 2 divided doses

● CAUTIONS Cardiac disorders · diabetes mellitus · elderly · history of bipolar depression · history of seizures · history of urinary retention · hypotension · psychoses (may aggravate psychotic symptoms) · susceptibility to angle-closure glaucoma

● INTERACTIONS → Appendix 1 (mirtazapine).

● SIDE-EFFECTS
▸ Common or very common Abnormal dreams · agitation (on withdrawal) · anxiety · anxiety (on withdrawal) · arthralgia · confusion · dizziness · dizziness (on withdrawal) · drowsiness · dry mouth · fatigue · headache (on withdrawal) · increased appetite · insomnia · myalgia ·

nausea (on withdrawal) · oedema · postural hypotension · tremor · vomiting (on withdrawal) · weight gain
▶ **Uncommon** Hallucinations · mania · movement disorders · syncope
▶ **Rare** Aggression · myoclonus · pancreatitis
▶ **Frequency not known** Angle-closure glaucoma · blood disorders · convulsions · dysarthria · hypersalivation · hyponatraemia · inappropriate secretion of antidiuretic hormone · sedation during initial treatment · Stevens-Johnson syndrome · suicidal behaviour · toxic epidermal necrolysis

● PREGNANCY Use with caution—limited experience; monitor neonate for withdrawal effects.

● BREAST FEEDING Present in milk; use only if potential benefit outweighs risk.

● HEPATIC IMPAIRMENT Use with caution. Discontinue if jaundice occurs.

● RENAL IMPAIRMENT Clearance reduced by 30% if eGFR less than 40 mL/minute/1.73 m^2; clearance reduced by 50% if eGFR less than 10 mL/minute/1.73 m^2.

● TREATMENT CESSATION Nausea, vomiting, dizziness, agitation, anxiety, and headache are most common features of withdrawal if treatment stopped abruptly or if dose reduced markedly; dose should be reduced over several weeks.

● DIRECTIONS FOR ADMINISTRATION Orodispersible tablet (*Zispin SolTab* ®) should be placed on the tongue, allowed to disperse and swallowed.

● PATIENT AND CARER ADVICE Counselling on administration of orodispersible tablet advised.
Blood Disorders Patients should be advised to report any fever, sore throat, stomatitis or other signs of infection during treatment. Blood count should be performed and the drug stopped immediately if blood dyscrasia suspected.

● MEDICINAL FORMS
There can be variation in the licensing of different medicines containing the same drug. Forms available from special-order manufacturers include: capsule, oral suspension, oral solution

Tablet
CAUTIONARY AND ADVISORY LABELS 2, 25
▶ Mirtazapine (Non-proprietary)
Mirtazapine 15 mg Mirtazapine 15mg tablets | 28 tablet PoM £17.75 DT price = £1.19
Mirtazapine 30 mg Mirtazapine 30mg tablets | 28 tablet PoM £17.50 DT price = £1.21
Mirtazapine 45 mg Mirtazapine 45mg tablets | 28 tablet PoM £13.18 DT price = £1.51

Orodispersible tablet
CAUTIONARY AND ADVISORY LABELS 2
EXCIPIENTS: May contain Aspartame
▶ Mirtazapine (Non-proprietary)
Mirtazapine 15 mg Mirtazapine 15mg orodispersible tablets | 30 tablet PoM £19.19 DT price = £1.57
Mirtazapine 30 mg Mirtazapine 30mg orodispersible tablets | 30 tablet PoM £19.19 DT price = £1.47
Mirtazapine 45 mg Mirtazapine 45mg orodispersible tablets | 30 tablet PoM £19.19 DT price = £2.10
▶ Zispin SolTab (Merck Sharp & Dohme Ltd)
Mirtazapine 15 mg Zispin SolTab 15mg orodispersible tablets | 30 tablet PoM £15.06 DT price = £1.57
Mirtazapine 30 mg Zispin SolTab 30mg orodispersible tablets | 30 tablet PoM £15.06 DT price = £1.47
Mirtazapine 45 mg Zispin SolTab 45mg orodispersible tablets | 30 tablet PoM £15.06 DT price = £2.10

Oral solution
CAUTIONARY AND ADVISORY LABELS 2
▶ Mirtazapine (Non-proprietary)
Mirtazapine 15 mg per 1 ml Mirtazapine 15mg/ml oral solution sugar free sugar-free | 66 ml PoM £51.05 DT price = £50.28

4

Nervous system

ANTIDEPRESSANTS ❭ TRICYCLIC ANTIDEPRESSANTS

Amitriptyline hydrochloride

● INDICATIONS AND DOSE

Abdominal pain or discomfort (in patients who have not responded to laxatives, loperamide, or antispasmodics)
▶ BY MOUTH
▶ Adult: Initially 5–10 mg daily, to be taken at night; increased in steps of 10 mg at least every 2 weeks as required; maximum 30 mg per day

Depressive illness (but not recommended)
▶ BY MOUTH
▶ Adult: Initially 75 mg daily in divided doses, alternatively initially 75 mg once daily, dose to be taken at bedtime, increased if necessary to 150–200 mg daily, dose to be increased gradually
▶ Elderly: Initially 30–75 mg daily in divided doses, alternatively initially 30–75 mg once daily, dose to be taken at bedtime, increased if necessary to 150–200 mg daily, dose to be increased gradually

Neuropathic pain
▶ BY MOUTH
▶ Adult: Initially 10 mg once daily, increased if necessary to 75 mg once daily, dose to be taken at night, dose to be increased gradually, higher doses to be given on specialist advice

Migraine prophylaxis
▶ BY MOUTH
▶ Adult: Initially 10 mg once daily, then increased if necessary to 50–75 mg once daily (max. per dose 150 mg), dose to be taken at night

● UNLICENSED USE Not licensed for use in neuropathic pain. Not licensed for use in migraine prophylaxis. Not licensed for use in abdominal pain or discomfort in patients who have not responded to laxatives, loperamide, or antispasmodics.

● CONTRA-INDICATIONS Acute porphyrias p. 918 · arrhythmias · during manic phase of bipolar disorder · heart block · immediate recovery period after myocardial infarction

● CAUTIONS Cardiovascular disease · chronic constipation · diabetes · epilepsy · history of bipolar disorder · history of psychosis · hyperthyroidism (risk of arrhythmias) · increased intra-ocular pressure · patients with a significant risk of suicide · phaeochromocytoma (risk of arrhythmias) · prostatic hypertrophy · susceptibility to angle-closure glaucoma · urinary retention

CAUTIONS, FURTHER INFORMATION
Treatment should be stopped if the patient enters a manic phase.

Elderly patients are particularly susceptible to many of the side-effects of tricyclic antidepressants; low initial doses should be used, with close monitoring, particularly for psychiatric and cardiac side-effects.

● INTERACTIONS → Appendix 1 (Antidepressants, tricyclic).

● SIDE-EFFECTS
▶ **Common or very common** Abdominal pain · fatigue · hypertension · mydriasis · oedema · palpitation · restlessness · stomatitis
▶ **Rare** Dysarthria · extrapyramidal symptoms · paralytic ileus · tremor
▶ **Very rare** Neuroleptic malignant syndrome · precipitation of angle-closure glaucoma
▶ **Frequency not known** Agitation · alopecia · anorexia · anxiety · arrhythmia · blurred vision · breast enlargement · changes in blood sugar · chills (on withdrawal) · confusion · constipation · convulsions · delusions · dizziness ·

drowsiness · dry mouth · ECG changes · galactorrhoea · gynaecomastia · haematological reactions · hallucinations · headache (on withdrawal) · heart block · hepatic reactions · hypomania · hyponatraemia · increased appetite · increased intra-ocular pressure · influenza-like symptoms (on withdrawal) · Insomnia (on withdrawal) · irritability · mania · movement disorders (on withdrawal) · myalgia (on withdrawal) · nausea · nausea (on withdrawal) · paraesthesia · photosensitivity · postural hypotension · pruritus · rash · sexual dysfunction · sleep disturbances · sudden death of patients with cardiac disease · suicidal behaviour · sweating · sweating (on withdrawal) · tachycardia · taste disturbance · tinnitus · urinary retention · urticaria · vivid dreams (on withdrawal) · vomiting · weight gain · weight loss

SIDE-EFFECTS, FURTHER INFORMATION

The patient should be encouraged to persist with treatment as some tolerance to these side-effects seems to develop. They are reduced if low doses are given initially and then gradually increased, but this must be balanced against the need to obtain a full therapeutic effect as soon as possible.

Overdose

Overdosage with amitriptyline is associated with a relatively high rate of fatality. Symptoms of overdosage may include dry mouth, coma of varying degree, hypotension, hypothermia, hyperreflexia, extensor plantar responses, convulsions, respiratory failure, cardiac conduction defects, and arrhythmias. Dilated pupils and urinary retention also occur. For details on the management of poisoning, see Tricyclic and related antidepressants, under Emergency treatment of poisoning p. 1194.

● **PREGNANCY** Use only if potential benefit outweighs risk.

● **BREAST FEEDING** The amount secreted into breast milk is too small to be harmful.

● **HEPATIC IMPAIRMENT** Sedative effects are increased in hepatic impairment. Avoid in severe liver disease.

● **TREATMENT CESSATION** Withdrawal effects may occur within 5 days of stopping treatment with antidepressant drugs; they are usually mild and self-limiting, but in some cases may be severe. The risk of withdrawal symptoms is increased if the antidepressant is stopped suddenly after regular administration for 8 weeks or more. The dose should preferably be reduced gradually over about 4 weeks, or longer if withdrawal symptoms emerge (6 months in patients who have been on long-term maintenance treatment). If possible tricyclic and related antidepressants should be withdrawn slowly.

● **PRESCRIBING AND DISPENSING INFORMATION** Limited quantities of tricyclic antidepressants should be prescribed at any one time because their cardiovascular and epileptogenic effects are dangerous in overdosage.

● **PATIENT AND CARER ADVICE**

Driving and skilled tasks
Drowsiness may affect the performance of skilled tasks (e.g. driving).
Effects of alcohol enhanced.

● **MEDICINAL FORMS**
There can be variation in the licensing of different medicines containing the same drug. Forms available from special-order manufacturers include: oral suspension, oral solution

Tablet

CAUTIONARY AND ADVISORY LABELS 2

▸ Amitriptyline hydrochloride (Non-proprietary)
  Amitriptyline hydrochloride 10 mg Amitriptyline 10mg tablets | 28 tablet [PoM] £1.23 DT price = £0.76
  Amitriptyline hydrochloride 25 mg Amitriptyline 25mg tablets | 28 tablet [PoM] £1.13 DT price = £0.78
  Amitriptyline hydrochloride 50 mg Amitriptyline 50mg tablets | 28 tablet [PoM] £3.60 DT price = £0.92

Oral solution

CAUTIONARY AND ADVISORY LABELS 2

▸ Amitriptyline hydrochloride (Non-proprietary)
  Amitriptyline hydrochloride 2 mg per 1 ml Amitriptyline 10mg/5ml oral solution sugar free sugar-free | 150 ml [PoM] £22.60–£129.25
  Amitriptyline hydrochloride 5 mg per 1 ml Amitriptyline 25mg/5ml oral solution sugar free sugar-free | 150 ml [PoM] £18.00 DT price = £18.00
  Amitriptyline hydrochloride 10 mg per 1 ml Amitriptyline 50mg/5ml oral solution sugar free sugar-free | 150 ml [PoM] £19.20 DT price = £19.20

Amitriptyline with perphenazine

The properties listed below are those particular to the combination only. For the properties of the components please consider, amitriptyline hydrochloride p. 341, perphenazine p. 356.

● **INDICATIONS AND DOSE**

Depression with anxiety
▸ BY MOUTH
▸ Adult: 1 tablet 3 times a day, an additional tablet may be taken at bedtime when required

● **LESS SUITABLE FOR PRESCRIBING** Less suitable for prescribing.

● **MEDICINAL FORMS**
There can be variation in the licensing of different medicines containing the same drug.

Tablet

CAUTIONARY AND ADVISORY LABELS 2

▸ Triptafen (AMCo)
  Perphenazine 2 mg, Amitriptyline hydrochloride 25 mg Triptafen tablets | 100 tablet [PoM] £33.13

Clomipramine hydrochloride

● **INDICATIONS AND DOSE**

Depressive illness
▸ BY MOUTH
▸ Adult: Initially 10 mg daily, then increased if necessary to 30–150 mg daily in divided doses, dose to be increased gradually, alternatively increased if necessary to 30–150 mg once daily, dose to be taken at bedtime; maximum 250 mg per day
▸ Elderly: Initially 10 mg daily, then increased to 30–75 mg daily, dose to be increased carefully over approximately 10 days

Phobic and obsessional states
▸ BY MOUTH
▸ Adult: Initially 25 mg daily, then increased to 100–150 mg daily, dose to be increased gradually over 2 weeks; maximum 250 mg per day
▸ Elderly: Initially 10 mg daily, then increased to 100–150 mg daily, dose to be increased gradually over 2 weeks; maximum 250 mg per day

Adjunctive treatment of cataplexy associated with narcolepsy
▸ BY MOUTH
▸ Adult: Initially 10 mg daily, dose to be gradually increased until satisfactory response; increased if necessary to 10–75 mg daily

● **CONTRA-INDICATIONS** Acute porphyrias p. 918 · arrhythmias · during the manic phase of bipolar disorder · heart block · immediate recovery period after myocardial infarction

● **CAUTIONS** Cardiovascular disease · chronic constipation · diabetes · epilepsy · history of bipolar disorder · history of psychosis · hyperthyroidism (risk of arrhythmias) ·

increased intra-ocular pressure · patients with a significant risk of suicide · phaeochromocytoma (risk of arrhythmias) · prostatic hypertrophy · susceptibility to angle-closure glaucoma · urinary retention

CAUTIONS, FURTHER INFORMATION
Treatment should be stopped if the patient enters a manic phase.

Elderly patients are particularly susceptible to many of the side-effects of tricyclic antidepressants; low initial doses should be used, with close monitoring, particularly for psychiatric and cardiac side-effects.

● INTERACTIONS → Appendix 1 (antidepressants, tricyclic).

● SIDE-EFFECTS

▶ **Common or very common** Abdominal pain · aggression · diarrhoea · fatigue · flushing · hypertension · impaired memory · muscle hypertonia · muscle weakness · mydriasis · myoclonus · restlessness · yawning

▶ **Rare** Dysarthria · extrapyramidal symptoms · paralytic ileus · tremor

▶ **Very rare** Allergic alveolitis · neuroleptic malignant syndrome · precipitation of angle-closure glaucoma

▶ **Frequency not known** Agitation · alopecia · anorexia · anxiety · arrhythmias · blurred vision · breast enlargement · changes in blood sugar · chills (on withdrawal) · confusion · constipation · convulsions · delusions · dizziness · dry mouth · ECG changes · galactorrhoea · gynaecomastia · haematological reactions · hallucinations · headache (on withdrawal) · heart block · hepatic reactions · hypomania · hyponatraemia · increased appetite · influenza-like symptoms (on withdrawal) · insomnia (on withdrawal) · irritability · mania · movement disorders (on withdrawal) · myalgia (on withdrawal) · nausea · nausea (on withdrawal) · paraesthesia · photosensitivity · postural hypotension · pruritus · rash · sexual dysfunction · sleep disturbances · sudden death of patients with cardiac disease · suicidal behaviour · sweating · sweating (on withdrawal) · tachycardia · taste disturbance · tinnitus · urinary retention · urticaria · vivid dreams (on withdrawal) · vomiting · weight gain · weight loss

SIDE-EFFECTS, FURTHER INFORMATION
The patient should be encouraged to persist with treatment as some tolerance to these side-effects seems to develop. They are reduced if low doses are given initially and then gradually increased, but this must be balanced against the need to obtain a full therapeutic effect as soon as possible.

Overdose
Tricyclic and related antidepressants cause dry mouth, coma of varying degree, hypotension, hypothermia, hyperreflexia, extensor plantar responses, convulsions, respiratory failure, cardiac conduction defects, and arrhythmias. Dilated pupils and urinary retention also occur. For details on the management of poisoning see Tricyclic and related antidepressants under Emergency treatment of poisoning p. 1194.

● PREGNANCY Neonatal withdrawal symptoms reported if used during third trimester.

● BREAST FEEDING The amount secreted into breast milk is too small to be harmful.

● HEPATIC IMPAIRMENT Sedative effects are increased in hepatic impairment. Avoid in severe liver disease.

● TREATMENT CESSATION Withdrawal effects may occur within 5 days of stopping treatment with antidepressant drugs; they are usually mild and self-limiting, but in some cases may be severe. The risk of withdrawal symptoms is increased if the antidepressant is stopped suddenly after regular administration for 8 weeks or more. The dose should preferably be reduced gradually over about 4 weeks, or longer if withdrawal symptoms emerge (6 months in patients who have been on long-term maintenance

treatment). If possible tricyclic and related antidepressants should be withdrawn slowly.

● PRESCRIBING AND DISPENSING INFORMATION Limited quantities of tricyclic antidepressants should be prescribed at any one time because their cardiovascular and epileptogenic effects are dangerous in overdosage.

● PATIENT AND CARER ADVICE
Driving and skilled tasks
Drowsiness may affect the performance of skilled tasks (e.g. driving).
Effects of alcohol enhanced.

● MEDICINAL FORMS
There can be variation in the licensing of different medicines containing the same drug. Forms available from special-order manufacturers include: oral suspension, oral solution

Capsule
CAUTIONARY AND ADVISORY LABELS 2
▶ Clomipramine hydrochloride (Non-proprietary)
Clomipramine hydrochloride 10 mg Clomipramine 10mg capsules | 28 capsule [PoM] £6.72 DT price = £1.26
Clomipramine hydrochloride 25 mg Clomipramine 25mg capsules | 28 capsule [PoM] £9.36 DT price = £1.50
Clomipramine hydrochloride 50 mg Clomipramine 50mg capsules | 28 capsule [PoM] £11.76 DT price = £1.83

Dosulepin hydrochloride
(Dothiepin hydrochloride)

● INDICATIONS AND DOSE
Depressive illness (particularly where sedation is required) (initiated by a specialist)
▶ BY MOUTH
▶ Adult: Initially 75 mg daily in divided doses, alternatively initially 75 mg once daily, dose to be taken at bedtime, increased if necessary to 150 mg daily, doses to be increased gradually; up to 225 mg daily in some circumstances (e.g. hospital use)
▶ Elderly: Initially 50–75 mg daily in divided doses, alternatively initially 50–75 mg once daily, dose to be taken at bedtime, increased if necessary to 75–150 mg daily, doses to be increased gradually; up to 225 mg daily in some circumstances (e.g. hospital use)

● CONTRA-INDICATIONS Acute porphyrias p. 918 · arrhythmias · during the manic phase of bipolar disorder · heart block · immediate recovery period after myocardial infarction

● CAUTIONS Cardiovascular disease · chronic constipation · diabetes · epilepsy · history of bipolar disorder · history of psychosis · hyperthyroidism (risk of arrhythmias) · increased intra-ocular pressure · patients with a significant risk of suicide · phaeochromocytoma (risk of arrhythmias) · prostatic hypertrophy · susceptibility to angle-closure glaucoma · urinary retention

CAUTIONS, FURTHER INFORMATION
Treatment should be stopped if the patient enters a manic phase.

Elderly patients are particularly susceptible to many of the side-effects of tricyclic antidepressants; low initial doses should be used, with close monitoring, particularly for psychiatric and cardiac side-effects.

● INTERACTIONS → Appendix 1 (antidepressants, tricyclic).

● SIDE-EFFECTS
▶ **Rare** Dysarthria · extrapyramidal symptoms · paralytic ileus · tremor
▶ **Very rare** Neuroleptic malignant syndrome · precipitation of angle-closure glaucoma
▶ **Frequency not known** Agitation · alopecia · anorexia · anxiety · arrhythmias · blurred vision · breast enlargement · changes in blood sugar · chills (on withdrawal) · confusion ·

constipation · convulsions · delusions · dizziness · dry mouth · ECG changes · galactorrhoea · gynaecomastia · haematological reactions · hallucinations · headache (on withdrawal) · heart block · hepatic reactions · hypomania · hyponatraemia · increased appetite · increased intraocular pressure · influenza-like symptoms (on withdrawal) · insomnia (on withdrawal) · irritability · mania · movement disorders (on withdrawal) · myalgia (on withdrawal) · nausea · nausea (on withdrawal) · paraesthesia · photosensitivity · postural hypotension · pruritus · rash · sexual dysfunction · sleep disturbances · sudden death of patients with cardiac disease · suicidal behaviour · sweating · sweating (on withdrawal) · tachycardia · taste disturbance · tinnitus · urinary retention · urticaria · vivid dreams (on withdrawal) · vomiting · weight gain · weight loss

SIDE-EFFECTS, FURTHER INFORMATION
The patient should be encouraged to persist with treatment as some tolerance to these side-effects seems to develop. They are reduced if low doses are given initially and then gradually increased, but this must be balanced against the need to obtain a full therapeutic effect as soon as possible.

Overdose
Overdosage with dosulepin is associated with a relatively high rate of fatality.

Tricyclic and related antidepressants cause dry mouth, coma of varying degree, hypotension, hypothermia, hyperreflexia, extensor plantar responses, convulsions, respiratory failure, cardiac conduction defects, and arrhythmias. Dilated pupils and urinary retention also occur. For details on the management of poisoning see Tricyclic and related antidepressants under Emergency treatment of poisoning p. 1194.

● PREGNANCY Use only if potential benefit outweighs risk.
● BREAST FEEDING The amount secreted into breast milk is too small to be harmful.
● HEPATIC IMPAIRMENT Sedative effects are increased in hepatic impairment. Avoid in severe liver disease.
● TREATMENT CESSATION Withdrawal effects may occur within 5 days of stopping treatment with antidepressant drugs; they are usually mild and self-limiting, but in some cases may be severe. The risk of withdrawal symptoms is increased if the antidepressant is stopped suddenly after regular administration for 8 weeks or more. The dose should preferably be reduced gradually over about 4 weeks, or longer if withdrawal symptoms emerge. (6 months in patients who have been on long-term maintenance treatment). If possible tricyclic and related antidepressants should be withdrawn slowly.
● PRESCRIBING AND DISPENSING INFORMATION Limited quantities of tricyclic antidepressants should be prescribed at any one time because their cardiovascular and epileptogenic effects are dangerous in overdosage.

A maximum prescription equivalent to 2 weeks' supply of 75 mg daily should be considered in patients with increased risk factors for suicide at initiation of treatment, during any dose adjustment, and until improvement occurs.
● PATIENT AND CARER ADVICE
Driving and skilled tasks
Drowsiness may affect the performance of skilled tasks (e.g. driving).

Effects of alcohol enhanced.
● LESS SUITABLE FOR PRESCRIBING Dosulepin hydrochloride is less suitable for prescribing.

● MEDICINAL FORMS
There can be variation in the licensing of different medicines containing the same drug. Forms available from special-order manufacturers include: oral suspension, oral solution
Tablet
CAUTIONARY AND ADVISORY LABELS 2
▸ Dosulepin hydrochloride (Non-proprietary)
   Dosulepin hydrochloride 75 mg Dosulepin 75mg tablets | 28 tablet PoM £2.15 DT price = £1.42
▸ Prothiaden (Teofarma)
   Dosulepin hydrochloride 75 mg Prothiaden 75mg tablets | 28 tablet PoM £2.97 DT price = £1.42
Capsule
CAUTIONARY AND ADVISORY LABELS 2
▸ Dosulepin hydrochloride (Non-proprietary)
   Dosulepin hydrochloride 25 mg Dosulepin 25mg capsules | 28 capsule PoM £3.00 DT price = £1.28
▸ Prothiaden (Teofarma)
   Dosulepin hydrochloride 25 mg Prothiaden 25mg capsules | 28 capsule PoM £1.70 DT price = £1.28

Doxepin

● INDICATIONS AND DOSE
Depressive illness (particularly where sedation is required)
▸ BY MOUTH
▸ Adult: Initially 75 mg daily in divided doses, alternatively 75 mg once daily, adjusted according to response, dose to taken at bedtime; maintenance 25–300 mg daily, doses above 100 mg given in 3 divided doses
▸ Elderly: Start with lower doses and adjust according to response

● CONTRA-INDICATIONS Acute porphyrias p. 918 · arrhythmias · during manic phase of bipolar disorder · heart block · immediate recovery period after myocardial infarction
● CAUTIONS Cardiovascular disease · chronic constipation · diabetes · epilepsy · history of bipolar disorder · history of psychosis · hyperthyroidism (risk of arrhythmias) · increased intra-ocular pressure · patients with significant risk of suicide · phaeochromocytoma (risk of arrhythmias) · prostatic hypertrophy · susceptibility to angle-closure glaucoma · urinary retention

CAUTIONS, FURTHER INFORMATION
Treatment should be stopped if the patient enters a manic phase.

Elderly patients are particularly susceptible to many of the side-effects of tricyclic antidepressants; low initial doses should be used, with close monitoring, particularly for psychiatric and cardiac side-effects.
● INTERACTIONS → Appendix 1 (antidepressants, tricyclic).
● SIDE-EFFECTS
▸ **Common or very common** Agitation · anxiety · confusion · dizziness · drowsiness · irritability · paraesthesia · sleep disturbances
▸ **Rare** Dysarthria · extrapyramidal symptoms · paralytic ileus · tremor
▸ **Very rare** Neuroleptic malignant syndrome · precipitation of angle-closure glaucoma
▸ **Frequency not known** Abdominal pain · alopecia · anorexia · arrhythmia · blurred vision · breast enlargement · changes in blood sugar · chills (on withdrawal) · constipation · convulsions · delusions · diarrhoea · dry mouth · ECG changes · flushing · galactorrhoea · gynaecomastia · haematological reactions · hallucinations · headache (on withdrawal) · heart block · hepatic reactions · hypomania · hyponatraemia · increased appetite · influenza-like symptoms (on withdrawal) · insomnia (on withdrawal) · mania · movement disorders (on withdrawal) · myalgia (on

withdrawal) · nausea · nausea (on withdrawal) · oedema · photosensitivity · postural hypotension · pruritus · rash · sexual dysfunction · stomatitis · sudden death of patients with cardiac disease · suicidal behaviour · sweating · sweating (on withdrawal) · tachycardia · taste disturbance · tinnitus · urinary retention · urticaria · vivid dreams (on withdrawal) · vomiting · weight gain · weight loss

SIDE-EFFECTS, FURTHER INFORMATION
The patient should be encouraged to persist with treatment as some tolerance to these side-effects seems to develop. They are reduced if low doses are given initially and then gradually increased, but this must be balanced against the need to obtain a full therapeutic effect as soon as possible.

Overdose
Tricyclic and related antidepressants cause dry mouth, coma of varying degree, hypotension, hypothermia, hyperreflexia, extensor plantar responses, convulsions, respiratory failure, cardiac conduction defects, and arrhythmias. Dilated pupils and urinary retention also occur. For details on the management of poisoning see Tricyclic and related antidepressants under Emergency treatment of poisoning p. 1194.

● PREGNANCY Use with caution—limited information available.

● BREAST FEEDING The amount secreted into breast milk is too small to be harmful. Accumulation of metabolite may cause sedation and respiratory depression in neonate.

● HEPATIC IMPAIRMENT Sedative effects are increased in hepatic impairment. Avoid in severe liver disease.

● RENAL IMPAIRMENT Use with caution.

● TREATMENT CESSATION Withdrawal effects may occur within 5 days of stopping treatment with antidepressant drugs; they are usually mild and self-limiting, but in some cases may be severe. The risk of withdrawal symptoms is increased if the antidepressant is stopped suddenly after regular administration for 8 weeks or more. The dose should preferably be reduced gradually over about 4 weeks, or longer if withdrawal symptoms emerge (6 months in patients who have been on long-term maintenance treatment). If possible tricyclic and related antidepressants should be withdrawn slowly.

● PRESCRIBING AND DISPENSING INFORMATION Limited quantities of tricyclic antidepressants should be prescribed at any one time because their cardiovascular and epileptogenic effects are dangerous in overdosage.

● PATIENT AND CARER ADVICE
Driving and skilled tasks
Drowsiness may affect performance of skilled tasks (e.g. driving).
Effects of alcohol enhanced.

● MEDICINAL FORMS
There can be variation in the licensing of different medicines containing the same drug. Forms available from special-order manufacturers include: capsule, oral suspension, oral solution

Capsule
CAUTIONARY AND ADVISORY LABELS 2
▸ Doxepin (Non-proprietary)
Doxepin (as Doxepin hydrochloride) 25 mg Doxepin 25mg capsules | 28 capsule PoM £48.00–£97.00 DT price = £97.00
Doxepin (as Doxepin hydrochloride) 50 mg Doxepin 50mg capsules | 28 capsule PoM £84.00–£154.00 DT price = £154.00

Imipramine hydrochloride

● INDICATIONS AND DOSE
Depressive illness
▸ BY MOUTH
▸ Adult: Initially up to 75 mg daily in divided doses, then increased to 150–200 mg daily, up to 150 mg may be given as a single dose at bedtime, dose to be increased gradually
▸ Elderly: Initially 10 mg daily, increased to 30–50 mg daily, dose to be increased gradually

Depressive illness in hospital patients
▸ BY MOUTH
▸ Adult: Initially up to 75 mg daily in divided doses, dose to be increased gradually, increased to up to 300 mg daily in divided doses

Nocturnal enuresis
▸ BY MOUTH
▸ Child 6-7 years: 25 mg once daily, to be taken at bedtime, initial period of treatment (including gradual withdrawal) 3 months—full physical examination before further course
▸ Child 8-10 years: 25–50 mg once daily, to be taken at bedtime, initial period of treatment (including gradual withdrawal) 3 months—full physical examination before further course
▸ Child 11-17 years: 50–75 mg once daily, to be taken at bedtime, initial period of treatment (including gradual withdrawal) 3 months—full physical examination before further course

● CONTRA-INDICATIONS Immediate recovery period after myocardial infarction (in adults) · Acute porphyrias p. 918 · arrhythmia · during the manic phase of bipolar disorder · heart block

● CAUTIONS Cardiovascular disease · chronic constipation · diabetes · epilepsy · history of bipolar disorder · history of psychosis · hyperthyroidism (risk of arrhythmias) · increased intra-ocular pressure (in adults) · patients with a significant risk of suicide · phaeochromocytoma (risk of arrhythmias) · prostatic hypertrophy (in adults) · susceptibility to angle-closure glaucoma · urinary retention

CAUTIONS, FURTHER INFORMATION
Treatment should be stopped if the patient enters a manic phase.

Elderly patients are particularly susceptible to many of the side-effects of tricyclic antidepressants; low initial doses should be used, with close monitoring, particularly for psychiatric and cardiac side-effects.

● INTERACTIONS → Appendix 1 (antidepressants tricyclic).

● SIDE-EFFECTS
▸ **Common or very common** Fatigue · flushing · headache · palpitation · restlessness
▸ **Rare** Extrapyramidal symptoms · paralytic ileus
▸ **Very rare** Abdominal pain · aggression · allergic alveolitis · cardiac decompensation · diarrhoea (in children) · hypertension · mydriasis · myoclonus · neuroleptic malignant syndrome · oedema · peripheral vasospasm · precipitation of angle-closure glaucoma · stomatitis
▸ **Frequency not known** Agitation · alopecia · anorexia · anxiety · arrhythmia · blurred vision · breast enlargement · changes in blood sugar · chills (on withdrawal) · confusion · constipation · convulsions · delusions · dizziness · drowsiness · dry mouth · dysarthria · ECG changes · galactorrhoea · gynaecomastia · haematologial reactions · hallucinations · headache (on withdrawal) · heart block · hepatic reactions · hypomania · hyponatraemia · increased appetite · influenza-like symptoms (on withdrawal) · insomnia (on withdrawal) · irritability · mania · movement disorders (on withdrawal) · myalgia (on withdrawal) ·

nausea · nausea (on withdrawal) · paraesthesia · photosensitivity · postural hypotension · pruritus · rash · sexual dysfunction · sleep disturbances · sudden death of patients with cardiac disease · suicidal behaviour · sweating · sweating (on withdrawal) · tachycardia · taste disturbance · tinnitus · tremor · urinary retention · urticaria · vivid dreams (on withdrawal) · vomiting · weight gain · weight loss

SIDE-EFFECTS, FURTHER INFORMATION
▶ In adults The patient should be encouraged to persist with treatment as some tolerance to these side-effects seems to develop. They are reduced if low doses are given initially and then gradually increased, but this must be balanced against the need to obtain a full therapeutic effect as soon as possible.

Overdose
Tricyclic and related antidepressants cause dry mouth, coma of varying degree, hypotension, hypothermia, hyperreflexia, extensor plantar responses, convulsions, respiratory failure, cardiac conduction defects, and arrhythmias. Dilated pupils and urinary retention also occur. For details on the management of poisoning see Tricyclic and related antidepressants under Emergency treatment of poisoning p. 1194.

● PREGNANCY Colic, tachycardia, dyspnoea, irritability, muscle spasms, respiratory depression and withdrawal symptoms reported in neonates when used in the third trimester.

● BREAST FEEDING The amount secreted into breast milk is too small to be harmful.

● HEPATIC IMPAIRMENT Sedative effects are increased in hepatic impairment. Avoid in severe liver disease.

● RENAL IMPAIRMENT Use with caution in severe impairment.

● TREATMENT CESSATION Withdrawal effects may occur within 5 days of stopping treatment with antidepressant drugs; they are usually mild and self-limiting, but in some cases may be severe. The risk of withdrawal symptoms is increased if the antidepressant is stopped suddenly after regular administration for 8 weeks or more. The dose should preferably be reduced gradually over about 4 weeks, or longer if withdrawal symptoms emerge (6 months in patients who have been on long-term maintenance treatment). If possible tricyclic antidepressants should be withdrawn slowly.

● PRESCRIBING AND DISPENSING INFORMATION Limited quantities of tricyclic antidepressants should be prescribed at any one time because their cardiovascular and epileptogenic effects are dangerous in overdosage.

● PATIENT AND CARER ADVICE
Medicines for Children leaflet: Imipramine www.medicinesforchildren.org.uk/imipramine
Driving and skilled tasks
Drowsiness may affect the performance of skilled tasks (e.g. driving).
Effects of alcohol enhanced.

● MEDICINAL FORMS
There can be variation in the licensing of different medicines containing the same drug. Forms available from special-order manufacturers include: oral suspension, oral solution

Tablet
CAUTIONARY AND ADVISORY LABELS 2
▶ Imipramine hydrochloride (Non-proprietary)
Imipramine hydrochloride **10 mg** Imipramine 10mg tablets | 28 tablet [PoM] £1.17 DT price = £1.05
Imipramine hydrochloride **25 mg** Imipramine 25mg tablets | 28 tablet [PoM] £1.16 DT price = £1.05

Oral solution
CAUTIONARY AND ADVISORY LABELS 2
▶ Imipramine hydrochloride (Non-proprietary)
Imipramine hydrochloride **5 mg per 1 ml** Imipramine 25mg/5ml oral solution sugar free sugar-free | 150 ml [PoM] £39.31

Lofepramine

● INDICATIONS AND DOSE
Depressive illness
▶ BY MOUTH
▸ Adult: 140–210 mg daily in divided doses
▸ Elderly: May respond to lower doses

● CONTRA-INDICATIONS Acute porphyrias p. 918 · arrhythmias · during the manic phase of bipolar disorder · heart block · immediate recovery period after myocardial infarction

● CAUTIONS Cardiovascular disease · chronic constipation · diabetes · epilepsy · history of bipolar disorder · history of psychosis · hyperthyroidism (risk of arrhythmias) · increased intra-ocular pressure · patients with a significant risk of suicide · phaeochromocytoma (risk of arrhythmias) · prostatic hypertrophy · susceptibility to angle-closure glaucoma · urinary retention

CAUTIONS, FURTHER INFORMATION
Treatment should be stopped if the patient enters a manic phase.
Elderly patients are particularly susceptible to many of the side-effects of tricyclic antidepressants; low initial doses should be used, with close monitoring, particularly for psychiatric and cardiac side-effects.

● INTERACTIONS → Appendix 1 (antidepressants, tricyclic).

● SIDE-EFFECTS
▶ **Common or very common** Agitation · anxiety · confusion · dizziness · irritability · paraesthesia · postural hypotension · sleep disturbances
▶ **Rare** Extrapyramidal symptoms · paralytic ileus
▶ **Very rare** Neuroleptic malignant syndrome · precipitation of angle-closure glaucoma
▶ **Frequency not known** Alopecia · anorexia · arrhythmias · blurred vision · breast enlargement · changes in blood sugar · chills (on withdrawal) · constipation · convulsions · delusions · diarrhoea · drowsiness · dry mouth · dysarthria · ECG changes · galactorrhoea · gynaecomastia · haematological reactions · hallucinations · headache · headache (on withdrawal) · heart block · hepatic reactions · hypomania · hyponatraemia · increased appetite · influenza-like symptoms (on withdrawal) · insomnia (on withdrawal) · mania · movement disorders (on withdrawal) · myalgia (on withdrawal) · nausea · nausea (on withdrawal) · oedema · photosensitivity · pruritus · rash · sexual dysfunction · sudden death of patients with cardiac disease · suicidal behaviour · sweating · sweating (on withdrawal) · tachycardia · taste disturbance · tinnitus · tremor · urinary retention · urticaria · vivid dreams (on withdrawal) · vomiting · weight gain · weight loss

SIDE-EFFECTS, FURTHER INFORMATION
The patient should be encouraged to persist with treatment as some tolerance to these side-effects seems to develop. They are reduced if low doses are given initially and then gradually increased, but this must be balanced against the need to obtain a full therapeutic effect as soon as possible.

Overdose
Tricyclic and related antidepressants cause dry mouth, coma of varying degree, hypotension, hypothermia, hyperreflexia, extensor plantar responses, convulsions, respiratory failure, cardiac conduction defects, and arrhythmias. Dilated pupils and urinary retention also occur. Lofepramine is associated with the lowest risk of

fatality in overdosage, in comparison with other tricyclic antidepressant drugs. For details on the management of poisoning see Tricyclic and related antidepressants under Emergency treatment of poisoning p. 1194.

- PREGNANCY Neonatal withdrawal symptoms and respiratory depression reported if used during third trimester.
- BREAST FEEDING The amount secreted into breast milk is too small to be harmful.
- HEPATIC IMPAIRMENT Sedative effects are increased in hepatic impairment. Avoid in severe liver disease.
- RENAL IMPAIRMENT Avoid in severe impairment.
- TREATMENT CESSATION Withdrawal effects may occur within 5 days of stopping treatment with antidepressant drugs; they are usually mild and self-limiting, but in some cases may be severe. The risk of withdrawal symptoms is increased if the antidepressant is stopped suddenly after regular administration for 8 weeks or more. The dose should preferably be reduced gradually over about 4 weeks, or longer if withdrawal symptoms emerge (6 months in patients who have been on long-term maintenance treatment). If possible tricyclic and related antidepressants should be withdrawn slowly.
- PRESCRIBING AND DISPENSING INFORMATION Limited quantities of tricyclic antidepressants should be prescribed at any one time because their cardiovascular and epileptogenic effects are dangerous in overdosage.
- PATIENT AND CARER ADVICE
  Driving and skilled tasks
  Drowsiness may affect the performance of skilled tasks (e.g. driving).
  Effects of alcohol enhanced.
- MEDICINAL FORMS
  There can be variation in the licensing of different medicines containing the same drug. Forms available from special-order manufacturers include: oral suspension, oral solution
  Tablet
  CAUTIONARY AND ADVISORY LABELS 2
  ▸ Lofepramine (Non-proprietary)
  Lofepramine (as Lofepramine hydrochloride) 70 mg Lofepramine 70mg tablets | 56 tablet [PoM] £59.97 DT price = £13.45
  Oral suspension
  CAUTIONARY AND ADVISORY LABELS 2
  ▸ Lofepramine (Non-proprietary)
  Lofepramine (as Lofepramine hydrochloride) 14 mg per 1 ml Lofepramine 70mg/5ml oral suspension sugar free sugar-free | 150 ml [PoM] £25.22 DT price = £22.22
  ▸ Lomont (Rosemont Pharmaceuticals Ltd)
  Lofepramine (as Lofepramine hydrochloride) 14 mg per 1 ml Lomont 70mg/5ml oral suspension sugar-free | 150 ml [PoM] £22.22 DT price = £22.22

Nortriptyline

- INDICATIONS AND DOSE
  Depressive illness
  ▸ BY MOUTH
  ▸ Adult: To be initiated at a low dose, then increased if necessary to 75–100 mg daily in divided doses, alternatively increased if necessary to 75–100 mg once daily; maximum 150 mg per day
  ▸ Elderly: To be initiated at a low dose, then increased if necessary to 30–50 mg daily in divided doses
  Neuropathic pain
  ▸ BY MOUTH
  ▸ Adult: Initially 10 mg once daily, to be taken at night, increased if necessary to 75 mg daily, dose to be increased gradually; higher doses to be given under specialist supervision

- UNLICENSED USE Not licensed for use in neuropathic pain.
- CONTRA-INDICATIONS Acute porphyrias p. 918 · arrhythmias · during the manic phase of bipolar disorder · heart block · immediate recovery period after myocardial infarction
- CAUTIONS Cardiovascular disease · chronic constipation · diabetes · epilepsy · history of bipolar disorder · history of psychosis · hyperthyroidism (risk of arrhythmias) · increased intra-ocular pressure · patients with a significant risk of suicide · phaeochromocytoma (risk of arrhythmias) · prostatic hypertrophy · susceptibility to angle-closure glaucoma · urinary retention
  CAUTIONS, FURTHER INFORMATION
  Treatment should be stopped if the patient enters a manic phase.
  Elderly patients are particularly susceptible to many of the side-effects of tricyclic antidepressants; low initial doses should be used, with close monitoring, particularly for psychiatric and cardiac side-effects.
- INTERACTIONS → Appendix 1 (antidepressants, tricyclic).
- SIDE-EFFECTS
  ▸ **Common or very common** Fatigue · hypertension · mydriasis · restlessness
  ▸ **Rare** Extrapyramidal symptoms · paralytic ileus
  ▸ **Very rare** Neuroleptic malignant syndrome · precipitation of angle-closure glaucoma
  ▸ **Frequency not known** Abdominal pain · agitation · alopecia · anorexia · anxiety · arrhythmia · blurred vision · breast enlargement · changes in blood sugar · chills (on withdrawal) · confusion · constipation · convulsions · delusions · diarrhoea · dizziness · drowsiness · dry mouth · dysarthria · ECG changes · flushing · galactorrhoea · gynaecomastia · haematological reactions · hallucinations · headache (on withdrawal) · heart block · hepatic reactions · hypomania · hyponatraemia · increased appetite · influenza-like symptoms (on withdrawal) · insomnia (on withdrawal) · irritability · mania · movement disorders (on withdrawal) · myalgia (on withdrawal) · nausea · nausea (on withdrawal) · oedema · paraesthesia · photosensitivity · postural hypotension · pruritus · rash · sexual dysfunction · sleep disturbances · stomatitis · sudden death of patients with cardiac disease · suicidal behaviour · sweating · sweating (on withdrawal) · tachycardia · taste disturbance · tinnitus · tremor · urinary retention · urticaria · vivid dreams (on withdrawal) · vomiting · weight gain · weight loss
  SIDE-EFFECTS, FURTHER INFORMATION
  The patient should be encouraged to persist with treatment as some tolerance to these side-effects seems to develop. They are reduced if low doses are given initially and then gradually increased, but this must be balanced against the need to obtain a full therapeutic effect as soon as possible.
  Overdose
  Tricyclic and related antidepressants cause dry mouth, coma of varying degree, hypotension, hypothermia, hyperreflexia, extensor plantar responses, convulsions, respiratory failure, cardiac conduction defects, and arrhythmias. Dilated pupils and urinary retention also occur. For details on the management of poisoning see Tricyclic and related antidepressants under Emergency treatment of poisoning p. 1194.
- PREGNANCY Use only if potential benefit outweighs risk.
- BREAST FEEDING The amount secreted into breast milk is too small to be harmful.
- HEPATIC IMPAIRMENT Sedative effects are increased in hepatic impairment. Avoid in severe liver disease.

4

Nervous system

Nervous system

4

- **MONITORING REQUIREMENTS**
  ▶ Manufacturer advises plasma-nortriptyline concentration monitoring if dose above 100 mg daily, but evidence of practical value uncertain.
- **TREATMENT CESSATION** Withdrawal effects may occur within 5 days of stopping treatment with antidepressant drugs; they are usually mild and self-limiting, but in some cases may be severe. The risk of withdrawal symptoms is increased if the antidepressant is stopped suddenly after regular administration for 8 weeks or more. The dose should preferably be reduced gradually over about 4 weeks, or longer if withdrawal symptoms emerge (6 months in patients who have been on long-term maintenance treatment). If possible tricyclic and related antidepressants should be withdrawn slowly.
- **PRESCRIBING AND DISPENSING INFORMATION** Limited quantities of tricyclic antidepressants should be prescribed at any one time because their cardiovascular and epileptogenic effects are dangerous in overdosage.
- **PATIENT AND CARER ADVICE** Drowsiness may affect the performance of skilled tasks (e.g. driving). Effects of alcohol enhanced.

- **MEDICINAL FORMS**
  There can be variation in the licensing of different medicines containing the same drug. Forms available from special-order manufacturers include: oral suspension, oral solution

  Tablet
  CAUTIONARY AND ADVISORY LABELS 2
  ▶ Nortriptyline (Non-proprietary)
  Nortriptyline (as Nortriptyline hydrochloride) 10 mg Nortriptyline 10mg tablets | 100 tablet [PoM] £34.51-£68.41 DT price = £56.76
  Nortriptyline (as Nortriptyline hydrochloride) 25 mg Nortriptyline 25mg tablets | 100 tablet [PoM] £56.11-£111.06 DT price = £64.57

Trimipramine

- **INDICATIONS AND DOSE**

Depressive illness (particularly where sedation required)
  ▶ BY MOUTH
  ▶ Adult: Initially 50–75 mg daily in divided doses, alternatively initially 50–75 mg once daily, dose to be taken at bedtime, increased if necessary to 150–300 mg daily
  ▶ Elderly: Initially 10–25 mg 3 times a day, maintenance 75–150 mg daily

- **CONTRA-INDICATIONS** Acute porphyrias p. 918 · arrhythmias · during the manic phase of bipolar disorder · heart block · immediate recovery period after myocardial infarction
- **CAUTIONS** Cardiovascular disease · chronic constipation · diabetes · epilepsy · history of bipolar disorder · history of psychosis · hyperthyroidism (risk of arrhythmias) · increased intra-ocular pressure · patients with a significant risk of suicide · phaeochromocytoma (risk of arrhythmias) · prostatic hypertrophy · susceptibility to angle-closure glaucoma · urinary retention
  CAUTIONS, FURTHER INFORMATION
  Treatment should be stopped if the patient enters a manic phase.
  Elderly patients are particularly susceptible to many of the side-effects of tricyclic antidepressants; low initial doses should be used, with close monitoring, particularly for psychiatric and cardiac side-effects.
- **INTERACTIONS** → Appendix 1 (antidepressants, tricyclic).
- **SIDE-EFFECTS**
- **Rare** Paralytic ileus
- **Very rare** Neuroleptic malignant syndrome · precipitation of angle-closure glaucoma

▶ **Frequency not known** Agitation · alopecia · anorexia · anxiety · arrhythmia · blurred vision · breast enlargement · changes in blood sugar · chills (on withdrawal) · confusion · constipation · convulsions · delusions · dizziness · dry mouth · dysarthria · ECG changes · extrapyramidal symptoms · galactorrhoea · gynaecomastia · haematological reactions · hallucinations · headache (on withdrawal) · heart block · hepatic reactions · hypomania · hyponatraemia · increased appetite · influenza-like symptoms (on withdrawal) · Insomnia (on withdrawal) · irritability · mania · movement disorders (on withdrawal) · myalgia (on withdrawal) · nausea · nausea (on withdrawal) · paraesthesia · photosensitivity · postural hypotension · pruritus · rash · sexual dysfunction · sleep disturbances · sudden death of patients with cardiac disease · suicidal behaviour · sweating · sweating (on withdrawal) · tachycardia · taste disturbance · tinnitus · tremor · urinary retention · urticaria · vivid dreams (on withdrawal) · vomiting · weight gain · weight loss

SIDE-EFFECTS, FURTHER INFORMATION
The patient should be encouraged to persist with treatment as some tolerance to these side-effects seems to develop. They are reduced if low doses are given initially and then gradually increased, but this must be balanced against the need to obtain a full therapeutic effect as soon as possible.

Overdose
Tricyclic and related antidepressants cause dry mouth, coma of varying degree, hypotension, hypothermia, hyperreflexia, extensor plantar responses, convulsions, respiratory failure, cardiac conduction defects, and arrhythmias. Dilated pupils and urinary retention also occur. For details on the management of poisoning see Tricyclic and related antidepressants under Emergency treatment of poisoning p. 1194.

- **PREGNANCY** Use only if potential benefit outweighs risk.
- **BREAST FEEDING** The amount secreted into breast milk is too small to be harmful.
- **HEPATIC IMPAIRMENT** Sedative effects are increased in hepatic impairment. Avoid in severe liver disease.
- **TREATMENT CESSATION** Withdrawal effects may occur within 5 days of stopping treatment with antidepressant drugs; they are usually mild and self-limiting, but in some cases may be severe. The risk of withdrawal symptoms is increased if the antidepressant is stopped suddenly after regular administration for 8 weeks or more. The dose should preferably be reduced gradually over about 4 weeks, or longer if withdrawal symptoms emerge (6 months in patients who have been on long-term maintenance treatment). If possible tricyclic and related antidepressants should be withdrawn slowly.
- **PRESCRIBING AND DISPENSING INFORMATION** Limited quantities of tricyclic antidepressants should be prescribed at any one time because their cardiovascular and epileptogenic effects are dangerous in overdosage.
- **PATIENT AND CARER ADVICE**
  Driving and skilled tasks
  Drowsiness may affect the performance of skilled tasks (e.g. driving).
  Effects of alcohol enhanced.

- **MEDICINAL FORMS**
  There can be variation in the licensing of different medicines containing the same drug. Forms available from special-order manufacturers include: oral suspension, oral solution
  Tablet
  CAUTIONARY AND ADVISORY LABELS 2
  ▶ Trimipramine (Non-proprietary)
  Trimipramine (as Trimipramine maleate) 10 mg Trimipramine 10mg tablets | 28 tablet [PoM] £146.33 DT price = £132.12 | 84 tablet [PoM] no price available

Trimipramine (as Trimipramine maleate) 25 mg Trimipramine 25mg tablets | 28 tablet [PoM] £163.32 DT price = £147.45 | 84 tablet [PoM] no price available

Capsule

CAUTIONARY AND ADVISORY LABELS 2
▶ Trimipramine (Non-proprietary)
Trimipramine (as Trimipramine maleate) 50 mg Trimipramine 50mg capsules | 28 capsule [PoM] £156.00 DT price = £150.00

OTHER ANTIDEPRESSANTS

Vortioxetine   17.5.2016

● DRUG ACTION Vortioxetine inhibits the re-uptake of serotonin (5-HT) and is an antagonist at 5-HT$_3$ and an agonist at 5-HT$_{1A}$ receptors. This multimodal activity appears to be associated with antidepressant and anxiolytic-like effects.

● INDICATIONS AND DOSE

Major depression
▶ BY MOUTH
▶ **Adult:** Initially 10 mg once daily; adjusted according to response to 5–20 mg once daily
▶ **Elderly:** Initially 5 mg once daily; increased if necessary up to 20 mg once daily

● CAUTIONS Bleeding disorders · cirrhosis of the liver (risk of hyponatraemia) · elderly (risk of hyponatraemia) · history of mania (discontinue if patient entering manic phase) · history of seizures · unstable epilepsy

CAUTIONS, FURTHER INFORMATION
▶ Seizures Discontinue treatment in patients who develop seizures or if there is an increase in seizure frequency.
▶ Elderly Manufacturer advises caution when treating elderly patients with doses over 10 mg daily—limited information.

● INTERACTIONS → Appendix 1 (vortioxetine).

● SIDE-EFFECTS
▶ **Common or very common** Abnormal dreams · constipation · diarrhoea · dizziness · nausea · pruritus · vomiting
▶ **Uncommon** Flushing · night sweats
▶ **Rare** Bleeding disorders
▶ **Frequency not known** Neuroleptic malignant syndrome—discontinue (potentially fatal) · serotonin syndrome · sexual dysfunction (with 20 mg dose only)

● PREGNANCY Manufacturer advises avoid unless potential benefit outweighs risk—toxicity in *animal* studies. If used during the later stages of pregnancy, there is a risk of neonatal withdrawal symptoms and persistent pulmonary hypertension in the newborn.

● BREAST FEEDING Manufacturer advises avoid—present in milk in *animal* studies.

● HEPATIC IMPAIRMENT Manufacturer advises caution in severe impairment—no information available.

● RENAL IMPAIRMENT Manufacturer advises caution in severe impairment—limited information available.

● TREATMENT CESSATION Manufacturer advises treatment can be stopped abruptly, without need for gradual dose reduction.

● PATIENT AND CARER ADVICE
Driving and skilled tasks
Manufacturer advises patients and carers should be counselled on the effects on driving and performance of skilled tasks, especially when starting treatment or changing the dose.

● NATIONAL FUNDING/ACCESS DECISIONS
NICE technology appraisals (TAs)
▶ Vortioxetine for treating major depressive episodes (November 2015) NICE TA367
Vortioxetine is recommended as an option for treating major depressive episodes in adults whose condition has responded inadequately to 2 antidepressants within the current episode.

Patients currently receiving vortioxetine whose disease does not meet the above criteria should be able to continue treatment until they and their clinician consider it appropriate to stop.
www.nice.org.uk/TA367

● MEDICINAL FORMS
There can be variation in the licensing of different medicines containing the same drug.
Tablet
▶ Brintellix (Lundbeck Ltd) ▼
Vortioxetine (as Vortioxetine hydrobromide) 5 mg Brintellix 5mg tablets | 28 tablet [PoM] £27.72
Vortioxetine (as Vortioxetine hydrobromide) 10 mg Brintellix 10mg tablets | 28 tablet [PoM] £27.72
Vortioxetine (as Vortioxetine hydrobromide) 20 mg Brintellix 20mg tablets | 28 tablet [PoM] £27.72

3.5 Inappropriate sexual behaviour

ANTIPSYCHOTICS › FIRST-GENERATION
352

Benperidol

● INDICATIONS AND DOSE
Control of deviant antisocial sexual behaviour
▶ BY MOUTH
▶ **Adult:** 0.25–1.5 mg daily in divided doses, adjusted according to response, for debilitated patients, use elderly dose
▶ **Elderly:** Initially 0.125–0.75 mg daily in divided doses, adjusted according to response

● CONTRA-INDICATIONS CNS depression · comatose states · phaeochromocytoma

● CAUTIONS Risk factors for stroke

● PREGNANCY Extrapyramidal effects and withdrawal syndrome have been reported occasionally in the neonate when antipsychotic drugs are taken during the third trimester of pregnancy. Following maternal use of antipsychotic drugs in the third trimester, neonates should be monitored for symptoms including agitation, hypertonia, hypotonia, tremor, drowsiness, feeding problems, and respiratory distress.

● BREAST FEEDING There is limited information available on the short- and long-term effects of antipsychotic drugs on the breast-fed infant. *Animal* studies indicate possible adverse effects of antipsychotic medicines on the developing nervous system. Chronic treatment with antipsychotic drugs whilst breast-feeding should be avoided unless absolutely necessary.

● HEPATIC IMPAIRMENT Can precipitate coma.

● RENAL IMPAIRMENT Start with small doses in severe renal impairment because of increased cerebral sensitivity.

● MONITORING REQUIREMENTS Manufacturer advises regular blood counts and liver function tests during long-term treatment.

● PRESCRIBING AND DISPENSING INFORMATION The proprietary name *Benquil* ® has been used for benperidol tablets.

4

Nervous system

● MEDICINAL FORMS
There can be variation in the licensing of different medicines containing the same drug. Forms available from special-order manufacturers include: oral suspension

Tablet
CAUTIONARY AND ADVISORY LABELS 2
▸ Benperidol (Non-proprietary)
Benperidol 250 microgram Benperidol 250microgram tablets | 112 tablet [PoM] £117.31 DT price = £117.31
▸ Anquil (ProStrakan Ltd)
Benperidol 250 microgram Anquil 250microgram tablets | 112 tablet [PoM] £117.31 DT price = £117.31

3.6 Psychoses and schizophrenia

Psychoses and related disorders

Advice of Royal College of Psychiatrists on doses of antipsychotic drugs above BNF upper limit

Unless otherwise stated, doses in the BNF are licensed doses—any higher dose is therefore **unlicensed**

- Consider alternative approaches including adjuvant therapy and newer or second-generation antipsychotic drugs such as clozapine.
- Bear in mind risk factors, including obesity; particular caution is indicated in older patients, especially those over 70.
- Consider potential for drug interactions—see interactions: Appendix 1 (antipsychotics).
- Carry out ECG to exclude untoward abnormalities such as prolonged QT interval; repeat ECG periodically and reduce dose if prolonged QT interval or other adverse cardiac abnormality develops.
- Increase dose slowly and not more often than once weekly.
- Carry out regular pulse, blood pressure, and temperature checks; ensure that patient maintains adequate fluid intake.
- Consider high-dose therapy to be for limited period and review regularly; abandon if no improvement after 3 months (return to standard dosage).

Important: When prescribing an antipsychotic for administration on an emergency basis, the intramuscular dose should be **lower** than the corresponding oral dose (owing to absence of first-pass effect), particularly if the patient is very active (increased blood flow to muscle considerably increases the rate of absorption). The prescription should specify the dose for **each route** and should **not** imply that the same dose can be given by mouth or by intramuscular injection. The dose of antipsychotic for emergency use should be reviewed at least **daily**.

Antipsychotic drugs

Antipsychotic drugs are also known as 'neuroleptics' and (misleadingly) as 'major tranquillisers'.

In the short term they are used to calm disturbed patients whatever the underlying psychopathology, which may be schizophrenia, brain damage, mania, toxic delirium, or agitated depression. Antipsychotic drugs are used to alleviate severe anxiety but this too should be a short-term measure.

Schizophrenia

The aim of treatment is to alleviate the suffering of the patient (and carer) and to improve social and cognitive functioning. Many patients require life-long treatment with antipsychotic medication. Antipsychotic drugs relieve positive psychotic symptoms such as thought disorder, hallucinations, and delusions, and prevent relapse; they are usually less effective on negative symptoms such as apathy and social withdrawal. In many patients, negative symptoms

persist between episodes of treated positive symptoms, but earlier treatment of psychotic illness may protect against the development of negative symptoms over time. Patients with acute schizophrenia generally respond better than those with chronic symptoms.

Long-term treatment of a patient with a definitive diagnosis of schizophrenia is usually required after the first episode of illness in order to prevent relapses. Doses that are effective in acute episodes should generally be continued as prophylaxis.

First-generation antipsychotic drugs

The first-generation antipsychotic drugs act predominantly by blocking dopamine D_2 receptors in the brain. First-generation antipsychotic drugs are not selective for any of the four dopamine pathways in the brain and so can cause a range of side-effects, particularly extrapyramidal symptoms and elevated prolactin. The **phenothiazine** derivatives can be divided into 3 main groups:

- *Group* 1: chlorpromazine hydrochloride p. 353, levomepromazine p. 403, and promazine hydrochloride p. 371, generally characterised by pronounced sedative effects and moderate antimuscarinic and extrapyramidal side-effects.
- *Group* 2: pericyazine p. 355, generally characterised by moderate sedative effects, but fewer extrapyramidal side-effects than groups 1 or 3.
- *Group* 3: fluphenazine decanoate p. 359, perphenazine p. 356, prochlorperazine p. 357, and trifluoperazine p. 358, generally characterised by fewer sedative and antimuscarinic effects, but more pronounced extrapyramidal side-effects than groups 1 and 2.

Butyrophenones (benperidol p. 349 and haloperidol p. 354) resemble the group 3 phenothiazines in their clinical properties. **Thioxanthenes** (flupentixol p. 354 and zuclopenthixol p. 358) have moderate sedative, antimuscarinic effects, and extrapyramidal effects. **Diphenylbutylpiperidines** (pimozide p. 356) and the **substituted benzamides** (sulpiride p. 357) have reduced sedative, antimuscarinic, and extrapyramidal effects.

Second-generation antipsychotic drugs

The second-generation antipsychotic drugs (sometimes referred to as atypical antipsychotic drugs) act on a range of receptors in comparison to first-generation antipsychotic drugs and have more distinct clinical profiles, particularly with regard to side-effects.

Prescribing for the elderly

The balance of risks and benefit should be considered before prescribing antipsychotic drugs for elderly patients. In elderly patients with dementia, antipsychotic drugs are associated with a small increased risk of mortality and an increased risk of stroke or transient ischaemic attack. Furthermore, elderly patients are particularly susceptible to postural hypotension and to hyper- and hypothermia in hot or cold weather.

It is recommended that:

- Antipsychotic drugs should not be used in elderly patients to treat mild to moderate psychotic symptoms.
- Initial doses of antipsychotic drugs in elderly patients should be reduced (to half the adult dose or less), taking into account factors such as the patient's weight, co-morbidity, and concomitant medication.
- Treatment should be reviewed regularly.

Side effects of antipsychotic drugs

Side-effects caused by antipsychotic drugs are common and contribute significantly to non-adherence to therapy.

Extrapyramidal symptoms occur most frequently with the piperazine phenothiazines (fluphenazine, perphenazine, prochlorperazine, and trifluoperazine), the butyrophenones (benperidol and haloperidol), and the first-generation depot preparations. They are easy to recognise but cannot be predicted accurately because they depend on the dose, the type of drug, and on individual susceptibility.

Extrapyramidal symptoms consist of:

- *parkinsonian symptoms* (including tremor), which may occur more commonly in adults or the elderly and may appear gradually;
- *dystonia* (abnormal face and body movements) and *dyskinesia*, which occur more commonly in children or young adults and appear after only a few doses;
- *akathisia* (restlessness), which characteristically occurs after large initial doses and may resemble an exacerbation of the condition being treated;
- *tardive dyskinesia* (rhythmic, involuntary movements of tongue, face, and jaw), which usually develops on long-term therapy or with high dosage, but it may develop on short-term treatment with low doses—short-lived tardive dyskinesia may occur after withdrawal of the drug.

Parkinsonian symptoms remit if the drug is withdrawn and may be suppressed by the administration of antimuscarinic drugs. However, routine administration of such drugs is not justified because not all patients are affected and they may unmask or worsen tardive dyskinesia.

Tardive dyskinesia is the most serious manifestation of extrapyramidal symptoms; it is of particular concern because it may be irreversible on withdrawing therapy and treatment is usually ineffective. In children, tardive dyskinesia is more likely to occur when the antipsychotic drug is withdrawn. However, some manufacturers suggest that drug withdrawal at the earliest signs of tardive dyskinesia (fine vermicular movements of the tongue) may halt its full development. Tardive dyskinesia occurs fairly frequently, especially in the elderly, and treatment must be carefully and regularly reviewed.

Hyperprolactinaemia

Most antipsychotic drugs, both first- and second-generation, increase prolactin concentration to some extent because dopamine inhibits prolactin release. Aripiprazole reduces prolactin because it is a dopamine-receptor partial agonist. Risperidone, amisulpride, and first-generation antipsychotic drugs are most likely to cause symptomatic hyperprolactinaemia. The clinical symptoms of hyperprolactinaemia include sexual dysfunction, reduced bone mineral density, menstrual disturbances, breast enlargement, and galactorrhoea.

Sexual dysfunction

Sexual dysfunction is one of the main causes of non-adherence to antipsychotic medication; physical illness, psychiatric illness, and substance misuse are contributing factors. Antipsychotic-induced sexual dysfunction is caused by more than one mechanism. Reduced dopamine transmission and hyperprolactinaemia decrease libido; antimuscarinic effects can cause disorders of arousal; and alpha$_1$-adrenoceptor antagonists are associated with erection and ejaculation problems in men. Risperidone and haloperidol commonly cause sexual dysfunction. If sexual dysfunction is thought to be antipsychotic-induced, dose reduction or switching medication should be considered.

Cardiovascular side-effects

Antipsychotic drugs have been associated with cardiovascular side-effects such as tachycardia, arrhythmias, and hypotension. QT-interval prolongation is a particular concern with pimozide and haloperidol. There is also a higher probability of QT-interval prolongation in patients using any intravenous antipsychotic drug, or any antipsychotic drug or combination of antipsychotic drugs with doses exceeding the recommended maximum. Cases of sudden death have occurred.

Hyperglycaemia

Hyperglycaemia and sometimes diabetes can occur with antipsychotic drugs, particularly clozapine, olanzapine,

quetiapine, and risperidone. All antipsychotic drugs may cause weight gain, but the risk and extent varies. Clozapine and olanzapine commonly cause weight gain.

Hypotension and interference with temperature regulation

Hypotension and interference with temperature regulation are dose-related side-effects that are liable to cause dangerous falls and hypothermia or hyperthermia in the elderly. Clozapine, chlorpromazine, lurasidone, and quetiapine can cause postural hypotension (especially during initial dose titration) which may be associated with syncope or reflex tachycardia in some patients.

Neuroleptic malignant syndrome

Neuroleptic malignant syndrome (hyperthermia, fluctuating level of consciousness, muscle rigidity, and autonomic dysfunction with pallor, tachycardia, labile blood pressure, sweating, and urinary incontinence) is a rare but potentially fatal side-effect of all antipsychotic drugs. Discontinuation of the antipsychotic drug is essential because there is no proven effective treatment, but bromocriptine and dantrolene have been used. The syndrome, which usually lasts for 5–7 days after drug discontinuation, may be unduly prolonged if depot preparations have been used.

Blood dyscrasias

Perform blood counts if unexplained infection or fever develops.

Choice

There is little meaningful difference in efficacy between each of the antipsychotic drugs (other than clozapine p. 363), and response and tolerability to each antipsychotic drug varies. There is no first-line antipsychotic drug which is suitable for all patients. Choice of antipsychotic medication is influenced by the patient's medication history, the degree of sedation required (although tolerance to this usually develops), and consideration of individual patient factors such as risk of extrapyramidal side-effects, weight gain, impaired glucose tolerance, QT-interval prolongation, or the presence of negative symptoms.

Negative symptoms

Second generation antipsychotic drugs may be better at treating the negative symptoms of schizophrenia.

Extrapyramidal side-effects

Second-generation antipsychotic drugs should be prescribed if extrapyramidal side-effects are a particular concern. Of these, aripiprazole p. 362, clozapine, olanzapine p. 365, and quetiapine p. 367 are least likely to cause extrapyramidal side-effects. Although amisulpride p. 361 is a dopamine-receptor antagonist, extrapyramidal side-effects are less common than with the first-generation antipsychotic drugs because amisulpride selectively blocks mesolimbic dopamine receptors, and extrapyramidal symptoms are caused by blockade of the striatal dopamine pathway.

QT interval

Aripiprazole has negligible effect on the QT interval. Other antipsychotic drugs with a reduced tendency to prolong QT interval include amisulpride, clozapine, flupentixol p. 354, fluphenazine decanoate p. 359, olanzapine, perphenazine p. 356, prochlorperazine p. 357, risperidone p. 368, and sulpiride p. 357.

Diabetes

Schizophrenia is associated with insulin resistance and diabetes; the risk of diabetes is increased in patients with schizophrenia who take antipsychotic drugs. First-generation antipsychotic drugs are less likely to cause diabetes than second-generation antipsychotic drugs, and of the first-generation antipsychotic drugs, fluphenazine decanoate and haloperidol p. 354 are lowest risk. Amisulpride and aripiprazole have the lowest risk of diabetes of the second-generation antipsychotic drugs. Amisulpride,

Nervous system

aripiprazole, haloperidol, sulpiride, and trifluoperazine p. 358 are least likely to cause weight gain.

Sexual dysfunction and prolactin
The antipsychotic drugs with the lowest risk of sexual dysfunction are aripiprazole and quetiapine. Olanzapine may be considered if sexual dysfunction is judged to be secondary to hyperprolactinaemia. Hyperprolactinaemia is usually not clinically significant with aripiprazole, clozapine, olanzapine, and quetiapine treatment. When changing from other antipsychotic drugs, a reduction in prolactin concentration may increase fertility.

Patients should receive an antipsychotic drug for 4–6 weeks before it is deemed ineffective. Prescribing more than one antipsychotic drug at a time should be avoided except in exceptional circumstances (e.g. clozapine augmentation or when changing medication during titration) because of the increased risk of adverse effects such as extrapyramidal symptoms, QT-interval prolongation, and sudden cardiac death.

Clozapine is licensed for the treatment of schizophrenia in patients unresponsive to, or intolerant of, other antipsychotic drugs. Clozapine should be introduced if schizophrenia is not controlled despite the sequential use of two or more antipsychotic drugs (one of which should be a second-generation antipsychotic drug), each for at least 6–8 weeks. If symptoms do not respond adequately to an optimised dose of clozapine, plasma-clozapine concentration should be checked before adding a second antipsychotic drug to augment clozapine; allow 8–10 weeks' treatment to assess response. Patients must be registered with a clozapine patient monitoring service.

Monitoring
Full blood count, urea and electrolytes, and liver function test monitoring is required at the start of therapy with antipsychotic drugs, and then annually thereafter.

Blood lipids and weight should be measured at baseline, at 3 months (weight should be measured at frequent intervals during the first 3 months), and then yearly.

Fasting blood glucose should be measured at baseline, at 4–6 months, and then yearly.

Before initiating antipsychotic drugs, an ECG may be required, particularly if physical examination identifies cardiovascular risk factors, if there is a personal history of cardiovascular disease, or if the patient is being admitted as an inpatient.

Blood pressure monitoring is advised before starting therapy and frequently during dose titration of antipsychotic drugs.

Other uses
Some antipsychotic drugs can be used for the treatment of nausea and vomiting, choreas, and motor tics. Chlorpromazine hydrochloride p. 353 and haloperidol can be used for intractable hiccup. Benperidol p. 349 is used in deviant antisocial sexual behaviour but its value is not established.

Psychomotor agitation should be investigated for an underlying cause; it can be managed with low doses of chlorpromazine hydrochloride p. 353 or haloperidol p. 354 used for short periods. Antipsychotic drugs can be used with caution for the short-term treatment of severe agitation and restlessness in the elderly.

Equivalent doses of oral antipsychotics
These equivalences are intended **only** as an approximate guide; individual dosage instructions should **also** be checked; patients should be carefully monitored after **any** change in medication. Equivalent daily dose of antipsychotic drug:
- Chlorpromazine 100 mg
- Clozapine 50 mg
- Haloperidol 2–3 mg
- Pimozide 2 mg

- Risperidone 0.5–1 mg
- Sulpiride 200 mg
- Trifluoperazine 5 mg

Important:These equivalences must **not** be extrapolated beyond the maximum dose for the drug. Higher doses require careful titration in specialist units and the equivalences shown here may not be appropriate.

Dosage
After an initial period of stabilisation, in most patients, the total daily oral dose can be given as a single dose. The Royal College of Psychiatrists has published advice on doses of antipsychotic drugs above BNF upper limit.

Antipsychotic depot injections
Long-acting depot injections are used for maintenance therapy especially when compliance with oral treatment is unreliable. However, depot injections of conventional antipsychotics may give rise to a higher incidence of extrapyramidal reactions than oral preparations; extrapyramidal reactions occur less frequently with second-generation antipsychotic depot preparations, such as risperidone p. 368 and olanzapine embonate p. 370.

Choice
There is no clear-cut division in the use of the conventional antipsychotics, but zuclopenthixol p. 358 may be suitable for the treatment of agitated or aggressive patients whereas flupentixol decanoate p. 359 can cause over-excitement in such patients. Zuclopenthixol decanoate p. 361 may be more effective in preventing relapses than other conventional antipsychotic depot preparations. The incidence of extrapyramidal reactions is similar for the conventional antipsychotics.

Equivalent doses of depot antipsychotics

Antipsychotic drug/interval	Dosage (mg)
Flupentixol decanoate / 2 weeks	40
Fluphenazine decanoate / 2 weeks	25
Haloperidol (as decanoate) / 4 weeks	100
Zuclopenthixol decanoate / 2 weeks	200

Important:These equivalences must **not** be extrapolated beyond the maximum dose for the drug

These equivalences are intended **only** as an approximate guide; individual dosage instructions should also be checked; patients should be carefully monitored after any change in medication.

Dosage
Individual responses to neuroleptic drugs are variable and to achieve optimum effect, dosage and dosage interval must be titrated according to the patient's response.

ANTIPSYCHOTICS

Antipsychotic drugs

- CAUTIONS Blood dyscrasias · cardiovascular disease · conditions predisposing to seizures · depression · epilepsy · history of jaundice · myasthenia gravis · Parkinson's disease (may be exacerbated) (in adults) · photosensitisation (may occur with higher dosages) · prostatic hypertrophy (in adults) · severe respiratory disease · susceptibility to angle-closure glaucoma

  CAUTIONS, FURTHER INFORMATION
  ‣ Cardiovascular disease An ECG may be required, particularly if physical examination identifies cardiovascular risk factors, personal history of cardiovascular disease, or if the patient is being admitted as an inpatient.

- INTERACTIONS → Appendix 1 (antipsychotics).
Increased risk of toxicity with myelosuppressive drugs.
- SIDE-EFFECTS
▶ **Rare** Neuroleptic malignant syndrome—discontinue (potentially fatal)
▶ **Very rare** Precipitation of angle-closure glaucoma
▶ **Frequency not known** Agitation · agranulocytosis · akathisia · antimuscarinic symptoms · apathy · blood dyscrasias · blurred vision · cardiovascular side-effects · confusion · constipation · contact sensitisation · convulsions · corneal and lens opacities · diabetes · difficulty with micturition · dizziness · drowsiness · dry mouth · dystonia · excitement · extrapyramidal symptoms · gastro-intestinal disturbances · headache · hyperglycaemia · hyperprolactineamia · hypotension (dose related) · insomnia · interference with temperature regulation (dose related) · jaundice (including cholestatic) · leucopenia · nasal congestion · parkinsonian symptoms · photosensitisation · purplish pigmentation of the conjunctiva · purplish pigmentation of the cornea · purplish pigmentation of the retina · purplish pigmentation of the skin · rashes · sexual dysfunction · tardive dyskinesia · venous thromboembolism · weight gain

Overdose
Phenothiazines cause less depression of consciousness and respiration than other sedatives. Hypotension, hypothermia, sinus tachycardia, and arrhythmias may complicate poisoning. For details on the management of poisoning see Antipsychotics under Emergency treatment of poisoning p. 1194.

- PREGNANCY Extrapyramidal effects and withdrawal syndrome have been reported occasionally in the neonate when antipsychotic drugs are taken during the third trimester of pregnancy. Following maternal use of antipsychotic drugs in the third trimester, neonates should be monitored for symptoms including agitation, hypertonia, hypotonia, tremor, drowsiness, feeding problems, and respiratory distress.
- BREAST FEEDING There is limited information available on the short- and long-term effects of antipsychotic drugs on the breast-fed infant. *Animal studies* indicate possible adverse effects of antipsychotic medicines on the developing nervous system. Chronic treatment with antipsychotic drugs whilst breast-feeding should be avoided unless absolutely necessary. Phenothiazine derivatives are sometimes used in breast-feeding women for short-term treatment of nausea and vomiting.
- MONITORING REQUIREMENTS
▶ It is advisable to monitor prolactin concentration at the start of therapy, at 6 months, and then yearly. Patients taking antipsychotic drugs not normally associated with symptomatic hyperprolactinaemia should be considered for prolactin monitoring if they show symptoms of hyperprolactinaemia (such as breast enlargement and galactorrhoea).
▶ Patients with schizophrenia should have physical health monitoring (including cardiovascular disease risk assessment) at least once per year.
▶ In children Regular clinical monitoring of endocrine function should be considered when children are taking an antipsychotic drug known to increase prolactin levels; this includes measuring weight and height, assessing sexual maturation, and monitoring menstrual function.
- TREATMENT CESSATION There is a high risk of relapse if medication is stopped after 1–2 years. Withdrawal of antipsychotic drugs after long-term therapy should always be gradual and closely monitored to avoid the risk of acute withdrawal syndromes or rapid relapse. Patients should be monitored for 2 years after withdrawal of antipsychotic medication for signs and symptoms of relapse.

- PATIENT AND CARER ADVICE
As photosensitisation may occur with higher dosages, patients should avoid direct sunlight.

Driving and skilled tasks
Drowsiness may affect performance of skilled tasks (e.g. driving or operating machinery), especially at start of treatment; effects of alcohol are enhanced.

ANTIPSYCHOTICS › FIRST-GENERATION

📖 352

Chlorpromazine hydrochloride

- INDICATIONS AND DOSE

Schizophrenia and other psychoses | Mania | Short-term adjunctive management of severe anxiety | Psychomotor agitation, excitement, and violent or dangerously impulsive behaviour
▶ BY MOUTH
▶ Adult: Initially 25 mg 3 times a day, adjusted according to response, alternatively initially 75 mg once daily, adjusted according to response, dose to be taken at night; maintenance 75–300 mg daily, increased if necessary up to 1 g daily, this dose may be required in psychoses; use a third to half adult dose in the elderly or debilitated patients
▶ BY RECTUM
▶ Adult: 100 mg every 6–8 hours, dose expressed as chlorpromazine base

Intractable hiccup
▶ BY MOUTH
▶ Adult: 25–50 mg 3–4 times a day

Relief of acute symptoms of psychoses (under expert supervision)
▶ BY DEEP INTRAMUSCULAR INJECTION
▶ Adult: 25–50 mg every 6–8 hours

Nausea and vomiting of terminal illness (where other drugs have failed or are not available)
▶ BY MOUTH
▶ Child 1–5 years: 500 micrograms/kg every 4–6 hours; maximum 40 mg per day
▶ Child 6–11 years: 500 micrograms/kg every 4–6 hours; maximum 75 mg per day
▶ Child 12–17 years: 10–25 mg every 4–6 hours
▶ Adult: 10–25 mg every 4–6 hours
▶ BY DEEP INTRAMUSCULAR INJECTION
▶ Child 1–5 years: 500 micrograms/kg every 6–8 hours; maximum 40 mg per day
▶ Child 6–11 years: 500 micrograms/kg every 6–8 hours; maximum 75 mg per day
▶ Child 12–17 years: Initially 25 mg, then 25–50 mg every 3–4 hours until vomiting stops
▶ Adult: Initially 25 mg, then 25–50 mg every 3–4 hours until vomiting stops
▶ BY RECTUM
▶ Adult: 100 mg every 6–8 hours

DOSE ADJUSTMENTS DUE TO INTERACTIONS
Dose adjustment may be necessary if smoking started or stopped during treatment.

DOSE EQUIVALENCE AND CONVERSION
For equivalent therapeutic effect 100 mg chlorpromazine base given *rectally* as a suppository ≡ 20–25 mg chlorpromazine hydrochloride *by intramuscular injection* ≡ 40–50 mg of chlorpromazine base or hydrochloride given *by mouth*.

- UNLICENSED USE Rectal route is not licensed.
- CONTRA-INDICATIONS CNS depression · comatose states · hypothyroidism · phaeochromocytoma
- CAUTIONS Diabetes

- SIDE-EFFECTS
  SIDE-EFFECTS, FURTHER INFORMATION
  ▸ Acute dystonic reactions Phenothiazines can induce acute dystonic reactions such as facial and skeletal muscle spasms and oculogyric crises; children (especially girls, young women, and those under 10 kg) are particularly susceptible.
- HEPATIC IMPAIRMENT Can precipitate coma; phenothiazines are hepatotoxic.
- RENAL IMPAIRMENT Start with small doses in severe renal impairment because of increased cerebral sensitivity.
- MONITORING REQUIREMENTS
  ▸ With intramuscular use Patients should remain supine, with blood pressure monitoring for 30 minutes after intramuscular injection.
- HANDLING AND STORAGE Owing to the risk of contact sensitisation, pharmacists, nurses, and other health workers should avoid direct contact with chlorpromazine; tablets should not be crushed and solutions should be handled with care.

- MEDICINAL FORMS
  There can be variation in the licensing of different medicines containing the same drug. Forms available from special-order manufacturers include: tablet, capsule, oral suspension, oral solution, suppository
  Tablet
  CAUTIONARY AND ADVISORY LABELS 2, 11
  ▸ Chlorpromazine hydrochloride (Non-proprietary)
  Chlorpromazine hydrochloride 25 mg Chlorpromazine 25mg tablets | 28 tablet [PoM] £4.92 DT price = £1.84
  Chlorpromazine hydrochloride 50 mg Chlorpromazine 50mg tablets | 28 tablet [PoM] £5.28 DT price = £1.73
  Chlorpromazine hydrochloride 100 mg Chlorpromazine 100mg tablets | 28 tablet [PoM] £5.70 DT price = £1.85
  Oral solution
  CAUTIONARY AND ADVISORY LABELS 2, 11
  ▸ Chlorpromazine hydrochloride (Non-proprietary)
  Chlorpromazine hydrochloride 5 mg per 1 ml Chlorpromazine 25mg/5ml syrup | 150 ml [PoM] £2.35 DT price = £2.35
  Chlorpromazine 25mg/5ml oral solution sugar free sugar-free | 150 ml [PoM] £2.35
  Chlorpromazine 25mg/5ml oral solution | 150 ml [PoM] £2.35 DT price = £2.35
  Chlorpromazine hydrochloride 20 mg per 1 ml Chlorpromazine 100mg/5ml oral solution | 150 ml [PoM] £5.50 DT price = £5.50
  Solution for injection
  ▸ Largactil (Sanofi)
  Chlorpromazine hydrochloride 25 mg per 1 ml Largactil 50mg/2ml solution for injection ampoules | 10 ampoule [PoM] £7.51

  ◖ 352 ▸

Flupentixol

(Flupenthixol)

- INDICATIONS AND DOSE

Schizophrenia and other psychoses, particularly with apathy and withdrawal but not mania or psychomotor hyperactivity
▸ BY MOUTH
▸ Adult: Initially 3–9 mg twice daily, adjusted according to response, for debilitated patients, use elderly dose; maximum 18 mg per day
▸ Elderly: Initially 0.75–4.5 mg twice daily, adjusted according to response

Depressive illness
▸ BY MOUTH
▸ Adult: Initially 1 mg once daily, dose to be taken in the morning, increased if necessary to 2 mg after 1 week, doses above 2 mg to be given in divided doses, last dose to be taken before 4 pm; discontinue if no response after 1 week at maximum dosage; maximum 3 mg per day

▸ Elderly: Initially 500 micrograms daily, dose to be taken in the morning, then increased if necessary to 1 mg after 1 week, doses above 1 mg to be given in divided doses, last dose to be taken before 4 pm; discontinue if no response after 1 week at maximum dosage; maximum 1.5 mg per day

- CONTRA-INDICATIONS Circulatory collapse · CNS depression · comatose states · excitable patients · impaired consciousness · overactive patients · phaeochromocytoma
- CAUTIONS Acute porphyrias p. 918 · cardiac disorders · cardiovascular disease · cerebral arteriosclerosis · diabetes · elderly · parkinsonism · QT-interval prolongation · senile confusional states
- INTERACTIONS Avoid concomitant administration of drugs that prolong QT interval.
- SIDE-EFFECTS Asthenia · dyspnoea · hypersalivation · myalgia · sudden death · torsade de pointes
  SIDE-EFFECTS, FURTHER INFORMATION
  Less sedating but extrapyramidal symptoms frequent.
- PREGNANCY Avoid unless potential benefit outweighs risk.
- BREAST FEEDING Present in breast milk—avoid.
- HEPATIC IMPAIRMENT Can precipitate coma. Consider serum-flupentixol concentration monitoring in hepatic impairment.
- RENAL IMPAIRMENT Start with small doses of antipsychotic drugs in severe renal impairment because of increased cerebral sensitivity. Manufacturer advises caution in renal failure.
- PATIENT AND CARER ADVICE Although drowsiness may occur, can also have an alerting effect so should not be taken in the evening.

- MEDICINAL FORMS
  There can be variation in the licensing of different medicines containing the same drug. Forms available from special-order manufacturers include: oral suspension, oral solution
  Tablet
  CAUTIONARY AND ADVISORY LABELS 2
  ▸ Depixol (Flupentixol dihydrochloride) (Lundbeck Ltd)
  Flupentixol (as Flupentixol dihydrochloride) 3 mg Depixol 3mg tablets | 100 tablet [PoM] £13.92 DT price = £13.92
  ▸ Fluanxol (Lundbeck Ltd)
  Flupentixol (as Flupentixol dihydrochloride)
  500 microgram Fluanxol 500microgram tablets | 60 tablet [PoM] £2.88 DT price = £2.88
  Flupentixol (as Flupentixol dihydrochloride) 1 mg Fluanxol 1mg tablets | 60 tablet [PoM] £4.86 DT price = £4.86

  ◖ 352 ▸

Haloperidol

- INDICATIONS AND DOSE

Nausea and vomiting
▸ BY INTRAMUSCULAR INJECTION
▸ Adult: 1–2 mg

Nausea and vomiting in palliative care
▸ BY MOUTH
▸ Adult: Initially 1.5 mg 1–2 times a day, increased if necessary to 5–10 mg daily in divided doses
▸ BY CONTINUOUS SUBCUTANEOUS INFUSION
▸ Adult: 5–15 mg, to be administered over 24 hours
▸ BY SUBCUTANEOUS INFUSION
▸ Adult: 2.5–10 mg/24 hours

Schizophrenia | Psychoses | Mania and hypomania | Organic brain damage (depending on symptoms)
▸ BY MOUTH
▸ Adult: Initially 2–20 mg once daily, alternatively initially 2–20 mg daily in divided doses; maintenance 1–3 mg 3 times a day, adjusted according to response, daily maximum to be given in divided doses, for

debilitated patients, use elderly dose; maximum 20 mg per day
‣ Elderly: Initially 1–10 mg once daily, alternatively initially 1–10 mg daily in divided doses; maintenance 1–3 mg 3 times a day, adjusted according to response, daily maximum to be given in divided doses; maximum 20 mg per day
▸ BY INTRAMUSCULAR INJECTION
‣ Adult: Initially 2–5 mg, repeated if necessary, repeated dose given according to response and tolerability, for debilitated patients, use elderly dose; maximum 12 mg per day
‣ Elderly: Initially 1–2.5 mg, repeated if necessary, repeated dose given according to response and tolerability; maximum 12 mg per day

Agitation and restlessness in the elderly
▸ BY MOUTH
‣ Elderly: Initially 0.75–1.5 mg 2–3 times a day, adjusted according to response, if necessary

Management of mental or behavioural problems such as aggression, hyperactivity and self-mutilation in patients with intellectual disabilities and in patients with organic brain damage (depending on symptoms) | Gilles de la Tourette syndrome | Severe tics | Intractable hiccup | Adjunct to short-term management of moderate to severe psychomotor agitation, excitement and, violent or dangerously impulsive behaviour
▸ BY MOUTH
‣ Adult: Initially 1.5–3 mg 2–3 times a day, alternatively initially 3–5 mg 2–3 times a day, higher dose in severely affected or resistant patients; maintenance 0.5–1 mg 3 times a day, increased if necessary to 2–3 mg 3 times a day, once symptoms are controlled, gradually reduce dose to the lowest effective maintenance dose, for debilitated patients, use elderly dose
‣ Elderly: Initially 0.75–1.5 mg 2–3 times a day, alternatively initially 1.5–2.5 mg 2–3 times a day, higher dose in severely affected or resistant patients; maintenance 0.5–1 mg 3 times a day, increased if necessary to 2–3 mg 3 times a day, once symptoms are controlled, gradually reduce dose to the lowest effective maintenance dose

Restlessness and confusion in palliative care
▸ BY MOUTH
‣ Adult: 2 mg, then 2 mg every 2 hours if required
▸ BY SUBCUTANEOUS INJECTION
‣ Adult: 2.5 mg, then 2.5 mg every 2 hours if required
▸ BY SUBCUTANEOUS INFUSION
‣ Adult: 5–15 mg/24 hours
DOSE ADJUSTMENTS DUE TO INTERACTIONS
Dose adjustment may be necessary if smoking started or stopped during treatment.

● UNLICENSED USE BNF doses for schizophrenia, psychoses, mania, hypomania, and organic brain damage differ from those in product literature.

IMPORTANT SAFETY INFORMATION
When prescribing, dispensing or administering for mental health disorders, check that this injection is the correct preparation—this preparation is usually used in hospital for the rapid control of an *acute episode* and should **not** be confused with depot preparations which are usually used in the community or clinics for *maintenance* treatment.

● CONTRA-INDICATIONS Bradycardia · CNS depression · comatose states · lesions of the basal ganglia · Parkinson's disease · phaeochromocytoma · QT-interval prolongation

● CAUTIONS Arteriosclerosis · hypocalcaemia · hypokalaemia · hypomagnesaemia · metabolic disturbances · subarachnoid haemorrhage · thyrotoxicosis
● INTERACTIONS Avoid concomitant administration of drugs that prolong QT interval.
● SIDE-EFFECTS
▸ Common or very common Depression · weight loss
▸ Uncommon Dyspnoea · oedema
▸ Rare Bronchospasm · hypoglycaemia · inappropriate antidiuretic hormone secretion · photosensitivity reactions · pigmentation
▸ Frequency not known Hypertension · Stevens-Johnson syndrome · sweating · toxic epidermal necrolysis
SIDE-EFFECTS, FURTHER INFORMATION
Less sedating and fewer antimuscarinic or hypotensive symptoms.
● PREGNANCY Avoid unless benefits outweigh risks.
● HEPATIC IMPAIRMENT Can precipitate coma.
● RENAL IMPAIRMENT Start with small doses in severe renal impairment because of increased cerebral sensitivity.
● MONITORING REQUIREMENTS Baseline ECG required before treatment—assess need for further ECGs during treatment on an individual basis.

● MEDICINAL FORMS
There can be variation in the licensing of different medicines containing the same drug. Forms available from special-order manufacturers include: oral suspension, oral solution
Tablet
CAUTIONARY AND ADVISORY LABELS 2
▸ Haloperidol (Non-proprietary)
Haloperidol 500 microgram Haloperidol 500microgram tablets | 28 tablet [PoM] £1.10–£20.05
Haloperidol 1.5 mg Haloperidol 1.5mg tablets | 28 tablet [PoM] £5.99 DT price = £2.12
Haloperidol 5 mg Haloperidol 5mg tablets | 28 tablet [PoM] £3.80 DT price = £3.06
Haloperidol 10 mg Haloperidol 10mg tablets | 28 tablet [PoM] £12.99 DT price = £12.87
Haloperidol 20 mg Haloperidol 20mg tablets | 28 tablet [PoM] £21.97–£22.00 DT price = £21.98
Capsule
CAUTIONARY AND ADVISORY LABELS 2
▸ Serenace (Teva UK Ltd)
Haloperidol 500 microgram Serenace 500microgram capsules | 30 capsule [PoM] £1.18 DT price = £1.18
Oral solution
CAUTIONARY AND ADVISORY LABELS 2
▸ Haloperidol (Non-proprietary)
Haloperidol 1 mg per 1 ml Haloperidol 5mg/5ml oral solution sugar free sugar-free | 100 ml [PoM] £35.99 DT price = £6.45 sugar-free | 500 ml [PoM] £32.20
Haloperidol 2 mg per 1 ml Haloperidol 10mg/5ml oral solution sugar free sugar-free | 100 ml [PoM] £46.75 DT price = £7.10 sugar-free | 500 ml [PoM] £35.50
▸ Haldol (Janssen-Cilag Ltd)
Haloperidol 2 mg per 1 ml Haldol 2mg/ml oral solution sugar-free | 100 ml [PoM] £4.45 DT price = £7.10
Solution for injection
▸ Haloperidol (Non-proprietary)
Haloperidol 5 mg per 1 ml Haloperidol 5mg/1ml solution for injection ampoules | 10 ampoule [PoM] £35.00

⟵ 352

Pericyazine
(Periciazine)

● INDICATIONS AND DOSE
Schizophrenia | Psychoses
▸ BY MOUTH
‣ Adult: Initially 75 mg daily in divided doses, then increased in steps of 25 mg every 1 week, adjusted according to response; maximum 300 mg per day

continued →

4

Nervous system

Nervous system

4

▸ Elderly: Initially 15–30 mg daily in divided doses, then increased in steps of 25 mg every 1 week, adjusted according to response; maximum 300 mg per day

Short-term adjunctive management of severe anxiety, psychomotor agitation, and violent or dangerously impulsive behaviour
▸ BY MOUTH
▸ Adult: Initially 15–30 mg daily in 2 divided doses, adjusted according to response, larger dose to be taken at bedtime
▸ Elderly: Initially 5–10 mg daily in 2 divided doses, adjusted according to response, larger dose to be taken at bedtime

● CONTRA-INDICATIONS CNS depression · comatose states · phaeochromocytoma
● SIDE-EFFECTS
▸ **Common or very common** Hypotension (when treatment initiated)
▸ **Frequency not known** Respiratory depression
SIDE-EFFECTS, FURTHER INFORMATION
More sedating.
● HEPATIC IMPAIRMENT Can precipitate coma; phenothiazines are hepatotoxic.
● RENAL IMPAIRMENT Avoid in renal impairment.

● MEDICINAL FORMS
There can be variation in the licensing of different medicines containing the same drug. Forms available from special-order manufacturers include: oral suspension, oral solution
Tablet
CAUTIONARY AND ADVISORY LABELS 2
▸ Pericyazine (Non-proprietary)
Pericyazine 2.5 mg Pericyazine 2.5mg tablets | 84 tablet PoM £16.95 DT price = £16.23
Pericyazine 10 mg Pericyazine 10mg tablets | 84 tablet PoM £40.94 DT price = £40.47
Oral solution
CAUTIONARY AND ADVISORY LABELS 2
▸ Pericyazine (Non-proprietary)
Pericyazine 2 mg per 1 ml Pericyazine 10mg/5ml oral solution | 100 ml PoM £46.00–£46.01 DT price = £46.01

⧫ 352

Perphenazine

● INDICATIONS AND DOSE
Schizophrenia and other psychoses | Mania | Short-term adjunctive management of anxiety | Severe psychomotor agitation, excitement, and violent or dangerously impulsive behaviour | Severe nausea and vomiting unresponsive to other anti-emetics
▸ BY MOUTH
▸ Adult: Initially 4 mg 3 times a day, adjusted according to response; maximum 24 mg per day
▸ Elderly: Initially 1–2 mg 3 times a day; maximum 12 mg per day

● CONTRA-INDICATIONS Agitation in the elderly · CNS depression · comatose states · phaeochromocytoma · restlessness in the elderly
● CAUTIONS Hypothyroidism
● SIDE-EFFECTS
▸ **Rare** Systemic lupus erythematosus
▸ **Frequency not known** Dystonic reactions
SIDE-EFFECTS, FURTHER INFORMATION
Less sedating.
▸ Acute dystonic reactions Phenothiazines can all induce acute dystonic reactions such as facial and skeletal muscle spasms and oculogyric crises; children (especially girls, young women, and those under 10 kg) are particularly susceptible.

● HEPATIC IMPAIRMENT Can precipitate coma; phenothiazines are hepatotoxic.
● RENAL IMPAIRMENT Start with small doses in severe renal impairment because of increased cerebral sensitivity.

● MEDICINAL FORMS
There can be variation in the licensing of different medicines containing the same drug. Forms available from special-order manufacturers include: tablet, oral suspension

⧫ 352

Pimozide

● INDICATIONS AND DOSE
Schizophrenia
▸ BY MOUTH
▸ Adult: Initially 2 mg daily, adjusted according to response, then increased in steps of 2–4 mg at intervals of not less than 1 week; usual dose 2–20 mg daily
▸ Elderly: Initially 1 mg daily, adjusted according to response, increased in steps of 2–4 mg at intervals of not less than 1 week; usual dose 2–20 mg daily
Monosymptomatic hypochondriacal psychosis | Paranoid psychosis
▸ BY MOUTH
▸ Adult: Initially 4 mg daily, adjusted according to response, then increased in steps of 2–4 mg at intervals of not less than 1 week; maximum 16 mg per day
▸ Elderly: Initially 2 mg daily, adjusted according to response, increased in steps of 2–4 mg at intervals of not less than 1 week; maximum 16 mg per day

● CONTRA-INDICATIONS CNS depression · comatose states · history of arrhythmias · history or family history of congenital QT prolongation · phaeochromocytoma
● SIDE-EFFECTS
▸ **Rare** Hyponatraemia
▸ **Frequency not known** Glycosuria · serious arrhythmias
SIDE-EFFECTS, FURTHER INFORMATION
Less sedating.
● HEPATIC IMPAIRMENT Can precipitate coma.
● RENAL IMPAIRMENT Start with small doses in severe renal impairment because of increased cerebral sensitivity.
● MONITORING REQUIREMENTS
▸ ECG monitoring Following reports of sudden unexplained death, an ECG is recommended before treatment. It is also recommended that patients taking pimozide should have an annual ECG (if the QT interval is prolonged, treatment should be reviewed and either withdrawn or dose reduced under close supervision) and that pimozide should not be given with other antipsychotic drugs (including depot preparations), tricyclic antidepressants or other drugs which prolong the QT interval, such as certain antimalarials, antiarrhythmic drugs and certain antihistamines and should not be given with drugs which cause electrolyte disturbances (especially diuretics).

● MEDICINAL FORMS
There can be variation in the licensing of different medicines containing the same drug. Forms available from special-order manufacturers include: oral suspension
Tablet
CAUTIONARY AND ADVISORY LABELS 2
▸ Pimozide (Non-proprietary)
Pimozide 1 mg Orap 1mg tablets | 100 tablet PoM no price available
Pimozide 4 mg Pimozide 4mg tablets | 100 tablet PoM no price available
▸ Orap (Eumedica Pharmaceuticals)
Pimozide 4 mg Orap 4mg tablets | 100 tablet PoM £40.31

Nervous system

4

Prochlorperazine

● **INDICATIONS AND DOSE**

Schizophrenia and other psychoses | Mania
▶ BY MOUTH
▶ Adult: 12.5 mg twice daily for 7 days, dose to be adjusted at intervals of 4–7 days according to response; usual dose 75–100 mg daily
▶ BY DEEP INTRAMUSCULAR INJECTION
▶ Adult: 12.5–25 mg 2–3 times a day

Short-term adjunctive management of severe anxiety
▶ BY MOUTH
▶ Adult: 15–20 mg daily in divided doses; maximum 40 mg per day

Nausea and vomiting, acute attack
▶ BY MOUTH
▶ Adult: Initially 20 mg, then 10 mg after 2 hours
▶ BY DEEP INTRAMUSCULAR INJECTION
▶ Adult: 12.5 mg as required, to be followed if necessary after 6 hours by an oral dose

Nausea and vomiting, prevention
▶ BY MOUTH
▶ Adult: 5–10 mg 2–3 times a day
▶ BY DEEP INTRAMUSCULAR INJECTION
▶ Adult: 12.5 mg as required, to be followed if necessary after 6 hours by an oral dose

Prevention and treatment of nausea and vomiting
▶ BY MOUTH
▶ Child 1–11 years (body-weight 10 kg and above): 250 micrograms/kg 2–3 times a day
▶ Child 12–17 years: 5–10 mg up to 3 times a day if required
▶ BY INTRAMUSCULAR INJECTION
▶ Child 2–4 years: 1.25–2.5 mg up to 3 times a day if required
▶ Child 5–11 years: 5–6.25 mg up to 3 times a day if required
▶ Child 12–17 years: 12.5 mg up to 3 times a day if required

Labyrinthine disorders
▶ BY MOUTH
▶ Adult: 5 mg 3 times a day, increased if necessary to 30 mg daily in divided doses, dose to be increased gradually, then reduced to 5–10 mg daily, dose is reduced after several weeks

Nausea and vomiting in previously diagnosed migraine
▶ BY MOUTH USING BUCCAL TABLET
▶ Child 12–17 years: 3–6 mg twice daily, tablets to be placed high between upper lip and gum and left to dissolve
▶ Adult: 3–6 mg twice daily, tablets to be placed high between upper lip and gum and left to dissolve

DOSE EQUIVALENCE AND CONVERSION
Doses are expressed as prochlorperazine maleate or mesilate; 1 mg prochlorperazine maleate ≡ 1 mg prochlorperazine mesilate.

● **UNLICENSED USE**
▶ With intramuscular use in children Injection not licensed for use in children.
▶ With buccal use in children Buccal tablets not licensed for use in children.

● **CONTRA-INDICATIONS** Avoid oral route in child under 10 kg · children (in psychotic disorders) · CNS depression · comatose states · phaeochromocytoma

● **CAUTIONS** Elderly (in adults) · hypotension (more likely after intramuscular injection)

● **SIDE-EFFECTS** Dystonic reactions · respiratory depression may occur in susceptible patients

SIDE-EFFECTS, FURTHER INFORMATION
▶ Acute dystonic reactions Phenothiazines can all induce acute dystonic reactions such as facial and skeletal muscle spasms and oculogyric crises; children (especially girls, young women, and those under 10 kg) are particularly susceptible.

● **HEPATIC IMPAIRMENT** Can precipitate coma; phenothiazines are hepatotoxic.

● **RENAL IMPAIRMENT** Start with small doses in severe renal impairment because of increased cerebral sensitivity.

● **DIRECTIONS FOR ADMINISTRATION**
▶ With buccal use Buccal tablets are placed high between upper lip and gum and left to dissolve.

● **PATIENT AND CARER ADVICE**
▶ With buccal use Patients or carers should be given advice on how to administer prochlorperazine buccal tablets.

● **MEDICINAL FORMS**
There can be variation in the licensing of different medicines containing the same drug.

Tablet
CAUTIONARY AND ADVISORY LABELS 2
▶ Prochlorperazine (Non-proprietary)
  Prochlorperazine maleate 5 mg Prochlorperazine 5mg tablets | 28 tablet [PoM] £2.75 DT price = £0.93 | 84 tablet [PoM] £5.95
▶ Stemetil (Sanofi)
  Prochlorperazine maleate 5 mg Stemetil 5mg tablets | 28 tablet [PoM] £1.98 DT price = £0.93 | 84 tablet [PoM] £5.94

Buccal tablet
CAUTIONARY AND ADVISORY LABELS 2
▶ Prochlorperazine (Non-proprietary)
  Prochlorperazine maleate 3 mg Prochlorperazine 3mg buccal tablets | 50 tablet [PoM] £35.94–£43.13 DT price = £41.68
▶ Buccastem (Alliance Pharmaceuticals Ltd)
  Prochlorperazine maleate 3 mg Buccastem M 3mg tablets | 8 tablet [P] £3.66

Oral solution
CAUTIONARY AND ADVISORY LABELS 2
▶ Stemetil (Sanofi)
  Prochlorperazine mesilate 1 mg per 1 ml Stemetil 5mg/5ml syrup | 100 ml [PoM] £3.34 DT price = £3.34

Solution for injection
▶ Prochlorperazine (Non-proprietary)
  Prochlorperazine mesilate 12.5 mg per 1 ml Prochlorperazine 12.5mg/1ml solution for injection ampoules | 10 ampoule [PoM] no price available DT price = £5.23
▶ Stemetil (Sanofi)
  Prochlorperazine mesilate 12.5 mg per 1 ml Stemetil 12.5mg/1ml solution for injection ampoules | 10 ampoule [PoM] £5.23 DT price = £5.23

Sulpiride

● **INDICATIONS AND DOSE**

Schizophrenia with predominantly negative symptoms
▶ BY MOUTH
▶ Adult: 200–400 mg twice daily; maximum 800 mg per day
▶ Elderly: Lower initial dose to be given, increased gradually according to response

Schizophrenia with mainly positive symptoms
▶ BY MOUTH
▶ Adult: 200–400 mg twice daily; maximum 2.4 g per day
▶ Elderly: Lower initial dose to be given, increased gradually according to response

● **CONTRA-INDICATIONS** CNS depression · comatose states · phaeochromocytoma

● **CAUTIONS** Aggressive patients (even low doses may aggravate symptoms) · agitated patients (even low doses may aggravate symptoms) · excited patients (even low doses may aggravate symptoms)

● **SIDE-EFFECTS** Hepatitis

- HEPATIC IMPAIRMENT Can precipitate coma.
- RENAL IMPAIRMENT Start with small doses in severe renal impairment because of increased cerebral sensitivity.
- MONITORING REQUIREMENTS Sulpiride does not affect blood pressure to the same extent as other antipsychotic drugs and so blood pressure monitoring is not mandatory for this drug.
- PRESCRIBING AND DISPENSING INFORMATION Flavours of oral liquid formulations may include lemon and aniseed.

- MEDICINAL FORMS
There can be variation in the licensing of different medicines containing the same drug. Forms available from special-order manufacturers include: oral suspension, oral solution

Tablet
CAUTIONARY AND ADVISORY LABELS 2
▸ Sulpiride (Non-proprietary)
Sulpiride 200 mg Sulpiride 200mg tablets | 30 tablet [PoM] £7.84 DT price = £3.96
Sulpiride 400 mg Sulpiride 400mg tablets | 30 tablet [PoM] £18.80 DT price = £18.80
▸ Dolmatil (Sanofi)
Sulpiride 200 mg Dolmatil 200mg tablets | 100 tablet [PoM] £6.00
Sulpiride 400 mg Dolmatil 400mg tablets | 100 tablet [PoM] £19.00

Oral solution
CAUTIONARY AND ADVISORY LABELS 2
▸ Sulpiride (Non-proprietary)
Sulpiride 40 mg per 1 ml Sulpiride 200mg/5ml oral solution sugar free sugar-free | 150 ml [PoM] £27.00 DT price = £25.38
▸ Sulpor (Rosemont Pharmaceuticals Ltd)
Sulpiride 40 mg per 1 ml Sulpor 200mg/5ml oral solution sugar-free | 150 ml [PoM] £25.38 DT price = £25.38

⌐ 352

Trifluoperazine

- **INDICATIONS AND DOSE**

Schizophrenia and other psychoses | Short-term adjunctive management of psychomotor agitation, excitement, and violent or dangerously impulsive behaviour
▸ BY MOUTH
▸ Adult: Initially 5 mg twice daily, increased by 5 mg daily after 1 week, then at intervals of 3 days, according to response
▸ Elderly: Initially up to 2.5 mg twice daily, increased by 5 mg daily after 1 week, then at intervals of 3 days, according to response

Short-term adjunctive management of severe anxiety
▸ BY MOUTH
▸ Adult: 2–4 mg daily in divided doses, increased if necessary to 6 mg daily
▸ Elderly: Up to 2 mg daily in divided doses, increased if necessary to 6 mg daily

Severe nausea and vomiting
▸ BY MOUTH
▸ Adult: 2–4 mg daily in divided doses; maximum 6 mg per day

- CONTRA-INDICATIONS CNS depression · comatose states · phaeochromocytoma
- SIDE-EFFECTS Anorexia · dystonic reactions · muscle weakness
  SIDE-EFFECTS, FURTHER INFORMATION
  Extrapyramidal symptoms are more frequent, especially at doses exceeding 6 mg daily.
  Phenothiazines can all induce acute dystonic reactions such as facial and skeletal muscle spasms and oculogyric crises.
- HEPATIC IMPAIRMENT Can precipitate coma; phenothiazines are hepatotoxic.

- RENAL IMPAIRMENT Start with small doses in severe renal impairment because of increased cerebral sensitivity.
- MONITORING REQUIREMENTS Trifluoperazine does not affect blood pressure to the same extent as other antipsychotic drugs and so blood pressure monitoring is not mandatory for this drug.

- MEDICINAL FORMS
There can be variation in the licensing of different medicines containing the same drug.

Tablet
CAUTIONARY AND ADVISORY LABELS 2
▸ Trifluoperazine (Non-proprietary)
Trifluoperazine (as Trifluoperazine hydrochloride) 1 mg Stelazine 1mg tablets | 50 tablet [PoM] no price available
Trifluoperazine 1mg tablets | 112 tablet [PoM] £54.00 DT price = £54.00
Trifluoperazine (as Trifluoperazine hydrochloride) 5 mg Stelazine 5mg tablets | 50 tablet [PoM] no price available
Trifluoperazine 5mg tablets | 112 tablet [PoM] £123.20 DT price = £123.20

Oral solution
CAUTIONARY AND ADVISORY LABELS 2
▸ Trifluoperazine (Non-proprietary)
Trifluoperazine (as Trifluoperazine hydrochloride) 200 microgram per 1 ml Trifluoperazine 1mg/5ml oral solution sugar free sugar-free | 200 ml [PoM] £102.53 DT price = £102.53
Trifluoperazine (as Trifluoperazine hydrochloride) 1 mg per 1 ml Trifluoperazine 5mg/5ml oral solution sugar free sugar-free | 150 ml [PoM] £25.50 DT price = £25.50

⌐ 352

Zuclopenthixol

- **INDICATIONS AND DOSE**

Schizophrenia and other psychoses
▸ BY MOUTH
▸ Adult: Initially 20–30 mg daily in divided doses, increased if necessary up to 150 mg daily; usual maintenance 20–50 mg daily (max. per dose 40 mg), for debilitated patients, use elderly dose
▸ Elderly: Initially 5–15 mg daily in divided doses, increased if necessary up to 150 mg daily; usual maintenance 20–50 mg daily (max. per dose 40 mg)

- CONTRA-INDICATIONS Apathetic states · CNS depression · comatose states · phaeochromocytoma · withdrawn states
- CAUTIONS Avoid in Acute porphyrias p. 918
- SIDE-EFFECTS Urinary frequency · urinary incontinence · weight loss (less common than weight gain)
- HEPATIC IMPAIRMENT Halve dose. Can precipitate coma. Consider serum-level monitoring in patients with hepatic impairment.
- RENAL IMPAIRMENT Halve dose in renal failure; smaller starting doses used in severe renal impairment because of increased cerebral sensitivity.

- MEDICINAL FORMS
There can be variation in the licensing of different medicines containing the same drug.

Tablet
CAUTIONARY AND ADVISORY LABELS 2
▸ Clopixol (Zuclopenthixol) (Lundbeck Ltd)
Zuclopenthixol (as Zuclopenthixol dihydrochloride) 2 mg Clopixol 2mg tablets | 100 tablet [PoM] £3.14 DT price = £3.14
Zuclopenthixol (as Zuclopenthixol dihydrochloride) 10 mg Clopixol 10mg tablets | 100 tablet [PoM] £8.06 DT price = £8.06
Zuclopenthixol (as Zuclopenthixol dihydrochloride) 25 mg Clopixol 25mg tablets | 100 tablet [PoM] £16.13 DT price = £16.13

Drops
▸ Zuclopenthixol (Non-proprietary)
Zuclopenthixol (as Zuclopenthixol dihydrochloride) 20 mg per 1 ml Ciatyl-Z 20mg/ml oral drops | 30 ml [PoM] no price available

Zuclopenthixol acetate

▶ 352

● INDICATIONS AND DOSE

Short-term management of acute psychosis | Short-term management of mania | Short-term management of exacerbation of chronic psychosis

▶ BY DEEP INTRAMUSCULAR INJECTION

▸ Adult: 50−150 mg, then 50−150 mg after 2−3 days if required, (1 additional dose may be needed 1−2 days after the first injection); maximum cumulative dose 400 mg in 2 weeks and maximum 4 injections; maximum duration of treatment 2 weeks—if maintenance treatment necessary change to an oral antipsychotic 2−3 days after last injection, or to a longer acting antipsychotic depot injection given concomitantly with last injection of zuclopenthixol acetate; to be administered into the gluteal muscle or lateral thigh

▸ Elderly: 50−100 mg, then 50−100 mg after 2−3 days if required, (1 additional dose may be needed 1−2 days after the first injection); maximum cumulative dose 400 mg in 2 weeks and maximum 4 injections; maximum duration of treatment 2 weeks—if maintenance treatment necessary change to an oral antipsychotic 2−3 days after last injection, or to a longer acting antipsychotic depot injection given concomitantly with last injection of zuclopenthixol acetate; to be administered into the gluteal muscle or lateral thigh

> **IMPORTANT SAFETY INFORMATION**
> When prescribing, dispensing, or administering, check that this is the correct preparation—this preparation is usually used in hospital for an *acute episode* and should **not** be confused with depot preparations which are usually used in the community or clinics for *maintenance* treatment.

● CONTRA-INDICATIONS CNS depression · comatose states · phaeochromocytoma

● CAUTIONS Avoid in Acute porphyrias p. 918

● HEPATIC IMPAIRMENT Can precipitate coma.

● RENAL IMPAIRMENT Start with small doses in severe renal impairment because of increased cerebral sensitivity.

● MEDICINAL FORMS
There can be variation in the licensing of different medicines containing the same drug.
Solution for injection
▸ Clopixol Acuphase (Lundbeck Ltd)
Zuclopenthixol acetate 50 mg per 1 ml Clopixol Acuphase 50mg/1ml solution for injection ampoules | 5 ampoule [PoM] £24.21
DT price = £24.21

ANTIPSYCHOTICS > FIRST-GENERATION (DEPOT INJECTIONS)

▶ 352

Flupentixol decanoate

(Flupenthixol Decanoate)

● INDICATIONS AND DOSE

Maintenance in schizophrenia and other psychoses

▶ BY DEEP INTRAMUSCULAR INJECTION

▸ Adult: Test dose 20 mg, dose to be injected into the upper outer buttock or lateral thigh, then 20−40 mg after at least 7 days, then 20−40 mg every 2−4 weeks, adjusted according to response, usual maintenance dose 50 mg every 4 weeks to 300 mg every 2 weeks; maximum 400 mg per week

▸ Elderly: Dose is initially quarter to half adult dose

● CONTRA-INDICATIONS Children · CNS depression · comatose states · excitable patients · overactive patients · phaeochromocytoma

● CAUTIONS An alternative antipsychotic may be necessary if symptoms such as aggression or agitation appear · avoid in Acute porphyrias p. 918 · diabetes · when transferring from oral to depot therapy, the dose by mouth should be reduced gradually

● SIDE-EFFECTS Erythema · hyperglycaemia · mood elevating effect · nodules · pain at injection site · swelling

SIDE-EFFECTS, FURTHER INFORMATION
If the dose needs to be reduced to alleviate side-effects, it is important to recognise that the plasma-drug concentration may not fall for some time after reducing the dose, therefore it may be a month or longer before side-effects subside.
    Less sedating but extrapyramidal symptoms frequent.

● HEPATIC IMPAIRMENT Can precipitate coma.

● RENAL IMPAIRMENT Start with small doses in severe renal impairment because of increased cerebral sensitivity.

● MONITORING REQUIREMENTS Treatment requires careful monitoring for optimum effect.

● DIRECTIONS FOR ADMINISTRATION In general not more than 2−3mL of oily injection should be administered at any one site. Correct injection technique (including use of z-track technique) and rotation of injection sites are essential. When initiating therapy with sustained-release preparations of conventional antipsychotics, patients should first be given a small test-dose as undesirable side-effects are prolonged.

● MEDICINAL FORMS
There can be variation in the licensing of different medicines containing the same drug.
Solution for injection
▸ Flupentixol decanoate (Non-proprietary)
Flupentixol decanoate 100 mg per 1 ml Flupentixol 100mg/1ml solution for injection ampoules | 10 ampoule [PoM] no price available
Flupentixol decanoate 200 mg per 1 ml Flupentixol 200mg/1ml solution for injection ampoules | 5 ampoule [PoM] no price available
▸ Depixol (Flupentixol decanoate) (Lundbeck Ltd)
Flupentixol decanoate 20 mg per 1 ml Depixol 40mg/2ml solution for injection ampoules | 10 ampoule [PoM] £25.39
Depixol 20mg/1ml solution for injection ampoules | 10 ampoule [PoM] £15.17
Flupentixol decanoate 100 mg per 1 ml Depixol Conc 100mg/1ml solution for injection ampoules | 10 ampoule [PoM] £62.51
Flupentixol decanoate 200 mg per 1 ml Depixol Low Volume 200mg/1ml solution for injection ampoules | 5 ampoule [PoM] £97.59
▸ Psytixol (Mylan Ltd)
Flupentixol decanoate 20 mg per 1 ml Psytixol 40mg/2ml solution for injection ampoules | 10 ampoule [PoM] £25.38
Psytixol 20mg/1ml solution for injection ampoules | 10 ampoule [PoM] £15.16
Flupentixol decanoate 100 mg per 1 ml Psytixol 50mg/0.5ml solution for injection ampoules | 10 ampoule [PoM] £34.12
Psytixol 100mg/1ml solution for injection ampoules | 10 ampoule [PoM] £62.50
Flupentixol decanoate 200 mg per 1 ml Psytixol 200mg/1ml solution for injection ampoules | 5 ampoule [PoM] £97.58

▶ 352

Fluphenazine decanoate

● INDICATIONS AND DOSE

Maintenance in schizophrenia and other psychoses

▶ BY DEEP INTRAMUSCULAR INJECTION

▸ Adult: Test dose 12.5 mg, dose to be administered into the gluteal muscle, then 12.5−100 mg after 4−7 days, then 12.5−100 mg every 14−35 days, adjusted according to response continued →

▸ **Elderly:** Test dose 6.25 mg, dose to be administered into the gluteal muscle, then 12.5–100 mg after 4–7 days, then 12.5–100 mg every 14–35 days, adjusted according to response

DOSE ADJUSTMENTS DUE TO INTERACTIONS
Dose adjustment may be necessary if smoking started or stopped during treatment.

● **CONTRA-INDICATIONS** Children · CNS depression · comatose states · marked cerebral atherosclerosis · phaeochromocytoma

● **CAUTIONS** QT-interval prolongation · when transferring from oral to depot therapy, the dose by mouth should be reduced gradually

● **INTERACTIONS** Avoid concomitant drugs that prolong QT interval.

● **SIDE-EFFECTS** Erythema · inappropriate antidiuretic hormone secretion · nodules · oedema · pain at injection site · swelling · systemic lupus erythematosus
SIDE-EFFECTS, FURTHER INFORMATION
Less sedating and fewer antimuscarinic or hypotensive symptoms, but extrapyramidal symptoms, particularly dystonic reactions and akathisia, more frequent. Extrapyramidal symptoms usually appear a few hours after injection and continue for about 2 days but may be delayed.
    If the dose needs to be reduced to alleviate side-effects, it is important to recognise that the plasma-drug concentration may not fall for some time after reducing the dose, therefore it may be a month or longer before side-effects subside.

● **HEPATIC IMPAIRMENT** Avoid in hepatic failure. Can precipitate coma; phenothiazines are hepatotoxic.

● **RENAL IMPAIRMENT** Start with small doses of antipsychotic drugs in severe renal impairment because of increased cerebral sensitivity. Manufacturer advises caution. Avoid in renal failure.

● **MONITORING REQUIREMENTS** Treatment requires careful monitoring for optimum effect.

● **DIRECTIONS FOR ADMINISTRATION** In general not more than 2–3 mL of oily injection should be administered at any one site. Correct injection technique (including use of z-track technique) and rotation of injection sites are essential. When initiating therapy with sustained-release preparations of conventional antipsychotics, patients should first be given a small test-dose as undesirable side-effects are prolonged.

● **MEDICINAL FORMS**
There can be variation in the licensing of different medicines containing the same drug.
Solution for injection
EXCIPIENTS: May contain Sesame oil
▸ Modecate (Sanofi)
   Fluphenazine decanoate 25 mg per 1 ml Modecate 50mg/2ml solution for injection ampoules | 5 ampoule [PoM] £22.22
   Modecate 25mg/1ml solution for injection ampoules | 10 ampoule [PoM] £22.55 DT price = £22.55
   Modecate 12.5mg/0.5ml solution for injection ampoules | 5 ampoule [PoM] £6.51
   Fluphenazine decanoate 100 mg per 1 ml Modecate Concentrate 100mg/1ml solution for injection ampoules | 5 ampoule [PoM] £43.73 DT price = £43.73
   Modecate Concentrate 50mg/0.5ml solution for injection ampoules | 10 ampoule [PoM] £44.73

Haloperidol decanoate

● **INDICATIONS AND DOSE**
Maintenance in schizophrenia and other psychoses
▸ BY DEEP INTRAMUSCULAR INJECTION
▸ **Adult:** Initially 50 mg every 4 weeks, increased in steps of 50 mg if required, increased if necessary up to 300 mg every 4 weeks, higher doses may be needed in some patients, dose to be administered into gluteal muscle, if 2-weekly administration preferred, doses should be halved
▸ **Elderly:** Initially 12.5–25 mg every 4 weeks, if 2-weekly administration preferred, doses should be halved

DOSE ADJUSTMENTS DUE TO INTERACTIONS
Dose adjustment may be necessary if smoking started or stopped during treatment.

IMPORTANT SAFETY INFORMATION
When prescribing, dispensing or administering, check that this is the correct preparation—this preparation is used for *maintenance* treatment and should **not** be used for the rapid control of an *acute episode*.

● **CONTRA-INDICATIONS** Bradycardia · children · CNS depression · comatose states · lesions of the basal ganglia · Parkinson's disease · phaeochromocytoma · QT-interval prolongation

● **CAUTIONS** Arteriosclerosis · hypocalcaemia · hypokalaemia · hypomagnesaemia · metabolic disturbances · subarachnoid haemorrhage · thyrotoxicosis · when transferring from oral to depot therapy, the dose by mouth should be reduced gradually

● **INTERACTIONS** Avoid concomitant administration of drugs that prolong QT interval.

● **SIDE-EFFECTS**
▸ **Common or very common** Depression · weight loss
▸ **Uncommon** Dyspnoea · oedema
▸ **Rare** Bronchospasm · hypoglycaemia · inappropriate antidiuretic hormone secretion · photosensitivity reactions · pigmentation
▸ **Frequency not known** Erythema · hypertension · nodules · pain may occur at injection site · Stevens-Johnson syndrome · sweating · swelling · toxic epidermal necrolysis
SIDE-EFFECTS, FURTHER INFORMATION
Less sedating and fewer antimuscarinic or hypotensive symptoms.

● **PREGNANCY** Avoid unless benefits outweigh risk.

● **HEPATIC IMPAIRMENT** Can precipitate coma.

● **RENAL IMPAIRMENT** Start with small doses in severe renal impairment because of increased cerebral sensitivity.

● **MONITORING REQUIREMENTS**
▸ Treatment requires careful monitoring for optimum effect.
▸ Baseline ECG required before treatment—assess need for further ECGs during treatment on an individual basis.

● **DIRECTIONS FOR ADMINISTRATION** In general not more than 2–3 mL of oily injection should be administered at any one site. Correct injection technique (including use of z-track technique) and rotation of injection sites are essential. When initiating therapy with sustained-release preparations of conventional antipsychotics, patients should first be given a small test-dose as undesirable side-effects are prolonged.

● MEDICINAL FORMS
There can be variation in the licensing of different medicines containing the same drug.

Solution for injection
EXCIPIENTS: May contain Benzyl alcohol, sesame oil
▸ Haldol decanoate (Janssen-Cilag Ltd)
Haloperidol (as Haloperidol decanoate) 50 mg per 1 ml Haldol decanoate 50mg/1ml solution for injection ampoules | 5 ampoule PoM £19.06
Haloperidol (as Haloperidol decanoate) 100 mg per 1 ml Haldol decanoate 100mg/1ml solution for injection ampoules | 5 ampoule PoM £25.26

▶ 352

Zuclopenthixol decanoate

● INDICATIONS AND DOSE
Maintenance in schizophrenia and paranoid psychoses
▸ BY DEEP INTRAMUSCULAR INJECTION
▸ Adult: Test dose 100 mg, dose to be administered into the upper outer buttock or lateral thigh, followed by 200–500 mg after at least 7 days, then 200–500 mg every 1–4 weeks, adjusted according to response, higher doses of more than 500mg can be used; do not exceed 600 mg weekly
▸ Elderly: A quarter to half usual starting dose to be used

IMPORTANT SAFETY INFORMATION
When prescribing, dispensing, or administering, check that this is the correct preparation—this preparation is used for *maintenance* treatment and should **not** be used for the short-term management of an *acute episode*.

● CONTRA-INDICATIONS Children · CNS depression · comatose states · phaeochromocytoma
● CAUTIONS Avoid in Acute porphyrias p. 918 · QT interval prolongation · when transferring from oral to depot therapy, the dose by mouth should be reduced gradually
● INTERACTIONS Avoid concomitant use of drugs that prolong QT interval.
● SIDE-EFFECTS Erythema · nodules · pain at injection site · swelling
SIDE-EFFECTS, FURTHER INFORMATION
If the dose needs to be reduced to alleviate side-effects, it is important to recognise that the plasma-drug concentration may not fall for some time after reducing the dose, therefore it may be a month or longer before side-effects subside.
● HEPATIC IMPAIRMENT Can precipitate coma.
● RENAL IMPAIRMENT Start with small doses in severe renal impairment because of increased cerebral sensitivity.
● MONITORING REQUIREMENTS Treatment requires careful monitoring for optimum effect.
● DIRECTIONS FOR ADMINISTRATION In general not more than 2–3 mL of oily injection should be administered at any one site. Correct injection technique (including use of z-track technique) and rotation of injection sites are essential. When initiating therapy with sustained-release preparations of conventional antipsychotics, patients should first be given a small test-dose as undesirable side-effects are prolonged.

● MEDICINAL FORMS
There can be variation in the licensing of different medicines containing the same drug.

Solution for injection
▸ Clopixol (Zuclopenthixol decanoate) (Lundbeck Ltd)
Zuclopenthixol decanoate 200 mg per 1 ml Clopixol 200mg/1ml solution for injection ampoules | 10 ampoule PoM £31.51 DT price = £31.51

Zuclopenthixol decanoate 500 mg per 1 ml Clopixol Conc 500mg/1ml solution for injection ampoules | 5 ampoule PoM £37.18 DT price = £37.18

ANTIPSYCHOTICS ⟩ SECOND-GENERATION

▶ 352

Amisulpride

● DRUG ACTION Amisulpride is a selective dopamine receptor antagonist with high affinity for mesolimbic D_2 and D_3 receptors.

● INDICATIONS AND DOSE
Acute psychotic episode in schizophrenia
▸ BY MOUTH
▸ Adult: 400–800 mg daily in 2 divided doses, adjusted according to response; maximum 1.2 g per day
Schizophrenia with predominantly negative symptoms
▸ BY MOUTH
▸ Adult: 50–300 mg daily

● CONTRA-INDICATIONS CNS depression · comatose states · phaeochromocytoma · prolactin-dependent tumours
● SIDE-EFFECTS
▸ **Common or very common** Anxiety
▸ **Uncommon** Bradycardia
● PREGNANCY Avoid.
● BREAST FEEDING Avoid—no information available.
● RENAL IMPAIRMENT Halve dose if eGFR 30–60 mL/minute/1.73 m². Use one-third dose if eGFR 10–30 mL/minute/1.73 m². No information available if eGFR less than 10 mL/minute/1.73 m².
● MONITORING REQUIREMENTS Amisulpride does not affect blood pressure to the same extent as other antipsychotic drugs and so blood pressure monitoring is not mandatory for this drug.
● PRESCRIBING AND DISPENSING INFORMATION Flavours of oral liquid formulations may include caramel.

● MEDICINAL FORMS
There can be variation in the licensing of different medicines containing the same drug. Forms available from special-order manufacturers include: oral suspension, oral solution

Tablet
CAUTIONARY AND ADVISORY LABELS 2
▸ Amisulpride (Non-proprietary)
Amisulpride 50 mg Amisulpride 50mg tablets | 60 tablet PoM £27.00 DT price = £2.73
Amisulpride 100 mg Amisulpride 100mg tablets | 60 tablet PoM £51.27 DT price = £4.08
Amisulpride 200 mg Amisulpride 200mg tablets | 60 tablet PoM £66.00 DT price = £7.22
Amisulpride 400 mg Amisulpride 400mg tablets | 60 tablet PoM £132.00 DT price = £35.20
▸ Solian (Sanofi)
Amisulpride 50 mg Solian 50 tablets | 60 tablet PoM £22.76 DT price = £2.73
Amisulpride 100 mg Solian 100 tablets | 60 tablet PoM £35.29 DT price = £4.08
Amisulpride 200 mg Solian 200 tablets | 60 tablet PoM £58.99 DT price = £7.22
Amisulpride 400 mg Solian 400 tablets | 60 tablet PoM £117.97 DT price = £35.20

Oral solution
CAUTIONARY AND ADVISORY LABELS 2
▸ Amisulpride (Non-proprietary)
Amisulpride 100 mg per 1 ml Amisulpride 100mg/ml oral solution sugar free sugar-free | 60 ml PoM £36.00 DT price = £35.68
▸ Solian (Sanofi)
Amisulpride 100 mg per 1 ml Solian 100mg/ml oral solution sugar-free | 60 ml PoM £33.76 DT price = £35.68

4

Nervous system

Aripiprazole

- **DRUG ACTION** Aripiprazole is a dopamine D_2 partial agonist with weak $5\text{-}HT_{1a}$ partial agonism and $5\text{-}HT_{2A}$ receptor antagonism.

● INDICATIONS AND DOSE

Maintenance in schizophrenia in patients stabilised with oral aripiprazole
- ▶ INITIALLY BY INTRAMUSCULAR INJECTION
- ▶ Adult: 400 mg every 1 month, to be injected into the gluteal muscle, minimum of 26 days between injections, for dose adjustment due to side effects or concomitant use of interacting drugs, consult product literature and (by mouth) 10–20 mg daily continued for 14 consecutive days after the first injection, for missed depot doses consult product literature

Schizophrenia
- ▶ BY MOUTH
- ▶ Adult: 10–15 mg once daily; usual dose 15 mg once daily (max. per dose 30 mg once daily), for dose adjustments due to concomitant use of interacting drugs—consult product literature

Treatment and recurrence prevention of mania
- ▶ BY MOUTH
- ▶ Adult: 15 mg once daily, increased if necessary up to 30 mg once daily, for dose adjustments due to concomitant use of interacting drugs—consult product literature

Control of agitation and disturbed behaviour in schizophrenia
- ▶ BY INTRAMUSCULAR INJECTION
- ▶ Adult: Initially 5.25–15 mg for 1 dose, alternatively usual dose 9.75 mg for 1 dose, followed by 5.25–15 mg after 2 hours if required, maximum 3 injections daily; maximum daily combined oral and parenteral dose 30 mg, for dose adjustments due to concomitant use of interacting drugs—consult product literature

> **IMPORTANT SAFETY INFORMATION**
> When prescribing, dispensing, or administering, check that the correct preparation is used—the preparation usually used in hospital for the rapid control of an *acute episode* (solution for injection containing aripiprazole 7.5 mg/mL) should **not** be confused with depot preparations (aripiprazole 400-mg vial with solvent), which are usually used in the community or clinics for *maintenance treatment*.

- **CONTRA-INDICATIONS** CNS depression · comatose state · phaeochromocytoma
- **CAUTIONS**
  GENERAL CAUTIONS
  Cerebrovascular disease · elderly (reduce initial dose)
  SPECIFIC CAUTIONS
  - ▶ With intramuscular use When transferring from oral to depot therapy, the dose by mouth should be reduced gradually
- **SIDE-EFFECTS**
  GENERAL SIDE-EFFECTS
  - ▶ **Common or very common** Anxiety · hypersalivation · malaise
  - ▶ **Uncommon** Depression · dry mouth
  - ▶ **Frequency not known** Alopecia · anorexia · bradycardia · hepatitis · hyponatraemia · infection · laryngospasm · myalgia · oedema · oropharyngeal spasm · pancreatitis · pathological gambling · respiratory disorders · rhabdomyolysis · suicidal ideation · sweating · urinary disorders

SPECIFIC SIDE-EFFECTS
- ▶ With intramuscular use Erythema · nodules · pain at injection site · swelling
SIDE-EFFECTS, FURTHER INFORMATION
- ▶ With intramuscular use If the dose needs to be reduced to alleviate side-effects, it is important to recognise that the plasma-drug concentration may not fall for some time after reducing the dose of the *depot injection*, therefore it may be a month or longer before side-effects subside.
- **PREGNANCY** Use only if potential benefit outweighs risk.
- **BREAST FEEDING** Manufacturer advises avoid—present in milk.
- **HEPATIC IMPAIRMENT** Use with caution in severe impairment (oral treatment preferred to intramuscular administration).
- **MONITORING REQUIREMENTS**
  - ▶ Aripiprazole does not affect blood pressure to the same extent as other antipsychotic drugs and so blood pressure monitoring is not mandatory for this drug.
  - ▶ With intramuscular use Treatment requires careful monitoring for optimum effect.
- **DIRECTIONS FOR ADMINISTRATION**
  - ▶ With oral use Orodispersible tablets should be placed on the tongue and allowed to dissolve, or be dispersed in water and swallowed.
  - ▶ With intramuscular use Correct injection technique (including the use of z-track technique) and rotation of injection sites are essential.
- **PATIENT AND CARER ADVICE**
  - ▶ With oral use Patients or carers should be given advice on how to administer aripiprazole orodispersible tablets.

- **MEDICINAL FORMS**
  There can be variation in the licensing of different medicines containing the same drug. Forms available from special-order manufacturers include: oral solution

Tablet
CAUTIONARY AND ADVISORY LABELS 2
- ▶ Aripiprazole (Non-proprietary)
  Aripiprazole 5 mg Aripiprazole 5mg tablets | 28 tablet [PoM] £96.04 DT price = £5.79
  Aripiprazole 10 mg Aripiprazole 10mg tablets | 28 tablet [PoM] £96.04 DT price = £5.79
  Aripiprazole 15 mg Aripiprazole 15mg tablets | 28 tablet [PoM] £96.04 DT price = £5.72
  Aripiprazole 30 mg Aripiprazole 30mg tablets | 28 tablet [PoM] £192.08 DT price = £103.07
- ▶ Abilify (Otsuka Pharmaceuticals (U.K.) Ltd)
  Aripiprazole 5 mg Abilify 5mg tablets | 28 tablet [PoM] £96.04 DT price = £5.79
  Aripiprazole 10 mg Abilify 10mg tablets | 28 tablet [PoM] £96.04 DT price = £5.79
  Aripiprazole 15 mg Abilify 15mg tablets | 28 tablet [PoM] £96.04 DT price = £5.72
  Aripiprazole 30 mg Abilify 30mg tablets | 28 tablet [PoM] £192.08 DT price = £103.07

Orodispersible tablet
CAUTIONARY AND ADVISORY LABELS 2
EXCIPIENTS: May contain Aspartame
- ▶ Aripiprazole (Non-proprietary)
  Aripiprazole 10 mg Aripiprazole 10mg orodispersible tablets sugar free sugar-free | 28 tablet [PoM] £91.24 DT price = £87.05
  Aripiprazole 15 mg Aripiprazole 15mg orodispersible tablets sugar free sugar-free | 28 tablet [PoM] £91.24 DT price = £87.05
- ▶ Abilify (Otsuka Pharmaceuticals (U.K.) Ltd)
  Aripiprazole 10 mg Abilify 10mg orodispersible tablets sugar-free | 28 tablet [PoM] £96.04 DT price = £87.05
  Aripiprazole 15 mg Abilify 15mg orodispersible tablets sugar-free | 28 tablet [PoM] £96.04 DT price = £87.05

Oral solution
CAUTIONARY AND ADVISORY LABELS 2
- ▶ Aripiprazole (Non-proprietary)
  Aripiprazole 1 mg per 1 ml Aripiprazole 1mg/ml oral solution | 150 ml [PoM] no price available DT price = £102.90

▸ Abilify (Otsuka Pharmaceuticals (U.K.) Ltd)
Aripiprazole 1 mg per 1 ml Abilify 1mg/ml oral solution |
150 ml [PoM] £102.90 DT price = £102.90

Solution for injection

▸ Abilify (Otsuka Pharmaceuticals (U.K.) Ltd)
Aripiprazole 7.5 mg per 1 ml Abilify 9.75mg/1.3ml solution for
injection vials | 1 vial [PoM] £3.43

Powder and solvent for suspension for injection

▸ Abilify Maintena (Otsuka Pharmaceuticals (U.K.) Ltd)
Aripiprazole 400 mg Abilify Maintena 400mg powder and solvent
for prolonged-release suspension for injection pre-filled syringes |
1 pre-filled disposable injection [PoM] £220.41
Abilify Maintena 400mg powder and solvent for prolonged-release
suspension for injection vials | 1 vial [PoM] £220.41

⏐▶ 352

⏐ Clozapine

● DRUG ACTION Clozapine is a dopamine D_1, dopamine D_2,
5-HT_{2A}, alpha$_1$-adrenoceptor, and muscarinic-receptor
antagonist.

● INDICATIONS AND DOSE

**Schizophrenia in patients unresponsive to, or intolerant
of, conventional antipsychotic drugs**

▸ BY MOUTH

▸ Adult 18–59 years: 12.5 mg 1–2 times a day for day 1,
then 25–50 mg for day 2, then increased, if tolerated,
in steps of 25–50 mg daily, dose to be increased
gradually over 14–21 days, increased to up to 300 mg
daily in divided doses, larger dose to be taken at night,
up to 200 mg daily may be taken as a single dose at
bedtime; increased in steps of 50–100 mg 1–2 times a
week if required, it is preferable to increase once a
week; usual dose 200–450 mg daily, max. 900 mg per
day, if restarting after interval of more than 48 hours,
12.5 mg once or twice on first day (but may be feasible
to increase more quickly than on initiation)—extreme
caution if previous respiratory or cardiac arrest with
initial dosing

▸ Adult 60 years and over: 12.5 mg once daily for day 1,
then increased to 25–37.5 mg for day 2, then increased,
if tolerated, in steps of up to 25 mg daily, dose to be
increased gradually over 14–21 days, increased to up to
300 mg daily in divided doses, larger dose at to be taken
night, up to 200 mg daily may be taken as a single dose
at bedtime; increased in steps of 50–100 mg 1–2 times
a week if required, it is preferable to increase once a
week; usual dose 200–450 mg daily, max. 900 mg per
day, if restarting after interval of more than 48 hours,
12.5 mg once or twice on first day (but may be feasible
to increase more quickly than on initiation)—extreme
caution if previous respiratory or cardiac arrest with
initial dosing

Psychosis in Parkinson's disease

▸ BY MOUTH

▸ Adult: 12.5 mg once daily, dose to be taken at bedtime,
then increased in steps of 12.5 mg up to twice weekly,
adjusted according to response; usual dose 25–37.5 mg
once daily, dose to be taken at bedtime; increased in
steps of 12.5 mg once weekly, this applies only in
exceptional cases, increased if necessary up to 100 mg
daily in 1–2 divided doses; Usual maximum
50 mg/24 hours

DOSE ADJUSTMENTS DUE TO INTERACTIONS
Dose adjustment may be necessary if smoking started or
stopped during treatment.

● CONTRA-INDICATIONS Alcoholic and toxic psychoses ·
bone-marrow disorders · coma · drug intoxication · history
of agranulocytosis · history of circulatory collapse · history
of neutropenia · paralytic ileus · severe cardiac disorders
(e.g. myocarditis) · severe CNS depression · uncontrolled
epilepsy

● CAUTIONS Age over 60 years · prostatic hypertrophy ·
susceptibility to angle-closure glaucoma · taper off other
antipsychotics before starting

CAUTIONS, FURTHER INFORMATION

▸ Agranulocytosis Neutropenia and potentially fatal
agranulocytosis reported. Leucocyte and differential blood
counts must be normal before starting; monitor counts
every week for 18 weeks then at least every 2 weeks and if
clozapine continued and blood count stable after 1 year at
least every 4 weeks (and 4 weeks after discontinuation); if
leucocyte count below 3000 /mm^3 or if absolute neutrophil
count below 1500 /mm^3 discontinue permanently and refer
to haematologist. Patients who have a low white blood cell
count because of benign ethnic neutropenia may be
started on clozapine with the agreement of a
haematologist. Avoid drugs which depress leucopoiesis;
patients should report immediately symptoms of infection,
especially influenza-like illness.

▸ Myocarditis and cardiomyopathy Fatal myocarditis (most
commonly in first 2 months) and cardiomyopathy
reported.

● Perform physical examination and take full medical
history before starting

● Specialist examination required if cardiac abnormalities
or history of heart disease found—clozapine initiated
only in absence of severe heart disease and if benefit
outweighs risk

● Persistent tachycardia especially in first 2 months
should prompt observation for other indicators for
myocarditis or cardiomyopathy

● If myocarditis or cardiomyopathy suspected clozapine
should be stopped and patient evaluated urgently by
cardiologist

● Discontinue permanently in clozapine-induced
myocarditis or cardiomyopathy

▸ Intestinal obstruction Impairment of intestinal peristalsis,
including constipation, intestinal obstruction, faecal
impaction, and paralytic ileus, (including fatal cases)
reported. Clozapine should be used with caution in
patients receiving drugs that may cause constipation (e.g.
antimuscarinic drugs) or in those with a history of colonic
disease or lower abdominal surgery. It is essential that
constipation is recognised and actively treated.

● INTERACTIONS Avoid concomitant use of clozapine with
drugs that have a substantial potential for causing
agranulocytosis.

● SIDE-EFFECTS

▸ **Common or very common** Anorexia · constipation ·
hypersalivation · malaise · speech disorders · urinary
incontinence

▸ **Uncommon** Agranulocytosis

▸ **Rare** Circulatory collapse · dysphagia · hepatitis ·
myocarditis · pancreatitis · pericarditis · pneumonia ·
pulmonary aspiration

▸ **Very rare** Cardiomyopathy · hypercholesterolaemia ·
hypertriglyceridaemia · interstitial nephritis · intestinal
obstruction (including fatal cases) · myocardial infarction ·
obsessive compulsive disorder · parotid gland enlargement
· respiratory depression

▸ **Frequency not known** Hepatic disorders · hepatic failure ·
muscle disorders · renal failure

SIDE-EFFECTS, FURTHER INFORMATION

▸ Hypersalivation Hypersalivation associated with clozapine
therapy can be treated with hyoscine hydrobromide
[unlicensed indication], provided that the patient is not at
particular risk from the additive antimuscarinic side-
effects of hyoscine and clozapine.

● PREGNANCY Use with caution.

● BREAST FEEDING Avoid.

4

Nervous system

- HEPATIC IMPAIRMENT Avoid in symptomatic liver disease. Avoid in progressive liver disease. Avoid in hepatic failure. Monitor hepatic function regularly.
- RENAL IMPAIRMENT Avoid in severe impairment.
- MONITORING REQUIREMENTS
  ▶ Monitor leucocyte and differential blood counts. Clozapine requires differential white blood cell monitoring weekly for 18 weeks, then fortnightly for up to one year, and then monthly as part of the clozapine patient monitoring service.
  ▶ Close medical supervision during initiation (risk of collapse because of hypotension and convulsions).
  ▶ Blood lipids and weight should be measured at baseline, at 3 months (weight should be measured at frequent intervals during the first 3 months), and then yearly with antipsychotics. Patients taking clozapine require more frequent monitoring of these parameters: every 3 months for the first year, then yearly.
  ▶ Fasting blood glucose should be measured at baseline, at 4–6 months, and then yearly. Patients taking clozapine should have fasting blood glucose tested at baseline, after one months' treatment, then every 4–6 months.
  ▶ Patient, prescriber, and supplying pharmacist must be registered with the appropriate Patient Monitoring Service—it takes several days to do this.
- TREATMENT CESSATION On planned withdrawal reduce dose over 1–2 weeks to avoid risk of rebound psychosis. If abrupt withdrawal necessary observe patient carefully.
- DIRECTIONS FOR ADMINISTRATION Shake oral suspension well for 90 seconds when dispensing or if visibly settled and stand for 24 hours before use; otherwise shake well for 10 seconds before use. May be diluted with water.
- PRESCRIBING AND DISPENSING INFORMATION Clozapine has been used for psychosis in Parkinson's disease in children aged 16 years and over.
- PATIENT AND CARER ADVICE Patients or carers should be given advice on how to administer clozapine oral suspension.

- MEDICINAL FORMS
  There can be variation in the licensing of different medicines containing the same drug. Forms available from special-order manufacturers include: oral suspension, oral solution

Tablet
CAUTIONARY AND ADVISORY LABELS 2, 10
  ▶ Clozaril (Novartis Pharmaceuticals UK Ltd)
  Clozapine 25 mg Clozaril 25mg tablets | 28 tablet [PoM] £2.95 | 84 tablet [PoM] £6.30 (Hospital only) | 100 tablet [PoM] £7.50 (Hospital only)
  Clozapine 100 mg Clozaril 100mg tablets | 28 tablet [PoM] £11.76 | 84 tablet [PoM] £25.21 (Hospital only) | 100 tablet [PoM] £30.01 (Hospital only)
  ▶ Denzapine (Britannia Pharmaceuticals Ltd)
  Clozapine 25 mg Denzapine 25mg tablets | 84 tablet [PoM] £16.64 | 100 tablet [PoM] £19.80
  Clozapine 100 mg Denzapine 100mg tablets | 84 tablet [PoM] £66.53 | 100 tablet [PoM] £79.20
  ▶ Zaponex (Teva UK Ltd)
  Clozapine 25 mg Zaponex 25mg tablets | 84 tablet [PoM] £8.28 | 500 tablet [PoM] £48.39
  Clozapine 100 mg Zaponex 100mg tablets | 84 tablet [PoM] £33.88 | 500 tablet [PoM] £196.43

Oral suspension
CAUTIONARY AND ADVISORY LABELS 2, 10
  ▶ Denzapine (Britannia Pharmaceuticals Ltd)
  Clozapine 50 mg per 1 ml Denzapine 50mg/ml oral suspension sugar-free | 100 ml [PoM] £39.60

Lurasidone hydrochloride

- DRUG ACTION Lurasidone is a dopamine D_2, 5-HT_{2A}, 5-HT_7, alpha$_{2A}$- and alpha$_{2C}$- adrenoceptor antagonist, and is a partial agonist at 5-HT_{1a} receptors.

- INDICATIONS AND DOSE
Schizophrenia
  ▶ BY MOUTH
  ▶ Adult: Initially 37 mg once daily, increased if necessary up to 148 mg once daily
Schizophrenia when given with concomitant moderate CYP3A4 inhibitors (e.g. diltiazem, erythromycin, fluconazole, and verapamil)
  ▶ BY MOUTH
  ▶ Adult: Initially 18.5 mg once daily (max. per dose 74 mg once daily)

- CAUTIONS High doses in elderly · susceptibility to QT-interval prolongation
- INTERACTIONS Contra-indicated with concomitant use of potent CYP3A4 inhibitors and potent CYP3A4 inducers. Caution with concomitant use of drugs that prolong the QT interval.
- SIDE-EFFECTS
  ▶ **Common or very common** Anxiety · musculoskeletal stiffness
  ▶ **Uncommon** Catatonia · decreased appetite · dysarthria · dysuria · hot flush · myalgia · nightmares
  ▶ **Frequency not known** Angina · AV block · bradycardia · dysphagia · panic attacks · pruritus · suicidal behaviour · vertigo
- PREGNANCY Use only if potential benefit outweighs risk—limited information available.
- HEPATIC IMPAIRMENT Initially 18.5 mg once daily, up to max. 74 mg once daily in moderate impairment. Use with caution in severe impairment—initially 18.5 mg once daily, up to max. 37 mg once daily.
- RENAL IMPAIRMENT Initially 18.5 mg once daily, up to max. 74 mg once daily if eGFR less than 50 mL/minute/1.73 m². Manufacturer advises use only if potential benefit outweighs risk if eGFR less than 15 mL/minute/1.73 m².
- DIRECTIONS FOR ADMINISTRATION Patients on doses higher than 111 mg once daily whose treatment is interrupted for longer than 3 days should restart on 111 mg once daily and titrate to usual dose; for all other doses, restart on usual dose.

- MEDICINAL FORMS
  There can be variation in the licensing of different medicines containing the same drug.
Tablet
CAUTIONARY AND ADVISORY LABELS 2, 21, 25
  ▶ Latuda (Sunovion Pharmaceuticals Europe Ltd) ▼
  Lurasidone (as Lurasidone hydrochloride) 18.5 mg Latuda 18.5mg tablets | 28 tablet [PoM] £90.72
  Lurasidone (as Lurasidone hydrochloride) 37 mg Latuda 37mg tablets | 28 tablet [PoM] £90.72
  Lurasidone (as Lurasidone hydrochloride) 74 mg Latuda 74mg tablets | 28 tablet [PoM] £90.72

4

Olanzapine

F 352

- DRUG ACTION Olanzapine is a dopamine D_1, D_2, D_4, 5-HT_2, histamine- 1-, and muscarinic-receptor antagonist.

INDICATIONS AND DOSE

Schizophrenia | Combination therapy for mania

▸ BY MOUTH
  ▸ Adult: 10 mg daily, adjusted according to response, usual dose 5–20 mg daily, doses greater than 10 mg daily only after reassessment, when one or more factors present that might result in slower metabolism (e.g. female gender, elderly, non-smoker) consider lower initial dose and more gradual dose increase; maximum 20 mg per day

Preventing recurrence in bipolar disorder

▸ BY MOUTH
  ▸ Adult: 10 mg daily, adjusted according to response, usual dose 5–20 mg daily, doses greater than 10 mg daily only after reassessment, when one or more factors present that might result in slower metabolism (e.g. female gender, elderly, non-smoker) consider lower initial dose and more gradual dose increase; maximum 20 mg per day

Monotherapy for mania

▸ BY MOUTH
  ▸ Adult: 15 mg daily, adjusted according to response, usual dose 5–20 mg daily, doses greater than 15 mg daily only after reassessment, when one or more factors present that might result in slower metabolism (e.g. female gender, elderly, non-smoker) consider lower initial dose and more gradual dose increase; maximum 20 mg per day

Control of agitation and disturbed behaviour in schizophrenia or mania

▸ BY INTRAMUSCULAR INJECTION
  ▸ Adult: Initially 5–10 mg for 1 dose; usual dose 10 mg for 1 dose, followed by 5–10 mg after 2 hours if required, maximum 3 injections daily for 3 days; maximum daily combined oral and parenteral dose 20 mg, when one or more factors present that might result in slower metabolism (e.g. female gender, elderly, non-smoker) consider lower initial dose and more gradual dose increase
  ▸ Elderly: Initially 2.5–5 mg, followed by 2.5–5 mg after 2 hours if required, maximum 3 injections daily for 3 days; maximum daily combined oral and parenteral dose 20 mg, when one or more factors present that might result in slower metabolism (e.g. female gender, elderly, non-smoker) consider lower initial dose and more gradual dose increase

DOSE ADJUSTMENTS DUE TO INTERACTIONS

Dose adjustment may be necessary if smoking started or stopped during treatment.

CONTRA-INDICATIONS

▸ With intramuscular use Acute myocardial infarction · bradycardia · recent heart surgery · severe hypotension · sick sinus syndrome · unstable angina

CAUTIONS Bone-marrow depression · diabetes mellitus (risk of exacerbation or ketoacidosis) · hypereosinophilic disorders · low leucocyte count · low neutrophil count · myeloproliferative disease · paralytic ileus

CAUTIONS, FURTHER INFORMATION

▸ CNS and respiratory depression
▸ With intramuscular use Blood pressure, pulse and respiratory rate should be monitored for at least 4 hours after intramuscular injection, particularly in those also receiving a benzodiazepine or another antipsychotic (leave at least one hour between administration of olanzapine intramuscular injection and parenteral benzodiazepines).

SIDE-EFFECTS

GENERAL SIDE-EFFECTS

▸ **Common or very common** Arthralgia · hypercholesterolaemia · hypertriglyceridaemia · increased appetite · malaise · oedema
▸ **Uncommon** Alopecia · amnesia · bradycardia · epistaxis
▸ **Rare** Hepatitis · pancreatitis · rhabdomyolysis

SPECIFIC SIDE-EFFECTS

▸ With intramuscular use Hypoventilation · sinus pause

PREGNANCY Use only if potential benefit outweighs risk; neonatal lethargy, tremor, and hypertonia reported when used in third trimester.

BREAST FEEDING Avoid—present in milk.

HEPATIC IMPAIRMENT Consider initial dose of 5 mg daily.

RENAL IMPAIRMENT Consider initial dose of 5 mg daily.

MONITORING REQUIREMENTS

▸ Blood lipids and weight should be measured at baseline, at 3 months (weight should be measured at frequent intervals during the first 3 months), and then yearly with antipsychotic drugs. Patients taking olanzapine require more frequent monitoring of these parameters: every 3 months for the first year, then yearly.
▸ Fasting blood glucose should be measured at baseline, at 4–6 months, and then yearly. Patients taking olanzapine should have fasting blood glucose tested at baseline, after one months' treatment, then every 4–6 months.

DIRECTIONS FOR ADMINISTRATION Olanzapine orodispersible tablet may be placed on the tongue and allowed to dissolve, or dispersed in water, orange juice, apple juice, milk, or coffee.

PRESCRIBING AND DISPENSING INFORMATION

▸ With intramuscular use When prescribing, dispensing, or administering, check that this injection is the correct preparation—this preparation is usually used in hospital for the rapid control of an *acute episode* and should **not** be confused with depot preparations which are usually used in the community or clinics for *maintenance* treatment.

PATIENT AND CARER ADVICE Patients or carers should be given advice on how to administer orodispersible tablets.

MEDICINAL FORMS

There can be variation in the licensing of different medicines containing the same drug. Forms available from special-order manufacturers include: oral suspension, oral solution

Tablet

CAUTIONARY AND ADVISORY LABELS 2

▸ Olanzapine (Non-proprietary)
  Olanzapine 2.5 mg Olanzapine 2.5mg tablets | 28 tablet [PoM] £21.85 DT price = £0.86
  Olanzapine 5 mg Olanzapine 5mg tablets | 28 tablet [PoM] £43.70 DT price = £0.94
  Olanzapine 7.5 mg Olanzapine 7.5mg tablets | 28 tablet £65.55 DT price = £1.11 | 56 tablet [PoM] £131.10
  Olanzapine 10 mg Olanzapine 10mg tablets | 28 tablet [PoM] £87.40 DT price = £1.13
  Olanzapine 15 mg Olanzapine 15mg tablets | 28 tablet [PoM] £119.18 DT price = £1.31
  Olanzapine 20 mg Olanzapine 20mg tablets | 28 tablet [PoM] £158.90 DT price = £1.53
▸ Zalasta (Consilient Health Ltd)
  Olanzapine 2.5 mg Zalasta 2.5mg tablets | 28 tablet [PoM] £18.57 DT price = £0.86
  Olanzapine 5 mg Zalasta 5mg tablets | 28 tablet [PoM] £37.14 DT price = £0.94
  Olanzapine 7.5 mg Zalasta 7.5mg tablets | 56 tablet [PoM] £111.43
  Olanzapine 10 mg Zalasta 10mg tablets | 28 tablet [PoM] £74.29 DT price = £1.13
  Olanzapine 15 mg Zalasta 15mg tablets | 28 tablet [PoM] £101.30 DT price = £1.31
  Olanzapine 20 mg Zalasta 20mg tablets | 28 tablet [PoM] £135.06 DT price = £1.53

4

Nervous system

▸ Zyprexa (Eli Lilly and Company Ltd)
Olanzapine 2.5 mg Zyprexa 2.5mg tablets | 28 tablet [PoM] £21.85
DT price = £0.86
Olanzapine 5 mg Zyprexa 5mg tablets | 28 tablet [PoM] £43.70 DT
price = £0.94
Olanzapine 7.5 mg Zyprexa 7.5mg tablets | 56 tablet [PoM] £131.10
Olanzapine 10 mg Zyprexa 10mg tablets | 28 tablet [PoM] £87.40 DT
price = £1.13
Olanzapine 15 mg Zyprexa 15mg tablets | 28 tablet [PoM] £119.18
DT price = £1.31
Olanzapine 20 mg Zyprexa 20mg tablets | 28 tablet [PoM] £158.90
DT price = £1.53

Orodispersible tablet
CAUTIONARY AND ADVISORY LABELS 2
EXCIPIENTS: May contain Aspartame
▸ Olanzapine (Non-proprietary)
Olanzapine 5 mg Olanzapine 5mg orodispersible tablets sugar free
sugar-free | 28 tablet [PoM] £40.86 DT price = £1.79
Olanzapine 5mg orodispersible tablets | 28 tablet [PoM] £4.99 DT
price = £2.54
Olanzapine 10 mg Olanzapine 10mg orodispersible tablets |
28 tablet [PoM] £5.99 DT price = £2.81
Olanzapine 10mg orodispersible tablets sugar free sugar-free |
28 tablet [PoM] £74.29 DT price = £2.41
Olanzapine 15 mg Olanzapine 15mg orodispersible tablets sugar free
sugar-free | 28 tablet [PoM] £111.44 DT price = £2.99
Olanzapine 15mg orodispersible tablets | 28 tablet [PoM] £6.99 DT
price = £3.20
Olanzapine 20 mg Olanzapine 20mg orodispersible tablets sugar
free sugar-free | 28 tablet [PoM] £148.57 DT price = £4.46
Olanzapine 20mg orodispersible tablets | 28 tablet [PoM] £7.99 DT
price = £4.32
▸ Arkolamyl (Mylan Ltd)
Olanzapine 5 mg Arkolamyl 5mg orodispersible tablets sugar-free |
28 tablet [PoM] £48.07 DT price = £1.79
Olanzapine 10 mg Arkolamyl 10mg orodispersible tablets sugar-free
| 28 tablet [PoM] £87.40 DT price = £2.41
Olanzapine 15 mg Arkolamyl 15mg orodispersible tablets sugar-free
| 28 tablet [PoM] £131.10 DT price = £2.99
Olanzapine 20 mg Arkolamyl 20mg orodispersible tablets sugar-free
| 28 tablet [PoM] £174.79 DT price = £4.46
▸ Zalasta (Consilient Health Ltd)
Olanzapine 5 mg Zalasta 5mg orodispersible tablets sugar-free |
28 tablet [PoM] £40.85 DT price = £1.79
Olanzapine 10 mg Zalasta 10mg orodispersible tablets sugar-free |
28 tablet [PoM] £74.29 DT price = £2.41
Olanzapine 15 mg Zalasta 15mg orodispersible tablets sugar-free |
28 tablet [PoM] £111.43 DT price = £2.99
Olanzapine 20 mg Zalasta 20mg orodispersible tablets sugar-free |
28 tablet [PoM] £148.57 DT price = £4.46

Oral lyophilisate
▸ Zyprexa Velotabs (Eli Lilly and Company Ltd)
Olanzapine 5 mg Zyprexa 5mg Velotabs sugar-free | 28 tablet [PoM]
£48.07 DT price = £48.07
Olanzapine 10 mg Zyprexa 10mg Velotabs sugar-free |
28 tablet [PoM] £87.40 DT price = £87.40
Olanzapine 15 mg Zyprexa 15mg Velotabs sugar-free |
28 tablet [PoM] £131.10 DT price = £131.10
Olanzapine 20 mg Zyprexa 20mg Velotabs sugar-free |
28 tablet [PoM] £174.79 DT price = £174.79

⌐ 352

Paliperidone

● DRUG ACTION Paliperidone is a metabolite of risperidone.

● INDICATIONS AND DOSE

**Maintenance in schizophrenia in patients previously
responsive to paliperidone or risperidone**
▸ BY DEEP INTRAMUSCULAR INJECTION
▸ Adult: 150 mg for 1 dose on day 1, then 100 mg for
1 dose on day 8, to be injected into the deltoid muscle,
dose subsequently adjusted at monthly intervals
according to response; maintenance 75 mg once a
month, alternatively maintenance 25–150 mg once a
month, following the second dose, monthly
maintenance doses can be administered into either the

deltoid or gluteal muscle, for missed doses see product
literature

**Schizophrenia | Psychotic or manic symptoms of
schizoaffective disorder**
▸ BY MOUTH
▸ Adult: 6 mg once daily, dose to be taken in the
morning, then adjusted in steps of 3 mg if required,
dose to be adjusted over at least 5 days; usual dose
3–12 mg daily

● CAUTIONS
GENERAL CAUTIONS
Cataract surgery (risk of intraoperative floppy iris
syndrome) · elderly patients with dementia · elderly
patients with risk factors for stroke · predisposition to
gastro-intestinal obstruction · prolactin-dependent
tumours
SPECIFIC CAUTIONS
▸ With intramuscular use When transferring from oral to depot
therapy, the dose by mouth should be reduced gradually

● SIDE-EFFECTS
GENERAL SIDE-EFFECTS
▸ **Common or very common** Anxiety · appetite changes ·
arthralgia · depression · epistaxis · hypertension · infection
· malaise · myalgia · oedema · respiratory disorders · sleep
disorders · toothache · urinary disorders
▸ **Uncommon** Alopecia · elevated plasma-cholesterol
concentrations · elevated plasma-triglyceride
concentrations · hypoaesthesia · paraesthesia · taste
disturbances · tinnitus · visual disorders
▸ **Rare** Inappropriate antidiuretic hormone secretion ·
intestinal obstruction · intra-operative floppy iris
syndrome · pancreatitis · pulmonary embolism ·
rhabdomyolysis
SPECIFIC SIDE-EFFECTS
▸ With intramuscular use Erythema · nodules · pain at injection
site · swelling
SIDE-EFFECTS, FURTHER INFORMATION
▸ With intramuscular use If the dose needs to be reduced to
alleviate side-effects, it is important to recognise that the
plasma-drug concentration may not fall for some time
after reducing the dose, therefore it may be a month or
longer before side-effects subside.

● PREGNANCY Use only if potential benefit outweighs risk—
toxicity in *animal* studies; if discontinuation during
pregnancy is necessary, withdraw gradually.

● BREAST FEEDING Avoid—present in milk.

● HEPATIC IMPAIRMENT Caution in severe impairment—no
information available.

● RENAL IMPAIRMENT
▸ With oral use Initially 3 mg once daily if eGFR
50–80 mL/minute/1.73 m^2 (max. 6 mg once daily). Initially
1.5 mg once daily if eGFR 10–50 mL/minute/1.73 m^2 (max.
3 mg once daily).
Avoid if eGFR less than 10 mL/minute/1.73 m^2.
▸ With intramuscular use Initial dose 100 mg on day 1 and then
75 mg on day 8 if eGFR 50–80 mL/minute/1.73 m^2;
recommended maintenance dose 50 mg (range 25–100 mg)
monthly if eGFR 50–80 mL/minute/1.73 m^2.
Avoid if eGFR less than 50 mL/minute/1.73 m^2.

● MONITORING REQUIREMENTS
▸ With intramuscular use Treatment requires careful
monitoring for optimum effect.

● DIRECTIONS FOR ADMINISTRATION
▸ With intramuscular use Correct injection technique
(including the use of z-track technique) and rotation of
injection sites are essential.
▸ With oral use Always take with breakfast or always take on
an empty stomach.

● PATIENT AND CARER ADVICE
▸ With oral use Patients or carers should be given advice on how to administer paliperidone tablets.

Missed doses
▸ With intramuscular use For missed doses see product literature.

● MEDICINAL FORMS
There can be variation in the licensing of different medicines containing the same drug.

Modified-release tablet
CAUTIONARY AND ADVISORY LABELS 2, 25
▸ Paliperidone (Non-proprietary)
Paliperidone 3 mg Paliperidone 3mg modified-release tablets | 28 tablet [PoM] no price available
Paliperidone 6 mg Paliperidone 6mg modified-release tablets | 28 tablet [PoM] no price available
Paliperidone 9 mg Paliperidone 9mg modified-release tablets | 28 tablet [PoM] no price available
▸ Invega (Janssen-Cilag Ltd)
Paliperidone 3 mg Invega 3mg modified-release tablets | 28 tablet [PoM] £97.28
Paliperidone 6 mg Invega 6mg modified-release tablets | 28 tablet [PoM] £97.28
Paliperidone 9 mg Invega 9mg modified-release tablets | 28 tablet [PoM] £145.92

Suspension for injection
▸ Xeplion (Janssen-Cilag Ltd)
Paliperidone palmitate 100 mg per 1 ml Xeplion 150mg/1.5ml suspension for injection pre-filled syringes | 1 pre-filled disposable injection [PoM] £392.59
Xeplion 75mg/0.75ml suspension for injection pre-filled syringes | 1 pre-filled disposable injection [PoM] £244.90
Xeplion 100mg/1ml suspension for injection pre-filled syringes | 1 pre-filled disposable injection [PoM] £314.07
Xeplion 50mg/0.5ml suspension for injection pre-filled syringes | 1 pre-filled disposable injection [PoM] £183.92

⚑ 352

Quetiapine

● DRUG ACTION Quetiapine is a dopamine D_1, dopamine D_2, 5-HT_2, alpha$_1$-adrenoceptor, and histamine-1 receptor antagonist.

● INDICATIONS AND DOSE

Schizophrenia
▸ BY MOUTH USING IMMEDIATE-RELEASE MEDICINES
▸ Adult: 25 mg twice daily for day 1, then 50 mg twice daily for day 2, then 100 mg twice daily for day 3, then 150 mg twice daily for day 4, then, adjusted according to response, usual dose 300–450 mg daily in 2 divided doses, the rate of dose titration may need to be slower and the daily dose lower in elderly patients; maximum 750 mg per day
▸ BY MOUTH USING MODIFIED-RELEASE MEDICINES
▸ Adult: 300 mg once daily for day 1, then 600 mg once daily for day 2, then, adjusted according to response, usual dose 600 mg once daily, maximum dose under specialist supervision; maximum 800 mg per day
▸ Elderly: Initially 50 mg once daily, adjusted according to response. adjusted in steps of 50 mg daily

Treatment of mania in bipolar disorder
▸ BY MOUTH USING IMMEDIATE-RELEASE MEDICINES
▸ Adult: 50 mg twice daily for day 1, then 100 mg twice daily for day 2, then 150 mg twice daily for day 3, then 200 mg twice daily for day 4, then adjusted in steps of up to 200 mg daily, adjusted according to response, usual dose 400–800 mg daily in 2 divided doses, the rate of dose titration may need to be slower and the daily dose lower in elderly patients; maximum 800 mg per day

▸ BY MOUTH USING MODIFIED-RELEASE MEDICINES
▸ Adult: 300 mg once daily for day 1, then 600 mg once daily for day 2, then, adjusted according to response, usual dose 400–800 mg once daily
▸ Elderly: Initially 50 mg once daily, adjusted according to response. adjusted in steps of 50 mg daily

Treatment of depression in bipolar disorder
▸ BY MOUTH USING IMMEDIATE-RELEASE MEDICINES
▸ Adult: 50 mg once daily for day 1, dose to be taken at bedtime, then 100 mg once daily for day 2, then 200 mg once daily for day 3, then 300 mg once daily for day 4, then, adjusted according to response; usual dose 300 mg once daily, the rate of dose titration may need to be slower and the daily dose lower in elderly patients; maximum 600 mg per day
▸ BY MOUTH USING MODIFIED-RELEASE MEDICINES
▸ Adult: 50 mg once daily for day 1, dose to be taken at bedtime, then 100 mg once daily for day 2, then 200 mg once daily for day 3, then 300 mg once daily for day 4, then, adjusted according to response; usual dose 300 mg once daily; maximum 600 mg per day

Prevention of mania and depression in bipolar disorder
▸ BY MOUTH USING IMMEDIATE-RELEASE MEDICINES
▸ Adult: Continue at the dose effective for treatment of bipolar disorder and adjust to lowest effective dose; usual dose 300–800 mg daily in 2 divided doses
▸ BY MOUTH USING MODIFIED-RELEASE MEDICINES
▸ Adult: Continue at the dose effective for treatment of bipolar disorder and adjust to lowest effective dose; usual dose 300–800 mg once daily

Adjunctive treatment of major depression
▸ BY MOUTH USING MODIFIED-RELEASE MEDICINES
▸ Adult: 50 mg once daily for 2 days, dose to be taken at bedtime, then 150 mg once daily for 2 days, then, adjusted according to response, usual dose 150–300 mg once daily
▸ Elderly: Initially 50 mg once daily for 3 days, then increased if necessary to 100 mg once daily for 4 days, then adjusted in steps of 50 mg, adjusted according to response, usual dose 50–300 mg once daily, dose of 300 mg should not be reached before day 22 of treatment

DOSE EQUIVALENCE AND CONVERSION
Patients can be switched from immediate-release to modified-release tablets at the equivalent daily dose; to maintain clinical response, dose titration may be required.

● CAUTIONS Cerebrovascular disease · elderly · patients at risk of aspiration pneumonia · treatment of depression in patients under 25 years (increased risk of suicide)

● SIDE-EFFECTS
▸ **Common or very common** Asthenia · dysarthria · dyspnoea · elevated plasma-cholesterol concentrations · elevated plasma-triglyceride concentrations · increased appetite · irritability · peripheral oedema · sleep disorders
▸ **Uncommon** Hyponatraemia · hypothyroidism · restless legs syndrome · rhinitis
▸ **Rare** Hepatitis · pancreatitis
▸ **Very rare** Angioedema · inappropriate secretion of antidiuretic hormone · rhabdomyolysis · Stevens-Johnson syndrome
▸ **Frequency not known** Suicidal behaviour (particularly on initiation) · toxic epidermal necrolysis

● PREGNANCY Use only if potential benefit outweighs risk.

● BREAST FEEDING Manufacturer advises avoid.

● HEPATIC IMPAIRMENT For *immediate-release tablets*, initially 25 mg daily, increased daily in steps of 25–50 mg. For *modified-release tablets*, initially 50 mg daily, increased daily in steps of 50 mg.

4

Nervous system

● MEDICINAL FORMS
There can be variation in the licensing of different medicines containing the same drug. Forms available from special-order manufacturers include: oral suspension, oral solution

Tablet

CAUTIONARY AND ADVISORY LABELS 2

▸ Quetiapine (Non-proprietary)
Quetiapine (as Quetiapine fumarate) 25 mg Quetiapine 25mg tablets | 60 tablet [PoM] £38.05 DT price = £1.11
Quetiapine (as Quetiapine fumarate) 100 mg Quetiapine 100mg tablets | 60 tablet [PoM] £107.45 DT price = £1.79
Quetiapine (as Quetiapine fumarate) 150 mg Quetiapine 150mg tablets | 60 tablet [PoM] £107.45 DT price = £2.27
Quetiapine (as Quetiapine fumarate) 200 mg Quetiapine 200mg tablets | 60 tablet [PoM] £107.45 DT price = £2.50
Quetiapine (as Quetiapine fumarate) 300 mg Quetiapine 300mg tablets | 60 tablet [PoM] £170.00 DT price = £3.20

▸ Seroquel (AstraZeneca UK Ltd)
Quetiapine (as Quetiapine fumarate) 25 mg Seroquel 25mg tablets | 60 tablet [PoM] £40.50 DT price = £1.11
Quetiapine (as Quetiapine fumarate) 100 mg Seroquel 100mg tablets | 60 tablet [PoM] £113.10 DT price = £1.79
Quetiapine (as Quetiapine fumarate) 200 mg Seroquel 200mg tablets | 60 tablet [PoM] £113.10 DT price = £2.50
Quetiapine (as Quetiapine fumarate) 300 mg Seroquel 300mg tablets | 60 tablet [PoM] £170.00 DT price = £3.20

Modified-release tablet

CAUTIONARY AND ADVISORY LABELS 2, 23, 25

▸ Atrolak XL (Accord Healthcare Ltd)
Quetiapine (as Quetiapine fumarate) 50 mg Atrolak XL 50mg tablets | 60 tablet [PoM] £67.65 DT price = £67.66
Quetiapine (as Quetiapine fumarate) 200 mg Atrolak XL 200mg tablets | 60 tablet [PoM] £113.09 DT price = £113.10
Quetiapine (as Quetiapine fumarate) 300 mg Atrolak XL 300mg tablets | 60 tablet [PoM] £169.99 DT price = £170.00
Quetiapine (as Quetiapine fumarate) 400 mg Atrolak XL 400mg tablets | 60 tablet [PoM] £226.19 DT price = £226.20

▸ Biquelle XL (Aspire Pharma Ltd)
Quetiapine (as Quetiapine fumarate) 50 mg Biquelle XL 50mg tablets | 60 tablet [PoM] £29.45 DT price = £67.66
Quetiapine (as Quetiapine fumarate) 150 mg Biquelle XL 150mg tablets | 60 tablet [PoM] £49.45 DT price = £113.10
Quetiapine (as Quetiapine fumarate) 200 mg Biquelle XL 200mg tablets | 60 tablet [PoM] £49.45 DT price = £113.10
Quetiapine (as Quetiapine fumarate) 300 mg Biquelle XL 300mg tablets | 60 tablet [PoM] £74.45 DT price = £170.00
Quetiapine (as Quetiapine fumarate) 400 mg Biquelle XL 400mg tablets | 60 tablet [PoM] £98.95 DT price = £226.20

▸ Ebesque XL (DB Ashbourne Ltd)
Quetiapine (as Quetiapine fumarate) 50 mg Ebesque XL 50mg tablets | 60 tablet [PoM] £31.80 DT price = £67.66
Quetiapine (as Quetiapine fumarate) 200 mg Ebesque XL 200mg tablets | 60 tablet [PoM] £53.16 DT price = £113.10
Quetiapine (as Quetiapine fumarate) 300 mg Ebesque XL 300mg tablets | 60 tablet [PoM] £79.90 DT price = £170.00
Quetiapine (as Quetiapine fumarate) 400 mg Ebesque XL 400mg tablets | 60 tablet [PoM] £106.31 DT price = £226.20

▸ Mintreleq XL (CEB Pharma Ltd)
Quetiapine (as Quetiapine fumarate) 50 mg Mintreleq XL 50mg tablets | 60 tablet [PoM] £29.45 DT price = £67.66
Quetiapine (as Quetiapine fumarate) 150 mg Mintreleq XL 150mg tablets | 60 tablet [PoM] £49.45 DT price = £113.10
Quetiapine (as Quetiapine fumarate) 200 mg Mintreleq XL 200mg tablets | 60 tablet [PoM] £49.45 DT price = £113.10
Quetiapine (as Quetiapine fumarate) 300 mg Mintreleq XL 300mg tablets | 60 tablet [PoM] £74.45 DT price = £170.00
Quetiapine (as Quetiapine fumarate) 400 mg Mintreleq XL 400mg tablets | 60 tablet [PoM] £98.95 DT price = £226.20

▸ Psyquet XL (Sandoz Ltd)
Quetiapine (as Quetiapine fumarate) 50 mg Psyquet XL 50mg tablets | 60 tablet [PoM] £27.97 DT price = £67.66
Quetiapine (as Quetiapine fumarate) 150 mg Psyquet XL 150mg tablets | 60 tablet [PoM] £46.97 DT price = £113.10
Quetiapine (as Quetiapine fumarate) 200 mg Psyquet XL 200mg tablets | 60 tablet [PoM] £46.97 DT price = £113.10
Quetiapine (as Quetiapine fumarate) 300 mg Psyquet XL 300mg tablets | 60 tablet [PoM] £70.72 DT price = £170.00
Quetiapine (as Quetiapine fumarate) 400 mg Psyquet XL 400mg tablets | 60 tablet [PoM] £93.99 DT price = £226.20

▸ Seroquel XL (AstraZeneca UK Ltd)
Quetiapine (as Quetiapine fumarate) 50 mg Seroquel XL 50mg tablets | 60 tablet [PoM] £67.66 DT price = £67.66
Quetiapine (as Quetiapine fumarate) 150 mg Seroquel XL 150mg tablets | 60 tablet [PoM] £113.10 DT price = £113.10
Quetiapine (as Quetiapine fumarate) 200 mg Seroquel XL 200mg tablets | 60 tablet [PoM] £113.10 DT price = £113.10
Quetiapine (as Quetiapine fumarate) 300 mg Seroquel XL 300mg tablets | 60 tablet [PoM] £170.00 DT price = £170.00
Quetiapine (as Quetiapine fumarate) 400 mg Seroquel XL 400mg tablets | 60 tablet [PoM] £226.20 DT price = £226.20

▸ Sondate XL (Teva UK Ltd)
Quetiapine (as Quetiapine fumarate) 50 mg Sondate XL 50mg tablets | 60 tablet [PoM] £25.16 DT price = £67.66
Quetiapine (as Quetiapine fumarate) 150 mg Sondate XL 150mg tablets | 60 tablet [PoM] £46.95 DT price = £113.10
Quetiapine (as Quetiapine fumarate) 200 mg Sondate XL 200mg tablets | 60 tablet [PoM] £42.26 DT price = £113.10
Quetiapine (as Quetiapine fumarate) 300 mg Sondate XL 300mg tablets | 60 tablet [PoM] £63.64 DT price = £170.00
Quetiapine (as Quetiapine fumarate) 400 mg Sondate XL 400mg tablets | 60 tablet [PoM] £84.58 DT price = £226.20

▸ Tenprolide XL (Actavis UK Ltd)
Quetiapine (as Quetiapine fumarate) 50 mg Tenprolide XL 50mg tablets | 60 tablet [PoM] £67.66 DT price = £67.66
Quetiapine (as Quetiapine fumarate) 200 mg Tenprolide XL 200mg tablets | 60 tablet [PoM] £113.10 DT price = £113.10
Quetiapine (as Quetiapine fumarate) 300 mg Tenprolide XL 300mg tablets | 60 tablet [PoM] £170.00 DT price = £170.00
Quetiapine (as Quetiapine fumarate) 400 mg Tenprolide XL 400mg tablets | 60 tablet [PoM] £226.20 DT price = £226.20

▸ Zaluron XL (Fontus Health Ltd)
Quetiapine (as Quetiapine fumarate) 50 mg Zaluron XL 50mg tablets | 60 tablet [PoM] £27.96 DT price = £67.66
Quetiapine (as Quetiapine fumarate) 150 mg Zaluron XL 150mg tablets | 60 tablet [PoM] £46.96 DT price = £113.10
Quetiapine (as Quetiapine fumarate) 200 mg Zaluron XL 200mg tablets | 60 tablet [PoM] £46.96 DT price = £113.10
Quetiapine (as Quetiapine fumarate) 300 mg Zaluron XL 300mg tablets | 60 tablet [PoM] £70.71 DT price = £170.00
Quetiapine (as Quetiapine fumarate) 400 mg Zaluron XL 400mg tablets | 60 tablet [PoM] £93.98 DT price = £226.20

◤ 352

Risperidone

● DRUG ACTION Risperidone is a dopamine D_2, 5-HT_{2A}, alpha$_1$-adrenoceptor, and histamine-1 receptor antagonist.

● INDICATIONS AND DOSE

Schizophrenia and other psychoses in patients tolerant to risperidone by mouth and taking oral risperidone up to 4 mg daily

▸ BY DEEP INTRAMUSCULAR INJECTION
▸ Adult: Initially 25 mg every 2 weeks, to be administered into the deltoid or gluteal muscle, adjusted in steps of 12.5 mg (max. per dose 50 mg every 2 weeks) at intervals of at least 4 weeks, during initiation risperidone by mouth may need to be continued for 4–6 weeks; risperidone by mouth may also be used during dose adjustment of depot injection

Schizophrenia and other psychoses in patients tolerant to risperidone by mouth and taking oral risperidone over 4 mg daily

▸ BY DEEP INTRAMUSCULAR INJECTION
▸ Adult: Initially 37.5 mg every 2 weeks, adjusted in steps of 12.5 mg (max. per dose 50 mg every 2 weeks) at intervals of at least 4 weeks, during initiation risperidone by mouth may need to be continued for 4–6 weeks; risperidone by mouth may also be used during dose adjustment of depot injection

Acute and chronic psychosis

▸ BY MOUTH
▸ Adult: 2 mg daily in 1–2 divided doses for day 1, then 4 mg daily in 1–2 divided doses for day 2, slower

titration is appropriate in some patients, usual dose 4–6 mg daily, doses above 10 mg daily only if benefit considered to outweigh risk; maximum 16 mg per day
▸ Elderly: Initially 500 micrograms twice daily, then increased in steps of 500 micrograms twice daily, increased to 1–2 mg twice daily

Mania
▸ BY MOUTH
▸ Adult: Initially 2 mg once daily, then increased in steps of 1 mg daily if required; usual dose 1–6 mg daily
▸ Elderly: Initially 500 micrograms twice daily, then increased in steps of 500 micrograms twice daily, increased to 1–2 mg twice daily

Short-term treatment (up to 6 weeks) of persistent aggression in patients with moderate to severe Alzheimer's dementia unresponsive to non-pharmacological interventions and when there is a risk of harm to self or others
▸ BY MOUTH
▸ Adult: Initially 250 micrograms twice daily, then increased in steps of 250 micrograms twice a day on alternate days, adjusted according to response; usual dose 500 micrograms twice daily (max. per dose 1 mg twice daily)

● CAUTIONS
GENERAL CAUTIONS
Avoid in Acute porphyrias p. 918 · cataract surgery (risk of intra-operative floppy iris syndrome) · dehydration · dementia with Lewy bodies · prolactin-dependent tumours
SPECIFIC CAUTIONS
▸ With intramuscular use When transferring from oral to depot therapy, the dose by mouth should be reduced gradually

● SIDE-EFFECTS
GENERAL SIDE-EFFECTS
▸ **Common or very common** Anxiety · appetite changes · arthralgia · depression · epistaxis · hypertension · infection · malaise · myalgia · oedema · respiratory disorders · sleep disorders · toothache · urinary disorders
▸ **Uncommon** Alopecia · elevated plasma-cholesterol concentrations · elevated plasma-triglyceride concentrations · hypoaesthesia · paraesthesia · taste disturbances · tinnitus · visual disorders
▸ **Rare** Inappropriate antidiuretic hormone secretion · intestinal obstruction · intra-operative floppy iris syndrome · pancreatitis · pulmonary embolism · rhabdomyolysis
SPECIFIC SIDE-EFFECTS
▸ With intramuscular use Erythema · nodules · pain at injection site · swelling
SIDE-EFFECTS, FURTHER INFORMATION
▸ With intramuscular use If the dose needs to be reduced to alleviate side-effects, it is important to recognise that the plasma-drug concentration may not fall for some time after reducing the dose, therefore it may be a month or longer before side-effects subside.

● PREGNANCY Use only if potential benefit outweighs risk.
● BREAST FEEDING Use only if potential benefit outweighs risk—small amount present in milk.

● HEPATIC IMPAIRMENT
▸ With intramuscular use If an oral dose of at least 2 mg daily tolerated, 25 mg as a depot injection can be given every 2 weeks.
▸ With oral use Initial and subsequent oral doses should be halved.

● RENAL IMPAIRMENT Initial and subsequent oral doses should be halved.

● MONITORING REQUIREMENTS
▸ With intramuscular use Treatment requires careful monitoring for optimum effect.

● DIRECTIONS FOR ADMINISTRATION
▸ With oral use Orodispersible tablets should be placed on the tongue, allowed to dissolve and swallowed. Oral liquid may be diluted with any non-alcoholic drink, except tea.
▸ With intramuscular use Correct injection technique (including the use of z-track technique) and rotation of injection sites are essential.

● PATIENT AND CARER ADVICE
▸ With oral use Patients or carers should be given advice on how to administer risperidone orodispersible tablets and oral liquid (counselling on use of dose syringe advised).

● MEDICINAL FORMS
There can be variation in the licensing of different medicines containing the same drug. Forms available from special-order manufacturers include: oral solution

Tablet
CAUTIONARY AND ADVISORY LABELS 2
▸ Risperidone (Non-proprietary)
Risperidone 500 microgram Risperidone 500microgram tablets | 20 tablet [PoM] £6.18 DT price = £0.82
Risperidone 1 mg Risperidone 1mg tablets | 20 tablet [PoM] £1.02 DT price = £0.81 | 60 tablet [PoM] £25.07
Risperidone 2 mg Risperidone 2mg tablets | 60 tablet [PoM] £60.10 DT price = £1.37
Risperidone 3 mg Risperidone 3mg tablets | 60 tablet [PoM] £88.38 DT price = £1.67
Risperidone 4 mg Risperidone 4mg tablets | 60 tablet [PoM] £116.67 DT price = £1.94
Risperidone 6 mg Risperidone 6mg tablets | 28 tablet [PoM] £82.50 DT price = £3.86 | 60 tablet [PoM] no price available
▸ Risperdal (Janssen-Cilag Ltd)
Risperidone 500 microgram Risperdal 500microgram tablets | 20 tablet [PoM] £5.08 DT price = £0.82
Risperidone 1 mg Risperdal 1mg tablets | 20 tablet [PoM] £8.36 DT price = £0.81 | 60 tablet [PoM] £17.56
Risperidone 2 mg Risperdal 2mg tablets | 60 tablet [PoM] £34.62 DT price = £1.37
Risperidone 3 mg Risperdal 3mg tablets | 60 tablet [PoM] £50.91 DT price = £1.67
Risperidone 4 mg Risperdal 4mg tablets | 60 tablet [PoM] £67.20 DT price = £1.94
Risperidone 6 mg Risperdal 6mg tablets | 28 tablet [PoM] £67.88 DT price = £3.86

Orodispersible tablet
CAUTIONARY AND ADVISORY LABELS 2
EXCIPIENTS: May contain Aspartame
▸ Risperidone (Non-proprietary)
Risperidone 500 microgram Risperidone 500microgram orodispersible tablets sugar free sugar-free | 28 tablet [PoM] £23.88 DT price = £23.86
Risperidone 1 mg Risperidone 1mg orodispersible tablets sugar free sugar-free | 28 tablet [PoM] £21.09 DT price = £21.07
Risperidone 2 mg Risperidone 2mg orodispersible tablets sugar free sugar-free | 28 tablet [PoM] £38.79 DT price = £38.77
Risperidone 3 mg Risperidone 3mg orodispersible tablets sugar free sugar-free | 28 tablet [PoM] £33.50 DT price = £33.50
Risperidone 4 mg Risperidone 4mg orodispersible tablets sugar free sugar-free | 28 tablet [PoM] £37.95 DT price = £37.95
▸ Risperdal Quicklet (Janssen-Cilag Ltd)
Risperidone 500 microgram Risperdal Quicklet 500microgram orodispersible tablets sugar-free | 28 tablet [PoM] £8.23 DT price = £23.86
Risperidone 1 mg Risperdal Quicklet 1mg orodispersible tablets sugar-free | 28 tablet [PoM] £13.86 DT price = £21.07
Risperidone 2 mg Risperdal Quicklet 2mg orodispersible tablets sugar-free | 28 tablet [PoM] £26.12 DT price = £38.77
Risperidone 3 mg Risperdal Quicklet 3mg orodispersible tablets sugar-free | 28 tablet [PoM] £28.99 DT price = £33.50
Risperidone 4 mg Risperdal Quicklet 4mg orodispersible tablets sugar-free | 28 tablet [PoM] £37.34 DT price = £37.95

Oral solution
CAUTIONARY AND ADVISORY LABELS 2
▸ Risperidone (Non-proprietary)
Risperidone 1 mg per 1 ml Risperidone 1mg/ml oral solution sugar free sugar-free | 100 ml [PoM] £61.15 DT price = £4.49

▸ Risperdal (Janssen-Cilag Ltd)
Risperidone 1 mg per 1 ml Risperdal 1mg/ml oral solution sugar-free | 100 ml [PoM] £37.01 DT price = £4.49

Powder and solvent for suspension for injection
▸ Risperdal Consta (Janssen-Cilag Ltd)
Risperidone 25 mg Risperdal Consta 25mg powder and solvent for suspension for injection vials | 1 vial [PoM] £79.69
Risperidone 37.5 mg Risperdal Consta 37.5mg powder and solvent for suspension for injection vials | 1 vial [PoM] £111.32
Risperidone 50 mg Risperdal Consta 50mg powder and solvent for suspension for injection vials | 1 vial [PoM] £142.76

ANTIPSYCHOTICS › SECOND-GENERATION (DEPOT INJECTIONS)

See under individual antipsychotics, second-generation monographs above for details of other depot injections

[☞ 352]

Olanzapine embonate

(Olanzapine pamoate)

● INDICATIONS AND DOSE

Maintenance in schizophrenia in patients tolerant to olanzapine by mouth (patients taking 10 mg oral olanzapine daily)
▸ BY DEEP INTRAMUSCULAR INJECTION
▸ Adult 18-75 years: Initially 210 mg every 2 weeks, alternatively initially 405 mg every 4 weeks, then maintenance 150 mg every 2 weeks, alternatively maintenance 300 mg every 4 weeks, maintenance dose to be started after 2 months of initial treatment, dose to be administered into the gluteal muscle, consult product literature if supplementation with oral olanzapine required

Maintenance in schizophrenia in patients tolerant to olanzapine by mouth (patients taking 15 mg oral olanzapine daily)
▸ BY DEEP INTRAMUSCULAR INJECTION
▸ Adult 18-75 years: Initially 300 mg every 2 weeks, then maintenance 210 mg every 2 weeks, alternatively maintenance 405 mg every 4 weeks, maintenance dose to be started after 2 months of initial treatment, dose to be administered into the gluteal muscle, consult product literature if supplementation with oral olanzapine required

Maintenance in schizophrenia in patients tolerant to olanzapine by mouth (patients taking 20 mg oral olanzapine daily)
▸ BY DEEP INTRAMUSCULAR INJECTION
▸ Adult: Initially 300 mg every 2 weeks, then maintenance 300 mg every 2 weeks (max. per dose 300 mg every 2 weeks), adjusted according to response, dose to be administered into the gluteal muscle, consult product literature if supplementation with oral olanzapine required

DOSE ADJUSTMENTS DUE TO INTERACTIONS
Dose adjustment may be necessary if smoking started or stopped during treatment.

IMPORTANT SAFETY INFORMATION
When prescribing, dispensing or administering, check that this is the correct preparation—this preparation is used for *maintenance* treatment and should **not** be used for the rapid control of an *acute* episode.

● CAUTIONS Bone-marrow depression · diabetes mellitus (risk of exacerbation or ketoacidosis) · hypereosinophilic disorders · low leucocyte count · low neutrophil count · myeloproliferative disease · paralytic ileus · when

transferring from oral to depot therapy, the dose by mouth should be reduced gradually

● SIDE-EFFECTS
▸ **Common or very common** Arthralgia · hypercholesterolaemia · hypertriglyceridaemia · increased appetite · malaise · oedema
▸ **Uncommon** Alopecia · amnesia · bradycardia · epistaxis
▸ **Rare** Hepatitis · pancreatitis · rhabdomyolysis
▸ **Frequency not known** Erythema · nodules · pain at injection site · swelling

SIDE-EFFECTS, FURTHER INFORMATION
If the dose needs to be reduced to alleviate side-effects, it is important to recognise that the plasma-drug concentration may not fall for some time after reducing the dose, therefore it may be a month or longer before side-effects subside.

Overdose
Post-injection reactions have been reported leading to signs and symptoms of overdose.

● PREGNANCY Use only if potential benefit outweighs risk; neonatal lethargy, tremor, and hypertonia reported when used in third trimester.

● BREAST FEEDING Avoid—present in milk.

● HEPATIC IMPAIRMENT Initially 150 mg every 4 weeks; increase with caution in moderate impairment.

● RENAL IMPAIRMENT Initially 150 mg every 4 weeks.

● MONITORING REQUIREMENTS
▸ Observe patient for at least 3 hours after injection.
▸ Treatment requires careful monitoring for optimum effect.
▸ Blood lipids and weight should be measured at baseline, at 3 months (weight should be measured at frequent intervals during the first 3 months), and then yearly with antipsychotic drugs. Patients taking olanzapine require more frequent monitoring of these parameters: every 3 months for the first year, then yearly.
▸ Fasting blood glucose should be measured at baseline, at 4–6 months, and then yearly. Patients taking olanzapine should have fasting blood glucose tested at baseline, after one months' treatment, then every 4–6 months.

● DIRECTIONS FOR ADMINISTRATION Correct injection technique (including use of z-track technique) and rotation of injection sites are essential.

● MEDICINAL FORMS
There can be variation in the licensing of different medicines containing the same drug.

Powder and solvent for suspension for injection
▸ Zypadhera (Eli Lilly and Company Ltd)
Olanzapine (as Olanzapine embonate monohydrate)
210 mg Zypadhera 210mg powder and solvent for suspension for injection vials | 1 vial [PoM] £142.76 (Hospital only)
Olanzapine (as Olanzapine embonate monohydrate)
300 mg Zypadhera 300mg powder and solvent for suspension for injection vials | 1 vial [PoM] £222.64 (Hospital only)
Olanzapine (as Olanzapine embonate monohydrate)
405 mg Zypadhera 405mg powder and solvent for suspension for injection vials | 1 vial [PoM] £285.52 (Hospital only)

4 Movement disorders

4.1 Dystonias and other involuntary movements

> **Drugs used for Dystonias and other involuntary movements not listed below** Chlorpromazine hydrochloride, p. 353 · Clonidine hydrochloride, p. 131 · Clozapine, p. 363 · Diazepam, p. 313 · Haloperidol, p. 354 · Orphenadrine hydrochloride, p. 375 · Pericyazine, p. 355 · Pramipexole, p. 387 · Prochlorperazine, p. 357 · Procyclidine hydrochloride, p. 376 · Ropinirole, p. 388 · Rotigotine, p. 390 · Trifluoperazine, p. 358 · Trihexyphenidyl hydrochloride, p. 376

ANTIPSYCHOTICS > FIRST-GENERATION

352

Promazine hydrochloride

● **INDICATIONS AND DOSE**

Short-term adjunctive management of psychomotor agitation
▸ BY MOUTH
▸ Adult: 100–200 mg 4 times a day

Agitation and restlessness in elderly
▸ BY MOUTH
▸ Elderly: 25–50 mg 4 times a day

● **CONTRA-INDICATIONS** CNS depression · comatose states · phaeochromocytoma
● **CAUTIONS** Cerebral arteriosclerosis
● **SIDE-EFFECTS** Haemolytic anaemia
● **HEPATIC IMPAIRMENT** Can precipitate coma; phenothiazines are hepatotoxic.
● **RENAL IMPAIRMENT** Start with small doses in severe renal impairment because of increased cerebral sensitivity.
● **LESS SUITABLE FOR PRESCRIBING** Promazine hydrochloride is less suitable for prescribing.

● **MEDICINAL FORMS**
There can be variation in the licensing of different medicines containing the same drug. Forms available from special-order manufacturers include: oral suspension, oral solution

Tablet
CAUTIONARY AND ADVISORY LABELS 2
▸ Promazine hydrochloride (Non-proprietary)
  Promazine hydrochloride 25 mg Promazine 25mg tablets | 100 tablet [PoM] £49.99
  Prazine 25mg tablets | 50 tablet [PoM] no price available
  Promazine hydrochloride 50 mg Promazine 50mg tablets | 100 tablet [PoM] £76.49

Oral solution
CAUTIONARY AND ADVISORY LABELS 2
▸ Promazine hydrochloride (Non-proprietary)
  Promazine hydrochloride 5 mg per 1 ml Promazine 25mg/5ml syrup | 150 ml [PoM] £13.00 DT price = £13.21
  Promazine 25mg/5ml oral solution | 150 ml [PoM] £13.41 DT price = £13.21
  Promazine hydrochloride 10 mg per 1 ml Promazine 50mg/5ml syrup | 150 ml [PoM] £15.00 DT price = £15.24
  Promazine 50mg/5ml oral solution | 150 ml [PoM] £15.47 DT price = £15.24

CNS STIMULANTS

Piracetam

● **INDICATIONS AND DOSE**

Adjunctive treatment of cortical myoclonus
▸ BY MOUTH
▸ Adult: Initially 7.2 g daily in 2–3 divided doses, then increased in steps of 4.8 g every 3–4 days, adjusted according to response, subsequently, attempts should be made to reduce dose of concurrent therapy; maximum 24 g per day

● **CONTRA-INDICATIONS** Cerebral haemorrhage · Huntington's chorea
● **CAUTIONS** Gastric ulcer · history of haemorrhagic stroke · increased risk of bleeding · major surgery · underlying disorders of haemostasis
● **INTERACTIONS** Caution with concomitant drugs that increase bleeding.
● **SIDE-EFFECTS**
▸ **Common or very common** Hyperkinesia · nervousness · weight gain
▸ **Uncommon** Abdominal pain · anxiety · asthenia · ataxia · confusion · depression · dermatitis · diarrhoea · drowsiness · haemorrhagic disorder · hallucination · headache · insomnia · nausea · pruritus · urticaria · vertigo · vomiting
● **PREGNANCY** Avoid.
● **BREAST FEEDING** Avoid.
● **HEPATIC IMPAIRMENT** Adjust dose if both hepatic and renal impairment.
● **RENAL IMPAIRMENT** Use two-thirds of normal dose if eGFR 50–80 mL/minute/1.73 m^2; use one-third of normal dose in 2 divided doses if eGFR 30–50 mL/minute/1.73 m^2; use one-sixth of normal dose as a single dose if eGFR 20–30 mL/minute/1.73 m^2. Avoid if eGFR less than 20 mL/minute/1.73 m^2.
● **TREATMENT CESSATION** Avoid abrupt withdrawal.
● **DIRECTIONS FOR ADMINISTRATION** Follow the oral solution with a glass of water (or soft drink) to reduce bitter taste.
● **PRESCRIBING AND DISPENSING INFORMATION** Piracetam has been used in children 16 years and over as adjunctive treatment for cortical myoclonus.

● **MEDICINAL FORMS**
There can be variation in the licensing of different medicines containing the same drug.

Tablet
CAUTIONARY AND ADVISORY LABELS 3
▸ Nootropil (UCB Pharma Ltd)
  Piracetam 800 mg Nootropil 800mg tablets | 90 tablet [PoM] £11.75
  Piracetam 1.2 gram Nootropil 1.2g tablets | 60 tablet [PoM] £10.97

Oral solution
CAUTIONARY AND ADVISORY LABELS 3
▸ Piracetam (Non-proprietary)
  Piracetam 333.3 mg per 1 ml Piracetam 333.3mg/ml oral solution sugar free sugar-free | 300 ml [PoM] no price available
▸ Nootropil (UCB Pharma Ltd)
  Piracetam 333.3 mg per 1 ml Nootropil 33% oral solution sugar-free | 300 ml [PoM] £16.31

4

Nervous system

Nervous system

4

MONOAMINE DEPLETING DRUGS

Tetrabenazine

- **INDICATIONS AND DOSE**

Movement disorders due to Huntington's chorea, hemiballismus, senile chorea, and related neurological conditions
▸ BY MOUTH
▸ Adult: Initially 25 mg 3 times a day, then increased, if tolerated, in steps of 25 mg every 3–4 days; maximum 200 mg per day
▸ Elderly: Lower initial dose may be necessary

Moderate to severe tardive dyskinesia
▸ BY MOUTH
▸ Adult: Initially 12.5 mg daily, dose to be gradually increased according to response

- **CONTRA-INDICATIONS** Depression · parkinsonism · phaeochromocytoma · prolactin-dependent tumours
- **CAUTIONS** Susceptibility to QT-interval prolongation
- **INTERACTIONS** → Appendix 1 (tetrabenazine). Caution with concomitant use of drugs that prolong QT interval.
- **SIDE-EFFECTS**
▸ **Common or very common** Anxiety · confusion · constipation · depression · diarrhoea · drowsiness · dysphagia · hypotension · insomnia · nausea · parkinsonism · vomiting
▸ **Uncommon** Altered consciousness level · extrapyramidal disorders · hyperthermia
▸ **Rare** Neuroleptic malignant syndrome
▸ **Very rare** Rhabdomyolysis
▸ **Frequency not known** Agitation · amnesia · ataxia · bradycardia · disorientation · dizziness · dry mouth · dyspepsia
- **PREGNANCY** Avoid unless essential—toxicity in *animal* studies.
- **BREAST FEEDING** Avoid.
- **HEPATIC IMPAIRMENT** Use half initial dose and slower titration in mild to moderate impairment. Use with caution in severe impairment.
- **RENAL IMPAIRMENT** Use with caution.
- **TREATMENT CESSATION** Avoid abrupt withdrawal.
- **PATIENT AND CARER ADVICE**
Driving and skilled tasks
May affect performance of skilled tasks (e.g. driving).
- **MEDICINAL FORMS**
There can be variation in the licensing of different medicines containing the same drug. Forms available from special-order manufacturers include: oral suspension

Tablet
CAUTIONARY AND ADVISORY LABELS 2
▸ Revocon (Sun Pharmaceuticals UK Ltd)
Tetrabenazine 25 mg Revocon 25mg tablets | 112 tablet [PoM] £100.00 DT price = £100.00
▸ Tetmodis (Beacon Pharmaceuticals Ltd)
Tetrabenazine 25 mg Tetmodis 25mg tablets | 112 tablet [PoM] £100.00 DT price = £100.00
▸ Xenazine (Alliance Pharmaceuticals Ltd)
Tetrabenazine 25 mg Xenazine 25 tablets | 112 tablet [PoM] £100.00 DT price = £100.00

MUSCLE RELAXANTS ⟩ PERIPHERALLY ACTING ⟩ NEUROTOXINS (BOTULINUM TOXINS)

Botulinum toxin type A

- **INDICATIONS AND DOSE**

Treatment of focal spasticity (including hand and wrist disability associated with stroke) (specialist use only) | Blepharospasm (specialist use only) | Hemifacial spasm (specialist use only) | Spasmodic torticollis (specialist use only) | Severe hyperhidrosis of the axillae (specialist use only) | Prophylaxis of headaches in adults with chronic migraine (specialist use only) | Temporary improvement of moderate to severe wrinkles between the eyebrows in adults under 65 years (specialist use only) | Ankle disability due to lower limb spasticity associated with stroke (specialist use only) | Management of bladder dysfunctions (specialist use only) | Temporary improvement of moderate to severe crow's feet (specialist use only)
▸ BY SUBCUTANEOUS INJECTION, OR BY INTRADERMAL INJECTION, OR BY INTRAMUSCULAR INJECTION
▸ Adult: (consult product literature)

DOSE EQUIVALENCE AND CONVERSION
Important: information is specific to each individual preparation.

- **CONTRA-INDICATIONS** Acute urinary retention (specific to use in bladder disorders only) · catheterisation difficulties (specific to use in bladder disorders only) · generalised disorders of muscle activity · infection at injection site · myasthenia gravis · presence of bladder calculi (specific to use in bladder disorders only) · urinary tract infection (specific to use in bladder disorders only)
- **CAUTIONS**
GENERAL CAUTIONS
Atrophy in target muscle · chronic respiratory disorder · elderly · excessive weakness in target muscle · history of aspiration · history of dysphagia · inflammation in target muscle · neurological disorders · neuromuscular disorders · off-label use (fatal adverse events reported)
SPECIFIC CAUTIONS
▸ When used for blepharospasm or hemifacial spasm Risk of angle-closure glaucoma
CAUTIONS, FURTHER INFORMATION
Neuromuscular or neurological disorders can lead to increased sensitivity and exaggerated muscle weakness including dysphagia and respiratory compromise.
▸ Blepharospasm or hemifacial spasm When used for blepharospasm and hemifacial spasm, reduced blinking can lead to corneal exposure, persistent epithelial defect and corneal ulceration (especially in those with VIIth nerve disorders)—careful testing of corneal sensation in previously operated eyes, avoidance of injection in lower lid area to avoid ectropion, and vigorous treatment of epithelial defect needed.
- **SIDE-EFFECTS**
GENERAL SIDE-EFFECTS
▸ **Common or very common** Excessive doses may paralyse distant muscles · increased electrophysiologic jitter in some distant muscles · influenza-like symptoms · misplaced injections may paralyse nearby muscle groups
▸ **Rare** Antibody formation (substantial deterioration in response) · arrhythmias · myocardial infarction · seizures
▸ **Very rare** Aspiration · dysphagia · dysphonia · exaggerated muscle weakness · respiratory disorders

SPECIFIC SIDE-EFFECTS
▸ **Common or very common**
▸ When used for axillary hyperhidrosis Abnormal skin odour · alopecia · hot flushes · non-axillary sweating · paraesthesia · pruritus · subcutaneous nodule
▸ When used for blepharospasm Dry eye · ecchymosis · facial oedema · irritation · keratitis · lacrimation · lagophthalmos · photophobia · ptosis
▸ When used for focal upper-limb spasticity associated with stroke Dysphagia · hypertonia · purpura
▸ When used for hemifacial spasm Dry eye · ecchymosis · facial oedema · irritation · keratitis · lacrimation · lagophthalmos · photophobia · ptosis
▸ When used for spasmodic torticollis Back pain · dizziness · drowsiness · dry mouth · dysphagia and pooling of saliva (occurs most frequently after injection into sternomastoid muscle) · headache · hypertonia · malaise · nausea · numbness · rhinitis · stiffness · weakness
▸ When used for temporary improvement of moderate to severe wrinkles between the eyebrows Facial oedema · headache · ptosis
▸ When used for axillary hyperhidrosis Pain in extremities
▸ **Uncommon**
▸ When used for axillary hyperhidrosis Joint pain · myalgia
▸ When used for blepharospasm Conjunctivitis · dermatitis · diplopia · dizziness · drooping · dry mouth · ectropion · entropion · facial weakness · headache · paraesthesia · tiredness · visual disturbances
▸ When used for focal upper-limb spasticity associated with stroke Amnesia · arthralgia · bursitis · cough · depression · dry mouth · dysaesthesia · haematoma · headache · insomnia · malaise · pain in extremities · paraesthesia · peripheral oedema · vertigo
▸ When used for focal upper-limb specificity associated with stroke Nausea
▸ When used for hemifacial spasm Conjunctivitis · dermatitis · diplopia · dizziness · drooping · dry mouth · ectropion · entropion · facial weakness · headache · paraesthesia · tiredness · visual disturbances
▸ When used for spasmodic torticollis Colitis · diarrhoea · diplopia · dyspnoea · eye pain · myalgia · ptosis · skeletal pain · sweating · tremor · voice alteration · vomiting
▸ When used for temporary improvement of moderate to severe wrinkles between the eyebrows Anxiety · asthenia · blepharitis · dizziness · dry mouth · dry skin · muscle cramp · nausea · paraesthesia · photosensitivity reactions · tinnitus · visual disturbances
▸ **Rare**
▸ When used for blepharospasm Eyelid bruising and swelling (minimised by applying gentle pressure at injection site immediately after injection)
▸ When used for hemifacial spasm Eyelid bruising and swelling (minimised by applying gentle pressure at injection site immediately after injection)
▸ **Very rare**
▸ When used for blepharospasm Angle-closure glaucoma · corneal epithelial defect · corneal perforation · corneal ulceration
▸ When used for hemifacial spasm Angle-closure glaucoma · corneal epithelial defect · corneal perforation · corneal ulceration
▸ **Frequency not known**
▸ When used for focal lower-limb spasticity associated with stroke Arthralgia · peripheral oedema · rash
● CONCEPTION AND CONTRACEPTION Avoid in women of child-bearing age unless using effective contraception.
● PREGNANCY Avoid unless essential—toxicity in *animal* studies (manufacturer of *Botox*® advise avoid).
● BREAST FEEDING Low risk of systemic absorption but avoid unless essential.
● PRESCRIBING AND DISPENSING INFORMATION Preparations are not interchangeable.

● PATIENT AND CARER ADVICE Patients and carers should be warned of the signs and symptoms of toxin spread, such as muscle weakness and breathing difficulties; they should be advised to seek immediate medical attention if swallowing, speech or breathing difficulties occur.
● NATIONAL FUNDING/ACCESS DECISIONS
NICE technology appraisals (TAs)
▸ Botulinum toxin type A for the prevention of headaches in adults with chronic migraine (June 2012) NICE TA260 Botulinum toxin type A is recommended as an option for the prophylaxis of headaches in adults with chronic migraine, (defined as headaches on at least 15 days per month, of which at least 8 days are with migraine), that has not responded to at least three prior pharmacological prophylaxis therapies and whose condition is appropriately managed for medication overuse.
www.nice.org.uk/TA260
Scottish Medicines Consortium (SMC) Decisions
The *Scottish Medicines Consortium* has advised (March 2011 and March 2013) that *Botox*® is **not** recommended for use within NHS Scotland for prophylaxis of headaches in adults with chronic migraine.
   The *Scottish Medicines Consortium* has advised that *Azzalure*® and *Vistabel*® (December 2010), and *Bocouture*® (February 2011) are **not** recommended for use within NHS Scotland.

● MEDICINAL FORMS
There can be variation in the licensing of different medicines containing the same drug.
Powder for solution for injection
▸ Azzalure (Galderma (UK) Ltd)
   Botulinum toxin type A 125 unit Azzalure 125unit powder for solution for injection vials | 1 vial [PoM] £64.00 | 2 vial [PoM] £128.00
▸ Bocouture (Merz Pharma UK Ltd)
   Botulinum toxin type A 50 unit Bocouture 50unit powder for solution for injection vials | 1 vial [PoM] £72.00
▸ Botox (Allergan Ltd)
   Botulinum toxin type A 50 unit Botox 50unit powder for solution for injection vials | 1 vial [PoM] £77.50
   Botulinum toxin type A 100 unit Botox 100unit powder for solution for injection vials | 1 vial [PoM] £138.20
   Botulinum toxin type A 200 unit Botox 200unit powder for solution for injection vials | 1 vial [PoM] £276.40
▸ Dysport (Ipsen Ltd)
   Botulinum toxin type A 300 unit Dysport 300unit powder for solution for injection vials | 1 vial [PoM] £92.40
   Botulinum toxin type A 500 unit Dysport 500unit powder for solution for injection vials | 2 vial [PoM] £308.00
▸ Xeomin (Merz Pharma UK Ltd)
   Botulinum toxin type A 50 unit Xeomin 50unit powder for solution for injection vials | 1 vial [PoM] £72.00
   Botulinum toxin type A 100 unit Xeomin 100unit powder for solution for injection vials | 1 vial [PoM] £129.90

Botulinum toxin type B

● INDICATIONS AND DOSE
Spasmodic torticollis (cervical dystonia) (specialist use only)
▸ BY INTRAMUSCULAR INJECTION
▸ Adult: Initially 5000–10 000 units, adjusted according to response, dose to be divided between 2–4 most affected muscles

DOSE EQUIVALENCE AND CONVERSION
Important: information specific to each individual preparation.

● CONTRA-INDICATIONS Neuromuscular disorders · neuromuscular junctional disorders
● CAUTIONS History of dysphagia or aspiration · off-label use (risk of toxin spread) · tolerance may occur

4

Nervous system

4

Nervous system

- SIDE-EFFECTS
- ▶ **Common or very common** Dry mouth · dyspepsia · dysphagia · dysphonia · headache · increased electrophysiologic jitter in some distant muscles · influenza-like symptoms · myasthenia · neck pain · taste disturbances · visual disturbances · worsening torticollis
- ▶ **Frequency not known** Aspiration pneumonia · constipation · exaggerated muscle weakness · malaise · ptosis · respiratory disorders · vomiting
- PREGNANCY Low risk of systemic absorption but avoid unless essential.
- BREAST FEEDING Low risk of systemic absorption but avoid unless essential.
- DIRECTIONS FOR ADMINISTRATION Injection may be diluted with sodium chloride 0.9%.
- PRESCRIBING AND DISPENSING INFORMATION **Important: not** interchangeable with other botulinum toxin preparations.
- PATIENT AND CARER ADVICE Patients should be warned of the signs and symptoms of toxin spread, such as muscle weakness and breathing difficulties; they should be advised to seek immediate medical attention if swallowing, speech or breathing difficulties occur.

- MEDICINAL FORMS
  There can be variation in the licensing of different medicines containing the same drug.
  Solution for injection
  ▶ NeuroBloc (Eisai Ltd)
  Botulinum toxin type B 5000 unit per 1 ml NeuroBloc 5,000units/1ml solution for injection vials | 1 vial [PoM] £148.27 (Hospital only)
  NeuroBloc 10,000units/2ml solution for injection vials | 1 vial [PoM] £197.69 (Hospital only)
  NeuroBloc 2,500units/0.5ml solution for injection vials | 1 vial [PoM] £111.20 (Hospital only)

NEUROPROTECTIVE DRUGS

Tafamidis

- INDICATIONS AND DOSE
  Treatment of transthyretin familial amyloid polyneuropathy (TTR-FAP) in patients with stage 1 symptomatic polyneuropathy to delay peripheral neurological impairment (initiated under specialist supervision)
  ▶ BY MOUTH
  ▶ Adult: 20 mg once daily

- SIDE-EFFECTS Abdominal pain · diarrhoea · urinary tract infection · vaginal infection
- CONCEPTION AND CONTRACEPTION Exclude pregnancy before treatment and ensure effective contraception during and for one month after stopping treatment.
- PREGNANCY Avoid (toxicity in *animal* studies).
- BREAST FEEDING Avoid—present in milk in *animal* studies.
- HEPATIC IMPAIRMENT Caution in severe impairment—no information available.
- PRESCRIBING AND DISPENSING INFORMATION Tafamidis should be prescribed in addition to standard treatment, but before liver transplantation; it should be discontinued in patients who undergo liver transplantation.

- MEDICINAL FORMS
  There can be variation in the licensing of different medicines containing the same drug.
  Capsule
  CAUTIONARY AND ADVISORY LABELS 25
  ▶ Vyndagel (Pfizer Ltd) ▼
  Tafamidis 20 mg Vyndagel 20mg capsules | 30 capsule [PoM] £10,685.00

4.2 Parkinson's disease

Parkinson's disease and related disorders

Parkinson's disease
In idiopathic Parkinson's disease, the progressive degeneration of pigmented neurones in the substantia nigra leads to a deficiency of the neurotransmitter dopamine. The resulting neurochemical imbalance in the basal ganglia causes the characteristic signs and symptoms of the illness. Drug therapy does not prevent disease progression, but it improves most patients' quality of life.

Patients with suspected Parkinson's disease should be referred to a specialist to confirm the diagnosis; the diagnosis should be reviewed every 6–12 months.

Features resembling those of Parkinson's disease can occur in diseases such as progressive supranuclear palsy and multiple system atrophy, but they do not normally show a sustained response to the drugs used in the treatment of idiopathic Parkinson's disease.

When initiating treatment, patients should be advised about its limitations and possible side-effects. About 5–10% of patients with Parkinson's disease respond poorly to treatment.

Treatment is usually not started until symptoms cause significant disruption of daily activities. **Levodopa, non-ergot-derived dopamine-receptor agonists**, or **monoamine-oxidase-B inhibitors** can be prescribed for initial treatment in early Parkinson's disease. Therapy with two or more antiparkinsonian drugs may be necessary as the disease progresses. Most patients eventually require levodopa and subsequently develop motor complications.

Elderly
Antiparkinsonian drugs can cause confusion in the elderly. It is particularly important to initiate treatment with low doses and to increase the dose gradually.

Dopaminergic drugs used in Parkinson's disease
Dopamine-receptor agonists
The dopamine-receptor agonists have a direct action on dopamine receptors. Initial treatment of Parkinson's disease is often with the dopamine-receptor agonists pramipexole p. 387, ropinirole p. 388, and rotigotine p. 390. The ergot-derived dopamine-receptor agonists bromocriptine p. 383, cabergoline p. 385, and pergolide p. 386 are rarely used because of the risk of fibrotic reactions.

When used alone, dopamine-receptor agonists cause fewer motor complications in long-term treatment compared with levodopa treatment but the overall motor performance improves slightly less. The dopamine-receptor agonists are associated with more psychiatric side-effects than levodopa.

Dopamine-receptor agonists are also used with levodopa in more advanced disease. If a dopamine-receptor agonist is added to levodopa therapy, the dose of levodopa needs to be reduced.

Apomorphine hydrochloride p. 382 is a potent dopamine-receptor agonist that is sometimes helpful in advanced disease for patients experiencing unpredictable 'off' periods with levodopa treatment. Apomorphine hydrochloride should be initiated in a specialist clinic. After an overnight withdrawal of oral antiparkinsonian medication to induce an 'off' episode, the threshold dose of apomorphine hydrochloride is determined. Oral antiparkinsonian medication is then restarted. The patient must be taught to self-administer apomorphine hydrochloride by subcutaneous injection into the lower abdomen or outer thigh at the first sign of an 'off' episode. Once treatment has been established it may be possible to gradually reduce other antiparkinsonian medications.

Levodopa

Levodopa, the amino-acid precursor of dopamine, acts by replenishing depleted striatal dopamine. It is given with an extracerebral **dopa-decarboxylase inhibitor**, which reduces the peripheral conversion of levodopa to dopamine, thereby limiting side-effects such as nausea, vomiting, and cardiovascular effects; additionally, effective brain-dopamine concentrations are achieved with lower doses of levodopa. The extracerebral dopa-decarboxylase inhibitors used with levodopa are benserazide (in co-beneldopa p. 379) and carbidopa (in co-careldopa p. 380).

Levodopa, in combination with a dopa-decarboxylase inhibitor, is useful in the elderly or frail, in patients with other significant illnesses, and in those with more severe symptoms. It is effective and well tolerated in the majority of patients.

Levodopa therapy should be initiated at a low dose and increased in small steps; the final dose should be as low as possible. Intervals between doses should be chosen to suit the needs of the individual patient.

Nausea and vomiting with co-beneldopa or co-careldopa are rarely dose-limiting and domperidone p. 394 can be useful in controlling these effects.

Levodopa treatment is associated with potentially troublesome motor complications including response fluctuations and dyskinesias. Response fluctuations are characterised by large variations in motor performance, with normal function during the 'on' period, and weakness and restricted mobility during the 'off' period. 'End-of-dose' deterioration with progressively shorter duration of benefit also occurs. Modified-release preparations may help with 'end-of-dose' deterioration or nocturnal immobility and rigidity. Motor complications are particularly problematic in young patients treated with levodopa.

Monoamine-oxidase-B inhibitors

Rasagiline p. 391 and selegiline hydrochloride p. 391 are monoamine-oxidase-B inhibitors used in Parkinson's disease. Early treatment with selegiline hydrochloride alone can delay the need for levodopa therapy.

Antimuscarinic drugs used in parkinsonism

Antimuscarinic drugs can be useful in drug-induced parkinsonism, but they are generally not used in idiopathic Parkinson's disease because they are less effective than dopaminergic drugs and they are associated with cognitive impairment.

The antimuscarinic drugs orphenadrine hydrochloride below, procyclidine hydrochloride p. 376, and trihexyphenidyl hydrochloride p. 376 reduce the symptoms of parkinsonism induced by antipsychotic drugs, but there is no justification for giving them routinely in the absence of parkinsonian side-effects. Tardive dyskinesia is not improved by antimuscarinic drugs and may be made worse.

In idiopathic Parkinson's disease, antimuscarinic drugs reduce tremor and rigidity but they have little effect on bradykinesia. They may be useful in reducing sialorrhoea.

There are no important differences between the antimuscarinic drugs, but some patients tolerate one better than another.

Procyclidine hydrochloride can be given parenterally and is effective emergency treatment for acute drug-induced dystonic reactions.

If treatment with an antimuscarinic is ineffective, intravenous diazepam p. 313 can be given for life-threatening acute drug-induced dystonic reactions.

Drugs used in essential tremor, chorea, tics, and related disorders

Tetrabenazine p. 372 is mainly used to control movement disorders in Huntington's chorea and related disorders. Tetrabenazine can also be prescribed for the treatment of tardive dyskinesia if switching or withdrawing the causative antipsychotic drug is not effective. It acts by depleting nerve endings of dopamine. It is effective in only a proportion of patients and its use may be limited by the development of depression.

Haloperidol p. 354 [unlicensed indication], olanzapine p. 365 [unlicensed indication], risperidone p. 368 [unlicensed indication], and quetiapine p. 367 [unlicensed indication], can also be used to suppress chorea in Huntington's disease.

Haloperidol can also improve motor tics and symptoms of Tourette syndrome and related choreas. Other treatments for Tourette syndrome include pimozide p. 356 [unlicensed indication] (**important**: ECG monitoring required), clonidine hydrochloride p. 131 [unlicensed indication], and sulpiride p. 357 [unlicensed indication]. Trihexyphenidyl hydrochloride in high dosage can also improve some movement disorders; it is sometimes necessary to build the dose up over many weeks. Chlorpromazine hydrochloride p. 353 and haloperidol are used to relieve intractable hiccup.

Propranolol hydrochloride p. 136 or another beta-adrenoceptor blocking drug may be useful in treating essential tremor or tremors associated with anxiety or thyrotoxicosis.

Primidone p. 305 in some cases provides relief from benign essential tremor; the dose is increased slowly to reduce side-effects.

Piracetam p. 371 is used as an adjunctive treatment for myoclonus of cortical origin. After an acute episode, attempts should be made every 6 months to decrease or discontinue treatment.

Riluzole p. 970 is used to extend life in patients with motor neurone disease who have amyotrophic lateral sclerosis.

Torsion dystonia and other involuntary movements

Treatment with botulinum toxin type A p. 372 can be considered after an acquired non-progressive brain injury if rapid-onset spasticity causes postural or functional difficulties.

ANTIMUSCARINICS

Orphenadrine hydrochloride

- DRUG ACTION Orphenadrine exerts its antiparkinsonian action by reducing the effects of the relative central cholinergic excess that occurs as a result of dopamine deficiency.

- INDICATIONS AND DOSE

Parkinsonism | Drug-induced extrapyramidal symptoms (but not tardive dyskinesia)
▸ BY MOUTH
▸ Adult: Initially 150 mg daily in divided doses, then increased in steps of 50 mg every 2–3 days, adjusted according to response; usual dose 150–300 mg daily in divided doses; maximum 400 mg per day
▸ Elderly: Preferably dose at lower end of range

- CONTRA-INDICATIONS Acute porphyrias p. 918 · gastro-intestinal obstruction · myasthenia gravis
- CAUTIONS Cardiovascular disease · elderly · hypertension · in patients susceptible to angle-closure glaucoma · liable to abuse · prostatic hypertrophy · psychotic disorders · pyrexia
- INTERACTIONS → Appendix 1 (antimuscarinics).

Many drugs have antimuscarinic effects; concomitant use of two or more such drugs can increase side-effects such as dry mouth, urine retention, and constipation. Concomitant use of other drugs with antimuscarinic effects can also lead to confusion in the elderly.

- SIDE-EFFECTS
  ► **Common or very common** Urinary retention
  ► **Uncommon** Drowsiness · impaired coordination · insomnia · seizures
  ► **Very rare** Angle-closure glaucoma
  ► **Frequency not known** Anxiety · blurred vision · confusion · constipation · dizziness · dry mouth · euphoria · hallucinations · impaired memory · nausea · rash · restlessness · tachycardia · vomiting
- PREGNANCY Caution.
- BREAST FEEDING Caution.
- HEPATIC IMPAIRMENT Use with caution.
- RENAL IMPAIRMENT Use with caution.
- TREATMENT CESSATION Avoid abrupt withdrawal in patients taking long-term treatment.
- PATIENT AND CARER ADVICE
  Driving and skilled tasks
  May affect performance of skilled tasks (e.g. driving).

- MEDICINAL FORMS
  There can be variation in the licensing of different medicines containing the same drug. Forms available from special-order manufacturers include: oral solution
  Tablet
  EXCIPIENTS: May contain Tartrazine
  ► Orphenadrine hydrochloride (Non-proprietary)
  Orphenadrine hydrochloride 50 mg Orphenadrine 50mg tablets | 100 tablet [PoM] £80.00 | 250 tablet [PoM] no price available
  Oral solution
  ► Orphenadrine hydrochloride (Non-proprietary)
  Orphenadrine hydrochloride 10 mg per 1 ml Orphenadrine 50mg/5ml oral solution sugar free sugar-free | 150 ml [PoM] £32.49 DT price = £32.87

Procyclidine hydrochloride

- DRUG ACTION Procyclidine exerts its antiparkinsonian action by reducing the effects of the relative central cholinergic excess that occurs as a result of dopamine deficiency.

- INDICATIONS AND DOSE

Parkinsonism | Extrapyramidal symptoms (but not tardive dyskinesia)
  ► BY MOUTH
  ► Adult: 2.5 mg 3 times a day, then increased in steps of 2.5–5 mg daily if required; increased if necessary up to 30 mg daily in 2–4 divided doses, to be increased at 2–3 day intervals. Maximum daily dose only to be used in exceptional circumstances; maximum 60 mg per day
  ► Elderly: Lower end of range preferable

Acute dystonia
  ► BY INTRAMUSCULAR INJECTION, OR BY INTRAVENOUS INJECTION
  ► Adult: 5–10 mg, occasionally, more than 10 mg, dose usually effective in 5–10 minutes but may need 30 minutes for relief
  ► Elderly: Lower end of range preferable

- CONTRA-INDICATIONS Gastro-intestinal obstruction · myasthenia gravis
- CAUTIONS Cardiovascular disease · elderly · hypertension · liable to abuse · prostatic hypertrophy · psychotic disorders · pyrexia · those susceptible to angle-closure glaucoma
- INTERACTIONS → Appendix 1 (antimuscarinics).

Many drugs have antimuscarinic effects; concomitant use of two or more such drugs can increase side-effects such as dry mouth, urine retention, and constipation. Concomitant use of other drugs with antimuscarinic effects can also lead to confusion in the elderly.

- SIDE-EFFECTS Angle-closure glaucoma · anxiety · blurred vision · confusion · constipation · dizziness · dry mouth · euphoria · gingivitis · hallucinations · impaired memory · nausea · rash · restlessness · tachycardia · urinary retention · vomiting
- PREGNANCY Use only if potential benefit outweighs risk.
- BREAST FEEDING No information available.
- HEPATIC IMPAIRMENT Use with caution.
- RENAL IMPAIRMENT Use with caution.
- TREATMENT CESSATION Avoid abrupt withdrawal in patients taking long-term treatment.
- PATIENT AND CARER ADVICE
  Driving and skilled tasks
  May affect performance of skilled tasks (e.g. driving).

- MEDICINAL FORMS
  There can be variation in the licensing of different medicines containing the same drug. Forms available from special-order manufacturers include: oral suspension, oral solution
  Tablet
  ► Procyclidine hydrochloride (Non-proprietary)
  Procyclidine hydrochloride 5 mg Procyclidine 5mg tablets | 28 tablet [PoM] £17.25 DT price = £11.97 | 100 tablet [PoM] £50.00 | 500 tablet [PoM] £255.00
  ► Kemadrin (Aspen Pharma Trading Ltd)
  Procyclidine hydrochloride 5 mg Kemadrin 5mg tablets | 100 tablet [PoM] £4.72 | 500 tablet [PoM] £23.62
  Oral solution
  ► Procyclidine hydrochloride (Non-proprietary)
  Procyclidine hydrochloride 500 microgram per 1 ml Procyclidine 2.5mg/5ml oral solution sugar free sugar-free | 150 ml [PoM] £6.22 DT price = £4.22
  Procyclidine hydrochloride 1 mg per 1 ml Procyclidine 5mg/5ml oral solution sugar free sugar-free | 150 ml [PoM] £11.54 DT price = £7.54
  ► Arpicolin (Rosemont Pharmaceuticals Ltd)
  Procyclidine hydrochloride 500 microgram per 1 ml Arpicolin 2.5mg/5ml oral solution sugar-free | 150 ml [PoM] £4.22 DT price = £4.22
  Procyclidine hydrochloride 1 mg per 1 ml Arpicolin 5mg/5ml oral solution sugar-free | 150 ml [PoM] £7.54 DT price = £7.54
  Solution for injection
  ► Procyclidine hydrochloride (Non-proprietary)
  Procyclidine hydrochloride 5 mg per 1 ml Procyclidine 10mg/2ml solution for injection ampoules | 5 ampoule [PoM] £60.00–£78.75 DT price = £72.18

Trihexyphenidyl hydrochloride

(Benzhexol hydrochloride)

- DRUG ACTION Trihexyphenidyl exerts its effects by reducing the effects of the relative central cholinergic excess that occurs as a result of dopamine deficiency.

- INDICATIONS AND DOSE

Parkinson's disease (if used in combination with co-careldopa or co-beneldopa)
  ► Adult: Maintenance 2–6 mg daily in divided doses, use not recommended because of toxicity in the elderly and the risk of aggravating dementia

Parkinsonism | Drug-induced extrapyramidal symptoms (but not tardive dyskinesia)
  ► BY MOUTH
  ► Adult: 1 mg daily, then increased in steps of 2 mg every 3–5 days, adjusted according to response; maintenance 5–15 mg daily in 3–4 divided doses, not recommended for use in Parkinson's disease because of toxicity in the

elderly and the risk of aggravating dementia; maximum 20 mg per day
▸ Elderly: Lower end of range preferable, not recommended for use in Parkinson's disease because of toxicity in the elderly and the risk of aggravating dementia

● CONTRA-INDICATIONS Gastro-intestinal obstruction · myasthenia gravis
● CAUTIONS Cardiovascular disease · elderly · hypertension · liable to abuse · prostatic hypertrophy · psychotic disorders · pyrexia · those susceptible to angle-closure glaucoma
● INTERACTIONS → Appendix 1 (antimuscarinics). Many drugs have antimuscarinic effects; concomitant use of two or more such drugs can increase side-effects such as dry mouth, urine retention, and constipation. Concomitant use of other drugs with antimuscarinic effects can also lead to confusion in the elderly.
● SIDE-EFFECTS
▸ Very rare Angle-closure glaucoma
▸ Frequency not known Anxiety · blurred vision · confusion · constipation · dizziness · dry mouth · euphoria · hallucinations · impaired memory · nausea · rash · restlessness · tachycardia · urinary retention · vomiting
● PREGNANCY Use only if potential benefit outweighs risk.
● BREAST FEEDING Avoid.
● HEPATIC IMPAIRMENT Use with caution.
● RENAL IMPAIRMENT Use with caution.
● TREATMENT CESSATION Avoid abrupt withdrawal in patients taking long-term treatment.
● DIRECTIONS FOR ADMINISTRATION Tablets should be taken with or after food.
● PATIENT AND CARER ADVICE
Driving and skilled tasks
May affect performance of skilled tasks (e.g. driving).

● MEDICINAL FORMS
There can be variation in the licensing of different medicines containing the same drug. Forms available from special-order manufacturers include: oral suspension, oral solution
Tablet
▸ Trihexyphenidyl hydrochloride (Non-proprietary)
Trihexyphenidyl hydrochloride 2 mg Trihexyphenidyl 2mg tablets | 84 tablet [PoM] £11.80 DT price = £5.51
Trihexyphenidyl hydrochloride 5 mg Trihexyphenidyl 5mg tablets | 84 tablet [PoM] £17.91 DT price = £17.91
Oral solution
EXCIPIENTS: May contain Propylene glycol
▸ Trihexyphenidyl hydrochloride (Non-proprietary)
Trihexyphenidyl hydrochloride 1 mg per 1 ml Trihexyphenidyl 5mg/5ml oral solution | 200 ml [PoM] £20.00–£24.00 DT price = £20.00

DOPAMINERGIC DRUGS > CATECHOL-O-METHYLTRANSFERASE INHIBITORS

Entacapone

● DRUG ACTION Entacapone prevents the peripheral breakdown of levodopa, by inhibiting catechol-*O*-methyltransferase, allowing more levodopa to reach the brain.

● INDICATIONS AND DOSE
Adjunct to co-beneldopa or co-careldopa in Parkinson's disease with 'end-of-dose' motor fluctuations (under expert supervision)
▸ BY MOUTH
▸ Adult: 200 mg, dose to be given with each dose of levodopa with dopa-decarboxylase inhibitor; maximum 2 g per day

● CONTRA-INDICATIONS History of neuroleptic malignant syndrome · history of non-traumatic rhabdomyolysis · phaeochromocytoma
● CAUTIONS Concurrent levodopa dose may need to be reduced by about 10–30% · ischaemic heart disease
● INTERACTIONS → Appendix 1 (entacapone). Avoid iron-containing products at the same time of day.
● SIDE-EFFECTS
▸ Common or very common Abdominal pain · abnormal dreams · confusion · constipation · diarrhoea · dizziness · dry mouth · dyskinesia · dystonia · fatigue · hallucinations · insomnia · ischaemic heart disease · nausea · sweating · urine may be coloured reddish-brown · vomiting
▸ Uncommon Myocardial infarction
▸ Rare Rash
▸ Very rare Agitation · anorexia · urticaria · weight loss
▸ Frequency not known Colitis · hepatitis · neuroleptic malignant syndrome · rhabdomyolysis · skin, hair, and nail discoloration
● PREGNANCY Avoid—no information available.
● BREAST FEEDING Avoid—present in milk in *animal* studies.
● HEPATIC IMPAIRMENT Avoid.
● TREATMENT CESSATION Avoid abrupt withdrawal.
● PATIENT AND CARER ADVICE Patient counselling is advised (may colour urine reddish-brown, concomitant iron containing products).

● MEDICINAL FORMS
There can be variation in the licensing of different medicines containing the same drug. Forms available from special-order manufacturers include: oral suspension, oral solution
Tablet
CAUTIONARY AND ADVISORY LABELS 14
▸ Entacapone (Non-proprietary)
Entacapone 200 mg Entacapone 200mg tablets | 30 tablet [PoM] £16.38 DT price = £5.20 | 100 tablet [PoM] £54.58
▸ Comtess (Orion Pharma (UK) Ltd)
Entacapone 200 mg Comtess 200mg tablets | 30 tablet [PoM] £17.24 DT price = £5.20 | 100 tablet [PoM] £57.45

Combinations available: *Carbidopa with entacapone and levodopa*, p. 378

Tolcapone

● DRUG ACTION Tolcapone prevents the peripheral breakdown of levodopa, by inhibiting catechol-*O*-methyltransferase, allowing more levodopa to reach the brain.

● INDICATIONS AND DOSE
Adjunct to co-beneldopa or co-careldopa in Parkinson's disease with 'end-of-dose' motor fluctuations if another inhibitor of peripheral catechol-O-methyltransferase inappropriate (under expert supervision)
▸ BY MOUTH
▸ Adult: 100 mg 3 times a day (max. per dose 200 mg 3 times a day) continuing beyond 3 weeks **only** if substantial improvement, leave 6 hours between each dose; first daily dose should be taken at the same time as levodopa with dopa-decarboxylase inhibitor, dose maximum only in exceptional circumstances

● CONTRA-INDICATIONS Phaeochromocytoma · previous history of hyperthermia · previous history of neuroleptic malignant syndrome · previous history of rhabdomyolysis · severe dyskinesia
● CAUTIONS Most patients receiving more than 600 mg levodopa daily require reduction of levodopa dose by about 30%

CAUTIONS, FURTHER INFORMATION
▸ **Hepatotoxicity** Potentially life-threatening hepatotoxicity including fulminant hepatitis reported rarely, usually in women and during the first 6 months, but late-onset liver injury also reported; discontinue if abnormal liver function tests or symptoms of liver disorder; do not re-introduce tolcapone once discontinued.

● INTERACTIONS → Appendix 1 (tolcapone).

● SIDE-EFFECTS
▸ **Common or very common** Abdominal pain · anorexia · chest pain · confusion · constipation · diarrhoea · dizziness · drowsiness · dyskinesia · dyspepsia · dystonia · excessive dreaming · hallucinations · headache · hepatotoxicity · nausea · sleep disturbances · sweating · syncope · urine discoloration · vomiting · xerostomia
▸ **Frequency not known** Neuroleptic malignant syndrome reported on dose reduction or withdrawal · rhabdomyolysis reported on dose reduction or withdrawal

● PREGNANCY Toxicity in *animal* studies—use only if potential benefit outweighs risk.

● BREAST FEEDING Avoid—present in milk in *animal* studies.

● HEPATIC IMPAIRMENT Avoid.

● RENAL IMPAIRMENT Caution if eGFR less than 30 mL/minute/1.73 m^2.

● MONITORING REQUIREMENTS Test liver function before treatment, and monitor every 2 weeks for first year, every 4 weeks for next 6 months and then every 8 weeks thereafter (restart monitoring schedule if dose increased).

● TREATMENT CESSATION Avoid abrupt withdrawal.

● PATIENT AND CARER ADVICE Patients should be told how to recognise signs of liver disorder and advised to seek immediate medical attention if symptoms such as anorexia, nausea, vomiting, fatigue, abdominal pain, dark urine, or pruritus develop.

● MEDICINAL FORMS
There can be variation in the licensing of different medicines containing the same drug.
Tablet
CAUTIONARY AND ADVISORY LABELS 14, 25
▸ Tasmar (Meda Pharmaceuticals Ltd)
Tolcapone 100 mg Tasmar 100mg tablets | 100 tablet [PoM] £95.20

DOPAMINERGIC DRUGS ⟩ DOPAMINE PRECURSORS

Carbidopa with entacapone and levodopa

The properties listed below are those particular to the combination only. For the properties of the components please consider, co-careldopa p. 380, entacapone p. 377.

● INDICATIONS AND DOSE

STALEVO® 100/25/200

Parkinson's disease and end-of-dose motor fluctuations not adequately controlled with levodopa and dopa-decarboxylase inhibitor treatment
▸ BY MOUTH
▸ Adult: 1 tablet for each dose; maximum 10 tablets per day

STALEVO® 125/31.25/200

Parkinson's disease and end-of-dose motor fluctuations not adequately controlled with levodopa and dopa-decarboxylase inhibitor treatment
▸ BY MOUTH
▸ Adult: 1 tablet for each dose; maximum 10 tablets per day

STALEVO® 150/37.5/200

Parkinson's disease and end-of-dose motor fluctuations not adequately controlled with levodopa and dopa-decarboxylase inhibitor treatment
▸ BY MOUTH
▸ Adult: 1 tablet for each dose; maximum 10 tablets per day

STALEVO® 175/43.75/200

Parkinson's disease and end-of-dose motor fluctuations not adequately controlled with levodopa and dopa-decarboxylase inhibitor treatment
▸ BY MOUTH
▸ Adult: 1 tablet for each dose; maximum 8 tablets per day

STALEVO® 200/50/200

Parkinson's disease and end-of-dose motor fluctuations not adequately controlled with levodopa and dopa-decarboxylase inhibitor treatment
▸ BY MOUTH
▸ Adult: 1 tablet for each dose; maximum 7 tablets per day

STALEVO® 50/12.5/200

Parkinson's disease and end-of-dose motor fluctuations not adequately controlled with levodopa and dopa-decarboxylase inhibitor treatment
▸ BY MOUTH
▸ Adult: 1 tablet for each dose; maximum 10 tablets per day

STALEVO® 75/18.75/200

Parkinson's disease and end-of-dose motor fluctuations not adequately controlled with levodopa and dopa-decarboxylase inhibitor treatment
▸ BY MOUTH
▸ Adult: 1 tablet for each dose; maximum 10 tablets per day

● PRESCRIBING AND DISPENSING INFORMATION Patients receiving standard-release co-careldopa or co-beneldopa alone, initiate *Stalevo*® at a dose that provides similar (or slightly lower) amount of levodopa.

Patients with dyskinesia or receiving more than 800 mg levodopa daily, introduce entacapone before transferring to *Stalevo*® (levodopa dose may need to be reduced by 10–30% initially).

Patients receiving entacapone and standard-release co-careldopa or co-beneldopa, initiate *Stalevo*® at a dose that provides similar (or slightly higher) amount of levodopa.

● PATIENT AND CARER ADVICE
Driving and skilled tasks
Sudden onset of sleep Excessive daytime sleepiness and sudden onset of sleep can occur with carbidopa with entacapone and levodopa.

Patients starting treatment with these drugs should be warned of the risk and of the need to exercise caution when driving or operating machinery. Those who have experienced excessive sedation or sudden onset of sleep should refrain from driving or operating machines until these effects have stopped occurring.

Management of excessive daytime sleepiness should focus on the identification of an underlying cause, such as depression or concomitant medication. Patients should be counselled on improving sleep behaviour.

● MEDICINAL FORMS
There can be variation in the licensing of different medicines
containing the same drug.

Tablet

CAUTIONARY AND ADVISORY LABELS 10, 14 ((urine reddish-brown)),
25

▸ Stalevo (Orion Pharma (UK) Ltd)

Carbidopa 25 mg, Levodopa 100 mg, Entacapone 200 mg Stalevo
100mg/25mg/200mg tablets | 30 tablet [PoM] £20.79 |
100 tablet [PoM] £69.31

**Carbidopa 18.75 mg, Levodopa 75 mg, Entacapone
200 mg** Stalevo 75mg/18.75mg/200mg tablets | 30 tablet [PoM]
£20.79 | 100 tablet [PoM] £69.31

**Carbidopa 37.5 mg, Levodopa 150 mg, Entacapone
200 mg** Stalevo 150mg/37.5mg/200mg tablets | 30 tablet [PoM]
£20.79 | 100 tablet [PoM] £69.31

Carbidopa 12.5 mg, Levodopa 50 mg, Entacapone 200 mg Stalevo
50mg/12.5mg/200mg tablets | 30 tablet [PoM] £20.79 |
100 tablet [PoM] £69.31

**Carbidopa 31.25 mg, Levodopa 125 mg, Entacapone
200 mg** Stalevo 125mg/31.25mg/200mg tablets | 30 tablet [PoM]
£20.79 | 100 tablet [PoM] £69.31

**Carbidopa 43.75 mg, Levodopa 175 mg, Entacapone
200 mg** Stalevo 175mg/43.75mg/200mg tablets | 30 tablet [PoM]
£20.79 | 100 tablet [PoM] £69.31

Carbidopa 50 mg, Entacapone 200 mg, Levodopa 200 mg Stalevo
200mg/50mg/200mg tablets | 30 tablet [PoM] £20.79 |
100 tablet [PoM] £69.31

Co-beneldopa

● INDICATIONS AND DOSE

Parkinson's disease

▸ BY MOUTH USING IMMEDIATE-RELEASE MEDICINES

▸ Adult: Initially 50 mg 3–4 times a day, then increased
in steps of 100 mg daily, dose to be increased once or
twice weekly according to response; maintenance
400–800 mg daily in divided doses

▸ Elderly: Initially 50 mg 1–2 times a day, then increased
in steps of 50 mg daily, dose to be increased every
3–4 days according to response

Parkinson's disease (in advanced disease)

▸ BY MOUTH USING IMMEDIATE-RELEASE MEDICINES

▸ Adult: Initially 100 mg 3 times a day, then increased in
steps of 100 mg daily, dose to be increased once or
twice weekly according to response; maintenance
400–800 mg daily in divided doses

**Parkinson's disease (patients not taking levodopa/dopa-
decarboxylase inhibitor therapy)**

▸ BY MOUTH USING MODIFIED-RELEASE MEDICINES

▸ Adult: Initially 1 capsule 3 times a day; maximum
6 capsules per day

**Parkinson's disease (patients transferring from
immediate-release levodopa/dopa-decarboxylase
inhibitor preparations)**

▸ BY MOUTH USING MODIFIED-RELEASE MEDICINES

▸ Adult: Initially 1 capsule substituted for every 100 mg
of levodopa and given at same dosage frequency,
increased every 2–3 days according to response;
average increase of 50% needed over previous levodopa
dose and titration may take up to 4 weeks,
supplementary dose of immediate-release *Madopar*®
may be needed with first morning dose; if response still
poor to total daily dose of *Madopar*® CR plus
Madopar® corresponding to 1.2 g levodopa—consider
alternative therapy.

DOSE EQUIVALENCE AND CONVERSION
Dose is expressed as levodopa.

IMPORTANT SAFETY INFORMATION

IMPULSE CONTROL DISORDERS

Treatment with levodopa is associated with impulse
control disorders, including pathological gambling,
binge eating, and hypersexuality. Patients and their
carers should be informed about the risk of impulse
control disorders. If the patient develops an impulse
control disorder, levodopa should be withdrawn or the
dose reduced until the symptoms resolve.

● CAUTIONS Cushing's syndrome · diabetes mellitus ·
endocrine disorders · history of convulsions · history of
myocardial infarction with residual arrhythmia · history of
peptic ulcer · hyperthyroidism · osteomalacia ·
phaeochromocytoma · psychiatric illness (avoid if severe
and discontinue if deterioration) · severe cardiovascular
disease · severe pulmonary disease · susceptibility to
angle-closure glaucoma

● INTERACTIONS → Appendix 1 (co-beneldopa, levodopa).

● SIDE-EFFECTS

▸ **Common or very common** Abnormal dreams · anorexia ·
anxiety · arrhythmias · chorea · confusion · dementia ·
depression · dizziness · drowsiness · dry mouth · dyskinesia
· dystonia · euphoria · fatigue · insomnia · nausea ·
palpitations · postural hypotension · psychosis · syncope ·
taste disturbances · vomiting

▸ **Uncommon** Ataxia · chest pain · constipation · diarrhoea ·
dysphagia · flatulence · hand tremor · hoarseness ·
hypersalivation · hypertension · malaise · muscle cramps, ·
oedema · reddish discoloration of the urine and other body
fluids · weakness · weight changes

▸ **Rare** Abdominal pain · activation of Horner's syndrome ·
activation of malignant melanoma · agitation ·
agranulocytosis · alopecia · blepharospasm · blurred vision
· bruxism · convulsions · diplopia · disorientation ·
duodenal ulcer · dyspepsia · dyspnoea · exanthema ·
flushing · gastro-intestinal bleeding · haemolytic anaemia ·
headache · Henoch-Schönlein purpura · hiccups ·
leucopenia · neuroleptic malignant syndrome (associated
with abrupt withdrawal) · non-haemolytic anaemia ·
oculogyric crisis · paraesthesia · phlebitis · priapism · pupil
dilatation · reduced mental acuity · sweating ·
thrombocytopenia · trismus · urinary incontinence ·
urinary retention

▸ **Very rare** Angle-closure glaucoma · suicidal ideation

▸ **Frequency not known** Compulsive behaviour

● PREGNANCY Caution in pregnancy—toxicity has occurred
in *animal* studies.

● BREAST FEEDING May suppress lactation; present in
milk—avoid.

● HEPATIC IMPAIRMENT Use with caution.

● RENAL IMPAIRMENT Use with caution.

● EFFECT ON LABORATORY TESTS False positive tests for
urinary ketones have been reported.

● TREATMENT CESSATION Avoid abrupt withdrawal (risk of
neuroleptic malignant syndrome and rhabdomyolysis).

● DIRECTIONS FOR ADMINISTRATION The dispersible tablets
can be dispersed in water or orange squash (not orange
juice) or swallowed whole.

● PRESCRIBING AND DISPENSING INFORMATION Co-
beneldopa is a mixture of benserazide hydrochloride and
levodopa in mass proportions corresponding to 1 part of
benserazide and 4 parts of levodopa.

When transferring patients from another
levodopa/dopa-decarboxylase inhibitor preparation, the
previous preparation should be discontinued 12 hours
before (although interval can be shorter).

When switching from modified-release levodopa to
dispersible co-beneldopa, reduce dose by approximately
30%.

Nervous system

4

When administered as an adjunct to other antiparkinsonian drugs, once therapeutic effect apparent, the other drugs may be reduced or withdrawn.

● PATIENT AND CARER ADVICE

Patients or carers should be given advice on how to administer co-beneldopa dispersible tablets.

Driving and skilled tasks

Sudden onset of sleep Excessive daytime sleepiness and sudden onset of sleep can occur with co-beneldopa.

Patients starting treatment with these drugs should be warned of the risk and of the need to exercise caution when driving or operating machinery. Those who have experienced excessive sedation or sudden onset of sleep should refrain from driving or operating machines until these effects have stopped occurring.

Management of excessive daytime sleepiness should focus on the identification of an underlying cause, such as depression or concomitant medication. Patients should be counselled on improving sleep behaviour.

● MEDICINAL FORMS

There can be variation in the licensing of different medicines containing the same drug. Forms available from special-order manufacturers include: oral suspension, oral solution

Dispersible tablet

CAUTIONARY AND ADVISORY LABELS 10, 14, 21

▸ Madopar (Roche Products Ltd)

Benserazide (as Benserazide hydrochloride) 12.5 mg, Levodopa 50 mg Madopar 50mg/12.5mg dispersible tablets sugar-free | 100 tablet [PoM] £5.90 DT price = £5.90

Benserazide (as Benserazide hydrochloride) 25 mg, Levodopa 100 mg Madopar 100mg/25mg dispersible tablets sugar-free | 100 tablet [PoM] £10.45 DT price = £10.45

Capsule

CAUTIONARY AND ADVISORY LABELS 10, 14, 21

▸ Co-beneldopa (Non-proprietary)

Benserazide (as Benserazide hydrochloride) 12.5 mg, Levodopa 50 mg Co-beneldopa 12.5mg/50mg capsules | 100 capsule [PoM] £4.71–£4.96 DT price = £4.96

Benserazide (as Benserazide hydrochloride) 25 mg, Levodopa 100 mg Co-beneldopa 25mg/100mg capsules | 100 capsule [PoM] £6.56–£6.91 DT price = £6.91

Benserazide (as Benserazide hydrochloride) 50 mg, Levodopa 200 mg Co-beneldopa 50mg/200mg capsules | 100 capsule [PoM] £11.19–£11.78 DT price = £11.78

▸ Madopar (Roche Products Ltd)

Benserazide (as Benserazide hydrochloride) 12.5 mg, Levodopa 50 mg Madopar 50mg/12.5mg capsules | 100 capsule [PoM] £4.96 DT price = £4.96

Benserazide (as Benserazide hydrochloride) 25 mg, Levodopa 100 mg Madopar 100mg/25mg capsules | 100 capsule [PoM] £6.91 DT price = £6.91

Benserazide (as Benserazide hydrochloride) 50 mg, Levodopa 200 mg Madopar 200mg/50mg capsules | 100 capsule [PoM] £11.78 DT price = £11.78

Modified-release capsule

CAUTIONARY AND ADVISORY LABELS 5, 10, 14, 25

▸ Madopar CR (Roche Products Ltd)

Benserazide (as Benserazide hydrochloride) 25 mg, Levodopa 100 mg Madopar CR capsules | 100 capsule [PoM] £12.77 DT price = £12.77

Co-careldopa

● INDICATIONS AND DOSE

Parkinson's disease

▸ BY MOUTH

▸ Adult: Initially 25/100 mg 3 times a day, then increased in steps of 12.5/50 mg once daily or on alternate days, alternatively increased in steps of 25/100 mg once daily or on alternate days, dose to be adjusted according to response; dose increased until 800 mg levodopa (with 200 mg carbidopa) daily in divided doses is reached, then maintenance up to 200/2000 mg daily in divided

doses, adjusted according to response, when co-careldopa is used, the total daily dose of carbidopa should be at least 70 mg. A lower dose may not achieve full inhibition of extracerebral dopa-decarboxylase, with a resultant increase in side-effects

Parkinson's disease—alternative regimen

▸ BY MOUTH

▸ Adult: Initially 12.5/50 mg 3–4 times a day, alternatively initially 10/100 mg 3–4 times a day, then increased in steps of 12.5/50 mg once daily or on alternate days, adjusted according to response, alternatively increased in steps of 10/100 mg once daily or on alternate days, adjusted according to response, dose increased until 800 mg levodopa (with up to 200 mg carbidopa) daily in divided doses is reached, then maintenance up to 200/2000 mg daily in divided doses, adjusted according to response, when co-careldopa is used, the total daily dose of carbidopa should be at least 70 mg. A lower dose may not achieve full inhibition of extracerebral dopa-decarboxylase, with a resultant increase in side-effects

DOSE EQUIVALENCE AND CONVERSION

The proportions are expressed in the form x/y where x and y are the strengths in milligrams of carbidopa and levodopa respectively.

2 tablets *Sinemet*® 12.5 mg/50 mg is equivalent to 1 tablet *Sinemet*® Plus 25 mg/100 mg.

CARAMET® CR

Parkinson's disease (patients not receiving levodopa/dopa-decarboxylase inhibitor preparations, expressed as levodopa)

▸ BY MOUTH USING MODIFIED-RELEASE TABLETS

▸ Adult: Initially 100–200 mg twice daily, dose to be given at least 6 hours apart; dose adjusted according to response at intervals of at least 2 days

Parkinson's disease (patients transferring from immediate-release levodopa/dopa-decarboxylase inhibitor preparations)

▸ BY MOUTH USING MODIFIED-RELEASE TABLETS

▸ Adult: Discontinue previous preparation at least 12 hours before first dose of *Caramet*®*CR*; substitute *Caramet*® *CR* to provide a similar amount of levodopa daily and extend dosing interval by 30–50%; dose then adjusted according to response at intervals of at least 2 days.

DUODOPA®

Severe Parkinson's disease inadequately controlled by other preparations

▸ Adult: Administered as intestinal gel, for use with enteral tube (consult product literature)

HALF SINEMET® CR

Parkinson's disease (for fine adjustment of Sinemet® CR dose)

▸ BY MOUTH

▸ Adult: (consult product literature)

SINEMET® CR

Parkinson's disease (patients not receiving levodopa/dopa-decarboxylase inhibitor therapy)

▸ BY MOUTH

▸ Adult: Initially 1 tablet twice daily, both dose and interval then adjusted according to response at intervals of not less than 3 days

Parkinson's disease (patients transferring from immediate-release levodopa/dopa-decarboxylase inhibitor preparations)

▸ BY MOUTH

▸ Adult: 1 tablet twice daily, dose can be substituted for a daily dose of levodopa 300–400 mg in immediate-release *Sinemet*® tablets (substitute *Sinemet*® *CR* to provide approximately 10% more levodopa per day and extend dosing interval by 30–50%); dose and interval then adjusted according to response at intervals of not less than 3 days.

IMPORTANT SAFETY INFORMATION
IMPULSE CONTROL DISORDERS
Treatment with levodopa is associated with impulse control disorders, including pathological gambling, binge eating, and hypersexuality. Patients and their carers should be informed about the risk of impulse control disorders. If the patient develops an impulse control disorder, levodopa should be withdrawn or the dose reduced until the symptoms resolve.

● CAUTIONS Cushing's syndrome · diabetes mellitus · endocrine disorders · history of convulsions · history of myocardial infarction with residual arrhythmia · history of peptic ulcer · hyperthyroidism · osteomalacia · phaeochromocytoma · psychiatric illness (avoid if severe and discontinue if deterioration) · severe cardiovascular disease · severe pulmonary disease · susceptibility to angle-closure glaucoma

● INTERACTIONS → Appendix 1 (co-careldopa, levodopa).

● SIDE-EFFECTS
▸ **Common or very common** Abnormal dreams · anorexia · anxiety · arrhythmias · chorea · confusion · dementia · depression · dizziness · drowsiness · dry mouth · dyskinesia · dystonia · euphoria · fatigue · insomnia · nausea · palpitations · postural hypotension · psychosis · syncope · taste disturbances · vomiting
▸ **Uncommon** Ataxia · chest pain · constipation · diarrhoea · dysphagia · flatulence · hand tremor · hoarseness · hypersalivation · hypertension · malaise · muscle cramps · oedema · reddish discoloration of the urine and other body fluids · weakness · weight changes
▸ **Rare** Abdominal pain · activation of Horner's syndrome · activation of malignant melanoma · agitation · agranulocytosis · alopecia · blepharospasm · blurred vision · bruxism · convulsions · diplopia · disorientation · duodenal ulcer · dyspepsia · dyspnoea · exanthema · flushing · gastro-intestinal bleeding · haemolytic anaemia · headache · Henoch-Schönlein purpura · hiccups · leucopenia · neuroleptic malignant syndrome (associated with abrupt withdrawal) · non-haemolytic anaemia · oculogyric crisis · paraesthesia · phlebitis · priapism · pupil dilatation · reduced mental acuity · sweating · thrombocytopenia · trismus · urinary incontinence · urinary retention
▸ **Very rare** Angle-closure glaucoma · suicidal ideation
▸ **Frequency not known** Compulsive behaviour

● PREGNANCY Use with caution—toxicity has occurred in *animal* studies.

● BREAST FEEDING May suppress lactation; present in milk—avoid.

● HEPATIC IMPAIRMENT Use with caution.

● RENAL IMPAIRMENT Use with caution.

● EFFECT ON LABORATORY TESTS False positive tests for urinary ketones have been reported.

● TREATMENT CESSATION Avoid abrupt withdrawal (risk of neuroleptic malignant syndrome and rhabdomyolysis).

● PRESCRIBING AND DISPENSING INFORMATION Co-careldopa is a mixture of carbidopa and levodopa; the proportions are expressed in the form x/y where x and y are the strengths in milligrams of carbidopa and levodopa respectively.

When transferring patients from another levodopa/dopa-decarboxylase inhibitor preparation, the previous preparation should be discontinued at least 12 hours before.

Co-careldopa 25/100 provides an adequate dose of carbidopa when low doses of levodopa are needed.

● PATIENT AND CARER ADVICE
Driving and skilled tasks
Sudden onset of sleep Excessive daytime sleepiness and sudden onset of sleep can occur with co-careldopa.

Patients starting treatment with these drugs should be warned of the risk and of the need to exercise caution when driving or operating machinery. Those who have experienced excessive sedation or sudden onset of sleep should refrain from driving or operating machines until these effects have stopped occurring.

Management of excessive daytime sleepiness should focus on the identification of an underlying cause, such as depression or concomitant medication. Patients should be counselled on improving sleep behaviour.

● MEDICINAL FORMS
There can be variation in the licensing of different medicines containing the same drug. Forms available from special-order manufacturers include: oral suspension, oral solution

Tablet
CAUTIONARY AND ADVISORY LABELS 10, 14
▸ Co-careldopa (Non-proprietary)
Carbidopa (as Carbidopa monohydrate) 10 mg, Levodopa 100 mg Co-careldopa 10mg/100mg tablets | 100 tablet [PoM] £9.38 DT price = £8.68
Carbidopa (as Carbidopa monohydrate) 25 mg, Levodopa 100 mg Co-careldopa 25mg/100mg tablets | 100 tablet [PoM] £26.99 DT price = £14.39
Carbidopa (as Carbidopa monohydrate) 25 mg, Levodopa 250 mg Co-careldopa 25mg/250mg tablets | 100 tablet [PoM] £35.00 DT price = £34.98
▸ Sinemet (Merck Sharp & Dohme Ltd)
Carbidopa (as Carbidopa monohydrate) 12.5 mg, Levodopa 50 mg Sinemet 12.5mg/50mg tablets | 90 tablet [PoM] £6.28 DT price = £6.28
Carbidopa (as Carbidopa monohydrate) 10 mg, Levodopa 100 mg Sinemet 10mg/100mg tablets | 100 tablet [PoM] £7.30 DT price = £8.68
Carbidopa (as Carbidopa monohydrate) 25 mg, Levodopa 250 mg Sinemet 25mg/250mg tablets | 100 tablet [PoM] £18.29 DT price = £34.98
▸ Sinemet Plus (Merck Sharp & Dohme Ltd)
Carbidopa (as Carbidopa monohydrate) 25 mg, Levodopa 100 mg Sinemet Plus 25mg/100mg tablets | 100 tablet [PoM] £12.88 DT price = £14.39

Modified-release tablet
CAUTIONARY AND ADVISORY LABELS 10, 14, 25
▸ Caramet CR (Teva UK Ltd)
Carbidopa (as Carbidopa monohydrate) 25 mg, Levodopa 100 mg Caramet 25mg/100mg CR tablets | 60 tablet [PoM] £11.47 DT price = £11.60
Carbidopa (as Carbidopa monohydrate) 50 mg, Levodopa 200 mg Caramet 50mg/200mg CR tablets | 60 tablet [PoM] £11.47 DT price = £11.60
▸ Half Sinemet CR (Merck Sharp & Dohme Ltd)
Carbidopa (as Carbidopa monohydrate) 25 mg, Levodopa 100 mg Half Sinemet CR 25mg/100mg tablets | 60 tablet [PoM] £11.60 DT price = £11.60
▸ Sinemet CR (Merck Sharp & Dohme Ltd)
Carbidopa (as Carbidopa monohydrate) 50 mg, Levodopa 200 mg Sinemet CR 50mg/200mg tablets | 60 tablet [PoM] £11.60 DT price = £11.60

Gel
CAUTIONARY AND ADVISORY LABELS 10, 14
▸ Duodopa (AbbVie Ltd)
Carbidopa (as Carbidopa monohydrate) 5 mg per 1 ml, Levodopa 20 mg per 1 ml Duodopa intestinal gel 100ml cassette | 1 bag [PoM] £77.00 | 7 bag [PoM] no price available

4

Nervous system

DOPAMINERGIC DRUGS > DOPAMINE RECEPTOR AGONISTS

Amantadine hydrochloride

- **DRUG ACTION** Amantadine is a weak dopamine agonist with modest antiparkinsonian effects.

- **INDICATIONS AND DOSE**

Parkinson's disease
- BY MOUTH
- Adult: 100 mg daily for 1 week, then increased to 100 mg twice daily, usually administered in conjunction with other treatment. Some patients may require higher doses; maximum 400 mg per day
- Elderly: 100 mg daily, adjusted according to response

Post-herpetic neuralgia
- BY MOUTH
- Adult: 100 mg twice daily for 14 days (continued for another 14 days if necessary)

Treatment of influenza A (but not recommended)
- BY MOUTH
- Adult: 100 mg daily 4–5 days

Prophylaxis of influenza A (but not recommended)
- BY MOUTH
- Adult: 100 mg daily usually for 6 weeks or with influenza vaccination for 2–3 weeks after vaccination

- **CONTRA-INDICATIONS** Epilepsy · history of gastric ulceration
- **CAUTIONS** Confused or hallucinatory states · congestive heart disease (may exacerbate oedema) · elderly · tolerance to the effects of amantadine may develop in Parkinson's disease
- **INTERACTIONS** → Appendix 1 (amantadine).
- **SIDE-EFFECTS**
- **Common or very common** Anorexia · anxiety · dizziness · dry mouth · gastro-intestinal disturbances · hallucinations · headache · impaired concentration · insomnia · lethargy · livedo reticularis · mood changes · myalgia · palpitation · peripheral oedema · postural hypotension · slurred speech · sweating
- **Uncommon** Confusion · movement disorders · neuroleptic malignant syndrome · psychosis · rash · seizure · tremor · urinary incontinence · urinary retention · visual disturbances
- **Frequency not known** Heart failure · leucopenia · photosensitisation
- **PREGNANCY** Avoid; toxicity in *animal* studies.
- **BREAST FEEDING** Avoid; present in milk; toxicity in infant reported.
- **HEPATIC IMPAIRMENT** Use with caution.
- **RENAL IMPAIRMENT** Reduce dose. Avoid if eGFR less than 15 mL/minute/1.73 m^2.
- **TREATMENT CESSATION** Avoid abrupt withdrawal in Parkinson's disease.
- **PATIENT AND CARER ADVICE**
Driving and skilled tasks
May affect performance of skilled tasks (e.g. driving).
- **NATIONAL FUNDING/ACCESS DECISIONS**
NICE technology appraisals (TAs)
- Oseltamivir, zanamivir, and amantadine for prophylaxis of influenza (September 2008) NICE TA158
Amantadine is **not** recommended for prophylaxis of influenza.
www.nice.org.uk/TA158

- Oseltamivir, zanamivir, and amantadine for treatment of influenza (February 2009) NICE TA168
Amantadine is **not** recommended for treatment of influenza.
www.nice.org.uk/TA168

- **MEDICINAL FORMS**
There can be variation in the licensing of different medicines containing the same drug. Forms available from special-order manufacturers include: tablet

Capsule
- Amantadine hydrochloride (Non-proprietary)
Amantadine hydrochloride 100 mg Amantadine 100mg capsules | 14 capsule PoM £10.25 | 56 capsule PoM £41.00 DT price = £41.00

Oral solution
- Amantadine hydrochloride (Non-proprietary)
Amantadine hydrochloride 10 mg per 1 ml Amantadine 50mg/5ml oral solution sugar free sugar-free | 150 ml PoM £136.74-£140.00 DT price = £137.16

Apomorphine hydrochloride

- **INDICATIONS AND DOSE**

Refractory motor fluctuations in Parkinson's disease ('off' episodes) inadequately controlled by co-beneldopa or co-careldopa or other dopaminergics (for capable and motivated patients) (under expert supervision)
- BY SUBCUTANEOUS INJECTION
- Adult: Initially 1 mg, dose to be administered at the first sign of 'off' episode, then 2 mg after 30 minutes, dose to be given if inadequate or no response following initial dose, thereafter increase dose at minimum 40-minute intervals until satisfactory response obtained, this determines threshold dose; usual dose 3–30 mg daily in divided doses (max. per dose 10 mg), subcutaneous infusion may be preferable in those requiring division of injections into more than 10 doses; maximum 100 mg per day

Refractory motor fluctuations in Parkinson's disease ('off' episodes) inadequately controlled by co-beneldopa or co-careldopa or other dopaminergics (in patients requiring division into more than 10 injections daily) (under expert supervision)
- BY CONTINUOUS SUBCUTANEOUS INFUSION
- Adult: Initially 1 mg/hour, adjusted according to response, then increased in steps of up to 500 micrograms/hour, dose to be increased at intervals not more often than every 4 hours; usual dose 1–4 mg/hour, alternatively usual dose 15–60 micrograms/kg/hour, change infusion site every 12 hours and give during waking hours only (tolerance may occur unless there is a 4-hour treatment-free period at night—24-hour infusions not recommended unless severe night time symptoms); intermittent bolus doses may be needed; maximum 100 mg per day

> **IMPORTANT SAFETY INFORMATION**
> IMPULSE CONTROL DISORDERS
> Treatment with dopamine-receptor agonists are associated with impulse control disorders, including pathological gambling, binge eating, and hypersexuality. Patients and their carers should be informed about the risk of impulse control disorders. There is no evidence that ergot- and non-ergot-derived dopamine-receptor agonists differ in their propensity to cause impulse control disorders, so switching between dopamine-receptor agonists to control these side-effects is not recommended. If the patient develops an impulse control disorder, the dopamine-receptor agonist or levodopa should be withdrawn or the dose reduced until the symptoms resolve.

- CONTRA-INDICATIONS Avoid if 'on' response to levodopa marred by severe dyskinesia or dystonia · dementia · psychosis · respiratory depression
- CAUTIONS Cardiovascular disease · history of postural hypotension (special care on initiation) · neuropsychiatric conditions · pulmonary disease · susceptibility to QT-interval prolongation
- INTERACTIONS → Appendix 1 (apomorphine).
- SIDE-EFFECTS
▸ **Common or very common** Confusion · drowsiness · hallucinations · nausea · sudden onset of sleep · vomiting · yawning
▸ **Uncommon** Dyskinesia during 'on' periods (may require discontinuation) · dyspnoea · haemolytic anaemia (with levodopa) · postural hypotension · rash · thrombocytopenia (with levodopa)
▸ **Rare** Eosinophilia
▸ **Frequency not known** Compulsive behaviour · dizziness · peripheral oedema
- ALLERGY AND CROSS-SENSITIVITY Contra-indicated if history of hypersensitivity to opioids.
- PREGNANCY Avoid unless clearly necessary.
- BREAST FEEDING No information available; may suppress lactation.
- HEPATIC IMPAIRMENT Avoid.
- RENAL IMPAIRMENT Use with caution.
- MONITORING REQUIREMENTS
▸ Monitor hepatic, haemopoietic, renal, and cardiovascular function.
▸ *With concomitant levodopa* test initially and every 6 months for haemolytic anaemia and thrombocytopenia (development calls for specialist haematological care with dose reduction and possible discontinuation).
- TREATMENT CESSATION Antiparkinsonian drug therapy should never be stopped abruptly as this carries a small risk of neuroleptic malignant syndrome.
- PATIENT AND CARER ADVICE
Driving and skilled tasks
Sudden onset of sleep Excessive daytime sleepiness and sudden onset of sleep can occur with dopamine-receptor agonists.

Patients starting treatment with these drugs should be warned of the risk and of the need to exercise caution when driving or operating machinery. Those who have experienced excessive sedation or sudden onset of sleep should refrain from driving or operating machines until these effects have stopped occurring.

Management of excessive daytime sleepiness should focus on the identification of an underlying cause, such as depression or concomitant medication. Patients should be counselled on improving sleep behaviour.
Drugs and driving Prescribers and other healthcare professionals should advise patients if treatment is likely to affect their ability to perform skilled tasks (e.g. driving). This applies especially to drugs with sedative effects; patients should be warned that these effects are increased by alcohol. General information about a patient's fitness to drive is available from the Driver and Vehicle Licensing Agency at www.dvla.gov.uk.

2015 legislation regarding driving whilst taking certain drugs, may also apply to apomorphine, see *Drugs and driving* under Guidance on prescribing p. 1.
Hypotensive reactions Hypotensive reactions can occur in some patients taking dopamine-receptor agonists; these can be particularly problematic during the first few days of treatment and care should be exercised when driving or operating machinery.

- MEDICINAL FORMS
There can be variation in the licensing of different medicines containing the same drug. Forms available from special-order manufacturers include: solution for injection, solution for infusion
Solution for injection
CAUTIONARY AND ADVISORY LABELS 10
EXCIPIENTS: May contain Sulfites
▸ APO-go (Britannia Pharmaceuticals Ltd)
Apomorphine hydrochloride 10 mg per 1 ml APO-go 50mg/5ml solution for injection ampoules | 5 ampoule [PoM] £73.11
APO-go 20mg/2ml solution for injection ampoules | 5 ampoule [PoM] £37.96
▸ APO-go Pen (Britannia Pharmaceuticals Ltd)
Apomorphine hydrochloride 10 mg per 1 ml APO-go PEN 30mg/3ml solution for injection | 5 pre-filled disposable injection [PoM] £123.91
Solution for infusion
CAUTIONARY AND ADVISORY LABELS 10
EXCIPIENTS: May contain Sulfites
▸ APO-go PFS (Britannia Pharmaceuticals Ltd)
Apomorphine hydrochloride 5 mg per 1 ml APO-go PFS 50mg/10ml solution for infusion pre-filled syringes | 5 pre-filled disposable injection [PoM] £73.11

Bromocriptine

- DRUG ACTION Bromocriptine is a stimulant of dopamine receptors in the brain; it also inhibits release of prolactin by the pituitary.

- INDICATIONS AND DOSE
Prevention of lactation
▸ BY MOUTH
▸ Adult: Initially 2.5 mg daily for 1 day, then 2.5 mg twice daily for 14 days

Suppression of lactation
▸ BY MOUTH
▸ Adult: Initially 2.5 mg daily for 2–3 days, then 2.5 mg twice daily for 14 days

Hypogonadism | Galactorrhoea | Infertility
▸ BY MOUTH
▸ Adult: Initially 1–1.25 mg daily, dose to be taken at bedtime, increase dose gradually; usual dose 7.5 mg daily in divided doses, increased if necessary up to 30 mg daily, usual dose in infertility without hyperprolactinaemia is 2.5 mg twice daily

Acromegaly
▸ BY MOUTH
▸ Adult: Initially 1–1.25 mg daily, dose to be taken at bedtime, then increased to 5 mg every 6 hours, increase dose gradually

Prolactinoma
▸ BY MOUTH
▸ Adult: Initially 1–1.25 mg daily, dose to be taken at bedtime, then increased to 5 mg every 6 hours, increase dose gradually. Occasionally patients may require up to 30 mg daily

Parkinson's disease
▸ BY MOUTH
▸ Adult: Initially 1–1.25 mg daily for 1 week, dose to be taken at night, then 2–2.5 mg daily for 1 week, dose to be taken at night, then 2.5 mg twice daily for 1 week, then 2.5 mg 3 times a day for 1 week, then increased in steps of 2.5 mg every 3–14 days, adjusted according to response; maintenance 10–30 mg daily

IMPORTANT SAFETY INFORMATION

FIBROTIC REACTIONS

Bromocriptine has been associated with pulmonary, retroperitoneal, and pericardial fibrotic reactions.

Exclude cardiac valvulopathy with echocardiography before starting treatment with these ergot derivatives for Parkinson's disease or chronic endocrine disorders (excludes suppression of lactation); it may also be appropriate to measure the erythrocyte sedimentation rate and serum creatinine and to obtain a chest X-ray. Patients should be monitored for dyspnoea, persistent cough, chest pain, cardiac failure, and abdominal pain or tenderness. If long-term treatment is expected, then lung-function tests may also be helpful.

IMPULSE CONTROL DISORDERS

Treatment with dopamine-receptor agonists are associated with impulse control disorders, including pathological gambling, binge eating, and hypersexuality. Patients and their carers should be informed about the risk of impulse control disorders. There is no evidence that ergot- and non-ergot-derived dopamine-receptor agonists differ in their propensity to cause impulse control disorders, so switching between dopamine-receptor agonists to control these side-effects is not recommended. If the patient develops an impulse control disorder, the dopamine-receptor agonist should be withdrawn or the dose reduced until the symptoms resolve.

● CONTRA-INDICATIONS Avoid in pre-eclampsia · cardiac valvulopathy (exclude before treatment) · hypertension in postpartum women or in puerperium

CONTRA-INDICATIONS, FURTHER INFORMATION

▸ Postpartum or puerperium Should not be used postpartum or in puerperium in women with high blood pressure, coronary artery disease, or symptoms (or history) of serious mental disorder; monitor blood pressure carefully (especially during first few days) in postpartum women. Very rarely hypertension, myocardial infarction, seizures or stroke (both sometimes preceded by severe headache or visual disturbances), and mental disorders have been reported in postpartum women given bromocriptine for lactation suppression—caution with antihypertensive therapy and avoid other ergot alkaloids. Discontinue immediately if hypertension, unremitting headache, or signs of CNS toxicity develop.

● CAUTIONS Acute porphyrias p. 918 · cardiovascular disease · history of peptic ulcer (particularly in acromegalic patients) · history of serious mental disorders (especially psychotic disorders) · Raynaud's syndrome

CAUTIONS, FURTHER INFORMATION

▸ Hyperprolactinemic patients In hyperprolactinaemic patients, the source of the hyperprolactinaemia should be established (i.e. exclude pituitary tumour before treatment).

● INTERACTIONS → Appendix 1 (bromocriptine). Tolerance may be reduced by alcohol.

● SIDE-EFFECTS

▸ **Common or very common** Constipation · headache · nasal congestion · nausea

▸ **Uncommon** Confusion (particularly with high doses) · dizziness · dry mouth · fatigue · hallucinations (particularly with high doses) · postural hypotension · psychomotor excitation (particularly with high doses) · vomiting

▸ **Rare** Abdominal pain · arrhythmia · bradycardia · diarrhoea · gastric ulcer · gastro-intestinal bleeding · insomnia · paraesthesia · psychosis · tachycardia · tinnitus · visual disturbances

▸ **Very rare** Neuroleptic malignant syndrome on withdrawal · vasospasm of fingers and toes (particularly in patients with Raynaud's syndrome)

▸ **Frequency not known** Allergic skin reactions · alopecia · cardiac valvulopathy · constrictive pericarditis · drowsiness · dyskinesia · hypersexuality · hyponatraemia · hypotension · increased libido · leg cramps · leucopenia · pathological gambling · pericardial effusion · peripheral oedema · pleural effusion · pleural fibrosis · pleuritis · pulmonary fibrosis · retroperitoneal fibrosis · reversible hearing loss · thrombocytopenia · urinary incontinence

SIDE-EFFECTS, FURTHER INFORMATION

▸ Gastro-intestinal bleeding Treatment should be withdrawn if gastro-intestinal bleeding occurs.

● ALLERGY AND CROSS-SENSITIVITY Bromocriptine should not be used in patients with hypersensitivity to ergot alkaloids.

● CONCEPTION AND CONTRACEPTION Caution—provide contraceptive advice if appropriate (oral contraceptives may increase prolactin concentration).

● BREAST FEEDING Suppresses lactation; avoid breast feeding for about 5 days if lactation prevention fails.

● HEPATIC IMPAIRMENT Dose reduction may be necessary.

● MONITORING REQUIREMENTS

▸ Specialist evaluation—monitor for pituitary enlargement, particularly during pregnancy; monitor visual field to detect secondary field loss in macroprolactinoma.

▸ Monitor for fibrotic disease.

▸ Monitor blood pressure for a few days after starting treatment and following dosage increase.

● TREATMENT CESSATION Antiparkinsonian drug therapy should never be stopped abruptly as this carries a small risk of neuroleptic malignant syndrome.

● PATIENT AND CARER ADVICE

Driving and skilled tasks

Sudden onset of sleep Excessive daytime sleepiness and sudden onset of sleep can occur with dopamine-receptor agonists.

Patients starting treatment with these drugs should be warned of the risk and of the need to exercise caution when driving or operating machinery. Those who have experienced excessive sedation or sudden onset of sleep should refrain from driving or operating machines until these effects have stopped occurring.

Management of excessive daytime sleepiness should focus on the identification of an underlying cause, such as depression or concomitant medication. Patients should be counselled on improving sleep behaviour.

Hypotensive reactions Hypotensive reactions can occur in some patients taking dopamine-receptor agonists; these can be particularly problematic during the first few days of treatment and care should be exercised when driving or operating machinery.

● MEDICINAL FORMS

There can be variation in the licensing of different medicines containing the same drug. Forms available from special-order manufacturers include: oral suspension

Tablet

CAUTIONARY AND ADVISORY LABELS 10, 21

▸ Bromocriptine (Non-proprietary)

Bromocriptine (as Bromocriptine mesilate) 1 mg Bromocriptine 1mg tablets | 100 tablet [PoM] £67.62 DT price = £67.62

Bromocriptine (as Bromocriptine mesilate) 2.5 mg Bromocriptine 2.5mg tablets | 30 tablet [PoM] £75.00 DT price = £74.77 | 100 tablet [PoM] £249.10

Capsule

CAUTIONARY AND ADVISORY LABELS 10, 21

▸ Parlodel (Meda Pharmaceuticals Ltd)

Bromocriptine (as Bromocriptine mesilate) 5 mg Parlodel 5mg capsules | 100 capsule [PoM] £37.57 DT price = £37.57

Bromocriptine (as Bromocriptine mesilate) 10 mg Parlodel 10mg capsules | 100 capsule [PoM] £69.50 DT price = £69.50

Cabergoline

- DRUG ACTION Cabergoline is a stimulant of dopamine receptors in the brain and it also inhibits release of prolactin by the pituitary.

- INDICATIONS AND DOSE

Prevention of lactation
▶ BY MOUTH
▶ Adult: 1 mg, to be taken as a single dose on the first day postpartum

Suppression of established lactation
▶ BY MOUTH
▶ Adult: 250 micrograms every 12 hours for 2 days

Hyperprolactinaemic disorders
▶ BY MOUTH
▶ Adult: Initially 500 micrograms once weekly, dose may be taken as a single dose or as 2 divided doses on separate days, then increased in steps of 500 micrograms every 1 month until optimal therapeutic response reached, increase dose following monthly monitoring of serum prolactin levels; usual dose 0.25–2 mg once weekly, usually 1 mg weekly; reduce initial dose and increase more gradually if patient intolerant, doses over 1 mg weekly to be given as divided dose; maximum 4.5 mg per week

Alone or as adjunct to co-beneldopa or co-careldopa in Parkinson's disease where dopamine-receptor agonists other than ergot derivative not appropriate
▶ BY MOUTH
▶ Adult: Initially 1 mg daily, then increased in steps of 0.5–1 mg every 7–14 days, concurrent dose of levodopa may be decreased gradually while dose of cabergoline is increased; maximum 3 mg per day

---

IMPORTANT SAFETY INFORMATION
FIBROTIC REACTIONS
Cabergoline has been associated with pulmonary, retroperitoneal, and pericardial fibrotic reactions.

Exclude cardiac valvulopathy with echocardiography before starting treatment with these ergot derivatives for Parkinson's disease or chronic endocrine disorders (excludes suppression of lactation); it may also be appropriate to measure the erythrocyte sedimentation rate and serum creatinine and to obtain a chest X-ray. Patients should be monitored for dyspnoea, persistent cough, chest pain, cardiac failure, and abdominal pain or tenderness. If long-term treatment is expected, then lung-function tests may also be helpful. Patients taking cabergoline should be regularly monitored for cardiac fibrosis by echocardiography (within 3–6 months of initiating treatment and subsequently at 6–12 month intervals).

IMPULSE CONTROL DISORDERS
Treatment with dopamine-receptor agonists are associated with impulse control disorders, including pathological gambling, binge eating, and hypersexuality. Patients and their carers should be informed about the risk of impulse control disorders. There is no evidence that ergot- and non-ergot-derived dopamine-receptor agonists differ in their propensity to cause impulse control disorders, so switching between dopamine-receptor agonists to control these side-effects is not recommended. If the patient develops an impulse control disorder, the dopamine-receptor agonist should be withdrawn or the dose reduced until the symptoms resolve.

- CONTRA-INDICATIONS Avoid in pre-eclampsia · cardiac valvulopathy (exclude before treatment) · history of pericardial fibrotic disorders · history of puerperal psychosis · history of pulmonary fibrotic disorders · history of retroperitoneal fibrotic disorders

- CAUTIONS Acute porphyrias p. 918 · cardiovascular disease · history of peptic ulcer (particularly in acromegalic patients) · history of serious mental disorders (especially psychotic disorders) · Raynaud's syndrome
CAUTIONS, FURTHER INFORMATION
▶ Hyperprolactinemic patients In hyperprolactinaemic patients, the source of the hyperprolactinaemia should be established (i.e. exclude pituitary tumour before treatment).

- INTERACTIONS → Appendix 1 (cabergoline). Tolerance may be reduced by alcohol.

- SIDE-EFFECTS
▶ **Common or very common** Abdominal pain · angina · breast pain · confusion · constipation · depression · dyspepsia · epigastric pain · gastritis · hallucinations · headache · nausea · syncope
▶ **Rare** Digital vasospasm · epistaxis · hot flushes · muscle weakness · palpitation · paraesthesia · transient hemianopia · vomiting
▶ **Frequency not known** Allergic skin reactions · alopecia · cardiac valvulopathy · constrictive pericarditis · drowsiness · dyskinesia · erythromelalgia · hypersexuality · hypotension · increased libido · leg cramps · pathological gambling · pericardial effusion · peripheral oedema · pleural effusion · pleural fibrosis · pleuritis · pulmonary fibrosis · retroperitoneal fibrosis
SIDE-EFFECTS, FURTHER INFORMATION
▶ Gastro-intestinal bleeding Treatment should be withdrawan if gastro-intestinal bleeding occurs.

- ALLERGY AND CROSS-SENSITIVITY Cabergoline should not be used in patients with hypersensitivity to ergot alkaloids.

- CONCEPTION AND CONTRACEPTION Exclude pregnancy before starting and perform monthly pregnancy tests during the amenorrhoeic period. Caution—advise non-hormonal contraception if pregnancy not desired. Discontinue 1 month before intended conception (ovulatory cycles persist for 6 months).

- PREGNANCY Discontinue if pregnancy occurs during treatment (specialist advice needed).

- BREAST FEEDING Suppresses lactation; avoid breast-feeding if lactation prevention fails.

- HEPATIC IMPAIRMENT Reduce dose in severe hepatic impairment.

- MONITORING REQUIREMENTS
▶ Monitor for fibrotic disorders.
▶ Monitor blood pressure for a few days after starting treatment and following dosage increase.

- TREATMENT CESSATION Antiparkinsonian drug therapy should never be stopped abruptly as this carries a small risk of neuroleptic malignant syndrome.

- PRESCRIBING AND DISPENSING INFORMATION Dispense in original container (contains desiccant).

- PATIENT AND CARER ADVICE

Driving and skilled tasks
Sudden onset of sleep Excessive daytime sleepiness and sudden onset of sleep can occur with dopamine-receptor agonists.

Patients starting treatment with these drugs should be warned of the risk and of the need to exercise caution when driving or operating machinery. Those who have experienced excessive sedation or sudden onset of sleep should refrain from driving or operating machines until these effects have stopped occurring.

Management of excessive daytime sleepiness should focus on the identification of an underlying cause, such as depression or concomitant medication. Patients should be counselled on improving sleep behaviour.

4

Nervous system

4

Nervous system

Hypotensive reactions Hypotensive reactions can occur in some patients taking dopamine-receptor agonists; these can be particularly problematic during the first few days of treatment and care should be exercised when driving or operating machinery.

● MEDICINAL FORMS
There can be variation in the licensing of different medicines containing the same drug.

Tablet
CAUTIONARY AND ADVISORY LABELS 10, 21
▸ Cabergoline (Non-proprietary)
  Cabergoline 500 microgram Cabergoline 500microgram tablets | 8 tablet [PoM] £34.99 DT price = £34.97
  Cabergoline 1 mg Cabergoline 1mg tablets | 20 tablet [PoM] £66.00 DT price = £64.25
  Cabergoline 2 mg Cabergoline 2mg tablets | 20 tablet [PoM] £73.14 DT price = £73.11
▸ Cabaser (Pfizer Ltd)
  Cabergoline 1 mg Cabaser 1mg tablets | 20 tablet [PoM] £83.00 DT price = £64.25
  Cabergoline 2 mg Cabaser 2mg tablets | 20 tablet [PoM] £83.00 DT price = £73.11
▸ Dostinex (Pfizer Ltd)
  Cabergoline 500 microgram Dostinex 500microgram tablets | 8 tablet [PoM] £30.04 DT price = £34.97

Pergolide

● INDICATIONS AND DOSE

Monotherapy in Parkinson's disease where dopamine-receptor agonists other than ergot derivative not appropriate
▸ BY MOUTH
▸ Adult: Initially 50 micrograms once daily for day 1, dose to be taken at bedtime, then 50 micrograms twice daily for days 2–4, then increased in steps of 100–250 micrograms daily, dose to be increased at intervals of 3–4 days, increased to 1.5 mg daily in 3 divided doses at day 28, then increased in steps of up to 250 micrograms every 3–4 days, this increase to be started after day 30; maintenance 2.1–2.5 mg daily; maximum 3 mg per day

Adjunctive therapy with co-beneldopa or co-careldopa in Parkinson's disease where dopamine-receptor agonists other than ergot derivative not appropriate
▸ BY MOUTH
▸ Adult: Initially 50 micrograms daily for 2 days, then increased in steps of 100–150 micrograms every 3 days, dose to be adjusted over next 12 days following initial dose and usually given in 3 divided doses, then increased in steps of 250 micrograms every 3 days, during pergolide titration, levodopa dose may be reduced cautiously; maximum 3 mg per day

IMPORTANT SAFETY INFORMATION
FIBROTIC REACTIONS
Pergolide has been associated with pulmonary, retroperitoneal, and pericardial fibrotic reactions.
  Exclude cardiac valvulopathy with echocardiography before starting treatment with pergolide; it may also be appropriate to measure the erythrocyte sedimentation rate and serum creatinine and to obtain a chest X-ray. Patients should be monitored for dyspnoea, persistent cough, chest pain, cardiac failure, and abdominal pain or tenderness. If long-term treatment is expected, then lung-function tests may also be helpful. Patients taking pergolide should be regularly monitored for cardiac fibrosis by echocardiography (within 3–6 months of initiating treatment and subsequently at 6–12 month intervals).

IMPULSE CONTROL DISORDERS
Treatment with dopamine-receptor agonists is associated with impulse control disorders, including pathological gambling, binge eating, and hypersexuality. Patients and their carers should be informed about the risk of impulse control disorders. There is no evidence that ergot- and non-ergot-derived dopamine-receptor agonists differ in their propensity to cause impulse control disorders, so switching between dopamine-receptor agonists to control these side-effects is not recommended. If the patient develops an impulse control disorder, the dopamine-receptor agonist or levodopa should be withdrawn or the dose reduced until the symptoms resolve.

● CONTRA-INDICATIONS Cardiac valvulopathy (exclude before treatment) · history of fibrotic disorders
● CAUTIONS Acute porphyrias p. 918 · arrhythmias · dyskinesia (may exacerbate) · hallucinations · history of confusion · psychosis · underlying cardiac disease
● INTERACTIONS → Appendix 1 (pergolide).
● SIDE-EFFECTS Abdominal pain · atrial premature contractions · compulsive behaviour · confusion · constipation · diarrhoea · diplopia · dizziness · drowsiness · dyskinesia · dyspepsia · dyspnoea · erythromelalgia · fever · hallucinations · hiccups · hypotension · insomnia · nausea · palpitation · rash · Raynaud's phenomenon · rhinitis · sudden onset of sleep · syncope · tachycardia · vomiting
● PREGNANCY Use only if potential benefit outweighs risk.
● BREAST FEEDING May suppress lactation.
● TREATMENT CESSATION Antiparkinsonian drug therapy should never be stopped abruptly as this carries a small risk of neuroleptic malignant syndrome.
● PATIENT AND CARER ADVICE
Driving and skilled tasks
Sudden onset of sleep Excessive daytime sleepiness and sudden onset of sleep can occur with dopamine-receptor agonists.
  Patients starting treatment with these drugs should be warned of the risk and of the need to exercise caution when driving or operating machinery. Those who have experienced excessive sedation or sudden onset of sleep should refrain from driving or operating machines until these effects have stopped occurring.
  Management of excessive daytime sleepiness should focus on the identification of an underlying cause, such as depression or concomitant medication. Patients should be counselled on improving sleep behaviour.
Hypotensive reactions Hypotensive reactions can occur in some patients taking dopamine-receptor agonists; these can be particularly problematic during the first few days of treatment and care should be exercised when driving or operating machinery.

● MEDICINAL FORMS
There can be variation in the licensing of different medicines containing the same drug.

Tablet
CAUTIONARY AND ADVISORY LABELS 10
▸ Pergolide (Non-proprietary)
  Pergolide (as Pergolide mesilate) 50 microgram Pergolide 50microgram tablets | 100 tablet [PoM] £32.09 DT price = £32.06
  Pergolide (as Pergolide mesilate) 250 microgram Pergolide 250microgram tablets | 100 tablet [PoM] £36.00–£39.00 DT price = £37.68
  Pergolide (as Pergolide mesilate) 1 mg Pergolide 1mg tablets | 100 tablet [PoM] £125.00–£135.00 DT price = £131.66

Pramipexole

INDICATIONS AND DOSE

Parkinson's disease, used alone or as an adjunct to co-beneldopa or co-careldopa

▶ BY MOUTH USING IMMEDIATE-RELEASE MEDICINES

▶ Adult: Initially 88 micrograms 3 times a day, if tolerated dose to be increased by doubling dose every 5–7 days, increased to 350 micrograms 3 times a day, then increased in steps of 180 micrograms 3 times a day if required, dose to be increased at weekly intervals, during dose titration and maintenance, levodopa dose may be reduced, maximum daily dose to be given in 3 divided doses; maximum 3.3 mg per day

▶ BY MOUTH USING MODIFIED-RELEASE MEDICINES

▶ Adult: Initially 260 micrograms once daily, dose to be increased by doubling dose every 5–7 days, increased to 1.05 mg once daily, then increased in steps of 520 micrograms every 1 week if required, during dose titration and maintenance, levodopa dose may be reduced according to response; maximum 3.15 mg per day

Moderate to severe restless legs syndrome

▶ BY MOUTH USING IMMEDIATE-RELEASE MEDICINES

▶ Adult: Initially 88 micrograms once daily, dose to be taken 2–3 hours before bedtime, dose to be increased by doubling dose every 4–7 days if necessary, repeat dose titration if restarting treatment after an interval of more than a few days; maximum 540 micrograms per day

DOSE EQUIVALENCE AND CONVERSION

Doses and strengths are stated in terms of pramipexole (base).

Equivalent strengths of pramipexole (base) in terms of pramipexole dihydrochloride monohydrate (salt) for immediate-release preparations are as follows:
88 micrograms base ≡ 125 micrograms salt;
180 micrograms base ≡ 250 micrograms salt;
350 micrograms base ≡ 500 micrograms salt;
700 micrograms base ≡ 1 mg salt.

Equivalent strengths of pramipexole (base) in terms of pramipexole dihydrochloride monohydrate (salt) for modified-release preparations are as follows:
260 micrograms base ≡ 375 micrograms salt;
520 micrograms base ≡ 750 micrograms salt;
1.05 mg base ≡ 1.5 mg salt;
1.57 mg base ≡ 2.25 mg salt;
2.1 mg base ≡ 3 mg salt;
2.62 mg base ≡ 3.75 mg salt;
3.15 mg base ≡ 4.5 mg salt.

IMPORTANT SAFETY INFORMATION
IMPULSE CONTROL DISORDERS

Treatment with dopamine-receptor agonists is associated with impulse control disorders, including pathological gambling, binge eating, and hypersexuality. Patients and their carers should be informed about the risk of impulse control disorders. There is no evidence that ergot- and non-ergot-derived dopamine-receptor agonists differ in their propensity to cause impulse control disorders, so switching between dopamine-receptor agonists to control these side-effects is not recommended. If the patient develops an impulse control disorder, the dopamine-receptor agonist should be withdrawn or the dose reduced until the symptoms resolve.

● CAUTIONS Psychotic disorders · risk of visual disorders (ophthalmological testing recommended) · severe cardiovascular disease

● INTERACTIONS → Appendix 1 (pramipexole).

● SIDE-EFFECTS

▶ **Common or very common** Confusion · constipation · decreased appetite · dizziness · drowsiness · dyskinesia · hallucinations · headache · hyperkinesia · hypotension · nausea · peripheral oedema · postural hypotension · restlessness · sleep disturbances · sudden onset of sleep · visual disturbances · vomiting · weight changes

▶ **Uncommon** Amnesia · binge eating · cardiac failure · compulsive behaviour · delusion · dyspnoea · hiccups · paranoia · pneumonia · pruritus · rash · syncope

▶ **Frequency not known** Paradoxical worsening of restless legs syndrome

● PREGNANCY Use only if potential benefit outweighs risk—no information available.

● BREAST FEEDING May suppress lactation; avoid—present in milk in *animal* studies.

● RENAL IMPAIRMENT For *immediate-release* tablets in Parkinson's disease, initially 88 micrograms twice daily (max. 1.57 mg daily in 2 divided doses) if eGFR 20–50 mL/minute/1.73 m^2; initially 88 micrograms once daily (max. 1.1 mg once daily) if eGFR less than 20 mL/minute/1.73 m^2. If renal function declines during treatment, reduce dose by the same percentage as the decline in eGFR. For *immediate-release* tablets in restless legs syndrome, reduce dose if eGFR less than 20 mL/minute/1.73 m^2. For *modified-release* tablets, initially 260 micrograms on alternate days if eGFR 30–50 mL/minute/1.73 m^2, increased to 260 micrograms once daily after 1 week, further increased if necessary by 260 micrograms daily at weekly intervals to max. 1.57 mg daily. For *modified-release* tablets, avoid if eGFR less than 30 mL/minute/1.73 m^2.

● MONITORING REQUIREMENTS Risk of postural hypotension (especially on initiation)—monitor blood pressure.

● TREATMENT CESSATION Antiparkinsonian drug therapy should never be stopped abruptly as this carries a small risk of neuroleptic malignant syndrome.

● PATIENT AND CARER ADVICE

Driving and skilled tasks
Sudden onset of sleep Excessive daytime sleepiness and sudden onset of sleep can occur with dopamine-receptor agonists.

Patients starting treatment with these drugs should be warned of the risk and of the need to exercise caution when driving or operating machinery. Those who have experienced excessive sedation or sudden onset of sleep should refrain from driving or operating machines until these effects have stopped occurring.

Management of excessive daytime sleepiness should focus on the identification of an underlying cause, such as depression or concomitant medication. Patients should be counselled on improving sleep behaviour.

Hypotensive reactions Hypotensive reactions can occur in some patients taking dopamine-receptor agonists; these can be particularly problematic during the first few days of treatment and care should be exercised when driving or operating machinery.

● MEDICINAL FORMS
There can be variation in the licensing of different medicines containing the same drug.

Tablet
CAUTIONARY AND ADVISORY LABELS 10
▶ Pramipexole (Non-proprietary)
Pramipexole (as Pramipexole dihydrochloride monohydrate)
88 microgram Pramipexole 88microgram tablets | 30 tablet [PoM]
£9.54 DT price = £1.89
Pramipexole (as Pramipexole dihydrochloride monohydrate)
180 microgram Pramipexole 180microgram tablets |
30 tablet [PoM] £17.19 DT price = £1.79 | 100 tablet [PoM] £19.09

4

Nervous system

Nervous system

4

Pramipexole (as Pramipexole dihydrochloride monohydrate)
350 microgram Pramipexole 350microgram tablets |
30 tablet [PoM] £38.20 DT price = £11.44 | 100 tablet [PoM] £38.23
Pramipexole (as Pramipexole dihydrochloride monohydrate)
700 microgram Pramipexole 700microgram tablets |
30 tablet [PoM] £76.40 DT price = £2.28 | 100 tablet [PoM] £254.69

▶ Mirapexin (Boehringer Ingelheim Ltd)

Pramipexole (as Pramipexole dihydrochloride monohydrate)
88 microgram Mirapexin 0.088mg tablets | 30 tablet [PoM] £11.24
DT price = £1.89
Pramipexole (as Pramipexole dihydrochloride monohydrate)
180 microgram Mirapexin 0.18mg tablets | 30 tablet [PoM] £22.49
DT price = £1.79 | 100 tablet [PoM] £74.95
Pramipexole (as Pramipexole dihydrochloride monohydrate)
350 microgram Mirapexin 0.35mg tablets | 30 tablet [PoM] £44.97
DT price = £11.44 | 100 tablet [PoM] £149.90
Pramipexole (as Pramipexole dihydrochloride monohydrate)
700 microgram Mirapexin 0.7mg tablets | 30 tablet [PoM] £89.94
DT price = £2.28 | 100 tablet [PoM] £299.82

▶ Oprymea (Consilient Health Ltd)

Pramipexole (as Pramipexole dihydrochloride monohydrate)
88 microgram Oprymea 0.088mg tablets | 30 tablet [PoM] £3.23 DT
price = £1.89
Pramipexole (as Pramipexole dihydrochloride monohydrate)
180 microgram Oprymea 0.18mg tablets | 30 tablet [PoM] £6.09 DT
price = £1.79 | 100 tablet [PoM] £15.46
Pramipexole (as Pramipexole dihydrochloride monohydrate)
350 microgram Oprymea 0.35mg tablets | 30 tablet [PoM] £32.47
DT price = £11.44 | 100 tablet [PoM] £108.23
Pramipexole (as Pramipexole dihydrochloride monohydrate)
700 microgram Oprymea 0.7mg tablets | 30 tablet [PoM] £18.26 DT
price = £2.28 | 100 tablet [PoM] £117.63

Modified-release tablet

CAUTIONARY AND ADVISORY LABELS 10, 25

▶ Pramipexole (Non-proprietary)

Pramipexole (as Pramipexole dihydrochloride monohydrate)
260 microgram Pramipexole 260microgram modified-release tablets
| 30 tablet [PoM] £30.87–£32.49 DT price = £32.49
Pramipexole (as Pramipexole dihydrochloride monohydrate)
520 microgram Pramipexole 520microgram modified-release tablets
| 30 tablet [PoM] £61.73–£64.98 DT price = £64.98
Pramipexole (as Pramipexole dihydrochloride monohydrate)
1.05 mg Pramipexole 1.05mg modified-release tablets |
30 tablet [PoM] £123.46–£129.96 DT price = £129.96
Pramipexole (as Pramipexole dihydrochloride monohydrate)
1.57 mg Pramipexole 1.57mg modified-release tablets |
30 tablet [PoM] £192.24–£202.36 DT price = £202.36
Pramipexole (as Pramipexole dihydrochloride monohydrate)
2.1 mg Pramipexole 2.1mg modified-release tablets | 30 tablet [PoM]
£246.91–£259.91 DT price = £259.91
Pramipexole (as Pramipexole dihydrochloride monohydrate)
2.62 mg Pramipexole 2.62mg modified-release tablets |
30 tablet [PoM] £320.41–£337.27 DT price = £337.27
Pramipexole (as Pramipexole dihydrochloride monohydrate)
3.15 mg Pramipexole 3.15mg modified-release tablets |
30 tablet [PoM] £370.38–£389.87 DT price = £389.87

▶ Mirapexin (Boehringer Ingelheim Ltd)

Pramipexole (as Pramipexole dihydrochloride monohydrate)
260 microgram Mirapexin 0.26mg modified-release tablets |
30 tablet [PoM] £32.49 DT price = £32.49
Pramipexole (as Pramipexole dihydrochloride monohydrate)
520 microgram Mirapexin 0.52mg modified-release tablets |
30 tablet [PoM] £64.98 DT price = £64.98
Pramipexole (as Pramipexole dihydrochloride monohydrate)
1.05 mg Mirapexin 1.05mg modified-release tablets | 30 tablet [PoM]
£129.96 DT price = £129.96
Pramipexole (as Pramipexole dihydrochloride monohydrate)
1.57 mg Mirapexin 1.57mg modified-release tablets |
30 tablet [PoM] £202.36 DT price = £202.36
Pramipexole (as Pramipexole dihydrochloride monohydrate)
2.1 mg Mirapexin 2.1mg modified-release tablets | 30 tablet [PoM]
£259.91 DT price = £259.91
Pramipexole (as Pramipexole dihydrochloride monohydrate)
2.62 mg Mirapexin 2.62mg modified-release tablets |
30 tablet [PoM] £337.27 DT price = £337.27
Pramipexole (as Pramipexole dihydrochloride monohydrate)
3.15 mg Mirapexin 3.15mg modified-release tablets | 30 tablet [PoM]
£389.87 DT price = £389.87

▶ Oprymea (Consilient Health Ltd)

Pramipexole (as Pramipexole dihydrochloride monohydrate)
260 microgram Oprymea 0.26mg modified-release tablets |
30 tablet [PoM] £25.56 DT price = £32.49
Pramipexole (as Pramipexole dihydrochloride monohydrate)
520 microgram Oprymea 0.52mg modified-release tablets |
30 tablet [PoM] £51.14 DT price = £64.98
Pramipexole (as Pramipexole dihydrochloride monohydrate)
1.05 mg Oprymea 1.05mg modified-release tablets | 30 tablet [PoM]
£102.28 DT price = £129.96
Pramipexole (as Pramipexole dihydrochloride monohydrate)
1.57 mg Oprymea 1.57mg modified-release tablets | 30 tablet [PoM]
£159.26 DT price = £202.36
Pramipexole (as Pramipexole dihydrochloride monohydrate)
2.1 mg Oprymea 2.1mg modified-release tablets | 30 tablet [PoM]
£204.56 DT price = £259.91
Pramipexole (as Pramipexole dihydrochloride monohydrate)
2.62 mg Oprymea 2.62mg modified-release tablets | 30 tablet [PoM]
£337.27 DT price = £337.27
Pramipexole (as Pramipexole dihydrochloride monohydrate)
3.15 mg Oprymea 3.15mg modified-release tablets | 30 tablet [PoM]
£389.87 DT price = £389.87

Ropinirole

● INDICATIONS AND DOSE

Parkinson's disease, either used alone or as adjunct to co-beneldopa or co-careldopa

▶ BY MOUTH USING IMMEDIATE-RELEASE MEDICINES

▶ Adult: Initially 750 micrograms daily in 3 divided doses,
then increased in steps of 750 micrograms daily, dose
to be increased at weekly intervals, increased to 3 mg
daily in 3 divided doses, then increased in steps of
1.5–3 mg daily, adjusted according to response, dose to
be increased at weekly intervals; usual dose 9–16 mg
daily in 3 divided doses, higher doses may be required if
used with levodopa, when administered as adjunct to
levodopa, concurrent dose of levodopa may be reduced
by approx. 20%, daily maximum dose to be given in
3 divided doses; maximum 24 mg per day

▶ BY MOUTH USING MODIFIED-RELEASE MEDICINES

▶ Adult: Initially 2 mg once daily for 1 week, then 4 mg
once daily, increased in steps of 2 mg at intervals of at
least 1 week, adjusted according to response, increased
to up to 8 mg once daily, dose to be increased further if
still no response; increased in steps of 2–4 mg at
intervals of at least 2 weeks if required; maximum
24 mg per day

Parkinson's disease in patients transferring from ropinirole immediate-release tablets

▶ BY MOUTH USING MODIFIED-RELEASE MEDICINES

▶ Adult: Initially ropinirole modified-release once daily
substituted for total daily dose equivalent of ropinirole
immediate-release tablets; if control not maintained
after switching, titrate dose, consider slower titration
in patients over 75 years, when administered as adjunct
to levodopa, concurrent dose of levodopa may
gradually be reduced by approx. 30%, if treatment
interrupted for 1 day or more, consider re-initiation
with immediate-release tablets

Moderate to severe restless legs syndrome

▶ BY MOUTH USING IMMEDIATE-RELEASE MEDICINES

▶ Adult: Initially 250 micrograms once daily for 2 days,
increased if tolerated to 500 micrograms once daily for
5 days, then increased if tolerated to 1 mg once daily
for 7 days, then increased in steps of 500 micrograms
daily, adjusted according to response, dose to be
increased at weekly intervals; usual dose 2 mg once
daily, doses to be taken at night, repeat dose titration if
restarting after interval of more than a few days;
maximum 4 mg per day

DOSE ADJUSTMENTS DUE TO INTERACTIONS
Dose adjustment may be necessary if smoking started or stopped during treatment.

● UNLICENSED USE Doses in the BNF may differ from those in product literature.

IMPORTANT SAFETY INFORMATION
IMPULSE CONTROL DISORDERS
Treatment with dopamine-receptor agonists is associated with impulse control disorders, including pathological gambling, binge eating, and hypersexuality. Patients and their carers should be informed about the risk of impulse control disorders. There is no evidence that ergot- and non-ergot-derived dopamine-receptor agonists differ in their propensity to cause impulse control disorders, so switching between dopamine-receptor agonists to control these side-effects is not recommended. If the patient develops an impulse control disorder, the dopamine-receptor agonist should be withdrawn or the dose reduced until the symptoms resolve.

● CAUTIONS Elderly · major psychotic disorders · severe cardiovascular disease (risk of hypotension—monitor blood pressure)
● INTERACTIONS → Appendix 1 (ropinirole).
● SIDE-EFFECTS
▶ **Common or very common** Abdominal pain · confusion · constipation · dizziness · drowsiness · dyskinesia · dyspepsia · fatigue · gastro-oesophageal reflux disease · hallucinations · hypotension · nausea · nervousness · peripheral oedema · sudden onset of sleep · syncope · vomiting
▶ **Uncommon** Compulsive behaviour · psychosis
▶ **Very rare** Hepatic disorders
▶ **Frequency not known** Paradoxical worsening of restless legs syndrome
● PREGNANCY Avoid unless potential benefit outweighs risk—toxicity in *animal* studies.
● BREAST FEEDING May suppress lactation—avoid.
● HEPATIC IMPAIRMENT Avoid—no information available.
● RENAL IMPAIRMENT Avoid if eGFR less than 30 mL/minute/1.73 m².
● TREATMENT CESSATION Antiparkinsonian drug therapy should never be stopped abruptly as this carries a small risk of neuroleptic malignant syndrome.
● PATIENT AND CARER ADVICE
Driving and skilled tasks
Sudden onset of sleep Excessive daytime sleepiness and sudden onset of sleep can occur with dopamine-receptor agonists.
    Patients starting treatment with these drugs should be warned of the risk and of the need to exercise caution when driving or operating machinery. Those who have experienced excessive sedation or sudden onset of sleep should refrain from driving or operating machines until these effects have stopped occurring.
    Management of excessive daytime sleepiness should focus on the identification of an underlying cause, such as depression or concomitant medication. Patients should be counselled on improving sleep behaviour.
Hypotensive reactions Hypotensive reactions can occur in some patients taking dopamine-receptor agonists; these can be particularly problematic during the first few days of treatment and care should be exercised when driving or operating machinery.

● NATIONAL FUNDING/ACCESS DECISIONS
Scottish Medicines Consortium (SMC) Decisions
The Scottish Medicines Consortium has advised (June 2006) that *Adartrel®* should be restricted for use in patients with a baseline score of 24 points or more on the International Restless Legs Scale.

● MEDICINAL FORMS
There can be variation in the licensing of different medicines containing the same drug. Forms available from special-order manufacturers include: oral suspension, oral solution, powder

Tablet
CAUTIONARY AND ADVISORY LABELS 10, 21
▶ Ropinirole (Non-proprietary)
Ropinirole (as Ropinirole hydrochloride)
250 microgram Ropinirole 250microgram tablets | 12 tablet [PoM] £4.13 DT price = £1.17
Ropinirole (as Ropinirole hydrochloride)
500 microgram Ropinirole 500microgram tablets | 28 tablet [PoM] £15.34 DT price = £1.81
Ropinirole (as Ropinirole hydrochloride) 1 mg Ropinirole 1mg tablets | 84 tablet [PoM] £16.33 DT price = £1.80
Ropinirole (as Ropinirole hydrochloride) 2 mg Ropinirole 2mg tablets | 28 tablet [PoM] £2.31-£26.97 DT price = £1.84 | 84 tablet [PoM] £33.35
Ropinirole (as Ropinirole hydrochloride) 5 mg Ropinirole 5mg tablets | 84 tablet [PoM] £69.68 DT price = £3.46
▶ Adartrel (GlaxoSmithKline Ltd)
Ropinirole (as Ropinirole hydrochloride) 250 microgram Adartrel 250microgram tablets | 12 tablet [PoM] £3.94 DT price = £1.17
Ropinirole (as Ropinirole hydrochloride) 500 microgram Adartrel 500microgram tablets | 28 tablet [PoM] £15.75 DT price = £1.81
Ropinirole (as Ropinirole hydrochloride) 2 mg Adartrel 2mg tablets | 28 tablet [PoM] £31.51 DT price = £1.84
▶ ReQuip (GlaxoSmithKline UK Ltd)
Ropinirole (as Ropinirole hydrochloride) 250 microgram ReQuip 250microgram tablets | 21 tablet [PoM] £5.70 | 42 tablet [PoM] no price available
Ropinirole (as Ropinirole hydrochloride) 500 microgram ReQuip 500microgram tablets | 42 tablet [PoM] no price available
Ropinirole (as Ropinirole hydrochloride) 1 mg ReQuip 1mg tablets | 21 tablet [PoM] no price available | 42 tablet [PoM] no price available | 84 tablet [PoM] £56.71 DT price = £1.80
Ropinirole (as Ropinirole hydrochloride) 2 mg ReQuip 2mg tablets | 63 tablet [PoM] no price available | 84 tablet [PoM] £113.44
Ropinirole (as Ropinirole hydrochloride) 5 mg ReQuip 5mg tablets | 84 tablet [PoM] £195.92 DT price = £3.46

Modified-release tablet
CAUTIONARY AND ADVISORY LABELS 10, 25
▶ Eppinix XL (DB Ashbourne Ltd)
Ropinirole (as Ropinirole hydrochloride) 2 mg Eppinix XL 2mg tablets | 28 tablet [PoM] £5.64 DT price = £12.54
Ropinirole (as Ropinirole hydrochloride) 3 mg Eppinix XL 3mg tablets | 28 tablet [PoM] £8.46
Ropinirole (as Ropinirole hydrochloride) 4 mg Eppinix XL 4mg tablets | 28 tablet [PoM] £11.29 DT price = £25.09
Ropinirole (as Ropinirole hydrochloride) 6 mg Eppinix XL 6mg tablets | 28 tablet [PoM] £15.32
Ropinirole (as Ropinirole hydrochloride) 8 mg Eppinix XL 8mg tablets | 28 tablet [PoM] £18.95 DT price = £42.11
▶ Ralnea XL (Consilient Health Ltd)
Ropinirole (as Ropinirole hydrochloride) 2 mg Ralnea XL 2mg tablets | 28 tablet [PoM] £10.65 DT price = £12.54
Ropinirole (as Ropinirole hydrochloride) 4 mg Ralnea XL 4mg tablets | 28 tablet [PoM] £21.32 DT price = £25.09
Ropinirole (as Ropinirole hydrochloride) 8 mg Ralnea XL 8mg tablets | 28 tablet [PoM] £35.79 DT price = £42.11
▶ Raponer XL (Actavis UK Ltd)
Ropinirole (as Ropinirole hydrochloride) 2 mg Raponer XL 2mg tablets | 28 tablet [PoM] £12.54 DT price = £12.54
Ropinirole (as Ropinirole hydrochloride) 4 mg Raponer XL 4mg tablets | 28 tablet [PoM] £25.09 DT price = £25.09
Ropinirole (as Ropinirole hydrochloride) 8 mg Raponer XL 8mg tablets | 28 tablet [PoM] £42.11 DT price = £42.11
▶ ReQuip XL (GlaxoSmithKline UK Ltd)
Ropinirole (as Ropinirole hydrochloride) 2 mg ReQuip XL 2mg tablets | 28 tablet [PoM] £12.54 DT price = £12.54
Ropinirole (as Ropinirole hydrochloride) 4 mg ReQuip XL 4mg tablets | 28 tablet [PoM] £25.09 DT price = £25.09

4

Nervous system

Ropinirole (as Ropinirole hydrochloride) 8 mg ReQuip XL 8mg tablets | 28 tablet [PoM] £42.11 DT price = £42.11
▸ Repinex XL (Aspire Pharma Ltd)
Ropinirole (as Ropinirole hydrochloride) 2 mg Repinex XL 2mg tablets | 28 tablet [PoM] £6.20 DT price = £12.54
Ropinirole (as Ropinirole hydrochloride) 4 mg Repinex XL 4mg tablets | 28 tablet [PoM] £12.50 DT price = £25.09
Ropinirole (as Ropinirole hydrochloride) 8 mg Repinex XL 8mg tablets | 28 tablet [PoM] £21.00 DT price = £42.11
▸ Spiroco XL (Teva UK Ltd)
Ropinirole (as Ropinirole hydrochloride) 2 mg Spiroco XL 2mg tablets | 28 tablet [PoM] £5.63 DT price = £12.54
Ropinirole (as Ropinirole hydrochloride) 4 mg Spiroco XL 4mg tablets | 28 tablet [PoM] £11.28 DT price = £25.09
Ropinirole (as Ropinirole hydrochloride) 8 mg Spiroco XL 8mg tablets | 28 tablet [PoM] £18.94 DT price = £42.11

Rotigotine

● **INDICATIONS AND DOSE**

Monotherapy in Parkinson's disease
▸ BY TRANSDERMAL APPLICATION USING PATCHES
▸ Adult: Initially 2 mg/24 hours, then increased in steps of 2 mg/24 hours every 1 week if required; maximum 8 mg/24 hours per day

Adjunctive therapy with co-beneldopa or co-careldopa in Parkinson's disease
▸ BY TRANSDERMAL APPLICATION USING PATCHES
▸ Adult: Initially 4 mg/24 hours, then increased in steps of 2 mg/24 hours every 1 week if required; maximum 16 mg/24 hours per day

Moderate to severe restless legs syndrome
▸ BY TRANSDERMAL APPLICATION USING PATCHES
▸ Adult: Initially 1 mg/24 hours, then increased in steps of 1 mg/24 hours every 1 week if required; maximum 3 mg/24 hours per day

---

IMPORTANT SAFETY INFORMATION
IMPULSE CONTROL DISORDERS

Treatment with dopamine-receptor agonists is associated with impulse control disorders, including pathological gambling, binge eating, and hypersexuality. Patients and their carers should be informed about the risk of impulse control disorders. There is no evidence that ergot- and non-ergot-derived dopamine-receptor agonists differ in their propensity to cause impulse control disorders, so switching between dopamine-receptor agonists to control these side-effects is not recommended. If the patient develops an impulse control disorder, the dopamine-receptor agonist should be withdrawn or the dose reduced until the symptoms resolve.

● CAUTIONS Avoid exposure of patch to heat · remove patch (aluminium-containing) before magnetic resonance imaging or cardioversion
● INTERACTIONS → Appendix 1 (rotigotine).
● SIDE-EFFECTS
▸ **Common or very common** Abnormal behaviour · abnormal thinking · aggression · application site reactions · confusion · constipation · dizziness · drowsiness · dry mouth · dyskinesia · dyspepsia · hallucinations · headache · hiccup · hypertension · malaise · nausea · palpitation · paranoia · peripheral oedema · postural hypotension · pruritus · psychosis · rash · sleep disturbances · sudden onset of sleep · sweating · syncope · vomiting · weight changes
▸ **Uncommon** Abdominal pain · atrial fibrillation · erectile dysfunction · hypotension · impulse control disorders · visual disturbances
▸ **Rare** Irritability · obsessive compulsive disorder · seizures · tachycardia

● PREGNANCY Avoid—no information available.
● BREAST FEEDING May suppress lactation; avoid—present in milk in *animal* studies.
● HEPATIC IMPAIRMENT Caution in severe impairment— no information available.
● MONITORING REQUIREMENTS Ophthalmic testing recommended.
● TREATMENT CESSATION Antiparkinsonian drug therapy should never be stopped abruptly as this carries a small risk of neuroleptic malignant syndrome.
● DIRECTIONS FOR ADMINISTRATION Apply patch to dry, non-irritated skin on torso, thigh, or upper arm, removing after 24 hours and siting replacement patch on a different area (avoid using the same area for 14 days).
● PATIENT AND CARER ADVICE
Driving and skilled tasks
Sudden onset of sleep Excessive daytime sleepiness and sudden onset of sleep can occur with dopamine-receptor agonists.
　Patients starting treatment with these drugs should be warned of the risk and of the need to exercise caution when driving or operating machinery. Those who have experienced excessive sedation or sudden onset of sleep should refrain from driving or operating machines until these effects have stopped occurring.
　Management of excessive daytime sleepiness should focus on the identification of an underlying cause, such as depression or concomitant medication. Patients should be counselled on improving sleep behaviour.
Hypotensive reactions Hypotensive reactions can occur in some patients taking dopamine-receptor agonists; these can be particularly problematic during the first few days of treatment and care should be exercised when driving or operating machinery.
● NATIONAL FUNDING/ACCESS DECISIONS
Scottish Medicines Consortium (SMC) Decisions
The *Scottish Medicines Consortium* has advised that *Neupro®* is accepted for restricted use for the treatment of advanced Parkinson's disease in combination with levodopa where the transdermal route would facilitate treatment (July 2007).
　The *Scottish Medicines Consortium* has advised that *Neupro®* is accepted as monotherapy for the treatment of early-stage idiopathic Parkinson's disease (June 2007).
　The *Scottish Medicines Consortium* has advised (April 2009) that rotigotine (*Neupro®*) is accepted for restricted use within NHS Scotland for the symptomatic treatment of moderate to severe idiopathic restless legs syndrome in adults with a baseline score of 15 points or more on the International Restless Legs Scale.

● MEDICINAL FORMS
There can be variation in the licensing of different medicines containing the same drug.
Transdermal patch
CAUTIONARY AND ADVISORY LABELS 10
▸ Neupro (UCB Pharma Ltd)
Rotigotine 1 mg per 24 hour Neupro 1mg/24hours transdermal patches | 28 patch [PoM] £77.24
Rotigotine 2 mg per 24 hour Neupro 2mg/24hours transdermal patches | 7 patch [PoM] no price available | 28 patch [PoM] £81.10 DT price = £81.10
Rotigotine 3 mg per 24 hour Neupro 3mg/24hours transdermal patches | 28 patch [PoM] £102.35
Rotigotine 4 mg per 24 hour Neupro 4mg/24hours transdermal patches | 7 patch [PoM] no price available | 28 patch [PoM] £123.60 DT price = £123.60
Rotigotine 6 mg per 24 hour Neupro 6mg/24hours transdermal patches | 7 patch [PoM] no price available | 28 patch [PoM] £149.93 DT price = £149.93
Rotigotine 8 mg per 24 hour Neupro 8mg/24hours transdermal patches | 7 patch [PoM] no price available | 28 patch [PoM] £149.93 DT price = £149.93

DOPAMINERGIC DRUGS > MONOAMINE-OXIDASE B INHIBITORS

Rasagiline

- **DRUG ACTION** Rasagiline is a monoamine-oxidase B inhibitor.

- ● **INDICATIONS AND DOSE**

Parkinson's disease, used alone or as adjunct to co-beneldopa or co-careldopa for 'end-of-dose' fluctuations
  - ▸ BY MOUTH
  - ▸ Adult: 1 mg daily

- **INTERACTIONS** → Appendix 1 (rasagiline).

- **SIDE-EFFECTS**
  - ▸ **Common or very common** Abnormal dreams · angina · anorexia · arthralgia · conjunctivitis · constipation · depression · dry mouth · dyspepsia · flatulence · hallucinations · headache · influenza-like symptoms · leucopenia · rash · rhinitis · skin carcinoma · urinary urgency · vertigo · weight loss
  - ▸ **Uncommon** Cerebrovascular accident · myocardial infarction

- **PREGNANCY** Use with caution.

- **BREAST FEEDING** Use with caution—may suppress lactation.

- **HEPATIC IMPAIRMENT** Use with caution in mild impairment. Avoid in moderate to severe impairment.

- **TREATMENT CESSATION** Avoid abrupt withdrawal.

- **MEDICINAL FORMS**
There can be variation in the licensing of different medicines containing the same drug. Forms available from special-order manufacturers include: oral suspension, oral solution

Tablet
  - ▸ Rasagiline (Non-proprietary)
  Rasagiline 1 mg Rasagiline 1mg tablets | 28 tablet PoM £70.72 DT price = £63.79
  - ▸ Azilect (Teva UK Ltd)
  Rasagiline 1 mg Azilect 1mg tablets | 28 tablet PoM £70.72 DT price = £63.79

Selegiline hydrochloride

- **DRUG ACTION** Selegiline is a monoamine-oxidase-B inhibitor.

- ● **INDICATIONS AND DOSE**

Parkinson's disease, used alone or as adjunct to co-beneldopa or co-careldopa to reduce 'end of dose' deterioration | Symptomatic parkinsonism
  - ▸ BY MOUTH USING IMMEDIATE-RELEASE MEDICINES
  - ▸ Adult: Initially 5 mg once daily for 2–4 weeks, then increased if tolerated to 10 mg daily, dose to be taken in the morning
  - ▸ BY MOUTH USING ORAL LYOPHILISATE
  - ▸ Adult: 1.25 mg once daily, dose to be taken before breakfast

DOSE EQUIVALENCE AND CONVERSION
1.25-mg oral lyophilisate is equivalent to 10-mg tablet. Patients receiving 10 mg conventional selegiline hydrochloride tablets can be switched to oral lyophilisates (*Zelapar*®) 1.25 mg.

- **CONTRA-INDICATIONS** Active duodenal ulceration · active gastric ulceration · avoid or use with great caution in postural hypotension (when used in combination with levodopa)

- **CAUTIONS** Angina · arrhythmias · avoid in Acute porphyrias p. 918 · duodenal ulceration · gastric ulceration · history of hepatic dysfunction · patients predisposed to

confusion and psychosis · psychosis · uncontrolled hypertension

- **INTERACTIONS** → Appendix 1 (selegiline).
Avoid with drugs that increase blood pressure.

- **SIDE-EFFECTS**
  - ▸ **Common or very common** Arthralgia · bradycardia · confusion · constipation · depression · diarrhoea · dizziness · dry mouth · fatigue · hair loss · headache · hypertension · hypotension · impaired balance · mouth ulcers · movement disorders · muscle cramps · myalgia · myopathy · nasal congestion · nausea · psychosis · sleeping disorders · stomatitis · sweating · tremor
  - ▸ **Uncommon** Agitation · angina · ankle oedema · anxiety · arrhythmias · blurred vision · dyspnoea · leucocytopenia · loss of appetite · micturition difficulties · palpitation · postural hypotension · skin reactions · supraventricular tachycardia · thrombocytopenia
  - ▸ **Frequency not known** Hypersexuality

  SIDE-EFFECTS, FURTHER INFORMATION
  Side-effects of levodopa may be increased—concurrent levodopa dosage can be reduced by 10–30% in steps of 10% every 3–4 days.

- **PREGNANCY** Avoid—no information available.

- **BREAST FEEDING** Avoid—no information available.

- **HEPATIC IMPAIRMENT** Use with caution in severe impairment.

- **RENAL IMPAIRMENT** Use with caution in severe impairment.

- **TREATMENT CESSATION** Avoid abrupt withdrawal.

- **DIRECTIONS FOR ADMINISTRATION** Oral lyophilisates should be placed on the tongue and allowed to dissolve. Advise patient not to drink, rinse, or wash mouth out for 5 minutes after taking the tablet.

- **PATIENT AND CARER ADVICE**
Patients or carers should be advised on how to administer selegiline hydrochloride oral lyophilisates.

Driving and skilled tasks
Counselling advised on driving.

Drugs and driving Prescribers and other healthcare professionals should advise patients if treatment is likely to affect their ability to perform skilled tasks (e.g. driving). This applies especially to drugs with sedative effects; patients should be warned that these effects are increased by alcohol. General information about a patient's fitness to drive is available from the Driver and Vehicle Licensing Agency at www.dvla.gov.uk.
  2015 legislation regarding driving whilst taking certain drugs, may also apply to selegiline, see *Drugs and driving* under Guidance on prescribing p. 1.

- **MEDICINAL FORMS**
There can be variation in the licensing of different medicines containing the same drug. Forms available from special-order manufacturers include: oral solution

Tablet
  - ▸ Selegiline hydrochloride (Non-proprietary)
  Selegiline hydrochloride 5 mg Selegiline 5mg tablets | 60 tablet PoM £28.08 DT price = £26.50
  Selegiline hydrochloride 10 mg Selegiline 10mg tablets | 30 tablet PoM £27.20 DT price = £9.50
  - ▸ Eldepryl (Orion Pharma (UK) Ltd)
  Selegiline hydrochloride 5 mg Eldepryl 5mg tablets | 100 tablet PoM £16.52
  Selegiline hydrochloride 10 mg Eldepryl 10mg tablets | 100 tablet PoM £32.23

Oral lyophilisate
EXCIPIENTS: May contain Aspartame
  - ▸ Zelapar (Teva UK Ltd)
  Selegiline hydrochloride 1.25 mg Zelapar 1.25mg oral lyophilisates sugar-free | 30 tablet PoM £43.16

5 Nausea and labyrinth disorders

Nausea and labyrinth disorders

Drug treatment

Antiemetics should be prescribed only when the cause of vomiting is known because otherwise they may delay diagnosis, particularly in children. Antiemetics are unnecessary and sometimes harmful when the cause can be treated, such as in diabetic ketoacidosis, or in digoxin p. 98 or antiepileptic overdose.

If antiemetic drug treatment is indicated, the drug is chosen according to the aetiology of vomiting.

Antihistamines are effective against nausea and vomiting resulting from many underlying conditions. There is no evidence that any one antihistamine is superior to another but their duration of action and incidence of adverse effects (drowsiness and antimuscarinic effects) differ.

The **phenothiazines** are dopamine antagonists and act centrally by blocking the chemoreceptor trigger zone. They are of considerable value for the prophylaxis and treatment of nausea and vomiting associated with diffuse neoplastic disease, radiation sickness, and the emesis caused by drugs such as opioids, general anaesthetics, and cytotoxics. Prochlorperazine p. 357, perphenazine p. 356, and trifluoperazine p. 358 are less sedating than chlorpromazine hydrochloride p. 353; severe dystonic reactions sometimes occur with phenothiazines, especially in children. Some phenothiazines are available as rectal suppositories, which can be useful in patients with persistent vomiting or with severe nausea; prochlorperazine can also be administered as a buccal tablet which is placed between the upper lip and the gum.

Other antipsychotic drugs including haloperidol p. 354 and levomepromazine p. 403 are used for the relief of nausea and vomiting in terminal illness.

Metoclopramide hydrochloride p. 395 is an effective antiemetic and its activity closely resembles that of the phenothiazines. Metoclopramide hydrochloride also acts directly on the gastro-intestinal tract and it may be superior to the phenothiazines for emesis associated with gastroduodenal, hepatic, and biliary disease.

Domperidone p. 394 acts at the chemoreceptor trigger zone; it is licensed only for the relief of nausea and vomiting. It has the advantage over metoclopramide hydrochloride and the phenothiazines of being less likely to cause central effects such as sedation and dystonic reactions because it does not readily cross the blood-brain barrier. In Parkinson's disease, it can be used to treat nausea caused by dopaminergic drugs.

Granisetron p. 397 and ondansetron p. 397 are of value in the management of nausea and vomiting in patients receiving cytotoxics and in postoperative nausea and vomiting. Palonosetron p. 399 is licensed for prevention of nausea and vomiting associated with moderately or highly emetogenic cytotoxic chemotherapy. Palonosetron is also available in combination with netupitant, a neurokinin 1-receptor antagonist, for the prevention of acute and delayed nausea and vomiting associated with moderately emetogenic chemotherapy and highly emetogenic cisplatin-based chemotherapy.

Dexamethasone p. 610 has antiemetic effects and it is used in vomiting associated with cancer chemotherapy. It can be used alone or with metoclopramide hydrochloride, prochlorperazine, lorazepam p. 308, or a 5HT$_3$-receptor antagonist.

Aprepitant p. 396 and fosaprepitant p. 396 are neurokinin 1-receptor antagonists licensed for the prevention of acute and delayed nausea and vomiting associated with cisplatin-based cytotoxic chemotherapy; they are given with dexamethasone and a 5HT$_3$-receptor antagonist.

Nabilone p. 394 is a synthetic cannabinoid with antiemetic properties. It may be used for nausea and vomiting caused by cytotoxic chemotherapy that is unresponsive to conventional antiemetics.

Vomiting during pregnancy

Nausea in the first trimester of pregnancy is generally mild and does not require drug therapy. On rare occasions if vomiting is severe, short-term treatment with an antihistamine, such as **promethazine**, may be required. Prochlorperazine or metoclopramide hydrochloride are alternatives. If symptoms do not settle in 24 to 48 hours then specialist opinion should be sought. Hyperemesis gravidarum is a more serious condition, which requires regular antiemetic therapy, intravenous fluid and electrolyte replacement and sometimes nutritional support. Supplementation with thiamine p. 938 must be considered in order to reduce the risk of Wernicke's encephalopathy.

Postoperative nausea and vomiting

The incidence of postoperative nausea and vomiting depends on many factors including the anaesthetic used, and the type and duration of surgery. Other risk factors include female sex, non-smokers, a history of postoperative nausea and vomiting or motion sickness, and intraoperative and postoperative use of opioids. Therapy to prevent postoperative nausea and vomiting should be based on the assessed risk of postoperative nausea and vomiting in each patient. Drugs used include **5HT$_3$-receptor antagonists**, droperidol p. 402, dexamethasone, some **phenothiazines** (e.g. prochlorperazine), and **antihistamines** (e.g. cyclizine p. 393). A combination of two or more antiemetic drugs that have different mechanisms of action is often indicated in those at high risk of postoperative nausea and vomiting or where postoperative vomiting presents a particular danger (e.g. in some types of surgery). When a prophylactic antiemetic drug has failed, postoperative nausea and vomiting should be treated with one or more drugs from a different class.

Motion sickness

Antiemetics should be given to prevent motion sickness rather than after nausea or vomiting develop. The most effective drug for the prevention of motion sickness is hyoscine hydrobromide p. 401. The sedating antihistamines are slightly less effective against motion sickness, but are generally better tolerated than hyoscine. If a sedative effect is desired **promethazine** is useful, but generally a slightly less sedating antihistamine such as cyclizine or cinnarizine p. 400 is preferred. Domperidone, metoclopramide hydrochloride, 5HT$_3$-receptor antagonists, and the phenothiazines (except the antihistamine phenothiazine promethazine) are **ineffective** in motion sickness.

Other vestibular disorders

Management of vestibular diseases is aimed at treating the underlying cause as well as treating symptoms of the balance disturbance and associated nausea and vomiting. Vertigo and nausea associated with Ménière's disease and middle-ear surgery can be difficult to treat.

Betahistine dihydrochloride p. 403 is an analogue of histamine and is claimed to reduce endolymphatic pressure by improving the microcirculation. Betahistine dihydrochloride is licensed for vertigo, tinnitus, and hearing loss associated with Ménière's disease.

A **diuretic** alone or combined with salt restriction may provide some benefit in vertigo associated with Ménière's disease; **antihistamines** (such as cinnarizine), and **phenothiazines** (such as prochlorperazine) are also used.

Where possible, prochlorperazine should be reserved for the treatment of acute symptoms.

Cytotoxic chemotherapy, palliative care, and migraine

Antiemetics have a role in the management of nausea and vomiting induced by cytotoxic chemotherapy, in palliative care, and associated with migraine.

> **Drugs used for Nausea and labyrinth disorders not listed below** Paracetamol with metoclopramide, p. 431 · Promethazine hydrochloride, p. 264

ANTIEMETICS AND ANTINAUSEANTS ›
ANTIHISTAMINES

▌Cyclizine

- ● **INDICATIONS AND DOSE**

Nausea | Vomiting | Vertigo | Motion sickness | Labyrinthine disorders
- ▸ BY MOUTH
- ▸ Adult: 50 mg up to 3 times a day, for motion sickness, take 1–2 hours before departure
- ▸ BY INTRAVENOUS INJECTION, OR BY INTRAMUSCULAR INJECTION
- ▸ Adult: 50 mg 3 times a day

Nausea and vomiting of known cause | Nausea and vomiting associated with vestibular disorders and palliative care
- ▸ BY MOUTH, OR BY INTRAVENOUS INJECTION
- ▸ Child 1 month–5 years: 0.5–1 mg/kg up to 3 times a day (max. per dose 25 mg), intravenous injection to be given over 3–5 minutes, for motion sickness, take 1–2 hours before departure
- ▸ Child 6–11 years: 25 mg up to 3 times a day, intravenous injection to be given over 3–5 minutes, for motion sickness, take 1–2 hours before departure
- ▸ Child 12–17 years: 50 mg up to 3 times a day, intravenous injection to be given over 3–5 minutes, for motion sickness, take 1–2 hours before departure
- ▸ BY RECTUM
- ▸ Child 2–5 years: 12.5 mg up to 3 times a day
- ▸ Child 6–11 years: 25 mg up to 3 times a day
- ▸ Child 12–17 years: 50 mg up to 3 times a day
- ▸ BY CONTINUOUS INTRAVENOUS INFUSION, OR BY SUBCUTANEOUS INFUSION
- ▸ Child 1–23 months: 3 mg/kg, dose to be given over 24 hours
- ▸ Child 2–5 years: 50 mg, dose to be given over 24 hours
- ▸ Child 6–11 years: 75 mg, dose to be given over 24 hours
- ▸ Child 12–17 years: 150 mg, dose to be given over 24 hours

Nausea and vomiting associated with palliative care
- ▸ BY SUBCUTANEOUS INFUSION
- ▸ Adult: 150 mg, dose to be given over 24 hours
- ▸ BY MOUTH
- ▸ Adult: 50 mg up to 3 times a day

- ● UNLICENSED USE
- ▸ In children Tablets not licensed for use in children under 6 years. Injection not licensed for use in children.
- ● CONTRA-INDICATIONS Avoid in Acute porphyrias p. 918 (some antihistamines are thought to be safe) · neonate (due to significant antimuscarinic activity)
- ● CAUTIONS Epilepsy · glaucoma (in children) · may counteract haemodynamic benefits of opioids · neuromuscular disorders—increased risk of transient paralysis with intravenous use · prostatic hypertrophy (in adults) · pyloroduodenal obstruction · severe heart

failure—may cause fall in cardiac output and associated increase in heart rate, mean arterial pressure and pulmonary wedge pressure · susceptibility to angle-closure glaucoma (in adults) · urinary retention
- ● INTERACTIONS → Appendix 1 (antihistamines).
- ● SIDE-EFFECTS
  GENERAL SIDE-EFFECTS
- ▸ **Common or very common** Drowsiness
- ▸ **Rare** Anaphylaxis · angioedema · angle-closure glaucoma · arrhythmias · blood disorders · bronchospasm · confusion · convulsions · depression · dizziness · extrapyramidal effects · hypersensitivity reactions · hypotension · liver dysfunction · palpitation · paradoxical stimulation (especially with high doses in children) (in children) · paradoxical stimulation (especially with high doses in the elderly) (in adults) · photosensitivity reactions · rashes · sleep disturbances · tremor
- ▸ **Frequency not known** Antimuscarinic effects · blurred vision · dry mouth · gastro-intestinal disturbances · hallucinations · headache · hypertension · movement disorders · oculogyric crisis · paraesthesia · psychomotor impairment · tachycardia · transient speech disorders · twitching · urinary retention
  SPECIFIC SIDE-EFFECTS
- ▸ **Rare**
- ▸ With intravenous use Transient paralysis
- ▸ **Frequency not known**
- ▸ With subcutaneous use Local irritation
  SIDE-EFFECTS, FURTHER INFORMATION
  Children and elderly patients are more susceptible to side-effects.

  Drowsiness is a significant side-effect with most of the older antihistamines although paradoxical stimulation may occur rarely, especially with high doses or in children and the elderly. Drowsiness may diminish after a few days of treatment and is considerably less of a problem with the newer antihistamines.
- ● PREGNANCY Manufacturer advises avoid; however, there is no evidence of teratogenicity. The use of sedating antihistamines in the latter part of the third trimester may cause adverse effects in neonates such as irritability, paradoxical excitability, and tremor.
- ● BREAST FEEDING No information available. Most antihistamines are present in breast milk in varying amounts; although not known to be harmful, most manufacturers advise avoiding their use in mothers who are breast-feeding.
- ● HEPATIC IMPAIRMENT Avoid in severe liver disease—increased risk of coma.
- ● DIRECTIONS FOR ADMINISTRATION For administration *by mouth*, tablets may be crushed.
  Mixing and compatibility for the use of syringe drivers in palliative care Cyclizine may precipitate at concentrations above 10 mg/mL or in the presence of sodium chloride 0.9% *or* as the concentration of diamorphine relative to cyclizine increases; mixtures of diamorphine and cyclizine are also likely to precipitate after 24 hours.
- ● PATIENT AND CARER ADVICE
  Driving and skilled tasks
  Drowsiness may affect performance of skilled tasks (e.g. cycling, driving); effects of alcohol enhanced.

4

Nervous system

● MEDICINAL FORMS
There can be variation in the licensing of different medicines containing the same drug. Forms available from special-order manufacturers include: oral suspension, oral solution, suppository

Tablet
CAUTIONARY AND ADVISORY LABELS 2
▸ Cyclizine (Non-proprietary)
  Cyclizine hydrochloride 50 mg Cyclizine 50mg tablets | 100 tablet P £15.62 DT price = £7.94

Solution for injection
▸ Cyclizine (Non-proprietary)
  Cyclizine lactate 50 mg per 1 ml Cyclizine 50mg/1ml solution for injection ampoules | 5 ampoule PoM £13.54 DT price = £13.54

ANTIEMETICS AND ANTINAUSEANTS ›
CANNIBINOIDS

Nabilone

● INDICATIONS AND DOSE
Nausea and vomiting caused by cytotoxic chemotherapy, unresponsive to conventional antiemetics (preferably in hospital setting) (under close medical supervision)
▸ BY MOUTH
▸ Adult: Initially 1 mg twice daily, increased if necessary to 2 mg twice daily throughout each cycle of cytotoxic therapy and, if necessary, for 48 hours after the last dose of each cycle, the first dose should be taken the night before initiation of cytotoxic treatment and the second dose 1–3 hours before the first dose of cytotoxic drug, daily dose maximum should be given in 3 divided doses; maximum 6 mg per day

● CAUTIONS Adverse effects on mental state can persist for 48–72 hours after stopping · elderly · heart disease · history of psychiatric disorder · hypertension
● SIDE-EFFECTS
▸ **Common or very common** Ataxia · concentration difficulties · drowsiness · dry mouth · dysphoria · euphoria · headache · hypotension · nausea · sleep disturbance · vertigo · visual disturbance
▸ **Frequency not known** Abdominal pain · confusion · decreased appetite · decreased coordination · depression · disorientation · hallucinations · psychosis · tachycardia · tremors

SIDE-EFFECTS, FURTHER INFORMATION
Drowsiness and dizziness occur frequently with standard doses.
● PREGNANCY Avoid unless essential.
● BREAST FEEDING Avoid—no information available.
● HEPATIC IMPAIRMENT Avoid in severe impairment.
● PATIENT AND CARER ADVICE
Driving and skilled tasks
Drowsiness may affect performance of skilled tasks (e.g. driving).
  Effects of alcohol enhanced.
  For information on 2015 legislation regarding driving whilst taking certain controlled drugs, including nabilone, see *Drugs and driving* under Guidance on prescribing p. 1.
Behavioural effects Patients should be made aware of possible changes of mood and other adverse behavioural effects.

● MEDICINAL FORMS
There can be variation in the licensing of different medicines containing the same drug. Forms available from special-order manufacturers include: capsule

Capsule
CAUTIONARY AND ADVISORY LABELS 2
▸ Nabilone (Non-proprietary)
  Nabilone 1 mg Nabilone 1mg capsules | 20 capsule PoM £196.00 CD2

ANTIEMETICS AND ANTINAUSEANTS ›
DOPAMINE RECEPTOR ANTAGONISTS

Domperidone

● INDICATIONS AND DOSE
Relief of nausea and vomiting
▸ BY MOUTH
▸ Child (body-weight up to 35 kg): 250 micrograms/kg up to 3 times a day; maximum 750 micrograms/kg per day
▸ Child 12–17 years (body-weight 35 kg and above): 10 mg up to 3 times a day; maximum 30 mg per day
▸ Adult (body-weight 35 kg and above): 10 mg up to 3 times a day; maximum 30 mg per day

Gastro-intestinal pain in palliative care
▸ BY MOUTH
▸ Adult: 10 mg 3 times a day, before meals

IMPORTANT SAFETY INFORMATION
MHRA/CHM ADVICE—DOMPERIDONE: RISK OF CARDIAC SIDE-EFFECTS—RESTRICTED INDICATION, NEW CONTRA-INDICATIONS, REDUCED DOSE AND DURATION OF USE
The benefits and risks of domperidone have been reviewed. As domperidone is associated with a small increased risk of serious cardiac side-effects, the following restrictions to indication, dose and duration of treatment have been made, and new contra-indications added:
● Domperidone should only be used for the relief of the symptoms of nausea and vomiting;
● Domperidone should be used at the lowest effective dose for the shortest possible duration (max. treatment duration should not normally exceed 1 week);
● Domperidone is contra-indicated for use in conditions where cardiac conduction is, or could be impaired, or where there is underlying cardiac disease, when administered concomitantly with drugs that prolong the QT interval or potent CYP3A4 inhibitors, and in severe hepatic impairment;
● The recommended dose in adults and adolescents over 12 years and over 35 kg is 10 mg up to 3 times daily;
● The recommended dose in children under 35 kg is 250 micrograms/kg up to 3 times daily;
● Oral liquid formulations should be given via an appropriately designed, graduated oral syringe to ensure dose accuracy.
This advice does not apply to unlicensed uses of domperidone (e.g. palliative care).

● CONTRA-INDICATIONS Cardiac disease · conditions where cardiac conduction is, or could be, impaired (in adults) · gastro-intestinal haemorrhage (in children) · if increased gastrointestinal motility harmful (in adults) · mechanical obstruction (in children) · mechanical perforation (in children) · predisposition to cardiac conduction disorders (in children) · prolactinoma
● CAUTIONS Children · if there are cardiac concerns, obtain ECG before and during treatment (in children) · patients over 60 years—increased risk of ventricular arrhythmia (in adults)

- INTERACTIONS → Appendix 1 (domperidone).
Contra-indicated with concomitant use of drugs that
prolong the QT interval.
Contra-indicated with concomitant use of potent CYP3A4
inhibitors.
- SIDE-EFFECTS
▸ **Common or very common** Drowsiness · dry mouth · malaise
▸ **Uncommon** Anxiety · breast pain · decreased libido ·
diarrhoea · galactorrhoea · headache · pruritus · rash
▸ **Frequency not known** Agitation · amenorrhoea ·
convulsions · extrapyramidal disorders · gynaecomastia ·
nervousness · oculogyric crisis · QT-interval prolongation ·
sudden cardiac death · urinary retention · ventricular
arrhythmias
- PREGNANCY Use only if potential benefit outweighs risk.
- BREAST FEEDING Amount too small to be harmful.
- HEPATIC IMPAIRMENT Avoid in moderate or severe
impairment.
- RENAL IMPAIRMENT Reduce frequency.
- PATIENT AND CARER ADVICE
Arrhythmia Patients and their carers should be told how to
recognise signs of arrhythmia and advised to seek medical
attention if symptoms such as palpitation or syncope
develop.

- MEDICINAL FORMS
There can be variation in the licensing of different medicines
containing the same drug. Forms available from special-order
manufacturers include: oral suspension

Tablet
CAUTIONARY AND ADVISORY LABELS 22
▸ Domperidone (Non-proprietary) ▼
   Domperidone (as Domperidone maleate) 10 mg Domperidone
   10mg tablets | 30 tablet [PoM] £2.71 DT price = £1.19 |
   100 tablet [PoM] £9.04 DT price = £3.97
▸ Motilium (Zentiva) ▼
   Domperidone (as Domperidone maleate) 10 mg Motilium 10mg
   tablets | 30 tablet [PoM] DT price = £1.19 | 100 tablet [PoM]
   £9.04 DT price = £3.97

Oral suspension
CAUTIONARY AND ADVISORY LABELS 22
▸ Domperidone (Non-proprietary) ▼
   Domperidone 1 mg per 1 ml Domperidone 5mg/5ml oral suspension
   sugar free sugar-free | 200 ml [PoM] £13.43 DT price = £13.43

Metoclopramide hydrochloride

- INDICATIONS AND DOSE
**Symptomatic treatment of nausea and vomiting including
that associated with acute migraine | Delayed (but not
acute) chemotherapy-induced nausea and vomiting |
Radiotherapy-induced nausea and vomiting | Prevention
of postoperative nausea and vomiting**
▸ BY MOUTH, OR BY INTRAMUSCULAR INJECTION, OR BY SLOW
INTRAVENOUS INJECTION
▸ Adult (body-weight up to 60 kg): Up to
500 micrograms/kg daily in 3 divided doses, when
administered by slow intravenous injection, to be given
over at least 3 minutes
▸ Adult (body-weight 60 kg and above): 10 mg up to 3 times
a day, when administered by slow intravenous
injection, to be given over at least 3 minutes

Hiccup in palliative care
▸ BY MOUTH, OR BY INTRAMUSCULAR INJECTION, OR BY
SUBCUTANEOUS INJECTION
▸ Adult: 10 mg every 6–8 hours

Nausea and vomiting in palliative care
▸ BY MOUTH
▸ Adult: 10 mg 3 times a day
▸ BY SUBCUTANEOUS INFUSION
▸ Adult: 30–100 mg/24 hours

IMPORTANT SAFETY INFORMATION
MHRA/CHM ADVICE—METOCLOPRAMIDE: RISK OF NEUROLOGICAL
ADVERSE EFFECTS—RESTRICTED DOSE AND DURATION OF USE
(AUGUST 2013)
The benefits and risks of metoclopramide have been
reviewed by the European Medicines Agency's
Committee on Medicinal Products for Human Use, which
concluded that the risk of neurological effects such as
extrapyramidal disorders and tardive dyskinesia
outweigh the benefits in long-term or high-dose
treatment. To help minimise the risk of potentially
serious neurological adverse effects, the following
restrictions to indications, dose, and duration of use
have been made:
- In adults over 18 years, metoclopramide should only
be used for prevention of postoperative nausea and
vomiting, radiotherapy-induced nausea and vomiting,
delayed (but not acute) chemotherapy-induced nausea
and vomiting, and symptomatic treatment of nausea
and vomiting, including that associated with acute
migraine (where it may also be used to improve
absorption of oral analgesics);
- Metoclopramide should only be prescribed for short-
term use (up to 5 days);
- Usual dose is 10 mg, repeated up to 3 times daily; max.
daily dose is 500 micrograms/kg;
- Intravenous doses should be administered as a slow
bolus over at least 3 minutes;
- Oral liquid formulations should be given via an
appropriately designed, graduated oral syringe to
ensure dose accuracy.
This advice does not apply to unlicensed uses of
metoclopramide (e.g. palliative care).

- CONTRA-INDICATIONS 3–4 days after gastrointestinal
surgery · gastro-intestinal haemorrhage · gastro-intestinal
obstruction · gastro-intestinal perforation ·
phaeochromocytoma
- CAUTIONS Asthma · atopic allergy · bradycardia · cardiac
conduction disturbances · children · elderly · epilepsy · may
mask underlying disorders such as cerebral irritation ·
Parkinson's disease · uncorrected electrolyte imbalance ·
young adults (15–19 years old)
- INTERACTIONS → Appendix 1 (metoclopramide).
Caution with concomitant use of other drugs affecting
cardiac conduction.
- SIDE-EFFECTS
GENERAL SIDE-EFFECTS
▸ **Common or very common** Extrapyramidal effects
(especially in children and young adults (15–19 years old))
· galactorrhoea · gynaecomastia · hyperprolactinaemia ·
menstrual changes
▸ **Very rare** Depression · methaemoglobinaemia (more
severe in G6PD deficiency) · neuroleptic malignant
syndrome
▸ **Frequency not known** Anxiety · confusion · diarrhoea ·
dizziness · drowsiness · dyspnoea · hypotension · oedema ·
pruritus · rash · restlessness · tardive dyskinesia on
prolonged administration · tremor · urticaria · visual
disturbances
SPECIFIC SIDE-EFFECTS
▸ **Very rare**
▸ With intravenous use Cardiac conduction abnormalities
SIDE-EFFECTS, FURTHER INFORMATION
Metoclopramide can induce acute dystonic reactions
involving facial and skeletal muscle spasms and oculogyric
crises. These dystonic effects are more common in the
young (especially girls and young women) and the very
old; they usually occur shortly after starting treatment
with metoclopramide and subside within 24 hours of

4 Nervous system

stopping it. Injection of an antiparkinsonian drug such as procyclidine will abort dystonic attacks.

- PREGNANCY Not known to be harmful.
- BREAST FEEDING Small amount present in milk; avoid.
- HEPATIC IMPAIRMENT Reduce dose.
- RENAL IMPAIRMENT Avoid or use small dose in severe impairment; increased risk of extrapyramidal reactions.
- DIRECTIONS FOR ADMINISTRATION Oral liquid preparation to be given via a graduated oral dosing syringe.
- PATIENT AND CARER ADVICE Counselling on use of pipette advised with oral solution.

- MEDICINAL FORMS
There can be variation in the licensing of different medicines containing the same drug. Forms available from special-order manufacturers include: oral solution

Tablet
▸ Metoclopramide hydrochloride (Non-proprietary)
  Metoclopramide hydrochloride 10 mg Metoclopramide 10mg tablets | 28 tablet (PoM) £1.23 DT price = £0.75
▸ Maxolon (AMCo)
  Metoclopramide hydrochloride 10 mg Maxolon 10mg tablets | 84 tablet (PoM) £5.24

Oral solution
▸ Metoclopramide hydrochloride (Non-proprietary)
  Metoclopramide hydrochloride 1 mg per 1 ml Metoclopramide 5mg/5ml oral solution sugar free sugar-free | 150 ml (PoM) £19.77 DT price = £19.77

Solution for injection
▸ Metoclopramide hydrochloride (Non-proprietary)
  Metoclopramide hydrochloride 5 mg per 1 ml Metoclopramide 10mg/2ml solution for injection ampoules | 5 ampoule (PoM) £1.31 | 10 ampoule (PoM) £3.50 DT price = £3.18
▸ Maxolon (AMCo)
  Metoclopramide hydrochloride 5 mg per 1 ml Maxolon 10mg/2ml solution for injection ampoules | 12 ampoule (PoM) £3.21

Combinations available: *Paracetamol with metoclopramide,* p. 431

ANTIEMETICS AND ANTINAUSEANTS ›
NEUROKININ RECEPTOR ANTAGONISTS

Aprepitant

- INDICATIONS AND DOSE

Adjunct to dexamethasone and a 5HT3-receptor antagonist in preventing nausea and vomiting associated with moderately and highly emetogenic chemotherapy
▸ BY MOUTH
▸ Adult: Initially 125 mg, dose to be taken 1 hour before chemotherapy, then 80 mg once daily for 2 days, consult product literature for dose of concomitant corticosteroid and 5HT$_3$-antagonist

- CONTRA-INDICATIONS Acute porphyrias p. 918
- INTERACTIONS → Appendix 1 (aprepitant).
- SIDE-EFFECTS
▸ **Common or very common** Anorexia · asthenia · constipation · diarrhoea · dizziness · dyspepsia · headache · hiccups
▸ **Uncommon** Abdominal pain · abnormal dreams · acne · anaemia · anxiety · bradycardia · chills · colitis · confusion · conjunctivitis · cough · drowsiness · dry mouth · duodenal ulcer · dysuria · euphoria · flatulence · flushing · haematuria · hyperglycaemia · hyponatraemia · myalgia · neutropenia · oedema · palpitations · pharyngitis · photosensitivity · polyuria · pruritus · rash · sneezing · stomatitis · sweating · taste disturbance · thirst · tinnitus · weight changes
▸ **Frequency not known** Dysarthria · dyspnoea · insomnia · Stevens-Johnson syndrome · urticaria · visual disturbances
- CONCEPTION AND CONTRACEPTION Effectiveness of hormonal contraceptives reduced—effective non-

hormonal methods of contraception necessary during treatment and for 2 months after stopping aprepitant.

- PREGNANCY Avoid unless potential benefit outweighs risk—no information available.
- BREAST FEEDING Avoid—present in milk in *animal* studies.
- HEPATIC IMPAIRMENT Caution in moderate to severe impairment.

- MEDICINAL FORMS
There can be variation in the licensing of different medicines containing the same drug. Forms available from special-order manufacturers include: oral suspension

Capsule
▸ Emend (Merck Sharp & Dohme Ltd)
  Aprepitant 80 mg Emend 80mg capsules | 2 capsule (PoM) £31.61
  Aprepitant 125 mg Emend 125mg capsules | 1 capsule (PoM) no price available | 5 capsule (PoM) £79.03
▸ Emend (Merck Sharp & Dohme Ltd)
  Emend 125mg and 80mg capsules | 3 capsule (PoM) £47.42

Fosaprepitant

- DRUG ACTION Fosaprepitant is a prodrug of aprepitant.

- INDICATIONS AND DOSE

Adjunct to dexamethasone and a 5HT3-receptor antagonist in preventing nausea and vomiting associated with moderately and highly emetogenic chemotherapy
▸ BY INTRAVENOUS INFUSION
▸ Adult: 150 mg, dose to be administered over 20–30 minutes and given 30 minutes before chemotherapy on day 1 of cycle only, consult product literature for dose of concomitant corticosteroid and 5HT$_3$-receptor antagonist

- CONTRA-INDICATIONS Acute porphyrias p. 918
- INTERACTIONS → Appendix 1 (fosaprepitant).
- SIDE-EFFECTS
▸ **Common or very common** Anorexia · asthenia · constipation · diarrhoea · dizziness · dyspepsia · headache · hiccups
▸ **Uncommon** Abdominal pain · abnormal dreams · acne · anaemia · anxiety · bradycardia · chills · colitis · confusion · conjunctivitis · cough · drowsiness · dry mouth · duodenal ulcer · dysuria · euphoria · flatulence · flushing · haematuria · hyperglycaemia · hyponatraemia · myalgia · neutropenia · oedema · palpitations · pharyngitis · photosensitivity · polyuria · pruritus · rash · sneezing · stomatitis · sweating · taste disturbance · thirst · tinnitus · weight changes
▸ **Frequency not known** Dysarthria · dyspnoea · insomnia · Stevens-Johnson syndrome · urticaria · visual disturbances
- CONCEPTION AND CONTRACEPTION Effectiveness of hormonal contraceptives reduced—effective non-hormonal methods of contraception necessary during treatment and for 2 months after stopping fosaprepitant.
- PREGNANCY Avoid unless potential benefit outweighs risk—no information available.
- BREAST FEEDING Avoid—present in milk in *animal* studies.
- HEPATIC IMPAIRMENT Caution in moderate to severe impairment.
- DIRECTIONS FOR ADMINISTRATION For *intravenous infusion* (*Ivemend* ®), give intermittently in Sodium chloride 0.9%; reconstitute each 150-mg vial with 5 mL sodium chloride 0.9% gently without shaking to avoid foaming, then dilute in 145 mL infusion fluid; give over 20–30 minutes.
- NATIONAL FUNDING/ACCESS DECISIONS
Scottish Medicines Consortium (SMC) Decisions
The *Scottish Medicines Consortium* has advised (January 2011) that fosaprepitant (*Ivemend* ®) is accepted for restricted use within NHS Scotland for the prevention of acute and delayed nausea and vomiting associated with highly emetogenic cisplatin-based chemotherapy.

● MEDICINAL FORMS
There can be variation in the licensing of different medicines containing the same drug.
Powder for solution for infusion
▸ Ivemend (Merck Sharp & Dohme Ltd)
Fosaprepitant (as Fosaprepitant dimeglumine) 150 mg Ivemend 150mg powder for solution for infusion vials | 1 vial [PoM] £47.42

ANTIEMETICS AND ANTINAUSEANTS ›
SEROTONIN (5HT3) RECEPTOR ANTAGONISTS

Granisetron

● DRUG ACTION Granisetron is a specific $5HT_3$-receptor antagonist which blocks $5HT_3$ receptors in the gastro-intestinal tract and in the CNS.

● INDICATIONS AND DOSE

Nausea and vomiting induced by cytotoxic chemotherapy for planned duration of 3–5 days where oral antiemetics cannot be used
▸ BY TRANSDERMAL APPLICATION USING PATCHES
▸ Adult: Apply 3.1 mg/24 hours, apply patch to clean, dry, non-irritated, non-hairy skin on upper arm (or abdomen if upper arm cannot be used) 24–48 hours before treatment, patch may be worn for up to 7 days; remove at least 24 hours after completing chemotherapy

Prevention of postoperative nausea and vomiting
▸ BY INTRAVENOUS INJECTION
▸ Adult: 1 mg, to be administered before induction of anaesthesia, dose to be diluted to 5 mL and given over 30 seconds

Treatment of postoperative nausea and vomiting
▸ BY INTRAVENOUS INJECTION
▸ Adult: 1 mg, dose to be diluted to 5 mL and given over 30 seconds; maximum 3 mg per day

Management of nausea and vomiting induced by cytotoxic chemotherapy or radiotherapy
▸ BY MOUTH
▸ Adult: 1–2 mg, to be taken within 1 hour before start of treatment, then 2 mg daily in 1–2 divided doses for up to 1 week following treatment, when intravenous route also used, maximum combined total dose 9 mg in 24 hours
▸ BY INTRAVENOUS INJECTION, OR BY INTRAVENOUS INFUSION
▸ Adult: 10–40 micrograms/kg (max. per dose 3 mg), to be given 5 minutes before start of treatment, dose may be repeated if necessary, further maintenance doses must not be given less than 10 minutes apart, for intravenous injection, each 1 mg granisetron diluted to 5 mL and given over not less than 30 seconds, for intravenous infusion, to be given over 5 minutes; maximum 9 mg per day

● CAUTIONS Subacute intestinal obstruction · susceptibility to QT-interval prolongation (including electrolyte disturbances)

● INTERACTIONS → Appendix 1 ($5HT_3$-receptor Antagonists). Caution with concomitant use of drugs that prolong QT interval.

● SIDE-EFFECTS
GENERAL SIDE-EFFECTS
▸ **Common or very common** Constipation · diarrhoea · headache · insomnia
▸ **Uncommon** Extrapyramidal reactions · QT-interval prolongation · rash
SPECIFIC SIDE-EFFECTS
▸ **Uncommon**
▸ With transdermal use Application-site reactions

● PREGNANCY Manufacturer advises avoid.

● BREAST FEEDING Avoid—no information available.

● HEPATIC IMPAIRMENT Manufacturer advises use with caution.

● DIRECTIONS FOR ADMINISTRATION
▸ With intravenous use For *intravenous infusion*, give intermittently in Glucose 5% or Sodium Chloride 0.9%; dilute up to 3 mL in 20–50 mL infusion fluid; give over 5 minutes.

● PATIENT AND CARER ADVICE
▸ With transdermal use Patients should be advised not to expose the site of the patch to sunlight during use and for 10 days after removal.

● MEDICINAL FORMS
There can be variation in the licensing of different medicines containing the same drug.
Tablet
▸ Granisetron (Non-proprietary)
Granisetron (as Granisetron hydrochloride) 1 mg Granisetron 1mg tablets | 10 tablet [PoM] £51.20 DT price = £33.99
Granisetron (as Granisetron hydrochloride) 2 mg Granisetron 2mg tablets | 5 tablet [PoM] no price available DT price = £52.39
▸ Kytril (Roche Products Ltd)
Granisetron (as Granisetron hydrochloride) 1 mg Kytril 1mg tablets | 10 tablet [PoM] £52.39 DT price = £33.99
Granisetron (as Granisetron hydrochloride) 2 mg Kytril 2mg tablets | 5 tablet [PoM] £52.39 DT price = £52.39
Solution for injection
▸ Granisetron (Non-proprietary)
Granisetron (as Granisetron hydrochloride) 1 mg per 1 ml Granisetron 3mg/3ml concentrate for solution for injection ampoules | 5 ampoule [PoM] £24.00
Granisetron 1mg/1ml concentrate for solution for injection ampoules | 5 ampoule [PoM] £8.00
Transdermal patch
▸ Sancuso (ProStrakan Ltd)
Granisetron 3.1 mg per 24 hour Sancuso 3.1mg/24hours transdermal patches | 1 patch [PoM] £56.00

Ondansetron

● DRUG ACTION Ondansetron is a specific $5HT_3$-receptor antagonist which blocks $5HT_3$ receptors in the gastro-intestinal tract and in the CNS.

● INDICATIONS AND DOSE

Moderately emetogenic chemotherapy or radiotherapy
▸ BY MOUTH
▸ Adult: Initially 8 mg, dose to be taken 1–2 hours before treatment, then 8 mg every 12 hours for up to 5 days
▸ BY RECTUM
▸ Adult: Initially 16 mg, dose to be taken 1–2 hours before treatment, then 16 mg daily for up to 5 days
▸ INITIALLY BY INTRAMUSCULAR INJECTION, OR BY SLOW INTRAVENOUS INJECTION
▸ Adult: Initially 8 mg, dose to be administered immediately before treatment, then (by mouth) 8 mg every 12 hours for up to 5 days, alternatively (by rectum) 16 mg daily for up to 5 days
▸ INITIALLY BY INTRAMUSCULAR INJECTION, OR BY INTRAVENOUS INFUSION
▸ Elderly: Initially 8 mg, dose to be administered immediately before treatment, intravenous infusion to be given over at least 15 minutes, then (by mouth) 8 mg every 12 hours for up to 5 days, alternatively (by rectum) 16 mg daily for up to 5 days continued →

4

Nervous system

Severely emetogenic chemotherapy (consult product literature for dose of concomitant corticosteroid)
▶ BY MOUTH
▶ Adult: 24 mg, dose to be taken 1–2 hours before treatment, then 8 mg every 12 hours for up to 5 days
▶ BY RECTUM
▶ Adult: 16 mg, dose to be administered 1–2 hours before treatment, then 16 mg daily for up to 5 days
▶ INITIALLY BY INTRAMUSCULAR INJECTION, OR BY SLOW INTRAVENOUS INJECTION
▶ Adult: Initially 8 mg, dose to be administered immediately before treatment, followed by (by intramuscular injection or by slow intravenous injection) 8 mg every 4 hours if required for 2 doses, alternatively, followed by (by continuous intravenous infusion) 1 mg/hour for up to 24 hours, then (by mouth) 8 mg every 12 hours for up to 5 days, alternatively (by rectum) 16 mg daily for up to 5 days
▶ INITIALLY BY INTRAMUSCULAR INJECTION
▶ Adult 65-74 years: Initially 8 mg, to be given immediately before treatment, followed by (by intramuscular injection) 8 mg every 4 hours if required for 2 doses, alternatively, followed by (by continuous intravenous infusion) 1 mg/hour for up to 24 hours, then (by mouth) 8 mg every 12 hours for up to 5 days, alternatively (by rectum) 16 mg daily for up to 5 days
▶ INITIALLY BY INTRAVENOUS INFUSION
▶ Adult: Initially 16 mg, immediately before treatment (over at least 15 minutes), followed by (by intramuscular injection or by slow intravenous injection) 8 mg every 4 hours if required for 2 doses, then (by mouth) 8 mg every 12 hours for up to 5 days, alternatively (by rectum) 16 mg daily for up to 5 days
▶ Adult 65-74 years: Initially 8–16 mg, immediately before treatment (over at least 15 minutes), followed by (by intramuscular injection or by intravenous infusion) 8 mg every 4 hours if required for 2 doses, then (by mouth) 8 mg every 12 hours for up to 5 days, alternatively (by rectum) 16 mg daily for up to 5 days
▶ Adult 75 years and over: Initially 8 mg, immediately before treatment (over at least 15 minutes), followed by (by intravenous infusion) 8 mg every 4 hours if required for 2 doses, then (by mouth) 8 mg every 12 hours for up to 5 days, alternatively (by rectum) 16 mg daily for up to 5 days

Prevention of postoperative nausea and vomiting
▶ INITIALLY BY MOUTH
▶ Adult: 16 mg, dose to be taken 1 hour before anaesthesia, alternatively (by intramuscular injection or by slow intravenous injection) 4 mg, dose to be administered at induction of anaesthesia

Treatment of postoperative nausea and vomiting
▶ BY INTRAMUSCULAR INJECTION, OR BY SLOW INTRAVENOUS INJECTION
▶ Adult: 4 mg for 1 dose

● CONTRA-INDICATIONS Congenital long QT syndrome
● CAUTIONS Adenotonsillar surgery · subacute intestinal obstruction · susceptibility to QT-interval prolongation (including electrolyte disturbances)
● INTERACTIONS → Appendix 1 (5HT₃-receptor Antagonists). Caution with concomitant use of drugs that prolong QT interval.
● SIDE-EFFECTS
GENERAL SIDE-EFFECTS
▶ **Common or very common** Constipation · flushing · headache · injection site-reactions
▶ **Uncommon** Arrhythmias · bradycardia · chest pain · hiccups · hypotension · movement disorders · seizures

SPECIFIC SIDE-EFFECTS
▶ **Rare**
▶ With intravenous use Dizziness · transient visual disturbances
▶ **Very rare**
▶ With intravenous use Transient blindness
▶ **Frequency not known**
▶ With rectal use Rectal irritation
● PREGNANCY No information available; avoid unless potential benefit outweighs risk.
● BREAST FEEDING Present in milk in *animal* studies—avoid.
● HEPATIC IMPAIRMENT Maximum 8 mg daily in moderate or severe impairment.
● DIRECTIONS FOR ADMINISTRATION
▶ With intravenous use For *intravenous infusion* (*Zofran*®), give continuously or intermittently in Glucose 5% or Glucose 5% with Potassium chloride 0.3% or Sodium chloride 0.9% or Sodium chloride 0.9% with Potassium chloride 0.3% or Mannitol 10% or Ringers solution; for intermittent infusion, dilute the required dose in 50–100 mL of infusion fluid and give over at least 15 minutes.
▶ With oral use Orodispersible films and lyophilisates should be placed on the tongue, allowed to disperse and swallowed.
● PRESCRIBING AND DISPENSING INFORMATION Flavours of oral liquid formulations may include strawberry.
● PATIENT AND CARER ADVICE Patients or carers should be given advice on how to administer orodispersible films and lyophilisates.
● MEDICINAL FORMS
There can be variation in the licensing of different medicines containing the same drug. Forms available from special-order manufacturers include: oral suspension, oral solution
Tablet
▶ Ondansetron (Non-proprietary)
Ondansetron (as Ondansetron hydrochloride) 4 mg Ondansetron 4mg tablets | 10 tablet [PoM] £25.46 DT price = £1.22 | 30 tablet £76.38
Ondansetron (as Ondansetron hydrochloride) 8 mg Ondansetron 8mg tablets | 10 tablet [PoM] £47.99 DT price = £2.34
▶ Ondemet (Alliance Pharmaceuticals Ltd)
Ondansetron (as Ondansetron hydrochloride) 4 mg Ondemet 4mg tablets | 30 tablet [PoM] £81.15
Ondansetron (as Ondansetron hydrochloride) 8 mg Ondemet 8mg tablets | 10 tablet [PoM] £54.36 DT price = £2.34 (Hospital only)
▶ Zofran (Novartis Pharmaceuticals UK Ltd)
Ondansetron (as Ondansetron hydrochloride) 4 mg Zofran 4mg tablets | 30 tablet [PoM] £107.91
Ondansetron (as Ondansetron hydrochloride) 8 mg Zofran 8mg tablets | 10 tablet [PoM] £71.94 DT price = £2.34
Orodispersible tablet
▶ Ondansetron (Non-proprietary)
Ondansetron 4 mg Ondansetron 4mg orodispersible tablets | 10 tablet [PoM] £43.46 DT price = £43.09
Ondansetron 8 mg Ondansetron 8mg orodispersible tablets | 10 tablet [PoM] £85.43 DT price = £85.43
Orodispersible film
▶ Setofilm (Norgine Pharmaceuticals Ltd)
Ondansetron 4 mg Setofilm 4mg orodispersible films sugar-free | 10 film [PoM] £28.50
Ondansetron 8 mg Setofilm 8mg orodispersible films sugar-free | 10 film [PoM] £57.00
Oral solution
▶ Ondansetron (Non-proprietary)
Ondansetron (as Ondansetron hydrochloride) 800 microgram per 1 ml Ondansetron 4mg/5ml oral solution sugar free sugar-free | 50 ml [PoM] £38.08 DT price = £38.02
▶ Demorem (Kappin Ltd)
Ondansetron (as Ondansetron hydrochloride) 800 microgram per 1 ml Demorem 4mg/5ml oral solution sugar-free | 50 ml [PoM] £38.19 DT price = £38.02

▶ Zofran (Novartis Pharmaceuticals UK Ltd)
**Ondansetron (as Ondansetron hydrochloride) 800 microgram
per 1 ml** Zofran 4mg/5ml syrup sugar-free | 50 ml [PoM] £35.97 DT
price = £38.02

Oral lyophilisate
EXCIPIENTS: May contain Aspartame
▶ Zofran Melt (Novartis Pharmaceuticals UK Ltd)
Ondansetron 4 mg Zofran Melt 4mg oral lyophilisates sugar-free |
10 tablet [PoM] £35.97 DT price = £35.97
Ondansetron 8 mg Zofran Melt 8mg oral lyophilisates sugar-free |
10 tablet [PoM] £71.94 DT price = £71.94

Solution for injection
▶ Ondansetron (Non-proprietary)
**Ondansetron (as Ondansetron hydrochloride) 2 mg per
1 ml** Ondansetron 8mg/4ml solution for injection ampoules |
5 ampoule [PoM] £58.45
Ondansetron 4mg/2ml solution for injection ampoules |
5 ampoule [PoM] £28.47 | 10 ampoule [PoM] £7.50
▶ Zofran Flexi-amp (Novartis Pharmaceuticals UK Ltd)
**Ondansetron (as Ondansetron hydrochloride) 2 mg per
1 ml** Zofran Flexi-amp 8mg/4ml solution for injection |
5 ampoule [PoM] £59.95
Zofran Flexi-amp 4mg/2ml solution for injection | 5 ampoule [PoM]
£29.97

Suppository
▶ Zofran (Novartis Pharmaceuticals UK Ltd)
Ondansetron 16 mg Zofran 16mg suppositories |
1 suppository [PoM] £14.39

Palonosetron

● DRUG ACTION Palonosetron is a specific $5HT_3$-receptor
antagonist which blocks $5HT_3$ receptors in the gastro-
intestinal tract and in the CNS.

● INDICATIONS AND DOSE

Moderately emetogenic chemotherapy
▶ INITIALLY BY MOUTH
▶ Adult: 500 micrograms, dose to be taken 1 hour before
treatment, alternatively (by intravenous injection)
250 micrograms for 1 dose, dose to be administered
over 30 seconds, 30 minutes before treatment

Severely emetogenic chemotherapy
▶ BY INTRAVENOUS INJECTION
▶ Adult: 250 micrograms for 1 dose, dose to be
administered over 30 seconds, 30 minutes before
treatment

● CAUTIONS History of constipation · intestinal obstruction ·
susceptibility to QT-interval prolongation (including
electrolyte disturbances)

● INTERACTIONS → Appendix 1 ($5HT_3$-receptor Antagonists).
Caution with concomitant use of drugs that prolong QT
interval.

● SIDE-EFFECTS
▶ **Common or very common** Constipation · diarrhoea ·
dizziness · headache
▶ **Uncommon** Abdominal pain · amblyopia · anorexia ·
anxiety · arrhythmia · arthralgia · asthenia · atrioventricular
block · bradycardia · changes in blood pressure · dry mouth
· dyspepsia · dyspnoea · electrolyte disturbance · euphoria ·
extrasystoles · eye irritation · eye swelling · flatulence ·
glycosuria · hiccups · hyperglycaemia · influenza-like
symptoms · insomnia · motion sickness · myalgia ·
myocardial ischaemia · peripheral neuropathy · rash ·
tachycardia · tinnitus · urinary retention

● PREGNANCY Avoid—no information available.

● BREAST FEEDING Avoid—no information available.

● PATIENT AND CARER ADVICE

Driving and skilled tasks
Dizziness or drowsiness may affect performance of skilled
tasks (e.g. driving).

● MEDICINAL FORMS
There can be variation in the licensing of different medicines
containing the same drug.

Capsule
▶ Aloxi (Sinclair IS Pharma Plc)
**Palonosetron (as Palonosetron hydrochloride)
500 microgram** Aloxi 500microgram capsules | 1 capsule [PoM]
£55.89

Solution for injection
▶ Aloxi (Sinclair IS Pharma Plc)
**Palonosetron (as Palonosetron hydrochloride) 50 microgram per
1 ml** Aloxi 250micrograms/5ml solution for injection vials |
1 vial [PoM] £55.89

Palonosetron with netupitant   20.6.2016

The properties listed below are those particular to the
combination only. For the properties of the components
please consider, palonosetron above

● INDICATIONS AND DOSE

Moderately emetogenic chemotherapy | Highly emetogenic cisplatin-based chemotherapy
▶ BY MOUTH
▶ Adult: 1 capsule, to be taken approximately 1 hour
before the start of each chemotherapy cycle

● CAUTIONS Patients over 75 years

● INTERACTIONS → Appendix 1 ($5HT_3$-receptor Antagonists,
netupitant).

● SIDE-EFFECTS
▶ **Common or very common** Fatigue
▶ **Uncommon** Alopecia · blood disorders · cardiomyopathy ·
conduction disorder · decreased appetite · urticaria ·
vertigo
▶ **Rare** Back pain · blurred vision · conjunctivitis · cystitis ·
dysphagia · hypoaesthesia · hypokalaemia · non-cardiac
chest pain · psychosis (acute) · sleep disorder

● CONCEPTION AND CONTRACEPTION Manufacturer
recommends exclude pregnancy before treatment in
females of childbearing age; ensure effective
contraception during treatment and for one month after
treatment.

● PREGNANCY Manufacturer advises avoid—toxicity in
animal studies.

● BREAST FEEDING Manufacturer advises avoid during
treatment and for 1 month after last dose—no information
available.

● HEPATIC IMPAIRMENT Manufacturer advises caution in
severe impairment.

● NATIONAL FUNDING/ACCESS DECISIONS

Scottish Medicines Consortium (SMC) Decisions
The *Scottish Medicines Consortium* (December 2015) has
advised that palonosetron in combination with netupitant
(*Akynzeo*®) is accepted for restricted use within NHS
Scotland for the prevention of acute and delayed nausea
and vomiting associated with highly emetogenic cisplatin-
based cancer chemotherapy.

● MEDICINAL FORMS
There can be variation in the licensing of different medicines
containing the same drug.

Capsule
CAUTIONARY AND ADVISORY LABELS 25
▶ Akynzeo (Chugai Pharma UK Ltd) ▼
**Palonosetron (as Palonosetron hydrochloride) 500 microgram,
Netupitant 300 mg** Akynzeo 300mg/0.5mg capsules |
1 capsule [PoM] £69.00 (Hospital only)

Nervous system

4

ANTIHISTAMINES > SEDATING ANTIHISTAMINES

Cinnarizine

- **INDICATIONS AND DOSE**

Relief of symptoms of vestibular disorders, such as vertigo, tinnitus, nausea, and vomiting in Ménière's disease
▸ BY MOUTH
  - Child 5-11 years: 15 mg 3 times a day
  - Child 12-17 years: 30 mg 3 times a day
  - Adult: 30 mg 3 times a day

Motion sickness
▸ BY MOUTH
  - Child 5-11 years: Initially 15 mg, dose to be taken 2 hours before travel, then 7.5 mg every 8 hours if required, dose to be taken during journey
  - Child 12-17 years: Initially 30 mg, dose to be taken 2 hours before travel, then 15 mg every 8 hours if required, dose to be taken during journey
  - Adult: Initially 30 mg, dose to be taken 2 hours before travel, then 15 mg every 8 hours if required, dose to be taken during journey

- **CONTRA-INDICATIONS** Avoid in Acute porphyrias p. 918 (some antihistamines are thought to be safe)
- **CAUTIONS** Epilepsy · glaucoma (in children) · Parkinson's disease (in adults) · prostatic hypertrophy (in adults) · pyloroduodenal obstruction · susceptibility to angle-closure glaucoma (in adults) · urinary retention
- **SIDE-EFFECTS**
▸ **Common or very common** Drowsiness
▸ **Rare** Anaphylaxis · angioedema · angle-closure glaucoma · arrhythmias · blood disorders · bronchospasm · confusion · convulsions · depression · dizziness · extrapyramidal effects · hypersensitivity reactions · hypotension · lichen planus · liver dysfunction · lupus-like skin reactions · palpitation · paradoxical stimulation (especially with high doses in children) (in children) · paradoxical stimulation (especially with high doses in the elderly) (in adults) · photosensitivity reactions · rashes · sleep disturbances · sweating · tremor · weight gain
▸ **Frequency not known** Antimuscarinic effects · blurred vision · dry mouth · gastro-intestinal disturbances · headache · psychomotor impairment · urinary retention
SIDE-EFFECTS, FURTHER INFORMATION
Children and the elderly are more susceptible to side-effects.
Drowsiness is a significant side-effect with most of the older antihistamines although paradoxical stimulation may occur rarely, especially with high doses or in children and the elderly. Drowsiness may diminish after a few days of treatment and is considerably less of a problem with the newer antihistamines.
- **PREGNANCY** Manufacturer advises avoid; however, there is no evidence of teratogenicity. The use of sedating antihistamines in the latter part of the third trimester may cause adverse effects in neonates such as irritability, paradoxical excitability, and tremor.
- **BREAST FEEDING** Most antihistamines are present in breast milk in varying amounts; although not known to be harmful, most manufacturers advise avoiding their use in mothers who are breast-feeding.
- **HEPATIC IMPAIRMENT** Avoid in severe liver disease—increased risk of coma.
- **RENAL IMPAIRMENT** Use with caution—no information available.

- **PATIENT AND CARER ADVICE**
Driving and skilled tasks
Drowsiness may affect performance of skilled tasks (e.g. cycling, driving); sedating effects enhanced by alcohol.

- **MEDICINAL FORMS**
There can be variation in the licensing of different medicines containing the same drug. Forms available from special-order manufacturers include: oral suspension
Tablet
CAUTIONARY AND ADVISORY LABELS 2
▸ Cinnarizine (Non-proprietary)
  Cinnarizine 15 mg Boots Motion Sickness15mg tablets | 15 tablet Ⓟ no price available
  Cinnarizine 15mg tablets | 84 tablet Ⓟ £15.40 DT price = £5.31
▸ Mylan (Mylan Ltd)
  Cinnarizine 15 mg Mylan Travel Sickness 15mg tablets | 15 tablet Ⓟ £2.50
▸ Stugeron (McNeil Products Ltd, Janssen-Cilag Ltd)
  Cinnarizine 15 mg Stugeron 15mg tablets | 15 tablet Ⓟ £1.84 | 100 tablet Ⓟ £4.18

Cinnarizine with dimenhydrinate

The properties listed below are those particular to the combination only. For the properties of the components please consider, cinnarizine above.

- **INDICATIONS AND DOSE**
Vertigo
▸ BY MOUTH
  - Adult: 1 tablet 3 times a day

- **MEDICINAL FORMS**
There can be variation in the licensing of different medicines containing the same drug.
Tablet
CAUTIONARY AND ADVISORY LABELS 2, 21
▸ Arlevert (Hampton Pharmaceuticals Ltd)
  Cinnarizine 20 mg, Dimenhydrinate 40 mg Arlevert tablets | 100 tablet ⓅⓄⓂ £24.00

Promethazine teoclate

- **INDICATIONS AND DOSE**
Nausea | Vomiting | Labyrinthine disorders
▸ BY MOUTH
  - Child 5-9 years: 12.5–37.5 mg daily
  - Child 10-17 years: 25–75 mg daily; maximum 100 mg per day
  - Adult: 25–75 mg daily; maximum 100 mg per day
Motion sickness prevention (acts longer than promethazine hydrochloride)
▸ BY MOUTH
  - Child 5-9 years: 12.5 mg once daily, dose to be taken at bedtime on night before travel or 1–2 hours before travel
  - Child 10-17 years: 25 mg once daily, dose to be taken at bedtime on night before travel or 1–2 hours before travel
  - Adult: 25 mg once daily, dose to be taken at bedtime on night before travel or 1–2 hours before travel
Motion sickness treatment (acts longer than promethazine hydrochloride)
▸ BY MOUTH
  - Child 5-9 years: 12.5 mg, dose to be taken at onset of motion sickness, then 12.5 mg daily for 2 days, dose to be taken at bedtime
  - Child 10-17 years: 25 mg, dose to be taken at onset of motion sickness, then 25 mg once daily for 2 days, dose to be taken at bedtime

> Adult: 25 mg, dose to be taken at onset of motion sickness, then 25 mg once daily for 2 days, dose to be taken at bedtime

---

IMPORTANT SAFETY INFORMATION

MHRA/CHM ADVICE (MARCH 2008 AND FEBRUARY 2009) OVER-THE-COUNTER COUGH AND COLD MEDICINES FOR CHILDREN

Children under 6 years should not be given over-the-counter cough and cold medicines containing promethazine.

● CAUTIONS Acute porphyrias p. 918 · asthma · bronchiectasis · bronchitis · epilepsy · prostatic hypertrophy (in adults) · pyloroduodenal obstruction · Reye's syndrome · severe coronary artery disease · susceptibility to angle-closure glaucoma · urinary retention
● INTERACTIONS → Appendix 1 (antihistamines).
● SIDE-EFFECTS
> Rare Anaphylaxis · angioedema · angle-closure glaucoma · arrhythmias · blood disorders · bronchospasm · confusion · convulsions · depression · dizziness · extrapyramidal effects · hypersensitivity reactions · hypotension · liver dysfunction · palpitation · photosensitivity reactions · rashes · sleep disturbances · tremor
> Frequency not known Antimuscarinic effects · blurred vision · drowsiness · dry mouth · gastro-intestinal disturbances · headache · psychomotor impairment · restlessness · urinary retention

SIDE-EFFECTS, FURTHER INFORMATION

Children and the elderly are more susceptible to side-effects.

Drowsiness is a significant side-effect with most of the older antihistamines although paradoxical stimulation may occur rarely, especially with high doses or in children and the elderly. Drowsiness may diminish after a few days of treatment and is considerably less of a problem with the newer antihistamines.

● PREGNANCY Most manufacturers of antihistamines advise avoiding their use during pregnancy; however, there is no evidence of teratogenicity. Use in the latter part of the third trimester may cause adverse effects in neonates such as irritability, paradoxical excitability, and tremor.
● BREAST FEEDING Most antihistamines are present in breast milk in varying amounts; although not known to be harmful, most manufacturers advise avoiding their use in mothers who are breast-feeding.
● HEPATIC IMPAIRMENT Avoid in severe liver disease—increased risk of coma.
● RENAL IMPAIRMENT Use with caution.
● PATIENT AND CARER ADVICE

Driving and skilled tasks

Drowsiness may affect performance of skilled tasks (e.g. cycling or driving); sedating effects enhanced by alcohol.

● MEDICINAL FORMS
There can be variation in the licensing of different medicines containing the same drug.

Tablet

CAUTIONARY AND ADVISORY LABELS 2
> Avomine (Manx Healthcare Ltd)
  Promethazine teoclate 25 mg Avomine 25mg tablets | 10 tablet [P] £1.13 | 28 tablet [P] £3.13 DT price = £3.13

ANTIMUSCARINICS

F 703

Hyoscine hydrobromide

(Scopolamine hydrobromide)

● INDICATIONS AND DOSE

Motion sickness
> BY MOUTH
> Child 4–9 years: 75–150 micrograms, dose to be taken up to 30 minutes before the start of journey, then 75–150 micrograms every 6 hours if required; maximum 450 micrograms per day
> Child 10–17 years: 150–300 micrograms, dose to be taken up to 30 minutes before the start of journey, then 150–300 micrograms every 6 hours if required; maximum 900 micrograms per day
> Adult: 150–300 micrograms, dose to be taken up to 30 minutes before the start of journey, then 150–300 micrograms every 6 hours if required; maximum 900 micrograms per day
> BY TRANSDERMAL APPLICATION
> Child 10–17 years: Apply 1 patch, apply behind ear 5–6 hours before journey, then apply 1 patch after 72 hours if required, remove old patch and site replacement patch behind the other ear
> Adult: Apply 1 patch, apply behind ear 5–6 hours before journey, then apply 1 patch after 72 hours if required, remove old patch and site replacement patch behind the other ear

Hypersalivation associated with clozapine therapy
> BY MOUTH
> Adult: 300 micrograms up to 3 times a day; maximum 900 micrograms per day

Excessive respiratory secretion (in palliative care)
> BY SUBCUTANEOUS INJECTION
> Adult: 400 micrograms every 4 hours as required, hourly use is occasionally necessary, particularly in excessive respiratory secretions
> BY CONTINUOUS SUBCUTANEOUS INFUSION
> Adult: 1.2–2 mg/24 hours

Bowel colic in palliative care
> BY SUBCUTANEOUS INJECTION
> Adult: 400 micrograms every 4 hours as required, hourly use is occasionally necessary
> BY SUBCUTANEOUS INFUSION
> Adult: 1.2–2 mg/24 hours

Bowel colic pain in palliative care
> BY MOUTH USING SUBLINGUAL TABLETS
> Adult: 300 micrograms 3 times a day, as *Kwells*®.

Premedication
> BY SUBCUTANEOUS INJECTION, OR BY INTRAMUSCULAR INJECTION
> Adult: 200–600 micrograms, to be administered 30–60 minutes before induction of anaesthesia

● UNLICENSED USE Not licensed for hypersalivation associated with clozapine therapy.

IMPORTANT SAFETY INFORMATION

Antimuscarininc drugs used for premedication to general anaesthesia should only be administered by, or under the direct supervision of, personnel experienced in their use.

● CAUTIONS Epilepsy

CAUTIONS, FURTHER INFORMATION
> Anticholinergic syndrome
> With systemic use In some patients, especially the elderly,

hyoscine may cause the central anticholinergic syndrome (excitement, ataxia, hallucinations, behavioural abnormalities, and drowsiness).

- PREGNANCY Use only if potential benefit outweighs risk. Injection may depress neonatal respiration.
- BREAST FEEDING Amount too small to be harmful.
- HEPATIC IMPAIRMENT Use with caution.
- RENAL IMPAIRMENT Use with caution.
- DIRECTIONS FOR ADMINISTRATION
  ▸ With transdermal use in children *Patch* applied to hairless area of skin behind ear; if less than whole patch required **either** cut with scissors along full thickness ensuring membrane is not peeled away **or** cover portion to prevent contact with skin.
  ▸ With oral use in children For administration by *mouth*, injection solution may be given orally.
- PRESCRIBING AND DISPENSING INFORMATION Flavours of chewable tablet formulations may include raspberry.
- PATIENT AND CARER ADVICE
  ▸ With transdermal use Explain accompanying instructions to patient and in particular emphasise advice to wash hands after handling and to wash application site after removing, and to use one patch at a time.

Driving and skilled tasks
  ▸ With transdermal use Drowsiness may persist for up to 24 hours or longer after removal of patch; effects of alcohol enhanced.

- MEDICINAL FORMS
  There can be variation in the licensing of different medicines containing the same drug. Forms available from special-order manufacturers include: oral suspension, oral solution

Tablet
CAUTIONARY AND ADVISORY LABELS 2
  ▸ Hyoscine hydrobromide (Non-proprietary)
  Hyoscine hydrobromide 300 microgram Hyoscine hydrobromide 300microgram tablets | 12 tablet P no price available DT price = £1.67
  ▸ Kwells (Bayer Plc)
  Hyoscine hydrobromide 150 microgram Kwells Kids 150microgram tablets | 12 tablet P £1.67 DT price = £1.67
  Hyoscine hydrobromide 300 microgram Kwells 300microgram tablets | 12 tablet P £1.67 DT price = £1.67

Chewable tablet
CAUTIONARY AND ADVISORY LABELS 2, 24
  ▸ Joy-Rides (Forest Laboratories UK Ltd)
  Hyoscine hydrobromide 150 microgram Joy-rides 150microgram chewable tablets sugar-free | 12 tablet P £1.55

Solution for injection
  ▸ Hyoscine hydrobromide (Non-proprietary)
  Hyoscine hydrobromide 400 microgram per 1 ml Hyoscine hydrobromide 400micrograms/1ml solution for injection ampoules | 10 ampoule PoM £25.00–£43.84 DT price = £42.85
  Hyoscine hydrobromide 600 microgram per 1 ml Hyoscine hydrobromide 600micrograms/1ml solution for injection ampoules | 10 ampoule PoM £46.70 DT price = £45.64

Transdermal patch
CAUTIONARY AND ADVISORY LABELS 19
  ▸ Scopoderm (Novartis Consumer Health UK Ltd)
  Hyoscine 1 mg per 72 hour Scopoderm 1.5mg patches | 2 patch P £4.52 DT price = £4.52

ANTIPSYCHOTICS > FIRST-GENERATION

⚑ 352

Droperidol

- DRUG ACTION Droperidol is a butyrophenone, structurally related to haloperidol, which blocks dopamine receptors in the chemoreceptor trigger zone.

- INDICATIONS AND DOSE

Prevention and treatment of postoperative nausea and vomiting
  ▸ BY INTRAVENOUS INJECTION
  ▸ Adult: 0.625–1.25 mg, dose to be given 30 minutes before end of surgery, then 0.625–1.25 mg every 6 hours as required
  ▸ Elderly: 625 micrograms, dose to be given 30 minutes before end of surgery, then 625 micrograms every 6 hours as required

Prevention of nausea and vomiting caused by opioid analgesics in postoperative patient-controlled analgesia (PCA)
  ▸ BY INTRAVENOUS INJECTION
  ▸ Adult: 15–50 micrograms of droperidol for every 1 mg of morphine in PCA, reduce dose in elderly; maximum 5 mg per day

- CONTRA-INDICATIONS Bradycardia · CNS depression · comatose states · hypokalaemia · hypomagnesaemia · phaeochromocytoma · QT-interval prolongation
- CAUTIONS Chronic obstructive pulmonary disease · electrolyte disturbances · history of alcohol abuse · respiratory failure
- INTERACTIONS → Appendix 1 (droperidol).
  Avoid concomitant administration of drugs that prolong QT interval.
- SIDE-EFFECTS Anxiety · cardiac arrest · hallucinations · inappropriate antidiuretic hormone secretion
- BREAST FEEDING Limited information available—avoid repeated administration.
- HEPATIC IMPAIRMENT In postoperative nausea and vomiting, max. 625 micrograms repeated every 6 hours as required.
  For nausea and vomiting caused by opioid analgesics in postoperative patient-controlled analgesia, reduce dose.
- RENAL IMPAIRMENT In postoperative nausea and vomiting, max. 625 micrograms repeated every 6 hours as required.
  For nausea and vomiting caused by opioid analgesics in postoperative patient-controlled analgesia, reduce dose.
- MONITORING REQUIREMENTS Continuous pulse oximetry required if risk of ventricular arrhythmia—continue for 30 minutes following administration.

- MEDICINAL FORMS
  There can be variation in the licensing of different medicines containing the same drug. Forms available from special-order manufacturers include: capsule, oral suspension, oral solution

Solution for injection
  ▸ Xomolix (ProStrakan Ltd)
  Droperidol 2.5 mg per 1 ml Xomolix 2.5mg/1ml solution for injection ampoules | 10 ampoule PoM £39.40

🔎 352

Levomepromazine

(Methotrimeprazine)

● **INDICATIONS AND DOSE**

Pain in palliative care (reserved for distressed patients with severe pain unresponsive to other measures)
▶ BY CONTINUOUS SUBCUTANEOUS INFUSION, OR BY INTRAMUSCULAR INJECTION, OR BY INTRAVENOUS INJECTION
  ▹ Adult: Seek specialist advice

Restlessness and confusion in palliative care
▶ BY CONTINUOUS SUBCUTANEOUS INFUSION
  ▹ Child 1–11 years: 0.35–3 mg/kg, to be administered over 24 hours
  ▹ Child 12–17 years: 12.5–200 mg, to be administered over 24 hours
▶ BY MOUTH
  ▹ Adult: 6 mg every 2 hours as required
▶ BY SUBCUTANEOUS INJECTION
  ▹ Adult: 6.25 mg every 2 hours as required
▶ BY SUBCUTANEOUS INFUSION
  ▹ Adult: Initially 12.5–50 mg/24 hours, titrated according to response (doses greater than 100 mg/24 hours should be given under specialist supervision)

Nausea and vomiting in palliative care
▶ BY CONTINUOUS INTRAVENOUS INFUSION, OR BY SUBCUTANEOUS INFUSION
  ▹ Child 1 month–11 years: 100–400 micrograms/kg, to be administered over 24 hours
  ▹ Child 12–17 years: 5–25 mg, to be administered over 24 hours
▶ BY MOUTH
  ▹ Adult: 6 mg once daily, dose to be taken at bedtime, increased if necessary to 12.5–25 mg twice daily
▶ BY SUBCUTANEOUS INJECTION
  ▹ Adult: 6.25 mg once daily, dose to be given at bedtime, increased if necessary to 12.5–25 mg twice daily
▶ BY SUBCUTANEOUS INFUSION
  ▹ Adult: 5–25 mg/24 hours, sedation can limit the dose

Schizophrenia (bed patients)
▶ BY MOUTH
  ▹ Adult: Initially 100–200 mg daily in 3 divided doses, increased if necessary to 1 g daily

Schizophrenia
▶ BY MOUTH
  ▹ Adult: Initially 25–50 mg daily in divided doses, dose can be increased as necessary

● CONTRA-INDICATIONS CNS depression · comatose states · phaeochromocytoma
● CAUTIONS Diabetes · patients receiving large initial doses should remain supine
  CAUTIONS, FURTHER INFORMATION
  ▶ In adults Risk of postural hypotension; not recommended for ambulant patients over 50 years unless risk of hypotensive reaction assessed.
● SIDE-EFFECTS Raised erythrocyte sedimentation rate
● HEPATIC IMPAIRMENT Can precipitate coma; phenothiazines are hepatotoxic.
● RENAL IMPAIRMENT Start with small doses in severe renal impairment because of increased cerebral sensitivity.
● DIRECTIONS FOR ADMINISTRATION
  ▶ With subcutaneous use in children For administration by *subcutaneous infusion* dilute with a suitable volume of Sodium Chloride 0.9%.

● MEDICINAL FORMS
  There can be variation in the licensing of different medicines containing the same drug. Forms available from special-order manufacturers include: oral suspension, oral solution
  Tablet
  CAUTIONARY AND ADVISORY LABELS 2
  ▶ Levomepromazine (Non-proprietary)
    Levomepromazine maleate 100 mg Nozinan 100mg tablets | 100 tablet [PoM] no price available
  ▶ Nozinan (Sanofi)
    Levomepromazine maleate 25 mg Nozinan 25mg tablets | 84 tablet [PoM] £20.26 DT price = £20.26
  Solution for injection
  ▶ Levomepromazine (Non-proprietary)
    Levomepromazine hydrochloride 25 mg per 1 ml Levomepromazine 25mg/1ml solution for injection ampoules | 10 ampoule [PoM] £20.13 DT price = £20.13
  ▶ Nozinan (Sanofi)
    Levomepromazine hydrochloride 25 mg per 1 ml Nozinan 25mg/1ml solution for injection ampoules | 10 ampoule [PoM] £20.13 DT price = £20.13

5.1   Meniere's disease

HISTAMINE ANALOGUES

Betahistine dihydrochloride

● **INDICATIONS AND DOSE**

Vertigo, tinnitus and hearing loss associated with Ménière's disease
▶ BY MOUTH
  ▹ Adult: Initially 16 mg 3 times a day, dose preferably taken with food; maintenance 24–48 mg daily

● CONTRA-INDICATIONS Phaeochromocytoma
● CAUTIONS Asthma · history of peptic ulcer
● INTERACTIONS → Appendix 1 (betahistine).
● SIDE-EFFECTS Gastro-intestinal disturbances · headache · pruritus · rashes
● PREGNANCY Avoid unless clearly necessary—no information available.
● BREAST FEEDING Use only if potential benefit outweighs risk—no information available.

● MEDICINAL FORMS
  There can be variation in the licensing of different medicines containing the same drug. Forms available from special-order manufacturers include: oral suspension, oral solution
  Tablet
  CAUTIONARY AND ADVISORY LABELS 21
  ▶ Betahistine dihydrochloride (Non-proprietary)
    Betahistine dihydrochloride 8 mg Betahistine 8mg tablets | 84 tablet [PoM] £10.50 DT price = £1.12 | 120 tablet [PoM] £13.50
    Betahistine dihydrochloride 16 mg Betahistine 16mg tablets | 84 tablet [PoM] £17.19 DT price = £1.30
  ▶ Serc (BGP Products Ltd)
    Betahistine dihydrochloride 8 mg Serc 8mg tablets | 120 tablet [PoM] £9.04
    Betahistine dihydrochloride 16 mg Serc 16mg tablets | 84 tablet [PoM] £12.65 DT price = £1.30

6   Pain

Analgesics

Drugs used for pain

The non-opioid drugs, paracetamol p. 406 and aspirin p. 109 (and other NSAIDs), are particularly suitable for pain in musculoskeletal conditions, whereas the opioid analgesics

4

Nervous system

are more suitable for moderate to severe pain, particularly of visceral origin.

Pain in sickle-cell disease

The pain of mild sickle-cell crises is managed with paracetamol, a NSAID, codeine phosphate p. 413, or dihydrocodeine tartrate p. 415. Severe crises may require the use of morphine p. 421 or diamorphine hydrochloride p. 415; concomitant use of a NSAID may potentiate analgesia and allow lower doses of the opioid to be used. Pethidine hydrochloride p. 426 should be avoided if possible because accumulation of a neurotoxic metabolite can precipitate seizures; the relatively short half-life of pethidine hydrochloride necessitates frequent injections.

Dental and orofacial pain

Analgesics should be used judiciously in dental care as a **temporary** measure until the cause of the pain has been dealt with.

Dental pain of inflammatory origin, such as that associated with pulpitis, apical infection, localised osteitis or pericoronitis is usually best managed by treating the infection, providing drainage, restorative procedures, and other local measures. Analgesics provide temporary relief of pain (usually for about 1 to 7 days) until the causative factors have been brought under control. In the case of pulpitis, intra-osseous infection or abscess, reliance on analgesics alone is usually inappropriate.

Similarly the pain and discomfort associated with acute problems of the oral mucosa (e.g. acute herpetic gingivostomatitis, erythema multiforme) may be relieved by benzydamine hydrochloride mouthwash or spray p. 1058 until the cause of the mucosal disorder has been dealt with. However, where a patient is febrile, the antipyretic action of paracetamol or ibuprofen p. 987 is often helpful.

The *choice* of an analgesic for dental purposes should be based on its suitability for the patient. Most dental pain is relieved effectively by non-steroidal anti-inflammatory drugs (NSAIDs). NSAIDs that are used for dental pain include ibuprofen, diclofenac sodium p. 980, and aspirin. Paracetamol has analgesic and antipyretic effects but no anti-inflammatory effect.

Opioid analgesics such as dihydrocodeine tartrate act on the central nervous system and are traditionally used for *moderate to severe pain*. However, opioid analgesics are relatively ineffective in dental pain and their side-effects can be unpleasant. Paracetamol, ibuprofen, or aspirin are adequate for most cases of dental pain and an opioid is rarely required.

Combining a non-opioid with an opioid analgesic can provide greater relief of pain than either analgesic given alone. However, this applies only when an adequate dose of each analgesic is used. Most combination analgesic preparations have not been shown to provide greater relief of pain than an adequate dose of the non-opioid component given alone. Moreover, combination preparations have the disadvantage of an increased number of side-effects.

Any analgesic given before a dental procedure should have a low risk of increasing postoperative bleeding. In the case of pain after the dental procedure, taking an analgesic before the effect of the local anaesthetic has worn off can improve control. Postoperative analgesia with ibuprofen or aspirin is usually continued for about 24 to 72 hours.

Temporomandibular dysfunction can be related to anxiety in some patients who may clench or grind their teeth (bruxism) during the day or night. The muscle spasm (which appears to be the main source of pain) may be treated empirically with an overlay appliance which provides a free sliding occlusion and may also interfere with grinding. In addition, diazepam p. 313, which has muscle relaxant as well as anxiolytic properties, may be helpful but it should only be prescribed on a short-term basis during the acute phase. Analgesics such as aspirin or ibuprofen may also be required.

Dysmenorrhoea

Use of an oral contraceptive prevents the pain of dysmenorrhoea which is generally associated with ovulatory cycles. If treatment is necessary paracetamol or a NSAID will generally provide adequate relief of pain. The vomiting and severe pain associated with dysmenorrhoea in women with endometriosis may call for an antiemetic (in addition to an analgesic). Antispasmodics (such as alverine citrate p. 78) have been advocated for dysmenorrhoea but the antispasmodic action does not generally provide significant relief.

Non-opioid analgesics and compound analgesic preparations

Aspirin is indicated for headache, transient musculoskeletal pain, dysmenorrhoea, and pyrexia. In inflammatory conditions, most physicians prefer anti-inflammatory treatment with another NSAID which may be better tolerated and more convenient for the patient. Aspirin is used increasingly for its antiplatelet properties. Aspirin tablets or dispersible aspirin tablets are adequate for most purposes as they act rapidly.

Gastric irritation may be a problem; it is minimised by taking the dose after food. Enteric-coated preparations are available, but have a slow onset of action and are therefore unsuitable for single-dose analgesic use (though their prolonged action may be useful for night pain).

Aspirin interacts significantly with a number of other drugs and its interaction with warfarin sodium p. 126 is a **special hazard**.

Paracetamol is similar in efficacy to aspirin, but has no demonstrable anti-inflammatory activity; it is less irritant to the stomach and for that reason is now generally preferred to aspirin, particularly in the elderly. **Overdosage** with paracetamol is particularly dangerous as it may cause hepatic damage which is sometimes not apparent for 4 to 6 days.

Nefopam hydrochloride p. 408 may have a place in the relief of persistent pain unresponsive to other non-opioid analgesics. It causes little or no respiratory depression, but sympathomimetic and antimuscarinic side-effects may be troublesome.

Non-steroidal anti-inflammatory analgesics (NSAIDs) are particularly useful for the treatment of patients with chronic disease accompanied by pain and inflammation. Some of them are also used in the short-term treatment of mild to moderate pain including transient musculoskeletal pain but paracetamol is now often preferred, particularly in the elderly. They are also suitable for the relief of pain in *dysmenorrhoea* and to treat pain caused by *secondary bone tumours*, many of which produce lysis of bone and release prostaglandins. Selective inhibitors of cyclo-oxygenase-2 may be used in preference to non-selective NSAIDs for patients at high risk of developing serious gastro-intestinal side-effects. Several NSAIDs are also used for postoperative analgesia.

A non-opioid analgesic administered by intrathecal infusion (**ziconotide** (*Prialt*®), available from Eisai) is licensed for the treatment of chronic severe pain; ziconotide can be used by a hospital specialist as an adjunct to opioid analgesics.

Compound analgesic preparations

Compound analgesic preparations that contain a simple analgesic (such as aspirin p. 109 or paracetamol p. 406) with an opioid component reduce the scope for effective titration of the individual components in the management of pain of varying intensity.

Compound analgesic preparations containing paracetamol or aspirin with a *low dose* of an opioid analgesic (e.g. 8 mg of codeine phosphate per compound tablet) are commonly used, but the advantages have not been substantiated. The low dose of the opioid may be enough to cause opioid side-effects (in particular, constipation) and can complicate the treatment of **overdosage** yet may not provide significant additional relief of pain.

A *full dose* of the opioid component (e.g. 60 mg codeine phosphate) in compound analgesic preparations effectively augments the analgesic activity but is associated with the full range of opioid side-effects (including nausea, vomiting, severe constipation, drowsiness, respiratory depression, and risk of dependence on long-term administration).

Important: the elderly are particularly susceptible to opioid side-effects and should receive lower doses.

In general, when assessing pain, it is necessary to weigh up carefully whether there is a need for a non-opioid and an opioid analgesic to be taken simultaneously.

Caffeine is a weak stimulant that is often included, in small doses, in analgesic preparations. It is claimed that the addition of caffeine may enhance the analgesic effect, but the alerting effect, mild habit-forming effect and possible provocation of headache may not always be desirable. Moreover, in excessive dosage or on withdrawal caffeine may itself induce headache.

Co-proxamol tablets (dextropropoxyphene in combination with paracetamol) are no longer licensed because of safety concerns, particularly toxicity in overdose. Co-proxamol tablets [unlicensed] may still be prescribed for patients who find it difficult to change, because alternatives are not effective or suitable.

Opioid analgesics

Opioid analgesics are usually used to relieve moderate to severe pain particularly of visceral origin. Repeated administration may cause dependence and tolerance, but this is no deterrent in the control of pain in terminal illness. Regular use of a potent opioid may be appropriate for certain cases of chronic non-malignant pain; treatment should be supervised by a specialist and the patient should be assessed at regular intervals.

Strong opioids

Morphine p. 421 remains the most valuable opioid analgesic for severe pain although it frequently causes nausea and vomiting. It is the standard against which other opioid analgesics are compared. In addition to relief of pain, morphine also confers a state of euphoria and mental detachment.

Morphine is the opioid of choice for the oral treatment of *severe pain in palliative care*. It is given regularly every 4 hours (or every 12 or 24 hours as modified-release preparations).

Buprenorphine p. 409 has both opioid agonist and antagonist properties and may precipitate withdrawal symptoms, including pain, in patients dependent on other opioids. It has abuse potential and may itself cause dependence. It has a much longer duration of action than morphine and sublingually is an effective analgesic for 6 to 8 hours. Unlike most opioid analgesics, the effects of buprenorphine are only partially reversed by naloxone hydrochloride p. 1204.

Dipipanone hydrochloride used alone is less sedating than morphine but the only preparation available contains an antiemetic and is therefore not suitable for regular regimens in palliative care.

Diamorphine hydrochloride (heroin) p. 415 is a powerful opioid analgesic. It may cause less nausea and hypotension than morphine. In *palliative care* the greater solubility of diamorphine hydrochloride allows effective doses to be injected in smaller volumes and this is important in the emaciated patient.

Alfentanil p. 1177, fentanyl p. 416 and remifentanil p. 1178 are used by injection for intra-operative analgesia; fentanyl is available in a transdermal drug delivery system as a self-adhesive patch which is changed every 72 hours.

Methadone hydrochloride p. 456 is less sedating than morphine and acts for longer periods. In prolonged use, methadone hydrochloride should not be administered more often than twice daily to avoid the risk of accumulation and opioid overdosage. Methadone hydrochloride may be used instead of morphine in the occasional patient who experiences excitation (or exacerbation of pain) with morphine.

Oxycodone hydrochloride p. 424 has an efficacy and side-effect profile similar to that of morphine. It is used primarily for control of *pain in palliative care*.

Papaveretum p. 426 is rarely used; morphine is easier to prescribe and less prone to error with regard to the strength and dose.

Pentazocine p. 426 has both agonist and antagonist properties and precipitates withdrawal symptoms, including pain in patients dependent on other opioids. By injection it is more potent than dihydrocodeine tartrate p. 415 or codeine phosphate, but hallucinations and thought disturbances may occur. It is not recommended and, in particular, should be avoided after myocardial infarction as it may increase pulmonary and aortic blood pressure as well as cardiac work.

Pethidine hydrochloride p. 426 produces prompt but short-lasting analgesia; it is less constipating than morphine, but even in high doses is a less potent analgesic. It is not suitable for severe continuing pain. It is used for analgesia in labour; however, other opioids, such as morphine or diamorphine hydrochloride, are often preferred for obstetric pain.

Tapentadol p. 427 produces analgesia by two mechanisms. It is an opioid-receptor agonist and it also inhibits noradrenaline reuptake. Nausea, vomiting, and constipation are less likely to occur with tapentadol than with other strong opioid analgesics.

Tramadol hydrochloride p. 427 produces analgesia by two mechanisms: an opioid effect and an enhancement of serotonergic and adrenergic pathways. It has fewer of the typical opioid side-effects (notably, less respiratory depression, less constipation and less addiction potential); psychiatric reactions have been reported.

Weak opioids

Codeine phosphate can be used for the relief of mild to moderate pain where other painkillers such as paracetamol or ibuprofen p. 987 have proved ineffective.

Dihydrocodeine tartrate has an analgesic efficacy similar to that of codeine phosphate. Higher doses may provide some additional pain relief but this may be at the cost of more nausea and vomiting.

Meptazinol p. 421 is claimed to have a low incidence of repiratory depression. It has a reported length of action of 2 to 7 hours with onset within 15 minutes.

Postoperative analgesia

A combination of opioid and non-opioid analgesics is used to treat postoperative pain. The use of intra-operative opioids affects the prescribing of postoperative analgesics. A postoperative opioid analgesic should be given with care since it may potentiate any residual respiratory depression.

Morphine is used most widely. Tramadol hydrochloride is not as effective in severe pain as other opioid analgesics. Buprenorphine may antagonise the analgesic effect of previously administered opioids and is generally not recommended. Pethidine hydrochloride is generally not recommended for postoperative pain because it is metabolised to norpethidine which may accumulate, particularly in renal impairment; norpethidine stimulates the central nervous system and may cause convulsions.

Opioids are also given epidurally [unlicensed route] in the postoperative period but are associated with side-effects such as pruritus, urinary retention, nausea and vomiting; respiratory depression can be delayed, particularly with morphine p. 421.

4

Nervous system

Patient-controlled analgesia (PCA) can be used to relieve postoperative pain—consult individual hospital protocols.

Pain management and opioid dependence

Although caution is necessary, patients who are dependent on opioids or have a history of drug dependence may be treated with opioid analgesics when there is a clinical need. Treatment with opioid analgesics in this patient group should normally be carried out with the advice of specialists. However, doctors do not require a special licence to prescribe opioid analgesics to patients with opioid dependence for relief of pain due to organic disease or injury.

> **Drugs used for Pain not listed below** Dexibuprofen, p. 978 · Diclofenac potassium, p. 980 · Fenoprofen, p. 985 · Levomepromazine, p. 403 · Mefenamic acid, p. 992

ANALGESICS > NON-OPIOID

Paracetamol
5.5.2016

(Acetaminophen)

● **INDICATIONS AND DOSE**

Mild to moderate pain | Pyrexia
▸ BY MOUTH
▹ Adult: 0.5–1 g every 4–6 hours; maximum 4 g per day
▸ BY INTRAVENOUS INFUSION
▹ Adult (body-weight up to 50 kg): 15 mg/kg every 4–6 hours, dose to be administered over 15 minutes; maximum 60 mg/kg per day
▹ Adult (body-weight 50 kg and above): 1 g every 4–6 hours, dose to be administered over 15 minutes; maximum 4 g per day
▸ BY RECTUM
▹ Adult: 0.5–1 g every 4–6 hours; maximum 4 g per day

Mild to moderate pain in patients with risk factors for hepatotoxicity | Pyrexia in patients with risk factors for hepatotoxicity
▸ BY INTRAVENOUS INFUSION
▹ Adult (body-weight up to 50 kg): 15 mg/kg every 4–6 hours, dose to be administered over 15 minutes; maximum 60 mg/kg per day
▹ Adult (body-weight 50 kg and above): 1 g every 4–6 hours, dose to be administered over 15 minutes; maximum 3 g per day

Pain | Pyrexia with discomfort
▸ BY MOUTH
▹ Child 3-5 months: 60 mg every 4–6 hours; maximum 4 doses per day
▹ Child 6 months-1 year: 120 mg every 4–6 hours; maximum 4 doses per day
▹ Child 2-3 years: 180 mg every 4–6 hours; maximum 4 doses per day
▹ Child 4-5 years: 240 mg every 4–6 hours; maximum 4 doses per day
▹ Child 6-7 years: 240–250 mg every 4–6 hours; maximum 4 doses per day
▹ Child 8-9 years: 360–375 mg every 4–6 hours; maximum 4 doses per day
▹ Child 10-11 years: 480–500 mg every 4–6 hours; maximum 4 doses per day
▹ Child 12-15 years: 480–750 mg every 4–6 hours; maximum 4 doses per day
▹ Child 16-17 years: 0.5–1 g every 4–6 hours; maximum 4 doses per day
▸ BY RECTUM
▹ Child 3-11 months: 60–125 mg every 4–6 hours as required; maximum 4 doses per day
▹ Child 1-4 years: 125–250 mg every 4–6 hours as required; maximum 4 doses per day

▹ Child 5-11 years: 250–500 mg every 4–6 hours as required; maximum 4 doses per day
▹ Child 12-17 years: 500 mg every 4–6 hours

Post-immunisation pyrexia in infants
▸ BY MOUTH
▹ Child 2-3 months: 60 mg for 1 dose, then 60 mg after 4–6 hours if required, (dose can be repeated twice for meningococcal B vaccine)
▹ Child 4 months: 60 mg for 1 dose, then 60 mg after 4–6 hours; maximum 4 doses per day

PANADOL OA®

Mild to moderate pain | Pyrexia
▸ BY MOUTH
▹ Adult: 1 g up to 4 times a day, dose not to be taken more often than every 4 hours

● UNLICENSED USE
▸ In children Paracetamol oral suspension 500 mg/5 mL not licensed for use in children under 16 years. Not licensed for use in children under 2 months by mouth; under 3 months by rectum. [EvGr] Second further dose for post-immunisation pyrexia in infants 2–3 months for meningococcal B vaccine not licensed. ⟨E⟩ Intravenous infusion not licensed in pre-term neonates. Intravenous infusion dose not licensed in children and neonates with body-weight under 10 kg.

● CAUTIONS Before administering, check when paracetamol last administered and cumulative paracetamol dose over previous 24 hours · body-weight under 50 kg · chronic alcohol consumption · chronic dehydration · chronic malnutrition · hepatocellular insufficiency · long-term use (especially in those who are malnourished)

CAUTIONS, FURTHER INFORMATION
[EvGr] Some patients may be at increased risk of experiencing toxicity at therapeutic doses, particularly those with a body-weight under 50 kg and those with risk factors for hepatotoxicity. Clinical judgement should be used to adjust the dose of oral and intravenous paracetamol in these patients. ⟨E⟩
[EvGr] Co-administration of enzyme-inducing antiepileptic medications may increase toxicity; doses should be reduced. ⟨E⟩

● INTERACTIONS → Appendix 1 (paracetamol).

● SIDE-EFFECTS
GENERAL SIDE-EFFECTS
▸ **Rare** Acute generalised exanthematous pustulosis · malaise · skin reactions · Stevens-Johnson syndrome · toxic epidermal necrolysis
▸ **Frequency not known** Blood disorders · leucopenia · neutropenia · thrombocytopenia
SPECIFIC SIDE-EFFECTS
▸ **Rare**
▸ With intravenous use Flushing · tachycardia
▸ **Frequency not known**
▸ With intravenous use Hypotension
Overdose
Important: liver damage and less frequently renal damage can occur following overdose.

Nausea and vomiting, the only early features of poisoning, usually settle within 24 hours. Persistence beyond this time, often associated with the onset of right subcostal pain and tenderness, usually indicates development of hepatic necrosis.

For specific details on the management of poisoning, see Paracetamol, under Emergency treatment of poisoning p. 1194

● PREGNANCY Not known to be harmful.

● BREAST FEEDING Amount too small to be harmful.

● HEPATIC IMPAIRMENT Dose-related toxicity—avoid large doses.

4
Nervous system

- **RENAL IMPAIRMENT**
- In adults Increase infusion dose interval to every 6 hours if eGFR less than 30 mL/minute/1.73 m^2.
- In children Increase infusion dose interval to every 6 hours if estimated glomerular filtration rate less than 30 mL/minute/1.73 m^2.
- **DIRECTIONS FOR ADMINISTRATION**
- With intravenous use For *intravenous infusion (Perfalgan®)*, give in Glucose 5% *or* Sodium Chloride 0.9%; dilute to a concentration of not less than 1 mg/mL and use within an hour; may also be given undiluted. For children under 33 kg, use 50 mL-vial.
- **PRESCRIBING AND DISPENSING INFORMATION** BP directs that when Paediatric Paracetamol Oral Suspension or Paediatric Paracetamol Mixture is prescribed Paracetamol Oral Suspension 120 mg/5 mL should be dispensed.
- **PATIENT AND CARER ADVICE**
  Medicines for Children leaflet: Paracetamol for mild-to-moderate pain www.medicinesforchildren.org.uk/paracetamol-for-mildtomoderate-pain
- **PROFESSION SPECIFIC INFORMATION**
  Dental practitioners' formulary
  Paracetamol Tablets may be prescribed.
  Paracetamol Soluble Tablets 500 mg may be prescribed.
  Paracetamol Oral Suspension may be prescribed.
- **EXCEPTIONS TO LEGAL CATEGORY** Paracetamol capsules or tablets can be sold to the public provided packs contain no more than 32 capsules or tablets; pharmacists can sell multiple packs up to a total quantity of 100 capsules or tablets in justifiable circumstances.

- **MEDICINAL FORMS**
  There can be variation in the licensing of different medicines containing the same drug. Forms available from special-order manufacturers include: oral suspension, oral solution, suppository

Tablet
CAUTIONARY AND ADVISORY LABELS 29 (does not apply to 1 g tablet), 30
- Paracetamol (Non-proprietary)
  Paracetamol 500 mg Paracetamol 500mg caplets | 32 tablet P £0.38 DT price = £0.74 | 100 tablet PoM £3.18 DT price = £2.31
  Paracetamol 500mg tablets | 32 tablet P £1.24 DT price = £0.74 | 100 tablet PoM £3.18 DT price = £2.31 | 1000 tablet PoM £25.63 | 5000 tablet PoM no price available
- Mandanol (M & A Pharmachem Ltd)
  Paracetamol 500 mg Mandanol 500mg caplets | 32 tablet P £0.20 DT price = £0.74
  Mandanol 500mg tablets | 100 tablet PoM £0.33 DT price = £2.31
- Panadol (GlaxoSmithKline Consumer Healthcare)
  Paracetamol 500 mg Panadol Advance 500mg tablets | 32 tablet P £1.74 DT price = £0.74

Effervescent tablet
CAUTIONARY AND ADVISORY LABELS 29, 30
- Paracetamol (Non-proprietary)
  Paracetamol 500 mg Paracetamol 500mg soluble tablets | 60 tablet P no price available | 60 tablet PoM £5.00 | 100 tablet GSL £44.28 DT price = £7.54 | 100 tablet P no price available DT price = £7.54

Soluble tablet
CAUTIONARY AND ADVISORY LABELS 13, 29, 30
- Paracetamol (Non-proprietary)
  Paracetamol 120 mg Paracetamol 120mg soluble tablets sugar free sugar-free | 16 tablet GSL no price available
- Brands may include Disprol

Orodispersible tablet
CAUTIONARY AND ADVISORY LABELS 30
- Calpol Fastmelts (McNeil Products Ltd)
  Paracetamol 250 mg Calpol Six Plus Fastmelts 250mg tablets sugar-free | 12 tablet P £2.28 sugar-free | 24 tablet P £3.59

Capsule
CAUTIONARY AND ADVISORY LABELS 29, 30
- Paracetamol (Non-proprietary)
  Paracetamol 500 mg Paracetamol 500mg capsules | 16 capsule P £0.55 | 32 capsule P £1.21 DT price = £1.00 | 100 capsule PoM £8.20 DT price = £3.13

Oral suspension
CAUTIONARY AND ADVISORY LABELS 30
- Paracetamol (Non-proprietary)
  Paracetamol 24 mg per 1 ml Paracetamol 120mg/5ml oral suspension paediatric | 100 ml P £0.72 | 500 ml P £3.14 DT price = £3.12
  Paracetamol 120mg/5ml oral suspension paediatric sugar free sugar-free | 100 ml P £2.40 DT price = £1.23 sugar-free | 200 ml P £2.72 sugar-free | 500 ml P £6.80 sugar-free | 1000 ml P £13.60
  Paracetamol 50 mg per 1 ml Paracetamol 250mg/5ml oral suspension | 100 ml P £1.25 DT price = £1.13 | 500 ml P £6.25
  Paracetamol 250mg/5ml oral suspension sugar free sugar-free | 100 ml P £2.75 sugar-free | 200 ml P £1.99 DT price = £1.97 sugar-free | 500 ml P £8.25 sugar-free | 1000 ml P £16.50
  Paracetamol 100 mg per 1 ml Paracetamol 500mg/5ml oral suspension sugar free sugar-free | 150 ml PoM £24.00 DT price = £24.00
- Calpol (McNeil Products Ltd)
  Paracetamol 24 mg per 1 ml Calpol Infant 120mg/5ml suspension | 200 ml P £3.35
  Calpol Infant 120mg/5ml oral suspension sugar free sugar-free | 200 ml P £3.35
  Paracetamol 50 mg per 1 ml Calpol Six Plus 250mg/5ml oral suspension | 200 ml P £3.88
  Calpol Six Plus 250mg/5ml oral suspension sugar free sugar-free | 100 ml P £2.40 sugar-free | 200 ml P £3.88 DT price = £1.97
- Mandanol (M & A Pharmachem Ltd)
  Paracetamol 24 mg per 1 ml Mandanol Infant paracetamol 120mg/5ml oral suspension sugar-free | 200 ml P £1.05
  Paracetamol 50 mg per 1 ml Mandanol 6+ paracetamol 250mg/5ml oral suspension sugar-free | 100 ml P £0.90 sugar-free | 200 ml P £1.10 DT price = £1.97

Oral solution
CAUTIONARY AND ADVISORY LABELS 30
- Paracetamol (Non-proprietary)
  Paracetamol 24 mg per 1 ml Paracetamol 120mg/5ml oral solution paediatric sugar free sugar-free | 500 ml P £2.86 DT price = £2.86 sugar-free | 2000 ml P £27.20
  Paracetamol 100 mg per 1 ml Paracetamol 500mg/5ml oral solution sugar free sugar-free | 200 ml PoM £18.00

Solution for infusion
CAUTIONARY AND ADVISORY LABELS 30
- Paracetamol (Non-proprietary)
  Paracetamol 10 mg per 1 ml Paracetamol 500mg/50ml solution for infusion vials | 10 vial PoM £11.00
  Paracetamol 1g/100ml solution for infusion vials | 10 vial PoM £12.00
- Perfalgan (Bristol-Myers Squibb Pharmaceuticals Ltd)
  Paracetamol 10 mg per 1 ml Perfalgan 1g/100ml solution for infusion vials | 12 vial PoM £14.96
  Perfalgan 500mg/50ml solution for infusion vials | 12 vial PoM £13.60

Suppository
CAUTIONARY AND ADVISORY LABELS 30
- Paracetamol (Non-proprietary)
  Paracetamol 80 mg Paracetamol 80mg suppositories | 10 suppository P £10.00
  Paracetamol 120 mg Paracetamol 120mg suppositories | 10 suppository P £11.26 DT price = £11.26
  Paracetamol 125 mg Paracetamol 125mg suppositories | 10 suppository P £15.00 DT price = £13.80
  Paracetamol 240 mg Paracetamol 240mg suppositories | 10 suppository P £22.01 DT price = £22.01
  Paracetamol 250 mg Paracetamol 250mg suppositories | 10 suppository P £15.00 DT price = £27.60
  Paracetamol 500 mg Paracetamol 500mg suppositories | 10 suppository P £36.50 DT price = £36.50
  Paracetamol 1 gram Paracetamol 1g suppositories | 10 suppository P no price available | 12 suppository P no price available
- Alvedon (Intrapharm Laboratories Ltd)
  Paracetamol 60 mg Alvedon 60mg suppositories | 10 suppository P £11.95 DT price = £11.95
  Paracetamol 125 mg Alvedon 125mg suppositories | 10 suppository P £13.80 DT price = £13.80
  Paracetamol 250 mg Alvedon 250mg suppositories | 10 suppository P £27.60 DT price = £27.60

Nervous system

4

Paracetamol with tramadol

The properties listed below are those particular to the combination only. For the properties of the components please consider, paracetamol p. 406, tramadol hydrochloride p. 427.

- ● **INDICATIONS AND DOSE**

  Moderate to severe pain
  ▸ BY MOUTH
  ▸ Child 12–17 years: 2 tablets up to every 6 hours; maximum 8 tablets per day
  ▸ Adult: 2 tablets up to every 6 hours; maximum 8 tablets per day

- ● **MEDICINAL FORMS**
  There can be variation in the licensing of different medicines containing the same drug.

  Tablet
  CAUTIONARY AND ADVISORY LABELS 2, 25, 29, 30
  ▸ Paracetamol with tramadol (Non-proprietary)
  Tramadol hydrochloride 37.5 mg, Paracetamol 325 mg Tramadol 37.5mg / Paracetamol 325mg tablets | 60 tablet PoM £9.68 DT price = £9.22 CD3
  ▸ Tramacet (Grunenthal Ltd)
  Tramadol hydrochloride 37.5 mg, Paracetamol 325 mg Tramacet 37.5mg/325mg tablets | 60 tablet PoM £9.68 DT price = £9.22 CD3

  Effervescent tablet
  CAUTIONARY AND ADVISORY LABELS 2, 13, 29, 30
  ELECTROLYTES: May contain Sodium
  ▸ Tramacet (Grunenthal Ltd)
  Tramadol hydrochloride 37.5 mg, Paracetamol 325 mg Tramacet 37.5mg/325mg effervescent tablets sugar-free | 60 tablet PoM £9.68 DT price = £9.68 CD3

ANALGESICS ⟩ NON-OPIOID, CENTRALLY ACTING

Nefopam hydrochloride

- ● **INDICATIONS AND DOSE**

  Moderate pain
  ▸ BY MOUTH
  ▸ Adult: Initially 60 mg 3 times a day, adjusted according to response; usual dose 30–90 mg 3 times a day
  ▸ Elderly: Initially 30 mg 3 times a day, adjusted according to response; usual dose 30–90 mg 3 times a day

- ● **CONTRA-INDICATIONS** Convulsive disorders · not indicated for myocardial infarction
- ● **CAUTIONS** Elderly · urinary retention
- ● **INTERACTIONS** → Appendix 1 (nefopam).
- ● **SIDE-EFFECTS**
  ▸ **Common or very common** Dry mouth · lightheadedness · nausea · nervousness · urinary retention
  ▸ **Uncommon** Blurred vision · confusion · drowsiness · hallucinations · headache · insomnia · sweating · tachycardia · vomiting
  ▸ **Frequency not known** May colour urine (pink)
- ● **PREGNANCY** No information available—avoid unless no safer treatment.
- ● **HEPATIC IMPAIRMENT** Caution.
- ● **RENAL IMPAIRMENT** Caution.

- ● **MEDICINAL FORMS**
  There can be variation in the licensing of different medicines containing the same drug. Forms available from special-order manufacturers include: oral suspension

  Tablet
  CAUTIONARY AND ADVISORY LABELS 2, 14
  ▸ Nefopam hydrochloride (Non-proprietary)
  Nefopam hydrochloride 30 mg Nefopam 30mg tablets | 90 tablet PoM £55.00–£66.60 DT price = £57.75

ANALGESICS ⟩ NON-STEROIDAL ANTI-INFLAMMATORY DRUGS

Aspirin with codeine

The properties listed below are those particular to the combination only. For the properties of the components please consider, aspirin p. 109, codeine phosphate p. 413.

- ● **INDICATIONS AND DOSE**

  Mild to moderate pain | Pyrexia
  ▸ BY MOUTH
  ▸ Adult: 1–2 tablets every 4–6 hours as required, dose to be dispersed in water; maximum 8 tablets per day

- ● **PRESCRIBING AND DISPENSING INFORMATION** When co-codaprin tablets or dispersible tablets are prescribed and no strength is stated, tablets or dispersible tablets, respectively, containing codeine phosphate 8 mg and aspirin 400 mg should be dispensed.
- ● **LESS SUITABLE FOR PRESCRIBING** Aspirin with codeine is less suitable for prescribing.
- ● **EXCEPTIONS TO LEGAL CATEGORY** Aspirin with codeine can be sold to the public provided packs contain no more than 32 capsules or tablets; pharmacists can sell multiple packs up to a total quantity of 100 capsules or tablets in justifiable circumstances.
- ● **MEDICINAL FORMS**
  There can be variation in the licensing of different medicines containing the same drug.

  Tablet
  ▸ Aspirin with codeine (Non-proprietary)
  Codeine phosphate 8 mg, Aspirin 400 mg Boots Aspirin and Codeine tablets | 32 tablet P no price available Schedule 5 (CD Inv)

  Dispersible tablet
  CAUTIONARY AND ADVISORY LABELS 13, 21, 32
  ▸ Aspirin with codeine (Non-proprietary)
  Codeine phosphate 8 mg, Aspirin 400 mg Co-codaprin 8mg/400mg dispersible tablets | 100 tablet PoM £97.55 DT price = £90.53 Schedule 5 (CD Inv)

ANALGESICS ⟩ OPIOIDS

Opioids

- ● **CONTRA-INDICATIONS** Acute respiratory depression · comatose patients · head injury (opioid analgesics interfere with pupillary responses vital for neurological assessment) · raised intracranial pressure (opioid analgesics interfere with pupillary responses vital for neurological assessment) · risk of paralytic ileus
- ● **CAUTIONS** Adrenocortical insufficiency (reduced dose is recommended) · asthma (avoid during an acute attack) · convulsive disorders · debilitated patients (reduced dose is recommended) (in adults) · diseases of the biliary tract · elderly (reduced dose is recommended) (in adults) · hypotension · hypothyroidism (reduced dose is recommended) · impaired respiratory function (avoid in chronic obstructive pulmonary disease) · inflammatory bowel disorders · myasthenia gravis · obstructive bowel disorders · prostatic hypertrophy (in adults) · shock · urethral stenosis (in adults)

  CAUTIONS, FURTHER INFORMATION
  ▸ Dependence Repeated use of opioid analgesics is associated with the development of psychological and physical dependence; although this is rarely a problem with therapeutic use, caution is advised if prescribing for patients with a history of drug dependence.
  ▸ Palliative care In the control of pain in terminal illness, the cautions listed should not necessarily be a deterrent to the use of opioid analgesics.

- INTERACTIONS → Appendix 1 (opioid analgesics).
- SIDE-EFFECTS
▶ **Common or very common** Biliary spasm · bradycardia · confusion · constipation · dependence · difficulty in micturition · dizziness · drowsiness · dry mouth · dysphoria · euphoria · flushing · hallucinations · headache · hypotension (larger doses) · miosis · mood changes · muscle rigidity (larger doses) · nausea (particularly in initial stages) · oedema · palpitation · postural hypotension · pruritus · rash · respiratory depression (larger doses) · sexual dysfunction · sleep disturbances · sweating · tachycardia · ureteric spasm · urinary retention · urticaria · vertigo · visual disturbances · vomiting (particularly in initial stages)
▶ **Frequency not known** Adrenal insufficiency (long-term use) · hyperalgesia (long-term use) · hypogonadism (long-term use)

SIDE-EFFECTS, FURTHER INFORMATION
▶ **Hypogonadism and adrenal insufficiency** Long-term use of opioid analgesics can cause hypogonadism and adrenal insufficiency in both males and females. This is thought to be dose related and can lead to amenorrhoea, reduced libido, infertility, depression, and erectile dysfunction.
▶ **Hyperalgesia** Long-term use of opioid analgesics has also been associated with a state of abnormal pain sensitivity (hyperalgesia). Pain associated with hyperalgesia is usually distinct from pain associated with disease progression or breakthrough pain, and is often more diffuse and less defined. Treatment of hyperalgesia involves reducing the dose of opioid medication or switching therapy; cases of suspected hyperalgesia should be referred to a specialist pain team.
▶ **Respiratory depression** Respiratory depression is a major concern with opioid analgesics; neonates (particularly if pre-term) may be more susceptible. It may be treated by artificial ventilation or be reversed by naloxone.
▶ **Dependence and withdrawal** Psychological dependence rarely occurs when opioids are used therapeutically (e.g. for pain relief) but tolerance can develop during long-term treatment.
Overdose
Opioids (narcotic analgesics) cause coma, respiratory depression, and pinpoint pupils. For details on the management of poisoning, see Opioids, under Emergency treatment of poisoning p. 1194 and consider the specific antidote, naloxone hydrochloride p. 1204.

- PREGNANCY Respiratory depression and withdrawal symptoms can occur in the neonate if opioid analgesics are used during delivery; also gastric stasis and inhalation pneumonia has been reported in the mother if opioid analgesics are used during labour.
- HEPATIC IMPAIRMENT Avoid use or reduce dose; may precipitate coma in patients with hepatic impairment.
- TREATMENT CESSATION Avoid abrupt withdrawal after long-term treatment; they should be withdrawn gradually to avoid abstinence symptoms.
- PATIENT AND CARER ADVICE
Driving and skilled tasks
Drowsiness may affect performance of skilled tasks (e.g. driving); effects of alcohol enhanced. Driving at the start of therapy with opioid analgesics, and following dose changes, should be avoided.
  For information on 2015 legislation regarding driving whilst taking certain controlled drugs, including opioids, see *Drugs and driving* under Guidance on prescribing p. 1.

⌐ 408
Buprenorphine
- DRUG ACTION Buprenorphine is an opioid-receptor partial agonist (it has opioid agonist and antagonist properties).

- INDICATIONS AND DOSE
Moderate to severe pain
▶ BY SUBLINGUAL ADMINISTRATION
▹ Child (body-weight 16-25 kg): 100 micrograms every 6–8 hours
▹ Child (body-weight 25-37.5 kg): 100–200 micrograms every 6–8 hours
▹ Child (body-weight 37.5-50 kg): 200–300 micrograms every 6–8 hours
▹ Child (body-weight 50 kg and above): 200–400 micrograms every 6–8 hours
▹ Adult: 200–400 micrograms every 6–8 hours
▶ BY INTRAMUSCULAR INJECTION, OR BY SLOW INTRAVENOUS INJECTION
▹ Child 6 months-11 years: 3–6 micrograms/kg every 6–8 hours (max. per dose 9 micrograms/kg)
▹ Child 12-17 years: 300–600 micrograms every 6–8 hours
▹ Adult: 300–600 micrograms every 6–8 hours
Premedication
▶ BY SUBLINGUAL ADMINISTRATION
▹ Adult: 400 micrograms
▶ BY INTRAMUSCULAR INJECTION
▹ Adult: 300 micrograms
Intra-operative analgesia
▶ BY SLOW INTRAVENOUS INJECTION
▹ Adult: 300–450 micrograms
Adjunct in the treatment of opioid dependence
▶ BY SUBLINGUAL ADMINISTRATION
▹ Adult: Initially 0.8–4 mg for 1 dose on the first day, adjusted in steps of 2–4 mg daily if required; usual dose 12–24 mg daily; maximum 32 mg per day

DOSE EQUIVALENCE AND CONVERSION
For opioid substitution therapy, in patients taking methadone who want to switch to buprenorphine, the dose of methadone should be reduced to a maximum of 30 mg daily before starting buprenorphine treatment. If the dose of methadone is over 10 mg daily, buprenorphine can be started at a dose of 4 mg daily and titrated according to requirements; if the methadone dose is below 10 mg daily, buprenorphine can be started at a dose of 2 mg daily.

BUTRANS®
Moderate, non-malignant pain unresponsive to non-opioid analgesics
▶ BY TRANSDERMAL APPLICATION USING PATCHES
▹ Adult: Initially 5 micrograms/hour up to every 7 days, dose adjustments—when starting, analgesic effect should not be evaluated until the system has been worn for 72 hours (to allow for gradual increase in plasma-buprenorphine concentration)—if necessary, dose should be adjusted at intervals of at least 3 days using a patch of the next strength or a combination of 2 patches applied in different places (applied at *same time* to avoid confusion). Maximum 2 patches can be used at any one time

HAPOCTASIN®
Moderate to severe chronic cancer pain in patients who have not previously received strong opioid analgesic | Severe pain unresponsive to non-opioid analgesics in patients who have not previously received strong opioid analgesic
▶ BY TRANSDERMAL APPLICATION USING PATCHES
▹ Adult: Initially 35 micrograms/hour up to every 72 hours, dose adjustment—when starting,   continued →

analgesic effect should not be evaluated until the system has been worn for 24 hours (to allow for gradual increase in plasma-buprenorphine concentration)—if necessary, dose should be adjusted at intervals of no longer than 72 hours using a patch of the next strength or using 2 patches of the same strength (applied at *same time* to avoid confusion). Maximum 2 patches can be used at any one time, for breakthrough pain, consider 200–400 micrograms buprenorphine sublingually

Moderate to severe chronic cancer pain in patients who have previously received strong opioid analgesic | Severe pain unresponsive to non-opioid analgesics in patients who have previously received strong opioid analgesic
▸ BY TRANSDERMAL APPLICATION USING PATCHES
▸ Adult: The initial dose should be based on previous 24-hour opioid requirement, consult product literature, dose adjustment—when starting, analgesic effect should not be evaluated until the system has been worn for 24 hours (to allow for gradual increase in plasma-buprenorphine concentration)—if necessary, dose should be adjusted at intervals of no longer than 72 hours using a patch of the next strength or using 2 patches of the same strength (applied at *same time* to avoid confusion). Maximum 2 patches can be used at any one time, for breakthrough pain, consider 200–400 micrograms buprenorphine sublingually

PHARMACOKINETICS
For *Hapoctasin*®: It may take approximately 25 hours for the plasma-buprenorphine concentration to decrease by 50% after patch is removed.

TRANSTEC®

Moderate to severe chronic cancer pain in patients who have not previously received strong opioid analgesic | Severe pain unresponsive to non-opioid analgesics in patients who have not previously received strong opioid analgesic
▸ BY TRANSDERMAL APPLICATION USING PATCHES
▸ Adult: Initially 35 micrograms/hour up to every 96 hours, dose adjustment—when starting, analgesic effect should not be evaluated until the system has been worn for 24 hours (to allow for gradual increase in plasma-buprenorphine concentration)—if necessary, dose should be adjusted at intervals of no longer than 96 hours using a patch of the next strength or using 2 patches of the same strength (applied at *same time* to avoid confusion). Maximum 2 patches can be used at any one time, for breakthrough pain, consider 200–400 micrograms buprenorphine sublingually

Moderate to severe chronic cancer pain in patients who have previously received strong opioid analgesic | Severe pain unresponsive to non-opioid analgesics in patients who have previously received strong opioid analgesic
▸ BY TRANSDERMAL APPLICATION USING PATCHES
▸ Adult: The initial dose should be based on previous 24-hour opioid requirement, consult product literature, dose adjustment—when starting, analgesic effect should not be evaluated until the system has been worn for 24 hours (to allow for gradual increase in plasma-buprenorphine concentration)—if necessary, dose should be adjusted at intervals of no longer than 96 hours using a patch of the next strength or using 2 patches of the same strength (applied at *same time* to avoid confusion). Maximum 2 patches can be used at any one time, for breakthrough pain, consider 200–400 micrograms buprenorphine sublingually

PHARMACOKINETICS
For *Transtec*®: It may take approximately 30 hours for the plasma-buprenorphine concentration to decrease by 50% after patch is removed.

● UNLICENSED USE
▸ With oral use in children Sublingual tablets not licensed for use in children under 6 years.
▸ With intramuscular use or intravenous use in children Injection not licensed for use in children under 6 months.

● CAUTIONS
GENERAL CAUTIONS
Impaired consciousness
SPECIFIC CAUTIONS
▸ With transdermal use Other opioids should not be administered within 24 hours of patch removal (long duration of action) (in adults)
▸ When used for adjunct in the treatment of opioid dependence Hepatitis B infection (in adults) · hepatitis C infection (in adults) · pre-existing liver enzyme abnormalities (in adults)

● INTERACTIONS Caution with concomitant use of hepatotoxic drugs.

● SIDE-EFFECTS
▸ **Common or very common** Abdominal pain · agitation · anorexia · anxiety · asthenia · diarrhoea · dyspepsia · dyspnoea · fatigue · mild withdrawal symptoms in patients dependent on opioids · paraesthesia · vasodilatation
▸ **Uncommon** Angina (in adults) · cough · depersonalisation · dry eye · dry skin · dysarthria · flatulence · hypertension · hypoaesthesia · hypoxia · impaired memory · influenza-like symptoms · muscle cramp · myalgia · pyrexia · restlessness · rhinitis · rigors · syncope · taste disturbance · tinnitus · tremor · wheezing
▸ **Rare** Diverticulitis (in children) · dysphagia · impaired concentration · paralytic ileus · psychosis
▸ **Very rare** Hiccups · hyperventilation · muscle fasciculation · retching
▸ **Frequency not known** Hepatic necrosis · hepatitis

SIDE-EFFECTS, FURTHER INFORMATION
▸ Fever or external heat
▸ With transdermal use in adults Monitor patients using patches for increased side-effects if fever present (increased absorption possible); avoid exposing application site to external heat (may also increase absorption).

Overdose
The effects of buprenorphine are only partially reversed by naloxone.

TRANSTEC®

SIDE-EFFECTS, FURTHER INFORMATION
In view of the long duration of action, patients who have severe side-effects should be monitored for up to 30 hours after removing patch.

HAPOCTASIN®

SIDE-EFFECTS, FURTHER INFORMATION
In view of the long duration of action, patients who have severe side-effects should be monitored for up to 25 hours after removing patch.

● BREAST FEEDING Present in low levels in breast milk. Neonates should be monitored for drowsiness, adequate weight gain, and developmental milestones.

● RENAL IMPAIRMENT Avoid use or reduce dose; opioid effects increased and prolonged and increased cerebral sensitivity occurs.

● PRE-TREATMENT SCREENING Documentation of viral hepatitis status is recommended before commencing therapy for opioid dependence.

● MONITORING REQUIREMENTS Monitor liver function; when used in opioid dependence baseline liver function test is recommended before commencing therapy, and regular liver function tests should be performed throughout treatment.

- DIRECTIONS FOR ADMINISTRATION
▸ With sublingual use in children For administration by *mouth*, tablets may be halved.

TRANSTEC® Apply patch to dry, non-irritated, non-hairy skin on upper torso, removing after no longer than 96 hours and siting replacement patch on a different area (avoid same area for at least 6 days).

HAPOCTASIN® Apply patch to dry, non-irritated, non-hairy skin on upper torso, removing after no longer than 72 hours and siting replacement patch on a different area (avoid same area for at least 7 days).

BUTRANS® Apply patch to dry, non-irritated, non-hairy skin on upper torso, removing after 7 days and siting replacement patch on a different area (avoid same area for at least 3 weeks).

- PRESCRIBING AND DISPENSING INFORMATION Transdermal buprenorphine patches are not suitable for acute pain or in those patients whose analgesic requirements are changing rapidly because the long time to steady state prevents rapid titration of the dose.

    Transdermal patches are available as 72-hourly, 96-hourly and 7-day formulations; prescribers and dispensers must ensure that the correct preparation is prescribed and dispensed. Preparations that should be applied up to every 72 hours include *Hapoctasin*®. Preparations that should be applied up to every 96 hours include *Transtec*®. Preparations that should be applied up to every 7 days include *BuTrans*®.

- PATIENT AND CARER ADVICE Patients or carers should be given advice on how to administer buprenorphine transdermal patches.

- NATIONAL FUNDING/ACCESS DECISIONS

NICE technology appraisals (TAs)
▸ Methadone and buprenorphine for the management of opioid dependence (January 2007) NICE TA114
Oral methadone and buprenorphine are recommended for maintenance therapy in the management of opioid dependence. Patients should be committed to a supportive care programme including a flexible dosing regimen administered under supervision for at least 3 months, until compliance is assured. Selection of methadone or buprenorphine should be made on a case-by-case basis, but methadone should be prescribed if both drugs are equally suitable.
www.nice.org.uk/TA114

- MEDICINAL FORMS
There can be variation in the licensing of different medicines containing the same drug.

Sublingual tablet
CAUTIONARY AND ADVISORY LABELS 2, 26
▸ Buprenorphine (Non-proprietary)
Buprenorphine (as Buprenorphine hydrochloride)
200 microgram Buprenorphine 200microgram sublingual tablets sugar free sugar-free | 50 tablet [PoM] £6.05 DT price = £5.04 [CD3]
Buprenorphine (as Buprenorphine hydrochloride)
400 microgram Buprenorphine 400microgram sublingual tablets sugar free sugar-free | 7 tablet [PoM] £1.60 DT price = £1.60 [CD3]
Buprenorphine (as Buprenorphine hydrochloride)
2 mg Buprenorphine 2mg sublingual tablets sugar free sugar-free | 7 tablet [PoM] £18.50 DT price = £1.57 [CD3]
Buprenorphine (as Buprenorphine hydrochloride)
8 mg Buprenorphine 8mg sublingual tablets sugar free sugar-free | 7 tablet [PoM] £52.00 DT price = £2.87 [CD3]
▸ Gabup (Martindale Pharmaceuticals Ltd)
Buprenorphine (as Buprenorphine hydrochloride)
400 microgram Gabup 0.4mg sublingual tablets sugar-free | 7 tablet [PoM] £1.60 DT price = £1.60 [CD3]
Buprenorphine (as Buprenorphine hydrochloride) 1 mg Gabup 1mg sublingual tablets sugar-free | 7 tablet [PoM] £2.00 [CD3]
Buprenorphine (as Buprenorphine hydrochloride) 2 mg Gabup 2mg sublingual tablets sugar-free | 7 tablet [PoM] £2.12 DT price = £1.57 [CD3]

Buprenorphine (as Buprenorphine hydrochloride) 4 mg Gabup 4mg sublingual tablets sugar-free | 7 tablet [PoM] £3.90 [CD3]
Buprenorphine (as Buprenorphine hydrochloride) 6 mg Gabup 6mg sublingual tablets sugar-free | 7 tablet [PoM] £4.10 [CD3]
Buprenorphine (as Buprenorphine hydrochloride) 8 mg Gabup 8mg sublingual tablets sugar-free | 7 tablet [PoM] £4.13 DT price = £2.87 [CD3]
▸ Natzon (Morningside Healthcare Ltd)
Buprenorphine (as Buprenorphine hydrochloride)
400 microgram Natzon 0.4mg sublingual tablets sugar-free | 7 tablet [PoM] £1.60 DT price = £1.60 [CD3]
Buprenorphine (as Buprenorphine hydrochloride) 2 mg Natzon 2mg sublingual tablets sugar-free | 7 tablet [PoM] £6.35 DT price = £1.57 [CD3]
Buprenorphine (as Buprenorphine hydrochloride) 8 mg Natzon 8mg sublingual tablets sugar-free | 7 tablet [PoM] £19.05 DT price = £2.87 [CD3]
▸ Prefibin (Sandoz Ltd)
Buprenorphine (as Buprenorphine hydrochloride)
400 microgram Prefibin 0.4mg sublingual tablets sugar-free | 7 tablet [PoM] £1.60 DT price = £1.60 [CD3]
Buprenorphine (as Buprenorphine hydrochloride) 2 mg Prefibin 2mg sublingual tablets sugar-free | 7 tablet [PoM] £5.38 DT price = £1.57 [CD3]
Buprenorphine (as Buprenorphine hydrochloride) 8 mg Prefibin 8mg sublingual tablets sugar-free | 7 tablet [PoM] £16.15 DT price = £2.87 [CD3]
▸ Subutex (RB Pharmaceuticals Ltd)
Buprenorphine (as Buprenorphine hydrochloride)
400 microgram Subutex 0.4mg sublingual tablets sugar-free | 7 tablet [PoM] £1.60 DT price = £1.60 [CD3]
Buprenorphine (as Buprenorphine hydrochloride) 2 mg Subutex 2mg sublingual tablets sugar-free | 7 tablet [PoM] £6.35 DT price = £1.57 [CD3]
Buprenorphine (as Buprenorphine hydrochloride) 8 mg Subutex 8mg sublingual tablets sugar-free | 7 tablet [PoM] £19.05 DT price = £2.87 [CD3]
▸ Temgesic (RB Pharmaceuticals Ltd)
Buprenorphine (as Buprenorphine hydrochloride)
200 microgram Temgesic 200microgram sublingual tablets sugar-free | 50 tablet [PoM] £5.04 DT price = £5.04 [CD3]
Buprenorphine (as Buprenorphine hydrochloride)
400 microgram Temgesic 400microgram sublingual tablets sugar-free | 50 tablet [PoM] £10.07 DT price = £10.07 [CD3]
▸ Tephine (Sandoz Ltd)
Buprenorphine (as Buprenorphine hydrochloride)
200 microgram Tephine 200microgram sublingual tablets sugar-free | 50 tablet [PoM] £4.27 DT price = £5.04 [CD3]
Buprenorphine (as Buprenorphine hydrochloride)
400 microgram Tephine 400microgram sublingual tablets sugar-free | 50 tablet [PoM] £8.54 DT price = £10.07 [CD3]

Solution for injection
▸ Temgesic (RB Pharmaceuticals Ltd)
Buprenorphine (as Buprenorphine hydrochloride)
300 microgram per 1 ml Temgesic 300micrograms/1ml solution for injection ampoules | 5 ampoule [PoM] £2.46 [CD3]

Transdermal patch
CAUTIONARY AND ADVISORY LABELS 2
▸ BuTrans (Napp Pharmaceuticals Ltd)
Buprenorphine 5 microgram per 1 hour BuTrans 5micrograms/hour transdermal patches | 4 patch [PoM] £17.60 DT price = £17.60 [CD3]
Buprenorphine 10 microgram per 1 hour BuTrans 10micrograms/hour transdermal patches | 4 patch [PoM] £31.55 DT price = £31.55 [CD3]
Buprenorphine 15 microgram per 1 hour BuTrans 15micrograms/hour transdermal patches | 4 patch [PoM] £49.15 [CD3]
Buprenorphine 20 microgram per 1 hour BuTrans 20micrograms/hour transdermal patches | 4 patch [PoM] £57.46 DT price = £57.46 [CD3]
▸ Hapoctasin (Actavis UK Ltd)
Buprenorphine 35 microgram per 1 hour Hapoctasin 35micrograms/hour transdermal patches | 4 patch [PoM] £9.48 DT price = £15.80 [CD3]
Buprenorphine 52.5 microgram per 1 hour Hapoctasin 52.5micrograms/hour transdermal patches | 4 patch [PoM] £14.23 DT price = £23.71 [CD3]
Buprenorphine 70 microgram per 1 hour Hapoctasin 70micrograms/hour transdermal patches | 4 patch [PoM] £18.96 DT price = £31.60 [CD3]

4

Nervous system

▸ Transtec (Napp Pharmaceuticals Ltd)
Buprenorphine 35 microgram per 1 hour Transtec
35micrograms/hour transdermal patches | 4 patch [PoM] £15.80 DT
price = £15.80 [CD3]
Buprenorphine 52.5 microgram per 1 hour Transtec
52.5micrograms/hour transdermal patches | 4 patch [PoM] £23.71 DT
price = £23.71 [CD3]
Buprenorphine 70 microgram per 1 hour Transtec
70micrograms/hour transdermal patches | 4 patch [PoM] £31.60 DT
price = £31.60 [CD3]

☞ 408

Co-codamol

● **INDICATIONS AND DOSE**

Mild to moderate pain (using co-codamol 8/500 preparations only)
▸ BY MOUTH
▸ Adult: 8/500–16/1000 mg every 4–6 hours as required;
maximum 64/4000 mg per day

Mild to moderate pain (using co-codamol 15/500 preparations only)
▸ BY MOUTH
▸ Adult: 15/500–30/1000 mg every 4–6 hours as required;
maximum 120/4000 mg per day

Severe pain (using co-codamol 30/500 preparations only)
▸ BY MOUTH
▸ Adult: 30/500–60/1000 mg every 4–6 hours as required;
maximum 240/4000 mg per day

KAPAKE® 15/500

Mild to moderate pain
▸ BY MOUTH
▸ Adult: 2 tablets every 4–6 hours as required; maximum
8 tablets per day

SOLPADOL® CAPLETS

Severe pain
▸ BY MOUTH
▸ Adult: 2 tablets every 4–6 hours as required; maximum
8 tablets per day

SOLPADOL® CAPSULES

Severe pain
▸ BY MOUTH
▸ Adult: 2 capsules every 4–6 hours as required;
maximum 8 capsules per day

SOLPADOL® EFFERVESCENT TABLETS

Severe pain
▸ BY MOUTH USING EFFERVESCENT TABLETS
▸ Adult: 2 tablets every 4–6 hours as required, tablets to
be dispersed in water; maximum 8 tablets per day

● CONTRA-INDICATIONS Acute ulcerative colitis · antibiotic-
associated colitis · conditions where abdominal distention
develops · conditions where inhibition of peristalsis should
be avoided · known ultra-rapid codeine metabolisers

● CAUTIONS Acute abdomen · alcohol dependence · avoid
abrupt withdrawal after long-term treatment · cardiac
arrhythmias · chronic alcoholism · chronic dehydration ·
chronic malnutrition · convulsive disorders · gallstones ·
hepatocellular insufficiency

CAUTIONS, FURTHER INFORMATION
▸ Variation in metabolism The capacity to metabolise codeine
to morphine can vary considerably between individuals;
there is a marked increase in morphine toxicity in patients
who are ultra-rapid codeine metabolisers (CYP2D6 ultra-
rapid metabolisers) and a reduced therapeutic effect in
poor codeine metabolisers.

● INTERACTIONS → Appendix 1 (paracetamol).

● SIDE-EFFECTS Abdominal pain · anorexia · blood disorders
· depression (with larger doses) · hypothermia · leucopenia

· malaise · muscle fasciculation · neutropenia · pancreatitis
· seizures · thrombocytopenia

Overdose
Important: liver damage (and less frequently renal
damage) following overdosage with paracetamol.

● BREAST FEEDING Avoid—although amount of codeine
usually too small to be harmful, mothers vary considerably
in their capacity to metabolise codeine—risk of morphine
overdose in infant.

● HEPATIC IMPAIRMENT Dose-related toxicity with
paracetamol—avoid large doses.

● RENAL IMPAIRMENT Reduce dose or avoid codeine;
increased and prolonged effect; increased cerebral
sensitivity.

● PRESCRIBING AND DISPENSING INFORMATION Co-codamol
is a mixture of codeine phosphate and paracetamol; the
proportions are expressed in the form x/y, where x and y
are the strengths in milligrams of codeine phosphate and
paracetamol respectively.

When co-codamol tablets, dispersible (or effervescent)
tablets, or capsules are prescribed and **no strength is
stated**, tablets, dispersible (or effervescent) tablets, or
capsules, respectively, containing codeine phosphate 8 mg
and paracetamol 500 mg should be dispensed.

The Drug Tariff allows tablets of co-codamol labelled
'dispersible' to be dispensed against an order for
'effervescent' and *vice versa.*

● LESS SUITABLE FOR PRESCRIBING Co-codamol is less
suitable for prescribing.

● EXCEPTIONS TO LEGAL CATEGORY Co-codamol 8/500 can
be sold to the public in certain circumstances; for
exemptions see *Medicines, Ethics and Practice,* London,
Pharmaceutical Press (always consult latest edition).

● MEDICINAL FORMS
There can be variation in the licensing of different medicines
containing the same drug. Forms available from special-order
manufacturers include: oral suspension, oral solution
Tablet
CAUTIONARY AND ADVISORY LABELS 2 (does not apply to the 8/500
tablet), 29, 30
▸ Co-codamol (Non-proprietary)
Codeine phosphate 8 mg, Paracetamol 500 mg Co-codamol
8mg/500mg tablets | 32 tablet [P] £1.02 Schedule 5 (CD Inv) |
100 tablet [PoM] £3.93 DT price = £3.07 Schedule 5 (CD Inv) |
500 tablet [PoM] £17.00 Schedule 5 (CD Inv) | 1000 tablet [PoM]
£34.00 Schedule 5 (CD Inv)
Co-codamol 8mg/500mg caplets | 32 tablet [P] £1.20 Schedule 5 (CD
Inv)
Codeine phosphate 15 mg, Paracetamol 500 mg Co-codamol
15mg/500mg tablets | 100 tablet [PoM] £15.00 DT price =
£9.58 Schedule 5 (CD Inv)
Codeine phosphate 30 mg, Paracetamol 500 mg Co-codamol
30mg/500mg caplets | 100 tablet [PoM] £9.00 DT price =
£4.17 Schedule 5 (CD Inv)
Co-codamol 30mg/500mg tablets | 30 tablet [PoM] £2.45 DT price =
£1.25 Schedule 5 (CD Inv) | 100 tablet [PoM] £11.00 DT price =
£4.17 Schedule 5 (CD Inv)
▸ Codipar (AMCo)
Codeine phosphate 15 mg, Paracetamol 500 mg Codipar
15mg/500mg tablets | 100 tablet [PoM] £8.25 DT price =
£9.58 Schedule 5 (CD Inv)
▸ Kapake (Galen Ltd)
Codeine phosphate 30 mg, Paracetamol 500 mg Kapake
30mg/500mg tablets | 100 tablet [PoM] £6.04 DT price =
£4.17 Schedule 5 (CD Inv)
▸ Migraleve Yellow (McNeil Products Ltd)
Codeine phosphate 8 mg, Paracetamol 500 mg Migraleve Yellow
tablets | 16 tablet [PoM] no price available Schedule 5 (CD Inv)
▸ Solpadol (Sanofi)
Codeine phosphate 30 mg, Paracetamol 500 mg Solpadol
30mg/500mg caplets | 30 tablet [PoM] £2.02 DT price =
£1.25 Schedule 5 (CD Inv) | 100 tablet [PoM] £6.74 DT price =
£4.17 Schedule 5 (CD Inv)

▸ Zapain (AMCo)

  Codeine phosphate 30 mg, Paracetamol 500 mg Zapain
  30mg/500mg tablets | 100 tablet PoM £3.03 DT price =
  £4.17 Schedule 5 (CD Inv)

Effervescent tablet

CAUTIONARY AND ADVISORY LABELS 2 (does not apply to the 8/500
tablet), 13, 29, 30
EXCIPIENTS: May contain Aspartame
ELECTROLYTES: May contain Sodium
▸ Co-codamol (Non-proprietary)

  Codeine phosphate 8 mg, Paracetamol 500 mg Co-codamol
  8mg/500mg effervescent tablets | 32 tablet P £2.24 DT price =
  £2.25 Schedule 5 (CD Inv) | 100 tablet PoM £12.97 DT price =
  £7.03 Schedule 5 (CD Inv)

  Codeine phosphate 30 mg, Paracetamol 500 mg Co-codamol
  30mg/500mg effervescent tablets | 32 tablet PoM £5.40 DT price =
  £2.58 Schedule 5 (CD Inv) | 100 tablet PoM £19.20 DT price =
  £8.06 Schedule 5 (CD Inv)

▸ Codipar (AMCo)

  Codeine phosphate 15 mg, Paracetamol 500 mg Codipar
  15mg/500mg effervescent tablets sugar-free | 100 tablet PoM £8.25
  DT price = £8.25 Schedule 5 (CD Inv)

▸ Paracodol (Bayer Plc)

  Codeine phosphate 8 mg, Paracetamol 500 mg Paracodol
  8mg/500mg effervescent tablets | 32 tablet P no price available DT
  price = £2.25 Schedule 5 (CD Inv)

▸ Solpadol (Sanofi)

  Codeine phosphate 30 mg, Paracetamol 500 mg Solpadol
  30mg/500mg effervescent tablets | 32 tablet PoM £2.59 DT price =
  £2.58 Schedule 5 (CD Inv) | 100 tablet PoM £8.90 DT price =
  £8.06 Schedule 5 (CD Inv)

▸ Tylex (UCB Pharma Ltd)

  Codeine phosphate 30 mg, Paracetamol 500 mg Tylex
  30mg/500mg effervescent tablets | 100 tablet PoM £9.06 DT price =
  £8.06 Schedule 5 (CD Inv)

Capsule

CAUTIONARY AND ADVISORY LABELS 2 (does not apply to the 8/500
capsule), 29, 30
EXCIPIENTS: May contain Sulfites
▸ Co-codamol (Non-proprietary)

  Codeine phosphate 8 mg, Paracetamol 500 mg Co-codamol
  8mg/500mg capsules | 100 capsule PoM £14.48 DT price =
  £12.63 Schedule 5 (CD Inv)

  Codeine phosphate 30 mg, Paracetamol 500 mg Co-codamol
  30mg/500mg capsules | 100 capsule PoM £15.00 DT price =
  £3.04 Schedule 5 (CD Inv)

▸ Codipar (AMCo)

  Codeine phosphate 15 mg, Paracetamol 500 mg Codipar
  15mg/500mg capsules | 100 capsule PoM £7.25 DT price =
  £7.25 Schedule 5 (CD Inv)

▸ Kapake (Galen Ltd)

  Codeine phosphate 30 mg, Paracetamol 500 mg Kapake
  30mg/500mg capsules | 100 capsule PoM £6.04 DT price =
  £3.04 Schedule 5 (CD Inv)

▸ Paracodol (Bayer Plc)

  Codeine phosphate 8 mg, Paracetamol 500 mg Paracodol
  8mg/500mg capsules | 20 capsule P £1.71 Schedule 5 (CD Inv) |
  32 capsule P £2.69 DT price = £4.04 Schedule 5 (CD Inv)

▸ Solpadol (Sanofi)

  Codeine phosphate 30 mg, Paracetamol 500 mg Solpadol
  30mg/500mg capsules | 100 capsule PoM £6.74 DT price =
  £3.04 Schedule 5 (CD Inv)

▸ Tylex (UCB Pharma Ltd)

  Codeine phosphate 30 mg, Paracetamol 500 mg Tylex
  30mg/500mg capsules | 100 capsule PoM £7.93 DT price =
  £3.04 Schedule 5 (CD Inv)

▸ Zapain (AMCo)

  Codeine phosphate 30 mg, Paracetamol 500 mg Zapain
  30mg/500mg capsules | 100 capsule PoM £3.85 DT price =
  £3.04 Schedule 5 (CD Inv)

Codeine phosphate

◀ 408

● INDICATIONS AND DOSE

Acute diarrhoea
▸ BY MOUTH
▸ Child 12-17 years: 30 mg 3–4 times a day; usual dose
  15–60 mg 3–4 times a day
▸ Adult: 30 mg 3–4 times a day; usual dose 15–60 mg
  3–4 times a day

Mild to moderate pain
▸ BY MOUTH
▸ Adult: 30–60 mg every 4 hours if required; maximum
  240 mg per day
▸ BY INTRAMUSCULAR INJECTION
▸ Adult: 30–60 mg every 4 hours if required

Short-term treatment of acute moderate pain
▸ BY MOUTH, OR BY INTRAMUSCULAR INJECTION
▸ Child 12-17 years: 30–60 mg every 6 hours if required for
  maximum 3 days; maximum 240 mg per day

Dry or painful cough
▸ BY MOUTH USING LINCTUS
▸ Adult: 15–30 mg 3–4 times a day

IMPORTANT SAFETY INFORMATION
MHRA/CHM ADVICE (JULY 2013) CODEINE FOR ANALGESIA:
RESTRICTED USE IN CHILDREN DUE TO REPORTS OF MORPHINE
TOXICITY
Codeine should only be used to relieve acute moderate
pain in children older than 12 years and only if it cannot
be relieved by other painkillers such as paracetamol or
ibuprofen alone. A significant risk of serious and life-
threatening adverse reactions has been identified in
children with obstructive sleep apnoea who received
codeine after tonsillectomy or adenoidectomy:

● in children aged 12–18 years, the maximum daily dose
  of codeine should not exceed 240 mg. Doses may be
  taken up to four times a day at intervals of no less than
  6 hours. The lowest effective dose should be used and
  duration of treatment should be limited to 3 days
● codeine is contra-indicated in all children (under
  18 years) who undergo the removal of tonsils or
  adenoids for the treatment of obstructive sleep apnoea
● codeine is not recommended for use in children whose
  breathing may be compromised, including those with
  neuromuscular disorders, severe cardiac or respiratory
  conditions, respiratory infections, multiple trauma or
  extensive surgical procedures
● codeine is contra-indicated in patients of any age who
  are known to be ultra-rapid metabolisers of codeine
  (CYP2D6 ultra-rapid metabolisers)
● codeine should not be used in breast-feeding mothers
  because it can pass to the baby through breast milk
● parents and carers should be advised on how to
  recognise signs and symptoms of morphine toxicity,
  and to stop treatment and seek medical attention if
  signs or symptoms of toxicity occur (including reduced
  consciousness, lack of appetite, somnolence,
  constipation, respiratory depression, 'pin-point'
  pupils, nausea, vomiting)

MHRA/CHM ADVICE (APRIL 2015) CODEINE FOR COUGH AND COLD:
RESTRICTED USE IN CHILDREN
Do not use codeine in children under 12 years as it is
associated with a risk of respiratory side effects. Codeine
is not recommended for adolescents (12–18 years) who
have problems with breathing. When prescribing or
dispensing codeine-containing medicines for cough and
cold, consider that codeine is contra-indicated in:

● children younger than 12 years old

4

Nervous system

- patients of any age known to be CYP2D6 ultra-rapid metabolisers
- breastfeeding mothers

- CONTRA-INDICATIONS Acute ulcerative colitis · antibiotic-associated colitis · children under 18 years who undergo the removal of tonsils or adenoids for the treatment of obstructive sleep apnoea · conditions where abdominal distension develops · conditions where inhibition of peristalsis should be avoided · known ultra-rapid codeine metabolisers
- CAUTIONS Acute abdomen · cardiac arrhythmias · gallstones · not recommended for adolescents aged 12–18 years with breathing problems

CAUTIONS, FURTHER INFORMATION
▸ Variation in metabolism The capacity to metabolise codeine to morphine can vary considerably between individuals; there is a marked increase in morphine toxicity in patients who are ultra-rapid codeine metabolisers (CYP2D6 ultra-rapid metabolisers) and a reduced therapeutic effect in poor codeine metabolisers.

- SIDE-EFFECTS Abdominal pain · anorexia · antidiuretic effect · hypothermia · malaise · muscle fasciculation · pancreatitis · seizures
- BREAST FEEDING Avoid—although amount usually too small to be harmful, mothers vary considerably in their capacity to metabolise codeine—risk of morphine overdose in infant.
- RENAL IMPAIRMENT Avoid use or reduce dose; opioid effects increased and prolonged, and increased cerebral sensitivity occurs.
- PRESCRIBING AND DISPENSING INFORMATION BP directs that when Diabetic Codeine Linctus is prescribed, Codeine Linctus formulated with a vehicle appropriate for administration to diabetics, whether or not labelled 'Diabetic Codeine Linctus', shall be dispensed or supplied.
- PATIENT AND CARER ADVICE
Medicines for Children leaflet: Codeine phosphate for pain www.medicinesforchildren.org.uk/codeine-phosphate-pain-0

- MEDICINAL FORMS
There can be variation in the licensing of different medicines containing the same drug. Forms available from special-order manufacturers include: oral suspension, oral solution, solution for injection

Tablet
CAUTIONARY AND ADVISORY LABELS 2
▸ Codeine phosphate (Non-proprietary)
Codeine phosphate 15 mg Codeine 15mg tablets | 28 tablet [PoM] £1.90 DT price = £0.94 Schedule 5 (CD Inv) | 30 tablet [PoM] no price available Schedule 5 (CD Inv) | 100 tablet [PoM] £6.60 DT price = £3.36 Schedule 5 (CD Inv) | 500 tablet [PoM] no price available Schedule 5 (CD Inv)
Codeine phosphate 30 mg Codeine 30mg tablets | 28 tablet [PoM] £2.50 DT price = £1.10 Schedule 5 (CD Inv) | 30 tablet [PoM] no price available Schedule 5 (CD Inv) | 100 tablet [PoM] £5.68 DT price = £3.93 Schedule 5 (CD Inv) | 500 tablet [PoM] no price available Schedule 5 (CD Inv)
Codeine phosphate 60 mg Codeine 60mg tablets | 28 tablet [PoM] £5.95 DT price = £1.84 Schedule 5 (CD Inv)

Oral solution
CAUTIONARY AND ADVISORY LABELS 2
▸ Codeine phosphate (Non-proprietary)
Codeine phosphate 3 mg per 1 ml Codeine 15mg/5ml linctus sugar free sugar-free | 200 ml [P] £1.87 DT price = £1.63 Schedule 5 (CD Inv) sugar-free | 2000 ml [P] £16.30 Schedule 5 (CD Inv) Codeine 15mg/5ml linctus | 200 ml [P] £1.84 DT price = £1.84 Schedule 5 (CD Inv) | 2000 ml [P] no price available Schedule 5 (CD Inv)
Codeine phosphate 5 mg per 1 ml Codeine 25mg/5ml oral solution | 500 ml [PoM] £6.46 DT price = £6.46 Schedule 5 (CD Inv)
▸ Galcodine (Thornton & Ross Ltd)
Codeine phosphate 3 mg per 1 ml Galcodine 15mg/5ml linctus sugar-free | 2000 ml [P] £9.90 Schedule 5 (CD Inv)

Solution for injection
▸ Codeine phosphate (Non-proprietary)
Codeine phosphate 60 mg per 1 ml Codeine 60mg/1ml solution for injection ampoules | 10 ampoule [PoM] £23.70–£25.70 [CD2]
Combinations available: *Aspirin with codeine*, p. 408

▸ 408

Co-dydramol

- INDICATIONS AND DOSE
Mild to moderate pain (using co-dydramol 10/500 preparations only)
▸ BY MOUTH
▸ Adult: 10/500–20/1000 mg every 4–6 hours as required; maximum 80/4000 mg per day
Severe pain (using co-dydramol 20/500 preparations only)
▸ BY MOUTH
▸ Adult: 20/500–40/1000 mg every 4–6 hours as required; maximum 160/4000 mg per day
Severe pain (using co-dydramol 30/500 preparations only)
▸ BY MOUTH
▸ Adult: 30/500–60/1000 mg every 4–6 hours as required; maximum 240/4000 mg per day

DOSE EQUIVALENCE AND CONVERSION
A mixture of dihydrocodeine tartrate and paracetamol; the proportions are expressed in the form x/y, where x and y are the strengths in milligrams of dihydrocodeine and paracetamol respectively.

- CAUTIONS Alcohol dependence · before administering, check when paracetamol last administered and cumulative paracetamol dose over previous 24 hours · chronic alcoholism · chronic dehydration · chronic malnutrition · hepatocellular insufficiency · pancreatitis · severe cor pulmonale
- INTERACTIONS → Appendix 1 (paracetamol).
- SIDE-EFFECTS Abdominal pain · acute generalised exanthematous pustulosis · blood disorders · leucopenia · malaise · neutropenia · pancreatitis · paraesthesia · paralytic ileus · skin reactions · Stevens-Johnson syndrome · thrombocytopenia · toxic epidermal necrolysis
Overdose
Important: liver damage (and less frequently renal damage) following overdosage with paracetamol.
- BREAST FEEDING Amount of dihydrocodeine too small to be harmful but use only if potential benefit outweighs risk.
- HEPATIC IMPAIRMENT Dose-related toxicity with paracetamol—avoid large doses.
- RENAL IMPAIRMENT Reduce dose or avoid dihydrocodeine; increased and prolonged effect; increased cerebral sensitivity.
- PRESCRIBING AND DISPENSING INFORMATION When co-dydramol tablets are prescribed and **no strength is stated**, tablets containing dihydrocodeine tartrate 10 mg and paracetamol 500 mg should be dispensed.
- LESS SUITABLE FOR PRESCRIBING Co-dydramol is less suitable for prescribing.

- MEDICINAL FORMS
There can be variation in the licensing of different medicines containing the same drug. Forms available from special-order manufacturers include: oral suspension, oral solution

Tablet
CAUTIONARY AND ADVISORY LABELS 2 (does not apply to the 10/500 tablet), 29, 30
▸ Co-dydramol (Non-proprietary)
Dihydrocodeine tartrate 10 mg, Paracetamol 500 mg Co-dydramol 10mg/500mg tablets | 30 tablet [PoM] £3.30 DT price = £0.89 Schedule 5 (CD Inv) | 100 tablet [PoM] £11.00 DT price = £2.97 Schedule 5 (CD Inv) | 500 tablet [PoM] £16.35 Schedule 5 (CD Inv)

F 408

Diamorphine hydrochloride

10.6.2016

(Heroin hydrochloride)

● INDICATIONS AND DOSE

Acute pain

▶ BY INTRAMUSCULAR INJECTION, OR BY SUBCUTANEOUS INJECTION
▸ Adult: 5 mg every 4 hours if required
▶ BY SLOW INTRAVENOUS INJECTION
▸ Adult: 1.25–2.5 mg every 4 hours if required

Acute pain (heavier, well-muscled patients)

▶ BY INTRAMUSCULAR INJECTION, OR BY SUBCUTANEOUS INJECTION
▸ Adult: Up to 10 mg every 4 hours if required
▶ BY SLOW INTRAVENOUS INJECTION
▸ Adult: 2.5–5 mg every 4 hours if required

Chronic pain not currently treated with a strong opioid analgesic

▶ BY SUBCUTANEOUS INJECTION, OR BY INTRAMUSCULAR INJECTION
▸ Adult: Initially 2.5–5 mg every 4 hours, adjusted according to response
▶ BY SUBCUTANEOUS INFUSION
▸ Adult: Initially 5–10 mg, adjusted according to response, dose to be administered over 24 hours

Acute pulmonary oedema

▶ BY SLOW INTRAVENOUS INJECTION
▸ Adult: 2.5–5 mg, dose to be administered at a rate of 1 mg/minute

Myocardial infarction

▶ BY SLOW INTRAVENOUS INJECTION
▸ Adult: 5 mg, followed by 2.5–5 mg if required, dose to be administered at a rate of 1–2 mg/minute
▸ Elderly: 2.5 mg, followed by 1.25–2.5 mg if required, dose to be administered at a rate of 1–2 mg/minute

Myocardial infarction (frail patients)

▶ BY SLOW INTRAVENOUS INJECTION
▸ Adult: 2.5 mg, followed by 1.25–2.5 mg if required, dose to be administered at a rate of 1–2 mg/minute

● CONTRA-INDICATIONS Delayed gastric emptying · phaeochromocytoma
● CAUTIONS CNS depression · severe cor pulmonale · severe diarrhoea · toxic psychosis
● SIDE-EFFECTS Anorexia · asthenia · myocardial infarction · raised intracranial pressure · syncope · taste disturbance
● BREAST FEEDING Therapeutic doses unlikely to affect infant; withdrawal symptoms in infants of dependent mothers; breast-feeding not best method of treating dependence in offspring.
● RENAL IMPAIRMENT Avoid use or reduce dose; opioid effects increased and prolonged and increased cerebral sensitivity occurs.

● MEDICINAL FORMS
There can be variation in the licensing of different medicines containing the same drug. Forms available from special-order manufacturers include: solution for injection, powder for solution for injection

Powder for solution for injection

▸ Diamorphine hydrochloride (Non-proprietary)
Diamorphine hydrochloride 5 mg Diamorphine 5mg powder for solution for injection vials | 5 vial [PoM] £15.00 [CD2]
Diamorphine 5mg powder for solution for injection ampoules | 5 ampoule [PoM] £11.36 DT price = £11.36 [CD2]
Diamorphine hydrochloride 10 mg Diamorphine 10mg powder for solution for injection ampoules | 5 ampoule [PoM] £15.10 DT price = £13.61 [CD2]
Diamorphine 10mg powder for solution for injection vials | 5 vial [PoM] £19.00 [CD2]

Diamorphine hydrochloride 30 mg Diamorphine 30mg powder for solution for injection ampoules | 5 ampoule [PoM] £14.79 DT price = £13.33 [CD2]
Diamorphine 30mg powder for solution for injection vials | 5 vial [PoM] £21.00 [CD2]
Diamorphine hydrochloride 100 mg Diamorphine 100mg powder for solution for injection vials | 5 vial [PoM] £54.00 [CD2]
Diamorphine 100mg powder for solution for injection ampoules | 5 ampoule [PoM] £42.39 DT price = £42.39 [CD2]
Diamorphine hydrochloride 500 mg Diamorphine 500mg powder for solution for injection vials | 5 vial [PoM] £190.00–£235.00 DT price = £209.00 [CD2]
Diamorphine 500mg powder for solution for injection ampoules | 5 ampoule [PoM] £187.70 DT price = £187.70 [CD2]

F 408

Dihydrocodeine tartrate

● INDICATIONS AND DOSE

Moderate to severe pain

▶ BY MOUTH USING IMMEDIATE-RELEASE MEDICINES
▸ Child 4–11 years: 0.5–1 mg/kg every 4–6 hours (max. per dose 30 mg)
▸ Child 12–17 years: 30 mg every 4–6 hours
▸ Adult: 30 mg every 4–6 hours as required
▶ BY DEEP SUBCUTANEOUS INJECTION, OR BY INTRAMUSCULAR INJECTION
▸ Adult: Up to 50 mg every 4–6 hours if required

Chronic severe pain

▶ BY MOUTH USING MODIFIED-RELEASE MEDICINES
▸ Child 12–17 years: 60–120 mg every 12 hours
▸ Adult: 60–120 mg every 12 hours

DF118 FORTE®

Severe pain

▶ BY MOUTH
▸ Child 12–17 years: 40–80 mg 3 times a day; maximum 240 mg per day
▸ Adult: 40–80 mg 3 times a day; maximum 240 mg per day

● UNLICENSED USE
▸ In children Most preparations not licensed for use in children under 4 years.
● CAUTIONS Pancreatitis · severe cor pulmonale
● SIDE-EFFECTS Abdominal pain · diarrhoea · paraesthesia · paralytic ileus · seizures
● BREAST FEEDING Use only if potential benefit outweighs risk.
● RENAL IMPAIRMENT Avoid use or reduce dose; opioid effects increased and prolonged and increased cerebral sensitivity occurs.
● PROFESSION SPECIFIC INFORMATION

Dental practitioners' formulary
Dihydrocodeine tablets 30 mg may be prescribed.

● MEDICINAL FORMS
There can be variation in the licensing of different medicines containing the same drug. Forms available from special-order manufacturers include: oral suspension, oral solution

Tablet
CAUTIONARY AND ADVISORY LABELS 2
▸ Dihydrocodeine tartrate (Non-proprietary)
Dihydrocodeine tartrate 30 mg Dihydrocodeine 30mg tablets | 28 tablet [PoM] £1.75 DT price = £1.20 Schedule 5 (CD Inv) | 30 tablet [PoM] £1.56 Schedule 5 (CD Inv) | 100 tablet [PoM] £6.81 DT price = £4.29 Schedule 5 (CD Inv) | 500 tablet [PoM] £23.75 Schedule 5 (CD Inv)
▸ DF 118 (Martindale Pharmaceuticals Ltd)
Dihydrocodeine tartrate 40 mg DF 118 Forte 40mg tablets | 100 tablet [PoM] £9.78 DT price = £9.78 Schedule 5 (CD Inv)

4

Nervous system

Modified-release tablet

CAUTIONARY AND ADVISORY LABELS 2, 25

▸ DHC Continus (Napp Pharmaceuticals Ltd)

Dihydrocodeine tartrate 60 mg DHC Continus 60mg tablets | 56 tablet [PoM] £5.20 DT price = £5.20 Schedule 5 (CD Inv)

Dihydrocodeine tartrate 90 mg DHC Continus 90mg tablets | 56 tablet [PoM] £8.66 DT price = £8.66 Schedule 5 (CD Inv)

Dihydrocodeine tartrate 120 mg DHC Continus 120mg tablets | 56 tablet [PoM] £10.95 DT price = £10.95 Schedule 5 (CD Inv)

Oral solution

CAUTIONARY AND ADVISORY LABELS 2

▸ Dihydrocodeine tartrate (Non-proprietary)

Dihydrocodeine tartrate 2 mg per 1 ml Dihydrocodeine 10mg/5ml oral solution | 150 ml [PoM] £7.16 DT price = £7.12 Schedule 5 (CD Inv)

Solution for injection

▸ Dihydrocodeine tartrate (Non-proprietary)

Dihydrocodeine tartrate 50 mg per 1 ml Dihydrocodeine 50mg/1ml solution for injection ampoules | 10 ampoule [PoM] £91.14 DT price = £91.14 [CD2]

F 408

Dipipanone hydrochloride with cyclizine

● INDICATIONS AND DOSE

Acute pain

▸ BY MOUTH

▸ Adult: Initially 1 tablet every 6 hours, then increased if necessary up to 3 tablets every 6 hours, dose to be increased gradually

● CAUTIONS Diabetes mellitus · palliative care (not recommended) · phaeochromocytoma

● SIDE-EFFECTS Psychosis · raised intracranial pressure · restlessness

● BREAST FEEDING No information available.

● RENAL IMPAIRMENT Avoid use or reduce dose; opioid effects increased and prolonged and increased cerebral sensitivity occurs.

● MEDICINAL FORMS
There can be variation in the licensing of different medicines containing the same drug.

Tablet

▸ Dipipanone hydrochloride with cyclizine (Non-proprietary)

Dipipanone hydrochloride 10 mg, Cyclizine hydrochloride 30 mg Dipipanone 10mg / Cyclizine 30mg tablets | 50 tablet [PoM] £353.06 DT price = £353.06 [CD2]

F 408

Fentanyl

● INDICATIONS AND DOSE

Chronic intractable pain not currently treated with a strong opioid analgesic

▸ BY TRANSDERMAL APPLICATION

▸ Child 16-17 years: Initially 12 micrograms/hour every 72 hours, alternatively initially 25 micrograms/hour every 72 hours, when starting, evaluation of the analgesic effect should not be made before the system has been worn for 24 hours (to allow for the gradual increase in plasma-fentanyl concentration)—previous analgesic therapy should be phased out gradually from time of first patch application, dose should be adjusted at 48–72 hour intervals in steps of 12–25 micrograms/hour if necessary, more than one patch may be used at a time (but applied at the same time to avoid confusion)—consider additional or alternative analgesic therapy if dose required exceeds 300 micrograms/hour (important: it takes 17 hours or more for the plasma-fentanyl concentration to decrease by 50%— replacement opioid therapy should be initiated at a low dose and increased gradually)

▸ Adult: Initially 12 micrograms/hour every 72 hours, alternatively initially 25 micrograms/hour every 72 hours, when starting, evaluation of the analgesic effect should not be made before the system has been worn for 24 hours (to allow for the gradual increase in plasma-fentanyl concentration)—previous analgesic therapy should be phased out gradually from time of first patch application, dose should be adjusted at 48–72 hour intervals in steps of 12–25 micrograms/hour if necessary, more than one patch may be used at a time (but applied at the same time to avoid confusion)—consider additional or alternative analgesic therapy if dose required exceeds 300 micrograms/hour (important: it takes 17 hours or more for the plasma-fentanyl concentration to decrease by 50%— replacement opioid therapy should be initiated at a low dose and increased gradually)

Chronic intractable pain currently treated with a strong opioid analgesic

▸ BY TRANSDERMAL APPLICATION

▸ Child 2-17 years: Initial dose based on previous 24-hour opioid requirement (consult product literature), for evaluating analgesic efficacy and dose increments, see under *Chronic intractable pain not currently treated with a strong opioid analgesic*, for conversion from long term oral morphine to transdermal fentanyl, see *Pain management with opioids* p. 21.

▸ Adult: Initial dose based on previous 24-hour opioid requirement (consult product literature), for evaluating analgesic efficacy and dose increments, see under *Chronic intractable pain not currently treated with a strong opioid analgesic*, for conversion from long term oral morphine to transdermal fentanyl, see *Pain management with opioids* p. 21.

Spontaneous respiration: analgesia and enhancement of anaesthesia, during operation

▸ BY SLOW INTRAVENOUS INJECTION

▸ Adult: Initially 50–100 micrograms (max. per dose 200 micrograms), dose maximum on specialist advice, then 25–50 micrograms as required

▸ BY INTRAVENOUS INFUSION

▸ Adult: 3–4.8 micrograms/kg/hour, adjusted according to response

Assisted ventilation: analgesia and enhancement of anaesthesia during operation

▸ BY SLOW INTRAVENOUS INJECTION

▸ Adult: Initially 300–3500 micrograms, then 100–200 micrograms as required

▸ BY INTRAVENOUS INFUSION

▸ Adult: Initially 10 micrograms/kg, dose to be given over 10 minutes, then 6 micrograms/kg/hour, adjusted according to response, may require up to 180 micrograms/kg/hour during cardiac surgery

Assisted ventilation: analgesia and respiratory depression in intensive care

▸ BY SLOW INTRAVENOUS INJECTION

▸ Adult: Initially 300–3500 micrograms, then 100–200 micrograms as required

▸ BY INTRAVENOUS INFUSION

▸ Adult: Initially 10 micrograms/kg, dose to be given over 10 minutes, then 6 micrograms/kg/hour, adjusted according to response, may require up to 180 micrograms/kg/hour during cardiac surgery

Breakthrough pain in patients receiving opioid therapy for chronic cancer pain

▸ BY BUCCAL ADMINISTRATION USING LOZENGES

▸ Child 16-17 years: Initially 200 micrograms, dose to be given over 15 minutes, then 200 micrograms after 15 minutes if required, no more than 2 dose units for each pain episode; if adequate pain relief not achieved with 1 dose unit for consecutive breakthrough pain

episodes, increase the strength of the dose unit until adequate pain relief achieved with 4 lozenges or less daily, if more than 4 episodes of breakthrough pain each day, adjust background analgesia
‣ Adult: Initially 200 micrograms, dose to be given over 15 minutes, then 200 micrograms after 15 minutes if required, no more than 2 dose units for each pain episode; if adequate pain relief not achieved with 1 dose unit for consecutive breakthrough pain episodes, increase the strength of the dose unit until adequate pain relief achieved with 4 lozenges or less daily, if more than 4 episodes of breakthrough pain each day, adjust background analgesia
▸ BY BUCCAL ADMINISTRATION USING BUCCAL FILMS
‣ Adult: Initially 200 micrograms, adjusted according to response, consult product literature for information on dose adjustments, maximum 1.2 mg per episode of breakthrough pain; leave at least 4 hours between treatment of episodes of breakthrough pain, if more than 4 episodes of breakthrough pain each day occur on more than 4 consecutive days, adjust background analgesia

DOSE EQUIVALENCE AND CONVERSION
Fentanyl films are **not bioequivalent** to other fentanyl preparations.
Fentanyl preparations for the treatment of breakthrough pain are not interchangeable; if patients are switched from another fentanyl-containing preparation, a new dose titration is required.

DOSES AT EXTREMES OF BODY-WEIGHT
To avoid excessive dosage in obese patients, weight-based doses may need to be calculated on the basis of ideal bodyweight.

ABSTRAL®
Breakthrough pain in patients receiving opioid therapy for chronic cancer pain
▸ BY MOUTH USING SUBLINGUAL TABLETS
‣ Adult: Initially 100 micrograms, then 100 micrograms after 15–30 minutes if required, dose to be adjusted according to response—consult product literature, no more than 2 dose units 15–30 minutes apart, for each pain episode; max. 800 micrograms per episode of breakthrough pain; leave at least 2 hours between treatment of episodes of breakthrough pain, if more than 4 episodes of breakthrough pain each day, adjust background analgesia

EFFENTORA®
Breakthrough pain in patients receiving opioid therapy for chronic cancer pain
▸ BY MOUTH USING SUBLINGUAL TABLETS
‣ Adult: Initially 100 micrograms, then 100 micrograms after 30 minutes if required, dose to be adjusted according to response—consult product literature, no more than 2 dose units for each pain episode; max. 800 micrograms per episode of breakthrough pain; leave at least 4 hours between treatment of episodes of breakthrough pain during titration

INSTANYL®
Breakthrough pain in patients receiving opioid therapy for chronic cancer pain
▸ BY INTRANASAL ADMINISTRATION
‣ Adult: Initially 50 micrograms, dose to be administered into one nostril, then 50 micrograms after 10 minutes if required, dose to be adjusted according to response, maximum 2 sprays for each pain episode and minimum 4 hours between treatment of each pain episode, if more than 4 breakthrough pain episodes daily, adjust background analgesia

PECFENT®
Breakthrough pain in patients receiving opioid therapy for chronic cancer pain
▸ BY INTRANASAL ADMINISTRATION
‣ Adult: Initially 100 micrograms, adjusted according to response, dose to be administered into one nostril only, maximum 2 sprays for each pain episode and minimum 4 hours between treatment of each pain episode, if more than 4 breakthrough pain episodes daily, adjust background analgesia

RECIVIT® SUBLINGUAL TABLETS
Breakthrough pain in patients receiving opioid therapy for chronic cancer pain
▸ BY MOUTH
‣ Adult: Initially 133 micrograms, then 133 micrograms after 15–30 minutes (max. per dose 800 micrograms), dose to be repeated only if necessary. Consult product literature for dose adjustments, no more than 2 dose units, 15-30 minutes apart, for each pain episode, maximum of 800 micrograms per episode of breakthrough pain, if more than 4 episodes of breakthrough pain each day, adjust background analgesia; maximum 4 doses per day

DOSE EQUIVALENCE AND CONVERSION
Fentanyl preparations for the treatment of breakthrough pain are not interchangeable; if patients are switched from another fentanyl-containing preparation, a new dose titration is required.

● CAUTIONS
GENERAL CAUTIONS
Cerebral tumour · diabetes mellitus (with *Actiq*® lozenges) · impaired consciousness
SPECIFIC CAUTIONS
▸ With buccal use Mucositis—absorption from oral preparations may be increased, caution during dose titration
CAUTIONS, FURTHER INFORMATION
▸ With transdermal use Transdermal fentanyl patches are not suitable for acute pain or in those patients whose analgesic requirements are changing rapidly because the long time to steady state prevents rapid titration of the dose. Risk of fatal respiratory depression, particularly in patients not previously treated with a strong opioid analgesic; manufacturer recommends use only in opioid tolerant patients.
▸ With intravenous use Repeated intra-operative doses should be given with care since the resulting respiratory depression can persist postoperatively and occasionally it may become apparent for the first time postoperatively when monitoring of the patient might be less intensive.

● SIDE-EFFECTS
GENERAL SIDE-EFFECTS
▸ **Common or very common** Abdominal pain · aesthenia · anorexia · anxiety · appetite changes · application-site reactions · diarrhoea · dyspepsia · dyspnoea · gastro-oesophageal reflux disease · hypertension · myoclonus · paraesthesia · pharyngitis · rhinitis · stomatitis · tremor · vasodilation
▸ **Uncommon** Amnesia · arthralgia · blood disorders · chills · depressed level of consciousness · dysgeusia · flatulence · hypoventilation · ileus · impaired concentration · impaired coordination · loss of consciousness · malaise · parosmia · pyrexia · seizures · speech disorder · thirst · thrombocytopenia
▸ **Rare** Hiccups
▸ **Very rare** Apnoea · arrhythmia · ataxia · bladder pain · delusions · haemoptysis

SPECIFIC SIDE-EFFECTS
► **Common or very common**
► With intravenous use Myoclonic movements
► **Uncommon**
► With intravenous use Laryngospasm
► **Rare**
► With intravenous use Asystole · insomnia

SIDE-EFFECTS, FURTHER INFORMATION
► Fever or external heat Monitor patients using patches for increased side-effects if fever present (increased absorption possible); avoid exposing application site to external heat, for example a hot bath or sauna (may also increase absorption).
► Muscle rigidity Intravenous administration of fentanyl can cause muscle rigidity, particularly of the chest wall or jaw; this can be managed by the use of neuromuscular blocking drugs.

● BREAST FEEDING Monitor infant for opioid-induced side-effects.

● RENAL IMPAIRMENT Avoid use or reduce dose; opioid effects increased and prolonged and increased cerebral sensitivity occurs.

● DIRECTIONS FOR ADMINISTRATION
► With transdermal use For *patches*, apply to dry, non-irritated, non-irradiated, non-hairy skin on torso or upper arm, removing after 72 hours and siting replacement patch on a different area (avoid using the same area for several days).
► With intravenous use in adults For *intravenous infusion* (*Sublimaze*), give continuously or intermittently in Glucose 5% or Sodium Chloride 0.9%.
► With buccal For buccal films, moisten mouth, place film on inner lining of cheek (pink side to cheek), hold for at least 5 seconds until it sticks, and leave to dissolve (15–30 minutes); if more than 1 film required do not overlap, but use another area of the mouth. Avoid liquids for 5 minutes after application; avoid food until the film has dissolved.
► With buccal use Patients should be advised to place the lozenge in the mouth against the cheek and move it around the mouth using the applicator; each lozenge should be sucked over a 15 minute period. In patients with a dry mouth, water may be used to moisten the buccal mucosa. Patients with diabetes should be advised each lozenge contains approximately 2 g glucose.
INSTANYL® Patient should sit or stand during administration.
EFFENTORA® Place tablet between cheek and gum and leave to dissolve; if more than 1 tablet required, place second tablet on the other side of the mouth; tablet may alternatively be placed under the tongue (sublingually).

● PRESCRIBING AND DISPENSING INFORMATION
► With transdermal use Prescriptions for fentanyl patches can be written to show the strength in terms of the release rate and it is acceptable to write *'Fentanyl 25 patches'* to prescribe patches that release fentanyl 25 micrograms per hour. The dosage should be expressed in terms of the interval between applying a patch and replacing it with a new one, e.g. *'one patch to be applied every 72 hours'*. The total quantity of patches to be supplied should be written in words and figures.

● PATIENT AND CARER ADVICE
Medicines for Children leaflet: Fentanyl lozenges for pain www. medicinesforchildren.org.uk/fentanyl-lozenges-for-pain
Medicines for Children leaflet: Fentanyl patches for pain www. medicinesforchildren.org.uk/fentanyl-patches-for-pain
► With transdermal use Patients and carers should be informed about safe use, including correct administration and disposal, strict adherence to dosage instructions, and the symptoms and signs of opioid overdosage. Patches should be removed immediately in case of breathing difficulties, marked drowsiness, confusion, dizziness, or impaired speech, and patients and carers should seek prompt medical attention.
Patients or carers should be given advice on how to administer fentanyl buccal films or fentanyl lozenges.
Patients or carers should be given advice on how to administer fentanyl nasal spray.
INSTANYL® Avoid concomitant use of other nasal preparations.
Patients or carers should be given advice on how to administer *Instanyl*® spray.
PECFENT® Avoid concomitant use of other nasal preparations.
Patients or carers should be given advice on how to administer *PecFent*® spray.
EFFENTORA® Patients or carers should be given advice on how to administer *Effentora*® buccal tablets.
Patients should be advised not to eat or drink until the tablet is completely dissolved; after 30 minutes, if any remnants remain, they may be swallowed with a glass of water. Patients with a dry mouth should be advised to drink water to moisten the buccal mucosa before administration of the tablets; if appropriate effervescence does not occur, a switch of therapy may be advised.
ABSTRAL® Patients should be advised not to eat or drink until the tablet is completely dissolved.
In patients with a dry mouth, the buccal mucosa may be moistened with water before administration of tablet.
RECIVIT® SUBLINGUAL TABLETS Patients should be advised not to eat or drink until the tablet is completely dissolved; after 30 minutes, if any remnants remain, they may be swallowed. In patients with a dry mouth, the buccal mucosa may be moistened with water before administration of tablet.

● NATIONAL FUNDING/ACCESS DECISIONS
INSTANYL®
Scottish Medicines Consortium (SMC) Decisions
The *Scottish Medicines Consortium* has advised that *Instanyl*® nasal spray should be restricted for use within NHS Scotland for the management of breakthrough pain in adult patients using opioid therapy for chronic cancer pain, when other short-acting opioids are unsuitable.
PECFENT®
Scottish Medicines Consortium (SMC) Decisions
The *Scottish Medicines Consortium* has advised (September 2008) that *PecFent*® nasal spray should be restricted for use within NHS Scotland for the management of breakthrough pain in adult patients using opioid therapy for chronic cancer pain, when other short-acting opioids are unsuitable.
EFFENTORA®
Scottish Medicines Consortium (SMC) Decisions
The *Scottish Medicines Consortium* has advised that *Effentora*® buccal tablets should be restricted for the management of breakthrough pain in adult patients using opioid therapy for chronic cancer pain, when other short acting opioids are unsuitable.
ABSTRAL®
Scottish Medicines Consortium (SMC) Decisions
The *Scottish Medicines Consortium* has advised (January 2009) that *Abstral*® sublingual tablets should be restricted for the management of breakthrough pain in adult patients using opioid therapy for chronic cancer pain, when other short acting opioids are unsuitable.

• MEDICINAL FORMS
There can be variation in the licensing of different medicines containing the same drug. Forms available from special-order manufacturers include: solution for injection, infusion, solution for infusion

Sublingual tablet
CAUTIONARY AND ADVISORY LABELS 2, 26
▶ Abstral (ProStrakan Ltd)

Fentanyl (as Fentanyl citrate) 100 microgram Abstral 100microgram sublingual tablets sugar-free | 10 tablet [PoM] £49.99 [CD2] sugar-free | 30 tablet [PoM] £149.70 [CD2]
Fentanyl (as Fentanyl citrate) 200 microgram Abstral 200microgram sublingual tablets sugar-free | 10 tablet [PoM] £49.99 [CD2] sugar-free | 30 tablet [PoM] £149.70 [CD2]
Fentanyl (as Fentanyl citrate) 300 microgram Abstral 300microgram sublingual tablets sugar-free | 10 tablet [PoM] £49.99 [CD2] sugar-free | 30 tablet [PoM] £149.70 [CD2]
Fentanyl (as Fentanyl citrate) 400 microgram Abstral 400microgram sublingual tablets sugar-free | 10 tablet [PoM] £49.99 [CD2] sugar-free | 30 tablet [PoM] £149.70 [CD2]
Fentanyl (as Fentanyl citrate) 600 microgram Abstral 600microgram sublingual tablets sugar-free | 30 tablet [PoM] £149.70 [CD2]
Fentanyl (as Fentanyl citrate) 800 microgram Abstral 800microgram sublingual tablets sugar-free | 30 tablet [PoM] £149.70 [CD2]
▶ Recivit (Grunenthal Ltd)

Fentanyl (as Fentanyl citrate) 133 microgram Recivit 133microgram sublingual tablets sugar-free | 30 tablet [PoM] £127.20 [CD2]
Fentanyl (as Fentanyl citrate) 267 microgram Recivit 267microgram sublingual tablets sugar-free | 30 tablet [PoM] £127.20 [CD2]
Fentanyl (as Fentanyl citrate) 400 microgram Recivit 400microgram sublingual tablets sugar-free | 30 tablet [PoM] £127.20 [CD2]
Fentanyl (as Fentanyl citrate) 533 microgram Recivit 533microgram sublingual tablets sugar-free | 30 tablet [PoM] £127.20 [CD2]
Fentanyl (as Fentanyl citrate) 800 microgram Recivit 800microgram sublingual tablets sugar-free | 30 tablet [PoM] £127.20 [CD2]

Buccal tablet
CAUTIONARY AND ADVISORY LABELS 2
ELECTROLYTES: May contain Sodium
▶ Effentora (Teva UK Ltd)

Fentanyl (as Fentanyl citrate) 100 microgram Effentora 100microgram buccal tablets sugar-free | 4 tablet [PoM] £19.96 [CD2] sugar-free | 28 tablet [PoM] £139.72 DT price = £139.72 [CD2]
Fentanyl (as Fentanyl citrate) 200 microgram Effentora 200microgram buccal tablets sugar-free | 4 tablet [PoM] £19.96 [CD2] sugar-free | 28 tablet [PoM] £139.72 DT price = £139.72 [CD2]
Fentanyl (as Fentanyl citrate) 400 microgram Effentora 400microgram buccal tablets sugar-free | 4 tablet [PoM] £19.96 [CD2] sugar-free | 28 tablet [PoM] £139.72 DT price = £139.72 [CD2]
Fentanyl (as Fentanyl citrate) 600 microgram Effentora 600microgram buccal tablets sugar-free | 4 tablet [PoM] £19.96 [CD2] sugar-free | 28 tablet [PoM] £139.72 DT price = £139.72 [CD2]
Fentanyl (as Fentanyl citrate) 800 microgram Effentora 800microgram buccal tablets sugar-free | 4 tablet [PoM] £19.96 [CD2] sugar-free | 28 tablet [PoM] £139.72 DT price = £139.72 [CD2]

Lozenge
CAUTIONARY AND ADVISORY LABELS 2
EXCIPIENTS: May contain Propylene glycol
▶ Actiq (Teva UK Ltd)

Fentanyl (as Fentanyl citrate) 200 microgram Actiq 200microgram lozenges with integral oromucosal applicator | 3 lozenge [PoM] £21.05 [CD2] | 30 lozenge [PoM] £210.41 [CD2]
Fentanyl (as Fentanyl citrate) 400 microgram Actiq 400microgram lozenges with integral oromucosal applicator | 3 lozenge [PoM] £21.05 [CD2] | 30 lozenge [PoM] £210.41 [CD2]
Fentanyl (as Fentanyl citrate) 600 microgram Actiq 600microgram lozenges with integral oromucosal applicator | 3 lozenge [PoM] £21.05 [CD2] | 30 lozenge [PoM] £210.41 [CD2]
Fentanyl (as Fentanyl citrate) 800 microgram Actiq 800microgram lozenges with integral oromucosal applicator | 3 lozenge [PoM] £21.05 [CD2] | 30 lozenge [PoM] £210.41 [CD2]
Fentanyl (as Fentanyl citrate) 1.2 mg Actiq 1.2mg lozenges with integral oromucosal applicator | 3 lozenge [PoM] £21.05 [CD2] | 30 lozenge [PoM] £210.41 [CD2]

Fentanyl (as Fentanyl citrate) 1.6 mg Actiq 1.6mg lozenges with integral oromucosal applicator | 3 lozenge [PoM] £21.05 [CD2] | 30 lozenge [PoM] £210.41 [CD2]

Solution for injection
▶ Fentanyl (Non-proprietary)

Fentanyl (as Fentanyl citrate) 50 microgram per 1 ml Fentanyl 100micrograms/2ml solution for injection ampoules | 10 ampoule [PoM] £13.95 [CD2]
Fentanyl 500micrograms/10ml solution for injection ampoules | 10 ampoule [PoM] £12.50 [CD2]
▶ Sublimaze (Janssen-Cilag Ltd)

Fentanyl (as Fentanyl citrate) 50 microgram per 1 ml Sublimaze 500micrograms/10ml solution for injection ampoules | 5 ampoule [PoM] £6.53 [CD2]

Solution for infusion
▶ Fentanyl (Non-proprietary)

Fentanyl (as Fentanyl citrate) 50 microgram per 1 ml Fentanyl 2.5mg/50ml solution for infusion vials | 1 vial [PoM] £5.00 [CD2]

Transdermal patch
CAUTIONARY AND ADVISORY LABELS 2
▶ Fentanyl (Non-proprietary)

Fentanyl 12 microgram per 1 hour Fentanyl 12micrograms/hour transdermal patches | 5 patch [PoM] £12.59 DT price = £12.59 [CD2]
Fentanyl 25 microgram per 1 hour Fentanyl 25micrograms/hour transdermal patches | 5 patch [PoM] £17.99 DT price = £17.99 [CD2]
Fentanyl 50 microgram per 1 hour Fentanyl 50micrograms/hour transdermal patches | 5 patch [PoM] £35.91 DT price = £33.66 [CD2]
Fentanyl 75 microgram per 1 hour Fentanyl 75micrograms/hour transdermal patches | 5 patch [PoM] £50.12 DT price = £46.99 [CD2]
Fentanyl 100 microgram per 1 hour Fentanyl 100micrograms/hour transdermal patches | 5 patch [PoM] £61.72 DT price = £57.86 [CD2]
▶ Durogesic DTrans (Janssen-Cilag Ltd)

Fentanyl 12 microgram per 1 hour Durogesic DTrans 12micrograms transdermal patches | 5 patch [PoM] £12.59 DT price = £12.59 [CD2]
Fentanyl 25 microgram per 1 hour Durogesic DTrans 25micrograms transdermal patches | 5 patch [PoM] £17.99 DT price = £17.99 [CD2]
Fentanyl 50 microgram per 1 hour Durogesic DTrans 50micrograms transdermal patches | 5 patch [PoM] £33.66 DT price = £33.66 [CD2]
Fentanyl 75 microgram per 1 hour Durogesic DTrans 75micrograms transdermal patches | 5 patch [PoM] £46.99 DT price = £46.99 [CD2]
Fentanyl 100 microgram per 1 hour Durogesic DTrans 100micrograms transdermal patches | 5 patch [PoM] £57.86 DT price = £57.86 [CD2]
▶ Fencino (DB Ashbourne Ltd)

Fentanyl 12 microgram per 1 hour Fencino 12micrograms/hour transdermal patches | 5 patch [PoM] £8.46 DT price = £12.59 [CD2]
Fentanyl 25 microgram per 1 hour Fencino 25micrograms/hour transdermal patches | 5 patch [PoM] £12.10 DT price = £17.99 [CD2]
Fentanyl 50 microgram per 1 hour Fencino 50micrograms/hour transdermal patches | 5 patch [PoM] £22.62 DT price = £33.66 [CD2]
Fentanyl 75 microgram per 1 hour Fencino 75micrograms/hour transdermal patches | 5 patch [PoM] £31.54 DT price = £46.99 [CD2]
Fentanyl 100 microgram per 1 hour Fencino 100micrograms/hour transdermal patches | 5 patch [PoM] £38.88 DT price = £57.86 [CD2]
▶ Fentalis (Sandoz Ltd)

Fentanyl 25 microgram per 1 hour Fentalis Reservoir 25micrograms/hour transdermal patches | 5 patch [PoM] £22.89 DT price = £17.99 [CD2]
Fentanyl 50 microgram per 1 hour Fentalis Reservoir 50micrograms/hour transdermal patches | 5 patch [PoM] £42.77 DT price = £33.66 [CD2]
Fentanyl 75 microgram per 1 hour Fentalis Reservoir 75micrograms/hour transdermal patches | 5 patch [PoM] £59.62 DT price = £46.99 [CD2]
Fentanyl 100 microgram per 1 hour Fentalis Reservoir 100micrograms/hour transdermal patches | 5 patch [PoM] £73.49 DT price = £57.86 [CD2]
▶ Matrifen (Teva UK Ltd)

Fentanyl 12 microgram per 1 hour Matrifen 12micrograms/hour transdermal patches | 5 patch [PoM] £7.52 DT price = £12.59 [CD2]
Fentanyl 25 microgram per 1 hour Matrifen 25micrograms/hour transdermal patches | 5 patch [PoM] £10.76 DT price = £17.99 [CD2]
Fentanyl 50 microgram per 1 hour Matrifen 50micrograms/hour transdermal patches | 5 patch [PoM] £20.12 DT price = £33.66 [CD2]
Fentanyl 75 microgram per 1 hour Matrifen 75micrograms/hour transdermal patches | 5 patch [PoM] £28.06 DT price = £46.99 [CD2]
Fentanyl 100 microgram per 1 hour Matrifen 100micrograms/hour transdermal patches | 5 patch [PoM] £34.59 DT price = £57.86 [CD2]

Nervous system

4

▸ Mezolar Matrix (Sandoz Ltd)

Fentanyl 12 microgram per 1 hour Mezolar Matrix 12micrograms/hour transdermal patches | 5 patch [PoM] £7.53 DT price = £12.59 [CD2]

Fentanyl 25 microgram per 1 hour Mezolar Matrix 25micrograms/hour transdermal patches | 5 patch [PoM] £10.77 DT price = £17.99 [CD2]

Fentanyl 37.5 microgram per 1 hour Mezolar Matrix 37.5microgram/hour transdermal patches | 5 patch [PoM] £15.46 [CD2]

Fentanyl 50 microgram per 1 hour Mezolar Matrix 50micrograms/hour transdermal patches | 5 patch [PoM] £20.13 DT price = £33.66 [CD2]

Fentanyl 75 microgram per 1 hour Mezolar Matrix 75micrograms/hour transdermal patches | 5 patch [PoM] £28.07 DT price = £46.99 [CD2]

Fentanyl 100 microgram per 1 hour Mezolar Matrix 100micrograms/hour transdermal patches | 5 patch [PoM] £34.60 DT price = £57.86 [CD2]

▸ Mylafent (Mylan Ltd)

Fentanyl 12 microgram per 1 hour Mylafent 12micrograms/hour transdermal patches | 5 patch [PoM] £7.53 DT price = £12.59 [CD2]

Fentanyl 25 microgram per 1 hour Mylafent 25micrograms/hour transdermal patches | 5 patch [PoM] £10.77 DT price = £17.99 [CD2]

Fentanyl 50 microgram per 1 hour Mylafent 50micrograms/hour transdermal patches | 5 patch [PoM] £20.13 DT price = £33.66 [CD2]

Fentanyl 75 microgram per 1 hour Mylafent 75micrograms/hour transdermal patches | 5 patch [PoM] £28.07 DT price = £46.99 [CD2]

Fentanyl 100 microgram per 1 hour Mylafent 100micrograms/hour transdermal patches | 5 patch [PoM] £34.60 DT price = £57.86 [CD2]

▸ Opiodur (Pfizer Ltd)

Fentanyl 12 microgram per 1 hour Opiodur 12micrograms/hour transdermal patches | 5 patch [PoM] £8.48 DT price = £12.59 [CD2]

Fentanyl 25 microgram per 1 hour Opiodur 25micrograms/hour transdermal patches | 5 patch [PoM] £12.12 DT price = £17.99 [CD2]

Fentanyl 50 microgram per 1 hour Opiodur 50micrograms/hour transdermal patches | 5 patch [PoM] £22.64 DT price = £33.66 [CD2]

Fentanyl 75 microgram per 1 hour Opiodur 75micrograms/hour transdermal patches | 5 patch [PoM] £31.56 DT price = £46.99 [CD2]

Fentanyl 100 microgram per 1 hour Opiodur 100micrograms/hour transdermal patches | 5 patch [PoM] £38.90 DT price = £57.86 [CD2]

▸ Osmanil (Zentiva)

Fentanyl 12 microgram per 1 hour Osmanil 12micrograms/hour transdermal patches | 5 patch [PoM] £18.11 DT price = £12.59 [CD2]

Fentanyl 25 microgram per 1 hour Osmanil 25micrograms/hour transdermal patches | 5 patch [PoM] £26.94 DT price = £17.99 [CD2]

Fentanyl 50 microgram per 1 hour Osmanil 50micrograms/hour transdermal patches | 5 patch [PoM] £50.32 DT price = £33.66 [CD2]

Fentanyl 75 microgram per 1 hour Osmanil 75micrograms/hour transdermal patches | 5 patch [PoM] £70.15 DT price = £46.99 [CD2]

Fentanyl 100 microgram per 1 hour Osmanil 100micrograms/hour transdermal patches | 5 patch [PoM] £86.46 DT price = £57.86 [CD2]

▸ Tilofyl (Tillomed Laboratories Ltd)

Fentanyl 25 microgram per 1 hour Tilofyl 25micrograms/hour transdermal patches | 5 patch [PoM] £27.00 DT price = £17.99 [CD2]

Fentanyl 50 microgram per 1 hour Tilofyl 50micrograms/hour transdermal patches | 5 patch [PoM] £51.00 DT price = £33.66 [CD2]

Fentanyl 75 microgram per 1 hour Tilofyl 75micrograms/hour transdermal patches | 5 patch [PoM] £71.00 DT price = £46.99 [CD2]

Fentanyl 100 microgram per 1 hour Tilofyl 100micrograms/hour transdermal patches | 5 patch [PoM] £88.00 DT price = £57.86 [CD2]

▸ Victanyl (Actavis UK Ltd)

Fentanyl 12 microgram per 1 hour Victanyl 12micrograms/hour transdermal patches | 5 patch [PoM] £12.58 DT price = £12.59 [CD2]

Fentanyl 25 microgram per 1 hour Victanyl 25micrograms/hour transdermal patches | 5 patch [PoM] £25.89 DT price = £17.99 [CD2]

Fentanyl 50 microgram per 1 hour Victanyl 50micrograms/hour transdermal patches | 5 patch [PoM] £48.36 DT price = £33.66 [CD2]

Fentanyl 75 microgram per 1 hour Victanyl 75micrograms/hour transdermal patches | 5 patch [PoM] £67.41 DT price = £46.99 [CD2]

Fentanyl 100 microgram per 1 hour Victanyl 100micrograms/hour transdermal patches | 5 patch [PoM] £83.09 DT price = £57.86 [CD2]

▸ Yemex (Sandoz Ltd)

Fentanyl 12 microgram per 1 hour Yemex 12micrograms/hour transdermal patches | 5 patch [PoM] £12.59 DT price = £12.59 [CD2]

Fentanyl 25 microgram per 1 hour Yemex 25micrograms/hour transdermal patches | 5 patch [PoM] £17.99 DT price = £17.99 [CD2]

Fentanyl 50 microgram per 1 hour Yemex 50micrograms/hour transdermal patches | 5 patch [PoM] £33.66 DT price = £33.66 [CD2]

Fentanyl 75 microgram per 1 hour Yemex 75micrograms/hour transdermal patches | 5 patch [PoM] £46.99 DT price = £46.99 [CD2]

Fentanyl 100 microgram per 1 hour Yemex 100micrograms/hour transdermal patches | 5 patch [PoM] £57.86 DT price = £57.86 [CD2]

Spray

CAUTIONARY AND ADVISORY LABELS 2

▸ Instanyl (Takeda UK Ltd)

Fentanyl (as Fentanyl citrate) 50 microgram per 1 dose Instanyl 50micrograms/dose nasal spray | 6 dose [PoM] £35.70 [CD2] | 10 dose [PoM] £59.50 [CD2] | 20 dose [PoM] £119.00 [CD2]

Fentanyl (as Fentanyl citrate) 100 microgram per 1 dose Instanyl 100micrograms/dose nasal spray | 6 dose [PoM] £35.70 [CD2] | 10 dose [PoM] £59.50 [CD2] | 20 dose [PoM] £119.00 [CD2]

Fentanyl (as Fentanyl citrate) 200 microgram per 1 dose Instanyl 200micrograms/dose nasal spray | 6 dose [PoM] £35.70 [CD2] | 10 dose [PoM] £59.50 [CD2] | 20 dose [PoM] £119.00 [CD2]

▸ PecFent (ProStrakan Ltd)

Fentanyl (as Fentanyl citrate) 100 microgram per 1 dose PecFent 100micrograms/dose nasal spray | 8 dose [PoM] £36.48 [CD2] | 32 dose [PoM] £145.92 [CD2]

Fentanyl (as Fentanyl citrate) 400 microgram per 1 dose PecFent 400micrograms/dose nasal spray | 8 dose [PoM] £36.48 [CD2] | 32 dose [PoM] £145.92 [CD2]

Ϝ 408

Hydromorphone hydrochloride

● **INDICATIONS AND DOSE**

Severe pain in cancer

▸ BY MOUTH USING IMMEDIATE-RELEASE MEDICINES

▸ Child 12–17 years: 1.3 mg every 4 hours, dose to be increased if necessary according to severity of pain

▸ Adult: 1.3 mg every 4 hours, dose to be increased if necessary according to severity of pain

▸ BY MOUTH USING MODIFIED-RELEASE MEDICINES

▸ Child 12–17 years: 4 mg every 12 hours, dose to be increased if necessary according to severity of pain

▸ Adult: 4 mg every 12 hours, dose to be increased if necessary according to severity of pain

● CONTRA-INDICATIONS Acute abdomen

● CAUTIONS Pancreatitis · toxic psychosis

● SIDE-EFFECTS

▸ **Common or very common** Abdominal pain · anorexia · anxiety

▸ **Uncommon** Agitation · diarrhoea · dysgeusia · dyskinesia · myoclonus · paraesthesia · paralytic ileus · peripheral oedema · seizures · tremor

● BREAST FEEDING Avoid—no information available.

● RENAL IMPAIRMENT Avoid use or reduce dose; opioid effects increased and prolonged and increased cerebral sensitivity occurs.

● DIRECTIONS FOR ADMINISTRATION For *immediate-release* capsules, swallow whole capsule or sprinkle contents on soft food. For *modified-release* capsules, swallow whole or open capsule and sprinkle contents on soft cold food (swallow the pellets within the capsule whole; do not crush or chew).

● PATIENT AND CARER ADVICE Patients or carers should be given advice on how to administer hydromorphone hydrochloride capsules and modified-release capsules.

● MEDICINAL FORMS
There can be variation in the licensing of different medicines containing the same drug. Forms available from special-order manufacturers include: oral solution

Capsule

CAUTIONARY AND ADVISORY LABELS 2

▸ Palladone (Napp Pharmaceuticals Ltd)

Hydromorphone hydrochloride 1.3 mg Palladone 1.3mg capsules | 56 capsule [PoM] £8.82 [CD2]

Hydromorphone hydrochloride 2.6 mg Palladone 2.6mg capsules | 56 capsule [PoM] £17.64 [CD2]

Modified-release capsule
CAUTIONARY AND ADVISORY LABELS 2
▸ Palladone SR (Napp Pharmaceuticals Ltd)
Hydromorphone hydrochloride 2 mg Palladone SR 2mg capsules |
56 capsule [PoM] £20.98 [CD2]
Hydromorphone hydrochloride 4 mg Palladone SR 4mg capsules |
56 capsule [PoM] £28.75 [CD2]
Hydromorphone hydrochloride 8 mg Palladone SR 8mg capsules |
56 capsule [PoM] £56.08 [CD2]
Hydromorphone hydrochloride 16 mg Palladone SR 16mg capsules
| 56 capsule [PoM] £106.53 [CD2]
Hydromorphone hydrochloride 24 mg Palladone SR 24mg capsules
| 56 capsule [PoM] £159.82 [CD2]

▶ 408

Meptazinol

● INDICATIONS AND DOSE

**Moderate to severe pain, including post-operative pain
and renal colic**
▸ BY MOUTH
▸ Adult: 200 mg every 3–6 hours as required
▸ BY INTRAMUSCULAR INJECTION
▸ Adult: 75–100 mg every 2–4 hours if required
▸ BY SLOW INTRAVENOUS INJECTION
▸ Adult: 50–100 mg every 2–4 hours if required

Obstetric analgesia
▸ BY INTRAMUSCULAR INJECTION
▸ Adult: 2 mg/kg, usual dose 100–150 mg

● CONTRA-INDICATIONS Myocardial infarction ·
phaeochromocytoma
● SIDE-EFFECTS Abdominal pain · can induce withdrawal
symptoms in patients dependent on opioids · diarrhoea ·
dyspepsia · hypothermia

Overdose
Effects only partially reversed by naloxone.
● BREAST FEEDING Use only if potential benefit outweighs
risk.
● RENAL IMPAIRMENT Avoid use or reduce dose; opioid
effects increased and prolonged and increased cerebral
sensitivity occurs.

● MEDICINAL FORMS
There can be variation in the licensing of different medicines
containing the same drug.
Tablet
CAUTIONARY AND ADVISORY LABELS 2
▸ Meptid (Almirall Ltd)
Meptazinol (as Meptazinol hydrochloride) 200 mg Meptid 200mg
tablets | 112 tablet [PoM] £22.11 DT price = £22.11
Solution for injection
▸ Meptid (Almirall Ltd)
**Meptazinol (as Meptazinol hydrochloride) 100 mg per
1 ml** Meptid 100mg/1ml solution for injection ampoules |
10 ampoule [PoM] £19.21

▶ 408

Morphine

● INDICATIONS AND DOSE

Pain
▸ BY SUBCUTANEOUS INJECTION
▸ Child 1-5 months: Initially 100–200 micrograms/kg
every 6 hours, adjusted according to response
▸ Child 6 months-1 year: Initially 100–200 micrograms/kg
every 4 hours, adjusted according to response
▸ Child 2-11 years: Initially 200 micrograms/kg every
4 hours, adjusted according to response
▸ Child 12-17 years: Initially 2.5–10 mg every 4 hours,
adjusted according to response

▸ INITIALLY BY INTRAVENOUS INJECTION
▸ Child 1-5 months: 100 micrograms/kg every 6 hours,
adjusted according to response, dose to be
administered over at least 5 minutes, alternatively (by
intravenous injection) initially 100 micrograms/kg,
dose to be administered over at least 5 minutes,
followed by (by continuous intravenous infusion)
10–30 micrograms/kg/hour, adjusted according to
response
▸ Child 6 months-11 years: 100 micrograms/kg every
4 hours, adjusted according to response, dose to be
administered over at least 5 minutes, alternatively (by
intravenous injection) initially 100 micrograms/kg,
dose to be administered over at least 5 minutes,
followed by (by continuous intravenous infusion)
20–30 micrograms/kg/hour, adjusted according to
response
▸ Child 12-17 years: 5 mg every 4 hours, adjusted
according to response, dose to be administered over at
least 5 minutes, alternatively (by intravenous
injection) initially 5 mg, dose to be administered over
at least 5 minutes, followed by (by continuous
intravenous infusion) 20–30 micrograms/kg/hour,
adjusted according to response
▸ BY MOUTH, OR BY RECTUM
▸ Child 1-2 months: Initially 50–100 micrograms/kg every
4 hours, adjusted according to response
▸ Child 3-5 months: 100–150 micrograms/kg every
4 hours, adjusted according to response
▸ Child 6-11 months: 200 micrograms/kg every 4 hours,
adjusted according to response
▸ Child 1 year: Initially 200–300 micrograms/kg every
4 hours, adjusted according to response
▸ Child 2-11 years: Initially 200–300 micrograms/kg every
4 hours (max. per dose 10 mg), adjusted according to
response
▸ Child 12-17 years: Initially 5–10 mg every 4 hours,
adjusted according to response

Acute pain
▸ BY SUBCUTANEOUS INJECTION, OR BY INTRAMUSCULAR
INJECTION
▸ Adult: Initially 10 mg every 4 hours, adjusted according
to response, subcutaneous injection not suitable for
oedematous patients, dose can be given more
frequently during titration, use dose for elderly in frail
patients
▸ Elderly: Initially 5 mg every 4 hours, adjusted according
to response, subcutaneous injection not suitable for
oedematous patients, dose can be given more
frequently during titration
▸ BY SLOW INTRAVENOUS INJECTION
▸ Adult: Initially 5 mg every 4 hours, adjusted according
to response, dose can be adjusted more frequently
during titration, reduced dose recommended in frail
and elderly patients

Chronic pain
▸ BY MOUTH, OR BY SUBCUTANEOUS INJECTION, OR BY
INTRAMUSCULAR INJECTION
▸ Adult: Initially 5–10 mg every 4 hours, adjusted
according to response, subcutaneous injection not
suitable for oedematous patients
▸ BY RECTUM
▸ Adult: Initially 15–30 mg every 4 hours, adjusted
according to response

Pain (with modified-release 12-hourly preparations)
▸ BY MOUTH USING MODIFIED-RELEASE MEDICINES
▸ Adult: Every 12 hours, dose adjusted according to daily
morphine requirements, dosage requirements should
be reviewed if the brand is altered   continued →

4

Nervous system

Pain (with modified-release 24-hourly preparations)
▸ BY MOUTH USING MODIFIED-RELEASE MEDICINES
▸ Adult: Every 24 hours, dose adjusted according to daily morphine requirements, dosage requirements should be reviewed if the brand is altered

Pain management in palliative care (starting dose for opioid-naïve patients)
▸ BY MOUTH
▸ Adult: 20–30 mg daily in divided doses, using immediate-release preparation 4-hourly or a 12-hourly modified-release preparation, for management of breakthrough pain and other general advice, see *Pain management with opioids* p. 21.

Pain management in palliative care (starting dose for patients being switched from a regular weak opioid)
▸ BY MOUTH
▸ Adult: 40–60 mg daily in divided doses, using immediate-release preparation 4-hourly or 12-hourly modified-release preparation, for management of breakthrough pain and other general advice, see *Pain management with opioids* p. 21.

Pain in palliative care (following initial titration)
▸ BY MOUTH USING IMMEDIATE-RELEASE MEDICINES
▸ Adult: Usual dose 30 mg every 4 hours; up to 200 mg every 4 hours, higher dose may be required for some patients (occasionally more is needed); for management of breakthrough pain and other general advice, see *Pain management with opioids* p. 21.
▸ BY MOUTH USING MODIFIED-RELEASE MEDICINES
▸ Adult: Usual dose 100 mg every 12 hours; up to 600 mg every 12 hours, higher dose may be required for some patients (occasionally more is needed); for management of breakthrough pain and other general advice, see *Pain management with opioids* p. 21.

Cough in terminal disease
▸ BY MOUTH
▸ Adult: Initially 5 mg every 4 hours

Premedication
▸ BY SUBCUTANEOUS INJECTION, OR BY INTRAMUSCULAR INJECTION
▸ Adult: Up to 10 mg, dose to be administered 60–90 minutes before operation

Patient controlled analgesia (PCA)
▸ BY INTRAVENOUS INFUSION
▸ Adult: (consult local protocol)

Myocardial infarction
▸ BY SLOW INTRAVENOUS INJECTION
▸ Adult: 5–10 mg, followed by 5–10 mg if required, dose to be administered at a rate of 1–2 mg/minute, use dose for elderly in frail patients
▸ Elderly: 2.5–5 mg, followed by 2.5–5 mg if required, dose to be administered at a rate of 1–2 mg/minute

Acute pulmonary oedema
▸ BY SLOW INTRAVENOUS INJECTION
▸ Adult: 5–10 mg, dose to be administered at a rate of 2 mg/minute, use dose for elderly in frail patients
▸ Elderly: 2.5–5 mg, dose to be administered at a rate of 2 mg/minute

Dyspnoea at rest in palliative care
▸ BY MOUTH
▸ Adult: Initially 5 mg every 4 hours, to be given in carefully titrated doses

DOSE EQUIVALENCE AND CONVERSION
The doses stated refer equally to morphine hydrochloride and sulfate.

● UNLICENSED USE
▸ With oral use in children *Oramorph* ® solution not licensed for use in children under 1 year. *Sevredol* ® tablets not

licensed for use in children under 3 years. *Oramorph* ® unit dose vials not licensed for use in children under 6 years.
▸ With rectal use in children Suppositories are not licensed for use in children.

● CONTRA-INDICATIONS Acute abdomen · delayed gastric emptying · heart failure secondary to chronic lung disease · phaeochromocytoma

● CAUTIONS Cardiac arrhythmias · pancreatitis · severe cor pulmonale

● SIDE-EFFECTS Abdominal pain · agitation · amenorrhoea · anorexia · asthenia · bronchospasm · delirium · disorientation · dyspepsia · exacerbation of pancreatitis · excitation · hypertension · hypothermia · inhibition of cough reflex · malaise · muscle fasciculation · myoclonus · nystagmus · paraesthesia · paralytic ileus · raised intracranial pressure · restlessness · rhabdomyolysis · seizures · syncope · taste disturbance

● BREAST FEEDING Therapeutic doses unlikely to affect infant.

● RENAL IMPAIRMENT Avoid use or reduce dose; opioid effects increased and prolonged; increased cerebral sensitivity.

● DIRECTIONS FOR ADMINISTRATION
▸ With intravenous use in children For *continuous intravenous infusion*, dilute with Glucose 5% or 10% or Sodium Chloride 0.9%.
▸ With oral use For *modified release capsules*—swallow whole or open capsule and sprinkle contents on soft food.

● PRESCRIBING AND DISPENSING INFORMATION Modified-release preparations are available as 12-hourly or 24-hourly formulations; prescribers must ensure that the correct preparation is prescribed. Preparations that should be given 12-hourly include *Filnarine* ® SR, *MST Continus* ®, *Morphgesic* ® SR and *Zomorph* ®. Preparations that should be given 24-hourly include *MXL* ®.
 Prescriptions must specify the 'form'.
▸ With oral use Do not confuse modified-release 12-hourly preparations with 24-hourly preparations.
▸ With rectal use Both the strength of the suppositories and the morphine salt contained in them must be specified by the prescriber.

● PATIENT AND CARER ADVICE
Medicines for Children leaflet: Morphine for pain www.medicinesforchildren.org.uk/morphine-for-pain
▸ With oral use Patients or carers should be given advice on how to administer morphine modified-release capsules.

● EXCEPTIONS TO LEGAL CATEGORY
Morphine Oral Solutions Prescription-only medicines or schedule 2 controlled drug. The proportion of morphine hydrochloride may be altered when specified by the prescriber; if above 13 mg per 5 mL the solution becomes a schedule 2 controlled drug. It is usual to adjust the strength so that the dose volume is 5 or 10 mL.
 Oral solutions of morphine can be prescribed by writing the formula:
 Morphine hydrochloride 5 mg
 Chloroform water to 5 mL

● MEDICINAL FORMS
There can be variation in the licensing of different medicines containing the same drug. Forms available from special-order manufacturers include: capsule, oral solution, solution for injection, infusion, solution for infusion, suppository
Tablet
CAUTIONARY AND ADVISORY LABELS 2
▸ Sevredol (Napp Pharmaceuticals Ltd)
 Morphine sulfate 10 mg Sevredol 10mg tablets | 56 tablet [PoM] £5.31 DT price = £5.31 [CD2]
 Morphine sulfate 20 mg Sevredol 20mg tablets | 56 tablet [PoM] £10.61 DT price = £10.61 [CD2]
 Morphine sulfate 50 mg Sevredol 50mg tablets | 56 tablet [PoM] £28.02 DT price = £28.02 [CD2]

Modified-release tablet

CAUTIONARY AND ADVISORY LABELS 2, 25

▸ MST Continus (Napp Pharmaceuticals Ltd)

Morphine sulfate 5 mg MST Continus 5mg tablets | 60 tablet [PoM] £3.29 DT price = £3.29 [CD2]

Morphine sulfate 10 mg MST Continus 10mg tablets | 60 tablet [PoM] £5.20 DT price = £5.20 [CD2]

Morphine sulfate 15 mg MST Continus 15mg tablets | 60 tablet [PoM] £9.10 DT price = £9.10 [CD2]

Morphine sulfate 30 mg MST Continus 30mg tablets | 60 tablet [PoM] £12.47 DT price = £12.47 [CD2]

Morphine sulfate 60 mg MST Continus 60mg tablets | 60 tablet [PoM] £24.32 DT price = £24.32 [CD2]

Morphine sulfate 100 mg MST Continus 100mg tablets | 60 tablet [PoM] £38.50 DT price = £38.50 [CD2]

Morphine sulfate 200 mg MST Continus 200mg tablets | 60 tablet [PoM] £81.34 DT price = £81.34 [CD2]

▸ Morphgesic SR (AMCo)

Morphine sulfate 10 mg Morphgesic SR 10mg tablets | 60 tablet [PoM] £3.85 DT price = £5.20 [CD2]

Morphine sulfate 30 mg Morphgesic SR 30mg tablets | 60 tablet [PoM] £9.24 DT price = £12.47 [CD2]

Morphine sulfate 60 mg Morphgesic SR 60mg tablets | 60 tablet [PoM] £18.04 DT price = £24.32 [CD2]

Morphine sulfate 100 mg Morphgesic SR 100mg tablets | 60 tablet [PoM] £28.54 DT price = £38.50 [CD2]

Modified-release capsule

CAUTIONARY AND ADVISORY LABELS 2

▸ MXL (Napp Pharmaceuticals Ltd)

Morphine sulfate 30 mg MXL 30mg capsules | 28 capsule [PoM] £10.91 [CD2]

Morphine sulfate 60 mg MXL 60mg capsules | 28 capsule [PoM] £14.95 [CD2]

Morphine sulfate 90 mg MXL 90mg capsules | 28 capsule [PoM] £22.04 [CD2]

Morphine sulfate 120 mg MXL 120mg capsules | 28 capsule [PoM] £29.15 [CD2]

Morphine sulfate 150 mg MXL 150mg capsules | 28 capsule [PoM] £36.43 [CD2]

Morphine sulfate 200 mg MXL 200mg capsules | 28 capsule [PoM] £46.15 [CD2]

▸ Zomorph (ProStrakan Ltd)

Morphine sulfate 10 mg Zomorph 10mg modified-release capsules | 60 capsule [PoM] £3.47 DT price = £3.47 [CD2]

Morphine sulfate 30 mg Zomorph 30mg modified-release capsules | 60 capsule [PoM] £8.30 DT price = £8.30 [CD2]

Morphine sulfate 60 mg Zomorph 60mg modified-release capsules | 60 capsule [PoM] £16.20 DT price = £16.20 [CD2]

Morphine sulfate 100 mg Zomorph 100mg modified-release capsules | 60 capsule [PoM] £21.80 [CD2]

Morphine sulfate 200 mg Zomorph 200mg modified-release capsules | 60 capsule [PoM] £43.60 DT price = £43.60 [CD2]

Modified-release granules

CAUTIONARY AND ADVISORY LABELS 2, 13

▸ MST Continus (Napp Pharmaceuticals Ltd)

Morphine sulfate 20 mg MST Continus Suspension 20mg granules sachets sugar-free | 30 sachet [PoM] £24.58 [CD2]

Morphine sulfate 30 mg MST Continus Suspension 30mg granules sachets sugar-free | 30 sachet [PoM] £25.54 [CD2]

Morphine sulfate 60 mg MST Continus Suspension 60mg granules sachets sugar-free | 30 sachet [PoM] £51.09 [CD2]

Morphine sulfate 100 mg MST Continus Suspension 100mg granules sachets sugar-free | 30 sachet [PoM] £85.15 [CD2]

Morphine sulfate 200 mg MST Continus Suspension 200mg granules sachets sugar-free | 30 sachet [PoM] £170.30 [CD2]

Oral solution

CAUTIONARY AND ADVISORY LABELS 2

▸ Morphine (Non-proprietary)

Morphine sulfate 2 mg per 1 ml Morphine sulfate 10mg/5ml oral solution unit dose vials sugar free sugar-free | 1 unit dose [PoM] no price available Schedule 5 (CD Inv)

Morphine sulfate 10mg/5ml oral solution | 100 ml [PoM] £1.82 Schedule 5 (CD Inv) | 300 ml [PoM] £5.45 DT price = £5.45 Schedule 5 (CD Inv) | 500 ml [PoM] £9.08 Schedule 5 (CD Inv)

▸ Oramorph (Boehringer Ingelheim Ltd)

Morphine sulfate 2 mg per 1 ml Oramorph 10mg/5ml oral solution | 100 ml [PoM] £1.89 Schedule 5 (CD Inv) | 300 ml [PoM] £5.45 DT price = £5.45 Schedule 5 (CD Inv) | 500 ml [PoM] £8.50 Schedule 5 (CD Inv)

Morphine sulfate 20 mg per 1 ml Oramorph 20mg/ml concentrated oral solution sugar-free | 30 ml [PoM] £4.98 [CD2] sugar-free | 120 ml [PoM] £19.50 DT price = £19.50 [CD2]

Solution for injection

▸ Morphine (Non-proprietary)

Morphine sulfate 1 mg per 1 ml Morphine sulfate 5mg/5ml solution for injection ampoules | 10 ampoule [PoM] £35.90 [CD2] Morphine sulfate 1mg/1ml solution for injection ampoules | 10 ampoule [PoM] £26.10 [CD2] Morphine sulfate 10mg/10ml solution for injection ampoules | 10 ampoule [PoM] £30.00–£38.00 [CD2]

Morphine sulfate 10 mg per 1 ml Morphine sulfate 10mg/1ml solution for injection ampoules | 10 ampoule [PoM] £9.36 DT price = £9.36 [CD2]

Morphine sulfate 15 mg per 1 ml Morphine sulfate 15mg/1ml solution for injection ampoules | 10 ampoule [PoM] £8.95 DT price = £8.95 [CD2]

Morphine sulfate 20 mg per 1 ml Morphine sulfate 20mg/1ml solution for injection ampoules | 10 ampoule [PoM] £51.69 [CD2]

Morphine sulfate 30 mg per 1 ml Morphine sulfate 30mg/1ml solution for injection ampoules | 10 ampoule [PoM] £9.04 DT price = £8.84 [CD2] Morphine sulfate 60mg/2ml solution for injection ampoules | 5 ampoule [PoM] £10.07 [CD2]

Solution for infusion

▸ Morphine (Non-proprietary)

Morphine sulfate 1 mg per 1 ml Morphine sulfate 50mg/50ml solution for infusion vials | 1 vial [PoM] £5.25–£5.78 [CD2] | 10 vial [PoM] £28.90 [CD2]

Morphine sulfate 2 mg per 1 ml Morphine sulfate 100mg/50ml solution for infusion vials | 1 vial [PoM] £6.48 [CD2] | 10 vial [PoM] £57.60 [CD2]

Suppository

CAUTIONARY AND ADVISORY LABELS 2

▸ Morphine (Non-proprietary)

Morphine sulfate 10 mg Morphine sulfate 10mg suppositories | 12 suppository [PoM] £18.34 [CD2]

Morphine sulfate 15 mg Morphine sulfate 15mg suppositories | 12 suppository [PoM] £16.48 DT price = £16.48 [CD2]

Morphine sulfate 30 mg Morphine sulfate 30mg suppositories | 12 suppository [PoM] £18.60 DT price = £18.60 [CD2]

Morphine with cyclizine

The properties listed below are those particular to the combination only. For the properties of the components please consider, morphine p. 421, cyclizine p. 393.

● **INDICATIONS AND DOSE**

CYCLIMORPH-10®

Moderate to severe pain (short-term use only)

▸ BY SUBCUTANEOUS INJECTION, OR BY INTRAMUSCULAR INJECTION, OR BY INTRAVENOUS INJECTION

▸ Adult: 1 mL, do not repeat dose more often than every 4 hours; maximum 3 doses per day

CYCLIMORPH-15®

Moderate to severe pain (short-term use only)

▸ BY SUBCUTANEOUS INJECTION, OR BY INTRAMUSCULAR INJECTION, OR BY INTRAVENOUS INJECTION

▸ Adult: 1 mL, do not repeat dose more often than every 4 hours; maximum 3 doses per day

● CAUTIONS Myocardial infarction (cyclizine may aggravate severe heart failure and counteract the haemodynamic benefits of opioids) · not recommended in palliative care

● MEDICINAL FORMS
There can be variation in the licensing of different medicines containing the same drug.

Solution for injection

▸ Cyclimorph (AMCo)

Morphine tartrate 15 mg per 1 ml, Cyclizine tartrate 50 mg per 1 ml Cyclimorph 15 solution for injection 1ml ampoules | 5 ampoule [PoM] £9.12 [CD2]

Morphine tartrate 10 mg per 1 ml, Cyclizine tartrate 50 mg per 1 ml Cyclimorph 10 solution for injection 1ml ampoules | 5 ampoule [PoM] £8.77 [CD2]

Nervous system

4

4

Nervous system

Oxycodone hydrochloride

⌐ 408

- **INDICATIONS AND DOSE**

Postoperative pain | Severe pain | Moderate to severe pain in palliative care

▸ BY MOUTH USING IMMEDIATE-RELEASE MEDICINES
▸ Adult: Initially 5 mg every 4–6 hours, dose to be increased if necessary according to severity of pain, some patients may require higher doses than the maximum daily dose; maximum 400 mg per day
▸ BY MOUTH USING MODIFIED-RELEASE MEDICINES
▸ Adult: Initially 10 mg every 12 hours (max. per dose 200 mg every 12 hours), dose to be increased if necessary according to severity of pain, some patients might require higher doses than the maximum daily dose
▸ BY SLOW INTRAVENOUS INJECTION
▸ Adult: 1–10 mg every 4 hours as required
▸ BY INTRAVENOUS INFUSION
▸ Adult: Initially 2 mg/hour, adjusted according to response
▸ BY SUBCUTANEOUS INJECTION
▸ Adult: Initially 5 mg every 4 hours as required
▸ BY SUBCUTANEOUS INFUSION
▸ Adult: Initially 7.5 mg/24 hours, adjusted according to response

Patient controlled analgesia (PCA)

▸ BY INTRAVENOUS INFUSION
▸ Adult: (consult local protocol)

DOSE EQUIVALENCE AND CONVERSION
2 mg oral oxycodone is approximately equivalent to 1 mg parenteral oxycodone.

- **CONTRA-INDICATIONS** Acute abdomen · chronic constipation · cor pulmonale · delayed gastric emptying
- **CAUTIONS** Pancreatitis · toxic psychosis
- **SIDE-EFFECTS**
▸ **Common or very common** Abdominal pain · anorexia · anxiety · asthenia · bronchospasm · chills · diarrhoea · dyspepsia · dyspnoea · impaired cough reflex
▸ **Uncommon** Agitation · amenorrhoea · amnesia · belching · cholestasis · dehydration · disorientation · dry skin · dysphagia · flatulence · gastritis · hiccups · hypoaesthesia · hypotonia · malaise · muscle fasciculation · paraesthesia · paralytic ileus · pyrexia · restlessness · seizures · speech disorder · supraventricular tachycardia · syncope · taste disturbance · thirst · tremor · vasodilatation
- **BREAST FEEDING** Present in milk—avoid.
- **HEPATIC IMPAIRMENT** Max. initial dose 2.5 mg every 6 hours in patients not currently treated with an opioid with mild impairment. Avoid in moderate to severe impairment.
- **RENAL IMPAIRMENT** Max. initial dose 2.5 mg every 6 hours in patients not currently treated with an opioid with mild to moderate impairment. Opioid effects increased and prolonged and increased cerebral sensitivity occurs.
  Avoid if eGFR less than 10 mL/minute/1.73 m^2.
- **DIRECTIONS FOR ADMINISTRATION**
▸ With intravenous use For intravenous infusion (*Oxynorm*®), give continuously or intermittently in Glucose 5% or Sodium chloride 0.9%; dilute to a concentration of 1 mg/mL.
- **NATIONAL FUNDING/ACCESS DECISIONS**

Scottish Medicines Consortium (SMC) Decisions
The *Scottish Medicines Consortium* has advised (October 2004 and November 2010) that *OxyNorm*® injection is restricted for use within NHS Scotland for patients with cancer who have difficulty in tolerating morphine or diamorphine.

- **MEDICINAL FORMS**
There can be variation in the licensing of different medicines containing the same drug. Forms available from special-order manufacturers include: oral solution, solution for infusion

Modified-release tablet
CAUTIONARY AND ADVISORY LABELS 2, 25
▸ Abtard (DB Ashbourne Ltd)
Oxycodone hydrochloride 5 mg Abtard 5mg modified-release tablets | 28 tablet PoM £6.26 DT price = £12.52 CD2
Oxycodone hydrochloride 10 mg Abtard 10mg modified-release tablets | 56 tablet PoM £12.52 DT price = £25.04 CD2
Oxycodone hydrochloride 15 mg Abtard 15mg modified-release tablets | 56 tablet PoM £19.06 DT price = £38.12 CD2
Oxycodone hydrochloride 20 mg Abtard 20mg modified-release tablets | 56 tablet PoM £25.04 DT price = £50.08 CD2
Oxycodone hydrochloride 30 mg Abtard 30mg modified-release tablets | 56 tablet PoM £38.11 DT price = £76.23 CD2
Oxycodone hydrochloride 40 mg Abtard 40mg modified-release tablets | 56 tablet PoM £50.09 DT price = £100.19 CD2
Oxycodone hydrochloride 60 mg Abtard 60mg modified-release tablets | 56 tablet PoM £76.24 DT price = £152.49 CD2
Oxycodone hydrochloride 80 mg Abtard 80mg modified-release tablets | 56 tablet PoM £100.19 DT price = £200.39 CD2
▸ Carexil (Sandoz Ltd)
Oxycodone hydrochloride 5 mg Carexil 5mg modified-release tablets | 28 tablet PoM £6.26 DT price = £12.52 CD2
Oxycodone hydrochloride 10 mg Carexil 10mg modified-release tablets | 56 tablet PoM £12.52 DT price = £25.04 CD2
Oxycodone hydrochloride 20 mg Carexil 20mg modified-release tablets | 56 tablet PoM £25.04 DT price = £50.08 CD2
Oxycodone hydrochloride 40 mg Carexil 40mg modified-release tablets | 56 tablet PoM £60.11 DT price = £100.19 CD2
Oxycodone hydrochloride 80 mg Carexil 80mg modified-release tablets | 56 tablet PoM £120.23 DT price = £200.39 CD2
▸ Longtec (Qdem Pharmaceuticals Ltd)
Oxycodone hydrochloride 5 mg Longtec 5mg modified-release tablets | 28 tablet PoM £6.26 DT price = £12.52 CD2
Oxycodone hydrochloride 10 mg Longtec 10mg modified-release tablets | 56 tablet PoM £12.52 DT price = £25.04 CD2
Oxycodone hydrochloride 15 mg Longtec 15mg modified-release tablets | 56 tablet PoM £19.06 DT price = £38.12 CD2
Oxycodone hydrochloride 20 mg Longtec 20mg modified-release tablets | 56 tablet PoM £25.04 DT price = £50.08 CD2
Oxycodone hydrochloride 30 mg Longtec 30mg modified-release tablets | 56 tablet PoM £38.11 DT price = £76.23 CD2
Oxycodone hydrochloride 40 mg Longtec 40mg modified-release tablets | 56 tablet PoM £50.09 DT price = £100.19 CD2
Oxycodone hydrochloride 60 mg Longtec 60mg modified-release tablets | 56 tablet PoM £76.24 DT price = £152.49 CD2
Oxycodone hydrochloride 80 mg Longtec 80mg modified-release tablets | 56 tablet PoM £100.19 DT price = £200.39 CD2
Oxycodone hydrochloride 120 mg Longtec 120mg modified-release tablets | 56 tablet PoM £152.51 DT price = £305.02 CD2
▸ Oxeltra (Wockhardt UK Ltd)
Oxycodone hydrochloride 5 mg Oxeltra 5mg modified-release tablets | 28 tablet PoM £11.27 DT price = £12.52 CD2
Oxycodone hydrochloride 10 mg Oxeltra 10mg modified-release tablets | 56 tablet PoM £22.54 DT price = £25.04 CD2
Oxycodone hydrochloride 15 mg Oxeltra 15mg modified-release tablets | 56 tablet PoM £34.31 DT price = £38.12 CD2
Oxycodone hydrochloride 20 mg Oxeltra 20mg modified-release tablets | 56 tablet PoM £45.07 DT price = £50.08 CD2
Oxycodone hydrochloride 30 mg Oxeltra 30mg modified-release tablets | 56 tablet PoM £68.61 DT price = £76.23 CD2
Oxycodone hydrochloride 40 mg Oxeltra 40mg modified-release tablets | 56 tablet PoM £90.17 DT price = £100.19 CD2
Oxycodone hydrochloride 60 mg Oxeltra 60mg modified-release tablets | 56 tablet PoM £137.24 DT price = £152.49 CD2
Oxycodone hydrochloride 80 mg Oxeltra 80mg modified-release tablets | 56 tablet PoM £180.35 DT price = £200.39 CD2
▸ OxyContin (Napp Pharmaceuticals Ltd)
Oxycodone hydrochloride 5 mg OxyContin 5mg modified-release tablets | 28 tablet PoM £12.52 DT price = £12.52 CD2
Oxycodone hydrochloride 10 mg OxyContin 10mg modified-release tablets | 56 tablet PoM £25.04 DT price = £25.04 CD2
Oxycodone hydrochloride 15 mg OxyContin 15mg modified-release tablets | 56 tablet PoM £38.12 DT price = £38.12 CD2
Oxycodone hydrochloride 20 mg OxyContin 20mg modified-release tablets | 56 tablet PoM £50.08 DT price = £50.08 CD2

4

Nervous system

Oxycodone hydrochloride 30 mg OxyContin 30mg modified-release tablets | 56 tablet [PoM] £76.23 DT price = £76.23 [CD2]

Oxycodone hydrochloride 40 mg OxyContin 40mg modified-release tablets | 56 tablet [PoM] £100.19 DT price = £100.19 [CD2]

Oxycodone hydrochloride 60 mg OxyContin 60mg modified-release tablets | 56 tablet [PoM] £152.49 DT price = £152.49 [CD2]

Oxycodone hydrochloride 80 mg OxyContin 80mg modified-release tablets | 56 tablet [PoM] £200.39 DT price = £200.39 [CD2]

Oxycodone hydrochloride 120 mg OxyContin 120mg modified-release tablets | 56 tablet [PoM] £305.02 DT price = £305.02 [CD2]

▸ Oxylan (Chanelle Medical UK Ltd)

Oxycodone hydrochloride 5 mg Oxylan 5mg modified-release tablets | 28 tablet [PoM] £12.50 DT price = £12.52 [CD2]

Oxycodone hydrochloride 10 mg Oxylan 10mg modified-release tablets | 56 tablet [PoM] £24.99 DT price = £25.04 [CD2]

Oxycodone hydrochloride 20 mg Oxylan 20mg modified-release tablets | 56 tablet [PoM] £49.98 DT price = £50.08 [CD2]

Oxycodone hydrochloride 40 mg Oxylan 40mg modified-release tablets | 56 tablet [PoM] £99.98 DT price = £100.19 [CD2]

Oxycodone hydrochloride 80 mg Oxylan 80mg modified-release tablets | 56 tablet [PoM] £199.97 DT price = £200.39 [CD2]

▸ Reltebon (Actavis UK Ltd)

Oxycodone hydrochloride 5 mg Reltebon 5mg modified-release tablets | 28 tablet [PoM] £6.26 DT price = £12.52 [CD2]

Oxycodone hydrochloride 10 mg Reltebon 10mg modified-release tablets | 56 tablet [PoM] £12.52 DT price = £25.04 [CD2]

Oxycodone hydrochloride 15 mg Reltebon 15mg modified-release tablets | 56 tablet [PoM] £19.06 DT price = £38.12 [CD2]

Oxycodone hydrochloride 20 mg Reltebon 20mg modified-release tablets | 56 tablet [PoM] £25.04 DT price = £50.08 [CD2]

Oxycodone hydrochloride 30 mg Reltebon 30mg modified-release tablets | 56 tablet [PoM] £38.11 DT price = £76.23 [CD2]

Oxycodone hydrochloride 40 mg Reltebon 40mg modified-release tablets | 56 tablet [PoM] £50.09 DT price = £100.19 [CD2]

Oxycodone hydrochloride 60 mg Reltebon 60mg modified-release tablets | 56 tablet [PoM] £76.24 DT price = £152.49 [CD2]

Oxycodone hydrochloride 80 mg Reltebon 80mg modified-release tablets | 56 tablet [PoM] £100.19 DT price = £200.39 [CD2]

▸ Zomestine (Accord Healthcare Ltd)

Oxycodone hydrochloride 5 mg Zomestine 5mg modified-release tablets | 28 tablet [PoM] £5.01 DT price = £12.52 [CD2]

Oxycodone hydrochloride 10 mg Zomestine 10mg modified-release tablets | 56 tablet [PoM] £10.02 DT price = £25.04 [CD2]

Oxycodone hydrochloride 20 mg Zomestine 20mg modified-release tablets | 56 tablet [PoM] £20.03 DT price = £50.08 [CD2]

Oxycodone hydrochloride 40 mg Zomestine 40mg modified-release tablets | 56 tablet [PoM] £40.08 DT price = £100.19 [CD2]

Oxycodone hydrochloride 80 mg Zomestine 80mg modified-release tablets | 56 tablet [PoM] £80.16 DT price = £200.39 [CD2]

Capsule

CAUTIONARY AND ADVISORY LABELS 2

▸ Lynlor (Actavis UK Ltd)

Oxycodone hydrochloride 5 mg Lynlor 5mg capsules | 56 capsule [PoM] £6.86 DT price = £11.43 [CD2]

Oxycodone hydrochloride 10 mg Lynlor 10mg capsules | 56 capsule [PoM] £13.72 DT price = £22.86 [CD2]

Oxycodone hydrochloride 20 mg Lynlor 20mg capsules | 56 capsule [PoM] £27.43 DT price = £45.71 [CD2]

▸ OxyNorm (Napp Pharmaceuticals Ltd)

Oxycodone hydrochloride 5 mg OxyNorm 5mg capsules | 56 capsule [PoM] £11.43 DT price = £11.43 [CD2]

Oxycodone hydrochloride 10 mg OxyNorm 10mg capsules | 56 capsule [PoM] £22.86 DT price = £22.86 [CD2]

Oxycodone hydrochloride 20 mg OxyNorm 20mg capsules | 56 capsule [PoM] £45.71 DT price = £45.71 [CD2]

▸ Shortec (Qdem Pharmaceuticals Ltd)

Oxycodone hydrochloride 5 mg Shortec 5mg capsules | 56 capsule [PoM] £6.86 DT price = £11.43 [CD2]

Oxycodone hydrochloride 10 mg Shortec 10mg capsules | 56 capsule [PoM] £13.72 DT price = £22.86 [CD2]

Oxycodone hydrochloride 20 mg Shortec 20mg capsules | 56 capsule [PoM] £27.43 DT price = £45.71 [CD2]

Oral solution

CAUTIONARY AND ADVISORY LABELS 2

▸ Oxycodone hydrochloride (Non-proprietary)

Oxycodone hydrochloride 1 mg per 1 ml Oxycodone 5mg/5ml oral solution sugar free sugar-free | 250 ml [PoM] £9.71 DT price = £9.71 [CD2]

Oxycodone hydrochloride 10 mg per 1 ml Oxycodone 10mg/ml oral solution sugar free sugar-free | 120 ml [PoM] £46.63 DT price = £46.63 [CD2]

▸ OxyNorm (Napp Pharmaceuticals Ltd)

Oxycodone hydrochloride 1 mg per 1 ml OxyNorm liquid 5mg/5ml oral solution sugar-free | 250 ml [PoM] £9.71 DT price = £9.71 [CD2]

Oxycodone hydrochloride 10 mg per 1 ml OxyNorm 10mg/ml concentrate oral solution sugar-free | 120 ml [PoM] £46.63 DT price = £46.63 [CD2]

Solution for injection

▸ Oxycodone hydrochloride (Non-proprietary)

Oxycodone hydrochloride 10 mg per 1 ml Oxycodone 20mg/2ml solution for injection ampoules | 5 ampoule [PoM] £16.00 DT price = £16.00 [CD2]

Oxycodone 10mg/1ml solution for injection ampoules | 5 ampoule [PoM] £8.00 DT price = £8.00 [CD2]

Oxycodone hydrochloride 50 mg per 1 ml Oxycodone 50mg/1ml solution for injection ampoules | 5 ampoule [PoM] £70.10 DT price = £70.10 [CD2]

▸ OxyNorm (Napp Pharmaceuticals Ltd)

Oxycodone hydrochloride 10 mg per 1 ml OxyNorm 10mg/1ml solution for injection ampoules | 5 ampoule [PoM] £8.00 DT price = £8.00 [CD2]

OxyNorm 20mg/2ml solution for injection ampoules | 5 ampoule [PoM] £16.00 DT price = £16.00 [CD2]

Oxycodone hydrochloride 50 mg per 1 ml OxyNorm 50mg/1ml solution for injection ampoules | 5 ampoule [PoM] £70.10 DT price = £70.10 [CD2]

▌ Oxycodone with naloxone

The properties listed below are those particular to the combination only. For the properties of the components please consider, oxycodone hydrochloride p. 424, naloxone hydrochloride p. 1204.

● **INDICATIONS AND DOSE**

Severe pain requiring opioid analgesia in patients not currently treated with opioid analgesics

▸ BY MOUTH

▸ Adult: Initially 10/5 mg every 12 hours (max. per dose 40/20 mg every 12 hours), dose to be increased according to response; patients already receiving opioid analgesics can start with a higher dose

Second-line treatment of symptomatic severe to very severe idiopathic restless legs syndrome after failure of dopaminergic therapy

▸ BY MOUTH

▸ Adult: Initially 5/2.5 mg every 12 hours, adjusted weekly according to response, usual dose 10/5 mg every 12 hours; maximum 60/30 mg per day

DOSE EQUIVALENCE AND CONVERSION

Dose quantities are expressed in the form x/y where x and y are the strengths in milligrams of oxycodone and naloxone respectively.

● **MEDICINAL FORMS**

There can be variation in the licensing of different medicines containing the same drug. Forms available from special-order manufacturers include: oral suspension

Modified-release tablet

CAUTIONARY AND ADVISORY LABELS 2, 25

▸ Targinact (Napp Pharmaceuticals Ltd)

Naloxone hydrochloride 2.5 mg, Oxycodone hydrochloride 5 mg Targinact 5mg/2.5mg modified-release tablets | 28 tablet [PoM] £21.16 DT price = £21.16 [CD2]

Naloxone hydrochloride 5 mg, Oxycodone hydrochloride 10 mg Targinact 10mg/5mg modified-release tablets | 56 tablet [PoM] £42.32 DT price = £42.32 [CD2]

Naloxone hydrochloride 10 mg, Oxycodone hydrochloride 20 mg Targinact 20mg/10mg modified-release tablets | 56 tablet [PoM] £84.62 DT price = £84.62 [CD2]

Naloxone hydrochloride 20 mg, Oxycodone hydrochloride 40 mg Targinact 40mg/20mg modified-release tablets | 56 tablet [PoM] £169.28 [CD2]

4

Nervous system

Papaveretum

▼ 408

● INDICATIONS AND DOSE

Postoperative analgesia | Severe chronic pain
▸ BY SUBCUTANEOUS INJECTION, OR BY INTRAMUSCULAR
  INJECTION
▸ Adult: 7.7–15.4 mg every 4 hours if required
▸ Elderly: Initially 7.7 mg every 4 hours if required
▸ BY INTRAVENOUS INJECTION
▸ Adult: Use 25 to 50% of the corresponding
  subcutaneous/intramuscular dose

Premedication
▸ BY INTRAVENOUS INJECTION
▸ Adult: Use 25 to 50% of the corresponding
  subcutaneous/intramuscular dose

IMPORTANT SAFETY INFORMATION
Do **not** confuse with papaverine.

● CONTRA-INDICATIONS Heart failure secondary to chronic
  lung disease · phaeochromocytoma
● CAUTIONS Supraventricular tachycardia
● SIDE-EFFECTS Hypothermia
● BREAST FEEDING Therapeutic doses unlikely to affect
  infant.
● RENAL IMPAIRMENT Avoid use or reduce dose; opioid
  effects increased and prolonged and increased cerebral
  sensitivity occurs.
● PRESCRIBING AND DISPENSING INFORMATION The name
  Omnopon® was formerly used for papaveretum
  preparations.
    Papaveretum is a mixture of 253 parts of morphine
  hydrochloride, 23 parts of papaverine hydrochloride and
  20 parts of codeine hydrochloride.
● LESS SUITABLE FOR PRESCRIBING Papaveretum is less
  suitable for prescribing.

● MEDICINAL FORMS
There can be variation in the licensing of different medicines
containing the same drug. Forms available from special-order
manufacturers include: solution for injection
Solution for injection
▸ Papaveretum (Non-proprietary)
  Papaveretum 15.4 mg per 1 ml Papaveretum 15.4mg/1ml solution
  for injection ampoules | 10 ampoule [PoM] £48.96 [CD2]

Pentazocine

▼ 408

● INDICATIONS AND DOSE

Moderate to severe pain
▸ BY MOUTH
▸ Adult: 50 mg every 3–4 hours, dose to be taken
  preferably after food, usual dose 25–100 mg every
  3–4 hours; maximum 600 mg per day

Moderate pain
▸ BY SUBCUTANEOUS INJECTION, OR BY INTRAMUSCULAR
  INJECTION, OR BY INTRAVENOUS INJECTION
▸ Adult: 30 mg every 3–4 hours as required; maximum
  360 mg per day

Severe pain
▸ BY SUBCUTANEOUS INJECTION, OR BY INTRAMUSCULAR
  INJECTION, OR BY INTRAVENOUS INJECTION
▸ Adult: 45–60 mg every 3–4 hours as required;
  maximum 360 mg per day

● CONTRA-INDICATIONS Acute porphyrias p. 918 · heart
  failure secondary to chronic lung disease · patients
  dependent on opioids (can precipitate withdrawal)

● CAUTIONS Arterial hypertension · cardiac arrhythmias ·
  myocardial infarction · pancreatitis · phaeochromocytoma ·
  pulmonary hypertension
● SIDE-EFFECTS Abdominal pain · blood disorders · chills ·
  disorientation · hypertension · hypothermia · myalgia ·
  paraesthesia · raised intracranial pressure · seizures ·
  syncope · toxic epidermal necrolysis · tremor
Overdose
Effects only partially reversed by naloxone.
● BREAST FEEDING Use with caution—limited information
  available.
● RENAL IMPAIRMENT Avoid use or reduce dose; opioid
  effects increased and prolonged and increased cerebral
  sensitivity occurs.
● LESS SUITABLE FOR PRESCRIBING Pentazocine is less
  suitable for prescribing.

● MEDICINAL FORMS
There can be variation in the licensing of different medicines
containing the same drug.
Tablet
CAUTIONARY AND ADVISORY LABELS 2, 21
▸ Pentazocine (Non-proprietary)
  Pentazocine hydrochloride 25 mg Pentazocine 25mg tablets |
  28 tablet [PoM] £24.27 DT price = £24.27 [CD3]
Capsule
CAUTIONARY AND ADVISORY LABELS 2, 21
▸ Pentazocine (Non-proprietary)
  Pentazocine hydrochloride 50 mg Pentazocine 50mg capsules |
  28 capsule [PoM] £28.54 [CD3]
Solution for injection
▸ Pentazocine (Non-proprietary)
  Pentazocine (as Pentazocine lactate) 30 mg per 1 ml Pentazocine
  60mg/2ml solution for injection ampoules | 10 ampoule [PoM] £32.14
  DT price = £32.14 [CD3]

Pethidine hydrochloride

▼ 408

(Meperidine)

● INDICATIONS AND DOSE

Acute pain
▸ BY MOUTH
▸ Adult: 50–150 mg every 4 hours
▸ BY SUBCUTANEOUS INJECTION, OR BY INTRAMUSCULAR
  INJECTION
▸ Adult: 25–100 mg, then 25–100 mg after 4 hours, for
  debilitated patients use dose described for elderly
  patients
▸ Elderly: Initially 25 mg, then 25–100 mg after 4 hours
▸ BY SLOW INTRAVENOUS INJECTION
▸ Adult: 25–50 mg, then 25–50 mg after 4 hours, for
  debilitated patients use dose described for elderly
  patients
▸ Elderly: Initially 25 mg, then 25–50 mg after 4 hours

Obstetric analgesia
▸ BY SUBCUTANEOUS INJECTION, OR BY INTRAMUSCULAR
  INJECTION
▸ Adult: 50–100 mg, then 50–100 mg after 1–3 hours if
  required; maximum 400 mg per day

Premedication
▸ BY INTRAMUSCULAR INJECTION
▸ Adult: 25–100 mg, dose to be given 1 hour before
  operation, for debilitated patients use dose described
  for elderly patients
▸ Elderly: 25 mg, dose to be given 1 hour before
  operation

Postoperative pain

‣ BY SUBCUTANEOUS INJECTION, OR BY INTRAMUSCULAR INJECTION

‣ Adult: 25–100 mg every 2–3 hours if required, for debilitated patients use dose described for elderly patients

‣ Elderly: Initially 25 mg every 2–3 hours if required

● CONTRA-INDICATIONS Phaeochromocytoma

● CAUTIONS Accumulation of metabolites may result in neurotoxicity · cardiac arrhythmias · not suitable for severe continuing pain · severe cor pulmonale

● SIDE-EFFECTS Hypothermia · restlessness · tremor

Overdose
Convulsions reported in overdosage.

● BREAST FEEDING Present in milk but not known to be harmful.

● RENAL IMPAIRMENT Avoid use or reduce dose; opioid effects increased and prolonged and increased cerebral sensitivity occurs.

● MEDICINAL FORMS
There can be variation in the licensing of different medicines containing the same drug. Forms available from special-order manufacturers include: capsule, oral solution, solution for injection

Tablet
CAUTIONARY AND ADVISORY LABELS 2
‣ Pethidine hydrochloride (Non-proprietary)
Pethidine hydrochloride 50 mg Pethidine 50mg tablets | 50 tablet PoM £49.92 DT price = £49.92 CD2

Solution for injection
‣ Pethidine hydrochloride (Non-proprietary)
Pethidine hydrochloride 10 mg per 1 ml Pethidine 50mg/5ml solution for injection ampoules | 10 ampoule PoM £52.91 CD2
Pethidine hydrochloride 50 mg per 1 ml Pethidine 50mg/1ml solution for injection ampoules | 10 ampoule PoM £4.97 DT price = £4.97 CD2
Pethidine 100mg/2ml solution for injection ampoules | 10 ampoule PoM £4.66 DT price = £4.66 CD2

F 408

Tapentadol

● INDICATIONS AND DOSE

Moderate to severe acute pain which can be managed only with opioid analgesics

‣ BY MOUTH USING IMMEDIATE-RELEASE MEDICINES

‣ Adult: Initially 50 mg every 4–6 hours, adjusted according to response, maximum 700 mg in the first 24 hours, during the first 24 hours of treatment, an additional dose of 50 mg may be taken 1 hour after the initial dose, if pain control not achieved; maximum 600 mg per day

Severe chronic pain

‣ BY MOUTH USING MODIFIED-RELEASE MEDICINES

‣ Adult: Initially 50 mg every 12 hours, adjusted according to response; maximum 500 mg per day

● SIDE-EFFECTS Abdominal discomfort · anxiety · ataxia · decreased appetite · diarrhoea · dysarthria · dyspepsia · hypoaesthesia · malaise · muscle spasms · paraesthesia · seizures · tremor · weight loss

● BREAST FEEDING Avoid—no information available.

● HEPATIC IMPAIRMENT For *immediate-release tablets*, initial max. daily dose 150 mg; for *modified-release tablets*, initial max. daily dose 50 mg.

● RENAL IMPAIRMENT Manufacturer advises no dose adjustment needed in mild or moderate impairment. Avoid in severe impairment; opioid effects increased and prolonged and increased cerebral sensitivity occurs.

● NATIONAL FUNDING/ACCESS DECISIONS

Scottish Medicines Consortium (SMC) Decisions
The *Scottish Medicines Consortium* has advised (May 2011) that tapentadol (*Palexia® SR*) is accepted for restricted use within NHS Scotland for the management of severe chronic pain in adult patients, which can be adequately managed only with opioid analgesics, when morphine sulfate modified-release has failed to provide adequate pain control or is not tolerated.

● MEDICINAL FORMS
There can be variation in the licensing of different medicines containing the same drug.

Tablet
CAUTIONARY AND ADVISORY LABELS 2
‣ Palexia (Grunenthal Ltd)
Tapentadol (as Tapentadol hydrochloride) 50 mg Palexia 50mg tablets | 28 tablet PoM £12.46 DT price = £12.46 CD2 | 56 tablet PoM £24.91 CD2
Tapentadol (as Tapentadol hydrochloride) 75 mg Palexia 75mg tablets | 28 tablet PoM £18.68 DT price = £18.68 CD2 | 56 tablet PoM £37.37 CD2

Modified-release tablet
CAUTIONARY AND ADVISORY LABELS 2, 25
‣ Palexia SR (Grunenthal Ltd)
Tapentadol (as Tapentadol hydrochloride) 50 mg Palexia SR 50mg tablets | 28 tablet PoM £12.46 DT price = £12.46 CD2 | 56 tablet PoM £24.91 CD2
Tapentadol (as Tapentadol hydrochloride) 100 mg Palexia SR 100mg tablets | 56 tablet PoM £49.82 DT price = £49.82 CD2
Tapentadol (as Tapentadol hydrochloride) 150 mg Palexia SR 150mg tablets | 56 tablet PoM £74.73 DT price = £74.73 CD2
Tapentadol (as Tapentadol hydrochloride) 200 mg Palexia SR 200mg tablets | 56 tablet PoM £99.64 DT price = £99.64 CD2
Tapentadol (as Tapentadol hydrochloride) 250 mg Palexia SR 250mg tablets | 56 tablet PoM £124.55 DT price = £124.55 CD2

Oral solution
CAUTIONARY AND ADVISORY LABELS 2
EXCIPIENTS: May contain Propylene glycol
‣ Palexia (Grunenthal Ltd)
Tapentadol (as Tapentadol hydrochloride) 20 mg per 1 ml Palexia 20mg/ml oral solution sugar-free | 100 ml PoM £17.80 DT price = £17.80 CD2 sugar-free | 200 ml PoM £35.60 CD2

F 408

Tramadol hydrochloride

● INDICATIONS AND DOSE

Moderate to severe pain

‣ BY INTRAMUSCULAR INJECTION, OR BY INTRAVENOUS INJECTION, OR BY INTRAVENOUS INFUSION

‣ Adult: 50–100 mg every 4–6 hours, intravenous injection to be given over 2–3 minutes

Moderate to severe acute pain

‣ BY MOUTH USING IMMEDIATE-RELEASE MEDICINES

‣ Child 12–17 years: Initially 100 mg, then 50–100 mg every 4–6 hours; usual maximum 400 mg per day

‣ Adult: Initially 100 mg, then 50–100 mg every 4–6 hours; usual maximum 400 mg per day

Moderate to severe chronic pain

‣ BY MOUTH USING IMMEDIATE-RELEASE MEDICINES

‣ Child 12–17 years: Initially 50 mg, then adjusted according to response; usual maximum 400 mg per day

‣ Adult: Initially 50 mg, then adjusted according to response; usual maximum 400 mg per day

Postoperative pain

‣ BY INTRAVENOUS INJECTION

‣ Adult: Initially 100 mg, then 50 mg every 10–20 minutes if required up to total maximum 250 mg (including initial dose) in first hour, then 50–100 mg every 4–6 hours, intravenous injection to be given over 2–3 minutes; maximum 600 mg per day

continued →

4

Nervous system

Moderate to severe pain (with modified-release 12-hourly preparations)

▶ BY MOUTH USING MODIFIED-RELEASE MEDICINES
▸ Child 12–17 years: 50–100 mg twice daily, increased if necessary to 150–200 mg twice daily, doses exceeding the usual maximum not generally required; Usual maximum 400 micrograms/24 hours
▸ Adult: 50–100 mg twice daily, increased if necessary to 150–200 mg twice daily, doses exceeding the usual maximum not generally required; Usual maximum 400 mg/24 hours

Moderate to severe pain (with modified-release 24-hourly preparations)

▶ BY MOUTH USING MODIFIED-RELEASE MEDICINES
▸ Child 12–17 years: Initially 100–150 mg once daily, increased if necessary up to 400 mg once daily; Usual maximum 400 mg/24 hours
▸ Adult: Initially 100–150 mg once daily, increased if necessary up to 400 mg once daily; Usual maximum 400 mg/24 hours

ZYDOL® XL

Moderate to severe pain

▶ BY MOUTH USING MODIFIED-RELEASE TABLETS
▸ Child 12–17 years: Initially 150 mg once daily, increased if necessary up to 400 mg once daily
▸ Adult: Initially 150 mg once daily, increased if necessary up to 400 mg once daily

● CONTRA-INDICATIONS Acute intoxication with alcohol · acute intoxication with analgesics · acute intoxication with hypnotics · acute intoxication with opioids · not suitable for narcotic withdrawal treatment · uncontrolled epilepsy

● CAUTIONS Excessive bronchial secretions · history of epilepsy—use tramadol only if compelling reasons · impaired consciousness · not suitable as a substitute in opioid-dependent patients · not suitable in some types of general anaesthesia · susceptibility to seizures—use tramadol only if compelling reasons

  CAUTIONS, FURTHER INFORMATION
▸ General anaesthesia Not recommended for analgesia during potentially light planes of general anaesthesia (possibly increased intra-operative recall reported).

● SIDE-EFFECTS
▶ **Common or very common** Malaise
▶ **Uncommon** Diarrhoea · flatulence · gastritis · retching
▶ **Rare** Abnormal coordination · anorexia · anxiety · bronchospasm · changes in appetite · delirium · dyspnoea · hypertension · muscle weakness · nightmares · paraesthesia · seizures · syncope · tremor · wheezing
▶ **Frequency not known** Blood disorders · hypoglycaemia · speech disorders

● PREGNANCY Embryotoxic in *animal* studies—manufacturers advise avoid.

● BREAST FEEDING Amount probably too small to be harmful, but manufacturer advises avoid.

● HEPATIC IMPAIRMENT Caution (avoid for *oral drops*) in severe impairment.

● RENAL IMPAIRMENT Avoid use or reduce dose; opioid effects increased and prolonged and increased cerebral sensitivity occurs. Caution (avoid for *oral drops*) in severe impairment.

● DIRECTIONS FOR ADMINISTRATION Tramadol hydrochloride *orodispersible tablets* should be sucked and then swallowed. May also be dispersed in water. Some tramadol hydrochloride modified-release capsule preparations may be opened and the contents swallowed immediately without chewing—check individual preparations.
  For *intravenous infusion*, dilute in Glucose 5% or Sodium Chloride 0.9%.

● PRESCRIBING AND DISPENSING INFORMATION Modified-release preparations are available as 12-hourly or 24-hourly formulations. Non-proprietary preparations of modified-release tramadol may be available as either 12-hourly or 24-hourly formulations; prescribers and dispensers must ensure that the correct formulation is prescribed and dispensed. Branded preparations that should be given 12-hourly include *Invodol® SR*, *Mabron®*, *Maneo®*, *Marol®*, *Maxitram® SR*, *Oldaram®*, *Tilodol® SR*, *Tramquel® SR*, *Tramulief® SR*, *Zamadol® SR*, *Zeridame® SR* and *Zydol SR®*. Preparations that should be given 24-hourly include *Tradorec XL®*, *Zamadol®* 24hr, and *Zydol XL®*.

● PATIENT AND CARER ADVICE
Patients or carers should be given advice on how to administer tramadol hydochloride orodispersible tablets. Medicines for Children leaflet: Tramadol for pain www.medicinesforchildren.org.uk/tramadol-for-pain

● MEDICINAL FORMS
There can be variation in the licensing of different medicines containing the same drug. Forms available from special-order manufacturers include: oral suspension

Soluble tablet
CAUTIONARY AND ADVISORY LABELS 2, 13
▸ Zydol (Grunenthal Ltd)
  Tramadol hydrochloride 50 mg Zydol 50mg soluble tablets sugar-free | 20 tablet [PoM] £2.79 [CD3] sugar-free | 100 tablet [PoM] £13.33 DT price = £13.33 [CD3]

Orodispersible tablet
CAUTIONARY AND ADVISORY LABELS 2
▸ Tramadol hydrochloride (Non-proprietary)
  Tramadol hydrochloride 50 mg Tramadol 50mg orodispersible tablets sugar free sugar-free | 60 tablet [PoM] no price available [CD3]
▸ Zamadol Melt (Meda Pharmaceuticals Ltd)
  Tramadol hydrochloride 50 mg Zamadol Melt 50mg tablets sugar-free | 60 tablet [PoM] £7.12 [CD3]

Modified-release tablet
CAUTIONARY AND ADVISORY LABELS 2, 25
▸ Tramadol hydrochloride (Non-proprietary)
  Tramadol hydrochloride 50 mg Tramadol 50mg modified-release tablets | 60 tablet [PoM] no price available DT price = £4.60 [CD3]
  Tramadol hydrochloride 100 mg Tramadol 100mg modified-release tablets | 60 tablet [PoM] £44.80 [CD3]
  Tramadol hydrochloride 150 mg Tramadol 150mg modified-release tablets | 60 tablet [PoM] £57.85 [CD3]
  Tramadol hydrochloride 200 mg Tramadol 200mg modified-release tablets | 30 tablet [PoM] no price available [CD3] | 60 tablet [PoM] £69.60 [CD3]
  Tramadol hydrochloride 300 mg Tramadol 300mg modified-release tablets | 30 tablet [PoM] no price available [CD3]
  Tramadol hydrochloride 400 mg Tramadol 400mg modified-release tablets | 28 tablet [PoM] no price available [CD3] | 30 tablet [PoM] no price available [CD3]
▸ Invodol SR (Ennogen Healthcare Ltd)
  Tramadol hydrochloride 100 mg Invodol SR 100mg tablets | 60 tablet [PoM] £14.61 [CD3]
  Tramadol hydrochloride 150 mg Invodol SR 150mg tablets | 60 tablet [PoM] £21.91 [CD3]
  Tramadol hydrochloride 200 mg Invodol SR 200mg tablets | 60 tablet [PoM] £29.22 [CD3]
▸ Mabron (Morningside Healthcare Ltd)
  Tramadol hydrochloride 100 mg Mabron 100mg modified-release tablets | 60 tablet [PoM] £18.26 [CD3]
  Tramadol hydrochloride 150 mg Mabron 150mg modified-release tablets | 60 tablet [PoM] £27.39 [CD3]
  Tramadol hydrochloride 200 mg Mabron 200mg modified-release tablets | 60 tablet [PoM] £36.52 [CD3]
▸ Maneo (Mylan Ltd)
  Tramadol hydrochloride 100 mg Maneo 100mg modified-release tablets | 60 tablet [PoM] £6.95 [CD3]
  Tramadol hydrochloride 150 mg Maneo 150mg modified-release tablets | 60 tablet [PoM] £10.40 [CD3]
  Tramadol hydrochloride 200 mg Maneo 200mg modified-release tablets | 60 tablet [PoM] £14.20 [CD3]

‣ Marol (Teva UK Ltd)

Tramadol hydrochloride 100 mg Marol 100mg modified-release tablets | 60 tablet [PoM] £6.94 [CD3]

Tramadol hydrochloride 150 mg Marol 150mg modified-release tablets | 60 tablet [PoM] £10.39 [CD3]

Tramadol hydrochloride 200 mg Marol 200mg modified-release tablets | 60 tablet [PoM] £14.19 [CD3]

‣ Oldaram (Ranbaxy (UK) Ltd)

Tramadol hydrochloride 100 mg Oldaram 100mg modified-release tablets | 60 tablet [PoM] £18.80 [CD3]

Tramadol hydrochloride 150 mg Oldaram 150mg modified-release tablets | 60 tablet [PoM] £28.21 [CD3]

Tramadol hydrochloride 200 mg Oldaram 200mg modified-release tablets | 60 tablet [PoM] £37.62 [CD3]

‣ Tilodol SR (Sandoz Ltd)

Tramadol hydrochloride 100 mg Tilodol SR 100mg tablets | 60 tablet [PoM] £15.52 [CD3]

Tramadol hydrochloride 150 mg Tilodol SR 150mg tablets | 60 tablet [PoM] £23.28 [CD3]

Tramadol hydrochloride 200 mg Tilodol SR 200mg tablets | 60 tablet [PoM] £31.04 [CD3]

‣ Tradorec XL (Paladin Labs Europe Ltd)

Tramadol hydrochloride 100 mg Tradorec XL 100mg tablets | 30 tablet [PoM] £14.10 [CD3]

Tramadol hydrochloride 200 mg Tradorec XL 200mg tablets | 30 tablet [PoM] £14.98 [CD3]

Tramadol hydrochloride 300 mg Tradorec XL 300mg tablets | 30 tablet [PoM] £22.47 [CD3]

‣ Tramulief SR (AMCo)

Tramadol hydrochloride 100 mg Tramulief SR 100mg tablets | 60 tablet [PoM] £6.98 [CD3]

Tramadol hydrochloride 150 mg Tramulief SR 150mg tablets | 60 tablet [PoM] £10.48 [CD3]

Tramadol hydrochloride 200 mg Tramulief SR 200mg tablets | 60 tablet [PoM] £14.28 [CD3]

‣ Zamadol 24hr (Meda Pharmaceuticals Ltd)

Tramadol hydrochloride 150 mg Zamadol 24hr 150mg modified-release tablets | 28 tablet [PoM] £10.70 [CD3]

Tramadol hydrochloride 200 mg Zamadol 24hr 200mg modified-release tablets | 28 tablet [PoM] £14.26 [CD3]

Tramadol hydrochloride 300 mg Zamadol 24hr 300mg modified-release tablets | 28 tablet [PoM] £21.39 [CD3]

Tramadol hydrochloride 400 mg Zamadol 24hr 400mg modified-release tablets | 28 tablet [PoM] £28.51 [CD3]

‣ Zeridame SR (Actavis UK Ltd)

Tramadol hydrochloride 100 mg Zeridame SR 100mg tablets | 60 tablet [PoM] £17.21 [CD3]

Tramadol hydrochloride 150 mg Zeridame SR 150mg tablets | 60 tablet [PoM] £25.82 [CD3]

Tramadol hydrochloride 200 mg Zeridame SR 200mg tablets | 60 tablet [PoM] £34.43 [CD3]

‣ Zydol SR (Grunenthal Ltd)

Tramadol hydrochloride 50 mg Zydol SR 50mg tablets | 60 tablet [PoM] £4.60 DT price = £4.60 [CD3]

Tramadol hydrochloride 100 mg Zydol SR 100mg tablets | 60 tablet [PoM] £18.26 [CD3]

Tramadol hydrochloride 150 mg Zydol SR 150mg tablets | 60 tablet [PoM] £27.39 [CD3]

Tramadol hydrochloride 200 mg Zydol SR 200mg tablets | 60 tablet [PoM] £36.52 [CD3]

‣ Zydol XL (Grunenthal Ltd)

Tramadol hydrochloride 150 mg Zydol XL 150mg tablets | 30 tablet [PoM] £12.18 [CD3]

Tramadol hydrochloride 200 mg Zydol XL 200mg tablets | 30 tablet [PoM] £17.98 [CD3]

Tramadol hydrochloride 300 mg Zydol XL 300mg tablets | 30 tablet [PoM] £24.94 [CD3]

Tramadol hydrochloride 400 mg Zydol XL 400mg tablets | 30 tablet [PoM] £32.47 [CD3]

Capsule

CAUTIONARY AND ADVISORY LABELS 2

‣ Tramadol hydrochloride (Non-proprietary)

Tramadol hydrochloride 50 mg Tramadol 50mg capsules | 30 capsule [PoM] £4.71 DT price = £0.89 [CD3] | 100 capsule [PoM] £14.40 DT price = £2.97 [CD3]

‣ Zamadol (Meda Pharmaceuticals Ltd)

Tramadol hydrochloride 50 mg Zamadol 50mg capsules | 100 capsule [PoM] £8.00 DT price = £2.97 [CD3]

‣ Zydol (Grunenthal Ltd)

Tramadol hydrochloride 50 mg Zydol 50mg capsules | 30 capsule [PoM] £2.29 DT price = £0.89 [CD3] | 100 capsule [PoM] £7.63 DT price = £2.97 [CD3]

Modified-release capsule

CAUTIONARY AND ADVISORY LABELS 2, 25

‣ Tramadol hydrochloride (Non-proprietary)

Tramadol hydrochloride 50 mg Tramadol 50mg modified-release capsules | 60 capsule [PoM] £7.75 DT price = £7.24 [CD3]

Tramadol hydrochloride 100 mg Tramadol 100mg modified-release capsules | 60 capsule [PoM] £15.43 DT price = £14.47 [CD3]

Tramadol hydrochloride 150 mg Tramadol 150mg modified-release capsules | 60 capsule [PoM] £23.35 DT price = £21.71 [CD3]

Tramadol hydrochloride 200 mg Tramadol 200mg modified-release capsules | 60 capsule [PoM] £31.22 DT price = £28.93 [CD3]

‣ Maxitram SR (Chiesi Ltd)

Tramadol hydrochloride 50 mg Maxitram SR 50mg capsules | 60 capsule [PoM] £4.55 DT price = £7.24 [CD3]

Tramadol hydrochloride 100 mg Maxitram SR 100mg capsules | 60 capsule [PoM] £12.14 DT price = £14.47 [CD3]

Tramadol hydrochloride 150 mg Maxitram SR 150mg capsules | 60 capsule [PoM] £18.21 DT price = £21.71 [CD3]

Tramadol hydrochloride 200 mg Maxitram SR 200mg capsules | 60 capsule [PoM] £24.28 DT price = £28.93 [CD3]

‣ Tramquel SR (Beechmere Pharmaceuticals Ltd)

Tramadol hydrochloride 50 mg Tramquel SR 50mg capsules | 60 capsule [PoM] £7.24 DT price = £7.24 [CD3]

Tramadol hydrochloride 100 mg Tramquel SR 100mg capsules | 60 capsule [PoM] £14.47 DT price = £14.47 [CD3]

Tramadol hydrochloride 150 mg Tramquel SR 150mg capsules | 60 capsule [PoM] £21.71 DT price = £21.71 [CD3]

Tramadol hydrochloride 200 mg Tramquel SR 200mg capsules | 60 capsule [PoM] £28.93 DT price = £28.93 [CD3]

‣ Zamadol SR (Meda Pharmaceuticals Ltd)

Tramadol hydrochloride 50 mg Zamadol SR 50mg capsules | 60 capsule [PoM] £7.24 DT price = £7.24 [CD3]

Tramadol hydrochloride 100 mg Zamadol SR 100mg capsules | 60 capsule [PoM] £14.47 DT price = £14.47 [CD3]

Tramadol hydrochloride 150 mg Zamadol SR 150mg capsules | 60 capsule [PoM] £21.71 DT price = £21.71 [CD3]

Tramadol hydrochloride 200 mg Zamadol SR 200mg capsules | 60 capsule [PoM] £28.93 DT price = £28.93 [CD3]

Oral drops

CAUTIONARY AND ADVISORY LABELS 2, 13

‣ Tramadol hydrochloride (Non-proprietary)

Tramadol (as Tramadol hydrochloride) 100 mg per 1 ml Tramadol 100mg/ml oral drops | 10 ml [PoM] £3.50 DT price = £3.50 [CD3]

Solution for injection

‣ Tramadol hydrochloride (Non-proprietary)

Tramadol hydrochloride 50 mg per 1 ml Tramadol 100mg/2ml solution for injection ampoules | 5 ampoule [PoM] £4.90–£4.92 [CD3] | 10 ampoule [PoM] £10.00 [CD3]

‣ Zamadol (Meda Pharmaceuticals Ltd)

Tramadol hydrochloride 50 mg per 1 ml Zamadol 100mg/2ml solution for injection ampoules | 5 ampoule [PoM] £5.49 [CD3]

‣ Zydol (Grunenthal Ltd)

Tramadol hydrochloride 50 mg per 1 ml Zydol 100mg/2ml solution for injection ampoules | 5 ampoule [PoM] £4.00 [CD3]

Combinations available: _Paracetamol with tramadol_, p. 408

6.1 Headache

Drugs used for Headache not listed below Clonidine hydrochloride, p. 131 · Sumatriptan, p. 436 · Verapamil hydrochloride, p. 150

ANTIHISTAMINES > SEDATING ANTIHISTAMINES

Pizotifen

● **INDICATIONS AND DOSE**

Prevention of vascular headache | Prevention of classical migraine | Prevention of common migraine | Prevention of cluster headache

▸ BY MOUTH

▸ Adult: Initially 500 micrograms once daily, then increased to 1.5 mg once daily, dose to be increased gradually and taken at night, alternatively increased to 1.5 mg daily in 3 divided doses, doses to be increased gradually; increased if necessary up to 4.5 mg daily (max. per dose 3 mg), this dose is rarely necessary

Prophylaxis of migraine

▸ BY MOUTH

▸ Child 5–17 years: Initially 500 micrograms once daily, dose to be taken at night, then increased to up to 1.5 mg daily in divided doses, dose to be increased gradually, max. single dose (at night) 1 mg

● **UNLICENSED USE**

▸ In children 1.5 mg tablets not licensed for use in children.

● **CAUTIONS** Avoid abrupt withdrawal · history of epilepsy · susceptibility to angle-closure glaucoma · urinary retention

● **INTERACTIONS** → Appendix 1 (pizotifen).

● **SIDE-EFFECTS**

▸ **Common or very common** Dizziness · drowsiness · dry mouth · increased appetite · nausea · weight gain

▸ **Uncommon** Constipation

▸ **Rare** Aggression · anxiety · arthralgia · depression · hallucination · insomnia · myalgia · paraesthesia

▸ **Very rare** Rash (in adults) · seizures · urticaria (in adults)

▸ **Frequency not known** Hepatitis · jaundice · muscle cramps

● **PREGNANCY** Avoid unless potential benefit outweighs risk.

● **BREAST FEEDING** Amount probably too small to be harmful, but manufacturer advises avoid.

● **HEPATIC IMPAIRMENT** Use with caution.

● **RENAL IMPAIRMENT** Use with caution.

● **PATIENT AND CARER ADVICE**

Medicines for Children leaflet: Pizotifen to prevent migraine headaches www.medicinesforchildren.org.uk/pizotifen-to-prevent-migraine-headaches

Driving and skilled tasks

Drowsiness may affect performance of skilled tasks (e.g. driving); effects of alcohol enhanced.

● **MEDICINAL FORMS**

There can be variation in the licensing of different medicines containing the same drug. Forms available from special-order manufacturers include: oral suspension, oral solution

Tablet

CAUTIONARY AND ADVISORY LABELS 2

▸ Pizotifen (Non-proprietary)

Pizotifen (as Pizotifen hydrogen malate)

500 microgram Pizotifen 500microgram tablets | 28 tablet PoM £9.56 DT price = £3.56

Pizotifen (as Pizotifen hydrogen malate) 1.5 mg Pizotifen 1.5mg tablets | 28 tablet PoM £14.74 DT price = £3.70

6.1a Migraine

Migraine

Treatment of acute migraine

Treatment of a migraine attack should be guided by response to previous treatment and the severity of the attacks. A **simple analgesic** such as aspirin p. 109, paracetamol p. 406 (preferably in a soluble or dispersible form) or a NSAID is often effective; concomitant **antiemetic** treatment may be required. If treatment with an analgesic is inadequate, an attack may be treated with a specific antimigraine compound such as a **$5HT_1$-receptor agonist** ('triptan'). **Ergot alkaloids** are rarely required now; oral preparations are associated with many side-effects and should be avoided in cerebrovascular or cardiovascular disease.

Excessive use of acute treatments for migraine (opioid and non-opioid analgesics, $5HT_1$-receptor agonists, and ergotamine) is associated with medication-overuse headache (analgesic-induced headache); therefore, increasing consumption of these medicines needs careful management.

Analgesics

Most migraine headaches respond to analgesics such as aspirin or paracetamol but because peristalsis is often reduced during migraine attacks the medication may not be sufficiently well absorbed to be effective; dispersible or effervescent preparations are therefore preferred. Compound preparations containing analgesics and antiemetics are available.

The NSAID tolfenamic acid p. 432 is licensed specifically for the treatment of an acute attack of migraine; diclofenac potassium p. 980, flurbiprofen p. 986, and ibuprofen p. 987 are also licensed for use in migraine.

$5HT_1$-receptor agonists

A $5HT_1$-receptor agonist is of considerable value in the treatment of an acute migraine attack. The $5HT_1$-receptor agonists ('triptans') act on the 5HT (serotonin) 1B/1D receptors and they are therefore sometimes referred to as $5HT_{1B/1D}$-receptor agonists. A $5HT_1$-receptor agonist may be used during the established headache phase of an attack and is the preferred treatment in those who fail to respond to conventional analgesics.

The $5HT_1$-receptor agonists available for treating migraine are almotriptan p. 433, eletriptan p. 434, frovatriptan p. 434, naratriptan p. 435, rizatriptan p. 435, sumatriptan p. 436, and zolmitriptan p. 437. If a patient does not respond to one $5HT_1$-receptor agonist, an alternative 5HT1-receptor agonist should be tried. For patients who have prolonged attacks that frequently recur despite treatment with a 5HT1-receptor agonist, combination therapy with a NSAID such as naproxen can be considered. Sumatriptan or zolmitriptan are also used to treat cluster headache.

Ergot Alkaloids

The value of ergotamine tartrate p. 433 for migraine is limited by difficulties in absorption and by its side-effects, particularly nausea, vomiting, abdominal pain, and muscular cramps; it is best avoided. The recommended doses of ergotamine tartrate preparations should **not** be exceeded and treatment should **not** be repeated at intervals of less than 4 days.

To avoid habituation the frequency of administration of ergotamine tartrate should be limited to **no more than** twice a month. It should **never** be prescribed prophylactically but in the management of cluster headache a low dose is occasionally given for 1 to 2 weeks [unlicensed indication].

Antiemetics

Antiemetics, such as metoclopramide hydrochloride p. 395 or domperidone p. 394, or phenothiazine and antihistamine antiemetics, relieve the nausea associated with migraine attacks. Antiemetics may be given by intramuscular injection or rectally if vomiting is a problem. Metoclopramide hydrochloride and domperidone have the added advantage of promoting gastric emptying and normal peristalsis; a single dose should be given at the onset of symptoms. Oral analgesic preparations containing metoclopramide hydrochloride are a convenient alternative.

Prophylaxis of migraine

Where migraine attacks are frequent, possible provoking factors such as stress, irregular life-style (e.g. lack of sleep), or chemical triggers (e.g. alcohol and nitrates) should be sought; combined oral contraceptives may also provoke migraine.

Preventive treatment for migraine should be considered for patients who:

- suffer at least two attacks a month;
- suffer an increasing frequency of headaches;
- suffer significant disability despite suitable treatment for migraine attacks;
- cannot take suitable treatment for migraine attacks.

Prophylaxis is also necessary in some rare migraine subtypes and those at risk of migrainous infarction.

The beta-blockers propranolol hydrochloride p. 136, atenolol p. 138, metoprolol tartrate p. 140, nadolol p. 135, and timolol maleate p. 137 are all effective. Propranolol hydrochloride is the most commonly used.

Tricyclic antidepressants [unlicensed indication], topiramate p. 301, sodium valproate p. 298 [unlicensed indication], valproic acid p. 323 [unlicensed indication], and gabapentin p. 287 [unlicensed indication] are also effective for preventing migraine.

Pizotifen p. 430 is an antihistamine and a serotonin-receptor antagonist, structurally related to the tricyclic antidepressants. It is of limited value and may cause weight gain.

Botulinum toxin type A is licensed for the prophylaxis of headaches in adults with chronic migraine.

Cluster headache and the trigeminal autonomic cephalalgias

Cluster headache rarely responds to standard analgesics. Sumatriptan given by subcutaneous injection is the drug of choice for the *treatment* of cluster headache. If an injection is unsuitable, sumatriptan nasal spray or zolmitriptan nasal spray [both unlicensed use] may be used. Alternatively, 100% oxygen at a rate of 10–15 litres/minute for 10–20 minutes is useful in aborting an attack.

Prophylaxis of cluster headache is considered if the attacks are frequent, last over 3 weeks, or if they cannot be treated effectively. Verapamil hydrochloride p. 150 or lithium [both unlicensed use] are used for prophylaxis.

Prednisolone p. 614 can be used for short-term prophylaxis of episodic cluster headache [unlicensed use] either as monotherapy, or in combination with verapamil hydrochloride during verapamil titration.

Ergotamine tartrate, used on an intermittent basis is an alternative for patients with short bouts, but it should not be used for prolonged periods.

The other trigeminal autonomic cephalalgias, paroxysmal hemicrania (sensitive to indometacin p. 989), and short-lasting unilateral neuralgiform headache attacks with conjunctival injection and tearing, are seen rarely and are best managed by a specialist.

> **Drugs used for Migraine not listed below** Amitriptyline hydrochloride, p. 341 · Botulinum toxin type A, p. 372 · Clonidine hydrochloride, p. 131 · Trifluoperazine, p. 358

ANALGESICS > NON-OPIOID

Paracetamol with isometheptene

The properties listed below are those particular to the combination only. For the properties of the components please consider, paracetamol p. 406.

- ● **INDICATIONS AND DOSE**
  Treatment of acute attacks of migraine
  ▸ BY MOUTH
  ▸ Adult: 2 capsules, dose to be taken at onset of attack, followed by 1 capsule every 1 hour if required, maximum of 5 capsules in 12 hours

- ● PATIENT AND CARER ADVICE Patient counselling is advised (dosage).

- ● LESS SUITABLE FOR PRESCRIBING Isometheptene with paracetamol is less suitable for prescribing (more effective treatments available).

- ● MEDICINAL FORMS
  There can be variation in the licensing of different medicines containing the same drug.
  Capsule
  CAUTIONARY AND ADVISORY LABELS 30
  ▸ Midrid (DHP Healthcare Ltd)
  Isometheptene mucate 65 mg, Paracetamol 325 mg Midrid 325mg/65mg capsules | 30 capsule [PoM] £7.50

Paracetamol with metoclopramide

The properties listed below are those particular to the combination only. For the properties of the components please consider, paracetamol p. 406, metoclopramide hydrochloride p. 395.

- ● **INDICATIONS AND DOSE**
  Acute migraine
  ▸ BY MOUTH USING TABLETS
  ▸ Adult: 2 tablets, to be taken at the onset of attack, followed by 2 tablets every 4 hours if required; maximum 6 tablets per day
  ▸ BY MOUTH USING EFFERVESCENT POWDER SACHETS
  ▸ Adult: 2 sachets, to be taken at the onset of attack, followed by 2 sachets every 4 hours if required, sachets to be dissolved in a quarter tumblerful of water; maximum 6 sachets per day

  > IMPORTANT SAFETY INFORMATION
  > Metoclopramide can cause **severe extrapyramidal effects**, particularly in young adults.

- ● CAUTIONS Treatment should not exceed 3 months due to risk of tardive dyskinesia

- ● MEDICINAL FORMS
  There can be variation in the licensing of different medicines containing the same drug.
  Tablet
  CAUTIONARY AND ADVISORY LABELS 17, 30
  ▸ Paramax (Zentiva)
  Metoclopramide hydrochloride 5 mg, Paracetamol 500 mg Paramax tablets | 42 tablet [PoM] £9.64 DT price = £9.64
  Effervescent powder
  CAUTIONARY AND ADVISORY LABELS 13, 17, 30
  ▸ Paramax (Zentiva)
  Metoclopramide hydrochloride 5 mg, Paracetamol 500 mg Paramax sachets sugar-free | 42 sachet [PoM] £12.52 DT price = £12.52

4

Nervous system

ANALGESICS › NON-STEROIDAL ANTI-INFLAMMATORY DRUGS

Aspirin with metoclopramide

The properties listed below are those particular to the combination only. For the properties of the components please consider, aspirin p. 109, metoclopramide hydrochloride p. 395.

● INDICATIONS AND DOSE

Acute migraine
▶ BY MOUTH
▶ Adult: 1 sachet, sachet to be mixed in water, and dose to be taken at the start of the attack, then 1 sachet after 2 hours if required; maximum 3 sachets per day

IMPORTANT SAFETY INFORMATION

Metoclopramide can cause **severe extrapyramidal effects**, particularly in children and young adults.

● CAUTIONS Treatment should not exceed 3 months due to risk of tardive dyskinesia

● PRESCRIBING AND DISPENSING INFORMATION Flavours of oral powder formulations may include lemon.

● MEDICINAL FORMS
There can be variation in the licensing of different medicines containing the same drug.
Powder
CAUTIONARY AND ADVISORY LABELS 13, 21, 32
EXCIPIENTS: May contain Aspartame
▶ MigraMax (Zentiva)
Metoclopramide hydrochloride 10 mg, Aspirin DL-Lysine **900 mg** MigraMax oral powder sachets sugar-free | 6 sachet [PoM] £6.61 DT price = £6.61

Tolfenamic acid

● INDICATIONS AND DOSE

Treatment of acute migraine
▶ BY MOUTH
▶ Adult: 200 mg, dose to be taken at onset, then 200 mg after 1–2 hours if required

● CONTRA-INDICATIONS Active gastro-intestinal bleeding · active gastro-intestinal ulceration · history of gastro-intestinal bleeding related to previous NSAID therapy · history of gastro-intestinal haemorrhage (two or more distinct episodes) · history of gastro-intestinal perforation related to previous NSAID therapy · history of recurrent gastro-intestinal ulceration (two or more distinct episodes) · severe heart failure

● CAUTIONS Allergic disorders · cardiac impairment (NSAIDs may impair renal function) · cerebrovascular disease · coagulation defects · connective-tissue disorders · Crohn's disease (may be exacerbated) · elderly (risk of serious side-effects and fatalities) · heart failure · ischaemic heart disease · peripheral arterial disease · risk factors for cardiovascular events · ulcerative colitis (may be exacerbated) · uncontrolled hypertension

● INTERACTIONS → Appendix 1 (NSAIDs).

● SIDE-EFFECTS
▶ Rare Alveolitis · aseptic meningitis (patients with connective-tissue disorders such as systemic lupus erythematosus may be especially susceptible) · hepatic damage · interstitial fibrosis associated with NSAIDs can lead to renal failure · pancreatitis · papillary necrosis associated with NSAIDs can lead to renal failure · pulmonary eosinophilia · Stevens-Johnson syndrome · toxic epidermal necrolysis

▶ Frequency not known Angioedema · blood disorders · bronchospasm · colitis (induction of or exacerbation of) · confusion · Crohn's disease (induction of or exacerbation of) · depression · diarrhoea · dizziness · drowsiness · dysuria (most commonly in men) · euphoria · fluid retention (rarely precipitating congestive heart failure) · gastro-intestinal bleeding · gastro-intestinal discomfort · gastro-intestinal disturbances · gastro-intestinal ulceration · haematuria · hallucination · headache · hearing disturbances · hypersensitivity reactions · insomnia · malaise · nausea · nervousness · paraesthesia · photosensitivity · raised blood pressure · rashes · renal failure (especially in patients with pre-existing renal impairment) · tinnitus · tremor · vertigo · visual disturbances

SIDE-EFFECTS, FURTHER INFORMATION
▶ Serious side-effects For information about cardiovascular and gastro-intestinal side-effects, and a possible exacerbation of symptoms in asthma, see Non-steroidal anti-inflammatory drugs p. 975.

● ALLERGY AND CROSS-SENSITIVITY Contra-indicated in patients with a history of hypersensitivity to aspirin or any other NSAID—which includes those in whom attacks of asthma, angioedema, urticaria or rhinitis have been precipitated by aspirin or any other NSAID.

● CONCEPTION AND CONTRACEPTION Caution—long-term use of some NSAIDs is associated with reduced female fertility, which is reversible on stopping treatment.

● PREGNANCY Avoid unless the potential benefit outweighs the risk. Avoid during the third trimester (risk of closure of fetal ductus arteriosus *in utero* and possibly persistent pulmonary hypertension of the newborn); onset of labour may be delayed and duration may be increased.

● BREAST FEEDING Amount too small to be harmful. Use with caution during breast-feeding.

● HEPATIC IMPAIRMENT Use with caution; there is an increased risk of gastro-intestinal bleeding and fluid retention. Avoid in severe liver disease.

● RENAL IMPAIRMENT The lowest effective dose should be used for the shortest possible duration. Avoid if possible or use with caution. In renal impairment monitor renal function; sodium and water retention may occur and renal function may deteriorate, possibly leading to renal failure.

● MEDICINAL FORMS
There can be variation in the licensing of different medicines containing the same drug.
Tablet
CAUTIONARY AND ADVISORY LABELS 21
▶ Tolfenamic acid (Non-proprietary)
Tolfenamic acid **200 mg** Tolfenamic acid 200mg tablets | 10 tablet [PoM] £19.25 DT price = £19.25
▶ Clotam Rapid (Galen Ltd)
Tolfenamic acid **200 mg** Clotam Rapid 200mg tablets | 10 tablet [PoM] £12.75 DT price = £19.25

ANTIHISTAMINES › SEDATING ANTIHISTAMINES

Paracetamol with buclizine hydrochloride and codeine phosphate

The properties listed below are those particular to the combination only. For the properties of the components please consider, paracetamol p. 406, codeine phosphate p. 413.

● INDICATIONS AND DOSE

MIGRALEVE®

Acute migraine
▶ BY MOUTH
▶ Child 12–14 years: Initially 1 tablet, (pink tablet) to be taken at onset of attack, or if it is imminent, followed

by 1 tablet every 4 hours if required, (yellow tablet) to be taken following initial dose; maximum 1 pink and 3 yellow tablets in 24 hours

▸ Child 15–17 years: Initially 2 tablets, (pink tablets) to be taken at onset of attack or if it is imminent, followed by 2 tablets every 4 hours if required, (yellow tablets) to be taken following initial dose; maximum 2 pink and 6 yellow tablets in 24 hours

▸ Adult: Initially 2 tablets, (pink tablets) to be taken at onset of attack or if it is imminent, followed by 2 tablets every 4 hours if required, (yellow tablets) to be taken following initial dose; maximum 2 pink and 6 yellow tablets in 24 hours

● LESS SUITABLE FOR PRESCRIBING
MIGRALEVE® *Migraleve*® is less suitable for prescribing.

● MEDICINAL FORMS
There can be variation in the licensing of different medicines containing the same drug.
Tablet
CAUTIONARY AND ADVISORY LABELS 2, 17, 30
▸ Migraleve Pink (McNeil Products Ltd)
Buclizine hydrochloride 6.25 mg, Codeine phosphate 8 mg, Paracetamol 500 mg Migraleve Pink tablets | 32 tablet PoM no price available Schedule 5 (CD Inv) | 48 tablet PoM £3.97 Schedule 5 (CD Inv)
CAUTIONARY AND ADVISORY LABELS 2, 17, 30
▸ Migraleve (McNeil Products Ltd)
Migraleve tablets | 48 tablet PoM £3.64 Schedule 5 (CD Inv)

ERGOT ALKALOIDS

Ergotamine tartrate

● INDICATIONS AND DOSE
Management of cluster headache
▸ BY MOUTH USING TABLETS
▸ Adult: 1 mg once daily for 6 nights in 7; occasionally given for 1–2 weeks, dose to be taken at night

● UNLICENSED USE Not licensed for the management of cluster headache.

● CONTRA-INDICATIONS Acute porphyrias p. 918 · coronary heart disease · hyperthyroidism · inadequately controlled hypertension · obliterative vascular disease · peripheral vascular disease · Raynaud's syndrome · sepsis · severe hypertension · temporal arteritis

● CAUTIONS Anaemia · cardiac disease · dependence · elderly · risk of peripheral vasospasm

● INTERACTIONS → Appendix 1 (ergot alkaloids).

● SIDE-EFFECTS
▸ **Common or very common** Abdominal pain · dizziness · nausea · vomiting
▸ **Uncommon** Cyanosis · diarrhoea · hypoaesthesia · pain in extremities · paraesthesia · peripheral vasoconstriction · weakness in extremities
▸ **Rare** Arrhythmias · bradycardia · dyspnoea · ergotism (including absence of pulse and numbness in extremities) · increased blood pressure · intestinal ischaemia · myalgia · rash · tachycardia · urticaria
▸ **Very rare** Gangrene · heart-valve fibrosis · myocardial infarction · myocardial ischaemia
▸ **Frequency not known** Anxiety · arthralgia · blood disorders · blurred vision · cerebral ischaemia · confusion · constipation · depression · drowsiness · dry mouth · extrapyramidal effects · hallucinations · renal artery spasm · seizures · sleep disturbances · thrombosis · tremor · urinary retention

● PREGNANCY Avoid; oxytocic effect on the uterus.

● BREAST FEEDING Avoid; ergotism may occur in infant; repeated doses may inhibit lactation.

● HEPATIC IMPAIRMENT Avoid in severe impairment—risk of toxicity increased.

● RENAL IMPAIRMENT Avoid; risk of renal vasoconstriction.

● PATIENT AND CARER ADVICE
Peripheral vasospasm Warn patient to stop treatment immediately if numbness or tingling of extremities develops and to contact doctor.

● LESS SUITABLE FOR PRESCRIBING Ergotamine tartrate is less suitable for prescribing.

● MEDICINAL FORMS
There can be variation in the licensing of different medicines containing the same drug.
No licensed medicines listed.

Ergotamine tartrate with caffeine hydrate and cyclizine hydrochloride

The properties listed below are those particular to the combination only. For the properties of the components please consider, ergotamine tartrate above, cyclizine p. 393.

● INDICATIONS AND DOSE
Treatment of acute migraine and migraine variants unresponsive to analgesics
▸ BY MOUTH
▸ Adult: 1 tablet, to be taken at onset, followed by 0.5–1 tablet after 30 minutes, then 0.5–1 tablet every 30 minutes if required, max. 3 tablets in 24 hours, max. 4 tablets per attack, max. 6 tablets in one week

● PATIENT AND CARER ADVICE Patient counselling is advised for cyclizine hydrochloride with caffeine hydrate and ergotamine tartrate tablets (dosage).

● LESS SUITABLE FOR PRESCRIBING Cyclizine hydrochloride with caffeine hydrate and ergotamine tartrate (*Migril*®) is less suitable for prescribing.

● MEDICINAL FORMS
There can be variation in the licensing of different medicines containing the same drug.
Tablet
CAUTIONARY AND ADVISORY LABELS 2, 18
▸ Migril (Wockhardt UK Ltd)
Ergotamine tartrate 2 mg, Cyclizine hydrochloride 50 mg, Caffeine hydrate 100 mg Migril tablets | 100 tablet PoM £51.00

TRIPTANS

Almotriptan

● INDICATIONS AND DOSE
Treatment of acute migraine
▸ BY MOUTH
▸ Adult: 12.5 mg, dose to be taken as soon as possible after onset, followed by 12.5 mg after 2 hours if required, dose to be taken only if migraine recurs (patient not responding to initial dose should not take second dose for same attack); maximum 25 mg per day

● UNLICENSED USE Not licensed for use in elderly.

● CONTRA-INDICATIONS Coronary vasospasm · ischaemic heart disease · peripheral vascular disease · previous cerebrovascular accident · previous myocardial infarction · previous transient ischaemic attack · Prinzmetal's angina · severe hypertension · uncontrolled hypertension

● CAUTIONS Conditions which predispose to coronary artery disease · elderly

● INTERACTIONS → Appendix 1 (5HT$_1$ agonists).

● SIDE-EFFECTS
▸ **Common or very common** Drowsiness · transient increase in blood pressure
▸ **Uncommon** Bone pain · chest pain · diarrhoea · dry mouth · dyspepsia · headache · myalgia · palpitation · paraesthesia · tinnitus
▸ **Very rare** Myocardial infarction · tachycardia
▸ **Frequency not known** Dizziness · fatigue · feeling of weakness · flushing · nausea · seizures · vomiting
SIDE-EFFECTS, FURTHER INFORMATION
Sensations of tingling, heat, heaviness, pressure, or tightness of any part of the body may occur (including throat and chest—discontinue if intense, may be due to coronary vasoconstriction or to anaphylaxis).

● ALLERGY AND CROSS-SENSITIVITY Caution in patients with sensitivity to sulfonamides.
● PREGNANCY There is limited experience of using 5HT₁-receptor agonists during pregnancy; manufacturers advise that they should be avoided unless the potential benefit outweighs the risk.
● BREAST FEEDING Present in milk in *animal* studies—withhold breast-feeding for 24 hours.
● HEPATIC IMPAIRMENT Caution in mild to moderate impairment. Avoid in severe impairment.
● RENAL IMPAIRMENT Max. 12.5 mg in 24 hours if eGFR less than 30 mL/minute/1.73 m².

● MEDICINAL FORMS
There can be variation in the licensing of different medicines containing the same drug.
Tablet
CAUTIONARY AND ADVISORY LABELS 3
▸ Almotriptan (Non-proprietary)
Almotriptan (as Almotriptan hydrogen malate)
12.5 mg Almotriptan 12.5mg tablets | 3 tablet [PoM] £9.07 | 6 tablet [PoM] £18.14 DT price = £18.14 | 9 tablet [PoM] £27.21
▸ Almogran (Almirall Ltd)
Almotriptan (as Almotriptan hydrogen malate) 12.5 mg Almogran 12.5mg tablets | 3 tablet [PoM] £9.07 | 6 tablet [PoM] £18.14 DT price = £18.14 | 9 tablet [PoM] £27.20

Eletriptan

● INDICATIONS AND DOSE
Treatment of acute migraine
▸ BY MOUTH
▸ Adult: 40 mg, followed by 40 mg after 2 hours if required, dose to be taken only if migraine recurs (patient not responding to initial dose should not take second dose for same attack); increased if necessary to 80 mg, dose to be taken for subsequent attacks if 40 mg dose inadequate; maximum 80 mg per day

● UNLICENSED USE Not licensed for use in elderly.
● CONTRA-INDICATIONS Arrhythmias · coronary vasospasm · heart failure · ischaemic heart disease · peripheral vascular disease · previous cerebrovascular accident · previous myocardial infarction · previous transient ischaemic attack · Prinzmetal's angina · severe hypertension · uncontrolled hypertension
● CAUTIONS Conditions which predispose to coronary artery disease · elderly
● INTERACTIONS → Appendix 1 (5HT₁ agonists).
● SIDE-EFFECTS
▸ **Common or very common** Abdominal pain · chills · drowsiness · dry mouth · dyspepsia · headache · myalgia · myasthenia · palpitation · pharyngitis · rhinitis · sweating · tachycardia
▸ **Uncommon** Agitation · anorexia · arthralgia · confusion · depersonalisation · depression · diarrhoea · dysarthria · dyspnoea · euphoria · glossitis · hypertonia · insomnia ·

movement disorders · oedema · photophobia · pruritus · rash · stupor · taste disturbance · thirst · tinnitus · tremor · urinary frequency · visual disturbances · yawning
▸ **Rare** Asthma · bradycardia · constipation · lymphadenopathy · menorrhagia · oesophagitis · syncope
▸ **Frequency not known** Dizziness · fatigue · feeling of weakness · flushing · hypertension · ischaemic colitis · nausea · vomiting
SIDE-EFFECTS, FURTHER INFORMATION
Sensations of tingling, heat, heaviness, pressure, or tightness of any part of the body may occur (including throat and chest—discontinue if intense, may be due to coronary vasoconstriction or to anaphylaxis).

● PREGNANCY There is limited experience of using 5HT₁-receptor agonists during pregnancy; manufacturers advise that they should be avoided unless the potential benefit outweighs the risk.
● BREAST FEEDING Present in milk—avoid breast-feeding for 24 hours.
● HEPATIC IMPAIRMENT Avoid in severe impairment.
● RENAL IMPAIRMENT Reduce initial dose to 20 mg; maximum 40 mg in 24 hours. Avoid if eGFR less than 30 mL/minute/1.73 m².

● MEDICINAL FORMS
There can be variation in the licensing of different medicines containing the same drug.
Tablet
CAUTIONARY AND ADVISORY LABELS 3
▸ Relpax (Pfizer Ltd)
Eletriptan (as Eletriptan hydrobromide) 20 mg Relpax 20mg tablets | 6 tablet [PoM] £22.50 DT price = £22.50
Eletriptan (as Eletriptan hydrobromide) 40 mg Relpax 40mg tablets | 6 tablet [PoM] £22.50 DT price = £22.50

Frovatriptan

● INDICATIONS AND DOSE
Treatment of acute migraine
▸ BY MOUTH
▸ Adult: 2.5 mg, dose to be taken as soon as possible after onset, followed by 2.5 mg after 2 hours if required, dose to be taken only if migraine recurs (patient not responding to initial dose should not take second dose for same attack); maximum 5 mg per day

● UNLICENSED USE Not licensed for use in elderly.
● CONTRA-INDICATIONS Coronary vasospasm · ischaemic heart disease · peripheral vascular disease · previous cerebrovascular attack · previous myocardial infarction · previous transient ischaemic attack · Prinzmetal's angina · severe hypertension · uncontrolled hypertension
● CAUTIONS Conditions which predispose to coronary artery disease · elderly
● INTERACTIONS → Appendix 1 (5HT₁ agonists).
● SIDE-EFFECTS
▸ **Common or very common** Abdominal pain · drowsiness · dry mouth · dyspepsia · headache · paraesthesia · sweating · visual disturbances
▸ **Uncommon** Agitation · anxiety · arthralgia · asthenia · confusion · dehydration · depersonalisation · depression · diarrhoea · dysphagia · flatulence · hypertension · impaired concentration · insomnia · laryngitis · micturition disorders · muscle stiffness · nervousness · palpitation · pharyngitis · pruritus · rhinitis · sinusitis · tachycardia · taste disturbances · thirst · tinnitus · tremor · vertigo
▸ **Rare** Abnormal dreams · amnesia · bilirubinaemia · bradycardia · breast tenderness · constipation · epistaxis · gastro-oesophageal reflux · hiccup · hypertonia · hyperventilation · hypocalcaemia · hypoglycaemia ·

hypotonia · irritable bowel syndrome · peptic ulcer · purpura · pyrexia · stomatitis · urticaria
‣ **Frequency not known** Dizziness · fatigue · feeling of weakness · flushing · nausea · vomiting
SIDE-EFFECTS, FURTHER INFORMATION
Sensations of tingling, heat, heaviness, pressure, or tightness of any part of the body may occur (including throat and chest—discontinue if intense, may be due to coronary vasoconstriction or to anaphylaxis).

● PREGNANCY There is limited experience of using $5HT_1$-receptor agonists during pregnancy; manufacturers advise that they should be avoided unless the potential benefit outweighs the risk.

● BREAST FEEDING Present in milk in *animal* studies—withhold breast-feeding for 24 hours.

● HEPATIC IMPAIRMENT Avoid in severe impairment.

● MEDICINAL FORMS
There can be variation in the licensing of different medicines containing the same drug.
Tablet
CAUTIONARY AND ADVISORY LABELS 3
‣ Frovatriptan (Non-proprietary)
**Frovatriptan (as Frovatriptan succinate monohydrate)
2.5 mg** Frovatriptan 2.5mg tablets | 6 tablet [PoM] £15.84–£16.67 DT price = £16.50
‣ Migard (A. Menarini Farmaceutica Internazionale SRL)
**Frovatriptan (as Frovatriptan succinate monohydrate)
2.5 mg** Migard 2.5mg tablets | 6 tablet [PoM] £16.67 DT price = £16.50

Naratriptan

● **INDICATIONS AND DOSE**

Treatment of acute migraine
‣ BY MOUTH
‣ Adult: 2.5 mg, followed by 2.5 mg after at least 4 hours if required, to be taken only if migraine recurs (patient not responding to initial dose should not take second dose for same attack); maximum 5 mg per day

● UNLICENSED USE Not licensed for use in elderly.

● CONTRA-INDICATIONS Coronary vasospasm · ischaemic heart disease · moderate or severe hypertension · peripheral vascular disease · previous cerebrovascular accident · previous myocardial infarction · previous transient ischaemic attack · Prinzmetal's angina · uncontrolled hypertension

● CAUTIONS Conditions which predispose to coronary artery disease · elderly

● INTERACTIONS → Appendix 1 ($5HT_1$ agonists).

● SIDE-EFFECTS
‣ **Uncommon** Bradycardia · palpitation · tachycardia · visual disturbance
‣ **Rare** Ischaemic colitis · pruritus · rash
‣ **Frequency not known** Dizziness · fatigue · feeling of weakness · flushing · nausea · vomiting
SIDE-EFFECTS, FURTHER INFORMATION
Sensations of tingling, heat, heaviness, pressure, or tightness of any part of the body may occur (including throat and chest—discontinue if intense, may be due to coronary vasoconstriction or to anaphylaxis).

● ALLERGY AND CROSS-SENSITIVITY Caution in patients with sensitivity to sulfonamides.

● PREGNANCY There is limited experience of using $5HT_1$-receptor agonists during pregnancy; manufacturers advise that they should be avoided unless the potential benefit outweighs the risk.

● BREAST FEEDING Withhold breast-feeding for 24 hours.

● HEPATIC IMPAIRMENT Max. 2.5 mg in 24 hours in moderate impairment. Avoid if severe.

● RENAL IMPAIRMENT Max. 2.5 mg in 24 hours. Avoid if eGFR less than 15 mL/minute/1.73 m^2.

● PATIENT AND CARER ADVICE
Driving and skilled tasks
Drowsiness may affect performance of skilled tasks (e.g. driving).

● MEDICINAL FORMS
There can be variation in the licensing of different medicines containing the same drug.
Tablet
CAUTIONARY AND ADVISORY LABELS 3
‣ Naratriptan (Non-proprietary)
Naratriptan (as Naratriptan hydrochloride) 2.5 mg Naratriptan 2.5mg tablets | 6 tablet [PoM] £25.00 DT price = £1.81 | 12 tablet [PoM] £46.64
‣ Naramig (GlaxoSmithKline UK Ltd)
Naratriptan (as Naratriptan hydrochloride) 2.5 mg Naramig 2.5mg tablets | 6 tablet [PoM] £24.55 DT price = £1.81

Rizatriptan

● **INDICATIONS AND DOSE**

Treatment of acute migraine
‣ BY MOUTH
‣ Adult: 10 mg, dose to be taken as soon as possible after onset, followed by 10 mg after 2 hours if required, dose to be taken only if migraine recurs (patient not responding to initial dose should not take second dose for same attack); maximum 20 mg per day

● UNLICENSED USE Not licensed for use in elderly.

● CONTRA-INDICATIONS Coronary vasospasm · ischaemic heart disease · peripheral vascular disease · previous cerebrovascular accident · previous myocardial infarction · previous transient ischaemic attack · Prinzmetal's angina · severe hypertension · uncontrolled hypertension

● CAUTIONS Conditions which predispose to coronary artery disease · elderly

● INTERACTIONS → Appendix 1 ($5HT_1$ agonists).

● SIDE-EFFECTS
‣ **Common or very common** Decreased alertness · diarrhoea · drowsiness · dry mouth · dyspnoea · headache · palpitation · paraesthesia · pharyngeal discomfort · sweating · tachycardia · tremor
‣ **Uncommon** Arrhythmias · ataxia · blurred vision · confusion · dyspepsia · hypertension · insomnia · muscle weakness · myalgia · nervousness · pruritus · taste disturbances · thirst · urticaria · vertigo
‣ **Rare** Bradycardia · syncope
‣ **Frequency not known** Dizziness · fatigue · feeling of weakness · flushing · nausea · seizures · toxic epidermal necrolysis · vomiting
SIDE-EFFECTS, FURTHER INFORMATION
Sensations of tingling, heat, heaviness, pressure, or tightness of any part of the body may occur (including throat and chest—discontinue if intense, may be due to coronary vasoconstriction or to anaphylaxis).

● PREGNANCY There is limited experience of using $5HT_1$-receptor agonists during pregnancy; manufacturers advise that they should be avoided unless the potential benefit outweighs the risk.

● BREAST FEEDING Present in milk in *animal* studies—withhold breast-feeding for 24 hours.

● HEPATIC IMPAIRMENT Reduce dose to 5 mg in mild to moderate impairment. Avoid in severe impairment.

● RENAL IMPAIRMENT Reduce dose to 5 mg in mild to moderate impairment. Avoid in severe impairment.

4

Nervous system

- DIRECTIONS FOR ADMINISTRATION Rizatriptan orodispersible tablets should be placed on the tongue, allowed to disperse and swallowed. Rizatriptan oral lyophilisates should be placed on the tongue and allowed to dissolve.
- PATIENT AND CARER ADVICE
Patients or carers should be given advice on how to administer rizatriptan orodispersible tablets and oral lyophilisates.
Driving and skilled tasks
Drowsiness may affect performance of skilled tasks (e.g. driving).

- MEDICINAL FORMS
There can be variation in the licensing of different medicines containing the same drug.
Tablet
CAUTIONARY AND ADVISORY LABELS 3
▸ Rizatriptan (Non-proprietary)
Rizatriptan (as Rizatriptan benzoate) 5 mg Rizatriptan 5mg tablets | 3 tablet [PoM] £13.37 | 6 tablet [PoM] £26.74 DT price = £26.74
Rizatriptan (as Rizatriptan benzoate) 10 mg Rizatriptan 10mg tablets | 3 tablet [PoM] £13.37 DT price = £1.54 | 6 tablet [PoM] £26.74
▸ Maxalt (Merck Sharp & Dohme Ltd)
Rizatriptan (as Rizatriptan benzoate) 5 mg Maxalt 5mg tablets | 6 tablet [PoM] £26.74 DT price = £26.74
Rizatriptan (as Rizatriptan benzoate) 10 mg Maxalt 10mg tablets | 3 tablet [PoM] £13.37 DT price = £1.54 | 6 tablet [PoM] £26.74
Orodispersible tablet
CAUTIONARY AND ADVISORY LABELS 3
EXCIPIENTS: May contain Aspartame
▸ Rizatriptan (Non-proprietary)
Rizatriptan (as Rizatriptan benzoate) 10 mg Rizatriptan 10mg orodispersible tablets sugar free | 3 tablet [PoM] £13.37 DT price = £2.19 sugar-free | 6 tablet [PoM] £26.74
Oral lyophilisate
CAUTIONARY AND ADVISORY LABELS 3
EXCIPIENTS: May contain Aspartame
▸ Maxalt Melt (Merck Sharp & Dohme Ltd)
Rizatriptan (as Rizatriptan benzoate) 10 mg Maxalt Melt 10mg oral lyophilisates sugar-free | 3 tablet [PoM] £13.37 DT price = £13.37 sugar-free | 6 tablet [PoM] £26.74 DT price = £26.74 sugar-free | 12 tablet [PoM] £53.48

Sumatriptan

- INDICATIONS AND DOSE
Treatment of acute migraine
▸ BY MOUTH
▸ Adult: Initially 50–100 mg for 1 dose, followed by 50–100 mg after at least 2 hours if required, to be taken only if migraine recurs (patient not responding to initial dose should not take second dose for same attack); maximum 300 mg per day
▸ BY SUBCUTANEOUS INJECTION
▸ Adult: Initially 6 mg for 1 dose, followed by 6 mg after at least 1 hour if required, to be taken only if migraine recurs (patient not responding to initial dose should not take second dose for same attack), dose to be administered using an auto-injector; not for intravenous injection which may cause coronary vasospasm and angina; maximum 12 mg per day
▸ BY INTRANASAL ADMINISTRATION
▸ Adult 18–65 years: Initially 10–20 mg, to be administered into one nostril, followed by 10–20 mg after at least 2 hours if required, to be taken only if migraine recurs (patient not responding to initial dose should not take second dose for same attack); maximum 40 mg per day

Treatment of acute cluster headache
▸ BY SUBCUTANEOUS INJECTION
▸ Adult: Initially 6 mg for 1 dose, followed by 6 mg after at least 1 hour if required, to be taken only if headache recurs (patient not responding to initial dose should not take second dose for same attack), dose to be administered using an auto-injector; not for intravenous injection which may cause coronary vasospasm and angina; maximum 12 mg per day
▸ BY INTRANASAL ADMINISTRATION
▸ Adult 18–65 years: Initially 10–20 mg, dose to be administered into one nostril, followed by 10–20 mg after at least 2 hours if required, to be taken only if headache recurs (patient not responding to initial dose should not take second dose for same attack); maximum 40 mg per day

- UNLICENSED USE Not licensed for use in elderly.
- CONTRA-INDICATIONS Coronary vasospasm · ischaemic heart disease · mild uncontrolled hypertension · moderate and severe hypertension · peripheral vascular disease · previous cerebrovascular accident · previous myocardial infarction · previous transient ischaemic attack · Prinzmetal's angina
- CAUTIONS Conditions which predispose to coronary artery disease · elderly · history of seizures · mild, controlled hypertension · pre-existing cardiac disease · risk factors for seizures
- INTERACTIONS → Appendix 1 ($5HT_1$ agonists).
- SIDE-EFFECTS
GENERAL SIDE-EFFECTS
▸ Common or very common Dizziness · drowsiness · dyspnoea · fatigue · flushing · myalgia · nausea · sensory disturbances · transient increase in blood pressure · vomiting · weakness
▸ Frequency not known Arrhythmias · angina · anxiety · arthralgia · bradycardia · diarrhoea · dystonia · hypersensitivity reactions · hypotension · ischaemic colitis · myocardial infarction · neck stiffness · nystagmus · palpitation · Raynaud's syndrome · seizures · sweating · tachycardia · transient ischaemic ECG changes · tremor · visual disturbances
SPECIFIC SIDE-EFFECTS
▸ Common or very common
▸ With intranasal use Dysgeusia · epistaxis
SIDE-EFFECTS, FURTHER INFORMATION
Sensations of tingling, heat, heaviness, pressure, or tightness of any part of the body may occur (including throat and chest—discontinue if intense, may be due to coronary vasoconstriction or to anaphylaxis).
- ALLERGY AND CROSS-SENSITIVITY Caution in patients with sensitivity to sulfonamides.
- PREGNANCY There is limited experience of using $5HT_1$-receptor agonists during pregnancy; manufacturers advise that they should be avoided unless the potential benefit outweighs the risk.
- BREAST FEEDING Present in milk but amount probably too small to be harmful; withhold breast-feeding for 12 hours after treatment.
- HEPATIC IMPAIRMENT Reduce oral dose to 25–50 mg. Avoid in severe impairment.
- RENAL IMPAIRMENT Use with caution.
- PATIENT AND CARER ADVICE
Driving and skilled tasks
Drowsiness may affect performance of skilled tasks (e.g. driving).
- EXCEPTIONS TO LEGAL CATEGORY
▸ With oral use Sumatriptan 50 mg tablets can be sold to the public to treat previously diagnosed migraine; max. daily dose 100 mg.

● MEDICINAL FORMS
There can be variation in the licensing of different medicines containing the same drug.

Tablet
CAUTIONARY AND ADVISORY LABELS 3, 10
▸ Sumatriptan (Non-proprietary)
  Sumatriptan (as Sumatriptan succinate) 50 mg Sumatriptan 50mg tablets | 6 tablet [PoM] £22.56 DT price = £1.20
  Sumatriptan (as Sumatriptan succinate) 100 mg Sumatriptan 100mg tablets | 6 tablet [PoM] £36.47 DT price = £1.47
▸ Imigran (GlaxoSmithKline UK Ltd, Forest Laboratories UK Ltd)
  Sumatriptan (as Sumatriptan succinate) 50 mg Imigran Radis 50mg tablets | 6 tablet [PoM] £23.90 DT price = £1.20
  Imigran 50mg tablets | 6 tablet [PoM] £31.85 DT price = £1.20
  Imigran Recovery 50mg tablets | 2 tablet [P] £4.76
  Sumatriptan (as Sumatriptan succinate) 100 mg Imigran 100mg tablets | 6 tablet [PoM] £51.48 DT price = £1.47
  Imigran Radis 100mg tablets | 6 tablet [PoM] £42.90 DT price = £1.47
▸ Migraitan (Bristol Laboratories Ltd)
  Sumatriptan (as Sumatriptan succinate) 50 mg Migraitan 50mg tablets | 2 tablet [P] £4.24

Solution for injection
CAUTIONARY AND ADVISORY LABELS 3, 10
▸ Sumatriptan (Non-proprietary)
  Sumatriptan (as Sumatriptan succinate) 12 mg per 1 ml Sumatriptan 6mg/0.5ml solution for injection pre-filled pen | 2 pre-filled disposable injection [PoM] £39.50 DT price = £39.50
▸ Imigran Subject (GlaxoSmithKline UK Ltd)
  Sumatriptan (as Sumatriptan succinate) 12 mg per 1 ml Imigran Subject 6mg/0.5ml solution for injection syringe refill pack | 2 pre-filled disposable injection [PoM] £40.41 DT price = £40.41
  Imigran Subject 6mg/0.5ml solution for injection pre-filled syringes with device | 2 pre-filled disposable injection [PoM] £42.47 DT price = £42.47

Spray
CAUTIONARY AND ADVISORY LABELS 3, 10
▸ Imigran (GlaxoSmithKline UK Ltd)
  Sumatriptan 100 mg per 1 ml Imigran 10mg nasal spray | 2 unit dose [PoM] £11.80 DT price = £11.80
  Sumatriptan 200 mg per 1 ml Imigran 20mg nasal spray | 2 unit dose [PoM] £14.16 | 6 unit dose [PoM] £35.39 DT price = £35.39

Zolmitriptan

● INDICATIONS AND DOSE
Treatment of acute migraine
▸ BY MOUTH
▸ Adult: 2.5 mg, followed by 2.5 mg after at least 2 hours if required, dose to be taken only if migraine recurs, then increased if necessary to 5 mg, dose to be taken only for subsequent attacks in patients not achieving satisfactory relief with 2.5 mg dose; maximum 10 mg per day
▸ BY INTRANASAL ADMINISTRATION
▸ Adult: 5 mg, dose to be administered as soon as possible after onset into one nostril only, followed by 5 mg after at least 2 hours if required, dose to be administered only if migraine recurs; maximum 10 mg per day

Treatment of acute cluster headache
▸ BY INTRANASAL ADMINISTRATION
▸ Adult: 5 mg, dose to be administered as soon as possible after onset into one nostril only, followed by 5 mg after at least 2 hours if required, dose to be administered only if migraine recurs; maximum 10 mg per day

DOSE ADJUSTMENTS DUE TO INTERACTIONS
Max. 5 mg in 24 hours with concomitant cimetidine, fluvoxamine, moclobemide, or quinolone antibiotics.

DOSE EQUIVALENCE AND CONVERSION
1 spray of *Zomig*® nasal spray = 5 mg zolmitriptan.

● UNLICENSED USE Not licensed for use in elderly. Not licensed for treatment of cluster headaches.

● CONTRA-INDICATIONS Arrhythmias associated with accessory cardiac conduction pathways · coronary vasospasm · ischaemic heart disease · previous cerebrovascular accident · previous myocardial infarction · Prinzmetal's angina · severe hypertension · transient ischaemic attack · uncontrolled hypertension · Wolff-Parkinson-White syndrome

● CAUTIONS Conditions which predispose to coronary artery disease · elderly · should not be taken within 24 hours of any other 5HT₁-receptor agonist

● INTERACTIONS → Appendix 1 (5HT₁ agonists).

● SIDE-EFFECTS
GENERAL SIDE-EFFECTS
▸ **Common or very common** Abdominal pain · drowsiness · dry mouth · dysphagia · headache · muscle weakness · myalgia · palpitation · paraesthesia
▸ **Uncommon** Polyuria · tachycardia · transient increase in blood pressure
▸ **Rare** Urticaria
▸ **Very rare** Angina · gastro-intestinal infarction · ischaemic colitis · myocardial infarction · splenic infarction
▸ **Frequency not known** Dizziness · fatigue · feeling of weakness · flushing
SPECIFIC SIDE-EFFECTS
▸ With intranasal use Epistaxis · taste disturbance
SIDE-EFFECTS, FURTHER INFORMATION
Sensations of tingling, heat, heaviness, pressure, or tightness of any part of the body may occur (including throat and chest—discontinue if intense, may be due to coronary vasoconstriction or to anaphylaxis).

● PREGNANCY There is limited experience of using 5HT₁-receptor agonists during pregnancy; manufacturers advise that they should be avoided unless the potential benefit outweighs the risk.

● BREAST FEEDING Use with caution—present in milk in *animal* studies.

● HEPATIC IMPAIRMENT Max. 5 mg in 24 hours in moderate or severe impairment.

● DIRECTIONS FOR ADMINISTRATION Zolmitriptan orodispersible tablets should be placed on the tongue, allowed to disperse and swallowed.

● PATIENT AND CARER ADVICE Patients or carers should be given advice on how to administer zolmitriptan orodispersible tablets.

● MEDICINAL FORMS
There can be variation in the licensing of different medicines containing the same drug.

Tablet
▸ Zolmitriptan (Non-proprietary)
  Zolmitriptan 2.5 mg Zolmitriptan 2.5mg tablets | 6 tablet [PoM] £16.20 DT price = £1.55 | 12 tablet [PoM] £3.42
  Zolmitriptan 5 mg Zolmitriptan 5mg tablets | 6 tablet [PoM] £3.60 | 12 tablet [PoM] £7.20
▸ Zomig (AstraZeneca UK Ltd)
  Zolmitriptan 2.5 mg Zomig 2.5mg tablets | 6 tablet [PoM] £23.94 DT price = £1.55

Orodispersible tablet
EXCIPIENTS: May contain Aspartame
▸ Zolmitriptan (Non-proprietary)
  Zolmitriptan 2.5 mg Zolmitriptan 2.5mg orodispersible tablets sugar free sugar-free | 6 tablet [PoM] £1.58 DT price = £1.43
  Zolmitriptan 5 mg Zolmitriptan 5mg orodispersible tablets sugar free sugar-free | 6 tablet [PoM] £11.49 DT price = £11.11
▸ Zomig Rapimelt (AstraZeneca UK Ltd)
  Zolmitriptan 2.5 mg Zomig Rapimelt 2.5mg orodispersible tablets sugar-free | 6 tablet [PoM] £23.99 DT price = £1.43
  Zolmitriptan 5 mg Zomig Rapimelt 5mg orodispersible tablets sugar-free | 6 tablet [PoM] £23.94 DT price = £11.11

Spray
▸ Zomig (AstraZeneca UK Ltd)
  Zolmitriptan 50 mg per 1 ml Zomig 5mg/0.1ml nasal spray 0.1ml unit dose | 6 unit dose [PoM] £36.50 DT price = £36.50

6.2 Neuropathic pain

Neuropathic pain

Overview and management

Neuropathic pain, which occurs as a result of damage to neural tissue, includes *phantom limb pain*, *compression neuropathies*, *peripheral neuropathies* (e.g. due to diabetes, chronic excessive alcohol intake, HIV infection, chemotherapy, idiopathic neuropathy), *trauma*, *central pain* (e.g. pain following stroke, spinal cord injury, and syringomyelia), and *postherpetic neuralgia* (peripheral nerve damage following acute herpes zoster infection (shingles)). The pain may occur in an area of sensory deficit and is sometimes accompanied by pain that is evoked by a non-noxious stimulus (allodynia).

Trigeminal neuralgia is also caused by dysfunction of neural tissue, but its management is distinct from other forms of neuropathic pain.

Neuropathic pain is generally managed with a **tricyclic antidepressant** or with certain **antiepileptic drugs**. Amitriptyline hydrochloride p. 341 [unlicensed indication] and pregabalin p. 295 are effective treatments for neuropathic pain. Amitriptyline hydrochloride and pregabalin can be used in combination if the patient has an inadequate response to either drug at the maximum tolerated dose.

Nortriptyline p. 347 [unlicensed indication] may be better tolerated than amitriptyline hydrochloride.

Gabapentin p. 287 is also effective for the treatment of neuropathic pain.

Neuropathic pain may respond to **opioid analgesics**. There is evidence of efficacy for tramadol hydrochloride p. 427, morphine p. 421, and oxycodone hydrochloride p. 424; however, treatment with morphine or oxycodone hydrochloride should be initiated only under specialist supervision. Tramadol hydrochloride can be prescribed when other treatments have been unsuccessful, while the patient is waiting for assessment by a specialist.

Patients with localised pain who are unable to take oral medicines may benefit from **topical local anaesthetic preparations**, such as lidocaine hydrochloride medicated plasters p. 1187, while awaiting specialist review.

Capsaicin below is licensed for neuropathic pain (but the intense burning sensation during initial treatment may limit use). Capsaicin 0.075% cream is licensed for the symptomatic relief of *postherpetic neuralgia*. A self-adhesive patch containing capsaicin 8% is licensed for the treatment of peripheral neuropathic pain in non-diabetic patients. It should be used under specialist supervision.

A corticosteroid may help to relieve pressure in compression neuropathy and thereby reduce pain.

Neuromodulation by spinal cord stimulation may be of benefit in some patients. Many patients with chronic neuropathic pain require multidisciplinary management, including physiotherapy and psychological support.

Trigeminal neuralgia

Surgery may be the treatment of choice in many patients; a neurological assessment will identify those who stand to benefit. Carbamazepine p. 283 taken during the acute stages of trigeminal neuralgia, reduces the frequency and severity of attacks. It is very effective for the severe pain associated with trigeminal neuralgia and (less commonly) glossopharyngeal neuralgia. Blood counts and electrolytes should be monitored when high doses are given. Small doses should be used initially to reduce the incidence of side-effects e.g. dizziness. Some cases respond to phenytoin p. 294; the drug may be given by intravenous infusion (possibly as fosphenytoin sodium p. 286) in a crisis (specialist use only).

Chronic facial pain

Chronic oral and facial pain including *persistent idiopathic facial pain* (also termed 'atypical facial pain') and *temporomandibular dysfunction* (previously termed temporomandibular joint pain dysfunction syndrome) may call for prolonged use of analgesics or for other drugs. **Tricyclic antidepressants** may be useful for facial pain [unlicensed indication], but are not on the Dental Practitioners' List. Disorders of this type require specialist referral and psychological support to accompany drug treatment. Patients on long-term therapy need to be monitored both for progress and for side-effects.

> **Drugs used for Neuropathic pain not listed below**
> Amantadine hydrochloride, p. 382

ANALGESICS > PLANT ALKALOIDS

Capsaicin

● **INDICATIONS AND DOSE**

AXSAIN®

Post-herpetic neuralgia

▶ TO THE SKIN
▸ **Adult:** Apply 3–4 times a day, dose to be applied sparingly; **important; after** lesions have healed, not more often than every 4 hours

Painful diabetic neuropathy (under expert supervision)

▶ TO THE SKIN
▸ **Adult:** Apply 3–4 times a day for 8 weeks then review, dose to be applied sparingly, not more often than every 4 hours

QUTENZA®

Peripheral neuropathic pain in non-diabetic patients (under the supervision of a physician)

▶ BY TRANSDERMAL APPLICATION USING PATCHES
▸ **Adult:** (consult product literature)

ZACIN®

Symptomatic relief in osteoarthritis

▶ TO THE SKIN
▸ **Adult:** Apply 4 times a day, dose to be applied sparingly, not more often than every 4 hours

● **CAUTIONS**

GENERAL CAUTIONS
Avoid contact with broken skin · avoid contact with inflamed skin

SPECIFIC CAUTIONS
▸ With topical use Avoid contact with eyes · avoid hot shower or bath just before or after application (burning sensation enhanced) · avoid inhalation of vapours · not to be used under tight bandages
▸ With transdermal use Avoid contact with the face, scalp or in proximity to mucous membranes · avoid holding near eyes or mucous membranes · recent cardiovascular events · uncontrolled hypertension

● **SIDE-EFFECTS**
▸ **Common or very common**
▸ With topical use Transient burning sensation during initial treatment (particularly if too much used or if administered less than 3–4 times daily)
▸ With transdermal use Application site reactions · erythema · pruritus · transient burning
▸ **Uncommon**
▸ With transdermal use Burning sensation · cough · dysgeusia · eye irritation · first degree AV block · hypertension · hypoaesthesia · muscle spasm · nausea · pain in extremities

· palpitations · peripheral oedema · pruritus · tachycardia · throat irritation

▶ **Rare**

▶ With topical use Cough · eye irritation · sneezing

▶ **Frequency not known**

▶ With topical use Dyspnoea · exacerbation of asthma

● MONITORING REQUIREMENTS

▶ With transdermal use Monitor blood pressure during treatment procedure.

● HANDLING AND STORAGE

▶ With topical use Wash hands immediately after use (or wash hands 30 minutes after application if hands treated).

▶ With transdermal use Nitrile gloves to be worn while handling patches and cleaning treatment areas (latex gloves do not provide adequate protection).

● NATIONAL FUNDING/ACCESS DECISIONS

QUTENZA®

Scottish Medicines Consortium (SMC) Decisions

The *Scottish Medicines Consortium* has advised (January 2011) that capsaicin 179 mg (8%) patch (*Qutenza*®) is accepted for restricted use in NHS Scotland for the treatment of postherpetic neuralgia in patients who have not achieved adequate pain relief from, or who have not tolerated conventional first and second line treatments. Treatment should be under the supervision of a specialist in pain management.

● MEDICINAL FORMS

There can be variation in the licensing of different medicines containing the same drug. Forms available from special-order manufacturers include: cream

Cream

EXCIPIENTS: May contain Benzyl alcohol, cetostearyl alcohol (including cetyl and stearyl alcohol)

▶ Axsain (Teva UK Ltd)
Capsaicin 750 microgram per 1 gram Axsain 0.075% cream | 45 gram [PoM] £14.58 DT price = £14.58

▶ Zacin (Teva UK Ltd)
Capsaicin 250 microgram per 1 gram Zacin 0.025% cream | 45 gram [PoM] £17.71 DT price = £17.71

Cutaneous patch

EXCIPIENTS: May contain Butylated hydroxyanisole

▶ Qutenza (Astellas Pharma Ltd)
Capsaicin 179 mg Qutenza 179mg cutaneous patches | 1 patch [PoM] £210.00

7 Sleep disorders

7.1 Insomnia

Hypnotics and anxiolytics

Overview

Most anxiolytics ('sedatives') will induce sleep when given at night and most hypnotics will sedate when given during the day. Prescribing of these drugs is widespread but dependence (both physical and psychological) and tolerance occur. This may lead to difficulty in withdrawing the drug after the patient has been taking it regularly for more than a few weeks. Hypnotics and anxiolytics should therefore be reserved for short courses to alleviate acute conditions after causal factors have been established.

Benzodiazepines are the most commonly used anxiolytics and hypnotics; they act at benzodiazepine receptors which are associated with gamma-aminobutyric acid (GABA) receptors. Older drugs such as meprobamate p. 316 and barbiturates are **not** recommended—they have more side-effects and interactions than benzodiazepines and are much more dangerous in overdosage.

Benzodiazepine indications

● Benzodiazepines are indicated for the short-term relief (two to four weeks only) of anxiety that is severe, disabling, or causing the patient unacceptable distress, occurring alone or in association with insomnia or short-term psychosomatic, organic, or psychotic illness.

● The use of benzodiazepines to treat short-term 'mild' anxiety is inappropriate.

● Benzodiazepines should be used to treat insomnia only when it is severe, disabling, or causing the patient extreme distress.

Dependence and withdrawal

Withdrawal of a benzodiazepine should be gradual because abrupt withdrawal may produce confusion, toxic psychosis, convulsions, or a condition resembling delirium tremens. The benzodiazepine withdrawal syndrome may develop at any time up to 3 weeks after stopping a long-acting benzodiazepine, but may occur within a day in the case of a short-acting one. It is characterised by insomnia, anxiety, loss of appetite and of body-weight, tremor, perspiration, tinnitus, and perceptual disturbances. Some symptoms may be similar to the original complaint and encourage further prescribing; some symptoms may continue for weeks or months after stopping benzodiazepines.

Benzodiazepine withdrawal should be flexible and carried out at a reduction rate that is tolerable for the patient. The rate should depend on the initial dose of benzodiazepine, duration of use, and the patient's clinical response. Short-term users of benzodiazepines (2–4 weeks only) can usually taper off within 2–4 weeks. However, long-term users should be withdrawn over a much longer period of several months or more.

A suggested protocol for withdrawal for prescribed long-term benzodiazepine patients is as follows:

● Transfer patient stepwise, one dose at a time over about a week, to an equivalent daily dose of diazepam preferably taken at night.

● Reduce diazepam dose, usually by 1–2 mg every 2–4 weeks (in patients taking high doses of benzodiazepines, initially it may be appropriate to reduce the dose by up to one-tenth every 1–2 weeks). If uncomfortable withdrawal symptoms occur, maintain this dose until symptoms lessen.

● Reduce diazepam dose further, if necessary in smaller steps; steps of 500 micrograms may be appropriate towards the end of withdrawal. Then stop completely.

● For long-term patients, the period needed for complete withdrawal may vary from several months to a year or more.

Approximate equivalent doses, diazepam 5 mg
≡ alprazolam 250 micrograms
≡ clobazam 10 mg
≡ clonazepam 250 micrograms
≡ flurazepam 7.5–15 mg
≡ chlordiazepoxide 12.5 mg
≡ loprazolam 0.5–1 mg
≡ lorazepam 500 micrograms
≡ lormetazepam 0.5–1 mg
≡ nitrazepam 5 mg
≡ oxazepam 10 mg
≡ temazepam 10 mg

Withdrawal symptoms for long-term users usually resolve within 6–18 months of the last dose. Some patients will recover more quickly, others may take longer. The addition of beta-blockers, antidepressants and antipsychotics should be **avoided** where possible.

Counselling can be of considerable help both during and after the taper.

4

Nervous system

Hypnotics

Before a hypnotic is prescribed the cause of the insomnia should be established and, where possible, underlying factors should be treated. However, it should be noted that some patients have unrealistic sleep expectations, and others understate their alcohol consumption which is often the cause of the insomnia. Short-acting hypnotics are preferable in patients with sleep onset insomnia, when sedation the following day is undesirable, or when prescribing for elderly patients. Long-acting hypnotics are indicated in patients with poor sleep maintenance (e.g. early morning waking) that causes daytime effects, when an anxiolytic effect is needed during the day, or when sedation the following day is acceptable.

Transient insomnia may occur in those who normally sleep well and may be due to extraneous factors such as noise, shift work, and jet lag. If a hypnotic is indicated one that is rapidly eliminated should be chosen, and only one or two doses should be given.

Short-term insomnia is usually related to an emotional problem or serious medical illness. It may last for a few weeks and may recur; a hypnotic can be useful but should not be given for more than three weeks (preferably only one week). Intermittent use is desirable with omission of some doses. A short-acting drug is usually appropriate.

Chronic insomnia is rarely benefited by hypnotics and is sometimes due to mild dependence caused by injudicious prescribing of hypnotics. Psychiatric disorders such as anxiety, depression, and abuse of drugs and alcohol are common causes. Sleep disturbance is very common in depressive illness and early wakening is often a useful pointer. The underlying psychiatric complaint should be treated, adapting the drug regimen to alleviate insomnia. For example, clomipramine hydrochloride p. 342 or mirtazapine p. 340 prescribed for depression will also help to promote sleep if taken at night. Other causes of insomnia include daytime cat-napping and physical causes such as pain, pruritus, and dyspnoea.

Hypnotics should **not** be prescribed indiscriminately and routine prescribing is undesirable. They should be reserved for short courses in the acutely distressed. Tolerance to their effects develops within 3 to 14 days of continuous use and long-term efficacy cannot be assured. A major drawback of long-term use is that withdrawal can cause rebound insomnia and a withdrawal syndrome.

Where prolonged administration is unavoidable hypnotics should be discontinued as soon as feasible and the patient warned that sleep may be disturbed for a few days before normal rhythm is re-established; broken sleep with vivid dreams may persist for several weeks.

Elderly

Benzodiazepines and the Z–drugs should be avoided in the elderly, because the elderly are at greater risk of becoming ataxic and confused, leading to falls and injury.

Dental patients

Some anxious patients may benefit from the use of hypnotics during dental procedures such as temazepam p. 443 or diazepam p. 313. Temazepam is preferred when it is important to minimise any residual effect the following day.

Benzodiazepines

Benzodiazepines used as hypnotics include nitrazepam p. 442 and flurazepam p. 441 which have a prolonged action and may give rise to residual effects on the following day; repeated doses tend to be cumulative.

Loprazolam p. 441, lormetazepam p. 442, and temazepam act for a shorter time and they have little or no hangover effect. Withdrawal phenomena are more common with the short-acting benzodiazepines.

If insomnia is associated with daytime anxiety then the use of a long-acting benzodiazepine anxiolytic such as diazepam given as a single dose at night may effectively treat both symptoms.

Zaleplon, zolpidem, and zopiclone

Zaleplon p. 445, zolpidem tartrate p. 446 and zopiclone p. 446 are non-benzodiazepine hypnotics (sometimes referred to as Z-drugs), but they act at the benzodiazepine receptor. They are not licensed for long-term use; dependence has been reported in a small number of patients. Zolpidem tartrate and zopiclone have a short duration of action; zaleplon is very short acting.

Chloral and derivatives

There is no convincing evidence that they are particularly useful in the elderly and their role as hypnotics is now very limited.

Clomethiazole

Clomethiazole p. 444 may be a useful hypnotic for elderly patients because of its freedom from hangover but, as with all hypnotics, routine administration is undesirable and dependence occurs.

Antihistamines

Some **antihistamines** such as promethazine hydrochloride p. 264 are on sale to the public for occasional insomnia; their prolonged duration of action can often cause drowsiness the following day. The sedative effect of antihistamines may diminish after a few days of continued treatment; antihistamines are associated with headache, psychomotor impairment and antimuscarinic effects.

Alcohol

Alcohol is a poor hypnotic because the diuretic action interferes with sleep during the latter part of the night. Alcohol also disturbs sleep patterns, and so can worsen sleep disorders.

Melatonin

Melatonin p. 445 is a pineal hormone; it is licensed for the short-term treatment of insomnia in adults over 55 years.

Anxiolytics

Benzodiazepine anxiolytics can be effective in alleviating anxiety states. Although these drugs are sometimes prescribed for stress-related symptoms, unhappiness, or minor physical disease, their use in such conditions is inappropriate. Benzodiazepine anxiolytics should not be used as sole treatment for chronic anxiety, and they are not appropriate for treating depression or chronic psychosis. In bereavement, psychological adjustment may be inhibited by benzodiazepines.

Anxiolytic benzodiazepine treatment should be limited to the lowest possible dose for the shortest possible time. Dependence is particularly likely in patients with a history of alcohol or drug abuse and in patients with marked personality disorders.

Some antidepressant drugs are licensed for use in anxiety and related disorders. Some antipsychotic drugs, in low doses, are also sometimes used in severe anxiety for their sedative action, but long-term use should be avoided because of the risk of adverse effects. The use of antihistamines (e.g. hydroxyzine hydrochloride p. 262) for their sedative effect in anxiety is not appropriate.

Beta-adrenoceptor blocking drugs do not affect psychological symptoms of anxiety, such as worry, tension, and fear, but they do reduce autonomic symptoms, such as palpitation and tremor; they do not reduce non-autonomic symptoms, such as muscle tension. Beta-blockers are therefore indicated for patients with predominantly somatic symptoms; this, in turn, may prevent the onset of worry and fear.

Benzodiazepines

Benzodiazepines are indicated for the *short-term relief of severe anxiety*; long-term use should be avoided. Diazepam, alprazolam p. 312, chlordiazepoxide hydrochloride p. 313, and clobazam p. 306 have a sustained action. Shorter-acting compounds such as lorazepam p. 308 and oxazepam p. 315 may be preferred in patients with hepatic impairment but they carry a greater risk of withdrawal symptoms.

In *panic disorders* (with or without agoraphobia) resistant to antidepressant therapy, a benzodiazepine may be used; alternatively, a benzodiazepine may be used as short-term adjunctive therapy at the start of antidepressant treatment to prevent the initial worsening of symptoms.

Diazepam or lorazepam are very occasionally administered intravenously for the *control of panic attacks*. This route is the most rapid but the procedure is not without risk and should be used only when alternative measures have failed. The intramuscular route has no advantage over the oral route.

Buspirone

Buspirone hydrochloride p. 311 is thought to act at specific serotonin (5HT$_{1A}$) receptors. Response to treatment may take up to 2 weeks. It does not alleviate the symptoms of benzodiazepine withdrawal. Therefore a patient taking a benzodiazepine still needs to have the benzodiazepine withdrawn gradually; it is advisable to do this before starting buspirone hydrochloride. The dependence and abuse potential of buspirone hydrochloride is low; it is, however, licensed for short-term use only (but specialists occasionally use it for several months).

Meprobamate

Meprobamate p. 316 is **less effective** than the benzodiazepines, more hazardous in overdosage, and can also induce dependence. It is **not** recommended.

Barbiturates

The intermediate-acting **barbiturates** have a place only in the treatment of severe intractable insomnia in patients **already taking** barbiturates; they should be **avoided** in the elderly. Intermediate-acting barbiturate preparations containing amobarbital sodium, butobarbital, and secobarbital sodium are available on a named patient basis.

The long-acting barbiturate phenobarbital is still sometimes of value in epilepsy but its use as a sedative is unjustified.

The very short-acting barbiturate thiopental sodium p. 308 is used in anaesthesia.

Increased hostility and aggression after barbiturates and alcohol usually indicates intoxication.

HYPNOTICS, SEDATIVES AND ANXIOLYTICS > BENZODIAZEPINES

🗲 312

Flurazepam

● **INDICATIONS AND DOSE**

Insomnia (short-term use)
▸ BY MOUTH
▸ Adult: 15–30 mg once daily, dose to be taken at bedtime, for debilitated patients, use elderly dose
▸ Elderly: 15 mg once daily, dose to be taken at bedtime

● CONTRA-INDICATIONS Not for use alone to treat chronic psychosis · not for use alone to treat depression (or anxiety associated with depression) · respiratory depression
● CAUTIONS Acute porphyrias p. 918 · hypoalbuminaemia · marked personality disorder · muscle weakness
  CAUTIONS, FURTHER INFORMATION
▸ Paradoxical effects A paradoxical increase in hostility and aggression may be reported by patients taking benzodiazepines. The effects range from talkativeness and excitement to aggressive and antisocial acts. Adjustment of the dose (up or down) sometimes attenuates the

impulses. Increased anxiety and perceptual disorders are other paradoxical effects.

● SIDE-EFFECTS
▸ **Common or very common** Amnesia · ataxia (especially in the elderly) · confusion (especially in the elderly) · dependence · drowsiness the next day · lightheadedness the next day · muscle weakness · paradoxical increase in aggression
▸ **Uncommon** Changes in libido · dizziness · dysarthria · gastro-intestinal disturbances · gynaecomastia · headache · hypotension · incontinence · salivation changes · slurred speech · tremor · urinary retention · vertigo · visual disturbances
▸ **Rare** Apnoea · blood disorders · jaundice · respiratory depression · skin reactions
● BREAST FEEDING Benzodiazepines are present in milk, and should be avoided if possible during breast-feeding.
● HEPATIC IMPAIRMENT Start with smaller initial doses or reduce dose. Can precipitate coma. If treatment is necessary, benzodiazepines with shorter half-lives (such as temazepam or oxazepam) are safer.
  Avoid in severe impairment.
● RENAL IMPAIRMENT Start with small doses in severe impairment.
● PATIENT AND CARER ADVICE
  Driving and skilled tasks
  May impair judgement and increase reaction time, and so affect ability to drive or operate machinery; they increase the effects of alcohol. Moreover the hangover effects of a night dose may impair driving on the following day.
● NATIONAL FUNDING/ACCESS DECISIONS
  NHS restrictions Flurazepam capsules are not prescribable under the NHS.

● MEDICINAL FORMS
  There can be variation in the licensing of different medicines containing the same drug.
  Capsule
  CAUTIONARY AND ADVISORY LABELS 19
  ▸ Dalmane (Meda Pharmaceuticals Ltd)
    Flurazepam (as Flurazepam hydrochloride) 15 mg Dalmane 15mg capsules | 30 capsule PoM £6.73 CD4-1
    Flurazepam (as Flurazepam hydrochloride) 30 mg Dalmane 30mg capsules | 30 capsule PoM £8.63 CD4-1

🗲 312

Loprazolam

● **INDICATIONS AND DOSE**

Insomnia (short-term use)
▸ BY MOUTH
▸ Adult: 1 mg once daily, then increased to 1.5–2 mg once daily if required, dose to be taken at bedtime, for debilitated patients, use elderly dose
▸ Elderly: 0.5–1 mg once daily, dose to be taken at bedtime

● CONTRA-INDICATIONS Not for use alone to treat chronic psychosis · not for use alone to treat depression (or anxiety associated with depression) · respiratory depression
● CAUTIONS Acute porphyrias p. 918 · hypoalbuminaemia · marked personality disorder · muscle weakness
  CAUTIONS, FURTHER INFORMATION
▸ Paradoxical effects A paradoxical increase in hostility and aggression may be reported by patients taking benzodiazepines. The effects range from talkativeness and excitement to aggressive and antisocial acts. Adjustment of the dose (up or down) sometimes attenuates the impulses. Increased anxiety and perceptual disorders are other paradoxical effects.

- SIDE-EFFECTS
▸ **Common or very common** Amnesia · ataxia (especially in the elderly) · confusion (especially in the elderly) · dependence · drowsiness the next day · lightheadedness the next day · muscle weakness · paradoxical increase in aggression
▸ **Uncommon** Changes in libido · dizziness · dysarthria · gastro-intestinal disturbances · gynaecomastia · headache · hypotension · incontinence · salivation changes · slurred speech · tremor · urinary retention · vertigo · visual disturbances
▸ **Rare** Apnoea · blood disorders · jaundice · respiratory depression · skin reactions
- BREAST FEEDING Benzodiazepines are present in milk, and should be avoided if possible during breast-feeding.
- HEPATIC IMPAIRMENT Start with smaller initial doses or reduce dose. Can precipitate coma. If treatment is necessary, benzodiazepines with shorter half-lives (such as temazepam or oxazepam) are safer.
   Avoid in severe impairment.
- RENAL IMPAIRMENT Start with small doses in severe impairment.
- PATIENT AND CARER ADVICE
Driving and skilled tasks
May impair judgement and increase reaction time, and so affect ability to drive or operate machinery; they increase the effects of alcohol. Moreover the hangover effects of a night dose may impair driving on the following day.

- MEDICINAL FORMS
There can be variation in the licensing of different medicines containing the same drug.
Tablet
CAUTIONARY AND ADVISORY LABELS 19
▸ Loprazolam (Non-proprietary)
   Loprazolam (as Loprazolam mesilate) 1 mg Loprazolam 1mg tablets | 28 tablet [PoM] £18.00 DT price = £18.00 [CD4-1]

 ⌀ 312

Lormetazepam

- INDICATIONS AND DOSE
Insomnia (short-term use)
▸ BY MOUTH
▸ Adult: 0.5–1.5 mg once daily, dose to be taken at bedtime, for debilitated patients, use elderly dose
▸ Elderly: 500 micrograms once daily, dose to be taken at bedtime

- CONTRA-INDICATIONS Not for use alone to treat chronic psychosis · not for use alone to treat depression (or anxiety associated with depression) · respiratory depression
- CAUTIONS Acute porphyrias p. 918 · hypoalbuminaemia · marked personality disorder · muscle weakness
   CAUTIONS, FURTHER INFORMATION
▸ Paradoxical effects A paradoxical increase in hostility and aggression may be reported by patients taking benzodiazepines. The effects range from talkativeness and excitement to aggressive and antisocial acts. Adjustment of the dose (up or down) sometimes attenuates the impulses. Increased anxiety and perceptual disorders are other paradoxical effects.
- SIDE-EFFECTS
▸ **Common or very common** Amnesia · ataxia (especially in the elderly) · confusion (especially in the elderly) · dependence · drowsiness the next day · lightheadedness the next day · muscle weakness · paradoxical increase in aggression
▸ **Uncommon** Changes in libido · dizziness · dysarthria · gastro-intestinal disturbances · gynaecomastia · headache · hypotension · incontinence · salivation changes · slurred

speech · tremor · urinary retention · vertigo · visual disturbances
▸ **Rare** Apnoea · blood disorders · jaundice · respiratory depression · skin reactions
- BREAST FEEDING Benzodiazepines are present in milk, and should be avoided if possible during breast-feeding.
- HEPATIC IMPAIRMENT Start with smaller initial doses or reduce dose. Can precipitate coma. If treatment is necessary, benzodiazepines with shorter half-lives (such as temazepam or oxazepam) are safer.
   Avoid in severe impairment.
- RENAL IMPAIRMENT Start with small doses in severe impairment.
- PATIENT AND CARER ADVICE
Driving and skilled tasks
May impair judgement and increase reaction time, and so affect ability to drive or operate machinery; they increase the effects of alcohol. Moreover the hangover effects of a night dose may impair driving on the following day.

- MEDICINAL FORMS
There can be variation in the licensing of different medicines containing the same drug. Forms available from special-order manufacturers include: oral suspension
Tablet
CAUTIONARY AND ADVISORY LABELS 19
▸ Lormetazepam (Non-proprietary)
   Lormetazepam 500 microgram Lormetazepam 500microgram tablets | 30 tablet [PoM] £64.17 DT price = £15.25 [CD4-1]
   Lormetazepam 1 mg Lormetazepam 1mg tablets | 30 tablet [PoM] £48.83 DT price = £11.16 [CD4-1]

 ⌀ 312

Nitrazepam

- INDICATIONS AND DOSE
Insomnia (short-term use)
▸ BY MOUTH
▸ Adult: 5–10 mg daily, dose to be taken at bedtime, for debilitated patients, use elderly dose
▸ Elderly: 2.5–5 mg daily, dose to be taken at bedtime

- CONTRA-INDICATIONS Not for use alone to treat chronic psychosis · not for use alone to treat depression (or anxiety associated with depression) · respiratory depression
- CAUTIONS Acute porphyrias p. 918 · hypoalbuminaemia · marked personality disorder · muscle weakness
   CAUTIONS, FURTHER INFORMATION
▸ Paradoxical effects A paradoxical increase in hostility and aggression may be reported by patients taking benzodiazepines. The effects range from talkativeness and excitement to aggressive and antisocial acts. Adjustment of the dose (up or down) sometimes attenuates the impulses. Increased anxiety and perceptual disorders are other paradoxical effects.
- SIDE-EFFECTS
▸ **Common or very common** Amnesia · ataxia (especially in the elderly) · confusion (especially in the elderly) · dependence · drowsiness the next day · lightheadedness the next day · muscle weakness · paradoxical increase in aggression
▸ **Uncommon** Changes in libido · dizziness · dysarthria · gastro-intestinal disturbances · gynaecomastia · headache · hypotension · incontinence · salivation changes · slurred speech · tremor · urinary retention · vertigo · visual disturbances
▸ **Rare** Apnoea · blood disorders · jaundice · respiratory depression · skin reactions
- BREAST FEEDING Benzodiazepines are present in milk, and should be avoided if possible during breast-feeding.
- HEPATIC IMPAIRMENT Start with smaller initial doses or reduce dose. Can precipitate coma. If treatment is

4

Nervous system

necessary, benzodiazepines with shorter half-lives (such as temazepam or oxazepam) are safer.

Avoid in severe impairment.

- RENAL IMPAIRMENT Start with small doses in severe impairment.
- PATIENT AND CARER ADVICE

Driving and skilled tasks

May impair judgement and increase reaction time, and so affect ability to drive or operate machinery; they increase the effects of alcohol. Moreover the hangover effects of a night dose may impair driving on the following day.

- MEDICINAL FORMS

There can be variation in the licensing of different medicines containing the same drug. Forms available from special-order manufacturers include: oral suspension

Tablet

CAUTIONARY AND ADVISORY LABELS 19

- Nitrazepam (Non-proprietary)

  Nitrazepam 5 mg Nitrazepam 5mg tablets | 28 tablet [PoM] £10.55 DT price = £1.26 [CD4-1] | 500 tablet [PoM] £24.82 [CD4-1]

- Mogadon (Meda Pharmaceuticals Ltd)

  Nitrazepam 5 mg Mogadon 5mg tablets | 30 tablet [PoM] £5.76 [CD4-1]

Oral suspension

CAUTIONARY AND ADVISORY LABELS 19

- Nitrazepam (Non-proprietary)

  Nitrazepam 500 microgram per 1 ml Nitrazepam 2.5mg/5ml oral suspension | 70 ml [PoM] £114.00 DT price = £114.00 [CD4-1]

▶ 312

Temazepam

- INDICATIONS AND DOSE

Insomnia (short-term use)

▶ BY MOUTH

- Adult: 10–20 mg once daily, alternatively 30–40 mg once daily, higher dose range only to be administered in exceptional circumstances, dose to be taken at bedtime, for debilitated patients, use elderly dose
- Elderly: 10 mg once daily, alternatively 20 mg once daily, higher dose only to be administered in exceptional circumstances, dose to be taken at bedtime

Conscious sedation for dental procedures

▶ BY MOUTH

- Adult: 15–30 mg, to be administered 30–60 minutes before procedure

Premedication before surgery or investigatory procedures

▶ BY MOUTH

- Adult: 10–20 mg, to be taken 1–2 hours before procedure, alternatively 30 mg, to be taken 1–2 hours before procedure, higher alternate dose only administered in exceptional circumstances
- Elderly: 10 mg, to be taken 1–2 hours before procedure, alternatively 20 mg, to be taken 1–2 hours before procedure, higher alternate dose only administered in exceptional circumstances

- UNLICENSED USE Temazepam doses in BNF may differ from those in product literature.

  Not licensed for conscious sedation for dental procedures.

- CONTRA-INDICATIONS CNS depression · compromised airway · hyperkinesis · not for use alone to treat chronic psychosis · not for use alone to treat depression (or anxiety associated with depression) · obsessional state · phobic states · respiratory depression

- CAUTIONS Hypoalbuminaemia · muscle weakness · organic brain changes · personality disorder (within the fearful group—dependent, avoidant, obsessive-compulsive)—may increase risk of dependence

CAUTIONS, FURTHER INFORMATION

▶ **Paradoxical effects** A paradoxical increase in hostility and aggression may be reported by patients taking benzodiazepines. The effects range from talkativeness and excitement to aggressive and antisocial acts. Adjustment of the dose (up or down) sometimes attenuates the impulses. Increased anxiety and perceptual disorders are other paradoxical effects.

- SIDE-EFFECTS

▶ **Common or very common** Amnesia · ataxia (especially in the elderly) · confusion (especially in the elderly) · dependence · drowsiness the next day · lightheadedness the next day · muscle weakness · paradoxical increase in aggression

▶ **Uncommon** Changes in libido · dizziness · dysarthria · gastro-intestinal disturbances · gynaecomastia · headache · hypotension · incontinence · salivation changes · slurred speech · tremor · urinary retention · vertigo · visual disturbances

▶ **Rare** Apnoea · blood disorders · jaundice · skin reactions

▶ **Frequency not known** Respiratory depression (may be marked when used for sedation; facilities for its treatment are essential)

- BREAST FEEDING Benzodiazepines are present in milk, and should be avoided if possible during breast-feeding.

- HEPATIC IMPAIRMENT Start with smaller initial doses or reduce dose. Can precipitate coma. Avoid in severe impairment.

  If treatment is necessary, benzodiazepines with shorter half-lives are safer.

- RENAL IMPAIRMENT Start with small doses in severe impairment.

- PATIENT AND CARER ADVICE

Driving and skilled tasks

May impair judgement and increase reaction time, and so affect ability to drive or operate machinery; they increase the effects of alcohol. Moreover the hangover effects of a night dose may impair driving on the following day.

Patients given sedatives and analgesics during minor outpatient procedures should be very carefully warned about the risks of undertaking skilled tasks (e.g. driving) afterwards. Responsible persons should be available to take patients home afterwards. The dangers of taking alcohol should be emphasised.

- PROFESSION SPECIFIC INFORMATION

Dental practitioners' formulary

Temazepam Tablets and Oral Solution may be prescribed.

- MEDICINAL FORMS

There can be variation in the licensing of different medicines containing the same drug. Forms available from special-order manufacturers include: oral suspension, oral solution

Tablet

CAUTIONARY AND ADVISORY LABELS 19

- Temazepam (Non-proprietary)

  Temazepam 10 mg Temazepam 10mg tablets | 28 tablet [PoM] £35.00 DT price = £3.80 [CD3] | 500 tablet [PoM] £624.82 [CD3]

  Temazepam 20 mg Temazepam 20mg tablets | 28 tablet [PoM] £35.00 DT price = £4.04 [CD3] | 250 tablet [PoM] £307.94 [CD3]

Oral solution

CAUTIONARY AND ADVISORY LABELS 19

- Temazepam (Non-proprietary)

  Temazepam 2 mg per 1 ml Temazepam 10mg/5ml oral solution sugar free sugar-free | 300 ml [PoM] £121.08 DT price = £119.30 [CD3]

Nervous system

4

HYPNOTICS, SEDATIVES AND ANXIOLYTICS ›
NON-BENZODIAZEPINE HYPNOTICS AND SEDATIVES

Chloral hydrate

● INDICATIONS AND DOSE

Insomnia (short-term use) using Chloral Mixture, BP 2000
▸ BY MOUTH USING ORAL SOLUTION
▸ Adult: 0.5–2 g daily, dose to be taken at bedtime

Insomnia (short-term use), using chloral hydrate 143.3 mg/5 ml oral solution
▸ BY MOUTH USING ORAL SOLUTION
▸ Adult: 15–30 mL, alternatively 430–860 mg once daily, dose to be taken with water or milk at bedtime; maximum 70 mL per day; maximum 2 g per day

Insomnia (short-term use), using chloral betaine 707 mg (≡ 414 mg chloral hydrate) tablets
▸ BY MOUTH USING TABLETS
▸ Adult: 1–2 tablets, alternatively 414–828 mg once daily, dose to be taken with water or milk at bedtime; maximum 4 tablets per day; maximum 2 g per day

● CONTRA-INDICATIONS Acute porphyrias p. 918 · gastritis · severe cardiac disease

● CAUTIONS Avoid contact with mucous membranes · avoid contact with skin · avoid prolonged use (and abrupt withdrawal thereafter) · reduce dose in debilitated · reduce dose in elderly

● INTERACTIONS → Appendix 1 (anxiolytics and hypnotics).

● SIDE-EFFECTS Abdominal distention · delirium (especially on abrupt withdrawal) · dependence · excitement · flatulence · gastric irritation · headache · ketonuria · nausea · rash · tolerance · vomiting

● PREGNANCY Avoid.

● BREAST FEEDING Risk of sedation in infant—avoid.

● HEPATIC IMPAIRMENT Reduce dose in mild to moderate impairment. Can precipitate coma. Avoid in severe impairment.

● RENAL IMPAIRMENT Avoid in severe impairment.

● DIRECTIONS FOR ADMINISTRATION
▸ With oral use For administration *by mouth* dilute liquid with plenty of water or juice to mask unpleasant taste.

● PRESCRIBING AND DISPENSING INFORMATION Flavours of oral liquid formulations may include black currant.
 When prepared extemporaneously, the BP states Chloral Mixture, BP 2000 consists of chloral hydrate 500 mg/5 mL in a suitable vehicle.

● PATIENT AND CARER ADVICE
Driving and skilled tasks
Drowsiness may persist the next day and affect performance of skilled tasks (e.g. driving); effects of alcohol enhanced.

● LESS SUITABLE FOR PRESCRIBING Chloral hydrate is less suitable for prescribing in insomnia.

● MEDICINAL FORMS
There can be variation in the licensing of different medicines containing the same drug. Forms available from special-order manufacturers include: oral solution

Tablet
CAUTIONARY AND ADVISORY LABELS 19, 27
▸ Chloral hydrate (Non-proprietary)
 Cloral betaine 707 mg Cloral betaine 707mg tablets | 30 tablet PoM £68.00–£138.59 DT price = £138.59

Oral solution
CAUTIONARY AND ADVISORY LABELS 1 (paediatric solution only), 19 (solution other than paediatric only), 27
▸ Chloral hydrate (Non-proprietary)
 Chloral hydrate 28.66 mg per 1 ml Chloral hydrate 143.3mg/5ml oral solution BP | 150 ml PoM £120.00–£244.26 DT price = £244.26

Clomethiazole
(Chlormethiazole)

● INDICATIONS AND DOSE

Severe insomnia (short-term use)
▸ BY MOUTH USING CAPSULES
▸ Elderly: 192–384 mg once daily, dose to be taken at bedtime
▸ BY MOUTH USING ORAL SOLUTION
▸ Elderly: 5–10 mL once daily, dose to be taken at bedtime

Restlessness and agitation
▸ BY MOUTH USING CAPSULES
▸ Elderly: 192 mg 3 times a day
▸ BY MOUTH USING ORAL SOLUTION
▸ Elderly: 5 mL 3 times a day

Alcohol withdrawal
▸ BY MOUTH USING CAPSULES
▸ Adult: Initially 2–4 capsules, to be repeated if necessary after some hours. 9–12 capsules daily in 3–4 divided doses on day 1 (first 24 hours), then 6–8 capsules daily in 3–4 divided doses on day 2, then 4–6 capsules daily in 3–4 divided doses on day 3, dose then to be gradually reduced over days 4–6, total duration of treatment for no more than 9 days
▸ BY MOUTH USING ORAL SOLUTION
▸ Adult: Initially 10–20 mL, to be repeated if necessary after some hours, then 45–60 mL daily in 3–4 divided doses on day 1 (first 24 hours), then 30–40 mL daily in 3–4 divided doses on day 2, then 20–30 mL daily in 3–4 divided doses on day 3, dose then to be gradually reduced over days 4–6, total duration of treatment for no more than 9 days

● CONTRA-INDICATIONS Acute pulmonary insufficiency · alcohol-dependent patients who continue to drink

● CAUTIONS Avoid prolonged use (and abrupt withdrawal thereafter) · cardiac disease (confusional state may indicate hypoxia) · chronic pulmonary insufficiency · elderly · excessive sedation may occur (particularly with higher doses); · history of drug abuse · marked personality disorder · respiratory disease (confusional state may indicate hypoxia) · sleep apnoea syndrome

● INTERACTIONS → Appendix 1 (anxiolytics and hypnotics).

● SIDE-EFFECTS
▸ **Common or very common** Conjunctival irritation · headache · increased bronchial secretions · increased nasopharyngeal secretions · nasal congestion · nasal irritation
▸ **Rare** Alterations in liver enzymes · anaphylaxis · bullous eruption · confusion · dependence · gastro-intestinal disturbances · paradoxical excitement · rash · urticaria

● PREGNANCY Avoid if possible—especially during the first and third trimesters.

● BREAST FEEDING Use only if benefit outweighs risk—present in breast milk but effects unknown.

● HEPATIC IMPAIRMENT Reduce dose. Can precipitate coma.

● RENAL IMPAIRMENT Start with small doses in severe impairment. Increased cerebral sensitivity.

● PATIENT AND CARER ADVICE

Driving and skilled tasks
Drowsiness may persist the next day and affect performance of skilled tasks (e.g. driving); effects of alcohol enhanced.

● MEDICINAL FORMS
There can be variation in the licensing of different medicines containing the same drug.

Capsule
CAUTIONARY AND ADVISORY LABELS 19
▸ Clomethiazole (Non-proprietary)
   Clomethiazole 192 mg Clomethiazole 192mg capsules | 60 capsule PoM £32.80 DT price = £31.40

Oral solution
CAUTIONARY AND ADVISORY LABELS 19
EXCIPIENTS: May contain Alcohol
▸ Clomethiazole (Non-proprietary)
   Clomethiazole (as Clomethiazole edisilate) 50 mg per 1 ml Clomethiazole 31.5mg/ml oral solution sugar free sugar-free | 300 ml PoM £30.00

Melatonin

● INDICATIONS AND DOSE

Insomnia (short-term use)
▸ BY MOUTH USING MODIFIED-RELEASE TABLETS
▸ Adult 55 years and over: 2 mg once daily for up to 13 weeks, dose to be taken 1–2 hours before bedtime

● CAUTIONS Autoimmune disease (manufacturer advises avoid—no information available)
● INTERACTIONS → Appendix 1 (melatonin).
● SIDE-EFFECTS
▸ **Uncommon** Abdominal pain · abnormal dreams · anxiety · chest pain · dizziness · dry mouth · dry skin · dyspepsia · glycosuria · headache · hypertension · irritability · malaise · mouth ulceration · nausea · nervousness · proteinuria · pruritus · rash · restlessness · weight gain
▸ **Rare** Aggression · angina · arthritis · electrolyte disturbances · flatulence · gastritis · haematuria · halitosis · hot flushes · hypertriglyceridaemia · impaired memory · increased libido · lacrimation · leucopenia · mood changes · muscle spasm · nail disorder · palpitation · paraesthesia · polyuria · priapism · prostatitis · restless legs syndrome · salivation · syncope · thirst · thrombocytopenia · visual disturbances · vomiting
▸ **Frequency not known** Galactorrhoea · mouth oedema · tongue oedema
● PREGNANCY No information available—avoid.
● BREAST FEEDING Present in milk—avoid.
● HEPATIC IMPAIRMENT Clearance reduced—avoid.
● RENAL IMPAIRMENT No information available—use with caution.

● MEDICINAL FORMS
There can be variation in the licensing of different medicines containing the same drug.
Modified-release tablet
CAUTIONARY AND ADVISORY LABELS 2, 21, 25
▸ Circadin (Flynn Pharma Ltd)
   Melatonin 2 mg Circadin 2mg modified-release tablets | 30 tablet PoM £15.39 DT price = £15.39

Zaleplon

● INDICATIONS AND DOSE

Insomnia (short-term use)
▸ BY MOUTH
▸ Adult: 10 mg daily for up to 2 weeks, dose to be taken at bedtime or after going to bed if difficulty falling asleep
▸ Elderly: 5 mg daily for up to 2 weeks, dose to be taken at bedtime or after going to bed if difficulty falling asleep

● CONTRA-INDICATIONS Marked neuromuscular respiratory weakness · sleep apnoea syndrome · unstable myasthenia gravis
● CAUTIONS Avoid prolonged use (risk of tolerance and withdrawal symptoms) · depression (risk of suicidal ideation) · history of alcohol abuse · history of drug abuse · muscle weakness · myasthenia gravis · respiratory insufficiency (avoid if severe)
● INTERACTIONS → Appendix 1 (anxiolytics and hypnotics).
● SIDE-EFFECTS
▸ **Common or very common** Amnesia · drowsiness · dysmenorrhea · paraesthesia
▸ **Uncommon** Anorexia · asthenia · confusion · depersonalisation · depression · disturbances of hearing · disturbances of smell · disturbances of speech · disturbances of vision · dizziness · hallucinations · impaired concentration · incoordination · nausea · photosensitivity
▸ **Frequency not known** Paradoxical effects · sleep-walking
SIDE-EFFECTS, FURTHER INFORMATION
▸ **Paradoxical effects** A paradoxical increase in hostility and aggression may be reported. The effects range from talkativeness and excitement to aggressive and antisocial acts. Adjustment of the dose (up or down) sometimes attenuates the impulses. Increased anxiety and perceptual disorders are other paradoxical effects. Increased hostility and aggression after barbiturates and alcohol usually indicates intoxication.
● PREGNANCY Use only if necessary and restrict to occasional short-term use. Risk of withdrawal symptoms in neonate if used in late pregnancy.
● BREAST FEEDING Present in milk but amount probably too small to be harmful.
● HEPATIC IMPAIRMENT Reduce dose to 5 mg. Can precipitate coma. Avoid if severe impairment.
● RENAL IMPAIRMENT Avoid in severe impairment.
● PATIENT AND CARER ADVICE Patients should be advised not to take a second dose during a single night.
● NATIONAL FUNDING/ACCESS DECISIONS
NICE technology appraisals (TAs)
▸ **Zaleplon, zolpidem, and zopiclone for the short-term management of insomnia (April 2004)** NICE TA77
Zaleplon is recommended for the short-term management of severe insomnia that interferes with normal daily life, and should be prescribed for short periods of time only.
www.nice.org.uk/TA77

● MEDICINAL FORMS
There can be variation in the licensing of different medicines containing the same drug.
No licensed medicines listed.

Zolpidem tartrate

● INDICATIONS AND DOSE

Insomnia (short-term use)
▸ BY MOUTH
▸ Adult: 10 mg daily for up to 4 weeks, dose to be taken at bedtime, for debilitated patients, use elderly dose
▸ Elderly: 5 mg daily for up to 4 weeks, dose to be taken at bedtime

● CONTRA-INDICATIONS Acute respiratory depression · marked neuromuscular respiratory weakness · obstructive sleep apnoea · psychotic illness · severe respiratory depression · unstable myasthenia gravis

● CAUTIONS Avoid prolonged use (and abrupt withdrawal thereafter) · depression · elderly · history of alcohol abuse · history of drug abuse · muscle weakness · myasthenia gravis

● INTERACTIONS → Appendix 1 (anxiolytics and hypnotics).

● SIDE-EFFECTS Agitation · amnesia · asthenia · ataxia · changes in libido · confusion · dependence · depression · diarrhoea · diplopia · dizziness · drowsiness · falls · hallucination · headache · memory disturbances · muscular weakness · nausea · nightmares · paradoxical effects · perceptual disturbances · skin reactions · sleep-walking · tremor · vomiting

SIDE-EFFECTS, FURTHER INFORMATION
▸ Paradoxical effects A paradoxical increase in hostility and aggression may be reported. The effects range from talkativeness and excitement to aggressive and antisocial acts. Adjustment of the dose (up or down) sometimes attenuates the impulses. Increased anxiety and perceptual disorders are other paradoxical effects. Increased hostility and aggression after barbiturates and alcohol usually indicates intoxication.

● PREGNANCY Avoid regular use (risk of neonatal withdrawal symptoms); high doses during late pregnancy or labour may cause neonatal hypothermia, hypotonia, and respiratory depression.

● BREAST FEEDING Small amounts present in milk—avoid.

● HEPATIC IMPAIRMENT Reduce dose to 5 mg. Can precipitate coma. Avoid if severe impairment.

● RENAL IMPAIRMENT Use with caution.

● PATIENT AND CARER ADVICE

Driving and skilled tasks
Drowsiness may persist the next day—leave at least 8 hours between taking zolpidem and performing skilled tasks (e.g. driving, or operating machinery); effects of alcohol and other CNS depressants enhanced.

● NATIONAL FUNDING/ACCESS DECISIONS

NICE technology appraisals (TAs)
▸ Zaleplon, zolpidem, and zopiclone for the short-term management of insomnia (April 2004) NICE TA77
Zolpidem is recommended for the short-term management of severe insomnia that interferes with normal daily life, and should be prescribed for short periods of time only.
www.nice.org.uk/TA77

● MEDICINAL FORMS
There can be variation in the licensing of different medicines containing the same drug.
Tablet
CAUTIONARY AND ADVISORY LABELS 19
▸ Zolpidem tartrate (Non-proprietary)
Zolpidem tartrate 5 mg Zolpidem 5mg tablets | 28 tablet PoM £3.08 DT price = £1.24 CD4-1
Zolpidem tartrate 10 mg Zolpidem 10mg tablets | 28 tablet PoM £4.48 DT price = £1.16 CD4-1 | 30 tablet PoM £4.48 CD4-1

▸ Stilnoct (Sanofi)
Zolpidem tartrate 5 mg Stilnoct 5mg tablets | 28 tablet PoM £1.10 DT price = £1.24 CD4-1
Zolpidem tartrate 10 mg Stilnoct 10mg tablets | 28 tablet PoM £1.00 DT price = £1.16 CD4-1

Zopiclone

● INDICATIONS AND DOSE

Insomnia (short-term use)
▸ BY MOUTH
▸ Adult: 7.5 mg once daily for up to 4 weeks, dose to be taken at bedtime
▸ Elderly: Initially 3.75 mg once daily for up to 4 weeks, dose to be taken at bedtime, increased if necessary to 7.5 mg daily

Insomnia (short-term use) in patients with chronic pulmonary insufficiency
▸ BY MOUTH
▸ Adult: Initially 3.75 mg once daily for up to 4 weeks, dose to be taken at bedtime, increased if necessary to 7.5 mg daily

● CONTRA-INDICATIONS Marked neuromuscular respiratory weakness · respiratory failure · severe sleep apnoea syndrome · unstable myasthenia gravis

● CAUTIONS Avoid prolonged use (risk of tolerance and withdrawal symptoms) · chronic pulmonary insufficiency (increased risk of respiratory depression) · elderly · history of drug abuse · muscle weakness · myasthenia gravis (avoid if unstable) · psychiatric illness

● INTERACTIONS → Appendix 1 (anxiolytics and hypnotics).

● SIDE-EFFECTS
▸ Common or very common Taste disturbance
▸ Uncommon Dizziness · drowsiness · dry mouth · headache · nausea · vomiting
▸ Rare Amnesia · confusion · depression · hallucinations · nightmares
▸ Very rare Incoordination · light headedness
▸ Frequency not known Paradoxical effects · sleep-walking

SIDE-EFFECTS, FURTHER INFORMATION
▸ Paradoxical effects A paradoxical increase in hostility and aggression may be reported. The effects range from talkativeness and excitement to aggressive and antisocial acts. Adjustment of the dose (up or down) sometimes attenuates the impulses. Increased anxiety and perceptual disorders are other paradoxical effects. Increased hostility and aggression after barbiturates and alcohol usually indicates intoxication.

● PREGNANCY Not recommended (risk of neonatal withdrawal symptoms). Use during late pregnancy or labour may cause neonatal hypothermia, hypotonia, and respiratory depression.

● BREAST FEEDING Present in milk—avoid.

● HEPATIC IMPAIRMENT Reduce dose to 3.75 mg in mild to moderate impairment, dose can be increased with caution if necessary. Avoid in severe impairment—can precipitate encephalopathy.

● RENAL IMPAIRMENT Start with reduced dose of 3.75 mg. Increased cerebral sensitivity.

● PATIENT AND CARER ADVICE

Driving and skilled tasks
Drowsiness may persist the next day and affect performance of skilled tasks (e.g. driving); effects of alcohol enhanced.

● NATIONAL FUNDING/ACCESS DECISIONS

NICE technology appraisals (TAs)

▶ **Zaleplon, zolpidem and zopiclone for the short-term management of insomnia (April 2004)** NICE TA77
Zopiclone is recommended for the short-term management of severe insomnia that interferes with normal daily life, and should be prescribed for short periods of time only.
www.nice.org.uk/TA77

● MEDICINAL FORMS
There can be variation in the licensing of different medicines containing the same drug. Forms available from special-order manufacturers include: oral suspension, oral solution

Tablet
CAUTIONARY AND ADVISORY LABELS 19, 25
▶ Zopiclone (Non-proprietary)
Zopiclone 3.75 mg Zopiclone 3.75mg tablets | 28 tablet [PoM] £2.50 DT price = £1.17 [CD4-1]
Zopiclone 7.5 mg Zopiclone 7.5mg tablets | 28 tablet [PoM] £3.75 DT price = £1.18 [CD4-1]
▶ Zimovane (Sanofi)
Zopiclone 3.75 mg Zimovane LS 3.75mg tablets | 28 tablet [PoM] £2.24 DT price = £1.17 [CD4-1]
Zopiclone 7.5 mg Zimovane 7.5mg tablets | 28 tablet [PoM] £3.26 DT price = £1.18 [CD4-1]

7.2 Narcolepsy

Drugs used for Narcolepsy not listed below
Dexamfetamine sulfate, p. 319 · Methylphenidate hydrochloride, p. 318

CENTRAL NERVOUS SYSTEM DEPRESSANTS

Sodium oxybate

● DRUG ACTION A central nervous system depressant.

● INDICATIONS AND DOSE

Narcolepsy with cataplexy (under expert supervision)
▶ BY MOUTH
▶ Adult: Initially 2.25 g daily, dose to be taken on retiring and 2.25 g after 2.5–4 hours, then increased in steps of 1.5 g daily in 2 divided doses, dose adjusted according to response at intervals of 1–2 weeks; dose titration should be repeated if restarting after interval of more than 14 days, maximum 9 g daily in 2 divided doses

● CONTRA-INDICATIONS Major depression · succinic semi-aldehyde dehydrogenase deficiency

● CAUTIONS Body mass index of 40 kg/m^2 or greater (higher risk of sleep apnoea) · elderly · epilepsy · heart failure (high sodium content) · history of depression · history of drug abuse · hypertension (high sodium content) · respiratory disorders · risk of discontinuation effects including rebound cataplexy and withdrawal symptoms

● INTERACTIONS → Appendix 1 (sodium oxybate).
If sodium oxybate and sodium valproate or valproic acid used concomitantly, reduce initial dose of sodium oxybate to 1.8 g on retiring and repeat 2.5–4 hours later.

● SIDE-EFFECTS
▶ **Common or very common** Abdominal pain · anorexia · anxiety · arthralgia · asthenia · back pain · blurred vision · confusion · depression · diarrhoea · disorientation · dizziness · drowsiness · dyspnoea · headache · hypertension · hypoaesthesia · impaired attention · muscle spasm · nasal congestion · nausea · nocturnal enuresis · palpitation · paraesthesia · peripheral oedema · rash · sleep disorders · sleep paralysis · sleep walking · sweating · taste disturbance · tremor · urinary incontinence · vertigo · vomiting

▶ **Uncommon** Agitation · amnesia · faecal incontinence · hallucination · myoclonus · paranoia · psychosis · restless legs syndrome · suicidal behaviour
▶ **Frequency not known** Dependence · euphoria · respiratory depression · seizures · sleep apnoea · suicidal ideation · urticaria

● PREGNANCY Avoid.

● BREAST FEEDING No information available.

● HEPATIC IMPAIRMENT Halve initial dose.

● RENAL IMPAIRMENT Caution—contains 3.96 mmol Na$^+$ per mL.

● DIRECTIONS FOR ADMINISTRATION Dilute each dose with 60 mL water; prepare both doses before retiring. Observe the same time interval (2–3 hours) each night between the last meal and the first dose.

● PATIENT AND CARER ADVICE
Patients or carers should be given advice on how to administer sodium oxybate oral solution.

Driving and skilled tasks
Leave at least 6 hours between taking sodium oxybate and performing skilled tasks (e.g. driving or operating machinery); effects of alcohol and other CNS depressants enhanced.

● MEDICINAL FORMS
There can be variation in the licensing of different medicines containing the same drug.

Oral solution
CAUTIONARY AND ADVISORY LABELS 13, 19
ELECTROLYTES: May contain Sodium
▶ Xyrem (UCB Pharma Ltd)
Sodium oxybate 500 mg per 1 ml Xyrem 500mg/ml oral solution sugar-free | 180 ml [PoM] £360.00 DT price = £360.00 [CD2]

CNS STIMULANTS > CENTRALLY ACTING SYMPATHOMIMETICS

Modafinil

● INDICATIONS AND DOSE

Excessive sleepiness associated with narcolepsy with or without cataplexy
▶ BY MOUTH
▶ Adult: Initially 200 mg daily in 2 divided doses, dose to be taken in the morning and at noon, alternatively initially 200 mg once daily, dose to be taken in the morning, adjusted according to response to 200–400 mg daily in 2 divided doses, alternatively adjusted according to response to 200–400 mg once daily
▶ Elderly: Initially 100 mg daily

● CONTRA-INDICATIONS Arrhythmia · history of clinically significant signs of CNS stimulant-induced mitral valve prolapse (including ischaemic ECG changes, chest pain and arrhythmias) · history of cor pulmonale · history of left ventricular hypertrophy · moderate uncontrolled hypertension · severe uncontrolled hypertension

● CAUTIONS History of alcohol abuse · history of depression · history of drug abuse · history of mania · history of psychosis · possibility of dependence

● INTERACTIONS → Appendix 1 (modafinil).

● SIDE-EFFECTS
▶ **Common or very common** Abdominal pain · anxiety · appetite changes · asthenia · chest pain · confusion · constipation · depression · diarrhoea · dizziness · drowsiness · dry mouth · dyspepsia · gastrointestinal disturbances · headache · nausea · palpitation · paraesthesia · sleep disturbances · tachycardia · vasodilatation · visual disturbances

Nervous system

4

▸ **Uncommon** Abnormal dreams · acne · aggression · agitation · amnesia · arrhythmia · arthralgia · bradycardia · decreased libido · dry eye · dyskinesia · dysphagia · dyspnoea · emotional lability · eosinophilia · epistaxis · flatulence · glossitis · hypercholesterolaemia · hyperglycaemia · hypertension · hypertonia · hypotension · leucopenia · menstrual disturbances · migraine · mouth ulcers · muscle cramps · myalgia · myasthenia · peripheral oedema · pruritus · rash · reflux · rhinitis · sinusitis · suicidal ideation · sweating · taste disturbance · thirst · tremor · urinary frequency · vomiting · weight changes
▸ **Rare** Hallucinations · mania · psychosis
▸ **Frequency not known** Multi-organ hypersensitivity reaction · psychiatric symptoms · Stevens-Johnson syndrome · toxic epidermal necrolysis

SIDE-EFFECTS, FURTHER INFORMATION
▸ Rash Discontinue treatment if rash develops.
▸ Psychiatric symptoms Discontinue treatment if psychiatric symptoms develop.

● PREGNANCY Avoid.

● BREAST FEEDING Avoid—present in milk in *animal* studies.

● HEPATIC IMPAIRMENT Halve dose in severe impairment.

● RENAL IMPAIRMENT Use with caution—limited information available.

● PRE-TREATMENT SCREENING ECG required before initiation.

● MONITORING REQUIREMENTS Monitor blood pressure and heart rate in hypertensive patients.

● MEDICINAL FORMS
There can be variation in the licensing of different medicines containing the same drug. Forms available from special-order manufacturers include: oral suspension, oral solution

Tablet
▸ Modafinil (Non-proprietary)
Modafinil 100 mg Modafinil 100mg tablets | 30 tablet [PoM] £52.60
DT price = £8.56
Modafinil 200 mg Modafinil 200mg tablets | 30 tablet [PoM]
£105.21 DT price = £14.71
▸ Provigil (Teva UK Ltd)
Modafinil 100 mg Provigil 100mg tablets | 30 tablet [PoM] £52.60
DT price = £8.56
Modafinil 200 mg Provigil 200mg tablets | 30 tablet [PoM] £105.21
DT price = £14.71

8   Substance dependence

Substance dependence

Guidance on treatment of drug misuse

The UK health departments have produced guidance on the treatment of drug misuse in the UK. *Drug Misuse and Dependence: UK Guidelines on Clinical Management* (2007) is available at www.nta.nhs.uk/uploads/clinical_guidelines_2007. pdf.

Alcohol dependence

Excessive drinking of alcoholic beverages over a prolonged period of time can result in an alcohol withdrawal syndrome on abrupt cessation of, or marked reduction in, drinking. The presence and severity of alcohol dependence can be assessed by *The Severity of Alcohol Dependence Questionnaire (SADQ)*; other assessment questionnaires are also available.

Acute alcohol withdrawal

People with moderate dependence can generally be treated in a community setting unless they are under 18 years of age, or are at high-risk of severe reactions or treatment failure. People with severe dependence should undergo withdrawal in an inpatient setting; withdrawal in severely dependent

patients without medical support may lead to seizures, delirium tremens, and death. Long-acting benzodiazepines, usually chlordiazepoxide hydrochloride p. 313, are used to attenuate alcohol withdrawal symptoms. In primary care, fixed-dose reducing regimens are usually used, whilst a symptom-triggered flexible regimen is used in hospital or other settings where continued assessment and monitoring is carried out for 24–48 hours, usually followed by a fixed 5-day reducing dose schedule (sometimes it may be necessary to continue treatment for up to 10 days). Patients with decompensated liver disease should be treated under specialist supervision.

Carbamazepine p. 283 [unlicensed indication] is sometimes used as an alternative treatment in acute alcohol withdrawal when benzodiazepines are contra-indicated or not tolerated. Clomethiazole p. 444 is licensed for use in acute alcohol withdrawal, but benzodiazepines are preferred. It should only be used in an inpatient setting and should not be prescribed if the patient is liable to continue drinking alcohol.

Patients with marked agitation or hallucinations and those at risk of delirium tremens (characterised by delirium, hallucinations, tremor, and disorientation) may be prescribed antipsychotic drugs, such as haloperidol p. 354 or olanzapine p. 365 [unlicensed indication], as adjunctive therapy to benzodiazepines; antipsychotics should not be used alone because they do not treat alcohol withdrawal and may lower the seizure threshold. Delirium tremens is a medical emergency that requires specialist inpatient care.

If a patient taking a benzodiazepine as part of a withdrawal regimen develops alcohol withdrawal seizures, a fast-acting benzodiazepine (such as intravenous lorazepam p. 308 [unlicensed indication] or rectal diazepam p. 313) should be prescribed; thereafter an increase in the dose of oral benzodiazepine should be considered to prevent further seizures from occurring.

Alcohol dependence

Acamprosate calcium p. 451 and naltrexone hydrochloride p. 452 are effective treatments for relapse prevention in patients with alcohol dependence; disulfiram p. 451 is an alternative. Disulfiram should only be used in patients in whom acamprosate calcium and naltrexone hydrochloride are not suitable, or if the patient prefers disulfiram. Nalmefene p. 452 is licensed for the reduction of alcohol consumption in patients with alcohol dependence who have a high drinking risk level, without physical withdrawal symptoms, and who do not require immediate detoxification.

Patients with alcohol dependence are at risk of developing Wernicke's encephalopathy; patients at high-risk are those who are malnourished, at risk of malnourishment, or have decompensated liver disease. Parenteral thiamine (as *Pabrinex*®) p. 938 should be prescribed for treatment of suspected or confirmed Wernicke's encephalopathy, and for prophylaxis in alcohol dependent patients attending hospital for acute treatment (including treatment unrelated to alcohol dependence); parenteral prophylaxis may also be considered for high-risk patients being treated in primary care. High-dose oral thiamine should be prescribed following parenteral treatment until cognitive function is maximised. In primary care, prophylactic high-dose oral thiamine should be prescribed during acute withdrawal of alcohol, before planned withdrawal, and for patients not undergoing withdrawal but who are at high-risk of developing Wernicke's encephalopathy.

Patients with chronic alcohol-related pancreatitis who have symptoms of steatorrhoea or who have poor nutritional status due to exocrine pancreatic insufficiency should be prescribed **pancreatic enzyme supplements**; supplements are not indicated when pain is the only symptom.

Corticosteroids are used in patients with severe acute alcohol-related hepatitis.

Drugs used in alcohol dependence
Acamprosate
Acamprosate calcium, in combination with counselling, may be helpful for maintaining abstinence in alcohol-dependent patients. It is useful for patients who are concerned that strong cravings will result in relapse. It should be initiated as soon as possible *after* abstinence has been achieved and continued for 1 year; treatment should be maintained if the patient has a temporary relapse but stopped if the patient returns to regular or excessive drinking that persists 4–6 weeks after starting treatment. Acamprosate calcium is not effective in all patients, so efficacy should be regularly assessed.

Disulfiram
Disulfiram gives rise to an extremely unpleasant systemic reaction after the ingestion of even a small amount of alcohol because it causes accumulation of acetaldehyde in the body; it is only effective if taken daily. Symptoms can occur within 10 minutes of ingesting alcohol and include flushing of the face, throbbing headache, palpitation, tachycardia, nausea, vomiting, and, with large doses of alcohol, arrhythmias, hypotension, and collapse; these reactions can last several hours. Small amounts of alcohol such as those included in many oral medicines may be sufficient to precipitate a reaction—even toiletries and mouthwashes that contain alcohol should be avoided.

Nalmefene
Nalmefene should only be prescribed in conjunction with continuous psychosocial support focused on treatment adherence and reducing alcohol consumption. Nalmefene is not recommended for patients aiming to achieve immediate abstinence.

Naltrexone
Naltrexone hydrochloride is an opioid-receptor antagonist, but is useful as an adjunct in the treatment of alcohol dependence after a successful withdrawal. Treatment should be initiated by a specialist and continued under specialist supervision. Naltrexone hydrochloride should be stopped if drinking continues for 4–6 weeks after starting treatment.

Nicotine dependence
Smoking cessation interventions are a cost-effective way of reducing ill health and prolonging life. Smokers should be advised to stop and offered help with follow-up when appropriate. If possible, smokers should have access to smoking cessation services for behavioural support.

Therapy to aid smoking cessation is chosen according to the smoker's likely adherence, availability of counselling and support, previous experience of smoking-cessation aids, contra-indications and adverse effects of the preparations, and the smoker's preferences. **Nicotine replacement therapy**, bupropion hydrochloride p. 453, and varenicline p. 455 are effective aids to smoking cessation. The use of nicotine replacement therapy in an individual who is already accustomed to nicotine introduces few new risks and it is widely accepted that there are no circumstances in which it is safer to smoke than to use nicotine replacement therapy.

Some patients benefit from having more than one type of nicotine replacement therapy prescribed, such as a combination of transdermal and oral preparations. The combination of nicotine replacement therapy with varenicline p. 455 or bupropion hydrochloride is not recommended.

Concomitant medication
Cigarette smoking increases the metabolism of some medicines by stimulating the hepatic enzyme CYP1A2. When smoking is discontinued, the dose of these drugs, in particular theophylline p. 250, cinacalcet p. 906, ropinirole p. 388, and some antipsychotics (including clozapine p. 363, olanzapine p. 365, chlorpromazine hydrochloride p. 353, and

haloperidol p. 354, may need to be reduced. Regular monitoring for adverse effects is advised.

Drugs used in nicotine dependence
Bupropion hydrochloride has been used as an antidepressant. Its mode of action in smoking cessation is not clear and may involve an effect on noradrenaline and dopamine neurotransmission.

Nicotine replacement therapy
Nicotine replacement therapy can be used in place of cigarettes after abrupt cessation of smoking, or alternatively to reduce the amount of cigarettes used in advance of making a quit attempt. Nicotine replacement therapy can also be used to minimise passive smoking, and to treat cravings and reduce compensatory smoking after enforced abstinence in smoke-free environments. Smokers who find it difficult to achieve abstinence should consult a healthcare professional for advice.

Choice
Nicotine patches p. 453 are a prolonged-release formulation and are applied for 16 hours (with the patch removed overnight) or for 24 hours. If patients experience strong cravings for cigarettes on waking, a 24-hour patch may be more suitable. Immediate-release nicotine preparations (gum, lozenges, sublingual tablets, inhalator, nasal spray, and oral spray) are used whenever the urge to smoke occurs or to prevent cravings.

The choice of nicotine replacement preparation depends largely on patient preference, and should take into account what preparations, if any, have been tried before. Patients with a high level of nicotine dependence, or who have failed with nicotine replacement therapy previously, may benefit from using a combination of an immediate-release preparation and patches to achieve abstinence.

Side-effects of specific nicotine preparations
Mild local reactions at the beginning of treatment are common because of the irritant effect of nicotine. Oral preparations and *inhalation cartridges* can cause irritation of the throat, *gum*, *lozenges*, and *oral spray* can cause increased salivation, and *patches* can cause minor skin irritation. The *nasal spray* commonly causes coughing, nasal irritation, epistaxis, sneezing, and watery eyes; the *oral spray* can cause watery eyes and blurred vision.

Gastro-intestinal disturbances are common and may be caused by swallowed nicotine. Nausea, vomiting, dyspepsia, and hiccup occur most frequently. Ulcerative stomatitis has also been reported. Dry mouth is a common side-effect of *lozenges*, *patches*, *oral spray*, and *sublingual tablets*. *Lozenges* cause diarrhoea, constipation, dysphagia, oesophagitis, gastritis, mouth ulcers, bloating, flatulence, and less commonly, taste disturbance, thirst, gingival bleeding, and halitosis. The *oral spray* may also cause abdominal pain, flatulence, and taste disturbance.

Palpitations may occur with nicotine replacement therapy and rarely *patches* and *oral spray* can cause arrhythmia. *Patches*, *lozenges*, and *oral spray* can cause chest pain. The *inhalator* can very rarely cause reversible atrial fibrillation.

Paraesthesia is a common side-effect of *oral spray*. Abnormal dreams can occur with *patches*; removal of the patch before bed may help. *Lozenges* and *oral spray* may cause rash and hot flushes. Sweating and myalgia can occur with *patches* and *oral spray*; the *patches* can also cause arthralgia.

Opioid dependence
The management of opioid dependence requires medical, social, and psychological treatment; access to a multidisciplinary team is recommended. Treatment for opioid dependence should be initiated under the supervision of an appropriately qualified prescriber.

Untreated heroin dependence shows early withdrawal symptoms within 8 hours, with peak symptoms at

36–72 hours; symptoms subside substantially after 5 days. Methadone hydrochloride p. 456 or buprenorphine p. 409 withdrawal occurs later, with longer-lasting symptoms.

Opioid substitution therapy
Methadone hydrochloride and buprenorphine are used as substitution therapy in opioid dependence. Substitute medication should be commenced with a short period of stabilisation, followed by either a withdrawal regimen or by maintenance treatment. Maintenance treatment enables patients to achieve stability, reduces drug use and crime, and improves health; it should be regularly reviewed to ensure the patient continues to derive benefit. The prescriber should monitor for signs of toxicity, and the patient should be told to be aware of warning signs of toxicity on initiation and during titration.

A withdrawal regimen after stabilisation with methadone hydrochloride or buprenorphine should be attempted only after careful consideration. Enforced withdrawal is ineffective for sustained abstinence, and it increases the risk of patients relapsing and subsequently overdosing because of loss of tolerance. Complete withdrawal from opioids usually takes up to 4 weeks in an inpatient or residential setting, and up to 12 weeks in a community setting. If abstinence is not achieved, illicit drug use is resumed, or the patient cannot tolerate withdrawal, the withdrawal regimen should be stopped and maintenance therapy should be resumed at the optimal dose. Following successful withdrawal treatment, further support and monitoring to maintain abstinence should be provided for a period of at least 6 months.

Missed doses
Patients who miss 3 days or more of their regular prescribed dose of opioid maintenance therapy are at risk of overdose because of loss of tolerance. Consider reducing the dose in these patients.

If the patient misses 5 or more days of treatment, an assessment of illicit drug use is also recommended before restarting substitution therapy; this is particularly important for patients taking buprenorphine because of the risk of precipitated withdrawal.

Buprenorphine
Buprenorphine is preferred by some patients because it is less sedating than methadone hydrochloride; for this reason it may be more suitable for employed patients or those undertaking other skilled tasks such as driving. Buprenorphine is safer than methadone hydrochloride when used in conjunction with other sedating drugs, and has fewer drug interactions. Dose reductions may be easier than with methadone hydrochloride because the withdrawal symptoms are milder, and patients generally require fewer adjunctive medications; there is also a lower risk of overdose. Buprenorphine can be given on alternate days in higher doses and it requires a shorter drug-free period than methadone hydrochloride before induction with naltrexone hydrochloride p. 452 for prevention of relapse.

Patients dependent on high doses of opioids may be at increased risk of precipitated withdrawal. Precipitated withdrawal can occur in any patient if buprenorphine p. 409 is administered when other opioid agonist drugs are in circulation. Precipitated opioid withdrawal, if it occurs, starts within 1–3 hours of the first buprenorphine dose and peaks at around 6 hours. Non-opioid adjunctive therapy, such as lofexidine hydrochloride p. 458, may be required if symptoms are severe.

To reduce the risk of precipitated withdrawal, the first dose of buprenorphine should be given when the patient is exhibiting signs of withdrawal, or 6–12 hours after the last use of heroin (or other short-acting opioid), or 24–48 hours after the last dose of methadone hydrochloride p. 456. It is possible to titrate the dose of buprenorphine within one week—more rapidly than with methadone hydrochloride

therapy—but care is still needed to avoid toxicity or precipitated withdrawal; dividing the dose on the first day may be useful.

A combination preparation containing buprenorphine with naloxone (Suboxone®) p. 457 can be prescribed for patients when there is a risk of dose diversion for parenteral administration; the naloxone hydrochloride component precipitates withdrawal if the preparation is injected, but it has little effect when the preparation is taken sublingually.

Methadone
Methadone hydrochloride, a long-acting opioid agonist, is usually administered in a single daily dose as methadone hydrochloride oral solution 1 mg/mL. Patients with a long history of opioid misuse, those who typically abuse a variety of sedative drugs and alcohol, and those who experience increased anxiety during withdrawal of opioids may prefer methadone hydrochloride to buprenorphine because it has a more pronounced sedative effect.

Methadone hydrochloride is initiated at least 8 hours after the last heroin dose, provided that there is objective evidence of withdrawal symptoms. A supplementary dose on the first day may be considered if there is evidence of persistent opioid withdrawal symptoms. Because of the long half-life, plasma concentrations progressively rise during initial treatment even if the patient remains on the same daily dose (it takes 3–10 days for plasma concentrations to reach steady-state in patients on a stable dose); a dose tolerated on the first day of treatment may become a toxic dose on the third day as cumulative toxicity develops. Thus, titration to the optimal dose in methadone hydrochloride maintenance treatment may take several weeks.

Opioid substitution during pregnancy
Acute withdrawal of opioids should be avoided in pregnancy because it can cause fetal death. Opioid substitution therapy is recommended during pregnancy because it carries a lower risk to the fetus than continued use of illicit drugs. If a woman who is stabilised on methadone hydrochloride or buprenorphine for treatment of opioid dependence becomes pregnant, therapy should be continued [buprenorphine is not licensed for use in pregnancy]. Many pregnant patients choose a withdrawal regimen, but withdrawal during the first trimester should be avoided because it is associated with an increased risk of spontaneous miscarriage. Withdrawal of methadone hydrochloride or buprenorphine should be undertaken gradually during the second trimester, with dose reductions made every 3–5 days. If illicit drug use occurs, the patient should be re-stabilised at the optimal maintenance dose and consideration should be given to stopping the withdrawal regimen.

Further withdrawal of methadone hydrochloride or buprenorphine in the third trimester is not recommended because maternal withdrawal, even if mild, is associated with fetal distress, stillbirth, and the risk of neonatal mortality. Drug metabolism can be increased in the third trimester; it may be necessary to either increase the dose of methadone hydrochloride or change to twice-daily consumption (or a combination of both strategies) to prevent withdrawal symptoms from developing.

The neonate should be monitored for respiratory depression and signs of withdrawal if the mother is prescribed high doses of opioid substitute.

Signs of neonatal withdrawal from opioids usually develop 24–72 hours after delivery but symptoms may be delayed for up to 14 days, so monitoring may be required for several weeks. Symptoms include a high-pitched cry, rapid breathing, hungry but ineffective suckling, and excessive wakefulness; severe, but rare symptoms include hypertonicity and convulsions.

Opioid substitution during breastfeeding
Doses of methadone and buprenorphine should be kept as low as possible in breast-feeding mothers. Increased

sleepiness, breathing difficulties, or limpness in breast-fed babies of mothers taking opioid substitutes should be reported urgently to a healthcare professional.

Adjunctive therapy and symptomatic treatment
Adjunctive therapy may be required for the management of opioid withdrawal symptoms. Loperamide hydrochloride p. 59 may be used for the control of diarrhoea; mebeverine hydrochloride p. 78 for controlling stomach cramps; paracetamol p. 406 and **non-steroidal anti-inflammatory drugs** for muscular pains and headaches; metoclopramide hydrochloride p. 395 or prochlorperazine p. 357 may be useful for nausea or vomiting. Topical **rubefacients** can be helpful for relieving muscle pain associated with methadone hydrochloride withdrawal. If a patient is suffering from insomnia, short-acting **benzodiazepines** or zopiclone p. 446 may be prescribed, but because of the potential for abuse, prescriptions should be limited to a short course of a few days only. If anxiety or agitation is severe, specialist advice should be sought.

Lofexidine
Lofexidine hydrochloride may alleviate some of the physical symptoms of opioid withdrawal by attenuating the increase in adrenergic neurotransmission that occurs during opioid withdrawal. Lofexidine hydrochloride can be prescribed as an adjuvant to opioid substitution therapy, initiated either at the same time as the opioid substitute or during withdrawal of the opioid substitute. Alternatively, lofexidine hydrochloride may be prescribed instead of an opioid substitute in patients who have mild or uncertain dependence (including young people), and those with a short history of illicit drug use.

Opioid-receptor antagonists
Patients dependant on opioids can be given a supply of naloxone hydrochloride to be used in case of accidental overdose.
   Naltrexone hydrochloride p. 452 precipitates withdrawal symptoms in opioid-dependent subjects. Because the effects of opioid-receptor agonists are blocked by naltrexone hydrochloride, it is prescribed as an aid to prevent relapse in formerly opioid-dependent patients.

Opioid dependence in children

In younger patients (under 18 years), the harmful effects of drug misuse are more often related to acute intoxication than to dependence, so substitution therapy is usually inappropriate. Maintenance treatment with opioid substitution therapy is therefore controversial in young people; however, it may be useful for the older adolescent who has a history of opioid use to undergo a period of stabilisation with buprenorphine or methadone hydrochloride before starting a withdrawal regimen.

8.1 Alcohol dependence

ALDEHYDE DEHYDROGENASE INHIBITORS

Disulfiram

● INDICATIONS AND DOSE

Adjunct in the treatment of alcohol dependence (under expert supervision)
▸ BY MOUTH
▸ Adult: 200 mg daily, increased if necessary up to 500 mg daily

● UNLICENSED USE Disulfiram doses in BNF may differ from those in product literature.

● CONTRA-INDICATIONS Cardiac failure · coronary artery disease · history of cerebrovascular accident · hypertension · psychosis · severe personality disorder · suicide risk
● CAUTIONS Alcohol challenge **not** recommended on routine basis (if considered essential—specialist units only with resuscitation facilities) · avoid in Acute porphyrias p. 918 · diabetes mellitus · epilepsy · respiratory disease
▸ INTERACTIONS → Appendix 1 (disulfiram).
Disulfiram gives rise to an extremely unpleasant systemic reaction after the ingestion of even a small amount of alcohol. Ensure that alcohol is not consumed for at least 24 hours before initiating treatment and should be avoided for at least 1 week after stopping treatment.
● SIDE-EFFECTS
▸ Common or very common Drowsiness · fatigue · halitosis · nausea · reduced libido · vomiting
▸ Rare Allergic dermatitis · depression · hepatic cell damage · mania · paranoia · peripheral neuritis · psychotic reactions · schizophrenia
● PREGNANCY High concentrations of acetaldehyde which occur in presence of alcohol may be teratogenic; avoid in first trimester.
● BREAST FEEDING Avoid—no information available.
● HEPATIC IMPAIRMENT Use with caution.
● RENAL IMPAIRMENT Use with caution.
● PRE-TREATMENT SCREENING Before initiating disulfiram, prescribers should evaluate the patient's suitability for treatment, because some patient factors, for example memory impairment or social circumstances, make compliance to treatment or abstinence from alcohol difficult.
● MONITORING REQUIREMENTS During treatment with disulfiram, patients should be monitored at least every 2 weeks for the first 2 months, then each month for the following 4 months, and at least every 6 months thereafter.
● PATIENT AND CARER ADVICE Patient counselling is advised (alcohol reaction).

● MEDICINAL FORMS
There can be variation in the licensing of different medicines containing the same drug.
Tablet
CAUTIONARY AND ADVISORY LABELS 2
▸ Disulfiram (Non-proprietary)
   Disulfiram 200 mg Disulfiram 200mg tablets | 50 tablet [PoM] £91.73 DT price = £91.73
   Disulfiram 250 mg Antabuse 250mg tablets | 100 tablet [PoM] no price available

GAMMA-AMINOBUTYRIC ACID ANALOGUES AND DERIVATIVES

Acamprosate calcium

● INDICATIONS AND DOSE

Maintenance of abstinence in alcohol-dependent patients
▸ BY MOUTH
▸ Adult 18–65 years (body-weight up to 60 kg): 666 mg once daily at breakfast and 333 mg twice daily at midday and at night
▸ Adult 18–65 years (body-weight 60 kg and above): 666 mg 3 times a day

● CAUTIONS Continued alcohol abuse (risk of treatment failure)
● SIDE-EFFECTS
▸ Common or very common Abdominal pain · diarrhoea · flatulence · frigidity · impotence · maculopapular rash · nausea · pruritus · vomiting

4

Nervous system

- **Very rare** Angioedema · hypersensitivity reactions · urticaria
- **Frequency not known** Fluctuation in libido · vesiculo-bullous skin reactions
- PREGNANCY Manufacturer advises avoid unless potential benefit outweighs risk.
- BREAST FEEDING Avoid.
- HEPATIC IMPAIRMENT Avoid if severe.
- RENAL IMPAIRMENT Avoid if serum-creatinine greater than 120 micromol/litre.
- PRESCRIBING AND DISPENSING INFORMATION Acamprosate calcium has been used for the maintenance of abstinence in alcohol dependence in children aged 16 years and over.
- MEDICINAL FORMS
  There can be variation in the licensing of different medicines containing the same drug.
  Gastro-resistant tablet
  CAUTIONARY AND ADVISORY LABELS 21, 25
  ELECTROLYTES: May contain Calcium
  ‣ Acamprosate calcium (Non-proprietary)
  Acamprosate calcium 333 mg Acamprosate 333mg gastro-resistant tablets | 168 tablet PoM £28.80–£29.37 DT price = £28.80
  ‣ Campral EC (Merck Serono Ltd)
  Acamprosate calcium 333 mg Campral EC 333mg tablets | 168 tablet PoM £28.80 DT price = £28.80

OPIOID RECEPTOR ANTAGONISTS

Nalmefene

- INDICATIONS AND DOSE
  Reduction of alcohol consumption in patients with alcohol dependence who have a high drinking risk level without physical withdrawal symptoms, and who do not require immediate detoxification
  ‣ BY MOUTH
  ‣ Adult: 18 mg daily if required, taken on each day there is a risk of drinking alcohol, preferably taken 1–2 hours before the anticipated time of drinking, if a dose has not been taken before drinking alcohol, 1 dose should be taken as soon as possible; maximum 18 mg per day

- CONTRA-INDICATIONS Recent history of acute alcohol withdrawal syndrome · recent or current opioid use
- CAUTIONS Continued treatment for more than 1 year · history of seizure disorders (including alcohol withdrawal seizures) · psychiatric illness
- INTERACTIONS → Appendix 1 (nalmefene).
  Avoid concomitant use of opioids—discontinue treatment 1 week before anticipated use of opioids; if emergency analgesia is required during treatment, an increased dose of opioid analgesic may be necessary (monitor for opioid intoxication).
- SIDE-EFFECTS
  ‣ **Common or very common** Confusion · decreased appetite · decreased libido · disturbance in attention · dizziness · dry mouth · headache · hyperhidrosis · hypoaesthesia · malaise · muscle spasms · nausea · palpitation · paraesthesia · restlessness · sleep disorders · somnolence · tachycardia · tremor · vomiting · weight loss
  ‣ **Frequency not known** Dissociation · hallucinations
- PREGNANCY Manufacturer advises avoid—toxicity in *animal* studies.
- BREAST FEEDING Manufacturer advises avoid—present in milk in *animal* studies.
- HEPATIC IMPAIRMENT Use with caution—avoid in severe impairment.
- RENAL IMPAIRMENT Use with caution—avoid in severe impairment.

- PRE-TREATMENT SCREENING Before initiating treatment, prescribers should evaluate the patient's clinical status, alcohol dependence, and level of alcohol consumption. Nalmefene should only be prescribed for patients who continue to have a high drinking risk level two weeks after the initial assessment.
- MONITORING REQUIREMENTS During treatment, patients should be monitored regularly and the need for continued treatment assessed.
- NATIONAL FUNDING/ACCESS DECISIONS
  NICE technology appraisals (TAs)
  ‣ **Nalmefene for reducing alcohol consumption in people with alcohol dependence (November 2014)** NICE TA325
  Nalmefene is recommended within its marketing authorisation, as an option for reducing alcohol consumption, for patients with alcohol dependence:
  - who have a high drinking risk level (defined as alcohol consumption of more than 60 g per day for men and more than 40 g per day for women, according to the World Health Organization's drinking risk levels) without physical withdrawal symptoms, **and**
  - who do not require immediate detoxification.
  The marketing authorisation states that nalmefene should:
  - only be prescribed in conjunction with continuous psychosocial support focused on treatment adherence and reducing alcohol consumption, **and**
  - be initiated only in patients who continue to have a high drinking risk level 2 weeks after initial assessment.
  www.nice.org.uk/TA325

- MEDICINAL FORMS
  There can be variation in the licensing of different medicines containing the same drug.
  Tablet
  CAUTIONARY AND ADVISORY LABELS 25
  ‣ Selincro (Lundbeck Ltd) ▼
  Nalmefene (as Nalmefene hydrochloride) 18 mg Selincro 18mg tablets | 14 tablet PoM £42.42 DT price = £42.42 | 28 tablet PoM £84.84

Naltrexone hydrochloride

- DRUG ACTION Naltrexone is an opioid-receptor antagonist.

- INDICATIONS AND DOSE
  Adjunct to prevent relapse in formerly opioid-dependent patients (who have remained opioid-free for at least 7–10 days) (initiated under specialist supervision)
  ‣ BY MOUTH
  ‣ Adult: Initially 25 mg daily, then increased to 50 mg daily, total weekly dose may be divided and given on 3 days of the week for improved compliance (e.g. 100 mg on Monday and Wednesday, and 150 mg on Friday); maximum 350 mg per week
  Adjunct to prevent relapse in formerly alcohol-dependent patients (initiated under specialist supervision)
  ‣ BY MOUTH
  ‣ Adult: 25 mg once daily on the first day, then increased if tolerated to 50 mg daily

- UNLICENSED USE 25 mg dose for adjunct to prevent relapse in formerly alcohol-dependent patients is an unlicensed dose.
- CONTRA-INDICATIONS Patients currently dependent on opioids
- INTERACTIONS Avoid concomitant use of opioids but increased dose of opioid analgesic may be required for pain (monitor for opioid intoxication).

- SIDE-EFFECTS
▶ **Common or very common** Joint and muscle pain · abdominal pain · anxiety · chest pain · chills · constipation · decreased potency · delayed ejaculation · diarrhoea · dizziness · headache · increased energy · increased lacrimation · increased sweating · increased thirst · irritability · mood swings · nausea · rash · reduced appetite · sleep disorders · urinary retention · vomiting
▶ **Rare** Depression · hepatic dysfunction · speech disorders · suicidal ideation · tinnitus
▶ **Very rare** Exanthema · hallucinations · idiopathic thrombocytopenia · tremor

- PREGNANCY Use only if benefit outweighs risk.

- BREAST FEEDING Avoid—potential toxicity.

- HEPATIC IMPAIRMENT Avoid in acute hepatitis, hepatic failure, or severe impairment.

- RENAL IMPAIRMENT Avoid in severe impairment.

- PRE-TREATMENT SCREENING Test for opioid dependence with naloxone before treatment.

- MONITORING REQUIREMENTS Liver function tests needed before and during treatment.

- PATIENT AND CARER ADVICE Patients should be warned that an attempt to overcome the blockade of opioid receptors by overdosing could result in acute opioid intoxication.

- NATIONAL FUNDING/ACCESS DECISIONS
  NICE technology appraisals (TAs)
▶ **Naltrexone for the management of opioid dependence (January 2007)** NICE TA115
  Naltrexone is recommended for the prevention of relapse in formerly opioid-dependent patients who are motivated to remain in a supportive care abstinence programme. Naltrexone should be administered under supervision and its effectiveness in preventing opioid misuse reviewed regularly.
  www.nice.org.uk/TA115

- MEDICINAL FORMS
  There can be variation in the licensing of different medicines containing the same drug. Forms available from special-order manufacturers include: capsule, oral suspension, oral solution
  Tablet
  ▶ Naltrexone hydrochloride (Non-proprietary)
    Naltrexone hydrochloride 50 mg Naltrexone 50mg tablets | 28 tablet [PoM] £23.00 DT price = £22.34
  ▶ Adepend (AOP Orphan Pharmaceuticals AG)
    Naltrexone hydrochloride 50 mg Adepend 50mg tablets | 28 tablet [PoM] £47.43 DT price = £22.34
  ▶ Nalorex (Bristol-Myers Squibb Pharmaceuticals Ltd)
    Naltrexone hydrochloride 50 mg Nalorex 50mg tablets | 28 tablet [PoM] £22.34 DT price = £22.34
  ▶ Opizone (Genus Pharmaceuticals Ltd)
    Naltrexone hydrochloride 50 mg Opizone 50mg tablets | 28 tablet [PoM] £19.55 DT price = £22.34

8.2 Nicotine dependence

ANTIDEPRESSANTS > SEROTONIN AND NORADRENALINE RE-UPTAKE INHIBITORS

Bupropion hydrochloride

(Amfebutamone hydrochloride)

- INDICATIONS AND DOSE

To aid smoking cessation in combination with motivational support in nicotine-dependent patients
▶ BY MOUTH
▶ Adult: Initially 150 mg daily for 6 days, then 150 mg twice daily (max. per dose 150 mg), minimum 8 hours

between doses; period of treatment 7–9 weeks, start treatment 1–2 weeks before target stop date, discontinue if abstinence not achieved at 7 weeks, consider maximum 150 mg daily in patients with risk factors for seizures; maximum 300 mg per day
▶ Elderly: 150 mg daily for 7–9 weeks, start treatment 1–2 weeks before target stop date, discontinue if abstinence not achieved at 7 weeks; maximum 150 mg per day

- CONTRA-INDICATIONS Acute alcohol withdrawal · acute benzodiazepine withdrawal · bipolar disorder · CNS tumour · eating disorders · history of seizures · severe hepatic cirrhosis

- CAUTIONS Alcohol abuse · diabetes · elderly · history of head trauma · predisposition to seizures (prescribe only if benefit clearly outweighs risk)

- INTERACTIONS → Appendix 1 (bupropion).
  Caution with concomitant use of drugs that lower seizure threshold.

- SIDE-EFFECTS
▶ **Common or very common** Agitation · anxiety · depression · dizziness · dry mouth · fever · gastro-intestinal disturbances · headache · impaired concentration · insomnia (reduced by avoiding dose at bedtime) · pruritus · rash · sweating · taste disturbance · tremor
▶ **Uncommon** Anorexia · asthenia · chest pain · confusion · flushing · hypertension · tachycardia · tinnitus · visual disturbances
▶ **Rare** Abnormal dreams · ataxia · blood-glucose changes · depersonalisation · dystonia · exacerbation of psoriasis · hallucinations · hepatitis · hostility · impaired memory · incoordination · irritability · jaundice · palpitation · paraesthesia · postural hypotension · seizures · Stevens-Johnson syndrome · twitching · urinary frequency · urinary retention · vasodilatation
▶ **Very rare** Aggression · delusions · paranoid ideation · restlessness
▶ **Frequency not known** Suicidal ideation

- PREGNANCY Avoid—no information available.

- BREAST FEEDING Present in milk—avoid.

- HEPATIC IMPAIRMENT Reduce dose to 150 mg daily. Avoid in severe hepatic cirrhosis.

- RENAL IMPAIRMENT Reduce dose to 150 mg daily.

- MONITORING REQUIREMENTS Measure blood pressure before and during treatment.

- PATIENT AND CARER ADVICE
  Driving and skilled tasks
  May impair performance of skilled tasks (e.g. driving).

- MEDICINAL FORMS
  There can be variation in the licensing of different medicines containing the same drug.
  Modified-release tablet
  CAUTIONARY AND ADVISORY LABELS 25
  ▶ Zyban (GlaxoSmithKline UK Ltd)
    Bupropion hydrochloride 150 mg Zyban 150mg modified-release tablets | 60 tablet [PoM] £41.76 DT price = £41.76

NICOTINIC RECEPTOR AGONISTS

Nicotine

- INDICATIONS AND DOSE

Nicotine replacement therapy in individuals who smoke fewer than 20 cigarettes each day
▶ BY MOUTH USING CHEWING GUM
▶ Adult: 2 mg as required, chew 1 piece of gum when the urge to smoke occurs or to prevent continued →

cravings, if attempting smoking cessation, treatment should continue for 3 months before reducing the dose
▸ BY SUBLINGUAL ADMINISTRATION USING SUBLINGUAL TABLETS
▸ Adult: 1 tablet every 1 hour, increased to 2 tablets every 1 hour if required, if attempting smoking cessation, treatment should continue for up to 3 months before reducing the dose; maximum 40 tablets per day

Nicotine replacement therapy in individuals who smoke more than 20 cigarettes each day or who require more than 15 pieces of 2-mg strength gum each day
▸ BY MOUTH USING CHEWING GUM
▸ Adult: 4 mg as required, chew 1 piece of gum when the urge to smoke occurs or to prevent cravings, individuals should not exceed 15 pieces of 4-mg strength gum daily, if attempting smoking cessation, treatment should continue for 3 months before reducing the dose

Nicotine replacement therapy in individuals who smoke more than 20 cigarettes each day
▸ BY SUBLINGUAL ADMINISTRATION USING SUBLINGUAL TABLETS
▸ Adult: 2 tablets every 1 hour, if attempting smoking cessation, treatment should continue for up to 3 months before reducing the dose; maximum 40 tablets per day

Nicotine replacement therapy
▸ BY INHALATION USING INHALATOR
▸ Adult: As required, the cartridges can be used when the urge to smoke occurs or to prevent cravings, individuals should not exceed 12 cartridges of the 10-mg strength daily, or 6 cartridges of the 15-mg strength daily
▸ BY MOUTH USING LOZENGES
▸ Adult: 1 lozenge every 1–2 hours as required, one lozenge should be used when the urge to smoke occurs, individuals who smoke less than 20 cigarettes each day should usually use the lower-strength lozenges; individuals who smoke more than 20 cigarettes each day and those who fail to stop smoking with the low-strength lozenges should use the higher-strength lozenges; If attempting smoking cessation, treatment should continue for 6–12 weeks before attempting a reduction in dose; maximum 15 lozenges per day
▸ BY MOUTH USING OROMUCOSAL SPRAY
▸ Adult: 1–2 sprays as required, individuals can spray in the mouth when the urge to smoke occurs or to prevent cravings, individuals should not exceed 2 sprays per episode (up to 4 sprays every hour); maximum 64 sprays per day
▸ BY INTRANASAL ADMINISTRATION USING NASAL SPRAY
▸ Adult: 1 spray as required, individuals can spray into each nostril when the urge to smoke occurs, up to twice every hour for 16 hours daily, if attempting smoking cessation, treatment should continue for 8 weeks before reducing the dose; maximum 64 sprays per day
▸ BY TRANSDERMAL APPLICATION USING PATCHES
▸ Adult: Individuals who smoke more than 10 cigarettes daily should apply a high-strength patch daily for 6–8 weeks, followed by the medium-strength patch for 2 weeks, and then the low-strength patch for the final 2 weeks; individuals who smoke fewer than 10 cigarettes daily can usually start with the medium-strength patch for 6–8 weeks followed by the low-strength patch for 2–4 weeks; a slower titration schedule can be used in individuals who are not ready to quit but want to reduce cigarette consumption before a quit attempt; if abstinence is not achieved, or if withdrawal symptoms are experienced, the strength of the patch used should be maintained or increased until the patient is stabilised; individuals using the high-strength patch who experience excessive side-effects, that do not resolve within a few days, should

change to a medium-strength patch for the remainder of the initial period and then use the low-strength patch for 2–4 weeks

● UNLICENSED USE All preparations are licensed for adults and children over 12 years (with the exception of *Nicotinell*® lozenges which are licensed for children under 18 years only when recommended by a doctor).
● CAUTIONS
GENERAL CAUTIONS
Diabetes mellitus—blood-glucose concentration should be monitored closely when initiating treatment · haemodynamically unstable patients hospitalised with cerebrovascular accident · haemodynamically unstable patients hospitalised with myocardial infarction · haemodynamically unstable patients hospitalised with severe arrhythmias · phaeochromocytoma · uncontrolled hyperthyroidism
SPECIFIC CAUTIONS
▸ When used by inhalation Bronchospastic disease · chronic throat disease · obstructive lung disease
▸ With intranasal use Bronchial asthma (may exacerbate)
▸ With oral use Gastritis (can be aggravated by swallowed nicotine) · oesophagitis (can be aggravated by swallowed nicotine) · peptic ulcers (can be aggravated by swallowed nicotine)
▸ With oral (topical) use *gum* may also stick to and damage dentures
▸ With transdermal use *patches* should not be placed on broken skin · patients with skin disorders
CAUTIONS, FURTHER INFORMATION
Most warnings for nicotine replacement therapy also apply to continued cigarette smoking, but the risk of continued smoking outweighs any risks of using nicotine preparations.
　Specific cautions for individual preparations are usually related to the local effect of nicotine.
● INTERACTIONS → Appendix 1 (nicotine).
● SIDE-EFFECTS
▸ **Common or very common** Bloating · blurred vision · constipation · coughing · diarrhoea · dry mouth · dyspepsia · dysphagia · epistaxis · flatulence · gastritis · gastro-intestinal disturbances (may be caused by swallowed nicotine) · hiccup · increased salivation · irritation of the throat · mild local reactions at the beginning of treatment are common because of the irritant effect of nicotine · minor skin irritation · mouth ulcers · nasal irritation · nausea · oesophagitis · paraesthesia · sneezing · vomiting · watery eyes
▸ **Uncommon** Gingival bleeding · halitosis · thirst
▸ **Rare** Arrhythmia
▸ **Very rare** Reversible atrial fibrillation
▸ **Frequency not known** Abdominal pain · abnormal dreams (may occur with patches, removal of the patch before bed may help) · arthralgia · chest pain · flatulence · hot flushes · myalgia · palpitations · rash · sweating · taste disturbance · ulcerative stomatitis
SIDE-EFFECTS, FURTHER INFORMATION
Side-effects listed have been reported with use of various nicotine replacement therapy preparations. See *Nicotine replacement therapy*, under Substance dependence p. 448 for further details on individual preparations.
▸ Nicotine withdrawal Some systemic effects occur on initiation of therapy, particularly if the patient is using high-strength preparations; however, the patient may confuse side-effects of the nicotine-replacement preparation with nicotine withdrawal symptoms.
　Common symptoms of nicotine withdrawal include malaise, headache, dizziness, sleep disturbance, coughing, influenza–like symptoms, depression, irritability, increased appetite, weight gain, restlessness, anxiety,

drowsiness, aphthous ulcers, decreased heart rate, and impaired concentration.

- **PREGNANCY** The use of nicotine replacement therapy in pregnancy is preferable to the continuation of smoking, but should be used only if smoking cessation without nicotine replacement fails. Intermittent therapy is preferable to patches but avoid liquorice-flavoured nicotine products. Patches are useful, however, if the patient is experiencing pregnancy-related nausea and vomiting. If patches are used, they should be removed before bed.

- **BREAST FEEDING** Nicotine is present in milk; however, the amount to which the infant is exposed is small and less hazardous than second-hand smoke. Intermittent therapy is preferred.

- **HEPATIC IMPAIRMENT** Use with caution in moderate to severe hepatic impairment.

- **RENAL IMPAIRMENT** Use with caution in severe renal impairment.

- **DIRECTIONS FOR ADMINISTRATION** Acidic beverages, such as coffee or fruit juice, may decrease the absorption of nicotine through the buccal mucosa and should be avoided for 15 minutes before the use of oral nicotine replacement therapy.
  Administration by transdermal patch Patches should be applied on waking to dry, non-hairy skin on the hip, trunk, or upper arm and held in position for 10–20 seconds to ensure adhesion; place next patch on a different area and avoid using the same site for several days.
  Administration by nasal spray Initially 1 spray should be used in both nostrils but when withdrawing from therapy, the dose can be gradually reduced to 1 spray in 1 nostril.
  Administration by oral spray The oral spray should be released into the mouth, holding the spray as close to the mouth as possible and avoiding the lips. The patient should not inhale while spraying and avoid swallowing for a few seconds after use. If using the oral spray for the first time, or if unit not used for 2 or more days, prime the unit before administration.
  Administration by sublingual tablet Each tablet should be placed under the tongue and allowed to dissolve.
  Administration by lozenge Slowly allow each lozenge to dissolve in the mouth; periodically move the lozenge from one side of the mouth to the other. Lozenges last for 10–30 minutes, depending on their size.
  Administration by inhalation Insert the cartridge into the device and draw in air through the mouthpiece; each session can last for approximately 5 minutes. The amount of nicotine from 1 puff of the cartridge is less than that from a cigarette, therefore it is necessary to inhale more often than when smoking a cigarette. A single 10 mg cartridge lasts for approximately 20 minutes of intense use; a single 15 mg cartridge lasts for approximately 40 minutes of intense use.
  Administration by medicated chewing gum Chew the gum until the taste becomes strong, then rest it between the cheek and gum; when the taste starts to fade, repeat this process. One piece of gum lasts for approximately 30 minutes.

- **PRESCRIBING AND DISPENSING INFORMATION** Flavours of chewing gum and lozenges may include mint, freshfruit, freshmint, icy white, or cherry.

- **PATIENT AND CARER ADVICE** Patient or carers should be given advice on how to administer nicotine chewing gum, inhalators, lozenges, sublingual tablets, oral spray, nasal spray and patches.

- **MEDICINAL FORMS**
  There can be variation in the licensing of different medicines containing the same drug.

Sublingual tablet
CAUTIONARY AND ADVISORY LABELS 26
▸ Nicotine (Non-proprietary)
  Nicotine (as Nicotine cyclodextrin complex) 2 mg sublingual tablets sugar-free | 100 tablet [GSL] no price available DT price = £13.12
▸ Brands may include Nicorette Microtab

Orodispersible film
▸ NiQuitin (Omega Pharma Ltd)
  Nicotine 2.5 mg NiQuitin Strips Mint 2.5mg oral films sugar-free | 15 film [GSL] £3.51 sugar-free | 60 film [GSL] £10.85

Lozenge
EXCIPIENTS: May contain Aspartame
ELECTROLYTES: May contain Sodium
▸ Nicotine (Non-proprietary)
  Nicotine (as Nicotine bitartrate) 1 mg lozenges sugar-free | 96 lozenge [GSL] no price available DT price = £9.12
  Nicotine (as Nicotine bitartrate) 2 mg lozenges sugar-free | 96 lozenge [GSL] no price available
▸ Brands may include NiQuitin, Nicorette, Nicotinell

Medicated chewing-gum
▸ Nicotine (Non-proprietary)
  Nicotine 2 mg medicated chewing gum sugar-free | [GSL] no price available
  Nicotine 4 mg medicated chewing gum sugar-free | [GSL] no price available
▸ Brands may include NiQuitin, Nicorette, Nicorette Icy White, Nicotinell

Inhalation vapour
▸ Nicotine (Non-proprietary)
  Nicotine 15 mg Inhalator | 4 cartridge [GSL] no price available DT price = £4.27 | 20 cartridge [GSL] no price available DT price = £15.11
▸ Brands may include Nicorette

Transdermal patch
▸ Nicotine (Non-proprietary)
  Nicotine 7 mg per 24 hour transdermal patches | 7 patch [GSL] no price available
  Nicotine 10 mg per 16 hour patches | 7 patch [GSL] no price available DT price = £10.37
  Nicotine 14 mg per 24 hour transdermal patches | 7 patch [GSL] no price available
  Nicotine 15 mg per 16 hour patches | 7 patch [GSL] no price available DT price = £10.37
  Nicotine 21 mg per 24 hour transdermal patches | 7 patch [GSL] no price available DT price = £9.97
  Nicotine 25 mg per 16 hour patches | 7 patch [GSL] no price available DT price = £10.37
▸ Brands may include NiQuitin, NiQuitin Clear, Nicorette invisi, Nicotinell TTS

Spray
EXCIPIENTS: May contain Ethanol
▸ Nicotine (Non-proprietary)
  Nicotine 500 microgram per 1 actuation 10mg/ml nasal spray | 10 ml [GSL] no price available DT price = £13.80
▸ Brands may include Nicorette, Nicorette QuickMist

Varenicline

- **DRUG ACTION** Varenicline is a selective nicotine-receptor partial agonist.

- **INDICATIONS AND DOSE**

To aid smoking cessation
▸ BY MOUTH
▸ Adult: Initially 500 micrograms once daily for 3 days, increased to 500 micrograms twice daily for 4 days, then 1 mg twice daily for 11 weeks; reduced if not tolerated to 500 micrograms twice daily, usually to be started 1–2 weeks before target stop date but can be started up to a maximum of 5 weeks before continued →

4

Nervous system

target stop date, 12-week course can be repeated in abstinent individuals to reduce risk of relapse

IMPORTANT SAFETY INFORMATION

MHRA/CHM ADVICE: SUICIDAL BEHAVIOUR AND VARENICLINE
Patients should be advised to discontinue treatment and seek prompt medical advice if they develop agitation, depressed mood, or suicidal thoughts. Patients with a history of psychiatric illness should be monitored closely while taking varenicline.

● CAUTIONS Conditions that may lower seizure threshold · history of cardiovascular disease · history of psychiatric illness (may exacerbate underlying illness including depression) · predisposition to seizures

● SIDE-EFFECTS
▶ **Common or very common** Taste disturbance · abnormal dreams · appetite changes · dizziness · drowsiness · dry mouth · gastro-intestinal disturbances · headache · sleep disorders
▶ **Uncommon** Acne · anxiety · aphthous stomatitis · arthralgia · asthenia · atrial fibrillation · chest pain · depression · dysarthria · dysuria · eye pain · gingival pain · hallucinations · hypertension · hypertonia · hypoaesthesia · impaired temperature regulation · incoordination · lacrimation · menorrhagia · mood swings · muscle spasm · palpitation · panic attack · pruritus · rash · restlessness · seizure · sexual dysfunction · sweating · tachycardia · thirst · tinnitus · tremor · vaginal discharge · visual disturbances · weight gain
▶ **Rare** Cerebrovascular accident
▶ **Frequency not known** Aggression · diabetes mellitus · hyperglycaemia · irrational behaviour · myocardial infarction · psychosis · sleep-walking · Stevens-Johnson syndrome · suicidal ideation

● PREGNANCY Avoid—toxicity in *animal* studies.

● BREAST FEEDING Avoid—present in milk in *animal* studies.

● RENAL IMPAIRMENT If eGFR less than 30 mL/minute/1.73 m^2, initial dose 500 micrograms once daily, increased after 3 days to 1 mg once daily.

● TREATMENT CESSATION Risk of relapse, irritability, depression, and insomnia on discontinuation; consider dose tapering on completion of 12-week course.

● NATIONAL FUNDING/ACCESS DECISIONS
NICE technology appraisals (TAs)
▶ **Varenicline for smoking cessation (July 2007)** NICE TA123 Varenicline is recommended, within its licensed indications, as an option for smokers who have expressed a desire to quit smoking; it should normally be prescribed only as part of a programme of behavioural support.
www.nice.org.uk/TA123

● MEDICINAL FORMS
There can be variation in the licensing of different medicines containing the same drug.
Tablet
CAUTIONARY AND ADVISORY LABELS 3
▶ Champix (Pfizer Ltd) ▼
Varenicline (as Varenicline tartrate) 500 microgram Champix 0.5mg tablets | 11 tablet PoM no price available | 56 tablet PoM £54.60 DT price = £54.60
Varenicline (as Varenicline tartrate) 1 mg Champix 1mg tablets | 14 tablet PoM no price available | 28 tablet PoM £27.30 DT price = £27.30 | 56 tablet PoM £54.60
▶ Champix (Pfizer Ltd) ▼
Champix 0.5mg/1mg 2 week treatment initiation pack | 25 tablet PoM £27.30 DT price = £27.30
Champix 0.5mg/1mg 4 week treatment initiation pack | 53 tablet PoM £54.60

8.3 Opioid dependence

ANALGESICS ⟩ OPIOIDS

F 408

| **Methadone hydrochloride**

● INDICATIONS AND DOSE
Severe pain
▶ BY MOUTH, OR BY SUBCUTANEOUS INJECTION, OR BY INTRAMUSCULAR INJECTION
▶ Adult: 5–10 mg every 6–8 hours, adjusted according to response, on prolonged use not to be given more frequently than every 12 hours
Adjunct in treatment of opioid dependence
▶ BY MOUTH USING ORAL SOLUTION
▶ Adult: Initially 10–30 mg daily, increased in steps of 5–10 mg daily if required until no signs of withdrawal nor evidence of intoxication, dose to be increased in the first week, then increased every few days as necessary up to usual dose, maximum weekly dose increase of 30 mg; usual dose 60–120 mg daily
Adjunct in treatment of opioid dependence if tolerance low or not known
▶ BY MOUTH USING ORAL SOLUTION
▶ Adult: Initially 10–20 mg daily, increased in steps of 5–10 mg daily if required until no signs of withdrawal nor evidence of intoxication, dose to be increased in the first week, then increased every few days as necessary up to usual dose, maximum weekly dose increase of 30 mg; usual dose 60–120 mg daily
Adjunct in treatment of opioid dependence if tolerance high (under expert supervision)
▶ BY MOUTH USING ORAL SOLUTION
▶ Adult: Initially up to 40 mg daily, increased in steps of 5–10 mg daily if required until no signs of withdrawal nor evidence of intoxication, dose to be increased in the first week, then increased every few days as necessary up to usual dose, maximum weekly dose increase of 30 mg; usual dose 60–120 mg daily
Cough in terminal disease
▶ INITIALLY BY MOUTH USING LINCTUS
▶ Adult: 1–2 mg every 4–6 hours, (by mouth) reduced to 1–2 mg twice daily, use twice daily frequency if prolonged use

DOSE EQUIVALENCE AND CONVERSION
See p. 409 for dose adjustments in opioid substitution therapy, for patients taking methadone who want to switch to buprenorphine.

● UNLICENSED USE Methadone hydrochloride doses for opioid dependence in the BNF may differ from those in the product literature.

IMPORTANT SAFETY INFORMATION
Methadone oral solution 1 mg/mL is 2½ times the strength of Methadone Linctus (2 mg/5mL). Many preparations of Methadone oral solution are licensed for opioid drug addiction only but some are also licensed for analgesia in severe pain.

● CONTRA-INDICATIONS Phaeochromocytoma
● CAUTIONS Family history of sudden death (ECG monitoring recommended) · history of cardiac conduction abnormalities

CAUTIONS, FURTHER INFORMATION
▶ QT-interval prolongation Patients with the following risk factors for QT-interval prolongation should be carefully monitored while taking methadone: heart or liver disease, electrolyte abnormalities, or concomitant treatment with

drugs that can prolong QT interval; patients requiring more than 100 mg daily should also be monitored.

- SIDE-EFFECTS Dry eyes · dysmenorrhoea · hyperprolactinaemia · hypothermia · QT-interval prolongation · raised intracranial pressure · restlessness · torsade de pointes

  SIDE-EFFECTS, FURTHER INFORMATION
  Methadone is a long-acting opioid therefore effects may be cumulative.

  Methadone, even in low doses is a **special hazard** for children; non-dependent adults are also at risk of toxicity; dependent adults are at risk if tolerance is incorrectly assessed during induction.

  Overdose
  Methadone has a very long duration of action; patients may need to be monitored for long periods following large overdoses.

- BREAST FEEDING Withdrawal symptoms in infant; breast-feeding permissible during maintenance but dose should be as low as possible and infant monitored to avoid sedation (high doses of methadone carry an increased risk of sedation and respiratory depression in the neonate).

- RENAL IMPAIRMENT Avoid use or reduce dose; opioid effects increased and prolonged and increased cerebral sensitivity occurs.

- TREATMENT CESSATION Avoid abrupt withdrawal.

- DIRECTIONS FOR ADMINISTRATION Syrup preserved with hydroxybenzoate (parabens) esters may be incompatible with methadone hydrochloride.

- PRESCRIBING AND DISPENSING INFORMATION Flavours of oral liquid formulations may include tolu.

  METHADOSE® The final strength of the methadone mixture to be dispensed to the patient must be specified on the prescription.

  Important—care is required in prescribing and dispensing the **correct strength** since any confusion could lead to an overdose; this preparation should be dispensed only **after dilution** as appropriate with *Methadose*® Diluent (life of diluted solution 3 months) and is for drug dependent persons.

- NATIONAL FUNDING/ACCESS DECISIONS

  NICE technology appraisals (TAs)
  ► Methadone and buprenorphine for the management of opioid dependence (January 2007) NICE TA114
  Oral methadone and buprenorphine are recommended for maintenance therapy in the management of opioid dependence. Patients should be committed to a supportive care programme including a flexible dosing regimen administered under supervision for at least 3 months, until compliance is assured. Selection of methadone or buprenorphine should be made on a case-by-case basis, but methadone should be prescribed if both drugs are equally suitable.
  www.nice.org.uk/TA114

- LESS SUITABLE FOR PRESCRIBING Methadone linctus is less suitable for prescribing for cough in terminal disease (has a tendency to accumulate).

- MEDICINAL FORMS
  There can be variation in the licensing of different medicines containing the same drug. Forms available from special-order manufacturers include: tablet, capsule, oral suspension, oral solution, solution for injection

  Tablet
  CAUTIONARY AND ADVISORY LABELS 2
  ► Physeptone (Martindale Pharmaceuticals Ltd)
  Methadone hydrochloride 5 mg Physeptone 5mg tablets | 50 tablet [PoM] £2.41 DT price = £2.41 [CD2]

Oral solution
CAUTIONARY AND ADVISORY LABELS 2
► Methadone hydrochloride (Non-proprietary)
Methadone hydrochloride 1 mg per 1 ml Methadone 1mg/ml oral solution | 100 ml [PoM] £1.10–£1.23 DT price = £1.11 [CD2] | 500 ml [PoM] £6.18 DT price = £5.55 [CD2] | 2500 ml [PoM] £27.50–£32.10 [CD2]
Methadone 1mg/ml oral solution sugar free sugar-free | 50 ml [PoM] £1.04 DT price = £1.04 [CD2] sugar-free | 100 ml [PoM] £2.08 DT price = £2.08 [CD2] sugar-free | 500 ml [PoM] £6.30 DT price = £6.30 [CD2] sugar-free | 2500 ml [PoM] £31.50–£32.50 [CD2]
► Methadose (Rosemont Pharmaceuticals Ltd)
Methadone hydrochloride 10 mg per 1 ml Methadose 10mg/ml oral solution concentrate sugar-free | 150 ml [PoM] £12.01 [CD2]
Methadone hydrochloride 20 mg per 1 ml Methadose 20mg/ml oral solution concentrate sugar-free | 150 ml [PoM] £24.02 [CD2]
► Metharose (Rosemont Pharmaceuticals Ltd)
Methadone hydrochloride 1 mg per 1 ml Metharose 1mg/ml oral solution sugar free sugar-free | 500 ml [PoM] £6.82 DT price = £6.30 [CD2]
► Physeptone (Martindale Pharmaceuticals Ltd)
Methadone hydrochloride 1 mg per 1 ml Physeptone 1mg/ml mixture | 100 ml [PoM] £1.08 DT price = £1.11 [CD2] | 500 ml [PoM] £5.46 DT price = £5.55 [CD2] | 2500 ml [PoM] £27.29 [CD2]
Physeptone 1mg/ml mixture sugar free sugar-free | 100 ml [PoM] £1.08 DT price = £2.08 [CD2] sugar-free | 500 ml [PoM] £6.30 DT price = £6.30 [CD2] sugar-free | 2500 ml [PoM] £27.29 [CD2]

Solution for injection
► Methadone hydrochloride (Non-proprietary)
Methadone hydrochloride 10 mg per 1 ml Methadone 35mg/3.5ml solution for injection ampoules | 10 ampoule [PoM] £13.92 DT price = £12.87 [CD2]
Methadone hydrochloride 25 mg per 1 ml Methadone 50mg/2ml solution for injection ampoules | 10 ampoule [PoM] no price available [CD2]
Methadone hydrochloride 50 mg per 1 ml Methadone 50mg/1ml solution for injection ampoules | 10 ampoule [PoM] no price available [CD2]
► Physeptone (Martindale Pharmaceuticals Ltd)
Methadone hydrochloride 10 mg per 1 ml Physeptone 35mg/3.5ml solution for injection ampoules | 10 ampoule [PoM] £12.87 DT price = £12.87 [CD2]
Physeptone 50mg/5ml solution for injection ampoules | 10 ampoule [PoM] £13.88 DT price = £13.88 [CD2]
Physeptone 10mg/1ml solution for injection ampoules | 10 ampoule [PoM] £6.49 DT price = £6.49 [CD2] | 100 ampoule [PoM] £62.10 [CD2]
Physeptone 20mg/2ml solution for injection ampoules | 10 ampoule [PoM] £11.17 DT price = £11.17 [CD2]
Methadone hydrochloride 25 mg per 1 ml Physeptone 50mg/2ml solution for injection ampoules | 10 ampoule [PoM] £15.06 [CD2]
Methadone hydrochloride 50 mg per 1 ml Physeptone 50mg/1ml solution for injection ampoules | 10 ampoule [PoM] £15.06 [CD2]

OPIOID RECEPTOR ANTAGONISTS

Buprenorphine with naloxone

The properties listed below are those particular to the combination only. For the properties of the components please consider, buprenorphine p. 409, naloxone hydrochloride p. 1204.

- INDICATIONS AND DOSE

  Adjunct in the treatment of opioid dependence (dose expressed as buprenorphine)
  ► BY SUBLINGUAL ADMINISTRATION
  ► Adult: Initially 2–4 mg once daily, an additional dose of 2–4 mg may be administered on day 1 depending on the individual patient's requirement, increased in steps of 2–8 mg, adjusted according to response, total weekly dose may be divided and given on alternate days or 3 times weekly; maximum 24 mg per day

- NATIONAL FUNDING/ACCESS DECISIONS

  Scottish Medicines Consortium (SMC) Decisions
  The *Scottish Medicines Consortium* has advised (February 2007) that Suboxone® should be restricted for use in patients in whom methadone is not suitable.

4

Nervous system

Nervous system

4

● MEDICINAL FORMS
There can be variation in the licensing of different medicines containing the same drug.

Sublingual tablet

CAUTIONARY AND ADVISORY LABELS 2, 26

▸ Suboxone (Indivior UK Ltd)

Naloxone (as Naloxone hydrochloride) 500 microgram, Buprenorphine (as Buprenorphine hydrochloride) 2 mg Suboxone 2mg/500microgram sublingual tablets sugar-free | 28 tablet PoM £25.40 DT price = £25.40 CD3

Naloxone (as Naloxone hydrochloride) 2 mg, Buprenorphine (as Buprenorphine hydrochloride) 8 mg Suboxone 8mg/2mg sublingual tablets sugar-free | 28 tablet PoM £76.19 DT price = £76.19 CD3

SYMPATHOMIMETICS › ALPHA₂-ADRENOCEPTOR AGONISTS

Lofexidine hydrochloride

● DRUG ACTION Lofexidine is an alpha₂-adrenergic agonist.

● INDICATIONS AND DOSE

Management of symptoms of opioid withdrawal

▸ BY MOUTH

▸ Adult: Initially 800 micrograms daily in divided doses, increased in steps of 400–800 micrograms daily (max. per dose 800 micrograms) as required recommended duration of treatment 7–10 days if no opioid use (but longer may be required); maximum 2.4 mg per day

● CAUTIONS Bradycardia · cerebrovascular disease · depression · history of QT prolongation · hypotension (monitor pulse rate and blood pressure) · metabolic disturbances · recent myocardial infarction · severe coronary insufficiency

● INTERACTIONS → Appendix 1 (lofexidine).
Caution with concomitant administration of drugs that prolong QT interval.

● SIDE-EFFECTS Bradycardia · dizziness · drowsiness · dry mucous membranes · hypotension · QT-interval prolongation

● PREGNANCY Use only if benefit outweighs risk—no information available.

● BREAST FEEDING Use only if benefit outweighs risk—no information available.

● RENAL IMPAIRMENT Caution in chronic impairment.

● MONITORING REQUIREMENTS Monitoring of blood pressure and pulse rate is recommended on initiation, for at least 72 hours or until a stable dose is achieved, and on discontinuation.

● TREATMENT CESSATION Treatment should be withdrawn gradually over 2–4 days (or longer) to reduce the risk of rebound hypertension and associated symptoms.

● PRESCRIBING AND DISPENSING INFORMATION Lofexidine has been used in children over 12 years in the management of symptoms of opioid withdrawal.

● PATIENT AND CARER ADVICE The patient should take part of the dose at bedtime to offset insomnia associated with opioid withdrawal.

● MEDICINAL FORMS
There can be variation in the licensing of different medicines containing the same drug.

Tablet

CAUTIONARY AND ADVISORY LABELS 2

▸ BritLofex (Britannia Pharmaceuticals Ltd)

Lofexidine hydrochloride 200 microgram BritLofex 200microgram tablets | 60 tablet PoM £61.79

Chapter 5
Infection

1 Amoebic infection

Drugs used for Amoebic infection not listed below
Metronidazole, p. 492 · Tinidazole, p. 493

ANTIPROTOZOALS

Diloxanide furoate

● **INDICATIONS AND DOSE**

Chronic amoebiasis | Acute amoebiasis as adjunct to metronidazole or tinidazole
▸ BY MOUTH
▸ Child 12-17 years: 500 mg 3 times a day for 10 days
▸ Adult: 500 mg 3 times a day for 10 days

● UNLICENSED USE
▸ In children Not licensed for use in children under 25 kg body-weight.
● SIDE-EFFECTS Flatulence · pruritus · urticaria · vomiting
● PREGNANCY Manufacturer advises avoid—no information available.
● BREAST FEEDING Manufacturer advises avoid.

● MEDICINAL FORMS
There can be variation in the licensing of different medicines containing the same drug. Forms available from special-order manufacturers include: oral suspension, oral solution
Tablet
CAUTIONARY AND ADVISORY LABELS 9
▸ Diloxanide furoate (Non-proprietary)
  Diloxanide furoate 500 mg Diloxanide 500mg tablets | 30 tablet [PoM] £93.50

Mepacrine hydrochloride

● **INDICATIONS AND DOSE**

Giardiasis
▸ BY MOUTH
▸ Adult: 100 mg every 8 hours for 5–7 days

● UNLICENSED USE Not licensed for use in giardiasis.
● CAUTIONS Avoid in psoriasis · elderly · history of psychosis
● INTERACTIONS → Appendix 1 (mepacrine).
● SIDE-EFFECTS Yellow discoloration of skin (on prolonged treatment) · aplastic anaemia (on prolonged treatment) · blue/black discoloration of nails · blue/black discoloration of palate · chronic dermatoses (on prolonged treatment) · CNS stimulation (with large doses) · corneal deposits with visual disturbances · dizziness · gastro-intestinal disturbances · headache · hepatitis (on prolonged treatment) · nausea (with large doses) · severe exfoliative dermatitis (on prolonged treatment) · transient acute toxic psychosis (with large doses) · vomiting (with large doses) · yellow discoloration of urine (on prolonged treatment)
● HEPATIC IMPAIRMENT Use with caution.

● MEDICINAL FORMS
There can be variation in the licensing of different medicines containing the same drug. Forms available from special-order manufacturers include: tablet

2 Bacterial infection

Antibacterials, principles of therapy

Choice of a suitable drug

Before selecting an antibacterial the clinician must first consider two factors— the patient and the known or likely causative organism. Factors related to the patient which must be considered include history of allergy, renal and hepatic function, susceptibility to infection (i.e. whether immunocompromised), ability to tolerate drugs by mouth, severity of illness, ethnic origin, age, whether taking other medication and, if female, whether pregnant, breast-feeding or taking an oral contraceptive.

The known or likely organism and its antibacterial sensitivity, in association with the above factors, will suggest one or more antibacterials, the final choice depending on the microbiological, pharmacological, and toxicological properties.

An example of a rational approach to the selection of an

antibacterial is treatment of a urinary-tract infection in a patient complaining of nausea and symptoms of a urinary-tract infection in early pregnancy. The organism is reported as being resistant to ampicillin p. 499 but sensitive to nitrofurantoin p. 535 (can cause nausea), gentamicin p. 471 (can be given only by injection and best avoided in pregnancy), tetracycline p. 515 (causes dental discoloration) and trimethoprim p. 521 (folate antagonist therefore theoretical teratogenic risk), and cefalexin p. 476. The safest antibiotics in pregnancy are the penicillins and cephalosporins; therefore, cefalexin would be indicated for this patient.

The principles involved in selection of an antibacterial must allow for a number of variables including changing renal and hepatic function, increasing bacterial resistance, and information on side-effects. Duration of therapy, dosage, and route of administration depend on site, type and severity of infection and response.

Antibacterial policies

Local policies often limit the antibacterials that may be used to achieve reasonable economy consistent with adequate cover, and to reduce the development of resistant organisms. A policy may indicate a range of drugs for general use, and permit other drugs only on the advice of the microbiologist or physician responsible for the control of infectious diseases.

Before starting therapy

The following precepts should be considered before starting:

- Viral infections should not be treated with antibacterials. However, antibacterials may be used to treat secondary bacterial infection (e.g. bacterial pneumonia secondary to influenza);
- Samples should be taken for culture and sensitivity testing; 'blind' antibacterial prescribing for unexplained pyrexia usually leads to further difficulty in establishing the diagnosis;
- Knowledge of **prevalent organisms** and their current sensitivity is of great help in choosing an antibacterial before bacteriological confirmation is available. Generally, narrow-spectrum antibacterials are preferred to broad-spectrum antibacterials unless there is a clear clinical indication (e.g. life-threatening sepsis);
- The **dose** of an antibacterial varies according to a number of factors including age, weight, hepatic function, renal function, and severity of infection. The prescribing of the so-called 'standard' dose in serious infections may result in failure of treatment or even death of the patient; therefore it is important to prescribe a dose appropriate to the condition. An inadequate dose may also increase the likelihood of antibacterial resistance. On the other hand, for an antibacterial with a narrow margin between the toxic and therapeutic dose (e.g. an aminoglycoside) it is also important to avoid an excessive dose and the concentration of the drug in the plasma may need to be monitored;
- The **route** of administration of an antibacterial often depends on the severity of the infection. Life-threatening infections require intravenous therapy. Antibacterials that are well absorbed may be given by mouth even for some serious infections. Parenteral administration is also appropriate when the oral route cannot be used (e.g. because of vomiting) or if absorption is inadequate. Whenever possible, painful intramuscular injections should be avoided in children;
- **Duration** of therapy depends on the nature of the infection and the response to treatment. Courses should not be unduly prolonged because they encourage resistance, they may lead to side-effects and they are costly. However, in certain infections such as tuberculosis or osteomyelitis it may be necessary to treat for prolonged periods. Conversely a single dose of an antibacterial may cure uncomplicated urinary-tract infections. The prescription for an antibacterial should specify the duration of treatment or the date when treatment is to be reviewed.

Superinfection

In general, broad-spectrum antibacterial drugs such as the cephalosporins are more likely to be associated with adverse reactions related to the selection of resistant organisms e.g. *fungal infections* or *antibiotic-associated colitis* (pseudomembranous colitis); other problems associated with superinfection include vaginitis and pruritus ani.

Therapy

When the pathogen has been isolated treatment may be changed to a more appropriate antibacterial if necessary. If no bacterium is cultured the antibacterial can be continued or stopped on clinical grounds.

Notifiable diseases

Doctors must notify the Proper Officer of the local authority (usually the consultant in communicable disease control) when attending a patient suspected of suffering from any of the diseases listed below; a form is available from the Proper Officer.

Anthrax	Mumps
Botulism	Paratyphoid fever
Brucellosis	Plague
Cholera	Poliomyelitis, acute
Diarrhoea (infectious bloody)	Rabies
Diphtheria	Rubella
Encephalitis, acute	SARS
Food poisoning	Scarlet fever
Haemolytic uraemic syndrome	Smallpox
Haemorrhagic fever (viral)	Streptococcal disease (Group A,
Hepatitis, viral	invasive)
Legionnaires' disease	Tetanus
Leprosy	Tuberculosis
Malaria	Typhoid fever
Measles	Typhus
Meningitis	Whooping cough
Meningococcal septicaemia	Yellow fever

Note It is good practice for doctors to also inform the consultant in communicable disease control of instances of other infections (e.g. psittacosis) where there could be a public health risk.

Antibacterials, use for prophylaxis

Prevention of recurrence of rheumatic fever

- Phenoxymethylpenicillin p. 497 *or* sulfadiazine p. 512.

Prevention of secondary case of invasive group A streptococcal infection

- Phenoxymethylpenicillin.

Patients who are penicillin allergic, *either* erythromycin p. 488 *or* azithromycin p. 486 [unlicensed indication].

For details of those who should receive chemoprophylaxis contact a consultant in communicable disease control (or a consultant in infectious diseases or the local Public Health England Laboratory).

Prevention of secondary case of meningococcal meningitis

- Ciprofloxacin p. 506 *or* rifampicin p. 527 *or* i/m ceftriaxone p. 480 [unlicensed indication].

For details of those who should receive chemoprophylaxis contact a consultant in communicable disease control (or a consultant in infectious diseases or the local Public Health England laboratory). Unless there has been direct exposure of the mouth or nose to infectious droplets from a patient with meningococcal disease who has received less than 24 hours of antibacterial treatment, healthcare workers do not generally require chemoprophylaxis.

Prevention of secondary case of *Haemophilus influenzae* type b disease

- Rifampicin *or* (if rifampicin cannot be used) i/m or i/v ceftriaxone [unlicensed indication].

For details of those who should receive chemoprophylaxis contact a consultant in communicable disease control (or a consultant in infectious diseases or the local Public Health England laboratory). Unless there has been direct exposure of the mouth or nose to infectious droplets from a patient with meningococcal disease who has received less than 24 hours of antibacterial treatment, healthcare workers do not generally require chemoprophylaxis.

Within 4 weeks of illness onset in an index case with confirmed or suspected invasive *Haemophilus influenzae* type b disease, give antibacterial prophylaxis to all household contacts if there is a vulnerable individual in the household. Also, give antibacterial prophylaxis to the index case if they are in contact with vulnerable household contacts or if they are under 10 years of age. Vulnerable individuals include the immunocompromised, those with asplenia, or children under 10 years of age. If there are 2 or more cases of invasive *Haemophilus influenzae* type b disease within 120 days in a pre-school or primary school, antibacterial prophylaxis should also be given to all room contacts (including staff). Also see immunisation against *Haemophilus influenzae* type b disease.

Prevention of secondary case of diphtheria in non-immune patient

- Erythromycin (*or* another macrolide e.g. azithromycin *or* clarithromycin p. 487).

Treat for further 10 days if nasopharyngeal swabs positive after first 7 days' treatment.

Prevention of pertussis

- Clarithromycin (*or* azithromycin *or* erythromycin).

Within 3 weeks of onset of cough in the index case, give antibacterial prophylaxis to all close contacts if amongst them there is at least one unimmunised or partially immunised child under 1 year of age, *or* if there is at least one individual who has not received a pertussis-containing vaccine more than 1 week and less than 5 years ago (so long as that individual lives or works with children under 4 months of age, is pregnant at over 32 weeks gestation, or is a healthcare worker who works with children under 1 year of age or with pregnant women).

Prevention of pneumococcal infection in asplenia or in patients with sickle-cell disease

- Phenoxymethylpenicillin.

If penicillin-allergic, erythromycin.

Antibacterial prophylaxis is not fully reliable. Antibacterial prophylaxis may be discontinued in children over 5 years of age with sickle-cell disease who have received pneumococcal immunisation and who do not have a history of severe pneumococcal infection.

Prevention of tuberculosis in susceptible close contacts or those who have become tuberculin positive

- Isoniazid p. 532 *or* isoniazid + rifampicin *or* (if isoniazid-resistant tuberculosis in patients under 35 years) rifampicin.

For details of those who should receive chemoprophylaxis contact the lead clinician for local tuberculosis services (or a consultant in communicable disease control).

Prevention of infection from animal and human bites

- Co-amoxiclav p. 501 alone (*or* doxycycline p. 513 + metronidazole p. 492 if penicillin-allergic).

Cleanse wound thoroughly. For tetanus-prone wound, give human tetanus immunoglobulin p. 1133 (with a tetanus-containing vaccine if necessary, according to immunisation history and risk of infection).

Consider rabies prophylaxis for bites from animals in endemic countries. Assess risk of blood-borne viruses (including HIV, hepatitis B and C) and give appropriate prophylaxis to prevent viral spread.

Antibacterial prophylaxis recommended for wounds less than 48–72 hours old when the risk of infection is high (e.g. bites from humans or cats; bites to the hand, foot, face, or genital area; bites involving oedema, crush or puncture injury, or other moderate to severe injury; wounds that cannot be debrided adequately; patients with diabetes mellitus, cirrhosis, asplenia, prosthetic joints or valves, or those who are immunocompromised). Give antibacterial prophylaxis for up to 5 days.

Prevention of early-onset neonatal infection

- i/v benzylpenicillin sodium p. 496 (or i/v clindamycin p. 485 if history of allergy to penicillins).

Give intrapartum prophylaxis to women with group B streptococcal colonisation, bacteriuria, or infection in the current pregnancy, or to women who had a previous baby with an invasive group B streptococcal infection. Consider prophylaxis for women in preterm labour if there is prelabour rupture of membranes or if intrapartum rupture of membranes lasting more than 18 hours is suspected.

Prevention of infection in gastro-intestinal procedures

Operations on stomach or oesophagus

- Single dose of i/v gentamicin p. 471 *or* i/v cefuroxime p. 478 *or* i/v co-amoxiclav (additional intra-operative or postoperative doses may be given for prolonged procedures or if there is major blood loss).

Intravenous antibacterial prophylaxis should be given up to 30 minutes before the procedure.

Add i/v teicoplanin p. 482 (*or* vancomycin p. 484) if high risk of meticillin-resistant *Staphylococcus aureus*.

Open biliary surgery

- Single dose of i/v cefuroxime + i/v metronidazole *or* i/v gentamicin + i/v metronidazole *or* i/v co-amoxiclav alone (additional intra-operative or postoperative doses may be given for prolonged procedures or if there is major blood loss).

Intravenous antibacterial prophylaxis should be given up to 30 minutes before the procedure.

Where i/v metronidazole is suggested, it may alternatively be given by suppository but to allow adequate absorption, it should be given 2 hours before surgery.

Add i/v teicoplanin (*or* vancomycin) if high risk of meticillin-resistant *Staphylococcus aureus*.

5

Infection

Resections of colon and rectum for carcinoma, and resections in inflammatory bowel disease, and appendicectomy

• Single dose of i/v gentamicin + i/v metronidazole or i/v cefuroxime + i/v metronidazole or i/v co-amoxiclav alone (additional intra-operative or postoperative doses may be given for prolonged procedures or if there is major blood loss).

Intravenous antibacterial prophylaxis should be given up to 30 minutes before the procedure.

Where i/v metronidazole p. 492 is suggested, it may alternatively be given by suppository but to allow adequate absorption, it should be given 2 hours before surgery.

Add i/v teicoplanin p. 482 (or vancomycin p. 484) if high risk of meticillin-resistant *Staphylococcus aureus*.

Endoscopic retrograde cholangiopancreatography

• Single dose of i/v gentamicin p. 471 or oral or i/v ciprofloxacin p. 506.

Intravenous antibacterial prophylaxis should be given up to 30 minutes before the procedure.

Prophylaxis recommended if pancreatic pseudocyst, immunocompromised, history of liver transplantation, or risk of incomplete biliary drainage. For biliary complications following liver transplantation, add i/v amoxicillin p. 498 or i/v teicoplanin (or vancomycin).

Percutaneous endoscopic gastrostomy or jejunostomy

• Single dose of i/v co-amoxiclav p. 501 or i/v cefuroxime p. 478.

Intravenous antibacterial prophylaxis should be given up to 30 minutes before the procedure.

Use single dose of i/v teicoplanin (or vancomycin) if history of allergy to penicillins or cephalosporins, or if high risk of meticillin-resistant *Staphylococcus aureus*.

Prevention of infection in orthopaedic surgery

Joint replacement including hip and knee

• Single dose of i/v cefuroxime alone or i/v flucloxacillin p. 503 + i/v gentamicin (additional intra-operative or postoperative doses may be given for prolonged procedures or if there is major blood loss).

Intravenous antibacterial prophylaxis should be given up to 30 minutes before the procedure.

If history of allergy to penicillins or to cephalosporins or if high risk of meticillin-resistant *Staphylococcus aureus*, use single dose of i/v teicoplanin (or vancomycin) + i/v gentamicin (additional intra-operative or postoperative doses may be given for prolonged procedures or if there is major blood loss).

Closed fractures

• Single dose of i/v cefuroxime or i/v flucloxacillin (additional intra-operative or postoperative doses may be given for prolonged procedures or if there is major blood loss).

Intravenous antibacterial prophylaxis should be given up to 30 minutes before the procedure.

If history of allergy to penicillins or to cephalosporins or if high risk of meticillin-resistant *Staphylococcus aureus*, use single dose of i/v teicoplanin (or vancomycin) (additional intra-operative or postoperative doses may be given for prolonged procedures or if there is major blood loss).

Open fractures

• Use i/v co-amoxiclav alone or i/v cefuroxime + i/v metronidazole (or i/v clindamycin p. 485 alone if history of allergy to penicillins or to cephalosporins).

Add i/v teicoplanin (or vancomycin) if high risk of meticillin-resistant *Staphylococcus aureus*. Start prophylaxis within 3 hours of injury and continue until soft tissue closure (max. 72 hours).

At first debridement also use a single dose of i/v cefuroxime + i/v metronidazole + i/v gentamicin or i/v co-amoxiclav + i/v gentamicin (or i/v clindamycin + i/v gentamicin if history of allergy to penicillins or to cephalosporins).

At time of skeletal stabilisation and definitive soft tissue closure use a single dose of i/v gentamicin + i/v teicoplanin (or vancomycin) (intravenous antibacterial prophylaxis should be given up to 30 minutes before the procedure).

High lower-limb amputation

• Use i/v co-amoxiclav alone or i/v cefuroxime + i/v metronidazole.

Intravenous antibacterial prophylaxis should be given up to 30 minutes before the procedure.

Continue antibacterial prophylaxis for at least 2 doses after procedure (max. duration of prophylaxis 5 days). If history of allergy to penicillin or to cephalosporins, or if high risk of meticillin-resistant *Staphylococcus aureus*, use i/v teicoplanin (or vancomycin) + i/v gentamicin + i/v metronidazole.

Where i/v metronidazole is suggested, it may alternatively be given by suppository but to allow adequate absorption, it should be given 2 hours before surgery.

Prevention of infection in urological procedures

Transrectal prostate biopsy

• Single dose of oral ciprofloxacin + oral metronidazole or i/v gentamicin + i/v metronidazole (additional intra-operative or postoperative doses may be given for prolonged procedures or if there is major blood loss).

Intravenous antibacterial prophylaxis should be given up to 30 minutes before the procedure.

Use single dose of i/v gentamicin + i/v metronidazole if high risk of meticillin-resistant *Staphylococcus aureus* (additional intra-operative or postoperative doses of antibacterial may be given for prolonged procedures or if there is major blood loss).

Where i/v metronidazole is suggested, it may alternatively be given by suppository but to allow adequate absorption, it should be given 2 hours before surgery.

Transurethral resection of prostate

• Single dose of oral ciprofloxacin or i/v gentamicin or i/v cefuroxime (additional intra-operative or postoperative doses may be given for prolonged procedures or if there is major blood loss).

Intravenous antibacterial prophylaxis should be given up to 30 minutes before the procedure.

Use single dose of i/v gentamicin if high risk of meticillin-resistant *Staphylococcus aureus* (additional intra-operative or postoperative doses may be given for prolonged procedures or if there is major blood loss).

Prevention of infection in obstetric and gynaecological surgery

Caesarean section

• Single dose of i/v cefuroxime (additional intra-operative or postoperative doses may be given for prolonged procedures or if there is major blood loss).

Intravenous antibacterial prophylaxis should be given up to 30 minutes before the procedure.

Substitute i/v clindamycin if history of allergy to penicillins or cephalosporins. Add i/v teicoplanin (or vancomycin) if high risk of meticillin-resistant *Staphylococcus aureus*.

Hysterectomy

• Single dose of i/v cefuroxime + i/v metronidazole or i/v gentamicin + i/v metronidazole or i/v co-amoxiclav alone (additional intra-operative or postoperative doses may be given for prolonged procedures or if there is major blood loss).

Intravenous antibacterial prophylaxis should be given up to 30 minutes before the procedure.

Use single dose of i/v gentamicin + i/v metronidazole or add i/v teicoplanin (or vancomycin) to other regimens if high risk of meticillin-resistant *Staphylococcus aureus* (additional intra-operative or postoperative doses may be given for prolonged procedures or if there is major blood loss).

Where i/v metronidazole is suggested, it may alternatively be given by suppository but to allow adequate absorption, it should be given 2 hours before surgery.

Termination of pregnancy

• Single dose of oral metronidazole (additional intra-operative or postoperative doses may be given for prolonged procedures or if there is major blood loss).

If genital chlamydial infection cannot be ruled out, give doxycycline p. 513 postoperatively.

Prevention of infection in cardiology procedures

Cardiac pacemaker insertion

• Single dose of i/v cefuroxime alone or i/v flucloxacillin + i/v gentamicin or i/v teicoplanin (or vancomycin) + i/v gentamicin (additional intra-operative or postoperative doses may be given for prolonged procedures or if there is major blood loss).

Intravenous antibacterial prophylaxis should be given up to 30 minutes before the procedure.

Use single dose of i/v teicoplanin (or vancomycin) + i/v cefuroxime or i/v teicoplanin (or vancomycin) + i/v gentamicin if high risk of meticillin-resistant *Staphylococcus aureus* (additional intra-operative or postoperative doses may be given for prolonged procedures or if there is major blood loss).

Prevention of infection in vascular surgery

Reconstructive arterial surgery of abdomen, pelvis or legs

• Single dose of i/v cefuroxime p. 478 alone or i/v flucloxacillin p. 503 + i/v gentamicin p. 471 (additional intra-operative or postoperative doses may be given for prolonged procedures or if there is major blood loss).

Intravenous antibacterial prophylaxis should be given up to 30 minutes before the procedure.

Add i/v metronidazole p. 492 for patients at risk from anaerobic infections including those with diabetes, gangrene, or undergoing amputation. Use single dose of i/v teicoplanin p. 482 (or vancomycin p. 484) + i/v gentamicin if history of allergy to penicillins or cephalosporins, or if high risk of meticillin-resistant *Staphylococcus aureus* (additional intra-operative or postoperative doses may be given for prolonged procedures or if there is major blood loss).

Prevention of endocarditis

NICE guidance: Antimicrobial prophylaxis against infective endocarditis in adults and children undergoing interventional procedures (March 2008)

• Antibacterial prophylaxis and chlorhexidine mouthwash are **not** recommended for the prevention of endocarditis in patients undergoing dental procedures.

Antibacterial prophylaxis is **not** recommended for the prevention of endocarditis in patients undergoing procedures of the:

▸ upper and lower respiratory tract (including ear, nose, and throat procedures and bronchoscopy);

▸ genito-urinary tract (including urological, gynaecological, and obstetric procedures);

▸ upper and lower gastro-intestinal tract.

Whilst these procedures can cause bacteraemia, there is no clear association with the development of infective endocarditis. Prophylaxis may expose patients to the adverse effects of antimicrobials when the evidence of benefit has not been proven.

Any infection in patients at risk of endocarditis should be investigated promptly and treated appropriately to reduce the risk of endocarditis.

If patients at risk of endocarditis are undergoing a gastro-intestinal or genito-urinary tract procedure at a site where infection is suspected, they should receive appropriate antibacterial therapy that includes cover against organisms that cause endocarditis.

Patients at risk of endocarditis should be:

▸ advised to maintain good oral hygiene;

▸ told how to recognise signs of infective endocarditis, and advised when to seek expert advice.

Patients at risk of endocarditis include those with valve replacement, acquired valvular heart disease with stenosis or regurgitation, structural congenital heart disease (including surgically corrected or palliated structural conditions, but excluding isolated atrial septal defect, fully repaired ventricular septal defect, fully repaired patent ductus arteriosus, and closure devices considered to be endothelialised); hypertrophic cardiomyopathy, or a previous episode of infective endocarditis.

Dermatological procedures

Advice of a Working Party of the British Society for Antimicrobial Chemotherapy is that patients who undergo dermatological procedures do not require antibacterial prophylaxis against endocarditis.

The British Association of Dermatologists Therapy Guidelines and Audit Subcommittee advise that such dermatological procedures include skin biopsies and excision of moles or of malignant lesions.

Joint prostheses and dental treatment

Advice of a Working Party of the British Society for Antimicrobial Chemotherapy is that patients with prosthetic joint implants (including total hip replacements) do not require antibiotic prophylaxis for dental treatment. The Working Party considers that it is unacceptable to expose patients to the adverse effects of antibiotics when there is no evidence that such prophylaxis is of any benefit, but that those who develop any intercurrent infection require prompt treatment with antibiotics to which the infecting organisms are sensitive.

The Working Party has commented that joint infections have rarely been shown to follow dental procedures and are even more rarely caused by oral streptococci.

Immunosuppression and indwelling intraperitoneal catheters

Advice of a Working Party of the British Society for Antimicrobial Chemotherapy is that patients who are immunosuppressed (including transplant patients) and patients with indwelling intraperitoneal catheters do not require antibiotic prophylaxis for dental treatment provided there is no other indication for prophylaxis.

The Working Party has commented that there is little evidence that dental treatment is followed by infection in immunosuppressed and immunodeficient patients nor is there evidence that dental treatment is followed by infection in patients with indwelling intraperitoneal catheters.

5

Infection

Blood infections, bacterial

Antibacterial therapy for septicaemia: community-acquired

- A broad-spectrum antipseudomonal penicillin (e.g. piperacillin with tazobactam p. 495, ticarcillin with clavulanic acid p. 496) *or* a broad-spectrum cephalosporin (e.g. cefuroxime p. 478)
- If meticillin-resistant *Staphylococcus aureus* suspected, add vancomycin p. 484 (*or* teicoplanin p. 482).
- If anaerobic infection suspected, add metronidazole p. 492 to broad-spectrum cephalosporin.
- If other resistant micro-organisms suspected, use a more broad-spectrum beta-lactam antibacterial (e.g. meropenem p. 475).

Antibacterial therapy for septicaemia: hospital-acquired

- A broad-spectrum antipseudomonal beta-lactam antibacterial (e.g. piperacillin with tazobactam, ticarcillin with clavulanic acid, ceftazidime p. 480, imipenem with cilastatin p. 474, *or* meropenem)
- If meticillin-resistant *Staphylococcus aureus* suspected, add vancomycin (*or* teicoplanin).
- If anaerobic infection suspected, add metronidazole to broad-spectrum cephalosporin

Septicaemia related to vascular catheter

- Vancomycin (*or* teicoplanin)
- If Gram-negative sepsis suspected, especially in the immunocompromised, add a broad-spectrum antipseudomonal beta-lactam.
- Consider removing vascular catheter, particularly if infection caused by *Staphylococcus aureus*, pseudomonas, or *Candida* species.

Meningococcal septicaemia

If meningococcal disease suspected, a single dose of benzylpenicillin sodium p. 496 should be given before urgent transfer to hospital, so long as this does not delay the transfer; cefotaxime p. 479 may be an alternative in penicillin allergy; chloramphenicol p. 517 may be used if history of immediate hypersensitivity reaction to penicillin or to cephalosporins.

- Benzylpenicillin sodium or cefotaxime (*or* ceftriaxone p. 480)
- *If history of immediate hypersensitivity reaction to penicillin or to cephalosporins,* chloramphenicol
- To eliminate nasopharyngeal carriage, ciprofloxacin p. 506, or rifampicin p. 527, or ceftriaxone may be used.

Cardiovascular system infections, bacterial

Antibacterial therapy for endocarditis: initial 'blind' therapy

- *Native valve endocarditis*, amoxicillin p. 498 (*or* ampicillin p. 499)
- Consider adding low-dose gentamicin p. 471
- If penicillin-allergic, or if meticillin-resistant *Staphylococcus aureus* suspected, or if severe sepsis, use vancomycin p. 484 + low-dose gentamicin
- If severe sepsis with risk factors for Gram-negative infection, use vancomycin + meropenem p. 475
- *If prosthetic valve endocarditis,* vancomycin + rifampicin p. 527 + low-dose gentamicin

Antibacterial therapy for native-valve endocarditis caused by staphylococci

- Flucloxacillin p. 503
- *Suggested duration of treatment* 4 weeks (at least 6 weeks if secondary lung abscess or osteomyelitis also present)
- *If penicillin-allergic or if meticillin-resistant Staphylococcus aureus,* vancomycin + rifampicin
- *Suggested duration of treatment* 4 weeks (at least 6 weeks if secondary lung abscess or osteomyelitis also present)

Antibacterial therapy for prosthetic valve endocarditis caused by staphylococci

- Flucloxacillin + rifampicin + low-dose gentamicin
- *Suggested duration of treatment* at least 6 weeks; review need to continue gentamicin at 2 weeks—seek specialist advice if gentamicin considered necessary beyond 2 weeks
- *If penicillin-allergic or if meticillin-resistant Staphylococcus aureus,* vancomycin + rifampicin + low-dose gentamicin
- *Suggested duration of treatment* at least 6 weeks; review need to continue gentamicin at 2 weeks—seek specialist advice if gentamicin considered necessary beyond 2 weeks

Antibacterial therapy for endocarditis caused by fully-sensitive streptococci

- Benzylpenicillin sodium p. 496
- *Suggested duration of treatment* 4–6 weeks (6 weeks for prosthetic valve endocarditis)
- *If penicillin-allergic,* vancomycin (*or* teicoplanin p. 482) + low-dose gentamicin
- *Suggested duration of treatment* 4–6 weeks (stop gentamicin after 2 weeks)

Antibacterial therapy for endocarditis caused by less-sensitive streptococci

- Benzylpenicillin sodium + low-dose gentamicin
- *Suggested duration of treatment* 4–6 weeks (6 weeks for prosthetic valve endocarditis); review need to continue gentamicin at 2 weeks—seek specialist advice if gentamicin considered necessary beyond 2 weeks; stop gentamicin at 2 weeks if micro-organisms moderately sensitive to penicillin
- *If penicillin-allergic or highly penicillin-resistant,* vancomycin (*or* teicoplanin) + low-dose gentamicin
- *Suggested duration of treatment* 4–6 weeks (6 weeks for prosthetic valve endocarditis); review need to continue gentamicin at 2 weeks—seek specialist advice if gentamicin considered necessary beyond 2 weeks; stop gentamicin at 2 weeks if micro-organisms moderately sensitive to penicillin

Antibacterial therapy for endocarditis caused by enterococci

- Amoxicillin (*or* ampicillin) + low dose gentamicin *or* benzylpenicillin sodium + low-dose gentamicin
- *Suggested duration of treatment* 4–6 weeks (6 weeks for prosthetic valve endocarditis); review need to continue gentamicin at 2 weeks—seek specialist advice if gentamicin considered necessary beyond 2 weeks
- *If penicillin-allergic or penicillin-resistant,* vancomycin (*or* teicoplanin) + low-dose gentamicin
- *Suggested duration of treatment* 4–6 weeks (6 weeks for prosthetic valve endocarditis); review need to continue gentamicin at 2 weeks—seek specialist advice if gentamicin considered necessary beyond 2 weeks
- If gentamicin resistant, amoxicillin (*or* ampicillin)
- Add streptomycin p. 472 (if susceptible) for 2 weeks
- *Suggested duration of treatment* at least 6 weeks

Antibacterial therapy for endocarditis caused by *Haemophilus, Actinobacillus, Cardiobacterium, Eikenella,* and *Kingella* species ('HACEK' micro-organisms)

- Amoxicillin (*or* ampicillin) + low-dose gentamicin
▸ *Suggested duration of treatment* 4 weeks (6 weeks for prosthetic valve endocarditis); stop gentamicin after 2 weeks
- *If* amoxicillin-*resistant*, ceftriaxone p. 480 (*or* cefotaxime p. 479) + low-dose gentamicin
▸ *Suggested duration of treatment* 4 weeks (6 weeks for prosthetic valve endocarditis); stop gentamicin after 2 weeks

Central nervous system infections, bacterial

Antibacterial therapy for meningitis: initial empirical therapy

- Transfer patient to hospital urgently.
- If *meningococcal disease* (meningitis with non-blanching rash or meningococcal septicaemia) suspected, benzylpenicillin sodium p. 496 should be given before transfer to hospital, so long as this does not delay the transfer. If a patient with suspected bacterial meningitis without non-blanching rash cannot be transferred to hospital urgently, benzylpenicillin sodium should be given before the transfer. Cefotaxime p. 479 may be an alternative in penicillin allergy; chloramphenicol p. 517 may be used if history of immediate hypersensitivity reaction to penicillin or to cephalosporins.
- In hospital, consider adjunctive treatment with dexamethasone p. 610 (particularly if pneumococcal meningitis suspected in adults), preferably starting before or with first dose of antibacterial, but no later than 12 hours after starting antibacterial; avoid dexamethasone in septic shock, meningococcal septicaemia, or if immunocompromised, or in meningitis following surgery.

In hospital, if aetiology unknown

- *Adult and child* 3 *months*–50 *years,* cefotaxime (*or* ceftriaxone p. 480)
▸ Consider adding vancomycin p. 484 if prolonged or multiple use of other antibacterials in the last 3 months, or if travelled, in the last 3 months, to areas outside the UK with highly penicillin- and cephalosporin-resistant pneumococci.
▸ *Suggested duration of treatment* at least 10 days
- *Adult over* 50 *years* cefotaxime (*or* ceftriaxone) + amoxicillin p. 498 (*or* ampicillin p. 499)
▸ Consider adding vancomycin if prolonged or multiple use of other antibacterials in the last 3 months, or if travelled, in the last 3 months, to areas outside the UK with highly penicillin- and cephalosporin-resistant pneumococci.
▸ *Suggested duration of treatment* at least 10 days

Antibacterial therapy for meningitis caused by meningococci

- Benzylpenicillin sodium *or* cefotaxime (*or* ceftriaxone)
▸ *Suggested duration of treatment* 7 days.
- *If history of immediate hypersensitivity reaction to penicillin or to cephalosporins,* chloramphenicol
▸ *Suggested duration of treatment* 7 days.

Antibacterial therapy for meningitis caused by pneumococci

- Cefotaxime (*or* ceftriaxone)
▸ Consider adjunctive treatment with dexamethasone, preferably starting before or with first dose of antibacterial, but no later than 12 hours after starting antibacterial (may reduce penetration of vancomycin into cerebrospinal fluid).
▸ If micro-organism penicillin-sensitive, replace cefotaxime with benzylpenicillin sodium.
▸ If micro-organism highly penicillin- and cephalosporin-resistant, add vancomycin and if necessary rifampicin p. 527.
▸ *Suggested duration of antibacterial treatment* 14 days

Antibacterial therapy for meningitis caused by *Haemophilus influenzae*

- Cefotaxime (*or* ceftriaxone)
▸ Consider adjunctive treatment with dexamethasone, preferably starting before or with first dose of antibacterial, but no later than 12 hours after starting antibacterial.
▸ *Suggested duration of antibacterial treatment* 10 days.
▸ For *H. influenzae* type b give rifampicin for 4 days before hospital discharge to those under 10 years of age or to those in contact with vulnerable household contacts
- *If history of immediate hypersensitivity reaction to penicillin or to cephalosporins, or if micro-organism resistant to cefotaxime,* chloramphenicol
▸ Consider adjunctive treatment with dexamethasone, preferably starting before or with first dose of antibacterial, but no later than 12 hours after starting antibacterial.
▸ *Suggested duration of antibacterial treatment* 10 days.
▸ For *H. influenzae* type b give rifampicin for 4 days before hospital discharge to those under 10 years of age or to those in contact with vulnerable household contacts

Antibacterial therapy for meningitis caused by Listeria

- Amoxicillin (*or* ampicillin) + gentamicin p. 471
▸ *Suggested duration of treatment* 21 days.
▸ Consider stopping gentamicin after 7 days.
- *If history of immediate hypersensitivity reaction to penicillin,* co-trimoxazole p. 511
▸ *Suggested duration of treatment* 21 days.

Ear infections, bacterial

Antibacterial therapy for otitis externa

For topical treatments, consider *Otitis externa,* under Ear p. 1039.

Consider systemic antibacterial if spreading cellulitis or patient systemically unwell.

- Flucloxacillin p. 503
▸ *If penicillin-allergic,* clarithromycin p. 487 (*or* azithromycin p. 486 *or* erythromycin p. 488)
▸ *If pseudomonas suspected,* ciprofloxacin p. 506 (*or* an aminoglycoside)

Antibacterial therapy for otitis media

Many infections caused by viruses. Most uncomplicated cases resolve without antibacterial treatment. In children without systemic features, antibacterial treatment may be started after 72 hours if no improvement. Consider earlier treatment if deterioration, if systemically unwell, if at high risk of serious complications (e.g. in immunosuppression,

cystic fibrosis), if mastoiditis present, or in children under 2 years of age with bilateral otitis media.
• Amoxicillin p. 498 (or ampicillin p. 499)
▸ Consider co-amoxiclav p. 501 if no improvement after 48 hours.
▸ In severe infection, initial parenteral therapy with co-amoxiclav or cefuroxime p. 478.
▸ *Suggested duration of treatment* 5 days (longer if severely ill).
• *If penicillin-allergic*, clarithromycin (or azithromycin or erythromycin)
▸ *Suggested duration of treatment* 5 days (longer if severely ill)

Eye infections, bacterial

Antibacterial therapy for purulent conjuctivitis

• Chloramphenicol eye drops p. 1018.

Gastro-intestinal system infections, bacterial

Antibacterial therapy for gastro-enteritis

Frequently self-limiting and may not be bacterial.
• Antibacterial not usually indicated

Antibacterial therapy for campylobacter enteritis

Frequently self-limiting; treat if immunocompromised or if severe infection.
• Clarithromycin p. 487 (or azithromycin p. 486 or erythromycin p. 488)
• *Alternative*, ciprofloxacin p. 506
▸ Strains with decreased sensitivity to ciprofloxacin isolated frequently

Antibacterial therapy for salmonella (non-typhoid)

Treat invasive or severe infection. Do not treat less severe infection unless there is a risk of developing invasive infection (e.g. immunocompromised patients, those with haemoglobinopathy, or children under 6 months of age).
• Ciprofloxacin or cefotaxime p. 479

Antibacterial therapy for shigellosis

Antibacterial not indicated for mild cases.
• Ciprofloxacin or azithromycin
• *Alternatives if micro-organism sensitive*, amoxicillin p. 498 or trimethoprim p. 521

Antibacterial therapy for typhoid fever

Infections from Middle-East, South Asia, and South-East Asia may be multiple-antibacterial-resistant and sensitivity should be tested.
• Cefotaxime (or ceftriaxone p. 480)
▸ azithromycin may be an alternative in mild or moderate disease caused by multiple-antibacterial-resistant organisms.
• *Alternative if micro-organism sensitive*, ciprofloxacin

Antibacterial therapy for *Clostridium difficile* infection

• *For first episode of mild to moderate infection*, oral metronidazole p. 492
▸ *Suggested duration of treatment* 10–14 days

• *For second or subsequent episode of infection, for severe infection, for infection not responding to* metronidazole, *or in patients intolerant of* metronidazole, oral vancomycin p. 484
▸ For severe infection in patients with multiple co-morbidities who are receiving treatment with other antibacterials, or for second or subsequent episode of infection, fidaxomicin p. 518 can replace vancomycin
▸ *Suggested duration of treatment* 10–14 days
• *For infection not responding to* vancomycin *or* fidaxomicin, *for life-threatening infection, or in patients with ileus*, oral vancomycin + i/v metronidazole
▸ For infection not responding to vancomycin in patients without life-threatening infection or ileus, fidaxomicin can be used instead of vancomycin + metronidazole
▸ *Suggested duration of treatment* 10–14 days

Antibacterial therapy for biliary-tract infection

• Ciprofloxacin or gentamicin p. 471 or a cephalosporin

Antibacterial therapy for peritonitis

• A cephalosporin + metronidazole or gentamicin + metronidazole or gentamicin + clindamycin p. 485 or piperacillin with tazobactam p. 495 alone

Antibacterial therapy for peritonitis: peritoneal dialysis-associated

• Vancomycin (or teicoplanin p. 482) + ceftazidime p. 480 added to dialysis fluid or vancomycin added to dialysis fluid + ciprofloxacin by mouth
▸ *Suggested duration of treatment* 14 days or longer

Genital system infections, bacterial

Antibacterial therapy for bacterial vaginosis

• Oral metronidazole p. 492
▸ *Suggested duration of treatment* 5–7 days (or high-dose metronidazole as a single dose)
• *Alternatively*, topical metronidazole for 5 days or topical clindamycin p. 485 for 7 days

Antibacterial therapy for uncomplicated genital chlamydial infection, non-gonococcal urethritis, and non-specific genital infection

Contact tracing recommended.
• Azithromycin p. 486 or doxycycline p. 513
▸ *Suggested duration of treatment* azithromycin as a single dose or doxycycline for 7 days
• *Alternatively*, erythromycin p. 488.
▸ *Suggested duration of treatment* 14 days

Antibacterial therapy for gonorrhoea: uncomplicated

Contact tracing recommended. Consider chlamydia co-infection. Choice of alternative antibacterial regimen depends on locality where infection acquired.
• Azithromycin + i/m ceftriaxone p. 480
▸ *Suggested duration of treatment* is a single-dose of each antibacterial
• *Alternatively, when parenteral administration is not possible*, cefixime p. 479 + azithromycin
▸ *Suggested duration of treatment* is a single-dose of each antibacterial

- *Alternatively, if micro-organism is sensitive to a quinolone,* ciprofloxacin p. 506 + azithromycin
▹ *Suggested duration of treatment* is a single-dose of each antibacterial
- *Pharyngeal infection,* azithromycin + i/m ceftriaxone
▹ *Suggested duration of treatment* is a single-dose of each antibacterial

Antibacterial therapy for pelvic inflammatory disease

Contact tracing recommended.
- Doxycycline + metronidazole + single-dose of i/m ceftriaxone *or* ofloxacin p. 510 + metronidazole
▹ *Suggested duration of treatment* 14 days (except i/m ceftriaxone).
▹ In severely ill patients initial treatment with doxycycline + i/v ceftriaxone + i/v metronidazole, then switch to oral treatment with doxycycline + metronidazole to complete 14 days' treatment

Antibacterial therapy for early syphilis (infection of less than 2 years)

Contact tracing recommended.
- Benzathine benzylpenicillin [unlicensed]
▹ *Suggested duration of treatment* single-dose (repeat dose after 7 days for women in the third trimester of pregnancy)
- *Alternatively,* doxycycline or erythromycin
▹ *Suggested duration of treatment* 14 days

Antibacterial therapy for late latent syphilis (asymptomatic infection of more than 2 years)

Contact tracing recommended.
- Benzathine benzylpenicillin [unlicensed]
▹ *Suggested duration of treatment* once weekly for 2 weeks
- *Alternatively,* doxycycline
▹ *Suggested duration of treatment* 28 days

Asymptomatic contacts of patients with infectious syphilis

- Doxycycline
▹ *Suggested duration of treatment* 14 days

Musculoskeletal system infections, bacterial

Antibacterial therapy for osteomyelitis

Seek specialist advice if chronic infection or prostheses present.
- Flucloxacillin p. 503
▹ Consider adding fusidic acid p. 519 or rifampicin p. 527 for initial 2 weeks.
▹ *Suggested duration of treatment* 6 weeks for acute infection
- *If penicillin-allergic,* clindamycin p. 485
▹ Consider adding fusidic acid or rifampicin for initial 2 weeks.
▹ *Suggested duration of treatment* 6 weeks for acute infection
- *If meticillin-resistant Staphylococcus aureus suspected,* vancomycin p. 484 (*or* teicoplanin p. 482)
▹ Consider adding fusidic acid or rifampicin for initial 2 weeks.
▹ *Suggested duration of treatment* 6 weeks for acute infection

Antibacterial therapy for septic arthritis

Seek specialist advice if prostheses present.
- Flucloxacillin
▹ *Suggested duration of treatment* 4–6 weeks (longer if infection complicated).
- *If penicillin-allergic,* clindamycin
▹ *Suggested duration of treatment* 4–6 weeks (longer if infection complicated).
- *If meticillin-resistant Staphylococcus aureus suspected,* vancomycin (*or* teicoplanin)
▹ *Suggested duration of treatment* 4–6 weeks (longer if infection complicated).
- *If gonococcal arthritis or Gram-negative infection suspected,* cefotaxime p. 479 (*or* ceftriaxone p. 480)
▹ *Suggested duration of treatment* 4–6 weeks (longer if infection complicated; treat gonococcal infection for 2 weeks).

Nose infections, bacterial

Antibacterial therapy for sinusitis

Antibacterial should usually be used only for persistent symptoms and purulent discharge lasting at least 7 days or if severe symptoms. Also, consider antibacterial for those at high risk of serious complications (e.g. in immunosuppression, cystic fibrosis).
- Amoxicillin p. 498 (or ampicillin p. 499) *or* doxycycline p. 513 *or* clarithromycin p. 487 (*or* azithromycin p. 486 *or* erythromycin p. 488)
▹ *Suggested duration of treatment* 7 days.
▹ Consider oral co-amoxiclav p. 501 if no improvement after 48 hours.
▹ In severe infection, initial parenteral therapy with co-amoxiclav or cefuroxime p. 478 may be required.

Oral bacterial infections

Antibacterial drugs

Antibacterial drugs should only be prescribed for the *treatment* of oral infections on the basis of defined need. They may be used in conjunction with (but not as an alternative to) other appropriate measures, such as providing drainage or extracting a tooth.

The 'blind' prescribing of an antibacterial for unexplained pyrexia, cervical lymphadenopathy, or facial swelling can lead to difficulty in establishing the diagnosis. In severe oral infections, a sample should always be taken for bacteriology.

Oral infections which may require antibacterial treatment include acute periapical or periodontal abscess, cellulitis, acutely created oral-antral communication (and acute sinusitis), severe pericoronitis, localised osteitis, acute necrotising ulcerative gingivitis, and destructive forms of chronic periodontal disease. Most of these infections are readily resolved by the early establishment of drainage and removal of the cause (typically an infected necrotic pulp). Antibacterials may be required if treatment has to be delayed, in immunocompromised patients, or in those with conditions such as diabetes or Paget's disease. Certain rarer infections including bacterial sialadenitis, osteomyelitis, actinomycosis, and infections involving fascial spaces such as Ludwig's angina, require antibiotics and specialist hospital care.

Antibacterial drugs may also be useful after dental surgery in some cases of spreading infection. Infection may spread to involve local lymph nodes, to fascial spaces (where it can cause airway obstruction), or into the bloodstream (where it can lead to cavernous sinus thrombosis and other serious

5

Infection

complications). Extension of an infection can also lead to maxillary sinusitis; osteomyelitis is a complication, which usually arises when host resistance is reduced.

If the oral infection fails to respond to antibacterial treatment within 48 hours the antibacterial should be changed, preferably on the basis of bacteriological investigation. Failure to respond may also suggest an incorrect diagnosis, lack of essential additional measures (such as drainage), poor host resistance, or poor patient compliance.

Combination of a penicillin (or a macrolide) with metronidazole p. 492 may sometimes be helpful for the treatment of severe oral infections or oral infections that have not responded to initial antibacterial treatment.

Penicillins

Phenoxymethylpenicillin p. 497 is effective for dentoalveolar abscess.

Broad-spectrum penicillins

Amoxicillin p. 498 is as effective as phenoxymethylpenicillin but is better absorbed; however, it may encourage emergence of resistant organisms.

Like phenoxymethylpenicillin, amoxicillin is ineffective against bacteria that produce beta-lactamases.

Amoxicillin may be useful for short course oral regimens. Co-amoxiclav p. 501 is active against beta-lactamase-producing bacteria that are resistant to amoxicillin. Co-amoxiclav may be used for severe dental infection with spreading cellulitis or dental infection not responding to first-line antibacterial treatment.

Cephalosporins

The cephalosporins offer little advantage over the penicillins in dental infections, often being less active against anaerobes. Infections due to oral streptococci (often termed viridans streptococci) which become resistant to penicillin are usually also resistant to cephalosporins. This is of importance in the case of patients who have had rheumatic fever and are on long-term penicillin therapy. Cefalexin p. 476 and cefradine p. 477 have been used in the treatment of oral infections.

Tetracyclines

In adults, tetracyclines can be effective against oral anaerobes but the development of resistance (especially by oral streptococci) has reduced their usefulness for the treatment of acute oral infections; they may still have a role in the treatment of destructive (refractory) forms of periodontal disease. Doxycycline p. 513 has a longer duration of action than tetracycline p. 515 or oxytetracycline p. 515 and need only be given once daily; it is reported to be more active against anaerobes than some other tetracyclines.

Doxycycline may have a role in the treatment of recurrent aphthous ulceration, or as an adjunct to gingival scaling and root planing for periodontitis.

Macrolides

The macrolides are an alternative for oral infections in penicillin-allergic patients or where a beta-lactamase producing organism is involved. However, many organisms are now resistant to macrolides or rapidly develop resistance; their use should therefore be limited to short courses.

Clindamycin

Clindamycin p. 485 should not be used routinely for the treatment of oral infections because it may be no more effective than penicillins against anaerobes and there may be cross-resistance with erythromycin p. 488-resistant bacteria. Clindamycin can be used for the treatment of dentoalveolar abscess that has not responded to penicillin or to metronidazole.

Metronidazole and tinidazole

Metronidazole is an alternative to a penicillin for the treatment of many oral infections where the patient is allergic to penicillin or the infection is due to beta-lactamase-producing anaerobes. It is the drug of first choice for the treatment of acute necrotising ulcerative gingivitis (Vincent's infection) and pericoronitis; amoxicillin is a suitable alternative. For these purposes metronidazole for 3 days is sufficient, but the duration of treatment may need to be longer in pericoronitis. Tinidazole p. 493 is licensed for the treatment of acute ulcerative gingivitis.

Respiratory system infections, bacterial

Antibacterial therapy for *Haemophilus influenzae* epiglottitis

- Cefotaxime p. 479 (*or* ceftriaxone p. 480)
- *If history of immediate hypersensitivity reaction to penicillin or to cephalosporins*, chloramphenicol p. 517

Antibacterial therapy for chronic bronchitis: acute exacerbations

Treat if increase in sputum purulence accompanied by an increase in sputum volume or increase in dyspnoea.

- Amoxicillin p. 498 (*or* ampicillin p. 499) *or* a tetracycline p. 515
- ▸ Some pneumococci and *Haemophilus influenzae* strains tetracycline-resistant; approx. 20% *H. influenzae* strains amoxicillin-resistant
- ▸ *Suggested duration of treatment* 5 days; longer treatment may be necessary in severely ill patients
- *Alternative*, clarithromycin p. 487 (*or* azithromycin p. 486 *or* erythromycin p. 488)
- ▸ *Suggested duration of treatment* 5 days; longer treatment may be necessary in severely ill patients

Antibacterial therapy for pneumonia: low-severity community-acquired

- Amoxicillin (*or* ampicillin)
- ▸ Pneumococci with decreased penicillin sensitivity being isolated, but not yet common in UK.
- ▸ If atypical pathogens suspected, add clarithromycin (*or* azithromycin *or* erythromycin).
- ▸ If staphylococci suspected (e. g. in influenza or measles), add flucloxacillin p. 503.
- ▸ *Suggested duration of treatment* 7 days (14–21 days for infections caused by staphylococci)
- *Alternatives*, doxycycline p. 513 or clarithromycin (*or* azithromycin *or* erythromycin)
- ▸ *Suggested duration of treatment* 7 days (14–21 days for infections caused by staphylococci)

Antibacterial therapy for pneumonia: moderate-severity community-acquired

- Amoxicillin (*or* ampicillin) + clarithromycin (*or* azithromycin *or* erythromycin) *or* doxycycline alone
- ▸ Pneumococci with decreased penicillin sensitivity being isolated, but not yet common in UK.
- ▸ If meticillin-resistant *Staphylococcus aureus* suspected, add vancomycin p. 484 (*or* teicoplanin p. 482).
- ▸ *Suggested duration of treatment* 7 days (14–21 days for infections caused by staphylococci)

Antibacterial therapy for pneumonia: high-severity community-acquired

- Benzylpenicillin sodium p. 496 + clarithromycin (*or* azithromycin *or* erythromycin) *or* benzylpenicillin sodium + doxycycline
- ▸ If meticillin-resistant *Staphylococcus aureus* suspected, add vancomycin (*or* teicoplanin).
- ▸ *Suggested duration of treatment* 7–10 days (may extend treatment to 14–21 days in some cases e.g. if staphylococci suspected)
- *If life-threatening infection, or if Gram-negative infection suspected, or if co-morbidities present, or if living in long-term residential or nursing home*, co-amoxiclav p. 501 + clarithromycin (*or* azithromycin *or* erythromycin)
- ▸ If meticillin-resistant *Staphylococcus aureus* suspected, add vancomycin (*or* teicoplanin)
- ▸ *Suggested duration of treatment* 7–10 days (may extend treatment to 14–21 days in some cases e.g. if staphylococci or Gram-negative enteric bacilli suspected)
- *Alternatives if life-threatening infection, or if Gram-negative infection suspected, or if co-morbidities present, or if living in long-term residential or nursing home*, cefuroxime p. 478 + clarithromycin (*or* azithromycin *or* erythromycin) *or* cefotaxime (*or* ceftriaxone) + clarithromycin (*or* azithromycin *or* erythromycin)
- ▸ If meticillin-resistant *Staphylococcus aureus* suspected, add vancomycin (*or* teicoplanin).
- ▸ *Suggested duration of treatment* 7–10 days (may extend treatment to 14–21 days in some cases e.g. if staphylococci or Gram-negative enteric bacilli suspected)

Antibacterial therapy for pneumonia possibly caused by atypical pathogens

- Clarithromycin (*or* azithromycin *or* erythromycin)
- ▸ If high-severity Legionella infection, add rifampicin p. 527 for the first few days.
- ▸ *Suggested duration of treatment* 14 days (usually 7–10 days for Legionella)
- *Alternative if Legionella infection suspected*, a quinolone
- ▸ If high-severity Legionella infection, add clarithromycin (*or* azithromycin *or* erythromycin) or rifampicin for the first few days.
- ▸ *Suggested duration of treatment* usually 7–10 days
- *Alternative for chlamydial or mycoplasma infections*, doxycycline
- ▸ *Suggested duration of treatment* 14 days

Antibacterial therapy for pneumonia: hospital-acquired

- *Early-onset infection* less than 5 days after admission to hospital), co-amoxiclav *or* cefuroxime
- ▸ If life-threatening infection, or if history of antibacterial treatment in the last 3 months, or if resistant micro-organisms suspected, treat as for late-onset hospital-acquired pneumonia.
- ▸ *Suggested duration of treatment* 7 days
- *Late-onset infection* (more than 5 days after admission to hospital), an antipseudomonal penicillin (e.g. piperacillin with tazobactam p. 495) *or* a broad-spectrum cephalosporin (e.g. ceftazidime p. 480) *or* another antipseudomonal beta-lactam *or* a quinolone (e.g. ciprofloxacin p. 506)
- ▸ If meticillin-resistant *Staphylococcus aureus* suspected, add vancomycin.
- ▸ For severe illness caused by *Pseudomonas aeruginosa*, consider adding an aminoglycoside.
- ▸ *Suggested duration of treatment* 7 days (longer if *Pseudomonas aeruginosa* confirmed)

Skin infections, bacterial

Antibacterial therapy for impetigo: small areas of skin infected

Seek local microbiology advice before using topical treatment in hospital.

- Topical fusidic acid p. 519
- ▸ *Suggested duration of treatment* 7 days is usually adequate (max. 10 days).
- *Alternatively, if meticillin-resistant Staphylococcus aureus*, topical mupirocin p. 1076
- ▸ *Suggested duration of treatment* 7 days is usually adequate (max. 10 days).

Impetigo: widespread infection

- Oral flucloxacillin p. 503
- ▸ If streptococci suspected in severe infection, add phenoxymethylpenicillin p. 497.
- ▸ *Suggested duration of treatment* 7 days.
- *If penicillin-allergic*, oral clarithromycin p. 487 (*or* azithromycin p. 486 *or* erythromycin p. 488)
- ▸ *Suggested duration of treatment* 7 days.

Antibacterial therapy for erysipelas

- Phenoxymethylpenicillin *or* benzylpenicillin sodium p. 496
- ▸ If severe infection, replace phenoxymethylpenicillin or benzylpenicillin sodium with high-dose flucloxacillin
- ▸ *Suggested duration of treatment* at least 7 days.
- *If penicillin-allergic*, clindamycin p. 485 *or* clarithromycin (*or* azithromycin *or* erythromycin)
- ▸ *Suggested duration of treatment* at least 7 days

Antibacterial therapy for cellulitis

- Flucloxacillin (high-dose)
- ▸ If streptococcal infection confirmed, replace flucloxacillin with phenoxymethylpenicillin *or* benzylpenicillin sodium
- ▸ If Gram-negative bacteria or anaerobes suspected, use broad-spectrum antibacterials.
- *If penicillin-allergic*, clindamycin *or* clarithromycin (*or* azithromycin *or* erythromycin) *or* vancomycin p. 484 (*or* teicoplanin p. 482)
- ▸ If Gram-negative bacteria suspected, use broad-spectrum antibacterials.

Antibacterial therapy for animal and human bites

Cleanse wound thoroughly. For tetanus-prone wound, give human tetanus immunoglobulin p. 1133 (with a tetanus-containing vaccine if necessary, according to immunisation history and risk of infection). Consider rabies prophylaxis for bites from animals in endemic countries. Assess risk of blood-borne viruses (including HIV, hepatitis B and C) and give appropriate prophylaxis to prevent viral spread.

- Co-amoxiclav p. 501
- *If penicillin-allergic*, doxycycline p. 513 + metronidazole p. 492

Antibacterial therapy for mastitis during breast-feeding

Treat if severe, if systemically unwell, if nipple fissure present, if symptoms do not improve after 12–24 hours of effective milk removal, or if culture indicates infection.

- Flucloxacillin, *if penicillin-allergic*, erythromycin
- ▸ Continue breast-feeding or expressing milk during treatment.
- ▸ *Suggested duration of treatment* 10–14 days.

Aminoglycosides

Overview

These include amikacin p. 471, gentamicin p. 471, neomycin sulfate p. 472, streptomycin p. 472, and tobramycin p. 473. All are bactericidal and active against some Gram-positive and many Gram-negative organisms. Amikacin, gentamicin, and tobramycin are also active against *Pseudomonas aeruginosa*; streptomycin is active against *Mycobacterium tuberculosis* and is now almost entirely reserved for tuberculosis.

The aminoglycosides are not absorbed from the gut (although there is a risk of absorption in inflammatory bowel disease and liver failure) and must therefore be given by injection for systemic infections.

Gentamicin is the aminoglycoside of choice in the UK and is used widely for the treatment of serious infections. It has a broad spectrum but is inactive against anaerobes and has poor activity against haemolytic streptococci and pneumococci. When used for the 'blind' therapy of undiagnosed serious infections it is usually given in conjunction with a penicillin or metronidazole p. 492 (or both). Gentamicin is used together with another antibiotic for the treatment of endocarditis. Streptomycin may be used as an alternative in gentamicin-resistant enterococcal endocarditis.

Loading and maintenance doses of gentamicin may be calculated on the basis of the patient's weight and renal function (e.g. using a nomogram); adjustments are then made according to serum-gentamicin concentrations. High doses are occasionally indicated for serious infections, especially in the neonate, in the patient with cystic fibrosis, or in the immunocompromised patient. Whenever possible treatment should not exceed 7 days.

Amikacin is more stable than gentamicin to enzyme inactivation. Amikacin is used in the treatment of serious infections caused by gentamicin-resistant Gram-negative bacilli.

Tobramycin has similar activity to gentamicin. It is slightly more active against *Ps. aeruginosa* but shows less activity against certain other Gram-negative bacteria. Tobramycin can be administered by nebuliser or by inhalation of powder on a cyclical basis (28 days of tobramycin followed by a 28-day tobramycin-free interval) for the treatment of chronic pulmonary *Ps. aeruginosa* infection in cystic fibrosis; however, resistance may develop and some patients do not respond to treatment.

Neomycin sulfate is too toxic for parenteral administration and can only be used for infections of the skin or mucous membranes or to reduce the bacterial population of the colon prior to bowel surgery or in hepatic failure. Oral administration may lead to malabsorption. Small amounts of neomycin sulfate may be absorbed from the gut in patients with hepatic failure and, as these patients may also be uraemic, cumulation may occur with resultant ototoxicity.

Once daily dosage

Once daily administration of aminoglycosides is more convenient, provides adequate serum concentrations, and in many cases has largely superseded *multiple daily dose regimens* (given in 2–3 divided doses during the 24 hours). Local guidelines on dosage and serum concentrations should be consulted. A once-daily, high-dose regimen of an aminoglycoside should be avoided in patients with endocarditis due to Gram-positive bacteria, HACEK endocarditis, burns of more than 20% of the total body surface area, or creatinine clearance less than 20 mL/minute. There is insufficient evidence to recommend a once daily, high-dose regimen of an aminoglycoside in pregnancy.

Serum concentrations

Serum concentration monitoring avoids both excessive and subtherapeutic concentrations thus preventing toxicity and ensuring efficacy. Serum-aminoglycoside concentrations should be monitored in patients receiving parenteral aminoglycosides and **must** be determined in the elderly, in obesity, and in cystic fibrosis, or if high doses are being given, or if there is renal impairment.

Aminoglycosides (by injection)

- **CONTRA-INDICATIONS** Myasthenia gravis (aminoglycosides may impair neuromuscular transmission)
- **CAUTIONS** Care must be taken with dosage (the main side-effects of the aminoglycosides are dose-related) · conditions characterised by muscular weakness (aminoglycosides may impair neuromuscular transmission) · if possible, dehydration should be corrected before starting an aminoglycoside · whenever possible, parenteral treatment should not exceed 7 days
- **INTERACTIONS** → Appendix 1 (aminoglycosides). If possible, aminoglycosides should not be given with potentially ototoxic drugs (e.g. cisplatin). Administration of an aminoglycoside and of an ototoxic diuretic (e.g. furosemide) should be separated by as long a period as practicable.
- **SIDE-EFFECTS**
  ▸ **Rare** Antibiotic-associated colitis · electrolyte disturbances · hypocalcaemia · hypokalaemia · hypomagnesaemia on prolonged therapy · nausea · peripheral neuropathy · stomatitis · vomiting
  ▸ **Very rare** Blood disorders · CNS effects · convulsions · encephalopathy · headache
  ▸ **Frequency not known** Auditory damage · impaired neuromuscular transmission · irreversible ototoxicity · nephrotoxicity · transient myasthenic syndrome in patients with normal neuromuscular function with large doses given during surgery · vestibular damage

  SIDE-EFFECTS, FURTHER INFORMATION
  ▸ Nephrotoxicity
  ▸ In adults Occurs most commonly in the elderly; therefore, monitoring is particularly important in these patients, who may require reduced doses.
  ▸ In children Occurs most commonly in children with renal failure.
- **PREGNANCY** There is a risk of auditory or vestibular nerve damage in the infant when aminoglycosides are used in the second and third trimesters of pregnancy. The risk is greatest with streptomycin. The risk is probably very small with gentamicin and tobramycin, but their use should be avoided unless essential.

  If given during pregnancy, serum-aminoglycoside concentration monitoring is essential.
- **RENAL IMPAIRMENT** If there is impairment of renal function, the interval between doses must be increased; if the renal impairment is severe, the dose itself should be reduced as well. Excretion of aminoglycosides is principally via the kidney and accumulation occurs in renal impairment.

  Ototoxicity and nephrotoxicity occur commonly in patients with renal failure. Serum-aminoglycoside concentrations **must** be monitored in patients with renal impairment; earlier and more frequent measurement of aminoglycoside concentration may be required.
  ▸ In adults A once-daily, high-dose regimen of an aminoglycoside should be avoided in patients with a creatinine clearance less than 20 mL/minute.
  ▸ In children A once-daily, high-dose regimen of an aminoglycoside should be avoided in children over

1 month of age with a creatinine clearance less than 20 mL/minute/1.73 m^2.

- MONITORING REQUIREMENTS
▸ Serum concentrations Serum concentration monitoring avoids both excessive and subtherapeutic concentrations thus preventing toxicity and ensuring efficacy.

Serum-aminoglycoside concentrations should be measured in all patients receiving parenteral aminoglycosides and **must** be determined in obesity, if high doses are being given and in cystic fibrosis.
▸ In adults Serum aminoglycoside concentrations **must** be determined in the elderly. In patients with normal renal function, aminoglycoside concentrations should be measured after 3 or 4 doses of a multiple daily dose regimen and after a dose change. For multiple daily dose regimens, blood samples should be taken approximately 1 hour after intramuscular or intravenous administration ('peak' concentration) and also just before the next dose ('trough' concentration). If the pre-dose ('trough') concentration is high, the interval between doses must be increased. If the post-dose ('peak') concentration is high, the dose must be decreased. For once daily dose regimens, consult local guidelines on serum concentration monitoring.
▸ In children In children with normal renal function, aminoglycoside concentrations should be measured after 3 or 4 doses of a multiple daily dose regimen. Blood samples should be taken just before the next dose is administered ('trough' concentration). If the pre-dose ('trough') concentration is high, the interval between doses must be increased. For multiple daily dose regimens, blood samples should also be taken approximately 1 hour after intramuscular or intravenous administration ('peak' concentration). If the post-dose ('peak') concentration is high, the dose must be decreased.
▸ Renal function should be assessed before starting an aminoglycoside and during treatment.
▸ Auditory and vestibular function should also be monitored during treatment.

🗏 470

Amikacin

- INDICATIONS AND DOSE

Serious Gram-negative infections resistant to gentamicin (multiple daily dose regimen)
▸ BY INTRAMUSCULAR INJECTION, OR BY SLOW INTRAVENOUS INJECTION, OR BY INTRAVENOUS INFUSION
▸ Adult: 15 mg/kg daily in 2 divided doses, increased to 22.5 mg/kg daily in 3 divided doses for up to 10 days, higher dose to be used in severe infections; maximum 1.5 g per day; maximum 15 g per course

Serious Gram-negative infections resistant to gentamicin (once daily dose regimen)
▸ BY INTRAVENOUS INFUSION
▸ Adult: Initially 15 mg/kg (max. per dose 1.5 g once daily), dose to be adjusted according to serum-amikacin concentration; maximum 15 g per course

DOSES AT EXTREMES OF BODY-WEIGHT
To avoid excessive dosage in obese patients, use ideal weight for height to calculate dose and monitor serum-amikacin concentration closely

- SIDE-EFFECTS
▸ **Uncommon** Rash

- MONITORING REQUIREMENTS
▸ *Multiple daily dose regimen*: one-hour ('peak') serum concentration should not exceed 30 mg/litre; pre-dose ('trough') concentration should be less than 10 mg/litre.
▸ *Once daily dose regimen*: pre-dose ('trough') concentration should be less than 5 mg/litre.

- DIRECTIONS FOR ADMINISTRATION For *intravenous infusion* (*Amikin®*); intermittent in Glucose 5% *or* Sodium chloride 0.9%. To be given over 30 minutes.
- PRESCRIBING AND DISPENSING INFORMATION Once daily dose regime not to be used for endocarditis, febrile neutropenia, or meningitis. Consult local guidelines.

- MEDICINAL FORMS
There can be variation in the licensing of different medicines containing the same drug.
Solution for injection
▸ Amikacin (Non-proprietary)
Amikacin (as Amikacin sulfate) 250 mg per 1 ml Amikacin 500mg/2ml solution for injection vials | 5 vial [PoM] £60.00
▸ Amikin (Bristol-Myers Squibb Pharmaceuticals Ltd)
Amikacin (as Amikacin sulfate) 50 mg per 1 ml Amikin 100mg/2ml solution for injection vials | 5 vial [PoM] £10.33

🗏 470

Gentamicin

- INDICATIONS AND DOSE

Gram-positive bacterial endocarditis or HACEK endocarditis (in combination with other antibacterials)
▸ BY INTRAMUSCULAR INJECTION, OR BY SLOW INTRAVENOUS INJECTION, OR BY INTRAVENOUS INFUSION
▸ Adult: 1 mg/kg every 12 hours, intravenous injection to be administered over at least 3 minutes, to be given in a multiple daily dose regimen

Septicaemia | Meningitis and other CNS infections | Biliary-tract infection | Acute pyelonephritis | Endocarditis | Pneumonia in hospital patients | Adjunct in listerial meningitis | Prostatitis
▸ BY INTRAVENOUS INFUSION, OR BY SLOW INTRAVENOUS INJECTION, OR BY INTRAMUSCULAR INJECTION
▸ Adult: 3–5 mg/kg daily in 3 divided doses, to be given in a multiple daily dose regimen, divided doses to be given every 8 hours, intravenous injection to be administered over at least 3 minutes
▸ BY INTRAVENOUS INFUSION
▸ Adult: Initially 5–7 mg/kg, subsequent doses adjusted according to serum-gentamicin concentration, to be given in a once daily dose regimen

CNS infections (administered on expert advice)
▸ BY INTRATHECAL INJECTION
▸ Adult: 1 mg daily, increased if necessary to 5 mg daily, seek specialist advice

Surgical prophylaxis
▸ BY SLOW INTRAVENOUS INJECTION
▸ Adult: 1.5 mg/kg, intravenous injection to be administered over at least 3 minutes, administer dose up to 30 minutes before the procedure, dose may be repeated every 8 hours for high-risk procedures; up to 3 further doses may be given

Surgical prophylaxis (including joint replacement surgery)
▸ BY INTRAVENOUS INFUSION
▸ Adult: 5 mg/kg for 1 dose, administer dose up to 30 minutes before the procedure

DOSES AT EXTREMES OF BODY-WEIGHT
▸ With intramuscular use or intravenous use To avoid excessive dosage in obese patients, use ideal weight for height to calculate dose and monitor serum-gentamicin concentration closely.

- SIDE-EFFECTS
▸ **Uncommon** Rash

- MONITORING REQUIREMENTS
▸ With intramuscular use or intravenous use For multiple daily dose regimen, one-hour ('peak') serum concentration should be 5–10 mg/litre; pre-dose ('trough') concentration should be less than 2 mg/litre.

For multiple daily dose regimen in endocarditis, one-hour ('peak') serum concentration should be 3–5 mg/litre;

pre-dose ('trough') concentration should be less than 1 mg/litre. Serum-gentamicin concentration should be measured after 3 or 4 doses, then at least every 3 days and after a dose change (more frequently in renal impairment).
▶ With intravenous use For once-daily dose regimen, consult local guidelines on monitoring serum-gentamicin concentration.

● DIRECTIONS FOR ADMINISTRATION
▶ With intrathecal use For *intrathecal* injection, use preservative-free intrathecal preparations only.
▶ With intravenous use For *intravenous infusion* (Cidomycin®); *Gentamicin paediatric injection,* Beacon; *Gentamicin injection* Hospira), give intermittently *or* via drip tubing in Glucose 5% or Sodium Chloride 0.9%. Suggested volume for intermittent infusion 50–100 ml given over 20–30 minutes (given over 60 minutes for once daily dose regimen).

● PRESCRIBING AND DISPENSING INFORMATION
▶ With intravenous use Local guidelines may vary in the dosing advice provided for once daily administration.
▶ With intrathecal use Only preservative-free intrathecal preparation should be used.

● MEDICINAL FORMS
There can be variation in the licensing of different medicines containing the same drug.
Solution for injection
▶ Gentamicin (Non-proprietary)
    Gentamicin (as Gentamicin sulfate) 5 mg per 1 ml Gentamicin Intrathecal 5mg/1ml solution for injection ampoules | 5 ampoule [PoM] £22.50 (Hospital only)
    Gentamicin (as Gentamicin sulfate) 10 mg per 1 ml Gentamicin 20mg/2ml solution for injection ampoules | 5 ampoule [PoM] £11.25 Gentamicin Paediatric 20mg/2ml solution for injection vials | 5 vial [PoM] £11.25
    Gentamicin (as Gentamicin sulfate) 40 mg per 1 ml Gentamicin 80mg/2ml solution for injection vials | 5 vial [PoM] £20.00 Gentamicin 80mg/2ml solution for injection ampoules | 5 ampoule [PoM] £6.88 | 10 ampoule [PoM] £10.00
▶ Cidomycin (Sanofi)
    Gentamicin (as Gentamicin sulfate) 40 mg per 1 ml Cidomycin Adult Injectable 80mg/2ml solution for injection vials | 5 vial [PoM] £6.88
    Cidomycin Adult Injectable 80mg/2ml solution for injection ampoules | 5 ampoule [PoM] £6.88
Infusion
▶ Gentamicin (Non-proprietary)
    Gentamicin (as Gentamicin sulfate) 1 mg per 1 ml Gentamicin 80mg/80ml infusion bags | 20 bag [PoM] £39.00
    Gentamicin (as Gentamicin sulfate) 3 mg per 1 ml Gentamicin 240mg/80ml infusion bags | 20 bag [PoM] £119.00 Gentamicin 360mg/120ml infusion bags | 20 bag [PoM] £169.00

Neomycin sulfate

● INDICATIONS AND DOSE
Bowel sterilisation before surgery
▶ BY MOUTH
▶ Adult: 1 g every 1 hour for 4 hours, then 1 g every 4 hours for 2–3 days

Hepatic coma
▶ BY MOUTH
▶ Adult: Up to 4 g daily in divided doses usually for 5–7 days

● CONTRA-INDICATIONS Intestinal obstruction · myasthenia gravis (aminoglycosides may impair neuromuscular transmission)
● CAUTIONS Avoid prolonged use
CAUTIONS, FURTHER INFORMATION
Although neomycin is associated with the same cautions as other aminoglycosides it is generally considered too toxic for systemic use.
● INTERACTIONS → Appendix 1 (aminoglycosides).

● SIDE-EFFECTS
▶ **Uncommon** Rash
▶ **Frequency not known** Impaired intestinal absorption with steatorrhoea and diarrhoea · increased salivation
SIDE-EFFECTS, FURTHER INFORMATION
Although neomycin is associated with the same side effects as other aminoglycosides it is generally considered too toxic for systemic use and is poorly absorbed after oral administration.
● PREGNANCY There is a risk of auditory or vestibular nerve damage in the infant when aminoglycosides are used in the second and third trimesters of pregnancy.
● HEPATIC IMPAIRMENT Absorbed from gastro-intestinal tract in liver disease—increased risk of ototoxicity.
● RENAL IMPAIRMENT Avoid–risk of ototoxicity and nephrotoxicity.
● MONITORING REQUIREMENTS Renal function should be assessed before starting an aminoglycoside and during treatment. Auditory and vestibular function should also be monitored during treatment.

● MEDICINAL FORMS
There can be variation in the licensing of different medicines containing the same drug. Forms available from special-order manufacturers include: oral solution, cream
Tablet
▶ Neomycin sulfate (Non-proprietary)
    Neomycin sulfate 500 mg Neomycin sulfate 500mg tablets | 100 tablet [PoM] £34.69 DT price = £34.69
Oral solution
▶ Neomycin sulfate (Non-proprietary)
    Neomycin sulfate 25 mg per 1 ml Neo-Fradin 125mg/5ml oral solution | 480 ml [PoM] no price available

📖 470

Streptomycin

● INDICATIONS AND DOSE
Tuberculosis, resistant to other treatment, in combination with other drugs
▶ BY DEEP INTRAMUSCULAR INJECTION
▶ Adult: 15 mg/kg daily (max. per dose 1 g), reduce dose in those under 50 kg and those over 40 years

Adjunct to doxycycline in brucellosis (administered on expert advice)
▶ BY DEEP INTRAMUSCULAR INJECTION
▶ Adult: (consult local protocol)

Enterococcal endocarditis
▶ Adult: (consult local protocol)

● UNLICENSED USE Use in tuberculosis is an unlicensed indication.

> IMPORTANT SAFETY INFORMATION
> Side-effects increase after a cumulative dose of 100 g, which should only be exceeded in exceptional circumstances.

● SIDE-EFFECTS
▶ **Common or very common** Rash
▶ **Frequency not known** Hypersensitivity reactions · paraesthesia of mouth
● RENAL IMPAIRMENT Should preferably be avoided. If essential, use with great care and consider dose reduction.
● MONITORING REQUIREMENTS
▶ One-hour ('peak') concentration should be 15–40 mg/litre; pre-dose ('trough') concentration should be less than 5 mg/litre (less than 1 mg/litre in renal impairment or in those over 50 years).

● MEDICINAL FORMS
There can be variation in the licensing of different medicines containing the same drug. Forms available from special-order manufacturers include: powder for solution for injection

Tobramycin

⏺ **INDICATIONS AND DOSE**

Septicaemia | Meningitis and other CNS infections | Biliary-tract infection | Acute pyelonephritis or prostatitis | Pneumonia in hospital patients

▸ BY INTRAMUSCULAR INJECTION, OR BY SLOW INTRAVENOUS INJECTION, OR BY INTRAVENOUS INFUSION

▸ Adult: 3 mg/kg daily in 3 divided doses; increased if necessary up to 5 mg/kg daily in 3–4 divided doses, increased dose used in severe infection; dose to be reduced back to 3 mg/kg as soon as clinically indicated

Urinary-tract infection

▸ BY INTRAMUSCULAR INJECTION

▸ Adult: 2–3 mg/kg for 1 dose

Chronic *Pseudomonas aeruginosa* infection in patients with cystic fibrosis

▸ BY INHALATION OF NEBULISED SOLUTION

▸ Adult: 300 mg every 12 hours for 28 days, subsequent courses repeated after 28-day interval without tobramycin nebuliser solution

▸ BY INHALATION OF POWDER

▸ Adult: 112 mg every 12 hours for 28 days, subsequent courses repeated after 28-day interval without tobramycin inhalation powder

DOSES AT EXTREMES OF BODY-WEIGHT

To avoid excessive dosage in obese patients, use ideal weight for height to calculate parenteral dose and monitor serum-tobramycin concentration closely.

⏺ CAUTIONS

▸ When used by inhalation Severe haemoptysis—risk of further haemorrhage

⏺ SIDE-EFFECTS

▸ **Uncommon**

▸ With intramuscular use or intravenous use Rash

▸ **Frequency not known**

▸ When used by inhalation Bronchospasm · cough (more frequent by inhalation of powder) · dysphonia · epistaxis · haemoptysis · laryngitis · mouth ulcers · pharyngitis · salivary hypersecretion · taste disturbances

⏺ MONITORING REQUIREMENTS

▸ With intramuscular use or intravenous use One-hour ('peak') serum concentration should not exceed 10 mg/litre; pre-dose ('trough') concentration should be less than 2 mg/litre.

▸ When used by inhalation Measure lung function before and after initial dose of tobramycin and monitor for bronchospasm; if bronchospasm occurs in a patient not using a bronchodilator, repeat test using bronchodilator. Monitor renal function before treatment and then annually.

⏺ DIRECTIONS FOR ADMINISTRATION

▸ With intravenous use For *intravenous infusion* (Nebcin®); intermittent or via drip tubing in Glucose 5% or Sodium chloride 0.9%. For adult intermittent infusion suggested volume 50–100 mL given over 20–60 minutes.

▸ When used by inhalation Other inhaled drugs should be administered before tobramycin.

⏺ PATIENT AND CARER ADVICE

▸ When used by inhalation Patient counselling is advised for Tobramycin dry powder for inhalation (administration).

⏺ NATIONAL FUNDING/ACCESS DECISIONS

▸ **NICE technology appraisals (TAs)**

▸ Tobramycin by dry powder inhalation for pseudomonal lung infection in cystic fibrosis (March 2013) NICE TA276

▸ When used by inhalation Tobramycin dry powder for inhalation is recommended for chronic pulmonary infection caused by *Pseudomonas aeruginosa* in patients

with cystic fibrosis only if there is an inadequate response to colistimethate sodium, or if colistimethate sodium cannot be used because of contra-indications or intolerance. The manufacturer must provide tobramycin dry powder for inhalation at the discount agreed as part of the patient access scheme to primary, secondary and tertiary care in the NHS. Patients currently receiving tobramycin dry powder for inhalation can continue treatment until they and their clinician consider it appropriate to stop.
www.nice.org.uk/TA276

⏺ MEDICINAL FORMS
There can be variation in the licensing of different medicines containing the same drug. Forms available from special-order manufacturers include: oral solution

Solution for injection

▸ Tobramycin (Non-proprietary)
Tobramycin (as Tobramycin sulfate) 40 mg per 1 ml Tobramycin 40mg/1ml solution for injection vials | 10 vial PoM £37.00 | 10 vial PoM £37.00 (Hospital only)
Tobramycin 80mg/2ml solution for injection vials | 5 vial PoM £20.80 | 10 vial PoM £37.72 | 10 vial PoM £47.00 (Hospital only)
Tobramycin 240mg/6ml solution for injection vials | 1 vial PoM £19.20

▸ Nebcin (Flynn Pharma Ltd)
Tobramycin (as Tobramycin sulfate) 40 mg per 1 ml Nebcin 80mg/2ml solution for injection vials | 1 vial PoM £5.37

Inhalation powder

▸ Tobi Podhaler (Novartis Pharmaceuticals UK Ltd)
Tobramycin 28 mg Tobi Podhaler 28mg inhalation powder capsules with device | 56 capsule PoM £447.50 | 224 capsule PoM £1,790.00

Nebuliser liquid

▸ Bramitob (Chiesi Ltd)
Tobramycin 75 mg per 1 ml Bramitob 300mg/4ml nebuliser solution 4ml ampoules | 56 ampoule PoM £1,187.00

▸ TOBI (Novartis Pharmaceuticals UK Ltd)
Tobramycin 60 mg per 1 ml Tobi 300mg/5ml nebuliser solution 5ml ampoules | 56 ampoule PoM £1,305.92 DT price = £1,305.92

▸ Tymbrineb (Teva UK Ltd)
Tobramycin 60 mg per 1 ml Tymbrineb 300mg/5ml nebuliser solution 5ml ampoules | 56 ampoule PoM £1,127.84 DT price = £1,305.92

ANTIBACTERIALS ⟩ CARBAPENEMS

Carbapenems

Overview

The carbapenems are beta-lactam antibacterials with a broad-spectrum of activity which includes many Gram-positive and Gram-negative bacteria, and anaerobes; **imipenem** (imipenem with cilastatin p. 474) and meropenem p. 475 have good activity against *Pseudomonas aeruginosa*. The carbapenems are not active against meticillin-resistant *Staphylococcus aureus* and *Enterococcus faecium*.

Imipenem (imipenem with cilastatin) and meropenem are used for the treatment of severe hospital-acquired infections and polymicrobial infections including septicaemia, hospital-acquired pneumonia, intra-abdominal infections, skin and soft-tissue infections, and complicated urinary-tract infections.

Ertapenem p. 474 is licensed for treating abdominal and gynaecological infections and for community-acquired pneumonia, but it is not active against atypical respiratory pathogens and it has limited activity against penicillin-resistant pneumococci. It is also licensed for treating foot infections of the skin and soft tissue in patients with diabetes. Unlike the other carbapenems, ertapenem is not active against *Pseudomonas* or against *Acinetobacter spp*.

Imipenem is partially inactivated in the kidney by enzymatic activity and is therefore administered in

5

Infection

Infection

5

combination with **cilastatin** (imipenem with cilastatin), a specific enzyme inhibitor, which blocks its renal metabolism. Meropenem and ertapenem are stable to the renal enzyme which inactivates imipenem and therefore can be given without cilastatin.

Side-effects of imipenem with cilastatin are similar to those of other beta-lactam antibiotics. Meropenem has less seizure-inducing potential and can be used to treat central nervous system infection.

Ertapenem

● **INDICATIONS AND DOSE**

Abdominal infections | Acute gynaecological infections | Community-acquired pneumonia
▸ BY INTRAVENOUS INFUSION
▸ Adult: 1 g once daily

Diabetic foot infections of the skin and soft-tissue
▸ BY INTRAVENOUS INFUSION
▸ Adult: 1 g once daily

Surgical prophylaxis, colorectal surgery
▸ BY INTRAVENOUS INFUSION
▸ Adult: 1 g for 1 dose, dose to be completed within 1 hour before surgery

● CAUTIONS CNS disorders—risk of seizures · elderly
● INTERACTIONS → Appendix 1 (ertapenem).
● SIDE-EFFECTS
▸ **Common or very common** Diarrhoea · headache · injection-site reactions · nausea · pruritus · raised platelet count · rash (also reported with eosinophilia and systemic symptoms) · vomiting
▸ **Uncommon** Abdominal pain · anorexia · antibiotic-associated colitis · asthenia · bradycardia · chest pain · confusion · constipation · dizziness · dry mouth · dyspepsia · dyspnoea · hypotension · melaena · oedema · petechiae · pharyngeal discomfort · raised glucose · seizures · sleep disturbances · taste disturbances
▸ **Rare** Agitation · anxiety · arrhythmia · blood disorders · cholecystitis · cough · depression · dysphagia · electrolyte disturbances · haemorrhage · hypoglycaemia · increase in blood pressure · jaundice · liver disorder · muscle cramp · nasal congestion · neutropenia · pelvic peritonitis · renal impairment · scleral disorder · syncope · thrombocytopenia · tremor · wheezing
▸ **Frequency not known** Dyskinesia · hallucinations
● ALLERGY AND CROSS-SENSITIVITY Avoid if history of **immediate hypersensitivity** reaction to beta-lactam antibacterials.
    Use with caution in patients with sensitivity to beta-lactam antibacterials.
● PREGNANCY Manufacturer advises avoid unless potential benefit outweighs risk.
● BREAST FEEDING Present in milk—manufacturer advises avoid.
● RENAL IMPAIRMENT
▸ With intravenous use Risk of seizures; max. 500 mg daily if eGFR less than 30 mL/minute/1.73 m^2.
● DIRECTIONS FOR ADMINISTRATION For *intravenous infusion* (*Invanz*®), give intermittently *in* Sodium chloride 0.9%. Reconstitute 1 g with 10 mL Water for injections *or* Sodium chloride 0.9%; dilute requisite dose in infusion fluid to a final concentration not exceeding 20 mg/mL; give over 30 minutes; incompatible with glucose solutions.

● MEDICINAL FORMS
There can be variation in the licensing of different medicines containing the same drug.
Powder for solution for infusion
ELECTROLYTES: May contain Sodium
▸ Invanz (Merck Sharp & Dohme Ltd)
    Ertapenem (as Ertapenem sodium) 1 gram Invanz 1g powder for solution for infusion vials | 1 vial [PoM] £31.65

Imipenem with cilastatin

● **INDICATIONS AND DOSE**

Aerobic and anaerobic Gram-positive and Gram-negative infections (not indicated for CNS infections) | Hospital-acquired septicaemia
▸ BY INTRAVENOUS INFUSION
▸ Adult: 500 mg every 6 hours, alternatively 1 g every 8 hours

Infection caused by *Pseudomonas* or other less sensitive organisms | Empirical treatment of infection in febrile patients with neutropenia | Life-threatening infection
▸ BY INTRAVENOUS INFUSION
▸ Adult: 1 g every 6 hours
DOSE EQUIVALENCE AND CONVERSION
Dose expressed in terms of imipenem.

● CAUTIONS CNS disorders · epilepsy
● INTERACTIONS → Appendix 1 (imipenem with cilastatin).
● SIDE-EFFECTS
▸ **Common or very common** Diarrhoea · eosinophilia · nausea (may reduce rate of infusion) · rash · vomiting
▸ **Uncommon** Confusion · dizziness · drowsiness · hallucinations · hypotension · leucopenia · myoclonic activity · seizures · thrombocytopenia · thrombocytosis
▸ **Rare** Acute renal failure · anaphylactic reactions · antibiotic-associated colitis · encephalopathy · hearing loss · hepatitis · paraesthesia · polyuria · Stevens-Johnson syndrome · taste disturbances · tooth, tongue or urine discoloration · toxic epidermal necrolysis · tremor
▸ **Very rare** Abdominal pain · aggravation of myasthenia gravis · asthenia · cyanosis · dyspnoea · flushing · glossitis · haemolytic anaemia · headache · heartburn · hyperhidrosis · hypersalivation · hyperventilation · palpitation · polyarthralgia · tachycardia · tinnitus
▸ **Frequency not known** Neurotoxicity (at high dose, renal failure, CNS disease)
● ALLERGY AND CROSS-SENSITIVITY Avoid if history of **immediate hypersensitivity** reaction to beta-lactam antibacterials.
    Use with caution in patients with sensitivity to beta-lactam antibacterials.
● PREGNANCY Manufacturer advises avoid unless potential benefit outweighs risk (toxicity in *animal* studies).
● BREAST FEEDING Present in milk but unlikely to be absorbed.
● RENAL IMPAIRMENT Risk of CNS side-effects; reduce dose if eGFR less than 70 mL/minute/1.73 m^2— consult product literature.
● EFFECT ON LABORATORY TESTS Positive Coombs' test.
● DIRECTIONS FOR ADMINISTRATION For *intravenous infusion* dilute to a concentration of 5 mg (as imipenem)/mL in Sodium chloride 0.9%; give up to 500 mg (as imipenem) over 20–30 minutes, give dose greater than 500 mg (as imipenem) over 40–60 minutes.

● MEDICINAL FORMS
There can be variation in the licensing of different medicines containing the same drug.
Powder for solution for infusion
ELECTROLYTES: May contain Sodium
▸ Imipenem with cilastatin (Non-proprietary)

Cilastatin (as Cilastatin sodium) 500 mg, Imipenem (as Imipenem monohydrate) 500 mg Imipenem 500mg / Cilastatin 500mg powder for solution for infusion vials | 1 vial P̲o̲M̲ £12.00 (Hospital only) | 5 vial P̲o̲M̲ £60.00 (Hospital only) | 10 vial P̲o̲M̲ £75.45–£120.00
▸ Primaxin I.V. (Merck Sharp & Dohme Ltd)

Cilastatin (as Cilastatin sodium) 500 mg, Imipenem (as Imipenem monohydrate) 500 mg Primaxin IV 500mg powder for solution for infusion vials | 1 vial P̲o̲M̲ £12.00

Meropenem

● INDICATIONS AND DOSE

Aerobic and anaerobic Gram-positive and Gram-negative infections | Hospital-acquired septicaemia
▸ BY INTRAVENOUS INFUSION, OR BY INTRAVENOUS INJECTION
▸ Adult: 0.5–1 g every 8 hours

Exacerbations of chronic lower respiratory-tract infection in cystic fibrosis
▸ BY INTRAVENOUS INFUSION, OR BY INTRAVENOUS INJECTION
▸ Adult: 2 g every 8 hours

Meningitis
▸ BY INTRAVENOUS INFUSION, OR BY INTRAVENOUS INJECTION
▸ Adult: 2 g every 8 hours

Endocarditis (in combination with another antibacterial)
▸ BY INTRAVENOUS INFUSION, OR BY INTRAVENOUS INJECTION
▸ Adult: 2 g every 8 hours

● UNLICENSED USE Not licensed for use in endocarditis.

● INTERACTIONS → Appendix 1 (meropenem).

● SIDE-EFFECTS
▸ **Common or very common** Abdominal pain · diarrhoea · disturbances in liver function tests · headache · nausea · pruritus · rash · thrombocythaemia · vomiting
▸ **Uncommon** Eosinophilia · leucopenia · paraesthesia · thrombocytopenia
▸ **Rare** Convulsions
▸ **Frequency not known** Antibiotic-associated colitis · haemolytic anaemia · Stevens-Johnson syndrome · toxic epidermal necrolysis

● ALLERGY AND CROSS-SENSITIVITY Avoid if history of **immediate hypersensitivity** reaction to beta-lactam antibacterials.
Use with caution in patients with sensitivity to beta-lactam antibacterials.

● PREGNANCY Use only if potential benefit outweighs risk—no information available.

● BREAST FEEDING Unlikely to be absorbed (however, manufacturer advises avoid).

● HEPATIC IMPAIRMENT

Monitoring
Monitor liver function in hepatic impairment.

● RENAL IMPAIRMENT Use normal dose every 12 hours if eGFR 26–50 mL/minute/1.73 m^2. Use half normal dose every 12 hours if eGFR 10–25 mL/minute/1.73 m^2. Use half normal dose every 24 hours if eGFR less than 10 mL/minute/1.73 m^2.

● EFFECT ON LABORATORY TESTS Positive Coombs' test.

● DIRECTIONS FOR ADMINISTRATION *Intravenous injection* to be administered over 5 minutes.
For *intravenous infusion* (Meronem®), give intermittently in Glucose 5% *or* Sodium chloride 0.9%.
Dilute dose in infusion fluid to a final concentration of 1–20 mg/mL; give over 15–30 minutes.

● MEDICINAL FORMS
There can be variation in the licensing of different medicines containing the same drug.
Powder for solution for injection
ELECTROLYTES: May contain Sodium
▸ Meropenem (Non-proprietary)

Meropenem (as Meropenem trihydrate) 500 mg Meropenem 500mg powder for solution for injection vials | 10 vial P̲o̲M̲ £76.90–£90.00
Meropenem (as Meropenem trihydrate) 1 gram Meropenem 1g powder for solution for injection vials | 10 vial P̲o̲M̲ £153.50–£206.28 | 10 vial P̲o̲M̲ £171.90–£206.28 (Hospital only)
▸ Meronem (AstraZeneca UK Ltd)

Meropenem (as Meropenem trihydrate) 500 mg Meronem 500mg powder for solution for injection vials | 10 vial P̲o̲M̲ £103.14
Meropenem (as Meropenem trihydrate) 1 gram Meronem 1g powder for solution for injection vials | 10 vial P̲o̲M̲ £206.28

ANTIBACTERIALS > CEPHALOSPORINS

Cephalosporins

Overview

The cephalosporins are broad-spectrum antibiotics which are used for the treatment of septicaemia, pneumonia, meningitis, biliary-tract infections, peritonitis, and urinary-tract infections. The pharmacology of the cephalosporins is similar to that of the penicillins, excretion being principally renal. Cephalosporins penetrate the cerebrospinal fluid poorly unless the meninges are inflamed; cefotaxime p. 479 and ceftriaxone p. 480 are suitable cephalosporins for infections of the CNS (e.g meningitis).

The principal side-effect of the cephalosporins is hypersensitivity and about 0.5–6.5% of penicillin-sensitive patients will also be allergic to the cephalosporins. If a cephalosporin is essential in patients with a history of immediate hypersensitivity to penicillin, because a suitable alternative antibacterial is not available, then cefixime p. 479, cefotaxime, ceftazidime p. 480, ceftriaxone, or cefuroxime p. 478 can be used with caution; cefaclor p. 477, cefadroxil p. 476, cefalexin p. 476, cefradine p. 477, and ceftaroline fosamil p. 482 should be avoided.

The orally active 'first generation' cephalosporins, cefalexin, cefradine, and cefadroxil and the 'second generation' cephalosporin, cefaclor, have a similar antimicrobial spectrum. They are useful for urinary-tract infections which do not respond to other drugs or which occur in pregnancy, respiratory-tract infections, otitis media, sinusitis, and skin and soft-tissue infections. Cefaclor has good activity against *H. influenzae*. Cefadroxil has a long duration of action and can be given twice daily; it has poor activity against *H. influenzae*. **Cefuroxime axetil**, an ester of the 'second generation' cephalosporin cefuroxime, has the same antibacterial spectrum as the parent compound; it is poorly absorbed and needs to be given with food to maximise absorption.

Cefixime is an orally active 'third generation' cephalosporin. It has a longer duration of action than the other cephalosporins that are active by mouth. It is only licensed for acute infections.

Cefuroxime is a 'second generation' cephalosporin that is less susceptible than the earlier cephalosporins to inactivation by beta-lactamases. It is, therefore, active against certain bacteria which are resistant to the other drugs and has greater activity against *Haemophilus influenzae*.

Cefotaxime, ceftazidime and ceftriaxone are 'third generation' cephalosporins with greater activity than the 'second generation' cephalosporins against certain Gram-negative bacteria. However, they are less active than cefuroxime against Gram-positive bacteria, most notably *Staphylococcus aureus*. Their broad antibacterial spectrum

5

Infection

may encourage superinfection with resistant bacteria or fungi.

Ceftazidime has good activity against pseudomonas. It is also active against other Gram-negative bacteria.

Ceftriaxone has a longer half-life and therefore needs to be given only once daily. Indications include serious infections such as septicaemia, pneumonia, and meningitis. The calcium salt of ceftriaxone forms a precipitate in the gall bladder which may rarely cause symptoms but these usually resolve when the antibiotic is stopped.

Ceftaroline fosamil is a 'fifth generation' cephalosporin with bactericidal activity similar to cefotaxime; however, ceftaroline fosamil has an extended spectrum of activity against Gram-positive bacteria that includes meticillin-resistant *Staphylococcus aureus* and multi-drug resistant *Streptococcus pneumoniae*. Ceftaroline fosamil is licensed for the treatment of community-acquired pneumonia and complicated skin and soft-tissue infections, but there is no experience of its use in pneumonia caused by meticillin-resistant *S. aureus*.

Cephalosporins

- INTERACTIONS → Appendix 1 (cephalosporins).

- SIDE-EFFECTS
▶ **Rare** Antibiotic-associated colitis
▶ **Frequency not known** Abdominal discomfort · agranulocytosis · allergic reactions · anaphylaxis · aplastic anaemia · blood disorders · confusion · diarrhoea · disturbances in liver enzymes · dizziness · eosinophilia · haemolytic anaemia · hallucinations · headache · hyperactivity · hypertonia · leucopenia · nausea · nervousness · pruritus · rashes · reversible interstitial nephritis · serum sickness-like reactions with rashes, fever and arthralgia · sleep disturbances · Stevens-Johnson syndrome · thrombocytopenia · toxic epidermal necrolysis · transient cholestatic jaundice · transient hepatitis · urticaria · vomiting

SIDE-EFFECTS, FURTHER INFORMATION
▶ Antibiotic-associated colitis Antibiotic-associated colitis may occur more commonly with second- and third-generation cephalosporins.

- ALLERGY AND CROSS-SENSITIVITY Contra-indicated in patients with cephalosporin hypersensitivity.
▶ Cross-sensitivity with other beta-lactam antibacterials About 0.5–6.5% of penicillin-sensitive patients will also be allergic to the cephalosporins. Patients with a history of **immediate hypersensitivity** to penicillin and other beta-lactams should not receive a cephalosporin. Cephalosporins should be used with caution in patients with sensitivity to penicillin and other beta-lactams.

- EFFECT ON LABORATORY TESTS False positive urinary glucose (if tested for reducing substances). False positive Coombs' test.

ANTIBACTERIALS > CEPHALOSPORINS, FIRST-GENERATION

◤ above

Cefadroxil

- INDICATIONS AND DOSE

Susceptible infections due to sensitive Gram-positive and Gram-negative bacteria
▶ BY MOUTH
▶ Child 6–17 years (body-weight up to 40 kg): 0.5 g twice daily
▶ Child 6–17 years (body-weight 40 kg and above): 0.5–1 g twice daily
▶ Adult: 0.5–1 g twice daily

Skin infections | Soft-tissue infections | Uncomplicated urinary-tract infections
▶ BY MOUTH
▶ Child 6–17 years (body-weight 40 kg and above): 1 g once daily
▶ Adult: 1 g daily

- PREGNANCY Not known to be harmful.

- BREAST FEEDING Present in milk in low concentration, but appropriate to use.

- RENAL IMPAIRMENT
▶ In adults 1 g initially, then 500 mg every 12 hours if eGFR 26–50 mL/minute/1.73 m². 1 g initially, then 500 mg every 24 hours if eGFR 11–26 mL/minute/1.73 m². 1 g initially, then 500 mg every 36 hours if eGFR less than 11 mL/minute/1.73 m².
▶ In children Reduce dose if estimated glomerular filtration rate less than 50 mL/minute/1.73 m².

- MEDICINAL FORMS
There can be variation in the licensing of different medicines containing the same drug.
Capsule
CAUTIONARY AND ADVISORY LABELS 9
▶ Cefadroxil (Non-proprietary)
Cefadroxil (as Cefadroxil monohydrate) 500 mg Cefadroxil 500mg capsules | 20 capsule [PoM] £22.38 DT price = £22.38 | 100 capsule [PoM] £111.90

◤ above

Cefalexin

(Cephalexin)

- INDICATIONS AND DOSE

Susceptible infections due to sensitive Gram-positive and Gram-negative bacteria
▶ BY MOUTH
▶ Child 1–11 months: 12.5 mg/kg twice daily, alternatively 125 mg twice daily
▶ Child 1–4 years: 12.5 mg/kg twice daily, alternatively 125 mg 3 times a day
▶ Child 5–11 years: 12.5 mg/kg twice daily, alternatively 250 mg 3 times a day
▶ Child 12–17 years: 500 mg 2–3 times a day
▶ Adult: 250 mg every 6 hours, alternatively 500 mg every 8–12 hours; increased to 1–1.5 g every 6–8 hours, increased dose to be used for severe infections

Serious susceptible infections due to sensitive Gram-positive and Gram-negative bacteria
▶ BY MOUTH
▶ Child 1 month–11 years: 25 mg/kg 2–4 times a day (max. per dose 1 g 4 times a day)
▶ Child 12–17 years: 1–1.5 g 3–4 times a day

Prophylaxis of recurrent urinary-tract infection
▶ BY MOUTH
▶ Child: 12.5 mg/kg once daily (max. per dose 125 mg), dose to be taken at night
▶ Adult: 125 mg once daily, dose to be taken at night

- PREGNANCY Not known to be harmful.

- BREAST FEEDING Present in milk in low concentration, but appropriate to use.

- RENAL IMPAIRMENT
▶ In adults Max. 3 g daily if eGFR 40–50 mL/minute/1.73 m². Max. 1.5 g daily if eGFR 10–40 mL/minute/1.73 m². Max. 750 mg daily if eGFR less than 10 mL/minute/1.73 m².
▶ In children Reduce dose in moderate impairment.

- PATIENT AND CARER ADVICE
Medicines for Children leaflet: Cefalexin for bacterial infections www.medicinesforchildren.org.uk/cefalexin-bacterial-infections-0

- **PROFESSION SPECIFIC INFORMATION**

Dental practitioners' formulary
Cefalexin Capsules may be prescribed. Cefalexin Tablets may be prescribed. Cefalexin Oral Suspension may be prescribed.

- **MEDICINAL FORMS**
There can be variation in the licensing of different medicines containing the same drug.

Tablet
CAUTIONARY AND ADVISORY LABELS 9
▸ Cefalexin (Non-proprietary)
Cefalexin 250 mg Cefalexin 250mg tablets | 28 tablet PoM £5.02 DT price = £1.95 | 100 tablet PoM £4.93
Cefalexin 500 mg Cefalexin 500mg tablets | 21 tablet PoM £5.88 DT price = £1.98
▸ Ceporex (Co-Pharma Ltd)
Cefalexin 250 mg Ceporex 250mg tablets | 28 tablet PoM £4.02 DT price = £1.95 | 100 tablet PoM £13.74
Cefalexin 500 mg Ceporex 500mg tablets | 28 tablet PoM £7.85 | 100 tablet PoM £26.90
▸ Keflex (Flynn Pharma Ltd)
Cefalexin 250 mg Keflex 250mg tablets | 28 tablet PoM £1.60 DT price = £1.95
Cefalexin 500 mg Keflex 500mg tablets | 21 tablet PoM £2.08 DT price = £1.98

Capsule
CAUTIONARY AND ADVISORY LABELS 9
▸ Cefalexin (Non-proprietary)
Cefalexin 250 mg Cefalexin 250mg capsules | 28 capsule PoM £4.01 DT price = £1.22 | 100 capsule PoM £5.01
Cefalexin 500 mg Cefalexin 500mg capsules | 21 capsule PoM £5.88 DT price = £1.40 | 100 capsule PoM £9.43
▸ Ceporex (Co-Pharma Ltd)
Cefalexin 250 mg Ceporex 250mg capsules | 28 capsule PoM £4.02 DT price = £1.22 | 100 capsule PoM £13.74
Cefalexin 500 mg Ceporex 500mg capsules | 28 capsule PoM £7.85 | 100 capsule PoM £26.90
▸ Keflex (Flynn Pharma Ltd)
Cefalexin 250 mg Keflex 250mg capsules | 28 capsule PoM £1.46 DT price = £1.22
Cefalexin 500 mg Keflex 500mg capsules | 21 capsule PoM £1.98 DT price = £1.40

Oral suspension
CAUTIONARY AND ADVISORY LABELS 9
▸ Cefalexin (Non-proprietary)
Cefalexin 25 mg per 1 ml Cefalexin 125mg/5ml oral suspension sugar free sugar-free | 100 ml PoM no price available Cefalexin 125mg/5ml oral suspension | 100 ml PoM £4.90 DT price = £2.03
Cefalexin 50 mg per 1 ml Cefalexin 250mg/5ml oral suspension sugar free sugar-free | 100 ml PoM no price available Cefalexin 250mg/5ml oral suspension | 100 ml PoM £5.25 DT price = £1.75
Cefalexin 100 mg per 1 ml Cefalexin 500mg/5ml oral suspension | 100 ml PoM no price available
▸ Ceporex (Co-Pharma Ltd)
Cefalexin 25 mg per 1 ml Ceporex 125mg/5ml syrup | 100 ml PoM £1.43 DT price = £2.03
Cefalexin 50 mg per 1 ml Ceporex 250mg/5ml syrup | 100 ml PoM £2.87 DT price = £1.75
Cefalexin 100 mg per 1 ml Ceporex 500mg/5ml syrup | 100 ml PoM £5.57
▸ Keflex (Flynn Pharma Ltd)
Cefalexin 25 mg per 1 ml Keflex 125mg/5ml oral suspension | 100 ml PoM £0.84 DT price = £2.03
Cefalexin 50 mg per 1 ml Keflex 250mg/5ml oral suspension | 100 ml PoM £1.40 DT price = £1.75

◤ 476

Cefradine
(Cephradine)

- **INDICATIONS AND DOSE**

Susceptible infections due to sensitive Gram-positive and Gram-negative bacteria | Surgical prophylaxis
▸ BY MOUTH
▸ Child 7–11 years: 25–50 mg/kg daily in 2–4 divided doses
▸ Child 12–17 years: 250–500 mg 4 times a day, alternatively 0.5–1 g twice daily; increased if necessary up to 1 g 4 times a day, increased dose may be used in severe infections
▸ Adult: 250–500 mg 4 times a day, alternatively 0.5–1 g twice daily; increased if necessary up to 1 g 4 times a day, increased dose may be used in severe infections

- **UNLICENSED USE** Not licensed for use in children for prevention of *Staphylococcus aureus* lung infection in cystic fibrosis.
- **PREGNANCY** Not known to be harmful.
- **BREAST FEEDING** Present in milk in low concentration, but appropriate to use.
- **RENAL IMPAIRMENT**
▸ In adults Use half normal dose if eGFR 5–20 mL/minute/1.73 m². Use one-quarter normal dose if eGFR less than 5 mL/minute/1.73 m².
▸ In children Reduce dose if estimated glomerular filtration rate less than 20 mL/minute/1.73 m².
- **PROFESSION SPECIFIC INFORMATION**

Dental practitioners' formulary
Cefradine Capsules may be prescribed.

- **MEDICINAL FORMS**
There can be variation in the licensing of different medicines containing the same drug.

Capsule
CAUTIONARY AND ADVISORY LABELS 9
▸ Cefradine (Non-proprietary)
Cefradine 250 mg Cefradine 250mg capsules | 20 capsule PoM £6.00 DT price = £1.83 | 100 capsule PoM no price available
Cefradine 500 mg Cefradine 500mg capsules | 20 capsule PoM £8.75 DT price = £2.70 | 100 capsule PoM no price available
▸ Nicef (Co-Pharma Ltd)
Cefradine 250 mg Nicef 250mg capsules | 20 capsule PoM £3.55 DT price = £1.83 | 100 capsule PoM £9.39
Cefradine 500 mg Nicef 500mg capsules | 20 capsule PoM £5.58 DT price = £2.70 | 100 capsule PoM £33.72

ANTIBACTERIALS ❯ CEPHALOSPORINS, SECOND-GENERATION

◤ 476

Cefaclor

- **INDICATIONS AND DOSE**

Susceptible infections due to sensitive Gram-positive and Gram-negative bacteria
▸ BY MOUTH USING IMMEDIATE-RELEASE MEDICINES
▸ Child 1–11 months: 20 mg/kg daily in 3 divided doses, alternatively 62.5 mg 3 times a day
▸ Child 1–4 years: 20 mg/kg daily in 3 divided doses, alternatively 125 mg 3 times a day
▸ Child 5–11 years: 20 mg/kg daily in 3 divided doses, usual max. 1 g daily, alternatively 250 mg 3 times a day
▸ Child 12–17 years: 250 mg 3 times a day; maximum 4 g per day
▸ Adult: 250 mg 3 times a day; maximum 4 g per day
▸ BY MOUTH USING MODIFIED-RELEASE MEDICINES
▸ Child 12–17 years: 375 mg every 12 hours, dose to be taken with food

continued →

▸ **Adult:** 375 mg every 12 hours, dose to be taken with food

Severe susceptible infections due to sensitive Gram-positive and Gram-negative bacteria
▸ BY MOUTH USING IMMEDIATE-RELEASE MEDICINES
▸ **Child 1–11 months:** 40 mg/kg daily in 3 divided doses, usual max. 1 g daily, alternatively 125 mg 3 times a day
▸ **Child 1–4 years:** 40 mg/kg daily in 3 divided doses, usual max. 1 g daily, alternatively 250 mg 3 times a day
▸ **Child 5–11 years:** 40 mg/kg daily in 3 divided doses, usual max. 1 g daily
▸ **Child 12–17 years:** 500 mg 3 times a day; maximum 4 g per day
▸ **Adult:** 500 mg 3 times a day; maximum 4 g per day

Pneumonia
▸ BY MOUTH USING MODIFIED-RELEASE TABLETS
▸ **Child 12–17 years:** 750 mg every 12 hours, dose to be taken with food
▸ **Adult:** 750 mg every 12 hours, dose to be taken with food

Lower urinary-tract infections
▸ BY MOUTH USING MODIFIED-RELEASE MEDICINES
▸ **Child 12–17 years:** 375 mg every 12 hours, dose to be taken with food
▸ **Adult:** 375 mg every 12 hours, dose to be taken with food

Asymptomatic carriage of *Haemophilus influenzae* **or mild exacerbations in cystic fibrosis**
▸ BY MOUTH USING IMMEDIATE-RELEASE MEDICINES
▸ **Child 1–11 months:** 125 mg every 8 hours
▸ **Child 1–6 years:** 250 mg 3 times a day
▸ **Child 7–17 years:** 500 mg 3 times a day

● SIDE-EFFECTS
SIDE-EFFECTS, FURTHER INFORMATION
▸ Skin reactions Cefaclor is associated with protracted skin reactions, especially in children.
● PREGNANCY Not known to be harmful.
● BREAST FEEDING Present in milk in low concentration, but appropriate to use.
● RENAL IMPAIRMENT No dose adjustment required. Manufacturer advises caution.

● MEDICINAL FORMS
There can be variation in the licensing of different medicines containing the same drug.
Modified-release tablet
CAUTIONARY AND ADVISORY LABELS 9, 21, 25
▸ Distaclor MR (Flynn Pharma Ltd)
 Cefaclor (as Cefaclor monohydrate) 375 mg Distaclor MR 375mg tablets | 14 tablet [PoM] £9.10 DT price = £9.10
Capsule
CAUTIONARY AND ADVISORY LABELS 9
▸ Cefaclor (Non-proprietary)
 Cefaclor (as Cefaclor monohydrate) 250 mg Cefaclor 250mg capsules | 21 capsule [PoM] no price available DT price = £6.80
 Cefaclor (as Cefaclor monohydrate) 500 mg Cefaclor 500mg capsules | 50 capsule [PoM] no price available
▸ Distaclor (Flynn Pharma Ltd)
 Cefaclor (as Cefaclor monohydrate) 500 mg Distaclor 500mg capsules | 21 capsule [PoM] £7.50 DT price = £7.50
▸ Keftid (Co-Pharma Ltd)
 Cefaclor (as Cefaclor monohydrate) 250 mg Keftid 250mg capsules | 21 capsule [PoM] £6.80 DT price = £6.80
 Cefaclor (as Cefaclor monohydrate) 500 mg Keftid 500mg capsules | 50 capsule [PoM] £31.99
Oral suspension
CAUTIONARY AND ADVISORY LABELS 9
▸ Cefaclor (Non-proprietary)
 Cefaclor (as Cefaclor monohydrate) 25 mg per 1 ml Cefaclor 125mg/5ml oral suspension sugar free sugar-free | 100 ml [PoM] £5.16 DT price = £5.16

Cefaclor 125mg/5ml oral suspension | 100 ml [PoM] no price available
 Cefaclor (as Cefaclor monohydrate) 50 mg per 1 ml Cefaclor 250mg/5ml oral suspension | 100 ml [PoM] no price available
▸ Distaclor (Flynn Pharma Ltd)
 Cefaclor (as Cefaclor monohydrate) 25 mg per 1 ml Distaclor 125mg/5ml oral suspension | 100 ml [PoM] £4.13
 Cefaclor (as Cefaclor monohydrate) 50 mg per 1 ml Distaclor 250mg/5ml oral suspension | 100 ml [PoM] £8.26
▸ Keftid (Co-Pharma Ltd)
 Cefaclor (as Cefaclor monohydrate) 25 mg per 1 ml Keftid 125mg/5ml oral suspension sugar-free | 100 ml [PoM] £5.16 DT price = £5.16
 Cefaclor (as Cefaclor monohydrate) 50 mg per 1 ml Keftid 250mg/5ml oral suspension sugar-free | 100 ml [PoM] £10.32 DT price = £10.32

◤ 476

Cefuroxime

● INDICATIONS AND DOSE

Susceptible infections due to Gram-positive and Gram-negative bacteria
▸ BY MOUTH
▸ **Child 3 months–1 year:** 10 mg/kg twice daily (max. per dose 125 mg)
▸ **Child 2–11 years:** 15 mg/kg twice daily (max. per dose 250 mg)
▸ **Child 12–17 years:** 250 mg twice daily, dose may be doubled in severe lower respiratory-tract infections or if pneumonia is suspected
▸ **Adult:** 250 mg twice daily, dose may be doubled in severe lower respiratory-tract infections or if pneumonia is suspected
▸ BY INTRAVENOUS INFUSION, OR BY INTRAVENOUS INJECTION, OR BY INTRAMUSCULAR INJECTION
▸ **Child:** 20 mg/kg every 8 hours (max. per dose 750 mg); increased to 50–60 mg/kg every 6–8 hours (max. per dose 1.5 g), increased dose used for severe infection and cystic fibrosis
▸ **Adult:** 750 mg every 6–8 hours; increased if necessary up to 1.5 g every 6–8 hours, increased dose used for severe infections

Lyme disease
▸ BY MOUTH
▸ **Adult:** 500 mg twice daily for 14–21 days (for 28 days in Lyme arthritis)

Lower urinary-tract infection
▸ BY MOUTH
▸ **Child 12–17 years:** 125 mg twice daily
▸ **Adult:** 125 mg twice daily

Pyelonephritis
▸ BY MOUTH
▸ **Adult:** 250 mg twice daily

Surgical prophylaxis
▸ INITIALLY BY INTRAVENOUS INJECTION
▸ **Adult:** 1.5 g, to be administered up to 30 minutes before the procedure, then (by intravenous injection or by intramuscular injection) 750 mg every 8 hours if required for up to 3 doses (in high risk procedures)

Open fractures, prophylaxis
▸ BY INTRAVENOUS INFUSION, OR BY INTRAVENOUS INJECTION
▸ **Adult:** 1.5 g every 8 hours until soft tissue closure (maximum duration 72 hours)

● UNLICENSED USE Duration of treatment in Lyme disease is unlicensed.
● PREGNANCY Not known to be harmful.
● BREAST FEEDING Present in milk in low concentration, but appropriate to use.

- RENAL IMPAIRMENT
▸ In adults Use parenteral dose of 750 mg twice daily if eGFR 10–20 mL/minute/1.73 m². Use parenteral dose of 750 mg once daily if eGFR less than 10 mL/minute/1.73 m².
▸ In children Reduce parenteral dose if estimated glomerular filtration rate less than 20 mL/minute/1.73 m².
- DIRECTIONS FOR ADMINISTRATION Single doses over 750 mg should be administered by the intravenous route only.
▸ With intravenous use in children Displacement value may be significant when reconstituting injection, consult local guidelines. For intermittent intravenous infusion, dilute reconstituted solution further in glucose 5% or sodium chloride 0.9%; give over 30 minutes.
▸ With intravenous use in adults For *intravenous infusion* (*Zinacef*®), give intermittently or via drip tubing in *Glucose* 5% or Sodium chloride 0.9%. Dissolve initially in water for injections (at least 2 mL for each 250 mg, 15 mL for 1.5 g); suggested volume 50–100 mL given over 30 minutes.

- MEDICINAL FORMS
There can be variation in the licensing of different medicines containing the same drug. Forms available from special-order manufacturers include: solution for injection, infusion

Tablet
CAUTIONARY AND ADVISORY LABELS 9, 21, 25
▸ Cefuroxime (Non-proprietary)
  Cefuroxime (as Cefuroxime axetil) 250 mg Cefuroxime 250mg tablets | 14 tablet PoM £17.72 DT price = £17.72
▸ Zinnat (GlaxoSmithKline UK Ltd)
  Cefuroxime (as Cefuroxime axetil) 125 mg Zinnat 125mg tablets | 14 tablet PoM £4.56 DT price = £4.56
  Cefuroxime (as Cefuroxime axetil) 250 mg Zinnat 250mg tablets | 14 tablet PoM £9.11 DT price = £17.72

Oral suspension
CAUTIONARY AND ADVISORY LABELS 9, 21
EXCIPIENTS: May contain Aspartame, sucrose
▸ Zinnat (GlaxoSmithKline UK Ltd)
  Cefuroxime (as Cefuroxime axetil) 25 mg per 1 ml Zinnat 125mg/5ml oral suspension | 70 ml PoM £5.20

Powder for injection
ELECTROLYTES: May contain Sodium
▸ Cefuroxime (Non-proprietary)
  Cefuroxime (as Cefuroxime sodium) 250 mg Cefuroxime 250mg powder for injection vials | 10 vial PoM £9.25
  Cefuroxime (as Cefuroxime sodium) 750 mg Cefuroxime 750mg powder for injection vials | 1 vial PoM £2.52 | 10 vial PoM £25.20
  Cefuroxime (as Cefuroxime sodium) 1.5 gram Cefuroxime 1.5g powder for injection vials | 1 vial PoM £5.05 | 10 vial PoM £50.50
▸ Zinacef (GlaxoSmithKline UK Ltd)
  Cefuroxime (as Cefuroxime sodium) 250 mg Zinacef 250mg powder for injection vials | 5 vial PoM £4.70
  Cefuroxime (as Cefuroxime sodium) 750 mg Zinacef 750mg powder for injection vials | 5 vial PoM £11.72 (Hospital only)
  Cefuroxime (as Cefuroxime sodium) 1.5 gram Zinacef 1.5g powder for injection vials | 1 vial PoM £4.70

ANTIBACTERIALS > CEPHALOSPORINS, THIRD-GENERATION

F 476

Cefixime

- INDICATIONS AND DOSE

Acute infections due to sensitive Gram-positive and Gram-negative bacteria
▸ BY MOUTH
▸ Child 6-11 months: 75 mg daily
▸ Child 1-4 years: 100 mg daily
▸ Child 5-9 years: 200 mg daily
▸ Child 10-17 years: 200–400 mg daily, alternatively 100–200 mg twice daily
▸ Adult: 200–400 mg daily in 1–2 divided doses

Uncomplicated gonorrhoea
▸ BY MOUTH
▸ Adult: 400 mg for 1 dose

- UNLICENSED USE Use of cefixime for uncomplicated gonorrhoea is an unlicensed indication.
- PREGNANCY Not known to be harmful.
- BREAST FEEDING Manufacturer advises avoid unless essential—no information available.
- RENAL IMPAIRMENT
▸ In adults Reduce dose if eGFR less than 20 mL/minute/1.73 m² (max. 200 mg once daily).
▸ In children Reduce dose if estimated glomerular filtration rate less than 20 mL/minute/1.73 m².

- MEDICINAL FORMS
There can be variation in the licensing of different medicines containing the same drug.
Tablet
CAUTIONARY AND ADVISORY LABELS 9
▸ Suprax (Sanofi)
  Cefixime 200 mg Suprax 200mg tablets | 7 tablet PoM £13.23 DT price = £13.23

F 476

Cefotaxime

- INDICATIONS AND DOSE

Uncomplicated gonorrhoea
▸ BY INTRAMUSCULAR INJECTION
▸ Adult: 500 mg for 1 dose

Infections due to sensitive Gram-positive and Gram-negative bacteria | Surgical prophylaxis | Haemophilus epiglottitis
▸ BY INTRAMUSCULAR INJECTION, OR BY INTRAVENOUS INJECTION, OR BY INTRAVENOUS INFUSION
▸ Adult: 1 g every 12 hours

Severe susceptible infections due to sensitive Gram-positive and Gram-negative bacteria | Meningitis
▸ BY INTRAMUSCULAR INJECTION, OR BY INTRAVENOUS INJECTION, OR BY INTRAVENOUS INFUSION
▸ Adult: 8 g daily in 4 divided doses, increased if necessary to 12 g daily in 3–4 divided doses, intramuscular doses over 1 g should be divided between more than one site

Emergency treatment of suspected bacterial meningitis or meningococcal disease, before urgent transfer to hospital, in patients who cannot be given benzylpenicillin (e.g. because of an allergy)
▸ BY INTRAVENOUS INJECTION, OR BY INTRAMUSCULAR INJECTION
▸ Child 1 month-11 years: 50 mg/kg for 1 dose
▸ Child 12-17 years: 1 g for 1 dose
▸ Adult: 1 g for 1 dose

- SIDE-EFFECTS
▸ **Rare** Arrhythmias (following rapid injection)
- PREGNANCY Not known to be harmful.
- BREAST FEEDING Present in milk in low concentration, but appropriate to use.
- RENAL IMPAIRMENT
▸ In adults If eGFR less than 5 mL/minute/1.73 m², initial dose of 1 g then use half normal dose.
▸ In children Usual initial dose, then use half normal dose if estimated glomerular filtration rate less than 5 mL/minute/1.73 m².
- DIRECTIONS FOR ADMINISTRATION
▸ With intravenous use in children Displacement value may be significant, consult local guidelines. For intermittent *intravenous infusion* dilute in glucose 5% *or* sodium

5

Infection

chloride 0.9%; administer over 20–60 minutes; incompatible with alkaline solutions.

▸ With intravenous use in adults For *intravenous infusion*, give intermittently *in* Glucose 5% *or* Sodium chloride 0.9%. Suggested volume 40–100 mL given over 20–60 minutes; incompatible with alkaline solutions.

● MEDICINAL FORMS
There can be variation in the licensing of different medicines containing the same drug.
Powder for solution for injection

▸ Cefotaxime (Non-proprietary)
Cefotaxime (as Cefotaxime sodium) 500 mg Cefotaxime 500mg powder for solution for injection vials | 1 vial [PoM] £1.50 | 10 vial [PoM] £25.50-£30.00
Cefotaxime (as Cefotaxime sodium) 1 gram Cefotaxime 1g powder for solution for injection vials | 1 vial [PoM] £3.00 | 10 vial [PoM] £35.00
Cefotaxime (as Cefotaxime sodium) 2 gram Cefotaxime 2g powder for solution for injection vials | 1 vial [PoM] £8.00 | 10 vial [PoM] £37.50

▪ 476

Ceftazidime

● INDICATIONS AND DOSE

Prophylaxis for transurethral resection of prostate
▸ BY INTRAVENOUS INJECTION, OR BY INTRAVENOUS INFUSION, OR BY DEEP INTRAMUSCULAR INJECTION
▸ Adult: 1 g, single dose to be administered up to 30 minutes before procedure and may be repeated if necessary when catheter removed

Pseudomonal lung infection in cystic fibrosis
▸ BY INTRAVENOUS INFUSION, OR BY INTRAVENOUS INJECTION, OR BY DEEP INTRAMUSCULAR INJECTION
▸ Adult: 100–150 mg/kg daily in 3 divided doses; maximum 9 g per day

Complicated urinary-tract infection
▸ BY INTRAVENOUS INJECTION, OR BY INTRAVENOUS INFUSION, OR BY DEEP INTRAMUSCULAR INJECTION
▸ Adult 18-79 years: 1–2 g every 8–12 hours
▸ Adult 80 years and over: 1–2 g every 8–12 hours; maximum 3 g per day

Septicaemia | Hospital-acquired pneumonia
▸ BY INTRAVENOUS INFUSION, OR BY INTRAVENOUS INJECTION, OR BY DEEP INTRAMUSCULAR INJECTION
▸ Adult 18-79 years: 2 g every 8 hours
▸ Adult 80 years and over: 2 g every 8 hours; maximum 3 g per day

Febrile neutropenia
▸ BY INTRAVENOUS INFUSION, OR BY INTRAVENOUS INJECTION, OR BY DEEP INTRAMUSCULAR INJECTION
▸ Adult 18-79 years: 2 g every 8 hours
▸ Adult 80 years and over: 2 g every 8 hours; maximum 3 g per day

Meningitis
▸ BY INTRAVENOUS INFUSION, OR BY INTRAVENOUS INJECTION, OR BY DEEP INTRAMUSCULAR INJECTION
▸ Adult 18-79 years: 2 g every 8 hours
▸ Adult 80 years and over: 2 g every 8 hours; maximum 3 g per day

Susceptible infections due to sensitive Gram-positive and Gram-negative bacteria
▸ BY INTRAVENOUS INFUSION, OR BY INTRAVENOUS INJECTION, OR BY DEEP INTRAMUSCULAR INJECTION
▸ Adult 18-79 years: 1–2 g every 8 hours
▸ Adult 80 years and over: 1–2 g every 8 hours; maximum 3 g per day

● SIDE-EFFECTS Paraesthesia · taste disturbances
● PREGNANCY Not known to be harmful.

● BREAST FEEDING Present in milk in low concentration, but appropriate to use.
● HEPATIC IMPAIRMENT Manufacturer advises caution in severe impairment.
● RENAL IMPAIRMENT Reduce dose if eGFR less than 50 mL/minute/1.73 m^2—consult product literature.
● DIRECTIONS FOR ADMINISTRATION Intramuscular administration used when intravenous administration not possible; single doses over 1 g by intravenous route only.
▸ With intravenous use For *intravenous infusion* give intermittently *or via* drip tubing *in* Glucose 5% or 10% *or* Sodium chloride 0.9%. Dissolve 2 g initially in 10 mL (3 g in 15 mL) infusion fluid. For *Fortum*® dilute further to a concentration of 40 mg/mL. For *Kefadim*® dilute further to a concentration of 20 mg/mL. Give over up to 30 minutes.

● MEDICINAL FORMS
There can be variation in the licensing of different medicines containing the same drug. Forms available from special-order manufacturers include: infusion, solution for infusion
Powder for solution for injection
ELECTROLYTES: May contain Sodium

▸ Ceftazidime (Non-proprietary)
Ceftazidime (as Ceftazidime pentahydrate) 500 mg Ceftazidime 500mg powder for solution for injection vials | 1 vial [PoM] £4.70
Ceftazidime (as Ceftazidime pentahydrate) 1 gram Ceftazidime 1g powder for solution for injection vials | 1 vial [PoM] £11.40 | 5 vial [PoM] £39.55 | 10 vial [PoM] £13.90
Ceftazidime (as Ceftazidime pentahydrate) 2 gram Ceftazidime 2g powder for solution for injection vials | 1 vial [PoM] £22.10 | 5 vial [PoM] £79.15 | 10 vial [PoM] £27.70
▸ Fortum (GlaxoSmithKline UK Ltd)
Ceftazidime (as Ceftazidime pentahydrate) 500 mg Fortum 500mg powder for solution for injection vials | 1 vial [PoM] £4.40 (Hospital only)
Ceftazidime (as Ceftazidime pentahydrate) 1 gram Fortum 1g powder for solution for injection vials | 1 vial [PoM] £8.79 (Hospital only)
Ceftazidime (as Ceftazidime pentahydrate) 2 gram Fortum 2g powder for solution for injection vials | 1 vial [PoM] £17.59 (Hospital only)
Ceftazidime (as Ceftazidime pentahydrate) 3 gram Fortum 3g powder for solution for injection vials | 1 vial [PoM] £25.76 (Hospital only)

▪ 476

Ceftriaxone

15.6.2016

● INDICATIONS AND DOSE

Community-acquired pneumonia | Hospital-acquired pneumonia | Intra-abdominal infections | Complicated urinary-tract infections | Acute exacerbations of chronic obstructive pulmonary disease
▸ BY INTRAVENOUS INFUSION, OR BY INTRAVENOUS INJECTION, OR BY DEEP INTRAMUSCULAR INJECTION
▸ Adult: 1–2 g once daily, 2 g dose to be used for hospital-acquired pneumonia and severe cases

Complicated skin and soft tissue infections | Infections of bones and joints
▸ BY INTRAVENOUS INFUSION, OR BY INTRAVENOUS INJECTION, OR BY DEEP INTRAMUSCULAR INJECTION
▸ Adult: 2 g once daily

Suspected bacterial infection in neutropenic patients
▸ BY INTRAVENOUS INFUSION, OR BY INTRAVENOUS INJECTION, OR BY DEEP INTRAMUSCULAR INJECTION
▸ Adult: 2–4 g once daily, doses at the higher end of the recommended range used in severe cases

Bacterial meningitis | Bacterial endocarditis
▸ BY INTRAVENOUS INFUSION, OR BY INTRAVENOUS INJECTION, OR BY DEEP INTRAMUSCULAR INJECTION
▸ Adult: 2–4 g once daily, doses at the higher end of the recommended range used in severe cases

▸ BY INTRAVENOUS INFUSION
▸ Child 1 month–11 years (body-weight up to 50 kg): 80–100 mg/kg once daily, 100 mg/kg once daily dose should be used for bacterial endocarditis; maximum 4 g per day
▸ Child 9–11 years (body-weight 50 kg and above): 2–4 g once daily, doses at the higher end of the recommended range used in severe cases
▸ Child 12–17 years: 2–4 g once daily, doses at the higher end of the recommended range used in severe cases
▸ BY INTRAVENOUS INJECTION
▸ Child 9–11 years (body-weight 50 kg and above): 2–4 g once daily, doses at the higher end of the recommended range used in severe cases
▸ Child 12–17 years: 2–4 g once daily, doses at the higher end of the recommended range used in severe cases
▸ BY DEEP INTRAMUSCULAR INJECTION
▸ Child 1 month–11 years (body-weight up to 50 kg): 80–100 mg/kg once daily, 100 mg/kg once daily dose should be used for bacterial endocarditis; maximum 4 g per day
▸ Child 9–11 years (body-weight 50 kg and above): 2–4 g once daily, doses at the higher end of the recommended range used in severe cases
▸ Child 12–17 years: 2–4 g once daily, doses at the higher end of the recommended range used in severe cases

Surgical prophylaxis
▸ BY INTRAVENOUS INFUSION, OR BY INTRAVENOUS INJECTION, OR BY DEEP INTRAMUSCULAR INJECTION
▸ Adult: 2 g for 1 dose, dose to be administered 30–90 minutes before procedure

Uncomplicated gonorrhoea | Pelvic inflammatory disease
▸ BY DEEP INTRAMUSCULAR INJECTION
▸ Adult: 500 mg for 1 dose

Syphilis
▸ BY INTRAVENOUS INFUSION, OR BY INTRAVENOUS INJECTION, OR BY DEEP INTRAMUSCULAR INJECTION
▸ Adult: 0.5–1 g once daily for 10–14 days, dose can be increased to 2 g once daily for neurosyphilis

Disseminated Lyme borreliosis (early [Stage II] and late [Stage III])
▸ BY INTRAVENOUS INFUSION, OR BY INTRAVENOUS INJECTION, OR BY DEEP INTRAMUSCULAR INJECTION
▸ Adult: 2 g once daily for 14–21 days, the recommended treatment durations vary and national or local guidelines should be taken into consideration

Prevention of secondary case of meningococcal meningitis
▸ BY INTRAMUSCULAR INJECTION
▸ Adult: 250 mg for 1 dose

Prevention of secondary case of *Haemophilus influenzae* type b disease
▸ BY INTRAMUSCULAR INJECTION, OR BY INTRAVENOUS INJECTION
▸ Adult: 1 g daily for 2 days

Acute otitis media
▸ BY INTRAMUSCULAR INJECTION
▸ Adult: 1–2 g for 1 dose, dose can be given for 3 days if severely ill or previous therapy failed

● UNLICENSED USE [EvGr] Not licensed for prophylaxis of *Haemophilus influenzae* type b disease. ⟨E⟩ Not licensed for prophylaxis of meningococcal meningitis.
▸ In children [EvGr] Not licensed for congenital gonococcal conjunctivitis. Not licensed for use in children under 12 years of age for uncomplicated gonorrhoea. Not licensed for use in children for pelvic inflammatory disease. ⟨E⟩
[EvGr] Dose not licensed for treatment of pelvic inflammatory disease in adults over 18 years. ⟨A⟩

● CONTRA-INDICATIONS Concomitant treatment with intravenous calcium (including total parenteral nutrition containing calcium) in neonates over 41 weeks corrected gestational age—risk of precipitation in urine and lungs (in neonates) · neonates less than 41 weeks corrected gestational age · neonates over 41 weeks corrected gestational age with jaundice, hypoalbuminaemia, acidosis, unconjugated hyperbilirubinaemia, or impaired bilirubin binding

● CAUTIONS
GENERAL CAUTIONS
History of hypercalciuria · history of kidney stones · use with caution in neonates
SPECIFIC CAUTIONS
▸ With intravenous use Concomitant treatment with intravenous calcium (including total parenteral nutrition containing calcium) (in adults)

● SIDE-EFFECTS
▸ **Common or very common** Calcium ceftriaxone precipitates in gall bladder—consider discontinuation if symptomatic · calcium ceftriaxone precipitates in urine (particularly in very young, dehydrated or those who are immobilised)—consider discontinuation if symptomatic
▸ **Rare** Pancreatitis · prolongation of prothrombin time

● PREGNANCY Not known to be harmful.

● BREAST FEEDING Present in milk in low concentration, but appropriate to use.

● HEPATIC IMPAIRMENT Reduce dose if both hepatic and severe renal impairment. Monitor plasma concentration if both hepatic and severe renal impairment.

● RENAL IMPAIRMENT Monitor plasma concentration if both hepatic and severe renal impairment. Use with caution in renal failure.
▸ In adults Reduce dose if eGFR less than 10 mL/minute/1.73 m^2 (max. 2 g daily).
▸ In children Max. 50 mg/kg daily (max. 2 g daily) in severe renal impairment.

● DIRECTIONS FOR ADMINISTRATION
▸ With intramuscular use or intravenous use Twice daily dosing may be considered for doses greater than 2 g daily.
▸ With intravenous use in children For *intravenous infusion* (preferred route), dilute reconstituted solution with Glucose 5% (or 10% in neonates) *or* Sodium Chloride 0.9%; give over at least 30 minutes (60 minutes in neonates—may displace bilirubin from serum albumin). Not to be given simultaneously with parenteral nutrition or infusion fluids containing calcium, even by different infusion lines; in children, may be infused sequentially with infusion fluids containing calcium if flush with sodium chloride 0.9% between infusions or give infusions by different infusion lines at different sites. Displacement value may be significant, consult local guidelines. For *intravenous injection*, give over 5 minutes; intravenous doses of 50 mg/kg or more in children under 12 years should be given by infusion.
▸ With intramuscular use in children For *intramuscular injection*, may be mixed with 1% Lidocaine Hydrochloride Injection to reduce pain at intramuscular injection site. Intramuscular injection should only be considered when the intravenous route is not possible or less appropriate. If administered by intramuscular injection, the lower end of the dose range should be used for the shortest time possible; volume depends on the age and size of the child, but doses over 1 g must be divided between more than one site. The maximum intramuscular dose is 2 g, doses greater than 2 g must be given by intravenous infusion or intravenous injection (see above). Displacement value may be significant, consult local guidelines.
▸ With intravenous use in adults For *intravenous infusion* (preferred route) (*Rocephin*®; *Ceftriaxone Injection*, Genus), give intermittently *or via* drip tubing *in* Glucose 5% or 10% *or* Sodium chloride 0.9%. Reconstitute 2-g vial with 40 mL infusion fluid. Give by intermittent infusion over at least

5

Infection

30 minutes. Not to be given simultaneously with total parenteral nutrition or infusion fluids containing calcium, even by different infusion lines. May be infused sequentially with infusion fluids containing calcium if flush with sodium chloride 0.9% between infusions or give infusions by different infusion lines at different sites. For *intravenous injection*, give over 5 minutes.

▸ With intramuscular use in adults For *intramuscular injection*, doses over 1 g must be divided between more than one site. The maximum intramuscular dose is 2 g, doses greater than 2 g must be given by intravenous administration. Displacement value may be significant, consult local guidelines.

● MEDICINAL FORMS
There can be variation in the licensing of different medicines containing the same drug. Forms available from special-order manufacturers include: infusion

Powder for solution for injection
ELECTROLYTES: May contain Sodium
▸ Ceftriaxone (Non-proprietary)
Ceftriaxone (as Ceftriaxone sodium) 250 mg Ceftriaxone 250mg powder for solution for injection vials | 1 vial PoM £1.80–£2.30 DT price = £2.40
Ceftriaxone (as Ceftriaxone sodium) 1 gram Ceftriaxone 1g powder for solution for injection vials | 1 vial PoM no price available DT price = £9.58 | 5 vial PoM £45.75 | 10 vial PoM £11.00
Ceftriaxone (as Ceftriaxone sodium) 2 gram Ceftriaxone 2g powder for solution for injection vials | 1 vial PoM £18.00 DT price = £19.18 | 10 vial PoM £21.00
▸ Rocephin (Roche Products Ltd)
Ceftriaxone (as Ceftriaxone sodium) 250 mg Rocephin 250mg powder for solution for injection vials | 1 vial PoM £2.40 DT price = £2.40
Ceftriaxone (as Ceftriaxone sodium) 1 gram Rocephin 1g powder for solution for injection vials | 1 vial PoM £9.58 DT price = £9.58
Ceftriaxone (as Ceftriaxone sodium) 2 gram Rocephin 2g powder for solution for injection vials | 1 vial PoM £19.18 DT price = £19.18

ANTIBACTERIALS > CEPHALOSPORINS, OTHER

⬧ 476

Ceftaroline fosamil

● INDICATIONS AND DOSE

Community-acquired pneumonia
▸ BY INTRAVENOUS INFUSION
▸ Adult: 600 mg every 12 hours for 5–7 days

Complicated skin infections | Complicated soft-tissue infections
▸ BY INTRAVENOUS INFUSION
▸ Adult: 600 mg every 12 hours for 5–14 days

● CAUTIONS Seizure disorders
● PREGNANCY Manufacturer advises avoid unless essential—no information available.
● BREAST FEEDING Manufacturer advises avoid—no information available.
● RENAL IMPAIRMENT 400 mg every 12 hours if eGFR 30–50 mL/minute/1.73 m². Manufacturer advises avoid if eGFR less than 30 mL/minute/1.73 m².
● DIRECTIONS FOR ADMINISTRATION For *intravenous infusion*, give intermittently *in* Glucose 5% *or* Sodium chloride 0.9%. Reconstitute 600 mg with 20 mL water for injections, then dilute with 250 mL infusion fluid (in fluid restriction, may be diluted with 50–100 mL infusion fluid); give over 60 minutes.
● NATIONAL FUNDING/ACCESS DECISIONS
Scottish Medicines Consortium (SMC) Decisions
The *Scottish Medicines Consortium*, has advised (Dec 2012) that ceftaroline fosamil (*Zinforo*®) is accepted for restricted use within NHS Scotland when meticillin–resistant *S. aureus* is suspected in complicated skin and soft-tissue infection and vancomycin cannot be used.

● MEDICINAL FORMS
There can be variation in the licensing of different medicines containing the same drug.
Powder for solution for infusion
▸ Zinforo (AstraZeneca UK Ltd) ▼
Ceftaroline fosamil (as Ceftaroline fosamil acetic acid solvate monohydrate) 600 mg Zinforo 600mg powder for concentrate for solution for infusion vials | 10 vial PoM £375.00

ANTIBACTERIALS > GLYCOPEPTIDE ANTIBACTERIALS

Teicoplanin

● DRUG ACTION The glycopeptide antibiotic teicoplanin has bactericidal activity against aerobic and anaerobic Gram-positive bacteria including multi-resistant staphylococci. However, there are reports of *Staphylococcus aureus* with reduced susceptibility to glycopeptides and increasing reports of glycopeptide-resistant enterococci. Teicoplanin is similar to vancomycin, but has a significantly longer duration of action, allowing once daily administration after the loading dose.

● INDICATIONS AND DOSE

***Clostridium difficile* infection**
▸ BY MOUTH
▸ Adult: 100–200 mg twice daily for 10–14 days

Serious infections caused by Gram-positive bacteria (e.g. complicated skin and soft-tissue infections, pneumonia)
▸ BY INTRAVENOUS INJECTION, OR BY INTRAVENOUS INFUSION, OR BY INTRAMUSCULAR INJECTION
▸ Adult (body-weight up to 70 kg): Initially 400 mg every 12 hours for 3 doses, followed by 400 mg once daily
▸ Adult (body-weight 70 kg and above): Initially 6 mg/kg every 12 hours for 3 doses, then 6 mg/kg once daily

Streptococcal or enterococcal endocarditis (in combination with another antibacterial)
▸ BY INTRAVENOUS INJECTION, OR BY INTRAVENOUS INFUSION
▸ Adult: Initially 10 mg/kg every 12 hours for 3–5 doses, then 10 mg/kg once daily, subsequent doses can be given by intramuscular injection

Bone and joint infections
▸ BY INTRAVENOUS INFUSION, OR BY INTRAVENOUS INJECTION
▸ Adult: Initially 12 mg/kg every 12 hours for 3–5 doses, then 12 mg/kg once daily subsequent doses can be given by intramuscular injection, increased risk of fever and rash with doses of 12 mg/kg

Surgical prophylaxis
▸ BY INTRAVENOUS INJECTION
▸ Adult: 400 mg, to be administered up to 30 minutes before the procedure

Surgical prophylaxis in open fractures
▸ BY INTRAVENOUS INFUSION
▸ Adult: 800 mg, to be administered up to 30 minutes before skeletal stabilisation and definitive soft-tissue closure

Peritonitis associated with peritoneal dialysis (added to dialysis fluid)
▸ BY INTRAPERITONEAL INFUSION
▸ Adult: (consult local protocol)
PHARMACOKINETICS
Teicoplanin should **not** be given by mouth for systemic infections because it is not absorbed significantly.

● UNLICENSED USE Not licensed for surgical prophylaxis. Teicoplanin doses in BNF may differ from those in product literature.
● INTERACTIONS → Appendix 1 (teicoplanin).
If other nephrotoxic or neurotoxic drugs given, monitor renal and auditory function on prolonged administration.

SIDE-EFFECTS
▶ **Common or very common** Pruritus · rash
▶ **Uncommon** Bronchospasm · diarrhoea · dizziness · eosinophilia · fever · headache · leucopenia · mild hearing loss · nausea · thrombocytopenia · thrombophlebitis · tinnitus · vestibular disorders · vomiting
▶ **Frequency not known** Exfoliative dermatitis · nephrotoxicity · renal failure · Stevens-Johnson syndrome · toxic epidermal necrolysis

SIDE-EFFECTS, FURTHER INFORMATION
▶ Nephrotoxicity Teicoplanin is associated with a lower incidence of nephrotoxicity than vancomycin.

● ALLERGY AND CROSS-SENSITIVITY Caution if history of vancomycin sensitivity.

● PREGNANCY Manufacturer advises use only if potential benefit outweighs risk.

● BREAST FEEDING No information available.

● RENAL IMPAIRMENT Use normal dose regimen on days 1–4, then use normal maintenance dose every 48 hours if eGFR 30–80 mL/minute/1.73 m^2 and use normal maintenance dose every 72 hours if eGFR less than 30 mL/minute/1.73 m^2. Plasma-teicoplanin concentration should be monitored during parenteral maintenance treatment. Also monitor renal and auditory function during prolonged treatment in renal impairment.

● MONITORING REQUIREMENTS
▶ With intramuscular use or intravenous use Plasma-teicoplanin concentration is not measured routinely because a relationship between plasma concentration and toxicity has not been established. However, the plasma-teicoplanin concentration can be used to optimise parenteral treatment in severe sepsis or burns, deep-seated staphylococcal infection (including bone and joint infection), endocarditis and in intravenous drug abusers. Pre-dose ('trough') concentrations should be greater than 15 mg/litre (greater than 20 mg/litre in endocarditis or deep-seated infection such as bone and joint infection), but less than 60 mg/litre.
▶ With intramuscular use or intravenous use Plasma-teicoplanin concentration should be measured in elderly patients.
▶ Blood counts and liver and kidney function tests required.

● DIRECTIONS FOR ADMINISTRATION
▶ With intravenous use For intravenous infusion (*Targocid* ®), give intermittently in Glucose 5% *or* Sodium chloride 0.9%; reconstitute initially with water for injections provided; infuse over 30 minutes. Continuous infusion not usually recommended.
▶ With oral use Injection can be used to prepare solution for oral administration.

● MEDICINAL FORMS
There can be variation in the licensing of different medicines containing the same drug. Forms available from special-order manufacturers include: solution for injection
Powder and solvent for solution for injection
ELECTROLYTES: May contain Sodium
▶ Targocid (Sanofi) ▼
 Teicoplanin 200 mg Targocid 200mg powder and solvent for solution for injection vials | 1 vial PoM £3.93
 Teicoplanin 400 mg Targocid 400mg powder and solvent for solution for injection vials | 1 vial PoM £7.32

Telavancin

● DRUG ACTION Telavancin is a glycopeptide antibacterial; it has bactericidal activity against aerobic and anaerobic Gram-positive bacteria including multi-resistant staphylococci. However, there are reports of *Staphylococcus aureus* with reduced susceptibility to glycopeptides. There are increasing reports of glycopeptide-resistant enterococci.

● INDICATIONS AND DOSE
Hospital-acquired pneumonia, known or suspected to be caused by meticillin-resistant *Staphylococcus aureus* when other antibacterials cannot be used
▶ BY INTRAVENOUS INFUSION
▶ Adult: 10 mg/kg once daily for 7–21 days

● CAUTIONS Conditions that predispose to renal impairment · predisposition to QT interval prolongation (including electrolyte disturbances, congenital long QT syndrome, uncompensated heart failure, severe left ventricular hypertrophy)

● INTERACTIONS → Appendix 1 (telavancin).
Use with caution if concomitant use with nephrotoxic drugs, drugs that prolong the QT interval or potentially ototoxic drugs.

● SIDE-EFFECTS
▶ **Common or very common** Acute renal failure · chills · constipation · diarrhoea · dizziness · fungal infection · headache · insomnia · malaise · nausea · pruritus · rash · taste disturbances · vomiting
▶ **Uncommon** Abdominal pain · agitation · altered sense of smell · angina · antibiotic-associated colitis · anxiety · arthralgia · atrial fibrillation · back pain · blood disorders · blurred vision · bradycardia · confusion · congestive cardiac failure · decreased appetite · depression · dry mouth · dyspepsia · dyspnoea · dysuria · electrolyte disturbances · erythema · eye irritation · flatulence · flushing · haematuria · hepatitis · hiccup · hyperhidrosis · hypertension · hypotension · increased INR · microalbuminuria · myalgia · nasal congestion · oedema · oliguria · oral hypoaesthesia · palpitation · paraesthesia · pharyngolaryngeal pain · phlebitis · pollakiuria · pyrexia · QT interval prolongation · sinus tachycardia · somnolence · supraventricular extrasystoles · tinnitus · tremor · urinary tract infection · urticaria · ventricular extrasystoles
▶ **Rare** Deafness
▶ **Frequency not known** Flushing of the upper body ('red man' syndrome) · non-cardiac chest pain

● ALLERGY AND CROSS-SENSITIVITY Use with caution in patients with vancomycin or teicoplanin sensitivity.

● CONCEPTION AND CONTRACEPTION Effective contraception required during treatment.

● PREGNANCY Avoid (teratogenic in *animal* studies).

● BREAST FEEDING Manufacturer advises avoid unless potential benefit outweighs risk—no information available.

● HEPATIC IMPAIRMENT Manufacturer advises caution in severe impairment—no information available.

● RENAL IMPAIRMENT In chronic renal failure, use 7.5 mg/kg once daily if eGFR 30–50 mL/minute/1.73 m^2. Avoid in acute renal failure—risk of mortality increased. In chronic renal failure, avoid if eGFR less than 30 mL/minute/1.73 m^2.

● MONITORING REQUIREMENTS Monitor renal function daily for at least the first 3–5 days, then every 2–3 days thereafter.

● DIRECTIONS FOR ADMINISTRATION For *intravenous infusion* (*Vibativ* ®). Avoid rapid infusion (can cause 'red man' syndrome). Give intermittently in Glucose 5% *or*

Sodium chloride 0.9%; reconstitute each 750 mg with 45 mL glucose 5%, sodium chloride 0.9%, or water for injections to produce a 15 mg/mL solution; for doses of 150–800 mg, dilute requisite dose in 100 to 250 mL infusion fluid; for doses outside this range, dilute to a final concentration of 0.6–8 mg/mL; give over at least 60 minutes.

● MEDICINAL FORMS
There can be variation in the licensing of different medicines containing the same drug.
Powder for solution for infusion
▸ Vibativ (Clinigen Healthcare Ltd) ▼
  Telavancin (as Telavancin hydrochloride) 750 mg Vibativ 750mg powder for solution for infusion vials | 1 vial PoM £645.00 (Hospital only)

Vancomycin

● DRUG ACTION The glycopeptide antibiotic vancomycin has bactericidal activity against aerobic and anaerobic Gram-positive bacteria including multi-resistant staphylococci. However, there are reports of *Staphylococcus aureus* with reduced susceptibility to glycopeptides. There are increasing reports of glycopeptide-resistant enterococci. Penetration into cerebrospinal fluid is poor.
▸ With intravenous use Vancomycin has a long duration of action and can therefore be given every 12 hours.

● INDICATIONS AND DOSE
Clostridium difficile infection
▸ BY MOUTH
▸ Adult: 125 mg 4 times a day for 10–14 days, dose may be increased if infection fails to respond or is life-threatening, increased if necessary up to 500 mg 4 times a day

Infections due to Gram-positive bacteria including endocarditis, osteomyelitis, septicaemia and soft-tissue infections
▸ BY INTRAVENOUS INFUSION
▸ Adult: 1–1.5 g every 12 hours
▸ Elderly: 500 mg every 12 hours, alternatively 1 g once daily

Surgical prophylaxis (when high risk of MRSA)
▸ BY INTRAVENOUS INFUSION
▸ Adult: 1 g for 1 dose

Peritonitis associated with peritoneal dialysis
▸ BY INTRAPERITONEAL ADMINISTRATION
▸ Adult: (consult local protocol)

PHARMACOKINETICS
Vancomycin should **not** be given by mouth for systemic infections because it is not absorbed significantly.

● UNLICENSED USE Vancomycin doses in BNF publications may differ from those in product literature. Use of vancomycin (added to dialysis fluid) for the treatment of peritonitis associated with peritoneal dialysis is an unlicensed route.

● CAUTIONS
GENERAL CAUTIONS
Avoid if history of deafness · elderly
SPECIFIC CAUTIONS
▸ With oral use Systemic absorption may follow oral administration especially in inflammatory bowel disorders or following multiple doses

● INTERACTIONS → Appendix 1 (vancomycin).

● SIDE-EFFECTS
▸ **Common or very common**
▸ With intravenous use Blood disorders, including neutropenia (usually after 1 week or cumulative dose of 25 g) ·

interstitial nephritis · nephrotoxicity · ototoxicity (discontinue if tinnitus occurs) · renal failure
▸ **Rare**
▸ With intravenous use Agranulocytosis · thrombocytopenia
▸ **Frequency not known**
▸ With intravenous use Anaphylaxis · cardiac arrest on rapid infusion · chills · dyspnoea · eosinophilia · exfoliative dermatitis · fever · flushing of the upper body ('red man' syndrome) · nausea · pain and muscle spasm of back and chest · phlebitis (irritant to tissue) · pruritus · rashes · severe hypotension on rapid infusion · shock on rapid infusion · Stevens-Johnson syndrome · toxic epidermal necrolysis · urticaria · vasculitis · wheezing
SIDE-EFFECTS, FURTHER INFORMATION
▸ Nephrotoxicity Vancomycin is associated with a higher incidence of nephrotoxicity than teicoplanin.

● ALLERGY AND CROSS-SENSITIVITY Caution if teicoplanin sensitivity.

● PREGNANCY Manufacturer advises use only if potential benefit outweighs risk.
  Plasma-vancomycin concentration monitoring essential to reduce risk of fetal toxicity.

● BREAST FEEDING Present in milk—significant absorption following oral administration unlikely.

● RENAL IMPAIRMENT Reduce dose. In renal impairment monitor plasma-vancomycin concentration and renal function regularly. Also monitor auditory function.

● MONITORING REQUIREMENTS
▸ All patients require plasma-vancomycin measurement (after 3 or 4 doses if renal function normal, earlier if renal impairment).
▸ With intravenous use Pre-dose ('trough') concentration should be 10–15 mg/litre (15–20 mg/litre for endocarditis or less sensitive strains of meticillin-resistant *Staphylococcus aureus* or for complicated infections caused by *S. aureus*). An initial loading dose, by intravenous infusion, may be considered—consult local guidelines.
▸ All patients require blood counts, urinalysis, and renal function tests.
▸ Monitor auditory function in elderly.

● DIRECTIONS FOR ADMINISTRATION
▸ With intravenous use Avoid rapid infusion (risk of anaphylactoid reactions) and rotate infusion sites.
▸ With intravenous use For *intravenous infusion* (*Vancocin®*), give intermittently in Glucose 5% or Sodium chloride 0.9%; reconstitute each 500 mg with 10 mL water for injections and dilute with infusion fluid to a concentration of up to 5 mg/mL (10 mg/mL in fluid restriction but increased risk of infusion-related effects); give over at least 60 minutes (rate not to exceed 10 mg/minute for doses over 500 mg); use continuous infusion only if intermittent not feasible.
▸ With oral use Injection can be used to prepare solution for oral administration; flavouring syrups may be added to the solution at the time of administration.

● MEDICINAL FORMS
There can be variation in the licensing of different medicines containing the same drug. Forms available from special-order manufacturers include: oral suspension, oral solution, pastille, solution for injection, infusion
Capsule
CAUTIONARY AND ADVISORY LABELS 9
▸ Vancomycin (Non-proprietary)
  Vancomycin (as Vancomycin hydrochloride) 125 mg Vancomycin 125mg capsules | 28 capsule PoM £132.47 DT price = £132.47
  Vancomycin (as Vancomycin hydrochloride) 250 mg Vancomycin 250mg capsules | 28 capsule PoM £140.08 DT price = £140.08
▸ Vancocin Matrigel (Flynn Pharma Ltd)
  Vancomycin (as Vancomycin hydrochloride) 125 mg Vancocin Matrigel 125mg capsules | 28 capsule PoM £88.31 DT price = £132.47

Powder for solution for infusion

▸ Vancomycin (Non-proprietary)

Vancomycin (as Vancomycin hydrochloride) 500 mg Vancomycin 500mg powder for solution for infusion vials | 1 vial PoM £7.25 (Hospital only) | 1 vial PoM £7.25
Vancomycin 500mg powder for concentrate for solution for infusion vials | 1 vial PoM £8.50
Vancomycin (as Vancomycin hydrochloride) 1 gram Vancomycin 1g powder for solution for infusion vials | 1 vial PoM £14.50 (Hospital only) | 1 vial PoM £17.25
Vancomycin 1g powder for concentrate for solution for infusion vials | 1 vial PoM £17.25

▸ Vancocin (Flynn Pharma Ltd)

Vancomycin (as Vancomycin hydrochloride) 500 mg Vancocin 500mg powder for solution for infusion vials | 1 vial PoM £6.25
Vancomycin (as Vancomycin hydrochloride) 1 gram Vancocin 1g powder for solution for infusion vials | 1 vial PoM £12.50

ANTIBACTERIALS ⟩ LINCOSAMIDES

Clindamycin

● **DRUG ACTION** Clindamycin is active against Gram-positive cocci, including streptococci and penicillin-resistant staphylococci, and also against many anaerobes, especially *Bacteroides fragilis*. It is well concentrated in bone and excreted in bile and urine.

● **INDICATIONS AND DOSE**

Staphylococcal bone and joint infections such as osteomyelitis | Peritonitis | Intra-abdominal sepsis | Meticillin-resistant *Staphylococcus aureus* (MRSA) in bronchiectasis, bone and joint infections, and skin and soft-tissue infections | Erysipelas or cellulitis in penicillin-allergic patients (alternative to macrolides)

▸ BY MOUTH

▸ Child: 3–6 mg/kg 4 times a day (max. per dose 450 mg)

▸ Adult: 150–300 mg every 6 hours; increased if necessary up to 450 mg every 6 hours if required, increased dose used in severe infection

▸ BY DEEP INTRAMUSCULAR INJECTION, OR BY INTRAVENOUS INFUSION

▸ Adult: 0.6–2.7 g daily in 2–4 divided doses; increased if necessary up to 4.8 g daily, increased dose used in life-threatening infection, single doses above 600 mg to be administered by intravenous infusion only, single doses by intravenous infusion not to exceed 1.2 g

Treatment of mild to moderate pneumocystis pneumonia (in combination with primaquine)

▸ BY MOUTH

▸ Adult: 600 mg every 8 hours

Treatment of falciparum malaria (to be given with or following quinine)

▸ BY MOUTH

▸ Child: 7–13 mg/kg every 8 hours (max. per dose 450 mg) for 7 days

▸ Adult: 450 mg every 8 hours for 7 days

● **UNLICENSED USE**

▸ In adults Not licensed for treatment of mild to moderate pneumocystis infection.

Not licensed for treatment of falciparum malaria.

● **CONTRA-INDICATIONS** Diarrhoeal states

● **CAUTIONS** Avoid in Acute porphyrias p. 918 · middle-aged and elderly women, especially after an operation (antibiotic-associated colitis more common)

● **INTERACTIONS** → Appendix 1 (clindamycin).

● **SIDE-EFFECTS**

▸ With intramuscular use Abscess · induration · pain

▸ With intravenous use Thrombophlebitis

▸ With systemic use Abdominal discomfort · anaphylactoid reactions · antibiotic-associated colitis · diarrhoea (discontinue treatment) · eosinophilia · exfoliative

dermatitis · jaundice · leucopenia · nausea · oesophageal ulcers · oesophagitis · polyarthritis · pruritus · rash · Stevens-Johnson syndrome · taste disturbances · thrombocytopenia · toxic epidermal necrolysis · urticaria · vesiculobullous dermatitis · vomiting

● SIDE-EFFECTS, FURTHER INFORMATION

▸ Antibiotic-associated colitis Clindamycin has been associated with antibiotic-associated colitis, which may be fatal. Although antibiotic-associated colitis can occur with most antibacterials, it occurs more frequently with clindamycin. Patients should therefore discontinue treatment immediately if diarrhoea develops.

● PREGNANCY Not known to be harmful.

● BREAST FEEDING Amount probably too small to be harmful but bloody diarrhoea reported in 1 infant.

● MONITORING REQUIREMENTS

▸ Monitor liver and renal function if treatment exceeds 10 days.

▸ In children Monitor liver and renal function in infants.

● DIRECTIONS FOR ADMINISTRATION

▸ With intravenous use Avoid rapid intravenous administration.

▸ With intravenous use in children For *intravenous infusion*, dilute to a concentration of not more than 18 mg/mL with Glucose 5% *or* Sodium Chloride 0.9%; give over 10–60 minutes at a max. rate of 20 mg/kg/hour.

▸ With intravenous use in adults For *intravenous infusion* (*Dalacin* ® *C Phosphate*), give continuously *or* intermittently *in* Glucose 5% *or* Sodium Chloride 0.9%; dilute to not more than 18 mg/mL and give over 10–60 minutes at a rate not exceeding 30 mg/minute (1.2 g over at least 60 minutes; higher doses by continuous infusion).

● PATIENT AND CARER ADVICE Capsules should be swallowed with a glass of water. Patients and their carers should be advised to discontinue immediately and contact doctor if diarrhoea develops.

● PROFESSION SPECIFIC INFORMATION

Dental practitioners' formulary
Clindamycin capsules may be prescribed.

● MEDICINAL FORMS
There can be variation in the licensing of different medicines containing the same drug. Forms available from special-order manufacturers include: oral suspension, oral solution

Capsule

CAUTIONARY AND ADVISORY LABELS 9, 27

▸ Clindamycin (Non-proprietary)

Clindamycin (as Clindamycin hydrochloride) 150 mg Clindamycin 150mg capsules | 24 capsule PoM £48.00 DT price = £12.00 | 100 capsule PoM £60.00
Clindamycin (as Clindamycin hydrochloride) 300 mg Clindamycin 300mg capsules | 30 capsule PoM £38.96 DT price = £37.46

▸ Dalacin C (Pfizer Ltd)

Clindamycin (as Clindamycin hydrochloride) 75 mg Dalacin C 75mg capsules | 24 capsule PoM £7.45 DT price = £7.45
Clindamycin (as Clindamycin hydrochloride) 150 mg Dalacin C 150mg capsules | 24 capsule PoM £13.72 DT price = £12.00 | 100 capsule PoM £55.08

Solution for injection

EXCIPIENTS: May contain Benzyl alcohol

▸ Clindamycin (Non-proprietary)

Clindamycin (as Clindamycin phosphate) 150 mg per 1 ml Clindamycin 600mg/4ml solution for injection ampoules | 5 ampoule PoM £61.75
Clindamycin 300mg/2ml solution for injection ampoules | 5 ampoule PoM £28.50–£31.01

▸ Dalacin C (Pfizer Ltd)

Clindamycin (as Clindamycin phosphate) 150 mg per 1 ml Dalacin C Phosphate 300mg/2ml solution for injection ampoules | 5 ampoule PoM £31.01
Dalacin C Phosphate 600mg/4ml solution for injection ampoules | 5 ampoule PoM £61.75

Macrolides

Overview

The macrolides have an antibacterial spectrum that is similar but not identical to that of penicillin; they are thus an alternative in penicillin-allergic patients. They are active against many-penicillin-resistant staphylococci, but some are now also resistant to the macrolides.

Indications for the macrolides include campylobacter enteritis, respiratory infections (including pneumonia, whooping cough, Legionella, chlamydia, and mycoplasma infection), and skin infections.

Erythromycin p. 488 is also used in the treatment of early syphilis, uncomplicated genital chlamydial infection, and non-gonococcal urethritis. Erythromycin has poor activity against *Haemophilus influenzae*. Erythromycin causes nausea, vomiting, and diarrhoea in some patients; in mild to moderate infections this can be avoided by giving a lower dose, but if a more serious infection, such as Legionella pneumonia, is suspected higher doses are needed.

Azithromycin below is a macrolide with slightly less activity than erythromycin against Gram-positive bacteria, but enhanced activity against some Gram-negative organisms including *H. influenzae*. Plasma concentrations are very low, but tissue concentrations are much higher. It has a long tissue half-life and once daily dosage is recommended. Azithromycin is also used in the treatment of uncomplicated genital chlamydial infection, non-gonococcal urethritis, uncomplicated gonorrhoea, typhoid [unlicensed indication], and trachoma [unlicensed indication].

Clarithromycin p. 487 is an erythromycin derivative with slightly greater activity than the parent compound. Tissue concentrations are higher than with erythromycin. It is given twice daily. Clarithromycin is also used in regimens for *Helicobacter pylori* eradication.

Telithromycin p. 490 is a ketolide derivative of erythromycin with an antibacterial spectrum similar to that of other macrolides and it is also active against penicillin- and erythromycin-resistant *Streptococcus pneumoniae*.

Erythromycin, azithromycin, and clarithromycin have a role in the treatment of Lyme disease p. 524.

Spiramycin is also a macrolide which is used for the treatment of toxoplasmosis.

Macrolides

- **CAUTIONS** Electrolyte disturbances (predisposition to QT interval prolongation) · may aggravate myasthenia gravis · predisposition to QT interval prolongation
- **SIDE-EFFECTS**
- **Common or very common** Abdominal discomfort · diarrhoea · nausea · vomiting
- **Uncommon** Cholestatic jaundice · hepatotoxicity · rash
- **Rare** Antibiotic-associated colitis · arrhythmias · pancreatitis · QT interval prolongation · Stevens-Johnson syndrome · toxic epidermal necrolysis
- **Frequency not known**
- With intravenous use Local tenderness · phlebitis · reversible hearing loss (sometimes with tinnitus) can occur after large doses
- With oral use Reversible hearing loss (sometimes with tinnitus) can occur after large doses

SIDE-EFFECTS, FURTHER INFORMATION
Gastro-intestinal side-effects are mild and less frequent with azithromycin and clarithromycin than with erythromycin.

Azithromycin

above

- **INDICATIONS AND DOSE**

Prevention of secondary case of invasive group A streptococcal infection in patients who are allergic to penicillin
▸ BY MOUTH
- Child 6 months–11 years: 12 mg/kg once daily (max. per dose 500 mg) for 5 days
- Child 12–17 years: 500 mg once daily for 5 days
- Adult: 500 mg once daily for 5 days

Respiratory-tract infections, otitis media, skin and soft-tissue infections
▸ BY MOUTH
- Child 6 months–17 years: 10 mg/kg once daily (max. per dose 500 mg) for 3 days
- Child 6 months–17 years (body-weight 15–25 kg): 200 mg once daily for 3 days
- Child 6 months–17 years (body-weight 26–35 kg): 300 mg once daily for 3 days
- Child 6 months–17 years (body-weight 36–45 kg): 400 mg once daily for 3 days
- Child 6 months–17 years (body-weight 46 kg and above): 500 mg once daily for 3 days
- Adult: 500 mg once daily for 3 days, alternatively initially 500 mg once daily for 1 day, then 250 mg once daily for 4 days

Uncomplicated genital chlamydial infections | Non-gonococcal urethritis
▸ BY MOUTH
- Child 12–17 years: 1 g for 1 dose
- Adult: 1 g for 1 dose

Uncomplicated gonorrhoea
▸ BY MOUTH
- Adult: 1 g for 1 dose

Lyme disease (under expert supervision)
▸ BY MOUTH
- Adult: 500 mg once daily for 7–10 days

Mild to moderate typhoid due to multiple-antibacterial resistant organisms
▸ BY MOUTH
- Adult: 500 mg once daily for 7 days

Community-acquired pneumonia, low to moderate severity
▸ BY MOUTH
- Adult: 500 mg once daily for 3 days, alternatively initially 500 mg once daily for 1 day, then 250 mg once daily for 4 days

Community-acquired pneumonia, high severity
▸ INITIALLY BY INTRAVENOUS INFUSION
- Adult: Initially 500 mg once daily for at least 2 days, then (by mouth) 500 mg once daily for a total duration of 7–10 days

Antibacterial prophylaxis for insertion of intra-uterine device
▸ BY MOUTH
- Adult: 1 g for 1 dose

- **UNLICENSED USE**
- In children Not licensed for typhoid fever or prophylaxis of group A streptococcal infection.
- In adults Oral azithromycin not licensed for trachoma which results from chronic infection with *Chlamydia trachomatis*.

  Not licensed for uncomplicated gonorrhoea, mild or moderate typhoid due to multiple-antibacterial-resistant organisms, Lyme disease, or prophylaxis of group A streptococcal infection. Not licensed for community-acquired pneumonia (high severity) when oral treatment continues for more than 3 days.

- **INTERACTIONS** → Appendix 1 (macrolides). Caution with concomitant use of drugs that prolong the QT interval.
- **SIDE-EFFECTS**
  - **Common or very common** Anorexia · arthralgia · disturbances in taste · disturbances in vision · dizziness · dyspepsia · flatulence · headache · malaise · paraesthesia · reversible hearing loss (sometimes with tinnitus) after long-term therapy ·
  - **Uncommon** Anxiety · chest pain · constipation · gastritis · hypoaesthesia · leucopenia · oedema · photosensitivity · sleep disturbances
  - **Rare** Agitation
  - **Frequency not known** Acute renal failure · convulsions · haemolytic anaemia · interstitial nephritis · smell disturbances · syncope · thrombocytopenia · tongue discoloration
- **PREGNANCY** Manufacturers advise use only if adequate alternatives not available.
- **BREAST FEEDING** Present in milk; use only if no suitable alternatives.
- **HEPATIC IMPAIRMENT** Manufacturers advise avoid in severe liver disease–no information available.
- **RENAL IMPAIRMENT**
  - In adults Use with caution if eGFR less than 10 mL/minute/1.73 m^2.
  - In children Use with caution if estimated glomerular filtration rate less than 10 mL/minute/1.73 m^2.
- **DIRECTIONS FOR ADMINISTRATION** For *intravenous infusion* (*Zedbac*®), give intermittently *in* Glucose 5% *or* Sodium Chloride 0.9%. Reconstitute 500 mg with 4.8 mL water for injections to produce a 100 mg/mL solution, then dilute 5 mL of solution with infusion fluid to a final concentration of 1 or 2 mg/mL; give the 1 mg/mL solution over 3 hours *or* give the 2 mg/mL solution over 1 hour.
- **PRESCRIBING AND DISPENSING INFORMATION** Flavours of oral liquid formulations may include cherry or banana.
- **PATIENT AND CARER ADVICE**
  Medicines for Children leaflet: Azithromycin for bacterial infections www.medicinesforchildren.org.uk/azithromycin-bacterial-infections-0
- **PROFESSION SPECIFIC INFORMATION**
  Dental practitioners' formulary
  Azithromycin Capsules may be prescribed. Azithromycin Tablets may be prescribed. Azithromycin Oral Suspension 200 mg/5 mL may be prescribed.
- **EXCEPTIONS TO LEGAL CATEGORY** Azithromycin tablets can be sold to the public for the treatment of confirmed, asymptomatic *Chlamydia trachomatis* genital infection in those over 16 years of age, and for the epidemiological treatment of their sexual partners, subject to maximum single dose of 1 g, maximum daily dose 1 g, and a pack size of 1 g.
- **MEDICINAL FORMS**
  There can be variation in the licensing of different medicines containing the same drug. Forms available from special-order manufacturers include: oral suspension

Tablet
CAUTIONARY AND ADVISORY LABELS 5, 9
  - Azithromycin (Non-proprietary)
    Azithromycin 250 mg Azithromycin 250mg tablets | 4 tablet PoM £10.11 DT price = £1.38 | 6 tablet PoM £14.46
    Azithromycin 500 mg Azithromycin 500mg tablets | 3 tablet PoM £9.80 DT price = £1.34

Capsule
CAUTIONARY AND ADVISORY LABELS 5, 9, 23
  - Azithromycin (Non-proprietary)
    Azithromycin (as Azithromycin dihydrate) 250 mg Azithromycin 250mg capsules | 4 capsule PoM £10.10 | 6 capsule PoM £15.15 DT price = £15.13
  - Zithromax (Pfizer Ltd)
    Azithromycin (as Azithromycin dihydrate) 250 mg Zithromax 250mg capsules | 4 capsule PoM £7.16 | 6 capsule PoM £10.74 DT price = £15.13

Oral suspension
CAUTIONARY AND ADVISORY LABELS 5, 9
  - Azithromycin (Non-proprietary)
    Azithromycin 40 mg per 1 ml Azithromycin 200mg/5ml oral suspension | 15 ml PoM £6.18 DT price = £4.06 | 30 ml PoM £11.04 DT price = £11.04
  - Zithromax (Pfizer Ltd)
    Azithromycin 40 mg per 1 ml Zithromax 200mg/5ml oral suspension | 15 ml PoM £4.06 DT price = £4.06 | 22.5 ml PoM £6.10 DT price = £6.10 | 30 ml PoM £11.04 DT price = £11.04

Powder for solution for infusion
ELECTROLYTES: May contain Sodium
  - Zedbac (Aspire Pharma Ltd)
    Azithromycin (as Azithromycin dihydrate) 500 mg Zedbac 500mg powder for solution for infusion vials | 1 vial PoM £9.50 (Hospital only)

◤ 486

Clarithromycin

- **INDICATIONS AND DOSE**

Respiratory-tract infections | Mild to moderate skin and soft-tissue infections | Otitis media
- BY MOUTH USING IMMEDIATE-RELEASE MEDICINES
  - Child 1 month–11 years (body-weight up to 8 kg): 7.5 mg/kg twice daily
  - Child 1 month–11 years (body-weight 8–11 kg): 62.5 mg twice daily
  - Child 1 month–11 years (body-weight 12–19 kg): 125 mg twice daily
  - Child 1 month–11 years (body-weight 20–29 kg): 187.5 mg twice daily
  - Child 1 month–11 years (body-weight 30–40 kg): 250 mg twice daily
  - Child 12–17 years: 250 mg twice daily usually for 7–14 days, increased to 500 mg twice daily, if required in severe infections (e.g. pneumonia)
  - Adult: 250 mg twice daily usually for 7–14 days, increased to 500 mg twice daily, if required in severe infections (e.g. pneumonia)
- BY MOUTH USING MODIFIED-RELEASE MEDICINES
  - Child 12–17 years: 500 mg once daily usually for 7–14 days, increased to 1 g once daily, if required in severe infections (e.g. pneumonia)
  - Adult: 500 mg once daily usually for 7–14 days, increased to 1 g once daily, if required in severe infections (e.g. pneumonia)
- BY INTRAVENOUS INFUSION
  - Adult: 500 mg every 12 hours maximum duration 5 days, switch to oral route when appropriate, to be administered into a large proximal vein

Lyme disease
- BY MOUTH
  - Child 12–17 years: 500 mg twice daily for 14–21 days
  - Adult: 500 mg twice daily for 14–21 days

Prevention of pertussis
- BY MOUTH
  - Child 1 month–11 years (body-weight up to 8 kg): 7.5 mg/kg twice daily for 7 days
  - Child 1 month–11 years (body-weight 8–11 kg): 62.5 mg twice daily for 7 days
  - Child 1 month–11 years (body-weight 12–19 kg): 125 mg twice daily for 7 days
continued →

5

Infection

- Child 1 month–11 years (body-weight 20–29 kg): 187.5 mg twice daily for 7 days
- Child 1 month–11 years (body-weight 30–40 kg): 250 mg twice daily for 7 days
- Child 12-17 years: 500 mg twice daily for 7 days
- Adult: 500 mg twice daily for 7 days

***Helicobacter pylori* eradication in combination with a proton pump inhibitor and amoxicillin**
▸ BY MOUTH
- Adult: 500 mg twice daily

***Helicobacter pylori* eradication in combination with a proton pump inhibitor and metronidazole**
▸ BY MOUTH
- Adult: 250 mg twice daily

- UNLICENSED USE Tablets not licensed for use in children under 12 years; oral suspension not licensed for use in infants under 6 months.
  Intravenous infusion not licensed for use in children under 12 years.
- INTERACTIONS → Appendix 1 (macrolides).
  Caution with concomitant use of drugs that prolong the QT interval.
- SIDE-EFFECTS
▸ **Common or very common** Dyspepsia · headache · hyperhidrosis · insomnia · taste disturbances
▸ **Uncommon** Anorexia · anxiety · blood disorders · chest pain · constipation · dizziness · dry mouth · flatulence · gastritis · glossitis · hepatic dysfunction including jaundice · leucopenia · malaise · myalgia · stomatitis · tinnitus · tremor
▸ **Frequency not known** Abnormal dreams · confusion · convulsions · depression · hypoglycaemia · interstitial nephritis · myopathy · paraesthesia · psychotic disorders · renal failure · smell disturbances · tongue discoloration · tooth discoloration
- PREGNANCY Manufacturer advises avoid, particularly in the first trimester, unless potential benefit outweighs risk.
- BREAST FEEDING Manufacturer advises avoid unless potential benefit outweighs risk—present in milk.
- HEPATIC IMPAIRMENT Avoid in severe impairment if renal impairment also present.
- RENAL IMPAIRMENT
▸ In adults Use half normal dose if eGFR less than 30 mL/minute/1.73 m ^{2}, max. duration 14 days.
▸ In children Use half normal dose if estimated glomerular filtration rate less than 30 mL/minute/1.73 m ^{2}, max. duration 14 days. Avoid if severe hepatic impairment also present.
▸ With oral use in adults Avoid *Klaricid XL* ® or clarithromycin m/r preparations if eGFR less than 30 mL/minute/1.73 m ^{2}.
▸ With oral use in children Avoid *Klaricid XL* ® or clarithromyin m/r preparations if estimated glomerular filtration rate less than 30 mL/minute/1.73 m ^{2}.
- DIRECTIONS FOR ADMINISTRATION
▸ With intravenous use in children For intermittent intravenous infusion dilute reconstituted solution further in Glucose 5% *or* Sodium chloride 0.9% to a concentration of 2 mg/mL; give into large proximal vein over 60 minutes.
▸ With intravenous use in adults For *intravenous infusion* (*Klaricid* ® *I.V.*), give intermittently in Glucose 5% or Sodium Chloride 0.9%; dissolve initially in water for injections (500 mg in 10 mL) then dilute to a concentration of 2 mg/mL; give over 60 minutes.
- PATIENT AND CARER ADVICE
  Medicines for Children leaflet: Clarithromycin for bacterial infections www.medicinesforchildren.org.uk/clarithromycin-bacterial-infections

- PROFESSION SPECIFIC INFORMATION
  Dental practitioners' formulary
  Clarithromycin Tablets may be prescribed.
  Clarithromycin Oral Suspension may be prescribed.

- MEDICINAL FORMS
  There can be variation in the licensing of different medicines containing the same drug.
  Tablet
  CAUTIONARY AND ADVISORY LABELS 9
  ▸ Clarithromycin (Non-proprietary)
    Clarithromycin 250 mg Clarithromycin 250mg tablets | 14 tablet [PoM] £10.50 DT price = £1.40
    Clarithromycin 500 mg Clarithromycin 500mg tablets | 14 tablet [PoM] £21.50 DT price = £2.35
  Modified-release tablet
  CAUTIONARY AND ADVISORY LABELS 9, 21, 25
  ▸ Clarie XL (Teva UK Ltd)
    Clarithromycin 500 mg Clarie XL 500mg tablets | 7 tablet [PoM] £6.72 DT price = £6.72 | 14 tablet [PoM] £13.23
  ▸ Klaricid XL (BGP Products Ltd)
    Clarithromycin 500 mg Klaricid XL 500mg tablets | 7 tablet [PoM] £6.72 DT price = £6.72 | 14 tablet [PoM] £13.23
  Granules
  CAUTIONARY AND ADVISORY LABELS 9, 13
  ▸ Klaricid (BGP Products Ltd)
    Clarithromycin 250 mg Klaricid Adult 250mg granules sachets | 14 sachet [PoM] £11.68
  Oral suspension
  CAUTIONARY AND ADVISORY LABELS 9
  ▸ Clarithromycin (Non-proprietary)
    Clarithromycin 25 mg per 1 ml Clarithromycin 125mg/5ml oral suspension | 70 ml [PoM] £11.99 DT price = £3.87
    Clarithromycin 50 mg per 1 ml Clarithromycin 250mg/5ml oral suspension | 70 ml [PoM] £21.75 DT price = £5.74
  ▸ Klaricid (BGP Products Ltd)
    Clarithromycin 25 mg per 1 ml Klaricid Paediatric 125mg/5ml oral suspension | 70 ml [PoM] £5.26 DT price = £3.87 | 100 ml [PoM] £9.04
    Clarithromycin 50 mg per 1 ml Klaricid Paediatric 250mg/5ml oral suspension | 70 ml [PoM] £10.51 DT price = £5.74
  Powder for solution for infusion
  ELECTROLYTES: May contain Sodium
  ▸ Clarithromycin (Non-proprietary)
    Clarithromycin 500 mg Clarithromycin 500mg powder for solution for infusion vials | 1 vial [PoM] £11.25 DT price = £9.45
    Clarithromycin 500mg powder for concentrate for solution for infusion vials | 1 vial [PoM] £8.98 DT price = £9.45
  ▸ Klaricid (BGP Products Ltd)
    Clarithromycin 500 mg Klaricid IV 500mg powder for solution for infusion vials | 1 vial [PoM] £9.45 DT price = £9.45

◸ 486

Erythromycin

- INDICATIONS AND DOSE

Susceptible infections in patients with penicillin hypersensitivity (e.g. respiratory-tract infections (including Legionella infection), skin and oral infections, and campylobacter enteritis)
▸ BY MOUTH
- Child 1 month–1 year: 125 mg 4 times a day, total daily dose may alternatively be given in two divided doses, increased to 250 mg 4 times a day, dose increase may be used in severe infections
- Child 2–7 years: 250 mg 4 times a day, total daily dose may alternatively be given in two divided doses, increased to 500 mg 4 times a day, dose increase may be used in severe infections
- Child 8–17 years: 250–500 mg 4 times a day, total daily dose may alternatively be given in two divided doses, increased to 500–1000 mg 4 times a day, dose increase may be used in severe infections
- Adult: 250–500 mg 4 times a day, total daily dose may alternatively be given in two divided doses, increased

to 500–1000 mg 4 times a day, dose increase may be used in severe infections
- BY INTRAVENOUS INFUSION
- Child: 12.5 mg/kg every 6 hours (max. per dose 1 g)
- Adult: 6.25 mg/kg every 6 hours, for mild infections when oral treatment not possible. increased to 12.5 mg/kg every 6 hours, dose increase may be used in severe infections

Lyme disease (under expert supervision)
- BY MOUTH
- Adult: 500 mg 4 times a day for 14–21 days

Early syphilis
- BY MOUTH
- Adult: 500 mg 4 times a day for 14 days

Uncomplicated genital chlamydia | Non-gonococcal urethritis
- BY MOUTH
- Adult: 500 mg twice daily for 14 days

Chronic prostatitis
- BY MOUTH
- Adult: 250–500 mg 4 times a day, total daily dose may alternatively be given in two divided doses, increased to 4 g daily in divided doses, dose increase may be used in severe infections
- BY INTRAVENOUS INFUSION
- Adult: 6.25 mg/kg every 6 hours, for mild infections when oral treatment is not possible, increased to 12.5 mg/kg every 6 hours, dose increase may be used in severe infections

Prevention and treatment of pertussis
- BY MOUTH
- Child 1 month-1 year: 125 mg 4 times a day, total daily dose may alternatively be given in two divided doses, increased to 250 mg 4 times a day, dose increase may be used in severe infections
- Child 2-7 years: 250 mg 4 times a day, total daily dose may alternatively be given in two divided doses, increased to 500 mg 4 times a day, dose increase may be used in severe infections
- Child 8-17 years: 250–500 mg 4 times a day, total daily dose may alternatively be given in two divided doses, increased to 500–1000 mg 4 times a day, dose increase may be used in severe infections
- Adult: (consult local protocol)

Prevention of secondary case of diphtheria in non-immune patient
- BY MOUTH
- Child 1 month-1 year: 125 mg every 6 hours for 7 days, treat for further 10 days if nasopharyngeal swabs positive after first 7 days' treatment
- Child 2-7 years: 250 mg every 6 hours for 7 days, treat for further 10 days if nasopharyngeal swabs positive after first 7 days' treatment
- Child 8-17 years: 500 mg every 6 hours for 7 days, treat for further 10 days if nasopharyngeal swabs positive after first 7 days' treatment
- Adult: 500 mg every 6 hours for 7 days, treat for further 10 days if nasopharyngeal swabs positive after first 7 days' treatment

Prevention of secondary case of invasive group A streptococcal infection in penicillin allergic patients
- BY MOUTH
- Child 1 month-1 year: 125 mg every 6 hours for 10 days
- Child 2-7 years: 250 mg every 6 hours for 10 days
- Child 8-17 years: 250–500 mg every 6 hours for 10 days
- Adult: 250–500 mg every 6 hours for 10 days

Prevention of pneumococcal infection in asplenia or in patients with sickle-cell disease (if penicillin-allergic)
- BY MOUTH
- Child 1 month-1 year: 125 mg twice daily, antibiotic prophylaxis is not fully reliable
- Child 2-7 years: 250 mg twice daily, antibiotic prophylaxis is not fully reliable. It may be discontinued in those over 5 years of age with sickle-cell disease who have received pneumococcal immunisation and who do not have a history of severe pneumococcal infection
- Child 8-17 years: 500 mg twice daily, antibiotic prophylaxis is not fully reliable. It may be discontinued in those with sickle-cell disease who have received pneumococcal immunisation and who do not have a history of severe pneumococcal infection
- Adult: 500 mg twice daily, antibiotic prophylaxis is not fully reliable. It may be discontinued in those with sickle-cell disease who have received pneumococcal immunisation and who do not have a history of severe pneumococcal infection

Prevention of recurrence of rheumatic fever
- BY MOUTH
- Child 1 month-1 year: 125 mg twice daily
- Child 2-17 years: 250 mg twice daily

Rosacea
- BY MOUTH
- Adult: 500 mg twice daily courses usually last 6–12 weeks and are repeated intermittently

Acne
- BY MOUTH
- Adult: 500 mg twice daily

- ● CAUTIONS Avoid in Acute porphyrias p. 918 · neonate under 2 weeks (risk of hypertrophic pyloric stenosis) (in neonates)
- ● INTERACTIONS → Appendix 1 (macrolides). Caution with concomitant use of drugs that prolong the QT interval.
- ● PREGNANCY Not known to be harmful.
- ● BREAST FEEDING Only small amounts in milk—not known to be harmful.
- ● HEPATIC IMPAIRMENT May cause idiosyncratic hepatotoxicity.
- ● RENAL IMPAIRMENT
  - In adults Max. 1.5 g daily in severe renal impairment (ototoxicity).
  - In children Reduce dose in severe renal impairment (ototoxicity).
- ● DIRECTIONS FOR ADMINISTRATION
  - With intravenous use in children Dilute reconstituted solution further in glucose 5% (neutralised with Sodium bicarbonate) or sodium chloride 0.9% to a concentration of 1–5 mg/mL; give over 20–60 minutes. Concentration of up to 10 mg/mL may be used in fluid-restriction if administered via a central venous catheter.
  - With intravenous use in adults For *intravenous infusion* (as lactobionate), give intermittently *in* Glucose 5% (neutralised with sodium bicarbonate) *or* Sodium chloride 0.9%; dissolve initially in water for injections (1 g in 20 mL) then dilute to a concentration of 1–5 mg/mL; give over 20–60 minutes.
- ● PRESCRIBING AND DISPENSING INFORMATION Flavours of oral liquid formulations may include banana.
- ● PATIENT AND CARER ADVICE
  Medicines for Children leaflet: Erythromycin for bacterial infections www.medicinesforchildren.org.uk/erythromycin-for-bacterial-infections

5 Infection

● PROFESSION SPECIFIC INFORMATION

Dental practitioners' formulary
Erythromycin tablets e/c may be prescribed. Erythromycin ethyl succinate oral suspension may be prescribed. Erythromycin stearate tablets may be prescribed. Erythromycin ethyl succinate tablets may be prescribed.

● MEDICINAL FORMS
There can be variation in the licensing of different medicines containing the same drug.

Tablet
CAUTIONARY AND ADVISORY LABELS 9
▸ Erythromycin (Non-proprietary)
Erythromycin (as Erythromycin ethyl succinate)
500 mg Erythromycin ethyl succinate 500mg tablets |
28 tablet [PoM] £15.95–£19.50 DT price = £10.78
▸ Erythrocin (AMCo)
Erythromycin (as Erythromycin stearate) 250 mg Erythrocin 250 tablets | 100 tablet [PoM] £18.20 DT price = £18.20
Erythromycin (as Erythromycin stearate) 500 mg Erythrocin 500 tablets | 100 tablet [PoM] £36.40 DT price = £36.40
▸ Erythrolar (Ennogen Pharma Ltd)
Erythromycin (as Erythromycin stearate) 250 mg Erythrolar 250mg tablets | 100 tablet [PoM] £22.80 DT price = £18.20
Erythromycin (as Erythromycin stearate) 500 mg Erythrolar 500mg tablets | 100 tablet [PoM] £45.60 DT price = £36.40
▸ Erythroped A (AMCo)
Erythromycin (as Erythromycin ethyl succinate)
500 mg Erythroped A 500mg tablets | 28 tablet [PoM] £10.78 DT price = £10.78

Gastro-resistant tablet
CAUTIONARY AND ADVISORY LABELS 5, 9, 25
▸ Erythromycin (Non-proprietary)
Erythromycin 250 mg Erythromycin 250mg gastro-resistant tablets | 28 tablet [PoM] £3.00 DT price = £1.44 | 500 tablet [PoM] £28.57

Gastro-resistant capsule
CAUTIONARY AND ADVISORY LABELS 5, 9, 25
▸ Erythromycin (Non-proprietary)
Erythromycin 250 mg Erythromycin 250mg gastro-resistant capsules | 28 capsule [PoM] no price available DT price = £5.61 | 30 capsule [PoM] no price available
▸ Erymax (Teva UK Ltd)
Erythromycin 250 mg Erymax 250mg gastro-resistant capsules | 28 capsule [PoM] £5.61 DT price = £5.61 | 112 capsule [PoM] £22.44
▸ Tiloryth (Tillomed Laboratories Ltd)
Erythromycin 250 mg Tiloryth 250mg gastro-resistant capsules | 30 capsule [PoM] £5.65 | 100 capsule [PoM] £18.66

Oral suspension
CAUTIONARY AND ADVISORY LABELS 9
▸ Erythromycin (Non-proprietary)
Erythromycin (as Erythromycin ethyl succinate) 25 mg per
1 ml Erythromycin ethyl succinate 125mg/5ml oral suspension | 100 ml [PoM] £4.05 DT price = £4.04
Erythromycin ethyl succinate 125mg/5ml oral suspension sugar free sugar-free | 100 ml [PoM] £4.05 DT price = £3.31
Erythromycin (as Erythromycin ethyl succinate) 50 mg per
1 ml Erythromycin ethyl succinate 250mg/5ml oral suspension | 100 ml [PoM] £6.38 DT price = £6.36
Erythromycin ethyl succinate 250mg/5ml oral suspension sugar free sugar-free | 100 ml [PoM] £7.99 DT price = £4.76
Erythromycin (as Erythromycin ethyl succinate) 100 mg per
1 ml Erythromycin ethyl succinate 500mg/5ml oral suspension | 100 ml [PoM] £11.24 DT price = £11.24
Erythromycin ethyl succinate 500mg/5ml oral suspension sugar free sugar-free | 100 ml [PoM] no price available DT price = £12.99
▸ Erythroped (AMCo)
Erythromycin (as Erythromycin ethyl succinate) 25 mg per
1 ml Erythroped PI SF 125mg/5ml oral suspension sugar-free | 140 ml [PoM] £3.06
Erythromycin (as Erythromycin ethyl succinate) 50 mg per
1 ml Erythroped SF 250mg/5ml oral suspension sugar-free | 140 ml [PoM] £5.95
Erythromycin (as Erythromycin ethyl succinate) 100 mg per
1 ml Erythroped Forte SF 500mg/5ml oral suspension sugar-free | 140 ml [PoM] £10.56

Powder for solution for infusion
▸ Erythromycin (Non-proprietary)
Erythromycin (as Erythromycin lactobionate)
1 gram Erythromycin 1g powder for solution for infusion vials | 1 vial [PoM] £22.92

Telithromycin

● DRUG ACTION The ketolide telithromycin is a derivative of erythromycin. The antibacterial spectrum of telithromycin is similar to that of macrolides and it is also active against penicillin- and erythromycin-resistant *Streptococcus pneumoniae*.

● INDICATIONS AND DOSE

Treatment of sinusitis or exacerbations of chronic bronchitis if caused by organisms resistant to beta-lactam antibacterials and other macrolides, or if conventional treatment is contra-indicated
▸ BY MOUTH
▹ Adult: 800 mg once daily for 5 days

Treatment of community-acquired pneumonia if caused by organisms resistant to beta-lactam antibacterials and other macrolides, or if conventional treatment is contra-indicated
▸ BY MOUTH
▹ Adult: 800 mg once daily for 7–10 days

Treatment of beta-haemolytic streptococcal pharyngitis if caused by organisms resistant to beta-lactam antibacterials and other macrolides, or if conventional treatment is contra-indicated | Treatment of beta-haemolytic streptococcal tonsillitis if caused by organisms resistant to beta-lactam antibacterials and other macrolides, or if conventional treatment is contra-indicated
▸ BY MOUTH
▹ Child 12–17 years: 800 mg once daily for 5 days
▹ Adult: 800 mg once daily for 5 days

● CONTRA-INDICATIONS Congenital history of QT interval prolongation (if not excluded by ECG) · family history of QT interval prolongation (if not excluded by ECG) · history of telithromycin-associated hepatitis · history of telithromycin-associated jaundice · myasthenia gravis · prolongation of QT interval

● CAUTIONS Avoid in Acute porphyrias p. 918 · bradycardia—risk of QT interval prolongation · coronary heart disease—risk of QT interval prolongation · hypokalaemia—risk of QT interval prolongation · hypomagnesaemia—risk of QT interval prolongation · ventricular arrhythmias—risk of QT interval prolongation

● INTERACTIONS → Appendix 1 (telithromycin). Caution with concomitant use of drugs that prolong the QT interval.

● SIDE-EFFECTS
▸ **Common or very common** Abdominal pain · diarrhoea · dizziness · flatulence · headache · nausea · taste disturbances · vomiting
▸ **Uncommon** Anorexia · blurred vision · constipation · drowsiness · eosinophilia · flushing · hepatitis · insomnia · nervousness · palpitations · pruritus · rash · stomatitis · urticaria
▸ **Rare** Arrhythmias · cholestatic jaundice · diplopia · hypotension · paraesthesia · transient loss of consciousness
▸ **Very rare** Altered sense of smell · antibiotic-associated colitis · erythema multiforme · muscle cramp
▸ **Frequency not known** Arthralgia · confusion · hallucinations · pancreatitis

● PREGNANCY Toxicity in *animal* studies—manufacturer advises use only if potential benefit outweighs risk.

- BREAST FEEDING Manufacturer advises avoid—present in milk in *animal* studies.
- HEPATIC IMPAIRMENT Manufacturer advises caution.
- RENAL IMPAIRMENT Manufacturer advises avoid if possible if eGFR less than 30 mL/minute/1.73 m^2—if no alternative, use alternating daily doses of 800 mg and 400 mg, starting with 800 mg dose.
- PATIENT AND CARER ADVICE

  Driving and skilled tasks
  Visual disturbances or transient loss of consciousness may affect performance of skilled tasks (e.g. driving); effects may occur after the first dose. Administration at bedtime may reduce these side-effects. Patients should be advised not to drive or operate machinery if affected.
  Hepatic disorders Counselling on hepatic disorders is advised. Patients should be told how to recognise signs of liver disorder, and advised to discontinue treatment and seek prompt medical attention if symptoms such as anorexia, nausea, vomiting, abdominal pain, jaundice, or dark urine develop.

- MEDICINAL FORMS
  There can be variation in the licensing of different medicines containing the same drug.
  No licensed medicines listed.

ANTIBACTERIALS > MONOBACTAMS

Aztreonam

- DRUG ACTION Aztreonam is a monocyclic beta-lactam ('monobactam') antibiotic with an antibacterial spectrum limited to Gram-negative aerobic bacteria including *Pseudomonas aeruginosa*, *Neisseria meningitidis*, and *Haemophilus influenzae*; it should not be used alone for 'blind' treatment since it is not active against Gram-positive organisms. Aztreonam is also effective against *Neisseria gonorrhoeae* (but not against concurrent chlamydial infection).

- INDICATIONS AND DOSE
  Gram-negative infections including *Pseudomonas aeruginosa*, *Haemophilus influenzae*, and *Neisseria meningitidis*
  ▸ BY DEEP INTRAMUSCULAR INJECTION, OR BY INTRAVENOUS INFUSION, OR BY INTRAVENOUS INJECTION
  ▸ Adult: 1 g every 8 hours, alternatively 2 g every 12 hours, single doses over 1 g intravenous route only
  Severe gram-negative infections including *Pseudomonas aeruginosa*, *Haemophilus influenzae*, *Neisseria meningitidis*, and lung infections in cystic fibrosis
  ▸ BY INTRAVENOUS INFUSION, OR BY INTRAVENOUS INJECTION
  ▸ Adult: 2 g every 6–8 hours
  Gonorrhoea | Cystitis
  ▸ BY INTRAMUSCULAR INJECTION
  ▸ Adult: 1 g for 1 single dose
  Urinary-tract infections
  ▸ BY DEEP INTRAMUSCULAR INJECTION, OR BY INTRAVENOUS INFUSION, OR BY INTRAVENOUS INJECTION
  ▸ Adult: 0.5–1 g every 8–12 hours
  Chronic pulmonary *Pseudomonas aeruginosa* infection in patients with cystic fibrosis
  ▸ BY INHALATION OF NEBULISED SOLUTION
  ▸ Adult: 75 mg 3 times a day for 28 days, doses to be administered at least 4 hours apart, subsequent courses repeated after 28-day interval without aztreonam nebuliser solution

- CAUTIONS
  ▸ When used by inhalation Haemoptysis— risk of further haemorrhage
- INTERACTIONS → Appendix 1 (aztreonam).

- SIDE-EFFECTS
  GENERAL SIDE-EFFECTS
  Bronchospasm · rash
  SPECIFIC SIDE-EFFECTS
  ▸ **Rare**
  ▸ With systemic use Antibiotic-associated colitis · asthenia · blood disorders · breast tenderness · chest pain · confusion · diplopia · dizziness · dyspnoea · gastro-intestinal bleeding · halitosis · headache · hepatitis · hypotension · insomnia · jaundice · myalgia · neutropenia · paraesthesia · seizures · thrombocytopenia · tinnitus
  ▸ **Frequency not known**
  ▸ When used by inhalation Arthralgia · cough · haemoptysis · pharyngolaryngeal pain · pyrexia · rhinorrhoea · wheezing
  ▸ With systemic use Abdominal pain · diarrhoea · erythema multiforme · flushing · mouth ulcers · nausea · taste disturbances · toxic epidermal necrolysis · vomiting
- ALLERGY AND CROSS-SENSITIVITY Contra-indicated in aztreonam hypersensitivity.
  Use with caution in patients with hypersensitivity to other beta-lactam antibiotics (although aztreonam may be less likely than other beta-lactams to cause hypersensitivity in penicillin-sensitive patients).
- PREGNANCY
  ▸ With systemic use No information available; manufacturer of injection advises avoid.
  ▸ When used by inhalation No information available; manufacturer of powder for nebuliser solution advises avoid unless essential.
- BREAST FEEDING Amount in milk probably too small to be harmful.
- HEPATIC IMPAIRMENT
  ▸ With systemic use Use injection with caution. Monitor liver function.
- RENAL IMPAIRMENT
  ▸ With systemic use If eGFR 10–30 mL/minute/1.73 m^2, usual initial dose of injection, then half normal dose. If eGFR less than 10 mL/minute/1.73 m^2, usual initial dose of injection, then one-quarter normal dose.
- MONITORING REQUIREMENTS
  ▸ When used by inhalation Measure lung function before and after initial dose of aztreonam and monitor for bronchospasm.
- DIRECTIONS FOR ADMINISTRATION For *intravenous injection*, give over 3–5 minutes.
  ▸ With intravenous use For *intravenous infusion (Azactam ®)*, give intermittently in Glucose 5% *or* Sodium chloride 0.9%. Dissolve initially in water for injections (1 g per 3 mL) then dilute to a concentration of less than 20 mg/mL; to be given over 20–60 minutes.
  ▸ When used by inhalation Other inhaled drugs should be administered before aztreonam; a bronchodilator should be administered before each dose.
- NATIONAL FUNDING/ACCESS DECISIONS
  Scottish Medicines Consortium (SMC) Decisions
  The *Scottish Medicines Consortium* has advised (December 2014) that aztreonam powder for nebuliser solution (*Cayston ®*) is accepted for restricted use within NHS Scotland when inhaled colistimethate sodium and inhaled tobramycin are not tolerated or are not providing satisfactory therapeutic benefit (measured as ≥2% decline in forced expiratory volume in 1 second).

- MEDICINAL FORMS
  There can be variation in the licensing of different medicines containing the same drug.
  Powder for solution for injection
  ▸ Azactam (Bristol-Myers Squibb Pharmaceuticals Ltd)
  Aztreonam 1 gram Azactam 1g powder for solution for injection vials | 1 vial [PoM] £9.40 (Hospital only)
  Aztreonam 2 gram Azactam 2g powder for solution for injection vials | 1 vial [PoM] £18.82 (Hospital only)

5

Infection

5

Infection

Powder and solvent for nebuliser solution

▶ Cayston (Gilead Sciences International Ltd)
Aztreonam (as Aztreonam lysine) 75 mg Cayston 75mg powder and solvent for nebuliser solution vials with Altera Nebuliser Handset | 84 vial [PoM] £2,181.53

ANTIBACTERIALS > NITROIMIDAZOLE DERIVATIVES

Metronidazole

● **DRUG ACTION** Metronidazole is an antimicrobial drug with high activity against anaerobic bacteria and protozoa.

● **INDICATIONS AND DOSE**

Anaerobic infections
▶ BY MOUTH
▶ Child 1 month: 7.5 mg/kg every 12 hours usually treated for 7 days (for 10–14 days in *Clostridium difficile* infection)
▶ Child 2 months-11 years: 7.5 mg/kg every 8 hours (max. per dose 400 mg) usually treated for 7 days (for 10–14 days in *Clostridium difficile* infection)
▶ Child 12-17 years: 400 mg every 8 hours usually treated for 7 days (for 10–14 days in *Clostridium difficile* infection)
▶ Adult: 400 mg every 8 hours, alternatively 500 mg every 8 hours usually treated for 7 days (for 10–14 days in *Clostridium difficile* infection)
▶ BY RECTUM
▶ Child 1-11 months: 125 mg 3 times a day for 3 days, then 125 mg twice daily, for usual total treatment duration of 7 days
▶ Child 1-4 years: 250 mg 3 times a day for 3 days, then 250 mg twice daily, for usual total treatment duration of 7 days
▶ Child 5-9 years: 500 mg 3 times a day for 3 days, then 500 mg twice daily, for usual total treatment duration of 7 days
▶ Child 10-17 years: 1 g 3 times a day for 3 days, then 1 g twice daily, for usual total treatment duration of 7 days
▶ Adult: 1 g 3 times a day for 3 days, then 1 g twice daily, for usual total treatment duration of 7 days
▶ BY INTRAVENOUS INFUSION
▶ Adult: 500 mg every 8 hours usually treated for 7 days (for 10–14 days in *Clostridium difficile* infection), to be given over 20 minutes

***Helicobacter pylori* eradication; in combination with clarithromycin and esomeprazole; or in combination with clarithromycin and lansoprazole; or in combination with amoxicillin and lansoprazole; or in combination with clarithromycin and omeprazole; or in combination with clarithromycin and pantoprazole; or in combination with clarithromycin and rabeprazole**
▶ BY MOUTH
▶ Adult: 400 mg twice daily

***Helicobacter pylori* eradication; in combination with amoxicillin and omeprazole**
▶ BY MOUTH
▶ Adult: 400 mg 3 times a day

***Helicobacter pylori* eradication failure (two-week regimen comprising a proton pump inhibitor plus tripotassium dicitratobismuthate plus tetracycline)**
▶ BY MOUTH
▶ Adult: 400–500 mg 3 times a day for 2 weeks

Fistulating Crohn's disease
▶ BY MOUTH
▶ Adult: 10–20 mg/kg daily in divided doses, usual dose 400–500 mg 3 times a day usually given for 1 month but no longer than 3 months because of concerns about peripheral neuropathy

Leg ulcers and pressure sores
▶ BY MOUTH
▶ Adult: 400 mg every 8 hours for 7 days

Bacterial vaginosis (notably *Gardnerella vaginalis* infection)
▶ BY MOUTH
▶ Adult: 400–500 mg twice daily for 5–7 days, alternatively 2 g for 1 dose

Bacterial vaginosis
▶ BY VAGINA USING VAGINAL GEL
▶ Adult: 1 applicatorful daily for 5 days, dose to be administered at night
DOSE EQUIVALENCE AND CONVERSION
1 applicatorful delivers a 5 g dose of metronidazole 0.75%.

Pelvic inflammatory disease
▶ BY MOUTH
▶ Adult: 400 mg twice daily for 14 days

Acute ulcerative gingivitis
▶ BY MOUTH
▶ Child 1-2 years: 50 mg every 8 hours for 3 days
▶ Child 3-6 years: 100 mg every 12 hours for 3 days
▶ Child 7-9 years: 100 mg every 8 hours for 3 days
▶ Child 10-17 years: 200–250 mg every 8 hours for 3 days
▶ Adult: 200–250 mg every 8 hours for 3 days

Acute oral infections
▶ BY MOUTH
▶ Child 1-2 years: 50 mg every 8 hours for 3–7 days
▶ Child 3-6 years: 100 mg every 12 hours for 3–7 days
▶ Child 7-9 years: 100 mg every 8 hours for 3–7 days
▶ Child 10-17 years: 200–250 mg every 8 hours for 3–7 days
▶ Adult: 200 mg every 8 hours for 3–7 days

Surgical prophylaxis
▶ BY MOUTH
▶ Adult: 400–500 mg, to be administered 2 hours before surgery, then 400–500 mg every 8 hours if required for up to 3 doses (in high-risk procedures)
▶ BY RECTUM
▶ Adult: 1 g, to be administered 2 hours before surgery, then 1 g every 8 hours if required for up to 3 doses (in high-risk procedures)
▶ BY INTRAVENOUS INFUSION
▶ Adult: 500 mg, to be administered up to 30 minutes before the procedure (if rectal administration inappropriate), then 500 mg every 8 hours if required for up to 3 further doses (in high-risk procedures)

Invasive intestinal amoebiasis | Extra-intestinal amoebiasis (including liver abscess)
▶ BY MOUTH
▶ Child 1-2 years: 200 mg 3 times a day for 5 days in intestinal infection (for 5–10 days in extra-intestinal infection)
▶ Child 3-6 years: 200 mg 4 times a day for 5 days in intestinal infection (for 5–10 days in extra-intestinal infection)
▶ Child 7-9 years: 400 mg 3 times a day for 5 days in intestinal infection (for 5–10 days in extra-intestinal infection)
▶ Child 10-17 years: 800 mg 3 times a day for 5 days in intestinal infection (for 5–10 days in extra-intestinal infection)
▶ Adult: 800 mg 3 times a day for 5 days in intestinal infection (for 5–10 days in extra-intestinal infection)

Urogenital trichomoniasis
▶ BY MOUTH
▶ Child 1-2 years: 50 mg 3 times a day for 7 days
▶ Child 3-6 years: 100 mg twice daily for 7 days
▶ Child 7-9 years: 100 mg 3 times a day for 7 days
▶ Child 10-17 years: 200 mg 3 times a day for 7 days, alternatively 400–500 mg twice daily for 5–7 days, alternatively 2 g for 1 dose

- Adult: 200 mg 3 times a day for 7 days, alternatively 400–500 mg twice daily for 5–7 days, alternatively 2 g for 1 dose

Giardiasis
▸ BY MOUTH
- Child 1-2 years: 500 mg once daily for 3 days
- Child 3-6 years: 600–800 mg once daily for 3 days
- Child 7-9 years: 1 g once daily for 3 days
- Child 10-17 years: 2 g once daily for 3 days, alternatively 400 mg 3 times a day for 5 days, alternatively 500 mg twice daily for 7–10 days
- Adult: 2 g once daily for 3 days, alternatively 400 mg 3 times a day for 5 days, alternatively 500 mg twice daily for 7–10 days

Established case of tetanus
▸ BY INTRAVENOUS INFUSION
- Adult: (consult product literature)

● UNLICENSED USE
▸ With systemic use in adults Metronidazole doses in the BNF may differ from those in product literature.

● CAUTIONS
▸ With vaginal use Not recommended during menstruation · some systemic absorption may occur with vaginal gel

● INTERACTIONS
▸ With systemic use → Appendix 1 (metronidazole). Caution—disulfiram-like reaction with alcohol.

● SIDE-EFFECTS
▸ Very rare
▸ With systemic use Arthralgia · ataxia · darkening of urine · dizziness · drowsiness · erythema multiforme · headache · hepatitis · jaundice · leucopenia (on prolonged or intensive therapy) · myalgia · pancreatitis · pancytopenia · peripheral neuropathy (on prolonged or intensive therapy) · pruritus · psychotic disorders · rash · thrombocytopenia · transient epileptiform seizures (on prolonged or intensive therapy) · visual disturbances
▸ Frequency not known
▸ With systemic use Anorexia · aseptic meningitis · furred tongue · gastro-intestinal disturbances · nausea · optic neuropathy · oral mucositis · taste disturbances · vomiting
▸ With vaginal use Abnormal vaginal discharge · local irritation · pelvic discomfort · vaginal candidiasis

● PREGNANCY
▸ With systemic use Manufacturer advises avoidance of high-dose regimens; use only if potential benefit outweighs risk.

● BREAST FEEDING
▸ With systemic use Significant amount in milk; manufacturer advises avoid large single doses though otherwise compatible; may give milk a bitter taste.

● HEPATIC IMPAIRMENT
▸ With systemic use In severe liver disease reduce total daily dose to one-third, and give once daily. Use with caution in hepatic encephalopathy.

● MONITORING REQUIREMENTS
▸ With systemic use Clinical and laboratory monitoring advised if treatment exceeds 10 days.

● DIRECTIONS FOR ADMINISTRATION
▸ With intravenous use For *intravenous infusion*, give over 20–30 minutes.

● PRESCRIBING AND DISPENSING INFORMATION
▸ With systemic use Metronidazole is well absorbed orally and the intravenous route is normally reserved for severe infections. Metronidazole by the rectal route is an effective alternative to the intravenous route when oral administration is not possible.

● PATIENT AND CARER ADVICE
Medicines for Children leaflet: Metronidazole for bacterial infections www.medicinesforchildren.org.uk/metronidazole-for-bacterial-infections

● PROFESSION SPECIFIC INFORMATION
Dental practitioners' formulary
Metronidazole Tablets may be prescribed. Metronidazole Oral Suspension may be prescribed.

● MEDICINAL FORMS
There can be variation in the licensing of different medicines containing the same drug. Forms available from special-order manufacturers include: oral solution

Tablet
CAUTIONARY AND ADVISORY LABELS 4, 9, 21, 25, 27
▸ Metronidazole (Non-proprietary)
Metronidazole 200 mg Metronidazole 200mg tablets | 21 tablet [PoM] £11.66 DT price = £1.40 | 250 tablet [PoM] £19.69
Metronidazole 400 mg Metronidazole 400mg tablets | 21 tablet [PoM] £7.95 DT price = £1.03
Metronidazole 500 mg Metronidazole 500mg tablets | 21 tablet [PoM] £37.82 DT price = £37.82
▸ Flagyl (Zentiva)
Metronidazole 200 mg Flagyl 200mg tablets | 21 tablet [PoM] £4.49 DT price = £1.40
Metronidazole 400 mg Flagyl 400mg tablets | 14 tablet [PoM] £6.34

Oral suspension
CAUTIONARY AND ADVISORY LABELS 4, 9
▸ Metronidazole (Non-proprietary)
Metronidazole (as Metronidazole benzoate) 40 mg per 1 ml Metronidazole 200mg/5ml oral suspension | 100 ml [PoM] £32.93 DT price = £32.93

Infusion
ELECTROLYTES: May contain Sodium
▸ Metronidazole (Non-proprietary)
Metronidazole 5 mg per 1 ml Metronidazole 500mg/100ml infusion 100ml bags | 20 bag [PoM] £62.00
Metronidazole 500mg/100ml infusion 100ml Macoflex bags | 1 bag [PoM] no price available | 60 bag [PoM] no price available

Suppository
CAUTIONARY AND ADVISORY LABELS 4, 9
▸ Flagyl (Zentiva)
Metronidazole 500 mg Flagyl 500mg suppositories | 10 suppository [PoM] £15.18
Metronidazole 1 gram Flagyl 1g suppositories | 10 suppository [PoM] £23.06

Vaginal gel
EXCIPIENTS: May contain Disodium edetate, hydroxybenzoates (parabens), propylene glycol
▸ Metronidazole (Non-proprietary)
Metronidazole 7.5 mg per 1 gram Metronidazole 0.75% vaginal gel | 40 gram [PoM] no price available
▸ Zidoval (Meda Pharmaceuticals Ltd)
Metronidazole 7.5 mg per 1 gram Zidoval 0.75% vaginal gel | 40 gram [PoM] £4.31

Tinidazole

● DRUG ACTION Tinidazole is an antimicrobial drug with high activity against anaerobic bacteria and protozoa; it has a longer duration of action than metronidazole.

● INDICATIONS AND DOSE
Anaerobic infections
▸ BY MOUTH
- Adult: Initially 2 g, followed by 1 g daily usually for 5–6 days, alternatively 500 mg twice daily usually for 5–6 days

Bacterial vaginosis | Acute ulcerative gingivitis
▸ BY MOUTH
- Adult: 2 g for 1 single dose

Abdominal surgery prophylaxis
▸ BY MOUTH
- Adult: 2 g for 1 single dose, to be administered approximately 12 hours before surgery continued →

Intestinal amoebiasis
▸ BY MOUTH
▸ Child 1 month–11 years: 50–60 mg/kg once daily (max. per dose 2 g) for 3 days
▸ Child 12–17 years: 2 g once daily for 2–3 days
▸ Adult: 2 g once daily for 2–3 days

Amoebic involvement of liver
▸ BY MOUTH
▸ Child 1 month–11 years: 50–60 mg/kg once daily (max. per dose 2 g) for 5 days
▸ Child 12–17 years: 1.5–2 g once daily for 3–6 days
▸ Adult: 1.5–2 g once daily for 3–6 days

Urogenital trichomoniasis | Giardiasis
▸ BY MOUTH
▸ Child 1 month–11 years: 50–75 mg/kg (max. per dose 2 g) for 1 single dose, dose may be repeated once if necessary
▸ Child 12–17 years: 2 g for 1 single dose, dose may be repeated once if necessary
▸ Adult: 2 g for 1 single dose

***Helicobacter pylori* eradication**
▸ BY MOUTH
▸ Adult: (consult local protocol)

● CAUTIONS Avoid in Acute porphyrias p. 918
● INTERACTIONS → Appendix 1 (tinidazole). Caution—disulfiram-like reaction with alcohol.
● SIDE-EFFECTS
▸ **Common or very common** Anorexia · furred tongue · gastro-intestinal disturbances · nausea · oral mucositis · taste disturbances · vomiting
▸ **Very rare** Arthralgia · ataxia · darkening of urine · dizziness · drowsiness · erythema multiforme · headache · hepatitis · jaundice · leucopenia (on prolonged or intensive therapy) · myalgia · pancreatitis · pancytopenia · peripheral neuropathy (on prolonged or intensive therapy) · pruritus · psychotic disorders · rash · thrombocytopenia · transient epileptiform seizures (on prolonged or intensive therapy) · visual disturbances
▸ **Frequency not known** Aseptic meningitis · optic neuropathy
● PREGNANCY Manufacturer advises avoid in first trimester.
● BREAST FEEDING Present in milk—manufacturer advises avoid breast-feeding during and for 3 days after stopping treatment.
● MONITORING REQUIREMENTS Clinical and laboratory monitoring advised if treatment exceeds 10 days.

● MEDICINAL FORMS
There can be variation in the licensing of different medicines containing the same drug.
Tablet
CAUTIONARY AND ADVISORY LABELS 4, 9, 21, 25
▸ Fasigyn (Pfizer Ltd)
Tinidazole 500 mg Fasigyn 500mg tablets | 16 tablet [PoM] £11.04
DT price = £11.04

ANTIBACTERIALS ❭ PENICILLINS

Penicillins

Benzylpenicillin and phenoxymethylpenicillin

Benzylpenicillin sodium p. 496 (Penicillin G) remains an important and useful antibiotic but is inactivated by bacterial beta-lactamases. It is effective for many streptococcal (including pneumococcal), gonococcal, and meningococcal infections and also for anthrax, diphtheria, gas-gangrene, leptospirosis, and treatment of Lyme disease. Pneumococci, meningococci, and gonococci which have decreased sensitivity to penicillin have been isolated;

benzylpenicillin sodium is no longer the drug of first choice for pneumococcal meningitis. Although benzylpenicillin sodium is effective in the treatment of tetanus, metronidazole p. 492 is preferred. Benzylpenicillin is inactivated by gastric acid and absorption from the gastro-intestinal tract is low; therefore it must be given by injection.

Benzathine benzylpenicillin is used for the treatment of early syphilis and late latent syphilis; it is given by intramuscular injection.

Phenoxymethylpenicillin p. 497 (Penicillin V) has a similar antibacterial spectrum to benzylpenicillin sodium, but is less active. It is gastric acid-stable, so is suitable for oral administration. It should not be used for serious infections because absorption can be unpredictable and plasma concentrations variable. It is indicated principally for respiratory-tract infections in children, for streptococcal tonsillitis, and for continuing treatment after one or more injections of benzylpenicillin sodium when clinical response has begun. It should not be used for meningococcal or gonococcal infections. Phenoxymethylpenicillin is used for prophylaxis against streptococcal infections following rheumatic fever and against pneumococcal infections following splenectomy or in sickle-cell disease.

Penicillinase-resistant penicillins

Most staphylococci are now resistant to benzylpenicillin because they produce penicillinases. Flucloxacillin p. 503, however, is not inactivated by these enzymes and is thus effective in infections caused by penicillin-resistant staphylococci, which is the sole indication for its use. Flucloxacillin is acid-stable and can, therefore, be given by mouth as well as by injection. Flucloxacillin is well absorbed from the gut.

Temocillin p. 504 is active against Gram-negative bacteria and is stable against a wide range of beta-lactamases. It should be reserved for the treatment of infections caused by beta-lactamase-producing strains of Gram-negative bacteria, including those resistant to third-generation cephalosporins. Temocillin is not active against *Pseudomonas aeruginosa* or *Acinetobacter* spp.

Broad-spectrum penicillins

Ampicillin p. 499 is active against certain Gram-positive and Gram-negative organisms but is inactivated by penicillinases including those produced by *Staphylococcus aureus* and by common Gram-negative bacilli such as *Escherichia coli*. Almost all staphylococci, approx. 60% of *E. coli* strains and approx. 20% of *Haemophilus influenzae* strains are now resistant. The likelihood of resistance should therefore be considered before using ampicillin for the 'blind' treatment of infections; in particular, it should not be used for hospital patients without checking sensitivity.

Ampicillin is well excreted in the bile and urine. It is principally indicated for the treatment of exacerbations of chronic bronchitis and middle ear infections, both of which may be due to *Streptococcus pneumoniae* and *H. influenzae*, and for urinary-tract infections.

Ampicillin can be given by mouth but less than half the dose is absorbed, and absorption is further decreased by the presence of food in the gut.

Maculopapular rashes commonly occur with ampicillin (and amoxicillin p. 498) but are not usually related to true penicillin allergy. They almost always occur in patients with glandular fever; broad-spectrum penicillins should not therefore be used for 'blind' treatment of a sore throat. The risk of rash is also increased in patients with acute or chronic lymphocytic leukaemia or in cytomegalovirus infection.

Amoxicillin is a derivative of ampicillin and has a similar antibacterial spectrum. It is better absorbed than ampicillin when given by mouth, producing higher plasma and tissue concentrations; unlike ampicillin, absorption is not affected by the presence of food in the stomach. Amoxicillin may also be used for the treatment of Lyme disease [not licensed].

Co-amoxiclav p. 501 consists of amoxicillin with the betalactamase inhibitor clavulanic acid. Clavulanic acid itself has no significant antibacterial activity but, by inactivating beta-lactamases, it makes the combination active against beta-lactamase-producing bacteria that are resistant to amoxicillin. These include resistant strains of *Staph. aureus*, *E. coli*, and *H. influenzae*, as well as many *Bacteroides* and *Klebsiella* spp. Co-amoxiclav should be reserved for infections likely, or known, to be caused by amoxicillin-resistant beta-lactamase-producing strains.

A combination of ampicillin with flucloxacillin (as co-fluampicil p. 500) is available to treat infections involving either streptococci or staphylococci (e.g. cellulitis).

Antipseudomonal penicillins

Piperacillin, a ureidopenicillin, is only available in combination with the beta-lactamase inhibitor tazobactam. **Ticarcillin**, a carboxypenicillin, is only available in combination with the beta-lactamase inhibitor clavulanic acid. Both preparations have a broad spectrum of activity against a range of Gram-positive and Gram-negative bacteria, and anaerobes. Piperacillin with tazobactam below has activity against a wider range of Gram-negative organisms than ticarcillin with clavulanic acid p. 496 and it is more active against *Pseudomonas aeruginosa*. These antibacterials are not active against MRSA. They are used in the treatment of septicaemia, hospital-acquired pneumonia, and complicated infections involving the urinary tract, skin and soft tissues, or intra-abdomen. For severe pseudomonas infections these antipseudomonal penicillins can be given with an aminoglycoside (e.g. gentamicin p. 471) since they have a synergistic effect.

Mecillinams

Pivmecillinam hydrochloride p. 502 has significant activity against many Gram-negative bacteria including *Escherichia coli*, klebsiella, enterobacter, and salmonellae. It is not active against *Pseudomonas aeruginosa* or enterococci. Pivmecillinam hydrochloride is hydrolysed to mecillinam, which is the active drug.

Penicillins

- DRUG ACTION The penicillins are bactericidal and act by interfering with bacterial cell wall synthesis. They diffuse well into body tissues and fluids, but penetration into the cerebrospinal fluid is poor except when the meninges are inflamed. They are excreted in the urine in therapeutic concentrations.
- CAUTIONS History of allergy
- INTERACTIONS → Appendix 1 (penicillins).
- SIDE-EFFECTS
- **Common or very common** Anaphylaxis · angioedema · diarrhoea · fever · hypersensitivity reactions · joint pains · rashes · serum sickness-like reaction · urticaria
- **Rare** Cerebral irritation · CNS toxicity (including convulsions) · coagulation disorders · encephalopathy · haemolytic anaemia · interstitial nephritis · leucopenia · thrombocytopenia
- **Frequency not known** Antibiotic-associated colitis
  SIDE-EFFECTS, FURTHER INFORMATION
- CNS toxicity A rare but serious toxic effect of the penicillins is encephalopathy due to cerebral irritation. This may result from excessively high doses or in patients with severe renal failure. The penicillins should **not** be given by intrathecal injection because they can cause encephalopathy which may be fatal.
- Diarrhoea Diarrhoea frequently occurs during oral penicillin therapy. It is most common with broad-

spectrum penicillins, which can also cause antibiotic-associated colitis.
- ALLERGY AND CROSS-SENSITIVITY The most important side-effect of the penicillins is hypersensitivity which causes rashes and anaphylaxis and can be fatal. Allergic reactions to penicillins occur in 1–10% of exposed individuals; anaphylactic reactions occur in fewer than 0.05% of treated patients. Patients with a history of atopic allergy (e.g. asthma, eczema, hay fever) are at a higher risk of anaphylactic reactions to penicillins. Individuals with a history of anaphylaxis, urticaria, or rash immediately after penicillin administration are at risk of immediate hypersensitivity to a penicillin; these individuals should not receive a penicillin. Individuals with a history of a minor rash (i.e. non-confluent, non-pruritic rash restricted to a small area of the body) or a rash that occurs more than 72 hours after penicillin administration are probably not allergic to penicillin and in these individuals a penicillin should not be withheld unnecessarily for serious infections; the possibility of an allergic reaction should, however, be borne in mind. Other beta-lactam antibiotics (including cephalosporins) can be used in these patients.

Patients who are allergic to one penicillin will be allergic to all because the hypersensitivity is related to the basic penicillin structure. Patients with a history of immediate hypersensitivity to penicillins may also react to the cephalosporins and other beta-lactam antibiotics, they should not receive these antibiotics. If a penicillin (or another beta-lactam antibiotic) is essential in an individual with immediate hypersensitivity to penicillin then specialist advice should be sought on hypersensitivity testing or using a beta-lactam antibiotic with a different structure to the penicillin that caused the hypersensitivity.

ANTIBACTERIALS > PENICILLINS, ANTIPSEUDOMONAL WITH BETA-LACTAMASE INHIBITOR
☞ above

Piperacillin with tazobactam

- INDICATIONS AND DOSE

Hospital-acquired pneumonia | Septicaemia | Complicated infections involving the urinary-tract | Complicated infections involving the skin | Complicated infections involving the soft-tissues
- ► BY INTRAVENOUS INFUSION
- ► Adult: 4.5 g every 8 hours; increased if necessary to 4.5 g every 6 hours, increased frequency may be used for severe infections

Infections in neutropenic patients
- ► BY INTRAVENOUS INFUSION
- ► Adult: 4.5 g every 6 hours

- CAUTIONS High doses may lead to hypernatraemia (owing to sodium content of preparations)
- SIDE-EFFECTS
- **Common or very common** Nausea · vomiting
- **Uncommon** Constipation · dyspepsia · headache · hypotension · injection-site reactions · insomnia · jaundice · stomatitis
- **Rare** Abdominal pain · eosinophilia · hepatitis
- **Very rare** Hypoglycaemia · hypokalaemia · pancytopenia · Steven-Johnson syndrome · toxic epidermal necrolysis
- PREGNANCY Manufacturers advise use only if potential benefit outweighs risk.
- BREAST FEEDING Trace amount in milk, but appropriate to use.
- RENAL IMPAIRMENT Max. 4.5 g every 8 hours if eGFR 20–40 mL/minute/1.73 m^2. Max. 4.5 g every 12 hours if eGFR less than 20 mL/minute/1.73 m^2.

5

Infection

● EFFECT ON LABORATORY TESTS False-positive urinary glucose (if tested for reducing substances).

● DIRECTIONS FOR ADMINISTRATION For *intravenous infusion*, give intermittently in Glucose 5% or Sodium chloride 0.9%. Reconstitute initially (2.25 g in 10 mL, 4.5 g in 20 mL) with water for injections, or glucose 5% (*Tazocin®* brand only), or sodium chloride 0.9%, then dilute to 50–150 mL with infusion fluid; give over 30 minutes.

● PRESCRIBING AND DISPENSING INFORMATION Dose expressed as a combination of piperacillin and tazobactam (both as sodium salts) in a ratio of 8:1.

● MEDICINAL FORMS
There can be variation in the licensing of different medicines containing the same drug. Forms available from special-order manufacturers include: infusion

Powder for solution for injection
ELECTROLYTES: May contain Sodium
▸ Piperacillin with tazobactam (Non-proprietary)
  Tazobactam (as Tazobactam sodium) 250 mg, Piperacillin (as Piperacillin sodium) 2 gram Piperacillin 2g / Tazobactam 250mg powder for solution for injection vials | 1 vial [PoM] £7.96 DT price = £7.91 (Hospital only) | 1 vial [PoM] £6.50–£7.91 DT price = £7.91 | 10 vial [PoM] £10.31–£60.80
  Tazobactam (as Tazobactam sodium) 500 mg, Piperacillin (as Piperacillin sodium) 4 gram Piperacillin 4g / Tazobactam 500mg powder for solution for injection vials | 1 vial [PoM] £15.77–£15.79 (Hospital only) | 1 vial [PoM] £12.90
▸ Tazocin (Pfizer Ltd)
  Tazobactam (as Tazobactam sodium) 250 mg, Piperacillin (as Piperacillin sodium) 2 gram Tazocin 2.25g powder for solution for injection vials | 1 vial [PoM] £7.65 DT price = £7.91
  Tazobactam (as Tazobactam sodium) 500 mg, Piperacillin (as Piperacillin sodium) 4 gram Tazocin 4.5g powder for solution for injection vials | 1 vial [PoM] £15.17 (Hospital only)

F 495

Ticarcillin with clavulanic acid

● INDICATIONS AND DOSE
Infections due to *Pseudomonas* and *Proteus* spp.
▸ BY INTRAVENOUS INFUSION
▸ Adult: 3.2 g every 6–8 hours; increased if necessary to 3.2 g every 4 hours, increased frequency used for more severe infections

● CAUTIONS High doses may lead to hypernatraemia (owing to sodium content of preparations)
CAUTIONS, FURTHER INFORMATION
▸ Cholestatic jaundice Cholestatic jaundice is possibly associated with clavulanic acid. An epidemiological study has shown that the risk of acute liver toxicity was about 6 times greater with co-amoxiclav (amoxicillin, clavulanic acid) than with amoxicillin. Cholestatic jaundice is more common in patients above the age of 65 years and in men; these reactions have only rarely been reported in children. Jaundice is usually self-limiting and very rarely fatal. The duration of treatment should be appropriate to the indication and should not usually exceed 14 days.

● SIDE-EFFECTS Eosinophilia · haemorrhagic cystitis (more frequent in children) · hypokalaemia · injection-site reactions · nausea · Stevens-Johnson syndrome · toxic epidermal necrolysis · vomiting

● PREGNANCY Not known to be harmful.

● BREAST FEEDING Trace amounts in milk, but appropriate to use.

● HEPATIC IMPAIRMENT Manufacturer advises caution in severe impairment.

● RENAL IMPAIRMENT Reduce dose to 3.2 g every eight hours if eGFR 30–60 mL/minute/1.73 m^2; 1.6 g every eight hours if eGFR 10–30 mL/minute/1.73 m^2; 1.6 g every twelve hours if eGFR less than 10 mL/minute/1.73 m^2.

Accumulation of electrolytes contained in preparation can occur in patients with renal failure.

● EFFECT ON LABORATORY TESTS False-positive urinary glucose (if tested for reducing substances).

● DIRECTIONS FOR ADMINISTRATION For *intravenous infusion* (*Timentin®*), give intermittently in Glucose 5%. Suggested volume (depending on dose) 100–150 mL; give over 30–40 minutes.

● PRESCRIBING AND DISPENSING INFORMATION Dose is expressed as a combination of ticarcillin (as sodium salt) and clavulanic acid (as potassium salt) in a ratio of 15:1.

● MEDICINAL FORMS
There can be variation in the licensing of different medicines containing the same drug.
Powder for solution for infusion
ELECTROLYTES: May contain Potassium, sodium
▸ Timentin (GlaxoSmithKline UK Ltd)
  Clavulanic acid (as Potassium clavulanate) 200 mg, Ticarcillin (as Ticarcillin sodium) 3 gram Timentin 3.2g powder for solution for infusion vials | 4 vial [PoM] £21.32

ANTIBACTERIALS ⟩ PENICILLINS, BETA-LACTAMASE SENSITIVE

F 495

Benzylpenicillin sodium
(Penicillin G)

● INDICATIONS AND DOSE
Mild to moderate susceptible infections | Throat infections | Otitis media | Cellulitis | Pneumonia
▸ BY INTRAMUSCULAR INJECTION, OR BY SLOW INTRAVENOUS INJECTION, OR BY INTRAVENOUS INFUSION
▸ Adult: 0.6–1.2 g every 6 hours, dose may be increased if necessary in more serious infections (consult product literature), single doses over 1.2 g to be given by intravenous route only

Endocarditis (in combination with other antibacterial if necessary)
▸ BY SLOW INTRAVENOUS INJECTION, OR BY INTRAVENOUS INFUSION
▸ Adult: 1.2 g every 4 hours, increased if necessary to 2.4 g every 4 hours, dose may be increased in infections such as enterococcal endocarditis

Anthrax (in combination with other antibacterials)
▸ BY SLOW INTRAVENOUS INJECTION, OR BY INTRAVENOUS INFUSION
▸ Adult: 2.4 g every 4 hours

Intrapartum prophylaxis against group B streptococcal infection
▸ BY SLOW INTRAVENOUS INJECTION, OR BY INTRAVENOUS INFUSION
▸ Adult: Initially 3 g for 1 dose, then 1.5 g every 4 hours until delivery

Meningitis | Meningococcal disease
▸ BY SLOW INTRAVENOUS INJECTION, OR BY INTRAVENOUS INFUSION
▸ Adult: 2.4 g every 4 hours
▸ BY INTRAVENOUS INFUSION
▸ Child: 50 mg/kg every 4–6 hours (max. per dose 2.4 g every 4 hours)

Suspected meningococcal disease (meningitis with non-blanching rash or meningococcal septicaemia) prior to urgent transfer to hospital
▸ BY INTRAVENOUS INJECTION, OR BY INTRAMUSCULAR INJECTION
  ▸ Child 1–11 months: 300 mg, administer as single dose prior to urgent transfer to hospital so long as does not delay transfer
  ▸ Child 1–9 years: 600 mg, administer as single dose prior to urgent transfer to hospital so long as does not delay transfer
  ▸ Child 10–17 years: 1.2 g, administer as single dose prior to urgent transfer to hospital so long as does not delay transfer
  ▸ Adult: 1.2 g, administer as single dose prior to urgent transfer to hospital so long as does not delay transfer

Suspected bacterial meningitis without non-blanching rash where patient cannot be transferred to hospital urgently
▸ BY INTRAVENOUS INJECTION, OR BY INTRAMUSCULAR INJECTION
  ▸ Child 1–11 months: 300 mg, administer as single dose prior to transfer to hospital
  ▸ Child 1–9 years: 600 mg, administer as single dose prior to transfer to hospital
  ▸ Child 10–17 years: 1.2 g, administer as single dose prior to transfer to hospital
  ▸ Adult: 1.2 g, administer as single dose prior to transfer to hospital

● UNLICENSED USE Benzylpenicillin doses in the BNF may differ from those in product literature.

> IMPORTANT SAFETY INFORMATION
> Intrathecal injection of benzylpenicillin is **not** recommended.

● CAUTIONS Accumulation of sodium from injection can occur with high doses
● PREGNANCY Not known to be harmful.
● BREAST FEEDING Trace amounts in milk, but appropriate to use.
● RENAL IMPAIRMENT
Accumulation of sodium from injection can occur in renal failure.
  High doses may cause neurotoxicity, including cerebral irritation, convulsions, or coma.
▸ In adults Reduce dose—consult product literature.
▸ In children Estimated glomerular filtration rate 10–50 mL/minute/1.73 m², use normal dose every 8–12 hours. Estimated glomerular filtration rate less than 10 mL/minute/1.73 m² use normal dose every 12 hours.
● EFFECT ON LABORATORY TESTS False-positive urinary glucose (if tested for reducing substances).
● DIRECTIONS FOR ADMINISTRATION
▸ With intravenous use in children Intravenous route recommended in neonates and infants. For *intravenous infusion*, dilute with Glucose 5% or Sodium Chloride 0.9%; give over 15–30 minutes. Longer administration time is particularly important when using doses of 50 mg/kg (or greater) to avoid CNS toxicity.
▸ With intravenous use in adults For *intravenous infusion* (Crystapen ®), give intermittently in Glucose 5% or Sodium chloride 0.9%; suggested volume 100 mL given over 30–60 minutes. Continuous infusion not usually recommended.

● MEDICINAL FORMS
There can be variation in the licensing of different medicines containing the same drug. Forms available from special-order manufacturers include: infusion
Powder for solution for injection
ELECTROLYTES: May contain Sodium
▸ Benzylpenicillin sodium (Non-proprietary)
  Benzylpenicillin sodium 600 mg Benzylpenicillin 600mg powder for solution for injection vials | 2 vial PoM £4.67 DT price = £4.67 | 25 vial PoM £58.37–£58.38
  Benzylpenicillin sodium 1.2 gram Benzylpenicillin 1.2g powder for solution for injection vials | 25 vial PoM £78.64 DT price = £78.64

F 495

Phenoxymethylpenicillin
(Penicillin V)

● INDICATIONS AND DOSE
Oral infections | Tonsillitis | Otitis media | Erysipelas | Cellulitis
▸ BY MOUTH
  ▸ Child 1–11 months: 62.5 mg 4 times a day; increased if necessary up to 12.5 mg/kg 4 times a day
  ▸ Child 1–5 years: 125 mg 4 times a day; increased if necessary up to 12.5 mg/kg 4 times a day
  ▸ Child 6–11 years: 250 mg 4 times a day; increased if necessary up to 12.5 mg/kg 4 times a day
  ▸ Child 12–17 years: 500 mg 4 times a day; increased if necessary up to 1 g 4 times a day
  ▸ Adult: 500 mg every 6 hours, increased if necessary up to 1 g every 6 hours

Prevention of recurrence of rheumatic fever
▸ BY MOUTH
  ▸ Child 1 month–5 years: 125 mg twice daily
  ▸ Child 6–17 years: 250 mg twice daily
  ▸ Adult: 250 mg twice daily

Prevention of secondary case of invasive group A streptococcal infection
▸ BY MOUTH
  ▸ Child 1–11 months: 62.5 mg every 6 hours for 10 days
  ▸ Child 1–5 years: 125 mg every 6 hours for 10 days
  ▸ Child 6–11 years: 250 mg every 6 hours for 10 days
  ▸ Child 12–17 years: 250–500 mg every 6 hours for 10 days
  ▸ Adult: 250–500 mg every 6 hours for 10 days

Prevention of pneumococcal infection in asplenia or in patients with sickle-cell disease
▸ BY MOUTH
  ▸ Child 1–11 months: 62.5 mg twice daily
  ▸ Child 1–4 years: 125 mg twice daily
  ▸ Child 5–17 years: 250 mg twice daily
  ▸ Adult: 250 mg twice daily

● UNLICENSED USE Phenoxymethylpenicillin doses in the BNF may differ from product literature.
● PREGNANCY Not known to be harmful.
● BREAST FEEDING Trace amounts in milk, but appropriate to use.
● EFFECT ON LABORATORY TESTS False-positive urinary glucose (if tested for reducing substances).
● PATIENT AND CARER ADVICE
Medicines for Children leaflet: Penicillin V for bacterial infections www.medicinesforchildren.org.uk/penicillin-v-for-bacterial-infections
Medicines for Children leaflet: Penicillin V for prevention of pneumococcal infection www.medicinesforchildren.org.uk/penicillin-v-for-prevention-of-pneumococcal-infection
● PROFESSION SPECIFIC INFORMATION
Dental practitioners' formulary
Phenoxymethylpenicillin Tablets may be prescribed.
  Phenoxymethylpenicillin Oral Solution may be prescribed.

5

Infection

5

Infection

● MEDICINAL FORMS
There can be variation in the licensing of different medicines containing the same drug.

Tablet
CAUTIONARY AND ADVISORY LABELS 9, 23
▶ Phenoxymethylpenicillin (Non-proprietary)
Phenoxymethylpenicillin (as Phenoxymethylpenicillin potassium)
250 mg Phenoxymethylpenicillin 250mg tablets | 28 tablet [PoM]
£5.00 DT price = £0.91

Oral solution
CAUTIONARY AND ADVISORY LABELS 9, 23
▶ Phenoxymethylpenicillin (Non-proprietary)
Phenoxymethylpenicillin (as Phenoxymethylpenicillin potassium)
25 mg per 1 ml Phenoxymethylpenicillin 125mg/5ml oral solution |
100 ml £80.00 DT price = £14.73
Phenoxymethylpenicillin 125mg/5ml oral solution sugar free sugar-
free | 100 ml [PoM] £25.00 DT price = £16.02
Phenoxymethylpenicillin (as Phenoxymethylpenicillin potassium)
50 mg per 1 ml Phenoxymethylpenicillin 250mg/5ml oral solution |
100 ml [PoM] £80.00 DT price = £14.66
Phenoxymethylpenicillin 250mg/5ml oral solution sugar free sugar-
free | 100 ml [PoM] £35.00 DT price = £16.02

ANTIBACTERIALS › PENICILLINS, BROAD-SPECTRUM

◀ 495

Amoxicillin

(Amoxycillin)

● INDICATIONS AND DOSE

Susceptible infections (including urinary-tract infections, otitis media, sinusitis, uncomplicated community acquired pneumonia, salmonellosis, oral infections)
▶ BY MOUTH
▶ Child 1-11 months: 125 mg 3 times a day; increased if necessary up to 30 mg/kg 3 times a day
▶ Child 1-4 years: 250 mg 3 times a day; increased if necessary up to 30 mg/kg 3 times a day
▶ Child 5-11 years: 500 mg 3 times a day; increased if necessary up to 30 mg/kg 3 times a day (max. per dose 1 g)
▶ Child 12-17 years: 500 mg 3 times a day; increased if necessary up to 1 g 3 times a day, use increased dose in severe infections
▶ Adult: 500 mg every 8 hours, increased if necessary to 1 g every 8 hours, increased dose used in severe infections
▶ BY INTRAMUSCULAR INJECTION
▶ Adult: 500 mg every 8 hours
▶ BY INTRAVENOUS INJECTION, OR BY INTRAVENOUS INFUSION
▶ Adult: 500 mg every 8 hours, increased to 1 g every 6 hours, use increased dose in severe infections

Lyme disease (under expert supervision)
▶ BY MOUTH
▶ Child 5-17 years: 500 mg 3 times a day for 14–21 days (for 28 days in Lyme arthritis)
▶ Adult: 500 mg 3 times a day for 14–21 days (for 28 days in Lyme arthritis)

Anthrax (treatment and post-exposure prophylaxis)
▶ BY MOUTH
▶ Child (body-weight up to 20 kg): 80 mg/kg daily in 3 divided doses
▶ Child (body-weight 20 kg and above): 500 mg 3 times a day
▶ Adult: 500 mg 3 times a day

Dental abscess (short course)
▶ BY MOUTH
▶ Adult: 3 g, then 3 g after 8 hours

Urinary-tract infections (short course)
▶ BY MOUTH
▶ Adult: 3 g, then 3 g after 10–12 hours

Listerial meningitis (in combination with another antibiotic)
▶ BY INTRAVENOUS INFUSION
▶ Adult: 2 g every 4 hours

Endocarditis (in combination with another antibiotic if necessary)
▶ BY INTRAVENOUS INFUSION
▶ Adult: 2 g every 4 hours

Prevention of pneumococcal infection in asplenia or in patients with sickle-cell disease—if cover also needed for *Haemophilus influenzae*
▶ BY MOUTH
▶ Child 1 month-4 years: 125 mg twice daily
▶ Child 5-11 years: 250 mg twice daily
▶ Child 12-17 years: 500 mg twice daily

***Helicobacter pylori* eradication in combination with metronidazole and omeprazole**
▶ BY MOUTH
▶ Adult: 500 mg 3 times a day

***Helicobacter pylori* eradication in combination with clarithromycin and esomeprazole; or in combination with clarithromycin and lansoprazole; or in combination with metronidazole and lansoprazole; or in combination with clarithromycin and omeprazole; or in combination with clarithromycin and pantoprazole; or in combination with clarithromycin and rabeprazole**
▶ BY MOUTH
▶ Adult: 1 g twice daily

● UNLICENSED USE Amoxicillin doses in BNF Publications may differ from those in product literature.
● CAUTIONS
GENERAL CAUTIONS
Acute lymphocytic leukaemia (increased risk of erythematous rashes) · chronic lymphocytic leukaemia (increased risk of erythematous rashes) · cytomegalovirus infection (increased risk of erythematous rashes) · glandular fever (erythematous rashes common) · maintain adequate hydration with high doses (particularly during parenteral therapy)
SPECIFIC CAUTIONS
▶ With intravenous use Accumulation of sodium can occur with high parenteral doses
● SIDE-EFFECTS
▶ Common or very common Nausea · vomiting
SIDE-EFFECTS, FURTHER INFORMATION
▶ Rash If rash occurs, discontinue treatment.
● PREGNANCY Not known to be harmful.
● BREAST FEEDING Trace amount in milk, but appropriate to use.
● RENAL IMPAIRMENT Reduce dose in severe impairment; rashes more common. Risk of crystalluria with high doses (particularly during parenteral therapy).
▶ With intravenous use Accumulation of sodium from injection can occur in patients with renal failure.
● DIRECTIONS FOR ADMINISTRATION
▶ With intravenous use in children Displacement value may be significant when reconstituting injection, consult local guidelines. Dilute intravenous injection to a concentration of 50 mg/mL (100 mg/mL for neonates). May be further diluted with Glucose 5% *or* Glucose 10% *or* Sodium chloride 0.9% *or* 0.45% for intravenous infusion. Give intravenous infusion over 30 minutes when using doses over 30 mg/kg.
▶ With intravenous use in adults For *intravenous infusion* (*Amoxil®*), give intermittently *in* Glucose 5% *or* Sodium chloride 0.9%. Reconstituted solutions diluted and given without delay; suggested volume 100 mL given over 30–60 minutes or *givevia* drip tubing *in* Glucose 5% *or*

Sodium chloride 0.9%; continuous infusion not usually recommended.

● PRESCRIBING AND DISPENSING INFORMATION Flavours of oral liquid formulations and sachets may include peach, strawberry, or lemon.

● PATIENT AND CARER ADVICE
Medicines for Children leaflet: Amoxicillin for bacterial infections www.medicinesforchildren.org.uk/amoxicillin-bacterial-infections-0
   Patient counselling is advised for Amoxicillin (*Amoxil®*) paediatric suspension (use of pipette).

● PROFESSION SPECIFIC INFORMATION

Dental practitioners' formulary
Amoxicillin capsules may be prescribed.
   Amoxicillin sachets may be prescribed as Amoxicillin Oral Powder.
   Amoxicillin Oral Suspension may be prescribed.

● MEDICINAL FORMS
There can be variation in the licensing of different medicines containing the same drug.

Capsule
CAUTIONARY AND ADVISORY LABELS 9
▸ Amoxicillin (Non-proprietary)
Amoxicillin (as Amoxicillin trihydrate) 250 mg Amoxicillin 250mg capsules | 15 capsule [PoM] £5.00 DT price = £0.73 | 21 capsule [PoM] £5.00 DT price = £1.02 | 500 capsule [PoM] £120.00
Amoxicillin (as Amoxicillin trihydrate) 500 mg Amoxicillin 500mg capsules | 15 capsule [PoM] £7.50 DT price = £0.91 | 21 capsule [PoM] £15.00 DT price = £1.27 | 100 capsule [PoM] £75.00
▸ Amoxil (GlaxoSmithKline UK Ltd)
Amoxicillin (as Amoxicillin trihydrate) 250 mg Amoxil 250mg capsules | 21 capsule [PoM] £3.38 DT price = £1.02
Amoxicillin (as Amoxicillin trihydrate) 500 mg Amoxil 500mg capsules | 21 capsule [PoM] £6.77 DT price = £1.27

Oral suspension
CAUTIONARY AND ADVISORY LABELS 9
EXCIPIENTS: May contain Sucrose
▸ Amoxicillin (Non-proprietary)
Amoxicillin (as Amoxicillin trihydrate) 25 mg per 1 ml Amoxicillin 125mg/5ml oral suspension sugar free sugar-free | 100 ml [PoM] £25.00 DT price = £1.02
Amoxicillin 125mg/5ml oral suspension | 100 ml [PoM] £25.00 DT price = £0.97
Amoxicillin (as Amoxicillin trihydrate) 50 mg per 1 ml Amoxicillin 250mg/5ml oral suspension sugar free sugar-free | 100 ml [PoM] £35.00 DT price = £1.18
Amoxicillin 250mg/5ml oral suspension | 100 ml [PoM] £35.00 DT price = £1.15
▸ Amoxil (GlaxoSmithKline UK Ltd)
Amoxicillin (as Amoxicillin trihydrate) 100 mg per 1 ml Amoxil 125mg/1.25ml paediatric oral suspension | 20 ml [PoM] £3.18 DT price = £3.18

Powder for solution for injection
ELECTROLYTES: May contain Sodium
▸ Amoxicillin (Non-proprietary)
Amoxicillin (as Amoxicillin sodium) 250 mg Amoxicillin 250mg powder for solution for injection vials | 10 vial [PoM] £4.65–£4.80
Amoxicillin (as Amoxicillin sodium) 500 mg Amoxicillin 500mg powder for solution for injection vials | 10 vial [PoM] £8.55–£9.60 DT price = £5.48
Amoxicillin (as Amoxicillin sodium) 1 gram Amoxicillin 1g powder for solution for injection vials | 1 vial [PoM] £1.92 | 10 vial [PoM] £16.50 DT price = £10.96
▸ Amoxil (GlaxoSmithKline UK Ltd)
Amoxicillin (as Amoxicillin sodium) 500 mg Amoxil 500mg powder for solution for injection vials | 10 vial [PoM] £5.48 DT price = £5.48
Amoxicillin (as Amoxicillin sodium) 1 gram Amoxil 1g powder for solution for injection vials | 10 vial [PoM] £10.96 DT price = £10.96

Powder
CAUTIONARY AND ADVISORY LABELS 9, 13
▸ Amoxicillin (Non-proprietary)
Amoxicillin (as Amoxicillin trihydrate) 3 gram Amoxicillin 3g oral powder sachets sugar free sugar-free | 2 sachet [PoM] £15.00 DT price = £9.98

▸ Amoxil (GlaxoSmithKline UK Ltd)
Amoxicillin (as Amoxicillin trihydrate) 3 gram Amoxil 3g oral powder sachets sucrose free sugar-free | 2 sachet [PoM] £2.99 DT price = £9.98

◀ 495

Ampicillin

● INDICATIONS AND DOSE

Susceptible infections (including bronchitis, urinary-tract infections, otitis media, sinusitis, uncomplicated community-acquired pneumonia, salmonellosis)
▸ BY MOUTH
▸ Child 1–11 months: 125 mg 4 times a day; increased if necessary up to 30 mg/kg 4 times a day
▸ Child 1–4 years: 250 mg 4 times a day; increased if necessary up to 30 mg/kg 4 times a day
▸ Child 5–11 years: 500 mg 4 times a day; increased if necessary up to 30 mg/kg 4 times a day (max. per dose 1 g)
▸ Child 12–17 years: 500 mg 4 times a day; increased if necessary to 1 g 4 times a day, use increased dose in severe infection
▸ Adult: 0.5–1 g every 6 hours
▸ BY INTRAVENOUS INJECTION, OR BY INTRAVENOUS INFUSION
▸ Adult: 500 mg every 4–6 hours
▸ BY INTRAMUSCULAR INJECTION
▸ Adult: 500 mg every 4–6 hours

Endocarditis (in combination with another antibiotic if necessary) | Listerial meningitis (in combination with another antibiotic)
▸ BY INTRAVENOUS INFUSION
▸ Adult: 2 g every 4 hours

● UNLICENSED USE Ampicillin doses in BNF may differ from those in product literature.

● CAUTIONS
GENERAL CAUTIONS
Acute lymphocytic leukaemia (increased risk of erythematous rashes) · chronic lymphocytic leukaemia (increased risk of erythematous rashes) · cytomegalovirus infection (increased risk of erythematous rashes) · glandular fever (erythematous rashes common)
SPECIFIC CAUTIONS
▸ With intravenous use Accumulation of electrolytes contained in parenteral preparations can occur with high doses

● SIDE-EFFECTS
▸ **Common or very common** Nausea · vomiting
SIDE-EFFECTS, FURTHER INFORMATION
▸ Rash If rash occurs, discontinue treatment.

● PREGNANCY Not known to be harmful.

● BREAST FEEDING Trace amounts in milk, but appropriate to use.

● RENAL IMPAIRMENT
▸ In adults Reduce dose if eGFR less than 10 mL/minute/1.73 m^2; rashes more common.
▸ In children If estimated glomerular filtration rate less than 10 mL/minute/1.73 m^2 reduce dose or frequency; rashes more common.
▸ With intravenous use Accumulation of electrolytes contained in parenteral preparations can occur in patients with renal failure.

● DIRECTIONS FOR ADMINISTRATION
▸ With oral use Administer at least 30 minutes before food.
▸ With intravenous use in children Displacement value may be significant when reconstituting injection, consult local guidelines. Dilute intravenous injection to a concentration of 50–100 mg/mL. May be further diluted with glucose 5% or 10% *or* sodium chloride 0.9% or 0.45% for infusion. Give

over 30 minutes when using doses of greater than 50 mg/kg to avoid CNS toxicity including convulsions.
▸ With intravenous use in adults For *intravenous infusion* (*Penbritin*®), give intermittently *in* Glucose 5% *or* Sodium chloride 0.9%. Reconstituted solutions diluted and given without delay; suggested volume 100 mL given over 30–60 minutes *via* drip tubing *in* Glucose 5% *or* Sodium chloride 0.9%. Continuous infusion not usually recommended.

● PATIENT AND CARER ADVICE
Medicines for Children leaflet: Ampicillin for bacterial infection www.medicinesforchildren.org.uk/ampicillin-bacterial-infection

● MEDICINAL FORMS
There can be variation in the licensing of different medicines containing the same drug.

Capsule
CAUTIONARY AND ADVISORY LABELS 9, 23
▸ Ampicillin (Non-proprietary)
   Ampicillin 250 mg Ampicillin 250mg capsules | 28 capsule [PoM] £25.00 DT price = £5.48
   Ampicillin 500 mg Ampicillin 500mg capsules | 28 capsule [PoM] £35.00 DT price = £29.92
▸ Penbritin (Chemidex Pharma Ltd)
   Ampicillin 250 mg Penbritin 250mg capsules | 28 capsule [PoM] £2.10 DT price = £5.48
   Ampicillin 500 mg Penbritin 500mg capsules | 28 capsule [PoM] £5.28 DT price = £29.92

Oral suspension
CAUTIONARY AND ADVISORY LABELS 9, 23
▸ Ampicillin (Non-proprietary)
   Ampicillin 25 mg per 1 ml Ampicillin 125mg/5ml oral suspension | 100 ml [PoM] £29.86 DT price = £29.86
   Ampicillin 50 mg per 1 ml Ampicillin 250mg/5ml oral suspension | 100 ml [PoM] £38.86 DT price = £38.86

Powder for solution for injection
▸ Ampicillin (Non-proprietary)
   Ampicillin (as Ampicillin sodium) 500 mg Ampicillin 500mg powder for solution for injection vials | 10 vial [PoM] £78.30 DT price = £78.30

F 495

Co-fluampicil

● INDICATIONS AND DOSE
Mixed infections involving beta-lactamase-producing staphylococci
▸ BY MOUTH
▸ Child 1 month-9 years: 125/125 mg every 6 hours
▸ Child 10-17 years: 250/250 mg every 6 hours
▸ Adult: 250/250 mg every 6 hours
▸ BY INTRAMUSCULAR INJECTION, OR BY SLOW INTRAVENOUS INJECTION, OR BY INTRAVENOUS INFUSION
▸ Adult: 250/250 mg every 6 hours

Severe mixed infections involving beta-lactamase-producing staphylococci
▸ BY MOUTH
▸ Child 1 month-9 years: 250/250 mg every 6 hours
▸ Adult: 500/500 mg every 6 hours
▸ BY INTRAMUSCULAR INJECTION, OR BY SLOW INTRAVENOUS INJECTION, OR BY INTRAVENOUS INFUSION
▸ Adult: 500/500 mg every 6 hours

IMPORTANT SAFETY INFORMATION
HEPATIC DISORDERS
Cholestatic jaundice and hepatitis may occur very rarely, up to two months after treatment with flucloxacillin has been stopped. Administration for more than 2 weeks and increasing age are risk factors. Healthcare professionals are reminded that:
● flucloxacillin should not be used in patients with a history of hepatic dysfunction associated with flucloxacillin;

● flucloxacillin should be used with caution in patients with hepatic impairment;
● careful enquiry should be made about hypersensitivity reactions to beta-lactam antibacterials.

● CAUTIONS
GENERAL CAUTIONS
Acute lymphocytic leukaemia (increased risk of erythematous rashes) · chronic lymphocytic leukaemia (increased risk of erythematous rashes) · cytomegalovirus infection (increased risk of erythematous rashes) · glandular fever (erythematous rashes common)
SPECIFIC CAUTIONS
▸ With intravenous use Accumulation of electrolytes contained in parenteral preparations can occur with high doses

● SIDE-EFFECTS
▸ **Common or very common** Gastro-intestinal disturbances · nausea · vomiting
▸ **Very rare** Cholestatic jaundice · hepatitis
SIDE-EFFECTS, FURTHER INFORMATION
▸ Rash If rash occurs, discontinue treatment.

● PREGNANCY Not known to be harmful.

● BREAST FEEDING Trace amount in milk, but appropriate to use.

● HEPATIC IMPAIRMENT Use with caution.

● RENAL IMPAIRMENT
▸ In adults Reduce dose if eGFR less than 10 mL/minute/1.73 m^2; rashes more common.
▸ In children Reduce dose or frequency if estimated glomerular filtration rate less than 10 mL/minute/1.73 m^2; rashes more common.
▸ With intravenous use Accumulation of electrolytes contained in parenteral preparations can occur in patients with renal failure.

● EFFECT ON LABORATORY TESTS False-positive urinary glucose (if tested for reducing substances).

● DIRECTIONS FOR ADMINISTRATION For *intravenous infusion* (*Magnapen*®), give intermittently *in* Glucose 5% *or* Sodium chloride 0.9%. Reconstituted solutions diluted and given without delay; suggested volume 100 mL given over 30–60 minutes. *Via* drip tubing *in* Glucose 5% *or* Sodium chloride 0.9%.

● PRESCRIBING AND DISPENSING INFORMATION Dose expressed as a combination of equal parts by mass of flucloxacillin and ampicillin.

● MEDICINAL FORMS
There can be variation in the licensing of different medicines containing the same drug.
Capsule
CAUTIONARY AND ADVISORY LABELS 9, 22
▸ Co-fluampicil (Non-proprietary)
   Ampicillin (as Ampicillin trihydrate) 250 mg, Flucloxacillin (as Flucloxacillin sodium) 250 mg Co-fluampicil 250mg/250mg capsules | 28 capsule [PoM] £10.31 DT price = £2.21 | 100 capsule [PoM] £13.41-£42.99

Oral suspension
CAUTIONARY AND ADVISORY LABELS 9, 22
▸ Co-fluampicil (Non-proprietary)
   Ampicillin (as Ampicillin trihydrate) 25 mg per 1 ml, Flucloxacillin (as Flucloxacillin magnesium) 25 mg per 1 ml Co-fluampicil 125mg/125mg/5ml oral suspension | 100 ml [PoM] £23.93 DT price = £23.93

Powder for solution for injection
ELECTROLYTES: May contain Sodium
▸ Co-fluampicil (Non-proprietary)
   Ampicillin (as Ampicillin sodium) 250 mg, Flucloxacillin (as Flucloxacillin sodium) 250 mg Co-fluampicil 250mg/250mg powder for solution for injection vials | 10 vial [PoM] £13.33

ANTIBACTERIALS > PENICILLINS, BROAD-SPECTRUM WITH BETA-LACTAMASE INHIBITOR

🔖 495

Co-amoxiclav

● **INDICATIONS AND DOSE**

Infections due to beta-lactamase-producing strains (where amoxicillin alone not appropriate), including respiratory tract infections, bone and joint infections, genito-urinary and abdominal infections, cellulitis and animal bites

▸ BY MOUTH USING TABLETS
▸ Child 12-17 years: 250/125 mg every 8 hours; increased to 500/125 mg every 8 hours, increased dose used for severe infection
▸ Adult: 250/125 mg every 8 hours; increased to 500/125 mg every 8 hours, increased dose used for severe infection
▸ BY INTRAVENOUS INJECTION, OR BY INTRAVENOUS INFUSION
▸ Child 1-2 months: 30 mg/kg every 12 hours
▸ Child 3 months-17 years: 30 mg/kg every 8 hours (max. per dose 1.2 g every 8 hours)
▸ Adult: 1.2 g every 8 hours

Infections due to beta-lactamase-producing strains (where amoxicillin alone not appropriate) including respiratory-tract infections, bone and joint infections, genito-urinary and abdominal infections, cellulitis, animal bites (doses for 125/31 suspension)

▸ BY MOUTH USING ORAL SUSPENSION
▸ Child 1-11 months: 0.25 mL/kilogram 3 times a day, dose doubled in severe infection
▸ Child 1-5 years: 0.25 mL/kilogram 3 times a day, alternatively 5 mL 3 times a day, dose doubled in severe infection

Infections due to beta-lactamase-producing strains (where amoxicillin alone not appropriate) including respiratory-tract infections, bone and joint infections, genito-urinary and abdominal infections, cellulitis, animal bites (doses for 250/62 suspension)

▸ BY MOUTH USING ORAL SUSPENSION
▸ Child 6-11 years: 0.15 mL/kilogram 3 times a day, alternatively 5 mL 3 times a day, dose doubled in severe infection

Infections due to beta-lactamase-producing strains (where amoxicillin alone not appropriate) including respiratory-tract infections, bone and joint infections, genito-urinary and abdominal infections, cellulitis, animal bites (doses for 400/57 suspension)

▸ BY MOUTH USING ORAL SUSPENSION
▸ Child 2 months-1 year: 0.15 mL/kilogram twice daily, doubled in severe infection
▸ Child 2-6 years (body-weight 13-21 kg): 2.5 mL twice daily, doubled in severe infection
▸ Child 7-12 years (body-weight 22-40 kg): 5 mL twice daily, doubled in severe infection
▸ Child 12-17 years (body-weight 41 kg and above): 10 mL twice daily; increased if necessary to 10 mL 3 times a day, increased frequency to be used in severe infection
▸ Adult: 10 mL twice daily; increased if necessary to 10 mL 3 times a day, increased frequency to be used in severe infection

Severe dental infection with spreading cellulitis | Dental infection not responding to first-line antibacterial

▸ BY MOUTH USING TABLETS
▸ Child 12-17 years: 250/125 mg every 8 hours for 5 days
▸ Adult: 250/125 mg every 8 hours for 5 days

Surgical prophylaxis

▸ BY INTRAVENOUS INJECTION, OR BY INTRAVENOUS INFUSION
▸ Adult: 1.2 g, to be administered up to 30 minutes before the procedure, then 1.2 g every 8 hours for up to 2-3 further doses in high risk procedures

DOSE EQUIVALENCE AND CONVERSION
Doses are expressed as co-amoxiclav.
A mixture of amoxicillin (as the trihydrate or as the sodium salt) and clavulanic acid (as potassium clavulanate); the proportions are expressed in the form x/y where x and y are the strengths in milligrams of amoxicillin and clavulanic acid respectively.

● CONTRA-INDICATIONS History of co-amoxiclav-associated jaundice or hepatic dysfunction · history of penicillin-associated jaundice or hepatic dysfunction

● CAUTIONS
GENERAL CAUTIONS
Acute lymphocytic leukaemia (increased risk of erythematous rashes) · chronic lymphocytic leukaemia (increased risk of erythematous rashes) · cytomegalovirus infection (increased risk of erythematous rashes) · glandular fever (erythematous rashes common) · maintain adequate hydration with high doses (particularly during parental therapy)

SPECIFIC CAUTIONS
▸ With intravenous use Accumulation of electrolytes contained in parenteral preparations can occur with high doses

CAUTIONS, FURTHER INFORMATION
▸ Cholestatic jaundice Cholestatic jaundice can occur either during or shortly after the use of co-amoxiclav. An epidemiological study has shown that the risk of acute liver toxicity was about 6 times greater with co-amoxiclav than with amoxicillin. Cholestatic jaundice is more common in patients above the age of 65 years and in men; these reactions have only rarely been reported in children. Jaundice is usually self-limiting and very rarely fatal. The duration of treatment should be appropriate to the indication and should not usually exceed 14 days.

● SIDE-EFFECTS
GENERAL SIDE-EFFECTS
▸ **Common or very common** Cholestatic jaundice · hepatitis · nausea · vomiting
▸ **Rare** Dizziness · headache · prolongation of bleeding time
▸ **Frequency not known** Exfoliative dermatitis · Steven-Johnson syndrome · toxic epidermal necrolysis · vasculitis

SPECIFIC SIDE-EFFECTS
▸ **Rare**
▸ With intravenous use Phlebitis at injection site
▸ With oral use Superficial staining of teeth with suspension

SIDE-EFFECTS, FURTHER INFORMATION
▸ Rash If rash occurs, discontinue treatment.

● PREGNANCY Not known to be harmful.

● BREAST FEEDING Trace amount in milk, but appropriate to use.

● HEPATIC IMPAIRMENT
Monitoring
Monitor liver function in liver disease.

● RENAL IMPAIRMENT
Risk of crystalluria with high doses (particularly during parenteral therapy).
▸ With oral use in adults *Co-amoxiclav* 250/125 *tablets or* 500/125 *tablets*: if eGFR 10–30 mL/minute/1.73 m^2, one 250/125 strength tablet every 12 hours or one 500/125 strength tablet every 12 hours; if eGFR less than 10 mL/minute/1.73 m^2, one 250/125 strength tablet every 24 hours or one 500/125 strength tablet every 24 hours.

5

Infection

5

Infection

Co-amoxiclav 400/57 *suspension* : avoid if eGFR less than 30 mL/minute/1.73 m².

▸ With intravenous use Accumulation of electrolytes contained in parenteral preparations can occur in patients with renal failure.

▸ With intravenous use in adults *Co-amoxiclav injection* (expressed as co-amoxiclav): if eGFR 10–30 mL/minute/1.73 m², 1.2 g initially, then 600 mg every 12 hours; if eGFR less than 10 mL/minute/1.73 m², 1.2 g initially, then 600 mg every 24 hours.

▸ With oral use in children *Co-amoxiclav* 125/31 *suspension*, 250/62 *suspension*, 250/125 *tablets, or* 500/125 *tablets* : use normal dose every 12 hours if estimated glomerular filtration rate 10–30 mL/minute/1.73 m². Use the normal dose recommended for mild or moderate infections every 12 hours if estimated glomerular filtration rate less than 10 mL/minute/1.73 m². *Co-amoxiclav* 400/57 *suspension* : avoid if estimated glomerular filtration rate less than 30 mL/minute/1.73 m².

▸ With intravenous use in children *Co-amoxiclav injection* : use normal initial dose and then use half normal dose every 12 hours if estimated glomerular filtration rate 10–30 mL/minute/1.73 m²; use normal initial dose and then use half normal dose every 24 hours if estimated glomerular filtration rate less than 10 mL/minute/1.73 m².

● DIRECTIONS FOR ADMINISTRATION

▸ With intravenous use in children For *intravenous infusion*, dilute reconstituted solution to a concentration of 10 mg/mL with Sodium Chloride 0.9%; give intermittently over 30–40 minutes. For *intravenous injection*, administer over 3–4 minutes.

▸ With intravenous use in adults For *intravenous infusion* (*Augmentin®*), give intermittently in Sodium chloride 0.9%. Reconstitute 600 mg initially with 10 mL water for injections, then dilute with 50 mL infusion fluid; reconstitute 1.2 g initially with 20 mL water for injections, then dilute with 100 mL infusion fluid; give over 30–40 minutes. For *intravenous injection*, administer over 3–4 minutes. *Via* drip tubing in Sodium chloride 0.9%.

● PRESCRIBING AND DISPENSING INFORMATION Doses are expressed as co-amoxiclav: a mixture of amoxicillin (as the trihydrate or as the sodium salt) and clavulanic acid (as potassium clavulanate); the proportions are expressed in the form x/y where x and y are the strengths in milligrams of amoxicillin and clavulanic acid respectively.

▸ With oral use Flavours of oral liquid formulations may include raspberry and orange.

● PATIENT AND CARER ADVICE

Medicines for Children leaflet: Co-amoxiclav for bacterial infections www.medicinesforchildren.org.uk/co-amoxiclav-bacterial-infections-0

● PROFESSION SPECIFIC INFORMATION

Dental practitioners' formulary
Co-amoxiclav 250/125 Tablets may be prescribed.
Co-amoxiclav 125/31 Suspension may be prescribed.
Co-amoxiclav 250/62 Suspension may be prescribed.

● MEDICINAL FORMS
There can be variation in the licensing of different medicines containing the same drug. Forms available from special-order manufacturers include: infusion

Tablet
CAUTIONARY AND ADVISORY LABELS 9
▸ Co-amoxiclav (Non-proprietary)
Clavulanic acid (as Potassium clavulanate) 125 mg, Amoxicillin (as Amoxicillin trihydrate) 250 mg Co-amoxiclav 250mg/125mg tablets | 21 tablet PoM £7.00 DT price = £2.42 | 100 tablet PoM no price available
Clavulanic acid (as Potassium clavulanate) 125 mg, Amoxicillin (as Amoxicillin trihydrate) 500 mg Co-amoxiclav 500mg/125mg tablets | 21 tablet PoM £15.00 DT price = £2.38

Clavulanic acid (as Potassium clavulanate) 125 mg, Amoxicillin (as Amoxicillin trihydrate) 875 mg Co-amoxiclav 875mg/125mg tablets | 14 tablet PoM £18.00 DT price = £8.60
▸ Augmentin (GlaxoSmithKline UK Ltd)
Clavulanic acid (as Potassium clavulanate) 125 mg, Amoxicillin (as Amoxicillin trihydrate) 250 mg Augmentin 375mg tablets | 21 tablet PoM £5.03 DT price = £2.42
Clavulanic acid (as Potassium clavulanate) 125 mg, Amoxicillin (as Amoxicillin trihydrate) 500 mg Augmentin 625mg tablets | 21 tablet PoM £9.60 DT price = £2.38

Oral suspension
CAUTIONARY AND ADVISORY LABELS 9
EXCIPIENTS: May contain Aspartame
▸ Co-amoxiclav (Non-proprietary)
Clavulanic acid (as Potassium clavulanate) 6.25 mg per 1 ml, Amoxicillin (as Amoxicillin trihydrate) 25 mg per 1 ml Co-amoxiclav 125mg/31mg/5ml oral suspension | 100 ml PoM £5.00 DT price = £5.00
Co-amoxiclav 125mg/31mg/5ml oral suspension sugar free sugar-free | 100 ml PoM £25.00 DT price = £1.79
Clavulanic acid (as Potassium clavulanate) 12.5 mg per 1 ml, Amoxicillin (as Amoxicillin trihydrate) 50 mg per 1 ml Co-amoxiclav 250mg/62mg/5ml oral suspension | 100 ml PoM £5.00 DT price = £5.00
Co-amoxiclav 250mg/62mg/5ml oral suspension sugar free sugar-free | 100 ml PoM £35.00 DT price = £1.62
Clavulanic acid (as Potassium clavulanate) 11.4 mg per 1 ml, Amoxicillin (as Amoxicillin trihydrate) 80 mg per 1 ml Co-amoxiclav 400mg/57mg/5ml oral suspension sugar free sugar-free | 35 ml PoM £4.13 DT price = £4.13 sugar-free | 70 ml PoM £6.97 DT price = £5.79
▸ Augmentin (GlaxoSmithKline UK Ltd)
Clavulanic acid (as Potassium clavulanate) 6.25 mg per 1 ml, Amoxicillin (as Amoxicillin trihydrate) 25 mg per 1 ml Augmentin 125/31 SF oral suspension sugar-free | 100 ml PoM £3.54 DT price = £1.79
Clavulanic acid (as Potassium clavulanate) 12.5 mg per 1 ml, Amoxicillin (as Amoxicillin trihydrate) 50 mg per 1 ml Augmentin 250/62 SF oral suspension sugar-free | 100 ml PoM £3.60 DT price = £1.62
▸ Augmentin-Duo (GlaxoSmithKline UK Ltd)
Clavulanic acid (as Potassium clavulanate) 11.4 mg per 1 ml, Amoxicillin (as Amoxicillin trihydrate) 80 mg per 1 ml Augmentin-Duo 400/57 oral suspension sugar-free | 35 ml PoM £4.13 DT price = £4.13 sugar-free | 70 ml PoM £5.79 DT price = £5.79

Powder for solution for injection
ELECTROLYTES: May contain Potassium, sodium
▸ Co-amoxiclav (Non-proprietary)
Clavulanic acid (as Potassium clavulanate) 100 mg, Amoxicillin (as Amoxicillin sodium) 500 mg Co-amoxiclav 500mg/100mg powder for solution for injection vials | 10 vial PoM £11.39–£14.90
Clavulanic acid (as Potassium clavulanate) 200 mg, Amoxicillin (as Amoxicillin sodium) 1000 mg Co-amoxiclav 1000mg/200mg powder for solution for injection vials | 10 vial PoM £29.70
▸ Augmentin Intravenous (GlaxoSmithKline UK Ltd)
Clavulanic acid (as Potassium clavulanate) 100 mg, Amoxicillin (as Amoxicillin sodium) 500 mg Augmentin Intravenous 600mg powder for solution for injection vials | 10 vial PoM £10.60
Clavulanic acid (as Potassium clavulanate) 200 mg, Amoxicillin (as Amoxicillin sodium) 1000 mg Augmentin Intravenous 1.2g powder for solution for injection vials | 10 vial PoM £10.60

ANTIBACTERIALS › PENICILLINS, MECILLINAM-TYPE

⌐ 495

Pivmecillinam hydrochloride

● INDICATIONS AND DOSE

Acute uncomplicated cystitis
▸ BY MOUTH
▸ Child (body-weight 40 kg and above): Initially 400 mg for 1 dose, then 200 mg every 8 hours for 3 days
▸ Adult (body-weight 40 kg and above): Initially 400 mg for 1 dose, then 200 mg every 8 hours for 3 days

Chronic or recurrent bacteriuria
▸ BY MOUTH
▹ Child (body-weight 40 kg and above): 400 mg every 6–8 hours
▹ Adult (body-weight 40 kg and above): 400 mg every 6–8 hours

Urinary-tract infections
▸ BY MOUTH
▹ Child (body-weight up to 40 kg): 5–10 mg/kg every 6 hours, alternatively 20–40 mg/kg daily in 3 divided doses

● UNLICENSED USE Not licensed for use in children under 3 months.

● CONTRA-INDICATIONS Carnitine deficiency · gastro-intestinal obstruction · infants under 3 months · oesophageal strictures

● CAUTIONS Avoid in Acute porphyrias p. 918

● SIDE-EFFECTS
▸ **Common or very common** Abdominal pain · dizziness · headache · nausea · vomiting
▸ **Frequency not known** Mouth ulcers · oesophagitis · reduced serum and total body carnitine (especially with long-term or repeated use)

● PREGNANCY Not known to be harmful, but manufacturer advises avoid.

● BREAST FEEDING Trace amount in milk, but appropriate to use.

● MONITORING REQUIREMENTS Liver and renal function tests required in long-term use.

● EFFECT ON LABORATORY TESTS False-positive urinary glucose (if tested for reducing substances).

● DIRECTIONS FOR ADMINISTRATION Tablets should be swallowed whole with plenty of fluid during meals while sitting or standing.

● PATIENT AND CARER ADVICE Patient counselling is advised on administration of pivmecillinam hydrochloride tablets (posture).

● MEDICINAL FORMS
There can be variation in the licensing of different medicines containing the same drug. Forms available from special-order manufacturers include: oral suspension
Tablet
CAUTIONARY AND ADVISORY LABELS 9, 21, 27
▹ Selexid (LEO Pharma)
Pivmecillinam hydrochloride 200 mg Selexid 200mg tablets | 10 tablet [PoM] £4.50 DT price = £4.50

ANTIBACTERIALS › PENICILLINS, PENICILLINASE-RESISTANT

⬛ Flucloxacillin

● INDICATIONS AND DOSE
Infections due to beta-lactamase-producing staphylococci including otitis externa | Adjunct in pneumonia | Adjunct in impetigo | Adjunct in cellulitis
▸ BY MOUTH
▹ Child 1 month-1 year: 62.5–125 mg 4 times a day
▹ Child 2-9 years: 125–250 mg 4 times a day
▹ Child 10-17 years: 250–500 mg 4 times a day
▹ Adult: 250–500 mg 4 times a day
▸ BY INTRAMUSCULAR INJECTION
▹ Adult: 250–500 mg every 6 hours
▸ BY SLOW INTRAVENOUS INJECTION, OR BY INTRAVENOUS INFUSION
▹ Adult: 0.25–2 g every 6 hours

Endocarditis (in combination with other antibacterial if necessary)
▸ BY SLOW INTRAVENOUS INJECTION, OR BY INTRAVENOUS INFUSION
▹ Adult (body-weight up to 85 kg): 8 g daily in 4 divided doses
▹ Adult (body-weight 85 kg and above): 12 g daily in 6 divided doses

Osteomyelitis
▸ BY SLOW INTRAVENOUS INJECTION, OR BY INTRAVENOUS INFUSION
▹ Adult: Up to 8 g daily in 3–4 divided doses

Surgical prophylaxis
▸ INITIALLY BY SLOW INTRAVENOUS INJECTION, OR BY INTRAVENOUS INFUSION
▹ Adult: 1–2 g, to be administered up to 30 minutes before the procedure, then (by mouth or by intramuscular injection or by slow intravenous injection or by intravenous infusion) 500 mg every 6 hours if required for up to 4 further doses in high risk procedures

Staphylococcal lung infection in cystic fibrosis
▸ BY MOUTH
▹ Child: 25 mg/kg 4 times a day (max. per dose 1 g), alternatively 100 mg/kg daily in 3 divided doses; maximum 4 g per day

Prevention of _Staphylococcus aureus_ lung infection in cystic fibrosis—primary prevention
▸ BY MOUTH
▹ Child 1 month-3 years: 125 mg twice daily

Prevention of _Staphylococcus aureus_ lung infection in cystic fibrosis—secondary prevention
▸ BY MOUTH
▹ Child: 50 mg/kg twice daily (max. per dose 1 g twice daily)

● UNLICENSED USE Flucloxacillin doses in the BNF may differ from those in product literature.

┌───┐
│ IMPORTANT SAFETY INFORMATION
│ HEPATIC DISORDERS
│ Cholestatic jaundice and hepatitis may occur very rarely, up to two months after treatment with flucloxacillin has been stopped. Administration for more than 2 weeks and increasing age are risk factors. Healthcare professionals are reminded that:
│ ● flucloxacillin should not be used in patients with a history of hepatic dysfunction associated with flucloxacillin
│ ● flucloxacillin should be used with caution in patients with hepatic impairment
│ ● careful enquiry should be made about hypersensitivity reactions to beta-lactam antibacterials
└───┘

● CAUTIONS
▸ With intravenous use Accumulation of electrolytes can occur with high doses · risk of kernicterus in jaundiced neonates when high doses given parenterally

● SIDE-EFFECTS
▸ **Common or very common** Gastrointestinal disturbances
▸ **Very rare** Cholestatic jaundice · hepatitis

● PREGNANCY Not known to be harmful.

● BREAST FEEDING Trace amounts in milk, but appropriate to use.

● HEPATIC IMPAIRMENT Use with caution.

● RENAL IMPAIRMENT
▸ In adults Reduce dose if eGFR less than 10 mL/minute/1.73 m^2.
▸ In children Use normal dose every 8 hours if estimated glomerular filtration rate less than 10 mL/minute/1.73 m^2.

5

Infection

5

Infection

▸ With intravenous use Accumulation of electrolytes can occur in patients with renal failure.

● EFFECT ON LABORATORY TESTS False-positive urinary glucose (if tested for reducing substances).

● DIRECTIONS FOR ADMINISTRATION

▸ With intravenous use in children For *intravenous infusion*, dilute reconstituted solution *in* Glucose 5% *or* Sodium Chloride 0.9% and give intermittently over 30–60 minutes.

▸ With intravenous use in adults For *intravenous infusion* (*Floxapen*®), give intermittently *in* Glucose 5% *or* Sodium chloride 0.9%; suggested volume 100 mL given over 30–60 minutes. *via* drip tubing *in* Glucose 5% *or* Sodium chloride 0.9%; continuous infusion not usually recommended.

● PATIENT AND CARER ADVICE
Medicines for Children leaflet: Flucloxacillin for bacterial infections www.medicinesforchildren.org.uk/flucloxacillin-for-bacterial-infections

● MEDICINAL FORMS
There can be variation in the licensing of different medicines containing the same drug. Forms available from special-order manufacturers include: infusion

Capsule
CAUTIONARY AND ADVISORY LABELS 9, 23
▸ Flucloxacillin (Non-proprietary)
Flucloxacillin (as Flucloxacillin sodium) 250 mg Flucloxacillin 250mg capsules | 20 capsule [PoM] £3.58 | 28 capsule [PoM] £5.00 DT price = £1.29 | 100 capsule [PoM] £17.80 | 500 capsule [PoM] £52.14
Flucloxacillin (as Flucloxacillin sodium) 500 mg Flucloxacillin 500mg capsules | 20 capsule [PoM] £7.50 | 28 capsule [PoM] £10.50 DT price = £2.19 | 100 capsule [PoM] £37.50

Oral solution
CAUTIONARY AND ADVISORY LABELS 9, 23
▸ Flucloxacillin (Non-proprietary)
Flucloxacillin (as Flucloxacillin sodium) 25 mg per 1 ml Flucloxacillin 125mg/5ml oral solution | 100 ml [PoM] £21.87 DT price = £5.10
Flucloxacillin 125mg/5ml oral solution sugar free sugar-free | 100 ml [PoM] £31.41 DT price = £22.58
Flucloxacillin (as Flucloxacillin sodium) 50 mg per 1 ml Flucloxacillin 250mg/5ml oral solution sugar free sugar-free | 100 ml [PoM] £38.94 DT price = £27.23
Flucloxacillin 250mg/5ml oral solution | 100 ml [PoM] £28.72 DT price = £26.04

Powder for solution for injection
▸ Flucloxacillin (Non-proprietary)
Flucloxacillin (as Flucloxacillin sodium) 250 mg Flucloxacillin 250mg powder for solution for injection vials | 10 vial [PoM] £10.43–£12.25
Flucloxacillin (as Flucloxacillin sodium) 500 mg Flucloxacillin 500mg powder for solution for injection vials | 10 vial [PoM] £20.85–£24.50
Flucloxacillin (as Flucloxacillin sodium) 1 gram Flucloxacillin 1g powder for solution for injection vials | 10 vial [PoM] £41.75–£49.00

⏷ 495

Temocillin

● INDICATIONS AND DOSE

Septicaemia | Urinary-tract infections | Lower respiratory-tract infections caused by susceptible Gram-negative bacteria
▸ BY INTRAMUSCULAR INJECTION, OR BY INTRAVENOUS INJECTION, OR BY INTRAVENOUS INFUSION
▸ Adult: 1–2 g every 12 hours, give over 3–4 minutes when administered by intravenous injection

● CAUTIONS Accumulation of sodium from injection can occur with high doses

● PREGNANCY Not known to be harmful.

● BREAST FEEDING Trace amounts in milk.

● RENAL IMPAIRMENT 1 g every 12 hours if eGFR 30–60 mL/minute/1.73 m². 1 g every 24 hours if eGFR

10–30 mL/minute/1.73 m². 1 g every 48 hours *or* 500 mg every 24 hours if eGFR less than 10 mL/minute/1.73 m². Accumulation of sodium from injection can occur in patients with renal failure.

● EFFECT ON LABORATORY TESTS False-positive urinary glucose (if tested for reducing substances).

● DIRECTIONS FOR ADMINISTRATION For *intravenous infusion* (*Negaban*®), give intermittently in Glucose 5% or 10% *or* Sodium chloride 0.9%. Reconstitute 1 g with 10 mL water for injections then dilute with 50–150 mL infusion fluid; give over 30–40 minutes.

● MEDICINAL FORMS
There can be variation in the licensing of different medicines containing the same drug.
Powder for solution for injection
ELECTROLYTES: May contain Sodium
▸ Negaban (Eumedica Pharmaceuticals)
Temocillin (as Temocillin sodium) 1 gram Negaban 1g powder for solution for injection vials | 1 vial [PoM] £25.45

ANTIBACTERIALS > POLYMYXINS

Colistimethate sodium

(Colistin sulfomethate sodium)

● DRUG ACTION The polymyxin antibiotic, colistimethate sodium (colistin sulfomethate sodium), is active against Gram-negative organisms including *Pseudomonas aeruginosa*, *Acinetobacter baumanii*, and *Klebsiella pneumoniae*. It is not absorbed by mouth and thus needs to be given by injection for a systemic effect.

● INDICATIONS AND DOSE

Gram-negative infections resistant to other antibacterials, including those caused by *Pseudomonas aeruginosa*, *Acinetobacter baumanii* and *Klebsiella pneumoniae*
▸ BY SLOW INTRAVENOUS INJECTION, OR BY INTRAVENOUS INFUSION
▸ Adult (body-weight up to 60 kg): 50 000–75 000 units/kg daily in 3 divided doses, to be administered into a totally implantable venous access device when giving via slow intravenous injection
▸ Adult (body-weight 60 kg and above): 1–2 million units every 8 hours, to be administered into a totally implantable venous access device when giving via slow intravenous injection; maximum 6 million units per day

Adjunct to standard antibacterial therapy for *Pseudomonas aeruginosa* infection in cystic fibrosis
▸ BY INHALATION OF NEBULISED SOLUTION
▸ Adult: 1–2 million units twice daily, adjusted according to response, increased to 2 million units 3 times daily for subsequent respiratory isolates of *Pseudomonas aeruginosa*
▸ BY INHALATION OF POWDER
▸ Adult: 1.66 million units twice daily

PROMIXIN®

Gram-negative infections resistant to other antibacterials, including those caused by *Pseudomonas aeruginosa*, *Acinetobacter baumanii* , *Klebsiella pneumoniae*
▸ BY SLOW INTRAVENOUS INJECTION, OR BY INTRAVENOUS INFUSION
▸ Adult: 9 million units daily in 2–3 divided doses, to be administered into a totally implantable venous access device when giving via slow intravenous injection, an initial loading dose of 9 million units (up to max. 12 million units, if adequate renal function) should be

used in those who are critically ill, consult product literature for details

PROMIXIN®

Management of chronic pulmonary infections due to *Pseudomonas aeruginosa* in patients with cystic fibrosis
▸ BY INHALATION OF NEBULISED SOLUTION
▸ Child 2-17 years: 1–2 million units 2–3 times a day, for specific advice on administration using nebulisers—consult product literature; maximum 6 million units per day
▸ Adult: 1–2 million units 2–3 times a day, for specific advice on administration using nebulisers—consult product literature; maximum 6 million units per day

● CONTRA-INDICATIONS Myasthenia gravis
● CAUTIONS
GENERAL CAUTIONS
Acute porphyrias p. 918
SPECIFIC CAUTIONS
▸ When used by inhalation Severe haemoptysis—risk of further haemorrhage
● INTERACTIONS → Appendix 1 (polymyxins).
● SIDE-EFFECTS
▸ Common or very common
▸ When used by inhalation Bronchospasm · cough · dysphonia · nausea · sore mouth · Sore throat · taste disturbances · vomiting
▸ Uncommon
▸ When used by inhalation Hypersalivation · thirst
▸ Rare
▸ With intravenous use Vasomotor instability
▸ Frequency not known
▸ With intravenous use Apnoea · confusion · headache · muscle weakness · nephrotoxicity · neurotoxicity reported especially with excessive doses · perioral paraesthesia · peripheral paraesthesia · psychosis · rash · slurred speech · vertigo · visual disturbances
SIDE-EFFECTS, FURTHER INFORMATION
▸ Dose-related side-effects The major adverse effects are dose-related neurotoxicity and nephrotoxicity.
● PREGNANCY
▸ When used by inhalation Clinical use suggests probably safe.
▸ With intravenous use Use only if potential benefit outweighs risk.
● BREAST FEEDING Present in milk but poorly absorbed from gut; manufacturers advise avoid (or use only if potential benefit outweighs risk).
● RENAL IMPAIRMENT
▸ With intravenous use Reduce dose.
▸ With intravenous use In renal impairment, monitor plasma colistimethate sodium concentration during parenteral treatment—consult product literature. Recommended 'peak' plasma colistimethate sodium concentration (approx. 1 hour after intravenous injection or infusion) 5–15 mg/litre; pre-dose ('trough') concentration 2–6 mg/litre.
● MONITORING REQUIREMENTS
▸ With intravenous use Monitor renal function.
▸ When used by inhalation Measure lung function before and after initial dose of colistimethate sodium and monitor for bronchospasm; if bronchospasm occurs in a patient not using a bronchodilator, repeat test using a bronchodilator before the dose of colistimethate sodium.
● DIRECTIONS FOR ADMINISTRATION
▸ When used by inhalation Other inhaled drugs should be administered before colistimethate sodium. For *nebulisation* administer required dose in 2–4 mL of sodium chloride 0.9% (or water for injections) or a 1:1 mixture of sodium chloride 0.9% and water for injection.

▸ With intravenous use For *intravenous infusion* (Colomycin®, Promixin®), give intermittently in Sodium chloride 0.9% (or Glucose 5% for Promixin® brand only); dilute with 50 mL infusion fluid and give over 30 minutes.
COLOMYCIN® Colomycin® Injection may be used for nebulisation; administer required dose in 2–4 mL of sodium chloride 0.9%, (or water for injections) or a 1:1 mixture of sodium chloride 0.9% and water for injection.
● PRESCRIBING AND DISPENSING INFORMATION
Colistimethate sodium is included in some preparations for topical application.
● PATIENT AND CARER ADVICE
▸ When used by inhalation Patient should be advised to rinse mouth with water after each dose of dry powder inhalation.
● NATIONAL FUNDING/ACCESS DECISIONS
NICE technology appraisals (TAs)
▸ **Colistimethate sodium by dry powder inhalation for pseudomonal lung infection in cystic fibrosis (March 2013)**
NICE TA276
Colistimethate sodium dry powder for inhalation is recommended for chronic pulmonary infection caused by *Pseudomonas aeruginosa* in patients with cystic fibrosis who would benefit from continued treatment, but do not tolerate the drug in its nebulised form. The manufacturer must provide colistimethate sodium dry powder for inhalation at the discount agreed as part of the patient access scheme to primary, secondary and tertiary care in the NHS. Patients currently receiving colistimethate sodium dry powder for inhalation can continue treatment until they and their clinician consider it appropriate to stop.
www.nice.org.uk/TA276

● MEDICINAL FORMS
There can be variation in the licensing of different medicines containing the same drug.
Powder for solution for injection
ELECTROLYTES: May contain Sodium
▸ Colistimethate sodium (Non-proprietary)
Colistimethate sodium 1000000 unit Colistimethate 1million unit powder for solution for injection vials | 10 vial [PoM] £18.00 | 10 vial [PoM] £16.79 (Hospital only)
▸ Colomycin (Forest Laboratories UK Ltd)
Colistimethate sodium 1000000 unit Colomycin 1million unit powder for solution for injection vials | 10 vial [PoM] £18.00
Colistimethate sodium 2000000 unit Colomycin 2million unit powder for solution for injection vials | 10 vial [PoM] £32.40
▸ Promixin (Profile Pharma Ltd)
Colistimethate sodium 1000000 unit Promixin 1million unit powder for solution for injection vials | 10 vial [PoM] £30.00 (Hospital only)
Powder for nebuliser solution
▸ Promixin (Profile Pharma Ltd)
Colistimethate sodium 1000000 unit Promixin 1million unit powder for nebuliser solution unit dose vials | 30 unit dose [PoM] £168.00

ANTIBACTERIALS ˃ QUINOLONES

Quinolones

Overview
Nalidixic acid p. 509 and norfloxacin p. 509 are effective in uncomplicated urinary-tract infections.

Ciprofloxacin p. 506 is active against both Gram-positive and Gram-negative bacteria. It is particularly active against Gram-negative bacteria, including salmonella, shigella, campylobacter, neisseria, and pseudomonas. Ciprofloxacin has only moderate activity against Gram-positive bacteria such as *Streptococcus pneumoniae* and *Enterococcus faecalis*; it should not be used for pneumococcal pneumonia. It is

Infection

5

active against chlamydia and some mycobacteria. Most anaerobic organisms are not susceptible. Ciprofloxacin can be used for respiratory tract infections (but not for pneumococcal pneumonia), urinary-tract infections, infections of the gastro-intestinal system (including typhoid fever), bone and joint infections, gonorrhoea and septicaemia caused by sensitive organisms.

Ofloxacin p. 510 is used for urinary-tract infections, lower respiratory-tract infections, gonorrhoea, and non-gonococcal urethritis and cervicitis.

Levofloxacin p. 508 is active against Gram-positive and Gram-negative organisms. It has greater activity against pneumococci than ciprofloxacin. Levofloxacin is licensed for the treatment of acute sinusitis, acute exacerbations of chronic bronchitis, and community-acquired pneumonia, but it should only be considered for these infections when first-line treatment cannot be used or is ineffective. Levofloxacin is also licensed for the treatment of urinary-tract infections.

Although ciprofloxacin, levofloxacin, moxifloxacin p. 508, and ofloxacin are licensed for skin and soft-tissue infections, many staphylococci are resistant to the quinolones and their use should be avoided in MRSA infections.

Moxifloxacin should be reserved for the treatment of sinusitis, community-acquired pneumonia, exacerbations of chronic bronchitis, mild to moderate pelvic inflammatory disease, or complicated skin and soft-tissue infections which have failed to respond to other antibacterials or for patients who cannot be treated with other antibacterials. It has been associated with QT interval prolongation and life-threatening hepatotoxicity. Moxifloxacin is active against Gram-positive and Gram-negative organisms. It has greater activity against Gram-positive organisms, including pneumococci, than ciprofloxacin. Moxifloxacin is not active against *Pseudomonas aeruginosa* or meticillin-resistant *Staphylococcus aureus* (MRSA).

Quinolones

IMPORTANT SAFETY INFORMATION
The CSM has warned that quinolones may induce **convulsions** in patients with or without a history of convulsions; taking NSAIDs at the same time may also induce them.

TENDON DAMAGE
Tendon damage (including rupture) has been reported rarely in patients receiving quinolones. Tendon rupture may occur within 48 hours of starting treatment; cases have also been reported several months after stopping a quinolone. Healthcare professionals are reminded that:
- quinolones are contra-indicated in patients with a history of tendon disorders related to quinolone use;
- patients over 60 years of age are more prone to tendon damage;
- the risk of tendon damage is increased by the concomitant use of corticosteroids;
- if tendinitis is suspected, the quinolone should be discontinued immediately.

● CONTRA-INDICATIONS History of tendon disorders related to quinolone use
● CAUTIONS Can prolong the QT interval · children or adolescents (arthropathy has developed in weight-bearing joints in young *animals*) · conditions that predispose to seizures · exposure to excessive sunlight should be avoided (discontinue if photosensitivity occurs) · G6PD deficiency · history of epilepsy · myasthenia gravis (risk of exacerbation)

CAUTIONS, FURTHER INFORMATION
▶ In children Quinolones cause arthropathy in the weight-bearing joints of immature *animals* and are therefore generally not recommended in children and growing adolescents. However, the significance of this effect in humans is uncertain and in some specific circumstances short-term use of either ciprofloxacin or nalidixic acid may be justified in children.
● INTERACTIONS → Appendix 1 (quinolones).
● SIDE-EFFECTS
▶ **Common or very common** Diarrhoea · dizziness · headache · nausea · vomiting
▶ **Uncommon** Abdominal pain · anorexia · anxiety · arthralgia · asthenia · blood disorders · confusion · depression · disturbances in taste · disturbances in vision · dyspepsia · eosinophilia · hallucinations · leucopenia · myalgia · rash · sleep disturbances · thrombocytopenia · tremor
▶ **Rare** Antibiotic-associated colitis · convulsions · disturbances in hearing · disturbances in smell · dyspnoea · hepatic dysfunction · hepatitis · hypotension · interstitial nephritis · jaundice · photosensitivity · psychoses · renal failure · symptoms of peripheral neuropathy (sometimes irreversible) · tendon damage · tendon inflammation · vasculitis
▶ **Very rare** Stevens-Johnson syndrome · toxic epidermal necrolysis
SIDE-EFFECTS, FURTHER INFORMATION
The drug should be **discontinued** if psychiatric, neurological, or hypersensitivity reactions (including severe rash) occur.
● ALLERGY AND CROSS-SENSITIVITY Use of quinolones contra-indicated in quinolone hypersensitivity.
● PREGNANCY Avoid in pregnancy—shown to cause arthropathy in *animal* studies; safer alternatives are available.

⬏ above

Ciprofloxacin

● INDICATIONS AND DOSE
Fistulating Crohn's disease
▶ BY MOUTH
▶ Adult: 500 mg twice daily
Respiratory-tract infections
▶ BY MOUTH
▶ Adult: 500–750 mg twice daily
▶ BY INTRAVENOUS INFUSION
▶ Adult: 400 mg every 8–12 hours, to be given over 60 minutes
Pseudomonal lower respiratory-tract infection in cystic fibrosis
▶ BY MOUTH
▶ Adult: 750 mg twice daily
Urinary-tract infections
▶ BY MOUTH
▶ Adult: 250–750 mg twice daily
▶ BY INTRAVENOUS INFUSION
▶ Adult: 400 mg every 8–12 hours, to be given over 60 minutes
Acute uncomplicated cystitis in women
▶ BY MOUTH
▶ Adult: 250 mg twice daily for 3 days
Acute or chronic prostatitis
▶ BY MOUTH
▶ Adult: 500 mg twice daily for 28 days
▶ BY INTRAVENOUS INFUSION
▶ Adult: 400 mg every 8–12 hours, to be given over 60 minutes

Gonorrhoea
▶ BY MOUTH
  ▸ Adult: 500 mg for 1 dose

Most other infections
▶ BY MOUTH
  ▸ Adult: Initially 500 mg twice daily; increased to 750 mg twice daily, in severe or deep-seated infection
▶ BY INTRAVENOUS INFUSION
  ▸ Adult: 400 mg every 8–12 hours, to be given over 60 minutes

Surgical prophylaxis
▶ BY MOUTH
  ▸ Adult: 750 mg, to be taken 60 minutes before procedure

Anthrax (treatment and post-exposure prophylaxis)
▶ BY MOUTH
  ▸ Adult: 500 mg twice daily
▶ BY INTRAVENOUS INFUSION
  ▸ Adult: 400 mg every 12 hours, to be given over 60 minutes

Prevention of secondary case of meningococcal meningitis
▶ BY MOUTH
  ▸ Child 1 month-4 years: 30 mg/kg (max. per dose 125 mg) for 1 dose
  ▸ Child 5-11 years: 250 mg for 1 dose
  ▸ Child 12-17 years: 500 mg for 1 dose
  ▸ Adult: 500 mg for 1 dose

● UNLICENSED USE Not licensed for use in children under 1 year of age. Not licensed for use in children for prophylaxis of meningococcal meningitis.
● CAUTIONS Acute myocardial infarction (risk factor for QT interval prolongation) · avoid excessive alkalinity of urine (risk of crystalluria) · bradycardia (risk factor for QT interval prolongation) · congenital long QT syndrome (risk factor for QT interval prolongation) · electrolyte disturbances (risk factor for QT interval prolongation) · ensure adequate fluid intake (risk of crystalluria) · heart failure with reduced left ventricular ejection fraction (risk factor for QT interval prolongation) · history of symptomatic arrhythmias (risk factor for QT interval prolongation)
● INTERACTIONS Caution if concomitant use with other drugs known to prolong the QT interval.
● SIDE-EFFECTS
▶ Common or very common
  ▸ With intravenous use Flatulence · pain at injection site · phlebitis at injection site
  ▸ With oral use Flatulence
▶ Rare Abnormal dreams · chest pain · dysphagia · dyspnoea · erythema nodosum · hot flushes · hyperglycaemia · hypoglycaemia · oedema · pancreatitis · sweating · syncope · tachycardia
▶ Very rare Intracranial hypertension · movement disorders · tenosynovitis · tinnitus · vasculitis (in children)
▶ Frequency not known Peripheral neuropathy · polyneuropathy
● PREGNANCY A single dose of ciprofloxacin may be used for the prevention of a secondary case of meningococcal meningitis.
● BREAST FEEDING Amount too small to be harmful but manufacturer advises avoid.
● RENAL IMPAIRMENT
  ▸ With oral use in adults Give 250–500 mg every 12 hours if eGFR 30–60 mL/minute/1.73 m^2 (every 24 hours if eGFR less than 30 mL/minute/1.73 m^2).
  ▸ With intravenous use in adults Give (200 mg over 30 minutes), 200–400 mg every 12 hours if eGFR 30–60 mL/minute/1.73m^2 (every 24 hours if eGFR less than 30 mL/minute/1.73 m^2).

  ▸ With oral use in children Reduce dose if estimated glomerular filtration rate less than 30 mL/minute/1.73 m^2—consult product literature.
● PRESCRIBING AND DISPENSING INFORMATION Flavours of oral liquid formulations may include strawberry.
● PATIENT AND CARER ADVICE
Driving and skilled tasks
May impair performance of skilled tasks (e.g. driving); effects enhanced by alcohol.
Medicines for Children leaflet: Ciprofloxacin for bacterial infections www.medicinesforchildren.org.uk/ciprofloxacin-bacterial-infections-0

● MEDICINAL FORMS
There can be variation in the licensing of different medicines containing the same drug. Forms available from special-order manufacturers include: oral suspension

Tablet
CAUTIONARY AND ADVISORY LABELS 7, 9, 25
  ▸ Ciprofloxacin (Non-proprietary)
  Ciprofloxacin (as Ciprofloxacin hydrochloride)
  100 mg Ciprofloxacin 100mg tablets | 6 tablet [PoM] £4.50 DT price = £1.86
  Ciprofloxacin (as Ciprofloxacin hydrochloride)
  250 mg Ciprofloxacin 250mg tablets | 10 tablet [PoM] £7.25 DT price = £0.75 | 20 tablet [PoM] £11.20 | 100 tablet [PoM] no price available
  Ciprofloxacin (as Ciprofloxacin hydrochloride)
  500 mg Ciprofloxacin 500mg tablets | 10 tablet [PoM] £14.00 DT price = £0.92 | 20 tablet [PoM] £21.23 | 100 tablet [PoM] no price available
  Ciprofloxacin (as Ciprofloxacin hydrochloride)
  750 mg Ciprofloxacin 750mg tablets | 10 tablet [PoM] £20.00 DT price = £8.00 | 20 tablet [PoM] no price available
  ▸ Ciproxin (Bayer Plc)
  Ciprofloxacin (as Ciprofloxacin hydrochloride) 250 mg Ciproxin 250mg tablets | 10 tablet [PoM] £6.59 DT price = £0.75
  Ciprofloxacin (as Ciprofloxacin hydrochloride) 500 mg Ciproxin 500mg tablets | 10 tablet [PoM] £12.49 DT price = £0.92
  Ciprofloxacin (as Ciprofloxacin hydrochloride) 750 mg Ciproxin 750mg tablets | 10 tablet [PoM] £17.78 DT price = £8.00

Oral suspension
CAUTIONARY AND ADVISORY LABELS 7, 9, 25
  ▸ Ciproxin (Bayer Plc)
  Ciprofloxacin 50 mg per 1 ml Ciproxin 250mg/5ml oral suspension | 100 ml [PoM] £19.80 DT price = £19.80

Infusion
  ▸ Ciprofloxacin (Non-proprietary)
  Ciprofloxacin (as Ciprofloxacin lactate) 2 mg per 1 ml Ciprofloxacin 200mg/100ml infusion bags | 10 bag [PoM] £100.00
  Ciprofloxacin 400mg/200ml infusion bags | 10 bag [PoM] £200.00 | 15 bag [PoM] £64.35

Solution for infusion
ELECTROLYTES: May contain Sodium
  ▸ Ciprofloxacin (Non-proprietary)
  Ciprofloxacin (as Ciprofloxacin lactate) 2 mg per 1 ml Ciprofloxacin 200mg/100ml solution for infusion vials | 1 vial [PoM] £14.45
  Ciprofloxacin 400mg/200ml solution for infusion vials | 1 vial £19.79 (Hospital only) | 1 vial [PoM] £19.59
  Ciprofloxacin 100mg/50ml solution for infusion vials | 1 vial [PoM] £7.57
  ▸ Ciproxin (Bayer Plc)
  Ciprofloxacin (as Ciprofloxacin lactate) 2 mg per 1 ml Ciproxin Infusion 100mg/50ml solution for infusion bottles | 1 bottle [PoM] £7.61 (Hospital only)
  Ciproxin Infusion 400mg/200ml solution for infusion bottles | 5 bottle [PoM] £114.23 (Hospital only)
  Ciproxin Infusion 200mg/100ml solution for infusion bottles | 5 bottle [PoM] £75.06 (Hospital only)

Levofloxacin

● INDICATIONS AND DOSE

Acute sinusitis
▸ BY MOUTH
- Adult: 500 mg once daily for 10–14 days

Acute exacerbation of chronic bronchitis
▸ BY MOUTH
- Adult: 500 mg once daily for 7–10 days

Community-acquired pneumonia
▸ BY MOUTH
- Adult: 500 mg 1–2 times a day for 7–14 days
▸ BY INTRAVENOUS INFUSION
- Adult: 500 mg 1–2 times a day, to be given over at least 60 minutes

Urinary-tract infections
▸ BY MOUTH
- Adult: 500 mg once daily for 7–14 days

Urinary-tract infections (uncomplicated infection)
▸ BY MOUTH
- Adult: 250 mg once daily for 3 days

Complicated urinary-tract infections
▸ BY INTRAVENOUS INFUSION
- Adult: 500 mg once daily, to be given over at least 60 minutes

Chronic prostatitis
▸ BY MOUTH
- Adult: 500 mg once daily for 28 days
▸ BY INTRAVENOUS INFUSION
- Adult: 500 mg once daily, to be given over at least 60 minutes

Complicated skin infections | Complicated soft-tissue infections
▸ BY MOUTH
- Adult: 500 mg 1–2 times a day for 7–14 days
▸ BY INTRAVENOUS INFUSION
- Adult: 500 mg 1–2 times a day, to be given over at least 60 minutes

Inhalation of anthrax (treatment and post-exposure prophylaxis)
▸ BY MOUTH
- Adult: 500 mg once daily for 8 weeks
▸ BY INTRAVENOUS INFUSION
- Adult: 500 mg once daily, to be given over at least 60 minutes

● CAUTIONS Acute myocardial infarction (risk factor for QT interval prolongation) · bradycardia (risk factor for QT interval prolongation) · congenital long QT syndrome (risk factor for QT interval prolongation) · electrolyte disturbances (risk factor for QT interval prolongation) · heart failure with reduced left ventricular ejection fraction (risk factor for QT interval prolongation) · history of psychiatric illness · history of symptomatic arrhythmias (risk factor for QT interval prolongation) · risk factors for QT interval prolongation

● INTERACTIONS Caution if concomitant use with other drugs known to prolong the QT interval.

● SIDE-EFFECTS
▸ **Common or very common** Constipation · flatulence · hyperhidrosis
▸ **Uncommon** Dyspnoea
▸ **Rare** Abnormal dreams · hypoglycaemia · palpitation · tachycardia · tinnitus
▸ **Frequency not known**
▸ With intravenous use Transient hypotension
▸ With oral use or intravenous use Benign intracranial hypertension · extrapyramidal symptoms · hyperglycaemia · peripheral neuropathy · pneumonitis · potentially life-threatening hepatic failure · rhabdomyolysis · stomatitis · syncope

● BREAST FEEDING Manufacturer advises avoid.

● RENAL IMPAIRMENT Usual initial dose, then use half normal dose if eGFR 20–50 mL/minute/1.73 m^2; consult product literature if eGFR less than 20 mL/minute/1.73 m^2.

● PATIENT AND CARER ADVICE

Driving and skilled tasks
May impair performance of skilled tasks (e.g. driving).

● MEDICINAL FORMS
There can be variation in the licensing of different medicines containing the same drug.

Tablet
CAUTIONARY AND ADVISORY LABELS 6, 9, 25
▸ Levofloxacin (Non-proprietary)
  Levofloxacin (as Levofloxacin hemihydrate) 250 mg Levofloxacin 250mg tablets | 5 tablet [PoM] £7.23 | 10 tablet [PoM] £14.45 DT price = £10.90
  Levofloxacin (as Levofloxacin hemihydrate) 500 mg Levofloxacin 500mg tablets | 5 tablet [PoM] £12.93 | 10 tablet [PoM] £25.85 DT price = £17.24
▸ Evoxil (Beacon Pharmaceuticals Ltd)
  Levofloxacin (as Levofloxacin hemihydrate) 250 mg Evoxil 250mg tablets | 5 tablet [PoM] £7.23 | 10 tablet [PoM] £14.45 DT price = £10.90
  Levofloxacin (as Levofloxacin hemihydrate) 500 mg Evoxil 500mg tablets | 10 tablet [PoM] £13.00 DT price = £17.24
▸ Tavanic (Sanofi)
  Levofloxacin (as Levofloxacin hemihydrate) 250 mg Tavanic 250mg tablets | 5 tablet [PoM] £7.23 | 10 tablet [PoM] £14.45 DT price = £10.90
  Levofloxacin (as Levofloxacin hemihydrate) 500 mg Tavanic 500mg tablets | 5 tablet [PoM] £12.93 | 10 tablet [PoM] £25.85 DT price = £17.24

Infusion
▸ Levofloxacin (Non-proprietary)
  Levofloxacin (as Levofloxacin hemihydrate) 5 mg per 1 ml Levofloxacin 500mg/100ml infusion bags | 20 bag [PoM] £502.00

Solution for infusion
ELECTROLYTES: May contain Sodium
▸ Levofloxacin (Non-proprietary)
  Levofloxacin (as Levofloxacin hemihydrate) 5 mg per 1 ml Levofloxacin 500mg/100ml solution for infusion vials | 1 vial [PoM] £25.00
  Levofloxacin 500mg/100ml solution for infusion bottles | 10 bottle [PoM] £224.00
▸ Evoxil (Beacon Pharmaceuticals Ltd)
  Levofloxacin (as Levofloxacin hemihydrate) 5 mg per 1 ml Evoxil 500mg/100ml solution for infusion vials | 1 vial [PoM] £26.40

Moxifloxacin

● INDICATIONS AND DOSE

Sinusitis
▸ BY MOUTH
- Adult: 400 mg once daily for 7 days

Community-acquired pneumonia
▸ BY MOUTH
- Adult: 400 mg once daily for 7–14 days
▸ BY INTRAVENOUS INFUSION
- Adult: 400 mg once daily for 7–14 days, to be given over 60 minutes

Exacerbations of chronic bronchitis
▸ BY MOUTH
- Adult: 400 mg once daily for 5–10 days

Mild to moderate pelvic inflammatory disease
▸ BY MOUTH
- Adult: 400 mg once daily for 14 days

Complicated skin and soft-tissue infections which have failed to respond to other antibacterials or for patients who cannot be treated with other antibacterials
▶ BY MOUTH
▹ Adult: 400 mg once daily for 7–21 days
▶ BY INTRAVENOUS INFUSION
▹ Adult: 400 mg once daily for 7–21 days, to be given over 60 minutes

● CONTRA-INDICATIONS Acute myocardial infarction (risk factor for QT interval prolongation) · bradycardia (risk factor for QT interval prolongation) · congenital long QT syndrome (risk factor for QT interval prolongation) · electrolyte disturbances (risk factor for QT interval prolongation) · heart failure with reduced left ventricular ejection fraction (risk factor for QT interval prolongation) · history of symptomatic arrhythmias (risk factor for QT interval prolongation)

● INTERACTIONS → Appendix 1 (quinolones).
Avoid concomitant use with other drugs known to prolong the QT interval.

● SIDE-EFFECTS
▶ **Common or very common** Angina · arrhythmias · constipation · flatulence · gastritis · hyperlipidaemia · palpitation · sweating · vasodilatation
▶ **Uncommon** Dyspnoea
▶ **Rare** Abnormal dreams · amnesia · dysphagia · hyperglycaemia · hypertension · hyperuricaemia · incoordination · myopathy · oedema · peripheral neuropathy · stomatitis · syncope
▶ **Very rare** Potentially life-threatening hepatic failure · rhabdomyolysis
▶ **Frequency not known**
▶ With intravenous use Pain at injection site · phlebitis at injection site

● BREAST FEEDING Manufacturer advises avoid—present in milk in *animal* studies.

● HEPATIC IMPAIRMENT Manufacturer advises avoid in severe impairment.

● PATIENT AND CARER ADVICE
Driving and skilled tasks
May impair performance of skilled tasks (e.g. driving).

● MEDICINAL FORMS
There can be variation in the licensing of different medicines containing the same drug.
Tablet
CAUTIONARY AND ADVISORY LABELS 6, 9
▹ Moxifloxacin (Non-proprietary)
Moxifloxacin (as Moxifloxacin hydrochloride)
400 mg Moxifloxacin 400mg tablets | 5 tablet [PoM] £11.81 DT price = £10.29
▹ Avelox (Bayer Plc)
Moxifloxacin (as Moxifloxacin hydrochloride) 400 mg Avelox 400mg tablets | 5 tablet [PoM] £12.43 DT price = £10.29
Infusion
▹ Moxifloxacin (Non-proprietary)
Moxifloxacin (as Moxifloxacin hydrochloride) 1.6 mg per 1 ml Avelox I.V. 400mg/250ml infusion bags | 1 bag [PoM] no price available
Solution for infusion
ELECTROLYTES: May contain Sodium
▹ Moxifloxacin (Non-proprietary)
Moxifloxacin (as Moxifloxacin hydrochloride) 1.6 mg per 1 ml Moxifloxacin 400mg/250ml solution for infusion bottles | 1 bottle [PoM] £39.95
▹ Avelox (Bayer Plc)
Moxifloxacin (as Moxifloxacin hydrochloride) 1.6 mg per 1 ml Avelox 400mg/250ml solution for infusion bottles | 1 bottle [PoM] £39.95 (Hospital only) | 5 bottle [PoM] £199.75 (Hospital only)

☞ 506

Nalidixic acid

● INDICATIONS AND DOSE
Urinary-tract infections
▶ BY MOUTH
▹ Adult: 900 mg every 6 hours for 7 days, then reduced to 600 mg every 6 hours for prolonged therapy in chronic infections

● CAUTIONS Acute myocardial infarction (risk factor for QT interval prolongation) · avoid in Acute porphyrias p. 918 · bradycardia (risk factor for QT interval prolongation) · congenital long QT syndrome (risk factor for QT interval prolongation) · electrolyte disturbances (risk factor for QT interval prolongation) · heart failure with reduced left ventricular ejection fraction (risk factor for QT interval prolongation) · history of symptomatic arrhythmias (risk factor for QT interval prolongation)

● INTERACTIONS Caution if concomitant use with other drugs known to prolong the QT interval.

● SIDE-EFFECTS Cranial nerve palsy · increased intracranial pressure · metabolic acidosis · peripheral neuropathy · toxic psychosis

● BREAST FEEDING Risk to infant very small but one case of haemolytic anaemia reported.

● HEPATIC IMPAIRMENT Manufacturer advises caution in liver disease.

● RENAL IMPAIRMENT Use with caution; avoid if eGFR less than 20 mL/minute/1.73 m^2.

● MONITORING REQUIREMENTS Monitor blood counts, renal and liver function if treatment exceeds 2 weeks.

● EFFECT ON LABORATORY TESTS False positive urinary glucose (if tested for reducing substances).

● PRESCRIBING AND DISPENSING INFORMATION Flavours of oral liquid formulations may include raspberry and strawberry.

● MEDICINAL FORMS
There can be variation in the licensing of different medicines containing the same drug.
No licensed medicines listed.

☞ 506

Norfloxacin

● INDICATIONS AND DOSE
Lower urinary-tract infections
▶ BY MOUTH
▹ Adult: 400 mg twice daily for 7–10 days (for 3 days for uncomplicated infections in women)
Chronic relapsing lower urinary-tract infections
▶ BY MOUTH
▹ Adult: 400 mg twice daily for up to 12 weeks; reduced to 400 mg once daily, if adequate suppression within first 4 weeks
Chronic prostatitis
▶ BY MOUTH
▹ Adult: 400 mg twice daily for 28 days

● CAUTIONS Acute myocardial infarction (risk factor for QT interval prolongation) · bradycardia (risk factor for QT interval prolongation) · congenital long QT syndrome (risk factor for QT interval prolongation) · electrolyte disturbances (risk factor for QT interval prolongation) · heart failure with reduced left ventricular ejection fraction (risk factor for QT interval prolongation) · history of symptomatic arrhythmias (risk factor for QT interval prolongation)

● INTERACTIONS Caution if concomitant use with other drugs known to prolong the QT interval.

5

Infection

● SIDE-EFFECTS
▸ **Common or very common** Epiphora · tinnitus
▸ **Rare** Pancreatitis
▸ **Very rare** Arrhythmias
▸ **Frequency not known** Exfoliative dermatitis · polyneuropathy

● BREAST FEEDING No information available—manufacturer advises avoid.

● RENAL IMPAIRMENT Use 400 mg once daily if eGFR less than 30 mL/minute/1.73 m^2.

● PATIENT AND CARER ADVICE
Driving and skilled tasks
May impair performance of skilled tasks (e.g. driving).

● MEDICINAL FORMS
There can be variation in the licensing of different medicines containing the same drug.
Tablet
CAUTIONARY AND ADVISORY LABELS 7, 9, 23
▸ Norfloxacin (Non-proprietary)
Norfloxacin 400 mg Norfloxacin 400mg tablets | 14 tablet [PoM] no price available

[F 506]

Ofloxacin

● INDICATIONS AND DOSE
Urinary-tract infections
▸ BY MOUTH
▸ Adult: 200–400 mg daily, preferably taken in the morning; increased if necessary to 400 mg twice daily, in upper urinary tract infections

Complicated urinary-tract infection
▸ BY INTRAVENOUS INFUSION
▸ Adult: 200 mg daily, increased if necessary to 400 mg twice daily, dose increased for severe or complicated infections, to be given over at least 30 minutes for each 200 mg

Acute or chronic prostatitis
▸ BY MOUTH
▸ Adult: 200 mg twice daily for 28 days

Lower respiratory-tract infections
▸ BY MOUTH
▸ Adult: 400 mg daily, dose preferably taken in the morning, then increased if necessary to 400 mg twice daily
▸ BY INTRAVENOUS INFUSION
▸ Adult: 200 mg twice daily, increased to 400 mg twice daily, dose to be increased for severe or complicated infections, to be given over at least 30 minutes for each 200 mg

Skin and soft-tissue infections
▸ BY MOUTH
▸ Adult: 400 mg twice daily
▸ BY INTRAVENOUS INFUSION
▸ Adult: 400 mg twice daily, to be given over at least 30 minutes for each 200 mg

Uncomplicated gonorrhoea
▸ BY MOUTH
▸ Adult: 400 mg as a single dose

Uncomplicated genital chlamydial infection | Non-gonococcal urethritis
▸ BY MOUTH
▸ Adult: 400 mg daily for 7 days, dose may be taken as a single daily dose or in divided doses

Pelvic inflammatory disease
▸ BY MOUTH
▸ Adult: 400 mg twice daily for 14 days

Septicaemia
▸ BY INTRAVENOUS INFUSION
▸ Adult: 200 mg twice daily, increased if necessary to 400 mg twice daily, dose to be increased for severe or complicated infections, to be given over at least 30 minutes for each 200 mg

● CAUTIONS Acute myocardial infarction (risk factor for QT interval prolongation) · bradycardia (risk factor for QT interval prolongation) · congenital long QT syndrome (risk factor for QT interval prolongation) · electrolyte disturbances (risk factor for QT interval prolongation) · heart failure with reduced left ventricular ejection fraction (risk factor for QT interval prolongation) · history of psychiatric illness · history of symptomatic arrhythmias (risk factor for QT interval prolongation)

● INTERACTIONS Caution if concomitant use with other drugs known to prolong the QT interval.

● SIDE-EFFECTS
▸ **Common or very common** Cough · eye irritation · nasopharyngitis
▸ **Rare** Abnormal dreams · arrhythmias · bronchospasm · dyspnoea · hot flushes · hyperhidrosis
▸ **Very rare** Extrapyramidal symptoms · neuropathy · tinnitus
▸ **Frequency not known** Changes in blood sugar · hypotension · local reactions · myopathy · pneumonitis · rhabdomyolysis · thrombophlebitis

● BREAST FEEDING Amount probably too small to be harmful but manufacturer advises avoid.

● HEPATIC IMPAIRMENT Use with caution; elimination may be reduced in severe impairment.

● RENAL IMPAIRMENT Usual initial dose, then use half normal dose if eGFR 20–50 mL/minute/1.73 m^2; 100 mg every 24 hours if eGFR less than 20 mL/minute/1.73 m^2

● PATIENT AND CARER ADVICE
Driving and skilled tasks
May affect performance of skilled tasks (e.g. driving); effects enhanced by alcohol.

● MEDICINAL FORMS
There can be variation in the licensing of different medicines containing the same drug. Forms available from special-order manufacturers include: oral suspension, oral solution
Tablet
CAUTIONARY AND ADVISORY LABELS 6, 9, 11
▸ Ofloxacin (Non-proprietary)
Ofloxacin 200 mg Ofloxacin 200mg tablets | 10 tablet [PoM] £6.75 DT price = £6.61
Ofloxacin 400 mg Ofloxacin 400mg tablets | 5 tablet [PoM] £12.80 DT price = £12.22 | 10 tablet [PoM] £24.26
▸ Tarivid (Sanofi)
Ofloxacin 200 mg Tarivid 200mg tablets | 10 tablet [PoM] £7.53 DT price = £6.61 | 20 tablet [PoM] £15.05
Ofloxacin 400 mg Tarivid 400mg tablets | 5 tablet [PoM] £7.52 DT price = £12.22 | 10 tablet [PoM] £14.99
Solution for infusion
▸ Tarivid (Sanofi)
Ofloxacin (as Ofloxacin hydrochloride) 2 mg per 1 ml Tarivid 200mg/100ml solution for infusion bottles | 1 bottle [PoM] £16.16

Co-trimoxazole

- **DRUG ACTION** Sulfamethoxazole and trimethoprim are used in combination (as **co-trimoxazole**) because of their synergistic activity (the importance of the sulfonamides has decreased as a result of increasing bacterial resistance and their replacement by antibacterials which are generally more active and less toxic).

- **INDICATIONS AND DOSE**

Treatment of susceptible infections
- BY MOUTH
  - Child 6 weeks–5 months: 120 mg twice daily, alternatively 24 mg/kg twice daily
  - Child 6 months–5 years: 240 mg twice daily, alternatively 24 mg/kg twice daily
  - Child 6–11 years: 480 mg twice daily, alternatively 24 mg/kg twice daily
  - Child 12–17 years: 960 mg twice daily
  - Adult: 960 mg twice daily
- BY INTRAVENOUS INFUSION
  - Adult: 960 mg every 12 hours, increased to 1.44 g every 12 hours, increased dose used in severe infection

Treatment of *Pneumocystis jirovecii* (*Pneumocystis carinii*) infections (undertaken where facilities for appropriate monitoring available—consult microbiologist and product literature)
- BY MOUTH, OR BY INTRAVENOUS INFUSION
  - Child: 120 mg/kg daily in 2–4 divided doses for 14–21 days, oral route preferred for children
  - Adult: 120 mg/kg daily in 2–4 divided doses for 14–21 days

Prophylaxis of *Pneumocystis jirovecii* (*Pneumocystis carinii*) infections
- BY MOUTH
  - Child: 450 mg/m² twice daily (max. per dose 960 mg twice daily) for 3 days of the week (either consecutively or on alternate days), dose regimens may vary, consult local guidelines
  - Adult: 960 mg once daily, reduced if not tolerated to 480 mg once daily, alternatively 960 mg once daily on alternate days, alternate day dose to be given 3 times weekly, alternatively 960 mg twice a day on alternate days, alternate day dose to be given 3 times weekly

DOSE EQUIVALENCE AND CONVERSION
480 mg of co-trimoxazole consists of sulfamethoxazole 400 mg and trimethoprim 80 mg.

- **UNLICENSED USE** Not licensed for *Burkholderia cepacia* infections in cystic fibrosis. Not licensed for *Stenotrophomonas maltophilia* infections.
- In children Not licensed for use in children under 6 weeks.

IMPORTANT SAFETY INFORMATION
RESTRICTIONS ON THE USE OF CO-TRIMOXAZOLE
Co-trimoxazole is the drug of choice in the prophylaxis and treatment of *Pneumocystis jirovecii* (*Pneumocystis carinii*) pneumonia; it is also indicated for nocardiasis, *Stenotrophomonas maltophilia* infection [unlicensed indication], and toxoplasmosis. It should only be considered for use in acute exacerbations of chronic bronchitis and infections of the urinary tract when there is bacteriological evidence of sensitivity to co-trimoxazole and good reason to prefer this combination to a single antibacterial; similarly it should only be used in acute otitis media in children when there is good reason to prefer it. Co-trimoxazole is also used for the treatment of infections caused by *Burkholderia cepacia* in cystic fibrosis [unlicensed indication].

- **CONTRA-INDICATIONS** Acute porphyrias p. 918
- **CAUTIONS** Asthma · avoid in blood disorders (unless under specialist supervision) · avoid in infants under 6 weeks (except for treatment or prophylaxis of pneumocystis pneumonia) because of the risk of kernicterus · elderly (increased risk of serious side-effects) (in adults) · G6PD deficiency (risk of haemolytic anaemia) · maintain adequate fluid intake · predisposition to folate deficiency · predisposition to hyperkalaemia (in adults)
- **INTERACTIONS** → Appendix 1 (trimethoprim, sulfamethoxazole).
- **SIDE-EFFECTS**
  - **Common or very common** Diarrhoea · headache · hyperkalaemia · nausea · rash
  - **Uncommon** Vomiting
  - **Rare** Agranulocytosis · bone marrow depression
  - **Very rare** Anorexia · antibiotic-associated colitis · arthralgia · aseptic meningitis · ataxia · blood disorders · convulsions · cough · depression · eosinophilia · glossitis · hallucinations · hepatic necrosis · hypoglycaemia · hyponatraemia · interstitial nephritis · jaundice · leucopenia · liver damage · megaloblastic anaemia · myalgia · myocarditis · pancreatitis · peripheral neuropathy · photosensitivity · pulmonary infiltrates · renal disorders · shortness of breath · Stevens-Johnson syndrome · stomatitis · systemic lupus erythematosus · thrombocytopenia · tinnitus · toxic epidermal necrolysis · uveitis · vasculitis · vertigo
  - **Frequency not known** Rhabdomyolysis reported in HIV-infected patients

SIDE-EFFECTS, FURTHER INFORMATION
- Blood disorders or rash Co-trimoxazole is associated with rare but serious side effects. Discontinue immediately if blood disorders (including leucopenia, thrombocytopenia, megaloblastic anaemia, eosinophilia) or rash (including Stevens-Johnson syndrome, toxic epidermal necrolysis, photosensitivity) develop.

- **PREGNANCY** Teratogenic risk in first trimester (trimethoprim a folate antagonist). Neonatal haemolysis and methaemoglobinaemia in third trimester; fear of increased risk of kernicterus in neonates appears to be unfounded.
- **BREAST FEEDING** Small risk of kernicterus in jaundiced infants and of haemolysis in G6PD-deficient infants (due to sulfamethoxazole).
- **HEPATIC IMPAIRMENT** Manufacturer advises avoid in severe liver disease.
- **RENAL IMPAIRMENT**
  - In adults Use half normal dose if eGFR 15–30 mL/minute/1.73 m². Avoid if eGFR less than 15 mL/minute/1.73 m² and if plasma-sulfamethoxazole concentration cannot be monitored.
  - In children Use half normal dose if estimated glomerular filtration rate 15–30 mL/minute/1.73 m². Avoid if estimated glomerular filtration rate less than 15 mL/minute/1.73 m² and if plasma-sulfamethoxazole concentration cannot be monitored.
- **MONITORING REQUIREMENTS**
  - In children Plasma concentration monitoring may be required with high doses; seek expert advice.
  - Monitor blood counts on prolonged treatment.
- **DIRECTIONS FOR ADMINISTRATION**
  - With intravenous use in children For intermittent *intravenous infusion*, may be further diluted in glucose 5% and 10% or sodium chloride 0.9%. Dilute contents of 1 ampoule (5 mL) to 125 mL, 2 ampoules (10 mL) to 250 mL or 3 ampoules (15 mL) to 500 mL; suggested duration of infusion 60–90 minutes (but may be adjusted according to fluid requirements); if fluid restriction necessary, 1 ampoule (5 mL) may be diluted with 75 mL glucose 5% and the

5

Infection

required dose infused over max. 60 minutes; check container for haze or precipitant during administration. In severe fluid restriction may be given undiluted via a central venous line.

▸ With intravenous use in adults For *intravenous infusion* (Septrin® *for infusion*), give intermittently *in* Glucose 5% or 10% *or* Sodium chloride 0.9%. Dilute contents of 1 ampoule (5 mL) to 125 mL, 2 ampoules (10 mL) to 250 mL or 3 ampoules (15 mL) to 500 mL; suggested duration of infusion 60–90 minutes (but may be adjusted according to fluid requirements); if fluid restriction necessary, 1 ampoule (5 mL) may be diluted with 75 mL glucose 5% and infused over max. 60 minutes.

● PRESCRIBING AND DISPENSING INFORMATION Co-trimoxazole is a mixture of trimethoprim and sulfamethoxazole (sulphamethoxazole) in the proportions of 1 part to 5 parts.

Flavours of oral liquid formulations may include banana, or vanilla.

● MEDICINAL FORMS
There can be variation in the licensing of different medicines containing the same drug.
Tablet
CAUTIONARY AND ADVISORY LABELS 9
▸ Co-trimoxazole (Non-proprietary)
Trimethoprim 80 mg, Sulfamethoxazole 400 mg Co-trimoxazole 80mg/400mg tablets | 28 tablet PoM £23.00 DT price = £2.50 | 100 tablet PoM £9.89–£10.91
Trimethoprim 160 mg, Sulfamethoxazole 800 mg Co-trimoxazole 160mg/800mg tablets | 100 tablet PoM £23.40–£23.46 DT price = £23.46
Oral suspension
CAUTIONARY AND ADVISORY LABELS 9
▸ Co-trimoxazole (Non-proprietary)
Trimethoprim 8 mg per 1 ml, Sulfamethoxazole 40 mg per 1 ml Co-trimoxazole 40mg/200mg/5ml oral suspension sugar free sugar-free | 100 ml PoM £9.95
Trimethoprim 16 mg per 1 ml, Sulfamethoxazole 80 mg per 1 ml Co-trimoxazole 80mg/400mg/5ml oral suspension | 100 ml PoM £10.95
Solution for infusion
EXCIPIENTS: May contain Alcohol, propylene glycol, sulfites
ELECTROLYTES: May contain Sodium
▸ Co-trimoxazole (Non-proprietary)
Trimethoprim 16 mg per 1 ml, Sulfamethoxazole 80 mg per 1 ml Co-trimoxazole 80mg/400mg/5ml solution for infusion ampoules | 10 ampoule PoM £35.00
▸ Septrin (Aspen Pharma Trading Ltd)
Trimethoprim 16 mg per 1 ml, Sulfamethoxazole 80 mg per 1 ml Septrin for Infusion 80mg/400mg/5ml solution for infusion ampoules | 10 ampoule PoM £17.76

Sulfadiazine

(Sulphadiazine)

● DRUG ACTION Sulfadiazine is a short-acting sulphonamide with bacteriostatic activity against a broad spectrum of organisms. The importance of the sulfonamides has decreased as a result of increasing bacterial resistance and their replacement by antibacterials which are generally more active and less toxic.

● INDICATIONS AND DOSE
Prevention of rheumatic fever recurrence
▸ BY MOUTH
▸ Adult (body-weight up to 30 kg): 500 mg daily
▸ Adult (body-weight 30 kg and above): 1 g daily

● UNLICENSED USE Not licensed for use in toxoplasmosis.
● CONTRA-INDICATIONS Acute porphyrias p. 918
● CAUTIONS Asthma · avoid in blood disorders (unless under specialist supervision) · elderly · G6PD deficiency (risk of haemolytic anaemia) · maintain adequate fluid intake ·

predisposition to folate deficiency · predisposition to hyperkalaemia

● INTERACTIONS → Appendix 1 (sulfonamides).
● SIDE-EFFECTS
▸ **Common or very common** Diarrhoea · headache · hyperkalaemia · nausea · rash
▸ **Uncommon** Vomiting
▸ **Rare** Agranulocytosis · bone marrow depression
▸ **Very rare** Anorexia · antibiotic-associated colitis · arthralgia · aseptic meningitis · ataxia · blood disorders · convulsions · cough · depression · eosinophilia · glossitis · hallucinations · hepatic necrosis · hypoglycaemia · hyponatraemia · interstitial nephritis · jaundice · leucopenia · liver damage · megaloblastic anaemia · myalgia · myocarditis · pancreatitis · peripheral neuropathy · photosensitivity · pulmonary infiltrates · renal disorders · shortness of breath · Stevens-Johnson syndrome · stomatitis · systemic lupus erythematosus · thrombocytopenia · tinnitus · toxic epidermal necrolysis · uveitis · vasculitis · vertigo
▸ **Frequency not known** Benign intracranial hypertension · hypothyroidism · optic neuropathy · rhabdomyolysis reported in HIV-infected patients

SIDE-EFFECTS, FURTHER INFORMATION
▸ Blood disorders or rash Discontinue immediately if blood disorders (including leucopenia, thrombocytopenia, megaloblastic anaemia, eosinophilia) or rash (including Stevens-Johnson syndrome, toxic epidermal necrolysis, photosensitivity) develop.

● PREGNANCY Risk of neonatal haemolysis and methaemoglobinaemia in third trimester; fear of increased risk of kernicterus in neonates appears to be unfounded.
● BREAST FEEDING Small risk of kernicterus in jaundiced infants and of haemolysis in G6PD-deficient infants.
● HEPATIC IMPAIRMENT Use with caution in mild to moderate impairment; avoid in severe impairment.
● RENAL IMPAIRMENT Use with caution in mild to moderate impairment; avoid in severe impairment; high risk of crystalluria.
● MONITORING REQUIREMENTS Monitor blood counts on prolonged treatment.

● MEDICINAL FORMS
There can be variation in the licensing of different medicines containing the same drug. Forms available from special-order manufacturers include: oral suspension
Tablet
CAUTIONARY AND ADVISORY LABELS 9, 27
▸ Sulfadiazine (Non-proprietary)
Sulfadiazine 500 mg Sulfadiazine 500mg tablets | 56 tablet PoM £85.55 DT price = £81.99

ANTIBACTERIALS ˃ TETRACYCLINES AND RELATED DRUGS

Tetracyclines

Overview

The tetracyclines are broad-spectrum antibiotics whose value has decreased owing to increasing bacterial resistance. They remain, however, the treatment of choice for infections caused by chlamydia (trachoma, psittacosis, salpingitis, urethritis, and lymphogranuloma venereum), rickettsia (including Q-fever), brucella (doxycycline p. 513 with either streptomycin p. 472 or rifampicin p. 527), and the spirochaete, *Borrelia burgdorferi* (See Lyme disease). They are also used in respiratory and genital mycoplasma infections, in acne, in destructive (refractory) periodontal disease, in exacerbations of chronic bronchitis (because of their activity against *Haemophilus influenzae*), and for leptospirosis in penicillin hypersensitivity (as an alternative to erythromycin p. 488).

Tetracyclines have a role in the management of meticillin-resistant *Staphylococcus aureus* (MRSA) infection.

Microbiologically, there is little to choose between the various tetracyclines, the only exception being minocycline p. 515 which has a broader spectrum; it is active against *Neisseria meningitidis* and has been used for meningococcal prophylaxis but is no longer recommended because of side-effects including dizziness and vertigo. Compared to other tetracyclines, minocycline is associated with a greater risk of lupus-erythematosus-like syndrome. Minocycline sometimes causes irreversible pigmentation.

Tetracyclines

- **CONTRA-INDICATIONS** Children under 12 years (deposition in growing bone and teeth, by binding to calcium, causes staining and occasionally dental hypoplasia)
- **CAUTIONS** Myasthenia gravis (muscle weakness may be increased) · systemic lupus erythematosus (may be exacerbated)
- **INTERACTIONS** → Appendix 1 (tetracyclines). Antacids, and aluminium, calcium, iron, magnesium and zinc salts decrease the absorption of tetracyclines. Use with caution in those receiving potentially hepatotoxic drugs.
- **SIDE-EFFECTS**
- ▸ **Rare** Anaphylaxis · angioedema · blood disorders · exfoliative dermatitis · hepatotoxicity · hypersensitivity reactions · pancreatitis · pericarditis · photosensitivity (particularly with demeclocycline) · rash · Stevens-Johnson syndrome · urticaria
- ▸ **Frequency not known** Antibiotic-associated colitis · benign intracranial hypertension · bulging fontanelles (in infants) · diarrhoea · dysphagia · headache · nausea · oesophageal irritation · visual disturbances · vomiting
- ▸ SIDE-EFFECTS, FURTHER INFORMATION
- ▸ Benign intracranial hypertension and visual disturbances may indicate benign intracranial hypertension (discontinue treatment).
- **PREGNANCY** Should **not** be given to pregnant women; effects on skeletal development have been documented in the first trimester in *animal* studies. Administration during the second or third trimester may cause discoloration of the child's teeth, and maternal hepatotoxicity has been reported with large parenteral doses.
- **BREAST FEEDING** Should **not** be given to women who are breast-feeding (although absorption and therefore discoloration of teeth in the infant is probably usually prevented by chelation with calcium in milk).
- **HEPATIC IMPAIRMENT** Should be avoided or used with caution in patients with hepatic impairment.

▸ above

Demeclocycline hydrochloride

- **INDICATIONS AND DOSE**

Susceptible infections (e.g. chlamydia, rickettsia and mycoplasma)
- ▸ BY MOUTH
- ▸ Adult: 150 mg 4 times a day, alternatively 300 mg twice daily

Treatment of hyponatraemia resulting from inappropriate secretion of antidiuretic hormone, if fluid restriction alone does not restore sodium concentration or is not tolerable
- ▸ BY MOUTH
- ▸ Adult: Initially 0.9–1.2 g daily in divided doses, maintenance 600–900 mg daily

- **CAUTIONS** Photosensitivity more common than with other tetracyclines
- **INTERACTIONS** Milk reduces absorption.
- **SIDE-EFFECTS** Acute renal failure · reversible nephrogenic diabetes insipidus
- **HEPATIC IMPAIRMENT** Max. 1 g daily in divided doses.
- **RENAL IMPAIRMENT** May exacerbate renal failure and should **not** be given to patients with renal impairment.
- **PATIENT AND CARER ADVICE** Patients should be advised to avoid exposure to sunlight or sun lamps.

- MEDICINAL FORMS
  There can be variation in the licensing of different medicines containing the same drug. Forms available from special-order manufacturers include: oral suspension, oral solution

Tablet
- ▸ Demeclocycline hydrochloride (Non-proprietary)
  Demeclocycline hydrochloride 150 mg Demeclocycline 150mg tablets | 100 tablet [PoM] no price available

Capsule
CAUTIONARY AND ADVISORY LABELS 7, 9, 11, 23
- ▸ Demeclocycline hydrochloride (Non-proprietary)
  Demeclocycline hydrochloride 150 mg Demeclocycline 150mg capsules | 28 capsule [PoM] £160.89 DT price = £160.89

▸ above

Doxycycline

- **INDICATIONS AND DOSE**

Susceptible infections (e.g. chlamydia, rickettsia and mycoplasma)
- ▸ BY MOUTH USING IMMEDIATE-RELEASE MEDICINES
- ▸ Child 12–17 years: Initially 200 mg daily for 1 dose, then maintenance 100 mg once daily
- ▸ Adult: Initially 200 mg daily for 1 dose, then maintenance 100 mg once daily

Severe infections (including refractory urinary-tract infections)
- ▸ BY MOUTH USING IMMEDIATE-RELEASE MEDICINES
- ▸ Child 12–17 years: 200 mg daily
- ▸ Adult: 200 mg once daily

Acne
- ▸ BY MOUTH USING IMMEDIATE-RELEASE MEDICINES
- ▸ Child 12–17 years: 100 mg once daily
- ▸ Adult: 100 mg once daily

Rosacea
- ▸ BY MOUTH USING IMMEDIATE-RELEASE MEDICINES
- ▸ Adult: 100 mg once daily

Papulopustular facial rosacea (without ocular involvement)
- ▸ BY MOUTH USING MODIFIED-RELEASE MEDICINES
- ▸ Adult: 40 mg once daily for 16 weeks, dose to be taken in the morning, consider discontinuing treatment if no response after 6 weeks

Early syphilis
- ▸ BY MOUTH USING IMMEDIATE-RELEASE MEDICINES
- ▸ Child 12–17 years: 100 mg twice daily for 14 days
- ▸ Adult: 100 mg twice daily for 14 days

Late latent syphilis
- ▸ BY MOUTH USING IMMEDIATE-RELEASE MEDICINES
- ▸ Child 12–17 years: 100 mg twice daily for 28 days
- ▸ Adult: 100 mg twice daily for 28 days

Neurosyphilis
- ▸ BY MOUTH USING IMMEDIATE-RELEASE MEDICINES
- ▸ Adult: 200 mg twice daily for 28 days

Uncomplicated genital chlamydia | Non-gonococcal urethritis
- ▸ BY MOUTH USING IMMEDIATE-RELEASE MEDICINES
- ▸ Child 12–17 years: 100 mg twice daily for 7 days
- ▸ Adult: 100 mg twice daily for 7 days   continued →

Pelvic inflammatory disease
▸ BY MOUTH USING IMMEDIATE-RELEASE MEDICINES
‣ Child 12–17 years: 100 mg twice daily for 14 days
‣ Adult: 100 mg twice daily for 14 days
Lyme disease (under expert supervision)
▸ BY MOUTH USING IMMEDIATE-RELEASE MEDICINES
‣ Child 12–17 years: 100 mg twice daily for 10–14 days (for 28 days in Lyme arthritis)
‣ Adult: 100 mg twice daily for 10–14 days (for 28 days in Lyme arthritis)
Anthrax (treatment or post-exposure prophylaxis)
▸ BY MOUTH USING IMMEDIATE-RELEASE MEDICINES
‣ Child 12–17 years: 100 mg twice daily
‣ Adult: 100 mg twice daily
Prophylaxis of malaria
▸ BY MOUTH USING IMMEDIATE-RELEASE MEDICINES
‣ Child 12–17 years: 100 mg once daily, to be started 1–2 days before entering endemic area and continued for 4 weeks after leaving, can be used for up to 2 years
‣ Adult: 100 mg once daily, to be started 1–2 days before entering endemic area and continued for 4 weeks after leaving, can be used for up to 2 years
Adjunct to quinine in treatment of _Plasmodium falciparum_ malaria
▸ BY MOUTH USING IMMEDIATE-RELEASE MEDICINES
‣ Child 12–17 years: 200 mg daily for 7 days
‣ Adult: 200 mg daily for 7 days
Periodontitis (as an adjunct to gingival scaling and root planing)
▸ BY MOUTH USING IMMEDIATE-RELEASE MEDICINES
‣ Child 12–17 years: 20 mg twice daily for 3 months
‣ Adult: 20 mg twice daily for 3 months

● UNLICENSED USE Not licensed for use in children under 12 years. Doxycycline doses in BNF Publications may differ from those in product literature. Not licensed for severe recurrent aphthous ulceration. Not licensed for malaria prophylaxis during pregnancy. Not licensed for treatment or post-exposure prophylaxis of anthrax.
‣ In adults Immediate-release doxycycline not licensed for treatment of rosacea.
● CAUTIONS Alcohol dependence
● INTERACTIONS The metabolism of doxycycline may be influenced by antiepileptics.
● SIDE-EFFECTS Anorexia · anxiety · dry mouth · flushing · fungal superinfection (when used for periodontitis) · tinnitus
● PREGNANCY When travel to malarious areas is unavoidable during pregnancy, doxycycline can be used for malaria prophylaxis if other regimens are unsuitable, and if the entire course of doxycycline can be completed before 15 weeks' gestation.
● RENAL IMPAIRMENT Use with caution (avoid excessive doses).
● MONITORING REQUIREMENTS When used for periodontitis, monitor for superficial fungal infection, particularly if predisposition to oral candidiasis.
● DIRECTIONS FOR ADMINISTRATION Capsules and Tablets should be swallowed whole with plenty of fluid, while sitting or standing. Capsules should be taken during meals.
● PATIENT AND CARER ADVICE Counselling on administration advised (posture).
Photosensitivity Patients should be advised to avoid exposure to sunlight or sun lamps.
● PROFESSION SPECIFIC INFORMATION

Dental practitioners' formulary
Doxycycline Capsules 100 mg may be prescribed.
    Dispersible tablets may be prescribed as Dispersible Doxycycline Tablets.
    Tablets may be prescribed as Doxycycline Tablets 20 mg.

● MEDICINAL FORMS
There can be variation in the licensing of different medicines containing the same drug. Forms available from special-order manufacturers include: oral suspension, oral solution
Tablet
CAUTIONARY AND ADVISORY LABELS 6, 11, 27
‣ Periostat (Alliance Pharmaceuticals Ltd)
Doxycycline (as Doxycycline hyclate) 20 mg Periostat 20mg tablets | 56 tablet [PoM] £17.30 DT price = £17.30
Dispersible tablet
CAUTIONARY AND ADVISORY LABELS 6, 9, 11, 13
‣ Vibramycin-D (Pfizer Ltd)
Doxycycline (as Doxycycline monohydrate) 100 mg Vibramycin-D 100mg dispersible tablets sugar-free | 8 tablet [PoM] £4.91 DT price = £4.91
Capsule
CAUTIONARY AND ADVISORY LABELS 6, 9, 11, 27
‣ Doxycycline (Non-proprietary)
Doxycycline (as Doxycycline hyclate) 50 mg Doxycycline 50mg capsules | 28 capsule [PoM] £4.00 DT price = £1.30
Doxycycline (as Doxycycline hyclate) 100 mg Doxycycline 100mg capsules | 8 capsule [PoM] £3.00 DT price = £0.88 | 50 capsule [PoM] £19.00
‣ Vibrox (Kent Pharmaceuticals Ltd)
Doxycycline (as Doxycycline hyclate) 100 mg Vibrox 100mg capsules | 8 capsule [PoM] £3.97 DT price = £0.88 | 14 capsule £4.48 | 50 capsule [PoM] £10.65
Modified-release capsule
CAUTIONARY AND ADVISORY LABELS 6, 11, 27
‣ Efracea (Galderma (UK) Ltd)
Doxycycline (as Doxycycline monohydrate) 40 mg Efracea 40mg modified-release capsules | 14 capsule [PoM] £7.99 DT price = £7.99 | 56 capsule [PoM] £21.71

F 513

Lymecycline

● INDICATIONS AND DOSE

Susceptible infections (e.g. chlamydia, rickettsia and mycoplasma)
▸ BY MOUTH
‣ Child 12–17 years: 408 mg twice daily, increased to 1.224–1.632 g daily, (in severe infection)
‣ Adult: 408 mg twice daily, increased to 1.224–1.632 g daily, (in severe infection)
Acne
▸ BY MOUTH
‣ Child 12–17 years: 408 mg daily for at least 8 weeks
‣ Adult: 408 mg daily for at least 8 weeks

● RENAL IMPAIRMENT May exacerbate renal failure and should **not** be given to patients with renal impairment.

● MEDICINAL FORMS
There can be variation in the licensing of different medicines containing the same drug.
Capsule
CAUTIONARY AND ADVISORY LABELS 6, 9
‣ Lymecycline (Non-proprietary)
Lymecycline 408 mg Lymecycline 408mg capsules | 28 capsule [PoM] £8.11 DT price = £7.23 | 56 capsule [PoM] £16.22
‣ Tetralysal (Galderma (UK) Ltd)
Lymecycline 408 mg Tetralysal 300 capsules | 28 capsule [PoM] £6.95 DT price = £7.23 | 56 capsule [PoM] £11.53

Minocycline

F 513

- **INDICATIONS AND DOSE**

Susceptible infections (e.g. chlamydia, rickettsia and mycoplasma)
‣ BY MOUTH USING IMMEDIATE-RELEASE MEDICINES
‣ Child 12–17 years: 100 mg twice daily
‣ Adult: 100 mg twice daily

Acne
‣ BY MOUTH USING IMMEDIATE-RELEASE MEDICINES
‣ Child 12–17 years: 100 mg once daily, alternatively 50 mg twice daily
‣ Adult: 100 mg once daily, alternatively 50 mg twice daily
‣ BY MOUTH USING MODIFIED-RELEASE MEDICINES
‣ Child 12–17 years: 100 mg daily
‣ Adult: 100 mg daily

Prophylaxis of asymptomatic meningococcal carrier state (but no longer recommended)
‣ BY MOUTH USING IMMEDIATE-RELEASE MEDICINES
‣ Adult: 100 mg twice daily for 5 days, minocycline treatment is usually followed by administration of rifampicin

- **CAUTIONS** Systemic lupus erythematosus
- **SIDE-EFFECTS**
‣ **Rare** Acute renal failure · alopecia · anorexia · hyperaesthesia · impaired hearing · paraesthesia · pigmentation (sometimes irreversible) · tinnitus
‣ **Very rare** Discoloration of conjunctiva · discoloration of sweat · discoloration of tears · systemic lupus erythematosus
‣ **Frequency not known** Dizziness (more common in women) · vertigo (more common in women)
- **RENAL IMPAIRMENT** Use with caution (avoid excessive doses).
- **MONITORING REQUIREMENTS** If treatment continued for longer than 6 months, monitor every 3 months for hepatotoxicity, pigmentation and for systemic lupus erythematosus—discontinue if these develop or if pre-existing systemic lupus erythematosus worsens.
- **DIRECTIONS FOR ADMINISTRATION** Tablets or capsules should be swallowed whole with plenty of fluid while sitting or standing.
- **PATIENT AND CARER ADVICE** Counselling on administration advised (posture).
- **LESS SUITABLE FOR PRESCRIBING** Less suitable for prescribing (compared with other tetracyclines, minocycline is associated with a greater risk of lupus-erythematosus-like syndrome; it sometimes causes irreversible pigmentation).

- **MEDICINAL FORMS**
There can be variation in the licensing of different medicines containing the same drug. Forms available from special-order manufacturers include: oral suspension, oral solution
Tablet
CAUTIONARY AND ADVISORY LABELS 6, 9
‣ Minocycline (Non-proprietary)
  Minocycline (as Minocycline hydrochloride) 50 mg Minocycline 50mg tablets | 28 tablet [PoM] £8.50 DT price = £6.19
  Minocycline (as Minocycline hydrochloride) 100 mg Minocycline 100mg tablets | 28 tablet [PoM] £14.50 DT price = £14.01
Capsule
CAUTIONARY AND ADVISORY LABELS 6, 9
‣ Aknemin (Almirall Ltd)
  Minocycline (as Minocycline hydrochloride) 50 mg Aknemin 50 capsules | 56 capsule [PoM] £15.27 DT price = £15.27
  Minocycline (as Minocycline hydrochloride) 100 mg Aknemin 100mg capsules | 28 capsule [PoM] £13.09 DT price = £13.09

Modified-release capsule
CAUTIONARY AND ADVISORY LABELS 6, 25
‣ Minocycline (Non-proprietary)
  Minocycline (as Minocycline hydrochloride) 100 mg Minocycline 100mg modified-release capsules | 56 capsule [PoM] £24.00 DT price = £20.08
‣ Acnamino MR (Almus Pharmaceuticals Ltd, Dexcel-Pharma Ltd)
  Minocycline (as Minocycline hydrochloride) 100 mg Acnamino MR 100mg capsules | 56 capsule [PoM] £21.14 DT price = £20.08
‣ Minocin MR (Meda Pharmaceuticals Ltd)
  Minocycline (as Minocycline hydrochloride) 100 mg Minocin MR 100mg capsules | 56 capsule [PoM] £20.08 DT price = £20.08

Oxytetracycline

F 513

- **INDICATIONS AND DOSE**

Susceptible infections (e.g. chlamydia, rickettsia and mycoplasma)
‣ BY MOUTH
‣ Child 12–17 years: 250–500 mg 4 times a day
‣ Adult: 250–500 mg 4 times a day

Rosacea
‣ BY MOUTH
‣ Adult: 500 mg twice daily usually for 6–12 weeks (course may be repeated intermittently)

Acne
‣ BY MOUTH
‣ Child 12–17 years: 500 mg twice daily for at least 3 months, if there is no improvement after the first 3 months another oral antibacterial should be used, maximum improvement usually occurs after 4 to 6 months but in more severe cases treatment may need to be continued for 2 years or longer
‣ Adult: 500 mg twice daily for at least 3 months, if there is no improvement after the first 3 months another oral antibacterial should be used, maximum improvement usually occurs after 4 to 6 months but in more severe cases treatment may need to be continued for 2 years or longer

- **INTERACTIONS** Milk reduces absorption.
- **RENAL IMPAIRMENT** May exacerbate renal failure and should **not** be given to patients with renal impairment.
- **PROFESSION SPECIFIC INFORMATION**

Dental practitioners' formulary
Oxytetracycline Tablets may be prescribed.

- **MEDICINAL FORMS**
There can be variation in the licensing of different medicines containing the same drug. Forms available from special-order manufacturers include: oral suspension
Tablet
CAUTIONARY AND ADVISORY LABELS 7, 9, 23
‣ Oxytetracycline (Non-proprietary)
  Oxytetracycline (as Oxytetracycline dihydrate)
  250 mg Oxytetracycline 250mg tablets | 28 tablet [PoM] £12.50 DT price = £0.91 | 1000 tablet [PoM] no price available

Tetracycline

F 513

- **INDICATIONS AND DOSE**

Susceptible infections (e.g. chlamydia, rickettsia, mycoplasma)
‣ BY MOUTH
‣ Child 12–17 years: 250 mg 4 times a day, increased if necessary to 500 mg 3–4 times a day, increased dose used in severe infections
‣ Adult: 250 mg 4 times a day, increased if necessary to 500 mg 3–4 times a day, increased dose used in severe infections

continued →

5

Infection

Rosacea

▸ BY MOUTH

▸ Adult: 500 mg twice daily usually for 6–12 weeks (course may be repeated intermittently)

Acne

▸ BY MOUTH

▸ Child 12-17 years: 500 mg twice daily for at least 3 months, if there is no improvement after the first 3 months another oral antibacterial should be used, maximum improvement usually occurs after 4 to 6 months but in more severe cases treatment may need to be continued for 2 years or longer

▸ Adult: 500 mg twice daily for at least 3 months, if there is no improvement after the first 3 months another oral antibacterial should be used, maximum improvement usually occurs after 4 to 6 months but in more severe cases treatment may need to be continued for 2 years or longer

Diabetic diarrhoea in autonomic neuropathy

▸ BY MOUTH

▸ Adult: 250 mg for 2 or 3 doses

Non-gonococcal urethritis

▸ BY MOUTH

▸ Child 12-17 years: 500 mg 4 times a day for 7–14 days (21 days if failure or relapse after first course)

▸ Adult: 500 mg 4 times a day for 7–14 days (21 days if failure or relapse after first course)

***Helicobacter pylori* eradication failure in combination with a proton pump inhibitor, tripotassium dicitratobismuthate, and metronidazole**

▸ BY MOUTH

▸ Adult: 500 mg 4 times a day for 2 weeks

● UNLICENSED USE Not licensed for treatment of diabetic diarrhoea in *autonomic neuropathy*.

● INTERACTIONS Milk reduces absorption.

● SIDE-EFFECTS Acute renal failure · skin discoloration

● HEPATIC IMPAIRMENT Max. 1 g daily in divided doses.

● RENAL IMPAIRMENT May exacerbate renal failure and should **not** be given to patients with renal impairment.

● DIRECTIONS FOR ADMINISTRATION Tablets should be swallowed whole with plenty of fluid while sitting or standing.

● PATIENT AND CARER ADVICE Counselling on administration advised.

● PROFESSION SPECIFIC INFORMATION

Dental practitioners' formulary
Tetracycline Tablets may be prescribed.

● MEDICINAL FORMS
There can be variation in the licensing of different medicines containing the same drug. Forms available from special-order manufacturers include: capsule, oral solution

Tablet
CAUTIONARY AND ADVISORY LABELS 7, 9, 23

▸ Tetracycline (Non-proprietary)
Tetracycline hydrochloride 250 mg Tetracycline 250mg tablets | 28 tablet [PoM] £25.65 DT price = £2.04

Tigecycline

● DRUG ACTION Tigecycline is a glycylcycline antibacterial structurally related to the tetracyclines. Tigecycline is active against Gram-positive and Gram-negative bacteria, including tetracycline-resistant organisms, and some anaerobes. It is also active against meticillin-resistant *Staphylococcus aureus* and vancomycin-resistant enterococci, but *Pseudomonas aeruginosa* and many strains of *Proteus spp* are resistant to tigecycline.

● INDICATIONS AND DOSE

Treatment of complicated skin and soft-tissue infections and complicated abdominal infections caused by multiple-antibacterial resistant organisms when other antibacterials cannot be used

▸ BY INTRAVENOUS INFUSION

▸ Adult: Initially 100 mg, then 50 mg every 12 hours for 5–14 days, not recommended for the treatment of foot infections in patients with diabetes

● CAUTIONS Cholestasis

● INTERACTIONS → Appendix 1 (tigecycline).

● SIDE-EFFECTS

▸ **Common or very common** Abdominal pain · anorexia · bilirubinaemia · diarrhoea · dizziness · dyspepsia · headache · hypoglycaemia · injection-site reactions · nausea · prolonged activated partial thromboplastin time · prolonged prothrombin time · pruritus · rash · vomiting

▸ **Uncommon** Cholestatic jaundice · hypoproteinaemia · pancreatitis

▸ **Frequency not known** Antibiotic-associated colitis · hepatic failure · Stevens-Johnson syndrome · thrombocytopenia

SIDE-EFFECTS, FURTHER INFORMATION
Side-effects similar to those of the tetracyclines can potentially occur.

● ALLERGY AND CROSS-SENSITIVITY Contra-indicated in patients hypersensitive to tetracyclines.

● PREGNANCY Tetracyclines should **not** be given to pregnant women; effects on skeletal development have been documented in the first trimester in *animal* studies. Administration during the second or third trimester may cause discoloration of the child's teeth, and maternal hepatotoxicity has been reported with large parenteral doses.

● BREAST FEEDING Manufacturer advises caution—present in milk in *animal* studies.

● HEPATIC IMPAIRMENT Initially 100 mg then 25 mg every 12 hours in severe hepatic impairment.

● DIRECTIONS FOR ADMINISTRATION For *intravenous infusion* (*Tygacil®*), give intermittently *in* Glucose 5% *or* Sodium Chloride 0.9%. Reconstitute each vial with 5.3 mL infusion fluid to produce a 10 mg/mL solution; dilute requisite dose in 100 mL infusion fluid; give over 30–60 minutes.

● MEDICINAL FORMS
There can be variation in the licensing of different medicines containing the same drug.

Powder for solution for infusion

▸ Tygacil (Pfizer Ltd)
Tigecycline 50 mg Tygacil 50mg powder for solution for infusion vials | 10 vial [PoM] £323.10 (Hospital only)

ANTIBACTERIALS > OTHER

Chloramphenicol

- **DRUG ACTION** Chloramphenicol is a potent broad-spectrum antibiotic.

- **INDICATIONS AND DOSE**

Life threatening infections particularly those caused by *Haemophilus infuenzae* | **Typhoid fever**
  ▸ BY MOUTH, OR BY INTRAVENOUS INJECTION, OR BY INTRAVENOUS INFUSION
  ▸ Adult: 12.5 mg/kg every 6 hours, in exceptional cases dose can be doubled for severe infections such as septicaemia and meningitis, providing high doses reduced as soon as clinically indicated

- **CONTRA-INDICATIONS** Acute porphyrias p. 918
- **CAUTIONS** Avoid repeated courses and prolonged treatment
- **INTERACTIONS** → Appendix 1 (chloramphenicol).
- **SIDE-EFFECTS** Blood disorders · depression · diarrhoea · dry mouth · erythema multiforme · glossitis · headache · nausea · nocturnal haemoglobinuria · optic neuritis · peripheral neuritis · reversible and irreversible aplastic anaemia (with reports of resulting leukaemia) · stomatitis · urticaria · vomiting

  SIDE-EFFECTS, FURTHER INFORMATION
  Associated with serious haematological side-effects when given systemically and should therefore be reserved for the treatment of life-threatening infections.
- **PREGNANCY** Manufacturer advises avoid; neonatal 'grey-baby syndrome' if used in third trimester.
- **BREAST FEEDING** Manufacturer advises avoid; use another antibiotic; may cause bone-marrow toxicity in infant; concentration in milk usually insufficient to cause 'grey syndrome'.
- **HEPATIC IMPAIRMENT** Reduce dose.
  Avoid if possible—increased risk of bone-marrow depression.
  Monitor plasma-chloramphenicol concentration in hepatic impairment.
- **RENAL IMPAIRMENT** Avoid in severe renal impairment unless no alternative; dose-related depression of haematopoiesis.
- **MONITORING REQUIREMENTS**
  ▸ Plasma concentration monitoring preferred in the elderly.
  ▸ Recommended peak plasma concentration (approx. 2 hours after administration by mouth, intravenous injection or infusion) 10–25 mg/litre; pre-dose ('trough') concentration should not exceed 15 mg/litre.
  ▸ Blood counts required before and periodically during treatment.
- **DIRECTIONS FOR ADMINISTRATION** For *intravenous infusion* (*Kemicetine*®), give intermittently or via drip tubing in Glucose 5% or Sodium chloride 0.9%.

- **MEDICINAL FORMS**
  There can be variation in the licensing of different medicines containing the same drug.
  Capsule
  ▸ Chloramphenicol (Non-proprietary)
    Chloramphenicol 250 mg Chloramphenicol 250mg capsules | 60 capsule [PoM] £377.00 DT price = £377.00
  Powder for solution for injection
  ELECTROLYTES: May contain Sodium
  ▸ Kemicetine (Pfizer Ltd)
    Chloramphenicol (as Chloramphenicol sodium succinate)
    1 gram Kemicetine 1g powder for solution for injection vials | 1 vial [PoM] £1.39

Daptomycin

- **DRUG ACTION** Daptomycin is a lipopeptide antibacterial with a spectrum of activity similar to vancomycin but its efficacy against enterococci has not been established. It needs to be given with other antibacterials for mixed infections involving Gram-negative bacteria and some anaerobes.

- **INDICATIONS AND DOSE**

Complicated skin and soft-tissue infections caused by Gram-positive bacteria, including meticillin-resistant *Staphylococcus aureus* **(MRSA)**
  ▸ BY SLOW INTRAVENOUS INJECTION, OR BY INTRAVENOUS INFUSION
  ▸ Adult: 4 mg/kg once daily; increased to 6 mg/kg once daily, increase dose only if associated with *Staphylococcus aureus* bacteraemia

Staphylococcal endocarditis caused by organisms resistant to vancomycin or in patients intolerant of vancomycin (in combination with other antibacterials)
  ▸ BY SLOW INTRAVENOUS INJECTION, OR BY INTRAVENOUS INFUSION
  ▸ Adult: 6 mg/kg once daily

- **UNLICENSED USE** Not licensed for use in left-sided endocarditis.
- **INTERACTIONS** → Appendix 1 (daptomycin).
  Monitor creatine kinase more frequently than weekly during treatment if receiving another drug known to cause myopathy (preferably avoid concomitant use).
- **SIDE-EFFECTS**
  ▸ **Common or very common** Abdominal pain · anaemia · anxiety · arthralgia · asthenia · constipation · diarrhoea · dizziness · flatulence · headache · hypertension · hypotension · injection-site reactions · insomnia · nausea · pruritus · rash · vomiting
  ▸ **Uncommon** Anorexia · arrhythmias · dyspepsia · electrolyte disturbances · eosinophilia · flushing · glossitis · hyperglycaemia · muscle effects · muscle weakness · myalgia · myositis · paraesthesia · renal failure · taste disturbance · thrombocythaemia · tremor
  ▸ **Rare** Jaundice · rhabdomyolysis
  ▸ **Frequency not known** Antibiotic-associated colitis · elevated creatine kinase · eosinophilic pneumonia · peripheral neuropathy · syncope · wheezing

  SIDE-EFFECTS, FURTHER INFORMATION
  ▸ Muscle effects If unexplained muscle pain, tenderness, weakness, or cramps develop during treatment, measure creatine kinase every 2 days; discontinue if unexplained muscular symptoms and creatine elevated markedly.
- **PREGNANCY** Manufacturer advises use only if potential benefit outweighs risk—no information available.
- **BREAST FEEDING** Present in milk in small amount, but absorption from gastrointestinal tract negligible.
- **HEPATIC IMPAIRMENT** Manufacturer advises caution in severe hepatic impairment—no information available.
- **RENAL IMPAIRMENT** Use normal dose every 48 hours if eGFR less than 30 mL/minute/1.73 m². If eGFR less than 80 mL/minute/1.73 m², monitor renal function, and monitor creatine kinase before treatment and then at least weekly during treatment.
- **MONITORING REQUIREMENTS** Monitor creatine kinase before treatment and then weekly during treatment (more frequently if creatine kinase elevated more than 5 times upper limit of normal before treatment).
- **EFFECT ON LABORATORY TESTS** Interference with assay for prothrombin time and INR—take blood sample immediately before daptomycin dose.

● DIRECTIONS FOR ADMINISTRATION For *intravenous infusion* (*Cubicin*®), give intermittently in Sodium chloride 0.9%; reconstitute with sodium chloride 0.9% (350 mg in 7 mL, 500 mg in 10 mL); gently rotate vial without shaking; allow to stand for at least 10 minutes then rotate gently to dissolve; dilute requisite dose in 50 mL infusion fluid and give over 30 minutes. For *intravenous injection*, give over 2 minutes.

● NATIONAL FUNDING/ACCESS DECISIONS

Scottish Medicines Consortium (SMC) Decisions
The *Scottish Medicines Consortium* has advised (February 2008) that daptomycin (*Cubicin*®) is accepted for restricted use within NHS Scotland for the treatment of MRSA bacteraemia associated with right-sided endocarditis or with complicated skin and soft-tissue infections.

● MEDICINAL FORMS
There can be variation in the licensing of different medicines containing the same drug.
Powder for solution for infusion
▸ Cubicin (Merck Sharp & Dohme Ltd)
   Daptomycin 350 mg Cubicin 350mg powder for concentrate for solution for infusion vials | 1 vial [PoM] £62.00
   Daptomycin 500 mg Cubicin 500mg powder for concentrate for solution for infusion vials | 1 vial [PoM] £88.57 (Hospital only)

Fidaxomicin

● DRUG ACTION Fidaxomicin is a macrocyclic antibacterial that is poorly absorbed from the gastro-intestinal tract, and, therefore, it should not be used to treat systemic infections.

● INDICATIONS AND DOSE
Clostridium difficile infection
▸ BY MOUTH
▸ Adult: 200 mg every 12 hours for 10 days, limited clinical data is available on the use of fidaxomicin in severe or life-threatening *Clostridium difficile* infection

● CAUTIONS Inflammatory bowel disease · severe or life-threatening *C. difficile* infection
● INTERACTIONS → Appendix 1 (fidaxomicin).
● SIDE-EFFECTS
▸ **Common or very common** Constipation · nausea · vomiting
▸ **Uncommon** Abdominal distension · decreased appetite · dizziness · dry mouth · flatulence · headache · taste disturbance
● ALLERGY AND CROSS-SENSITIVITY Use with caution in macrolide hypersensitivity.
● PREGNANCY Manufacturer advises avoid—no information available.
● BREAST FEEDING Manufacturer advises avoid—no information available.
● HEPATIC IMPAIRMENT Manufacturer advises caution in moderate to severe impairment—no information available.
● RENAL IMPAIRMENT Manufacturer advises caution in severe impairment—no information available.
● NATIONAL FUNDING/ACCESS DECISIONS

Scottish Medicines Consortium (SMC) Decisions
The *Scottish Medicines Consortium* has advised (June 2012) that fidaxomicin (*Dificlir*®) is accepted for restricted use within NHS Scotland to treat the first recurrence of *C. difficile* infection, on the advice of a microbiologist or specialist in infectious diseases.

● MEDICINAL FORMS
There can be variation in the licensing of different medicines containing the same drug.
Tablet
CAUTIONARY AND ADVISORY LABELS 9
▸ Dificlir (Astellas Pharma Ltd) ▼
   Fidaxomicin 200 mg Dificlir 200mg tablets | 20 tablet [PoM] £1,350.00

Fosfomycin

● DRUG ACTION Fosfomycin, a phosphonic acid antibacterial, is active against a range of Gram-positive and Gram-negative bacteria including *Staphylococcus aureus* and Enterobacteriaceae.

● INDICATIONS AND DOSE
Uncomplicated lower urinary-tract infections caused by multiple-antibacterial resistant organisms when other antibacterials cannot be used
▸ BY MOUTH
▸ Adult (female): 3 g for 1 dose.
▸ Adult (male): 3 g for 1 dose, then 3 g after 3 days.
Osteomyelitis when first-line treatments are inappropriate or ineffective | Hospital-acquired lower respiratory-tract infections when first-line treatments are inappropriate or ineffective
▸ BY INTRAVENOUS INFUSION
▸ Adult: 12–24 g daily in 2–3 divided doses (max. per dose 8 g), use the high-dose regimen in severe infection suspected or known to be caused by less sensitive organisms
Complicated urinary-tract infections when first-line treatment ineffective or inappropriate
▸ BY INTRAVENOUS INFUSION
▸ Adult: 12–16 g daily in 2–3 divided doses (max. per dose 8 g)
Bacterial meningitis when first-line treatment ineffective or inappropriate
▸ BY INTRAVENOUS INFUSION
▸ Adult: 16–24 g daily in 3–4 divided doses (max. per dose 8 g), use the high-dose regimen in severe infection suspected or known to be caused by less sensitive organisms

● UNLICENSED USE Oral preparations containing fosfomycin are not marketed in the UK and use of these preparations is unlicensed.
● CAUTIONS
▸ With intravenous use Cardiac insufficiency · elderly (high doses) · hyperaldosteronism · hypernatraemia · hypertension · pulmonary oedema
● INTERACTIONS → Appendix 1 (fosfomycin).
● SIDE-EFFECTS
GENERAL SIDE-EFFECTS
▸ **Common or very common** Gastro-intestinal disturbances · rash
▸ **Uncommon** Diarrhoea · nausea · vomiting
▸ **Frequency not known** Abdominal pain
SPECIFIC SIDE-EFFECTS
▸ **Uncommon**
▸ With intravenous use Decreased appetite · dyspnoea · fatigue · headache · hypernatraemia · hypokalaemia · taste disturbances · vertigo
▸ **Rare**
▸ With intravenous use Aplastic anaemia · blood disorders · eosinophilia
▸ **Very rare**
▸ With intravenous use Fatty liver · visual impairment

▶ **Frequency not known**
▶ With intravenous use Antibiotic-associated colitis · bronchospasm · confusion · hepatitis · jaundice · tachycardia

● PREGNANCY Manufacturer advises use only if potential benefit outweighs risk.

● BREAST FEEDING Manufacturer advises use only if potential benefit outweighs risk—present in milk.

● RENAL IMPAIRMENT
▶ With oral use Avoid *oral* treatment if eGFR less than 10 mL/minute/1.73 m^2.
▶ With intravenous use Use *intravenous* treatment with caution if eGFR 40–80 mL/minute/1.73 m^2 and consult product literature for dose if eGFR less than 40 mL/minute/1.73 m^2.

● MONITORING REQUIREMENTS
▶ With intravenous use Monitor electrolytes and fluid balance.

● DIRECTIONS FOR ADMINISTRATION For *intravenous infusion* (*Fomicyt* ®), give intermittently *in* Glucose 5% *or* 10% *or* Water for Injections; reconstitute each 2-g vial with 50 mL infusion fluid; give 2 g over 15 minutes.

● PRESCRIBING AND DISPENSING INFORMATION Doses expressed as fosfomycin base.
▶ With oral use Although oral preparations containing fosfomycin are not marketed in the UK, they can be used, on the advice of a microbiologist, for the treatment of uncomplicated lower urinary tract infections caused by multiple-antibacterial resistant organisms when other antibacterials cannot be used.

● NATIONAL FUNDING/ACCESS DECISIONS
Scottish Medicines Consortium (SMC) Decisions
The *Scottish Medicines Consortium* has advised (February 2015) that Fosfomycin (*Fomicyt* ®) is accepted for restricted use within NHS Scotland; initiation should be restricted to microbiologists or infectious disease specialists.

● MEDICINAL FORMS
There can be variation in the licensing of different medicines containing the same drug. Forms available from special-order manufacturers include: capsule

Capsule
▶ Fosfomycin (Non-proprietary)
Fosfomycin calcium 500 mg Fosfocina 500mg capsules | 24 capsule [PoM] no price available

Granules
CAUTIONARY AND ADVISORY LABELS 9, 13, 23
▶ Fosfomycin (Non-proprietary)
Fosfomycin (as Fosfomycin trometamol) 3 gram Monurol 3g granules sachets | 1 sachet [PoM] no price available
Fosfomycin 3g granules sachets | 1 sachet [PoM] £75.45

Oral suspension
▶ Fosfomycin (Non-proprietary)
Fosfomycin calcium 50 mg per 1 ml Fosfocina 250mg/5ml oral suspension | 120 ml [PoM] no price available

Powder for solution for infusion
ELECTROLYTES: May contain Sodium
▶ Fomicyt (Nordic Pharma Ltd)
Fosfomycin (as Fosfomycin sodium) 2 gram Fomicyt 2g powder for solution for infusion vials | 10 vial [PoM] £150.00
Fosfomycin (as Fosfomycin sodium) 4 gram Fomicyt 4g powder for solution for infusion vials | 10 vial [PoM] £300.00

Fusidic acid

● DRUG ACTION Fusidic acid and its salts are narrow-spectrum antibiotics used for staphylococcal infections.

● INDICATIONS AND DOSE
Staphylococcal skin infection
▶ BY MOUTH USING TABLETS
▶ Child 12–17 years: 250 mg every 12 hours for 5–10 days
▶ Adult: 250 mg every 12 hours for 5–10 days

▶ TO THE SKIN
▶ Child: Apply 3–4 times a day usually for 7 days
▶ Adult: Apply 3–4 times a day

Penicillin-resistant staphylococcal infection including osteomyelitis | Staphylococcal endocarditis in combination with other antibacterials
▶ BY MOUTH USING ORAL SUSPENSION
▶ Child 1–11 months: 15 mg/kg 3 times a day
▶ Child 1–4 years: 250 mg 3 times a day
▶ Child 5–11 years: 500 mg 3 times a day
▶ Child 12–17 years: 750 mg 3 times a day
▶ Adult: 750 mg 3 times a day
▶ BY MOUTH USING TABLETS
▶ Child 12–17 years: 500 mg every 8 hours, increased to 1 g every 8 hours, increased dose can be used for severe infections
▶ Adult: 500 mg every 8 hours, increased to 1 g every 8 hours, increased dose can be used for severe infections

DOSE EQUIVALENCE AND CONVERSION
▶ With oral use Fusidic acid is incompletely absorbed and doses recommended for suspension are proportionately higher than those for sodium fusidate tablets.

● CAUTIONS
▶ With topical use Avoid contact of cream or ointment with eyes
CAUTIONS, FURTHER INFORMATION
▶ Avoiding resistance
▶ With topical use To avoid the development of resistance, fusidic acid should not be used for longer than 10 days and local microbiology advice should be sought before using it in hospital.

● INTERACTIONS → Appendix 1 (fusidic acid).

● SIDE-EFFECTS
▶ **Common or very common**
▶ With oral use Abdominal pain · diarrhoea · dizziness · drowsiness · dyspepsia · nausea · vomiting
▶ **Uncommon**
▶ With oral use Anorexia · headache · malaise · pruritus · rash
▶ **Rare**
▶ With topical use Hypersensitivity reactions
▶ Frequency not known
▶ With oral use Acute renal failure (usually with jaundice) · blood disorders · reversible jaundice especially after high dosage (withdraw therapy if persistent)

● PREGNANCY
▶ With oral use Not known to be harmful; manufacturer advises use only if potential benefit outweighs risk.

● BREAST FEEDING
▶ With oral use Present in milk—manufacturer advises caution.

● HEPATIC IMPAIRMENT
▶ With oral use Impaired biliary excretion; possibly increased risk of hepatotoxicity; avoid or reduce dose.
   Elimination may be reduced in hepatic impairment or biliary disease or biliary obstruction.
   Monitor liver function in hepatic impairment.

● MONITORING REQUIREMENTS
▶ With oral use Monitor liver function with high doses or on prolonged therapy.

● PRESCRIBING AND DISPENSING INFORMATION Flavours of oral liquid formulations may include banana and orange.

● PROFESSION SPECIFIC INFORMATION
Dental practitioners' formulary
▶ With topical use May be prescribed as Sodium Fusidate ointment.

5

Infection

- MEDICINAL FORMS

There can be variation in the licensing of different medicines containing the same drug.

Tablet

CAUTIONARY AND ADVISORY LABELS 9

▸ Fucidin (Sodium fusidate) (LEO Pharma)

Sodium fusidate 250 mg Fucidin 250mg tablets | 10 tablet [PoM] £6.02 DT price = £6.02 | 100 tablet [PoM] £54.99

Oral suspension

CAUTIONARY AND ADVISORY LABELS 9, 21

▸ Fucidin (Fusidic acid) (LEO Pharma)

Fusidic acid 50 mg per 1 ml Fucidin 250mg/5ml oral suspension | 50 ml [PoM] £6.73

Cream

EXCIPIENTS: May contain Butylated hydroxyanisole, cetostearyl alcohol (including cetyl and stearyl alcohol)

▸ Fusidic acid (Non-proprietary)

Fusidic acid 20 mg per 1 gram Fusidic acid 2% cream | 15 gram [PoM] £1.92 DT price = £1.92 | 30 gram [PoM] £3.59 DT price = £3.59

▸ Fucidin (Fusidic acid) (LEO Pharma)

Fusidic acid 20 mg per 1 gram Fucidin 20mg/g cream | 15 gram [PoM] £1.92 DT price = £1.92 | 30 gram [PoM] £3.59 DT price = £3.59

Ointment

EXCIPIENTS: May contain Cetostearyl alcohol (including cetyl and stearyl alcohol), wool fat and related substances including lanolin

▸ Fucidin (Sodium fusidate) (LEO Pharma)

Sodium fusidate 20 mg per 1 gram Fucidin 20mg/g ointment | 15 gram [PoM] £2.68 DT price = £2.68 | 30 gram [PoM] £4.55 DT price = £4.55

Linezolid

- DRUG ACTION Linezolid, an oxazolidinone antibacterial, is active against Gram-positive bacteria including meticillin-resistant *Staphylococcus aureus* (MRSA), and glycopeptide-resistant enterococci. Resistance to linezolid can develop with prolonged treatment or if the dose is less than that recommended. Linezolid is **not** active against common Gram-negative organisms; it must be given in combination with other antibacterials for mixed infections that also involve Gram-negative organisms.

- INDICATIONS AND DOSE

Pneumonia (when other antibacterials e.g. a glycopeptide, such as vancomycin, cannot be used) (initiated under specialist supervision) | Complicated skin and soft-tissue infections caused by Gram-positive bacteria, when other antibacterials cannot be used (initiated under specialist supervision)

▸ BY MOUTH

▸ Adult: 600 mg every 12 hours usually for 10–14 days (maximum duration of treatment 28 days)

▸ BY INTRAVENOUS INFUSION

▸ Adult: 600 mg every 12 hours

IMPORTANT SAFETY INFORMATION

CHM ADVICE (OPTIC NEUROPATHY)

Severe optic neuropathy may occur rarely, particularly if linezolid is used for longer than 28 days. The CHM recommends that:

- patients should be warned to report symptoms of visual impairment (including blurred vision, visual field defect, changes in visual acuity and colour vision) immediately;
- patients experiencing new visual symptoms (regardless of treatment duration) should be evaluated promptly, and referred to an ophthalmologist if necessary;
- visual function should be monitored regularly if treatment is required for longer than 28 days.

BLOOD DISORDERS

Haematopoietic disorders (including thrombocytopenia, anaemia, leucopenia, and pancytopenia) have been reported in patients receiving linezolid. It is recommended that full blood counts are monitored weekly. Close monitoring is recommended in patients who:

- receive treatment for more than 10–14 days;
- have pre-existing myelosuppression;
- are receiving drugs that may have adverse effects on haemoglobin, blood counts, or platelet function;
- have severe renal impairment.

If significant myelosuppression occurs, treatment should be stopped unless it is considered essential, in which case intensive monitoring of blood counts and appropriate management should be implemented.

- CAUTIONS Acute confusional states · bipolar depression · carcinoid tumour · elderly (increased risk of blood disorders) · history of seizures · phaeochromocytoma · schizophrenia · thyrotoxicosis · uncontrolled hypertension

CAUTIONS, FURTHER INFORMATION

▸ Close observation Unless close observation and blood pressure monitoring possible, linezolid should be avoided in uncontrolled hypertension, phaeochromocytoma, carcinoid tumour, thyrotoxicosis, bipolar depression, schizophrenia, or acute confusional states.

- INTERACTIONS → Appendix 1 (MAOIs).

▸ **Monoamine oxidase inhibition** Linezolid is a reversible, non-selective monoamine oxidase inhibitor (MAOI). Patients should avoid consuming large amounts of tyramine-rich foods (such as mature cheese, yeast extracts, undistilled alcoholic beverages, and fermented soya bean products). In addition, linezolid should not be given with another MAOI or within 2 weeks of stopping another MAOI. Unless close observation and blood-pressure monitoring is possible, avoid in those receiving SSRIs, 5HT$_1$ agonists ('triptans'), tricyclic antidepressants, sympathomimetics, dopaminergics, buspirone, pethidine and possibly other opioid analgesics.

- SIDE-EFFECTS

GENERAL SIDE-EFFECTS

▸ **Common or very common** Diarrhoea · eosinophilia · headache · nausea · taste disturbances · vomiting

▸ **Uncommon** Abdominal pain · blurred vision · constipation · diaphoresis · dizziness · dry mouth · dyspepsia · electrolyte disturbances · fatigue · fever · gastritis · glossitis · hypertension · hypoaesthesia · insomnia · leucopenia · pancreatitis · paraesthesia · polyuria · pruritus · rash · stomatitis · thirst · thrombocytopenia · tinnitus · tongue discoloration

▸ **Rare** Renal failure · tachycardia · transient ischaemic attacks

▸ **Frequency not known** Anaemia · antibiotic-associated colitis · convulsions · hyponatraemia · lactic acidosis · optic neuropathy reported on prolonged therapy · pancytopenia · peripheral neuropathy reported on prolonged therapy · Stevens-Johnson syndrome · tooth discoloration · toxic epidermal necrolysis

SPECIFIC SIDE-EFFECTS

▸ **Uncommon**

▸ With intravenous use Injection-site reactions

- PREGNANCY Manufacturer advises use only if potential benefit outweighs risk—no information available.

- BREAST FEEDING Manufacturer advises avoid—present in milk in *animal* studies.

- HEPATIC IMPAIRMENT In severe hepatic impairment manufacturer advises use only if potential benefit outweighs risk.

- RENAL IMPAIRMENT Manufacturer advises metabolites may accumulate if eGFR less than 30 mL/minute/1.73 m^2.
- MONITORING REQUIREMENTS Monitor full blood count (including platelet count) weekly.
- DIRECTIONS FOR ADMINISTRATION Infusion to be administered over 30–120 minutes.
- PRESCRIBING AND DISPENSING INFORMATION Flavours of oral liquid formulations may include orange.
- PATIENT AND CARER ADVICE Patients should be advised to read the patient information leaflet given with linezolid.

- MEDICINAL FORMS
There can be variation in the licensing of different medicines containing the same drug.

Tablet
CAUTIONARY AND ADVISORY LABELS 9, 10
- Linezolid (Non-proprietary)
  Linezolid 600 mg Linezolid 600mg tablets | 10 tablet PoM £228.86–£445.00
- Zyvox (Pfizer Ltd)
  Linezolid 600 mg Zyvox 600mg tablets | 10 tablet PoM £445.00

Oral suspension
CAUTIONARY AND ADVISORY LABELS 9, 10
EXCIPIENTS: May contain Aspartame
- Zyvox (Pfizer Ltd)
  Linezolid 20 mg per 1 ml Zyvox 100mg/5ml granules for oral suspension | 150 ml PoM £222.50

Infusion
EXCIPIENTS: May contain Glucose
ELECTROLYTES: May contain Sodium
- Linezolid (Non-proprietary)
  Linezolid 2 mg per 1 ml Linezolid 600mg/300ml infusion bags | 10 bag PoM £445.00 (Hospital only)
- Zyvox (Pfizer Ltd)
  Linezolid 2 mg per 1 ml Zyvox 600mg/300ml infusion bags | 10 bag PoM £445.00

Trimethoprim

- INDICATIONS AND DOSE

Urinary-tract infections | Respiratory tract infections
▶ BY MOUTH
- Child 4–5 weeks: 4 mg/kg twice daily (max. per dose 200 mg)
- Child 6 weeks–5 months: 4 mg/kg twice daily (max. per dose 200 mg), alternatively 25 mg twice daily
- Child 6 months–5 years: 4 mg/kg twice daily (max. per dose 200 mg), alternatively 50 mg twice daily
- Child 6–11 years: 4 mg/kg twice daily (max. per dose 200 mg), alternatively 100 mg twice daily
- Child 12–17 years: 200 mg twice daily
- Adult: 200 mg twice daily

Prophylaxis of urinary-tract infection (considered for recurrent infection, significant urinary-tract anomalies, or significant kidney damage)
▶ BY MOUTH
- Child 4–5 weeks: 2 mg/kg once daily (max. per dose 100 mg), dose to be taken at night
- Child 6 weeks–5 months: 2 mg/kg once daily (max. per dose 100 mg), dose to be taken at night, alternatively 12.5 mg once daily, dose to be taken at night
- Child 6 months–5 years: 2 mg/kg once daily (max. per dose 100 mg), dose to be taken at night, alternatively 25 mg once daily, dose to be taken at night
- Child 6–11 years: 2 mg/kg once daily (max. per dose 100 mg), dose to be taken at night, alternatively 50 mg once daily, dose to be taken at night
- Child 12–17 years: 100 mg once daily, dose to be taken at night
- Adult: 100 mg once daily, dose to be taken at night

Treatment of mild to moderate *Pneumocystis jirovecii* (*Pneumocystis carinii*) pneumonia in patients who cannot tolerate co-trimoxazole (in combination with dapsone)
▶ BY MOUTH
- Child: 5 mg/kg every 6–8 hours
- Adult: 5 mg/kg every 6–8 hours

Acne resistant to other antibacterials
▶ BY MOUTH
- Adult: 300 mg twice daily

Prostatitis
▶ BY MOUTH
- Adult: (consult product literature)

Shigellosis | Invasive salmonella infection
▶ BY MOUTH
- Adult: (consult product literature)

- UNLICENSED USE Not licensed for treatment of pneumocystis pneumonia. Not licensed for use in children under 6 weeks.
  Not licensed for treatment of acne resistant to other antibacterials.
- CONTRA-INDICATIONS Blood dyscrasias
- CAUTIONS Elderly · Acute porphyrias p. 918 · neonates (specialist supervision required) · predisposition to folate deficiency
- INTERACTIONS → Appendix 1 (trimethoprim).
- SIDE-EFFECTS
- **Rare** Allergic reactions · anaphylaxis · angioedema · erythema multiforme · photosensitivity · toxic epidermal necrolysis
- **Frequency not known** Aseptic meningitis · depression of haematopoiesis · gastro-intestinal disturbances · hyperkalaemia · nausea · pruritus · rashes · uveitis (in adults) · vomiting

  SIDE-EFFECTS, FURTHER INFORMATION
  Trimethoprim has side-effects similar to co-trimoxazole but they are less severe and occur less frequently.
- PREGNANCY Teratogenic risk in first trimester (folate antagonist). Manufacturers advise avoid during pregnancy.
- BREAST FEEDING Present in milk—short-term use not known to be harmful.
- RENAL IMPAIRMENT
- In adults Use half normal dose after 3 days if eGFR 15–30 mL/minute/1.73 m^2. Use half normal dose if eGFR less than 15 mL/minute/1.73 m^2.
- In children Use half normal dose after 3 days if estimated glomerular filtration rate 15–30 mL/minute/1.73 m^2. Use half normal dose if estimated glomerular filtration rate less than 15 mL/minute/1.73 m^2. Monitor plasma-trimethoprim concentration if eGFR less than 10 mL/minute/1.73 m^2.
- MONITORING REQUIREMENTS Manufacturer recommends blood counts on long-term therapy (but evidence of practical value unsatisfactory).
- PATIENT AND CARER ADVICE
  Medicines for Children leaflet: Trimethoprim for bacterial infections www.medicinesforchildren.org.uk/trimethoprim-for-bacterial-infections
  Blood disorders On long-term treatment, patients and their carers should be told how to recognise signs of blood disorders and advised to seek immediate medical attention if symptoms such as fever, sore throat, rash, mouth ulcers, purpura, bruising or bleeding develop.

- MEDICINAL FORMS
There can be variation in the licensing of different medicines containing the same drug. Forms available from special-order manufacturers include: oral suspension, oral solution

Tablet

CAUTIONARY AND ADVISORY LABELS 9
▸ Trimethoprim (Non-proprietary)
Trimethoprim 100 mg Trimethoprim 100mg tablets | 28 tablet [PoM] £9.99 DT price = £1.68
Trimethoprim 200 mg Trimethoprim 200mg tablets | 6 tablet [PoM] £2.15 DT price = £1.03 | 14 tablet [PoM] £9.99 DT price = £2.40

Oral suspension

CAUTIONARY AND ADVISORY LABELS 9
▸ Trimethoprim (Non-proprietary)
Trimethoprim 10 mg per 1 ml Trimethoprim 50mg/5ml oral suspension sugar free sugar-free | 100 ml [PoM] £15.00 DT price = £1.72
▸ Monotrim (Chemidex Pharma Ltd)
Trimethoprim 10 mg per 1 ml Monotrim 50mg/5ml oral suspension sugar-free | 100 ml [PoM] £1.77 DT price = £1.72

ANTIMYCOBACTERIALS > RIFAMYCINS

Rifabutin

- INDICATIONS AND DOSE
Prophylaxis of *Mycobacterium avium* complex infections in immunosuppressed patients with low CD4 count
▸ BY MOUTH
▸ Adult: 300 mg once daily, also consult product literature

Treatment of non-tuberculous mycobacterial disease, in combination with other drugs
▸ BY MOUTH
▸ Adult: 450–600 mg once daily for up to 6 months after cultures negative

Treatment of pulmonary tuberculosis, in combination with other drugs
▸ BY MOUTH
▸ Adult: 150–450 mg once daily for at least 6 months

- CAUTIONS Acute porphyrias p. 918 · discolours soft contact lenses
- INTERACTIONS → Appendix 1 (rifamycins).
- SIDE-EFFECTS
▸ **Common or very common** Anaemia · blood disorders · leucopenia · myalgia · nausea · pyrexia · rash · thrombocytopenia
▸ **Uncommon** Arthralgia · body secretions coloured orange-red · bronchospasm · corneal deposits · eosinophilia · hypersensitivity reactions · jaundice · raised liver enzymes · saliva coloured orange-red · skin coloured orange-red · urine coloured orange-red · uveitis (especially following high doses or concomitant use with drugs that increase plasma concentration) · vomiting
▸ **Rare** Haemolysis
▸ **Frequency not known** Chest pain · dyspnoea · hepatitis · influenza-like symptoms
SIDE-EFFECTS, FURTHER INFORMATION
Discontinue permanently if serious side-effects develop.
- ALLERGY AND CROSS-SENSITIVITY Contra-indicated in patients with rifamycin hypersensitivity.
- CONCEPTION AND CONTRACEPTION
Important Rifabutin induces hepatic enzymes and the effectiveness of hormonal contraceptives is reduced; alternative family planning advice should be offered.
- PREGNANCY Manufacturer advises avoid—no information available.
- BREAST FEEDING Manufacturer advises avoid—no information available.

- HEPATIC IMPAIRMENT Reduce dose in severe impairment. In patients with pre-existing liver disease or hepatic impairment monitor liver function regularly and particularly frequently in the first 2 months; blood counts should also be monitored in these patients.
- RENAL IMPAIRMENT Use half normal dose if eGFR less than 30 mL/minute/1.73 m^2.
- MONITORING REQUIREMENTS
▸ *Renal function* should be checked before treatment.
▸ *Hepatic function* should be checked before treatment. If there is no evidence of liver disease (and pre-treatment liver function is normal), further checks are only necessary if the patient develops fever, malaise, vomiting, jaundice or unexplained deterioration during treatment. However, hepatic function should be monitored on prolonged therapy.
▸ Blood counts should be monitored on prolonged therapy.
▸ Those with alcohol dependence should have frequent checks of hepatic function, particularly in the first 2 months. Blood counts should also be monitored in these patients.
- PRESCRIBING AND DISPENSING INFORMATION If treatment interruption occurs, re-introduce with low dosage and increase gradually.
- PATIENT AND CARER ADVICE
Soft contact lenses Patients or their carers should be advised that rifabutin discolours soft contact lenses.
Hepatic disorders Patients or their carers should be told how to recognise signs of liver disorder, and advised to discontinue treatment and seek immediate medical attention if symptoms such as persistent nausea, vomiting, malaise or jaundice develop.
- MEDICINAL FORMS
There can be variation in the licensing of different medicines containing the same drug. Forms available from special-order manufacturers include: oral suspension, oral solution

Capsule

CAUTIONARY AND ADVISORY LABELS 8, 14
▸ Mycobutin (Pfizer Ltd)
Rifabutin 150 mg Mycobutin 150mg capsules | 30 capsule [PoM] £90.38

Rifaximin

- DRUG ACTION Rifaximin is a rifamycin that is poorly absorbed from the gastro-intestinal tract, and, therefore, should not be used to treat systemic infections.

- INDICATIONS AND DOSE
Travellers' diarrhoea that is not associated with fever, bloody diarrhoea, blood or leucocytes in the stool, or 8 or more unformed stools in the previous 24 hours
▸ BY MOUTH
▸ Adult: 200 mg every 8 hours for 3 days
Reduction in recurrence of hepatic encephalopathy
▸ BY MOUTH
▸ Adult: 550 mg twice daily

- CONTRA-INDICATIONS Intestinal obstruction
- INTERACTIONS → Appendix 1 (rifaximin).
Rifamycins interactions in Appendix 1 do not apply to rifaximin.
- SIDE-EFFECTS
▸ **Common or very common** Abdominal pain · depression · diarrhoea · dizziness · dyspnoea · flatulence · headache · muscle spasm · nausea · pruritus · rash · vomiting
▸ **Uncommon** Anorexia · antibiotic-associated colitis · anxiety · blood disorders · convulsions · dry mouth · dysuria · glycosuria · hyperkalaemia · hypoaesthesia · influenza-like symptoms · memory impairment · paraesthesia ·

peripheral oedema · polymenorrhoea · polyuria · sleep disturbances · taste disturbances

▸ **Rare** Blood pressure changes · constipation

▸ **Frequency not known** Syncope

● ALLERGY AND CROSS-SENSITIVITY Contra-indicated if history of rifamycin hypersensitivity.

● PREGNANCY Manufacturer advises avoid—toxicity in *animal* studies.

● BREAST FEEDING Unlikely to be present in milk in significant amounts, but manufacturer advises avoid.

● HEPATIC IMPAIRMENT Manufacturer advises caution when used for hepatic encephalopathy in patients with severe hepatic impairment.

● PRESCRIBING AND DISPENSING INFORMATION Not recommended for diarrhoea associated with invasive organisms such as *Campylobacter* and *Shigella*.

● NATIONAL FUNDING/ACCESS DECISIONS

NICE technology appraisals (TAs)
▸ **Rifaximin for preventing episodes of overt hepatic encephalopathy (March 2015)** NICE TA337
Rifaximin is recommended, within its marketing authorisation, as an option for reducing the recurrence of episodes of overt hepatic encephalopathy in adults.
www.nice.org.uk/TA337

● MEDICINAL FORMS
There can be variation in the licensing of different medicines containing the same drug.

Tablet
CAUTIONARY AND ADVISORY LABELS 14 (Targaxan® brand only), 9 (Xifaxantan® brand only)
▸ Rifaximin (Non-proprietary)
Rifaximin 200 mg Normix 200mg tablets | 12 tablet no price available
Rifaximin 550 mg Xifaxan 550mg tablets | 60 tablet [PoM] no price available
▸ Targaxan (Norgine Pharmaceuticals Ltd)
Rifaximin 550 mg Targaxan 550mg tablets | 56 tablet [PoM] £259.23 DT price = £259.23
▸ Xifaxanta (Norgine Pharmaceuticals Ltd)
Rifaximin 200 mg Xifaxanta 200mg tablets | 9 tablet [PoM] £15.15 DT price = £15.15

Oral suspension
▸ Rifaximin (Non-proprietary)
Rifaximin 20 mg per 1 ml Normix 100mg/5ml granules for oral suspension | 100 ml [PoM] no price available

2.1 Anthrax

Anthrax

Treatment and post-exposure prophylaxis

Inhalation or *gastro-intestinal anthrax* should be treated initially with either ciprofloxacin p. 506 or, in patients over 12 years, doxycycline p. 513 [unlicensed indication] combined with one or two other antibacterials (such as amoxicillin p. 498, benzylpenicillin sodium p. 496, chloramphenicol p. 517, clarithromycin p. 487, clindamycin p. 485, imipenem with cilastatin p. 474, rifampicin p. 527 [unlicensed indication], and vancomycin p. 484). When the condition improves and the sensitivity of the *Bacillus anthracis* strain is known, treatment may be switched to a single antibacterial. Treatment should continue for 60 days because germination may be delayed.

Cutaneous anthrax should be treated with either ciprofloxacin [unlicensed indication] or doxycycline [unlicensed indication] for 7 days. Treatment may be switched to amoxicillin if the infecting strain is susceptible. Treatment may need to be extended to 60 days if exposure is due to aerosol. A combination of antibacterials for 14 days is

recommended for cutaneous anthrax with systemic features, extensive oedema, or lesions of the head or neck.

Ciprofloxacin or doxycycline may be given for *post-exposure prophylaxis*. If exposure is confirmed, antibacterial prophylaxis should continue for 60 days. Antibacterial prophylaxis may be switched to amoxicillin after 10–14 days if the strain of *B. anthracis* is susceptible. Vaccination against anthrax may allow the duration of antibacterial prophylaxis to be shortened.

2.2 Leprosy

Leprosy

Management

Advice from a member of the Panel of Leprosy Opinion is essential for the treatment of leprosy (Hansen's disease). Details can be obtained from the Hospital for Tropical Diseases, London (telephone (020) 3456 7890).

The World Health Organization has made recommendations to overcome the problem of dapsone p. 524 resistance and to prevent the emergence of resistance to other antileprotic drugs. Drugs recommended are dapsone, rifampicin p. 527, and clofazimine below. Other drugs with significant activity against *Mycobacterium leprae* include ofloxacin p. 510, minocycline p. 515 and clarithromycin p. 487, but none of these are as active as rifampicin; at present they should be reserved as second-line drugs for leprosy.

A three-drug regimen is recommended for *multibacillary leprosy* (lepromatous, borderline-lepromatous, and borderline leprosy) and a two-drug regimen for *paucibacillary leprosy* (borderline-tuberculoid, tuberculoid, and indeterminate).

Multibacillary leprosy should be treated with a combination of rifampicin, dapsone and clofazimine for at least 2 years. Treatment should be continued unchanged during both type I (reversal) or type II (erythema nodosum leprosum) reactions. During reversal reactions neuritic pain or weakness can herald the rapid onset of permanent nerve damage. Treatment with prednisolone p. 614 should be instituted at once. Mild type II reactions may respond to aspirin. Severe type II reactions may require corticosteroids; thalidomide p. 845 [unlicensed] is also useful in patients who have become corticosteroid dependent, but it should be used only under **specialist supervision**. Thalidomide is teratogenic and, therefore, contra-indicated in pregnancy; it must **not** be given to women of child-bearing potential unless they comply with a pregnancy prevention programme. Increased doses of clofazimine are also useful.

Paucibacillary leprosy should be treated with rifampicin and dapsone for 6 months. If treatment is interrupted the regimen should be recommenced where it was left off to complete the full course.

Neither the multibacillary nor the paucibacillary antileprosy regimen is sufficient to treat tuberculosis.

ANTIMYCOBACTERIALS

Clofazimine

● INDICATIONS AND DOSE

Multibacillary leprosy in combination with rifampicin and dapsone (3-drug regimen)
▸ BY MOUTH
▸ Adult: 300 mg once a month, (supervised administration) and 50 mg daily, (self-administered), alternatively 100 mg once daily on alternate days, (self-administered) continued →

5

Infection

Lepromatous lepra reactions
▶ BY MOUTH
▶ Adult: Increased to 300 mg daily for max. 3 months

Severe type II (erythema nodosum leprosum) reactions
▶ BY MOUTH
▶ Adult: Increased to 100 mg 3 times a day for the first month (with subsequent reductions), may take 4–6 weeks to attain full effect

● CAUTIONS Avoid if persistent abdominal pain and diarrhoea · may discolour soft contact lenses
● SIDE-EFFECTS Abdominal pain · acne-like eruptions · anorexia · bowel obstruction · brownish-black discoloration of lesions and skin including areas exposed to light · dimmed vision · dry eyes · dry skin · elevation of blood sugar · eosinophilic enteropathy · headache · lymphadenopathy · macular corneal pigmentation · nausea · photosensitivity · pruritus · rash · red discoloration of body fluids · red discoloration of faeces · red discoloration of urine · reversible hair discoloration · splenic infarction · subepithelial corneal pigmentation · tiredness · vomiting (hospitalise if persistent) · weight loss
● PREGNANCY Use with caution.
● BREAST FEEDING May alter colour of milk; skin discoloration of infant.
● HEPATIC IMPAIRMENT Use with caution.
● RENAL IMPAIRMENT Use with caution.

● MEDICINAL FORMS
There can be variation in the licensing of different medicines containing the same drug. Forms available from special-order manufacturers include: capsule
Capsule
CAUTIONARY AND ADVISORY LABELS 8, 14, 21
▶ Clofazimine (Non-proprietary)
 Clofazimine 50 mg Lamprene 50mg capsules | 100 capsule [PoM] no price available

Dapsone

● INDICATIONS AND DOSE
Multibacillary leprosy in combination with rifampicin and clofazimine (3-drug regimen) | Paucibacillary leprosy in combination with rifampicin (2-drug regimen)
▶ BY MOUTH
▶ Adult (body-weight up to 35 kg): 50 mg daily, alternatively 1–2 mg/kg daily, may be self-administered
▶ Adult (body-weight 35 kg and above): 100 mg daily, may be self-administered

Dermatitis herpetiformis
▶ BY MOUTH
▶ Adult: (consult product literature or local protocols)

Treatment of mild to moderate *Pneumocystis jirovecii* (*Pneumocystis carinii*) pneumonia (in combination with trimethoprim)
▶ BY MOUTH
▶ Adult: 100 mg once daily

Prophylaxis of *Pneumocystis jirovecii* (*Pneumocystis carinii*) pneumonia
▶ BY MOUTH
▶ Adult: 100 mg daily

● UNLICENSED USE Not licensed for treatment of pneumocystis (*P. jirovecii*) pneumonia.
● CAUTIONS Anaemia (treat severe anaemia before starting) · avoid in Acute porphyrias p. 918 · cardiac disease · G6PD deficiency · pulmonary disease · susceptibility to haemolysis
● INTERACTIONS → Appendix 1 (dapsone).

● SIDE-EFFECTS
▶ **Rare** Stevens-Johnson syndrome · toxic epidermal necrolysis
▶ **Frequency not known** Agranulocytosis · allergic dermatitis · anorexia · dapsone syndrome · haemolysis · headache · hepatitis · insomnia · methaemoglobinaemia · nausea · neuropathy · psychosis · tachycardia · vomiting
SIDE-EFFECTS, FURTHER INFORMATION
▶ Dapsone syndrome If dapsone syndrome occurs (rash with fever and eosinophilia)—discontinue immediately (may progress to exfoliative dermatitis, hepatitis, hypoalbuminaemia, psychosis and death).
  Side-effects are dose-related and uncommon at doses used for leprosy.
● PREGNANCY Folic acid p. 886 (higher dose) should be given to mother throughout pregnancy; neonatal haemolysis and methaemoglobinaemia reported in third trimester.
● BREAST FEEDING Haemolytic anaemia; although significant amount in milk, risk to infant very small unless infant is G6PD deficient.
● PATIENT AND CARER ADVICE
Blood disorders On long-term treatment, patients and their carers should be told how to recognise signs of blood disorders and advised to seek immediate medical attention if symptoms such as fever, sore throat, rash, mouth ulcers, purpura, bruising or bleeding develop.

● MEDICINAL FORMS
There can be variation in the licensing of different medicines containing the same drug. Forms available from special-order manufacturers include: oral suspension, oral solution
Tablet
CAUTIONARY AND ADVISORY LABELS 8
▶ Dapsone (Non-proprietary)
 Dapsone 50 mg Dapsone 50mg tablets | 28 tablet [PoM] £64.77 DT price = £21.12
 Dapsone 100 mg Dapsone 100mg tablets | 28 tablet [PoM] £117.80 DT price = £104.60

2.3 Lyme disease

Lyme disease

Treatment

Lyme disease should generally be treated by those experienced in its management. Doxycycline p. 513, amoxicillin p. 498 [unlicensed indication] or cefuroxime p. 478 (as cefuroxime axetil) are the antibacterials of choice for *early Lyme disease* or *Lyme arthritis*. If these antibacterials are contra-indicated, a **macrolide** (e.g. clarithromycin p. 487) can be used for early Lyme disease. Intravenous administration of ceftriaxone p. 480, cefotaxime p. 479, or benzylpenicillin sodium p. 496 is recommended for Lyme disease associated with cardiac or neurological complications. The duration of treatment is usually 2–4 weeks; Lyme arthritis may require further treatment.

2.4 Methicillin-resistant staphylococcus aureus

MRSA

Management

Infection from *Staphylococcus aureus* strains resistant to meticillin [now discontinued] (meticillin-resistant *Staph. aureus*, MRSA) and to flucloxacillin p. 503 can be difficult to manage. Treatment is guided by the sensitivity of the infecting strain.

Rifampicin p. 527 or fusidic acid p. 519 should **not** be used alone because resistance may develop rapidly. A **tetracycline** alone or a combination of rifampicin and fusidic acid can be used for *skin* and *soft-tissue infections* caused by MRSA; clindamycin p. 485 alone is an alternative. A **glycopeptide** (e.g. vancomycin p. 484) can be used for severe skin and soft-tissue infections associated with MRSA; if a glycopeptide is unsuitable, linezolid p. 520 can be used on expert advice. As linezolid is **not** active against Gram-negative organisms, it can be used for mixed skin and soft-tissue infections only when other treatments are not available; linezolid must be given with other antibacterials if the infection also involves Gram-negative organisms. A combination of a glycopeptide and fusidic acid *or* a glycopeptide and rifampicin can be considered for skin and soft-tissue infections that have failed to respond to a single antibacterial.

Tigecycline p. 516 and daptomycin p. 517 are licensed for the treatment of complicated skin and soft-tissue infections involving MRSA.

A **tetracycline** or clindamycin can be used for *bronchiectasis* caused by MRSA. A **glycopeptide** can be used for *pneumonia* associated with MRSA; if a glycopeptide is unsuitable, linezolid can be used on expert advice. Linezolid must be given with other antibacterials if the infection also involves Gram-negative organisms.

A **tetracycline** can be used for *urinary-tract infections* caused by MRSA; trimethoprim p. 521 or nitrofurantoin p. 535 are alternatives. A **glycopeptide** can be used for urinary-tract infections that are severe or resistant to other antibacterials.

A **glycopeptide** can be used for *septicaemia* associated with MRSA.

See the management of *endocarditis, osteomyelitis,* or *septic arthritis* associated with MRSA.

Prophylaxis with vancomycin or teicoplanin p. 482 (alone or in combination with another antibacterial active against other pathogens) is appropriate for patients undergoing surgery if:

- there is a history of MRSA colonisation or infection without documented eradication;
- there is a risk that the patient's MRSA carriage has recurred;
- the patient comes from an area with a high prevalence of MRSA.

See eradication of nasal carriage of MRSA in Nose p. 1044.

2.5 Tuberculosis

Tuberculosis

Treatment phases, overview

Tuberculosis is treated in two phases—an *initial phase* using 4 drugs and a *continuation phase* using 2 drugs in fully sensitive cases. Treatment requires specialised knowledge and supervision, particularly where the disease involves resistant organisms or non-respiratory organs.

There are two regimens recommended for the treatment of tuberculosis in the UK; variations occur in other countries. Either the unsupervised regimen or the supervised regimen should be used; the two regimens should **not** be used concurrently. Compliance with therapy is a major determinant of its success.

Initial phase

The concurrent use of 4 drugs during the initial phase is designed to reduce the bacterial population as rapidly as possible and to prevent the emergence of drug-resistant bacteria. The drugs are best given as combination preparations unless one of the components cannot be given because of resistance or intolerance. The treatment of choice for the initial phase is the daily use of isoniazid p. 532, rifampicin p. 527, pyrazinamide p. 533 and ethambutol hydrochloride p. 532. Treatment should be started without waiting for culture results if clinical features or histology results are consistent with tuberculosis; treatment should be continued even if initial culture results are negative. The initial phase drugs should be continued for 2 months. Where a positive culture for *M. tuberculosis* has been obtained, but susceptibility results are not available after 2 months, treatment with rifampicin, isoniazid, pyrazinamide and ethambutol hydrochloride should be continued until full susceptibility is confirmed, even if this is for longer than 2 months.

Streptomycin p. 472 is rarely used in the UK but it may be used in the initial phase of treatment if resistance to isoniazid has been established before therapy is commenced.

Continuation phase

After the initial phase, treatment is continued for a further 4 months with rifampicin with isoniazid p. 529 (preferably given as a combination preparation). Longer treatment is necessary for meningitis, direct spinal cord involvement, and for resistant organisms which may also require modification of the regimen.

Unsupervised treatment

The unsupervised treatment regimen should be used for patients who are likely to take antituberculous drugs reliably **without supervision**. Patients who are unlikely to comply with daily administration of antituberculous drugs should be treated with the regimen described under Supervised Treatment.

Pregnancy and breast-feeding

The standard unsupervised 6-month treatment regimen may be used during pregnancy. Streptomycin should not be given in pregnancy.

The standard unsupervised 6-month treatment regimen may be used during breast-feeding.

Supervised treatment

Drug administration needs to be **fully supervised** (directly observed therapy, DOT) in patients who cannot comply reliably with the treatment regimen. These patients are given isoniazid, rifampicin, pyrazinamide and ethambutol hydrochloride (or streptomycin) 3 times a week under supervision for the first 2 months followed by isoniazid and rifampicin 3 times a week for a further 4 months.

Immunocompromised patients

Multi-resistant *Mycobacterium tuberculosis* may be present in immunocompromised patients. The organism should always be cultured to confirm its type and drug sensitivity. Confirmed *M. tuberculosis* infection sensitive to first-line drugs should be treated with a standard 6-month regimen; after completing treatment, patients should be closely monitored. The regimen may need to be modified if infection is caused by resistant organisms, and specialist advice is needed.

Specialist advice should be sought about tuberculosis treatment or chemoprophylaxis in a HIV-positive individual; care is required in choosing the regimen and in avoiding potentially serious interactions. Starting antiretroviral treatment in the first 2 months of antituberculosis treatment increases the risk of immune reconstitution syndrome.

Infection may also be caused by other mycobacteria e.g. *M. avium* complex in which case specialist advice on management is needed.

5

Infection

Recommended dosage for standard unsupervised 6-month treatment

Rifampicin with isoniazid and pyrazinamide	Adult: ▸ body-weight up to 40 kg: 3 tablets daily for 2 months (initial phase), use *Rifater*® Tablets, preferably taken before breakfast; ▸ body-weight 40-49 kg: 4 tablets daily for 2 months (initial phase), use *Rifater*® Tablets, preferably taken before breakfast; ▸ body-weight 50-64 kg: 5 tablets daily for 2 months (initial phase), use *Rifater*® Tablets, preferably taken before breakfast; ▸ body-weight 65 kg and above: 6 tablets daily for 2 months (initial phase), use *Rifater*® Tablets, preferably taken before breakfast
Ethambutol hydrochloride	Adult: 15 mg/kg once daily for 2 months (initial phase)
Rifampicin with isoniazid	Adult: ▸ body-weight up to 50 kg: 450/300 mg daily for 4 months (continuation phase after 2-month initial phase), use *Rifinah*® *150/100* Tablets, preferably taken before breakfast; ▸ body-weight 50 kg and above: 600/300 mg daily for 4 months (continuation phase after 2-month initial phase), use *Rifinah*® *300/150* Tablets, preferably taken before breakfast
or (if combination preparations not appropriate):	
Isoniazid	Child: 10 mg/kg once daily (max. per dose 300 mg) for 6 months (initial and continuation phases) Adult: 300 mg daily for 6 months (initial and continuation phases)
Rifampicin	Child: ▸ body-weight up to 50 kg: 15 mg/kg once daily for 6 months (initial and continuation phases); maximum 450 mg per day; ▸ body-weight 50 kg and above: 15 mg/kg once daily for 6 months (initial and continuation phases); maximum 600 mg per day Adult: ▸ body-weight up to 50 kg: 450 mg once daily for 6 months (initial and continuation phases); ▸ body-weight 50 kg and above: 600 mg once daily for 6 months (initial and continuation phases)
Pyrazinamide	Child: ▸ body-weight up to 50 kg: 35 mg/kg once daily for 2 months (initial phase); maximum 1.5 g per day; ▸ body-weight 50 kg and above: 35 mg/kg once daily for 2 months (initial phase); maximum 2 g per day Adult: ▸ body-weight up to 50 kg: 1.5 g once daily for 2 months (initial phase); ▸ body-weight 50 kg and above: 2 g once daily for 2 months (initial phase)
Ethambutol hydrochloride	Child: 20 mg/kg once daily for 2 months (initial phase) Adult: 15 mg/kg once daily for 2 months (initial phase)

Recommended dosage for intermittent supervised 6-month treatment

Isoniazid	Child: 15 mg/kg 3 times a week (max. per dose 900 mg) for 6 months (initial and continuation phases) Adult: 15 mg/kg 3 times a week (max. per dose 900 mg) for 6 months (initial and continuation phases)
Rifampicin	Child: 15 mg/kg 3 times a week (max. per dose 900 mg) for 6 months (initial and continuation phases) Adult: 600-900 mg 3 times a week for 6 months (initial and continuation phases)
Pyrazinamide	Child: ▸ body-weight up to 50 kg: 50 mg/kg 3 times a week (max. per dose 2 g 3 times a week) for 2 months (initial phase) ▸ body-weight 50 kg and above: 50 mg/kg 3 times a week (max. per dose 2.5 g 3 times a week) for 2 months (initial phase) Adult: ▸ body-weight up to 50 kg: 2 g 3 times a week for 2 months (initial phase); ▸ body-weight 50 kg and above: 2.5 g 3 times a week for 2 months (initial phase)
Ethambutol hydrochloride	Child: 30 mg/kg 3 times a week for 2 months (initial phase) Adult: 30 mg/kg 3 times a week for 2 months (initial phase)

Corticosteroids

In meningeal or pericardial tuberculosis, a corticosteroid should be started at the same time as antituberculosis therapy.

Prevention of tuberculosis

Some individuals may develop tuberculosis owing to reactivation of previously latent disease. Chemoprophylaxis may be required in those who have evidence of latent tuberculosis and are receiving treatment with immunosuppressants (including cytotoxics and possibly long-term treatment with systemic corticosteroids). In these cases, chemoprophylaxis involves use of either isoniazid alone for 6 months or of isoniazid and rifampicin for 3 months; longer chemoprophylaxis is not recommended.

See prevention of tuberculosis in susceptible close contacts or those who have become tuberculin-positive. See advice on immunisation against tuberculosis.

Treatment failure

Major causes of treatment failure are incorrect prescribing by the physician and inadequate compliance by the patient. Monthly tablet counts and urine examination (rifampicin imparts an orange-red coloration) may be useful indicators of compliance with treatment. Avoid both excessive and inadequate dosage. Treatment should be supervised by a specialist physician.

Antituberculosis drugs

Isoniazid is cheap and highly effective. Like rifampicin it should always be included in any antituberculous regimen unless there is a specific contra-indication.

Rifampicin, a rifamycin, is a key component of any antituberculous regimen. Like isoniazid it should always be included unless there is a specific contra-indication.

During the first two months ('initial phase') of rifampicin administration transient disturbance of liver function with elevated serum transaminases is common but generally does not require interruption of treatment. Occasionally more serious liver toxicity requires a change of treatment particularly in those with pre-existing liver disease.

On intermittent treatment six toxicity syndromes have been recognised—influenza-like, abdominal, and respiratory symptoms, shock, renal failure, and thrombocytopenic purpura—and can occur in 20 to 30% of patients.

Rifabutin p. 522, another rifamycin, is indicated for *prophylaxis* against *M. avium* complex infections in patients with a low CD4 count; it is also licensed for the *treatment* of non-tuberculous mycobacterial disease and pulmonary tuberculosis.

Pyrazinamide is a bactericidal drug only active against intracellular dividing forms of *Mycobacterium tuberculosis*; it exerts its main effect only in the first two or three months. It is particularly useful in tuberculous meningitis because of good meningeal penetration. It is not active against *M. bovis*.

Ethambutol hydrochloride is included in a treatment regimen if isoniazid resistance is suspected; it can be omitted if the risk of resistance is low.

Streptomycin [unlicensed] is now rarely used in the UK except for resistant organisms.

Drug-resistant tuberculosis should be treated by a specialist physician with experience in such cases, and where appropriate facilities for infection-control exist. Second-line drugs available for infections caused by resistant organisms, or when first-line drugs cause unacceptable side-effects, include **aminosalicylic acid p. 530**, **amikacin p. 471**, **capreomycin p. 531**, **cycloserine p. 531**, newer macrolides (e.g. **azithromycin p. 486** and **clarithromycin p. 487**), **moxifloxacin p. 508** and protionamide (prothionamide; no longer on UK market). **Bedaquiline p. 530** and **delamanid p. 531** are licensed for the treatment of multiple-drug

resistant pulmonary tuberculosis. Bedaquiline has a long half-life.

Management of tuberculosis in children

Children are given isoniazid p. 532, rifampicin below, pyrazinamide p. 533, and ethambutol hydrochloride p. 532 for the first 2 months followed by isoniazid and rifampicin during the next 4 months. However, care is needed in young children receiving ethambutol hydrochloride because of the difficulty in testing eyesight and in obtaining reports of visual symptoms.

ANTIMYCOBACTERIALS > RIFAMYCINS

Rifampicin

● INDICATIONS AND DOSE

Brucellosis in combination with other antibacterials | Legionnaires disease in combination with other antibacterials | Serious staphylococcal infections in combination with other antibacterials
▸ BY MOUTH, OR BY INTRAVENOUS INFUSION
▸ Child 1–11 months: 5–10 mg/kg twice daily
▸ Child 1–17 years: 10 mg/kg twice daily (max. per dose 600 mg)
▸ Adult: 0.6–1.2 g daily in 2–4 divided doses

Endocarditis in combination with other drugs
▸ BY MOUTH, OR BY INTRAVENOUS INFUSION
▸ Adult: 0.6–1.2 g daily in 2–4 divided doses

Tuberculosis, in combination with other drugs (intermittent supervised 6-month treatment) (under expert supervision)
▸ BY MOUTH
▸ Child: 15 mg/kg 3 times a week (max. per dose 900 mg) for 6 months (initial and continuation phases)
▸ Adult: 600–900 mg 3 times a week for 6 months (initial and continuation phases)

Tuberculosis, in combination with other drugs (standard unsupervised 6-month treatment)
▸ BY MOUTH
▸ Child (body-weight up to 50 kg): 15 mg/kg once daily for 6 months (initial and continuation phases); maximum 450 mg per day
▸ Child (body-weight 50 kg and above): 15 mg/kg once daily for 6 months (initial and continuation phases); maximum 600 mg per day
▸ Adult (body-weight up to 50 kg): 450 mg once daily for 6 months (initial and continuation phases)
▸ Adult (body-weight 50 kg and above): 600 mg once daily for 6 months (initial and continuation phases)

Prevention of tuberculosis in susceptible close contacts or those who have become tuberculin positive, in combination with isoniazid
▸ BY MOUTH
▸ Child 1 month–11 years (body-weight up to 50 kg): 15 mg/kg daily for 3 months; maximum 450 mg per day
▸ Child 1 month–11 years (body-weight 50 kg and above): 15 mg/kg daily for 3 months; maximum 600 mg per day
▸ Child 12–17 years (body-weight up to 50 kg): 450 mg daily for 3 months
▸ Child 12–17 years (body-weight 50 kg and above): 600 mg daily for 3 months
▸ Adult (body-weight up to 50 kg): 450 mg daily for 3 months
▸ Adult (body-weight 50 kg and above): 600 mg daily for 3 months continued →

Prevention of tuberculosis in susceptible close contacts or those who have become tuberculin positive, who are isoniazid-resistant

▶ BY MOUTH
▶ Child 1 month–11 years (body-weight up to 50 kg): 15 mg/kg daily for 6 months; maximum 450 mg per day
▶ Child 1 month–11 years (body-weight 50 kg and above): 15 mg/kg daily for 6 months; maximum 600 mg per day
▶ Child 12–17 years (body-weight up to 50 kg): 450 mg daily for 6 months
▶ Child 12–17 years (body-weight 50 kg and above): 600 mg daily for 6 months

Prevention of tuberculosis in susceptible close contacts or those who have become tuberculin positive, who are isoniazid-resistant and under 35 years

▶ BY MOUTH
▶ Adult 18–34 years (body-weight up to 50 kg): 450 mg daily for 6 months
▶ Adult 18–34 years (body-weight 50 kg and above): 600 mg daily for 6 months

Prevention of secondary case of _Haemophilus influenzae_ type b disease

▶ BY MOUTH
▶ Child 1–2 months: 10 mg/kg once daily for 4 days
▶ Child 3 months–11 years: 20 mg/kg once daily (max. per dose 600 mg) for 4 days
▶ Child 12–17 years: 600 mg once daily for 4 days
▶ Adult: 600 mg once daily for 4 days

Prevention of secondary case of meningococcal meningitis

▶ BY MOUTH
▶ Child 1–11 months: 5 mg/kg every 12 hours for 2 days
▶ Child 1–11 years: 10 mg/kg every 12 hours (max. per dose 600 mg), for 2 days
▶ Child 12–17 years: 600 mg every 12 hours for 2 days
▶ Adult: 600 mg every 12 hours for 2 days

Multibacillary leprosy in combination with dapsone and clofazimine (3-drug regimen) | Paucibacillary leprosy in combination with dapsone (2-drug regimen)

▶ BY MOUTH
▶ Adult (body-weight up to 35 kg): 450 mg once a month, supervised administration
▶ Adult (body-weight 35 kg and above): 600 mg once a month, supervised administration

● UNLICENSED USE Not licensed for use in children for pruritus due to cholestasis.
● CONTRA-INDICATIONS Acute porphyrias p. 918 · jaundice
● CAUTIONS Discolours soft contact lenses
● INTERACTIONS → Appendix 1 (rifamycins). Rifampicin induces hepatic enzymes which accelerate the metabolism of several drugs including oestrogens, corticosteroids, phenytoin, sulfonylureas, and anticoagulants.
● SIDE-EFFECTS
GENERAL SIDE-EFFECTS
Acute renal failure · adrenal insufficiency · alterations of liver function · anorexia · antibiotic-associated colitis · body secretions coloured orange-red · collapse and shock · diarrhoea · disseminated intravascular coagulation · drowsiness · eosinophilia · exfoliative dermatitis · flushing · gastro-intestinal symptoms · haemolytic anaemia · headache · influenza-like symptoms (with chills, fever, dizziness, bone pain) · jaundice · leucopenia · menstrual disturbances · muscular weakness · myopathy · nausea · oedema · pemphigoid reactions · psychoses · rashes · respiratory symptoms · saliva coloured orange-red · shortness of breath · Stevens-Johnson syndrome ·

thrombocytopenic purpura · toxic epidermal necrolysis · urine coloured orange-red · urticaria · vomiting
SPECIFIC SIDE-EFFECTS
▶ With intravenous use Thrombophlebitis reported if infusion used for prolonged period
SIDE-EFFECTS, FURTHER INFORMATION
Discontinue permanently if serious side-effects develop.
▶ Intermittent therapy Side-effects that mainly occur with intermittent therapy include influenza-like symptoms (with chills, fever, dizziness, bone pain), respiratory symptoms (including shortness of breath), collapse and shock, haemolytic anaemia, thrombocytopenic purpura, disseminated intravascular coagulation, and acute renal failure

● ALLERGY AND CROSS-SENSITIVITY Contra-indicated in patients with rifamycin hypersensitivity.
● CONCEPTION AND CONTRACEPTION
Important Effectiveness of hormonal contraceptives is reduced and alternative family planning advice should be offered.
● PREGNANCY Manufacturers advise very high doses teratogenic in _animal_ studies in first trimester; risk of neonatal bleeding may be increased in third trimester.
● BREAST FEEDING Amount too small to be harmful.
● HEPATIC IMPAIRMENT Avoid or do not exceed 8 mg/kg daily. Impaired elimination. In patients with pre-existing liver disease or hepatic impairment, monitor liver function regularly and particularly frequently in the first 2 months; blood counts should also be monitored in these patients.
● RENAL IMPAIRMENT
▶ In children Use with caution if doses above 10 mg/kg daily.
▶ In adults Use with caution if dose above 600 mg daily.
● MONITORING REQUIREMENTS
▶ _Renal function_ should be checked before treatment.
▶ _Hepatic function_ should be checked before treatment. If there is no evidence of liver disease (and pre-treatment liver function is normal), further checks are only necessary if the patient develops fever, malaise, vomiting, jaundice or unexplained deterioration during treatment. However, liver function should be monitored on prolonged therapy.
▶ Blood counts should be monitored in patients on prolonged therapy.
▶ In adults Those with alcohol dependence should have frequent checks of hepatic function, particularly in the first 2 months. Blood counts should also be monitored in these patients.
● DIRECTIONS FOR ADMINISTRATION
▶ With intravenous use in adults For _intravenous infusion_ (_Rifadin_®), give intermittently in Glucose 5% _or_ Sodium chloride 0.9%; reconstitute with solvent provided then dilute with 500 mL infusion fluid; give over 2–3 hours.
▶ With intravenous use in children Displacement value may be significant, consult local reconstitution guidelines; reconstitute with solvent provided. May be further diluted with Glucose 5% _or_ Sodium chloride 0.9% to a final concentration of 1.2 mg/mL. Infuse over 2–3 hours.
● PRESCRIBING AND DISPENSING INFORMATION If treatment interruption occurs, re-introduce with low dosage and increase gradually.
Flavours of syrup may include raspberry.
▶ With oral use in children In general, doses should be rounded up to facilitate administration of suitable volumes of liquid or an appropriate strength of tablet. Doses may also need to be recalculated to allow for weight gain in younger children.
● PATIENT AND CARER ADVICE
Medicines for Children leaflet: Rifampicin for meningococcal prophylaxis www.medicinesforchildren.org.uk/ rifampicin-for-meningococcal-prophylaxis

Medicines for Children leaflet: Rifampicin for the treatment of tuberculosis www.medicinesforchildren.org.uk/rifampicin-for-treatment-of-tuberculosis

Soft contact lenses Patients or their carers should be advised that rifampicin discolours soft contact lenses.

Hepatic disorders Patients or their carers should be told how to recognise signs of liver disorder, and advised to discontinue treatment and seek immediate medical attention if symptoms such as persistent nausea, vomiting, malaise or jaundice develop.

● MEDICINAL FORMS
There can be variation in the licensing of different medicines containing the same drug. Forms available from special-order manufacturers include: oral suspension, oral solution

Capsule
CAUTIONARY AND ADVISORY LABELS 8, 14, 23
▸ Rifampicin (Non-proprietary)
Rifampicin 150 mg Rifampicin 150mg capsules | 100 capsule [PoM] £44.84 DT price = £38.48
Rifampicin 300 mg Rifampicin 300mg capsules | 100 capsule [PoM] £103.25 DT price = £87.77
▸ Rifadin (Sanofi)
Rifampicin 150 mg Rifadin 150mg capsules | 100 capsule [PoM] £18.32 DT price = £38.48
Rifampicin 300 mg Rifadin 300mg capsules | 100 capsule [PoM] £36.63 DT price = £87.77
▸ Rimactane (Sandoz Ltd)
Rifampicin 300 mg Rimactane 300mg capsules | 60 capsule [PoM] £25.92

Oral suspension
CAUTIONARY AND ADVISORY LABELS 8, 14, 23
EXCIPIENTS: May contain Sucrose
▸ Rifadin (Sanofi)
Rifampicin 20 mg per 1 ml Rifadin 100mg/5ml syrup | 120 ml [PoM] £4.27

Powder and solvent for solution for injection
▸ Rifampicin (Non-proprietary)
Rifampicin 300 mg RIFA parenteral 300mg powder and solvent for solution for injection vials | 1 vial [PoM] no price available

Powder and solvent for solution for infusion
ELECTROLYTES: May contain Sodium
▸ Rifadin (Sanofi)
Rifampicin 600 mg Rifadin 600mg powder and solvent for solution for infusion vials | 1 vial [PoM] £9.20

Rifampicin with ethambutol, isoniazid and pyrazinamide

The properties listed below are those particular to the combination only. For the properties of the components please consider, rifampicin p. 527, ethambutol hydrochloride p. 532, isoniazid p. 532, pyrazinamide p. 533.

● INDICATIONS AND DOSE
Initial treatment of tuberculosis
▸ BY MOUTH
▸ Adult (body-weight 30–39 kg): 2 tablets daily for 2 months (initial phase)
▸ Adult (body-weight 40–54 kg): 3 tablets daily for 2 months (initial phase)
▸ Adult (body-weight 55–69 kg): 4 tablets daily for 2 months (initial phase)
▸ Adult (body-weight 70 kg and above): 5 tablets daily for 2 months (initial phase)

DOSE EQUIVALENCE AND CONVERSION
Tablet quantities refer to the number of *Voractiv*® Tablets which should be taken. Each *Voractiv*® Tablet contains ethambutol hydrochloride 275 mg, isoniazid 75 mg, pyrazinamide 400 mg and rifampicin 150 mg.

● CAUTIONS
CAUTIONS, FURTHER INFORMATION
▸ **Peripheral neuropathy** The risk of peripheral neuropathy may be increased by high doses of isoniazid; pyridoxine should, therefore, be considered for those receiving *Voractiv*® 5 tablets daily.

● MEDICINAL FORMS
There can be variation in the licensing of different medicines containing the same drug.
Tablet
CAUTIONARY AND ADVISORY LABELS 8, 14, 22
▸ Voractiv (Thornton & Ross Ltd)
Isoniazid 75 mg, Rifampicin 150 mg, Ethambutol hydrochloride 275 mg, Pyrazinamide 400 mg Voractiv tablets | 60 tablet [PoM] £39.50

Rifampicin with isoniazid

The properties listed below are those particular to the combination only. For the properties of the components please consider, rifampicin p. 527, isoniazid p. 532.

● INDICATIONS AND DOSE
Treatment of tuberculosis (continuation phase)
▸ BY MOUTH
▸ Adult (body-weight up to 50 kg): 450/300 mg daily for 4 months (continuation phase after 2-month initial phase), use *Rifinah*® 150/100 Tablets, preferably taken before breakfast.
▸ Adult (body-weight 50 kg and above): 600/300 mg daily for 4 months (continuation phase after 2-month initial phase), use *Rifinah*® 300/150 Tablets, preferably taken before breakfast.

DOSE EQUIVALENCE AND CONVERSION
Rifinah® Tablets contain rifampicin and isoniazid; the proportions are expressed in the form x/y where x and y are the strengths in milligrams of rifampicin and isoniazid respectively.
Each *Rifinah*® 150/100 Tablet contains rifampicin 150 mg and isoniazid 100 mg.
Each *Rifinah*® 300/150 Tablet contains rifampicin 300 mg and isoniazid 150 mg.

● MEDICINAL FORMS
There can be variation in the licensing of different medicines containing the same drug.
Tablet
CAUTIONARY AND ADVISORY LABELS 8, 14, 23
▸ Rifinah (Sanofi)
Isoniazid 100 mg, Rifampicin 150 mg Rifinah 150mg/100mg tablets | 84 tablet [PoM] £19.09
Isoniazid 150 mg, Rifampicin 300 mg Rifinah 300mg/150mg tablets | 56 tablet [PoM] £25.22

Rifampicin with isoniazid and pyrazinamide

The properties listed below are those particular to the combination only. For the properties of the components please consider, rifampicin p. 527, isoniazid p. 532, pyrazinamide p. 533.

● INDICATIONS AND DOSE
Initial unsupervised treatment of tuberculosis (in combination with ethambutol)
▸ BY MOUTH
▸ Adult (body-weight up to 40 kg): 3 tablets daily for 2 months (initial phase), use *Rifater*® Tablets, preferably taken before breakfast. continued →

5

Infection

▶ Adult (body-weight 40–49 kg): 4 tablets daily for 2 months (initial phase), use *Rifater* Tablets, preferably taken before breakfast.
▶ Adult (body-weight 50–64 kg): 5 tablets daily for 2 months (initial phase), use *Rifater* Tablets, preferably taken before breakfast.
▶ Adult (body-weight 65 kg and above): 6 tablets daily for 2 months (initial phase), use *Rifater* Tablets, preferably taken before breakfast.

DOSE EQUIVALENCE AND CONVERSION
Tablet quantities refer to the number of *Rifater* Tablets which should be taken. Each *Rifater* Tablet contains isoniazid 50 mg, pyrazinamide 300 mg and rifampicin 120 mg.

● MEDICINAL FORMS
There can be variation in the licensing of different medicines containing the same drug.
Tablet
CAUTIONARY AND ADVISORY LABELS 8, 14, 22
▶ Rifater (Sanofi)
 Isoniazid 50 mg, Rifampicin 120 mg, Pyrazinamide 300 mg Rifater tablets | 100 tablet [PoM] £26.34

ANTIMYCOBACTERIALS > OTHER

Aminosalicylic acid

● INDICATIONS AND DOSE
Multiple-drug resistant tuberculosis, in combination with other drugs
▶ BY MOUTH
▶ Adult: 4 g every 8 hours for a usual treatment duration of 24 months; maximum 12 g per day
Desensitisation regimen
▶ BY MOUTH
▶ Adult: (consult product literature)

● CAUTIONS Peptic ulcer
● SIDE-EFFECTS
▶ **Common or very common** Abdominal pain · bloating · diarrhoea · nausea · rash · vestibular syndrome · vomiting
▶ **Uncommon** Anorexia
▶ **Rare** Gastrointestinal bleeding · hypothyroidism · jaundice · malabsorption syndrome · metallic taste · peptic ulcer · urticaria
▶ **Very rare** Agranulocytosis · anaemia · crystalluria · dizziness · headache · hypoglycaemia · leucopenia · methemoglobinaemia · peripheral neuropathy · purpura · tendon pain · thrombocytopenia · visual abnormalities · weight loss
▶ **Frequency not known** Hepatitis · hypersensitivity
● PREGNANCY Manufacturer advises avoid unless essential—toxicity in *animal* studies (highest risk during first trimester).
● BREAST FEEDING Present in milk—manufacturer advises avoid.
● HEPATIC IMPAIRMENT Use with caution.
● RENAL IMPAIRMENT Use with caution in mild to moderate impairment. Avoid in severe impairment due to accumulation of inactive metabolites.
● MONITORING REQUIREMENTS
▶ Monitor for hypersensitivity reaction during the first 3 months of treatment—for desensitisation dosing regimen consult product literature.
▶ Monitor liver function—discontinue immediately if signs or symptoms of hepatic toxicity (including rash, fever and gastrointestinal disturbance).

● DIRECTIONS FOR ADMINISTRATION Disperse granules in orange or tomato juice and take immediately (granules will not dissolve, ensure all granules are swallowed). Granules can be sprinkled on apple sauce or yoghurt for administration.
● PATIENT AND CARER ADVICE Patients should be advised that the skeletons of the granules may be seen in the stools. Counselling advised on administration.

● MEDICINAL FORMS
There can be variation in the licensing of different medicines containing the same drug.
Gastro-resistant granules
CAUTIONARY AND ADVISORY LABELS 9, 25
▶ Aminosalicylic acid (Non-proprietary)
 Aminosalicylic acid 1 gram per 1 gram Paser gastro-resistant granules 4g sachets sugar-free | 30 sachet [PoM] no price available
▶ Granupas (Lucane Pharma Ltd)
 Aminosalicylic acid 1 gram per 1 gram Granupas gastro-resistant granules 4g sachets sugar-free | 30 sachet [PoM] £331.00

Bedaquiline

● INDICATIONS AND DOSE
Multiple-drug resistant pulmonary tuberculosis, in combination with other drugs
▶ BY MOUTH
▶ Adult: Initially 400 mg once daily for 2 weeks, then 200 mg 3 times a week for 22 weeks, intervals of at least 48 hours between each dose, continue appropriate combination therapy after bedaquiline

● CONTRA-INDICATIONS QTc interval more than 500 milliseconds (derived using Fridericia's formula) · ventricular arrhythmia
● CAUTIONS Hypothyroidism · QTc interval (derived using Fridericia's formula) 450–500 milliseconds—discontinue if QTc interval more than 500 milliseconds · risk factors for QT interval prolongation (e.g. electrolyte disturbances, heart failure with reduced left ventricular ejection fraction, history of symptomatic arrhythmias (avoid if ventricular arrhythmia present), bradycardia, congenital long QT syndrome)
● INTERACTIONS → Appendix 1 (bedaquiline). Caution with concomitant use of hepatotoxic drugs.
● SIDE-EFFECTS Arthralgia · diarrhoea · dizziness · headache · myalgia · nausea · QT interval prolongation · vomiting
SIDE-EFFECTS, FURTHER INFORMATION
▶ Syncope If syncope occurs, obtain ECG.
● PREGNANCY Manufacturer advises avoid unless potential benefit outweighs risk.
● BREAST FEEDING Manufacturer advises avoid—present in milk in *animal* studies.
● HEPATIC IMPAIRMENT Manufacturer advises caution in moderate impairment; avoid in severe impairment—no information available. Avoid concomitant use of hepatotoxic drugs unless essential.
● RENAL IMPAIRMENT Manufacturer advises caution if eGFR less than 30 mL/minute/1.73 m^2.
● MONITORING REQUIREMENTS
▶ Determine serum potassium, calcium, and magnesium before starting treatment (correct if abnormal)—remeasure if QT prolongation occurs during treatment.
▶ Obtain ECG before starting treatment, and then at least monthly during treatment or more frequently if concomitant use with other drugs known to prolong the QT interval.
▶ Monitor liver function before starting treatment and then at least monthly during treatment—discontinue treatment if severe abnormalities in liver function tests.

● PATIENT AND CARER ADVICE
Missed doses
If a dose is missed during the first two weeks of treatment, the missed dose should not be taken and the next dose should be taken at the usual time; if a dose is missed during weeks 3–24 of treatment, the missed dose should be taken as soon as possible and then the usual regimen resumed.

Driving and skilled tasks
Dizziness may affect performance of skilled tasks (e.g. driving)

● MEDICINAL FORMS
There can be variation in the licensing of different medicines containing the same drug.
Tablet
CAUTIONARY AND ADVISORY LABELS　4, 8, 21
▸ Sirturo (Janssen-Cilag Ltd)　▼
　Bedaquiline (as Bedaquiline fumarate) 100 mg Sirturo 100mg tablets | 188 tablet [PoM] £18,700.00

Capreomycin

● INDICATIONS AND DOSE
Tuberculosis resistant to first-line drugs, in combination with other drugs
▸ BY DEEP INTRAMUSCULAR INJECTION
▸ Adult: 1 g daily (max. per dose 20 mg/kg) for 2–4 months, then reduced to 1 g 2–3 times a week

● CAUTIONS　Auditory impairment
● INTERACTIONS　→ Appendix 1 (capreomycin).
● SIDE-EFFECTS　Induration at injection site · changes in liver function tests · electrolyte disturbances · hearing loss with tinnitus and vertigo · hypersensitivity reactions · leucocytosis · leucopenia · nephrotoxicity · neuromuscular block after large doses · pain at injection site · rashes · thrombocytopenia · urticaria
● PREGNANCY　Manufacturer advises use only if potential benefit outweighs risk—teratogenic in *animal* studies.
● BREAST FEEDING　Manufacturer advises caution—no information available.
● HEPATIC IMPAIRMENT　Use with caution.
● RENAL IMPAIRMENT　Reduce dose—consult product literature. Nephrotoxic; ototoxic.
● MONITORING REQUIREMENTS　Monitor renal, hepatic, auditory, and vestibular function and electrolytes.
● MEDICINAL FORMS
There can be variation in the licensing of different medicines containing the same drug.
Powder for solution for injection
▸ Capreomycin (Non-proprietary)
　Capreomycin (as Capreomycin sulfate) 1 gram Capreomycin 1g powder for solution for injection vials | 1 vial [PoM] £28.61

Cycloserine

● INDICATIONS AND DOSE
Tuberculosis resistant to first-line drugs, in combination with other drugs
▸ BY MOUTH
▸ Adult: Initially 250 mg every 12 hours for 2 weeks, then increased if necessary up to 500 mg every 12 hours, dose to be increased according to blood concentration and response

PHARMACOKINETICS
Cycloserine penetrates the CNS.

● CONTRA-INDICATIONS　Alcohol dependence · depression · epilepsy · psychotic states · severe anxiety
● INTERACTIONS　→ Appendix 1 (cycloserine).
● SIDE-EFFECTS　Allergic dermatitis · changes in liver function tests · confusion · convulsions · depression · dizziness · drowsiness · headache · heart failure at high doses · megaloblastic anaemia · psychosis · rashes · tremor · vertigo

SIDE-EFFECTS, FURTHER INFORMATION
▸ CNS toxicity　Discontinue or reduce dose if symptoms of CNS toxicity occur.
▸ Rashes or allergic dermatitis　Discontinue or reduce dose if rashes or allergic dermatitis develops.
● PREGNANCY　Manufacturer advises use only if potential benefit outweighs risk—crosses the placenta.
● BREAST FEEDING　Present in milk—amount too small to be harmful.
● RENAL IMPAIRMENT　Increase interval between doses if creatinine clearance less than 50 mL/minute. Monitor blood-cycloserine concentration if creatinine clearance less than 50 mL/minute.
● MONITORING REQUIREMENTS
▸ Blood concentration monitoring required especially in renal impairment or if dose exceeds 500 mg daily or if signs of toxicity; blood concentration should not exceed 30 mg/litre.
▸ Monitor haematological, renal, and hepatic function.
● MEDICINAL FORMS
There can be variation in the licensing of different medicines containing the same drug.
Capsule
CAUTIONARY AND ADVISORY LABELS　2, 8
▸ Cycloserine (Non-proprietary)
　Cycloserine 250 mg Cycloserine 250mg capsules | 100 capsule [PoM] £402.63 DT price = £402.63

Delamanid

● INDICATIONS AND DOSE
Multiple-drug resistant pulmonary tuberculosis, in combination with other drugs
▸ BY MOUTH
▸ Adult: 100 mg twice daily for 24 weeks, continue appropriate combination therapy after delamanid

● CONTRA-INDICATIONS　QTc interval more than 500 milliseconds (derived using Fridericia's formula) · serum albumin less than 28 g/litre
● CAUTIONS　Risk factors for QT interval prolongation (e.g. electrolyte disturbances, acute myocardial infarction, heart failure with reduced left ventricular ejection fraction, severe hypertension, left ventricular hypertrophy, bradycardia, congenital long QT syndrome, history of symptomatic arrhythmias)
● INTERACTIONS　→ Appendix 1 (delamanid).
Caution when concomitant use with other drugs known to prolong the QT interval.
Contra-indicated with concomitant use of potent CYP3A4 inducers.
● SIDE-EFFECTS
▸ **Common or very common**　Abdominal pain · acne · agitation · anxiety · chest pain · cough · decreased appetite · depression · dermatitis · dyspepsia · dyspnoea · earache · haemoptysis · headache · hyperhidrosis · hyperlipidaemia · hypertension · hypokalaemia · hypotension · insomnia · malaise · nausea · oropharyngeal pain · osteochondrosis · palpitation · peripheral neuropathy · photophobia · psychiatric disorder · QT interval prolongation · reticulocytosis · tinnitus · tremor · vomiting

5

Infection

▸ **Uncommon** Arrhythmias · balance disorder · dehydration · dysphagia · herpes zoster · hypocalcaemia · leucopenia · nocturia · rash · thrombocytopenia · urinary retention

● CONCEPTION AND CONTRACEPTION Effective contraception required during treatment.

● PREGNANCY Manufacturer advises avoid—toxicity in *animal* studies.

● BREAST FEEDING Manufacturer advises avoid—present in milk in *animal* studies.

● HEPATIC IMPAIRMENT Manufacturer advises avoid in moderate to severe impairment.

● RENAL IMPAIRMENT Manufacturer advises avoid in severe impairment—no information available.

● MONITORING REQUIREMENTS
▸ Monitor serum albumin and electrolytes before starting treatment and then during treatment—discontinue treatment if serum albumin less than 28 g/litre.
▸ Obtain ECG before starting treatment and then monthly during treatment (more frequently if serum albumin 28–34 g/litre, or if concomitant use of potent CYP3A4 inhibitors, or if risk factors for QT interval prolongation, or if QTc interval 450–500 milliseconds in men or 470–500 milliseconds in women)—discontinue treatment if QTc interval more than 500 milliseconds (derived using Fridericia's formula).

● HANDLING AND STORAGE Dispense in original container (contains desiccant).

● MEDICINAL FORMS
There can be variation in the licensing of different medicines containing the same drug.
Tablet
CAUTIONARY AND ADVISORY LABELS 8, 21
▸ Deltyba (Otsuka Novel Products GmbH) ▼
Delamanid 50 mg Deltyba 50mg tablets | 48 tablet [PoM] £1,250.00

Ethambutol hydrochloride

● INDICATIONS AND DOSE
Tuberculosis, in combination with other drugs (standard unsupervised 6-month treatment)
▸ BY MOUTH
▸ Child: 20 mg/kg once daily for 2 months (initial phase)
▸ Adult: 15 mg/kg once daily for 2 months (initial phase)
Tuberculosis, in combination with other drugs (intermittent supervised 6-month treatment) (under expert supervision)
▸ BY MOUTH
▸ Child: 30 mg/kg 3 times a week for 2 months (initial phase)
▸ Adult: 30 mg/kg 3 times a week for 2 months (initial phase)

● CONTRA-INDICATIONS Optic neuritis · poor vision
● CAUTIONS Elderly · young children
CAUTIONS, FURTHER INFORMATION
▸ Understanding warnings Patients who cannot understand warnings about visual side-effects should, if possible, be given an alternative drug. In particular, ethambutol should be used with caution in children until they are at least 5 years old and capable of reporting symptomatic visual changes accurately.

● INTERACTIONS → Appendix 1 (ethambutol).

● SIDE-EFFECTS
▸ **Rare** Pruritus · rash · thrombocytopenia · urticaria
▸ **Frequency not known** Colour blindness · loss of visual acuity · optic neuritis · peripheral neuritis · red/green colour blindness · restriction of visual fields · visual disturbances

SIDE-EFFECTS, FURTHER INFORMATION
▸ Ocular toxicity Ocular toxicity is more common where excessive dosage is used or if the patient's renal function is impaired. Early discontinuation of the drug is almost always followed by recovery of eyesight.

● PREGNANCY Not known to be harmful.
● BREAST FEEDING Amount too small to be harmful.
● RENAL IMPAIRMENT
▸ In adults If creatinine clearance less than 30 mL/minute, use 15–25 mg/kg (max. 2.5 g) 3 times a week.
▸ In children If creatinine clearance less than 30 mL/minute/1.73 m², use 15–25 mg/kg (max. 2.5 g) 3 times a week. Risk of optic nerve damage. Should preferably be avoided in patients with renal impairment. If creatinine clearance less than 30 mL/minute, monitor plasma-ethambutol concentration.

● MONITORING REQUIREMENTS
▸ 'Peak' concentration (2–2.5 hours after dose) should be 2–6 mg/litre (7–22 micromol/litre); 'trough' (pre-dose) concentration should be less than 1 mg/litre (4 micromol/litre).
▸ Renal function should be checked before treatment.
▸ Visual acuity should be tested by Snellen chart before treatment with ethambutol.
▸ In children In young children, routine ophthalmological monitoring recommended.

● PATIENT AND CARER ADVICE
Medicines for Children leaflet: Ethambutol for the treatment of tuberculosis www.medicinesforchildren.org.uk/ethambutol-for-the-treatment-of-tuberculosis
Ocular toxicity The earliest features of ocular toxicity are subjective and patients should be advised to discontinue therapy immediately if they develop deterioration in vision and promptly seek further advice.

● MEDICINAL FORMS
There can be variation in the licensing of different medicines containing the same drug. Forms available from special-order manufacturers include: oral suspension, oral solution
Tablet
CAUTIONARY AND ADVISORY LABELS 8
▸ Ethambutol hydrochloride (Non-proprietary)
Ethambutol hydrochloride 100 mg Ethambutol 100mg tablets | 56 tablet [PoM] £11.51 DT price = £11.51
Ethambutol hydrochloride 400 mg Ethambutol 400mg tablets | 56 tablet [PoM] £42.74 DT price = £42.74

Combinations available: *Rifampicin with ethambutol, isoniazid and pyrazinamide,* p. 529

Isoniazid

● INDICATIONS AND DOSE
Tuberculosis, in combination with other drugs (standard unsupervised 6-month treatment)
▸ BY MOUTH, OR BY INTRAMUSCULAR INJECTION, OR BY INTRAVENOUS INJECTION
▸ Child: 10 mg/kg once daily (max. per dose 300 mg) for 6 months (initial and continuation phases)
▸ Adult: 300 mg daily for 6 months (initial and continuation phases)
Tuberculosis, in combination with other drugs (intermittent supervised 6-month treatment) (under expert supervision)
▸ BY MOUTH, OR BY INTRAMUSCULAR INJECTION, OR BY INTRAVENOUS INJECTION
▸ Child: 15 mg/kg 3 times a week (max. per dose 900 mg) for 6 months (initial and continuation phases)
▸ Adult: 15 mg/kg 3 times a week (max. per dose 900 mg) for 6 months (initial and continuation phases)

Prevention of tuberculosis in susceptible close contacts or those who have become tuberculin positive

▶ BY MOUTH, OR BY INTRAMUSCULAR INJECTION, OR BY INTRAVENOUS INJECTION

▶ Child 1 month–11 years: 10 mg/kg daily (max. per dose 300 mg) for 6 months, alternatively 10 mg/kg daily (max. per dose 300 mg) for 3 months, to be taken in combination with rifampicin

▶ Child 12–17 years: 300 mg daily for 6 months, alternatively 300 mg daily for 3 months, to be taken in combination with rifampicin

▶ Adult: 300 mg daily for 6 months, alternatively 300 mg daily for 3 months, to be taken in combination with rifampicin

● CONTRA-INDICATIONS Drug-induced liver disease

● CAUTIONS Acute porphyrias p. 918 · alcohol dependence · diabetes mellitus · epilepsy · history of psychosis · HIV infection · malnutrition · slow acetylator status (increased risk of side-effects)

CAUTIONS, FURTHER INFORMATION

▶ Peripheral neuropathy Peripheral neuropathy is more likely to occur where there are pre-existing risk factors such as diabetes, alcohol dependence, chronic renal failure, pregnancy, malnutrition and HIV infection. In patients at increased risk of peripheral neuropathy, pyridoxine hydrochloride p. 937 should be given prophylactically from the start of treatment.

● INTERACTIONS → Appendix 1 (isoniazid).
When used with tyramine or histamine rich foods, tachycardia, palpitation, hypotension, flushing, headache, dizziness, and sweating reported.

● SIDE-EFFECTS

▶ **Common or very common** Peripheral neuropathy

▶ **Rare** Hepatitis · psychotic episodes

▶ **Frequency not known** Agranulocytosis · aplastic anaemia · blood disorders · constipation · convulsions · difficulty with micturition · dry mouth · fever · gynaecomastia · haemolytic anaemia · hearing loss (in patients with end-stage renal impairment) · hyperglycaemia · hyperreflexia · hypersensitivity reactions · interstitial pneumonitis · nausea · optic neuritis · pancreatitis · pellagra · peripheral neuritis with high doses · purpura · Stevens-Johnson syndrome · systemic lupus erythematosus-like syndrome · tinnitus (in patients with end-stage renal impairment) · vertigo · vomiting

SIDE-EFFECTS, FURTHER INFORMATION

▶ Hepatitis Hepatitis more common in those aged over 35 years.

● PREGNANCY Not known to be harmful; prophylactic pyridoxine recommended.

● BREAST FEEDING Theoretical risk of convulsions and neuropathy; prophylactic pyridoxine advisable in mother. In breast-feeding, monitor infant for possible toxicity.

● HEPATIC IMPAIRMENT Use with caution. In patients with pre-existing liver disease or hepatic impairment monitor liver function regularly and particularly frequently in the first 2 months.

● RENAL IMPAIRMENT Risk of ototoxicity and peripheral neuropathy; prophylactic pyridoxine hydrochloride p. 937 recommended.

● MONITORING REQUIREMENTS

▶ Renal function should be checked before treatment.

▶ Hepatic function should be checked before treatment. If there is no evidence of liver disease (and pre-treatment liver function is normal), further checks are only necessary if the patient develops fever, malaise, vomiting, jaundice or unexplained deterioration during treatment.

▶ In adults Those with alcohol dependence should have frequent checks of hepatic function, particularly in the first 2 months.

● PRESCRIBING AND DISPENSING INFORMATION

▶ With oral use in children In general, doses should be rounded up to facilitate administration of suitable volumes of liquid or an appropriate strength of tablet.

▶ In children Doses may need to be recalculated to allow for weight gain in younger children.

● PATIENT AND CARER ADVICE
Medicines for Children leaflet: Isoniazid for latent tuberculosis www.medicinesforchildren.org.uk/ isoniazid-for-latent-tuberculosis
Medicines for Children leaflet: Isoniazid for treatment of tuberculosis www.medicinesforchildren.org.uk/ isoniazid-for-the-treatment-of-tuberculosis
Hepatic disorders Patients or their carers should be told how to recognise signs of liver disorder, and advised to discontinue treatment and seek immediate medical attention if symptoms such as persistent nausea, vomiting, malaise or jaundice develop.

● MEDICINAL FORMS
There can be variation in the licensing of different medicines containing the same drug. Forms available from special-order manufacturers include: oral suspension, oral solution

Tablet
CAUTIONARY AND ADVISORY LABELS 8, 22

▶ Isoniazid (Non-proprietary)
Isoniazid 50 mg Isoniazid 50mg tablets | 56 tablet [PoM] £19.24 DT price = £19.24
Isoniazid 100 mg Isoniazid 100mg tablets | 28 tablet [PoM] £19.24 DT price = £19.24
Isoniazid 300 mg Isoniazid 300mg tablets | 30 tablet [PoM] no price available

Solution for injection

▶ Isoniazid (Non-proprietary)
Isoniazid 20 mg per 1 ml Tebesium-S 100mg/5ml solution for injection ampoules | 12 ampoule [PoM] no price available
Isoniazid 25 mg per 1 ml Isoniazid 50mg/2ml solution for injection ampoules | 10 ampoule [PoM] £299.16

Combinations available: *Rifampicin with ethambutol, isoniazid and pyrazinamide,* p. 529 · *Rifampicin with isoniazid,* p. 529 · *Rifampicin with isoniazid and pyrazinamide,* p. 529

Pyrazinamide

● INDICATIONS AND DOSE

Tuberculosis, in combination with other drugs (standard unsupervised 6-month treatment)

▶ BY MOUTH

▶ Child (body-weight up to 50 kg): 35 mg/kg once daily for 2 months (initial phase); maximum 1.5 g per day

▶ Child (body-weight 50 kg and above): 35 mg/kg once daily for 2 months (initial phase); maximum 2 g per day

▶ Adult (body-weight up to 50 kg): 1.5 g once daily for 2 months (initial phase)

▶ Adult (body-weight 50 kg and above): 2 g once daily for 2 months (initial phase)

Tuberculosis, in combination with other drugs (intermittent supervised 6-month treatment) (under expert supervision)

▶ BY MOUTH

▶ Child (body-weight up to 50 kg): 50 mg/kg 3 times a week (max. per dose 2 g 3 times a week) for 2 months (initial phase)

▶ Child (body-weight 50 kg and above): 50 mg/kg 3 times a week (max. per dose 2.5 g 3 times a week) for 2 months (initial phase)

▶ Adult (body-weight up to 50 kg): 2 g 3 times a week for 2 months (initial phase) continued →

▸ Adult (body-weight 50 kg and above): 2.5 g 3 times a week for 2 months (initial phase)

● CONTRA-INDICATIONS Acute attack of gout (in adults)
● CAUTIONS Diabetes · gout (in adults)
● INTERACTIONS → Appendix 1 (pyrazinamide).
● SIDE-EFFECTS Anorexia · arthralgia · dysuria · fever · flushing (in adults) · hepatomegaly · hepatotoxicity · jaundice · liver failure · nausea · photosensitivity · rash · sideroblastic anaemia · splenomegaly · thrombocytopenia · vomiting
● PREGNANCY Manufacturer advises use only if potential benefit outweighs risk.
● BREAST FEEDING Amount too small to be harmful.
● HEPATIC IMPAIRMENT Idiosyncratic hepatotoxicity more common; avoid in severe hepatic impairment. In patients with pre-existing liver disease or hepatic impairment monitor liver function regularly and particularly frequently in the first 2 months.
● RENAL IMPAIRMENT
▸ In adults 25–30 mg/kg 3 times a week if eGFR less than 30 mL/minute/1.73 m^2.
▸ In children If estimated glomerular filtration rate less than 30 mL/minute/1.73 m^2, use 25–30 mg/kg 3 times a week. Monitor for gout in renal impairment.
● MONITORING REQUIREMENTS
▸ *Renal function* should be checked before treatment.
▸ *Hepatic function* should be checked before treatment. If there is no evidence of liver disease (and pre-treatment liver function is normal), further checks are only necessary if the patient develops fever, malaise, vomiting, jaundice or unexplained deterioration during treatment.
▸ In adults Those with alcohol dependence should have frequent checks of hepatic function, particularly in the first 2 months.
● PRESCRIBING AND DISPENSING INFORMATION
▸ In children In general, doses should be rounded up to facilitate administration of suitable volumes of liquid or an appropriate strength of tablet. Doses may also need to be recalculated to allow for weight gain in younger children.
● PATIENT AND CARER ADVICE
Medicines for Children leaflet: Pyrazinamide for treatment of tuberculosis www.medicinesforchildren.org.uk/pyrazinamide-for-tuberculosis
Hepatic disorders Patients or their carers should be told how to recognise signs of liver disorder, and advised to discontinue treatment and seek immediate medical attention if symptoms such as persistent nausea, vomiting, malaise or jaundice develop.

● MEDICINAL FORMS
There can be variation in the licensing of different medicines containing the same drug. Forms available from special-order manufacturers include: oral suspension, oral solution

Tablet
CAUTIONARY AND ADVISORY LABELS 8
▸ Pyrazinamide (Non-proprietary)
Pyrazinamide 500 mg Pyrazinamide 500mg tablets | 30 tablet [PoM] £31.35-£38.34 | 50 tablet [PoM] £52.25
▸ Zinamide (Thornton & Ross Ltd)
Pyrazinamide 500 mg Zinamide 500mg tablets | 30 tablet [PoM] £31.35

Combinations available: *Rifampicin with ethambutol, isoniazid and pyrazinamide,* p. 529 · *Rifampicin with isoniazid and pyrazinamide,* p. 529

2.6 Urinary tract infections

Urinary-tract infections

Overview

Urinary-tract infection is more common in women than in men; when it occurs in men there is frequently an underlying abnormality of the renal tract. Recurrent episodes of infection are an indication for radiological investigation especially in children in whom untreated pyelonephritis may lead to permanent kidney damage.

Escherichia coli is the most common cause of urinary-tract infection; *Staphylococcus saprophyticus* is also common in sexually active young women. Less common causes include Proteus and Klebsiella spp. *Pseudomonas aeruginosa* infections usually occur in the hospital setting and may be associated with functional or anatomical abnormalities of the renal tract. *Staphylococcus epidermidis* and *Enterococcus faecalis* infection may complicate catheterisation or instrumentation.

A specimen of urine should be collected for culture and sensitivity testing before starting antibacterial therapy;
● in men;
● in pregnant women;
● in children under 3 years of age;
● in patients with suspected upper urinary-tract infection;
● complicated infection, or recurrent infection;
● if resistant organisms are suspected;
● if urine dipstick testing gives a single positive result for leucocyte esterase or nitrite;
● if clinical symptoms are not consistent with results of dipstick testing.

Treatment should not be delayed while waiting for results. The antibacterial chosen should reflect current local bacterial sensitivity to antibacterials.

Antibacterial therapy for lower urinary-tract infections

Uncomplicated lower urinary-tract infections often respond to trimethoprim p. 521 or nitrofurantoin p. 535, *or alternatively,* amoxicillin p. 498, ampicillin p. 499 or oral cephalosporin.

Suggested duration of treatment is 7 days, but a short course (e.g. 3 days) is usually adequate for uncomplicated urinary-tract infections in women.

Infections caused by fully sensitive bacteria respond to amoxicillin.

Widespread bacterial resistance to ampicillin, amoxicillin, and trimethoprim has been reported. Alternatives for resistant organisms include co-amoxiclav p. 501 (amoxicillin with clavulanic acid), an oral cephalosporin, nitrofurantoin, pivmecillinam hydrochloride p. 502, or a quinolone.

Fosfomycin [unlicensed] can be used, on the advice of a microbiologist, for the treatment of uncomplicated lower urinary-tract infections caused by multiple-antibacterial resistant organisms when other antibacterials cannot be used.

Long-term low dose therapy may be required in selected patients to prevent *recurrence of infection*; indications include frequent relapses and significant kidney damage. Trimethoprim, nitrofurantoin and cefalexin p. 476 have been recommended for long-term therapy.

Methenamine hippurate p. 535 (hexamine hippurate) should **not** generally be used because it requires an acidic urine for its antimicrobial activity and it is ineffective for upper urinary-tract infections; it may, however, have a role in the prophylaxis and treatment of chronic or recurrent uncomplicated lower urinary-tract infections.

Antibacterial therapy for upper urinary-tract infections

Acute pyelonephritis can lead to septicaemia and is treated initially by injection of a broad-spectrum antibacterial such as a cephalosporin (e.g. cefuroxime p. 478) or a quinolone if the patient is severely ill; gentamicin p. 471 can also be used.

Suggested duration of treatment is 10–14 days (longer treatment may be necessary in complicated pyelonephritis).

Prostatitis can be difficult to cure and requires treatment for several weeks with an antibacterial which penetrates prostatic tissue such as some of the quinolones (ciprofloxacin p. 506 *or* ofloxacin p. 510), or *alternatively*, trimethoprim.

Suggested duration of treatment is 28 days.

Where infection is localised and associated with an indwelling *catheter*, a bladder instillation is often effective.

Pregnancy

Urinary-tract infection in pregnancy may be asymptomatic and requires prompt treatment to prevent progression to acute pyelonephritis. Penicillins and cephalosporins are suitable for treating urinary-tract infection during pregnancy. Nitrofurantoin may also be used but it should be avoided at term. Sulfonamides and quinolones should be avoided during pregnancy; trimethoprim should also preferably be avoided particularly in the first trimester.

Renal impairment

In renal failure antibacterials normally excreted by the kidney accumulate with resultant toxicity unless the dose is reduced. This applies especially to the aminoglycosides which should be used with great caution; tetracyclines, methenamine hippurate, and nitrofurantoin should be avoided altogether.

Urinary-tract infections in children

Urinary-tract infections in children require prompt antibacterial treatment to minimise the risk of renal scarring. Uncomplicated 'lower' urinary-tract infections in *children over* 3 *months of age* can be treated with trimethoprim, nitrofurantoin, a first generation cephalosporin (e.g. cefalexin), or amoxicillin for 3 days; children should be reassessed if they continue to be unwell 24–48 hours after the initial assessment. Amoxicillin should only be used if the organism causing the infection is sensitive to it.

Acute pyelonephritis in children over 3 months of age can be treated with a first generation cephalosporin or co-amoxiclav for 7–10 days. If the patient is severely ill, then the infection is best treated initially by injection of a broad-spectrum antibacterial such as cefotaxime p. 479 or co-amoxiclav; gentamicin is an alternative.

Children under 3 *months of age* should be transferred to hospital and treated initially with intravenous antibacterial drugs such as ampicillin with gentamicin, or cefotaxime alone, until the infection responds; full doses of oral antibacterials are then given for a further period.

Recurrent episodes of infection are an indication for imaging tests. *Antibacterial prophylaxis* with low doses of trimethoprim or nitrofurantoin may be considered for children with recurrent infection, significant urinary-tract anomalies, or significant kidney damage.

ANTIBACTERIALS

Methenamine hippurate

(Hexamine hippurate)

● **INDICATIONS AND DOSE**

Prophylaxis and long-term treatment of chronic or recurrent uncomplicated lower urinary-tract infections
▸ BY MOUTH
  ▸ Adult: 1 g every 12 hours

Prophylaxis and long-term treatment of chronic or recurrent uncomplicated lower urinary-tract infections in patients with catheters
▸ BY MOUTH
  ▸ Adult: 1 g every 8–12 hours

● **CONTRA-INDICATIONS** Gout · metabolic acidosis · severe dehydration

● **INTERACTIONS** → Appendix 1 (methenamine). Caution—avoid concurrent administration with sulfonamides (risk of crystalluria) or urinary alkalinising agents.

● **SIDE-EFFECTS** Bladder irritation · gastro-intestinal disturbances · rash

● **PREGNANCY** Use with caution.

● **BREAST FEEDING** Amount too small to be harmful.

● **HEPATIC IMPAIRMENT** Avoid.

● **RENAL IMPAIRMENT** Avoid if eGFR less than 10 mL/minute/1.73 m^2—risk of hippurate crystalluria.

● **LESS SUITABLE FOR PRESCRIBING** Methenamine (hexamine) hippurate should **not** generally be used because it requires an acidic urine for its antimicrobial activity and it is ineffective for upper urinary-tract infections; it may, however, have a role in the prophylaxis and treatment of chronic or recurrent uncomplicated lower urinary-tract infections. It is considered less suitable for prescribing.

● **MEDICINAL FORMS**
There can be variation in the licensing of different medicines containing the same drug.
Tablet
CAUTIONARY AND ADVISORY LABELS 9
  ▸ Hiprex (Meda Pharmaceuticals Ltd)
    Methenamine hippurate 1 gram Hiprex 1g tablets | 60 tablet Ⓟ
    £19.74 DT price = £19.74

Nitrofurantoin

● **INDICATIONS AND DOSE**

Acute uncomplicated urinary-tract infections
▸ BY MOUTH USING IMMEDIATE-RELEASE MEDICINES
  ▸ Child 3 months–11 years: 750 micrograms/kg 4 times a day for 3–7 days
  ▸ Child 12–17 years: 50 mg 4 times a day for 3–7 days
  ▸ Adult: 50 mg 4 times a day for 3–7 days, dose to be taken with food
▸ BY MOUTH USING MODIFIED-RELEASE MEDICINES
  ▸ Child 12–17 years: 100 mg twice daily, dose to be taken with food
  ▸ Adult: 100 mg twice daily, dose to be taken with food

Severe chronic recurrent urinary-tract infections
▸ BY MOUTH USING IMMEDIATE-RELEASE MEDICINES
  ▸ Child 12–17 years: 100 mg 4 times a day for 3–7 days
  ▸ Adult: 100 mg 4 times a day for 7 days, dose to be taken with food, reduce dose or discontinue treatment if severe nausea occurs continued →

5

Infection

Prophylaxis of urinary-tract infection (considered for recurrent infection, significant urinary-tract anomalies, or significant kidney damage)
▸ BY MOUTH USING IMMEDIATE-RELEASE MEDICINES
  ▹ Child 3 months-11 years: 1 mg/kg once daily, dose to be taken at night
  ▹ Child 12-17 years: 50–100 mg once daily, dose to be taken at night
  ▹ Adult: 50–100 mg once daily, dose to be taken at night
Genito-urinary surgical prophylaxis
▸ BY MOUTH USING MODIFIED-RELEASE MEDICINES
  ▹ Adult: 100 mg twice daily on day of procedure and for 3 days after

● CONTRA-INDICATIONS Acute porphyrias p. 918 · G6PD deficiency · infants less than 3 months old
● CAUTIONS Anaemia · diabetes mellitus · electrolyte imbalance · folate deficiency · pulmonary disease · susceptibility to peripheral neuropathy · urine may be coloured yellow or brown · vitamin B deficiency
● INTERACTIONS → Appendix 1 (nitrofurantoin).
● SIDE-EFFECTS
  ▸ **Rare** Agranulocytosis · aplastic anaemia · arthralgia · benign intracranial hypertension · blood disorders · cholestatic jaundice · erythema multiforme · exfoliative dermatitis · hepatitis · pancreatitis · thrombocytopenia · transient alopecia
  ▸ **Frequency not known** Acute pulmonary reactions · anaphylaxis · angioedema · anorexia · chronic pulmonary reactions (pulmonary fibrosis reported; possible association with lupus erythematosus-like syndrome) · diarrhoea · hypersensitivity reactions · nausea · peripheral neuropathy · pruritus · rash · sialadenitis · urticaria · vomiting
● PREGNANCY Avoid at term—may produce neonatal haemolysis.
● BREAST FEEDING Avoid; only small amounts in milk but enough to produce haemolysis in G6PD-deficient infants.
● HEPATIC IMPAIRMENT Use with caution; cholestatic jaundice and chronic active hepatitis reported.
● RENAL IMPAIRMENT Risk of peripheral neuropathy; antibacterial efficacy depends on renal secretion of the drug into urinary tract.
  ▸ In adults Avoid if eGFR less than 45 mL/minute/1.73 m²; may be used with caution if eGFR 30–44 mL/minute/1.73 m² as a short-course only (3 to 7 days), to treat uncomplicated lower urinary-tract infection caused by suspected or proven multidrug resistant bacteria and only if potential benefit outweighs risk.
  ▸ In children Avoid if estimated glomerular filtration rate less than 45 mL/minute/1.73 m² ; may be used with caution if estimated glomerular filtration rate 30–44 mL/minute/1.73 m² as a short-course only (3 to 7 days), to treat uncomplicated lower urinary-tract infection caused by suspected or proven multidrug resistant bacteria and only if potential benefit outweighs risk.
● MONITORING REQUIREMENTS On long-term therapy, monitor liver function and monitor for pulmonary symptoms, especially in the elderly (discontinue if deterioration in lung function).
● EFFECT ON LABORATORY TESTS False positive urinary glucose (if tested for reducing substances).
● PATIENT AND CARER ADVICE
  Medicines for Children leaflet: Nitrofurantoin for urinary tract infections www.medicinesforchildren.org.uk/nitrofurantoin-for-urinary-tract-infections

● MEDICINAL FORMS
  There can be variation in the licensing of different medicines containing the same drug. Forms available from special-order manufacturers include: oral solution
Tablet
CAUTIONARY AND ADVISORY LABELS 9, 14, 21
  ▸ Nitrofurantoin (Non-proprietary)
    Nitrofurantoin 50 mg Nitrofurantoin 50mg tablets | 28 tablet [PoM] £35.00 DT price = £7.42 | 100 tablet [PoM] £111.89
    Nitrofurantoin 100 mg Nitrofurantoin 100mg tablets | 28 tablet [PoM] £13.28 DT price = £2.60 | 100 tablet [PoM] £45.00
  ▸ Genfura (Genesis Pharmaceuticals Ltd)
    Nitrofurantoin 50 mg Genfura 50mg tablets | 28 tablet [PoM] £14.40 DT price = £7.42
    Nitrofurantoin 100 mg Genfura 100mg tablets | 28 tablet [PoM] £10.62 DT price = £2.60 | 100 tablet [PoM] £37.92
Capsule
CAUTIONARY AND ADVISORY LABELS 9, 14, 21
  ▸ Nitrofurantoin (Non-proprietary)
    Nitrofurantoin 50 mg Nitrofurantoin 50mg capsules | 30 capsule [PoM] £15.42 DT price = £15.42
    Nitrofurantoin 100 mg Nitrofurantoin 100mg capsules | 30 capsule [PoM] £10.42 DT price = £10.42
Modified-release capsule
CAUTIONARY AND ADVISORY LABELS 9, 14, 21, 25
  ▸ Macrobid (AMCo)
    Nitrofurantoin 100 mg Macrobid 100mg modified-release capsules | 14 capsule [PoM] £9.50 DT price = £9.50
Oral suspension
CAUTIONARY AND ADVISORY LABELS 9, 14, 21
  ▸ Nitrofurantoin (Non-proprietary)
    Nitrofurantoin 5 mg per 1 ml Nitrofurantoin 25mg/5ml oral suspension sugar free sugar-free | 300 ml [PoM] £446.95 DT price = £446.95

3 Fungal infection

Antifungals, systemic use

Common fungal infections

The systemic treatment of common fungal infections is outlined below; specialist treatment is required in most forms of systemic or disseminated fungal infections. Local treatment is suitable for a number of fungal infections (genital, bladder, eye, ear, oropharynx, and skin).

Aspergillosis

Aspergillosis most commonly affects the respiratory tract but in severely immunocompromised patients, invasive forms can affect the heart, brain, and skin. Voriconazole p. 544 is the treatment of choice for aspergillosis; liposomal amphotericin p. 539 is an alternative first-line treatment when voriconazole cannot be used. Caspofungin p. 538, itraconazole p. 542, or posaconazole p. 543 can be used in patients who are refractory to, or intolerant of voriconazole and liposomal amphotericin. Itraconazole is also used for the treatment of chronic pulmonary aspergillosis or as an adjunct in the treatment of allergic bronchopulmonary aspergillosis [unlicensed indication].

Candidiasis

Many superficial candidal infections including infections of the skin are treated locally; widespread or intractable infection requires systemic antifungal treatment. Vaginal candidiasis may be treated with locally acting antifungals or with fluconazole p. 540 given by mouth; for resistant organisms in adults, itraconazole can be given by mouth.

Oropharyngeal candidiasis generally responds to topical therapy; fluconazole is given by mouth for unresponsive infections; it is effective and is reliably absorbed. Itraconazole may be used for infections that do not respond to fluconazole. Topical therapy may not be adequate in immunocompromised patients and an oral triazole antifungal is preferred.

For *invasive or disseminated candidiasis*, an **echinocandin** can be used. Fluconazole is an alternative for *Candida albicans* infection in clinically stable patients who have not received an azole antifungal recently. Amphotericin is an alternative when an echinocandin or fluconazole cannot be used, however, amphotericin should be considered for the initial treatment of CNS candidiasis. Voriconazole can be used for infections caused by fluconazole-resistant *Candida* spp. when oral therapy is required, or in patients intolerant of amphotericin or an echinocandin. In refractory cases, flucytosine p. 545 can be used with intravenous amphotericin.

Cryptococcosis

Cryptococcosis is uncommon but infection in the immunocompromised, especially in HIV-positive patients, can be life-threatening; cryptococcal meningitis is the most common form of fungal meningitis. The treatment of choice in cryptococcal meningitis is amphotericin by intravenous infusion and flucytosine by intravenous infusion for 2 weeks, followed by fluconazole by mouth for 8 weeks or until cultures are negative. In cryptococcosis, fluconazole is sometimes given alone as an alternative in HIV-positive patients with mild, localised infections or in those who cannot tolerate amphotericin. Following successful treatment, fluconazole can be used for prophylaxis against relapse until immunity recovers.

Histoplasmosis

Histoplasmosis is rare in temperate climates; it can be life-threatening, particularly in HIV-infected persons. Itraconazole can be used for the treatment of immunocompetent patients with indolent non-meningeal infection, including chronic pulmonary histoplasmosis. Amphotericin by intravenous infusion is used for the initial treatment of fulminant or severe infections, followed by a course of itraconazole by mouth. Following successful treatment, itraconazole can be used for prophylaxis against relapse until immunity recovers.

Skin and nail infections

Mild localised fungal infections of the skin (including tinea corporis, tinea cruris, and tinea pedis) respond to topical therapy. Systemic therapy is appropriate if topical therapy fails, if many areas are affected, or if the site of infection is difficult to treat such as in infections of the nails (onychomycosis) and of the scalp (tinea capitis). Oral imidazole or triazole antifungals (particularly itraconazole) and terbinafine p. 1079 are used more frequently than griseofulvin p. 545 because they have a broader spectrum of activity and require a shorter duration of treatment.

Tinea capitis is treated systemically; additional topical application of an antifungal may reduce transmission. Griseofulvin is used for tinea capitis in adults and children; it is effective against infections caused by *Trichophyton tonsurans* and *Microsporum spp.* Terbinafine is used for tinea capitis caused by *T. tonsurans* [unlicensed indication]. The role of terbinafine in the management of *Microsporum* infections is uncertain.

Pityriasis versicolor may be treated with itraconazole by mouth if topical therapy is ineffective; fluconazole by mouth is an alternative. Oral terbinafine is **not** effective for pityriasis versicolor.

Antifungal treatment may not be necessary in asymptomatic patients with tinea infection of the nails. If treatment is necessary, a systemic antifungal is more effective than topical therapy. Terbinafine and itraconazole have largely replaced griseofulvin for the systemic treatment of *onychomycosis*, particularly of the toenail; terbinafine is considered to be the drug of choice. Itraconazole can be administered as intermittent 'pulse' therapy. Topical

antifungals also have a role in the treatment of onychomycosis.

Immunocompromised patients

Immunocompromised patients are at particular risk of fungal infections and may receive antifungal drugs prophylactically; oral triazole antifungals are the drugs of choice for prophylaxis. Fluconazole is more reliably absorbed than itraconazole, but fluconazole is not effective against *Aspergillus* spp. Itraconazole is preferred in patients at risk of invasive aspergillosis. Posaconazole can be used for prophylaxis in patients who are undergoing haematopoietic stem cell transplantation or receiving chemotherapy for acute myeloid leukaemia and myelodysplastic syndrome, if they are intolerant of fluconazole or itraconazole. Micafungin p. 538 can be used for prophylaxis of candidiasis in patients undergoing haematopoietic stem cell transplantation when fluconazole, itraconazole or posaconazole cannot be used.

Amphotericin by intravenous infusion or caspofungin is used for the empirical *treatment* of serious fungal infections; caspofungin is not effective against fungal infections of the CNS.

Triazole antifungals

Triazole antifungal drugs have a role in the prevention and systemic treatment of fungal infections.

Fluconazole is very well absorbed after oral administration. It also achieves good penetration into the cerebrospinal fluid to treat fungal meningitis. Fluconazole is excreted largely unchanged in the urine and can be used to treat candiduria.

Itraconazole is active against a wide range of dermatophytes. Itraconazole capsules require an acid environment in the stomach for optimal absorption. Itraconazole has been associated with liver damage and should be avoided or used with caution in patients with liver disease; fluconazole is less frequently associated with hepatotoxicity.

Posaconazole is licensed for the treatment of invasive fungal infections unresponsive to conventional treatment.

Voriconazole is a broad-spectrum antifungal drug which is licensed for use in life-threatening infections.

Imidazole antifungals

The imidazole antifungals include clotrimazole p. 1076, econazole nitrate p. 1076, ketoconazole p. 751, p. 1077, and tioconazole p. 1078. They are used for the local treatment of vaginal candidiasis and for dermatophyte infections. Miconazole p. 1061 can be used locally for oral infections; it is also effective in intestinal infections. Systemic absorption may follow use of miconazole oral gel and may result in significant drug interactions.

Polyene antifungals

The polyene antifungals include amphotericin p. 539 and nystatin p. 1062; neither drug is absorbed when given by mouth. Nystatin is used for oral, oropharyngeal, and perioral infections by local application in the mouth. Nystatin is also used for *Candida albicans* infection of the skin.

Amphotericin by intravenous infusion is used for the treatment of systemic fungal infections and is active against most fungi and yeasts. It is highly protein bound and penetrates poorly into body fluids and tissues. When given parenterally amphotericin is toxic and side-effects are common. Lipid formulations of amphotericin (*Abelcet*® and *AmBisome*®) are significantly less toxic and are recommended when the conventional formulation of amphotericin is contra-indicated because of toxicity, especially nephrotoxicity or when response to conventional amphotericin is inadequate; lipid formulations are more expensive.

Echinocandin antifungals

The echinocandin antifungals include anidulafungin below, caspofungin below and micafungin below. They are only active against *Aspergillus* spp. and *Candida* spp.; however, anidulafungin and micafungin are not used for the treatment of aspergillosis. Echinocandins are not effective against fungal infections of the CNS.

Other antifungals

Flucytosine p. 545 is used with amphotericin in a synergistic combination. Bone marrow depression can occur which limits its use, particularly in HIV-positive patients; weekly blood counts are necessary during prolonged therapy. Resistance to flucytosine can develop during therapy and sensitivity testing is essential before and during treatment. Flucytosine has a role in the treatment of systemic candidiasis and cryptococcal meningitis.

Griseofulvin p. 545 is effective for widespread or intractable dermatophyte infections but has been superseded by newer antifungals, particularly for nail infections. It is the drug of choice for trichophyton infections in children. Duration of therapy is dependent on the site of the infection and may extend to a number of months.

Terbinafine p. 1079 is the drug of choice for fungal nail infections and is also used for ringworm infections where oral treatment is considered appropriate.

ANTIFUNGALS > ECHINOCANDIN ANTIFUNGALS

Anidulafungin

● **INDICATIONS AND DOSE**

Invasive candidiasis

▶ BY INTRAVENOUS INFUSION
▶ Adult: Initially 200 mg once daily for 1 day, then 100 mg once daily

● **SIDE-EFFECTS**

▶ **Common or very common** Coagulopathy · convulsion · diarrhoea · flushing · headache · hypokalaemia · nausea · pruritus · raised serum creatinine · rash · vomiting
▶ **Uncommon** Abdominal pain · cholestasis · hyperglycaemia · hypertension · injection-site pain · urticaria
▶ **Frequency not known** Bronchospasm · dyspnoea · hepatitis · hypotension

● **PREGNANCY** Manufacturer advises avoid—no information available.

● **BREAST FEEDING** Manufacturer advises avoid unless potential benefit outweighs risk—present in milk in *animal* studies.

● **DIRECTIONS FOR ADMINISTRATION** For *intravenous infusion* (*Ecalta* ®), give intermittently *in* Glucose 5% *or* Sodium chloride 0.9%. Reconstitute each 100 mg with 30 mL water for injections and allow up to 5 minutes for reconstitution; dilute dose in infusion fluid to a concentration of 770 micrograms/mL; give at a rate not exceeding 1.1 mg/minute. Follow product information if using stock supplied with ethanol solvent.

● MEDICINAL FORMS
There can be variation in the licensing of different medicines containing the same drug.
Powder for solution for infusion
▶ Ecalta (Pfizer Ltd)
  Anidulafungin 100 mg Ecalta 100mg powder for concentrate for solution for infusion vials | 1 vial [PoM] £299.99 (Hospital only)

Caspofungin

● **INDICATIONS AND DOSE**

Invasive aspergillosis | **Invasive candidiasis** | **Empirical treatment of systemic fungal infections in patients with neutropenia**

▶ BY INTRAVENOUS INFUSION
▶ Adult (body-weight up to 81 kg): 70 mg once daily for 1 day, then 50 mg once daily
▶ Adult (body-weight 81 kg and above): 70 mg once daily

● INTERACTIONS → Appendix 1 (caspofungin).

● SIDE-EFFECTS

▶ **Common or very common** Arthralgia · diarrhoea · dyspnoea · headache · hypokalaemia · injection-site reactions · nausea · pruritus · rash · sweating · vomiting
▶ **Uncommon** Abdominal pain · anaemia · anorexia · anxiety · arrhythmia · ascites · blurred vision · bronchospasm · chest pain · cholestasis · constipation · cough · disorientation · dizziness · dry mouth · dyspepsia · dysphagia · erythema multiforme · fatigue · flatulence · flushing · heart failure · hepatic dysfunction · hyperglycaemia · hypertension · hypoaesthesia · hypocalcaemia · hypomagnesaemia · hypotension · leucopenia · metabolic acidosis · muscular weakness · myalgia · palpitation · paraesthesia · renal failure · sleep disturbances · taste disturbances · thrombocytopenia · thrombophlebitis · tremor
▶ **Frequency not known** Adult respiratory distress syndrome · anaphylaxis

● PREGNANCY Manufacturer advises avoid unless essential—toxicity in *animal* studies.

● BREAST FEEDING Present in milk in *animal* studies—manufacturer advises avoid.

● HEPATIC IMPAIRMENT 70 mg on first day then 35 mg once daily in moderate impairment. No information available for severe impairment.

● DIRECTIONS FOR ADMINISTRATION For *intravenous infusion* (*Cancidas* ®), give intermittently *in* Sodium chloride 0.9%. Allow vial to reach room temperature; initially reconstitute each vial with 10.5 mL water for injections, mixing gently to dissolve then dilute requisite dose in 250 mL infusion fluid (35- or 50-mg doses may be diluted in 100 ml infusion fluid if necessary); give over 60 minutes; incompatible with glucose solutions.

● MEDICINAL FORMS
There can be variation in the licensing of different medicines containing the same drug.
Powder for solution for infusion
▶ Cancidas (Merck Sharp & Dohme Ltd)
  Caspofungin (as Caspofungin acetate) 50 mg Cancidas 50mg powder for solution for infusion vials | 1 vial [PoM] £327.67
  Caspofungin (as Caspofungin acetate) 70 mg Cancidas 70mg powder for solution for infusion vials | 1 vial [PoM] £416.78

Micafungin

● **INDICATIONS AND DOSE**

Invasive candidiasis

▶ BY INTRAVENOUS INFUSION
▶ Adult (body-weight up to 40 kg): 2 mg/kg once daily for at least 14 days; increased if necessary to 4 mg/kg once daily, increase dose if response inadequate
▶ Adult (body-weight 40 kg and above): 100 mg once daily for at least 14 days; increased if necessary to 200 mg once daily, increase dose if response inadequate

Oesophageal candidiasis

▶ BY INTRAVENOUS INFUSION
▶ Adult (body-weight up to 40 kg): 3 mg/kg once daily
▶ Adult (body-weight 40 kg and above): 150 mg once daily

Prophylaxis of candidiasis in patients undergoing bone-marrow transplantation or who are expected to become neutropenic for over 10 days
▸ BY INTRAVENOUS INFUSION
▸ Adult (body-weight up to 40 kg): 1 mg/kg once daily continue for at least 7 days after neutrophil count is in desirable range
▸ Adult (body-weight 40 kg and above): 50 mg once daily continue for at least 7 days after neutrophil count is in desirable range

● INTERACTIONS → Appendix 1 (micafungin).
Caution with concomitant use of other hepatotoxic drugs.
● SIDE-EFFECTS
▸ **Common or very common** Abdominal pain · anaemia · diarrhoea · fever · headache · hypocalcaemia · hypokalaemia · hypomagnesaemia · leucopenia · nausea · phlebitis · rash · vomiting
▸ **Uncommon** Anorexia · anxiety · blood pressure changes · bradycardia · cholestasis · confusion · constipation · dizziness · dyspepsia · dyspnoea · eosinophilia · flushing · hepatitis · hepatomegaly · hyperhidrosis · hyperkalaemia · hyponatraemia · hypophosphataemia · palpitation · pancytopenia · pruritus · sleep disturbances · tachycardia · taste disturbances · thrombocytopenia · tremor
▸ **Rare** Haemolytic anaemia
▸ **Frequency not known** Disseminated intravascular coagulation · hepatotoxicity (potentially life-threatening) · renal failure · Stevens-Johnson syndrome · toxic epidermal necrolysis
● PREGNANCY Manufacturer advises avoid unless essential—toxicity in *animal* studies.
● BREAST FEEDING Manufacturer advises use only if potential benefit outweighs risk—present in milk in *animal* studies.
● HEPATIC IMPAIRMENT Use with caution in mild to moderate impairment. Avoid in severe impairment.
● RENAL IMPAIRMENT Use with caution; renal function may deteriorate.
● MONITORING REQUIREMENTS
▸ Monitor renal function.
▸ Monitor liver function—discontinue if significant and persistent abnormalities in liver function tests develop.
● DIRECTIONS FOR ADMINISTRATION For *intravenous infusion* (*Mycamine*®), give intermittently in Glucose 5% or Sodium chloride 0.9%. Reconstitute each vial with 5 mL infusion fluid; gently rotate vial, without shaking, to dissolve; dilute requisite dose with infusion fluid to 100 mL (final concentration of 0.5–2 mg/mL); protect infusion from light; give over 60 minutes.

● MEDICINAL FORMS
There can be variation in the licensing of different medicines containing the same drug.
Powder for solution for infusion
▸ Mycamine (Astellas Pharma Ltd)
   Micafungin (as Micafungin sodium) 50 mg Mycamine 50mg powder for solution for infusion vials | 1 vial [PoM] £196.08
   Micafungin (as Micafungin sodium) 100 mg Mycamine 100mg powder for solution for infusion vials | 1 vial [PoM] £341.00

ANTIFUNGALS › POLYENE ANTIFUNGALS

Amphotericin
(Amphotericin B)

● INDICATIONS AND DOSE
ABELCET®

Severe invasive candidiasis | Severe systemic fungal infections in patients not responding to conventional amphotericin or to other antifungal drugs or where toxicity or renal impairment precludes conventional amphotericin, including invasive aspergillosis, cryptococcal meningitis and disseminated cryptococcosis in HIV patients
▸ BY INTRAVENOUS INFUSION
▸ Adult: Test dose 1 mg, to be given over 15 minutes, then 5 mg/kg once daily for at least 14 days

AMBISOME®

Severe systemic or deep mycoses where toxicity (particularly nephrotoxicity) precludes use of conventional amphotericin | Suspected or proven infection in febrile neutropenic patients unresponsive to broad-spectrum antibacterials
▸ BY INTRAVENOUS INFUSION
▸ Adult: Test dose 1 mg, to be given over 10 minutes, then 3 mg/kg once daily; maximum 5 mg/kg per day

Aspergillosis
▸ BY INTRAVENOUS INFUSION
▸ Adult: Test dose 1 mg, to be given over 10 minutes, then 3 mg/kg once daily; maximum 5 mg/kg per day

Visceral leishmaniasis (unresponsive to the antimonial alone)
▸ BY INTRAVENOUS INFUSION
▸ Adult: 1–3 mg/kg daily for 10–21 days to a cumulative dose of 21–30 mg/kg, alternatively 3 mg/kg for 5 consecutive days, followed by 3 mg/kg after 6 days for 1 dose

FUNGIZONE®

Systemic fungal infections
▸ BY INTRAVENOUS INFUSION
▸ Adult: Test dose 1 mg, to be given over 20–30 minutes, then 250 micrograms/kg daily, gradually increased over 2–4 days, increased if tolerated to 1 mg/kg daily, max. (severe infection) 1.5 mg/kg daily or on alternate days. Prolonged treatment usually necessary; if interrupted for longer than 7 days recommence at 250 micrograms/kg daily and increase gradually

● UNLICENSED USE
AMBISOME® Use at the maximum dose of 5 mg/kg once daily is an unlicensed dose.
● CAUTIONS Avoid rapid infusion (risk of arrhythmias) · when given parenterally, toxicity common (close supervision necessary and close observation required for at least 30 minutes after test dose)
CAUTIONS, FURTHER INFORMATION
▸ Anaphylaxis Anaphylaxis can occur with any intravenous amphotericin product and a test dose is advisable before the first infusion; the patient should be carefully observed for at least 30 minutes after the test dose. Prophylactic antipyretics or hydrocortisone should only be used in patients who have previously experienced acute adverse reactions (in whom continued treatment with amphotericin is essential).
● INTERACTIONS → Appendix 1 (amphotericin).
Caution—corticosteroids (avoid except to control reactions).

5

Infection

5

Infection

- SIDE-EFFECTS
‣ **Common or very common** Abdominal pain · abnormal liver function (discontinue treatment) · anaemia · arrhythmias · blood disorders · blood pressure changes · cardiovascular effects · chest pain · diarrhoea · disturbances in renal function · dyspnoea · electrolyte disturbances · febrile reactions · headache · hypokalaemia · hypomagnesaemia · nausea · rash · renal tubular acidosis · thrombocytopenia · vomiting
‣ **Uncommon** Anaphylactoid reactions · bronchospasm · convulsions · diplopia · encephalopathy · hearing loss · neurological disorders · peripheral neuropathy · tremor
‣ **Frequency not known** Anorexia · arthralgia · myalgia · Stevens-Johnson syndrome · toxic epidermal necrolysis
- PREGNANCY Not known to be harmful but manufacturers advise avoid unless potential benefit outweighs risk.
- BREAST FEEDING No information available.
- RENAL IMPAIRMENT Use only if no alternative; nephrotoxicity may be reduced with use of lipid formulation.
- MONITORING REQUIREMENTS Hepatic and renal function tests, blood counts, and plasma electrolyte (including plasma-potassium and magnesium concentration) monitoring required.
- DIRECTIONS FOR ADMINISTRATION
ABELCET® **Amphotericin (lipid complex)**
  For *intravenous infusion*, give intermittently *in* Glucose 5%. Allow suspension to reach room temperature, shake gently to ensure no yellow settlement, withdraw requisite dose (using 17-19 gauge needle) into one or more 20-mL syringes; replace needle on syringe with a 5-micron filter needle provided (fresh needle for each syringe) and dilute to a concentration of 1 mg/mL (2 mg/mL can be used in fluid restriction and in children); preferably give *via* an infusion pump at a rate of 2.5 mg/kg/hour (initial test dose of 1 mg over 15 minutes); an in-line filter (pore size no less than 15 micron) may be used; do not use sodium chloride or other electrolyte solutions, flush existing intravenous line with glucose 5% or use separate line.
AMBISOME® **Amphotericin (liposomal)**
  For *intravenous infusion* (*AmBisome*®), give intermittently *in* Glucose 5% or 10%. Reconstitute each vial with 12 mL water for injections and shake vigorously to produce a preparation containing 4 mg/mL; withdraw requisite dose from vial and introduce into infusion fluid through the 5 micron filter provided to produce a final concentration of 0.2–2 mg/mL; infuse over 30–60 minutes, or if non-anaphylactic infusion-related reactions occur infuse over 2 hours (initial test dose of 1 mg over 10 minutes); an in-line filter (pore size no less than 1 micron) may be used; incompatible with sodium chloride solutions, flush existing intravenous line with glucose 5% or 10%, or use separate line.
FUNGIZONE® **Amphotericin (as sodium deoxycholate complex)**
  For *intravenous infusion* (*Fungizone*®), give intermittently *in* Glucose 5%. Reconstitute each vial with 10 mL water for injections and shake immediately to produce a 5 mg/mL colloidal solution; dilute further in infusion fluid to a concentration of 100 micrograms/mL; pH of the glucose must not be below 4.2 (check each container—consult product literature for details of the buffer); infuse over 2–4 hours, or longer if not tolerated (initial test dose of 1 mg over 20–30 minutes); begin infusion immediately after dilution; protect from light; incompatible with sodium chloride solutions, flush existing intravenous line with glucose 5% or use separate line; an in-line filter (pore size no less than 1 micron) may be used.
- PRESCRIBING AND DISPENSING INFORMATION Different preparations of intravenous amphotericin vary in their pharmacodynamics, pharmacokinetics, dosage, and

administration; these preparations should **not** be considered interchangeable. To avoid confusion, prescribers should specify the brand to be dispensed.

- MEDICINAL FORMS
  There can be variation in the licensing of different medicines containing the same drug.
  Powder for solution for infusion
  EXCIPIENTS: May contain Sucrose
  ELECTROLYTES: May contain Sodium
  ‣ AmBisome (Gilead Sciences International Ltd)
    Amphotericin B liposomal 50 mg AmBisome 50mg powder for solution for infusion vials | 10 vial [PoM] £821.87
  ‣ Fungizone (Bristol-Myers Squibb Pharmaceuticals Ltd)
    Amphotericin B 50 mg Fungizone 50mg powder for solution for infusion vials | 1 vial [PoM] £3.88
  Suspension for infusion
  ELECTROLYTES: May contain Sodium
  ‣ Abelcet (Teva UK Ltd)
    Amphotericin B (as Amphotericin B phospholipid complex) 5 mg per 1 ml Abelcet 100mg/20ml concentrate for suspension for infusion vials | 10 vial [PoM] £775.04 (Hospital only)

ANTIFUNGALS > TRIAZOLE ANTIFUNGALS

Fluconazole

- INDICATIONS AND DOSE
Candidal balanitis
‣ BY MOUTH
‣ Child 16-17 years: 150 mg for 1 dose
‣ Adult: 150 mg for 1 dose
Vaginal candidiasis
‣ BY MOUTH
‣ Child 16-17 years: 150 mg for 1 dose
‣ Adult: 150 mg for 1 dose
Vulvovaginal candidiasis (recurrent)
‣ BY MOUTH
‣ Adult: Initially 150 mg every 72 hours for 3 doses, then 150 mg once weekly for 6 months
Mucosal candidiasis (except genital)
‣ BY MOUTH, OR BY INTRAVENOUS INFUSION
‣ Child 1 month-11 years: 3–6 mg/kg, dose to be given on first day, then 3 mg/kg daily (max. per dose 100 mg) for 7–14 days in oropharyngeal candidiasis (max. 14 days except in severely immunocompromised patients); for 14–30 days in other mucosal infections (e.g. oesophagitis, candiduria, non-invasive bronchopulmonary infections)
‣ Child 12-17 years: 50 mg daily for 7–14 days in oropharyngeal candidiasis (max. 14 days except in severely immunocompromised patients); for 14–30 days in other mucosal infections (e.g. oesophagitis, candiduria, non-invasive bronchopulmonary infections); increased to 100 mg daily, increased dose only for unusually difficult infections
‣ BY MOUTH
‣ Adult: 50 mg daily given for 7–14 days in oropharyngeal candidiasis (max. 14 days except in severely immunocompromised patients); for 14 days in atrophic oral candidiasis associated with dentures; for 14–30 days in other mucosal infections (e.g. oesophagitis, candiduria, non-invasive bronchopulmonary infections); increased to 100 mg daily, increased dose only for unusually difficult infections
Tinea pedis, corporis, cruris, pityriasis versicolor | Dermal candidiasis
‣ BY MOUTH
‣ Adult: 50 mg daily for 2–4 weeks (for up to 6 weeks in tinea pedis); max. duration of treatment 6 weeks

Invasive candidal infections (including candidaemia and disseminated candidiasis) and cryptococcal infections (including meningitis)
▸ BY MOUTH, OR BY INTRAVENOUS INFUSION
▸ Child: 6–12 mg/kg daily (max. per dose 800 mg), treatment continued according to response (at least 8 weeks for cryptococcal meningitis)
▸ Adult: 400 mg, dose to be given on first day, then 200–400 mg daily (max. per dose 800 mg once daily), treatment continued according to response (at least 8 weeks for cryptococcal meningitis), maximum dose for use in severe infections

Prevention of fungal infections in immunocompromised patients
▸ BY MOUTH, OR BY INTRAVENOUS INFUSION
▸ Child: 3–12 mg/kg daily (max. per dose 400 mg), commence treatment before anticipated onset of neutropenia and continue for 7 days after neutrophil count in desirable range, dose given according to extent and duration of neutropenia
▸ Adult: 50–400 mg daily, commence treatment before anticipated onset of neutropenia and continue for 7 days after neutrophil count in desirable range, dose adjusted according to risk

Prevention of fungal infections in immunocompromised patients (for patients with high risk of systemic infections e.g. following bone-marrow transplantation)
▸ BY MOUTH, OR BY INTRAVENOUS INFUSION
▸ Adult: 400 mg daily, commence treatment before anticipated onset of neutropenia and continue for 7 days after neutrophil count in desirable range

Prevention of relapse of cryptococcal meningitis in HIV-infected patients after completion of primary therapy
▸ BY MOUTH, OR BY INTRAVENOUS INFUSION
▸ Adult: 200 mg daily

● CONTRA-INDICATIONS Acute porphyrias p. 918
● CAUTIONS Susceptibility to QT interval prolongation
● INTERACTIONS → Appendix 1 (antifungals, triazole); in general, fluconazole interactions in Appendix 1 relate to multiple-dose treatment.
Caution with concomitant use of hepatotoxic drugs.
● SIDE-EFFECTS
▸ **Common or very common** Abdominal discomfort · diarrhoea · flatulence · headache · nausea · rash
▸ **Uncommon** Alopecia · anaphylaxis · angioedema (in children) · dizziness · dyspepsia · hepatic disorders · hyperlipidaemia · hypersensitivity reactions (in adults) · pruritus · seizures · Stevens-Johnson syndrome · taste disturbance · toxic epidermal necrolysis · vomiting
▸ **Frequency not known** Hypokalaemia · leucopenia · thrombocytopenia

SIDE-EFFECTS, FURTHER INFORMATION
If rash occurs, discontinue treatment (or monitor closely if infection invasive or systemic); severe cutaneous reactions are more likely in patients with AIDS.

● PREGNANCY Manufacturer advises avoid—multiple congenital abnormalities reported with long-term high doses.
● BREAST FEEDING Present in milk but amount probably too small to be harmful.
● HEPATIC IMPAIRMENT Toxicity with related drugs.
● RENAL IMPAIRMENT
▸ In adults Usual initial dose then halve subsequent doses if eGFR less than 50 mL/minute/1.73 m^2.
▸ In children Usual initial dose then halve subsequent doses if estimated glomerular filtration rate less than 50 mL/minute/1.73 m^2.

● MONITORING REQUIREMENTS Monitor liver function with high doses or extended courses—discontinue if signs or symptoms of hepatic disease (risk of hepatic necrosis).
● DIRECTIONS FOR ADMINISTRATION
▸ With intravenous use in children For *intravenous infusion*, give over 10–30 minutes; do not exceed an infusion rate of 5–10 mL/minute.
● PRESCRIBING AND DISPENSING INFORMATION Flavours of oral liquid formulations may include orange.
● PROFESSION SPECIFIC INFORMATION
Dental practitioners' formulary
Fluconazole Capsules 50 mg may be prescribed.
Fluconazole Oral Suspension 50 mg/5 mL may be prescribed.
● EXCEPTIONS TO LEGAL CATEGORY Fluconazole capsules can be sold to the public for vaginal candidiasis and associated candidal balanitis in those aged 16–60 years, in a container or packaging containing not more than 150 mg and labelled to show a max. dose of 150 mg.

● MEDICINAL FORMS
There can be variation in the licensing of different medicines containing the same drug.
Capsule
CAUTIONARY AND ADVISORY LABELS 9 (50 mg and 200 mg strengths only)
▸ Fluconazole (Non-proprietary)
Fluconazole 50 mg Fluconazole 50mg capsules | 7 capsule [PoM] £5.00 DT price = £0.86
Fluconazole 150 mg Boots Pharmacy Thrush 150mg capsules | 1 capsule [P] no price available DT price = £0.81
Lloydspharmacy Thrush Oral 150mg capsules | 1 capsule [P] no price available DT price = £0.81
Fluconazole 150mg capsules | 1 capsule [PoM] £8.50 DT price = £0.81 | 1 capsule [P] no price available DT price = £0.81
Galpharm Single Dose Thrush Treatment 150mg capsules | 1 capsule [P] no price available DT price = £0.81
Fluconazole 200 mg Fluconazole 200mg capsules | 7 capsule [PoM] £12.50 DT price = £6.05
▸ Canesten (fluconazole) (Bayer Plc)
Fluconazole 150 mg Canesten 150mg capsules | 1 capsule [P] £6.33 DT price = £0.81
▸ Diflucan (Pfizer Ltd)
Fluconazole 50 mg Diflucan 50mg capsules | 7 capsule [PoM] £16.61 DT price = £0.86
Fluconazole 150 mg Diflucan 150mg capsules | 1 capsule [PoM] £7.12 DT price = £0.81
Fluconazole 200 mg Diflucan 200mg capsules | 7 capsule [PoM] £66.42 DT price = £6.05

Oral suspension
CAUTIONARY AND ADVISORY LABELS 9
▸ Fluconazole (Non-proprietary)
Fluconazole 10 mg per 1 ml Fluconazole 50mg/5ml oral suspension | 35 ml [PoM] £20.51 DT price = £20.51
▸ Diflucan (Pfizer Ltd)
Fluconazole 10 mg per 1 ml Diflucan 50mg/5ml oral suspension | 35 ml [PoM] £16.61 DT price = £20.51
Fluconazole 40 mg per 1 ml Diflucan 200mg/5ml oral suspension | 35 ml [PoM] £66.42 DT price = £66.42

Solution for infusion
ELECTROLYTES: May contain Sodium
▸ Fluconazole (Non-proprietary)
Fluconazole 2 mg per 1 ml Fluconazole 100mg/50ml solution for infusion bottles | 5 bottle [PoM] £12.60
Fluconazole 200mg/100ml solution for infusion vials | 1 vial [PoM] £29.28
Fluconazole 50mg/25ml solution for infusion vials | 1 vial [PoM] £7.31–£7.32
▸ Diflucan (Pfizer Ltd)
Fluconazole 2 mg per 1 ml Diflucan 200mg/100ml solution for infusion vials | 1 vial [PoM] £29.28

Itraconazole

● **INDICATIONS AND DOSE**

Vulvovaginal candidiasis
▸ BY MOUTH
▹ Adult: 200 mg twice daily for 1 day

Vulvovaginal candidiasis (recurrent)
▸ BY MOUTH
▹ Adult: 50–100 mg daily for 6 months

Oral or oesophageal candidiasis that has not responded to fluconazole
▸ BY MOUTH USING ORAL SOLUTION
▹ Adult: 100–200 mg twice daily for 2 weeks (continue for another 2 weeks if no response; the higher dose should not be used for longer than 2 weeks if no signs of improvement)

Oral or oesophageal candidiasis in HIV-positive or other immunocompromised patients
▸ BY MOUTH USING ORAL SOLUTION
▹ Adult: 200 mg daily in 1–2 divided doses for 1 week (continue for another week if no response)

Systemic candidiasis where other antifungal drugs inappropriate or ineffective
▸ BY MOUTH
▹ Adult: 100–200 mg once daily
▸ BY INTRAVENOUS INFUSION
▹ Adult: 200 mg every 12 hours for 2 days, then 200 mg once daily for max. 12 days

Systemic candidiasis (invasive or disseminated) where other antifungal drugs inappropriate or ineffective
▸ BY MOUTH
▹ Adult: 200 mg twice daily

Pityriasis versicolor
▸ BY MOUTH
▹ Adult: 200 mg once daily for 7 days

Tinea pedis | Tinea manuum
▸ BY MOUTH
▹ Adult: 100 mg once daily for 30 days, alternatively 200 mg twice daily for 7 days

Tinea corporis | Tinea cruris
▸ BY MOUTH
▹ Adult: 100 mg once daily for 15 days, alternatively 200 mg once daily for 7 days

Onychomycosis
▸ BY MOUTH
▹ Adult: 200 mg once daily for 3 months, alternatively 200 mg twice daily for 7 days, subsequent courses repeated after 21-day intervals; fingernails 2 courses, toenails 3 courses

Aspergillosis
▸ BY MOUTH
▹ Adult: 200 mg twice daily

Systemic aspergillosis where other antifungal drugs inappropriate or ineffective
▸ BY INTRAVENOUS INFUSION
▹ Adult: 200 mg every 12 hours for 2 days, then 200 mg once daily for max. 12 days

Histoplasmosis
▸ BY MOUTH
▹ Adult: 200 mg 3 times a day for 3 days, then 200 mg 1–2 times a day
▸ BY INTRAVENOUS INFUSION
▹ Adult: 200 mg every 12 hours for 2 days, then 200 mg once daily for max. 12 days

Systemic cryptococcosis including cryptococcal meningitis where other antifungal drugs inappropriate or ineffective
▸ BY MOUTH
▹ Adult: 200 mg once daily, dose increased in invasive or disseminated disease and in cryptococcal meningitis, increased to 200 mg twice daily
▸ BY INTRAVENOUS INFUSION
▹ Adult: 200 mg every 12 hours for 2 days, then 200 mg once daily for max. 12 days

Maintenance in HIV-infected patients to prevent relapse of underlying fungal infection and prophylaxis in neutropenia when standard therapy inappropriate
▸ BY MOUTH
▹ Adult: 200 mg once daily, then increased to 200 mg twice daily, dose increased only if low plasma-itraconazole concentration

Prophylaxis of deep fungal infections (when standard therapy inappropriate) in patients with haematological malignancy or undergoing bone-marrow transplantation who are expected to become neutropenic
▸ BY MOUTH USING ORAL SOLUTION
▹ Adult: 5 mg/kg daily in 2 divided doses, to be started before transplantation or before chemotherapy (taking care to avoid interaction with cytotoxic drugs) and continued until neutrophil count recovers, safety and efficacy not established in elderly patients

● **UNLICENSED USE** Itraconazole doses in BNF may differ from those in product literature.

┌───┐
IMPORTANT SAFETY INFORMATION
HEART FAILURE
Following reports of heart failure, caution is advised when prescribing itraconazole to patients at high risk of heart failure. Those at risk include:
● patients receiving high doses and longer treatment courses;
● older adults and those with cardiac disease;
● patients with chronic lung disease (including chronic obstructive pulmonary disease) associated with pulmonary hypertension;
● patients receiving treatment with negative inotropic drugs, e.g. calcium channel blockers.
Itraconazole should be avoided in patients with ventricular dysfunction or a history of heart failure unless the infection is serious.
└───┘

● **CONTRA-INDICATIONS** Acute porphyrias p. 918
● **CAUTIONS** Active liver disease · history of hepatotoxicity with other drugs · susceptibility to congestive heart failure
● **INTERACTIONS** → Appendix 1 (antifungals, triazole).
● **SIDE-EFFECTS**
GENERAL SIDE-EFFECTS
▸ **Common or very common** Abdominal pain · diarrhoea · dyspnoea · headache · hepatitis · hypokalaemia · nausea · rash · taste disturbances · vomiting
▸ **Uncommon** Constipation · dizziness · dyspepsia · flatulence · menstrual disorder · myalgia · oedema · peripheral neuropathy (discontinue treatment)
▸ **Rare** Alopecia · deafness · erectile dysfunction · heart failure · hypertriglyceridaemia · leucopenia · pancreatitis · photosensitivity · Stevens-Johnson syndrome · tinnitus · toxic epidermal necrolysis · urinary frequency · visual disturbances
▸ **Frequency not known** Arthralgia · blood pressure changes · confusion · drowsiness · hepatotoxicity · renal impairment · thrombocytopenia · tremor
SPECIFIC SIDE-EFFECTS
▸ With intravenous use Hyperglycaemia

SIDE-EFFECTS, FURTHER INFORMATION
‣ **Hepatotoxicity** Potentially life-threatening hepatotoxicity reported very rarely—discontinue if signs of hepatitis develop.
● **CONCEPTION AND CONTRACEPTION** Ensure effective contraception during treatment and until the next menstrual period following end of treatment.
● **PREGNANCY** Manufacturer advises use only in life-threatening situations (toxicity at high doses in *animal* studies).
● **BREAST FEEDING** Small amounts present in milk—may accumulate; manufacturer advises avoid.
● **HEPATIC IMPAIRMENT** Dose reduction may be necessary. Use only if potential benefit outweighs risk of hepatotoxicity.
● **RENAL IMPAIRMENT** Risk of congestive heart failure.
‣ With oral use Bioavailability of oral formulations possibly reduced.
‣ With intravenous use Use intravenous infusion with caution if eGFR 30–80 mL/minute/1.73 m^2; avoid intravenous infusion if eGFR less than 30 mL/minute/1.73 m^2.
● **MONITORING REQUIREMENTS**
‣ Absorption reduced in AIDS and neutropenia (monitor plasma-itraconazole concentration and increase dose if necessary).
‣ Monitor liver function if treatment continues for longer than one month, if receiving other hepatotoxic drugs, if history of hepatotoxicity with other drugs, or in hepatic impairment.
● **DIRECTIONS FOR ADMINISTRATION** For *intravenous infusion* (*Sporanox®*), give intermittently in Sodium Chloride 0.9%; dilute 250 mg in 50 mL infusion fluid and infuse only 60 mL through an in-line filter (0.2 micron) over 60 minutes.
For *oral liquid*, do not take with food; swish around mouth and swallow, do not rinse afterwards.
● **PRESCRIBING AND DISPENSING INFORMATION** Flavours of oral liquid formulations may include cherry.
● **PATIENT AND CARER ADVICE** Patients should be told how to recognise signs of liver disorder and advised to seek prompt medical attention if symptoms such as anorexia, nausea, vomiting, fatigue, abdominal pain or dark urine develop.
Patients or carers should be given advice on how to administer itraconazole oral liquid.

● **MEDICINAL FORMS**
There can be variation in the licensing of different medicines containing the same drug. Forms available from special-order manufacturers include: oral suspension, oral solution

Capsule
CAUTIONARY AND ADVISORY LABELS 5, 9, 21, 25
‣ Itraconazole (Non-proprietary)
Itraconazole 100 mg Itraconazole 100mg capsules | 15 capsule [PoM] £21.50 DT price = £3.64 | 60 capsule [PoM] £56.21
Itraconazole 100mg Capsules | 15 capsule [PoM] £4.04 DT price = £3.64
‣ Sporanox (Janssen-Cilag Ltd)
Itraconazole 100 mg Sporanox-Pulse 100mg capsules | 28 capsule [PoM] £25.72
Sporanox 100mg capsules | 4 capsule [PoM] £3.67 | 15 capsule [PoM] £13.77 DT price = £3.64 | 60 capsule [PoM] £55.10

Oral solution
CAUTIONARY AND ADVISORY LABELS 9, 23
‣ Itraconazole (Non-proprietary)
Itraconazole 10 mg per 1 ml Itraconazole 50mg/5ml oral solution sugar free sugar-free | 150 ml [PoM] £58.34 DT price = £58.34
‣ Sporanox (Janssen-Cilag Ltd)
Itraconazole 10 mg per 1 ml Sporanox 50mg/5ml oral solution sugar-free | 150 ml [PoM] £58.34 DT price = £58.34

Solution for infusion
EXCIPIENTS: May contain Propylene glycol
‣ Sporanox (Janssen-Cilag Ltd)
Itraconazole 10 mg per 1 ml Sporanox I.V. 250mg/25ml solution for infusion ampoules and diluent | 1 ampoule [PoM] £79.71

Posaconazole

● **INDICATIONS AND DOSE**

Invasive aspergillosis in patients who are refractory to, or intolerant of voriconazole and liposomal amphotericin | Fusariosis either unresponsive to, or in patients intolerant of, amphotericin | Chromoblastomycosis and mycetoma either unresponsive to, or in patients intolerant of, itraconazole | Coccidioidomycosis either unresponsive to, or in patients intolerant of, amphotericin, itraconazole, or fluconazole
‣ BY MOUTH USING ORAL SUSPENSION
‣ Adult: 400 mg twice daily, to be taken with food, alternatively 200 mg 4 times a day, dose if food not tolerated
‣ BY MOUTH USING TABLETS
‣ Adult: 300 mg twice daily on first day, then 300 mg once daily

Oropharyngeal candidiasis (severe infection or in immunocompromised patients only)
‣ BY MOUTH USING ORAL SUSPENSION
‣ Adult: 200 mg on first day, then 100 mg once daily for 13 days, dose to be taken with food

Prophylaxis of invasive fungal infections in patients undergoing bone-marrow transplantation or receiving chemotherapy for acute myeloid leukaemia and myelodysplastic syndrome who are expected to become neutropenic, and who are intolerant of fluconazole or itraconazole
‣ BY MOUTH USING ORAL SUSPENSION
‣ Adult: 200 mg 3 times a day start before transplantation or before chemotherapy and continued until neutrophil count recovers, dose to be taken with food
‣ BY MOUTH USING TABLETS
‣ Adult: 300 mg twice daily on first day, then 300 mg once daily start before transplantation or before chemotherapy and continued until neutrophil count recovers

DOSE EQUIVALENCE AND CONVERSION
Posaconazole oral suspension is **not** interchangeable with tablets on a milligram-for-milligram basis.

PHARMACOKINETICS
Posaconazole oral suspension has to be administered 2 to 4 times daily and must be taken with food (preferably a high fat meal) or nutritional supplement to ensure adequate exposure for systemic effects. Where possible, tablets should be used in preference to suspension because tablets have a higher bioavailability.

● **UNLICENSED USE** Tablets not licensed for oropharyngeal candidiasis.
● **CONTRA-INDICATIONS** Acute porphyrias p. 918
● **CAUTIONS** Body-weight over 120 kg—risk of treatment failure possibly increased · body-weight under 60 kg—risk of side effects increased · bradycardia · cardiomyopathy · history of QT interval prolongation · symptomatic arrhythmias
● **INTERACTIONS** → Appendix 1 (antifungals, triazole). Caution with concomitant use with other drugs known to cause QT-interval prolongation.

5

Infection

- **SIDE-EFFECTS**
  - ▸ **Common or very common** Abdominal pain · anaemia · anorexia · blood disorders · constipation · diarrhoea · dizziness · drowsiness · dry mouth · dyspepsia · electrolyte disturbances · fatigue · fever · flatulence · gastro-intestinal disturbances · headache · nausea · neutropenia · paraesthesia · pruritus · rash · thrombocytopenia · vomiting
  - ▸ **Uncommon** Alopecia · aphasia · arrhythmias · bradycardia · changes in blood pressure · convulsions · cough · gastro-oesophageal reflux · hepatic disorders · hiccups · hyperglycaemia · insomnia · menstrual disorders · mouth ulcers · musculoskeletal pain · neuropathy · oedema · palpitation · pancreatitis · renal failure · tachycardia · tremor · vasculitis · visual disturbances
  - ▸ **Rare** Adrenal insufficiency · breast pain · cardiac failure · depression · encephalopathy · hearing impairment · ileus · myocardial infarction · pneumonitis · psychosis · Stevens-Johnson syndrome · stroke · syncope · thrombosis
- **CONCEPTION AND CONTRACEPTION** Manufacturer recommends effective contraception during treatment.
- **PREGNANCY** Manufacturer advises avoid unless potential benefit outweighs risk; toxicity in *animal* studies.
- **BREAST FEEDING** Manufacturer advises avoid—present in milk in *animal* studies.
- **HEPATIC IMPAIRMENT** Manufacturer advises caution. Monitor liver function in hepatic impairment.
- **MONITORING REQUIREMENTS**
  - ▸ Monitor electrolytes (including potassium, magnesium, and calcium) before and during therapy.
  - ▸ Monitor liver function before and during therapy.
- **PRESCRIBING AND DISPENSING INFORMATION** Flavours of oral liquid formulations may include cherry.

- **MEDICINAL FORMS**
  There can be variation in the licensing of different medicines containing the same drug.

  Gastro-resistant tablet
  CAUTIONARY AND ADVISORY LABELS 3, 9, 25
  - ▸ Noxafil (Merck Sharp & Dohme Ltd)
    Posaconazole 100 mg Noxafil 100mg gastro-resistant tablets | 24 tablet PoM £596.96 | 96 tablet PoM £2,387.85

  Oral suspension
  CAUTIONARY AND ADVISORY LABELS 3, 9, 21
  - ▸ Noxafil (Merck Sharp & Dohme Ltd)
    Posaconazole 40 mg per 1 ml Noxafil 40mg/ml oral suspension | 105 ml PoM £491.20 (Hospital only)

Voriconazole

- **INDICATIONS AND DOSE**

  Invasive aspergillosis | Serious infections caused by *Scedosporium* spp., *Fusarium* spp., or invasive fluconazole-resistant *Candida* spp. (including *C. krusei*)
  - ▸ BY MOUTH
    - ▸ Adult (body-weight up to 40 kg): Initially 200 mg every 12 hours for 2 doses, then 100 mg every 12 hours, increased if necessary to 150 mg every 12 hours
    - ▸ Adult (body-weight 40 kg and above): Initially 400 mg every 12 hours for 2 doses, then 200 mg every 12 hours, increased if necessary to 300 mg every 12 hours
  - ▸ BY INTRAVENOUS INFUSION
    - ▸ Adult: Initially 6 mg/kg every 12 hours for 2 doses, then 4 mg/kg every 12 hours; reduced if not tolerated to 3 mg/kg every 12 hours; for max. 6 months

- **CONTRA-INDICATIONS** Acute porphyrias p. 918
- **CAUTIONS** Avoid exposure to sunlight · bradycardia · cardiomyopathy · electrolyte disturbances · history of QT interval prolongation · patients at risk of pancreatitis · symptomatic arrhythmias

- **INTERACTIONS** → Appendix 1 (antifungals, triazole). Caution with concomitant use with other drugs that prolong QT interval.
- **SIDE-EFFECTS**
  GENERAL SIDE-EFFECTS
  - ▸ **Common or very common** Abdominal pain · acute renal failure · agitation · alopecia · altered perception · anaemia · anxiety · asthenia · blood disorders · blurred vision · cheilitis · chest pain · confusion · depression · diarrhoea · dizziness · haematuria · hallucinations · headache · hypoglycaemia · hypokalaemia · hypotension · influenza-like symptoms · jaundice · leucopenia · nausea · oedema · pancytopenia · paraesthesia · photophobia · photosensitivity · pruritus · rash · respiratory distress syndrome · sinusitis · thrombocytopenia · tremor · visual disturbances · vomiting
  - ▸ **Uncommon** Adrenocortical insufficiency · arrhythmias · arthritis · ataxia · blepharitis · cholecystitis · constipation · duodenitis · dyspepsia · flushing · fulminant hepatic failure · gingivitis · glossitis · hepatitis · hypersensitivity reactions · hypoaesthesia · hyponatraemia · nystagmus · optic neuritis · pancreatitis · psoriasis · QT interval prolongation · raised serum cholesterol · scleritis · Stevens-Johnson syndrome · syncope
  - ▸ **Rare** Convulsions · discoid lupus erythematosus · extrapyramidal effects · hearing disturbances · hyperthyroidism · hypertonia · hypothyroidism · insomnia · optic atrophy · pseudomembranous colitis · pseudoporphyria · retinal haemorrhage · taste disturbances (more common with oral suspension) · tinnitus · toxic epidermal necrolysis
  - ▸ **Frequency not known** On long term treatment, squamous cell carcinoma of skin (particularly in presence of phototoxicity) · periostitis (particularly in transplant patients)
  SPECIFIC SIDE-EFFECTS
  - ▸ **Common or very common**
  - ▸ With intravenous use Injection-site reactions
  SIDE-EFFECTS, FURTHER INFORMATION
  - ▸ Hepatotoxicity Hepatitis, cholestasis, and fulminant hepatic failure usually occur in the first 10 days; risk of hepatotoxicity increased in patients with haematological malignancy. Consider treatment discontinuation if severe abnormalities in liver function tests.
  - ▸ Phototoxicity Phototoxicity occurs commonly. If phototoxicity occurs, consider treatment discontinuation; if treatment is continued, monitor for pre-malignant skin lesions and squamous cell carcinoma, and discontinue treatment if they occur.
- **CONCEPTION AND CONTRACEPTION** Effective contraception required during treatment.
- **PREGNANCY** Toxicity in *animal* studies—manufacturer advises avoid unless potential benefit outweighs risk.
- **BREAST FEEDING** Manufacturer advises avoid—no information available.
- **HEPATIC IMPAIRMENT** In mild to moderate hepatic cirrhosis use usual initial dose then halve maintenance dose. No information available for severe hepatic cirrhosis—manufacturer advises use only if potential benefit outweighs risk.
- **RENAL IMPAIRMENT** Intravenous vehicle may accumulate if eGFR less than 50 mL/minute/1.73 m^2—use intravenous infusion only if potential benefit outweighs risk, and monitor renal function; alternatively, use tablets or oral suspension (no dose adjustment required).
- **MONITORING REQUIREMENTS**
  - ▸ Monitor renal function.
  - ▸ Monitor liver function before starting treatment, then at least weekly for 1 month, and then monthly during treatment.

- DIRECTIONS FOR ADMINISTRATION For *intravenous infusion*, reconstitute each 200 mg with 19 mL Water for Injections *or* Sodium Chloride 0.9% to produce a 10 mg/mL solution; dilute dose to concentration of 0.5–5 mg/mL with Glucose 5% or Sodium Chloride 0.9% and give intermittently at a rate not exceeding 3 mg/kg/hour.
- PRESCRIBING AND DISPENSING INFORMATION Flavours of oral liquid formulations may include orange.
- PATIENT AND CARER ADVICE Patients and their carers should be advised to keep the alert card with them at all times.

  Patients and their carers should be told how to recognise symptoms of liver disorder, and advised to seek immediate medical attention if symptoms such as persistent nausea, vomiting, malaise or jaundice develop.

  Patients and their carers should be advised that patients should avoid intense or prolonged exposure to direct sunlight, and to avoid the use of sunbeds. In sunlight, patients should cover sun-exposed areas of skin and use a sunscreen with a high sun protection factor. Patients should seek medical attention if they experience sunburn or a severe skin reaction following exposure to light or sun.

- MEDICINAL FORMS
  There can be variation in the licensing of different medicines containing the same drug.

  Tablet
  CAUTIONARY AND ADVISORY LABELS 9, 11, 23
  ▸ VFEND (Pfizer Ltd)
  Voriconazole 50 mg VFEND 50mg tablets | 28 tablet [PoM] £275.68
  Voriconazole 200 mg VFEND 200mg tablets | 28 tablet [PoM] £1,102.74

  Oral suspension
  CAUTIONARY AND ADVISORY LABELS 9, 11, 23
  ▸ VFEND (Pfizer Ltd)
  Voriconazole 40 mg per 1 ml VFEND 40mg/ml oral suspension | 75 ml [PoM] £551.37

  Powder for solution for infusion
  EXCIPIENTS: May contain Sulfobutylether beta cyclodextrin sodium
  ELECTROLYTES: May contain Sodium
  ▸ VFEND (Pfizer Ltd)
  Voriconazole 200 mg VFEND 200mg powder for solution for infusion vials | 1 vial [PoM] £77.14 (Hospital only)

  Powder and solvent for solution for infusion
  EXCIPIENTS: May contain Sulfobutylether beta cyclodextrin sodium
  ELECTROLYTES: May contain Sodium
  ▸ VFEND (Pfizer Ltd)
  Voriconazole 200 mg VFEND 200mg powder and solvent for solution for infusion vials | 1 vial [PoM] £77.14 (Hospital only)

ANTIFUNGALS > OTHER

Flucytosine

- **INDICATIONS AND DOSE**
  Systemic yeast and fungal infections | Adjunct to amphotericin in severe systemic candidiasis and in other severe or long-standing infections
  ▸ BY INTRAVENOUS INFUSION
  ▸ Adult: Usual dose 200 mg/kg daily in 4 divided doses usually for not more than 7 days, alternatively 100–150 mg/kg daily in 4 divided doses, lower dose may be sufficient for extremely sensitive organisms
  Cryptococcal meningitis (adjunct to amphotericin)
  ▸ BY INTRAVENOUS INFUSION
  ▸ Adult: 100 mg/kg daily in 4 divided doses for 2 weeks

- UNLICENSED USE Use in cryptococcal meningitis for 2 weeks is an unlicensed duration.
- CAUTIONS Blood disorders · elderly
- INTERACTIONS → Appendix 1 (flucytosine).

- SIDE-EFFECTS
  ▸ **Common or very common** Diarrhoea · nausea · rashes · vomiting
  ▸ **Uncommon** Alterations in liver function tests · cardiotoxicity · confusion · convulsions · hallucinations · headache · sedation · toxic epidermal necrolysis · vertigo
  ▸ **Frequency not known** Aplastic anaemia · blood disorders · hepatic necrosis · hepatitis · leucopenia · thrombocytopenia

- PREGNANCY Teratogenic in *animal* studies; manufacturer advises use only if potential benefit outweighs risk.
- BREAST FEEDING Manufacturer advises avoid.
- RENAL IMPAIRMENT Use 50 mg/kg every 12 hours if creatinine clearance 20–40 mL/minute; use 50 mg/kg every 24 hours if creatinine clearance 10–20 mL/minute; use initial dose of 50 mg/kg if creatinine clearance less than 10 mL/minute and then adjust dose according to plasma-flucytosine concentration. In renal impairment liver- and kidney-function tests and blood counts required weekly.

- MONITORING REQUIREMENTS
  ▸ For plasma concentration monitoring, blood should be taken shortly before starting the next infusion; plasma concentration for optimum response 25–50 mg/litre (200–400 micromol/litre)—should not be allowed to exceed 80 mg/litre (620 micromol/litre).
  ▸ Liver- and kidney-function tests and blood counts required (weekly in blood disorders).
- DIRECTIONS FOR ADMINISTRATION For *intravenous infusion*, give over 20–40 minutes.

- MEDICINAL FORMS
  There can be variation in the licensing of different medicines containing the same drug. Forms available from special-order manufacturers include: oral solution
  Solution for infusion
  ELECTROLYTES: May contain Sodium
  ▸ Ancotil (Meda Pharmaceuticals Ltd)
  Flucytosine 10 mg per 1 ml Ancotil 2.5g/250ml solution for infusion bottles | 5 bottle [PoM] £151.67 (Hospital only)

Griseofulvin

- **INDICATIONS AND DOSE**
  Dermatophyte infections of the skin, scalp, hair and nails where topical therapy has failed or is inappropriate
  ▸ BY MOUTH
  ▸ Adult: 500 mg daily, alternatively increased if necessary to 1 g daily, for severe infections; reduce dose when response occurs, daily dose may be taken once daily or in divided doses
  Tinea capitis caused by *Trichophyton tonsurans*
  ▸ BY MOUTH
  ▸ Adult: 1 g once daily, alternatively 1 g daily in divided doses

- UNLICENSED USE Griseofulvin doses in BNF may differ from those in product literature.
- CONTRA-INDICATIONS Acute porphyrias p. 918 · systemic lupus erythematosus (risk of exacerbation)
- INTERACTIONS → Appendix 1 (griseofulvin).
- SIDE-EFFECTS
  ▸ **Rare** Erythema multiforme · toxic epidermal necrolysis
  ▸ **Very rare** Headache
  ▸ **Frequency not known** Abdominal pain · agitation · confusion · depression · diarrhoea · dizziness · dyspepsia · fatigue · glossitis · hepatotoxicity · impaired coordination · impaired hearing · leucopenia · menstrual disturbances · nausea · peripheral neuropathy · photosensitivity · rash · renal failure · sleep disturbances · systemic lupus erythematosus · taste disturbances · vomiting

5

Infection

- CONCEPTION AND CONTRACEPTION Effective contraception required during and for at least 1 month after administration to women (important: effectiveness of oral contraceptives may be reduced, additional contraceptive precautions e.g. barrier method, required). Men should avoid fathering a child during and for at least 6 months after administration
- PREGNANCY Avoid (fetotoxicity and teratogenicity in *animals*).
- BREAST FEEDING Avoid—no information available.
- HEPATIC IMPAIRMENT Avoid in severe liver disease.
- PATIENT AND CARER ADVICE
Driving and skilled tasks
May impair performance of skilled tasks (e.g. driving); effects of alcohol enhanced.

- MEDICINAL FORMS
There can be variation in the licensing of different medicines containing the same drug. Forms available from special-order manufacturers include: oral suspension
Tablet
CAUTIONARY AND ADVISORY LABELS 9, 21
▸ Griseofulvin (Non-proprietary)
Griseofulvin 125 mg Griseofulvin 125mg tablets | 100 tablet [PoM] £96.67 DT price = £96.67
Griseofulvin 500 mg Griseofulvin 500mg tablets | 90 tablet [PoM] £99.00 | 100 tablet [PoM] £90.34 DT price = £100.17

3.1 Pneumocystis pneumonia

Pneumocystis pneumonia

Overview
Pneumonia caused by *Pneumocystis jirovecii* (*Pneumocystis carinii*) occurs in immunosuppressed patients; it is a common cause of pneumonia in AIDS. Pneumocystis pneumonia should generally be treated by those experienced in its management. Blood gas measurement is used to assess disease severity.

Treatment
Mild to moderate disease
Co-trimoxazole p. 511 in high dosage is the drug of choice for the treatment of mild to moderate pneumocystis pneumonia.

Atovaquone below is licensed for the treatment of mild to moderate pneumocystis infection in patients who cannot tolerate co-trimoxazole. A combination of dapsone p. 524 with trimethoprim p. 521 is given by mouth for the treatment of mild to moderate disease [unlicensed indication].

A combination of clindamycin p. 485 and primaquine p. 562 by mouth is used in the treatment of mild to moderate disease [unlicensed indication]; this combination is associated with considerable toxicity.

Severe disease
Co-trimoxazole in high dosage, given by mouth or by intravenous infusion, is the drug of choice for the treatment of severe pneumocystis pneumonia. Pentamidine isetionate p. 547 given by intravenous infusion is an alternative for patients who cannot tolerate co-trimoxazole, or who have not responded to it. Pentamidine isetionate is a potentially toxic drug that can cause severe hypotension during or immediately after infusion.

Corticosteroid treatment can be lifesaving in those with severe pneumocystis pneumonia.

Adjunctive therapy
In moderate to severe infections associated with HIV infection, prednisolone p. 614 is given by mouth for 5 days (alternatively, hydrocortisone p. 612 may be given

parenterally); the dose is then reduced to complete 21 days of treatment. Corticosteroid treatment should ideally be started at the same time as the anti-pneumocystis therapy and certainly no later than 24–72 hours afterwards. The corticosteroid should be withdrawn before anti-pneumocystis treatment is complete.

Prophylaxis
Prophylaxis against pneumocystis pneumonia should be given to all patients with a history of the infection. Prophylaxis against pneumocystis pneumonia should also be considered for severely immunocompromised patients. Prophylaxis should continue until immunity recovers sufficiently. It should not be discontinued if the patient has oral candidiasis, continues to lose weight, or is receiving cytotoxic therapy or long-term immunosuppressant therapy.

Co-trimoxazole by mouth is the drug of choice for prophylaxis against pneumocystis pneumonia. It is given daily or on alternate days (3 times a week); the dose may be reduced to improve tolerance.

Inhaled pentamidine isetionate is better tolerated than parenteral pentamidine isetionate. Intermittent inhalation of pentamidine isetionate is used for prophylaxis against pneumocystis pneumonia in patients unable to tolerate co-trimoxazole. It is effective but patients may be prone to extrapulmonary infection. Alternatively, dapsone can be used. Atovaquone has also been used for prophylaxis [unlicensed indication].

ANTIPROTOZOALS

Atovaquone

- INDICATIONS AND DOSE
Treatment of mild to moderate *Pneumocystis jirovecii* (*Pneumocystis carinii*) pneumonia in patients intolerant of co-trimoxazole
▸ BY MOUTH
▸ Adult: 750 mg twice daily for 21 days, dose to be taken with food, particularly high fat food
Prophylaxis against pneumocystis pneumonia
▸ BY MOUTH
▸ Adult: 750 mg twice daily

- UNLICENSED USE Not licensed for prophylaxis against pneumocystis pneumonia.
- CAUTIONS Other causes of pulmonary disease should be sought and treated · elderly · initial diarrhoea and difficulty in taking with food may reduce absorption (and require alternative therapy)
- INTERACTIONS → Appendix 1 (atovaquone).
- SIDE-EFFECTS Anaemia · diarrhoea · fever · headache · hyponatraemia · insomnia · nausea · neutropenia · pruritus · rash · Stevens-Johnson syndrome · vomiting
- PREGNANCY Manufacturer advises avoid unless potential benefit outweighs risk—no information available.
- BREAST FEEDING Manufacturer advises avoid.
- HEPATIC IMPAIRMENT Manufacturer advises caution. Monitor more closely in hepatic impairment.
- RENAL IMPAIRMENT Manufacturer advises caution. Monitor more closely in renal impairment.
- PRESCRIBING AND DISPENSING INFORMATION Flavours of oral liquid formulations may include tutti-frutti.

- MEDICINAL FORMS
There can be variation in the licensing of different medicines containing the same drug.
Oral suspension
CAUTIONARY AND ADVISORY LABELS 21
▸ Wellvone (GlaxoSmithKline UK Ltd)
Atovaquone 150 mg per 1 ml Wellvone 750mg/5ml oral suspension sugar-free | 226 ml [PoM] £486.37

Pentamidine isetionate

INDICATIONS AND DOSE

Treatment of *Pneumocystis jirovecii* (*Pneumocystis carinii*) pneumonia (specialist use only)
▶ BY INTRAVENOUS INFUSION
▸ Adult: 4 mg/kg once daily for at least 14 days

Prophylaxis of *Pneumocystis jirovecii* (*Pneumocystis carinii*) pneumonia (specialist use only)
▶ BY INHALATION OF NEBULISED SOLUTION
▸ Adult: 300 mg every 4 weeks, alternatively 150 mg every 2 weeks, using suitable equipment—consult product literature

Visceral leishmaniasis (specialist use only)
▶ BY DEEP INTRAMUSCULAR INJECTION
▸ Adult: 3–4 mg/kg once daily on alternate days, maximum total of 10 injections, course may be repeated if necessary

Cutaneous leishmaniasis (specialist use only)
▶ BY DEEP INTRAMUSCULAR INJECTION
▸ Adult: 3–4 mg/kg 1–2 times a week until condition resolves

Trypanosomiasis (specialist use only)
▶ BY DEEP INTRAMUSCULAR INJECTION, OR BY INTRAVENOUS INFUSION
▸ Adult: 4 mg/kg once daily or on alternate days for a total of 7–10 injections

- UNLICENSED USE Not licensed for primary prevention of *Pneumocystis jirovecii* (*Pneumocystis carinii*) pneumonia by inhalation of nebulised solution.
- CAUTIONS Anaemia · bradycardia · coronary heart disease · history of ventricular arrhythmias · hyperglycaemia · hypertension · hypoglycaemia · hypokalaemia · hypomagnesaemia · hypotension · leucopenia · risk of severe hypotension following administration · thrombocytopenia
- INTERACTIONS → Appendix 1 (pentamidine isetionate). Caution with concomitant use of other drugs that prolong the QT interval.
- SIDE-EFFECTS
GENERAL SIDE-EFFECTS
Abnormal liver-function tests · acute renal failure · anaemia · arrhythmias (can be severe and sometimes fatal) · azotaemia · dizziness · flushing · hyperglycaemia · hyperkalaemia · hypocalcaemia · hypoglycaemia (can be severe and sometimes fatal) · hypotension (can be severe and sometimes fatal) · leucopenia · nausea · pancreatitis (can be severe and sometimes fatal) · rash · Stevens-Johnson syndrome · syncope · taste disturbances · thrombocytopenia · vomiting
SPECIFIC SIDE-EFFECTS
▸ When used by inhalation Bronchoconstriction (may be prevented by prior use of bronchodilators) · cough · shortness of breath
▸ With intramuscular or intravenous use Injection site reactions (muscle necrosis, discomfort, pain, induration, abscess formation)
- PREGNANCY Manufacturer advises avoid unless essential.
- BREAST FEEDING Manufacturer advises avoid unless essential—no information available.
- HEPATIC IMPAIRMENT Manufacturer advises caution.
- RENAL IMPAIRMENT Reduce intravenous dose for pneumocystis pneumonia if creatinine clearance less than 10 mL/minute: in *life-threatening infection*, use 4 mg/kg once daily for 7–10 days, then 4 mg/kg on alternate days to complete course of at least 14 doses; in *less severe infection*, use 4 mg/kg on alternate days for at least 14 doses.

- MONITORING REQUIREMENTS
▶ Monitor blood pressure before starting treatment, during administration, and at regular intervals, until treatment concluded.
▶ Carry out laboratory monitoring according to product literature.
- DIRECTIONS FOR ADMINISTRATION Patient should be lying down when receiving drug parenterally. Direct intravenous injection should be avoided whenever possible and **never** given rapidly; intramuscular injections should be deep and preferably given into the buttock. For *intravenous infusion*, reconstitute 300 mg with 3–5 mL Water for Injections (displacement value may be significant), then dilute required dose with 50–250 mL Glucose 5% *or* Sodium Chloride 0.9%; give over at least 60 minutes.
  Powder for injection (dissolved in water for injection) may be used for nebulisation.
- HANDLING AND STORAGE Pentamidine isetionate is toxic and personnel should be adequately protected during handling and administration—consult product literature.
- MEDICINAL FORMS
There can be variation in the licensing of different medicines containing the same drug.
Powder for solution for injection
▸ Pentacarinat (Sanofi)
  Pentamidine isetionate 300 mg Pentacarinat 300mg powder for solution for injection vials | 5 vial PoM £158.86

4 Helminth infection

Helminth infections

Specialist centres
Advice on prophylaxis and treatment of helminth infections is available from the following specialist centres:

Birmingham	(0121) 424 0357
Scotland	Contact local Infectious Diseases Unit
Liverpool	(0151) 705 3100
London	0845 155 5000 (treatment)

Drugs for threadworms
Anthelmintics are effective in threadworm (pinworms, *Enterobius vermicularis*) infections, but their use needs to be combined with hygienic measures to break the cycle of auto-infection. All members of the family require treatment.
  Adult threadworms do not live for longer than 6 weeks and for development of fresh worms, ova must be swallowed and exposed to the action of digestive juices in the upper intestinal tract. Direct multiplication of worms does not take place in the large bowel. Adult female worms lay ova on the perianal skin which causes pruritus; scratching the area then leads to ova being transmitted on fingers to the mouth, often via food eaten with unwashed hands. Washing hands and scrubbing nails before each meal and after each visit to the toilet is essential. A bath taken immediately after rising will remove ova laid during the night.
  Mebendazole p. 549 is the drug of choice for treating threadworm infection in patients of all ages over 6 months. It is given as a single dose; as reinfection is very common, a second dose may be given after 2 weeks.

Ascaricides (common roundworm infections)
Mebendazole is effective against *Ascaris lumbricoides* and is generally considered to be the drug of choice.
  Levamisole p. 549 [unlicensed] (available from 'special-order' manufacturers or specialist importing companies) is

5

Infection

an alternative when mebendazole cannot be used. It is very well tolerated.

Drugs for tapeworm infections

Taenicides

Niclosamide [unlicensed] (available from 'special-order' manufacturers or specialist importing companies) is the most widely used drug for tapeworm infections and side-effects are limited to occasional gastro-intestinal upset, lightheadedness, and pruritus; it is not effective against larval worms. Fears of developing cysticercosis in *Taenia solium* infections have proved unfounded. All the same, an antiemetic can be given before treatment and a laxative can be given 2 hours after niclosamide.

Praziquantel p. 550 [unlicensed] (available from 'special-order' manufacturers or specialist importing companies) is as effective as niclosamide.

Hydatid disease

Cysts caused by *Echinococcus granulosus* grow slowly and asymptomatic patients do not always require treatment. Surgical treatment remains the method of choice in many situations. Albendazole below [unlicensed] (available from 'special-order' manufacturers or specialist importing companies) is used in conjunction with surgery to reduce the risk of recurrence or as primary treatment in inoperable cases. Alveolar echinococcosis due to *E. multilocularis* is usually fatal if untreated. Surgical removal with albendazole cover is the treatment of choice, but where effective surgery is impossible, repeated cycles of albendazole (for a year or more) may help. Careful monitoring of liver function is particularly important during drug treatment.

Drugs for hookworms

Hookworms (ancylostomiasis, necatoriasis) live in the upper small intestine and draw blood from the point of their attachment to their host. An iron-deficiency anaemia may occur and, if present, effective treatment of the infection requires not only expulsion of the worms but treatment of the anaemia.

Mebendazole has a useful broad-spectrum activity, and is effective against hookworms. Albendazole [unlicensed] (available from 'special-order' manufacturers or specialist importing companies) is an alternative. Levamisole is also is also effective in children.

Schistosomicides (bilharziasis)

Adult *Schistosoma haematobium* worms live in the genito-urinary veins and adult *S. mansoni* in those of the colon and mesentery. *S. japonicum* is more widely distributed in veins of the alimentary tract and portal system.

Praziquantel [unlicensed] is available from Merck Serono (*Cysticide*®) and is effective against all human schistosomes. No serious adverse effects have been reported. Of all the available schistosomicides, it has the most attractive combination of effectiveness, broad-spectrum activity, and low toxicity.

Filaricides

Diethylcarbamazine [unlicensed] (available from 'special-order' manufacturers or specialist importing companies) is effective against microfilariae and adults of *Loa loa*, *Wuchereria bancrofti*, and *Brugia malayi*. To minimise reactions, treatment in adults and children over 1 month, is commenced with a dose of diethylcarbamazine citrate on the first day and increased gradually over 3 days. Length of treatment varies according to infection type, and usually gives a radical cure for these infections. Close medical supervision is necessary particularly in the early phase of treatment.

In heavy infections there may be a febrile reaction, and in heavy *Loa loa* infection there is a small risk of encephalopathy. In such cases specialist advice should be sought, and treatment must be given under careful in-patient supervision and stopped at the first sign of cerebral involvement.

Ivermectin p. 549 [unlicensed] (available from 'special-order' manufacturers or specialist importing companies) is very effective in *onchocerciasis* and it is now the drug of choice; reactions are usually slight. Diethylcarbamazine or suramin should no longer be used for *onchocerciasis* because of their toxicity.

Drugs for cutaneous larva migrans (creeping eruption)

Dog and cat hookworm larvae may enter human skin where they produce slowly extending itching tracks usually on the foot. Single tracks can be treated with topical tiabendazole (no commercial preparation available). Multiple infections respond to ivermectin, albendazole or **tiabendazole** (thiabendazole) by mouth [all unlicensed] (available from 'special-order' manufacturers or specialist importing companies).

Drugs for strongyloidiasis

Adult *Strongyloides stercoralis* live in the gut and produce larvae which penetrate the gut wall and invade the tissues, setting up a cycle of auto-infection. Ivermectin [unlicensed] (available from 'special-order' manufacturers or specialist importing companies) is the treatment of choice for chronic *Strongyloides* infection in adults and children over 5 years. Albendazole [unlicensed] (available from 'special order' manufacturers or specialist importing companies) is an alternative given to adults and children over 2 years.

ANTHELMINTICS

Albendazole

- **INDICATIONS AND DOSE**

Chronic *Strongyloides* infection
▶ BY MOUTH
- Adult: 400 mg twice daily for 3 days, dose may be repeated after 3 weeks if necessary

Hydatid disease, in conjunction with surgery to reduce the risk of recurrence or as primary treatment in inoperable cases
▶ BY MOUTH
- Adult: (consult product literature)

Hookworm infections
▶ BY MOUTH
- Adult: 400 mg for 1 dose

- **UNLICENSED USE** Albendazole is an unlicensed drug.
- **INTERACTIONS** → Appendix 1 (albendazole).

- **MEDICINAL FORMS**
There can be variation in the licensing of different medicines containing the same drug. Forms available from special-order manufacturers include: tablet, chewable tablet, oral suspension

Tablet
CAUTIONARY AND ADVISORY LABELS 9
▶ Albendazole (Non-proprietary)
  Albendazole 400 mg Eskazole 400mg tablets | 60 tablet [PoM] no price available

Chewable tablet
CAUTIONARY AND ADVISORY LABELS 9
▶ Albendazole (Non-proprietary)
  Albendazole 200 mg Zentel 200mg chewable tablets | 6 tablet [PoM] no price available
  Albendazole 400 mg Zentel 400mg chewable tablets | 1 tablet [PoM] no price available | 3 tablet [PoM] no price available

Diethylcarbamazine

- **INDICATIONS AND DOSE**
Wuchereria bancrofti infections | Brugia malayi infections
▶ BY MOUTH
▸ Adult: Initially 1 mg/kg daily on the first day, then increased to 6 mg/kg daily in divided doses, dose to be increased gradually over 3 days
Loa loa infections
▶ BY MOUTH
▸ Adult: Initially 1 mg/kg daily on the first day, then increased to 6 mg/kg daily in divided doses, dose to be increased gradually over 3 days; maximum 9 mg/kg per day

- **UNLICENSED USE** Diethylcarbamazine is an unlicensed drug.
- **INTERACTIONS** → Appendix 1 (diethylcarbamazine).

- **MEDICINAL FORMS**
There can be variation in the licensing of different medicines containing the same drug.
No licensed medicines listed.

Ivermectin

- **INDICATIONS AND DOSE**
Chronic Strongyloides infection
▶ BY MOUTH
▸ Adult: 200 micrograms/kg daily for 2 days
Onchocerciasis
▶ BY MOUTH
▸ Adult: 150 micrograms/kg for 1 dose, retreatment at intervals of 6 to 12 months may be required depending on symptoms
Scabies, in combination with topical drugs, for the treatment of hyperkeratotic (crusted or 'Norwegian') scabies that does not respond to topical treatment alone
▶ BY MOUTH
▸ Adult: 200 micrograms/kg for 1 dose, further doses of 200 micrograms/kg may be required

- **UNLICENSED USE** Ivermectin is an unlicensed drug.
- **INTERACTIONS** → Appendix 1 (ivermectin).
- **SIDE-EFFECTS** Aggravation of itching · aggravation of rash

- **MEDICINAL FORMS**
There can be variation in the licensing of different medicines containing the same drug. Forms available from special-order manufacturers include: tablet
Tablet
▸ Ivermectin (Non-proprietary)
Ivermectin 3 mg Stromectol 3mg tablets | 4 tablet P͟o͟M͟ no price available | 20 tablet P͟o͟M͟ no price available

Levamisole

- **INDICATIONS AND DOSE**
Roundworm infections
▶ BY MOUTH
▸ Adult: 120–150 mg for 1 dose

- **UNLICENSED USE** Not licensed.
- **CONTRA-INDICATIONS** Blood disorders
- **CAUTIONS** Epilepsy · Sjögren's syndrome
- **INTERACTIONS** → Appendix 1 (levamisole).
- **SIDE-EFFECTS** Arthralgia (on *prolonged treatment*) · blood disorders (on *prolonged treatment*) · convulsions (on *prolonged treatment*) · diarrhoea · dizziness · headache · influenza-like syndrome (on *prolonged treatment*) ·

insomnia (on *prolonged treatment*) · myalgia (on *prolonged treatment*) · nausea · rash (on *prolonged treatment*) · taste disturbances (on *prolonged treatment*) · vasculitis (on *prolonged treatment*) · vomiting
- **PREGNANCY** Embryotoxic in *animal* studies, avoid if possible.
- **BREAST FEEDING** No information available.
- **HEPATIC IMPAIRMENT** Use with caution—dose adjustment may be necessary.

- **MEDICINAL FORMS**
There can be variation in the licensing of different medicines containing the same drug. Forms available from special-order manufacturers include: tablet
Tablet
CAUTIONARY AND ADVISORY LABELS 4
▸ Ergamisol (Imported (Belgium))
Levamisole (as Levamisole hydrochloride) 50 mg Ergamisol 50mg tablets | 20 tablet P͟o͟M͟ no price available

Mebendazole

- **INDICATIONS AND DOSE**
Threadworm infections
▶ BY MOUTH
▸ Child 6 months–17 years: 100 mg for 1 dose, if reinfection occurs, second dose may be needed after 2 weeks
▸ Adult: 100 mg for 1 dose, if reinfection occurs, second dose may be needed after 2 weeks
Whipworm infections | Hookworm infections
▶ BY MOUTH
▸ Child 1–17 years: 100 mg twice daily for 3 days
▸ Adult: 100 mg twice daily for 3 days
Roundworm infections
▶ BY MOUTH
▸ Child 1 year: 100 mg twice daily for 3 days
▸ Child 2–17 years: 100 mg twice daily for 3 days, alternatively 500 mg for 1 dose
▸ Adult: 100 mg twice daily for 3 days, alternatively 500 mg for 1 dose

- **UNLICENSED USE** Not licensed for use in children under 2 years.
▸ In adults Treatment of roundworm infections with mebendazole 500 mg as a single dose is an unlicensed dose.
- **INTERACTIONS** → Appendix 1 (mebendazole).
- **SIDE-EFFECTS**
▸ **Common or very common** Abdominal pain
▸ **Uncommon** Diarrhoea · flatulence
▸ **Rare** Alopecia · convulsions · dizziness · hepatitis · neutropenia · rash · Stevens-Johnson syndrome · toxic epidermal necrolysis · urticaria
- **PREGNANCY** Manufacturer advises avoid—toxicity in *animal* studies.
- **BREAST FEEDING** Amount present in milk too small to be harmful but manufacturer advises avoid.
- **PRESCRIBING AND DISPENSING INFORMATION** Flavours of oral liquid formulations may include banana.
- **PATIENT AND CARER ADVICE**
Medicines for Children leaflet: Mebendazole for worm infections www.medicinesforchildren.org.uk/mebendazole-for-worm-infections
- **EXCEPTIONS TO LEGAL CATEGORY** Mebendazole tablets can be sold to the public if supplied for oral use in the treatment of enterobiasis in adults and children over 2 years provided its container or package is labelled to show a max. single dose of 100 mg and it is supplied in a container or package containing not more than 800 mg.

5

Infection

● MEDICINAL FORMS

There can be variation in the licensing of different medicines containing the same drug.

Chewable tablet

▸ Mebendazole (Non-proprietary)

Mebendazole 100 mg Boots Threadworm Treatment 100mg chewable tablets sugar-free | 4 tablet P no price available

▸ Ovex (McNeil Products Ltd)

Mebendazole 100 mg Ovex 100mg chewable tablets sugar-free | 1 tablet P £2.03 sugar-free | 4 tablet P £4.74

▸ Vermox (Janssen-Cilag Ltd)

Mebendazole 100 mg Vermox 100mg chewable tablets sugar-free | 6 tablet PoM £1.34 DT price = £1.34

Oral suspension

▸ Ovex (McNeil Products Ltd)

Mebendazole 20 mg per 1 ml Ovex 100mg/5ml oral suspension | 30 ml P £6.03 DT price = £1.55

▸ Vermox (Janssen-Cilag Ltd)

Mebendazole 20 mg per 1 ml Vermox 100mg/5ml oral suspension | 30 ml PoM £1.55 DT price = £1.55

Praziquantel

● INDICATIONS AND DOSE

Tapeworm infections (*Taenia solium*)

▸ BY MOUTH

▸ Adult: 5–10 mg/kg for 1 dose, to be taken after a light breakfast

Tapeworm infections (*Hymenolepis nana*)

▸ BY MOUTH

▸ Adult: 25 mg/kg for 1 dose, to be taken after a light breakfast

Schistosoma haematobium worm infections | Schistosoma mansoni worm infections

▸ BY MOUTH

▸ Adult: 20 mg/kg, followed by 20 mg/kg after 4–6 hours

Schistosoma japonicum worm infections

▸ BY MOUTH

▸ Adult: 20 mg/kg 3 times a day for 1 day

● UNLICENSED USE Praziquantel is an unlicensed drug.

● INTERACTIONS → Appendix 1 (praziquantel).

● MEDICINAL FORMS

There can be variation in the licensing of different medicines containing the same drug. Forms available from special-order manufacturers include: tablet

Tablet

▸ Praziquantel (Non-proprietary)

Praziquantel 150 mg Cesol 150mg tablets | 6 tablet PoM no price available

Praziquantel 600 mg Biltricide 600mg tablets | 6 tablet PoM no price available

▸ Cysticide (Imported (Germany))

Praziquantel 500 mg Cysticide 500mg tablets | 90 tablet PoM no price available

5 Protozoal infection

Antiprotozoal drugs

Amoebicides

Metronidazole p. 492 is the drug of choice for *acute invasive amoebic dysentery* since it is very effective against vegetative forms of *Entamoeba histolytica* in ulcers. Tinidazole p. 493 is also effective. Metronidazole and tinidazole are also active against amoebae which may have migrated to the liver. Treatment with metronidazole (or tinidazole) is followed by a 10-day course of diloxanide furoate p. 459.

Diloxanide furoate is the drug of choice for asymptomatic patients with *E. histolytica* cysts in the faeces; metronidazole and tinidazole are relatively ineffective. Diloxanide furoate is relatively free from toxic effects and the usual course is of 10 days, given alone for chronic infections or following metronidazole or tinidazole treatment.

For *amoebic abscesses* of the liver metronidazole is effective; tinidazole is an alternative. Aspiration of the abscess is indicated where it is suspected that it may rupture or where there is no improvement after 72 hours of metronidazole; the aspiration may need to be repeated. Aspiration aids penetration of metronidazole and, for abscesses with more than 100 mL of pus, if carried out in conjunction with drug therapy, may reduce the period of disability.

Diloxanide furoate is not effective against hepatic amoebiasis, but a 10-day course should be given at the completion of metronidazole or tinidazole treatment to destroy any amoebae in the gut.

Trichomonacides

Metronidazole is the treatment of choice for *Trichomonas vaginalis* infection. Contact tracing is recommended and sexual contacts should be treated simultaneously. If metronidazole is ineffective, tinidazole may be tried.

Antigiardial drugs

Metronidazole is the treatment of choice for *Giardia lamblia* infections. Alternative treatments are tinidazole or mepacrine hydrochloride p. 459.

Leishmaniacides

Cutaneous leishmaniasis frequently heals spontaneously but if skin lesions are extensive or unsightly, treatment is indicated, as it is in visceral leishmaniasis (kala-azar). Leishmaniasis should be treated under specialist supervision.

Sodium stibogluconate p. 551, an organic pentavalent antimony compound, is used for visceral leishmaniasis. The dosage varies with different geographical regions and expert advice should be obtained. Some early non-inflamed lesions of cutaneous leishmaniasis can be treated with intralesional injections of sodium stibogluconate under specialist supervision.

Amphotericin p. 539 is used with or after an antimony compound for visceral leishmaniasis unresponsive to the antimonial alone; side-effects may be reduced by using liposomal amphotericin (*AmBisome®*). *Abelcet®*, a lipid formulation of amphotericin is also likely to be effective but less information is available.

Pentamidine isetionate p. 547 has been used in antimony-resistant visceral leishmaniasis, but although the initial response is often good, the relapse rate is high; it is associated with serious side-effects. Other treatments include paromomycin [unlicensed] (available from 'special-order' manufacturers or specialist importing companies).

Trypanocides

The prophylaxis and treatment of trypanosomiasis is difficult and differs according to the strain of organism. Expert advice should therefore be obtained.

Drugs for toxoplasmosis

Most infections caused by *Toxoplasma gondii* are self-limiting, and treatment is not necessary. Exceptions are patients with eye involvement (toxoplasma choroidoretinitis), and those who are immunosuppressed. Toxoplasmic encephalitis is a common complication of AIDS. The treatment of choice is a combination of pyrimethamine p. 563 and sulfadiazine p. 512, given for several weeks (expert advice **essential**). Pyrimethamine is a folate antagonist, and adverse reactions to this combination are relatively common (folinic acid supplements and weekly blood counts needed). Alternative regimens use combinations of pyrimethamine with clindamycin p. 485 or clarithromycin p. 487 or azithromycin p. 486. Long-term secondary prophylaxis is required after treatment of toxoplasmosis in immunocompromised patients; prophylaxis should continue until immunity recovers.

If toxoplasmosis is acquired in pregnancy, transplacental infection may lead to severe disease in the fetus; specialist advice should be sought on management. Spiramycin [unlicensed] (available from 'special-order' manufacturers or specialist importing companies) may reduce the risk of transmission of maternal infection to the fetus.

5.1 Leishmaniasis

ANTIPROTOZOALS

Sodium stibogluconate

- **INDICATIONS AND DOSE**
  Visceral leishmaniasis (specialist use only)
  ▸ BY INTRAVENOUS INJECTION, OR BY INTRAMUSCULAR INJECTION
  ▸ Adult: 20 mg/kg daily for 28 days
  Cutaneous leishmaniasis (specialist use only)
  ▸ BY INTRAVENOUS INJECTION, OR BY INTRAMUSCULAR INJECTION
  ▸ Adult: 20 mg/kg daily for 20 days

- CAUTIONS Heart disease (withdraw if conduction disturbances occur) · mucocutaneous disease · predisposition to QT interval prolongation · treat intercurrent infection (e.g. pneumonia)
  CAUTIONS, FURTHER INFORMATION
  ▸ Mucocutaneous disease Successful treatment of mucocutaneous leishmaniasis may induce severe inflammation around the lesions (may be life-threatening if pharyngeal or tracheal involvement)—may require corticosteroid.

- INTERACTIONS → Appendix 1 (sodium stibogluconate). Caution with concomitant use of drugs that prolong QT interval.

- SIDE-EFFECTS
  ▸ Rare Bleeding from gums · bleeding from nose · fever · flushing · jaundice · rash · substernal pain · sweating · vertigo
  ▸ Frequency not known Abdominal pain · anaphylaxis · anorexia · arthralgia · coughing · diarrhoea · ECG changes · headache · lethargy · myalgia · nausea · pain on intramuscular injection · pain on intravenous administration · pancreatitis · thrombosis on intravenous administration · vomiting

- PREGNANCY Manufacturer advises use only if potential benefit outweighs risk.

- BREAST FEEDING Amount probably too small to be harmful.

- HEPATIC IMPAIRMENT Use with caution.

- RENAL IMPAIRMENT Avoid in significant impairment.

- MONITORING REQUIREMENTS Monitor ECG before and during treatment.

- DIRECTIONS FOR ADMINISTRATION Intravenous injections must be given slowly over 5 minutes (to reduce risk of local thrombosis) and stopped if coughing or substernal pain occur. Injection should be filtered immediately before administration using a filter of 5 microns or less.

- MEDICINAL FORMS
  There can be variation in the licensing of different medicines containing the same drug.
  Solution for injection
  ▸ Pentostam (GlaxoSmithKline UK Ltd)
  Antimony pentavalent (as Sodium stibogluconate) 100 mg per 1 ml Pentostam 10g/100ml solution for injection vials | 1 vial PoM £66.43

5.2 Malaria

Antimalarials

Artemether with lumefantrine

Artemether with lumefantrine p. 558 is licensed for the *treatment of acute non-complicated falciparum malaria*.

Chloroquine

Chloroquine p. 560 is used for the *prophylaxis of malaria* in areas of the world where the *risk of chloroquine-resistant falciparum malaria is still low*. It is also used with proguanil hydrochloride p. 562 when chloroquine-resistant falciparum malaria is present but this regimen may not give optimal protection (see recommended regimens for prophylaxis against malaria in Malaria, prophylaxis p. 552).

Chloroquine is **no longer recommended** for the *treatment of falciparum malaria* owing to widespread resistance, nor is it recommended if the infective species is *not known* or if the infection is *mixed*; in these cases treatment should be with quinine p. 564, *Malarone®*, or *Riamet®*. It is still recommended for the *treatment of non-falciparum malaria*.

Mefloquine

Mefloquine p. 561 is used for the *prophylaxis of malaria* in areas of the world where there is a *high risk of chloroquine-resistant falciparum malaria* (for details, see Recommended regimens for prophylaxis against malaria in Malaria, prophylaxis p. 552).

Mefloquine is now rarely used for the *treatment of falciparum malaria* because of increased resistance. It is rarely used for the *treatment of non-falciparum malaria* because better tolerated alternatives are available. Mefloquine should not be used for treatment if it has been used for prophylaxis.

Piperaquine with artenimol

Artenimol with piperaquine phosphate p. 559 is not recommended for the first-line treatment of acute uncomplicated falciparum malaria because there is limited experience of its use in travellers who usually reside in areas where malaria is not endemic. Piperaquine has a long half-life.

Primaquine

Primaquine p. 562 is used to eliminate the liver stages of *P. vivax* or *P. ovale* following chloroquine treatment.

Proguanil

Proguanil hydrochloride is used (usually *with chloroquine*, but occasionally *alone*) for the *prophylaxis of malaria*, (for details, see Recommended regimens for prophylaxis against malaria p. 552).

Proguanil hydrochloride used alone is not suitable for the *treatment of malaria*; however, *Malarone®* (a combination of atovaquone with proguanil hydrochloride p. 559) is licensed for the treatment of acute uncomplicated falciparum malaria. *Malarone®* is also used for the *prophylaxis of falciparum malaria* in areas of *widespread mefloquine or chloroquine resistance*. *Malarone®* is also used as an alternative to mefloquine or doxycycline p. 513. *Malarone®* is

5

Infection

particularly suitable for short trips to highly chloroquine-resistant areas because it needs to be taken only for 7 days after leaving an endemic area.

Pyrimethamine

Pyrimethamine p. 563 should not be used alone, but is used with sulfadoxine.

Pyrimethamine with sulfadoxine p. 563 is not recommended for the *prophylaxis of malaria*, but can be used in the *treatment of falciparum malaria with (or following) quinine*.

Quinine

Quinine is not suitable for the *prophylaxis of malaria*.

Quinine is used for the *treatment of falciparum malaria* or if the infective species is *not known* or if the infection is mixed (for details see Malaria, treatment p. 557).

Tetracyclines

Doxycycline is used in adults and children over 12 years for the *prophylaxis of malaria* in areas of *widespread mefloquine* or *chloroquine resistance*. Doxycycline is also used as an alternative to mefloquine or *Malarone*® (for details, see Recommended regimens for prophylaxis against malaria p. 553).

Malaria, prophylaxis

Prophylaxis

The recommendations on prophylaxis reflect guidelines agreed by UK malaria specialists; the advice is aimed at residents of the UK who travel to endemic areas. The choice of drug for a particular individual should take into account:

- risk of exposure to malaria
- extent of drug resistance
- efficacy of the recommended drugs
- side-effects of the drugs
- patient-related factors (e.g. age, pregnancy, renal or hepatic impairment, compliance with prophylactic regimen)

Protection against bites
Prophylaxis is not absolute, and breakthrough infection can occur with any of the drugs recommended. Personal protection against being bitten is very important. Mosquito nets impregnated with permethrin p. 1082 provide the most effective barrier protection against insects; mats and vaporised insecticides are also useful. Diethyltoluamide (DEET) 20–50% in lotions, sprays, or roll-on formulations is safe and effective when applied to the skin of adults and children over 2 months of age. It can also be used during pregnancy and breast-feeding. The duration of protection varies according to the concentration of DEET and is longest for DEET 50%. When sunscreen is also required, DEET should be applied after the sunscreen. DEET reduces the SPF of sunscreen, so a sunscreen of SPF 30-50 should be applied. Long sleeves and trousers worn after dusk also provide protection against bites.

Length of prophylaxis
In order to determine tolerance and to establish habit, prophylaxis should generally be started one week (2–3 weeks in the case of mefloquine p. 561) before travel into an endemic area; *Malarone*® or doxycycline p. 513 prophylaxis should be started 1–2 days before travel. Prophylaxis should be continued for **4 weeks after leaving** (except for *Malarone*® prophylaxis which should be stopped 1 week after leaving). For extensive journeys across different regions, the traveller must be protected in all areas of risk.

In those requiring long-term prophylaxis, chloroquine p. 560 and proguanil hydrochloride p. 562 may be used for periods of over 5 years. Mefloquine is licensed for up to

1 year (although, if it is tolerated in the short term, there is no evidence of harm when it is used for up to 3 years). Doxycycline can be used for up to 2 years. *Malarone*® can be used for up to 1 year. Prophylaxis with mefloquine, doxycycline, or *Malarone*® may be considered for longer durations if it is justified by the risk of exposure to malaria. Specialist advice should be sought for long-term prophylaxis.

Return from malarial region
It is important to be aware that **any illness** that occurs within 1 year and **especially within 3 months of return might be malaria** even if all recommended precautions against malaria were taken. Travellers should be **warned** of this and told that if they develop any illness **particularly within 3 months** of their return they should go **immediately** to a doctor and specifically mention their exposure to malaria.

Epilepsy
Both chloroquine and mefloquine are unsuitable for malaria prophylaxis in individuals with a history of epilepsy. In areas *without chloroquine resistance* proguanil alone is recommended; in areas *with chloroquine resistance*, doxycycline or *Malarone*® may be considered.

Asplenia
Asplenic individuals (or those with severe splenic dysfunction) are at particular risk of severe malaria. If travel to malarious areas is unavoidable, rigorous precautions are required against contracting the disease.

Renal impairment
Avoidance (or dosage reduction) of proguanil hydrochloride is recommended since it is excreted by the kidneys. *Malarone*® should not be used for prophylaxis in patients with estimated glomerular filtration rate less than 30 mL/minute/1.73m². Chloroquine is only partially excreted by the kidneys and reduction of the dose for prophylaxis is not required except in severe impairment. Mefloquine is considered to be appropriate to use in renal impairment and does not require dosage reduction. Doxycycline is also considered to be appropriate.

Pregnancy
Travel to malarious areas should be avoided during pregnancy; if travel is unavoidable, effective prophylaxis must be used. Chloroquine and proguanil hydrochloride can be given in the usual doses during pregnancy, but these drugs are not appropriate for most areas because their effectiveness has declined, particularly in Sub-Saharan Africa; in the case of proguanil hydrochloride, folic acid p. 886 (dosed as a pregnancy at 'high-risk' of neural tube defects) should be given for at least the first trimester. The centres listed (see Malaria, treatment p. 557) should be consulted for advice on prophylaxis in chloroquine-resistant areas. Although the manufacturer advises that mefloquine should not be used during pregnancy, particularly in the first trimester, unless the potential benefit outweighs the risk, studies of mefloquine in pregnancy (including use in the first trimester) indicate that it can be considered for travel to chloroquine-resistant areas. Doxycycline is contra-indicated during pregnancy; however, it can be used for malaria prophylaxis if other regimens are unsuitable, and if the entire course of doxycycline can be completed before 15 weeks' gestation [unlicensed]. *Malarone*® should be avoided during pregnancy, however, it can be considered during the second and third trimesters if there is no suitable alternative.

Breast-feeding
Prophylaxis is required in **breast-fed infants**; although antimalarials are present in milk, the amounts are too variable to give reliable protection.

Key to recommended regimens for prophylaxis against malaria

Codes for regimens	Details of regimens for prophylaxis against malaria
1	Chemoprophylaxis not recommended, but avoid mosquito bites and consider malaria if fever presents
2	Chloroquine only
3	Chloroquine with proguanil
4	Atovaquone with proguanil hydrochloride or doxycycline or mefloquine
5	Atovaquone with proguanil hydrochloride or doxycycline

Specific recommendations

Country	Comments on risk of malaria and regional or seasonal variation	Codes for regimens
Afghanistan	Risk below 2000 m from May–November	3
	Low risk below 2000 m from December–April	1
Algeria	Very low risk in Illizi department only	1
Andaman and Nicobar Islands (India)	Risk present	1
Angola	High risk	4
Argentina	Low risk in low altitude areas of Salta provinces bordering Bolivia and in Chaco, Corrientes, and Misiones provinces close to border with Paraguay and Brazil	2
	No risk in Iguaçu Falls and areas other than those above	1
Armenia	No risk	1
Azerbaijan	Low to no risk	1
Bangladesh	High risk in Chittagong Hill Tract districts (but not Chittagong city)	4
	Low to no risk in Chittagong city and other areas, except Chittagong Hill Tract districts	1
Belize	Low risk in rural areas	2
	No risk in Belize district (including Belize city and islands)	1
Benin	High risk	4
Bhutan	Risk in southern belt districts, along border with India: Chukha, Geyleg-phug, Samchi, Samdrup Jonkhar, and Shemgang	3
	Low to no risk in areas other than those above	1
Bolivia	High risk in Amazon basin	4
	Risk in rural areas below 2500 m (other than above)	2
	No risk above 2500 m	1
Botswana	High risk from November–June in northern half, including Okavango Delta area	4
	Low risk from July–October in northern half; low to no risk all year in southern half	1
Brazil	Risk in Amazon basin, including city of Manaus	4
	Very low risk in areas other than those above, and no risk in Iguaçu Falls	1
Brunei Darussalam	Very low risk	1
Burkina Faso	High risk	4
Burundi	High risk	4
Cambodia	High risk, with widespread chloroquine and mefloquine resistance, in western provinces bordering Thailand	5
	High risk in areas other than those above and below	4
	Very low risk in Angkor Wat and Lake Tonle Sap, including Siem Reap; no risk in Phnom Penh	1
Cameroon	High risk	4
Cape Verde	Very low risk on island of Santiago (Sao Tiago) and Boa Vista	1
Central African Republic	High risk	4
Chad	High risk	4
China	High risk in Yunnan and Hainan provinces	4
	Very low risk in areas other than those above and below	1
	No risk in Hong Kong	–
Colombia	High risk in rural areas below 1600 m	4
	Low to no risk above 1600 m and in Cartagena	1

Key to recommended regimens for prophylaxis against malaria

Codes for regimens	Details of regimens for prophylaxis against malaria
1	Chemoprophylaxis not recommended, but avoid mosquito bites and consider malaria if fever presents
2	Chloroquine only
3	Chloroquine with proguanil
4	Atovaquone with proguanil hydrochloride or doxycycline or mefloquine
5	Atovaquone with proguanil hydrochloride or doxycycline

Specific recommendations

Country	Comments on risk of malaria and regional or seasonal variation	Codes for regimens
Comoros	High risk	4
Congo	High risk	4
Costa Rica	Risk in Limon province (but not city of Limon)	2
	Very low risk in areas other than those above	1
Cote d'Ivoire (Ivory Coast)	High risk	4
Democratic Republic of the Congo	High risk	4
Djibouti	High risk	4
Dominican Republic	Risk in all areas except cities of Santiago and Santo Domingo	2
	Cities of Santiago and Santo Domingo	1
East Timor (Timor-Leste)	High risk	4
Ecuador	Risk in areas below 1500 m including coastal provinces and Amazon basin (no risk in Galapagos islands or city of Guayaquil)	4
Egypt	No risk	1
El Salvador	Low risk in rural areas of Santa Ana, Ahuachapán, and La Unión provinces in western part of country; low to no risk in other areas	1
Equatorial Guinea	High risk	4
Eritrea	High risk below 2200 m	4
Ethiopia	High risk below 2000 m	4
French Guiana	High risk (particularly in border areas) except city of Cayenne or Devil's Island (Ile du Diable)	4
	No risk in city of Cayenne or Devil's Island (Ile du Diable)	1
Gabon	High risk	4
Gambia	High risk	4
Georgia	Very low risk in rural south east from June–October	1
Ghana	High risk	4
Guatemala	Low risk below 1500 m	2
	No risk in Guatemala City, Antigua, or Lake Atitlan	–
Guinea	High risk	4
Guinea-Bissau	High risk	4
Guyana	High risk in all interior regions	4
	Very low risk in Georgetown and coastal region	1
Haiti	Risk present	2
Honduras	Risk below 1000 m and in Roatán and other Bay Islands (no risk in San Pedro Sula or Tegucigalpa)	2
India	High risk in states of Assam and Orissa, districts of East Godavari, Srikakulam, Vishakhapatnam, and Vizianagaram in the state of Andhra Pradesh, and districts of Balaghat, Dindori, Mandla, and Seoni in the state of Madhya Pradesh	4
	Risk in areas other than those above or below (including Goa, Andaman and Nicobar islands)	1
	No risk in Lakshadweep islands	–
Indonesia	High risk in Lombok and Irian Jaya (Papua)	4
	Risk in areas other than those above or below	3
	Very low risk in Bali, and cities on islands of Java and Sumatra	1
	No risk in city of Jakarta	–

Country	Comments on risk of malaria and regional or seasonal variation	Codes for regimens
Indonesia (Borneo)	High risk	4
Iran	Risk from March-November in rural south eastern provinces and in north, along Azerbaijan border in Ardabil, and near Turkmenistan border in North Khorasan	3
	Low to no risk in areas other than those above	1
Iraq	Very low risk from May-November in rural northern area below 1500 m	1
Kenya	High risk below 2500 m (except city of Nairobi)	4
	Very low risk in the highlands above 2500 m and in city of Nairobi	1
Kyrgyzstan	Very low risk from June-October in southwest areas bordering Tajikistan and Uzbekistan	1
Laos	High risk along the border with Myanmar in the provinces of Bokeo and Louang Namtha, and along the border with Thailand in the province of Champasak and Saravan	5
	High risk in areas other than those above or below	4
	Low to no risk in city of Vientiane	1
Liberia	High risk	4
Libya	No risk	1
Madagascar	High risk	4
Malawi	High risk	4
Malaysia	Risk in inland forested areas of peninsular Malaysia	4
	Very low risk in rest of peninsular Malaysia, including Cameron Highlands and city of Kuala Lumpur	1
Malaysia (Borneo)	High risk in inland areas of eastern Sabah and in inland, forested areas of Sarawak	4
	Very low risk in areas other than those above, including coastal areas of Sabah and Sarawak	1
Mali	High risk	4
Mauritania	High risk all year in southern provinces, and from July-October in the northern provinces	4
	Low risk from November-June in the northern provinces	1
Mauritius	No risk	1
Mayotte	Risk present	4
Mexico	Low risk in Oaxaca and Chiapas	2
	Very low risk in areas other than those above	1
Mozambique	High risk	4
Myanmar	High risk (but not in cities of Mandalay and Yangon)	5
	No risk in cities of Mandalay and Yangon	1
Namibia	High risk all year in regions of Caprivi Strip, Kavango, and Kunene river, and from November-June in northern third of country	4
	Low to no risk in areas other than those above; low risk from July-October in northern third of country	1
Nepal	Risk below 1500 m, particularly in Terai district	3
	No risk in city of Kathmandu and on typical Himalayan treks	1
Nicaragua	Low risk (except Managua)	2
	Very low risk in Managua	1
Niger	High risk	4
Nigeria	High risk	4
North Korea	Very low risk in some southern areas	1
Pakistan	Risk below 2000 m	3
	Low to no risk above 2000 m	1
Panama	Risk east of Canal Zone	3
	Low risk west of Canal Zone	2
	No risk in Panama City or Canal Zone itself	1
Papua New Guinea	High risk below 1800 m	4
	Low to no risk above 1800 m	1
Paraguay	Low risk in departments of Alto Paraná and Caaguazú	2
	Very low risk in areas other than those above	1

Infection

5

Key to recommended regimens for prophylaxis against malaria

Codes for regimens	Details of regimens for prophylaxis against malaria
1	Chemoprophylaxis not recommended, but avoid mosquito bites and consider malaria if fever presents
2	Chloroquine only
3	Chloroquine with proguanil
4	Atovaquone with proguanil hydrochloride or doxycycline or mefloquine
5	Atovaquone with proguanil hydrochloride or doxycycline

Specific recommendations

Country	Comments on risk of malaria and regional or seasonal variation	Codes for regimens
Peru	High risk in Amazon basin along border with Brazil, particularly in Loreto province	4
	Risk in rural areas below 2000 m (other than those above and below) including in Amazon basin along border with Bolivia	2
	No risk in city of Lima and coastal region south of Chiclayo	1
Philippines	Risk in rural areas below 600 m and on islands of Luzon, Mindanao, Mindoro, and Palawan	3
	No risk in cities or on islands of Boracay, Bohol, Catanduanes, Cebu, or Leyte	1
Rwanda	High risk	4
São Tomé and Principe	High risk	4
Saudi Arabia	Risk in south-western provinces along border with Yemen, including below 2000 m in Asir province	3
	No risk in cities of Jeddah, Makkah (Mecca), Medina, Riyadh, or Ta'if, or above 2000 m in Asir province	1
Senegal	High risk	4
Sierra Leone	High risk	4
Solomon Islands	High risk	4
Somalia	High risk	4
South Africa	Moderate risk from September–May in low altitude areas of Mpumalanga and Limpopo, which border Mozambique and Zimbabwe (including Kruger National Park)	4
	Low risk in north-east KwaZulu-Natal	1
	Low risk in areas bordering those above	1
South Korea	Very low risk in northern areas, in Gangwon-do and Gyeonggi-do provinces, and Incheon city (towards Demilitarized Zone)	1
South Sudan	High risk	4
Sri Lanka	Low risk north of Vavuniya	1
	Very low risk in areas other than those above and below	1
	No risk in Colombo or Kandy	-
Sudan	High risk in central and southern areas; risk also present in rest of country (except Khartoum)	4
	Very low risk in Khartoum	1
Suriname	High risk (except coastal districts or city of Paramaribo)	4
	Very low risk in coastal districts; no risk in city of Paramaribo	1
Swaziland	High risk in northern and eastern regions bordering Mozambique and South Africa, including all of Lubombo district and Big Bend, Mhlume, Simunye, and Tshaneni regions	4
	Very low risk in the areas other than those above	1
Syria	Very low risk in small, remote foci of El Hasakah	1
Tajikistan	Risk below 2000 m from June–October	3
	Low risk below 2000 m from November–May	1
Tanzania	High risk below 1800 m; risk also in Zanzibar	4
Thailand	High risk, with chloroquine and mefloquine resistance, in rural forested borders with Cambodia, Laos, and Myanmar	5
	Very low risk in areas other than those above, including Kanchanaburi (Kwai Bridge); no risk in cities of Bangkok, Chiang Mai, Chiang Rai, Koh Phangan, Koh Samui, and Pattaya	1

Country	Comments on risk of malaria and regional or seasonal variation	Codes for regimens
Togo	High risk	4
Turkey	Low risk from May–October along the border plain with Syria, around Adana and east of Adana	2
	Very low risk from November–April along the border plain with Syria, around Adana and east of Adana; very low risk all year in rest of country	1
Uganda	High risk	4
Uzbekistan	Very low risk in extreme south-east	1
Vanuatu	Risk present	4
Venezuela	High risk in all areas south of, and including, the Orinoco river and Angel Falls	4
	Risk in rural areas of Apure, Monagas, Sucre, and Zulia states	3
	No risk in city of Caracas or on Margarita Island	1
Vietnam	Risk in rural areas, and in southern provinces of Tay Ninh, Lam Dong, Dac Lac, Gia Lai, and Kon Tum	5
	Very low risk in Mekong river delta until border area with Cambodia; no risk in large cities (including Ho Chi Minh (Saigon) and Hanoi), Red river delta, and coastal areas north of Nha Trang and Phu Quoc Island	1
Western Sahara	No risk	1
Yemen	Risk below 2000 m	3
	Very low risk on Socrota Island; no risk above 2000 m, including Sana'a city	1
Zambia	High risk	4
Zimbabwe	High risk all year in Zambezi valley, and from November–June in areas below 1200 m	4
	Low risk from July–October in areas below 1200 m; very low risk all year in Harare and Bulawayo	1

Anticoagulants
Travellers taking warfarin sodium p. 126 should begin chemoprophylaxis 2–3 weeks before departure. The INR should be stable before departure. It should be measured before starting chemoprophylaxis, 7 days after starting, and after completing the course. For prolonged stays, the INR should be checked at regular intervals.

Standby treatment
Travellers visiting remote, malarious areas for prolonged periods should carry standby treatment if they are likely to be more than 24 hours away from medical care. Self-medication should be **avoided** if medical help is accessible.

In order to avoid excessive self-medication, the traveller should be provided with **written instructions** that urgent medical attention should be sought if fever (38°C or more) develops 7 days (or more) after arriving in a malarious area and that self-treatment is indicated if medical help is not available within 24 hours of fever onset.

In view of the continuing emergence of resistant strains and of the different regimens required for different areas expert advice should be sought on the best treatment course for an individual traveller. A drug used for chemoprophylaxis should not be considered for standby treatment for the same traveller.

Specific recommendations
Where a journey requires two regimens, the regimen for the higher risk area should be used for the whole journey. Those travelling to remote or little-visited areas may require expert advice. See *Recommended regimens for prophylaxis against malaria.*

Important
Settled immigrants (or long-term visitors) to the UK may be unaware that **any immunity they may have acquired while living in malarious areas is lost rapidly** after migration to the UK, or that any non-malarious areas where they lived previously **may now be malarious**.

Malaria, treatment

Advice for healthcare professionals

A number of specialist centres are able to provide advice on specific problems.

PHE (Public Health England) Malaria Reference Laboratory (020) 7637 0248 (fax) (prophylaxis only) www.malaria-reference.co.uk

National Travel Health Network and Centre 0845 602 6712

Travel Medicine Team, Health Protection Scotland (registered users of Travax only) www.travax.nhs.uk (for registered users of the NHS Travax website only) (0141) 300 1100 (weekdays 2–4 p.m. only)

Birmingham (0121) 424 2358
Liverpool (0151) 705 3100
London 0845 155 5000 (treatment)
Oxford (01865) 225 430

Advice for travellers

Hospital for Tropical Diseases Travel Healthline (020) 7950 7799 www.fitfortravel.nhs.uk

WHO advice on international travel and health www.who.int/ith

National Travel Health Network and Centre (NaTHNaC) www.nathnac.org/travel/index.htm

Treatment of malaria

Recommendations on the treatment of malaria reflect guidelines agreed by UK malaria specialists.

If the infective species is **not known**, or if the infection is **mixed**, initial treatment should be as for *falciparum malaria* with quinine p. 564, *Malarone*® (atovaquone with proguanil hydrochloride p. 559), or *Riamet*® (artemether with lumefantrine p. 558). Falciparum malaria can progress rapidly in unprotected individuals and antimalarial treatment should be considered in those with features of

5

Infection

severe malaria and possible exposure, even if the initial blood tests for the organism are negative.

Falciparum malaria (treatment)

Falciparum malaria (malignant malaria) is caused by *Plasmodium falciparum*. In most parts of the world *P. falciparum* is now resistant to chloroquine p. 560 which should not therefore be given for treatment.

Quinine, *Malarone*® (atovaquone with proguanil hydrochloride), or *Riamet*® (artemether with lumefantrine) can be given *by mouth* if the patient can swallow and retain tablets and there are no serious manifestations (e.g. impaired consciousness); quinine should be given *by intravenous infusion* if the patient is seriously ill or unable to take tablets. Mefloquine p. 561 is now rarely used for treatment because of concerns about resistance.

Oral quinine is given by mouth for 5–7 days, together with or followed by either doxycycline p. 513 for 7 days or clindamycin p. 485 for 7 days [unlicensed].

If the parasite is likely to be sensitive, pyrimethamine with sulfadoxine p. 563 as a single dose [unlicensed] may be given (instead of either clindamycin or doxycycline) together with, or after, a course of quinine.

Alternatively, *Malarone*®, or *Riamet*® may be given instead of quinine. It is not necessary to give clindamycin, doxycycline, or pyrimethamine with sulfadoxine after *Malarone*® or *Riamet*® treatment.

If the patient is seriously ill or unable to take tablets, or if more than 2% of red blood cell are parasitized, quinine should be given by *intravenous infusion* [unlicensed] (until patient can swallow tablets to complete the 7-day course *together with* or *followed by either* doxycycline or clindamycin).

Specialist advice should be sought in difficult cases (e.g. very high parasite count, deterioration on optimal doses of quinine, infection acquired in quinine-resistant areas of south east Asia) because intravenous **artesunate** may be available for 'named-patient' use.

Pregnancy

Falciparum malaria is particularly dangerous in pregnancy, especially in the last trimester. The adult treatment doses or oral and intravenous quinine (including the loading dose) can safely be given to pregnant women. Clinamycin should be given after quinine [unlicensed indication]. Doxycycline should be avoided in pregnancy (affects teeth and skeletal development); pyrimethamine with sulfadoxine, *Malarone*®, and *Riamet*® are also best avoided until more information is available. Specialist advice should be sought in difficult cases (e.g. very high parasite count, deterioration on optimal doses of quinine, infection acquired in quinine-resistant areas of south east Asia) because intravenous artesunate may be available for 'named patient' use.

Non-falciparum malaria (treatment)

Non-falciparum malaria is usually caused by *Plasmodium vivax* and less commonly by *P. ovale* and *P. malariae*. *P. knowlesi* is also present in the Asia-Pacific region. Chloroquine is the drug of choice for the treatment of non-falciparum malaria (but chloroquine-resistant *P. vivax* has been reported in the Indonesian archipelago, the Malay Peninsula, including Myanmar, and eastward to Southern Vietnam).

For the treatment of chloroquine-resistant non-falciparum malaria, *Malarone*® [unlicensed indication], quinine, or *Riamet*® [unlicensed indication] can be used; as with chloroquine, primaquine p. 562 should be given for radical cure.

Chloroquine alone is adequate for *P. malariae* and *P. knowlesi* infections but in the case of *P. vivax* and *P. ovale*, a *radical cure* (to destroy parasites in the liver and thus prevent relapses) is required. This is achieved with primaquine [unlicensed] given after chloroquine, with the dose dependent on the infecting organism. For a radical

cure, primaquine [unlicensed] is then given for 14 days, with the dose also dependent on the infecting organism.

Parenteral

Parenteral If the patient is unable to take oral therapy, quinine can be given by intravenous infusion [unlicensed], changed to oral chloroquine as soon as the patient's condition permits.

Pregnancy

The adult treatment doses of chloroquine can be given for non-falciparum malaria. In the case of *P.vivax* or *P.ovale*, however, the radical cure with primaquine should be **postponed** until the pregnancy is over; instead chloroquine should be continued, given weekly during the pregnancy.

ANTIPROTOZOALS > ANTIMALARIALS

Artemether with lumefantrine

- **INDICATIONS AND DOSE**

Treatment of acute uncomplicated falciparum malaria | Treatment of chloroquine-resistant non-falciparum malaria

▸ BY MOUTH

▸ Adult (body-weight 35 kg and above): Initially 4 tablets, followed by 4 tablets for 5 doses each given at 8, 24, 36, 48 and 60 hours (total 24 tablets over 60 hours)

- UNLICENSED USE Use in treatment of non-falciparum malaria is an unlicensed indication.

- CONTRA-INDICATIONS Family history of congenital QT interval prolongation · family history of sudden death · history of arrhythmias · history of clinically relevant bradycardia · history of congestive heart failure accompanied by reduced left ventricular ejection fraction

- CAUTIONS Avoid in Acute porphyrias p. 918 · electrolyte disturbances

- INTERACTIONS → Appendix 1 (artemether with lumefantrine).
Caution if concomitant use with other drugs known to cause QT-interval prolongation.

- SIDE-EFFECTS
▸ **Common or very common** Abdominal pain · anorexia · arthralgia · asthenia · cough · diarrhoea · dizziness · headache · myalgia · nausea · palpitation · paraesthesia · prolonged QT interval · pruritus · rash · sleep disturbances · vomiting
▸ **Uncommon** Ataxia · clonus · hypoaesthesia

- PREGNANCY Toxicity in *animal* studies with artemether. Manufacturer advises use only if potential benefit outweighs risk.

- BREAST FEEDING Manufacturer advises avoid breastfeeding for at least 1 week after last dose. Present in milk in *animal* studies.

- HEPATIC IMPAIRMENT Manufacturer advises caution in severe impairment.

- RENAL IMPAIRMENT Manufacturer advises caution in severe impairment. In severe renal impairment monitor ECG and plasma potassium concentration.

- MONITORING REQUIREMENTS Monitor patients unable to take food (greater risk of recrudescence).

- DIRECTIONS FOR ADMINISTRATION Tablets may be crushed just before administration.

- PATIENT AND CARER ADVICE

Driving and skilled tasks

Dizziness may affect performance of skilled tasks (e.g. driving).

● MEDICINAL FORMS
There can be variation in the licensing of different medicines containing the same drug.

Tablet
CAUTIONARY AND ADVISORY LABELS 21
▸ Riamet (Novartis Pharmaceuticals UK Ltd)
    Artemether 20 mg, Lumefantrine 120 mg Riamet tablets | 24 tablet PoM £22.50

Artenimol with piperaquine phosphate

(Piperaquine tetraphosphate with dihydroartemisinin)

● INDICATIONS AND DOSE

Treatment of uncomplicated falciparum malaria
▸ BY MOUTH
▸ Child 6 months–17 years (body-weight 7–12 kg): 0.5 tablet once daily for 3 days, max. 2 courses in 12 months; second course given at least 2 months after first course
▸ Child 6 months–17 years (body-weight 13–23 kg): 1 tablet once daily for 3 days, max. 2 courses in 12 months; second course given at least 2 months after first course
▸ Child 6 months–17 years (body-weight 24–35 kg): 2 tablets once daily for 3 days, max. 2 courses in 12 months; second course given at least 2 months after first course
▸ Child 6 months–17 years (body-weight 36–74 kg): 3 tablets once daily for 3 days, max. 2 courses in 12 months; second course given at least 2 months after first course
▸ Child 6 months–17 years (body-weight 75–99 kg): 4 tablets once daily for 3 days, max. 2 courses in 12 months; second course given at least 2 months after first course
▸ Adult (body-weight 36–74 kg): 3 tablets once daily for 3 days, max. 2 courses in 12 months; second course given at least 2 months after first course
▸ Adult (body-weight 75–99 kg): 4 tablets once daily for 3 days, max. 2 courses in 12 months; second course given at least 2 months after first course

● CONTRA-INDICATIONS Acute myocardial infarction · bradycardia · congenital long QT syndrome · electrolyte disturbances · family history of sudden death · heart failure with reduced left ventricular ejection fraction · history of symptomatic arrhythmias · left ventricular hypertrophy · risk factors for QT interval prolongation · severe hypertension

● INTERACTIONS → Appendix 1 (artenimol with piperaquine).
Piperaquine has a long half-life; there is a potential for drug interactions to occur for up to 3 months after treatment has been stopped.
Concomitant use with other drugs known to prolong the QT interval contra-indicated.

● SIDE-EFFECTS
▸ **Common or very common** Abdominal pain (in children) · anaemia · blood disorders (in children) · conjunctivitis (in children) · cough (in children) · diarrhoea (in children) · headache (in adults) · irregular heart rate (in children) · leucopenia (in children) · malaise · QT interval prolonged · rash (in children) · tachycardia (in adults) · thrombocytopenia (in children) · vomiting (in children)
▸ **Uncommon** Abdominal pain (in adults) · acanthosis (in children) · anorexia (in adults) · arrhythmias · arthralgia · bradycardia (in adults) · convulsions · cough (in adults) · diarrhoea (in adults) · dizziness (in adults) · headache (in children) · heart murmur (in children) · hepatitis · hepatomegaly · influenza-like symptoms · jaundice (in children) · myalgia (in adults) · nausea · pruritus (in adults) · stomatitis (in children) · vomiting (in adults)

● PREGNANCY Teratogenic in *animal* studies—manufacturer advises use only if other antimalarials cannot be used.

● BREAST FEEDING Manufacturer advises avoid—present in milk in *animal* studies.

● HEPATIC IMPAIRMENT No information available in moderate to severe impairment. Manufacturer advises monitor ECG and plasma-potassium concentration in moderate to severe hepatic impairment.

● RENAL IMPAIRMENT No information available in moderate to severe impairment. Manufacturer advises monitor ECG and plasma-potassium concentration in moderate to severe renal impairment.

● MONITORING REQUIREMENTS
▸ Consider obtaining ECG in all patients before third dose and 4–6 hours after third dose. If QT$_C$ interval more than 500 milliseconds, discontinue treatment and monitor ECG for a further 24–48 hours.
▸ Obtain ECG as soon as possible after starting treatment then continue monitoring in those taking medicines that increase plasma-piperaquine concentration, in children who are vomiting, in females, or in the elderly.

● DIRECTIONS FOR ADMINISTRATION Tablets to be taken at least 3 hours before and at least 3 hours after food. Tablets may be crushed and mixed with water immediately before administration.

● PATIENT AND CARER ADVICE Patients or carers should be given advice on how to administer tablets containing piperaquine phosphate with artenimol.

● MEDICINAL FORMS
There can be variation in the licensing of different medicines containing the same drug.

Tablet
▸ Eurartesim (Sigma-Tau Pharma Ltd) ▼
    Artenimol 40 mg, Piperaquine phosphate 320 mg Eurartesim 320mg/40mg tablets | 12 tablet PoM £40.00

Atovaquone with proguanil hydrochloride

● INDICATIONS AND DOSE

MALARONE®

Prophylaxis of falciparum malaria, particularly where resistance to other antimalarial drugs suspected
▸ BY MOUTH
▸ Adult (body-weight 41 kg and above): 1 tablet daily, to be started 1–2 days before entering endemic area and continued for 1 week after leaving

Treatment of acute uncomplicated falciparum malaria | Treatment of non-falciparum malaria
▸ BY MOUTH
▸ Adult: 4 tablets once daily for 3 days

● UNLICENSED USE Not licensed for treatment of non-falciparum malaria.

● CAUTIONS Diarrhoea or vomiting (reduced absorption of atovaquone) · efficacy not evaluated in cerebral or complicated malaria (including hyperparasitaemia, pulmonary oedema or renal failure)

● INTERACTIONS → Appendix 1 (proguanil, atovaquone).

● SIDE-EFFECTS
▸ **Common or very common** Abdominal pain · abnormal dreams · anorexia · cough · depression · diarrhoea · dizziness · fever · headache · insomnia · nausea · pruritus · rash · vomiting
▸ **Uncommon** Anxiety · blood disorders · hair loss · hyponatraemia · palpitation · stomatitis

Infection

5

▶ **Frequency not known** Cholestasis · hallucinations · hepatitis · mouth ulcers · photosensitivity · seizures · Stevens-Johnson syndrome · tachycardia · vasculitis

● PREGNANCY Manufacturer advises avoid unless essential.

● BREAST FEEDING Use only if no suitable alternative available.

● RENAL IMPAIRMENT Avoid for malaria prophylaxis (and if possible for malaria treatment) if eGFR less than 30 mL/minute/1.73m².

● PATIENT AND CARER ADVICE Warn travellers about **importance** of avoiding mosquito bites, **importance** of taking prophylaxis regularly, and **importance** of immediate visit to doctor if ill within 1 year and **especially** within 3 months of return.

● NATIONAL FUNDING/ACCESS DECISIONS

NHS restrictions Drugs for malaria prophylaxis not prescribable on the NHS; health authorities may investigate circumstances under which antimalarials prescribed.

● MEDICINAL FORMS
There can be variation in the licensing of different medicines containing the same drug.

Tablet
CAUTIONARY AND ADVISORY LABELS 21
▶ Malarone (GlaxoSmithKline UK Ltd)
Proguanil hydrochloride 25 mg, Atovaquone 62.5 mg Malarone Paediatric tablets │ 12 tablet [PoM] £6.26
Proguanil hydrochloride 100 mg, Atovaquone 250 mg Malarone tablets │ 12 tablet [PoM] £25.21 DT price = £25.21

Chloroquine

● INDICATIONS AND DOSE

Active rheumatoid arthritis (administered on expert advice) │ Systemic and discoid lupus erythematosus (administered on expert advice)
▶ BY MOUTH
▶ Adult: 150 mg daily; maximum 2.5 mg/kg per day

Prophylaxis of malaria
▶ INITIALLY BY MOUTH USING SYRUP
▶ Child 6 weeks–5 months (body-weight 4.5–7 kg): 50 mg once weekly, started 1 week before entering endemic area and continued for 4 weeks after leaving
▶ Child 6–11 months (body-weight 8–10 kg): 75 mg once weekly, started 1 week before entering endemic area and continued for 4 weeks after leaving
▶ Child 1–2 years (body-weight 11–14 kg): 100 mg once weekly, started 1 week before entering endemic area and continued for 4 weeks after leaving
▶ Child 3–4 years (body-weight 15–16.4 kg): 125 mg once weekly, started 1 week before entering endemic area and continued for 4 weeks after leaving
▶ Child 4–7 years (body-weight 16.5–24 kg): 150 mg once weekly, alternatively (by mouth using tablets) 155 mg once weekly, started 1 week before entering endemic area and continued for 4 weeks after leaving
▶ Child 8–13 years (body-weight 25–44 kg): 225 mg once weekly, alternatively (by mouth using tablets) 232.5 mg once weekly, started 1 week before entering endemic area and continued for 4 weeks after leaving
▶ INITIALLY BY MOUTH USING TABLETS
▶ Child 14–17 years (body-weight 45 kg and above): 310 mg once weekly, alternatively (by mouth using syrup) 300 mg once weekly, started 1 week before entering endemic area and continued for 4 weeks after leaving
▶ Adult (body-weight 45 kg and above): 310 mg once weekly, alternatively (by mouth using syrup) 300 mg once weekly, started 1 week before entering endemic area and continued for 4 weeks after leaving

Treatment of non-falciparum malaria
▶ BY MOUTH
▶ Child: Initially 10 mg/kg (max. per dose 620 mg), then 5 mg/kg after 6–8 hours (max. per dose 310 mg), then 5 mg/kg daily (max. per dose 310 mg) for 2 days
▶ Adult: Initially 620 mg, then 310 mg after 6–8 hours, then 310 mg daily for 2 days, approximate total cumulative dose of 25 mg/kg of base

***P. vivax* or *P. ovale* infection during pregnancy while radical cure is postponed**
▶ BY MOUTH
▶ Adult: 310 mg once weekly

DOSE EQUIVALENCE AND CONVERSION
Doses expressed as chloroquine base. Chloroquine base 150 mg = chloroquine sulfate 200 mg = chloroquine phosphate 250 mg (approx).

DOSES AT EXTREMES OF BODY-WEIGHT
▶ With oral use in adults In active rheumatoid arthritis and systemic and discoid lupus erythematosus, to avoid excessive dosage in obese patients, the daily maximum dose should be calculated on the basis of ideal body weight.

● UNLICENSED USE Chloroquine doses for the treatment and prophylaxis of malaria in BNF publications may differ from those in product literature.

┌───┐
IMPORTANT SAFETY INFORMATION
▶ In adults
Ocular toxicity is unlikely if the dose of chloroquine phosphate does not exceed 4 mg/kg daily (equivalent to chloroquine base approx. 2.5 mg/kg daily).
└───┘

● CAUTIONS Acute porphyrias p. 918 elderly · G6PD deficiency · long-term therapy (regular ophthalmic examination recommended by manufacturers) · may aggravate myasthenia gravis · may exacerbate psoriasis · neurological disorders, especially epilepsy (avoid for prophylaxis of malaria if history of epilepsy) · severe gastro-intestinal disorders

CAUTIONS, FURTHER INFORMATION
▶ Screening for ocular toxicity
▶ In adults A review group convened by the Royal College of Ophthalmologists has updated guidelines for screening to prevent ocular toxicity on long-term treatment with chloroquine and hydroxychloroquine (*Hydroxychloroquine and Ocular Toxicity: Recommendations on Screening* 2009). Chloroquine should be considered (for treating chronic inflammatory conditions) **only** if other drugs have failed. All patients taking chloroquine should receive ocular examination according to a protocol arranged locally between the prescriber and the ophthalmologist.

● INTERACTIONS → Appendix 1 (chloroquine).
Avoid concurrent therapy with hepatotoxic drugs.

● SIDE-EFFECTS
GENERAL SIDE-EFFECTS
▶ **Common or very common** Gastro-intestinal disturbances · headache · pruritus · rashes · skin reactions
▶ **Uncommon** Convulsions · discoloration of mucous membranes · discoloration of nails · discoloration of skin · ECG changes · hair depigmentation · hair loss · keratopathy · ototoxicity · retinal damage · visual changes
▶ **Rare** Acute generalised exanthematous pustulosis · agranulocytosis · angioedema · aplastic anaemia · blood disorders · bone marrow suppression · cardiomyopathy · emotional disturbances · exfoliative dermatitis · hepatic damage · hypersensitivity reactions · mental changes · myopathy · neuromyopathy · photosensitivity · psychosis · Stevens-Johnson syndrome · thrombocytopenia · urticaria
▶ **Frequency not known** Bronchospasm (in children) · diffuse parenchymal lung disease · drug rash with eosinophilia

and systemic symptoms · extrapyramidal symptoms (associated with use in malaria) · hypotension · visual disturbances

SIDE-EFFECTS, FURTHER INFORMATION

▸ **Malaria prophylaxis and treatment** Serious skin reactions, ECG changes, visual effects, ototoxicity, blood disorders, mental changes, myopathies and hepatic damage are not usually associated with malaria prophylaxis or treatment.

Overdose

Chloroquine is very toxic in overdosage; overdosage is extremely hazardous and difficult to treat. Urgent advice from the National Poisons Information Service is essential. Life-threatening features include arrhythmias (which can have a very rapid onset) and convulsions (which can be intractable).

● PREGNANCY Benefit of use in prophylaxis and treatment in malaria outweighs risk. For rheumatoid disease, it is not necessary to withdraw an antimalarial drug during pregnancy if the disease is well controlled.

● BREAST FEEDING Present in breast milk and breast-feeding should be avoided when used to treat rheumatic disease. Amount in milk probably too small to be harmful when used for malaria.

● HEPATIC IMPAIRMENT Use with caution in moderate to severe impairment.

● RENAL IMPAIRMENT Only partially excreted by the kidneys and reduction of the dose is not required for prophylaxis of malaria except in severe impairment. For rheumatoid arthritis and lupus erythematosus, reduce dose. Manufacturers advise caution.

● MONITORING REQUIREMENTS

▸ In adults Manufacturers recommend regular ophthalmological examination but the evidence of practical value is unsatisfactory.

▸ In children Ophthalmic examination with long-term therapy.

● PATIENT AND CARER ADVICE Warn travellers going to malarious areas about **importance** of avoiding mosquito bites, **importance** of taking prophylaxis regularly, and **importance** of immediate visit to doctor if ill within 1 year and **especially** within 3 months of return.

● NATIONAL FUNDING/ACCESS DECISIONS

NHS restrictions Drugs for malaria prophylaxis not prescribable on the NHS; health authorities may investigate circumstances under which antimalarials prescribed.

● EXCEPTIONS TO LEGAL CATEGORY Can be sold to the public provided it is licensed and labelled for the prophylaxis of malaria.

● MEDICINAL FORMS
There can be variation in the licensing of different medicines containing the same drug. Forms available from special-order manufacturers include: oral solution

Tablet
CAUTIONARY AND ADVISORY LABELS 5
▸ Avloclor (Alliance Pharmaceuticals Ltd)
Chloroquine phosphate 250 mg Avloclor 250mg tablets | 20 tablet PoM £7.95 DT price = £7.95

Oral solution
CAUTIONARY AND ADVISORY LABELS 5
▸ Malarivon (Wallace Manufacturing Chemists Ltd)
Chloroquine phosphate 16 mg per 1 ml Malarivon 80mg/5ml syrup | 75 ml PoM £30.00

Chloroquine with proguanil

The properties listed below are those particular to the combination only. For the properties of the components please consider, chloroquine p. 560, proguanil hydrochloride p. 562.

● INDICATIONS AND DOSE

Prophylaxis of malaria
▸ BY MOUTH
▸ Adult: (consult product literature)

● EXCEPTIONS TO LEGAL CATEGORY Can be sold to the public provided it is licensed and labelled for the prophylaxis of malaria.

● MEDICINAL FORMS
There can be variation in the licensing of different medicines containing the same drug.
Tablet
▸ Paludrine/Avloclor (Alliance Pharmaceuticals Ltd)
Paludrine/Avloclor tablets anti-malarial travel pack | 112 tablet P £13.50

Mefloquine

● INDICATIONS AND DOSE

Treatment of malaria
▸ BY MOUTH
▸ Adult: (consult product literature)

Prophylaxis of malaria
▸ BY MOUTH
▸ Child (body-weight 5–15 kg): 62.5 mg once weekly, dose to be started 2–3 weeks before entering endemic area and continued for 4 weeks after leaving
▸ Child (body-weight 16–24 kg): 125 mg once weekly, dose to be started 2–3 weeks before entering endemic area and continued for 4 weeks after leaving
▸ Child (body-weight 25–44 kg): 187.5 mg once weekly, dose to be started 2–3 weeks before entering endemic area and continued for 4 weeks after leaving
▸ Child (body-weight 45 kg and above): 250 mg once weekly, dose to be started 2–3 weeks before entering endemic area and continued for 4 weeks after leaving
▸ Adult (body-weight 45 kg and above): 250 mg once weekly, dose to be started 2–3 weeks before entering endemic area and continued for 4 weeks after leaving

● UNLICENSED USE Mefloquine doses in BNF Publications may differ from those in product literature.

▸ In children Not licensed for use in children under 5 kg body-weight and under 3 months.

● CONTRA-INDICATIONS Avoid for prophylaxis if history of psychiatric disorders (including depression) or convulsions · avoid for standby treatment if history of convulsions · history of blackwater fever

● CAUTIONS Cardiac conduction disorders · epilepsy (avoid for prophylaxis) · not recommended in infants under 3 months (5 kg) (in children) · traumatic brain injury

CAUTIONS, FURTHER INFORMATION

▸ Neuropsychiatric reactions Mefloquine is associated with potentially serious neuropsychiatric reactions. Abnormal dreams, insomnia, anxiety, and depression occur commonly. Psychosis, suicidal ideation, and suicide have also been reported. Psychiatric symptoms such as nightmares, acute anxiety, depression, restlessness, or confusion should be regarded as potentially prodromal for a more serious event. If neuropsychiatric symptoms occur, patients should be advised to discontinue mefloquine and to seek immediate medical attention so that mefloquine can be replaced with an alternative antimalarial. Adverse reactions may occur and persist up to several months after

5

Infection

discontinuation because mefloquine has a long half-life. Mefloquine is contra-indicated for malaria prophylaxis in those with a history of psychiatric disorders or convulsions.

- INTERACTIONS → Appendix 1 (mefloquine).
- SIDE-EFFECTS
  ▶ **Common or very common** Abdominal pain · diarrhoea · dizziness · headache · nausea · neuropsychiatric reactions · pruritus · visual disturbances · vomiting
  ▶ **Very rare** Optic neuropathy
  ▶ **Frequency not known** Alopecia · amnesia · anorexia · arrhythmias · arthralgia · ataxia · blood disorders · bradycardia · cataract · chest pain · confusion · drowsiness · dyspepsia · dyspnoea · encephalopathy · fever · flushing · hepatic failure · hyperhidrosis · hypertension · hypotension · leucocytosis · leucopenia · malaise · motor neuropathies · muscle weakness · myalgia · oedema · palpitation · panic attacks · pneumonitis · rash · seizures · sensory neuropathies · speech disturbances · Stevens-Johnson syndrome · syncope · tachycardia · thrombocytopenia · tremor · vestibular disorders
- ALLERGY AND CROSS-SENSITIVITY Contra-indicated in patients with hypersensitivity to quinine.
- CONCEPTION AND CONTRACEPTION Manufacturer advises adequate contraception during prophylaxis and for 3 months after stopping (teratogenicity in *animal* studies).
- PREGNANCY Manufacturer advises avoid (particularly in the first trimester) unless the potential benefit outweighs the risk; however, studies of mefloquine in pregnancy (including use in the first trimester) indicate that it can be considered for travel to chloroquine-resistant areas.
- BREAST FEEDING Present in milk but risk to infant minimal.
- HEPATIC IMPAIRMENT Elimination may be prolonged; avoid in severe impairment.
- RENAL IMPAIRMENT Manufacturer advises caution.
- DIRECTIONS FOR ADMINISTRATION Tablet may be crushed and mixed with food such as jam or honey just before administration.
- PATIENT AND CARER ADVICE
  Driving and skilled tasks
  Dizziness or a disturbed sense of balance may affect performance of skilled tasks (e.g. driving); effects may occur and persist up to several months after stopping mefloquine.
  Inform travellers about adverse reactions of mefloquine and, if they occur, to seek medical advice on alternative antimalarials before the next dose is due. Also warn travellers about **importance** of avoiding mosquito bites, **importance** of taking prophylaxis regularly, and **importance** of immediate visit to doctor if ill within 1 year and especially within 3 months of return.
- NATIONAL FUNDING/ACCESS DECISIONS
  NHS restrictions Drugs for malaria prophylaxis not prescribable on the NHS; health authorities may investigate circumstances under which antimalarials prescribed.

- MEDICINAL FORMS
  There can be variation in the licensing of different medicines containing the same drug.
  Tablet
  CAUTIONARY AND ADVISORY LABELS 21, 27
  ▶ Lariam (Roche Products Ltd)
  Mefloquine (as Mefloquine hydrochloride) 250 mg Lariam 250mg tablets | 8 tablet [PoM] £14.53

Primaquine

- INDICATIONS AND DOSE

Adjunct in the treatment of non-falciparum malaria caused by P.vivax infection
▶ BY MOUTH
▶ Adult: 30 mg daily for 14 days

Adjunct in the treatment of non-falciparum malaria caused by P.ovale infection
▶ BY MOUTH
▶ Adult: 15 mg daily for 14 days

Adjunct in the treatment of non-falciparum malaria caused by P.vivax infection in patients with mild G6PD deficiency (administered on expert advice) | Adjunct in the treatment of non-falciparum malaria caused by P.ovale infection in patients with mild G6PD deficiency (administered on expert advice)
▶ BY MOUTH
▶ Adult: 45 mg once weekly for 8 weeks

Treatment of mild to moderate pneumocystis infection (in combination with clindamycin)
▶ BY MOUTH
▶ Adult: 30 mg daily, this combination is associated with considerable toxicity

- UNLICENSED USE Not licensed.
- CAUTIONS G6PD deficiency · systemic diseases associated with granulocytopenia (e.g. juvenile idiopathic arthritis, rheumatoid arthritis, lupus erythematosus)
- INTERACTIONS → Appendix 1 (primaquine).
- SIDE-EFFECTS
  ▶ **Common or very common** Abdominal pain · anorexia · nausea · vomiting
  ▶ **Uncommon** Haemolytic anaemia especially in G6PD deficiency · leucopenia · methaemoglobinaemia
- PREGNANCY Risk of neonatal haemolysis and methaemoglobinaemia in third trimester.
- BREAST FEEDING No information available; theoretical risk of haemolysis in G6PD-deficient infants.
- PRE-TREATMENT SCREENING Before starting primaquine, blood should be tested for glucose-6-phosphate dehydrogenase (G6PD) activity since the drug can cause haemolysis in G6PD-deficient patients. Specialist advice should be obtained in G6PD deficiency.

- MEDICINAL FORMS
  There can be variation in the licensing of different medicines containing the same drug. Forms available from special-order manufacturers include: oral suspension
  Tablet
  ▶ Primaquine (Non-proprietary)
  Primaquine (as Primaquine phosphate) 15 mg Primaquine 15mg tablets | 100 tablet [PoM] no price available

Proguanil hydrochloride

- INDICATIONS AND DOSE

Prophylaxis of malaria
▶ BY MOUTH
▶ Child 4–11 weeks (body-weight up to 6 kg): 25 mg once daily, dose to be started 1 week before entering endemic area and continued for 4 weeks after leaving
▶ Child 3–11 months (body-weight 6–9 kg): 50 mg once daily, dose to be started 1 week before entering endemic area and continued for 4 weeks after leaving
▶ Child 1–3 years (body-weight 10–15 kg): 75 mg once daily, dose to be started 1 week before entering endemic area and continued for 4 weeks after leaving

- Child 4-7 years (body-weight 16-24 kg): 100 mg once daily, dose to be started 1 week before entering endemic area and continued for 4 weeks after leaving
- Child 8-12 years (body-weight 25-44 kg): 150 mg once daily, dose to be started 1 week before entering endemic area and continued for 4 weeks after leaving
- Child 13-17 years (body-weight 45 kg and above): 200 mg once daily, dose to be started 1 week before entering endemic area and continued for 4 weeks after leaving
- Adult: 200 mg once daily, dose to be started 1 week before entering endemic area and continued for 4 weeks after leaving

- UNLICENSED USE Proguanil doses in BNF Publications may differ from those in product literature.
- INTERACTIONS → Appendix 1 (proguanil).
- SIDE-EFFECTS
- **Common or very common** Constipation · diarrhoea · mild gastric intolerance
- **Very rare** Cholestasis · hair loss · skin reactions · vasculitis
- **Frequency not known** Mouth ulcers · stomatitis
- PREGNANCY Benefit of prophylaxis in malaria outweighs risk. Adequate folate supplements should be given to mother.
- BREAST FEEDING Amount in milk probably too small to be harmful when used for malaria prophylaxis.
- RENAL IMPAIRMENT
- In children Use half normal dose if estimated glomerular filtration rate 20-60 mL/minute/1.73m². Use one-quarter normal dose on alternate days if estimated glomerular filtration rate 10-20 mL/minute/1.73m². Use one-quarter normal dose once weekly if estimated glomerular filtration rate less than 10 mL/minute/1.73m²; increased risk of haematological toxicity in severe impairment.
- In adults 100 mg once daily if eGFR 20-60 mL/minute/1.73m². 50 mg on alternate days if eGFR 10-20 mL/minute/1.73m². 50 mg once weekly if eGFR less than 10 mL/minute/1.73m²; increased risk of haematological toxicity in severe impairment.
- DIRECTIONS FOR ADMINISTRATION Tablet may be crushed and mixed with food such as milk, jam, or honey just before administration.
- PATIENT AND CARER ADVICE Warn travellers about **importance** of avoiding mosquito bites, **importance** of taking prophylaxis regularly, and **importance** of immediate visit to doctor if ill within 1 year and **especially** within 3 months of return.
- NATIONAL FUNDING/ACCESS DECISIONS
  NHS restrictions Drugs for malaria prophylaxis not prescribable on the NHS; health authorities may investigate circumstances under which antimalarials prescribed.
- EXCEPTIONS TO LEGAL CATEGORY Can be sold to the public provided it is licensed and labelled for the prophylaxis of malaria.
- MEDICINAL FORMS
  There can be variation in the licensing of different medicines containing the same drug. Forms available from special-order manufacturers include: oral suspension, oral solution
  Tablet
  CAUTIONARY AND ADVISORY LABELS 21
  - Paludrine (Alliance Pharmaceuticals Ltd)
    Proguanil hydrochloride 100 mg Paludrine 100mg tablets | 98 tablet Ⓟ £11.95 DT price = £11.95

Pyrimethamine

- ● INDICATIONS AND DOSE
  Toxoplasmosis in pregnancy (in combination with sulfadiazine and folinic acid)
  - BY MOUTH
  - Adult: 50 mg once daily until delivery
  Malaria
  - BY MOUTH
  - Adult: No dose stated because not recommended alone

- CAUTIONS History of seizures—avoid large loading doses · predisposition to folate deficiency
- INTERACTIONS → Appendix 1 (pyrimethamine).
- SIDE-EFFECTS
- **Common or very common** Anaemia (with high doses) · blood disorders (with high doses) · diarrhoea · dizziness · headache · leucopenia (with high doses) · nausea · rash · thrombocytopenia (with high doses) · vomiting
- **Uncommon** Abnormal skin pigmentation · fever
- **Very rare** Buccal ulceration · colic · convulsions
- PREGNANCY Theoretical teratogenic risk in *first trimester* (folate antagonist). Adequate folate supplements should be given to the mother.
- BREAST FEEDING Significant amount in milk—avoid administration of other folate antagonists to infant. Avoid breast-feeding during toxoplasmosis treatment.
- HEPATIC IMPAIRMENT Manufacturer advises caution.
- RENAL IMPAIRMENT Manufacturer advises caution.
- MONITORING REQUIREMENTS Blood counts required with prolonged treatment.
- LESS SUITABLE FOR PRESCRIBING Pyrimethamine should not be used alone for malaria, but is used with sulfadoxine.

- MEDICINAL FORMS
  There can be variation in the licensing of different medicines containing the same drug. Forms available from special-order manufacturers include: oral suspension
  Tablet
  - Daraprim (GlaxoSmithKline UK Ltd)
    Pyrimethamine 25 mg Daraprim 25mg tablets | 30 tablet PoM £13.00

Pyrimethamine with sulfadoxine

- ● INDICATIONS AND DOSE
  Adjunct to quinine in treatment of Plasmodium falciparum malaria
  - BY MOUTH
  - Child 1 month-4 years (body-weight 5 kg and above): 12.5/250 mg for 1 dose
  - Child 5-6 years: 25/500 mg for 1 dose
  - Child 7-9 years: 37.5/750 mg for 1 dose
  - Child 10-13 years: 50/1000 mg for 1 dose
  - Child 14-17 years: 75/1500 mg for 1 dose
  - Adult: 75/1500 mg for 1 dose
  Malaria prophylaxis
  - BY MOUTH
  - Adult: Not recommended by UK malaria experts
  DOSE EQUIVALENCE AND CONVERSION
  Dose quantities are expressed in the form x/y where x and y are the strengths in milligrams of pyrimethamine and sulfadoxine respectively.

- UNLICENSED USE Not licensed for use in children of body-weight under 5 kg.
- CONTRA-INDICATIONS Acute porphyrias p. 918
- CAUTIONS Asthma · avoid in blood disorders (unless under specialist supervision) · avoid in infants under 6 weeks ·

elderly · G6PD deficiency · history of seizures—avoid large loading doses · not recommended for prophylaxis (severe side-effects on long-term use) · predisposition to folate deficiency · predisposition to hyperkalaemia (in adults)

● INTERACTIONS → Appendix 1 (pyrimethamine, sulfonamides).

● SIDE-EFFECTS

▸ **Common or very common** Diarrhoea · headache · hyperkalaemia · nausea · rash

▸ **Uncommon** Vomiting

▸ **Very rare** Anorexia · antibiotic-associated colitis · arthralgia · aseptic meningitis · ataxia · blood disorders · convulsions · cough · depression · eosinophilia · glossitis · hallucinations · hepatic necrosis · hypoglycaemia · hyponatraemia · interstitial nephritis · jaundice · leucopenia · liver damage · megaloblastic anaemia · myalgia · myocarditis · pancreatitis · peripheral neuropathy · photosensitivity · renal disorders · rhabdomyolysis reported in HIV-infected patients · shortness of breath · Stevens-Johnson syndrome · stomatitis · systemic lupus erythematosus · thrombocytopenia · tinnitus · toxic epidermal necrolysis · uveitis · vasculitis · vertigo

▸ **Frequency not known** Allergic alveolitis · eosinophilic alveolitis · pulmonary infiltrates

SIDE-EFFECTS, FURTHER INFORMATION

Discontinue immediately if blood disorders or rash occur. Discontinue if cough or shortness of breath occur.

● ALLERGY AND CROSS-SENSITIVITY Contra-indicated in patients with sulfonamide allergy.

● PREGNANCY Possible teratogenic risk in *first trimester* (pyrimethamine a folate antagonist); in *third trimester*— risk of neonatal haemolysis and methaemoglobinaemia. Fear of increased risk of kernicterus in neonates appears to be unfounded.

● BREAST FEEDING Small risk of kernicterus in jaundiced infants; risk of haemolysis in G6PD-deficient infants (due to sulfadoxine).

● MONITORING REQUIREMENTS Monitor blood counts on prolonged treatment.

● PRESCRIBING AND DISPENSING INFORMATION Also known as *Fansidar®*.

● PATIENT AND CARER ADVICE Patients should be advised to maintain adequate fluid intake.

● MEDICINAL FORMS
There can be variation in the licensing of different medicines containing the same drug.
No licensed medicines listed.

Quinine

● INDICATIONS AND DOSE

Nocturnal leg cramps

▸ BY MOUTH

▸ Adult: 200–300 mg once daily, to be taken at bedtime

Non-falciparum malaria

▸ BY INTRAVENOUS INFUSION

▸ Adult: 10 mg/kg every 8 hours (max. per dose 700 mg), infused over 4 hours, given if patient is unable to take oral therapy. Changed to oral chloroquine as soon as the patient's condition permits

Falciparum malaria

▸ BY MOUTH

▸ Child: 10 mg/kg every 8 hours (max. per dose 600 mg) for 7 days, together with or followed by either doxycycline (in children over 12 years), or clindamycin

▸ Adult: 600 mg every 8 hours for 5–7 days, the quinine should be given together with or followed by either doxycycline or clindamycin

▸ BY INTRAVENOUS INFUSION

▸ Adult: Loading dose 20 mg/kg (max. per dose 1.4 g), infused over 4 hours, the loading dose of 20 mg/kg should **not** be used if the patient has received quinine or mefloquine during the previous 12 hours, then maintenance 10 mg/kg every 8 hours (max. per dose 700 mg) until patient can swallow tablets to complete the 7-day course, maintenance dose to be given 8 hours after the start of the loading dose and infused over 4 hours, the quinine should be given together with or followed by either doxycycline or clindamycin

Falciparum malaria (in intensive care unit)

▸ BY INTRAVENOUS INFUSION

▸ Adult: Loading dose 7 mg/kg, infused over 30 minutes, followed immediately by maintenance 10 mg/kg, infused over 4 hours, then maintenance 10 mg/kg every 8 hours (max. per dose 700 mg) until patient can swallow tablets to complete the 7-day course, maintenance dose to be given 8 hours after the start of the loading dose and infused over 4 hours, the quinine should be given together with or followed by either doxycycline or clindamycin

DOSE EQUIVALENCE AND CONVERSION

When using quinine for malaria, doses are valid for quinine hydrochloride, dihydrochloride, and sulfate; they are **not valid** for quinine bisulfate which contains a correspondingly smaller amount of quinine. Quinine (anhydrous base) 100 mg = quinine bisulfate 169 mg; quinine dihydrochloride 122 mg; quinine hydrochloride 122 mg; and quinine sulfate 121 mg. Quinine bisulfate 300 mg tablets are available but provide less quinine than 300 mg of the dihydrochloride, hydrochloride, or sulfate.

● UNLICENSED USE Injection not licensed.

● CONTRA-INDICATIONS Haemoglobinuria · myasthenia gravis · optic neuritis · tinnitus

● CAUTIONS Atrial fibrillation (monitor ECG during parenteral treatment) · cardiac disease (monitor ECG during parenteral treatment) · conduction defects (monitor ECG during parenteral treatment) · elderly (monitor ECG during parenteral treatment) (in adults) · G6PD deficiency · heart block (monitor ECG during parenteral treatment)

● INTERACTIONS → Appendix 1 (quinine).

● SIDE-EFFECTS Agitation · tinnitus · abdominal pain · acute renal failure · angioedema · blood disorders · cardiovascular effects · cinchonism · confusion · diarrhoea · dyspnoea · flushed skin · headache · hearing impairment · hot skin · hypersensitivity reactions · hypoglycaemia (especially after parenteral administration) · intravascular coagulation · muscle weakness · nausea · photosensitivity · rashes · temporary blindness · thrombocytopenia · vertigo · visual disturbances · vomiting

Overdose

Quinine is very toxic in overdosage; life-threatening features include arrhythmias (which can have a very rapid onset) and convulsions (which can be intractable).
   For details on the management of poisoning, see Emergency treatment of poisoning p. 1194.

● PREGNANCY High doses are teratogenic in *first trimester*, but in malaria benefit of treatment outweighs risk.

● BREAST FEEDING Present in milk but not known to be harmful.

● HEPATIC IMPAIRMENT

▸ With intravenous use For treatment of malaria in severe impairment, reduce intravenous maintenance dose to 5–7 mg/kg of quinine salt.

- ● RENAL IMPAIRMENT
- ▶ With intravenous use For treatment of malaria in severe impairment, reduce parenteral maintenance dose to 5–7 mg/kg of quinine salt.
- ● MONITORING REQUIREMENTS
- ▶ With intravenous use Monitor blood glucose and electrolyte concentration during parenteral treatment.
- ▶ In adults Patients taking quinine for nocturnal leg cramps should be monitored closely during the early stages for adverse effects as well as for benefit.
- ● DIRECTIONS FOR ADMINISTRATION
- ▶ With intravenous use in children For *intravenous infusion*, dilute to a concentration of 2 mg/mL (max. 30 mg/mL in fluid restriction) with Glucose 5% *or* Sodium Chloride 0.9% and give over 4 hours.
- ▶ With intravenous use in adults For *intravenous infusion*, give continuously in Glucose 5% or Sodium Chloride 0.9%. To be given over 4 hours.
- ● PRESCRIBING AND DISPENSING INFORMATION Intravenous injection of quinine is so hazardous that it has been superseded by infusion.

- ● MEDICINAL FORMS
There can be variation in the licensing of different medicines containing the same drug. Forms available from special-order manufacturers include: capsule, oral suspension, oral solution, solution for infusion

Tablet
- ▶ Quinine (Non-proprietary)
  Quinine sulfate 200 mg Quinine sulfate 200mg tablets | 28 tablet [PoM] £6.05 DT price = £1.67
  Quinine bisulfate 300 mg Quinine bisulfate 300mg tablets | 28 tablet [PoM] £4.80 DT price = £1.91
  Quinine sulfate 300 mg Quinine sulfate 300mg tablets | 28 tablet [PoM] £5.05 DT price = £1.97 | 500 tablet [PoM] no price available

6 Viral infection

6.1 Hepatitis

Hepatitis

Overview

Treatment for viral hepatitis should be initiated by a specialist. The management of uncomplicated acute viral hepatitis is largely symptomatic. Early treatment of acute hepatitis C with interferon alfa p. 839 [unlicensed indication] may reduce the risk of chronic infection. Hepatitis B and hepatitis C viruses are major causes of chronic hepatitis. Active or passive immunisation against hepatitis A and B infections can be given.

Chronic hepatitis B

Peginterferon alfa p. 567 is an option for the initial treatment of chronic hepatitis B and may be preferable to interferon alfa. The use of peginterferon alfa and interferon alfa is limited by a response rate of 30–40% and relapse is frequent. Treatment should be discontinued if no improvement occurs after 4 months. The manufacturers of peginterferon alfa-2a and interferon alfa contraindicate use in decompensated liver disease, but low doses can be used with great caution in these patients. Although interferon alfa is contra-indicated in patients receiving immunosuppressant treatment (or who have received it recently), cautious use of peginterferon alfa-2a may be justified in some cases.

Entecavir p. 566 or tenofovir disoproxil p. 591 are options for the initial treatment of chronic hepatitis B. If the response is inadequate after 6–9 months of treatment, a change in treatment should be considered. Other drugs that

are licensed for the treatment of chronic hepatitis B include adefovir dipivoxil p. 567, lamivudine p. 590, or telbivudine p. 566.

Entecavir alone, tenofovir disoproxil alone, or a combination of lamivudine with either adefovir dipivoxil or tenofovir disoproxil can be used in patients with decompensated liver disease.

If drug-resistant hepatitis B virus emerges during treatment, another antiviral drug to which the virus is sensitive should be added. Hepatitis B viruses with reduced susceptibility to lamivudine have emerged following extended therapy. Adefovir dipivoxil or tenofovir disoproxil can be given with lamivudine in lamivudine-resistant chronic hepatitis B; telbivudine or entecavir should not be used because cross-resistance can occur.

If there is no toxicity or loss in efficacy, treatment with adefovir dipivoxil, entecavir, lamivudine, telbivudine, or tenofovir disoproxil is usually continued until 6 months after adequate seroconversion has occurred. Treatment is usually continued long-term in patients with decompensated liver disease.

Tenofovir disoproxil, or a combination of tenofovir disoproxil with either emtricitabine p. 589 or lamivudine may be used with other antiretrovirals, as part of 'highly active antiretroviral therapy' in patients who require treatment for both HIV and chronic hepatitis B. If patients infected with both HIV and chronic hepatitis B only require treatment for chronic hepatitis B, they should receive antivirals that are not active against HIV, such as peginterferon alfa or adefovir dipivoxil. Treatment may be continued long-term, even if adequate seroconversion occurs. Management of these patients should be coordinated between HIV and hepatology specialists.

Chronic hepatitis C

Before starting treatment, the genotype of the infecting hepatitis C virus should be determined and the viral load measured as this may affect the choice and duration of treatment. A combination of ribavirin p. 569 and peginterferon alfa is used for the treatment of chronic hepatitis C. The combination of ribavirin and interferon alfa is less effective than the combination of peginterferon alfa and ribavirin. Peginterferon alfa alone should be used if ribavirin is contra-indicated or not tolerated. Ribavirin monotherapy is ineffective.

Boceprevir p. 573 and telaprevir p. 574 are protease inhibitors that inhibit the replication of hepatitis C virus genotype 1, but they are less effective against other genotypes of the virus. Monotherapy is not recommended because there is a high likelihood of resistance developing. Either boceprevir or telaprevir is licensed for use in combination with ribavirin and peginterferon alfa for the treatment of chronic hepatitis C infection of genotype 1 in patients with compensated liver disease; these combinations are more effective than dual therapy with ribavirin and peginterferon alfa. However, triple therapy is associated with a higher incidence and greater severity of anaemia than dual therapy. Neutropenia seems to be more frequent during treatment with regimens containing boceprevir than with those containing telaprevir. Rash is a particular concern with telaprevir, and to a lesser extent with boceprevir.

Daclatasvir p. 568 is licensed for use in combination with sofosbuvir p. 571 for the treatment of chronic hepatitis C infection of genotypes 1 or 4, with or without compensated cirrhosis; the addition of ribavirin should be considered for patients with advanced liver disease or with other negative prognostic factors, such as prior treatment experience. It is also licensed in combination with sofosbuvir and ribavirin for the treatment of chronic hepatitis C infection of genotype 3 in patients who are treatment experienced, with or without compensated cirrhosis, and in combination with peginterferon alfa and ribavirin for the treatment of chronic

5

Infection

hepatitis C infection of genotype 4. Daclatasvir must not be given as monotherapy.

Ombitasvir with paritaprevir and ritonavir p. 569 (*Viekirax*®), is licensed for use in combination with dasabuvir p. 575, with or without ribavirin, for the treatment of chronic hepatitis C infection of genotype 1 in patients with or without compensated cirrhosis; it is also licensed for use in combination with ribavirin for the treatment of chronic hepatitis C infection of genotype 4 with or without compensated cirrhosis.

Sofosbuvir is a pro-drug of a nucleoside inhibitor that is effective against hepatitis C virus polymerase NS5B. It is licensed for use in combination with ribavirin, with or without peginterferon alfa, for the treatment of chronic hepatitis C infection of genotypes 1, 2, 3, 4, 5, or 6, in patients with compensated liver disease. Sofosbuvir monotherapy is not recommended because it is less effective than combination therapy.

Ledipasvir is licensed for use in combination with sofosbuvir (sofosbuvir with ledipasvir p. 572), with or without ribavirin, for the treatment of chronic hepatitis C infections of genotypes 1, 3, 4, 5 or 6.

Simeprevir p. 573 is licensed for use in combination with ribavirin and peginterferon alfa for the treatment of chronic hepatitis C infection of genotype 1 or 4; regimens containing peginterferon alfa-2b are less effective than those containing peginterferon alfa-2a. Simeprevir may also be used in combination with sofosbuvir, with or without ribavirin, for the urgent treatment of chronic hepatitis C infection of genotypes 1 or 4 only when peginterferon alfa cannot be used because of intolerance or contra-indications. Simeprevir monotherapy is not recommended.

6.2 Hepatitis infections

6.2a Chronic hepatitis B

> **Drugs used for Chronic hepatitis B not listed below**
> Interferon alfa, p. 839 · Lamivudine, p. 590 · Tenofovir disoproxil, p. 591

ANTIVIRALS 〉 NUCLEOSIDE ANALOGUES

Entecavir

● **INDICATIONS AND DOSE**

Chronic hepatitis B in patients with compensated liver disease (with evidence of viral replication, and histologically documented active liver inflammation or fibrosis) not previously treated with nucleoside analogues
▸ BY MOUTH
▹ Adult: 500 micrograms once daily

Chronic hepatitis B in patients with compensated liver disease (with evidence of viral replication, and histologically documented active liver inflammation or fibrosis) and lamivudine-resistance
▸ BY MOUTH
▹ Adult: 1 mg once daily, consider other treatment if inadequate response after 6 months

Chronic hepatitis B in patients with decompensated liver disease
▸ BY MOUTH
▹ Adult: 1 mg once daily

● **CAUTIONS** HIV infection—risk of HIV resistance in patients not receiving 'highly active antiretroviral therapy' · lamivudine-resistant chronic hepatitis B—risk of entecavir resistance

CAUTIONS, FURTHER INFORMATION
Discontinue if deterioration in liver function, hepatic steatosis, progressive hepatomegaly or unexplained lactic acidosis.

● **SIDE-EFFECTS**
▸ **Common or very common** Diarrhoea · dizziness · dyspepsia · fatigue · headache · nausea · raised serum amylase · raised serum lipase · sleep disturbances · vomiting
▸ **Uncommon** Alopecia · rash · thrombocytopenia

● **CONCEPTION AND CONTRACEPTION** Effective contraception required during treatment.

● **PREGNANCY** Toxicity in *animal* studies—manufacturer advises use only if potential benefit outweighs risk.

● **BREAST FEEDING** Manufacturer advises avoid—present in milk in *animal* studies.

● **RENAL IMPAIRMENT** Reduce dose if eGFR less than 50 mL/minute/1.73 m^2. Consult product literature.

● **MONITORING REQUIREMENTS** Monitor liver function tests every 3 months, and viral markers for hepatitis B every 3–6 months during treatment (continue monitoring for at least 1 year after discontinuation—recurrent hepatitis may occur on discontinuation).

● **DIRECTIONS FOR ADMINISTRATION** To be taken at least 2 hours before or 2 hours after food.

● **PRESCRIBING AND DISPENSING INFORMATION** Flavours of oral liquid formulations may include orange.

● **PATIENT AND CARER ADVICE** Patients or carers should be counselled on the administration of entecavir tablets and oral solution.

● **NATIONAL FUNDING/ACCESS DECISIONS**
NICE technology appraisals (TAs)
▸ **Entecavir for chronic hepatitis B (August 2008)** NICE TA153 Entecavir is an option for the treatment of chronic hepatitis B.
www.nice.org.uk/TA153

● **MEDICINAL FORMS**
There can be variation in the licensing of different medicines containing the same drug.
Tablet
▸ Baraclude (Bristol-Myers Squibb Pharmaceuticals Ltd)
   Entecavir (as Entecavir monohydrate) 500 microgram Baraclude 0.5mg tablets | 30 tablet PoM £363.26
   Entecavir (as Entecavir monohydrate) 1 mg Baraclude 1mg tablets | 30 tablet PoM £363.26
Oral solution
▸ Baraclude (Bristol-Myers Squibb Pharmaceuticals Ltd)
   Entecavir (as Entecavir monohydrate) 50 microgram per 1 ml Baraclude 0.05mg/ml oral solution sugar-free | 210 ml PoM £423.80

Telbivudine

● **INDICATIONS AND DOSE**

Chronic hepatitis B infection with compensated liver disease, evidence of viral replication, and histologically documented active liver inflammation or fibrosis, when other treatment is not appropriate
▸ BY MOUTH
▹ Adult: 600 mg once daily

● **CAUTIONS** Lamivudine-resistant chronic hepatitis B—risk of telbivudine resistance

CAUTIONS, FURTHER INFORMATION
Discontinue if deterioration in liver function, hepatic steatosis, progressive hepatomegaly or unexplained lactic acidosis.

● **INTERACTIONS** → Appendix 1 (telbivudine).

- SIDE-EFFECTS
  - ▶ **Common or very common** Abdominal pain · cough · diarrhoea · dizziness · fatigue · headache · nausea · raised serum amylase · raised serum lipase · rash
  - ▶ **Uncommon** Arthralgia · myalgia · myopathy (discontinue treatment) · peripheral neuropathy · taste disturbance
  - ▶ **Rare** Lactic acidosis · rhabdomyolysis
- PREGNANCY Manufacturer advises use only if potential benefit outweighs risk.
- BREAST FEEDING Manufacturer advises avoid—present in milk in *animal* studies.
- RENAL IMPAIRMENT 600 mg every 48 hours if eGFR 30–49 mL/minute/1.73 m^2; 600 mg every 72 hours if eGFR less than 30 mL/minute/1.73 m^2.
- MONITORING REQUIREMENTS Monitor liver function tests every 3 months and viral markers of hepatitis B every 3–6 months during treatment (continue monitoring for at least 1 year after discontinuation—recurrent hepatitis may occur on discontinuation).
- PATIENT AND CARER ADVICE
  Muscle effects and peripheral neuropathy Patients should be advised to promptly report unexplained muscle pain, tenderness, or weakness, or numbness, tingling or burning sensations.
- NATIONAL FUNDING/ACCESS DECISIONS
  NICE technology appraisals (TAs)
  ▶ **Telbivudine for chronic hepatitis B (August 2008)** NICE TA154 Telbivudine is not recommended for the treatment of chronic hepatitis B. Patients currently receiving telbivudine can continue treatment until they and their clinician consider it appropriate to stop.
  www.nice.org.uk/TA154
- MEDICINAL FORMS
  There can be variation in the licensing of different medicines containing the same drug.
  Tablet
  ▶ Sebivo (Novartis Pharmaceuticals UK Ltd)
    Telbivudine 600 mg Sebivo 600mg tablets | 28 tablet PoM
    £290.33

ANTIVIRALS > NUCLEOTIDE ANALOGUES

Adefovir dipivoxil

- INDICATIONS AND DOSE
  Chronic hepatitis B infection with either compensated liver disease with evidence of viral replication, and histologically documented active liver inflammation and fibrosis, when other treatment not appropriate or decompensated liver disease in combination with another antiviral for chronic hepatitis B that has no cross-resistance to adefovir
  ▶ BY MOUTH
  ▶ Adult: 10 mg once daily
- CAUTIONS Elderly
  CAUTIONS, FURTHER INFORMATION
  Discontinue if deterioration in liver function, hepatic steatosis, progressive hepatomegaly or unexplained lactic acidosis.
- SIDE-EFFECTS Abdominal pain · asthenia · diarrhoea · dyspepsia · flatulence · headache · hypophosphataemia · nausea · pancreatitis · pruritus · rash · renal failure · vomiting
- CONCEPTION AND CONTRACEPTION Effective contraception required during treatment.
- PREGNANCY Toxicity in *animal* studies—manufacturer advises use only if potential benefit outweighs risk.

- BREAST FEEDING Manufacturer advises avoid—no information available.
- RENAL IMPAIRMENT 10 mg every 48 hours if eGFR 30–50 mL/minute/1.73 m^2; 10 mg every 72 hours if eGFR 10–30 mL/minute/1.73 m^2. No information available if eGFR less than 10 mL/minute/1.73 m^2. Monitor renal function more frequently in patients with renal impairment.
- MONITORING REQUIREMENTS
  ▶ Monitor liver function tests every 3 months, and viral markers for hepatitis B every 3–6 months during treatment (continue monitoring for at least 1 year after discontinuation—recurrent hepatitis may occur on discontinuation).
  ▶ Monitor renal function before treatment then every 3 months, more frequently in patients receiving nephrotoxic drugs.
- MEDICINAL FORMS
  There can be variation in the licensing of different medicines containing the same drug.
  Tablet
  ▶ Hepsera (Gilead Sciences International Ltd)
    Adefovir dipivoxil 10 mg Hepsera 10mg tablets | 30 tablet PoM
    £252.22

IMMUNOSTIMULANTS > INTERFERONS

Peginterferon alfa

- DRUG ACTION Polyethylene glycol-conjugated ('pegylated') derivatives of interferon alfa (peginterferon alfa-2a and peginterferon alfa-2b) are available; pegylation increases the persistence of the interferon in the blood.
- INDICATIONS AND DOSE
  PEGASYS®
  Combined with ribavirin for chronic hepatitis C | Monotherapy for chronic hepatitis C if ribavirin not tolerated or contra-indicated | Monotherapy for chronic hepatitis B
  ▶ BY SUBCUTANEOUS INJECTION
  ▶ Adult: (consult product literature)
  VIRAFERONPEG®
  Combined with ribavirin for chronic hepatitis C | Combined with ribavirin and boceprevir for chronic hepatitis C infection of genotype 1 in patients with compensated liver disease | Monotherapy for chronic hepatitis C if ribavirin not tolerated or contra-indicated
  ▶ BY SUBCUTANEOUS INJECTION
  ▶ Adult: (consult product literature)
- CONTRA-INDICATIONS
  CONTRA-INDICATIONS, FURTHER INFORMATION
  For contra-indications consult product literature.
- CAUTIONS
  CAUTIONS, FURTHER INFORMATION
  For cautions consult product literature.
- INTERACTIONS → Appendix 1 (interferons).
- SIDE-EFFECTS
  ▶ **Common or very common** Anorexia · diarrhoea · influenza-like symptoms · lethargy · nausea
  ▶ **Frequency not known** Alopecia · arrhythmias · cardiovascular problems · coma (usually with high doses in the elderly) · confusion · depression · hepatotoxicity · hyperglycaemia · hypersensitivity reactions · hypertension · hypertriglyceridaemia (sometimes severe) · hypotension · myelosuppression (particularly affecting granulocyte counts) · nephrotoxicity · ocular side-effects · palpitation ·

Infection

5

psoriasiform rash · seizures (usually with high doses in the elderly) · suicidal behaviour · thyroid abnormalities

SIDE-EFFECTS, FURTHER INFORMATION

For information on side effects consult product literature.

● CONCEPTION AND CONTRACEPTION Effective contraception required during treatment—consult product literature.

● PREGNANCY Manufacturers recommend avoid unless potential benefit outweighs risk (toxicity in *animal* studies).

● BREAST FEEDING Manufacturers advise avoid—no information available.

● HEPATIC IMPAIRMENT Avoid in severe impairment. Close monitoring required in mild to moderate hepatic impairment.

● RENAL IMPAIRMENT Reduce dose in moderate to severe impairment. For information on peginterferon alfa use in renal impairment consult product literature. Close monitoring required in renal impairment.

● MONITORING REQUIREMENTS Monitoring of lipid concentration is recommended.

● NATIONAL FUNDING/ACCESS DECISIONS

NICE technology appraisals (TAs)

▸ Peginterferon alfa and ribavirin for mild chronic hepatitis C (August 2006 and September 2010) NICE TA200
The combination of peginterferon alfa and ribavirin can be used for treating mild chronic hepatitis C in patients over 18 years. Alternatively, treatment can be delayed until the disease has reached a moderate stage ('watchful waiting'). Peginterferon alfa alone can be used if ribavirin is contra-indicated or not tolerated.
www.nice.org.uk/TA200

▸ Peginterferon alfa, interferon alfa, and ribavirin for moderate to severe chronic hepatitis C (January 2004 and September 2010) NICE TA200
The combination of peginterferon alfa and ribavirin should be used for treating moderate to severe chronic hepatitis C in patients aged over 18 years:
  ● not previously treated with interferon alfa or peginterferon alfa;
  ● treated previously with interferon alfa alone or in combination with ribavirin;
  ● whose condition did not respond to peginterferon alfa alone or to a combination of peginterferon alfa and ribavirin, or responded but subsequently relapsed;
  ● co-infected with HIV.
Peginterferon alfa alone should be used if ribavirin is contra-indicated or not tolerated. Interferon alfa for either monotherapy or combined therapy should be used only if neutropenia and thrombocytopenia are a particular risk. Patients receiving interferon alfa may be switched to peginterferon alfa.
www.nice.org.uk/TA200

● MEDICINAL FORMS
There can be variation in the licensing of different medicines containing the same drug.
Solution for injection
EXCIPIENTS: May contain Benzyl alcohol
▸ Pegasys (Roche Products Ltd)
Peginterferon alfa-2a 180 microgram per 1 ml Pegasys 90micrograms/0.5ml solution for injection pre-filled syringes | 1 pre-filled disposable injection PoM £76.51
Peginterferon alfa-2a 270 microgram per 1 ml Pegasys 135micrograms/0.5ml solution for injection pre-filled syringes | 1 pre-filled disposable injection PoM £107.76
Pegasys 135micrograms/0.5ml solution for injection pre-filled pen | 1 pre-filled disposable injection PoM £107.76
Peginterferon alfa-2a 360 microgram per 1 ml Pegasys 180micrograms/0.5ml solution for injection pre-filled syringes | 4 pre-filled disposable injection PoM £497.60
Pegasys 180micrograms/0.5ml solution for injection pre-filled pen | 4 pre-filled disposable injection PoM £497.60

Powder and solvent for solution for injection
▸ ViraferonPeg (Merck Sharp & Dohme Ltd)
Peginterferon alfa-2b 50 microgram ViraferonPeg 50microgram powder and solvent for solution for injection pre-filled disposable devices | 1 pre-filled disposable injection PoM £66.46
Peginterferon alfa-2b 80 microgram ViraferonPeg 80microgram powder and solvent for solution for injection pre-filled disposable devices | 1 pre-filled disposable injection PoM £106.34
Peginterferon alfa-2b 100 microgram ViraferonPeg 100microgram powder and solvent for solution for injection pre-filled disposable devices | 1 pre-filled disposable injection PoM £132.92
Peginterferon alfa-2b 120 microgram ViraferonPeg 120microgram powder and solvent for solution for injection pre-filled disposable devices | 1 pre-filled disposable injection PoM £159.51
Peginterferon alfa-2b 150 microgram ViraferonPeg 150microgram powder and solvent for solution for injection pre-filled disposable devices | 1 pre-filled disposable injection PoM £199.38

6.2b Chronic hepatitis C

Drugs used for Chronic hepatitis C not listed below
Interferon alfa, p. 839 · Peginterferon alfa, p. 567

ANTIVIRALS ⟩ NON-STRUCTURAL PROTEIN 5A INHIBITORS

Daclatasvir
22.3.2016

● DRUG ACTION Daclatasvir is an inhibitor of the multifunctional protein NS5A, which is an essential component of the hepatitis C virus replication process.

● INDICATIONS AND DOSE
In combination with sofosbuvir for the treatment of chronic hepatitis C infection of genotypes 1 or 4, with or without compensated cirrhosis | In combination with sofosbuvir and ribavirin for the treatment of chronic hepatitis C infection of genotype 3 in patients who are treatment experienced, with or without compensated cirrhosis | In combination with peginterferon alfa and ribavirin for the treatment of chronic hepatitis C infection of genotype 4
▸ BY MOUTH
▸ Adult: Usual dose 60 mg once daily (for duration of treatment consult product literature)

DOSE ADJUSTMENTS DUE TO INTERACTIONS
Reduce dose to 30 mg once daily with concomitant use of potent CYP3A4 inhibitors (e.g. atazanavir boosted with ritonavir, boceprevir, clarithromycin, cobicistat, itraconazole, ketoconazole, posaconazole, telaprevir, telithromycin, and voriconazole).
Increase dose to 90 mg once daily with concomitant use of moderate CYP3A4 inducers (e.g. efavirenz).

● CAUTIONS Decompensated liver disease · hepatitis B virus co-infection · human immunodeficiency virus co-infection · organ transplant patients · retreatment—efficacy not established in patients with prior exposure to a NS5A inhibitor

● INTERACTIONS → Appendix 1 (daclatasvir).

● SIDE-EFFECTS
▸ **Common or very common** Abdominal pain · alopecia · anaemia · anxiety · arthralgia · blurred vision · constipation · cough · decreased appetite · depression · diarrhoea · disturbance in attention · dizziness · dry mouth · dry skin · dyspnoea · flatulence · gastro-oesophageal reflux · headache · hot flush · insomnia · irritability · lymphopenia · malaise · migraine · myalgia · nasal congestion · nausea · neutropenia · pruritus · pyrexia · rash · reduced visual acuity · vomiting

SIDE-EFFECTS, FURTHER INFORMATION
Side-effects listed are reported when daclatasvir is used in combination with sofosbuvir with or without ribavirin *or* with ribavirin and peginterferon alfa.

- CONCEPTION AND CONTRACEPTION Highly effective contraception required during and for 5 weeks after treatment.
- PREGNANCY Manufacturer advises avoid (toxicity in *animal* studies).
- BREAST FEEDING Manufacturer advises avoid—present in milk in *animal* studies.
- PATIENT AND CARER ADVICE
Missed doses
If a dose is more than 20 hours late, the missed dose should not be taken and the next dose should be taken at the normal time.
Driving and skilled tasks
May affect performance of skilled tasks (e.g. driving)
- NATIONAL FUNDING/ACCESS DECISIONS
NICE technology appraisals (TAs)
▶ Daclatasvir for treating chronic hepatitis C (November 2015) NICE TA364
Daclatasvir in combination with sofosbuvir or peginterferon alfa, and with/without ribavirin, is recommended as an option for the treatment of chronic hepatitis C infection of genotypes 1, 3 or 4 in adults, depending on the level of fibrosis **and** only if the manufacturer provides daclatasvir at the same price or lower than agreed with the Commercial Medicines Unit.
www.nice.org.uk/TA364
Scottish Medicines Consortium (SMC) Decisions
The *Scottish Medicines Consortium* has advised (November 2014) that daclatasvir (*Daklinza*®) is accepted for restricted use within NHS Scotland for the treatment of chronic hepatitis C virus infection in patients with significant fibrosis (Metavir score F3–F4) or compensated cirrhosis.

- MEDICINAL FORMS
There can be variation in the licensing of different medicines containing the same drug.
Tablet
CAUTIONARY AND ADVISORY LABELS 25
▶ Daklinza (Bristol-Myers Squibb Pharmaceuticals Ltd) ▼
Daclatasvir (as Daclatasvir dihydrochloride) 30 mg Daklinza 30mg tablets | 28 tablet PoM £8,172.61
Daclatasvir (as Daclatasvir dihydrochloride) 60 mg Daklinza 60mg tablets | 28 tablet PoM £8,172.61

Ombitasvir with paritaprevir and ritonavir
29.3.2016

The properties listed below are those particular to the combination only. For the properties of the components please consider, ritonavir p. 596.

- INDICATIONS AND DOSE
Chronic hepatitis C of genotype 1 (in combination with dasabuvir, with or without ribavirin) | Chronic hepatitis C of genotype 4 (in combination with ribavirin)
▶ BY MOUTH
▶ Adult: 2 tablets once daily for duration of treatment consult product literature, to be taken with food

- CONTRA-INDICATIONS HIV co-infection without suppressive antiretroviral therapy
- CAUTIONS Retreatment—efficacy not established
- INTERACTIONS → Appendix 1 (ombitasvir, paritaprevir, ritonavir).

- SIDE-EFFECTS
▶ **Common or very common** Anaemia · asthenia · fatigue · insomnia · nausea
▶ **Frequency not known** Transient hyperbilirubinemia
SIDE-EFFECTS, FURTHER INFORMATION
Side-effects listed are reported when ombitasvir with paritaprevir and ritonavir is used in combination with dasabuvir, with or without ribavirin.

- CONCEPTION AND CONTRACEPTION For women of child-bearing potential, exclude pregnancy before initiation of treatment; effective contraception should be used during treatment.
- PREGNANCY Manufacturer advises avoid—toxicity in *animal* studies.
- BREAST FEEDING Manufacturer advises avoid—present in milk in *animal* studies.
- HEPATIC IMPAIRMENT Manufacturer advises avoid in moderate or severe impairment.
- PATIENT AND CARER ADVICE
Missed doses
If a dose is more than 12 hours late, the missed dose should not be taken and the next dose should be taken at the normal time.
- NATIONAL FUNDING/ACCESS DECISIONS
NICE technology appraisals (TAs)
▶ Ombitasvir with paritaprevir and ritonavir with or without dasabuvir for treating chronic hepatitis C NICE TA365
Ombitasvir with paritaprevir and ritonavir with or without dasabuvir is recommended, within its marketing authorisation, as an option for treating genotype 1 or 4 chronic hepatitis C in adults, only if the manufacturer provides it with the discount agreed in the patient access scheme.
www.nice.org.uk/guidance/ta365

- MEDICINAL FORMS
There can be variation in the licensing of different medicines containing the same drug.
Tablet
CAUTIONARY AND ADVISORY LABELS 21, 25
EXCIPIENTS: May contain Propylene glycol
▶ Viekirax (AbbVie Ltd) ▼
Ombitasvir 12.5 mg, Ritonavir 50 mg, Paritaprevir 75 mg Viekirax 12.5mg/75mg/50mg tablets | 56 tablet PoM £10,733.33

ANTIVIRALS › NUCLEOSIDE ANALOGUES

Ribavirin
(Tribavirin)

- INDICATIONS AND DOSE
Bronchiolitis
▶ BY INHALATION OF AEROSOL, OR BY INHALATION OF NEBULISED SOLUTION
▶ Child 1-23 months: Inhale a solution containing 20 mg/mL for 12–18 hours for at least 3 days, maximum of 7 days, to be administered via small particle aerosol generator
Life-threatening RSV, parainfluenza virus, and adenovirus infection in immunocompromised children (administered on expert advice)
▶ BY INTRAVENOUS INFUSION
▶ Child: 33 mg/kg for 1 dose, to be administered over 15 minutes, then 16 mg/kg every 6 hours for 4 days, then 8 mg/kg every 8 hours for 3 days
continued →

5

Infection

COPEGUS® TABLETS

Chronic hepatitis C (in combination with direct acting antivirals, or interferon alfa 2a, or peginterferon alfa 2a with or without direct acting antivirals)
▸ BY MOUTH
▸ Adult (body-weight up to 75 kg): 400 mg, dose to be taken in the morning and 600 mg, dose to be taken in the evening
▸ Adult (body-weight 75 kg and above): 600 mg twice daily

Chronic hepatitis C (in combination with peginterferon alfa 2b with or without direct acting antivirals)
▸ BY MOUTH
▸ Adult (body-weight up to 65 kg): 400 mg twice daily
▸ Adult (body-weight 65-80 kg): 400 mg, to be taken in the morning and 600 mg, to be taken in the evening
▸ Adult (body-weight 81-105 kg): 600 mg twice daily
▸ Adult (body-weight 106 kg and above): 600 mg, to be taken in the morning and 800 mg, to be taken in the evening

Chronic hepatitis C genotype 2 or 3 (not previously treated), or patients infected with HIV and hepatitis C (in combination with peginterferon alfa)
▸ BY MOUTH
▸ Adult: Usual dose 400 mg twice daily

REBETOL® CAPSULES

Chronic hepatitis C (in combination with interferon alfa 2b, or peginterferon alfa 2b with or without boceprevir)
▸ BY MOUTH
▸ Adult (body-weight up to 65 kg): 400 mg twice daily
▸ Adult (body-weight 65-80 kg): 400 mg, dose to be taken in the morning and 600 mg, dose to be taken in the evening
▸ Adult (body-weight 81-104 kg): 600 mg twice daily
▸ Adult (body-weight 105 kg and above): 600 mg, dose to be taken in the morning and 800 mg, dose to be taken in the evening

REBETOL® ORAL SOLUTION

Chronic hepatitis C (in combination with interferon alfa 2b, or peginterferon alfa 2b with or without boceprevir)
▸ BY MOUTH
▸ Adult (body-weight up to 65 kg): 400 mg twice daily
▸ Adult (body-weight 65-80 kg): 400 mg daily, dose to be taken in the morning and 600 mg daily, dose to be taken in the evening
▸ Adult (body-weight 81-104 kg): 600 mg twice daily
▸ Adult (body-weight 105 kg and above): 600 mg daily, dose to be taken in the morning and 800 mg daily, dose to be taken in the evening

● UNLICENSED USE
▸ When used by inhalation in children Inhalation licensed for use in children (age range not specified by manufacturer).
▸ With intravenous use in children Intravenous preparation not licensed.

● CONTRA-INDICATIONS
▸ With systemic use Active severe psychiatric condition (in children) · autoimmune disease (in children) · autoimmune hepatitis (in children) · consult product literature for specific contra-indications when ribavirin p. 569 used in combination with other medicinal products · haemoglobinopathies · history of severe psychiatric condition (in children) · severe cardiac disease (in adults) · severe debilitating medical conditions · severe, uncontrolled cardiac disease in children with chronic hepatitis C (in children) · unstable or uncontrolled cardiac disease in previous 6 months (in adults)

● CAUTIONS
▸ When used by inhalation Maintain standard supportive respiratory and fluid management therapy

▸ With systemic use Anaemia (haemoglobin concentration should be monitored during the treatment and corrective action taken) (in adults) · cardiac disease (assessment including ECG recommended before and during treatment—discontinue if deterioration) · consult product literature for specific cautions when ribavirin p. 569 used in combination with other medicinal products · gout (in adults) · haemolysis (haemoglobin concentration should be monitored during the treatment and corrective action taken) (in adults) · patients with a transplant—risk of rejection · risk of growth retardation in children, the reversibility of which is uncertain—if possible, consider starting treatment after pubertal growth spurt (in children) · severe dental disorders (in adults) · severe ocular disorders (in adults) · severe periodontal disorders (in adults) · severe psychiatric effects (in adults)

● INTERACTIONS → Appendix 1 (ribavirin).

● SIDE-EFFECTS
▸ When used by inhalation Bacterial pneumonia · haemolysis · non-specific anaemia · pneumothorax · worsening respiration
▸ With oral use Abdominal pain · abnormal dreams · acne · alopecia · angina (in adults) · anorexia (in adults) · anxiety · aplastic anaemia · arrhythmias · arthralgia · asthenia (in children) · ataxia · bipolar disorders (in adults) · breast pain · cardiomyopathy · cerebral haemorrhage (in adults) · cerebral ischaemia (in adults) · changes in blood pressure · cheilitis · chest pain · colitis · constipation · cough · dehydration · depression · diabetes (in adults) · diarrhoea · dizziness · dry eyes · dry mouth · dry skin · dyspepsia · dysphagia · dysphonia (in children) · dyspnoea · earache · endocarditis (in adults) · epistaxis (in children) · eye pain · flatulence · flushing · gastro-intestinal bleeding · gastroesophageal reflux (in children) · gingival bleeding (in adults) · gingivitis · glossitis · growth retardation (including decrease in height and weight) (in children) · haemolytic anaemia (anaemia may be improved by epoetin) · hallucination (in children) · headache · hearing impairment · hearing loss (in adults) · hyperaesthesia · hyperglycaemia · hyperkinesia (in children) · hypertonia · hypertriglyceridaemia · hyperuricaemia · hypoaesthesia · hypocalcaemia · impaired concentration and memory · increased sweating · influenza-like symptoms · interstitial pneumonitis · leucopenia · loose stools (in children) · lymphadenopathy · malaise (in adults) · mania (in adults) · menstrual disturbance · micturition disorders · mood disorders (in children) · mouth ulcers · musculoskeletal pain · myalgia · myocardial infarction · myositis (in adults) · nasal congestion · nausea · neutropenia · optic neuropathy · oral candidiasis · pallor (in children) · palpitation · pancreatitis · panic attack (in children) · paraesthesia · peptic ulcer · pericarditis · peripheral ischaemia (in children) · peripheral neuropathy · peripheral oedema · photosensitivity · prostatitis (in adults) · pruritus · psoriasis · psychotic disorders · pulmonary embolism · rash · renal failure · respiratory infections · retinal detachment (in adults) · retinal haemorrhage (in adults) · rhabdomyolysis (in adults) · rheumatoid arthritis · sarcoidosis · seizures · sexual dysfunction · sinus congestion · skin discoloration · sleep disturbances · sore throat · Stevens-Johnson syndrome · stomatitis · stroke (in children) · suicidal ideation (more frequent in children) · syncope · systemic lupus erythematosus · tachycardia · tachypnoea (in children) · taste disturbance · testicular pain (in children) · thrombocytopenia · thrombocytopenia purpura (in adults) · thyroid disorders · tinnitus · tongue pigmentation (in adults) · tooth disorder (in children) · toxic epidermal necrolysis · tremor (in adults) · urinary tract infections · vaculitis (in children) · vertigo (in children) · virilism (in children) · vision loss (in adults) · visual disturbances · vomiting · weight loss · wheezing

SIDE-EFFECTS, FURTHER INFORMATION
Side effects listed are reported when oral ribivirin is used in combination with peginterferon alfa or interferon alfa, consult product literature for details.

- **CONCEPTION AND CONTRACEPTION**
  - With systemic use Exclude pregnancy before treatment in females of childbearing age. Effective contraception essential during treatment and for 4 months after treatment in females and for 7 months after treatment in males of childbearing age. Routine monthly pregnancy tests recommended. Condoms must be used if partner of male patient is pregnant (ribavirin excreted in semen).
  - When used by inhalation Women planning pregnancy should avoid exposure to aerosol.
- **PREGNANCY** Avoid; teratogenicity in *animal* studies.
  - When used by inhalation Pregnant women should avoid exposure to aerosol.
- **BREAST FEEDING** Avoid—no information available.
- **HEPATIC IMPAIRMENT** No dosage adjustment required. Avoid oral ribavirin in severe hepatic dysfunction or decompensated cirrhosis.
- **RENAL IMPAIRMENT** Plasma-ribavirin concentration increased.
  - In adults Manufacturer advises avoid oral ribavirin unless essential if eGFR less than 50 mL/minute/1.73 m²—monitor haemoglobin concentration closely.
  - In children Manufacturer advises avoid oral ribavirin if estimated glomerular filtration rate less than 50 mL/minute/1.73 m²—monitor haemoglobin concentration closely. Manufacturer advises use intravenous preparation with caution if estimated glomerular filtration rate less than 30 mL/minute/1.73 m².
- **MONITORING REQUIREMENTS**
  - When used by inhalation Monitor electrolytes closely. Monitor equipment for precipitation.
  - With systemic use Determine full blood count, platelets, electrolytes, glucose, serum creatinine, liver function tests and uric acid before starting treatment and then on weeks 2 and 4 of treatment, then as indicated clinically—adjust dose if adverse reactions or laboratory abnormalities develop (consult product literature).
  - With systemic use in children Test thyroid function before treatment and then every 3 months.
- **PRESCRIBING AND DISPENSING INFORMATION** Flavours of oral liquid formulations may include bubble-gum.
- **NATIONAL FUNDING/ACCESS DECISIONS**

  NICE technology appraisals (TAs)
  - Peginterferon alfa and ribavirin for mild chronic hepatitis C (August 2006 and September 2010) NICE TA200
  - In adults The combination of peginterferon alfa and ribavirin can be used for treating mild chronic hepatitis C in patients over 18 years. Alternatively, treatment can be delayed until the disease has reached a moderate stage ('watchful waiting').
  www.nice.org.uk/TA200
  - Peginterferon alfa, interferon alfa, and ribavirin for moderate to severe chronic hepatitis C (January 2004 and September 2010) NICE TA200
  - In adults The combination of peginterferon alfa and ribavirin should be used for treating moderate to severe chronic hepatitis C in patients aged over 18 years:.
    - not previously treated with interferon alfa or peginterferon alfa;
    - treated previously with interferon alfa alone or in combination with ribavirin;
    - whose condition did not respond to peginterferon alfa alone or to a combination of peginterferon alfa and ribavirin, or responded but subsequently relapsed;
    - co-infected with HIV.
  Peginterferon alfa alone should be used if ribavirin is contra-indicated or not tolerated. Interferon alfa for either

monotherapy or combined therapy should be used only if neutropenia and thrombocytopenia are a particular risk. Patients receiving interferon alfa may be switched to peginterferon alfa.
www.nice.org.uk/TA200

- **LESS SUITABLE FOR PRESCRIBING** Ribavirin inhalation is less suitable for prescribing.
- **MEDICINAL FORMS**
  There can be variation in the licensing of different medicines containing the same drug. No licensed solution for injection listed

Tablet
CAUTIONARY AND ADVISORY LABELS 21
- Ribavirin (Non-proprietary)
  Ribavirin 200 mg Ribavirin 200mg tablets | 42 tablet [PoM] £92.50 | 112 tablet [PoM] £246.55 | 168 tablet [PoM] £369.98
- Copegus (Roche Products Ltd)
  Ribavirin 200 mg Copegus 200mg tablets | 42 tablet [PoM] £92.50 | 112 tablet [PoM] £246.65 | 168 tablet [PoM] £369.98
  Ribavirin 400 mg Copegus 400mg tablets | 56 tablet [PoM] £246.65

Capsule
CAUTIONARY AND ADVISORY LABELS 21
- Ribavirin (Non-proprietary)
  Ribavirin 200 mg Ribavirin 200mg capsules | 84 capsule [PoM] £160.69 | 140 capsule [PoM] £267.81 | 168 capsule [PoM] £321.38
- Rebetol (Merck Sharp & Dohme Ltd)
  Ribavirin 200 mg Rebetol 200mg capsules | 84 capsule [PoM] £160.69 | 140 capsule [PoM] £267.81 | 168 capsule [PoM] £321.38

Oral solution
CAUTIONARY AND ADVISORY LABELS 21
- Rebetol (Merck Sharp & Dohme Ltd)
  Ribavirin 40 mg per 1 ml Rebetol 40mg/ml oral solution | 100 ml [PoM] £67.08

ANTIVIRALS > NUCLEOTIDE ANALOGUES

Sofosbuvir

- **INDICATIONS AND DOSE**

  In combination with ribavirin (Copegus®), with or without peginterferon alfa, for chronic hepatitis C infection of genotypes 1, 3, 4, 5, or 6 in patients with compensated liver disease | In combination with ribavirin (Copegus®) for chronic hepatitis C infection of genotype 2 in patients with compensated liver disease | In combination with daclatasvir for chronic hepatitis C infection of genotype 1, 3, or 4
  - BY MOUTH
    - Adult: 400 mg once daily, for duration of treatment consult product literature

- **CAUTIONS**
  CAUTIONS, FURTHER INFORMATION
  In chronic hepatitis C of genotype 1, 4, 5, or 6, only use sofosbuvir with ribavirin in those with intolerance or contra-indications to peginterferon alfa who require urgent treatment.
- **INTERACTIONS** → Appendix 1 (sofosbuvir).
- **SIDE-EFFECTS** Abdominal discomfort · agitation · alopecia · anaemia · anxiety · arthralgia · asthenia · blurred vision · chest pain · constipation · cough · decreased appetite · depression · diarrhoea · disturbance in attention · dizziness · dry mouth · dyspnoea · gastro-oesophageal reflux · headache · influenza-like symptoms · insomnia · irritability · memory impairment · migraine · myalgia · nausea · neutropenia · rash · vomiting · weight loss
  SIDE-EFFECTS, FURTHER INFORMATION
  Side-effects listed are reported when sofosbuvir is used in combination with ribavirin *or* with ribavirin and peginterferon alfa.
- **PREGNANCY** Manufacturer advises avoid.

- BREAST FEEDING Manufacturer advises avoid—metabolites present in milk in *animal* studies.
- RENAL IMPAIRMENT Safety and efficacy not established if eGFR less than 30 mL/minute/1.73 m^2—accumulation may occur.
- PRESCRIBING AND DISPENSING INFORMATION Dispense in original container (contains desiccant).
- PATIENT AND CARER ADVICE

Missed doses
If a dose is more than 18 hours late, the missed dose should not be taken and the next dose should be taken at the normal time.

- NATIONAL FUNDING/ACCESS DECISIONS

NICE technology appraisals (TAs)

▶ **Sofosbuvir for treating chronic hepatitis C (February 2015)** NICE TA330
Sofosbuvir in combination with peginterferon alfa and ribavirin is an option for treating adults with chronic hepatitis C infection:
  - of genotype 1
  - of genotype 3 with cirrhosis (treatment naive patients)
  - of genotype 3 that has not adequately responded to interferon-based treatment
  - of genotype 4, 5, or 6 with cirrhosis
Sofosbuvir in combination with ribavirin is an option for treating adults with chronic hepatitis C infection:
  - of genotype 2 who are intolerant to *or* ineligible for interferon (treatment naive patients)
  - of genotype 2 that has not adequately responded to interferon-based treatment
  - of genotype 3 with cirrhosis who are intolerant to *or* ineligible for interferon (treatment naive patients)
  - of genotype 3 with cirrhosis that has not adequately responded to interferon-based treatment
www.nice.org.uk/TA330

▶ **Sofosbuvir for treating chronic hepatitis C (February 2015)** NICE TA330
Sofosbuvir in combination with ribavirin is not recommended for the treatment of adults with chronic hepatitis C infection of genotypes 1, 4, 5, or 6.
www.nice.org.uk/TA330

Scottish Medicines Consortium (SMC) Decisions
The *Scottish Medicines Consortium* has advised (June 2014) that sofosbuvir (*Sovaldi*®) is accepted for use within NHS Scotland for the treatment of chronic hepatitis C infection of genotypes 1 to 6; its use in combination with ribavirin as dual therapy for chronic hepatitis C infection of either genotype 2 (in treatment naive patients) or genotype 3 is restricted to those who cannot use peginterferon alfa because of intolerance or contra-indications.

- MEDICINAL FORMS
There can be variation in the licensing of different medicines containing the same drug.

Tablet
CAUTIONARY AND ADVISORY LABELS 21, 25
▶ Sovaldi (Gilead Sciences International Ltd) ▼
  Sofosbuvir 400 mg Sovaldi 400mg tablets | 28 tablet [PoM]
  £11,660.98

Sofosbuvir with ledipasvir

25.4.2016

The properties listed below are those particular to the combination only. For the properties of the components please consider, sofosbuvir p. 571.

- DRUG ACTION Sofosbuvir is a nucleotide analogue inhibitor and ledipasvir is an HCV inhibitor; they reduce viral load by inhibiting hepatitis C virus RNA replication.

- INDICATIONS AND DOSE

Chronic hepatitis C of genotypes 1, 4, 5 or 6 in patients with or without compensated cirrhosis (with or without ribavirin) | Chronic hepatitis C of genotypes 1, 4, 5 or 6 in post-liver transplant patients, with or without compensated cirrhosis (with or without ribavirin) | Chronic hepatitis C of genotypes 1, 4, 5 or 6 in patients with decompensated cirrhosis, irrespective of transplant status (with or without ribavirin) | In combination with ribavirin for chronic hepatitis C infection of genotype 3 in patients with compensated cirrhosis or prior treatment failure
  ▶ BY MOUTH
  ▶ Adult: 1 tablet once daily, for duration of treatment consult product literature

- CAUTIONS Retreatment following treatment failure—efficacy not established
- INTERACTIONS → Appendix 1 (sofosbuvir, ledipasvir)
- SIDE-EFFECTS
  ▶ **Common or very common** Headache · malaise
- BREAST FEEDING Manufacturer advises avoid—present in milk in *animal* studies.
- PRESCRIBING AND DISPENSING INFORMATION Dispense in original container (contains desiccant).
- PATIENT AND CARER ADVICE

Missed doses
If a dose is more than 18 hours late, the missed dose should not be taken and the next dose should be taken at the normal time.
Vomiting If vomiting occurs within 5 hours of administration, an additional dose should be taken.

- NATIONAL FUNDING/ACCESS DECISIONS

NICE technology appraisals (TAs)

▶ **Ledipasvir with sofosbuvir for the treatment of chronic hepatitis C (November 2015)** NICE TA363
Ledipasvir with sofosbuvir is recommended as an option for treating adults with chronic hepatitis C infection:
  - of genotype 1 without cirrhosis (treatment naive patients)—8 weeks' treatment
  - of genotype 1 or 4 with cirrhosis (treatment naive patients)—12 weeks' treatment
  - of genotype 1 or 4 without cirrhosis (or with cirrhosis but only if the person has a low risk of the disease getting worse) that has not responded adequately to previous treatment—12 weeks' treatment
In addition, ledipasvir with sofosbuvir is only recommended in patients with cirrhosis for the durations mentioned above if the following criteria are met:
  - Child-Pugh class A
  - platelet count of 75 000/mm^3 or more
  - no features of portal hypertension
  - no history of an HCV-associated decompensation episode
  - not previously treated with an NS5A inhibitor
Patients whose treatment with ledipasvir with sofosbuvir is not recommended in this NICE guidance, but was started within the NHS before this guidance was published, should be able to continue treatment until they and their clinician consider it appropriate to stop.
www.nice.org.uk/TA363

Scottish Medicines Consortium (SMC) Decisions

The *Scottish Medicines Consortium* has advised (March and September 2015) that *Harvoni*® (ledipasvir with sofosbuvir) is accepted for restricted use within NHS Scotland for the treatment of chronic hepatitis C infection of genotypes 1, 3 and 4 only, in patients who are ineligible for, or unable to tolerate, interferon.

● MEDICINAL FORMS

There can be variation in the licensing of different medicines containing the same drug.

Tablet

▸ Harvoni (Gilead Sciences International Ltd) ▼
Ledipasvir 90 mg, Sofosbuvir 400 mg Harvoni 90mg/400mg tablets | 28 tablet PoM £12,993.33

ANTIVIRALS > PROTEASE INHIBITORS

Boceprevir

● INDICATIONS AND DOSE

Chronic hepatitis C infection of genotype 1 in patients with compensated liver disease (in combination with ribavirin and peginterferon alfa)

▸ BY MOUTH
▸ Adult: 800 mg 3 times a day, for duration of treatment consult product literature

DOSE ADJUSTMENTS DUE TO INTERACTIONS

Appendix 1 (boceprevir).

Caution with concomitant use of other drugs known to prolong QT interval.

● CONTRA-INDICATIONS Autoimmune hepatitis

● CAUTIONS Coagulopathy · hypoalbuminaemia · low platelets · predisposition to QT interval prolongation

CAUTIONS, FURTHER INFORMATION

▸ Low platelets, hypoalbuminaemia, or coagulopathy Not recommended in patients with low platelets, hypoalbuminaemia, or coagulopathy—if initiated in these patients monitor closely for signs of infection, worsening liver impairment and anaemia (increased risk of severe morbidity and mortality).

● SIDE-EFFECTS

▸ **Common or very common** Abdominal pain · agitation · alopecia · amnesia · anaemia · anxiety · arthralgia · asthenia · blood pressure changes · changes in libido · constipation · cough · decreased appetite · depression · diarrhoea · disturbances in smell · disturbances in taste · dizziness · dry eyes · dry mouth · dyspnoea · erectile dysfunction · flatulence · gastro-oesophageal reflux · haemorrhoids · headache · hyperglycaemia · hyperhidrosis · hypertriglyceridaemia · hyperuricaemia · hypoaesthesia · hypothyroidism · influenza-like symptoms · insomnia · leucopenia · mouth ulcers · muscle spasms · myalgia · nausea · palpitation · pancytopenia · paraesthesia · peripheral oedema · polyuria · pruritus · psoriasis · rash · stomatitis · syncope · thrombocytopenia · tinnitus · tooth disorder · tremor · visual disturbances · vomiting · weight loss

▸ **Uncommon** Amenorrhoea · arrhythmias · colitis · conjunctival haemorrhage · dysphagia · dysphonia · dysuria · eye pain · flushing · gingivitis · gout · hearing impairment · homicidal ideation · hyperaesthesia · hyperbilirubinaemia · hypercalcaemia · hypersalivation · hyperthyroidism · hypokalaemia · increased lacrimation · menorrhagia · pallor · pancreatitis · photophobia · photosensitivity · retinal ischaemia · retinopathy · skin ulceration · suicidal ideation · tongue discoloration · venous thromboembolism

▸ **Rare** Acute myocardial infarction · aspermia · bipolar disorder · cholecystitis · coronary artery disease · encephalopathy · hallucinations · pericarditis · pleural fibrosis · respiratory failure · sarcoidosis · thyroid neoplasms

▸ **Frequency not known** Rash with eosinophilia and systemic symptoms · Stevens-Johnson syndrome

SIDE-EFFECTS, FURTHER INFORMATION

Side-effects listed are reported when boceprevir is used in combination with ribavirin and peginterferon alfa.

● PREGNANCY Manufacturer advises avoid.

● BREAST FEEDING Manufacturer advises avoid; present in milk in *animal* studies.

● MONITORING REQUIREMENTS Monitor full blood count before starting treatment and then on weeks 2, 4, 8, and 12 of treatment, then as indicated clinically.

● PATIENT AND CARER ADVICE

Missed doses

If a dose is more than 6 hours late, the missed dose should not be taken and the next dose should be taken at the normal time.

● NATIONAL FUNDING/ACCESS DECISIONS

NICE technology appraisals (TAs)

▸ Boceprevir for chronic hepatitis C infection of genotype 1 (April 2012) NICE TA253

Boceprevir in combination with ribavirin and peginterferon alfa is an option for the treatment of chronic hepatitis C infection of genotype 1 in adults with compensated liver disease:

● who have not been treated previously;
● in whom previous treatment (e.g. with peginterferon alfa in combination with ribavirin) has failed.

www.nice.org.uk/TA253

● MEDICINAL FORMS

There can be variation in the licensing of different medicines containing the same drug.

Capsule

CAUTIONARY AND ADVISORY LABELS 21

▸ Victrelis (Merck Sharp & Dohme Ltd) ▼
Boceprevir 200 mg Victrelis 200mg capsules | 336 capsule PoM £2,800.00

Simeprevir

● INDICATIONS AND DOSE

In combination with ribavirin and peginterferon alfa for chronic hepatitis C infection of genotype 1 or 4 | In combination with sofosbuvir (with or without ribavirin) for urgent treatment of chronic hepatitis C infection of genotype 1 or 4 when peginterferon alfa cannot be used because of intolerance or contra-indications

▸ BY MOUTH
▸ Adult: 150 mg once daily (for duration of treatment consult product literature)

● CAUTIONS Consider alternative treatment in presence of NS3 Q80K polymorphism—efficacy of simeprevir is reduced · patients of East Asian origin

● INTERACTIONS → Appendix 1 (simeprevir).

● SIDE-EFFECTS Constipation · dyspnoea · fatigue (in combination with sofosbuvir) · headache (in combination with sofosbuvir) · insomnia (in combination with sofosbuvir) · nausea · photosensitivity · pruritus · raised bilirubin concentration · rash

SIDE-EFFECTS, FURTHER INFORMATION

▸ Rash Monitor for deterioration if mild or moderate; discontinue if severe.

● CONCEPTION AND CONTRACEPTION Effective contraception essential during treatment.

● PREGNANCY Manufacturer advises use only if potential benefit outweighs risk—toxicity in *animal* studies.

Infection

5

- BREAST FEEDING Manufacturer advises avoid—present in plasma of breast-fed *animals*.
- HEPATIC IMPAIRMENT Manufacturer advises caution in moderate to severe impairment—elimination reduced in severe impairment. Manufacturer advises caution in decompensated cirrhosis—elimination reduced in severe impairment.
- RENAL IMPAIRMENT Manufacturer advises caution if eGFR less than 30 mL/minute/1.73 m^2—elimination may be reduced.
- PRE-TREATMENT SCREENING Test for NS3 Q80K polymorphism before combination treatment with ribavirin and peginterferon alfa in patients with chronic hepatitis C infection of genotype 1a. Consider testing for NS3 Q80K polymorphism before combination treatment with sofosbuvir (with or without ribavirin) in patients with chronic hepatitis C infection of genotype 1a.
- PATIENT AND CARER ADVICE
  Missed doses
  If a dose is more than 12 hours late, the missed dose should not be taken and the next dose should be taken at the normal time.
- NATIONAL FUNDING/ACCESS DECISIONS
  NICE technology appraisals (TAs)
  ▶ Simeprevir in combination with peginterferon alfa and ribavirin for treating genotypes 1 and 4 chronic hepatitis C (February 2015) NICE TA331
  Simeprevir in combination with peginterferon alfa and ribavirin, is recommended within its marketing authorisation, as an option for the treatment of chronic hepatitis C infection of genotype 1 and 4 in adults.
  www.nice.org.uk/TA331

- MEDICINAL FORMS
  There can be variation in the licensing of different medicines containing the same drug.
  Capsule
  CAUTIONARY AND ADVISORY LABELS 11, 21
  ▶ Olysio (Janssen-Cilag Ltd) ▼
  Simeprevir (as Simeprevir sodium) 150 mg Olysio 150mg capsules | 7 capsule [PoM] £1,866.50

Telaprevir

- INDICATIONS AND DOSE

In combination with ribavirin and peginterferon alfa in chronic hepatitis C infection of genotype 1 in patients with compensated liver disease
  ▶ BY MOUTH
  ▶ Adult: 1.125 g every 12 hours, alternatively 750 mg every 8 hours, for duration of treatment consult product literature

- CAUTIONS Bradycardia · congenital or family history of QT interval prolongation · electrolyte disturbances · family history of sudden death · heart failure with reduced left ventricular ejection fraction · hypoalbuminaemia · low platelets · prolongation of QT interval
  CAUTIONS, FURTHER INFORMATION
  ▶ Low platelets or hypoalbuminaemia Not recommended in patients with low platelets or hypoalbuminaemia—if initiated in these patients monitor closely for signs of infection, worsening liver impairment, and anaemia (increased risk of severe morbidity and mortality).
- INTERACTIONS → Appendix 1 (telaprevir). Caution in concomitant use with other drugs known to prolong QT interval.
- SIDE-EFFECTS
  ▶ **Common or very common** Anaemia · anal fissure · diarrhoea · eczema · haemorrhoids · hyperbilirubinaemia ·

hyperuricaemia · hypokalaemia · hypothyroidism · lymphopenia · nausea · peripheral oedema · pruritus · rash · syncope · taste disturbances · thrombocytopenia · vomiting
  ▶ **Uncommon** Gout · proctitis · retinopathy · urticaria
  ▶ **Rare** Stevens-Johnson syndrome · toxic epidermal necrolysis
  SIDE-EFFECTS, FURTHER INFORMATION
  Side-effects listed are reported when telaprevir is used in combination with ribavirin and peginterferon alfa.
  ▶ Rash Rash occurs very commonly. If rash mild or moderate, may continue without interruption, but monitor for deterioration. If moderate rash deteriorates, consider permanent discontinuation of telaprevir; if rash does not improve within 7 days of discontinuation, suspend ribavirin. If severe rash or if rash accompanied by blistering or mucosal ulceration, discontinue telaprevir permanently; if rash does not improve within 7 days of discontinuation, consider discontinuation of ribavirin and peginterferon alfa. If serious rash, or if severe rash deteriorates, or if rash accompanied by systemic symptoms, discontinue telaprevir, ribavirin, and peginterferon alfa permanently.
- CONCEPTION AND CONTRACEPTION Effectiveness of hormonal contraceptives reduced during treatment and for 2 months after stopping telaprevir—effective non-hormonal methods of contraception necessary during this time.
- PREGNANCY Manufacturer advises avoid.
- BREAST FEEDING Manufacturer advises avoid—present in milk in *animal* studies.
- HEPATIC IMPAIRMENT Manufacturer advises avoid in moderate to severe impairment.
- MONITORING REQUIREMENTS Monitor full blood count, platelets, electrolytes, serum creatinine, uric acid, and liver and thyroid function tests before starting treatment and then on weeks 2, 4, 8, and 12 of treatment, then as indicated clinically.
- PRESCRIBING AND DISPENSING INFORMATION Dispense in original container (contains desiccant).
- PATIENT AND CARER ADVICE
  Patients should be told to seek immediate medical attention if a rash develops or if an existing rash worsens.
  Missed doses
  If a dose is more than 6 hours late with the 12 hourly regimen (or more than 4 hours late with the 8 hourly regimen), the missed dose should not be taken and the next dose should be taken at the normal time.
- NATIONAL FUNDING/ACCESS DECISIONS
  NICE technology appraisals (TAs)
  ▶ Telaprevir for chronic hepatitis C infection of genotype 1 (April 2012) NICE TA252
  Telaprevir in combination with ribavirin and peginterferon alfa is an option for the treatment of chronic hepatitis C infection of genotype 1 in adults with compensated liver disease:
  - who have not been treated previously;
  - in whom previous treatment (e.g. with peginterferon alfa in combination with ribavirin) has failed.
  www.nice.org.uk/TA252

- MEDICINAL FORMS
  There can be variation in the licensing of different medicines containing the same drug.
  Tablet
  CAUTIONARY AND ADVISORY LABELS 21
  ▶ Incivo (Janssen-Cilag Ltd) ▼
  Telaprevir 375 mg Incivo 375mg tablets | 42 tablet [PoM] £1,866.50

ANTIVIRALS > OTHER

Dasabuvir

29.3.2016

- **DRUG ACTION** Dasabuvir is a non-nucleoside inhibitor of hepatitis C virus polymerase NS5B, which is an essential component of the hepatitis C virus replication process.

- **INDICATIONS AND DOSE**

Chronic hepatitis C infection of genotype 1, in combination with other antiviral drugs (ombitasvir with paritaprevir and ritonavir, with or without ribavirin)
  ▶ BY MOUTH
  ▶ Adult: 250 mg twice daily for details of duration of treatment, consult product literature, dose to be taken in the morning and evening

- **CONTRA-INDICATIONS** HIV co-infection without suppressive antiretroviral therapy
- **CAUTIONS** Retreatment—efficacy not established
- **INTERACTIONS** → Appendix 1 (dasabuvir)
- **SIDE-EFFECTS**
- **Common or very common** Anaemia · asthenia · fatigue · insomnia · nausea
  SIDE-EFFECTS, FURTHER INFORMATION
  Side-effects listed are reported when dasabuvir is used in combination with *Viekirax*® (ombitasvir with paritaprevir and ritonavir), with or without ribavirin.
- **PREGNANCY** Manufacturer advises avoid—no information available.
- **BREAST FEEDING** Manufacturer advises avoid—present in milk in *animal* studies.
- **HEPATIC IMPAIRMENT** Manufacturer advises avoid in moderate to severe impairment.
- **PATIENT AND CARER ADVICE**
  Missed doses
  If a dose is more than 6 hours late, the missed dose should not be taken and the next dose should be taken at the normal time.
- **NATIONAL FUNDING/ACCESS DECISIONS**
  NICE technology appraisals (TAs)
  ▶ Ombitasvir with paritaprevir and ritonavir with or without dasabuvir for treating chronic hepatitis C (November 2015) NICE TA365
  Dasabuvir, in combination with ombitasvir with paritaprevir and ritonavir p. 569, is recommended, within its marketing authorisation, as an option for treating genotype 1 or 4 chronic hepatitis C in adults only if the manufacturer provides it with the discount agreed in the patient access scheme.
  www.nice.org.uk/guidance/ta365

- **MEDICINAL FORMS**
  There can be variation in the licensing of different medicines containing the same drug.
  Tablet
  CAUTIONARY AND ADVISORY LABELS 3, 21, 25
  ▶ Exviera (AbbVie Ltd) ▼
  Dasabuvir (as Dasabuvir sodium monohydrate) 250 mg Exviera 250mg tablets | 56 tablet [PoM] £933.33

6.3 Herpesvirus infections

Herpesvirus infections

Herpes simplex and varicella–zoster infection

The two most important herpesvirus pathogens are herpes simplex virus (herpesvirus hominis) and varicella–zoster virus.

Herpes simplex infections

Herpes infection of the mouth and lips and in the eye is generally associated with herpes simplex virus serotype 1 (HSV-1); other areas of the skin may also be infected, especially in immunodeficiency. Genital infection is most often associated with HSV-2 and also HSV-1. Treatment of herpes simplex infection should start as early as possible and usually within 5 days of the appearance of the infection.

In individuals with good immune function, mild infection of the eye (ocular herpes) and of the lips (herpes labialis or cold sores) is treated with a topical antiviral drug. Primary herpetic gingivostomatitis is managed by changes to diet and with analgesics. Severe infection, neonatal herpes infection or infection in immunocompromised individuals requires treatment with a systemic antiviral drug. Primary or recurrent genital herpes simplex infection is treated with an antiviral drug given by mouth. Persistence of a lesion or recurrence in an immunocompromised patient may signal the development of resistance.

Specialist advice should be sought for systemic treatment of herpes simplex infection in pregnancy.

Varicella-zoster infections

Regardless of immune function and the use of any immunoglobulins, neonates with *chickenpox* should be treated with a parenteral antiviral to reduce the risk of severe disease. Oral therapy in children is not recommended as absorption is variable. Chickenpox in otherwise healthy children between 1 month and 12 years is usually mild and antiviral treatment is not usually required.

Chickenpox is more severe in adolescents and adults than in children; antiviral treatment started within 24 hours of the onset of rash may reduce the duration and severity of symptoms in otherwise healthy adults and adolescents. Antiviral treatment is generally recommended in immunocompromised patients and those at special risk (e.g. because of severe cardiovascular or respiratory disease or chronic skin disorder); in such cases, an antiviral is given for 10 days with at least 7 days of parenteral treatment.

Pregnant women who develop severe chickenpox may be at risk of complications, especially varicella pneumonia. Specialist advice should be sought for the treatment of chickenpox during pregnancy.

Those who have been exposed to chickenpox and are at special risk of complications may require prophylaxis with varicella-zoster immunoglobulin (see under Disease Specific Immunoglobulins).

In *herpes zoster* (shingles) systemic antiviral treatment can reduce the severity and duration of pain, reduce complications, and reduce viral shedding. Treatment with the antiviral should be started within 72 hours of the onset of rash and is usually continued for 7–10 days. Immunocompromised patients at high risk of disseminated or severe infection should be treated with a parenteral antiviral drug.

Chronic pain which persists after the rash has healed (postherpetic neuralgia) requires specific management.

Choice

Aciclovir p. 576 is active against herpesviruses but does not eradicate them. Uses of aciclovir include systemic treatment of varicella–zoster and the systemic and topical treatment of herpes simplex infections of the skin and mucous membranes. It is used by mouth for severe herpetic stomatitis. Aciclovir eye ointment is used for herpes simplex infections of the eye; it is combined with systemic treatment for ophthalmic zoster.

Famciclovir p. 578, a prodrug of penciclovir, is similar to aciclovir and is licensed for use in herpes zoster and genital herpes.

Valaciclovir p. 579 is an ester of aciclovir, licensed for herpes zoster and herpes simplex infections of the skin and mucous membranes (including genital herpes); it is also licensed for preventing cytomegalovirus disease following

Infection

5

solid organ transplantation. Famciclovir or valaciclovir are suitable alternatives to aciclovir for oral lesions associated with herpes zoster. Valaciclovir once daily may reduce the risk of transmitting genital herpes to heterosexual partners—specialist advice should be sought.

Foscarnet sodium p. 581 is used for mucocutaneous herpes simplex virus infection unresponsive to aciclovir in immunocompromised patients; it is toxic and can cause renal impairment.

Inosine pranobex below has been used by mouth for herpes simplex infections; its effectiveness remains unproven.

Cytomegalovirus infection

Ganciclovir p. 580 is related to aciclovir but it is more active against cytomegalovirus (CMV); it is also much more toxic than aciclovir and should therefore be prescribed only when the potential benefit outweighs the risks. Ganciclovir is administered by intravenous infusion for the *initial treatment* of CMV infection. Ganciclovir causes profound myelosuppression when given with zidovudine p. 592; the two should not normally be given together particularly during initial ganciclovir therapy. The likelihood of ganciclovir resistance increases in patients with a high viral load or in those who receive the drug over a long duration.

Valaciclovir is licensed for prevention of cytomegalovirus disease following renal transplantation.

Valganciclovir p. 581 is an ester of ganciclovir which is licensed for the *initial treatment* and *maintenance treatment* of CMV retinitis in AIDS patients. Valganciclovir is also licensed for preventing CMV disease following solid organ transplantation from a cytomegalovirus-positive donor.

Foscarnet sodium is also active against cytomegalovirus; it is toxic and can cause renal impairment.

See local treatment of CMV retinitis.

ANTIVIRALS > INOSINE COMPLEXES

Inosine pranobex

(Inosine acedoben dimepranol)

- ● **INDICATIONS AND DOSE**

Mucocutaneous herpes simplex
- ▶ BY MOUTH
- ▶ Adult: 1 g 4 times a day for 7–14 days

Adjunctive treatment of genital warts
- ▶ BY MOUTH
- ▶ Adult: 1 g 3 times a day for 14–28 days

Subacute sclerosing panencephalitis
- ▶ BY MOUTH
- ▶ Adult: 50–100 mg/kg daily in 6 divided doses

- ● CAUTIONS History of gout · history of hyperuricaemia
- ● SIDE-EFFECTS
- ▶ **Common or very common** Reversible increase in serum uric acid · reversible increase in urinary uric acid
- ▶ **Uncommon** Arthralgia · epigastric discomfort · fatigue · headache · itching · nausea · rashes · vertigo · vomiting
- ▶ **Rare** Anxiety · constipation · diarrhoea · polyuria · sleep disturbances
- ● PREGNANCY Manufacturer advises avoid.
- ● RENAL IMPAIRMENT Manufacturer advises caution; metabolised to uric acid.
- ● LESS SUITABLE FOR PRESCRIBING Inosine pranobex is less suitable for prescribing.

- ● MEDICINAL FORMS
  There can be variation in the licensing of different medicines containing the same drug.
  Tablet
  CAUTIONARY AND ADVISORY LABELS 9
  - ▶ Imunovir (KoRa Healthcare)
    Inosine acedoben dimepranol 500 mg Imunovir 500mg tablets | 100 tablet [PoM] £39.50

ANTIVIRALS > NUCLEOSIDE ANALOGUES

Aciclovir

(Acyclovir)

- ● **INDICATIONS AND DOSE**

Herpes simplex, suppression
- ▶ BY MOUTH
- ▶ Child 12-17 years: 400 mg twice daily, alternatively 200 mg 4 times a day; increased to 400 mg 3 times a day, dose may be increased if recurrences occur on standard suppressive therapy or for suppression of genital herpes during late pregnancy (from 36 weeks gestation), therapy interrupted every 6–12 months to reassess recurrence frequency—consider restarting after two or more recurrences
- ▶ Adult: 400 mg twice daily, alternatively 200 mg 4 times a day; increased to 400 mg 3 times a day, dose may be increased if recurrences occur on standard suppressive therapy or for suppression of genital herpes during late pregnancy (from 36 weeks gestation), therapy interrupted every 6–12 months to reassess recurrence frequency—consider restarting after two or more recurrences

Herpes simplex, prophylaxis in the immunocompromised
- ▶ BY MOUTH
- ▶ Child 1-23 months: 100–200 mg 4 times a day
- ▶ Child 2-17 years: 200–400 mg 4 times a day
- ▶ Adult: 200–400 mg 4 times a day
- ▶ BY INTRAVENOUS INFUSION
- ▶ Adult: 5 mg/kg every 8 hours

Herpes simplex, treatment (non-genital)
- ▶ BY MOUTH
- ▶ Adult: 200 mg 5 times a day usually for 5 days (longer if new lesions appear during treatment or if healing incomplete)

Herpes simplex, treatment (non-genital) in immunocompromised or if absorption impaired
- ▶ BY MOUTH
- ▶ Adult: 400 mg 5 times a day usually for 5 days (longer if new lesions appear during treatment or if healing incomplete)

Herpes simplex, treatment
- ▶ BY MOUTH
- ▶ Child 1-23 months: 100 mg 5 times a day usually for 5 days (longer if new lesions appear during treatment or if healing incomplete)
- ▶ Child 2-17 years: 200 mg 5 times a day usually for 5 days (longer if new lesions appear during treatment or if healing incomplete)

Herpes simplex, treatment, in immunocompromised or if absorption impaired
- ▶ BY MOUTH
- ▶ Child 1-23 months: 200 mg 5 times a day usually for 5 days (longer if new lesions appear during treatment or if healing incomplete)
- ▶ Child 2-17 years: 400 mg 5 times a day usually for 5 days (longer if new lesions appear during treatment or if healing incomplete)

5

Infection

Genital herpes simplex, treatment of first episode
▶ BY MOUTH
▶ Adult: 200 mg 5 times a day, alternatively 400 mg 3 times a day both courses usually for 5 days (longer if new lesions appear during treatment or if healing incomplete)

Genital herpes simplex, treatment of first episode, in immunocompromised or HIV-positive
▶ BY MOUTH
▶ Adult: 400 mg 5 times a day for 7–10 days (longer if new lesions appear during treatment or if healing incomplete)

Severe genital herpes simplex, treatment, initial infection | Treatment of herpes simplex in the immunocompromised
▶ BY INTRAVENOUS INFUSION
▶ Adult: Initially 5 mg/kg every 8 hours usually for 5 days, alternatively 10 mg/kg every 8 hours for at least 14 days in encephalitis (at least 21 days if also immunocompromised)—confirm cerebrospinal fluid negative for herpes simplex virus before stopping treatment, higher dose to be used only if resistant organisms suspected or in simplex encephalitis

Genital herpes simplex, treatment of recurrent infection
▶ BY MOUTH
▶ Adult: 800 mg 3 times a day for 2 days, alternatively 200 mg 5 times a day for 5 days, alternatively 400 mg 3 times a day for 3–5 days

Genital herpes simplex, treatment of recurrent infection in immunocompromised or HIV-positive patients
▶ BY MOUTH
▶ Adult: 400 mg 3 times a day for 5–10 days

Varicella zoster (chickenpox), treatment | Herpes zoster (shingles), treatment
▶ BY MOUTH
▶ Child 1-23 months: 200 mg 4 times a day for 5 days
▶ Child 2-5 years: 400 mg 4 times a day for 5 days
▶ Child 6-11 years: 800 mg 4 times a day for 5 days
▶ Child 12-17 years: 800 mg 5 times a day for 7 days
▶ Adult: 800 mg 5 times a day for 7 days
▶ BY INTRAVENOUS INFUSION
▶ Adult: 5 mg/kg every 8 hours usually for 5 days

Varicella zoster (chickenpox), treatment in immunocompromised | Herpes zoster (shingles), treatment in immunocompromised
▶ BY INTRAVENOUS INFUSION
▶ Adult: 10 mg/kg every 8 hours usually for 5 days

Herpes zoster (shingles), treatment in immunocompromised
▶ BY MOUTH
▶ Child 1-23 months: 200 mg 4 times a day continued for 2 days after crusting of lesions
▶ Child 2-5 years: 400 mg 4 times a day continued for 2 days after crusting of lesions
▶ Child 6-11 years: 800 mg 4 times a day continued for 2 days after crusting of lesions
▶ Child 12-17 years: 800 mg 5 times a day continued for 2 days after crusting of lesions
▶ Adult: 800 mg 5 times a day continued for 2 days after crusting of lesions

Herpes zoster, treatment in encephalitis | Varicella zoster, treatment in encephalitis
▶ BY INTRAVENOUS INFUSION
▶ Adult: 10 mg/kg every 8 hours given for 10–14 days in encephalitis, possibly longer if also immunocompromised or if severe infection

Varicella zoster (chickenpox), attenuation of infection if varicella-zoster immunoglobulin not indicated
▶ BY MOUTH
▶ Child: 10 mg/kg 4 times a day for 7 days, to be started 1 week after exposure
▶ Adult: 10 mg/kg 4 times a day for 7 days, to be started 1 week after exposure

DOSES AT EXTREMES OF BODY-WEIGHT
▶ With intravenous use To avoid excessive dosage in obese patients parenteral dose should be calculated on the basis of ideal weight for height.

● UNLICENSED USE Tablets and suspension not licensed for suppression of herpes simplex or for treatment of herpes zoster in children (age range not specified by manufacturer).
   Intravenous infusion not licensed for herpes zoster in children under 18 years.
▶ With oral use Aciclovir doses in BNF may differ from those in product literature. Attenuation of chickenpox is an unlicensed indication.

● CAUTIONS Elderly (risk of neurological reactions) · maintain adequate hydration (especially with infusion or high doses)

● INTERACTIONS → Appendix 1 (aciclovir).

● SIDE-EFFECTS
▶ Common or very common
▶ With systemic use Abdominal pain · diarrhoea · fatigue · headache · nausea · photosensitivity · pruritus · rash · urticaria · vomiting
▶ Very rare
▶ With intravenous use Agitation · fever · psychosis · severe local inflammation (sometimes leading to ulceration) · tremors
▶ With systemic use Acute renal failure · anaemia · ataxia · confusion · convulsions · dizziness · drowsiness · dysarthria · dyspnoea · hallucinations · hepatitis · jaundice · leucopenia · neurological reactions · thrombocytopenia

● PREGNANCY
▶ With systemic use Not known to be harmful—manufacturers advise use only when potential benefit outweighs risk.

● BREAST FEEDING Significant amount in milk after systemic administration—not known to be harmful but manufacturer advises caution.

● RENAL IMPAIRMENT
▶ With intravenous use in adults Use normal intravenous dose every 12 hours if eGFR 25–50 mL/minute/1.73 m^2 (every 24 hours if eGFR 10–25 mL/minute/1.73 m^2). Consult product literature for intravenous dose if eGFR less than 10 mL/minute/1.73 m^2.
▶ With oral use in adults For herpes zoster, use normal oral dose every 8 hours if eGFR 10–25 mL/minute/1.73 m^2 (every 12 hours if eGFR less than 10 mL/minute/1.73 m^2). For herpes simplex, use normal oral dose every 12 hours if eGFR less than 10 mL/minute/1.73 m^2.
▶ With intravenous use in children Use normal intravenous dose every 12 hours if estimated glomerular filtration rate 25–50 mL/minute/1.73m^2 (every 24 hours if estimated glomerular filtration rate 10–25 mL/minute/1.73m^2). Consult product literature for intravenous dose if estimated glomerular filtration rate less than 10 mL/minute/1.73m^2.
▶ With oral use in children For herpes zoster, use normal oral dose every 8 hours if estimated glomerular filtration rate 10–25 mL/minute/1.73m^2 (every 12 hours if estimated glomerular filtration rate less than 10 mL/minute/1.73m^2). For herpes simplex, use normal dose every 12 hours if estimated glomerular filtration rate less than 10 mL/minute/1.73^2.

5

Infection

‣ With systemic use Risk of neurological reactions increased. Maintain adequate hydration (especially during renal impairment).

● DIRECTIONS FOR ADMINISTRATION
‣ With intravenous use in children For *intravenous infusion*, reconstitute to 25 mg/mL with Water for Injections or Sodium Chloride 0.9% then dilute to concentration of 5 mg/mL with Sodium Chloride 0.9% or Sodium Chloride and Glucose and give over 1 hour; alternatively, may be administered in a concentration of 25 mg/mL using a suitable infusion pump and central venous access and given over 1 hour.
‣ With intravenous use in adults For *intravenous infusion Zovirax IV®*, *Aciclovir IV*(Genus), give intermittently *in* Sodium chloride 0.9% *or* Sodium chloride and glucose; initially reconstitute to 25 mg/mL in water for injection or sodium chloride 0.9% then dilute to not more than 5 mg/mL with the infusion fluid; to be given over 1 hour; alternatively, may be administered in a concentration of 25 mg/mL using a suitable infusion pump and given over 1 hour; for *Aciclovir IV* (Hospira) dilute to not more than 5 mg/mL with infusion fluid; give over 1 hour.

● PRESCRIBING AND DISPENSING INFORMATION Flavours of oral liquid preparations may include banana, or orange.

● PATIENT AND CARER ADVICE
Medicines for Children leaflet: Aciclovir (oral) for viral infections
‣ With oral use in children www.medicinesforchildren.org.uk/aciclovir-for-viral-infections

● PROFESSION SPECIFIC INFORMATION
Dental practitioners' formulary
Aciclovir Tablets 200 mg or 800 mg may be prescribed.
Aciclovir Oral Suspension 200 mg/5mL may be prescribed.

● MEDICINAL FORMS
There can be variation in the licensing of different medicines containing the same drug.

Tablet
CAUTIONARY AND ADVISORY LABELS 9
‣ Aciclovir (Non-proprietary)
Aciclovir 200 mg Aciclovir 200mg tablets | 25 tablet [PoM] £10.00 DT price = £1.44
Aciclovir 400 mg Aciclovir 400mg tablets | 56 tablet [PoM] £15.00 DT price = £3.20
Aciclovir 800 mg Aciclovir 800mg tablets | 35 tablet [PoM] £20.00 DT price = £3.48

Dispersible tablet
CAUTIONARY AND ADVISORY LABELS 9
‣ Aciclovir (Non-proprietary)
Aciclovir 200 mg Aciclovir 200mg dispersible tablets | 25 tablet [PoM] £17.50 DT price = £1.77
Aciclovir 400 mg Aciclovir 400mg dispersible tablets | 56 tablet [PoM] £20.00 DT price = £11.95
Aciclovir 800 mg Aciclovir 800mg dispersible tablets | 35 tablet [PoM] £65.00 DT price = £10.96
‣ Zovirax (GlaxoSmithKline UK Ltd)
Aciclovir 200 mg Zovirax 200mg dispersible tablets | 25 tablet [PoM] £2.85 DT price = £1.77
Aciclovir 800 mg Zovirax 800mg dispersible tablets | 35 tablet [PoM] £10.50 DT price = £10.96

Oral suspension
CAUTIONARY AND ADVISORY LABELS 9
‣ Aciclovir (Non-proprietary)
Aciclovir 40 mg per 1 ml Aciclovir 200mg/5ml oral suspension sugar free sugar-free | 125 ml [PoM] £35.76 DT price = £35.76
Aciclovir 80 mg per 1 ml Aciclovir 400mg/5ml oral suspension sugar free sugar-free | 100 ml [PoM] £39.47 DT price = £39.47
‣ Zovirax (GlaxoSmithKline UK Ltd)
Aciclovir 40 mg per 1 ml Zovirax 200mg/5ml oral suspension sugar-free | 125 ml [PoM] £29.56 DT price = £35.76
Aciclovir 80 mg per 1 ml Zovirax Double Strength 400mg/5ml oral suspension sugar-free | 100 ml [PoM] £33.02 DT price = £39.47

Solution for infusion
ELECTROLYTES: May contain Sodium
‣ Aciclovir (Non-proprietary)
Aciclovir (as Aciclovir sodium) 25 mg per 1 ml Aciclovir 1g/40ml solution for infusion vials | 1 vial [PoM] £40.00
Aciclovir 500mg/20ml solution for infusion vials | 5 vial [PoM] £100.00
Aciclovir 250mg/10ml solution for infusion vials | 5 vial [PoM] £50.00

Powder for solution for infusion
ELECTROLYTES: May contain Sodium
‣ Aciclovir (Non-proprietary)
Aciclovir (as Aciclovir sodium) 250 mg Aciclovir 250mg powder for solution for infusion vials | 5 vial [PoM] £45.66
‣ Zovirax (GlaxoSmithKline UK Ltd)
Aciclovir (as Aciclovir sodium) 250 mg Zovirax I.V. 250mg powder for solution for infusion vials | 5 vial [PoM] £16.70
Aciclovir (as Aciclovir sodium) 500 mg Zovirax I.V. 500mg powder for solution for infusion vials | 5 vial [PoM] £17.00

Famciclovir

● INDICATIONS AND DOSE
Herpes zoster infection, treatment
‣ BY MOUTH
‣ Adult: 500 mg 3 times a day for 7 days, alternatively 750 mg 1–2 times a day for 7 days

Herpes zoster infection, treatment in immunocompromised patients
‣ BY MOUTH
‣ Adult: 500 mg 3 times a day for 10 days, continue for 2 days after crusting of lesions

Genital herpes, suppression
‣ BY MOUTH
‣ Adult: 250 mg twice daily, therapy to be interrupted every 6–12 months to reassess recurrence frequency—consider restarting after two or more recurrences

Genital herpes, suppression in immunocompromised or HIV-positive patients
‣ BY MOUTH
‣ Adult: 500 mg twice daily, therapy to be interrupted every 6–12 months to reassess recurrence frequency—consider restarting after two or more recurrences

Genital herpes infection, treatment of first episode
‣ BY MOUTH
‣ Adult: 250 mg 3 times a day for 5 days or longer if new lesions appear during treatment or if healing incomplete

Genital herpes infection, treatment of first episode in immunocompromised or HIV-positive patients
‣ BY MOUTH
‣ Adult: 500 mg twice daily for 10 days

Genital herpes infection, treatment of recurrent infection
‣ BY MOUTH
‣ Adult: 125 mg twice daily for 5 days, alternatively 1 g twice daily for 1 day

Genital herpes infection, treatment of recurrent infections in immunocompromised or HIV-positive patients
‣ BY MOUTH
‣ Adult: 500 mg twice daily for 5–10 days

Herpes simplex infection (non-genital), treatment in immunocompromised patients
‣ BY MOUTH
‣ Adult: 500 mg twice daily for 7 days

● UNLICENSED USE Famciclovir doses in BNF may differ from those in product literature.
● INTERACTIONS → Appendix 1 (famciclovir).
● SIDE-EFFECTS
‣ **Common or very common** Headache · nausea · vomiting
‣ **Rare** Confusion

▸ **Very rare** Dizziness · drowsiness · hallucinations · jaundice · rash · Stevens-Johnson syndrome · thrombocytopenia

▸ **Frequency not known** Constipation · abdominal pain · diarrhoea · fatigue · fever · pruritus · sweating

● **PREGNANCY** Manufacturers advise avoid unless potential benefit outweighs risk.

● **BREAST FEEDING** No information available—present in milk in *animal* studies.

● **HEPATIC IMPAIRMENT** Usual dose in well compensated liver disease (information not available on decompensated).

● **RENAL IMPAIRMENT** Reduce dose; consult product literature.

● **PRESCRIBING AND DISPENSING INFORMATION** Famciclovir is a pro-drug of penciclovir.

● **MEDICINAL FORMS**
There can be variation in the licensing of different medicines containing the same drug. Forms available from special-order manufacturers include: tablet

Tablet
CAUTIONARY AND ADVISORY LABELS 9

▸ Famciclovir (Non-proprietary)
Famciclovir 125 mg Famciclovir 125mg tablets | 10 tablet PoM £37.12 DT price = £35.95
Famciclovir 250 mg Famciclovir 250mg tablets | 15 tablet PoM £111.35 | 21 tablet PoM | £155.87 DT price = £153.84 | 56 tablet PoM £407.60–£409.49
Famciclovir 500 mg Famciclovir 500mg tablets | 14 tablet PoM £207.86 DT price = £158.31 | 30 tablet PoM £305.83–£445.28

▸ Famvir (Novartis Pharmaceuticals UK Ltd)
Famciclovir 125 mg Famvir 125mg tablets | 10 tablet PoM £53.45 DT price = £35.95
Famciclovir 250 mg Famvir 250mg tablets | 15 tablet PoM £160.34 | 21 tablet PoM £187.04 DT price = £153.84 | 56 tablet PoM £598.56
Famciclovir 500 mg Famvir 500mg tablets | 14 tablet PoM £249.43 DT price = £158.31 | 30 tablet PoM £641.21

Valaciclovir

● **INDICATIONS AND DOSE**

Herpes zoster infection, treatment
▸ BY MOUTH
▸ Adult: 1 g 3 times a day for 7 days

Herpes zoster infection, treatment in immunocompromised patients
▸ BY MOUTH
▸ Adult: 1 g 3 times a day for at least 7 days and continued for 2 days after crusting of lesions

Herpes simplex, treatment of first infective episode
▸ BY MOUTH
▸ Adult: 500 mg twice daily for 5 days (longer if new lesions appear during treatment or healing is incomplete)

Herpes simplex infections treatment of first episode in immunocompromised or HIV-positive patients
▸ BY MOUTH
▸ Adult: 1 g twice daily for 10 days

Herpes simplex, treatment of recurrent infections
▸ BY MOUTH
▸ Adult: 500 mg twice daily for 3–5 days

Treatment of recurrent herpes simplex infections in immunocompromised or HIV-positive patients
▸ BY MOUTH
▸ Adult: 1 g twice daily for 5–10 days

Herpes labialis treatment
▸ BY MOUTH
▸ Child 12-17 years: Initially 2 g, then 2 g after 12 hours
▸ Adult: Initially 2 g, then 2 g after 12 hours

Herpes simplex, suppression of infections
▸ BY MOUTH
▸ Adult: 500 mg daily in 1–2 divided doses, therapy to be interrupted every 6–12 months to reassess recurrence frequency—consider restarting after two or more recurrences

Herpes simplex, suppression of infections in immunocompromised or HIV-positive patients
▸ BY MOUTH
▸ Adult: 500 mg twice daily, therapy to be interrupted every 6–12 months to reassess recurrence frequency—consider restarting after two or more recurrences

Genital herpes, reduction of transmission (administered on expert advice)
▸ BY MOUTH
▸ Adult: 500 mg once daily, to be taken by the infected partner

Prevention of cytomegalovirus disease following solid organ transplantation when valganciclovir or ganciclovir cannot be used
▸ BY MOUTH
▸ Adult: 2 g 4 times a day usually for 90 days, preferably starting within 72 hours of transplantation

● **CAUTIONS** Elderly (risk of neurological reactions) · maintain adequate hydration (especially with high doses)

● **INTERACTIONS** → Appendix 1 (valaciclovir).

● **SIDE-EFFECTS**

▸ **Very rare** Acute renal failure · anaemia · ataxia · confusion · convulsions · dizziness · drowsiness · dysarthria · dyspnoea · hallucinations · hepatitis · jaundice · leucopenia · neurological reactions · thrombocytopenia

▸ **Frequency not known** Abdominal pain · diarrhoea · fatigue · headache · nausea · photosensitivity · pruritus · rash · urticaria · vomiting

SIDE-EFFECTS, FURTHER INFORMATION

▸ **Neurological reactions** Neurological reactions (including dizziness, confusion, hallucinations, convulsions, ataxia, dysarthria, and drowsiness) more frequent with higher doses.

● **PREGNANCY** Not known to be harmful—manufacturers advise use only when potential benefit outweighs risk.

● **BREAST FEEDING** Significant amount in milk after systemic administration—not known to be harmful but manufacturer advises caution.

● **HEPATIC IMPAIRMENT** Manufacturer advises caution with high doses used for herpes labialis and prevention of cytomegalovirus disease—no information available.

● **RENAL IMPAIRMENT**

▸ In adults For *herpes zoster*, 1 g every 12 hours if eGFR 30–50 mL/minute/1.73 m^2 (1 g every 24 hours if eGFR 10– 30 mL/minute/1.73 m^2; 500 mg every 24 hours if eGFR less than 10 mL/minute/1.73 m^2). For *treatment of herpes simplex*, 500 mg (1 g in immunocompromised or HIV-positive patients) every 24 hours if eGFR less than 30 mL/minute/1.73 m^2. For *treatment of herpes labialis*, if eGFR 30–50 mL/minute/1.73 m^2, initially 1 g, then 1 g 12 hours after initial dose (if eGFR 10–30 mL/minute/1.73 m^2, initially 500 mg, then 500 mg 12 hours after initial dose; if eGFR less than 10 mL/minute/1.73 m^2, 500 mg as a single dose). For *suppression of herpes simplex*, 250 mg (500 mg in immunocompromised or HIV-positive patients) every 24 hours if eGFR less than 30 mL/minute/1.73 m^2. For *reduction of genital herpes transmission*, 250 mg every 24 hours if eGFR less than 15 mL/minute/1.73 m^2. Reduce dose according to eGFR for *cytomegalovirus prophylaxis* following solid organ transplantation (consult product literature).

5

Infection

▸ In children For *herpes zoster*, 1 g every 12 hours if estimated glomerular filtration rate 30–50 mL/minute/1.73 m^2 (1 g every 24 hours if estimated glomerular filtration rate 10–30 mL/minute/1.73 m^2; 500 mg every 24 hours if estimated glomerular filtration rate less than 10 mL/minute/1.73 m^2). For *treatment of herpes simplex*, 500 mg (1 g in immunocompromised or HIV-positive children) every 24 hours if estimated glomerular filtration rate less than 30 mL/minute/1.73 m^2. For *treatment of herpes labialis*, if estimated glomerular filtration rate 30–50 mL/minute/1.73 m^2, initially 1 g, then 1 g 12 hours after initial dose (if estimated glomerular filtration rate 10–30 mL/minute/1.73 m^2, initially 500 mg, then 500 mg 12 hours after initial dose; if estimated glomerular filtration rate less than 10 mL/minute/1.73 m^2, 500 mg as a single dose). For *suppression of herpes simplex*, 250 mg (500 mg in immunocompromised or HIV-positive children) every 24 hours if estimated glomerular filtration rate less than 30 mL/minute/1.73 m^2. Reduce dose according to estimated glomerular filtration rate for *cytomegalovirus prophylaxis* following solid organ transplantation (consult product literature). Maintain adequate hydration.

● PRESCRIBING AND DISPENSING INFORMATION Valaciclovir is a pro-drug of aciclovir.

● MEDICINAL FORMS
There can be variation in the licensing of different medicines containing the same drug. Forms available from special-order manufacturers include: oral suspension
Tablet
CAUTIONARY AND ADVISORY LABELS 9
▸ Valaciclovir (Non-proprietary)
Valaciclovir (as Valaciclovir hydrochloride) 500 mg Valaciclovir 500mg tablets | 10 tablet [PoM] £20.59 DT price = £3.04 | 42 tablet [PoM] £86.30
▸ Valtrex (GlaxoSmithKline UK Ltd)
Valaciclovir (as Valaciclovir hydrochloride) 250 mg Valtrex 250mg tablets | 60 tablet [PoM] £123.28 DT price = £123.28
Valaciclovir (as Valaciclovir hydrochloride) 500 mg Valtrex 500mg tablets | 10 tablet [PoM] £20.59 DT price = £3.04 | 42 tablet [PoM] £86.30

6.3a Cytomegalovirus infections

ANTIVIRALS > NUCLEOSIDE ANALOGUES

Ganciclovir

● INDICATIONS AND DOSE
Prevention of cytomegalovirus disease during immunosuppressive therapy following organ transplantation
▸ BY INTRAVENOUS INFUSION
▸ Adult: 5 mg/kg every 12 hours for 7–14 days

Treatment of life-threatening or sight-threatening cytomegalovirus infections in immunocompromised patients only
▸ BY INTRAVENOUS INFUSION
▸ Adult: Initially 5 mg/kg every 12 hours for 14–21 days, followed by maintenance 6 mg/kg daily on 5 days of the week, alternatively 5 mg/kg daily until adequate recovery of immunity, maintenance only for patients at risk of relapse of retinitis, if retinitis progresses initial induction treatment may be repeated

● CONTRA-INDICATIONS Abnormally low haemoglobin count (consult product literature) · abnormally low neutrophil count (consult product literature) · abnormally low platelet count (consult product literature)
● CAUTIONS Children (possible risk of long-term carcinogenic or reproductive toxicity) · ensure adequate

hydration · history of cytopenia · potential carcinogen · potential teratogen · radiotherapy · vesicant
● INTERACTIONS → Appendix 1 (ganciclovir). Increased risk of myelosuppression with other myelosuppressive drugs—consult product literature.
● SIDE-EFFECTS
▸ **Common or very common** Abdominal pain · abnormal thinking · anaemia · anorexia · anxiety · arthralgia · chest pain · confusion · constipation · convulsions · cough · depression · dermatitis · diarrhoea · dizziness · dyspepsia · dysphagia · dyspnoea · ear pain · eye pain · fatigue · flatulence · headache · hepatic dysfunction · infection · injection-site reactions · insomnia · leucopenia · macular oedema · myalgia · nausea · night sweats · pancytopenia · peripheral neuropathy · pruritus · pyrexia · renal impairment · retinal detachment · taste disturbance · thrombocytopenia · vitreous floaters · vomiting · weight loss
▸ **Uncommon** Alopecia · anaphylactic reactions · arrhythmias · disturbances in hearing and vision · haematuria · hypotension · male infertility · mouth ulcers · pancreatitis · psychosis · tremor
● ALLERGY AND CROSS-SENSITIVITY Contra-indicated in patients hypersensitive to valganciclovir, aciclovir, or valaciclovir.
● CONCEPTION AND CONTRACEPTION Ensure effective contraception during treatment and barrier contraception for men during and for at least 90 days after treatment.
● PREGNANCY Avoid—teratogenic risk.
● BREAST FEEDING Avoid—no information available.
● RENAL IMPAIRMENT Reduce dose if eGFR less than 70 mL/minute/1.73 m^2; consult product literature.
● MONITORING REQUIREMENTS Monitor full blood count closely (severe deterioration may require correction and possibly treatment interruption).
● DIRECTIONS FOR ADMINISTRATION Infuse into vein with adequate flow preferably using plastic cannula. For *intravenous infusion* (Cymevene®) give intermittently in Glucose 5% or Sodium chloride 0.9%. Reconstitute initially in water for injections (500 mg/10 mL then dilute to not more than 10 mg/m with infusion fluid (usually 100 mL); give over 1 hour.
● HANDLING AND STORAGE
Caution in handling Ganciclovir is toxic and personnel should be adequately protected during handling and administration; if solution comes into contact with skin or mucosa, wash off immediately with soap and water.

● MEDICINAL FORMS
There can be variation in the licensing of different medicines containing the same drug.
Powder for solution for infusion
ELECTROLYTES: May contain Sodium
▸ Cymevene (Roche Products Ltd)
Ganciclovir (as Ganciclovir sodium) 500 mg Cymevene 500mg powder for solution for infusion vials | 5 vial [PoM] £148.83

Valganciclovir

● **INDICATIONS AND DOSE**

Cytomegalovirus retinitis, induction and maintenance treatment in patients with AIDS

▸ BY MOUTH

▸ Adult: Initially 900 mg twice daily for 21 days, then 900 mg daily, induction regimen may be repeated if retinitis progresses

Prevention of cytomegalovirus disease following solid organ transplantation from a cytomegalovirus positive donor

▸ BY MOUTH

▸ Adult: 900 mg daily for 100 days (for 100–200 days following kidney transplantation), to be started within 10 days of transplantation

DOSE EQUIVALENCE AND CONVERSION
Oral valganciclovir 900 mg twice daily is equivalent to intravenous ganciclovir 5 mg/kg twice daily.

● CONTRA-INDICATIONS Abnormally low haemoglobin count (consult product literature) · abnormally low neutrophil count (consult product literature) · abnormally low platelet count (consult product literature)

● CAUTIONS Children (possible risk of long-term carcinogenic or reproductive toxicity) · history of cytopenia · potential carcinogen · potential teratogen · radiotherapy

● INTERACTIONS → Appendix 1 (valganciclovir).

● SIDE-EFFECTS

▸ **Common or very common** Abdominal pain · abnormal thinking · anaemia · anorexia · anxiety · arthralgia · chest pain · confusion · constipation · convulsions · cough · depression · dermatitis · diarrhoea · dizziness · dyspepsia · dysphagia · dyspnoea · ear pain · eye pain · fatigue · flatulence · headache · hepatic dysfunction · infection · insomnia · leucopenia · macular oedema · myalgia · nausea · night sweats · pancytopenia · peripheral neuropathy · pruritus · pyrexia · renal impairment · retinal detachment · taste disturbance · thrombocytopenia · vitreous floaters · vomiting · weight loss

▸ **Uncommon** Alopecia · anaphylactic reactions · arrhythmias · disturbances in hearing · disturbances in vision · haematuria · hypotension · male infertility · mouth ulcers · pancreatitis · psychosis · tremor

● ALLERGY AND CROSS-SENSITIVITY Contra-indicated in patients hypersensitive to ganciclovir, aciclovir, or valaciclovir.

● CONCEPTION AND CONTRACEPTION Ensure effective contraception during treatment and barrier contraception for men during and for at least 90 days after treatment.

● PREGNANCY Avoid—teratogenic risk.

● BREAST FEEDING Avoid—no information available.

● RENAL IMPAIRMENT Reduce dose, consult product literature.

● MONITORING REQUIREMENTS Monitor full blood count closely (severe deterioration may require correction and possibly treatment interruption).

● PRESCRIBING AND DISPENSING INFORMATION Valganciclovir is a pro-drug of ganciclovir.
Flavours of oral liquid formulations may include tutti-frutti.

● HANDLING AND STORAGE
Caution in handling Valganciclovir is a potential teratogen and carcinogen and caution is advised when handling the powder, reconstituted solution, or broken tablets; if these come into contact with skin or mucosa, wash off immediately with water; avoid inhalation of powder.

● MEDICINAL FORMS
There can be variation in the licensing of different medicines containing the same drug. Forms available from special-order manufacturers include: oral suspension, oral solution

Tablet
CAUTIONARY AND ADVISORY LABELS 21
▸ Valcyte (Roche Products Ltd)
Valganciclovir (as Valganciclovir hydrochloride) 450 mg Valcyte 450mg tablets | 60 tablet P̲o̲M̲ £1,081.46

Oral solution
CAUTIONARY AND ADVISORY LABELS 21
▸ Valcyte (Roche Products Ltd)
Valganciclovir (as Valganciclovir hydrochloride) 50 mg per 1 ml Valcyte 50mg/ml oral solution sugar-free | 100 ml P̲o̲M̲ £230.32

ANTIVIRALS > OTHER

Foscarnet sodium

● **INDICATIONS AND DOSE**

Cytomegalovirus disease

▸ BY INTRAVENOUS INFUSION

▸ Adult: Initially 60 mg/kg every 8 hours for 2–3 weeks, alternatively initially 90 mg/kg every 12 hours for 2–3 weeks, then maintenance 60 mg/kg daily, then increased if tolerated to 90–120 mg/kg daily, if disease progresses on maintenance dose, repeat induction regimen

Mucocutaneous herpes simplex virus infections unresponsive to aciclovir in immunocompromised patients

▸ BY INTRAVENOUS INFUSION

▸ Adult: 40 mg/kg every 8 hours for 2–3 weeks or until lesions heal

● UNLICENSED USE Licensed for CMV retinitis in AIDS patients only. Foscarnet doses in BNF may differ from those in product literature.

● CAUTIONS Ensure adequate hydration

● INTERACTIONS → Appendix 1 (foscarnet).

● SIDE-EFFECTS

▸ **Common or very common** Abdominal pain · acute renal failure · aggression · agitation · anaemia · anorexia · anxiety · changes in blood pressure · changes in ECG · confusion · constipation · convulsions · depression · diarrhoea · dizziness · dyspepsia · dysuria · electrolyte disturbances · genital irritation and ulceration (due to high concentrations excreted in urine) · granulocytopenia · headache · hepatic dysfunction · hypocalcaemia · hypokalaemia · hypomagnesaemia · leucopenia · malaise · myalgia · nausea (reduce infusion rate) · neurological disorders · oedema · palpitation · pancreatitis · paraesthesia (reduce infusion rate) · polyuria · pruritus · rash · renal impairment · thrombocytopenia · thrombophlebitis if given undiluted by peripheral vein · tremor · vomiting

▸ **Uncommon** Acidosis

▸ **Frequency not known** Diabetes insipidus · myasthenia · myositis · oesophageal ulceration · rhabdomyolysis · ventricular arrhythmias

● CONCEPTION AND CONTRACEPTION Men should avoid fathering a child during and for 6 months after treatment.

● PREGNANCY Manufacturer advises avoid.

● BREAST FEEDING Avoid—present in milk in *animal* studies.

● RENAL IMPAIRMENT Reduce dose; consult product literature.

● MONITORING REQUIREMENTS
▸ Monitor electrolytes, particularly calcium and magnesium.
▸ Monitor serum creatinine every second day during induction and every week during maintenance.

5

Infection

Infection

5

- DIRECTIONS FOR ADMINISTRATION Avoid rapid infusion. For *intravenous infusion* (*Foscavir*®), give intermittently *in* Glucose 5% or Sodium Chloride 0.9%; dilute to a concentration of 12 mg/mL for infusion into peripheral vein (undiluted solution *via* central venous line only); infuse over at least 1 hour (infuse doses greater than 60 mg/kg over 2 hours).

- MEDICINAL FORMS
  There can be variation in the licensing of different medicines containing the same drug.
  Solution for infusion
  ELECTROLYTES: May contain Sodium
  ▸ Foscavir (Clinigen Healthcare Ltd)
    Foscarnet sodium 24 mg per 1 ml Foscavir 6g/250ml solution for infusion bottles | 1 bottle PoM £119.85 (Hospital only)

6.4 HIV infection

HIV infection

Overview

There is no cure for infection caused by the human immunodeficiency virus (HIV) but a number of drugs slow or halt disease progression. Drugs for HIV infection (antiretrovirals) may be associated with serious side-effects. Although antiretrovirals increase life expectancy considerably and decrease the risk of complications associated with premature ageing, mortality and morbidity remain slightly higher than in uninfected individuals. Treatment should be undertaken only by those experienced in their use.

Principles of treatment

Treatment aims to prevent the mortality and morbidity associated with chronic HIV infection whilst minimising drug toxicity. Although it should be started before the immune system is irreversibly damaged, the need for early drug treatment should be balanced against the risk of toxicity. Commitment to treatment and strict adherence over many years are required; the regimen chosen should take into account convenience and patient tolerance. The development of drug resistance is reduced by using a combination of drugs; such combinations should have synergistic or additive activity while ensuring that their toxicity is not additive. It is recommended that viral sensitivity to antiretroviral drugs is established before starting treatment or before switching drugs if the infection is not responding.

Treatment also reduces the risk of HIV transmission to sexual partners, but the risk is not eliminated completely; this risk and strategies to reduce HIV transmission should be discussed with patients and their sexual partners.

Initiation of treatment

The optimum time for initiating antiretroviral treatment depends primarily on the CD4 cell count. The timing and choice of treatment should also take account of clinical symptoms, comorbidities, and the possible effect of antiretroviral drugs on factors such as the risk of cardiovascular events. Treatment includes a combination of drugs known as 'highly active antiretroviral therapy'. Treatment of HIV-1 is initiated with 2 nucleoside reverse transcriptase inhibitors and *either* a non-nucleoside reverse transcriptase inhibitor, *or* a boosted protease inhibitor, *or* an integrase inhibitor; the regimens of choice contain tenofovir disoproxil p. 591 and emtricitabine p. 589 with *either* efavirenz p. 585 *or* ritonavir p. 596-boosted atazanavir p. 593, *or* ritonavir-boosted darunavir p. 594, *or* raltegravir p. 584. Alternative regimens contain abacavir p. 587 and lamivudine p. 590 with *either* lopinavir with

ritonavir p. 595, *or* ritonavir-boosted fosamprenavir p. 594, *or* nevirapine p. 586, *or* rilpivirine p. 587. Patients who require treatment for both HIV and chronic hepatitis B should be treated with antivirals active against both diseases.

Switching therapy

Deterioration of the condition (including clinical and virological changes) may require a change in therapy. The choice of an alternative regimen depends on factors such as the response to previous treatment, tolerance and the possibility of cross-resistance.

Pregnancy

Treatment of HIV infection in pregnancy aims to reduce the risk of toxicity to the fetus (although information on the teratogenic potential of most antiretroviral drugs is limited), to minimise the viral load and disease progression in the mother, and to prevent transmission of infection to the neonate. **All treatment options require careful assessment by a specialist.** Combination antiretroviral therapy maximises the chance of preventing transmission and represents optimal therapy for the mother. However, it may be associated with a greater risk of preterm delivery. Pregnancies in HIV-positive women and babies born to them should be reported prospectively to the National Study of HIV in Pregnancy and Childhood at www.ucl.ac.uk/nshpc/ **and** to the Antiretroviral Pregnancy Registry at www.apregistry.com.

Breast-feeding

Breast-feeding by HIV-positive mothers may cause HIV infection in the infant and should be avoided.

Post-exposure prophylaxis

Prophylaxis with antiretroviral drugs [unlicensed indication] may be appropriate following exposure to HIV-contaminated material. Immediate expert advice should be sought in such cases; national guidelines on post-exposure prophylaxis for healthcare workers have been developed (by the Chief Medical Officer's Expert Advisory Group on AIDS), www.gov.uk/dh and local ones may also be available. Antiretrovirals for prophylaxis are chosen on the basis of efficacy and potential for toxicity. Prompt prophylaxis with antiretroviral drugs [unlicensed indication] is also appropriate following potential sexual exposure to HIV; recommendations have been developed by the British Association for Sexual Health and HIV, www.bashh.org.

Drugs for HIV infection

Zidovudine p. 592, a nucleoside reverse transcriptase inhibitor (or 'nucleoside analogue'), was the first anti-HIV drug to be introduced. Other nucleoside reverse transcriptase inhibitors include abacavir, didanosine p. 589, emtricitabine, lamivudine, stavudine p. 590, and tenofovir disoproxil.

The protease inhibitors include atazanavir, darunavir, fosamprenavir (a pro-drug of amprenavir), indinavir p. 595, lopinavir (available as lopinavir with ritonavir), ritonavir, saquinavir p. 596, and tipranavir p. 597. Indinavir is rarely used in the treatment of HIV-infection because it is associated with nephrolithiasis. Ritonavir in low doses boosts the activity of atazanavir, darunavir, fosamprenavir, indinavir, lopinavir (available as lopinavir with ritonavir), saquinavir, and tipranavir increasing the persistence of plasma concentrations of these drugs; at such a low dose, ritonavir has no intrinsic antiviral activity. The protease inhibitors are metabolised by cytochrome P450 enzyme systems and therefore have a significant potential for drug interactions. Protease inhibitors are associated with lipodystrophy and metabolic effects.

The non-nucleoside reverse transcriptase inhibitors efavirenz, etravirine p. 585, nevirapine, and rilpivirine are used in the treatment of HIV-1 infection, but not against the subtype HIV-2, a subtype that is rare in the UK. Nevirapine is associated with a high incidence of rash (including Stevens-Johnson syndrome) and occasionally fatal hepatitis. Rash is also associated with efavirenz and etravirine but it is usually milder. Psychiatric or CNS disturbances are common with efavirenz; CNS disturbances are often self-limiting and can be reduced by taking the dose at bedtime (especially in the first 2–4 weeks of treatment). Efavirenz has also been associated with an increased plasma-cholesterol concentration. Etravirine is used in regimens containing a boosted protease inhibitor for HIV infection resistant to other non-nucleoside reverse transcriptase inhibitors and protease inhibitors.

Enfuvirtide below, which inhibits the fusion of HIV to the host cell, is licensed for managing infection that has failed to respond to a regimen of other antiretroviral drugs; enfuvirtide should be combined with other potentially active antiretroviral drugs.

Maraviroc p. 597 is an antagonist of the CCR5 chemokine receptor. It is licensed for patients exclusively infected with CCR5-tropic HIV.

Dolutegravir p. 584 and raltegravir are inhibitors of HIV integrase. They are licensed for the treatment of HIV infection in combination with other antiretroviral drugs.

Elvitegravir is also an inhibitor of HIV integrase that is only available as a component of a fixed-dose combination product (tenofovir with cobicistat, elvitegravir and emtricitabine p. 591). Cobicistat p. 597 is a pharmacokinetic enhancer that boosts the concentrations of other antiretrovirals, but it has no antiretroviral activity itself.

Immune reconstitution syndrome

Improvement in immune function as a result of antiretroviral treatment may provoke a marked inflammatory reaction against residual opportunistic organisms; these reactions may occur within the first few weeks or months of initiating treatment. Autoimmune disorders (such as Graves' disease) have also been reported many months after initiation of treatment.

Lipodystrophy syndrome

Metabolic effects associated with antiretroviral treatment include *fat redistribution, insulin resistance*, and *dyslipidaemia*; collectively these have been termed *lipodystrophy syndrome*. The usual risk factors for cardiovascular disease should be taken into account before starting antiretroviral therapy and patients should be advised about lifestyle changes to reduce their cardiovascular risk. Plasma lipids and blood glucose should be measured before starting antiretroviral therapy, after 3–6 months of treatment, and then annually.

Fat redistribution (with loss of subcutaneous fat, increased abdominal fat, 'buffalo hump' and breast enlargement) is associated with regimens containing protease inhibitors and nucleoside reverse transcriptase inhibitors. Stavudine (especially in combination with didanosine), and to a lesser extent zidovudine, are associated with a higher risk of lipoatrophy and should be used only if alternative regimens are not suitable.

Dyslipidaemia is associated with antiretroviral treatment, particularly with protease inhibitors. Protease inhibitors and some nucleoside reverse transcriptase inhibitors are associated with insulin resistance and hyperglycaemia. Of the protease inhibitors, atazanavir and darunavir may be less likely to cause dyslipidaemia, while saquinavir and atazanavir may be less likely to impair glucose tolerance.

Osteonecrosis

Osteonecrosis has been reported in patients with advanced HIV disease or following long-term exposure to combination antiretroviral therapy.

HIV infection in children

HIV disease in children has a different natural progression to adults. Children infected with HIV should be managed within a formal paediatric HIV clinical network by specialists with access to guidelines and information on antiretroviral drugs for children.

ANTIVIRALS ⟩ HIV-FUSION INHIBITORS

Enfuvirtide

● DRUG ACTION Enfuvirtide inhibits the fusion of HIV to the host cell.

● INDICATIONS AND DOSE

HIV infection in combination with other antiretroviral drugs for resistant infection or for patients intolerant to other antiretroviral regimens
▸ BY SUBCUTANEOUS INJECTION
▸ Adult: 90 mg twice daily

● INTERACTIONS → Appendix 1 (enfuvirtide).

● SIDE-EFFECTS

▸ **Common or very common** Acne · anorexia · anxiety · asthenia · conjunctivitis · diabetes mellitus · dry skin · erythema · gastro-oesophageal reflux disease · haematuria · hypertriglyceridaemia · impaired concentration · influenza-like illness · injection-site reactions · irritability · lymphadenopathy · myalgia · nightmares · pancreatitis · peripheral neuropathy · pneumonia · renal calculi · sinusitis · skin papilloma · tremor · vertigo · weight loss
▸ **Uncommon** Hypersensitivity reactions
▸ **Frequency not known** Osteonecrosis

SIDE-EFFECTS, FURTHER INFORMATION
▸ Hypersensitivity reactions Hypersensitivity reactions including rash, fever, nausea, vomiting, chills, rigors, low blood pressure, respiratory distress, glomerulonephritis, and raised liver enzymes reported; discontinue immediately if any signs or symptoms of systemic hypersensitivity develop and do not rechallenge.
▸ Osteonecrosis For further information see HIV infection p. 582.

● PREGNANCY Manufacturer advises use only if potential benefit outweighs risk.

● HEPATIC IMPAIRMENT Manufacturer advises caution— no information available; chronic hepatitis B or C (possibly greater risk of hepatic side-effects).

● DIRECTIONS FOR ADMINISTRATION For *subcutaneous injection*, reconstitute with 1.1 mL Water for Injections and allow to stand (for up to 45 minutes) to dissolve; do **not** shake or invert vial.

● PATIENT AND CARER ADVICE
Hypersensitivity reactions Patients or carers should be told how to recognise signs of hypersensitivity, and advised to discontinue treatment and seek immediate medical attention if symptoms develop.

● MEDICINAL FORMS
There can be variation in the licensing of different medicines containing the same drug.
Powder and solvent for solution for injection
ELECTROLYTES: May contain Sodium
▸ Fuzeon (Roche Products Ltd)
Enfuvirtide 108 mg Fuzeon 108mg powder and solvent for solution for injection vials | 60 vial PoM £1,081.57

5

Infection

Dolutegravir

20.11.2016

- **DRUG ACTION** Dolutegravir is an inhibitor of HIV integrase.

- **INDICATIONS AND DOSE**

HIV infection without resistance to other inhibitors of HIV integrase, in combination with other antiretroviral drugs
  ▸ BY MOUTH
  ▸ Adult: 50 mg once daily

HIV infection in patients where resistance to other inhibitors of HIV integrase suspected, in combination with other antiretroviral drugs
  ▸ BY MOUTH
  ▸ Adult: 50 mg twice daily, dose to be taken with food

HIV infection in combination with other antiretroviral drugs (with concomitant carbamazepine, efavirenz, etravirine (without boosted protease inhibitors, but see also Interactions), fosphenytoin, phenobarbital, phenytoin, primidone, nevirapine, oxcarbazepine, St John's wort, rifampicin, or tipranavir)
  ▸ BY MOUTH
  ▸ Adult: 50 mg twice daily, avoid concomitant use with these drugs if resistance to other inhibitors of HIV integrase suspected

- **INTERACTIONS** → Appendix 1 (dolutegravir).
  Caution—avoid concomitant use with etravirine, unless used in combination with atazanavir, darunavir, or lopinavir.

- **SIDE-EFFECTS**
  ▸ **Common or very common** Abdominal pain · abnormal dreams · diarrhoea · dizziness · fatigue · flatulence · headache · insomnia · nausea · pruritus · raised creatine kinase · rash · vomiting
  ▸ **Uncommon** Hepatitis · hypersensitivity reactions
  ▸ **Frequency not known** Osteonecrosis
    SIDE-EFFECTS, FURTHER INFORMATION
  ▸ Hypersensitivity reactions Hypersensitivity reactions (including severe rash, or rash accompanied by fever, malaise, arthralgia, myalgia, blistering, oral lesions, conjunctivitis, angioedema, eosinophilia, or raised liver enzymes) reported uncommonly. Discontinue immediately if any sign or symptoms of hypersensitivity reactions develop.
  ▸ Osteonecrosis For further information see HIV infection p. 582.

- **PREGNANCY** Manufacturer advises use only if potential benefit outweighs risk.

- **HEPATIC IMPAIRMENT** Manufacturer advises caution in severe impairment—no information available.

- **DIRECTIONS FOR ADMINISTRATION** Avoid antacids 6 hours before or 2 hours after taking dolutegravir.

- **PATIENT AND CARER ADVICE**
  Missed doses
  If a dose is more than 20 hours late on the once daily regimen (or more than 8 hours late on the twice daily regimen), the missed dose should not be taken and the next dose should be taken at the normal time.
    Patients or carers should be given advice on how to administer dolutegravir tablets.

- **MEDICINAL FORMS**
  There can be variation in the licensing of different medicines containing the same drug.
  Tablet
  ▸ Tivicay (ViiV Healthcare UK Ltd) ▼
    Dolutegravir (as Dolutegravir sodium) 50 mg Tivicay 50mg tablets | 30 tablet [PoM] £498.75

  Combinations available: *Abacavir with dolutegravir and lamivudine*, p. 588

Raltegravir

- **DRUG ACTION** Raltegravir is an inhibitor of HIV integrase.

- **INDICATIONS AND DOSE**

HIV infection in combination with other antiretroviral drugs
  ▸ BY MOUTH USING TABLETS
  ▸ Adult: 400 mg twice daily

DOSE EQUIVALENCE AND CONVERSION
The bioavailability of *Isentress*® chewable tablets is higher than that of the 'standard' 400 mg tablets; the chewable tablets are **not** interchangeable with the 'standard' tablets on a milligram-for-milligram basis.

- **CAUTIONS** Psychiatric illness (may exacerbate underlying illness including depression) · risk factors for myopathy · risk factors for rhabdomyolysis

- **INTERACTIONS** → Appendix 1 (raltegravir).

- **SIDE-EFFECTS**
  ▸ **Common or very common** Abdominal pain · abnormal dreams · asthenia · depression · diarrhoea · dizziness · dyspepsia · flatulence · headache · hyperactivity · hypertriglyceridaemia · insomnia · nausea · rash · vomiting
  ▸ **Uncommon** Acne · alopecia · anaemia · anxiety · appetite changes · arthralgia · bradycardia · carpal tunnel syndrome · chest pain · chills · confusion · constipation · drowsiness · dry mouth · dry skin · dysphonia · epistaxis · erectile dysfunction · flushing · gastritis · gingivitis · glossitis · gynaecomastia · hepatitis · hyperhidrosis · hypertension · impaired memory and attention · lipodystrophy · Lipodystrophy Syndrome · menopausal symptoms · myalgia · nasal congestion · neutropenia · nocturia · oedema · osteopenia · pain on swallowing · palpitation · pancreatitis · peptic ulcer · peripheral neuropathy · polydipsia · pruritus · pyrexia · rash with eosinophilia and systemic symptoms · rectal bleeding · renal failure · rhabdomyolysis · skin papilloma · Stevens-Johnson syndrome · suicidal ideation · taste disturbances · thrombocytopenia · tinnitus · tremor · ventricular extrasystoles · visual disturbances
  ▸ **Frequency not known** Osteonecrosis
    SIDE-EFFECTS, FURTHER INFORMATION
  ▸ Rash Rash occurs commonly. Discontinue if severe rash or rash accompanied by fever, malaise, arthralgia, myalgia, blistering, mouth ulceration, conjunctivitis, angioedema, hepatitis, or eosinophilia.
  ▸ Lipodystrophy syndrome For further information see HIV infection p. 582.
  ▸ Osteonecrosis For further information see HIV infection p. 582.

- **PREGNANCY** Manufacturer advises avoid—toxicity in *animal* studies.

- **HEPATIC IMPAIRMENT** Manufacturer advises caution in severe impairment—no information available. Use with caution in patients with chronic hepatitis B or C (at greater risk of hepatic side-effects).

- **PRESCRIBING AND DISPENSING INFORMATION** Dispense raltegravir chewable tablets in original container (contains desiccant).

- **NATIONAL FUNDING/ACCESS DECISIONS**

Scottish Medicines Consortium (SMC) Decisions
The *Scottish Medicines Consortium* has advised (April 2010) that raltegravir (*Isentress*®) is accepted for restricted use within NHS Scotland for the treatment of HIV infection when non-nucleoside reverse transcriptase inhibitors or protease inhibitors cannot be used because of intolerance, drug interactions, or resistance.

- **MEDICINAL FORMS**
There can be variation in the licensing of different medicines containing the same drug.
Tablet
CAUTIONARY AND ADVISORY LABELS 25
▸ Isentress (Merck Sharp & Dohme Ltd)
  Raltegravir 400 mg Isentress 400mg tablets | 60 tablet [PoM] £471.41

ANTIVIRALS > NON-NUCLEOSIDE REVERSE TRANSCRIPTASE INHIBITORS

Efavirenz

- **INDICATIONS AND DOSE**

HIV infection in combination with other antiretroviral drugs
▸ BY MOUTH USING CAPSULES
▸ Adult: 600 mg once daily
▸ BY MOUTH USING TABLETS
▸ Adult: 600 mg once daily
▸ BY MOUTH USING ORAL SOLUTION
▸ Adult: 720 mg once daily

DOSE EQUIVALENCE AND CONVERSION
The bioavailability of *Sustiva*® oral solution is lower than that of the capsules and tablets; the oral solution is **not** interchangeable with either capsules or tablets on a milligram-for-milligram basis.

- **UNLICENSED USE** Opening capsules and adding contents to food is an unlicensed method of administration.
- **CAUTIONS** Acute porphyrias p. 918 · elderly · history of psychiatric disorders · history of seizures
- **INTERACTIONS** → Appendix 1 (efavirenz).
- **SIDE-EFFECTS**
▸ **Common or very common** Abdominal pain · abnormal dreams · anxiety · depression · diarrhoea · dizziness · fatigue · headache · impaired concentration · nausea · pruritus · rash · sleep disturbances · Stevens-Johnson syndrome · vomiting
▸ **Uncommon** Amnesia · ataxia · blurred vision · convulsions · flushing · gynaecomastia · hepatitis · hypersensitivity · mania · pancreatitis · psychosis · suicidal ideation · tinnitus · tremor · vertigo
▸ **Rare** Hepatic failure · photosensitivity · suicide
▸ **Frequency not known** Lipodystrophy syndrome · osteonecrosis · raised serum cholesterol
  SIDE-EFFECTS, FURTHER INFORMATION
▸ Rash Rash, usually in the first 2 weeks, is the most common side-effect; discontinue if severe rash with blistering, desquamation, mucosal involvement or fever; if rash mild or moderate, may continue without interruption—usually resolves within 1 month.
▸ CNS effects Administration at bedtime especially in first 2–4 weeks reduces CNS effects.
▸ Lipodystrophy syndrome For further information see HIV infection p. 582.
▸ Osteonecrosis For further information see HIV infection p. 582.
▸ Immune Reconstitution Syndrome For further information see HIV infection p. 582.

- **PREGNANCY** Reports of neural tube defects when used in first trimester.
- **HEPATIC IMPAIRMENT** Greater risk of hepatic side-effects in chronic hepatitis B or C. Avoid in moderate to severe impairment. In mild liver disease, monitor for dose related side-effects (e.g. CNS effects) and monitor liver function.
- **RENAL IMPAIRMENT** Manufacturer advises caution in severe renal failure—no information available.
- **MONITORING REQUIREMENTS** Monitor liver function if receiving other hepatotoxic drugs.
- **DIRECTIONS FOR ADMINISTRATION** Capsules may be opened and contents added to food (contents have a peppery taste).
- **PRESCRIBING AND DISPENSING INFORMATION** Flavours of oral liquid formulations may include strawberry and mint.
- **PATIENT AND CARER ADVICE**
Psychiatric disorders Patients or their carers should be advised to seek immediate medical attention if symptoms such as severe depression, psychosis or suicidal ideation occur.

- **MEDICINAL FORMS**
There can be variation in the licensing of different medicines containing the same drug.
Tablet
CAUTIONARY AND ADVISORY LABELS 23
▸ Efavirenz (Non-proprietary)
  Efavirenz 600 mg Efavirenz 600mg tablets | 30 tablet [PoM] £190.26–£200.27 | 30 tablet [PoM] £90.43 (Hospital only)
▸ Sustiva (Bristol-Myers Squibb Pharmaceuticals Ltd)
  Efavirenz 600 mg Sustiva 600mg tablets | 30 tablet [PoM] £200.27 (Hospital only)
Capsule
CAUTIONARY AND ADVISORY LABELS 23
▸ Sustiva (Bristol-Myers Squibb Pharmaceuticals Ltd)
  Efavirenz 50 mg Sustiva 50mg capsules | 30 capsule [PoM] £16.73 (Hospital only)
  Efavirenz 100 mg Sustiva 100mg capsules | 30 capsule [PoM] £33.41 (Hospital only)
  Efavirenz 200 mg Sustiva 200mg capsules | 90 capsule [PoM] £200.27 (Hospital only)

Combinations available: *Tenofovir with efavirenz and emtricitabine,* p. 592

Etravirine

- **INDICATIONS AND DOSE**

HIV infection resistant to other non-nucleoside reverse transcriptase inhibitor and protease inhibitors in combination with other antiretroviral drugs (including a boosted protease inhibitor)
▸ BY MOUTH
▸ Adult: 200 mg twice daily, to be taken after food

- **CONTRA-INDICATIONS** Acute porphyrias p. 918
- **INTERACTIONS** → Appendix 1 (etravirine).
- **SIDE-EFFECTS**
▸ **Common or very common** Abdominal pain · anaemia · diabetes · flatulence · gastritis · gastro-oesophageal reflux · hyperlipidaemia · hypertension · Lipodystrophy Syndrome · myocardial infarction · nausea · peripheral neuropathy · rash · renal failure
▸ **Uncommon** Angina · blurred vision · bronchospasm · drowsiness · dry mouth · gynaecomastia · haematemesis · hepatitis · malaise · pancreatitis · sweating
▸ **Rare** Stevens-Johnson syndrome
▸ **Very rare** Toxic epidermal necrolysis
▸ **Frequency not known** Haemorrhagic stroke · hypersensitivity reactions · osteonecrosis

Infection

5

SIDE-EFFECTS, FURTHER INFORMATION
▸ **Hypersensitivity reactions** Rash, usually in the second week, is the most common side-effect and appears more frequently in females. Life-threatening hypersensitivity reactions reported usually during week 3–6 of treatment and characterised by rash, eosinophilia, and systemic symptoms (including fever, general malaise, myalgia, arthralgia, blistering, oral lesions, conjunctivitis, and hepatitis). Discontinue permanently if hypersensitivity reaction or severe rash develop. If rash mild or moderate (without signs of hypersensitivity reaction), may continue without interruption—usually resolves within 2 weeks.
▸ **Lipodystrophy** For further information see HIV infection p. 582.
▸ **Osteonecrosis** For further information see HIV infection p. 582.
● **HEPATIC IMPAIRMENT** Manufacturer advises caution in moderate impairment; avoid in severe impairment— no information available; greater risk of hepatic side-effects in chronic hepatitis B or C.
● **DIRECTIONS FOR ADMINISTRATION** Patients with swallowing difficulties may disperse tablets in a glass of water just before administration.
● **PRESCRIBING AND DISPENSING INFORMATION** Dispense in original container (contains desiccant).
● **PATIENT AND CARER ADVICE**
Missed doses
If a dose is more than 6 hours late, the missed dose should not be taken and the next dose should be taken at the normal time.
Hypersensitivity reactions Patients or carers should be told how to recognise hypersensitivity reactions and advised to seek immediate medical attention if hypersensitivity reaction or severe rash develop.

● **MEDICINAL FORMS**
There can be variation in the licensing of different medicines containing the same drug.
Tablet
CAUTIONARY AND ADVISORY LABELS 21
▸ Intelence (Janssen-Cilag Ltd)
Etravirine 25 mg Intelence 25mg tablets | 120 tablet PoM £75.32
Etravirine 100 mg Intelence 100mg tablets | 120 tablet PoM £301.27
Etravirine 200 mg Intelence 200mg tablets | 60 tablet PoM £301.27

Nevirapine

● **INDICATIONS AND DOSE**
HIV infection in combination with other antiretroviral drugs (initial dose)
▸ BY MOUTH USING IMMEDIATE-RELEASE MEDICINES
▸ Adult: Initially 200 mg once daily for first 14 days, initial dose titration using 'immediate-release' preparation should not exceed 28 days; if rash occurs and is not resolved within 28 days, alternative treatment should be sought. If treatment interrupted for more than 7 days, restart using the lower dose of the 'immediate-release' preparation for the first 14 days as for new treatment

HIV infection in combination with other antiretroviral drugs (maintenance dose following initial dose titration if no rash present)
▸ BY MOUTH USING IMMEDIATE-RELEASE MEDICINES
▸ Adult: 200 mg twice daily
▸ BY MOUTH USING MODIFIED-RELEASE MEDICINES
▸ Adult: 400 mg once daily

● **CONTRA-INDICATIONS** Acute porphyrias p. 918 · post-exposure prophylaxis

● **CAUTIONS** Females (at greater risk of hepatic side effects) · high CD4 cell count (at greater risk of hepatic side effects)
CAUTIONS, FURTHER INFORMATION
▸ **Hepatic effects** Patients with chronic hepatitis B or C, high CD4 cell count, and women are at increased risk of hepatic side effects—if plasma HIV-1 RNA detectable, manufacturer advises avoid in women with CD4 cell count greater than 250 cells/mm^3 or in men with CD4 cell count greater than 400 cells/mm^3 unless potential benefit outweighs risk.
● **INTERACTIONS** → Appendix 1 (nevirapine).
● **SIDE-EFFECTS**
▸ **Common or very common** Abdominal pain · diarrhoea · fatigue · fever · granulocytopenia · headache · hepatitis · hypersensitivity reactions (may involve hepatic reactions and rash) · nausea · rash · Stevens-Johnson syndrome · toxic epidermal necrolysis · vomiting
▸ **Uncommon** Anaemia · arthralgia · myalgia
▸ **Frequency not known** Osteonecrosis
SIDE-EFFECTS, FURTHER INFORMATION
▸ **Hepatic effects** Potentially life-threatening hepatotoxicity including fatal fulminant hepatitis reported usually in first 6 weeks; discontinue permanently if abnormalities in liver function tests accompanied by hypersensitivity reaction (rash, fever, arthralgia, myalgia, lymphadenopathy, hepatitis, renal impairment, eosinophilia, granulocytopenia); suspend if severe abnormalities in liver function tests but no hypersensitivity reaction— discontinue permanently if significant liver function abnormalities recur; monitor patient closely if mild to moderate abnormalities in liver function tests with no hypersensitivity reaction.
▸ **Rash** Rash, usually in first 6 weeks, is most common side-effect; incidence reduced if introduced at low dose and dose increased gradually (after 14 days). Discontinue permanently if severe rash or if rash accompanied by blistering, oral lesions, conjunctivitis, facial oedema, general malaise or hypersensitivity reactions; if rash mild or moderate may continue without interruption but dose should not be increased until rash resolves.
▸ **Osteonecrosis** For more information see HIV infection p. 582.
● **HEPATIC IMPAIRMENT** Manufacturer advises avoid modified-release preparation—no information available; use 'immediate-release' preparation with caution in moderate impairment and avoid in severe impairment. Use with caution in patients with chronic hepatitis B or C (at greater risk of hepatic side effects).
● **RENAL IMPAIRMENT** Manufacturer advises avoid modified-release preparation—no information available.
● **MONITORING REQUIREMENTS**
▸ **Hepatic disease** Close monitoring of liver function required during first 18 weeks; monitor liver function before treatment then every 2 weeks for 2 months then after 1 month and then regularly.
▸ **Rash** Monitor closely for skin reactions during first 18 weeks.
● **PATIENT AND CARER ADVICE**
Missed doses
If a dose is more than 8 hours late with the 'immediate-release' preparation (or more than 12 hours late with the modified-release preparation), the missed dose should not be taken and the next dose should be taken at the usual time.
Hypersensitivity reactions Patients or carers should be told how to recognise hypersensitivity reactions and advised to discontinue treatment and seek immediate medical attention if severe skin reaction, hypersensitivity reactions, or symptoms of hepatitis develop.

- MEDICINAL FORMS
There can be variation in the licensing of different medicines containing the same drug.

Tablet
▶ Nevirapine (Non-proprietary)
  Nevirapine 200 mg Nevirapine 200mg tablets | 60 tablet [PoM] £28.60–£170.00
▶ Viramune (Boehringer Ingelheim Ltd)
  Nevirapine 200 mg Viramune 200mg tablets | 14 tablet [PoM] £39.67 | 60 tablet [PoM] £170.00

Modified-release tablet
CAUTIONARY AND ADVISORY LABELS 25
▶ Viramune (Boehringer Ingelheim Ltd)
  Nevirapine 100 mg Viramune 100mg modified-release tablets | 90 tablet [PoM] £127.50 (Hospital only)
  Nevirapine 400 mg Viramune 400mg modified-release tablets | 30 tablet [PoM] £170.00 (Hospital only)

Oral suspension
▶ Viramune (Boehringer Ingelheim Ltd)
  Nevirapine (as Nevirapine hemihydrate) 10 mg per 1 ml Viramune 50mg/5ml oral suspension | 240 ml [PoM] £50.40

Rilpivirine

- INDICATIONS AND DOSE

HIV infection in combination with other antiretroviral drugs in patients not previously treated with antiretroviral therapy and if plasma HIV-1 RNA concentration less than 100 000 copies/mL
▶ BY MOUTH
▶ Adult: 25 mg once daily

- INTERACTIONS → Appendix 1 (rilpivirine).
Caution if concomitant use with drugs that prolong QT interval.

- SIDE-EFFECTS Abdominal pain · abnormal dreams · anorexia · depression · dizziness · dry mouth · headache · hyperlipidaemia · Lipodystrophy Syndrome · malaise · nausea · osteonecrosis · raised serum amylase · raised serum lipase · rash · sleep disturbances · vomiting

SIDE-EFFECTS, FURTHER INFORMATION
▶ Lipodystrophy For further information see HIV infection p. 582.
▶ Osteonecrosis For further information see HIV infection p. 582.

- PREGNANCY Manufacturer advises avoid unless essential— no information available.

- HEPATIC IMPAIRMENT Manufacturer advises caution in moderate impairment; avoid in severe impairment— no information available; greater risk of hepatic side-effects in chronic hepatitis B or C.

- RENAL IMPAIRMENT Manufacturer advises caution in severe impairment.

- DIRECTIONS FOR ADMINISTRATION Avoid antacids 2 hours before or 4 hours after taking rilpivirine.

- PATIENT AND CARER ADVICE
Missed doses
If a dose is more than 12 hours late, the missed dose should not be taken and the next dose should be taken at the normal time.
   Patients or carers should be given advice on how to administer rilpivirine tablets.

- MEDICINAL FORMS
There can be variation in the licensing of different medicines containing the same drug.

Tablet
CAUTIONARY AND ADVISORY LABELS 21, 25
▶ Edurant (Janssen-Cilag Ltd) ▼
  Rilpivirine (as Rilpivirine hydrochloride) 25 mg Edurant 25mg tablets | 30 tablet [PoM] £200.27

Combinations available: *Tenofovir with emtricitabine and rilpivirine*, p. 592

ANTIVIRALS > NUCLEOSIDE REVERSE TRANSCRIPTASE INHIBITORS

Nucleoside reverse transcriptase inhibitors

- CAUTIONS Alcohol abuse (increased risk of lactic acidosis) · obese women (increased risk of lactic acidosis) · patients at risk of lactic acidosis

CAUTIONS, FURTHER INFORMATION
▶ Lactic acidosis Life-threatening lactic acidosis associated with hepatomegaly and hepatic steatosis has been reported with nucleoside reverse transcriptase inhibitors. They should be used with caution in patients with hepatomegaly, hepatitis (especially hepatitis C treated with interferon alfa and ribavirin), liver-enzyme abnormalities and with other risk factors for liver disease and hepatic steatosis. Treatment with the nucleoside reverse transcriptase inhibitor should be **discontinued** in case of symptomatic hyperlactataemia, lactic acidosis, progressive hepatomegaly or rapid deterioration of liver function.

- SIDE-EFFECTS Abdominal pain · anaemia · anorexia · arthralgia · blood disorders · cough · diarrhoea · dizziness · dyspnoea · fatigue · fever · flatulence · gastro-intestinal disturbances · headache · insomnia · lactic acidosis · lipodystrophy (Lipodystrophy Syndrome) · liver damage · metabolic effects · myalgia · nausea · neutropenia · osteonecrosis · pancreatitis · rash · thrombocytopenia · urticaria · vomiting

SIDE-EFFECTS, FURTHER INFORMATION
▶ Lipodystrophy syndrome For further information see HIV infection p. 582.
▶ Osteonecrosis For further information see HIV infection p. 582.

- PREGNANCY Mitochondrial dysfunction has been reported in infants exposed to nucleoside reverse transcriptase inhibitors in utero; the main effects include haematological, metabolic, and neurological disorders; all infants whose mothers received nucleoside reverse transcriptase inhibitors during pregnancy should be monitored for relevant signs or symptoms.

- HEPATIC IMPAIRMENT Use with caution in patients with chronic hepatitis B or C (greater risk of hepatic side-effects).

◀ above

Abacavir

- INDICATIONS AND DOSE

HIV infection in combination with other antiretroviral drugs
▶ BY MOUTH
▶ Adult: 600 mg daily in 1–2 divided doses

- CAUTIONS HIV load greater than 100 000 copies/mL · patients at high risk of cardiovascular disease (especially if 10-year cardiovascular risk greater than 20%)

- INTERACTIONS → Appendix 1 (abacavir).

- SIDE-EFFECTS
- ▶ **Very rare** Stevens-Johnson syndrome · toxic epidermal necrolysis
- ▶ **Frequency not known** Hypersensitivity reactions
  SIDE-EFFECTS, FURTHER INFORMATION
- ▶ Hypersensitivity reactions Life-threatening hypersensitivity reactions reported—characterised by fever or rash and possibly nausea, vomiting, diarrhoea, abdominal pain, dyspnoea, cough, lethargy, malaise, headache, and myalgia; less frequently mouth ulceration, oedema, hypotension, sore throat, acute respiratory distress syndrome, anaphylaxis, paraesthesia, arthralgia, conjunctivitis, lymphadenopathy, lymphocytopenia and renal failure; rarely myolysis; laboratory abnormalities may include raised liver function tests and creatine kinase; symptoms usually appear in the first 6 weeks, but may occur at any time.

  Discontinue immediately if any symptom of hypersensitivity develops and do not rechallenge (risk of more severe hypersensitivity reaction); discontinue if hypersensitivity cannot be ruled out, even when other diagnoses possible—if rechallenge necessary it must be carried out in hospital setting; if abacavir is stopped for any reason other than hypersensitivity, exclude hypersensitivity reaction as the cause and rechallenge only if medical assistance is readily available; care needed with concomitant use of drugs which cause skin toxicity.

- ALLERGY AND CROSS-SENSITIVITY Caution—increased risk of hypersensitivity reaction in presence of HLA-B*5701 allele.
- HEPATIC IMPAIRMENT Monitor closely in mild impairment (combination preparations not recommended as reduced abacavir dose may be required). Avoid in moderate impairment unless essential—close monitoring recommended. Avoid in severe impairment.
- RENAL IMPAIRMENT Manufacturer advises avoid in end-stage renal disease.
- PRE-TREATMENT SCREENING Test for HLA-B*5701 allele before treatment or if restarting treatment and HLA-B*5701 status not known.
- MONITORING REQUIREMENTS Monitor for symptoms of hypersensitivity reaction every 2 weeks for 2 months.
- PRESCRIBING AND DISPENSING INFORMATION Flavours of oral liquid formulations may include banana, or strawberry.
- PATIENT AND CARER ADVICE Patients should be provided with an alert card and advised to keep it with them at all times.

  Patients and their carers should be told the importance of regular dosing (intermittent therapy may increase the risk of sensitisation), how to recognise signs of hypersensitivity, and advised to seek immediate medical attention if symptoms develop or before re-starting treatment.

- MEDICINAL FORMS
  There can be variation in the licensing of different medicines containing the same drug.
  Tablet
  - ▶ Ziagen (ViiV Healthcare UK Ltd)
    Abacavir (as Abacavir sulfate) 300 mg Ziagen 300mg tablets | 60 tablet [PoM] £177.60
  Oral solution
  EXCIPIENTS: May contain Propylene glycol
  - ▶ Ziagen (ViiV Healthcare UK Ltd)
    Abacavir (as Abacavir sulfate) 20 mg per 1 ml Ziagen 20mg/ml oral solution sugar-free | 240 ml [PoM] £47.36

Abacavir with dolutegravir and lamivudine

The properties listed below are those particular to the combination only. For the properties of the components please consider, abacavir p. 587, lamivudine p. 590, dolutegravir p. 584.

- INDICATIONS AND DOSE
  HIV infection
  - ▶ BY MOUTH
    - ▶ Adult (body-weight 40 kg and above): 1 tablet once daily
- RENAL IMPAIRMENT Avoid *Triumeq®* if eGFR less than 50 mL/minute/1.73 m^2 (consult product literature).
- PATIENT AND CARER ADVICE
  Missed doses
  If a dose is more than 20 hours late, the missed dose should not be taken and the next dose should be taken at the normal time.
- MEDICINAL FORMS
  There can be variation in the licensing of different medicines containing the same drug.
  Tablet
  - ▶ Triumeq (ViiV Healthcare UK Ltd) ▼
    Dolutegravir (as Dolutegravir sodium) 50 mg, Lamivudine 300 mg, Abacavir (as Abacavir sulfate) 600 mg Triumeq 50mg/600mg/300mg tablets | 30 tablet [PoM] £798.16

Abacavir with lamivudine

The properties listed below are those particular to the combination only. For the properties of the components please consider, abacavir p. 587, lamivudine p. 590.

- INDICATIONS AND DOSE
  HIV infection in combination with other antiretrovirals
  - ▶ BY MOUTH
    - ▶ Adult (body-weight 40 kg and above): 1 tablet once daily
- RENAL IMPAIRMENT Avoid *Kivexa®* if eGFR less than 50 mL/minute/1.73 m^2 (consult product literature).
- MEDICINAL FORMS
  There can be variation in the licensing of different medicines containing the same drug.
  Tablet
  - ▶ Abacavir with lamivudine (Non-proprietary)
    Lamivudine 300 mg, Abacavir (as Abacavir sulfate) 600 mg Abacavir 600mg / Lamivudine 300mg tablets | 30 tablet [PoM] £194.62
  - ▶ Kivexa (ViiV Healthcare UK Ltd)
    Lamivudine 300 mg, Abacavir (as Abacavir sulfate) 600 mg Kivexa 600mg/300mg tablets | 30 tablet [PoM] £299.41

Abacavir with lamivudine and zidovudine

The properties listed below are those particular to the combination only. For the properties of the components please consider, abacavir p. 587, lamivudine p. 590, zidovudine p. 592.

- INDICATIONS AND DOSE
  HIV infection (use only if patient is stabilised for 6–8 weeks on the individual components in the same proportions)
  - ▶ BY MOUTH
    - ▶ Adult: 1 tablet twice daily

- RENAL IMPAIRMENT Avoid *Trizivir*® if eGFR less than 50 mL/minute/1.73 m² (consult product literature).

- MEDICINAL FORMS
There can be variation in the licensing of different medicines containing the same drug.
Tablet
▸ Trizivir (ViiV Healthcare UK Ltd)
   Lamivudine 150 mg, Abacavir (as Abacavir sulfate) 300 mg, Zidovudine 300 mg Trizivir tablets | 60 tablet [PoM] £432.70

☞ 587

Didanosine

(ddI; DDI)

- INDICATIONS AND DOSE

HIV infection in combination with other antiretroviral drugs
▸ BY MOUTH
▸ Adult (body-weight up to 60 kg): 250 mg daily in 1–2 divided doses
▸ Adult (body-weight 60 kg and above): 400 mg daily in 1–2 divided doses

- CAUTIONS History of pancreatitis (preferably avoid, otherwise extreme caution) · hyperuricaemia · peripheral neuropathy

- INTERACTIONS → Appendix 1 (didanosine).
Antacids in tablet formulation might affect absorption of other drugs—give at least 2 hours apart.

- SIDE-EFFECTS Acute renal failure · alopecia · anaphylactic reactions · diabetes mellitus · dry eyes · dry mouth · hyperuricaemia (suspend if raised significantly) · hypoglycaemia · liver failure · non-cirrhotic portal hypertension · optic nerve changes · pancreatitis (less common in children) · parotid gland enlargement · peripheral neuropathy (switch to another antiretroviral if peripheral neuropathy develops) · retinal changes · rhabdomyolysis · sialadenitis

SIDE-EFFECTS, FURTHER INFORMATION
▸ Pancreatitis Suspend treatment if serum lipase raised (even if asymptomatic) or if symptoms of pancreatitis develop; discontinue if pancreatitis confirmed. Whenever possible avoid concomitant treatment with other drugs known to cause pancreatic toxicity (e.g. intravenous pentamidine isetionate); monitor closely if concomitant therapy unavoidable. Since significant elevations of triglycerides cause pancreatitis monitor closely if elevated.

- PREGNANCY Manufacturer advises use only if potential benefit outweighs risk.

- HEPATIC IMPAIRMENT Insufficient information. In hepatic impairment, monitor for toxicity.

- RENAL IMPAIRMENT Reduce dose if eGFR less than 60 mL/minute/1.73 m²; consult product literature.

- MONITORING REQUIREMENTS Ophthalmological examination (including visual acuity, colour vision, and dilated fundus examination) recommended annually or if visual changes occur.

- DIRECTIONS FOR ADMINISTRATION Capsules should be swallowed whole and taken at least 2 hours before or 2 hours after food.
   With chewable tablets, to ensure sufficient antacid, each dose to be taken as at least 2 tablets chewed thoroughly, crushed or dispersed in water; clear apple juice may be added for flavouring; tablets to be taken 2 hours after lopinavir with ritonavir capsules and oral solution or atazanavir with ritonavir.

- PATIENT AND CARER ADVICE Patients or carers should be given advice on how to administer didanosine capsules and chewable tablets.

- MEDICINAL FORMS
There can be variation in the licensing of different medicines containing the same drug.
Chewable tablet
CAUTIONARY AND ADVISORY LABELS 23
EXCIPIENTS: May contain Aspartame
▸ Videx (Bristol-Myers Squibb Pharmaceuticals Ltd)
   Didanosine 25 mg Videx 25mg chewable dispersible tablets sugar-free | 60 tablet [PoM] £25.06 (Hospital only)
Gastro-resistant capsule
CAUTIONARY AND ADVISORY LABELS 25
▸ Videx EC (Bristol-Myers Squibb Pharmaceuticals Ltd)
   Didanosine 125 mg Videx EC 125mg capsules | 30 capsule [PoM] £48.18 (Hospital only)
   Didanosine 200 mg Videx EC 200mg capsules | 30 capsule [PoM] £77.09 (Hospital only)
   Didanosine 250 mg Videx EC 250mg capsules | 30 capsule [PoM] £96.37 (Hospital only)
   Didanosine 400 mg Videx EC 400mg capsules | 30 capsule [PoM] £154.19 (Hospital only)

☞ 587

Emtricitabine

(FTC)

- INDICATIONS AND DOSE

HIV infection in combination with other antiretroviral drugs
▸ BY MOUTH USING CAPSULES
▸ Adult: 200 mg once daily
▸ BY MOUTH USING ORAL SOLUTION
▸ Adult: 240 mg once daily

DOSE EQUIVALENCE AND CONVERSION
240 mg oral solution ≡ 200 mg capsule; where appropriate the capsule may be used instead of the oral solution.

- INTERACTIONS → Appendix 1 (emtricitabine).

- SIDE-EFFECTS Abnormal dreams · hyperpigmentation · pruritus

- HEPATIC IMPAIRMENT On discontinuation, monitor patients with hepatitis B (risk of exacerbation of hepatitis).

- RENAL IMPAIRMENT Reduce dose if eGFR less than 50 mL/minute/1.73 m²; consult product literature.

- PRESCRIBING AND DISPENSING INFORMATION Flavours of oral liquid formulations may contain candy.

- PATIENT AND CARER ADVICE
Missed doses
If a dose is more than 12 hours late, the missed dose should not be taken and the next dose should be taken at the normal time.

- MEDICINAL FORMS
There can be variation in the licensing of different medicines containing the same drug.
Capsule
▸ Emtriva (Gilead Sciences International Ltd)
   Emtricitabine 200 mg Emtriva 200mg capsules | 30 capsule [PoM] £138.98
Oral solution
ELECTROLYTES: May contain Sodium
▸ Emtriva (Gilead Sciences International Ltd)
   Emtricitabine 10 mg per 1 ml Emtriva 10mg/ml oral solution sugar-free | 170 ml [PoM] £39.53

5

Infection

Lamivudine

☞ 587

(3TC)

- **INDICATIONS AND DOSE**

EPIVIR® ORAL SOLUTION

HIV infection in combination with other antiretroviral drugs
▸ BY MOUTH
▸ Adult: 150 mg every 12 hours, alternatively 300 mg once daily

EPIVIR® TABLETS

HIV infection in combination with other antiretroviral drugs
▸ BY MOUTH
▸ Adult: 150 mg every 12 hours, alternatively 300 mg once daily

ZEFFIX®

Chronic hepatitis B infection either with compensated liver disease (with evidence of viral replication and histology of active liver inflammation or fibrosis) when first-line treatments cannot be used, or (in combination with another antiviral drug without cross-resistance to lamivudine) with decompensated liver disease
▸ BY MOUTH
▸ Adult: 100 mg once daily, patients receiving lamivudine for concomitant HIV infection should continue to receive lamivudine in a dose appropriate for HIV infection

- **CAUTIONS** Recurrent hepatitis in patients with chronic hepatitis B may occur on discontinuation of lamivudine
- **INTERACTIONS** → Appendix 1 (lamivudine).
- **SIDE-EFFECTS** Alopecia · muscle disorders · nasal symptoms · peripheral neuropathy · rhabdomyolysis
- **BREAST FEEDING** Can be used with caution in women infected with chronic hepatitis B alone, providing that adequate measures are taken to prevent hepatitis B infection in infants.
- **RENAL IMPAIRMENT** Reduce dose if eGFR less than 50 mL/minute/1.73 m²; consult product literature.
- **MONITORING REQUIREMENTS** When treating chronic hepatitis B with lamivudine, monitor liver function tests every 3 months, and viral markers of hepatitis B every 3–6 months, more frequently in patients with advanced liver disease or following transplantation (monitoring to continue for at least 1 year after discontinuation—recurrent hepatitis may occur on discontinuation).
- **PRESCRIBING AND DISPENSING INFORMATION** Flavours of oral liquid formulations may include banana and strawberry.

- **MEDICINAL FORMS**
There can be variation in the licensing of different medicines containing the same drug.

Tablet
▸ Epivir (ViiV Healthcare UK Ltd)
  Lamivudine 150 mg Epivir 150mg tablets | 60 tablet [PoM] £121.82
  Lamivudine 300 mg Epivir 300mg tablets | 30 tablet [PoM] £133.89
▸ Zeffix (GlaxoSmithKline UK Ltd)
  Lamivudine 100 mg Zeffix 100mg tablets | 28 tablet [PoM] £78.09
  DT price = £67.75
Oral solution
EXCIPIENTS: May contain Sucrose
▸ Epivir (ViiV Healthcare UK Ltd)
  Lamivudine 10 mg per 1 ml Epivir 50mg/5ml oral solution | 240 ml [PoM] £33.16

Stavudine

☞ 587

(d4T)

- **INDICATIONS AND DOSE**

HIV infection in combination with other antiretroviral drugs when no suitable alternative available and when prescribed for shortest period possible
▸ BY MOUTH
▸ Adult (body-weight up to 60 kg): 30 mg every 12 hours, to be taken preferably at least 1 hour before food
▸ Adult (body-weight 60 kg and above): 40 mg every 12 hours, to be taken preferably at least 1 hour before food

- **CAUTIONS** Excessive alcohol intake · higher risk of lactic acidosis than other nucleoside reverse transcriptase inhibitors (especially when used in combination with didanosine)—use only if alternative regimens are not suitable · history of pancreatitis · history of peripheral neuropathy
- **INTERACTIONS** → Appendix 1 (stavudine).
  Caution with concomitant use of isoniazid—risk of peripheral neuropathy.
  Caution with concomitant use with other drugs associated with pancreatitis.
- **SIDE-EFFECTS**
▸ **Common or very common** Abnormal dreams · cognitive dysfunction · depression · drowsiness · peripheral neuropathy (switch to another antiretroviral if peripheral neuropathy develops) · pruritus
▸ **Uncommon** Anxiety · gynaecomastia
- **PREGNANCY** Manufacturer advises use only if potential benefit outweighs risk.
- **RENAL IMPAIRMENT** Use half normal dose every 12 hours if eGFR 25–50 mL/minute/1.73 m². Use half normal dose every 24 hours if eGFR less than 25 mL/minute/1.73 m². Risk of peripheral neuropathy.
- **PRESCRIBING AND DISPENSING INFORMATION** Flavours of oral liquid formulations may include cherry.
- **LESS SUITABLE FOR PRESCRIBING** Stavudine (especially in combination with didanosine) is associated with a higher risk of lipoatrophy and should be used only if alternative regimens are not suitable; it is considered to be less suitable for prescribing.

- **MEDICINAL FORMS**
There can be variation in the licensing of different medicines containing the same drug.
Capsule
▸ Zerit (Bristol-Myers Squibb Pharmaceuticals Ltd)
  Stavudine 20 mg Zerit 20mg capsules | 56 capsule [PoM] £139.46 (Hospital only)
  Stavudine 30 mg Zerit 30mg capsules | 56 capsule [PoM] £146.25 (Hospital only)
  Stavudine 40 mg Zerit 40mg capsules | 56 capsule [PoM] £150.66 (Hospital only)
Oral solution
▸ Zerit (Bristol-Myers Squibb Pharmaceuticals Ltd)
  Stavudine 1 mg per 1 ml Zerit 1mg/ml oral solution | 200 ml [PoM] £22.94 (Hospital only)

🠶 587

Tenofovir disoproxil

● **INDICATIONS AND DOSE**

HIV infection in combination with other antiretroviral drugs | Chronic hepatitis B infection with compensated liver disease (with evidence of viral replication, and histologically documented active liver inflammation or fibrosis) | Chronic hepatitis B infection with decompensated liver disease
▸ BY MOUTH
▸ Adult: 245 mg once daily

DOSE EQUIVALENCE AND CONVERSION
7.5 scoops of granules contains approx. 245 mg tenofovir disoproxil (as fumarate).

● **INTERACTIONS** → Appendix 1 (tenofovir).
Use with caution if concomitant or recent use of nephrotoxic drugs.

● **SIDE-EFFECTS**
▸ **Rare** Nephrogenic diabetes insipidus · proximal renal tubulopathy · renal failure
▸ **Frequency not known** Hypophosphataemia · reduced bone density

● **RENAL IMPAIRMENT** *Granules*: 132 mg once daily if eGFR 30–50 mL/minute/1.73 m^2; 66 mg once daily if eGFR 20–30 mL/minute/1.73 m^2; 33 mg once daily if eGFR 10–20 mL/minute/1.73 m^2. *Tablets*: 245 mg every 2 days if eGFR 30–50 mL/minute/1.73 m^2; 245 mg every 3–4 days if eGFR 10–30 mL/minute/1.73 m^2. Monitor renal function—interrupt treatment if further deterioration.

● **MONITORING REQUIREMENTS**
▸ Test renal function and serum phosphate before treatment, then every 4 weeks (more frequently if at increased risk of renal impairment) for 1 year and then every 3 months, interrupt treatment if renal function deteriorates or serum phosphate decreases.
▸ When treating chronic hepatitis B with tenofovir, monitor liver function tests every 3 months and viral markers for hepatitis B every 3–6 months during treatment (continue monitoring for at least 1 year after discontinuation—recurrent hepatitis may occur on discontinuation).

● **DIRECTIONS FOR ADMINISTRATION** *Granules*: mix 1 scoop of granules with 1 tablespoon of soft food (e.g. yoghurt, apple sauce) and take immediately without chewing. Do **not** mix granules with liquids.

● **PATIENT AND CARER ADVICE**

Missed doses
If a dose is more than 12 hours late, the missed dose should not be taken and the next dose should be taken at the normal time.
 Patients or carers should be given advice on how to administer tenofovir granules.

● **NATIONAL FUNDING/ACCESS DECISIONS**

NICE technology appraisals (TAs)
▸ **Tenofovir disoproxil for the treatment of chronic hepatitis B (July 2009)** NICE TA173
Tenofovir is an option for the treatment of chronic hepatitis B.
www.nice.org.uk/TA173

● **MEDICINAL FORMS**
There can be variation in the licensing of different medicines containing the same drug.

Tablet
CAUTIONARY AND ADVISORY LABELS 21
▸ Viread (Gilead Sciences International Ltd)
 Tenofovir disoproxil (as Tenofovir disoproxil fumarate) **123 mg** Viread 123mg tablets | 30 tablet PoM £102.60
 Tenofovir disoproxil (as Tenofovir disoproxil fumarate) **163 mg** Viread 163mg tablets | 30 tablet PoM £135.98

 Tenofovir disoproxil (as Tenofovir disoproxil fumarate) **204 mg** Viread 204mg tablets | 30 tablet PoM £170.19
 Tenofovir disoproxil (as Tenofovir disoproxil fumarate) **245 mg** Viread 245mg tablets | 30 tablet PoM £204.39

Granules
CAUTIONARY AND ADVISORY LABELS 21
▸ Viread (Gilead Sciences International Ltd)
 Tenofovir disoproxil (as Tenofovir disoproxil fumarate) **33 mg per 1 gram** Viread 33mg/g granules | 60 gram PoM £54.50

Tenofovir with cobicistat, elvitegravir and emtricitabine

The properties listed below are those particular to the combination only. For the properties of the components please consider, tenofovir disoproxil above, emtricitabine p. 589, cobicistat p. 597.

● **INDICATIONS AND DOSE**

HIV infection
▸ BY MOUTH
▸ Adult: 1 tablet once daily

● **INTERACTIONS** → Appendix 1 (cobicistat, elvitegravir, emtricitabine, tenofovir).

● **SIDE-EFFECTS**
▸ **Uncommon** Depression and suicidal ideation (in patients with a history of psychiatric illness)

● **CONCEPTION AND CONTRACEPTION** Women of child-bearing potential should use effective contraception during treatment (if using a hormonal contraceptive, it must contain norgestimate as the progestogen and at least 30 micrograms ethinylestradiol).

● **PREGNANCY** Manufacturer advises use only if potential benefit outweighs risk.

● **HEPATIC IMPAIRMENT** Avoid *Stribild*® in severe impairment.

● **RENAL IMPAIRMENT** If eGFR less than 90 mL/minute/1.73 m^2, only *initiate Stribild*® if other treatments cannot be used (avoid *initiating Stribild*® if eGFR less than 70 mL/minute/1.73 m^2); if eGFR less than 70 mL/minute/1.73 m^2, only *continue Stribild*® if potential benefit outweighs risk (discontinue *Stribild*® if eGFR less than 50 mL/minute/1.73 m^2).

● **MONITORING REQUIREMENTS** Test urine glucose before treatment, then every 4 weeks for 1 year and then every 3 months.

● **DIRECTIONS FOR ADMINISTRATION** Avoid antacids 4 hours before or 4 hours after taking *Stribild*®.

● **PRESCRIBING AND DISPENSING INFORMATION** Dispense in original container (contains desiccant).

● **PATIENT AND CARER ADVICE**

Missed doses
If a dose is more than 18 hours late, the missed dose should not be taken and the next dose should be taken at the normal time.
 Patients or carers should be given advice on how to administer *Stribild*®.

● **MEDICINAL FORMS**
There can be variation in the licensing of different medicines containing the same drug.

Tablet
CAUTIONARY AND ADVISORY LABELS 21
▸ Stribild (Gilead Sciences International Ltd) ▼
 Cobicistat 150 mg, Elvitegravir 150 mg, Emtricitabine 200 mg, Tenofovir disoproxil (as Tenofovir disoproxil fumarate) **245 mg** Stribild 150mg/150mg/200mg/245mg tablets | 30 tablet PoM £879.51

5

Infection

Tenofovir with efavirenz and emtricitabine

The properties listed below are those particular to the combination only. For the properties of the components please consider, tenofovir disoproxil p. 591, efavirenz p. 585, emtricitabine p. 589.

- **INDICATIONS AND DOSE**

HIV infection stabilised on antiretroviral therapy for more than 3 months
- ▸ BY MOUTH
  - ▸ Adult: 1 tablet once daily

- **HEPATIC IMPAIRMENT** Manufacturer of *Atripla*® advises caution in mild impairment; avoid *Atripla*® in moderate to severe impairment.
- **RENAL IMPAIRMENT** Avoid *Atripla*® if eGFR less than 50 mL/minute/1.73 m².
- **PATIENT AND CARER ADVICE**

Missed doses
If a dose is more than 12 hours late, the missed dose should not be taken and the next dose should be taken at the normal time.

- **MEDICINAL FORMS**
There can be variation in the licensing of different medicines containing the same drug.
Tablet
CAUTIONARY AND ADVISORY LABELS 23, 25
- ▸ Atripla (Gilead Sciences International Ltd)
  Emtricitabine 200 mg, Tenofovir disoproxil (as Tenofovir disoproxil fumarate) 245 mg, Efavirenz 600 mg Atripla 600mg/200mg/245mg tablets | 30 tablet PoM £532.87

Tenofovir with emtricitabine

The properties listed below are those particular to the combination only. For the properties of the components please consider, tenofovir disoproxil p. 591, emtricitabine p. 589.

- **INDICATIONS AND DOSE**

HIV infection in combination with other antiretroviral drugs
- ▸ BY MOUTH
  - ▸ Adult: 1 tablet once daily

- **RENAL IMPAIRMENT** Use normal dose of *Truvada*® every 2 days if eGFR 30–50 mL/minute/1.73 m². Avoid *Truvada*® if eGFR less than 30 mL/minute/1.73 m².
- **DIRECTIONS FOR ADMINISTRATION** Patients with swallowing difficulties may disperse tablet in half a glass of water, orange juice, or grape juice (but bitter taste).
- **PATIENT AND CARER ADVICE**

Missed doses
If a dose is more than 12 hours late, the missed dose should not be taken and the next dose should be taken at the normal time.
Patients or carers should be given advice on how to administer emtricitabine with tenofovir tablets.

- **MEDICINAL FORMS**
There can be variation in the licensing of different medicines containing the same drug.
Tablet
CAUTIONARY AND ADVISORY LABELS 21
- ▸ Truvada (Gilead Sciences International Ltd)
  Emtricitabine 200 mg, Tenofovir disoproxil (as Tenofovir disoproxil fumarate) 245 mg Truvada tablets | 30 tablet PoM £355.73

Tenofovir with emtricitabine and rilpivirine

The properties listed below are those particular to the combination only. For the properties of the components please consider, tenofovir disoproxil p. 591, emtricitabine p. 589, rilpivirine p. 587.

- **INDICATIONS AND DOSE**

HIV infection in patients with plasma HIV-1 RNA concentration less than 100 000 copies/mL
- ▸ BY MOUTH
  - ▸ Adult: 1 tablet once daily

- **HEPATIC IMPAIRMENT** Manufacturer of *Eviplera*® advises caution in moderate impairment; avoid *Eviplera*® in severe impairment.
- **RENAL IMPAIRMENT** Avoid *Eviplera*® if eGFR less than 50 mL/minute/1.73 m².
- **DIRECTIONS FOR ADMINISTRATION** Avoid antacids 2 hours before or 4 hours after taking *Eviplera*®.
- **PATIENT AND CARER ADVICE**

Missed doses
If a dose is more than 12 hours late, the missed dose should not be taken and the next dose should be taken at the normal time.
Patients or carers should be given advice on how to administer *Eviplera*®.

- **MEDICINAL FORMS**
There can be variation in the licensing of different medicines containing the same drug.
Tablet
CAUTIONARY AND ADVISORY LABELS 21, 25
- ▸ Eviplera (Gilead Sciences International Ltd) ▼
  Rilpivirine (as Rilpivirine hydrochloride) 25 mg, Emtricitabine 200 mg, Tenofovir disoproxil (as Tenofovir disoproxil fumarate) 245 mg Eviplera 200mg/25mg/245mg tablets | 30 tablet PoM £525.95

▸ 587

Zidovudine

(Azidothymidine; AZT)

- **INDICATIONS AND DOSE**

HIV infection in combination with other antiretroviral drugs
- ▸ BY MOUTH
  - ▸ Adult: 250–300 mg twice daily

Prevention of maternal-fetal HIV transmission
- ▸ BY MOUTH, OR BY INTRAVENOUS INFUSION
  - ▸ Adult: Seek specialist advice (combination therapy preferred) (consult local protocol)

HIV infection in combination with other antiretroviral drugs in patients temporarily unable to take zidovudine by mouth
- ▸ BY INTRAVENOUS INFUSION
  - ▸ Adult: 0.8–1 mg/kg every 4 hours usually for not more than 2 weeks, dose approximating to 1.2–1.5 mg/kg every 4 hours by mouth

- **CONTRA-INDICATIONS** Abnormally low haemoglobin concentration (consult product literature) · abnormally low neutrophil counts (consult product literature) · Acute porphyrias p. 918
- **CAUTIONS** Elderly · risk of haematological toxicity particularly with high dose and advanced disease · vitamin B_{12} deficiency (increased risk of neutropenia)
- **INTERACTIONS** → Appendix 1 (zidovudine). Increased risk of toxicity with nephrotoxic and myelosuppressive drugs—for further details consult product literature.

- SIDE-EFFECTS Anaemia (may require transfusion) · anxiety · chest pain · convulsions · depression · dizziness · drowsiness · gynaecomastia · influenza-like symptoms · loss of mental acuity · myopathy · neuropathy · paraesthesia · pigmentation of nails · pigmentation of oral mucosa · pigmentation of skin · pruritus · sweating · taste disturbance · urinary frequency

  SIDE-EFFECTS, FURTHER INFORMATION
  ‣ Anaemia and myelosuppression If anaemia or myelosuppression occur, reduce dose or interrupt treatment according to product literature, or consider other treatment
  ‣ Lipoatrophy Zidovudine is associated with a higher risk of lipoatrophy than other antiretrovirals and should be used only if alternative regimens are not suitable.
- HEPATIC IMPAIRMENT Accumulation may occur.
- RENAL IMPAIRMENT Reduce oral dose to 300–400 mg daily in divided doses or intravenous dose to 1 mg/kg 3–4 times daily if eGFR is less than 10 mL/minute/1.73 m².
- MONITORING REQUIREMENTS Monitor full blood count after 4 weeks of treatment, then every 3 months.
- DIRECTIONS FOR ADMINISTRATION
  ‣ With intravenous use For *intermittent intravenous infusion*, dilute to a concentration of 2 mg/mL or 4 mg/mL with Glucose 5% and give over 1 hour.
- PRESCRIBING AND DISPENSING INFORMATION The abbreviation AZT which is sometimes used for zidovudine has also been used for another drug.

- MEDICINAL FORMS
  There can be variation in the licensing of different medicines containing the same drug.

  Capsule
  ‣ Zidovudine (Non-proprietary)
  Zidovudine 100 mg Zidovudine 100mg capsules | 60 capsule PoM £40.41
  Zidovudine 250 mg Zidovudine 250mg capsules | 60 capsule PoM £96.36
  ‣ Retrovir (ViiV Healthcare UK Ltd)
  Zidovudine 100 mg Retrovir 100mg capsules | 100 capsule PoM £88.86
  Zidovudine 250 mg Retrovir 250mg capsules | 40 capsule PoM £88.86

  Oral solution
  ‣ Retrovir (ViiV Healthcare UK Ltd)
  Zidovudine 10 mg per 1 ml Retrovir 50mg/5ml oral solution sugar-free | 200 ml PoM £17.78

  Solution for infusion
  ‣ Retrovir (ViiV Healthcare UK Ltd)
  Zidovudine 10 mg per 1 ml Retrovir IV 200mg/20ml concentrate for solution for infusion vials | 5 vial PoM £44.61

Zidovudine with lamivudine

The properties listed below are those particular to the combination only. For the properties of the components please consider, zidovudine p. 592, lamivudine p. 590.

- INDICATIONS AND DOSE
  HIV infection in combination with other antiretroviral drugs
  ‣ BY MOUTH
  ‣ Adult: 1 tablet twice daily

- RENAL IMPAIRMENT Avoid if eGFR less than 50 mL/minute/1.73 m² (consult product literature).
- DIRECTIONS FOR ADMINISTRATION
  COMBIVIR® TABLETS Tablets may be crushed and mixed with semi-solid food or liquid just before administration.

- MEDICINAL FORMS
  There can be variation in the licensing of different medicines containing the same drug.

  Tablet
  ‣ Zidovudine with lamivudine (Non-proprietary)
  Lamivudine 150 mg, Zidovudine 300 mg Zidovudine 300mg / Lamivudine 150mg tablets | 60 tablet PoM £70.61-£285.11
  ‣ Combivir (ViiV Healthcare UK Ltd)
  Lamivudine 150 mg, Zidovudine 300 mg Combivir 150mg/300mg tablets | 60 tablet PoM £255.10

ANTIVIRALS > PROTEASE INHIBITORS, HIV

Protease inhibitors

- CONTRA-INDICATIONS Acute porphyrias p. 918
- CAUTIONS Diabetes · haemophilia (increased risk of bleeding)
- SIDE-EFFECTS Abdominal pain · anaemia · anaphylaxis · anorexia · blood disorders · diarrhoea · dizziness · fatigue · flatulence · gastro-intestinal disturbances · headache · hepatic dysfunction · hypersensitivity reactions · lipodystrophy · Lipodystrophy Syndrome · metabolic effects · myalgia · myositis · nausea · neutropenia · osteonecrosis · pancreatitis · paraesthesia · pruritus · rash · rhabdomyolysis · sleep disturbances · Stevens-Johnson syndrome · taste disturbances · thrombocytopenia · vomiting

  SIDE-EFFECTS, FURTHER INFORMATION
  ‣ Lipodystrophy Syndrome For further information see HIV infection p. 582.
  ‣ Osteonecrosis For further information see HIV infection p. 582.
- HEPATIC IMPAIRMENT Use with caution in patients with chronic hepatitis B or C (increased risk of hepatic side-effects).

Atazanavir

- INDICATIONS AND DOSE
  HIV infection in combination with other antiretroviral drugs—with low-dose ritonavir
  ‣ BY MOUTH
  ‣ Adult: 300 mg once daily

  HIV infection in combination with other antiretroviral drugs—with cobicistat
  ‣ BY MOUTH
  ‣ Adult: 300 mg daily

- CAUTIONS Cardiac conduction disorders · electrolyte disturbances · predisposition to QT interval prolongation
- INTERACTIONS → Appendix 1 (atazanavir).
  Caution if concomitant use with drugs that prolong PR interval.
  Caution with concomitant use of drugs that prolong QT interval.
- SIDE-EFFECTS
  ‣ Uncommon Abnormal dreams · alopecia · amnesia · anxiety · arthralgia · chest pain · cholelithiasis · depression · disorientation · dry mouth · dyspnoea · gynaecomastia · haematuria · hypertension · increased appetite · mouth ulcers · nephrolithiasis · peripheral neuropathy · proteinuria · syncope · torsade de pointes · urinary frequency · weight changes
  ‣ Rare Abnormal gait · cholecystitis · hepatosplenomegaly · oedema · palpitation

  SIDE-EFFECTS, FURTHER INFORMATION
  ‣ Rash Mild to moderate rash occurs commonly, usually within the first 3 weeks of therapy. Severe rash occurs less

5

Infection

frequently and may be accompanied by systemic symptoms. Discontinue if severe rash develops.

- PREGNANCY Theoretical risk of hyperbilirubinaemia in neonate if used at term.
  In pregnancy, monitor viral load and plasma-atazanavir concentration during third trimester.
- HEPATIC IMPAIRMENT Manufacturer advises caution in mild impairment; avoid in moderate to severe impairment.
- MEDICINAL FORMS
  There can be variation in the licensing of different medicines containing the same drug.
  Capsule
  CAUTIONARY AND ADVISORY LABELS 5, 21
  ▸ Reyataz (Bristol-Myers Squibb Pharmaceuticals Ltd)
  Atazanavir (as Atazanavir sulfate) 150 mg Reyataz 150mg capsules | 60 capsule [PoM] £303.38 (Hospital only)
  Atazanavir (as Atazanavir sulfate) 200 mg Reyataz 200mg capsules | 60 capsule [PoM] £303.38 (Hospital only)
  Atazanavir (as Atazanavir sulfate) 300 mg Reyataz 300mg capsules | 30 capsule [PoM] £303.38 (Hospital only)

▸ 593

Darunavir

- INDICATIONS AND DOSE

HIV infection in combination with other antiretroviral drugs in patients previously treated with antiretroviral therapy—with low-dose ritonavir
▸ BY MOUTH
▸ Adult: 600 mg twice daily, alternatively 800 mg once daily, once daily dose only to be used if no resistance to darunavir, if plasma HIV-RNA concentration less than 100 000 copies/mL, and if CD4 cell count greater than 100 cells × 10^6/ litre

HIV infection in combination with other antiretroviral drugs in patients previously treated with antiretroviral therapy—with cobicistat
▸ BY MOUTH
▸ Adult: 800 mg once daily, dose appropriate if no resistance to darunavir, if plasma HIV-RNA concentration less than 100 000 copies/mL, and if CD4 cell count greater than 100 cells × 10^6/litre

HIV infection in combination with other antiretroviral drugs in patients not previously treated with antiretroviral therapy—with low-dose ritonavir
▸ BY MOUTH
▸ Adult: 800 mg once daily

HIV infection in combination with other antiretroviral drugs in patients not previously treated with antiretroviral therapy—with cobicistat
▸ BY MOUTH
▸ Adult: 800 mg once daily

- INTERACTIONS → Appendix 1 (darunavir).
- SIDE-EFFECTS
▸ **Common or very common** Peripheral neuropathy · rash
▸ **Uncommon** Abnormal dreams · acne · alopecia · angina · anxiety · arthralgia · conjunctival hyperaemia · cough · depression · dry eyes · dry mouth · dyspnoea · dysuria · eczema · erectile dysfunction · flushing · gynaecomastia · hypertension · hypothyroidism · increased appetite · increased sweating · memory impairment · myocardial infarction · nail discoloration · nephrolithiasis · osteoporosis · peripheral oedema · polyuria · pyrexia · QT interval prolongation · reduced libido · renal failure · severe skin rash · Stevens-Johnson syndrome · stomatitis · tachycardia · throat irritation · toxic epidermal necrolysis · weight changes
▸ **Rare** Bradycardia · confusion · convulsions · haematemesis · palpitation · rhinorrhoea · seborrhoeic dermatits · syncope · visual disturbances

SIDE-EFFECTS, FURTHER INFORMATION
▸ **Rash** Mild to moderate rash occurs commonly, usually within the first 4 weeks of therapy and resolves without stopping treatment. Severe skin rash (including Stevens-Johnson syndrome and toxic epidermal necrolysis) occurs less frequently and may be accompanied by fever, malaise, arthralgia, myalgia, oral lesions, conjunctivitis, hepatitis, or eosinophilia; treatment should be stopped if severe rash develops.

- ALLERGY AND CROSS-SENSITIVITY Use with caution in patients with sulfonamide sensitivity.
- PREGNANCY Manufacturer advises use only if potential benefit outweighs risk; if required, use the twice daily dose regimen.
- HEPATIC IMPAIRMENT Manufacturer advises caution in mild to moderate impairment; avoid in severe impairment—no information available.
- MONITORING REQUIREMENTS Monitor liver function before and during treatment.
- PRESCRIBING AND DISPENSING INFORMATION Flavours of oral liquid formulations may include strawberry.
- PATIENT AND CARER ADVICE
  Missed doses
  If a dose is more than 6 hours late on the twice daily regimen (or more than 12 hours late on the once daily regimen), the missed dose should not be taken and the next dose should be taken at the normal time.

- MEDICINAL FORMS
  There can be variation in the licensing of different medicines containing the same drug.
  Tablet
  CAUTIONARY AND ADVISORY LABELS 21
  ▸ Prezista (Janssen-Cilag Ltd)
  Darunavir (as Darunavir ethanolate) 75 mg Prezista 75mg tablets | 480 tablet [PoM] £446.70
  Darunavir (as Darunavir ethanolate) 150 mg Prezista 150mg tablets | 240 tablet [PoM] £446.70
  Darunavir (as Darunavir ethanolate) 400 mg Prezista 400mg tablets | 60 tablet [PoM] £297.80
  Darunavir (as Darunavir ethanolate) 600 mg Prezista 600mg tablets | 60 tablet [PoM] £446.70
  Darunavir (as Darunavir ethanolate) 800 mg Prezista 800mg tablets | 30 tablet [PoM] £297.80
  Oral suspension
  CAUTIONARY AND ADVISORY LABELS 21
  ▸ Prezista (Janssen-Cilag Ltd)
  Darunavir (as Darunavir ethanolate) 100 mg per 1 ml Prezista 100mg/ml oral suspension sugar-free | 200 ml [PoM] £248.17

▸ 593

Fosamprenavir

- DRUG ACTION Fosamprenavir is a pro-drug of amprenavir.

- INDICATIONS AND DOSE

HIV infection in combination with other antiretroviral drugs—with low-dose ritonavir
▸ BY MOUTH
▸ Adult: 700 mg twice daily

DOSE EQUIVALENCE AND CONVERSION
700 mg fosamprenavir is equivalent to approximately 600 mg amprenavir.

- INTERACTIONS → Appendix 1 (fosamprenavir).
- SIDE-EFFECTS
▸ **Rare** Stevens-Johnson syndrome
▸ **Frequency not known** Rash
SIDE-EFFECTS, FURTHER INFORMATION
▸ **Rash** Rash may occur, usually in the second week of therapy; discontinue permanently if severe rash with systemic or allergic symptoms or, mucosal involvement; if rash mild or moderate, may continue without

interruption—usually resolves within 2 weeks and may respond to antihistamines.

- PREGNANCY Toxicity in *animal* studies; manufacturer advises use only if potential benefit outweighs risk.
- HEPATIC IMPAIRMENT Reduce dose to 450 mg twice daily in moderate impairment; reduce dose to 300 mg twice daily in severe impairment. Manufacturer advises caution in mild impairment.
- DIRECTIONS FOR ADMINISTRATION In adults, oral suspension should be taken on an empty stomach.
- PRESCRIBING AND DISPENSING INFORMATION Flavours of oral liquid formulations may include grape, bubblegum, or peppermint.
- PATIENT AND CARER ADVICE Patients or carers should be given advice on how to administer fosamprenavir oral suspension.

- MEDICINAL FORMS
There can be variation in the licensing of different medicines containing the same drug.
Tablet
▸ Telzir (ViiV Healthcare UK Ltd)
 Fosamprenavir (as Fosamprenavir calcium) 700 mg Telzir 700mg tablets | 60 tablet PoM £220.13
Oral suspension
EXCIPIENTS: May contain Propylene glycol
▸ Telzir (ViiV Healthcare UK Ltd)
 Fosamprenavir (as Fosamprenavir calcium) 50 mg per 1 ml Telzir 50mg/ml oral suspension | 225 ml PoM £58.70

`F 593`

Indinavir

- **INDICATIONS AND DOSE**

HIV infection in combination with nucleoside reverse transcriptase inhibitors
▸ BY MOUTH
▸ Adult: Seek specialist advice

- CAUTIONS Ensure adequate hydration (risk of nephrolithiasis) · patients at high risk of cardiovascular disease (especially if 10-year cardiovascular risk greater than 20%) · patients at risk of nephrolithiasis (monitor for nephrolithiasis)
- INTERACTIONS → Appendix 1 (indinavir).
- SIDE-EFFECTS Alopecia · crystalluria · dry mouth · dry skin · dysuria · haematuria · haemolytic anaemia · hyperpigmentation · hypoaesthesia · interstitial nephritis (with medullary calcification and cortical atrophy in asymptomatic severe leucocyturia) · nephrolithiasis (may require interruption or discontinuation) · paronychia · proteinuria · pyelonephritis
- PREGNANCY Toxicity in *animal* studies; manufacturer advises use only if potential benefit outweighs risk; theoretical risk of hyperbilirubinaemia and renal stones in neonate if used at term.
- HEPATIC IMPAIRMENT Reduce dose in mild to moderate impairment. Not studied in severe impairment. Increased risk of nephrolithiasis.
- RENAL IMPAIRMENT Use with caution. In patients with renal impairment, monitor for nephrolithiasis.
- DIRECTIONS FOR ADMINISTRATION Administer 1 hour before or 2 hours after a meal; may be administered with a low-fat light meal; in combination with didanosine tablets, allow 1 hour between each drug (antacids in didanosine tablets reduce absorption of indinavir); in combination with low-dose ritonavir, give with food.
- PRESCRIBING AND DISPENSING INFORMATION Dispense in original container (contains desiccant).
- PATIENT AND CARER ADVICE Patients or carers should be given advice on how to administer indinavir capsules.

- LESS SUITABLE FOR PRESCRIBING Indinavir is rarely used in the treatment of HIV-infection because it is associated with nephrolithiasis; it is considered to be less suitable for prescribing.

- MEDICINAL FORMS
There can be variation in the licensing of different medicines containing the same drug.
Capsule
CAUTIONARY AND ADVISORY LABELS 27
▸ Crixivan (Merck Sharp & Dohme Ltd)
 Indinavir (as Indinavir sulfate) 200 mg Crixivan 200mg capsules | 360 capsule PoM £181.02
 Indinavir (as Indinavir sulfate) 400 mg Crixivan 400mg capsules | 180 capsule PoM £181.02

`F 593`

Lopinavir with ritonavir

- **INDICATIONS AND DOSE**

HIV infection in combination with other antiretroviral drugs
▸ BY MOUTH USING TABLETS
▸ Adult: 400/100 mg twice daily, alternatively 800/200 mg once daily, once daily dose to be used only in adults with a HIV strain that has less than 3 mutations to protease inhibitors
▸ BY MOUTH USING ORAL SOLUTION
▸ Adult: 5 mL twice daily, to be taken with food, oral solution contains 400 mg lopinavir, 100 mg ritonavir/5 mL

- CAUTIONS Cardiac conduction disorders · pancreatitis · patients at high risk of cardiovascular disease (especially if 10-year cardiovascular risk greater than 20%) · structural heart disease
- INTERACTIONS → Appendix 1 (lopinavir, ritonavir). Caution if concomitant use with drugs that prolong QT or PR interval.
- SIDE-EFFECTS
▸ **Common or very common** Amenorrhoea · anxiety · arthralgia · colitis · hypertension · menorrhagia · neuropathy · night sweats · sexual dysfunction · weight changes
▸ **Uncommon** Abnormal dreams · alopecia · AV block · cerebrovascular accident · convulsions · deep vein thrombosis · dry mouth · gastro-intestinal ulcer · haematuria · myocardial infarction · nephritis · rectal bleeding · stomatitis · tinnitus · tremor · visual disturbances
 SIDE-EFFECTS, FURTHER INFORMATION
▸ Pancreatitis Signs and symptoms suggestive of pancreatitis (including raised serum lipase) should be evaluated—discontinue if pancreatitis diagnosed
- PREGNANCY Avoid oral solution due to high propylene glycol content; use tablets only if potential benefit outweighs risk (toxicity in *animal* studies).
- HEPATIC IMPAIRMENT Avoid oral solution due to propylene glycol content; manufacturer advises avoid tablets in severe impairment.
- RENAL IMPAIRMENT Avoid oral solution due to high propylene glycol content. Use tablets with caution in severe impairment.
- MONITORING REQUIREMENTS Monitor liver function before and during treatment.
- PATIENT AND CARER ADVICE Oral solution tastes bitter.

MEDICINAL FORMS
There can be variation in the licensing of different medicines containing the same drug.

Tablet
CAUTIONARY AND ADVISORY LABELS 25
▸ Kaletra (AbbVie Ltd)
Ritonavir 25 mg, Lopinavir 100 mg Kaletra 100mg/25mg tablets | 60 tablet [PoM] £76.85
Ritonavir 50 mg, Lopinavir 200 mg Kaletra 200mg/50mg tablets | 120 tablet [PoM] £285.41

Oral solution
CAUTIONARY AND ADVISORY LABELS 21
EXCIPIENTS: May contain Alcohol, propylene glycol
▸ Kaletra (AbbVie Ltd)
Ritonavir 20 mg per 1 ml, Lopinavir 80 mg per 1 ml Kaletra 80mg/20mg/1ml oral solution | 300 ml [PoM] £307.39

⟟ 593

Ritonavir

● INDICATIONS AND DOSE

HIV infection in combination with other antiretroviral drugs (high-dose ritonavir)
▸ BY MOUTH
▹ Adult: Initially 300 mg every 12 hours for 3 days, increased in steps of 100 mg every 12 hours over not longer than 14 days; increased to 600 mg every 12 hours

Low-dose booster to increase effect of other protease inhibitors
▸ BY MOUTH
▹ Adult: 100–200 mg 1–2 times a day

● CAUTIONS Cardiac conduction disorders · pancreatitis · structural heart disease
● INTERACTIONS → Appendix 1 (ritonavir). Caution if concomitant use with drugs that prolong PR interval.
● SIDE-EFFECTS
▸ Common or very common Acne · anxiety · arthralgia · blood pressure changes · blurred vision · confusion · cough · decreased blood thyroxine concentration · fever · flushing · gastro-intestinal haemorrhage · menorrhagia · mouth ulcers · oedema · peripheral neuropathy · pharyngitis · renal impairment · seizures · syncope
▸ Uncommon Electrolyte disturbances · myocardial infarction
▸ Rare Toxic epidermal necrolysis
SIDE-EFFECTS, FURTHER INFORMATION
▸ Pancreatitis Signs and symptoms suggestive of pancreatitis (including raised serum lipase) should be evaluated—discontinue if pancreatitis diagnosed.
● PREGNANCY Only use low-dose booster to increase the effect of other protease inhibitors.
● HEPATIC IMPAIRMENT Avoid in decompensated liver disease; in severe impairment without decompensation, use 'booster' doses with caution (avoid treatment doses).
● DIRECTIONS FOR ADMINISTRATION Bitter taste of oral solution can be masked by mixing with chocolate milk; do not mix with water, measuring cup must be dry.
● PATIENT AND CARER ADVICE Patients or carers should be given advice on how to administer ritonavir oral solution.

● MEDICINAL FORMS
There can be variation in the licensing of different medicines containing the same drug.

Tablet
CAUTIONARY AND ADVISORY LABELS 21, 25
▸ Norvir (AbbVie Ltd)
Ritonavir 100 mg Norvir 100mg tablets | 30 tablet [PoM] £19.44

Oral solution
CAUTIONARY AND ADVISORY LABELS 21
EXCIPIENTS: May contain Alcohol, propylene glycol
▸ Norvir (AbbVie Ltd)
Ritonavir 80 mg per 1 ml Norvir 80mg/ml oral solution sugar-free | 450 ml [PoM] £403.20

⟟ 593

Saquinavir

● INDICATIONS AND DOSE

HIV infection in combination with other antiretrovirals in patients previously treated with antiretroviral therapy—with low-dose ritonavir
▸ BY MOUTH
▹ Adult: 1 g every 12 hours

HIV infection in combination with other antiretrovirals in patients not previously treated with antiretroviral therapy—with low-dose ritonavir
▸ BY MOUTH
▹ Adult: 500 mg every 12 hours for 7 days, then increased to 1 g every 12 hours

● CONTRA-INDICATIONS Bradycardia · congenital QT prolongation · electrolyte disturbances · heart failure with reduced left ventricular ejection fraction · history of symptomatic arrhythmias · predisposition to cardiac arrhythmias
● INTERACTIONS → Appendix 1 (saquinavir). Caution with concomitant use of garlic (avoid garlic capsules—reduces plasma-saquinavir concentration). Contra-indicated if concomitant use of drugs that prolong QT or PR interval. Contra-indicated if concomitant use of drugs that increase plasma-saquinavir concentration (avoid unless no alternative treatment available).
● SIDE-EFFECTS
▸ Common or very common Alopecia · changes in libido · dry mouth · dyspnoea · increased appetite · peripheral neuropathy
▸ Uncommon Convulsions · mucosal ulceration · renal impairment · visual impairment
● HEPATIC IMPAIRMENT Manufacturer advises caution in moderate impairment; avoid in decompensated liver disease.
● RENAL IMPAIRMENT Use with caution if eGFR less than 30 mL/minute/1.73 m^2.
● MONITORING REQUIREMENTS Monitor ECG before starting treatment (do not initiate treatment if QT interval over 450 milliseconds); if baseline QT interval less than 450 milliseconds, monitor ECG during treatment (particularly 10 days after starting treatment in patients not previously treated with antiretroviral therapy)—discontinue if QT interval increases over 480 milliseconds, if QT interval more than 20 milliseconds above baseline, if prolongation of PR interval, or if arrhythmias occur.
● PATIENT AND CARER ADVICE
Arrhythmias Patients should be told how to recognise signs of arrhythmia and advised to seek medical attention if symptoms such as palpitation or syncope develop.

● MEDICINAL FORMS
There can be variation in the licensing of different medicines containing the same drug.
Tablet
CAUTIONARY AND ADVISORY LABELS 21
▸ Invirase (Roche Products Ltd)
Saquinavir (as Saquinavir mesilate) 500 mg Invirase 500mg tablets | 120 tablet [PoM] £251.26

◄ 593

Tipranavir

- **INDICATIONS AND DOSE**

HIV infection resistant to other protease inhibitors, in combination with other antiretroviral drugs in patients previously treated with antiretrovirals–with low-dose ritonavir
▸ BY MOUTH USING CAPSULES
▸ Adult: 500 mg twice daily

DOSE EQUIVALENCE AND CONVERSION
The bioavailability of tipranavir oral solution is higher than that of the capsules; the oral solution is not interchangeable with the capsules on a milligram-for-milligram basis.

- CAUTIONS Patients at risk of increased bleeding from trauma, surgery or other pathological conditions
- INTERACTIONS → Appendix 1 (tipranavir).
Caution with concomitant use of drugs that increase risk of bleeding.
- SIDE-EFFECTS
▸ **Rare** Dehydration
▸ **Frequency not known** Anorexia · dyspnoea · influenza-like symptoms · peripheral neuropathy · photosensitivity · renal impairment
SIDE-EFFECTS, FURTHER INFORMATION
▸ Hepatotoxicity Potentially life-threatening hepatotoxicity reported. Discontinue if signs or symptoms of hepatitis develop or if liver-function abnormality develops (consult product literature).
- PREGNANCY Manufacturer advises use only if potential benefit outweighs risk—toxicity in *animal* studies.
- HEPATIC IMPAIRMENT Manufacturer advises caution in mild impairment; avoid in moderate or severe impairment—no information available.
- MONITORING REQUIREMENTS Monitor liver function before treatment then every 2 weeks for 1 month, then every 3 months.
- PRESCRIBING AND DISPENSING INFORMATION Flavours of oral liquid formulations may include toffee and mint.
- PATIENT AND CARER ADVICE Patients or carers should be told to observe the oral solution for crystallisation; the bottle should be replaced if more than a thin layer of crystals form (doses should continue to be taken at the normal time until the bottle is replaced).

- MEDICINAL FORMS
There can be variation in the licensing of different medicines containing the same drug.
Capsule
CAUTIONARY AND ADVISORY LABELS 5, 21
EXCIPIENTS: May contain Ethanol
▸ Aptivus (Boehringer Ingelheim Ltd)
Tipranavir 250 mg Aptivus 250mg capsules | 120 capsule PoM £441.00
Oral solution
CAUTIONARY AND ADVISORY LABELS 5, 21
EXCIPIENTS: May contain Vitamin e
▸ Aptivus (Boehringer Ingelheim Ltd)
Tipranavir 100 mg per 1 ml Aptivus 100mg/ml oral solution sugar-free | 95 ml PoM £129.65

ANTIVIRALS › OTHER

Maraviroc

- DRUG ACTION Maraviroc is an antagonist of the CCR5 chemokine receptor.

- **INDICATIONS AND DOSE**

CCR5-tropic HIV infection in combination with other antiretroviral drugs in patients previously treated with antiretrovirals
▸ BY MOUTH
▸ Adult: 300 mg twice daily

- CAUTIONS Cardiovascular disease
- INTERACTIONS → Appendix 1 (maraviroc).
- SIDE-EFFECTS
▸ **Common or very common** Abdominal pain · anaemia · anorexia · depression · diarrhoea · flatulence · headache · insomnia · malaise · nausea · rash
▸ **Uncommon** Myositis · proteinuria · renal failure · seizures
▸ **Rare** Angina · granulocytopenia · hepatitis · pancytopenia · Stevens-Johnson syndrome · toxic epidermal necrolysis
▸ **Frequency not known** Eosinophilia · fever · hepatic reactions · hypersensitivity reactions · osteonecrosis · rash
SIDE-EFFECTS, FURTHER INFORMATION
▸ Osteonecrosis For further information see HIV infection p. 582.
- PREGNANCY Manufacturer advises use only if potential benefit outweighs risk—toxicity in *animal* studies.
- HEPATIC IMPAIRMENT Manufacturer advises caution in hepatic impairment, including patients with chronic hepatitis B or C.
- RENAL IMPAIRMENT If eGFR less than 80 mL/minute/1.73 m², consult product literature.
- NATIONAL FUNDING/ACCESS DECISIONS
Scottish Medicines Consortium (SMC) Decisions
The *Scottish Medicines Consortium* has advised (March 2008) that maraviroc (*Celsentri*®) is **not** recommended for use within NHS Scotland.

- MEDICINAL FORMS
There can be variation in the licensing of different medicines containing the same drug.
Tablet
▸ Celsentri (ViiV Healthcare UK Ltd)
Maraviroc 150 mg Celsentri 150mg tablets | 60 tablet PoM £441.27
Maraviroc 300 mg Celsentri 300mg tablets | 60 tablet PoM £441.27

PHARMACOKINETIC ENHANCERS

Cobicistat

- **INDICATIONS AND DOSE**

Pharmacokinetic enhancer used to increase the effect of atazanavir or darunavir
▸ BY MOUTH
▸ Adult: 150 mg once daily

- INTERACTIONS → Appendix 1 (cobicistat).
- PREGNANCY Manufacturer advises avoid unless essential.
- HEPATIC IMPAIRMENT Manufacturer advises avoid in severe impairment—no information available.
- RENAL IMPAIRMENT No dose adjustment required; inhibits tubular secretion of creatinine; when any co-administered drug requires dose adjustment based on renal function, avoid initiating cobicistat if eGFR less than 70 mL/minute/1.73 m².

5

Infection

5

Infection

- ● PRESCRIBING AND DISPENSING INFORMATION Dispense in original container (contains desiccant).
- ● PATIENT AND CARER ADVICE
Missed doses
If a dose is more than 12 hours late, the missed dose should not be taken and the next dose should be taken at the normal time.

- ● MEDICINAL FORMS
There can be variation in the licensing of different medicines containing the same drug.
Tablet
CAUTIONARY AND ADVISORY LABELS 21
▸ Tybost (Gilead Sciences International Ltd) ▼
Cobicistat 150 mg Tybost 150mg tablets | 30 tablet PoM £21.38

Combinations available: *Tenofovir with cobicistat, elvitegravir and emtricitabine,* p. 591

6.5 Influenza

Influenza

Management
Oseltamivir below and zanamivir p. 600 are most effective for the treatment of influenza if started within a few hours of the onset of symptoms; they are licensed for use within 48 hours of the first symptoms. In otherwise healthy individuals they reduce the duration of symptoms by about 1–1.5 days. Oseltamivir or zanamivir can reduce the risk of complications from influenza in the elderly and in patients with chronic disease.

Oseltamivir and zanamivir are licensed for post-exposure prophylaxis of influenza when influenza is circulating in the community. Oseltamivir should be given within 48 hours of exposure to influenza while zanamivir should be given within 36 hours of exposure to influenza. However, in patients with severe influenza or in those who are immunocompromised, antivirals may still be effective after this time if viral shedding continues [unlicensed use]. Oseltamivir and zanamivir are also licensed for use in exceptional circumstances (e.g. when vaccination does not cover the infecting strain) to prevent influenza in an epidemic.

There is evidence that some strains of influenza A virus have reduced susceptibility to oseltamivir, but may retain susceptibility to zanamivir. Resistance to oseltamivir may be greater in severely immunocompromised patients.

Zanamivir should be reserved for patients who are severely immunocompromised, or when oseltamivir cannot be used, or when resistance to oseltamivir is suspected. For those unable to use the dry powder for inhalation, zanamivir is available as a solution that can be administered by nebuliser or intravenously [unlicensed].

Amantadine hydrochloride p. 382 is licensed for prophylaxis and treatment of influenza A but it is no longer recommended.

Information on pandemic influenza, avian influenza, and swine influenza may be found at www.gov.uk/phe.

Immunisation against influenza is recommended for persons at high risk, and to reduce transmission of infection.

Oseltamivir in children under 1 year of age
Data on the use of oseltamivir in children under 1 year of age is limited. Furthermore, oseltamivir may be ineffective in neonates because they may not be able to metabolise oseltamivir to its active form. However, oseltamivir can be used (under specialist supervision) for the treatment or post-exposure prophylaxis of influenza in children under 1 year of age. The Department of Health has advised (May 2009) that during a pandemic, treatment with oseltamivir can be

overseen by healthcare professionals experienced in assessing children.

ANTIVIRALS > NEURAMINIDASE INHIBITORS

Oseltamivir

- ● DRUG ACTION Reduces replication of influenza A and B viruses by inhibiting viral neuraminidase.

- ● INDICATIONS AND DOSE
Prevention of influenza
▸ BY MOUTH
▸ Child 1–11 months: 3 mg/kg once daily for 10 days for post-exposure prophylaxis
▸ Child 1–12 years (body-weight 10–15 kg): 30 mg once daily for 10 days for post-exposure prophylaxis; for up to 6 weeks during an epidemic
▸ Child 1–12 years (body-weight 15–23 kg): 45 mg once daily for 10 days for post-exposure prophylaxis; for up to 6 weeks during an epidemic
▸ Child 1–12 years (body-weight 23–40 kg): 60 mg once daily for 10 days for post-exposure prophylaxis; for up to 6 weeks during an epidemic
▸ Child 1–12 years (body-weight 40 kg and above): 75 mg once daily for 10 days for post-exposure prophylaxis; for up to 6 weeks during an epidemic
▸ Child 13–17 years: 75 mg once daily for 10 days for post-exposure prophylaxis; for up to 6 weeks during an epidemic
▸ Adult: 75 mg once daily for 10 days for post-exposure prophylaxis; for up to 6 weeks during an epidemic
Treatment of influenza
▸ BY MOUTH
▸ Child 1–11 months: 3 mg/kg twice daily for 5 days
▸ Child 1–12 years (body-weight 10–15 kg): 30 mg twice daily for 5 days
▸ Child 1–12 years (body-weight 15–23 kg): 45 mg twice daily for 5 days
▸ Child 1–12 years (body-weight 23–40 kg): 60 mg twice daily for 5 days
▸ Child 1–12 years (body-weight 40 kg and above): 75 mg twice daily for 5 days
▸ Child 13–17 years: 75 mg twice daily for 5 days
▸ Adult: 75 mg twice daily for 5 days

- ● UNLICENSED USE Not licensed for use in premature infants.
- ● SIDE-EFFECTS
▸ **Common or very common** Abdominal pain · dyspepsia · headache · nausea · vomiting
▸ **Uncommon** Altered consciousness (usually in children and adolescents) · arrhythmias · convulsions · eczema · rash
▸ **Rare** Gastro-intestinal bleeding · hepatitis · neuropsychiatric disorders (usually in children and adolescents) · Stevens-Johnson syndrome · thrombocytopenia · toxic epidermal necrolysis · visual disturbances
- ● PREGNANCY Although safety data are limited, oseltamivir can be used in women who are pregnant when the potential benefit outweighs the risk (e.g. during a pandemic). Use only if potential benefit outweighs risk (e.g. during a pandemic).
- ● BREAST FEEDING Although safety data are limited, oseltamivir can be used in women who are breast-feeding when the potential benefit outweighs the risk (e.g. during a pandemic). Oseltamivir is the preferred drug in women who are breast-feeding. Amount probably too small to be harmful; use only if potential benefit outweighs risk (e.g. during a pandemic).

● RENAL IMPAIRMENT
▸ In adults For *treatment*, use 30 mg twice daily if eGFR
30–60 mL/minute/1.73 m^2 (30 mg once daily if eGFR
10–30 mL/minute/1.73 m^2). For *prevention*, use 30 mg once
daily if eGFR 30–60 mL/minute/1.73 m^2 (30 mg every
48 hours if eGFR 10–30 mL/minute/1.73 m^2). Avoid for
treatment and *prevention* if eGFR less than
10 mL/minute/1.73 m^2.
▸ In children For *treatment*, use 40% of normal dose twice
daily if estimated glomerular filtration rate
30–60 mL/minute/1.73 m^2 (40% of normal dose once daily
if estimated glomerular filtration rate
10–30 mL/minute/1.73 m^2). For *prevention*, use 40% of
normal dose once daily if estimated glomerular filtration
rate 30–60 mL/minute/1.73 m^2 (40% of normal dose every
48 hours if estimated glomerular filtration rate
10–30 mL/minute/1.73 m^2). Avoid for *treatment* and
prevention if estimated glomerular filtration rate less than
10 mL/minute/1.73 m^2.

● DIRECTIONS FOR ADMINISTRATION If suspension not
available, capsules can be opened and the contents mixed
with a small amount of sweetened food, such as sugar
water or chocolate syrup, just before administration.

● PRESCRIBING AND DISPENSING INFORMATION Flavours of
oral liquid formulations may include tutti-frutti.

● PATIENT AND CARER ADVICE
Medicines for Children leaflet: Oseltamivir for influenza (flu)
www.medicinesforchildren.org.uk/oseltamivir-for-influenza

● NATIONAL FUNDING/ACCESS DECISIONS
NICE technology appraisals (TAs)
▸ Oseltamivir, zanamivir, and amantadine for prophylaxis of
influenza (September 2008) NICE TA158
Oseltamivir is **not** a substitute for vaccination, which
remains the most effective way of preventing illness from
influenza.
  ● Oseltamivir is **not** recommended for seasonal
    prophylaxis against influenza.
  ● When influenza is circulating in the community,
    oseltamivir s an option recommended (in accordance
    with UK licensing) for post-exposure prophylaxis in at-
    risk patients who are not effectively protected by
    influenza vaccine, and who have been in close contact
    with someone suffering from influenza-like illness in the
    same household or residential setting. Oseltamivir
    should be given within 48 hours of exposure to
    influenza. (National surveillance schemes, including
    those run by Public Health England, should be used to
    indicate when influenza is circulating in the
    community.)
  ● During local outbreaks of influenza-like illness, when
    there is a high level of certainty that influenza is
    present, oseltamivir may be used for post-exposure
    prophylaxis in at-risk patients (regardless of influenza
    vaccination) living in long-term residential or nursing
    homes.
At risk patients include those aged over 65 years *or* those
who have one or more of the following conditions:
  ● chronic respiratory disease (including asthma and
    chronic obstructive pulmonary disease);
  ● chronic heart disease;
  ● chronic renal disease;
  ● chronic liver disease;
  ● chronic neurological disease;
  ● immunosuppression;
  ● diabetes mellitus.
The Department of Health in England has advised
(November 2010 and April 2011) that 'at risk patients' also
includes patients under 65 years of age who are at risk of
developing medical complications from influenza
(treatment only) or women who are pregnant.

This guidance does not cover the circumstances of a
pandemic, an impending pandemic, or a widespread
epidemic of a new strain of influenza to which there is
little or no immunity in the community.
www.nice.org.uk/TA158
▸ Oseltamivir, zanamivir, and amantadine for treatment of
influenza (February 2009) NICE TA168
Oseltamivir is **not** a substitute for vaccination, which
remains the most effective way of preventing illness from
influenza.
  ● When influenza is circulating in the community,
    oseltamiviris an option recommended (in accordance
    with UK licensing) for the treatment of influenza in at-
    risk patients who can start treatment within 48 hours of
    the onset of symptoms. (National surveillance schemes,
    including those run by Public Health England, should be
    used to indicate when influenza is circulating in the
    community.)
  ● During local outbreaks of influenza-like illness, when
    there is a high level of certainty that influenza is
    present, oseltamivir may be used for treatment in at-risk
    patients living in long-term residential or nursing
    homes.
At risk patients include those aged over 65 years *or* those
who have one or more of the following conditions:
  ● chronic respiratory disease (including asthma and
    chronic obstructive pulmonary disease);
  ● chronic heart disease;
  ● chronic renal disease;
  ● chronic liver disease;
  ● chronic neurological disease;
  ● immunosuppression;
  ● diabetes mellitus.
The Department of Health in England has advised
(November 2010 and April 2011) that 'at risk patients' also
includes patients under 65 years of age who are at risk of
developing medical complications from influenza
(treatment only) or women who are pregnant.
This guidance does not cover the circumstances of a
pandemic, an impending pandemic, or a widespread
epidemic of a new strain of influenza to which there is
little or no immunity in the community.
www.nice.org.uk/TA168
NHS restrictions   Except for the treatment and
prophylaxis of influenza as indicated in the NICE
guidance; endorse prescription 'SLS'.

● MEDICINAL FORMS
There can be variation in the licensing of different medicines
containing the same drug. Forms available from special-order
manufacturers include: oral suspension, oral solution
Capsule
CAUTIONARY AND ADVISORY LABELS 9
▸ Tamiflu (Roche Products Ltd)
   Oseltamivir (as Oseltamivir phosphate) 30 mg Tamiflu 30mg
   capsules | 10 capsule PoM £7.71
   Oseltamivir (as Oseltamivir phosphate) 45 mg Tamiflu 45mg
   capsules | 10 capsule PoM £15.41
   Oseltamivir (as Oseltamivir phosphate) 75 mg Tamiflu 75mg
   capsules | 10 capsule PoM £15.41
Oral suspension
CAUTIONARY AND ADVISORY LABELS 9
EXCIPIENTS: May contain Sorbitol
▸ Tamiflu (Roche Products Ltd)
   Oseltamivir (as Oseltamivir phosphate) 6 mg per 1 ml Tamiflu
   6mg/ml oral suspension sugar-free | 65 ml PoM £10.27
Oral solution
CAUTIONARY AND ADVISORY LABELS 9
▸ Oseltamivir (Non-proprietary)
   **Oseltamivir (as Oseltamivir phosphate) 15 mg per
   1 ml** Oseltamivir 15mg/ml oral solution sugar free sugar-free |
   20 ml PoM £10.00

5

Infection

5

Infection

Zanamivir

- **DRUG ACTION** Reduces replication of influenza A and B viruses by inhibiting viral neuraminidase.

- **INDICATIONS AND DOSE**
Post-exposure prophylaxis of influenza
▸ BY INHALATION OF POWDER
▸ Child 5–17 years: 10 mg once daily for 10 days
▸ Adult: 10 mg once daily for 10 days
Prevention of influenza during an epidemic
▸ BY INHALATION OF POWDER
▸ Child 5–17 years: 10 mg once daily for up to 28 days
▸ Adult: 10 mg once daily for up to 28 days
Treatment of influenza
▸ BY INHALATION OF POWDER
▸ Child 5–17 years: 10 mg twice daily for 5 days (for up to 10 days if resistance to oseltamivir suspected)
▸ Adult: 10 mg twice daily for 5 days (for up to 10 days if resistance to oseltamivir suspected)

- **UNLICENSED USE** Use of zanamivir for up to 10 days if resistance to oseltamivir suspected is an unlicensed duration.

- **CAUTIONS** Asthma · chronic pulmonary disease · uncontrolled chronic illness
  CAUTIONS, FURTHER INFORMATION
  ▸ Asthma and chronic pulmonary disease Risk of bronchospasm—short-acting bronchodilator should be available.
    Avoid in severe asthma unless close monitoring possible and appropriate facilities available to treat bronchospasm.

- **SIDE-EFFECTS**
- **Common or very common** Rash
- **Uncommon** Angioedema · bronchospasm · dyspnoea · urticaria
- **Rare** Neuropsychiatric disorders (in children) · neuropsychiatric disorders (especially in children and adolescents) (in adults) · Stevens-Johnson syndrome · toxic epidermal necrolysis

- **PREGNANCY** Although safety data are limited, zanamivir can be used in women who are pregnant when the potential benefit outweighs the risk (e.g. during a pandemic). Use only if potential benefit outweighs risk (e.g. during a pandemic).

- **BREAST FEEDING** Although safety data are limited, zanamivir can be used in women who are breast-feeding when the potential benefit outweighs the risk (e.g. during a pandemic). Amount probably too small to be harmful; use only if potential benefit outweighs risk (e.g. during a pandemic).

- **DIRECTIONS FOR ADMINISTRATION** Other inhaled drugs should be administered before zanamivir.

- **PRESCRIBING AND DISPENSING INFORMATION** Except for the treatment and prophylaxis of influenza as indicated in the NICE guidance; endorse prescription 'SLS'.

- **NATIONAL FUNDING/ACCESS DECISIONS**
  NICE technology appraisals (TAs)
  ▸ Oseltamivir, zanamivir, and amantadine for prophylaxis of influenza (September 2008) NICE TA158
  Zanamivir is **not** a substitute for vaccination, which remains the most effective way of preventing illness from influenza.
  - Zanamivir is **not** recommended for seasonal prophylaxis against influenza.
  - When influenza is circulating in the community, zanamivir is an option recommended (in accordance with UK licensing) for post-exposure prophylaxis in at-risk patients who are not effectively protected by influenza vaccine, and who have been in close contact

with someone suffering from influenza-like illness in the same household or residential setting. anamivir should be given within 36 hours of exposure to influenza. (National surveillance schemes, including those run by Public Health England, should be used to indicate when influenza is circulating in the community).
- During local outbreaks of influenza-like illness, when there is a high level of certainty that influenza is present, zanamivir may be used for post-exposure prophylaxis in at-risk patients (regardless of influenza vaccination) living in long-term residential or nursing homes.
At risk patients include those aged over 65 years or those who have one or more of the following conditions:
- chronic respiratory disease (including asthma and chronic obstructive pulmonary disease);
- chronic heart disease;
- chronic renal disease;
- chronic liver disease;
- chronic neurological disease;
- immunosuppression;
- diabetes mellitus.
The Department of Health in England has advised (November 2010 and April 2011) that 'at risk patients' also includes patients under 65 years of age who are at risk of developing medical complications from influenza (treatment only) or women who are pregnant.
  This guidance does not cover the circumstances of a pandemic, an impending pandemic, or a widespread epidemic of a new strain of influenza to which there is little or no immunity in the community.
www.nice.org.uk/TA158
▸ **Oseltamivir, zanamivir, and amantadine for treatment of influenza (February 2009)** NICE TA168
Zanamivir is **not** a substitute for vaccination, which remains the most effective way of preventing illness from influenza.
- When influenza is circulating in the community, zanamivir is an option recommended (in accordance with UK licensing) for the treatment of influenza in at-risk patients who can start treatment within 48 hours (within 36 hours for zanamivir in children) of the onset of symptoms. (National surveillance schemes, including those run by Public Health England, should be used to indicate when influenza is circulating in the community.)
- During local outbreaks of influenza-like illness, when there is a high level of certainty that influenza is present, zanamivir may be used for treatment in at-risk patients living in long-term residential or nursing homes.
At risk patients include those aged over 65 years or those who have one or more of the following conditions:
- chronic respiratory disease (including asthma and chronic obstructive pulmonary disease);
- chronic heart disease;
- chronic renal disease;
- chronic liver disease;
- chronic neurological disease;
- immunosuppression;
- diabetes mellitus.
The Department of Health in England has advised (November 2010 and April 2011) that 'at risk patients' also includes patients under 65 years of age who are at risk of developing medical complications from influenza (treatment only) or women who are pregnant.
  This guidance does not cover the circumstances of a pandemic, an impending pandemic, or a widespread epidemic of a new strain of influenza to which there is little or no immunity in the community.
www.nice.org.uk/TA168

● MEDICINAL FORMS
There can be variation in the licensing of different medicines
containing the same drug.

Inhalation powder
▸ Relenza (GlaxoSmithKline UK Ltd)
Zanamivir 5 mg Relenza 5mg inhalation powder blisters with
Diskhaler | 20 blister PoM £16.36

6.6 Respiratory syncytial virus

Respiratory syncytial virus

Management in adults

Ribavirin p. 569 inhibits a wide range of DNA and RNA
viruses. It is given by mouth for the treatment of chronic
hepatitis C infection, in double therapy with peginterferon
alfa p. 567, interferon alfa p. 839, or sofosbuvir p. 571, or in
triple therapy with peginterferon alfa and one protease
inhibitor (i.e. boceprevir p. 573, telaprevir p. 574 or
simeprevir p. 573) or sofosbuvir. Ribavirin is also effective in
Lassa fever [unlicensed indication].

Management in children

Ribavirin is licensed for administration by inhalation for the
treatment of severe bronchiolitis caused by the respiratory
syncytial virus (RSV) in infants, especially when they have
other serious diseases. However, there is no evidence that
ribavirin produces clinically relevant benefit in RSV
bronchiolitis.

Palivizumab is a monoclonal antibody licensed for
preventing serious lower respiratory-tract disease caused by
respiratory syncytial virus in children at high risk of the
disease; it should be prescribed under specialist supervision
and on the basis of the likelihood of hospitalisation.
Palivizumab is recommended for:

● children under 9 months of age with chronic lung disease
(defined as requiring oxygen for at least 28 days from
birth) and who were born preterm;

● children under 6 months of age with haemodynamically
significant, acyanotic congenital heart disease who were
born preterm.

Palivizumab should be considered for:

● children under 2 years of age with severe combined
immunodeficiency syndrome;

● children under 1 year of age who require long-term
ventilation;

● children 1–2 years of age who require long-term
ventilation and have an additional co-morbidity (including
cardiac disease or pulmonary hypertension).

For details of the preterm age groups included in the
recommendations, see *Immunisation against Infectious
Disease* (2006), available at www.gov.uk/dh.

Chapter 6
Endocrine system

CONTENTS

1 Antidiuretic hormone disorders

Posterior pituitary hormones and antagonists

Posterior pituitary hormones

Diabetes insipidus

Vasopressin p. 605 (antidiuretic hormone, ADH) is used in the treatment of *pituitary* ('cranial') *diabetes insipidus* as is its analogue desmopressin p. 603. Dosage is tailored to produce a slight diuresis every 24 hours to avoid water intoxication. Treatment may be required for a limited period only in diabetes insipidus following trauma or pituitary surgery.

Desmopressin is more potent and has a longer duration of action than vasopressin; unlike vasopressin it has no vasoconstrictor effect. It is given by mouth or intranasally for maintenance therapy, and by injection in the postoperative period or in unconscious patients. Desmopressin is also used in the differential diagnosis of diabetes insipidus. Following a dose intramuscularly or intranasally, restoration of the ability to concentrate urine after water deprivation confirms a diagnosis of cranial diabetes insipidus. Failure to respond occurs in nephrogenic diabetes insipidus.

In *nephrogenic* and *partial pituitary diabetes insipidus* benefit may be gained from the paradoxical antidiuretic effect of thiazides.

Carbamazepine p. 283 is sometimes useful in partial pituitary diabetes insipidus [unlicensed]; it may act by sensitising the renal tubules to the action of remaining endogenous vasopressin.

Other uses

Desmopressin is also used to boost factor VIII concentration in mild to moderate haemophilia and in von Willebrand's disease; it is also used to test fibrinolytic response. Desmopressin may also have a role in nocturnal enuresis.

Vasopressin infusion is used to control variceal bleeding in portal hypertension, prior to more definitive treatment and with variable results. Terlipressin acetate, a derivative of vasopressin with reportedly less pressor and antidiuretic activity, is used similarly.

Oxytocin p. 744, another posterior pituitary hormone, is indicated in obstetrics.

Antidiuretic hormone antagonists

Demeclocycline hydrochloride p. 513 can be used in the treatment of hyponatraemia resulting from inappropriate secretion of antidiuretic hormone, if fluid restriction alone does not restore sodium concentration or is not tolerable. Demeclocycline hydrochloride is thought to act by directly blocking the renal tubular effect of antidiuretic hormone.

Tolvaptan p. 605 is a vasopressin V_2-receptor antagonist licensed for the treatment of hyponatraemia secondary to syndrome of inappropriate antidiuretic hormone secretion; treatment duration with tolvaptan is determined by the underlying disease and its treatment.

Rapid correction of hyponatraemia during tolvaptan therapy can cause osmotic demyelination, leading to serious neurological events; close monitoring of serum sodium concentration and fluid balance is essential.

1.1 Diabetes insipidus

> **Drugs used for Diabetes insipidus not listed below**
> Chlortalidone, p. 213

PITUITARY AND HYPOTHALAMIC HORMONES AND ANALOGUES > VASOPRESSIN AND ANALOGUES

Desmopressin

● DRUG ACTION Desmopressin is an analogue of vasopressin.

● INDICATIONS AND DOSE

Diabetes insipidus, treatment

▶ BY MOUTH
  ‣ Child 1-23 months: Initially 10 micrograms 2–3 times a day, adjusted according to response; usual dose 30–150 micrograms daily
  ‣ Child 2-11 years: Initially 50 micrograms 2–3 times a day, adjusted according to response; usual dose 100–800 micrograms daily
  ‣ Child 12-17 years: Initially 100 micrograms 2–3 times a day, adjusted according to response; usual dose 0.2–1.2 mg daily
  ‣ Adult: Initially 100 micrograms 3 times a day; maintenance 100–200 micrograms 3 times a day; usual dose 0.2–1.2 mg daily
▶ BY SUBLINGUAL ADMINISTRATION
  ‣ Child 2-17 years: Initially 60 micrograms 3 times a day, adjusted according to response; usual dose 40–240 micrograms 3 times a day
  ‣ Adult: Initially 60 micrograms 3 times a day, adjusted according to response; usual dose 40–240 micrograms 3 times a day
▶ BY INTRANASAL ADMINISTRATION
  ‣ Child 1-23 months: Initially 2.5–5 micrograms 1–2 times a day, adjusted according to response
  ‣ Child 2-11 years: Initially 5–20 micrograms 1–2 times a day, adjusted according to response
  ‣ Child 12-17 years: Initially 10–20 micrograms 1–2 times a day, adjusted according to response
  ‣ Adult: 10–40 micrograms daily in 1–2 divided doses
▶ BY SUBCUTANEOUS INJECTION, OR BY INTRAVENOUS INJECTION, OR BY INTRAMUSCULAR INJECTION
  ‣ Adult: 1–4 micrograms daily

Primary nocturnal enuresis

▶ BY MOUTH
  ‣ Child 5-17 years: 200 micrograms once daily, only increased to 400 micrograms if lower dose not effective; withdraw for at least 1 week for reassessment after 3 months, dose to be taken at bedtime, limit fluid intake from 1 hour before to 8 hours after administration
  ‣ Adult 18-65 years: 200 micrograms once daily, only increased to 400 micrograms if lower dose not effective; withdraw for at least 1 week for reassessment after 3 months, dose to be taken at bedtime, limit fluid intake from 1 hour before to 8 hours after administration
▶ BY SUBLINGUAL ADMINISTRATION
  ‣ Child 5-17 years: 120 micrograms once daily, increased if necessary to 240 micrograms once daily, dose to be taken at bedtime, limit fluid intake from 1 hour before to 8 hours after administration, dose to be increased only if lower dose not effective, reassess after 3 months by withdrawing treatment for at least 1 week
  ‣ Adult 18-65 years: 120 micrograms once daily, increased if necessary to 240 micrograms once daily, dose to be taken at bedtime, limit fluid intake from 1 hour before to 8 hours after administration, dose to be increased only if lower dose not effective, reassess after 3 months by withdrawing treatment for at least 1 week

Postoperative polyuria or polydipsia

▶ BY MOUTH
  ‣ Adult: Dose to be adjusted according to urine osmolality

Polyuria or polydipsia after hypophysectomy

▶ BY SUBLINGUAL ADMINISTRATION
  ‣ Adult: Dose to be adjusted according to urine osmolality

Diabetes insipidus, diagnosis (water deprivation test)

▶ BY INTRANASAL ADMINISTRATION
  ‣ Adult: 20 micrograms, limit fluid intake to 500 mL from 1 hour before to 8 hours after administration
▶ BY INTRAMUSCULAR INJECTION, OR BY SUBCUTANEOUS INJECTION
  ‣ Adult: 2 micrograms for 1 dose, limit fluid intake to 500 mL from 1 hour before to 8 hours after administration

Nocturia associated with multiple sclerosis (when other treatments have failed)

▶ BY INTRANASAL ADMINISTRATION
  ‣ Adult 18-65 years: 10–20 micrograms once daily, to be taken at bedtime, dose not to be repeated within 24 hours, limit fluid intake from 1 hour before to 8 hours after administration

Renal function testing

▶ BY INTRANASAL ADMINISTRATION
  ‣ Adult: 40 micrograms, empty bladder at time of administration and limit fluid intake to 500 mL from 1 hour before until 8 hours after administration to avoid fluid overload
▶ BY SUBCUTANEOUS INJECTION, OR BY INTRAMUSCULAR INJECTION
  ‣ Adult: 2 micrograms, empty bladder at time of administration and restrict fluid intake to 500 mL from 1 hour before until 8 hours after administration to avoid fluid overload

Mild to moderate haemophilia and von Willebrand's disease

▶ BY INTRANASAL ADMINISTRATION
  ‣ Adult: 300 micrograms every 12 hours if required, one 150 microgram spray into each nostril, 30 minutes before surgery or when bleeding, dose may alternatively be repeated at intervals of at least 3 days, if self-administered
▶ BY INTRAVENOUS INFUSION, OR BY SUBCUTANEOUS INJECTION
  ‣ Adult: 300 nanograms/kg for 1 dose, to be administered immediately before surgery or after trauma; may be repeated at intervals of 12 hours

Fibrinolytic response testing

▶ BY INTRANASAL ADMINISTRATION
  ‣ Adult: 300 micrograms, blood to be sampled after 1 hour for fibrinolytic activity, one 150 microgram spray to be administered into each nostril
▶ BY SUBCUTANEOUS INJECTION, OR BY INTRAVENOUS INJECTION
  ‣ Adult: 300 nanograms/kg for 1 dose, blood to be sampled after 20 minutes for fibrinolytic activity

Lumbar-puncture-associated headache

▶ BY INTRAMUSCULAR INJECTION, OR BY SUBCUTANEOUS INJECTION
  ‣ Adult: (consult product literature)

● UNLICENSED USE
  ▶ In children Consult product literature for individual preparations. Oral use of *DDAVP* intravenous injection is not licensed.

● CONTRA-INDICATIONS Cardiac insufficiency · conditions treated with diuretics · polydipsia in alcohol dependence · psychogenic polydipsia

6

Endocrine system

● CAUTIONS

GENERAL CAUTIONS

Asthma · avoid fluid overload · cardiovascular disease (not indicated for nocturnal enuresis or nocturia) · conditions which might be aggravated by water retention · cystic fibrosis · elderly (avoid for nocturnal enuresis and nocturia in those over 65 years) (in adults) · epilepsy · heart failure · hypertension (not indicated for nocturnal enuresis or nocturia) · migraine · nocturia—limit fluid intake to minimum from 1 hour before dose until 8 hours afterwards · nocturnal enuresis—limit fluid intake to minimum from 1 hour before dose until 8 hours afterwards

SPECIFIC CAUTIONS

▸ With intranasal use Should not be given intranasally for nocturnal enuresis due to an increased incidence of side-effects

● INTERACTIONS → Appendix 1 (desmopressin).

● SIDE-EFFECTS

GENERAL SIDE-EFFECTS

Allergic reactions · emotional disturbance in children · epistaxis · fluid retention · headache · hyponatraemia (in more serious cases with convulsions) on administration without restricting fluid intake · nasal congestion · nausea · stomach pain · vomiting

SPECIFIC SIDE-EFFECTS

▸ With intranasal use Rhinitis

SIDE-EFFECTS, FURTHER INFORMATION

▸ Hyponatraemic convulsions The risk of hyponatraemic convulsions can be minimised by keeping to the recommended starting doses and by avoiding concomitant use of drugs which increase secretion of vasopressin (e.g. tricyclic antidepressants).

● PREGNANCY Small oxytocic effect in third trimester; increased risk of pre-eclampsia.

● BREAST FEEDING Amount too small to be harmful.

● RENAL IMPAIRMENT Use with caution; antidiuretic effect may be reduced.

● MONITORING REQUIREMENTS In *nocturia*, periodic blood pressure and weight checks are needed to monitor for fluid overload.

● DIRECTIONS FOR ADMINISTRATION *DDVAP*® and *Desmotabs*® tablets may be crushed.
DDAVP® intranasal solution may be diluted with Sodium Chloride 0.9% to a concentration of 10 micrograms/mL.
DDAVP® injection may be administered orally. Desmopressin oral lyophilisates are for sublingual administration.
For *intravenous infusion* (*DDVAP*®, *Octim*®), give intermittently in Sodium chloride 0.9%; dilute with 50 mL and give over 20 minutes.

● PRESCRIBING AND DISPENSING INFORMATION Oral, intranasal, intravenous, subcutaneous and intramuscular doses are expressed as desmopressin acetate; sublingual doses are expressed as desmopressin base.
Children requiring an intranasal dose of less than 10 micrograms should be given *DDAVP*® intranasal solution.

● PATIENT AND CARER ADVICE

Medicines for Children leaflet: Desmopressin for bedwetting www.medicinesforchildren.org.uk/desmopressin-bedwetting-0
Hyponatraemic convulsions Patients being treated for primary nocturnal enuresis should be warned to avoid fluid overload (including during swimming) and to stop taking desmopressin during an episode of vomiting or diarrhoea (until fluid balance normal).

● MEDICINAL FORMS

There can be variation in the licensing of different medicines containing the same drug. Forms available from special-order manufacturers include: capsule, oral suspension, oral solution, spray, nasal drops

Tablet

▸ Desmopressin (Non-proprietary)

Desmopressin acetate 100 microgram Desmopressin 100microgram tablets | 90 tablet [PoM] £76.62 DT price = £62.88
Desmopressin acetate 200 microgram Desmopressin 200microgram tablets | 30 tablet [PoM] £35.23 DT price = £7.58 | 90 tablet [PoM] £87.50

▸ DDAVP (Ferring Pharmaceuticals Ltd)

Desmopressin acetate 100 microgram DDAVP 0.1mg tablets | 90 tablet [PoM] £44.12 DT price = £62.88
Desmopressin acetate 200 microgram DDAVP 0.2mg tablets | 90 tablet [PoM] £88.23

▸ Desmotabs (Ferring Pharmaceuticals Ltd)

Desmopressin acetate 200 microgram Desmotabs 0.2mg tablets | 30 tablet [PoM] £29.43 DT price = £7.58

Oral solution

▸ Desmopressin (Non-proprietary)

Desmopressin (as Desmopressin acetate) 360 microgram per 1 ml Desmopressin 360micrograms/ml oral solution | 15 ml [PoM] £30.00

Oral lyophilisate

CAUTIONARY AND ADVISORY LABELS 26

▸ Desmopressin (Non-proprietary)

Desmopressin (as Desmopressin acetate) 120 microgram Desmopressin 120microgram oral lyophilisates sugar free sugar-free | 30 tablet [PoM] no price available DT price = £30.34
Desmopressin (as Desmopressin acetate) 240 microgram Desmopressin 240microgram oral lyophilisates sugar free sugar-free | 30 tablet [PoM] no price available DT price = £60.68

▸ DDAVP (Ferring Pharmaceuticals Ltd)

Desmopressin (as Desmopressin acetate) 60 microgram DDAVP Melt 60microgram oral lyophilisates sugar-free | 100 tablet [PoM] £50.53 DT price = £50.53
Desmopressin (as Desmopressin acetate) 120 microgram DDAVP Melt 120microgram oral lyophilisates sugar-free | 100 tablet [PoM] £101.07 DT price = £101.07
Desmopressin (as Desmopressin acetate) 240 microgram DDAVP Melt 240microgram oral lyophilisates sugar-free | 100 tablet [PoM] £202.14

▸ DesmoMelt (Ferring Pharmaceuticals Ltd)

Desmopressin (as Desmopressin acetate) 120 microgram DesmoMelt 120microgram oral lyophilisates sugar-free | 30 tablet [PoM] £30.34 DT price = £30.34
Desmopressin (as Desmopressin acetate) 240 microgram DesmoMelt 240microgram oral lyophilisates sugar-free | 30 tablet [PoM] £60.68 DT price = £60.68

Solution for injection

▸ DDAVP (Ferring Pharmaceuticals Ltd)

Desmopressin acetate 4 microgram per 1 ml DDAVP 4micrograms/1ml solution for injection ampoules | 10 ampoule [PoM] £13.16

▸ Octim (Ferring Pharmaceuticals Ltd)

Desmopressin acetate 15 microgram per 1 ml Octim 15micrograms/1ml solution for injection ampoules | 10 ampoule [PoM] £192.20

Spray

▸ Desmopressin (Non-proprietary)

Desmopressin acetate 2.5 microgram per 1 dose Minirin 2.5micrograms/dose nasal spray | 50 dose [PoM] no price available
Desmopressin acetate 10 microgram per 1 dose Desmopressin 10micrograms/dose nasal spray | 60 dose [PoM] £30.00 DT price = £12.41

▸ Desmospray (Ferring Pharmaceuticals Ltd)

Desmopressin acetate 2.5 microgram per 1 dose Desmospray 2.5micrograms/dose nasal spray | 50 dose [PoM] no price available
Desmopressin acetate 10 microgram per 1 dose Desmospray 10micrograms/dose nasal spray | 60 dose [PoM] £25.02 DT price = £12.41

▸ Octim (Ferring Pharmaceuticals Ltd)

Desmopressin acetate 150 microgram per 1 dose Octim 150micrograms/dose nasal spray | 25 dose [PoM] £576.60

Nasal drops

▸ DDAVP (Ferring Pharmaceuticals Ltd)
Desmopressin acetate 100 microgram per 1 ml DDAVP
100micrograms/ml intranasal solution | 2.5 ml PoM £9.72 DT price =
£9.72

Vasopressin

● **INDICATIONS AND DOSE**

Pituitary diabetes insipidus
▸ BY INTRAMUSCULAR INJECTION, OR BY SUBCUTANEOUS
  INJECTION
▸ Adult: 5–20 units every 4 hours

Initial control of oesophageal variceal bleeding
▸ BY INTRAVENOUS INFUSION
▸ Adult: 20 units, dose to be administered over
  15 minutes

● CONTRA-INDICATIONS Chronic nephritis (until reasonable
  blood nitrogen concentrations attained) · vascular disease
  (especially disease of coronary arteries) unless extreme
  caution

● CAUTIONS Asthma · avoid fluid overload · conditions which
  might be aggravated by water retention · epilepsy · heart
  failure · hypertension · migraine

● SIDE-EFFECTS
▸ **Rare** Gangrene
▸ **Frequency not known** Abdominal cramps · anaphylaxis ·
  anginal attacks · belching · constriction of coronary
  arteries · desire to defaecate · fluid retention · headache ·
  hypersensitivity reactions · myocardial ischaemia · nausea ·
  pallor · peripheral ischaemia · sweating · tremor · vertigo ·
  vomiting

● PREGNANCY Oxytocic effect in third trimester.

● BREAST FEEDING Not known to be harmful.

● DIRECTIONS FOR ADMINISTRATION
▸ With intravenous use For *intravenous infusion* (argipressin),
  give intermittently in Glucose 5%; suggested
  concentration 20 units/100mL given over 15 minutes.

● MEDICINAL FORMS
  There can be variation in the licensing of different medicines
  containing the same drug.
  Solution for injection
  ▸ Vasopressin (Non-proprietary)
    Argipressin 20 unit per 1 ml Argipressin 20units/1ml solution for
    injection ampoules | 10 ampoule PoM £800.00 (Hospital only)

1.2 Syndrome of inappropriate antidiuretic hormone secretion

DIURETICS ❯ SELECTIVE VASOPRESSIN
V₂-RECEPTOR ANTAGONISTS

Tolvaptan

● DRUG ACTION Tolvaptan is a vasopressin V_2-receptor
  antagonist.

● **INDICATIONS AND DOSE**

JINARC ®

**Autosomal dominant polycystic kidney disease in adults
with CKD stage 1 to 3 at initiation of treatment with
evidence of rapidly progressing disease (initiated by a
specialist)**
▸ BY MOUTH
▸ Adult: Initially 60 mg daily in 2 divided doses for at
  least a week, 45 mg in the morning before breakfast,
  and then 15 mg taken 8 hours later; increased to 90 mg
  daily in 2 divided doses for at least a week, 60 mg in the
  morning before breakfast, and then 30 mg taken
  8 hours later, then increased if tolerated to 120 mg
  daily in 2 divided doses, 90 mg in the morning before
  breakfast, and then 30 mg taken 8 hours later, dose
  titration should be performed cautiously; patients may
  down-titrate to lower doses based on tolerability

SAMSCA®

**Treatment of hyponatraemia secondary to syndrome of
inappropriate antidiuretic hormone secretion**
▸ BY MOUTH
▸ Adult: 15 mg once daily, increased if necessary up to
  60 mg daily; treatment duration is determined by the
  underlying disease and its treatment

● CONTRA-INDICATIONS Anuria · hypernatraemia ·
  hypovolaemic hyponatraemia · impaired perception of
  thirst · volume depletion

● CAUTIONS Alcoholism (increased risk of demyelination
  syndrome if rapid correction of hyponatraemia) · diabetes
  mellitus · ensure adequate fluid intake · hypoxia (increased
  risk of demyelination syndrome if rapid correction of
  hyponatraemia) · malnutrition (increased risk of
  demyelination syndrome if rapid correction of
  hyponatraemia) · pseudohyponatraemia associated with
  diabetes mellitus (exclude before treatment)

● INTERACTIONS → Appendix 1 (tolvaptan).
  Avoid concomitant drugs that increase serum-sodium
  concentration.

● SIDE-EFFECTS
▸ **Common or very common** Constipation · decreased appetite
  · dehydration · dry mouth · ecchymosis · fever ·
  hyperglycaemia · hyperkalaemia · increased blood
  creatinine · malaise · nausea · neurological disturbance
  (following rapid correction of hyponatraemia) · postural
  hypotension · pruritus · thirst · urinary frequency
▸ **Uncommon** Renal impairment · taste disturbance
▸ **Frequency not known** Dizziness · hepatic impairment
  (discontinue) · hypernatraemia · hyperuricaemia ·
  hypoglycaemia · syncope

  SIDE-EFFECTS, FURTHER INFORMATION
▸ Hepatic impairment Discontinue and perform liver-function
  tests promptly if symptoms of hepatic impairment
  (anorexia, nausea, vomiting, fatigue, abdominal pain,
  jaundice, dark urine, pruritus).

6

Endocrine system

Endocrine system

6

- PREGNANCY Avoid—toxicity in *animal* studies.
- BREAST FEEDING Avoid—present in milk in *animal* studies.
- HEPATIC IMPAIRMENT Use with caution in severe impairment—no information available.
- RENAL IMPAIRMENT No information available in severe impairment.
- MONITORING REQUIREMENTS
  ▸ Monitor for dehydration in patients who are fluid-restricted.
  ▸ Monitor serum-sodium concentration and fluid balance no later than 6 hours after initiating treatment and every 6 hours during the first 1–2 days of treatment and until dose stabilised. Discontinue if rapid rise in serum-sodium concentration (greater than 12 mmol/litre in 24 hours or 18 mmol/litre in 48 hours).
- PATIENT AND CARER ADVICE For *Jinarc®*, morning dose to be taken 30 minutes before food, second dose can be taken with or without food.
- NATIONAL FUNDING/ACCESS DECISIONS

NICE technology appraisals (TAs)
▸ **Tolvaptan for treating autosomal dominant polycystic kidney disease (October 2015)** NICE TA358
Tolvaptan (*Jinarc®*) is recommended as an option for the treatment of autosomal dominant polycystic kidney disease in adults if:
- the patient has chronic kidney disease stage 2 or 3 at the start of treatment *and*
- there is evidence of rapidly progressing disease
- **and** the manufacturer provides tolvaptan with the discount agreed in the patient access scheme
Patients currently receiving tolvaptan (*Jinarc®*) whose disease does not meet the above criteria should be able to continue treatment until they and their clinician consider it appropriate to stop.
www.nice.org.uk/guidance/TA358

- MEDICINAL FORMS
There can be variation in the licensing of different medicines containing the same drug.

Tablet
▸ Jinarc (Otsuka Pharmaceuticals (U.K.) Ltd) ▼
  Tolvaptan 15 mg Jinarc 15mg tablets | 7 tablet PoM £302.05
  Tolvaptan 30 mg Jinarc 30mg tablets | 7 tablet PoM £302.05
  Tolvaptan 45 mg Jinarc 45mg tablets | 7 tablet PoM no price available
  Tolvaptan 60 mg Jinarc 60mg tablets | 7 tablet PoM no price available
  Tolvaptan 90 mg Jinarc 90mg tablets | 7 tablet PoM no price available
▸ Samsca (Otsuka Pharmaceuticals (U.K.) Ltd)
  Tolvaptan 15 mg Samsca 15mg tablets | 10 tablet PoM £746.80
  Tolvaptan 30 mg Samsca 30mg tablets | 10 tablet PoM £746.80
▸ Jinarc (Otsuka Pharmaceuticals (U.K.) Ltd) ▼
  Jinarc 45mg tablets and Jinarc 15mg tablets | 56 tablet PoM £1,208.20
  Jinarc 60mg tablets and Jinarc 30mg tablets | 56 tablet PoM £1,208.20
  Jinarc 90mg tablets and Jinarc 30mg tablets | 56 tablet PoM £1,208.20

2 Corticosteroid responsive conditions

CORTICOSTEROIDS

Corticosteroids, general use

Overview

Dosages of corticosteroids vary widely in different diseases and in different patients. If the use of a corticosteroid can save or prolong life, as in exfoliative dermatitis, pemphigus, acute leukaemia or acute transplant rejection, high doses may need to be given, because the complications of therapy are likely to be less serious than the effects of the disease itself.

When long-term corticosteroid therapy is used in some chronic diseases, the adverse effects of treatment may become greater than the disabilities caused by the disease. To minimise side-effects the maintenance dose should be kept as low as possible.

When potentially less harmful measures are ineffective corticosteroids are used topically for the treatment of inflammatory conditions of the skin. Corticosteroids should be avoided or used only under specialist supervision in psoriasis.

Corticosteroids are used both topically (by rectum) and systemically (by mouth or intravenously) in the management of ulcerative colitis and Crohn's disease. They are also included in locally applied creams for haemorrhoids.

Use can be made of the mineralocorticoid activity of fludrocortisone acetate p. 612 to treat postural hypotension in autonomic neuropathy.

High-dose corticosteroids should be avoided for the management of septic shock. However, there is evidence that administration of lower doses of hydrocortisone p. 612 and fludrocortisone acetate is of benefit in adrenocortical insufficiency resulting from septic shock.

Dexamethasone p. 610 and betamethasone p. 610 have little if any mineralocorticoid action and their long duration of action makes them particularly suitable for suppressing corticotropin secretion in congenital adrenal hyperplasia where the dose should be tailored to clinical response and by measurement of adrenal androgens and 17-hydroxyprogesterone. In common with all glucocorticoids their suppressive action on the hypothalamic- pituitary-adrenal axis is greatest and most prolonged when they are given at night. In most individuals a single dose of dexamethasone at night, is sufficient to inhibit corticotropin secretion for 24 hours. This is the basis of the 'overnight dexamethasone suppression test' for diagnosing Cushing's syndrome.

Betamethasone and dexamethasone are also appropriate for conditions where water retention would be a disadvantage.

A corticosteroid may be used in the management of raised intracranial pressure or cerebral oedema that occurs as a result of malignancy (see Prescribing in palliative care p. 21); high doses of betamethasone or dexamethasone are generally used. However, a corticosteroid should not be used for the management of head injury or stroke because it is unlikely to be of benefit and may even be harmful.

In acute hypersensitivity reactions, such as angioedema of the upper respiratory tract and anaphylaxis, corticosteroids are indicated as an adjunct to emergency treatment with adrenaline/epinephrine p. 205. In such cases hydrocortisone (as sodium succinate) by intravenous injection may be required.

Corticosteroids are preferably used by inhalation in the management of asthma but systemic therapy in association with bronchodilators is required for the emergency treatment of severe acute asthma.

Corticosteroids may also be useful in conditions such as autoimmune hepatitis, rheumatoid arthritis and sarcoidosis; they may also lead to remissions of acquired haemolytic anaemia, and some cases of the nephrotic syndrome (particularly in children) and thrombocytopenic purpura.

Corticosteroids can improve the prognosis of serious conditions such as systemic lupus erythematosus, temporal arteritis, and polyarteritis nodosa; the effects of the disease process may be suppressed and symptoms relieved, but the underlying condition is not cured, although it may ultimately remit. It is usual to begin therapy in these conditions at fairly high dose, and then to reduce the dose to the lowest commensurate with disease control.

For other references to the use of corticosteroids see: Prescribing in Palliative Care, immunosuppression, rheumatic diseases, eye, otitis externa allergic rhinitis, and aphthous ulcers.

Side-effects

Overdosage or prolonged use can exaggerate some of the normal physiological actions of corticosteroids leading to mineralocorticoid and glucocorticoid side-effects.

Mineralocorticoid side effects

- hypertension
- sodium retention
- water retention
- potassium loss
- calcium loss

Mineralocorticoid side effects are most marked with fludrocortisone, but are significant with hydrocortisone, corticotropin, and tetracosactide. Mineralocorticoid actions are negligible with the high potency glucocorticoids, betamethasone and dexamethasone, and occur only slightly with methylprednisolone, prednisolone, and triamcinolone.

Glucocorticoid side effects

- diabetes
- osteoporosis, which is a danger, particularly in the elderly, as it can result in osteoporotic fractures for example of the hip or vertebrae;
- in addition high doses are associated with avascular necrosis of the femoral head.
- Muscle wasting (proximal myopathy) can also occur.
- Corticosteroid therapy is also weakly linked with peptic ulceration and perforation.
- Psychiatric reactions may also occur.

Managing side-effects

Side-effects can be minimised by using lowest effective dose for minimum period possible. The suppressive action of a corticosteroid on cortisol secretion is least when it is given as a single dose in the morning. In an attempt to reduce pituitary-adrenal suppression further, the total dose for two days can sometimes be taken as a single dose on alternate days; alternate-day administration has not been very successful in the management of asthma. Pituitary-adrenal suppression can also be reduced by means of intermittent therapy with short courses. In some conditions it may be possible to reduce the dose of corticosteroid by adding a small dose of an immunosuppressive drug.

Whenever possible *local treatment* with creams, intra-articular injections, inhalations, eye-drops, or enemas should be used in preference to *systemic treatment*.

Inhaled corticosteroids have considerably fewer systemic effects than oral corticosteroids, but adverse effects including adrenal suppression have been reported. Use of other corticosteroid therapy (including topical) or concurrent use of drugs which inhibit corticosteroid metabolism should be taken into account when assessing systemic risk. In children, growth restriction associated with systemic corticosteroid therapy does not seem to occur with recommended doses of inhaled therapy; although initial growth velocity may be reduced, there appears to be no effect on achieving normal adult height. Large-volume spacer devices should be used for administering inhaled corticosteroids in children under 15 years; they are also useful in older children and adults, particularly if high doses are required. Spacer devices increase airway deposition and reduce oropharyngeal deposition.

Corticosteroids, replacement therapy

Overview

The adrenal cortex normally secretes hydrocortisone p. 612 (cortisol) which has glucocorticoid activity and weak mineralocorticoid activity. It also secretes the mineralocorticoid aldosterone.

In deficiency states, physiological replacement is best achieved with a combination of hydrocortisone and the mineralocorticoid fludrocortisone acetate p. 612; hydrocortisone alone does not usually provide sufficient mineralocorticoid activity for complete replacement.

In *Addison's disease* or following adrenalectomy, hydrocortisone by mouth is usually required. This is given in 2 doses, the larger in the morning and the smaller in the evening, mimicking the normal diurnal rhythm of cortisol secretion. The optimum daily dose is determined on the basis of clinical response. Glucocorticoid therapy is supplemented by fludrocortisone acetate.

In *acute adrenocortical insufficiency*, hydrocortisone is given intravenously (preferably as sodium succinate) every 6 to 8 hours in sodium chloride intravenous infusion 0.9% p. 901.

In *hypopituitarism*, glucocorticoids should be given as in adrenocortical insufficiency, but since production of aldosterone is also regulated by the renin-angiotensin system a mineralocorticoid is not usually required. Additional replacement therapy with levothyroxine sodium p. 699 and sex hormones should be given as indicated by the pattern of hormone deficiency.

Glucocorticoid therapy

Glucocorticoid and mineralocorticoid activity

In comparing the relative potencies of corticosteroids in terms of their anti-inflammatory (glucocorticoid) effects it should be borne in mind that high glucocorticoid activity in itself is of no advantage unless it is accompanied by relatively low mineralocorticoid activity (see Disadvantages of Corticosteroids). The mineralocorticoid activity of fludrocortisone acetate p. 612 is so high that its anti-inflammatory activity is of no clinical relevance.

Equivalent anti-inflammatory doses of corticosteroids
This table takes no account of mineralocorticoid effects, nor does it take account of variations in duration of action
Prednisolone 5 mg
≡ Betamethasone 750 micrograms
≡ Deflazacort 6 mg
≡ Dexamethasone 750 micrograms
≡ Hydrocortisone 20 mg
≡ Methylprednisolone 4 mg
≡ Prednisone 5 mg
≡ Triamcinolone 4 mg

6

Endocrine system

The relatively high mineralocorticoid activity of hydrocortisone p. 612, and the resulting fluid retention, makes it unsuitable for disease suppression on a long-term basis. However, hydrocortisone can be used for adrenal replacement therapy. Hydrocortisone is used on a short-term basis by intravenous injection for the emergency management of some conditions. The relatively moderate anti-inflammatory potency of hydrocortisone also makes it a useful topical corticosteroid for the management of inflammatory skin conditions because side-effects (both topical and systemic) are less marked.

Prednisolone p. 614 and prednisone p. 615 have predominantly glucocorticoid activity. Prednisolone is the corticosteroid most commonly used by mouth for long-term disease suppression.

Betamethasone p. 610 and dexamethasone p. 610 have very high glucocorticoid activity in conjunction with insignificant mineralocorticoid activity. This makes them particularly suitable for high-dose therapy in conditions where fluid retention would be a disadvantage.

Betamethasone and dexamethasone also have a long duration of action and this, coupled with their lack of mineralocorticoid action makes them particularly suitable for conditions which require suppression of corticotropin (corticotrophin) secretion (e.g. congenital adrenal hyperplasia).

Some esters of betamethasone and of beclometasone dipropionate p. 39 (beclometasone) exert a considerably more marked topical effect (e.g. on the skin or the lungs) than when given by mouth; use is made of this to obtain topical effects whilst minimising systemic side-effects (e.g. for skin applications and asthma inhalations).

Deflazacort p. 610 has a high glucocorticoid activity; it is derived from prednisolone.

Corticosteroids (systemic)

- **CONTRA-INDICATIONS** Avoid injections containing benzyl alcohol in neonates · avoid live virus vaccines in those receiving immunosuppressive doses (serum antibody response diminished) · systemic infection (unless specific therapy given)

CONTRA-INDICATIONS, FURTHER INFORMATION
▸ With intra-articular use or intradermal use or intralesional use For further information on contra-indications associated with intra-articular, intradermal and intralesional preparations, consult product literature.

- **CAUTIONS** Congestive heart failure · diabetes mellitus (including a family history of) · diverticulitis · epilepsy · glaucoma (including a family history of or susceptibility to) · history of steroid myopathy · history of tuberculosis or X-ray changes (frequent monitoring required) · hypertension · hypothyroidism · infection (particularly untreated) · myasthenia gravis · ocular herpes simplex (risk of corneal perforation) · osteoporosis (in children) · osteoporosis (post-menopausal women and the elderly at special risk) (in adults) · peptic ulcer · psychiatric reactions · recent intestinal anastomoses · recent myocardial infarction (rupture reported) · severe affective disorders (particularly if history of steroid-induced psychosis) · should not be used long-term · thromboembolic disorders · ulcerative colitis

CAUTIONS, FURTHER INFORMATION
▸ With intra-articular use or intradermal use or intralesional use For further information on cautions associated with intra-articular, intradermal and intralesional preparations, consult product literature.

- **INTERACTIONS** → Appendix 1 (corticosteroids).

- **SIDE-EFFECTS**
GENERAL SIDE-EFFECTS
Abdominal distension · acute pancreatitis · aggravation of epilepsy · aggravation of schizophrenia · amenorrhoea · anaphylaxis (in children) · bruising · candidiasis · congestive heart failure · corneal thinning · Cushing's syndrome (with moon face, striae and acne) · dyspepsia · ecchymoses · exacerbation of ophthalmic fungal disease · exacerbation of ophthalmic viral disease · exophthalmos · facial erythema · glaucoma · headache · hiccups · hirsutism · hypercholesterolaemia · hyperglycaemia · hyperhidrosis · hyperlipidaemia · hypersensitivity reactions (in children) · impaired healing · increased appetite · increased intra-ocular pressure · increased intracranial pressure with papilloedema (usually after withdrawal) (in children) · increased susceptibility to and severity of infection · insomnia · leucocytosis · long bone fractures · malaise · menstrual irregularities · muscle weakness · myocardial rupture following recent myocardial infarction · nausea · negative calcium balance · negative nitrogen balance · oesophageal ulceration · papilloedema (in adults) · petechiae · posterior subcapsular cataracts · potassium loss · psychological dependence · reactivation of dormant tuberculosis · scleral thinning · skin atrophy · sodium retention · suppression of growth (in children) · telangiectasia · tendon rupture · thromboembolism · urticaria · vertebral fractures · vertigo · water retention · weight gain

SPECIFIC SIDE-EFFECTS
▸ With intra-articular use Flushing · may affect the hyaline cartilage

SIDE-EFFECTS, FURTHER INFORMATION
▸ With intra-articular use or intradermal use or intralesional use in adults For further information on side-effects associated with intra-articular, intradermal and intralesional preparations, consult product literature.

Side effects can be managed by choice of route and duration of course. For further detail see Corticosteroids, general use p. 606

▸ Adrenal suppression During prolonged therapy with corticosteroids, particularly with systemic use, adrenal atrophy develops and can persist for years after stopping. Abrupt withdrawal after a prolonged period can lead to acute adrenal insufficiency, hypotension, or death.

To compensate for a diminished adrenocortical response caused by prolonged corticosteroid treatment, any significant intercurrent illness, trauma, or surgical procedure requires a temporary increase in corticosteroid dose, or if already stopped, a temporary reintroduction of corticosteroid treatment. To avoid a precipitous fall in blood pressure during anaesthesia or in the immediate postoperative period, anaesthetists **must** know whether a patient is taking or has been taking a corticosteroid. A suitable regimen for corticosteroid replacement, in patients who have taken more than 10 mg prednisolone daily (or equivalent) within 3 months of surgery, is:
- Minor surgery under general anaesthesia—usual oral corticosteroid dose on the morning of surgery or hydrocortisone (usually the sodium succinate) intravenously at induction; the usual oral corticosteroid dose is recommended after surgery.
- Moderate or major surgery—usual oral corticosteroid dose on the morning of surgery and hydrocortisone intravenously at induction, followed by hydrocortisone 3 times a day by intravenous injection for 24 hours after moderate surgery or for 48–72 hours after major surgery; the usual pre-operative oral corticosteroid dose is recommened on stopping hydrocortisone injections.

Patients on long-term corticosteroid treatment should carry a steroid treatment card which gives guidance on minimising risk and provides details of prescriber, drug, dosage and duration of treatment.

▸ Infections Prolonged courses of corticosteroids increase susceptibility to infections and severity of infections; clinical presentation of infections may also be atypical. Serious infections e.g. *septicaemia* and *tuberculosis* may reach an advanced stage before being recognised, and *amoebiasis* or *strongyloidiasis* may be activated or exacerbated (exclude before initiating a corticosteroid in those at risk or with suggestive symptoms). Fungal or viral *ocular infections* may also be exacerbated.

▸ Chickenpox Unless they have had chickenpox, patients receiving oral or parenteral corticosteroids for purposes other than replacement should be regarded as being *at risk of severe chickenpox* (see Steroid Treatment Card). Manifestations of fulminant illness include pneumonia, hepatitis and disseminated intravascular coagulation; rash is not necessarily a prominent feature.

Passive immunisation with varicella–zoster immunoglobulin is needed for exposed non–immune patients receiving systemic corticosteroids or for those who have used them within the previous 3 months. Confirmed chickenpox warrants specialist care and urgent treatment. Corticosteroids should not be stopped and dosage may need to be increased.

Topical, inhaled or rectal corticosteroids are less likely to be associated with an increased risk of severe chickenpox.

▸ Measles Patients taking corticosteroids should be advised to take particular care to avoid exposure to measles and to seek immediate medical advice if exposure occurs. Prophylaxis with intramuscular normal immunoglobulin may be needed.

▸ Psychiatric reactions Systemic corticosteroids, particularly in high doses, are linked to psychiatric reactions including euphoria, nightmares, insomnia, irritability, mood lability, suicidal thoughts, psychotic reactions, and behavioural disturbances. A serious paranoid state or depression with risk of suicide can be induced, particularly in patients with a history of mental disorder. These reactions frequently subside on reducing the dose or discontinuing the corticosteroid but they may also require specific management. Patients should be advised to seek medical advice if psychiatric symptoms (especially depression and suicidal thoughts) occur and they should also be alert to the rare possibility of such reactions during withdrawal of corticosteroid treatment.

Systemic corticosteroids should be prescribed with care in those predisposed to psychiatric reactions, including those who have previously suffered corticosteroid–induced psychosis, or who have a personal or family history of psychiatric disorders.

● PREGNANCY The benefit of treatment with corticosteroids during pregnancy outweighs the risk. Corticosteroid cover is required during labour. Following a review of the data on the safety of systemic corticosteroids used in pregnancy and breast-feeding the CSM (May 1998) concluded that corticosteroids vary in their ability to cross the placenta but there is no convincing evidence that systemic corticosteroids increase the incidence of congenital abnormalities such as cleft palate or lip. When administration is prolonged or repeated during pregnancy, systemic corticosteroids increase the risk of intra-uterine growth restriction; there is no evidence of intra-uterine growth restriction following short-term treatment (e.g. prophylactic treatment for neonatal respiratory distress syndrome). Any adrenal suppression in the neonate following prenatal exposure usually resolves spontaneously after birth and is rarely clinically important.

Pregnant women with fluid retention should be monitored closely when given systemic corticosteroids.

● BREAST FEEDING The benefit of treatment with corticosteroids during breast-feeding outweighs the risk.

● HEPATIC IMPAIRMENT The plasma-drug concentration may be increased (particularly on systemic use). Oral and parenteral use should be undertaken with caution.

● RENAL IMPAIRMENT Use by oral and injectable routes should be undertaken with caution.

● MONITORING REQUIREMENTS
▸ In children The height and weight of children receiving prolonged treatment with corticosteroids should be monitored annually; if growth is slowed, referral to a paediatrician should be considered.

● EFFECT ON LABORATORY TESTS Suppression of skin test reactions.

● TREATMENT CESSATION
▸ In adults Abrupt withdrawal after a prolonged period can lead to acute adrenal insufficiency, hypotension or death. Withdrawal can also be associated with fever, myalgia, arthralgia, rhinitis, conjunctivitis, painful itchy skin nodules and weight loss. The magnitude and speed of dose reduction in corticosteroid withdrawal should be determined on a case–by–case basis, taking into consideration the underlying condition that is being treated, and individual patient factors such as the likelihood of relapse and the duration of corticosteroid treatment. *Gradual* withdrawal of systemic corticosteroids should be considered in those whose disease is unlikely to relapse and have:
● received more than 40 mg prednisolone (or equivalent) daily for more than 1 week;
● been given repeat doses in the evening;
● received more than 3 weeks' treatment;
● recently received repeated courses (particularly if taken for longer than 3 weeks);
● taken a short course within 1 year of stopping long-term therapy;
● other possible causes of adrenal suppression.

Systemic corticosteroids may be stopped abruptly in those whose disease is unlikely to relapse *and* who have received treatment for 3 weeks or less *and* who are not included in the patient groups described above.

During corticosteroid withdrawal the dose may be reduced rapidly down to physiological doses (equivalent to prednisolone 7.5 mg daily) and then reduced more slowly. Assessment of the disease may be needed during withdrawal to ensure that relapse does not occur.

▸ In children The magnitude and speed of dose reduction in corticosteroid withdrawal should be determined on a case–by–case basis, taking into consideration the underlying condition that is being treated, and individual patient factors such as the likelihood of relapse and the duration of corticosteroid treatment. *Gradual* withdrawal of systemic corticosteroids should be considered in those whose disease is unlikely to relapse and have:
● received more than 40 mg prednisolone (or equivalent) daily for more than 1 week *or* 2 mg/kg daily for 1 week *or* 1 mg/kg daily for 1 month;
● been given repeat doses in the evening;
● received more than 3 weeks' treatment;
● recently received repeated courses (particularly if taken for longer than 3 weeks);
● taken a short course within 1 year of stopping long-term therapy;
● other possible causes of adrenal suppression.

Systemic corticosteroids may be stopped abruptly in those whose disease is unlikely to relapse *and* who have received treatment for 3 weeks or less *and* who are not included in the patient groups described above.

During corticosteroid withdrawal the dose may be reduced rapidly down to physiological doses (equivalent to prednisolone 2–2.5 mg/m^2 daily) and then reduced more slowly. Assessment of the disease may be needed during withdrawal to ensure that relapse does not occur.

Endocrine system

6

● PATIENT AND CARER ADVICE

Advice for patients Patients on long-term corticosteroid treatment should carry a Steroid Treatment Card which gives guidance on minimising risk and provides details of prescriber, drug, dosage and duration of treatment.

A patient information leaflet should be supplied to every patient when a systemic corticosteroid is prescribed. Patients should especially be advised of the following:

- **Immunosuppression** Prolonged courses of corticosteroids can increase susceptibility to infection and serious infections can go unrecognised. Unless already immune, patients are at risk of severe **chickenpox** and should avoid close contact with people who have chickenpox or shingles. Similarly, precautions should also be taken against contracting **measles**;
- **Adrenal suppression** If the corticosteroid is given for longer than 3 weeks, treatment must not be stopped abruptly. Adrenal suppression can last for a year or more after stopping treatment and the patient must mention the course of corticosteroid when receiving treatment for any illness or injury;
- **Mood and behaviour changes** Corticosteroid treatment, especially with high doses, can alter mood and behaviour early in treatment—the patient can become confused, irritable and suffer from delusion and suicidal thoughts. These effects can also occur when corticosteroid treatment is being withdrawn. Medical advice should be sought if worrying psychological changes occur;
- **Other serious effects** Serious gastro-intestinal, musculoskeletal, and ophthalmic effects which require medical help can also occur.

Steroid treatment cards Steroid treatment cards should be issued where appropriate. Consider giving a 'steroid card' to support communication of the risks associated with treatment, and specific written advice to consider corticosteroid replacement during an episode of stress, such as severe intercurrent illness or an operation, to patients using greater than maximum licensed doses of inhaled corticosteroids. Steroid treatment cards are available for purchase from:

3M Security Print and Systems Limited, Gorse Street, Chadderton, Oldham, OL9 9QH

Tel: 0845 610 1112

GP practices can obtain supplies through their Local Area Team Stores. NHS Trusts can order supplies from www.nhsforms.co.uk or by emailing nhsforms@mmm.com.

In **Scotland**, steroid treatment cards can be obtained from APS Group Scotland by emailing stockorders.dppas@theapsgroup.com or by fax on 0131 629 9967.

F 608

Betamethasone

● INDICATIONS AND DOSE

Suppression of inflammatory and allergic disorders | Congenital adrenal hyperplasia

▸ BY MOUTH

- Adult: Usual dose 0.5–5 mg daily

▸ BY INTRAMUSCULAR INJECTION, OR BY SLOW INTRAVENOUS INJECTION, OR BY INTRAVENOUS INFUSION

- Adult: 4–20 mg, repeated up to 4 times in 24 hours

● PREGNANCY Readily crosses the placenta. Transient effect on fetal movements and heart rate.

● DIRECTIONS FOR ADMINISTRATION For *intravenous infusion* (as sodium phosphate) (*Betnesol®*), give continuously or intermittently *or via* drip tubing *in* Glucose 5% *or* Sodium chloride 0.9%.

● PATIENT AND CARER ADVICE Patient counselling is advised for betamethasone soluble tablets (steroid card).

● MEDICINAL FORMS

There can be variation in the licensing of different medicines containing the same drug.

Soluble tablet

CAUTIONARY AND ADVISORY LABELS 10, 13, 21 (not for use as mouthwash for oral ulceration)

▸ Betamethasone (Non-proprietary)

Betamethasone (as Betamethasone sodium phosphate) 500 microgram Betamethasone 500microgram soluble tablets sugar free sugar-free | 100 tablet [PoM] £42.60 DT price = £42.04

Solution for injection

CAUTIONARY AND ADVISORY LABELS 10

▸ Betamethasone (Non-proprietary)

Betamethasone (as Betamethasone sodium phosphate) 4 mg per 1 ml Betamethasone 4mg/1ml solution for injection ampoules | 5 ampoule [PoM] £13.06

F 608

Deflazacort

● INDICATIONS AND DOSE

Suppression of inflammatory and allergic disorders

▸ BY MOUTH

- Adult: Maintenance 3–18 mg daily

Suppression of inflammatory and allergic disorders (acute disorders)

▸ BY MOUTH

- Adult: Initially up to 120 mg daily

Inflammatory and allergic disorders

▸ BY MOUTH

- Child 1 month–11 years: 0.25–1.5 mg/kg once daily or on alternate days; increased if necessary up to 2.4 mg/kg daily (max. per dose 120 mg), in emergency situations
- Child 12–17 years: 3–18 mg once daily or on alternate days; increased if necessary up to 2.4 mg/kg daily (max. per dose 120 mg), in emergency situations

● RENAL IMPAIRMENT Use with caution.

● PATIENT AND CARER ADVICE Patient counselling is advised for deflazacort tablets (steroid card).

● MEDICINAL FORMS

There can be variation in the licensing of different medicines containing the same drug. Forms available from special-order manufacturers include: tablet

Tablet

CAUTIONARY AND ADVISORY LABELS 5, 10

▸ Calcort (Sanofi)

Deflazacort 6 mg Calcort 6mg tablets | 60 tablet [PoM] £15.82

F 608

Dexamethasone

6.6.2016

● INDICATIONS AND DOSE

Suppression of inflammatory and allergic disorders

▸ BY MOUTH

- Adult: 0.5–10 mg daily

Mild croup

▸ BY MOUTH

- Child: 150 micrograms/kg for 1 dose

Severe croup (or mild croup that might cause complications)

▸ INITIALLY BY MOUTH

- Child: Initially 150 micrograms/kg for 1 dose, to be given before transfer to hospital, then (by mouth or by intravenous injection) 150 micrograms/kg, then (by mouth or by intravenous injection) 150 micrograms/kg after 12 hours if required

Diagnosis of Cushing's disease | Congenital adrenal hyperplasia
▶ BY MOUTH
  ▸ Adult: 0.5–10 mg daily
▶ BY INTRAMUSCULAR INJECTION, OR BY SLOW INTRAVENOUS INJECTION, OR BY INTRAVENOUS INFUSION
  ▸ Adult: 0.4–20 mg

Overnight dexamethasone suppression test
▶ BY MOUTH
  ▸ Adult: 1 mg for 1 dose, to be given at night

Adjunctive treatment of bacterial meningitis (starting before or with first dose of antibacterial)
▶ BY INTRAVENOUS INJECTION
  ▸ Adult: 8.3 mg every 6 hours for 4 days

Symptom control of anorexia (in palliative care)
  ▸ Adult: 2–4 mg daily

Obstruction due to tumour (dysphagia in palliative care)
  ▸ Adult: 8 mg daily

Bronchospasm or partial obstruction (dyspnoea in palliative care)
  ▸ Adult: 4–8 mg daily

Nausea and vomiting (adjunct in palliative care)
▶ BY MOUTH
  ▸ Adult: 8–16 mg daily

Headaches due to raised intracranial pressure (in palliative care)
  ▸ Adult: 16 mg daily for 4–5 days, then reduced to 4–6 mg daily, reduce dose if possible. To be given before 6pm to reduce the risk of insomnia

Pain due to nerve compression (in palliative care)
  ▸ Adult: 8 mg daily

Cerebral oedema associated with malignancy
▶ BY MOUTH
  ▸ Adult: 0.5–10 mg daily

Cerebral oedema
▶ INITIALLY BY INTRAVENOUS INJECTION
  ▸ Adult: Initially 8–16 mg for 1 dose, then (by intramuscular injection or by intravenous injection) 5 mg every 6 hours until adequate response achieved then taper-off gradually, use the 3.8 mg/mL injection preparation for this dose

Cerebral oedema associated with malignancy
▶ INITIALLY BY INTRAVENOUS INJECTION
  ▸ Adult: Initially 8.3 mg for 1 dose, then (by intramuscular injection) 3.3 mg every 6 hours as required for 2–4 days, subsequently, reduce dose gradually and stop over 5–7 days, use the 3.3 mg/mL injection preparation for this dose

● UNLICENSED USE
▶ With intravenous use Consult product literature; not licensed for use in bacterial meningitis.

● SIDE-EFFECTS
▶ With intravenous use Perineal irritation may follow intravenous administration of the phosphate ester

● PREGNANCY Dexamethasone readily crosses the placenta.

● DIRECTIONS FOR ADMINISTRATION
▶ With oral use in children For administration *by mouth* tablets may be dispersed in water or injection solution given by mouth.
▶ With intravenous use in adults For *intravenous infusion* (*Dexamethasone*, Hospira) give continuously *or* intermittently *or via* drip tubing *in* Glucose 5% *or* Sodium Chloride 0.9%.

● PRESCRIBING AND DISPENSING INFORMATION
▶ With systemic use Dexamethasone 3.8 mg/mL Injection has replaced Dexamethasone 4 mg/mL Injection. All dosage recommendations for intravenous, intramuscular,

intrarticular use or local infiltration; are given in units of dexamethasone base.

● PATIENT AND CARER ADVICE
  Medicines for Children leaflet: Dexamethasone for croup
  www.medicinesforchildren.org.uk/dexamethasone-croup-0
▶ With systemic use Patient counselling is advised for dexamethasone tablet, oral solution and injection (steroid card).

● MEDICINAL FORMS
  There can be variation in the licensing of different medicines containing the same drug. Forms available from special-order manufacturers include: capsule, oral suspension, oral solution

Tablet
CAUTIONARY AND ADVISORY LABELS 10, 21
▶ Dexamethasone (Non-proprietary)
  Dexamethasone 500 microgram Dexamethasone 500microgram tablets | 28 tablet [PoM] £54.48 DT price = £54.09 | 30 tablet [PoM] £64.82
  Dexamethasone 2 mg Dexamethasone 2mg tablets | 50 tablet [PoM] £49.04 DT price = £49.00 | 100 tablet [PoM] £98.08 | 500 tablet [PoM] £490.00

Soluble tablet
▶ Dexamethasone (Non-proprietary)
  Dexamethasone (as Dexamethasone sodium phosphate) 2 mg Dexamethasone 2mg soluble tablets sugar free sugar-free | 50 tablet [PoM] £30.00
  Dexamethasone (as Dexamethasone sodium phosphate) 4 mg Dexamethasone 4mg soluble tablets sugar free sugar-free | 50 tablet [PoM] £60.00
  Dexamethasone (as Dexamethasone sodium phosphate) 8 mg Dexamethasone 8mg soluble tablets sugar free sugar-free | 50 tablet [PoM] £120.00

Oral solution
CAUTIONARY AND ADVISORY LABELS 10, 21
▶ Dexamethasone (Non-proprietary)
  Dexamethasone (as Dexamethasone sodium phosphate) 400 microgram per 1 ml Dexamethasone 2mg/5ml oral solution sugar free sugar-free | 75 ml [PoM] no price available sugar-free | 150 ml [PoM] £42.30 DT price = £42.30
  Dexamethasone (as Dexamethasone sodium phosphate) 2 mg per 1 ml Dexamethasone 10mg/5ml oral solution sugar free sugar-free | 50 ml [PoM] £24.50–£24.95 sugar-free | 150 ml [PoM] £101.40 DT price = £94.44
  Dexamethasone (as Dexamethasone sodium phosphate) 4 mg per 1 ml Dexamethasone 20mg/5ml oral solution sugar free sugar-free | 50 ml [PoM] £49.50
▶ Dexsol (Rosemont Pharmaceuticals Ltd)
  Dexamethasone (as Dexamethasone sodium phosphate) 400 microgram per 1 ml Dexsol 2mg/5ml oral solution sugar-free | 75 ml [PoM] £21.15 sugar-free | 150 ml [PoM] £42.30 DT price = £42.30
▶ Martapan (Martindale Pharmaceuticals Ltd)
  Dexamethasone (as Dexamethasone sodium phosphate) 400 microgram per 1 ml Martapan 2mg/5ml oral solution sugar-free | 150 ml [PoM] £42.30 DT price = £42.30

Solution for injection
CAUTIONARY AND ADVISORY LABELS 10
▶ Dexamethasone (Non-proprietary)
  Dexamethasone (as Dexamethasone sodium phosphate) 3.3 mg per 1 ml Dexamethasone 6.6mg/2ml solution for injection vials | 5 vial [PoM] £24.00
  Dexamethasone 6.6mg/2ml solution for injection ampoules | 5 ampoule [PoM] £11.00
  Dexamethasone 3.3mg/1ml solution for injection ampoules | 5 ampoule [PoM] £12.00 | 10 ampoule [PoM] £12.00
  Dexamethasone (as Dexamethasone sodium phosphate) 3.8 mg per 1 ml Dexamethasone 3.8mg/1ml solution for injection vials | 10 vial [PoM] £19.99 DT price = £19.99

6

Endocrine system

6

Endocrine system

Fluorocortisone acetate ☞ 608

● INDICATIONS AND DOSE

Neuropathic postural hypotension
▸ BY MOUTH
▸ Adult: 100–400 micrograms daily

Mineralocorticoid replacement in adrenocortical insufficiency
▸ BY MOUTH
▸ Adult: 50–300 micrograms once daily

Adrenocortical insufficiency resulting from septic shock (in combination with hydrocortisone)
▸ BY MOUTH
▸ Adult: 50 micrograms daily

● UNLICENSED USE Not licensed for use in neuropathic postural hypotension.

● HEPATIC IMPAIRMENT Monitor patient closely in hepatic impairment.

● MEDICINAL FORMS
There can be variation in the licensing of different medicines containing the same drug. Forms available from special-order manufacturers include: capsule, oral suspension

Tablet
CAUTIONARY AND ADVISORY LABELS 10
▸ Fludrocortisone acetate (Non-proprietary)
Fludrocortisone acetate 100 microgram Fludrocortisone 100microgram tablets | 30 tablet PoM £30.00 DT price = £30.00

Hydrocortisone ☞ 608

● INDICATIONS AND DOSE

Thyrotoxic crisis (thyroid storm)
▸ BY INTRAVENOUS INJECTION
▸ Adult: 100 mg every 6 hours, to be administered as sodium succinate

Adrenocortical insufficiency resulting from septic shock
▸ BY INTRAVENOUS INJECTION
▸ Adult: 50 mg every 6 hours, given in combination with fludrocortisone

Acute hypersensitivity reactions such as angioedema of the upper respiratory tract and anaphylaxis (adjunct to adrenaline)
▸ BY INTRAVENOUS INJECTION
▸ Adult: 100–300 mg, to be administered as sodium succinate

Corticosteroid replacement, in patients who have taken more than 10 mg prednisolone daily (or equivalent) within 3 months of minor surgery under general anaesthesia
▸ BY INTRAVENOUS INJECTION, OR BY INTRAVENOUS INFUSION
▸ Adult: Initially 25–50 mg, to be administered at induction of surgery, the patient's usual oral corticosteroid dose is recommenced after surgery

Corticosteroid replacement, in patients who have taken more than 10 mg prednisolone daily (or equivalent) within 3 months of moderate or major surgery
▸ BY INTRAVENOUS INJECTION, OR BY INTRAVENOUS INFUSION
▸ Adult: Initially 25–50 mg, to be administered at induction of surgery (following usual oral corticosteroid dose on the morning of surgery), followed by 25–50 mg 3 times a day for 24 hours after moderate surgery and for 48–72 hours after major surgery

Adrenocortical insufficiency in Addison's disease or following adrenalectomy
▸ BY MOUTH USING IMMEDIATE-RELEASE MEDICINES
▸ Adult: 20–30 mg daily in 2 divided doses, the larger dose to be given in the morning and the smaller in the evening, mimicking the normal diurnal rhythm of cortisol secretion, the optimum daily dose is determined on the basis of clinical response

Adrenocortical insufficiency
▸ BY INTRAMUSCULAR INJECTION, OR BY SLOW INTRAVENOUS INJECTION, OR BY INTRAVENOUS INFUSION
▸ Adult: 100–500 mg 3–4 times a day or when required

Severe inflammatory bowel disease
▸ BY SLOW INTRAVENOUS INJECTION, OR BY INTRAVENOUS INFUSION
▸ Adult: 100–500 mg 3–4 times a day or when required

Replacement in adrenocortical insufficiency
▸ BY MOUTH USING MODIFIED-RELEASE MEDICINES
▸ Adult: 20–30 mg once daily, adjusted according to response, dose to be taken in the morning
▸ BY MOUTH USING IMMEDIATE-RELEASE MEDICINES
▸ Adult: 20–30 mg daily in divided doses, adjusted according to response

Ulcerative colitis | Proctitis | Proctosigmoiditis
▸ BY RECTUM USING RECTAL FOAM
▸ Adult: Initially 1 metered application 1–2 times a day for 2–3 weeks, then reduced to 1 metered application once daily on alternate days, to be inserted into the rectum

Acute hypersensitivity reactions | Angioedema
▸ BY INTRAMUSCULAR INJECTION, OR BY INTRAVENOUS INJECTION
▸ Child 1–5 months: Initially 25 mg 3 times a day, adjusted according to response
▸ Child 6 months–5 years: Initially 50 mg 3 times a day, adjusted according to response
▸ Child 6–11 years: Initially 100 mg 3 times a day, adjusted according to response
▸ Child 12–17 years: Initially 200 mg 3 times a day, adjusted according to response

Severe acute asthma | Life-threatening acute asthma
▸ BY INTRAVENOUS INJECTION
▸ Child 1 month–1 year: 4 mg/kg every 6 hours (max. per dose 100 mg), alternatively 25 mg every 6 hours until conversion to oral prednisolone is possible, dose given, preferably, as sodium succinate
▸ Child 2–4 years: 4 mg/kg every 6 hours (max. per dose 100 mg), alternatively 50 mg every 6 hours until conversion to oral prednisolone is possible, dose given, preferably, as sodium succinate
▸ Child 5–11 years: 4 mg/kg every 6 hours (max. per dose 100 mg), alternatively 100 mg every 6 hours until conversion to oral prednisolone is possible, dose given, preferably, as sodium succinate
▸ Child 12–17 years: 4 mg/kg every 6 hours (max. per dose 100 mg), alternatively 100 mg every 6 hours until conversion to oral prednisolone is possible, dose given, preferably, as sodium succinate
▸ Adult: 100 mg every 6 hours until conversion to oral prednisolone is possible, dose given, preferably, as sodium succinate

DOSE EQUIVALENCE AND CONVERSION
▸ With oral use in adults When switching from immediate-release hydrocortisone tablets to modified release *Plenadren* ® use same total daily dose. Bioavailability of *Plenadren* ® lower than immediate release tablets—monitor clinical response.

● CONTRA-INDICATIONS
▸ With rectal use Bowel perforation · extensive fistulas · intestinal obstruction · recent intestinal anastomoses

- CAUTIONS
- ▸ With rectal use Systemic absorption may occur
- SIDE-EFFECTS
- ▸ With intravenous use Phosphate ester associated with pain and paraesthesia (particularly in the perineal region)
- ▸ With rectal use Local irritation
- DIRECTIONS FOR ADMINISTRATION
- ▸ With intravenous use in children For *intravenous administration*, dilute with Glucose 5% or Sodium Chloride 0.9%. For *intermittent infusion* give over 20–30 minutes.
- ▸ With intravenous use in adults For *intravenous infusion* (*SoluCortef* ®), give continuously *or* intermittently *or via* drip tubing *in* Glucose 5% *or* Sodium chloride 0.9%.
- PATIENT AND CARER ADVICE
- ▸ With systemic use Patient counselling is advised for hydrocortisone tablets and injections (steroid card).
- LESS SUITABLE FOR PRESCRIBING
- ▸ With intravenous use Hydrocortisone as the sodium phosphate is less suitable for prescribing as paraesthesia and pain (particularly in the perineal region) may follow intravenous injection.
- EXCEPTIONS TO LEGAL CATEGORY
- ▸ With intramuscular use or intravenous use Prescription only medicine restriction does not apply where administration is for saving life in emergency.

- MEDICINAL FORMS
  There may be variation in the licensing of different medicines containing the same drug. Forms available from special-order manufacturers include: capsule, oral suspension, oral solution

Tablet
CAUTIONARY AND ADVISORY LABELS 10, 21
- ▸ Hydrocortisone (Non-proprietary)
  Hydrocortisone 10 mg Hydrocortisone 10mg tablets │ 30 tablet [PoM] £113.00 DT price = £76.07
  Hydrocortisone 20 mg Hydrocortisone 20mg tablets │ 30 tablet [PoM] £100.86 DT price = £101.40

Modified-release tablet
CAUTIONARY AND ADVISORY LABELS 10, 22, 25
- ▸ Plenadren (Shire Pharmaceuticals Ltd)
  Hydrocortisone 5 mg Plenadren 5mg modified-release tablets │ 50 tablet [PoM] £242.50
  Hydrocortisone 20 mg Plenadren 20mg modified-release tablets │ 50 tablet [PoM] £400.00

Solution for injection
CAUTIONARY AND ADVISORY LABELS 10
- ▸ Hydrocortisone (Non-proprietary)
  Hydrocortisone (as Hydrocortisone sodium phosphate) 100 mg per 1 ml Hydrocortisone sodium phosphate 100mg/1ml solution for injection ampoules │ 5 ampoule [PoM] £8.33
  Hydrocortisone sodium phosphate 500mg/5ml solution for injection ampoules │ 5 ampoule [PoM] £36.45

Powder for solution for injection
- ▸ Solu-Cortef (Pfizer Ltd)
  Hydrocortisone (as Hydrocortisone sodium succinate) 100 mg Solu-Cortef 100mg powder for solution for injection vials │ 10 vial [PoM] £9.17

Powder and solvent for solution for injection
CAUTIONARY AND ADVISORY LABELS 10
- ▸ Solu-Cortef (Pfizer Ltd)
  Hydrocortisone (as Hydrocortisone sodium succinate) 100 mg Solu-Cortef 100mg powder and solvent for solution for injection vials │ 1 vial [PoM] £1.16 DT price = £1.16

Foam
EXCIPIENTS: May contain Cetostearyl alcohol (including cetyl and stearyl alcohol), hydroxybenzoates (parabens), propylene glycol
- ▸ Colifoam (Meda Pharmaceuticals Ltd)
  Hydrocortisone acetate 100 mg per 1 gram Colifoam 10% aerosol │ 14 dose [PoM] £9.33 DT price = £9.33

⧫ 608

Methylprednisolone

- INDICATIONS AND DOSE

Suppression of inflammatory and allergic disorders │ Cerebral oedema associated with malignancy
- ▸ BY MOUTH
- ▸ Adult: Usual dose 2–40 mg daily
- ▸ BY INTRAMUSCULAR INJECTION, OR BY SLOW INTRAVENOUS INJECTION, OR BY INTRAVENOUS INFUSION
- ▸ Adult: Initially 10–500 mg

Treatment of graft rejection reactions
- ▸ BY INTRAVENOUS INFUSION
- ▸ Adult: Up to 1 g daily for up to 3 days

DEPO-MEDRONE®

Suppression of inflammatory and allergic disorders
- ▸ BY DEEP INTRAMUSCULAR INJECTION
- ▸ Adult: 40–120 mg, then 40–120 mg after 2–3 weeks if required, to be injected into the gluteal muscle

- CAUTIONS
- ▸ With intravenous use Rapid intravenous administration of large doses associated with cardiovascular collapse
- DIRECTIONS FOR ADMINISTRATION
- ▸ With intravenous use For *intravenous infusion* (as sodium succinate) (*Solu-Medrone* ®), give continuously *or* intermittently *or via* drip tubing in Glucose 5% *or* Sodium chloride 0.9%. Reconstitute initially with water for injections; doses up to 250 mg should be given over at least 5 minutes, high doses over at least 30 minutes.
- PATIENT AND CARER ADVICE Patient counselling is advised for methylprednisolone tablets and injections (steroid card).

- MEDICINAL FORMS
  There can be variation in the licensing of different medicines containing the same drug. Forms available from special-order manufacturers include: oral suspension

Tablet
CAUTIONARY AND ADVISORY LABELS 10, 21
- ▸ Medrone (Pfizer Ltd)
  Methylprednisolone 2 mg Medrone 2mg tablets │ 30 tablet [PoM] £3.88
  Methylprednisolone 4 mg Medrone 4mg tablets │ 30 tablet [PoM] £6.19
  Methylprednisolone 16 mg Medrone 16mg tablets │ 30 tablet [PoM] £17.17
  Methylprednisolone 100 mg Medrone 100mg tablets │ 20 tablet [PoM] £48.32

Powder and solvent for solution for injection
CAUTIONARY AND ADVISORY LABELS 10
- ▸ Methylprednisolone (Non-proprietary)
  Methylprednisolone (as Methylprednisolone sodium succinate) 500 mg Methylprednisolone sodium succinate 500mg powder and solvent for solution for injection vials │ 1 vial [PoM] £9.60
  Methylprednisolone (as Methylprednisolone sodium succinate) 1 gram Methylprednisolone sodium succinate 1g powder and solvent for solution for injection vials │ 1 vial [PoM] £17.30
- ▸ Solu-Medrone (Pfizer Ltd)
  Methylprednisolone (as Methylprednisolone sodium succinate) 40 mg Solu-Medrone 40mg powder and solvent for solution for injection vials │ 1 vial [PoM] £1.58
  Methylprednisolone (as Methylprednisolone sodium succinate) 125 mg Solu-Medrone 125mg powder and solvent for solution for injection vials │ 1 vial [PoM] £4.75
  Methylprednisolone (as Methylprednisolone sodium succinate) 500 mg Solu-Medrone 500mg powder and solvent for solution for injection vials │ 1 vial [PoM] £9.60
  Methylprednisolone (as Methylprednisolone sodium succinate) 1 gram Solu-Medrone 1g powder and solvent for solution for injection vials │ 1 vial [PoM] £17.30
  Methylprednisolone (as Methylprednisolone sodium succinate) 2 gram Solu-Medrone 2g powder and solvent for solution for injection vials │ 1 vial [PoM] £32.86

6

Endocrine system

6

Endocrine system

Suspension for injection
CAUTIONARY AND ADVISORY LABELS 10
- Depo-Medrone (Pfizer Ltd)
  Methylprednisolone acetate 40 mg per 1 ml Depo-Medrone
  40mg/1ml suspension for injection vials | 1 vial [PoM] £3.44 DT price
  = £3.44 | 10 vial [PoM] £34.04
  Depo-Medrone 80mg/2ml suspension for injection vials | 1 vial [PoM]
  £6.18 DT price = £6.18 | 10 vial [PoM] £61.39
  Depo-Medrone 120mg/3ml suspension for injection vials |
  1 vial [PoM] £8.96 DT price = £8.96 | 10 vial [PoM] £88.81

                                                              ⮞ 608

Prednisolone

- **INDICATIONS AND DOSE**

Acute exacerbation of chronic obstructive pulmonary disease (if increased breathlessness interferes with daily activities)
- BY MOUTH
- Adult: 30 mg daily for 7–14 days

Severe croup (before transfer to hospital) | Mild croup that might cause complications (before transfer to hospital)
- BY MOUTH
- Child: 1–2 mg/kg

Mild to moderate acute asthma (when oral corticosteroid taken for more than a few days) | Severe or life-threatening acute asthma (when oral corticosteroid taken for more than a few days)
- BY MOUTH
- Child 1 month-11 years: 2 mg/kg once daily (max. per dose 60 mg) for up to 3 days, longer if necessary

Mild to moderate acute asthma | Severe or life-threatening acute asthma
- BY MOUTH
- Child 1 month-11 years: 1–2 mg/kg once daily (max. per dose 40 mg) for up to 3 days, longer if necessary
- Child 12-17 years: 40–50 mg daily for at least 5 days
- Adult: 40–50 mg daily for at least 5 days

Suppression of inflammatory and allergic disorders
- BY MOUTH
- Adult: Initially 10–20 mg daily, dose preferably taken in the morning after breakfast, can often be reduced within a few days but may need to be continued for several weeks or months; maintenance 2.5–15 mg daily, higher doses may be needed; cushingoid side-effects increasingly likely with doses above 7.5 mg daily
- BY INTRAMUSCULAR INJECTION
- Adult: 25–100 mg 1–2 times a week, as prednisolone acetate

Suppression of inflammatory and allergic disorders (initial dose in severe disease)
- BY MOUTH
- Adult: Initially up to 60 mg daily, dose preferably taken in the morning after breakfast, can often be reduced within a few days but may need to be continued for several weeks or months

Idiopathic thrombocytopenic purpura
- BY MOUTH
- Adult: 1 mg/kg daily, gradually reduce dose over several weeks

Ulcerative colitis | Crohn's disease
- BY MOUTH
- Adult: Initially 20–40 mg daily until remission occurs, followed by reducing doses, up to 60 mg daily, may be used in some cases, doses preferably taken in the morning after breakfast

Neuritic pain or weakness heralding rapid onset of permanent nerve damage (during reversal reactions multibacillary leprosy)
- BY MOUTH
- Adult: Initially 40–60 mg daily, dose to be instituted at once

Generalised myasthenia gravis (when given on alternate days)
- BY MOUTH
- Adult: Initially 10 mg once daily on alternate days, then increased in steps of 10 mg once daily on alternate days, increased to 1–1.5 mg/kg once daily on alternate days (max. per dose 100 mg)

Generalised myasthenia gravis in ventilated patients (when given on alternate days)
- BY MOUTH
- Adult: Initially 1.5 mg/kg once daily on alternate days (max. per dose 100 mg)

Generalised myasthenia gravis (when giving daily)
- BY MOUTH
- Adult: Initially 5 mg daily, increased in steps of 5 mg daily. maintenance 60–80 mg daily, alternatively maintenance 0.75–1 mg/kg daily, ventilated patients may be started on 1.5 mg/kg (max. 100 mg) on alternate days

Ocular myasthenia
- BY MOUTH
- Adult: Usual dose 10–40 mg once daily on alternate days, reduce to minimum effective dose

Reduction in rate of joint destruction in moderate to severe rheumatoid arthritis of less than 2 years' duration
- BY MOUTH
- Adult: 7.5 mg daily

Polymyalgia rheumatica
- BY MOUTH
- Adult: 10–15 mg daily until remission of disease activity; maintenance 7.5–10 mg daily, reduce gradually to maintenance dose. Many patients require treatment for at least 2 years and in some patients it may be necessary to continue long term low-dose corticosteroid treatment

Giant cell (temporal) arteritis
- BY MOUTH
- Adult: 40–60 mg daily until remission of disease activity, the higher dose being used if visual symptoms occur; maintenance 7.5–10 mg daily, reduce gradually to maintenance dose. Many patients require treatment for at least 2 years and in some patients it may be necessary to continue long term low-dose corticosteroid treatment

Polyarteritis nodosa | Polymyositis | Systemic lupus erythematosus
- BY MOUTH
- Adult: Initially 60 mg daily, to be reduced gradually; maintenance 10–15 mg daily

Anorexia (symptom control in palliative care)
- BY MOUTH
- Adult: 15–30 mg daily

Pneumocystis pneumonia in moderate to severe infections associated with HIV infection
- BY MOUTH
- Adult: 50–80 mg daily for 5 days, the dose is then reduced to complete 21 days of treatment, corticosteroid treatment should ideally be started at the same time as the anti-pneumocystis therapy and certainly no later than 24–72 hours afterwards. The corticosteroid should be withdrawn before anti-pneumocystis treatment is complete

Short-term prophylaxis of episodic cluster headache as monotherapy or in combination with verapamil during verapamil titration

▶ BY MOUTH

▶ Adult: 60–100 mg once daily for 2–5 days, then reduced in steps of 10 mg every 2–3 days until prednisolone is discontinued

Proctitis

▶ BY RECTUM USING RECTAL FOAM

▶ Adult: 1 metered application 1–2 times a day for 2 weeks, continued for further 2 weeks if good response, to be inserted into the rectum, 1 metered application contains 20 mg prednisolone

▶ BY RECTUM USING SUPPOSITORIES

▶ Adult: 5 mg twice daily, to be inserted in to the rectum morning and night, after a bowel movement

Distal ulcerative colitis

▶ BY RECTUM USING RECTAL FOAM

▶ Adult: 1 metered application 1–2 times a day for 2 weeks, continued for further 2 weeks if good response, to be inserted into the rectum, 1 metered application contains 20 mg prednisolone

Rectal complications of Crohn's disease

▶ BY RECTUM USING SUPPOSITORIES

▶ Adult: 5 mg twice daily, to be inserted in to the rectum morning and night, after a bowel movement

Rectal and rectosigmoidal ulcerative colitis | Rectal and rectosigmoidal Crohn's disease

▶ BY RECTUM USING ENEMA

▶ Adult: 20 mg daily for 2–4 weeks, continued if response good, to be used at bedtime

● CONTRA-INDICATIONS

▶ With rectal use Bowel perforation · extensive fistulas · intestinal obstruction · recent intestinal anastomoses

● CAUTIONS

▶ With rectal use Systemic absorption may occur with rectal preparations

▶ With systemic use Duchenne's muscular dystrophy (possible transient rhabdomyolysis and myoglobinuria following strenuous physical activity)

● PREGNANCY As it crosses the placenta 88% of prednisolone is inactivated.

▶ With systemic use Pregnant women with fluid retention should be monitored closely.

● BREAST FEEDING Prednisolone appears in small amounts in breast milk but maternal doses of up to 40 mg daily are unlikely to cause systemic effects in the infant.

▶ With systemic use Infant should be monitored for adrenal suppression if mother is taking a dose higher than 40 mg.

● PATIENT AND CARER ADVICE

Medicines for Children leaflet: Prednisolone for asthma www.medicinesforchildren.org.uk/prednisolone-for-asthma

▶ With oral use Patient counselling is advised for prednisolone tablets (steroid card).

● MEDICINAL FORMS

There can be variation in the licensing of different medicines containing the same drug. Forms available from special-order manufacturers include: oral suspension, oral solution, enema

Tablet

CAUTIONARY AND ADVISORY LABELS 10, 21

▶ Prednisolone (Non-proprietary)

Prednisolone 1 mg Prednisolone 1mg tablets | 28 tablet PoM £4.00 DT price = £0.78 | 100 tablet PoM no price available

Prednisolone 2.5 mg Prednisolone 2.5mg tablets | 28 tablet PoM £0.68

Prednisolone 5 mg Prednisolone 5mg tablets | 28 tablet PoM £11.00 DT price = £0.88 | 100 tablet PoM no price available

Prednisolone 10 mg Prednisolone 10mg tablets | 28 tablet PoM £2.72

Prednisolone 20 mg Prednisolone 20mg tablets | 28 tablet PoM £5.43

Prednisolone 25 mg Prednisolone 25mg tablets | 56 tablet PoM £75.00 DT price = £75.00

Prednisolone 30 mg Prednisolone 30mg tablets | 28 tablet PoM £8.15

▶ Pevanti (AMCo)

Prednisolone 2.5 mg Pevanti 2.5mg tablets | 30 tablet PoM £1.42 DT price = £1.42

Prednisolone 5 mg Pevanti 5mg tablets | 30 tablet PoM £0.95

Prednisolone 10 mg Pevanti 10mg tablets | 30 tablet PoM £1.90 DT price = £1.90

Prednisolone 20 mg Pevanti 20mg tablets | 30 tablet PoM £3.80 DT price = £3.80

Prednisolone 25 mg Pevanti 25mg tablets | 56 tablet PoM £40.00 DT price = £75.00

Soluble tablet

CAUTIONARY AND ADVISORY LABELS 10, 13, 21

▶ Prednisolone (Non-proprietary)

Prednisolone (as Prednisolone sodium phosphate)

5 mg Prednisolone 5mg soluble tablets | 30 tablet PoM £75.00 DT price = £53.48

Gastro-resistant tablet

CAUTIONARY AND ADVISORY LABELS 5, 10, 25

▶ Prednisolone (Non-proprietary)

Prednisolone 1 mg Prednisolone 1mg gastro-resistant tablets | 30 tablet PoM £1.60

Prednisolone 2.5 mg Prednisolone 2.5mg gastro-resistant tablets | 28 tablet PoM £15.45 DT price = £1.26 | 30 tablet PoM £6.15 | 100 tablet PoM £4.96

Prednisolone 5 mg Prednisolone 5mg gastro-resistant tablets | 28 tablet PoM £13.50 DT price = £1.31 | 30 tablet PoM £6.29 | 100 tablet PoM £5.18

▶ Deltacortril Enteric (Alliance Pharmaceuticals Ltd)

Prednisolone 2.5 mg Deltacortril 2.5mg gastro-resistant tablets | 30 tablet PoM £1.16

Prednisolone 5 mg Deltacortril 5mg gastro-resistant tablets | 30 tablet PoM £1.19

▶ Dilacort (Crescent Pharma Ltd)

Prednisolone 2.5 mg Dilacort 2.5mg gastro-resistant tablets | 28 tablet PoM £1.39 DT price = £1.26

Prednisolone 5 mg Dilacort 5mg gastro-resistant tablets | 28 tablet PoM £1.45 DT price = £1.31

Oral solution

▶ Prednisolone (Non-proprietary)

Prednisolone 1 mg per 1 ml Prednisolone 5mg/5ml oral solution unit dose | 10 unit dose PoM £11.41 DT price = £11.41

Prednisolone 10 mg per 1 ml Prednisolone 10mg/ml oral solution sugar free sugar-free | 30 ml PoM £55.00–£55.50

Suspension for injection

▶ Deltastab (AMCo)

Prednisolone acetate 25 mg per 1 ml Deltastab 25mg/1ml suspension for injection ampoules | 10 ampoule PoM £68.72

Foam

▶ Prednisolone (Non-proprietary)

Prednisolone (as Prednisolone sodium metasulfobenzoate) 20 mg per 1 application Prednisolone 20mg/application foam enema | 14 dose PoM £78.00 DT price = £78.00

Suppository

▶ Prednisolone (Non-proprietary)

Prednisolone (as Prednisolone sodium phosphate)

5 mg Prednisolone sodium phosphate 5mg suppositories | 10 suppository PoM £38.63 DT price = £37.89

Enema

▶ Predsol (Focus Pharmaceuticals Ltd)

Prednisolone sodium phosphate 200 microgram per 1 ml Predsol 20mg/100ml retention enema | 7 enema PoM £7.50 DT price = £7.50

◀ 608

Prednisone

● INDICATIONS AND DOSE

Moderate to severe rheumatoid arthritis

▶ BY MOUTH USING MODIFIED-RELEASE MEDICINES

▶ Adult: 10–20 mg daily, adjusted according to response, dose to be take at bedtime

- **HEPATIC IMPAIRMENT** Monitor patient closely in hepatic impairment.
- **PATIENT AND CARER ADVICE** Patient counselling is advised for prednisone tablets (steroid card).

- **MEDICINAL FORMS**
There can be variation in the licensing of different medicines containing the same drug.
Modified-release tablet
CAUTIONARY AND ADVISORY LABELS 10, 21, 25
  ‣ Lodotra (Napp Pharmaceuticals Ltd)
  Prednisone 1 mg Lodotra 1mg modified-release tablets | 30 tablet PoM £26.70
  Prednisone 2 mg Lodotra 2mg modified-release tablets | 30 tablet PoM £26.70 | 100 tablet PoM £89.00
  Prednisone 5 mg Lodotra 5mg modified-release tablets | 30 tablet PoM £26.70 | 100 tablet PoM £89.00

⬆ 608

Triamcinolone acetonide

- **INDICATIONS AND DOSE**
Suppression of inflammatory and allergic disorders
  ‣ BY DEEP INTRAMUSCULAR INJECTION
  ‣ Adult: 40 mg (max. per dose 100 mg), repeated if necessary, dose given for depot effect, to be administered into gluteal muscle; repeated at intervals according to patient's response

- **CAUTIONS** High dosage (may cause proximal myopathy), avoid in chronic therapy
- **PATIENT AND CARER ADVICE** Patient counselling is advised for triamcinolone acetonide injection (steroid card).

- **MEDICINAL FORMS**
There can be variation in the licensing of different medicines containing the same drug.
Suspension for injection
CAUTIONARY AND ADVISORY LABELS 10
EXCIPIENTS: May contain Benzyl alcohol
  ‣ Kenalog (Bristol-Myers Squibb Pharmaceuticals Ltd)
  Triamcinolone acetonide 40 mg per 1 ml Kenalog Intra-articular / Intramuscular 40mg/1ml suspension for injection vials | 5 vial PoM £7.45 DT price = £7.45
  ‣ Triesence (Alcon Laboratories (UK) Ltd)
  Triamcinolone acetonide 40 mg per 1 ml Triesence 40mg/1ml suspension for injection vials | 1 vial PoM £44.90

2.1 Cushing's syndrome and disease

Cushing's Syndrome

Management

Most types of *Cushing's syndrome* are treated surgically, that which occasionally accompanies carcinoma of the bronchus is not usually amenable to surgery. Metyrapone p. 617 has been found helpful in controlling the symptoms of the disease; it is also used in other forms of Cushing's syndrome to prepare the patient for surgery.

The dosages of metyrapone used are either low, and tailored to cortisol production, or high, in which case corticosteroid replacement therapy is also needed.

Ketoconazole below may have a direct effect on corticotropic tumour cells in patients with Cushing's disease. It is used under specialist supervision for treatment of endogenous Cushing's syndrome.

Drugs used for Cushing's syndrome and disease not listed below; Pasireotide, p. 836

ENZYME INHIBITORS

Ketoconazole

- **DRUG ACTION** An imidazole derivative which acts as a potent inhibitor of cortisol and aldosterone synthesis by inhibiting the activity of 17α-hydroxylase, 11-hydroxylation steps and at higher doses the cholesterol side-chain cleavage enzyme. It also inhibits the activity of adrenal C17-20 lyase enzymes resulting in androgen synthesis inhibition, and may have a direct effect on corticotropic tumour cells in patients with Cushing's disease.

- **INDICATIONS AND DOSE**
Endogenous Cushing's syndrome (specialist use only)
  ‣ BY MOUTH
  ‣ Adult: Initially 400–600 mg daily in 2–3 divided doses, increased to 800–1200 mg daily; maintenance 400–800 mg daily in 2–3 divided doses, for dose titrations in patients with established dose, adjustments in adrenal insufficiency, or concomitant corticosteroid replacement therapy, consult product literature; maximum 1200 mg per day

IMPORTANT SAFETY INFORMATION
CHMP ADVICE: KETOCONAZOLE (JULY 2013)
The CHMP has recommended that the marketing authorisation for oral ketoconazole to treat fungal infections should be suspended. The CHMP concluded that the risk of hepatotoxicity associated with oral ketoconazole is greater than the benefit in treating fungal infections. Doctors should review patients who are being treated with oral ketoconazole for fungal infections, with a view to stopping treatment or choosing an alternative treatment. Patients with a prescription of oral ketoconazole for fungal infections should be referred back to their doctors.

Oral ketoconazole for Cushing's syndrome and topical products containing ketoconazole are not affected by this advice.

- **CONTRA-INDICATIONS** Acquired QTc prolongation · avoid concomitant use of hepatotoxic drugs · congenital QTc prolongation
- **CAUTIONS** Risk of adrenal insufficiency
- **INTERACTIONS** → Appendix 1 (antifungals, imidazole).
- **SIDE-EFFECTS**
  ‣ **Common or very common** Abdominal pain · adrenal insufficiency · diarrhoea · hepatic enzymes increased · nausea · pruritus · rash · vomiting
  ‣ **Uncommon** Alopecia · dizziness · headache · malaise · somnolence · thrombocytopenia · urticaria
  ‣ **Rare** Hepatic failure · hepatitis · jaundice · liver damage
  ‣ **Very rare** Pyrexia
  ‣ **Frequency not known** Alcohol intolerance · anorexia · arthralgia · azoospermia · dermatitis · dry mouth · dysgeusia · dyspepsia · epistaxis · erectile dysfunction · erythema · flatulence · gynaecomastia · hot flush · increased appetite · insomnia · menstrual disorder · myalgia · nervousness · paraesthesia · peripheral oedema · photophobia · photosensitivity · raised intracranial pressure · reduced testosterone concentrations · tongue discoloration · xeroderma
  SIDE-EFFECTS, FURTHER INFORMATION
  ‣ Hepatotoxicity Potentially life-threatening hepatotoxicity reported rarely.
- **CONCEPTION AND CONTRACEPTION** Effective contraception must be used in women of child-bearing potential.

- PREGNANCY Manufacturer advises avoid—teratogenic in *animal* studies.
- BREAST FEEDING Manufacturer advises avoid—present in breast milk.
- HEPATIC IMPAIRMENT Avoid in acute or chronic impairment. Do not initiate treatment if liver enzymes greater than 2 times the normal upper limit.
- MONITORING REQUIREMENTS
- ► Monitor ECG before and one week after initiation, and then as clinically indicated thereafter.
- ► Adrenal insufficiency Monitor adrenal function within one week of initiation, then regularly thereafter. When cortisol levels are normalised or close to target and effective dose established, monitor every 3–6 months as there is a risk of autoimmune disease development or exacerbation after normalisation of cortisol levels. If symptoms suggestive of adrenal insufficiency such as fatigue, anorexia, nausea, vomiting, hypotension, hyponatraemia, hyperkalaemia, and/or hypoglycaemia occur, measure cortisol levels and discontinue treatment temporarily (can be resumed thereafter at lower dose) or reduce dose and if necessary, initiate corticosteroid substitution.
- ► Hepatotoxicity Monitor liver function before initiation of treatment, then weekly for 1 month after initiation, then monthly for 6 months—more frequently if dose adjusted or abnormal liver function detected. Reduce dose if liver enzymes increase less than 3 times the normal upper limit—consult product literature; if liver enzymes are raised to 3 times or greater the normal upper limit, discontinue treatment permanently.
- PATIENT AND CARER ADVICE
Patients or their carers should be told how to recognise signs of liver disorder, and advised to discontinue treatment and seek prompt medical attention if symptoms such as anorexia, nausea, vomiting, fatigue, jaundice, abdominal pain, or dark urine develop. Patients or their carers should also be told how to recognise signs of adrenal insufficiency.
Driving and skilled tasks
Dizziness and somnolence may affect the performance of skilled tasks (e.g. driving).
- MEDICINAL FORMS
There can be variation in the licensing of different medicines containing the same drug. Forms available from special-order manufacturers include: oral suspension
Tablet
CAUTIONARY AND ADVISORY LABELS 2, 5, 21
- ► Ketoconazole (Non-proprietary) ▼
  Ketoconazole 200 mg Ketoconazole 200mg tablets | 60 tablet PoM £480.00

Metyrapone

- DRUG ACTION Metyrapone is a competitive inhibitor of 11β-hydroxylation in the adrenal cortex; the resulting inhibition of cortisol (and to a lesser extent aldosterone) production leads to an increase in ACTH production which, in turn, leads to increased synthesis and release of cortisol precursors. Metyrapone may be used as a test of anterior pituitary function.

- INDICATIONS AND DOSE
Differential diagnosis of ACTH-dependent Cushing's syndrome (specialist supervision in hospital)
- ► BY MOUTH
- ► Adult: 750 mg every 4 hours for 6 doses

Management of Cushing's syndrome (specialist supervision in hospital)
- ► BY MOUTH
- ► Adult: Usual dose 0.25–6 g daily, dose to be tailored to cortisol production, dose is either low, and tailored to cortisol production, or high, in which case corticosteroid replacement therapy is also needed

Resistant oedema due to increased aldosterone secretion in cirrhosis, nephrotic syndrome, and congestive heart failure (with glucocorticoid replacement therapy) (specialist supervision in hospital)
- ► BY MOUTH
- ► Adult: 3 g daily in divided doses

- CONTRA-INDICATIONS Adrenocortical insufficiency
- CAUTIONS Avoid in Acute porphyrias p. 918 · gross hypopituitarism (risk of precipitating acute adrenal failure) · hypertension on long-term administration · hypothyroidism (delayed response)
- INTERACTIONS Many drugs interfere with diagnostic estimation of steroids.
- SIDE-EFFECTS
- ► **Rare** Abdominal pain · allergic skin reactions · hirsutism · hypoadrenalism
- ► **Frequency not known** Dizziness · headache · hypotension · nausea · sedation · vomiting
- PREGNANCY Avoid (may impair biosynthesis of fetal-placental steroids).
- BREAST FEEDING Avoid—no information available.
- HEPATIC IMPAIRMENT Use with caution in hepatic impairment (delayed response).
- PATIENT AND CARER ADVICE
Driving and skilled tasks
Drowsiness may affect the performance of skilled tasks (e.g. driving).
- MEDICINAL FORMS
There can be variation in the licensing of different medicines containing the same drug.
Capsule
CAUTIONARY AND ADVISORY LABELS 21
- ► Metopirone (HRA Pharma UK Ltd)
  Metyrapone 250 mg Metopirone 250mg capsules | 100 capsule PoM £363.66

3 Diabetes mellitus and hypoglycaemia

3.1 Diabetes mellitus

Diabetes

Overview

Diabetes mellitus occurs because of a lack of insulin or resistance to its action. It is diagnosed by measuring fasting or random blood-glucose concentration (and occasionally by oral glucose tolerance test). Although there are many subtypes, the two principal classes of diabetes are type 1 diabetes and type 2 diabetes.

Type 1 diabetes, (formerly referred to as insulin-dependent diabetes mellitus (IDDM)), occurs as a result of a deficiency of insulin following autoimmune destruction of pancreatic beta cells. Patients with type 1 diabetes require administration of insulin.

Type 2 diabetes, (formerly referred to as non-insulin-dependent diabetes (NIDDM)), is due to reduced secretion of insulin or to peripheral resistance to the action of insulin or

Endocrine system

6

to a combination of both. Although patients may be controlled on diet alone, many also require oral antidiabetic drugs or insulin (or both) to maintain satisfactory control. In overweight individuals, type 2 diabetes may be prevented by losing weight and increasing physical activity; use of the anti-obesity drug orlistat p. 82 may be considered in obese patients.

Treatment of diabetes

Treatment of all forms of diabetes should be aimed at alleviating symptoms and minimising the risk of long-term complications; tight control of diabetes is essential.

Diabetes is a strong risk factor for cardiovascular disease. Other risk factors for cardiovascular disease such as smoking, hypertension, obesity, and hyperlipidaemia should be addressed. Cardiovascular risk in patients with diabetes can be further reduced by the use of an ACE inhibitor, low-dose aspirin p. 109 and a lipid-regulating drug.

Prevention of diabetic complications

Optimal glycaemic control in both type 1 diabetes and type 2 diabetes reduces, in the long term, the risk of microvascular complications including retinopathy, development of proteinuria and to some extent neuropathy. However, a temporary deterioration in established diabetic retinopathy may occur when normalising blood-glucose concentration. (ACE inhibitors and angiotensin-II receptor antagonists may also have a role in the management of diabetic nephropathy).

A measure of the total glycosylated (or glycated) haemoglobin (HbA_1) or a specific fraction (HbA_{1c}) provides a good indication of glycaemic control over the previous 2–3 months. Overall it is ideal to aim for an HbA_{1c} (glycosylated haemoglobin) concentration of 48–59 mmol/mol or less (reference range 20–42 mmol/mol) but this cannot always be achieved and for those using insulin there is a significantly increased risk of disabling hypoglycaemia; in those at risk of arterial disease, the aim should be to maintain the HbA_{1c} concentration at 48 mmol/mol or less. HbA_{1c} should be measured every 3–6 months.

Measurement of HbA_{1c}

HbA_{1c} values are expressed in *mmol of glycosylated haemoglobin per mol of haemoglobin (mmol/mol)*, a standardised unit specific for HbA_{1c} created by the International Federation of Clinical Chemistry and Laboratory Medicine (IFCC). HbA_{1c} values were previously aligned to the assay used in the Diabetes Control and Complications Trial (DCCT) and expressed as a percentage.

Equivalent values	
IFCC-HbA$_{1c}$ (mmol/mol)	DCCT-HbA$_{1c}$(%)
42	6.0
48	6.5
53	7.0
59	7.5
64	8.0
75	9.0

Laboratory measurement of serum-fructosamine concentration is technically simpler and cheaper than the measurement of HbA_{1c} and can be used to assess control over short periods of time, particularly when HbA_{1c} monitoring is invalid (e.g. disturbed erythrocyte turnover or abnormal haemoglobin type).

Tight control of blood pressure in hypertensive patients with type 2 diabetes reduces mortality and protects visual acuity (by reducing considerably the risks of maculopathy and retinal photocoagulation).

Driving

Drivers with diabetes may be required to notify the Driver and Vehicle Licensing Agency (DVLA) of their condition depending on their treatment, the type of licence, and whether they have diabetic complications. Detailed guidance on eligibility to drive, and precautions required, is available from the DVLA (www.gov.uk/government/publications/at-a-glance).

Drivers need to be particularly careful to avoid hypoglycaemia and should be warned of the problems. Drivers treated with insulin should normally check their blood-glucose concentration before driving and, on long journeys, at 2-hour intervals as specified by DVLA guidance; depending on the type of licence, monitoring may also be necessary for drivers taking oral antidiabetic drugs which carry a risk of hypoglycaemia (e.g. sulfonylureas, nateglinide p. 632, repaglinide p. 633). Drivers treated with insulin should ensure that a supply of sugar is always available in the vehicle and they should avoid driving if their meal is delayed. If hypoglycaemia occurs, or warning signs develop, the driver should:

- stop the vehicle in a safe place;
- switch off the ignition and move from the driver's seat;
- eat or drink a suitable source of sugar;
- wait until 45 minutes after blood glucose has returned to normal, before continuing journey.

Diabetic nephropathy

Regular review of diabetic patients should include an annual test for urinary protein (using *Albustix*®) and serum creatinine measurement. If the urinary protein test is negative, the urine should be test for microalbuminuria (the earliest sign of nephropathy). If reagent strip tests (*Micral-Test II*® or *Microbumintest*®) are used and prove positive, the result should be confirmed by laboratory analysis of a urine sample. Provided there are no contra-indications, all diabetic patients with nephropathy causing proteinurea or with established microalbuminuria (at least 3 positive tests) should be treated with an ACE inhibitor or an angiotensin-II receptor antagonist even if the blood pressure is normal; in any case, to minimise the risk of renal deterioration, blood pressure should be carefully controlled. Patients with diabetic nephropathy are particularly susceptible to developing hyperkalaemia and should not be given an ACE inhibitor together with an angiotensin-II receptor antagonist.

ACE inhibitors can potentiate the hypoglycaemic effect of insulin and oral antidiabetic drugs; this effect is more likely during the first weeks of combined treatment and in patients with renal impairment.

See also treatment of hypertension in diabetes.

Diabetic neuropathy

Optimal diabetic control is beneficial for the management of *painful neuropathy* in patients with type 1 diabetes. Paracetamol p. 406 or a non-steroidal anti-inflammatory drug such as ibuprofen p. 987 may relieve *mild to moderate pain*.

Duloxetine p. 336 is effective for the treatment of painful diabetic neuropathy; amitriptyline hydrochloride p. 341 [unlicensed use] can be used if duloxetine is ineffective or unsuitable. Nortriptyline p. 347 [unlicensed use] may be better tolerated than amitriptyline hydrochloride p. 341. If treatment with amitriptyline hydrochloride or duloxetine p. 336 is inadequate, treatment with pregabalin p. 295 should be tried. Combination therapy of duloxetine or amitriptyline hydrochloride with pregabalin can be used if monotherapy at the maximum tolerated dose does not control symptoms.

Neuropathic pain may respond to opioid analgesics. There is evidence of efficacy for tramadol hydrochloride p. 427, morphine p. 421, and oxycodone hydrochloride p. 424;

however treatment with morphine or oxycodone hydrochloride should be initiated only under specialist supervision. Tramadol hydrochloride can be prescribed while the patient is waiting for assessment by a specialist if other treatments have been unsuccessful.

Gabapentin p. 287 and carbamazepine p. 283 are sometimes used for the treatment of neuropathic pain. Capsaicin cream 0.075% p. 438 is licensed for painful diabetic neuropathy and may have some effect, but it produces an intense burning sensation during the initial treatment period.

In *autonomic neuropathy* diabetic diarrhoea can often be managed by **tetracyline** [unlicensed use], otherwise codeine phosphate p. 413 is the best drug, but other antidiarrhoeal preparations can be tried. Erythromycin p. 488 (especially when given intravenously) may be beneficial for gastroparesis [unlicensed use] but this needs confirmation.

In *neuropathic postural hypotension* increased salt intake and the use of the mineralcorticoid fludrocortisone acetate p. 612 [unlicensed use] may help by increasing plasma volume, but uncomfortable oedema is a common side-effect. Fludrocortisone can also be combined with flurbiprofen p. 986 and ephedrine hydrochloride p. 248 [both unlicensed]. Midodrine [unlicensed], an alpha agonist, may also be useful in postural hypotension.

Gustatory sweating can be treated with an antimuscarinic such as propantheline bromide p. 78; side-effects are common. See the management of hyperhidrosis (Antiperspirants p. 1106).

In some patients with *neuropathic oedema*, ephedrine hydrochloride [unlicensed use] offers effective relief.

See also the management of erectile dysfunction.

Diabetic ketoacidosis

Management

The management of diabetic ketoacidosis involves the replacement of fluid and electrolytes and the administration of insulin. Guidelines for the Management of Diabetic Ketoacidosis in Adults, published by the Joint British Diabetes Societies Inpatient Care Group (available at www.diabetes.org.uk/About_us/What-we-say/Specialist-care-for-children-and-adults-and-complications/The-Management-of-Diabetic-Ketoacidosis-in-Adults), should be followed.

- To restore circulating volume if systolic blood pressure is below 90 mmHg (adjusted for age, sex, and medication as appropriate), give 500 mL **sodium chloride 0.9%** by intravenous infusion over 10–15 minutes; repeat if blood pressure remains below 90 mmHg and seek senior medical advice.
- When blood pressure is over 90 mmHg, **sodium chloride 0.9%** should be given by intravenous infusion at a rate that replaces deficit and provides maintenance; see guideline or suggested regimen.
- Include **potassium chloride** in the fluids unless anuria is suspected; adjust according to plasma-potassium concentration (measure at 60 minutes, 2 hours, and 2 hourly thereafter; measure hourly if outside the normal range).
- Start an intravenous insulin infusion: **soluble insulin** should be diluted (and **mixed thoroughly**) with **sodium chloride 0.9%** intravenous infusion to a concentration of 1 unit/mL; infuse at a fixed rate of 0.1 units/kg/hour.
- Established subcutaneous therapy with long-acting insulin analogues (insulin detemir p. 643 or insulin glargine p. 643) should be continued during treatment of diabetic ketoacidosis.
- Monitor blood-ketone and blood-glucose concentrations hourly and adjust the insulin infusion rate accordingly. Blood-ketone concentration should fall by at least

0.5 mmol/litre/hour and blood-glucose concentration should fall by at least 3 mmol/litre/hour.
- Once blood-glucose concentration falls below 14 mmol/litre, **glucose 10%** should be given by intravenous infusion (into a large vein through a large-gauge needle) at a rate of 125 mL/hour, in addition to the **sodium chloride 0.9% infusion**.
- Continue insulin infusion until blood-ketone concentration is below 0.3 mmol/litre, blood pH is above 7.3 *and* the patient is able to eat and drink; ideally give subcutaneous fast-acting insulin and a meal, and stop the insulin infusion 1 hour later.

The management of hyperosmolar hyperglycaemic state or hyperosmolar hyperglycaemic nonketotic coma is similar to that of diabetic ketoacidosis, although lower rates of insulin infusion are usually necessary and slower rehydration may be required.

Insulins and anti-diabetic drugs

Insulins

Insulin plays a key role in the regulation of carbohydrate, fat, and protein metabolism. It is a polypeptide hormone of complex structure. There are differences in the amino-acid sequence of animal insulins, human insulins and the human insulin analogues. Insulin may be extracted from pork pancreas and purified by crystallisation; it may also be extracted from beef pancreas, but beef insulins are now rarely used. Human sequence insulin may be produced semisynthetically by enzymatic modification of porcine insulin (emp) or biosynthetically by recombinant DNA technology using bacteria (crb, prb) or yeast (pyr).

All insulin preparations are to a greater or lesser extent immunogenic in man but immunological resistance to insulin action is uncommon. Preparations of human sequence insulin should theoretically be less immunogenic, but no real advantage has been shown in trials.

Insulin is inactivated by gastro-intestinal enzymes, and must therefore be given by injection; the subcutaneous route is ideal in most circumstances. Insulin is usually injected into the upper arms, thighs, buttocks, or abdomen; absorption from a limb site may be increased if the limb is used in strenuous exercise after the injection. Generally subcutaneous insulin injections cause few problems; lipodystrophy may occur but can be minimised by using different injection sites in rotation. Local allergic reactions are rare.

Insulin is needed by all patients with ketoacidosis, and it is likely to be needed by most patients with:

- rapid onset of symptoms;
- substantial loss of weight;
- weakness;
- ketonuria;
- a first-degree relative who has type 1 diabetes.

Insulin is also needed for type 2 diabetes when other methods have failed to achieve good control, and temporarily in the presence of intercurrent illness or peri-operatively. Pregnant women with type 2 diabetes may be treated with insulin when diet alone fails. Antidiabetic drugs have a role in the management of diabetes in pregnancy.

Safe and Effective Use of Insulin in Hospitalised Patients (March 2010)

NHS diabetes guidance available at www.diabetes.nhs.uk.

Management of diabetes with insulin

The aim of treatment is to achieve the best possible control of blood-glucose concentration without making the patient obsessional and to avoid disabling hypoglycaemia; close co-operation is needed between the patient and the medical team because good control reduces the risk of complications.

6

Endocrine system

Insulin preparations can be divided into 3 types:

- those of **short** duration which have a relatively rapid onset of action, namely soluble insulin and the rapid-acting insulin analogues, insulin glulisine p. 645, insulin aspart p. 645, and insulin lispro p. 646;
- those with an **intermediate** action, e.g. isophane insulin p. 641; and
- those whose action is slower in onset and lasts for **long** periods, e.g. protamine zinc insulin p. 644, insulin detemir p. 643, and insulin glargine p. 643.

The duration of action of a particular type of insulin varies considerably from one patient to another, and needs to be assessed individually.

Mixtures of insulin preparations may be required and appropriate combinations have to be determined for the individual patient. Treatment should be started with a short-acting insulin (e.g. soluble insulin) or a rapid-acting insulin analogue (e.g. insulin aspart) given before meals with intermediate-acting or long-acting insulin once or twice daily. Alternatively, for those who have difficulty with, or prefer not to use, multiple injection regimens, a mixture of premixed short-acting insulin or rapid-acting insulin analogue with an intermediate-acting or long-acting insulin (most commonly in a proportion of 30% soluble insulin and 70% isophane insulin) can be given once or twice daily. The dose of short-acting or rapid-acting insulin (or the proportion of the short-acting soluble insulin component in premixed insulin) can be increased in those with excessive postprandial hyperglycaemia. The dose of insulin is increased gradually according to the patient's individual requirements, taking care to avoid troublesome hypoglycaemic reactions.

Insulin requirements may be increased by infection, stress, accidental or surgical trauma, and during puberty. Requirements may be decreased in those with certain endocrine disorders (e.g. Addison's disease, hypopituitarism), or in coeliac disease.

Examples of recommended insulin regimens

- Multiple injection regimen: short-acting insulin or rapid-acting insulin analogue, before meals. With intermediate-acting or long-acting insulin, once or twice daily;
- Short-acting insulin or rapid-acting insulin analogue mixed with intermediate-acting or long-acting insulin, once or twice daily (before meals);
- Intermediate-acting or long-acting insulin, once or twice daily. With or without short-acting insulin or rapid-acting insulin before meals;
- Continuous subcutaneous insulin infusion.

Hypoglycaemia

Loss of warning of hypoglycaemia among insulin-treated patients can be a serious hazard, especially for drivers and those in dangerous occupations. Very tight control of diabetes lowers the blood-glucose concentration needed to trigger hypoglycaemic symptoms; an increase in the frequency of hypoglycaemic episodes may reduce the warning symptoms experienced by the patient. Beta-blockers can also blunt hypoglycaemic awareness (and also delay recovery).

To restore the warning signs, episodes of hypoglycaemia must be minimised; this involves appropriate adjustment of insulin type, dose and frequency together with suitable timing and quantity of meals and snacks.

Some patients have reported loss of hypoglycaemia warning after transfer to human insulin. Clinical studies do not confirm that human insulin decreases hypoglycaemia awareness. If a patient believes that human insulin is responsible for the loss of warning it is reasonable to revert to animal insulin and essential to educate the patient about avoiding hypoglycaemia. Great care should be taken to specify whether a human or an animal preparation is required.

Few patients are now treated with beef insulins; when undertaking conversion from beef to human insulin, the total dose should be reduced by about 10% with careful monitoring for the first few days. When changing between pork and human-sequence insulins, a dose change is not usually needed, but careful monitoring is still advised.

Diabetes and surgery

Perioperative control of blood-glucose concentrations in patients with type 1 diabetes is achieved via an adjustable, continuous, intravenous infusion of insulin. Detailed local protocols should be available to all healthcare professionals involved in the treatment of these patients; in general, the following steps should be followed:

- give an injection of the patient's usual insulin on the night before the operation;
- early on the day of the operation, start an intravenous infusion of glucose containing potassium chloride (provided that the patient is not hyperkalaemic) and infuse at a constant rate appropriate to the patient's fluid requirements (usually 125 mL per hour); make up a solution of soluble insulin in sodium chloride 0.9% and infuse intravenously using a syringe pump piggy-backed to the intravenous infusion. Glucose and potassium infusions, and insulin infusions should be made up according to locally agreed protocols;
- the rate of the insulin infusion should be adjusted according to blood-glucose concentration (frequent monitoring necessary) in line with locally agreed protocols. Other factors affecting the rate of infusion include the patient's volume depletion, cardiac function, and age.

Protocols should include specific instructions on how to manage resistant cases (such as patients who are in shock or severely ill or those receiving corticosteroids or sympathomimetics) and those with hypoglycaemia.

If a syringe pump is not available, soluble insulin should be added to the intravenous infusion of glucose p. 903 and potassium chloride p. 917 (provided the patient is not hyperkalaemic), and the infusion run at the rate appropriate to the patient's fluid requirements (usually 125 mL per hour) with the insulin dose adjusted according to blood-glucose concentration in line with locally agreed protocols.

Once the patient starts to eat and drink, give subcutaneous insulin before breakfast and stop intravenous insulin 30 minutes later; the dose may need to be 10–20% more than usual if the patient is still in bed or unwell. If the patient was not previously receiving insulin, an appropriate initial dose is 30–40 units daily in four divided doses using soluble insulin before meals and intermediate-acting insulin at bedtime and the dose adjusted from day to day. Patients with hyperglycaemia often relapse after conversion back to subcutaneous insulin calling for one of the following approaches:

- additional doses of soluble insulin at any of the four injection times (before meals or bedtime) or
- temporary addition of intravenous insulin infusion (while continuing the subcutaneous regimen) until blood-glucose concentration is satisfactory or
- complete reversion to the intravenous regimen (especially if the patient is unwell).

Short-acting insulins

Soluble insulin is a short-acting form of insulin. For maintenance regimens it is usual to inject it 15 to 30 minutes before meals.

Soluble insulin is the most appropriate form of insulin for use in diabetic emergencies e.g. diabetic ketoacidosis (see Diabetic ketoacidosis p. 619) and at the time of surgery. It can be given intravenously and intramuscularly, as well as subcutaneously.

When injected subcutaneously, soluble insulin has a rapid onset of action (30 to 60 minutes), a peak action between 2 and 4 hours, and a duration of action of up to 8 hours.

When injected intravenously, soluble insulin has a very short half-life of only about 5 minutes and its effect disappears within 30 minutes.

The rapid-acting human insulin analogues, insulin aspart p. 645, insulin glulisine p. 645, and insulin lispro p. 646 have a faster onset and shorter duration of action than soluble insulin; as a result, compared to soluble insulin, fasting and preprandial blood-glucose concentrations are a little higher, postprandial blood-glucose concentration is a little lower, and hypoglycaemia occurs slightly less frequently. Subcutaneous injection of insulin analogues may be convenient for those who wish to inject shortly before or, when necessary, shortly after a meal. They can also help those susceptible to hypoglycaemia before lunch and those who eat late in the evening and are prone to nocturnal hypoglycaemia. They can also be administered by subcutaneous infusion. Insulin aspart and insulin lispro can be administered intravenously and can be used as alternatives to soluble insulin for diabetic emergencies and at the time of surgery.

Intermediate- and long-acting insulins

When given by subcutaneous injection, intermediate- and long-acting insulins have an onset of action of approximately 1–2 hours, a maximal effect at 4–12 hours, and a duration of 16–42 hours. Some are given twice daily in conjunction with short-acting (soluble) insulin, and others are given once daily, particularly in elderly patients. Soluble insulin can be mixed with intermediate and long-acting insulins (except insulin detemir p. 643, insulin glargine p. 643, and insulin degludec p. 642) in the syringe, essentially retaining the properties of the two components, although there may be some blunting of the initial effect of the soluble insulin component (especially on mixing with protamine zinc insulin p. 644).

Isophane insulin p. 641 is a suspension of insulin with protamine; it is of particular value for initiation of twice-daily insulin regimens. Patients usually mix isophane with soluble insulin but ready-mixed preparations may be appropriate (biphasic isophane insulin p. 641, biphasic insulin aspart p. 642, or biphasic insulin lispro p. 642).

Insulin zinc suspension p. 643 (30% amorphous, 70% crystalline) has a more prolonged duration of action.

Protamine zinc insulin is usually given once daily with short-acting (soluble) insulin. It has the drawback of binding with the soluble insulin when mixed in the same syringe and is now rarely used.

Insulin glargine and insulin detemir are both long-acting human insulin analogues with a prolonged duration of action; insulin glargine is given once daily and insulin detemir is given once or twice daily. NICE (December 2002) has recommended that insulin glargine should be available as an option for patients with type 1 diabetes.

NICE (May 2009) has recommended that, if insulin is required in patients with type 2 diabetes, insulin detemir or insulin glargine may be considered for those:

- who require assistance with injecting insulin *or*
- whose lifestyle is significantly restricted by recurrent symptomatic hypoglycaemia *or*
- who would otherwise need twice-daily basal insulin injections in combination with oral antidiabetic drugs *or*
- who cannot use the device needed to inject isophane insulin.

Insulin detemir is also licensed as add-on therapy in patients receiving treatment with liraglutide p. 631.

Insulin degludec is a long-acting human insulin analogue for once daily subcutaneous administration.

Hypodermic equipment

Patients should be advised on the safe disposal of lancets, single-use syringes, and needles. Suitable arrangements for the safe disposal of contaminated waste must be made before these products are prescribed for patients who are carriers of infectious diseases.

Lancets, **needles**, **syringes**, and **accessories** are listed under Hypodermic Equipment in Part IXA of the Drug Tariff (Part III of the Northern Ireland Drug Tariff, Part 3 of the Scottish Drug Tariff). The drug Tariffs can be access online at:

- National Health Service Drug Tariff for England and Wales: www.ppa.org.uk/ppa/edt_intro.htm
- Health and Personal Social Services for Northern Ireland Drug Tariff: www.dhsspsni.gov.uk/pas-tariff
- Scottish Drug Tariff: www.isdscotland.org/Health-Topics/Prescribing-and-Medicines/Scottish-Drug-Tariff/

Antidiabetic drugs

Oral antidiabetic drugs are used for the treatment of type 2 diabetes mellitus. They should be prescribed only if the patient fails to respond adequately to at least 3 months' restriction of energy and carbohydrate intake and an increase in physical activity. They should be used to augment the effect of diet and exercise, and not to replace them.

For patients not adequately controlled by diet and oral hypoglycaemic drugs, insulin may be added to the treatment regimen or substituted for oral therapy. When insulin is added to oral therapy, it is generally given at bedtime as isophane or long-acting insulin, and when insulin replaces an oral regimen it may be given as twice-daily injections of a biphasic insulin (or isophane insulin p. 641 mixed with soluble insulin), or a multiple injection regimen. Weight gain and hypoglycaemia may be complications of insulin therapy but weight gain may be reduced if the insulin is given in combination with metformin hydrochloride p. 624.

Pregnancy and breast-feeding

During pregnancy, women with *pre-existing diabetes* can be treated with metformin hydrochloride [unlicensed use], either alone or in combination with insulin. Metformin hydrochloride can be continued, or glibenclamide p. 637 resumed, during breast-feeding for those with pre-existing diabetes. Women with *gestational diabetes* may be treated, with or without concomitant insulin, with glibenclamide from 11 weeks gestation (after organogenesis) [unlicensed use] or with metformin [unlicensed use]. Women with gestational diabetes should discontinue hypoglycaemic treatment after giving birth.

Sulfonylureas

The sulfonylureas act mainly by augmenting insulin secretion and consequently are effective only when some residual pancreatic beta-cell activity is present; during long-term administration they also have an extrapancreatic action. All may cause hypoglycaemia but this is uncommon and usually indicates excessive dosage. Sulfonylurea-induced hypoglycaemia may persist for many hours and must always be treated in hospital.

Sulfonylureas are considered for patients who are not overweight, or in whom metformin hydrochloride is contra-indicated or not tolerated. Several sulfonylureas are available and choice is determined by side-effects and the duration of action as well as the patient's age and renal function. Glibenclamide, a long-acting sulfonylurea, is associated with a greater risk of hypoglycaemia; for this reason it should be avoided in the elderly, and shorter-acting alternatives, such as gliclazide p. 637 or tolbutamide p. 639, should be used instead.

When the combination of strict diet and sulfonylurea treatment fails, other options include:

- combining with metformin;
- combining with pioglitazone;
- combining with alogliptin, linagliptin, saxagliptin, sitagliptin, or vildagliptin;
- combining with canagliflozin, dapagliflozin or empagliflozin;
- combining with exenatide, liraglutide, or lixisenatide;
- combining with acarbose, which may have a small beneficial effect, but flatulence can be a problem;
- combining with bedtime isophane insulin but weight gain and hypoglycaemia can occur.

Insulin therapy should be instituted temporarily during intercurrent illness (such as myocardial infarction, coma, infection, and trauma). Sulfonylureas should be omitted on the morning of surgery; insulin is required because of the ensuing hyperglycaemia in these circumstances.

Biguanides

Metformin hydrochloride, the only available biguanide, has a different mode of action from the sulfonylureas, and is not interchangeable with them.

Metformin hydrochloride is the drug of first choice in overweight patients in whom strict dieting has failed to control diabetes, if appropriate it may also be considered as an option in patients who are not overweight. It is also used when diabetes is inadequately controlled with sulfonylurea treatment. When the combination of strict diet and metformin hydrochloride treatment fails, other options include:

- combining with a sulfonylurea;
- combining with pioglitazone p. 639;
- combining with repaglinide p. 633 or nateglinide p. 632;
- combining with alogliptin p. 625, linagliptin p. 626, saxagliptin p. 626, sitagliptin p. 627, or vildagliptin p. 628;
- combining with canagliflozin p. 633, dapagliflozin p. 634 or empagliflozin p. 636;
- combining with exenatide p. 630, liraglutide p. 631, or lixisenatide p. 632;
- combining with acarbose p. 623, which may have a small beneficial effect, but flatulence can be a problem;
- combining with insulin but weight gain and hypoglycaemia can be problems (weight gain minimised if insulin given at night).

Insulin treatment is almost always required in medical and surgical emergencies; insulin should also be substituted before elective surgery (omit metformin hydrochloride on the morning of surgery and give insulin if required).

Hypoglycaemia does not usually occur with metformin hydrochloride; other advantages are the lower incidence of weight gain and lower plasma-insulin concentration. It does not exert a hypoglycaemic action in non-diabetic subjects unless given in overdose.

Metformin hydrochloride is used for the symptomatic management of polycystic ovary syndrome [unlicensed indication]; however, treatment should be initiated by a specialist. Metformin hydrochloride improves insulin sensitivity, may aid weight reduction, helps to normalise menstrual cycle (increasing the rate of spontaneous ovulation), and may improve hirsutism.

Other antidiabetic drugs

Use of acarbose is usually reserved for when other oral hypoglycaemics are not tolerated or are contra-indicated. Postprandial hyperglycaemia in type 1 diabetes can be reduced by acarbose, but it has been little used for this purpose. Flatulence deters some from using acarbose although this side-effect tends to decrease with time.

Nateglinide and repaglinide stimulate insulin secretion. Both drugs have a rapid onset of action and short duration of activity, and should be administered shortly before each main meal. Repaglinide may be given as monotherapy for

patients who are not overweight or for those in whom metformin hydrochloride is contra-indicated or not tolerated, or it may be given in combination with metformin hydrochloride. Nateglinide is licensed only for use with metformin hydrochloride.

Pioglitazone can be used alone or in combination with metformin hydrochloride or with a sulfonylurea (if metformin hydrochloride inappropriate), or with both; the combination of pioglitazone plus metformin hydrochloride is preferred to pioglitazone plus sulfonylurea, particularly for obese patients. Inadequate response to a combination of metformin hydrochloride and sulfonylurea may indicate failing insulin release; the introduction of pioglitazone has a limited role in these circumstances and the initiation of insulin is often more appropriate. Pioglitazone is also licensed in combination with insulin, in patients who have not achieved adequate glycaemic control with insulin alone, when metformin hydrochloride is inappropriate. Blood-glucose control may deteriorate temporarily when pioglitazone is substituted for an oral antidiabetic drug that is being used in combination with another. Long-term benefits of pioglitazone have not yet been demonstrated. NICE (May 2009) has recommended that, when glycaemic control is inadequate with existing treatment, pioglitazone can be added to:

- a sulfonylurea, if metformin hydrochloride is contra-indicated or not tolerated;
- metformin, if risks of hypoglycaemia with sulfonylurea are unacceptable or a sulfonylurea is contra-indicated or not tolerated;
- a combination of metformin hydrochloride and a sulfonylurea, if insulin is unacceptable because of lifestyle or other personal issues, or because the patient is obese.

NICE has recommended that treatment with pioglitazone is continued only if HbA1c concentration is reduced by at least 0.5 percentage points within 6 months of starting treatment.

Linagliptin is licensed for use in type 2 diabetes as monotherapy (if metformin hydrochloride inappropriate), or in combination with metformin hydrochloride (when treatment with metformin hydrochloride alone fails to achieve adequate glycaemic control), or both metformin hydrochloride and a sulfonylurea (when dual therapy with these drugs fails to achieve adequate glycaemic control). Linagliptin may also be used in combination with insulin (with or without metformin hydrochloride) when a stable dose of insulin has not provided adequate glycaemic control.

Saxagliptin and vildagliptin are licensed for use in type 2 diabetes as monotherapy (if metformin hydrochloride inappropriate), or in combination with metformin hydrochloride or a sulfonylurea (if metformin hydrochloride inappropriate), or pioglitazone p. 639 (when treatment with either metformin hydrochloride p. 624 or a sulfonylurea or pioglitazone fails to achieve adequate glycaemic control), and also in combination with both metformin hydrochloride and a sulfonylurea (when dual therapy with these drugs fails to achieve adequate glycaemic control). The combination of either saxagliptin p. 626 or vildagliptin p. 628, and insulin (with or without metformin hydrochloride) is also licensed for use when a stable dose of insulin has not provided adequate glycaemic control.

Alogliptin p. 625 is also licensed for use as triple therapy in combination with metformin hydrochloride and either pioglitazone or insulin.

NICE (May 2009) has recommended that, when glycaemic control is inadequate with existing treatment:

- sitagliptin or vildagliptin (instead of a sulfonylurea) can be added to metformin, if there is a significant risk of hypoglycaemia or if a sulfonylurea is contra-indicated or not tolerated;
- sitagliptin or vildagliptin can be added to a sulfonylurea, if metformin is contra-indicated or not tolerated;

- sitagliptin can be added to both metformin and a sulfonylurea, if insulin is unacceptable because of lifestyle or other personal issues, or because the patient is obese.

NICE has recommended that treatment with sitagliptin p. 627 or vildagliptin is continued only if HbA$_{1c}$ concentration is reduced by at least 0.5 percentage points within 6 months of starting treatment.

Treatment with exenatide p. 630, liraglutide p. 631, and lixisenatide p. 632 is associated with the prevention of weight gain and possible promotion of weight loss which can be beneficial in overweight patients. They are given by subcutaneous injection for the treatment of type 2 diabetes mellitus.

Exenatide is licensed in combination with metformin hydrochloride or a sulfonylurea, or both, or with pioglitazone, or with both metformin hydrochloride and pioglitazone, in patients who have not achieved adequate glycaemic control with these drugs alone or in combination; standard-release exenatide is also licensed in combination with basal insulin alone or with metformin hydrochloride or pioglitazone (or both).

NICE (May 2009) has recommended that, when glycaemic control is inadequate with metformin hydrochloride and sulfonylurea treatment, the addition of standard-release exenatide may be considered if the patient has:

- a body mass index of 35 kg/m^2 or over and is of European descent (with appropriate adjustment for other ethnic groups) and weight-related psychological or medical problems or
- a body mass index less than 35 kg/m^2, and insulin would be unacceptable for occupational reasons or weight loss would benefit other significant obesity-related comorbidities.

NICE has recommended that treatment with standard release exenatide is continued only if HbA$_{1c}$ concentration is reduced by at least 1 percentage point and a weight loss of at least 3% is achieved within 6 months of starting treatment.

Albiglutide p. 629 is licensed for the treatment of type 2 diabetes mellitus, either alone (if metformin hydrochloride inappropriate) or in combination with insulin or other antidiabetic drugs (if existing treatment fails to achieve adequate glycaemic control).

Dulaglutide p. 629 is licensed for the treatment of type 2 diabetes mellitus, alone (if metformin is inappropriate) or in combination with other antidiabetic drugs in patients who have not achieved adequate glycaemic control with these drugs.

Liraglutide is licensed for the treatment of type 2 diabetes mellitus in combination with metformin hydrochloride or a sulfonylurea, or both, in patients who have not achieved adequate glycaemic control with these drugs alone or in combination. Liraglutide is also licensed for use in combination with basal insulin or both metformin hydrochloride and pioglitazone when dual therapy with these drugs fails to achieve adequate glycaemic control.

Lixisenatide is licensed for the treatment of type 2 diabetes mellitus in combination with oral antidiabetic drugs (e.g. metformin hydrochloride, pioglitazone, or a sulfonylurea) or basal insulin, or both, when adequate glycaemic control has not been achieved with these drugs; lixisenatide should not be used in combination with both basal insulin and a sulfonylurea because of an increased risk of hypoglycaemia.

Canagliflozin p. 633 and dapagliflozin p. 634, and empagliflozin p. 636 are licensed for use in type 2 diabetes as monotherapy (if metformin hydrochloride inappropriate), or in combination with insulin or other antidiabetic drugs (if existing treatment fails to achieve adequate glycaemic control). Dapagliflozin is not recommended in combination with pioglitazone.

BLOOD GLUCOSE LOWERING DRUGS > ALPHA GLUCOSIDASE INHIBITORS

Acarbose

- **DRUG ACTION** Acarbose, an inhibitor of intestinal alpha glucosidases, delays the digestion and absorption of starch and sucrose; it has a small but significant effect in lowering blood glucose.

- **INDICATIONS AND DOSE**

Diabetes mellitus inadequately controlled by diet or by diet with oral antidiabetic drugs

▶ BY MOUTH

▶ Adult: Initially 50 mg daily, then increased to 50 mg 3 times a day for 6–8 weeks, then increased if necessary to 100 mg 3 times a day (max. per dose 200 mg 3 times a day)

- **CONTRA-INDICATIONS** Hernia · inflammatory bowel disease · predisposition to partial intestinal obstruction · previous abdominal surgery

- **CAUTIONS** May enhance hypoglycaemic effects of insulin and sulfonylureas (hypoglycaemic episodes may be treated with oral glucose but not with sucrose)

- **INTERACTIONS** → Appendix 1 (antidiabetics).

- **SIDE-EFFECTS**

▶ **Common or very common** Abdominal distention and pain · diarrhoea (may need to reduce dose or withdraw) · flatulence · soft stools

▶ **Rare** Abnormal liver function tests · nausea · skin reactions

▶ **Very rare** Hepatitis · ileus · jaundice · oedema

SIDE-EFFECTS, FURTHER INFORMATION

▶ Antacids Antacids unlikely to be beneficial for treating side effects.

- **PREGNANCY** Avoid.

- **BREAST FEEDING** Avoid.

- **HEPATIC IMPAIRMENT** Avoid.

- **RENAL IMPAIRMENT** Avoid if eGFR less than 25 mL/minute/1.73 m^2.

- **MONITORING REQUIREMENTS** Monitor liver function.

- **DIRECTIONS FOR ADMINISTRATION** Tablets should be chewed with first mouthful of food or swallowed whole with a little liquid immediately before food.

- **PATIENT AND CARER ADVICE** Antacids unlikely to be beneficial for treating side-effects. To counteract possible hypoglycaemia, patients receiving insulin or a sulfonylurea as well as acarbose need to carry glucose (not sucrose—acarbose interferes with sucrose absorption). Patients should be given advice on how to administer acarbose tablets.

- **MEDICINAL FORMS**
There can be variation in the licensing of different medicines containing the same drug.
Tablet
▶ Acarbose (Non-proprietary)
  Acarbose 50 mg Acarbose 50mg tablets | 90 tablet [PoM] £11.70 DT price = £11.36
  Acarbose 100 mg Acarbose 100mg tablets | 90 tablet [PoM] £19.30 DT price = £18.82
▶ Glucobay (Bayer Plc)
  Acarbose 50 mg Glucobay 50mg tablets | 90 tablet [PoM] £7.35 DT price = £11.36
  Acarbose 100 mg Glucobay 100mg tablets | 90 tablet [PoM] £13.50 DT price = £18.82

6

Endocrine system

BLOOD GLUCOSE LOWERING DRUGS >
BIGUANIDES

Metformin hydrochloride

- DRUG ACTION Metformin exerts its effect mainly by decreasing gluconeogenesis and by increasing peripheral utilisation of glucose; since it acts only in the presence of endogenous insulin it is effective only if there are some residual functioning pancreatic islet cells.

● **INDICATIONS AND DOSE**

Diabetes mellitus
▸ BY MOUTH USING IMMEDIATE-RELEASE MEDICINES
▸ Child 10–17 years (specialist use only): Initially 500 mg once daily, dose to be adjusted according to response at intervals of at least 1 week, maximum daily dose to be given in 2–3 divided doses; maximum 2 g per day
▸ Adult: Initially 500 mg once daily for at least 1 week, dose to be taken with breakfast, then 500 mg twice daily for at least 1 week, dose to be taken with breakfast and evening meal, then 500 mg 3 times a day, dose to be taken with breakfast, lunch and evening meal; maximum 2 g per day
▸ BY MOUTH USING MODIFIED-RELEASE MEDICINES
▸ Adult: Initially 500 mg once daily, then increased if necessary up to 2 g once daily, dose increased gradually, every 10–15 days, dose to be taken with evening meal, alternatively increased to 1 g twice daily, dose to be taken with meals, alternative dose only to be used if control not achieved with once daily dose regimen. If control still not achieved then change to standard release tablets

Polycystic ovary syndrome
▸ BY MOUTH USING IMMEDIATE-RELEASE MEDICINES
▸ Adult: Initially 500 mg once daily for 1 week, dose to be taken with breakfast, then 500 mg twice daily for 1 week, dose to be taken with breakfast and evening meal, then 1.5–1.7 g daily in 2–3 divided doses

● UNLICENSED USE
▸ In adults Doses in the BNF may differ from those in the product literature. Not licensed for polycystic ovary syndrome.
▸ In children Not licensed for use in children under 10 years.
● CONTRA-INDICATIONS Ketoacidosis · use of general anaesthesia (suspend metformin on the morning of surgery and restart when renal function returns to baseline)
  CONTRA-INDICATIONS, FURTHER INFORMATION
▸ Iodine-containing X-ray contrast media Intravascular administration of iodinated contrast agents can cause renal failure, which can increase the risk of lactic acidosis with metformin. Suspend metformin prior to the test; restart no earlier than 48 hours after the test if renal function has returned to baseline.
● CAUTIONS Can provoke lactic acidosis
● INTERACTIONS → Appendix 1 (antidiabetics).
● SIDE-EFFECTS
▸ Common or very common Abdominal pain · anorexia · diarrhoea (usually transient) · nausea · taste disturbance · vomiting
▸ Rare Decreased vitamin-B_{12} absorption · erythema · lactic acidosis (withdraw treatment) · pruritus · urticaria
▸ Frequency not known Hepatitis
  SIDE-EFFECTS, FURTHER INFORMATION
▸ Gastro-intestinal effects Gastro-intestinal side-effects are initially common with metformin, and may persist in some patients, particularly when very high doses are given. A slow increase in dose may improve tolerability.

● PREGNANCY Can be used in pregnancy for both pre-existing and gestational diabetes. Women with gestational diabetes should discontinue treatment after giving birth.
● BREAST FEEDING May be used during breast-feeding in women with pre-existing diabetes.
● HEPATIC IMPAIRMENT Withdraw if tissue hypoxia likely.
● RENAL IMPAIRMENT Use with caution in renal impairment— increased risk of lactic acidosis.
  Lactic acidosis Withdraw or interrupt treatment in those at risk of tissue hypoxia or sudden deterioration in renal function, such as those with dehydration, severe infection, shock, sepsis, acute heart failure, respiratory failure or hepatic impairment, or those who have recently had a myocardial infarction.
▸ In adults NICE (clinical guideline 87 (May 2009): Type 2 diabetes: The management of type 2 diabetes) recommends that the dose should be reviewed if eGFR less than 45 mL/minute/1.73 m^2 and to avoid if eGFR less than 30 mL/minute/1.73 m^2.
▸ In children Avoid in significant renal impairment.
● MONITORING REQUIREMENTS Determine renal function before treatment and at least annually (at least twice a year in patients with additional risk factors for renal impairment, or if deterioration suspected).
● PRESCRIBING AND DISPENSING INFORMATION
▸ In adults Patients taking up to 2 g daily of the standard-release metformin may start with the same daily dose of metformin modified release; not suitable if dose of standard-release tablets more than 2 g daily.
● PATIENT AND CARER ADVICE
  Medicines for Children leaflet: Metformin for diabetes www.medicinesforchildren.org.uk/metformin-diabetes
● NATIONAL FUNDING/ACCESS DECISIONS
  GLUCOPHAGE® SR
  Scottish Medicines Consortium (SMC) Decisions
  The *Scottish Medicines Consortium* has advised (September 2009) that *Glucophage® SR* is accepted for restricted use within NHS Scotland for the treatment of type 2 diabetes mellitus in adult patients who are intolerant of standard-release metformin, and in whom the prolonged-release tablet allows the use of a dose of metformin not previously tolerated, or in patients for whom a once daily preparation offers a clinically significant benefit.

● MEDICINAL FORMS
  There can be variation in the licensing of different medicines containing the same drug. Forms available from special-order manufacturers include: capsule, oral suspension, oral solution

Tablet
CAUTIONARY AND ADVISORY LABELS 21
▸ Metformin hydrochloride (Non-proprietary)
  Metformin hydrochloride 500 mg Metformin 500mg tablets | 28 tablet [PoM] £1.55 DT price = £0.86 | 84 tablet [PoM] £3.81 | 500 tablet [PoM] £16.96
  Metformin hydrochloride 850 mg Metformin 850mg tablets | 56 tablet [PoM] £2.48 DT price = £1.30 | 60 tablet [PoM] no price available | 300 tablet [PoM] £10.00
▸ Glucophage (Merck Serono Ltd)
  Metformin hydrochloride 500 mg Glucophage 500mg tablets | 84 tablet [PoM] £2.88
  Metformin hydrochloride 850 mg Glucophage 850mg tablets | 56 tablet [PoM] £3.20 DT price = £1.30

Modified-release tablet
CAUTIONARY AND ADVISORY LABELS 21, 25
▸ Metformin hydrochloride (Non-proprietary)
  Metformin hydrochloride 500 mg Metformin 500mg modified-release tablets | 28 tablet [PoM] £2.66 | 56 tablet [PoM] £5.32 DT price = £5.32
  Metformin hydrochloride 1 gram Metformin 1g modified-release tablets | 28 tablet [PoM] £4.79 | 56 tablet [PoM] £9.00 DT price = £8.52

‣ Bolamyn SR (Teva UK Ltd)
Metformin hydrochloride 500 mg Bolamyn SR 500mg tablets |
28 tablet PoM £3.20 | 56 tablet PoM £6.40 DT price = £5.32
Metformin hydrochloride 1 gram Bolamyn SR 1000mg tablets |
28 tablet PoM £5.06 | 56 tablet PoM £10.13 DT price = £8.52

‣ Diagemet XL (Genus Pharmaceuticals Ltd)
Metformin hydrochloride 500 mg Diagemet XL 500mg tablets |
28 tablet PoM £1.49 | 56 tablet PoM £2.97 DT price = £5.32

‣ Glucient SR (Consilient Health Ltd)
Metformin hydrochloride 500 mg Glucient SR 500mg tablets |
28 tablet PoM £2.51 | 56 tablet PoM £5.03 DT price = £5.32
Metformin hydrochloride 750 mg Glucient SR 750mg tablets |
28 tablet PoM £3.20
Metformin hydrochloride 1 gram Glucient SR 1000mg tablets |
28 tablet PoM £4.26 | 56 tablet PoM £8.52 DT price = £8.52

‣ Glucophage SR (Merck Serono Ltd)
Metformin hydrochloride 500 mg Glucophage SR 500mg tablets |
28 tablet PoM £2.66 | 56 tablet PoM £5.32 DT price = £5.32
Metformin hydrochloride 750 mg Glucophage SR 750mg tablets |
28 tablet PoM £3.20 | 56 tablet PoM £6.40 DT price = £6.40
Metformin hydrochloride 1 gram Glucophage SR 1000mg tablets |
28 tablet PoM £4.26 | 56 tablet PoM £8.52 DT price = £8.52

‣ Metabet SR (Morningside Healthcare Ltd)
Metformin hydrochloride 500 mg Metabet SR 500mg tablets |
28 tablet PoM £3.07 | 56 tablet PoM £6.14 DT price = £5.32
Metformin hydrochloride 1 gram Metabet SR 1000mg tablets |
28 tablet PoM £5.33 | 56 tablet PoM £10.66 DT price = £8.52

‣ Sukkarto SR (Morningside Healthcare Ltd)
Metformin hydrochloride 500 mg Sukkarto SR 500mg tablets |
56 tablet PoM £3.46 DT price = £5.32
Metformin hydrochloride 1 gram Sukkarto SR 1000mg tablets |
56 tablet PoM £5.54 DT price = £8.52

Oral solution
CAUTIONARY AND ADVISORY LABELS 21
▸ Metformin hydrochloride (Non-proprietary)
Metformin hydrochloride 100 mg per 1 ml Metformin 500mg/5ml
oral solution sugar free sugar-free | 100 ml PoM £15.00 sugar-free
| 150 ml PoM £60.00 DT price = £17.24

Powder
▸ Metformin hydrochloride (Non-proprietary)
Metformin hydrochloride 1 gram Metformin 1g oral powder sachets
sugar free sugar-free | 30 sachet PoM no price available

Combinations available: *Alogliptin with metformin,* below ·
Canagliflozin with metformin, p. 634 · *Dapagliflozin with
metformin,* p. 635 · *Empagliflozin with metformin,* p. 636 ·
Linagliptin with metformin, p. 626 · *Pioglitazone with
metformin,* p. 640 · *Saxagliptin with metformin,* p. 628 ·
Sitagliptin with metformin, p. 629 · *Vildagliptin with
metformin,* p. 629

BLOOD GLUCOSE LOWERING DRUGS ›
DIPEPTIDYLPEPTIDASE-4 INHIBITORS (GLIPTINS)

Alogliptin

● DRUG ACTION Inhibits dipeptidylpeptidase-4 to increase
insulin secretion and lower glucagon secretion.

● INDICATIONS AND DOSE

**Type 2 diabetes mellitus as dual therapy in combination
with either metformin, pioglitazone, a sulfonylurea, or
insulin (when treatment with these drugs alone fails to
achieve adequate glycaemic control), or as triple therapy
in combination with metformin and either pioglitazone
or insulin**
▸ BY MOUTH
▸ Adult: 25 mg once daily

DOSE ADJUSTMENTS DUE TO INTERACTIONS
Dose of concomitant sulfonylurea or insulin may need to
be reduced.
Caution with use in combination with both metformin
and pioglitazone—risk of hypoglycaemia (dose of
metformin or pioglitazone may need to be reduced).

● CONTRA-INDICATIONS Ketoacidosis

● CAUTIONS History of pancreatitis · not recommended in
moderate to severe heart failure (limited experience)

● INTERACTIONS → Appendix 1 (antidiabetics).

● SIDE-EFFECTS

▸ **Common or very common** Abdominal pain · gastro-
oesophageal reflux · headache · nasopharyngitis · pruritus ·
rash · upper respiratory-tract infection

▸ **Frequency not known** Angioedema · hepatic impairment ·
pancreatitis · Stevens-Johnson syndrome · urticaria

SIDE-EFFECTS, FURTHER INFORMATION
▸ Pancreatitis Discontinue if symptoms of acute pancreatitis
(persistent, severe abdominal pain).

● ALLERGY AND CROSS-SENSITIVITY Contra-indicated if
history of serious hypersensitivity to dipeptidylpeptidase-
4 inhibitors.

● PREGNANCY Manufacturer advises avoid—no information
available.

● BREAST FEEDING Avoid—present in milk in *animal* studies.

● HEPATIC IMPAIRMENT Manufacturer advises avoid in
severe impairment—no information available.

● RENAL IMPAIRMENT Reduce dose to 12.5 mg once daily if
eGFR 30–50 mL/minute/1.73 m^2. Reduce dose to 6.25 mg
once daily if eGFR less than 30 mL/minute/1.73 m^2. Use
with caution if eGFR less than 30 mL/minute/1.73 m^2.

● MONITORING REQUIREMENTS Determine renal function
before treatment and periodically thereafter.

● MEDICINAL FORMS
There can be variation in the licensing of different medicines
containing the same drug.
Tablet
▸ Alogliptin (Non-proprietary) ▼
  Alogliptin (as Alogliptin benzoate) 6.25 mg Alogliptin 6.25mg
  tablets | 28 tablet PoM no price available DT price = £26.60
  Alogliptin (as Alogliptin benzoate) 12.5 mg Alogliptin 12.5mg
  tablets | 28 tablet PoM no price available DT price = £26.60
  Alogliptin (as Alogliptin benzoate) 25 mg Alogliptin 25mg tablets
  | 28 tablet PoM no price available DT price = £26.60
▸ Vipidia (Takeda UK Ltd) ▼
  Alogliptin (as Alogliptin benzoate) 6.25 mg Vipidia 6.25mg tablets
  | 28 tablet PoM £26.60 DT price = £26.60
  Alogliptin (as Alogliptin benzoate) 12.5 mg Vipidia 12.5mg tablets
  | 28 tablet PoM £26.60 DT price = £26.60
  Alogliptin (as Alogliptin benzoate) 25 mg Vipidia 25mg tablets |
  28 tablet PoM £26.60 DT price = £26.60

Alogliptin with metformin

The properties listed below are those particular to the
combination only. For the properties of the components
please consider, alogliptin above, metformin hydrochloride
p. 624.

● INDICATIONS AND DOSE

**Type 2 diabetes mellitus not controlled by metformin
alone or by metformin in combination with either
pioglitazone or insulin**
▸ BY MOUTH
▸ Adult: 1 tablet twice daily, based on patient's current
metformin dose

● INTERACTIONS Dose of concomitant sulfonylurea or
insulin may need to be reduced.
Caution with use in combination with both metformin and
pioglitazone—risk of hypoglycaemia (dose of metformin or
pioglitazone may need to be reduced).

6

Endocrine system

● MEDICINAL FORMS
There can be variation in the licensing of different medicines containing the same drug.

Tablet
CAUTIONARY AND ADVISORY LABELS 21
▸ Alogliptin with metformin (Non-proprietary) ▼
Alogliptin (as Alogliptin benzoate) 12.5 mg, Metformin hydrochloride 1 gram Alogliptin 12.5mg / Metformin 1g tablets | 56 tablet [PoM] no price available DT price = £26.60
▸ Vipdomet (Takeda UK Ltd) ▼
Alogliptin (as Alogliptin benzoate) 12.5 mg, Metformin hydrochloride 1 gram Vipdomet 12.5mg/1000mg tablets | 56 tablet [PoM] £26.60 DT price = £26.60

Linagliptin

● DRUG ACTION Inhibits dipeptidylpeptidase-4 to increase insulin secretion and lower glucagon secretion.

● INDICATIONS AND DOSE

Type 2 diabetes mellitus as monotherapy (if metformin inappropriate), or in combination with metformin (when treatment with metformin alone fails to achieve adequate glycaemic control), or both metformin and a sulfonylurea (when dual therapy with these drugs fails to achieve adequate glycaemic control) | Type 2 diabetes mellitus in combination with insulin (with or without metformin) when a stable dose of insulin has not provided adequate glycaemic control
▸ BY MOUTH
▸ Adult: 5 mg once daily

DOSE ADJUSTMENTS DUE TO INTERACTIONS
Dose of concomitant sulfonylurea or insulin may need to be reduced.

● INTERACTIONS → Appendix 1 (antidiabetics).
● SIDE-EFFECTS
▸ Uncommon Cough · nasopharyngitis
▸ **Frequency not known** Pancreatitis
 SIDE-EFFECTS, FURTHER INFORMATION
▸ Pancreatitis Discontinue if symptoms of acute pancreatitis (persistent, severe abdominal pain).
● PREGNANCY Avoid—no information available.
● BREAST FEEDING Avoid—present in milk in *animal* studies.
● NATIONAL FUNDING/ACCESS DECISIONS
Scottish Medicines Consortium (SMC) Decisions
The *Scottish Medicines Consortium* has advised that linagliptin (*Trajenta* ®) is accepted for restricted use within NHS Scotland for the treatment of type 2 diabetes mellitus as monotherapy when both metformin and a sulfonylurea are inappropriate (January 2013), and in combination with metformin when addition of a sulfonylurea is inappropriate (December 2011).

● MEDICINAL FORMS
There can be variation in the licensing of different medicines containing the same drug.

Tablet
▸ Trajenta (Boehringer Ingelheim Ltd)
Linagliptin 5 mg Trajenta 5mg tablets | 28 tablet [PoM] £33.26 DT price = £33.26

Linagliptin with metformin

The properties listed below are those particular to the combination only. For the properties of the components please consider, linagliptin above, metformin hydrochloride p. 624.

● INDICATIONS AND DOSE

Type 2 diabetes mellitus not controlled by metformin alone or by metformin in combination with either a sulfonylurea or insulin
▸ BY MOUTH
▸ Adult: 1 tablet twice daily, based on patient's current metformin dose

● INTERACTIONS Dose of concomitant sulfonylurea or insulin may need to be reduced.
● NATIONAL FUNDING/ACCESS DECISIONS
Scottish Medicines Consortium (SMC) Decisions
The *Scottish Medicines Consortium* has advised (May 2015) that linagliptin plus metformin combination tablets (*Jentadueto* ®) are accepted for restricted use within NHS Scotland for the treatment of adult patients with type 2 diabetes mellitus in combination with insulin, as an adjunct to diet and exercise to improve glycaemic control when a combination of insulin and metformin alone is inadequate. It is restricted to use in the treatment of patients for whom a combination of linagliptin and metformin is an appropriate choice of therapy and the fixed doses are considered appropriate.

● MEDICINAL FORMS
There can be variation in the licensing of different medicines containing the same drug.

Tablet
CAUTIONARY AND ADVISORY LABELS 21
▸ Jentadueto (Boehringer Ingelheim Ltd) ▼
Linagliptin 2.5 mg, Metformin hydrochloride 850 mg Jentadueto 2.5mg/850mg tablets | 56 tablet [PoM] £33.26
Linagliptin 2.5 mg, Metformin hydrochloride 1000 mg Jentadueto 2.5mg/1000mg tablets | 56 tablet [PoM] £33.26

Saxagliptin

● DRUG ACTION Inhibits dipeptidylpeptidase-4 to increase insulin secretion and lower glucagon secretion.

● INDICATIONS AND DOSE

Type 2 diabetes mellitus as monotherapy (if metformin inappropriate), or in combination with metformin or a sulfonylurea (if metformin inappropriate), or pioglitazone (when treatment with either metformin or a sulfonylurea or pioglitazone fails to achieve adequate glycaemic control), and also in combination with both metformin and a sulfonylurea (when dual therapy with these drugs fails to achieve adequate glycaemic control) | Type 2 diabetes mellitus in combination with insulin (with or without metformin) when a stable dose of insulin has not provided adequate glycaemic control
▸ BY MOUTH
▸ Adult: 5 mg once daily

DOSE ADJUSTMENTS DUE TO INTERACTIONS
Dose of concomitant sulfonylurea or insulin may need to be reduced.

● CAUTIONS Elderly
● INTERACTIONS → Appendix 1 (antidiabetics).
● SIDE-EFFECTS
▸ **Common or very common** Dizziness · dyspepsia · fatigue · gastritis · gastroenteritis · headache · hypoglycaemia · myalgia · nasopharyngitis · peripheral oedema · sinusitis · upper respiratory tract infection · urinary tract infection · vomiting

▶ **Uncommon** Anaphylaxis · arthralgia · dyslipidaemia · erectile dysfunction · hypersensitivity reactions · hypertriglyceridaemia · pancreatitis
▶ **Frequency not known** Rash

SIDE-EFFECTS, FURTHER INFORMATION
▶ Pancreatitis Discontinue if symptoms of acute pancreatitis (persistent, severe abdominal pain).

● ALLERGY AND CROSS-SENSITIVITY Contra-indicated if patient has a history of serious hypersensitivity to dipeptidylpeptidase-4 inhibitors.

● PREGNANCY Avoid unless essential—toxicity in *animal* studies.

● BREAST FEEDING Avoid—present in milk in *animal* studies.

● HEPATIC IMPAIRMENT Use with caution in moderate impairment. Avoid in severe impairment.

● RENAL IMPAIRMENT Reduce dose to 2.5 mg once daily in moderate to severe impairment. Use with caution in severe impairment.

● MONITORING REQUIREMENTS Determine renal function before treatment and periodically thereafter.

● NATIONAL FUNDING/ACCESS DECISIONS

Scottish Medicines Consortium (SMC) Decisions
The *Scottish Medicines Consortium* has advised that saxagliptin (*Onglyza* ®) is accepted for restricted use within NHS Scotland for the treatment of type 2 diabetes mellitus as triple therapy in combination with metformin and a sulfonylurea, as an alternative to existing dipeptidyl peptidase-4 inhibitors, when treatment with metformin and a sulfonylurea is inadequate (November 2013).

● MEDICINAL FORMS
There can be variation in the licensing of different medicines containing the same drug.

Tablet
▶ Onglyza (AstraZeneca UK Ltd)
Saxagliptin (as Saxagliptin hydrochloride) 2.5 mg Onglyza 2.5mg tablets | 28 tablet [PoM] £31.60 DT price = £31.60
Saxagliptin (as Saxagliptin hydrochloride) 5 mg Onglyza 5mg tablets | 28 tablet [PoM] £31.60 DT price = £31.60

Saxagliptin with metformin

The properties listed below are those particular to the combination only. For the properties of the components please consider, saxagliptin p. 626, metformin hydrochloride p. 624.

● INDICATIONS AND DOSE

Type 2 diabetes mellitus not controlled by metformin alone or by metformin in combination with either a sulfonylurea or insulin
▶ BY MOUTH
▶ Adult: 1 tablet twice daily, based on patient's current metformin dose

● INTERACTIONS Dose of concomitant sulfonylurea or insulin may need to be reduced.

● NATIONAL FUNDING/ACCESS DECISIONS

Scottish Medicines Consortium (SMC) Decisions
The *Scottish Medicines Consortium* has advised (May 2013) that *Komboglyze*® is accepted for restricted use within NHS Scotland for the treatment of type 2 diabetes mellitus in patients unable to achieve adequate glycaemic control with metformin alone and when the addition of a sulfonylurea is inappropriate.

● MEDICINAL FORMS
There can be variation in the licensing of different medicines containing the same drug.

Tablet
CAUTIONARY AND ADVISORY LABELS 21
▶ Komboglyze (AstraZeneca UK Ltd)
Saxagliptin (as Saxagliptin hydrochloride) 2.5 mg, Metformin hydrochloride 850 mg Komboglyze 2.5mg/850mg tablets | 56 tablet [PoM] £31.60 DT price = £31.60
Saxagliptin (as Saxagliptin hydrochloride) 2.5 mg, Metformin hydrochloride 1 gram Komboglyze 2.5mg/1000mg tablets | 56 tablet [PoM] £31.60 DT price = £31.60

Sitagliptin

● DRUG ACTION Inhibits dipeptidylpeptidase-4 to increase insulin secretion and lower glucagon secretion.

● INDICATIONS AND DOSE

Type 2 diabetes mellitus as monotherapy (if metformin inappropriate), or in combination with metformin or a sulfonylurea (if metformin inappropriate), or pioglitazone (when treatment with either metformin or a sulfonylurea or pioglitazone fails to achieve adequate glycaemic control), and also in combination with both metformin and sulfonylurea (when dual therapy with these drugs fails to achieve adequate glycaemic control) | Type 2 diabetes mellitus in combination with both metformin and pioglitazone when dual therapy with these drugs fails to achieve adequate glycaemic control, and may also be used in combination with insulin (with or without metformin) when a stable dose of insulin has not provided adequate glycaemic control
▶ BY MOUTH
▶ Adult: 100 mg once daily

DOSE ADJUSTMENTS DUE TO INTERACTIONS
Dose of concomitant sulfonylurea or insulin may need to be reduced.

● CONTRA-INDICATIONS Ketoacidosis

● INTERACTIONS → Appendix 1 (antidiabetics).

● SIDE-EFFECTS
▶ **Common or very common** Gastro-intestinal disturbances · nasopharyngitis · pain · peripheral oedema · upper respiratory tract infection
▶ **Uncommon** Anorexia · dizziness · drowsiness · dry mouth · headache · hypoglycaemia · osteoarthritis
▶ **Frequency not known** Cutaneous vasculitis · pancreatitis · rash · Stevens-Johnson syndrome

SIDE-EFFECTS, FURTHER INFORMATION
▶ Pancreatitis Discontinue if symptoms of acute pancreatitis (persistent, severe abdominal pain).

● PREGNANCY Avoid—toxicity in *animal* studies.

● BREAST FEEDING Avoid—present in milk in *animal* studies.

● RENAL IMPAIRMENT Reduce dose to 50 mg once daily if eGFR 30–50 mL/minute/1.73 m^2. Reduce dose to 25 mg once daily if eGFR less than 30 mL/minute/1.73 m^2.

● NATIONAL FUNDING/ACCESS DECISIONS

Scottish Medicines Consortium (SMC) Decisions
The *Scottish Medicines Consortium* has advised (June 2010) that *Januvia* ® is accepted for restricted use within NHS Scotland as monotherapy, to improve glycaemic control in patients with type 2 diabetes mellitus, for whom both metformin and sulfonylureas are not appropriate.

6

Endocrine system

Endocrine system

6

● MEDICINAL FORMS
There can be variation in the licensing of different medicines containing the same drug. Forms available from special-order manufacturers include: oral solution

Tablet
▸ Januvia (Merck Sharp & Dohme Ltd)
Sitagliptin (as Sitagliptin phosphate) 25 mg Januvia 25mg tablets | 28 tablet [PoM] £33.26 DT price = £33.26
Sitagliptin (as Sitagliptin phosphate) 50 mg Januvia 50mg tablets | 28 tablet [PoM] £33.26 DT price = £33.26
Sitagliptin (as Sitagliptin phosphate) 100 mg Januvia 100mg tablets | 28 tablet [PoM] £33.26 DT price = £33.26

Sitagliptin with metformin

The properties listed below are those particular to the combination only. For the properties of the components please consider, sitagliptin p. 627, metformin hydrochloride p. 624.

● INDICATIONS AND DOSE
Type 2 diabetes mellitus not controlled by metformin alone or by metformin in combination with either a sulfonylurea or pioglitazone or insulin
▸ BY MOUTH
▸ Adult: 1 tablet twice daily

● INTERACTIONS Dose of concomitant sulfonylurea or insulin may need to be reduced.

● NATIONAL FUNDING/ACCESS DECISIONS
Scottish Medicines Consortium (SMC) Decisions
The *Scottish Medicines Consortium* has advised (July 2008) that *Janumet* ® is accepted for restricted use within NHS Scotland for the treatment of type 2 diabetes mellitus when the addition of a sulfonylurea to metformin is not appropriate; it is also accepted for use in NHS Scotland in combination with a sulfonylurea in patients inadequately controlled on maximum tolerated doses of metformin and a sulfonylurea.

● MEDICINAL FORMS
There can be variation in the licensing of different medicines containing the same drug.

Tablet
CAUTIONARY AND ADVISORY LABELS 21
▸ Janumet (Merck Sharp & Dohme Ltd)
Sitagliptin (as Sitagliptin phosphate) 50 mg, Metformin hydrochloride 1 gram Janumet 50mg/1000mg tablets | 56 tablet [PoM] £33.26 DT price = £33.26

Vildagliptin

● DRUG ACTION Inhibits dipeptidylpeptidase-4 to increase insulin secretion and lower glucagon secretion.

● INDICATIONS AND DOSE
Type 2 diabetes mellitus as monotherapy (if metformin inappropriate) | Type 2 diabetes mellitus in combination with metformin or pioglitazone (when treatment with either metformin or pioglitazone fails to achieve adequate glycaemic control) | Type 2 diabetes mellitus in combination with both metformin and a sulfonylurea (when dual therapy with these drugs fails to achieve adequate glycaemic control) | Type 2 diabetes mellitus in combination with insulin (with or without metformin) when a stable dose of insulin has not provided adequate glycaemic control
▸ BY MOUTH
▸ Adult: 50 mg twice daily

Type 2 diabetes mellitus in combination with sulfonylurea (if metformin inappropriate)
▸ BY MOUTH
▸ Adult: 50 mg daily, dose to be taken in the morning

DOSE ADJUSTMENTS DUE TO INTERACTIONS
Dose of concomitant sulfonylurea or insulin may need to be reduced.

● CONTRA-INDICATIONS Ketoacidosis
● CAUTIONS Manufacturer advises avoid in severe heart failure—no information available
● INTERACTIONS → Appendix 1 (antidiabetics).
● SIDE-EFFECTS
▸ **Common or very common** Asthenia · dizziness · headache · nausea · peripheral oedema · tremor
▸ **Uncommon** Arthralgia · constipation · hypoglycaemia
▸ **Rare** Hepatic dysfunction
▸ **Very rare** Nasopharyngitis · upper respiratory tract infection
▸ **Frequency not known** Bullous skin reactions · exfoliative skin reactions · pancreatitis
SIDE-EFFECTS, FURTHER INFORMATION
▸ Pancreatitis Discontinue if symptoms of acute pancreatitis (persistent, severe abdominal pain).
▸ Liver toxicity Rare reports of liver dysfunction; discontinue if jaundice or other signs of liver dysfunction occur.
● PREGNANCY Avoid—toxicity in *animal* studies.
● BREAST FEEDING Avoid—present in milk in *animal* studies.
● HEPATIC IMPAIRMENT Avoid.
● RENAL IMPAIRMENT Reduce dose to 50 mg once daily if eGFR less than 50 mL/minute/1.73 m^2.
● MONITORING REQUIREMENTS Monitor liver function before treatment and every 3 months for first year and periodically thereafter.
● PATIENT AND CARER ADVICE
Liver toxicity Patients should be advised to seek prompt medical attention if symptoms such as nausea, vomiting, abdominal pain, fatigue, and dark urine develop.
● NATIONAL FUNDING/ACCESS DECISIONS
Scottish Medicines Consortium (SMC) Decisions
The *Scottish Medicines Consortium* has advised that vildagliptin (*Galvus* ®) is accepted for restricted use within NHS Scotland for the treatment of type 2 diabetes mellitus as monotherapy when treatment with metformin or a sulfonylurea is inappropriate (December 2012), and in combination with metformin when addition of a sulfonylurea is inappropriate (March 2008), and in combination with a sulfonylurea if metformin is inappropriate (September 2009), and also as triple therapy in combination with metformin and a sulfonylurea, as an alternative to existing dipeptidyl peptidase-4 inhibitors, when treatment with metformin and a sulfonylurea is inadequate (November 2013).

● MEDICINAL FORMS
There can be variation in the licensing of different medicines containing the same drug.
Tablet
▸ Galvus (Novartis Pharmaceuticals UK Ltd)
Vildagliptin 50 mg Galvus 50mg tablets | 56 tablet [PoM] £33.35 DT price = £33.35

Vildagliptin with metformin

The properties listed below are those particular to the combination only. For the properties of the components please consider, vildagliptin p. 628, metformin hydrochloride p. 624.

- **INDICATIONS AND DOSE**

Type 2 diabetes mellitus not controlled by metformin alone or by metformin in combination with either a sulfonylurea or insulin
- ▸ BY MOUTH
- ▸ Adult: 1 tablet twice daily, based on patient's current metformin dose

- **INTERACTIONS** Dose of concomitant sulfonylurea or insulin may need to be reduced.
- **NATIONAL FUNDING/ACCESS DECISIONS**

Scottish Medicines Consortium (SMC) Decisions
The *Scottish Medicines Consortium* has advised (June 2008) that *Eucreas* ® is accepted for restricted use within NHS Scotland for the treatment of type 2 diabetes mellitus in patients unable to achieve adequate glycaemic control with metformin alone or those already treated with vildagliptin and metformin as separate tablets.

- **MEDICINAL FORMS**
There can be variation in the licensing of different medicines containing the same drug.
Tablet
CAUTIONARY AND ADVISORY LABELS 21
- ▸ Eucreas (Novartis Pharmaceuticals UK Ltd)
  Vildagliptin 50 mg, Metformin hydrochloride 850 mg Eucreas 50mg/850mg tablets | 60 tablet [PoM] £35.68 DT price = £35.68
  Vildagliptin 50 mg, Metformin hydrochloride 1 gram Eucreas 50mg/1000mg tablets | 60 tablet [PoM] £35.68 DT price = £35.68

BLOOD GLUCOSE LOWERING DRUGS >
GLUCAGON-LIKE PEPTIDE-1 RECEPTOR AGONISTS

Albiglutide
1.6.2016

- **DRUG ACTION** Albiglutide is a GLP-1 (glucagon-like peptide-1) receptor agonist that augments glucose-dependent insulin secretion, and slows gastric emptying.

- **INDICATIONS AND DOSE**

Type 2 diabetes mellitus as monotherapy when treatment with metformin is considered inappropriate | Type 2 diabetes mellitus in combination with basal insulin and other oral glucose lowering agents
- ▸ BY SUBCUTANEOUS INJECTION
- ▸ Adult: 30 mg once weekly, increased if necessary up to 50 mg once weekly, to be administered on the same day each week

DOSE ADJUSTMENTS DUE TO INTERACTIONS
Dose of concomitant insulin or drugs that stimulate insulin secretion may need to be reduced.

- **CONTRA-INDICATIONS** Severe gastrointestinal disease—no information available
- **CAUTIONS** History of pancreatitis · moderate to severe heart failure—no information available
- **INTERACTIONS** → Appendix 1 (antidiabetics)
- **SIDE-EFFECTS**
- ▸ **Common or very common** Atrial fibrillation · constipation · diarrhoea · dyspepsia · gastro-oesophageal reflux disease · hypoglycaemia · injection site reactions · nausea · vomiting
- ▸ **Uncommon** Intestinal obstruction · pancreatitis (discontinue treatment)
- **CONCEPTION AND CONTRACEPTION** Manufacturer recommends effective contraception in women of

childbearing potential. Discontinue treatment at least one month before a planned pregnancy.
- **PREGNANCY** Manufacturer advises avoid—toxicity in *animal* studies.
- **BREAST FEEDING** Manufacturer advises avoid—no information available.
- **RENAL IMPAIRMENT** Manufacturer advises avoid if eGFR less than 30 mL/minute/1.73 m².
- **HANDLING AND STORAGE** Store at 2–8°C. May be stored at temperatures up to 30°C for up to 4 weeks.
- **PATIENT AND CARER ADVICE**
Patients or carers should be given advice on how to administer albiglutide injection.
Acute pancreatitis Patients should be told how to recognise signs and symptoms of acute pancreatitis and advised to seek medical attention if symptoms such as persistent, severe abdominal pain develop.

Missed doses
If a dose is missed it should be administered as soon as possible within 3 days; if more than 3 days have passed, the missed dose should not be taken and the next dose should be taken at the normal time.

- **NATIONAL FUNDING/ACCESS DECISIONS**

Scottish Medicines Consortium (SMC) Decisions
The *Scottish Medicines Consortium* has advised (January 2016) that albiglutide (*Eperzan* ®) is accepted for restricted use for treating adults with type 2 diabetes to improve glycaemic control in combination with other glucose-lowering medicines when these, together with diet and exercise, do not provide adequate glycaemic control. It is restricted to use as an alternative once weekly GLP-1 mimetic for use in combination with oral anti-diabetic agents as a third-line pre-insulin treatment option.

- **MEDICINAL FORMS**
There can be variation in the licensing of different medicines containing the same drug.
Powder and solvent for solution for injection
- ▸ Eperzan (GlaxoSmithKline UK Ltd) ▼
  Albiglutide 30 mg Eperzan 30mg powder and solvent for solution for injection pre-filled pen | 4 pre-filled disposable injection [PoM] £71.00
  Albiglutide 50 mg Eperzan 50mg powder and solvent for solution for injection pre-filled pen | 4 pre-filled disposable injection [PoM] £71.00

Dulaglutide
14.6.2016

- **DRUG ACTION** Dulaglutide is a long-acting glucagon-like peptide 1 (GLP-1) receptor agonist that augments glucose-dependent insulin secretion, and slows gastric emptying.

- **INDICATIONS AND DOSE**

Type 2 diabetes mellitus as monotherapy if metformin inappropriate
- ▸ BY SUBCUTANEOUS INJECTION
- ▸ Adult: 0.75 mg once weekly

Type 2 diabetes mellitus in combination with insulin or other antidiabetic drugs (if existing treatment fails to achieve adequate glycaemic control)
- ▸ BY SUBCUTANEOUS INJECTION
- ▸ Adult: 1.5 mg once weekly

DOSE ADJUSTMENTS DUE TO INTERACTIONS
Dose of concomitant insulin or drugs that stimulate insulin secretion may need to be reduced.

- **CONTRA-INDICATIONS** Severe gastro-intestinal disease—no information available
- **CAUTIONS** Congestive heart failure—no information available
- **INTERACTIONS** → Appendix 1 (antidiabetics)

6

Endocrine system

- SIDE-EFFECTS
- **Common or very common** Abdominal distention, · abdominal pain · atrioventricular block · constipation · decreased appetite · diarrhoea · dyspepsia · fatigue · flatulence · gastro-oesophageal reflux disease · nausea · sinus tachycardia · vomiting
- **Rare** Acute pancreatitis (discontinue treatment)
- PREGNANCY Manufacturer advises avoid—toxicity in *animal* studies.
- BREAST FEEDING Manufacturer advises avoid— no information available.
- RENAL IMPAIRMENT Manufacturer advises avoid in severe impairment and end stage renal disease—no information available.
- HANDLING AND STORAGE **Refrigerated storage** is usually necessary (2 °C – 8 °C). Once in use, may be stored unrefrigerated for up to 14 days at a temperature not above 30 °C.
- PATIENT AND CARER ADVICE
Patients or carers should be given advice on how to administer dulaglutide injection.
Acute pancreatitis Patients should be told how to recognise signs and symptoms of acute pancreatitis and advised to seek medical attention if symptoms such as persistent, severe abdominal pain develop.
Missed doses
If a dose is missed, it should be administered as soon as possible only if there are at least 3 days until the next scheduled dose; if less than 3 days remain before the next scheduled dose, the missed dose should not be taken and the next dose should be taken at the normal time.
- NATIONAL FUNDING/ACCESS DECISIONS
Scottish Medicines Consortium (SMC) Decisions
The *Scottish Medicines Consortium* has advised (January 2016) that dulaglutide (*Trulicity* ®) is accepted for restricted use for treating adults with type 2 diabetes to improve glycaemic control as add-on therapy in combination with other glucose-lowering medicines, when these, together with diet and exercise, do not provide adequate glycaemic control. It is restricted to use as part of a triple therapy in people with inadequate glycaemic control on 2 oral anti-diabetic medicines, as an alternative GLP-1 mimetic option.
- MEDICINAL FORMS
There can be variation in the licensing of different medicines containing the same drug.
Solution for injection
- Trulicity (Eli Lilly and Company Ltd) ▼
Dulaglutide 1.5 mg per 1 ml Trulicity 0.75mg/0.5ml solution for injection pre-filled pen | 4 pre-filled disposable injection PoM £73.25
Dulaglutide 3 mg per 1 ml Trulicity 1.5mg/0.5ml solution for injection pre-filled pen | 4 pre-filled disposable injection PoM £73.25

Exenatide

- DRUG ACTION Binds to, and activates, the GLP-1 (glucagon-like peptide-1) receptor to increase insulin secretion, suppresses glucagon secretion, and slows gastric emptying.

- INDICATIONS AND DOSE
Type 2 diabetes mellitus in combination with metformin or a sulfonylurea, or both, or with pioglitazone, or with both metformin and pioglitazone, in patients who have not achieved adequate glycaemic control with these drugs alone or in combination
- BY SUBCUTANEOUS INJECTION USING IMMEDIATE-RELEASE MEDICINES
- Adult: Initially 5 micrograms twice daily for at least 1 month, then increased if necessary up to

10 micrograms twice daily, dose to be taken within 1 hour before 2 main meals (at least 6 hours apart)
- BY SUBCUTANEOUS INJECTION USING MODIFIED-RELEASE MEDICINES
- Adult: 2 mg once weekly

Type 2 diabetes mellitus in combination with basal insulin alone or with metformin or pioglitazone (or both)
- BY SUBCUTANEOUS INJECTION USING IMMEDIATE-RELEASE MEDICINES
- Adult: Initially 5 micrograms twice daily for at least 1 month, then increased if necessary up to 10 micrograms twice daily, dose to be taken within 1 hour before 2 main meals (at least 6 hours apart)

DOSE ADJUSTMENTS DUE TO INTERACTIONS
Dose of concomitant sulfonylurea may need to be reduced.

PHARMACOKINETICS
Effect of *modified-release* exenatide injection (*Bydureon* ®) may persist for 10 weeks after discontinuation.

- CONTRA-INDICATIONS Ketoacidosis · severe gastro-intestinal disease
- CAUTIONS Elderly · may cause weight loss greater than 1.5 kg weekly · pancreatitis
- INTERACTIONS → Appendix 1 (antidiabetics).
Other drugs administered orally may need to be taken at least 1 hour before or 4 hours after exenatide injection, or taken with a meal when exenatide is not administered, to minimise possible interference with absorption.
- SIDE-EFFECTS
- **Common or very common** Abdominal pain and distension · agitation · antibody formation · asthenia · decreased appetite · diarrhoea · dizziness · dyspepsia · gastro-intestinal disturbances · gastro-oesophageal reflux disease · headache · hypoglycaemia · increased sweating · injection-site reactions · nausea · vomiting · weight loss
- **Uncommon** Pancreatitis
- **Rare** Alopecia
- **Very rare** Anaphylactic reactions
- **Frequency not known** Angioedema · constipation · dehydration · drowsiness · eructation · flatulence · pruritus · rash · renal impairment · taste disturbance · urticaria
SIDE-EFFECTS, FURTHER INFORMATION
- Pancreatitis Severe pancreatitis (sometimes fatal), including haemorrhagic or necrotising pancreatitis, has been reported rarely; discontinue permanently if pancreatitis is diagnosed.
- CONCEPTION AND CONTRACEPTION Women of child-bearing age should use effective contraception during treatment with modified-release exenatide and for 12 weeks after discontinuation.
- PREGNANCY Avoid—toxicity in *animal* studies.
- BREAST FEEDING Avoid—no information available.
- RENAL IMPAIRMENT For *standard-release* injection, use with caution if eGFR 30–50 mL/minute/1.73 m². For *standard-release* injection, avoid if eGFR less than 30 mL/minute/1.73 m². For *modified-release* injection, avoid if eGFR less than 50 mL/minute/1.73 m².
- PATIENT AND CARER ADVICE
Patients changing from standard-release to modified-release exenatide formulation may experience initial transient increase in blood glucose.
Some oral medications should be taken at least 1 hour before or 4 hours after exenatide injection—consult product literature for details.
Patients or their carers should be told how to recognise signs and symptoms of pancreatitis and advised to seek prompt medical attention if symptoms such as abdominal pain, nausea, and vomiting develop.

6

Missed doses

If a dose of the immediate-release medicine is missed, continue with the next scheduled dose—do not administer **after** a meal.

• NATIONAL FUNDING/ACCESS DECISIONS

NICE technology appraisals (TAs)

▸ **Exenatide modified-release for the treatment of type 2 diabetes mellitus (February 2012)** NICE TA248

Modified-release exenatide in triple therapy regimens (in combination with metformin and a sulphonylurea, or metformin and a thiazolidinedione) is recommended for the treatment of type 2 diabetes, only when glycaemic control is inadequate and the patient has:

• a body mass index (BMI) $\geq$35 kg/m^2 (in those of European descent, with appropriate adjustment for other ethnic groups) and weight-related psychological or medical problems, *or*

• a BMI < 35 kg/m^2, and insulin would be unacceptable for occupational reasons, or weight loss would benefit other significant obesity-related comorbidities.

Treatment with modified-release exenatide in a triple therapy regimen should be continued only if HbA$_{1c}$ concentration is reduced by at least 1 percentage point and a weight loss of at least 3% is achieved within 6 months of starting treatment.

Modified-release exenatide in dual therapy regimens (in combination with metformin or a sulphonylurea) is recommended only if:

• treatment with metformin or a sulphonylurea is contra-indicated or not tolerated, *and*

• treatment with thiazolidinediones and dipeptidylpeptidase-4 inhibitors is contra-indicated or not tolerated.

Modified-release exenatide in a dual therapy regimen should be continued only if HbA$_{1c}$ concentration is reduced by at least 1 percentage point within 6 months of starting treatment.
www.nice.org.uk/TA248

Scottish Medicines Consortium (SMC) Decisions

The *Scottish Medicines Consortium* has advised (June 2007) that standard-release exenatide (*Byetta*®) is accepted for restricted use within NHS Scotland for the treatment of type 2 diabetes in combination with metformin or sulphonylurea (or both), as an alternative to treatment with insulin in patients where treatment with metformin or sulfonylurea (or both) at maximally tolerated doses has been inadequate, and treatment with insulin would be the next option.

The *Scottish Medicines Consortium* has also advised (February 2011) that standard-release exenatide (*Byetta*®) is accepted for restricted use within NHS Scotland for the treatment of type 2 diabetes in combination with metformin and pioglitazone as a third-line pre-insulin treatment option.

The *Scottish Medicines Consortium* has advised (December 2011) that modified-release exenatide (*Bydureon*®) is accepted for restricted use within NHS Scotland for the treatment of type 2 diabetes as a third-line treatment option.

• MEDICINAL FORMS
There can be variation in the licensing of different medicines containing the same drug.

Solution for injection
CAUTIONARY AND ADVISORY LABELS 10
▸ Byetta (AstraZeneca UK Ltd)
 Exenatide 250 microgram per 1 ml Byetta 10micrograms/0.04ml solution for injection 2.4ml pre-filled disposable devices | 1 pre-filled disposable injection [PoM] £68.24 DT price = £68.24
 Byetta 5micrograms/0.02ml solution for injection 1.2ml pre-filled disposable devices | 1 pre-filled disposable injection [PoM] £68.24 DT price = £68.24

Powder and solvent for suspension for injection
CAUTIONARY AND ADVISORY LABELS 10
▸ Bydureon (AstraZeneca UK Ltd)
 Exenatide 2 mg Bydureon 2mg powder and solvent for prolonged-release suspension for injection pre-filled pen | 4 pre-filled disposable injection [PoM] £73.36
 Bydureon 2mg powder and solvent for suspension for prolonged-release injection vials | 4 vial [PoM] £73.36

Liraglutide

1.6.2016

• DRUG ACTION Liraglutide binds to, and activates, the GLP-1 (glucagon-like peptide-1) receptor to increase insulin secretion, suppresses glucagon secretion, and slows gastric emptying.

• INDICATIONS AND DOSE

Type 2 diabetes mellitus in combination with metformin or a sulfonylurea, or both, in patients who have not achieved adequate glycaemic control with these drugs alone or in combination | Type 2 diabetes mellitus in combination with basal insulin or both metformin and pioglitazone when dual therapy with these drugs fails to achieve adequate glycaemic control
▸ BY SUBCUTANEOUS INJECTION
▸ Adult: Initially 0.6 mg once daily for at least 1 week, then increased to 1.2 mg once daily for at least 1 week, then increased if necessary up to 1.8 mg once daily

DOSE ADJUSTMENTS DUE TO INTERACTIONS
Dose of concomitant insulin or sulfonylurea may need to be reduced.

• CONTRA-INDICATIONS Diabetic gastroparesis · inflammatory bowel disease · ketoacidosis · moderate to severe congestive heart failure—no information available

• CAUTIONS History of pancreatitis · mild congestive heart failure—limited experience · thyroid disease

• INTERACTIONS → Appendix 1 (antidiabetics).

• SIDE-EFFECTS
▸ **Common or very common** Abdominal pain and distension · bronchitis · constipation · decreased appetite · diarrhoea · dizziness · dyspepsia · flatulence · gastritis · gastro-intestinal disturbances · gastro-oesophageal reflux disease · headache · hypoglycaemia · injection site reactions · malaise · nasopharyngitis · nausea · tachycardia · vomiting
▸ **Uncommon** Acute renal failure · dehydration · renal impairment
▸ **Very rare** Acute pancreatitis
▸ **Frequency not known** Goitre · increased blood calcitonin · thyroid neoplasm

SIDE-EFFECTS, FURTHER INFORMATION
▸ Pancreatitis Discontinue if symptoms of acute pancreatitis (persistent, severe abdominal pain).

• PREGNANCY Manufacturer advises avoid—toxicity in *animal* studies (recommendation also supported by primary literature).

• BREAST FEEDING Avoid—no information available.

• HEPATIC IMPAIRMENT Manufacturer advises avoid—limited experience.

• RENAL IMPAIRMENT Manufacturer advises avoid if eGFR less than 30 mL/minute/1.73 m^2—limited experience.

• HANDLING AND STORAGE Store in a refrigerator (2°C–8°C); after first use can be stored below 30°C, discard 1 month after first use.

• PATIENT AND CARER ADVICE Patients or carers should be given advice on how to administer liraglutide injection. Acute pancreatitis Patients should be told how to recognise signs and symptoms of acute pancreatitis and advised to seek immediate medical attention if symptoms such as persistent, severe abdominal pain develop.

- **MEDICINAL FORMS**
There can be variation in the licensing of different medicines containing the same drug.
Solution for injection
▸ Liraglutide (Non-proprietary)
Liraglutide 6 mg per 1 ml Liraglutide 6mg/ml solution for injection 3ml pre-filled disposable devices | 2 pre-filled disposable injection PoM no price available DT price = £78.48 | 3 pre-filled disposable injection PoM no price available
▸ Victoza (Novo Nordisk Ltd)
Liraglutide 6 mg per 1 ml Victoza 6mg/ml solution for injection 3ml pre-filled pen | 2 pre-filled disposable injection PoM £78.48 DT price = £78.48 | 3 pre-filled disposable injection PoM £117.72

Combinations available: *Insulin degludec with liraglutide,* p. 642

Lixisenatide

- **DRUG ACTION** Binds to, and activates, the GLP-1 (glucagon-like peptide-1) receptor to increase insulin secretion, suppresses glucagon secretion, and slows gastric emptying.

- **INDICATIONS AND DOSE**

Type 2 diabetes mellitus in combination with oral antidiabetic drugs (e.g. metformin, pioglitazone, or a sulfonylurea) or basal insulin, or both, when adequate glycaemic control has not been achieved with these drugs
▸ BY SUBCUTANEOUS INJECTION
▸ Adult: Initially 10 micrograms once daily for 14 days, then increased to 20 micrograms once daily, dose to be taken within 1 hour before the first meal of the day or the evening meal

DOSE ADJUSTMENTS DUE TO INTERACTIONS
Dose of concomitant sulfonylurea or insulin may need to be reduced.

- **CONTRA-INDICATIONS** Ketoacidosis · severe gastro-intestinal disease
- **INTERACTIONS** → Appendix 1 (antidiabetics). Other drugs administered orally may need to be taken at least 1 hour before or 4 hours after lixisenatide injection, or taken with a meal when lixisenatide is not administered, to minimise possible interference with absorption.
- **SIDE-EFFECTS**
▸ **Common or very common** Diarrhoea · dizziness · drowsiness · dyspepsia · headache · hypoglycaemia · injection-site reactions · nausea · palpitation · vomiting
▸ **Uncommon** Tachycardia · urticaria
SIDE-EFFECTS, FURTHER INFORMATION
▸ Pancreatitis Discontinue if symptoms of acute pancreatitis (persistent, severe abdominal pain).
- **CONCEPTION AND CONTRACEPTION** Women of child-bearing age should use effective contraception.
- **PREGNANCY** Avoid—toxicity in *animal* studies.
- **BREAST FEEDING** Avoid—no information available.
- **RENAL IMPAIRMENT** Use with caution if eGFR 30–50 mL/minute/1.73 m^2. Avoid if eGFR less than 30 mL/minute/1.73 m^2—no information available.
- **PATIENT AND CARER ADVICE**
Some oral medications should be taken at least 1 hour before or 4 hours after lixisenatide injection—consult product literature for details.
Missed doses
If a dose is missed, inject within 1 hour before the next meal—do not administer **after** a meal.

- **NATIONAL FUNDING/ACCESS DECISIONS**
Scottish Medicines Consortium (SMC) Decisions
The *Scottish Medicines Consortium* has advised (August 2013) that lixisenatide (*Lyxumia*®) is accepted for restricted use within NHS Scotland for the treatment of type 2 diabetes in combination with oral antidiabetic drugs or basal insulin (or both), when adequate glycaemic control has not been achieved with these drugs; use is restricted to patients in whom a GLP-1 agonist is appropriate, as an alternative to an existing GLP-1 agonist (exenatide or liraglutide).

- **MEDICINAL FORMS**
There can be variation in the licensing of different medicines containing the same drug.
Solution for injection
CAUTIONARY AND ADVISORY LABELS 10
▸ Lyxumia (Sanofi) ▼
Lixisenatide 50 microgram per 1 ml Lyxumia 10micrograms/0.2ml solution for injection 3ml pre-filled pen | 1 pre-filled disposable injection PoM £31.67 DT price = £31.67
Lixisenatide 100 microgram per 1 ml Lyxumia 20micrograms/0.2ml solution for injection 3ml pre-filled pen | 1 pre-filled disposable injection PoM no price available | 1 pre-filled disposable injection PoM £57.93 DT price = £57.93
▸ Lyxumia (Sanofi) ▼
Lyxumia 10micrograms/20micrograms treatment initiation pack | 2 pre-filled disposable injection PoM £57.93

BLOOD GLUCOSE LOWERING DRUGS ›
MEGLITINIDES

Nateglinide

- **DRUG ACTION** Nateglinide stimulates insulin secretion.

- **INDICATIONS AND DOSE**

Type 2 diabetes mellitus in combination with metformin when metformin alone inadequate
▸ BY MOUTH
▸ Adult: Initially 60 mg 3 times a day (max. per dose 180 mg), adjusted according to response, to be taken within 30 minutes before main meals

- **CONTRA-INDICATIONS** Ketoacidosis
- **CAUTIONS** Debilitated patients · elderly · malnourished patients
CAUTIONS, FURTHER INFORMATION
Substitute insulin during intercurrent illness (such as myocardial infarction, coma, infection, and trauma) and during surgery (omit nateglinide on morning of surgery and recommence when eating and drinking normally).
- **INTERACTIONS** → Appendix 1 (antidiabetics).
- **SIDE-EFFECTS** Hypersensitivity reactions · hypoglycaemia · pruritus · rashes · urticaria
- **PREGNANCY** Avoid—toxicity in *animal* studies.
- **BREAST FEEDING** Avoid—present in milk in *animal* studies.
- **HEPATIC IMPAIRMENT** Caution in moderate hepatic impairment. Avoid in severe impairment—no information available.
- **PATIENT AND CARER ADVICE**
Driving and skilled tasks
Drivers need to be particularly careful to avoid hypoglycaemia and should be warned of the problems.

- **MEDICINAL FORMS**
There can be variation in the licensing of different medicines containing the same drug.
Tablet
▸ Starlix (Novartis Pharmaceuticals UK Ltd)
Nateglinide 60 mg Starlix 60mg tablets | 84 tablet PoM £26.12 DT price = £26.12

Nateglinide 120 mg Starlix 120mg tablets | 84 tablet PoM £29.76
DT price = £29.76
Nateglinide 180 mg Starlix 180mg tablets | 84 tablet PoM £29.76
DT price = £29.76

Repaglinide

- DRUG ACTION Repaglinide stimulates insulin secretion.

- **INDICATIONS AND DOSE**

Type 2 diabetes mellitus (as monotherapy or in combination with metformin when metformin alone inadequate)
▶ BY MOUTH
▸ Adult 18–74 years: Initially 500 micrograms (max. per dose 4 mg), adjusted according to response, dose to be taken within 30 minutes before main meals and adjusted at intervals of 1–2 weeks; maximum 16 mg per day
▸ Adult 75 years and over: Not recommended

Type 2 diabetes mellitus (as monotherapy or in combination with metformin when metformin alone inadequate), if transferring from another oral antidiabetic drug
▶ BY MOUTH
▸ Adult 18–74 years: Initially 1 mg (max. per dose 4 mg), adjusted according to response, dose to be taken within 30 minutes before main meals and adjusted at intervals of 1–2 weeks; maximum 16 mg per day
▸ Adult 75 years and over: Not recommended

- CONTRA-INDICATIONS Ketoacidosis
- CAUTIONS Debilitated patients · malnourished patients
  CAUTIONS, FURTHER INFORMATION
  Substitute insulin during intercurrent illness (such as myocardial infarction, coma, infection, and trauma) and during surgery (omit repaglinide on morning of surgery and recommence when eating and drinking normally).
- INTERACTIONS → Appendix 1 (antidiabetics).
- SIDE-EFFECTS
▶ **Common or very common** Abdominal pain · constipation · diarrhoea · nausea · vomiting
▶ **Rare** Hypersensitivity reactions · hypoglycaemia · pruritus · rashes · urticaria · vasculitis · visual disturbances
- PREGNANCY Avoid.
- BREAST FEEDING Avoid—present in milk in *animal* studies.
- HEPATIC IMPAIRMENT Avoid in severe liver disease.
- RENAL IMPAIRMENT Use with caution.
- PATIENT AND CARER ADVICE
  Driving and skilled tasks
  Drivers need to be particularly careful to avoid hypoglycaemia and should be warned of the problems.

- MEDICINAL FORMS
  There can be variation in the licensing of different medicines containing the same drug.
  Tablet
  ▸ Repaglinide (Non-proprietary)
  Repaglinide 500 microgram Repaglinide 500microgram tablets | 30 tablet PoM £3.92 | 90 tablet PoM £11.76 DT price = £9.03
  Repaglinide 1 mg Repaglinide 1mg tablets | 30 tablet PoM £3.92 | 90 tablet PoM £11.76 DT price = £10.84
  Repaglinide 2 mg Repaglinide 2mg tablets | 90 tablet PoM £28.00 DT price = £5.88
  ▸ Enyglid (Consilient Health Ltd)
  Repaglinide 500 microgram Enyglid 0.5mg tablets | 30 tablet PoM £3.33 | 90 tablet PoM £9.99 DT price = £9.03
  Repaglinide 1 mg Enyglid 1mg tablets | 30 tablet PoM £3.33 | 90 tablet PoM £9.99 DT price = £10.84
  Repaglinide 2 mg Enyglid 2mg tablets | 90 tablet PoM £9.99 DT price = £5.88

▸ Prandin (Novo Nordisk Ltd)
  Repaglinide 500 microgram Prandin 0.5mg tablets | 30 tablet PoM £3.92 | 90 tablet PoM £11.76 DT price = £9.03
  Repaglinide 1 mg Prandin 1mg tablets | 30 tablet PoM £3.92 | 90 tablet PoM £11.76 DT price = £10.84
  Repaglinide 2 mg Prandin 2mg tablets | 90 tablet PoM £11.76 DT price = £5.88

BLOOD GLUCOSE LOWERING DRUGS › SODIUM GLUCOSE CO-TRANSPORTER 2 INHIBITORS

Canagliflozin

- DRUG ACTION Reversibly inhibits sodium-glucose co-transporter 2 (SGLT2) in the renal proximal convoluted tubule to reduce glucose reabsorption and increase urinary glucose excretion.

- **INDICATIONS AND DOSE**

Type 2 diabetes mellitus as monotherapy (if metformin inappropriate) | Type 2 diabetes mellitus in combination with insulin or other antidiabetic drugs (if existing treatment fails to achieve adequate glycaemic control)
▶ BY MOUTH
▸ Adult: 100 mg once daily; increased if tolerated to 300 mg once daily if required, dose to be taken preferably before breakfast

DOSE ADJUSTMENTS DUE TO INTERACTIONS
Dose of concomitant insulin or drugs that stimulate insulin secretion may need to be reduced.

> IMPORTANT SAFETY INFORMATION
> MHRA/CHM ADVICE (JUNE 2015): RISK OF DIABETIC KETOACIDOSIS WITH SODIUM-GLUCOSE CO-TRANSPORTER 2 INHIBITORS (CANAGLIFLOZIN, DAPAGLIFLOZIN OR EMPAGLIFLOZIN)
> Serious and potentially life-threatening cases of diabetic ketoacidosis (DKA) have been reported in patients taking the SGLT2 inhibitor canagliflozin for type 2 diabetes. To minimise the risk of such effects when treating patients with a SGLT2 inhibitor, the European Medicines Agency has issued the following advice:
> • Test for raised ketones in patients presenting with symptoms of DKA, even if plasma glucose levels are near-normal; omitting this test could delay diagnosis of DKA.
> • Discontinue treatment if DKA is suspected.
> • If DKA is confirmed, take appropriate measures to correct the DKA and monitor glucose levels.
> • Patients should be advised on how to recognise the signs and symptoms of DKA such as nausea, vomiting, anorexia, abdominal pain, excessive thirst, difficulty breathing, confusion, unusual fatigue, or sleepiness, and to seek prompt medical attention if symptoms of DKA develop.

- CONTRA-INDICATIONS Ketoacidosis
- CAUTIONS Cardiovascular disease (risk of hypotension) · elderly (risk of hypotension) · elevated haematocrit · history of hypotension
  CAUTIONS, FURTHER INFORMATION
  ▸ Volume depletion Correct hypovolaemia before starting treatment.
- INTERACTIONS → Appendix 1 (antidiabetics).
- SIDE-EFFECTS
▶ **Common or very common** Constipation · dyslipidaemia · genital infection · hypoglycaemia (in combination with insulin or sulfonylurea) · nausea · polyuria · raised haematocrit · thirst · urinary frequency · urinary-tract infection
▶ **Uncommon** Dehydration · dizziness · hypovolaemia · postural hypotension · raised serum creatinine · raised serum urea · rash · syncope

Endocrine system

SIDE-EFFECTS, FURTHER INFORMATION

‣ Volume depletion Consider interrupting treatment if volume depletion occurs.
● PREGNANCY Avoid—toxicity in *animal* studies.
● BREAST FEEDING Avoid—present in milk in *animal* studies.
● HEPATIC IMPAIRMENT Manufacturer advises avoid in severe impairment—no information available.
● RENAL IMPAIRMENT Reduce dose to 100 mg once daily if eGFR falls persistently below 60 mL/minute/1.73 m^2 and existing canagliflozin treatment tolerated. Avoid initiation if eGFR less than 60 mL/minute/1.73 m^2. Avoid if eGFR less than 45 mL/minute/1.73 m^2. Monitor renal function at least twice a year in moderate impairment.
● MONITORING REQUIREMENTS Determine renal function before treatment and at least annually thereafter, and before initiation of concomitant drugs that reduce renal function and periodically thereafter.
● PATIENT AND CARER ADVICE Patients should be advised to report symptoms of volume depletion including postural hypotension and dizziness. Patients should be informed of the signs and symptoms of diabetic ketoacidosis, see MHRA advice.
● NATIONAL FUNDING/ACCESS DECISIONS

NICE technology appraisals (TAs)

‣ Canagliflozin in combination therapy for treating type 2 diabetes (June 2014) NICE TA315
Canagliflozin in a dual therapy regimen in combination with metformin is recommended for the treatment of type 2 diabetes, only if a sulfonylurea is contra-indicated or not tolerated *or* the patient has a significant risk of hypoglycaemia.

Canagliflozin in a triple therapy regimen is an option for the treatment of type 2 diabetes in combination with metformin and a sulfonylurea *or* metformin and a thiazolidinedione.

Canagliflozin in combination with insulin (alone or with other antidiabetic drugs) is an option for the treatment of type 2 diabetes.

Patients currently receiving canagliflozin in a dual or triple therapy regimen that is not recommended according to the above criteria should have the option to continue treatment until they and their clinician consider it appropriate to stop.
www.nice.org.uk/TA315

Scottish Medicines Consortium (SMC) Decisions
The *Scottish Medicines Consortium* has advised (May 2014) that canagliflozin (*Invokana*®) is accepted for restricted use within NHS Scotland for the treatment of type 2 diabetes in combination with metformin as dual therapy, or in combination with metformin and standard of care as triple therapy, or in combination with insulin and standard of care. Standard of care refers to any antidiabetic drugs that are indicated to be prescribed in combination with metformin or insulin for the treatment of type 2 diabetes.

● MEDICINAL FORMS
There can be variation in the licensing of different medicines containing the same drug.
Tablet
‣ Invokana (Janssen-Cilag Ltd) ▼
  Canagliflozin (as Canagliflozin hemihydrate) 100 mg Invokana 100mg tablets | 30 tablet [PoM] £39.20 DT price = £39.20
  Canagliflozin (as Canagliflozin hemihydrate) 300 mg Invokana 300mg tablets | 30 tablet [PoM] £39.20 DT price = £39.20

Canagliflozin with metformin

The properties listed below are those particular to the combination only. For the properties of the components please consider, canagliflozin p. 633, metformin hydrochloride p. 624.

● INDICATIONS AND DOSE

Type 2 diabetes mellitus not controlled by metformin alone or by metformin in combination with insulin or other antidiabetic drugs
‣ BY MOUTH
‣ Adult: 1 tablet twice daily, dose based on patient's current metformin dose, daily dose of metformin should not exceed 2 g

DOSE ADJUSTMENTS DUE TO INTERACTIONS
Dose of concomitant insulin or drugs that stimulate insulin secretion may need to be reduced.

● RENAL IMPAIRMENT Avoid if eGFR less than 60 mL/minute/1.73 m^2.
● NATIONAL FUNDING/ACCESS DECISIONS

Scottish Medicines Consortium (SMC) Decisions
The *Scottish Medicines Consortium* has advised (December 2014) that *Vokanamet*® is accepted for restricted use within NHS Scotland in patients with type 2 diabetes mellitus for whom a combination of canagliflozin and metformin is an appropriate choice of therapy.

● MEDICINAL FORMS
There can be variation in the licensing of different medicines containing the same drug.
Tablet
CAUTIONARY AND ADVISORY LABELS 21
‣ Vokanamet (Janssen-Cilag Ltd) ▼
  Canagliflozin (as Canagliflozin hemihydrate) 50 mg, Metformin hydrochloride 850 mg Vokanamet 50mg/850mg tablets | 60 tablet [PoM] £39.20 DT price = £39.20
  Canagliflozin (as Canagliflozin hemihydrate) 50 mg, Metformin hydrochloride 1 gram Vokanamet 50mg/1000mg tablets | 60 tablet [PoM] £39.20 DT price = £39.20

Dapagliflozin

● DRUG ACTION Reversibly inhibits sodium-glucose co-transporter 2 (SGLT2) in the renal proximal convoluted tubule to reduce glucose reabsorption and increase urinary glucose excretion.

● INDICATIONS AND DOSE

Type 2 diabetes mellitus as monotherapy (if metformin inappropriate) | Type 2 diabetes mellitus in combination with insulin or other antidiabetic drugs (if existing treatment fails to achieve adequate glycaemic control)
‣ BY MOUTH
‣ Adult 18–74 years: 10 mg once daily
‣ Adult 75 years and over: Initiation not recommended

DOSE ADJUSTMENTS DUE TO INTERACTIONS
Dose of concomitant insulin or drugs that stimulate insulin secretion may need to be reduced.

IMPORTANT SAFETY INFORMATION
MHRA/CHM ADVICE (JUNE 2015): RISK OF DIABETIC KETOACIDOSIS WITH SODIUM-GLUCOSE CO-TRANSPORTER 2 INHIBITORS (CANAGLIFLOZIN, DAPAGLIFLOZIN OR EMPAGLIFLOZIN)
Serious and potentially life-threatening cases of diabetic ketoacidosis (DKA) have been reported in patients taking the SGLT2 inhibitor dapagliflozin for type 2 diabetes. To minimise the risk of such effects when treating patients with a SGLT2 inhibitor, the European Medicines Agency has issued the following advice:

- Test for raised ketones in patients presenting with symptoms of DKA, even if plasma glucose levels are near-normal; omitting this test could delay diagnosis of DKA.
- Discontinue treatment if DKA is suspected.
- If DKA is confirmed, take appropriate measures to correct the DKA and monitor glucose levels.
- Patients should be advised on how to recognise the signs and symptoms of DKA such as nausea, vomiting, anorexia, abdominal pain, excessive thirst, difficulty breathing, confusion, unusual fatigue, or sleepiness, and to seek prompt medical attention if symptoms of DKA develop.

- CONTRA-INDICATIONS Ketoacidosis
- CAUTIONS Cardiovascular disease (risk of hypotension) · elderly (risk of hypotension) · electrolyte disturbances · hypotension · raised haematocrit
  CAUTIONS, FURTHER INFORMATION
  ‣ Volume depletion Correct hypovolaemia before starting treatment.
- INTERACTIONS → Appendix 1 (antidiabetics).
- SIDE-EFFECTS
  ‣ Common or very common Back pain · constipation · dyslipidaemia · dysuria · genital infection · hypoglycaemia (in combination with insulin or sulphonylurea) · polyuria · sweating · thirst · urinary-tract infection
  ‣ Uncommon Dehydration · dizziness · hypotension · hypovolaemia · nausea · nocturia · raised serum creatinine · raised serum urea · rash
  SIDE-EFFECTS, FURTHER INFORMATION
  ‣ Volume depletion Consider interrupting treatment if volume depletion occurs.
- PREGNANCY Avoid—toxicity in *animal* studies.
- BREAST FEEDING Avoid—present in milk in *animal* studies.
- HEPATIC IMPAIRMENT Initial dose 5 mg daily in severe impairment, increased according to response.
- RENAL IMPAIRMENT Avoid if eGFR less than 60 mL/minute/1.73 m² (ineffective).
- MONITORING REQUIREMENTS Determine renal function before treatment and at least annually thereafter.
- PATIENT AND CARER ADVICE Patients should be informed of the signs and symptoms of diabetic ketoacidosis, see MHRA advice.
- NATIONAL FUNDING/ACCESS DECISIONS
  NICE technology appraisals (TAs)
  ‣ Dapagliflozin in combination therapy for treating type 2 diabetes (June 2013) NICE TA288
  Dapagliflozin in a dual therapy regimen in combination with metformin is recommended for the treatment of type 2 diabetes, only if glycaemic control is inadequate, and the patient has a significant risk of hypoglycaemia or if a sulfonylurea is contra-indicated or not tolerated.
  Dapagliflozin in combination with insulin (alone or with other antidiabetic drugs) is an option for the treatment of type 2 diabetes.
  Dapagliflozin in combination with metformin and a sulfonylurea as triple therapy is not recommended for the treatment of type 2 diabetes except as part of a clinical trial.
  Patients currently receiving dapagliflozin in a dual or triple therapy regimen that is not recommended according to the above criteria should have the option to continue treatment until they and their clinician consider it appropriate to stop.
  www.nice.org.uk/TA288
  Scottish Medicines Consortium (SMC) Decisions
  The *Scottish Medicines Consortium* has advised that dapagliflozin (*Forxiga*®) is accepted for restricted use

within NHS Scotland for the treatment of type 2 diabetes in combination with metformin, when treatment with metformin alone is inadequate and a sulfonylurea is inappropriate (December 2012), or in combination with insulin when treatment with insulin alone is inadequate (February 2014).

- MEDICINAL FORMS
  There can be variation in the licensing of different medicines containing the same drug.
  Tablet
  ‣ Forxiga (AstraZeneca UK Ltd) ▼
  Dapagliflozin 5 mg Forxiga 5mg tablets | 28 tablet [PoM] £36.59 DT price = £36.59
  Dapagliflozin 10 mg Forxiga 10mg tablets | 28 tablet [PoM] £36.59 DT price = £36.59

Dapagliflozin with metformin

The properties listed below are those particular to the combination only. For the properties of the components please consider, dapagliflozin p. 634, metformin hydrochloride p. 624.

- INDICATIONS AND DOSE

Type 2 diabetes mellitus not controlled by metformin alone or by metformin in combination with insulin or other antidiabetic drugs
  ‣ BY MOUTH
  ‣ Adult 18-74 years: 1 tablet twice daily, based on patient's current metformin dose
  ‣ Adult 75 years and over: Initiation not recommended

- INTERACTIONS Dose of concomitant insulin or drugs that stimulate insulin secretion may need to be reduced.
- HEPATIC IMPAIRMENT Avoid.
- NATIONAL FUNDING/ACCESS DECISIONS
  Scottish Medicines Consortium (SMC) Decisions
  The *Scottish Medicines Consortium* has advised (July 2014) that dapagliflozin plus metformin (*Xigduo*®) is accepted for restricted use within NHS Scotland in patients for whom a combination of dapagliflozin and metformin is an appropriate choice of therapy i.e when metformin alone does not provide adequate glycaemic control and a sulfonylurea is inappropriate, *or* in combination with insulin, when insulin and metformin does not provide adequate control, *or* in combination with a sulphonylurea, when a sulfonylurea and metformin does not provide adequate control.

- MEDICINAL FORMS
  There can be variation in the licensing of different medicines containing the same drug.
  Tablet
  CAUTIONARY AND ADVISORY LABELS 21
  ‣ Xigduo (AstraZeneca UK Ltd) ▼
  Dapagliflozin 5 mg, Metformin hydrochloride 850 mg Xigduo 5mg/850mg tablets | 56 tablet [PoM] £36.59 DT price = £36.59
  Dapagliflozin 5 mg, Metformin hydrochloride 1 gram Xigduo 5mg/1000mg tablets | 56 tablet [PoM] £36.59 DT price = £36.59

6

Endocrine system

Empagliflozin

- **DRUG ACTION** Reversibly inhibits sodium-glucose co-transporter 2 (SGLT2) in the renal proximal convoluted tubule to reduce glucose reabsorption and increase urinary glucose excretion.

- **INDICATIONS AND DOSE**

Type 2 diabetes mellitus as monotherapy (if metformin inappropriate) | Type 2 diabetes mellitus in combination with insulin or other antidiabetic drugs (if existing treatment fails to achieve adequate glycaemic control)
  - ▸ BY MOUTH
  - ▸ Adult 18–84 years: 10 mg once daily, increased to 25 mg once daily if necessary and if tolerated
  - ▸ Adult 85 years and over: Initiation not recommended
  DOSE ADJUSTMENTS DUE TO INTERACTIONS
  Dose of concomitant insulin or drugs that stimulate insulin secretion may need to be reduced.

IMPORTANT SAFETY INFORMATION

MHRA/CHM ADVICE (JUNE 2015): RISK OF DIABETIC KETOACIDOSIS WITH SODIUM-GLUCOSE CO-TRANSPORTER 2 INHIBITORS (CANAGLIFLOZIN, DAPAGLIFLOZIN OR EMPAGLIFLOZIN)
Serious and potentially life-threatening cases of diabetic ketoacidosis (DKA) have been reported in patients taking the SGLT2 inhibitor empagliflozin for type 2 diabetes. To minimise the risk of such effects when treating patients with a SGLT2 inhibitor, the European Medicines Agency has issued the following advice:
- Test for raised ketones in patients presenting with symptoms of DKA, even if plasma glucose levels are near-normal; omitting this test could delay diagnosis of DKA.
- Discontinue treatment if DKA is suspected.
- If DKA is confirmed, take appropriate measures to correct the DKA and monitor glucose levels.
- Patients should be advised on how to recognise the signs and symptoms of DKA such as nausea, vomiting, anorexia, abdominal pain, excessive thirst, difficulty breathing, confusion, unusual fatigue, or sleepiness, and to seek prompt medical attention if symptoms of DKA develop.

- **CONTRA-INDICATIONS** Diabetic ketoacidosis

- **CAUTIONS** Cardiovascular disease (increased risk of volume depletion) · complicated urinary tract infections—consider temporarily interrupting treatment · concomitant antihypertensive therapy (increased risk of volume depletion) · elderly patients aged over 75 years (increased risk of volume depletion) · heart failure · history of hypotension (increased risk of volume depletion) · patients at increased risk of volume depletion · predisposition to fluid disturbances e.g. gastro-intestinal illness, concomitant use of diuretics (increased risk of volume depletion)
  CAUTIONS, FURTHER INFORMATION
  - ▸ Volume depletion Correct hypovolaemia before starting treatment. Consider interrupting treatment if volume depletion occurs.

- **INTERACTIONS** → Appendix 1 (antidiabetics).

- **SIDE-EFFECTS**
  - ▸ **Common or very common** Genital infection · hypoglycaemia (in combination with insulin or sulfonylurea) · polyuria · pruritus · urinary tract infection
  - ▸ **Uncommon** Dysuria · volume depletion

- **PREGNANCY** Manufacturer advises avoid—toxicity in *animal* studies.

- **BREAST FEEDING** Manufacturer advises avoid—present in milk in *animal* studies.

- **HEPATIC IMPAIRMENT** Manufacturer advises avoid in severe impairment—no information available.

- **RENAL IMPAIRMENT** Reduce dose to 10 mg once daily if eGFR falls persistently below 60 mL/minute/1.73 m². Avoid initiation if eGFR below 60 mL/minute/1.73 m². Avoid if eGFR is persistently below 45 mL/minute/1.73 m².

- **MONITORING REQUIREMENTS** Determine renal function before treatment and before initiation of concomitant drugs that may reduce renal function, then at least annually thereafter.

- **PATIENT AND CARER ADVICE** Patients should be informed of the signs and symptoms of diabetic ketoacidosis, see MHRA advice.

- **NATIONAL FUNDING/ACCESS DECISIONS**
  NICE technology appraisals (TAs)
  - ▸ **Empagliflozin in combination therapy for treating type 2 diabetes (March 2015)** NICE TA336
  Empagliflozin in a dual therapy regimen in combination with metformin is an option for the treatment of type 2 diabetes, only if:
    - a sulfonylurea is contra-indicated or not tolerated, **or**
    - the patient is at significant risk of hypoglycaemia or its consequences.
  Empagliflozin in a triple therapy regimen is an option for the treatment of type 2 diabetes in combination with:
    - metformin and a sulfonylurea **or**
    - metformin and a thiazolidinedione.
  Empagliflozin in combination with insulin with or without other antidiabetic drugs is an option for the treatment of type 2 diabetes.
    Patients currently receiving empagliflozin whose disease does not meet the above criteria should have the option to continue treatment until they and their clinician consider it appropriate to stop.
  www.nice.org.uk/TA336

- **MEDICINAL FORMS**
  There can be variation in the licensing of different medicines containing the same drug.
  Tablet
  - ▸ Jardiance (Boehringer Ingelheim Ltd) ▼
    Empagliflozin 10 mg Jardiance 10mg tablets | 28 tablet [PoM]
    £36.59 DT price = £36.59
    Empagliflozin 25 mg Jardiance 25mg tablets | 28 tablet [PoM]
    £36.59 DT price = £36.59

Empagliflozin with metformin

25.4.2016

The properties listed below are those particular to the combination only. For the properties of the components please consider, empagliflozin above, metformin hydrochloride p. 624.

- **INDICATIONS AND DOSE**

Type 2 diabetes mellitus not controlled by metformin alone or by metformin in combination with other antidiabetic drugs or insulin
  - ▸ BY MOUTH
  - ▸ Adult 18–84 years: 5/850–5/1000 mg twice daily, based on patient's current metformin dose, increased if necessary to 12.5/850–12.5/1000 mg twice daily
  - ▸ BY MOUTH
  - ▸ Adult 85 years and over: Initiation not recommended
  DOSE ADJUSTMENTS DUE TO INTERACTIONS
  Dose of concomitant insulin or drugs that stimulate insulin secretion may need to be reduced.
  DOSE EQUIVALENCE AND CONVERSION
  The proportions are expressed in the form "x"/"y" where "x" and "y" are the strengths in milligrams of empagliflozin and metformin respectively.

● NATIONAL FUNDING/ACCESS DECISIONS
Scottish Medicines Consortium (SMC) Decisions
The *Scottish Medicines Consortium* has advised (October 2015) that *Synjardy*® (empagliflozin with metformin) is accepted for restricted use within NHS Scotland in patients for whom a fixed dose combination of empagliflozin and metformin is an appropriate choice of therapy *or* when use of a sulfonylurea is considered inappropriate.

● MEDICINAL FORMS
There can be variation in the licensing of different medicines containing the same drug.
Tablet
CAUTIONARY AND ADVISORY LABELS 21
  ▸ Synjardy (Boehringer Ingelheim Ltd) ▼
    Empagliflozin 12.5 mg, Metformin hydrochloride 850 mg Synjardy 12.5mg/850mg tablets | 56 tablet PoM £36.59
    Empagliflozin 5 mg, Metformin hydrochloride 850 mg Synjardy 5mg/850mg tablets | 56 tablet PoM £36.59
    Empagliflozin 12.5 mg, Metformin hydrochloride 1 gram Synjardy 12.5mg/1000mg tablets | 56 tablet PoM £36.59
    Empagliflozin 5 mg, Metformin hydrochloride 1 gram Synjardy 5mg/1000mg tablets | 56 tablet PoM £36.59

BLOOD GLUCOSE LOWERING DRUGS ⟩
SULFONYLUREAS

Sulfonylureas

● DRUG ACTION The sulfonylureas act mainly by augmenting insulin secretion and consequently are effective only when some residual pancreatic beta-cell activity is present; during long-term administration they also have an extrapancreatic action.

● CONTRA-INDICATIONS Presence of ketoacidosis
● CAUTIONS Can encourage weight gain (should be prescribed only if poor control and symptoms persist despite adequate attempts at dieting) · elderly · G6PD deficiency
● SIDE-EFFECTS
▸ **Uncommon** Hypoglycaemia
▸ **Rare** Agranulocytosis · aplastic anaemia · blood disorders · cholestatic jaundice · haemolytic anaemia · hepatic failure · hepatitis · leucopenia · pancytopenia · thrombocytopenia
▸ **Frequency not known** Allergic skin reactions (usually in the first 6–8 weeks of therapy) · constipation · diarrhoea · disturbance in liver function · erythema multiforme (usually in the first 6–8 weeks of therapy) · exfoliative dermatitis (usually in the first 6–8 weeks of therapy) · fever (usually in the first 6–8 weeks of therapy) · gastro-intestinal disturbances · hypersensitivity reactions (usually in the first 6–8 weeks of therapy) · jaundice (usually in the first 6–8 weeks of therapy) · nausea · vomiting

SIDE-EFFECTS, FURTHER INFORMATION
▸ Hypoglycaemia This is uncommon and usually indicates excessive dosage. Sulfonylurea-induced hypoglycaemia may persist for many hours and must always be treated in hospital.

● HEPATIC IMPAIRMENT Sulfonylureas should be avoided or a reduced dose should be used in severe hepatic impairment, because there is an increased risk of hypoglycaemia. Jaundice may occur.
● RENAL IMPAIRMENT Sulfonylureas should be used with care in those with mild to moderate renal impairment, because of the hazard of hypoglycaemia. Care is required to use the lowest dose that adequately controls blood glucose. Avoid where possible in severe renal impairment.
● PATIENT AND CARER ADVICE
Driving and skilled tasks
Driving Drivers need to be particularly careful to avoid hypoglycaemia and should be warned of the problems.

The risk of hypoglycaemia associated with sulfonylureas should be discussed with the patient, especially when concomitant glucose-lowering drugs are prescribed.

↗ above

Glibenclamide

● INDICATIONS AND DOSE
Type 2 diabetes mellitus
▸ BY MOUTH
▸ Adult: Initially 5 mg daily, adjusted according to response, dose to be taken with or immediately after breakfast; maximum 15 mg per day

● UNLICENSED USE Not licensed for use in breast feeding women with pre-existing diabetes. Not licensed for use in gestational diabetes.
● CONTRA-INDICATIONS Avoid where possible in Acute porphyrias p. 918
● INTERACTIONS → Appendix 1 (antidiabetics).
● PREGNANCY The use of sulfonylureas in pregnancy should generally be avoided because of the risk of neonatal hypoglycaemia; however, glibenclamide can be used during the second and third trimesters of pregnancy in women with gestational diabetes.
● BREAST FEEDING Glibenclamide can be used during breast-feeding in women with pre-existing diabetes.

● MEDICINAL FORMS
There can be variation in the licensing of different medicines containing the same drug. Forms available from special-order manufacturers include: oral suspension, oral solution
Tablet
  ▸ Glibenclamide (Non-proprietary)
    Glibenclamide 2.5 mg Glibenclamide 2.5mg tablets | 28 tablet PoM £7.21 DT price = £6.95
    Glibenclamide 5 mg Glibenclamide 5mg tablets | 28 tablet PoM £19.99 DT price = £0.85

↗ above

Gliclazide

● INDICATIONS AND DOSE
Type 2 diabetes mellitus
▸ BY MOUTH USING IMMEDIATE-RELEASE MEDICINES
▸ Adult: Initially 40–80 mg daily, adjusted according to response, increased if necessary up to 160 mg once daily, dose to be taken with breakfast, doses higher than 160 mg to be given in divided doses; maximum 320 mg per day
▸ BY MOUTH USING MODIFIED-RELEASE MEDICINES
▸ Adult: Initially 30 mg daily, dose to be taken with breakfast, adjust dose according to response every 4 weeks (after 2 weeks if no decrease in blood glucose); maximum 120 mg per day

DOSE EQUIVALENCE AND CONVERSION
Gliclazide modified release 30 mg may be considered to be approximately equivalent in therapeutic effect to standard formulation gliclazide 80 mg.

● CONTRA-INDICATIONS Avoid where possible in Acute porphyrias p. 918
● INTERACTIONS → Appendix 1 (antidiabetics).
● PREGNANCY The use of sulfonylureas in pregnancy should generally be avoided because of the risk of neonatal hypoglycaemia.
● BREAST FEEDING Avoid—theoretical possibility of hypoglycaemia in the infant.
● RENAL IMPAIRMENT If necessary, gliclazide which is principally metabolised in the liver, can be used in renal impairment but careful monitoring of blood-glucose concentration is essential.

Endocrine system

6

● MEDICINAL FORMS
There can be variation in the licensing of different medicines containing the same drug. Forms available from special-order manufacturers include: oral suspension

Tablet
▸ Gliclazide (Non-proprietary)
Gliclazide 40 mg Gliclazide 40mg tablets | 28 tablet [PoM] £3.66 DT price = £3.36
Gliclazide 80 mg Gliclazide 80mg tablets | 28 tablet [PoM] £12.74 DT price = £0.85 | 60 tablet [PoM] £19.85
▸ Diamicron (Servier Laboratories Ltd)
Gliclazide 80 mg Diamicron 80mg tablets | 60 tablet [PoM] £4.38
▸ Zicron (Bristol Laboratories Ltd)
Gliclazide 40 mg Zicron 40mg tablets | 28 tablet [PoM] £3.36 DT price = £3.36

Modified-release tablet
CAUTIONARY AND ADVISORY LABELS 25
▸ Gliclazide (Non-proprietary)
Gliclazide 30 mg Gliclazide 30mg modified-release tablets | 28 tablet [PoM] £4.00 DT price = £2.81 | 56 tablet [PoM] £8.00
▸ Bilxona (Actavis UK Ltd)
Gliclazide 30 mg Bilxona 30mg modified-release tablets | 28 tablet [PoM] £1.63 DT price = £2.81 | 56 tablet [PoM] £3.27
Gliclazide 60 mg Bilxona 60mg modified-release tablets | 28 tablet [PoM] £3.27 DT price = £4.77 | 56 tablet [PoM] £6.55
▸ Dacadis MR (Mylan Ltd)
Gliclazide 30 mg Dacadis MR 30mg tablets | 28 tablet [PoM] £2.81 DT price = £2.81 | 56 tablet [PoM] £5.62
▸ Diamicron MR (Servier Laboratories Ltd)
Gliclazide 30 mg Diamicron 30mg MR tablets | 28 tablet [PoM] £2.81 DT price = £2.81 | 56 tablet [PoM] £5.62
▸ Edicil MR (Teva UK Ltd)
Gliclazide 30 mg Edicil MR 30mg tablets | 28 tablet [PoM] £2.62 DT price = £2.81 | 56 tablet [PoM] £5.24
▸ Laaglyda MR (Consilient Health Ltd)
Gliclazide 60 mg Laaglyda MR 60mg tablets | 28 tablet [PoM] £4.77 DT price = £4.77
▸ Nazdol MR (Consilient Health Ltd)
Gliclazide 30 mg Nazdol MR 30mg tablets | 28 tablet [PoM] £2.35 DT price = £2.81 | 56 tablet [PoM] £4.92
▸ Vamju (AMCo)
Gliclazide 30 mg Vamju 30mg modified-release tablets | 28 tablet [PoM] £1.64 DT price = £2.81 | 56 tablet [PoM] £3.28
Gliclazide 60 mg Vamju 60mg modified-release tablets | 28 tablet [PoM] £3.28 DT price = £4.77
▸ Ziclaseg (Lupin (Europe) Ltd)
Gliclazide 30 mg Ziclaseg 30mg modified-release tablets | 28 tablet [PoM] £2.38 DT price = £2.81 | 56 tablet [PoM] £4.77

◀ 637

Glimepiride

● INDICATIONS AND DOSE
Type 2 diabetes mellitus
▸ BY MOUTH
▸ Adult: Initially 1 mg daily, adjusted according to response, then increased in steps of 1 mg every 1–2 weeks, increased to 4 mg daily, dose to be taken shortly before or with first main meal, the daily dose may be increased further, in exceptional circumstances; maximum 6 mg per day

● CAUTIONS
CAUTIONS, FURTHER INFORMATION
▸ Porphyria Sulfonylureas should be avoided where possible in Acute porphyrias p. 918 but glimepiride is thought to be safe.
● INTERACTIONS → Appendix 1 (antidiabetics).
● SIDE-EFFECTS Hyponatraemia
● PREGNANCY The use of sulfonylureas in pregnancy should generally be avoided because of the risk of neonatal hypoglycaemia.
● BREAST FEEDING Avoid—theoretical possibility of hypoglycaemia in the infant.

● MONITORING REQUIREMENTS Manufacturer recommends regular hepatic and haematological monitoring but limited evidence of clinical value.

● MEDICINAL FORMS
There can be variation in the licensing of different medicines containing the same drug. Forms available from special-order manufacturers include: oral suspension, oral solution

Tablet
▸ Glimepiride (Non-proprietary)
Glimepiride 1 mg Glimepiride 1mg tablets | 30 tablet [PoM] £4.33 DT price = £0.85
Glimepiride 2 mg Glimepiride 2mg tablets | 30 tablet [PoM] £7.13 DT price = £1.76
Glimepiride 3 mg Glimepiride 3mg tablets | 30 tablet [PoM] £10.75 DT price = £0.92
Glimepiride 4 mg Glimepiride 4mg tablets | 30 tablet [PoM] £14.24 DT price = £1.06
▸ Amaryl (Zentiva)
Glimepiride 3 mg Amaryl 3mg tablets | 30 tablet [PoM] £10.75 DT price = £0.92

◀ 637

Glipizide

● INDICATIONS AND DOSE
Type 2 diabetes mellitus
▸ BY MOUTH
▸ Adult: Initially 2.5–5 mg daily, adjusted according to response, dose to be taken shortly before breakfast or lunch, doses up to 15 mg may be given as a single dose, higher doses to be given in divided doses; maximum 20 mg per day

● CAUTIONS
CAUTIONS, FURTHER INFORMATION
▸ Porphyria Sulfonylureas should be avoided where possible in Acute porphyrias p. 918 but glipizide is thought to be safe.
● INTERACTIONS → Appendix 1 (antidiabetics).
● SIDE-EFFECTS
▸ **Rare** Photosensitivity
▸ **Frequency not known** Dizziness · drowsiness · hyponatraemia
● PREGNANCY The use of sulfonylureas in pregnancy should generally be avoided because of the risk of neonatal hypoglycaemia.
● BREAST FEEDING Avoid—theoretical possibility of hypoglycaemia in the infant.
● HEPATIC IMPAIRMENT Avoid if the patient has both renal and hepatic impairment.
● RENAL IMPAIRMENT Avoid if the patient has both renal and hepatic impairment.

● MEDICINAL FORMS
There can be variation in the licensing of different medicines containing the same drug.

Tablet
▸ Glipizide (Non-proprietary)
Glipizide 5 mg Glipizide 5mg tablets | 28 tablet [PoM] £2.61 DT price = £2.36 | 56 tablet [PoM] £13.44
▸ Minodiab (Pfizer Ltd)
Glipizide 5 mg Minodiab 5mg tablets | 28 tablet [PoM] £1.26 DT price = £2.36

Tolbutamide

- **INDICATIONS AND DOSE**

Type 2 diabetes mellitus
▶ BY MOUTH
▶ Adult: 0.5–1.5 g daily in divided doses, dose to be taken with or immediately after meals, alternatively 0.5–1.5 g once daily, dose to be taken with or immediately after breakfast; maximum 2 g per day

- **CONTRA-INDICATIONS** Avoid where possible in Acute porphyrias p. 918
- **INTERACTIONS** → Appendix 1 (antidiabetics).
- **SIDE-EFFECTS** Headache · tinnitus
- **PREGNANCY** The use of sulfonylureas in pregnancy should generally be avoided because of the risk of neonatal hypoglycaemia.
- **BREAST FEEDING** The use of sulfonylureas in breast-feeding should be avoided because there is a theoretical possibility of hypoglycaemia in the infant.
- **RENAL IMPAIRMENT** If necessary, the short-acting drug tolbutamide can be used in renal impairment but careful monitoring of blood-glucose concentration is essential.

- **MEDICINAL FORMS**
There can be variation in the licensing of different medicines containing the same drug. Forms available from special-order manufacturers include: oral suspension

Tablet
▶ Tolbutamide (Non-proprietary)
Tolbutamide 500 mg Tolbutamide 500mg tablets | 28 tablet [PoM] £42.50 DT price = £11.12 | 112 tablet [PoM] £57.28

BLOOD GLUCOSE LOWERING DRUGS ›
THIAZOLIDINEDIONES

Pioglitazone

- **DRUG ACTION** The thiazolidinedione, pioglitazone, reduces peripheral insulin resistance, leading to a reduction of blood-glucose concentration.

- **INDICATIONS AND DOSE**

Type 2 diabetes mellitus (alone or combined with metformin or a sulfonylurea, or with both, or with insulin)
▶ BY MOUTH
▶ Adult: Initially 15–30 mg once daily, adjusted according to response to 45 mg once daily, in elderly patients, initiate with lowest possible dose and increase gradually; review treatment after 3–6 months and regularly thereafter

DOSE ADJUSTMENTS DUE TO INTERACTIONS
Dose of concomitant sulfonylurea or insulin may need to be reduced.

IMPORTANT SAFETY INFORMATION
MHRA/CHM ADVICE: PIOGLITAZONE CARDIOVASCULAR SAFETY (DECEMBER 2007 AND JANUARY 2011)
Incidence of heart failure is increased when pioglitazone is combined with insulin especially in patients with predisposing factors e.g. previous myocardial infarction. Patients who take pioglitazone should be closely monitored for signs of heart failure; treatment should be discontinued if any deterioration in cardiac status occurs.
Pioglitazone should not be used in patients with heart failure or a history of heart failure.

PIOGLITAZONE: RISK OF BLADDER CANCER (JULY 2011)
The European Medicines Agency has advised that there is a small increased risk of bladder cancer associated with pioglitazone use. However, in patients who respond adequately to treatment, the benefits of pioglitazone continue to outweigh the risks.
Pioglitazone should not be used in patients with active bladder cancer or a past history of bladder cancer, or in those who have uninvestigated macroscopic haematuria. Pioglitazone should be used with caution in elderly patients as the risk of bladder cancer increases with age.
Before initiating treatment with pioglitazone, patients should be assessed for risk factors of bladder cancer (including age, smoking status, exposure to certain occupational or chemotherapy agents, or previous radiation therapy to the pelvic region) and any macroscopic haematuria should be investigated. The safety and efficacy of pioglitazone should be reviewed after 3–6 months and pioglitazone should be stopped in patients who do not respond adequately to treatment.
Patients already receiving treatment with pioglitazone should be assessed for risk factors of bladder cancer and treatment should be reviewed after 3–6 months, as above.
Patients should be advised to report promptly any haematuria, dysuria, or urinary urgency during treatment.

- **CONTRA-INDICATIONS** History of heart failure · previous or active bladder cancer · uninvestigated macroscopic haematuria
- **CAUTIONS** Avoid in Acute porphyrias p. 918 · cardiovascular disease or in combination with insulin (risk of heart failure) · elderly (increased risk of heart failure, fractures, and bladder cancer) · increased risk of bone fractures, particularly in women · risk factors for bladder cancer
CAUTIONS, FURTHER INFORMATION
Substitute insulin during peri-operative period (omit pioglitazone on morning of surgery and recommence when eating and drinking normally).
- **INTERACTIONS** → Appendix 1 (antidiabetics).
- **SIDE-EFFECTS**
▶ **Common or very common** Anaemia · arthralgia · dizziness · gastro-intestinal disturbances · haematuria · headache · hypoaesthesia · impotence · oedema · vertigo · visual disturbances · weight gain
▶ **Uncommon** Altered blood lipids · bladder cancer · fatigue · hypoglycaemia · insomnia · proteinuria · sweating
▶ **Rare** Liver dysfunction
SIDE-EFFECTS, FURTHER INFORMATION
▶ Liver toxicity Rare reports of liver dysfunction; discontinue if jaundice occurs.
- **PREGNANCY** Avoid—toxicity in *animal* studies.
- **BREAST FEEDING** Avoid—present in milk in *animal* studies.
- **HEPATIC IMPAIRMENT** Avoid.
- **MONITORING REQUIREMENTS** Monitor liver function before treatment and periodically thereafter.
- **PATIENT AND CARER ADVICE**
Liver toxicity Patients should be advised to seek immediate medical attention if symptoms such as nausea, vomiting, abdominal pain, fatigue and dark urine develop.
- **NATIONAL FUNDING/ACCESS DECISIONS**
Scottish Medicines Consortium (SMC) Decisions
The *Scottish Medicines Consortium* accepts use of pioglitazone (February 2007) with metformin and a sulfonylurea, for patients (especially if overweight) whose glycaemic control is inadequate despite the use of 2 oral hypoglycaemic drugs and who are unable or unwilling to

take insulin; treatment should be initiated and monitored by an experienced diabetes physician.

- MEDICINAL FORMS

There can be variation in the licensing of different medicines containing the same drug. Forms available from special-order manufacturers include: oral suspension

Tablet

‣ Pioglitazone (Non-proprietary)

Pioglitazone (as Pioglitazone hydrochloride) 15 mg Pioglitazone 15mg tablets | 28 tablet [PoM] £25.83 DT price = £10.12
Pioglitazone (as Pioglitazone hydrochloride) 30 mg Pioglitazone 30mg tablets | 28 tablet [PoM] £35.89 DT price = £9.90
Pioglitazone (as Pioglitazone hydrochloride) 45 mg Pioglitazone 45mg tablets | 28 tablet [PoM] £39.55 DT price = £30.46

‣ Actos (Takeda UK Ltd)

Pioglitazone (as Pioglitazone hydrochloride) 15 mg Actos 15mg tablets | 28 tablet [PoM] £25.83 DT price = £10.12
Pioglitazone (as Pioglitazone hydrochloride) 30 mg Actos 30mg tablets | 28 tablet [PoM] £35.89 DT price = £9.90
Pioglitazone (as Pioglitazone hydrochloride) 45 mg Actos 45mg tablets | 28 tablet [PoM] £39.55 DT price = £30.46

‣ Diabiom (Tillomed Laboratories Ltd)

Pioglitazone (as Pioglitazone hydrochloride) 15 mg Diabiom 15mg tablets | 28 tablet [PoM] £26.00 DT price = £10.12
Pioglitazone (as Pioglitazone hydrochloride) 30 mg Diabiom 30mg tablets | 28 tablet [PoM] £36.00 DT price = £9.90
Pioglitazone (as Pioglitazone hydrochloride) 45 mg Diabiom 45mg tablets | 28 tablet [PoM] £40.00 DT price = £30.46

‣ Glidipion (Actavis UK Ltd)

Pioglitazone (as Pioglitazone hydrochloride) 15 mg Glidipion 15mg tablets | 28 tablet [PoM] £25.83 DT price = £10.12
Pioglitazone (as Pioglitazone hydrochloride) 30 mg Glidipion 30mg tablets | 28 tablet [PoM] £35.89 DT price = £9.90
Pioglitazone (as Pioglitazone hydrochloride) 45 mg Glidipion 45mg tablets | 28 tablet [PoM] £39.55 DT price = £30.46

Pioglitazone with metformin

The properties listed below are those particular to the combination only. For the properties of the components please consider, pioglitazone p. 639, metformin hydrochloride p. 624.

- INDICATIONS AND DOSE

Type 2 diabetes not controlled by metformin alone
▶ BY MOUTH
▶ Adult: 1 tablet twice daily, titration with the individual components (pioglitazone and metformin) desirable before initiation

- MEDICINAL FORMS

There can be variation in the licensing of different medicines containing the same drug.

Tablet
CAUTIONARY AND ADVISORY LABELS 21
▶ Competact (Takeda UK Ltd)

Pioglitazone (as Pioglitazone hydrochloride) 15 mg, Metformin hydrochloride 850 mg Competact 15mg/850mg tablets | 56 tablet [PoM] £35.89 DT price = £35.89

INSULINS

Insulins ⚑

- SIDE-EFFECTS
▶ **Common or very common** Fat hypertrophy at injection site · local reactions at injection site · transient oedema
▶ **Rare** Hypersensitivity reactions · rash · urticaria

Overdose
Overdose causes hypoglycaemia.

- PREGNANCY During pregnancy, insulin requirements may alter and doses should be assessed frequently by an experienced diabetes physician. The dose of insulin

generally needs to be increased in the second and third trimesters of pregnancy.

- BREAST FEEDING

During breast-feeding, insulin requirements may alter and doses should be assessed frequently by an experienced diabetes physician.

- HEPATIC IMPAIRMENT Insulin requirements may be decreased in patients with hepatic impairment.

- RENAL IMPAIRMENT Insulin requirements may decrease in patients with renal impairment and therefore dose reduction may be necessary. The compensatory response to hypoglycaemia is impaired in renal impairment.

- MONITORING REQUIREMENTS
▶ Many patients now monitor their own blood-glucose concentrations; all carers and children need to be trained to do this.
▶ Since blood-glucose concentration varies substantially throughout the day, 'normoglycaemia' cannot always be achieved throughout a 24-hour period without causing damaging hypoglycaemia.
▶ In adults It is therefore best to recommend that patients should maintain a blood-glucose concentration of between 4 and 9 mmol/litre for most of the time (4–7 mmol/litre before meals and less than 9 mmol/litre after meals).
▶ In children It is therefore best to recommend that children should maintain a blood-glucose concentration of between 4 and 10 mmol/litre for most of the time (4–8 mmol/litre before meals and less than 10 mmol/litre after meals).

While accepting that on occasions, for brief periods, the blood-glucose concentration will be above these values; strenuous efforts should be made to prevent it from falling below 4 mmol/litre. Patients using multiple injection regimens should understand how to adjust their insulin dose according to their carbohydrate intake. With fixed-dose insulin regimens, the carbohydrate intake needs to be regulated, and should be distributed throughout the day to match the insulin regimen. The intake of energy and of simple and complex carbohydrates should be adequate to allow normal growth and development but obesity must be avoided.

- DIRECTIONS FOR ADMINISTRATION Insulin is generally given by *subcutaneous injection*; the injection site should be rotated to prevent lipodystrophy. Injection devices ('pens'), which hold the insulin in a cartridge and meter the required dose, are convenient to use. Insulin syringes (for use with needles) are required for insulins not available in cartridge form, but are less popular with children and carers. For intensive insulin regimens multiple subcutaneous injections (3 or more times daily) are usually recommended.

- PRESCRIBING AND DISPENSING INFORMATION

Units The word 'unit' should **not** be abbreviated.
Show container to patient or carer and confirm the expected version is dispensed.

- PATIENT AND CARER ADVICE

Driving and skilled tasks
Driving Drivers need to be particularly careful to avoid hypoglycaemia and should be warned of the problems.
Insulin Passport Insulin Passports and patient information booklets should be offered to patients receiving insulin. The Insulin Passport provides a record of the patient's current insulin preparations and contains a section for emergency information. The patient information booklet provides advice on the safe use of insulin. They are available for purchase from:

3M Security Print and Systems Limited
Gorse Street, Chadderton
Oldham
OL9 9QH
Tel: 0845 610 1112

GP practices can obtain supplies through their Local Area Team stores.

NHS Trusts can order supplies from www.nhsforms.co.uk or by emailing nhsforms@mmm.com. Further information is available at www.npsa.nhs.uk.

Hypoglycaemia Hypoglycaemia is a potential problem with insulin therapy. All patients must be carefully instructed on how to avoid it; this involves appropriate adjustment of insulin type, dose and frequency together with suitable timing and quantity of meals and snacks.

INSULINS > INTERMEDIATE-ACTING

F 640

Biphasic isophane insulin

(Biphasic Isophane Insulin Injection— intermediate acting)

● **INDICATIONS AND DOSE**

Diabetes mellitus
▸ BY SUBCUTANEOUS INJECTION
▸ Child: According to requirements
▸ Adult: According to requirements

● INTERACTIONS → Appendix 1 (antidiabetics).

● SIDE-EFFECTS Protamine may cause allergic reactions

● PRESCRIBING AND DISPENSING INFORMATION A sterile buffered suspension of either porcine or human insulin complexed with protamine sulfate (or another suitable protamine) in a solution of insulin of the same species.

Check product container—the proportions of the two components should be checked carefully (the order in which the proportions are stated may not be the same in other countries).

● MEDICINAL FORMS
There can be variation in the licensing of different medicines containing the same drug.

Suspension for injection
▸ Humulin M3 (Eli Lilly and Company Ltd)
Insulin human (as Insulin soluble human) 30 unit per 1 ml, Insulin human (as Insulin isophane human) 70 unit per 1 ml Humulin M3 100units/ml suspension for injection 3ml cartridges | 5 cartridge [PoM] £19.08
Humulin M3 100units/ml suspension for injection 10ml vials | 1 vial [PoM] £15.68
▸ Humulin M3 KwikPen (Eli Lilly and Company Ltd)
Insulin human (as Insulin soluble human) 30 unit per 1 ml, Insulin human (as Insulin isophane human) 70 unit per 1 ml Humulin M3 KwikPen 100units/ml suspension for injection 3ml pre-filled pen | 5 pre-filled disposable injection [PoM] £21.70
▸ Hypurin Porcine 30/70 Mix (Wockhardt UK Ltd)
Insulin porcine (as Insulin soluble porcine) 30 unit per 1 ml, Insulin porcine (as Insulin isophane porcine) 70 unit per 1 ml Hypurin Porcine 30/70 Mix 100units/ml suspension for injection 3ml cartridges | 5 cartridge [PoM] £37.80
Hypurin Porcine 30/70 Mix 100units/ml suspension for injection 10ml vials | 1 vial [PoM] £25.20
▸ Insuman Comb 15 (Sanofi)
Insulin human (as Insulin soluble human) 15 unit per 1 ml, Insulin human (as Insulin isophane human) 85 unit per 1 ml Insuman Comb 15 100units/ml suspension for injection 3ml cartridges | 5 cartridge [PoM] £17.50
▸ Insuman Comb 25 (Sanofi)
Insulin human (as Insulin soluble human) 25 unit per 1 ml, Insulin human (as Insulin isophane human) 75 unit per 1 ml Insuman Comb 25 100units/ml suspension for injection 5ml vials | 1 vial [PoM] £5.61
Insuman Comb 25 100units/ml suspension for injection 3ml cartridges | 5 cartridge [PoM] £17.50
▸ Insuman Comb 25 SoloStar (Sanofi)
Insulin human (as Insulin soluble human) 25 unit per 1 ml, Insulin human (as Insulin isophane human) 75 unit per 1 ml Insuman Comb 25 100units/ml suspension for injection 3ml pre-filled SoloStar pen | 5 pre-filled disposable injection [PoM] £19.80

▸ Insuman Comb 50 (Sanofi)
Insulin human (as Insulin isophane human) 50 unit per 1 ml, Insulin human (as Insulin soluble human) 50 unit per 1 ml Insuman Comb 50 100units/ml suspension for injection 3ml cartridges | 5 cartridge [PoM] £17.50

F 640

Isophane insulin

(Isophane Insulin Injection; Isophane Protamine Insulin Injection; Isophane Insulin (NPH)— intermediate acting)

● **INDICATIONS AND DOSE**

Diabetes mellitus
▸ BY SUBCUTANEOUS INJECTION
▸ Child: According to requirements
▸ Adult: According to requirements

● INTERACTIONS → Appendix 1 (antidiabetics).

● SIDE-EFFECTS Protamine may cause allergic reactions

● PREGNANCY Recommended where longer-acting insulins are needed.

● PRESCRIBING AND DISPENSING INFORMATION A sterile suspension of bovine or porcine insulin or of human insulin in the form of a complex obtained by the addition of protamine sulfate or another suitable protamine.

● MEDICINAL FORMS
There can be variation in the licensing of different medicines containing the same drug.

Suspension for injection
▸ Humulin I (Eli Lilly and Company Ltd)
Insulin human (as Insulin isophane human) 100 unit per 1 ml Humulin I 100units/ml suspension for injection 10ml vials | 1 vial [PoM] £15.68
Humulin I 100units/ml suspension for injection 3ml cartridges | 5 cartridge [PoM] £19.08
▸ Humulin I KwikPen (Eli Lilly and Company Ltd)
Insulin human (as Insulin isophane human) 100 unit per 1 ml Humulin I KwikPen 100units/ml suspension for injection 3ml pre-filled pen | 5 pre-filled disposable injection [PoM] £21.70
▸ Hypurin Bovine Isophane (Wockhardt UK Ltd)
Insulin bovine (as Insulin isophane bovine) 100 unit per 1 ml Hypurin Bovine Isophane 100units/ml suspension for injection 10ml vials | 1 vial [PoM] £27.72
Hypurin Bovine Isophane 100units/ml suspension for injection 3ml cartridges | 5 cartridge [PoM] £41.58
▸ Hypurin Porcine Isophane (Wockhardt UK Ltd)
Insulin porcine (as Insulin isophane porcine) 100 unit per 1 ml Hypurin Porcine Isophane 100units/ml suspension for injection 10ml vials | 1 vial [PoM] £25.20
Hypurin Porcine Isophane 100units/ml suspension for injection 3ml cartridges | 5 cartridge [PoM] £37.80
▸ Insulatard (Novo Nordisk Ltd)
Insulin human (as Insulin isophane human) 100 unit per 1 ml Insulatard 100units/ml suspension for injection 10ml vials | 1 vial [PoM] £7.48
▸ Insulatard InnoLet (Novo Nordisk Ltd)
Insulin human (as Insulin isophane human) 100 unit per 1 ml Insulatard InnoLet 100units/ml suspension for injection 3ml pre-filled pen | 5 pre-filled disposable injection [PoM] £20.40
▸ Insulatard Penfill (Novo Nordisk Ltd)
Insulin human (as Insulin isophane human) 100 unit per 1 ml Insulatard Penfill 100units/ml suspension for injection 3ml cartridges | 5 cartridge [PoM] £22.90
▸ Insuman Basal (Sanofi)
Insulin human (as Insulin isophane human) 100 unit per 1 ml Insuman Basal 100units/ml suspension for injection 5ml vials | 1 vial [PoM] £5.61
Insuman Basal 100units/ml suspension for injection 3ml cartridges | 5 cartridge [PoM] £17.50
▸ Insuman Basal SoloStar (Sanofi)
Insulin human (as Insulin isophane human) 100 unit per 1 ml Insuman Basal 100units/ml suspension for injection 3ml pre-filled SoloStar pen | 5 pre-filled disposable injection [PoM] £19.80

6

Endocrine system

6

Endocrine system

INSULINS › INTERMEDIATE-ACTING COMBINED WITH RAPID-ACTING

📖 640

Biphasic insulin aspart

(Intermediate-acting insulin)

- ● **INDICATIONS AND DOSE**

Diabetes mellitus
- ▸ BY SUBCUTANEOUS INJECTION
  - ▸ **Child:** Administer up to 10 minutes before or soon after a meal, according to requirements
  - ▸ **Adult:** Administer up to 10 minutes before or soon after a meal, according to requirements

- ● INTERACTIONS → Appendix 1 (antidiabetics).
- ● SIDE-EFFECTS Protamine may cause allergic reactions
- ● PRESCRIBING AND DISPENSING INFORMATION Check product container—the proportions of the two components should be checked carefully (the order in which the proportions are stated may not be the same in other countries).

- ● MEDICINAL FORMS
  There can be variation in the licensing of different medicines containing the same drug.
  Suspension for injection
  - ▸ NovoMix 30 FlexPen (Novo Nordisk Ltd)
    Insulin aspart 30 unit per 1 ml, Insulin aspart (as Insulin aspart protamine) 70 unit per 1 ml NovoMix 30 FlexPen 100units/ml suspension for injection 3ml pre-filled pen | 5 pre-filled disposable injection PoM £29.89
  - ▸ NovoMix 30 Penfill (Novo Nordisk Ltd)
    Insulin aspart 30 unit per 1 ml, Insulin aspart (as Insulin aspart protamine) 70 unit per 1 ml NovoMix 30 Penfill 100units/ml suspension for injection 3ml cartridges | 5 cartridge PoM £28.79

📖 640

Biphasic insulin lispro

(Intermediate-acting insulin)

- ● **INDICATIONS AND DOSE**

Diabetes mellitus
- ▸ BY SUBCUTANEOUS INJECTION
  - ▸ **Child:** Administer up to 15 minutes before or soon after a meal, according to requirements
  - ▸ **Adult:** Administer up to 15 minutes before or soon after a meal, according to requirements

- ● CAUTIONS Children under 12 years (use only if benefit likely compared to soluble insulin)
- ● INTERACTIONS → Appendix 1 (antidiabetics).
- ● SIDE-EFFECTS Protamine may cause allergic reactions
- ● PRESCRIBING AND DISPENSING INFORMATION Check product container—the proportions of the two components should be checked carefully (the order in which the proportions are stated may not be the same in other countries).

- ● MEDICINAL FORMS
  There can be variation in the licensing of different medicines containing the same drug.
  Suspension for injection
  - ▸ Humalog Mix25 (Eli Lilly and Company Ltd)
    Insulin lispro 25 unit per 1 ml, Insulin lispro (as Insulin lispro protamine) 75 unit per 1 ml Humalog Mix25 100units/ml suspension for injection 10ml vials | 1 vial PoM £16.61
    Humalog Mix25 100units/ml suspension for injection 3ml cartridges | 5 cartridge PoM £29.46
  - ▸ Humalog Mix25 KwikPen (Eli Lilly and Company Ltd)
    Insulin lispro 25 unit per 1 ml, Insulin lispro (as Insulin lispro protamine) 75 unit per 1 ml Humalog Mix25 KwikPen 100units/ml

suspension for injection 3ml pre-filled pen | 5 pre-filled disposable injection PoM £30.98
- ▸ Humalog Mix50 (Eli Lilly and Company Ltd)
  Insulin lispro 50 unit per 1 ml, Insulin lispro (as Insulin lispro protamine) 50 unit per 1 ml Humalog Mix50 100units/ml suspension for injection 3ml cartridges | 5 cartridge PoM £29.46
- ▸ Humalog Mix50 KwikPen (Eli Lilly and Company Ltd)
  Insulin lispro 50 unit per 1 ml, Insulin lispro (as Insulin lispro protamine) 50 unit per 1 ml Humalog Mix50 KwikPen 100units/ml suspension for injection 3ml pre-filled pen | 5 pre-filled disposable injection PoM £30.98

INSULINS › LONG-ACTING

📖 640

Insulin degludec

(Recombinant human insulin analogue—long acting)

- ● **INDICATIONS AND DOSE**

Diabetes mellitus
- ▸ BY SUBCUTANEOUS INJECTION
  - ▸ **Child 1-17 years:** Dose to be given according to requirements
  - ▸ **Adult:** Dose to be given according to requirements

- ● INTERACTIONS → Appendix 1 (antidiabetics).
- ● PREGNANCY Evidence of the safety of long-acting insulin analogues in pregnancy is limited, therefore isophane insulin is recommended where longer-acting insulins are needed; insulin detemir may also be considered.
- ● PRESCRIBING AND DISPENSING INFORMATION Insulin degludec (*Tresiba®*) is available in strengths of 100 units/mL (allows 1-unit dose adjustment) and 200 units/mL (allows 2-unit dose adjustment)—ensure correct strength prescribed.

- ● MEDICINAL FORMS
  There can be variation in the licensing of different medicines containing the same drug.
  Solution for injection
  - ▸ Tresiba FlexTouch (Novo Nordisk Ltd) ▼
    Insulin human (as Insulin degludec) 100 unit per 1 ml Tresiba FlexTouch 100units/ml solution for injection 3ml pre-filled pen | 5 pre-filled disposable injection PoM £72.00
    Insulin human (as Insulin degludec) 200 unit per 1 ml Tresiba FlexTouch 200units/ml solution for injection 3ml pre-filled pen | 3 pre-filled disposable injection PoM £86.40
  - ▸ Tresiba Penfill (Novo Nordisk Ltd) ▼
    Insulin human (as Insulin degludec) 100 unit per 1 ml Tresiba Penfill 100units/ml solution for injection 3ml cartridges | 5 cartridge PoM £72.00

Insulin degludec with liraglutide

2.6.2016

The properties listed below are those particular to the combination only. For the properties of the components please consider, insulin degludec above, liraglutide p. 631.

- ● **INDICATIONS AND DOSE**

As add-on to oral antidiabetics in type 2 diabetes mellitus not controlled by oral antidiabetics alone
- ▸ BY SUBCUTANEOUS INJECTION
  - ▸ **Adult:** Initially 10 dose-steps once daily, adjusted according to response; maximum 50 dose-steps per day

When transferring from basal insulin in type 2 diabetes mellitus not controlled by oral antidiabetics in combination with basal insulin
- ▸ BY SUBCUTANEOUS INJECTION
  - ▸ **Adult:** Initially 16 dose-steps once daily, adjusted according to response; maximum 50 dose-steps per day

- ● INTERACTIONS Dose of concomitant sulfonylurea may need to be reduced.

- **PATIENT AND CARER ADVICE** Counselling advised on administration. Show container to patient and confirm that patient is expecting the version dispensed.
- **NATIONAL FUNDING/ACCESS DECISIONS**

Scottish Medicines Consortium (SMC) Decisions
The *Scottish Medicines Consortium* has advised (October 2015) that insulin degludec with liraglutide (*Xultophy®*) is accepted for restricted use within NHS Scotland for the treatment of type 2 diabetes mellitus to improve glycaemic control in combination with oral glucose-lowering medicinal products when these alone or combined with a GLP-1 receptor agonist or with basal insulin do not provide adequate glycaemic control.

- **MEDICINAL FORMS**
There can be variation in the licensing of different medicines containing the same drug.

Solution for injection
- Xultophy (Novo Nordisk Ltd) ▼
  Insulin human (as Insulin degludec) 100 unit per 1 ml, Liraglutide 3.6 mg per 1 ml Xultophy 100units/ml / 3.6mg/ml solution for injection 3ml pre-filled pen | 3 pre-filled disposable injection PoM £95.53

▶ 640

Insulin detemir

(Recombinant human insulin analogue—long acting)

- **INDICATIONS AND DOSE**

Diabetes mellitus
▶ BY SUBCUTANEOUS INJECTION
- Child 2-17 years: According to requirements
- Adult: According to requirements

- **INTERACTIONS** → Appendix 1 (antidiabetics).
- **PREGNANCY** Evidence of the safety of long-acting insulin analogues in pregnancy is limited, therefore isophane insulin p. 641 is recommended where longer-acting insulins are needed; insulin detemir may also be considered where longer-acting insulins are needed.

- **MEDICINAL FORMS**
There can be variation in the licensing of different medicines containing the same drug.

Solution for injection
- Levemir FlexPen (Novo Nordisk Ltd)
  Insulin human (as Insulin detemir) 100 unit per 1 ml Levemir FlexPen 100units/ml solution for injection 3ml pre-filled pen | 5 pre-filled disposable injection PoM £42.00
- Levemir InnoLet (Novo Nordisk Ltd)
  Insulin human (as Insulin detemir) 100 unit per 1 ml Levemir InnoLet 100units/ml solution for injection 3ml pre-filled pen | 5 pre-filled disposable injection PoM £44.85
- Levemir Penfill (Novo Nordisk Ltd)
  Insulin human (as Insulin detemir) 100 unit per 1 ml Levemir Penfill 100units/ml solution for injection 3ml cartridges | 5 cartridge PoM £42.00

▶ 640

Insulin glargine

(Recombinant human insulin analogue—long acting)

- **INDICATIONS AND DOSE**

Diabetes mellitus
▶ BY SUBCUTANEOUS INJECTION
- Child 2-17 years: According to requirements
- Adult: According to requirements

TOUJEO®

Diabetes mellitus
▶ BY SUBCUTANEOUS INJECTION
- Adult: According to requirements

- **INTERACTIONS** → Appendix 1 (antidiabetics).
- **PREGNANCY** Evidence of the safety of long-acting insulin analogues in pregnancy is limited, therefore isophane insulin is recommended where longer-acting insulins are needed; insulin detemir may also be considered.
- **PRESCRIBING AND DISPENSING INFORMATION** Products containing insulin glargine are not identical and although there should be no important differences in terms of safety and efficacy, when prescribing biological products it is good practice to use the brand name see *Biosimilar medicines*, under Guidance on prescribing p. 1. Dose adjustments and close metabolic monitoring is recommended if switching between insulin glargine preparations.
- **NATIONAL FUNDING/ACCESS DECISIONS**

Scottish Medicines Consortium (SMC) Decisions
The *Scottish Medicines Consortium* has advised that *Lantus®* preparations (April 2013) and *Toujeo®* (August 2015) are accepted for restricted use within NHS Scotland for the treatment of type 1 diabetes:
- in those who are at risk of or experience unacceptable frequency or severity of nocturnal hypoglycaemia on attempting to achieve better hypoglycaemic control during treatment with other insulins
- as a once daily insulin therapy for patients who require a carer to administer their insulin
It is **not** recommended for routine use in patients with type 2 diabetes unless they suffer from recurrent episodes of hypoglycaemia or require assistance with their insulin injections.

- **MEDICINAL FORMS**
There can be variation in the licensing of different medicines containing the same drug.

Solution for injection
- Abasaglar (Eli Lilly and Company Ltd) ▼
  Insulin human (as Insulin glargine) 100 unit per 1 ml Abasaglar 100units/ml solution for injection 3ml cartridges | 5 cartridge PoM £35.28
- Abasaglar KwikPen (Eli Lilly and Company Ltd) ▼
  Insulin human (as Insulin glargine) 100 unit per 1 ml Abasaglar KwikPen 100units/ml solution for injection 3ml pre-filled pen | 5 pre-filled disposable injection PoM £35.28
- Lantus (Sanofi)
  Insulin human (as Insulin glargine) 100 unit per 1 ml Lantus 100units/ml solution for injection 3ml cartridges | 5 cartridge PoM £41.50
  Lantus 100units/ml solution for injection 10ml vials | 1 vial PoM £30.68
- Lantus SoloStar (Sanofi)
  Insulin human (as Insulin glargine) 100 unit per 1 ml Lantus 100units/ml solution for injection 3ml pre-filled SoloStar pen | 5 pre-filled disposable injection PoM £41.50
- Toujeo (Sanofi)
  Insulin human (as Insulin glargine) 300 unit per 1 ml Toujeo 300units/ml solution for injection 1.5ml pre-filled SoloStar pen | 3 pre-filled disposable injection PoM £33.13

▶ 640

Insulin zinc suspension

(Insulin zinc suspension (mixed)—long acting)

- **INDICATIONS AND DOSE**

Diabetes mellitus
▶ BY SUBCUTANEOUS INJECTION
- Child: According to requirements
- Adult: According to requirements

- **INTERACTIONS** → Appendix 1 (antidiabetics).

6

Endocrine system

- PREGNANCY Evidence of the safety of long-acting insulin analogues in pregnancy is limited, therefore isophane insulin p. 641 is recommended where longer-acting insulins are needed; insulin detemir p. 643 may also be considered.

- PRESCRIBING AND DISPENSING INFORMATION A sterile neutral suspension of bovine and/or porcine insulin or of human insulin in the form of a complex obtained by the addition of a suitable zinc salt; consists of rhombohedral crystals (10–40 microns) and of particles of no uniform shape (not exceeding 2 microns).

- MEDICINAL FORMS
There can be variation in the licensing of different medicines containing the same drug.
Suspension for injection
‣ Hypurin Bovine Lente (Wockhardt UK Ltd)
Insulin bovine (as Insulin zinc suspension mixed bovine) 100 unit per 1 ml Hypurin Bovine Lente 100units/ml suspension for injection 10ml vials | 1 vial PoM £27.72

⟋ 640

Protamine zinc insulin

(Protamine zinc insulin injection—long acting)

- INDICATIONS AND DOSE
Diabetes mellitus
▸ BY SUBCUTANEOUS INJECTION
‣ Child: According to requirements
‣ Adult: According to requirements

- INTERACTIONS → Appendix 1 (antidiabetics).
- SIDE-EFFECTS Protamine may cause allergic reactions
- PREGNANCY Evidence of the safety of long-acting insulin analogues in pregnancy is limited, therefore isophane insulin p. 641 is recommended where longer-acting insulins are needed; insulin detemir p. 643 may also be considered.
- PRESCRIBING AND DISPENSING INFORMATION A sterile suspension of insulin in the form of a complex obtained by the addition of a suitable protamine and zinc chloride; this preparation was included in BP 1980 but is not included in BP 1988.

- MEDICINAL FORMS
There can be variation in the licensing of different medicines containing the same drug.
Suspension for injection
▸ Hypurin Bovine Protamine Zinc (Wockhardt UK Ltd)
Insulin bovine (as Insulin protamine zinc bovine) 100 unit per 1 ml Hypurin Bovine Protamine Zinc 100units/ml suspension for injection 10ml vials | 1 vial PoM £27.72

INSULINS > RAPID-ACTING

⟋ 640

Insulin

(Insulin Injection; Neutral Insulin; Soluble Insulin—short acting)

- INDICATIONS AND DOSE
Diabetes mellitus
▸ BY SUBCUTANEOUS INJECTION, OR BY INTRAMUSCULAR INJECTION, OR BY INTRAVENOUS INJECTION, OR BY INTRAVENOUS INFUSION
‣ Adult: According to requirements
Diabetic ketoacidosis | Diabetes during surgery
▸ BY INTRAVENOUS INFUSION
‣ Adult: (consult local protocol)

- INTERACTIONS → Appendix 1 (antidiabetics).

- DIRECTIONS FOR ADMINISTRATION Short-acting injectable insulins can be given by continuous subcutaneous infusion using a portable infusion pump. This device delivers a continuous basal insulin infusion and patient-activated bolus doses at meal times. This technique can be useful for patients who suffer recurrent hypoglycaemia or marked morning rise in blood-glucose concentration despite optimised multiple-injection regimens. Patients on subcutaneous insulin infusion must be highly motivated, able to monitor their blood-glucose concentration, and have expert training, advice and supervision from an experienced healthcare team. Some insulin preparations are not recommended for use in subcutaneous insulin infusion pumps—may precipitate in catheter or needle—consult product literature.

▸ With intravenous use For *intravenous infusion* give continuously in Sodium chloride 0.9%. Adsorbed to some extent by plastic infusion set; ensure insulin is not injected into 'dead space' of injection port of the infusion bag.

- PRESCRIBING AND DISPENSING INFORMATION A sterile solution of insulin (i.e. bovine or porcine) or of human insulin; pH 6.6–8.0.
- NATIONAL FUNDING/ACCESS DECISIONS
NICE technology appraisals (TAs)
▸ **Continuous subcutaneous insulin infusion for the treatment of diabetes mellitus (type 1) (July 2008)** NICE TA151
Continuous subcutaneous insulin infusion is recommended as an option in adults and children over 12 years with type 1 diabetes:
  • who suffer repeated or unpredictable hypoglycaemia, whilst attempting to achieve optimal glycaemic control with multiple-injection regimens, **or**
  • whose glycaemic control remains inadequate (HbA$_{1c}$ over 8.5% [69 mmol/mol]) despite optimised multiple-injection regimens (including the use of long-acting insulin analogues where appropriate).
Continuous subcutaneous insulin infusion is also recommended as an option for children under 12 years with type 1 diabetes for whom multiple-injection regimens are considered impractical or inappropriate. Children on insulin pumps should undergo a trial of multiple-injection therapy between the ages of 12 and 18 years.
www.nice.org.uk/TA151

- MEDICINAL FORMS
There can be variation in the licensing of different medicines containing the same drug. Forms available from special-order manufacturers include: solution for injection, solution for infusion
Solution for injection
▸ Insulin (Non-proprietary)
Insulin human 100 unit per 1 ml Humulin R 100units/ml solution for injection 10ml vials | 1 vial PoM no price available
Insulin human 500 unit per 1 ml Humulin R 500units/ml solution for injection 20ml vials | 1 vial PoM no price available
▸ Actrapid (Novo Nordisk Ltd)
Insulin human (as Insulin soluble human) 100 unit per 1 ml Actrapid 100units/ml solution for injection 10ml vials | 1 vial PoM £7.48
▸ Humulin S (Eli Lilly and Company Ltd)
Insulin human (as Insulin soluble human) 100 unit per 1 ml Humulin S 100units/ml solution for injection 10ml vials | 1 vial PoM £15.68
Humulin S 100units/ml solution for injection 3ml cartridges | 5 cartridge PoM £19.08
▸ Hypurin Bovine Neutral (Wockhardt UK Ltd)
Insulin bovine (as Insulin soluble bovine) 100 unit per 1 ml Hypurin Bovine Neutral 100units/ml solution for injection 10ml vials | 1 vial PoM £27.72
Hypurin Bovine Neutral 100units/ml solution for injection 3ml cartridges | 5 cartridge PoM £41.58

› Hypurin Porcine Neutral (Wockhardt UK Ltd)
**Insulin porcine (as Insulin soluble porcine) 100 unit per
1 ml** Hypurin Porcine Neutral 100units/ml solution for injection 10ml
vials | 1 vial [PoM] £25.20
Hypurin Porcine Neutral 100units/ml solution for injection 3ml
cartridges | 5 cartridge [PoM] £37.80
› Insuman Infusat (Sanofi)
Insulin human 100 unit per 1 ml Insuman Infusat 100units/ml
solution for injection 3.15ml cartridges | 5 cartridge [PoM] £250.00
Insuman Infusat 100units/ml solution for injection 10ml vials |
3 vial [PoM] £250.00
› Insuman Rapid (Sanofi)
**Insulin human (as Insulin soluble human) 100 unit per
1 ml** Insuman Rapid 100units/ml solution for injection 3ml cartridges
| 5 cartridge [PoM] £17.50

◤ 640

Insulin aspart

(Recombinant human insulin analogue—short acting)

● INDICATIONS AND DOSE
Diabetes mellitus
▶ BY SUBCUTANEOUS INJECTION
› Child 2-17 years: Administer immediately before meals
or when necessary shortly after meals, according to
requirements
› Adult: Administer immediately before meals or when
necessary shortly after meals, according to
requirements
▶ BY SUBCUTANEOUS INFUSION, OR BY INTRAVENOUS INFUSION,
OR BY INTRAVENOUS INJECTION
› Child 2-17 years: According to requirements
› Adult: According to requirements

● UNLICENSED USE
▶ In children Not licensed for use in children under 2 years.
● INTERACTIONS → Appendix 1 (antidiabetics).
● PREGNANCY Not known to be harmful—may be used
during pregnancy.
● BREAST FEEDING Not known to be harmful—may be used
during lactation.
● DIRECTIONS FOR ADMINISTRATION Short-acting injectable
insulins can be given by continuous subcutaneous infusion
using a portable infusion pump. This device delivers a
continuous basal insulin infusion and patient-activated
bolus doses at meal times. This technique can be useful for
patients who suffer recurrent hypoglycaemia or marked
morning rise in blood-glucose concentration despite
optimised multiple-injection regimens. Patients on
subcutaneous insulin infusion must be highly motivated,
able to monitor their blood-glucose concentration, and
have expert training, advice and supervision from an
experienced healthcare team.
▶ With intravenous use in adults For *intravenous infusion*, give
continuously in Glucose 5% or Sodium chloride 0.9%;
dilute to 0.05-1 unit/mL with infusion fluid; absorbed to
some extent by plastics of infusion set.
▶ With intravenous use in children For *intravenous infusion*,
dilute to a concentration of 0.05–1 unit/mL with Glucose
5% or Sodium Chloride 0.9% and mix thoroughly; insulin
may be adsorbed by plastics, flush giving set with 5 mL of
infusion fluid containing insulin.
● NATIONAL FUNDING/ACCESS DECISIONS
NICE technology appraisals (TAs)
▶ **Continuous subcutaneous insulin infusion for the treatment of
diabetes mellitus (type 1) (July 2008)** NICE TA151
Continuous subcutaneous insulin infusion is
recommended as an option in adults and children over
12 years with type 1 diabetes:

● who suffer repeated or unpredictable hypoglycaemia,
whilst attempting to achieve optimal glycaemic control
with multiple-injection regimens, **or**
● whose glycaemic control remains inadequate (HbA$_{1c}$
over 8.5% [69 mmol/mol]) despite optimised multiple-
injection regimens (including the use of long-acting
insulin analogues where appropriate).
Continuous subcutaneous insulin infusion is also
recommended as an option for children under 12 years
with type 1 diabetes for whom multiple-injection regimens
are considered impractical or inappropriate. Children on
insulin pumps should undergo a trial of multiple-injection
therapy between the ages of 12 and 18 years.
www.nice.org.uk/TA151

● MEDICINAL FORMS
There can be variation in the licensing of different medicines
containing the same drug.
Solution for injection
▶ NovoRapid (Novo Nordisk Ltd)
Insulin aspart 100 unit per 1 ml NovoRapid 100units/ml solution for
injection 10ml vials | 1 vial [PoM] £14.08
▶ NovoRapid FlexPen (Novo Nordisk Ltd)
Insulin aspart 100 unit per 1 ml NovoRapid FlexPen 100units/ml
solution for injection 3ml pre-filled pen | 5 pre-filled disposable
injection [PoM] £30.60
▶ NovoRapid FlexTouch (Novo Nordisk Ltd)
Insulin aspart 100 unit per 1 ml NovoRapid FlexTouch 100units/ml
solution for injection 3ml pre-filled pen | 5 pre-filled disposable
injection [PoM] £32.13
▶ NovoRapid Penfill (Novo Nordisk Ltd)
Insulin aspart 100 unit per 1 ml NovoRapid Penfill 100units/ml
solution for injection 3ml cartridges | 5 cartridge [PoM] £28.31
▶ NovoRapid PumpCart (Novo Nordisk Ltd)
Insulin aspart 100 unit per 1 ml NovoRapid PumpCart 100units/ml
solution for injection 1.6ml cartridges | 5 cartridge [PoM] £15.10

◤ 640

Insulin glulisine

(Recombinant human insulin analogue—short acting)

● INDICATIONS AND DOSE
Diabetes mellitus
▶ BY SUBCUTANEOUS INJECTION
› Child: Administer immediately before meals or when
necessary shortly after meals, according to
requirements
› Adult: Administer immediately before meals or when
necessary shortly after meals, according to
requirements
▶ BY SUBCUTANEOUS INFUSION, OR BY INTRAVENOUS INFUSION
› Child: According to requirements
› Adult: According to requirements

● UNLICENSED USE
▶ In children Not licensed for children under 6 years.
● INTERACTIONS → Appendix 1 (antidiabetics).
● DIRECTIONS FOR ADMINISTRATION Short-acting injectable
insulins can be given by continuous subcutaneous infusion
using a portable infusion pump. This device delivers a
continuous basal insulin infusion and patient-activated
bolus doses at meal times. This technique can be useful for
patients who suffer recurrent hypoglycaemia or marked
morning rise in blood-glucose concentration despite
optimised multiple-injection regimens. Patients on
subcutaneous insulin infusion must be highly motivated,
able to monitor their blood-glucose concentration, and
have expert training, advice and supervision from an
experienced healthcare team.
▶ With intravenous use in adults For *intravenous infusion*
(*Apidra*®), give continuously in Sodium chloride 0.9%;
dilute to 1 unit/mL with infusion fluid; use a co-extruded

polyolefin/polyamide plastic infusion bag with a dedicated infusion line.

● NATIONAL FUNDING/ACCESS DECISIONS

NICE technology appraisals (TAs)

▶ Continuous subcutaneous insulin infusion for the treatment of diabetes mellitus (type 1) (July 2008) NICE TA151
Continuous subcutaneous insulin infusion is recommended as an option in adults and children over 12 years with type 1 diabetes:

● who suffer repeated or unpredictable hypoglycaemia, whilst attempting to achieve optimal glycaemic control with multiple-injection regimens, **or**

● whose glycaemic control remains inadequate (HbA$_{1c}$ over 8.5% [69 mmol/mol]) despite optimised multiple-injection regimens (including the use of long-acting insulin analogues where appropriate).

Continuous subcutaneous insulin infusion is also recommended as an option for children under 12 years with type 1 diabetes for whom multiple-injection regimens are considered impractical or inappropriate. Children on insulin pumps should undergo a trial of multiple-injection therapy between the ages of 12 and 18 years.
www.nice.org.uk/TA151

Scottish Medicines Consortium (SMC) Decisions

The *Scottish Medicines Consortium* has advised (October 2008) that *Apidra*® is accepted for restricted use within NHS Scotland for the treatment of adults and children over 6 years with diabetes mellitus in whom the use of a short-acting insulin analogue is appropriate.

● MEDICINAL FORMS
There can be variation in the licensing of different medicines containing the same drug.

Solution for injection

▶ Apidra (Sanofi)
Insulin glulisine 100 unit per 1 ml Apidra 100units/ml solution for injection 10ml vials | 1 vial [PoM] £16.00
Apidra 100units/ml solution for injection 3ml cartridges | 5 cartridge [PoM] £28.30

▶ Apidra SoloStar (Sanofi)
Insulin glulisine 100 unit per 1 ml Apidra 100units/ml solution for injection 3ml pre-filled SoloStar pen | 5 pre-filled disposable injection [PoM] £28.30

⬛ ☞ 640

Insulin lispro

(Recombinant human insulin analogue—short acting)

● INDICATIONS AND DOSE

Diabetes mellitus

▶ BY SUBCUTANEOUS INJECTION

▶ Child 2–17 years: Administer shortly before meals or when necessary shortly after meals, according to requirements

▶ Adult: Administer shortly before meals or when necessary shortly after meals, according to requirements

▶ BY SUBCUTANEOUS INFUSION, OR BY INTRAVENOUS INFUSION, OR BY INTRAVENOUS INJECTION

▶ Child 2–17 years: According to requirements

▶ Adult: According to requirements

● UNLICENSED USE

▶ In children Not licensed for use in children under 2 years.

● CAUTIONS Children under 12 years (use only if benefit likely compared to soluble insulin)

● INTERACTIONS → Appendix 1 (antidiabetics).

● PREGNANCY Not known to be harmful—may be used during pregnancy.

● BREAST FEEDING Not known to be harmful—may be used during lactation.

● DIRECTIONS FOR ADMINISTRATION Short-acting injectable insulins can be given by continuous subcutaneous infusion using a portable infusion pump. This device delivers a continuous basal insulin infusion and patient-activated bolus doses at meal times. This technique can be useful for patients who suffer recurrent hypoglycaemia or marked morning rise in blood-glucose concentration despite optimised multiple-injection regimens (see also NICE guidance, below). Patients on subcutaneous insulin infusion must be highly motivated, able to monitor their blood-glucose concentration, and have expert training, advice and supervision from an experienced healthcare team.

▶ With intravenous use in adults For *intravenous infusion* give continuously in Glucose 5% or Sodium chloride 0.9%. Adsorbed to some extent by plastics of infusion set.

▶ With intravenous use in children For *intravenous infusion*, dilute to a concentration of 0.1–1 unit/mL with Glucose 5% or Sodium Chloride 0.9% and mix thoroughly; insulin may be adsorbed by plastics, flush giving set with 5 mL of infusion fluid containing insulin.

● NATIONAL FUNDING/ACCESS DECISIONS

NICE technology appraisals (TAs)

▶ Continuous subcutaneous insulin infusion for the treatment of diabetes mellitus (type 1) (July 2008) NICE TA151
Continuous subcutaneous insulin infusion is recommended as an option in adults and children over 12 years with type 1 diabetes:

● who suffer repeated or unpredictable hypoglycaemia, whilst attempting to achieve optimal glycaemic control with multiple-injection regimens, **or**

● whose glycaemic control remains inadequate (HbA$_{1c}$ over 8.5% [69 mmol/mol]) despite optimised multiple-injection regimens (including the use of long-acting insulin analogues where appropriate).

Continuous subcutaneous insulin infusion is also recommended as an option for children under 12 years with type 1 diabetes for whom multiple-injection regimens are considered impractical or inappropriate. Children on insulin pumps should undergo a trial of multiple-injection therapy between the ages of 12 and 18 years.
www.nice.org.uk/TA151

● MEDICINAL FORMS
There can be variation in the licensing of different medicines containing the same drug.

Solution for injection

▶ Humalog (Eli Lilly and Company Ltd)
Insulin lispro 100 unit per 1 ml Humalog 100units/ml solution for injection 10ml vials | 1 vial [PoM] £16.61
Humalog 100units/ml solution for injection 3ml cartridges | 5 cartridge [PoM] £28.31

▶ Humalog KwikPen (Eli Lilly and Company Ltd)
Insulin lispro 100 unit per 1 ml Humalog KwikPen 100units/ml solution for injection 3ml pre-filled pen | 5 pre-filled disposable injection [PoM] £29.46
Insulin lispro 200 unit per 1 ml Humalog KwikPen 200units/ml solution for injection 3ml pre-filled pen | 5 pre-filled disposable injection [PoM] £58.92

3.1a Diabetes, diagnosis and monitoring

Diabetes mellitus, diagnostic and monitoring devices

Urinalysis

Reagent strips are available for measuring for glucose in the urine. Tests for ketones by patients are rarely required unless they become unwell—see Blood Monitoring.

Meters and test strips

Meter (all [NHS])	Type of monitoring	Compatible test strips	Test strip net price	Sensitivity range (mmol/litre)	Manufacturer
Accu-Chek® Active	Blood glucose	Active®	50 strip = £9.95	0.6–33.3 mmol/litre	Roche Diabetes Care Ltd
Accu-Chek® Advantage Meter no longer available	Blood glucose	Advantage Plus®	50 strip = £0.00	0.6–33.3 mmol/litre	Roche Diabetes Care Ltd
Accu-Chek® Aviva	Blood glucose	Aviva®	50 strip = £15.79	0.6–33.3 mmol/litre	Roche Diabetes Care Ltd
Accu-Chek® Aviva Expert	Blood glucose	Aviva®	50 strip = £15.79	0.6–33.3 mmol/litre	Roche Diabetes Care Ltd
Accu-Chek® Compact Plus Meter no longer available	Blood glucose	Compact®	3 × 17 strips = £16.22	0.6–33.3 mmol/litre	Roche Diabetes Care Ltd
Accu-Chek® Mobile	Blood glucose	Mobile®	100 device = £32.48	0.3–33.3 mmol/litre	Roche Diabetes Care Ltd
Accu-Chek® Aviva Nano	Blood glucose	Aviva®	50 strip = £15.79	0.6–33.3 mmol/litre	Roche Diabetes Care Ltd
BGStar® Free of charge from diabetes healthcare professionals	Blood glucose	BGStar®	50 strip = £14.73	1.1–33.3 mmol/litre	Sanofi
Breeze 2®	Blood glucose	Breeze 2®	50 strip = £15.00	0.6–33.3 mmol/litre	Bayer Plc
CareSens N® Free of charge from diabetes healthcare professionals	Blood glucose	CareSens N®	50 strip = £12.75	1.1–33.3 mmol/litre	Spirit Healthcare Ltd
Contour®	Blood glucose	Contour®	50 strip = £9.95	0.6–33.3 mmol/litre	Bayer Diagnostics Manufacturing Ltd
Contour® XT	Blood glucose	Contour® Next	50 strip = £15.04	0.6–33.3 mmol/litre	Bayer Diagnostics Manufacturing Ltd
Element®	Blood glucose	Element®	50 strip = £9.89	0.55–33.3 mmol/litre	Neon Diagnostics Ltd
FreeStyle® Meter no longer available	Blood glucose	FreeStyle®	50 strip = £15.81	1.1–27.8 mmol/litre	Abbott Laboratories Ltd
FreeStyle Freedom® Meter no longer available	Blood glucose	FreeStyle®	50 strip = £15.81	1.1–27.8 mmol/litre	Abbott Laboratories Ltd
FreeStyle Freedom Lite®	Blood glucose	FreeStyle Lite®	50 strip = £15.80	1.1–27.8 mmol/litre	Abbott Laboratories Ltd
FreeStyle InsuLinx®	Blood glucose	FreeStyle Lite®	50 strip = £15.80	1.1–27.8 mmol/litre	Abbott Laboratories Ltd
FreeStyle Lite®	Blood glucose	FreeStyle Lite®	50 strip = £15.80	1.1–27.8 mmol/litre	Abbott Laboratories Ltd
FreeStyle Mini® Meter no longer available	Blood glucose	FreeStyle®	50 strip = £15.81	1.1–27.8 mmol/litre	Abbott Laboratories Ltd
FreeStyle Optium®	Blood glucose	FreeStyle Optium®	50 strip = £15.71	1.1–27.8 mmol/litre	Abbott Laboratories Ltd
FreeStyle Optium®	Blood ketones	FreeStyle Optium® β-ketone	10 strip = £21.14	0–8.0 mmol/litre	Abbott Laboratories Ltd
FreeStyle Optium Neo®	Blood glucose	FreeStyle Optium®	50 strip = £15.71	1.1–27.8 mmol/litre	Abbott Laboratories Ltd
FreeStyle Optium Neo®	Blood ketones	FreeStyle Optium® β-ketone	10 strip = £21.14	0–8.0 mmol/litre	Abbott Laboratories Ltd
GlucoDock® module For use with iPhone®, iPod touch®, and iPad®	Blood glucose	GlucoDock®	50 strip = £14.90	1.1–33.3 mmol/litre	Medisana Healthcare (UK) Ltd
GlucoLab®	Blood glucose	GlucoLab®	50 strip = £9.89	0.55–33.3 mmol/litre	Neon Diagnostics Ltd

Meter (all NHS)	Type of monitoring	Compatible test strips	Test strip net price	Sensitivity range (mmol/litre)	Manufacturer
GlucoMen® GM	Blood glucose	GlucoMen® GM	50 strip = £9.95	0.6–33.3 mmol/litre	A Menarini Diagnostics Ltd
GlucoMen® LX	Blood glucose	GlucoMen® LX Sensor	50 strip = £15.59	1.1–33.3 mmol/litre	A Menarini Diagnostics Ltd
GlucoMen® LX Plus	Blood glucose	GlucoMen® LX Sensor	50 strip = £15.59	1.1–33.3 mmol/litre	A Menarini Diagnostics Ltd
GlucoMen® LX Plus	Blood ketones	GlucoMen® LX Ketone	10 strip = £20.84	0–0.8 mmol/litre	A Menarini Diagnostics Ltd
GlucoMen® Visio	Blood glucose	GlucoMen® Visio Sensor	50 strip = £15.75	1.1–33.3 mmol/litre	A Menarini Diagnostics Ltd
GlucoRx® Free of charge from diabetes healthcare professionals	Blood glucose	GlucoRx®	50 strip = £9.45	1.1–33.3 mmol/litre	GlucoRx Ltd
GlucoRx Nexus® Free of charge from diabetes healthcare professionals	Blood glucose	GlucoRx Nexus®	50 strip = £9.95	1.1–33.3 mmol/litre	GlucoRx Ltd
Glucotrend® Meter no longer available	Blood glucose	Active®	50 strip = £9.95	0.6–33.3 mmol/litre	Roche Diabetes Care Ltd
iBGStar®	Blood glucose	BGStar®	50 strip = £14.73	1.1–33.3 mmol/litre	Sanofi
IME-DC®	Blood glucose	IME-DC®	50 strip = £14.10	1.1–33.3 mmol/litre	Arctic Medical Ltd
Mendor Discreet®	Blood glucose	Mendor Discreet®	50 strip = £14.75	1.1–33.3 mmol/litre	SpringMed Solutions Ltd
Microdot®+ Free of charge from diabetes healthcare professionals	Blood glucose	Microdot®+	50 strip = £9.49	1.1–29.2 mmol/litre	Cambridge Sensors Ltd
MyGlucoHealth®	Blood glucose	MyGlucoHealth®	50 strip = £15.50	0.6–33.3 mmol/litre	Entra Health Systems Ltd
Omnitest® 3	Blood glucose	Omnitest® 3	50 strip = £9.89	0.6–33.3 mmol/litre	B.Braun Medical Ltd
One Touch Ultra® Meter no longer available	Blood glucose	One Touch Ultra®	50 strip = £9.99	1.1–33.3 mmol/litre	LifeScan
One Touch Ultra 2® Free of charge from diabetes healthcare professionals	Blood glucose	One Touch Ultra®	50 strip = £9.99	1.1–33.3 mmol/litre	LifeScan
One Touch UltraEasy® Free of charge from diabetes healthcare professionals	Blood glucose	One Touch Ultra®	50 strip = £9.99	1.1–33.3 mmol/litre	LifeScan
One Touch UltraSmart® Free of charge from diabetes healthcare professionals	Blood glucose	One Touch Ultra®	50 strip = £9.99	1.1–33.3 mmol/litre	LifeScan
One Touch® VerioPro Free of charge from diabetes healthcare professionals	Blood glucose	One Touch® Verio	50 strip = £15.12	1.1–33.3 mmol/litre	LifeScan
One Touch® Vita Free of charge from diabetes healthcare professionals	Blood glucose	One Touch® Vita	50 strip = £15.07	1.1–33.3 mmol/litre	LifeScan
SD CodeFree®	Blood glucose	SD CodeFree®	50 strip = £6.99	0.6–33.3 mmol/litre	SD Biosensor Inc
Sensocard Plus® Meter no longer available	Blood glucose	Sensocard®	50 strip = £16.30	1.1–33.3 mmol/litre	BBI Healthcare Ltd

Meter (all [NHS])	Type of monitoring	Compatible test strips	Test strip net price	Sensitivity range (mmol/litre)	Manufacturer
SuperCheck2® Free of charge from diabetes healthcare professionals	Blood glucose	SuperCheck2®	50 strip = £8.49	1.1–33.3 mmol/litre	Apollo Medical Technologies Ltd
TRUEone® All-in-one test strips and meter	Blood glucose	TRUEone®	50 strip = £14.99	1.1–33.3 mmol/litre	Nipro Diagnostics (UK) Ltd
TRUEresult® Free of charge from diabetes healthcare professionals	Blood glucose	TRUEresult®	50 strip = £14.99	1.1–33.3 mmol/litre	Nipro Diagnostics (UK) Ltd
TRUEresult twist® Free of charge from diabetes healthcare professionals	Blood glucose	TRUEresult®	50 strip = £14.99	1.1–33.3 mmol/litre	Nipro Diagnostics (UK) Ltd
TRUEtrack® Free of charge from diabetes healthcare professionals	Blood glucose	TRUEtrack®	50 strip = £14.99	1.1–33.3 mmol/litre	Nipro Diagnostics (UK) Ltd
TRUEyou mini®	Blood glucose	TRUEyou®	50 strip = £9.92	1.1–33.3 mmol/litre	Nipro Diagnostics (UK) Ltd
WaveSense JAZZ® Free of charge from	Blood glucose	WaveSense JAZZ®	50 strip = £9.87	1.1–33.3 mmol/litre	AgaMatrix Europe Ltd

Microalbuminuria can be detected with *Micral-Test II* ® but this should be followed by confirmation in the laboratory, since false positive results are common.

Blood monitoring

Blood glucose monitoring using a meter gives a direct measure of the glucose concentration at the time of the test and can detect hypoglycaemia as well as hyperglycaemia. Patients should be properly trained in the use of blood glucose monitoring systems and to take appropriate action on the results obtained. Inadequate understanding of the normal fluctuations in blood glucose can lead to confusion and inappropriate action.

Patients using multiple injection regimens should understand how to adjust their insulin dose according to their carbohydrate intake. With fixed-dose insulin regimens, the carbohydrate intake needs to be regulated, and should be distributed throughout the day to match the insulin regimen.

Self-monitoring of blood-glucose concentration is appropriate for patients with type 2 diabetes:

- who are treated with insulin;
- who are treated with oral hypoglycaemic drugs e.g. sulfonylureas, to provide information on hypoglycaemia;
- to monitor changes in blood-glucose concentration resulting from changes in lifestyle or medication, and during intercurrent illness;
- to ensure safe blood-glucose concentration during activities, including driving.

In the UK blood-glucose concentration is expressed in mmol/litre and Diabetes UK advises that these units should be used for self-monitoring of blood glucose. In other European countries units of mg/100 mL (or mg/dL) are commonly used.

It is advisable to check that the meter is pre-set in the correct units.

If the patient is unwell and diabetic ketoacidosis is suspected, blood **ketones** should be measured according to local guidelines. Patients and their carers should be trained in the use of blood ketone monitoring systems and to take appropriate action on the results obtained, including when to seek medical attention.

Oral glucose tolerance test

The oral glucose tolerance test p. 903 is used mainly for diagnosis of impaired glucose tolerance; it is not recommended or necessary for routine diagnostic use when severe symptoms of hyperglycaemia are present. In patients who have less severe symptoms and blood glucose levels that do not establish or exclude diabetes (e.g. impaired fasting glycaemia), an oral glucose tolerance test may be required. It is also used to establish the presence of gestational diabetes. The oral glucose tolerance test generally involves giving anhydrous glucose by mouth to the fasting patient, and measuring blood-glucose concentrations at intervals.

The appropriate amount of glucose should be given with 200–300 mL fluid. Anhydrous glucose may alternatively be given as 113 mL *Polycal* ® with extra fluid to administer a total volume of 200–300 mL, or as *Rapilose* ® *OGTT* oral solution.

Blood monitoring test strips

● BLOOD GLUCOSE TESTING STRIPS

Active testing strips (Roche Diabetes Care Ltd)
50 strip · NHS indicative price = £9.95 · Drug Tariff (Part IXr)

Advocate Redi-Code+ testing strips (Diabetes Care Technology Ltd)
50 strip · NHS indicative price = £9.95 · Drug Tariff (Part IXr)

AutoSense testing strips (Advance Diagnostic Products (NI) Ltd)
25 strip · NHS indicative price = £4.50 · Drug Tariff (Part IXr)

Aviva testing strips (Roche Diabetes Care Ltd)
50 strip · NHS indicative price = £15.79 · Drug Tariff (Part IXr)

BGStar testing strips (Sanofi)
50 strip · NHS indicative price = £14.73 · Drug Tariff (Part IXr)

Betachek C50 cassette (National Diagnostic Products)
100 device · NHS indicative price = £29.98 · Drug Tariff (Part IXr)

Betachek G5 testing strips (National Diagnostic Products)
50 strip · NHS indicative price = £14.19 · Drug Tariff (Part IXr)

Betachek Visual testing strips (National Diagnostic Products)
50 strip · NHS indicative price = £6.80 · Drug Tariff (Part IXr)

Breeze 2 testing discs (Bayer Plc)
50 strip · NHS indicative price = £15.00 · Drug Tariff (Part IXr)

CareSens N testing strips (Spirit Healthcare Ltd)
50 strip · NHS indicative price = £12.75 · Drug Tariff (Part IXr)

6

Endocrine system

Compact testing strips (Roche Diabetes Care Ltd)
51 strip · NHS indicative price = £16.22 · Drug Tariff (Part IXr)

Contour Next testing strips (Bayer Diagnostics Manufacturing Ltd)
50 strip · NHS indicative price = £15.04 · Drug Tariff (Part IXr)

Contour TS testing strips (Bayer Diagnostics Manufacturing Ltd)
50 strip · NHS indicative price = £9.50 · Drug Tariff (Part IXr)

Contour testing strips (Bayer Diagnostics Manufacturing Ltd)
50 strip · NHS indicative price = £9.95 · Drug Tariff (Part IXr)

Dario Lite testing strips (LabStyle Innovations Ltd)
50 strip · NHS indicative price = £9.95 · Drug Tariff (Part IXr)

Dario testing strips (LabStyle Innovations Ltd)
50 strip · NHS indicative price = £14.95 · Drug Tariff (Part IXr)

Diastix testing strips (Bayer Diagnostics Manufacturing Ltd)
50 strip · NHS indicative price = £2.89 · Drug Tariff (Part IXr)

Element testing strips (Neon Diagnostics Ltd)
50 strip · NHS indicative price = £9.89 · Drug Tariff (Part IXr)

Finetest Lite testing strips (Neon Diagnostics Ltd)
50 strip · NHS indicative price = £7.86 · Drug Tariff (Part IXr)

FreeStyle Lite testing strips (Abbott Laboratories Ltd)
50 strip · NHS indicative price = £15.80 · Drug Tariff (Part IXr)

FreeStyle Optium testing strips (Abbott Laboratories Ltd)
50 strip · NHS indicative price = £15.71 · Drug Tariff (Part IXr)

FreeStyle testing strips (Abbott Laboratories Ltd)
50 strip · NHS indicative price = £15.81 · Drug Tariff (Part IXr)

GluNEO testing strips (Neon Diagnostics Ltd)
50 strip · NHS indicative price = £9.89 · Drug Tariff (Part IXr)

GlucoDock testing strips (Medisana Healthcare (UK) Ltd)
50 strip · NHS indicative price = £14.90 · Drug Tariff (Part IXr)

GlucoLab testing strips (Neon Diagnostics Ltd)
50 strip · NHS indicative price = £9.89 · Drug Tariff (Part IXr)

GlucoMen GM testing strips (A Menarini Diagnostics Ltd)
50 strip · NHS indicative price = £9.95 · Drug Tariff (Part IXr)

GlucoMen LX Sensor testing strips (A Menarini Diagnostics Ltd)
50 strip · NHS indicative price = £15.59 · Drug Tariff (Part IXr)

GlucoMen Sensor testing strips (A Menarini Diagnostics Ltd)
50 strip · NHS indicative price = £14.83 · Drug Tariff (Part IXr)

GlucoMen Visio testing strips (A Menarini Diagnostics Ltd)
50 strip · NHS indicative price = £15.75 · Drug Tariff (Part IXr)

GlucoMen areo Sensor testing strips (A Menarini Diagnostics Ltd)
50 strip · NHS indicative price = £9.95 · Drug Tariff (Part IXr)

GlucoNavii testing strips (Neon Diagnostics Ltd)
50 strip · NHS indicative price = £8.95 · Drug Tariff (Part IXr)

GlucoRx GO testing strips (GlucoRx Ltd)
50 strip · NHS indicative price = £9.95 · Drug Tariff (Part IXr)

GlucoRx HCT Glucose testing strips (GlucoRx Ltd)
50 strip · NHS indicative price = £13.95 · Drug Tariff (Part IXr)

GlucoRx Nexus testing strips (GlucoRx Ltd)
50 strip · NHS indicative price = £9.95 · Drug Tariff (Part IXr)

GlucoRx Original testing strips (GlucoRx Ltd)
50 strip · NHS indicative price = £9.45 · Drug Tariff (Part IXr)

GlucoZen.auto testing strips (GlucoZen Ltd)
50 strip · NHS indicative price = £7.64 · Drug Tariff (Part IXr)

Glucoflex-R testing strips (Bio-Diagnostics Ltd)
50 strip · NHS indicative price = £6.75 · Drug Tariff (Part IXr)

IME-DC testing strips (Arctic Medical Ltd)
50 strip · NHS indicative price = £14.10 · Drug Tariff (Part IXr)

MODZ testing strips (Modz Oy)
50 strip · NHS indicative price = £14.00 · Drug Tariff (Part IXr)

Medi-Test Glucose testing strips (BHR Pharmaceuticals Ltd)
50 strip · NHS indicative price = £2.33 · Drug Tariff (Part IXr)

MediSense SoftSense testing strips (Abbott Laboratories Ltd)
50 strip · NHS indicative price = £15.05 · Drug Tariff (Part IXr)

MediTouch 2 testing strips (Medisana Healthcare (UK) Ltd)
50 strip · NHS indicative price = £12.49 · Drug Tariff (Part IXr)

MediTouch testing strips (Medisana Healthcare (UK) Ltd)
50 strip · NHS indicative price = £14.90 · Drug Tariff (Part IXr)

Mendor Discreet testing strips (SpringMed Solutions Ltd)
50 strip · NHS indicative price = £14.75 · Drug Tariff (Part IXr)

Microdot+ testing strips (Cambridge Sensors Ltd)
50 strip · NHS indicative price = £9.49 · Drug Tariff (Part IXr)

Mission Glucose testing strips (Spirit Healthcare Ltd)
50 strip · NHS indicative price = £2.29 · Drug Tariff (Part IXr)

Mobile cassette (Roche Diabetes Care Ltd)
100 device · NHS indicative price = £32.48 · Drug Tariff (Part IXr)

Myglucohealth testing strips (Entra Health Systems Ltd)
50 strip · NHS indicative price = £15.50 · Drug Tariff (Part IXr)

Mylife Pura testing strips (Ypsomed Ltd)
50 strip · NHS indicative price = £9.50 · Drug Tariff (Part IXr)

Mylife Unio testing strips (Ypsomed Ltd)
50 strip · NHS indicative price = £9.50 · Drug Tariff (Part IXr)

Omnitest 3 testing strips (B.Braun Medical Ltd)
50 strip · NHS indicative price = £9.89 · Drug Tariff (Part IXr)

On-Call Advanced testing strips (Point Of Care Testing Ltd)
50 strip · NHS indicative price = £13.65 · Drug Tariff (Part IXr)

OneTouch Select Plus testing strips (LifeScan)
50 strip · NHS indicative price = £9.99 · Drug Tariff (Part IXr)

OneTouch Ultra testing strips (LifeScan)
50 strip · NHS indicative price = £9.99 · Drug Tariff (Part IXr)

OneTouch Verio testing strips (LifeScan)
50 strip · NHS indicative price = £15.12 · Drug Tariff (Part IXr)

OneTouch Vita testing strips (LifeScan)
50 strip · NHS indicative price = £15.07 · Drug Tariff (Part IXr)

Performa testing strips (Roche Diabetes Care Ltd)
50 strip · NHS indicative price = £9.95 · Drug Tariff (Part IXr)

SD CodeFree testing strips (SD Biosensor Inc)
50 strip · NHS indicative price = £6.99 · Drug Tariff (Part IXr)

SURESIGN Resure testing strips (Ciga Healthcare Ltd)
50 strip · NHS indicative price = £9.99 · Drug Tariff (Part IXr)

Sensocard testing strips (BBI Healthcare Ltd)
50 strip · NHS indicative price = £16.30 · Drug Tariff (Part IXr)

SuperCheck 2 testing strips (Apollo Medical Technologies Ltd)
50 strip · NHS indicative price = £8.49 · Drug Tariff (Part IXr)

SuperCheck Plus testing strips (Apollo Medical Technologies Ltd)
50 strip · NHS indicative price = £9.45 · Drug Tariff (Part IXr)

TEE2 testing strips (Spirit Healthcare Ltd)
50 strip · NHS indicative price = £7.75 · Drug Tariff (Part IXr)

TRUEone testing strips (Nipro Diagnostics (UK) Ltd)
50 strip · NHS indicative price = £14.99 · Drug Tariff (Part IXr)

TRUEresult testing strips (Nipro Diagnostics (UK) Ltd)
50 strip · NHS indicative price = £14.99 · Drug Tariff (Part IXr)

TRUEyou testing strips (Nipro Diagnostics (UK) Ltd)
50 strip · NHS indicative price = £9.92 · Drug Tariff (Part IXr)

TrueTrack System testing strips (Nipro Diagnostics (UK) Ltd)
50 strip · NHS indicative price = £14.99 · Drug Tariff (Part IXr)

WaveSense JAZZ Duo testing strips (AgaMatrix Europe Ltd)
50 strip · NHS indicative price = £9.95 · Drug Tariff (Part IXr)

WaveSense JAZZ testing strips (AgaMatrix Europe Ltd)
50 strip · NHS indicative price = £9.87 · Drug Tariff (Part IXr)

eBchek testing strips (IRASCO Ltd)
50 strip · NHS indicative price = £15.89 · Drug Tariff (Part IXr)

iHealth testing strips (Technomed Ltd)
50 strip · NHS indicative price = £9.49 · Drug Tariff (Part IXr)

palmdoc iCare Advanced Solo testing strips (Palmdoc Ltd)
50 strip · NHS indicative price = £13.50 · Drug Tariff (Part IXr)

palmdoc iCare Advanced testing strips (Palmdoc Ltd)
50 strip · NHS indicative price = £9.70 · Drug Tariff (Part IXr)

palmdoc testing strips (Palmdoc Ltd)
50 strip · NHS indicative price = £9.40 · Drug Tariff (Part IXr)

● BLOOD KETONES TESTING STRIPS

FreeStyle Optium beta-ketone testing strips (Abbott Laboratories Ltd) | 10 strip · NHS indicative price = £21.14 · Drug Tariff (Part IXr)

GlucoMen LX beta-ketone testing strips (A Menarini Diagnostics Ltd) | 10 strip · NHS indicative price = £20.84 · Drug Tariff (Part IXr)

GlucoRx HCT Ketone testing strips (GlucoRx Ltd) | 10 strip · NHS indicative price = £14.95 · Drug Tariff (Part IXr)

Hypodermic insulin injection pens

● HYPODERMIC INSULIN INJECTION PENS

AUTOPEN® 24

Autopen®24 (for use with Sanofi- Aventis 3-mL insulin cartridges), allowing 1-unit dosage adjustment, max. 21 units (single-unit version) or 2-unit dosage adjustment, max. 42 units (2- unit version).

Autopen 24 hypodermic insulin injection pen reusable for 3ml cartridge 1 unit dial up / range 1-21 units (Owen Mumford Ltd)
1 device · NHS indicative price = £16.47 · Drug Tariff (Part IXa)

Autopen 24 hypodermic insulin injection pen reusable for 3ml cartridge 2 unit dial up / range 2-42 units (Owen Mumford Ltd)
1 device · NHS indicative price = £16.47 · Drug Tariff (Part IXa)

AUTOPEN® CLASSIC

Autopen® *Classic* (for use with Lilly and Wockhardt 3-mL insulin cartridges), allowing 1-unit dosage adjustment, max. 21 units (single-unit version) or 2-unit dosage adjustment, max. 42 units (2-unit version).

Autopen Classic hypodermic insulin injection pen reusable for 3ml cartridge 1 unit dial up / range 1-21 units (Owen Mumford Ltd)
1 device · NHS indicative price = £16.72 · Drug Tariff (Part IXa)

Autopen Classic hypodermic insulin injection pen reusable for 3ml cartridge 2 unit dial up / range 2-42 units (Owen Mumford Ltd)
1 device · NHS indicative price = £16.72 · Drug Tariff (Part IXa)

CLIKSTAR®

For use with *Lantus*®, *Apidra*®, and *Insuman*® 3-mL insulin cartridges; allowing 1-unit dose adjustment, max. 80 units.

ClikSTAR hypodermic insulin injection pen reusable for 3ml cartridge 1 unit dial up / range 1-80 units (Sanofi)
1 device · NHS indicative price = £25.00 · Drug Tariff (Part IXa)

ClikSTAR hypodermic insulin injection pen reusable for 3ml cartridge 1 unit dial up / range 1-80 units (Sanofi)
1 device · NHS indicative price = £25.00 · Drug Tariff (Part IXa)

HUMAPEN® LUXURA HD

For use with *Humulin*® and *Humalog*® 3-mL cartridges; allowing 0.5-unit dosage adjustment, max. 30 units.

HumaPen Luxura HD hypodermic insulin injection pen reusable for 3ml cartridge 0.5 unit dial up / range 1-30 units (Eli Lilly and Company Ltd)
1 device · NHS indicative price = £26.82 · Drug Tariff (Part IXa)

NOVOPEN® 4

For use with *Penfill*® 3-mL insulin cartridges; allowing 1-unit dosage adjustment, max. 60 units.

NovoPen 4 hypodermic insulin injection pen reusable for 3ml cartridge 1 unit dial up / range 1-60 units (Novo Nordisk Ltd)
1 device · NHS indicative price = £26.86 · Drug Tariff (Part IXa)

NovoPen 4 hypodermic insulin injection pen reusable for 3ml cartridge 1 unit dial up / range 1-60 units (Novo Nordisk Ltd)
1 device · NHS indicative price = £26.86 · Drug Tariff (Part IXa)

Needle free Insulin delivery systems

● NEEDLE FREE INSULIN DELIVERY SYSTEMS

INSUJET®

For use with any 10-mL vial or 3-mL cartridge of insulin, allowing 1-unit dosage adjustment, max 40 units.
Available as *starter set* (*InsuJet*® device, nozzle cap, nozzle and piston, 1 × 10-mL adaptor, 1 × 3-mL adaptor, 1 cartridge cap removal key), *nozzle pack* (15 nozzles), *cartridge adaptor pack* (15 adaptors), or *vial adaptor pack* (15 adaptors).

InsuJet starter set (Spirit Healthcare Ltd)
1 pack · NHS indicative price = £90.00 · Drug Tariff (Part IXa)

Urinanalysis reagent strips

● PRESCRIBING AND DISPENSING INFORMATION
Other reagent strips available for urinalysis
Include: *Combur-3 Test*® (glucose and protein—Roche Diagnostics); *Clinitek Microalbumin*® (albumin and creatinine—Siemens); *Ketodiastix*® (glucose and ketones—Bayer Diagnostics); *Medi-Test Combi 2*® (glucose and protein—BHR); *Micral-Test II*®, used to detect microalbuminuria but this should be followed by confirmation in the laboratory—false positive results are common (albumin—Roche Diagnostics); *Microbustix*® (albumin and creatinine—Siemens); *Uristix*® (glucose and protein—Siemens).

These reagent strips are not prescribable under National Health Service (NHS).

● URINE GLUCOSE TESTING STRIPS

Diastix testing strips (Bayer Diagnostics Manufacturing Ltd)
50 strip · NHS indicative price = £2.89 · Drug Tariff (Part IXr)

Medi-Test Glucose testing strips (BHR Pharmaceuticals Ltd)
50 strip · NHS indicative price = £2.33 · Drug Tariff (Part IXr)

Mission Glucose testing strips (Spirit Healthcare Ltd)
50 strip · NHS indicative price = £2.29 · Drug Tariff (Part IXr)

● URINE PROTEIN TESTING STRIPS

Albustix testing strips (Siemens Medical Solutions Diagnostics Ltd)
50 strip · NHS indicative price = £4.10 · Drug Tariff (Part IXr)

Medi-Test Protein 2 testing strips (BHR Pharmaceuticals Ltd)
50 strip · NHS indicative price = £3.27 · Drug Tariff (Part IXr)

● URINE KETONES TESTING STRIPS

GlucoRx KetoRx Sticks 2GK testing strips (GlucoRx Ltd)
50 strip · NHS indicative price = £2.25 · Drug Tariff (Part IXr)

Ketostix testing strips (Bayer Diagnostics Manufacturing Ltd)
50 strip · NHS indicative price = £3.06 · Drug Tariff (Part IXr)

Mission Ketone testing strips (Spirit Healthcare Ltd)
50 strip · NHS indicative price = £2.50 · Drug Tariff (Part IXr)

3.2 Hypoglycaemia

Hypoglycaemia

Treatment of hypoglycaemia

Initially glucose 10–20 g is given by mouth either in liquid form or as granulated sugar or sugar lumps. Approximately 10 g of glucose is available from non-diet versions of *Lucozade*® *Energy Original* 55 mL, *Coca-Cola*® 100 mL, *Ribena*® *Blackcurrant* 19 mL (to be diluted), 2 teaspoons of sugar, and also from 3 sugar lumps. Proprietary products of quick-acting carbohydrate (e.g. *GlucoGel*®, *Dextrogel*®, *GSF-Syrup*®, *Rapilose*® gel) are available on prescription for the patient to keep to hand in case of hypoglycaemia. If necessary this may be repeated in 10–15 minutes. After initial treatment, a snack providing sustained availability of carbohydrate (e.g. a sandwich, fruit, milk, or biscuits) or the next meal, if it is due, can prevent blood-glucose concentration from falling again.

Hypoglycaemia which causes unconsciousness is an emergency. Glucagon p. 652, a polypeptide hormone produced by the alpha cells of the islets of Langerhans, increases plasma-glucose concentration by mobilising glycogen stored in the liver. In hypoglycaemia, if sugar cannot be given by mouth, glucagon can be given by injection. Carbohydrates should be given as soon as possible to restore liver glycogen; glucagon is not appropriate for chronic hypoglycaemia. Glucagon may be issued to close relatives of insulin-treated patients for emergency use in hypoglycaemic attacks. It is often advisable to prescribe on an 'if necessary' basis to hospitalised insulin-treated patients, so that it may be given rapidly by the nurses during

6

Endocrine system

an hypoglycaemic emergency. If not effective in 10 minutes intravenous glucose should be given.

Alternatively, glucose **intravenous infusion 20%** may be given intravenously into a large vein through a large-gauge needle; care is required since this concentration is irritant especially if extravasation occurs. Glucose intravenous infusion 10% may also be used but larger volumes are needed. Glucose intravenous infusion 50% is not recommended because of the higher risk of extravasation injury and because administration is difficult. Close monitoring is necessary in the case of an overdose with a long-acting insulin because further administration of glucose may be required. Patients whose hypoglycaemia is caused by an oral antidiabetic drug should be transferred to hospital because the hypoglycaemic effects of these drugs may persist for many hours.

See also, emergency management of hypoglycaemia in dental practice for further advice.

Chronic hypoglycaemia

Diazoxide below, administered by mouth, is useful in the management of patients with chronic hypoglycaemia from excess endogenous insulin secretion, either from an islet cell tumour or islet cell hyperplasia. It has no place in the management of acute hypoglycaemia.

GLYCOGENOLYTIC HORMONES

Glucagon

● **INDICATIONS AND DOSE**

Insulin-induced hypoglycaemia

▸ BY SUBCUTANEOUS INJECTION, OR BY INTRAMUSCULAR INJECTION

▹ Child 1 month-1 year: 500 micrograms
▹ Child 2-17 years (body-weight up to 25 kg): 500 micrograms, if no response within 10 minutes intravenous glucose must be given
▹ Child 2-17 years (body-weight 25 kg and above): 1 mg, if no response within 10 minutes intravenous glucose must be given
▹ Adult: 1 mg, if no response within 10 minutes intravenous glucose must be given

Beta-blocker poisoning (cardiogenic shock unresponsive to atropine)

▸ INITIALLY BY INTRAVENOUS INJECTION

▹ Child: 50–150 micrograms/kg (max. per dose 10 mg), to be administered in glucose 5% (with precautions to protect the airway in case of vomiting), followed by (by intravenous infusion) 50 micrograms/kg/hour
▹ Adult: 2–10 mg, to be administered in glucose 5% (with precautions to protect the airway in case of vomiting), followed by (by intravenous infusion) 50 micrograms/kg/hour

Diagnostic aid

▸ BY INTRAVENOUS INJECTION, OR BY INTRAMUSCULAR INJECTION

▹ Adult: (consult product literature)

DOSE EQUIVALENCE AND CONVERSION
1 unit of glucagon = 1 mg of glucagon.

● UNLICENSED USE Dose and indication for cardiogenic shock unresponsive to atropine in beta-blocker overdose not licensed.
▹ In children Unlicensed for growth hormone test and hyperinsulinism.
● CONTRA-INDICATIONS Phaeochromocytoma
● CAUTIONS Glucagonoma · ineffective in chronic hypoglycaemia, starvation, and adrenal insufficiency · insulinoma · when used in the diagnosis of growth hormone secretion, delayed hypoglycaemia may result—

deaths reported (ensure a meal is eaten before discharge) (in children)
● SIDE-EFFECTS
▸ Rare Hypersensitivity reactions
▸ Frequency not known Abdominal pain (in adults) · diarrhoea (in children) · hypokalaemia · hypotension (in adults) · nausea · vomiting
● DIRECTIONS FOR ADMINISTRATION
▸ With intravenous use in children When administered by *continuous intravenous infusion*, do not add to infusion fluids containing calcium—precipitation may occur.
● PATIENT AND CARER ADVICE
Medicines for Children leaflet: Glucagon for hypoglycaemia www. medicinesforchildren.org.uk/glucagon-for-hypoglycaemia
● EXCEPTIONS TO LEGAL CATEGORY Prescription-only medicine restriction does not apply where administration is for saving life in emergency.

● MEDICINAL FORMS
There can be variation in the licensing of different medicines containing the same drug.
Powder and solvent for solution for injection
▸ GlucaGen Hypokit (Novo Nordisk Ltd)
Glucagon hydrochloride 1 mg GlucaGen Hypokit 1mg powder and solvent for solution for injection | 1 vial [PoM] £11.52 DT price = £11.52

3.2a Chronic hypoglycaemia

THIAZIDE DERIVATIVES

Diazoxide

● **INDICATIONS AND DOSE**

Chronic intractable hypoglycaemia

▸ BY MOUTH

▹ Adult: Initially 5 mg/kg daily in 2–3 divided doses, adjusted according to response; maintenance 3–8 mg/kg daily in 2–3 divided doses

● CAUTIONS Aortic coarctation · aortic stenosis · arteriovenous shunt · heart failure · hyperuricaemia · impaired cardiac circulation · impaired cerebral circulation
● INTERACTIONS → Appendix 1 (diazoxide).
● SIDE-EFFECTS Taste disturbance · abdominal pain · anaemia · anorexia (prolonged use) · bleeding · constipation · decreased libido · dermatitis · diarrhoea · dizziness · dyspnoea · eosinophilia · extrapyramidal effects · galactorrhoea · headache · heart failure · hyperglycaemia · hyperosmolar non-ketotic coma · hypertrichosis · hyperuricaemia (prolonged use) · hypotension · ileus · lacrimation · leucopenia · lichenoid eruption · musculoskeletal pain · nausea · pancreatitis · pruritus · pulmonary hypertension · raised serum creatinine · raised serum urea · reversible nephritic syndrome · sodium and fluid retention · thrombocytopenia · tinnitus · transient cataracts · visual disturbances · vomiting
● PREGNANCY Use only if essential; alopecia and hypertrichosis reported in neonates with prolonged use; may inhibit uterine activity during labour.
● BREAST FEEDING Manufacturer advises avoid—no information available.
● RENAL IMPAIRMENT Dose reduction may be required.
● MONITORING REQUIREMENTS
▸ Monitor blood pressure.
▸ Monitor white cell and platelet count during prolonged use.

● MEDICINAL FORMS
There can be variation in the licensing of different medicines containing the same drug. Forms available from special-order manufacturers include: capsule, oral suspension, oral solution

Tablet
▸ Eudemine (Focus Pharmaceuticals Ltd)
  Diazoxide 50 mg Eudemine 50mg tablets | 100 tablet PoM £46.45

Capsule
▸ Diazoxide (Non-proprietary)
  Diazoxide 25 mg Proglycem 25 capsules | 100 capsule PoM no price available

Oral suspension
▸ Diazoxide (Non-proprietary)
  Diazoxide 50 mg per 1 ml Proglycem 250mg/5ml oral suspension | 30 ml PoM no price available DT price = £126.47

---

4 Disorders of bone metabolism

Bone metabolism

Osteoporosis

Osteoporosis occurs most commonly in postmenopausal women and in those taking long-term oral corticosteroids (glucocorticosteroids). Other risk factors for osteoporosis include low body weight, cigarette smoking, excess alcohol intake, lack of physical activity, family history of osteoporosis, and early menopause.

Those at risk of osteoporosis should maintain an adequate intake of **calcium and vitamin D** and any deficiency should be corrected by increasing dietary intake or taking supplements.

Elderly patients, especially those who are housebound or live in residential or nursing homes, are at increased risk of calcium and vitamin D deficiency and may benefit from supplements. Reversible secondary causes of osteoporosis such as hyperthyroidism, hyperparathyroidism, osteomalacia or hypogonadism should be excluded, in both men and women, before treatment for osteoporosis is initiated.

Also see: calcium, phosphorus, vitamin D and oestrogens in postmenopausal osteoporosis.

Postmenopausal osteoporosis

The **bisphosphonates** (alendronic acid and risedronate) are effective for preventing postmenopausal osteoporosis. **Hormone replacement therapy** (HRT) is an option when other therapies are contra-indicated, cannot be tolerated, or if there is a lack of response. The CSM has advised that HRT should **not** be considered first-line therapy for long-term prevention of osteoporosis in women over 50 years of age. HRT is of most benefit for the prophylaxis of postmenopausal osteoporosis if started early in menopause and continued for up to 5 years, but bone loss resumes (possibly at an accelerated rate) on stopping HRT. Women of Afro-Caribbean origin appear to be less susceptible to osteoporosis than those who are white or of Asian origin.

Postmenopausal osteoporosis may be *treated* with a **bisphosphonate**. The bisphosphonates (such as alendronate and risedronate) decrease the risk of vertebral fracture; alendronate and risedronate have also been shown to reduce non-vertebral fractures. If bisphosphonates are unsuitable calcitriol p. 941 or **strontium ranelate** may be considered. Calcitonin (salmon) p. 660 is no longer recommended for the treatment of postmenopausal osteoporosis as the benefits are outweighed by the risk of malignancy associated with long-term use. Calcitonin (salmon) [unlicensed indication] has been used for pain relief for up to 3 months after a vertebral fracture when other analgesics were ineffective, but the benefits of treatment should be balanced against the risks. **Teriparatide** has been introduced for the treatment of postmenopausal osteoporosis.

Raloxifene hydrochloride p. 680 is licensed for the *prophylaxis* and *treatment* of vertebral fractures in postmenopausal women.

Corticosteroid-induced osteoporosis

To reduce the risk of osteoporosis doses of oral corticosteroids should be as low as possible and courses of treatment as short as possible. The risk of osteoporosis may be related to cumulative dose of corticosteroids; even intermittent courses can therefore increase the risk. The greatest rate of bone loss occurs during the first 6–12 months of corticosteroid use and so early steps to prevent the development of osteoporosis are important. Long-term use of high-dose inhaled corticosteroids may also contribute to corticosteroid-induced osteoporosis.

Patients taking (or who are likely to take) an oral corticosteroid for 3 months or longer should be assessed and where necessary given prophylactic treatment; those aged over 65 years are at greater risk. Patients taking oral corticosteroids who have sustained a low trauma fracture should receive treatment for osteoporosis. The therapeutic options for *prophylaxis* and *treatment* of corticosteroid-induced osteoporosis are the same:

● a bisphosphonate;
● Calcitriol [unlicensed indication];
● hormone replacement (HRT in women, testosterone in men [unlicensed indication]).

Calcitonin and parathyroid hormone

Calcitonin is involved with parathyroid hormone in the regulation of bone turnover and hence in the maintenance of calcium balance and homoeostasis. Calcitonin (salmon) (synthetic or recombinant salmon calcitonin) is used to lower the plasma-calcium concentration in patients with hypercalcaemia associated with malignancy.

Calcitonin (salmon) is also licensed for treatment of Paget's disease of bone when other treatments are ineffective or inappropriate; it is also licensed for the prevention of acute bone loss due to sudden immobility. Calcitonin (salmon) is no longer recommended for the prevention or treatment of postmenopausal osteoporosis because the benefits are outweighed by the risk of malignancy associated with long-term use.

Teriparatide p. 661 (a recombinant fragment of parathyroid hormone) is used for the treatment of postmenopausal osteoporosis, osteoporosis in men at increased risk of fracture, and corticosteroid-induced osteoporosis.

Cinacalcet p. 906 is licensed for the treatment of hypercalcaemia in parathyroid carcinoma.

Bisphosphonates

Bisphosphonates have an important role in the prophylaxis and treatment of osteoporosis and corticosteroid-induced osteoporosis; alendronic acid p. 655 or risedronate sodium p. 658 are considered the drugs of choice for these conditions.

Bisphosphonates are also used in the treatment of *Paget's disease*, hypercalcaemia of malignancy, and in bone metastases in breast cancer.

Strontium ranelate

Strontium ranelate treatment has been associated with an increased risk of serious cardiovascular disease, including myocardial infarction, and the risk should be assessed before treatment and regularly during treatment. Strontium ranelate should be initiated only by specialists for the treatment of severe osteoporosis in postmenopausal women or men at high risk of fracture for whom other treatments are contra-indicated or not tolerated.

6

Endocrine system

ANABOLIC STEROIDS

Nandrolone

- **INDICATIONS AND DOSE**

Osteoporosis in postmenopausal women (but not recommended)
  - ▸ BY DEEP INTRAMUSCULAR INJECTION
  - ▸ Adult (female): 50 mg every 3 weeks.

- CONTRA-INDICATIONS Acute porphyrias p. 918 · male breast cancer · prostate cancer
- CAUTIONS Cardiac impairment · diabetes mellitus · epilepsy · hypertension · migraine · skeletal metastases (risk of hypercalcaemia)
- INTERACTIONS → Appendix 1 (anabolic steroids).
- SIDE-EFFECTS Abnormal liver-function tests (with high doses) · acne · amenorrhoea · inhibition of spermatogenesis · liver tumours (with prolonged treatment with anabolic steroids) · premature epiphyseal closure · sodium retention with oedema · virilisation (with high doses including voice changes—sometimes irreversible)
- HEPATIC IMPAIRMENT Use in severe hepatic impairment only if benefit outweighs risk.
- RENAL IMPAIRMENT Use with caution—may cause sodium and water retention.
- MONITORING REQUIREMENTS Monitor skeletal maturation in young patients.
- LESS SUITABLE FOR PRESCRIBING Nandrolone injection is less suitable for prescribing.

- MEDICINAL FORMS
There can be variation in the licensing of different medicines containing the same drug.
Solution for injection
EXCIPIENTS: May contain Arachis (peanut) oil, benzyl alcohol
  - ▸ Deca-Durabolin (Aspen Pharma Trading Ltd)
    Nandrolone decanoate 50 mg per 1 ml Deca-Durabolin 50mg/1ml solution for injection ampoules | 1 ampoule [PoM] £3.17 [CD4-2]

BISPHOSPHONATES

Bisphosphonates

- DRUG ACTION Bisphosphonates are adsorbed onto hydroxyapatite crystals in bone, slowing both their rate of growth and dissolution, and therefore reducing the rate of bone turnover.

IMPORTANT SAFETY INFORMATION

MHRA/CHM ADVICE: BISPHOSPHONATES: ATYPICAL FEMORAL FRACTURES (JUNE 2011)
Atypical femoral fractures have been reported rarely with bisphosphonate treatment, mainly in patients receiving long-term treatment for osteoporosis.

The need to continue bisphosphonate treatment for osteoporosis should be re-evaluated periodically based on an assessment of the benefits and risks of treatment for individual patients, particularly after 5 or more years of use.

Patients should be advised to report any thigh, hip, or groin pain during treatment with a bisphosphonate.

Discontinuation of bisphosphonate treatment in patients suspected to have an atypical femoral fracture should be considered after an assessment of the benefits and risks of continued treatment.

MHRA/CHM ADVICE: BISPHOSPHONATES: OSTEONECROSIS OF THE JAW (NOVEMBER 2009) AND INTRAVENOUS BISPHOSPHONATES: OSTEONECROSIS OF THE JAW—FURTHER MEASURES TO MINIMISE RISK (JULY 2015)
The risk of osteonecrosis of the jaw is substantially greater for patients receiving intravenous bisphosphonates in the treatment of cancer than for patients receiving oral bisphosphonates for osteoporosis or Paget's disease.

Risk factors for developing osteonecrosis of the jaw that should be considered are: potency of bisphosphonate (highest for zoledronate), route of administration, cumulative dose, duration and type of malignant disease, concomitant treatment, smoking, comorbid conditions, and history of dental disease.

All patients should have a dental check-up (and any necessary remedial work should be performed) before bisphosphonate treatment, or as soon as possible after starting treatment. Patients should also maintain good oral hygiene, receive routine dental check-ups, and report any oral symptoms such as dental mobility, pain, or swelling, non-healing sores or discharge to a doctor and dentist during treatment.

Before prescribing an intravenous bisphosphonate, patients should be given a patient reminder card and informed of the risk of osteonecrosis of the jaw. Advise patients to tell their doctor if they have any problems with their mouth or teeth before starting treatment, and if the patient wears dentures, they should make sure their dentures fit properly. Patients should tell their doctor and dentist that they are receiving an intravenous bisphosphonate if they need dental treatment or dental surgery.

Guidance for dentists in primary care is included in *Oral Health Management of Patients Prescribed Bisphosphonates: Dental Clinical Guidance*, Scottish Dental Clinical Effectiveness Programme, April 2011 (available at www.sdcep.org.uk).

MHRA/CHM ADVICE: BISPHOSPHONATES: OSTEONECROSIS OF THE EXTERNAL AUDITORY CANAL (DECEMBER 2015)
Benign idiopathic osteonecrosis of the external auditory canal has been reported very rarely with bisphosphonate treatment, mainly in patients receiving long-term therapy (2 years or longer).

The possibility of osteonecrosis of the external auditory canal should be considered in patients receiving bisphosphonates who present with ear symptoms, including chronic ear infections, or suspected cholesteatoma.

Risk factors for developing osteonecrosis of the external auditory canal include: steroid use, chemotherapy, infection, an ear operation, or cotton-bud use.

Patients should be advised to report any ear pain, discharge from the ear, or an ear infection during treatment with a bisphosphonate.

- PATIENT AND CARER ADVICE
Atypical femoral fractures Patients should be advised to report any thigh, hip, or groin pain during treatment with a bisphosphonate.
Osteonecrosis of the jaw During bisphosphonate treatment patients should maintain good oral hygiene, receive routine dental check-ups, and report any oral symptoms.
Osteonecrosis of the external auditory canal Patients should be advised to report any ear pain, discharge from ear or an ear infection during treatment with a bisphosphonate.

◄ 654

Alendronic acid

10.6.2016

(Alendronate)

● INDICATIONS AND DOSE

Treatment of postmenopausal osteoporosis
▸ BY MOUTH
  ▸ Adult (female): 10 mg daily, alternatively 70 mg once weekly.

Treatment of osteoporosis in men
▸ BY MOUTH
  ▸ Adult (male): 10 mg daily.

Prevention and treatment of corticosteroid-induced osteoporosis in postmenopausal women not receiving hormone replacement therapy
▸ BY MOUTH
  ▸ Adult (female): 10 mg daily.

● CONTRA-INDICATIONS Abnormalities of oesophagus · hypocalcaemia · other factors which delay emptying (e.g. stricture or achalasia)

● CAUTIONS Active gastro-intestinal bleeding · atypical femoral fractures · duodenitis · dysphagia · exclude other causes of osteoporosis · gastritis · history (within 1 year) of ulcers · surgery of the upper gastro-intestinal tract · symptomatic oesophageal disease · ulcers · upper gastro-intestinal disorders

● INTERACTIONS → Appendix 1 (bisphosphonates).

● SIDE-EFFECTS
▸ **Common or very common** Abdominal distension · abdominal pain · alopecia · asthenia · constipation · diarrhoea · dizziness · dyspepsia · flatulence · headache · joint swelling · musculoskeletal pain · oesophageal reactions · peripheral oedema · pruritus · regurgitation · vertigo
▸ **Uncommon** Dysgeusia · episcleritis · erythema · gastritis · malaise (on initiation) · melena · myalgia (on initiation) · nausea · rash · scleritis · uveitis · vomiting
▸ **Rare** Atypical femoral fractures with long-term use · fever (on initiation) · hypocalcaemia · osteonecrosis of the jaw · photosensitivity · severe skin reactions · Stevens-Johnson syndrome · toxic epidermal necrolysis
▸ **Very rare** Osteonecrosis of the external auditory canal

SIDE-EFFECTS, FURTHER INFORMATION
▸ Oesophageal reactions Severe oesophageal reactions (oesophagitis, oesophageal ulcers, oesophageal stricture and oesophageal erosions) have been reported; patients should be advised to stop taking the tablets and to seek medical attention if they develop symptoms of oesophageal irritation such as dysphagia, new or worsening heartburn, pain on swallowing or retrosternal pain.

● PREGNANCY Avoid.

● BREAST FEEDING Manufacturer advises avoid—no information available.

● RENAL IMPAIRMENT Avoid if eGFR less than 35 mL/minute/1.73 m^2.

● MONITORING REQUIREMENTS Correct disturbances of calcium and mineral metabolism (e.g. vitamin-D deficiency, hypocalcaemia) before starting treatment. Monitor serum-calcium concentration during treatment.

● DIRECTIONS FOR ADMINISTRATION Tablets should be swallowed whole and oral solution should be swallowed as a single 100 mL dose. Doses should be taken with plenty of water while sitting or standing, on an empty stomach at least 30 minutes before breakfast (or another oral medicine); patient should stand or sit upright for at least 30 minutes after administration.

● PATIENT AND CARER ADVICE Patients or their carers should be given advice on how to administer alendronic acid tablets and oral solution.
Oesophageal reactions Patients (or their carers) should be advised to stop taking alendronic acid and to seek medical attention if they develop symptoms of oesophageal irritation such as dysphagia, new or worsening heartburn, pain on swallowing or retrosternal pain.

● NATIONAL FUNDING/ACCESS DECISIONS

NICE technology appraisals (TAs)
▸ Alendronate, etidronate, risedronate, raloxifene and strontium ranelate for the primary prevention of osteoporotic fragility fractures in postmenopausal women (October 2008) NICE TA160
  Alendronate is recommended as a treatment option for the primary prevention of osteoporotic fractures in the following susceptible postmenopausal women:
  ● Women over 70 years who have an independent risk factor for fracture (parental history of hip fracture, alcohol intake of 4 or more units per day, or rheumatoid arthritis) *or* an indicator of low bone mineral density (body mass index under 22 kg/m^2, ankylosing spondylitis, Crohn's disease, prolonged immobility, untreated premature menopause, or rheumatoid arthritis) **and** confirmed osteoporosis.
  ● Women aged 65–69 years who have an independent risk factor for fracture and confirmed osteoporosis.
  ● Women under 65 years who have an independent risk factor for fracture and at least one additional indicator of low bone mineral density and confirmed osteoporosis.
  www.nice.org.uk/TA160
▸ Alendronate, etidronate, risedronate, raloxifene, strontium ranelate, and teriparatide for the secondary prevention of osteoporotic fragility fractures in postmenopausal women (October 2008) NICE TA161
  This guideline recommends treatment options for the secondary prevention of osteoporotic fractures in postmenopausal women with confirmed osteoporosis who have also sustained a clinically apparent osteoporotic fracture.
  Alendronate is recommended as a treatment option for the secondary prevention of osteoporotic fractures in susceptible postmenupausal women.
  www.nice.org.uk/TA161

Scottish Medicines Consortium (SMC) Decisions
The *Scottish Medicines Consortium* has advised (April 2016) that alendronic acid (*Binosto*®) is accepted for restricted use within NHS Scotland for the treatment of postmenopausal osteoporosis where alendronic acid is the appropriate treatment choice, but the patient is unable to swallow tablets.

● MEDICINAL FORMS
There can be variation in the licensing of different medicines containing the same drug. Forms available from special-order manufacturers include: oral solution

Tablet
▸ Alendronic acid (Non-proprietary)
  Alendronic acid (as Alendronate sodium) 10 mg Alendronic acid 10mg tablets | 28 tablet [PoM] £3.25 DT price = £1.78
  Alendronic acid (as Alendronate sodium) 70 mg Alendronic acid 70mg tablets | 4 tablet [PoM] £22.80 DT price = £0.79
▸ Fosamax (Merck Sharp & Dohme Ltd)
  Alendronic acid (as Alendronate sodium) 10 mg Fosamax 10mg tablets | 28 tablet [PoM] £23.12 DT price = £1.78
  Alendronic acid (as Alendronate sodium) 70 mg Fosamax Once Weekly 70mg tablets | 4 tablet [PoM] £22.80 DT price = £0.79

Effervescent tablet
▸ Binosto (Internis Pharmaceuticals Ltd)
  Alendronic acid (as Alendronate sodium) 70 mg Binosto 70mg effervescent tablets sugar-free | 4 tablet [PoM] £22.80 DT price = £22.80

Oral solution

▸ Alendronic acid (Non-proprietary)
  Alendronic acid 700 microgram per 1 ml Alendronic acid 70mg/100ml oral solution unit dose sugar free sugar-free | 4 unit dose PoM £27.36 DT price = £27.36

Alendronic acid with colecalciferol

The properties listed below are those particular to the combination only. For the properties of the components please consider, alendronic acid p. 655, colecalciferol p. 941.

● **INDICATIONS AND DOSE**

Treatment of postmenopausal osteoporosis in women at risk of vitamin D deficiency

▸ BY MOUTH

▸ Adult (female): 1 tablet once weekly.

● **DIRECTIONS FOR ADMINISTRATION** Tablets should be swallowed whole with plenty of water while sitting or standing; to be taken on an empty stomach at least 30 minutes before breakfast (or another oral medicine); patient should stand or sit upright for at least 30 minutes after taking tablet.

● **PATIENT AND CARER ADVICE** Patients or carers should be given advice on how to administer alendronic acid with colecalciferol tablets.

● MEDICINAL FORMS
There can be variation in the licensing of different medicines containing the same drug.
Tablet
▸ Fosavance (Merck Sharp & Dohme Ltd)
  Colecalciferol 70 microgram, Alendronic acid (as Alendronate sodium) 70 mg Fosavance tablets | 4 tablet PoM £22.80 DT price = £22.80

F 654

Ibandronic acid

● **INDICATIONS AND DOSE**

Reduction of bone damage in bone metastases in breast cancer

▸ INITIALLY BY MOUTH

▸ Adult: 50 mg daily, alternatively (by intravenous infusion) 6 mg every 3–4 weeks

Hypercalcaemia of malignancy

▸ BY INTRAVENOUS INFUSION

▸ Adult: 2–4 mg as a single infusion, dose to be adjusted according to serum calcium concentration

Treatment of postmenopausal osteoporosis

▸ INITIALLY BY MOUTH

▸ Adult (female): 150 mg once a month, alternatively (by intravenous injection) 3 mg every 3 months, to be administered over 15–30 seconds.

● CONTRA-INDICATIONS
GENERAL CONTRA-INDICATIONS
Hypocalcaemia
SPECIFIC CONTRA-INDICATIONS
▸ With oral use Abnormalities of the oesophagus · other factors which delay emptying (e.g. stricture or achalasia)

● CAUTIONS Atypical femoral fractures · cardiac disease (avoid fluid overload)

● INTERACTIONS → Appendix 1 (bisphosphonates).

● SIDE-EFFECTS
GENERAL SIDE-EFFECTS
▸ **Common or very common** Abdominal pain · asthenia · bone pain · chills · diarrhoea · dyspepsia · fever · gastritis · headache · hypocalcaemia · hypophosphataemia · influenza-like symptoms · muscle pain · nausea · pharyngitis · rash · vomiting

▸ **Rare** Anaemia · angioedema · atypical femoral fractures · bronchospasm · hypersensitivity reactions · injection-site reactions · pruritus · urticaria

▸ **Very rare** Osteonecrosis of the external auditory canal · osteonecrosis of the jaw
SPECIFIC SIDE-EFFECTS
▸ **Common or very common**
▸ With oral use Severe oesophageal reactions (discontinue)

● PREGNANCY Avoid.

● BREAST FEEDING Avoid—present in milk in *animal* studies.

● RENAL IMPAIRMENT
▸ With intravenous use When used for bone metastases, if eGFR 30–50 mL/minute/1.73 m^2 reduce dose to 4 mg and infuse over 1 hour; if eGFR less than 30 mL/minute/1.73 m^2 reduce dose to 2 mg and infuse over 1 hour.
▸ With oral use When used for bone metastases, if eGFR 30–50 mL/minute/1.73 m^2 reduce dose to 50 mg on alternative days; if eGFR less than 30 mL/minute/1.73 m^2 reduce dose to 50 mg once weekly. When used for postmenopausal osteoporosis, avoid if eGFR less than 30 mL/minute/1.73 m^2.

● MONITORING REQUIREMENTS Monitor renal function and serum calcium, phosphate and magnesium.

● DIRECTIONS FOR ADMINISTRATION Tablets should be swallowed whole with plenty of water while sitting or standing; to be taken on an empty stomach at least 30 minutes (for most ibandronic acid tablets, 50 mg) or 1 hour (for *Bonviva* ® tablets, 150 mg) before first food or drink (other than water) of the day, or another oral medicine; patient should stand or sit upright for at least 1 hour after taking tablet.
For *intravenous infusion* (*Bondronat*®), give intermittently in Glucose 5% or Sodium chloride 0.9%; dilute requisite dose in 500 mL infusion fluid and give over 1–2 hours.

● PATIENT AND CARER ADVICE A patient reminder card should be provided to patients receiving intravenous ibandronic acid (risk of osteonecrosis of the jaw).
Patients or carers should be given advice on how to administer ibandronic acid tablets.
Oesophageal reactions Patients and carers should be advised to stop tablets and seek medical attention for symptoms of oesophageal irritation such as dysphagia, pain on swallowing, retrosternal pain, or heartburn.

● MEDICINAL FORMS
There can be variation in the licensing of different medicines containing the same drug.
Tablet
▸ Ibandronic acid (Non-proprietary)
  Ibandronic acid (as Ibandronic sodium monohydrate)
  50 mg Ibandronic acid 50mg tablets | 28 tablet PoM £174.51 DT price = £13.49
  Ibandronic acid (as Ibandronic sodium monohydrate)
  150 mg Ibandronic acid 150mg tablets | 1 tablet PoM £17.48 DT price = £1.20 | 3 tablet PoM £52.44
▸ Bondronat (Roche Products Ltd)
  Ibandronic acid (as Ibandronic sodium monohydrate)
  50 mg Bondronat 50mg tablets | 28 tablet PoM £183.69 DT price = £13.49
▸ Bonviva (Roche Products Ltd)
  Ibandronic acid (as Ibandronic sodium monohydrate)
  150 mg Bonviva 150mg tablets | 1 tablet PoM £18.40 DT price = £1.20
▸ Iasibon (Aspire Pharma Ltd)
  Ibandronic acid (as Ibandronic sodium monohydrate)
  50 mg Iasibon 50mg tablets | 28 tablet PoM £174.50 DT price = £13.49
▸ Quodixor (Aspire Pharma Ltd)
  Ibandronic acid (as Ibandronic sodium monohydrate)
  150 mg Quodixor 150mg tablets | 1 tablet PoM £18.40 DT price = £1.20

Solution for injection
▸ Ibandronic acid (Non-proprietary)
Ibandronic acid (as Ibandronic sodium monohydrate) 1 mg per 1 ml Ibandronic acid 3mg/3ml solution for injection pre-filled syringes | 1 pre-filled disposable injection PoM £65.20–£68.64
▸ Bonviva (Roche Products Ltd)
Ibandronic acid (as Ibandronic sodium monohydrate) 1 mg per 1 ml Bonviva 3mg/3ml solution for injection pre-filled syringes | 1 pre-filled disposable injection PoM £68.64

Solution for infusion
▸ Ibandronic acid (Non-proprietary)
Ibandronic acid (as Ibandronic sodium monohydrate) 1 mg per 1 ml Ibandronic acid 2mg/2ml solution for infusion vials | 1 vial PoM £89.36 (Hospital only)
Ibandronic acid 6mg/6ml solution for infusion vials | 1 vial PoM £183.68 (Hospital only) | 1 vial PoM £165.32
▸ Bondronat (Roche Products Ltd)
Ibandronic acid (as Ibandronic sodium monohydrate) 1 mg per 1 ml Bondronat 2mg/2ml concentrate for solution for infusion vials | 1 vial PoM £89.36 (Hospital only)
Bondronat 6mg/6ml concentrate for solution for infusion vials | 1 vial PoM £183.69

☞ 654

Pamidronate disodium

(Formerly called aminohydroxypropylidenediphosphonate disodium (APD))

● **INDICATIONS AND DOSE**

Hypercalcaemia of malignancy
▸ BY INTRAVENOUS INFUSION
▸ Adult: 15–60 mg, to be given (via cannula in a relatively large vein) as a single infusion or in divided doses over 2–4 days, dose adjusted according to serum calcium concentration; maximum 90 mg per course

Osteolytic lesions and bone pain in bone metastases associated with breast cancer or multiple myeloma
▸ BY INTRAVENOUS INFUSION
▸ Adult: 90 mg every 4 weeks, to be administered via cannula in a relatively large vein, dose may alternatively be administered every 3 weeks, to coincide with chemotherapy in breast cancer

Paget's disease of bone
▸ BY INTRAVENOUS INFUSION
▸ Adult: 30 mg every 1 week for a 6 week course (total dose 180 mg), alternatively initially 30 mg once weekly for 1 week, then increased to 60 mg every 2 weeks (max. per dose 60 mg) for a 6 week course (total dose 210 mg), to be administered via cannula in a relatively large vein, course may be repeated every 6 months; maximum 360 mg per course

● CAUTIONS Atypical femoral fractures · cardiac disease (especially in elderly) · ensure adequate hydration · previous thyroid surgery (risk of hypocalcaemia)

● INTERACTIONS → Appendix 1 (bisphosphonates). Avoid concurrent use with other bisphosphonates.

● SIDE-EFFECTS
▸ **Common or very common** Abdominal pain · anaemia · anorexia · arthralgia · bone pain · constipation · diarrhoea · drowsiness · fever · headache · hypertension · hypomagnesaemia · hypophosphataemia · influenza- like symptoms (sometimes accompanied by malaise, rigors, fatigue and flushes) · insomnia · lymphocytopenia · myalgia · nausea · paraesthesia · rash · symptomatic hypocalcaemia · tetany · thrombocytopenia · vomiting
▸ **Rare** Acute renal failure · agitation · atypical femoral fractures · confusion · conjunctivitis · deterioration of renal disease · dizziness · dyspepsia · haematuria · hallucinations · hyperkalaemia · hypernatraemia · hypokalaemia · hypotension · isolated cases of seizures · lethargy ·

leucopenia · muscle cramps · osteonecrosis of the jaw · other ocular symptoms · pruritus
▸ **Very rare** Osteonecrosis of the external auditory canal
▸ **Frequency not known** Atrial fibrillation · injection-site reactions · reactivation of herpes simplex · reactivation of herpes zoster

SIDE-EFFECTS, FURTHER INFORMATION
▸ Calcium and vitamin D supplements Oral supplements are advised to minimise potential risk of hypocalcaemia for those with mainly lytic bone metastases or multiple myeloma at risk of calcium or vitamin D deficiency (e.g. through malabsorption or lack of exposure to sunlight) and in those with Paget's disease.

● PREGNANCY Avoid—toxicity in *animal* studies.

● BREAST FEEDING Avoid.

● HEPATIC IMPAIRMENT Caution in severe hepatic impairment—no information available.

● RENAL IMPAIRMENT Max. infusion rate 20 mg/hour. Avoid if eGFR less than 30 mL/minute/1.73 m^2, except in life-threatening hypercalcaemia if benefit outweighs risk. If renal function deteriorates in patients with bone metastases, withhold dose until serum creatinine returns to within 10% of baseline value.

● MONITORING REQUIREMENTS
▸ Monitor serum electrolytes, calcium and phosphate—possibility of convulsions due to electrolyte changes.
▸ Assess renal function before each dose.

● DIRECTIONS FOR ADMINISTRATION
▸ With intravenous use For *slow intravenous infusion* (*Aredia®*; *Pamidronate disodium*, Hospira, Medac, Wockhardt), give intermittently in Glucose 5% or Sodium chloride 0.9%; give at a rate not exceeding 1 mg/minute; not to be given with infusion fluids containing calcium. For *Aredia®*, reconstitute initially with water for injections (15 mg in 5 mL, 30 mg or 90 mg in 10 mL), then dilute with infusion fluid to a concentration of not more than 90 mg in 250 mL. For *Pamidronate disodium* (Medac, Hospira, Wockhardt) dilute with infusion fluid to a concentration of not more than 90 mg in 250 mL

● PATIENT AND CARER ADVICE
A patient reminder card should be provided (risk of osteonecrosis of the jaw).

Driving and skilled tasks
Patients should be warned against performing skilled tasks (e.g. cycling, driving or operating machinery) immediately after treatment (somnolence or dizziness can occur).

● MEDICINAL FORMS
There can be variation in the licensing of different medicines containing the same drug.

Solution for infusion
▸ Pamidronate disodium (Non-proprietary)
Pamidronate disodium 3 mg per 1 ml Pamidronate disodium 15mg/5ml solution for infusion vials | 1 vial PoM £27.50 (Hospital only) | 5 vial PoM £149.15
Pamidronate disodium 30mg/10ml solution for infusion vials | 1 vial PoM £55.00 (Hospital only) | 1 vial PoM £59.66
Pamidronate disodium 60mg/20ml solution for infusion vials | 1 vial PoM £110.00 (Hospital only)
Pamidronate disodium 90mg/30ml solution for infusion vials | 1 vial PoM £165.00 (Hospital only)
Pamidronate disodium 6 mg per 1 ml Pamidronate disodium 60mg/10ml solution for infusion vials | 1 vial PoM £115.25
Pamidronate disodium 9 mg per 1 ml Pamidronate disodium 90mg/10ml solution for infusion vials | 1 vial PoM £170.45
Pamidronate disodium 15 mg per 1 ml Pamidronate disodium 60mg/4ml solution for infusion ampoules | 1 ampoule PoM £119.32
Pamidronate disodium 15mg/1ml solution for infusion ampoules | 4 ampoule PoM £119.32
Pamidronate disodium 90mg/6ml solution for infusion ampoules | 1 ampoule PoM £170.46
Pamidronate disodium 30mg/2ml solution for infusion ampoules | 2 ampoule PoM £119.32

6

Endocrine system

Risedronate sodium

☞ 654

● INDICATIONS AND DOSE

Paget's disease of bone
▶ BY MOUTH
▶ Adult: 30 mg daily for 2 months, course may be repeated if necessary after at least 2 months

Treatment of postmenopausal osteoporosis to reduce risk of vertebral or hip fractures
▶ BY MOUTH
▶ Adult (female): 5 mg daily, alternatively 35 mg once weekly.

Prevention of osteoporosis (including corticosteroid-induced osteoporosis) in postmenopausal women
▶ BY MOUTH
▶ Adult (female): 5 mg daily.

Treatment of osteoporosis in men at high risk of fractures
▶ BY MOUTH
▶ Adult (male): 35 mg once weekly.

● CONTRA-INDICATIONS Hypocalcaemia
● CAUTIONS Atypical femoral fractures · oesophageal abnormalities · other factors which delay transit or emptying (e.g. stricture or achalasia
● INTERACTIONS → Appendix 1 (bisphosphonates).
● SIDE-EFFECTS
▶ **Common or very common** Abdominal pain · constipation · diarrhoea · dyspepsia · headache · musculoskeletal pain · nausea
▶ **Uncommon** Duodenitis · dysphagia · gastritis · oesophageal ulcer · oesophagitis · uveitis
▶ **Rare** Atypical femoral fractures · glossitis · oesophageal stricture
▶ **Very rare** Osteonecrosis of the external auditory canal
▶ **Frequency not known** Cutaneous vasculitis · gastroduodenal ulceration · hair loss · hepatic disorders · osteonecrosis of the jaw · Stevens-Johnson syndrome · toxic epidermal necrolysis
● PREGNANCY Avoid.
● BREAST FEEDING Avoid.
● RENAL IMPAIRMENT Avoid if eGFR less than 30 mL/minute/1.73 m^2.
● MONITORING REQUIREMENTS
▶ Correct hypocalcaemia before starting.
▶ Correct other disturbances of bone and mineral metabolism (e.g. vitamin- D deficiency) at onset of treatment.
● DIRECTIONS FOR ADMINISTRATION Swallow tablets whole with full glass of water; on rising, take on an empty stomach at least 30 minutes before first food or drink of the day **or**, if taking at any other time of the day, avoid food and drink for at least 2 hours before or after risedronate (particularly avoid calcium-containing products e.g. milk; also avoid iron and mineral supplements and antacids); stand or sit upright for at least 30 minutes; do not take tablets at bedtime or before rising.
● PATIENT AND CARER ADVICE Patients or carers should be given advice on how to administer risedronate sodium tablets.
Oesophageal reactions Patients should be advised to stop taking the tablets and seek medical attention if they develop symptoms of oesophageal irritation such as dysphagia, pain on swallowing, retrosternal pain, or heartburn.
● NATIONAL FUNDING/ACCESS DECISIONS

NICE technology appraisals (TAs)
▶ Alendronate, etidronate, risedronate, raloxifene and strontium ranelate for the primary prevention of osteoporotic

fragility fractures in postmenopausal women (October 2008) NICE TA160
▶ With oral use **Risedronate** is recommended as an alternative for women:
  ● in whom alendronate is contra-indicated or not tolerated **and**
  ● who comply with particular combinations of bone mineral density measurement, age, and independent risk factors for fracture, as indicated in the full NICE guidance.
www.nice.org.uk/TA160
▶ Alendronate, etidronate, risedronate, raloxifene, strontium ranelate, and teriparatide for the secondary prevention of osteoporotic fragility fractures in postmenopausal women (October 2008) NICE TA161
▶ With oral use This guideline recommends treatment options for the secondary prevention of osteoporotic fractures in postmenopausal women with confirmed osteoporosis who have also sustained a clinically apparent osteoporotic fracture. **Risedronate** is are recommended as an alternative for women:
  ● in whom alendronate is contra-indicated or not tolerated **and**
  ● who comply with particular combinations of bone mineral density measurement, age, and independent risk factors for fracture (parental history of hip fracture, alcohol intake of 4 or more units per day, or rheumatoid arthritis, as indicated in the full NICE guidance.
www.nice.org.uk/TA161

● MEDICINAL FORMS
There can be variation in the licensing of different medicines containing the same drug. Forms available from special-order manufacturers include: oral suspension, oral solution
Tablet
▶ Risedronate sodium (Non-proprietary)
  Risedronate sodium 5 mg Risedronate sodium 5mg tablets | 28 tablet [PoM] £24.78 DT price = £18.87
  Risedronate sodium 30 mg Risedronate sodium 30mg tablets | 28 tablet [PoM] £143.95 DT price = £143.89
  Risedronate sodium 35 mg Risedronate sodium 35mg tablets | 4 tablet [PoM] £19.12 DT price = £0.88
▶ Actonel (Warner Chilcott UK Ltd)
  Risedronate sodium 5 mg Actonel 5mg tablets | 28 tablet [PoM] £17.99 DT price = £18.87
  Risedronate sodium 30 mg Actonel 30mg tablets | 28 tablet [PoM] £143.95 DT price = £143.89
  Risedronate sodium 35 mg Actonel Once a Week 35mg tablets | 4 tablet [PoM] £19.12 DT price = £0.88
  Actonel 35mg tablets | 4 tablet [PoM] no price available DT price = £0.88

Risedronate with calcium carbonate and colecalciferol

The properties listed below are those particular to the combination only. For the properties of the components please consider, risedronate sodium above, calcium carbonate p. 906, colecalciferol p. 941.

● INDICATIONS AND DOSE

Treatment of postmenopausal osteoporosis to reduce risk of vertebral or hip fractures
▶ BY MOUTH
▶ Adult: 1 tablet once weekly on day 1 of the weekly cycle, followed by 1 sachet daily on days 2–6 of the weekly cycle

● DIRECTIONS FOR ADMINISTRATION Tablets should be swallowed whole with plenty of water while sitting or standing; to be taken on an empty stomach at least 30 minutes before breakfast (or another oral medicine); patient should stand or sit upright for at least 30 minutes after taking tablet. Granules should be stirred into a glass of water and after dissolution complete taken immediately.

- **PRESCRIBING AND DISPENSING INFORMATION** *Actonel Combi*® effervescent granules contain calcium carbonate 2.5 g (calcium 1 g or Ca^{2+} 25 mmol) and colecalciferol 22 micrograms (880 units)/sachet.

- **PATIENT AND CARER ADVICE** Patients or carers should be given advice on how to administer calcium carbonate with colecalciferol and risedronate tablets and granules.

- **MEDICINAL FORMS** There can be variation in the licensing of different medicines containing the same drug.
  Tablet/Granules
  ▸ Actonel Combi (Warner Chilcott UK Ltd)
    Actonel Combi 35mg tablets and 1000mg/880unit effervescent granules sachets | 4 week supply [PoM] £19.12

☞ 654

Sodium clodronate

- **INDICATIONS AND DOSE**

Osteolytic lesions, hypercalcaemia and bone pain associated with skeletal metastases in patients with breast cancer or multiple myeloma
▸ BY MOUTH
  ▸ Adult: 1.6 g daily in 1–2 divided doses, then increased if necessary up to 3.2 g daily in 2 divided doses

LORON 520®

Osteolytic lesions, hypercalcaemia and bone pain associated with skeletal metastases in patients with breast cancer or multiple myeloma
▸ BY MOUTH
  ▸ Adult: Initially 2 tablets daily in 1–2 divided doses, increased if necessary up to 4 tablets daily

- **CONTRA-INDICATIONS** Acute gastro-intestinal inflammatory conditions

- **CAUTIONS** Atypical femoral fractures · maintain adequate fluid intake during treatment

- **INTERACTIONS** → Appendix 1 (bisphosphonates). Renal dysfunction reported in patients receiving concomitant NSAIDs.

- **SIDE-EFFECTS**
▸ **Common or very common** Bronchospasm · diarrhoea · nausea · skin reactions · vomiting
▸ **Rare** Atypical femoral fractures
▸ **Very rare** Osteonecrosis of the external auditory canal · osteonecrosis of the jaw
▸ **Frequency not known** Renal impairment · uveitis

- **PREGNANCY** Avoid.

- **BREAST FEEDING** Manufacturer advises avoid—no information available.

- **RENAL IMPAIRMENT** Max. initial dose 1200 mg daily if eGFR 30-50 mL/minute/1.73m². Use half normal dose if eGFR 10–30 mL/minute/1.73 m². Avoid if eGFR less than 10 mL/minute/1.73 m².

- **MONITORING REQUIREMENTS** Monitor renal function, serum calcium and serum phosphate before and during treatment.

- **DIRECTIONS FOR ADMINISTRATION** Avoid food for 2 hours before and 1 hour after treatment, particularly calcium-containing products e.g. milk; also avoid iron and mineral supplements and antacids; maintain adequate fluid intake.

- **PATIENT AND CARER ADVICE** Patients or carers should be given advice on how to administer sodium clodronate capsules and tablets.

- **MEDICINAL FORMS** There can be variation in the licensing of different medicines containing the same drug.
  Tablet
  CAUTIONARY AND ADVISORY LABELS 10
  ▸ Sodium clodronate (Non-proprietary)
    Sodium clodronate 800 mg Sodium clodronate 800mg tablets | 60 tablet [PoM] £116.72 DT price = £146.43
  ▸ Bonefos (Bayer Plc)
    Sodium clodronate 800 mg Bonefos 800mg tablets | 60 tablet [PoM] £146.43 DT price = £146.43
  ▸ Clasteon (Beacon Pharmaceuticals Ltd)
    Sodium clodronate 800 mg Clasteon 800mg tablets | 60 tablet [PoM] £146.43 DT price = £146.43
  ▸ Loron (Intrapharm Laboratories Ltd)
    Sodium clodronate 520 mg Loron 520mg tablets | 60 tablet [PoM] £152.59 DT price = £152.59
  Capsule
  ▸ Sodium clodronate (Non-proprietary)
    Sodium clodronate 400 mg Sodium clodronate 400mg capsules | 30 capsule [PoM] £40.49 | 120 capsule [PoM] £161.97 DT price = £139.83
  ▸ Bonefos (Bayer Plc)
    Sodium clodronate 400 mg Bonefos 400mg capsules | 120 capsule [PoM] £139.83 DT price = £139.83
  ▸ Clasteon (Beacon Pharmaceuticals Ltd)
    Sodium clodronate 400 mg Clasteon 400mg capsules | 30 capsule [PoM] £34.96 | 120 capsule [PoM] £139.83 DT price = £139.83

☞ 654

Zoledronic acid

- **INDICATIONS AND DOSE**

ACLASTA®

Treatment of Paget's disease of bone
▸ BY INTRAVENOUS INFUSION
  ▸ Adult: 5 mg as a single dose, to be administered over at least 15 minutes, at least 500 mg elemental calcium twice daily (with vitamin D) for at least 10 days is recommended following infusion

Treatment of postmenopausal osteoporosis and osteoporosis in men (including corticosteroid-induced osteoporosis)
▸ BY INTRAVENOUS INFUSION
  ▸ Adult: 5 mg once yearly as a single dose, to be administered over at least 15 minutes, in patients with a recent low-trauma hip fracture, the dose should be given 2 or more weeks following hip fracture repair; before first infusion give 50000–125000 units of vitamin D

ZOMETA® INFUSION

Reduction of bone damage in advanced malignancies involving bone
▸ BY INTRAVENOUS INFUSION
  ▸ Adult: 4 mg every 3–4 weeks, to be administered over at least 15 minutes, calcium 500 mg daily and vitamin D 400 units daily should also be taken

Hypercalcaemia of malignancy
▸ BY INTRAVENOUS INFUSION
  ▸ Adult: 4 mg for 1 dose, to be administered over at least 15 minutes

- **CAUTIONS** Atypical femoral fractures · cardiac disease (avoid fluid overload) · concomitant medicines that affect renal function

- **INTERACTIONS** → Appendix 1 (bisphosphonates).

- **SIDE-EFFECTS**
▸ **Common or very common** Anaemia · arthralgia · atrial fibrillation · bone pain · conjunctivitis · dizziness · fever · gastro-intestinal disturbances · headache · hypophosphataemia · influenza- like symptoms · myalgia · renal impairment · rigors

6

Endocrine system

▸ **Uncommon** Angioedema · anorexia · anxiety · asthenia · blurred vision · chest pain · cough · dry mouth · dyspnoea · haematuria · hypersensitivity reactions · hypertension · hypokalaemia · hypomagnesaemia · hypotension · injection-site reactions · lethargy · leucopenia · muscle cramps · paraesthesia · peripheral oedema · proteinuria · pruritus · rash · sleep disturbance · stomatitis · sweating · taste disturbance · thrombocytopenia · tremor · urinary frequency · weight gain

▸ **Rare** Acute renal failure · atypical femoral fractures · bradycardia · confusion · hyperkalaemia · hypernatraemia · osteonecrosis of the jaw · pancytopenia

▸ **Very rare** Episcleritis · osteonecrosis of the external auditory canal · uveitis

● SIDE-EFFECTS, FURTHER INFORMATION

▸ **Renal function** Renal impairment and renal failure have been reported; ensure patient is hydrated before each dose and assess renal function.

● CONCEPTION AND CONTRACEPTION Contra-indicated in women of child-bearing potential.

● PREGNANCY Avoid—toxicity in *animal* studies.

● BREAST FEEDING Avoid—no information available.

● HEPATIC IMPAIRMENT Caution in severe hepatic impairment—limited information available.

● RENAL IMPAIRMENT In advanced malignancies involving bone, if eGFR 50–60 mL/minute/1.73 m^2 reduce dose to 3.5 mg every 3–4 weeks; if eGFR 40–50 mL/minute/1.73 m^2 reduce dose to 3.3 mg every 3–4 weeks; if eGFR 30–40 mL/minute/1.73 m^2 reduce dose to 3 mg every 3–4 weeks; if renal function deteriorates in patients with bone metastases, withhold dose until serum creatinine returns to within 10% of baseline value. Avoid in tumour-induced hypercalcaemia if serum creatinine above 400 micromol/litre. Avoid in advanced malignancies involving bone if eGFR less than 30 mL/minute/1.73 m^2 (or if serum creatinine greater than 265 micromol/litre).

Avoid in Paget's disease, treatment of postmenopausal osteoporosis and osteoporosis in men if eGFR less than 35 mL/minute/1.73 m^2.

● MONITORING REQUIREMENTS

▸ Correct disturbances of calcium metabolism (e.g. vitamin D deficiency, hypocalcaemia) before starting. Monitor serum electrolytes, calcium, phosphate and magnesium.

▸ Monitor renal function in patients at risk, such as those with pre-existing renal impairment, those of advanced age, those taking concomitant nephrotoxic drugs or diuretics, or those who are dehydrated.

● DIRECTIONS FOR ADMINISTRATION For *intravenous infusion* (*Zometa*®), give intermittently in Glucose 5% *or* Sodium chloride 0.9%; dilute requisite dose according to product literature; infuse over at least 15 minutes; administer as a single intravenous solution in a separate infusion line.

● PATIENT AND CARER ADVICE A patient reminder card should be provided (risk of osteonecrosis of the jaw).

● NATIONAL FUNDING/ACCESS DECISIONS

ZOMETA® INFUSION

Scottish Medicines Consortium (SMC) Decisions
The *Scottish Medicines Consortium* has advised (May 2003) that for the prevention of skeletal related events *Zometa*® is accepted for restricted use within NHS Scotland for the treatment of patients with breast cancer and multiple myeloma if prescribed by an oncologist.

ACLASTA®

Scottish Medicines Consortium (SMC) Decisions
The *Scottish Medicines Consortium* has advised (February 2008) that in postmenopausal women *Aclasta*® is accepted for restricted use within the NHS Scotland for the treatment of osteoporosis in those for whom oral treatment options for osteoporosis are inappropriate and when initiated by a specialist.

● MEDICINAL FORMS
There can be variation in the licensing of different medicines containing the same drug.

Infusion

▸ Aclasta (Novartis Pharmaceuticals UK Ltd)
Zoledronic acid (as Zoledronic acid monohydrate) 50 microgram per 1 ml Aclasta 5mg/100ml infusion bottles | 1 bottle PoM
£253.38

▸ Zometa (Novartis Pharmaceuticals UK Ltd)
Zoledronic acid (as Zoledronic acid monohydrate) 40 microgram per 1 ml Zometa 4mg/100ml infusion bottles | 1 bottle PoM
£174.14

Solution for infusion

▸ Zometa (Novartis Pharmaceuticals UK Ltd)
Zoledronic acid (as Zoledronic acid monohydrate) 800 microgram per 1 ml Zometa 4mg/5ml solution for infusion vials | 1 vial PoM £174.14

CALCIUM REGULATING DRUGS 〉 BONE RESORPTION INHIBITORS

Calcitonin (salmon)

(Salcatonin)

● INDICATIONS AND DOSE

Hypercalcaemia of malignancy

▸ BY SUBCUTANEOUS INJECTION, OR BY INTRAMUSCULAR INJECTION

▸ Adult: 100 units every 6–8 hours (max. per dose 400 units every 6–8 hours), adjusted according to response

▸ BY INTRAVENOUS INFUSION

▸ Adult: Up to 10 units/kg, in severe or emergency cases, to be administered by slow intravenous infusion over at least 6 hours

Paget's disease of bone

▸ BY SUBCUTANEOUS INJECTION, OR BY INTRAMUSCULAR INJECTION

▸ Adult: 100 units daily, adjusted according to response for maximum 3 months (6 months in exceptional circumstances), a minimum dosage regimen of 50 units three times a week has been shown to achieve clinical and biochemical improvement

Prevention of acute bone loss due to sudden immobility

▸ BY SUBCUTANEOUS INJECTION, OR BY INTRAMUSCULAR INJECTION

▸ Adult: Initially 100 units daily in 1–2 divided doses, then reduced to 50 units daily at the start of mobilisation, usual duration of treatment is 2 weeks; maximum 4 weeks

● CONTRA-INDICATIONS Hypocalcaemia

● CAUTIONS Heart failure · history of allergy (skin test advised) · risk of malignancy—avoid prolonged use (use lowest effective dose for shortest possible time)

● SIDE-EFFECTS

▸ **Common or very common** Abdominal pain · diarrhoea · dizziness · fatigue · flushing · headache · malignancy (with long-term use) · musculoskeletal pain · nausea · taste disturbances · vomiting

▸ **Uncommon** Cough · hypersensitivity reactions · hypertension · injection-site reactions · oedema · polyuria · pruritus · rash · visual disturbances

▸ **Frequency not known** Tremor

● PREGNANCY Avoid unless potential benefit outweighs risk (toxicity in *animal* studies).

● BREAST FEEDING Avoid; inhibits lactation in *animals*.

● RENAL IMPAIRMENT Use with caution.

● DIRECTIONS FOR ADMINISTRATION

▸ With intravenous use For *intravenous infusion* (*Miacalcic*®), give intermittently in Sodium chloride 0.9%. Diluted solution given without delay. Dilute in 500 mL give over at least 6 hours; glass or hard plastic containers should not be used; some loss of potency on dilution and administration.

● MEDICINAL FORMS
There can be variation in the licensing of different medicines containing the same drug.
Solution for injection
▸ Miacalcic (Novartis Pharmaceuticals UK Ltd)
  Calcitonin (salmon) 50 unit per 1 ml Miacalcic 50units/1ml solution for injection ampoules | 5 ampoule [PoM] £17.10
  Calcitonin (salmon) 100 unit per 1 ml Miacalcic 100units/1ml solution for injection ampoules | 5 ampoule [PoM] £34.21
  Calcitonin (salmon) 200 unit per 1 ml Miacalcic 400units/2ml multidose solution for injection vials | 1 vial [PoM] £24.60

Strontium ranelate

● DRUG ACTION Stimulates bone formation and reduces bone resorption.

● INDICATIONS AND DOSE

Treatment of severe osteoporosis in postmenopausal women or men at high risk of fracture for whom other treatments are contra-indicated or not tolerated (initiated under specialist supervision)
▸ BY MOUTH
▸ Adult: 2 g once daily, dose to be taken in water, preferably at bedtime

● CONTRA-INDICATIONS Cerebrovascular disease · current or previous venous thromboembolic event · ischaemic heart disease · peripheral arterial disease · temporary or prolonged immobilisation · uncontrolled hypertension

● CAUTIONS Predisposition to cardiovascular disease—assess risk before and every 6–12 months during treatment

● INTERACTIONS → Appendix 1 (strontium ranelate).

● SIDE-EFFECTS
▸ **Common or very common** Dermatitis · diarrhoea · eczema · headache · myocardial infarction · nausea · venous thromboembolism
▸ **Very rare** Angioedema · hypersensitivity reactions · pruritus · rash · urticaria
▸ **Frequency not known** Abdominal pain · alopecia · bone marrow suppression · constipation · dyspepsia · flatulence · gastro-oesophageal reflux · peripheral oedema · stomatitis · vomiting

SIDE-EFFECTS, FURTHER INFORMATION
▸ Severe allergic reactions Severe allergic reactions, including drug rash with eosinophilia and systemic symptoms (DRESS), have been reported in patients taking strontium ranelate. DRESS starts with rash, fever, swollen glands, and increased white cell count, and it can affect the liver, kidneys and lungs; DRESS can also be fatal. Treatment with strontium ranelate should not be restarted.

● RENAL IMPAIRMENT Avoid if eGFR less than 30 mL/minute/1.73 m^2.

● EFFECT ON LABORATORY TESTS Interferes with colorimetric measurements of calcium in blood and urine.

● DIRECTIONS FOR ADMINISTRATION Avoid food for 2 hours before and after taking granules, particularly calcium-containing products e.g. milk; also preferably avoid concomitant antacids containing aluminium and magnesium hydroxides for 2 hours after taking granules.

● PATIENT AND CARER ADVICE
Patients or carers should be given advice on how to administer strontium ranelate granules.
Severe allergic reactions Patients should be advised to stop taking strontium ranelate and consult their doctor immediately if skin rash develops.

● NATIONAL FUNDING/ACCESS DECISIONS
NICE technology appraisals (TAs)
▸ Alendronate, etidronate, risedronate, raloxifene and strontium ranelate for the primary prevention of osteoporotic fragility fractures in postmenopausal women (October 2008) NICE TA160
Strontium ranelate is recommended as an alternative for women:
  ● in whom alendronate and risedronate are contra-indicated or not tolerated **and**
  ● who comply with particular combinations of bone mineral density measurement, age, and independent risk factors for fracture, as indicated in the full NICE guidance.
www.nice.org.uk/TA160

▸ Alendronate, etidronate, risedronate, raloxifene, strontium ranelate, and teriparatide for the secondary prevention of osteoporotic fragility fractures in postmenopausal women (October 2008) NICE TA161
This guideline recommends treatment options for the secondary prevention of osteoporotic fractures in postmenopausal women with confirmed osteoporosis who have also sustained a clinically apparent osteoporotic fracture.
Strontium ranelate is recommended as an alternative for women:
  ● in whom alendronate and risedronate are contra-indicated or not tolerated **and**
  ● who comply with particular combinations of bone mineral density measurement, age, and independent risk factors for fracture, as indicated in the full NICE guidance.
www.nice.org.uk/TA161

● MEDICINAL FORMS
There can be variation in the licensing of different medicines containing the same drug.
Granules
CAUTIONARY AND ADVISORY LABELS 5, 13
EXCIPIENTS: May contain Aspartame
▸ Protelos (Servier Laboratories Ltd) ▼
  Strontium ranelate 2 gram Protelos 2g granules sachets sugar-free | 28 sachet [PoM] £27.08 DT price = £27.08

CALCIUM REGULATING DRUGS › PARATHYROID HORMONES AND ANALOGUES

Teriparatide

● INDICATIONS AND DOSE

Treatment of osteoporosis in postmenopausal women and in men at increased risk of fractures | Treatment of corticosteroid-induced osteoporosis
▸ BY SUBCUTANEOUS INJECTION
▸ Adult: 20 micrograms daily for maximum duration of treatment 24 months (course not to be repeated)

● CONTRA-INDICATIONS Bone metastases · hyperparathyroidism · metabolic bone diseases · Paget's disease · pre-existing hypercalcaemia · previous radiation therapy to the skeleton · skeletal malignancies · unexplained raised alkaline phosphatase

● SIDE-EFFECTS
▸ **Common or very common** Anaemia · arthralgia · asthenia · depression · dizziness · dyspnoea · fatigue · gastro-intestinal disorders · haemorrhoids · headache · increased sweating · muscle cramps · myalgia · nausea · palpitation · reflux · sciatica · vertigo
▸ **Uncommon** Hypercalcaemia · injection-site reactions · urinary disorders
▸ **Rare** Hypersensitivity reactions

● PREGNANCY Avoid.

6

Endocrine system

- BREAST FEEDING Avoid.
- RENAL IMPAIRMENT Caution in moderate impairment; avoid if severe.
- NATIONAL FUNDING/ACCESS DECISIONS

NICE technology appraisals (TAs)
- Alendronate, etidronate, risedronate, raloxifene, strontium ranelate, and teriparatide for the secondary prevention of osteoporotic fragility fractures in postmenopausal women (October 2008) NICE TA161

This guideline recommends treatment options for the secondary prevention of osteoporotic fractures in postmenopausal women with confirmed osteoporosis who have also sustained a clinically apparent osteoporotic fracture.

Teriparatide is recommended as an alternative for women:
- in whom alendronate or risedronate, *or* strontium ranelate are contra-indicated or not tolerated, **or** where treatment with alendronate or risedronate has been unsatisfactory (indicated by another fragility fracture and a decline in bone mineral density despite treatment for 1 year) **and**
- who comply with particular combinations of bone mineral density measurement, age, and number of fractures, as indicated in the full NICE guidance.
www.nice.org.uk/TA161

Scottish Medicines Consortium (SMC) Decisions
The *Scottish Medicines Consortium* has advised (December 2003) that the use of teriparatide (*Forsteo* ®) in postmenopausal women should be restricted to the treatment of established (severe) osteoporosis and should be initiated by specialists experienced in the treatment of osteoporosis.

- MEDICINAL FORMS
There can be variation in the licensing of different medicines containing the same drug.
Solution for injection
- Forsteo (Eli Lilly and Company Ltd)
  Teriparatide 250 microgram per 1 ml Forsteo 20micrograms/80microlitres solution for injection 2.4ml pre-filled disposable devices | 1 pre-filled disposable injection PoM £271.88

DRUGS AFFECTING BONE STRUCTURE AND MINERALISATION > MONOCLONAL ANTIBODIES

Denosumab

- DRUG ACTION Denosumab is a human monoclonal antibody that inhibits osteoclast formation, function, and survival, thereby decreasing bone resorption.

- INDICATIONS AND DOSE
PROLIA®

Treatment of osteoporosis in postmenopausal women and in men at increased risk of fractures | Treatment of bone loss associated with hormone ablation in men with prostate cancer at increased risk of fractures
- BY SUBCUTANEOUS INJECTION
- Adult: 60 mg every 6 months, supplement with calcium and vitamin D

XGEVA®

Prevention of skeletal related events in patients with bone metastases from solid tumours
- BY SUBCUTANEOUS INJECTION
- Adult: 120 mg every 4 weeks, supplementation of at least Calcium 500 mg and vitamin D 400 units daily should also be taken unless hypercalcaemia is present

Treatment of giant cell tumour of bone that is unresectable or where surgical resection is likely to result in severe morbidity in adults and skeletally mature adolescents
- BY SUBCUTANEOUS INJECTION
- Adult: 120 mg every 4 weeks, give additional dose on days 8 and 15 of the first month of treatment only, supplementation of at least Calcium 500 mg and vitamin D 400 units daily should also be taken unless hypercalcaemia is present

IMPORTANT SAFETY INFORMATION
MHRA/CHM ADVICE: DENOSUMAB: ATYPICAL FEMORAL FRACTURES (FEBRUARY 2013)
Atypical femoral fractures have been reported rarely in patients receiving denosumab for the long-term treatment (2.5 or more years) of postmenopausal osteoporosis.

Patients should be advised to report any new or unusual thigh, hip, or groin pain during treatment with denosumab.

Discontinuation of denosumab in patients suspected to have an atypical femoral fracture should be considered after an assessment of the benefits and risks of continued treatment.

MHRA/CHM ADVICE: DENOSUMAB: MINIMISING THE RISK OF OSTEONECROSIS OF THE JAW; MONITORING FOR HYPOCALCAEMIA—UPDATED RECOMMENDATIONS (SEPTEMBER 2014) AND DENOSUMAB: OSTEONECROSIS OF THE JAW—FURTHER MEASURES TO MINIMISE RISK (JULY 2015)
Denosumab is associated with a risk of osteonecrosis of the jaw (ONJ) and with a risk of hypocalcaemia.
Osteonecrosis of the jaw
Osteonecrosis of the jaw is a well-known and common side-effect in patients receiving denosumab 120 mg for cancer. Risk factors include smoking, old age, poor oral hygiene, invasive dental procedures (including tooth extractions, dental implants, oral surgery), comorbidity (including dental disease, anaemia, coagulopathy, infection), advanced cancer, previous treatment with bisphosphonates, and concomitant treatments (including chemotherapy, anti-angiogenic biologics, corticosteroids, and radiotherapy to head and neck). The following precautions are now recommended to reduce the risk of ONJ:
Denosumab 120 mg (cancer indication)
- A dental examination and appropriate preventative dentistry before starting treatment are now recommended for all patients
- Do not start denosumab in patients with a dental or jaw condition requiring surgery, or in patients who have unhealed lesions from dental or oral surgery
Denosumab 60 mg (osteoporosis indication)
- Check for ONJ risk factors before starting treatment. A dental examination and appropriate preventative dentistry are now recommended for patients with risk factors

All patients should be given a patient reminder card and informed of the risk of ONJ. Advise patients to tell their doctor if they have any problems with their mouth or teeth before starting treatment, if they wear dentures they should make sure their dentures fit properly before starting treatment, to maintain good oral hygiene, receive routine dental check-ups during treatment, and immediately report any oral symptoms such as dental mobility, pain, swelling, non-healing sores or discharge to a doctor and dentist. Patients should tell their doctor and dentist that they are receiving denosumab if they need dental treatment or dental surgery.
Hypocalcaemia
Denosumab is associated with a risk of hypocalcaemia. This risk increases with the degree of renal impairment.

Hypocalcaemia usually occurs in the first weeks of denosumab treatment, but it can also occur later in treatment.

Plasma-calcium concentration monitoring is recommended for denosumab 120 mg (cancer indication):
- before the first dose
- within two weeks after the initial dose
- if suspected symptoms of hypocalcaemia occur
- consider monitoring more frequently in patients with risk factors for hypocalcaemia (e.g. severe renal impairment, creatinine clearance less than 30 mL/minute)

Plasma-calcium concentration monitoring is recommended for denosumab 60 mg (osteoporosis indication):
- before each dose
- within two weeks after the initial dose in patients with risk factors for hypocalcaemia (e.g. severe renal impairment, creatinine clearance less than 30 mL/minute)
- if suspected symptoms of hypocalcaemia occur

All patients should be advised to report symptoms of hypocalcaemia to their doctor (e.g. muscle spasms, twitches, cramps, numbness or tingling in the fingers, toes, or around the mouth).

- CONTRA-INDICATIONS Hypocalcaemia
  XGEVA® Unhealed lesions from dental or oral surgery
- CAUTIONS Atypical femoral fractures · hypocalcaemia · osteonecrosis of the jaw—consider temporary interruption of treatment if occurs
- SIDE-EFFECTS
  ▶ **Common or very common** Abdominal discomfort · cataracts · constipation · diarrhoea · dyspnoea · eczema · hypocalcaemia (fatal cases reported) · hypophosphataemia · musculoskeletal pain · osteonecrosis of the jaw · pain in extremity · rash · sciatica · sweating · upper respiratory tract infection · urinary tract infection
  ▶ **Uncommon** Cellulitis (seek prompt medical attention) · diverticulitis · ear infection · skin infections (seek prompt medical attention)
  ▶ **Rare** Atypical femoral fractures · osteonecrosis of the jaw
- CONCEPTION AND CONTRACEPTION Ensure effective contraception in women of child-bearing potential, during treatment and for at least 5 months after stopping treatment.
- PREGNANCY Avoid—toxicity in *animal* studies; risk of toxicity increases with each trimester—advise women who become pregnant during treatment to enrol in the manufacturer's Pregnancy Surveillance Programme (consult product literature).
- BREAST FEEDING Avoid (if women do decide to breast-feed during treatment, they should enrol in the manufacturer's Lactation Surveillance Programme—consult product literature.
- RENAL IMPAIRMENT Increased risk of hypocalcaemia if eGFR less than 30 mL/minute/1.73 m^2.
- MONITORING REQUIREMENTS Correct hypocalcaemia and vitamin D deficiency before starting. Monitor plasma-calcium concentration during therapy.
- PATIENT AND CARER ADVICE A patient reminder card should be provided (risk of osteonecrosis of the jaw). Atypical femoral fractures Patients should be advised to report any new or unusual thigh, hip, or groin pain during treatment with denosumab.
  Osteonecrosis of the jaw All patients should be informed to maintain good oral hygiene, receive routine dental check-ups, and immediately report any oral symptoms such as dental mobility, pain, or swelling to a doctor and dentist.

Hypocalaemia All patients should be advised to report symptoms of hypocalcaemia to their doctor (e.g. muscle spasms, twitches, cramps, numbness or tingling in the fingers, toes, or around the mouth).

- NATIONAL FUNDING/ACCESS DECISIONS

NICE technology appraisals (TAs)
▶ **Denosumab for the prevention of osteoporotic fractures in postmenopausal women (October 2010)** NICE TA204
Denosumab is recommended as a treatment option for the *primary prevention* of osteoporotic fragility fractures in postmenopausal women at increased risk of fractures:
- who are unable to comply with the special instructions for administering alendronate and risedronate, or have an intolerance of, or a contra-indication to, those treatments **and**
- who comply with particular combinations of bone mineral density measurement, age, and independent risk factors for fracture, as indicated in the full NICE guidance.

Denosumab is recommended as a treatment option for the *secondary prevention* of osteoporotic fragility fractures only in postmenopausal women at increased risk of fractures who are unable to comply with the special instructions for administering alendronate and risedronate, or have an intolerance of, or a contra-indication to, those treatments.
www.nice.org.uk/TA204

▶ **Denosumab for the prevention of skeletal-related events in adults with bone metastases from solid tumours (October 2012)** NICE TA265
Denosumab is recommended for the prevention of skeletal-related events in adults with bone metastases from breast cancer and from solid tumours other than prostate if:
- bisphosphonates would otherwise be prescribed, **and**
- the manufacturer provides denosumab with the discount agreed in the patient access scheme.

Denosumab is **not** recommended for preventing skeletal-related events in adults with bone metastases from prostate cancer.

Patients with bone metastases from solid tumours currently receiving denosumab whose disease does not meet the above criteria can continue treatment until they and their clinician consider it appropriate to stop.
www.nice.org.uk/TA265

PROLIA®

Scottish Medicines Consortium (SMC) Decisions
The *Scottish Medicines Consortium* has advised (November 2010) that denosumab (*Prolia*®) is accepted for restricted use within NHS Scotland for the treatment of osteoporosis in postmenopausal women at increased risk of fractures who have a bone mineral density T-score <-2.5 and ≥-4.0 and for whom bisphosphonates are unsuitable.

- MEDICINAL FORMS
There can be variation in the licensing of different medicines containing the same drug.
Solution for injection
▶ Prolia (Amgen Ltd)
  Denosumab 60 mg per 1 ml Prolia 60mg/1ml solution for injection pre-filled syringes | 1 pre-filled disposable injection PoM £183.00 DT price = £183.00
▶ Xgeva (Amgen Ltd) ▼
  Denosumab 70 mg per 1 ml Xgeva 120mg/1.7ml solution for injection vials | 1 vial PoM £309.86

Endocrine system

6

5 Dopamine responsive conditions

DOPAMINERGIC DRUGS > DOPAMINE RECEPTOR AGONISTS

Dopamine-receptor agonists

Overview

Bromocriptine p. 383 is used for the treatment of galactorrhoea, and for the treatment of prolactinomas (when it reduces both plasma prolactin concentration and tumour size). Bromocriptine also inhibits the release of growth hormone and is sometimes used in the treatment of acromegaly, but somatostatin analogues (such as octreotide p. 835) are more effective.

Cabergoline p. 385 has similar side-effects to bromocriptine, however patients intolerant of bromocriptine may be able to tolerate cabergoline (and *vice versa*).

Quinagolide below has actions and uses similar to those of ergot-derived dopamine agonists, but its side-effects differ slightly.

Suppression of lactation

Although bromocriptine and cabergoline are licensed to suppress lactation, they are **not** recommended for routine suppression (or for the relief of symptoms of postpartum pain and engorgement) that can be adequately treated with simple analgesics and breast support. If a dopamine-receptor agonist is required, cabergoline is preferred. Quinagolide is not licensed for the suppression of lactation.

Quinagolide

- DRUG ACTION Quinagolide is a non-ergot dopamine D_2 agonist.

- INDICATIONS AND DOSE
Hyperprolactinaemia
  ▸ BY MOUTH
  ▸ Adult: Initially 25 micrograms once daily for 3 days, dose to be taken at bedtime, increased in steps of 25 micrograms every 3 days; usual dose 75–150 micrograms daily, for doses higher than 300 micrograms daily increase in steps of 75–150 micrograms at intervals of not less than 4 weeks

- UNLICENSED USE Not licensed for the suppression of lactation.

- CAUTIONS Acute porphyrias p. 918 · history of psychotic illness · history of serious mental disorders
  CAUTIONS, FURTHER INFORMATION
  ▸ Hyperprolactinemic patients In hyperprolactinaemic patients, the source of the hyperprolactinaemia should be established (i.e. exclude pituitary tumour before treatment).

- INTERACTIONS → Appendix 1 (quinagolide). Tolerance may be reduced by alcohol.

- SIDE-EFFECTS
  ▸ Common or very common Abdominal pain · anorexia · constipation or diarrhoea · dizziness · fatigue · flushing · headache · hypotension · insomnia · nasal congestion · nausea · oedema · syncope · vomiting
  ▸ Very rare Psychosis
  SIDE-EFFECTS, FURTHER INFORMATION
  ▸ Gastro-intestinal bleeding Treatment should be withdrawn if gastro-intestinal bleeding occurs.

- ALLERGY AND CROSS-SENSITIVITY Quinagolide should not be used in patients with hypersensitivity to quinagolide (does not apply to hypersensitivity to ergot alkaloids).

- CONCEPTION AND CONTRACEPTION Advise non-hormonal contraception if pregnancy not desired.

- PREGNANCY Discontinue when pregnancy confirmed unless medical reason for continuing (specialist advice needed).

- BREAST FEEDING Suppresses lactation.

- HEPATIC IMPAIRMENT Avoid—no information available.

- RENAL IMPAIRMENT Avoid—no information available.

- MONITORING REQUIREMENTS Monitor blood pressure for a few days after starting treatment and following dosage increase.

- PATIENT AND CARER ADVICE
Driving and skilled tasks
Sudden onset of sleep Excessive daytime sleepiness and sudden onset of sleep can occur with dopamine-receptor agonists.

Patients starting treatment with these drugs should be warned of the risk and of the need to exercise caution when driving or operating machinery. Those who have experienced excessive sedation or sudden onset of sleep should refrain from driving or operating machines until these effects have stopped occurring.

Management of excessive daytime sleepiness should focus on the identification of an underlying cause, such as depression or concomitant medication. Patients should be counselled on improving sleep behaviour.
Hypotensive reactions Hypotensive reactions can be disturbing in some patients during the first few days of treatment with dopamine-receptor agonists, particular care should be exercised when driving or operating machinery.

- MEDICINAL FORMS
There can be variation in the licensing of different medicines containing the same drug.
Tablet
CAUTIONARY AND ADVISORY LABELS 10, 21
  ▸ Quinagolide (Non-proprietary)
    Quinagolide (as Quinagolide hydrochloride)
    75 microgram Quinagolide 75microgram tablets | 30 tablet [PoM] no price available
  ▸ Norprolac (Ferring Pharmaceuticals Ltd)
    Quinagolide (as Quinagolide hydrochloride)
    25 microgram Norprolac 25microgram tablets | 3 tablet [PoM] no price available
    Quinagolide (as Quinagolide hydrochloride)
    50 microgram Norprolac 50microgram tablets | 3 tablet [PoM] no price available
    Quinagolide (as Quinagolide hydrochloride)
    75 microgram Norprolac 75microgram tablets | 30 tablet [PoM] £27.00
  ▸ Norprolac (Ferring Pharmaceuticals Ltd)
    Norprolac tablets starter pack | 6 tablet [PoM] £4.50

6 Gonadotrophin responsive conditions

Gonadotrophins

Drugs affecting gonadotrophins

Danazol p. 670 is licensed for the treatment of *endometriosis* and for the relief of severe pain and tenderness in *benign fibrocystic breast disease* where other measures have proved unsatisfactory. It may also be effective in the long-term management of *hereditary angioedema* [unlicensed indication].

Cetrorelix below and ganirelix below are luteinising hormone releasing hormone antagonists, which inhibit the release of gonadotrophins (luteinising hormone and follicle stimulating hormone). They are used in the treatment of infertility by assisted reproductive techniques.

Gonadorelin analogues

Gonadorelin analogues are used in the treatment of endometriosis, precocious puberty, infertility, male hypersexuality with severe sexual deviation, anaemia due to uterine fibroids (together with iron supplementation), breast cancer, prostate cancer and before intra-uterine surgery. Use of leuprorelin acetate and triptorelin for 3 to 4 months before surgery reduces the uterine volume, fibroid size and associated bleeding. For women undergoing hysterectomy or myomectomy, a vaginal procedure is made more feasible following the use of a gonadorelin analogue.

Breast pain (mastalgia)

Once any serious underlying cause for breast pain has been ruled out, most women will respond to reassurance and reduction in dietary fat; withdrawal of an oral contraceptive or of hormone replacement therapy may help to resolve the pain.

Mild, non-cyclical breast pain is treated with simple analgesics; moderate to severe pain, cyclical pain or symptoms that persist for longer than 6 months may require specific drug treatment.

Danazol is licensed for the relief of severe pain and tenderness in benign fibrocystic breast disease which has not responded to other treatment.

Tamoxifen p. 837 may be a useful adjunct in the treatment of mastalgia [unlicensed indication] especially when symptoms can definitely be related to cyclic oestrogen production; it may be given on the days of the cycle when symptoms are predicted.

Treatment for breast pain should be reviewed after 6 months and continued if necessary. Symptoms recur in about 50% of women within 2 years of withdrawal of therapy but may be less severe.

PITUITARY AND HYPOTHALAMIC HORMONES AND ANALOGUES > ANTI-GONADOTROPHIN-RELEASING HORMONES

Cetrorelix

● **INDICATIONS AND DOSE**

Adjunct in the treatment of female infertility (initiated under specialist supervision)
▸ BY SUBCUTANEOUS INJECTION
▸ Adult (female): 250 micrograms once daily, dose to be administered in the morning, starting on day 5 or 6 of ovarian stimulation with gonadotrophins (or each evening starting on day 5 of ovarian stimulation), continue throughout administration of gonadotrophin including day of ovulation induction (or evening before ovulation induction), dose to be injected into the lower abdominal wall.

● **SIDE-EFFECTS**
▸ **Common or very common** Headache · injection site reactions · nausea
▸ **Rare** Hypersensitivity reactions
● **PREGNANCY** Avoid in confirmed pregnancy.
● **BREAST FEEDING** Avoid.
● **HEPATIC IMPAIRMENT** Avoid in moderate or severe liver impairment.
● **RENAL IMPAIRMENT** Avoid in moderate or severe renal impairment.

● **MEDICINAL FORMS**
There can be variation in the licensing of different medicines containing the same drug.
Powder and solvent for solution for injection
▸ Cetrotide (Merck Serono Ltd)
Cetrorelix (as Cetrorelix acetate) 250 microgram Cetrotide 250microgram powder and solvent for solution for injection vials | 1 vial [PoM] £22.61

Ganirelix

● **INDICATIONS AND DOSE**

Adjunct in the treatment of female infertility (initiated under specialist supervision)
▸ BY SUBCUTANEOUS INJECTION
▸ Adult: 250 micrograms once daily, dose to be administered in the morning (or each afternoon) starting on day 5 or day 6 of ovarian stimulation with gonadotrophins, continue throughout administration of gonadotrophins including day of ovulation induction (if administering in afternoon, give last dose in afternoon before ovulation induction), dose to be injected preferably into the upper leg (rotate injection sites to prevent lipoatrophy)

● **SIDE-EFFECTS**
▸ **Very rare** Facial oedema · hypersensitivity reactions · rash
▸ **Frequency not known** Dyspnoea · headache · injection-site reactions · malaise · nausea
● **PREGNANCY** Avoid in confirmed pregnancy—toxicity in *animal* studies.
● **BREAST FEEDING** Avoid—no information available.
● **HEPATIC IMPAIRMENT** Avoid in moderate or severe hepatic impairment.
● **RENAL IMPAIRMENT** Avoid in moderate to severe renal impairment.

● **MEDICINAL FORMS**
There can be variation in the licensing of different medicines containing the same drug.
Solution for injection
▸ Orgalutran (Merck Sharp & Dohme Ltd)
Ganirelix 500 microgram per 1 ml Orgalutran 250micrograms/0.5ml solution for injection pre-filled syringes | 1 pre-filled disposable injection [PoM] £21.48

PITUITARY AND HYPOTHALAMIC HORMONES AND ANALOGUES > GONADOTROPIN-RELEASING HORMONES

Buserelin

● **DRUG ACTION** Administration of gonadorelin analogues produces an initial phase of stimulation; continued administration is followed by down-regulation of gonadotrophin-releasing hormone receptors, thereby reducing the release of gonadotrophins (follicle stimulating hormone and luteinising hormone) which in turn leads to inhibition of androgen and oestrogen production.

● **INDICATIONS AND DOSE**

Endometriosis
▸ BY INTRANASAL ADMINISTRATION
▸ Adult: 300 micrograms 3 times a day maximum duration of treatment 6 months (do not repeat), to be started on days 1 or 2 of menstruation; administer one 150 microgram spray into each nostril continued →

Endocrine system

6

Pituitary desensitisation before induction of ovulation by gonadotrophins for in vitro fertilisation (under expert supervision)
▸ BY SUBCUTANEOUS INJECTION
▸ Adult: 200–500 micrograms once daily, increased if necessary up to 500 micrograms twice daily, starting in early follicular phase (day 1) or, after exclusion of pregnancy, in midluteal phase (day 21) and continued until down-regulation achieved (usually 1–3 weeks) then maintained during gonadotrophin administration (stopping gonadotrophin and buserelin on administration of chorionic gonadotrophin at appropriate stage of follicular development)
▸ BY INTRANASAL ADMINISTRATION
▸ Adult: 150–300 micrograms 4 times a day, (150 micrograms equivalent to one spray), to be administered during waking hours. Start in early follicular phase (day 1) or, after exclusion of pregnancy, in the midluteal phase (day 21) and continued until down-regulation achieved (usually about 2–3 weeks) then maintained during gonadotrophin administration (stopping gonadotrophin and buserelin on administration of chorionic gonadotrophin at appropriate stage of follicular development)

Advanced prostate cancer
▸ INITIALLY BY SUBCUTANEOUS INJECTION
▸ Adult: 500 micrograms every 8 hours for 7 days, then (by intranasal administration) 200 micrograms 6 times a day, (a single 100 microgram spray to be administered into each nostril)

● CONTRA-INDICATIONS
▸ When used for endometriosis Hormone dependent tumours · undiagnosed vaginal bleeding · use longer than 6 months (do not repeat)
▸ When used for pituitary desensitisation Hormone dependent tumours · undiagnosed vaginal bleeding
● CAUTIONS Depression · diabetes · hypertension · patients with metabolic bone disease (decrease in bone mineral density can occur) · polycystic ovarian disease
● SIDE-EFFECTS
GENERAL SIDE-EFFECTS
Abdominal pain · acne · altered blood lipids · anaphylaxis · anxiety · arthralgia · asthma · bleeding associated with fibroid degeneration (when treating uterine fibroids) · breakthrough bleeding · breast tenderness · changes in appetite · changes in breast size · changes in scalp and body hair · concentration disturbances · constipation · decrease in trabecular bone density · depression · diarrhoea · dizziness · drowsiness · dry eyes · dry skin · dyspareunia · fatigue · gynaecomastia · hair loss · headache · hearing disturbances · hot flushes · hypersensitivity reactions · hypertension · increased sweating · increased thirst · initially withdrawal bleeding · lactation · leucopenia · leucorrhoea · local reactions at injection site · loss of libido · memory disturbances · menopausal-like symptoms · migraine · mood changes · musculoskeletal pain · musculoskeletal weakness · myalgia · nausea · nervousness · oedema of the face and extremities · ovarian cysts (may require withdrawal) · palpitation · paraesthesia · pruritus · rash · reduced glucose tolerance · sexual dysfunction · sleep disturbances · splitting nails · thrombocytopenia · urticaria · vaginal dryness · visual disturbances · vomiting · weight changes
SPECIFIC SIDE-EFFECTS
▸ With intranasal use Altered sense of taste and smell · nasal irritation · nose bleeds

SIDE-EFFECTS, FURTHER INFORMATION
▸ Tumour flare
▸ When used for Advanced prostate cancer During the initial stage (1–2 weeks) increased production of testosterone may be associated with progression of prostate cancer. In susceptible patients this tumour 'flare' may cause spinal cord compression, ureteric obstruction or increased bone pain.
● CONCEPTION AND CONTRACEPTION Non-hormonal, barrier methods of contraception should be used during entire treatment period. Pregnancy should be excluded before treatment, the first injection should be given during menstruation or shortly afterwards or use barrier contraception for 1 month beforehand.
● PREGNANCY Avoid.
● BREAST FEEDING Avoid.
● DIRECTIONS FOR ADMINISTRATION
▸ With intranasal use Avoid use of nasal decongestants before and for at least 30 minutes after treatment.
▸ With subcutaneous use Rotate injection site to prevent atrophy and nodule formation.
● PATIENT AND CARER ADVICE Patients or carers should be given advice on how to administer buserelin nasal spray.

● MEDICINAL FORMS
There can be variation in the licensing of different medicines containing the same drug.
Solution for injection
▸ Suprecur (Sanofi)
Buserelin (as Buserelin acetate) 1 mg per 1 ml Suprecur 5.5mg/5.5ml solution for injection vials | 2 vial [PoM] £33.02
▸ Suprefact (Sanofi)
Buserelin (as Buserelin acetate) 1 mg per 1 ml Suprefact 5.5mg/5.5ml solution for injection vials | 2 vial [PoM] £34.37
Spray
▸ Suprecur (Sanofi)
Buserelin (as Buserelin acetate) 150 microgram per 1 dose Suprecur 150micrograms/dose nasal spray | 168 dose [PoM] £105.16
▸ Suprefact (Sanofi)
Buserelin (as Buserelin acetate) 100 microgram per 1 dose Suprefact 100micrograms/dose nasal spray | 336 dose [PoM] £122.24

Goserelin

● DRUG ACTION Administration of gonadorelin analogues produces an initial phase of stimulation; continued administration is followed by down-regulation of gonadotrophin-releasing hormone receptors, thereby reducing the release of gonadotrophins (follicle stimulating hormone and luteinising hormone) which in turn leads to inhibition of androgen and oestrogen production.

● INDICATIONS AND DOSE
ZOLADEX LA®

Locally advanced prostate cancer as an alternative to surgical castration | Adjuvant treatment to radiotherapy or radical prostatectomy in patients with high-risk localised or locally advanced prostate cancer | Neoadjuvant treatment prior to radiotherapy in patients with high-risk localised or locally advanced prostate cancer | Metastatic prostate cancer
▸ BY SUBCUTANEOUS INJECTION
▸ Adult: 10.8 mg every 12 weeks, to be administered into the anterior abdominal wall

ZOLADEX®

Locally advanced prostate cancer as an alternative to surgical castration | Adjuvant treatment to radiotherapy or radical prostatectomy in patients with high-risk localised or locally advanced prostate cancer | Neoadjuvant treatment prior to radiotherapy in patients with high-risk localised or locally advanced prostate cancer | Metastatic prostate cancer | Advanced breast cancer | Oestrogen-receptor-positive early breast cancer

▸ BY SUBCUTANEOUS INJECTION

▸ Adult: 3.6 mg every 28 days, to be administered into the anterior abdominal wall

Endometriosis

▸ BY SUBCUTANEOUS INJECTION

▸ Adult: 3.6 mg every 28 days maximum duration of treatment 6 months (do not repeat), to be administered into the anterior abdominal wall

Endometrial thinning before intra-uterine surgery

▸ BY SUBCUTANEOUS INJECTION

▸ Adult: 3.6 mg, dose may be repeated after 28 days if uterus is large or to allow flexible surgical timing, to be administered into the anterior abdominal wall

Before surgery in women who have anaemia due to uterine fibroids

▸ BY SUBCUTANEOUS INJECTION

▸ Adult: 3.6 mg every 28 days maximum duration of treatment 3 months, to be given with supplementary iron, to be administered into the anterior abdominal wall

Pituitary desensitisation before induction of ovulation by gonadotrophins for in vitro fertilisation (after exclusion of pregnancy) (under expert supervision)

▸ BY SUBCUTANEOUS INJECTION

▸ Adult: 3.6 mg, dose given to achieve pituitary down-regulation (usually 1–3 weeks) then gonadotrophin is administered (stopping gonadotrophin on administration of chorionic gonadotrophin at appropriate stage of follicular development), to be administered into the anterior abdominal wall

● CONTRA-INDICATIONS Undiagnosed vaginal bleeding · use longer than 6 months in endometriosis (do not repeat)

● CAUTIONS Depression · diabetes · hypertension · patients with metabolic bone disease (decrease in bone mineral density can occur) · polycystic ovarian disease · risk of spinal cord compression in men · risk of ureteric obstruction in men

● SIDE-EFFECTS

▸ Rare Hypercalcaemia (in women)

▸ **Frequency not known** Anaphylaxis · arthralgia · asthma · breast tenderness · changes in blood pressure · changes in breast size · changes in scalp and body hair · decrease in trabecular bone density · depression · dizziness · dyspareunia (when used for gynaecological conditions) · gastro-intestinal disturbances · gynaecomastia · headache · heart failure (when used for prostate or breast cancer) · hot flushes · hypersensitivity reactions · increased sweating · local reactions at injection site · loss of libido · menopausal-like symptoms · migraine · mood changes · musculoskeletal pain (when used for gynaecological conditions) · musculoskeletal weakness (when used for gynaecological conditions) · myalgia · myocardial infarction (when used for prostate or breast cancer) · oedema of the face and extremities (when used for gynaecological conditions) · ovarian cysts (may require withdrawal) · palpitation (when used for gynaecological conditions) · paraesthesia · paraesthesia · pruritus · rash · sexual dysfunction · sleep disorders · urticaria · vaginal bleeding · vaginal dryness · visual disturbances · weight change · withdrawal bleeding

SIDE-EFFECTS, FURTHER INFORMATION

▸ Tumour flare (when used for prostate cancer) During the initial stage (1–2 weeks) increased production of testosterone may be associated with progression of prostate cancer. In susceptible patients this tumour 'flare' may cause spinal cord compression, ureteric obstruction or increased bone pain.

● CONCEPTION AND CONTRACEPTION Non-hormonal, barrier methods of contraception should be used during entire treatment period. Pregnancy should be excluded before treatment, the first injection should be given during menstruation or shortly afterwards or use barrier contraception for 1 month beforehand.

● PREGNANCY Avoid.

● BREAST FEEDING Avoid.

● MONITORING REQUIREMENTS Men at risk of tumour 'flare' should be monitored closely during the first month of therapy for prostate cancer.

● DIRECTIONS FOR ADMINISTRATION Rotate injection site to prevent atrophy and nodule formation.

● MEDICINAL FORMS
There can be variation in the licensing of different medicines containing the same drug.

Implant

▸ Zoladex (AstraZeneca UK Ltd)
Goserelin (as Goserelin acetate) 3.6 mg Zoladex 3.6mg implant SafeSystem pre-filled syringes | 1 pre-filled disposable injection [PoM] £65.00 DT price = £65.00

▸ Zoladex LA (AstraZeneca UK Ltd)
Goserelin (as Goserelin acetate) 10.8 mg Zoladex LA 10.8mg implant SafeSystem pre-filled syringes | 1 pre-filled disposable injection [PoM] £235.00 DT price = £235.00

Leuprorelin acetate

● DRUG ACTION Administration of gonadorelin analogues produces an initial phase of stimulation; continued administration is followed by down-regulation of gonadotrophin-releasing hormone receptors, thereby reducing the release of gonadotrophins (follicle stimulating hormone and luteinising hormone) which in turn leads to inhibition of androgen and oestrogen production.

● INDICATIONS AND DOSE

PROSTAP 3 DCS®

Locally advanced prostate cancer as an alternative to surgical castration | Adjuvant treatment to radiotherapy or radical prostatectomy in patients with high-risk localised or locally advanced prostate cancer | Metastatic prostate cancer

▸ BY SUBCUTANEOUS INJECTION

▸ Adult: 11.25 mg every 3 months

Endometriosis

▸ BY INTRAMUSCULAR INJECTION

▸ Adult: Initially 11.25 mg for 1 dose, dose to be given as a single dose in first 5 days of menstrual cycle, then 11.25 mg every 3 months for maximum 6 months (course not to be repeated)

PROSTAP SR DCS®

Locally advanced prostate cancer as an alternative to surgical castration | Adjuvant treatment to radiotherapy or radical prostatectomy in patients with high-risk localised or locally advanced prostate cancer | Metastatic prostate cancer

▸ BY SUBCUTANEOUS INJECTION, OR BY INTRAMUSCULAR INJECTION

▸ Adult: 3.75 mg every 1 month   continued →

6

Endocrine system

Endocrine system

6

Endometriosis
▶ BY SUBCUTANEOUS INJECTION, OR BY INTRAMUSCULAR INJECTION
▸ Adult: Initially 3.75 mg for 1 dose, dose to be given as a single dose in first 5 days of menstrual cycle, then 3.75 mg every 1 month for maximum 6 months (course not to be repeated)

Endometrial thinning before intra-uterine surgery
▶ BY SUBCUTANEOUS INJECTION, OR BY INTRAMUSCULAR INJECTION
▸ Adult: Initially 3.75 mg for 1 dose, dose to be given as a single dose between day 3 and 5 of menstrual cycle, 5–6 weeks before surgery

Reduction of size of uterine fibroids and of associated bleeding before surgery
▶ BY SUBCUTANEOUS INJECTION, OR BY INTRAMUSCULAR INJECTION
▸ Adult: Initially 3.75 mg every 1 month usually for 3–4 months (maximum 6 months)

- CONTRA-INDICATIONS
  GENERAL CONTRA-INDICATIONS
  Undiagnosed vaginal bleeding
  SPECIFIC CONTRA-INDICATIONS
  ▸ When used for endometriosis Use longer than 6 months (do not repeat)
- CAUTIONS Diabetes · family history of osteoporosis · patients with metabolic bone disease (decrease in bone mineral density can occur) · risk of spinal cord compression in men with prostate cancer · risk of ureteric obstruction in men with prostate cancer
- INTERACTIONS Caution with chronic use of other drugs which reduce bone density including alcohol and tobacco.
- SIDE-EFFECTS Alteration of glucose tolerance · altered blood lipids · anaphylaxis · anorexia · asthma · breast tenderness (males and females) · changes in blood pressure · changes in breast size · changes in scalp and body hair · chills · decrease in trabecular bone density · depression · diarrhoea · dizziness · dyspareunia · fatigue · fever · gastro-intestinal disturbances · headache · hot flushes · hypersensitivity reactions · increased sweating · jaundice · leucopenia · local reactions at injection site · loss of libido · menopausal-like symptoms · migraine · mood changes · musculoskeletal pain · musculoskeletal weakness · nausea · palpitation · paraesthesia · paralysis · pruritus · pulmonary embolism · rash · sexual dysfunction · sleep disturbances · spinal fracture · thrombocytopenia · urticaria · vaginal bleeding · vaginal dryness · visual disturbances · vomiting · weight changes

  SIDE-EFFECTS, FURTHER INFORMATION
  ▸ Tumour flare in prostate cancer In prostate cancer, during the initial stage (1–2 weeks) increased production of testosterone may be associated with progression of prostate cancer. In susceptible patients this tumour 'flare' may cause spinal cord compression, ureteric obstruction or increased bone pain.
- CONCEPTION AND CONTRACEPTION Non-hormonal, barrier methods of contraception should be used during entire treatment period. Pregnancy should be excluded before treatment, the first injection should be given during menstruation or shortly afterwards or use barrier contraception for 1 month beforehand.
- PREGNANCY Avoid—teratogenic in *animal* studies.
- BREAST FEEDING Avoid.
- MONITORING REQUIREMENTS
  ▸ Monitor liver function.
  ▸ Men at risk of tumour 'flare' should be monitored closely during the first month of therapy.
- DIRECTIONS FOR ADMINISTRATION Rotate injection site to prevent atrophy and nodule formation.

- MEDICINAL FORMS
  There can be variation in the licensing of different medicines containing the same drug.
  Powder and solvent for suspension for injection
  ▸ Prostap 3 DCS (Takeda UK Ltd)
    Leuprorelin acetate 11.25 mg Prostap 3 DCS 11.25mg powder and solvent for suspension for injection pre-filled syringes | 1 pre-filled disposable injection [PoM] £225.72 DT price = £225.72
  ▸ Prostap SR DCS (Takeda UK Ltd)
    Leuprorelin acetate 3.75 mg Prostap SR DCS 3.75mg powder and solvent for suspension for injection pre-filled syringes | 1 pre-filled disposable injection [PoM] £75.24 DT price = £75.24

| Nafarelin

- DRUG ACTION Administration of gonadorelin analogues produces an initial phase of stimulation; continued administration is followed by down-regulation of gonadotrophin-releasing hormone receptors, thereby reducing the release of gonadotrophins (follicle stimulating hormone and luteinising hormone) which in turn leads to inhibition of androgen and oestrogen production.

- INDICATIONS AND DOSE
Endometriosis
▶ BY INTRANASAL ADMINISTRATION
▸ Adult (female): 200 micrograms twice daily for maximum 6 months (do not repeat), one spray in one nostril in the morning, and one spray in the other nostril in the evening (starting on days 2–4 of menstruation).

Pituitary desensitisation before induction of ovulation by gonadotrophins for in vitro fertilisation (under expert supervision)
▶ BY INTRANASAL ADMINISTRATION
▸ Adult: 400 micrograms twice daily, one spray in each nostril, to be started in early follicular phase (day 2) or, after exclusion of pregnancy, in midluteal phase (day 21) and continued until down regulation achieved (usually within 4 weeks) then maintained (usually for 8–12 days) during gonadotrophin administration (stopping gonadotrophin and nafarelin on administration of chorionic gonadotrophin at follicular maturity), discontinue if down-regulation not achieved within 12 weeks

- CONTRA-INDICATIONS Undiagnosed vaginal bleeding · use longer than 6 months in the treatment of endometriosis (do not repeat)
- CAUTIONS Patients with metabolic bone disease (decrease in bone mineral density can occur)
- SIDE-EFFECTS Acne · anaphylaxis · asthma · changes in breast size · changes in scalp and body hair · decrease in trabecular bone density · dyspareunia · headache · hot flushes · hypersensitivity reactions · hypertension · increased sweating · irritation of the nasal mucosa · loss of libido · menopausal-like symptoms · migraine · mood changes · musculoskeletal pain · musculoskeletal weakness · oedema of the face and extremities · ovarian cysts (may require withdrawal) · palpitation · paraesthesia · pruritus · rash · urticaria · vaginal dryness · visual disturbances · weight changes

  SIDE-EFFECTS, FURTHER INFORMATION
  ▸ Menopausal-like symptoms These effects can be reduced by hormone replacement (e.g. with an oestrogen and a progestogen or with tibolone).
- CONCEPTION AND CONTRACEPTION Non-hormonal, barrier methods of contraception should be used during entire treatment period. Pregnancy should be excluded before treatment, the first dose should be given during

menstruation or shortly afterwards or use barrier contraception for 1 month beforehand.

● PREGNANCY Avoid.

● BREAST FEEDING Avoid.

● DIRECTIONS FOR ADMINISTRATION Avoid use of nasal decongestants before and for at least 30 minutes after treatment; repeat dose if sneezing occurs during or immediately after administration.

● PATIENT AND CARER ADVICE Patients or carers should be given advice on how to administer nafarelin nasal spray.

● MEDICINAL FORMS
There can be variation in the licensing of different medicines containing the same drug.

Spray
CAUTIONARY AND ADVISORY LABELS 10
▸ Synarel (Pfizer Ltd)
   Nafarelin (as Nafarelin acetate) 200 microgram per 1 dose Synarel 200micrograms/dose nasal spray | 60 dose [PoM] £52.43

Triptorelin

● DRUG ACTION Administration of gonadorelin analogues produces an initial phase of stimulation; continued administration is followed by down-regulation of gonadotrophin-releasing hormone receptors, thereby reducing the release of gonadotrophins (follicle stimulating hormone and luteinising hormone) which in turn leads to inhibition of androgen and oestrogen production.

● INDICATIONS AND DOSE
DECAPEPTYL® SR 11.25MG

Locally advanced non-metastatic prostate cancer as an alternative to surgical castration | Metastatic prostate cancer | Adjuvant treatment to radiotherapy in high-risk localised or locally advanced prostate cancer | Neoadjuvant treatment prior to radiotherapy in patients with high-risk localised or locally advanced prostate cancer | Adjuvant treatment to radical prostatectomy in patients with locally advanced prostate cancer at high risk of disease progression
▸ BY INTRAMUSCULAR INJECTION
▸ Adult: 11.25 mg every 3 months

Endometriosis
▸ BY INTRAMUSCULAR INJECTION
▸ Adult: 11.25 mg every 3 months for maximum 6 months (not to be repeated), to be started during first 5 days of menstrual cycle

DECAPEPTYL® SR 22.5MG

Locally advanced non-metastatic prostate cancer as an alternative to surgical castration | Metastatic prostate cancer | Adjuvant treatment to radiotherapy in high-risk localised or locally advanced prostate cancer | Neoadjuvant treatment prior to radiotherapy in patients with high-risk localised or locally advanced prostate cancer | Adjuvant treatment to radical prostatectomy in patients with locally advanced prostate cancer at high risk of disease progression
▸ BY INTRAMUSCULAR INJECTION
▸ Adult: 22.5 mg every 6 months

DECAPEPTYL® SR 3MG

Locally advanced non-metastatic prostate cancer as an alternative to surgical castration | Metastatic prostate cancer | Adjuvant treatment to radiotherapy in high-risk localised or locally advanced prostate cancer | Neoadjuvant treatment prior to radiotherapy in patients with high-risk localised or locally advanced prostate cancer | Adjuvant treatment to radical prostatectomy in patients with locally advanced prostate cancer at high risk of disease progression
▸ BY INTRAMUSCULAR INJECTION
▸ Adult: 3 mg every 4 weeks

Endometriosis
▸ BY INTRAMUSCULAR INJECTION
▸ Adult: 3 mg every 4 weeks maximum duration of 6 months (not to be repeated), to be started during first 5 days of menstrual cycle

Reduction in size of uterine fibroids
▸ BY INTRAMUSCULAR INJECTION
▸ Adult: 3 mg every 4 weeks for at least 3 months, maximum duration of treatment 6 months (not to be repeated), to be started during first 5 days of menstrual cycle

GONAPEPTYL DEPOT®

Advanced prostate cancer
▸ BY SUBCUTANEOUS INJECTION, OR BY DEEP INTRAMUSCULAR INJECTION
▸ Adult: 3.75 mg every 4 weeks

Endometriosis | Reduction in size of uterine fibroids
▸ BY SUBCUTANEOUS INJECTION, OR BY DEEP INTRAMUSCULAR INJECTION
▸ Adult: 3.75 mg every 4 weeks maximum duration of 6 months (not to be repeated), to be started during first 5 days of menstrual cycle

SALVACYL®

Male hypersexuality with severe sexual deviation
▸ BY INTRAMUSCULAR INJECTION
▸ Adult: 11.25 mg every 12 weeks

● CONTRA-INDICATIONS In endometriosis do not use for longer than 6 months (do not repeat) · undiagnosed vaginal bleeding
SALVACYL® Severe osteoporosis

● CAUTIONS
GENERAL CAUTIONS
Patients with metabolic bone disease (decrease in bone mineral density can occur)
SPECIFIC CAUTIONS
▸ When used for prostate cancer Risk factors for osteoporosis · risk of spinal cord compression in men · risk of ureteric obstruction in men
SALVACYL® Increased risk of sensitivity to restored testosterone if treatment interrupted—consider administration of an antiandrogen before stopping treatment · transient increase in serum testosterone occurs on initiation—consider administration of an anti-androgen

● SIDE-EFFECTS
GENERAL SIDE-EFFECTS
Anaphylaxis · arthralgia · asthenia · asthma · breast tenderness (males and females) · changes in blood pressure · changes in breast size · changes in scalp and body hair · depression · gastro-intestinal disturbances · headache · hot flushes · hypersensitivity reactions · increased sweating · local reactions at injection site · mood changes · ovarian cysts (may require withdrawal) · paraesthesia · pruritus · rash · urticaria · visual disturbances · weight changes

6

Endocrine system

SPECIFIC SIDE-EFFECTS

► When used for endometriosis Decrease in trabecular bone density · dyspareunia · loss of libido · menopausal-like symptoms · migraine · musculoskeletal pain · musculoskeletal weakness · oedema of the face and extremities · palpitation · vaginal dryness · withdrawal bleeding (may occur in the first month of treatment)

► When used for gonadotrophin-dependent precocious puberty Decrease in trabecular bone density · dyspareunia · loss of libido · menopausal-like symptoms · migraine · musculoskeletal pain · musculoskeletal weakness · oedema of the face and extremities · palpitation · vaginal dryness · withdrawal bleeding (may occur in the first month of treatment)

► When used for male hypersexuality with severe sexual deviation Decrease in trabecular bone density · dyspareunia · loss of libido · migraine · musculoskeletal pain · musculoskeletal weakness · oedema of the face and extremities · palpitation

► When used for prostate cancer Dizziness · dry mouth · hair loss · increased dysuria · myalgia · peripheral oedema · sexual dysfunction · sleep disorders

► When used for reduction in size of uterine fibroids Bleeding associated with fibroid degeneration · decrease in trabecular bone density · dyspareunia · loss of libido · menopausal-like symptoms · migraine · musculoskeletal pain · musculoskeletal weakness · oedema of the face and extremities · palpitation · vaginal dryness · withdrawal bleeding (may occur in the first month of treatment)

SIDE-EFFECTS, FURTHER INFORMATION

► Tumour flare in prostate cancer During the initial stage (1–2 weeks) increased production of testosterone may be associated with progression of prostate cancer. In susceptible patients this tumour 'flare' may cause spinal cord compression, ureteric obstruction or increased bone pain.

● CONCEPTION AND CONTRACEPTION Non-hormonal, barrier methods of contraception should be used during entire treatment period. Pregnancy should be excluded before treatment, the first injection should be given during menstruation or shortly afterwards or use barrier contraception for 1 month beforehand.

● PREGNANCY Avoid.

● BREAST FEEDING Avoid.

● MONITORING REQUIREMENTS

► When used for Prostate cancer Men at risk of tumour 'flare' should be monitored closely during the first month of therapy.

● DIRECTIONS FOR ADMINISTRATION Rotate injection site to prevent atrophy and nodule formation.

● PRESCRIBING AND DISPENSING INFORMATION

DECAPEPTYL® SR 11.25MG Each vial includes an overage to allow accurate administration of an 11.25 mg dose.

DECAPEPTYL® SR 22.5MG Each vial includes an overage to allow accurate administration of a 22.5 mg dose.

DECAPEPTYL® SR 3MG Each vial includes an overage to allow accurate administration of 3 mg dose.

● MEDICINAL FORMS
There can be variation in the licensing of different medicines containing the same drug.

Powder and solvent for suspension for injection

► Decapeptyl SR (Ipsen Ltd)
Triptorelin (as Triptorelin acetate) 3 mg Decapeptyl SR 3mg powder and solvent for suspension for injection vials | 1 vial £69.00

Triptorelin (as Triptorelin acetate) 11.25 mg Decapeptyl SR 11.25mg powder and solvent for suspension for injection vials | 1 vial [PoM] £207.00

Triptorelin (as Triptorelin embonate) 22.5 mg Decapeptyl SR 22.5mg powder and solvent for suspension for injection vials | 1 vial [PoM] £414.00

► Gonapeptyl Depot (Ferring Pharmaceuticals Ltd)
Triptorelin (as Triptorelin acetate) 3.75 mg Gonapeptyl Depot 3.75mg powder and solvent for suspension for injection pre-filled disposable devices | 1 pre-filled disposable injection [PoM] £81.69

► Salvacyl (Ipsen Ltd)
Triptorelin (as Triptorelin embonate) 11.25 mg Salvacyl 11.25mg powder and solvent for suspension for injection vials | 1 vial [PoM] £248.00

6.1   Hereditary angioedema

PITUITARY AND HYPOTHALAMIC HORMONES AND ANALOGUES > ANTI-GONADOTROPHIN-RELEASING HORMONES

Danazol

● DRUG ACTION Danazol inhibits pituitary gonadotrophins; it combines androgenic activity with antioestrogenic and antiprogestogenic activity.

● INDICATIONS AND DOSE

Endometriosis
► BY MOUTH
► Adult: 200–800 mg daily in up to 4 divided doses usually for 3–6 months, dose to be adjusted to achieve amenorrhoea, in women of child-bearing potential, treatment should start during menstruation, preferably on day 1

Severe pain and tenderness in benign fibrocystic breast disease not responding to other treatment
► BY MOUTH
► Adult: 300 mg daily in divided doses usually for 3–6 months, in women of child-bearing potential, treatment should start during menstruation, preferably on day 1

Hereditary angioedema
► BY MOUTH
► Adult: Initially 100–200 mg daily, dose to be reduced according to response, in women of child-bearing potential, treatment should start during menstruation, preferably on day 1

● UNLICENSED USE Not licensed for use in hereditary angioedema.

● CONTRA-INDICATIONS Acute porphyrias p. 918 · androgen-dependent tumours · thromboembolic disease · undiagnosed genital bleeding

● CAUTIONS Cardiac impairment (avoid if severe) · diabetes mellitus · elderly · epilepsy · history of thrombosis or thromboembolic disease · hypertension · lipoprotein disorder · migraine · polycythaemia

● INTERACTIONS → Appendix 1 (danazol).

● SIDE-EFFECTS

► **Rare** Benign hepatic adenomata · cholestatic jaundice · clitoral hypertrophy · pancreatitis · peliosis hepatis

► **Frequency not known** Acne · androgenic effects · anxiety · backache · changes in libido · dizziness · eosinophilia · epigastric pain · exfoliative dermatitis · fatigue · fever · flushing and reduction in breast size · hair loss · headache · headache (may indicate benign intracranial hypertension) · hirsutism · insulin resistance · joint pain · joint swelling · leucopenia · menstrual disturbances · mood changes · musculo-skeletal spasm · nausea · nervousness · oedema · oily skin · pleuritic pain · rashes · reversible erythrocytosis · reversible polycythaemia · skin reactions · temporary alteration in lipoproteins and other metabolic changes · thrombocytopenia · thrombotic events · vaginal dryness · vaginal irritation · vertigo · visual disturbances (may indicate benign intracranial hypertension) · voice changes · weight gain

SIDE-EFFECTS, FURTHER INFORMATION
▸ Virilisation Withdraw if virilisation effects occur—may be irreversible on continued use.
● CONCEPTION AND CONTRACEPTION Ensure patients with amenorrhoea are not pregnant. Non-hormonal contraceptive methods should be used, if appropriate.
● PREGNANCY Avoid; has weak androgenic effects and virilisation of female fetus reported.
● BREAST FEEDING No data available but avoid because of possible androgenic effects in infant.
● HEPATIC IMPAIRMENT Caution in hepatic impairment (avoid if severe).
● RENAL IMPAIRMENT Caution in renal impairment (avoid if severe).

● MEDICINAL FORMS
There can be variation in the licensing of different medicines containing the same drug. Forms available from special-order manufacturers include: capsule

Capsule
▸ Danazol (Non-proprietary)
Danazol 100 mg Danazol 100mg capsules | 28 capsule PoM £18.40 CD4-2
Danazol 200 mg Danazol 200mg capsules | 56 capsule PoM £30.27-£66.20 CD4-2
▸ Danol (Sanofi)
Danazol 100 mg Danol 100mg capsules | 60 capsule PoM £16.38 DT price = £16.38 CD4-2
Danazol 200 mg Danol 200mg capsules | 60 capsule PoM £32.43 DT price = £32.43 CD4-2

7 Hypothalamic and anterior pituitary hormone related disorders

Hypothalamic and anterior pituitary hormones

Anterior pituitary hormones
Corticotrophins
Tetracosactide below (tetracosactrin), an analogue of corticotropin (ACTH), is used to test adrenocortical function; failure of the plasma cortisol concentration to rise after administration of tetracosactide indicates adrenocortical insufficiency.

Both corticotropin and tetracosactide were formerly used as alternatives to corticosteroids in conditions such as Crohn's disease or rheumatoid arthritis; their value was limited by the variable and unpredictable therapeutic response and by the waning of their effect with time.

Gonadotrophins
Follicle-stimulating hormone (FSH) and luteinising hormone (LH) together, follicle-stimulating hormone alone (as in **follitropin**), or chorionic gonadotrophin p. 673, are used in the treatment of infertility in women with proven hypopituitarism or who have not responded to clomifene citrate p. 693, or in superovulation treatment for assisted conception (such as in vitro fertilisation).

The gonadotrophins are also occasionally used in the treatment of hypogonadotrophic hypogonadism and associated oligospermia. There is no justification for their use in primary gonadal failure.

Chorionic gonadotrophin has also been used in delayed puberty in the male to stimulate endogenous testosterone production, but has little advantage over testosterone.

Growth hormone
Growth hormone is used to treat deficiency of the hormone in children and in adults. In children it is used in Prader-Willi syndrome, Turner syndrome, chronic renal insufficiency, short children considered small for gestational age at birth, and short stature homeobox-containing gene (SHOX) deficiency.

Growth hormone of human origin (HGH; somatotrophin) has been replaced by a growth hormone of human sequence, somatropin p. 676, produced using recombinant DNA technology.

Mecasermin, a human insulin-like growth factor-I (rhIGF-I), is licensed to treat growth failure in children and adolescents with severe primary insulin-like growth factor-I deficiency.

Hypothalamic hormones
Gonadorelin p. 672 when injected intravenously in normal subjects leads to a rapid rise in plasma concentrations of both luteinising hormone (LH) and follicle-stimulating hormone (FSH). It has not proved to be very helpful, however, in distinguishing hypothalamic from pituitary lesions. **Gonadorelin analogues** are indicated in endometriosis and infertility and in breast and prostate cancer.

7.1 Adrenocortical function testing

PITUITARY AND HYPOTHALAMIC HORMONES AND ANALOGUES › CORTICOTROPHINS

Tetracosactide
(Tetracosactrin)

● INDICATIONS AND DOSE
Diagnosis of adrenocortical insufficiency (diagnostic 30-minute test)
▸ BY INTRAVENOUS INJECTION, OR BY INTRAMUSCULAR INJECTION
▸ Adult: 250 micrograms for 1 dose
Diagnosis of adrenocortical insufficiency (diagnostic 5-hour test)
▸ BY INTRAMUSCULAR INJECTION USING DEPOT INJECTION
▸ Adult: 1 mg for 1 dose
Alternative to corticosteroids in conditions such as Crohn's disease or rheumatoid arthritis (formerly used but value was limited by the variable and unpredictable therapeutic response and by the waning of effect with time)
▸ BY INTRAMUSCULAR INJECTION USING DEPOT INJECTION
▸ Adult: Initially 1 mg daily, alternatively initially 1 mg every 12 hours, (in acute cases), then reduced to 1 mg every 2–3 days, followed by 1 mg once weekly, alternatively 500 micrograms every 2–3 days

● CONTRA-INDICATIONS Acute psychosis · adrenogenital syndrome · allergic disorders · asthma · avoid injections containing benzyl alcohol in neonates · Cushing's syndrome · infectious diseases · peptic ulcer · primary adrenocortical insufficiency · refractory heart failure
● CAUTIONS Active infectious diseases (should not be used unless disease-specific therapy is being given) · active systemic diseases (should not be used unless adequate disease-specific therapy is being given) · diabetes mellitus · diverticulitis · history of asthma · history of atopic allergy · history of eczema · history of hayfever · history of hypersensitivity · hypertension · latent amoebiasis (may become activated) · latent tuberculosis

(may become activated) · myasthenia gravis · ocular herpes simplex · osteoporosis · predisposition to thromboembolic · pscyhological disturbances may be triggered · recent intestinal anastomosis · reduced immune response (should not be used unless adequate disease-specific therapy is being given) · ulcerative colitis

CAUTIONS, FURTHER INFORMATION

▸ Risk of anaphylaxis Should only be administered under medical supervision.
  Consult product literature.

▸ Hypertension Patients already receiving medication for moderate to severe hypertension must have their dosage adjusted if treatment started.

▸ Diabetes mellitus Patients already receiving medication for diabetes mellitus must have their dosage adjusted if treatment started.

● INTERACTIONS → Appendix 1 (corticosteroids).

● SIDE-EFFECTS Abdominal distention · abscess · acne · anaphylactic shock · angioneurotic oedema · aseptic necrosis of femoral and humeral heads · benign intracranial pressure increased with papilloedema · calcium deficiency · cardiac disorders · convulsions · Cushing's syndrome · decreased carbohydrate tolerance · dizziness · dysponea · ecchymosis · erythema · euphoria · fluid retention · flushing · glaucoma · growth retardation · headache · hirsutism · hyperglycaemia · hyperhidrosis · hypersensitivity reactions (tend to be more severe in patients susceptible to allergies, especially asthma) · hypertension · hypokalaemia · hypokalaemic alkalosis · impaired healing · increased appetite · increased intraocular pressure · infection susceptibility increased · insomnia · irregular menstruation · leukocytosis · malaise · manifestations of latent diabetes mellitus · mood swings · muscle atrophy · muscular weakness · myopathy · nausea · necrotising vasculitis · negative nitrogen balance · osteoporosis · pancreatitis · pathological fracture of long bones · peptic ulcer · personality changes · petechiae · posterior subcapsular cataracts · pruritus · psychotic manifestations · Quincke's oedema · secondary adrenocortical unresponsiveness · secondary pituitary unresponsiveness · severe depression · skin atrophy · skin hyperpigmentation · skin reactions at injection site · sodium retention · spinal compression fractures · tendon rupture · thromboembolism · ulcerative oesophagitis · urticaria · vertigo · vomiting · weight increase

● ALLERGY AND CROSS-SENSITIVITY Contra-indicated in patients with history of hypersensitivity to tetracosactide/corticotrophins or excipients.

● PREGNANCY Avoid (but may be used diagnostically if essential).

● BREAST FEEDING Avoid (but may be used diagnostically if essential).

● HEPATIC IMPAIRMENT An enhanced effect of tetracosactide therapy may occur in patients with cirrhosis of the liver. Use with caution in hepatic impairment. Monitor hepatic function closely during treatment.

● RENAL IMPAIRMENT Use with caution in patients with renal impairment.

● EFFECT ON LABORATORY TESTS May suppress skin test reactions.
  Post administration total plasma cortisol levels during 30-minute test for diagnosis of adrenocotical insufficiency might be misleading due to altered cortisol binding globulin levels in some special clinical situations including, patients on oral contraceptives, post-operative patients, critical illness, severe liver disease and nephrotic syndrome.

● MEDICINAL FORMS
There can be variation in the licensing of different medicines containing the same drug.
Solution for injection
▸ Synacthen (Mallinckrodt Specialty Pharmaceuticals Ireland Ltd)
  Tetracosactide acetate 250 microgram per 1 ml Synacthen 250micrograms/1ml solution for injection ampoules |
  1 ampoule PoM £38.00
Suspension for injection
EXCIPIENTS: May contain Benzyl alcohol
▸ Synacthen Depot (Mallinckrodt Specialty Pharmaceuticals Ireland Ltd)
  Tetracosactide acetate 1 mg per 1 ml Synacthen Depot 1mg/1ml suspension for injection ampoules | 1 ampoule PoM £346.28

7.2 Assessment of pituitary function

PITUITARY AND HYPOTHALAMIC HORMONES AND ANALOGUES › GONADOTROPIN-RELEASING HORMONES

Gonadorelin

(Gonadotrophin-releasing hormone; GnRH; LH–RH)

● **INDICATIONS AND DOSE**

Assessment of pituitary function
▸ BY SUBCUTANEOUS INJECTION, OR BY INTRAVENOUS INJECTION
▸ Adult: 100 micrograms for 1 dose

● CAUTIONS Pituitary adenoma

● SIDE-EFFECTS Abdominal pain · headache · hypersensitivity reaction on repeated administration of large doses · increased menstrual bleeding · irritation at injection site · nausea

● PREGNANCY Avoid.

● BREAST FEEDING Avoid.

● MEDICINAL FORMS
There can be variation in the licensing of different medicines containing the same drug.
Powder and solvent for solution for injection
EXCIPIENTS: May contain Benzyl alcohol
▸ Gonadorelin (Non-proprietary)
  Gonadorelin (as Gonadorelin hydrochloride)
  100 microgram Gonadorelin 100microgram powder and solvent for solution for injection vials | 1 vial PoM £75.00 (Hospital only)

7.3 Gonadotrophin replacement therapy

GONADOTROPHINS

Choriogonadotropin alfa

(Human chorionic gonadotropin)

● **INDICATIONS AND DOSE**

Treatment of infertility in women with proven hypopituitarism or who have not responded to clomifene | Superovulation treatment for assisted conception (such as in vitro fertilisation)
▸ BY SUBCUTANEOUS INJECTION
▸ Adult (female): Adjusted according to response.

● CONTRA-INDICATIONS Active thromboembolic disorders · ectopic pregnancy in previous 3 months · hypothalamus malignancy · mammary malignancy · ovarian enlargement or cyst (unless caused by polycystic ovarian disease) · ovarian malignancy · pituitary malignancy · uterine malignancy

- CAUTIONS Acute porphyrias p. 918
- SIDE-EFFECTS Abdominal pain · breast pain · depression · diarrhoea · ectopic pregnancy · headache · injection-site reactions · irritability · nausea · ovarian hyperstimulation syndrome · ovarian torsion · tiredness · vomiting

- MEDICINAL FORMS
  There can be variation in the licensing of different medicines containing the same drug.
  Solution for injection
  ▸ Ovitrelle (Merck Serono Ltd)
    Choriogonadotropin alfa 500 microgram per 1 ml Ovitrelle 250micrograms/0.5ml solution for injection pre-filled syringes | 1 pre-filled disposable injection PoM £31.38 CD4-2
    Ovitrelle 250micrograms/0.5ml solution for injection pre-filled pen | 1 pre-filled disposable injection PoM £31.38 CD4-2

Chorionic gonadotrophin

(Human chorionic gonadotrophin; HCG)

- DRUG ACTION A preparation of a glycoprotein fraction secreted by the placenta and obtained from the urine of pregnant women having the action of the pituitary luteinising hormone.

- INDICATIONS AND DOSE
  Treatment of infertility in women with proven hypopituitarism or who have not responded to clomifene | Superovulation treatment for assisted conception (such as in vitro fertilisation)
  ▸ BY INTRAMUSCULAR INJECTION, OR BY SUBCUTANEOUS INJECTION
  ▸ Adult (female): Adjusted according to response.

- CONTRA-INDICATIONS Androgen-dependent tumours
- CAUTIONS Asthma · cardiac impairment · epilepsy · migraine · prepubertal boys (risk of premature epiphyseal closure or precocious puberty)
- SIDE-EFFECTS Gynaecomastia · headache · local reactions · may aggravate ovarian hyperstimulation · mood changes · multiple pregnancy · oedema (particularly in males—reduce dose) · tiredness
- RENAL IMPAIRMENT Use with caution.

- MEDICINAL FORMS
  There can be variation in the licensing of different medicines containing the same drug.
  Powder and solvent for solution for injection
  ▸ Choragon (Ferring Pharmaceuticals Ltd)
    Chorionic gonadotrophin human 5000 unit Choragon 5,000unit powder and solvent for solution for injection ampoules | 3 ampoule PoM £9.77 CD4-2
  ▸ Pregnyl (Merck Sharp & Dohme Ltd)
    Chorionic gonadotrophin human 1500 unit Pregnyl 1,500unit powder and solvent for solution for injection ampoules | 1 ampoule PoM £2.12 CD4-2
    Chorionic gonadotrophin human 5000 unit Pregnyl 5,000unit powder and solvent for solution for injection ampoules | 1 ampoule PoM £3.15 CD4-2

Corifollitropin alfa

- INDICATIONS AND DOSE
  Controlled ovarian stimulation in combination with a gonadotrophin-releasing hormone antagonist
  ▸ BY SUBCUTANEOUS INJECTION
  ▸ Adult (body-weight up to 60 kg): 100 micrograms
  ▸ Adult (body-weight 60 kg and above): 150 micrograms

- CONTRA-INDICATIONS History of ovarian hyperstimulation syndrome · ovarian enlargement or cyst · polycystic ovarian syndrome · tumours of breast · tumours of hypothalamus · tumours of ovaries · tumours of pituitary · tumours of uterus · vaginal bleeding of unknown cause
- CAUTIONS Acute porphyrias p. 918 · risk factors for thromboembolism · risk of ovarian hyperstimulation syndrome
- SIDE-EFFECTS
  ▸ Common or very common Breast pain · fatigue · headache · nausea · ovarian hyperstimulation · pelvic pain
  ▸ Uncommon Abdominal distension and pain · constipation · diarrhoea · dizziness · ovarian torsion · vomiting
  ▸ Frequency not known Ectopic pregnancy · miscarriage · multiple pregnancies
- BREAST FEEDING Avoid.
- RENAL IMPAIRMENT Avoid.

- MEDICINAL FORMS
  There can be variation in the licensing of different medicines containing the same drug.
  Solution for injection
  ▸ Elonva (Merck Sharp & Dohme Ltd)
    Corifollitropin alfa 200 microgram per 1 ml Elonva 100micrograms/0.5ml solution for injection pre-filled syringes | 1 pre-filled disposable injection PoM £638.00
    Corifollitropin alfa 300 microgram per 1 ml Elonva 150micrograms/0.5ml solution for injection pre-filled syringes | 1 pre-filled disposable injection PoM £638.00

Follitropin alfa

(Recombinant human follicle stimulating hormone)

- INDICATIONS AND DOSE
  Infertility in women with proven hypopituitarism or who have not responded to clomifene | Superovulation treatment for assisted conception (such as in vitro fertilisation)
  ▸ BY SUBCUTANEOUS INJECTION
  ▸ Adult (female): Adjusted according to response.
  Hypogonadotrophic hypogonadism
  ▸ BY SUBCUTANEOUS INJECTION
  ▸ Adult (male): (consult product literature).

- CONTRA-INDICATIONS Ovarian cysts (not caused by polycystic ovarian syndrome) · ovarian enlargement (not caused by polycystic ovarian syndrome) · tumours of breast · tumours of hypothalamus · tumours of ovaries · tumours of pituitary · tumours of prostate · tumours of testes · tumours of uterus · vaginal bleeding of unknown cause
- CAUTIONS Acute porphyrias p. 918 · history of tubal disease
- SIDE-EFFECTS
  ▸ Common or very common Fever · gastro-intestinal disturbances · headache · hypersensitivity reactions · injection site reactions · joint pain · ovarian hyperstimulation · varicocele
  ▸ Very rare Exacerbation or aggravation of asthma · thromboembolism
  ▸ Frequency not known Acne · gynaecomastia · increased risk of miscarriage · increased risk of multiple pregnancy · weight gain
- PREGNANCY Avoid.
- BREAST FEEDING Avoid.
- PRESCRIBING AND DISPENSING INFORMATION Products containing follitropin alfa are not identical and although theoretically there should be no important differences in terms of safety and efficacy, when prescribing biological

products it is good practice to use the brand name, see *Biosimilar medicines*, under Guidance on prescribing p. 1.

● PATIENT AND CARER ADVICE

Patient advice required around conception and contraception Patients planning to conceive should be warned that there is a risk of multiple pregnancy.

● MEDICINAL FORMS

There can be variation in the licensing of different medicines containing the same drug.

Solution for injection

▸ Bemfola (Finox Biotech UK) ▼

Follitropin alfa 600 unit per 1 ml Bemfola 225units/0.375ml solution for injection pre-filled pen | 1 pre-filled disposable injection PoM £70.50
Bemfola 300units/0.5ml solution for injection pre-filled pen | 1 pre-filled disposable injection PoM £94.00
Bemfola 150units/0.25ml solution for injection pre-filled pen | 1 pre-filled disposable injection PoM £47.00
Bemfola 75units/0.125ml solution for injection pre-filled pen | 1 pre-filled disposable injection PoM £23.50
Bemfola 450units/0.75ml solution for injection pre-filled pen | 1 pre-filled disposable injection PoM £141.00

▸ Gonal-f (Merck Serono Ltd)

Follitropin alfa 600 unit per 1 ml Gonal-f 900units/1.5ml solution for injection pre-filled pen | 1 pre-filled disposable injection PoM £282.00
Gonal-f 300units/0.5ml solution for injection pre-filled pen | 1 pre-filled disposable injection PoM £94.00
Gonal-f 450units/0.75ml solution for injection pre-filled pen | 1 pre-filled disposable injection PoM £141.00

▸ Ovaleap (Teva UK Ltd) ▼

Follitropin alfa 600 unit per 1 ml Ovaleap 450units/0.75ml solution for injection cartridges | 1 cartridge PoM £112.80
Ovaleap 900units/1.5ml solution for injection cartridges | 1 cartridge PoM £225.60
Ovaleap 300units/0.5ml solution for injection cartridges | 1 cartridge PoM £75.20

Powder and solvent for solution for injection

▸ Gonal-f (Merck Serono Ltd)

Follitropin alfa 75 unit Gonal-f 75unit powder and solvent for solution for injection vials | 1 vial PoM £21.02
Follitropin alfa 450 unit Gonal-f 450unit powder and solvent for solution for injection vials | 1 vial PoM £126.10
Follitropin alfa 1050 unit Gonal-f 1,050unit powder and solvent for solution for injection vials | 1 vial PoM £294.22

Follitropin alfa with lutropin alfa

The properties listed below are those particular to the combination only. For the properties of the components please consider, follitropin alfa p. 673, lutropin alfa p. 675.

● INDICATIONS AND DOSE

Infertility in women with proven hypopituitarism or who have not responded to clomifene | Superovulation treatment for assisted conception (such as in vitro fertilisation)

▸ BY SUBCUTANEOUS INJECTION

▸ Adult (female): Adjusted according to response.

● MEDICINAL FORMS

There can be variation in the licensing of different medicines containing the same drug.

Powder and solvent for solution for injection

ELECTROLYTES: May contain Sodium

▸ Pergoveris (Merck Serono Ltd)

Lutropin alfa 75 unit, Follitropin alfa 150 unit Pergoveris 150unit/75unit powder and solvent for solution for injection vials | 1 vial PoM £60.29 | 10 vial PoM £602.90

Follitropin beta

(Recombinant human follicle stimulating hormone)

● INDICATIONS AND DOSE

Infertility in women with proven hypopituitarism or who have not responded to clomifene | Superovulation treatment for assisted conception (such as in vitro fertilisation)

▸ BY INTRAMUSCULAR INJECTION, OR BY SUBCUTANEOUS INJECTION

▸ Adult (female): Adjusted according to response.

Hypogonadotrophic hypogonadism

▸ BY INTRAMUSCULAR INJECTION, OR BY SUBCUTANEOUS INJECTION

▸ Adult (male): (consult product literature).

● CONTRA-INDICATIONS Ovarian cysts (not caused by polycystic ovarian syndrome) · ovarian enlargement (not caused by polycystic ovarian syndrome) · tumours of breast · tumours of hypothalamus · tumours of ovaries · tumours of pituitary · tumours of prostate · tumours of testes · tumours of uterus · vaginal bleeding of unknown cause

● CAUTIONS Acute porphyrias p. 918 · history of tubal disease

● SIDE-EFFECTS

▸ **Common or very common** Fever · gastro-intestinal disturbances · headache · hypersensitivity reactions · injection site reactions · joint pain · ovarian hyperstimulation

▸ **Very rare** Thromboembolism

▸ **Frequency not known** Acne · gynaecomastia · increased risk of miscarriage · increased risk of multiple pregnancy · weight gain

● PREGNANCY Avoid.

● BREAST FEEDING Avoid.

● DIRECTIONS FOR ADMINISTRATION Cartridges and vials are used for subcutaneous administration; vials are used for intramuscular injection.

● PATIENT AND CARER ADVICE

Patient advice required around conception and contraception Patients planning to conceive should be warned that there is a risk of multiple pregnancy.

● MEDICINAL FORMS

There can be variation in the licensing of different medicines containing the same drug.

Solution for injection

EXCIPIENTS: May contain Neomycin, streptomycin

▸ Puregon (Merck Sharp & Dohme Ltd)

Follitropin beta 100 unit per 1 ml Puregon 50units/0.5ml solution for injection vials | 1 vial PoM £18.03
Follitropin beta 200 unit per 1 ml Puregon 100units/0.5ml solution for injection vials | 1 vial PoM £36.06
Follitropin beta 833 unit per 1 ml Puregon 900units/1.08ml solution for injection cartridges | 1 cartridge PoM £292.23
Puregon 600units/0.72ml solution for injection cartridges | 1 cartridge PoM £194.82
Puregon 300units/0.36ml solution for injection cartridges | 1 cartridge PoM £97.41

Lutropin alfa

(Recombinant human luteinising hormone)

- **INDICATIONS AND DOSE**

Treatment of infertility in women with proven hypopituitarism or who have not responded to clomifene (in conjunction with follicle-stimulating hormone) | Superovulation treatment for assisted conception (such as in vitro fertilisation) (in conjunction with follicle-stimulating hormone)
- ▶ BY SUBCUTANEOUS INJECTION
- ▶ Adult (female): Adjusted according to response.

- **CONTRA-INDICATIONS** Mammary carcinoma · ovarian carcinoma · ovarian enlargement or cyst (unless caused by polycystic ovarian disease) · tumours of hypothalamus · tumours of pituitary · undiagnosed vaginal bleeding · uterine carcinoma
- **CAUTIONS** Acute porphyrias p. 918
- **SIDE-EFFECTS** Abdominal pain · adnexal torsion · breast pain · ectopic pregnancy · haemoperitoneum · headache · injection-site reactions · nausea · ovarian cyst · ovarian hyperstimulation syndrome · pelvic pain · somnolence · thromboembolism · vomiting

- **MEDICINAL FORMS**
There can be variation in the licensing of different medicines containing the same drug.
Powder and solvent for solution for injection
- ▶ Luveris (Merck Serono Ltd)
Lutropin alfa 75 unit Luveris 75unit powder and solvent for solution for injection vials | 1 vial [PoM] £31.38

Menotrophin

- **INDICATIONS AND DOSE**

Infertility in women with proven hypopituitarism or who have not responded to clomifene | Superovulation treatment for assisted conception (such as in vitro fertilisation)
- ▶ BY SUBCUTANEOUS INJECTION, OR BY DEEP INTRAMUSCULAR INJECTION
- ▶ Adult (female): Adjusted according to response.

Hypogonadotrophic hypogonadism
- ▶ BY DEEP INTRAMUSCULAR INJECTION, OR BY SUBCUTANEOUS INJECTION
- ▶ Adult (male): (consult product literature).

- **CONTRA-INDICATIONS** Ovarian cysts (not caused by polycystic ovarian syndrome) · ovarian enlargement (not caused by polycystic ovarian syndrome) · tumours of breast · tumours of hypothalamus · tumours of ovaries · tumours of pituitary · tumours of prostate · tumours of testes · tumours of uterus · vaginal bleeding of unknown cause
- **CAUTIONS** Acute porphyrias p. 918 · history of tubal disease
- **SIDE-EFFECTS**
- ▶ Very rare Thromboembolism
- ▶ Frequency not known Acne · fever · gastro-intestinal disturbances · gynaecomastia · headache · hypersensitivity reactions · increased risk of multiple pregnancy and miscarriage · injection site reactions · joint pain · ovarian hyperstimulation · weight gain
- **PREGNANCY** Avoid.
- **BREAST FEEDING** Avoid.
- **PRESCRIBING AND DISPENSING INFORMATION**
Menotrophin is purified extract of human post-menopausal urine containing follicle-stimulating hormone (FSH) and luteinising hormone (LH) in a ratio of 1:1.

- **PATIENT AND CARER ADVICE**
Patient advice required around conception and contraception
Patients planning to conceive should be warned that there is a risk of multiple pregnancy.

- **MEDICINAL FORMS**
There can be variation in the licensing of different medicines containing the same drug.
Powder and solvent for solution for injection
- ▶ Menopur (Ferring Pharmaceuticals Ltd)
Menotrophin 75 unit Menopur 75unit powder and solvent for solution for injection vials | 1 vial [PoM] £16.38 | 10 vial [PoM] £163.80
Menotrophin 150 unit Menopur 150unit powder and solvent for solution for injection vials | 5 vial [PoM] £163.80 | 10 vial [PoM] £327.60
Menotrophin 600 unit Menopur 600unit powder and solvent for solution for injection vials | 1 vial [PoM] £131.04
Menotrophin 1200 unit Menopur 1,200unit powder and solvent for solution for injection vials | 1 vial [PoM] £262.08
- ▶ Merional (IBSA Farmaceutici Italia Srl)
Menotrophin 75 unit Merional 75unit powder and solvent for solution for injection vials | 10 vial [PoM] £279.00
Menotrophin 150 unit Merional 150unit powder and solvent for solution for injection vials | 10 vial [PoM] £558.00

Urofollitropin

- **INDICATIONS AND DOSE**

Infertility in women with proven hypopituitarism or who have not responded to clomifene | Superovulation treatment for assisted conception (such as in vitro fertilisation)
- ▶ BY SUBCUTANEOUS INJECTION, OR BY DEEP INTRAMUSCULAR INJECTION
- ▶ Adult (female): Adjusted according to response.

- **CONTRA-INDICATIONS** Ovarian cysts (not caused by polycystic ovarian syndrome) · tumours of breast · tumours of hypothalamus · tumours of ovaries · tumours of pituitary · tumours of prostate · tumours of testes · tumours of uterus · vaginal bleeding of unknown cause
- **CAUTIONS** Acute porphyrias p. 918
- **SIDE-EFFECTS**
- ▶ Very rare Thromboembolism
- ▶ Frequency not known Fever · gastro-intestinal disturbances · headache · hypersensitivity reactions · increased risk of miscarriage · increased risk of multiple pregnancy · injection site reactions · joint pain · ovarian hyperstimulation
- **PREGNANCY** Avoid.
- **BREAST FEEDING** Avoid.
- **PRESCRIBING AND DISPENSING INFORMATION**
Urofollitropin is purified extract of human post-menopausal urine containing follicle-stimulating hormone (FSH).
- **PATIENT AND CARER ADVICE**
Patient advice required around conception and contraception
Patients planning to conceive should be warned that there is a risk of multiple pregnancy.

- **MEDICINAL FORMS**
There can be variation in the licensing of different medicines containing the same drug.
Powder and solvent for solution for injection
- ▶ Bravelle (Ferring Pharmaceuticals Ltd)
Follicle stimulating hormone human (as Urofollitropin)
75 unit Bravelle 75unit powder and solvent for solution for injection vials | 10 vial [PoM] £270.00
- ▶ Fostimon (IBSA Farmaceutici Italia Srl)
Follicle stimulating hormone human (as Urofollitropin)
75 unit Fostimon 75unit powder and solvent for solution for injection vials | 10 vial [PoM] £279.00

6

Endocrine system

Follicle stimulating hormone human (as Urofollitropin)
150 unit Fostimon 150unit powder and solvent for solution for injection vials | 10 vial [PoM] £558.00

7.4 Growth hormone disorders

PITUITARY AND HYPOTHALAMIC HORMONES
AND ANALOGUES > GROWTH HORMONE
RECEPTOR ANTAGONISTS

Pegvisomant

- DRUG ACTION Pegvisomant is a genetically modified analogue of human growth hormone and is a highly selective growth hormone receptor antagonist.

- INDICATIONS AND DOSE

Treatment of acromegaly in patients with inadequate response to surgery, radiation, or both, and to treatment with somatostatin analogues (initiated by a specialist)
▶ BY SUBCUTANEOUS INJECTION
▶ Adult: Initially 80 mg for 1 dose, followed by 10 mg daily, then increased in steps of 5 mg daily, adjusted according to response; maximum 30 mg per day

- CAUTIONS Diabetes mellitus (adjustment of antidiabetic therapy may be necessary) · liver disease
- SIDE-EFFECTS
▶ Uncommon Bleeding tendency · leucocytosis · leucopenia · thrombocytopenia
▶ Frequency not known Abdominal distension · arthralgia · asthenia · constipation · diarrhoea · dizziness · drowsiness · dyspepsia · elevated liver enzymes · fatigue · flatulence · headache · hypercholesterolaemia · hyperglycaemia · hypertension · hypoglycaemia · influenza-like syndrome · injection- site reactions · myalgia · nausea · pruritus · rash · sleep disturbances · sweating · tremor · vomiting · weight gain

SIDE-EFFECTS, FURTHER INFORMATION
▶ Injection-site reactions Rotate injection sites to avoid lipohypertrophy.

- CONCEPTION AND CONTRACEPTION Possible increase in female fertility.
- PREGNANCY Avoid.
- BREAST FEEDING Avoid.
- MONITORING REQUIREMENTS Monitor liver enzymes every 4–6 weeks for 6 months or if symptoms of hepatitis develop.

- MEDICINAL FORMS
There can be variation in the licensing of different medicines containing the same drug.
Powder and solvent for solution for injection
▶ Somavert (Pfizer Ltd)
Pegvisomant 10 mg Somavert 10mg powder and solvent for solution for injection vials | 30 vial [PoM] £1,500.00 (Hospital only)
Pegvisomant 15 mg Somavert 15mg powder and solvent for solution for injection vials | 30 vial [PoM] £2,250.00 (Hospital only)
Pegvisomant 20 mg Somavert 20mg powder and solvent for solution for injection vials | 1 vial [PoM] £100.00 (Hospital only) | 30 vial [PoM] £3,000.00 (Hospital only)
Pegvisomant 25 mg Somavert 25mg powder and solvent for solution for injection vials | 30 vial [PoM] £3,750.00 (Hospital only)
Pegvisomant 30 mg Somavert 30mg powder and solvent for solution for injection vials | 30 vial [PoM] £4,500.00 (Hospital only)

PITUITARY AND HYPOTHALAMIC HORMONES
AND ANALOGUES > HUMAN GROWTH HORMONES

Somatropin

(Recombinant Human Growth Hormone)

- INDICATIONS AND DOSE

Gonadal dysgenesis (Turner syndrome)
▶ BY SUBCUTANEOUS INJECTION
▶ Adult: 1.4 mg/m^2 daily, alternatively 45–50 micrograms/kg daily

Deficiency of growth hormone
▶ BY SUBCUTANEOUS INJECTION
▶ Adult: Initially 150–300 micrograms daily, then increased if necessary up to 1 mg daily, dose to be increased gradually, use minimum effective dose (requirements may decrease with age)
DOSE EQUIVALENCE AND CONVERSION
Dose formerly expressed in units; somatropin 1 mg ≡ 3 units.

- CONTRA-INDICATIONS Evidence of tumour activity (complete antitumour therapy and ensure intracranial lesions inactive before starting) · not to be used after renal transplantation · severe obesity in Prader-Willi syndrome · severe respiratory impairment in Prader-Willi syndrome
- CAUTIONS Diabetes mellitus (adjustment of antidiabetic therapy may be necessary) · disorders of the epiphysis of the hip (monitor for limping) · history of malignant disease · hypothyroidism—manufacturers recommend periodic thyroid function tests but limited evidence of clinical value · initiation of treatment close to puberty not recommended in child born small for corrected gestational age · papilloedema · relative deficiencies of other pituitary hormones · resolved intracranial hypertension (monitor closely) · Silver-Russell syndrome
- INTERACTIONS → Appendix 1 (somatropin).
- SIDE-EFFECTS Antibody formation · arthralgia · benign intracranial hypertension · carpal tunnel syndrome · fluid retention (peripheral oedema) · headache · hyperglycaemia · hypoglycaemia · hypothyroidism · insulin resistance · leukaemia in children with growth hormone deficiency · myalgia · nausea · papilloedema · paraesthesia · reactions at injection site · visual problems · vomiting
SIDE-EFFECTS, FURTHER INFORMATION
▶ Papilloedema Funduscopy for papilloedema recommended if severe or recurrent headache, visual problems, nausea and vomiting occur—if papilloedema confirmed consider benign intracranial hypertension (rare cases reported).
- PREGNANCY Discontinue if pregnancy occurs—no information available.
- BREAST FEEDING No information available. Absorption from milk unlikely.
- DIRECTIONS FOR ADMINISTRATION Rotate subcutaneous injection sites to prevent lipoatrophy.
SAIZEN® SOLUTION FOR INJECTION For use by subcutaneous injection.
NUTROPINAQ® For use by subcutaneous injection.
OMNITROPE® For use by subcutaneous injection.
NORDITROPIN® PREPARATIONS For use by subcutaneous injection.
ZOMACTON® For use by subcutaneous injection.
GENOTROPIN® PREPARATIONS For use by subcutaneous injection.
SAIZEN® POWDER AND SOLVENT FOR SOLUTION FOR INJECTION For use by subcutaneous injection.
HUMATROPE® Cartridges for use by subcutaneous injection.

- **PRESCRIBING AND DISPENSING INFORMATION** Medicinal products containing somatropin are not identical and although there should be no important differences in terms of safety and efficacy, when prescribing biological products it is good practice to use the brand name, see *Biosimilar medicines*, under Guidance on prescribing p. 1.

SAIZEN® SOLUTION FOR INJECTION For use with *cool.click*® needle-free autoinjector device or *easypod*® autoinjector device (non-NHS but available free of charge from clinics).

NUTROPINAQ® For use with *NutropinAq*® Pen device (non-NHS but available free of charge from clinics).

OMNITROPE® For use with *Omnitrope Pen 5*® and *Omnitrope Pen 10*® devices (non-NHS but available free of charge from clinics).

NORDITROPIN® PREPARATIONS Cartridges are for use with appropriate *NordiPen*® device (non-NHS but available free of charge from clinics).

Multidose disposable prefilled pens for use with *NovoFine*® or *NovoTwist*® needles.

ZOMACTON® 4 mg vial for use with *ZomaJet 2*® *Vision* needle-free device (non-NHS but available free of charge from clinics) or with needles and syringes.

10 mg vial for use with *ZomaJet Vision X*® needle-free device (non-NHS but available free of charge from clinics) or with needles and syringes.

GENOTROPIN® PREPARATIONS Cartridges are for use with *Genotropin*® Pen device (non-NHS but available free of charge from clinics).

SAIZEN® POWDER AND SOLVENT FOR SOLUTION FOR INJECTION For use with *one. click*® autoinjector device or *cool.click*® needle-free autoinjector device or *easypod*® autoinjector device (non-NHS but available free of charge from clinics).

- **NATIONAL FUNDING/ACCESS DECISIONS**

NICE technology appraisals (TAs)

▸ **Somatropin for the treatment of growth failure in children (May 2010)** NICE TA188
Somatropin is recommended for children with growth failure who:
- have growth-hormone deficiency
- have Turner syndrome
- have Prader-Willi syndrome
- have chronic renal insufficiency
- are born small for gestational age with subsequent growth failure at 4 years of age or later
- have short stature homeobox-containing gene (SHOX) deficiency.

Treatment should be discontinued if growth velocity increases by less than 50% from baseline in the first year of treatment.
www.nice.org.uk/TA188

▸ **Somatropin for adults with growth hormone deficiency (August 2003)** NICE TA64
Somatropin is recommended in adults **only** if the following 3 criteria are fulfilled:
- Severe growth hormone deficiency, established by an appropriate method,
- Impaired quality of life, measured by means of a specific questionnaire,
- Already receiving treatment for another pituitary hormone deficiency.

Somatropin treatment should be discontinued if the quality of life has not improved sufficiently by 9 months.

Severe growth hormone deficiency developing after linear growth is complete but before the age of 25 years should be treated with growth hormone; treatment should continue until adult peak bone mass has been achieved. Treatment for adult-onset growth hormone deficiency should be stopped only when the patient and the patient's

physician consider it appropriate.
Treatment with somatropin should be initiated and managed by a physician with expertise in growth hormone disorders; maintenance treatment can be prescribed in the community under a shared-care protocol.
www.nice.org.uk/TA64

- **MEDICINAL FORMS**
There can be variation in the licensing of different medicines containing the same drug.

Solution for injection
EXCIPIENTS: May contain Benzyl alcohol
▸ Norditropin NordiFlex (Novo Nordisk Ltd)
  Somatropin (epr) 3.3 mg per 1 ml Norditropin NordiFlex 5mg/1.5ml solution for injection pre-filled pen | 1 pre-filled disposable injection PoM £115.90 CD4-2
  Somatropin (epr) 6.7 mg per 1 ml Norditropin NordiFlex 10mg/1.5ml solution for injection pre-filled pen | 1 pre-filled disposable injection PoM £231.80 CD4-2
  Somatropin (epr) 10 mg per 1 ml Norditropin NordiFlex 15mg/1.5ml solution for injection pre-filled pen | 1 pre-filled disposable injection PoM £347.70 CD4-2
▸ Norditropin SimpleXx (Novo Nordisk Ltd)
  Somatropin (epr) 3.3 mg per 1 ml Norditropin SimpleXx 5mg/1.5ml solution for injection cartridges | 1 cartridge PoM £106.35 CD4-2
  Somatropin (epr) 6.7 mg per 1 ml Norditropin SimpleXx 10mg/1.5ml solution for injection cartridges | 1 cartridge PoM £212.70 CD4-2
  Somatropin (epr) 10 mg per 1 ml Norditropin SimpleXx 15mg/1.5ml solution for injection cartridges | 1 cartridge PoM £319.05 CD4-2
▸ NutropinAq (Ipsen Ltd)
  Somatropin (rbe) 5 mg per 1 ml NutropinAq 10mg/2ml solution for injection cartridges | 1 cartridge PoM £203.00 CD4-2 | 3 cartridge PoM £609.00 CD4-2
▸ Omnitrope Pen (Sandoz Ltd)
  Somatropin (rbe) 3.333 mg per 1 ml Omnitrope Pen 5 5mg/1.5ml solution for injection cartridges | 5 cartridge PoM £368.74 CD4-2
  Somatropin (rbe) 6.667 mg per 1 ml Omnitrope Pen 10 10mg/1.5ml solution for injection cartridges | 5 cartridge PoM £737.49 CD4-2
▸ Omnitrope SurePal (Sandoz Ltd)
  Somatropin (rbe) 3.333 mg per 1 ml Omnitrope SurePal 5 5mg/1.5ml solution for injection cartridges | 5 cartridge PoM £368.74 CD4-2
  Somatropin (rbe) 6.667 mg per 1 ml Omnitrope SurePal 10 10mg/1.5ml solution for injection cartridges | 5 cartridge PoM £737.49 CD4-2
  Somatropin (rbe) 10 mg per 1 ml Omnitrope SurePal 15 15mg/1.5ml solution for injection cartridges | 5 cartridge PoM £1,106.22 CD4-2
▸ Saizen (Merck Serono Ltd)
  Somatropin (rmc) 5.825 mg per 1 ml Saizen 6mg/1.03ml solution for injection cartridges | 1 cartridge PoM £139.08 CD4-2
  Somatropin (rmc) 8 mg per 1 ml Saizen 20mg/2.5ml solution for injection cartridges | 1 cartridge PoM £463.60 CD4-2
  Saizen 12mg/1.5ml solution for injection cartridges | 1 cartridge PoM £278.16 CD4-2

Powder and solvent for solution for injection
EXCIPIENTS: May contain Benzyl alcohol
▸ Genotropin (Pfizer Ltd)
  Somatropin (rbe) 5.3 mg Genotropin 5.3mg powder and solvent for solution for injection cartridges | 1 cartridge PoM £92.15 CD4-2
  Somatropin (rbe) 12 mg Genotropin 12mg powder and solvent for solution for injection cartridges | 1 cartridge PoM £208.65 CD4-2
▸ Genotropin GoQuick (Pfizer Ltd)
  Somatropin (rbe) 5.3 mg Genotropin GoQuick 5.3mg powder and solvent for solution for injection pre-filled disposable devices | 1 pre-filled disposable injection PoM £92.15 CD4-2
  Somatropin (rbe) 12 mg Genotropin GoQuick 12mg powder and solvent for solution for injection pre-filled disposable devices | 1 pre-filled disposable injection PoM £208.65 CD4-2
▸ Genotropin MiniQuick (Pfizer Ltd)
  Somatropin (rbe) 200 microgram Genotropin MiniQuick 200microgram powder and solvent for solution for injection pre-filled disposable devices | 7 pre-filled disposable injection PoM £24.35 CD4-2
  Somatropin (rbe) 400 microgram Genotropin MiniQuick 400microgram powder and solvent for solution for injection pre-filled disposable devices | 7 pre-filled disposable injection PoM £48.68 CD4-2

6

Endocrine system

Somatropin (rbe) 600 microgram Genotropin MiniQuick 600microgram powder and solvent for solution for injection pre-filled disposable devices | 7 pre-filled disposable injection [PoM] £73.03 [CD4-2]

Somatropin (rbe) 800 microgram Genotropin MiniQuick 800microgram powder and solvent for solution for injection pre-filled disposable devices | 7 pre-filled disposable injection [PoM] £97.37 [CD4-2]

Somatropin (rbe) 1 mg Genotropin MiniQuick 1mg powder and solvent for solution for injection pre-filled disposable devices | 7 pre-filled disposable injection [PoM] £121.71 [CD4-2]

Somatropin (rbe) 1.2 mg Genotropin MiniQuick 1.2mg powder and solvent for solution for injection pre-filled disposable devices | 7 pre-filled disposable injection [PoM] £146.06 [CD4-2]

Somatropin (rbe) 1.4 mg Genotropin MiniQuick 1.4mg powder and solvent for solution for injection pre-filled disposable devices | 7 pre-filled disposable injection [PoM] £170.39 [CD4-2]

Somatropin (rbe) 1.6 mg Genotropin MiniQuick 1.6mg powder and solvent for solution for injection pre-filled disposable devices | 7 pre-filled disposable injection [PoM] £194.74 [CD4-2]

Somatropin (rbe) 1.8 mg Genotropin MiniQuick 1.8mg powder and solvent for solution for injection pre-filled disposable devices | 7 pre-filled disposable injection [PoM] £219.08 [CD4-2]

Somatropin (rbe) 2 mg Genotropin MiniQuick 2mg powder and solvent for solution for injection pre-filled disposable devices | 7 pre-filled disposable injection [PoM] £243.42 [CD4-2]

▸ **Humatrope** (Eli Lilly and Company Ltd)

Somatropin (rbe) 6 mg Humatrope 6mg powder and solvent for solution for injection cartridges | 1 cartridge [PoM] £108.00 [CD4-2]

Somatropin (rbe) 12 mg Humatrope 12mg powder and solvent for solution for injection cartridges | 1 cartridge [PoM] £216.00 [CD4-2]

Somatropin (rbe) 24 mg Humatrope 24mg powder and solvent for solution for injection cartridges | 1 cartridge [PoM] £432.00 [CD4-2]

▸ **Saizen** (Merck Serono Ltd)

Somatropin (rmc) 8 mg Saizen 8mg click.easy powder and solvent for solution for injection vials | 1 vial [PoM] £185.44 [CD4-2]

▸ **Zomacton** (Ferring Pharmaceuticals Ltd)

Somatropin (rbe) 4 mg Zomacton 4mg powder and solvent for solution for injection vials | 1 vial [PoM] £79.69 [CD4-2]

Somatropin (rbe) 10 mg Zomacton 10mg powder and solvent for solution for injection vials | 1 vial [PoM] £199.23 [CD4-2]

8 Sex hormone responsive conditions

Sex hormones

Oestrogens and HRT

Oestrogens are necessary for the development of female secondary sexual characteristics; they also stimulate myometrial hypertrophy with endometrial hyperplasia.

In terms of oestrogenic activity *natural oestrogens* (estradiol p. 682 (oestradiol), estrone (oestrone), and estriol p. 753 (oestriol)) have a more appropriate profile for hormone replacement therapy (HRT) than *synthetic oestrogens* (ethinylestradiol p. 685 (ethinyloestradiol) and mestranol). Tibolone p. 686 has oestrogenic, progestogenic and weak androgenic activity.

Oestrogen therapy is given cyclically or continuously for a number of gynaecological conditions. If long-term therapy is required in women with a uterus, a progestogen should normally be added to reduce the risk of cystic hyperplasia of the endometrium (or of endometriotic foci in women who have had a hysterectomy) and possible transformation to cancer.

Oestrogens are no longer used to suppress lactation because of their association with thromboembolism.

Hormone replacement therapy

Hormone replacement therapy (HRT) with small doses of an oestrogen (together with a progestogen in women with a uterus) is appropriate for alleviating menopausal symptoms such as vaginal atrophy or vasomotor instability. Oestrogen

given systemically in the perimenopausal and postmenopausal period or tibolone given in the postmenopausal period also diminish postmenopausal osteoporosis but other drugs are preferred. Menopausal atrophic vaginitis may respond to a short course of a topical vaginal oestrogen preparation used for a few weeks and repeated if necessary.

Systemic therapy with an oestrogen or drugs with oestrogenic properties alleviates the symptoms of oestrogen deficiency such as vasomotor symptoms. Tibolone combines oestrogenic and progestogenic activity with weak androgenic activity; it is given continuously, without cyclical progestogen.

HRT may be used in women with early natural or surgical menopause (before age 45 years), since they are at high risk of osteoporosis. For early menopause, HRT can be given until the approximate age of natural menopause (i.e. until age 50 years). Alternatives to HRT should be considered if osteoporosis is the main concern.

Clonidine hydrochloride p. 131 may be used to reduce vasomotor symptoms in women who cannot take an oestrogen, but clonidine hydrochloride may cause unacceptable side-effects.

HRT increases the risk of venous thromboembolism, stroke, endometrial cancer (reduced by a progestogen), breast cancer, and ovarian cancer; there is an increased risk of coronary heart disease in women who start combined HRT more than 10 years after menopause. For details of these risks see HRT Risk table.

The minimum effective dose of HRT should be used for the shortest duration. Treatment should be reviewed at least annually and for osteoporosis alternative treatments considered. HRT does not prevent coronary heart disease or protect against a decline in cognitive function and it should not be prescribed for these purposes. Experience of treating women over 65 years with HRT is limited.

For the treatment of menopausal symptoms the benefits of short-term HRT outweigh the risks in the majority of women, especially in those aged under 60 years.

Risk of breast cancer

It is estimated that using all types of HRT, including tibolone, increases the risk of breast cancer within 1–2 years of initiating treatment. The increased risk is related to the duration of HRT use (but not to the age at which HRT is started) and this excess risk disappears within 5 years of stopping. Radiological detection of breast cancer can be made more difficult as mammographic density can increase with HRT use; tibolone has only a limited effect on mammographic density.

Risk of endometrial cancer

The increased risk of endometrial cancer depends on the dose and duration of oestrogen-only HRT. In women with a uterus, the addition of a progestogen cyclically (for at least 10 days per 28-day cycle) reduces the additional risk of endometrial cancer; this additional risk is eliminated if a progestogen is given continuously. However, this should be weighed against the increased risk of breast cancer.

Risk of ovarian cancer

Long-term use of combined HRT or oestrogen-only HRT is associated with a small increased risk of ovarian cancer; this excess risk disappears within a few years of stopping.

Risk of venous thromboembolism

Women using combined or oestrogen-only HRT are at an increased risk of deep vein thrombosis and of pulmonary embolism especially in the first year of use. In women who have predisposing factors (such as a personal or family history of deep vein thrombosis or pulmonary embolism, severe varicose veins, obesity, trauma, or prolonged bed-rest) it is prudent to review the need for HRT, as in some cases the risks of HRT may exceed the benefits. Travel involving prolonged immobility further increases the risk of deep vein thrombosis.

Risk of stroke
Risk of stroke increases with age, therefore older women have a greater absolute risk of stroke. Combined HRT or oestrogen-only HRT slightly increases the risk of stroke. Tibolone increases the risk of stroke about 2.2 times from the first year of treatment.

Risk of coronary heart disease
HRT does not prevent coronary heart disease and should not be prescribed for this purpose. There is an increased risk of coronary heart disease in women who start combined HRT more than 10 years after menopause. Although very little information is available on the risk of coronary heart disease in younger women who start HRT close to the menopause, studies suggest a lower relative risk compared with older women.

Choice
The choice of HRT for an individual depends on an overall balance of indication, risk, and convenience. A woman with a uterus normally requires oestrogen with cyclical progestogen for the last 12 to 14 days of the cycle or a preparation which involves continuous administration of an oestrogen and a progestogen (or one which provides both oestrogenic and progestogenic activity in a single preparation). Continuous combined preparations or tibolone are **not suitable** for use in the perimenopause or within 12 months of the last menstrual period; women who use such preparations may bleed irregularly in the early stages of treatment—if bleeding continues endometrial abnormality should be ruled out and consideration given to changing to cyclical HRT.

An oestrogen alone is suitable for continuous use in women without a uterus. However, in endometriosis, endometrial foci may remain despite hysterectomy and the addition of a progestogen should be considered in these circumstances.

An oestrogen may be given by mouth or by transdermal administration, which avoids first-pass metabolism.

Surgery
Major surgery under general anaesthesia, including orthopaedic and vascular leg surgery, is a predisposing factor for venous thromboembolism and it may be prudent to stop HRT 4–6 weeks before surgery; it should be restarted only after full mobilisation. If HRT is continued or if discontinuation is not possible (e.g. in non-elective surgery), prophylaxis with unfractionated or low molecular weight heparin and graduated compression hosiery is advised.

Reasons to stop HRT
Hormone replacement therapy should be stopped (pending investigation and treatment), if any of the following occur:
* sudden severe chest pain (even if not radiating to left arm);
* sudden breathlessness (or cough with blood-stained sputum);
* unexplained swelling or severe pain in calf of one leg;
* severe stomach pain;
* serious neurological effects including unusual severe, prolonged headache especially if first time or getting progressively worse or sudden partial or complete loss of vision or sudden disturbance of hearing or other perceptual disorders or dysphasia or bad fainting attack or collapse or first unexplained epileptic seizure or weakness, motor disturbances, very marked numbness suddenly affecting one side or one part of body;
* hepatitis, jaundice, liver enlargement;
* blood pressure above systolic 160 mmHg or diastolic 95 mmHg;
* prolonged immobility after surgery or leg injury;
* detection of a risk factor which contra-indicates treatment

Ethinylestradiol
Ethinylestradiol p. 685 (ethinyloestradiol) is licensed for short-term treatment of symptoms of oestrogen deficiency, for osteoporosis prophylaxis if other drugs cannot be used and for the treatment of female hypogonadism and menstrual disorders.

Ethinylestradiol is occasionally used under **specialist supervision** for the management of *hereditary haemorrhagic telangiectasia* (but evidence of benefit is limited). It is also used licensed for the palliative treatment of prostate cancer.

Raloxifene
Raloxifene hydrochloride p. 680 is licensed for the treatment and prevention of *postmenopausal osteoporosis*; unlike hormone replacement therapy, raloxifene hydrochloride does not reduce menopausal vasomotor symptoms.

Progestogens and progesterone receptor modulators
There are two main groups of progestogen, progesterone and its analogues (dydrogesterone and medroxyprogesterone acetate p. 733) and testosterone analogues (norethisterone p. 691 and norgestrel). The newer progestogens (desogestrel p. 728, norgestimate, and gestodene) are all derivatives of norgestrel; levonorgestrel p. 729 is the active isomer of norgestrel and has twice its potency. Progesterone p. 692 and its analogues are less androgenic than the testosterone derivatives and neither progesterone nor dydrogesterone causes virilisation.

Where endometriosis requires drug treatment, it may respond to a progestogen, e.g. norethisterone, administered on a continuous basis. Danazol p. 670 and gonadorelin analogues are also available.

Although oral progestogens have been used widely for menorrhagia they are relatively ineffective compared with tranexamic acid p. 99 or, particularly where dysmenorrhoea is also a factor, mefenamic acid p. 992; the levonorgestrel-releasing intra-uterine system may be particularly useful for women also requiring contraception. Oral progestogens have also been used for severe dysmenorrhoea, but where contraception is also required in younger women the best choice is a combined oral contraceptive.

Progestogens have also been advocated for the alleviation of premenstrual symptoms, but no convincing physiological basis for such treatment has been shown.

Progestogens have been used for the prevention of miscarriage in women with a history of recurrent miscarriage but there is no evidence of benefit and they are **not** recommended for this purpose. In pregnant women with antiphospholipid antibody syndrome who have suffered recurrent miscarriage, administration of low-dose aspirin p. 109 and a prophylactic dose of a low molecular weight heparin may decrease the risk of fetal loss (use under specialist supervision only).

Hormone replacement therapy
In women with a uterus a progestogen needs to be added to long-term oestrogen therapy for hormone replacement, to prevent cystic hyperplasia of the endometrium and possible transformation to cancer; it can be added on a cyclical or a continuous basis. Combined packs incorporating suitable progestogen tablets are available.

Oral contraception
Desogestrel, gestodene, levonorgestrel, norethisterone, and norgestimate are used in combined oral contraceptives and in progestogen-only contraceptives.

Cancer
Progestogens also have a role in neoplastic disease.

HRT Risks

Risk	Age range (years)	Background incidence per 1000 women in Europe not using HRT		Additional cases per 1000 women using oestrogen only HRT (estimated)		Additional cases per 1000 women using combined (oestrogen-progesterone) HRT (estimated)	
		Over 5 years	Over 10 years	For 5 years' use	For 10 years' use	For 5 years' use	For 10 years' use
Breast cancer[1]	50-59	10	20	2	6	6	24
	60-69	15	30	3	9	9	36
Endometrial cancer[2,3]	50-59	2	4	4	32	NS	NS
	60-69	3	6	6	48	NS	NS
Ovarian cancer	50-59	2	4	<1	1	<1	1
	60-69	3	6	<1	2	<1	2
Venous thromboembolism[4,5]	50-59	5	–	2	–	7	–
	60-69	8	–	2	–	10	–
Stroke[6]	50-59	4	–	1	–	1	–
	60-69	9	–	3	–	3	–
Coronary heart disease[7,8]	70-79	29-44	–	NS	–	15	–

Where background incidence or additional cases have not been included in the table, this indicates a lack of available data. NS indicates a non-significant difference. Taken from MHRA/CHM (*Drug Safety* 2007; 1 (2): 2-6) available at www.gov.uk/drug-safety-update

1 Tibolone increases the risk of breast cancer but to a lesser extent than with combined HRT.
2 Evidence suggests an increased risk of endometrial cancer with tibolone. After 2.7 years of use (in women of average age 68 years), 1 extra case of endometrial hyperplasia and 4 extra cases of endometrial cancer were diagnosed compared with placebo users.
3 The risk of endometrial cancer cannot be reliably estimated in those using combined HRT because the addition of progestogen for at least 10 days per 28-day cycle greatly reduces the additional risk, and addition of a daily progestogen eliminates the additional risk. The risk of endometrial cancer in women who have not used HRT increases with body mass index (BMI); the increased risk of endometrial cancer in users of oestrogen-only HRT or tibolone is more apparent in women who are not overweight.
4 Limited data does not suggest an increased risk of thromboembolism with tibolone compared with combined HRT or women not taking HRT.
5 Although the level of risk of thromboembolism associated with non-oral routes of administration of HRT has not been established, it may be lower for the transdermal route.
6 Tibolone increases the risk of stroke about 2.2 times from the first year of treatment; risk of stroke is age-dependent and therefore the absolute risk of stroke with tibolone increases with age.
7 Increased risk of coronary heart disease in women who start combined HRT more than 10 years after menopause.
8 There is insufficient data to draw a conclusion on the risk of coronary heart disease with tibolone.

Progesterone receptor modulators

Ulipristal acetate p. 727 is a progesterone receptor modulator with a partial progesterone antagonist effect. Ulipristal acetate is used in the pre-operative treatment of moderate to severe symptoms of uterine fibroids; it is also used as an hormonal emergency contraceptive.

8.1 Female sex hormone responsive conditions

CALCIUM REGULATING DRUGS > BONE RESORPTION INHIBITORS

Raloxifene hydrochloride

● INDICATIONS AND DOSE

Treatment and prevention of postmenopausal osteoporosis
▸ BY MOUTH
▸ Adult: 60 mg once daily

● CONTRA-INDICATIONS Cholestasis · endometrial cancer · history of venous thromboembolism · undiagnosed uterine bleeding

● CAUTIONS Avoid in Acute porphyrias p. 918 · breast cancer (manufacturer advises avoid during treatment for breast cancer) · history of oestrogen-induced hypertriglyceridaemia (monitor serum triglycerides) · risk

factors for stroke · risk factors for venous thromboembolism (discontinue if prolonged immobilisation)

● INTERACTIONS → Appendix 1 (raloxifene).

● SIDE-EFFECTS
▸ **Common or very common** Hot flushes · influenza-like symptoms · leg cramps · peripheral oedema
▸ **Uncommon** Thrombophlebitis · venous thromboembolism
▸ **Rare** Arterial thromboembolism · breast discomfort · gastro-intestinal disturbances · headache · hypertension · migraine · rashes · thrombocytopenia

● HEPATIC IMPAIRMENT Avoid.

● RENAL IMPAIRMENT Caution in mild to moderate impairment. Avoid in severe impairment.

● NATIONAL FUNDING/ACCESS DECISIONS

NICE technology appraisals (TAs)
▸ Alendronate, etidronate, risedronate, raloxifene and strontium ranelate for the primary prevention of osteoporotic fragility fractures in postmenopausal women (October 2008) NICE TA160
Raloxifene is not recommended as a treatment option in postmenopausal women for primary prevention of osteoporotic fractures.
www.nice.org.uk/TA160
▸ Alendronate, etidronate, risedronate, raloxifene, strontium ranelate and teriparatide for the secondary prevention of osteoporotic fragility fractures in postmenopausal women (October 2008) NICE TA161
This guideline recommends treatment options for the secondary prevention of osteoporotic fractures in

postmenopausal women with confirmed osteoporosis who have also sustained a clinically apparent osteoporotic fracture.

Raloxifene is recommended as an alternative treatment option for women:

- in whom alendronate and risedronate are contra-indicated or not tolerated **and**
- who comply with particular combinations of bone mineral density measurement, age, and independent risk factors for fracture, as indicated in the full NICE guidance (available at www.nice.org.uk/TA161).
www.nice.org.uk/TA161

● MEDICINAL FORMS
There can be variation in the licensing of different medicines containing the same drug.

Tablet
▸ Raloxifene hydrochloride (Non-proprietary)
Raloxifene hydrochloride 60 mg Raloxifene 60mg tablets | 28 tablet PoM £17.06 DT price = £3.89 | 84 tablet PoM £56.61
▸ Evirex (Somex Pharma)
Raloxifene hydrochloride 60 mg Evirex 60mg tablets | 28 tablet PoM £5.10 DT price = £3.89
▸ Evista (Daiichi Sankyo UK Ltd)
Raloxifene hydrochloride 60 mg Evista 60mg tablets | 28 tablet PoM £17.06 DT price = £3.89
▸ Ostiral (Lupin (Europe) Ltd)
Raloxifene hydrochloride 60 mg Ostiral 60mg tablets | 28 tablet PoM £14.50 DT price = £3.89
▸ Razylan (Aspire Pharma Ltd)
Raloxifene hydrochloride 60 mg Razylan 60mg tablets | 28 tablet PoM £17.06 DT price = £3.89

OESTROGENS

Conjugated oestrogens (equine)

● INDICATIONS AND DOSE
PREMARIN® TABLETS

Menopausal symptoms
▸ BY MOUTH
▸ Adult: 0.3–1.25 mg daily continuously; with cyclical progestogen for 12–14 days of each cycle in women with a uterus

Osteoporosis prophylaxis
▸ BY MOUTH
▸ Adult: 0.625–1.25 mg daily continuously; with cyclical progestogen for 12–14 days of each cycle in women with a uterus

● CONTRA-INDICATIONS Active arterial thromboembolic disease (e.g. angina or myocardial infarction) · active thrombophlebitis · Dubin-Johnson syndromes (or monitor closely) · history of breast cancer · history of recurrent venous thromboembolism (unless already on anticoagulant treatment) · liver disease (where liver function tests have failed to return to normal) · oestrogen-dependent cancer · recent arterial thromboembolic disease (e.g. angina or myocardial infarction) · Rotor syndromes (or monitor closely) · thrombophilic disorder · undiagnosed vaginal bleeding · untreated endometrial hyperplasia · venous thromboembolism

● CAUTIONS Acute porphyrias p. 918 · diabetes (increased risk of heart disease) · factors predisposing to thromboembolism · history of breast nodules (closely monitor breast status—risk of breast cancer) · history of endometrial hyperplasia · history of fibrocystic disease (closely monitor breast status—risk of breast cancer) · hypophyseal tumours · increased risk of gall-bladder disease reported · migraine · migraine-like headaches · presence of antiphospholipid antibodies (increased risk of thrombotic events) · risk factors for oestrogen-dependent

tumours (e.g. breast cancer in first-degree relative) · risk of breast cancer

CAUTIONS, FURTHER INFORMATION
▸ Risk of breast cancer It is estimated that using *all* types of HRT, including tibolone, increases the risk of breast cancer within 1–2 years of initiating treatment. The increased risk is related to the duration of HRT use (but not to the age at which HRT is started) and this excess risk disappears within 5 years of stopping.

   Radiological detection of breast cancer can be made more difficult as mammographic density can increase with HRT use.
▸ Risk of endometrial cancer The increased risk of endometrial cancer depends on the dose and duration of oestrogen-only HRT.

   In women with a uterus, the addition of a progestogen cyclically (for at least 10 days per 28-day cycle) reduces the additional risk of endometrial cancer; this additional risk is eliminated if a progestogen is given continuously. However, this should be weighed against the increased risk of breast cancer.
▸ Risk of ovarian cancer Long-term use of combined HRT or oestrogen-only HRT is associated with a small increased risk of ovarian cancer. This excess risk disappears within a few years of stopping.
▸ Risk of venous thromboembolism Women using combined or oestrogen-only HRT are at an increased risk of deep vein thrombosis and of pulmonary embolism especially in the first year of use.

   In *women who have predisposing factors* (such as a personal or family history of deep vein thrombosis or pulmonary embolism, severe varicose veins, obesity, trauma, or prolonged bed-rest) it is prudent to review the need for HRT, as in some cases the risks of HRT may exceed the benefits.

   Travel involving prolonged immobility further increases the risk of deep vein thrombosis.
▸ Risk of stroke Risk of stroke increases with age, therefore older women have a greater absolute risk of stroke. Combined HRT or oestrogen-only HRT slightly increases the risk of stroke.
▸ Risk of coronary heart disease HRT does not prevent coronary heart disease and should not be prescribed for this purpose. There is an increased risk of coronary heart disease in women who start combined HRT more than 10 years after menopause. Although very little information is available on the risk of coronary heart disease in younger women who start HRT close to the menopause, studies suggest a lower relative risk compared with older women.
▸ Other conditions The product literature advises caution in other conditions including hypertension, renal disease, asthma, epilepsy, sickle-cell disease, melanoma, otosclerosis, multiple sclerosis, and systemic lupus erythematosus (but care required if antiphospholipid antibodies present). Evidence for caution in these conditions is unsatisfactory and many women with these conditions may stand to benefit from HRT.

● INTERACTIONS → Appendix 1 (oestrogens).

● SIDE-EFFECTS Abdominal bloating · abdominal cramps · altered blood lipids (may lead to pancreatitis, rashes and chloasma) · breast enlargement · breast tenderness · changes in libido · cholestatic jaundice · contact lenses may irritate · depression · dizziness · fluid retention · glucose intolerance · headache · headache (on vigorous exercise) · leg cramps (rule out venous thrombosis) · migraine · mood changes · nausea · premenstrual-like syndrome · prolonged exposure to unopposed oestrogens may increase risk of developing endometrial cancer · sodium retention · symptoms of endometriosis may be exacerbated · uterine fibroids may increase in size · vaginal candidiasis · vomiting · weight changes

SIDE-EFFECTS, FURTHER INFORMATION

▸ Withdrawal bleeding Cyclical HRT (where a progestogen is taken for 12–14 days of each 28-day oestrogen treatment cycle) usually results in *regular withdrawal bleeding* towards the end of the progestogen. The aim of continuous combined HRT (where a combination of oestrogen and progestogen is taken, usually in a single tablet, throughout each 28-day treatment cycle) is to avoid bleeding, but *irregular bleeding* may occur during the early treatment stages (if it continues endometrial abnormality should be excluded and consideration given to cyclical HRT instead).

● CONCEPTION AND CONTRACEPTION HRT does **not** provide contraception and a woman is considered potentially fertile for 2 years after her last menstrual period if she is under 50 years, and for 1 year if she is over 50 years. A woman who is under 50 years and free of all risk factors for venous and arterial disease can use a low-oestrogen combined oral contraceptive pill to provide both relief of menopausal symptoms and contraception; it is recommended that the oral contraceptive be stopped at 50 years of age since there are more suitable alternatives. If any potentially fertile woman needs HRT, non-hormonal contraceptive measures (such as condoms) are necessary. Measurement of follicle-stimulating hormone can help to determine fertility, but high measurements alone (particularly in women aged under 50 years) do not necessarily preclude the possibility of becoming pregnant.

● PREGNANCY Not known to be harmful.

● BREAST FEEDING Avoid until weaning or for 6 months after birth (adverse effects on lactation).

● HEPATIC IMPAIRMENT Avoid in active liver disease including disorders of hepatic excretion (e.g. Dubin-Johnson or Rotor syndromes), infective hepatitis (until liver function returns to normal), and liver tumours.

● MEDICINAL FORMS
There can be variation in the licensing of different medicines containing the same drug.
Tablet
▸ Premarin (Pfizer Ltd)
Conjugated oestrogens 300 microgram Premarin 0.3mg tablets | 84 tablet [PoM] £6.07 DT price = £6.07
Conjugated oestrogens 625 microgram Premarin 0.625mg tablets | 84 tablet [PoM] £4.02 DT price = £4.02
Conjugated oestrogens 1.25 mg Premarin 1.25mg tablets | 84 tablet [PoM] £3.58 DT price = £3.58

Combinations available: *Conjugated oestrogens with medroxyprogesterone*, p. 687 · *Conjugated oestrogens with norgestrel*, p. 687

Estradiol

● INDICATIONS AND DOSE
BEDOL®

Menopausal symptoms | Osteoporosis prophylaxis
▸ BY MOUTH
▸ Adult: 2 mg daily, started on day 1–5 of menstruation (or at any time if cycles have ceased or are infrequent), to be taken with cyclical progestogen for 12–14 days of each cycle in women with a uterus

CLIMAVAL®

Menopausal symptoms (if patient has had a hysterectomy)
▸ BY MOUTH
▸ Adult: 1–2 mg daily

ELLESTE SOLO® MX

Menopausal symptoms
▸ BY TRANSDERMAL APPLICATION
▸ Adult: Apply 1 patch twice weekly continuously, started within 5 days of onset of menstruation (or at any time if cycles have ceased or are infrequent), to be used with cyclical progestogen for 12–14 days of each cycle in women with a uterus, initiate therapy with *MX* 40, subsequently adjust according to response

Osteoporosis prophylaxis
▸ BY TRANSDERMAL APPLICATION
▸ Adult: Apply 1 patch twice weekly continuously, started within 5 days of onset of menstruation (or at any time if cycles have ceased or are infrequent), to be used with cyclical progestogen for 12–14 days of each cycle in women with a uterus, initiate therapy with *MX* 80, subsequently adjust according to response

ELLESTE-SOLO® 1-MG

Menopausal symptoms
▸ BY MOUTH
▸ Adult: 1 mg daily, starting on day 1 of menstruation (or at any time if cycles have ceased or are infrequent), to be taken with cyclical progestogen for 12–14 days of each cycle in women with a uterus

ELLESTE-SOLO® 2-MG

Menopausal symptoms not controlled with lower strength | Osteoporosis prophylaxis
▸ BY MOUTH
▸ Adult: 2 mg daily, started on day 1 of menstruation (or at any time if cycles have ceased or are infrequent), to be given with cyclical progestogen for 12–14 days of each cycle in women with a uterus

ESTRADERM MX®

Menopausal symptoms
▸ BY TRANSDERMAL APPLICATION
▸ Adult: Apply 1 patch twice weekly continuously, started within 5 days of onset of menstruation (or at any time if cycles have ceased or are infrequent), to be used with cyclical progestogen for at least 12 days of each cycle in women with a uterus, initiate therapy with *MX*25 for first 3 months; subsequently adjust according to response

Osteoporosis prophylaxis
▸ BY TRANSDERMAL APPLICATION
▸ Adult: Apply 1 patch twice weekly continuously, started within 5 days of onset of menstruation (or at any time if cycles have ceased or are infrequent), to be used with cyclical progestogen for at least 12 days of each cycle in women with a uterus, initiate therapy with *MX*50; subsequently adjust according to response

ESTRADOT®

Menopausal symptoms
▸ BY TRANSDERMAL APPLICATION
▸ Adult: Apply 1 patch twice weekly continuously, to be used with cyclical progestogen for 12–14 days of each cycle in women with a uterus, initiate therapy with 25 *patch* for 3 months; subsequently adjust according to response

Osteoporosis prophylaxis
▸ BY TRANSDERMAL APPLICATION
▸ Adult: Apply 1 patch twice weekly continuously, to be used with cyclical progestogen for 12–14 days of each cycle in women with a uterus, initiate therapy with 50 *patch*; subsequently adjust according to response

EVOREL®

Menopausal symptoms | Osteoporosis prophylaxis
▶ BY TRANSDERMAL APPLICATION
▶ Adult: Apply 1 patch twice weekly continuously, started within 5 days of onset of menstruation (or at any time if cycles have ceased or are infrequent), to be used with cyclical progestogen for 12–14 days of each cycle in women with a uterus, therapy should be initiated with *Evorel* 50 patch; subsequently adjust according to response; dose may be reduced to *Evorel* 25 patch after first month if necessary for menopausal symptoms **only**

FEMSEVEN®

Menopausal symptoms | Osteoporosis prophylaxis
▶ BY TRANSDERMAL APPLICATION
▶ Adult: Apply 1 patch once weekly continuously, to be used with cyclical progestogen for 12–14 days of each cycle in women with a uterus, initiate therapy with *FemSeven* 50 patches for the first few months, subsequently adjust according to response

OESTROGEL®

Menopausal symptoms
▶ TO THE SKIN
▶ Adult: Apply 1.5 mg once daily continuously, increased if necessary up to 3 mg after 1 month continuously, to be applied over an area twice that of the template provided, starting within 5 days of menstruation (or anytime if cycles have ceased or are infrequent), to be used with cyclical progestogen for at least 12 days of each cycle in women with a uterus

Osteoporosis prophylaxis
▶ TO THE SKIN
▶ Adult: Apply 1.5 mg once daily continuously, to be applied over an area twice that of the template provided, starting within 5 days of menstruation (or anytime if cycles have ceased or are infrequent), to be used with cyclical progestogen for at least 12 days of each cycle in women with a uterus

DOSE EQUIVALENCE AND CONVERSION
For *Oestrogel*®: 2 measures is equivalent to estradiol 1.5 mg.

PROGYNOVA®

Menopausal symptoms
▶ BY MOUTH
▶ Adult: 1–2 mg daily continuously, to be started on day 1 of menstruation (or at any time if cycles have ceased or are infrequent), to be taken with cyclical progestogen for 12–14 days of each cycle in women with a uterus

Osteoporosis prophylaxis
▶ BY MOUTH
▶ Adult: 2 mg daily continuously, to be taken with cyclical progestogen for 12–14 days of each cycle in women with a uterus

PROGYNOVA® TS

Menopausal symptoms | Osteoporosis prophylaxis
▶ BY TRANSDERMAL APPLICATION
▶ Adult: Apply 1 patch once weekly continuously, alternatively apply 1 patch once weekly for 3 weeks, followed by a 7-day patch-free interval (cyclical), to be used with cyclical progestogen for 12–14 days of each cycle in women with a uterus, initiate therapy with *Progynova TS* 50, subsequently adjust according to response, women receiving *Progynova TS* 100 patches for menopausal symptoms may continue with this strength for osteoporosis prophylaxis

SANDRENA®

Menopausal symptoms
▶ TO THE SKIN
▶ Adult: Apply 1 mg once daily, to be applied over area 1–2 times size of hand; in women with a uterus, dose may be adjusted after 2–3 cycles to lowest effective dose; usual dose 0.5–1.5 mg daily

ZUMENON®

Menopausal symptoms
▶ BY MOUTH
▶ Adult: Initially 1 mg daily, to be started within 5 days of onset of menstruation (or any time if cycles have ceased or are infrequent), increased if necessary to 2 mg daily, to be taken with a cyclical progestogen for 12–14 days of each cycle in women with a uterus

Osteoporosis prophylaxis
▶ BY MOUTH
▶ Adult: 2 mg daily, to be taken with a cyclical progestogen for 12–14 days of each cycle in women with a uterus

● CONTRA-INDICATIONS Active arterial thromboembolic disease (e.g. angina or myocardial infarction) · active thrombophlebitis · Dubin-Johnson syndrome (or monitor closely) · history of breast cancer · history of recurrent venous thromboembolism (unless already on anticoagulant treatment) · oestrogen-dependent cancer · recent arterial thromboembolic disease (e.g. angina or myocardial infarction) · Rotor syndrome (or monitor closely) · thrombophilic disorder · undiagnosed vaginal bleeding · untreated endometrial hyperplasia · venous thromboembolism

● CAUTIONS Acute porphyrias p. 918 · diabetes (increased risk of heart disease) · history of breast nodules—closely monitor breast status (risk of breast cancer) · history of endometrial hyperplasia; factors predisposing to thromboembolism · history of fibrocystic disease—closely monitor breast status (risk of breast cancer) · hypophyseal tumours · increased risk of gall-bladder disease · migraine (or migraine-like headaches) · presence of antiphospholipid antibodies (increased risk of thrombotic events) · prolonged exposure to unopposed oestrogens may increase risk of developing endometrial cancer · risk factors for oestrogen-dependent tumours (e.g. breast cancer in first-degree relative) · symptoms of endometriosis may be exacerbated · uterine fibroids may increase in size

CAUTIONS, FURTHER INFORMATION
▶ Risk of breast cancer It is estimated that using *all* types of HRT increases the risk of breast cancer within 1–2 years of initiating treatment. The increased risk is related to the duration of HRT use (but not to the age at which HRT is started) and this excess risk disappears within 5 years of stopping.
  Radiological detection of breast cancer can be made more difficult as mammographic density can increase with HRT use.
▶ Risk of endometrial cancer The increased risk of endometrial cancer depends on the dose and duration of oestrogen-only HRT.
  In women with a uterus, the addition of a progestogen cyclically (for at least 10 days per 28-day cycle) reduces the additional risk of endometrial cancer; this additional risk is eliminated if a progestogen is given continuously. However, this should be weighed against the increased risk of breast cancer.
▶ Risk of ovarian cancer Long-term use of combined HRT or oestrogen-only HRT is associated with a small increased

6

Endocrine system

risk of ovarian cancer. This excess risk disappears within a few years of stopping.

▸ Risk of venous thromboembolism Women using combined or oestrogen-only HRT are at an increased risk of deep vein thrombosis and of pulmonary embolism especially in the first year of use.

In *women who have predisposing factors* (such as a personal or family history of deep vein thrombosis or pulmonary embolism, severe varicose veins, obesity, trauma, or prolonged bed-rest) it is prudent to review the need for HRT, as in some cases the risks of HRT may exceed the benefits.

Travel involving prolonged immobility further increases the risk of deep vein thrombosis.

▸ Risk of stroke Risk of stroke increases with age, therefore older women have a greater absolute risk of stroke. Combined HRT or oestrogen-only HRT slightly increases the risk of stroke.

▸ Risk of coronary heart disease HRT does not prevent coronary heart disease and should not be prescribed for this purpose. There is an increased risk of coronary heart disease in women who start combined HRT more than 10 years after menopause. Although very little information is available on the risk of coronary heart disease in younger women who start HRT close to the menopause, studies suggest a lower relative risk compared with older women.

▸ Other conditions The product literature advises caution in other conditions including hypertension, renal disease, asthma, epilepsy, sickle-cell disease, melanoma, otosclerosis, multiple sclerosis, and systemic lupus erythematosus (but care required if antiphospholipid antibodies present). Evidence for caution in these conditions is unsatisfactory and many women with these conditions may stand to benefit from HRT.

● INTERACTIONS → Appendix 1 (oestrogens).

● SIDE-EFFECTS

GENERAL SIDE-EFFECTS

Abdominal bloating · abdominal cramps · altered blood lipids (may lead to pancreatitis, rashes and chloasma) · breast enlargement · breast tenderness · changes in libido · cholestatic jaundice · contact lenses may irritate · depression · dizziness · fluid retention · glucose intolerance · headache · headache (on vigorous exercise) · leg cramps (rule out venous thrombosis) · migraine · mood changes · nausea · premenstrual-like syndrome · sodium retention · vaginal candidiasis · vomiting · weight changes

SPECIFIC SIDE-EFFECTS

▸ With transdermal use Cause contact sensitisation (possible severe hypersensitivity reaction on continued exposure)

SIDE-EFFECTS, FURTHER INFORMATION

▸ Withdrawal bleeding Cyclical HRT (where a progestogen is taken for 12–14 days of each 28-day oestrogen treatment cycle) usually results in *regular withdrawal bleeding* towards the end of the progestogen. The aim of continuous combined HRT (where a combination of oestrogen and progestogen is taken, usually in a single tablet, throughout each 28-day treatment cycle) is to avoid bleeding, but *irregular bleeding* may occur during the early treatment stages (if it continues endometrial abnormality should be excluded and consideration given to cyclical HRT instead).

● CONCEPTION AND CONTRACEPTION HRT does **not** provide contraception and a woman is considered potentially fertile for 2 years after her last menstrual period if she is under 50 years, and for 1 year if she is over 50 years. A woman who is under 50 years and free of all risk factors for venous and arterial disease can use a low-oestrogen combined oral contraceptive pill to provide both relief of menopausal symptoms and contraception; it is recommended that the oral contraceptive be stopped at 50 years of age since there are more suitable alternatives.

If any potentially fertile woman needs HRT, non-hormonal contraceptive measures (such as condoms) are necessary. Measurement of follicle-stimulating hormone can help to determine fertility, but high measurements alone (particularly in women aged under 50 years) do not necessarily preclude the possibility of becoming pregnant.

● PREGNANCY Not known to be harmful.

● BREAST FEEDING Avoid; adverse effects on lactation.

● HEPATIC IMPAIRMENT Avoid in active liver disease including disorders of hepatic excretion (e.g. Dubin-Johnson or Rotor syndromes), infective hepatitis (until liver function returns to normal), and liver tumours.

● MONITORING REQUIREMENTS

▸ History of breast nodules or fibrocystic disease—closely monitor breast status (risk of breast cancer.

▸ The endometrial safety of long-term or repeated use of topical vaginal oestrogens is uncertain; treatment should be reviewed at least annually, with special consideration given to any symptoms of endometrial hyperplasia or carcinoma.

● DIRECTIONS FOR ADMINISTRATION

▸ With transdermal use Patch should be removed after 3–4 days (or once a week in case of 7-day patch) and replaced with fresh patch on slightly different site; recommended sites: clean, dry, unbroken areas of skin on trunk below waistline; not to be applied on or near breasts or under waistband. If patch falls off in bath allow skin to cool before applying new patch.

● PATIENT AND CARER ADVICE

▸ With transdermal use Patient counselling is advised for estradiol patches (administration).

▸ With topical use Patient counselling is advised for estradiol gels (administration).

OESTROGEL® ▸ With topical use Apply gel to clean, dry, intact skin such as arms, shoulders or inner thighs and allow to dry for 5 minutes before covering with clothing. Not to be applied on or near breasts or on vulval region. Avoid skin contact with another person (particularly male) and avoid other skin products or washing the area for at least 1 hour after application.

SANDRENA® ▸ With topical use Apply gel to intact areas of skin such as lower trunk or thighs, using right and left sides on alternate days. Wash hands after application. Not to be applied on the breasts or face and avoid contact with eyes. Allow area of application to dry for 5 minutes and do not wash area for at least 1 hour.

● MEDICINAL FORMS
There can be variation in the licensing of different medicines containing the same drug.

Tablet
▸ Bedol (ReSource Medical UK Ltd)
Estradiol 2 mg Bedol 2mg tablets | 84 tablet [PoM] £5.07
▸ Climaval (Novartis Pharmaceuticals UK Ltd)
Estradiol valerate 2 mg Climaval 2mg tablets | 28 tablet [PoM] £3.53
▸ Elleste Solo (Meda Pharmaceuticals Ltd)
Estradiol 1 mg Elleste Solo 1mg tablets | 84 tablet [PoM] £5.06
Estradiol 2 mg Elleste Solo 2mg tablets | 84 tablet [PoM] £5.06
▸ Progynova (Bayer Plc)
Estradiol valerate 1 mg Progynova 1mg tablets | 84 tablet [PoM] £7.30
Estradiol valerate 2 mg Progynova 2mg tablets | 84 tablet [PoM] £7.30
▸ Zumenon (BGP Products Ltd)
Estradiol 1 mg Zumenon 1mg tablets | 84 tablet [PoM] £6.89
Estradiol 2 mg Zumenon 2mg tablets | 84 tablet [PoM] £6.89

Transdermal patch
▸ Elleste Solo MX (Meda Pharmaceuticals Ltd)
Estradiol 40 microgram per 24 hour Elleste Solo MX 40 transdermal patches | 8 patch [PoM] £5.19
Estradiol 80 microgram per 24 hour Elleste Solo MX 80 transdermal patches | 8 patch [PoM] £5.99

> Estraderm MX (Merus Labs Luxco S.a R.L.)

Estradiol 25 microgram per 24 hour Estraderm MX 25 patches |
8 patch [PoM] £5.50 | 24 patch [PoM] £16.46

Estradiol 50 microgram per 24 hour Estraderm MX 50 patches |
8 patch [PoM] £5.51 | 20 patch [PoM] no price available (Hospital
only) | 24 patch [PoM] £16.46

Estradiol 75 microgram per 24 hour Estraderm MX 75 patches |
8 patch [PoM] £6.42 | 24 patch [PoM] £19.27

Estradiol 100 microgram per 24 hour Estraderm MX 100 patches |
8 patch [PoM] £6.66 | 24 patch [PoM] £19.99

> Estradot (Novartis Pharmaceuticals UK Ltd)

Estradiol 25 microgram per 24 hour Estradot
25micrograms/24hours patches | 8 patch [PoM] £5.99

Estradiol 37.5 microgram per 24 hour Estradot
37.5micrograms/24hours patches | 8 patch [PoM] £6.00

Estradiol 50 microgram per 24 hour Estradot
50micrograms/24hours patches | 8 patch [PoM] £6.02

Estradiol 75 microgram per 24 hour Estradot
75micrograms/24hours patches | 8 patch [PoM] £7.00

Estradiol 100 microgram per 24 hour Estradot
100micrograms/24hours patches | 8 patch [PoM] £7.27

> Evorel (Janssen-Cilag Ltd)

Estradiol 25 microgram per 24 hour Evorel 25 patches |
8 patch [PoM] £3.42

Estradiol 50 microgram per 24 hour Evorel 50 patches |
4 patch [PoM] no price available | 8 patch [PoM] £3.88 |
24 patch [PoM] £11.66

Estradiol 75 microgram per 24 hour Evorel 75 patches |
8 patch [PoM] £4.12

Estradiol 100 microgram per 24 hour Evorel 100 patches |
8 patch [PoM] £4.28

> FemSeven (Teva UK Ltd)

Estradiol 50 microgram per 24 hour FemSeven 50 patches |
4 patch [PoM] £6.04 | 12 patch [PoM] £18.02

Estradiol 75 microgram per 24 hour FemSeven 75 patches |
4 patch [PoM] £6.98

Estradiol 100 microgram per 24 hour FemSeven 100 patches |
4 patch [PoM] £7.28

> Progynova TS (Bayer Plc)

Estradiol 50 microgram per 24 hour Progynova TS
50micrograms/24hours transdermal patches | 12 patch [PoM] £18.90

Estradiol 100 microgram per 24 hour Progynova TS
100micrograms/24hours transdermal patches | 12 patch [PoM]
£20.70

Gel

EXCIPIENTS: May contain Propylene glycol

> Oestrogel (Besins Healthcare (UK) Ltd)

Estradiol 600 microgram per 1 gram Oestrogel Pump-Pack 0.06%
gel | 80 gram [PoM] £4.80 DT price = £4.80

> Sandrena (Orion Pharma (UK) Ltd)

Estradiol (as Estradiol hemihydrate) 500 microgram Sandrena
500microgram gel sachets | 28 sachet [PoM] £5.08 DT price = £5.08

Estradiol (as Estradiol hemihydrate) 1 mg Sandrena 1mg gel
sachets | 28 sachet [PoM] £5.85 DT price = £5.85 | 91 sachet [PoM]
£17.57

Combinations available: *Estradiol with drospirenone*, p. 688 ·
Estradiol with dydrogesterone, p. 688 · *Estradiol with
levonorgestrel*, p. 689 · *Estradiol with medroxyprogesterone*,
p. 689 · *Estradiol with norethisterone*, p. 689 · *Estradiol with
norgestrel*, p. 691

Estradiol with estriol and estrone

The properties listed below are those particular to the
combination only. For the properties of the components
please consider, estradiol p. 682, estriol p. 753.

● INDICATIONS AND DOSE

Menopausal symptoms | Osteoporosis prophylaxis

▸ BY MOUTH

▸ Adult: 1–2 tablets daily continuously or cyclically
(21 days out of 28), started within 5 days of onset of
menstruation (or at any time if cycles have ceased or
are infrequent), to be taken with cyclical progestogen
for 12–14 days of each cycle in women with a uterus

● MEDICINAL FORMS

There can be variation in the licensing of different medicines
containing the same drug.

Tablet

▸ Hormonin (AMCo)

**Estriol 270 microgram, Estradiol 600 microgram, Estrone
1.4 mg** Hormonin tablets | 84 tablet [PoM] £7.93

Ethinylestradiol

(Ethinyloestradiol)

● INDICATIONS AND DOSE

**Short-term treatment of symptoms of oestrogen
deficiency | Osteoporosis prophylaxis if other drugs
cannot be used**

▸ BY MOUTH

▸ Adult (female): 10–50 micrograms daily for 21 days,
repeated after 7-day tablet-free period, to be given
with progestogen for 12–14 days per cycle in women
with intact uterus.

Female hypogonadism

▸ BY MOUTH

▸ Adult (female): 10–50 micrograms daily usually on
cyclical basis, initial oestrogen therapy should be
followed by combined oestrogen and progestogen
therapy.

Menstrual disorders

▸ BY MOUTH

▸ Adult (female): 20–50 micrograms daily from day 5 to
25 of each cycle, to be given with progestogen, added
either throughout the cycle or from day 15 to 25.

Palliative treatment of prostate cancer

▸ BY MOUTH

▸ Adult (male): 0.15–1.5 mg daily.

● CONTRA-INDICATIONS Active or recent arterial
thromboembolic disease (e.g. angina or myocardial
infarction) · active thrombophlebitis · Acute porphyrias
p. 918 · Dubin-Johnson and Rotor syndromes (or monitor
closely) · gallstones · heart disease associated with
pulmonary hypertension · heart disease associated with
risk of embolus · history during pregnancy of cholestatic
jaundice · history during pregnancy of chorea · history
during pregnancy of pemphigoid gestationis · history
during pregnancy of pruritus · history of breast cancer ·
history of haemolytic uraemic syndrome · liver disease
(where liver function tests have failed to return to normal)
· migraine with aura · oestrogen-dependent cancer ·
sclerosing treatment for varicose veins · severe or multiple
risk factors for arterial disease · severe or multiple risk
factors for venous thromboembolism · systemic lupus
erythematosus with (or unknown) antiphospholipid
antibodies · thrombophilic disorder · transient cerebral
ischaemic attacks without headaches · undiagnosed
vaginal bleeding · untreated endometrial hyperplasia ·
venous thromboembolism, or history of recurrent venous
thromboembolism (unless already on anticoagulant
treatment)

● CAUTIONS Active trophoblastic disease (until return to
normal of urine- and plasma-gonadotrophin
concentration)—seek specialist advice · cardiovascular
disease (sodium retention with oedema,
thromboembolism) · Crohn's disease · diabetes (increased
risk of heart disease) · gene mutations associated with
breast cancer (e.g. BRCA 1) · history of breast nodules or
fibrocystic disease—closely monitor breast status (risk of
breast cancer) · history of endometrial hyperplasia · history
of severe depression (especially if induced by hormonal
contraceptive) · hyperprolactinaemia (seek specialist
advice) · hypophyseal tumours · increased risk of gall-

6

Endocrine system

bladder disease · inflammatory bowel disease · migraine (migraine-like headaches) · personal or family history of hypertriglyceridaemia (increased risk of pancreatitis) · presence of antiphospholipid antibodies (increased risk of thrombotic events) · prolonged exposure to unopposed oestrogens may increase risk of developing endometrial cancer · risk factors for arterial disease · risk factors for migraine · risk factors for oestrogen-dependent tumours (e.g. breast cancer in first-degree relative) · risk factors for venous thromboembolism · sickle-cell disease · undiagnosed breast mass

CAUTIONS, FURTHER INFORMATION
▶ **Other conditions** The product literature advises caution in other conditions including hypertension, renal disease, asthma, epilepsy, sickle-cell disease, melanoma, otosclerosis, multiple sclerosis, and systemic lupus erythematosus (but care required if antiphospholipid antibodies present, see above). Evidence for caution in these conditions is unsatisfactory and many women with these conditions may stand to benefit from HRT.
▶ **Risk of venous thromboembolism** Use with **caution** if any of following factors present but **avoid** if two or more factors present:
  ● *family history of venous thromboembolism* in first-degree relative aged under 45 years (avoid if known prothrombotic coagulation abnormality e.g. factor V Leiden or antiphospholipid antibodies (including lupus anticoagulant));
  ● *obesity*—body mass index ≥30 kg/m² (avoid if body mass index ≥35 kg/m² unless no suitable alternative); (In adolescents, caution if obese according to BMI (adjusted for age and gender); in those who are markedly obese, avoid unless no suitable alternative);
  ● *long-term immobilisation* e.g. in a wheelchair (avoid if confined to bed or leg in plaster cast);
  ● *history of superficial thrombophlebitis;*
  ● *age* over 35 years (avoid if over 50 years);
  ● *smoking.*
▶ **Risk factors for arterial disease** Use with **caution** if any one of following factors present but **avoid** if two or more factors present:
  ● *family history of arterial disease* in first degree relative aged under 45 years (avoid if atherogenic lipid profile);
  ● *diabetes mellitus* (avoid if diabetes complications present);
  ● *hypertension*—blood pressure above *systolic* 140 *mmHg* or *diastolic* 90 *mmHg* (avoid if blood pressure above *systolic* 160 *mmHg* or *diastolic* 95 *mmHg*); (In adolescents, avoid if blood pressure very high);
  ● *smoking* (avoid if smoking 40 or more cigarettes daily);
  ● *age* over 35 years (avoid if over 50 years);
  ● *obesity* (avoid if body mass index ≥35 kg/m² unless no suitable alternative); (In adolescents, caution if obese according to BMI (adjusted for age and gender); in those who are markedly obese, avoid unless no suitable alternative);
  ● *migraine without aura* (avoid if *migraine with aura* (focal symptoms), *or* severe migraine frequently lasting over 72 hours despite treatment, *or* migraine treated with ergot derivatives).
▶ **Migraine** Women should report any increase in headache frequency or onset of focal symptoms (discontinue immediately and refer urgently to neurology expert if focal neurological symptoms not typical of aura persist for more than 1 hour).
● INTERACTIONS → Appendix 1 (oestrogens).
● SIDE-EFFECTS
▶ **Rare** Gallstones · systemic lupus erythematosus
▶ **Frequency not known** Abdominal bloating · abdominal cramps · absence of withdrawal bleeding · altered blood lipids (may lead to pancreatitis) · amenorrhoea after discontinuation · breast enlargement · breast secretion ·

breast tenderness · cervical erosion · changes in libido · changes in lipid metabolism · changes in vaginal discharge · chloasma · cholestatic jaundice · chorea · contact lenses may irritate · depression · dizziness · feminising effects · fluid retention · glucose intolerance · headache · hepatic tumours · hypertension · irritability · leg cramps (rule out venous thrombosis) · liver impairment · migraine · mood changes · nausea · nervousness · photosensitivity · premenstrual-like syndrome · rashes · reduced menstrual loss · skin reactions · sodium retention · symptoms of endometriosis may be exacerbated · thrombosis (more common when factor V Leiden present or in blood groups A, B, and AB) · uterine fibroids may increase in size · vaginal candidiasis · visual disturbances · vomiting · weight changes · 'spotting' in early cycles

SIDE-EFFECTS, FURTHER INFORMATION
▶ **Withdrawal bleeding** Cyclical HRT (where a progestogen is taken for 12–14 days of each 28-day oestrogen treatment cycle) usually results in regular withdrawal bleeding towards the end of the progestogen. The aim of continuous combined HRT (where a combination of oestrogen and progestogen is taken, usually in a single tablet, throughout each 28-day treatment cycle) is to avoid bleeding, but irregular bleeding may occur during the early treatment stages (if it continues endometrial abnormality should be excluded and consideration given to cyclical HRT instead).
● PREGNANCY Not known to be harmful.
● BREAST FEEDING Avoid until weaning or for 6 months after birth (adverse effects on lactation).
● HEPATIC IMPAIRMENT Avoid.
● MEDICINAL FORMS
There can be variation in the licensing of different medicines containing the same drug. Forms available from special-order manufacturers include: tablet, capsule, oral suspension
Tablet
▶ Ethinylestradiol (Non-proprietary)
  Ethinylestradiol 10 microgram Ethinylestradiol 10microgram tablets | 21 tablet PoM £200.00 DT price = £200.00
  Ethinylestradiol 50 microgram Ethinylestradiol 50microgram tablets | 21 tablet PoM £200.00 DT price = £200.00
  Ethinylestradiol 1 mg Ethinylestradiol 1mg tablets | 28 tablet PoM £200.00 DT price = £200.00

NORETYNODREL DERIVATIVES

Tibolone

● INDICATIONS AND DOSE
Short-term treatment of symptoms of oestrogen deficiency (including women being treated with gonadotrophin releasing hormone analogues) | Osteoporosis prophylaxis in women at high risk of fractures when other prophylaxis contra-indicated or not tolerated
▶ BY MOUTH
▶ Adult: 2.5 mg daily

● CONTRA-INDICATIONS Active or recent arterial thromboembolic disease (e.g. angina or myocardial infarction) · active thrombophlebitis · Acute porphyrias p. 918 · Dubin-Johnson and Rotor syndrome (or monitor closely) · history of breast cancer · history of cardiovascular disease · history of cerebrovascular disease · history of recurrent venous thromboembolism (unless already on anticoagulant treatment) · history of thromboembolism · history of thrombophlebitis · hormone-dependent tumours · liver disease (where liver function tests have failed to return to normal) · oestrogen-dependent cancer · thrombophilic disorder · uninvestigated or undiagnosed vaginal bleeding · untreated endometrial hyperplasia · venous thromboembolism

- CAUTIONS Acute porphyrias p. 918 · diabetes (increased risk of heart disease) · epilepsy · factors predisposing to thromboembolism · history of breast nodules—closely monitor breast status (risk of breast cancer) · history of endometrial hyperplasia · history of fibrocystic disease—closely monitor breast status (risk of breast cancer) · history of liver disease · hypertriglyceridaemia · hypophyseal tumours · migraine (or migraine-like headaches) · presence of antiphospholipid antibodies (increased risk of thrombotic events) · prolonged exposure to unopposed oestrogens may increase risk of developing endometrial cancer · risk factors for oestrogen-dependent tumours (e.g. breast cancer in first-degree relative) · risk of stroke

  CAUTIONS, FURTHER INFORMATION
  ▸ Other conditions The product literature advises caution in other conditions including hypertension, renal disease, asthma, epilepsy, sickle-cell disease, melanoma, otosclerosis, multiple sclerosis, and systemic lupus erythematosus (but care required if antiphospholipid antibodies present). Evidence for caution in these conditions is unsatisfactory and many women with these conditions may stand to benefit from HRT.

- INTERACTIONS → Appendix 1 (tibolone).

- SIDE-EFFECTS
  ▸ **Common or very common** Abdominal pain · facial hair · leucorrhoea · vaginal bleeding · weight changes
  ▸ **Rare** Amnesia
  ▸ **Frequency not known** Arthralgia · breast cancer · depression · dizziness · gastro-intestinal disturbances · headache · increased risk of gall-bladder disease · migraine · myalgia · oedema · pruritus · rash · seborrhoeic dermatitis · symptoms of endometriosis may be exacerbated · uterine fibroids may increase in size · visual disturbances

  SIDE-EFFECTS, FURTHER INFORMATION
  ▸ Vaginal bleeding Investigate for endometrial cancer if bleeding continues beyond 6 months or after stopping treatment.
  ▸ Reasons to withdraw treatment Withdraw treatment if signs of thromboembolic disease, abnormal liver function tests, or signs of cholestatic jaundice.

- PREGNANCY Avoid; toxicity in *animal* studies.

- BREAST FEEDING Avoid.

- HEPATIC IMPAIRMENT Avoid in acute liver disease or if history of liver disease and liver function tests not returned to normal.

- RENAL IMPAIRMENT Patients with renal impairment should be closely monitored (risk of fluid retention).

- PRESCRIBING AND DISPENSING INFORMATION Unsuitable for use in the premenopause (unless being treated with gonadotrophin-releasing hormone analogue) and as (or with) an oral contraceptive.
  Also unsuitable for use within 12 months of last menstrual period (may cause irregular bleeding).
  If transferring from cyclical HRT, start at end of regimen; if transferring from continuous-combined HRT, start at any time.

- MEDICINAL FORMS
  There can be variation in the licensing of different medicines containing the same drug.
  Tablet
  ▸ Tibolone (Non-proprietary)
  Tibolone 2.5 mg Tibolone 2.5mg tablets | 28 tablet [PoM] £10.36–£10.95 DT price = £10.36 | 84 tablet [PoM] £31.08–£32.63
  ▸ Livial (Merck Sharp & Dohme Ltd)
  Tibolone 2.5 mg Livial 2.5mg tablets | 28 tablet [PoM] £10.36 DT price = £10.36 | 84 tablet [PoM] £31.08

OESTROGENS COMBINED WITH PROGESTOGENS

Conjugated oestrogens with medroxyprogesterone

The properties listed below are those particular to the combination only. For the properties of the components please consider, conjugated oestrogens (equine) p. 681, medroxyprogesterone acetate p. 733.

- INDICATIONS AND DOSE
  PREMIQUE®
  Menopausal symptoms in women with a uterus | Osteoporosis prophylaxis in women with a uterus
  ▸ BY MOUTH
  ▸ Adult: 1 tablet daily continuously
  PREMIQUE® LOW DOSE TABLETS
  Menopausal symptoms in women with a uterus
  ▸ BY MOUTH
  ▸ Adult: 1 tablet daily continuously

- INTERACTIONS → Appendix 1 (oestrogens, progestogens).

- MEDICINAL FORMS
  There can be variation in the licensing of different medicines containing the same drug.
  Tablet
  ▸ Premique (Pfizer Ltd)
  Conjugated oestrogens 625 microgram, Medroxyprogesterone acetate 5 mg Premique 0.625mg/5mg tablets | 84 tablet [PoM] £10.61 DT price = £10.61
  Modified-release tablet
  ▸ Premique (Pfizer Ltd)
  Conjugated oestrogens 300 microgram, Medroxyprogesterone acetate 1.5 mg Premique Low Dose 0.3mg/1.5mg modified-release tablets | 84 tablet [PoM] £6.52 DT price = £6.52

Conjugated oestrogens with norgestrel

The properties listed below are those particular to the combination only. For the properties of the components please consider, conjugated oestrogens (equine) p. 681.

- INDICATIONS AND DOSE
  PREMPAK C® 0.625
  Menopausal symptoms in women with a uterus | Osteoporosis prophylaxis in women with a uterus
  ▸ BY MOUTH
  ▸ Adult: 1 tablet daily continuously, maroon tablet to taken and started on day 1 of menstruation (or at any time if cycles have ceased or are infrequent) and 1 tablet daily, brown tablet to be taken and started on days 17–28 of each 28-day treatment cycle, subsequent courses are repeated without interval
  PREMPAK C® 1.25
  Menopausal symptoms in women with a uterus (if symptoms not fully controlled with lower strength pack) | Osteoporosis prophylaxis in women with a uterus (if symptoms not fully controlled with lower strength pack)
  ▸ BY MOUTH
  ▸ Adult: 1 tablet daily continuously, (yellow tablet) to taken and started on day 1 of menstruation (or at any time if cycles have ceased or are infrequent) and 1 tablet daily, (brown tablet) to be taken and started on days 17–28 of each 28-day treatment cycle, subsequent courses are repeated without interval

6

Endocrine system

6

Endocrine system

● MEDICINAL FORMS
There can be variation in the licensing of different medicines containing the same drug.
Tablet
▸ Prempak-C (Pfizer Ltd)
Prempak-C 1.25mg/0.15mg tablets | 120 tablet [PoM] £7.40 DT price = £7.40
Prempak-C 0.625mg/0.15mg tablets | 120 tablet [PoM] £6.25 DT price = £6.25

Estradiol with drospirenone

The properties listed below are those particular to the combination only. For the properties of the components please consider, estradiol p. 682.

● INDICATIONS AND DOSE

Menopausal symptoms in women with a uterus whose last menstrual period occurred over 12 months previously | Osteoporosis prophylaxis in women with a uterus whose last menstrual period occurred over 12 months previously
▸ BY MOUTH
▸ Adult: 1 tablet daily continuously, if changing from cyclical HRT begin treatment the day after finishing oestrogen plus progestogen phase

● CAUTIONS Use with care if an increased concentration of potassium might be hazardous

● RENAL IMPAIRMENT Avoid if eGFR less than 30 mL/minute/1.73 m².

● MEDICINAL FORMS
There can be variation in the licensing of different medicines containing the same drug.
Tablet
▸ Angeliq (Bayer Plc)
Estradiol (as Estradiol hemihydrate) 1 mg, Drospirenone 2 mg Angeliq tablets | 84 tablet [PoM] £29.00

Estradiol with dydrogesterone

The properties listed below are those particular to the combination only. For the properties of the components please consider, estradiol p. 682.

● INDICATIONS AND DOSE
FEMOSTON® 1 MG/10 MG

Menopausal symptoms in women with a uterus
▸ BY MOUTH
▸ Adult: 1 tablet daily for 14 days, white tablet to be taken and started within 5 days of onset of menstruation (or any time if cycles have ceased or are infrequent), then 1 tablet daily for 14 days, grey tablet to be taken, subsequent courses repeated without interval, *Femoston®* 1 *mg*/10 *mg* given initially and *Femoston®* 2 *mg*/10 *mg* substituted if symptoms not controlled

Osteoporosis prophylaxis in women with a uterus
▸ BY MOUTH
▸ Adult: 1 tablet daily for 14 days, white tablet to be taken and started within 5 days of onset of menstruation (or any time if cycles have ceased or are infrequent), then 1 tablet daily for 14 days, grey tablet to be taken, subsequent courses repeated without interval

FEMOSTON® 2 MG/10 MG

Menopausal symptoms in women with a uterus
▸ BY MOUTH
▸ Adult: 1 tablet daily for 14 days, red tablet to be taken and started within 5 days of onset of menstruation (or

any time if cycles have ceased or are infrequent), then 1 tablet daily for 14 days, yellow tablet to be taken, subsequent courses repeated without interval, *Femoston®* 1 *mg*/10 *mg* given initially and *Femoston®* 2 *mg*/10 *mg* substituted if symptoms not controlled

Osteoporosis prophylaxis in women with a uterus
▸ BY MOUTH
▸ Adult: 1 tablet daily for 14 days, red tablet to be taken and started within 5 days of onset of menstruation (or any time if cycles have ceased or are infrequent), then 1 tablet daily for 14 days, yellow tablet to be taken, subsequent courses repeated without interval

FEMOSTON®-CONTI 0.5 MG/2.5MG

Menopausal symptoms in women with a uterus whose last menstrual period occurred over 12 months previously
▸ BY MOUTH
▸ Adult: 1 tablet daily continuously, if changing from cyclical HRT begin treatment the day after finishing oestrogen plus progestogen phase

FEMOSTON®-CONTI 1 MG/5MG

Menopausal symptoms in women with a uterus whose last menstrual period occurred over 12 months previously | Osteoporosis prophylaxis in women with a uterus whose last menstrual period occurred over 12 months previously
▸ BY MOUTH
▸ Adult: 1 tablet daily continuously, if changing from cyclical HRT begin treatment the day after finishing oestrogen plus progestogen phase

● CONTRA-INDICATIONS Acute porphyrias p. 918 · genital or breast cancer · history during pregnancy of idiopathic jaundice, severe pruritus, or pemphigoid gestationis · history of liver tumours · severe arterial disease · undiagnosed vaginal bleeding

● CAUTIONS Conditions that may worsen with fluid retention e.g. epilepsy, hypertension, migraine, asthma, or cardiac dysfunction · diabetes (progestogens can decrease glucose tolerance) · history of depression · in those susceptible to thromboembolism (particular caution with high dose)

● INTERACTIONS → Appendix 1 (progestogens).

● SIDE-EFFECTS Acne · alopecia · anaphylactoid reactions · bloating · breast tenderness · change in libido · depression · dizziness · drowsiness · fluid retention · headache · hirsutism · insomnia · jaundice · menstrual disturbances · nausea · premenstrual-like syndrome · pruritus · rash · skin reactions · urticaria · weight change

● HEPATIC IMPAIRMENT Avoid.

● RENAL IMPAIRMENT Use with caution.

● MEDICINAL FORMS
There can be variation in the licensing of different medicines containing the same drug.
Tablet
▸ Femoston-conti (BGP Products Ltd)
Dydrogesterone 2.5 microgram, Estradiol 500 microgram Femoston-conti 0.5mg/2.5mg tablets | 84 tablet [PoM] £24.43
Estradiol 1 mg, Dydrogesterone 5 mg Femoston-conti 1mg/5mg tablets | 84 tablet [PoM] £24.43 DT price = £24.43
▸ Femoston 1/10 (BGP Products Ltd)
Femoston 1/10mg tablets | 84 tablet [PoM] £16.16
▸ Femoston 2/10 (BGP Products Ltd)
Femoston 2/10mg tablets | 84 tablet [PoM] £16.16

Estradiol with levonorgestrel

The properties listed below are those particular to the combination only. For the properties of the components please consider, estradiol p. 682, levonorgestrel p. 729.

- **INDICATIONS AND DOSE**
FEMSEVEN CONTI®

Menopausal symptoms in women with a uterus whose last menstrual period occurred over 12 months previously
▸ BY TRANSDERMAL APPLICATION
▸ Adult: Apply 1 patch once weekly continuously
FEMSEVEN SEQUI®

Menopausal symptoms in women with a uterus
▸ BY TRANSDERMAL APPLICATION
▸ Adult: Apply 1 patch once weekly for 2 weeks, phase 1 patches to be applied, then apply 1 patch once weekly for 2 weeks, phase 2 patches to be applied, subsequent courses are repeated without interval

- **PATIENT AND CARER ADVICE** Patient counselling is advised for estradiol with levonorgestrel patches (application).

- **MEDICINAL FORMS**
There can be variation in the licensing of different medicines containing the same drug.
Transdermal patch
▸ FemSeven Conti (Teva UK Ltd)
Levonorgestrel 7 microgram per 24 hour, Estradiol 50 microgram per 24 hour FemSeven Conti patches | 4 patch PoM £15.48 | 12 patch PoM £44.12
▸ FemSeven Sequi Phase 2 (Teva UK Ltd)
Levonorgestrel 10 microgram per 24 hour, Estradiol 50 microgram per 24 hour FemSeven Sequi Phase 2 patches | 2 patch PoM no price available | 6 patch PoM no price available
▸ FemSeven Sequi (Teva UK Ltd)
FemSeven Sequi patches | 4 patch PoM £13.18 | 12 patch PoM £37.54

Estradiol with medroxyprogesterone

The properties listed below are those particular to the combination only. For the properties of the components please consider, estradiol p. 682, medroxyprogesterone acetate p. 733.

- **INDICATIONS AND DOSE**
INDIVINA® TABLETS

**Menopausal symptoms in women with a uterus whose last menstrual period occurred over 3 years previously |
Osteoporosis prophylaxis in women with a uterus whose last menstrual period occurred over 3 years previously**
▸ BY MOUTH
▸ Adult: Initially 1/2.5 mg daily taken continuously, adjust according to response, to be started at end of scheduled bleed if changing from cyclical HRT
TRIDESTRA®

**Menopausal symptoms in women with a uterus |
Osteoporosis prophylaxis in women with a uterus**
▸ BY MOUTH
▸ Adult: 1 tablet daily for 70 days, white tablet to be taken, then 1 tablet daily for 14 days, blue tablet to be taken, then 1 tablet daily for 7 days, yellow tablet to be taken, subsequent courses are repeated without interval

- **MEDICINAL FORMS**
There can be variation in the licensing of different medicines containing the same drug.
Tablet
▸ Indivina (Orion Pharma (UK) Ltd)
Estradiol valerate 1 mg, Medroxyprogesterone acetate 2.5 mg Indivina 1mg/2.5mg tablets | 84 tablet PoM £20.58 DT price = £20.58
Estradiol valerate 2 mg, Medroxyprogesterone acetate 5 mg Indivina 2mg/5mg tablets | 84 tablet PoM £20.58 DT price = £20.58
Estradiol valerate 1 mg, Medroxyprogesterone acetate 5 mg Indivina 1mg/5mg tablets | 84 tablet PoM £20.58 DT price = £20.58
▸ Tridestra (Orion Pharma (UK) Ltd)
Tridestra tablets | 91 tablet PoM £20.49

Estradiol with norethisterone

The properties listed below are those particular to the combination only. For the properties of the components please consider, estradiol p. 682, norethisterone p. 691.

- **INDICATIONS AND DOSE**
CLIMAGEST® 1-MG

Menopausal symptoms
▸ BY MOUTH
▸ Adult: 1 tablet daily for 16 days, grey tablet to be taken and started on day 1 of menstruation (or at any time if cycles have ceased or are infrequent), then 1 tablet daily for 12 days, white tablet to be taken, subsequent courses are repeated without interval
CLIMAGEST® 2-MG

Menopausal symptoms (if symptoms not controlled with lower strength)
▸ BY MOUTH
▸ Adult: 1 tablet daily for 16 days, blue tablet to be taken and started on day 1 of menstruation (or at any time if cycles have ceased or are infrequent), then 1 tablet daily for 12 days, white tablet to be taken, subsequent courses are repeated without interval
CLIMESSE®

**Menopausal symptoms in women with a uterus whose last menstrual period occurred over 12 months previously |
Osteoporosis prophylaxis in women with a uterus whose last menstrual period occurred over 12 months previously**
▸ BY MOUTH
▸ Adult: 1 tablet daily continuously
CLINORETTE®

**Menopausal symptoms in women with a uterus |
Osteoporosis prophylaxis in women with a uterus**
▸ BY MOUTH
▸ Adult: 1 tablet daily for 16 days, white tablets to be taken, starting on day 5 of menstruation (or at any time if cycles have ceased or are infrequent), then 1 tablet daily for 12 days, pink tablets to be taken, subsequent courses are repeated without interval
ELLESTE-DUET® 1-MG

Menopausal symptoms
▸ BY MOUTH
▸ Adult: 1 tablet daily for 16 days, white tablet to be taken and started on day 1 of menstruation (or at any time if cycles have ceased or are infrequent), then 1 tablet daily for 12 days, green tablets to be taken, subsequent courses are repeated without interval

continued →

6

Endocrine system

ELLESTE-DUET® 2-MG

Menopausal symptoms | Osteoporosis prophylaxis
▶ BY MOUTH
▶ Adult: 1 tablet daily for 16 days, orange tablet to be taken, to be started on day 1 of menstruation (or at any time if cycles have ceased or are infrequent), then 1 tablet daily for 12 days, grey tablet to be taken, subsequent courses are repeated without interval

ELLESTE-DUET® CONTI

Menopausal symptoms in women with a uterus whose last menstrual period occurred over 12 months previously | Osteoporosis prophylaxis in women with a uterus whose last menstrual period occurred over 12 months previously
▶ BY MOUTH
▶ Adult: 1 tablet daily continuous basis, if changing from cyclical HRT begin treatment at the end of scheduled bleed

EVOREL® CONTI

Menopausal symptoms in women with a uterus | Osteoporosis prophylaxis in women with a uterus
▶ BY TRANSDERMAL APPLICATION
▶ Adult: Apply 1 patch twice weekly continuously

EVOREL® SEQUI

Menopausal symptoms in women with a uterus | Osteoporosis prophylaxis in women with a uterus
▶ BY TRANSDERMAL APPLICATION
▶ Adult: Apply 1 patch twice weekly for 2 weeks, *Evorel*® 50 patch to be applied and started within 5 days of onset of menstruation (or at any time if cycles have ceased or are infrequent), then apply 1 patch twice weekly, *Evorel*® Conti patch to be applied, subsequent courses are repeated without interval.

KLIOFEM®

Menopausal symptoms in women with a uterus whose last menstrual period occurred over 12 months previously | Osteoporosis prophylaxis in women with a uterus whose last menstrual period occurred over 12 months previously
▶ BY MOUTH
▶ Adult: 1 tablet daily continuously, to be started at end of scheduled bleed if changing from cyclical HRT

KLIOVANCE®

Menopausal symptoms in women with a uterus whose last menstrual period occurred over 12 months previously | Osteoporosis prophylaxis in women with a uterus whose last menstrual period occurred over 12 months previously
▶ BY MOUTH
▶ Adult: 1 tablet daily continuously, to be started at end of scheduled bleed if changing from cyclical HRT

NOVOFEM®

Menopausal symptoms in women with a uterus | Osteoporosis prophylaxis in women with a uterus
▶ BY MOUTH
▶ Adult: 1 tablet daily for 16 days, red tablets to be taken, then 1 tablet daily for 12 days, white tablets to be taken, subsequent courses are repeated without interval; start treatment with red tablet at any time or if changing from cyclical HRT, start treatment the day after finishing oestrogen plus progestogen phase

NUVELLE® CONTINUOUS

Menopausal symptoms in women with a uterus whose last menstrual period occurred over 12 months previously | Osteoporosis prophylaxis in women with a uterus whose last menstrual period occurred over 12 months previously
▶ BY MOUTH
▶ Adult: 1 tablet daily continuously, if changing from cyclical HRT, start treatment the day after finishing oestrogen plus progestogen phase

TRISEQUENS®

Menopausal symptoms in women with a uterus | Osteoporosis prophylaxis in women with a uterus
▶ BY MOUTH
▶ Adult: 1 tablet daily for 12 days, blue tablets to be taken, followed by 1 tablet daily for 10 days, white tablet to be taken, then 1 tablet daily for 6 days, red tablet to be taken, subsequent courses are repeated without interval

● PATIENT AND CARER ADVICE
EVOREL® SEQUI Patients and carers should be advised on the application of *Evorel*® Sequi patches.

● MEDICINAL FORMS
There can be variation in the licensing of different medicines containing the same drug.

Tablet
▶ Climagest (Novartis Pharmaceuticals UK Ltd)
Climagest 2mg tablets | 28 tablet [PoM] £6.61 | 84 tablet [PoM] £19.22
▶ Clinorette (ReSource Medical UK Ltd)
Clinorette tablets | 84 tablet [PoM] £9.23
▶ Elleste Duet (Meda Pharmaceuticals Ltd)
Elleste Duet 1mg tablets | 84 tablet [PoM] £9.20
Elleste Duet 2mg tablets | 84 tablet [PoM] £9.20
▶ Elleste Duet Conti (Meda Pharmaceuticals Ltd)
Norethisterone acetate 1 mg, Estradiol 2 mg Elleste Duet Conti tablets | 84 tablet [PoM] £17.02
▶ Kliofem (Novo Nordisk Ltd)
Norethisterone acetate 1 mg, Estradiol 2 mg Kliofem tablets | 84 tablet [PoM] £11.43
▶ Kliovance (Novo Nordisk Ltd)
Norethisterone acetate 500 microgram, Estradiol 1 mg Kliovance tablets | 84 tablet [PoM] £13.20 DT price = £13.20
▶ Novofem (Novo Nordisk Ltd)
Novofem tablets | 84 tablet [PoM] £11.43
▶ Nuvelle Continuous (Bayer Plc)
Norethisterone acetate 1 mg, Estradiol 2 mg Nuvelle Continuous tablets | 84 tablet [PoM] £19.00
▶ Trisequens (Novo Nordisk Ltd)
Trisequens tablets | 84 tablet [PoM] £11.10

Transdermal patch
▶ Evorel Conti (Janssen-Cilag Ltd)
Estradiol 50 microgram per 24 hour, Norethisterone acetate 170 microgram per 24 hour Evorel Conti patches | 4 patch [PoM] no price available | 8 patch [PoM] £13.00 | 24 patch [PoM] £37.22 DT price = £37.22
▶ Evorel Sequi (Janssen-Cilag Ltd)
Evorel Sequi patches | 8 patch [PoM] £11.09

Estradiol with norgestrel

The properties listed below are those particular to the combination only. For the properties of the components please consider, estradiol p. 682.

● **INDICATIONS AND DOSE**

CYCLO-PROGYNOVA® 2MG TABLETS

Menopausal symptoms in women with a uterus | Osteoporosis prophylaxis in women with a uterus
▸ BY MOUTH
▸ Adult: 1 tablet daily for 11 days, white tablet to be taken; start on day 5 of menstruation (or at any time if cycles have ceased or are infrequent), then 1 tablet daily for 10 days, brown tablet to be taken, followed by a 7-day tablet free interval

● **MEDICINAL FORMS**
There can be variation in the licensing of different medicines containing the same drug.
Tablet
▸ Cyclo-Progynova (Meda Pharmaceuticals Ltd)
Cyclo-Progynova 2mg tablets | 21 tablet [PoM] £3.11

PROGESTOGENS

Norethisterone

● **INDICATIONS AND DOSE**

Endometriosis
▸ BY MOUTH
▸ Adult: 10–15 mg daily for 4–6 months or longer, to be started on day 5 of cycle; increased to 20–25 mg daily if required, dose only increased if spotting occurs and reduced once bleeding has stopped

Dysfunctional uterine bleeding (to arrest bleeding) | Menorrhagia (to arrest bleeding)
▸ BY MOUTH
▸ Adult: 5 mg 3 times a day for 10 days

Dysfunctional uterine bleeding (to prevent bleeding) | Menorrhagia (to prevent bleeding)
▸ BY MOUTH
▸ Adult: 5 mg twice daily, to be taken from day 19 to day 26 of cycle

Dysmenorrhoea
▸ BY MOUTH
▸ Adult: 5 mg 3 times a day for 3–4 cycles, to be taken from day 5–24 of cycle

Premenstrual syndrome (but not recommended)
▸ BY MOUTH
▸ Adult: 5 mg 2–3 times a day for several cycles, to be taken from day 19–26 of cycle

Postponement of menstruation
▸ BY MOUTH
▸ Females of childbearing potential: 5 mg 3 times a day, to be started 3 days before expected onset (menstruation occurs 2–3 days after stopping)

Breast cancer
▸ BY MOUTH
▸ Adult: 40 mg daily, increased if necessary to 60 mg daily

Short-term contraception
▸ BY DEEP INTRAMUSCULAR INJECTION
▸ Females of childbearing potential: 200 mg, to be administered within first 5 days of cycle or immediately after parturition (duration 8 weeks). To be injected into the gluteal muscle, then 200 mg after 8 weeks if required

Contraception
▸ BY MOUTH
▸ Females of childbearing potential: 350 micrograms daily, dose to be taken at same time each day, starting on day 1 of cycle then continuously, if administration delayed for 3 hours or more it should be regarded as a 'missed pill'

● **CONTRA-INDICATIONS**

GENERAL CONTRA-INDICATIONS
Avoid in patients with a history of liver tumours · breast cancer (unless progestogens are being used in the management of this condition) · genital cancer (unless progestogens are being used in the management of this condition) · history during pregnancy of idiopathic jaundice · history during pregnancy of pemphigoid gestationis (non-contraceptive indications) · history during pregnancy of severe pruritus (non-contraceptive indications) · when used as a contraceptive, history of breast cancer (can be used after 5 years if no evidence of disease and non-hormonal contraceptive methods unacceptable)

SPECIFIC CONTRA-INDICATIONS
▸ With oral use Acute porphyrias p. 918 · severe arterial disease · undiagnosed vaginal bleeding

● **CAUTIONS**

GENERAL CAUTIONS
Asthma · cardiac dysfunction · conditions that may worsen with fluid retention · diabetes (progestogens can decrease glucose tolerance—monitor patient closely) · epilepsy · history of depression · hypertension · migraine · susceptibility to thromboembolism (particular caution with high dose)

SPECIFIC CAUTIONS
▸ When used for contraception Active trophoblastic disease (until return to normal of urine- and plasma-gonadotrophin concentration)—seek specialist advice · arterial disease · functional ovarian cysts · history of jaundice in pregnancy · malabsorption syndromes · past ectopic pregnancy · sex-steroid dependent cancer · systemic lupus erythematosus with positive (or unknown) anti-phospholipid antibodies

with intramuscular use for contraception disturbances of lipid metabolism · history during pregnancy of deterioration of otosclerosis · history during pregnancy of pruritus · possible risk of breast cancer

CAUTIONS, FURTHER INFORMATION
▸ Use as a contraceptive in co-morbidities The product literature advises caution in patients with history of thromboembolism, hypertension, diabetes mellitus and migraine; evidence for caution in these conditions is unsatisfactory.
▸ Breast cancer risk with contraceptive use There is a small increase in the risk of having breast cancer diagnosed in women using, or who have recently used, a progestogen-only contraceptive pill; this relative risk may be due to an earlier diagnosis. The most important risk factor appears to be the age at which the contraceptive is stopped rather than the duration of use; the risk disappears gradually during the 10 years after stopping and there is no excess risk by 10 years. A possible small increase in the risk of breast cancer should be weighed against the benefits.

● **INTERACTIONS** → Appendix 1 (progestogens).
▸ With intramuscular use Effectiveness of parenteral progestogen-only contraceptives is not affected by antibacterials that do not induce liver enzymes. The effectiveness of norethisterone intramuscular injection is not affected by enzyme-inducing drugs and may be continued as normal during courses of these drugs.

6

Endocrine system

• SIDE-EFFECTS

GENERAL SIDE-EFFECTS

Acne · alopecia · anaphylactoid reactions · breast tenderness · change in libido · depression · disturbance of appetite · dizziness · fluid retention · headache · hirsutism · insomnia (non-contraceptive indications) · jaundice · menstrual disturbances · nausea · premenstrual-like syndrome · pruritus · rash · skin reactions · urticaria · vomiting · weight change

SPECIFIC SIDE-EFFECTS

▸ With intramuscular use Injection-site reactions

SIDE-EFFECTS, FURTHER INFORMATION

▸ Cervical cancer Use of injectable progestogen-only contraceptives may be associated with a small increased risk of cervical cancer, similar to that seen with combined oral contraceptives (use of combined oral contraceptives for 5 years or longer is associated with a small increased risk of cervical cancer; the risk diminishes after stopping and disappears by about 10 years). The risk of cervical cancer with other progestogen-only contraceptives is not yet known.

• PREGNANCY

▸ With oral use Masculinisation of female fetuses and other defects reported with non-contraceptive use.

• BREAST FEEDING Progestogen-only contraceptives do not affect lactation. Higher doses (used in malignant conditions) may suppress lactation and alter milk composition—use lowest effective dose.

▸ With intramuscular use Withhold breast-feeding for neonates with severe or persistent jaundice requiring medical treatment.

• HEPATIC IMPAIRMENT When used as a contraceptive; caution in severe liver disease and recurrent cholestatic jaundice, avoid in liver tumour. Avoid in non-contraceptive indications.

• RENAL IMPAIRMENT Use with caution in non-contraceptive indications.

• PATIENT AND CARER ADVICE

Missed oral contraceptive pill The following advice is recommended: 'If you forget a pill, take it as soon as you remember and carry on with the next pill at the right time. If the pill was more than 3 hours overdue you are not protected. Continue normal pill-taking but you must also use another method, such as the condom, for the next 2 days.'

The Faculty of Sexual and Reproductive Healthcare recommends emergency contraception if one or more progestogen-only contraceptive tablets are missed or taken more than 3 hours late and unprotected intercourse has occurred before 2 further tablets have been correctly taken.

Diarrhoea and vomiting with oral contraceptives Vomiting and persistent, severe diarrhoea can interfere with the absorption of oral progestogen-only contraceptives. If vomiting occurs within 2 hours of taking an oral progestogen-only contraceptive, another pill should be taken as soon as possible. If a replacement pill is not taken within 3 hours of the normal time for taking the progestogen-only pill, or in cases of persistent vomiting or very severe diarrhoea, additional precautions should be used during illness and for 2 days after recovery.

Starting routine for oral contraceptives One tablet daily, on a continuous basis, starting on day 1 of cycle and taken at the same time each day (if delayed by longer than 3 hours contraceptive protection may be lost). Additional contraceptive precautions are not required if norethisterone is started up to and including day 5 of the menstrual cycle; if started after this time, additional contraceptive precautions are required for 2 days.

Changing from a combined oral contraceptive Start on the day following completion of the combined oral contraceptive course without a break (or in the case of ED tablets omitting the inactive ones).

After childbirth Oral progestogen-only contraceptives can be started up to and including day 21 postpartum without the need for additional contraceptive precautions. If started more than 21 days postpartum, additional contraceptive precautions are required for 2 days.

Contraceptives by injection Full counselling backed by *patient information leaflet* required before administration—likelihood of menstrual disturbance and the potential for a delay in return to full fertility. Delayed return of fertility and irregular cycles may occur after discontinuation of treatment but there is no evidence of permanent infertility.

• MEDICINAL FORMS
There can be variation in the licensing of different medicines containing the same drug. Forms available from special-order manufacturers include: oral suspension

Tablet

▸ Norethisterone (Non-proprietary)
Norethisterone 5 mg Norethisterone 5mg tablets | 30 tablet [PoM] £4.50 DT price = £2.18

▸ Micronor (Janssen-Cilag Ltd)
Norethisterone 350 microgram Micronor 350microgram tablets | 84 tablet [PoM] £1.80 DT price = £1.80

▸ Noriday (Pfizer Ltd)
Norethisterone 350 microgram Noriday 350microgram tablets | 84 tablet [PoM] £2.10 DT price = £1.80

▸ Primolut N (Bayer Plc)
Norethisterone 5 mg Primolut N 5mg tablets | 30 tablet [PoM] £2.26 DT price = £2.18

▸ Utovlan (Pfizer Ltd)
Norethisterone 5 mg Utovlan 5mg tablets | 30 tablet [PoM] £1.40 DT price = £2.18 | 90 tablet [PoM] £4.21

Solution for injection

▸ Noristerat (Bayer Plc)
Norethisterone enantate 200 mg per 1 ml Noristerat 200mg/1ml solution for injection ampoules | 1 ampoule [PoM] £4.05

Combinations available: *Estradiol with norethisterone,* p. 689

Progesterone

• INDICATIONS AND DOSE

CRINONE® VAGINAL GEL

Infertility due to inadequate luteal phase

▸ BY VAGINA

▸ Adult: 1 applicatorful daily, to be started either after documented ovulation or on day 18–21 of cycle, in vitro fertilisation, daily application continued for 30 days after laboratory evidence of pregnancy

CYCLOGEST® PESSARIES

Premenstrual syndrome | Post-natal depression

▸ BY VAGINA, OR BY RECTUM

▸ Adult: 200–800 mg daily, doses above 200 mg to be given in 2 divided doses, for premenstrual syndrome start on day 12–14 and continue until onset of menstruation (but not recommended); rectally if barrier methods of contraception are used, in patients who have recently given birth or in those who suffer from vaginal infection or recurrent cystitis

GESTONE® SOLUTION FOR INJECTION

Dysfunctional uterine bleeding

▸ BY DEEP INTRAMUSCULAR INJECTION

▸ Adult: 5–10 mg daily for 5–10 days until 2 days before expected onset of menstruation, to be administered into buttocks

Recurrent miscarriage due to inadequate luteal phase (but not recommended) or following in vitro fertilisation or gamete intra-fallopian transfer

▶ BY DEEP INTRAMUSCULAR INJECTION

▶ Adult: 25–100 mg 2–7 times a week from day 15, or day of embryo or gamete transfer, until 8–16 weeks of pregnancy, to be administered into buttocks; maximum 200 mg per day

LUBION®

Supplementation of luteal phase during assisted reproductive technology (ART) treatment in women for whom vaginal preparations are inappropriate

▶ BY SUBCUTANEOUS INJECTION, OR BY INTRAMUSCULAR INJECTION

▶ Adult: 25 mg once daily from day of oocyte retrieval up to week 12 of pregnancy

UTROGESTAN® CAPSULES

Progestogenic opposition of oestrogen HRT

▶ BY MOUTH

▶ Adult: 200 mg once daily on days 15–26 of each 28-day oestrogen HRT cycle, alternatively 100 mg once daily on days 1–25 of each 28-day oestrogen HRT cycle

UTROGESTAN® VAGINAL CAPSULES

Supplementation of luteal phase during assisted reproductive technology (ART) cycles

▶ BY VAGINA

▶ Adult: 1 capsule 3 times a day from day of embryo transfer until at least week 7 of pregnancy up to week 12 of pregnancy

● CONTRA-INDICATIONS Acute porphyrias p. 918 · avoid in patients with a history of liver tumours · breast cancer (unless progestogens are being used in the management of this condition) · genital cancer (unless progestogens are being used in the management of this condition) · history during pregnancy of idiopathic jaundice · history during pregnancy of pemphigoid gestationis · history during pregnancy of severe pruritus · incomplete miscarriage · missed miscarriage · severe arterial disease · undiagnosed vaginal bleeding

● CAUTIONS Asthma · cardiac dysfunction · conditions that may worsen with fluid retention · diabetes (progestogens can decrease glucose tolerance—monitor patient closely) · epilepsy · history of depression · hypertension · migraine · susceptibility to thromboembolism (particular caution with high dose)

● INTERACTIONS → Appendix 1 (progestogens).

● SIDE-EFFECTS
GENERAL SIDE-EFFECTS
Acne · alopecia · anaphylactoid reactions · bloating · breast tenderness · change in libido · depression · dizziness · drowsiness · fluid retention · headache · hirsutism · insomnia · jaundice · menstrual disturbances · nausea · premenstrual-like syndrome · pruritus · rash · skin reactions · urticaria · weight change

SPECIFIC SIDE-EFFECTS

▶ With intramuscular use Injection-site reactions
▶ With rectal use Diarrhoea · flatulence · pain
▶ With subcutaneous use Injection-site reactions
▶ With vaginal use Local irritation

● PREGNANCY Not known to be harmful.

● BREAST FEEDING Avoid—present in milk.

● HEPATIC IMPAIRMENT Avoid in hepatic impairment. Avoid in active liver disease including disorders of hepatic excretion (e.g. Dublin-Johnson or Rotor Syndromes), infective hepatitis (until liver function returns to normal) and liver tumours.

● RENAL IMPAIRMENT Use with caution.

● DIRECTIONS FOR ADMINISTRATION
▶ With oral use Capsules should be taken at bedtime on an empty stomach.

● PATIENT AND CARER ADVICE
▶ With oral use Patient counselling is advised for progesterone capsules (administration).

● LESS SUITABLE FOR PRESCRIBING
▶ With vaginal use Progesterone pessaries are less suitable for prescribing.

● MEDICINAL FORMS
There can be variation in the licensing of different medicines containing the same drug.

Capsule
EXCIPIENTS: May contain Arachis (peanut) oil
▶ Utrogestan (Besins Healthcare (UK) Ltd)
Progesterone 100 mg Utrogestan 100mg capsules |
30 capsule PoM £5.13
Progesterone 200 mg Utrogestan 200mg vaginal capsules with applicators | 21 capsule PoM £21.00

Solution for injection
▶ Gestone (Nordic Pharma Ltd)
Progesterone 50 mg per 1 ml Gestone 50mg/1ml solution for injection ampoules | 10 ampoule PoM £45.00
Gestone 100mg/2ml solution for injection ampoules |
10 ampoule PoM £45.00
▶ Lubion (Pharmasure Ltd)
Progesterone 22.35 mg per 1 ml Lubion 25mg/1.119ml solution for injection vials | 7 vial PoM £56.00

Pessary
▶ Cyclogest (Actavis UK Ltd)
Progesterone 200 mg Cyclogest 200mg pessaries |
15 pessary PoM £8.95 DT price = £8.95
Progesterone 400 mg Cyclogest 400mg pessaries |
15 pessary PoM £12.96 DT price = £12.96

Vaginal gel
▶ Crinone (Merck Serono Ltd)
Progesterone 80 mg per 1 gram Crinone 8% progesterone vaginal gel | 15 unit dose PoM £30.83

8.1a Anti-oestrogens

OVULATION STIMULANTS

Clomifene citrate

(Clomiphene citrate)

● DRUG ACTION Anti-oestrogen which induces gonadotrophin release by occupying oestrogen receptors in the hypothalamus, thereby interfering with feedback mechanisms; chorionic gonadotrophin is sometimes used as an adjunct.

● INDICATIONS AND DOSE

Treatment of female infertility due to oligomenorrhoea or secondary amenorrhoea (e.g. associated with polycystic ovarian disease)

▶ BY MOUTH

▶ Adult (female): 50 mg daily for 5 days, to be started within about 5 days of onset of menstruation (preferably on 2nd day) or at any time (normally preceded by a progestogen induced withdrawal bleed) if cycles have ceased, followed by 100 mg daily if required for a further 5 days, this second course may be given in absence of ovulation; most patients who are going to respond will do so to first course, continued →

6

Endocrine system

6

Endocrine system

3 courses should constitute adequate therapeutic trial; long-term cyclical therapy not recommended.

> **IMPORTANT SAFETY INFORMATION**
> The CSM has recommended that clomifene should not normally be used for longer than 6 cycles (possibly increased risk of ovarian cancer).

- CONTRA-INDICATIONS Abnormal uterine bleeding of undetermined cause · hormone-dependent tumours · ovarian cysts
- CAUTIONS Ectopic pregnancy · incidence of multiple births increased (consider ultrasound monitoring) · ovarian hyperstimulation syndrome · polycystic ovary syndrome (cysts may enlarge during treatment, also risk of exaggerated response to usual doses) · uterine fibroids
- SIDE-EFFECTS Abdominal discomfort · breast tenderness · convulsions · depression · dizziness · endometriosis · hair loss · headache · hot flushes · insomnia · intermenstrual spotting · menorrhagia · nausea · ovarian hyperstimulation (withdraw) · rashes · visual disturbances (withdraw and initiate ophthalmological examination) · vomiting · weight gain
- CONCEPTION AND CONTRACEPTION Exclude pregnancy before treatment.
- PREGNANCY Possible effects on fetal development.
- BREAST FEEDING May inhibit lactation.
- HEPATIC IMPAIRMENT Avoid in severe liver disease.
- PATIENT AND CARER ADVICE
  Patient advice required around conception and contraception Patients planning to conceive should be warned that there is a risk of multiple pregnancy (*rarely* more than twins).

- MEDICINAL FORMS
  There can be variation in the licensing of different medicines containing the same drug.
  Tablet
  ▸ Clomifene citrate (Non-proprietary)
    Clomifene citrate 50 mg Clomifene 50mg tablets | 30 tablet [PoM] £21.74 DT price = £10.15
  ▸ Clomid (Sanofi)
    Clomifene citrate 50 mg Clomid 50mg tablets | 30 tablet [PoM] £10.15 DT price = £10.15

8.2 Male sex hormone responsive conditions

Androgens, anti-androgens and anabolic steroids

Androgens

Androgens cause masculinisation; they may be used as replacement therapy in castrated adults and in those who are hypogonadal due to either pituitary or testicular disease. In the normal male they inhibit pituitary gonadotrophin secretion and depress spermatogenesis. Androgens also have an anabolic action which led to the development of anabolic steroids.

Androgens are useless as a treatment of impotence and impaired spermatogenesis unless there is associated hypogonadism; they should not be given until the hypogonadism has been properly investigated. Treatment should be under expert supervision.

When given to patients with hypopituitarism they can lead to normal sexual development and potency but not to fertility. If fertility is desired, the usual treatment is with gonadotrophins or pulsatile gonadotrophin-releasing

hormone which will stimulate spermatogenesis as well as androgen production.

Intramuscular depot preparations of **testosterone esters** are preferred for replacement therapy. Testosterone enantate, propionate or undecanoate, or alternatively *Sustanon*®, which consists of a mixture of testosterone esters and has a longer duration of action, may be used.

Anti-androgens

Cyproterone acetate

Cyproterone acetate p. 696 is an anti-androgen used in the treatment of severe hypersexuality and sexual deviation in the male. It inhibits spermatogenesis and produces reversible infertility (but is not a male contraceptive); abnormal sperm forms are produced. Fully informed consent is recommended and an initial spermatogram. As hepatic tumours have been produced in *animal* studies, careful consideration should be given to the risk/benefit ratio before treatment. Cyproterone acetate is also licensed for use alone in patients with metastatic prostate cancer refractory to gonadorelin analogue therapy and has been used as an adjunct in prostatic cancer and in the treatment of acne and hirsutism in women.

Dutasteride and finasteride

Dutasteride p. 712 and finasteride p. 712 are alternatives to alpha-blockers particularly in men with a significantly enlarged prostate. Finasteride is also licensed for use with doxazosin p. 708 in the management of benign prostatic hyperplasia.

A low strength of finasteride is licensed for treating male-pattern baldness in men.

Anabolic steroids

Anabolic steroids have some androgenic activity but they cause less virilisation than androgens in women. They are used in the treatment of some *aplastic anaemias*. Anabolic steroids have been given for osteoporosis in women but they are no longer advocated for this purpose.

The protein-building properties of anabolic steroids have not proved beneficial in the clinical setting. Their use as body builders or tonics is unjustified; some athletes abuse them.

ANDROGENS

Androgens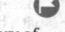

- CONTRA-INDICATIONS Breast cancer in males · history of liver tumours · hypercalcaemia · prostate cancer
- CAUTIONS Cardiac impairment · diabetes mellitus · elderly · epilepsy · hypertension · ischaemic heart disease · migraine · pre-pubertal boys (fusion of epiphyses is hastened and may result in short stature)—statural growth and sexual development should be monitored · skeletal metastases—risk of hypercalcaemia or hypercalciuria (if this occurs, treat appropriately and restart treatment once normal serum calcium concentration restored) · sleep apnoea · stop treatment or reduce dose if severe polycythaemia occurs · tumours—risk of hypercalcaemia or hypercalciuria (if this occurs, treat appropriately and restart treatment once normal serum calcium concentration restored)
- INTERACTIONS → Appendix 1 (testosterone).
- SIDE-EFFECTS
▸ **Common or very common** Acne · androgenic effects (to be assessed regularly in women) · anxiety · arthralgia · asthenia · changes in libido · cholestatic jaundice · depression · electrolyte disturbances · excessive duration of penile erection · excessive frequency of penile erection · gastro-intestinal bleeding · gynaecomastia · headache · hirsutism · hypercalcaemia · hypertension · increased bone

growth · irritability · male-pattern baldness · muscle cramps · nausea · nervousness · oedema · paraesthesia · polycythaemia · precocious sexual development in pre-pubertal males · premature closure of epiphyses in pre-pubertal males · prostate abnormalities · prostate cancer · pruritus · seborrhoea · sodium retention · suppression of virilism in women · vomiting · weight gain
▸ **Rare** Liver tumours
▸ **Frequency not known** Sleep apnoea
  SIDE-EFFECTS, FURTHER INFORMATION
▸ Polycythaemia Stop treatment or reduce dose if severe polycythaemia occurs.
● PREGNANCY Avoid—causes masculinisation of female fetus.
● BREAST FEEDING Avoid.
● HEPATIC IMPAIRMENT Avoid if possible—fluid retention and dose-related toxicity.
● RENAL IMPAIRMENT Caution—potential for fluid retention.
● MONITORING REQUIREMENTS
▸ Monitor haematocrit and haemoglobulin before treatment, every three months for the first year, and yearly thereafter.
▸ Monitor prostate and PSA in men over 45 years.
● PATIENT AND CARER ADVICE
  Androgenic effects in women Women should be advised to report any signs of virilisation e.g. deepening of the voice or hirsutism.

> ⚐ 694

Mesterolone

● INDICATIONS AND DOSE
Androgen deficiency | Male infertility associated with hypogonadism
▸ BY MOUTH
▸ Adult: 25 mg 3–4 times a day for several months, then maintenance 50–75 mg daily in divided doses

● MEDICINAL FORMS
There can be variation in the licensing of different medicines containing the same drug.
Tablet
▸ Pro-Viron (Bayer Plc)
  Mesterolone 25 mg Pro-Viron 25mg tablets | 30 tablet [PoM] £4.19 [CD4-2]

> ⚐ 694

Testosterone

● INDICATIONS AND DOSE
TESTIM®
Hypogonadism due to testosterone deficiency in men
▸ BY TRANSDERMAL APPLICATION
▸ Adult: Apply 50 mg once daily, subsequent application adjusted according to response; maximum 100 mg per day
DOSE EQUIVALENCE AND CONVERSION
One tube of 5 g contains 50 mg testosterone.
TESTOGEL®
Hypogonadism due to androgen deficiency in men
▸ BY TRANSDERMAL APPLICATION
▸ Adult: Apply 50 mg once daily; increased in steps of 25 mg, adjusted according to response; maximum 100 mg per day
DOSE EQUIVALENCE AND CONVERSION
One sachet of 5 g contains 50 mg of testosterone.

TOSTRAN®
Hypogonadism due to testosterone deficiency in men
▸ BY TRANSDERMAL APPLICATION
▸ Adult: Apply 60 mg once daily, subsequent application adjusted according to response; maximum 80 mg per day
DOSE EQUIVALENCE AND CONVERSION
1 g of gel contains 20 mg testosterone.

● SIDE-EFFECTS Allergic reactions · local irritation · suppression of spermatogenesis
● DIRECTIONS FOR ADMINISTRATION Avoid skin contact with gel application sites to prevent testosterone transfer to other people, especially pregnant women and children—consult product literature.
TESTOGEL® Apply thin layer of gel on clean, dry, healthy skin such as shoulders, arms or abdomen, immediately after sachet is opened. Not to be applied on genital area as high alcohol content may cause local irritation. Allow to dry for 3–5 minutes before dressing. Wash hands with soap and water after applying gel, avoid shower or bath for at least 6 hours.
TESTIM® Squeeze entire content of tube on to one palm and apply as a thin layer on clean, dry, healthy skin of shoulder or upper arm, preferably in the morning after washing or bathing (if 2 tubes required use 1 per shoulder or upper arm); rub in and allow to dry before putting on clothing to cover site; wash hands with soap after application; avoid washing application site for at least 6 hours.
TOSTRAN® Apply gel on clean, dry, intact skin of abdomen or both inner thighs, preferably in the morning. Gently rub in with a finger until dry before dressing. Wash hands with soap and water after applying gel; avoid washing application site for at least 2 hours. Not to be applied on genital area.
● PATIENT AND CARER ADVICE Patient or carer should be given advice on how to administer testosterone gel.

● MEDICINAL FORMS
There can be variation in the licensing of different medicines containing the same drug.
Gel
EXCIPIENTS: May contain Butylated hydroxytoluene, propylene glycol
▸ Testim (Ferring Pharmaceuticals Ltd)
  Testosterone 50 mg Testim 50mg/5g gel | 30 tube [PoM] £32.00 [CD4-2]
▸ Testogel (Besins Healthcare (UK) Ltd)
  Testosterone 50 mg Testogel 50mg/5g gel sachets | 30 sachet [PoM] £31.11 DT price = £31.11 [CD4-2]
▸ Tostran (ProStrakan Ltd)
  Testosterone 20 mg per 1 gram Tostran 2% gel | 60 gram [PoM] £28.67 [CD4-2]

> ⚐ 694

Testosterone decanoate, isocaproate, phenylpropionate and propionate

The properties listed below are those particular to the combination only. For the properties of the components please consider, testosterone propionate p. 696.

● INDICATIONS AND DOSE
Androgen deficiency
▸ BY DEEP INTRAMUSCULAR INJECTION
▸ Adult: 1 mL every 3 weeks

- MEDICINAL FORMS
There can be variation in the licensing of different medicines containing the same drug.
Solution for injection
EXCIPIENTS: May contain Arachis (peanut) oil, benzyl alcohol
▸ Sustanon (Aspen Pharma Trading Ltd)
  Testosterone propionate 30 mg per 1 ml, Testosterone isocaproate 60 mg per 1 ml, Testosterone phenylpropionate 60 mg per 1 ml, Testosterone decanoate 100 mg per 1 ml Sustanon 250mg/1ml solution for injection ampoules | 1 ampoule [PoM] £2.45 [CD4-2]

⊩ 694

Testosterone enantate

- INDICATIONS AND DOSE
Hypogonadism
▸ BY SLOW INTRAMUSCULAR INJECTION
▸ Adult: Initially 250 mg every 2–3 weeks; maintenance 250 mg every 3–6 weeks

Breast cancer
▸ BY SLOW INTRAMUSCULAR INJECTION
▸ Adult: 250 mg every 2–3 weeks

- UNLICENSED USE Not licensed for use in breast cancer.
- SIDE-EFFECTS Suppression of spermatogenesis

- MEDICINAL FORMS
There can be variation in the licensing of different medicines containing the same drug.
Solution for injection
▸ Testosterone enantate (Non-proprietary)
  Testosterone enantate 250 mg per 1 ml Testosterone enantate 250mg/1ml solution for injection ampoules | 3 ampoule [PoM] £72.50 DT price = £72.50 [CD4-2]

⊩ 694

Testosterone propionate

- INDICATIONS AND DOSE
Androgen deficiency
▸ BY INTRAMUSCULAR INJECTION
▸ Adult: 50 mg 2–3 times a week

Delayed puberty in males
▸ BY INTRAMUSCULAR INJECTION
▸ Adult: 50 mg once weekly

Breast cancer in women
▸ BY INTRAMUSCULAR INJECTION
▸ Adult: 100 mg 2–3 times a week

- SIDE-EFFECTS Suppression of spermatogenesis

- MEDICINAL FORMS
There can be variation in the licensing of different medicines containing the same drug. Forms available from special-order manufacturers include: solution for injection

⊩ 694

Testosterone undecanoate

- INDICATIONS AND DOSE
Androgen deficiency
▸ BY MOUTH
▸ Adult: 120–160 mg daily for 2–3 weeks; maintenance 40–120 mg daily

Hypogonadism
▸ BY DEEP INTRAMUSCULAR INJECTION
▸ Adult (male): 1 g every 10–14 weeks, to be given over 2 minutes, if necessary, second dose may be given after 6 weeks to achieve rapid steady state plasma testosterone levels and then every 10–14 weeks.

- SIDE-EFFECTS Suppression of spermatogenesis

- MEDICINAL FORMS
There can be variation in the licensing of different medicines containing the same drug.
Capsule
CAUTIONARY AND ADVISORY LABELS 21, 25
▸ Restandol (Merck Sharp & Dohme Ltd)
  Testosterone undecanoate 40 mg Restandol 40mg Testocaps | 30 capsule [PoM] £8.55 [CD4-2] | 60 capsule [PoM] £17.10 DT price = £17.10 [CD4-2]
Solution for injection
▸ Nebido (Bayer Plc)
  Testosterone undecanoate 250 mg per 1 ml Nebido 1000mg/4ml solution for injection vials | 1 vial [PoM] £87.11 DT price = £80.00 [CD4-2]

8.2a Male sex hormone antagonism

ANTI-ANDROGENS

Cyproterone acetate

- INDICATIONS AND DOSE
Hyper-sexuality in males | Sexual deviation in males
▸ BY MOUTH
▸ Adult: 50 mg twice daily, to be taken after food

Prevention of tumour flare with initial gonadorelin analogue therapy
▸ BY MOUTH
▸ Adult (male): 200 mg daily in 2–3 divided doses for 5–7 days before initiation of gonadorelin analogue, followed by 200 mg daily in 2–3 divided doses for 3–4 weeks after initiation of gonadorelin analogue; maximum 300 mg per day.

Long-term palliative therapy where gonadorelin analogues or orchidectomy contra-indicated, not tolerated, or where oral therapy preferred
▸ BY MOUTH
▸ Adult (male): 200–300 mg daily in 2–3 divided doses.

Hot flushes with gonadorelin analogue therapy or after orchidectomy
▸ BY MOUTH
▸ Adult (male): Initially 50 mg daily, then adjusted according to response to 50–150 mg daily in 1–3 divided doses.

- CONTRA-INDICATIONS In hypersexuality, Dubin-Johnson syndrome · in hypersexuality, history of thromboembolic disorders · in hypersexuality, liver-disease · in hypersexuality, malignant diseases · in hypersexuality, previous or existing liver tumours · in hypersexuality, Rotor syndrome · in hypersexuality, severe depression · in hypersexuality, severe diabetes (with vascular changes) · in hypersexuality, sickle-cell anaemia · in hypersexuality, wasting diseases · meningioma or history of meningioma
- CAUTIONS Diabetes mellitus · in prostate cancer, severe depression · in prostate cancer, sickle-cell anaemia · ineffective for male hypersexuality in chronic alcoholism (relevance to prostate cancer not known)
- SIDE-EFFECTS
▸ Rare Hypersensitivity reactions · osteoporosis · rash
▸ Frequency not known Breathlessness · changes in hair pattern · fatigue · gynaecomastia (rarely leading to galactorrhoea and benign breast nodules) · hepatic failure · hepatitis · hepatotoxicity · inhibition of spermatogenesis · jaundice · lassitude · reduced sebum production (may clear acne) · risk of recurrence of thromboembolic disease · weight changes

SIDE-EFFECTS, FURTHER INFORMATION
▸ Hepatotoxicity Direct hepatic toxicity including jaundice, hepatitis and hepatic failure have been reported (fatalities reported, usually after several months, at dosages of 100 mg and above). If hepatotoxicity is confirmed, cyproterone should normally be withdrawn unless the hepatotoxicity can be explained by another cause such as metastatic disease (in which case cyproterone should be continued only if the perceived benefit exceeds the risk).

● **HEPATIC IMPAIRMENT** Avoid (unless used for prostate cancer)—dose-related toxicity.

● **MONITORING REQUIREMENTS**
▸ Monitor blood counts initially and throughout treatment.
▸ Monitor adrenocortical function regularly.
▸ Monitor hepatic function regularly—liver function tests should be performed before and regularly during treatment and whenever symptoms suggestive of hepatotoxicity occur.

● **PATIENT AND CARER ADVICE**
  Driving and skilled tasks
  Fatigue and lassitude may impair performance of skilled tasks (e.g. driving).

● **MEDICINAL FORMS**
  There can be variation in the licensing of different medicines containing the same drug. Forms available from special-order manufacturers include: tablet, capsule, oral suspension, oral solution
  Tablet
  CAUTIONARY AND ADVISORY LABELS 21
    ▸ Cyproterone acetate (Non-proprietary)
    Cyproterone acetate 50 mg Cyproterone 50mg tablets | 56 tablet [PoM] £48.95 | 168 tablet [PoM] £87.00 DT price = £87.00
    Cyproterone acetate 100 mg Cyproterone 100mg tablets | 84 tablet [PoM] £132.57 DT price = £55.19
    ▸ Androcur (Bayer Plc)
    Cyproterone acetate 50 mg Androcur 50mg tablets | 56 tablet [PoM] £29.25
    ▸ Cyprostat (Bayer Plc)
    Cyproterone acetate 50 mg Cyprostat 50mg tablets | 168 tablet [PoM] £87.00 DT price = £87.00
    Cyproterone acetate 100 mg Cyprostat 100mg tablets | 84 tablet [PoM] £87.00 DT price = £55.19

9 Thyroid disorders

PITUITARY AND HYPOTHALAMIC HORMONES AND ANALOGUES ﹥THYROID STIMULATING HORMONES

Thyrotropin alfa

(Recombinant human thyroid stimulating hormone; rhTSH)

● DRUG ACTION Thyrotropin alfa is a recombinant form of thyrotrophin (thyroid stimulating hormone).

  ● **INDICATIONS AND DOSE**
  Detection of thyroid remnants and thyroid cancer in post-thyroidectomy patients, together with serum thyroglobulin testing (with or without radioiodine imaging) | To increase radio-iodine uptake for the ablation of thyroid remnant tissue in suitable post-thyroidectomy patients
    ▸ BY INTRAMUSCULAR INJECTION
    ▸ Adult: 900 micrograms every 24 hours for 2 doses, dose to be administered into the gluteal muscle, consult product literature for further information on indications and dose

● CAUTIONS Presence of thyroglobulin autoantibodies may give false negative results

● SIDE-EFFECTS
▸ **Common or very common** Dizziness · fatigue · headache · nausea · vomiting
▸ **Uncommon** Asthenia · back pain · influenza-like symptoms · paraesthesia · rash · urticaria
▸ **Rare** Diarrhoea
▸ **Very rare** Arthralgia · dyspnoea · flushing · hyperhidrosis · injection-site pain · injection-site pruritus · injection-site rash · injection-site reactions · myalgia · pain at site of metastases · palpitation · tremor

● ALLERGY AND CROSS-SENSITIVITY Contra-indicated if previous hypersensitivity to bovine or human thyrotrophin.

● PREGNANCY Avoid.

● BREAST FEEDING Avoid.

● MEDICINAL FORMS
  There can be variation in the licensing of different medicines containing the same drug.
  Powder for solution for injection
    ▸ Thyrogen (Genzyme Therapeutics Ltd)
    Thyrotropin alfa 900 microgram Thyrogen 900microgram powder for solution for injection vials | 2 vial [PoM] £583.04

9.1 Hyperthyroidism

Antithyroid drugs

Overview

Antithyroid drugs are used for hyperthyroidism either to prepare patients for thyroidectomy or for long-term management. In the UK carbimazole p. 698 is the most commonly used drug. Propylthiouracil p. 698 should be reserved for patients who are intolerant of carbimazole or for those who experience sensitivity reactions to carbimazole (sensitivity is not necessarily displayed to both drugs), and for whom other treatments are inappropriate. Both drugs act primarily by interfering with the synthesis of thyroid hormones.

Over-treatment with antithyroid drugs can result in the rapid development of hypothyroidism and should be avoided particularly during pregnancy because it can cause fetal goitre.

A combination of carbimazole with levothyroxine sodium p. 699 daily, may be used in a *blocking-replacement regimen*; therapy is usually given for 18 months. The blocking-replacement regimen is **not** suitable during pregnancy.

Iodine has been used as an adjunct to antithyroid drugs for 10 to 14 days before partial thyroidectomy; however, there is little evidence of a beneficial effect. Iodine should not be used for long-term treatment because its antithyroid action tends to diminish.

Radioactive sodium iodide (^{131}I) solution is used increasingly for the treatment of thyrotoxicosis at all ages, particularly where medical therapy or compliance is a problem, in patients with cardiac disease, and in patients who relapse after thyroidectomy.

Propranolol hydrochloride p. 136 is useful for rapid relief of thyrotoxic symptoms and may be used in conjunction with antithyroid drugs or as an adjunct to radioactive iodine. Beta-blockers are also useful in neonatal thyrotoxicosis and in supraventricular arrhythmias due to hyperthyroidism. Propranolol hydrochloride has been used in conjunction with iodine to prepare mildly thyrotoxic patients for surgery but it is preferable to make the patient euthyroid with carbimazole. Laboratory tests of thyroid function are not altered by beta-blockers. Most experience in treating

Endocrine system

6

thyrotoxicosis has been gained with propranolol hydrochloride but nadolol p. 135 is also used.

Thyrotoxic crisis ('thyroid storm') requires emergency treatment with intravenous administration of fluids, propranolol hydrochloride and hydrocortisone p. 612 (as sodium succinate), as well as oral iodine solution and carbimazole or propylthiouracil which may need to be administered by nasogastric tube.

Pregnancy

Radioactive iodine therapy is contra-indicated during pregnancy. Propylthiouracil and carbimazole can be given but the blocking-replacement regimen is **not** suitable. Rarely, carbimazole has been associated with congenital defects, including aplasia cutis of the neonate, therefore propylthiouracil remains the drug of choice during the first trimester of pregnancy. In the second trimester, consider switching to carbimazole because of the potential risk of hepatotoxicity with propylthiouracil. Both propylthiouracil and carbimazole cross the placenta and in high doses may cause fetal goitre and hypothyroidism—the lowest dose that will control the hyperthyroid state should be used (requirements in Graves' disease tend to fall during pregnancy).

> **Drugs used for Hyperthyroidism not listed below**
> Metoprolol tartrate, p. 140

ANTITHYROID DRUGS > SULFUR-CONTAINING IMIDAZOLES

| Carbimazole

- **● INDICATIONS AND DOSE**

Hyperthyroidism
▶ BY MOUTH
> Adult: 15–40 mg daily continue until the patient becomes euthyroid, usually after 4 to 8 weeks, higher doses should be prescribed under specialist supervision only, then reduced to 5–15 mg daily, reduce dose gradually, therapy usually given for 12 to 18 months

Hyperthyroidism (blocking-replacement regimen) in combination with levothyroxine
▶ BY MOUTH
> Adult: 40–60 mg daily, therapy usually given for 18 months

DOSE EQUIVALENCE AND CONVERSION
When substituting, carbimazole 1 mg is considered equivalent to propylthiouracil 10 mg but the dose may need adjusting according to response.

IMPORTANT SAFETY INFORMATION
NEUTROPENIA AND AGRANULOCYTOSIS
Doctors are reminded of the importance of recognising bone marrow suppression induced by carbimazole and the need to stop treatment promptly.

- Patient should be asked to report symptoms and signs suggestive of infection, especially sore throat.
- A white blood cell count should be performed if there is any clinical evidence of infection.
- Carbimazole should be stopped promptly if there is clinical or laboratory evidence of neutropenia.

- **● CONTRA-INDICATIONS** Severe blood disorders
- **● INTERACTIONS** → Appendix 1 (carbimazole).
- **● SIDE-EFFECTS**
- ▶ **Common or very common** Arthralgia · fever · headache · jaundice · malaise · mild gastro-intestinal disturbances · nausea · pruritus · rash · taste disturbance

- ▶ **Rare** Agranulocytosis · alopecia · bone marrow suppression · jaundice · myopathy · pancytopenia
  SIDE-EFFECTS, FURTHER INFORMATION
  Rashes and pruritus are common with carbimazole but they can be treated with antihistamines without discontinuing therapy; alternatively propylthiouracil can be substituted.

- **● PREGNANCY** Carbimazole can be given but the blocking-replacement regimen is **not** suitable. Rarely, carbimazole has been associated with congenital defects, including aplasia cutis of the neonate. Carbimazole cross the placenta and in high doses may cause fetal goitre and hypothyroidism—the lowest dose that will control the hyperthyroid state should be used (requirements in Graves' disease tend to fall during pregnancy).

- **● BREAST FEEDING** Present in breast milk but this does not preclude breast-feeding as long as neonatal development is closely monitored and the lowest effective dose is used. Amount in milk may be sufficient to affect neonatal thyroid function therefore lowest effective dose should be used.

- **● HEPATIC IMPAIRMENT** Use with caution in mild to moderate impairment. Avoid in severe impairment.

- **● PATIENT AND CARER ADVICE** Warn patient or carers to tell doctor **immediately** if sore throat, mouth ulcers, bruising, fever, malaise, or non-specific illness develops.

- **● MEDICINAL FORMS**
  There can be variation in the licensing of different medicines containing the same drug. Forms available from special-order manufacturers include: capsule, oral suspension, oral solution
  Tablet
  ▶ Carbimazole (Non-proprietary)
  Carbimazole 5 mg Carbimazole 5mg tablets | 100 tablet [PoM]
  £90.00 DT price = £78.83
  Carbimazole 20 mg Carbimazole 20mg tablets | 100 tablet [PoM]
  £240.00 DT price = £197.14

ANTITHYROID DRUGS > THIOURACILS

| Propylthiouracil

- **● INDICATIONS AND DOSE**

Hyperthyroidism
▶ BY MOUTH
> Adult: Initially 200–400 mg daily in divided doses until the patient becomes euthyroid, then reduced to 50–150 mg daily in divided doses, initial dose should be gradually reduced to the maintenance dose

DOSE EQUIVALENCE AND CONVERSION
When substituting, carbimazole 1 mg is considered equivalent to propylthiouracil 10 mg but the dose may need adjusting according to response.

- **● SIDE-EFFECTS**
- ▶ **Common or very common** Arthralgia · fever · headache · jaundice · leucopenia · malaise · mild gastro-intestinal disturbances · nausea · pruritus · rash · taste disturbance
- ▶ **Rare** Agranulocytosis · alopecia · aplastic anaemia · bone marrow suppression · cutaneous vasculitis · encephalopathy · hepatic disorders · hepatic failure · hepatic necrosis · hepatitis · hypoprothrombinaemia · jaundice · lupus erythematous-like syndromes · myopathy · nephritis · pancytopenia · thrombocytopenia
  SIDE-EFFECTS, FURTHER INFORMATION
- ▶ Hepatotoxicity Severe hepatic reactions have been reported, including fatal cases and cases requiring liver transplant—discontinue if significant liver-enzyme abnormalities develop.

- **● PREGNANCY** Propylthiouracil can be given but the blocking-replacement regimen is **not** suitable. Propylthiouracil crosses the placenta and in high doses may cause fetal goitre and hypothyroidism—the lowest dose that will control the hyperthyroid state should be used (requirements in Graves' disease tend to fall during pregnancy).

- BREAST FEEDING Present in breast milk but this does not preclude breast-feeding as long as neonatal development is closely monitored and the lowest effective dose is used. Amount in milk probably too small to affect infant; high doses may affect neonatal thyroid function.

  Monitor infant's thyroid status.

- HEPATIC IMPAIRMENT Reduce dose.

- RENAL IMPAIRMENT Use three-quarters normal dose if eGFR 10–50 mL/minute/1.73 m^2. Use half normal dose if eGFR less than 10 mL/minute/1.73 m^2.

- MONITORING REQUIREMENTS Monitor for hepatotoxicity.

- PATIENT AND CARER ADVICE Patients should be told how to recognise signs of liver disorder and advised to seek prompt medical attention if symptoms such as anorexia, nausea, vomiting, fatigue, abdominal pain, jaundice, dark urine, or pruritus develop.

- MEDICINAL FORMS
  There can be variation in the licensing of different medicines containing the same drug. Forms available from special-order manufacturers include: oral suspension, oral solution
  Tablet
  ▸ Propylthiouracil (Non-proprietary)
  Propylthiouracil 50 mg Propylthiouracil 50mg tablets | 56 tablet [PoM] £73.50 DT price = £57.72 | 100 tablet [PoM] £131.25

VITAMINS AND TRACE ELEMENTS

Iodide with iodine

- **INDICATIONS AND DOSE**
  Thyrotoxicosis (pre-operative)
  ▸ BY MOUTH USING ORAL SOLUTION
  ▸ Adult: 0.1–0.3 mL 3 times a day

- CAUTIONS Children · not for long-term treatment

- SIDE-EFFECTS Bronchitis · conjunctivitis · coryza-like symptoms · depression (on prolonged treatment) · goitre in infants of mothers taking iodides · headache · hypersensitivity reactions · impotence (on prolonged treatment) · insomnia (on prolonged treatment) · lacrimation · laryngitis · pain in salivary glands · rashes

- PREGNANCY Neonatal goitre and hypothyroidism.

- BREAST FEEDING Stop breast-feeding. Danger of neonatal hypothyroidism or goitre. Appears to be concentrated in milk.

- DIRECTIONS FOR ADMINISTRATION For oral solution, dilute well with milk or water.

- MEDICINAL FORMS
  There can be variation in the licensing of different medicines containing the same drug.
  Oral solution
  CAUTIONARY AND ADVISORY LABELS 27
  ▸ Iodide with iodine (Non-proprietary)
  Iodine 50 mg per 1 ml, Potassium iodide 100 mg per 1 ml Iodine aqueous oral solution | 500 ml [P] £9.58

9.2 Hypothyroidism

Thyroid hormones

Overview

Thyroid hormones are used in hypothyroidism (myxoedema), and also in diffuse non-toxic goitre,

Hashimoto's thyroiditis (lymphadenoid goitre), and thyroid carcinoma. Neonatal hypothyroidism requires prompt treatment for normal development. Levothyroxine sodium below (thyroxine sodium) is the treatment of choice for *maintenance* therapy.

In infants and children with congenital hypothyroidism and juvenile myxoedema, the dose of levothyroxine sodium should be titrated according to clinical response, growth assessment, and measurements of plasma thyroxine and thyroid-stimulating hormone.

Liothyronine sodium p. 700 has a similar action to levothyroxine sodium but is more rapidly metabolised and has a more rapid effect. Its effects develop after a few hours and disappear within 24 to 48 hours of discontinuing treatment. It may be used in *severe hypothyroid states* when a rapid response is desired.

Liothyronine sodium by intravenous injection is the treatment of choice in *hypothyroid coma*. Adjunctive therapy includes intravenous fluids, hydrocortisone p. 612, and treatment of infection; assisted ventilation is often required.

THYROID HORMONES

Levothyroxine sodium

(Thyroxine sodium)

- **INDICATIONS AND DOSE**
  Hypothyroidism
  ▸ BY MOUTH
  ▸ Adult 18–49 years: Initially 50–100 micrograms once daily; adjusted in steps of 25–50 micrograms every 3–4 weeks, adjusted according to response; maintenance 100–200 micrograms once daily, dose to be taken preferably at least 30 minutes before breakfast, caffeine-containing liquids (e.g. coffee, tea), or other medication
  ▸ Adult 50 years and over: Initially 25 micrograms once daily; adjusted in steps of 25 micrograms every 4 weeks, adjusted according to response; maintenance 50–200 micrograms once daily, dose to be taken preferably at least 30 minutes before breakfast, caffeine-containing liquids (e.g. coffee, tea), or other medication

  Hypothyroidism in patients with cardiac disease | Severe hypothyroidism
  ▸ BY MOUTH
  ▸ Adult: Initially 25 micrograms once daily; adjusted in steps of 25 micrograms every 4 weeks, adjusted according to response; maintenance 50–200 micrograms once daily, dose to be taken preferably at least 30 minutes before breakfast, caffeine-containing liquids (e.g. coffee, tea), or other medication

  Hyperthyroidism (blocking-replacement regimen) in combination with carbimazole
  ▸ BY MOUTH
  ▸ Adult: 50–150 micrograms daily therapy usually given for 18 months

- CONTRA-INDICATIONS Thyrotoxicosis

- CAUTIONS Cardiovascular disorders · diabetes insipidus · diabetes mellitus (dose of antidiabetic drugs including insulin may need to be increased) · elderly · hypertension · long-standing hypothyroidism · myocardial infarction · myocardial insufficiency · panhypopituitarism (initiate corticosteroid therapy before starting levothyroxine) · predisposition to adrenal insufficiency (initiate corticosteroid therapy before starting levothyroxine)

CAUTIONS, FURTHER INFORMATION
‣ Cardiovascular disorders Baseline ECG is valuable because changes induced by hypothyroidism can be confused with ischaemia.

● INTERACTIONS → Appendix 1 (thyroid hormones).

● SIDE-EFFECTS Anginal pain (usually at excessive dosage) · arrhythmias (usually at excessive dosage) · diarrhoea (usually at excessive dosage) · excitability (usually at excessive dosage) · fever · flushing · headache · heat intolerance · hypersensitivity reactions · insomnia (usually at excessive dosage) · muscle cramp · muscular weakness · oedema · palpitation (usually at excessive dosage) · pruritus · rash · restlessness (usually at excessive dosage) · sweating · tachycardia (usually at excessive dosage) · transient hair loss in children · tremor (usually at excessive dosage) · vomiting (usually at excessive dosage) · weight-loss

SIDE-EFFECTS, FURTHER INFORMATION
‣ Initial dosage in patients with cardiovascular disorders If metabolism increases too rapidly (causing diarrhoea, nervousness, rapid pulse, insomnia, tremors and sometimes anginal pain where there is latent myocardial ischaemia), reduce dose or withhold for 1–2 days and start again at a lower dose.

● PREGNANCY Levothyroxine requirement may increase during pregnancy. Levothyroxine may cross the placenta. Excessive or insufficient maternal thyroid hormones can be detrimental to fetus.

Assess maternal thyroid function before conception (if possible), at diagnosis of pregnancy, at antenatal booking, during both the second and third trimesters, and after delivery (more frequent monitoring required on initiation or adjustment of levothyroxine).

● BREAST FEEDING Amount too small to affect tests for neonatal hypothyroidism.

● MEDICINAL FORMS
There can be variation in the licensing of different medicines containing the same drug. Forms available from special-order manufacturers include: capsule, oral suspension, oral solution

Tablet
‣ Levothyroxine sodium (Non-proprietary)
Levothyroxine sodium anhydrous 25 microgram Levothyroxine sodium 25microgram tablets | 28 tablet [PoM] £4.00 DT price = £2.46 | 500 tablet [PoM] £56.25
Levothyroxine sodium 25microgram tablets lactose free | 100 tablet [PoM] no price available
Levothyroxine sodium anhydrous 50 microgram Levothyroxine sodium 50microgram tablets lactose free | 100 tablet [PoM] no price available
Levothyroxine sodium 50microgram tablets | 28 tablet [PoM] £3.00 DT price = £1.73 | 1000 tablet [PoM] £68.21
Levothyroxine sodium anhydrous 100 microgram Levothyroxine sodium 100microgram tablets lactose free | 100 tablet [PoM] no price available
Levothyroxine sodium 100microgram tablets | 28 tablet [PoM] £3.00 DT price = £1.73 | 1000 tablet [PoM] £68.57
‣ Eltroxin (AMCo)
Levothyroxine sodium anhydrous 25 microgram Eltroxin 25microgram tablets | 28 tablet [PoM] £2.54 DT price = £2.46
Levothyroxine sodium anhydrous 50 microgram Eltroxin 50microgram tablets | 28 tablet [PoM] £1.77 DT price = £1.73
Levothyroxine sodium anhydrous 100 microgram Eltroxin 100microgram tablets | 28 tablet [PoM] £1.78 DT price = £1.73

Capsule
‣ Levothyroxine sodium (Non-proprietary)
Levothyroxine sodium anhydrous 25 microgram Tirosint 25microgram capsules | 28 capsule [PoM] no price available
Levothyroxine sodium anhydrous 50 microgram Tirosint 50microgram capsules | 28 capsule [PoM] no price available
Levothyroxine sodium anhydrous 100 microgram Tirosint 100microgram capsules | 28 capsule [PoM] no price available

Oral solution
‣ Levothyroxine sodium (Non-proprietary)
Levothyroxine sodium anhydrous 5 microgram per 1 ml Levothyroxine sodium 25micrograms/5ml oral solution sugar free sugar-free | 100 ml [PoM] £95.00 DT price = £93.45
Levothyroxine sodium anhydrous 10 microgram per 1 ml Levothyroxine sodium 50micrograms/5ml oral solution sugar free sugar-free | 100 ml [PoM] £101.79 DT price = £97.52
Levothyroxine sodium anhydrous 20 microgram per 1 ml Levothyroxine sodium 100micrograms/5ml oral solution sugar free sugar-free | 100 ml [PoM] £165.00 DT price = £161.77

Liothyronine sodium
(L-Tri-iodothyronine sodium)

● INDICATIONS AND DOSE
Hypothyroidism
‣ BY MOUTH
‣ Adult: Initially 10–20 micrograms daily; increased to 60 micrograms daily in 2–3 divided doses, dose should be increased gradually, smaller initial doses given for the elderly

Hypothyroid coma
‣ BY SLOW INTRAVENOUS INJECTION
‣ Adult: 5–20 micrograms every 12 hours, increased to 5–20 micrograms every 4 hours if required, alternatively initially 50 micrograms for 1 dose, then 25 micrograms every 8 hours, reduced to 25 micrograms twice daily

DOSE EQUIVALENCE AND CONVERSION
20–25 micrograms of liothyronine sodium is equivalent to approximately 100 micrograms of levothyroxine sodium.
Brands without a UK licence may not be bioequivalent and dose adjustment may be necessary.

● CONTRA-INDICATIONS Thyrotoxicosis

● CAUTIONS Cardiovascular disorders · diabetes insipidus · diabetes mellitus (dose of antidiabetic drugs including insulin may need to be increased) · elderly · hypertension · long-standing hypothyroidism · myocardial infarction · myocardial insufficiency · panhypopituitarism (initiate corticosteroid therapy before starting liothyronine) · predisposition to adrenal insufficiency (initiate corticosteroid therapy before starting liothyronine)

CAUTIONS, FURTHER INFORMATION
‣ Cardiovascular disorders Baseline ECG is valuable because changes induced by hypothyroidism can be confused with ischaemia.

● INTERACTIONS → Appendix 1 (thyroid hormones).

● SIDE-EFFECTS Anginal pain (usually at excessive dosage) · arrhythmias (usually at excessive dosage) · diarrhoea (usually at excessive dosage) · excitability (usually at excessive dosage) · fever · flushing · headache · heat intolerance · hypersensitivity reactions · insomnia (usually at excessive dosage) · muscle cramp · muscular weakness · oedema · palpitation (usually at excessive dosage) · pruritus · rash · restlessness (usually at excessive dosage) · sweating · tachycardia (usually at excessive dosage) · tremor (usually at excessive dosage) · vomiting (usually at excessive dosage) · weight-loss

SIDE-EFFECTS, FURTHER INFORMATION
‣ Initial dosage in patients with cardiovascular disorders If metabolism increases too rapidly (causing diarrhoea, nervousness, rapid pulse, insomnia, tremors and sometimes anginal pain where there is latent myocardial ischaemia), reduce dose or withhold for 1–2 days and start again at a lower dose.

● PREGNANCY Liothyronine requirement may increase during pregnancy. Does not cross the placenta in

significant amounts. Excessive or insufficient maternal
thyroid hormones can be detrimental to fetus.

Assess maternal thyroid function before conception (if
possible), at diagnosis of pregnancy, at antenatal booking,
during both the second and third trimesters, and after
delivery (more frequent monitoring required on initiation
or adjustment of liothyronine).

● BREAST FEEDING Amount too small to affect tests for
neonatal hypothyroidism.

● PRESCRIBING AND DISPENSING INFORMATION
Switching to a different brand Patients switched to a different
brand should be monitored (particularly if pregnant or if
heart disease present) as brands without a UK licence may
not be bioequivalent. Pregnant women or those with heart
disease should undergo an early review of thyroid status,
and other patients should have thyroid function assessed if
experiencing a significant change in symptoms. If
liothyronine is continued long-term, thyroid function tests
should be repeated 1–2 months after any change in brand.

● MEDICINAL FORMS
There can be variation in the licensing of different medicines
containing the same drug. Forms available from special-order
manufacturers include: tablet, capsule, oral suspension, oral
solution, solution for injection

Tablet
▸ Liothyronine sodium (Non-proprietary)
   Liothyronine sodium 5 microgram Cytomel 5microgram tablets |
   100 tablet PoM no price available
   Liothyronine sodium 20 microgram Liothyronine 20microgram
   tablets | 28 tablet PoM £258.20 DT price = £258.20
   Liothyronine sodium 25 microgram Cytomel 25microgram tablets
   | 100 tablet PoM no price available

Powder for solution for injection
▸ Liothyronine sodium (Non-proprietary)
   Liothyronine sodium 20 microgram Liothyronine 20microgram
   powder for solution for injection vials | 5 vial PoM £1,425.00

Chapter 7
Genito-urinary system

CONTENTS

1 Bladder and urinary disorders

1.1 Urinary frequency, enuresis, and incontinence

Urinary frequency, enuresis and incontinence

Urinary frequency and incontinence

Incontinence in adults which arises from detrusor instability is managed by combining drug therapy with conservative methods for managing urge incontinence such as pelvic floor exercises and bladder training; stress incontinence is generally managed by non-drug methods. Duloxetine p. 336 can be added and is licensed for the treatment of moderate to severe stress incontinence in women; it may be more effective when used as an adjunct to pelvic floor exercises.

Antimuscarinic drugs reduce symptoms of urgency and urge incontinence and increase bladder capacity. Oxybutynin hydrochloride p. 704 also has a direct relaxant effect on urinary smooth muscle. Side-effects limit the use of oxybutynin hydrochloride, but they may be reduced by starting at a lower dose. A modified-release preparation of oxybutynin hydrochloride is effective and has fewer side-effects; a transdermal patch is also available. The efficacy and side-effects of tolterodine tartrate p. 706 are comparable to those of modified-release oxybutynin hydrochloride. Flavoxate hydrochloride p. 704 has less marked side-effects but it is also less effective. Darifenacin p. 703, fesoterodine fumarate p. 703, propiverine hydrochloride p. 706, solifenacin succinate p. 705, and trospium chloride p. 705 are newer antimuscarinic drugs licensed for urinary frequency, urgency, and incontinence. The need for continuing antimuscarinic drug therapy should be reviewed every 4–6 weeks until symptoms stabilise, and then every 6–12 months.

Propantheline bromide p. 78 and tricyclic antidepressants were used for urge incontinence but they are little used now because of their side-effects. The use of imipramine hydrochloride p. 345 is limited by its potential to cause cardiac side-effects.

Mirabegron p. 707, a selective beta$_3$ agonist, is licensed for the treatment of urinary frequency, urgency, and urge incontinence associated with overactive bladder syndrome.

Purified bovine collagen implant (*Contigen*®, Bard) is indicated for *urinary incontinence* caused by intrinsic sphincter deficiency (poor or non-functioning bladder outlet mechanism). The implant should be inserted only by surgeons or physicians trained in the technique for injection of the implant.

Nocturnal enuresis in children

Nocturnal enuresis is common in young children, but persists in a small proportion by 10 years of age. For children under 5 years, reassurance and advice on the management of nocturnal enuresis can be useful for some families. Treatment may be considered in children over 5 years depending on their maturity and motivation, the frequency of nocturnal enuresis, and the needs of the child and their family.

Initially, advice should be given on fluid intake, diet, toileting behaviour, and reward systems; for children who do not respond to this advice, further treatment may be necessary. An **enuresis alarm** should be first line treatment for motivated, well-supported children; alarms have a lower relapse rate than drug treatment when discontinued. Treatment should be reviewed after 4 weeks, and, if there are early signs of response, continued until a minimum of 2 weeks' uninterrupted dry nights have been achieved. If complete dryness is not achieved after 3 months, only continue if the condition is still improving and the child remains motivated to use the alarm. If initial alarm treatment is unsuccessful, consider combination treatment with **desmopressin p. 603**, or desmopressin alone if the alarm is no longer appropriate or desirable.

Desmopressin is given by oral or by sublingual administration. Desmopressin alone can be offered to children over 5 years of age if an alarm is inappropriate or undesirable, or when rapid or short-term results are the priority (for example to cover periods away from home); desmopressin alone can also be used if there has been a partial response to a combination of desmopressin and an alarm following initial treatment with an alarm. Treatment should be assessed after 4 weeks and continued for 3 months if there are signs of response. Desmopressin should be withdrawn at regular intervals (for 1 week every 3 months) for full reassessment. When stopping treatment with desmopressin, gradual withdrawal should be considered.

Nocturnal enuresis associated with daytime symptoms (overactive bladder) can be managed with antimuscarinic drugs (see Urinary incontinence) in combination with desmopressin. Treatment should be prescribed only after specialist assessment and should be continued for 3 months; the course can be repeated if necessary.

The tricyclic antidepressant imipramine hydrochloride may be considered for children who have not responded to all other treatments and have undergone specialist assessment, however, behavioural disturbances can occur and relapse is common after withdrawal. Treatment should not normally exceed 3 months unless a physical examination is made and the child is fully reassessed; toxicity following overdosage with tricyclics is of particular concern.

ANTIMUSCARINICS

Antimuscarinics (systemic)

- CONTRA-INDICATIONS Gastro-intestinal obstruction · intestinal atony · myasthenia gravis (but some antimuscarinics may be used to decrease muscarinic side-effects of anticholinesterases) · paralytic ileus · prostatic enlargement (in adults) · pyloric stenosis · severe ulcerative colitis · significant bladder outflow obstruction · toxic megacolon · urinary retention
- CAUTIONS Acute myocardial infarction (in adults) · arrhythmias (may be worsened) · autonomic neuropathy · cardiac insufficiency (due to association with tachycardia) · cardiac surgery (due to association with tachycardia) · children (increased risk of side-effects) (in children) · conditions characterised by tachycardia · congestive heart failure (may be worsened) · coronary artery disease (may be worsened) · diarrhoea · elderly (especially if frail) (in adults) · gastro-oesophageal reflux disease · hiatus hernia with reflux oesophagitis · hypertension · hyperthyroidism (due to association with tachycardia) · individuals susceptible to angle-closure glaucoma · prostatic hyperplasia (in adults) · pyrexia · ulcerative colitis
- INTERACTIONS → Appendix 1 (antimuscarinics). Many drugs have antimuscarinic effects; concomitant use of two or more such drugs can increase side-effects such as dry mouth, urine retention, and constipation. Concomitant use of other drugs with antimuscarinic effects can also lead to confusion in the elderly.
- SIDE-EFFECTS
- ▶ **Common or very common** Constipation · dilation of pupils with loss of accommodation · dry mouth · photophobia · reduced bronchial secretions · skin dryness · skin flushing · transient bradycardia (followed by tachycardia, palpitation and arrhythmias) · urinary retention · urinary urgency
- ▶ **Uncommon** Confusion (particularly in the elderly) · giddiness · nausea · vomiting
- ▶ **Very rare** Angle-closure glaucoma
- ▶ **Frequency not known** Angioedema · blurred vision · blurred vision · central nervous system stimulation · convulsion · diarrhoea · difficulty in micturition · disorientation · dizziness · drowsiness · dry eyes · euphoria · fatigue · flatulence · hallucinations · headache · impaired memory · palpitation · photosensitivity · rash · reduced sweating (may lead to heat sensations and fainting in hot environments or patients with fever) · restlessness · taste disturbances

- PATIENT AND CARER ADVICE
Driving and skilled tasks
Antimuscarinics can affect the performance of skilled tasks (e.g. driving).

ANTIMUSCARINICS > URINARY
◤ above

Darifenacin

- INDICATIONS AND DOSE
Urinary frequency | Urinary urgency | Incontinence
▶ BY MOUTH
▸ Adult: Initially 7.5 mg once daily, increased if necessary to 15 mg after 2 weeks

- SIDE-EFFECTS
- ▶ **Uncommon** Cough · dyspnoea · hypertension · impotence · insomnia · oedema · rhinitis · ulcerative stomatitis · vaginitis · weakness
- PREGNANCY Manufacturer advises avoid—toxicity in *animal* studies.
- BREAST FEEDING Present in milk in *animal* studies—manufacturer advises caution.
- HEPATIC IMPAIRMENT Max. 7.5 mg daily in moderate impairment. Avoid in severe impairment.
- PRESCRIBING AND DISPENSING INFORMATION The need for continuing therapy for urinary incontinence should be reviewed every 4–6 weeks until symptoms stabilise, and then every 6–12 months.

- MEDICINAL FORMS
There can be variation in the licensing of different medicines containing the same drug.
Modified-release tablet
CAUTIONARY AND ADVISORY LABELS 3, 25
▸ Darifenacin (Non-proprietary)
Darifenacin (as Darifenacin hydrobromide) 15 mg Darifenacin 15mg modified-release tablets | 28 tablet [PoM] no price available
▸ Emselex (Merus Labs Luxco S.a R.L.)
Darifenacin (as Darifenacin hydrobromide) 7.5 mg Emselex 7.5mg modified-release tablets | 28 tablet [PoM] £25.48 DT price = £25.48
Darifenacin (as Darifenacin hydrobromide) 15 mg Emselex 15mg modified-release tablets | 28 tablet [PoM] £25.48
◤ above

Fesoterodine fumarate

- INDICATIONS AND DOSE
Urinary frequency | Urinary urgency | Urge incontinence
▶ BY MOUTH
▸ Adult: 4 mg once daily, increased if necessary up to 8 mg once daily

DOSE ADJUSTMENTS DUE TO INTERACTIONS
Max. 4 mg daily with concomitant atazanavir, clarithromycin, indinavir, itraconazole, ritonavir, saquinavir, or telithromycin.
In patients with hepatic or renal impairment, consult product literature before concomitant use with amprenavir, aprepitant, atazanavir, clarithromycin, diltiazem, erythromycin, fluconazole, fosamprenavir, indinavir, itraconazole, ritonavir, saquinavir, telithromycin, verapamil, or grapefruit juice.

- SIDE-EFFECTS
- ▶ **Common or very common** Insomnia
- ▶ **Uncommon** Cough · nasal dryness · pharyngolaryngeal pain · vertigo
- PREGNANCY Manufacturer advises avoid—toxicity in *animal* studies.
- BREAST FEEDING Manufacturer advises avoid—no information available.

- HEPATIC IMPAIRMENT Manufacturer advises increase dose cautiously; max. 4 mg daily in moderate impairment. Avoid in severe impairment. Consult product literature before concomitant use of cytochrome P450 enzyme inhibitors.
- RENAL IMPAIRMENT Increase dose cautiously if eGFR 30–80 mL/minute/1.73m²; max. 4 mg daily if eGFR less than 30 mL/minute/1.73m². Consult product literature before concomitant use of cytochrome P450 enzyme inhibitors.
- PRESCRIBING AND DISPENSING INFORMATION The need for continuing therapy for urinary incontinence should be reviewed every 4–6 weeks until symptoms stabilise, and then every 6–12 months.
- NATIONAL FUNDING/ACCESS DECISIONS
Scottish Medicines Consortium (SMC) Decisions
The *Scottish Medicines Consortium* has advised (June 2008) that fesoterodine (*Toviaz* ®) is accepted for restricted use within NHS Scotland as a second-line treatment for overactive bladder syndrome.

- MEDICINAL FORMS
There can be variation in the licensing of different medicines containing the same drug.
Modified-release tablet
CAUTIONARY AND ADVISORY LABELS 3, 25
▸ Toviaz (Pfizer Ltd)
Fesoterodine fumarate 4 mg Toviaz 4mg modified-release tablets | 28 tablet [PoM] £25.78 DT price = £25.78
Fesoterodine fumarate 8 mg Toviaz 8mg modified-release tablets | 28 tablet [PoM] £25.78 DT price = £25.78

Flavoxate hydrochloride

▸ F 703

- INDICATIONS AND DOSE
Urinary frequency | Urinary incontinence | Dysuria | Urinary urgency | Bladder spasm due to catheterisation, cytoscopy, or surgery
▸ BY MOUTH
  ▸ Adult: 200 mg 3 times a day

- CONTRA-INDICATIONS Gastro-intestinal haemorrhage
- SIDE-EFFECTS Eosinophilia · erythema · leucopenia · pruritus · urticaria · vertigo
- PREGNANCY Manufacturer advises avoid unless no safer alternative.
- BREAST FEEDING Manufacturer advises caution—no information available.
- PRESCRIBING AND DISPENSING INFORMATION The need for continuing therapy for urinary incontinence should be reviewed every 4–6 weeks until symptoms stabilise, and then every 6–12 months.
- MEDICINAL FORMS
There can be variation in the licensing of different medicines containing the same drug. Forms available from special-order manufacturers include: oral suspension, oral solution
Tablet
CAUTIONARY AND ADVISORY LABELS 3
▸ Urispas (Recordati Pharmaceuticals Ltd)
Flavoxate hydrochloride 200 mg Urispas 200 tablets | 90 tablet [PoM] £11.67 DT price = £11.67

Oxybutynin hydrochloride

▸ F 703

- INDICATIONS AND DOSE
Urinary frequency | Urinary urgency | Urinary incontinence | Neurogenic bladder instability
▸ BY MOUTH USING IMMEDIATE-RELEASE MEDICINES
  ▸ Child 5–11 years: Initially 2.5–3 mg twice daily, increased to 5 mg 2–3 times a day
  ▸ Child 12–17 years: Initially 5 mg 2–3 times a day, increased if necessary up to 5 mg 4 times a day
  ▸ Adult: Initially 5 mg 2–3 times a day, increased if necessary up to 5 mg 4 times a day
  ▸ Elderly: Initially 2.5–3 mg twice daily, increased if tolerated to 5 mg twice daily, adjusted according to response
▸ BY MOUTH USING MODIFIED-RELEASE TABLETS
  ▸ Child 5–17 years: Initially 5 mg once daily, adjusted in steps of 5 mg every 1 week, adjusted according to response; maximum 15 mg per day
  ▸ Adult: Initially 5 mg once daily, increased in steps of 5 mg every 1 week, adjusted according to response; maximum 20 mg per day

Urinary frequency | Urinary urgency | Urinary incontinence
▸ BY TRANSDERMAL APPLICATION USING PATCHES
  ▸ Adult: Apply 1 patch twice weekly, patch is to be applied to clean, dry unbroken skin on abdomen, hip or buttock. Patch should be removed every 3–4 days and site replacement patch on a different area. The same area should be avoided for 7 days

Nocturnal enuresis associated with overactive bladder
▸ BY MOUTH USING IMMEDIATE-RELEASE MEDICINES
  ▸ Child 5–17 years: 2.5–3 mg twice daily, increased to 5 mg 2–3 times a day, last dose to be taken before bedtime
▸ BY MOUTH USING MODIFIED-RELEASE TABLETS
  ▸ Child 5–17 years: Initially 5 mg once daily, adjusted in steps of 5 mg every 1 week, adjusted according to response; maximum 15 mg per day

DOSE EQUIVALENCE AND CONVERSION
Patients taking immediate-release oxybutynin may be transferred to the nearest equivalent daily dose of *Lyrinel* ® XL

- UNLICENSED USE Not licensed for use in children under 5 years.
- CAUTIONS Acute porphyrias p. 918
- SIDE-EFFECTS
  GENERAL SIDE-EFFECTS
  ▸ **Uncommon** Anorexia · facial flushing
  ▸ **Rare** Night terrors
  ▸ **Frequency not known** Cognitive impairment (in adults)
  SPECIFIC SIDE-EFFECTS
  ▸ **Rare**
  ▸ With transdermal use Application site reactions with *patches*
- PREGNANCY Manufacturers advise avoid unless essential—toxicity in *animal* studies.
- BREAST FEEDING Manufacturers advise avoid—present in milk in *animal* studies.
- HEPATIC IMPAIRMENT Manufacturer advises caution.
- RENAL IMPAIRMENT Manufacturer advises caution.
- DIRECTIONS FOR ADMINISTRATION
  ▸ With transdermal use Apply patches to clean, dry, unbroken skin on abdomen, hip or buttock, remove after every 3–4 days and site replacement patch on a different area (avoid using same area for 7 days).

- PRESCRIBING AND DISPENSING INFORMATION
▸ In adults The need for continuing therapy for urinary incontinence should be reviewed every 4–6 weeks until symptoms stabilise, and then every 6–12 months.
▸ In children The need for therapy for urinary indications should be reviewed soon after it has been commenced and then at regular intervals; a response usually occurs within 6 months but may take longer.

- PATIENT AND CARER ADVICE
Medicines for Children leaflet: Oxybutynin for daytime urinary symptoms www.medicinesforchildren.org.uk/oxybutynin-for-daytime-urinary-symptoms
▸ With transdermal use Patients or carers should be given advice on how to administer oxybutynin transdermal patches.

- NATIONAL FUNDING/ACCESS DECISIONS
Scottish Medicines Consortium (SMC) Decisions
The *Scottish Medicines Consortium* has advised (July 2005) that *Kentera®* should be restricted for use in patients who benefit from oral oxybutynin but cannot tolerate its side-effects.

- MEDICINAL FORMS
There can be variation in the licensing of different medicines containing the same drug. Forms available from special-order manufacturers include: oral suspension, oral solution
Tablet
CAUTIONARY AND ADVISORY LABELS 3
▸ Oxybutynin hydrochloride (Non-proprietary)
Oxybutynin hydrochloride 2.5 mg Oxybutynin 2.5mg tablets | 56 tablet [PoM] £6.58 DT price = £1.44 | 84 tablet [PoM] £10.75
Oxybutynin hydrochloride 3 mg Oxybutynin 3mg tablets | 56 tablet [PoM] £16.80 DT price = £16.80
Oxybutynin hydrochloride 5 mg Oxybutynin 5mg tablets | 56 tablet [PoM] £14.00 DT price = £1.91 | 84 tablet [PoM] £20.77
▸ Cystrin (Zentiva)
Oxybutynin hydrochloride 5 mg Cystrin 5mg tablets | 84 tablet [PoM] £21.99
▸ Ditropan (Sanofi)
Oxybutynin hydrochloride 2.5 mg Ditropan 2.5mg tablets | 84 tablet [PoM] £1.60
Oxybutynin hydrochloride 5 mg Ditropan 5mg tablets | 84 tablet [PoM] £2.90
Modified-release tablet
CAUTIONARY AND ADVISORY LABELS 3, 25
▸ Lyrinel XL (Janssen-Cilag Ltd)
Oxybutynin hydrochloride 5 mg Lyrinel XL 5mg tablets | 30 tablet [PoM] £13.77 DT price = £13.77
Oxybutynin hydrochloride 10 mg Lyrinel XL 10mg tablets | 30 tablet [PoM] £27.54 DT price = £27.54
Oral solution
CAUTIONARY AND ADVISORY LABELS 3
▸ Oxybutynin hydrochloride (Non-proprietary)
Oxybutynin hydrochloride 500 microgram per 1 ml Oxybutynin 2.5mg/5ml oral solution sugar free sugar-free | 150 ml [PoM] £144.50–£167.40 DT price = £144.50
Oxybutynin hydrochloride 1 mg per 1 ml Oxybutynin 5mg/5ml oral solution sugar free sugar-free | 150 ml [PoM] £199.20–£234.36 DT price = £199.20
Transdermal patch
CAUTIONARY AND ADVISORY LABELS 3
▸ Kentera (Orion Pharma (UK) Ltd)
Oxybutynin 3.9 mg per 24 hour Kentera 3.9mg/24hours patches | 8 patch [PoM] £27.20 DT price = £27.20

F 703

Solifenacin succinate

- INDICATIONS AND DOSE
Urinary frequency | Urinary urgency | Urinary incontinence
▸ BY MOUTH
▸ Adult: 5 mg once daily, increased if necessary to 10 mg once daily

- DOSE ADJUSTMENTS DUE TO INTERACTIONS
Max. 5 mg daily with concomitant potent inhibitors of cytochrome P450 enzyme CYP3A4 (such as itraconazole, ketoconazole, or ritonavir).

- CONTRA-INDICATIONS Narrow-angle glaucoma
- CAUTIONS Neurogenic bladder disorder · susceptibility to QT-interval prolongation
- SIDE-EFFECTS
▸ **Uncommon** Gastro-oesophageal reflux · oedema
▸ **Frequency not known** Dysphonia · hepatic impairment · hyperkalaemia · muscle weakness · reduced appetite · torsade de pointes
- PREGNANCY Manufacturer advises caution—no information available.
- BREAST FEEDING Manufacturer advises avoid—present in milk in *animal* studies.
- HEPATIC IMPAIRMENT Max. 5 mg daily in moderate impairment. Avoid in moderate impairment in those already taking potent inhibitors of cytochrome P450 enzyme CYP3A4 (such as itraconazole, ketoconazole or ritonavir). Avoid in severe impairment.
- RENAL IMPAIRMENT Max. 5 mg daily if eGFR less than 30 mL/minute/1.73 m^2. Avoid if eGFR less than 30 mL/minute/1.73 m^2 in those already taking potent inhibitors of cytochrome P450 enzyme CYP3A4 (such as itraconazole, ketoconazole or ritonavir).
- PRESCRIBING AND DISPENSING INFORMATION The need for continuing therapy for urinary incontinence should be reviewed every 4–6 weeks until symptoms stabilise, and then every 6–12 months.

- MEDICINAL FORMS
There can be variation in the licensing of different medicines containing the same drug. Forms available from special-order manufacturers include: oral suspension, oral solution
Tablet
CAUTIONARY AND ADVISORY LABELS 3
▸ Vesicare (Astellas Pharma Ltd)
Solifenacin succinate 5 mg Vesicare 5mg tablets | 30 tablet [PoM] £27.62 DT price = £27.62
Solifenacin succinate 10 mg Vesicare 10mg tablets | 30 tablet [PoM] £35.91 DT price = £35.91

F 703

Trospium chloride

- INDICATIONS AND DOSE
Urinary frequency | Urinary urgency | Urinary incontinence
▸ BY MOUTH USING IMMEDIATE-RELEASE MEDICINES
▸ Adult: 20 mg twice daily, to be taken before food
▸ BY MOUTH USING MODIFIED-RELEASE MEDICINES
▸ Adult: 60 mg once daily

- SIDE-EFFECTS
▸ **Rare** Asthenia · chest pain · dyspnoea
▸ **Very rare** Arthralgia · myalgia
- PREGNANCY Manufacturer advises caution.
- BREAST FEEDING Manufacturer advises caution.
- HEPATIC IMPAIRMENT Manufacturer advises caution in mild to moderate impairment. Avoid in severe impairment.
- RENAL IMPAIRMENT Reduce dose to 20 mg once daily or 20 mg on alternate days if eGFR 10–30 mL/minute/1.73m^2. Use with caution. Avoid *Regurin® XL*.
- PRESCRIBING AND DISPENSING INFORMATION The need for continuing therapy for urinary incontinence should be reviewed every 4–6 weeks until symptoms stabilise, and then every 6–12 months.

7

Genito-urinary system

● MEDICINAL FORMS
There can be variation in the licensing of different medicines containing the same drug. Forms available from special-order manufacturers include: oral solution

Tablet
CAUTIONARY AND ADVISORY LABELS 23
▸ Trospium chloride (Non-proprietary)
  Trospium chloride 20 mg Trospium chloride 20mg tablets | 60 tablet PoM £26.00 DT price = £5.21
▸ Flotros (Galen Ltd)
  Trospium chloride 20 mg Flotros 20mg tablets | 60 tablet PoM £15.47 DT price = £5.21
▸ Regurin (Speciality European Pharma Ltd)
  Trospium chloride 20 mg Regurin 20mg tablets | 60 tablet PoM £26.00 DT price = £5.21
▸ Uraplex (Speciality European Pharma Ltd)
  Trospium chloride 20 mg Uraplex 20mg tablets | 60 tablet PoM £26.00 DT price = £5.21

Modified-release capsule
CAUTIONARY AND ADVISORY LABELS 23, 25
▸ Trospium chloride (Non-proprietary)
  Trospium chloride 60 mg Trospium chloride 60mg modified-release capsules | 28 capsule PoM no price available DT price = £23.05 | 30 capsule PoM no price available
▸ Regurin XL (Speciality European Pharma Ltd)
  Trospium chloride 60 mg Regurin XL 60mg capsules | 28 capsule PoM £23.05 DT price = £23.05

ANTIMUSCARINICS ⟩ OTHER

⌐ 703

Propiverine hydrochloride

● INDICATIONS AND DOSE
Urinary frequency, urgency and incontinence associated with overactive bladder
▸ BY MOUTH USING IMMEDIATE-RELEASE MEDICINES
▸ Adult: 15 mg 1–2 times a day, increased if necessary up to 15 mg 3 times a day
▸ BY MOUTH USING MODIFIED-RELEASE CAPSULES
▸ Adult: 30 mg once daily

Urinary frequency, urgency and incontinence associated with neurogenic bladder instability
▸ BY MOUTH USING IMMEDIATE-RELEASE MEDICINES
▸ Adult: 15 mg 3 times a day

● PREGNANCY Manufacturer advises avoid (restriction of skeletal development in *animals*).

● BREAST FEEDING Manufacturer advises avoid—present in milk in *animal* studies.

● HEPATIC IMPAIRMENT Avoid in moderate to severe impairment.

● RENAL IMPAIRMENT Max. daily dose 30 mg if eGFR less than 30 mL/minute/1.73m². Manufacturer advises caution in mild or moderate impairment.

● PRESCRIBING AND DISPENSING INFORMATION The need for continuing therapy for urinary incontinence should be reviewed every 4–6 weeks until symptoms stabilise, and then every 6–12 months.

● MEDICINAL FORMS
There can be variation in the licensing of different medicines containing the same drug.

Tablet
CAUTIONARY AND ADVISORY LABELS 3
▸ Detrunorm (AMCo)
  Propiverine hydrochloride 15 mg Detrunorm 15mg tablets | 56 tablet PoM £18.00 DT price = £18.00

Modified-release capsule
CAUTIONARY AND ADVISORY LABELS 3, 25
▸ Detrunorm XL (AMCo)
  Propiverine hydrochloride 30 mg Detrunorm XL 30mg capsules | 28 capsule PoM £24.45 DT price = £24.45
  Propiverine hydrochloride 45 mg Detrunorm XL 45mg capsules | 28 capsule PoM £27.00 DT price = £27.00

⌐ 703

Tolterodine tartrate

● INDICATIONS AND DOSE
Urinary frequency | Urinary urgency | Urinary incontinence
▸ BY MOUTH USING IMMEDIATE-RELEASE MEDICINES
▸ Adult: 2 mg twice daily, reduced if not tolerated to 1 mg twice daily
▸ BY MOUTH USING MODIFIED-RELEASE CAPSULES
▸ Adult: 4 mg once daily

DOSE EQUIVALENCE AND CONVERSION
Children stabilised on immediate-release tolterodine tartrate 2 mg twice daily may be transferred to modified-release tolterodine tartrate 4 mg once daily.

● CAUTIONS History of QT-interval prolongation

● INTERACTIONS Caution with concomitant use with other drugs known to prolong QT interval.

● SIDE-EFFECTS
▸ **Common or very common** Bronchitis · chest pain · fatigue · paraesthesia · peripheral oedema · sinusitis · vertigo · weight gain
▸ **Uncommon** Memory impairment
▸ **Frequency not known** Flushing

● PREGNANCY Manufacturer advises avoid—toxicity in *animal* studies.

● BREAST FEEDING Manufacturer advises avoid—no information available.

● HEPATIC IMPAIRMENT Reduce dose to 1 mg twice daily. Avoid modified-release preparations.

● RENAL IMPAIRMENT Reduce dose to 1 mg twice daily if eGFR less than 30 mL/minute/1.73m². Avoid modified-release preparations if eGFR less than 30 mL/minute/1.73m².

● PRESCRIBING AND DISPENSING INFORMATION The need for continuing therapy for urinary incontinence should be reviewed every 4–6 weeks until symptoms stabilise, and then every 6–12 months.

● MEDICINAL FORMS
There can be variation in the licensing of different medicines containing the same drug. Forms available from special-order manufacturers include: oral suspension, oral solution

Tablet
CAUTIONARY AND ADVISORY LABELS 3
▸ Tolterodine tartrate (Non-proprietary)
  Tolterodine tartrate 1 mg Tolterodine 1mg tablets | 56 tablet PoM £29.03 DT price = £1.95
  Tolterodine tartrate 2 mg Tolterodine 2mg tablets | 56 tablet PoM £30.56 DT price = £2.22
▸ Detrusitol (Pfizer Ltd)
  Tolterodine tartrate 1 mg Detrusitol 1mg tablets | 56 tablet PoM £29.03 DT price = £1.95
  Tolterodine tartrate 2 mg Detrusitol 2mg tablets | 56 tablet PoM £30.56 DT price = £2.22

Modified-release capsule
CAUTIONARY AND ADVISORY LABELS 3, 25
▸ Tolterodine tartrate (Non-proprietary)
  Tolterodine tartrate 2 mg Tolterodine 2mg modified-release capsules | 28 capsule PoM no price available
▸ Blerone XL (Zentiva)
  Tolterodine tartrate 4 mg Blerone XL 4mg capsules | 28 capsule PoM £25.78 DT price = £25.78
▸ Detrusitol XL (Pfizer Ltd)
  Tolterodine tartrate 4 mg Detrusitol XL 4mg capsules | 28 capsule PoM £25.78 DT price = £25.78
▸ Efflosomyl XL (Mylan Ltd)
  Tolterodine tartrate 4 mg Efflosomyl XL 4mg capsules | 28 capsule PoM £20.62 DT price = £25.78
▸ Inconex XL (Sandoz Ltd)
  Tolterodine tartrate 4 mg Inconex XL 4mg capsules | 28 capsule PoM £21.91 DT price = £25.78

▸ Mariosea XL (Teva UK Ltd)
Tolterodine tartrate 2 mg Mariosea XL 2mg capsules |
28 capsule [PoM] £11.59
Tolterodine tartrate 4 mg Mariosea XL 4mg capsules |
28 capsule [PoM] £12.88 DT price = £25.78
▸ Neditol XL (Aspire Pharma Ltd)
Tolterodine tartrate 2 mg Neditol XL 2mg capsules |
28 capsule [PoM] £11.60
Tolterodine tartrate 4 mg Neditol XL 4mg capsules |
28 capsule [PoM] £12.89 DT price = £25.78
▸ Preblacon XL (Actavis UK Ltd)
Tolterodine tartrate 4 mg Preblacon XL 4mg capsules |
28 capsule [PoM] £25.78 DT price = £25.78
▸ Santizor XL (Pfizer Ltd)
Tolterodine tartrate 4 mg Santizor XL 4mg capsules |
28 capsule [PoM] £25.78 DT price = £25.78

BETA₃-ADRENOCEPTOR AGONISTS

Mirabegron

● **INDICATIONS AND DOSE**
Urinary frequency, urgency, and urge incontinence
▸ BY MOUTH
▸ Adult: 50 mg once daily

● CONTRA-INDICATIONS Severe uncontrolled hypertension
(systolic blood pressure ≥180 mmHg or diastolic blood
pressure ≥110 mmHg)

● CAUTIONS History of QT-interval prolongation · stage 2
hypertension

● INTERACTIONS → Appendix 1 (mirabegron).
Caution with concomitant use with drugs that prolong the
QT interval.
▸ **Hepatic impairment**
With concomitant use of strong cytochrome P450
inhibitors such as itraconazole, ketoconazole, ritonavir, or
clarithromycin reduce dose to 25 mg once daily in mild
impairment, and avoid in moderate impairment.
▸ **Renal impairment**
With concomitant use of strong cytochrome P450
inhibitors such as itraconazole, ketoconazole, ritonavir, or
clarithromycin reduce dose to 25 mg once daily if eGFR
less than 30–89 mL/minute/1.73 m², and avoid if eGFR less
than 30 mL/minute/1.73 m².

● SIDE-EFFECTS
▸ **Common or very common** Tachycardia · urinary-tract
infection
▸ **Uncommon** Atrial fibrillation · dyspepsia · gastritis ·
hypertension · joint swelling · palpitation · pruritus · rash ·
vulvovaginal infection · vulvovaginal pruritus

● CONCEPTION AND CONTRACEPTION Contraception advised
in women of child-bearing potential.

● PREGNANCY Avoid—toxicity in *animal* studies.

● BREAST FEEDING Avoid—present in milk in *animal* studies.

● HEPATIC IMPAIRMENT Reduce dose to 25 mg once daily in
moderate impairment. Avoid in severe impairment—no
information available.

● RENAL IMPAIRMENT Reduce dose to 25 mg once daily if
eGFR 15–29 mL/minute/1.73 m². Avoid if eGFR less than
15 mL/minute/1.73 m²—no information available.

● MONITORING REQUIREMENTS Blood pressure should be
monitored before starting treatment and regularly during
treatment, especially in patients with pre-existing
hypertension.

● NATIONAL FUNDING/ACCESS DECISIONS
NICE technology appraisals (TAs)
▸ **Mirabegron for treating symptoms of overactive bladder (June
2013)** NICE TA290
Mirabegron is recommended as an option only for patients
in whom antimuscarinic drugs are ineffective, contra-

indicated, or not tolerated; patients currently receiving
mirabegron who do not meet these criteria should have the
option to continue until they and their clinician consider it
appropriate to stop.
www.nice.org.uk/TA290

● MEDICINAL FORMS
There can be variation in the licensing of different medicines
containing the same drug.
Modified-release tablet
CAUTIONARY AND ADVISORY LABELS 25
▸ Betmiga (Astellas Pharma Ltd) ▼
Mirabegron 25 mg Betmiga 25mg modified-release tablets |
30 tablet [PoM] £29.00 DT price = £29.00
Mirabegron 50 mg Betmiga 50mg modified-release tablets |
30 tablet [PoM] £29.00 DT price = £29.00

1.2 Urinary retention

Drugs for urinary retention

Overview

Acute retention is painful and is treated by catheterisation.
Chronic retention is painless and often long-standing.
Catheterisation is unnecessary unless there is deterioration
of renal function. After the cause has initially been
established and treated, drugs may be required to increase
detrusor muscle tone.
Benign prostatic hyperplasia is treated either surgically or
medically with alpha-blockers. Dutasteride p. 712 and
finasteride p. 712 are alternatives to alpha-blockers,
particularly in men with a significantly enlarged prostate.
Tadalafil p. 737, a phosphodiesterase type-5 inhibitor, may
also be used in the management of benign prostatic
hyperplasia.

Alpha-blockers

The alpha₁-selective alpha blockers, alfuzosin hydrochloride
below, doxazosin p. 708, indoramin p. 709, prazosin p. 709,
tamsulosin hydrochloride p. 710 and terazosin p. 711 relax
smooth muscle in benign prostatic hyperplasia producing an
increase in urinary flow-rate and an improvement in
obstructive symptoms.

Parasympathomimetics

The parasympathomimetic bethanechol chloride p. 712
increases detrusor muscle contraction. However, it has only
a limited role in the relief of urinary retention; its use has
been superseded by catheterisation.

ALPHA-ADRENOCEPTOR BLOCKERS

Alfuzosin hydrochloride

● **INDICATIONS AND DOSE**
Benign prostatic hyperplasia
▸ BY MOUTH USING IMMEDIATE-RELEASE MEDICINES
▸ Adult: 2.5 mg 3 times a day; maximum 10 mg per day
▸ Elderly: Initially 2.5 mg twice daily, adjusted according
to response; maximum 10 mg per day
▸ BY MOUTH USING MODIFIED-RELEASE MEDICINES
▸ Adult: 10 mg once daily

**Acute urinary retention associated with benign prostatic
hyperplasia**
▸ BY MOUTH USING MODIFIED-RELEASE TABLETS
▸ Elderly: 10 mg once daily for 2–3 days during
catheterisation and for one day after removal; max.
4 days

7

Genito-urinary system

- CONTRA-INDICATIONS Avoid if history micturition syncope · avoid if history of postural hypotension
- CAUTIONS Acute heart failure · concomitant antihypertensives (reduced dosage and specialist supervision may be required) · discontinue if angina worsens · elderly · history of QT-interval prolongation · patients undergoing cataract surgery (risk of intra-operative floppy iris syndrome)
- INTERACTIONS → Appendix 1 (alpha-blockers). Caution with concomitant use with other drugs known to prolong QT interval.
- SIDE-EFFECTS
- **Uncommon** Chest pain · flushes
- **Frequency not known** Angioedema · asthenia · blurred vision · cholestasis · depression · dizziness · drowsiness · dry mouth · erectile disorders (including priapism) · gastro-intestinal disturbances · headache · hypersensitivity · hypotension (notably postural hypotension) · intra-operative floppy iris syndrome · liver damage · oedema · palpitations · pruritus · rash · rhinitis · syncope · tachycardia

  SIDE-EFFECTS, FURTHER INFORMATION
- First dose effect First dose may cause collapse due to hypotensive effect (therefore should be taken on retiring to bed). Patient should be warned to lie down if symptoms such as dizziness, fatigue or sweating develop, and to remain lying down until they abate completely.
- HEPATIC IMPAIRMENT Initial dose 2.5 mg once daily, adjusted according to response to 2.5 mg twice daily in mild to moderate impairment—avoid if severe. Avoid modified-release preparations.
- RENAL IMPAIRMENT Initial dose 2.5 mg twice daily and adjust according to response. Manufacturers advise avoid use of modified-release preparations if eGFR less than 30 mL/minute/1.73 m^2 as limited experience.
- PATIENT AND CARER ADVICE
  Patient should be counselled on the first dose effect.

  Driving and skilled tasks
  May affect performance of skilled tasks e.g. driving.

- MEDICINAL FORMS
  There can be variation in the licensing of different medicines containing the same drug. Forms available from special-order manufacturers include: oral solution

Tablet
- Alfuzosin hydrochloride (Non-proprietary)
  Alfuzosin hydrochloride 2.5 mg Alfuzosin 2.5mg tablets | 60 tablet [PoM] £21.20 DT price = £2.32
- Xatral (Sanofi)
  Alfuzosin hydrochloride 2.5 mg Xatral 2.5mg tablets | 60 tablet [PoM] £20.37 DT price = £2.32

Modified-release tablet
CAUTIONARY AND ADVISORY LABELS 21, 25
- Alfuzosin hydrochloride (Non-proprietary)
  Alfuzosin hydrochloride 10 mg Alfuzosin 10mg modified-release tablets | 30 tablet [PoM] no price available DT price = £12.51
- Besavar XL (Zentiva)
  Alfuzosin hydrochloride 10 mg Besavar XL 10mg tablets | 30 tablet [PoM] £12.51 DT price = £12.51
- Fuzatal XL (Teva UK Ltd)
  Alfuzosin hydrochloride 10 mg Fuzatal XL 10mg tablets | 30 tablet [PoM] £12.76 DT price = £12.51
- Vasran XL (Ranbaxy (UK) Ltd)
  Alfuzosin hydrochloride 10 mg Vasran XL 10mg tablets | 30 tablet [PoM] £11.48 DT price = £12.51
- Xatral XL (Sanofi)
  Alfuzosin hydrochloride 10 mg Xatral XL 10mg tablets | 10 tablet [PoM] £4.17 | 30 tablet [PoM] £12.51 DT price = £12.51

Doxazosin

- INDICATIONS AND DOSE

Hypertension
- BY MOUTH USING IMMEDIATE-RELEASE MEDICINES
- Adult: Initially 1 mg once daily for 1–2 weeks, then increased to 2 mg once daily, then increased if necessary to 4 mg once daily; maximum 16 mg per day
- BY MOUTH USING MODIFIED-RELEASE MEDICINES
- Adult: Initially 4 mg once daily, dose can be adjusted after 4 weeks, then increased if necessary to 8 mg once daily

Benign prostatic hyperplasia
- BY MOUTH USING IMMEDIATE-RELEASE MEDICINES
- Adult: Initially 1 mg daily, dose may be doubled at intervals of 1–2 weeks according to response; usual maintenance 2–4 mg daily; maximum 8 mg per day
- BY MOUTH USING MODIFIED-RELEASE MEDICINES
- Adult: Initially 4 mg once daily, dose can be adjusted after 4 weeks, then increased if necessary to 8 mg once daily

DOSE ADJUSTMENTS DUE TO INTERACTIONS
Caution with concomitant antihypertensives in benign prostatic hyperplasia—reduced dosage and specialist supervision may be required.

DOSE EQUIVALENCE AND CONVERSION
Patients stabilised on immediate-release doxazosin can be transferred to the equivalent dose of modified-release doxazosin.

- CONTRA-INDICATIONS History of micturition syncope (in patients with benign prostatic hypertrophy) · history of postural hypotension · monotherapy in patients with overflow bladder or anuria
- CAUTIONS Care with initial dose (postural hypotension) · cataract surgery (risk of intra-operative floppy iris syndrome) · elderly · heart failure · pulmonary oedema due to aortic or mitral stenosis
- INTERACTIONS → Appendix 1 (alpha-blockers).
- SIDE-EFFECTS
- **Common or very common** Anxiety · back pain · coughing · dyspnoea · fatigue · influenza-like symptoms · myalgia · paraesthesia · sleep disturbance · vertigo
- **Uncommon** Agitation · angina · arthralgia · epistaxis · gout · hypoaesthesia · micturition disturbance · myocardial infarction · tinnitus · tremor · weight changes
- **Very rare** Abnormal ejaculation · alopecia · arrhythmias · bradycardia · bronchospasm · cholestasis · gynaecomastia · hepatitis · hot flushes · jaundice · leucopenia · thrombocytopenia
- **Frequency not known** Angioedema · asthenia · blurred vision · depression · dizziness · drowsiness · dry mouth · erectile disorders · gastro-intestinal disturbances · headache · hypersensitivity · hypotension · intra-operative floppy iris syndrome · oedema · palpitations · postural hypotension · priapism · pruritus · rash · rhinitis · syncope · tachycardia
- PREGNANCY No evidence of teratogenicity; manufacturers advise use only when potential benefit outweighs risk.
- BREAST FEEDING Accumulates in milk in *animal* studies—manufacturer advises avoid.
- HEPATIC IMPAIRMENT Use with caution. Manufacturer advises avoid in severe impairment—no information available.
- PATIENT AND CARER ADVICE
  Patient counselling is advised for doxazosin tablets (initial dose).

  Driving and skilled tasks
  May affect performance of skilled tasks e.g. driving.

● MEDICINAL FORMS
There can be variation in the licensing of different medicines containing the same drug. Forms available from special-order manufacturers include: capsule, oral suspension, oral solution

Tablet

▸ Doxazosin (Non-proprietary)
  Doxazosin (as Doxazosin mesilate) 1 mg Doxazosin 1mg tablets | 28 tablet [PoM] £10.56 DT price = £0.71
  Doxazosin (as Doxazosin mesilate) 2 mg Doxazosin 2mg tablets | 28 tablet [PoM] £14.08 DT price = £0.73
  Doxazosin (as Doxazosin mesilate) 4 mg Doxazosin 4mg tablets | 28 tablet [PoM] £14.08 DT price = £0.81

▸ Cardura (Pfizer Ltd)
  Doxazosin (as Doxazosin mesilate) 1 mg Cardura 1mg tablets | 28 tablet [PoM] £10.56 DT price = £0.71
  Doxazosin (as Doxazosin mesilate) 2 mg Cardura 2mg tablets | 28 tablet [PoM] £14.08 DT price = £0.73

▸ Doxadura (Discovery Pharmaceuticals)
  Doxazosin (as Doxazosin mesilate) 1 mg Doxadura 1mg tablets | 28 tablet [PoM] £0.71 DT price = £0.71
  Doxazosin (as Doxazosin mesilate) 2 mg Doxadura 2mg tablets | 28 tablet [PoM] £0.73 DT price = £0.73
  Doxazosin (as Doxazosin mesilate) 4 mg Doxadura 4mg tablets | 28 tablet [PoM] £0.80 DT price = £0.81

Modified-release tablet

CAUTIONARY AND ADVISORY LABELS   25

▸ Cardozin XL (Almus Pharmaceuticals Ltd)
  Doxazosin (as Doxazosin mesilate) 4 mg Cardozin XL 4mg tablets | 28 tablet [PoM] £6.33 DT price = £5.00

▸ Cardura XL (Pfizer Ltd)
  Doxazosin (as Doxazosin mesilate) 4 mg Cardura XL 4mg tablets | 28 tablet [PoM] £5.00 DT price = £5.00
  Doxazosin (as Doxazosin mesilate) 8 mg Cardura XL 8mg tablets | 28 tablet [PoM] £9.98 DT price = £9.98

▸ Doxadura XL (Discovery Pharmaceuticals)
  Doxazosin (as Doxazosin mesilate) 4 mg Doxadura XL 4mg tablets | 28 tablet [PoM] £4.50 DT price = £5.00

▸ Doxzogen XL (Mylan Ltd)
  Doxazosin (as Doxazosin mesilate) 4 mg Doxzogen XL 4mg tablets | 28 tablet [PoM] £5.70 DT price = £5.00

▸ Larbex XL (Teva UK Ltd)
  Doxazosin (as Doxazosin mesilate) 4 mg Larbex XL 4mg tablets | 28 tablet [PoM] £6.08 DT price = £5.00

▸ Raporsin XL (Actavis UK Ltd)
  Doxazosin (as Doxazosin mesilate) 4 mg Raporsin XL 4mg tablets | 28 tablet [PoM] £5.70 DT price = £5.00

▸ Slocinx XL (Zentiva)
  Doxazosin (as Doxazosin mesilate) 4 mg Slocinx XL 4mg tablets | 28 tablet [PoM] £5.96 DT price = £5.00

Indoramin

● INDICATIONS AND DOSE

Hypertension

▸ BY MOUTH
▸ **Adult:** Initially 25 mg twice daily, increased in steps of 25–50 mg every 2 weeks, maximum daily dose should be given in divided doses; maximum 200 mg per day

Benign prostatic hyperplasia

▸ BY MOUTH
▸ **Adult:** 20 mg twice daily, increased in steps of 20 mg every 2 weeks if required, increased if necessary up to 100 mg daily in divided doses
▸ **Elderly:** 20 mg daily may be adequate, dose to be taken at night

DOSE ADJUSTMENTS DUE TO INTERACTIONS
Caution with concomitant antihypertensives in benign prostatic hyperplasia—reduced dosage and specialist supervision may be required.

● CONTRA-INDICATIONS Established heart failure · history micturition syncope (when used for benign prostatic hyperplasia) · history of postural hypotension (when used for benign prostatic hyperplasia)

● CAUTIONS Cataract surgery (risk of intra-operative floppy iris syndrome) · control incipient heart failure before initiating indoramin · elderly · epilepsy (convulsions in *animal* studies) · history of depression · Parkinson's disease (extrapyramidal disorders reported)

● INTERACTIONS → Appendix 1 (alpha-blockers).
Avoid alcohol (enhances rate and extent of absorption).

● SIDE-EFFECTS
▸ **Common or very common** Sedation
▸ **Uncommon** Failure of ejaculation · fatigue · weight gain
▸ **Frequency not known** Angioedema · asthenia · blurred vision · depression · dizziness · drowsiness · dry mouth · erectile disorders · extrapyramidal disorders · gastro-intestinal disturbances · headache · hypersensitivity reactions · hypotension · incontinence · intra-operative floppy iris syndrome · oedema · palpitations · postural hypotension · priapism · pruritus · rash · rhinitis · syncope · tachycardia · urinary frequency

● PREGNANCY No evidence of teratogenicity; manufacturers advise use only when potential benefit outweighs risk.

● BREAST FEEDING No information available.

● HEPATIC IMPAIRMENT Manufacturer advises caution.

● RENAL IMPAIRMENT Manufacturer advises caution.

● PATIENT AND CARER ADVICE

Driving and skilled tasks
Drowsiness may affect performance of skilled tasks (e.g. driving); effects of alcohol may be enhanced.

● MEDICINAL FORMS
There can be variation in the licensing of different medicines containing the same drug.

Tablet

CAUTIONARY AND ADVISORY LABELS   2

▸ Indoramin (Non-proprietary)
  Indoramin hydrochloride 20 mg Indoramin 20mg tablets | 60 tablet [PoM] £13.30 DT price = £9.41
  Indoramin (as Indoramin hydrochloride) 25 mg Indoramin 25mg tablets | 84 tablet [PoM] £60.26 DT price = £60.26

▸ Doralese Tiltab (Chemidex Pharma Ltd)
  Indoramin hydrochloride 20 mg Doralese Tiltab 20mg tablets | 60 tablet [PoM] £11.44 DT price = £9.41

Prazosin

● INDICATIONS AND DOSE

Hypertension

▸ BY MOUTH
▸ **Adult:** Initially 500 micrograms 2–3 times a day for 3–7 days, the initial dose should be taken on retiring to bed at night to avoid collapse, increased to 1 mg 2–3 times a day for a further 3–7 days, then increased if necessary up to 20 mg daily in divided doses

Congestive heart failure (rarely used)

▸ BY MOUTH
▸ **Adult:** 500 micrograms 2–4 times a day, initial dose to be taken at bedtime, then increased to 4 mg daily in divided doses; maintenance 4–20 mg daily in divided doses

Raynaud's syndrome (but efficacy not established)

▸ BY MOUTH
▸ **Adult:** Initially 500 micrograms twice daily, initial dose to be taken at bedtime, dose may be increased after 3–7 days, then increased if necessary to 1–2 mg twice daily

Benign prostatic hyperplasia

▸ BY MOUTH
▸ **Adult:** Initially 500 micrograms twice daily for 3–7 days, subsequent doses should be adjusted according to response, maintenance 2 mg twice daily, initiate with lowest possible dose in elderly patients continued →

DOSE ADJUSTMENTS DUE TO INTERACTIONS
Caution with concomitant antihypertensives in benign prostatic hyperplasia—reduced dosage and specialist supervision may be required.

- **CONTRA-INDICATIONS** History of micturition syncope · history of postural hypotension · not recommended for congestive heart failure due to mechanical obstruction (e.g. aortic stenosis)
- **CAUTIONS** Cataract surgery (risk of intra-operative floppy iris syndrome) · elderly · first dose hypotension
- **INTERACTIONS** → Appendix 1 (alpha-blockers).
- **SIDE-EFFECTS**
  ▸ **Common or very common** Blurred vision · depression · dizziness · drowsiness · dry mouth · dyspnoea · gastro-intestinal disturbances · headache · nasal congestion · nervousness · oedema · palpitations · syncope · urinary frequency · vertigo · weakness
  ▸ **Uncommon** Arthralgia · epistaxis · eye disorders · insomnia · paraesthesia · pruritus · rash · sweating · tachycardia · tinnitus · urticaria
  ▸ **Rare** Alopecia · bradycardia · flushing · gynaecomastia · hallucinations · pancreatitis · priapism · urinary incontinence · vasculitis · worsening of narcolepsy
  ▸ **Frequency not known** Angioedema · asthenia · erectile disorders · hypersensitivity reactions · hypotension · intra-operative floppy iris syndrome · postural hypotension · rhinitis
- **PREGNANCY** No evidence of teratogenicity; manufacturers advise use only when potential benefit outweighs risk.
- **BREAST FEEDING** Present in milk, amount probably too small to be harmful; manufacturer advises use with caution.
- **HEPATIC IMPAIRMENT** Initially 500 micrograms daily; increased with caution.
- **RENAL IMPAIRMENT** Initially 500 micrograms daily in moderate to severe impairment; increased with caution.
- **PATIENT AND CARER ADVICE**
  Driving and skilled tasks
  May affect performance of skilled tasks e.g. driving. First dose effect First dose may cause collapse due to hypotensive effect (therefore should be taken on retiring to bed). Patients should be warned to lie down if symptoms such as dizziness, fatigue or sweating develop, and to remain lying down until they abate completely.

- **MEDICINAL FORMS**
  There can be variation in the licensing of different medicines containing the same drug. Forms available from special-order manufacturers include: tablet, oral suspension, oral solution
  Tablet
  ▸ Prazosin (Non-proprietary)
  Prazosin (as Prazosin hydrochloride) 2 mg Minipress 2mg tablets | 100 tablet [PoM] no price available
  Prazosin (as Prazosin hydrochloride) 5 mg Minipress 5mg tablets | 100 tablet [PoM] no price available
  ▸ Hypovase (Pfizer Ltd)
  Prazosin (as Prazosin hydrochloride) 500 microgram Hypovase 500microgram tablets | 60 tablet [PoM] £2.69 DT price = £2.69
  Prazosin (as Prazosin hydrochloride) 1 mg Hypovase 1mg tablets | 60 tablet [PoM] £3.46 DT price = £3.46

Tamsulosin hydrochloride

- **INDICATIONS AND DOSE**
  Benign prostatic hyperplasia
  ▸ BY MOUTH USING MODIFIED-RELEASE MEDICINES
  ▸ Adult: 400 micrograms once daily

- **CONTRA-INDICATIONS** History of micturition syncope · history of postural hypotension

- **CAUTIONS** Cataract surgery (risk of intra-operative floppy iris syndrome) · concomitant antihypertensives (reduced dosage and specialist supervision may be required) · elderly
- **INTERACTIONS** → Appendix 1 (alpha-blockers).
- **SIDE-EFFECTS** Angioedema · asthenia · blurred vision · depression · dizziness · drowsiness · dry mouth · erectile disorders · gastro-intestinal disturbances · headache · hypersensitivity reactions · hypotension (notably postural hypotension) · intra-operative floppy iris syndrome · oedema · palpitations · priapism · pruritus · rash · rhinitis · syncope · tachycardia
- **HEPATIC IMPAIRMENT** Avoid in severe impairment.
- **RENAL IMPAIRMENT** Use with caution if eGFR less than 10 mL/minute/1.73 m².
- **PATIENT AND CARER ADVICE**
  Driving and skilled tasks
  May affect performance of skilled tasks e.g. driving.
- **EXCEPTIONS TO LEGAL CATEGORY** Tamsulosin hydrochloride 400 microgram capsules can be sold to the public for the treatment of functional symptoms of benign prostatic hyperplasia in men aged 45–75 years to be taken for up to 6 weeks before clinical assessment by a doctor.

- **MEDICINAL FORMS**
  There can be variation in the licensing of different medicines containing the same drug.
  Modified-release tablet
  CAUTIONARY AND ADVISORY LABELS 25
  ▸ Tamsulosin hydrochloride (Non-proprietary)
  Tamsulosin hydrochloride 400 microgram Tamsulosin 400microgram modified-release tablets | 30 tablet [PoM] £10.47 DT price = £10.47
  ▸ Cositam XL (Consilient Health Ltd)
  Tamsulosin hydrochloride 400 microgram Cositam XL 400microgram tablets | 30 tablet [PoM] £8.89 DT price = £10.47
  ▸ Faramsil (Sandoz Ltd)
  Tamsulosin hydrochloride 400 microgram Faramsil 400microgram modified-release tablets | 30 tablet [PoM] £8.89 DT price = £10.47
  ▸ Flectone XL (Teva UK Ltd)
  Tamsulosin hydrochloride 400 microgram Flectone XL 400microgram tablets | 30 tablet [PoM] £9.95 DT price = £10.47
  ▸ Flomaxtra XL (Astellas Pharma Ltd)
  Tamsulosin hydrochloride 400 microgram Flomaxtra XL 400microgram tablets | 30 tablet [PoM] £10.47 DT price = £10.47
  Modified-release capsule
  CAUTIONARY AND ADVISORY LABELS 25
  ▸ Tamsulosin hydrochloride (Non-proprietary)
  Tamsulosin hydrochloride 400 microgram Tamsulosin 400microgram modified-release capsules | 30 capsule [PoM] £5.07 DT price = £4.05
  ▸ Contiflo XL (Ranbaxy (UK) Ltd)
  Tamsulosin hydrochloride 400 microgram Contiflo XL 400microgram capsules | 30 capsule [PoM] £7.44 DT price = £4.05
  ▸ Diffundox XL (Zentiva)
  Tamsulosin hydrochloride 400 microgram Diffundox XL 400microgram capsules | 30 capsule [PoM] £9.55 DT price = £4.05
  ▸ Flomax MR (Boehringer Ingelheim Self-Medication Division)
  Tamsulosin hydrochloride 400 microgram Flomax Relief MR 400microgram capsules | 14 capsule [P] £5.58 | 28 capsule [P] £10.55
  ▸ Galebon (Consilient Health Ltd)
  Tamsulosin hydrochloride 400 microgram Galebon 400microgram modified-release capsules | 30 capsule [PoM] £3.78 DT price = £4.05
  ▸ Losinate MR (Aspire Pharma Ltd)
  Tamsulosin hydrochloride 400 microgram Losinate MR 400microgram capsules | 30 capsule [PoM] £10.14 DT price = £4.05
  ▸ Pamsvax XL (Almus Pharmaceuticals Ltd, Actavis UK Ltd)
  Tamsulosin hydrochloride 400 microgram Pamsvax XL 400microgram capsules | 30 capsule [PoM] £1.28–£4.42 DT price = £4.05
  ▸ Petyme MR (Teva UK Ltd)
  Tamsulosin hydrochloride 400 microgram Petyme 400microgram MR capsules | 30 capsule [PoM] £4.06 DT price = £4.05

‣ Pinexel PR (Wockhardt UK Ltd)
Tamsulosin hydrochloride 400 microgram Pinexel PR
400microgram capsules | 30 capsule [PoM] £2.50 DT price = £4.05
‣ Prosurin XL (Mylan Ltd)
Tamsulosin hydrochloride 400 microgram Prosurin XL
400microgram capsules | 30 capsule [PoM] £4.28 DT price = £4.05
‣ Tabphyn MR (ProStrakan Ltd)
Tamsulosin hydrochloride 400 microgram Tabphyn MR
400microgram capsules | 30 capsule [PoM] £4.39 DT price = £4.05
‣ Tamfrex XL (Milpharm Ltd)
Tamsulosin hydrochloride 400 microgram Tamfrex XL
400microgram capsules | 30 capsule [PoM] no price available DT price
= £4.05
‣ Tamurex (Somex Pharma)
Tamsulosin hydrochloride 400 microgram Tamurex
400microgram modified-release capsules | 30 capsule [PoM] £3.50 DT
price = £4.05

Tamsulosin with dutasteride

The properties listed below are those particular to the
combination only. For the properties of the components
please consider, tamsulosin hydrochloride p. 710,
dutasteride p. 712.

● INDICATIONS AND DOSE

Benign prostatic hyperplasia
▶ BY MOUTH
▶ Adult (male): 1 capsule daily.

● PATIENT AND CARER ADVICE

Driving and skilled tasks
May affect performance of skilled tasks e.g. driving.

● MEDICINAL FORMS
There can be variation in the licensing of different medicines
containing the same drug.
Capsule
CAUTIONARY AND ADVISORY LABELS 25
‣ Combodart (GlaxoSmithKline UK Ltd)
**Tamsulosin hydrochloride 400 microgram, Dutasteride
500 microgram** Combodart 0.5mg/0.4mg capsules |
30 capsule [PoM] £19.80 DT price = £19.80

Tamsulosin with solifenacin

The properties listed below are those particular to the
combination only. For the properties of the components
please consider, tamsulosin hydrochloride p. 710, solifenacin
succinate p. 705.

● INDICATIONS AND DOSE

**Moderate to severe urinary frequency, urgency, and
obstructive symptoms associated with benign prostatic
hyperplasia when monotherapy ineffective**
▶ BY MOUTH
▶ Adult (male): 1 tablet daily.
DOSE ADJUSTMENTS DUE TO INTERACTIONS
Max. 1 *Vesomni*® tablet daily with concomitant potent
inhibitors of cytochrome P450 enzyme CYP3A4 (such as
itraconazole, ketoconazole, or ritonavir).

● HEPATIC IMPAIRMENT Max. 1 *Vesomni*® tablet daily in
moderate impairment.
● RENAL IMPAIRMENT Max. 1 *Vesomni*® tablet daily if eGFR
less than 30 mL/minute/1.73 m².

● MEDICINAL FORMS
There can be variation in the licensing of different medicines
containing the same drug.
Modified-release tablet
CAUTIONARY AND ADVISORY LABELS 3, 25
‣ Vesomni (Astellas Pharma Ltd)
**Tamsulosin hydrochloride 400 microgram, Solifenacin succinate
6 mg** Vesomni 6mg/0.4mg modified-release tablets | 30 tablet [PoM]
£27.62 DT price = £27.62

Terazosin

● INDICATIONS AND DOSE

Mild to moderate hypertension
▶ BY MOUTH
▶ Adult: 1 mg daily for 7 days, then increased if necessary
to 2 mg daily, dose should be taken at bedtime;
maintenance 2–10 mg once daily, doses above 20 mg
rarely improve efficacy
Benign prostatic hyperplasia
▶ BY MOUTH
▶ Adult: Initially 1 mg daily, dose should be taken at
bedtime, if necessary dose may be doubled at intervals
of 1–2 weeks according to response; maintenance
5–10 mg daily; maximum 10 mg per day

● CONTRA-INDICATIONS History of micturition syncope (in
benign prostatic hyperplasia) · history of postural
hypotension (in benign prostatic hyperplasia)
● CAUTIONS Cataract surgery (risk of intra-operative floppy
iris syndrome) · elderly · first dose
CAUTIONS, FURTHER INFORMATION
▶ First dose First dose may cause collapse due to hypotension
within 30–90 minutes, therefore should be taken on
retiring to bed; may also occur with rapid dose increase.
● INTERACTIONS → Appendix 1 (alpha-blockers).
● SIDE-EFFECTS Angioedema · asthenia · back pain · blurred
vision · decreased libido · depression · dizziness ·
drowsiness · dry mouth · dyspnoea · erectile disorders ·
gastro-intestinal disturbances · headache · hypersensitivity
reactions · hypotension · intra-operative floppy iris
syndrome · nervousness · oedema · pain in extremities ·
palpitations · paraesthesia · postural hypotension ·
priapism · pruritus · rash · rhinitis · syncope · tachycardia ·
thrombocytopenia · weight gain
● PREGNANCY No evidence of teratogenicity; manufacturers
advise use only when potential benefit outweighs risk.
● BREAST FEEDING No information available.
● PATIENT AND CARER ADVICE
Patient counselling is advised for terazosin tablets (initial
dose).
First dose effect First dose may cause collapse due to
hypotensive effect (therefore should be taken on retiring
to bed). Patient should be warned to lie down if symptoms
such as dizziness, fatigue or sweating develop, and to
remain lying down until they abate completely.

Driving and skilled tasks
May affect performance of skilled tasks e.g. driving.

● MEDICINAL FORMS
There can be variation in the licensing of different medicines
containing the same drug.
Tablet
▶ Terazosin (Non-proprietary)
Terazosin (as Terazosin hydrochloride) 2 mg Terazosin 2mg
tablets | 28 tablet [PoM] £2.70 DT price = £2.20
Terazosin (as Terazosin hydrochloride) 5 mg Terazosin 5mg
tablets | 28 tablet [PoM] £3.34 DT price = £2.60
Terazosin (as Terazosin hydrochloride) 10 mg Terazosin 10mg
tablets | 28 tablet [PoM] £8.11 DT price = £7.87

- Hytrin (AMCo)
  Terazosin (as Terazosin hydrochloride) 1 mg Hytrin 1mg tablets |
  7 tablet PoM no price available
  Terazosin (as Terazosin hydrochloride) 2 mg Hytrin 2mg tablets |
  14 tablet PoM no price available | 21 tablet PoM no price available
  | 28 tablet PoM £2.20 DT price = £2.20
  Terazosin (as Terazosin hydrochloride) 5 mg Hytrin 5mg tablets |
  7 tablet PoM no price available | 28 tablet PoM £4.13 DT price =
  £2.60
  Terazosin (as Terazosin hydrochloride) 10 mg Hytrin 10mg tablets
  | 28 tablet PoM £7.87 DT price = £7.87
- Hytrin (AMCo)
  Hytrin BPH tablets starter pack | 28 tablet PoM £10.97
  Hytrin tablets starter pack | 28 tablet PoM £13.00

CHOLINE ESTERS

Bethanechol chloride

- **INDICATIONS AND DOSE**
  Urinary retention
  ▶ BY MOUTH
  ▶ Adult: 10–25 mg 3–4 times a day, to be taken
    30 minutes before food

- **CONTRA-INDICATIONS** Bradycardia · cardiovascular
  disorders · conditions where increased motility of the
  gastro-intestinal tract could be harmful · conditions where
  increased motility of the urinary tract could be harmful ·
  epilepsy · heart block · hyperthyroidism · hypotension ·
  intestinal obstruction · obstructive airways disease ·
  parkinsonism · peptic ulcer · recent myocardial infarction ·
  urinary obstruction
- **CAUTIONS** Autonomic neuropathy (use lower initial dose)
- **INTERACTIONS** → Appendix 1 (parasympathomimetics).
- **SIDE-EFFECTS** Abdominal pain · bradycardia ·
  bronchoconstriction · diarrhoea · eructation · flushing ·
  headache · hypotension · increased lacrimation · increased
  salivation · increased sweating · nausea · rhinorrhoea ·
  vomiting
- **PREGNANCY** Manufacturer advises avoid—no information
  available.
- **BREAST FEEDING** Manufacturer advises avoid;
  gastrointestinal disturbances in infant reported.
- **LESS SUITABLE FOR PRESCRIBING** Less suitable for
  prescribing.

- **MEDICINAL FORMS**
  There can be variation in the licensing of different medicines
  containing the same drug. Forms available from special-order
  manufacturers include: oral suspension, oral solution
  Tablet
  CAUTIONARY AND ADVISORY LABELS 22
  ▶ Myotonine (Cheplapharm Arzneimittel GmbH)
    Bethanechol chloride 10 mg Myotonine 10mg tablets |
    100 tablet PoM £18.51
    Bethanechol chloride 25 mg Myotonine 25mg tablets |
    100 tablet PoM £27.26

5α-REDUCTASE INHIBITORS

Dutasteride

- **DRUG ACTION** A specific inhibitor of the enzyme 5α-
  reductase, which metabolises testosterone into the more
  potent androgen, dihydrotestosterone.

- **INDICATIONS AND DOSE**
  Benign prostatic hyperplasia
  ▶ BY MOUTH
  ▶ Adult: 500 micrograms daily, review treatment at
    3–6 months and then every 6–12 months (may require
    several months treatment before benefit is obtained)

- **INTERACTIONS** → Appendix 1 (dutasteride).
- **SIDE-EFFECTS** Breast enlargement · breast tenderness ·
  decreased libido · ejaculation disorders · impotence
- **CONCEPTION AND CONTRACEPTION** Dutasteride is excreted
  in semen and use of a condom is recommended if sexual
  partner is pregnant or likely to become pregnant.
- **HEPATIC IMPAIRMENT** Avoid in severe impairment—no
  information available.
- **EFFECT ON LABORATORY TESTS** May decrease serum
  concentration of prostate cancer markers such as prostate-
  specific antigen; reference values may need adjustment.
- **HANDLING AND STORAGE** Women of childbearing potential
  should avoid handling leaking capsules of dutasteride.
- **PATIENT AND CARER ADVICE** Cases of male breast cancer
  have been reported. Patients or their carers should be told
  to promptly report to their doctor any changes in breast
  tissue such as lumps, pain, or nipple discharge.

- **MEDICINAL FORMS**
  There can be variation in the licensing of different medicines
  containing the same drug. Forms available from special-order
  manufacturers include: oral solution
  Capsule
  CAUTIONARY AND ADVISORY LABELS 25
  ▶ Avodart (GlaxoSmithKline UK Ltd)
    Dutasteride 500 microgram Avodart 500microgram capsules |
    30 capsule PoM £14.60 DT price = £14.60

  Combinations available: *Tamsulosin with dutasteride*, p. 711

Finasteride

- **DRUG ACTION** A specific inhibitor of the enzyme 5α-
  reductase, which metabolises testosterone into the more
  potent androgen, dihydrotestosterone.

- **INDICATIONS AND DOSE**
  Benign prostatic hyperplasia
  ▶ BY MOUTH
  ▶ Adult: 5 mg daily, review treatment at 3–6 months and
    then every 6–12 months (may require several months
    treatment before benefit is obtained)
  Androgenetic alopecia in men
  ▶ BY MOUTH
  ▶ Adult: 1 mg daily

- **CAUTIONS** Obstructive uropathy
- **SIDE-EFFECTS** Breast enlargement · breast tenderness ·
  decreased libido · ejaculation disorders · face swelling ·
  hypersensitivity reactions · impotence · lip swelling · male
  breast cancer · pruritus · rash · testicular pain
- **CONCEPTION AND CONTRACEPTION** Finasteride is excreted
  in semen and use of a condom is recommended if sexual
  partner is pregnant or likely to become pregnant.
- **EFFECT ON LABORATORY TESTS** Decreases serum
  concentration of prostate cancer markers such as prostate-
  specific antigen; reference values may need adjustment.
- **HANDLING AND STORAGE** Women of childbearing potential
  should avoid handling crushed or broken tablets of
  finasteride.
- **PATIENT AND CARER ADVICE** Cases of male breast cancer
  have been reported. Patients or their carers should be told
  to promptly report to their doctor any changes in breast
  tissue such as lumps, pain, or nipple discharge.
- **NATIONAL FUNDING/ACCESS DECISIONS**
  NHS restrictions Finasteride is not prescribable under the
  NHS for the treatment of androgenetic alopecia in men.

● MEDICINAL FORMS
There can be variation in the licensing of different medicines containing the same drug. Forms available from special-order manufacturers include: oral suspension

Tablet

▸ Finasteride (Non-proprietary)
Finasteride 1 mg Finasteride 1mg tablets | 28 tablet [PoM] no price available
Finasteride 5 mg Finasteride 5mg tablets | 28 tablet [PoM] £11.85 DT price = £1.15

▸ Aindeem (Actavis UK Ltd)
Finasteride 1 mg Aindeem 1mg tablet | 28 tablet [PoM] £33.68 | 84 tablet [PoM] £88.40

▸ Propecia (Merck Sharp & Dohme Ltd)
Finasteride 1 mg Propecia 1mg tablets | 28 tablet [PoM] £33.68 | 84 tablet [PoM] £88.40

▸ Proscar (Merck Sharp & Dohme Ltd)
Finasteride 5 mg Proscar 5mg tablets | 28 tablet [PoM] £13.94 DT price = £1.15

1.3 Urological pain

Urological pain

Treatment

The acute pain of *ureteric colic* may be relieved with pethidine hydrochloride p. 426. **Diclofenac** by injection or as suppositories is also effective and compares favourably with pethidine hydrochloride; other non-steroidal anti-inflammatory drugs are occasionally given by injection.

Lidocaine hydrochloride **gel** p. 1187 is a useful topical application in *urethral pain* or to relieve the discomfort of catheterisation.

Alkalinisation of urine

Alkalinisation of urine can be undertaken with potassium citrate. The alkalinising action may relieve the discomfort of *cystitis* caused by lower urinary tract infections. Sodium bicarbonate p. 898 is used as a urinary alkalinising agent in some metabolic and renal disorders.

ALKALISING DRUGS

Citric acid with potassium citrate

● INDICATIONS AND DOSE

Relief of discomfort in mild urinary-tract infections | Alkalinisation of urine

▸ BY MOUTH USING ORAL SOLUTION
▸ Adult: 10 mL 3 times a day, diluted well with water

● CAUTIONS Cardiac disease · elderly

● INTERACTIONS → Appendix 1 (potassium salts).

● SIDE-EFFECTS Hyperkalaemia on prolonged high dosage · mild diuresis

● RENAL IMPAIRMENT Avoid in severe impairment. Close monitoring required in renal impairment—high risk of hyperkalaemia.

● PRESCRIBING AND DISPENSING INFORMATION When prepared extemporaneously, the BP states Potassium Citrate Mixture BP consists of potassium citrate 30%, citric acid monohydrate 5% in a suitable vehicle with a lemon flavour. Extemporaneous preparations should be recently prepared according to the following formula: potassium citrate 3 g, citric acid monohydrate 500 mg, syrup 2.5 mL, quillaia tincture 0.1 mL, lemon spirit 0.05 mL, double-strength chloroform water 3 mL, water to 10 mL. Contains about 28 mmol K$^+$/10 mL.

● EXCEPTIONS TO LEGAL CATEGORY Proprietary brands of potassium citrate are on sale to the public for the relief of discomfort in mild urinary-tract infections.

● MEDICINAL FORMS
There can be variation in the licensing of different medicines containing the same drug.

Oral solution
CAUTIONARY AND ADVISORY LABELS 27

▸ Citric acid with potassium citrate (Non-proprietary)
Citric acid monohydrate 50 mg per 1 ml, Potassium citrate 300 mg per 1 ml Potassium citrate mixture | 200 ml [GSL] £1.33 DT price = £1.33 | 200 ml [P] £1.33 DT price = £1.33

Sodium citrate

● INDICATIONS AND DOSE

Bladder washouts
▸ Adult: (consult product literature)

Relief of discomfort in mild urinary-tract infections
▸ BY MOUTH
▸ Adult: (consult product literature)

MICOLETTE®

Constipation
▸ BY RECTUM
▸ Child 3–17 years: 5–10 mL for 1 dose
▸ Adult: 5–10 mL for 1 dose

MICRALAX®

Constipation
▸ BY RECTUM
▸ Child 3–17 years: 5 mL for 1 dose
▸ Adult: 5 mL for 1 dose

RELAXIT®

Constipation
▸ BY RECTUM
▸ Child 1 month–2 years: 5 mL for 1 dose, insert only half the nozzle length
▸ Child 3–17 years: 5 mL for 1 dose
▸ Adult: 5 mL for 1 dose

● CONTRA-INDICATIONS
▸ With rectal use Acute gastro-intestinal conditions

● CAUTIONS
▸ With oral use Cardiac disease · elderly · hypertension · patients on a sodium-restricted diet
▸ With rectal use Debilitated patients (in adults) · sodium and water retention in susceptible individuals

● INTERACTIONS
▸ With oral use → Appendix 1 (sodium citrate).

● SIDE-EFFECTS
▸ With oral use Mild diuresis

● PREGNANCY
▸ With oral use Use with caution.

● RENAL IMPAIRMENT
▸ With oral use In patients with fluid retention, avoid preparations containing large amounts of sodium.

● PRESCRIBING AND DISPENSING INFORMATION Sodium citrate 300 mmol/litre (88.2 mg/mL) oral solution is licensed for use before general anaesthesia for caesarean section (available from Viridian).

● EXCEPTIONS TO LEGAL CATEGORY Proprietary brands of sodium citrate are on sale to the public for the relief of discomfort in mild urinary-tract infections.

7

Genito-urinary system

- MEDICINAL FORMS
There can be variation in the licensing of different medicines
containing the same drug. Forms available from special-order
manufacturers include: oral solution
Granules
▸ Sodium citrate (Non-proprietary)
  Sodium citrate 4 gram Cystitis Relief 4g oral granules sachets |
  6 sachet GSL £2.33
▸ Brands may include Cymalon (sodium citrate), Cystocalm
Oral solution
▸ Sodium citrate (Non-proprietary)
  Sodium citrate 88.23 mg per 1 ml Sodium citrate 0.3M oral solution
  | 30 ml PoM £39.60
  Sodium citrate 441.17mg/5ml oral solution | 30 ml PoM no price
  available
Enema
▸ Micolette Micro-enema (Pinewood Healthcare)
  Sodium citrate 90 mg per 1 ml Micolette Micro-enema 5ml |
  12 enema P £3.40
▸ Micralax Micro-enema (Focus Pharmaceuticals Ltd)
  Sodium citrate 90 mg per 1 ml Micralax Micro-enema 5ml |
  12 enema P £4.87
▸ Relaxit (Supra Enterprises Ltd)
  Sodium citrate 90 mg per 1 ml Relaxit Micro-enema 5ml |
  12 enema P £5.21
Irrigation solution
▸ Sodium citrate (Non-proprietary)
  Sodium citrate 3% irrigation solution 1litre bags | 1 bag no price
  available
Powder
▸ Sodium citrate (Non-proprietary)
  Sodium citrate 1 mg per 1 mg Sodium citrate powder |
  500 gram GSL £5.28 DT price = £5.28

TERPENES

Anethol with borneol, camphene, cineole, fenchone and pinene

- INDICATIONS AND DOSE
Urolithiasis for the expulsion of calculi
▸ BY MOUTH
▸ Adult: 1–2 capsules 3–4 times a day, to be taken before
  food

- LESS SUITABLE FOR PRESCRIBING Preparation is less
suitable for prescribing.

- MEDICINAL FORMS
There can be variation in the licensing of different medicines
containing the same drug.
Capsule
CAUTIONARY AND ADVISORY LABELS 25
▸ Rowatinex (Meadow Laboratories Ltd)
  **Cineole 3 mg, Anethol 4 mg, Fenchone 4 mg, Borneol 10 mg,
  Camphene 15 mg, Pinene 31 mg** Rowatinex capsules |
  50 capsule PoM £7.35

2 Bladder instillations and urological surgery

Bladder instillations and urological surgery

Bladder infection

Various solutions are available as irrigations or washouts.
  Aqueous chlorhexidine p. 1053 can be used in the
management of common infections of the bladder but it is
ineffective against most *Pseudomonas spp*. Solutions
containing chlorhexidine 1 in 5000 (0.02%) are used but they
may irritate the mucosa and cause burning and haematuria
(in which case they should be discontinued); sterile sodium
chloride **solution 0.9%** p. 901 (physiological saline) is
usually adequate and is preferred as a mechanical irrigant.
  Continuous bladder irrigation with amphotericin
50 micrograms/mL p. 539 may be of value in mycotic
infections in adults.

Dissolution of blood clots

Clot retention is usually treated by irrigation with sterile
sodium chloride solution 0.9% but sterile sodium citrate
solution for bladder irrigation 3% p. 713 may also be helpful.

Bladder cancer

Bladder instillations of doxorubicin hydrochloride p. 798 and
mitomycin p. 812 are used for recurrent superficial bladder
tumours. Such instillations reduce systemic side-effects;
adverse effects on the bladder (e.g. micturition disorders and
reduction in bladder capacity) may occur.
  Instillation of epirubicin hydrochloride p. 799 is used for
treatment and prophylaxis of certain forms of superficial
bladder cancer; instillation of doxorubicin hydrochloride is
also used for some papillary tumours.
  Instillation of **BCG** (bacillus calmette-guérin p. 841), a live
attenuated strain derived from *Mycobacterium bovis* is
licensed for the treatment of primary or recurrent bladder
carcinoma *in-situ* and for the prevention of recurrence
following transurethral resection.

Urological surgery

Glycine irrigation solution 1.5% p. 715 is the irrigant of
choice for transurethral resection of the prostate gland and
bladder tumours; sterile sodium chloride solution 0.9%
(physiological saline) is used for percutaneous renal surgery.

Maintenance of indwelling urinary catheters

The deposition which occurs in catheterised patients is
usually chiefly composed of phosphate and to minimise this
the catheter (if latex) should be changed at least as often as
every 6 weeks. If the catheter is to be left for longer periods a
silicone catheter should be used together with the
appropriate use of catheter maintenance solutions. Repeated
blockage usually indicates that the catheter needs to be
changed.

ANTISEPTICS AND DISINFECTANTS

Chlorhexidine with lidocaine

The properties listed below are those particular to the
combination only. For the properties of the components
please consider, chlorhexidine p. 1053, lidocaine
hydrochloride p. 1187.

- INDICATIONS AND DOSE
Urethral sounding and catheterisation
▸ BY URETHRAL APPLICATION
▸ Adult: 6–11 mL
Cystoscopy
▸ BY URETHRAL APPLICATION
▸ Adult: 11 mL, then 6–11 mL if required

- MEDICINAL FORMS
There can be variation in the licensing of different medicines
containing the same drug.
Gel
EXCIPIENTS: May contain Hydroxybenzoates (parabens)
▸ Instillagel (CliniMed Ltd)
  **Chlorhexidine gluconate 500 microgram per 1 ml, Lidocaine
  hydrochloride 20 mg per 1 ml** Instillagel gel | 60 ml P £14.05 DT
  price = £14.05 | 110 ml P £15.76 DT price = £15.76

IRRIGATING SOLUTIONS

Glycine

● **INDICATIONS AND DOSE**

Bladder irrigation during urological surgery | Irrigation for transurethral resection of the prostate gland and bladder tumours

▸ Adult: (consult product literature)

● **CAUTIONS**

CAUTIONS, FURTHER INFORMATION

▸ **Urological surgery** There is a high risk of fluid absorption from the irrigant used in endoscopic surgery within the urinary tract.

● **SIDE-EFFECTS** Haemolysis · hypervolaemia · renal failure

● **MEDICINAL FORMS**
There can be variation in the licensing of different medicines containing the same drug.
Irrigation solution
▸ Glycine (Non-proprietary)
  Glycine 1.5% irrigation solution 3litre Easyflow bags | 1 bag no price available
  Glycine 1.5% irrigation solution 1litre Flowfusor bottles | 1 bottle no price available
  Glycine 1.5% irrigation solution 1litre Easyflow bags | 1 bag no price available
  Glycine 1.5% irrigation solution 2litre Flowfusor bottles | 1 bottle no price available

UROLOGICAL ANTI-INFLAMMATORY DRUGS

Dimethyl sulfoxide

● **INDICATIONS AND DOSE**

Symptomatic relief in interstitial cystitis (Hunner's ulcer)
▸ BY INTRAVESICAL INSTILLATION
▸ Adult: 50 mL every 2 weeks retained for 15 minutes then voided by the patient, 50% solution is used and instilled into the bladder

● **INTERACTIONS** → Appendix 1 (dimethyl sulfoxide).

● **SIDE-EFFECTS** Bladder spasm · hypersensitivity

● **MONITORING REQUIREMENTS** Ophthalmic, renal and hepatic assessments at intervals of 6 months are required in long-term treatment.

● **MEDICINAL FORMS**
There can be variation in the licensing of different medicines containing the same drug. Forms available from special-order manufacturers include: cream

Catheter maintenance solutions

● **CATHETER MAINTENANCE SOLUTIONS**

OptiFlo R citric acid 6% catheter maintenance solution (Bard Ltd) | 50 ml · NHS indicative price = £3.56 · Drug Tariff (Part IXa) | 100 ml · NHS indicative price = £3.56 · Drug Tariff (Part IXa)

Uro-Tainer Twin Solutio R citric acid 6% catheter maintenance solution (B.Braun Medical Ltd) | 60 ml · NHS indicative price = £4.81 · Drug Tariff (Part IXa)

OptiFlo S saline 0.9% catheter maintenance solution (Bard Ltd) **Sodium chloride 9 mg per 1 ml** | 50 ml · NHS indicative price = £3.36 · Drug Tariff (Part IXa) | 100 ml · NHS indicative price = £3.36 · Drug Tariff (Part IXa)

Uro-Tainer M sodium chloride 0.9% catheter maintenance solution (B.Braun Medical Ltd) **Sodium chloride 9 mg per 1 ml** | 50 ml · No NHS indicative price available · Drug Tariff (Part IXa) | 100 ml · No NHS indicative price available · Drug Tariff (Part IXa)

Uro-Tainer sodium chloride 0.9% catheter maintenance solution (B.Braun Medical Ltd) **Sodium chloride 9 mg per 1 ml** | 50 ml · NHS indicative price = £3.51 · Drug Tariff (Part IXa) | 100 ml · NHS indicative price = £3.51 · Drug Tariff (Part IXa)

3 Contraception

Contraceptives, hormonal

Overview

The Fraser Guidelines (Department of Health Guidance (July 2004): Best practice guidance for doctors and other health professionals on the provision of advice and treatment to young people under 16 on contraception, sexual and reproductive health, available at www.tinyurl.com/bpg16) should be followed when prescribing contraception for women under 16 years. The UK Medical Eligibility Criteria for Contraceptive Use (available at www.fsrh.org) is published by the Faculty of Sexual and Reproductive Healthcare; it categorises the risks of using contraceptive methods with pre-existing medical conditions.

Hormonal contraception is the most effective method of fertility control, but can have major and minor side-effects, especially for certain groups of women. Hormonal contraception should only be used by adolescents after menarche.

Intra-uterine devices are a highly effective method of contraception but may produce undesirable local side-effects. They may be used in women of all ages irrespective of parity, but are less appropriate for those with an increased risk of pelvic inflammatory disease.

Barrier methods alone (condoms, diaphragms, and caps) are less effective but can be reliable for well-motivated couples if used in conjunction with a **spermicide**. Occasionally sensitivity reactions occur. A female condom (*Femidom* ®) is also available; it is pre-lubricated but does not contain a spermicide.

Combined hormonal contraceptives

Oral contraceptives containing an oestrogen and a progestogen ('combined oral contraceptives') are effective preparations for general use. Advantages of combined oral contraceptives include:
● reliable and reversible;
● reduced dysmenorrhoea and menorrhagia;
● reduced incidence of premenstrual tension;
● less symptomatic fibroids and functional ovarian cysts;
● less benign breast disease;
● reduced risk of ovarian and endometrial cancer;
● reduced risk of pelvic inflammatory disease.

Combined oral contraceptives containing a fixed amount of an oestrogen and a progestogen in each active tablet are termed 'monophasic'; those with varying amounts of the two hormones are termed 'phasic'. A transdermal patch and a vaginal ring, both containing an oestrogen with a progestogen, are also available.

Combined Oral Contraceptives Monophasic 21-day preparations

Oestrogen content	Progestogen content	Brand
Ethinylestradiol 20 micrograms	Desogestrel 150 micrograms	Gedarel® 20/150
Ethinylestradiol 20 micrograms	Desogestrel 150 micrograms	Mercilon®
Ethinylestradiol 20 micrograms	Gestodene 75 micrograms	Femodette®
Ethinylestradiol 20 micrograms	Gestodene 75 micrograms	Millinette® 20/75
Ethinylestradiol 20 micrograms	Gestodene 75 micrograms	Sunya 20/75®
Ethinylestradiol 20 micrograms	Norethisterone acetate 1 mg	Loestrin 20®
Ethinylestradiol 30 micrograms	Desogestrel 150 micrograms	Gedarel® 30/150
Ethinylestradiol 30 micrograms	Desogestrel 150 micrograms	Marvelon®
Ethinylestradiol 30 micrograms	Drospirenone 3 mg	Yasmin®
Ethinylestradiol 30 micrograms	Gestodene 75 micrograms	Femodene®
Ethinylestradiol 30 micrograms	Gestodene 75 micrograms	Katya 30/75®
Ethinylestradiol 30 micrograms	Gestodene 75 micrograms	Millinette® 30/75
Ethinylestradiol 30 micrograms	Levonorgestrel 150 micrograms	Levest®
Ethinylestradiol 30 micrograms	Levonorgestrel 150 micrograms	Microgynon 30®
Ethinylestradiol 30 micrograms	Levonorgestrel 150 micrograms	Ovranette®
Ethinylestradiol 30 micrograms	Levonorgestrel 150 micrograms	Rigevidon®
Ethinylestradiol 30 micrograms	Norethisterone acetate 1.5 mg	Loestrin 30®
Ethinylestradiol 35 micrograms	Norgestimate 250 micrograms	Cilest®
Ethinylestradiol 35 micrograms	Norethisterone 500 micrograms	Brevinor®
Ethinylestradiol 35 micrograms	Norethisterone 500 micrograms	Ovysmen®
Ethinylestradiol 35 micrograms	Norethisterone 1 mg	Norimin®
Mestranol 50 micrograms	Norethisterone 1 mg	Norinyl-1®

Combined Oral Contraceptives Monophasic 28-day preparations

Oestrogen content	Progestogen content	Brand
Ethinylestradiol 30 micrograms	Gestodene 75 micrograms	Femodene® ED
Ethinylestradiol 30 micrograms	Levonorgestrel 150 micrograms	Microgynon 30 ED®
Estradiol (as hemihydrate) 1.5 mg	Nomegestrol acetate 2.5 mg	Zoely®

Combined Oral Contraceptives Phasic 21-day preparations

Oestrogen content	Progestogen content	Brand
Ethinylestradiol 30 micrograms	Gestodene 50 micrograms	Triadene®
Ethinylestradiol 40 micrograms	Gestodene 70 micrograms	
Ethinylestradiol 30 micrograms	Gestodene 100 micrograms	
Ethinylestradiol 30 micrograms	Levonorgestrel 50 micrograms	Logynon®
Ethinylestradiol 40 micrograms	Levonorgestrel 75 micrograms	
Ethinylestradiol 30 micrograms	Levonorgestrel 125 micrograms	
Ethinylestradiol 30 micrograms	Levonorgestrel 50 micrograms	TriRegol®
Ethinylestradiol 40 micrograms	Levonorgestrel 75 micrograms	
Ethinylestradiol 30 micrograms	Levonorgestrel 125 micrograms	
Ethinylestradiol 35 micrograms	Norethisterone 500 micrograms	BiNovum®
Ethinylestradiol 35 micrograms	Norethisterone 1 mg	
Ethinylestradiol 35 micrograms	Norethisterone 500 micrograms	Synphase®
Ethinylestradiol 35 micrograms	Norethisterone 1 mg	
Ethinylestradiol 35 micrograms	Norethisterone 500 micrograms	

Combined Oral Contraceptives Phasic 28-day preparations

Oestrogen content	Progestogen content	Brand
Ethinylestradiol 30 micrograms	Levonorgestrel 50 micrograms	Logynon ED®
Ethinylestradiol 40 micrograms	Levonorgestrel 75 micrograms	
Ethinylestradiol 30 micrograms	Levonorgestrel 125 micrograms	
Estradiol valerate 3 mg		Qlaira®
Estradiol valerate 2 mg	Dienogest 2 mg	
Estradiol valerate 2 mg	Dienogest 3 mg	
Estradiol valerate 1 mg		

Choice

The majority of combined oral contraceptives contain ethinylestradiol p. 685 as the oestrogen component; mestranol and estradiol are also used. The ethinylestradiol content of combined oral contraceptives ranges from 20 to 40 micrograms. Generally a preparation with the lowest oestrogen and progestogen content which gives good cycle control and minimal side-effects in the individual woman is chosen. It is recommended that combined hormonal contraceptives are not continued beyond 50 years of age since more suitable alternatives exist.

- *Low strength preparations* (containing ethinylestradiol 20 micrograms) are particularly appropriate for women with risk factors for circulatory disease, provided a combined oral contraceptive is otherwise suitable.
- *Standard strength preparations* (containing ethinylestradiol 30 or 35 micrograms or in 30–40 microgram *phased* preparations) are appropriate for standard use. Phased preparations are generally reserved for women who *either* do not have withdrawal bleeding or who have breakthrough bleeding with monophasic products.

The progestogens ethinylestradiol with desogestrel p. 722, ethinylestradiol with drospirenone p. 722, and ethinylestradiol with gestodene p. 723 may be considered for women who have side-effects (such as acne, headache, depression, breast symptoms, and breakthrough bleeding) with other progestogens. Drospirenone, a derivative of spironolactone, has anti-androgenic and anti-mineralocorticoid activity; it should be used with care if an increased plasma-potassium concentration might be hazardous.

Dienogest with estradiol valerate p. 721 is in the combined oral contraceptive *Qlaira®*. Nomegestrol is the progestogen contained in the combined oral contraceptive *Zoely®*, in combination with estradiol.

The progestogen norelgestromin is combined with ethinylestradiol in a transdermal patch (*Evra®*). The vaginal contraceptive ring contains the progestogen etonogestrel combined with ethinylestradiol (*NuvaRing®*).

Surgery
Oestrogen-containing contraceptives should preferably be discontinued (and adequate alternative contraceptive arrangements made) 4 weeks before major elective surgery and all surgery to the legs or surgery which involves prolonged immobilisation of a lower limb; they should normally be recommenced at the first menses occurring at least 2 weeks after full mobilisation. A progestogen-only contraceptive may be offered as an alternative and the oestrogen-containing contraceptive restarted after mobilisation. When discontinuation of an oestrogen-containing contraceptive is not possible, e.g. after trauma or if a patient admitted for an elective procedure is still on an oestrogen-containing contraceptive, thromboprophylaxis (with unfractionated or low molecular weight heparin and graduated compression hosiery) is advised. These recommendations do not apply to minor surgery with short duration of anaesthesia, e.g. laparoscopic sterilisation or tooth extraction, or to women using oestrogen-free hormonal contraceptives.

Reason to stop immediately
Combined hormonal contraceptives or hormone replacement therapy (HRT) should be stopped (pending investigation and treatment), if any of the following occur:
- sudden severe chest pain (even if not radiating to left arm);
- sudden breathlessness (or cough with blood-stained sputum);
- unexplained swelling or severe pain in calf of one leg;
- severe stomach pain;
- serious neurological effects including unusual severe, prolonged headache especially if first time or getting progressively worse *or* sudden partial or complete loss of vision *or* sudden disturbance of hearing or other perceptual disorders *or* dysphasia *or* bad fainting attack or collapse *or* first unexplained epileptic seizure *or* weakness, motor disturbances, very marked numbness suddenly affecting one side or one part of body;
- hepatitis, jaundice, liver enlargement;
- blood pressure above systolic 160 mmHg or diastolic 95 mmHg; (in adolescents stop if blood pressure very high);
- prolonged immobility after surgery or leg injury;

- detection of a risk factor which contra-indicates treatment.

Progestogen-only contraceptives
Oral progestogen-only contraceptives
Oral progestogen-only preparations alter cervical mucus to prevent sperm penetration and may inhibit ovulation in some women; oral desogestrel-only preparations consistently inhibit ovulation and this is their primary mechanism of action. There is insufficient clinical trial evidence to compare the efficacy of oral progestogen-only contraceptives with each other or with combined hormonal contraceptives. Progestogen-only contraceptives offer a suitable alternative to combined hormonal contraceptives when oestrogens are contra-indicated (including those with venous thrombosis or a past history or predisposition to venous thromboembolism, heavy smokers, those with hypertension above systolic 160 mmHg or diastolic 95 mmHg, valvular heart disease, diabetes mellitus with complications, and migraine with aura).

Parenteral progestogen-only contraceptives
Medroxyprogesterone acetate (*Depo-Provera®*, *SAYANA PRESS®*) p. 733 is a long-acting progestogen given by injection; it is at least as effective as the combined oral preparations but because of its prolonged action it should never be given without *full counselling backed by the patient information leaflet*. It may be used as a short-term or long-term contraceptive for women who have been counselled about the likelihood of menstrual disturbance and the potential for a delay in return to full fertility. Delayed return of fertility and irregular cycles may occur after discontinuation of treatment but there is no evidence of permanent infertility. Troublesome bleeding has been reported in patients given medroxyprogesterone acetate in the immediate puerperium; delaying the first injection until 6 weeks after birth may minimise bleeding problems. If the woman is not breast-feeding, the first injection may be given within 5 days postpartum (she should be warned that the risk of troublesome bleeding may be increased).
- In adolescents, medroxyprogesterone acetate (*Depo-Provera®*, *SAYANA PRESS®*) should be used only when other methods of contraception are inappropriate;
- in all women, the benefits of using medroxyprogesterone acetate beyond 2 years should be evaluated against the risks;
- in women with risk factors for osteoporosis, a method of contraception other than medroxyprogesterone acetate should be considered.

Norethisterone enantate (*Noristerat®*) is a long-acting progestogen given as an oily injection which provides contraception for 8 weeks; it is used as short-term interim contraception e.g. before vasectomy becomes effective.

An **etonogestrel-releasing implant** (*Nexplanon®*) is also available. It is a highly effective long-acting contraceptive, consisting of a single flexible rod that is inserted subdermally into the lower surface of the upper arm and provides contraception for up to 3 years. The manufacturer advises that in heavier women, blood-etonogestrel concentrations are lower and therefore the implant may not provide effective contraception during the third year; they advise that earlier replacement may be considered in such patients—however, evidence to support this recommendation is lacking. Local reactions such as bruising and itching can occur at the insertion site. The contraceptive effect of etonogestrel is rapidly reversed on removal of the implant.

Intra-uterine progestogen-only device
The progestogen-only intra-uterine systems *Mirena®*, *Jaydess®* and *Levosert®* release levonorgestrel p. 729 directly into the uterine cavity. *Mirena®* is licensed for use as a contraceptive, for the treatment of primary menorrhagia and

for the prevention of endometrial hyperplasia during oestrogen replacement therapy. *Jaydess* ® and *Levosert* ® are licensed for contraception, and *Levosert* ® is additionally licensed for the treatment of menorrhagia. These may therefore be a contraceptive method of choice for women who have excessively heavy menses.

The effects of the progestogen-only intra-uterine system are mainly local and hormonal including prevention of endometrial proliferation, thickening of cervical mucus, and suppression of ovulation in some women (in some cycles). In addition to the progestogenic activity, the intra-uterine system itself may contribute slightly to the contraceptive effect. Return of fertility after removal is rapid and appears to be complete.

Advantages of the progestogen-only intra-uterine system over copper intra-uterine devices are that there may be an improvement in any dysmenorrhoea and a reduction in blood loss; there is also evidence that the frequency of pelvic inflammatory disease may be reduced (particularly in the youngest age groups who are most at risk).

In primary menorrhagia, menstrual bleeding is reduced significantly within 3–6 months of inserting the progestogen-only intra-uterine system, probably because it prevents endometrial proliferation. Another treatment should be considered if menorrhagia does not improve within this time.

Surgery
All progestogen-only contraceptives (including those given by injection) are suitable for use as an alternative to combined hormonal contraceptives before major elective surgery, before all surgery to the legs, or before surgery which involves prolonged immobilisation of a lower limb.

Emergency contraception

Hormonal methods
Hormonal emergency contraceptives include levonorgestrel and ulipristal acetate p. 727; either drug should be taken as soon as possible after unprotected intercourse to increase efficacy.

Levonorgestrel is effective if taken within 72 hours (3 days) of unprotected intercourse and may also be used between 72 and 96 hours after unprotected intercourse [unlicensed use], but efficacy decreases with time. Ulipristal acetate, a progesterone receptor modulator, is effective if taken within 120 hours (5 days) of unprotected intercourse.

Levonorgestrel is less effective than insertion of an intra-uterine device. Ulipristal acetate is as effective as levonorgestrel, but its efficacy compared to an intra-uterine device is not yet known.

Intra–uterine device
Insertion of an intra-uterine device is more effective than oral levonorgestrel for emergency contraception. A copper intra-uterine contraceptive device can be inserted up to 120 hours (5 days) after unprotected intercourse; sexually transmitted infections should be tested for and insertion of the device should usually be covered by antibacterial prophylaxis (e.g. azithromycin p. 486). If intercourse has occurred more than 5 days previously, the device can still be inserted up to 5 days after the earliest likely calculated ovulation (i.e. within the minimum period before implantation), regardless of the number of episodes of unprotected intercourse earlier in the cycle.

Contraceptives, interactions

Combined hormonal contraceptives interactions
The effectiveness of *combined* oral contraceptives, *progestogen-only* oral contraceptives, contraceptive patches, and vaginal rings can be considerably reduced by interaction with drugs that induce hepatic enzyme activity (e.g.

carbamazepine p. 283, eslicarbazepine acetate p. 285, nevirapine p. 586, oxcarbazepine p. 292, phenytoin p. 294, phenobarbital p. 304, primidone p. 305, ritonavir p. 596, St John's Wort, topiramate p. 301 and, above all, rifabutin p. 522 and rifampicin p. 527). A condom together with a long-acting method, such as an injectable contraceptive, may be more suitable for patients with HIV infection or at risk of HIV infection; advice on the possibility of interaction with antiretroviral drugs should be sought from HIV specialists.

Women taking combined hormonal contraceptives who require enzyme-inducing drugs should be advised to change to a contraceptive method that is unaffected by enzyme-inducers (e.g. some parenteral progestogen-only contraceptives, intra-uterine devices) for the duration of treatment and for 4 weeks after stopping. If a change in contraceptive method is undesirable or inappropriate the following options should be discussed:

- For a *short course (2 months or less) of an enzyme-inducing drug*, continue with a combined oral contraceptive providing ethinylestradiol 30 micrograms or more daily and use a 'tricycling' regimen (i.e. taking 3 packets of monophasic tablets without a break followed by a shortened tablet-free interval of 4 days [unlicensed use]). Additional contraceptive precautions should also be used whilst taking the enzyme-inducing drug and for 4 weeks after stopping. Another option (except for rifampicin or rifabutin) is to follow the advice for long-term courses.

For women using combined hormonal contraceptive patches or vaginal rings, additional contraceptive precautions are also required whilst taking the enzyme-inducing drug and for 4 weeks after stopping. If concomitant administration runs beyond the 3 weeks of patch or vaginal ring use, a new treatment cycle should be started immediately, without a patch-free or ring-free break.

- For a *long-term course (over 2 months) of an enzyme-inducing drug* (except rifampicin or rifabutin), adjust the dose of combined oral contraceptive to provide ethinylestradiol 50 micrograms or more daily [unlicensed use] and use a 'tricycling' regimen; continue for the duration of treatment with the enzyme-inducing drug and for 4 weeks after stopping.

If breakthrough bleeding occurs (and all other causes are ruled out) it is recommended that the dose of ethinylestradiol is increased by increments of 10 micrograms up to a maximum of 70 micrograms daily [unlicensed use], or to use additional precautions, or to change to a method unaffected by enzyme-inducing drugs.

Contraceptive patches and vaginal rings are not recommended for women taking enzyme-inducing drugs over a long period.

- For a *long-term course (over 2 months) of rifampicin or rifabutin*, an alternative method of contraception (such as an IUD) is **always** recommended because they are such potent enzyme-inducing drugs; the alternative method of contraception should be continued for 4 weeks after stopping the enzyme-inducing drug.

Antibacterials that do not induce liver enzymes
Latest recommendations are that no additional contraceptive precautions are required when *combined* oral contraceptives are used with antibacterials that do not induce liver enzymes, unless diarrhoea or vomiting occur. These recommendations should be discussed with the woman, who should also be advised that guidance in patient information leaflets may differ.

It is also currently recommended that no additional contraceptive precautions are required when contraceptive patches or vaginal rings are used with antibacterials that do not induce liver enzymes. There have been concerns that some antibacterials that do not induce liver enzymes (e.g. ampicillin p. 499, doxycycline p. 513) reduce the efficacy of *combined* oral contraceptives by impairing the bacterial flora responsible for recycling ethinylestradiol from the large bowel. However, there is a lack of evidence to support this interaction.

Oral progestogen-only contraceptives interactions

Effectiveness of oral progestogen-only preparations is not affected by antibacterials that do not induce liver enzymes. The efficacy of oral progestogen-only preparations is, however, reduced by enzyme-inducing drugs and an alternative contraceptive method, unaffected by the interacting drug, is recommended during treatment with an enzyme-inducing drug and for at least 4 weeks afterwards. For a short course of an enzyme-inducing drug, if a change in contraceptive method is undesirable or inappropriate, the progestogen-only oral method may be continued in combination with additional contraceptive precautions (e.g. barrier methods) for the duration of treatment with the enzyme-inducing drug and for 4 weeks after stopping.

Parenteral progestogen-only contraceptives interactions

Effectiveness of parenteral progestogen-only contraceptives is not affected by antibacterials that do not induce liver enzymes. The effectiveness of norethisterone intramuscular injection p. 691 and medroxyprogesterone acetate intramuscular and subcutaneous injections p. 733 is not affected by enzyme-inducing drugs and they may be continued as normal during courses of these drugs. However, effectiveness of the etonogestrel-releasing implant p. 732 may be reduced by enzyme-inducing drugs and an alternative contraceptive method, unaffected by the interacting drug, is recommended during treatment with the enzyme-inducing drug and for at least 4 weeks after stopping. For a short course of an enzyme-inducing drug, if a change in contraceptive method is undesirable or inappropriate, the implant may be continued in combination with additional contraceptive precautions (e.g. condom) for the duration of treatment with the enzyme-inducing drug and for 4 weeks after stopping it.

Hormonal emergency contraception interactions

The effectiveness of levonorgestrel p. 729, and possibly ulipristal acetate p. 727, is reduced in women taking enzyme-inducing drugs (and possibly for 4 weeks after stopping); a copper intra-uterine device can be offered instead. If the copper intra-uterine device is undesirable or inappropriate, the dose of levonorgestrel should be increased to a total of 3 mg taken as a single dose [unlicensed dose—advise women accordingly]. There is not need to increase the dose for emergency contraception if the patient is taking antibacterials that are not enzyme inducers.

Contraceptives, non-hormonal

Spermicidal contraceptives

Spermicidal contraceptives are useful additional safeguards but do **not** give adequate protection if used alone unless fertility is already significantly diminished. They have two components: a spermicide and a vehicle which itself may have some inhibiting effect on sperm activity. They are suitable for use with barrier methods, such as diaphragms or caps; however, spermicidal contraceptives are not generally recommended for use with condoms, as there is no evidence of any additional protection compared with non-spermicidal lubricants.

Spermicidal contraceptives are not suitable for use in those with or at high risk of sexually transmitted infections (including HIV); high frequency use of the spermicide nonoxinol p. 735 '9' has been associated with genital lesions, which may increase the risk of acquiring these infections.

Products such as petroleum jelly (*Vaseline*®), baby oil and oil-based vaginal and rectal preparations are likely to damage condoms and contraceptive diaphragms made from latex rubber, and may render them less effective as a barrier method of contraception and as a protection from sexually transmitted infections (including HIV).

Contraceptive devices

Intra-uterine devices

The intra-uterine device (IUD) is a suitable contraceptive for women of all ages irrespective of parity; however, it is less appropriate for those with an increased risk of pelvic inflammatory disease e.g. women under 25 years.

The most effective intra-uterine devices have at least 380 mm^2 of copper and have banded copper on the arms. Smaller devices have been introduced to minimise side-effects; these consist of a plastic carrier wound with copper wire or fitted with copper bands; some also have a central core of silver to prevent fragmentation of the copper.

Fertility declines with age and therefore a copper intra-uterine device which is fitted in a woman over the age of 40, may remain in the uterus until menopause.

A frameless, copper-bearing intra-uterine device (*Gyne Fix*®) is also available. It consists of a knotted, polypropylene thread with 6 copper sleeves; the device is anchored in the uterus by inserting the knot into the uterine fundus.

3.1   Contraception, combined

OESTROGENS COMBINED WITH PROGESTOGENS

Combined hormonal contraceptives

- CONTRA-INDICATIONS Acute porphyrias p. 918 · gallstones · heart disease associated with pulmonary hypertension or risk of embolus · history during pregnancy of cholestatic jaundice · history during pregnancy of chorea · history during pregnancy of pemphigoid gestationis · history during pregnancy of pruritus · history of breast cancer (but can be used after 5 years if no evidence of disease and non-hormonal methods unacceptable) · history of haemolytic uraemic syndrome · migraine with aura · personal history of venous or arterial thrombosis · sclerosing treatment for varicose veins · severe or multiple risk factors for arterial disease · severe or multiple risk factors for venous thromboembolism · systemic lupus erythematosus with (or unknown) antiphospholipid antibodies · transient cerebral ischaemic attacks without headaches · undiagnosed vaginal bleeding

- CAUTIONS Active trophoblastic disease (until return to normal of urine- and plasma-gonadotrophin concentration)—seek specialist advice · Crohn's disease · gene mutations associated with breast cancer (e.g. BRCA 1) · history of severe depression especially if induced by hormonal contraceptive · hyperprolactinaemia (seek specialist advice) · inflammatory bowel disease · migraine · personal or family history of hypertriglyceridaemia (increased risk of pancreatitis) · risk factors for arterial disease · risk factors for venous thromboembolism · sickle-cell disease · undiagnosed breast mass

  CAUTIONS, FURTHER INFORMATION
  ▸ Risk of venous thromboembolism   There is an increased risk of venous thromboembolic disease in users of combined hormonal contraceptives particularly during the first year and possibly after restarting combined hormonal contraceptives following a break of four weeks or more. This risk is considerably smaller than that associated with

pregnancy (about 60 cases of venous thromboembolic disease per 100 000 pregnancies). In all cases the risk of venous thromboembolism increases with age and in the presence of other risk factors, such as obesity. The risk also varies depending on the type of progestogen.

Provided that women are informed of the relative risks of venous thromboembolism and accept them, the choice of oral contraceptive is for the woman together with the prescriber jointly to make in light of her individual medical history and any contra-indications.

Combined hormonal contraceptives also slightly increase the risk of *arterial* thromboembolism; however, there is no evidence to suggest that this risk varies between different preparations.

▸ Risk factors for venous thromboembolism Use with **caution** if any of following factors present but **avoid** if two or more factors present:
- *family history of venous thromboembolism* in first-degree relative aged under 45 years (avoid contraceptive containing desogestrel or gestodene, *or* avoid if known prothrombotic coagulation abnormality e.g. factor V Leiden or antiphospholipid antibodies (including lupus anticoagulant));
- *obesity*; body mass index $\geq$ 30 kg/m^2 (avoid if body mass index $\geq$ 35 kg/m^2 unless no suitable alternative); (in adolescents, caution if obese according to BMI (adjusted for age and gender); in those who are markedly obese, avoid unless no suitable alternative);
- *long-term immobilisation* e.g. in a wheelchair (avoid if confined to bed or leg in plaster cast);
- *history of superficial thrombophlebitis*;
- *age* over 35 years (avoid if over 50 years);
- *smoking*.

Combined Hormonal Contraception and Risk of Venous Thromboembolism

Progestogen in Combined Hormonal Contraceptive	Estimated incidence per 10 000 women per year of use
Non-pregnant, not using combined hormonal contraception	2
Levonorgesterol[1]	5-7
Norgestimate[1]	5-7
Norethisterone[1]	5-7
Etonogestrel[1]	6-12
Norelgestromin[1]	6-12
Gestodene[1]	9-12
Desogestrel[1]	9-12
Drospirenone[1]	9-12
Dienogest[2]	Not known–insufficient data
Nomegestrol[2]	Not known–insufficient data

[1]Combined with ethinylestradiol [2]Combined with estradiol

▸ Risk factors for arterial disease Use with **caution** if any one of following factors present but **avoid** if two or more factors present:
- *family history of arterial disease* in first degree relative aged under 45 years (avoid if atherogenic lipid profile);
- *diabetes mellitus* (avoid if diabetes complications present);
- *hypertension*; blood pressure above *systolic* 140 *mmHg* or *diastolic* 90 *mmHg* (avoid if blood pressure above *systolic* 160 *mmHg* or *diastolic* 95 *mmHg*); (in adolescents, avoid if blood pressure very high);
- *smoking* (avoid if smoking 40 or more cigarettes daily);
- *age* over 35 years (avoid if over 50 years);

- *obesity* (avoid if body mass index $\geq$ 35 kg/m^2 unless no suitable alternative); (in adolescents, caution if obese according to BMI (adjusted for age and gender); in those who are markedly obese, avoid unless no suitable alternative);
- *migraine without aura* (avoid if *migraine with aura* (focal symptoms), *or* severe migraine frequently lasting over 72 hours despite treatment, *or* migraine treated with ergot derivatives).

▸ Migraine Women should report any increase in headache frequency or onset of focal symptoms (discontinue immediately and refer urgently to neurology expert if focal neurological symptoms not typical of aura persist for more than 1 hour).

Combined hormonal contraceptives should be stopped (pending investigation and treatment), if serious neurological effects occur, including unusual severe, prolonged headache especially if first time or getting progressively worse *or* sudden partial or complete loss of vision *or* sudden disturbance of hearing or other perceptual disorders *or* dysphasia *or* bad fainting attack or collapse *or* first unexplained epileptic seizure *or* weakness, motor disturbances, very marked numbness suddenly affecting one side or one part of body.

● INTERACTIONS → Appendix 1 (oestrogens, progestogens).

● SIDE-EFFECTS
▸ Rare Gallstones · systemic lupus erythematosus
▸ Frequency not known Abdominal cramps · absence of withdrawal bleeding · amenorrhoea after discontinuation · breast enlargement · breast secretion · breast tenderness · cervical erosion · changes in libido · changes in lipid metabolism · changes in vaginal discharge · chloasma · chorea · contact lenses may irritate · depression · fluid retention · headache · hepatic tumours · hypertension · irritability · leg cramps · liver impairment · nausea · nervousness · photosensitivity · reduced menstrual loss · skin reactions · thrombosis (more common when factor V Leiden present or in blood groups A, B, and AB) · visual disturbances · vomiting · 'spotting' in early cycles

SIDE-EFFECTS, FURTHER INFORMATION
▸ Breast cancer There is a small increase in the risk of having breast cancer diagnosed in women taking the combined oral contraceptive pill; this relative risk may be due to an earlier diagnosis. In users of combined oral contraceptive pills the cancers are more likely to be localised to the breast. The most important factor for diagnosing breast cancer appears to be the age at which the contraceptive is stopped rather than the duration of use; any increase in the rate of diagnosis diminishes gradually during the 10 years after stopping and disappears by 10 years.
▸ Cervical cancer Use of combined oral contraceptives for 5 years or longer is associated with a small increased risk of cervical cancer; the risk diminishes after stopping and disappears by about 10 years.

The possible small increase in the risk of breast cancer and cervical cancer should be weighed against the protective effect against cancers of the ovary and endometrium.

● PREGNANCY Not known to be harmful.

● BREAST FEEDING Avoid until weaning or for 6 months after birth (adverse effects on lactation).

● HEPATIC IMPAIRMENT Avoid in active liver disease including disorders of hepatic excretion (e.g. Dubin-Johnson or Rotor syndromes), infective hepatitis (until liver function returns to normal), liver tumours.

● DIRECTIONS FOR ADMINISTRATION
▸ With oral use Each tablet should be taken at approximately same time each day; if delayed, contraceptive protection may be lost. 21-*day combined preparations*, 1 tablet daily for 21 days; subsequent courses repeated after a 7-day interval (during which withdrawal bleeding occurs); if reasonably certain woman is not pregnant, first course can

be started on any day of cycle—if starting on day 6 of cycle or later, additional precautions (barrier methods) necessary during first 7 days. *Every day (ED) combined preparations*, 1 *active* tablet daily for 21 days, followed by 1 *inactive* tablet daily for 7 days; subsequent courses repeated without interval (withdrawal bleeding occurs when *inactive* tablets being taken); if reasonably certain woman is not pregnant, first course can be started on any day of cycle—if starting on day 6 of cycle or later, additional precautions (barrier methods) necessary during first 7 days.

Changing to combined preparation containing different progestogen If previous contraceptive used correctly, or pregnancy can reasonably be excluded, start the first active tablet of new brand immediately. See individual monographs for requirements of specific preparations.

Changing from progestogen-only tablet If previous contraceptive used correctly, or pregnancy can reasonably be excluded, start new brand immediately, additional precautions (barrier methods) necessary for first 7 days.

Secondary amenorrhoea (exclude pregnancy) Start any day, additional precautions (barrier methods) necessary during first 7 days (9 days for *Qlaira ®*).

After childbirth (not breast-feeding) Start 3 weeks after birth (increased risk of thrombosis if started earlier); later than 3 weeks postpartum additional precautions (barrier methods) necessary for first 7 days (9 days for *Qlaira ®*). After abortion or miscarriage Start same day.

● PATIENT AND CARER ADVICE

Missed doses

Missed pill The critical time for loss of contraceptive protection is when a pill is omitted at the *beginning* or *end* of a cycle (which lengthens the pill-free interval).

If a woman forgets to take a pill, it should be taken as soon as she remembers, and the next one taken at the normal time (even if this means taking 2 pills together). A missed pill is one that is 24 or more hours late. If a woman misses only one pill, she should take an active pill as soon as she remembers and then resume normal pill-taking. No additional precautions are necessary.

If a woman misses 2 or more pills (especially from the first 7 in a packet), she may not be protected. She should take an active pill as soon as she remembers and then resume normal pill-taking. In addition, she must either abstain from sex or use an additional method of contraception such as a condom for the next 7 days. If these 7 days run beyond the end of the packet, the next packet should be started at once, omitting the pill-free interval (or, in the case of *everyday* (ED) pills, omitting the 7 inactive tablets).

Emergency contraception is recommended if 2 or more combined oral contraceptive tablets are missed from the first 7 tablets in a packet and unprotected intercourse has occurred since finishing the last packet.

Travel Women taking oral contraceptives are at an increased risk of deep vein thrombosis during travel involving long periods of immobility (over 3 hours). The risk may be reduced by appropriate exercise during the journey and possibly by wearing graduated compression hosiery.

Diarrhoea and vomiting Vomiting and persistent, severe diarrhoea can interfere with the absorption of combined oral contraceptives. If vomiting occurs within 2 hours of taking a combined oral contraceptive another pill should be taken as soon as possible. In cases of persistent vomiting or severe diarrhoea lasting more than 24 hours, additional precautions should be used during and for 7 days after recovery. If the vomiting and diarrhoea occurs during the last 7 tablets, the next pill-free interval should be omitted (in the case of ED tablets the inactive ones should be omitted).

F 719

Dienogest with estradiol valerate

● INDICATIONS AND DOSE

Contraception with 28-day combined preparations | Menstrual symptoms with 28-day combined preparations

▶ BY MOUTH

▶ Females of childbearing potential: 1 active tablet once daily for 26 days, followed by 1 inactive tablet daily for 2 days, withdrawal bleeding may occur during the 2-day interval of *inactive* tablets, tablets should be taken at approximately the same time each day

● DIRECTIONS FOR ADMINISTRATION

● Changing to *Qlaira ®*: start the first active *Qlaira ®* tablet on the day after taking the last active tablet of the previous brand

● PATIENT AND CARER ADVICE

Missed doses

A missed pill for a patient taking *Qlaira ®* is one that is 12 hours or more late; for information on how to manage missed pills in women taking *Qlaira ®*, refer to product literature.

Diarrhoea and vomiting In cases of persistent vomiting or severe diarrhoea lasting more than 12 hours in women taking *Qlaira ®*, refer to product literature.

● MEDICINAL FORMS

There can be variation in the licensing of different medicines containing the same drug.

Tablet

▶ Dienogest with estradiol valerate (Non-proprietary)
Dienogest 2 mg, Estradiol valerate 2 mg Estradiol valerate 2mg / Dienogest 2mg tablets | 15 tablet PoM no price available
Estradiol valerate 2 mg, Dienogest 3 mg Estradiol valerate 2mg / Dienogest 3mg tablets | 51 tablet PoM no price available
▶ Qlaira (Bayer Plc)
Qlaira tablets | 84 tablet PoM £25.18

F 719

Estradiol with nomegestrol

● INDICATIONS AND DOSE

Contraception

▶ BY MOUTH

▶ Females of childbearing potential: 1 active tablet daily for 24 days, followed by 1 inactive tablet daily for 4 days, to be started on day 1 of cycle with first active tablet (withdrawal bleeding occurs when inactive tablets being taken); subsequent courses repeated without interval

● PREGNANCY Toxicity in *animal* studies.

● DIRECTIONS FOR ADMINISTRATION

● Changing to *Zoely ®*: start the first active *Zoely ®* tablet on the day after taking the last active tablet of the previous brand or, at the latest, the day after the tablet-free or inactive tablet interval of the previous brand

● PATIENT AND CARER ADVICE

Missed doses

A missed pill for a patient taking *Zoely ®* is one that is 12 hours or more late; for information on how to manage missed pills in women taking *Zoely ®*, refer to product literature.

Diarrhoea and vomiting In cases of persistent vomiting or severe diarrhoea lasting more than 12 hours in women taking *Zoely ®*, refer to product literature.

● MEDICINAL FORMS
There can be variation in the licensing of different medicines containing the same drug.

Tablet

▸ Zoely (Merck Sharp & Dohme Ltd) ▼
Estradiol (as Estradiol hemihydrate) 1.5 mg, Nomegestrol 2.5 mg Zoely 2.5mg/1.5mg tablets | 84 tablet PoM £19.80 DT price = £19.80

F 719

Ethinylestradiol with desogestrel

● INDICATIONS AND DOSE

Contraception with 21-day combined preparations | **Menstrual symptoms with 21-day combined preparations**

▸ BY MOUTH
▸ Females of childbearing potential: 1 tablet once daily for 21 days; subsequent courses repeated after 7-day interval, withdrawal bleeding occurs during the 7-day interval, if reasonably certain woman is not pregnant, first course can be started on any day of cycle—if starting on day 6 of cycle or later, additional precautions (barrier methods) necessary during first 7 days, tablets should be taken at approximately the same time each day

● MEDICINAL FORMS
There can be variation in the licensing of different medicines containing the same drug.

Tablet

▸ Ethinylestradiol with desogestrel (Non-proprietary)
Ethinylestradiol 20 microgram, Desogestrel 150 microgram Ethinylestradiol 20microgram / Desogestrel 150microgram tablets | 63 tablet PoM no price available
Ethinylestradiol 30 microgram, Desogestrel 150 microgram Ethinylestradiol 30microgram / Desogestrel 150microgram tablets | 63 tablet PoM no price available
▸ Alenini (Actavis UK Ltd)
Ethinylestradiol 20 microgram, Desogestrel 150 microgram Alenini 150microgram/20microgram tablets | 63 tablet PoM £8.44
▸ Alenvona (Actavis UK Ltd)
Ethinylestradiol 30 microgram, Desogestrel 150 microgram Alenvona 150microgram/30microgram tablets | 63 tablet PoM £6.45
▸ Bimizza (Morningside Healthcare Ltd)
Ethinylestradiol 20 microgram, Desogestrel 150 microgram Bimizza 150microgram/20microgram tablets | 63 tablet PoM £5.04
▸ Cimizt (Morningside Healthcare Ltd)
Ethinylestradiol 30 microgram, Desogestrel 150 microgram Cimizt 30microgram/150microgram tablets | 63 tablet PoM £3.80
▸ Gedarel (Consilient Health Ltd)
Ethinylestradiol 20 microgram, Desogestrel 150 microgram Gedarel 20microgram/150microgram tablets | 63 tablet PoM £5.08
Ethinylestradiol 30 microgram, Desogestrel 150 microgram Gedarel 30microgram/150microgram tablets | 63 tablet PoM £4.19
▸ Lestramyl (Mylan Ltd)
Ethinylestradiol 20 microgram, Desogestrel 150 microgram Lestramyl 20microgram/150microgram tablets | 63 tablet PoM £4.30
Ethinylestradiol 30 microgram, Desogestrel 150 microgram Lestramyl 30microgram/150microgram tablets | 63 tablet PoM £3.80
▸ Marvelon (Merck Sharp & Dohme Ltd)
Ethinylestradiol 30 microgram, Desogestrel 150 microgram Marvelon tablets | 63 tablet PoM £7.10
▸ Mercilon (Merck Sharp & Dohme Ltd)
Ethinylestradiol 20 microgram, Desogestrel 150 microgram Mercilon 150microgram/20microgram tablets | 63 tablet PoM £8.44

▸ Munalea (Lupin (Europe) Ltd)
Ethinylestradiol 20 microgram, Desogestrel 150 microgram Munalea 150microgram/20microgram tablets | 63 tablet PoM £6.45
Ethinylestradiol 30 microgram, Desogestrel 150 microgram Munalea 150microgram/30microgram tablets | 63 tablet PoM £7.67

F 719

Ethinylestradiol with drospirenone

● INDICATIONS AND DOSE

Contraception with 21-day combined preparations | **Menstrual symptoms with 21-day combined preparations**

▸ BY MOUTH
▸ Females of childbearing potential: 1 tablet once daily for 21 days; subsequent courses repeated after 7-day interval, withdrawal bleeding occurs during the 7-day interval

● MEDICINAL FORMS
There can be variation in the licensing of different medicines containing the same drug.

Tablet

▸ Ethinylestradiol with drospirenone (Non-proprietary)
Ethinylestradiol 20 microgram, Drospirenone 3 mg Yaz tablets | 84 tablet PoM no price available
Ethinylestradiol 30 microgram, Drospirenone 3 mg Ethinylestradiol 30microgram / Drospirenone 3mg tablets | 63 tablet PoM no price available
▸ Acondro (Mylan Ltd)
Ethinylestradiol 30 microgram, Drospirenone 3 mg Acondro 0.03mg/3mg tablets | 63 tablet PoM £8.35
▸ Cleosensa (Actavis UK Ltd)
Ethinylestradiol 30 microgram, Drospirenone 3 mg Cleosensa 0.03mg/3mg tablets | 63 tablet PoM £14.70
▸ Daylette (Consilient Health Ltd)
Ethinylestradiol 20 microgram, Drospirenone 3 mg Daylette 0.02mg/3mg tablets | 84 tablet PoM £10.50
▸ Dretine (Teva UK Ltd)
Ethinylestradiol 30 microgram, Drospirenone 3 mg Dretine 0.03mg/3mg tablets | 63 tablet PoM £8.30
▸ ELOINE (Bayer Plc)
Ethinylestradiol 20 microgram, Drospirenone 3 mg Eloine 0.02mg/3mg tablets | 84 tablet PoM £14.70
▸ Lucette (Consilient Health Ltd)
Ethinylestradiol 30 microgram, Drospirenone 3 mg Lucette 0.03mg/3mg tablets | 63 tablet PoM £9.35
▸ Yacella (Morningside Healthcare Ltd)
Ethinylestradiol 30 microgram, Drospirenone 3 mg Yacella 0.03mg/3mg tablets | 63 tablet PoM £8.30
▸ Yasmin (Bayer Plc)
Ethinylestradiol 30 microgram, Drospirenone 3 mg Yasmin tablets | 63 tablet PoM £14.70

F 719

Ethinylestradiol with etonogestrel

● INDICATIONS AND DOSE

Contraception | **Menstrual symptoms**

▸ BY VAGINA
▸ Females of childbearing potential: 1 unit, insert the ring into the vagina on day 1 of cycle and leave in for 3 weeks; remove ring on day 22; subsequent courses repeated after 7-day ring free interval (during which withdrawal bleeding occurs)

● DIRECTIONS FOR ADMINISTRATION
Changing method of contraception to vaginal ring
Changing from combined hormonal contraception Insert ring at the latest on the day after the usual tablet-free, patch-free, or inactive-tablet interval. If previous contraceptive used correctly, or pregnancy can reasonably be excluded, can switch to ring on any day of cycle.

Changing from progestogen-only method From an implant or intra-uterine progestogen-only device, insert ring on the day implant or intra-uterine progestogen-only device removed; from an injection, insert ring when next injection due; from oral preparation, first ring may be inserted on any day after stopping pill. For all methods additional precautions (barrier methods) should be used concurrently for first 7 days.

● PATIENT AND CARER ADVICE

Patients or carers should be given advice on how to administer vaginal ring.

Counselling The presence of the ring should be checked regularly.

Missed doses

Expulsion, delayed insertion or removal, or broken vaginal ring If the vaginal ring is expelled for *less than* 3 *hours*, rinse the ring with cool water and reinsert immediately; no additional contraception is needed.

If the ring remains outside the vagina for *more than* 3 *hours* or if the user does not know when the ring was expelled, contraceptive protection may be reduced:

● If ring expelled during week 1 or 2 of cycle, rinse ring with cool water and reinsert; use additional precautions (barrier methods) for next 7 days;

● If ring expelled during week 3 of cycle, either insert a new ring to start a new cycle *or* allow a withdrawal bleed and insert a new ring no later than 7 days after ring was expelled; latter option only available if ring was used continuously for at least 7 days before expulsion.

If insertion of a new ring at the start of a new cycle is delayed, contraceptive protection is lost. A new ring should be inserted as soon as possible; additional precautions (barrier methods) should be used for the first 7 days of the new cycle. If intercourse occurred during the extended ring-free interval, pregnancy should be considered.

No additional contraception is required if removal of the ring is delayed by up to 1 week (4 weeks of continuous use). The 7-day ring-free interval should be observed and subsequently a new ring should be inserted. Contraceptive protection may be reduced with continuous use of the ring for more than 4 weeks—pregnancy should be ruled out before inserting a new ring.

If the ring breaks during use, remove it and insert a new ring immediately; additional precautions (barrier methods) should be used for the first 7 days of the new cycle.

● MEDICINAL FORMS

There can be variation in the licensing of different medicines containing the same drug.

Vaginal delivery system

▸ Ethinylestradiol with etonogestrel (Non-proprietary)

  Ethinylestradiol 2.7 mg, Etonogestrel 11.7 mg Ethinylestradiol 2.7mg / Etonogestrel 11.7mg vaginal delivery system | 3 system [PoM] no price available

▸ NuvaRing (Merck Sharp & Dohme Ltd)

  Ethinylestradiol 2.7 mg, Etonogestrel 11.7 mg NuvaRing 0.12mg/0.015mg per day vaginal delivery system | 3 system [PoM] £29.70

▸ 719

Ethinylestradiol with gestodene

● INDICATIONS AND DOSE

Contraception with 21-day combined preparations | Menstrual symptoms with 21-day combined preparations

▸ BY MOUTH

▸ Females of childbearing potential: 1 tablet once daily for 21 days; subsequent courses repeated after 7-day interval, withdrawal bleeding occurs during the 7-day

interval, if reasonably certain woman is not pregnant, first course can be started on any day of cycle—if starting on day 6 of cycle or later, additional precautions (barrier methods) necessary during first 7 days, tablets should be taken at approximately the same time each day

Contraception with 28-day combined preparations | Menstrual symptoms with 28-day combined preparations

▸ BY MOUTH

▸ Females of childbearing potential: 1 active tablet once daily for 21 days, followed by 1 inactive tablet daily for 7 days; subsequent courses repeated without interval, withdrawal bleeding occurs during the 7-day interval of *inactive* tablets being taken, if reasonably certain woman is not pregnant, first course can be started on any day of cycle—if starting on day 6 of cycle or later, additional precautions (barrier methods) necessary during first 7 days, tablets should be taken at approximately the same time each day

● MEDICINAL FORMS

There can be variation in the licensing of different medicines containing the same drug.

Tablet

▸ Ethinylestradiol with gestodene (Non-proprietary)

  Ethinylestradiol 30 microgram, Gestodene
  50 microgram Ethinylestradiol 30microgram / Gestodene 50microgram tablets | 18 tablet [PoM] no price available
  Ethinylestradiol 40 microgram, Gestodene
  70 microgram Ethinylestradiol 40microgram / Gestodene 70microgram tablets | 15 tablet [PoM] no price available
  Ethinylestradiol 20 microgram, Gestodene
  75 microgram Ethinylestradiol 20microgram / Gestodene 75microgram tablets | 63 tablet [PoM] no price available
  Ethinylestradiol 30 microgram, Gestodene
  75 microgram Ethinylestradiol 30microgram / Gestodene 75microgram tablets | 63 tablet [PoM] no price available
  Ethinylestradiol 30 microgram, Gestodene
  100 microgram Ethinylestradiol 30microgram / Gestodene 100microgram tablets | 30 tablet [PoM] no price available

▸ Aidulan (Lupin (Europe) Ltd)

  Ethinylestradiol 30 microgram, Gestodene 75 microgram Aidulan 30microgram/75microgram tablets | 63 tablet [PoM] £6.04
  Ethinylestradiol 20 microgram, Gestodene 75 microgram Aidulan 20microgram/75microgram tablets | 63 tablet [PoM] £5.41

▸ Femodene (Bayer Plc)

  Ethinylestradiol 30 microgram, Gestodene
  75 microgram Femodene tablets | 63 tablet [PoM] £6.73

▸ Femodette (Bayer Plc)

  Ethinylestradiol 20 microgram, Gestodene
  75 microgram Femodette tablets | 63 tablet [PoM] £8.85

▸ Juliperla (Actavis UK Ltd)

  Ethinylestradiol 20 microgram, Gestodene
  75 microgram Juliperla 75microgram/20microgram tablets | 63 tablet [PoM] £5.41

▸ Katya (Stragen UK Ltd)

  Ethinylestradiol 30 microgram, Gestodene 75 microgram Katya 30/75 tablets | 63 tablet [PoM] £5.03

▸ Millinette (Consilient Health Ltd)

  Ethinylestradiol 30 microgram, Gestodene
  75 microgram Millinette 30microgram/75microgram tablets | 63 tablet [PoM] £4.12
  Ethinylestradiol 20 microgram, Gestodene
  75 microgram Millinette 20microgram/75microgram tablets | 63 tablet [PoM] £5.41

▸ Sofiperla (Actavis UK Ltd)

  Ethinylestradiol 30 microgram, Gestodene
  75 microgram Sofiperla 75microgram/30microgram tablets | 63 tablet [PoM] £4.12

▸ Sunya (Stragen UK Ltd)

  Ethinylestradiol 20 microgram, Gestodene 75 microgram Sunya 20/75 tablets | 63 tablet [PoM] £6.62

► 719

Ethinylestradiol with levonorgestrel

● INDICATIONS AND DOSE

Contraception with 21-day combined preparations | Menstrual symptoms with 21-day combined preparations

► BY MOUTH

► Females of childbearing potential: 1 tablet once daily for 21 days; subsequent courses repeated after 7-day interval, withdrawal bleeding occurs during the 7-day interval, if reasonably certain woman is not pregnant, first course can be started on any day of cycle—if starting on day 6 of cycle or later, additional precautions (barrier methods) necessary during first 7 days, tablets should be taken at approximately the same time each day

Contraception with 28-day combined preparations | Menstrual symptoms with 28-day combined preparations

► BY MOUTH

► Females of childbearing potential: 1 active tablet once daily for 21 days, followed by 1 inactive tablet once daily for 7 days, withdrawal bleeding occurs during the 7-day interval of *inactive* tablets being taken, if reasonably certain woman is not pregnant, first course can be started on any day of cycle—if starting on day 6 of cycle or later, additional precautions (barrier methods) necessary during first 7 days, tablets should be taken at approximately the same time each day. Subsequent courses repeated without interval

● MEDICINAL FORMS
There can be variation in the licensing of different medicines containing the same drug.

Tablet

► Ethinylestradiol with levonorgestrel (Non-proprietary)
Ethinylestradiol 30 microgram, Levonorgestrel
50 microgram Ethinylestradiol 30microgram / Levonorgestrel 50microgram tablets | 6 tablet [PoM] no price available | 18 tablet [PoM] no price available
Ethinylestradiol 40 microgram, Levonorgestrel
75 microgram Ethinylestradiol 40microgram / Levonorgestrel 75microgram tablets | 5 tablet [PoM] no price available | 15 tablet [PoM] no price available
Ethinylestradiol 30 microgram, Levonorgestrel
125 microgram Ethinylestradiol 30microgram / Levonorgestrel 125microgram tablets | 10 tablet [PoM] no price available | 30 tablet [PoM] no price available

► Elevin (MedRx Healthcare LLP)
Ethinylestradiol 30 microgram, Levonorgestrel
150 microgram Elevin 150microgram/30microgram tablets | 63 tablet [PoM] £29.25 DT price = £2.82

► Erlibelle (Actavis UK Ltd)
Ethinylestradiol 30 microgram, Levonorgestrel
150 microgram Erlibelle 30microgram/150microgram tablets | 63 tablet [PoM] £2.82 DT price = £2.82

► Levest (Morningside Healthcare Ltd)
Ethinylestradiol 30 microgram, Levonorgestrel
150 microgram Levest 150/30 tablets | 21 tablet [PoM] £0.85 (Hospital only) | 63 tablet [PoM] £1.80 DT price = £2.82

► Maexeni (Lupin (Europe) Ltd)
Ethinylestradiol 30 microgram, Levonorgestrel
150 microgram Maexeni 150microgram/30microgram tablets | 63 tablet [PoM] £2.82 DT price = £2.82

► Microgynon 30 (Bayer Plc)
Ethinylestradiol 30 microgram, Levonorgestrel
150 microgram Microgynon 30 tablets | 63 tablet [PoM] £2.82 DT price = £2.82

► Ovranette (Pfizer Ltd)
Ethinylestradiol 30 microgram, Levonorgestrel
150 microgram Ovranette 150microgram/30microgram tablets | 63 tablet [PoM] £2.20 DT price = £2.82

► Rigevidon (Consilient Health Ltd)
Ethinylestradiol 30 microgram, Levonorgestrel
150 microgram Rigevidon tablets | 63 tablet [PoM] £1.89 DT price = £2.82

► 719

Ethinylestradiol with norelgestromin

● INDICATIONS AND DOSE

Contraception | Menstrual symptoms

► BY TRANSDERMAL APPLICATION

► Females of childbearing potential: Apply 1 patch once weekly for 3 weeks, apply first patch on day 1 of cycle, change patch on days 8 and 15; remove third patch on day 22 and apply new patch after 7-day patch-free interval to start subsequent contraceptive cycle, subsequent courses repeated after a 7-day patch free interval (during which withdrawal bleeding occurs)

● DIRECTIONS FOR ADMINISTRATION Adhesives or bandages should not be used to hold patch in place. If no longer sticky do not reapply but use a new patch.

Changing to a transdermal combined hormonal contraceptive
Changing from combined oral contraception Apply patch on the first day of withdrawal bleeding; if no withdrawal bleeding within 5 days of taking last *active* tablet, rule out pregnancy before applying first patch. Unless patch is applied on first day of withdrawal bleeding, additional precautions (barrier methods) should be used concurrently for first 7 days.

Changing from progestogen-only method
● from an implant, apply first patch on the day implant removed
● from an injection, apply first patch when next injection due
● from oral progestogen, first patch may be applied on any day after stopping pill
For all methods additional precautions (barrier methods) should be used concurrently for first 7 days.

After childbirth (not breast-feeding) Start 4 weeks after birth; if started later than 4 weeks after birth additional precautions (barrier methods) should be used for first 7 days.

After abortion or miscarriage Before 20 weeks' gestation start immediately; no additional contraception required if started immediately. After 20 weeks' gestation start on day 21 after abortion or on the first day of first spontaneous menstruation; additional precautions (barrier methods) should be used for first 7 days after applying the patch.

● PATIENT AND CARER ADVICE
Patients and carers should be given advice on how to administer patches.

Missed doses
Delayed application or detached patch If a patch is partly detached for less than 24 hours, reapply to the same site or replace with a new patch immediately; no additional contraception is needed and the next patch should be applied on the usual 'change day'. If a patch remains detached for more than 24 hours or if the user is not aware when the patch became detached, then stop the current contraceptive cycle and start a new cycle by applying a new patch, giving a new 'Day 1'; an additional non-hormonal contraceptive must be used concurrently for the first 7 days of the new cycle.

If application of a new patch at the start of a new cycle is delayed, contraceptive protection is lost. A new patch should be applied as soon as remembered giving a new 'Day 1'; additional non-hormonal methods of contraception should be used for the first 7 days of the new cycle. If application of a patch in the middle of the cycle is delayed (i.e. the patch is not changed on day 8 or day 15):

- for up to 48 hours, apply a new patch immediately; next patch 'change day' remains the same and no additional contraception is required;
- for more than 48 hours, contraceptive protection may have been lost. Stop the current cycle and start a new 4-week cycle immediately by applying a new patch giving a new 'Day 1'; additional non-hormonal contraception should be used for the first 7 days of the new cycle.

If the patch is not removed at the end of the cycle (day 22), remove it as soon as possible and start the next cycle on the usual 'change day', the day after day 28; no additional contraception is required.

Travel Women using patches are at an increased risk of deep vein thrombosis during travel involving long periods of immobility (over 3 hours). The risk may be reduced by appropriate exercise during the journey and possibly by wearing graduated compression hosiery.

● NATIONAL FUNDING/ACCESS DECISIONS

Scottish Medicines Consortium (SMC) Decisions
The *Scottish Medicines Consortium* has advised (September 2003) that *Evra*® patches should be restricted for use in women who are likely to comply poorly with combined oral contraceptives.

● MEDICINAL FORMS
There can be variation in the licensing of different medicines containing the same drug.
Transdermal patch
▸ Evra (Janssen-Cilag Ltd)
Ethinylestradiol 33.9 microgram per 24 hour, Norelgestromin 203 microgram per 24 hour Evra transdermal patches | 9 patch [PoM] £19.51 DT price = £19.51

☞ 719

Ethinylestradiol with norethisterone

● INDICATIONS AND DOSE

Contraception with 21-day combined preparations | Menstrual symptoms with 21-day combined preparations
▸ BY MOUTH
▸ Females of childbearing potential: 1 tablet once daily for 21 days; subsequent courses repeated after 7-day interval, withdrawal bleeding occurs during the 7-day interval, if reasonably certain woman is not pregnant, first course can be started on any day of cycle—if starting on day 6 of cycle or later, additional precautions (barrier methods) necessary during first 7 days, tablets should be taken at approximately the same time each day

● MEDICINAL FORMS
There can be variation in the licensing of different medicines containing the same drug.
Tablet
▸ Ethinylestradiol with norethisterone (Non-proprietary)
Ethinylestradiol 35 microgram, Norethisterone
500 microgram Ethinylestradiol 35microgram / Norethisterone 500microgram tablets | 5 tablet [PoM] no price available | 7 tablet [PoM] no price available | 21 tablet [PoM] no price available
Ethinylestradiol 35 microgram, Norethisterone
750 microgram Ethinylestradiol 35microgram / Norethisterone 750microgram tablets | 21 tablet [PoM] no price available
Ethinylestradiol 35 microgram, Norethisterone
1 mg Ethinylestradiol 35microgram / Norethisterone 1mg tablets | 9 tablet [PoM] no price available | 21 tablet [PoM] no price available | 42 tablet [PoM] no price available

▸ Brevinor (Pfizer Ltd)
Ethinylestradiol 35 microgram, Norethisterone
500 microgram Brevinor 500microgram/35microgram tablets | 63 tablet [PoM] £1.99
▸ Loestrin 20 (Galen Ltd)
Ethinylestradiol 20 microgram, Norethisterone acetate
1 mg Loestrin 20 tablets | 63 tablet [PoM] £2.30
▸ Loestrin 30 (Galen Ltd)
Ethinylestradiol 30 microgram, Norethisterone acetate
1.5 mg Loestrin 30 tablets | 63 tablet [PoM] £3.32
▸ Norimin (Pfizer Ltd)
Ethinylestradiol 35 microgram, Norethisterone 1 mg Norimin 1mg/35microgram tablets | 63 tablet [PoM] £2.28 DT price = £2.28

☞ 719

Ethinylestradiol with norgestimate

● INDICATIONS AND DOSE

Contraception with 21-day combined preparations | Menstrual symptoms with 21-day combined preparations
▸ BY MOUTH
▸ Females of childbearing potential: 1 tablet once daily for 21 days; subsequent courses repeated after 7-day interval, withdrawal bleeding occurs during the 7-day interval, if reasonably certain woman is not pregnant, first course can be started on any day of cycle—if starting on day 6 of cycle or later, additional precautions (barrier methods) necessary during first 7 days, tablets should be taken at approximately the same time each day

● MEDICINAL FORMS
There can be variation in the licensing of different medicines containing the same drug.
Tablet
▸ Ethinylestradiol with norgestimate (Non-proprietary)
Ethinylestradiol 35 microgram, Norgestimate
250 microgram Ethinylestradiol 35microgram / Norgestimate 250microgram tablets | 63 tablet [PoM] no price available
▸ Cilest (Janssen-Cilag Ltd)
Ethinylestradiol 35 microgram, Norgestimate
250 microgram Cilest 35microgram/250microgram tablets | 63 tablet [PoM] £7.16 | 126 tablet [PoM] £14.32
▸ Cilique (Consilient Health Ltd)
Ethinylestradiol 35 microgram, Norgestimate
250 microgram Cilique 250microgram/35microgram tablets | 63 tablet [PoM] £4.65
▸ Lizinna (Morningside Healthcare Ltd)
Ethinylestradiol 35 microgram, Norgestimate
250 microgram Lizinna 250microgram/35microgram tablets | 63 tablet [PoM] £5.37

☞ 719

Norethisterone with mestranol

● INDICATIONS AND DOSE

Contraception | Menstrual symptoms
▸ BY MOUTH
▸ Females of childbearing potential: 1 tablet once daily for 21 days; subsequent courses repeated after 7-day interval, withdrawal bleeding can occur during the 7-day interval, if reasonably certain woman is not pregnant, first course can be started on any day of cycle—if starting on day 6 of cycle or later, additional precautions (barrier methods) necessary during first 7 days, tablets should be taken at the same time each day

● MEDICINAL FORMS
There can be variation in the licensing of different medicines containing the same drug.

Tablet
▸ Norinyl-1 (Pfizer Ltd)
Mestranol 50 microgram, Norethisterone 1 mg Norinyl-1 tablets | 63 tablet [PoM] £2.19 DT price = £2.19

3.2 Contraception, devices

Contraceptive devices not listed below Levonorgestrel, p. 729

CONTRACEPTIVE DEVICES

Intra-uterine contraceptive devices (copper)

● INDICATIONS AND DOSE
Contraception
▸ BY INTRA-UTERINE ADMINISTRATION
▸ Females of childbearing potential: (consult product literature)

IMPORTANT SAFETY INFORMATION
MHRA/CHM ADVICE (JUNE 2015) INTRA-UTERINE CONTRACEPTION: UTERINE PERFORATION—UPDATED INFORMATION ON RISK FACTORS
Uterine perforation most often occurs during insertion, but might not be detected until sometime later. The risk of uterine perforation is increased when the device is inserted up to 36 weeks postpartum or in patients who are breastfeeding. Before inserting an intra-uterine contraceptive device, inform patients that perforation occurs in approximately 1 in every 1000 insertions and signs and symptoms include:
● severe pelvic pain after insertion (worse than period cramps);
● pain or increased bleeding after insertion which continues for more than a few weeks;
● sudden changes in periods;
● pain during intercourse;
● unable to feel the threads.
Patients should be informed on how to check their threads and to arrange a check-up if threads cannot be felt, especially if they also have significant pain. Partial perforation may occur even if the threads can be seen; consider this if there is severe pain following insertion and perform an ultrasound.

● CONTRA-INDICATIONS Active trophoblastic disease (until return to normal of urine and plasma-gonadotrophin concentration) · distorted uterine cavity · established or marked immunosuppression · genital malignancy · medical diathermy · pelvic inflammatory disease · recent sexually transmitted infection (if not fully investigated and treated) · severe anaemia · small uterine cavity · unexplained uterine bleeding · Wilson's disease
● CAUTIONS Anaemia · anticoagulant therapy (avoid if possible) · diabetes · disease-induced immunosuppression (risk of infection—avoid if marked immunosuppression) · drug-induced immunosuppression (risk of infection—avoid if marked immunosuppression) · endometriosis · epilepsy (risk of seizure at time of insertion) · fertility problems · history of pelvic inflammatory disease · increased risk of expulsion if inserted before uterine involution · menorrhagia (progestogen intra-uterine system might be preferable) · nulliparity · severe cervical

stenosis · severe primary dysmenorrhoea · severely scarred uterus (including after endometrial resection) · young age
CAUTIONS, FURTHER INFORMATION
An intra-uterine device should not be removed in mid-cycle unless an additional contraceptive was used for the previous 7 days. If removal is essential post-coital contraception should be considered.
▸ Risk of infection The main excess risk of infection occurs in the first 20 days after insertion and is believed to be related to existing carriage of a sexually transmitted infection. Women are considered to be at a higher risk of sexually transmitted infections if:
● they are under 25 years old or
● they are over 25 years old and ● have a new partner or
● have had more than one partner in the past year or
● their regular partner has other partners.
In these women, pre-insertion screening (for chlamydia and, depending on sexual history and local prevalence of disease, Neisseria gonorrhoeae) should be performed. If results are unavailable at the time of fitting an intra-uterine device for emergency contraception, appropriate prophylactic antibacterial cover should be given. The woman should be advised to attend as an emergency if she experiences sustained pain during the next 20 days.
● SIDE-EFFECTS Allergy · bleeding (on insertion) · cervical perforation · displacement · dysmenorrhoea · expulsion · menorrhagia · occasionally epileptic seizure (on insertion) · pain (on insertion, alleviated by NSAID such as ibuprofen 30 minutes before insertion) · pelvic infection may be exacerbated · uterine perforation · vasovagal attack (on insertion)
SIDE-EFFECTS, FURTHER INFORMATION
▸ Presence of significant symptoms (especially pain) Advise the patient to seek medical attention promptly in case of significant symptoms.
● ALLERGY AND CROSS-SENSITIVITY Contra-indicated if patient has a copper allergy.
● PREGNANCY If an intra-uterine device fails and the woman wishes to continue to full-term the device should be removed in the first trimester if possible. Remove device; if pregnancy occurs, increased likelihood that it may be ectopic.
● BREAST FEEDING Not known to be harmful.
● MONITORING REQUIREMENTS Gynaecological examination before insertion, 6–8 weeks after insertion, then annually.
● DIRECTIONS FOR ADMINISTRATION The timing and technique of fitting an intra-uterine device are critical for its subsequent performance. The healthcare professional inserting (or removing) the device should be fully trained in the technique and should provide full counselling backed, where available, by the patient information leaflet. Devices should not be fitted during the heavy days of the period; they are best fitted after the end of menstruation and before the calculated time of implantation.
● PRESCRIBING AND DISPENSING INFORMATION
UT380 STANDARD® For uterine length 6.5–9 cm; replacement every 5 years.
NOVAPLUS T 380® AG 'Mini' size for minimum uterine length 5 cm; 'Normal' size for uterine length 6.5–9 cm; replacement every 5 years.
GYNEFIX® Suitable for all uterine sizes; replacement every 5 years.
UT380 SHORT® For uterine length 5–7 cm; replacement every 5 years.
NOVA-T® 380 For uterine length 6.5–9 cm; replacement every 5 years.
FLEXI-T®+ 380 For uterine length over 6 cm; replacement every 5 years.

NOVAPLUS T 380® CU *'Mini'* size for minimum uterine length 5 cm; *'Normal'* size for uterine length 6.5–9 cm; replacement every 5 years.

LOAD® 375 For uterine length over 7 cm; replacement every 5 years.

ANCORA® 375 CU For uterine length over 6.5 cm; replacement every 5 years.

T-SAFE® 380A QL For uterine length 6.5–9 cm; replacement every 10 years.

MULTILOAD® CU375 For uterine length 6–9 cm; replacement every 5 years.

MINI TT380® SLIMLINE For minimum uterine length 5 cm; replacement every 5 years.

COPPER T380 A® For uterine length 6.5–9 cm; replacement every 10 years.

TT380® SLIMLINE For uterine length 6.5–9 cm; replacement every 5 years.

NEO-SAFE® T380 For uterine length 6.5–9 cm; replacement every 5 years.

MULTI-SAFE® 375 For uterine length 6–9 cm; replacement every 5 years.

FLEXI-T® 300 For uterine length over 5 cm; replacement every 5 years.

● MEDICINAL FORMS
There can be variation in the licensing of different medicines containing the same drug.

Intra-uterine device
▸ Intra-uterine contraceptive devices (R.F. Medical Supplies Ltd, Farla Medical Ltd, Durbin Plc, Williams Medical Supplies Ltd, Bayer Plc, Organon Laboratories Ltd)
Copper T380 A intra-uterine contraceptive device | 1 device £8.95
Steriload intra-uterine contraceptive device | 1 device £9.65
Load 375 intra-uterine contraceptive device | 1 device £8.52
Novaplus T 380 Ag intra-uterine contraceptive device mini | 1 device £12.50
T-Safe 380A QL intra-uterine contraceptive device | 1 device £10.47
UT380 Standard intra-uterine contraceptive device | 1 device £11.22
Nova-T 380 intra-uterine contraceptive device | 1 device £15.20
Flexi-T+ 380 intra-uterine contraceptive device | 1 device £10.06
Mini TT380 Slimline intra-uterine contraceptive device | 1 device £12.46
Flexi-T 300 intra-uterine contraceptive device | 1 device £9.47
Multi-Safe 375 intra-uterine contraceptive device | 1 device £8.96
Multiload Cu375 intra-uterine contraceptive device | 1 device £9.24
Optima TCu 380A intra-uterine contraceptive device | 1 device £9.65
Novaplus T 380 Ag intra-uterine contraceptive device normal | 1 device £12.50
GyneFix intra-uterine contraceptive device | 1 device £27.11
Novaplus T 380 Cu intra-uterine contraceptive device mini | 1 device £10.95
TT380 Slimline intra-uterine contraceptive device | 1 device £12.46
Ancora 375 Cu intra-uterine contraceptive device | 1 device £7.95
Novaplus T 380 Cu intra-uterine contraceptive device normal | 1 device £10.95
Neo-Safe T380 intra-uterine contraceptive device | 1 device £13.31
UT380 Short intra-uterine contraceptive device | 1 device £11.22

Vaginal contraceptives

● SILICONE CONTRACEPTIVE DIAPHRAGMS

Milex arcing spring silicone diaphragm 60mm (Durbin Plc)
1 device · NHS indicative price = £9.31 · Drug Tariff (Part IXa)

Milex arcing spring silicone diaphragm 65mm (Durbin Plc)
1 device · NHS indicative price = £9.31 · Drug Tariff (Part IXa)

Milex arcing spring silicone diaphragm 70mm (Durbin Plc)
1 device · NHS indicative price = £9.31 · Drug Tariff (Part IXa)

Milex arcing spring silicone diaphragm 75mm (Durbin Plc)
1 device · NHS indicative price = £9.31 · Drug Tariff (Part IXa)

Milex arcing spring silicone diaphragm 80mm (Durbin Plc)
1 device · NHS indicative price = £9.31 · Drug Tariff (Part IXa)

Milex arcing spring silicone diaphragm 85mm (Durbin Plc)
1 device · NHS indicative price = £9.31 · Drug Tariff (Part IXa)

Milex arcing spring silicone diaphragm 90mm (Durbin Plc)
1 device · NHS indicative price = £9.31 · Drug Tariff (Part IXa)

Milex omniflex coil spring silicone diaphragm 60mm (Durbin Plc)
1 device · NHS indicative price = £9.31 · Drug Tariff (Part IXa)

Milex omniflex coil spring silicone diaphragm 65mm (Durbin Plc)
1 device · NHS indicative price = £9.31 · Drug Tariff (Part IXa)

Milex omniflex coil spring silicone diaphragm 70mm (Durbin Plc)
1 device · NHS indicative price = £9.31 · Drug Tariff (Part IXa)

Milex omniflex coil spring silicone diaphragm 75mm (Durbin Plc)
1 device · NHS indicative price = £9.31 · Drug Tariff (Part IXa)

Milex omniflex coil spring silicone diaphragm 80mm (Durbin Plc)
1 device · NHS indicative price = £9.31 · Drug Tariff (Part IXa)

Milex omniflex coil spring silicone diaphragm 85mm (Durbin Plc)
1 device · NHS indicative price = £9.31 · Drug Tariff (Part IXa)

Milex omniflex coil spring silicone diaphragm 90mm (Durbin Plc)
1 device · NHS indicative price = £9.31 · Drug Tariff (Part IXa)

Ortho All-Flex arcing spring silicone diaphragm 65mm (Janssen-Cilag Ltd)
1 device · NHS indicative price = £8.35 · Drug Tariff (Part IXa)

Ortho All-Flex arcing spring silicone diaphragm 70mm (Janssen-Cilag Ltd)
1 device · NHS indicative price = £8.35 · Drug Tariff (Part IXa)

Ortho All-Flex arcing spring silicone diaphragm 75mm (Janssen-Cilag Ltd)
1 device · NHS indicative price = £8.35 · Drug Tariff (Part IXa)

Ortho All-Flex arcing spring silicone diaphragm 80mm (Janssen-Cilag Ltd)
1 device · NHS indicative price = £8.35 · Drug Tariff (Part IXa)

● SILICONE CONTRACEPTIVE PESSARIES

FemCap 22mm (Durbin Plc)
1 device · NHS indicative price = £15.29 · Drug Tariff (Part IXa)

FemCap 26mm (Durbin Plc)
1 device · NHS indicative price = £15.29 · Drug Tariff (Part IXa)

FemCap 30mm (Durbin Plc)
1 device · NHS indicative price = £15.29 · Drug Tariff (Part IXa)

3.3 Contraception, emergency

> **Drugs used for Contraception, emergency not listed below** Intra-uterine contraceptive devices (copper), p. 726 · Levonorgestrel, p. 729

PROGESTERONE RECEPTOR MODULATORS

Ulipristal acetate

● DRUG ACTION Ulipristal acetate is a progesterone receptor modulator with a partial progesterone antagonist effect.

● INDICATIONS AND DOSE

Pre-operative and intermittent treatment of moderate to severe symptoms of uterine fibroids
▸ BY MOUTH
▸ Adult: 5 mg once daily for up to 3 months starting during the first week of menstruation, courses may be repeated if necessary, re-treatment should start no sooner than during the first week of the second menstruation following completion of the first course; max. 4 courses

Emergency contraception
▸ BY MOUTH
▸ Females of childbearing potential: 30 mg for 1 dose, to be taken as soon as possible after coitus, but no later than after 120 hours

- **CONTRA-INDICATIONS**

  GENERAL CONTRA-INDICATIONS

  Repeated use as an emergency contraceptive within a menstrual cycle

  SPECIFIC CONTRA-INDICATIONS

  ‣ When used for uterine fibroids Breast cancer · cervical cancer · ovarian cancer · undiagnosed vaginal bleeding · uterine cancer · vaginal bleeding not caused by uterine fibroids

- **CAUTIONS** Uncontrolled severe asthma

- **INTERACTIONS** → Appendix 1 (ulipristal).

  The effectiveness of ulipristal as an emergency contraceptive is possibly reduced in women taking enzyme-inducing drugs (and possibly for 4 weeks after stopping); a copper intra-uterine device can be offered instead. There is no need to increase the dose for emergency contraception if the patient is taking antibacterials that are not enzyme inducers.

- **SIDE-EFFECTS**

- ‣ **Common or very common**

- ‣ When used for emergency contraception Abdominal pain · back pain · diarrhoea · dizziness · fatigue · gastro-intestinal disturbances · headache · menstrual irregularities · muscle spasms · nausea · vomiting

- ‣ When used for uterine fibroids Abdominal pain · acne · breast pain · dizziness · endometrial thickening · headache · hot flushes · hyperhidrosis · malaise · menstrual disturbances · myalgia · nausea · oedema · ovarian cyst (including rupture) · pelvic pain · uterine haemorrhage

- ‣ **Uncommon**

- ‣ When used for emergency contraception Blurred vision · breast tenderness · dry mouth · hot flushes · pruritus · rash · tremor · uterine spasm

- ‣ When used for uterine fibroids Anxiety · constipation · dry mouth · dyspepsia · epistaxis · flatulence · urinary incontinence

- **CONCEPTION AND CONTRACEPTION** When ulipristal is given as an emergency contraceptive the effectiveness of combined hormonal and progestogen-only contraceptives may be reduced—additional precautions (barrier methods) required for 14 days for combined and parenteral progestogen-only hormonal contraceptives (16 days for *Qlaira*®) and 9 days for oral progestogen-only contraceptives. When ulipristal is given for uterine fibroids non-hormonal contraceptive methods (barrier methods or intra-uterine device) should be used both during treatment and for 12 days after stopping, if required.

- **PREGNANCY** Limited information available when used as an emergency contraceptive. Manufacturer advises avoid for uterine fibroids—no information available.

- **BREAST FEEDING** In emergency contraception manufacturer advises avoid for 1 week after administration—present in milk. When used for uterine fibroids, manufacturer advises avoid—no information available.

- **HEPATIC IMPAIRMENT**

- ‣ When used for Emergency contraception Manufacturer advises avoid in severe impairment—no information available.

- ‣ When used for Uterine fibroids Manufacturer advises avoid in moderate to severe impairment unless patient is closely monitored —no information available.

- **RENAL IMPAIRMENT**

- ‣ When used for Uterine fibroids Manufacturer advises avoid in severe impairment unless patient is closely monitored—no information available.

- **MONITORING REQUIREMENTS**

- ‣ When used for Uterine fibroids Periodic monitoring of the endometrium is recommended following repeated intermittent treatment.

- **PATIENT AND CARER ADVICE**

  Missed doses

- ‣ When used for Uterine fibroids If a dose is more than 12 hours late, the missed dose should not be taken and the next dose should be taken at the normal time.

  Treatment free intervals

- ‣ When used for Uterine fibroids The prescriber should explain the requirement for treatment free intervals.

- ‣ When used for Emergency contraception If vomiting occurs within 3 hours of taking a dose, a replacement dose should be given. When prescribing or supplying hormonal emergency contraception, women should be advised:

  - that their next period may be early or late;
  - that a barrier method of contraception needs to be used until the next period;
  - to seek medical attention promptly if any lower abdominal pain occurs because this could signify an ectopic pregnancy;
  - to return in 3 to 4 weeks if the subsequent menstrual bleed is abnormally light, heavy or brief, or is absent, or if she is otherwise concerned (if there is any doubt as to whether menstruation has occurred, a pregnancy test should be performed at least 3 weeks after unprotected intercourse).

- **MEDICINAL FORMS**

  There can be variation in the licensing of different medicines containing the same drug.

  Tablet

- ‣ Ellaone (HRA Pharma UK Ltd)

  Ulipristal acetate 30 mg EllaOne 30mg tablets | 1 tablet P £14.05

- ‣ Esmya (Gedeon Richter (UK) Ltd)

  Ulipristal acetate 5 mg Esmya 5mg tablets | 28 tablet PoM £114.13

3.4 Contraception, oral progestogen-only

> **Drugs used for Contraception, oral progestogen-only not listed below** Norethisterone, p. 691

PROGESTOGENS

Desogestrel

- **INDICATIONS AND DOSE**

  Contraception

  ▸ BY MOUTH

  ‣ Females of childbearing potential: 75 micrograms daily, dose to be taken at same time each day, starting on day 1 of cycle then continuously, if administration delayed for 12 hours or more it should be regarded as a 'missed pill'

- **CONTRA-INDICATIONS** Acute porphyrias p. 918 · history of breast cancer but can be used after 5 years if no evidence of disease and non-hormonal contraceptive methods unacceptable · severe arterial disease · undiagnosed vaginal bleeding

- **CAUTIONS** Active trophoblastic disease (until return to normal of urine- and plasma-gonadotrophin concentration)—seek specialist advice · arterial disease · functional ovarian cysts · history of jaundice in pregnancy · malabsorption syndromes · past ectopic pregnancy · sex-steroid dependent cancer · systemic lupus erythematosus with positive (or unknown) antiphospholipid antibodies

CAUTIONS, FURTHER INFORMATION
- Other conditions The product literature advises caution in patients with history of thromboembolism, hypertension, diabetes mellitus and migraine; evidence for caution in these conditions is unsatisfactory.

- INTERACTIONS → Appendix 1 (progestogens).

- SIDE-EFFECTS Breast discomfort · changes in libido · depression · disturbance of appetite · dizziness · headache · menstrual irregularities · nausea · skin disorders · vomiting

SIDE-EFFECTS, FURTHER INFORMATION
- Breast cancer There is a small increase in the risk of having breast cancer diagnosed in women using, or who have recently used, a progestogen-only contraceptive pill; this relative risk may be due to an earlier diagnosis. The most important risk factor appears to be the age at which the contraceptive is stopped rather than the duration of use; the risk disappears gradually during the 10 years after stopping and there is no excess risk by 10 years. A possible small increase in the risk of breast cancer should be weighed against the benefits.

- PREGNANCY Not known to be harmful.

- BREAST FEEDING Progestogen-only contraceptives do not affect lactation.

- HEPATIC IMPAIRMENT Caution in severe liver disease and recurrent cholestatic jaundice. Avoid in liver tumour.

- PATIENT AND CARER ADVICE
Missed doses
Missed pill The following advice is recommended: 'If you forget a pill, take it as soon as you remember and carry on with the next pill at the right time. If the pill was more than 12 hours overdue you are not protected. Continue normal pill-taking but you must also use another method, such as the condom, for the next 2 days'.

The Faculty of Sexual and Reproductive Healthcare recommends emergency contraception if one or more tablets are missed or taken more than 12 hours late and unprotected intercourse has occurred before 2 further tablets have been correctly taken.
Surgery All progestogen-only contraceptives are suitable for use as an alternative to combined hormonal contraceptives before major elective surgery, before all surgery to the legs, or before surgery which involves prolonged immobilisation of a lower limb.
Starting routine One tablet daily, on a continuous basis, starting on day 1 of cycle and taken at the same time each day (if delayed by longer than 12 hours contraceptive protection may be lost). Additional contraceptive precautions are not required if desogestrel is started up to and including day 5 of the menstrual cycle; if started after this time, additional contraceptive precautions are required for 2 days.
Changing from a combined oral contraceptive Start on the day following completion of the combined oral contraceptive course without a break (or in the case of ED tablets omitting the inactive ones).
After childbirth Oral progestogen-only contraceptives can be started up to and including day 21 postpartum without the need for additional contraceptive precautions. If started more than 21 days postpartum, additional contraceptive precautions are required for 2 days.
Diarrhoea and vomiting Vomiting and persistent, severe diarrhoea can interfere with the absorption of oral progestogen-only contraceptives. If vomiting occurs within 2 hours of taking desogestrel, another pill should be taken as soon as possible. If a replacement pill is not taken within 12 hours of the normal time for taking desogestrel, or in cases of persistent vomiting or very severe diarrhoea, additional precautions should be used during illness and for 2 days after recovery.

- NATIONAL FUNDING/ACCESS DECISIONS
Scottish Medicines Consortium (SMC) Decisions
The *Scottish Medicines Consortium* has advised (September 2003) that *Cerazette*® should be restricted for use in women who cannot tolerate oestrogen-containing contraceptives or in whom such preparations are contra-indicated.

- MEDICINAL FORMS
There can be variation in the licensing of different medicines containing the same drug.
Tablet
- Desogestrel (Non-proprietary)
Desogestrel 75 microgram Desogestrel 75microgram tablets | 84 tablet PoM £9.55 DT price = £2.30
- Aizea (Besins Healthcare (UK) Ltd)
Desogestrel 75 microgram Aizea 75microgram tablets | 84 tablet PoM £5.21 DT price = £2.30
- Cerazette (Merck Sharp & Dohme Ltd)
Desogestrel 75 microgram Cerazette 75microgram tablets | 84 tablet PoM £9.55 DT price = £2.30
- Cerelle (Consilient Health Ltd)
Desogestrel 75 microgram Cerelle 75microgram tablets | 84 tablet PoM £3.50 DT price = £2.30
- Desomono (MedRx Developments Ltd)
Desogestrel 75 microgram Desomono 75microgram tablets | 84 tablet PoM £7.49 DT price = £2.30
- Desorex (Somex Pharma)
Desogestrel 75 microgram Desorex 75microgram tablets | 84 tablet PoM £6.70 DT price = £2.30
- Feanolla (Lupin (Europe) Ltd)
Desogestrel 75 microgram Feanolla 75microgram tablets | 84 tablet PoM £7.37 DT price = £2.30
- Nacrez (Teva UK Ltd)
Desogestrel 75 microgram Nacrez 75microgram tablets | 84 tablet PoM £3.50 DT price = £2.30
- Zelleta (Morningside Healthcare Ltd)
Desogestrel 75 microgram Zelleta 75microgram tablets | 84 tablet PoM £3.35 DT price = £2.30

Levonorgestrel
18.2.2016

- INDICATIONS AND DOSE
Emergency contraception
- BY MOUTH
- Females of childbearing potential: 1.5 mg for 1 dose, taken as soon as possible after coitus, preferably within 12 hours but no later than after 72 hours

Contraception
- BY MOUTH
- Females of childbearing potential: 1 tablet daily starting on day 1 of the cycle then continuously, dose is to be taken at the same time each day, if administration delayed for 3 hours or more it should be regarded as a "missed pill"

JAYDESS® 13.5MG INTRA-UTERINE DEVICE
Contraception
- BY VAGINA
- Females of childbearing potential: Insert into uterine cavity within 7 days of onset of menstruation, or any time if replacement, or immediately after first-trimester termination; postpartum insertions should be delayed until at least 6 weeks after delivery (12 weeks if uterus involution is substantially delayed); effective for 3 years

LEVOSERT® 20MICROGRAMS/24HOURS INTRA-UTERINE DEVICE
Contraception | Menorrhagia
- BY INTRA-UTERINE ADMINISTRATION
- Females of childbearing potential: Insert into uterine cavity within 7 days of onset of menstruation, or any time if replacement, or immediately after first-trimester abortion; postpartum insertions continued →

should be delayed until at least 6 weeks after delivery; effective for 3 years

MIRENA®20MICROGRAMS/24HOURS INTRA-UTERINE DEVICE

Contraception | Menorrhagia
▶ BY INTRA-UTERINE ADMINISTRATION
▶ Females of childbearing potential: Insert into uterine cavity within 7 days of onset of menstruation, or any time if replacement, or any time if reasonably certain woman is not pregnant and there is no risk of conception (additional precautions (e.g. barrier methods) necessary for next 7 days), or immediately after first-trimester termination by curettage; postpartum insertions should be delayed until at least 4 weeks after delivery; effective for 5 years

Prevention of endometrial hyperplasia during oestrogen replacement therapy
▶ BY INTRA-UTERINE ADMINISTRATION
▶ Females of childbearing potential: Insert during last days of menstruation or withdrawal bleeding or at any time if amenorrhoeic; effective for 4 years

● UNLICENSED USE
▶ With oral use in children Consult product literature for licensing status of individual preparations.
▶ With vaginal use in children Not licensed for use in women under 18 years.

IMPORTANT SAFETY INFORMATION

MHRA/CHM ADVICE (JUNE 2015) INTRA-UTERINE CONTRACEPTION: UTERINE PERFORATION—UPDATED INFORMATION ON RISK FACTORS

Uterine perforation most often occurs during insertion, but might not be detected until sometime later. The risk of uterine perforation is increased when the device is inserted up to 36 weeks postpartum or in patients who are breastfeeding. Before inserting an intra-uterine contraceptive device, inform patients that perforation occurs in approximately 1 in every 1000 insertions and signs and symptoms include:
● severe pelvic pain after insertion (worse than period cramps);
● pain or increased bleeding after insertion which continues for more than a few weeks;
● sudden changes in periods;
● pain during intercourse;
● unable to feel the threads.
Patients should be informed on how to check their threads and to arrange a check-up if threads cannot be felt, especially if they also have significant pain. Partial perforation may occur even if the threads can be seen; consider this if there is severe pain following insertion and perform an ultrasound.

● CONTRA-INDICATIONS
▶ With intra-uterine use Active trophoblastic disease (until return to normal of urine- and plasma-gonadotrophin concentration) · acute cervicitis · acute vaginitis · distorted uterine cavity · established immunosuppression · genital malignancy · history of breast cancer but can be considered for a woman in long-term remission who has menorrhagia and requires effective contraception · infected abortion during the previous three months · marked immunosuppression · not suitable for emergency contraception · pelvic inflammatory disease · postpartum endometritis · recent sexually transmitted infection (if not fully investigated and treated) · severe anaemia · small uterine cavity · unexplained uterine bleeding
▶ With oral use Acute porphyrias p. 918
▶ When used for contraception With oral use for contraception history of breast cancer but can be used after 5 years if no evidence of disease and non-hormonal contraceptive

methods unacceptable · severe arterial disease · undiagnosed vaginal bleeding
● CAUTIONS
▶ With intra-uterine use Disease-induced immunosuppression (risk of infection—avoid if marked immunosuppression) · anaemia · anticoagulant therapy (avoid if possible) · diabetes · drug-induced immunosuppression (risk of infection—avoid if marked immunosuppression) · endometriosis · epilepsy (risk of seizure at time of insertion) · fertility problems · history of pelvic inflammatory disease · increased risk of expulsion if inserted before uterine involution · menorrhagia (progestogen intra-uterine system might be preferable) · nulliparity · severe cervical stenosis · severe primary dysmenorrhoea · severely scarred uterus (including after endometrial resection) · young age
▶ When used for contraception With oral use for contraception active trophoblastic disease (until return to normal of urine- and plasma-gonadotrophin concentration)—seek specialist advice · arterial disease · functional ovarian cysts · history of jaundice in pregnancy · malabsorption syndromes · past ectopic pregnancy · sex-steroid dependent cancer · systemic lupus erythematosus with positive (or unknown) antiphospholipid antibodies
▶ When used for emergency contraception With oral use for emergency contraception active trophoblastic disease (until return to normal of urine- and plasma-gonadotrophin concentration)—seek specialist advice · past ectopic pregnancy · severe malabsorption syndromes

CAUTIONS, FURTHER INFORMATION
An intra-uterine device should not be removed in mid-cycle unless an additional contraceptive was used for the previous 7 days. If removal is essential post-coital contraception should be considered.
▶ Risk of infection with intra-uterine devices The main excess risk of infection occurs in the first 20 days after insertion and is believed to be related to existing carriage of a sexually transmitted infection. Women are considered to be at a higher risk of sexually transmitted infections if:
● they are under 25 years old or
● they are over 25 years old and
● have a new partner or
● have had more than one partner in the past year or
● their regular partner has other partners.
   In these women, pre-insertion screening (for chlamydia and, depending on sexual history and local prevalence of disease, *Neisseria gonorrhoeae*) should be performed. If results are unavailable at the time of fitting an intra-uterine device for emergency contraception, appropriate prophylactic antibacterial cover should be given. The woman should be advised to attend *as an emergency* if she experiences sustained pain during the next 20 days.
▶ Use as a contraceptive in co-morbidities
▶ With oral use The product literature advises caution in patients with history of thromboembolism, hypertension, diabetes mellitus and migraine; evidence for caution in these conditions is unsatisfactory.

MIRENA®20MICROGRAMS/24HOURS INTRA-UTERINE DEVICE Advanced uterine atrophy
● INTERACTIONS → Appendix 1 (progestogens).
When used orally as an emergency contraceptive, the effectiveness of levonorgestrel is reduced in women taking enzyme-inducing drugs (and possibly for 4 weeks after stopping); a copper intra-uterine device can be offered instead. If the copper intra-uterine device is undesirable or inappropriate, the dose of levonorgestrel should be increased to a total of 3 mg taken as a single dose [unlicensed dose—advise women accordingly]. There is no need to increase the dose for emergency contraception if the patient is taking antibacterials that are not enzyme inducers.
With the progestogen-only intra-uterine device,

levonorgestrel is released close to the site of the main contraceptive action (on cervical mucus and endometrium) and therefore progestogenic side-effects and interactions are less likely; in particular, enzyme-inducing drugs are unlikely to significantly reduce the contraceptive effect of the progestogen-only intra-uterine system and additional contraceptive precautions are not required.

● SIDE-EFFECTS
  GENERAL SIDE-EFFECTS
▸ **Common or very common** Depression (sometimes severe) · headache · nausea
▸ **Frequency not known** Vomiting
  SPECIFIC SIDE-EFFECTS
▸ **Common or very common**
▸ With intra-uterine use Changes in the pattern and duration of menstrual bleeding (spotting or prolonged bleeding) · abdominal pain · acne · alopecia · back pain · breast pain · expulsion · hirsutism · migraine · nervousness · pelvic pain · peripheral oedema · salpingitis
▸ **Uncommon**
▸ With intra-uterine use Abdominal distension · cervicitis · eczema · pelvic inflammatory disease · pruritus · skin hyperpigmentation
▸ **Rare**
▸ With intra-uterine use Rash · uterine perforation
▸ **Frequency not known**
▸ With intra-uterine use Functional ovarian cysts (usually asymptomatic and usually resolve spontaneously—ultrasound monitoring recommended) · allergy · bleeding (on insertion) · cervical perforation · displacement · dysmenorrhoea · epileptic seizures (on insertion) · menorrhagia · pain (on insertion, alleviated by NSAID such as ibuprofen 30 minutes before insertion) · pelvic infection may be exacerbated · vasovagal attack (on insertion)
▸ With oral use Breast discomfort · breast tenderness · changes in libido · disturbances of appetite · dizziness · fatigue · menstrual irregularities · skin disorders
  SIDE-EFFECTS, FURTHER INFORMATION
▸ Breast cancer There is a small increase in the risk of having breast cancer diagnosed in women using, or who have recently used, a progestogen-only contraceptive pill; this relative risk may be due to an earlier diagnosis. The most important risk factor appears to be the age at which the contraceptive is stopped rather than the duration of use; the risk disappears gradually during the 10 years after stopping and there is no excess risk by 10 years. A possible small increase in the risk of breast cancer should be weighed against the benefits.

Although the progestogen-only intra-uterine system produces little systemic progestogenic activity, it is usually avoided for 5 years after any evidence of breast cancer. However, the system can be considered for a woman in long-term remission from breast cancer who has menorrhagia and requires effective contraception.
▸ With intra-uterine use Endometrial disorders should be ruled out before insertion and the patient should be fully counselled (and provided with a patient information leaflet). Improvement in progestogenic side-effects, such as mastalgia and in the bleeding pattern may often become very light or absent. Removal of the intra-uterine system should be considered if the patient experiences migraine or severe headache, jaundice, marked increase of blood pressure, or severe arterial disease.

● PREGNANCY
▸ With oral use Not known to be harmful.
▸ With vaginal use If an intra-uterine device fails and the woman wishes to continue to full-term the device should be removed in the first trimester if possible. Avoid; if pregnancy occurs remove intra-uterine system.

● BREAST FEEDING Progestogen-only contraceptives do not affect lactation.
● HEPATIC IMPAIRMENT Caution in severe liver disease and recurrent cholestatic jaundice. Avoid in liver tumour.
● MONITORING REQUIREMENTS
▸ With intra-uterine use Gynaecological examination before insertion, 4–6 weeks after insertion, then annually.
● DIRECTIONS FOR ADMINISTRATION
▸ With intra-uterine use *The doctor or nurse administering (or removing) the system should be fully trained in the technique and should provide full counselling reinforced by the patient information leaflet.*
● PRESCRIBING AND DISPENSING INFORMATION
▸ With intra-uterine use Levonorgestrel-releasing intra-uterine devices vary in licensed indication, duration of use and insertion technique—the MHRA recommends to prescribe and dispense by brand name to avoid inadvertent switching.
  MIRENA®20MICROGRAMS/24HOURS INTRA-UTERINE DEVICE When system is removed (and not immediately replaced) and pregnancy is not desired, remove during the first few days of menstruation, otherwise additional precautions (e.g. barrier methods) should be used for at least 7 days before removal.
  JAYDESS® 13.5MG INTRA-UTERINE DEVICE When system is removed (and not immediately replaced) and pregnancy is not desired, remove within 7 days of the onset of menstruation; additional precautions (e.g. barrier methods) should be used if the system is removed at some other time during the cycle and there is intercourse within 7 days.
  LEVONELLE® ONE STEP Can be sold to women over 16 years; when supplying emergency contraception to the public, pharmacists should refer to guidance issued by the Royal Pharmaceutical Society.
● PATIENT AND CARER ADVICE
  Missed doses
  When used as an oral contraceptive, the following advice is recommended 'If you forget a pill, take it as soon as you remember and carry on with the next pill at the right time. If the pill was more than 3 hours overdue you are not protected. Continue normal pill-taking but you must also use another method, such as the condom, for the next 2 days'.
  The Faculty of Sexual and Reproductive Healthcare recommends emergency contraception if one or more progestogen-only contraceptive tablets are missed or taken more than 3 hours late and unprotected intercourse has occurred before 2 further tablets have been correctly taken.
  Diarrhoea and vomiting with use as an oral contraceptive Vomiting and persistent, severe diarrhoea can interfere with the absorption of oral progestogen-only contraceptives. If vomiting occurs within 2 hours of taking an oral progestogen-only contraceptive, another pill should be taken as soon as possible. If a replacement pill is not taken within 3 hours of the normal time for taking the progestogen-only pill, or in cases of persistent vomiting or very severe diarrhoea, additional precautions should be used during illness and for 2 days after recovery.
  Starting routine
▸ With oral use for Contraception One tablet daily, on a continuous basis, starting on day 1 of cycle and taken at the same time each day (if delayed by longer than 3 hours contraceptive protection may be lost). Additional contraceptive precautions are not required if levonorgestrel is started up to and including day 5 of the menstrual cycle; if started after this time, additional contraceptive precautions are required for 2 days.
  Changing from a combined oral contraceptive Start on the day

following completion of the combined oral contraceptive course without a break (or in the case of ED tablets omitting the inactive ones).

After childbirth Oral progestogen-only contraceptives can be started up to and including day 21 postpartum without the need for additional contraceptive precautions. If started more than 21 days postpartum, additional contraceptive precautions are required for 2 days.

▸ **With intra-uterine use** Counsel women to seek medical attention promptly in case of significant symptoms, especially pain. Patient counselling advised. Patient information leaflet to be provided.

▸ **With oral use for Emergency contraception** If vomiting occurs within 2 hours of taking levonorgestrel, a replacement dose should be given.

▸ **With oral use for Emergency contraception**
  • When prescribing or supplying hormonal emergency contraception, women should be advised:
  • that their next period may be early or late;
  • that a barrier method of contraception needs to be used until the next period;
  • to seek medical attention promptly if any lower abdominal pain occurs because this could signify an ectopic pregnancy;
  • to return in 3 to 4 weeks if the subsequent menstrual bleed is abnormally light, heavy or brief, or is absent, or if she is otherwise concerned (if there is any doubt as to whether menstruation has occurred, a pregnancy test should be performed at least 3 weeks after unprotected intercourse).

• **EXCEPTIONS TO LEGAL CATEGORY** *Levonelle® One Step* can be sold to women over 16 years; when supplying emergency contraception to the public, pharmacists should refer to guidance issued by the Royal Pharmaceutical Society.

• **MEDICINAL FORMS**
There can be variation in the licensing of different medicines containing the same drug.

Tablet
▸ Levonorgestrel (Non-proprietary)
  Levonorgestrel 1.5 mg Levonorgestrel 1.5mg tablets | 1 tablet P
  £13.83 DT price = £5.20 | 1 tablet PoM £3.86–£5.20 DT price = £5.20
▸ Emerres (Morningside Healthcare Ltd)
  Levonorgestrel 1.5 mg Emerres Una 1.5mg tablets | 1 tablet P
  £13.83 DT price = £5.20
  Emerres 1.5mg tablets | 1 tablet PoM £3.65 DT price = £5.20
▸ Isteranda (Sandoz Ltd)
  Levonorgestrel 1.5 mg Isteranda 1.5mg tablets | 1 tablet PoM
  £5.20 DT price = £5.20
▸ Levonelle (Bayer Plc)
  Levonorgestrel 1.5 mg Levonelle 1500microgram tablets |
  1 tablet PoM £5.20 DT price = £5.20
  Levonelle One Step 1.5mg tablets | 1 tablet P £13.83 DT price =
  £5.20
▸ Norgeston (Bayer Plc)
  Levonorgestrel 30 microgram Norgeston 30microgram tablets |
  35 tablet PoM £0.92 DT price = £0.92
▸ Upostelle (Consilient Health Ltd)
  Levonorgestrel 1.5 mg Upostelle 1500microgram tablets |
  1 tablet PoM £3.75 DT price = £5.20

Intra-uterine device
▸ Jaydess (Bayer Plc) ▼
  Levonorgestrel 13.5 mg Jaydess 13.5mg intra-uterine device |
  1 device PoM £69.22
▸ Levosert (Allergan Ltd)
  Levonorgestrel 20 microgram per 24 hour Levosert
  20micrograms/24hours intra-uterine device | 1 device PoM £66.00
▸ Mirena (Bayer Plc)
  Levonorgestrel 20 microgram per 24 hour Mirena
  20micrograms/24hours intra-uterine device | 1 device PoM £88.00

3.5 Contraception, parenteral progestogen-only

> **Drugs used for Contraception, parenteral progestogen-only not listed below** Norethisterone, p. 691

PROGESTOGENS

Etonogestrel

2.6.2016

• **INDICATIONS AND DOSE**

Contraception (no hormonal contraceptive use in previous month)
▸ BY SUBDERMAL IMPLANTATION
▸ Females of childbearing potential: 1 implant inserted during first 5 days of cycle, implant should be removed within 3 years of insertion

Contraception (postpartum)
▸ BY SUBDERMAL IMPLANTATION
▸ Females of childbearing potential: 1 implant to be inserted 21–28 days after delivery, 1 implant to be inserted after 28 days postpartum in breast-feeding mothers, implant should be removed within 3 years of insertion

Contraception following abortion or miscarriage in the second trimester
▸ BY SUBDERMAL IMPLANTATION
▸ Females of childbearing potential: 1 implant to be inserted 21–28 days after abortion or miscarriage, implant should be removed within 3 years of insertion

Contraception following abortion or miscarriage in the first trimester
▸ BY SUBDERMAL IMPLANTATION
▸ Females of childbearing potential: 1 implant to be inserted within 5 days, implant should be removed within 3 years of insertion

Contraception (changing from other hormonal contraceptive)
▸ BY SUBDERMAL IMPLANTATION
▸ Females of childbearing potential: Implant should be removed within 3 years of insertion (consult product literature)

• **CONTRA-INDICATIONS** Acute porphyria · history of breast cancer but can be used after 5 years if no evidence of disease and non-hormonal contraceptive methods unacceptable · severe arterial disease · undiagnosed vaginal bleeding

• **CAUTIONS** Active trophoblastic disease (until return to normal of urine- and plasma-gonadotrophin concentration)—seek specialist advice · arterial disease · disturbances of lipid metabolism · history during pregnancy of deterioration of otosclerosis · history during pregnancy of pruritus · history of jaundice in pregnancy · malabsorption syndromes · possible risk of breast cancer · sex-steroid dependent cancer · systemic lupus erythematosus with positive (or unknown) antiphospholipid antibodies

• **INTERACTIONS** → Appendix 1 (progestogens). Effectiveness of parenteral progestogen-only contraceptives is not affected by antibacterials that do not induce liver enzymes. Effectiveness of the etonogestrel-releasing implant may be reduced by enzyme-inducing drugs and an alternative contraceptive method, unaffected by the interacting drug, is recommended during treatment with the enzyme-inducing drug and for at least 4 weeks after stopping. For a short course of an enzyme-inducing drug, if a change in contraceptive method is undesirable or inappropriate, the implant may be continued in combination with additional contraceptive precautions (e.g. condom) for the duration of treatment with the enzyme-inducing drug and for 4 weeks after stopping it.

● SIDE-EFFECTS Breast discomfort · changes in libido · depression · disturbance of appetite · dizziness · headache · injection-site reactions · menstrual irregularities · nausea · vomiting

SIDE-EFFECTS, FURTHER INFORMATION

▸ Cervical cancer Use of injectable progestogen-only contraceptives may be associated with a small increased risk of cervical cancer, similar to that seen with combined oral contraceptives. The risk of cervical cancer with other progestogen-only contraceptives is not yet known.

▸ Breast cancer There is a small increase in the risk of having breast cancer diagnosed in women using, or who have recently used, a progestogen-only contraceptive pill; this relative risk may be due to an earlier diagnosis. The most important risk factor appears to be the age at which the contraceptive is stopped rather than the duration of use; the risk disappears gradually during the 10 years after stopping and there is no excess risk by 10 years. A possible small increase in the risk of breast cancer should be weighed against the benefits.

● PREGNANCY Not known to be harmful, remove implant if pregnancy occurs.

● BREAST FEEDING Progestogen-only contraceptives do not affect lactation.

● DIRECTIONS FOR ADMINISTRATION The doctor or nurse administering (or removing) the system should be fully trained in the technique and should provide full counselling reinforced by the patient information leaflet.

● PATIENT AND CARER ADVICE Full counselling backed by patient information leaflet required before administration.

● MEDICINAL FORMS
There can be variation in the licensing of different medicines containing the same drug.

Implant

▸ Etonogestrel (Non-proprietary)
Etonogestrel 68 mg Etonogestrel 68mg implant | 1 device PoM no price available DT price = £83.43

▸ Nexplanon (Merck Sharp & Dohme Ltd)
Etonogestrel 68 mg Nexplanon 68mg implant | 1 device PoM £83.43 DT price = £83.43

Medroxyprogesterone acetate

● INDICATIONS AND DOSE

Dysfunctional uterine bleeding

▸ BY MOUTH

▸ Adult: 2.5–10 mg daily for 5–10 days, repeated for 2 cycles, begin treatment on day 16–21 of cycle

Secondary amenorrhoea

▸ BY MOUTH

▸ Adult: 2.5–10 mg daily for 5–10 days, repeated for 3 cycles, begin treatment on day 16–21 of cycle

Mild to moderate endometriosis

▸ BY MOUTH

▸ Adult: 10 mg 3 times a day for 90 consecutive days, begin treatment on day 1 of cycle

Progestogenic opposition of oestrogen HRT

▸ BY MOUTH

▸ Adult: 10 mg daily for the last 14 days of each 28-day oestrogen HRT cycle

Endometrial cancer | Renal cell cancer

▸ BY MOUTH

▸ Adult: 200–600 mg daily

Breast cancer

▸ BY MOUTH

▸ Adult: 0.4–1.5 g daily

Contraception

▸ BY DEEP INTRAMUSCULAR INJECTION

▸ Females of childbearing potential: 150 mg, to be administered within the first 5 days of cycle or within first 5 days after parturition (delay until 6 weeks after parturition if breast-feeding)

▸ BY SUBCUTANEOUS INJECTION

▸ Females of childbearing potential: 104 mg, to be administered within first 5 days of cycle or within 5 days postpartum (delay until 6 weeks postpartum if breast-feeding), injected into anterior thigh or abdomen, dose only suitable if no hormonal contraceptive use in previous month

Long-term contraception

▸ BY DEEP INTRAMUSCULAR INJECTION

▸ Females of childbearing potential: 150 mg every 12 weeks, to be administered within the first 5 days of cycle or within first 5 days after parturition (delay until 6 weeks after parturition if breast-feeding)

▸ BY SUBCUTANEOUS INJECTION

▸ Females of childbearing potential: 104 mg every 13 weeks, to be administered within first 5 days of cycle or within 5 days postpartum (delay until 6 weeks postpartum if breast-feeding), injected into anterior thigh or abdomen, dose only suitable if no hormonal contraceptive use in previous month

Contraception (when patient changing from other hormonal contraception)

▸ BY SUBCUTANEOUS INJECTION

▸ Females of childbearing potential: (consult product literature)

● CONTRA-INDICATIONS

GENERAL CONTRA-INDICATIONS

Acute porphyrias p. 918 · severe arterial disease · undiagnosed vaginal bleeding

SPECIFIC CONTRA-INDICATIONS

▸ With intramuscular use History of breast cancer but can be used after 5 years if no evidence of disease and non-hormonal contraceptive methods unacceptable

▸ With oral use Breast cancer (unless progestogens are being used in the management of this condition) · genital cancer (unless progestogens are being used in the management of this condition) · history of liver tumours

▸ With subcutaneous use History of breast cancer but can be used after 5 years if no evidence of disease and non-hormonal contraceptive methods unacceptable

● CAUTIONS

GENERAL CAUTIONS

Possible risk of breast cancer

SPECIFIC CAUTIONS

▸ With intramuscular use History during pregnancy in disturbances of lipid metabolism · history during pregnancy of deterioration of otosclerosis · history during pregnancy of pruritus

▸ With oral use Asthma · cardiac dysfunction · conditions that may worsen with fluid retention · diabetes (progestogens can decrease glucose tolerance—monitor patient closely) · epilepsy · history of depression · hypertension · migraine · susceptibility to thromboembolism (particular caution with high dose)

▸ With subcutaneous use History during pregnancy in disturbances of lipid metabolism · history during pregnancy of deterioration of otosclerosis · history during pregnancy of pruritus

7

Genito-urinary system

● INTERACTIONS → Appendix 1 (progestogens).

▸ With intramuscular use or subcutaneous use Effectiveness of parenteral progestogen-only contraceptives is not affected by antibacterials that do not induce liver enzymes. The effectiveness of medroxyprogesterone acetate intramuscular and subcutaneous injections is not affected by enzyme-inducing drugs and they may be continued as normal during courses of these drugs.

● SIDE-EFFECTS

GENERAL SIDE-EFFECTS

Breast discomfort · changes in libido · depression · dizziness · headache · indigestion · loss of vision during treatment (discontinue treatment if papilloedema or retinal vascular lesions) · menstrual irregularities · nausea · pruritus · vomiting · weight gain

SPECIFIC SIDE-EFFECTS

▸ **Rare**

▸ With intramuscular use Osteoporosis · osteoporotic fractures
▸ With subcutaneous use Osteoporosis · osteoporotic fractures

▸ **Frequency not known**

▸ With intramuscular use Disturbance of appetite · injection site-reactions · reduced bone mineral density · skin disorders

▸ With oral use Acne · adrenergic-like effects (when used for malignant disease) · alopecia · anaphylactoid reactions · bloating · breast tenderness · cervical erosions (when used for malignant disease) · confusion (when used for malignant disease) · congestive heart failure (when used for malignant disease) · constipation (when used for malignant disease) · diarrhoea (when used for malignant disease) · drowsiness · dry mouth (when used for malignant disease) · euphoria (when used for malignant disease) · fluid retention · galactorrhoea (when used for malignant disease) · glucocorticoid effects may lead to a cushingoid syndrome (with high doses for malignant disease) · hirsutism · hypercalcaemia (when used for malignant disease) · hyperpyrexia (when used for malignant disease) · hypertension (when used for malignant disease) · insomnia · jaundice · loss of concentration (when used for malignant disease) · nervousness (when used for malignant disease) · palpitation (when used for malignant disease) · premenstrual-like syndrome · raised platelet count (when used for malignant disease) · raised white blood cell count (when used for malignant disease) · rash · retinal thrombosis (when used for malignant disease) · skin reactions · tachycardia (when used for malignant disease) · urticaria · vision disorders (when used for malignant disease)

▸ With subcutaneous use Disturbance of appetite · injection site-reactions · reduced bone mineral density · skin disorders

SIDE-EFFECTS, FURTHER INFORMATION

▸ With intramuscular use or subcutaneous use Use of injectable progestogen-only contraceptives may be associated with a small increased risk of cervical cancer, similar to that seen with combined oral contraceptives. The risk of cervical cancer with other progestogen-only contraceptives is not yet known.

▸ With intramuscular use or subcutaneous use Reduction in bone mineral density occurs in the first 2–3 years of use then stabilises.

● CONCEPTION AND CONTRACEPTION

▸ With intramuscular use If interval between dose is greater than 12 weeks and 5 days (in long-term contraception), rule out pregnancy before next injection and advise patient to use additional contraceptive measures (e.g. barrier) for 14 days after the injection.

▸ With subcutaneous use If interval between dose is greater than 13 weeks and 7 days (in long-term contraception), rule out pregnancy before next injection.

● PREGNANCY

▸ With oral use Avoid—genital malformations and cardiac defects reported.

▸ With intramuscular use or subcutaneous use Not known to be harmful.

● BREAST FEEDING Present in milk—no adverse effects reported. Progestogen-only contraceptives do not affect lactation.

▸ With intramuscular use or subcutaneous use The manufacturers advise that in women who are breast-feeding, the first dose should be delayed until 6 weeks after birth; however, evidence suggests no harmful effect to infant if given earlier. The benefits of using medroxyprogesterone acetate in breast-feeding women outweigh any risks.

● HEPATIC IMPAIRMENT Avoid in liver tumour.

▸ With oral use Avoid in hepatic impairment.

▸ With intramuscular use or subcutaneous use Caution in severe liver disease and recurrent cholestatic jaundice.

● RENAL IMPAIRMENT

▸ When used for Mild to moderate endometriosis or Progestogenic opposition of oestrogen HRT or Dysfunctional uterine bleeding or Secondary amenorrhoea Use with caution.

● PATIENT AND CARER ADVICE

▸ With intramuscular use or subcutaneous use Full counselling backed by *patient information leaflet* required before administration—likelihood of menstrual disturbance and the potential for a delay in return to full fertility. Delayed return of fertility and irregular cycles may occur after discontinuation of treatment but there is no evidence of permanent infertility.

● MEDICINAL FORMS
There can be variation in the licensing of different medicines containing the same drug. Forms available from special-order manufacturers include: oral suspension, oral solution

Tablet

▸ Climanor (ReSource Medical UK Ltd)
  Medroxyprogesterone acetate 5 mg Climanor 5mg tablets | 28 tablet [PoM] £3.27

▸ Provera (Pfizer Ltd)
  Medroxyprogesterone acetate 2.5 mg Provera 2.5mg tablets | 30 tablet [PoM] £1.84 DT price = £1.84
  Medroxyprogesterone acetate 5 mg Provera 5mg tablets | 10 tablet [PoM] £1.23 DT price = £1.23 | 100 tablet [PoM] £12.32
  Medroxyprogesterone acetate 10 mg Provera 10mg tablets | 10 tablet [PoM] £2.47 | 90 tablet [PoM] £22.16 DT price = £22.16 | 100 tablet [PoM] £24.73
  Medroxyprogesterone acetate 100 mg Provera 100mg tablets | 60 tablet [PoM] £29.98 | 100 tablet [PoM] £49.94 DT price = £49.94
  Medroxyprogesterone acetate 200 mg Provera 200mg tablets | 30 tablet [PoM] £29.65 DT price = £29.65
  Medroxyprogesterone acetate 400 mg Provera 400mg tablets | 30 tablet [PoM] £58.67 DT price = £58.67

Suspension for injection

▸ Depo-Provera (Pfizer Ltd)
  Medroxyprogesterone acetate 150 mg per 1 ml Depo-Provera 150mg/1ml suspension for injection pre-filled syringes | 1 pre-filled disposable injection [PoM] £6.01 DT price = £6.01

▸ Sayana Press (Pfizer Ltd)
  Medroxyprogesterone acetate 160 mg per 1 ml Sayana Press 104mg/0.65 ml suspension for injection pre-filled disposable devices | 1 pre-filled disposable injection [PoM] £6.90

3.6 Contraception, spermicidal

SPERMICIDALS

Nonoxinol

- ● INDICATIONS AND DOSE

  Spermicidal contraceptive in conjunction with barrier methods of contraception such as diaphragms or caps
  - ▶ BY VAGINA
  - ▶ Females of childbearing potential: (consult product literature)

- ● SIDE-EFFECTS Genital lesions

  SIDE-EFFECTS, FURTHER INFORMATION
  High frequency use of the spermicide nonoxinol '9' has been associated with genital lesions, which may increase the risk of acquiring these infections.

- ● CONCEPTION AND CONTRACEPTION No evidence of harm to latex condoms and diaphragms.

- ● PREGNANCY Toxicity in *animal* studies.

- ● BREAST FEEDING Present in milk in *animal* studies.

- ● MEDICINAL FORMS
  There can be variation in the licensing of different medicines containing the same drug.

  Gel
  EXCIPIENTS: May contain Hydroxybenzoates (parabens), propylene glycol, sorbic acid
  - ▶ Gygel (Marlborough Pharmaceuticals Ltd)
    Nonoxinol-9 20 mg per 1 ml Gygel 2% contraceptive jelly |
    30 gram GSL £4.25 | 81 gram GSL £11.00

4   Erectile and ejaculatory conditions

4.1 Erectile dysfunction

Erectile dysfunction

Overview

Reasons for failure to produce a satisfactory erection include *psychogenic, vascular, neurogenic,* and *endocrine abnormalities*; impotence can also be drug-induced. Intracavernosal, urethral or topical application of vasoactive drugs under careful medical supervision are used for the management of erectile dysfunction. Intracavernosal or intraurethral preparations can also be used in the diagnosis of erectile dysfunction.

Erectile disorders may also be treated with drugs given by mouth which increase the blood flow to the penis. Drugs should be used with caution if the penis is deformed (e.g. in angulation, cavernosal fibrosis, and Peyronie's disease).

Priapism

If priapism occurs with alprostadil p. 739, treatment should not be delayed more than 6 hours and is as follows:

- Initial therapy by penile aspiration—using aseptic technique a 19–21 gauge butterfly needle inserted into the corpus cavernosum and 20–50 mL of blood aspirated; if necessary the procedure may be repeated on the opposite side.
- If initial aspiration is unsuccessful a second 19–21 gauge butterfly needle can be inserted into the opposite corpus cavernosum and sterile physiological saline introduced through the first needle and drained through the second.

- If aspiration and lavage of corpora are unsuccessful, *cautious* intracavernosal injection of a sympathomimetic with action on alpha-adrenergic receptors, continuously monitoring blood pressure and pulse (*extreme caution*: coronary heart disease, hypertension, cerebral ischaemia or if taking antidepressant) can be given.
- If necessary the sympathomimetic injections can be followed by further aspiration of blood through the same butterfly needle.
- If sympathomimetics unsuccessful, urgent surgical referral for management (possibly including shunt procedure).

Prescribing on the NHS

Some drug treatments for erectile dysfunction may only be prescribed on the NHS under certain circumstances; for details see the criteria listed in part XVIIIB of the Drug Tariff (Part XIb of the Northern Ireland Drug Tariff, Part 12 of the Scottish Drug Tariff). The Drug Tariffs can be accessed online at: National Health Service Drug Tariff for England and Wales: www.ppa.org.uk/ppa/edt_intro.htm

Health and Personal Social Services for Northern Ireland Drug Tariff: www.hscbusiness.hscni.net/services/2034.htm

Scottish Drug Tariff: www.isdscotland.org/Health-Topics/Prescribing-and-Medicines/Scottish-Drug-Tariff/

Alprostadil

Alprostadil (prostaglandin E_1) is given by intracavernosal injection, intraurethral application, or topical application for the management of erectile dysfunction (after exclusion of treatable medical causes). Intracavernosal or intraurethral preparations can also be used in the diagnosis of erectile dysfunction.

Phosphodiesterase type-5 inhibitors

Avanafil below, sildenafil p. 736, tadalafil p. 737 and vardenafil p. 738 are phosphodiesterase type-5 inhibitors licensed for the treatment of erectile dysfunction; they are not recommended for use with other treatments for erectile dysfunction. The patient should be assessed appropriately before prescribing avanafil, sildenafil, tadalafil or vardenafil. Since these drugs are given by mouth there is a potential for drug interactions.

Papaverine and phentolamine

Although not licensed the smooth muscle relaxant papaverine has also been given by intracavernosal injection for erectile dysfunction. Patients with neurological or psychogenic impotence are more sensitive to the effect of papaverine than those with vascular abnormalities. Phentolamine mesilate p. 167 is added if the response is inadequate [unlicensed indication].

Persistence of the erection for longer than 4 hours is an emergency.

PHOSPHODIESTERASE TYPE-5 INHIBITORS

Avanafil

- ● INDICATIONS AND DOSE

  Erectile dysfunction
  - ▶ BY MOUTH
  - ▶ Adult: Initially 100 mg, to be taken approximately 15–30 minutes before sexual activity, then adjusted according to response to 50–200 mg (max. per dose 200 mg), to be taken as a single dose as needed; maximum 1 dose per day

  Erectile dysfunction in patients on alpha-blocker therapy
  - ▶ BY MOUTH
  - ▶ Adult: Initially 50 mg, to be taken approximately 15–30 minutes before sexual activity, then continued →

adjusted according to response to 50–200 mg (max. per dose 200 mg), to be taken as a single dose as needed; maximum 1 dose per day

DOSE ADJUSTMENTS DUE TO INTERACTIONS
Max. 100 mg once every 48 hours with concomitant moderate inhibitors of cytochrome P450 enzyme CYP3A4 e.g. aprepitant, diltiazem, erythromycin, fluconazole, fosamprenavir, or verapamil.
Concomitant treatment with a phosphodiesterase type-5 inhibitor and an alpha-blocker can increase the risk of postural hypotension—initiate treatment with a phosphodiesterase type-5 inhibitor (at a low dose) only once the patient is stable on the alpha-blocker.

- **CONTRA-INDICATIONS** Avoid if systolic blood pressure below 90 mmHg (no information available) · blood pressure >170/100 mmHg · hereditary degenerative retinal disorders · history of non-arteritic anterior ischaemic optic neuropathy · life-threatening arrhythmia in previous 6 months · mild to severe heart failure · patients in whom vasodilation or sexual activity are inadvisable · recent history of myocardial infarction · recent history of stroke · recent unstable angina

- **CAUTIONS** Active peptic ulceration · anatomical deformation of the penis (e.g. angulation, cavernosal fibrosis, Peyronie's disease) · bleeding disorders · cardiovascular disease · left ventricular outflow obstruction · predisposition to priapism (e.g. in sickle-cell disease, multiple myeloma, or leukaemia)

- **INTERACTIONS** → Appendix 1 (avanafil). Avoid concomitant use of nitrates.

- **SIDE-EFFECTS**
  - **Common or very common** Back pain · dizziness · dyspepsia · flushing · headache · migraine · myalgia · nasal congestion · nausea · visual disturbances · vomiting
  - **Uncommon** Drowsiness · epistaxis · hypertension · hypotension · malaise · painful red eyes · palpitation · tachycardia
  - **Rare** Abdominal pain · diarrhoea · dry mouth · facial oedema · gastritis · genital irritation · gout · haematuria · hyperactivity · hyperbilirubinaemia · hypersensitivity reactions · increased serum creatinine · insomnia · muscle spasms · peripheral oedema · pollakiuria · priapism · rash · Stevens-Johnson syndrome · syncope · weight gain
  - **Frequency not known** Arrhythmia · myocardial infarction · non-arteritic anterior ischaemic optic neuropathy (stop drug if sudden visual impairment occurs) · retinal vascular occlusion · seizures · serious cardiovascular events · sudden hearing loss (discontinue drug and seek medical advice) · unstable angina

- **HEPATIC IMPAIRMENT** Use lowest effective initial dose in mild to moderate impairment, adjusted according to response. Manufacturer advises avoid in severe impairment—no information available.

- **RENAL IMPAIRMENT** Avoid if eGFR less than 30 mL/minute/1.73 m^2.

- **PATIENT AND CARER ADVICE** Onset of effect may be delayed if taken with food.

- **NATIONAL FUNDING/ACCESS DECISIONS**
  NHS restrictions *Spedra*® is not prescribable under the NHS for treatment of erectile dysfunction except in men who meet the criteria listed in part XVIIIB of the Drug Tariff (Part XIb of the Northern Ireland Drug Tariff, Part 12 of the Scottish Drug Tariff). The prescription must be endorsed 'SLS'. For more information see *Prices in the BNF*, under *How to use the BNF*.

- **MEDICINAL FORMS**
  There can be variation in the licensing of different medicines containing the same drug.
  Tablet
  - Spedra (A. Menarini Farmaceutica Internazionale SRL) ▼
    Avanafil 50 mg Spedra 50mg tablets | 4 tablet [PoM] £10.94 DT price = £10.94 | 8 tablet [PoM] £19.70 DT price = £19.70
    Avanafil 100 mg Spedra 100mg tablets | 4 tablet [PoM] £14.08 DT price = £14.08 | 8 tablet [PoM] £26.26 DT price = £26.26
    Avanafil 200 mg Spedra 200mg tablets | 4 tablet [PoM] £21.90 DT price = £21.90 | 8 tablet [PoM] £39.40 DT price = £39.40

Sildenafil

- **INDICATIONS AND DOSE**

Pulmonary arterial hypertension (initiated under specialist supervision)
- BY MOUTH
  - Adult: 20 mg 3 times a day
- BY INTRAVENOUS INJECTION
  - Adult: 10 mg 3 times a day, use intravenous route when the oral route is not appropriate

Erectile dysfunction
- BY MOUTH
  - Adult: Initially 50 mg, to be taken approximately 1 hour before sexual activity, adjusted according to response to 25–100 mg (max. per dose 100 mg) as required, to be taken as a single dose; maximum 1 dose per day

- **CONTRA-INDICATIONS**
  GENERAL CONTRA-INDICATIONS
  Hereditary degenerative retinal disorders · history of non-arteritic anterior ischaemic optic neuropathy · recent history of myocardial infarction · recent history of stroke
  SPECIFIC CONTRA-INDICATIONS
  - When used for erectile dysfunction Avoid if systolic blood pressure below 90 mmHg (no information available) · patients in whom vasodilation or sexual activity are inadvisable · recent unstable angina
  - When used for pulmonary arterial hypertension Sickle-cell anaemia

- **CAUTIONS**
  GENERAL CAUTIONS
  Active peptic ulceration · bleeding disorders · cardiovascular disease · left ventricular outflow obstruction
  SPECIFIC CAUTIONS
  - When used for erectile dysfunction Anatomical deformation of the penis (e.g. angulation, cavernosal fibrosis, Peyronie's disease) · predisposition to priapism (e.g. in sickle-cell disease, multiple myeloma, or leukaemia)
  - When used for pulmonary arterial hypertension Anatomical deformation of the penis · autonomic dysfunction · hypotension (avoid if systolic blood pressure below 90 mmHg) · intravascular volume depletion · predisposition to priapism · pulmonary veno-occlusive disease

- **INTERACTIONS** → Appendix 1 (sildenafil).

- **SIDE-EFFECTS**
  GENERAL SIDE-EFFECTS
  - **Common or very common** Back pain · dyspepsia · flushing · migraine · myalgia · nasal congestion · visual disturbances
  - **Frequency not known** Non-arteritic anterior ischaemic optic neuropathy (discontinue if sudden visual impairment occurs) · sudden hearing loss (advise patient to seek medical help)
  SPECIFIC SIDE-EFFECTS
  - **Common or very common**
  - When used for erectile dysfunction Nausea · dizziness · vomiting

▸ When used for pulmonary arterial hypertension Abdominal distension · alopecia · anaemia · anxiety · bronchitis · cellulitis · cough · diarrhoea · dry mouth · epistaxis · fever · gastritis · gastro-oesophageal reflux · haemorrhoids · headache · influenza-like symptoms · insomnia · limb pain · night sweats · oedema · painful red eyes · paraesthesia · photophobia · retinal haemorrhage · tremor · vertigo

▸ **Uncommon**

▸ When used for erectile dysfunction Chest pain · drowsiness · dry mouth · epistaxis · fatigue · hypertension · hypoaesthesia · hypotension · painful red eyes · palpitation · tachycardia · tinnitus · vertigo

▸ When used for pulmonary arterial hypertension Gynaecomastia · haematuria · penile haemorrhage · priapism

▸ **Rare**

▸ When used for erectile dysfunction Atrial fibrillation · cerebrovascular accident · facial oedema · hypersensitivity reactions · priapism · rash · Stevens-Johnson syndrome · syncope

▸ **Frequency not known**

▸ When used for erectile dysfunction Arrhythmia · myocardial infarction · seizures · unstable angina

▸ When used for pulmonary arterial hypertension Rash · retinal vascular occlusion

● PREGNANCY Use only if potential benefit outweighs risk— no evidence of harm in *animal* studies.

● BREAST FEEDING Manufacturer advises avoid—no information available.

● HEPATIC IMPAIRMENT In pulmonary arterial hypertension, if usual dose not tolerated, reduce *oral* dose to 20 mg twice daily and *intravenous* dose to 10 mg twice daily. For erectile dysfunction, use initial dose of 25 mg. Manufacturer advises avoid in severe impairment.

● RENAL IMPAIRMENT Use initial dose of 25 mg in erectile dysfunction if eGFR less than 30 mL/minute/1.73 m^2.
   In pulmonary hypertension, if usual dose not tolerated, reduce *oral* dose to 20 mg twice daily and *intravenous* dose to 10 mg twice daily..

● TREATMENT CESSATION

▸ When used for Pulmonary arterial hypertension Consider gradual withdrawal.

● PATIENT AND CARER ADVICE

▸ When used for Erectile dysfunction Onset of effect may be delayed if taken with food.

● NATIONAL FUNDING/ACCESS DECISIONS

Scottish Medicines Consortium (SMC) Decisions
The *Scottish Medicines Consortium* has advised (January 2010 and February 2011) that sildenafil tablets (*Revatio*®) should be initiated for patients with pulmonary arterial hypertension only by specialists in the Scottish Pulmonary Vascular Unit or other similar specialists and that sildenafil injection (*Revatio*®) should be prescribed only on the advice of specialists in the Scottish Pulmonary Vascular Unit or the Scottish Adult Congenital Cardiac Service.
NHS restrictions *Viagra*® is not prescribable under NHS for treatment of erectile dysfunction except in men who meet the criteria listed in part XVIIIB of the Drug Tariff (Part XIb of the Northern Ireland Drug Tariff, Part 12 of the Scottish Drug Tariff). The prescription must be endorsed 'SLS'. For more information see *Prices in the BNF*, under How to use the BNF.

● MEDICINAL FORMS
There can be variation in the licensing of different medicines containing the same drug. Forms available from special-order manufacturers include: oral suspension, oral solution

Tablet

▸ Sildenafil (Non-proprietary)
Sildenafil (as Sildenafil citrate) 25 mg Sildenafil 25mg tablets | 4 tablet PoM £17.45 DT price = £0.83 | 8 tablet PoM £33.19

Sildenafil (as Sildenafil citrate) 50 mg Sildenafil 50mg tablets | 4 tablet PoM £22.45 DT price = £0.91 | 8 tablet PoM £42.54
Sildenafil (as Sildenafil citrate) 100 mg Sildenafil 100mg tablets | 4 tablet PoM £24.25 DT price = £1.01 | 8 tablet PoM £48.25 | 12 tablet PoM £7.85

▸ Revatio (Pfizer Ltd)
Sildenafil (as Sildenafil citrate) 20 mg Revatio 20mg tablets | 90 tablet PoM £446.33

▸ Viagra (Pfizer Ltd)
Sildenafil (as Sildenafil citrate) 25 mg Viagra 25mg tablets | 4 tablet PoM £16.59 DT price = £0.83 | 8 tablet PoM £33.19
Sildenafil (as Sildenafil citrate) 50 mg Viagra 50mg tablets | 4 tablet PoM £21.27 DT price = £0.91 | 8 tablet PoM £42.54
Sildenafil (as Sildenafil citrate) 100 mg Viagra 100mg tablets | 4 tablet PoM £23.50 DT price = £1.01 | 8 tablet PoM £46.99

▸ Vizarsin (Consilient Health Ltd)
Sildenafil (as Sildenafil citrate) 25 mg Vizarsin 25mg tablets | 4 tablet PoM £14.10 DT price = £0.83
Sildenafil (as Sildenafil citrate) 50 mg Vizarsin 50mg tablets | 4 tablet PoM £18.07 DT price = £0.91
Sildenafil (as Sildenafil citrate) 100 mg Vizarsin 100mg tablets | 4 tablet PoM £19.97 DT price = £1.01

Chewable tablet
CAUTIONARY AND ADVISORY LABELS 24
EXCIPIENTS: May contain Aspartame

▸ Nipatra (AMCo)
Sildenafil (as Sildenafil citrate) 25 mg Nipatra 25mg chewable tablets sugar-free | 4 tablet PoM £1.05 sugar-free | 8 tablet PoM £2.10

Sildenafil (as Sildenafil citrate) 50 mg Nipatra 50mg chewable tablets sugar-free | 4 tablet PoM £1.03 sugar-free | 8 tablet PoM £2.06

Sildenafil (as Sildenafil citrate) 100 mg Nipatra 100mg chewable tablets sugar-free | 4 tablet PoM £1.11 sugar-free | 8 tablet PoM £2.22

Oral suspension

▸ Revatio (Pfizer Ltd)
Sildenafil (as Sildenafil citrate) 10 mg per 1 ml Revatio 10mg/ml oral suspension sugar-free | 112 ml PoM £186.75

Solution for injection

▸ Revatio (Pfizer Ltd)
Sildenafil (as Sildenafil citrate).8 mg per 1 ml Revatio 10mg/12.5ml solution for injection vials | 1 vial PoM £45.28

Tadalafil

● INDICATIONS AND DOSE

Pulmonary arterial hypertension (initiated under specialist supervision)

▸ BY MOUTH

▸ Adult: 40 mg once daily

Erectile dysfunction

▸ BY MOUTH

▸ Adult: Initially 10 mg once daily (max. per dose 20 mg), to be taken at least 30 minutes before sexual activity, subsequent doses adjusted according to response, the effect of intermittent dosing may persist for longer than 24 hours, daily dose of 10–20 mg not recommended; maximum 1 dose per day

Erectile dysfunction; for patients who anticipate sexual activity at least twice a week

▸ BY MOUTH

▸ Adult: 5 mg once daily, reduced to 2.5 mg once daily, adjusted according to response, the effect of intermittent dosing may persist for longer than 24 hours

Benign prostatic hyperplasia

▸ BY MOUTH

▸ Adult: 5 mg once daily

● CONTRA-INDICATIONS
GENERAL CONTRA-INDICATIONS
History of non-arteritic anterior ischaemic optic neuropathy

7

Genito-urinary system

SPECIFIC CONTRA-INDICATIONS
▸ When used for benign prostatic hyperplasia or erectile dysfunction Hypotension (avoid if systolic blood pressure below 90 mmHg) · mild to severe heart failure · myocardial infarction · patients in whom vasodilation or sexual activity are inadvisable · recent stroke · uncontrolled arrhythmias · uncontrolled hypertension · unstable angina
▸ When used for pulmonary arterial hypertension Acute myocardial infarction in past 90 days
● CAUTIONS
▸ When used for benign prostatic hyperplasia or erectile dysfunction Anatomical deformation of the penis (e.g. angulation, cavernosal fibrosis, Peyronie's disease) · cardiovascular disease · left ventricular outflow obstruction · predisposition to priapism (e.g. in sickle-cell disease, multiple myeloma, or leukaemia)
▸ When used for pulmonary arterial hypertension Anatomical deformation of the penis · aortic and mitral valve disease · congestive cardiomyopathy · coronary artery disease · hereditary degenerative retinal disorders · hypotension (avoid if systolic blood pressure below 90 mmHg) · left ventricular dysfunction · life-threatening arrhythmias · pericardial constriction · predisposition to priapism · pulmonary veno-occlusive disease · uncontrolled hypertension
● INTERACTIONS → Appendix 1 (tadalafil).
● SIDE-EFFECTS
GENERAL SIDE-EFFECTS
▸ **Common or very common** Back pain · dyspepsia · flushing · headache · myalgia · nausea · vomiting
▸ **Uncommon** Hypertension · tachycardia
▸ **Frequency not known** Arrhythmia · myocardial infarction · non-arteritic anterior ischaemic optic neuropathy (stop drug if sudden visual impairment occurs) · retinal vascular occlusion · sudden hearing loss (discontinue drug and seek medical advice) · unstable angina
SPECIFIC SIDE-EFFECTS
▸ **Common or very common**
▸ When used for benign prostatic hyperplasia or erectile dysfunction Dizziness · migraine · nasal congestion · visual disturbances
▸ When used for pulmonary arterial hypertension Blurred vision · chest pain · epistaxis · facial oedema · gastro-oesophageal reflux · hypotension · increased uterine bleeding · limb pain · nasopharyngitis · palpitation · rash
▸ **Uncommon**
▸ When used for benign prostatic hyperplasia or erectile dysfunction Epistaxis · hypotension · painful red eyes · palpitation
▸ When used for pulmonary arterial hypertension Amnesia · hyperhidrosis · priapism · seizures
▸ **Rare**
▸ When used for benign prostatic hyperplasia or erectile dysfunction Facial oedema · hypersensitivity reactions · priapism · rash · Stevens-Johnson syndrome · syncope
▸ **Frequency not known**
▸ When used for benign prostatic hyperplasia or erectile dysfunction Abdominal pain · increased sweating · seizures · serious cardiovascular events · transient amnesia
▸ When used for pulmonary arterial hypertension Stevens-Johnson syndrome · stroke · visual field defect
● PREGNANCY Manufacturer advises avoid.
● BREAST FEEDING Manufacturer advises avoid—present in milk in *animal* studies.
● HEPATIC IMPAIRMENT For pulmonary arterial hypertension use initial dose of 20 mg once daily in mild to moderate impairment. Use maximum dose of 10 mg in erectile dysfunction and benign prostatic hyperplasia. When used for pulmonary arterial hypertension, avoid in severe impairment. Manufacturer advises caution in severe impairment and for regular once-daily dosing in erectile

dysfunction and benign prostatic hyperplasia—no information available.
● RENAL IMPAIRMENT In pulmonary arterial hypertension for patients with mild to moderate impairment, initially use 20 mg once daily, increased to 40 mg once daily if tolerated. For erectile dysfunction and benign prostatic hyperplasia, maximum dose 10 mg if eGFR less than 30 mL/minute/1.73 m^2 (avoid regular once-daily dosing). In pulmonary arterial hypertension, avoid in severe impairment.
● NATIONAL FUNDING/ACCESS DECISIONS
Scottish Medicines Consortium (SMC) Decisions
The *Scottish Medicines Consortium* has advised (June 2012) that tadalafil (*Adcirca*®) should be initiated only by specialists in the Scottish Pulmonary Vascular Unit or other similar specialists.
NHS restrictions   *Cialis*® is not prescribable under the NHS for treatment of erectile dysfunction except in men who meet the criteria listed in part XVIIIB of the Drug Tariff (Part XIb of the Northern Ireland Drug Tariff, Part 12 of the Scottish Drug Tariff). The prescription must be endorsed 'SLS'. For more information see *Prices in the BNF*, under How to use the BNF.

● MEDICINAL FORMS
There can be variation in the licensing of different medicines containing the same drug.
Tablet
▸ Adcirca (Eli Lilly and Company Ltd)
  Tadalafil 20 mg Adcirca 20mg tablets | 56 tablet [PoM] £491.22
▸ Cialis (Eli Lilly and Company Ltd)
  Tadalafil 2.5 mg Cialis 2.5mg tablets | 28 tablet [PoM] £54.99 DT price = £54.99
  Tadalafil 5 mg Cialis 5mg tablets | 28 tablet [PoM] £54.99 DT price = £54.99
  Tadalafil 10 mg Cialis 10mg tablets | 4 tablet [PoM] £28.88 DT price = £28.88
  Tadalafil 20 mg Cialis 20mg tablets | 4 tablet [PoM] £28.88 DT price = £28.88 | 8 tablet [PoM] £57.76

Vardenafil

● INDICATIONS AND DOSE
Erectile dysfunction
▸ BY MOUTH USING TABLETS
▸ Adult: Initially 10 mg (max. per dose 20 mg), to be taken approximately 25–60 minutes before sexual activity, subsequent doses adjusted according to response, onset of effect may be delayed if taken with high-fat meal; maximum 1 dose per day
▸ BY MOUTH USING ORODISPERSIBLE TABLET
▸ Adult: 10 mg, to be taken approximately 25–60 minutes before sexual activity; maximum 10 mg per day
Erectile dysfunction (patients on alpha-blocker therapy)
▸ BY MOUTH USING TABLETS
▸ Adult: Initially 5 mg (max. per dose 20 mg), to be taken approximately 25–60 minutes before sexual activity, subsequent doses adjusted according to response, onset of effect may be delayed if taken with high-fat meal; maximum 1 dose per day
DOSE ADJUSTMENTS DUE TO INTERACTIONS
Concomitant treatment with phosphodiesterase type-5 inhibitor and an alpha-blocker can increase the risk of postural hypotension—initiate treatment with a phosphodiesterase type-5 inhibitor (at a low dose) only once the patient is stable on the alpha-blocker.
DOSE EQUIVALENCE AND CONVERSION
Levitra® 10 mg orodispersible tablets and *Levitra*® 10 mg film coated tablets are **not** bioequivalent.

- CONTRA-INDICATIONS Avoid if systolic blood pressure below 90 mmHg · hereditary degenerative retinal disorders · myocardial infarction · patients in whom vasodilation or sexual activity are inadvisable · previous history of non-arteritic anterior ischaemic optic neuropathy · recent stroke · unstable angina

- CAUTIONS Active peptic ulceration · anatomical deformation of the penis (e.g. angulation, cavernosal fibrosis, Peyronie's disease) · bleeding disorders · cardiovascular disease · elderly · left ventricular outflow obstruction · predisposition to priapism (e.g. in sickle-cell disease, multiple myeloma, or leukaemia) · susceptibility to prolongation of QT interval

- INTERACTIONS → Appendix 1 (vardenafil) Caution with concomitant use of drugs which prolong QT interval. Avoid concomitant use of nitrates.

- SIDE-EFFECTS
- **Common or very common** Back pain · dizziness · dyspepsia · flushing · headache · migraine · myalgia · nasal congestion · nausea · visual disturbances · vomiting
- **Uncommon** Drowsiness · dyspnoea · epistaxis · hypertension · hypotension · increased lacrimation · painful red eyes · palpitation · photosensitivity · tachycardia
- **Rare** Anxiety · facial oedema · hypersensitivity reactions · hypertonia · priapism · raised intra-ocular pressure · rash · Stevens-Johnson syndrome · syncope · transient amnesia
- **Frequency not known** Arrhythmia · myocardial infarction · non-arteritic anterior ischaemic optic neuropathy (stop drug if sudden visual impairment occurs) · retinal vascular occlusion · seizures · serious cardiovascular events · sudden hearing loss (discontinue drug and seek medical advice) · unstable angina

- HEPATIC IMPAIRMENT Initial dose 5 mg in mild to moderate impairment, increased subsequently according to response (max. 10 mg in moderate impairment). Manufacturer advises avoid in severe impairment.
  Orodispersible tablets not suitable for patients with moderate hepatic impairment.

- RENAL IMPAIRMENT Initial dose 5 mg if eGFR less than 30 mL/minute/1.73 m². Orodispersible tablets not suitable if eGFR less than 30 mL/minute/1.73 m².

- PRESCRIBING AND DISPENSING INFORMATION Orodispersible tablets not suitable for initiation of therapy in patients taking alpha-blockers.

- NATIONAL FUNDING/ACCESS DECISIONS
  Scottish Medicines Consortium (SMC) Decisions
  The *Scottish Medicines Consortium* has advised (September 2011) that vardenafil orodispersible tablets (*Levitra* ®) are accepted for restricted use within NHS Scotland for men for whom an orodispersible tablet is an appropriate formulation.
  NHS restrictions *Levitra* ® is not prescribable under the NHS for the treatment of erectile dysfunction except in men who meet the criteria listed in part XVIIIB of the Drug Tariff (Part XIb of the Northern Ireland Drug Tariff, Part 12 of the Scottish Drug Tariff). The prescription must be endorsed 'SLS'. For more information see *Prices in the BNF*, under How to use the BNF.

  LEVITRA® ORODISPERSIBLE TABLETS
  Scottish Medicines Consortium (SMC) Decisions
  The *Scottish Medicines Consortium* has advised (September 2011) that vardenafil orodispersible tablets (*Levitra* ®) are accepted for restricted use within NHS Scotland for men for whom an orodispersible tablet is an appropriate formulation.

- MEDICINAL FORMS
  There can be variation in the licensing of different medicines containing the same drug.
  Tablet
  ▸ Levitra (Bayer Plc)
  Vardenafil (as Vardenafil hydrochloride trihydrate) 5 mg Levitra 5mg tablets | 4 tablet [PoM] £7.56 DT price = £7.56 | 8 tablet [PoM] £15.12
  Vardenafil (as Vardenafil hydrochloride trihydrate) 10 mg Levitra 10mg tablets | 4 tablet [PoM] £14.08 DT price = £14.08 | 8 tablet [PoM] £28.16
  Vardenafil (as Vardenafil hydrochloride trihydrate) 20 mg Levitra 20mg tablets | 4 tablet [PoM] £23.48 DT price = £23.48 | 8 tablet [PoM] £46.96
  Orodispersible tablet
  EXCIPIENTS: May contain Aspartame
  ▸ Levitra (Bayer Plc)
  Vardenafil (as Vardenafil hydrochloride trihydrate) 10 mg Levitra 10mg orodispersible tablets sugar-free | 4 tablet [PoM] £17.88 DT price = £17.88

PROSTAGLANDIN ANALOGUES AND PROSTAMIDES > PROSTAGLANDINS, ERECTILE DYSFUNCTION

Alprostadil

- INDICATIONS AND DOSE
  Erectile dysfunction (initiated under specialist supervision)
  ▸ BY URETHRAL APPLICATION
  ▸ Adult: Initially 250 micrograms, adjusted according to response; usual dose 0.125–1 mg; maximum 2 doses per day; maximum 7 doses per week

  Aid to diagnosis of erectile dysfunction
  ▸ BY URETHRAL APPLICATION
  ▸ Adult: 500 micrograms for 1 dose

  Erectile dysfunction
  ▸ TO THE SKIN
  ▸ Adult: Apply 300 micrograms, to the tip of the penis, 5–30 minutes before sexual activity; max 1 dose in 24 hours not more than 2–3 times per week

  CAVERJECT®
  Erectile dysfunction
  ▸ BY INTRACAVERNOSAL INJECTION
  ▸ Adult: Initially 2.5 micrograms for 1 dose (first dose), followed by 5 micrograms for 1 dose (second dose), to be given if some response to first dose, alternatively 7.5 micrograms for 1 dose (second dose), to be given if no response to first dose, then increased in steps of 5–10 micrograms, to obtain a dose suitable for producing erection lasting not more than 1 hour; if no response to dose then next higher dose can be given within 1 hour, if there is a response the next dose should not be given for at least 24 hours; usual dose 5–20 micrograms (max. per dose 60 micrograms), maximum frequency of injection not more than 3 times per week with at least 24 hour interval between injections

  Erectile dysfunction associated with neurological dysfunction
  ▸ BY INTRACAVERNOSAL INJECTION
  ▸ Adult: Initially 1.25 micrograms for 1 dose (first dose), then 2.5 micrograms for 1 dose (second dose), then 5 micrograms for 1 dose (third dose), increased in steps of 5–10 micrograms, to obtain a dose suitable for producing erection lasting not more than 1 hour; if no response to dose then next higher dose can be given within 1 hour, if there is a response the next dose should not be given for at least 24 hours; usual dose 5–20 micrograms (max. per dose continued →

7

Genito-urinary system

7

Genito-urinary system

60 micrograms), maximum frequency of injection not more than 3 times per week with at least 24 hour interval between injections

Aid to diagnosis
▶ BY INTRACAVERNOSAL INJECTION
▶ Adult: 10–20 micrograms for 1 dose (consult product literature)

Aid to diagnosis where evidence of neurological dysfunction
▶ BY INTRACAVERNOSAL INJECTION
▶ Adult: Initially 5 micrograms (max. per dose 10 micrograms) for 1 dose, (consult product literature)

CAVERJECT® DUAL CHAMBER

Erectile dysfunction
▶ BY INTRACAVERNOSAL INJECTION
▶ Adult: Initially 2.5 micrograms for 1 dose (first dose), followed by 5 micrograms for 1 dose (second dose), to be given if some response to first dose, alternatively 7.5 micrograms for 1 dose (second dose), to be given if no response to first dose, then increased in steps of 5–10 micrograms, to obtain a dose suitable for producing erection lasting not more than 1 hour; if no response to dose then next higher dose can be given within 1 hour, if there is a response the next dose should not be given for at least 24 hours; usual dose 5–20 micrograms (max. per dose 60 micrograms), maximum frequency of injection not more than 3 times per week with at least 24 hour interval between injections

Erectile dysfunction associated with neurological dysfunction
▶ BY INTRACAVERNOSAL INJECTION
▶ Adult: Initially 1.25 micrograms for 1 dose (first dose), then 2.5 micrograms for 1 dose (second dose), then 5 micrograms for 1 dose (third dose), increased in steps of 5–10 micrograms, to obtain a dose suitable for producing erection lasting not more than 1 hour; if no response to dose then next higher dose can be given within 1 hour, if there is a response the next dose should not be given for at least 24 hours; usual dose 5–20 micrograms (max. per dose 60 micrograms), maximum frequency of injection not more than 3 times per week with at least 24 hour interval between injections

Aid to diagnosis
▶ BY INTRACAVERNOSAL INJECTION
▶ Adult: 10–20 micrograms for 1 dose (consult product literature)

Aid to diagnosis where evidence of neurological dysfunction
▶ BY INTRACAVERNOSAL INJECTION
▶ Adult: Initially 5 micrograms (max. per dose 10 micrograms) for 1 dose, (consult product literature)

VIRIDAL® DUO CONTINUATION PACK

Erectile dysfunction
▶ BY INTRACAVERNOSAL INJECTION
▶ Adult: Initially 5 micrograms, increased in steps of 2.5–5 micrograms, to obtain dose suitable for producing erection not lasting more than 1 hour; usual dose 10–20 micrograms (max. per dose 40 micrograms), maximum frequency of injection not more than 2–3 times per week with at least 24 hour interval between injections; reduce dose if erection lasts longer than 2 hours

Neurogenic erectile dysfunction
▶ BY INTRACAVERNOSAL INJECTION
▶ Adult: Initially 2.5 micrograms, increased in steps of 2.5–5 micrograms, to obtain dose suitable for producing erection not lasting more than 1 hour; usual

dose 10–20 micrograms (max. per dose 40 micrograms), maximum frequency of injection not more than 2–3 times per week with at least 24 hour interval between injections; reduce dose if erection lasts longer than 2 hours

VIRIDAL® DUO STARTER PACK

Neurogenic erectile dysfunction
▶ BY INTRACAVERNOSAL INJECTION
▶ Adult: Initially 2.5 micrograms, increased in steps of 2.5–5 micrograms, to obtain dose suitable for producing erection not lasting more than 1 hour; usual dose 10–20 micrograms (max. per dose 40 micrograms), maximum frequency of injection not more than 2–3 times per week with at least 24 hour interval between injections; reduce dose if erection lasts longer than 2 hours

Erectile dysfunction
▶ BY INTRACAVERNOSAL INJECTION
▶ Adult: Initially 5 micrograms, increased in steps of 2.5–5 micrograms, to obtain dose suitable for producing erection not lasting more than 1 hour; usual dose 10–20 micrograms (max. per dose 40 micrograms), maximum frequency of injection not more than 2–3 times per week with at least 24 hour interval between injections; reduce dose if erection lasts longer than 2 hours

● CONTRA-INDICATIONS
GENERAL CONTRA-INDICATIONS
Not for use in patients with penile implants or when sexual activity medically inadvisable (e.g. orthostatic hypotension, myocardial infarction, and syncope) · not for use with other agents for erectile dysfunction · predisposition to prolonged erection (as in thrombocythemia, polycythemia, sickle cell anaemia, multiple myeloma or leukaemia) · urethral application contra-indicated in balanitis · urethral application contra-indicated in severe curvature · urethral application contra-indicated in severe hypospadia · urethral application contra-indicated in urethral stricture · urethral application contra-indicated in urethritis

SPECIFIC CONTRA-INDICATIONS
▶ With topical use Balanitis · severe curvature · severe hypospadia · urethral stricture · urethritis

● CAUTIONS Anatomical deformations of penis (painful erection more likely)—follow up regularly to detect signs of penile fibrosis (consider discontinuation if angulation, cavernosal fibrosis or Peyronie's disease develop) · priapism (patients should be instructed to report any erection lasting 4 hours or longer)

● INTERACTIONS → Appendix 1 (alprostadil).

● SIDE-EFFECTS
▶ **Common or very common** Dizziness · haematoma · haemosiderin deposits · headache · hypertension · hypotension · influenza-like syndrome · injection site reactions · other localised pain (buttocks, leg, testicular, abdominal) · penile fibrosis · penile oedema · penile pain · penile rash · urethral bleeding · urethral burning
▶ **Uncommon** Abnormal ejaculation · asthenia · balantitis · dry mouth · haematuria · irritation · leg cramps · local reactions · micturition difficulties · mydriasis · nausea · pelvic pain · penile numbness or sensitivity · penile warmth · phimosis · priapism · pruritus · rapid pulse · scrotal erythema · scrotal oedema · scrotal pain · supraventricular extrasystole · sweating · syncope · testicular oedema · testicular thickening · urethral stenosis · vasodilatation
▶ **Rare** Anaphylaxis · erythema · hypersensitivity reactions · rash · urinary-tract infection · urticaria · vertigo

- CONCEPTION AND CONTRACEPTION
  - With urethral use If partner is pregnant, barrier contraception should be used. No evidence of harm to latex condoms and diaphragms.
  - With topical use Condoms should be used to avoid exposure to women of child-bearing age, pregnant or lactating women. No evidence of harm to latex condoms.
- DIRECTIONS FOR ADMINISTRATION
  - With intracavernosal use The first dose of the intracavernosal injection must be given by medically trained personnel; self-administration may only be undertaken after proper training.
  - With urethral use During initiation of treatment the urethral application should be used under medical supervision; self-administration may only be undertaken after proper training.
- PATIENT AND CARER ADVICE Patients should be instructed to report any erection lasting 4 hours or longer.
  - With topical use Counsel patients that condoms should be used to avoid local reactions and exposure of alprostadil to women of childbearing age, pregnant, or lactating women.
- NATIONAL FUNDING/ACCESS DECISIONS
  NHS restrictions *Caverject®*, *Viridal®Duo*, *Vitaros®* and *MUSE®* are not prescribable under the NHS for treatment of erectile dysfunction except in men who meet the criteria listed in part XVIIIB of the Drug Tariff (Part XIb of the Northern Ireland Drug Tariff, Part 12 of the Scottish Drug Tariff). The prescription must be endorsed 'SLS'. For more information see *Prices in the BNF*, under *How to use the BNF*.

- MEDICINAL FORMS
  There can be variation in the licensing of different medicines containing the same drug.

  Powder and solvent for solution for injection
  - Caverject (Pfizer Ltd)
    Alprostadil 5 microgram Caverject 5microgram powder and solvent for solution for injection vials | 1 vial [PoM] £7.73 DT price = £7.73
    Alprostadil 10 microgram Caverject 10microgram powder and solvent for solution for injection vials | 1 vial [PoM] £9.24 DT price = £9.24
    Alprostadil 20 microgram Caverject 20microgram powder and solvent for solution for injection vials | 1 vial [PoM] £11.94 DT price = £11.94
    Alprostadil 40 microgram Caverject 40microgram powder and solvent for solution for injection vials | 1 vial [PoM] £21.58 DT price = £21.58
  - Caverject Dual Chamber (Pfizer Ltd)
    Alprostadil 10 microgram Caverject Dual Chamber 10microgram powder and solvent for solution for injection | 2 pre-filled disposable injection [PoM] £14.70
    Alprostadil 20 microgram Caverject Dual Chamber 20microgram powder and solvent for solution for injection | 2 pre-filled disposable injection [PoM] £19.00
  - Viridal (UCB Pharma Ltd)
    Alprostadil 10 microgram Viridal Duo Starter Pack 10microgram powder and solvent for solution for injection cartridges with device | 2 cartridge [PoM] £20.13 (Hospital only)
    Viridal Duo Continuation Pack 10microgram powder and solvent for solution for injection cartridges | 2 cartridge [PoM] £16.55
    Alprostadil 20 microgram Viridal Duo Starter Pack 20microgram powder and solvent for solution for injection cartridges with device | 2 cartridge [PoM] £24.54 (Hospital only)
    Viridal Duo Continuation Pack 20microgram powder and solvent for solution for injection cartridges | 2 cartridge [PoM] £21.39
    Alprostadil 40 microgram Viridal Duo Starter Pack 40microgram powder and solvent for solution for injection cartridges with device | 2 cartridge [PoM] £29.83 (Hospital only)
    Viridal Duo Continuation Pack 40microgram powder and solvent for solution for injection cartridges | 2 cartridge [PoM] £27.22

  Cream
  - Vitaros (Takeda UK Ltd)
    Alprostadil 3 mg per 1 gram Vitaros 3mg/g cream | 4 applicator [PoM] £40.00

Stick
- Muse (Meda Pharmaceuticals Ltd)
  Alprostadil 250 microgram Muse 250microgram urethral sticks | 1 applicator [PoM] £11.30 DT price = £11.30 | 6 applicator [PoM] £67.79
  Alprostadil 500 microgram Muse 500microgram urethral sticks | 1 applicator [PoM] £11.30 DT price = £11.30 | 6 applicator [PoM] £67.79
  Alprostadil 1 mg Muse 1000microgram urethral sticks | 1 applicator [PoM] £11.56 DT price = £11.56 | 6 applicator [PoM] £65.67

SYMPATHOMIMETICS > VASOCONSTRICTOR

Adrenaline/epinephrine

- DRUG ACTION Acts on both alpha and beta receptors and increases both heart rate and contractility ($beta_1$ effects); it can cause peripheral vasodilation (a $beta_2$ effect) or vasoconstriction (an alpha effect).

- INDICATIONS AND DOSE

  Priapism associated with alprostadil, if aspiration and lavage of corpora are unsuccessful (alternative to phenylephrine or metaraminol)
  - BY INTRACAVERNOSAL INJECTION
  - Adult: 10–20 micrograms every 5–10 minutes, using a 20 microgram/mL solution, **Important:** if suitable strength of adrenaline not available may be specially prepared by diluting 0.1 mL of the adrenaline 1 in 1000 (1 mg/mL) injection to 5 mL with sodium chloride 0.9%, continuously monitor blood pressure and pulse; maximum 100 micrograms per course

- UNLICENSED USE The use of adrenaline for the treatment of priapism is an unlicensed indication.
- CAUTIONS Arteriosclerosis · arrhythmias · cerebrovascular disease · cor pulmonale · diabetes mellitus · elderly · hypercalcaemia · hyperreflexia · hypertension · hyperthyroidism · hypokalaemia · ischaemic heart disease · obstructive cardiomyopathy · occlusive vascular disease · organic brain damage · phaeochromocytoma · prostate disorders · psychoneurosis · severe angina · susceptibility to angle-closure glaucoma
- INTERACTIONS → Appendix 1 (sympathomimetics)
- SIDE-EFFECTS Angina · angle-closure glaucoma · anorexia · anxiety · arrhythmias · cold extremities · confusion · difficulty in micturition · dizziness · dry mouth · dyspnoea · headache · hyperglycaemia · hypersalivation · hypertension (risk of cerebral haemorrhage) · hypokalaemia · insomnia · metabolic acidosis · mydriasis · myocardial infarction · nausea · pallor · palpitation · psychosis · pulmonary oedema (on excessive dosage or extreme sensitivity) · restlessness · sweating · tachycardia · tissue necrosis at injection site · tissue necrosis of bowel · tissue necrosis of extremities · tissue necrosis of kidneys · tissue necrosis of liver · tremor · urinary retention · vomiting · weakness
- RENAL IMPAIRMENT Manufacturers advise use with caution in severe impairment.

- MEDICINAL FORMS
  There can be variation in the licensing of different medicines containing the same drug. Forms available from special-order manufacturers include: solution for injection
  Solution for injection
  EXCIPIENTS: May contain Sulfites
  - Adrenaline/epinephrine (Non-proprietary)
    Adrenaline (as Adrenaline acid tartrate) 1 mg per 1 ml Adrenaline (base) 5mg/5ml (1 in 1,000) solution for injection ampoules | 10 ampoule [PoM] £73.66
    Adrenaline (base) 500micrograms/0.5ml (1 in 1,000) solution for injection ampoules | 10 ampoule [PoM] £58.08-£58.41 DT price = £58.25
    Adrenaline (base) 1mg/1ml (1 in 1,000) solution for injection ampoules | 10 ampoule [PoM] £5.82 DT price = £5.81

7

Genito-urinary system

Metaraminol

- **INDICATIONS AND DOSE**

Priapism (alternative to intracavernosal injections of phenylephrine and adrenaline)
- ▶ BY INTRACAVERNOSAL INJECTION
- ▶ Adult: 1 mg every 15 minutes

- **UNLICENSED USE** Use for priapism is an unlicensed indication.
- **CONTRA-INDICATIONS** Hypertension
- **CAUTIONS** Associated with fatal hypertensive crises · cirrhosis · coronary vascular thrombosis · diabetes mellitus · elderly · extravasation at injection site may cause necrosis · following myocardial infarction · hypercapnia · hyperthyroidism · hypoxia · mesenteric vascular thrombosis · peripheral vascular thrombosis · Prinzmetal's variant angina · uncorrected hypovolaemia
- **INTERACTIONS** → Appendix 1 (sympathomimetics).
- **SIDE-EFFECTS** Angle-closure glaucoma · anorexia · anxiety · arrhythmias · bradycardia · confusion · dyspnoea · fatal ventricular arrhythmia reported in Laennec's cirrhosis · headache · hypertension · hypoxia · insomnia · nausea · palpitation · peripheral ischaemia · psychosis · tachycardia · tremor · urinary retention · vomiting · weakness
- **MONITORING REQUIREMENTS** Monitor blood pressure and rate of flow frequently.
- **DIRECTIONS FOR ADMINISTRATION** For *intracavernosal injection*, dilute 1 mg (0.1 mL of 10 mg/mL) metaraminol injection to 50 mL with Sodium chloride injection 0.9% and give carefully by slow injection into the corpora in 5 mL injections.

- **MEDICINAL FORMS**
There can be variation in the licensing of different medicines containing the same drug. Forms available from special-order manufacturers include: solution for injection
Solution for injection
- ▶ Metaraminol (Non-proprietary)
  Metaraminol (as Metaraminol tartrate) 10 mg per 1 ml Metaraminol 10mg/1ml solution for injection ampoules | 10 ampoule [PoM] £31.97

Phenylephrine hydrochloride

- **INDICATIONS AND DOSE**

Priapism associated with alprostadil, if aspiration and lavage of the corpora are unsuccessful (alternative to adrenaline or metaraminol)
- ▶ BY INTRACAVERNOSAL INJECTION
- ▶ Adult: 100–200 micrograms every 5–10 minutes, dose to be administered using a 200 micrograms/mL solution; maximum 1 mg per course

- **UNLICENSED USE** Use of phenylephrine hydrochloride injection in priapism is an unlicensed indication.
- **CONTRA-INDICATIONS** Hypertension
- **INTERACTIONS** → Appendix 1 (sympathomimetics). Phenylephrine may interact with systemically administered monoamine-oxidase inhibitors.
- **SIDE-EFFECTS** Arrhythmias · hypertension · palpitation · tachycardia
- **DIRECTIONS FOR ADMINISTRATION** For *intracavernosal injection*, if suitable strength of phenylephrine injection is not available, it may be specially prepared by diluting 0.1 mL of the phenylephrine 1% (10 mg/mL) injection to 5 mL with sodium chloride 0.9%.

- **MEDICINAL FORMS**
There can be variation in the licensing of different medicines containing the same drug. Forms available from special-order manufacturers include: solution for injection
Solution for injection
- ▶ Phenylephrine hydrochloride (Non-proprietary)
  Phenylephrine hydrochloride 10 mg per 1 ml Phenylephrine 10mg/1ml solution for injection ampoules | 10 ampoule [PoM] £99.12

4.2 Premature ejaculation

SELECTIVE SEROTONIN RE-UPTAKE INHIBITORS

Dapoxetine

- **DRUG ACTION** Dapoxetine is a short-acting selective serotonin re-uptake inhibitor.

- **INDICATIONS AND DOSE**

Premature ejaculation in men who meet all the following criteria: poor control over ejaculation, a history of premature ejaculation over the past 6 months, marked distress or interpersonal difficulty as a consequence of premature ejaculation, and an intravaginal ejaculatory latency time of less than two minutes
- ▶ BY MOUTH
- ▶ Adult: Initially 30 mg, to be taken approximately 1–3 hours before sexual activity, subsequent doses adjusted according to response; review treatment after 4 weeks (or 6 doses) and at least every 6 months thereafter, not recommended for adults 65 years and over; maximum 1 dose per day; maximum 60 mg per day

Premature ejaculation in men who meet all the following criteria: poor control over ejaculation, a history of premature ejaculation over the past 6 months, marked distress or interpersonal difficulty as a consequence of premature ejaculation, and an intravaginal ejaculatory latency time of less than two minutes (with concomitant aprepitant, clarithromycin, diltiazem, erythromycin, fluconazole, fosamprenavir, and verapamil)
- ▶ BY MOUTH
- ▶ Adult: Up to 30 mg, to be taken approximately 1–3 hours before sexual activity; review treatment after 4 weeks (or 6 doses) and at least every 6 months thereafter, not recommended for adults 65 years and over; maximum 1 dose per day

DOSE ADJUSTMENTS DUE TO INTERACTIONS
Max. single dose 30 mg with concomitant aprepitant, clarithromycin, diltiazem, erythromycin, fluconazole, fosamprenavir, and verapamil.
Use 60-mg dose with caution with concomitant potent inhibitors of cytochrome P450 enzyme CYP2D6.

- **CONTRA-INDICATIONS** History of bipolar disorder · history of mania · history of severe depression · history of syncope · significant cardiac disease · uncontrolled epilepsy
- **CAUTIONS** Bleeding disorders · epilepsy (discontinue if convulsions develop) · susceptibility to angle-closure glaucoma
- **INTERACTIONS** → Appendix 1 (dapoxetine). Caution with concomitant use of drugs that increase risk of bleeding.
- **SIDE-EFFECTS**
- ▶ **Common or very common** Abdominal distension · abdominal pain · abnormal dreams · agitation · anxiety · constipation · diarrhoea · dizziness · drowsiness · dry mouth · dyspepsia · flushing · headache · hypertension · impaired attention · irritability · malaise · nausea ·

paraesthesia · sexual dysfunction · sleep disturbances · sweating · tinnitus · tremor · visual disturbances · vomiting
► **Uncommon** Abnormal thoughts · bradycardia · bruxism · confusion · depression · eye pain · hypotension · mood disturbances · mydriasis · postural hypotension · pruritus · restlessness · sinus arrest · syncope · tachycardia · taste disturbances · vertigo
► **Rare** Defaecation urgency · sudden onset of sleep

SIDE-EFFECTS, FURTHER INFORMATION
Discontinue if psychiatric disorder develops.
   Avoid if postural hypotension occurs during test dose.

● HEPATIC IMPAIRMENT Avoid in moderate to severe impairment.

● RENAL IMPAIRMENT Use with caution if eGFR 30–80 mL/minute/1.73 m^2; avoid if eGFR less than 30 mL/minute/1.73 m^2.

● PRE-TREATMENT SCREENING Test for postural hypotension before starting treatment.

● PATIENT AND CARER ADVICE
Postural hypotension and syncope Patients should be advised to maintain hydration and to sit or lie down until prodromal symptoms such as nausea, dizziness, and sweating abate.

● MEDICINAL FORMS
There can be variation in the licensing of different medicines containing the same drug.
Tablet
CAUTIONARY AND ADVISORY LABELS 2, 25
► Dapoxetine (Non-proprietary)
   Dapoxetine 30 mg Dapoxetine 30mg tablets | 6 tablet [PoM] no price available
► Priligy (A. Menarini Farmaceutica Internazionale SRL)
   Dapoxetine 30 mg Priligy 30mg tablets | 3 tablet [PoM] £14.71 | 6 tablet [PoM] £26.48
   Dapoxetine 60 mg Priligy 60mg tablets | 3 tablet [PoM] £19.12 | 6 tablet [PoM] £34.42

5   Obstetrics

Obstetrics

Prostaglandins and oxytocics

Prostaglandins and oxytocics are used to induce abortion or induce or augment labour and to minimise blood loss from the placental site. They include oxytocin p. 744, carbetocin p. 745, ergometrine maleate p. 746, and the prostaglandins. All induce uterine contractions with varying degrees of pain according to the strength of contractions induced.

Induction of abortion
Gemeprost p. 748, a prostaglandin administered vaginally as pessaries, is suitable for the medical induction of late therapeutic abortion; gemeprost is also used to ripen the cervix before surgical abortion, particularly in primigravidas. The prostaglandin misoprostol p. 748 is given by mouth, buccally, sublingually, or vaginally, to induce medical abortion [unlicensed indication]; intravaginal use ripens the cervix before surgical abortion [unlicensed indication]. Extra-amniotic dinoprostone is rarely used nowadays.
   Pre-treatment with mifepristone p. 747 can facilitate the process of medical abortion. It sensitises the uterus to subsequent administration of a prostaglandin and, therefore, abortion occurs in a shorter time and with a lower dose of prostaglandin.

Induction and augmentation of labour
Dinoprostone is available as vaginal tablets, pessaries and vaginal gels for the induction of labour. The intravenous solution is rarely used; it is associated with more side-effects.

Oxytocin (*Syntocinon*®) is administered by slow intravenous infusion, using an infusion pump, to induce or augment labour, usually in conjunction with amniotomy. Uterine activity must be monitored carefully and hyperstimulation avoided. Large doses of oxytocin may result in excessive fluid retention.
   Misoprostol is given orally or vaginally for the induction of labour [unlicensed indication].
   NICE Guidance, Induction of labour (updated July 2008), available at www.nice.org.uk/guidance/CG70.

Prevention and treatment of haemorrhage
Bleeding due to incomplete miscarriage or abortion can be controlled with ergometrine maleate and oxytocin (*Syntometrine*®) given intramuscularly, the dose is adjusted according to the patient's condition and blood loss. This is commonly used before surgical evacuation of the uterus, particularly when surgery is delayed. Oxytocin and ergometrine maleate combined are more effective in early pregnancy than either drug alone.
   Active management of the third stage of labour reduces the risk of postpartum haemorrhage; oxytocin is given by intramuscular injection [unlicensed] on delivery of the anterior shoulder or, at the latest, immediately after the baby is delivered. Alternatively, ergometrine maleate with oxytocin (*Syntometrine*®) can be given by intramuscular injection in the absence of hypertension; oxytocin alone causes less nausea, vomiting, and hypertension than when given with ergometrine maleate.
   In excessive uterine bleeding, any placental products remaining in the uterus should be removed. Oxytocic drugs are used to treat postpartum haemorrhage caused by uterine atony; treatment options are as follows:

● oxytocin by slow intravenous injection, followed in severe cases by intravenous infusion of oxytocin at a rate that controls uterine atony *or*
● ergometrine by intramuscular injection *or*
● ergometrine by slow intravenous injection (use with caution—risk of hypertension) *or*
● ergometrine with oxytocin (*Syntometrine*®) by intramuscular injection

   Carboprost p. 746 has an important role in severe postpartum haemorrhage unresponsive to ergometrine maleate and oxytocin.
   Misoprostol [unlicensed] can be used in postpartum haemorrhage when oxytocin, ergometrine maleate, and carboprost are not available or are inappropriate.

Mifepristone

For termination of pregnancy, a single dose of mifepristone is followed by administration of a prostaglandin (gemeprost or misoprostol [unlicensed]).
   Guidelines of the Royal College of Obstetricians and Gynaecologists (November 2011) include [unlicensed] regimens for inducing medical abortion.

Myometrial relaxants

Tocolytic drugs postpone *premature labour* and they are used with the aim of reducing harm to the child. However, there is no satisfactory evidence that the use of these drugs reduces mortality. The greatest benefit is gained by using the delay to administer corticosteroid therapy or to implement other measures which improve perinatal health (including transfer to a unit with neonatal intensive care facility).
   The oxytocin receptor antagonist, atosiban p. 746, is licensed for the inhibition of uncomplicated premature labour *between 24 and 33 weeks* of gestation. Atosiban may be preferable to a beta$_2$ agonist because it has fewer side effects. The dihydropyridine calcium-channel blocker nifedipine p. 148 also has fewer side-effects than a beta$_2$ agonist.
   The beta$_2$ agonists salbutamol p. 233 and terbutaline sulfate p. 235 are licensed for inhibiting uncomplicated premature labour between 22 and 37 weeks of gestation to

permit a delay in delivery of up to 48 hours. Use of high-dose short acting beta$_2$ agonists in obstetric indications has been associated with serious, sometimes fatal cardiovascular events in the mother and fetus, particularly when used for a prolonged period of time. Oral therapy is no longer recommended and parenteral therapy should be restricted to a maximum duration of 48 hours, given under the supervision of a specialist, and with close monitoring.

Indometacin p. 989, a cyclo-oxygenase inhibitor, also inhibits labour [unlicensed indication] and it can be useful in situations where a beta$_2$ agonist is not appropriate; however, there are concerns about neonatal complications such as transient impairment of renal function and premature closure of ductus arteriosus.

5.1 Induction of labour

PROSTAGLANDINS AND OXYTOCICS

Dinoprostone

● **INDICATIONS AND DOSE**

PROPESS®

Cervical ripening and induction of labour at term

▶ BY VAGINA

▶ Adult: 1 pessary, insert pessary (in retrieval device) high into posterior fornix and remove when cervical ripening adequate; if oxytocin necessary, remove 30 minutes before oxytocin infusion; remove if cervical ripening inadequate after 24 hours (dose not to be repeated)

PROSTIN E2® VAGINAL GEL

Induction of labour

▶ BY VAGINA

▶ Adult: 1 mg, inserted high into the posterior fornix (avoid administration into the cervical canal), followed by 1–2 mg after 6 hours if required; maximum 3 mg per course

Induction of labour (unfavourable primigravida)

▶ BY VAGINA

▶ Adult: 2 mg, inserted high into the posterior fornix (avoid administration into the cervical canal), followed by 1–2 mg if required, after 6 hours; maximum 4 mg per course

PROSTIN E2® VAGINAL TABLETS

Induction of labour

▶ BY VAGINA

▶ Adult: 3 mg, inserted high into the posterior fornix, followed by 3 mg after 6–8 hours, to be given if labour not established; maximum 6 mg per course

DOSE EQUIVALENCE AND CONVERSION

Prostin E2 Vaginal Gel and *Vaginal Tablets* are not bioequivalent.

● **CONTRA-INDICATIONS** Active cardiac disease · active pulmonary disease · avoid extra-amniotic route in cervicitis or vaginitis · fetal distress · fetal malpresentation · grand multiparas · history of caesarean section · history of difficult or traumatic delivery · history of major uterine surgery · major cephalopelvic disproportion · multiple pregnancy · placenta praevia or unexplained vaginal bleeding during pregnancy · ruptured membranes · untreated pelvic infection

● **CAUTIONS** Effect of oxytocin enhanced · history of asthma · history of epilepsy · history of glaucoma and raised intra-ocular pressure · hypertension · risk factors for disseminated intravascular coagulation · uterine rupture · uterine scarring

● **INTERACTIONS** → Appendix 1 (prostaglandins).

● **SIDE-EFFECTS** Abruptio placenta · amniotic fluid embolism · backache · bronchospasm · cardiac arrest · diarrhoea · disseminated intravascular coagulation · fetal distress · fever · low Apgar scores · maternal hypertension · nausea · pulmonary embolism · rapid cervical dilation · severe uterine contractions · stillbirth or neonatal death · uterine hypercontractility with or without fetal bradycardia · uterine hypertonus · uterine rupture · vaginal symptoms (warmth, irritation, pain) · vomiting

● **HEPATIC IMPAIRMENT** Manufacturers advise avoid.

● **RENAL IMPAIRMENT** Manufacturers advise avoid.

● **MONITORING REQUIREMENTS**

▶ Monitor for disseminated intravascular coagulation after parturition.

▶ Monitor uterine activity and fetal status (particular care if history of uterine hypertony)

▶ Care needed in monitoring uterine activity when used in sequence following oxytocin.

● **PRESCRIBING AND DISPENSING INFORMATION** **Important:** Do not confuse dose of *Prostin E2* ® **vaginal gel** with that of *Prostin E2* ® **vaginal tablets**—not bioequivalent.

● **LESS SUITABLE FOR PRESCRIBING** Intravenous solution rarely used and is considered less suitable for prescribing. Extra-amniotic solution less commonly used and is considered less suitable for prescribing.

● **MEDICINAL FORMS**

There can be variation in the licensing of different medicines containing the same drug.

Pessary

▶ Prostin E2 (Pfizer Ltd)

Dinoprostone 3 mg Prostin E2 3mg vaginal tablets | 8 pessary PoM £106.23 (Hospital only)

Vaginal device

▶ Propess (Ferring Pharmaceuticals Ltd)

Dinoprostone 10 mg Propess 10mg vaginal delivery system | 5 device PoM £150.00

Vaginal gel

▶ Prostin E2 (Pfizer Ltd)

Dinoprostone 400 microgram per 1 ml Prostin E2 1mg vaginal gel | 2.5 ml PoM £13.28 (Hospital only)

Dinoprostone 800 microgram per 1 ml Prostin E2 2mg vaginal gel | 2.5 ml PoM £13.28 (Hospital only)

Oxytocin

● **INDICATIONS AND DOSE**

Induction of labour for medical reasons | Stimulation of labour in hypotonic uterine inertia

▶ BY INTRAVENOUS INFUSION

▶ Adult: Initially 0.001–0.004 unit/minute, not to be started for at least 6 hours after administration of vaginal prostaglandin, dose increased at intervals of at least 30 minutes until a maximum of 3–4 contractions occur every 10 minutes (0.01 units/minute is often adequate) up to max. 0.02 units/minute, if regular contractions not established after a total 5 units, stop induction attempt (may be repeated next day starting again at 0.001–0.004 units/minute)

Caesarean section

▶ BY SLOW INTRAVENOUS INJECTION

▶ Adult: 5 units immediately after delivery

Prevention of postpartum haemorrhage after delivery of placenta

▶ BY SLOW INTRAVENOUS INJECTION

▶ Adult: 5 units, if infusion previously used for induction or enhancement of labour, increase rate during third stage and for next few hours

▶ BY INTRAMUSCULAR INJECTION

▶ Adult: 10 units, can be used instead of oxytocin with ergometrine (*Syntometrine* ®).

Treatment of postpartum haemorrhage
▶ BY SLOW INTRAVENOUS INJECTION
▶ Adult: 5 units, repeated if necessary

Treatment of severe cases of postpartum haemorrhage (following intravenous injection)
▶ BY INTRAVENOUS INFUSION
▶ Adult: 40 units, given in 500 mL infusion fluid given at a rate sufficient to control uterine atony

Incomplete, inevitable, or missed miscarriage
▶ INITIALLY BY SLOW INTRAVENOUS INJECTION
▶ Adult: 5 units, followed by (by intravenous infusion) 0.02–0.04 unit/minute if required, the rate of infusion can be faster if necessary

● UNLICENSED USE Oxytocin doses in the BNF may differ from those in the product literature. Administration by Intramuscular injection is an unlicensed use.

IMPORTANT SAFETY INFORMATION
Prolonged intravenous administration at high doses with large volume of fluid (which is possible in inevitable or missed miscarriage or postpartum haemorrhage) may cause water intoxication with hyponatraemia. To avoid: use electrolyte-containing diluent (i.e. not glucose), increase oxytocin concentration to reduce fluid, restrict fluid intake by mouth; monitor fluid and electrolytes.

● CONTRA-INDICATIONS Any condition where spontaneous labour inadvisable · any condition where vaginal delivery inadvisable · avoid intravenous injection during labour · avoid prolonged administration in oxytocin-resistant uterine inertia · avoid rapid intravenous injection (may transiently reduce blood pressure) · fetal distress (discontinue immediately if this occurs) · hypertonic uterine contractions (discontinue immediately if this occurs) · severe cardiovascular disease · severe pre-eclamptic toxaemia

● CAUTIONS Avoid large infusion volumes and restrict fluid intake by mouth (risk of hyponatraemia and water-intoxication) · enhancement of labour—presence of borderline cephalopelvic disproportion (avoid if significant) · history of lower-uterine segment caesarean section · induction of labour—presence of borderline cephalopelvic disproportion (avoid if significant) · mild pregnancy-induced cardiac disease · mild pregnancy-induced hypertension · moderate pregnancy-induced cardiac disease · moderate pregnancy-induced hypertension · risk factors for disseminated intravascular coagulation · secondary uterine inertia · women over 35 years

● INTERACTIONS → Appendix 1 (oxytocin).
Effects enhanced by concomitant prostaglandins (very careful monitoring of uterine activity).
Caudal block anaesthesia (may enhance hypertensive effects of sympathomimetic vasopressors).

● SIDE-EFFECTS
▶ **Common or very common** Arrhythmia · headache · nausea · vomiting
▶ **Rare** Anaphylactoid reactions (with dyspnoea, hypotension, or shock) · disseminated intravascular coagulation · hyponatraemia associated with high doses with large infusion volumes of electrolyte-free fluid · rash · uterine hyperstimulation (usually with excessive doses—may cause fetal distress, asphyxia, and death, or may lead to hypertonicity, tetanic contractions, soft-tissue damage or uterine rupture) · uterine spasm (may occur at low doses) · water intoxication associated with high doses with large infusion volumes of electrolyte-free fluid

● SIDE-EFFECTS, FURTHER INFORMATION
Avoid rapid intravenous injection (may transiently reduce blood pressure).

Overdose
Placental abruption and amniotic fluid embolism reported on overdose.

● MONITORING REQUIREMENTS
▶ Careful monitoring of fetal heart rate and uterine motility essential for dose titration.
▶ Monitor for disseminated intravascular coagulation after parturition.

● DIRECTIONS FOR ADMINISTRATION For *intravenous infusion* (*Syntocinon®*), give continuously in Glucose 5% or Sodium chloride 0.9%. Preferably given *via* a variable-speed infusion pump in a concentration appropriate to the pump; if given by drip infusion for *induction* or *enhancement of labour*, dilute 5 units in 500 mL infusion fluid or for higher doses, 10 units in 500 mL; for *treatment of postpartum uterine haemorrhage* dilute 40 units in 500 mL; if high doses given for prolonged period (e.g. for inevitable or missed abortion or for postpartum haemorrhage), use low volume of an electrolyte-containing infusion fluid (not Glucose 5%) given at higher concentration than for induction or enhancement of labour; close attention to patient's fluid and electrolyte status essential.

● MEDICINAL FORMS
There can be variation in the licensing of different medicines containing the same drug. Forms available from special-order manufacturers include: infusion, solution for infusion
Solution for injection
▶ Oxytocin (Non-proprietary)
 Oxytocin 10 unit per 1 ml Oxytocin 10units/1ml concentrate for solution for infusion ampoules | 5 ampoule [PoM] £4.55–£4.67 | 10 ampoule [PoM] £9.00
▶ Syntocinon (Novartis Pharmaceuticals UK Ltd)
 Oxytocin 5 unit per 1 ml Syntocinon 5units/1ml solution for injection ampoules | 5 ampoule [PoM] £4.01 (Hospital only)
 Oxytocin 10 unit per 1 ml Syntocinon 10units/1ml solution for injection ampoules | 5 ampoule [PoM] £4.53 (Hospital only)

5.2 Postpartum haemorrhage

PROSTAGLANDINS AND OXYTOCICS

Carbetocin

● INDICATIONS AND DOSE
Prevention of uterine atony after caesarean section
▶ BY SLOW INTRAVENOUS INJECTION
▶ Adult: 100 micrograms for 1 dose, to be given over 1 minute, administer as soon as possible after delivery, preferably before removal of placenta

● CONTRA-INDICATIONS Eclampsia · epilepsy · pre-eclampsia
● CAUTIONS Asthma · cardiovascular disease (avoid if severe) · hyponatraemia · migraine
● SIDE-EFFECTS Abdominal pain · anaemia · back pain · chest pain · chills · dizziness · dyspnoea · feeling of warmth · flushing · headache · hypotension · metallic taste · nausea · pruritus · sweating · tachycardia · tremor · vomiting
● HEPATIC IMPAIRMENT Manufacturer advises avoid.
● RENAL IMPAIRMENT Manufacturer advises avoid.

7

Genito-urinary system

● MEDICINAL FORMS
There can be variation in the licensing of different medicines containing the same drug.
Solution for injection
▸ Pabal (Ferring Pharmaceuticals Ltd)
Carbetocin 100 microgram per 1 ml Pabal 100micrograms/1ml solution for injection ampoules | 5 ampoule PoM £88.20 (Hospital only)

Carboprost

● INDICATIONS AND DOSE
Postpartum haemorrhage due to uterine atony in patients unresponsive to ergometrine and oxytocin
▸ BY DEEP INTRAMUSCULAR INJECTION
▸ Adult: 250 micrograms at least every 15 minutes, repeated if necessary, total dose should not exceed 2 mg (8 doses)

● CONTRA-INDICATIONS Cardiac disease · pulmonary disease · untreated pelvic infection
● CAUTIONS Excessive dosage may cause uterine rupture · history of anaemia · history of asthma · history of diabetes · history of epilepsy · history of glaucoma · history of hypertension · history of hypotension · history of jaundice · history of raised intra-ocular pressure · uterine scars
● INTERACTIONS → Appendix 1 (prostaglandins).
● SIDE-EFFECTS Bronchospasm · cardiovascular collapse · chills · diaphoresis · diarrhoea · dizziness · dyspnoea · erythema at injection site · flushing · headache · hyperthermia · nausea · pain at injection site · pulmonary oedema · raised blood pressure · vomiting
● HEPATIC IMPAIRMENT Manufacturer advises avoid.
● RENAL IMPAIRMENT Manufacturer advises avoid.

● MEDICINAL FORMS
There can be variation in the licensing of different medicines containing the same drug.
Solution for injection
▸ Hemabate (Pfizer Ltd)
Carboprost (as Carboprost trometamol) 250 microgram per 1 ml Hemabate 250micrograms/1ml solution for injection ampoules | 10 ampoule PoM £182.01 (Hospital only)

Ergometrine maleate

● INDICATIONS AND DOSE
Postpartum haemorrhage caused by uterine atony
▸ BY INTRAMUSCULAR INJECTION, OR BY SLOW INTRAVENOUS INJECTION
▸ Adult: 250–500 micrograms

● CONTRA-INDICATIONS Eclampsia · first stage of labour · induction of labour · second stage of labour · sepsis · severe cardiac disease · severe hypertension · vascular disease
● CAUTIONS Acute porphyrias p. 918 · cardiac disease · hypertension · multiple pregnancy · risk of hypertension associated with intravenous administration
● INTERACTIONS → Appendix 1 (ergot alkaloids).
● SIDE-EFFECTS
▸ Common or very common Abdominal pain · arrhythmias · bradycardia · chest pain · dizziness · dyspnoea · headache · hypertension · nausea · palpitation · pulmonary oedema · rash · tinnitus · vasoconstriction · vomiting
▸ Very rare Myocardial infarction
● HEPATIC IMPAIRMENT Manufacturer advises caution in mild or moderate impairment. Manufacturer advises avoid in severe impairment.

● RENAL IMPAIRMENT Manufacturer advises caution in mild or moderate impairment. Manufacturer advises avoid in severe impairment.

● MEDICINAL FORMS
There can be variation in the licensing of different medicines containing the same drug.
Solution for injection
▸ Ergometrine maleate (Non-proprietary)
Ergometrine maleate 500 microgram per 1 ml Ergometrine 500micrograms/1ml solution for injection ampoules | 10 ampoule PoM £15.00

Ergometrine with oxytocin

The properties listed below are those particular to the combination only. For the properties of the components please consider, ergometrine maleate above, oxytocin p. 744.

● INDICATIONS AND DOSE
Active management of the third stage of labour | Postpartum haemorrhage caused by uterine atony
▸ BY INTRAMUSCULAR INJECTION
▸ Adult: 1 mL for one dose
▸ BY INTRAVENOUS INJECTION
▸ Adult: No longer recommended
Bleeding due to incomplete miscarriage or abortion
▸ BY INTRAMUSCULAR INJECTION
▸ Adult: Adjusted according to response to, the patient's condition and blood loss

● MEDICINAL FORMS
There can be variation in the licensing of different medicines containing the same drug.
Solution for injection
▸ Syntometrine (Alliance Pharmaceuticals Ltd)
Ergometrine maleate 500 microgram per 1 ml, Oxytocin 5 unit per 1 ml Syntometrine 500micrograms/1ml solution for injection ampoules | 5 ampoule PoM £7.87

5.3 Premature labour

OXYTOCIN RECEPTOR ANTAGONISTS

Atosiban

● INDICATIONS AND DOSE
Uncomplicated premature labour between 24 and 33 weeks of gestation
▸ INITIALLY BY INTRAVENOUS INJECTION
▸ Adult: Initially 6.75 mg over 1 minute, then (by intravenous infusion) 18 mg/hour for 3 hours, then (by intravenous infusion) reduced to 6 mg/hour for up to 45 hours. Maximum duration of treatment is 48 hours

● CONTRA-INDICATIONS Abruptio placenta · antepartum haemorrhage (requiring immediate delivery) · eclampsia · intra-uterine fetal death · intra-uterine infection · intra-uterine growth restriction with abnormal fetal heart rate · placenta praevia · premature rupture of membranes after 30 weeks' gestation · severe pre-eclampsia
● CAUTIONS Abnormal placental site · intra-uterine growth restriction
● SIDE-EFFECTS
▸ Common or very common Dizziness · headache · hot flushes · hyperglycaemia · hypotension · injection-site reaction · nausea · tachycardia · vomiting
▸ Uncommon Fever · insomnia · pruritus · rash
● HEPATIC IMPAIRMENT No information available.
● RENAL IMPAIRMENT No information available.

- MONITORING REQUIREMENTS Monitor blood loss after delivery.
- DIRECTIONS FOR ADMINISTRATION For *intravenous infusion* (*Tractocile*®) concentrate for intravenous infusion), give continuously *in* Glucose 5% *or* Sodium chloride 0.9%. Withdraw 10 mL infusion fluid from 100-mL bag and replace with 10 mL atosiban concentrate (7.5 mg/mL) to produce a final concentration of 750 micrograms/mL.

- MEDICINAL FORMS
  There can be variation in the licensing of different medicines containing the same drug.
  Solution for injection
  ▸ Atosiban (Non-proprietary)
  Atosiban (as Atosiban acetate) 7.5 mg per 1 ml Atosiban 6.75mg/0.9ml solution for injection vials | 1 vial [PoM] £18.41 (Hospital only)
  ▸ Tractocile (Ferring Pharmaceuticals Ltd)
  Atosiban (as Atosiban acetate) 7.5 mg per 1 ml Tractocile 6.75mg/0.9ml solution for injection vials | 1 vial [PoM] £18.41 (Hospital only)
  Solution for infusion
  ▸ Atosiban (Non-proprietary)
  Atosiban (as Atosiban acetate) 7.5 mg per 1 ml Atosiban 37.5mg/5ml concentrate for solution for infusion vials | 1 vial [PoM] £52.82 (Hospital only)
  Atosiban 37.5mg/5ml solution for infusion vials | 1 vial [PoM] £51.09
  ▸ Tractocile (Ferring Pharmaceuticals Ltd)
  Atosiban (as Atosiban acetate) 7.5 mg per 1 ml Tractocile 37.5mg/5ml solution for infusion vials | 1 vial [PoM] £52.82 (Hospital only)

5.4 Termination of pregnancy

PROGESTERONE RECEPTOR MODULATORS

Mifepristone

- DRUG ACTION Mifepristone, an antiprogestogenic steroid, sensitises the myometrium to prostaglandin-induced contractions and ripens the cervix.

● INDICATIONS AND DOSE

Cervical ripening before mechanical cervical dilatation for termination of pregnancy of up to 84 days gestation (under close medical supervision)
▸ BY MOUTH
▸ Adult: 200 mg for 1 dose, to be taken 36-48 hours before procedure

Labour induction in fetal death in utero where prostaglandin or oxytocin inappropriate (under close medical supervision)
▸ BY MOUTH
▸ Adult: 600 mg once daily for 2 days, if labour not started within 72 hours of first dose, another method should be used

Medical termination of intra-uterine pregnancy of up to 49 days gestation (under close medical supervision)
▸ BY MOUTH
▸ Adult: 600 mg for 1 dose, dose followed 36-48 hours later (unless abortion already complete) by gemeprost 1 mg by vagina *or* misoprostol 400 micrograms by mouth, alternatively 200 mg for 1 dose, dose followed 36-48 hours later (unless abortion already complete) by gemeprost 1 mg by vagina; observe for at least 3 hours (or until bleeding or pain at acceptable level); follow-up visit within 2 weeks to verify complete expulsion and to assess vaginal bleeding

Medical termination of intra-uterine pregnancy of 50-63 days gestation (under close medical supervision)
▸ BY MOUTH
▸ Adult: 600 mg for 1 dose, alternatively 200 mg for 1 dose, dose followed 36-48 hours later (unless abortion already complete) by gemeprost 1 mg by vagina; observe for at least 3 hours (or until bleeding or pain at acceptable level); follow-up visit within 2 weeks to verify complete expulsion and to assess vaginal bleeding

Termination of pregnancy of 13-24 weeks gestation (in combination with a prostaglandin) (under close medical supervision)
▸ BY MOUTH
▸ Adult: 600 mg for 1 dose, alternatively 200 mg for 1 dose, dose followed 36-48 hours later by gemeprost 1 mg by vagina every 3 hours up to max. 5 mg *or* misoprostol; if abortion does not occur, 24 hours after start of treatment repeat course of gemeprost 1 mg by vagina up to max. 5 mg; follow-up visit after appropriate interval to assess vaginal bleeding recommended

- CONTRA-INDICATIONS Acute porphyrias p. 918 · chronic adrenal failure · suspected ectopic pregnancy (use other specific means of termination) · uncontrolled severe asthma
- CAUTIONS Adrenal suppression (may require corticosteroid) · anticoagulant therapy · asthma (avoid if severe and uncontrolled) · existing cardiovascular disease · haemorrhagic disorders · history of endocarditis · prosthetic heart valve · risk factors for cardiovascular disease
- INTERACTIONS → Appendix 1 (mifepristone).
- SIDE-EFFECTS
  ▸ Common or very common Gastro-intestinal cramps · uterine contractions · vaginal bleeding (sometimes severe) may occur between administration of mifepristone and surgery (and rarely abortion may occur before surgery)
  ▸ Uncommon Hypersensitivity reactions · rash · urticaria
  ▸ Rare Chills · dizziness · fever · headache · hot flushes · hypotension · malaise
  ▸ Frequency not known Infections · toxic shock syndrome
- HEPATIC IMPAIRMENT Manufacturer advises avoid.
- RENAL IMPAIRMENT Manufacturer advises avoid.
- MONITORING REQUIREMENTS Careful monitoring of blood pressure and pulse essential for 3 hours after administration of gemeprost pessary (risk of profound hypotension).
- PRESCRIBING AND DISPENSING INFORMATION Supplied to NHS hospitals and premises approved under Abortion Act 1967.
- PATIENT AND CARER ADVICE Patient information leaflet to be provided.

- MEDICINAL FORMS
  There can be variation in the licensing of different medicines containing the same drug.
  Tablet
  CAUTIONARY AND ADVISORY LABELS 10
  ▸ Mifepristone (Non-proprietary)
  Mifepristone 200 mg Mifepristone 200mg tablets | 1 tablet [PoM] no price available (Hospital only)
  ▸ Mifegyne (Nordic Pharma Ltd)
  Mifepristone 200 mg Mifegyne 200mg tablets | 3 tablet [PoM] £52.66 (Hospital only)

7

Genito-urinary system

PROSTAGLANDINS AND OXYTOCICS

Gemeprost

● **INDICATIONS AND DOSE**

Cervical ripening prior to first trimester surgical abortion
▶ BY VAGINA
▸ Adult: 1 mg, dose to be inserted into posterior fornix 3 hours before surgery

Second trimester abortion
▶ BY VAGINA
▸ Adult: 1 mg every 3 hours for maximum 5 administrations, to be inserted into posterior fornix, second course may begin 24 hours after start of treatment (if treatment fails, pregnancy should be terminated by another method)

Second trimester intra-uterine death
▶ BY VAGINA
▸ Adult: 1 mg every 3 hours for maximum 5 administrations only, to be inserted into posterior fornix

Medical termination of intra-uterine pregnancy of up to 49 days gestation following mifepristone | Medical termination of intra-uterine pregnancy of 50–63 days gestation following mifepristone
▶ BY VAGINA
▸ Adult: 1 mg

Termination of pregnancy of 13–24 weeks gestation (in combination with a prostaglandin) following mifepristone
▶ BY VAGINA
▸ Adult: 1 mg every 3 hours, if abortion does not occur, 24 hours after start of treatment repeat course of gemeprost 1 mg by vagina up to max. 5 mg; follow-up visit after appropriate interval to assess vaginal bleeding recommended, careful monitoring of blood pressure and pulse essential for 3 hours after administration of gemeprost pessary (risk of profound hypotension); maximum 5 mg per course

● CONTRA-INDICATIONS Placenta praevia · unexplained vaginal bleeding · uterine scarring
● CAUTIONS Cardiovascular insufficiency · cervicitis · obstructive airways disease · raised intra-ocular pressure · vaginitis
● INTERACTIONS → Appendix 1 (prostaglandins).
● SIDE-EFFECTS Backache · chest pain · chills · coronary artery spasm · diarrhoea · dizziness · dyspnoea · flushing · headache · mild pyrexia · muscle weakness · myocardial infarction · nausea · palpitation · severe hypotension · uterine pain · uterine rupture (most commonly in multiparas or if history of uterine surgery or if given with intravenous oxytocics) · vaginal bleeding · vomiting
● RENAL IMPAIRMENT Manufacturer advises avoid.
● MONITORING REQUIREMENTS
▸ If used in combination with mifepristone, carefully monitor blood pressure and pulse for 3 hours.
▸ When used for second trimester intra-uterine death, monitor for coagulopathy during treatment.

● MEDICINAL FORMS
There can be variation in the licensing of different medicines containing the same drug.
Pessary
▸ Gemeprost (Non-proprietary)
  Gemeprost 1 mg Gemeprost 1mg pessaries | 5 pessary [PoM] no price available

Misoprostol

● DRUG ACTION Misoprostol acts as a potent uterine stimulant.

● **INDICATIONS AND DOSE**

Termination of pregnancy following mifepristone (gestation up to 49 days)
▶ BY MOUTH
▸ Adult: 400 micrograms for 1 dose, dose to be given 24–48 hours after mifepristone

Termination of pregnancy following mifepristone (gestation 50 to 63 days)
▶ INITIALLY BY VAGINA, OR BY BUCCAL ADMINISTRATION, OR BY SUBLINGUAL ADMINISTRATION
▸ Adult: 800 micrograms for 1 dose, dose to be given 24–48 hours after mifepristone, if abortion has not occurred 4 hours after first misoprostol dose a further dose may be given, (by mouth or by vagina) 400 micrograms for 1 dose

Termination of pregnancy following mifepristone (gestation of 9 to 13 weeks)
▶ INITIALLY BY VAGINA
▸ Adult: 800 micrograms for 1 dose, dose to be given 36–48 hours after mifepristone, followed by (by vagina or by mouth) 400 micrograms every 3 hours if required for a maximum of 4 doses

Termination of pregnancy following mifepristone (gestation of 13 to 24 weeks)
▶ INITIALLY BY VAGINA
▸ Adult: 800 micrograms for 1 dose, dose to be given 36–48 hours after mifepristone, followed by (by vagina or by mouth) 400 micrograms every 3 hours if required for a maximum of 4 doses, if abortion has not occurred 3 hours after the last dose of misoprostol, a further dose of mifepristone may be given, and misoprostol may be recommenced 12 hours later

● UNLICENSED USE Use of misoprostol for termination of pregnancy is an unlicensed use.
● CAUTIONS Conditions where hypotension might precipitate severe complications (e.g. cerebrovascular disease, cardiovascular disease) · inflammatory bowel disease
● INTERACTIONS → Appendix 1 (misoprostol)
● SIDE-EFFECTS
▶ **Common or very common** Diarrhoea
▶ **Frequency not known** Abdominal pain · abnormal vaginal bleeding · dizziness · dyspepsia · flatulence · intermenstrual bleeding · menorrhagia · nausea · postmenopausal bleeding · rashes · vomiting
● BREAST FEEDING Present in milk, but amount probably too small to be harmful.

● MEDICINAL FORMS
There can be variation in the licensing of different medicines containing the same drug.
Tablet
CAUTIONARY AND ADVISORY LABELS 21
▸ Misoprostol (Non-proprietary)
  Misoprostol 100 microgram Apo-Misoprostol 100microgram tablets | 100 tablet [PoM] no price available
  Misoprostol 200 microgram Misoprostol 200microgram vaginal tablets | 4 tablet [PoM] no price available (Hospital only)
▸ Cytotec (Pfizer Ltd)
  Misoprostol 200 microgram Cytotec 200microgram tablets | 56 tablet [PoM] no price available | 60 tablet [PoM] £10.03 DT price = £10.03
▸ Topogyne (Nordic Pharma Ltd)
  Misoprostol 400 microgram Topogyne 400microgram tablets | 16 tablet [PoM] £128.00 (Hospital only)

6 Vaginal and vulval conditions

Vaginal and vulval conditions

Management

Symptoms are often restricted to the vulva, but infections almost invariably involve the vagina which should also be treated. Applications to the vulva alone are likely to give only symptomatic relief without cure.

Aqueous medicated douches may disturb normal vaginal acidity and bacterial flora.

Topical anaesthetic agents give only symptomatic relief and may cause sensitivity reactions. They are indicated only in cases of pruritus where specific local causes have been excluded.

Systemic drugs are required in the treatment of infections such as gonorrhoea and syphilis.

Preparations for vaginal and vulval changes

Topical HRT for vaginal atrophy

A cream containing an oestrogen may be applied on a short-term basis to improve the vaginal epithelium in *menopausal atrophic vaginitis*. It is **important** to bear in mind that topical oestrogens should be used in the **smallest effective** amount to minimise systemic effects. Modified-release vaginal tablets and an impregnated vaginal ring are now also available.

The risk of endometrial hyperplasia and carcinoma is increased when *systemic* oestrogens are administered alone for prolonged periods. The endometrial safety of long-term or repeated use of *topical* vaginal oestrogens is uncertain; treatment should be reviewed at least annually, with special consideration given to any symptoms of endometrial hyperplasia or carcinoma.

Topical oestrogens are also used in postmenopausal women before vaginal surgery for prolapse when there is epithelial atrophy.

Non-hormonal preparations for vaginal atrophy

Several non-hormonal vaginal moisturisers are available and some are prescribable on the NHS (consult Drug Tariff).

Vaginal and vulval infections

Effective specific treatments are available for the common vaginal infections.

Fungal infections

Candidal vulvitis can be treated locally with cream, but is almost invariably associated with vaginal infection which should also be treated. *Vaginal candidiasis* is treated primarily with antifungal pessaries or cream inserted high into the vagina (including during menstruation). Single-dose preparations offer an advantage when compliance is a problem. Local irritation may occur on application of vaginal antifungal products.

Imidazole drugs (clotrimazole p. 750, econazole nitrate p. 750, fenticonazole nitrate p. 751, and miconazole p. 751) are effective against candida in short courses of 1 to 14 days according to the preparation used; treatment can be repeated if initial course fails to control symptoms or if symptoms recur. Vaginal applications may be supplemented with antifungal cream for vulvitis and to treat other superficial sites of infection.

Oral treatment of vaginal infection with fluconazole p. 540 or itraconazole p. 542 is also effective.

Vulvovaginal candidiasis in pregnancy

Vulvovaginal candidiasis is common during pregnancy and can be treated with vaginal application of an imidazole (such as clotrimazole), and a topical imidazole cream for vulvitis.

Pregnant women need a longer duration of treatment, usually about 7 days, to clear the infection. Oral antifungal treatment should be avoided during pregnancy.

Recurrent vulvovaginal candidiasis

Recurrence of vulvovaginal candidiasis is particularly likely if there are predisposing factors, such as antibacterial therapy, pregnancy, diabetes mellitus, or possibly oral contraceptive use. Reservoirs of infection may also lead to recontamination and should be treated; these include other skin sites such as the digits, nail beds, and umbilicus as well as the gastro-intestinal tract and the bladder. The partner may also be the source of reinfection and, if symptomatic, should be treated with a topical imidazole cream at the same time.

Treatment against candida may need to be extended for 6 months in recurrent vulvovaginal candidiasis.

Other infections

Trichomonal infections commonly involve the lower urinary tract as well as the genital system and need systemic treatment with metronidazole p. 492 or tinidazole p. 493.

Bacterial infections with Gram-negative organisms are particularly common in association with gynaecological operations and trauma. Metronidazole is effective against certain Gram-negative organisms, especially *Bacteroides* spp. and can be used prophylactically in gynaecological surgery.

Clindamycin below cream and metronidazole gel are indicated for bacterial vaginosis.

Vaginal preparations intended to restore normal acidity may prevent recurrence of vaginal infections and permit the re-establishment of the normal vaginal flora.

The antiviral drugs aciclovir p. 576, famciclovir p. 578, and valaciclovir p. 579 can be used in the treatment of genital infection due to *herpes simplex virus*, the HSV type 2 being a major cause of genital ulceration; they have a beneficial effect on virus shedding and healing, generally giving relief from pain and other symptoms.

6.1 Vaginal and vulval infections

6.1a Vaginal and vulval bacterial infections

> **Drugs used for Vaginal and vulval bacterial infections not listed below** Metronidazole, p. 492

ANTIBACTERIALS ❯ LINCOSAMIDES

Clindamycin

- ● **INDICATIONS AND DOSE**

  DALACIN® 2% CREAM

  Bacterial vaginosis
  - ▶ BY VAGINA
  - ▶ Adult: 1 applicatorful daily for 3–7 nights, dose to be administered at night

  DOSE EQUIVALENCE AND CONVERSION

  1 applicatorful delivers a 5 g dose of clindamycin 2%.

- ● SIDE-EFFECTS Cervicitis · irritation · vaginitis

  SIDE-EFFECTS, FURTHER INFORMATION

  Clindamycin 2% cream is poorly absorbed into the blood—low risk of systemic effects.

- ● CONCEPTION AND CONTRACEPTION Damages latex condoms and diaphragms.

7

Genito-urinary system

● MEDICINAL FORMS
There can be variation in the licensing of different medicines containing the same drug.

Cream
EXCIPIENTS: May contain Benzyl alcohol, cetostearyl alcohol (including cetyl and stearyl alcohol), polysorbates, propylene glycol
▸ Dalacin (Pfizer Ltd)
　Clindamycin (as Clindamycin phosphate) 20 mg per 1 gram Dalacin 2% cream | 40 gram PoM £10.86 DT price = £10.86

CARBOXYLIC ACIDS

Lactic acid

● INDICATIONS AND DOSE
BALANCE ACTIV RX® GEL

Prevention of bacterial vaginosis
▸ BY VAGINA
▸ Adult: 5 mL 1–2 times a week, insert the content of 1 tube (5 mL)

RELACTAGEL® GEL

Prevention of bacterial vaginosis
▸ BY VAGINA
▸ Adult: 5 mL daily for 2–3 nights after menstruation, insert the contents of one tube

● SIDE-EFFECTS
RELACTAGEL® GEL Mild irritation

● CONCEPTION AND CONTRACEPTION
RELACTAGEL® GEL Not recommended if trying to conceive.

● MEDICINAL FORMS
There can be variation in the licensing of different medicines containing the same drug.

Gel
EXCIPIENTS: May contain Propylene glycol
▸ Balance Activ (BBI Healthcare Ltd)
　Balance Activ BV vaginal pH correction gel | 7 device £5.25
　Balance Activ pessaries | 7 pessary £5.25
▸ Relactagel (KoRa Healthcare)
　Relactagel vaginal pH correction gel | 7 device £5.25

6.1b Vaginal and vulval fungal infections

ANTIFUNGALS ⟩ IMIDAZOLE ANTIFUNGALS

Clotrimazole

● INDICATIONS AND DOSE

Superficial sites of infection in vaginal and vulval candidiasis (dose for 1% or 2% cream)
▸ BY VAGINA USING CREAM
▸ Adult: Apply 2–3 times a day, to be applied to anogenital area

Vaginal candidiasis (dose for 10% intravaginal cream)
▸ BY VAGINA USING VAGINAL CREAM
▸ Adult: 5 g for 1 dose, one applicatorful to be inserted into the vagina at night, dose can be repeated once if necessary

Vaginal candidiasis
▸ BY VAGINA USING PESSARIES
▸ Adult: 200 mg for 3 nights, course can be repeated once if necessary, alternatively 100 mg for 6 nights, course can be repeated once if necessary, alternatively 500 mg for 1 night, dose can be repeated once if necessary

Recurrent vulvovaginal candidiasis
▸ BY VAGINA USING PESSARIES
▸ Adult: 500 mg every 1 week for 6 months, dose to be administered following topical imidazole for 10–14 days

● SIDE-EFFECTS Local irritation

● CONCEPTION AND CONTRACEPTION Cream and pessaries may damage latex condoms and diaphragms.

● PREGNANCY Pregnant women need a longer duration of treatment, usually about 7 days, to clear the infection. Oral antifungal treatment should be avoided during pregnancy.

● EXCEPTIONS TO LEGAL CATEGORY Brands for sale to the public include *Canesten*® Internal Cream.

● MEDICINAL FORMS
There can be variation in the licensing of different medicines containing the same drug.

Pessary
EXCIPIENTS: May contain Benzyl alcohol, cetostearyl alcohol (including cetyl and stearyl alcohol), polysorbates
▸ Clotrimazole (Non-proprietary)
　Clotrimazole 500 mg Clotrimazole 500mg pessaries | 1 pessary P £6.60 DT price = £2.91
▸ Canesten (clotrimazole) (Bayer Plc)
　Clotrimazole 100 mg Canesten 100mg pessaries | 6 pessary P £3.50 DT price = £3.50
　Clotrimazole 200 mg Canesten 200mg pessaries | 3 pessary P £3.10 DT price = £3.10
　Clotrimazole 500 mg Canesten 500mg Soft Gel pessaries | 1 pessary P £6.41 DT price = £2.91
　Canesten 500mg pessaries | 1 pessary P no price available DT price = £2.91
　Canesten Vaginal 500mg pessaries | 1 pessary PoM £2.00 DT price = £2.91

Cream
EXCIPIENTS: May contain Benzyl alcohol, cetostearyl alcohol (including cetyl and stearyl alcohol), polysorbates
▸ Clotrimazole (Non-proprietary)
　Clotrimazole 10 mg per 1 gram Clotrimazole 1% cream | 20 gram P £2.79 DT price = £1.04 | 50 gram P £5.45 DT price = £2.60
▸ Canesten (clotrimazole) (Bayer Plc)
　Clotrimazole 10 mg per 1 gram Canesten 1% cream | 20 gram P £2.14 DT price = £1.04 | 50 gram P £3.50 DT price = £2.60
　Canesten Antifungal 1% cream | 20 gram P £1.85 DT price = £1.04
　Clotrimazole 20 mg per 1 gram Canesten 2% thrush cream | 10 gram P no price available | 20 gram P £4.46 DT price = £4.46
　Clotrimazole 100 mg per 1 gram Canesten Internal 10% cream | 5 gram P £6.23 DT price = £6.23
　Canesten 10% VC cream | 5 gram PoM £4.50 DT price = £6.23

Econazole nitrate

● INDICATIONS AND DOSE
GYNO-PEVARYL® ONCE

Vaginal and vulval candidiasis
▸ BY VAGINA
▸ Adult: 1 pessary for 1 dose, pessary to be inserted at night, dose to be repeated once if necessary

GYNO-PEVARYL® CREAM

Vaginal and vulval candidiasis
▸ INITIALLY BY VAGINA USING VAGINAL CREAM
▸ Adult: 1 applicatorful daily for at least 14 days, dose to be inserted vaginally at night

GYNO-PEVARYL® PESSARY

Vaginal and vulval candidiasis
▸ BY VAGINA
▸ Adult: 1 pessary daily for 3 days, pessary to be inserted at night, course can be repeated once if necessary

● SIDE-EFFECTS Occasional local irritation

- CONCEPTION AND CONTRACEPTION Cream and pessaries damage latex condoms and diaphragms.
- PREGNANCY Pregnant women need a longer duration of treatment, usually about 7 days, to clear the infection.

- MEDICINAL FORMS
There can be variation in the licensing of different medicines containing the same drug.

Pessary
▸ Gyno-Pevaryl (Janssen-Cilag Ltd)
Econazole nitrate 150 mg Gyno-Pevaryl Once 150mg vaginal pessary | 1 pessary PoM £3.69
Gyno-Pevaryl 150mg vaginal pessaries | 3 pessary PoM £4.17

Cream
EXCIPIENTS: May contain Butylated hydroxyanisole, fragrances
▸ Gyno-Pevaryl (Janssen-Cilag Ltd)
Econazole nitrate 10 mg per 1 gram Gyno-Pevaryl 1% cream | 15 gram PoM £2.11 | 30 gram PoM £3.78

Fenticonazole nitrate

- INDICATIONS AND DOSE

Vaginal and vulva candidiasis
▸ BY VAGINA USING CAPSULES
- Adult: 200 mg daily for 3 days, alternatively 600 mg daily for 1 dose, to be inserted at night
▸ BY VAGINA USING CREAM
- Adult: 1 applicatorful twice daily for 3 days
DOSE EQUIVALENCE AND CONVERSION
▸ With topical use 1 applicatorful delivers a 5 g dose of fenticonazole 2 %.

- SIDE-EFFECTS Local irritation
- CONCEPTION AND CONTRACEPTION Intravaginal cream and vaginal capsules damage latex condoms and diaphragms.

- MEDICINAL FORMS
There can be variation in the licensing of different medicines containing the same drug.

Capsule
EXCIPIENTS: May contain Hydroxybenzoates (parabens)
▸ Gynoxin (Recordati Pharmaceuticals Ltd)
Fenticonazole nitrate 200 mg Gynoxin 200mg vaginal capsules | 3 capsule PoM £2.42
Fenticonazole nitrate 600 mg Gynoxin 600mg vaginal capsules | 1 capsule PoM £2.62

Cream
EXCIPIENTS: May contain Cetostearyl alcohol (including cetyl and stearyl alcohol), propylene glycol, wool fat and related substances including lanolin
▸ Gynoxin (Recordati Pharmaceuticals Ltd)
Fenticonazole nitrate 20 mg per 1 gram Gynoxin 2% vaginal cream | 30 gram PoM £3.74

Ketoconazole

- INDICATIONS AND DOSE

Vaginal and vulva candidiasis
▸ BY VAGINA USING CREAM
- Adult: Apply 1–2 times a day, to be applied to the anogenital area

- CAUTIONS Avoid contact with eyes
- INTERACTIONS → Appendix 1 (antifungals, imidazole).
- SIDE-EFFECTS Erythema · hypersensitivity reactions · itching · mild burning sensation · occasional local irritation
SIDE-EFFECTS, FURTHER INFORMATION
Treatment should be discontinued if side-effects are severe.

- CONCEPTION AND CONTRACEPTION Effect on latex condoms and diaphragms not yet known.

- NATIONAL FUNDING/ACCESS DECISIONS
NHS restrictions Ketoconazole cream is not prescribable on the NHS except for seborrhoeic dermatitis and pityriasis versicolor and endorsed 'SLS'.

- MEDICINAL FORMS
There can be variation in the licensing of different medicines containing the same drug.

Cream
EXCIPIENTS: May contain Cetostearyl alcohol (including cetyl and stearyl alcohol), polysorbates, propylene glycol
▸ Nizoral (Janssen-Cilag Ltd)
Ketoconazole 20 mg per 1 gram Nizoral 2% cream | 30 gram PoM £4.24 DT price = £4.24

Miconazole

- INDICATIONS AND DOSE

Vaginal and vulval candidiasis
▸ BY VAGINA USING CAPSULES
- Child: 1 capsule daily, ovule to be inserted at night as a single dose, dose can be repeated once if necessary
- Adult: 1 capsule daily, ovule to be inserted at night as a single dose, dose can be repeated once if necessary
▸ BY VAGINA USING CREAM
- Adult: Apply 1 applicatorful daily for 10 to 14 days, alternatively apply 1 applicatorful twice daily for 7 days, course can be repeated once if necessary

Superficial sites of infection in vaginal and vulval candidiasis | Vulvitis
▸ BY VAGINA USING CREAM
- Adult: Apply twice daily, apply to the anogenital area

- CAUTIONS Avoid in Acute porphyrias p. 918 · avoid intravaginal preparations (particularly those that require use of an applicator) in young girls who are not sexually active, unless there is no alternative
- INTERACTIONS → Appendix 1 (antifungals, imidazole).
- SIDE-EFFECTS
- **Common or very common** Nausea · rash · vomiting
- **Frequency not known** Occasional local irritation
- CONCEPTION AND CONTRACEPTION *Gyno-Daktarin®* damages latex condoms and diaphragms.
- PREGNANCY Pregnant women need a longer duration of treatment, usually about 7 days, to clear the infection.
- BREAST FEEDING Manufacturer advises caution—no information available.

- MEDICINAL FORMS
There can be variation in the licensing of different medicines containing the same drug.

Capsule
EXCIPIENTS: May contain Hydroxybenzoates (parabens)
▸ Gyno-Daktarin (Janssen-Cilag Ltd)
Miconazole nitrate 1.2 gram Gyno-Daktarin 1200mg vaginal capsules | 1 capsule PoM £2.94 DT price = £2.94

Cream
EXCIPIENTS: May contain Butylated hydroxyanisole
▸ Gyno-Daktarin (Janssen-Cilag Ltd)
Miconazole nitrate 20 mg per 1 gram Gyno-Daktarin 2% vaginal cream | 78 gram PoM £4.33

Genito-urinary system

7

6.2 Vaginal atrophy

OESTROGENS

Estradiol

● **INDICATIONS AND DOSE**

ESTRING®

Postmenopausal urogenital conditions (not suitable for vasomotor symptoms or osteoporosis prophylaxis)
▸ BY VAGINA
▸ Adult: To be inserted into upper third of vagina and worn continuously; replace after 3 months; max. duration of continuous treatment 2 years

VAGIFEM®

Improve the vaginal epithelium in menopausal atrophic vaginitis
▸ BY VAGINA
▸ Adult: 1 tablet daily for 2 weeks, then reduced to 1 tablet twice weekly

● **CONTRA-INDICATIONS** Active arterial thromboembolic disease (e.g. angina or myocardial infarction) · active thrombophlebitis · Dubin-Johnson syndrome (or monitor closely) · history of breast cancer · history of recurrent venous thromboembolism (unless already on anticoagulant treatment) · oestrogen-dependent cancer · recent arterial thromboembolic disease (e.g. angina or myocardial infarction) · Rotor syndrome (or monitor closely) · thrombophilic disorder · undiagnosed vaginal bleeding · untreated endometrial hyperplasia · venous thromboembolism

● **CAUTIONS** Acute porphyrias p. 918 · diabetes (increased risk of heart disease) · history of breast nodules—closely monitor breast status (risk of breast cancer) · history of endometrial hyperplasia; factors predisposing to thromboembolism · history of fibrocystic disease—closely monitor breast status (risk of breast cancer) · hypophyseal tumours · increased risk of gall-bladder disease · interrupt treatment periodically to assess need for continued treatment · migraine (or migraine-like headaches) · presence of antiphospholipid antibodies (increased risk of thrombotic events) · prolonged exposure to unopposed oestrogens may increase risk of developing endometrial cancer · risk factors for oestrogen-dependent tumours (e.g. breast cancer in first-degree relative) · symptoms of endometriosis may be exacerbated · uterine fibroids may increase in size

CAUTIONS, FURTHER INFORMATION
▸ Risk of breast cancer It is estimated that using *all* types of HRT increases the risk of breast cancer within 1–2 years of initiating treatment. The increased risk is related to the duration of HRT use (but not to the age at which HRT is started) and this excess risk disappears within 5 years of stopping.

Radiological detection of breast cancer can be made more difficult as mammographic density can increase with HRT use.
▸ Risk of endometrial cancer The increased risk of endometrial cancer depends on the dose and duration of oestrogen-only HRT.

In women with a uterus, the addition of a progestogen cyclically (for at least 10 days per 28-day cycle) reduces the additional risk of endometrial cancer; this additional risk is eliminated if a progestogen is given continuously. However, this should be weighed against the increased risk of breast cancer.
▸ Risk of ovarian cancer Long-term use of combined HRT or oestrogen-only HRT is associated with a small increased

risk of ovarian cancer. This excess risk disappears within a few years of stopping.
▸ Risk of venous thromboembolism Women using combined or oestrogen-only HRT are at an increased risk of deep vein thrombosis and of pulmonary embolism especially in the first year of use.

In *women who have predisposing factors* (such as a personal or family history of deep vein thrombosis or pulmonary embolism, severe varicose veins, obesity, trauma, or prolonged bed-rest) it is prudent to review the need for HRT, as in some cases the risks of HRT may exceed the benefits.

Travel involving prolonged immobility further increases the risk of deep vein thrombosis.
▸ Risk of stroke Risk of stroke increases with age, therefore older women have a greater absolute risk of stroke. Combined HRT or oestrogen-only HRT slightly increases the risk of stroke.
▸ Risk of coronary heart disease HRT does not prevent coronary heart disease and should not be prescribed for this purpose. There is an increased risk of coronary heart disease in women who start combined HRT more than 10 years after menopause. Although very little information is available on the risk of coronary heart disease in younger women who start HRT close to the menopause, studies suggest a lower relative risk compared with older women.
▸ Other conditions The product literature advises caution in other conditions including hypertension, renal disease, asthma, epilepsy, sickle-cell disease, melanoma, otosclerosis, multiple sclerosis, and systemic lupus erythematosus (but care required if antiphospholipid antibodies present). Evidence for caution in these conditions is unsatisfactory and many women with these conditions may stand to benefit from HRT.

● **INTERACTIONS** → Appendix 1 (oestrogens).

● **SIDE-EFFECTS** Abdominal bloating · abdominal cramps · altered blood lipids (may lead to pancreatitis, rashes and chloasma) · breast enlargement · breast tenderness · changes in libido · cholestatic jaundice · contact lenses may irritate · depression · dizziness · fluid retention · glucose intolerance · headache · headache (on vigorous exercise) · leg cramps (rule out venous thrombosis) · local irritation · migraine · mood changes · nausea · premenstrual-like syndrome · sodium retention · vaginal candidiasis · vomiting · weight changes

SIDE-EFFECTS, FURTHER INFORMATION
▸ Withdrawal bleeding Cyclical HRT (where a progestogen is taken for 12–14 days of each 28-day oestrogen treatment cycle) usually results in *regular withdrawal bleeding* towards the end of the progestogen. The aim of continuous combined HRT (where a combination of oestrogen and progestogen is taken, usually in a single tablet, throughout each 28-day treatment cycle) is to avoid bleeding, but *irregular bleeding* may occur during the early treatment stages (if it continues endometrial abnormality should be excluded and consideration given to cyclical HRT instead).

● **CONCEPTION AND CONTRACEPTION** HRT does **not** provide contraception and a woman is considered potentially fertile for 2 years after her last menstrual period if she is under 50 years, and for 1 year if she is over 50 years. A woman who is under 50 years and free of all risk factors for venous and arterial disease can use a low-oestrogen combined oral contraceptive pill to provide both relief of menopausal symptoms and contraception; it is recommended that the oral contraceptive be stopped at 50 years of age since there are more suitable alternatives. If any potentially fertile woman needs HRT, non-hormonal contraceptive measures (such as condoms) are necessary. Measurement of follicle-stimulating hormone can help to determine fertility, but high measurements alone (particularly in women aged under 50 years) do not necessarily preclude the possibility of becoming pregnant.

VAGIFEM® No evidence of damage to latex condoms and diaphragms.

- PREGNANCY Not known to be harmful.
- BREAST FEEDING Avoid; adverse effects on lactation.
- HEPATIC IMPAIRMENT Avoid in active liver disease including disorders of hepatic excretion (e.g. Dubin-Johnson or Rotor syndromes), infective hepatitis (until liver function returns to normal), and liver tumours.
- MONITORING REQUIREMENTS
- ▸ History of breast nodules or fibrocystic disease—closely monitor breast status (risk of breast cancer).
- ▸ The endometrial safety of long-term or repeated use of topical vaginal oestrogens is uncertain; treatment should be reviewed at least annually, with special consideration given to any symptoms of endometrial hyperplasia or carcinoma.

- MEDICINAL FORMS
There can be variation in the licensing of different medicines containing the same drug.

Pessary
- ▸ Vagifem (Novo Nordisk Ltd)
 Estradiol 10 microgram Vagifem 10microgram vaginal tablets | 24 pessary [PoM] £16.72 DT price = £16.72

Vaginal delivery system
CAUTIONARY AND ADVISORY LABELS 10
- ▸ Estring (Pfizer Ltd)
 Estradiol (as Estradiol hemihydrate) 7.5 microgram per 24 hour Estring 7.5micrograms/24hours vaginal delivery system | 1 device [PoM] £31.42

Estriol

- INDICATIONS AND DOSE

OVESTIN®

Improve the vaginal epithelium in menopausal atrophic vaginitis (short-term use)
- ▸ BY VAGINA
- ▸ Adult: Apply 1 applicatorful daily for 2–3 weeks, then reduced to 1 applicatorful twice weekly, discontinue every 2–3 months for 4 weeks to assess need for further treatment

Vaginal surgery for prolapse when there is epithelial atrophy in postmenopausal women (before surgery)
- ▸ BY VAGINA
- ▸ Adult: Apply 1 applicatorful daily for 2 weeks before surgery, resume 2 weeks after surgery

- CONTRA-INDICATIONS Active arterial thromboembolic disease (e.g. angina or myocardial infarction) · active thrombophlebitis · Dubin-Johnson syndrome (or monitor closely) · history of breast cancer · history of recurrent venous thromboembolism (unless already on anticoagulant treatment) · oestrogen-dependent cancer · recent arterial thromboembolic disease (e.g. angina or myocardial infarction) · Rotor syndrome (or monitor closely) · thrombophilic disorder · undiagnosed vaginal bleeding · untreated endometrial hyperplasia · venous thromboembolism

- CAUTIONS Acute porphyrias p. 918 · diabetes (increased risk of heart disease) · factors predisposing to thromboembolism · history of breast nodules—closely monitor breast status (risk of breast cancer) · history of endometrial hyperplasia · history of fibrocystic disease—closely monitor breast status (risk of breast cancer) · hypophyseal tumours · increased risk of gall-bladder disease · interrupt treatment periodically to assess need for continued treatment · migraine (or migraine-like headaches) · presence of antiphospholipid antibodies

(increased risk of thrombotic events) · prolonged exposure to unopposed oestrogens may increase risk of developing endometrial cancer · risk factors for oestrogen-dependent tumours (e.g. breast cancer in first-degree relative) · symptoms of endometriosis may be exacerbated · uterine fibroids may increase in size

CAUTIONS, FURTHER INFORMATION
- ▸ **Risk of breast cancer** It is estimated that using *all* types of HRT increases the risk of breast cancer within 1–2 years of initiating treatment. The increased risk is related to the duration of HRT use (but not to the age at which HRT is started) and this excess risk disappears within 5 years of stopping.

 Radiological detection of breast cancer can be made more difficult as mammographic density can increase with HRT use.
- ▸ **Risk of endometrial cancer** The increased risk of endometrial cancer depends on the dose and duration of oestrogen-only HRT.

 In women with a uterus, the addition of a progestogen cyclically (for at least 10 days per 28-day cycle) reduces the additional risk of endometrial cancer; this additional risk is eliminated if a progestogen is given continuously. However, this should be weighed against the increased risk of breast cancer.
- ▸ **Risk of ovarian cancer** Long-term use of combined HRT or oestrogen-only HRT is associated with a small increased risk of ovarian cancer. This excess risk disappears within a few years of stopping.
- ▸ **Risk of venous thromboembolism** Women using combined or oestrogen-only HRT are at an increased risk of deep vein thrombosis and of pulmonary embolism especially in the first year of use.

 In *women who have predisposing factors* (such as a personal or family history of deep vein thrombosis or pulmonary embolism, severe varicose veins, obesity, trauma, or prolonged bed-rest) it is prudent to review the need for HRT, as in some cases the risks of HRT may exceed the benefits.

 Travel involving prolonged immobility further increases the risk of deep vein thrombosis.
- ▸ **Risk of stroke** Risk of stroke increases with age, therefore older women have a greater absolute risk of stroke. Combined HRT or oestrogen-only HRT slightly increases the risk of stroke.
- ▸ **Risk of coronary heart disease** HRT does not prevent coronary heart disease and should not be prescribed for this purpose. There is an increased risk of coronary heart disease in women who start combined HRT more than 10 years after menopause. Although very little information is available on the risk of coronary heart disease in younger women who start HRT close to the menopause, studies suggest a lower relative risk compared with older women.
- ▸ **Other conditions** The product literature advises caution in other conditions including hypertension, renal disease, asthma, epilepsy, sickle-cell disease, melanoma, otosclerosis, multiple sclerosis, and systemic lupus erythematosus (but care required if antiphospholipid antibodies present). Evidence for caution in these conditions is unsatisfactory and many women with these conditions may stand to benefit from HRT.

- INTERACTIONS → Appendix 1 (oestrogens).
- SIDE-EFFECTS Abdominal bloating · abdominal cramps · altered blood lipids (may lead to pancreatitis, rashes and chloasma) · breast enlargement · breast tenderness · changes in libido · cholestatic jaundice · contact lenses may irritate · depression · dizziness · fluid retention · glucose intolerance · headache · leg cramps · local irritation · migraine · mood changes · nausea · premenstrual-like

syndrome · sodium retention · vaginal candidiasis · vomiting · weight changes

SIDE-EFFECTS, FURTHER INFORMATION

‣ **Leg Cramps** Venous thrombosis should be ruled out.
‣ **Withdrawal Bleeding** Cyclical HRT (where a progestogen is taken for 12–14 days of each 28-day oestrogen treatment cycle) usually results in *regular withdrawal bleeding* towards the end of the progestogen. The aim of continuous combined HRT (where a combination of oestrogen and progestogen is taken, usually in a single tablet, throughout each 28-day treatment cycle) is to avoid bleeding, but *irregular bleeding* may occur during the early treatment stages (if it continues endometrial abnormality should be excluded and consideration given to cyclical HRT instead).

● CONCEPTION AND CONTRACEPTION Effect on latex condoms and diaphragms not yet known.

● PREGNANCY Not known to be harmful.

● BREAST FEEDING Avoid; adverse effects on lactation.

● HEPATIC IMPAIRMENT Avoid in active liver disease including disorders of hepatic excretion (e.g. Dubin-Johnson or Rotor syndromes), infective hepatitis (until liver function returns to normal), and liver tumours.

● RENAL IMPAIRMENT Manufacturer advises caution in renal disease. Evidence for caution is unsatisfactory and many women with these conditions may stand to benefit from HRT.

● MONITORING REQUIREMENTS
‣ Closely monitor breast status if history of breast nodules or fibrocystic disease (risk of breast cancer).
‣ The endometrial safety of long-term or repeated use of topical vaginal oestrogens is uncertain; treatment should be reviewed at least annually, with special consideration given to any symptoms of endometrial hyperplasia or carcinoma.

● MEDICINAL FORMS
There can be variation in the licensing of different medicines containing the same drug.

Cream
EXCIPIENTS: May contain Arachis (peanut) oil, cetostearyl alcohol (including cetyl and stearyl alcohol), polysorbates
‣ Ovestin (Aspen Pharma Trading Ltd)
  Estriol 1 mg per 1 gram Ovestin 1mg cream | 15 gram [PoM] £4.45
  DT price = £4.45

Chapter 8
Immune system and malignant disease

CONTENTS

Immune system

1   Immune system disorders and transplantation

Immune response

Inflammatory bowel disease

Azathioprine p. 757, ciclosporin p. 758, mercaptopurine p. 806, and methotrexate p. 807 have a role in the treatment of inflammatory bowel disease.

Folic acid p. 886 should be given to reduce the possibility of methotrexate toxicity [unlicensed indication]. Folic acid is usually given weekly on a different day to the methotrexate; alternative regimens may be used in some settings.

Immunosuppressant therapy

Immunosuppressants are used to suppress rejection in organ transplant recipients and to treat a variety of chronic inflammatory and autoimmune diseases. Solid organ transplant patients are maintained on drug regimens, which may include antiproliferative drugs (azathioprine or mycophenolate mofetil p. 765), calcineurin inhibitors (ciclosporin or tacrolimus p. 761), corticosteroids, or sirolimus p. 760. Choice is dependent on the type of organ, time after transplantation, and clinical condition of the patient. Specialist management is required and other immunomodulators may be used to initiate treatment or to treat rejection.

Impaired immune responsiveness

Modification of tissue reactions caused by corticosteroids and other immunosuppressants may result in the rapid *spread of infection*. Corticosteroids may suppress clinical signs of infection and allow diseases such as septicaemia or tuberculosis to reach an advanced stage before being recognised—**important**: normal immunoglobulin administration should be considered as soon as possible after measles exposure, and varicella–zoster immunoglobulin (VZIG) is recommended for individuals who have significant chickenpox (varicella) exposure. Specialist advice should be sought on the use of live vaccines for those being treated with immunosuppressive drugs.

Antiproliferative immunosuppressants

Azathioprine is widely used for transplant recipients and it is also used to treat a number of auto-immune conditions, usually when corticosteroid therapy alone provides inadequate control. It is metabolised to mercaptopurine, and doses should be reduced when allopurinol p. 968 is given concurrently.

Mycophenolate mofetil is metabolised to mycophenolic acid which has a more selective mode of action than azathioprine.

There is evidence that compared with similar regimens incorporating azathioprine, mycophenolate mofetil reduces the risk of acute rejection episodes; the risk of opportunistic infections (particularly due to tissue-invasive cytomegalovirus) and the occurrence of blood disorders such as leucopenia may be higher.

Cyclophosphamide p. 793 is less commonly prescribed as an immunosuppressant.

Corticosteroids and other immunosuppressants

Prednisolone p. 614 is widely used in oncology. It has a marked antitumour effect in acute lymphoblastic leukaemia, Hodgkin's disease, and the non-Hodgkin lymphomas. It has a role in the palliation of symptomatic end-stage malignant disease when it may enhance appetite and produce a sense of well-being.

The corticosteroids are also powerful immunosuppressants. They are used to prevent organ transplant rejection, and in high dose to treat rejection episodes.

Ciclosporin a calcineurin inhibitor, is a potent immunosuppressant which is virtually non-myelotoxic but markedly nephrotoxic. It has an important role in organ and tissue transplantation, for prevention of graft rejection following bone marrow, kidney, liver, pancreas, heart, lung, and heart-lung transplantation, and for prophylaxis and treatment of graft-versus-host disease.

Tacrolimus is also a calcineurin inhibitor. Although not chemically related to ciclosporin it has a similar mode of action and side-effects, but the incidence of neurotoxicity appears to be greater; cardiomyopathy has also been reported. Disturbance of glucose metabolism also appears to be significant.

Sirolimus is a non-calcineurin inhibiting immunosuppressant licensed for renal transplantation.

Basiliximab p. 764 is used for prophylaxis of acute rejection in allogeneic renal transplantation. It is given with ciclosporin and corticosteroid immunosuppression regimens; its use should be confined to specialist centres.

Belatacept p. 766 is a fusion protein and co-stimulation blocker that prevents T-cell activation; it is licensed for prophylaxis of graft rejection in adults undergoing renal transplantation who are seropositive for the Epstein-Barr virus. It is used with interleukin-2 receptor antagonist induction, in combination with corticosteroids and a mycophenolic acid.

Antithymocyte immunoglobulin (rabbit) below is licensed for the prophylaxis of organ rejection in renal and heart allograft recipients and for the treatment of corticosteroid-resistant allograft rejection in renal transplantation. Tolerability is increased by pretreatment with an intravenous corticosteroid and antihistamine; an antipyretic drug such as paracetamol may also be beneficial.

NICE technology appraisals (TAs)

Immunosuppressive therapy for renal transplantation in adults (September 2004) Immunosuppressive therapy for renal transplantation in children and adolescents (April 2006) NICE TA85

For induction therapy in the prophylaxis of organ rejection, either basiliximab or daclizumab [discontinued] are options for combining with a calcineurin inhibitor. For each individual, ciclosporin or tacrolimus is chosen as the calcineurin inhibitor on the basis of side-effects.

Mycophenolate mofetil [mycophenolic acid also available but not licensed for use in children] is recommended as part of an immunosuppressive regimen only if:

- the calcineurin inhibitor is not tolerated, particularly if nephrotoxicity endangers the transplanted kidney; or
- there is very high risk of nephrotoxicity from the calcineurin inhibitor, requiring a reduction in the dose of the calcineurin inhibitor or its avoidance.

Sirolimus is recommended as a component of immunosuppressive regimen **only if** intolerance necessitates the withdrawal of a calcineurin inhibitor. These recommendations may not be consistent with the marketing authorisation of some of the products.
www.nice.org.uk/TA85

Immunosuppressive therapy for renal transplantation in children and adolescents (April 2006) NICE TA99

NICE has recommended that for induction therapy in the prophylaxis of organ rejection, either basiliximab or daclizumab [discontinued] are options for combining with a calcineurin inhibitor. For each individual, ciclosporin or tacrolimus is chosen as the calcineurin inhibitor on the basis of side-effects. Mycophenolate mofetil is recommended as part of an immunosuppressive regimen **only if**:

- the calcineurin inhibitor is not tolerated, particularly if nephrotoxicity endangers the transplanted kidney; or
- there is very high risk of nephrotoxicity from the calcineurin inhibitor, requiring a reduction in the dose of the calcineurin inhibitor or its avoidance.

Mycophenolic acid is not recommended as part of an immunosuppressive regimen for renal transplantation in children or adolescents.

Sirolimus [not licensed for use in children] is recommended as a component of immunosuppressive regimen **only if** intolerance necessitates the withdrawal of a calcineurin inhibitor.

These recommendations may not be consistent with the marketing authorisation of some of the products.
www.nice.org.uk/TA99

Drugs used for Immune system disorders and transplantation not listed below Chloroquine, p. 560 · Everolimus, p. 853 · Hydroxychloroquine sulfate, p. 950 · Rituximab, p. 783

Antithymocyte immunoglobulin (rabbit)

● **INDICATIONS AND DOSE**

Prophylaxis of organ rejection in heart allograft recipients
▶ BY INTRAVENOUS INFUSION
▶ Adult: 1–2.5 mg/kg daily for 3–5 days, to be given over at least 6 hours

Prophylaxis of organ rejection in renal allograft recipients
▶ BY INTRAVENOUS INFUSION
▶ Adult: 1–1.5 mg/kg daily for 3–9 days, to be given over at least 6 hours

Treatment of corticosteroid-resistant allograft rejection in renal transplantation
▶ BY INTRAVENOUS INFUSION
▶ Adult: 1.5 mg/kg daily for 7–14 days, to be given over at least 6 hours

DOSES AT EXTREMES OF BODY-WEIGHT
To avoid excessive dosage in obese patients, calculate dose on the basis of ideal body weight.

● CONTRA-INDICATIONS Infection

● SIDE-EFFECTS Anaphylaxis · cytokine release syndrome · diarrhoea · dysphagia · fever · hypotension · increased susceptibility to infection · increased susceptibility to malignancy · infusion-related reactions · lymphopenia · myalgia · nausea · neutropenia · pruritus · rash · serum sickness · shivering · thrombocytopenia · vomiting

SIDE-EFFECTS, FURTHER INFORMATION
Tolerability is increased by pretreatment with an intravenous corticosteroid and antihistamine; an antipyretic drug such as paracetamol may also be beneficial.

● PREGNANCY Manufacturer advises use only if potential benefit outweighs risk—no information available.

● BREAST FEEDING Manufacturer advises avoid—no information available.

● MONITORING REQUIREMENTS Monitor blood count.

● DIRECTIONS FOR ADMINISTRATION For *continuous intravenous infusion* (*Thymoglobuline®*) in Glucose 5% or Sodium chloride 0.9%; reconstitute each vial with 5 mL water for injections to produce a solution of 5 mg/mL; gently rotate to dissolve. Dilute requisite dose with infusion fluid to a total volume of 50–500 mL (usually 50 mL); begin infusion immediately after dilution; give through an in-line filter (pore size 0.22 micron); not to be given with unfractionated heparin and hydrocortisone in glucose infusion—precipitation reported.

● MEDICINAL FORMS
There can be variation in the licensing of different medicines containing the same drug.

Solution for infusion
▶ Antithymocyte immunoglobulin (rabbit) (Non-proprietary)
  Antithymocyte immunoglobulin (rabbit) 20 mg per 1 ml Grafalon 100mg/5ml concentrate for solution for infusion vials | 1 vial PoM no price available

Powder and solvent for solution for infusion
▶ Thymoglobulin (Sanofi)
  Antithymocyte immunoglobulin (rabbit) 25 mg Thymoglobuline 25mg powder and solvent for solution for infusion vials | 1 vial PoM £158.77 (Hospital only)

IMMUNOSUPPRESSANTS › ANTIMETABOLITES

Azathioprine

● **DRUG ACTION** Azathioprine is metabolised to mercaptopurine.

● **INDICATIONS AND DOSE**

Severe acute Crohn's disease | Maintenance of remission of Crohn's disease | Maintenance of remission of acute ulcerative colitis
▸ BY MOUTH
▸ Adult: 2–2.5 mg/kg daily, some patients may respond to lower doses

Rheumatoid arthritis that has not responded to other disease-modifying drugs | Severe systemic lupus erythematosus and other connective tissue disorders | Polymyositis in cases of corticosteroid resistance
▸ BY MOUTH
▸ Adult: Initially up to 2.5 mg/kg daily in divided doses, adjusted according to response, rarely more than 3 mg/kg daily; maintenance 1–3 mg/kg daily, consider withdrawal if no improvement within 3 months

Autoimmune conditions
▸ BY MOUTH, OR BY INTRAVENOUS INJECTION, OR BY INTRAVENOUS INFUSION
▸ Adult: 1–3 mg/kg daily, adjusted according to response, consider withdrawal if no improvement within 3 months, oral administration preferable, if not possible then can be given by intravenous injection (intravenous solution very irritant) *or* by intravenous infusion

Suppression of transplant rejection
▸ BY MOUTH, OR BY INTRAVENOUS INJECTION, OR BY INTRAVENOUS INFUSION
▸ Adult: 1–2.5 mg/kg daily, adjusted according to response, oral administration preferable, if not possible then can be given by intravenous injection (intravenous solution very irritant) *or* by intravenous infusion

Severe refractory eczema, normal or high TPMT activity
▸ BY MOUTH
▸ Adult: 1–3 mg/kg daily

Severe refractory eczema, intermediate TPMT activity
▸ BY MOUTH
▸ Adult: 0.5–1.5 mg/kg daily

Generalised myasthenia gravis
▸ BY MOUTH, OR BY INTRAVENOUS INJECTION, OR BY INTRAVENOUS INFUSION
▸ Adult: Initially 0.5–1 mg/kg daily, then increased to 2–2.5 mg/kg daily, dose is increased over 3–4 weeks, azathioprine is usually started at the same time as the corticosteroid and allows a lower maintenance dose of the corticosteroid to be used, oral administration preferable, if not possible then can be given by intravenous injection (intravenous solution very irritant) *or* by intravenous infusion

● **UNLICENSED USE** Azathioprine doses given in BNF for suppression of transplant rejection and autoimmune conditions may differ from those in product literature. Use for severe refractory eczema is unlicensed.

● **CONTRA-INDICATIONS**
▸ When used for severe refractory eczema Absent thiopurine methyltransferase (TPMT) activity · very low thiopurine methyltransferase (TPMT) activity

● **CAUTIONS** Reduce dose in elderly · reduced thiopurine methyltransferase activity

● **INTERACTIONS** → Appendix 1 (azathioprine).

● **SIDE-EFFECTS**
▸ **Rare** Hepatic veno-occlusive disease · lymphoma · pancreatitis · pneumonitis · red cell aplasia
▸ **Frequency not known** Arthralgia · cholestatic jaundice · colitis in patients also receiving corticosteroids · diarrhoea · dizziness · dose-related bone marrow suppression · fever · hair loss · herpes zoster infection · hypersensitivity reactions · hypotension · increased susceptibility to infections in patients also receiving corticosteroids · interstitial nephritis · liver impairment · malaise · myalgia · nausea · neutropenia · rash · rigors · thrombocytopenia · vomiting

SIDE-EFFECTS, FURTHER INFORMATION
▸ Red cell aplasia Cases of pure red cell aplasia have been reported with azathioprine; dose reduction or discontinuation should be considered under specialist supervision.
▸ Neutropenia and thrombocytopenia Usually resolved by reducing the dose.
▸ Hypersensitivity reactions Hypersensitivity reactions (including malaise, dizziness, vomiting, diarrhoea, fever, rigors, myalgia, arthralgia, rash, hypotension and interstitial nephritis) call for immediate withdrawal.
▸ Nausea, vomiting and diarrhoea Nausea, vomiting and diarrhoea may occur, usually starting early during the course of treatment, and in rheumatoid arthritis it may be appropriate to withdraw the drug.

● **ALLERGY AND CROSS-SENSITIVITY** Contra-indicated in hypersensitivity to mercaptopurine.

● **PREGNANCY** Transplant patients immunosuppressed with azathioprine should not discontinue it on becoming pregnant. However, there have been reports of premature birth and low birth-weight following exposure to azathioprine, particularly in combination with corticosteroids. Spontaneous abortion has been reported following maternal or paternal exposure. Azathioprine is teratogenic in *animal* studies. The use of azathioprine during pregnancy needs to be supervised in specialist units. Treatment should not generally be initiated during pregnancy.

● **BREAST FEEDING** Present in milk in low concentration. No evidence of harm in small studies—use if potential benefit outweighs risk.

● **HEPATIC IMPAIRMENT** Reduce dose. Monitor liver function.

● **RENAL IMPAIRMENT** Reduce dose.

● **PRE-TREATMENT SCREENING**
Thiopurine methyltransferase The enzyme thiopurine methyltransferase (TPMT) metabolises thiopurine drugs (azathioprine, mercaptopurine, tioguanine); the risk of myelosuppression is increased in patients with reduced activity of the enzyme, particularly for the few individuals in whom TPMT activity is undetectable. Consider measuring TPMT activity before starting azathioprine, mercaptopurine, or tioguanine therapy. Patients with absent TPMT activity should not receive thiopurine drugs; those with reduced TPMT activity may be treated under specialist supervision.

● **MONITORING REQUIREMENTS**
▸ Monitor for toxicity throughout treatment.
▸ Monitor full blood count weekly (more frequently with higher doses or if severe hepatic or renal impairment) for first 4 weeks (manufacturer advises weekly monitoring for 8 weeks but evidence of practical value unsatisfactory), thereafter reduce frequency of monitoring to at least every 3 months.
▸ Blood tests and monitoring for signs of myelosuppression are essential in long-term treatment.

● **DIRECTIONS FOR ADMINISTRATION** For *intravenous injection*, give over at least 1 minute (followed by 50 mL sodium chloride intravenous infusion). For *intravenous*

8

Immune system and malignant disease

infusion (*Imuran®*), give intermittently in Glucose 5% *or* Sodium Chloride 0.9%. Reconstitute 50 mg with 5–15 mL Water for Injections; dilute requisite dose to a volume of 20–200 mL with infusion fluid. Intravenous injection is alkaline and very irritant, intravenous route should therefore be used **only** if oral route not feasible.

● PATIENT AND CARER ADVICE

Bone marrow suppression Patients and their carers should be warned to report immediately any signs or symptoms of bone marrow suppression e.g. inexplicable bruising or bleeding, infection.

● MEDICINAL FORMS

There can be variation in the licensing of different medicines containing the same drug. Forms available from special-order manufacturers include: capsule, oral suspension, oral solution

Tablet

CAUTIONARY AND ADVISORY LABELS 21

▸ Azathioprine (Non-proprietary)
Azathioprine 25 mg Azathioprine 25mg tablets | 28 tablet [PoM] £8.41 DT price = £2.24 | 100 tablet [PoM] £33.26
Azathioprine 50 mg Azathioprine 50mg tablets | 56 tablet [PoM] £15.85 DT price = £2.43 | 100 tablet [PoM] £29.00

▸ Azapress (Ennogen Pharma Ltd)
Azathioprine 50 mg Azapress 50mg tablets | 56 tablet [PoM] £2.83 DT price = £2.43

▸ Imuran (Aspen Pharma Trading Ltd)
Azathioprine 25 mg Imuran 25mg tablets | 100 tablet [PoM] £10.99
Azathioprine 50 mg Imuran 50mg tablets | 100 tablet [PoM] £7.99

Powder for solution for injection

▸ Imuran (Aspen Pharma Trading Ltd)
Azathioprine 50 mg Imuran 50mg powder for solution for injection vials | 1 vial [PoM] £15.38

IMMUNOSUPPRESSANTS › CALCINEURIN INHIBITORS AND RELATED DRUGS

Ciclosporin

(Cyclosporin)

● DRUG ACTION Ciclosporin is a calcineurin inhibitor.

● INDICATIONS AND DOSE

Severe acute ulcerative colitis refractory to corticosteroid treatment

▸ BY CONTINUOUS INTRAVENOUS INFUSION

▸ Adult: 2 mg/kg, to be given over 24 hours, dose adjusted according to blood-ciclosporin concentration and response

Severe active rheumatoid arthritis when conventional second-line therapy inappropriate or ineffective (administered on expert advice)

▸ BY MOUTH

▸ Adult: Initially 2.5 mg/kg daily in 2 divided doses, increased if necessary up to 4 mg/kg daily after 6 weeks, if dose increases are necessary they should be made gradually, discontinue if response insufficient after 3 months, dose adjusted according to response for maintenance and treatment reviewed after 6 months (continue only if benefits outweigh risks)

Short-term treatment of severe atopic dermatitis where conventional therapy ineffective or inappropriate (administered on expert advice)

▸ BY MOUTH

▸ Adult: Initially 1.25 mg/kg twice daily (max. per dose 2.5 mg/kg twice daily) usual maximum duration of 8 weeks but may be used for longer under specialist supervision, if good initial response not achieved within 2 weeks, increase dose rapidly up to maximum

Short-term treatment of very severe atopic dermatitis where conventional therapy ineffective or inappropriate (administered on expert advice)

▸ BY MOUTH

▸ Adult: 2.5 mg/kg twice daily usual maximum duration of 8 weeks but may be used for longer under specialist supervision

Severe psoriasis where conventional therapy ineffective or inappropriate (administered on expert advice)

▸ BY MOUTH

▸ Adult: Initially 1.25 mg/kg twice daily (max. per dose 2.5 mg/kg twice daily), increased gradually to maximum if no improvement within 1 month, initial dose of 2.5 mg/kg twice daily justified if condition requires rapid improvement; discontinue if inadequate response after 3 months at the optimum dose; max. duration of treatment usually 1 year unless other treatments cannot be used

Organ transplantation (used alone)

▸ BY MOUTH

▸ Adult: 10–15 mg/kg, to be administered 4–12 hours before transplantation, followed by 10–15 mg/kg daily for 1–2 weeks postoperatively, then maintenance 2–6 mg/kg daily, reduce dose gradually to maintenance. Dose should be adjusted according to blood-ciclosporin concentration and renal function; dose is lower if given concomitantly with other immunosuppressant therapy (e.g. corticosteroids); if necessary one-third corresponding oral dose can be given by intravenous infusion over 2–6hours

Bone-marrow transplantation | Prevention and treatment of graft-versus-host disease

▸ INITIALLY BY INTRAVENOUS INFUSION

▸ Adult: 3–5 mg/kg daily, to be administered over 2–6 hours from day before transplantation to 2 weeks postoperatively, alternatively (by mouth) 12.5–15 mg/kg daily, then (by mouth) 12.5 mg/kg daily for 3-6 months and then tailed off (may take up to a year after transplantation)

Nephrotic syndrome

▸ BY MOUTH

▸ Adult: 5 mg/kg daily in 2 divided doses, for maintenance reduce to lowest effective dose according to proteinuria and serum creatinine measurements; discontinue after 3 months if no improvement in glomerulonephritis or glomerulosclerosis (after 6 months in membranous glomerulonephritis)

● UNLICENSED USE Not licensed for use in severe acute ulcerative colitis refractory to corticosteroid treatment

IMPORTANT SAFETY INFORMATION
Patients should be stabilised on a particular brand of oral ciclosporin because switching between formulations without close monitoring may lead to clinically important changes in blood-ciclosporin concentration.

● CONTRA-INDICATIONS Abnormal renal function (in non-transplant indications) · malignancy (in non-transplant indications) · uncontrolled hypertension (in non-transplant indications) · uncontrolled infections (in non-transplant indications) · use with tacrolimus specifically contra-indicated

● CAUTIONS Hyperuricaemia · in atopic dermatitis allow herpes simplex infections to clear before starting (if they occur during treatment withdraw if severe) · in atopic dermatitis and psoriasis discontinue if lymphoproliferative disorder develops · in atopic dermatitis *Staphylococcus aureus* skin infections—not absolute contra-indication providing controlled (but avoid erythromycin unless no other alternative) · in psoriasis treat patients with malignant or pre-malignant conditions of skin only after appropriate treatment (and if no other option)

- INTERACTIONS → Appendix 1 (ciclosporin).
For patients other than transplant recipients, preferably avoid other immunosuppressants (increased risk of infection and malignancies, including lymphoma and skin cancer).

- SIDE-EFFECTS
GENERAL SIDE-EFFECTS

▶ **Common or very common** Abdominal pain · anorexia · diarrhoea · fatigue · gingival hyperplasia · headache · hepatic dysfunction · hypercholesterolaemia · hyperkalaemia · hyperlipidaemia · hypertension · hypertrichosis · hyperuricaemia · hypomagnesaemia · muscle cramps · myalgia · nausea · paraesthesia · renal dysfunction (renal structural changes on long-term administration) · tremor · vomiting

▶ **Uncommon** Anaemia · oedema · signs of encephalopathy · thrombocytopenia · weight gain

▶ **Rare** Gynaecomastia · haemolytic uraemic syndrome · hyperglycaemia · menstrual disturbances · micro-angiopathic haemolytic anaemia · motor polyneuropathy · muscle weakness · myopathy · pancreatitis · visual disturbances secondary to benign intracranial hypertension

SPECIFIC SIDE-EFFECTS
▶ With intravenous use Anaphylaxis
SIDE-EFFECTS, FURTHER INFORMATION
▶ Visual disturbances Discontinue if visual disturbances secondary to benign intracranial hypertension occur.

- PREGNANCY Crosses placenta. There is less experience of ciclosporin in pregnancy but it does not appear to be any more harmful than azathioprine. The use of ciclosporin during pregnancy needs to be supervised in specialist units.

- BREAST FEEDING Present in milk—manufacturer advises avoid.

- HEPATIC IMPAIRMENT Dosage adjustment based on bilirubin and liver enzymes may be needed.

- RENAL IMPAIRMENT In patients with nephrotic syndrome and renal impairment initially 2.5 mg/kg daily. Reduce dose by 25–50% if serum creatinine more than 30% above baseline on more than one measurement.
    In rheumatoid arthritis, reduce dose if serum creatinine increases more than 30% above baseline in more than 1 measurement; if above 50%, reduce dose by 50% (even if within normal range) and discontinue if reduction not successful within 1 month.
    In psoriasis and atopic dermatitis, reduce dose by 25–50% if serum creatinine increases more than 30% above baseline (even if within normal range) and discontinue if reduction not successful within 1 month.

- PRE-TREATMENT SCREENING In psoriasis, exclude malignancies (including those of skin and cervix) before starting (biopsy any lesions not typical of psoriasis).

- MONITORING REQUIREMENTS
▶ Dermatological and physical examination, including blood pressure and renal function measurements required at least twice before starting treatment for psoriasis or atopic dermatitis.
▶ Monitor liver function.
▶ Monitor serum potassium especially in renal dysfunction (risk of hyperkalaemia).
▶ Monitor serum magnesium.
▶ Measure blood lipids before treatment and after the first month of treatment.
▶ In psoriasis and atopic dermatitis monitor serum creatinine every 2 weeks for first 3 months then every month.
▶ Investigate lymphadenopathy that persists despite

improvement in atopic dermatitis.
▶ Monitor kidney function—dose dependent increase in serum creatinine and urea during first few weeks may necessitate dose reduction in transplant patients (exclude rejection if kidney transplant) or discontinuation in non-transplant patients.
▶ Monitor blood pressure—discontinue if hypertension develops that cannot be controlled by antihypertensives.
▶ In long-term management of nephrotic syndrome, perform renal biopsies at yearly intervals.
▶ In rheumatoid arthritis measure serum creatinine at least twice before treatment. During treatment, monitor serum creatinine every 2 weeks for first 3 months, then every month for a further 3 months, then every 4–8 weeks depending on the stability of the disease, concomitant medication, and concomitant diseases (or more frequently if dose increased or concomitant NSAIDs introduced or increased).
▶ Monitor hepatic function if concomitant NSAIDs given.

- DIRECTIONS FOR ADMINISTRATION
▶ With oral use Mix solution with orange juice (or squash) or apple juice (to improve taste) or with water immediately before taking (and rinse with more to ensure total dose). Do not mix with grapefruit juice. With capsules and oral solution, total daily dose should be taken in 2 divided doses.
▶ With intravenous use For *intravenous infusion* (*Sandimmun®*), give intermittently *or* continuously in Glucose 5% *or* Sodium Chloride 0.9%; dilute to a concentration of 50 mg in 20–100 mL; give intermittent infusion over 2–6 hours; not to be used with PVC equipment. Observe patient for signs of anaphylaxis for at least 30 minutes after starting infusion and at frequent intervals thereafter.

- PRESCRIBING AND DISPENSING INFORMATION
Brand name prescribing Prescribing and dispensing of ciclosporin should be by brand name to avoid inadvertent switching. If it is necessary to switch a patient to a different brand of ciclosporin, the patient should be monitored closely for changes in blood-ciclosporin concentration, serum creatinine, blood pressure, and transplant function.
▶ With oral use *Sandimmun®* capsules and oral solution are available direct from Novartis for patients who cannot be transferred to a different oral preparation.

- HANDLING AND STORAGE Keep medicine measure away from other liquids (including water).

- PATIENT AND CARER ADVICE
Avoid excessive exposure to UV light, including sunlight. In psoriasis and atopic dermatitis, avoid use of UVB or PUVA.
▶ With oral use Patients and carers should be counselled on the administration of ciclosporin capsules and oral solution.

- MEDICINAL FORMS
There can be variation in the licensing of different medicines containing the same drug.
Capsule
EXCIPIENTS: May contain Ethanol, ethyl lactate, propylene glycol
▶ Ciclosporin (Non-proprietary)
Ciclosporin 25 mg Ciclosporin 25mg capsules | 30 capsule [PoM] no price available DT price = £18.37
Ciclosporin 50 mg Ciclosporin 50mg capsules | 30 capsule [PoM] no price available DT price = £35.97
Ciclosporin 100 mg Ciclosporin 100mg capsules | 30 capsule [PoM] no price available DT price = £68.28
▶ Capimune (Mylan Ltd)
Ciclosporin 25 mg Capimune 25mg capsules | 30 capsule [PoM] £13.05 DT price = £18.37
Ciclosporin 50 mg Capimune 50mg capsules | 30 capsule [PoM] £25.50 DT price = £35.97
Ciclosporin 100 mg Capimune 100mg capsules | 30 capsule [PoM] £48.50 DT price = £68.28

Immune system and malignant disease

▸ Capsorin (Morningside Healthcare Ltd)
Ciclosporin 25 mg Capsorin 25mg capsules | 30 capsule [PoM]
£13.05 DT price = £18.37
Ciclosporin 50 mg Capsorin 50mg capsules | 30 capsule [PoM]
£25.59 DT price = £35.97
Ciclosporin 100 mg Capsorin 100mg capsules | 30 capsule [PoM]
£48.89 DT price = £68.28

▸ Deximune (Dexcel-Pharma Ltd)
Ciclosporin 25 mg Deximune 25mg capsules | 30 capsule [PoM]
£13.06 DT price = £18.37
Ciclosporin 50 mg Deximune 50mg capsules | 30 capsule [PoM]
£25.60 DT price = £35.97
Ciclosporin 100 mg Deximune 100mg capsules | 30 capsule [PoM]
£48.90 DT price = £68.28

▸ Neoral (Novartis Pharmaceuticals UK Ltd)
Ciclosporin 10 mg Neoral 10mg capsules | 60 capsule [PoM] £18.25
DT price = £18.25
Ciclosporin 25 mg Neoral 25mg capsules | 30 capsule [PoM] £18.37
DT price = £18.37
Ciclosporin 50 mg Neoral 50mg capsules | 30 capsule [PoM] £35.97
DT price = £35.97
Ciclosporin 100 mg Neoral 100mg capsules | 30 capsule [PoM]
£68.28 DT price = £68.28

▸ Vanquoral (Teva UK Ltd)
Ciclosporin 10 mg Vanquoral 10mg capsules | 30 capsule [PoM]
£12.75 | 60 capsule [PoM] £12.75 DT price = £18.25
Ciclosporin 25 mg Vanquoral 25mg capsules | 30 capsule [PoM]
£13.05 DT price = £18.37
Ciclosporin 50 mg Vanquoral 50mg capsules | 30 capsule [PoM]
£25.59 DT price = £35.97
Ciclosporin 100 mg Vanquoral 100mg capsules | 30 capsule [PoM]
£48.89 DT price = £68.28

Oral solution
EXCIPIENTS: May contain Alcohol, propylene glycol
▸ Neoral (Novartis Pharmaceuticals UK Ltd)
Ciclosporin 100 mg per 1 ml Neoral 100mg/ml oral solution sugar-
free | 50 ml [PoM] £102.30

Solution for infusion
EXCIPIENTS: May contain Alcohol, polyoxyl castor oils
▸ Sandimmun (Novartis Pharmaceuticals UK Ltd)
Ciclosporin 50 mg per 1 ml Sandimmun 250mg/5ml concentrate for
solution for infusion ampoules | 10 ampoule [PoM] £110.05
Sandimmun 50mg/1ml concentrate for solution for infusion ampoules
| 10 ampoule [PoM] £23.23

Sirolimus

● DRUG ACTION Sirolimus is a non-calcineurin inhibiting
immunosuppressant.

● INDICATIONS AND DOSE

**Prophylaxis of organ rejection in kidney allograft
recipients**
▸ BY MOUTH
▸ Adult: Initially 6 mg for 1 dose, to be given after
surgery once wound has healed, then 2 mg once daily;
to be given in combination with ciclosporin and
corticosteroid for 2–3 months (sirolimus doses should
be given 4 hours after ciclosporin), ciclosporin should
then be withdrawn over 4–8 weeks (if not possible,
sirolimus should be discontinued and an alternate
immunosuppressive regimen used), dose to be adjusted
according to whole blood-sirolimus trough
concentration

DOSE EQUIVALENCE AND CONVERSION
The 500 microgram tablet is not bioequivalent to the
1 mg and 2 mg tablets. Multiples of 500 microgram tablets
should **not** be used as a substitute for other tablet
strengths.

● CAUTIONS Hyperlipidaemia · increased susceptibility to
infection (especially urinary-tract infection) · increased
susceptibility to lymphoma and other malignancies,
particularly of the skin (limit exposure to UV light)
● INTERACTIONS → Appendix 1 (sirolimus).

● SIDE-EFFECTS
▸ **Common or very common** Abdominal pain · acne · anaemia ·
arthralgia · ascites · constipation · diarrhoea · epistaxis ·
haemolytic uraemic syndrome · headache ·
hypercholesterolaemia · hyperglycaemia · hypertension ·
hypertriglyceridaemia · hypokalaemia ·
hypophosphataemia · impaired healing · leucopenia ·
lymphocele · nausea · neutropenia · oedema · osteonecrosis
· pleural effusion · pneumonitis · proteinuria · pyrexia · rash
· stomatitis · tachycardia · thrombocytopenia · thrombotic
thrombocytopenic purpura · venous thromboembolism
▸ **Uncommon** Nephrotic syndrome · pancreatitis ·
pancytopenia · pericardial effusion · pulmonary embolism ·
pulmonary haemorrhage
▸ **Rare** Alveolar proteinosis · anaphylactic reactions ·
angioedema · exfoliative dermatitis · hepatic necrosis ·
hypersensitivity reactions · hypersensitivity vasculitis ·
interstitial lung disease · lymphoedema
▸ **Frequency not known** Focal segmental glomerulosclerosis ·
reversible impairment of male fertility

● CONCEPTION AND CONTRACEPTION Effective
contraception must be used during treatment and for
12 weeks after stopping.
● PREGNANCY Avoid unless essential—toxicity in *animal*
studies.
● BREAST FEEDING Discontinue breast-feeding.
● HEPATIC IMPAIRMENT In severe impairment decrease dose
by 50% and monitor whole blood-sirolimus trough
concentration every 5–7 days until 3 consecutive
measurements have shown stable blood-sirolimus
concentration. Clearance reduced in mild to moderate
impairment. Monitor whole blood-sirolimus level closely
and consult local treatment protocol in hepatic
impairment.
● MONITORING REQUIREMENTS
▸ Monitor whole blood-sirolimus trough concentration
(Afro-Caribbean patients may require higher doses).
▸ Manufacturer advises pre-dose ('trough') whole blood-
sirolimus concentration (using **chromatographic** assay)
when used with ciclosporin should be
4–12 micrograms/litre (local treatment protocols may
differ); after withdrawal of ciclosporin pre-dose whole
blood-sirolimus concentration should be
12–20 micrograms/litre (local treatment protocols may
differ).
▸ Close monitoring of whole blood-sirolimus concentration
required if concomitant treatment with potent inducers or
inhibitors of metabolism and after discontinuing them, or
if ciclosporin dose reduced significantly or stopped.
▸ When changing between oral solution and tablets,
measurement of whole blood 'trough' sirolimus
concentration after 1–2 weeks is recommended.
▸ Therapeutic drug monitoring assays Sirolimus whole-blood
concentration is measured using either high performance
liquid chromatography (HPLC) or immunoassay. Switching
between different immunoassays or between an
immunoassay and HPLC can lead to clinically significant
differences in results and therefore incorrect dose
adjustments. Adjustment to the target therapeutic dose
range should be made with knowledge of the assay used
and corresponding reference range.
▸ Monitor kidney function when given with ciclosporin;
monitor lipids; monitor urine proteins.
● DIRECTIONS FOR ADMINISTRATION Food may affect
absorption (take at the same time with respect to food).
Sirolimus oral solution should be mixed with at least 60 mL
water or orange juice in a glass or plastic container
immediately before taking; refill container with at least
120 mL of water or orange juice and drink immediately (to
ensure total dose). Do not mix with any other liquids.

- PATIENT AND CARER ADVICE Patient or carers should be given advice on how to administer sirolimus.
  Patients should be advised to avoid excessive exposure to UV light.

- MEDICINAL FORMS
  There can be variation in the licensing of different medicines containing the same drug.
  Tablet
  ▸ Rapamune (Pfizer Ltd)
  Sirolimus 500 microgram Rapamune 0.5mg tablets | 30 tablet [PoM] £69.00 DT price = £69.00
  Sirolimus 1 mg Rapamune 1mg tablets | 30 tablet [PoM] £86.49 DT price = £86.49
  Sirolimus 2 mg Rapamune 2mg tablets | 30 tablet [PoM] £172.98 DT price = £172.98
  Oral solution
  EXCIPIENTS: May contain Ethanol
  ▸ Rapamune (Pfizer Ltd)
  Sirolimus 1 mg per 1 ml Rapamune 1mg/ml oral solution sugar-free | 60 ml [PoM] £162.41

Tacrolimus

- DRUG ACTION Tacrolimus is a calcineurin inhibitor.

- INDICATIONS AND DOSE
  ADOPORT®
  Prophylaxis of graft rejection following liver transplantation, starting 12 hours after transplantation
  ▸ BY MOUTH
  ▸ Adult: Initially 100–200 micrograms/kg daily in 2 divided doses
  Prophylaxis of graft rejection following kidney transplantation, starting within 24 hours of transplantation
  ▸ BY MOUTH
  ▸ Adult: Initially 200–300 micrograms/kg daily in 2 divided doses
  Prophylaxis of graft rejection following heart transplantation following antibody induction, starting within 5 days of transplantation
  ▸ BY MOUTH
  ▸ Adult: Initially 75 micrograms/kg daily in 2 divided doses
  Prophylaxis of graft rejection following heart transplantation without antibody induction, starting within 12 hours of transplantation
  ▸ BY MOUTH
  ▸ Adult: Initially 75 micrograms/kg daily in 2 divided doses
  Allograft rejection resistant to conventional immunosuppressive therapy
  ▸ BY MOUTH
  ▸ Adult: Seek specialist advice
  ADVAGRAF®
  Prophylaxis of graft rejection following liver transplantation, starting 12–18 hours after transplantation
  ▸ BY MOUTH
  ▸ Adult: Initially 100–200 micrograms/kg once daily, to be taken in the morning
  Prophylaxis of graft rejection following kidney transplantation, starting within 24 hours of transplantation
  ▸ BY MOUTH
  ▸ Adult: Initially 200–300 micrograms/kg once daily, to be taken in the morning

Allograft rejection resistant to conventional immunosuppressive therapy
▸ BY MOUTH
▸ Adult: Seek specialist advice
CAPEXION®
Prophylaxis of graft rejection following liver transplantation, starting 12 hours after transplantation
▸ BY MOUTH
▸ Adult: Initially 100–200 micrograms/kg daily in 2 divided doses
Prophylaxis of graft rejection following kidney transplantation, starting within 24 hours of transplantation
▸ BY MOUTH
▸ Adult: Initially 200–300 micrograms/kg daily in 2 divided doses
Prophylaxis of graft rejection following heart transplantation following antibody induction, starting within 5 days of transplantation
▸ BY MOUTH
▸ Adult: Initially 75 micrograms/kg daily in 2 divided doses
Prophylaxis of graft rejection following heart transplantation without antibody induction, starting within 12 hours of transplantation
▸ BY MOUTH
▸ Adult: Initially 75 micrograms/kg daily in 2 divided doses
Allograft rejection resistant to conventional immunosuppressive therapy
▸ BY MOUTH
▸ Adult: Seek specialist advice
ENVARSUS® MODIFIED-RELEASE TABLETS
Prophylaxis of graft rejection following liver transplantation, starting within 24 hours of transplantation
▸ BY MOUTH
▸ Adult: Initially 110–130 micrograms/kg once daily, to be taken in the morning
Prophylaxis of graft rejection following renal transplantation, starting within 24 hours of transplantation
▸ BY MOUTH
▸ Adult: Initially 170 micrograms/kg once daily, to be taken in the morning
Rejection therapy
▸ BY MOUTH
▸ Adult: Seek specialist advice
MODIGRAF®
Prophylaxis of graft rejection following liver transplantation, starting 12 hours after transplantation
▸ BY MOUTH
▸ Adult: Initially 100–200 micrograms/kg daily in 2 divided doses
Prophylaxis of graft rejection following kidney transplantation, starting within 24 hours of transplantation
▸ BY MOUTH
▸ Adult: Initially 200–300 micrograms/kg daily in 2 divided doses
Prophylaxis of graft rejection following heart transplantation following antibody induction, starting within 5 days of transplantation
▸ BY MOUTH
▸ Adult: Initially 75 micrograms/kg daily in 2 divided doses

continued →

8 Immune system and malignant disease

Prophylaxis of graft rejection following heart transplantation without antibody induction, starting within 12 hours of transplantation
▸ BY MOUTH
▸ Adult: Initially 75 micrograms/kg daily in 2 divided doses

Rejection therapy
▸ BY MOUTH
▸ Adult: Seek specialist advice

PROGRAF® CAPSULES

Prophylaxis of graft rejection following liver transplantation, starting 12 hours after transplantation
▸ BY MOUTH
▸ Adult: Initially 100–200 micrograms/kg daily in 2 divided doses

Prophylaxis of graft rejection following kidney transplantation, starting within 24 hours of transplantation
▸ BY MOUTH
▸ Adult: Initially 200–300 micrograms/kg daily in 2 divided doses

Prophylaxis of graft rejection following heart transplantation following antibody induction, starting within 5 days of transplantation
▸ BY MOUTH
▸ Adult: Initially 75 micrograms/kg daily in 2 divided doses

Prophylaxis of graft rejection following heart transplantation without antibody induction, starting within 12 hours of transplantation
▸ BY MOUTH
▸ Adult: Initially 75 micrograms/kg daily in 2 divided doses

Allograft rejection resistant to conventional immunosuppressive therapy
▸ BY MOUTH
▸ Adult: Seek specialist advice

PROGRAF® INFUSION

Prophylaxis of graft rejection following liver transplantation, starting 12 hours after transplantation when oral route not appropriate
▸ BY INTRAVENOUS INFUSION
▸ Adult: Initially 10–50 micrograms/kg daily for up to 7 days (then transfer to oral therapy), dose to be administered over 24 hours

Prophylaxis of graft rejection following kidney transplantation, starting within 24 hours of transplantation when oral route not appropriate
▸ BY INTRAVENOUS INFUSION
▸ Adult: Initially 50–100 micrograms/kg daily for up to 7 days (then transfer to oral therapy), dose to be administered over 24 hours

Prophylaxis of graft rejection following heart transplantation following antibody induction, starting within 5 days of transplantation
▸ BY INTRAVENOUS INFUSION
▸ Adult: Initially 10–20 micrograms/kg daily for up to 7 days (then transfer to oral therapy), dose to be administered over 24 hours

Prophylaxis of graft rejection following heart transplantation without antibody induction, starting within 12 hours of transplantation
▸ BY INTRAVENOUS INFUSION
▸ Adult: Initially 10–20 micrograms/kg daily for up to 7 days (then transfer to oral therapy), dose to be administered over 24 hours

Allograft rejection resistant to conventional immunosuppressive therapy
▸ BY CONTINUOUS INTRAVENOUS INFUSION
▸ Adult: Seek specialist advice (consult local protocol)

TACNI®

Prophylaxis of graft rejection following liver transplantation, starting 12 hours after transplantation
▸ BY MOUTH
▸ Adult: Initially 100–200 micrograms/kg daily in 2 divided doses

Prophylaxis of graft rejection following kidney transplantation, starting within 24 hours of transplantation
▸ BY MOUTH
▸ Adult: Initially 200–300 micrograms/kg daily in 2 divided doses

Prophylaxis of graft rejection following heart transplantation following antibody induction, starting within 5 days of transplantation
▸ BY MOUTH
▸ Adult: Initially 75 micrograms/kg daily in 2 divided doses

Prophylaxis of graft rejection following heart transplantation without antibody induction, starting within 12 hours of transplantation
▸ BY MOUTH
▸ Adult: Initially 75 micrograms/kg daily in 2 divided doses

Allograft rejection resistant to conventional immunosuppressive therapy
▸ BY MOUTH
▸ Adult: Seek specialist advice

VIVADEX®

Prophylaxis of graft rejection following liver transplantation, starting 12 hours after transplantation
▸ BY MOUTH
▸ Adult: Initially 100–200 micrograms/kg daily in 2 divided doses

Prophylaxis of graft rejection following kidney transplantation, starting within 24 hours of transplantation
▸ BY MOUTH
▸ Adult: Initially 200–300 micrograms/kg daily in 2 divided doses

Prophylaxis of graft rejection following heart transplantation following antibody induction, starting within 5 days of transplantation
▸ BY MOUTH
▸ Adult: Initially 75 micrograms/kg daily in 2 divided doses

Prophylaxis of graft rejection following heart transplantation without antibody induction, starting within 12 hours of transplantation
▸ BY MOUTH
▸ Adult: Initially 75 micrograms/kg daily in 2 divided doses

Allograft rejection resistant to conventional immunosuppressive therapy
▸ BY MOUTH
▸ Adult: Seek specialist advice

> **IMPORTANT SAFETY INFORMATION**
> MHRA/CHM ADVICE: ORAL TACROLIMUS PRODUCTS: PRESCRIBE AND DISPENSE BY BRAND NAME ONLY, TO MINIMISE THE RISK OF INADVERTENT SWITCHING BETWEEN PRODUCTS, WHICH HAS BEEN ASSOCIATED WITH REPORTS OF TOXICITY AND GRAFT REJECTION (JUNE 2012)
> Inadvertent switching between oral tacrolimus products has been associated with reports of toxicity and graft

rejection. To ensure maintenance of therapeutic response when a patient is stabilised on a particular brand, oral tacrolimus products should be prescribed and dispensed by brand name only.

- *Adoport®*, *Prograf®*, *Capexion®*, *Tacni®*, and *Vivadex®* are immediate-release capsules that are taken twice daily, once in the morning and once in the evening;
- *Modigraf®* granules are used to prepare an immediate-release oral suspension which is taken twice daily, once in the morning and once in the evening;
- *Advagraf®* is a prolonged-release capsule that is taken once daily in the morning.

Switching between tacrolimus brands requires careful supervision and therapeutic monitoring by an appropriate specialist.

Important: *Envarsus®* is not interchangeable with other oral tacrolimus containing products; the MHRA has advised (June 2012) that oral tacrolimus products should be prescribed and dispensed by brand only.

- CAUTIONS Increased risk of infections · lymphoproliferative disorders · malignancies · neurotoxicity · QT-interval prolongation · UV light (avoid excessive exposure to sunlight and sunlamps)
- INTERACTIONS → Appendix 1 (tacrolimus). Contra-indication—avoid concurrent administration with ciclosporin (care if patient has previously received ciclosporin).
- SIDE-EFFECTS
- **Common or very common** Acne · alopecia · anaemia · anorexia · anxiety · arthralgia · ascites · bile-duct abnormalities · bloating · blood disorders · cholestasis · confusion · constipation · depression · diarrhoea · dizziness · dyspepsia · dyspnoea · electrolyte disturbances · flatulence · gastro-intestinal inflammation · gastro-intestinal perforation · gastro-intestinal ulceration · haemorrhage · headache · hepatic dysfunction · hyperglycaemia · hyperkalaemia · hypertension · hyperuricaemia · hypokalaemia · impaired hearing · ischaemic events · jaundice · leucopenia · mood changes · muscle cramp · nausea · oedema · pancytopenia · paraesthesia · parenchymal lung disorders · peripheral neuropathy · photophobia · pleural effusion · psychosis · renal failure · renal impairment · renal tubular necrosis · seizures · sleep disturbances · sweating · tachycardia · thrombocytopenia · thromboembolic events · tinnitus · tremor · urinary abnormalities · visual disturbances · vomiting · weight changes
- **Uncommon** Amnesia · arrhythmia · cardiac arrest · cardiomyopathy · cataract · cerebrovascular accident · coagulation disorders · coma · dermatitis · dysmenorrhoea · encephalopathy · gastro-intestinal reflux disease · heart failure · hypertonia · hypoglycaemia · influenza-like symptoms · palpitation · pancreatitis · paralysis · paralytic ileus · peritonitis · photosensitivity · respiratory failure · speech disorder
- **Rare** Blindness · dehydration · hirsutism · pericardial effusion · posterior reversible encephalopathy syndrome · respiratory distress syndrome · thrombotic thrombocytopenic purpura · toxic epidermal necrolysis
- **Very rare** Haemorrhagic cystitis · myasthenia · Stevens-Johnson syndrome
- **Frequency not known** Agranulocytosis · haemolytic anaemia · pure red cell aplasia

SIDE-EFFECTS, FURTHER INFORMATION
- Cardiomyopathy Cardiomyopathy has been reported. Patients should be monitored by echocardiography for hypertrophic changes—consider dose reduction or discontinuation if these occur.
- ALLERGY AND CROSS-SENSITIVITY Contra-indicated if history of hypersensitivity to macrolides.

- CONCEPTION AND CONTRACEPTION Exclude pregnancy before treatment.
- PREGNANCY Avoid unless potential benefit outweighs risk—crosses the placenta and risk of premature delivery, intra-uterine growth restriction, and hyperkalaemia.
- BREAST FEEDING Avoid—present in breast milk (following systemic administration).
- HEPATIC IMPAIRMENT Dose reduction may be necessary in severe impairment.
- MONITORING REQUIREMENTS
- ▸ After initial dosing, and for maintenance treatment, tacrolimus doses should be adjusted according to whole-blood concentration. Monitor whole blood-tacrolimus trough concentration (especially during episodes of diarrhoea)—consult local treatment protocol for details.
- ▸ Monitor blood pressure, ECG (for hypertrophic changes—risk of cardiomyopathy), fasting blood-glucose concentration, haematological and neurological (including visual) and coagulation parameters, electrolytes, hepatic and renal function.
- DIRECTIONS FOR ADMINISTRATION For *intravenous infusion* (*Prograf®*); give continuously in Glucose 5% *or* Sodium Chloride 0.9%. Dilute concentrate in infusion fluid to a final concentration of 4–100 micrograms/mL; give over 24 hours. Tacrolimus is incompatible with PVC.
- PATIENT AND CARER ADVICE
Avoid excessive exposure to UV light including sunlight.
Driving and skilled tasks
May affect performance of skilled tasks (e.g. driving).
- NATIONAL FUNDING/ACCESS DECISIONS

Scottish Medicines Consortium (SMC) Decisions
The *Scottish Medicines Consortium* has advised (November 2010) that tacrolimus granules for oral suspension (*Modigraf®*) are accepted for restricted use within NHS Scotland in patients for whom tacrolimus is an appropriate choice of immunosuppressive therapy and where small changes (less than 500 micrograms) in dosing increments are required (such as, in paediatric patients) or in seriously ill patients who are unable to swallow tacrolimus capsules.

- MEDICINAL FORMS
There can be variation in the licensing of different medicines containing the same drug. Forms available from special-order manufacturers include: oral suspension, oral solution

Modified-release tablet
- ▸ Envarsus (Chiesi Ltd)
   Tacrolimus (as Tacrolimus monohydrate)
   750 microgram Envarsus 750microgram modified-release tablets | 30 tablet [PoM] £44.33
   Tacrolimus (as Tacrolimus monohydrate) 1 mg Envarsus 1mg modified-release tablets | 30 tablet [PoM] £59.10
   Tacrolimus (as Tacrolimus monohydrate) 4 mg Envarsus 4mg modified-release tablets | 30 tablet [PoM] £236.40

Capsule
CAUTIONARY AND ADVISORY LABELS 23
- ▸ Adoport (Sandoz Ltd)
   Tacrolimus 500 microgram Adoport 0.5mg capsules | 50 capsule [PoM] £42.92 DT price = £61.88
   Tacrolimus 750 microgram Adoport 0.75mg capsules | 50 capsule [PoM] £51.75
   Tacrolimus 1 mg Adoport 1mg capsules | 50 capsule [PoM] £55.69 DT price = £80.28 | 100 capsule [PoM] £111.36
   Tacrolimus 2 mg Adoport 2mg capsules | 50 capsule [PoM] £111.00
   Tacrolimus 5 mg Adoport 5mg capsules | 50 capsule [PoM] £205.74 DT price = £296.58
- ▸ Capexion (Mylan Ltd)
   Tacrolimus 500 microgram Capexion 0.5mg capsules | 50 capsule [PoM] £52.50 DT price = £61.88
   Tacrolimus 1 mg Capexion 1mg capsules | 50 capsule [PoM] £68.20 DT price = £80.28 | 100 capsule [PoM] £136.20
   Tacrolimus 5 mg Capexion 5mg capsules | 50 capsule [PoM] £252.00 DT price = £296.58

8

Immune system and malignant disease

8

Immune system and malignant disease

▸ Prograf (Astellas Pharma Ltd)
Tacrolimus 500 microgram Prograf 500microgram capsules | 50 capsule [PoM] £61.88 DT price = £61.88
Tacrolimus 1 mg Prograf 1mg capsules | 50 capsule [PoM] £80.28 DT price = £80.28 | 100 capsule [PoM] £160.54
Tacrolimus 5 mg Prograf 5mg capsules | 50 capsule [PoM] £296.58 DT price = £296.58

Modified-release capsule
CAUTIONARY AND ADVISORY LABELS 23, 25
▸ Advagraf (Astellas Pharma Ltd)
Tacrolimus (as Tacrolimus monohydrate)
500 microgram Advagraf 0.5mg modified-release capsules | 50 capsule [PoM] £35.79
Tacrolimus (as Tacrolimus monohydrate) 1 mg Advagraf 1mg modified-release capsules | 50 capsule [PoM] £71.59 | 100 capsule [PoM] £143.17
Tacrolimus (as Tacrolimus monohydrate) 3 mg Advagraf 3mg modified-release capsules | 50 capsule [PoM] £214.76
Tacrolimus (as Tacrolimus monohydrate) 5 mg Advagraf 5mg modified-release capsules | 50 capsule [PoM] £266.92

Granules
CAUTIONARY AND ADVISORY LABELS 13, 23
▸ Modigraf (Astellas Pharma Ltd)
Tacrolimus (as Tacrolimus monohydrate)
200 microgram Modigraf 0.2mg granules sachets sugar-free | 50 sachet [PoM] £71.30 DT price = £71.30
Tacrolimus (as Tacrolimus monohydrate) 1 mg Modigraf 1mg granules sachets sugar-free | 50 sachet [PoM] £356.65 DT price = £356.65

Solution for infusion
EXCIPIENTS: May contain Polyoxyl castor oils
▸ Prograf (Astellas Pharma Ltd)
Tacrolimus 5 mg per 1 ml Prograf 5mg/1ml solution for infusion ampoules | 10 ampoule [PoM] £584.51

IMMUNOSUPPRESSANTS > MONOCLONAL ANTIBODIES

Canakinumab

● DRUG ACTION Canakinumab is a recombinant human monoclonal antibody that selectively inhibits interleukin-1 beta receptor binding.

● INDICATIONS AND DOSE
Acute gout in patients whose condition has not responded adequately to treatment with NSAIDs or colchicine, or who are intolerant of them
▸ BY SUBCUTANEOUS INJECTION
▸ Adult: 150 mg for 1 dose, dose may be repeated at least 12 weeks after initial response if symptoms recur, patients who do not respond to initial dose should not be retreated

Treatment of cryopyrin-associated periodic syndromes, including severe forms of familial cold auto-inflammatory syndrome (or familial cold urticaria), Muckle-Wells syndrome, and neonatal-onset multisystem inflammatory disease (also known as chronic infantile neurological cutaneous and articular syndrome)
▸ BY SUBCUTANEOUS INJECTION
▸ Adult: (consult product literature)

● CONTRA-INDICATIONS Active infection · leucopenia · neutropenia
● CAUTIONS History of recurrent infection · latent and active tuberculosis · predisposition to infection
CAUTIONS, FURTHER INFORMATION
▸ Vaccinations Patients should receive all recommended vaccinations (including pneumococcal and inactivated influenza vaccine) before starting treatment; avoid live vaccines unless potential benefit outweighs risk—consult product literature for further information.
● INTERACTIONS → Appendix 1 (canakinumab).

Contra-indicated with concomitant use with tumour necrosis factor inhibitors (possible increased risk of infections).
● SIDE-EFFECTS
▸ **Common or very common** Back pain · increased susceptibility to infection (including serious infection) · injection-site reactions · malaise · neutropenia · vertigo
▸ **Uncommon** Gastro-oesophageal reflux
▸ **Frequency not known** Malignancy · vomiting
● CONCEPTION AND CONTRACEPTION Effective contraception required during treatment and for up to 3 months after last dose.
● PREGNANCY Manufacturer advises avoid unless potential benefit outweighs risk.
● BREAST FEEDING Consider if benefit outweighs risk—not known if present in human milk.
● HEPATIC IMPAIRMENT No information available.
● RENAL IMPAIRMENT Limited information available but manufacturer advises no dose adjustment required.
● PRE-TREATMENT SCREENING Patients should be evaluated for latent and active tuberculosis before starting treatment.
● MONITORING REQUIREMENTS
▸ Monitor full blood count including neutrophil count before starting treatment, 1–2 months after starting treatment, and periodically thereafter.
▸ Monitor for signs and symptoms of tuberculosis during and after treatment.
● MEDICINAL FORMS
There can be variation in the licensing of different medicines containing the same drug.
Powder for solution for injection
▸ Ilaris (Novartis Pharmaceuticals UK Ltd) ▼
Canakinumab 150 mg Ilaris 150mg powder for solution for injection vials | 1 vial [PoM] £9,927.80

IMMUNOSUPPRESSANTS > MONOCLONAL ANTIBODIES > ANTI-LYMPHOCYTE

Basiliximab

● DRUG ACTION Basiliximab is a monoclonal antibody that acts as an interleukin-2 receptor antagonist and prevents T-lymphocyte proliferation.

● INDICATIONS AND DOSE
Prophylaxis of acute rejection in allogeneic renal transplantation used in combination with ciclosporin and corticosteroid-containing immunosuppression regimens (specialist use only)
▸ BY INTRAVENOUS INJECTION, OR BY INTRAVENOUS INFUSION
▸ Adult: Initially 20 mg, administered within 2 hours before transplant surgery, followed by 20 mg after 4 days, dose to be administered after surgery, withhold second dose if severe hypersensitivity or graft loss occurs

● CAUTIONS Off-label use in cardiac transplantation—increased risk of serious cardiac side-effects
● INTERACTIONS → Appendix 1 (basiliximab).
● SIDE-EFFECTS Atrial flutter · cardiac arrest · cytokine release syndrome · palpitations · severe hypersensitivity reactions
● CONCEPTION AND CONTRACEPTION Adequate contraception must be used during treatment and for 16 weeks after last dose.
● PREGNANCY Manufacturer advises avoid—no information available.
● BREAST FEEDING Manufacturer advises avoid—no information available.

- DIRECTIONS FOR ADMINISTRATION For *intravenous infusion* (*Simulect*®) give intermittently in Glucose 5% or Sodium chloride 0.9%; reconstitute 10 mg with 2.5 mL water for injections then dilute to at least 25 mL with infusion fluid; reconstitute 20 mg with 5 mL water for injections then dilute to at least 50 mL with infusion fluid; give over 20-30 minutes.

- MEDICINAL FORMS
  There can be variation in the licensing of different medicines containing the same drug.
  Powder and solvent for solution for injection
  ‣ Simulect (Novartis Pharmaceuticals UK Ltd)
    Basiliximab 10 mg Simulect 10mg powder and solvent for solution for injection vials | 1 vial [PoM] £758.69 (Hospital only)
    Basiliximab 20 mg Simulect 20mg powder and solvent for solution for injection vials | 1 vial [PoM] £842.38 (Hospital only)

Belimumab

- INDICATIONS AND DOSE
  Adjunctive therapy in patients with active, autoantibody-positive systemic lupus erythematosus with a high degree of disease activity despite standard therapy
  ‣ BY INTRAVENOUS INFUSION
  ‣ Adult: 10 mg/kg every 2 weeks for 3 doses, then 10 mg/kg every 4 weeks, review treatment if no response within 6 months

- CAUTIONS Do not initiate until active infections controlled · history or development of malignancy · predisposition to infection
- INTERACTIONS → Appendix 1 (belimumab).
- SIDE-EFFECTS
- **Common or very common** Infusion-related reactions
- **Frequency not known** Depression · diarrhoea · hypersensitivity reactions · infections · insomnia · leucopenia · migraine · nausea · pain in extremities · pyrexia · vomiting
  SIDE-EFFECTS, FURTHER INFORMATION
  Infusion-related side-effects are reported commonly, including severe or life-threatening hypersensitivity and infusion reactions. Premedication with an antihistamine, with or without an antipyretic may be considered.
- CONCEPTION AND CONTRACEPTION Manufacturer advises adequate contraception during treatment and for at least 4 months after last dose.
- PREGNANCY Avoid unless essential.
- BREAST FEEDING Avoid—present in milk in *animal* studies.
- RENAL IMPAIRMENT Caution in severe impairment—no information available.
- MONITORING REQUIREMENTS Delay in the onset of acute hypersensitivity reactions has been observed; patients should remain under clinical supervision for several hours following at least the first 2 infusions.
- DIRECTIONS FOR ADMINISTRATION For *intravenous infusion* (*Benlysta*®), give intermittently in Sodium chloride 0.9%; reconstitute with water for injections (120 mg in 1.5 mL, 400 mg in 4.8 mL) to produce a solution containing 80 mg/mL; gently swirl vial for 60 seconds, then allow to stand; swirl vial (without shaking) for 60 seconds every 5 minutes until dissolved; dilute requisite dose with infusion fluid to a final volume of 250 mL and give over 1 hour.

- MEDICINAL FORMS
  There can be variation in the licensing of different medicines containing the same drug.
  Powder for solution for infusion
  ‣ Benlysta (GlaxoSmithKline UK Ltd) ▼
    Belimumab 120 mg Benlysta 120mg powder for concentrate for solution for infusion vials | 1 vial [PoM] £121.50 (Hospital only)
    Belimumab 400 mg Benlysta 400mg powder for concentrate for solution for infusion vials | 1 vial [PoM] £405.00 (Hospital only)

IMMUNOSUPPRESSANTS > PURINE SYNTHESIS INHIBITORS

Mycophenolate mofetil

- INDICATIONS AND DOSE
  Prophylaxis of acute rejection in renal transplantation (in combination with a corticosteroid and ciclosporin) (under expert supervision)
  ‣ BY MOUTH
  ‣ Adult: 1 g twice daily, to be started within 72 hours of transplantation
  ‣ BY INTRAVENOUS INFUSION
  ‣ Adult: 1 g twice daily for maximum 14 days, then transfer to oral therapy, to be started within 24 hours of transplantation
  Prophylaxis of acute rejection in cardiac transplantation (in combination with ciclosporin and corticosteroids) (under expert supervision)
  ‣ BY MOUTH
  ‣ Adult: 1.5 g twice daily, to be started within 5 days of transplantation
  Prophylaxis of acute rejection in hepatic transplantation (in combination with ciclosporin and corticosteroids) (under expert supervision)
  ‣ INITIALLY BY INTRAVENOUS INFUSION
  ‣ Adult: 1 g twice daily for 4 days, up to a maximum of 14 days, to be started within 24 hours of transplantation, then (by mouth) 1.5 g twice daily, the dose route should be changed as soon as is tolerated

  MYFORTIC®
  Renal transplantation
  ‣ BY MOUTH
  ‣ Adult: 720 mg twice daily, to be started within 72 hours of transplantation
  DOSE EQUIVALENCE AND CONVERSION
  For *Myfortic*®: Mycophenolic acid 720 mg is approximately equivalent to mycophenolate mofetil 1 g but avoid unnecessary switching because of pharmacokinetic differences.

- CAUTIONS Active serious gastro-intestinal disease (risk of haemorrhage, ulceration and perforation) · delayed graft function · elderly (increased risk of infection, gastro-intestinal haemorrhage and pulmonary oedema) · increased susceptibility to skin cancer (avoid exposure to strong sunlight) · risk of hypogammaglobulinaemia or bronchiectasis when used in combination with other immunosuppressants
  CAUTIONS, FURTHER INFORMATION
  ‣ Hypogammaglobulinaemia or bronchiectasis Measure serum immunoglobulin levels if recurrent infections develop, and consider bronchiectasis or pulmonary fibrosis if persistent respiratory symptoms such as cough and dyspnoea develop.
- INTERACTIONS → Appendix 1 (mycophenolate).
- **Live vaccines** Specialist advice should be sought for those being treated with immunosuppressive drugs.
- SIDE-EFFECTS
- **Common or very common** Abdominal pain · acne · agitation · alopecia · anaemia · anorexia · anxiety · arthralgia · blood

disorders · confusion · constipation · convulsions · cough · depression · disturbances of blood lipids · disturbances of electrolytes and blood lipids · dizziness · dyspnoea · flatulence · gastro-intestinal bleeding · gastro-intestinal inflammation · gastro-intestinal ulceration · gingival hyperplasia · headache · hepatitis · hyperglycaemia · hypertension · hypotension · infections · influenza-like syndrome · insomnia · jaundice · leucopenia · malignancy (particularly of the skin) · myasthenic syndrome · nausea · oedema · pancreatitis · pancytopenia · paraesthesia · rash · red cell aplasia · renal impairment · skin hypertrophy · stomatitis · tachycardia · taste disturbance · thrombocytopenia · tremor · vasodilatation · vomiting · weight loss

▶ **Frequency not known** Interstitial lung disease · intestinal villous atrophy · progressive multifocal leucoencephalopathy · pulmonary fibrosis

SIDE-EFFECTS, FURTHER INFORMATION
Cases of pure red cell aplasia have been reported with mycophenolate mofetil; dose reduction or discontinuation should be considered under specialist supervision.

● CONCEPTION AND CONTRACEPTION
Pregnancy prevention In females of child-bearing potential, exclude pregnancy immediately before and during treatment. Women should use 2 methods of effective contraception during treatment, and for 6 weeks after discontinuation. Men should use condoms during treatment and for at least 90 days after discontinuation of treatment; female partners of male patients should also use effective contraception during treatment and for 90 days after discontinuation.

MYFORTIC® Manufacturer advises that men should use condoms during treatment and for 13 weeks after last dose.

● PREGNANCY Avoid unless no suitable alternative—congenital malformations and spontaneous abortions reported.

● BREAST FEEDING Manufacturer advises avoid—present in milk in *animal* studies.

● RENAL IMPAIRMENT No data available in cardiac or hepatic transplant patients with renal impairment.

● MONITORING REQUIREMENTS Monitor full blood count every week for 4 weeks then twice a month for 2 months then every month in the first year (consider interrupting treatment if neutropenia develops).

● DIRECTIONS FOR ADMINISTRATION For *intravenous infusion* (*CellCept®*), give intermittently in Glucose 5%; reconstitute each 500-mg vial with 14 mL glucose 5% and dilute the contents of 2 vials in 140 mL infusion fluid; give over 2 hours.

● PATIENT AND CARER ADVICE
Bone marrow suppression Patients should be warned to report immediately any signs or symptoms of bone marrow suppression e.g. infection or inexplicable bruising or bleeding.

● MEDICINAL FORMS
There can be variation in the licensing of different medicines containing the same drug. Forms available from special-order manufacturers include: oral suspension

Tablet
▶ Mycophenolate mofetil (Non-proprietary)
Mycophenolate mofetil 500 mg Mycophenolate mofetil 500mg tablets | 50 tablet [PoM] £82.26 DT price = £8.05
▶ CellCept (Roche Products Ltd)
Mycophenolate mofetil 500 mg CellCept 500mg tablets | 50 tablet [PoM] £82.26 DT price = £8.05
▶ Myfenax (Teva UK Ltd)
Mycophenolate mofetil 500 mg Myfenax 500mg tablets | 50 tablet [PoM] £78.15 DT price = £8.05

Gastro-resistant tablet
CAUTIONARY AND ADVISORY LABELS 25
▶ Myfortic (Novartis Pharmaceuticals UK Ltd)
Mycophenolic acid (as Mycophenolate sodium) 180 mg Myfortic 180mg gastro-resistant tablets | 120 tablet [PoM] £96.72
Mycophenolic acid (as Mycophenolate sodium) 360 mg Myfortic 360mg gastro-resistant tablets | 120 tablet [PoM] £193.43

Capsule
▶ Mycophenolate mofetil (Non-proprietary)
Mycophenolate mofetil 250 mg Mycophenolate mofetil 250mg capsules | 100 capsule [PoM] £82.26 DT price = £82.26
▶ CellCept (Roche Products Ltd)
Mycophenolate mofetil 250 mg CellCept 250mg capsules | 100 capsule [PoM] £82.26 DT price = £82.26
▶ Myfenax (Teva UK Ltd)
Mycophenolate mofetil 250 mg Myfenax 250mg capsules | 100 capsule [PoM] £78.15 DT price = £82.26

Oral suspension
EXCIPIENTS: May contain Aspartame
▶ CellCept (Roche Products Ltd)
Mycophenolate mofetil 200 mg per 1 ml CellCept 1g/5ml oral suspension sugar-free | 175 ml [PoM] £115.16

Powder for solution for infusion
▶ CellCept (Roche Products Ltd)
Mycophenolate mofetil (as Mycophenolate mofetil hydrochloride) 500 mg CellCept 500mg powder for solution for infusion vials | 4 vial [PoM] £36.49

IMMUNOSUPPRESSANTS 〉 T-CELL ACTIVATION INHIBITORS

Belatacept

● INDICATIONS AND DOSE
Prophylaxis of graft rejection in adults undergoing renal transplantation who are seropositive for the Epstein-Barr virus
▶ BY INTRAVENOUS INFUSION
▶ Adult: (consult product literature)

● CAUTIONS Increased risk of acute graft rejection—with tapering of corticosteroid, particularly in patients with high immunologic risk · increased risk of infection · latent and active tuberculosis · risk factors for post-transplant lymphoproliferative disorder

● SIDE-EFFECTS
▶ **Common or very common** Anaemia · constipation · cough · dehydration · diarrhoea · headache · hypertension · hypophosphataemia · infection · leucopenia · malignancy · nausea · peripheral oedema · pyrexia · vomiting
▶ **Uncommon** Infusion related reactions · progressive multifocal leucoencephalopathy

SIDE-EFFECTS, FURTHER INFORMATION
Side effects are reported when used in combination with basiliximab, mycophenolate mofetil and corticosteroids.

● CONCEPTION AND CONTRACEPTION Adequate contraception must be used during treatment and for up to 8 weeks after last dose.

● PREGNANCY Use only if essential.

● BREAST FEEDING Avoid—no information available.

● PRE-TREATMENT SCREENING Patients should be evaluated for latent and active tuberculosis before starting treatment.

● MONITORING REQUIREMENTS Patients should be monitored for signs and symptoms of tuberculosis during and after treatment.

● PATIENT AND CARER ADVICE Patients should be advised to avoid excessive exposure to UV light including sunlight.

- MEDICINAL FORMS
There can be variation in the licensing of different medicines containing the same drug.
Powder for solution for infusion
  ▸ Nulojix (Bristol-Myers Squibb Pharmaceuticals Ltd)
  Belatacept 250 mg Nulojix 250mg powder for concentrate for solution for infusion vials | 1 vial [PoM] £354.52 (Hospital only) | 2 vial [PoM] £709.04 (Hospital only)

1.1 Multiple sclerosis

CHOLINERGIC RECEPTOR STIMULATING DRUGS

Fampridine

- INDICATIONS AND DOSE
Improvement of walking disability in multiple sclerosis (specialist use only)
  ▸ BY MOUTH
  ▸ Adult: 10 mg every 12 hours, discontinue treatment if no improvement within 2 weeks

- CONTRA-INDICATIONS History of seizures (discontinue treatment if seizures occur)
- CAUTIONS Atrioventricular conduction disorders · predisposition to seizures · sinoatrial conduction disorders · symptomatic cardiac rhythm disorders
- INTERACTIONS → Appendix 1 (fampridine). Caution in concomitant use of drugs that lower seizure threshold.
- SIDE-EFFECTS
  ▸ **Common or very common** Anxiety · back pain · constipation · dizziness · dyspepsia · dyspnoea · headache · insomnia · malaise · nausea · paraesthesia · pharyngolaryngeal pain · tremor · urinary tract infection · vomiting
  ▸ **Uncommon** Seizures
- PREGNANCY Avoid—toxicity in *animal* studies.
- BREAST FEEDING Avoid—no information available.
- RENAL IMPAIRMENT Avoid if eGFR less than 80 mL/minute/1.73 m^2.
- PRESCRIBING AND DISPENSING INFORMATION Dispense in original container (pack contains a desiccant) and discard any tablets remaining 7 days after opening.

- MEDICINAL FORMS
There can be variation in the licensing of different medicines containing the same drug. Forms available from special-order manufacturers include: capsule
Modified-release tablet
CAUTIONARY AND ADVISORY LABELS 23, 25
  ▸ Fampyra (Biogen Idec Ltd) ▼
  Fampridine 10 mg Fampyra 10mg modified-release tablets | 28 tablet [PoM] £181.00 | 56 tablet [PoM] £362.00

IMMUNOSTIMULANTS ⟩ INTERFERONS

Interferon beta

- INDICATIONS AND DOSE
AVONEX® INJECTION

For relapsing, remitting multiple sclerosis (characterised by at least two attacks of neurological dysfunction over the previous 2 or 3 years, followed by complete or incomplete recovery) who are able to walk unaided | For a single demyelinating event with an active inflammatory process (if severe enough to require intravenous corticosteroid and patient at high risk of developing multiple sclerosis)
  ▸ BY INTRAMUSCULAR INJECTION
  ▸ Adult: (consult product literature)

AVONEX® VIAL

For relapsing, remitting multiple sclerosis (characterised by at least two attacks of neurological dysfunction over the previous 2 or 3 years, followed by complete or incomplete recovery) who are able to walk unaided | For a single demyelinating event with an active inflammatory process (if severe enough to require intravenous corticosteroid and patient at high risk of developing multiple sclerosis)
  ▸ BY INTRAMUSCULAR INJECTION
  ▸ Adult: (consult product literature)

BETAFERON® INJECTION

For relapsing, remitting multiple sclerosis (characterised by at least two attacks of neurological dysfunction over the previous 2 or 3 years, followed by complete or incomplete recovery) who are able to walk unaided | For secondary progressive multiple sclerosis with active disease | For a single demyelinating event with an active inflammatory process (if severe enough to require intravenous corticosteroid and patient at high risk of developing multiple sclerosis)
  ▸ BY SUBCUTANEOUS INJECTION
  ▸ Adult: (consult product literature)

EXTAVIA®

For relapsing, remitting multiple sclerosis (characterised by at least two attacks of neurological dysfunction over the previous 2 or 3 years, followed by complete or incomplete recovery) who are able to walk unaided | For secondary progressive multiple sclerosis with active disease | For a single demyelinating event with an active inflammatory process (if severe enough to require intravenous corticosteroid and patient at high risk of developing multiple sclerosis)
  ▸ BY SUBCUTANEOUS INJECTION
  ▸ Adult: (consult product literature)

REBIF® CARTRIDGE

For relapsing, remitting multiple sclerosis (characterised by at least two attacks of neurological dysfunction over the previous 2 or 3 years, followed by complete or incomplete recovery) who are able to walk unaided | For a single demyelinating event with an active inflammatory process (if severe enough to require intravenous corticosteroid and patient at high risk of developing multiple sclerosis)
  ▸ BY SUBCUTANEOUS INJECTION
  ▸ Adult: (consult product literature) continued →

REBIF® PRE-FILLED PEN AND SYRINGE

For relapsing, remitting multiple sclerosis (characterised by at least two attacks of neurological dysfunction over the previous 2 or 3 years, followed by complete or incomplete recovery) who are able to walk unaided | For a single demyelinating event with an active inflammatory process (if severe enough to require intravenous corticosteroid and patient at high risk of developing multiple sclerosis)
▸ BY SUBCUTANEOUS INJECTION
▸ Adult: (consult product literature)

● CONTRA-INDICATIONS Decompensated liver disease · severe depressive illness

CONTRA-INDICATIONS, FURTHER INFORMATION
Consult product literature for further information on contra-indications.

● CAUTIONS History of cardiac disorders · history of depressive disorders (avoid in severe depression or in those with suicidal ideation) · history of seizures · history of severe myelosupression

CAUTIONS, FURTHER INFORMATION
Consult product literature for further information on cautions.

● SIDE-EFFECTS Alopecia · anaphylaxis · blood disorders · chills · confusion · convulsions · fever · hepatitis · hypersensitivity reactions · influenza-like symptoms (decreasing over time) · irritation at injection site (including inflammation, hypersensitivity, necrosis) · malaise · menstrual disorders · mood and personality changes · myalgia · nausea · nephrotic syndrome · suicide attempts · thrombotic microangiopathy · thyroid dysfunction · urticaria · vomiting

SIDE-EFFECTS, FURTHER INFORMATION
Also consult product literature for all side effects.

● CONCEPTION AND CONTRACEPTION Effective contraception required during treatment—consult product literature.

● PREGNANCY Avoid unless potential benefit outweighs risk (toxicity in *animal* studies).

● BREAST FEEDING Avoid—no information available.

● HEPATIC IMPAIRMENT Caution in severe hepatic impairment.

● RENAL IMPAIRMENT Caution in severe renal impairment.

● MONITORING REQUIREMENTS
▸ Monitor for signs of hepatic injury—hepatic failure has been reported rarely.
▸ Patients should be monitored for clinical features of thrombotic microangiopathy (TMA), including thrombocytopenia, new onset hypertension, fever, central nervous system symptoms (e.g. confusion and paresis), and impaired renal function. Any signs of TMA should be investigated fully and, if diagnosed, interferon beta should be stopped immediately and treatment for TMA promptly initiated (consult product literature for details).
▸ Patients should also be monitored for signs and symptoms of nephrotic syndrome, including oedema, proteinuria, and impaired renal function—monitor renal function periodically. If nephrotic syndrome develops, treat promptly and consider stopping interferon beta treatment.

● PRESCRIBING AND DISPENSING INFORMATION
REBIF® CARTRIDGE Cartridges for use with *RebiSmart*® auto-injector device.

BETAFERON® INJECTION An auto-injector device (*Betaject*® Light) is available from Bayer Schering.

EXTAVIA® An auto-injector device (*ExtaviPro*® 30G) is supplied as part of the *ExtaviPro*® 30G kit.

● NATIONAL FUNDING/ACCESS DECISIONS

NICE technology appraisals (TAs)
▸ Interferon beta and glatiramer for multiple sclerosis (January 2002) NICE TA32
Interferon beta and glatiramer acetate are **not** recommended for the treatment of multiple sclerosis in the NHS in England and Wales.

Patients who are currently receiving interferon beta or glatiramer acetate for multiple sclerosis, whether as routine therapy or as part of a clinical trial, should have the option to continue treatment until they and their consultant consider it appropriate to stop, having regard to the established criteria for withdrawal from treatment.
www.nice.org.uk/TA32

NHS restrictions
Provision of disease-modifying therapies for multiple sclerosis The Department of Health, the National Assembly for Wales, the Scottish Executive, the Northern Ireland Department of Health, Social Services & Public Safety, and the manufacturers have reached agreement on a risk-sharing scheme for the NHS supply of interferon beta and glatiramer acetate for multiple sclerosis. Health Service Circular (HSC 2002/004) explains how patients can participate in the scheme. It is available on the Department of Health website (www.dh.gov.uk).

● MEDICINAL FORMS
There can be variation in the licensing of different medicines containing the same drug.
Solution for injection
EXCIPIENTS: May contain Benzyl alcohol
▸ Avonex (Biogen Idec Ltd)
Interferon beta-1a 12 mega u per 1 ml Avonex 30micrograms/0.5ml (6million units) solution for injection pre-filled syringes | 4 pre-filled disposable injection [PoM] £654.00 | 12 pre-filled disposable injection [PoM] £1,962.00
Avonex 30micrograms/0.5ml (6million units) solution for injection pre-filled pen | 4 pre-filled disposable injection [PoM] £654.00 | 12 pre-filled disposable injection [PoM] £1,962.00
▸ Rebif (Merck Serono Ltd)
Interferon beta-1a 12 mega u per 1 ml Rebif 22micrograms/0.5ml (6million units) solution for injection 1.5ml cartridges | 4 cartridge [PoM] £613.52
Rebif 8.8micrograms/0.2ml (2.4million units) solution for injection pre-filled syringes | 6 pre-filled disposable injection [PoM] no price available
Rebif 8.8micrograms/0.2ml (2.4million units) solution for injection pre-filled pen | 6 pre-filled disposable injection [PoM] no price available
Rebif 22micrograms/0.5ml (6million units) solution for injection pre-filled pen | 6 pre-filled disposable injection [PoM] no price available | 12 pre-filled disposable injection [PoM] £613.52
Rebif 22micrograms/0.5ml (6million units) solution for injection pre-filled syringes | 6 pre-filled disposable injection [PoM] no price available | 12 pre-filled disposable injection [PoM] £613.52
Interferon beta-1a 24 mega u per 1 ml Rebif 44micrograms/0.5ml (12million units) solution for injection pre-filled pen | 12 pre-filled disposable injection [PoM] £813.21
Rebif 44micrograms/0.5ml (12million units) solution for injection pre-filled syringes | 12 pre-filled disposable injection [PoM] £813.21
Rebif 44micrograms/0.5ml (12million units) solution for injection 1.5ml cartridges | 4 cartridge [PoM] £813.21

Powder and solvent for solution for injection
▸ Betaferon (Bayer Plc)
Interferon beta-1b 300 microgram Betaferon 300microgram powder and solvent for solution for injection vials | 15 vial [PoM] £596.63 (Hospital only)
▸ Extavia (Novartis Pharmaceuticals UK Ltd)
Interferon beta-1b 300 microgram Extavia 300microgram powder and solvent for solution for injection vials | 15 vial [PoM] £596.63

Peginterferon beta-1a

- **DRUG ACTION** Peginterferon beta-1a is a polyethylene glycol-conjugated ('pegylated') derivative of interferon beta; pegylation increases the persistence of interferon in the blood.

- **INDICATIONS AND DOSE**

  Treatment of relapsing, remitting multiple sclerosis
  - ▸ BY SUBCUTANEOUS INJECTION
  - ▸ Adult: (consult product literature)

- **CONTRA-INDICATIONS** Severe depression · suicidal ideation
- **CAUTIONS** History of cardiac disorders · history of depressive disorders (avoid in severe depression or in those with suicidal ideation) · history of seizures · history of severe myelosupression

  CAUTIONS, FURTHER INFORMATION
  Consult product literature for further information about cautions.

- **SIDE-EFFECTS**

  SIDE-EFFECTS, FURTHER INFORMATION
  Consult product literature for information about side effects.

- **CONCEPTION AND CONTRACEPTION** Effective contraception required during treatment—consult product literature.
- **PREGNANCY** Do not initiate during pregnancy. Avoid unless potential benefit outweighs risk.
- **BREAST FEEDING** Avoid—no information available.
- **HEPATIC IMPAIRMENT** Caution in severe hepatic impairment.
- **RENAL IMPAIRMENT** Caution in severe renal impairment.
- **MONITORING REQUIREMENTS**
  - ▸ Monitor for signs of hepatic injury—hepatic failure has been reported rarely.
  - ▸ Thrombotic microangiopathy Patients should be monitored for clinical features of thrombotic microangiopathy (TMA), including thrombocytopenia, new onset hypertension, fever, central nervous system symptoms (e.g. confusion and paresis), and impaired renal function. Any signs of TMA should be investigated fully and, if diagnosed, interferon beta should be stopped immediately and treatment for TMA promptly initiated (consult product literature for details).
  - ▸ Nephrotic syndrome Patients should also be monitored for signs and symptoms of nephrotic syndrome, including oedema, proteinuria, and impaired renal function—monitor renal function periodically. If nephrotic syndrome develops, treat promptly and consider stopping interferon beta treatment.

- **MEDICINAL FORMS**
  There can be variation in the licensing of different medicines containing the same drug.

  Solution for injection
  - ▸ Plegridy (Biogen Idec Ltd) ▼
    Peginterferon beta-1a 126 microgram per 1 ml Plegridy 63micrograms/0.5ml solution for injection pre-filled pen | 1 pre-filled disposable injection PoM no price available
    Peginterferon beta-1a 188 microgram per 1 ml Plegridy 94micrograms/0.5ml solution for injection pre-filled pen | 1 pre-filled disposable injection PoM no price available
    Peginterferon beta-1a 250 microgram per 1 ml Plegridy 125micrograms/0.5ml solution for injection pre-filled pen | 2 pre-filled disposable injection PoM £654.00 | 6 pre-filled disposable injection PoM £1,962.00

IMMUNOSTIMULANTS ⟩ OTHER

Glatiramer acetate

- **DRUG ACTION** Glatiramer is an immunomodulating drug comprising synthetic polypeptides.

- **INDICATIONS AND DOSE**

  Treatment of initial symptoms in patients at high risk of developing multiple sclerosis (initiated under specialist supervision) | Reducing frequency of relapses in ambulatory patients with relapsing-remitting multiple sclerosis who have had at least 2 clinical relapses in the past 2 years (initiated under specialist supervision)
  - ▸ BY SUBCUTANEOUS INJECTION
  - ▸ Adult: 20 mg daily

- **CAUTIONS** Cardiac disorders
- **SIDE-EFFECTS**
  - ▸ **Common or very common** Anxiety · arthralgia · asthenia · back pain · chest pain · constipation · depression · dyspepsia · dyspnoea (may occur within minutes of injection) · flushing · headache · hypersensitivity reactions · hypertonia · influenza-like symptoms · injection-site reactions · lymphadenopathy · nausea · oedema · palpitation · rash · sweating · syncope · tachycardia · tremor
  - ▸ **Rare** Seizures
- **PREGNANCY** Manufacturer advises avoid—no information available.
- **BREAST FEEDING** Manufacturer advises caution—no information available.
- **RENAL IMPAIRMENT** No information available—manufacturer advises caution.
- **NATIONAL FUNDING/ACCESS DECISIONS**

  NICE technology appraisals (TAs)
  - ▸ **Interferon beta and glatiramer for multiple sclerosis (January 2002)** NICE TA32
    Interferon beta and glatiramer acetate are **not** recommended for the treatment of multiple sclerosis in the NHS in England and Wales.

    Patients who are currently receiving interferon beta or glatiramer acetate for multiple sclerosis, whether as routine therapy or as part of a clinical trial, should have the option to continue treatment until they and their consultant consider it appropriate to stop, having regard to the established criteria for withdrawal from treatment. www.nice.org.uk/TA32

  NHS restrictions
  Provision of disease-modifying therapies for multiple sclerosis The Department of Health, the National Assembly for Wales, the Scottish Executive, the Northern Ireland Department of Health, Social Services & Public Safety, and the manufacturers have reached agreement on a risk-sharing scheme for the NHS supply of interferon beta and glatiramer acetate for multiple sclerosis. Health Service Circular (HSC 2002/004) explains how patients can participate in the scheme. It is available on the Department of Health website (www.dh.gov.uk).

- **MEDICINAL FORMS**
  There can be variation in the licensing of different medicines containing the same drug.

  Solution for injection
  - ▸ Copaxone (Teva UK Ltd)
    Glatiramer acetate 20 mg per 1 ml Copaxone 20mg/1ml solution for injection pre-filled syringes | 28 pre-filled disposable injection PoM £513.95
    Glatiramer acetate 40 mg per 1 ml Copaxone 40mg/1ml solution for injection pre-filled syringes | 12 pre-filled disposable injection PoM £513.95

8

Immune system and malignant disease

Immune system and malignant disease

8

IMMUNOSUPPRESSANTS >
IMMUNOMODULATING DRUGS

Dimethyl fumarate

- **DRUG ACTION** Dimethyl fumarate has immunomodulatory and anti-inflammatory properties.

- **INDICATIONS AND DOSE**

Treatment of adults with relapsing-remitting multiple sclerosis (initiated by a specialist)
 ‣ BY MOUTH
 ‣ Adult: 120 mg twice daily for 7 days, then increased to 240 mg twice daily, for dose adjustment due to side effects—consult product literature

- **CAUTIONS** Reduced lymphocyte count · risk of serious infections (do not start treatment until resolved and consider suspending treatment if infection develops during treatment) · severe active gastro-intestinal disease

- **SIDE-EFFECTS** Abdominal pain · burning sensation · diarrhoea · dyspepsia · erythema · flushing (may be severe and indicate hypersensitivity) · gastritis · gastroenteritis · leucopenia · lymphopenia · nausea · proteinuria · pruritus · rash · vomiting

SIDE-EFFECTS, FURTHER INFORMATION
‣ Progressive multifocal leukoencephalopathy (PML) Severe prolonged lymphopenia reported, and patients are exposed to a potential risk of PML. Treatment should be stopped immediately if PML is suspected.

- **CONCEPTION AND CONTRACEPTION** Contraception required in women of child-bearing potential (consider non-hormonal methods).

- **PREGNANCY** Manufacturer advises avoid unless essential and potential benefit outweighs risk—toxicity in *animal* studies.

- **BREAST FEEDING** Manufacturer advises avoid.

- **HEPATIC IMPAIRMENT** Manufacturer advises caution in severe impairment.

- **RENAL IMPAIRMENT** Manufacturer advises caution in severe impairment.

- **MONITORING REQUIREMENTS**
‣ Monitor full blood count (including lymphocytes) before treatment (within 6 months before initiation), then every 6 to 12 months thereafter, and as clinically indicated.
‣ Monitor patient closely for features of progressive multifocal leukoencephalopathy (PML) (e.g. signs and symptoms of neurological dysfunction) and other opportunistic infections.
‣ Monitor renal and hepatic function before treatment, after 3 and 6 months of treatment, then every 6 to 12 months thereafter, and as clinically indicated.

- **PATIENT AND CARER ADVICE** Patient information leaflet should be provided. Counselling is advised on progressive multifocal leukoencephalopathy.

- **NATIONAL FUNDING/ACCESS DECISIONS**

NICE technology appraisals (TAs)
‣ Dimethyl fumarate for treating relapsing-remitting multiple sclerosis (August 2014) NICE TA320
Dimethyl fumarate is recommended for the treatment of active relapsing-remitting multiple sclerosis, only if:
 - the patient does not have highly active or rapidly evolving severe relapsing-remitting multiple sclerosis **and**
 - the manufacturer provides dimethyl fumarate with the discount agreed in the patient access scheme
Patients currently receiving dimethyl fumarate whose disease does not meet the above criteria should be able to continue treatment until they and their clinician consider it appropriate to stop.
www.nice.org.uk/TA320

- **MEDICINAL FORMS**
There can be variation in the licensing of different medicines containing the same drug.
Gastro-resistant capsule
CAUTIONARY AND ADVISORY LABELS 21, 25
 ‣ Tecfidera (Biogen Idec Ltd)
 Dimethyl fumarate 120 mg Tecfidera 120mg gastro-resistant capsules | 14 capsule [PoM] £343.00
 Dimethyl fumarate 240 mg Tecfidera 240mg gastro-resistant capsules | 56 capsule [PoM] £1,373.00

Fingolimod

- **DRUG ACTION** Fingolimod is an immunomodulating drug.

- **INDICATIONS AND DOSE**

Treatment of highly active relapsing-remitting multiple sclerosis in patients who have high disease activity despite treatment with at least one disease modifying therapy or in those with rapidly evolving severe relapsing-remitting multiple sclerosis (initiated under specialist supervision)
 ‣ BY MOUTH
 ‣ Adult: 500 micrograms once daily

IMPORTANT SAFETY INFORMATION
MHRA/CHM ADVICE: FINGOLIMOD—NOT RECOMMENDED FOR PATIENTS AT KNOWN RISK OF CARDIOVASCULAR EVENTS. ADVICE FOR EXTENDED MONITORING FOR THOSE WITH SIGNIFICANT BRADYCARDIA OR HEART BLOCK AFTER THE FIRST DOSE AND FOLLOWING TREATMENT INTERRUPTION (JANUARY 2013)
Fingolimod is known to cause transient bradycardias and heart block after the first dose. Fingolimod is not recommended in the following patient groups who are at high risk of cardiovascular events unless the anticipated benefits outweigh the potential risks, and advice from a cardiologist is sought before initiation:
 Patients with the following medical conditions:
 - 2nd degree Mobitz Type II or higher degree atrioventricular block, sick sinus syndrome, or sino-atrial heart block
 - significant QT prolongation (QT-interval greater than 470 milliseconds in women, or greater than 450 milliseconds in men)
 - history of symptomatic bradycardia or recurrent syncope, known ischaemic heart disease, cerebrovascular disease, history of myocardial infarction, congestive heart failure, history of cardiac arrest, uncontrolled hypertension, or severe sleep apnoea.
Patients receiving the following antiarrhythmic or heart-rate lowering drugs:
 - class Ia or class III antiarrhythmics
 - beta blockers
 - heart rate-lowering calcium channel blockers
 - other substances which may decrease heart rate (e.g. digoxin, anticholinesteratic drugs or pilocarpine).
All patients receiving fingolimod should be monitored at treatment initiation, (first dose monitoring), and after treatment interruption (see note below); monitoring should include:
 Pre-treatment
 - a 12-lead ECG and blood pressure measurement before starting
During the first 6 hours of treatment
 - continuous ECG monitoring for 6 hours
 - blood pressure and heart rate measurement every hour
After 6 hours of treatment
 - a further 12-lead ECG and blood pressure measurement
If heart rate at the end of the 6 hour period is at its lowest since fingolimod was first administered,

monitoring should be extended by at least 2 hours and until heart rate increases.

Extended monitoring, (at least overnight), should be performed in patients with evidence of clinically important cardiac effects during first dose monitoring. Monitoring in patients requiring pharmacological intervention for bradyarrhythmia-related symptoms during first dose monitoring should be extended at least overnight, and first dose monitoring should be repeated after the second dose.

Note

First dose monitoring as above **should be repeated** in all patients whose treatment is interrupted for:
• 1 day or more during the first 2 weeks of treatment
• more than 7 days during weeks 3 and 4 of treatment
• more than 2 weeks after one month of treatment
If the treatment interruption is of shorter duration than the above, repeated monitoring is not required and treatment should be continued with the next dose as planned.

● CONTRA-INDICATIONS Active infection · active malignancies (except cutaneous basal cell carcinoma) · immunosuppression

● CAUTIONS Check varicella zoster virus status—consult product literature for further information · chronic obstructive pulmonary disease · pulmonary fibrosis · risk of macular oedema · severe respiratory disease · susceptibility to QT-interval prolongation (including electrolyte disturbances)

CAUTIONS, FURTHER INFORMATION
▶ Washout period A washout period is recommended when switching treatment from some disease modifying therapies—consult product literature for further information.

● INTERACTIONS → Appendix 1 (fingolimod). Caution with concomitant use of drugs that prolong QT interval.

● SIDE-EFFECTS
▶ **Common or very common** Alopecia · AV block · back pain · blurred vision · bradycardia · bronchitis · cough · depression · diarrhoea · dizziness · dyspnoea · eczema · gastroenteritis · headache · herpes · hypertension · influenza · leucopenia · lymphopenia · malaise · migraine · paraesthesia · pruritus · sinusitis · tinea versicolor
▶ **Uncommon** Macular oedema · neutropenia · pneumonia
▶ **Frequency not known** Haemophagocytic syndrome · lymphoma · posterior reversible encephalopathy syndrome · progressive multifocal leukoencephalopathy

● CONCEPTION AND CONTRACEPTION Exclude pregnancy before treatment. Ensure effective contraception during and for at least 2 months after treatment.

● PREGNANCY Avoid (toxicity in *animal* studies).

● BREAST FEEDING Avoid.

● HEPATIC IMPAIRMENT Use with caution in mild to moderate impairment. Avoid in severe impairment.

● MONITORING REQUIREMENTS
▶ Eye examination recommended 3–4 months after initiation of treatment (and before initiation of treatment in patients with diabetes or history of uveitis).
▶ Monitor hepatic transaminases before treatment, then every 3 months for 1 year, then periodically thereafter.
▶ Monitor full blood count before treatment, at 3 months, then at least yearly thereafter and if signs of infection—interrupt treatment if lymphocyte count reduced—consult product literature.
▶ Monitor for signs and symptoms of haemophagocytic syndrome (including pyrexia, asthenia, hepato-splenomegaly and adenopathy—may be associated with hepatic failure and respiratory distress; also progressive

cytopenia, elevated serum-ferritin concentrations, hypertriglyceridaemia, hypofibrinogenaemia, coagulopathy, hepatic cytolysis, hyponatraemia)—initiate treatment immediately.

● NATIONAL FUNDING/ACCESS DECISIONS
NICE technology appraisals (TAs)
▶ Fingolimod for the treatment of highly active relapsing-remitting multiple sclerosis (April 2012) NICE TA254
Fingolimod is recommended as an option for the treatment of highly active relapsing-remitting multiple sclerosis in adults, only if:
• they have an unchanged or increased relapse rate or ongoing severe relapses compared with the previous year despite treatment with interferon beta, **and**
• the manufacturer provides fingolimod with the discount agreed as part of the patient access scheme
Patients currently receiving fingolimod whose disease does not meet the above criteria should be able to continue treatment until they and their clinician consider it appropriate to stop.
www.nice.org.uk/TA254

Scottish Medicines Consortium (SMC) Decisions
The *Scottish Medicines Consortium* has advised (August 2012) that fingolimod (*Gilenya®*) is accepted for restricted use within NHS Scotland as single disease modifying therapy in highly active relapsing-remitting multiple sclerosis despite treatment with interferon beta, with an unchanged or increased relapse rate or ongoing severe relapses, as compared to the previous year.

● MEDICINAL FORMS
There can be variation in the licensing of different medicines containing the same drug.
Capsule
▶ Gilenya (Novartis Pharmaceuticals UK Ltd) ▼
Fingolimod (as Fingolimod hydrochloride)
500 microgram Gilenya 0.5mg capsules | 7 capsule PoM £367.50 | 28 capsule PoM £1,470.00

IMMUNOSUPPRESSANTS > MONOCLONAL ANTIBODIES > ANTI-LYMPHOCYTE

Anti-lymphocyte monoclonal antibodies

● DRUG ACTION The anti-lymphocyte monoclonal antibodies cause lysis of B lymphocytes.

> IMPORTANT SAFETY INFORMATION
> All anti-lymphocyte monoclonal antibodies should be given under the supervision of an experienced specialist, in an environment where full resuscitation facilities are immediately available.

● SIDE-EFFECTS
▶ **Common or very common** Allergic reactions · angioedema · bronchospasm · chills · cytokine release syndrome · dyspnoea · fever · flushing · nausea · pruritus · rash · tumour pain · vomiting
▶ **Frequency not known** Cardiac events

SIDE-EFFECTS, FURTHER INFORMATION
▶ Infusion-related side-effects In rare cases infusion reactions may be fatal. Infusion-related side-effects occur predominantly during the first infusion. Patients should receive premedication before administration of anti-lymphocyte monoclonal antibodies to reduce these effects—consult product literature for details of individual regimens. The infusion may have to be stopped temporarily and the infusion-related effects treated—consult product literature for appropriate management. Evidence of pulmonary infiltration and features of tumour

lysis syndrome should be sought if infusion-related effects occur.

▸ Cytokine release syndrome Fatalities following **severe** cytokine release syndrome (characterised by severe dyspnoea) and associated with features of tumour lysis syndrome have occurred after infusions of anti-lymphocyte monoclonal antibodies. Patients with a high tumour burden as well as those with pulmonary insufficiency or infiltration are at increased risk and should be monitored **very closely** (and a slower rate of infusion considered).

● PRE-TREATMENT SCREENING All patients should be screened for hepatitis B before treatment.

● MONITORING REQUIREMENTS Patients should also be monitored for cytopenias—consult product literature for specific recommendations.

▶ 771

Alemtuzumab

● INDICATIONS AND DOSE

Treatment of adults with relapsing-remitting multiple sclerosis with active disease defined by clinical or imaging features
▸ BY INTRAVENOUS INFUSION
▸ Adult: (consult product literature)

● UNLICENSED USE Although no longer licensed for oncological and transplant indications, alemtuzumab is also available through a patient access programme for these indications.

> IMPORTANT SAFETY INFORMATION
> Alemtuzumab should be given under the care of a specialist with facilities for the management of hypersenstivity and anaphylactic reactions.

● CONTRA-INDICATIONS Human immunodeficiency virus
● CAUTIONS Hepatitis B carriers · hepatitis C carriers · in patients with active infection, a delay in initiation of alemtuzumab treatment should be considered until the infection is fully controlled · not recommended for inactive disease · not recommended for stable disease · patients should receive oral prophylaxis for herpes infection starting on the first day of treatment and continuing for at least a month following each treatment course · patients with previous autoimmune conditions other than multiple sclerosis · pretreatment before administration is required (consult product literature)

CAUTIONS, FURTHER INFORMATION
For full details of cautions, consult product literature.
▸ Autoimmune mediated conditions The risk of autoimmune mediated conditions may increase during treatment, including immune thrombocytopenic purpura, thyroid disorders, nephropathies, and cytopenias, and should be monitored for throughout the course of treatment (consult product literature).

● INTERACTIONS → Appendix 1 (alemtuzumab).

● SIDE-EFFECTS

SIDE-EFFECTS, FURTHER INFORMATION
For full side effects details (including monitoring and management) consult product literature

● CONCEPTION AND CONTRACEPTION Women of childbearing potential should use effective contraception during and for 4 months after treatment.

● PREGNANCY Manufacturer advises avoid unless potential benefit outweighs risk—toxicity in *animal* studies. Autoimmune thyroid disease during treatment may affect fetus (consult product literature).

● BREAST FEEDING Manufacturer advises avoid during and for 4 months after each treatment course unless potential benefit outweighs risk.

● PRE-TREATMENT SCREENING Screening patients at high risk of hepatitis B or C is recommended before treatment. All patients should be evaluated for active or latent tuberculosis before starting treatment.

● MONITORING REQUIREMENTS HPV screening should be carried out annually in female patients.

● PRESCRIBING AND DISPENSING INFORMATION All patients should receive oral prophylaxis for herpes infection starting on the first day of treatment and continuing for at least a month following each treatment course.

● PATIENT AND CARER ADVICE Patients should be provided with a patient alert card and patient guide.

● NATIONAL FUNDING/ACCESS DECISIONS
NICE technology appraisals (TAs)
▸ **Alemtuzumab for treating relapsing-remitting multiple sclerosis (May 2014)** NICE TA312
Alemtuzumab is recommended as an option, within its marketing authorisation, for treating adults with active relapsing-remitting multiple sclerosis.
www.nice.org.uk/TA312

● MEDICINAL FORMS
There can be variation in the licensing of different medicines containing the same drug.
Solution for infusion
▸ Lemtrada (Genzyme Therapeutics Ltd) ▼
Alemtuzumab 10 mg per 1 ml Lemtrada 12mg/1.2ml concentrate for solution for infusion vials | 1 vial PoM £7,045.00 (Hospital only)

▶ 771

Natalizumab

● DRUG ACTION Natalizumab is a monoclonal antibody that inhibits the migration of leucocytes into the central nervous system, hence reducing inflammation and demyelination.

● INDICATIONS AND DOSE

Highly active relapsing-remitting multiple sclerosis despite treatment with interferon beta or glatiramer acetate, or those patients with rapidly evolving severe relapsing-remitting multiple sclerosis (initiated under specialist supervision)
▸ BY INTRAVENOUS INFUSION
▸ Adult 18–65 years: 300 mg every 4 weeks, treatment should be discontinued if no response after 6 months

● CONTRA-INDICATIONS Active infection · active malignancies (except cutaneous basal cell carcinoma) · immunosuppression · progressive multifocal leucoencephalopathy

● CAUTIONS

CAUTIONS, FURTHER INFORMATION
▸ Progressive Multifocal Leucoencephalopathy Natalizumab is associated with an increased risk of opportunistic infection and progressive multifocal leucoencephalopathy (PML) caused by JC virus. The risk of developing PML increases with the presence of anti-JCV antibodies, previous use of immunosuppressant therapy, and treatment duration (especially beyond 2 years of treatment); the risk beyond 4 years of treatment is not known. Patients with all three risk factors should only be treated with natalizumab if the benefits of treatment outweigh the risks. Treatment should be suspended until PML has been excluded. If a patient develops an opportunistic infection or PML, natalizumab should be permanently discontinued.
For information on cautions consult product literature.

● INTERACTIONS → Appendix 1 (natalizumab).
Concurrent use of interferon beta or glatiramer acetate contra-indicated.

● SIDE-EFFECTS
▸ **Common or very common** Arthralgia · arthralgia (during infusion) · autoantibodies · dizziness (during infusion) · fatigue (during infusion) · headache (during infusion) · nasopharyngitis · nausea (during infusion) · pyrexia (during infusion) · rigors (during infusion) · urinary-tract infection · urticaria (during infusion) · vomiting (during infusion)
▸ **Uncommon** Hypersensitivity reactions (discontinue permanently) · Progressive Multifocal Leucoencephalopathy (PML)
▸ **Frequency not known** Flushing (during infusion) · increased risk of opportunistic infection · liver toxicity

SIDE-EFFECTS, FURTHER INFORMATION
▸ Progressive Multifocal Leucoencephalopathy If Progressive Multifocal Leucoencephalopathy (PML) is suspected, treatment should be suspended until PML has been excluded. If a patient develops an opportunistic infection or PML, natalizumab should be permanently discontinued.
▸ Liver toxicity Discontinue treatment if significant liver injury occurs.

● PREGNANCY Avoid unless essential—toxicity in *animal* studies.

● BREAST FEEDING Present in milk in *animal* studies—avoid.

● PRE-TREATMENT SCREENING
Progressive Multifocal Leucoencephalopathy A magnetic resonance image (MRI) scan is recommended before starting treatment with natalizumab.

Testing for serum anti-JCV antibodies before starting treatment or in those with unknown antibody status already receiving natalizumab is recommended and should be repeated every 6 months (consult product literature for full details).

● MONITORING REQUIREMENTS
▸ Monitor liver function.
▸ Progressive Multifocal Leucoencephalopathy A magnetic resonance image (MRI) scan is recommended annually. Patients should be monitored for new or worsening neurological symptoms, and for cognitive and psychiatric signs of PML.
▸ All patients should continue to be monitored for signs and symptoms that may be suggestive of PML for approximately 6 months following discontinuation of treatment.
▸ Hypersensitivity reactions Patients should be observed for hypersensitivity reactions, including anaphylaxis, during the infusion and for 1 hour after completion of the infusion.

● DIRECTIONS FOR ADMINISTRATION For *intravenous infusion* (*Tysabri®*), give intermittently in Sodium chloride 0.9%; dilute 300 mg in 100 mL infusion fluid; gently invert to mix, do not shake. Use within 8 hours of dilution and give over 1 hour.

● PATIENT AND CARER ADVICE A patient alert card should be provided.
Hypersensitivity reactions Patients should be told the importance of uninterrupted dosing, particularly in the early months of treatment (intermittent therapy may increase risk of sensitisation).
Progressive Multifocal Leucoencephalopathy Patients should be informed about the risks of PML before starting treatment with natalizumab and again after 2 years; they should be given an alert card which includes information about the symptoms of PML.
Liver toxicity Advise patients to seek immediate medical attention if symptoms such as jaundice or dark urine develop.

● NATIONAL FUNDING/ACCESS DECISIONS
NICE technology appraisals (TAs)
▸ **Natalizumab for the treatment of adults with highly active relapsing-remitting multiple sclerosis (August 2007)**
NICE TA127
Natalizumab is an option for the treatment only of rapidly evolving severe relapsing-remitting multiple sclerosis (RES). RES is defined by 2 or more disabling relapses in 1 year, and 1 or more gadolinium-enhancing lesions on brain magnetic resonance imaging (MRI) or a significant increase in T2 lesion load compared with a previous MRI. www.nice.org.uk/TA127

Scottish Medicines Consortium (SMC) Decisions
The *Scottish Medicines Consortium* has advised (August 2007) that natalizumab is accepted for restricted use as single disease-modifying therapy in highly active relapsing-remitting multiple sclerosis only in patients with rapidly evolving severe relapsing-remitting multiple sclerosis defined by 2 or more disabling relapses in 1 year and with 1 or more gadolinium-enhancing lesions on brain magnetic resonance imaging (MRI) or a significant increase in T2 lesion load compared with a previous MRI.

● MEDICINAL FORMS
There can be variation in the licensing of different medicines containing the same drug.
Solution for infusion
ELECTROLYTES: May contain Sodium
▸ Tysabri (Biogen Idec Ltd) ▾
Natalizumab 20 mg per 1 ml Tysabri 300mg/15ml concentrate for solution for infusion vials | 1 vial [PoM] no price available (Hospital only)

IMMUNOSUPPRESSANTS › PYRIMIDINE SYNTHESIS INHIBITORS

Teriflunomide

● DRUG ACTION Teriflunomide is a metabolite of leflunomide which has immunomodulating and anti-inflammatory properties.

● INDICATIONS AND DOSE
Treatment of relapsing-remitting multiple sclerosis (initiated under specialist supervision)
▸ BY MOUTH
▸ Adult: 14 mg once daily

● CONTRA-INDICATIONS Anaemia · leucopenia · neutropenia · serious infection · severe hypoproteinaemia · severe immunodeficiency · significantly impaired bone-marrow function · thrombocytopenia

● CAUTIONS Adult over 65 years · anaemia · dyspnoea— assess for interstitial lung disease and consider suspending treatment · hypoproteinaemia (avoid if severe) · impaired bone-marrow function (avoid if severe) · latent tuberculosis · leucopenia · persistent cough—assess for interstitial lung disease and consider suspending treatment · severe infection—delay or suspend treatment until resolved · significant alcohol consumption · signs or symptoms of serious skin reactions (including ulcerative stomatitis, Stevens-Johnson syndrome, and toxic epidermal necrolysis)—discontinue treatment · switching between other immunomodulating drugs · thrombocytopenia

● INTERACTIONS → Appendix 1 (teriflunomide).

● SIDE-EFFECTS
▸ **Common or very common** Acne · alopecia · anxiety · carpal tunnel syndrome · cystitis · diarrhoea · elevated liver enzymes · gastroenteritis · hyperaesthesia · hypertension · laryngitis · leucopenia · menorrhagia · musculoskeletal pain · myalgia · nausea · neuralgia · neutropenia · oral infection · paraesthesia · peripheral neuropathy ·

8

Immune system and malignant disease

pollakiuria · rash · respiratory tract infection · sciatica · tinea pedis · urinary tract infection · vomiting · weight loss
▶ **Uncommon** Anaemia · thrombocytopenia
▶ **Very rare** Interstitial lung disease · pancreatitis

SIDE-EFFECTS, FURTHER INFORMATION
▶ Accelerated elimination procedure **Important**: accelerated elimination procedure recommended following discontinuation due to serious adverse effects (consult product literature).
▶ Hepatic injury Discontinue treatment if signs or symptoms of hepatic injury, or if liver enzymes exceed 3 times the upper limit of reference range.

● CONCEPTION AND CONTRACEPTION Effective contraception essential for women of child-bearing potential during treatment and for up to 2 years after treatment. In patients undergoing treatment with teriflunomide that are planning to conceive, the accelerated elimination procedure should be used prior to conception. Use of non-oral contraception is recommended during the accelerated elimination procedure—consult product literature.
● PREGNANCY Avoid—toxicity in animal studies.
● BREAST FEEDING Present in milk in *animal* studies—manufacturer advises avoid.
● HEPATIC IMPAIRMENT Avoid in severe impairment.
● MONITORING REQUIREMENTS
▶ Monitor full blood count (including differential white cell count and platelet count) before treatment and as clinically indicated during treatment.
▶ Monitor blood pressure before treatment and periodically thereafter.
▶ Hepatic monitoring Monitor liver function before treatment and every 2 weeks for first 6 months then every 8 weeks thereafter or as clinically indicated (pre-existing liver disease may increase risk). Increase to weekly monitoring if alanine aminotransferase (ALT) is 2–3 times the upper limit of reference range; discontinue treatment if signs or symptoms of hepatic injury, or if liver enzymes exceed 3 times the upper limit of reference range.
● TREATMENT CESSATION
Accelerated elimination procedures To aid drug elimination in case of serious adverse effect or before conception, stop treatment and give *either* colestyramine p. 180 *or* charcoal, activated p. 1201. After the accelerated elimination procedure a plasma concentration of less than 20 micrograms/litre (measured on 2 occasions at least 14 days apart) and a waiting period of one and a half months are necessary before conception.
● NATIONAL FUNDING/ACCESS DECISIONS
NICE technology appraisals (TAs)
▶ Teriflunomide for treating relapsing-remitting multiple sclerosis (January 2014) NICE TA303
Teriflunomide is recommended for the treatment of adults with active relapsing-remitting multiple sclerosis (normally defined as 2 clinically significant relapses in the previous 2 years), in adults who:
- do not have highly active or rapidly evolving severe relapsing-remitting multiple sclerosis **and**
- the manufacturer provides teriflunomide with the discount agreed in the patient access scheme
www.nice.org.uk/TA303

Scottish Medicines Consortium (SMC) Decisions
The *Scottish Medicines Consortium* has advised (February 2014) that the use of teriflunomide (*Aubagio*)® in NHS Scotland is restricted to use in patients with relapsing-remitting multiple sclerosis who do not have highly active disease, and only as an alternative to treatment with interferon beta or glatiramer acetate.

● MEDICINAL FORMS
There can be variation in the licensing of different medicines containing the same drug.
Tablet
▶ Aubagio (Genzyme Therapeutics Ltd) ▼
Teriflunomide 14 mg Aubagio 14mg tablets | 28 tablet [PoM] £1,037.84

Malignant disease

1 Antibody responsive malignancy

ANTINEOPLASTIC DRUGS > MONOCLONAL ANTIBODIES

Bevacizumab

● DRUG ACTION Bevacizumab is a monoclonal antibody that inhibits vascular endothelial growth factor.

● INDICATIONS AND DOSE
Treatment of metastatic colorectal cancer in combination with fluoropyrimidine-based chemotherapy | First-line treatment of metastatic breast cancer in combination with paclitaxel when treatment with other chemotherapy, including taxanes or anthracyclines is not appropriate | First-line treatment of metastatic breast cancer in combination with capecitabine when treatment with other chemotherapy, including taxanes or anthracyclines is not appropriate (patients who have received adjuvant taxane or anthracycline-containing regimens in the previous 12 months should not be treated with bevacizumab in combination with capecitabine) | Advanced or metastatic renal cell carcinoma in combination with interferon alfa-2a | First-line treatment of unresectable advanced, metastatic or recurrent non-small cell lung cancer other than predominantly squamous cell histology (In combination with platinum-based chemotherapy) | First-line treatment of advanced (FIGO stages IIIB, IIIC and IV) epithelial ovarian, fallopian tube, or primary peritoneal cancer (in combination with carboplatin and paclitaxel) | First recurrence of platinum-sensitive epithelial ovarian, fallopian tube, or primary peritoneal cancer in patients who have not been treated previously with bevacizumab or other drugs that target vascular endothelial growth factor (in combination with carboplatin and gemcitabine)
▶ BY INTRAVENOUS INFUSION
▶ Adult: (consult local protocol)

IMPORTANT SAFETY INFORMATION
MHRA/CHM ADVICE: BEVACIZUMAB AND SUNITINIB: RISK OF OSTEONECROSIS OF THE JAW (JANUARY 2011)
Treatment with bevacizumab or sunitinib may be a risk factor for the development of osteonecrosis of the jaw.
Patients treated with bevacizumab or sunitinib, who have previously received bisphosphonates, or are treated concurrently with bisphosphonates, may be particularly at risk.
Dental examination and appropriate preventive dentistry should be considered before treatment with bevacizumab or sunitinib.
If possible, invasive dental procedures should be avoided in patients treated with bevacizumab or sunitinib who have previously received, or who are currently receiving, intravenous bisphosphonates.

- CAUTIONS Elective surgery (withhold treatment and avoid for at least 28 days after major surgery or until wound fully healed) · history of arterial thromboembolism · history of cardiovascular disease (increased risk of cardiovascular events, especially in the elderly) · history of hypertension (increased risk of proteinuria—discontinue if nephrotic syndrome) · increased risk of fistulas (discontinue permanently if tracheo-oesophageal or grade 4 fistula develops) · increased risk of haemorrhage · increased risk of tumour-associated haemorrhage · intra-abdominal inflammation (risk of gastro-intestinal perforation and gall bladder perforation · uncontrolled hypertension · untreated CNS metastases
- INTERACTIONS → Appendix 1 (bevacizumab).
- SIDE-EFFECTS Abdominal pain · alopecia · anaemia · anorexia · arterial thromboembolism · asthenia · bone marrow suppression · chest pain · congestive heart failure · constipation · dehydration · diarrhoea · drowsiness · dry skin · dysarthria · dyspnoea · exfoliative dermatitis · extravasation · eye disorders · fistulas · flushing · gall bladder perforation · gastro-intestinal perforation · haemorrhage · hand-foot syndrome · headache · hypersensitivity reactions · hypertension · hyperuricaemia · hypotension · hypoxia · impaired wound healing · infection · intestinal obstruction · lethargy · mucocutaneous bleeding · nausea · necrotising fasciitis (discontinue and initiate treatment promptly) · neutropenia · oral mucositis · osteonecrosis of the jaw · peripheral neuropathy · posterior reversible encephalopathy syndrome · proteinuria · pulmonary hypertension · pyrexia · rash · rhinitis · rigors · skin discoloration · supraventricular tachycardia · syncope · taste disturbances · thrombocytopenia · thromboembolism · tumour lysis syndrome · vomiting
- CONCEPTION AND CONTRACEPTION Effective contraception required during and for at least 6 months after treatment in women.
- PREGNANCY Avoid—toxicity in *animal* studies. See also *Pregnancy and reproductive function* in Cytotoxic drugs p. 787.
- BREAST FEEDING Manufacturer advises avoid breast-feeding during and for at least 6 months after treatment.
- MONITORING REQUIREMENTS
- Monitor for necrotising fasciitis (usually secondary to wound healing complications, gastro-intestinal perforation or fistula formation)—discontinue and initiate treatment promptly.
- Monitor blood pressure.
- Monitor for congestive heart failure.
- Monitor for posterior reversible encephalopathy syndrome (presenting as seizures, headache, altered mental status, visual disturbance or cortical blindness, with or without hypertension).
- Consider dental check-up before initiating treatment (risk of osteonecrosis of the jaw).
- NATIONAL FUNDING/ACCESS DECISIONS

NICE technology appraisals (TAs)
- Bevacizumab in combination with paclitaxel and carboplatin for the first-line treatment of advanced ovarian cancer (May 2013) NICE TA284
Bevacizumab in combination with paclitaxel and carboplatin is **not** recommended for the first-line treatment of advanced ovarian cancer (including fallopian tube and primary peritoneal cancer).
www.nice.org.uk/TA284

- Cetuximab, bevacizumab and panitumumab for the treatment of metastatic colorectal cancer after first-line chemotherapy (January 2012) NICE TA242
Bevacizumab in combination with non-oxaliplatin (fluoropyrimidine-based) chemotherapy is **not** recommended for the treatment of patients with metastatic colorectal cancer that has progressed after first-line chemotherapy; see also NICE guidance Bevacizumab and cetuximab for the treatment of metastatic colorectal cancer (January 2007).
www.nice.org.uk/TA242

- Bevacizumab in combination with gemcitabine and carboplatin for the treatment of the first recurrence of platinum-sensitive advanced ovarian cancer (May 2013) NICE TA285
Bevacizumab in combination with gemcitabine and carboplatin is **not** recommended within its marketing authorisation, that is, for the treatment of the first recurrence of platinum-sensitive advanced ovarian cancer (including fallopian tube and primary peritoneal cancer) that has not been previously treated with bevacizumab or other vascular endothelial growth factor (VEGF) inhibitors or VEGF receptor-targeted agents.
www.nice.org/TA285

- Bevacizumab in combination with capecitabine for the first-line treatment of metastatic breast cancer (August 2012) NICE TA263
Bevacizumab in combinations with capecitabine is **not** recommended within its marketing authorisation for the first-line treatment of metastatic breast cancer, that is, when treatment with other chemotherapy options including taxanes or anthracyclines is not considered appropriate, or when taxanes or anthracyclines have been used as part of adjuvant treatment in the previous 12 months.
www.nice.org.uk/TA263

- Bevacizumab in combination with a taxane for the first-line treatment of metastatic breast cancer (February 2011) NICE TA214
Bevacizumab in combination with a taxane is **not** recommended for the first-line treatment of metastatic breast cancer.
www.nice.org.uk/TA214

- Bevacizumab in combination with oxaliplatin and either fluorouracil plus folinic acid or capecitabine for the treatment of metastatic colorectal cancer (December 2010) NICE TA212
Bevacizumab in combination with oxaliplatin and either fluorouracil plus folinic acid or capecitabine is **not** recommended for the treatment of metastatic colorectal cancer.
www.nice.org.uk/TA212

- Bevacizumab and cetuximab for the treatment of metastatic colorectal cancer (January 2007) NICE TA118
Bevacizumab in combination with fluorouracil plus folinic acid, with or without irinotecan, is **not** recommended for the first-line treatment of metastatic colorectal cancer; see also NICE guidance Cetuximab, bevacizumab and panitumumab for the treatment of metastatic colorectal cancer after first-line chemotherapy.
www.nice.org.uk/TA118

- Bevacizumab (first-line), sorafenib (first and second-line), sunitinib (second-line) and temsirolimus (first-line) for the treatment of advanced or metastatic renal cell carcinoma (August 2009) NICE TA178
Bevacizumab, sorafenib, and temsirolimus are **not** recommended as first-line treatments for people with advanced or metastatic renal cell carcinoma. Sorafenib and sunitinib are not recommended as second-line treatments for people with advanced or metastatic renal cell carcinoma.
www.nice.org.uk/TA178

8

Immune system and malignant disease

8

Immune system and malignant disease

Scottish Medicines Consortium (SMC) Decisions
The *Scottish Medicines Consortium* has advised (April 2012)
that bevacizumab (*Avastin*®) is **not** recommended for use
within NHS Scotland for the first line treatment of patients
with metastatic breast cancer in whom treatment with
other chemotherapy options including taxanes or
anthracyclines is not considered appropriate.

The *Scottish Medicines Consortium* has advised (August
2015) that bevacizumab (*Avastin*®) is accepted for
restricted use within NHS Scotland in combination with
paclitaxel for the treatment of adult patients with
platinum-resistant recurrent epithelial ovarian, fallopian
tube, or primary peritoneal cancer who received no more
than two prior chemotherapy regimens and who have not
received prior therapy with bevacizumab or other vascular
endothelial growth factor (VEGF) inhibitors or VEGF
receptor-targeted agents.

The *Scottish Medicines Consortium* has advised (October
2015) that bevacizumab (*Avastin*®) is accepted for
restricted use within NHS Scotland in combination with
carboplatin and paclitaxel for the first-line treatment of
advanced FIGO stage IV epithelial ovarian, fallopian tube,
or primary peritoneal cancer.

● MEDICINAL FORMS
There can be variation in the licensing of different medicines
containing the same drug. Forms available from special-order
manufacturers include: solution for injection
Solution for infusion
▸ Avastin (Roche Products Ltd)
    Bevacizumab 25 mg per 1 ml Avastin 400mg/16ml solution for
    infusion vials | 1 vial PoM £924.40 (Hospital only)
    Avastin 100mg/4ml solution for infusion vials | 1 vial PoM £242.66
    (Hospital only)

Brentuximab vedotin

● INDICATIONS AND DOSE
**Treatment of relapsed or refractory CD-30 positive
Hodgkin's disease following autologous stem cell
transplant or following at least two prior therapies,
when autologous stem cell transplant or multi-agent
chemotherapy is not a treatment option | Relapsed or
refractory systemic anaplastic large cell lymphoma**
    ▸ BY INTRAVENOUS INFUSION
    ▸ Adult: (consult product literature)

● CAUTIONS Elevated BMI—risk of hyperglycaemia · high
tumour burden—risk of tumour lysis syndrome · rapidly
proliferating tumours—risk of tumour lysis syndrome
● INTERACTIONS → Appendix 1 (brentuximab vedotin).
● SIDE-EFFECTS
▸ **Common or very common** Anaphylaxis · arthralgia · back
pain · constipation · cough · demyelinating polyneuropathy
· diarrhoea · dizziness · dyspnoea · fatigue · hyperglycaemia
· infusion-related reactions · myalgia · peripheral
neuropathy · pruritus · rash
▸ **Uncommon** Stevens-Johnson syndrome
▸ **Frequency not known** Alopecia · bone-marrow suppression
· extravasation · hyperuricaemia · nausea · oral mucositis ·
progressive multifocal leucoencephalopathy ·
thromboembolism · tumour lysis syndrome · vomiting
● CONCEPTION AND CONTRACEPTION Effective
contraception required during treatment and for 6 months
after treatment in men and women.
● PREGNANCY Avoid unless potential benefit outweighs risk
(toxicity in *animal* studies).
● BREAST FEEDING Avoid—no information available.

● MONITORING REQUIREMENTS
▸ Monitor for symptoms of progressive multifocal
leucoencephalopathy (presenting as new or worsening
neurological, cognitive or behavioural signs or symptoms).
▸ Monitor for new or worsening abdominal pain—
investigate and withhold treatment if acute pancreatitis
suspected and discontinue if confirmed (fatal cases
reported).
▸ Monitor for pulmonary toxicity—treat symptoms
promptly.
▸ Routinely monitor hepatic function.
▸ Monitor for infusion-related (including anaphylactic)
reactions.
▸ Monitor for signs of peripheral neuropathy—consult
product literature for treatment adjustment.

● MEDICINAL FORMS
There can be variation in the licensing of different medicines
containing the same drug.
Powder for solution for infusion
ELECTROLYTES: May contain Sodium
▸ Adcetris (Takeda UK Ltd) ▼
    Brentuximab vedotin 50 mg Adcetris 50mg powder for concentrate
    for solution for infusion vials | 1 vial PoM £2,500.00

Catumaxomab

● INDICATIONS AND DOSE
**Treatment of malignant ascites in patients with epithelial
cell adhesion molecule (EpCAM) positive carcinomas,
where standard therapy is not available or no longer
feasible**
    ▸ BY INTRAPERITONEAL INFUSION
    ▸ Adult: (consult product literature)

● CAUTIONS Haemodynamic insufficiency ·
hypoproteinaemia · oedema
● INTERACTIONS → Appendix 1 (catumaxomab).
● SIDE-EFFECTS
▸ **Common or very common** Abdominal pain · anorexia ·
anxiety · arthralgia · cholangitis · constipation · cough ·
dehydration · diarrhoea · dizziness · dyspepsia · dyspnoea ·
electrolyte disturbances · flatulence · flushing · haematuria
· headache · hyperglycaemia · hypertension · hypotension ·
hypoxia · ileus · infection · insomnia · leucocyturia ·
myalgia · pleural effusion · proteinuria · rash · skin
reactions · sweating · tachycardia · vertigo
▸ **Uncommon** Acute renal failure · gastro-intestinal
haemorrhage · intestinal obstruction · seizures
▸ **Frequency not known** Alopecia · bone-marrow suppression
· extravasation · hyperuricaemia · infusion related side-
effects · nausea · oral mucositis · thromboembolism ·
tumour lysis syndrome · vomiting
SIDE-EFFECTS, FURTHER INFORMATION
▸ Infusion-related side-effects Infusion-related side-effects
have been reported with catumaxomab; premedication
with analgesics, antipyretics, or NSAIDs is recommended
by the manufacturer.
● CONCEPTION AND CONTRACEPTION Contraceptive advice
required, see *Pregnancy and reproductive function* in
Cytotoxic drugs p. 787.
● PREGNANCY Avoid—limited information available.
● BREAST FEEDING Avoid—limited information available.

- MEDICINAL FORMS
There can be variation in the licensing of different medicines containing the same drug.

Solution for infusion

▸ Removab (Neovii Biotech GmbH)

Catumaxomab 100 microgram per 1 ml Removab 50micrograms/0.5ml concentrate for solution for infusion pre-filled syringes | 1 pre-filled disposable injection PoM £2,550.00 (Hospital only)

Removab 10micrograms/0.1ml concentrate for solution for infusion pre-filled syringes | 1 pre-filled disposable injection PoM £510.00 (Hospital only)

Cetuximab

- INDICATIONS AND DOSE

Treatment of wild-type RAS metastatic colorectal cancer in patients with tumours expressing epidermal growth factor receptor, as combination therapy, or as monotherapy if oxaliplatin- and irinotecan-based therapy has failed or if irinotecan is not tolerated | **Treatment of locally advanced squamous cell cancer of the head and neck (in combination with radiotherapy)** | **Treatment of recurrent or metastatic squamous cell cancer of the head and neck (in combination with platinum-based chemotherapy)**

▸ BY INTRAVENOUS INFUSION

▸ Adult (initiated by a specialist): (consult product literature or local protocols)

IMPORTANT SAFETY INFORMATION

MHRA/CHM ADVICE: EPIDERMAL GROWTH FACTOR RECEPTOR (EGFR) INHIBITORS: SERIOUS CASES OF KERATITIS AND ULCERATIVE KERATITIS (MAY 2012)

Keratitis and ulcerative keratitis have been reported following treatment with epidermal growth factor receptor (EGFR) inhibitors for cancer (cetuximab, erlotinib, gefitinib and panitumumab). In rare cases, this has resulted in corneal perforation and blindness. Patients undergoing treatment with EGFR inhibitors who present with acute or worsening signs and symptoms suggestive of keratitis should be referred promptly to an opthalmology specialist. Treatment should be interupted or discontinued if ulcerative keratitis is diagnosed.

Patients must receive an antihistamine and a corticosteroid at least one hour before infusion. Resuscitation facilities should be available and treatment should be initiated by a specialist.

- CONTRA-INDICATIONS Combination of cetuximab with oxaliplatin-containing chemotherapy is contra-indicated in patients with metastatic colorectal cancer who have mutant or unknown *RAS* status · *RAS* mutated colorectal tumours (or if *RAS* tumour status unknown)
- CAUTIONS Cardiopulmonary disease · cardiovascular disease · history of keratitis · pulmonary disease— discontinue if interstitial lung disease · risk factors for keratitis · severe dry eye · ulcerative keratitis (including contact lens use)
- INTERACTIONS → Appendix 1 (cetuximab).
- SIDE-EFFECTS
▸ **Common or very common** Acne · aseptic meningitis · blepharitis · bronchospasm · chills · conjunctivitis · desquamation · diarrhoea · dizziness · dry skin · dyspnoea · fever · headache · hypertension · hypertrichosis · hypocalcaemia · hypomagnesaemia · hypotension · infusion-related reactions · keratitis · nail disorders · nausea · pruritus · rash · severe (sometimes fatal) hypersensitivity reactions (possibly delayed onset) · shock · skin reactions · urticaria · vomiting

▸ **Very rare** Stevens-Johnson syndrome · toxic epidermal necrolysis

- CONCEPTION AND CONTRACEPTION Contraceptive advice required, see *Pregnancy and reproductive function* in Cytotoxic drugs p. 787.
- PREGNANCY Use only if potential benefit outweighs risk— no information available. See also *Pregnancy and reproductive function* in Cytotoxic drugs p. 787.
- BREAST FEEDING Avoid breast-feeding during and for 2 months after treatment—no information available.
- PRE-TREATMENT SCREENING Evidence of non-mutated (wild-type) *RAS* status (at exons 2, 3 and 4 of *KRAS* and *NRAS*) is required before cetuximab is initiated for the treatment of metastatic colorectal cancer, and should be determined by an experienced laboratory using a validated test method.
- DIRECTIONS FOR ADMINISTRATION Resuscitation facilities should be available.
- NATIONAL FUNDING/ACCESS DECISIONS

NICE technology appraisals (TAs)

▸ **Cetuximab for the treatment of locally advanced squamous cell cancer of the head and neck (June 2008)** NICE TA145
Cetuximab in combination with radiotherapy is an option for the treatment of locally advanced squamous cell cancer of the head and neck in patients who have a Karnofsky performance status of 90% or greater and when all forms of platinum-based chemoradiotherapy treatment are contra-indicated.
www.nice.org.uk/TA145

▸ **Cetuximab for the treatment of recurrent or metastatic squamous cell cancer of the head and neck (June 2009)** NICE TA172
Cetuximab in combination with platinum-based chemotherapy is **not** recommended for the treatment of recurrent or metastatic squamous cell cancer of the head and neck.
www.nice.org.uk/TA172

▸ **Cetuximab for the first-line treatment of metastatic colorectal cancer (August 2009)** NICE TA176
Cetuximab in combination with fluorouracil, folinic acid and oxaliplatin is an option for the first-line treatment of metastatic colorectal cancer under the following circumstances:
  - the primary tumour has been resected or is potentially operable;
  - the metastatic disease is confined to the liver and is unresectable; and
  - the patient is fit to undergo surgery to resect the primary colorectal tumour and to undergo liver surgery if the metastases become resectable after treatment with cetuximab.
In patients unable to tolerate oxaliplatin, or in whom oxaliplatin is contra-indicated, cetuximab in combination with fluorouracil, folinic acid and irinotecan can be used as an alternative.
In addition, the manufacturer is required to rebate 16% of the amount of cetuximab used per patient when used in combination with fluorouracil, folinic acid, and oxaliplatin.
Patients who meet the above criteria should receive cetuximab for no more than 16 weeks. At 16 weeks, cetuximab should be stopped and the patient should be assessed for resection of liver metastases.
www.nice.org.uk/TA176

▸ **Cetuximab, bevacizumab and panitumumab for the treatment of metastatic colorectal cancer after first-line chemotherapy (January 2012)** NICE TA242
Cetuximab monotherapy or combination chemotherapy is **not** recommended for the treatment of patients with metastatic colorectal cancer that has progressed after first-line chemotherapy.
www.nice.org.uk/TA242

8

Immune system and malignant disease

Scottish Medicines Consortium (SMC) Decisions
The *Scottish Medicines Consortium* has advised (December 2014) that cetuximab (*Erbitux®*) is accepted for restricted use within NHS Scotland, in combination with irinotecan or oxaliplatin-based chemotherapy, for the treatment of RAS wild-type metastatic colorectal cancer in patients who have not previously received chemotherapy for their metastatic disease (first-line treatment).

● MEDICINAL FORMS
There can be variation in the licensing of different medicines containing the same drug.
Solution for infusion
▸ Erbitux (Merck Serono Ltd)
Cetuximab 5 mg per 1 ml Erbitux 100mg/20ml solution for infusion vials | 1 vial [PoM] £178.10 (Hospital only)
Erbitux 500mg/100ml solution for infusion vials | 1 vial [PoM] £890.50 (Hospital only)

Ipilimumab

● DRUG ACTION Ipilimumab causes T-cell activation.

● INDICATIONS AND DOSE
Treatment of unresectable or metastatic advanced melanoma
▸ BY INTRAVENOUS INFUSION
▸ Adult: (consult product literature)

● CAUTIONS
CAUTIONS, FURTHER INFORMATION
For full details consult product literature.
● INTERACTIONS → Appendix 1 (ipilimumab).
● SIDE-EFFECTS Infusion-related side-effects
SIDE-EFFECTS, FURTHER INFORMATION
For further information on side-effects, (including monitoring and management of side effects) consult product literature.
▸ Immune-related reactions A corticosteroid can be used after starting ipilimumab, to treat immune-related reactions.
● CONCEPTION AND CONTRACEPTION Use effective contraception.
● PREGNANCY Avoid unless potential benefit outweighs risk (toxicity in *animal* studies).
● BREAST FEEDING Discontinue breast-feeding—no information available.
● HEPATIC IMPAIRMENT Use with caution if plasma-bilirubin concentration greater than 3 times upper limit of normal range *or* if plasma-transaminase concentration 5 times or greater than the upper limit of normal range.
● MONITORING REQUIREMENTS For information on monitoring of side effects, consult product literature.
● PRESCRIBING AND DISPENSING INFORMATION Infusion-related side-effects have been reported; premedication with paracetamol and an antihistamine is recommended.
● NATIONAL FUNDING/ACCESS DECISIONS
NICE technology appraisals (TAs)
▸ **Ipilimumab for previously untreated advanced (unresectable or metastatic) melanoma (July 2014)** NICE TA319
Ipilimumab is recommended, within its marketing authorisation, as an option for treating adults with previously untreated advanced (unresectable or metastatic) melanoma, only if the manufacturer provides ipilimumab with the discount agreed in the patient access scheme.
www.nice.org.uk/TA319
▸ **Ipilimumab for previously treated advanced (unresectable or metastatic) melanoma (December 2012)** NICE TA268
Ipilimumab is recommended as an option for the treatment of advanced (unresectable or metastatic) melanoma in patients who have received prior therapy,

only if the manufacturer provides ipilimumab with the discount agreed in the patient access scheme.
www.nice.org.uk/TA268
Scottish Medicines Consortium (SMC) Decisions
The *Scottish Medicines Consortium* has advised (March 2013) that ipilimumab (*Yervoy®*) is accepted for restricted use within NHS Scotland for the treatment of advanced (unresectable or metastatic) melanoma in adults who have received prior therapy, only whilst ipilimumab is available at the price agreed in the patient access scheme.

● MEDICINAL FORMS
There can be variation in the licensing of different medicines containing the same drug.
Solution for infusion
ELECTROLYTES: May contain Sodium
▸ Yervoy (Bristol-Myers Squibb Pharmaceuticals Ltd) ▼
Ipilimumab 5 mg per 1 ml Yervoy 50mg/10ml concentrate for solution for infusion vials | 1 vial [PoM] £3,750.00 (Hospital only)
Yervoy 200mg/40ml concentrate for solution for infusion vials | 1 vial [PoM] £15,000.00 (Hospital only)

[F 771]

Obinutuzumab

● INDICATIONS AND DOSE
Treatment of previously untreated chronic lymphocytic leukaemia in patients for whom full-dose fludarabine-based therapy is unsuitable due to co-morbidities
▸ BY INTRAVENOUS INFUSION
▸ Adult: (consult product literature or local protocols)

● CONTRA-INDICATIONS
CONTRA-INDICATIONS, FURTHER INFORMATION
For obinutuzumab contra-indications, consult product literature.
● CAUTIONS
CAUTIONS, FURTHER INFORMATION
For full details on the cautions of obinutuzumab, consult product literature.
▸ Hepatitis B infection and reactivation Hepatitis B infection and reactivation (including fatal cases) have been reported in patients taking **obinutuzumab**. Patients with positive hepatitis B serology should be referred to a liver specialist for monitoring and initiation of antiviral therapy before treatment initiation; treatment should not be initiated in patients with evidence of current hepatitis B infection until the infection has been adequately treated. Patients should be closely monitored for clinical and laboratory signs of active hepatitis B infection during treatment and for up to a year following the last infusion (consult product literature).
● INTERACTIONS → Appendix 1 (obinutuzumab).
● SIDE-EFFECTS
SIDE-EFFECTS, FURTHER INFORMATION
For full side effect details for obinutuzumab (including monitoring and management), consult product literature.
● CONCEPTION AND CONTRACEPTION Use effective contraception during and for 18 months after treatment.
● PREGNANCY Avoid unless potential benefit outweighs risk of B-lymphocyte depletion in fetus.
● BREAST FEEDING Avoid breast-feeding during and for 18 months after treatment—present in milk in *animal* studies.
● MONITORING REQUIREMENTS Patients should be closely monitored for clinical and laboratory signs of active hepatitis B infection during treatment and for up to a year following the last infusion (consult product literature).
● PRESCRIBING AND DISPENSING INFORMATION Infusion related side-effects have been reported; Patients should receive premedication with paracetamol, an

antihistamine, and a corticosteroid before each dose—consult product literature for details.

● NATIONAL FUNDING/ACCESS DECISIONS

NICE technology appraisals (TAs)

▸ **Obinutuzumab in combination with chlorambucil for untreated chronic lymphocytic leukaemia (June 2015)** NICE TA343

Obinutuzumab, in combination with chlorambucil, is an option for untreated chronic lymphocytic leukaemia in patients who have comorbidities that make full-dose fludarabine-based therapy unsuitable for them, only if:
● bendamustine-based therapy is not suitable **and**
● the manufacturer provides obinutuzumab with the discount agreed in the patient access scheme.

Patients currently receiving obinutuzumab that is not recommended according to the above criteria should have the option to continue treatment until they and their clinician consider it appropriate to stop.
www.nice.org.uk/TA343

● MEDICINAL FORMS

There can be variation in the licensing of different medicines containing the same drug.

Solution for infusion

▸ Gazyvaro (Roche Products Ltd) ▼
Obinutuzumab 25 mg per 1 ml Gazyvaro 1000mg/40ml concentrate for solution for infusion vials | 1 vial PoM £3,312.00 (Hospital only)

                                                              ⏴ 771

Ofatumumab

● INDICATIONS AND DOSE

Treatment of chronic lymphocytic leukaemia (CLL) in patients refractory to fludarabine and alemtuzumab | Treatment of CLL in patients who have not received prior therapy and who are not eligible for fludarabine based therapy (in combination with chlorambucil or bendamustine)

▸ BY INTRAVENOUS INFUSION
▸ Adult: Premedication must be given 30 minutes to 2 hours before each dose—consult product literature for details

● CONTRA-INDICATIONS

CONTRA-INDICATIONS, FURTHER INFORMATION
For full details on the contra-indications for ofatumumab, consult product literature.

● CAUTIONS History of cardiac disease—monitor closely and discontinue treatment if cardiac arrhythmias occur

CAUTIONS, FURTHER INFORMATION
▸ Hepatitis B infection and reactivation Hepatitis B infection and reactivation (including fatal cases) have been reported in patients taking **ofatumumab**. Patients with positive hepatitis B serology should be referred to a liver specialist for monitoring and initiation of antiviral therapy before treatment initiation; treatment should not be initiated in patients with evidence of current hepatitis B infection until the infection has been adequately treated. Patients should be closely monitored for clinical and laboratory signs of active hepatitis B infection during treatment and for up to a year following the last infusion (consult product literature).

For full details about the cautions for ofatumumab, consult product literature

● INTERACTIONS → Appendix 1 (ofatumumab).

● SIDE-EFFECTS

SIDE-EFFECTS, FURTHER INFORMATION
Infusion-related side-effects (including cytokine release syndrome) have been reported with ofatumumab; premedication with paracetamol, an antihistamine, and a corticosteroid must be given—consult product literature.

For full details (including monitoring and management of side-effects) consult product literature.

● CONCEPTION AND CONTRACEPTION Use effective contraception during and for 12 months after treatment.

● PREGNANCY Avoid unless potential benefit outweighs risk.

● BREAST-FEEDING Discontinue breast-feeding during and for 12 months after treatment—no information available.

● RENAL IMPAIRMENT No information available for creatinine clearance less than 30 mL/minute.

● MONITORING REQUIREMENTS
▸ Monitor electrolytes (including potassium and magnesium) before and during administration and correct if abnormal.
▸ Patients must be monitored closely during each infusion for the onset of infusion reactions.

● NATIONAL FUNDING/ACCESS DECISIONS

NICE technology appraisals (TAs)

▸ **Ofatumumab for the treatment of chronic lymphocytic leukaemia refractory to fludarabine and alemtuzumab (October 2010)** NICE TA202

Ofatumumab is **not** recommended for the treatment of chronic lymphocytic leukaemia that is refractory to fludarabine and alemtuzumab.

Patients currently receiving ofatumumab for this condition should have the option to continue treatment until they and their clinician consider it appropriate to stop.
www.nice.org.uk/TA202

▸ **Ofatumumab in combination with chlorambucil or bendamustine for untreated chronic lymphocytic leukaemia (June 2015)** NICE TA344

Ofatumumab in combination with chlorambucil is an option for untreated chronic lymphocytic leukaemia only if:
● the person is ineligible for fludarabine-based therapy **and**
● bendamustine is not suitable **and**
● the manufacturer provides ofatumumab with the discount agreed in the patient access scheme.

Patients currently receiving ofatumumab that is not recommended according to the above criteria should have the option to continue treatment until they and their clinician consider it appropriate to stop.
www.nice.org.uk/TA344

Scottish Medicines Consortium (SMC) Decisions

The *Scottish Medicines Consortium* has advised (April 2015) that ofatumumab (*Arzerra*®) is accepted for restricted use within NHS Scotland for the treatment of chronic lymphocytic leukaemia in patients who have not received prior therapy and who are not eligible for fludarabine-based therapy. It is restricted to use in patients who would not be considered for bendamustine therapy and who would receive chlorambucil-based therapy.

● MEDICINAL FORMS
There can be variation in the licensing of different medicines containing the same drug.

Solution for infusion
ELECTROLYTES: May contain Sodium
▸ Arzerra (Novartis Pharmaceuticals UK Ltd)
Ofatumumab 20 mg per 1 ml Arzerra 100mg/5ml concentrate for solution for infusion vials | 3 vial PoM no price available (Hospital only)
Arzerra 1000mg/50ml concentrate for solution for infusion vials | 1 vial PoM £1,820.00 (Hospital only)

Panitumumab

- DRUG ACTION Panitumumab is a monoclonal antibody that binds to the epidermal growth factor receptor (EGFR).

● INDICATIONS AND DOSE

Treatment of non-mutated RAS metastatic colorectal cancer (combination therapy) | Treatment of non-mutated RAS metastatic colorectal cancer (monotherapy after failure of fluoropyrimidine-, oxaliplatin-, and irinotecan-containing chemotherapy regimens)
- ▶ BY INTRAVENOUS INFUSION
- ▶ Adult: (consult product literature)

IMPORTANT SAFETY INFORMATION

MHRA/CHM ADVICE: SEVERE SKIN REACTIONS
Severe skin reactions have been reported very commonly in patients treated with panitumumab. Patients receiving panitumumab who have severe skin reactions or develop worsening skin reactions should be monitored for the development of inflammatory or infectious sequelae (including cellulitis, sepsis, and necrotising fasciitis). Appropriate treatment should be promptly initiated and panitumumab withheld or discontinued.

MHRA/CHM ADVICE: EPIDERMAL GROWTH FACTOR RECEPTOR (EGFR) INHIBITORS: SERIOUS CASES OF KERATITIS AND ULCERATIVE KERATITIS (MAY 2012)
Keratitis and ulcerative keratitis have been reported following treatment with epidermal growth factor receptor (EGFR) inhibitors for cancer (cetuximab, erlotinib, gefitinib and panitumumab). In rare cases, this has resulted in corneal perforation and blindness. Patients undergoing treatment with EGFR inhibitors who present with acute or worsening signs and symptoms suggestive of keratitis should be referred promptly to an opthalmology specialist. Treatment should be interupted or discontinued if ulcerative keratitis is diagnosed.

- CONTRA-INDICATIONS Interstitial pulmonary disease · the combination of panitumumab with oxaliplatin-containing chemotherapy is contra-indicated in patients with mutant *RAS* metastatic colorectal cancer or for whom *RAS* status is unknown
- CAUTIONS History of keratitis · history of severe dry eye · history of ulcerative keratitis · pulmonary disease—discontinue if interstitial lung disease develops · risk factors for keratitis · risk factors for severe dry eye · risk factors for ulcerative keratitis (including contact lens use)
- INTERACTIONS → Appendix 1 (panitumumab).
- SIDE-EFFECTS
- ▶ **Common or very common** Anorexia · anxiety · back pain · biochemical disturbances · cellulitis · cheilitis · chills · cough · deep vein thrombosis · dyspepsia · dyspnoea · electrolyte disturbances · epistaxis · eyelash growth · flushing · folliculitis · gastro-oesophageal reflux disease · hyperhydrosis · insomnia · malaise · pain in extremities · peripheral oedema · pulmonary embolism · pyrexia · rectal haemorrhage · severe hypersensitivity reactions (possibly delayed) · urinary tract infection · weight loss
- ▶ **Uncommon** Bronchospasm · cyanosis · hirsutism · infusion-related reactions · nasal dryness
- ▶ **Rare** Keratitis · skin necrosis · Stevens-Johnson syndrome · toxic epidermal necrolysis
- ▶ **Frequency not known** Abdominal pain · acne · alopecia · bone-marrow suppression · conjunctivitis · constipation · dehydration · diarrhoea · dizziness · dry eyes · dry mouth · dry skin · erythema · extravasation · hand-foot syndrome · headache · hypertension · hypertrichosis · hyperuricaemia · hypocalcaemia · hypomagnesaemia · hypotension ·

increased lacrimation · interstitial lung disease · mucosal inflammation · nail disorders · nausea · ocular disorders · ocular hyperaemia · oral mucositis · pruritus · rash · skin reactions · tachycardia · thromboembolism · tumour lysis syndrome · vomiting
- CONCEPTION AND CONTRACEPTION Manufacturer advises effective contraception during and for 6 months after treatment.
- PREGNANCY Avoid (toxicity in *animal* studies). See also *Pregnancy and reproductive function* in Cytotoxic drugs p. 787.
- BREAST FEEDING Manufacturer advises avoid breastfeeding during and for 2 months after treatment.
- PRE-TREATMENT SCREENING Evidence of non-mutated *RAS* status (at exons 2, 3 and 4 of *KRAS* and *NRAS*) is required before panitumumab treatment is initiated, and should be determined by an experienced laboratory using a validated test method.
- MONITORING REQUIREMENTS
- ▶ Monitor for hypomagnesaemia.
- ▶ Monitor for hypocalcaemia.
- ▶ Monitor for dermatological reactions including Stevens-Johnson syndrome and toxic epidermal necrolysis (consult product literature).
- NATIONAL FUNDING/ACCESS DECISIONS
  NICE technology appraisals (TAs)
- ▶ **Cetuximab, bevacizumab and panitumumab for the treatment of metastatic colorectal cancer after first-line chemotherapy (January 2012)** NICE TA242
  Panitinumab monotherapy is **not** recommended for the treatment of patients with metastatic colorectal cancer that has progressed after first-line chemotherapy.
  www.nice.org.uk/TA242
- MEDICINAL FORMS
  There can be variation in the licensing of different medicines containing the same drug.
  Solution for infusion
  ELECTROLYTES: May contain Sodium
- ▶ Vectibix (Amgen Ltd)
  Panitumumab 20 mg per 1 ml Vectibix 400mg/20ml concentrate for solution for infusion vials | 1 vial POM £1,517.16 (Hospital only)
  Vectibix 100mg/5ml concentrate for solution for infusion vials | 1 vial POM £379.29 (Hospital only)

Pembrolizumab

1.6.2016

- DRUG ACTION Pembrolizumab is a monoclonal antibody, which binds to the programmed death-1 (PD-1) receptor, thereby potentiating an immune response to tumour cells.

● INDICATIONS AND DOSE

Treatment of unresectable or metastatic advanced melanoma
- ▶ BY INTRAVENOUS INFUSION
- ▶ Adult: 2 mg/kg every 3 weeks

- CAUTIONS Patients may need pretreatment to minimise the development of adverse reactions (consult product literature)
- INTERACTIONS → Appendix 1 (pembrolizumab).
- SIDE-EFFECTS
- ▶ **Common or very common** Abdominal pain · alopecia · arthritis · blood dyscrasia · changes in hair colour · chills · colitis · constipation · cough · decreased appetite · depigmentation · diarrhoea · dizziness · dry eye · dry mouth · dry skin · eczema · erythema · headache · hepatitis · influenza-like symptoms · infusion-related reactions · insomnia · malaise · musculoskeletal pain · myositis · nausea · oedema · peripheral neuropathy · pneumonitis ·

pruritus · pyrexia · rash · shortness of breath · taste disturbances · thyroid dysfunction · vomiting
▸ **Uncommon** Adrenal insufficiency · dermatitis · diabetes mellitus · electrolyte imbalance · epilepsy · hypertension · inflammation of the pituitary gland · lethargy · lichenoid keratosis · nephritis · pancreatitis · papule · psoriasis · tenosynovitis · uveitis
▸ **Rare** Guillain-Barré syndrome · myasthenic syndrome · small intestinal perforation

SIDE-EFFECTS, FURTHER INFORMATION
▸ Immune-related reactions Most immune-related adverse reactions are reversible and managed by temporarily stopping treatment and administration of a corticosteroid—consult product literature for further information.
▸ Infusion-related reactions Manufacturer advises to permanently discontinue treatment in patients with severe infusion reactions.
● CONCEPTION AND CONTRACEPTION Manufacturer recommends effective contraception during treatment and for at least 4 months after treatment in women of childbearing potential.
● PREGNANCY Manufacturer advises avoid unless potential benefit outweighs risk—no information available
● BREAST FEEDING Manufacturer advises avoid—no information available.
● MONITORING REQUIREMENTS Manufacturer advises monitor for signs and symptoms of infusion- and immune-related reactions.
● DIRECTIONS FOR ADMINISTRATION For *intravenous infusion* (*Keytruda®*), give intermittently in Sodium chloride 0.9% or Glucose 5%. Reconstitute each 50 mg vial with 2.3 mL water for injection, to produce a 25 mg/mL solution. Gently swirl without shaking to dissolve, and allow up to 5 minutes for the bubbles to clear. Withdraw the required volume and transfer into an intravenous bag containing infusion fluid to prepare a final concentration ranging from 1–10 mg/mL; give over 30 minutes.
● HANDLING AND STORAGE Manufacturer advises store in a refrigerator at 2–8°C.
● PATIENT AND CARER ADVICE Patients should be provided with an alert card and advised to keep it with them at all times.
● NATIONAL FUNDING/ACCESS DECISIONS
NICE technology appraisals (TAs)
▸ **Pembrolizumab for treating advanced melanoma after disease progression with ipilimumab (October 2015)** NICE TA357
Pembrolizumab is recommended as an option for treating advanced (unresectable or metastatic) melanoma only if:
● the disease has progressed with ipilimumab and, for BRAF V600 mutation-positive disease, a BRAF or MEK inhibitor **and**
● the manufacturer provides pembrolizumab with the discount agreed in the patient access scheme.
www.nice.org.uk/guidance/TA357
▸ **Pembrolizumab for advanced melanoma not previously treated with ipilimumab (November 2015)** NICE TA366
Pembrolizumab is recommended as an option for treating advanced (unresectable or metastatic) melanoma that has not been previously treated with ipilimumab, only if the manufacturer provides pembrolizumab with the discount agreed in the patient access scheme.
www.nice.org.uk/guidance/TA366

● MEDICINAL FORMS
There can be variation in the licensing of different medicines containing the same drug.
Powder for solution for infusion
CAUTIONARY AND ADVISORY LABELS 3
▸ Keytruda (Merck Sharp & Dohme Ltd) ▼
Pembrolizumab 50 mg Keytruda 50mg powder for concentrate for solution for infusion vials | 1 vial [PoM] £1,315.00 (Hospital only)

Pertuzumab

● DRUG ACTION Pertuzumab is a recombinant humanised monoclonal antibody, and acts by inhibiting human epidermal growth factor receptor 2 protein (HER2) dimerisation.

● INDICATIONS AND DOSE
Treatment of HER2-positive metastatic or locally recurrent unresectable breast cancer in combination with trastuzumab and docetaxel, in patients who have not received previous anti-HER2 therapy or chemotherapy (initiated by a specialist)
▸ BY INTRAVENOUS INFUSION
▸ Adult: (consult product literature)

● CAUTIONS Conditions that could impair left ventricular function · history of congestive heart failure · impaired left ventricular function · prior anthracycline exposure · radiotherapy to the chest area · recent myocardial infarction · serious cardiac arrhythmia · uncontrolled hypertension
● INTERACTIONS → Appendix 1 (pertuzumab).
● SIDE-EFFECTS
▸ **Common or very common** Anaemia · arthralgia · chills · constipation · cough · decreased appetite · diarrhoea · dizziness · dry skin · dyspepsia · dyspnoea · febrile neutropenia · headache · increased lacrimation · infusion-related reactions · insomnia · left ventricular dysfunction · leucopenia · malaise · myalgia · nail disorder · nasopharyngitis · neutropenia · oedema · pain · paronychia · peripheral neuropathy · pleural effusion · pruritus · pyrexia · rash · severe hypersensitivity reactions · taste disturbance · upper respiratory-tract infection
▸ **Uncommon** Interstitial lung disease
▸ **Frequency not known** Alopecia · bone-marrow suppression · extravasation · hyperuricaemia · nausea · oral mucositis · thromboembolism · tumour lysis syndrome · vomiting
SIDE-EFFECTS, FURTHER INFORMATION
Side effects mostly described for pertuzumab in combination with trastuzumab and docetaxel.
● CONCEPTION AND CONTRACEPTION Ensure effective contraception during and for six months after treatment in women of childbearing potential.
● PREGNANCY Avoid (toxicity in *animal* studies). Most cytotoxic drugs are teratogenic and should not be administered during pregnancy, especially during the first trimester. Considerable caution is necessary if a pregnant woman presents with cancer requiring chemotherapy, and specialist advice should always be sought.
● BREAST FEEDING Avoid—no information available.
● HEPATIC IMPAIRMENT Caution—no information available.
● RENAL IMPAIRMENT Caution in severe impairment—no information available.
● MONITORING REQUIREMENTS
▸ Assess for signs and symptoms of congestive heart failure (including left ventricular ejection fraction) before and during treatment—consult product literature, and withhold treatment if necessary.
▸ Monitor for febrile neutropenia.

- **DIRECTIONS FOR ADMINISTRATION** Resuscitation facilities should be available.

- **MEDICINAL FORMS**
There can be variation in the licensing of different medicines containing the same drug.
Solution for infusion
▸ Perjeta (Roche Products Ltd) ▼
Pertuzumab 30 mg per 1 ml Perjeta 420mg/14ml concentrate for solution for infusion vials | 1 vial [PoM] £2,395.00 (Hospital only)

Ramucirumab
31.5.2016

- **DRUG ACTION** Ramucirumab is a human monoclonal antibody that binds to the vascular endothelial growth factor receptor-2 (VEGFR-2), inhibiting VEGF-induced angiogenesis.

- **INDICATIONS AND DOSE**

Treatment of advanced gastric cancer or gastro-oesophageal junction adenocarcinoma, in combination with paclitaxel, in patients with disease progression after prior platinum and fluoropyrimidine chemotherapy
▸ BY INTRAVENOUS INFUSION
▸ Adult: 8 mg/kg on days 1 and 15 of a 28 day cycle, dose to be administered prior to paclitaxel infusion, consult product literature for dose adjustments due to side-effects and infusion-related reactions

Treatment of advanced gastric cancer or gastro-oesophageal junction adenocarcinoma, as monotherapy, in patients with disease progression after prior platinum or fluoropyrimidine chemotherapy, and for whom treatment in combination with paclitaxel is not appropriate
▸ BY INTRAVENOUS INFUSION
▸ Adult: 8 mg/kg every 2 weeks, consult product literature for dose adjustments due to side-effects and infusion-related reactions

Treatment of metastatic colorectal cancer, in combination with FOLFIRI (irinotecan, fluorouracil and folinic acid), in patients with disease progression on or, after, prior therapy with bevacizumab, oxaliplatin and a fluoropyrimidine
▸ BY INTRAVENOUS INFUSION
▸ Adult: 8 mg/kg every 2 weeks, dose to be administered prior to FOLFIRI administration, consult product literature for dose adjustments due to side-effects and infusion-related reactions

Treatment of locally advanced or metastatic non-small cell lung cancer, in combination with docetaxel, in patients with disease progression after platinum-based chemotherapy
▸ BY INTRAVENOUS INFUSION
▸ Adult: 10 mg/kg on day 1 of a 21 day cycle, dose to be administered prior to docetaxel infusion, consult product literature for dose adjustments due to side-effects and infusion-related reactions

- **CAUTIONS** Elective surgery—discontinue treatment for at least 4 weeks prior to surgery · hypertension—must be controlled before initiation · impaired wound healing—discontinue treatment until wound fully healed · pretreatment is recommended to minimise the development of adverse reactions (consult product literature) · risk of bleeding

- **INTERACTIONS** → Appendix 1 (ramucirumab).

- **SIDE-EFFECTS**
▸ **Common or very common** Abdominal pain · diarrhoea · epistaxis · gastro-intestinal haemorrhage · headache · hypertension · hypoalbuminaemia · hypokalaemia · hyponatraemia · leucopenia · malaise · mucosal

inflammation · neutropenia · palmar-plantar erthyrodysaesthesia syndrome · peripheral oedema · proteinuria · stomatitis · thrombocytopenia
▸ **Frequency not known** Arterial thromboembolic events (permanently discontinue if severe) · fistula (permanently discontinue) · gastro-intestinal perforation (permanently discontinue) · infusion-related reactions · intestinal obstruction · rash · sepsis (in combination with paclitaxel)

SIDE-EFFECTS, FURTHER INFORMATION
▸ Infusion-related reactions Infusion-related hypersensitivity reactions have been reported with ramucirumab, particularly during or following the first or second infusion; if the patient experiences a grade 1 or 2 infusion-related reaction, the manufacturer advises to reduce rate of infusion by 50% and give premedication for all subsequent infusions—consult product literature. Manufacturer advises to permanently discontinue treatment in the event of a grade 3 or 4 infusion-related reaction.

- **CONCEPTION AND CONTRACEPTION** Manufacturer advises effective contraception during treatment and for up to 3 months after treatment in women of childbearing potential.

- **PREGNANCY** Manufacturer advises avoid unless potential benefit outweighs risk—no information available.

- **BREAST FEEDING** Manufacturer advises discontinue breast-feeding during treatment and for at least 3 months after treatment—no information available.

- **HEPATIC IMPAIRMENT** Manufacturer advises caution in severe cirrhosis, cirrhosis with hepatic encephalopathy, cirrhosis with clinically significant ascites, or hepatorenal syndrome—use only if potential benefit outweighs risk of progressive hepatic failure.

- **MONITORING REQUIREMENTS** Manufacturer advises monitor for signs of infusion-related hypersensitivity reactions; monitor blood pressure prior to each infusion; monitor for development or worsening of proteinuria during treatment—consult product literature; monitor blood counts and coagulation parameters in patients at risk of bleeding.

- **DIRECTIONS FOR ADMINISTRATION** For *intravenous infusion* (*Cyramza®*), give intermittently *in* Sodium chloride 0.9%; dilute requisite dose with infusion fluid to final volume of 250 mL and invert gently to mix. Do not exceed a rate of 25 mg/minute, and give over approximately 60 minutes via an infusion pump using a separate infusion line with a protein sparing 0.22 micron filter.

- **PRESCRIBING AND DISPENSING INFORMATION** For *Cyramza®*, each 10 mL vial contains sodium 17 mg (equivalent to Na+ 0.74 mmol).

- **NATIONAL FUNDING/ACCESS DECISIONS**
NICE technology appraisals (TAs)
▸ Ramucirumab for treating advanced gastric cancer or gastro-oesophageal junction adenocarcinoma previously treated with chemotherapy (January 2016) NICE TA378
Ramucirumab alone or in combination with paclitaxel is **not** recommended for the treatment of advanced gastric cancer or gastro-oesophageal junction adenocarcinoma previously treated with chemotherapy.
    Patients whose treatment was started before this guidance was published, should have the option to continue treatment until they and their clinician consider it appropriate to stop.
www.nice.org.uk/TA378

- MEDICINAL FORMS
There can be variation in the licensing of different medicines containing the same drug.
Solution for infusion
ELECTROLYTES: May contain Sodium
▸ Cyramza (Eli Lilly and Company Ltd) ▼
Ramucirumab 10 mg per 1 ml Cyramza 100mg/10ml concentrate for solution for infusion vials | 1 vial [PoM] £500.00 (Hospital only)
Cyramza 500mg/50ml concentrate for solution for infusion vials | 1 vial [PoM] £2,500.00 (Hospital only)

⚑ 771

Rituximab

- INDICATIONS AND DOSE

Treatment of severe active rheumatoid arthritis in patients whose condition has not responded adequately to other disease-modifying antirheumatic drugs (including one or more tumour necrosis factor inhibitors) or who are intolerant of them (in combination with methotrexate)
▸ BY INTRAVENOUS INFUSION
▸ Adult: 1 g, then 1 g after 2 weeks, patients should receive premedication before each infusion (consult product literature for details)

Treatment of previously untreated stage III–IV follicular lymphoma (in combination with other chemotherapy) | Maintenance therapy in patients with follicular non-Hodgkin's lymphoma that has responded to induction therapy (in combination with other chemotherapy) | Treatment of diffuse large B-cell non-Hodgkin's lymphoma (in combination with other chemotherapy) | Treatment of chemotherapy-resistant or relapsed stage III–IV follicular non-Hodgkin's lymphoma | Previously untreated or relapsed chronic lymphocytic leukaemia | Induction of remission in patients with severe, active granulomatosis with polyangiitis (Wegener's) and microscopic polyangiitis (in combination with glucocorticoids)
▸ BY INTRAVENOUS INFUSION
▸ Adult: Patients should receive premedication before each dose (consult product literature for details) (consult product literature or local protocols)

- CONTRA-INDICATIONS Severe heart failure (when used to treat granulomatosis with polyangiitis or microscopic polyangiitis) · severe infection · severe, uncontrolled heart disease (when used to treat granulomatosis with polyangiitis or microscopic polyangiitis)
CONTRA-INDICATIONS, FURTHER INFORMATION
For full details on contra-indications, consult product literature.

- CAUTIONS
GENERAL CAUTIONS
History of cardiovascular disease; in adults exacerbation of angina, arrhythmia, and heart failure have been reported · patients receiving cardiotoxic chemotherapy; in adults exacerbation of angina, arrhythmia, and heart failure have been reported · transient hypotension occurs frequently during infusion (anti-hypertensives may need to be withheld for 12 hours before infusion)
SPECIFIC CAUTIONS
▸ When used for rheumatoid arthritis Predisposition to infection
CAUTIONS, FURTHER INFORMATION
▸ Hepatitis B infection and reactivation Hepatitis B infection and reactivation (including fatal cases) have been reported in patients taking **rituximab**. Patients with positive hepatitis B serology should be referred to a liver specialist for monitoring and initiation of antiviral therapy before treatment initiation; treatment should not be initiated in patients with evidence of current hepatitis B infection until the infection has been adequately treated. Patients should be closely monitored for clinical and laboratory signs of active hepatitis B infection during treatment and for up to a year following the last infusion (consult product literature).
For full details on cautions, consult product literature or local treatment protocol.

- INTERACTIONS → Appendix 1 (rituximab).

- SIDE-EFFECTS Abdominal pain · anaemia · antibody formation · aplastic anaemia · arthralgia · asthenia · blood disorders · depression · dyspepsia · headache · hypertension · hypotension · injection-site reactions · leucopenia · lupus erythematosus-like syndrome · migraine · muscle spasm · pancytopenia · paraesthesia · progressive multifocal leucoencephalopathy · pruritus · rhinitis · severe fatal skin reactions · severe skin reactions (permanently discontinue treatment if occurs) · sore throat · Stevens-Johnson syndrome (permanently discontinue treatment if occurs) · thrombocytopenia · toxic epidermal necrolysis (permanently discontinue treatment if occurs) · urticaria · worsening heart failure
SIDE-EFFECTS, FURTHER INFORMATION
Associated with infections, sometimes severe, including tuberculosis, septicaemia, and hepatitis B reactivation.
▸ Progressive multifocal leucoencephalopathy Progressive multifocal leucoencephalopathy (which is usually fatal or causes severe disability) has been reported in association with rituximab; patients should be monitored for cognitive, neurological, or psychiatric signs and symptoms. If progressive multifocal leucoencephalopathy is suspected, suspend treatment until it has been excluded.
For full details, including management of side-effects, consult product literature.

- CONCEPTION AND CONTRACEPTION Effective contraception (in both sexes) required during and for 12 months after treatment.

- PREGNANCY Avoid unless potential benefit to mother outweighs risk of B-lymphocyte depletion in fetus.

- BREAST FEEDING Avoid breast-feeding during and for 12 months after treatment.

- MONITORING REQUIREMENTS For full details on monitoring requirements consult product literature.

- DIRECTIONS FOR ADMINISTRATION
▸ With intravenous use For *intravenous infusion* (*MabThera*®), give intermittently in Glucose 5% or Sodium chloride 0.9%; dilute to 1-4 mg/mL and gently invert bag to avoid foaming.

- PATIENT AND CARER ADVICE
Alert card Patients treated for granulomatosis with polyangiitis and microscopic polyangiitis or rheumatoid arthritis should be provided with a patient alert card with each infusion.

- NATIONAL FUNDING/ACCESS DECISIONS
NICE technology appraisals (TAs)
▸ Rituximab in combination with glucocorticoids for treating anti-neutrophil cytoplasmic antibody-associated vasculitis (March 2014) NICE TA308
This NICE guidance was issued for rituximab by intravenous infusion. Rituximab, in combination with glucocorticoids, is recommended as an option for inducing remission in adults with anti-neutrophil cytoplasmic antibody [ANCA]-associated vasculitis (severely active granulomatosis with polyangiitis [Wegener's] and microscopic polyangiitis), only if:
- further cyclophosphamide treatment would exceed the maximum cumulative cyclophosphamide dose, **or**
- cyclophosphamide is contra-indicated or not tolerated, **or**
- the patient has not completed their family, and treatment with cyclophosphamide may materially affect their fertility, **or**

8

Immune system and malignant disease

- the disease has remained active or progressed despite a course of cyclophosphamide lasting 3–6 months **or**
- the patient has had uroepithelial malignancy.
www.nice.org.uk/TA308

▸ **Adalimumab, etanercept, infliximab, rituximab, and abatacept for the treatment of rheumatoid arthritis after the failure of a TNF inhibitor (August 2010)** NICE TA195
Rituximab, in combination with methotrexate, is an option for the treatment of severe active rheumatoid arthritis in adults who have had an inadequate response to, or are intolerant of, other disease-modifying antirheumatic drugs (DMARDs), including at least 1 tumour necrosis factor (TNF) inhibitor. Repeat courses of rituximab should be given no more frequently than every 6 months, and should only be continued if an adequate response is achieved and maintained.
www.nice.org.uk/TA195

▸ **Rituximab for the first-line treatment of stage III-IV follicular lymphoma (January 2012)** NICE TA243
This NICE guidance was issued for rituximab by intravenous infusion. Rituximab, in combination with:
- cyclophosphamide, vincristine and prednisolone (CVP);
- cyclophosphamide, doxorubicin, vincristine and prednisolone (CHOP);
- mitoxantrone, chlorambucil and prednisolone (MCP);
- cyclophosphamide, doxorubicin, etoposide, prednisolone and interferon-alfa (CHVPi); *or*
- chlorambucil
is recommended as an option for the treatment of symptomatic stage III and IV follicular lymphoma in previously untreated patients.
www.nice.org.uk/TA243

▸ **Rituximab for the treatment of relapsed or refractory stage III or IV follicular non-Hodgkin's lymphoma (February 2008)** NICE TA137
This NICE guidance was issued for rituximab by intravenous infusion. Rituximab, in combination with chemotherapy, is an option for the induction of remission in patients with relapsed stage III or IV follicular non-Hodgkin's lymphoma.
  Rituximab monotherapy as maintenance therapy is an option for the treatment of patients with relapsed stage III or IV follicular non-Hodgkin's lymphoma in remission induced with chemotherapy (with or without rituximab).
  Rituximab monotherapy is an option for the treatment of patients with relapsed or refractory stage III or IV follicular non-Hodgkin's lymphoma, when all alternative treatment options have been exhausted (that is, if there is resistance to or intolerance of chemotherapy).
www.nice.org.uk/TA137

▸ **Rituximab for the treatment of relapsed or refractory chronic lymphocytic leukaemia (July 2010)** NICE TA193
This NICE guidance was issued for rituximab by intravenous infusion. Rituximab in combination with fludarabine and cyclophosphamide is recommended as a treatment option for people with relapsed or refractory chronic lymphocytic leukaemia except when the condition:
- is refractory to fludarabine (that is, it has not responded to fludarabine, or has relapsed within 6 months of treatment), **or**
- has previously been treated with rituximab, unless it was in the context of a clinical trial, at a dose lower than the dose currently licensed for chronic lymphocytic leukaemia or with chemotherapy other than fludarabine and cyclophosphamide.
Rituximab in combination with fludarabine and cyclophosphamide is recommended only in the context of research for patients with relapsed or refractory chronic lymphocytic leukaemia that has previously been treated with rituximab, unless rituximab has been given as specified above.
www.nice.org.uk/TA193

▸ **Rituximab for the first-line maintenance treatment of follicular non-Hodgkin's lymphoma (June 2011)** NICE TA226
This NICE guidance was issued for rituximab by intravenous infusion. Rituximab maintenance therapy is recommended as an option for the treatment of people with follicular non-Hodgkins's lymphoma that has responded to first-line induction therapy with rituximab in combination with chemotherapy.
www.nice.org.uk/TA226

▸ **Rituximab for the first-line treatment of chronic lymphocytic leukaemia (July 2009)** NICE TA174
This NICE guidance was issued for rituximab by intravenous infusion. Rituximab, in combination with fludarabine and cyclophosphamide, is recommended as an option for the first-line treatment of chronic lymphocytic leukaemia.
www.nice.org.uk/TA174

▸ **Idelalisib for treating chronic lymphocytic leukaemia (October 2015)** NICE TA359
Rituximab, in combination with idelalisib, is recommended as an option for treatment in adults:
- who have untreated chronic lymphocytic leukaemia **or**
- who have chronic lymphocytic leukaemia when the disease has been treated but has relapsed within 24 months **and**
- if the manufacturer provides idelalisib with the discount agreed in the simple discount agreement.
Patients who are already receiving idelalisib should continue treatment until they or their clinician consider it appropriate to stop.
www.nice.org.uk/guidance/TA359

▸ **Rituximab for aggressive non-Hodgkin's lymphoma (September 2003)** NICE TA65
This NICE guidance was issued for rituximab by intravenous infusion. Rituximab, in combination with cyclophosphamide, doxorubicin, vincristine, and prednisolone, is recommended for first-line treatment of CD20-positive diffuse large-B-cell lymphoma at clinical stage II, III or IV.
  The use of rituximab for localised (stage I) disease should be limited to clinical trials.
www.nice.org.uk/TA65

Scottish Medicines Consortium (SMC) Decisions
The *Scottish Medicines Consortium* has advised (August 2013) that Rituximab (*MabThera*®) is accepted for restricted use within NHS Scotland, in combination with glucocorticoids for the induction of remission in adult patients with severe, active granulomatosis with polyangiitis (Wegener's) and microscopic polyangiitis. It is restricted to use in patients who have relapsed following treatment with cyclophosphamide or who are intolerant to or unable to receive cyclophosphamide.
  The *Scottish Medicines Consortium* has advised (June 2014) that subcutaneous rituximab (*MabThera*)® is accepted for restricted use within NHS Scotland, in accordance with UK licensing, except in the maintenance setting, where use is restricted to patients who have responded to induction therapy with rituximab plus chemotherapy.

● MEDICINAL FORMS
There can be variation in the licensing of different medicines containing the same drug.
Solution for infusion
▸ MabThera (Roche Products Ltd)
  Rituximab 10 mg per 1 ml MabThera 100mg/10ml concentrate for solution for infusion vials | 2 vial [PoM] £349.25
  MabThera 500mg/50ml concentrate for solution for infusion vials | 1 vial [PoM] £873.15

Siltuximab

- **DRUG ACTION** Siltuximab is a monoclonal antibody that inhibits interleukin-6 receptor binding.

  - **INDICATIONS AND DOSE**

  Treatment of multicentric Castleman's disease (MCD) in patients who are human immunodeficiency virus (HIV) negative and human herpesvirus-8 (HHV-8) negative
  - ▸ BY INTRAVENOUS INFUSION
  - ▸ Adult: 11 mg/kg every 3 weeks

- **CAUTIONS** Patients at increased risk of gastrointestinal perforation—promptly investigate those presenting with symptoms suggestive of gastrointestinal perforation · severe infection—withhold treatment until resolved · treat infection prior to treatment

  CAUTIONS, FURTHER INFORMATION
- ▸ Hypersensitivity reactions Infusion-related side-effects are reported commonly with siltuximab; resuscitation facilities should be available during treatment.
    Consult product literature for further information about siltuximab cautions.

- **INTERACTIONS** → Appendix 1 (siltuximab).
  Live vaccines should not be given concurrently or within 4 weeks before starting siltuximab treatment.

- **SIDE-EFFECTS**
- ▸ **Common or very common** Infusion related side effects
- ▸ **Frequency not known** Abdominal pain · anaphylaxis · hepatitis B reactivation · hypersensitivity reactions · hypertension · hypertriglyceridaemia · hypoglobulinaemia · increased haemoglobin levels · infections · localised oedema · maculopapular rash · nasopharyngitis · neutropenia · pruritus · renal impairment · thrombocytopenia · upper respiratory tract infection · weight gain

  SIDE-EFFECTS, FURTHER INFORMATION
- ▸ Infusion-related side effects Siltuximab therapy should be discontinued permanently in the event of a severe infusion-related reaction, anaphylaxis, a severe allergic reaction, or the occurrence of cytokine-release syndrome. Mild to moderate infusion-related reactions may improve by temporarily reducing the rate or stopping the infusion. When restarting treatment, a reduced infusion rate and the administration of antihistamines, paracetamol, and corticosteroids should be considered. Consider discontinuation of siltuximab if more than 2 doses are delayed due to treatment-related toxicities during the first 48 weeks—for full details consult product literature.

- **CONCEPTION AND CONTRACEPTION** Women of childbearing potential should use effective contraception during and for 3 months after treatment.

- **PREGNANCY** Manufacturer advises avoid unless potential benefit outweighs risk.

- **BREAST FEEDING** Manufacturer advises avoid—no information available.

- **HEPATIC IMPAIRMENT** Use with caution in hepatic impairment.

- **MONITORING REQUIREMENTS**
- ▸ Monitor neutrophil and platelet count, and haemoglobin levels prior to each dose of siltuximab treatment for the first 12 months and thereafter prior to every third dosing cycle. Consider delaying treatment if required neutrophil, platelet, and haemoglobin levels not achieved—consult product literature for details.
- ▸ Monitor for infection during treatment.

- **DIRECTIONS FOR ADMINISTRATION** For *intravenous infusion* (*Sylvant*®), give intermittently *in* Glucose 5%. Allow vials to reach room temperature over approximately 30 minutes, then reconstitute each 100 mg vial with 5.2 mL of water for injection, and each 400 mg vial with 20 mL of

water for injection, to produce a 20 mg/mL solution. Gently swirl without shaking to dissolve. Further dilute to 250 mL with glucose 5% and gently mix. Use within 6 hours of dilution and give over 60 minutes using an administration set lined with polyvinyl chloride or polyurethane, through a low-protein binding in-line 0.2 micron filter.

- **MEDICINAL FORMS**
  There can be variation in the licensing of different medicines containing the same drug.
  Powder for solution for infusion
  - ▸ Sylvant (Janssen-Cilag Ltd) ▼
    Siltuximab 100 mg Sylvant 100mg powder for concentrate for solution for infusion vials | 1 vial PoM £415.00 (Hospital only)
    Siltuximab 400 mg Sylvant 400mg powder for concentrate for solution for infusion vials | 1 vial PoM £1,661.00 (Hospital only)

Trastuzumab   24.2.2016

- **INDICATIONS AND DOSE**

  Treatment of early breast cancer which overexpresses human epidermal growth factor receptor-2 (HER2) (initiated by a specialist) | Treatment of metastatic breast cancer in patients with HER2-positive tumours who have not received chemotherapy for metastatic breast cancer and in whom anthracycline treatment is inappropriate (in combination with paclitaxel or docetaxel) (initiated by a specialist) | Treatment of metastatic breast cancer in postmenopausal patients with hormone-receptor positive HER2-positive tumours not previously treated with trastuzumab (in combination with an aromatase inhibitor) (initiated by a specialist)
  - ▸ BY INTRAVENOUS INFUSION, OR BY SUBCUTANEOUS INJECTION
  - ▸ Adult: (consult product literature or local protocols)

  Monotherapy for metastatic breast cancer in patients with tumours that overexpress HER2 who have received at least 2 chemotherapy regimens including, where appropriate, an anthracycline and a taxane (initiated by a specialist)
  - ▸ BY INTRAVENOUS INFUSION, OR BY SUBCUTANEOUS INJECTION
  - ▸ Adult: Women with oestrogen-receptor-positive breast cancer should also have received hormonal therapy (consult product literature or local protocols)

  Treatment of metastatic gastric cancer in patients with HER2-positive tumours who have not received treatment for metastatic gastric cancer (in combination with capecitabine or fluorouracil and cisplatin) (initiated by a specialist)
  - ▸ BY INTRAVENOUS INFUSION
  - ▸ Adult: (consult product literature or local protocols)

- **CONTRA-INDICATIONS** Severe dyspnoea at rest

- **CAUTIONS** Coronary artery disease · history of hypertension · symptomatic heart failure · uncontrolled arrhythmias

- **INTERACTIONS** → Appendix 1 (trastuzumab)
- ▸ Use with anthracyclines Cardiac function should be monitored closely on the concomitant use of trastuzumab with anthracyclines.

- **SIDE-EFFECTS** Acne · alopecia · alopecia · anaphylaxis · angioedema · anxiety · arthralgia · arthritis · asthenia · bone pain · bone-marrow suppression · cardiotoxicity · chest pain · chills · depression · dizziness · drowsiness · dry eye · dry skin · ecchymosis · extravasation · fever · gastro-intestinal symptoms · headache · hepatitis · hypersensitivity reactions · hypertension · hypertonia · hyperuricaemia · hypotension · increased lacrimation · infection · infusion-related side-effects (possibly delayed onset) · insomnia · leg cramps · malaise · mastitis · myalgia · nail disorders · nausea · oedema · oral mucositis ·

8

Immune system and malignant disease

paraesthesia · paresis · peripheral neuropathy · pruritus · pulmonary events (possibly delayed onset) · rash · sweating · taste disturbance · thromboembolism · tremor · tumour lysis syndrome · urticaria · vomiting · weight loss

- CONCEPTION AND CONTRACEPTION Contraceptive advice required, see *Pregnancy and reproductive function* in Cytotoxic drugs p. 787.
- PREGNANCY Manufacturer advises avoid—oligohydramnios reported. See also *Pregnancy and reproductive function* in Cytotoxic drugs p. 787.
- BREAST FEEDING Avoid breast-feeding during treatment and for 7 months afterwards.
- MONITORING REQUIREMENTS
▶ Cardiotoxicity Monitor cardiac function before and during treatment—for details of monitoring and managing cardiotoxicity, consult product literature.
- DIRECTIONS FOR ADMINISTRATION Resuscitation facilities should be available during administration of trastuzumab.
- PRESCRIBING AND DISPENSING INFORMATION When prescribing, dispensing or administering, check that this is the correct preparation—trastuzumab is **not** interchangeable with trastuzumab emtansine.
- NATIONAL FUNDING/ACCESS DECISIONS

NICE technology appraisals (TAs)
▶ **Lapatinib or trastuzumab in combination with an aromatase inhibitor for the first-line treatment of metastatic hormone-receptor-positive breast cancer that overexpresses HER2 (June 2012)** NICE TA257
Lapatinib or trastuzumab in combination with an aromatase inhibitor is **not** recommended for first-line treatment in postmenopausal women of metastatic hormone-receptor-positive breast cancer that overexpresses human epidermal growth factor receptor 2 (HER2).

Postmenopausal women currently receiving lapatinib or trastuzumab in combination with an aromatase inhibitor for this indication should have the option to continue treatment until they and their clinician consider it appropriate to stop.
www.nice.org.uk/TA257

▶ **Guidance on the use of trastuzumab for the treatment of advanced breast cancer (March 2002)** NICE TA34
Trastuzumab in combination with paclitaxel is recommended as an option for patients with tumours expressing human epidermal growth factor receptor 2 (HER2) scored at levels of 3+ who have not received chemotherapy for metastatic breast cancer, and in whom anthracycline treatment is inappropriate.

Trastuzumab monotherapy is recommended as an option for patients with tumours expressing HER2 scored at levels of 3+ who have received at least two chemotherapy regimens for metastatic breast cancer. Prior chemotherapy must have included at least an anthracycline and a taxane where these treatments are appropriate. It should also have included hormonal therapy in suitable oestrogen-receptor-positive patients.
www.nice.org.uk/TA34

▶ **Trastuzumab for the adjuvant treatment of early-stage HER2-positive breast cancer (August 2006)** NICE TA107
Trastuzumab, given at 3-week intervals for 1 year or until disease recurrence (whichever is the shorter period), is recommended as an option for women with early-stage HER2-positive breast cancer following surgery, chemotherapy (neoadjuvant or adjuvant) and radiotherapy (if applicable).
www.nice.org.uk/TA107

▶ **Trastuzumab for the treatment of HER2-positive metastatic gastric cancer (November 2010)** NICE TA208
Trastuzumab in combination with cisplatin and capecitabine or fluorouracil is recommended for human epidermal growth factor receptor-2-positive metastatic

adenocarcinoma of the stomach or gastro-oesophageal junction in patients who:
- have not received treatment for metastatic disease **and**
- have tumours expressing high levels of HER2 as defined by a positive immunohistochemistry score of 3.
www.nice.org.uk/TA208

Scottish Medicines Consortium (SMC) Decisions
The *Scottish Medicines Consortium* has advised (December 2013) that subcutaneous trastuzumab injection (*Herceptin®*) is accepted for restricted use within NHS Scotland for the treatment of adults with HER2 positive metastatic breast cancer and early breast cancer, when used within licensed indications excluding use in combination with an aromatase inhibitor for the treatment of postmenopausal patients with hormone-receptor positive metastatic breast cancer, not previously treated with trastuzumab.

The *Scottish Medicines Consortium* has advised (September 2015) that trastuzumab solution for infusion (*Herceptin®*) is accepted for restricted use within NHS Scotland in combination with capecitabine or fluorouracil and cisplatin for the treatment of patients with HER2 positive metastatic adenocarcinoma of the stomach or gastro-oesophageal junction, who have not received prior anti-cancer treatment for their metastatic disease. It is restricted to patients with metastatic gastric cancer whose tumours have HER2 over-expression, as determined by an accurate and validated assay.

- MEDICINAL FORMS
There can be variation in the licensing of different medicines containing the same drug.
Solution for injection
▶ Herceptin (Roche Products Ltd)
Trastuzumab 120 mg per 1 ml Herceptin 600mg/5ml solution for injection vials | 1 vial [PoM] £1,222.20 (Hospital only)
Powder for solution for infusion
▶ Herceptin (Roche Products Ltd)
Trastuzumab 150 mg Herceptin 150mg powder for solution for infusion vials | 1 vial [PoM] £407.40

Trastuzumab emtansine
15.4.2016

- DRUG ACTION Trastuzumab emtansine is an antibody-drug conjugate that contains trastuzumab covalently linked to DM1, a cytotoxic microtubule inhibitor.

- INDICATIONS AND DOSE
Monotherapy for the treatment of HER2-positive, unresectable, locally advanced or metastatic breast cancer, in adult patients who have previously received trastuzumab and a taxane separately or in combination (initiated by a specialist) | Monotherapy for the treatment of HER2-positive, unresectable, locally advanced or metastatic breast cancer, in adult patients who have developed disease recurrence during or within 6 months of completing adjuvant therapy (initiated by a specialist)
▶ BY INTRAVENOUS INFUSION
▶ Adult: (consult product literature or local protocols)

- CAUTIONS Dyspnoea at rest—increased risk of pulmonary events · history of congestive heart failure · patients over 75 years · peripheral neuropathy (temporarily discontinue treatment—consult product literature) · recent history of myocardial infarction · recent history of unstable angina · risk of left ventricular dysfunction—consult product literature for specific risks with trastuzumab treatment · serious arrhythmias
- INTERACTIONS → Appendix 1 (trastuzumab).
Caution with concomitant anticoagulant medication—increased risk of thrombocytopenia with haemorrhagic events.

- SIDE-EFFECTS
▶ **Common or very common** Abdominal pain · arthralgia · blurred vision · chills · conjunctivitis · constipation · cough · diarrhoea · dizziness · dry eye · dry mouth · dysgeusia · dyspepsia · dyspnoea · epistaxis · gingival bleeding · haemorrhage · hand-foot syndrome · headache · hypertension · hypokalaemia · increased lacrimation · infusion-related reactions · insomnia · left ventricular dysfunction · malaise · memory impairment · myalgia · nail disorder · peripheral neuropathy · peripheral oedema · pruritus · pyrexia · rash · thrombocytopenia · urinary tract infection · urticaria
▶ **Uncommon** Hepatic failure · hepatic toxicity · interstitial lung disease · nodular regenerative hyperplasia · pneumonitis · portal hypertension
▶ **Frequency not known** Alopecia · bone-marrow suppression · extravasation · hyperuricaemia · nausea · oral mucositis · thromboembolism · tumour lysis syndrome · vomiting

- CONCEPTION AND CONTRACEPTION Effective contraception must be used during and for 6 months after stopping treatment in women and men.

- PREGNANCY Manufacturer advises avoid—oligohydramnios reported with trastuzumab. See also Pregnancy and reproductive function in Cytotoxic drugs below.

- BREAST FEEDING Manufacturer advises avoid breast-feeding during and for 6 months after treatment.

- HEPATIC IMPAIRMENT Consult product literature for dose modification in cases of abnormal liver function tests. Consult product literature for initiating treatment and discontinuation in cases of abnormal liver function tests.

- RENAL IMPAIRMENT No information available—manufacturer advises caution in severe impairment.

- MONITORING REQUIREMENTS
▶ Monitor hepatic function before each dose.
▶ Monitor for signs and symptoms of neurotoxicity.
▶ Monitor closely for infusion-related and hypersensitivity reactions.
▶ Monitor platelet count before each dose and as clinically indicated (consult product literature for treatment modification in thrombocytopenia).
▶ Test cardiac function before treatment and regularly during treatment—delay or discontinue treatment in cases of left ventricular dysfunction.
▶ Monitor for dyspnoea, cough, fatigue and pulmonary infiltrates—discontinue if interstitial lung disease or pneumonitis confirmed (fatal cases reported).

- DIRECTIONS FOR ADMINISTRATION Resuscitation facilities should be available during administration of trastuzumab emtansine.

- PRESCRIBING AND DISPENSING INFORMATION When prescribing, dispensing or administering, check that this is the correct preparation— trastuzumab emtansine and trastuzumab are **not** interchangeable.

- NATIONAL FUNDING/ACCESS DECISIONS
  NICE technology appraisals (TAs)
▶ **Trastuzumab emtansine for treating HER2-positive, unresectable locally advanced or metastatic breast cancer after treatment with trastuzumab and a taxane (December 2015)** NICE TA371
  Trastuzumab emtansine is **not** recommended for treating adults with human epidermal growth factor 2 (HER2) positive, unresectable locally advanced or metastatic breast cancer previously treated with trastuzumab and a taxane.
  www.nice.org.uk/TA371
  Scottish Medicines Consortium (SMC) Decisions
  The *Scottish Medicines Consortium* has advised (September 2014) trastuzumab emtansine (*Kadcyla*®) is **not** recommended for use within NHS Scotland as

monotherapy for the treatment of adult patients with human epidermal growth factor type 2 (HER2)-positive, unresectable locally advanced or metastatic breast cancer who previously received trastuzumab and a taxane, separately or in combination.

- MEDICINAL FORMS
  There can be variation in the licensing of different medicines containing the same drug.
  Powder for solution for infusion
▶ Kadcyla (Roche Products Ltd) ▼
  Trastuzumab emtansine 100 mg Kadcyla 100mg powder for concentrate for solution for infusion vials | 1 vial [PoM] £1,641.01
  Trastuzumab emtansine 160 mg Kadcyla 160mg powder for concentrate for solution for infusion vials | 1 vial [PoM] £2,625.62

2 Cytotoxic responsive malignancy

Cytotoxic drugs

Overview

The chemotherapy of cancer is complex and should be confined to specialists in oncology. Cytotoxic drugs have both anti-cancer activity and the potential to damage normal tissue; most cytotoxic drugs are teratogenic. Chemotherapy may be given with a curative intent or it may aim to prolong life or to palliate symptoms. In an increasing number of cases chemotherapy may be combined with radiotherapy or surgery or both as either neoadjuvant treatment (initial chemotherapy aimed at shrinking the primary tumour, thereby rendering local therapy less destructive or more effective) or as adjuvant treatment (which follows definitive treatment of the primary disease, when the risk of subclinical metastatic disease is known to be high). All cytotoxic drugs cause side-effects and a balance has to be struck between likely benefit and acceptable toxicity.

Combinations of cytotoxic drugs, as continuous or pulsed cycles of treatment, are frequently more toxic than single drugs but have the advantage in certain tumours of enhanced response, reduced development of drug resistance and increased survival. However for some tumours, single-agent chemotherapy remains the treatment of choice.

Cytotoxic drugs fall into a number of classes, each with characteristic antitumour activity, sites of action, and toxicity. A knowledge of sites of metabolism and excretion is important because impaired drug handling as a result of disease is not uncommon and may result in enhanced toxicity.

Guidelines for handling cytotoxic drugs

- Trained personnel should reconstitute cytotoxics
- Reconstitution should be carried out in designated pharmacy areas
- Protective clothing (including gloves, gowns, and masks) should be worn
- The eyes should be protected and means of first aid should be specified
- Pregnant staff should avoid exposure to cytotoxic drugs (all females of child-bearing age should be informed of the reproductive hazard)
- Use local procedures for dealing with spillages and safe disposal of waste material, including syringes, containers, and absorbent material
- Staff exposure to cytotoxic drugs should be monitored

Intrathecal chemotherapy

A Health Service Circular (HSC 2008/001) provides guidance on the introduction of safe practice in NHS Trusts where intrathecal chemotherapy is administered; written local guidance covering all aspects of national guidance should be available.Support for training programmes is also available.

Copies, and further information may be obtained from:
Department of Health
PO Box 777
London
SE1 6XH
Fax: 01623 724524

It is also available from the Department of Health website (www.dh.gov.uk).

Safe systems for cytotoxic medicines

NHS cancer networks have been established across the UK to bring together all stakeholders in all sectors of care, to work collaboratively to plan and deliver high quality cancer services for a given population. NHS cancer networks have websites containing information on local chemotherapy services and treatment.

Safe systems requirements:

- cytotoxic drugs for the treatment of cancer should be given as part of a wider pathway of care coordinated by a multidisciplinary team
- cytotoxic drugs should be prescribed, dispensed, and administered only in the context of a written protocol or treatment plan
- injectable cytotoxic drugs should only be dispensed if they are prepared for administration
- oral cytotoxic medicines should be dispensed with clear directions for use

> **IMPORTANT SAFETY INFORMATION**
>
> RISK OF INCORRECT DOSING OF ORAL ANTI-CANCER MEDICINES
> The National Patient Safety Agency has advised (January 2008) that the prescribing and use of oral cytotoxic medicines should be carried out to the same standard as parenteral cytotoxic therapy.
> - non-specialists who prescribe or administer on-going oral cytotoxic medication should have access to written protocols and treatment plans, including guidance on the monitoring and treatment of toxicity;
> - staff dispensing oral cytotoxic medicines should confirm that the prescribed dose is appropriate for the patient. Patients should have written information that includes details of the intended oral anti-cancer regimen, the treatment plan, and arrangements for monitoring, taken from the original protocol from the initiating hospital. Staff dispensing oral cytotoxic medicines should also have access to this information, and to advice from an experienced cancer pharmacist in the initiating hospital.

Doses

Doses of cytotoxic drugs are determined using a variety of different methods including body-surface area or body-weight. Alternatively, doses may be fixed. Doses may be further adjusted following consideration of a patient's neutrophil count, renal and hepatic function, and history of previous adverse effects to the cytotoxic drug. Doses may also differ depending on whether a drug is used alone or in combination.

Because of the complexity of dosage regimens in the treatment of malignant disease, dose statements have been omitted from some of the drug entries in this chapter. However, even where dose statements have been provided, detailed specialist literature, individual hospital chemotherapy protocols, or local cancer networks should be consulted before prescribing, dispensing, or administering cytotoxic drugs.

Prescriptions should **not** be repeated except on the instructions of a specialist.

Side-effects of cytotoxic drugs

Side-effects common to most cytotoxic drugs are discussed below whilst side-effects characteristic of a particular drug or class of drugs (e.g. neurotoxicity with vinca alkaloids) are mentioned in the appropriate sections. Manufacturers' product literature, hospital-trust protocols, and cancer-network protocols should be consulted for full details of side-effects associated with individual drugs and specific chemotherapy regimes.

Many side-effects of cytotoxic drugs often do not occur at the time of administration, but days or weeks later. It is therefore important that patients and healthcare professionals can identify symptoms that cause concern and can contact an expert for advice. Toxicities should be accurately recorded using a recognised scoring system such as the Common Toxicity Criteria for Adverse Events (CTCAE) developed by the National Cancer Institute.

Extravasation of intravenous drugs

A number of cytotoxic drugs will cause severe local tissue necrosis if leakage into the extravascular compartment occurs. To reduce the risk of extravasation injury it is recommended that cytotoxic drugs are administered by appropriately trained staff. See information on the prevention and management of extravasation injury.

Oral mucositis

A sore mouth is a common complication of cancer chemotherapy; it is most often associated with fluorouracil p. 805, methotrexate p. 807, and the anthracyclines. It is best to prevent the complication. Good oral hygiene (rinsing the mouth frequently and effective brushing of the teeth with a soft brush 2–3 times daily) is probably beneficial. For fluorouracil p. 805, sucking ice chips during short infusions of the drug is also helpful.

Once a sore mouth has developed, treatment is much less effective. Saline mouthwashes should be used but there is no good evidence to support the use of antiseptic or anti-inflammatory mouthwashes. In general, mucositis is self-limiting but with poor oral hygiene it can be a focus for blood-borne infection.

Tumour lysis syndrome

Tumour lysis syndrome occurs secondary to spontaneous or treatment-related rapid destruction of malignant cells. Patients at risk of tumour lysis syndrome include those with non-Hodgkin's lymphoma (especially if high grade and bulky disease), Burkitt's lymphoma, acute lymphoblastic leukaemia and acute myeloid leukaemia (particularly if high white blood cell counts or bulky disease), and occasionally those with solid tumours. Pre-existing hyperuricaemia, dehydration, and renal impairment are also predisposing factors. Features include hyperkalaemia, hyperuricaemia (see below), and hyperphosphataemia with hypocalcaemia; renal damage and arrhythmias can follow. Early identification of patients at risk, and initiation of prophylaxis or therapy for tumour lysis syndrome, is essential.

Hyperuricaemia

Hyperuricaemia, which may be present in high-grade lymphoma and leukaemia, can be markedly worsened by chemotherapy and is associated with acute renal failure. Allopurinol p. 968 should be started 24 hours before treating such tumours and patients should be adequately hydrated. The dose of mercaptopurine p. 806 or azathioprine p. 757 should be reduced if allopurinol needs to be given concomitantly.

Rasburicase p. 828, a recombinant urate oxidase, is licensed for hyperuricaemia in patients with haematological malignancy. It rapidly reduces plasma-uric acid concentration and may be of particular value in preventing complications following treatment of leukaemias or bulky lymphomas.

Bone-marrow suppression

All cytotoxic drugs except vincristine sulfate p. 820 and bleomycin p. 811 cause bone-marrow suppression. This commonly occurs 7 to 10 days after administration, but is delayed for certain drugs, such as carmustine p. 792, lomustine p. 795, and melphalan p. 795. Peripheral blood counts must be checked before each treatment, and doses should be reduced or therapy delayed if bone-marrow has not recovered.

Cytotoxic drugs may be contra-indicated in patients with acute infection; any infection should be treated before, or when starting, cytotoxic drugs.

Fever in a neutropenic patient (neutrophil count less than 1.06×10^9/litre) requires immediate broad-spectrum antibacterial therapy. Appropriate bacteriological investigations should be conducted as soon as possible. Patients taking cytotoxic drugs who have signs or symptoms of infection should be advised to seek prompt medical attention. All patients should initially be investigated and treated under the supervision of the appropriate oncology or haematology specialist.

In selected patients, the duration and the severity of neutropenia can be reduced by the use of recombinant human granulocyte-colony stimulating factors.

Symptomatic anaemia is usually treated with red blood cell transfusions. For guidance on the use of erythropoietins in patients with cancer, see MHRA/CHM advice and NICE guidance.

See advice on the use of live vaccines in individuals with impaired immune response, see Vaccines.

Alopecia

Reversible hair loss is a common complication, although it varies in degree between drugs and individual patients. No pharmacological methods of preventing this are available.

Thromboembolism

Venous thromboembolism can be a complication of cancer itself, but chemotherapy increases the risk.

Pregnancy and reproductive function

Most cytotoxic drugs are teratogenic and should not be administered during pregnancy, especially during the first trimester. Considerable caution is necessary if a pregnant woman presents with cancer requiring chemotherapy, and specialist advice should always be sought.

Exclude pregnancy before treatment with cytotoxic drugs. Contraceptive advice should be given before cytotoxic therapy begins- women of childbearing age should use effective contraception during and after treatment.

Regimens that do not contain an alkylating drug or procarbazine may have less effect on fertility, but those with an alkylating drug or procarbazine carry the risk of causing permanent male sterility (there is no effect on potency). Pretreatment counselling and consideration of sperm storage may be appropriate. Women are less severely affected, though the span of reproductive life may be shortened by the onset of a premature menopause. No increase in fetal abnormalities or abortion rate has been recorded in patients who remain fertile after cytotoxic chemotherapy.

Nausea and vomiting

Nausea and vomiting cause considerable distress to many patients who receive chemotherapy and to a lesser extent abdominal radiotherapy, and may lead to refusal of further treatment; prophylaxis of nausea and vomiting is therefore extremely important. Symptoms may be acute (occurring within 24 hours of treatment), delayed (first occurring more than 24 hours after treatment), or anticipatory (occurring prior to subsequent doses). Delayed and anticipatory symptoms are more difficult to control than acute symptoms and require different management.

Patients vary in their susceptibility to drug-induced nausea and vomiting; those affected more often include women, patients under 50 years of age, anxious patients, and those who experience motion sickness. Susceptibility also increases with repeated exposure to the cytotoxic drug.

Drugs may be divided according to their emetogenic potential and some examples are given below, but the symptoms vary according to the dose, to other drugs administered and to the individual's susceptibility to emetogenic stimuli.

Mildly emetogenic treatment—fluorouracil, etoposide p. 814, methotrexate p. 807 (less than 100 mg/m², low dose in children), the vinca alkaloids, and abdominal radiotherapy.

Moderately emetogenic treatment—the taxanes, doxorubicin hydrochloride p. 798, intermediate and low doses of cyclophosphamide p. 793, mitoxantrone p. 800, and high doses of methotrexate ($0.1– 1.2$ g/m²).

Highly emetogenic treatment—cisplatin p. 813, dacarbazine p. 793, and high doses of cyclophosphamide.

Prevention of acute symptoms

For patients at *low risk of emesis*, pretreatment with dexamethasone p. 610 or lorazepam p. 308 may be used.

For patients at *high risk of emesis*, a 5HT3-receptor antagonist, usually given by mouth in combination with dexamethasone and the neurokinin receptor antagonist aprepitant p. 396 is effective.

Prevention of delayed symptoms

For delayed symptoms associated with moderately emetogenic chemotherapy, a combination of dexamethasone and 5HT$_3$-receptor antagonist is effective; for highly emetogenic chemotherapy, a combination of dexamethasone and aprepitant is effective. Metoclopramide hydrochloride p. 395 is also licensed for delayed chemotherapy-induced nausea and vomiting.

Prevention of anticipatory symptoms

Good symptom control is the best way to prevent anticipatory symptoms. Lorazepam can be helpful for its amnesic, sedative, and anxiolytic effects.

Treatment for cytotoxic-induced side effects

Anthracycline side-effects

Anthracycline-induced cardiotoxicity

The anthracycline cytotoxic drugs are associated with dose-related, cumulative, and potentially life-threatening cardiotoxic side-effects.

Anthracycline extravasation

Local guidelines for the management of extravasation should be followed or specialist advice sought.

See further information on the prevention and management of extravasation injury.

Chemotherapy-induced mucositis and myelosuppression

Folinic acid p. 827 (given as calcium folinate) is used to counteract the folate-antagonist action of methotrexate p. 807 and thus speed recovery from methotrexate-induced mucositis or myelosuppression ('folinic acid rescue').

Folinic acid is also used in the management of methotrexate overdose, together with other measures to maintain fluid and electrolyte balance, and to manage possible renal failure.

Folinic acid does not counteract the antibacterial activity of folate antagonists such as trimethoprim p. 521.

When folinic acid and fluorouracil p. 805 are used together in metastatic colorectal cancer the response-rate improves compared to that with fluorouracil alone.

The calcium salt of levofolinic acid p. 828, a single isomer of folinic acid, is also used for rescue therapy following methotrexate administration, for cases of methotrexate overdose, and for use with fluorouracil for colorectal cancer.

The dose of calcium levofolinate is generally half that of calcium folinate.

The disodium salts of folinic acid and levofolinic acid are also used for rescue therapy following methotrexate therapy, and for use with fluorouracil for colorectal cancer.

Urothelial toxicity

Haemorrhagic cystitis is a common manifestation of urothelial toxicity which occurs with the oxazaphosphorines, cyclophosphamide p. 793 and ifosfamide p. 794; it is caused by the metabolite acrolein. Mesna p. 827 reacts specifically with this metabolite in the urinary tract, preventing toxicity. Mesna is used routinely (preferably by mouth) in patients receiving ifosfamide, and in patients receiving cyclophosphamide by the intravenous route at a high dose (e.g. more than 2 g) or in those who experienced urothelial toxicity when given cyclophosphamide previously.

Anthracyclines and other cytotoxic antibiotics

Drugs in this group are widely used. Many cytotoxic antibiotics act as radiomimetics and simultaneous use of radiotherapy should be **avoided** because it may markedly increased toxicity. Daunorubicin p. 797, doxorubicin hydrochloride p. 798, epirubicin hydrochloride p. 799 and idarubicin hydrochloride p. 799 are anthracycline antibiotics. Mitoxantrone p. 800 is an anthracycline derivative.

Doxorubicin hydrochloride is available as both *conventional* and *liposomal* formulations. The different formulations vary in their licensed indications, pharmacokinetics, dosage and administration, and are not interchangeable. *Conventional* doxorubicin hydrochloride is used to treat the acute leukaemias, Hodgkin's and non-Hodgkin's lymphomas, paediatric malignancies, and some solid tumours including breast cancer.

Epirubicin hydrochloride is structurally related to doxorubicin hydrochloride and clinical trials suggest that it is as effective in the treatment of breast cancer.

Idarubicin hydrochloride has general properties similar to those of doxorubicin hydrochloride; it is mostly used in the treatment of haematological malignancies.

Daunorubicin also has general properties similar to those of doxorubicin hydrochloride.

Mitoxantrone is structurally related to doxorubicin hydrochloride.

Pixantrone p. 800 is licensed as monotherapy for the treatment of refractory or multiply relapsed aggressive non-Hodgkin B-cell lymphomas, although the benefits of using it as a fifth-line or greater chemotherapy in refractory patients has not been established.

Bleomycin p. 811 is given intravenously or intramuscularly to treat metastatic germ cell cancer and, in some regimens, non-Hodgkin's lymphoma.

Dactinomycin is principally used to treat paediatric cancers. Its side-effects are similar to those of doxorubicin, except that cardiac toxicity is not a problem.

Mitomycin p. 812 is given intravenously to treat upper gastrointestinal and breast cancers and by bladder instillation for superficial bladder tumours. It causes delayed bone marrow toxicity and therefore it is usually administered at 6-weekly intervals.

Vinca alkaloids

The vinca alkaloids, vinblastine sulfate p. 819, vincristine sulfate p. 820, and vindesine sulfate p. 820, are used to treat a variety of cancers including leukaemias, lymphomas, and some solid tumours (e.g. breast and lung cancer). Vinorelbine p. 821 is a semi-synthetic vinca alkaloid. See also, role of vinorelbine in the treatment of breast cancer.

Antimetabolites

Antimetabolites are incorporated into new nuclear material or combine irreversibly with cellular enzymes, preventing normal cellular division.

Alkylating drugs

Extensive experience is available with these drugs, which are among the most widely used in cancer chemotherapy. They act by damaging DNA, thus interfering with cell replication.

Cyclophosphamide is used mainly in combination with other agents for treating a wide range of malignancies, including some leukaemias, lymphomas, and solid tumours. It is given by mouth or intravenously; it is inactive until metabolised by the liver.

Ifosfamide is related to cyclophosphamide and is given intravenously.

Melphalan p. 795 is licensed for the treatment of multiple myeloma, polycythaemia vera, childhood neuroblastoma, advanced ovarian adenocarcinoma, and advanced breast cancer. However, in practice, melphalan is rarely used for ovarian adenocarcinoma; it is no longer used for advanced breast cancer. Melphalan is also licensed for regional arterial perfusion in localised malignant melanoma of the extremities and localised soft-tissue sarcoma of the extremities.

Lomustine p. 795 is a lipid-soluble nitrosourea and the drug is given at intervals of 4 to 6 weeks.

Carmustine p. 792 has similar activity to lomustine; it is given to patients with multiple myeloma, non-Hodgkin's lymphomas, and brain tumours. Carmustine implants are licensed for intralesional use in adults for the treatment of recurrent glioblastoma multiforme as an adjunct to surgery. Carmustine implants are also licensed for high-grade malignant glioma as adjunctive treatment to surgery and radiotherapy.

Estramustine phosphate p. 794 is a combination of an oestrogen and chlormethine used predominantly in prostate cancer. It is given by mouth and has both an antimitotic effect and (by reducing testosterone concentration) a hormonal effect.

Mitobronitol is occasionally used to treat chronic myeloid leukaemia; it is available on a named-patient basis from specialist importing companies.

ANTINEOPLASTIC DRUGS > ALKYLATING AGENTS

Bendamustine hydrochloride

- **INDICATIONS AND DOSE**

Treatment of chronic lymphocytic leukaemia | Treatment of non-Hodgkin's lymphoma | Treatment of multiple myeloma
▶ BY INTRAVENOUS INFUSION
▸ Adult: (consult local protocol)

- CONTRA-INDICATIONS Jaundice · low leucocyte count · low platelet count · major surgery less than 30 days before start of treatment · severe bone marrow suppression
- CAUTIONS Avoid in Acute porphyrias p. 918 · cardiac disorders—monitor serum potassium and ECG
- INTERACTIONS → Appendix 1 (bendamustine).
- SIDE-EFFECTS
▶ **Common or very common** Amenorrhoea · angina · anorexia · arrhythmias · chills · constipation · dehydration · diarrhoea · electrolyte disturbances · haemorrhage · hypertension · hypokalaemia · hypotension · infection · insomnia · malaise · pain · palpitation · pyrexia · respiratory dysfunction
▶ **Uncommon** Pericardial effusion
▶ **Rare** Acute circulatory failure · drowsiness · sweating · voice changes
▶ **Very rare** Anticholinergic syndrome · ataxia · cardiac failure · encephalitis · haemolysis · multiple organ failure · myocardial infarction · neurological disorders · paraesthesia · peripheral neuropathy · phlebitis · pulmonary fibrosis · tachycardia · taste disturbance

▶ **Frequency not known** Alopecia · bone-marrow suppression · extravasation · hyperuricaemia · male sterility · nausea · oral mucositis · premature menopause · secondary malignancy · Stevens-Johnson syndrome · thromboembolism · toxic epidermal necrolysis · tumour lysis syndrome · vomiting

SIDE-EFFECTS, FURTHER INFORMATION
▶ Secondary malignancy Prolonged use of alkylating drugs, particularly when combined with extensive irradiation, is associated with a marked increase in the incidence of acute non-lymphocytic leukaemia.

● CONCEPTION AND CONTRACEPTION Effective contraception is required during treatment in men or women, and for 6 months after treatment in men. See also *Pregnancy and reproductive function* in Cytotoxic drugs p. 787.

● PREGNANCY Avoid (teratogenic and mutagenic in *animal* studies). See also *Pregnancy and reproductive function* in Cytotoxic drugs p. 787.

● BREAST FEEDING Discontinue breast-feeding.

● HEPATIC IMPAIRMENT Consider a 30% dose reduction in moderate impairment. Avoid in severe impairment.

● RENAL IMPAIRMENT No information available on use in patients with creatinine clearance less than 10 mL/minute.

● NATIONAL FUNDING/ACCESS DECISIONS

NICE technology appraisals (TAs)
▶ **Bendamustine for the first-line treatment of chronic lymphocytic leukaemia (February 2011)** NICE TA216
Bendamustine is recommended as an option for the treatment of chronic lymphocytic leukaemia in patients for whom fludarabine combination chemotherapy is not appropriate.
www.nice.org.uk/TA216

Scottish Medicines Consortium (SMC) Decisions
The *Scottish Medicines Consortium* has advised (March 2011) that bendamustine (*Levact* ®) is accepted for restricted use within NHS Scotland for the treatment of chronic lymphocytic leukaemia in patients for whom fludarabine combination chemotherapy is not appropriate.

● MEDICINAL FORMS
There can be variation in the licensing of different medicines containing the same drug.

Powder for solution for infusion
▶ Bendamustine hydrochloride (Non-proprietary)
  Bendamustine hydrochloride 25 mg Bendamustine 25mg powder for concentrate for solution for infusion vials | 1 vial PoM £6.85–£65.98 | 5 vial PoM no price available
  Bendamustine hydrochloride 100 mg Bendamustine 100mg powder for concentrate for solution for infusion vials | 1 vial PoM £27.77–£262.02 | 5 vial PoM no price available
▶ Levact (Napp Pharmaceuticals Ltd)
  Bendamustine hydrochloride 25 mg Levact 25mg powder for concentrate for solution for infusion vials | 5 vial PoM £347.26 (Hospital only)
  Bendamustine hydrochloride 100 mg Levact 100mg powder for concentrate for solution for infusion vials | 5 vial PoM £1,379.04 (Hospital only)

Busulfan
(Busulphan)

● INDICATIONS AND DOSE
Chronic myeloid leukaemia, induction of remission
▶ BY MOUTH
▶ Adult: 60 micrograms/kg daily (max. per dose 4 mg); maintenance 0.5–2 mg daily

Conditioning treatment before haematopoietic progenitor cell transplantation
▶ BY MOUTH, OR BY INTRAVENOUS INFUSION
▶ Adult: (consult local protocol)

Conditioning treatment before haematopoietic progenitor cell transplantation in patients who are candidates for a reduced-intensity conditioning (RIC) regimen
▶ BY INTRAVENOUS INFUSION
▶ Adult: (consult local protocol)

DOSES AT EXTREMES OF BODY-WEIGHT
Dose may need to be calculated based on body surface area or adjusted ideal body weight in obese patients— consult product literature.

IMPORTANT SAFETY INFORMATION
RISKS OF INCORRECT DOSING OF ORAL ANTI-CANCER MEDICINES
See Cytotoxic drugs p. 787.

● CAUTIONS Avoid in Acute porphyrias p. 918 · high dose (antiepileptic prophylaxis required) · history of seizures (antiepileptic prophylaxis required) · ineffective once in blast crisis phase · previous progenitor cell transplant (increased risk of hepatic veno-occlusive disease) · previous radiation therapy (increased risk of hepatic veno-occlusive disease) · risk of second malignancy · three or more cycles of chemotherapy (increased risk of hepatic veno-occlusive disease)

● INTERACTIONS → Appendix 1 (busulfan).

● SIDE-EFFECTS

GENERAL SIDE-EFFECTS
▶ **Common or very common** Cardiac tamponade in thalassaemia · hepatic fibrosis · hepatic veno-occlusive disease · hepatotoxicity · hyperbilirubinaemia · jaundice · pneumonia · skin hyperpigmentation
▶ **Rare** Aplastic anaemia · seizures · visual disturbances
▶ **Very rare** Gynaecomastia · myasthenia gravis
▶ **Frequency not known** Alopecia · bone-marrow suppression · hyperuricaemia · irreversible bone-marrow aplasia · lung toxicity · male sterility · nausea · oral mucositis · premature menopause · secondary malignancy · thromboembolism · tumour lysis syndrome · vomiting

SPECIFIC SIDE-EFFECTS
▶ With intravenous use Extravasation

SIDE-EFFECTS, FURTHER INFORMATION
▶ Lung toxicity Discontinue if lung toxicity develops.
▶ Secondary malignancy Prolonged use of alkylating drugs, particularly when combined with extensive irradiation, is associated with a marked increase in the incidence of acute non-lymphocytic leukaemia.

● CONCEPTION AND CONTRACEPTION Manufacturers advise effective contraception during and for 6 months after treatment in men or women. See also *Pregnancy and reproductive function* in Cytotoxic drugs p. 787.

● PREGNANCY Avoid (teratogenic in *animals*). See also *Pregnancy and reproductive function* in Cytotoxic drugs p. 787.

● BREAST FEEDING Discontinue breast-feeding.

● HEPATIC IMPAIRMENT Manufacturer advises caution. In patients with hepatic impairment, manufacturer advises regular liver function tests—consult product literature.

8

Immune system and malignant disease

8

Immune system and malignant disease

- MONITORING REQUIREMENTS
▸ Monitor cardiac and liver function.
▸ Frequent blood tests are necessary because excessive myelosuppression may result in irreversible bone-marrow aplasia.

- MEDICINAL FORMS
There can be variation in the licensing of different medicines containing the same drug. Forms available from special-order manufacturers include: capsule, oral suspension, oral solution

Tablet
▸ Busulfan (Non-proprietary)
  Busulfan 2 mg Busulfan 2mg tablets | 25 tablet [PoM] £69.02

Solution for infusion
▸ Busilvex (Pierre Fabre Ltd)
  Busulfan 6 mg per 1 ml Busilvex 60mg/10ml concentrate for solution for infusion ampoules | 8 ampoule [PoM] £1,610.00 (Hospital only)

Carmustine

- INDICATIONS AND DOSE

Multiple myeloma | Non-Hodgkin's lymphomas | Brain tumours
▸ BY INTRAVENOUS INFUSION
▸ Adult: (consult product literature)

Recurrent glioblastoma multiforme as an adjunct to surgery | High-grade malignant glioma as adjunctive treatment to surgery and radiotherapy
▸ BY INTRALESIONAL IMPLANTATION
▸ Adult: (consult product literature)

- CAUTIONS Avoid in Acute porphyrias p. 918
- INTERACTIONS → Appendix 1 (carmustine).
- SIDE-EFFECTS

GENERAL SIDE-EFFECTS
Alopecia · bone-marrow suppression (delayed) · hyperuricaemia · irritant to tissues · male sterility · nausea · oral mucositis · premature menopause · secondary malignancy · thromboembolism · tumour lysis syndrome · vomiting
SPECIFIC SIDE-EFFECTS
▸ With intravenous use Pulmonary fibrosis (delayed) · renal damage (cumulative)
SIDE-EFFECTS, FURTHER INFORMATION
▸ Secondary malignancy Prolonged use of alkylating drugs, particularly when combined with extensive irradiation, is associated with a marked increase in the incidence of acute non-lymphocytic leukaemia.

- CONCEPTION AND CONTRACEPTION Manufacturer advises effective contraception during treatment in men or women. See also *Pregnancy and reproductive function* in Cytotoxic drugs p. 787.
- PREGNANCY Avoid (teratogenic and embryotoxic in *animals*). See also *Pregnancy and reproductive function* in Cytotoxic drugs p. 787.
- BREAST FEEDING Discontinue breast-feeding.
- NATIONAL FUNDING/ACCESS DECISIONS

NICE technology appraisals (TAs)
▸ Carmustine implants and temozolomide for the treatment of newly diagnosed high-grade glioma (June 2007) NICE TA121
Carmustine implants are an option for the treatment of newly diagnosed high-grade (Grade 3 or 4) glioma **only** for patients in whom at least 90% of the tumour has been resected. Carmustine implants should only be used within specialist centres.
www.nice.org.uk/TA121

- MEDICINAL FORMS
There can be variation in the licensing of different medicines containing the same drug.
Implant
▸ Gliadel (Eisai Ltd)
  Carmustine 7.7 mg Gliadel 7.7mg implant | 8 device [PoM] £5,203.00 (Hospital only)

Chlorambucil

- INDICATIONS AND DOSE

Some lymphomas and chronic leukaemias (used either alone or in combination therapy)
▸ BY MOUTH
▸ Adult: (consult local protocol)

IMPORTANT SAFETY INFORMATION
RISKS OF INCORRECT DOSING OF ORAL ANTI-CANCER MEDICINES
See Cytotoxic drugs p. 787.

- CAUTIONS Avoid in Acute porphyrias p. 918 · history of epilepsy (increased seizure risk)
- SIDE-EFFECTS
▸ **Uncommon** Skin rash
▸ **Very rare** Male sterility (in prepubertal and pubertal males)
▸ **Frequency not known** Alopecia · bone-marrow suppression · hyperuricaemia · nausea · oral mucositis · premature menopause · secondary malignancy · Stevens-Johnson syndrome · thromboembolism · toxic epidermal necrolysis · tumour lysis syndrome · vomiting
SIDE-EFFECTS, FURTHER INFORMATION
▸ Secondary malignancy Prolonged use of alkylating drugs, particularly when combined with extensive irradiation, is associated with a marked increase in the incidence of acute non-lymphocytic leukaemia.
▸ Skin reactions If a rash occurs further chlorambucil is contra-indicated and cyclophosphamide is substituted.

- CONCEPTION AND CONTRACEPTION Contraceptive advice required, see *Pregnancy and reproductive function* in Cytotoxic drugs p. 787.
- PREGNANCY Avoid. See also *Pregnancy and reproductive function* in Cytotoxic drugs p. 787.
- BREAST FEEDING Discontinue breast-feeding.
- HEPATIC IMPAIRMENT Manufacturer advises consider dose reduction in severe impairment—limited information available.
- NATIONAL FUNDING/ACCESS DECISIONS

NICE technology appraisals (TAs)
▸ Obinutuzumab in combination with chlorambucil for untreated chronic lymphocytic leukaemia (June 2015) NICE TA343
Obinutuzumab, in combination with chlorambucil, is an option for untreated chronic lymphocytic leukaemia in patients who have comorbidities that make full-dose fludarabine-based therapy unsuitable for them, only if:
● bendamustine-based therapy is not suitable **and**
● the manufacturer provides obinutuzumab with the discount agreed in the patient access scheme.
Patients currently receiving obinutuzumab that is not recommended according to the above criteria should have the option to continue treatment until they and their clinician consider it appropriate to stop.
www.nice.org.uk/TA343

▸ **Ofatumumab in combination with chlorambucil or bendamustine for untreated chronic lymphocytic leukaemia (June 2015) NICE TA344**

Ofatumumab in combination with chlorambucil is an option for untreated chronic lymphocytic leukaemia only if:

- the person is ineligible for fludarabine-based therapy **and**
- bendamustine is not suitable **and**
- the manufacturer provides ofatumumab with the discount agreed in the patient access scheme.

Patients currently receiving ofatumumab that is not recommended according to the above criteria should have the option to continue treatment until they and their clinician consider it appropriate to stop.

www.nice.org.uk/TA344

● MEDICINAL FORMS
There can be variation in the licensing of different medicines containing the same drug.

Tablet
▸ Chlorambucil (Non-proprietary)
Chlorambucil 2 mg Chlorambucil 2mg tablets | 25 tablet PoM
£42.87 DT price = £42.87

Cyclophosphamide

● **INDICATIONS AND DOSE**

Rheumatoid arthritis with severe systemic manifestations
▸ BY MOUTH
▸ Adult: 1–1.5 mg/kg daily

Severe systemic rheumatoid arthritis | Other connective tissue diseases (especially with active vasculitis)
▸ BY INTRAVENOUS INJECTION
▸ Adult: 0.5–1 g every 2 weeks, then reduced to 0.5–1 g every 1 month, frequency adjusted according to clinical response and haematological monitoring. To be given with prophylactic mesna

Used, mainly in combination with other agents for treating a wide range of malignancies, including some leukaemias, lymphomas, and solid tumours
▸ BY MOUTH, OR BY INTRAVENOUS INFUSION
▸ Adult: (consult local protocol)

● UNLICENSED USE Not licensed for rheumatoid arthritis with severe systemic manifestations.

> **IMPORTANT SAFETY INFORMATION**
> RISKS OF INCORRECT DOSING OF ORAL ANTI-CANCER MEDICINES
> See Cytotoxic drugs p. 787.

● CONTRA-INDICATIONS Haemorrhagic cystitis

● CAUTIONS Avoid in Acute porphyrias p. 918 · diabetes mellitus · previous or concurrent mediastinal irradiation—risk of cardiotoxicity

● INTERACTIONS → Appendix 1 (cyclophosphamide).

● SIDE-EFFECTS
GENERAL SIDE-EFFECTS
▸ **Common or very common** Anorexia · cardiotoxicity at high doses · disturbances of carbohydrate metabolism · inappropriate secretion of anti-diuretic hormone · interstitial pulmonary fibrosis · pancreatitis · pigmentation of nails · pigmentation of palms · pigmentation of soles · urothelial toxicity
▸ **Rare** Hepatotoxicity · renal dysfunction
▸ **Frequency not known** Alopecia · bone-marrow suppression · haemorrhagic cystitis · hyperuricaemia · male sterility · nausea · oral mucositis · premature menopause · secondary malignancy · thromboembolism · tumour lysis syndrome · vomiting

SPECIFIC SIDE-EFFECTS
▸ With intravenous use Extravasation
SIDE-EFFECTS, FURTHER INFORMATION
▸ **Haemorrhagic cystitis** A urinary metabolite of cyclophosphamide, acrolein, can cause haemorrhagic cystitis; this is a rare but serious complication; increased fluid intake for 24–48 hours after intravenous injection, can prevent this complication. When high-dose therapy (e.g. more than 2 g intravenously) is used or when the patient is considered to be at high risk of cystitis (e.g. because of pelvic irradiation), mesna (given initially intravenously then by mouth) can also help prevent cystitis.
▸ **Secondary malignancy** Prolonged use of alkylating drugs, particularly when combined with extensive irradiation, is associated with a marked increase in the incidence of acute non-lymphocytic leukaemia.

● CONCEPTION AND CONTRACEPTION Manufacturer advises effective contraception during and for at least 3 months after treatment in men or women. See also *Pregnancy and reproductive function* in Cytotoxic drugs p. 787.

● PREGNANCY Avoid. See also *Pregnancy and reproductive function* in Cytotoxic drugs p. 787.

● BREAST FEEDING Discontinue breast-feeding during and for 36 hours after stopping treatment.

● HEPATIC IMPAIRMENT Reduce dose—consult local treatment protocol for details.

● RENAL IMPAIRMENT Reduce dose if serum creatinine concentration greater than 120 micromol/litre.

● DIRECTIONS FOR ADMINISTRATION
▸ With intravenous use For *intravenous infusion* (cyclophosphamide injection; *Baxter*) give via drip tubing in Glucose 5% or Sodium chloride 0.9%; reconstitute 500 mg with 25 mL sodium chloride 0.9%; reconstitute 1 g with 50 mL sodium chloride 0.9%.

● MEDICINAL FORMS
There can be variation in the licensing of different medicines containing the same drug. Forms available from special-order manufacturers include: tablet, oral suspension, oral solution, solution for injection, solution for infusion

Tablet
CAUTIONARY AND ADVISORY LABELS 25, 27
▸ Cyclophosphamide (Non-proprietary)
Cyclophosphamide (as Cyclophosphamide monohydrate)
50 mg Cyclophosphamide 50mg tablets | 100 tablet PoM £139.00
DT price = £139.00
▸ Cytoxan (Imported (United States))
Cyclophosphamide 25 mg Cytoxan 25mg tablets | 100 tablet PoM
no price available

Powder for solution for injection
▸ Cyclophosphamide (Non-proprietary)
Cyclophosphamide (as Cyclophosphamide monohydrate)
500 mg Cyclophosphamide 500mg powder for solution for injection
vials | 1 vial PoM £9.66–£9.95
Cyclophosphamide (as Cyclophosphamide monohydrate)
1 gram Cyclophosphamide 1g powder for solution for injection vials |
1 vial PoM £17.06–£18.47
Cyclophosphamide (as Cyclophosphamide monohydrate)
2 gram Cyclophosphamide 2g powder for solution for injection vials
| 1 vial PoM £34.12

Dacarbazine

● **INDICATIONS AND DOSE**

Metastatic melanoma | Soft-tissue sarcomas (combination therapy) | Hodgkin's disease (combination therapy)
▸ BY INTRAVENOUS INFUSION, OR BY INTRAVENOUS INJECTION
▸ Adult: (consult local protocol)

● CAUTIONS Caution in handling—irritant to tissues

● INTERACTIONS → Appendix 1 (dacarbazine).

- SIDE-EFFECTS
  ▶ **Rare** Irritant to skin · irritant to tissues · liver necrosis due to hepatic vein thrombosis
  ▶ **Frequency not known** Alopecia · bone-marrow suppression · extravasation · hyperuricaemia · myelosuppression · oral mucositis · severe nausea · severe vomiting · tumour lysis syndrome · vomiting
- CONCEPTION AND CONTRACEPTION Ensure effective contraception during and for at least 6 months after treatment in men or women. See also *Pregnancy and reproductive function* in Cytotoxic drugs p. 787.
- PREGNANCY Avoid (carcinogenic and teratogenic in *animal* studies). See also *Pregnancy and reproductive function* in Cytotoxic drugs p. 787.
- BREAST FEEDING Discontinue breast-feeding.
- HEPATIC IMPAIRMENT Dose reduction may be required in combined renal and hepatic impairment. Avoid in severe impairment.
- RENAL IMPAIRMENT Dose reduction may be required in combined renal and hepatic impairment. Avoid in severe impairment.
- PRESCRIBING AND DISPENSING INFORMATION Dacarbazine is a component of a commonly used combination for Hodgkin's disease (ABVD—doxorubicin [previously *Adriamycin®*], bleomycin, vinblastine, and dacarbazine).

- MEDICINAL FORMS
  There can be variation in the licensing of different medicines containing the same drug.
  Powder for solution for injection
  ▶ Dacarbazine (Non-proprietary)
    Dacarbazine (as Dacarbazine citrate) 100 mg Dacarbazine 100mg powder for solution for injection vials | 10 vial [PoM] £90.00
    Dacarbazine (as Dacarbazine citrate) 200 mg Dacarbazine 200mg powder for solution for injection vials | 10 vial [PoM] £160.00
  Powder for solution for infusion
  ▶ Dacarbazine (Non-proprietary)
    Dacarbazine (as Dacarbazine citrate) 500 mg Dacarbazine 500mg powder for solution for infusion vials | 1 vial [PoM] £37.50
    Dacarbazine (as Dacarbazine citrate) 1 gram Dacarbazine 1g powder for solution for infusion vials | 1 vial [PoM] £70.00

Estramustine phosphate

- INDICATIONS AND DOSE
  Prostate cancer
  ▶ BY MOUTH
  ▶ Adult: Initially 560–840 mg daily in divided doses; maintenance 140–1400 mg daily in divided doses

IMPORTANT SAFETY INFORMATION
RISKS OF INCORRECT DOSING OF ORAL ANTI-CANCER MEDICINES
See Cytotoxic drugs p. 787.

- CONTRA-INDICATIONS Peptic ulceration · severe cardiovascular disease · thromboembolic disorders
- CAUTIONS Avoid in Acute porphyrias p. 918 · cardiovascular disease · cerebrovascular disease · conditions which might be aggravated by fluid retention (such as epilepsy or migraine) · congestive heart failure · diabetes · hypercalcaemia · hypertension
- INTERACTIONS → Appendix 1 (estramustine).
- SIDE-EFFECTS
  ▶ **Rare** Angioedema
  ▶ **Frequency not known** Alopecia · altered endocrine function · altered liver function · bone-marrow suppression · congestive heart failure · diarrhoea · gynaecomastia · hyperuricaemia · impotence · ischaemic heart disease · male sterility · myocardial infarction · nausea · oedema ·

oral mucositis · secondary malignancy · thromboembolism · tumour lysis syndrome · vomiting
  SIDE-EFFECTS, FURTHER INFORMATION
  ▶ Secondary malignancy Prolonged use of alkylating drugs, particularly when combined with extensive irradiation, is associated with a marked increase in the incidence of acute non-lymphocytic leukaemia.
- CONCEPTION AND CONTRACEPTION Men should use effective contraceptive methods during treatment. See also *Pregnancy and reproductive function* in Cytotoxic drugs p. 787.
- HEPATIC IMPAIRMENT Manufacturer advises caution. Avoid in severe impairment. In hepatic impairment, manufacturer advises regular liver function tests.
- RENAL IMPAIRMENT Manufacturer advises caution.
- DIRECTIONS FOR ADMINISTRATION Each dose should be taken not less than 1 hour before or 2 hours after meals and should not be taken with products containing calcium, magnesium or aluminium, including dairy products and antacid medication.
- PATIENT AND CARER ADVICE Patients should be given advice on how to administer estramustine capsules.

- MEDICINAL FORMS
  There can be variation in the licensing of different medicines containing the same drug.
  Capsule
  CAUTIONARY AND ADVISORY LABELS 5, 23
  ▶ Estracyt (Pfizer Ltd)
    Estramustine phosphate (as Estramustine sodium phosphate) 140 mg Estracyt 140mg capsules | 100 capsule [PoM] £171.28

Ifosfamide

- INDICATIONS AND DOSE
  Malignant disease
  ▶ BY INTRAVENOUS INFUSION
  ▶ Adult: (consult local protocol)

- CONTRA-INDICATIONS Acute infection · urinary-tract infection · urinary-tract obstruction · urothelial damage
- CAUTIONS Avoid in Acute porphyrias p. 918 · diabetes mellitus
- INTERACTIONS → Appendix 1 (ifosfamide).
- SIDE-EFFECTS
  ▶ **Common or very common** Confusion · disorientation · drowsiness · psychosis · renal toxicity (may lead to tubular dysfunction, Fanconi's syndrome, or diabetes insipidus) · restlessness · urothelial toxicity
  ▶ **Uncommon** Severe encephalopathy
  ▶ **Rare** Anorexia · constipation · convulsions · diarrhoea
  ▶ **Very rare** Jaundice · syndrome of inappropriate antidiuretic hormone secretion · thrombophlebitis
  ▶ **Frequency not known** Acute pancreatitis · alopecia · arrhythmias · bone-marrow suppression · extravasation · heart failure · hyperuricaemia · male sterility · nausea · oral mucositis · premature menopause · secondary malignancy · thromboembolism · tumour lysis syndrome · vomiting
  SIDE-EFFECTS, FURTHER INFORMATION
  ▶ Urothelial toxicity Mesna is routinely given with ifosfamide to reduce urothelial toxicity.
  ▶ Secondary malignancy Prolonged use of alkylating drugs, particularly when combined with extensive irradiation, is associated with a marked increase in the incidence of acute non-lymphocytic leukaemia.
- CONCEPTION AND CONTRACEPTION Manufacturer advises adequate contraception during and for at least 6 months after treatment in men or women. See also *Pregnancy and reproductive function* in Cytotoxic drugs p. 787.

8

Immune system and malignant disease

- PREGNANCY Avoid (teratogenic and carcinogenic in *animals*). See also *Pregnancy and reproductive function* in Cytotoxic drugs p. 787.
- BREAST FEEDING Discontinue breast-feeding.
- HEPATIC IMPAIRMENT Avoid.
- RENAL IMPAIRMENT Avoid if serum creatinine concentration greater than 120 micromol/litre.
- MONITORING REQUIREMENTS Ensure satisfactory electrolyte balance and renal function before each course (risk of tubular dysfunction, Fanconi's syndrome or diabetes insipidus if renal toxicity not treated promptly).

- MEDICINAL FORMS
There can be variation in the licensing of different medicines containing the same drug.
Powder for solution for injection
- Ifosfamide (Non-proprietary)
Ifosfamide 1 gram Ifosfamide 1g powder for concentrate for solution for injection vials | 1 vial [PoM] £91.32
Ifosfamide 2 gram Ifosfamide 2g powder for concentrate for solution for injection vials | 1 vial [PoM] £179.88

Lomustine

- DRUG ACTION Lomustine is a lipid-soluble nitrosourea.

- INDICATIONS AND DOSE
Hodgkin's disease resistant to conventional therapy | Malignant melanoma | Certain solid tumours
▸ BY MOUTH
▸ Adult: 120–130 mg/m^2 every 6–8 weeks, dose is for when lomustine is used alone

IMPORTANT SAFETY INFORMATION
RISKS OF INCORRECT DOSING OF ORAL ANTI-CANCER MEDICINES
See Cytotoxic drugs p. 787.

- CONTRA-INDICATIONS Coeliac disease
- CAUTIONS Avoid in Acute porphyrias p. 918
- INTERACTIONS → Appendix 1 (lomustine).
- SIDE-EFFECTS Alopecia · bone-marrow suppression (delayed) · hyperuricaemia · male sterility · nausea · oral mucositis · permanent bone marrow damage (with prolonged use) · premature menopause · secondary malignancy · thromboembolism · tumour lysis syndrome · vomiting
SIDE-EFFECTS, FURTHER INFORMATION
▸ Secondary malignancy Prolonged use of alkylating drugs, particularly when combined with extensive irradiation, is associated with a marked increase in the incidence of acute non-lymphocytic leukaemia.
- CONCEPTION AND CONTRACEPTION Manufacturer advises effective contraception during and for at least 6 months after treatment in men or women. See also *Pregnancy and reproductive function* in Cytotoxic drugs p. 787.
- PREGNANCY Avoid. See also *Pregnancy and reproductive function* in Cytotoxic drugs p. 787.
- BREAST FEEDING Discontinue breast-feeding.
- RENAL IMPAIRMENT Avoid in severe impairment.
- PRESCRIBING AND DISPENSING INFORMATION The brand name *CCNU*® has been used for lomustine capsules.

- MEDICINAL FORMS
There can be variation in the licensing of different medicines containing the same drug. Forms available from special-order manufacturers include: capsule
Capsule
▸ Lomustine (Non-proprietary)
Lomustine 10 mg CeeNU 10mg capsules | 20 capsule [PoM] no price available

Lomustine 40 mg Lomustine 40mg capsules | 20 capsule [PoM] £780.82
Lomustine 100 mg CeeNU 100mg capsules | 20 capsule [PoM] no price available

Melphalan

- INDICATIONS AND DOSE
Multiple myeloma
▸ BY MOUTH
▸ Adult: 150 micrograms/kg daily for 4 days, dose to be repeated every 6 weeks, dose may vary according to regimen
▸ BY INTRAVENOUS INJECTION, OR BY INTRAVENOUS INFUSION
▸ Adult: (consult product literature)
Polycythaemia vera
▸ BY MOUTH
▸ Adult: Initially 6–10 mg daily for 5-7 days, then reduced to 2–4 mg daily until satisfactory response, then reduced to 2–6 mg once weekly
Localised malignant melanoma of the extremities | Localised soft-tissue sarcoma of the extremities
▸ BY REGIONAL ARTERIAL PERFUSION
▸ Adult: (consult local protocol)

IMPORTANT SAFETY INFORMATION
RISKS OF INCORRECT DOSING OF ORAL ANTI-CANCER MEDICINES
See Cytotoxic drugs p. 787.

- CAUTIONS Avoid in Acute porphyrias p. 918
- INTERACTIONS → Appendix 1 (melphalan).
- SIDE-EFFECTS
GENERAL SIDE-EFFECTS
▸ Rare Interstitial pneumonitis · life threatening pulmonary fibrosis
▸ Frequency not known Alopecia · bone-marrow suppression (delayed) · hyperuricaemia · male sterility · nausea · oral mucositis · premature menopause · secondary malignancy · thromboembolism · tumour lysis syndrome · vomiting
SPECIFIC SIDE-EFFECTS
▸ With intravenous use Extravasation
SIDE-EFFECTS, FURTHER INFORMATION
▸ Secondary malignancy Prolonged use of alkylating drugs, particularly when combined with extensive irradiation, is associated with a marked increase in the incidence of acute non-lymphocytic leukaemia.
- CONCEPTION AND CONTRACEPTION Manufacturer advises adequate contraception during treatment in men or women. See also *Pregnancy and reproductive function* in Cytotoxic drugs p. 787.
- PREGNANCY Avoid. See also *Pregnancy and reproductive function* in Cytotoxic drugs p. 787.
- BREAST FEEDING Discontinue breast-feeding.
- RENAL IMPAIRMENT Reduce dose initially (consult product literature).
- MONITORING REQUIREMENTS Monitor full blood count before and throughout treatment.

- MEDICINAL FORMS
There can be variation in the licensing of different medicines containing the same drug.
Tablet
▸ Melphalan (Non-proprietary)
Melphalan 2 mg Melphalan 2mg tablets | 25 tablet [PoM] £45.38 DT price = £45.38
Powder and solvent for solution for injection
▸ Melphalan (Non-proprietary)
Melphalan (as Melphalan hydrochloride) 50 mg Melphalan 50mg powder and solvent for solution for injection vials | 1 vial [PoM] £137.37

8

Immune system and malignant disease

8

Immune system and malignant disease

Temozolomide

- DRUG ACTION Temozolomide is structurally related to dacarbazine.

INDICATIONS AND DOSE

Newly diagnosed glioblastoma multiforme in adults (in combination with radiotherapy) and subsequently as monotherapy | Second-line treatment of malignant glioma in adults
- BY MOUTH
- Adult: (consult product literature)

IMPORTANT SAFETY INFORMATION
RISKS OF INCORRECT DOSING OF ORAL ANTI-CANCER MEDICINES
See Cytotoxic drugs p. 787.

- CAUTIONS *Pneumocystis jirovecii* pneumonia—consult product literature for monitoring and prophylaxis requirements
- INTERACTIONS → Appendix 1 (temozolomide).
- SIDE-EFFECTS Alopecia · bone-marrow suppression · hyperuricaemia · nausea · oral mucositis · thromboembolism · tumour lysis syndrome · vomiting
  SIDE-EFFECTS, FURTHER INFORMATION
  For further information on side-effects consult product literature.
- CONCEPTION AND CONTRACEPTION Manufacturer advises adequate contraception during treatment. Men should avoid fathering a child during and for at least 6 months after treatment. See also *Pregnancy and reproductive function* in Cytotoxic drugs p. 787.
- PREGNANCY Avoid (teratogenic and embryotoxic in *animal* studies). See also *Pregnancy and reproductive function* in Cytotoxic drugs p. 787.
- BREAST FEEDING Discontinue breast-feeding.
- HEPATIC IMPAIRMENT Use with caution in severe impairment—no information available.
- RENAL IMPAIRMENT Manufacturer advises caution—no information available.
- MONITORING REQUIREMENTS
- Monitor liver function before treatment initiation, after each treatment cycle and midway through 42-day treatment cycles—consider the balance of benefits and risks of treatment if results are abnormal at any point (fatal liver injury reported).
- Monitor for myelodysplastic syndrome.
- Monitor for secondary malignancies.
- NATIONAL FUNDING/ACCESS DECISIONS
  NICE technology appraisals (TAs)
- **Temozolomide for the treatment of recurrent malignant glioma (brain cancer) (April 2001)** NICE TA23
  Temozolomide may be considered for the treatment of recurrent malignant glioma, which has not responded to first-line chemotherapy.
  www.nice.org/TA23
- **Carmustine implants and temozolomide for the treatment of newly diagnosed high-grade glioma (June 2007)** NICE TA121
  Temozolomide is an option for the treatment of newly diagnosed glioblastoma multiforme in patients with a WHO performance status of 0 or 1.
  www.nice.org.uk/TA121

- MEDICINAL FORMS
  There can be variation in the licensing of different medicines containing the same drug. Forms available from special-order manufacturers include: oral suspension
  Capsule
  CAUTIONARY AND ADVISORY LABELS 23, 25
- ▸ Temozolomide (Non-proprietary)
  Temozolomide 5 mg Temozolomide 5mg capsules | 5 capsule [PoM] £16.44 | 5 capsule [PoM] £17.30 (Hospital only)
  Temozolomide 20 mg Temozolomide 20mg capsules | 5 capsule [PoM] £67.88 | 5 capsule [PoM] £69.20 (Hospital only)
  Temozolomide 100 mg Temozolomide 100mg capsules | 5 capsule [PoM] £328.70 | 5 capsule [PoM] £346.00 (Hospital only)
  Temozolomide 140 mg Temozolomide 140mg capsules | 5 capsule [PoM] £465.00 | 5 capsule [PoM] £484.49 (Hospital only)
  Temozolomide 180 mg Temozolomide 180mg capsules | 5 capsule [PoM] £610.92 | 5 capsule [PoM] £622.80 (Hospital only)
  Temozolomide 250 mg Temozolomide 250mg capsules | 5 capsule [PoM] £814.00 | 5 capsule [PoM] £865.00 (Hospital only)
- ▸ Temodal (Merck Sharp & Dohme Ltd)
  Temozolomide 5 mg Temodal 5mg capsules | 5 capsule [PoM] £10.59 (Hospital only)
  Temozolomide 20 mg Temodal 20mg capsules | 5 capsule [PoM] £42.35 (Hospital only)
  Temozolomide 100 mg Temodal 100mg capsules | 5 capsule [PoM] £211.77 (Hospital only)
  Temozolomide 140 mg Temodal 140mg capsules | 5 capsule [PoM] £296.48 (Hospital only)
  Temozolomide 180 mg Temodal 180mg capsules | 5 capsule [PoM] £381.19 (Hospital only)
  Temozolomide 250 mg Temodal 250mg capsules | 5 capsule [PoM] £529.43 (Hospital only)
- ▸ Temomedac (medac UK)
  Temozolomide 5 mg Temomedac 5mg capsules | 5 capsule [PoM] £16.12
  Temozolomide 20 mg Temomedac 20mg capsules | 5 capsule [PoM] £64.49
  Temozolomide 100 mg Temomedac 100mg capsules | 5 capsule [PoM] £322.43
  Temozolomide 140 mg Temomedac 140mg capsules | 5 capsule [PoM] £451.40
  Temozolomide 180 mg Temomedac 180mg capsules | 5 capsule [PoM] £580.37
  Temozolomide 250 mg Temomedac 250mg capsules | 5 capsule [PoM] £806.08

Thiotepa

INDICATIONS AND DOSE

Conditioning treatment before haematopoietic stem cell transplantation in the treatment of haematological disease or solid tumours, in combination with other chemotherapy
- BY INTRAVENOUS INFUSION
- Adult: (consult local protocol)

- CAUTIONS Avoid in Acute porphyrias p. 918
- INTERACTIONS → Appendix 1 (thiotepa).
- SIDE-EFFECTS Alopecia · bone-marrow suppression · extravasation · hyperuricaemia · male sterility · nausea · oral mucositis · premature menopause · secondary malignancy · thromboembolism · tumour lysis syndrome · vomiting
  SIDE-EFFECTS, FURTHER INFORMATION
- Secondary malignancy Prolonged use of alkylating drugs, particularly when combined with extensive irradiation, is associated with a marked increase in the incidence of acute non-lymphocytic leukaemia.
- CONCEPTION AND CONTRACEPTION Contraceptive advice required, see *Pregnancy and reproductive function* in Cytotoxic drugs p. 787.
- PREGNANCY Avoid (teratogenic and embryotoxic in *animals*). See also *Pregnancy and reproductive function* in Cytotoxic drugs p. 787.

- BREAST FEEDING Discontinue breast-feeding.
- NATIONAL FUNDING/ACCESS DECISIONS

Scottish Medicines Consortium (SMC) Decisions
The *Scottish Medicines Consortium* has advised (June 2012) that thiotepa (*Tepadina* ®) is **not** recommended for use within NHS Scotland in combination with other chemotherapy as conditioning treatment in adults or children with haematological diseases, or solid tumours prior to haematopoietic stem cell transplantation.

- MEDICINAL FORMS
There can be variation in the licensing of different medicines containing the same drug.
Powder for solution for infusion
▸ Tepadina (Adienne Pharma & Biotech)
  Thiotepa 15 mg Tepadina 15mg powder for concentrate for solution for infusion vials | 1 vial PoM no price available
  Thiotepa 100 mg Tepadina 100mg powder for concentrate for solution for infusion vials | 1 vial PoM no price available

Treosulfan

- INDICATIONS AND DOSE

Ovarian cancer
▸ BY MOUTH, OR BY INTRAVENOUS INJECTION, OR BY INTRAVENOUS INFUSION, OR BY INTRAPERITONEAL INSTILLATION
▸ Adult: (consult product literature)

IMPORTANT SAFETY INFORMATION
RISKS OF INCORRECT DOSING OF ORAL ANTI-CANCER MEDICINES
See Cytotoxic drugs p. 787.

- CAUTIONS Avoid in Acute porphyrias p. 918
- SIDE-EFFECTS
▸ **Common or very common** Skin pigmentation
▸ **Rare** Allergic alveolitis · haemorrhagic cystitis · pulmonary fibrosis
▸ **Frequency not known** Alopecia · bone-marrow suppression · extravasation of intravenous drugs · hyperuricaemia · nausea · oral mucositis · premature menopause · secondary malignancy · thromboembolism · tumour lysis syndrome · vomiting

SIDE-EFFECTS, FURTHER INFORMATION
▸ Secondary malignancy Prolonged use of alkylating drugs, particularly when combined with extensive irradiation, is associated with a marked increase in the incidence of acute non-lymphocytic leukaemia.

- CONCEPTION AND CONTRACEPTION Contraceptive advice required, see *Pregnancy and reproductive function* in Cytotoxic drugs p. 787.
- PREGNANCY Avoid. See also *Pregnancy and reproductive function* in Cytotoxic drugs p. 787.
- BREAST FEEDING Discontinue breast-feeding.
- MEDICINAL FORMS
There can be variation in the licensing of different medicines containing the same drug.
Capsule
CAUTIONARY AND ADVISORY LABELS 25
▸ Treosulfan (Non-proprietary)
  Treosulfan 250 mg Treosulfan 250mg capsules | 100 capsule PoM £622.10-£653.20
Powder for solution for injection
▸ Treosulfan (Non-proprietary)
  Treosulfan 1 gram Treosulfan 1g powder for solution for injection vials | 5 vial PoM £269.17
  Treosulfan 5 gram Treosulfan 5g powder for solution for injection vials | 5 vial PoM £1,040.17

Daunorubicin

- INDICATIONS AND DOSE

Acute myelogenous leukaemia | Acute lymphocytic leukaemia
▸ BY INTRAVENOUS INFUSION
▸ Adult: (consult local protocol)

Advanced AIDS-related Kaposi's sarcoma (liposomal formulation only)
▸ BY INTRAVENOUS INFUSION
▸ Adult: (consult product literature)

- CONTRA-INDICATIONS Myocardial insufficiency · previous treatment with maximum cumulative doses of daunorubicin or other anthracycline · recent myocardial infarction · severe arrhythmia
- CAUTIONS Caution in handling—irritant to tissues
- INTERACTIONS → Appendix 1 (daunorubicin). Caution is necessary with concomitant use of cardiotoxic drugs, or drugs that reduce cardiac contractility. Cardiac function should be monitored closely on the concomitant use of anthracyclines with trastuzumab.
- SIDE-EFFECTS Alopecia · bone-marrow suppression · extravasation · hyperuricaemia · nausea · oral mucositis · thromboembolism · tumour lysis syndrome · vomiting

SIDE-EFFECTS, FURTHER INFORMATION
▸ Cardiotoxicity All anthracycline antibiotics have been associated with varying degrees of cardiac toxicity—this may be idiosyncratic and reversible, but is commonly related to total cumulative dose and is irreversible.

- CONCEPTION AND CONTRACEPTION Contraceptive advice required, see *Pregnancy and reproductive function* in Cytotoxic drugs p. 787.
- PREGNANCY Avoid (teratogenic and carcinogenic in *animal* studies). See also *Pregnancy and reproductive function* in Cytotoxic drugs p. 787.
- BREAST FEEDING Discontinue breast-feeding.
- HEPATIC IMPAIRMENT Reduce dose according to serum bilirubin concentration—consult local protocol for details. Avoid in severe impairment.
- RENAL IMPAIRMENT Reduce dose by 25% if serum creatinine 105–265 micromol/litre. Reduce dose by 50% if serum creatinine greater than 265 micromol/litre. Avoid in severe impairment.
- MONITORING REQUIREMENTS Cardiac monitoring essential.

- MEDICINAL FORMS
There can be variation in the licensing of different medicines containing the same drug.
Powder for solution for infusion
▸ Daunorubicin (Non-proprietary)
  Daunorubicin (as Daunorubicin hydrochloride)
  20 mg Daunorubicin 20mg powder for solution for infusion vials | 10 vial PoM £650.00 (Hospital only)
Emulsion for infusion
▸ DaunoXome (Galen Ltd)
  Daunorubicin (as Daunorubicin hydrochloride citrate)
  50 mg DaunoXome 50mg emulsion for infusion vials | 1 vial PoM £250.00

8

Immune system and malignant disease

Immune system and malignant disease

8

Doxorubicin hydrochloride

10.6.2016

- ● **INDICATIONS AND DOSE**

Acute leukaemias | Hodgkin's lymphoma | Non-Hodgkin's lymphoma | Some solid tumours including breast cancer
- ▸ BY INTRAVENOUS INJECTION
- ▸ Adult: (consult product literature)

Some papillary bladder tumours (bladder instillation) | Recurrent superficial bladder tumours (bladder instillation) | Transitional cell carcinoma (bladder instillation) | Carcinoma in situ (bladder instillation)
- ▸ BY INTRAVESICAL INSTILLATION
- ▸ Adult: (consult product literature)

CAELYX®

For AIDS-related Kaposi's sarcoma in patients with low CD4 count and extensive mucocutaneous or visceral disease | Advanced ovarian cancer when platinum-based chemotherapy has failed | Progressive multiple myeloma (in combination with bortezomib) in patients who have received at least one prior therapy and who have undergone or are unsuitable for bone-marrow transplantation | Monotherapy for metastatic breast cancer in patients with increased cardiac risk
- ▸ BY INTRAVENOUS INFUSION
- ▸ Adult: (consult product literature)

MYOCET®

For use with cyclophosphamide for metastatic breast cancer
- ▸ Adult: (consult product literature)

- ● CONTRA-INDICATIONS Consult product literature
- ● CAUTIONS Cardiac disease · caution in handling—irritant to tissues · consult product literature · elderly · hypertension · previous myocardial irradiation
- ● INTERACTIONS → Appendix 1 (doxorubicin). Caution is necessary with concomitant use of cardiotoxic drugs, or drugs that reduce cardiac contractility. Cardiac function should be monitored closely on the concomitant use of anthracyclines with trastuzumab.
- ● SIDE-EFFECTS
- ▸ **Common or very common** Dehydration · diarrhoea · red colouration of the urine
- ▸ **Uncommon** Supraventricular tachycardia (related to drug administration)
- ▸ **Frequency not known** Alopecia · bone-marrow suppression · cardiomyopathy (with higher cumulative doses) · consult product literature · extravasation · heart failure (potentially fatal) · hyperuricaemia · nausea · oral mucositis · renal damage · thromboembolism · tumour lysis syndrome · vomiting

SIDE-EFFECTS, FURTHER INFORMATION
- ▸ Extravasation Extravasation can cause severe tissue necrosis.
- ▸ Cardiomyopathy Higher cumulative doses are associated with cardiomyopathy and it is usual to limit total cumulative doses to 450 mg/m^2 because symptomatic and potentially fatal heart failure is common above this dose.
- ▸ Cardiotoxic Some evidence suggests that weekly low-dose administration may be less cardiotoxic.
- ▸ Liposomal formulations *Liposomal* formulations of doxorubicin may reduce the incidence of cardiotoxicity and lower the potential for local necrosis, but infusion reactions, sometimes severe, may occur. Hand-foot syndrome (painful, macular reddening skin eruptions) occurs commonly with liposomal doxorubicin and may be dose limiting. It can occur after 2–3 treatment cycles and may be prevented by cooling hands and feet and avoiding socks, gloves, or tight-fitting footwear for 4–7 days after treatment.

- ▸ Elevated bilirubin concentration Doxorubicin is largely excreted in the bile and an elevated bilirubin concentration is an indication for reducing the dose.
- ● CONCEPTION AND CONTRACEPTION Manufacturer advises effective contraception during and for at least 6 months after treatment in men or women.
- ● PREGNANCY Avoid (teratogenic and toxic in *animal* studies). See also *Pregnancy and reproductive function* in Cytotoxic drugs p. 787.
- ● BREAST FEEDING Discontinue breast-feeding.
- ● HEPATIC IMPAIRMENT Reduce dose according to bilirubin concentration—consult product literature or local treatment protocol for details. Avoid in severe impairment.
- ● RENAL IMPAIRMENT Consult product literature in severe impairment.
- ● MONITORING REQUIREMENTS Patients should be assessed before treatment, by echocardiography. Cardiac monitoring during treatment may assist in determining safe dosage.
- ● DIRECTIONS FOR ADMINISTRATION *Conventional* doxorubicin is given by injection into a fast-running infusion, commonly at 21-day intervals.
- ● PRESCRIBING AND DISPENSING INFORMATION Doxorubicin is available as both *conventional* and *liposomal* formulations. The different formulations vary in their licensed indications, pharmacokinetics, dosage and administration, and are not interchangeable.
- ● NATIONAL FUNDING/ACCESS DECISIONS

NICE technology appraisals (TAs)
- ▸ Topotecan, pegylated liposomal doxorubicin hydrochloride, paclitaxel, trabectedin and gemcitabine for treating recurrent ovarian cancer (April 2016) NICE TA389

Pegylated liposomal doxorubicin hydrochloride (PLDH) monotherapy or in combination with platinum, is recommended as an option for treating recurrent ovarian cancer.

PLDH, in combination with trabectedin, is **not** recommended for treating the first recurrence of platinum-sensitive ovarian cancer.

Patients currently receiving PLDH in combination with trabectedin should have the option to continue their treatment until they and their clinician consider it appropriate to stop.
www.nice.org.uk/TA389

- ● MEDICINAL FORMS
There can be variation in the licensing of different medicines containing the same drug. Forms available from special-order manufacturers include: solution for infusion

Solution for injection
- ▸ Doxorubicin hydrochloride (Non-proprietary)
  Doxorubicin hydrochloride 2 mg per 1 ml Doxorubicin 10mg/5ml solution for injection vials | 1 vial PoM £18.54 (Hospital only)
  Doxorubicin 50mg/25ml solution for injection Cytosafe vials | 1 vial PoM £103.00
  Doxorubicin 50mg/25ml solution for infusion vials | 1 vial PoM £103.00 (Hospital only)
  Doxorubicin 10mg/5ml solution for injection Cytosafe vials | 1 vial PoM £20.60
  Doxorubicin 10mg/5ml concentrate for solution for infusion vials | 1 vial PoM no price available
  Doxorubicin 10mg/5ml solution for infusion vials | 1 vial PoM £20.60 (Hospital only)
  Doxorubicin 50mg/25ml solution for injection vials | 1 vial PoM £92.70 (Hospital only)
  Doxorubicin 50mg/25ml concentrate for solution for infusion vials | 1 vial PoM no price available

Powder for solution for injection
- ▸ Doxorubin (medac UK)
  Doxorubicin hydrochloride 10 mg Doxorubin 10mg powder for solution for injection vials | 10 vial PoM £182.80
  Doxorubicin hydrochloride 50 mg Doxorubin 50mg powder for solution for injection vials | 10 vial PoM £914.00

Solution for infusion

▸ Doxorubicin hydrochloride (Non-proprietary)

Doxorubicin hydrochloride 2 mg per 1 ml Doxorubicin 200mg/100ml solution for injection Cytosafe vials | 1 vial PoM £412.00

Doxorubicin 200mg/100ml solution for infusion vials | 1 vial PoM £370.80–£412.00 (Hospital only)

Doxorubicin 200mg/100ml concentrate for solution for infusion vials | 1 vial PoM no price available

▸ Caelyx (Janssen-Cilag Ltd)

Doxorubicin hydrochloride (as Doxorubicin hydrochloride liposomal pegylated) 2 mg per 1 ml Caelyx 50mg/25ml concentrate for solution for infusion vials | 1 vial PoM £712.49

Caelyx 20mg/10ml concentrate for solution for infusion vials | 1 vial PoM £360.23

Powder and solvent for suspension for infusion

ELECTROLYTES: May contain Sodium

▸ Myocet (Teva UK Ltd)

Doxorubicin hydrochloride 50 mg Myocet 50mg powder and solvent for suspension for infusion vials | 2 vial PoM £912.26 (Hospital only)

Epirubicin hydrochloride

● INDICATIONS AND DOSE

Treatment of breast cancer | Treatment and prophylaxis of certain forms of superficial bladder cancer

▸ BY INTRAVENOUS INFUSION, OR BY INTRAVESICAL INSTILLATION

▸ Adult: (consult product literature or local protocols)

● CONTRA-INDICATIONS Bladder inflammation or contraction (when used as a bladder instillation) · catheterisation difficulties (when used as a bladder instillation) · haematuria (when used as a bladder instillation) · invasive tumours penetrating the bladder (when used as a bladder instillation) · myocardiopathy · previous treatment with maximum cumulative doses of epirubicin or other anthracycline · recent myocardial infarction · severe arrhythmia · severe myocardial insufficiency · unstable angina · urinary tract infections (when used as a bladder instillation)

● CAUTIONS Caution in handling—irritant to tissues

● INTERACTIONS → Appendix 1 (epirubicin).

Caution is necessary with concomitant use of cardiotoxic drugs, or drugs that reduce cardiac contractility. Cardiac function should be monitored closely on the concomitant use of anthracyclines with trastuzumab.

● SIDE-EFFECTS Alopecia · bone-marrow suppression · cardiotoxicity · extravasation · hyperpigmentation of nails · hyperpigmentation of oral mucosa · hyperpigmentation of skin · hyperuricaemia · nausea · oral mucositis · red colouration of the urine · thromboembolism · tumour lysis syndrome · vomiting

SIDE-EFFECTS, FURTHER INFORMATION

▸ Cardiotoxicity A maximum cumulative dose of 0.9–1 g/m² is recommended to help avoid cardiotoxicity.

● CONCEPTION AND CONTRACEPTION Contraceptive advice required, see *Pregnancy and reproductive function* in Cytotoxic drugs p. 787.

● PREGNANCY Avoid (carcinogenic in *animal* studies). See also *Pregnancy and reproductive function* in Cytotoxic drugs p. 787.

● BREAST FEEDING Discontinue breast-feeding.

● HEPATIC IMPAIRMENT Reduce dose according to bilirubin concentration—consult local treatment protocol for details. Avoid in severe impairment.

● RENAL IMPAIRMENT Dose reduction may be necessary in severe impairment.

● MEDICINAL FORMS

There can be variation in the licensing of different medicines containing the same drug. Forms available from special-order manufacturers include: solution for injection, solution for infusion

Solution for injection

▸ Epirubicin hydrochloride (Non-proprietary)

Epirubicin hydrochloride 2 mg per 1 ml Epirubicin 50mg/25ml solution for injection vials | 1 vial PoM £100.88

Epirubicin 10mg/5ml solution for injection vials | 1 vial PoM £21.24

▸ Pharmorubicin (Pfizer Ltd)

Epirubicin hydrochloride 2 mg per 1 ml Pharmorubicin 50mg/25ml solution for injection Cytosafe vials | 1 vial PoM £106.19

Pharmorubicin 10mg/5ml solution for injection Cytosafe vials | 1 vial PoM £21.24

Solution for infusion

▸ Epirubicin hydrochloride (Non-proprietary)

Epirubicin hydrochloride 2 mg per 1 ml Epirubicin 100mg/50ml solution for infusion vials | 1 vial PoM £169.92

Epirubicin 200mg/100ml solution for infusion vials | 1 vial PoM £386.16

▸ Pharmorubicin (Pfizer Ltd)

Epirubicin hydrochloride 2 mg per 1 ml Pharmorubicin 200mg/100ml solution for infusion Cytosafe vials | 1 vial PoM £386.16

Idarubicin hydrochloride

● INDICATIONS AND DOSE

Acute non-lymphocytic leukaemias monotherapy

▸ BY MOUTH

▸ Adult: 30 mg/m² daily for 3 days; maximum 400 mg/m² per course

Acute non-lymphocytic leukaemia in combination therapy

▸ BY MOUTH

▸ Adult: 15–30 mg/m² daily for 3 days; maximum 400 mg/m² per course

Advanced breast cancer after failure of first-line chemotherapy (not including anthracyclines)—monotherapy

▸ BY MOUTH

▸ Adult: 45 mg/m² for 1 dose, repeat treatment every 3–4 weeks, alternatively 15 mg/m² daily for 3 consecutive days, repeat treatment every 3–4 weeks; maximum 400 mg/m² per course

Acute leukaemias | Advanced breast cancer after failure of first-line chemotherapy (not including anthracyclines)

▸ BY INTRAVENOUS INJECTION

▸ Adult: (consult product literature)

> IMPORTANT SAFETY INFORMATION
> RISKS OF INCORRECT DOSING OF ORAL ANTI-CANCER MEDICINES
> See Cytotoxic drugs p. 787.

● CONTRA-INDICATIONS Previous treatment with maximum cumulative dose of idarubicin or other anthracycline · recent myocardial infarction · severe arrhythmias · severe myocardial insufficiency

● CAUTIONS Caution in handling—irritant to tissues

● INTERACTIONS → Appendix 1 (idarubicin).

Cardiac function should be monitored closely on the concomitant use of anthracyclines with trastuzumab.

● SIDE-EFFECTS

GENERAL SIDE-EFFECTS

▸ Common or very common Abdominal pain · cardiac disorders · diarrhoea · haemorrhage · rash · red pigmentation of the urine

▸ Uncommon Nail hyperpigmentation · skin hyperpigmentation

8

Immune system and malignant disease

▶ **Frequency not known** Alopecia · bone-marrow suppression · hyperuricaemia · nausea · oral mucositis · thromboembolism · tumour lysis syndrome · vomiting
SPECIFIC SIDE-EFFECTS

▶ With intravenous use Extravasation

● CONCEPTION AND CONTRACEPTION Contraceptive advice required, see *Pregnancy and reproductive function* in Cytotoxic drugs p. 787.

● PREGNANCY Avoid (teratogenic and toxic in *animal* studies). See also *Pregnancy and reproductive function* in Cytotoxic drugs p. 787.

● BREAST FEEDING Discontinue breast-feeding.

● HEPATIC IMPAIRMENT Reduce dose according to serum bilirubin concentration. Avoid in severe impairment.

● RENAL IMPAIRMENT Reduce dose. Avoid in severe impairment.

● MEDICINAL FORMS
There can be variation in the licensing of different medicines containing the same drug.
Capsule
CAUTIONARY AND ADVISORY LABELS 25
▶ Zavedos (Pfizer Ltd)
Idarubicin hydrochloride 5 mg Zavedos 5mg capsules | 1 capsule [PoM] £41.47
Idarubicin hydrochloride 10 mg Zavedos 10mg capsules | 1 capsule [PoM] £69.12
Powder for solution for injection
▶ Zavedos (Pfizer Ltd)
Idarubicin hydrochloride 5 mg Zavedos 5mg powder for solution for injection vials | 1 vial [PoM] £87.36
Idarubicin hydrochloride 10 mg Zavedos 10mg powder for solution for injection vials | 1 vial [PoM] £174.72

Mitoxantrone

(Mitozantrone)

● INDICATIONS AND DOSE

Metastatic breast cancer | Non-Hodgkin's lymphoma | Adult acute non-lymphocytic leukaemia | Non-resectable primary hepatocellular carcinoma
▶ BY INTRAVENOUS INFUSION
▶ Adult: (consult local protocol)

● CAUTIONS Intrathecal administration not recommended

● INTERACTIONS → Appendix 1 (mitoxantrone).
Caution is necessary with concomitant use of cardiotoxic drugs, or drugs that reduce cardiac contractility. Cardiac function should be monitored closely on the concomitant use of anthracyclines with trastuzumab.

● SIDE-EFFECTS Abdominal pain · alopecia · amenorrhoea · anorexia · anxiety · blue discoloration of nails · blue discoloration of skin · bone-marrow suppression · confusion · constipation · diarrhoea · dose-related cardiotoxicity · drowsiness · dyspnoea · extravasation · gastro-intestinal bleeding · hyperuricaemia · myelosuppression · nausea · oral mucositis · paraesthesia · thromboembolism · transient blue-green discoloration of urine · tumour lysis syndrome · vomiting
SIDE-EFFECTS, FURTHER INFORMATION

▶ Cardiotoxicity Cardiac examinations are recommended after a cumulative dose of 160 mg/m^2.

● CONCEPTION AND CONTRACEPTION Manufacturer advises effective contraception during and for at least 6 months after treatment in men or women.

● PREGNANCY Avoid. See also *Pregnancy and reproductive function* in Cytotoxic drugs p. 787.

● BREAST FEEDING Discontinue breast-feeding.

● HEPATIC IMPAIRMENT Use with caution—consult local treatment protocol.

● MEDICINAL FORMS
There can be variation in the licensing of different medicines containing the same drug.
Solution for infusion
▶ Mitoxantrone (Non-proprietary)
Mitoxantrone (as Mitoxantrone hydrochloride) 2 mg per 1 ml Mitoxantrone 20mg/10ml concentrate for solution for infusion vials | 1 vial [PoM] £121.85
▶ Onkotrone (Baxter Healthcare Ltd)
Mitoxantrone (as Mitoxantrone hydrochloride) 2 mg per 1 ml Onkotrone 20mg/10ml solution for infusion vials | 1 vial [PoM] no price available
Onkotrone 25mg/12.5ml solution for infusion vials | 1 vial [PoM] no price available

Pixantrone

● INDICATIONS AND DOSE

Treatment of refractory or multiply relapsed aggressive non-Hodgkin B-cell lymphomas (monotherapy)
▶ BY INTRAVENOUS INFUSION
▶ Adult: (consult product literature)

● CONTRA-INDICATIONS Active severe infection · risk factors for severe infection

● CAUTIONS Active cardiovascular disease · cardiac risk factors · caution in handling—irritant to tissues · concurrent radiotherapy to the mediastinal area · history of cardiovascular disease · previous radiotherapy to the mediastinal area · previous therapy with anthracenediones · previous therapy with anthracyclines

● INTERACTIONS → Appendix 1 (pixantrone).
Caution with concurrent use of cardiotoxic drugs - increased risk of cardiotoxicity.
Contra-indicated with concurrent immunisation with live virus vaccines.

● SIDE-EFFECTS

▶ **Common or very common** Abdominal pain · abnormal liver function tests · biochemical disturbances · bone pain · cardiac disorders · cardiac toxicity (during or following treatment) · chromaturia · conjunctivitis · constipation · cough · diarrhoea · drowsiness · dry mouth · dyspepsia · dyspnoea · electrolyte disturbances · haematuria · headache · hypotension · infection · loss of appetite · malaise · nail disorder · oedema · pallor · paraesthesia · proteinuria · pruritus · pyrexia · severe myelosuppression · skin discolouration · tachycardia · taste disturbances · vein discoloration · weight loss

▶ **Uncommon** Anxiety · arrhythmia · arthralgia · arthritis · dizziness · dry eye · keratitis · musculoskeletal pain · musculoskeletal weakness · night sweats · oesophagitis · oliguria · petechiae · pleural effusion · pneumonitis · rash · rectal haemorrhage · rhinorrhoea · skin ulcer · sleep disorder · spontaneous erection · tumour progression · vein disorder · vertigo

▶ **Frequency not known** Alopecia · bone-marrow suppression · extravasation · hyperuricaemia · nausea · oral mucositis · photosensitivity · thromboembolism · tumour lysis syndrome · vomiting

● CONCEPTION AND CONTRACEPTION Ensure effective contraception during and for at least 6 months after treatment in men or women.

● PREGNANCY Manufacturer advises avoid—toxicity in *animal* studies. See also *Pregnancy and reproductive function* in Cytotoxic drugs p. 787.

● BREAST FEEDING Manufacturer advises avoid—no information available.

● HEPATIC IMPAIRMENT No information available—manufacturer advises caution in mild to moderate impairment. Avoid in severe impairment.

- RENAL IMPAIRMENT No information available—manufacturer advises caution.
- MONITORING REQUIREMENTS
▶ Baseline investigations should include a full blood count, assessment of cardiac function measured by left ventricular ejection fraction, and measurement of serum concentrations of total bilirubin and total creatinine.
▶ Full blood count and cardiac function should be monitored throughout treatment.
- PATIENT AND CARER ADVICE
Photosensitivity Photosensitivity is a theoretical risk and patients should be advised to follow sun protection strategies.
- NATIONAL FUNDING/ACCESS DECISIONS
NICE technology appraisals (TAs)
▶ Pixantrone monotherapy for treating multiply relapsed or refractory aggressive non-Hodgkin's B-cell lymphoma (February 2014) NICE TA306
Pixantrone monotherapy is recommended as an option for treating adults with multiply relapsed or refractory aggressive non-Hodgkin's B-cell lymphoma in patients:
  - who have previously been treated with rituximab **and**
  - who are receiving third- or fourth-line treatment **and**
  - if the manufacturer provides pixantrone with the discount agreed in the patient access scheme.
www.nice.org.uk/TA306

- MEDICINAL FORMS
There can be variation in the licensing of different medicines containing the same drug.
Powder for solution for infusion
ELECTROLYTES: May contain Sodium
▶ Pixuvri (CTI Life Sciences Ltd) ▼
  Pixantrone (as Pixantrone dimaleate) 29 mg Pixuvri 29mg powder for concentrate for solution for infusion vials | 1 vial PoM no price available

ANTINEOPLASTIC DRUGS > ANTIMETABOLITES

Azacitidine

- DRUG ACTION Azacitidine is a pyrimidine analogue.

- INDICATIONS AND DOSE
Treatment of intermediate-2 and high-risk myelodysplastic syndromes, chronic myelomonocytic leukaemia, and acute myeloid leukaemia, in adults who are not eligible for haemotopoietic stem cell transplantation
▶ BY SUBCUTANEOUS INJECTION
▶ Adult: (consult local protocol)

- CONTRA-INDICATIONS Advanced malignant hepatic tumour
- CAUTIONS History of severe congestive heart failure · unstable cardiac disease (consider cardiopulmonary assessment before and during treatment) · unstable pulmonary disease (consider cardiopulmonary assessment before and during treatment)
- SIDE-EFFECTS
▶ **Common or very common** Abdominal pain · anorexia · anxiety · arthralgia · cerebral haemorrhage · constipation · diarrhoea · dizziness · drowsiness · dyspepsia · dyspnoea · gastro-intestinal disturbances · haematoma · haematuria · haemorrhage · headache · hypertension · hypokalaemia · hypotension · injection-site reactions · insomnia · myalgia · pneumonia · rash
▶ **Uncommon** Anaphylactic reactions · hypersensitivity reactions
▶ **Frequency not known** Alopecia · bone-marrow suppression · extravasation · hepatic coma · hepatic failure · hyperuricaemia · nausea · oral mucositis · renal failure · thromboembolism · tumour lysis syndrome · vomiting

- CONCEPTION AND CONTRACEPTION Manufacturer advises effective contraception during and for 3 months after treatment in men or women.
- PREGNANCY Avoid (toxicity in *animal* studies). See also *Pregnancy and reproductive function* in Cytotoxic drugs p. 787.
- BREAST FEEDING Discontinue breast-feeding.
- HEPATIC IMPAIRMENT Caution in severe impairment.
- RENAL IMPAIRMENT Delay next treatment cycle if serum-creatinine or blood urea nitrogen greater than twice baseline value and above the upper level of normal until values return to normal or baseline, and then reduce dose by 50% on the next treatment cycle. Reduce dose by 50% on the next treatment cycle if serum-bicarbonate concentration less than 20 mmol/litre.
- MONITORING REQUIREMENTS
▶ Monitor liver function tests, serum creatinine, and serum bicarbonate before initiation of treatment and before each treatment cycle.
▶ Monitor full blood count before initiation of treatment, before each treatment cycle, and as clinically indicated.
▶ Monitor for bleeding.
- NATIONAL FUNDING/ACCESS DECISIONS
NICE technology appraisals (TAs)
▶ Azacitidine for the treatment of myelodysplastic syndromes, chronic myelomonocytic leukaemia and acute myeloid leukaemia (March 2011) NICE TA218
Azacitidine is recommended in adults who are not eligible for haemotopoietic stem cell transplantation as an option for the treatment of intermediate-2 and high-risk myelodysplastic syndromes, chronic myelomonocytic leukaemia, or acute myeloid leukaemia.
www.nice.org.uk/TA218

- MEDICINAL FORMS
There can be variation in the licensing of different medicines containing the same drug.
Powder for suspension for injection
▶ Vidaza (Celgene Ltd)
  Azacitidine 100 mg Vidaza 100mg powder for suspension for injection vials | 1 vial PoM £321.00

Capecitabine

- DRUG ACTION Capecitabine is metabolised to fluorouracil.

- INDICATIONS AND DOSE
Stage III colon cancer, adjuvant following surgery (monotherapy)
▶ BY MOUTH
▶ Adult: 1.25 g/m^2 twice daily for 14 days, subsequent courses repeated after a 7-day interval, recommended duration of treatment is 6 months, adjust dose according to tolerability—consult product literature
Stage III colon cancer, adjuvant following surgery (combination therapy)
▶ BY MOUTH
▶ Adult: 0.8–1 g/m^2 twice daily for 14 days, subsequent courses repeated after a 7-day interval, recommended duration of treatment is 6 months, adjust dose according to tolerability—consult product literature
Metastatic colorectal cancer (monotherapy)
▶ BY MOUTH
▶ Adult: 1.25 g/m^2 twice daily for 14 days, subsequent courses repeated after a 7-day interval, adjust dose according to tolerability—consult product literature

continued →

8

Immune system and malignant disease

Metastatic colorectal cancer (combination therapy)
▶ BY MOUTH
▶ Adult: 0.8–1 g/m^2 twice daily for 14 days, subsequent courses repeated after a 7-day interval, adjust dose according to tolerability—consult product literature

Advanced gastric cancer (first-line treatment in combination with a platinum based regimen)
▶ BY MOUTH
▶ Adult: 0.8–1 g/m^2 twice daily for 14 days, subsequent courses repeated after a 7-day interval, alternatively 625 mg/m^2 twice daily given continuously, adjust dose according to tolerability—consult product literature

Locally advanced or metastatic breast cancer (second-line treatment as monotherapy after failure of a taxane and anthracycline regimen or where further anthracycline treatment is not indicated) | Locally advanced or metastatic breast cancer (second-line treatment, in combination with docetaxel, where previous therapy included an anthracycline)
▶ BY MOUTH
▶ Adult: 1.25 g/m^2 twice daily for 14 days, subsequent courses repeated after a 7-day interval, adjust dose according to tolerability—consult product literature

> IMPORTANT SAFETY INFORMATION
> RISKS OF INCORRECT DOSING OF ORAL ANTI-CANCER MEDICINES
> See Cytotoxic drugs p. 787.

● CONTRA-INDICATIONS Dihydropyrimidine dehydrogenase deficiency
● CAUTIONS Diabetes mellitus · diarrhoea or dehydration—consult product literature for guidance on dose modification and treatment interruption · electrolyte disturbances · history of angina pectoris · history of arrhythmias · history of significant cardiovascular disease · nervous system disease
● INTERACTIONS → Appendix 1 (capecitabine).
● SIDE-EFFECTS Alopecia · bone-marrow suppression · hyperuricaemia · nausea · oral mucositis · thromboembolism · tumour lysis syndrome · vomiting
SIDE-EFFECTS, FURTHER INFORMATION
For further information on side-effects, consult product literature.
● CONCEPTION AND CONTRACEPTION Contraceptive advice required, see *Pregnancy and reproductive function* in Cytotoxic drugs p. 787.
● PREGNANCY Avoid (teratogenic in *animal* studies). See also *Pregnancy and reproductive function* in Cytotoxic drugs p. 787.
● BREAST FEEDING Discontinue breast-feeding.
● HEPATIC IMPAIRMENT Manufacturer advises monitor liver function in mild to moderate impairment—consult product literature for guidance on treatment interruption; avoid in severe impairment.
● RENAL IMPAIRMENT Reduce starting dose of 1.25 g/m^2 to 75% if creatinine clearance 30–50 mL/minute. Avoid if creatinine clearance less than 30 mL/minute.
● MONITORING REQUIREMENTS
▶ Severe skin reactions Monitor for symptoms of severe skin reactions (including Stevens-Johnson syndrome and toxic epidermal necrolysis)—permanently discontinue treatment immediately if symptoms occur.
▶ Hand-foot syndrome Monitor for symptoms of hand-foot syndrome—interrupt treatment if significant syndrome occurs and refer to product literature.
▶ Monitor plasma-calcium concentration.
▶ Monitor for eye disorders (including keratitis and corneal disorders).

● NATIONAL FUNDING/ACCESS DECISIONS

NICE technology appraisals (TAs)
▶ **Bevacizumab in combination with capecitabine for the first-line treatment of metastatic breast cancer (August 2012)** NICE TA263
Bevacizumab in combinations with capecitabine is **not** recommended within its marketing authorisation for the first-line treatment of metastatic breast cancer, that is, when treatment with other chemotherapy options including taxanes or anthracyclines is not considered appropriate, or when taxanes or anthracyclines have been used as part of adjuvant treatment in the previous 12 months.
www.nice.org.uk/TA263
▶ **Bevacizumab in combination with oxaliplatin and either fluorouracil plus folinic acid or capecitabine for the treatment of metastatic colorectal cancer (December 2010)** NICE TA212
Bevacizumab in combination with oxaliplatin and either fluorouracil plus folinic acid or capecitabine is **not** recommended for the treatment of metastatic colorectal cancer.
www.nice.org.uk/TA212
▶ **Capecitabine for the treatment of advanced gastric cancer (July 2010)** NICE TA191
Capecitabine in combination with a platinum-based regimen is recommended for the first-line treatment of inoperable advanced gastric cancer.
www.nice.org.uk/TA191
▶ **Capecitabine and tegafur with uracil for metastatic colorectal cancer (May 2003)** NICE TA61
Capecitabine or tegafur with uracil [now discontinued] (in combination with folinic acid) is an option for the first-line treatment of metastatic colorectal cancer.
www.nice.org.uk/TA61
▶ **Capecitabine and oxaliplatin in the adjuvant treatment of stage III (Dukes' C) colon cancer (April 2006)** NICE TA100
Capecitabine alone *or* oxaliplatin combined with fluorouracil and folinic acid are options for adjuvant treatment following surgery for stage III (Dukes' C) colon cancer.
www.nice.org.uk/TA100

● MEDICINAL FORMS
There can be variation in the licensing of different medicines containing the same drug.
Tablet
CAUTIONARY AND ADVISORY LABELS 21
▶ Capecitabine (Non-proprietary)
Capecitabine 150 mg Capecitabine 150mg tablets | 60 tablet [PoM] £39.99
Capecitabine 300 mg Capecitabine 300mg tablets | 30 tablet [PoM] £39.99 | 60 tablet [PoM] £54.00
Capecitabine 500 mg Capecitabine 500mg tablets | 120 tablet [PoM] £265.00 | 120 tablet [PoM] £265.55 (Hospital only)
▶ Xeloda (Roche Products Ltd)
Capecitabine 150 mg Xeloda 150mg tablets | 60 tablet [PoM] £40.02
Capecitabine 500 mg Xeloda 500mg tablets | 120 tablet [PoM] £265.55

Cladribine

● INDICATIONS AND DOSE

LEUSTAT®

B-cell chronic lymphocytic leukaemia in patients who have failed to respond to standard regimens containing an alkylating agent | Hairy cell leukaemia
▶ BY INTRAVENOUS INFUSION
▶ Adult: (consult product literature or local protocols)

LITAK®
Hairy cell leukaemia
▶ BY SUBCUTANEOUS INJECTION
▶ Adult: (consult product literature or local protocols)

● CAUTIONS Use irradiated blood only
CAUTIONS, FURTHER INFORMATION
▶ Immunosuppressive effect of cladribine Cladribine has a potent and prolonged immunosuppressive effect. Patients treated with cladribine are more prone to serious bacterial, opportunistic fungal, and viral infections, and prophylactic therapy is recommended in those at risk. To prevent potentially fatal transfusion-related graft-versus-host reaction, only irradiated blood products should be administered. Prescribers should consult specialist literature when using highly immunosuppressive drugs.

● INTERACTIONS → Appendix 1 (cladribine).

● SIDE-EFFECTS Abdominal pain · acute renal failure (with high doses) · alopecia · anxiety · arthralgia · asthenia · bone-marrow suppression · chills · constipation · cough · diarrhoea · dizziness · dyspnoea · extravasation · flatulence · haemolytic anaemia · headache · hyperuricaemia · insomnia · malaise · myalgia · nausea · oedema · oral mucositis · pruritus · purpura · rash · severe myelosupression (with neutropenia, anaemia and thrombocytopenia) · severe neurotoxicity (with high doses) · sweating · tachycardia · thromboembolism · tumour lysis syndrome · vomiting

● CONCEPTION AND CONTRACEPTION Manufacturer advises that men should not father children during and for 6 months after treatment.

● PREGNANCY Avoid (teratogenic in *animal* studies). See also *Pregnancy and reproductive function* in Cytotoxic drugs p. 787.

● BREAST FEEDING Discontinue breast-feeding.

● HEPATIC IMPAIRMENT Regular monitoring recommended in hepatic impairment.

● RENAL IMPAIRMENT Regular monitoring recommended in renal impairment.

● DIRECTIONS FOR ADMINISTRATION *Litak®* for subcutaneous use only—no dilution required.

● MEDICINAL FORMS
There can be variation in the licensing of different medicines containing the same drug.
Solution for injection
▶ Litak (Lipomed GmbH)
   Cladribine 2 mg per 1 ml Litak 10mg/5ml solution for injection vials | 1 vial [PoM] £165.00 (Hospital only) | 5 vial [PoM] £820.00 (Hospital only)
Solution for infusion
▶ Leustat (Janssen-Cilag Ltd)
   Cladribine 1 mg per 1 ml Leustat 10mg/10ml solution for infusion vials | 1 vial [PoM] £159.70

Clofarabine

● INDICATIONS AND DOSE
Relapsed or refractory acute lymphoblastic leukaemia in patients who have received at least two previous regimens
▶ BY INTRAVENOUS INFUSION
▶ Adult 18-20 years: (consult local protocol)

● CAUTIONS Cardiac disease

● SIDE-EFFECTS Abdominal pain · agitation · alopecia · anxiety · arthralgia · bone-marrow suppression · cough · diarrhoea · dizziness · drowsiness · dyspnoea · extravasation · flushing · haematoma · haematuria · hand-foot (desquamative) syndrome · headache · hyperuricaemia

· hypotension · jaundice · myalgia · nausea · oedema · oral mucositis · pancreatitis · paraesthesia · pericardial effusion · peripheral neuropathy · pruritus · rash · restlessness · sweating · tachycardia · thromboembolism · tumour lysis syndrome · vomiting

● CONCEPTION AND CONTRACEPTION Contraceptive advice required, see *Pregnancy and reproductive function* in Cytotoxic drugs p. 787.

● PREGNANCY Manufacturer advises avoid (teratogenic in *animal* studies). See also *Pregnancy and reproductive function* in Cytotoxic drugs p. 787.

● BREAST FEEDING Discontinue breast-feeding.

● HEPATIC IMPAIRMENT Manufacturer advises caution in mild to moderate impairment. Avoid in severe impairment.

● RENAL IMPAIRMENT Manufacturer advises caution in mild to moderate impairment. Avoid in severe impairment.

● MEDICINAL FORMS
There can be variation in the licensing of different medicines containing the same drug.
Solution for infusion
ELECTROLYTES: May contain Sodium
▶ Evoltra (Sanofi) ▼
   Clofarabine 1 mg per 1 ml Evoltra 20mg/20ml concentrate for solution for infusion vials | 4 vial [PoM] £5,304.72 (Hospital only)

Cytarabine

● DRUG ACTION Cytarabine acts by interfering with pyrimidine synthesis.

● INDICATIONS AND DOSE
Induction of remission of acute myeloblastic leukaemia
▶ BY INTRAVENOUS INFUSION, OR BY INTRAVENOUS INJECTION, OR BY SUBCUTANEOUS INJECTION
▶ Adult: (consult local protocol)
Lymphomatous meningitis
▶ BY INTRATHECAL INJECTION
▶ Adult: (consult local protocol)

IMPORTANT SAFETY INFORMATION
Not all cytarabine preparations can be given by intrathecal injection—consult product literature.

● INTERACTIONS → Appendix 1 (cytarabine).

● SIDE-EFFECTS Alopecia · bone-marrow suppression · extravasation · hyperuricaemia · nausea · oral mucositis · thromboembolism · tumour lysis syndrome · vomiting

● CONCEPTION AND CONTRACEPTION Contraceptive advice required, see *Pregnancy and reproductive function* in Cytotoxic drugs p. 787.

● PREGNANCY Avoid (teratogenic in *animal* studies). See also *Pregnancy and reproductive function* in Cytotoxic drugs p. 787.

● BREAST FEEDING Discontinue breast-feeding.

● HEPATIC IMPAIRMENT Reduce dose—consult product literature.

● MONITORING REQUIREMENTS
▶ Haematological monitoring Cytarabine is a potent myelosuppressant and requires careful haematological monitoring.

● NATIONAL FUNDING/ACCESS DECISIONS
DEPOCYTE®
Scottish Medicines Consortium (SMC) Decisions
The *Scottish Medicines Consortium* has advised (July 2007) that liposomal cytarabine suspension (*DepoCyte®*) is not recommended for use within NHS Scotland for the intrathecal treatment of lymphomatous meningitis.

8

Immune system and malignant disease

● MEDICINAL FORMS
There can be variation in the licensing of different medicines containing the same drug. Forms available from special-order manufacturers include: solution for injection

Solution for injection
▸ Cytarabine (Non-proprietary)
Cytarabine 20 mg per 1 ml Cytarabine 500mg/25ml solution for injection vials | 1 vial [PoM] £19.50
Cytarabine 100mg/5ml solution for injection vials | 5 vial [PoM] £20.98–£30.00
Cytarabine 100 mg per 1 ml Cytarabine 500mg/5ml solution for injection vials | 5 vial [PoM] £100.00
Cytarabine 100mg/1ml solution for injection vials | 5 vial [PoM] £30.00
Cytarabine 2g/20ml solution for injection vials | 1 vial [PoM] £79.00
Cytarabine 1g/10ml solution for injection vials | 1 vial [PoM] £40.00

Suspension for injection
▸ DepoCyte (Napp Pharmaceuticals Ltd)
Cytarabine 10 mg per 1 ml DepoCyte 50mg/5ml suspension for injection vials | 1 vial [PoM] £1,223.75 (Hospital only)

Decitabine

● DRUG ACTION Decitabine is a pyrimidine analogue.

● INDICATIONS AND DOSE

Treatment of newly diagnosed acute myeloid leukaemia in patients over 65 years of age who are not candidates for standard induction chemotherapy
▸ BY INTRAVENOUS INFUSION
▸ Elderly: (consult local protocol)

● CAUTIONS History of severe congestive heart failure · history of unstable cardiac disease

● INTERACTIONS → Appendix 1 (decitabine).

● SIDE-EFFECTS
▸ **Common or very common** Diarrhoea · epistaxis · headache
▸ **Uncommon** Acute febrile neutrophilic dermatosis
▸ **Frequency not known** Alopecia · bone-marrow suppression · extravasation · hyperuricaemia · nausea · oral mucositis · thromboembolism · tumour lysis syndrome · vomiting

● CONCEPTION AND CONTRACEPTION Men must avoid fathering a child during and for 3 months after treatment.

● PREGNANCY Avoid (teratogenic in *animal* studies). See also *Pregnancy and reproductive function* in Cytotoxic drugs p. 787.

● BREAST FEEDING Discontinue breast-feeding.

● HEPATIC IMPAIRMENT Manufacturer advises caution—no information available.

● RENAL IMPAIRMENT Manufacturer advises caution if creatinine clearance less than 30 mL/minute—no information available.

● MEDICINAL FORMS
There can be variation in the licensing of different medicines containing the same drug.

Powder for solution for infusion
ELECTROLYTES: May contain Potassium, sodium
▸ Dacogen (Janssen-Cilag Ltd) ▼
Decitabine 50 mg Dacogen 50mg powder for concentrate for solution for infusion vials | 1 vial [PoM] £970.86

Fludarabine phosphate

● INDICATIONS AND DOSE

Initial treatment of advanced B-cell chronic lymphocytic leukaemia (CLL) or after first line treatment in patients with sufficient bone-marrow reserves
▸ BY MOUTH
▸ Adult: 40 mg/m^2 for 5 days every 28 days, usually given for 6 cycles

▸ BY INTRAVENOUS INJECTION, OR BY INTRAVENOUS INFUSION
▸ Adult: (consult product literature)

> IMPORTANT SAFETY INFORMATION
> RISKS OF INCORRECT DOSING OF ORAL ANTI-CANCER MEDICINES
> See Cytotoxic drugs p. 787.

● CONTRA-INDICATIONS Haemolytic anaemia

● CAUTIONS Increased susceptibility to skin cancer · worsening of existing skin cancer

CAUTIONS, FURTHER INFORMATION
Co-trimoxazole is used to prevent pneumocytis infection.
▸ Immunosuppression Fludarabine has a potent and prolonged immunosuppresive effect. Patients treated with fludarabine are more prone to serious bacterial, opportunistic fungal, and viral infections, and prophylactic therapy is recommended in those at risk. To prevent potentially fatal transfusion-related graft-versus-host reaction, only irradiated blood products should be administered. Prescribers should consult specialist literature when using highly immunosuppressive drugs.

● INTERACTIONS → Appendix 1 (fludarabine).

● SIDE-EFFECTS
▸ **Common or very common** Acute myeloid leukaemia · anorexia · chills · cough · diarrhoea · fever · immunosuppression · malaise · myelodysplastic syndrome · myelosupression (may be cumulative) · oedema · peripheral neuropathy · pneumonia · rash · visual disturbances · weakness
▸ **Uncommon** Autoimmune disorder · confusion · fibrosis · haemorrhage · immune-mediated haemolytic anaemia · neutropenia · pneumonitis · pulmonary toxicity · thrombocytopenia
▸ **Rare** Agitation · arrhythmia · blindness · coma · heart failure · optic neuropathy · seizures · skin cancer · Stevens-Johnson syndrome · toxic epidermal necrolysis
▸ **Frequency not known** Alopecia · bone-marrow suppression · extravasation · haemorrhagic cystitis · hyperuricaemia · nausea · oral mucositis · thromboembolism · tumour lysis syndrome · vomiting

● CONCEPTION AND CONTRACEPTION Manufacturer advises effective contraception during and for at least 6 months after treatment in men or women.

● PREGNANCY Avoid (embryotoxic and teratogenic in *animal* studies). See also *Pregnancy and reproductive function* in Cytotoxic drugs p. 787.

● BREAST FEEDING Discontinue breast-feeding.

● RENAL IMPAIRMENT Reduce dose by up to 50% if creatinine clearance 30–70 mL/minute. Avoid if creatinine clearance less than 30 mL/minute.

● MONITORING REQUIREMENTS
▸ Monitor for signs of haemolysis.
▸ Monitor for neurological toxicity.
▸ Assess creatinine clearance in patients over 65 years before treatment initiation.

● DIRECTIONS FOR ADMINISTRATION Concentrate for intravenous injection or infusion must be diluted before administration (consult product literature).

● NATIONAL FUNDING/ACCESS DECISIONS

NICE technology appraisals (TAs)
▸ **Fludarabine monotherapy for the first-line treatment of chronic lymphocytic leukaemia (February 2007)** NICE TA119
Fludarabine monotherapy is **not** recommended for the first-line treatment of chronic lymphocytic leukaemia.
www.nice.org.uk/TA119
▸ **Fludarabine for the treatment of B-cell chronic lymphocytic leukaemia (September 2001)** NICE TA29
Oral fludarabine is recommended for the second-line treatment of B-cell chronic lymphocytic leukaemia in

patients who have either failed, or are intolerant of, first line chemotherapy, and who would otherwise have received combination chemotherapy of either:

- cyclophosphamide, doxorubicin, vincristine and prednisolone (CHOP)
- cyclophosphamide, doxorubicin and prednisolone (CAP) or
- cyclophosphamide, vincristine and prednisolone (CVP)

Intravenous fludarabine should only be used when oral fludarabine is contra-indicated.
www.nice.org.uk/TA29

Scottish Medicines Consortium (SMC) Decisions

The *Scottish Medicines Consortium* has advised (October 2006) that fludarabine is accepted for restricted use for the treatment of B-cell chronic lymphocytic leukaemia (CLL) in patients with sufficient bone marrow reserves. First-line treatment should only be initiated in patients with advanced disease, Rai stages III/IV (Binet stage C), or Rai stages I/II (Binet stage A/B) where the patient has disease-related symptoms or evidence of progressive disease.

● MEDICINAL FORMS
There can be variation in the licensing of different medicines containing the same drug.

Tablet
▸ Fludara (Sanofi)
Fludarabine phosphate 10 mg Fludara 10mg tablets | 15 tablet PoM £302.48 (Hospital only) | 20 tablet PoM £403.31 (Hospital only)

Solution for injection
▸ Fludarabine phosphate (Non-proprietary)
Fludarabine phosphate 25 mg per 1 ml Fludarabine phosphate 50mg/2ml solution for injection vials | 1 vial PoM £117.75
Fludarabine phosphate 50mg/2ml concentrate for solution for injection vials | 1 vial PoM £156.00 (Hospital only) | 1 vial PoM £155.00

Powder for solution for injection
▸ Fludarabine phosphate (Non-proprietary)
Fludarabine phosphate 50 mg Fludarabine phosphate 50mg powder for solution for injection vials | 1 vial PoM £155.00 (Hospital only) | 1 vial PoM £155.00 | 5 vial PoM £735.35 (Hospital only)
▸ Fludara (Sanofi)
Fludarabine phosphate 50 mg Fludara 50mg powder for solution for injection vials | 5 vial PoM £735.34 (Hospital only)

Fluorouracil

● INDICATIONS AND DOSE
Treatment of some solid tumours including gastro-intestinal tract cancers and breast cancer | In combination with folinic acid in advanced colorectal cancer
▸ BY INTRAVENOUS INJECTION, OR BY INTRAVENOUS INFUSION, OR BY INTRA-ARTERIAL INFUSION
▸ Adult: (consult product literature)

● INTERACTIONS → Appendix 1 (fluorouracil).
● SIDE-EFFECTS
▸ **Rare** Cerebellar syndrome
▸ **Frequency not known** Alopecia · bone-marrow suppression · desquamative hand-foot syndrome (on prolonged infusion) · extravasation · hyperuricaemia · mucositis · myelosuppression · nausea · oral mucositis · thromboembolism · tumour lysis syndrome · vomiting
● CONCEPTION AND CONTRACEPTION Contraceptive advice required, see *Pregnancy and reproductive function* in Cytotoxic drugs p. 787.
● PREGNANCY Avoid (teratogenic). See also *Pregnancy and reproductive function* in Cytotoxic drugs p. 787.
● BREAST FEEDING Discontinue breast-feeding.
● HEPATIC IMPAIRMENT Manufacturer advises caution.

● HANDLING AND STORAGE Caution in handling—irritant to tissues.

● MEDICINAL FORMS
There can be variation in the licensing of different medicines containing the same drug.

Solution for injection
▸ Fluorouracil (Non-proprietary)
Fluorouracil (as Fluorouracil sodium) 25 mg per 1 ml Fluorouracil 500mg/20ml solution for injection vials | 10 vial PoM £64.00
Fluorouracil 250mg/10ml solution for injection vials | 5 vial PoM £20.00
Fluorouracil (as Fluorouracil sodium) 50 mg per 1 ml Fluorouracil 1g/20ml solution for injection vials | 1 vial PoM £12.80
Fluorouracil 500mg/10ml solution for injection vials | 1 vial PoM £6.40 | 5 vial PoM £32.00

Solution for infusion
▸ Fluorouracil (Non-proprietary)
Fluorouracil (as Fluorouracil sodium) 25 mg per 1 ml Fluorouracil 2.5g/100ml solution for infusion vials | 1 vial PoM £32.00
Fluorouracil (as Fluorouracil sodium) 50 mg per 1 ml Fluorouracil 5g/100ml solution for infusion vials | 1 vial PoM £64.00
Fluorouracil 2.5g/50ml solution for infusion vials | 1 vial PoM £32.00

Gemcitabine

10.6.2016

● INDICATIONS AND DOSE
First-line treatment for locally advanced or metastatic non-small cell lung cancer (as monotherpay in elderly patients and in palliative treatment; otherwise in combination with cisplatin) | Treatment of locally advanced or metastatic pancreatic cancer | Treatment of advanced or metastatic bladder cancer (in combination with cisplatin) | Treatment of locally advanced or metastatic epithelial ovarian cancer which has relapsed after a recurrence-free interval of at least 6 months following previous platinum-based therapy (in combination with carboplatin) | Treatment of metastatic breast cancer which has relapsed after previous chemotherapy including an anthracycline (in combination with paclitaxel)
▸ BY INTRAVENOUS INFUSION
▸ Adult: (consult local protocol)

● INTERACTIONS → Appendix 1 (gemcitabine).
● SIDE-EFFECTS
▸ **Rare** Haemolytic uraemic syndrome
▸ **Frequency not known** Alopecia · bone-marrow suppression · extravasation · hyperuricaemia · influenza-like symptoms · microangiopathic haemolytic anaemia · mild gastro-intestinal side-effects · musculoskeletal pain · nausea · oral mucositis · pulmonary toxicity · rash · renal impairment · thromboembolism · tumour lysis syndrome · vomiting
SIDE-EFFECTS, FURTHER INFORMATION
▸ Microangiopathic haemolytic anaemia Gemcitabine should be discontinued if signs of microangiopathic haemolytic anaemia occur.
● CONCEPTION AND CONTRACEPTION Manufacturer advises effective contraception during treatment. Men must avoid fathering a child during and for 6 months after treatment.
● PREGNANCY Avoid (teratogenic in *animal* studies). See *Pregnancy and reproductive function* in Cytotoxic drugs p. 787.
● BREAST FEEDING Discontinue breast-feeding.
● HEPATIC IMPAIRMENT Manufacturer advises caution.
● RENAL IMPAIRMENT Manufacturer advises caution.
● NATIONAL FUNDING/ACCESS DECISIONS

NICE technology appraisals (TAs)
▸ Gemcitabine for the treatment of pancreatic cancer (May 2001) NICE TA25
Gemcitabine is an option for first-line chemotherapy for patients with advanced or metastatic adenocarcinoma of

the pancreas and a Karnofsky score of at least 50 [Karnofsky score is a measure of the ability to perform ordinary tasks].

Gemcitabine is not recommended for patients who can have potentially curative surgery. There is insufficient evidence about its use for second-line treatment of pancreatic adenocarcinoma.
www.nice.org.uk/TA25

▸ **Gemcitabine for the treatment of metastatic breast cancer (January 2007)** NICE TA116
Gemcitabine, in combination with paclitaxel, is an option for the treatment of metastatic breast cancer **only** when docetaxel monotherapy or docetaxel plus capecitabine are also considered appropriate.
www.nice.org.uk/TA116

▸ **Bevacizumab in combination with gemcitabine and carboplatin for the treatment of the first recurrence of platinum-sensitive advanced ovarian cancer (May 2013)** NICE TA285
Bevacizumab in combination with gemcitabine and carboplatin is **not** recommended within its marketing authorisation, that is, for the treatment of the first recurrence of platinum-sensitive advanced ovarian cancer (including fallopian tube and primary peritoneal cancer) that has not been previously treated with bevacizumab or other vascular endothelial growth factor (VEGF) inhibitors or VEGF receptor-targeted agents.
www.nice.org/TA285

▸ **Paclitaxel as albumin-bound nanoparticles in combination with gemcitabine for previously untreated metastatic pancreatic cancer (October 2015)** NICE TA360
Gemcitabine in combination with albumin-bound paclitaxel (nab-paclitaxel, *Abraxane*®) is **not** recommended for the treatment of previously untreated metastatic adenocarcinoma of the pancreas.

Patients whose treatment was started before this guidance was published should continue treatment until they and their clinician consider it appropriate to stop.
www.nice.org.uk/TA360

▸ **Topotecan, pegylated liposomal doxorubicin hydrochloride, paclitaxel, trabectedin and gemcitabine for treating recurrent ovarian cancer (April 2016)** NICE TA389
Gemcitabine, in combination with carboplatin, is **not** recommended for treating the first recurrence of platinum-sensitive ovarian cancer.

Patient currently receiving gemcitabine in combination with carboplatin should have the option to continue their treatment until they and their clinician consider it appropriate to stop.
www.nice.org.uk/TA389

Scottish Medicines Consortium (SMC) Decisions
The *Scottish Medicines Consortium* has advised (November 2006) that gemcitabine is accepted for restricted use for the treatment of metastatic breast cancer, which has relapsed following previous chemotherapy including an anthracycline (unless contra-indicated).

● MEDICINAL FORMS
There can be variation in the licensing of different medicines containing the same drug.
Solution for infusion
▸ Gemcitabine (Non-proprietary)
Gemcitabine (as Gemcitabine hydrochloride)
200 mg Gemcitabine 200mg/5.3ml concentrate for solution for infusion vials | 1 vial [PoM] £25.00 (Hospital only)
Gemcitabine 200mg/5ml concentrate for solution for infusion vials | 1 vial [PoM] £6.40
Gemcitabine 200mg/2ml concentrate for solution for infusion vials | 1 vial [PoM] no price available
Gemcitabine (as Gemcitabine hydrochloride) 1 gram Gemcitabine 1g/26.3ml concentrate for solution for infusion vials | 1 vial [PoM] £125.00 (Hospital only)
Gemcitabine 1g/25ml concentrate for solution for infusion vials | 1 vial [PoM] £13.09

Gemcitabine 1g/10ml concentrate for solution for infusion vials | 1 vial [PoM] no price available
Gemcitabine (as Gemcitabine hydrochloride) 2 gram Gemcitabine 2g/50ml concentrate for solution for infusion vials | 1 vial [PoM] £26.86
Gemcitabine 2g/20ml concentrate for solution for infusion vials | 1 vial [PoM] no price available
Gemcitabine 2g/52.6ml concentrate for solution for infusion vials | 1 vial [PoM] £250.00 (Hospital only)
Powder for solution for infusion
▸ Gemcitabine (Non-proprietary)
Gemcitabine (as Gemcitabine hydrochloride)
200 mg Gemcitabine 200mg powder for solution for infusion vials | 1 vial [PoM] £32.00–£32.55 (Hospital only) | 1 vial [PoM] £32.00
Gemcitabine (as Gemcitabine hydrochloride) 1 gram Gemcitabine 1g powder for solution for infusion vials | 1 vial [PoM] £162.00–£162.76 (Hospital only) | 1 vial [PoM] £162.00
Gemcitabine (as Gemcitabine hydrochloride)
1.5 gram Gemcitabine 1.5g powder for solution for infusion vials | 1 vial [PoM] £231.93
Gemcitabine (as Gemcitabine hydrochloride) 2 gram Gemcitabine 2g powder for solution for infusion vials | 1 vial [PoM] £324.00 (Hospital only) | 1 vial [PoM] £324.00
▸ Gemzar (Eli Lilly and Company Ltd)
Gemcitabine (as Gemcitabine hydrochloride) 200 mg Gemzar 200mg powder for solution for infusion vials | 1 vial [PoM] £32.55 (Hospital only)
Gemcitabine (as Gemcitabine hydrochloride) 1 gram Gemzar 1g powder for solution for infusion vials | 1 vial [PoM] £162.76 (Hospital only)

Mercaptopurine

(6-Mercaptopurine)

● INDICATIONS AND DOSE

Severe acute Crohn's disease | Maintenance of remission of Crohn's disease | Ulcerative colitis
▸ BY MOUTH
▸ Adult: 1–1.5 mg/kg daily, some patients may respond to lower doses

Acute leukaemias | Chronic myeloid leukaemia
▸ BY MOUTH USING TABLETS
▸ Adult: Initially 2.5 mg/kg daily, adjusted according to response, alternatively initially 50–75 mg/m^2 daily, adjusted according to response
▸ BY MOUTH USING ORAL SUSPENSION
▸ Adult: Initially 25–75 mg/m^2 daily, adjusted according to response

DOSE EQUIVALENCE AND CONVERSION
Mercaptopurine tablets and *Xaluprine*® oral suspension are **not** bioequivalent, haematological monitoring is advised when switching formulations.

● UNLICENSED USE Not licensed for use in severe ulcerative colitis and Crohn's disease.

IMPORTANT SAFETY INFORMATION
RISKS OF INCORRECT DOSING OF ORAL ANTI-CANCER MEDICINES
See Cytotoxic drugs p. 787.

● CONTRA-INDICATIONS Absent thiopurine methyltransferase activity
● CAUTIONS Reduced thiopurine methyltransferase activity
CAUTIONS, FURTHER INFORMATION
▸ Thiopurine methyltransferase The enzyme thiopurine methyltransferase (TPMT) metabolises thiopurine drugs (azathioprine, mercaptopurine, tioguanine); the risk of myelosuppression is increased in patients with reduced activity of the enzyme, particularly for the few individuals in whom TPMT activity is undetectable. Patients with absent TPMT activity should not receive thiopurine drugs; those with reduced TPMT activity may be treated under specialist supervision.

- INTERACTIONS → Appendix 1 (mercaptopurine).
- SIDE-EFFECTS
- ▶ **Rare** Pancreatitis · transient oligospermia
- ▶ **Very rare** Intestinal ulceration · lymphoma
- ▶ **Frequency not known** Alopecia · anorexia · bone-marrow suppression · hepatotoxicity · hyperuricaemia · nausea · oral mucositis · thromboembolism · tumour lysis syndrome · vomiting

  SIDE-EFFECTS, FURTHER INFORMATION
- ▶ Gastro-intestinal side-effects Tioguanine has a lower incidence of gastrointestinal side-effects than mercaptopurine.
- CONCEPTION AND CONTRACEPTION Contraceptive advice required, see *Pregnancy and reproductive function* in Cytotoxic drugs p. 787.
- PREGNANCY Avoid (teratogenic). See also *Pregnancy and reproductive function* in Cytotoxic drugs p. 787.
- BREAST FEEDING Discontinue breast-feeding.
- HEPATIC IMPAIRMENT May need dose reduction.
- RENAL IMPAIRMENT Reduce dose.
- PRE-TREATMENT SCREENING Consider measuring thiopurine methyltransferase (TPMT) activity before starting mercaptopurine therapy.
- MONITORING REQUIREMENTS Monitor liver function.
- PRESCRIBING AND DISPENSING INFORMATION Flavours of oral liquid formulations may include raspberry.

- MEDICINAL FORMS
There can be variation in the licensing of different medicines containing the same drug. Forms available from special-order manufacturers include: tablet, capsule, oral suspension
Tablet
▶ Mercaptopurine (Non-proprietary)
  Mercaptopurine 50 mg Mercaptopurine 50mg tablets | 25 tablet [PoM] £49.15 DT price = £49.15
Oral suspension
EXCIPIENTS: May contain Aspartame
▶ Xaluprine (Nova Laboratories Ltd)
  Mercaptopurine 20 mg per 1 ml Xaluprine 20mg/ml oral suspension | 100 ml [PoM] £170.00

Methotrexate

- DRUG ACTION Methotrexate inhibits the enzyme dihydrofolate reductase, essential for the synthesis of purines and pyrimidines.

- INDICATIONS AND DOSE
Severe Crohn's disease
▶ BY INTRAMUSCULAR INJECTION
▶ Adult: Initially 25 mg once weekly until remission induced; maintenance 15 mg once weekly
Maintenance of remission of severe Crohn's disease
▶ BY MOUTH
▶ Adult: 10–25 mg once weekly
Moderate to severe active rheumatoid arthritis
▶ BY MOUTH
▶ Adult: 7.5 mg once weekly, adjusted according to response; maximum 20 mg per week
Severe active rheumatoid arthritis
▶ BY INTRAVENOUS INJECTION, OR BY INTRAMUSCULAR INJECTION, OR BY SUBCUTANEOUS INJECTION
▶ Adult: Initially 7.5 mg once weekly, then increased in steps of 2.5 mg once weekly, adjusted according to response; maximum 25 mg per week
Neoplastic diseases
▶ BY INTRAVENOUS INJECTION, OR BY INTRATHECAL INJECTION, OR BY INTRA-ARTERIAL INFUSION, OR BY INTRAMUSCULAR INJECTION, OR BY INTRAVENOUS INFUSION, OR BY MOUTH
▶ Adult: (consult product literature)

Severe psoriasis unresponsive to conventional therapy (specialist use only)
▶ BY MOUTH, OR BY INTRAMUSCULAR INJECTION, OR BY INTRAVENOUS INJECTION, OR BY SUBCUTANEOUS INJECTION
▶ Adult: Initially 2.5–10 mg once weekly, then increased in steps of 2.5–5 mg, adjusted according to response, dose to be adjusted at intervals of at least 1 week; usual dose 7.5–15 mg once weekly, stop treatment if inadequate response after 3 months at the optimum dose; maximum 30 mg per week

- UNLICENSED USE Not licensed for use in severe Crohn's disease.

> IMPORTANT SAFETY INFORMATION
> Note that the dose is a **weekly** dose. To avoid error with low-dose methotrexate, it is recommended that:
> - the patient is carefully advised of the **dose** and **frequency** and the reason for taking methotrexate and any other prescribed medicine (e.g. folic acid);
> - only one strength of methotrexate tablet (usually 2.5 mg) is prescribed and dispensed;
> - the prescription and the dispensing label clearly show the dose and frequency of methotrexate administration;
> - the patient is warned to report immediately the onset of any feature of blood disorders (e.g. sore throat, bruising, and mouth ulcers), liver toxicity (e.g. nausea, vomiting, abdominal discomfort, and dark urine), and respiratory effects (e.g. shortness of breath).

- CONTRA-INDICATIONS Active infection (in non-malignant conditions) · ascites · immunodeficiency syndromes (in non-malignant conditions) · significant pleural effusion
- CAUTIONS Acute porphyrias p. 918 · photosensitivity—psoriasis lesions aggravated by UV radiation (skin ulceration reported) · diarrhoea · extreme caution in blood disorders (avoid if severe) · peptic ulceration · risk of accumulation in pleural effusion or ascites—drain before treatment · ulcerative colitis · ulcerative stomatitis
  CAUTIONS, FURTHER INFORMATION
- ▶ Blood count Bone marrow suppression can occur abruptly; factors likely to increase toxicity include advanced age, renal impairment, and concomitant use with another anti-folate drug (e.g. trimethoprim). A clinically significant drop in white cell count or platelet count calls for immediate withdrawal of methotrexate and introduction of supportive therapy.
- ▶ Gastro-intestinal toxicity Withdraw treatment if stomatitis develops—may be first sign of gastro-intestinal toxicity.
- ▶ Liver toxicity Liver cirrhosis reported. Treatment should not be started or should be discontinued if any abnormality of liver function tests or liver biopsy is present or develops during therapy. Abnormalities can return to normal within 2 weeks after which treatment may be recommenced if judged appropriate.
- ▶ Pulmonary toxicity Pulmonary toxicity may be a special problem in rheumatoid arthritis (patient to seek medical attention if dyspnoea, cough or fever); monitor for symptoms at each visit—discontinue if pneumonitis suspected.
- INTERACTIONS → Appendix 1 (methotrexate). If aspirin or other NSAIDs are given concurrently the dose of methotrexate should be carefully monitored.
- SIDE-EFFECTS
- ▶ **Rare** Pneumonitis
- ▶ **Frequency not known** Abdominal discomfort · acne · alopecia · anaphylactic reactions · anorexia · arthralgia · blood disorders · changes in nail pigmentation · changes in skin pigmentation · chills · chronic pulmonary fibrosis · confusion · conjunctivitis · cystitis · diarrhoea · dizziness · drowsiness · dyspepsia · dysuria · ecchymosis · fever ·

furuncolosis · gastro-intestinal bleeding · gastro-intestinal ulceration · haematuria · headache · hepatotoxicity · hypotension · impotence · injection-site reactions · insomnia · interstitial pneumonitis · malaise · menstrual disturbances · mood changes · mucositis · myalgia · myelosuppresion · nausea · neurotoxicity · osteoporosis · paraesthesia · pericardial tamponade · pericarditis · photosensitivity · pleuritic pain · precipitation of diabetes · pruritus · pulmonary fibrosis · pulmonary oedema · rash · reduced libido · renal failure · Stevens-Johnson syndrome · telangiectasia · thrombosis · toxic epidermal necrolysis · toxic megacolon · urticaria · vaginitis · vasculitis · visual disturbance · vomiting

SIDE-EFFECTS, FURTHER INFORMATION
In patients taking methotrexate for non-malignant conditions who experience side-effects, folic acid given on a different day from the methotrexate, may help to reduce the frequency of such side-effects.

Withdraw treatment if stomatitis develops—may be first sign of gastro-intestinal toxicity.

Treatment with folinic acid (as calcium folinate) may be required in acute toxicity.

● CONCEPTION AND CONTRACEPTION Effective contraception required during and for at least 3 months after treatment in men or women.

● PREGNANCY Avoid (teratogenic; fertility may be reduced during therapy but this may be reversible).

● BREAST FEEDING Discontinue breast-feeding—present in milk.

● HEPATIC IMPAIRMENT When used for malignancy, avoid in severe hepatic impairment—consult local treatment protocol for details. Avoid with hepatic impairment in non-malignant conditions—dose-related toxicity.

● RENAL IMPAIRMENT Reduce dose. Risk of nephrotoxicity at high doses. Avoid in severe impairment.

● PRE-TREATMENT SCREENING Exclude pregnancy before treatment.

Patients should have full blood count and renal and liver function tests before starting treatment.

● MONITORING REQUIREMENTS
▶ In view of reports of blood dyscrasias (including fatalities) and liver cirrhosis with low-dose methotrexate patients should:
  ● have full blood count and renal and liver function tests repeated every 1–2 weeks until therapy stabilised, thereafter patients should be monitored every 2–3 months.
  ● be advised to report all symptoms and signs suggestive of infection, especially sore throat
▶ Local protocols for frequency of monitoring may vary.
▶ Treatment with folinic acid (as calcium folinate) may be required in acute toxicity.

● PRESCRIBING AND DISPENSING INFORMATION Folinic acid following methotrexate administration helps to prevent methotrexate-induced mucositis and myelosuppression.

● PATIENT AND CARER ADVICE
Patients and their carers should be warned to report immediately the onset of any feature of blood disorders (e.g. sore throat, bruising, and mouth ulcers), liver toxicity (e.g. nausea, vomiting, abdominal discomfort and dark urine), and respiratory effects (e.g. shortness of breath).

Patients should be advised to avoid self-medication with over-the-counter aspirin or ibuprofen.

Patients should be counselled on the dose, treatment booklet, and the use of NSAIDs.

Methotrexate treatment booklets Methotrexate treatment booklets should be issued where appropriate.

In **England**, **Wales**, and **Northern Ireland**, they are available for purchase from:
  Gorse Street, Chadderton
  Oldham
  OL9 9QH
  Tel: 0845 610 1112
GP practices can obtain supplies through their Local Area Team stores.
NHS Hospitals can order supplies from www.nhsforms.co.uk or by emailing nhsforms@mmm.com.
In **Scotland**, treatment booklets can be obtained by emailing stockorders.dppas@theapsgroup.com or by fax on 0131 629 9967.

These booklets include advice for adults taking oral methotrexate for inflammatory conditions, and a section for recording results of blood tests and dosage information.

● MEDICINAL FORMS
There can be variation in the licensing of different medicines containing the same drug. Forms available from special-order manufacturers include: oral suspension, oral solution, solution for injection

Tablet
▶ Methotrexate (Non-proprietary)
  Methotrexate 2.5 mg Methotrexate 2.5mg tablets | 24 tablet [PoM] £3.75 | 28 tablet [PoM] £3.82 DT price = £1.97 | 100 tablet [PoM] £14.19
  Methotrexate 10 mg Methotrexate 10mg tablets | 100 tablet [PoM] £57.21 DT price = £37.75
▶ Maxtrex (Pfizer Ltd)
  Methotrexate 2.5 mg Maxtrex 2.5mg tablets | 24 tablet [PoM] £2.39 | 100 tablet [PoM] £9.96
  Methotrexate 10 mg Maxtrex 10mg tablets | 100 tablet [PoM] £45.16 DT price = £37.75

Oral solution
▶ Methotrexate (Non-proprietary)
  Methotrexate (as Methotrexate sodium) 2 mg per 1 ml Methotrexate 2mg/ml oral solution sugar free sugar-free | 35 ml [PoM] £95.00–£114.00 DT price = £95.00 sugar-free | 65 ml [PoM] £125.00–£150.00 DT price = £125.00

Solution for injection
▶ Methotrexate (Non-proprietary)
  Methotrexate (as Methotrexate sodium) 2.5 mg per 1 ml Methotrexate 5mg/2ml solution for injection vials | 5 vial [PoM] £30.00
  Methotrexate (as Methotrexate sodium) 25 mg per 1 ml Methotrexate 1g/40ml solution for injection vials | 1 vial [PoM] £43.68 (Hospital only) | 1 vial [PoM] £44.57–£67.50 Methotrexate 500mg/20ml solution for injection vials | 1 vial [PoM] £38.30 (Hospital only) | 1 vial [PoM] £22.56–£48.00 Methotrexate 50mg/2ml solution for injection vials | 1 vial [PoM] £4.49 (Hospital only) | 1 vial [PoM] £3.00 | 5 vial [PoM] £35.00 Methotrexate 200mg/8ml solution for injection vials | 1 vial [PoM] £10.02
  Methotrexate (as Methotrexate sodium) 100 mg per 1 ml Methotrexate 1g/10ml solution for injection vials | 1 vial [PoM] £85.00
▶ Metoject PEN (medac UK)
  Methotrexate 50 mg per 1 ml Metoject PEN 30mg/0.6ml solution for injection pre-filled pen | 1 pre-filled disposable injection [PoM] £18.95 Metoject PEN 22.5mg/0.45ml solution for injection pre-filled pen | 1 pre-filled disposable injection [PoM] £18.45 Metoject PEN 12.5mg/0.25ml solution for injection pre-filled pen | 1 pre-filled disposable injection [PoM] £16.50 Metoject PEN 20mg/0.4ml solution for injection pre-filled pen | 1 pre-filled disposable injection [PoM] £17.84 Metoject PEN 17.5mg/0.35ml solution for injection pre-filled pen | 1 pre-filled disposable injection [PoM] £17.50 Metoject PEN 7.5mg/0.15ml solution for injection pre-filled pen | 1 pre-filled disposable injection [PoM] £14.85 Metoject PEN 10mg/0.2ml solution for injection pre-filled pen | 1 pre-filled disposable injection [PoM] £15.29 Metoject PEN 27.5mg/0.55ml solution for injection pre-filled pen | 1 pre-filled disposable injection [PoM] £18.89 Metoject PEN 25mg/0.5ml solution for injection pre-filled pen | 1 pre-filled disposable injection [PoM] £18.48 Metoject PEN 15mg/0.3ml solution for injection pre-filled pen | 1 pre-filled disposable injection [PoM] £16.57

▸ Zlatal (Nordic Pharma Ltd)
Methotrexate (as Methotrexate sodium) 25 mg per 1 ml Zlatal
17.5mg/0.7ml solution for injection pre-filled syringes | 1 pre-filled
disposable injection [PoM] £15.75
Zlatal 10mg/0.4ml solution for injection pre-filled syringes | 1 pre-
filled disposable injection [PoM] £13.77
Zlatal 25mg/1ml solution for injection pre-filled syringes | 1 pre-
filled disposable injection [PoM] £16.64
Zlatal 20mg/0.8ml solution for injection pre-filled syringes | 1 pre-
filled disposable injection [PoM] £16.06
Zlatal 12.5mg/0.5ml solution for injection pre-filled syringes | 1 pre-
filled disposable injection [PoM] £14.85
Zlatal 7.5mg/0.3ml solution for injection pre-filled syringes | 1 pre-
filled disposable injection [PoM] £13.37
Zlatal 22.5mg/0.9ml solution for injection pre-filled syringes | 1 pre-
filled disposable injection [PoM] £16.61
Zlatal 15mg/0.6ml solution for injection pre-filled syringes | 1 pre-
filled disposable injection [PoM] £14.92

Solution for infusion
▸ Methotrexate (Non-proprietary)
**Methotrexate (as Methotrexate sodium) 25 mg per
1 ml** Methotrexate 5g/200ml solution for infusion vials | 1 vial [PoM]
£200.57
**Methotrexate (as Methotrexate sodium) 100 mg per
1 ml** Methotrexate 5g/50ml solution for infusion vials | 1 vial [PoM]
£400.00

Nelarabine

● **INDICATIONS AND DOSE**

**T-cell acute lymphoblastic leukaemia and T-cell
lymphoblastic lymphoma in patients who have relapsed
or who are refractory after receiving at least two
previous regimens**
▸ BY INTRAVENOUS INFUSION
▸ Adult: (consult local protocol)

● CAUTIONS Previous or concurrent craniospinal irradiation
(increased risk of neurotoxicity) · previous or concurrent
intrathecal chemotherapy (increased risk of neurotoxicity)

● SIDE-EFFECTS
▸ **Common or very common** Neurotoxicity (discontinue)
▸ **Frequency not known** Abdominal pain · alopecia · amnesia ·
anorexia · arthralgia · asthenia · ataxia · benign and
malignant tumours · blurred vision · bone-marrow
suppression · confusion · constipation · cough ·
demyelination · diarrhoea · dizziness · drowsiness ·
dyspnoea · electrolyte disturbances · extravasation · fatigue
· headache · hyperuricaemia · hypoaesthesia · hypotension
· muscle weakness · myalgia · nausea · oedema · oral
mucositis · paraesthesia · peripheral neurological disorders
· pleural effusion · pyrexia · seizures · taste disturbance ·
thromboembolism · tremor · tumour lysis syndrome ·
vomiting · wheezing

● CONCEPTION AND CONTRACEPTION Manufacturer advises
effective contraception during and for at least 3 months
after treatment in men and women.

● PREGNANCY Avoid (toxicity in *animal* studies). See also
Pregnancy and reproductive function in Cytotoxic drugs
p. 787.

● BREAST FEEDING Discontinue breast-feeding.

● MONITORING REQUIREMENTS
▸ Neurotoxicity Close monitoring for neurological events is
strongly recommended—discontinue if neurotoxicty
occurs.

● PATIENT AND CARER ADVICE

Driving and skilled tasks
Drowsiness may affect performance of skilled tasks (e.g.
cycling or driving).

● NATIONAL FUNDING/ACCESS DECISIONS

Scottish Medicines Consortium (SMC) Decisions
The *Scottish Medicines Consortium* has advised (March
2008) that the use of nelarabine (*Atriance*®) within NHS

Scotland is restricted to bridging treatment before stem
cell transplantation.

● MEDICINAL FORMS
There can be variation in the licensing of different medicines
containing the same drug.
Solution for infusion
ELECTROLYTES: May contain Sodium
▸ Atriance (Novartis Pharmaceuticals UK Ltd) ▼
Nelarabine 5 mg per 1 ml Atriance 250mg/50ml solution for infusion
vials | 6 vial [PoM] £1,332.00

Pemetrexed

● DRUG ACTION Pemetrexed inhibits thymidylate
transferase and other folate-dependent enzymes.

● **INDICATIONS AND DOSE**

**Treatment of unresectable malignant pleural
mesothelioma which has not previously been treated
with chemotherapy (in combination with cisplatin) |
First-line treatment of locally advanced or metastatic
non-small cell lung cancer other than predominantly
squamous cell histology (in combination with cisplatin) |
Second-line treatment of locally advanced or metastatic
non-small cell lung cancer other than predominantly
squamous cell histology (monotherapy) | Maintenance
treatment in locally advanced or metastatic non-small
cell lung cancer other than predominantly squamous cell
histology that has not progressed immediately following
platinum-based chemotherapy (monotherapy)**
▸ BY INTRAVENOUS INFUSION
▸ Adult: (consult local protocol)

● CAUTIONS Diabetes · history of cardiovascular disease ·
prophylactic folic acid supplementation required (consult
product literature) · prophylactic vitamin B_{12}
supplementation required (consult product literature)

● INTERACTIONS → Appendix 1 (pemetrexed).
Caution with concomitant nephrotoxic drugs including
non-steroidal anti-inflammatory drugs (consult product
literature).

● SIDE-EFFECTS
▸ **Common or very common** Conjunctivitis · dehydration ·
gastro-intestinal disturbances · increased lacrimation ·
neuropathy · oedema · skin disorders
▸ **Uncommon** Arrhythmias · colitis · interstitial pneumonitis
▸ **Rare** Acute renal failure · hepatitis · peripheral ischaemia
▸ **Frequency not known** Alopecia · bone-marrow suppression
· extravasation · hyperuricaemia · nausea · oral mucositis ·
Stevens-Johnson syndrome · thromboembolism · toxic
epidermal necrolysis · tumour lysis syndrome · vomiting

● CONCEPTION AND CONTRACEPTION Manufacturer advises
effective contraception during treatment. Men must avoid
fathering a child during and for 6 months after treatment.

● PREGNANCY Avoid (toxicity in *animal* studies). See also
Pregnancy and reproductive function in Cytotoxic drugs
p. 787.

● BREAST FEEDING Discontinue breast-feeding.

● RENAL IMPAIRMENT Manufacturer advises avoid if
creatinine clearance less than 45 mL/minute—no
information available.

● NATIONAL FUNDING/ACCESS DECISIONS

NICE technology appraisals (TAs)
▸ Pemetrexed maintenance treatment following induction
therapy with pemetrexed and cisplatin for non-squamous
non-small-cell lung cancer (April 2014) NICE TA309
Pemetrexed is **not** recommended for the maintenance
treatment of locally advanced or metastatic non-squamous
non-small-cell lung cancer in patients whose disease has

8

Immune system and malignant disease

not progressed immediately following induction therapy with pemetrexed and cisplatin.
www.nice.org.uk/TA309

▶ **Pemetrexed for the treatment of non-small cell lung cancer (June 2010)** NICE TA190
Pemetrexed is an option for the maintenance treatment of locally advanced or metastatic non-small cell lung cancer other than predominantly squamous cell histology that has not progressed immediately following combination therapy of a platinum compound with either gemcitabine, paclitaxel, or docetaxel.
www.nice.org.uk/TA190

▶ **Pemetrexed for the treatment of non-small cell lung cancer (August 2007)** NICE TA124
Pemetrexed is **not** recommended for the treatment of locally advanced or metastatic non-small cell lung cancer which has previously been treated with chemotherapy.
www.nice.org.uk/TA124

▶ **Pemetrexed for the first-line treatment of non-small cell lung cancer (September 2009)** NICE TA181
Pemetrexed, in combination with cisplatin, is an option for the first-line treatment of locally advanced or metastatic non-small cell lung cancer only if the histology of the tumour has been confirmed as adenocarcinoma or large-cell carcinoma.
www.nice.org.uk/TA181

▶ **Pemetrexed for the treatment of malignant pleural mesothelioma (January 2008)** NICE TA135
Pemetrexed is an option for the treatment of malignant pleural mesothelioma only in patients who have a WHO performance status of 0 or 1 [WHO performance status is a measure of the ability to perform ordinary tasks], who are considered to have advanced disease and for whom surgical resection is considered inappropriate.
www.nice.org.uk/TA135

Scottish Medicines Consortium (SMC) Decisions
The *Scottish Medicines Consortium* has advised (August 2008) that pemetrexed (*Alimta ®*) is accepted for restricted use within NHS Scotland as monotherapy for the second-line treatment of locally advanced or metastatic non-small cell lung cancer without predominantly squamous cell histology; it is restricted for use in patients with good performance status who would otherwise be eligible for docetaxel treatment.

The *Scottish Medicines Consortium* has advised (January 2010) that pemetrexed (*Alimta ®*) is accepted for restricted use within NHS Scotland in combination with cisplatin for the first-line treatment of locally advanced or metastatic non-small cell lung cancer other than predominantly squamous cell histology; it is restricted to patients in whom the histology of the tumour has been confirmed as adenocarcinoma or large cell carcinoma.

The *Scottish Medicines Consortium* has advised (July 2005) that pemetrexed (*Alimta ®*) in combination with cisplatin is accepted for restricted use within NHS Scotland for previously untreated patients with stage III/IV unresectable malignant pleural mesothelioma.

● MEDICINAL FORMS
There can be variation in the licensing of different medicines containing the same drug.
Solution for infusion
▶ Pemetrexed (Non-proprietary)
Pemetrexed (as Pemetrexed ditrometamol) 25 mg per 1 ml Pemetrexed 100mg/4ml concentrate for solution for infusion vials | 1 vial PoM £140.00
Pemetrexed 500mg/20ml concentrate for solution for infusion vials | 1 vial PoM £700.00
Pemetrexed 1000mg/40ml concentrate for solution for infusion vials | 1 vial PoM £1,400.00

Powder for solution for infusion
ELECTROLYTES: May contain Sodium
▶ Alimta (Eli Lilly and Company Ltd)
Pemetrexed (as Pemetrexed disodium) 100 mg Alimta 100mg powder for concentrate for solution for infusion vials | 1 vial PoM £160.00 (Hospital only)
Pemetrexed (as Pemetrexed disodium) 500 mg Alimta 500mg powder for concentrate for solution for infusion vials | 1 vial PoM £800.00 (Hospital only)

Tegafur with gimeracil and oteracil

● DRUG ACTION Tegafur is a prodrug of fluorouracil. Gimeracil inhibits the degradation of fluorouracil and oteracil decreases the activity of fluorouracil in normal gastrointestinal mucosa.

● INDICATIONS AND DOSE
Treatment of advanced gastric cancer when used in combination with cisplatin
▶ BY MOUTH
▶ Adult: (consult local protocol)

> IMPORTANT SAFETY INFORMATION
> RISKS OF INCORRECT DOSING OF ORAL ANTI-CANCER MEDICINES
> See Cytotoxic drugs p. 787.

● CONTRA-INDICATIONS Dihydropyrimidine dehydrogenase deficiency

● INTERACTIONS → Appendix 1 (tegafur).

● SIDE-EFFECTS Alopecia · bone-marrow suppression · hyperuricaemia · nausea · neuropathy · ocular toxicity · oral mucositis · thromboembolism · tumour lysis syndrome · vomiting

● CONCEPTION AND CONTRACEPTION Manufacturer advises effective contraception during and for up to 6 months after treatment.

● PREGNANCY Avoid. See also *Pregnancy and reproductive function* in Cytotoxic drugs p. 787.

● BREAST FEEDING Discontinue breast-feeding.

● RENAL IMPAIRMENT Reduce dose if creatinine clearance 30–50 mL/minute—consult product literature. Manufacturer advises avoid if creatinine clearance less than 30 mL/minute.

● NATIONAL FUNDING/ACCESS DECISIONS
Scottish Medicines Consortium (SMC) Decisions
The *Scottish Medicines Consortium* has advised (August 2012) that tegafur with gimeracil and oteracil (*Teysuno ®*) is accepted for restricted use within NHS Scotland for the treatment of advanced gastric cancer, when given in combination with cisplatin, in patients who are unsuitable for an anthracycline, fluorouracil and platinum triplet first-line regimen.

● MEDICINAL FORMS
There can be variation in the licensing of different medicines containing the same drug.
Capsule
CAUTIONARY AND ADVISORY LABELS 23
▶ Teysuno (Nordic Pharma Ltd)
Gimeracil 4.35 mg, Oteracil (as Oteracil potassium) 11.8 mg, Tegafur 15 mg Teysuno 15mg/4.35mg/11.8mg capsules | 126 capsule PoM £279.72
Gimeracil 5.8 mg, Oteracil (as Oteracil potassium) 15.8 mg, Tegafur 20 mg Teysuno 20mg/5.8mg/15.8mg capsules | 84 capsule PoM £248.40

Tioguanine
(Thioguanine)

- **INDICATIONS AND DOSE**

Acute leukaemia | Chronic myeloid leukaemia
▶ BY MOUTH
▶ Adult: 100–200 mg/m^2 daily, can be given at various stages of treatment in short-term cycles

---

IMPORTANT SAFETY INFORMATION
RISKS OF INCORRECT DOSING OF ORAL ANTI-CANCER MEDICINES
See Cytotoxic drugs p. 787.

- CONTRA-INDICATIONS Absent thiopurine methyltransferase activity
- CAUTIONS Thiopurine methyltransferase status
  CAUTIONS, FURTHER INFORMATION
  ▶ Thiopurine methyltransferase The enzyme thiopurine methyltransferase (TPMT) metabolises thiopurine drugs (azathioprine, mercaptopurine, tioguanine); the risk of myelosuppression is increased in patients with reduced activity of the enzyme, particularly for the few individuals in whom TPMT activity is undetectable. Patients with absent TPMT activity should not receive thiopurine drugs; those with reduced TPMT activity may be treated under specialist supervision.
  ▶ Long-term therapy Long-term therapy is no longer recommended because of the high risk of liver toxicity.
- INTERACTIONS → Appendix 1 (tioguanine).
- SIDE-EFFECTS
  ▶ Rare Intestinal necrosis · intestinal perforation
  ▶ Frequency not known Alopecia · bone-marrow suppression · hepatotoxicity (discontinue) · hyperuricaemia · nausea · oral mucositis · stomatitis · thromboembolism · tumour lysis syndrome · vomiting
  SIDE-EFFECTS, FURTHER INFORMATION
  ▶ Gastro-intestinal side-effects Tioguanine has a lower incidence of gastrointestinal side-effects than mercaptopurine.
- CONCEPTION AND CONTRACEPTION Ensure effective contraception during treatment in men or women.
- PREGNANCY Avoid (teratogenicity reported when men receiving tioguanine have fathered children). See also *Pregnancy and reproductive function* in Cytotoxic drugs p. 787.
- BREAST FEEDING Discontinue breast-feeding.
- HEPATIC IMPAIRMENT Reduce dose.
- RENAL IMPAIRMENT Reduce dose.
- PRE-TREATMENT SCREENING Consider measuring thiopurine methyltransferase (TPMT) activity before starting tioguanine therapy.
- MONITORING REQUIREMENTS Monitor liver function weekly—discontinue if liver toxicity develops.

- MEDICINAL FORMS
  There can be variation in the licensing of different medicines containing the same drug. Forms available from special-order manufacturers include: capsule
  Tablet
  ▶ Tioguanine (Non-proprietary)
    Tioguanine 40 mg Tioguanine 40mg tablets | 25 tablet PoM £109.57

ANTINEOPLASTIC DRUGS > CYTOTOXIC ANTIBIOTICS AND RELATED SUBSTANCES

Bleomycin

- **INDICATIONS AND DOSE**

Squamous cell carcinoma | Metastatic germ cell cancer | Non-Hodgkin's lymphoma
▶ BY INTRAVENOUS INJECTION, OR BY LOCAL INFILTRATION, OR BY INTRA-ARTERIAL INFUSION, OR BY INTRAMUSCULAR INJECTION, OR BY INTRAVENOUS INFUSION
▶ Adult: (consult product literature or local protocols)

- CAUTIONS Caution in handling—irritant to tissues
- INTERACTIONS → Appendix 1 (bleomycin).
- SIDE-EFFECTS
  ▶ Common or very common Dermatological toxicity · mucositis
  ▶ Frequency not known Alopecia · chills (after drug administration) · extravasation · fever (after drug administration) · hypersensitivity reactions · hyperuricaemia · increased pigmentation particularly affecting the flexures and subcutaneous sclerotic plaques · less bone marrow suppression · nausea · oral mucositis · progressive pulmonary fibrosis (dose-related) · pulmonary toxicity · Raynaud's phenomenon · thromboembolism · tumour lysis syndrome · vomiting
  SIDE-EFFECTS, FURTHER INFORMATION
  ▶ Hypersensitivity reactions Hypersensitivity reactions manifest by chills and fevers commonly occur a few hours after drug administration and may be prevented by simultaneous administration of a corticosteroid, for example hydrocortisone intravenously.
  ▶ Progressive pulmonary fibrosis This is dose-related, occurring more commonly at cumulative doses greater than 300 000 units and in the elderly. Basal lung crepitations or suspicious chest X-ray changes are an indication to stop therapy with this drug.
  ▶ Respiratory failure Patients who have received extensive treatment with bleomycin (e.g. cumulative dose more than 100 000 units) may be at risk of developing respiratory failure if a general anaesthetic is given with high inspired oxygen concentrations. Anaesthetists should be warned of this.
- CONCEPTION AND CONTRACEPTION Contraceptive advice required, see *Pregnancy and reproductive function* in Cytotoxic drugs p. 787.
- PREGNANCY Avoid (teratogenic and carcinogenic in *animal* studies). See also *Pregnancy and reproductive function* in Cytotoxic drugs p. 787
- BREAST FEEDING Discontinue breast feeding.
- RENAL IMPAIRMENT Reduce dose by half if serum creatinine 177–354 micromol/litre; reduce dose further if serum-creatinine greater than 354 micromol/litre.
- PRESCRIBING AND DISPENSING INFORMATION To conform to the European Pharmacopoeia vials previously labelled as containing '15 units' of bleomycin are now labelled as containing 15 000 units. The amount of bleomycin in the vial has not changed.

- MEDICINAL FORMS
  There can be variation in the licensing of different medicines containing the same drug.
  Powder for solution for injection
  ▶ Bleo-Kyowa (ProStrakan Ltd)
    Bleomycin (as Bleomycin sulfate) 15000 unit Bleo-Kyowa 15,000unit powder for solution for injection vials | 10 vial PoM £190.60

8

Mitomycin

● **INDICATIONS AND DOSE**

Recurrent superficial bladder tumours (bladder instillation)
▸ BY INTRAVESICAL INSTILLATION
▸ Adult: (consult product literature or local protocols)

Upper gastro-intestinal cancers | Breast cancers
▸ BY INTRAVENOUS INJECTION
▸ Adult: (consult product literature or local protocols)

● CAUTIONS Caution in handling—irritant to tissues

● SIDE-EFFECTS
GENERAL SIDE-EFFECTS
Alopecia · bone marrow damage · bone-marrow suppression · hyperuricaemia · lung fibrosis · nausea · oral mucositis · renal damage · thromboembolism · tumour lysis syndrome · vomiting
SPECIFIC SIDE-EFFECTS
▸ With intravenous use Extravasation
SIDE-EFFECTS, FURTHER INFORMATION
▸ Bone-marrow toxicity Mitomycin is usually administered at 6-weekly intervals because it causes delayed bone-marrow toxicity. Prolonged use may result in a permanent effect.

● CONCEPTION AND CONTRACEPTION Contraceptive advice required, see *Pregnancy and reproductive function* in Cytotoxic drugs p. 787.

● PREGNANCY Avoid (teratogenic in *animal* studies). See also *Pregnancy and reproductive function* in Cytotoxic drugs p. 787.

● BREAST FEEDING Discontinue breast-feeding.

● MEDICINAL FORMS
There can be variation in the licensing of different medicines containing the same drug.
Powder for solution for injection
▸ Mitomycin-C (ProStrakan Ltd)
Mitomycin 2 mg Mitomycin-C Kyowa 2mg powder for solution for injection vials | 10 vial [PoM] £58.83
Mitomycin 10 mg Mitomycin-C Kyowa 10mg powder for solution for injection vials | 1 vial [PoM] £21.37
Mitomycin 20 mg Mitomycin-C Kyowa 20mg powder for solution for injection vials | 1 vial [PoM] £39.94
Mitomycin 40 mg Mitomycin-C Kyowa 40mg powder for solution for injection vials | 1 vial [PoM] £79.88

Pentostatin

● **INDICATIONS AND DOSE**

Hairy cell leukaemia (initiated in specialist centres)
▸ BY INTRAVENOUS INJECTION, OR BY INTRAVENOUS INFUSION
▸ Adult: To be given on alternate weeks (consult product literature)

● INTERACTIONS → Appendix 1 (pentostatin).

● SIDE-EFFECTS Alopecia · bone-marrow suppression · extravasation · hyperuricaemia · immunosuppression · myelosuppression · nausea · neurotoxicity (withhold or discontinue) · oral mucositis · severe rash (withhold treatment) · thromboembolism · tumour lysis syndrome · vomiting
SIDE-EFFECTS, FURTHER INFORMATION
Pentostatin can cause myelosuppression, immunosuppression, and a number of other side-effects that may be severe. Treatment should be withheld in patients who develop a severe rash, and withheld or discontinued in patients showing signs of neurotoxicity.

● CONCEPTION AND CONTRACEPTION Manufacturer advises that men should not father children during and for 6 months after treatment.

● PREGNANCY Avoid (teratogenic in *animal* studies). See also *Pregnancy and reproductive function* in Cytotoxic drugs p. 787.

● BREAST FEEDING Discontinue breast-feeding.

● HEPATIC IMPAIRMENT Manufacturer advises caution—limited information available.

● RENAL IMPAIRMENT Avoid if creatinine clearance less than 60 mL/minute.

● MEDICINAL FORMS
There can be variation in the licensing of different medicines containing the same drug.
Powder for solution for injection
▸ Nipent (Hospira UK Ltd)
Pentostatin 10 mg Nipent 10mg powder for solution for injection vials | 1 vial [PoM] £734.21 (Hospital only)

ANTINEOPLASTIC DRUGS > PLANT ALKALOIDS

Trabectedin
10.6.2016

● **INDICATIONS AND DOSE**

Treatment of advanced soft-tissue sarcoma when treatment with anthracyclines and ifosfamide has failed or is contra-indicated | Treatment of relapsed platinum-sensitive ovarian cancer (in combination with pegylated liposomal doxorubicin)
▸ BY INTRAVENOUS INFUSION
▸ Adult: (consult product literature or local protocols)

● CONTRA-INDICATIONS Elevated creatine phosphokinase (consult product literature)

● INTERACTIONS Caution in concomitant use with hepatotoxic drugs (avoid alcohol).

● SIDE-EFFECTS
▸ **Uncommon** Rhabdomyolysis (with raised creatine phosphokinase)
▸ **Rare** Hepatic failure (fatal cases reported)
▸ **Frequency not known** Abdominal pain · alopecia · anorexia · arthralgia · asthenia · back pain · bone-marrow suppression · constipation · cough · dehydration · diarrhoea · dizziness · dyspepsia · dyspnoea · extravasation · fatigue · flushing · headache · hepatobiliary disorders · hyperuricaemia · hypokalaemia · hypotension · increased blood creatine kinase · insomnia · myalgia · nausea · oedema · oral mucositis · paraesthesia · peripheral neuropathy · pyrexia · taste disturbance · thromboembolism · tumour lysis syndrome · vomiting
SIDE-EFFECTS, FURTHER INFORMATION
A corticosteroid, such as dexamethasone by intravenous infusion, must be given 30 minutes before therapy for its antiemetic and hepatoprotective effects (consult product literature).

● CONCEPTION AND CONTRACEPTION Effective contraception recommended during and for at least 3 months after treatment in women and during and for at least 5 months after treatment in men.

● PREGNANCY See *Pregnancy and reproductive function* in Cytotoxic drugs p. 787.

● BREAST FEEDING Manufacturer advises avoid breast-feeding and for 3 months after treatment.

● HEPATIC IMPAIRMENT Manufacturer advises caution in impairment—consider dose reduction. Avoid in patients with raised bilirubin. Monitor hepatic function closely in patients with hepatic impairment.

● RENAL IMPAIRMENT Avoid monotherapy if creatinine clearance less than 30 mL/minute. Avoid combination regimens if creatinine clearance less than 60 mL/minute.

- MONITORING REQUIREMENTS
▸ Specific haematological, renal and hepatic parameters must be monitored and within certain ranges prior to starting treatment and repeated weekly during the first 2 cycles and at least once between treatments in subsequent cycles—consult product literature for full details.
▸ Monitor for signs and symptoms of rhabdomyolysis (including myelotoxicity, severe liver function disorder, renal failure, muscle weakness or pain)—monitor creatine phosphokinase closely and discontinue treatment (consult product literature).

- NATIONAL FUNDING/ACCESS DECISIONS
NICE technology appraisals (TAs)
▸ **Trabectedin for the treatment of advanced soft tissue sarcoma (February 2010)** NICE TA185
Trabectedin is an option for advanced soft tissue sarcoma when treatment with anthracyclines and ifosfamide has failed, is inappropriate or is not tolerated. The cost of trabectedin for treatment after the fifth cycle is met by the manufacturer.
www.nice.org.uk/TA185
▸ **Topotecan, pegylated liposomal doxorubicin hydrochloride, paclitaxel, trabectedin and gemcitabine for treating recurrent ovarian cancer (April 2016)** NICE TA389
Trabectedin in combination with pegylated liposomal doxorubicin hydrochloride (PLDH) is **not** recommended for treating the first recurrence of platinum-sensitive ovarian cancer.
   Patients currently receiving trabectedin in combination with PLDH should have the option to continue their treatment until they or their clinician consider it appropriate to stop.
www.nice.org.uk/TA389

- MEDICINAL FORMS
There can be variation in the licensing of different medicines containing the same drug.
Powder for solution for infusion
▸ Yondelis (Pharma Mar, S.A.)
Trabectedin 250 microgram Yondelis 0.25mg powder for concentrate for solution for infusion vials | 1 vial [PoM] no price available (Hospital only)
Trabectedin 1 mg Yondelis 1mg powder for concentrate for solution for infusion vials | 1 vial [PoM] no price available (Hospital only)

ANTINEOPLASTIC DRUGS > PLATINUM COMPOUNDS

Carboplatin

10.6.2016

- INDICATIONS AND DOSE
Treatment of advanced ovarian cancer and lung cancer (particularly the small cell type)
▸ BY INTRAVENOUS INFUSION
▸ Adult: The dose of carboplatin is determined according to renal function rather than body surface area (consult product literature)

- INTERACTIONS → Appendix 1 (platinum compounds).
- SIDE-EFFECTS Alopecia · bone-marrow suppression · extravasation · hyperuricaemia · myelosuppression · nausea · nausea · nephrotoxicity · neurotoxicity · oral mucositis · ototoxicity · thromboembolism · tumour lysis syndrome · vomiting · vomiting

SIDE-EFFECTS, FURTHER INFORMATION
Carboplatin is better tolerated than cisplatin; nausea and vomiting are reduced in severity and nephrotoxicity, neurotoxicity, and ototoxicity are much less of a problem than with cisplatin. It is, however, more myelosuppressive than cisplatin.

- CONCEPTION AND CONTRACEPTION Contraceptive advice required, see *Pregnancy and reproductive function* in Cytotoxic drugs p. 787.
- PREGNANCY Avoid (teratogenic and embryotoxic in *animal* studies). See also *Pregnancy and reproductive function* in Cytotoxic drugs p. 787.
- BREAST FEEDING Discontinue breast-feeding.
- RENAL IMPAIRMENT Reduce dose. Avoid if creatinine clearance less than 20 mL/minute. Monitor haematological parameters in renal impairment. Monitor renal function in renal impairment.
- PRESCRIBING AND DISPENSING INFORMATION Carboplatin can be given in an outpatient setting.
- NATIONAL FUNDING/ACCESS DECISIONS
NICE technology appraisals (TAs)
▸ **Bevacizumab in combination with paclitaxel and carboplatin for the first-line treatment of advanced ovarian cancer (May 2013)** NICE TA284
Bevacizumab in combination with paclitaxel and carboplatin is **not** recommended for the first-line treatment of advanced ovarian cancer (including fallopian tube and primary peritoneal cancer).
www.nice.org.uk/TA284
▸ **Bevacizumab in combination with gemcitabine and carboplatin for the treatment of the first recurrence of platinum-sensitive advanced ovarian cancer (May 2013)** NICE TA285
Bevacizumab in combination with gemcitabine and carboplatin is **not** recommended within its marketing authorisation, that is, for the treatment of the first recurrence of platinum-sensitive advanced ovarian cancer (including fallopian tube and primary peritoneal cancer) that has not been previously treated with bevacizumab or other vascular endothelial growth factor (VEGF) inhibitors or VEGF receptor-targeted agents.
www.nice.org/TA285

- MEDICINAL FORMS
There can be variation in the licensing of different medicines containing the same drug.
Solution for infusion
▸ Carboplatin (Non-proprietary)
Carboplatin 10 mg per 1 ml Carboplatin 50mg/5ml concentrate for solution for infusion vials | 1 vial [PoM] £22.04 (Hospital only) | 1 vial [PoM] £20.00
Carboplatin 150mg/15ml concentrate for solution for infusion vials | 1 vial [PoM] £56.92 (Hospital only) | 1 vial [PoM] £50.00
Carboplatin 600mg/60ml concentrate for solution for infusion vials | 1 vial [PoM] £260.00
Carboplatin 600mg/60ml solution for infusion vials | 1 vial [PoM] £260.00
Carboplatin 450mg/45ml concentrate for solution for infusion vials | 1 vial [PoM] £168.85 (Hospital only) | 1 vial [PoM] £160.00
Carboplatin 450mg/45ml solution for infusion vials | 1 vial [PoM] £197.48
Carboplatin 150mg/15ml solution for infusion vials | 1 vial [PoM] £65.83
Carboplatin 50mg/5ml solution for infusion vials | 1 vial [PoM] £22.86

Cisplatin

- INDICATIONS AND DOSE
Treatment of testicular, lung, cervical, bladder, head and neck, and ovarian cancer (alone or in combination)
▸ BY INTRAVENOUS INFUSION
▸ Adult: (consult product literature)

- CAUTIONS

CAUTIONS, FURTHER INFORMATION
▸ Hydration Cisplatin requires intensive intravenous hydration and treatment may be complicated by severe nausea and vomiting.

- INTERACTIONS → Appendix 1 (platinum compounds).
- SIDE-EFFECTS Alopecia · bone-marrow suppression · extravasation · hyperuricaemia · hypomagnesaemia · myelosuppression · nephrotoxicity · oral mucositis · ototoxicity · peripheral neuropathy · severe nausea · severe vomiting · thromboembolism · tumour lysis syndrome
- CONCEPTION AND CONTRACEPTION Manufacturer advises effective contraception during and for at least 6 months after treatment in men or women.
- PREGNANCY Avoid (teratogenic and toxic in *animal* studies. See also *Pregnancy and reproductive function* in Cytotoxic drugs p. 787.
- BREAST FEEDING Discontinue breast-feeding.
- RENAL IMPAIRMENT Avoid if possible—nephrotoxic.
- MONITORING REQUIREMENTS
  ▶ Monitor full blood count.
  ▶ Monitor audiology.
  ▶ Monitor plasma electrolytes.
  ▶ Nephrotoxicity Monitoring of renal function is essential.
- DIRECTIONS FOR ADMINISTRATION Cisplatin is increasingly given in a day care setting.

- MEDICINAL FORMS
  There can be variation in the licensing of different medicines containing the same drug.
  Solution for infusion
  ▶ Cisplatin (Non-proprietary)
  Cisplatin 1 mg per 1 ml Cisplatin 50mg/50ml concentrate for solution for infusion vials | 1 vial [PoM] no price available
  Cisplatin 100mg/100ml solution for infusion vials | 1 vial [PoM] £50.22 (Hospital only) | 1 vial [PoM] £50.22–£55.64
  Cisplatin 10mg/10ml solution for infusion vials | 1 vial [PoM] £5.90 (Hospital only) | 1 vial [PoM] £5.90
  Cisplatin 50mg/50ml solution for infusion vials | 1 vial [PoM] £25.37 (Hospital only) | 1 vial [PoM] £25.37–£28.11
  Cisplatin 10mg/10ml concentrate for solution for infusion vials | 1 vial [PoM] no price available
  Cisplatin 100mg/100ml concentrate for solution for infusion vials | 1 vial [PoM] £50.22 (Hospital only) | 1 vial [PoM] no price available

Oxaliplatin

- INDICATIONS AND DOSE
  Treatment of metastatic colorectal cancer (in combination with fluorouracil and folinic acid) | Treatment of colon cancer after resection of the primary tumour (adjuvant treatment)
  ▶ BY INTRAVENOUS INFUSION
  ▶ Adult: (consult product literature)

- CONTRA-INDICATIONS Peripheral neuropathy with functional impairment
- INTERACTIONS → Appendix 1 (platinum compounds).
- SIDE-EFFECTS Alopecia · bone-marrow suppression · extravasation · gastro-intestinal disturbances · hyperuricaemia · myelosuppression · nausea · neurotoxicity (dose limiting) · ototoxicity · posterior reversible encephalopathy syndrome (associated with oxaliplatin combination chemotherapy) · sensory peripheral neuropathy (dose limiting) · thromboembolism · transient vision loss (reversible on discontinuation) · tumour lysis syndrome · vomiting
  SIDE-EFFECTS, FURTHER INFORMATION
  ▶ Respiratory symptoms If unexplained respiratory symptoms occur, oxaliplatin should be discontinued until investigations exclude interstitial lung disease and pulmonary fibrosis.
- CONCEPTION AND CONTRACEPTION Effective contraception required during and for 4 months after treatment in women and 6 months after treatment in men.

- PREGNANCY Manufacturer advises avoid—toxicity in *animal* studies. See also *Pregnancy and reproductive function* in Cytotoxic drugs p. 787.
- BREAST FEEDING Discontinue breast-feeding.
- RENAL IMPAIRMENT Reduce dose in mild to moderate impairment (consult product literature). Avoid if creatinine clearance less than 30 mL/minute.
- NATIONAL FUNDING/ACCESS DECISIONS
  NICE technology appraisals (TAs)
  ▶ **Capecitabine and oxaliplatin in the adjuvant treatment of stage III (Dukes' C) colon cancer (April 2006)** NICE TA100
  Capecitabine alone *or* oxaliplatin combined with fluorouracil and folinic acid are options for adjuvant treatment following surgery for stage III (Dukes' C) colon cancer.
  www.nice.org.uk/TA100
  ▶ **Irinotecan, oxaliplatin, and raltitrexed for advanced colorectal cancer (August 2005)** NICE TA93
  A combination of fluorouracil and folinic acid with either irinotecan or oxaliplatin are options for first-line treatment for advanced colorectal cancer.
  Irinotecan alone or fluorouracil and folinic acid with oxaliplatin are options for patients who require further treatment subsequently.
  www.nice.org.uk/TA93

- MEDICINAL FORMS
  There can be variation in the licensing of different medicines containing the same drug.
  Solution for infusion
  ▶ Oxaliplatin (Non-proprietary)
  Oxaliplatin 5 mg per 1 ml Oxaliplatin 100mg/20ml concentrate for solution for infusion vials | 1 vial [PoM] £330.00 (Hospital only) | 1 vial [PoM] £313.15
  Oxaliplatin 50mg/10ml concentrate for solution for infusion vials | 1 vial [PoM] £165.00 (Hospital only) | 1 vial [PoM] £156.75
  Oxaliplatin 200mg/40ml concentrate for solution for infusion vials | 1 vial [PoM] £627.00
  Powder for solution for infusion
  ▶ Oxaliplatin (Non-proprietary)
  Oxaliplatin 50 mg Oxaliplatin 50mg powder for solution for infusion vials | 1 vial [PoM] £150.00–£156.75
  Oxaliplatin 100 mg Oxaliplatin 100mg powder for solution for infusion vials | 1 vial [PoM] £299.50–£313.50

ANTINEOPLASTIC DRUGS > PODOPHYLLOTOXIN DERIVATIVES

Etoposide

- INDICATIONS AND DOSE
  Small cell carcinoma of the bronchus, the lymphomas and testicular cancer
  ▶ BY MOUTH
  ▶ Adult: 120–240 mg/m^2 daily for 5 days
  ▶ BY INTRAVENOUS INFUSION
  ▶ Adult: (consult product literature)

  IMPORTANT SAFETY INFORMATION
  RISKS OF INCORRECT DOSING OF ORAL ANTI-CANCER MEDICINES
  See Cytotoxic drugs p. 787.

- INTERACTIONS → Appendix 1 (etoposide).
- SIDE-EFFECTS Alopecia · bone-marrow suppression · hyperuricaemia · irritant to tissues · nausea · oral mucositis (more common if given with doxorubicin) · thromboembolism · tumour lysis syndrome · vomiting
- CONCEPTION AND CONTRACEPTION Contraceptive advice required, see *Pregnancy and reproductive function* in Cytotoxic drugs p. 787.

- **PREGNANCY** Avoid (teratogenic in *animal* studies). See also *Pregnancy and reproductive function* in Cytotoxic drugs p. 787.
- **BREAST FEEDING** Discontinue breast-feeding.
- **HEPATIC IMPAIRMENT** Avoid in severe impairment.
- **RENAL IMPAIRMENT** Consider dose reduction—consult local treatment protocol for details.
- **DIRECTIONS FOR ADMINISTRATION** Etoposide may be given orally or by slow intravenous infusion, the oral dose being double the intravenous dose. A preparation containing etoposide phosphate can be given by intravenous injection or infusion. Etoposide is usually given daily for 3–5 days and courses should not be repeated more frequently than at intervals of 21 days.

- **MEDICINAL FORMS**
There can be variation in the licensing of different medicines containing the same drug.
Capsule
CAUTIONARY AND ADVISORY LABELS 23
▸ Vepesid (Bristol-Myers Squibb Pharmaceuticals Ltd)
Etoposide 50 mg Vepesid 50mg capsules | 20 capsule PoM £99.82 (Hospital only)
Etoposide 100 mg Vepesid 100mg capsules | 10 capsule PoM £87.23 (Hospital only)
Powder for solution for injection
▸ Etopophos (Bristol-Myers Squibb Pharmaceuticals Ltd)
Etoposide (as Etoposide phosphate) 100 mg Etopophos 100mg powder for solution for injection vials | 10 vial PoM £261.68 (Hospital only)
Solution for infusion
▸ Etoposide (Non-proprietary)
Etoposide 20 mg per 1 ml Etoposide 100mg/5ml concentrate for solution for infusion vials | 1 vial PoM no price available (Hospital only) | 1 vial PoM £11.50 | 10 vial PoM £115.00
Etoposide 500mg/25ml concentrate for solution for infusion vials | 1 vial PoM £60.75 (Hospital only)
▸ Eposin (medac UK)
Etoposide 20 mg per 1 ml Eposin 500mg/25ml concentrate for solution for infusion vials | 1 vial PoM £67.50 (Hospital only)
Eposin 100mg/5ml concentrate for solution for infusion vials | 1 vial PoM £13.50 (Hospital only)

ANTINEOPLASTIC DRUGS ˃ TAXANES

Cabazitaxel

- **INDICATIONS AND DOSE**

Treatment of hormone refractory metastatic prostate cancer in patients who have previously been treated with a docetaxel-containing regimen (in combination with prednisone or prednisolone)
▸ BY INTRAVENOUS INFUSION
▸ Adult: (consult product literature or local protocols)

- **CAUTIONS** Avoid in Acute porphyrias p. 918
- **INTERACTIONS** → Appendix 1 (cabazitaxel).
- **SIDE-EFFECTS**
▸ **Common or very common** Hypersensitivity reactions
▸ **Frequency not known** Abdominal pain · alopecia · anxiety · arthralgia · atrial fibrillation · bone-marrow suppression · chest pain · chills · confusion · constipation · cough · dehydration · diarrhoea · dizziness · dry mouth · dry skin · dyspepsia · dyspnoea · electrolyte disturbances · erythema · extravasation · flushing · gastroesophageal reflux · haemorrhoids · headache · hyperglycaemia · hypertension · hyperuricaemia · hypoesthesia · hypotension · increased lacrimation · malaise · muscle spasm · myalgia · nausea · oedema · oral mucositis · paraesthesia · peripheral neuropathy · rectal haemorrhage · renal disorders (fatal cases of renal failure reported) · sciatica · tachycardia · taste disturbance · thromboembolism · tinnitus · tumour

lysis syndrome · urinary incontinence · urinary retention · vertigo · vomiting · weight changes
SIDE-EFFECTS, FURTHER INFORMATION
▸ Hypersensitivity reactions Routine premedication with a corticosteroid, an antihistamine, and a histamine H_2-receptor antagonist is recommended to prevent severe hypersensitivity reactions.
    For further information on side-effects, consult product literature.

- **CONCEPTION AND CONTRACEPTION** Ensure effective contraception during treatment (women) and for up to 6 months after treatment (men).
- **PREGNANCY** See also *Pregnancy and reproductive function* in Cytotoxic drugs p. 787.
- **BREAST FEEDING** Discontinue breast-feeding.
- **HEPATIC IMPAIRMENT** Avoid.
- **RENAL IMPAIRMENT** Use with caution if creatinine clearance less than 50 mL/minute.
- **MONITORING REQUIREMENTS** Monitor electrolytes—correct dehydration.
- **DIRECTIONS FOR ADMINISTRATION** Intravenous infusion incompatible with PVC.
- **NATIONAL FUNDING/ACCESS DECISIONS**
NICE technology appraisals (TAs)
▸ **Cabazitaxel for hormone-refractory metastatic prostate cancer previously treated with a docetaxel-containing regimen (May 2012)** NICE TA255
Cabazitaxel in combination with prednisone or prednisolone is not recommended for the treatment of hormone-refractory metastatic prostate cancer previously treated with a docetaxel-containing regimen.
    Patients currently receiving cabazitaxel in combination with prednisone or prednisolone for the treatment of hormone-refractory metastatic prostate cancer previously treated with a docetaxel-containing regimen should have the option to continue treatment until they and their clinicians consider it appropriate to stop.
www.nice.org.uk/TA255

- **MEDICINAL FORMS**
There can be variation in the licensing of different medicines containing the same drug.
Solution for infusion
EXCIPIENTS: May contain Ethanol
▸ Jevtana (Sanofi)
Cabazitaxel 40 mg per 1 ml JEVTANA 60mg/1.5ml concentrate and solvent for solution for infusion vials | 1 vial PoM £3,696.00 (Hospital only)

Docetaxel

● INDICATIONS AND DOSE

Adjuvant treatment of operable node-positive and operable node-negative breast cancer (in combination with doxorubicin and cyclophosphamide) | Initial chemotherapy of locally advanced or metastatic breast cancer (with doxorubicin) | Locally advanced or metastatic breast cancer where cytotoxic chemotherapy with an anthracycline or an alkylating drug has failed (monotherapy) | Locally advanced or metastatic breast cancer where cytotoxic chemotherapy with an anthracycline has failed (with capecitabine) | Initial chemotherapy of metastatic breast cancer which overexpresses human epidermal growth factor-2 (with trastuzumab) | Locally advanced or metastatic non-small cell lung cancer where previous chemotherapy has failed | Initial chemotherapy of unresectable, locally advanced or metastatic non-small cell lung cancer (with cisplatin) | Hormone-resistant metastatic prostate cancer (in combination with prednisone or prednisolone) | Initial treatment of metastatic gastric adenocarcinoma, including adenocarcinoma of the gastro-oesophageal junction (with cisplatin and fluorouracil) | Induction treatment of locally advanced squamous cell carcinoma of the head and neck (with cisplatin and fluorouracil)

▶ BY INTRAVENOUS INFUSION

▶ Adult: (consult product literature or local protocols)

● CAUTIONS Avoid in Acute porphyrias p. 918 · consult product literature

● INTERACTIONS → Appendix 1 (docetaxel).

● SIDE-EFFECTS Alopecia · bone-marrow suppression · cystoid macular oedema · extravasation · fatal respiratory disorders · gastro-intestinal toxicity · heart failure · hypersensitivity reactions · hyperuricaemia · nausea · oral mucositis · peripheral neurotoxicity · persistent fluid retention (commonly as leg oedema that worsens during treatment) can be resistant to treatment · severe skin reactions · thromboembolism · tumour lysis syndrome · vomiting

SIDE-EFFECTS, FURTHER INFORMATION

▶ Hypersensitivity reactions and fluid retention Pretreatment with dexamethasone by mouth is recommended for reducing fluid retention and hypersensitivity reactions (consult product literature).

Consult product literature for monitoring and management of side effects.

● CONCEPTION AND CONTRACEPTION Manufacturer advises effective contraception for men and women during treatment, and for at least 6 months after stopping treatment in men.

● PREGNANCY Avoid (toxicity in *animal* studies). See also *Pregnancy and reproductive function* in Cytotoxic drugs p. 787.

● BREAST FEEDING Discontinue breast-feeding.

● HEPATIC IMPAIRMENT Reduce dose according to liver enzymes (consult product literature). Avoid in severe impairment. Monitor liver function in hepatic impairment.

● NATIONAL FUNDING/ACCESS DECISIONS

NICE technology appraisals (TAs)

▶ **Docetaxel for the treatment of hormone-refractory metastatic prostate cancer (June 2006)** NICE TA101

Docetaxel is an option for hormone-refractory metastatic prostate cancer and a Karnofsky score of at least 60% [Karnofsky score is a measure of the ability to perform ordinary tasks].

www.nice.org.uk/TA101

▶ **Docetaxel for the adjuvant treatment of early node-positive breast cancer (September 2006)** NICE TA109

Docetaxel, when given concurrently with doxorubicin and cyclophosphamide (TAC regimen), is recommended as an option for the adjuvant treatment of women with early node-positive breast cancer.

www.nice.org.uk/TA109

Scottish Medicines Consortium (SMC) Decisions

The *Scottish Medicines Consortium* has advised that docetaxel (*Taxotere*®) in combination with cisplatin and fluorouracil is accepted for restricted use within NHS Scotland for the induction treatment of patients with unresectable (May 2007) and resectable (June 2008) locally advanced squamous cell carcinoma of the head and neck.

● MEDICINAL FORMS

There can be variation in the licensing of different medicines containing the same drug.

Solution for infusion

EXCIPIENTS: May contain Ethanol

▶ Docetaxel (Non-proprietary)

Docetaxel 10 mg per 1 ml Docetaxel 80mg/8ml concentrate for solution for infusion vials | 1 vial PoM £534.75 (Hospital only) | 1 vial PoM £534.75

Docetaxel 160mg/16ml concentrate for solution for infusion vials | 1 vial PoM £1,069.50 (Hospital only)

Docetaxel 20mg/2ml concentrate for solution for infusion vials | 1 vial PoM £162.75 (Hospital only)

Docetaxel 20 mg per 1 ml Docetaxel 80mg/4ml concentrate for solution for infusion vials | 1 vial PoM £530.00

Docetaxel 160mg/8ml concentrate for solution for infusion vials | 1 vial PoM no price available

Docetaxel 140mg/7ml concentrate for solution for infusion vials | 1 vial PoM £900.00

Docetaxel 20mg/1ml concentrate for solution for infusion vials | 1 vial PoM £160.00

▶ Taxceus (medac UK)

Docetaxel 20 mg per 1 ml Taxceus 80mg/4ml concentrate for solution for infusion vials | 1 vial PoM £508.01

Taxceus 20mg/1ml concentrate for solution for infusion vials | 1 vial PoM £154.61

Taxceus 140mg/7ml concentrate for solution for infusion vials | 1 vial PoM £720.10

▶ Taxotere (Sanofi)

Docetaxel 20 mg per 1 ml Taxotere 20mg/1ml concentrate for solution for infusion vials | 1 vial PoM £153.47 (Hospital only)

Taxotere 160mg/8ml concentrate for solution for infusion vials | 1 vial PoM £1,008.54 (Hospital only)

Taxotere 80mg/4ml concentrate for solution for infusion vials | 1 vial PoM £504.27 (Hospital only)

8

Immune system and malignant disease

Paclitaxel

1.6.2016

- **DRUG ACTION** Paclitaxel is a member of the taxane group of drugs.

- **INDICATIONS AND DOSE**

Treatment of ovarian cancer (advanced or residual disease following laparotomy) in combination with cisplatin (conventional paclitaxel only) | Treatment of metastatic ovarian cancer where platinum-containing therapy has failed (conventional paclitaxel only) | Treatment of locally advanced or metastatic breast cancer (in combination with other cytotoxics or alone if other cytotoxics have failed or are inappropriate) (conventional paclitaxel only) | Adjuvant treatment of node-positive breast cancer following treatment with anthracycline and cyclophosphamide (conventional paclitaxel only) | Treatment of non-small cell lung cancer (in combination with cisplatin) when surgery or radiotherapy not appropriate (conventional paclitaxel only) | Treatment of advanced AIDS-related Kaposi's sarcoma where liposomal anthracycline therapy has failed (conventional paclitaxel only) | First-line treatment of metastatic adenocarcinoma of the pancreas (in combination with gemcitabine) (conventional paclitaxel only) | Monotherapy of metastatic breast cancer when first-line treatment has failed and standard, anthracycline-containing therapy is not indicated (albumin-bound paclitaxel only) | In combination with gemcitabine for the first-line treatment of metastatic adenocarcinoma of the pancreas (albumin-bound paclitaxel only)

  ▸ BY INTRAVENOUS INFUSION
  ▸ Adult: (consult product literature or local protocols)

- **CAUTIONS** Avoid in Acute porphyrias p. 918 · consult product literature · patients aged over 75 years with metastatic adenocarcinoma of the pancreas

- **INTERACTIONS** → Appendix 1 (paclitaxel).

- **SIDE-EFFECTS**
▸ **Common or very common** Arrhythmia · arthralgia · febrile neutropenia · gastro-intestinal disorders · myalgia · peripheral neuropathy · sensory neuropathy · tachycardia
▸ **Rare** Bradycardia · cardiac arrest · congestive heart failure · left ventricular dysfunction
▸ **Frequency not known** Alopecia · arrhythmias (nearly always asymptomatic) · asymptomatic hypotension · bone-marrow suppression · bradycardia · cardiac conduction defects · extravasation · hypersensitivity reactions · hyperuricaemia · muscle pain · myelosuppression · nausea · neutropenia · oral mucositis · pneumonitis · Stevens-Johnson syndrome · thromboembolism · toxic epidermal necrolysis · tumour lysis syndrome · vomiting

SIDE-EFFECTS, FURTHER INFORMATION
▸ Hypersensitivity reactions Routine premedication with a corticosteroid, an antihistamine and a histamine H_2-receptor antagonist is recommended to prevent severe hypersensitivity reactions; hypersensitivity reactions may occur rarely despite premedication.

- **CONCEPTION AND CONTRACEPTION** Ensure effective contraception during and for at least 6 months after treatment in men or women.

- **PREGNANCY** Avoid (toxicity in *animal* studies). See also *Pregnancy and reproductive function* in Cytotoxic drugs p. 787.

- **BREAST FEEDING** Discontinue breast-feeding.

- **HEPATIC IMPAIRMENT** Avoid in severe impairment.

- **MONITORING REQUIREMENTS**
▸ Cardiac monitoring should be undertaken, particularly if

patients have underlying cardiac disease or previous exposure to anthracyclines.
▸ Patients should be monitored for signs and symptoms of pneumonitis and sepsis.

- **PRESCRIBING AND DISPENSING INFORMATION** Paclitaxel is available as both conventional and albumin-bound formulations. The different formulations vary in their licensed indications, pharmacokinetics, dosage and administration, and are not interchangeable. Prescribers should specify the brand to be dispensed.

- **NATIONAL FUNDING/ACCESS DECISIONS**

NICE technology appraisals (TAs)
▸ **Paclitaxel for ovarian cancer (January 2003)** NICE TA55
Either paclitaxel in combination with a platinum compound (cisplatin or carboplatin) *or* a platinum compound alone are alternatives for the first-line treatment of ovarian cancer (usually following surgery).
www.nice.org.uk/TA55
▸ **Paclitaxel for the adjuvant treatment of early node-positive breast cancer (September 2006)** NICE TA108
Paclitaxel, within its licensed indication, is **not** recommended for the adjuvant treatment of women with early node-positive breast cancer.
www.nice.org.uk/TA108
▸ **Bevacizumab in combination with paclitaxel and carboplatin for the first-line treatment of advanced ovarian cancer (May 2013)** NICE TA284
Bevacizumab in combination with paclitaxel and carboplatin is **not** recommended for the first-line treatment of advanced ovarian cancer (including fallopian tube and primary peritoneal cancer).
www.nice.org.uk/TA284
▸ **Paclitaxel as albumin-bound nanoparticles in combination with gemcitabine for previously untreated metastatic pancreatic cancer (October 2015)** NICE TA360
Albumin-bound paclitaxel (nab-paclitaxel, *Abraxane*®) with gemcitabine, within its licensed indication, is **not** recommended for the treatment of previously untreated metastatic adenocarcinoma of the pancreas.
  Patients whose treatment was started before this guidance was published should continue treatment until they and their clinician consider it appropriate to stop.
www.nice.org.uk/TA360
▸ **Topotecan, pegylated liposomal doxorubicin hydrochloride, paclitaxel, trabectedin and gemcitabine for treating recurrent ovarian cancer (April 2016)** NICE TA389
Paclitaxel, in combination with platinum or as monotherapy, is recommended as an option for treating recurrent ovarian cancer.
www.nice.org.uk/TA389

- **MEDICINAL FORMS**
There can be variation in the licensing of different medicines containing the same drug.

Solution for infusion
EXCIPIENTS: May contain Polyoxyl castor oils
▸ Paclitaxel (Non-proprietary)
  Paclitaxel 6 mg per 1 ml Paclitaxel 150mg/25ml concentrate for solution for infusion vials | 1 vial [PoM] £504.90–£561.00 (Hospital only) | 1 vial [PoM] £300.52
  Paclitaxel 30mg/5ml concentrate for solution for infusion vials | 1 vial [PoM] £112.31–£116.05 (Hospital only) | 1 vial [PoM] £105.84
  Paclitaxel 300mg/50ml concentrate for solution for infusion vials | 1 vial [PoM] £1,009.80–£1,122.00 (Hospital only) | 1 vial [PoM] £951.63
  Paclitaxel 100mg/16.7ml concentrate for solution for infusion vials | 1 vial [PoM] £336.60–£374.00 (Hospital only) | 1 vial [PoM] £317.21

Powder for suspension for infusion
ELECTROLYTES: May contain Sodium
▸ Abraxane (Celgene Ltd)
  Paclitaxel albumin 100 mg Abraxane 100mg powder for suspension for infusion vials | 1 vial [PoM] £246.00 (Hospital only)

8

Immune system and malignant disease

ANTINEOPLASTIC DRUGS > TOPOISOMERASE I INHIBITORS

Irinotecan hydrochloride

- DRUG ACTION Irinotecan inhibits topoisomerase I, an enzyme involved in DNA replication.

- ● INDICATIONS AND DOSE

Metastatic colorectal cancer in combination with fluorouracil and folinic acid or as monotherapy when treatment containing fluorouracil has failed | Treatment of epidermal growth factor receptor-expressing metastatic colorectal cancer after failure of chemotherapy that has included irinotecan (in combination with cetuximab) | First-line treatment of metastatic carcinoma of the colon or rectum (in combination with fluorouracil, folinic acid and bevacizumab) | First-line treatment of metastatic colorectal carcinoma (in combination with capecitabine with or without bevacizumab)
  - ▶ BY INTRAVENOUS INFUSION
  - ▶ Adult: (consult product literature or local protocols)

- ● CONTRA-INDICATIONS Bowel obstruction · chronic inflammatory bowel disease
- ● CAUTIONS Raised plasma-bilirubin concentration · risk factors for cardiac disease
- ● INTERACTIONS → Appendix 1 (irinotecan).
- ● SIDE-EFFECTS
  - ▶ **Uncommon** Interstitial pulmonary disease
  - ▶ **Frequency not known** Acute cholinergic syndrome (with early diarrhoea) and delayed diarrhoea (consult product literature) · alopecia · anorexia · asthenia · bone-marrow suppression · extravasation · gastro-intestinal effects (delayed diarrhoea requiring prompt treatment may follow irinotecan treatment) · hyperuricaemia · myelosuppression (dose limiting) · nausea · oral mucositis · thromboembolism · tumour lysis syndrome · vomiting
- ● CONCEPTION AND CONTRACEPTION Manufacturer advises effective contraception during and for up to 1 month after treatment in women and up to 3 months after treatment in men.
- ● PREGNANCY Avoid (teratogenic and toxic in *animal* studies). See also Pregnancy and reproductive function in Cytotoxic drugs p. 787.
- ● BREAST FEEDING Discontinue breast-feeding.
- ● HEPATIC IMPAIRMENT Avoid if plasma-bilirubin concentration greater than 3 times upper limit of normal range. Monitor closely for neutropenia if plasma-bilirubin concentration 1.5–3 times upper limit of normal range (consult product literature).
- ● RENAL IMPAIRMENT Manufacturer advises avoid—no information available.
- ● MONITORING REQUIREMENTS Monitor respiratory function.
- ● NATIONAL FUNDING/ACCESS DECISIONS

NICE technology appraisals (TAs)
  - ▶ **Irinotecan, oxaliplatin, and raltitrexed for advanced colorectal cancer (August 2005)** NICE TA93
  A combination of fluorouracil and folinic acid with either irinotecan or oxaliplatin are options for first-line treatment for advanced colorectal cancer.
  Irinotecan alone or fluorouracil and folinic acid with oxaliplatin are options for patients who require further treatment subsequently.
  www.nice.org.uk/TA93

- ● MEDICINAL FORMS
  There can be variation in the licensing of different medicines containing the same drug.
  Solution for infusion
  - ▶ Irinotecan hydrochloride (Non-proprietary)
    Irinotecan hydrochloride trihydrate 20 mg per 1 ml Irinotecan 500mg/25ml concentrate for solution for infusion vials | 1 vial [PoM] £601.25–£650.00 (Hospital only)
    Irinotecan 40mg/2ml concentrate for solution for infusion vials | 1 vial [PoM] £49.03–£53.00 (Hospital only) | 1 vial [PoM] £45.11–£50.35
    Irinotecan 300mg/15ml concentrate for solution for infusion vials | 1 vial [PoM] £390.00 (Hospital only) | 1 vial [PoM] £331.83–£390.00
    Irinotecan 100mg/5ml concentrate for solution for infusion vials | 1 vial [PoM] £120.25–£130.00 (Hospital only) | 1 vial [PoM] £110.62–£123.50
  - ▶ Campto (Pfizer Ltd)
    Irinotecan hydrochloride trihydrate 20 mg per 1 ml Campto 100mg/5ml concentrate for solution for infusion vials | 1 vial [PoM] £130.00 (Hospital only)
    Campto 40mg/2ml concentrate for solution for infusion vials | 1 vial [PoM] £53.00 (Hospital only)
    Campto 300mg/15ml concentrate for solution for infusion vials | 1 vial [PoM] £390.00 (Hospital only)

Topotecan

10.6.2016

- DRUG ACTION Topotecan inhibits topoisomerase I, an enzyme involved in DNA replication.

- ● INDICATIONS AND DOSE

Metastatic ovarian cancer when first-line or subsequent treatment has failed | Treatment of recurrent carcinoma of the cervix, after radiotherapy, and for patients with stage IVB disease (in combination with cisplatin)
  - ▶ BY INTRAVENOUS INFUSION
  - ▶ Adult: (consult product literature or local protocols)

Relapsed small-cell lung cancer when retreatment with the first-line regimen is considered inappropriate
  - ▶ BY INTRAVENOUS INFUSION, OR BY MOUTH
  - ▶ Adult: (consult product literature or local protocols)

> **IMPORTANT SAFETY INFORMATION**
> RISKS OF INCORRECT DOSING OF ORAL ANTI-CANCER MEDICINES
> See Cytotoxic drugs p. 787.

- ● SIDE-EFFECTS Alopecia · anorexia · asthenia · bone-marrow suppression · extravasation · gastro-intestinal effects · hyperuricaemia · myelosuppression (dose-limiting) · nausea · oral mucositis · thromboembolism · tumour lysis syndrome · vomiting
- ● CONCEPTION AND CONTRACEPTION Contraceptive advice required, see *Pregnancy and reproductive function* in Cytotoxic drugs p. 787.
- ● PREGNANCY Avoid (teratogenicity and fetal loss in *animal* studies). See also *Pregnancy and reproductive function* in Cytotoxic drugs p. 787.
- ● BREAST FEEDING Discontinue breast-feeding.
- ● HEPATIC IMPAIRMENT Avoid in severe impairment.
- ● RENAL IMPAIRMENT Reduce dose. Avoid infusion if creatinine clearance less than 20 mL/minute. Avoid oral route if creatinine clearance less than 60 mL/minute.
- ● NATIONAL FUNDING/ACCESS DECISIONS

NICE technology appraisals (TAs)
  - ▶ **Topotecan for the treatment of recurrent and stage IVB cervical cancer (October 2009)** NICE TA183
  Topotecan in combination with cisplatin is recommended as a treatment option for recurrent or stage IVB cervical cancer in patients who have not previously received cisplatin.
  www.nice.org.uk/TA183

▶ **Topotecan for the treatment of relapsed small-cell lung cancer (November 2009)** NICE TA184

Oral topotecan is recommended as an option for treatment in patients with relapsed small-cell lung cancer only if re-treatment with the first-line regimen is not considered appropriate, and the combination of cyclophosphamide, doxorubicin and vincristine is contra-indicated. Intravenous topotecan is not recommended for people with relapsed small-cell lung cancer.
www.nice.org.uk/TA184

▶ **Topotecan, pegylated liposomal doxorubicin hydrochloride, paclitaxel, trabectedin and gemcitabine for treating recurrent ovarian cancer (April 2016)** NICE TA389

Topotecan is **not** recommended for treating first recurrence of platinum-sensitive ovarian cancer, recurrent platinum-resistant ovarian cancer, or platinum-refractory ovarian cancer.

Patients currently receiving topotecan should have the option to continue their treatment until they or their clinician consider it appropriate to stop.
www.nice.org.uk/TA389

Scottish Medicines Consortium (SMC) Decisions
The *Scottish Medicines Consortium* has advised (November 2007) that topotecan (*Hycamtin*®) is accepted for restricted use in combination with cisplatin for treatment of recurrent carcinoma of the cervix after radiotherapy and for stage IVB disease; it is restricted to patients who have not previously received cisplatin treatment.

● MEDICINAL FORMS
There can be variation in the licensing of different medicines containing the same drug.

Capsule
CAUTIONARY AND ADVISORY LABELS 25
▶ Hycamtin (Novartis Pharmaceuticals UK Ltd)
Topotecan (as Topotecan hydrochloride)
250 microgram Hycamtin 0.25mg capsules | 10 capsule PoM £75.00
Topotecan (as Topotecan hydrochloride) 1 mg Hycamtin 1mg capsules | 10 capsule PoM £360.00

Solution for infusion
▶ Topotecan (Non-proprietary)
Topotecan (as Topotecan hydrochloride) 1 mg per 1 ml Topotecan 4mg/4ml concentrate for solution for infusion vials | 1 vial PoM £261.55 (Hospital only) | 1 vial PoM no price available | 5 vial PoM £1,453.10 (Hospital only)
Topotecan 1mg/1ml concentrate for solution for infusion vials | 1 vial PoM £87.88 (Hospital only) | 1 vial PoM no price available | 5 vial PoM £488.25 (Hospital only)

Powder for solution for infusion
▶ Hycamtin (Novartis Pharmaceuticals UK Ltd)
Topotecan (as Topotecan hydrochloride) 1 mg Hycamtin 1mg powder for concentrate for solution for infusion vials | 1 vial PoM £97.65
Topotecan (as Topotecan hydrochloride) 4 mg Hycamtin 4mg powder for concentrate for solution for infusion vials | 1 vial PoM £348.76
▶ Potactasol (Actavis UK Ltd)
Topotecan (as Topotecan hydrochloride) 1 mg Potactasol 1mg powder for concentrate for solution for infusion vials | 1 vial PoM £97.00 (Hospital only)
Topotecan (as Topotecan hydrochloride) 4 mg Potactasol 4mg powder for concentrate for solution for infusion vials | 1 vial PoM £290.00 (Hospital only)

ANTINEOPLASTIC DRUGS ⟩VINCA ALKALOIDS

Vinblastine sulfate

● INDICATIONS AND DOSE
Variety of cancers including leukaemias, lymphomas, and some solid tumours (e.g. breast and lung cancer)
▶ Adult: (consult product literature)

IMPORTANT SAFETY INFORMATION
Vinblastine is for **intravenous administration only**. Inadvertent intrathecal administration can cause severe neurotoxicity, which is usually fatal.

The National Patient Safety Agency has advised (August 2008) that adult and teenage patients treated in an adult or adolescent unit should receive their vinca alkaloid dose in a 50 mL minibag. Teenagers and children treated in a child unit may receive their vinca alkaloid dose in a syringe.

● CONTRA-INDICATIONS
CONTRA-INDICATIONS, FURTHER INFORMATION
Intrathecal injection **contra-indicated**.

● CAUTIONS Caution in handling—irritant to tissues

● INTERACTIONS → Appendix 1 (vinblastine).

● SIDE-EFFECTS Abdominal pain · alopecia · autonomic neuropathy · constipation · hyperuricaemia · loss of deep tendon reflexes · motor weakness · myelosuppression (dose-limiting) · nausea · neurotoxicity · oral mucositis · ototoxicity · peripheral neuropathy · peripheral paraesthesia · severe bronchospasm following administration (more commonly when used in combination with mitomycin-C) · severe local irritation (care must be taken to avoid extravasation) · thromboembolism · tumour lysis syndrome · vomiting
SIDE-EFFECTS, FURTHER INFORMATION
▶ Neurotoxicity Neurotoxicity, usually as peripheral or autonomic neuropathy, occurs with all vinca alkaloids; it occurs less often with vinblastine than with vincristine. Patients with neurotoxicity commonly have peripheral paraesthesia, loss of deep tendon reflexes, abdominal pain, and constipation; ototoxicity has been reported. If symptoms of neurotoxicity are severe, doses should be reduced.

Motor weakness can also occur and dose reduction or discontinuation of therapy may be appropriate if motor weakness increases. Recovery from neurotoxic effects is usually slow but complete.

● CONCEPTION AND CONTRACEPTION Contraceptive advice required, see *Pregnancy and reproductive function* in Cytotoxic drugs p. 787.

● PREGNANCY Avoid (limited experience suggests fetal harm; teratogenic in *animal* studies). See also *Pregnancy and reproductive function* in Cytotoxic drugs p. 787.

● BREAST FEEDING Discontinue breast-feeding.

● HEPATIC IMPAIRMENT Dose reduction may be necessary—consult local treatment protocol for details.

● MEDICINAL FORMS
There can be variation in the licensing of different medicines containing the same drug.
Solution for injection
▶ Vinblastine sulfate (Non-proprietary)
Vinblastine sulfate 1 mg per 1 ml Vinblastine 10mg/10ml solution for injection vials | 5 vial PoM £85.00

Vincristine sulfate

● INDICATIONS AND DOSE

Variety of cancers including leukaemias, lymphomas, and some solid tumours (e.g. breast and lung cancer)
▸ Adult: (consult local protocol)

IMPORTANT SAFETY INFORMATION

Vincristine injections are for **intravenous administration only**. Inadvertent intrathecal administration can cause severe neurotoxicity, which is usually fatal.

The National Patient Safety Agency has advised (August 2008) that adult and teenage patients treated in an adult or adolescent unit should receive their vinca alkaloid dose in a 50 mL minibag. Teenagers and children treated in a child unit may receive their vinca alkaloid dose in a syringe.

● CONTRA-INDICATIONS

CONTRA-INDICATIONS, FURTHER INFORMATION
Intrathecal injection **contra-indicated**.

● CAUTIONS Caution in handling—irritant to tissues · neuromuscular disease

● INTERACTIONS → Appendix 1 (vincristine).

● SIDE-EFFECTS
▸ Rare Diarrhoea · inappropriate secretion of antidiuretic hormone · intestinal necrosis · paralytic ileus · seizures · urinary retention
▸ Frequency not known Abdominal pain · alopecia · autonomic neuropathy · constipation · extravasation · eye disorders · hyperuricaemia · loss of deep tendon reflexes · motor weakness · muscle wasting · myelosuppression (negligible) · nausea · neurotoxicity · oral mucositis · ototoxicity · peripheral neuropathy · peripheral paraesthesia · severe bronchospasm following administration (more commonly when used in combination with mitomycin-C) · severe local irritation (care must be taken to avoid extravasation) · thromboembolism · tumour lysis syndrome · vomiting

SIDE-EFFECTS, FURTHER INFORMATION
▸ Neurotoxicity Neurotoxicity, usually as peripheral or autonomic neuropathy, occurs with all vinca alkaloids and is a limiting side-effect of vincristine. Patients with neurotoxicity commonly have peripheral paraesthesia, loss of deep tendon reflexes, abdominal pain, and constipation; ototoxicity has been reported. If symptoms of neurotoxicity are severe, doses should be reduced.

Motor weakness can also occur and dose reduction or discontinuation of therapy may be appropriate if motor weakness increases. Recovery from neurotoxic effects is usually slow but complete.

● CONCEPTION AND CONTRACEPTION Contraceptive advice required, see *Pregnancy and reproductive function* in Cytotoxic drugs p. 787.

● PREGNANCY Avoid (teratogenicity and fetal loss in *animal* studies). See also *Pregnancy and reproductive function* in Cytotoxic drugs p. 787.

● BREAST FEEDING Discontinue breast-feeding.

● HEPATIC IMPAIRMENT Dose reduction may be necessary—consult local treatment protocol for details.

● MEDICINAL FORMS
There can be variation in the licensing of different medicines containing the same drug.
Solution for injection
▸ Vincristine sulfate (Non-proprietary)
Vincristine sulfate 1 mg per 1 ml Vincristine 1mg/1ml solution for injection vials | 1 vial PoM £13.47 (Hospital only) | 5 vial PoM £67.35

Vincristine 2mg/2ml solution for injection vials | 1 vial PoM £26.66 (Hospital only) | 5 vial PoM £133.30
Vincristine 5mg/5ml solution for injection vials | 5 vial PoM £329.50

Vindesine sulfate

● INDICATIONS AND DOSE

Variety of cancers including leukaemias, lymphomas, and some solid tumours (e.g. breast and lung cancer)
▸ Adult: (consult product literature)

IMPORTANT SAFETY INFORMATION

Vindesine injections are for **intravenous administration only**. Inadvertent intrathecal administration can cause severe neurotoxicity, which is usually fatal.

The National Patient Safety Agency has advised (August 2008) that adult and teenage patients treated in an adult or adolescent unit should receive their vinca alkaloid dose in a 50 mL minibag. Teenagers and children treated in a child unit may receive their vinca alkaloid dose in a syringe.

● CONTRA-INDICATIONS

CONTRA-INDICATIONS, FURTHER INFORMATION
Intrathecal injection **contra-indicated**.

● CAUTIONS Caution in handling—irritant to tissues · neuromuscular disease

● INTERACTIONS → Appendix 1 (vindesine).

● SIDE-EFFECTS Alopecia · autonomic neuropathy · bone-marrow suppression · extravasation · hyperuricaemia · irritant to tissues · myelosuppression (dose-limiting) · nausea · neurotoxicity · oral mucositis · peripheral neuropathy · severe bronchospasm following administration (more commonly when used in combination with mitomycin-C) · severe local irritation (if extravasated) · thromboembolism · tumour lysis syndrome · vomiting

SIDE-EFFECTS, FURTHER INFORMATION
▸ Neurotoxicity Neurotoxicity, usually as peripheral or autonomic neuropathy; it occurs less often with vindesine than with vincristine. Patients with neurotoxicity commonly have peripheral paraesthesia, loss of deep tendon reflexes, abdominal pain, and constipation; ototoxicity has been reported. If symptoms of neurotoxicity are severe, doses should be reduced.

Motor weakness can also occur, and increasing motor weakness calls for dose reduction or discontinuation. Recovery from neurotoxic effects is usually slow but complete.

● CONCEPTION AND CONTRACEPTION Contraceptive advice required, see *Pregnancy and reproductive function* in Cytotoxic drugs p. 787.

● PREGNANCY Avoid (teratogenic in *animal* studies). See also *Pregnancy and reproductive function* in Cytotoxic drugs p. 787.

● BREAST FEEDING Discontinue breast-feeding.

● HEPATIC IMPAIRMENT Dose reduction may be necessary.

● MEDICINAL FORMS
There can be variation in the licensing of different medicines containing the same drug.
Powder for solution for injection
▸ Eldisine (Genus Pharmaceuticals Ltd)
Vindesine sulfate 5 mg Eldisine 5mg powder for solution for injection vials | 1 vial PoM £66.55 (Hospital only)

Vinflunine

● INDICATIONS AND DOSE

Treatment of advanced or metastatic transitional cell carcinoma of the urothelial tract after failure of a platinum-containing regimen (monotherapy)
▸ Adult: (consult local protocol)

IMPORTANT SAFETY INFORMATION

Vinflunine injections are for **intravenous administration only**. Inadvertent intrathecal administration can cause severe neurotoxicity, which is usually fatal.

The National Patient Safety Agency has advised (August 2008) that adult and teenage patients treated in an adult or adolescent unit should receive their vinca alkaloid dose in a 50 mL minibag. Teenagers and children treated in a child unit may receive their vinca alkaloid dose in a syringe.

● CONTRA-INDICATIONS
CONTRA-INDICATIONS, FURTHER INFORMATION
Intrathecal injection **contra-indicated**.
● CAUTIONS Cardiovascular disease · QT-interval prolongation (avoid hypokalaemia)
● INTERACTIONS → Appendix 1 (vinflunine)
Caution with concomitant use of drugs that prolong QT-interval.
● SIDE-EFFECTS
▸ Common or very common Anorexia · cutaneous reactions · dehydration · diarrhoea · dyspepsia · fatigue · hypertension · hypotension · insomnia · oedema · sweating · tachycardia · thrombosis
▸ Uncommon Increased weight · myocardial infarction · renal failure
▸ Frequency not known Alopecia · autonomic neuropathy · blurred vision · extravasation · hyperuricaemia · inappropriate anti-diuretic hormone secretion · myelosuppression (dose-limiting) · nausea · neurotoxicity · oral mucositis · peripheral neuropathy · QT-interval prolongation · severe bronchospasm following administration (more commonly when used in combination with mitomycin-C) · severe local irritation (if extravasated) · thromboembolism · tumour lysis syndrome · vomiting
SIDE-EFFECTS, FURTHER INFORMATION
▸ Neurotoxicity Neurotoxicity, usually as peripheral or autonomic neuropathy, occurs with all vinca alkaloids and is a limiting side-effect of vincristine. Patients with neurotoxicity commonly have peripheral paraesthesia, loss of deep tendon reflexes, abdominal pain, and constipation; ototoxicity has been reported. If symptoms of neurotoxicity are severe, doses should be reduced.

Motor weakness can also occur and dose reduction or discontinuation of therapy may be appropriate if motor weakness increases. Recovery from neurotoxic effects is usually slow but complete.
● CONCEPTION AND CONTRACEPTION Manufacturer advises effective contraception during and for up to 3 months after treatment.
● PREGNANCY Avoid unless essential—teratogenicity and embryotoxicity in *animal* studies. See also *Pregnancy and reproductive function* in Cytotoxic drugs p. 787.
● BREAST FEEDING Discontinue breast-feeding.
● HEPATIC IMPAIRMENT Reduce dose—consult product literature.
● RENAL IMPAIRMENT Reduce dose if creatinine clearance less than 60 mL/minute—consult product literature.

● NATIONAL FUNDING/ACCESS DECISIONS
NICE technology appraisals (TAs)
▸ Vinflunine for the treatment of advanced or metastatic transitional cell carcinoma of the urothelial tract (January 2013) NICE TA272
Vinflunine is **not** recommended for the treatment of advanced or metastatic transitional cell carcinoma of the urothelial tract that has progressed after treatment with platinum-based chemotherapy.
www.nice.org.uk/TA272
● MEDICINAL FORMS
There can be variation in the licensing of different medicines containing the same drug.
Solution for infusion
▸ Javlor (Pierre Fabre Ltd)
Vinflunine (as Vinflunine ditartrate) 25 mg per 1 ml Javlor 250mg/10ml concentrate for solution for infusion | 1 vial [PoM] £1,062.50
Javlor 50mg/2ml concentrate for solution for infusion | 1 vial [PoM] £212.50

Vinorelbine

● DRUG ACTION Vinorelbine is a semi-synthetic vinca alkaloid.

● INDICATIONS AND DOSE

Advanced breast cancer | Advanced non-small cell lung cancer
▸ BY MOUTH
▸ Adult: 60 mg/m^2 once weekly for 3 weeks, then increased if tolerated to 80 mg/m^2 once weekly (max. per dose 160 mg once weekly)
▸ BY INTRAVENOUS INJECTION, OR BY INTRAVENOUS INFUSION
▸ Adult: (consult product literature)

IMPORTANT SAFETY INFORMATION

Vinorelbine injections are for **intravenous administration only**. Inadvertent intrathecal administration can cause severe neurotoxicity, which is usually fatal.

The National Patient Safety Agency has advised (August 2008) that adult and teenage patients treated in an adult or adolescent unit should receive their vinca alkaloid dose in a 50 mL minibag. Teenagers and children treated in a child unit may receive their vinca alkaloid dose in a syringe.

RISKS OF INCORRECT DOSING OF ORAL ANTI-CANCER MEDICINES
See Cytotoxic drugs p. 787.

● CONTRA-INDICATIONS
▸ With oral use Concurrent radiotherapy if treating the liver · long-term oxygen therapy · previous significant surgical resection of small bowel · previous significant surgical resection of stomach
CONTRA-INDICATIONS, FURTHER INFORMATION
Intrathecal injection **contra-indicated**.
● CAUTIONS Caution in handling—irritant to tissues · ischaemic heart disease
● INTERACTIONS → Appendix 1 (vinorelbine).
● SIDE-EFFECTS
▸ Rare Pancreatitis
▸ Frequency not known Alopecia · autonomic neuropathy · extravasation · hyperuricaemia · hyponatraemia · inappropriate secretion of antidiuretic hormone · irritant to tissues · motor weakness · myelosuppression (dose-limiting) · nausea · neurotoxicity · oral mucositis · peripheral neuropathy · severe bronchospasm following administration of the vinca alkaloids (more commonly when used in combination with mitomycin-C) · severe

8

Immune system and malignant disease

Immune system and malignant disease

local irritation (if extravasated) · thromboembolism · tumour lysis syndrome · vomiting

SIDE-EFFECTS, FURTHER INFORMATION

▶ Neurotoxicity Neurotoxicity, usually as peripheral or autonomic neuropathy, occurs with all vinca alkaloids; it occurs less often with vinorelbine. Patients with neurotoxicity commonly have peripheral paraesthesia, loss of deep tendon reflexes, abdominal pain, and constipation; ototoxicity has been reported. If symptoms of neurotoxicity are severe, doses should be reduced.

Motor weakness can also occur, and increasing motor weakness calls for dose reduction or discontinuation of these drugs. Recovery from neurotoxic effects is usually slow but complete.

● CONCEPTION AND CONTRACEPTION Manufacturer advises effective contraception during and for 3 months after treatment; men must avoid fathering a child during and for at least 3 months after treatment.

● PREGNANCY Avoid unless essential (teratogenicity, and fetal loss in *animal* studies). See also *Pregnancy and reproductive function* in Cytotoxic drugs p. 787.

● BREAST FEEDING Discontinue breast-feeding.

● HEPATIC IMPAIRMENT

▶ With oral use Reduce *oral* dose in moderate impairment. Avoid *oral* use in severe impairment.

▶ With injectable use Reduce *intravenous dose* in severe impairment. Consult product literature.

● MEDICINAL FORMS
There can be variation in the licensing of different medicines containing the same drug.

Capsule
CAUTIONARY AND ADVISORY LABELS 21, 25
▶ Navelbine (Pierre Fabre Ltd)
Vinorelbine (as Vinorelbine tartrate) 20 mg Navelbine 20mg capsules | 1 capsule [PoM] £43.98 (Hospital only)
Vinorelbine (as Vinorelbine tartrate) 30 mg Navelbine 30mg capsules | 1 capsule [PoM] £65.98 (Hospital only)
Vinorelbine (as Vinorelbine tartrate) 80 mg Navelbine 80mg capsules | 1 capsule [PoM] £175.92 (Hospital only)

Solution for infusion
▶ Vinorelbine (Non-proprietary)
Vinorelbine (as Vinorelbine tartrate) 10 mg per 1 ml Vinorelbine 50mg/5ml concentrate for solution for infusion vials | 1 vial [PoM] £139.00 | 10 vial [PoM] £1,539.80
Vinorelbine 10mg/1ml concentrate for solution for infusion vials | 1 vial [PoM] £29.00 | 10 vial [PoM] £329.50
▶ Navelbine (Pierre Fabre Ltd)
Vinorelbine (as Vinorelbine tartrate) 10 mg per 1 ml Navelbine 10mg/1ml concentrate for solution for infusion vials | 10 vial [PoM] £297.45 (Hospital only)
Navelbine 50mg/5ml concentrate for solution for infusion vials | 10 vial [PoM] £1,399.79 (Hospital only)

ANTINEOPLASTIC DRUGS > OTHER

Arsenic trioxide

● INDICATIONS AND DOSE

Acute promyelocytic leukaemia in patients who have relapsed or failed to respond to previous treatment with a retinoid and chemotherapy
▶ BY INTRAVENOUS INFUSION
▶ Adult: (consult local protocol)

● CAUTIONS Hypokalaemia (correct before treatment) · hypomagnesaemia (correct before treatment) · previous treatment with anthracyclines (increased risk of QT interval prolongation)

● INTERACTIONS → Appendix 1 (arsenic trioxide). Avoid concomitant administration with drugs causing QT interval prolongation.

● SIDE-EFFECTS
▶ Common or very common Atrial fibrillation · atrial flutter · diarrhoea · fatigue · haemorrhage · hyperglycaemia · hypokalaemia · leucocyte activation syndrome · musculoskeletal pain · paraesthesia · pleuritic pain · QT interval prolongation
▶ Uncommon Abdominal pain · blurred vision · hypotension · oedema · pneumonitis · rash · renal failure · seizures · tachycardia · vasculitis
▶ Frequency not known Alopecia · bone-marrow suppression · extravasation · hyperuricaemia · nausea · oral mucositis · thromboembolism · tumour lysis syndrome · vomiting

SIDE-EFFECTS, FURTHER INFORMATION
▶ Leucocyte activation syndrome Signs and symptoms of leucocyte activation syndrome include unexplained fever, dyspnoea, weight gain, pulmonary infiltrates, pleural or pericardial effusions, with or without leucocytosis—treat with high dose corticosteroids, consult product literature.

● CONCEPTION AND CONTRACEPTION Manufacturer advises effective contraception during treatment in men and women.

● PREGNANCY Avoid (teratogenic and embryotoxic in *animal* studies). See also *Pregnancy and reproductive function* in Cytotoxic drugs p. 787.

● BREAST FEEDING Discontinue breast-feeding.

● HEPATIC IMPAIRMENT Manufacturer advises caution—limited information available.

● RENAL IMPAIRMENT Manufacturer advises caution—limited information available.

● MONITORING REQUIREMENTS ECG required before and during treatment—consult product literature.

● MEDICINAL FORMS
There can be variation in the licensing of different medicines containing the same drug.

Solution for infusion
▶ Trisenox (Teva UK Ltd)
Arsenic trioxide 1 mg per 1 ml Trisenox 10mg/10ml concentrate for solution for infusion ampoules | 10 ampoule [PoM] £2,920.00 (Hospital only)

Crisantaspase

● DRUG ACTION Crisantaspase is the enzyme asparaginase produced by *Erwinia chrysanthemi*.

● INDICATIONS AND DOSE

Acute lymphoblastic leukaemia
▶ BY INTRAMUSCULAR INJECTION, OR BY SUBCUTANEOUS INJECTION, OR BY INTRAVENOUS INJECTION
▶ Adult: (consult product literature)

● CONTRA-INDICATIONS History of pancreatitis related to asparaginase therapy

● SIDE-EFFECTS
▶ Common or very common Coagulation disorders · confusion · convulsions · diarrhoea · dizziness · drowsiness · headache · lethargy · liver dysfunction · neurotoxicity · pancreatitis
▶ Uncommon Anaphylaxis · changes in blood lipids · hyperglycaemia
▶ Rare CNS depression
▶ Very rare Abdominal pain · hypertension · myalgia
▶ Frequency not known Alopecia · bone-marrow suppression · extravasation · hyperuricaemia · nausea · oral mucositis · thromboembolism · tumour lysis syndrome · vomiting

● CONCEPTION AND CONTRACEPTION Contraceptive advice required, see *Pregnancy and reproductive function* in Cytotoxic drugs p. 787.

● PREGNANCY Avoid. See also, *Pregnancy and reproductive function* in Cytotoxic drugs p. 787.

● BREAST FEEDING Discontinue breast-feeding.

- DIRECTIONS FOR ADMINISTRATION Facilities for the management of anaphylaxis should be available.

- MEDICINAL FORMS
There can be variation in the licensing of different medicines containing the same drug.
  Powder for solution for injection
  ‣ Erwinase (EUSA Pharma Ltd)
    Crisantaspase 10000 unit Erwinase 10,000unit powder for solution for injection vials | 5 vial [PoM] £3,065.00

Eribulin

- INDICATIONS AND DOSE

  Treatment of locally advanced or metastatic breast cancer when the disease has progressed after treatment with at least 1 chemotherapy regimen for advanced disease
  ‣ BY INTRAVENOUS INJECTION
  ‣ Adult: Give on day 1 and day 8 of a 21-day cycle, previous therapy should have included an anthracycline and a taxane in either the adjuvant or metastatic setting unless the patient is unsuitable for these treatments (consult local protocol)

- CONTRA-INDICATIONS Congenital long QT syndrome
- CAUTIONS Bradyarrhythmias (increased susceptibility to QT-interval prolongation) · congestive heart failure (increased susceptibility to QT-interval prolongation) · electrolyte disturbances (increased susceptibility to QT-interval prolongation) · susceptibility to QT-interval prolongation
- INTERACTIONS → Appendix 1 (eribulin).
Caution with concomitant use of drugs that prolong QT-interval.
- SIDE-EFFECTS Alopecia · bone-marrow suppression · extravasation · hyperuricaemia · myelosuppression · nausea · oral mucositis · peripheral neuropathy · QT-interval prolongation · thromboembolism · tumour lysis syndrome · vomiting
  SIDE-EFFECTS, FURTHER INFORMATION
  For further information on side effects, consult product literature.
- CONCEPTION AND CONTRACEPTION Ensure effective contraception during and for up to 3 months after treatment in men or women.
- PREGNANCY Avoid unless essential (teratogenic in *animal* studies). See also *Pregnancy and reproductive function* in Cytotoxic drugs p. 787.
- BREAST FEEDING Discontinue breast-feeding.
- HEPATIC IMPAIRMENT Reduce dose.
- RENAL IMPAIRMENT Consider dose reduction if creatinine clearance less than 40 mL/minute.
- MONITORING REQUIREMENTS
‣ Monitor for signs of peripheral neuropathy—severe peripheral neurotoxicity requires treatment delay or dose reduction (consult product literature).
‣ ECG monitoring recommended in patients prescribed concomitant use of drugs that prolong the QT-interval or who are susceptible to QT-interval prolongation.
‣ Monitor electrolytes periodically.
- NATIONAL FUNDING/ACCESS DECISIONS

  NICE technology appraisals (TAs)
‣ **Eribulin for the treatment of locally advanced or metastatic breast cancer (April 2012)** NICE TA250
Eribulin is **not** recommended for the treatment of locally advanced or metastatic breast cancer that has progressed after at least two chemotherapy regimens for advanced disease.
www.nice.org.uk/TA250

Scottish Medicines Consortium (SMC) Decisions
The *Scottish Medicines Consortium* has advised (March 2016) that eribulin (*Halaven*®) is accepted for restricted use within NHS Scotland for the treatment of patients with locally advanced or metastatic breast cancer that has progressed after at least two prior chemotherapy regimens for advanced disease, which includes capecitabine if indicated.

- MEDICINAL FORMS
There can be variation in the licensing of different medicines containing the same drug.
  Solution for injection
  EXCIPIENTS: May contain Ethanol
  ‣ Halaven (Eisai Ltd)
    Eribulin.44 mg per 1 ml Halaven 0.88mg/2ml solution for injection vials | 1 vial [PoM] £361.00 (Hospital only) | 6 vial [PoM] £2,166.00 (Hospital only)
    Halaven 1.32mg/3ml solution for injection vials | 1 vial [PoM] £541.50 (Hospital only)

Hydroxycarbamide

(Hydroxyurea)

- INDICATIONS AND DOSE

  Treatment of chronic myeloid leukaemia | Treatment of cancer of the cervix in conjunction with radiotherapy | Polycythaemia
  ‣ BY MOUTH
  ‣ Adult: 20–30 mg/kg daily, alternatively 80 mg/kg every 3 days

  Sickle-cell disease —consult with a specialist centre
  ‣ BY MOUTH
  ‣ Adult: Initially 15 mg/kg daily, increased in steps of 2.5–5 mg/kg daily, dose to be increased every 12 weeks according to response; usual dose 15–30 mg/kg daily; maximum 35 mg/kg per day

  ---
  IMPORTANT SAFETY INFORMATION
  RISKS OF INCORRECT DOSING OF ORAL ANTI-CANCER MEDICINES
  See Cytotoxic drugs p. 787.

- CAUTIONS Leg ulcers (review treatment if cutaneous vasculitic ulcerations develop)
- INTERACTIONS → Appendix 1 (hydroxycarbamide).
- SIDE-EFFECTS
‣ **Common or very common** Headache · myelosuppression · skin reactions
‣ **Rare** Amenorrhoea (in sickle-cell disease) · fever (in sickle-cell disease)
‣ **Frequency not known** Alopecia · bleeding (in sickle-cell disease) · bone-marrow suppression · dizziness · hyperuricaemia · hypomagnesaemia (in sickle-cell disease) · nausea · oral mucositis · rash · reduced sperm count and activity · skin cancers (particularly in elderly patients) · thromboembolism · tumour lysis syndrome · vomiting
- CONCEPTION AND CONTRACEPTION Manufacturer advises effective contraception before and during treatment.
- PREGNANCY Avoid (teratogenic in *animal* studies). See also *Pregnancy and reproductive function* in Cytotoxic drugs p. 787.
- BREAST FEEDING Discontinue breast-feeding.
- HEPATIC IMPAIRMENT Manufacturer advises caution in mild to moderate impairment. Avoid in severe impairment, unless used for malignant conditions.
- RENAL IMPAIRMENT In sickle-cell disease, reduce initial dose by 50% if eGFR less than 60 mL/minute/1.73 m². In sickle-cell disease, avoid if eGFR less than 30 mL/minute/1.73 m².
  Use with caution in malignant disease.

8

Immune system and malignant disease

- MONITORING REQUIREMENTS
- ▶ Monitor renal and hepatic function before and during treatment.
- ▶ Monitor full blood count before treatment, and repeatedly throughout use; in sickle-cell disease monitor every 2 weeks for the first 2 months and then every 2 months thereafter (or every 2 weeks if on maximum dose).
- ▶ Patients receiving long-term therapy for malignant disease should be monitored for secondary malignancies.
- PATIENT AND CARER ADVICE Patients receiving long-term therapy with hydroxycarbamide should be advised to protect skin from sun exposure.

- MEDICINAL FORMS
  There can be variation in the licensing of different medicines containing the same drug. Forms available from special-order manufacturers include: capsule, oral suspension, oral solution

  Tablet
  - ▶ Siklos (Nordic Pharma Ltd)
    Hydroxycarbamide 100 mg Siklos 100mg tablets | 60 tablet [PoM] £100.00 DT price = £100.00
    Hydroxycarbamide 1 gram Siklos 1000mg tablets | 30 tablet [PoM] £500.00

  Capsule
  - ▶ Hydroxycarbamide (Non-proprietary)
    Hydroxycarbamide 500 mg Hydroxycarbamide 500mg capsules | 100 capsule [PoM] £86.00 DT price = £11.70
  - ▶ Droxia (Imported (United States))
    Hydroxycarbamide 300 mg Droxia 300mg capsules | 60 capsule [PoM] no price available
  - ▶ Hydrea (Bristol-Myers Squibb Pharmaceuticals Ltd)
    Hydroxycarbamide 500 mg Hydrea 500mg capsules | 100 capsule [PoM] £10.47 DT price = £11.70

Mitotane

- DRUG ACTION Mitotane selectively inhibits the activity of the adrenal cortex, necessitating corticosteroid replacement therapy.

- INDICATIONS AND DOSE

  Symptomatic treatment of advanced or inoperable adrenocortical carcinoma
  - ▶ BY MOUTH
  - ▶ Adult: Initially 2–3 g daily in 2–3 divided doses adjusted according to plasma-concentration monitoring, in severe illness initial dose can be increased up to 6 g daily, reduce dose or interrupt treatment if signs of toxicity, discontinue if inadequate response after 3 months

  > IMPORTANT SAFETY INFORMATION
  > RISKS OF INCORRECT DOSING OF ORAL ANTI-CANCER MEDICINES
  > See Cytotoxic drugs p. 787.

- CAUTIONS Avoid in Acute porphyrias p. 918 · risk of accumulation in overweight patients
- INTERACTIONS → Appendix 1 (mitotane).
- SIDE-EFFECTS
- ▶ **Common or very common** Anaemia · anorexia · asthenia · ataxia · cognitive impairment · confusion · diarrhoea · dizziness · drowsiness · endocrine side effects · epigastric discomfort · gastro-intestinal disturbances · gynaecomastia · headache · hypercholesterolaemia · hypertriglyceridaemia · hypogonadism · leucopenia · liver disorders · movement disorder · myasthenia · nausea · neuropathy · neurotoxicity · paraesthesia · prolonged bleeding time · rash · thrombocytopenia · thyroid disorders · vomiting
- ▶ **Rare** Flushing · haematuria · haemorrhagic cystitis · hypersalivation · hypertension · hypouricaemia · ocular

disorders · postural hypotension · proteinuria · pyrexia · visual disturbances
- ▶ **Frequency not known** Alopecia · bone-marrow suppression · hyperuricaemia · nausea · oral mucositis · thromboembolism · tumour lysis syndrome · vomiting
- CONCEPTION AND CONTRACEPTION Contraceptive advice required, see *Pregnancy and reproductive* function in Cytotoxic drugs p. 787.
- PREGNANCY Manufacturer advises avoid. See also *Pregnancy and reproductive function* in Cytotoxic drugs p. 787.
- BREAST FEEDING Discontinue breast-feeding.
- HEPATIC IMPAIRMENT Manufacturer advises caution in mild to moderate impairment. Avoid in severe impairment. In mild to moderate hepatic impairment, monitoring of plasma-mitotane concentration is recommended.
- RENAL IMPAIRMENT Manufacturer advises caution in mild to moderate impairment. Avoid in severe impairment. In mild to moderate renal impairment, monitoring of plasma-mitotane concentration is recommended.
- MONITORING REQUIREMENTS
- ▶ Plasma-mitotane concentration for optimum response 14–20 mg/litre.
- ▶ Monitor plasma-mitotane concentration—consult product literature.
- PRESCRIBING AND DISPENSING INFORMATION
  Corticosteroid replacement therapy Corticosteroid replacement therapy is necessary with treatment with mitotane. The dose of glucocorticoid should be increased in case of shock, trauma, or infection.
- PATIENT AND CARER ADVICE
  Patients should be warned to contact doctor immediately if injury, infection, or illness occurs (because of risk of acute adrenal insufficiency).
  Driving and skilled tasks
  Central nervous system toxicity may affect performance of skilled tasks (e.g. driving).

- MEDICINAL FORMS
  There can be variation in the licensing of different medicines containing the same drug.

  Tablet
  CAUTIONARY AND ADVISORY LABELS 2, 10, 21
  - ▶ Lysodren (HRA Pharma UK Ltd)
    Mitotane 500 mg Lysodren 500mg tablets | 100 tablet [PoM] £590.97

Procarbazine

- DRUG ACTION Procarbazine is a mild monoamine-oxidase inhibitor.

- INDICATIONS AND DOSE

  Hodgkin's lymphoma
  - ▶ BY MOUTH
  - ▶ Adult: (consult local protocol)

  > IMPORTANT SAFETY INFORMATION
  > RISKS OF INCORRECT DOSING OF ORAL ANTI-CANCER MEDICINES
  > See Cytotoxic drugs p. 787.

- CONTRA-INDICATIONS Pre-existing severe leucopenia · pre-existing severe thrombocytopenia
- CAUTIONS Cardiovascular disease · cerebrovascular disease · epilepsy · phaeochromocytoma · procarbazine is a mild monoamineoxidase inhibitor (dietary restriction is rarely considered necessary)
- INTERACTIONS → Appendix 1 (procarbazine).
  Alcohol ingestion may cause a disulfiram-like reaction.

● SIDE-EFFECTS
▶ **Common or very common** Loss of appetite
▶ **Frequency not known** Alopecia · bone-marrow suppression
· hypersensitivity rash (discontinue treatment) ·
hyperuricaemia · jaundice · myelosuppression · nausea ·
oral mucositis · thromboembolism · tumour lysis syndrome
· vomiting

● CONCEPTION AND CONTRACEPTION Contraceptive advice
required, see *Pregnancy and reproductive function* in
Cytotoxic drugs p. 787.

● PREGNANCY Avoid (teratogenic in *animal* studies and
isolated reports in humans). See also *Pregnancy and
reproductive function* in Cytotoxic drugs p. 787.

● BREAST FEEDING Discontinue breast-feeding.

● HEPATIC IMPAIRMENT Caution in mild to moderate
impairment. Avoid in severe impairment.

● RENAL IMPAIRMENT Caution in mild to moderate
impairment. Avoid in severe impairment.

● MEDICINAL FORMS
There can be variation in the licensing of different medicines
containing the same drug.
Capsule
CAUTIONARY AND ADVISORY LABELS 4
▶ Procarbazine (Non-proprietary)
Procarbazine (as Procarbazine hydrochloride)
50 mg Procarbazine 50mg capsules | 50 capsule PoM £339.95

Raltitrexed

● DRUG ACTION Raltitrexed is a thymidylate synthase
inhibitor.

● INDICATIONS AND DOSE
**Palliation of advanced colorectal cancer when fluorouracil
and folinic acid cannot be used**
▶ BY INTRAVENOUS INFUSION
▶ Adult: (consult local protocol)

● INTERACTIONS → Appendix 1 (raltitrexed).

● SIDE-EFFECTS Alopecia · bone-marrow suppression ·
extravasation · gastro-intestinal effects · hyperuricaemia ·
myelosuppression · nausea · oral mucositis ·
thromboembolism · tumour lysis syndrome · vomiting

● CONCEPTION AND CONTRACEPTION Ensure effective
contraception during and for at least 6 months after
treatment in men or women.

● PREGNANCY See *Pregnancy and reproductive function* in
Cytotoxic drugs p. 787.

● BREAST FEEDING Discontinue breast-feeding.

● HEPATIC IMPAIRMENT Caution in mild to moderate
impairment. Avoid in severe impairment.

● RENAL IMPAIRMENT Reduce dose and increase dosing
interval if creatinine clearance less than 65 mL/minute
(consult product literature). Avoid if creatinine clearance
less than 25 mL/minute.

● NATIONAL FUNDING/ACCESS DECISIONS
NICE technology appraisals (TAs)
▶ Irinotecan, oxaliplatin, and raltitrexed for advanced colorectal
cancer (August 2005) NICE TA93
Raltitrexed is **not** recommended for the treatment of
advanced colorectal cancer. Its use should be confined to
clinical studies.
www.nice.org.uk/TA93

● MEDICINAL FORMS
There can be variation in the licensing of different medicines
containing the same drug.
Powder for solution for infusion
▶ Tomudex (Hospira UK Ltd)
Raltitrexed 2 mg Tomudex 2mg powder for solution for infusion vials
| 1 vial PoM £175.00

RETINOID AND RELATED DRUGS

Bexarotene

● DRUG ACTION Bexarotene is an agonist at the retinoid X
receptor, which is involved in the regulation of cell
differentiation and proliferation. Bexarotene can cause
regression of cutaneous T-cell lymphoma.

● INDICATIONS AND DOSE
**Skin manifestations of cutaneous T-cell lymphoma
refractory to previous systemic treatment**
▶ BY MOUTH
▶ Adult: Initially 300 mg/m^2 once daily, adjusted
according to response, to be taken with a meal

> IMPORTANT SAFETY INFORMATION
> RISKS OF INCORRECT DOSING OF ORAL ANTI-CANCER MEDICINES
> See Cytotoxic drugs p. 787.

● CONTRA-INDICATIONS History of pancreatitis ·
hypervitaminosis A · uncontrolled hyperlipidaemia ·
uncontrolled hypothyroidism

● CAUTIONS Avoid in Acute porphyrias p. 918 ·
hyperlipidaemia · hypothyroidism

● INTERACTIONS → Appendix 1 (bexarotene).

● SIDE-EFFECTS Alopecia · bone-marrow suppression ·
headache · hyperlipidaemia · hyperuricaemia ·
hypothyroidism · immunosuppression · leucopenia ·
myelosuppression · nausea · oral mucositis · pruritus · rash
· thromboembolism · tumour lysis syndrome · vomiting

● ALLERGY AND CROSS-SENSITIVITY Caution—
hypersensitivity to retinoids.

● CONCEPTION AND CONTRACEPTION Manufacturer advises
effective contraception during and for at least 1 month
after treatment in men and women.

● PREGNANCY Avoid. See also *Pregnancy and reproductive
function* in Cytotoxic drugs p. 787.

● BREAST FEEDING Discontinue breast-feeding.

● HEPATIC IMPAIRMENT Avoid.

● NATIONAL FUNDING/ACCESS DECISIONS
Scottish Medicines Consortium (SMC) Decisions
The *Scottish Medicines Consortium* has advised (November
2002) that bexarotene is recommended for restricted use
as a second-line treatment for patients with advanced
cutaneous T-cell lymphoma.

● MEDICINAL FORMS
There can be variation in the licensing of different medicines
containing the same drug.
Capsule
▶ Targretin (Eisai Ltd)
Bexarotene 75 mg Targretin 75mg capsules | 100 capsule PoM
£937.50

Tretinoin

- **INDICATIONS AND DOSE**

Induction of remission in acute promyelocytic leukaemia (used in previously untreated patients as well as in those who have relapsed after standard chemotherapy or who are refractory to it)
▶ BY MOUTH
▸ Adult: 45 mg/m² daily in 2 divided doses maximum duration of treatment is 90 days, consult product literature for details of concomitant chemotherapy

- CAUTIONS Increased risk of thromboembolism during first month of treatment
- INTERACTIONS → Appendix 1 (retinoids).
- SIDE-EFFECTS Alopecia · anxiety · arrhythmias · benign intracranial hypertension · bone pain · cheilitis · chest pain · confusion · depression · dizziness · dry mucous membranes · dry skin · erythema · flushing · gastro-intestinal disturbances · genital ulceration · headache · hearing disturbances · hypercalcaemia · insomnia · oedema · pancreatitis · paraesthesia · pruritus · raised lipids · raised liver enzymes · raised serum creatinine · rash · retinoic acid syndrome · shivering · sweating · thromboembolism · visual disturbances

SIDE-EFFECTS, FURTHER INFORMATION
▸ Retinoic acid syndrome Fever, dyspnoea, acute respiratory distress, pulmonary infiltrates, pleural effusion, hyperleucocytosis, hypotension, oedema, weight gain, hepatic, renal and multi-organ failure requires immediate treatment—consult product literature.

- CONCEPTION AND CONTRACEPTION Effective contraception must be used for at least 1 month before oral treatment, during treatment and for at least 1 month after stopping (oral progestogen-only contraceptives not considered effective).
- PREGNANCY Teratogenic. See *Pregnancy and reproductive function* in Cytotoxic drugs p. 787.
- BREAST FEEDING Avoid (discontinue breast-feeding).
- HEPATIC IMPAIRMENT Reduce dose to 25 mg/m².
- RENAL IMPAIRMENT Reduce dose to 25 mg/m².
- MONITORING REQUIREMENTS Monitor haematological and coagulation profile, liver function, serum calcium and plasma lipids before and during treatment.
- PRESCRIBING AND DISPENSING INFORMATION Tretinoin is the acid form of vitamin A.

- MEDICINAL FORMS
There can be variation in the licensing of different medicines containing the same drug.
Capsule
CAUTIONARY AND ADVISORY LABELS 21, 25
▸ Tretinoin (Non-proprietary)
  Tretinoin 10 mg Tretinoin 10mg capsules | 100 capsule [PoM]
  £240.00 DT price = £240.00

2.1 Cytotoxic drug-induced side effects

ANTIDOTES AND CHELATORS ⟩ IRON CHELATORS

Dexrazoxane

- DRUG ACTION Dexrazoxane is an iron chelator.

- **INDICATIONS AND DOSE**
CARDIOXANE®

Prevention of chronic cumulative cardiotoxicity caused by doxorubicin or epirubicin treatment in advanced or metastatic breast cancer patients who have received a prior cumulative dose of 300 mg/m² of doxorubicin or a prior cumulative dose of 540 mg/m² of epirubicin when further anthracycline treatment is required
▶ BY INTRAVENOUS INFUSION
▸ Adult: Administer 10 times the doxorubicin-equivalent dose or 10 times the epirubicin-equivalent dose, dose to be given 30 minutes before anthracycline administration

SAVENE®
Anthracycline extravasation
▶ BY INTRAVENOUS INFUSION
▸ Adult: Initially 1 g/m² daily (max. per dose 2 g) for 2 days, then 500 mg/m² for 1 day, first dose to be given as soon as possible and within 6 hours after injury

- CAUTIONS Myelosuppression (effects may be additive to those of chemotherapy)
CARDIOXANE® Manufacturer advises caution in patients with heart failure—no information available · manufacturer advises caution in patients with myocardial infarction in previous 12 months—no information available · manufacturer advises caution in patients with symptomatic valvular heart disease—no information available · manufacturer advises caution in patients with uncontrolled angina—no information available
- INTERACTIONS → Appendix 1 (dexrazoxane).
- SIDE-EFFECTS
CARDIOXANE® ▸ **Common or very common** Anorexia · asthenia · diarrhoea · dizziness · dry mouth · dyspnoea · erythema · infection · malaise · nausea · oedema · paraesthesia · peripheral neuropathy · stomatitis · syncope · vomiting
▸ **Uncommon** Abdominal pain · acute myeloid leukaemia · constipation · cough · dyspepsia · headache · lymphoedema · nail disorder · reduced ejection fraction · tachycardia · thromboembolism (when given with cytotoxic drugs)
▸ **Frequency not known** Alopecia · anaemia · blood disorders · fatigue · injection-site reactions · leucopenia · phlebitis · pruritus · pyrexia · thrombocytopenia
SAVENE® ▸ **Common or very common** Alopecia · anaemia · anorexia · blood disorders · diarrhoea · dizziness · drowsiness · dry mouth · dyspnoea · erythema · fatigue · infection · injection-site reactions · leucopenia · malaise · nausea · oedema · peripheral neuropathy · peripheral oedema · phlebitis · pruritus · pyrexia · stomatitis · syncope · thrombocytopenia · tremor · vaginal haemorrhage · vomiting
▸ **Uncommon** Drowsiness · myalgia · thromboembolism (when given with cytotoxic drugs) · weight loss
- CONCEPTION AND CONTRACEPTION Ensure effective contraception during and for at least 3 months after treatment in men and women.

- PREGNANCY Avoid unless essential (toxicity in *animal* studies).
- BREAST FEEDING Discontinue breast-feeding.
- HEPATIC IMPAIRMENT

  CARDIOXANE® Manufacturer advises that if anthracycline dose is reduced, reduce the *Cardioxane*® dose by a similar ratio.

  SAVENE® Manufacturer advises avoid—no information available.
- RENAL IMPAIRMENT

  CARDIOXANE® Manufacturer advises reduce dose by 50% if creatinine clearance less than 40 mL/minute.

  SAVENE® Manufacturer advises avoid—risk of accumulation.
- MONITORING REQUIREMENTS
  ‣ Monitor full blood count.
  ‣ Monitor for cardiac toxicity.
  ‣ Monitor liver function.
- DIRECTIONS FOR ADMINISTRATION Local coolants such as ice packs should be removed at least 15 minutes before administration.

  CARDIOXANE® For *intravenous infusion*, give intermittently *in* Compound sodium lactate; reconstitute each vial with 25 mL water for injections and dilute each vial with 25–100 mL infusion fluid; give requisite dose over 15 minutes.

  SAVENE® For *intravenous infusion*, give intermittently *in* diluent; reconstitute each 500-mg vial with 25 mL of diluent; dilute requisite dose further in remaining diluent and give over 1–2 hours into a large vein in an area other than the one affected.
- MEDICINAL FORMS
  There can be variation in the licensing of different medicines containing the same drug.
  Powder for solution for infusion
  ‣ Cardioxane (Clinigen Healthcare Ltd)
    Dexrazoxane 500 mg Cardioxane 500mg powder for solution for infusion vials | 1 vial PoM £156.57
  Powder and solvent for solution for infusion
  ELECTROLYTES: May contain Potassium, sodium
  ‣ Savene (Clinigen Healthcare Ltd)
    Dexrazoxane 500 mg Savene 500mg powder for concentrate and solvent for solution for infusion vials | 10 vial PoM no price available

DETOXIFYING DRUGS > RECOMBINANT HUMAN KERATINOCYTE GROWTH FACTORS

Palifermin

- DRUG ACTION Palifermin is a human keratinocyte growth factor.

- INDICATIONS AND DOSE
  Management of oral mucositis in patients with haematological malignancies receiving myeloblative radiochemotherapy with autologous haematopoietic stem-cell support
  ‣ BY INTRAVENOUS INJECTION
  ‣ Adult: 60 micrograms/kg once daily for 3 doses (third dose given 24-48 hours before myeloblative therapy) then 3 further doses at least 24 hours after myeloblative therapy, and more than 4 days after most recent palifermin injection, starting on the same day as (but after) stem-cell infusion

- SIDE-EFFECTS Arthralgia · discoloration of the tongue · erythema · fever · oedema · oral paraesthesia · pruritus · rash · skin hyperpigmentation · taste disturbance · thickening of the tongue
- PREGNANCY Manufacturer advises avoid unless potential benefit outweighs risk—toxicity in *animal* studies.

- BREAST FEEDING Manufacturer advises avoid—no information available.
- MEDICINAL FORMS
  There can be variation in the licensing of different medicines containing the same drug.
  No licensed medicines listed.

DETOXIFYING DRUGS > UROPROTECTIVE DRUGS

Mesna

- INDICATIONS AND DOSE
  Cytotoxic induced urothelial toxicity
  ‣ BY MOUTH, OR BY INTRAVENOUS INJECTION
  ‣ Adult: Dose to be calculated according to oxazaphosphorine (cyclophosphamide or ifosfamide) treatment (consult product literature)

- SIDE-EFFECTS
  ‣ **Common or very common** Colic · depression · diarrhoea · fatigue · headache · hypotension · irritability · joint pains · limb pains · nausea · rash · tachycardia · vomiting
  ‣ **Rare** Hypersensitivity reactions (more common in patients with auto-immune disorders)
- ALLERGY AND CROSS-SENSITIVITY Contra-indicated if history of hypersensitivity to thiol-containing compounds.
- PREGNANCY Not known to be harmful. See also *Pregnancy and reproductive function* in Cytotoxic drugs p. 787.
- EFFECT ON LABORATORY TESTS False positive urinary ketones. False positive or false negative urinary erythrocytes.
- DIRECTIONS FOR ADMINISTRATION For oral administration of the injection, contents of ampoule are taken in a flavoured drink such as orange juice or cola which may be stored in a refrigerator for up to 24 hours in a sealed container.

- MEDICINAL FORMS
  There can be variation in the licensing of different medicines containing the same drug. Forms available from special-order manufacturers include: oral solution
  Tablet
  ‣ Mesna (Non-proprietary)
    Mesna 400 mg Mesna 400mg tablets | 10 tablet PoM £134.30-£134.40
    Mesna 600 mg Mesna 600mg tablets | 10 tablet PoM £190.60
  Solution for injection
  ‣ Mesna (Non-proprietary)
    Mesna 100 mg per 1 ml Mesna 1g/10ml solution for injection ampoules | 15 ampoule PoM £441.15
    Mesna 400mg/4ml solution for injection ampoules | 15 ampoule PoM £201.15

VITAMINS AND TRACE ELEMENTS > FOLATES

Folinic acid

- INDICATIONS AND DOSE
  Prevention of methotrexate-induced adverse effects
  ‣ BY INTRAMUSCULAR INJECTION, OR BY INTRAVENOUS INJECTION, OR BY INTRAVENOUS INFUSION
  ‣ Adult: 15 mg every 6 hours for 24 hours, to be started usually 12–24 hours after start of methotrexate infusion, dose may be continued by mouth, consult local treatment protocol for further information
  Suspected methotrexate overdosage
  ‣ BY INTRAVENOUS INJECTION, OR BY INTRAVENOUS INFUSION
  ‣ Adult: Initial dose equal to or exceeding dose of methotrexate, to be given at a maximum rate of 160 mg/minute, consult poisons information centres for advice on continuing management continued →

8

Immune system and malignant disease

Adjunct to fluorouracil in colorectal cancer
▸ BY SLOW INTRAVENOUS INJECTION
▸ Adult: (consult product literature)

SODIOFOLIN®

As an antidote to methotrexate
▸ BY INTRAMUSCULAR INJECTION, OR BY INTRAVENOUS INJECTION
▸ Adult: (consult product literature)

Adjunct to fluorouracil in colorectal cancer
▸ BY INTRAVENOUS INJECTION, OR BY INTRAVENOUS INFUSION
▸ Adult: (consult product literature)

● CONTRA-INDICATIONS Intrathecal injection
● CAUTIONS Avoid simultaneous administration of methotrexate · **not** indicated for pernicious anaemia or other megaloblastic anaemias caused by vitamin B_{12} deficiency
● INTERACTIONS → Appendix 1 (folates).
● SIDE-EFFECTS
▸ Rare Agitation (after high doses) · depression (after high doses) · insomnia (after high doses) · pyrexia (after parenteral use)
● PREGNANCY Not known to be harmful; benefit outweighs risk.
● BREAST FEEDING Presence in milk unknown but benefit outweighs risk.
● NATIONAL FUNDING/ACCESS DECISIONS

NICE technology appraisals (TAs)
▸ Bevacizumab in combination with oxaliplatin and either fluorouracil plus folinic acid or capecitabine for the treatment of metastatic colorectal cancer (December 2010) NICE TA212 Bevacizumab in combination with oxaliplatin and either fluorouracil plus folinic acid or capecitabine is not recommended for the treatment of metastatic colorectal cancer.
www.nice.org.uk/TA212

● MEDICINAL FORMS
There can be variation in the licensing of different medicines containing the same drug. Forms available from special-order manufacturers include: oral suspension, oral solution

Tablet
▸ Folinic acid (Non-proprietary)
 Folinic acid (as Calcium folinate) 15 mg Calcium folinate 15mg tablets | 10 tablet PoM £49.10 DT price = £49.11
▸ Refolinon (Pfizer Ltd)
 Folinic acid (as Calcium folinate) 15 mg Refolinon 15mg tablets | 30 tablet PoM £85.74

Solution for injection
▸ Folinic acid (Non-proprietary)
 Folinic acid (as Calcium folinate) 3 mg per 1 ml Calcium folinate 3mg/1ml solution for injection ampoules | 5 ampoule PoM £30.00
 Folinic acid (as Calcium folinate) 7.5 mg per 1 ml Calcium folinate 15mg/2ml solution for injection ampoules | 5 ampoule PoM £38.99-£39.00
 Folinic acid (as Calcium folinate) 10 mg per 1 ml Calcium folinate 50mg/5ml solution for injection vials | 1 vial PoM £18.44 (Hospital only) | 1 vial PoM £20.00
 Calcium folinate 300mg/30ml solution for injection vials | 1 vial PoM £89.95 (Hospital only) | 1 vial PoM £100.00
 Calcium folinate 100mg/10ml solution for injection vials | 1 vial PoM £34.94 (Hospital only) | 1 vial PoM £37.50
 Folinic acid (as Disodium folinate) 50 mg per 1 ml Disodium folinate 50mg/1ml solution for injection vials | 1 vial PoM £24.70
 Disodium folinate 200mg/4ml solution for injection vials | 1 vial PoM £80.40
▸ Refolinon (Pfizer Ltd)
 Folinic acid (as Calcium folinate) 3 mg per 1 ml Refolinon 30mg/10ml solution for injection ampoules | 5 ampoule PoM £23.12
▸ Sodiofolin (medac UK)
 Folinic acid (as Disodium folinate) 50 mg per 1 ml Sodiofolin 400mg/8ml solution for injection vials | 1 vial PoM £126.25 (Hospital only)
 Sodiofolin 100mg/2ml solution for injection vials | 1 vial PoM £35.09 (Hospital only)

Levofolinic acid

● DRUG ACTION Levofolinic acid is an isomer of folinic acid.

● INDICATIONS AND DOSE

Prevention of methotrexate-induced adverse effects
▸ BY INTRAMUSCULAR INJECTION, OR BY INTRAVENOUS INJECTION, OR BY INTRAVENOUS INFUSION
▸ Adult: Usual dose 7.5 mg every 6 hours for 10 doses, usually started 12–24 hours after beginning of methotrexate infusion

Suspected methotrexate overdosage
▸ BY INTRAVENOUS INFUSION, OR BY INTRAVENOUS INJECTION
▸ Adult: Initial dose at least 50% of the dose of methotrexate, intravenous infusion to be administered at a maximum rate of 160 mg/minute, consult poisons information centres for advice on continuing management

Adjunct to fluorouracil in colorectal cancer
▸ BY SLOW INTRAVENOUS INJECTION
▸ Adult: (consult product literature)

● CONTRA-INDICATIONS Intrathecal injection
● CAUTIONS Avoid simultaneous administration of methotrexate · **not** indicated for pernicious anaemia or other megaloblastic anaemias caused by vitamin B_{12} deficiency
● INTERACTIONS → Appendix 1 (folates).
● SIDE-EFFECTS
▸ Rare Agitation (after high doses) · depression (after high doses) · insomnia (after high doses) · pyrexia (after parenteral use)
● PREGNANCY Not known to be harmful; benefit outweighs risk.
● BREAST FEEDING Presence in milk unknown but benefit outweighs risk.

● MEDICINAL FORMS
There can be variation in the licensing of different medicines containing the same drug.
Solution for injection
▸ Isovorin (Pfizer Ltd)
 Levofolinic acid (as Calcium levofolinate) 10 mg per 1 ml Isovorin 175mg/17.5ml solution for injection vials | 1 vial PoM £81.33 (Hospital only)
 Isovorin 25mg/2.5ml solution for injection vials | 1 vial PoM £11.62 (Hospital only)

2.1a Hyperuricaemia associated with cytotoxic drugs

Drugs used for Hyperuricaemia associated with cytotoxic drugs not listed below Allopurinol, p. 968

DETOXIFYING DRUGS > URATE OXIDASES

Rasburicase

● INDICATIONS AND DOSE

Prophylaxis and treatment of acute hyperuricaemia, before and during initiation of chemotherapy, in patients with haematological malignancy and high tumour burden at risk of rapid lysis
▸ BY INTRAVENOUS INFUSION
▸ Adult: 200 micrograms/kg once daily for up to 7 days according to plasma-uric acid concentration

● CONTRA-INDICATIONS G6PD deficiency
● CAUTIONS Atopic allergies

- SIDE-EFFECTS
- ▶ **Common or very common** Fever
- ▶ **Uncommon** Anaphylaxis · bronchospasm · diarrhoea · haemolytic anaemia · headache · hypersensitivity reactions · methaemoglobinaemia · nausea · rash · vomiting

- PREGNANCY Manufacturer advises avoid—no information available.

- BREAST FEEDING Manufacturer advises avoid—no information available.

- MONITORING REQUIREMENTS Monitor closely for hypersensitivity.

- EFFECT ON LABORATORY TESTS May interfere with test for uric acid—consult product literature.

- DIRECTIONS FOR ADMINISTRATION For *intravenous infusion* (*Fasturtec*®), give intermittently in Sodium chloride 0.9%; reconstitute with solvent provided; gently swirl vial without shaking to dissolve; dilute requisite dose to 50 mL with infusion fluid and give over 30 minutes.

- MEDICINAL FORMS
  There can be variation in the licensing of different medicines containing the same drug.

  Powder and solvent for solution for infusion
  ▶ Fasturtec (Sanofi)
    Rasburicase 1.5 mg Fasturtec 1.5mg powder and solvent for solution for infusion vials | 3 vial [PoM] £208.39 (Hospital only)
    Rasburicase 7.5 mg Fasturtec 7.5mg powder and solvent for solution for infusion vials | 1 vial [PoM] £347.32 (Hospital only)

3 Hormone responsive malignancy

Breast cancer
1.6.2016

Description of condition

Breast cancer is the most common form of malignancy in women. The causes of breast cancer are complex and there are several risk factors. Established risk factors include age, early onset of menstruation, late menopause, greater age at first completed pregnancy, and a family history. The use of oral contraceptives and postmenopausal HRT are also associated with a small excess risk.

Non-invasive breast cancer, also known as ductal carcinoma *in situ*, is when the cancer remains localised in the ducts. However, in most cases, the cancer is invasive at the time of diagnosis, which means that malignant cells are liable to spread beyond the immediate area of the tumour. Invasive breast cancer, where malignant cells spread beyond the ducts, can be defined as early breast cancer (operable, primary, stage I/II), locally advanced disease (inoperable local, stage III) and advanced disease (metastatic, stage IV).

Aims of treatment

Reducing mortality, increasing progression-free and disease-free survival and improving quality of life are the main aims of the available treatments for breast cancer and are dependant on the stage of the disease.

Surgery and radiotherapy aim to remove the tumour mass, while adjuvant drug therapy aims to reduce the risk of recurrence and the risk of developing invasive disease. Advanced breast cancer is not curable and treatment aims to achieve remission, to prolong the disease free survival, to relieve symptoms and improve quality of life.

Treatment

The course of the disease and the therapeutic approach vary depending on the characteristics of the cancer; factors such as patient age and menopausal status, tumour size and

grade, involvement of axillary lymph nodes or skin, and presence of hormone receptors within the tumour may inform the extent and aggressiveness of the disease. The management of patients with breast cancer involves surgery, radiotherapy, drug therapy, or a combination of these.

Early and locally advanced breast cancer

EvGr For operable breast cancer, primary treatment is surgical using breast-conserving surgery or mastectomy, followed by adjuvant therapy to eradicate the micro-metastases that cause relapses. Radiotherapy is recommended after breast conserving surgery, as it reduces local recurrence rates. It is also used after mastectomy if there is a high risk of recurrence. Ⓐ

EvGr Drug therapy can be used after surgery (adjuvant therapy) or may be offered before surgery (neoadjuvant therapy) to achieve local tumour downsizing in order to make breast-conserving surgery possible. The choice of adjuvant therapy is determined by the safety and efficacy of the drugs, the oestrogen-receptor status, and the human epidermal growth factor 2 (HER2) status of the primary tumour. Ⓐ

EvGr Adjuvant chemotherapy or radiotherapy should be considered for all patients, irrespective of age, and it should be started as soon as clinically possible within 31 days of surgery. Ⓐ

EvGr A high-dose anthracycline-based chemotherapy regimen is usually preferred to a low-dose anthracycline-based regimen or to a non-anthracycline-based regimen. Choice of chemotherapy regimen is usually guided by local policy, Clinical Cancer Networks, and funding arrangements. Ⓐ

EvGr Adjuvant anthracycline-taxane combination chemotherapy should be considered in patients where the additional benefit outweighs risk. For patients with lymph node-positive breast cancer, docetaxel p. 816 can be added as part of an adjuvant chemotherapy regimen; paclitaxel p. 817 is not recommended. Ⓐ

EvGr Following surgery, tamoxifen p. 837, alone or in combination with chemotherapy, can be given to premenopausal women with oestrogen-receptor-positive early invasive breast cancer. If chemotherapy has not been selected, tamoxifen can be used in combination with ovarian ablation or suppression. Tamoxifen is not recommended for non-invasive (ductal carcinoma *in situ*) early breast cancer. Premenopausal women with oestrogen-receptor-positive breast cancer who decline chemotherapy may benefit from treatment with goserelin p. 666 or ovarian ablation. Ⓐ

EvGr For postmenopausal women with oestrogen-receptor-positive early invasive breast cancer, not considered to be low risk, an aromatase inhibitor, such as anastrozole p. 838 or letrozole p. 839, is first-line therapy. Tamoxifen is an alternative if an aromatase inhibitor is not tolerated or is contra-indicated. An aromatase inhibitor should be given as initial adjuvant therapy for 5 years, or by switching to an aromatase inhibitor after 2–3 years of tamoxifen for a total of 5 years. Postmenopausal women who have already received tamoxifen for 5 years may be considered for extended therapy (5 years) with letrozole. Ⓐ

EvGr Adjuvant trastuzumab p. 785 is recommended as an option in patients with HER2 positive breast cancer following surgery, chemotherapy (neoadjuvant or adjuvant) and radiotherapy. Trastuzumab should not be given concurrently with anthracycline-containing regimens (because of the risk of congestive heart failure) but it may be given either concurrently with taxane-based regimens or sequentially. Ⓐ

Advanced breast cancer

Treatment of advanced breast cancer depends on the patient's drug history, disease severity, and oestrogen receptor and HER2 status.

[EvGr] For the majority of patients with oestrogen-receptor-positive advanced breast cancer, endocrine therapy is first-line treatment. Aromatase inhibitors, such as anastrozole, letrozole and exemestane p. 839, may be offered to patients with no previous history of endocrine treatment or in those previously treated with tamoxifen. [A]

[EvGr] Tamoxifen should be considered as first-line treatment for pre- and perimenopausal women with oestrogen-receptor-positive breast cancer not previously treated with tamoxifen. Ovarian suppression is used in pre- and perimenopausal women who have had disease progression despite treatment with tamoxifen. [A]

[EvGr] In patients with advanced breast cancer that is imminently life-threatening or with visceral organ involvement, which requires early relief of symptoms, an anthracycline-based chemotherapy regimen is the preferred treatment. If anthracyclines are not suitable, the alternative is docetaxel monotherapy as first-line treatment, vinorelbine p. 821 or capecitabine p. 801 as second-line treatment or, for third-line treatment, whichever of the two drugs was not used second line. Gemcitabine p. 805 in combination with paclitaxel is recommended for the treatment of metastatic breast cancer only when docetaxel monotherapy or docetaxel with capecitabine are also considered appropriate. [A]

[EvGr] Trastuzumab is recommended for the treatment of HER2-positive advanced breast cancer. It is used in combination with paclitaxel in those who have not received chemotherapy for metastatic breast cancer and as monotherapy for patients who have received at least two chemotherapy regimens for metastatic breast cancer (see trastuzumab *National funding/access decisions*). [A]

Lapatinib p. 858 in combination with an aromatase inhibitor, fulvestrant p. 837, trastuzumab emtansine p. 786, and toremifene p. 838 are all licensed for use in patients with metastatic breast cancer, however their use is not recommended (see drug monographs for *Indications* and *National funding/access decisions*).

The gonadorelin analogue, goserelin is licensed for advanced breast cancer in pre- and perimenopausal women suitable for hormone manipulation. Some progestogen preparations, such as medroxyprogesterone acetate p. 733, norethisterone p. 691, megestrol acetate p. 836 are also licensed for the treatment of breast cancer (see drug monographs).

[EvGr] The use of bisphosphonates in patients with metastatic breast cancer may reduce pain and prevent skeletal complications of bone metastases. [A]

Familial breast cancer

Chemoprevention may be an option for patients who have been identified as having a high or moderate risk of developing breast cancer. The decision whether to consider or offer either tamoxifen p. 837 or raloxifene hydrochloride p. 680 [unlicensed indications] for 5 years is dependent on menopausal status and past history or risk of developing thromboembolic disease or endometrial cancer.

[EvGr] Tamoxifen [unlicensed indication] is recommended for pre- and postmenopausal women with or without uterus. Raloxifene hydrochloride [unlicensed indication] is recommended only for postmenopausal women with a uterus. Neither, tamoxifen nor raloxifene should be given to patients at high risk of developing breast cancer who have had a bilateral mastectomy. [A]

Breast cancer in men

Breast cancer in men is rare. Although, not fully understood, risk factors may be associated with sex hormone metabolism, including those acquired through liver disease or testicular trauma, environmental risk factors such as industrial exposure to heat, and genetic predisposition. Treatment is similar to that for women involving surgery, radiotherapy, drug therapy, or a combination of these.

Useful Resources

Early and locally advanced breast cancer: Diagnosis and treatment. National Institute for Health and Care Excellence. Clinical guideline 80. February 2009 (updated July 2014). www.nice.org.uk/guidance/cg80

Advanced breast cancer (update): Diagnosis and treatment. National Institute for Health and Care Excellence. Clinical guideline 81. July 2014. www.nice.org.uk/guidance/cg81

Treatment of primary breast cancer. Scottish Intercollegiate Guidelines Network. Clinical guideline 134. September 2013. www.sign.ac.uk/guidelines/fulltext/134/index.html

Prostate Cancer

31.5.2016

Description of condition

Prostate cancer is the most common form of cancer affecting men. The main risk factors are age (most cases being diagnosed in men over 65 years of age), ethnicity (more common in black African-Caribbean men), and a familial component. Prostate cancer is usually slow-growing and asymptomatic at diagnosis, however, the presenting symptoms of advanced disease are usually urinary outflow obstruction, or, pelvic or back pain due to bone metastases. Treatment decisions are guided by baseline prostate specific antigen (PSA) levels, tumour grade (Gleason score), the stage of the tumour, the patient's life expectancy (based on age and comorbid conditions), treatment morbidity, and patient preference.

Aims of treatment

In early or locally advanced prostate cancer, radical treatment aims to eliminate the malignancy. In metastatic disease, drug therapy is aimed at prolonging survival and reducing symptoms.

Drug treatment

Treatment options for patients with prostate cancer include active monitoring, radical prostatectomy, external beam radiotherapy, and brachytherapy. Hormone therapy (androgen deprivation or anti-androgens) is the primary treatment for metastatic prostate cancer, but is also increasingly being used for patients with locally advanced, non-metastatic disease.

In patients with localised prostate cancer, the choice of treatment is guided by whether the disease is considered low, intermediate, or high risk according to the Gleason score, the serum PSA level, and the tumour stage.

Localised or locally advanced prostate cancer

[EvGr] In patients with **low-risk localised prostate cancer**, and those at **intermediate risk** who decline radical treatments (prostatectomy or radiotherapy), active monitoring is a suitable option. This involves close monitoring to avoid unnecessary treatment until disease progression occurs (or until the patient requests treatment). [A]

[EvGr] In patients with **intermediate-risk** or **high-risk localised prostate cancer** (when there is a realistic prospect of long-term disease control) and in those with **locally advanced disease**, radical prostatectomy or radical radiotherapy should be offered. Other treatment options include a combination of radical radiotherapy and androgen deprivation therapy, consisting of 6 months of androgen deprivation therapy before, during or after prostate radiotherapy. Pelvic radiotherapy should be considered in those with locally advanced prostate cancer who have a higher than 15% risk of pelvic lymph node involvement and are to receive neoadjuvant hormonal therapy. [A]

EvGr Androgen deprivation therapy involves the use of a luteinising hormone-releasing hormone (LHRH) agonist (buserelin p. 665, goserelin p. 666, leuprorelin acetate p. 667, or triptorelin p. 669), or bilateral orchidectomy, which removes the supply of endogenous hormone. Androgen deprivation therapy may be continued for up to 3 years in patients with high-risk localised prostate cancer. ⟨A⟩

EvGr Patients should be informed about the side-effects of treatment, particularly urinary and sexual dysfunction, loss of fertility, radiation-induced enteropathy, and hot flushes. Although there is limited evidence, intermittent therapy may be considered for patients who are having long-term androgen deprivation therapy, to reduce drug toxicity. Tumour flare, due to an initial surge in testosterone concentrations, has been reported in the initial stages of treatment with androgen deprivation therapy and prophylactic anti-androgen therapy (such as cyproterone acetate p. 696) may be added. ⟨A⟩

EvGr Medroxyprogesterone acetate p. 733 [unlicensed indication] can be used, initially for up to 10 weeks, to manage troublesome hot flushes caused by long-term androgen suppression; cyproterone acetate is an alternative if medroxyprogesterone acetate is not effective or not tolerated. ⟨A⟩

EvGr Patients who experience a reduction in libido and loss of sexual function should have access to specialist erectile dysfunction services and be considered for treatment with a phosphodiesterase type-5 inhibitor. ⟨A⟩

EvGr Osteoporosis and fatigue may also be a problem with androgen deprivation therapy. A bisphosphonate can be offered to men who have osteoporosis; denosumab p. 662 is an alternative if bisphosphonates are not appropriate. Gynaecomastia can occur with long-term (longer than 6 months) bicalutamide p. 832 treatment. Prophylactic radiotherapy (within the first month of treatment), or weekly tamoxifen p. 837 [unlicensed indication], if radiotherapy is unsuccessful, can be considered. ⟨A⟩

Metastatic prostate cancer

EvGr Bilateral orchidectomy should be offered to all patients with **metastatic prostate cancer** as an alternative to continuous LHRH agonist treatment. Anti-androgen monotherapy with bicalutamide [unlicensed indication] can be offered to those who are willing to accept the adverse impact on overall survival and gynaecomastia in the hope of retaining sexual function. However, if satisfactory sexual function is not maintained, stop bicalutamide and start androgen deprivation therapy. ⟨A⟩

EvGr Abiraterone acetate below (in combination with prednisone p. 615 or prednisolone p. 614) and enzalutamide p. 832 are both recommended as options for the treatment of castration-resistant metastatic prostate cancer in patients whose disease has progressed during or after treatment with a docetaxel p. 816-containing chemotherapy regimen. ⟨A⟩

EvGr In patients who develop **hormone-relapsed metastatic tumour**, chemotherapy with docetaxel can be used. It is recommended to stop the treatment with docetaxel after 10 cycles, or if severe adverse events occurred, or if there is evidence of disease progression. ⟨A⟩

EvGr Abiraterone acetate (in combination with prednisone or prednisolone) is also recommended as an option for treating **metastatic hormone-relapsed prostate cancer** in patients who have no or mild symptoms after androgen deprivation therapy has failed, and before chemotherapy is indicated. ⟨A⟩

EvGr In patients with hormone-relapsed prostate cancer, a corticosteroid, such as dexamethasone p. 610, can be offered as third line therapy, after androgen deprivation therapy and anti-androgen therapy. ⟨A⟩

Useful Resources

Prostate cancer: diagnosis and treatment. National Institute for Health and Care Excellence. Clinical guideline 175. January 2014.
www.nice.org.uk/guidance/cg175

> **Drugs used for Hormone responsive malignancy not listed below** Ethinylestradiol, p. 685

ANTINEOPLASTIC DRUGS > ANTI-ANDROGENS

Abiraterone acetate
31.5.2016

● **INDICATIONS AND DOSE**

Metastatic castration-resistant prostate cancer in patients whose disease has progressed during or after treatment with a docetaxel-containing chemotherapy regimen (in combination with prednisone or prednisolone) | Metastatic castration-resistant prostate cancer in patients who are asymptomatic or mildly symptomatic after failure of androgen deprivation therapy in whom chemotherapy is not yet clinically indicated (in combination with prednisone or prednisolone)

▶ BY MOUTH
▶ Adult: 1 g once daily, for dose of concurrent prednisone or prednisolone—consult product literature

● CAUTIONS Diabetes (increased risk of hyperglycaemia—monitor blood sugar frequently) · history of cardiovascular disease

CAUTIONS, FURTHER INFORMATION
▶ Cardiovascular disease Correct hypertension and hypokalaemia before treatment (if significant risk of congestive heart failure, such as history of cardiac failure, uncontrolled hypertension or cardiac events, consult product literature for management and increased monitoring).

● INTERACTIONS → Appendix 1 (abiraterone).
Caution with concurrent chemotherapy—safety and efficacy not established.
Caution with concomitant use of drugs known to be associated with myopathy or rhabdomyolysis.

● SIDE-EFFECTS
▶ **Common or very common** Angina · arrhythmia · atrial fibrillation · diarrhoea · dyspepsia · fractures · haematuria · heart failure · hepatotoxicity · hypertension · hypertriglyceridaemia · hypokalaemia · peripheral oedema · rash · sepsis · tachycardia · urinary tract infection
▶ **Uncommon** Adrenal insufficiency · myopathy · rhabdomyolysis
▶ **Rare** Allergic alveolitis

● CONCEPTION AND CONTRACEPTION Men should use condoms if their partner is pregnant, and use condoms in combination with another effective contraceptive method if their partner is of child-bearing potential—toxicity in *animal* studies.

● HEPATIC IMPAIRMENT Use with caution in moderate impairment and only if benefit clearly outweighs risk. Avoid in severe impairment.

● RENAL IMPAIRMENT Use with caution in severe impairment—no information available.

● MONITORING REQUIREMENTS
▶ Monitor blood pressure, serum potassium concentration, and fluid balance before treatment, and at least monthly during treatment—consult product literature for management of hypertension, hypokalaemia and oedema.
▶ Monitor liver function before treatment, then every 2 weeks for the first 3 months of treatment, then monthly thereafter—interrupt treatment if serum alanine

Immune system and malignant disease

8

aminotransferase or aspartate aminotransferase greater than 5 times the upper limit (consult product literature for details of restarting treatment at a lower dose) and discontinue permanently if 20 times the upper limit.

● NATIONAL FUNDING/ACCESS DECISIONS

NICE technology appraisals (TAs)

▸ Abiraterone for castration-resistant metastatic prostate cancer previously treated with a docetaxel-containing regimen (June 2012) NICE TA259

Abiraterone in combination with prednisone or prednisolone is recommended as an option for the treatment of castration-resistant metastatic prostate cancer only if:

- their disease has progressed on or after one docetaxel-containing chemotherapy regimen, **and**
- the manufacturer provides abiraterone with the discount agreed in the patient access scheme.

Patients currently receiving abiraterone in combination with prednisone or prednisolone whose disease does not meet the first criteria should be able to continue therapy until they and their clinician consider it appropriate to stop.

www.nice.org.uk/TA259

▸ Abiraterone for treating metastatic hormone-relapsed prostate cancer before chemotherapy is indicated (April 2016) NICE TA387

Abiraterone, in combination with prednisone or prednisolone, is recommended as an option for treating metastatic hormone-relapsed prostate cancer in patients who have mild or no symptoms after androgen deprivation therapy has failed, and before chemotherapy is indicated. In addition, the manufacturer is required to rebate the cost of abiraterone from the 11th month until the end of treatment for patients who remain on treatment for more than 10 months.

www.nice.org.uk/TA387

Scottish Medicines Consortium (SMC) Decisions

The *Scottish Medicines Consortium* has advised (July 2012) that abiraterone (*Zytiga®*), in combination with prednisone or prednisolone, is accepted for restricted use within NHS Scotland for the treatment of metastatic castration-resistant prostate cancer in patients whose disease has progressed during or after treatment with docetaxel-containing chemotherapy regimen, and have received only one prior chemotherapy regimen.

● MEDICINAL FORMS
There can be variation in the licensing of different medicines containing the same drug.

Tablet

CAUTIONARY AND ADVISORY LABELS 23

▸ Zytiga (Janssen-Cilag Ltd) ▼
Abiraterone acetate 250 mg Zytiga 250mg tablets | 120 tablet [PoM] £2,930.00

Bicalutamide

● INDICATIONS AND DOSE

Locally advanced prostate cancer at high risk of disease progression either alone or as adjuvant treatment to prostatectomy or radiotherapy | Locally advanced, non-metastatic prostate cancer when surgical castration or other medical intervention inappropriate

▸ BY MOUTH
▸ Adult: 150 mg once daily

Advanced prostate cancer, in combination with gonadorelin analogue or surgical castration

▸ BY MOUTH
▸ Adult: 50 mg once daily, to be started at the same time as surgical castration or at least 3 days before gonadorelin therapy

● CAUTIONS Risk of photosensitivity—avoid excessive exposure to UV light and sunlight

● INTERACTIONS → Appendix 1 (bicalutamide).

● SIDE-EFFECTS

▸ **Common or very common** Abdominal pain · alopecia · anaemia · asthenia · breast tenderness · chest pain · cholestasis · constipation · decreased appetite · decreased libido · depression · dizziness · dry skin · dyspepsia · flatulence · gynaecomastia · haematuria · hepatotoxicity · hirsutism · hot flushes · impotence · jaundice · nausea · oedema · pruritus · rash · somnolence · weight gain

▸ **Uncommon** Angioedema · hypersensitivity reactions · interstitial lung disease · urticaria

▸ **Rare** Hepatic failure · photosensitivity reactions

● HEPATIC IMPAIRMENT Increased accumulation possible in moderate to severe impairment—manufacturer advises caution.

● MONITORING REQUIREMENTS Consider periodic liver function tests.

● PATIENT AND CARER ADVICE
Risk of photosensitivity Patients should be advised to consider the use of sunscreen.

● MEDICINAL FORMS
There can be variation in the licensing of different medicines containing the same drug. Forms available from special-order manufacturers include: oral suspension

Tablet

▸ Bicalutamide (Non-proprietary)
Bicalutamide 50 mg Bicalutamide 50mg tablets | 28 tablet [PoM] £128.00 DT price = £1.57
Bicalutamide 150 mg Bicalutamide 150mg tablets | 28 tablet [PoM] £240.00 DT price = £3.98

▸ Casodex (AstraZeneca UK Ltd)
Bicalutamide 50 mg Casodex 50mg tablets | 28 tablet [PoM] £119.79 DT price = £1.57
Bicalutamide 150 mg Casodex 150mg tablets | 28 tablet [PoM] £240.00 DT price = £3.98

Enzalutamide

27.4.2016

● INDICATIONS AND DOSE

Metastatic castration-resistant prostate cancer in patients whose disease has progressed during or after docetaxel therapy

▸ BY MOUTH
▸ Adult: 160 mg once daily, for dose adjustments due to side-effects, consult product literature

● CAUTIONS Alcoholism · bradycardia · brain injury · brain metastases · brain tumours · history of QT-interval prolongation · history or risk of seizure · recent cardiovascular disease · risk factors for QT-interval prolongation · stroke · uncontrolled hypertension

● INTERACTIONS → Appendix 1 (enzalutamide).
Caution with concurrent use of medication which may lower seizure threshold.
Caution with concurrent chemotherapy—safety and efficacy not established.
Caution with concomitant use of drugs that prolong QT interval.

● SIDE-EFFECTS

▸ **Common or very common** Anxiety · cognitive disorder · dry skin · falls · fractures · headache · hot flush · hypertension · memory impairment · neutropenia · pruritus · visual hallucinations

▸ **Uncommon** Leucopenia · seizure

● CONCEPTION AND CONTRACEPTION Men should use condoms during treatment and for 3 months after stopping treatment if their partner is pregnant, and use condoms in combination with another effective

contraceptive method if their partner is of child-bearing potential—toxicity in *animal* studies.
- **HEPATIC IMPAIRMENT** Manufacturer advises caution in moderate impairment. Avoid in severe impairment.
- **RENAL IMPAIRMENT** Caution in severe impairment—no information available.
- **NATIONAL FUNDING/ACCESS DECISIONS**

NICE technology appraisals (TAs)
▸ **Enzalutamide for treating metastatic hormone-relapsed prostate cancer before chemotherapy is indicated (January 2016)** NICE TA377
Enzalutamide is recommended as an option for treating metastatic hormone-relapsed prostate cancer in patients who have mild or no symptoms after androgen deprivation therapy has failed, and before chemotherapy is indicated, **and** only if the manufacturer provides enzalutamide with the discount agreed in the patient access scheme.
www.nice.org.uk/TA377
▸ **Enzalutamide for metastatic hormone relapsed prostate cancer previously treated with a docetaxel containing regimen (July 2014)** NICE TA316
Enzalutamide is recommended, within its marketing authorisation, as an option for treating metastatic hormone-relapsed prostate cancer in adults only if, their disease has progressed during or after docetaxel-containing chemotherapy, **and** the manufacturer provides enzalutamide with the discount agreed in the patient access scheme. This guidance does not cover the use of enzalutamide for metastatic hormone-relapsed prostate cancer previously treated with abiraterone.
www.nice.org.uk/TA316

- **MEDICINAL FORMS** There can be variation in the licensing of different medicines containing the same drug.

Capsule
CAUTIONARY AND ADVISORY LABELS 25
▸ Xtandi (Astellas Pharma Ltd) ▼
  Enzalutamide 40 mg Xtandi 40mg capsules | 112 capsule PoM
  £2,734.67

Flutamide

- **INDICATIONS AND DOSE**

Advanced prostate cancer | Metastatic prostate cancer refractory to gonadorelin analogue therapy (monotherapy)
▸ BY MOUTH
▸ Adult: 250 mg 3 times a day

- **CAUTIONS** Avoid excessive alcohol consumption · avoid in Acute porphyrias p. 918 · cardiac disease (oedema reported)
- **INTERACTIONS** → Appendix 1 (flutamide).
- **SIDE-EFFECTS** Blurred vision · chest pain · cholestatic jaundice · decreased libido · diarrhoea · dizziness · galactorrhoea · gastric pain · gynaecomastia · haemolytic anaemia · headache · hepatic encephalopathy · hepatic injury (occasionally causing fatality) · hepatic necrosis · hypertension · increased appetite · insomnia · lymphoedema · nausea · oedema · pruritus · rash · reduced sperm count · systemic lupus erythematosus-like syndrome · thirst · tiredness · transaminase abnormalities · vomiting
- **HEPATIC IMPAIRMENT** Use with caution (hepatotoxic).
- **MONITORING REQUIREMENTS** Liver function tests, monthly for first 4 months, periodically thereafter and at the first sign or symptom of liver disorder (e.g. pruritus, dark urine, persistent anorexia, jaundice, abdominal pain, unexplained influenza-like symptoms).

- **MEDICINAL FORMS** There can be variation in the licensing of different medicines containing the same drug.

Tablet
▸ Flutamide (Non-proprietary)
  Flutamide 250 mg Flutamide 250mg tablets | 84 tablet PoM
  £106.25 DT price = £105.18

OESTROGENS

Diethylstilbestrol

(Stilboestrol)

- **INDICATIONS AND DOSE**

Breast cancer in postmenopausal women
▸ BY MOUTH
▸ Adult: 10–20 mg daily
Prostate cancer
▸ BY MOUTH
▸ Adult: 1–3 mg daily

- **CAUTIONS** Cardiovascular disease
- **SIDE-EFFECTS** Arterial thrombosis · bone pain (in breast cancer) · feminising effects in men · fluid retention · gynaecomastia · hypercalcaemia (in breast cancer) · impotence · jaundice · nausea · sodium retention with oedema · thromboembolism · venous thrombosis · withdrawal bleeding
- **PREGNANCY** In first trimester, high doses associated with vaginal carcinoma, urogenital abnormalities, and reduced fertility in female offspring. Increased risk of hypospadias in male offspring.
- **HEPATIC IMPAIRMENT** Avoid. Avoid in active liver disease including disorders of hepatic excretion (e.g. Dubin-Johnson or Rotor syndromes), infective hepatitis (until liver function returns to normal), and liver tumours.

- **MEDICINAL FORMS** There can be variation in the licensing of different medicines containing the same drug.

Tablet
▸ Diethylstilbestrol (Non-proprietary)
  Diethylstilbestrol 1 mg Diethylstilbestrol 1mg tablets | 28 tablet PoM £123.00 DT price = £118.13
  Diethylstilbestrol 5 mg Diethylstilbestrol 5mg tablets | 28 tablet PoM £185.00–£208.00 DT price = £208.00

PITUITARY AND HYPOTHALAMIC HORMONES AND ANALOGUES ⟩ ANTI-GONADOTROPHIN-RELEASING HORMONES

Degarelix

- **INDICATIONS AND DOSE**

Advanced hormone-dependent prostate cancer
▸ BY SUBCUTANEOUS INJECTION
▸ Adult: Initially 240 mg, to be administered as 2 injections of 120 mg, then 80 mg every 28 days, dose to be administered into the abdominal region

- **CAUTIONS** Diabetes · susceptibility to QT-interval prolongation
- **INTERACTIONS** Avoid concomitant use of drugs that prolong QT interval.
- **SIDE-EFFECTS**
▸ **Common or very common** Asthenia · dizziness · drowsiness · headache · hot flushes · influenza-like symptoms · injection-site reactions · insomnia · nausea · night sweats · sweating · weight gain
▸ **Uncommon** Abdominal discomfort · alopecia · anaemia · anorexia · anxiety · atrio-ventricular block · constipation ·

8

Immune system and malignant disease

depression · diarrhoea · dry mouth · fainting · gynaecomastia · hypersensitivity reactions · hypertension · micturition urgency · musculoskeletal pain · oedema · pelvic pain · prostatitis · QT-interval prolongation · rash · renal impairment · sexual dysfunction · testicular pain · tinnitus · urticaria · vomiting

● HEPATIC IMPAIRMENT Manufacturer advises caution in severe impairment—no information available.

● RENAL IMPAIRMENT Manufacturer advises caution in severe impairment—no information available.

● MONITORING REQUIREMENTS Monitor bone density.

● MEDICINAL FORMS
There can be variation in the licensing of different medicines containing the same drug.

Powder and solvent for solution for injection
▶ Firmagon (Ferring Pharmaceuticals Ltd)
Degarelix (as Degarelix acetate) 80 mg Firmagon 80mg powder and solvent for solution for injection vials | 1 vial [PoM] £129.37
Degarelix (as Degarelix acetate) 120 mg Firmagon 120mg powder and solvent for solution for injection vials | 2 vial [PoM] £260.00

PITUITARY AND HYPOTHALAMIC HORMONES AND ANALOGUES › SOMATOSTATIN ANALOGUES

Somatostatin analogues, malignant disease

Overview

Lanreotide below, octreotide p. 835 and pasireotide p. 836 are analogues of the hypothalamic release-inhibiting hormone somatostatin. Lanreotide and octreotide are indicated for the relief of symptoms associated with neuroendocrine (particularly carcinoid) tumours and acromegaly. Additionally, lanreotide is licensed for the treatment of thyroid tumours and octreotide is also licensed for the prevention of complications following pancreatic surgery. Lanreotide (*Somatuline Autogel ®*) is also licensed for the treatment of unresectable locally advanced or metastatic gastroenteropancreatic neuroendocrine tumours of midgut, pancreatic or unknown origin where hindgut sites of origin have been excluded. Octreotide long-acting depot injection is licensed for treatment of advanced neuroendocrine tumours of the midgut, or treatment where primary origin is not known but non-midgut sites of origin have been excluded. Octreotide may also be valuable in reducing vomiting in palliative care and in stopping variceal bleeding [unlicensed indication]—see also vasopressin p. 605 and terlipressin acetate p. 81. Pasireotide is licensed for the treatment of Cushing's disease when surgery has failed or is inappropriate.

Somatostatin analogues

● CAUTIONS Diabetes mellitus (antidiabetic requirements may be reduced) · insulinoma (increased depth and duration of hypoglycaemia may occur—observe patients and monitor blood glucose levels when initiating treatment and changing doses) · may cause growth hormone-secreting pituitary tumour expansion during treatment (causing serious complications)

● SIDE-EFFECTS
▶ **Rare** Pancreatitis (shortly after administration)
▶ **Frequency not known** Abdominal pain · anorexia · bloating · diarrhoea · flatulence · gallstones (after long-term treatment) · gastro-intestinal disturbances · hyperglycaemia (with chronic administration) · hypoglycaemia · impaired postprandial glucose tolerance (with chronic administration) · irritation at the injection

site · nausea · pain at the injection site · steatorrhoea · vomiting

● MONITORING REQUIREMENTS
▶ Monitor for signs of tumour expansion (e.g. visual field defects).
▶ Ultrasound examination of the gallbladder is recommended before treatment and at intervals of 6–12 months during treatment.

● DIRECTIONS FOR ADMINISTRATION Injection sites should be rotated.

Lanreotide

● INDICATIONS AND DOSE

SOMATULINE AUTOGEL®

Acromegaly (if somatostatin analogue not given previously)
▶ BY DEEP SUBCUTANEOUS INJECTION
▶ Adult: Initially 60 mg every 28 days, adjusted according to response, (consult product literature), for patients treated previously with somatostatin analogue, consult product literature for initial dose, dose to be given in the gluteal region

Neuroendocrine (particularly carcinoid) tumours
▶ BY DEEP SUBCUTANEOUS INJECTION
▶ Adult: Initially 60–120 mg every 28 days, adjusted according to response, dose to be given in the gluteal region

Unresectable locally advanced or metastatic gastroenteropancreatic neuroendocrine tumours of midgut, pancreatic or unknown origin where hindgut sites of origin have been excluded
▶ BY DEEP SUBCUTANEOUS INJECTION
▶ Adult: 120 mg every 28 days

SOMATULINE LA®

Acromegaly and neuroendocrine (particularly carcinoid) tumours
▶ BY INTRAMUSCULAR INJECTION
▶ Adult: Initially 30 mg every 14 days, increased to 30 mg every 7–10 days, adjusted according to response

Thyroid tumours
▶ BY INTRAMUSCULAR INJECTION
▶ Adult: Initially 30 mg every 14 days, increased to 30 mg every 10 days, adjusted according to response

● CAUTIONS Cardiac disorders (including bradycardia) · patients with carcinoid tumours—exclude the presence of an obstructive intestinal tumour before treatment

● INTERACTIONS → Appendix 1 (lanreotide).

● SIDE-EFFECTS
▶ **Common or very common** Alopecia · biliary dilatation · bradycardia · constipation · dizziness · dyspepsia · headache · lethargy · malaise · musculoskeletal pain · myalgia · raised bilirubin
▶ **Uncommon** Hot flushes · insomnia
▶ **Rare** Hypothyroidism

● PREGNANCY Manufacturer advises use only if potential benefit outweighs risk.

● BREAST FEEDING Manufacturer advises caution—no information available.

● MONITORING REQUIREMENTS Monitor for hypothyroidism when clinically indicated.

● MEDICINAL FORMS
There can be variation in the licensing of different medicines containing the same drug.

Solution for injection

▸ Somatuline Autogel (Ipsen Ltd)

Lanreotide (as Lanreotide acetate) 120 mg per 1 ml Somatuline Autogel 60mg/0.5ml solution for injection pre-filled syringes with safety system | 1 pre-filled disposable injection [PoM] £551.00

Lanreotide (as Lanreotide acetate) 180 mg per 1 ml Somatuline Autogel 90mg/0.5ml solution for injection pre-filled syringes with safety system | 1 pre-filled disposable injection [PoM] £736.00

Lanreotide (as Lanreotide acetate) 240 mg per 1 ml Somatuline Autogel 120mg/0.5ml solution for injection pre-filled syringes with safety system | 1 pre-filled disposable injection [PoM] £937.00

Powder and solvent for suspension for injection

▸ Somatuline LA (Ipsen Ltd)

Lanreotide (as Lanreotide acetate) 30 mg Somatuline LA 30mg powder and solvent for suspension for injection vials | 1 vial [PoM] £323.00

📌 834

Octreotide

● INDICATIONS AND DOSE

Symptoms associated with carcinoid tumours with features of carcinoid syndrome, VIPomas, glucagonomas
▸ BY SUBCUTANEOUS INJECTION
▸ Adult: Initially 50 micrograms 1–2 times a day, adjusted according to response; increased to 200 micrograms 3 times a day, higher doses may be required exceptionally; maintenance doses are variable; in carcinoid tumours, discontinue after 1 week if no effect, if rapid response required, initial dose may be given by intravenous injection (with ECG monitoring and after dilution)

Acromegaly, short-term treatment before pituitary surgery or long-term treatment in those inadequately controlled by other treatment or until radiotherapy becomes fully effective
▸ BY SUBCUTANEOUS INJECTION
▸ Adult: 100–200 micrograms 3 times a day, discontinue if no improvement within 3 months

Prevention of complications following pancreatic surgery
▸ BY SUBCUTANEOUS INJECTION
▸ Adult: (consult product literature)

Test dose before use of depot preparation
▸ BY SUBCUTANEOUS INJECTION
▸ Adult: Test dose 50–100 micrograms for 1 dose, test dose should be given if subcutanous octreotide not previously given

Acromegaly | Neuroendocrine (particularly carcinoid) tumour adequately controlled by subcutaneous octreotide
▸ BY DEEP INTRAMUSCULAR INJECTION USING DEPOT INJECTION
▸ Adult: Initially 20 mg every 4 weeks for 3 months then adjusted according to response, increased if necessary up to 30 mg every 4 weeks, to be administered into the gluteal muscle, for *acromegaly*, start depot 1 day after the last dose of subcutaneous octreotide, for *neuroendocrine tumours*, continue subcutaneous octreotide for 2 weeks after first dose of depot octreotide

Advanced neuroendocrine tumours of the midgut, or tumours of unknown primary origin where non-midgut sites of origin have been excluded
▸ BY DEEP INTRAMUSCULAR INJECTION USING DEPOT INJECTION
▸ Adult: 30 mg every 4 weeks

Reduce intestinal secretions in palliative care | Reduce vomiting due to bowel obstruction in palliative care
▸ BY CONTINUOUS SUBCUTANEOUS INFUSION
▸ Adult: 0.25–0.5 mg/24 hours (max. per dose 0.75 mg/24 hours), occasionally doses higher than the maximum are sometimes required

● INTERACTIONS → Appendix 1 (octreotide).

● SIDE-EFFECTS Alopecia · arrhythmias · biliary colic (associated with abrupt withdrawal of subcutaneous octreotide) · bradycardia · dehydration · dizziness · dyspnoea · headache · hepatitis · pancreatitis (associated with abrupt withdrawal of subcutaneous octreotide) · rash

SIDE-EFFECTS, FURTHER INFORMATION
▸ Gastro-intestinal side-effects Administering non-depot injections of octreotide between meals and at bedtime may reduce gastro-intestinal side-effects.

● CONCEPTION AND CONTRACEPTION Effective contraception required during treatment.

● PREGNANCY Possible effect on fetal growth; manufacturer advises use only if potential benefit outweighs risk.

● BREAST FEEDING Manufacturer advises avoid—present in milk in *animal* studies.

● HEPATIC IMPAIRMENT Adjustment of maintenance dose of non-depot preparations may be necessary in patients with liver cirrhosis.

● MONITORING REQUIREMENTS
▸ Monitor thyroid function on long-term therapy.
▸ Monitor liver function.
▸ With intravenous use ECG monitoring required with intravenous administration.

● TREATMENT CESSATION Avoid abrupt withdrawal of short-acting subcutaneous octreotide (associated with biliary colic and pancreatitis).

● DIRECTIONS FOR ADMINISTRATION For *intravenous injection* or *intravenous infusion*, dilute with Sodium Chloride 0.9% to a concentration of 10–50%.

● MEDICINAL FORMS
There can be variation in the licensing of different medicines containing the same drug.

Solution for injection

▸ Octreotide (Non-proprietary)

Octreotide (as Octreotide acetate) 50 microgram per 1 ml Octreotide 50micrograms/1ml solution for injection pre-filled syringes | 5 pre-filled disposable injection [PoM] £15.85 Octreotide 50micrograms/1ml solution for injection vials | 5 vial [PoM] £14.87–£22.00 Octreotide 50micrograms/1ml solution for injection ampoules | 5 ampoule [PoM] £4.60–£18.60

Octreotide (as Octreotide acetate) 100 microgram per 1 ml Octreotide 100micrograms/1ml solution for injection ampoules | 5 ampoule [PoM] £7.24–£32.65 Octreotide 100micrograms/1ml solution for injection pre-filled syringes | 5 pre-filled disposable injection [PoM] £28.90 Octreotide 100micrograms/1ml solution for injection vials | 5 vial [PoM] £27.97–£32.65

Octreotide (as Octreotide acetate) 200 microgram per 1 ml Octreotide 1mg/5ml solution for injection vials | 1 vial [PoM] £65.00–£69.66

Octreotide (as Octreotide acetate) 500 microgram per 1 ml Octreotide 500micrograms/1ml solution for injection vials | 5 vial [PoM] £135.47–£158.25 Octreotide 500micrograms/1ml solution for injection pre-filled syringes | 5 pre-filled disposable injection [PoM] £135.47–£149.00 Octreotide 500micrograms/1ml solution for injection ampoules | 5 ampoule [PoM] £14.12–£169.35 DT price = £135.47

▸ Sandostatin (Novartis Pharmaceuticals UK Ltd)

Octreotide (as Octreotide acetate) 50 microgram per 1 ml Sandostatin 50micrograms/1ml solution for injection ampoules | 5 ampoule [PoM] £14.87

Octreotide (as Octreotide acetate) 100 microgram per 1 ml Sandostatin 100micrograms/1ml solution for injection ampoules | 5 ampoule [PoM] £27.97

Octreotide (as Octreotide acetate) 200 microgram per 1 ml Sandostatin 1mg/5ml solution for injection vials | 1 vial [PoM] £55.73

Octreotide (as Octreotide acetate) 500 microgram per 1 ml Sandostatin 500micrograms/1ml solution for injection ampoules | 5 ampoule [PoM] £135.47 DT price = £135.47

8

Immune system and malignant disease

Powder and solvent for suspension for injection

▶ Sandostatin LAR (Novartis Pharmaceuticals UK Ltd)

Octreotide (as Octreotide acetate) 10 mg Sandostatin LAR 10mg powder and solvent for suspension for injection vials | 1 vial [PoM] £549.71

Octreotide (as Octreotide acetate) 20 mg Sandostatin LAR 20mg powder and solvent for suspension for injection vials | 1 vial [PoM] £799.33

Octreotide (as Octreotide acetate) 30 mg Sandostatin LAR 30mg powder and solvent for suspension for injection vials | 1 vial [PoM] £998.41

F 834

Pasireotide

● **INDICATIONS AND DOSE**

Cushing's disease when surgery has failed or is inappropriate

▶ BY SUBCUTANEOUS INJECTION

▶ Adult: Initially 600 micrograms twice daily for 2 months, then increased if necessary to 900 micrograms twice daily, consider discontinuation if no response within 2 months, for dose adjustment due to side effects—consult product literature

● CAUTIONS Cardiac disorders (including bradycardia) · susceptibility to QT-interval prolongation (including electrolyte disturbances)

● INTERACTIONS → Appendix 1 (pasireotide). Caution with concomitant use of drugs that prolong QT interval.

● SIDE-EFFECTS Adrenal insufficiency · alopecia · anaemia · arthralgia · bradycardia · decreased appetite · fatigue · headache · hyperglycaemia · hypotension · myalgia · pruritus · QT-interval prolongation

● PREGNANCY Avoid—toxicity in *animal* studies.

● BREAST FEEDING Avoid—present in milk in *animal* studies.

● HEPATIC IMPAIRMENT Reduce initial dose to 300 micrograms twice daily (increased if necessary after 2 months to max. 600 micrograms twice daily) in moderate impairment. Avoid in severe impairment.

● MONITORING REQUIREMENTS

▶ Monitor liver function before treatment and after 1, 2, 4, 8, and 12 weeks of treatment.

▶ QT-interval prolongation Monitor ECG and electrolytes in patients susceptible to QT-prolongation before treatment, after one week, and periodically thereafter.

▶ Diabetes mellitus In diabetic patients, assess glycaemic status before treatment, weekly for the first 2–3 months of treatment, periodically thereafter, and 3 months after treatment is complete.

● MEDICINAL FORMS
There can be variation in the licensing of different medicines containing the same drug.

Solution for injection

▶ Signifor (Novartis Pharmaceuticals UK Ltd) ▼

Pasireotide (as Pasireotide diaspartate) 300 microgram per 1 ml Signifor 0.3mg/1ml solution for injection ampoules | 60 ampoule [PoM] £2,800.00

Pasireotide (as Pasireotide diaspartate) 600 microgram per 1 ml Signifor 0.6mg/1ml solution for injection ampoules | 60 ampoule [PoM] £3,240.00

Pasireotide (as Pasireotide diaspartate) 900 microgram per 1 ml Signifor 0.9mg/1ml solution for injection ampoules | 60 ampoule [PoM] £3,240.00

Powder and solvent for suspension for injection

▶ Signifor (Novartis Pharmaceuticals UK Ltd) ▼

Pasireotide (as Pasireotide pamoate) 20 mg Signifor 20mg powder and solvent for suspension for injection vials | 1 vial [PoM] £2,300.00

Pasireotide (as Pasireotide pamoate) 40 mg Signifor 40mg powder and solvent for suspension for injection vials | 1 vial [PoM] £2,300.00

Pasireotide (as Pasireotide pamoate) 60 mg Signifor 60mg powder and solvent for suspension for injection vials | 1 vial [PoM] £2,300.00

PROGESTOGENS

Megestrol acetate

● **INDICATIONS AND DOSE**

Treatment of breast cancer

▶ BY MOUTH

▶ Adult: 160 mg once daily

● CONTRA-INDICATIONS Acute porphyrias p. 918 · breast cancer (unless progestogens are being used in the management of this condition) · genital cancer (unless progestogens are being used in the management of this condition) · history during pregnancy of idiopathic jaundice · history during pregnancy of pemphigoid gestationis · history during pregnancy of severe pruritus · history of liver tumours · severe arterial disease · undiagnosed vaginal bleeding

● CAUTIONS Asthma · cardiac dysfunction · conditions that may worsen with fluid retention · diabetes (progestogens can decrease glucose tolerance—monitor patient closely) · epilepsy · history of depression · hypertension · migraine · susceptibility to thromboembolism (particular caution with high dose)

● INTERACTIONS → Appendix 1 (progestogens).

● SIDE-EFFECTS Acne · adrenal insufficiency · alopecia · anaphylactoid reactions · asthenia · bloating · breast tenderness · carpal tunnel syndrome · change in libido · constipation · Cushing's syndrome · depression · diarrhoea · dizziness · drowsiness · fluid retention · headache · hirsutism · indigestion · insomnia · jaundice · loss of vision during treatment (discontinue treatment if papilloedema or retinal vascular lesions) · menstrual disturbances · nausea · premenstrual-like syndrome · pruritus · rash · skin reactions · tumour flare (with or without hypercalcaemia) · urinary frequency · urticaria · vomiting · weight change · weight gain

● PREGNANCY Avoid. Reversible feminisation of male fetuses reported in *animal* studies. Risk of hypospadias in male fetuses and masculinisation of female fetuses.

● BREAST FEEDING Discontinue breast-feeding.

● HEPATIC IMPAIRMENT Manufacturer advises caution in severe impairment.

● MEDICINAL FORMS
There can be variation in the licensing of different medicines containing the same drug. Forms available from special-order manufacturers include: tablet, capsule, oral suspension

Tablet

▶ Megestrol acetate (Non-proprietary)

Megestrol acetate 40 mg Megestrol 40mg tablets | 100 tablet no price available

▶ Megace (Swedish Orphan Biovitrum Ltd)

Megestrol acetate 160 mg Megace 160mg tablets | 30 tablet [PoM] £19.52 DT price = £19.52

Oral suspension

▶ Megestrol acetate (Non-proprietary)

Megestrol acetate 40 mg per 1 ml Megestrol 200mg/5ml oral suspension | 240 ml [PoM] no price available | 480 ml [PoM] no price available

3.1　Hormone responsive breast cancer

ANTINEOPLASTIC DRUGS > ANTI-OESTROGENS

Fulvestrant

● INDICATIONS AND DOSE

Treatment of oestrogen-receptor-positive metastatic or locally advanced breast cancer in postmenopausal women in whom disease progresses or relapses while on, or after, other anti-oestrogen therapy
▶ BY DEEP INTRAMUSCULAR INJECTION
▶ Adult: 500 mg every 2 weeks for the first 3 doses, then 500 mg every 1 month, to be administered into the buttock

● SIDE-EFFECTS
▶ **Common or very common** Anorexia · asthenia · back pain · diarrhoea · headache · hot flushes · hypersensitivity reactions · injection-site reactions · nausea · rash · urinary-tract infections · venous thromboembolism · vomiting
▶ **Uncommon** Leucorrhoea · vaginal candidiasis · vaginal haemorrhage

● PREGNANCY Manufacturer advises avoid—increased incidence of fetal abnormalities and death in *animal* studies.

● BREAST FEEDING Manufacturer advises avoid—present in milk in *animal* studies.

● HEPATIC IMPAIRMENT Manufacturer advises caution in mild to moderate impairment. Avoid in severe impairment.

● RENAL IMPAIRMENT Manufacturer advises caution if creatinine clearance less than 30 mL/minute—no information available.

● DIRECTIONS FOR ADMINISTRATION 500 mg dose should be administered as one 250-mg injection (slowly over 1–2 minutes) into each buttock.

● MEDICINAL FORMS
There can be variation in the licensing of different medicines containing the same drug.
Solution for injection
▶ Faslodex (AstraZeneca UK Ltd)
Fulvestrant 50 mg per 1 ml Faslodex 250mg/5ml solution for injection pre-filled syringes | 2 pre-filled disposable injection PoM £522.41

Tamoxifen

● DRUG ACTION An anti-oestrogen which induces gonadotrophin release by occupying oestrogen receptors in the hypothalamus, thereby interfering with feedback mechanisms; chorionic gonadotrophin is sometimes used as an adjunct in the treatment of female infertility.

● INDICATIONS AND DOSE

Pre- and perimenopausal women with oestrogen-receptor-positive breast cancer not previously treated with tamoxifen
▶ BY MOUTH
▶ Adult: 20 mg daily

Anovulatory infertility
▶ BY MOUTH
▶ Adult: Initially 20 mg daily on days 2, 3, 4 and 5 of cycle, if necessary the daily dose may be increased to 40 mg then 80 mg for subsequent courses; if cycles irregular, start initial course on any day, with

subsequent course starting 45 days later or on day 2 of cycle if menstruation occurs

● CONTRA-INDICATIONS Treatment of infertility contra-indicated if personal or family history of idiopathic venous thromboembolism or genetic predisposition to thromboembolism

● CAUTIONS Porphyria

● INTERACTIONS → Appendix 1 (tamoxifen).

● SIDE-EFFECTS
▶ **Rare** Angioedema · bullous pemphigoid · cholestasis · fatty liver · hepatitis · hypersensitivity reactions · hypertriglyceridaemia · interstitial pneumonitis · neutropenia · Stevens-Johnson syndrome
▶ **Frequency not known** Alopecia · anaemia · cataracts · corneal changes · decreased platelet counts · endometrial changes · gastrointestinal disturbances · headache · hot flushes · hypercalcaemia if bony metastases · increased risk of thromboembolic events, especially when used with cytotoxics · leucopenia · light-headedness · liver enzyme changes · occasional cystic ovarian swellings in premenopausal women · occasionally oedema · pancreatitis · pruritus vulvae · rashes · retinopathy · suppression of menstruation in some premenopausal women · thrombocytopenia · thromboembolic events · tumour flare · uterine fibroids · vaginal bleeding · vaginal discharge · visual disturbances

SIDE-EFFECTS, FURTHER INFORMATION
▶ Endometrial changes Increased endometrial changes, including hyperplasia, polyps, cancer, and uterine sarcoma reported; prompt investigation required if abnormal vaginal bleeding including menstrual irregularities, vaginal discharge, and pelvic pain or pressure in those receiving (or who have received) tamoxifen.
▶ Risk of thromboembolism Tamoxifen can increase the risk of thromboembolism particularly during and immediately after major surgery or periods of immobility (consider interrupting treatment to initiate anticoagulant measures).

● CONCEPTION AND CONTRACEPTION Unless being used in the treatment of female infertility, effective contraception must be used during treatment and for 2 months after stopping. Patients being treated for infertility should be warned that there is a risk of multiple pregnancy (*rarely* more than twins).

● PREGNANCY Avoid—possible effects on fetal development.

● BREAST FEEDING Suppresses lactation. Avoid unless potential benefit outweighs risk.

● PATIENT AND CARER ADVICE
Endometrial changes Patients should be informed of the risk of endometrial cancer and told to report relevant symptoms promptly.
Thromboembolism Patients should be made aware of the symptoms of thromboembolism and advised to report sudden breathlessness and any pain in the calf of one leg.

● MEDICINAL FORMS
There can be variation in the licensing of different medicines containing the same drug. Forms available from special-order manufacturers include: oral suspension, oral solution
Tablet
▶ Tamoxifen (Non-proprietary)
Tamoxifen (as Tamoxifen citrate) 10 mg Tamoxifen 10mg tablets | 30 tablet PoM £37.99 DT price = £37.59
Tamoxifen (as Tamoxifen citrate) 20 mg Tamoxifen 20mg tablets | 30 tablet PoM £13.00 DT price = £2.75
Tamoxifen (as Tamoxifen citrate) 40 mg Tamoxifen 40mg tablets | 30 tablet PoM £33.51 DT price = £32.19
Oral suspension
▶ Tamoxifen (Non-proprietary)
Tamoxifen (as Tamoxifen citrate) 2 mg per 1 ml Tamoxifen 10mg/5ml oral suspension | 150 ml PoM no price available

8

Immune system and malignant disease

8

Immune system and malignant disease

Oral solution

▸ Tamoxifen (Non-proprietary)

Tamoxifen (as Tamoxifen citrate) 2 mg per 1 ml Tamoxifen 10mg/5ml oral solution sugar free sugar-free | 150 ml PoM no price available DT price = £29.61

▸ Soltamox (Rosemont Pharmaceuticals Ltd)

Tamoxifen (as Tamoxifen citrate) 2 mg per 1 ml Soltamox 10mg/5ml oral solution sugar-free | 150 ml PoM £29.61 DT price = £29.61

Toremifene

● INDICATIONS AND DOSE

Hormone-dependent metastatic breast cancer in postmenopausal women

▸ BY MOUTH

▸ Adult: 60 mg daily

● CONTRA-INDICATIONS Bradycardia · electrolyte disturbances (particularly uncorrected hypokalaemia) · endometrial hyperplasia · heart failure with reduced left-ventricular ejection fraction · history of arrhythmias · QT prolongation

● CAUTIONS Avoid in Acute porphyrias p. 918 · history of severe thromboembolic disease

● INTERACTIONS → Appendix 1 (toremifene). Avoid concomitant administration of drugs that prolong QT interval.

● SIDE-EFFECTS

▸ **Common or very common** Depression · dizziness · fatigue · hot flushes · nausea · oedema · rash · sweating · vaginal bleeding · vaginal discharge · vomiting

▸ **Uncommon** Anorexia · constipation · dyspnoea · endometrial hypertrophy · headache · increased weight · insomnia · thromboembolic events

▸ **Very rare** Alopecia · jaundice · transient corneal opacity

▸ **Frequency not known** Hypercalcaemia (especially if bone metastases and usually at beginning of treatment)

SIDE-EFFECTS, FURTHER INFORMATION

▸ Endometrial changes Increased endometrial changes, including hyperplasia, polyps and cancer reported. Abnormal vaginal bleeding including menstrual irregularities, vaginal discharge and symptoms such as pelvic pain or pressure should be promptly investigated.

● PREGNANCY Avoid.

● BREAST FEEDING Avoid.

● HEPATIC IMPAIRMENT Elimination decreased in hepatic impairment—avoid if severe.

● MEDICINAL FORMS
There can be variation in the licensing of different medicines containing the same drug.

Tablet

▸ Fareston (Orion Pharma (UK) Ltd)

Toremifene (as Toremifene citrate) 60 mg Fareston 60mg tablets | 30 tablet PoM £29.08

HORMONE ANTAGONISTS AND RELATED AGENTS > AROMATASE INHIBITORS

Anastrozole

● INDICATIONS AND DOSE

Adjuvant treatment of oestrogen-receptor-positive early invasive breast cancer in postmenopausal women | Adjuvant treatment of oestrogen-receptor-positive early breast cancer in postmenopausal women following 2–3 years of tamoxifen therapy | Advanced breast cancer in postmenopausal women which is oestrogen-receptor-positive or responsive to tamoxifen

▸ BY MOUTH

▸ Adult: 1 mg daily

● CONTRA-INDICATIONS Not for premenopausal women

● CAUTIONS Susceptibility to osteoporosis

● SIDE-EFFECTS

▸ **Very rare** Allergic reactions · anaphylaxis · angioedema

▸ **Frequency not known** Anorexia · arthralgia · arthritis · asthenia · bone fractures · bone pain · cutaneous vasculitis · diarrhoea · drowsiness · hair thinning · headache · hot flushes · nausea · rash · slight increases in total cholesterol levels · Stevens-Johnson syndrome · vaginal bleeding · vaginal dryness · vomiting

● PREGNANCY Avoid.

● BREAST FEEDING Avoid.

● HEPATIC IMPAIRMENT Avoid in moderate to severe impairment.

● RENAL IMPAIRMENT Avoid if creatinine clearance less than 20 mL/minute.

● PRE-TREATMENT SCREENING Laboratory test for menopause if doubt.

● MONITORING REQUIREMENTS

▸ Osteoporosis Assess bone mineral density before treatment and at regular intervals.

● PATIENT AND CARER ADVICE

Driving and skilled tasks
Asthenia and drowsiness may initially affect ability to drive or operate machinery.

● NATIONAL FUNDING/ACCESS DECISIONS

ARIMIDEX®

Scottish Medicines Consortium (SMC) Decisions
The *Scottish Medicines Consortium* has advised (August 2005 and October 2006) that anastrozole (*Arimidex*®) is accepted for restricted use within NHS Scotland, within the licensed indications, for early breast cancer and early invasive breast cancer.

● MEDICINAL FORMS
There can be variation in the licensing of different medicines containing the same drug.

Tablet

▸ Anastrozole (Non-proprietary)

Anastrozole 1 mg Anastrozole 1mg tablets | 28 tablet PoM £65.13 DT price = £1.27

▸ Arimidex (AstraZeneca UK Ltd)

Anastrozole 1 mg Arimidex 1mg tablets | 28 tablet PoM £68.56 DT price = £1.27

Exemestane

- **INDICATIONS AND DOSE**

Adjuvant treatment of oestrogen-receptor-positive early breast cancer in postmenopausal women following 2–3 years of tamoxifen therapy | Advanced breast cancer in postmenopausal women in whom anti-oestrogen therapy has failed
  ▶ BY MOUTH
  ▶ Adult: 25 mg daily

- **CONTRA-INDICATIONS** Not indicated for premenopausal women
- **INTERACTIONS** → Appendix 1 (exemestane).
- **SIDE-EFFECTS**
  ▶ **Common or very common** Abdominal pain · alopecia · anorexia · constipation · depression · dizziness · dyspepsia · fatigue · headache · hot flushes · insomnia · nausea · rash · sweating · vomiting
  ▶ **Uncommon** Asthenia · drowsiness · peripheral oedema
  ▶ **Rare** Leucopenia · thrombocytopenia
- **PREGNANCY** Avoid.
- **BREAST FEEDING** Avoid.
- **HEPATIC IMPAIRMENT** Manufacturer advises caution.
- **RENAL IMPAIRMENT** Manufacturer advises caution.
- **NATIONAL FUNDING/ACCESS DECISIONS**

Scottish Medicines Consortium (SMC) Decisions
The *Scottish Medicines Consortium* has advised (October 2005) that exemestane (*Aromasin®*) is accepted for restricted use within NHS Scotland as an adjuvant treatment in postmenopausal women with oestrogen-receptor-positive invasive early breast cancer, following 2–3 years of initial adjuvant tamoxifen therapy.

- **MEDICINAL FORMS**
There can be variation in the licensing of different medicines containing the same drug.
Tablet
CAUTIONARY AND ADVISORY LABELS 21
  ▶ Exemestane (Non-proprietary)
    Exemestane 25 mg Exemestane 25mg tablets | 30 tablet [PoM] £88.80 DT price = £8.65 | 90 tablet [PoM] no price available
  ▶ Aromasin (Pfizer Ltd)
    Exemestane 25 mg Aromasin 25mg tablets | 30 tablet [PoM] £88.80 DT price = £8.65

Letrozole

- **INDICATIONS AND DOSE**

First-line treatment in postmenopausal women with hormone-dependent advanced breast cancer | Adjuvant treatment of oestrogen-receptor-positive invasive early breast cancer in postmenopausal women | Advanced breast cancer in postmenopausal women (naturally or artificially induced menopause) in whom other anti-oestrogen therapy has failed | Extended adjuvant treatment of hormone-dependent invasive breast cancer in postmenopausal women who have received standard adjuvant tamoxifen therapy for 5 years | Neo-adjuvant treatment in postmenopausal women with localised hormone-receptor-positive, human epidermal growth factor-2 negative breast cancer where chemotherapy is not suitable and surgery not yet indicated
  ▶ BY MOUTH
  ▶ Adult: 2.5 mg daily

- **CONTRA-INDICATIONS** Not indicated for premenopausal women
- **CAUTIONS** Susceptibility to osteoporosis

- **SIDE-EFFECTS**
  ▶ **Common or very common** Abdominal pain · alopecia · anorexia · appetite increase · arthralgia · bone fracture · constipation · depression · diarrhoea · dizziness · dry skin · dyspepsia · fatigue · headache · hot flushes · hypercholesterolaemia · hypertension · increased sweating · musculoskeletal pain · nausea · osteoporosis · peripheral oedema · rash · vaginal bleeding · vomiting · weight changes
  ▶ **Uncommon** Anxiety · arthritis · blurred vision · breast pain · cardiac events · cataract · cerebrovascular events · cough · dysaesthesia · dyspnoea · eye irritation · general oedema · insomnia · leucopenia · memory impairment · mucosal dryness · palpitation · pruritus · pyrexia · stomatitis · tachycardia · taste disturbance · thrombophlebitis · tumour pain · urinary frequency · urinary-tract infection · urticaria · vaginal discharge
  ▶ **Rare** Arterial thrombosis · pulmonary embolism
  ▶ **Frequency not known** Hepatitis · toxic epidermal necrolysis
- **CONCEPTION AND CONTRACEPTION** Manufacturer advises effective contraception required until postmenopausal status fully established (return of ovarian function reported in postmenopausal women).
- **PREGNANCY** Avoid (isolated cases of birth defects reported).
- **BREAST FEEDING** Manufacturer advises avoid.
- **HEPATIC IMPAIRMENT** Manufacturer advises caution in severe impairment.
- **RENAL IMPAIRMENT** Manufacturer advises caution if creatinine clearance less than 10 mL/minute.
- **MONITORING REQUIREMENTS**
  ▶ **Osteoporosis** Assess bone mineral density before treatment and at regular intervals.
- **MEDICINAL FORMS**
There can be variation in the licensing of different medicines containing the same drug.
Tablet
  ▶ Letrozole (Non-proprietary)
    Letrozole 2.5 mg Letrozole 2.5mg tablets | 14 tablet [PoM] £49.90 DT price = £1.44 | 28 tablet [PoM] £73.24
  ▶ Femara (Novartis Pharmaceuticals UK Ltd)
    Letrozole 2.5 mg Femara 2.5mg tablets | 30 tablet [PoM] £90.92

4   Immunotherapy responsive malignancy

IMMUNOSTIMULANTS 〉 INTERFERONS

Interferon alfa

- **DRUG ACTION** Interferon alfa has shown some antitumour effect in certain lymphomas and solid tumours.

- **INDICATIONS AND DOSE**
INTRONA® PEN

Chronic myelogenous leukaemia (as monotherapy or in combination with cytarabine) | Hairy cell leukaemia | Follicular lymphoma | Lymph or liver metastases of carcinoid tumour | Chronic hepatitis B | Chronic hepatitis C | Adjunct to surgery in malignant melanoma | Maintenance of remission in multiple myeloma
  ▶ BY SUBCUTANEOUS INJECTION
  ▶ Adult: (consult local protocol)

continued →

8

Immune system and malignant disease

INTRONA® VIALS

Chronic myelogenous leukaemia (as monotherapy or in combination with cytarabine) | Hairy cell leukaemia | Follicular lymphoma | Lymph or liver metastases of carcinoid tumour | Chronic hepatitis B | Chronic hepatitis C | Adjunct to surgery in malignant melanoma | Maintenance of remission in multiple myeloma

▸ BY SUBCUTANEOUS INJECTION, OR BY INTRAVENOUS INFUSION

▸ Adult: (consult local protocol)

ROFERON-A®

Chronic myelogenous leukaemia | Hairy cell leukaemia | Chronic hepatitis B | Chronic hepatitis C | Adjunct to surgery in malignant melanoma | AIDS-related Kaposi's sarcoma | Advanced renal cell carcinoma | Progressive cutaneous T-cell lymphoma | Follicular non-Hodgkin's lymphoma

▸ BY SUBCUTANEOUS INJECTION

▸ Adult: (consult local protocol)

● CONTRA-INDICATIONS

CONTRA-INDICATIONS, FURTHER INFORMATION
For contra-indications consult product literature and local treatment protocol.

● CAUTIONS

CAUTIONS, FURTHER INFORMATION
For cautions consult product literature and local treatment protocol.

● INTERACTIONS → Appendix 1 (interferons).

● SIDE-EFFECTS

▸ **Common or very common** Anorexia · diarrhoea · influenza-like symptoms · lethargy · nausea

▸ **Frequency not known** Alopecia · arrhythmias · cardiovascular problems · coma (usually with high doses in the elderly) · confusion · depression · hepatotoxicity · hyperglycaemia · hypersensitivity reactions · hypertension · hypertriglyceridaemia (sometimes severe) · hypotension · myelosuppression (particularly affecting granulocyte counts) · nephrotoxicity · ocular side-effects · palpitation · psoriasiform rash · seizures (usually with high doses in the elderly). · suicidal behaviour · thyroid abnormalities

SIDE-EFFECTS, FURTHER INFORMATION
Consult product literature and local treatment protocols for information on side-effects.

● CONCEPTION AND CONTRACEPTION Effective contraception required during treatment—consult product literature.

● PREGNANCY Avoid unless potential benefit outweighs risk (toxicity in *animal* studies).

● BREAST FEEDING Unlikely to be harmful.

● HEPATIC IMPAIRMENT Avoid in severe hepatic impairment. Close monitoring required in mild to moderate hepatic impairment.

● RENAL IMPAIRMENT Avoid in severe renal impairment. Close monitoring required in mild to moderate renal impairment.

● MONITORING REQUIREMENTS Monitoring of lipid concentration is recommended.

● DIRECTIONS FOR ADMINISTRATION

ROFERON-A® *Roferon-A*® injection for subcutaneous injection.

INTRONA® VIALS *IntronA*® injection vials for subcutaneous injection or intravenous infusion.

● NATIONAL FUNDING/ACCESS DECISIONS

NICE technology appraisals (TAs)

▸ Peginterferon alfa, interferon alfa, and ribavirin for moderate to severe chronic hepatitis C (January 2004 and September 2010) NICE TA200
Interferon alfa for either monotherapy or combined therapy should be used only if neutropenia and thrombocytopenia are a particular risk. Patients receiving interferon alfa may be switched to peginterferon alfa.
www.nice.org.uk/TA200

● MEDICINAL FORMS
There can be variation in the licensing of different medicines containing the same drug.

Solution for injection
EXCIPIENTS: May contain Benzyl alcohol

▸ IntronA (Merck Sharp & Dohme Ltd)
Interferon alfa-2b 10 mega u per 1 ml IntronA 10million units/1ml solution for injection vials | 1 vial [PoM] no price available
IntronA 25million units/2.5ml solution for injection multidose vials | 1 vial [PoM] £103.94
Interferon alfa-2b 15 mega u per 1 ml IntronA 18million units/1.2ml solution for injection multidose pens | 1 pre-filled disposable injection [PoM] £74.83
Interferon alfa-2b 25 mega u per 1 ml IntronA 30million units/1.2ml solution for injection multidose pens | 1 pre-filled disposable injection [PoM] £124.72
Interferon alfa-2b 50 mega u per 1 ml IntronA 60million units/1.2ml solution for injection multidose pens | 1 pre-filled disposable injection [PoM] £249.45

▸ Roferon-A (Roche Products Ltd)
Interferon alfa-2a 6 mega u per 1 ml Roferon-A 3million units/0.5ml solution for injection pre-filled syringes | 1 pre-filled disposable injection [PoM] £14.20
Interferon alfa-2a 9 mega u per 1 ml Roferon-A 4.5million units/0.5ml solution for injection pre-filled syringes | 1 pre-filled disposable injection [PoM] £21.29
Interferon alfa-2a 12 mega u per 1 ml Roferon-A 6million units/0.5ml solution for injection pre-filled syringes | 1 pre-filled disposable injection [PoM] £28.37
Interferon alfa-2a 18 mega u per 1 ml Roferon-A 9million units/0.5ml solution for injection pre-filled syringes | 1 pre-filled disposable injection [PoM] £42.57

Interferon gamma-1b

(Immune interferon)

● INDICATIONS AND DOSE

To reduce the frequency of serious infection in chronic granulomatous disease

▸ BY SUBCUTANEOUS INJECTION

▸ Adult: 50 micrograms/m^2 3 times a week

To reduce the frequency of serious infection in severe malignant osteoporosis

▸ BY SUBCUTANEOUS INJECTION

▸ Adult: 50 micrograms/m^2 3 times a week

● CAUTIONS Arrhythmias · cardiac disease · congestive heart failure · ischaemia · seizure disorders (including seizures associated with fever)

● INTERACTIONS → Appendix 1 (interferons).
Avoid simultaneous administration of foreign proteins including immunological products (risk of exaggerated immune response).

● SIDE-EFFECTS

▸ **Common or very common** Abdominal pain · arthralgia · chills · depression · diarrhoea · fatigue · fever · headache · injection-site reactions · myalgia · nausea · rash · vomiting

▸ **Rare** Confusion · systemic lupus erythematosus

▸ **Frequency not known** Neutropenia · proteinuria · raised liver enzymes · thrombocytopenia

● CONCEPTION AND CONTRACEPTION Effective contraception required during treatment—consult product literature.

- PREGNANCY Manufacturers recommend avoid unless potential benefit outweighs risk (toxicity in *animal* studies).
- BREAST FEEDING Manufacturers advise avoid—no information available.
- HEPATIC IMPAIRMENT Manufacturer advises caution in severe impairment—risk of accumulation.
- RENAL IMPAIRMENT Manufacturer advises caution in severe impairment—risk of accumulation.
- MONITORING REQUIREMENTS Monitor before and during treatment: haematological tests (including full blood count, differential white cell count, and platelet count), blood chemistry tests (including renal and liver function tests) and urinalysis.

- MEDICINAL FORMS
There can be variation in the licensing of different medicines containing the same drug.
Solution for injection
  ‣ Immukin (Boehringer Ingelheim Ltd)
  Interferon gamma-1b (recombinant human) 200 microgram per 1 ml Immukin 100micrograms/0.5ml solution for injection vials | 6 vial [PoM] £450.00

IMMUNOSTIMULANTS › INTERLEUKINS

Aldesleukin

- DRUG ACTION Aldesleukin produces tumour shrinkage in a small proportion of patients, but it has not been shown to increase survival.

- INDICATIONS AND DOSE
Metastatic renal cell carcinoma (specialist use only)
  ‣ BY SUBCUTANEOUS INJECTION, OR BY INTRAVENOUS INFUSION
  ‣ Adult: (consult product literature)

- UNLICENSED USE Aldesleukin is not licensed for use in patients in whom all three of the following prognostic factors are present: performance status of Eastern Co-operative Oncology Group of 1 or greater, more than one organ with metastatic disease sites, and a period of less than 24 months between initial diagnosis of primary tumour and date of evaluation of treatment.
- CONTRA-INDICATIONS
  CONTRA-INDICATIONS, FURTHER INFORMATION
  Consult product literature for information about aldesleukin contra-indications.
- CAUTIONS
  CAUTIONS, FURTHER INFORMATION
  Consult product literature for information about aldesleukin cautions.
- INTERACTIONS → Appendix 1 (aldesleukin).
- SIDE-EFFECTS
  ‣ **Common or very common** Bone-marrow toxicity · CNS toxicity · hepatic toxicity · renal toxicity · thyroid toxicity
  ‣ **Frequency not known** Alopecia · bone-marrow suppression · extravasation · hyperuricaemia · nausea · oral mucositis · thromboembolism · tumour lysis syndrome · vomiting
  SIDE-EFFECTS, FURTHER INFORMATION
  Also consult product literature.
- CONCEPTION AND CONTRACEPTION Ensure effective contraception during treatment in men and women.
- PREGNANCY Use only if potential benefit outweighs risk (toxicity in *animal* studies). See also *Pregnancy and reproductive function* in Cytotoxic drugs p. 787.
- BREAST FEEDING Discontinue breast-feeding.
- DIRECTIONS FOR ADMINISTRATION Aldesleukin is now rarely given by intravenous infusion because of an increased risk of capillary leak syndrome, which can cause pulmonary oedema and hypotension.

- MEDICINAL FORMS
There can be variation in the licensing of different medicines containing the same drug.
Powder for solution for injection
  ‣ Proleukin (Novartis Pharmaceuticals UK Ltd)
  Aldesleukin 18 mega u Proleukin 18million unit powder for solution for injection vials | 1 vial [PoM] £112.00 | 10 vial [PoM] £1,036.00

IMMUNOSTIMULANTS › OTHER

Bacillus calmette-guérin

- DRUG ACTION Bacillus Calmette-Guérin is a live attenuated strain derived from *Mycobacterium bovis*.

- INDICATIONS AND DOSE
Bladder instillation for the treatment of primary or recurrent bladder carcinoma and for the prevention of recurrence following transurethral resection
  ‣ BY INTRAVESICAL INSTILLATION
  ‣ Adult: (consult product literature)

- CONTRA-INDICATIONS Fever of unknown origin · HIV infection · impaired immune response · severe haematuria · tuberculosis · urinary-tract infection
- CAUTIONS Bladder injury (delay administration until mucosal damage healed) · traumatic catheterisation (delay administration until mucosal damage healed) · urethral injury (delay administration until mucosal damage healed)
- SIDE-EFFECTS
  ‣ **Rare** Arthralgia · bladder contracture · hypersensitivity reactions · orchitis · rash · renal abscess · transient urethral obstruction
  ‣ **Frequency not known** Cystitis · dysuria · fever · haematuria · influenza-like syndrome · malaise · ocular symptoms · systemic BCG infection (with fatalities)—consult product literature · urinary frequency
- PREGNANCY Avoid.
- BREAST FEEDING Avoid.
- PRE-TREATMENT SCREENING Screen for active tuberculosis (contra-indicated if tuberculosis confirmed).

- MEDICINAL FORMS
There can be variation in the licensing of different medicines containing the same drug.
Powder for reconstitution for instillation
  ‣ ImmuCyst (Alliance Pharmaceuticals Ltd)
  Connaught strain Bacillus of Calmette-Guerin 81 mg ImmuCyst 81mg powder for reconstitution for instillation vials | 1 vial [PoM] £118.73 (Hospital only)
  ‣ OncoTICE (Merck Sharp & Dohme Ltd)
  TICE strain Bacillus of Calmette-Guerin 12.5 mg OncoTICE 12.5mg powder for reconstitution for instillation vials | 1 vial [PoM] £71.61 (Hospital only)

Histamine dihydrochloride

- INDICATIONS AND DOSE
Maintenance therapy, in combination with aldesleukin, in patients with acute myeloid leukaemia in first remission
  ‣ BY SUBCUTANEOUS INJECTION
  ‣ Adult: (consult local protocol)

- CONTRA-INDICATIONS
  CONTRA-INDICATIONS, FURTHER INFORMATION
  Consult product literature for information about histamine dihydrochloride contra-indications.
- CAUTIONS
  CAUTIONS, FURTHER INFORMATION
  Consult product literature for information about histamine dihydrochloride cautions.
- INTERACTIONS → Appendix 1 (histamine).

8

Immune system and malignant disease

● SIDE-EFFECTS

SIDE-EFFECTS, FURTHER INFORMATION
Consult product literature for side effects.

● CONCEPTION AND CONTRACEPTION Ensure effective contraception during treatment in men and women.

● PREGNANCY Manufacturer advises avoid—no information available.

● BREAST FEEDING Manufacturer advises avoid—no information available.

● HEPATIC IMPAIRMENT Increased risk of tachycardia and hypotension in moderate to severe impairment.

● RENAL IMPAIRMENT Increased risk of hypotension in severe impairment.

● NATIONAL FUNDING/ACCESS DECISIONS

Scottish Medicines Consortium (SMC) Decisions
The *Scottish Medicines Consortium* has advised (December 2010) that histamine dihydrochloride (*Ceplene*®) is **not** recommended for use within NHS Scotland.

● MEDICINAL FORMS
There can be variation in the licensing of different medicines containing the same drug.
No licensed medicines listed.

Mifamurtide

● INDICATIONS AND DOSE

Treatment of high-grade, resectable, non-metastatic osteosarcoma after complete surgical resection (in combination with chemotherapy)
▶ BY INTRAVENOUS INFUSION
▶ Adult: Infusion to be given over 1 hour (consult product literature or local protocols)

● UNLICENSED USE Not licensed for use in patients over 30 years of age at initial diagnosis.

● CAUTIONS Asthma—consider prophylactic bronchodilator therapy · chronic obstructive pulmonary disease—consider prophylactic bronchodilator therapy · history of autoimmune disease · history of collagen disease · history of inflammatory disease

● INTERACTIONS → Appendix 1 (mifamurtide).

● SIDE-EFFECTS Abdominal pain · alopecia · anaemia · anorexia · anxiety · blurred vision · confusion · constipation · cough · depression · diarrhoea · dizziness · drowsiness · dry skin · dyspepsia · dyspnoea · dysuria · epistaxis · flushing · gastro-intestinal disturbances · granulocytopenia · haematuria · haemoptysis · headache · hearing loss · hypertension · hypoaesthesia · hypokalaemia · hypotension · insomnia · leucopenia · musculoskeletal pain · nausea · oedema · palpitations · paraesthesia · phlebitis · pleural effusion · pollakiuria · rash · respiratory disorders · sweating · tachycardia · tachypnoea · thrombocytopenia · tinnitus · tremor · vertigo · vomiting

● CONCEPTION AND CONTRACEPTION Effective contraception required.

● PREGNANCY Avoid.

● BREAST FEEDING Avoid—no information available.

● HEPATIC IMPAIRMENT Use with caution—no information available.

● RENAL IMPAIRMENT Use with caution—no information available.

● MONITORING REQUIREMENTS
▶ Monitor renal function, hepatic function and clotting parameters.
▶ Monitor patients with history of venous thrombosis, vasculitis, or unstable cardiovascular disorders for persistent or worsening symptoms during administration—consult product literature.

● NATIONAL FUNDING/ACCESS DECISIONS

NICE technology appraisals (TAs)
▶ Mifamurtide for the treatment of osteosarcoma (October 2011) NICE TA235
Mifamurtide in combination with postoperative multi-agent chemotherapy is recommended (within its licensed indication), as an option for the treatment of high-grade resectable non-metastatic osteosarcoma after macroscopically complete surgical resection in children, adolescents and young adults and when mifamurtide is made available at a reduced cost to the NHS under the patient access scheme.
www.nice.org.uk/TA235

● MEDICINAL FORMS
There can be variation in the licensing of different medicines containing the same drug.
Powder for suspension for infusion
▶ Mepact (Takeda UK Ltd)
Mifamurtide 4 mg Mepact 4mg powder for suspension for infusion vials | 1 vial [PoM] no price available

IMMUNOSUPPRESSANTS ⟩THALIDOMIDE AND RELATED ANOLOGUES

Lenalidomide

9.5.2016

● DRUG ACTION Lenalidomide is an immunomodulating drug with anti-neoplastic, anti-angiogenic, and pro-erythropoietic properties.

● INDICATIONS AND DOSE

Multiple myeloma (newly diagnosed) in patients not eligible for transplant, given in combination with dexamethasone until disease progression
▶ BY MOUTH
▶ Adult: 25 mg once daily for 21 consecutive days of repeated 28-day cycles, for doses of dexamethasone, and dose adjustments due to side-effects, consult product literature

Multiple myeloma (newly diagnosed) in patients not eligible for transplant, given in combination with melphalan and prednisone followed by maintenance monotherapy
▶ BY MOUTH
▶ Adult: 10 mg once daily for 21 consecutive days of repeated 28-day cycles for up to 9 cycles, for doses of melphalan and prednisone, and dose adjustments due to side- effects, consult product literature

Multiple myeloma in patients who have received at least one prior therapy, given in combination with dexamethasone
▶ BY MOUTH
▶ Adult: 25 mg once daily for 21 consecutive days of repeated 28-day cycles, for doses of dexamethasone, and dose adjustments due to side-effects, consult product literature

Treatment of transfusion-dependent anaemia due to low- or intermediate-1-risk myelodysplastic syndromes (MDS) associated with an isolated deletion 5q cytogenetic abnormality when other treatment options are insufficient or inadequate
▶ BY MOUTH
▶ Adult: 10 mg once daily for 21 consecutive days of repeated 28-day cycles, for dose adjustments due to side-effects, consult product literature

● CAUTIONS High tumour burden—risk of tumour lysis syndrome · patients with risk factors for myocardial infarction

CAUTIONS, FURTHER INFORMATION

▶ Thromboembolism Risk factors for thromboembolism (such as smoking, hypertension, hyperlipidaemia) should be minimised and thromboprophylaxis should be considered in patients with multiple risk factors.

▶ Second primary malignancy Patients should be carefully evaluated before and during treatment with lenalidomide using routine cancer screening for occurrence of second primary malignancy and treatment should be instituted as indicated.

● INTERACTIONS → Appendix 1 (lenalidomide).
Use caution with concomitant drugs that increase the risk of thromboembolism.

● SIDE-EFFECTS

▶ **Common or very common** Abdominal pain · anaemia · arrhythmias · arthralgia · ataxia · atrial fibrillation · bacterial infections · bradycardia · cardiac failure · cataract · cerebrovascular events · chest pain · cholestasis · constipation · decreased appetite · deep vein thrombosis · dehydration · depression · diarrhoea · dizziness · dry mouth · dyspepsia · dysphagia · dyspnoea · electrolyte disturbances · falls · flu-like illness · fungal infections · haematoma · haematuria · haemorrhagic disorders · headache · hearing disturbances · hyperglycaemia · hyperhidrosis · hypertension · hypotension · hypothyroidism · insomnia · iron-overload · lethargy · leucopenia · malaise · mood changes · musculoskeletal disorders · myalgia · myocardial infarction · nausea · oedema · peripheral neuropathy · pneumonia · pruritus · pulmonary embolism · pyrexia · rash · renal failure · respiratory distress · respiratory tract infections · sepsis · severe neutropenia · sexual dysfunction · sinusitis · skin disorders · stomatitis · syncope · tachycardia · taste disturbance · thrombocytopenia · tremor · urinary incontinence · urinary retention · vasculitis · viral infections · visual disturbances · vomiting

▶ **Uncommon** Acquired Fanconi syndrome · angioedema · blindness · caecitis · clotting disorders · colitis · haemolysis · hepatic failure · ischaemia · secondary malignancies

▶ **Rare** Stevens-Johnson syndrome · toxic epidermal necrolysis · tumour lysis syndrome

▶ **Frequency not known** Cholestatic hepatitis · cytolytic hepatitis · interstitial pneumonitis · leukocytoclastic vasculitis · pancreatitis · toxic hepatitis

SIDE-EFFECTS, FURTHER INFORMATION

▶ Rash If rash occurs, treatment should be discontinued and only restarted following appropriate clinical evaluation. Discontinue permanently if angioedema, exfoliative or bullous rash, or if Stevens-Johnson syndrome or toxic epidermal necrolysis is suspected.
  For information on side effects consult product literature.

● CONCEPTION AND CONTRACEPTION For women of child-bearing potential, pregnancy must be excluded before starting treatment with lenalidomide (perform pregnancy test on initiation or within 3 days prior to initiation). Women must practise effective contraception at least 1 month before, during, and for at least 1 month after treatment, including during dose interruptions (oral combined hormonal contraceptives and copper-releasing intra-uterine devices not recommended) and men should use condoms during treatment, during dose interruption, and for at least 1 week after stopping if their partner is pregnant or is of childbearing potential and not using effective contraception. Patients, prescribers and pharmacists must comply with pregnancy prevention measures as specified in the manufacturer's Pregnancy Prevention Programme.

● PREGNANCY **Important: teratogenic risk.** Lenalidomide is structurally related to thalidomide and there is a risk of teratogenesis.

● BREAST FEEDING Discontinue breast-feeding—no information available.

● RENAL IMPAIRMENT Reduce dose in moderate to severe impairment—consult product literature.

● MONITORING REQUIREMENTS

▶ Monitor full blood count (including differential white cell count, platelet count, haemoglobin, and haematocrit) and liver function before treatment, then every week for the first 8 weeks, then monthly thereafter (reduce dose or interrupt treatment if neutropenia, thrombocytopenia or impaired liver function develop—consult product literature).

▶ Monitor for arterial or venous thromboembolism (if thromboembolic event occurs, discontinue lenalidomide and treat with standard anticoagulation therapy; lenalidomide may be restarted with continued anticoagulation therapy once thromboembolic event resolved—consult product literature).

▶ Monitor thyroid function.

▶ Monitor for signs and symptoms of peripheral neuropathy.

▶ Monitor visual ability regularly (risk of cataract).

▶ Hepatic disorders Liver function should be monitored particularly when there is history of, or concurrent viral liver infection, or when lenalidomide is combined with drugs known to be associated with liver dysfunction (e.g. paracetamol).

● PRESCRIBING AND DISPENSING INFORMATION Patient, prescriber, and supplying pharmacy must comply with a pregnancy prevention programme. Every prescription must be accompanied by a completed Prescription Authorisation Form.

● PATIENT AND CARER ADVICE
Thromboembolism Patients and their carers should be made aware of the symptoms of thromboembolism and advised to report sudden breathlessness, chest pain, or swelling of a limb.

Neutropenia and thrombocytopenia Patients and their carers should be made aware of the symptoms of neutropenia and advised to seek medical advice if symptoms suggestive of neutropenia (such as fever, sore throat) or of thrombocytopenia (such as bleeding) develop.

Patient advice required around conception and contraception
Pregnancy and contraception Patient counselling is advised for lenalidomide capsules (pregnancy and contraception).

● NATIONAL FUNDING/ACCESS DECISIONS

NICE technology appraisals (TAs)

▶ **Lenalidomide for treating myelodysplastic syndromes associated with an isolated deletion 5q cytogenetic abnormality (September 2014)** NICE TA322
Lenalidomide is recommended as an option, within its marketing authorisation, for treating transfusion-dependent anaemia caused by low or intermediate-1-risk myelodysplastic syndromes associated with an isolated deletion 5q cytogenetic abnormality when other therapeutic options are insufficient or inadequate, with the following condition:
  ● the drug cost of lenalidomide (excluding any related costs) for people who remain on treatment for more than 26 cycles (each of 28 days; normally a period of 2 years) will be met by the company.
www.nice.org.uk/TA322

▶ **Lenalidomide for the treatment of multiple myeloma (June 2009)** NICE TA171
Lenalidomide in combination with dexamethasone is an option for the treatment of multiple myeloma in patients who have received two or more prior therapies. The drug cost of lenalidomide will be met by the manufacturer for patients who remain on treatment for more than 26 cycles.
www.nice.org.uk/TA171

Scottish Medicines Consortium (SMC) Decisions
The *Scottish Medicines Consortium* has advised (April 2010) that lenalidomide, in combination with dexamethasone, is accepted for restricted use within NHS Scotland for patients with multiple myeloma who have received at least two prior therapies and (March 2014) for those who have received prior treatment with bortezomib and for whom thalidomide has not been tolerated or is contra-indicated.

The *Scottish Medicines Consortium* has advised (December 2015) that lenalidomide is accepted for restricted use within NHS Scotland for patients with previously untreated multiple myeloma who are not eligible for transplant and when thalidomide-containing regimens are unsuitable.

● MEDICINAL FORMS
There can be variation in the licensing of different medicines containing the same drug.

Capsule
CAUTIONARY AND ADVISORY LABELS 25
▸ Revlimid (Celgene Ltd) ▼
Lenalidomide 2.5 mg Revlimid 2.5mg capsules | 21 capsule PoM £3,426.00
Lenalidomide 5 mg Revlimid 5mg capsules | 21 capsule PoM £3,570.00
Lenalidomide 7.5 mg Revlimid 7.5mg capsules | 21 capsule PoM £3,675.00
Lenalidomide 10 mg Revlimid 10mg capsules | 21 capsule PoM £3,780.00
Lenalidomide 15 mg Revlimid 15mg capsules | 21 capsule PoM £3,969.00
Lenalidomide 20 mg Revlimid 20mg capsules | 21 capsule PoM £4,168.50
Lenalidomide 25 mg Revlimid 25mg capsules | 21 capsule PoM £4,368.00

Pomalidomide

● DRUG ACTION Pomalidomide is structurally related to thalidomide and has immunomodulatory properties and direct anti-myeloma tumoricidal activity.

● INDICATIONS AND DOSE
Treatment of relapsed and refractory multiple myeloma in patients who have received at least two prior treatment regimens, including both lenalidomide and bortezomib, and who have had disease progression during the last treatment (in combination with dexamethasone)
▸ BY MOUTH
▸ Adult: 4 mg once daily for 21 consecutive days of repeated 28–day cycles, for doses of dexamethasone and dose adjustment due to side effects—consult product literature

● CAUTIONS Cardiac disease · cardiac risk factors · high tumour burden—risk of tumour lysis syndrome · interstitial lung disease—discontinue if suspected · peripheral neuropathy
CAUTIONS, FURTHER INFORMATION
▸ Thromboembolism Risk factors for thromboembolism (such as smoking, hypertension, hyperlipidaemia) should be minimised. Thromboprophylaxis should be considered, particularly in patients with additional risk factors.
▸ Second primary malignancy Patients should be carefully evaluated before and during treatment with pomalidomide using routine cancer screening for occurrence of second primary malignancy and treatment should be instituted as indicated.

● INTERACTIONS → Appendix 1 (pomalidomide).
Use caution with concomitant drugs that increase the risk of bleeding or thromboembolism.

● SIDE-EFFECTS
▸ **Common or very common** Anaemia · bone pain · cardiac failure · confusion · constipation · cough · decreased appetite · diarrhoea · dizziness · dyspnoea · febrile neutropenia · hyperkalaemia · hyponatraemia · impaired consciousness · interstitial lung disease · leucopenia · malaise · muscle spasms · nasopharyngitis · nausea · neutropenia · neutropenic sepsis · pelvic pain · peripheral neuropathy · peripheral oedema · pneumonia · pruritus · pyrexia · rash · renal failure · respiratory tract infection · thrombocytopenia · thromboembolic events · tremor · urinary retention · vertigo · vomiting
▸ **Uncommon** Hepatitis
▸ **Frequency not known** Atrial fibrillation · pulmonary oedema

● CONCEPTION AND CONTRACEPTION For women of child-bearing potential, pregnancy must be excluded before starting treatment with pomalidomide (perform pregnancy test on initiation or within 3 days prior to initiation). Women must practise effective contraception at least 1 month before, during, and for at least 1 month after treatment, including during dose interruptions (oral combined hormonal contraceptives and copper-releasing intra-uterine devices not recommended) and men should use condoms during treatment, during dose interruption, and for at least 1 week after stopping if their partner is pregnant or is of childbearing potential and not using effective contraception. Patients, prescribers and pharmacists must comply with pregnancy prevention measures as specified in the manufacturer's Pregnancy Prevention Programme.

● PREGNANCY **Important: teratogenic risk.**

● BREAST FEEDING Avoid—present in milk in *animal* studies.

● HEPATIC IMPAIRMENT Manufacturer advises caution—no information available.

● RENAL IMPAIRMENT Manufacturer advises caution—no information available.

● MONITORING REQUIREMENTS
▸ Monitor full blood count before treatment, then every week for the first 8 weeks, then monthly thereafter (reduce dose or interrupt treatment if neutropenia or thrombocytopenia develop—consult product literature).
▸ Monitor for arterial or venous thromboembolism.
▸ Monitor for signs and symptoms of cardiac failure.
▸ Monitor for acute onset or unexplained worsening of respiratory symptoms.
▸ Monitor liver function for 6 months after initiation, then as clinically indicated.

● PRESCRIBING AND DISPENSING INFORMATION Patient, prescriber, and supplying pharmacy must comply with a pregnancy prevention programme. Every prescription must be accompanied by a completed Prescription Authorisation Form.

● PATIENT AND CARER ADVICE Patients and their carers should be made aware of the symptoms of thromboembolism and advised to report sudden breathlessness, chest pain, or swelling of a limb.
Patients and their carers should be made aware of the symptoms of neutropenia and advised to seek medical advice if symptoms suggestive of neutropenia (such as fever, sore throat) or of thrombocytopenia (such as bleeding) develop.

Patient advice required around conception and contraception
Patient counselling is advised for pomalidomide capsules (pregnancy and contraception).

● NATIONAL FUNDING/ACCESS DECISIONS

NICE technology appraisals (TAs)

▶ Pomalidomide for relapsed and refractory multiple myeloma previously treated with lenalidomide and bortezomib (March 2015) NICE TA338

Pomalidomide, in combination with dexamethasone, is **not** recommended for the treatment of relapsed and refractory multiple myeloma in adults who have had at least 2 previous treatments, including lenalidomide and bortezomib, and whose disease has progressed on the last therapy.

www.nice.org.uk/TA338

● MEDICINAL FORMS

There can be variation in the licensing of different medicines containing the same drug.

Capsule

CAUTIONARY AND ADVISORY LABELS 3, 25

EXCIPIENTS: May contain Propylene glycol

▶ Imnovid (Celgene Ltd) ▼

Pomalidomide 1 mg Imnovid 1mg capsules | 21 capsule [PoM]
£8,884.00

Pomalidomide 2 mg Imnovid 2mg capsules | 21 capsule [PoM]
£8,884.00

Pomalidomide 3 mg Imnovid 3mg capsules | 21 capsule [PoM]
£8,884.00

Pomalidomide 4 mg Imnovid 4mg capsules | 21 capsule [PoM]
£8,884.00

Thalidomide

● DRUG ACTION Thalidomide has immunomodulatory and anti-inflammatory activity.

● INDICATIONS AND DOSE

First-line treatment for untreated multiple myeloma, in patients aged 65 years and over, or for those not eligible for high-dose chemotherapy (for example, patients with significant co-morbidity such as cardiac risk factors) in combination with melphalan and prednisolone

▶ BY MOUTH

▶ Adult 18–75 years: 200 mg once daily for 6–week cycle for a maximum of 12 cycles, dose to be taken at bedtime

▶ Adult 76 years and over: 100 mg once daily for 6–week cycle for a maximum of 12 cycles, dose to be taken at bedtime

● CAUTIONS High tumour burden—risk of tumour lysis syndrome · patients aged 76 years and over—increased risk of serious side-effects

CAUTIONS, FURTHER INFORMATION

▶ Thromboembolism Risk factors for thromboembolism (such as smoking, hypertension, hyperlipidaemia) should be minimised. Thromboprophylaxis is recommended for at least the first 5 months of treatment, especially in patients with additional thrombotic risk factors.

▶ Second primary malignancy Patients should be carefully evaluated before and during treatment with thalidomide using routine cancer screening for occurrence of second primary malignancy and treatment should be instituted as indicated.

▶ Peripheral neuropathy Patients with pre-existing peripheral neuropathy should not be treated with thalidomide unless the potential clinical benefits outweigh the risk.

● INTERACTIONS Use caution with concomitant drugs that increase the risk of peripheral neuropathy or thromboembolism.

● SIDE-EFFECTS

▶ **Common or very common** Anaemia · asthenia · bradycardia · cardiac failure · confusion · constipation · deep vein thrombosis · depression · dizziness · drowsiness · dry mouth · dysaesthesia · dyspepsia · dyspnoea · interstitial lung disease · leucopenia · lymphopenia · neutropenia · paraesthesia · peripheral neuropathy · peripheral oedema · pneumonia · pulmonary embolism · pyrexia · skin reactions · Stevens-Johnson syndrome · syncope · thrombocytopenia · tremor · vomiting

▶ **Frequency not known** Atrial fibrillation · atrioventricular block · cerebrovascular events · convulsions · gastro-intestinal haemorrhage · gastro-intestinal perforation · hearing loss · hepatic disorders · hypothyroidism · intestinal obstruction · menstrual disorders · myocardial infarction · renal failure · second primary malignancy · sexual dysfunction · toxic epidermal necrolysis · worsening of Parkinson's disease symptoms

SIDE-EFFECTS, FURTHER INFORMATION

▶ Rash If rash occurs, treatment should be discontinued and only restarted following appropriate clinical evaluation.

▶ Peripheral neuropathy If symptoms suggestive of peripheral neuropathy develop (such as paraesthesia, abnormal coordination, or weakness) dose reduction, dose interruption, or treatment discontinuation may be necessary—consult product literature.

● CONCEPTION AND CONTRACEPTION For women of child-bearing potential, pregnancy must be excluded before starting treatment with thalidomide (perform pregnancy test on initiation or within 3 days prior to initiation). Women must practise effective contraception at least 1 month before, during, and for at least 1 month after treatment, including during dose interruptions (oral combined hormonal contraceptives and copper-releasing intra-uterine devices not recommended) and men should use condoms during treatment, during dose interruption, and for at least 1 week after stopping if their partner is pregnant or is of childbearing potential and not using effective contraception. Patients, prescribers and pharmacists must comply with pregnancy prevention measures as specified in the manufacturer's Pregnancy Prevention Programme.

● PREGNANCY **Important: teratogenic risk**.

● BREAST FEEDING Avoid—present in milk in *animal* studies.

● HEPATIC IMPAIRMENT Caution in severe impairment—no information available.

● RENAL IMPAIRMENT Caution in severe impairment—no information available.

● MONITORING REQUIREMENTS

▶ Monitor white blood cell count (including differential count) and platelet count (reduce dose or interrupt treatment if neutropenia or thrombocytopenia develop—consult product literature).

▶ Monitor for arterial or venous thromboembolism.

▶ Monitor patients for signs and symptoms of peripheral neuropathy.

▶ Hepatic disorder Liver function should be monitored, particularly when there is history of, or concurrent viral liver infection, or when thalidomide is combined with drugs known to be associated with liver dysfunction (e.g. paracetamol).

● PRESCRIBING AND DISPENSING INFORMATION Patient, prescriber, and supplying pharmacy must comply with a pregnancy prevention programme. Every prescription must be accompanied by a complete Prescription Authorisation Form.

● PATIENT AND CARER ADVICE Patients and their carers should be made aware of the symptoms of thromboembolism and advised to report sudden breathlessness, chest pain, or swelling of a limb.

Patients and their carers should be made aware of the symptoms of neutropenia and advised to seek medical advice if symptoms suggestive of neutropenia (such as fever, sore throat) or of thrombocytopenia (such as bleeding) develop.

Patients and their carers should be advised to seek

8

Immune system and malignant disease

medical advice if symptoms of peripheral neuropathy such as paraesthesia, abnormal coordination, or weakness develop.

Patient advice required around conception and contraception Patient counselling advised for thalidomide capsules (pregnancy and contraception).

● NATIONAL FUNDING/ACCESS DECISIONS

NICE technology appraisals (TAs)

▶ Bortezomib and thalidomide for the first-line treatment of multiple myeloma (July 2011) NICE TA228
Thalidomide in combination with an alkylating drug and a corticosteroid is recommended as an option for the first-line treatment of multiple myeloma in people for whom high-dose chemotherapy with stem cell transplantation is considered inappropriate.
www.nice.org.uk/TA228

● MEDICINAL FORMS
There can be variation in the licensing of different medicines containing the same drug. Forms available from special-order manufacturers include: tablet, oral suspension, oral solution
Capsule
CAUTIONARY AND ADVISORY LABELS 2
▶ Thalidomide (Non-proprietary)
Thalidomide 50 mg Thalidomide Celgene 50mg capsules | 28 capsule [PoM] £298.48
Thalidomide 50mg capsules | 28 capsule [PoM] no price available

5 Photodynamic therapy responsive malignancy

PHOTOSENSITISERS

Porfimer sodium

● DRUG ACTION Porfimer sodium accumulates in malignant tissue and is activated by laser light to produce a cytotoxic effect.

● INDICATIONS AND DOSE

Photodynamic therapy of non-small cell lung cancer and obstructing oesophageal cancer
▶ BY SLOW INTRAVENOUS INJECTION
▶ Adult: (consult product literature)

● CONTRA-INDICATIONS Acute porphyrias p. 918 · broncho-oesophageal fistula · tracheo-oesophageal fistula

● SIDE-EFFECTS Alopecia · bone-marrow suppression · constipation · extravasation · hyperuricaemia · nausea · oral mucositis · photosensitivity (sunscreens offer no protection) · thromboembolism · tumour lysis syndrome · vomiting

● PREGNANCY Manufacturer advises avoid unless essential.

● BREAST FEEDING No information available—manufacturer advises avoid.

● HEPATIC IMPAIRMENT Avoid in severe impairment.

● PATIENT AND CARER ADVICE
Photosensitivity Avoid exposure of skin and eyes to direct sunlight or bright indoor light for at least 30 days.

● MEDICINAL FORMS
There can be variation in the licensing of different medicines containing the same drug.
Powder for solution for injection
▶ Photofrin (Axcan Pharma Inc)
Porfimer sodium 15 mg Photofrin 15mg powder for solution for injection vials | 1 vial [PoM] no price available (Hospital only)
Porfimer sodium 75 mg Photofrin 75mg powder for solution for injection vials | 1 vial [PoM] no price available (Hospital only)

Temoporfin

● DRUG ACTION Temoporfin accumulates in malignant tissue and is activated by laser light to produce a cytotoxic effect.

● INDICATIONS AND DOSE

Photodynamic therapy of advanced head and neck squamous cell carcinoma refractory to, or unsuitable for, other treatments
▶ BY SLOW INTRAVENOUS INJECTION
▶ Adult: (consult product literature)

● CONTRA-INDICATIONS Acute porphyrias p. 918 · concomitant photosensitising treatment · diseases exacerbated by light · elective surgery · ophthalmic slit-lamp examination for 30 days after administration

● INTERACTIONS → Appendix 1 (temoporfin).

● SIDE-EFFECTS Alopecia · blistering · bone-marrow suppression · constipation · dysphagia · erythema · extravasation · facial pain · giddiness · haemorrhage · hyperpigmentation · hyperuricaemia · injection site pain · nausea · oedema · oral mucositis · photosensitivity (sunscreens ineffective) · scarring · skin necrosis · thromboembolism · trismus · tumour lysis syndrome · vomiting

● CONCEPTION AND CONTRACEPTION Manufacturer advises avoid pregnancy for at least 3 months after treatment.

● PREGNANCY Toxicity in *animal* studies. See also Pregnancy and reproductive function in Cytotoxic drugs p. 787.

● BREAST FEEDING Manufacturer advises avoid breastfeeding for at least 1 month after treatment—no information available.

● PATIENT AND CARER ADVICE
Photosensitivity Avoid exposure of skin and eyes to direct sunlight or bright indoor light for at least 15 days after administration.
Avoid prolonged exposure of injection site arm to direct sunlight for 6 months after administration.
If extravasation occurs protect area from light for at least 3 months.

● MEDICINAL FORMS
There can be variation in the licensing of different medicines containing the same drug.
Solution for injection
▶ Foscan (Biolitec Pharma Ltd)
Temoporfin 1 mg per 1 ml Foscan 3mg/3ml solution for injection vials | 1 vial [PoM] £1,800.00 (Hospital only)
Foscan 6mg/6ml solution for injection vials | 1 vial [PoM] £3,400.00 (Hospital only)

6   Targeted therapy responsive malignancy

ANTINEOPLASTIC DRUGS > PROTEIN KINASE INHIBITORS

Afatinib

- **DRUG ACTION** Afatinib is a protein kinase inhibitor.

● INDICATIONS AND DOSE

Treatment of locally advanced or metastatic non-small cell lung cancer with activating epidermal growth factor receptor (EGFR) mutations, in patients who have not previously been treated with EGFR tyrosine kinase inhibitor

▶ BY MOUTH
▶ Adult: 40 mg once daily; increased if tolerated to up to 50 mg once daily, dose increase may be considered after 3 weeks at initial dose; consult product literature for details on dosing and dose adjustment due to side effects

---

IMPORTANT SAFETY INFORMATION
RISKS OF INCORRECT DOSING OF ORAL ANTI-CANCER MEDICINES
See Cytotoxic drugs p. 787.

- **CAUTIONS** Cardiac risk factors · conditions which may affect left ventricular ejection fraction—consider cardiac monitoring, including assessment of left ventricular ejection fraction, at baseline and during treatment · diarrhoea—proactive management recommended (consult product literature) · exposure to sun (protect skin from exposure to sun) · history of keratitis · new pulmonary symptoms (including dyspnoea, cough, fever)—interrupt treatment until interstitial lung disease is excluded · severe dry eyes · signs and symptoms of keratitis—promptly refer to ophthalmologist for assessment · signs and symptoms of skin reaction—treat promptly and interrupt afatinib treatment if severe or if Stevens-Johnson syndrome suspected (consult product literature) · ulcerative keratitis · use of contact lenses · worsening pulmonary symptoms (including dyspnoea, cough, fever)—interrupt treatment until interstitial lung disease is excluded
- **INTERACTIONS** → Appendix 1 (afatinib).
- **SIDE-EFFECTS**
▶ **Common or very common** Acne · conjunctivitis · cystitis · decreased appetite · dehydration · diarrhoea · dry eyes · dry skin · dysgeusia · dyspepsia · epistaxis · hand-foot syndrome · hypokalaemia · muscle spasms · paronychia · pruritus · pyrexia · rash (see Cautions) · renal failure · rhinorrhoea · weight loss
▶ **Uncommon** Interstitial lung disease · keratitis
▶ **Frequency not known** Alopecia · bone-marrow suppression · hyperuricaemia · nausea · oral mucositis · thromboembolism · tumour lysis syndrome · vomiting
- **CONCEPTION AND CONTRACEPTION** Ensure effective contraception during and for at least one month after treatment in women of childbearing potential.
- **PREGNANCY** Manufacturer advises avoid. See also *Pregnancy and reproductive function* in Cytotoxic drugs p. 787.
- **BREAST FEEDING** Manufacturer advises avoid—present in milk in *animal* studies.
- **HEPATIC IMPAIRMENT** Monitor hepatic function regularly and consult product literature for dose adjustment in worsening liver function. Manufacturer advises avoid in severe hepatic impairment.

- **RENAL IMPAIRMENT** Manufacturer advises avoid in severe renal impairment.
- **DIRECTIONS FOR ADMINISTRATION** Tablets should be taken whole on an empty stomach. Food should not be consumed for at least 3 hours before and at least 1 hour after each dose.
  Giotrif® tablets may be dispersed in approximately 100 mL of noncarbonated water by stirring occasionally for up to 15 minutes (must not be crushed). The dispersion should be swallowed immediately, and the glass rinsed with the same volume of water which should also be swallowed. The dispersion can also be administered via a gastric tube.
- **PATIENT AND CARER ADVICE** Patient counselling advised (administration).

  Driving and skilled tasks
  Ocular adverse reactions may affect performance of skilled tasks e.g. driving.
- **NATIONAL FUNDING/ACCESS DECISIONS**

  NICE technology appraisals (TAs)
▶ **Afatinib for treating epidermal growth factor receptor mutation-positive locally advanced or metastatic non-small-cell lung cancer (April 2014)** NICE TA310
  Afatinib is recommended as an option, within its marketing authorisation, for treating locally advanced and metastatic non-small-cell lung cancer in adults:
  - whose tumour tests positive for the epidermal growth factor receptor tyrosine kinase (EGFR-TK) mutation, **and**
  - who have not previously had an EGFR-TK inhibitor, **and**
  - if the manufacturer provides afatinib with the discount agreed in the patient access scheme.
  www.nice.org.uk/TA310
- **MEDICINAL FORMS**
  There can be variation in the licensing of different medicines containing the same drug.

  Tablet
  CAUTIONARY AND ADVISORY LABELS 25
▶ Afatinib (Non-proprietary)
  Afatinib 20 mg Gilotrif 20mg tablets | 30 tablet [PoM] no price available
  Afatinib 30 mg Gilotrif 30mg tablets | 30 tablet [PoM] no price available
  Afatinib 40 mg Gilotrif 40mg tablets | 30 tablet [PoM] no price available
▶ Giotrif (Boehringer Ingelheim Ltd) ▼
  Afatinib 20 mg Giotrif 20mg tablets | 28 tablet [PoM] £2,023.28
  Afatinib 30 mg Giotrif 30mg tablets | 28 tablet [PoM] £2,023.28
  Afatinib 40 mg Giotrif 40mg tablets | 28 tablet [PoM] £2,023.28
  Afatinib 50 mg Giotrif 50mg tablets | 28 tablet [PoM] £2,023.28

Axitinib

- **DRUG ACTION** Axitinib is a tyrosine kinase inhibitor.

● INDICATIONS AND DOSE

Treatment of advanced renal cell carcinoma following failure of previous treatment with sunitinib or a cytokine (aldesleukin or interferon alfa)

▶ BY MOUTH
▶ Adult: (consult product literature)

IMPORTANT SAFETY INFORMATION
RISKS OF INCORRECT DOSING OF ORAL ANTI-CANCER MEDICINES
See Cytotoxic drugs p. 787.

- **CONTRA-INDICATIONS** Recent active gastro-intestinal bleeding · untreated brain metastases
- **CAUTIONS** Hypertension (blood pressure should be well-controlled before starting and monitored during treatment)

8

Immune system and malignant disease

- INTERACTIONS → Appendix 1 (axitinib).
- SIDE-EFFECTS
  ▸ **Common or very common** Abdominal pain · anal fistula · arthralgia · asthenia · cerebral haemorrhage · constipation · cough · decreased appetite · dehydration · diarrhoea · dizziness · dry skin · dysgeusia · dyspepsia · dysphonia · dyspnoea · erythema · fatigue · flatulence · gastro-intestinal haemorrhage · gastro-intestinal perforation · haemoptysis · haemorrhage · haemorrhoids · hand-foot syndrome · headache · hypercalcaemia · hyperkalaemia · hypertension · hyperthyroidism · hypothyroidism · myalgia · proteinuria · pruritus · rash · renal failure · tinnitus · weight loss
  ▸ **Uncommon** Hypertensive crisis · polycythaemia · posterior reversible encephalopathy syndrome
  ▸ **Frequency not known** Alopecia · bone-marrow suppression · hyperuricaemia · nausea · oral mucositis · thromboembolism · tumour lysis syndrome · vomiting
- CONCEPTION AND CONTRACEPTION Effective contraception required during and for up to 1 week after treatment.
- PREGNANCY Manufacturer advises avoid unless potential benefit outweighs risk (toxicity in *animal* studies). See also *Pregnancy and reproductive function* in Cytotoxic drugs p. 787.
- HEPATIC IMPAIRMENT Reduce starting dose in moderate impairment. Avoid in severe impairment—no information available.
- MONITORING REQUIREMENTS
  ▸ Monitor for thyroid dysfunction.
  ▸ Monitor haemoglobin or haematocrit before and during treatment.
  ▸ Monitor for symptoms of gastro-intestinal perforation.
  ▸ Monitor for symptoms of fistula.
  ▸ Monitor for proteinuria before and during treatment.
  ▸ Monitor liver function before and during treatment.
- NATIONAL FUNDING/ACCESS DECISIONS

  NICE technology appraisals (TAs)
  ▸ Axitinib for treating advanced renal cell carcinoma after failure of prior systemic treatment (February 2015) NICE TA333
  Axitinib is recommended as an option for treating adults with advanced renal cell carcinoma after failure of treatment with a first-line tyrosine kinase inhibitor or a cytokine, **only** if the company provides axitinib with the discount agreed in the patient access scheme.
  www.nice.org.uk/TA333

- MEDICINAL FORMS
  There can be variation in the licensing of different medicines containing the same drug.
  Tablet
  CAUTIONARY AND ADVISORY LABELS 25
  ▸ Inlyta (Pfizer Ltd) ▼
    Axitinib 1 mg Inlyta 1mg tablets | 56 tablet PoM £703.40 (Hospital only)
    Axitinib 3 mg Inlyta 3mg tablets | 56 tablet PoM £2,110.20 (Hospital only)
    Axitinib 5 mg Inlyta 5mg tablets | 56 tablet PoM £3,517.00 (Hospital only)
    Axitinib 7 mg Inlyta 7mg tablets | 56 tablet PoM £4,923.80 (Hospital only)

Bosutinib

- INDICATIONS AND DOSE

  Treatment of chronic, accelerated and blast phase Philadelphia chromosome-positive chronic myeloid leukaemia, in those previously treated with one or more tyrosine kinase inhibitors, and for whom imatinib, nilotinib and dasatinib are not clinically appropriate
  ▸ BY MOUTH
  ▸ Adult: 500 mg once daily, consult product literature for dose adjustment due to side effects, or incomplete haematologic response by week 8, or incomplete cytogenetic response by week 12

IMPORTANT SAFETY INFORMATION
RISKS OF INCORRECT DOSING OF ORAL ANTI-CANCER MEDICINES
See Cytotoxic drugs p. 787.

- CAUTIONS Cardiac disease · history of pancreatitis—withhold treatment if lipase elevated and abdominal symptoms occur · history of QT prolongation—monitor ECG and correct hypokalaemia and hypomagnesaemia before and during treatment · recent cardiac event—monitor ECG and correct hypokalaemia and hypomagnesaemia before and during treatment · risk factors for QT prolongation—monitor ECG and correct hypokalaemia and hypomagnesaemia before and during treatment · significant gastrointestinal disorder
- INTERACTIONS → Appendix 1 (bosutinib).
  Caution with concomitant use of drugs that prolong the QT interval (monitor ECG and correct hypokalaemia and hypomagnesaemia before and during treatment).
- SIDE-EFFECTS
  ▸ **Common or very common** Abdominal pain · abnormal liver function · acne · arthralgia · biochemical disturbances · cough · decreased appetite · dehydration · diarrhoea · dizziness · dysgeusia · dyspnoea · electrolyte disturbances · gastritis · headache · hepatotoxicity · infection · malaise · myalgia · oedema · pericardial effusion · pleural effusion · pruritus · pyrexia · QT prolongation · rash · renal failure · renal impairment · urticaria
  ▸ **Uncommon** Gastric haemorrhage · pancreatitis · pericarditis · pulmonary hypertension · pulmonary oedema · respiratory failure · tinnitus
  ▸ **Frequency not known** Alopecia · bone-marrow suppression · hyperuricaemia · nausea · oral mucositis · thromboembolism · tumour lysis syndrome · vomiting
- CONCEPTION AND CONTRACEPTION Effective contraception required during treatment in women.
- PREGNANCY Avoid—toxicity in *animal* studies. See also *Pregnancy and reproductive function* in Cytotoxic drugs p. 787.
- BREAST FEEDING Manufacturer advises avoid—no information available.
- HEPATIC IMPAIRMENT Caution—no information available.
- MONITORING REQUIREMENTS
  ▸ Monitor liver function before treatment initiation, then monthly for the first 3 months and thereafter as clinically indicated—consult product literature for management of raised transaminases.
  ▸ Monitor full blood count weekly for the first month and then monthly thereafter or as clinically indicated.
  ▸ Monitor for signs and symptoms of fluid retention (including pericardial effusion, pleural effusion and pulmonary oedema).

● NATIONAL FUNDING/ACCESS DECISIONS

NICE technology appraisals (TAs)

▶ **Bosutinib for previously treated chronic myeloid leukaemia (November 2013)** NICE TA299
Bosutinib is **not** recommended within its marketing authorisation for treating Philadelphia-chromosomepositive chronic myeloid leukaemia.
www.nice.org.uk/TA299

● MEDICINAL FORMS

There can be variation in the licensing of different medicines containing the same drug.

Tablet

CAUTIONARY AND ADVISORY LABELS 21

▶ Bosulif (Pfizer Ltd) ▼
Bosutinib 100 mg Bosulif 100mg tablets | 28 tablet P o M £859.17 (Hospital only)
Bosutinib 500 mg Bosulif 500mg tablets | 28 tablet P o M £3,436.67 (Hospital only)

Cabozantinib

● DRUG ACTION Cabozantinib is an inhibitor of several protein kinases.

● INDICATIONS AND DOSE

Treatment of progressive, unresectable locally advanced or metastatic medullary thyroid carcinoma

▶ BY MOUTH

▶ Adult: 140 mg once daily, for dose adjustment or treatment interruption due to side effects, consult product literature (closely monitor for first 8 weeks of therapy)

IMPORTANT SAFETY INFORMATION

RISKS OF INCORRECT DOSING OF ORAL ANTI-CANCER MEDICINES
See Cytotoxic drugs p. 787.

● CONTRA-INDICATIONS Reversible Posterior Leukoencephalopathy Syndrome

● CAUTIONS Hypertension—discontinue treatment if uncontrolled despite medical intervention · palmar-plantar erythrodysaesthesia syndrome—consider treatment interruption if severe and restart at a lower dose when resolved to grade 1 · patients at increased risk of fistulas—consult product literature · patients at increased risk of gastro-intestinal perforation—consult product literature · patients at increased risk of intra-abdominal abscess—consult product literature · patients at risk of haemorrhage (including tumour involvement of the trachea or bronchi)—discontinue if symptoms develop · patients at risk of thromboembolic events including myocardial infarction—discontinue if symptoms develop · risk of osteonecrosis of the jaw · susceptibility to QT-interval prolongation (e.g. cardiac disease, electrolyte disturbances, bradycardia, concomitant use of drugs that prolong the QT interval)—monitor ECG and electrolytes periodically

CAUTIONS, FURTHER INFORMATION

▶ Elective surgery Withhold treatment for at least 28 days before elective surgery and restart only if adequate wound healing—discontinue in patients with wound healing complications requiring medical intervention.

▶ Risk of osteonecrosis of the jaw Discontinue treatment at least 28 days before elective invasive dental procedures—monitor for symptoms before and during treatment and discontinue if osteonecrosis develops.

● INTERACTIONS → Appendix 1 (cabozantinib).
Caution with concomitant use of drugs which increase the risk of osteonecrosis of the jaw e.g. bisphosphonates. Caution with concomitant use of drugs that prolong the QT interval.

● SIDE-EFFECTS

▶ **Common or very common** Abdominal pain · abnormal hair growth · abscess · acne · alopecia · anal fissure · anxiety · arthralgia · aspiration · atrial fibrillation · blurred vision · cheilitis · chills · cholelithiasis · constipation · decreased appetite · dehydration · depression · diarrhoea · dizziness · dry skin · dysgeusia · dyspepsia · dysphagia · dysphonia · dysuria · erythema · face oedema · folliculitis · fungal infection · gastro-intestinal perforation · gastrointestinal haemorrhage · glossodynia · haematuria · haemorrhoids · hair colour changes · headache · hyperbilirubinaemia · hyperkeratosis · hypertension · hypoalbuminaemia · hypocalcaemia · hypokalaemia · hypophosphataemia · hypotension · hypothyroidism · impaired wound healing · lymphopenia · mucosal inflammation · muscle spasms · musculoskeletal chest pain · nausea · neutropenia · non-gastro-intestinal fistula · oropharyngeal pain · osteonecrosis of jaw · pallor · palmar-plantar erythrodysaesthesia syndrome · pancreatitis · paraesthesia · peripheral coldness · peripheral neuropathy · platelet disorders · pneumonia · proteinuria · pulmonary embolism · rash · respiratory tract haemorrhage · skin exfoliation · skin hypopigmentation · stomatitis · tinnitus · tremor · venous thrombosis · vomiting

▶ **Uncommon** Hypoacusis · acute renal failure · amenorrhoea · angina · arterial thrombosis · aspergilloma · ataxia · atelectasis · cataract · conjunctivitis · cyst · delirium · facial pain · gastro-intestinal fistula · hepatic encephalopathy · loss of consciousness · oesophagitis · pharyngeal oedema · pneumonitis · posterior reversible encephalopathy syndrome · rhabdomyolysis · skin ulcer · speech disorder · supraventricular tachycardia · telangiectasia · transient ischaemic attack · vaginal haemorrhage

▶ **Frequency not known** Bone-marrow suppression · hyperuricaemia · oral mucositis · thromboembolism · tumour lysis syndrome

● CONCEPTION AND CONTRACEPTION Patients and their sexual partners must use effective contraception (in addition to barrier method) during treatment and for at least 4 months after the last dose.

● PREGNANCY Manufacturer advises avoid unless potential benefit outweighs risk—toxicity in *animal* studies. See also *Pregnancy and reproductive function* in Cytotoxic drugs p. 787.

● BREAST FEEDING Manufacturer advises discontinue breast-feeding during treatment and for at least 4 months after the last dose.

● HEPATIC IMPAIRMENT Manufacturer advises avoid.

● RENAL IMPAIRMENT Manufacturer advises caution in renal impairment. Avoid in severe impairment.

● MONITORING REQUIREMENTS Monitor urine protein regularly and discontinue if nephrotic syndrome develops.

● PATIENT AND CARER ADVICE
Food should not be consumed for at least 2 hours before and at least 1 hour after each dose.
Driving and skilled tasks
Fatigue and weakness may affect performance of skilled tasks e.g. driving.

● MEDICINAL FORMS

There can be variation in the licensing of different medicines containing the same drug.

Capsule

CAUTIONARY AND ADVISORY LABELS 25

▶ Cometriq (Swedish Orphan Biovitrum Ltd) ▼
Cabozantinib (as Cabozantinib s-malate) 20 mg Cometriq 20mg capsules | 7 capsule P o M no price available | 21 capsule P o M no price available | 84 capsule P o M £4,800.00
Cabozantinib (as Cabozantinib s-malate) 80 mg Cometriq 80mg capsules | 7 capsule P o M no price available

▶ Cometriq (Swedish Orphan Biovitrum Ltd) ▼
Cometriq 20mg capsules and Cometriq 80mg capsules | 56 capsule P o M £4,800.00 | 112 capsule P o M £4,800.00

Crizotinib

● DRUG ACTION Crizotinib is a tyrosine kinase inhibitor.

● INDICATIONS AND DOSE

Treatment of previously treated anaplastic lymphoma kinase (ALK)-positive advanced non-small cell lung cancer

▶ BY MOUTH
▶ Adult: 250 mg twice daily, for dose adjustments due to side-effect, consult product literature

---

IMPORTANT SAFETY INFORMATION
RISKS OF INCORRECT DOSING OF ORAL ANTI-CANCER MEDICINES
See Cytotoxic drugs p. 787.

MHRA/CHM ADVICE (NOVEMBER 2015): RISK OF CARDIAC FAILURE
Severe, sometimes fatal cases of cardiac failure have been reported in patients treated with crizotinib. The MHRA has issued the following advice:
● Monitor all patients for signs and symptoms of heart failure (including dyspnoea, oedema, or rapid weight gain from fluid retention)
● Consider reducing the dose, or interrupting or stopping treatment if symptoms of heart failure occur

---

● CAUTIONS History of diverticulitis (risk of gastro-intestinal perforation—discontinue treatment if gastrointestinal perforation occurs) · metastases of gastrointestinal tract (risk of gastro-intestinal perforation—discontinue treatment if gastrointestinal perforation occurs) · patients with susceptibility to QT-prolongation (including bradycardia, history of cardiac disease, concomitant use of drugs that prolong QT interval, and electrolyte disturbances)—periodic renal monitoring required · risk of gastro-intestinal perforation—discontinue treatment if gastrointestinal perforation occurs · vision disorders reported—consider full ophthalmological evaluation if vision disorder worsens or persists

CAUTIONS, FURTHER INFORMATION
▶ Fatal interstitial lung disease and pneumonitis Fatal interstitial lung disease and pneumonitis reported (monitor patients with pulmonary symptoms, withdraw treatment if suspected, and permanently discontinue treatment if diagnosed).

● INTERACTIONS → Appendix 1 (crizotinib).
Caution with concomitant use of drugs that prolong QT interval—periodic renal monitoring required.
Caution with concomitant use of drugs which may cause gastrointestinal perforation—discontinue treatment if gastrointestinal perforation occurs.

● SIDE-EFFECTS
▶ Common or very common Bone-marrow suppression · bradycardia · cardiac failure · constipation · decreased appetite · diarrhoea · dizziness · dyspepsia · fatigue · hypophosphataemia · interstitial lung disease · nausea · neuropathy · oedema · pneumonitis · pneumonitis · QT-interval prolongation · rash · renal cyst · syncope · taste disturbance · vision disorder · vomiting
▶ Uncommon Gastrointestinal perforation (fatalities reported) · hepatotoxicity (including fatal hepatic failure)
▶ Frequency not known Alopecia · hyperuricaemia · oral mucositis · thromboembolism · tumour lysis syndrome

SIDE-EFFECTS, FURTHER INFORMATION
▶ Cardiac failure Consider reducing the dose, or interrupting or stopping treatment if symptoms of cardiac failure occur.

● CONCEPTION AND CONTRACEPTION Ensure effective contraception during and for at least 90 days after treatment.

● PREGNANCY Avoid (toxicity in *animal* studies). See also *Pregnancy and reproductive function* in Cytotoxic drugs p. 787.

● BREAST FEEDING Avoid—no information available.

● HEPATIC IMPAIRMENT Manufacturer advises caution in mild to moderate impairment. Avoid in severe impairment.

● RENAL IMPAIRMENT Reduce dose to 250 mg once daily in severe impairment not requiring peritoneal dialysis or hemodialysis, may be increased to 200 mg twice daily after at least 4 weeks, based on individual assessment of safety and tolerability.

● MONITORING REQUIREMENTS Monitor liver function once a week during the first 2 months of treatment, then at least monthly thereafter and as clinically indicated. Monitor ECG and electrolytes (correct if abnormal) in all patients before starting treatment, then periodically and as clinically indicated thereafter. Monitor for signs and symptoms of treatment emergent bradycardia (including syncope, dizziness and hypotension)—monitor blood pressure and heart rate regularly.

● PATIENT AND CARER ADVICE
Counsel all patients on the early signs and symptoms of gastrointestinal perforation—advice to seek immediate medical attention.

Driving and skilled tasks
Symptomatic bradycardia (including syncope, dizziness and hypotension), vision disorder and fatigue may affect performance of skilled tasks (e.g. driving or operating machinery).

● NATIONAL FUNDING/ACCESS DECISIONS

NICE technology appraisals (TAs)
▶ Crizotinib for previously treated non-small-cell lung cancer associated with an anaplastic lymphoma kinase fusion gene (September 2013) NICE TA296
Crizotinib is **not** recommended within its marketing authorisation, for treating adults with previously treated anaplastic-lymphoma-kinase-positive advanced non-small-cell lung cancer.
www.nice.org.uk/TA296

● MEDICINAL FORMS
There can be variation in the licensing of different medicines containing the same drug.
Capsule
CAUTIONARY AND ADVISORY LABELS 25
▶ Xalkori (Pfizer Ltd) ▼
Crizotinib 200 mg Xalkori 200mg capsules | 60 capsule PoM £4,689.00 (Hospital only)
Crizotinib 250 mg Xalkori 250mg capsules | 60 capsule PoM £4,689.00 (Hospital only)

Dabrafenib

● DRUG ACTION Dabrafenib is a BRAF kinase inhibitor.

● INDICATIONS AND DOSE

Monotherapy for the treatment of unresectable or metastatic melanoma with BRAF V600 mutation

▶ BY MOUTH
▶ Adult: 150 mg every 12 hours, for dose adjustments due to side effects consult product literature

---

IMPORTANT SAFETY INFORMATION
RISKS OF INCORRECT DOSING OF ORAL ANTI-CANCER MEDICINES
See Cytotoxic drugs p. 787.

● CONTRA-INDICATIONS BRAF wild-type melanoma · long QT syndrome · uncorrectable electrolyte abnormalities (including magnesium)

- CAUTIONS Pyrexia (interrupt treatment if ≥38.5°C and assess for signs and symptoms of infection—consult product literature)
- INTERACTIONS → Appendix 1 (dabrafenib). Contra-indicated with concomitant use of drugs that prolong the QT interval.
- SIDE-EFFECTS
▶ **Common or very common** Acrochordon · arthralgia · basal cell carcinoma · chills · constipation · cough · cutaneous squamous cell carcinoma · decrease in left ventricular ejection fraction · decreased appetite · diarrhoea · dry skin · erythema · hand-foot syndrome · headache · hyperglycaemia · hyperkeratosis · hypophosphataemia · influenza-like symptoms · keratosis · malaise · myalgia · papilloma · pruritus · pyrexia · rash · skin lesions
▶ **Uncommon** Nephritis · new primary melanoma · pancreatitis · panniculitis · QT-interval prolongation · renal failure · uveitis
▶ **Frequency not known** Alopecia · bone-marrow suppression · hyperuricaemia · nausea · oral mucositis · thromboembolism · tumour lysis syndrome · vomiting
SIDE-EFFECTS, FURTHER INFORMATION
▶ Pancreatitis Promptly investigate signs and symptoms of pancreatitis—consult product literature.
- CONCEPTION AND CONTRACEPTION Effective non-hormonal contraception required during and for one month after treatment in women of childbearing potential.
- PREGNANCY Manufacturer advises unless potential benefit outweighs risk (toxicity in *animal* studies). See also *Pregnancy and reproductive function* in Cytotoxic drugs p. 787.
- BREAST FEEDING Manufacturer advises avoid.
- HEPATIC IMPAIRMENT Manufacturer advises caution in moderate to severe impairment. Additional monitoring of ECG and electrolytes required in hepatic impairment—consult product literature.
- RENAL IMPAIRMENT Manufacturer advises caution in severe impairment—no information available.
- MONITORING REQUIREMENTS
▶ Assess for cutaneous squamous cell carcinoma and new primary melanoma before treatment, monthly during treatment, and for 6 months after discontinuation or until initiation of alternative treatment.
▶ Assess and monitor for non-cutaneous secondary or recurrent malignancy before, during, and for 6 months after discontinuation or until initiation of alternative treatment—consult product literature.
▶ Monitor serum creatinine and other signs of renal failure—consult product literature and interrupt dose as appropriate.
▶ Monitor for ophthalmologic reactions including uveitis and iritis.
▶ Monitor ECG and electrolytes (including magnesium) before and one month after treatment initiation and after each dose modification— consult product literature if abnormalities occur.
- PATIENT AND CARER ADVICE
Driving and skilled tasks
Ocular adverse reactions and fatigue may affect performance of skilled tasks e.g. driving.
- NATIONAL FUNDING/ACCESS DECISIONS
NICE technology appraisals (TAs)
▶ **Dabrafenib for treating unresectable or metastatic BRAF V600 mutation-positive melanoma (October 2014)** NICE TA321 Dabrafenib is recommended, within its marketing authorisation, as an option for treating unresectable or metastatic BRAF V600 mutation-positive melanoma only if the manufacturer provides dabrafenib with the discount agreed in the patient access scheme.
www.nice.org.uk/TA321

Scottish Medicines Consortium (SMC) Decisions
The *Scottish Medicines Consortium* has advised (February 2015) that dabrafenib (*Tafinlar*®) is accepted for restricted use within NHS Scotland for the treatment of unresectable or metastatic BRAFV600 mutation-positive melanoma in patients who have received no prior therapy.

- MEDICINAL FORMS
There can be variation in the licensing of different medicines containing the same drug.
Capsule
CAUTIONARY AND ADVISORY LABELS 23, 25
▶ Tafinlar (Novartis Pharmaceuticals UK Ltd) ▼
Dabrafenib (as Dabrafenib mesilate) 50 mg Tafinlar 50mg capsules | 28 capsule PoM £933.33 (Hospital only)
Dabrafenib (as Dabrafenib mesilate) 75 mg Tafinlar 75mg capsules | 28 capsule PoM £1,400.00 (Hospital only)

Dasatinib

- DRUG ACTION Dasatinib is a tyrosine kinase inhibitor.

- INDICATIONS AND DOSE
Chronic phase chronic myeloid leukaemia (consult product literature for details)
▶ BY MOUTH
▶ Adult: 100 mg once daily, then increased if necessary up to 140 mg once daily
Accelerated and blast phase chronic myeloid leukaemia (consult product literature for details) | Acute lymphoblastic leukaemia (consult product literature for details)
▶ BY MOUTH
▶ Adult: 140 mg once daily, then increased if necessary up to 180 mg once daily

---

IMPORTANT SAFETY INFORMATION
RISKS OF INCORRECT DOSING OF ORAL ANTI-CANCER MEDICINES
See Cytotoxic drugs p. 787.

- CAUTIONS Risk of cardiac dysfunction (monitor closely) · susceptibility to QT-interval prolongation (correct hypokalaemia or hypomagnesaemia before starting treatment)
CAUTIONS, FURTHER INFORMATION
▶ Pulmonary arterial hypertension Patients should be evaluated for signs and symptoms of underlying cardiopulmonary disease before starting treatment; echocardiography should be performed at the start of treatment in patients with symptoms of cardiac disease and considered for patients with risk factors for cardiac or pulmonary disease.
Treatment should be interrupted or the dose reduced in patients who develop dyspnoea or fatigue, while they are evaluated for common aetiologies (e.g. pleural effusion, pulmonary oedema, anaemia or lung infiltration); pulmonary arterial hypertension should be considered in the absence of these conditions, and if there is no improvement following dose reduction or interruption.
If pulmonary arterial hypertension is confirmed, dasatinib should be permanently discontinued.
- INTERACTIONS → Appendix 1 (dasatinib).
- SIDE-EFFECTS
▶ **Common or very common** Abdominal pain · acne · anorexia · arrhythmias · chest pain · CNS haemorrhage · colitis · congestive heart failure · constipation · cough · depression · dermatitis · diarrhoea · dizziness · dry skin · dyspepsia · dyspnoea · flushing · gastritis · gastro-intestinal haemorrhage · haemorrhage · headache · hypertension · influenza-like symptoms · insomnia · musculoskeletal pain · neuropathy · oedema (more common in patients over 65 years old) · palpitation · pleural effusion · pruritus ·

pulmonary hypertension · sweating · taste disturbance · tinnitus · urticaria · visual disturbances · weight changes
- **Uncommon** Amnesia · asthma · cholecystitis · cholestasis · drowsiness · erythema nodosum · gynaecomastia · hepatitis · hypersensitivity reactions · hypocalcaemia · hypotension · irregular menstruation · nail disorders · oesophagitis · pancreatitis · photosensitivity · pigmentation · proteinuria · rhabdomyolysis · seizures · syncope · thrombophlebitis · transient ischaemic attack · tremor · urinary frequency
- **Rare** Cor pulmonale
- **Frequency not known** Alopecia · bone-marrow suppression · hyperuricaemia · interstitial lung disease · nausea · oral mucositis · thromboembolism · thrombosis · tumour lysis syndrome · vomiting
- CONCEPTION AND CONTRACEPTION Effective contraception required during treatment.
- PREGNANCY Manufacturer advises avoid unless potential benefit outweighs risk—toxicity in *animal* studies. See also *Pregnancy and reproductive function* in Cytotoxic drugs p. 787.
- BREAST FEEDING Discontinue breast-feeding.
- HEPATIC IMPAIRMENT Manufacturer advises caution in hepatic impairment.
- NATIONAL FUNDING/ACCESS DECISIONS

NICE technology appraisals (TAs)
- Dasatinib, nilotinib and standard-dose imatinib for the first-line treatment of chronic myeloid leukaemia (April 2012) NICE TA251
  Dasatinib is **not** recommended for the first-line treatment of chronic phase Philadelphia-chromosome-positive CML.
  www.nice.org.uk/TA251
- Dasatinib, high dose imatinib and nilotinib for the treatment of imatinib-resistant chronic myeloid leukaemia (CML), and dasatinib and nilotinib for people with CML for whom treatment with imatinib has failed because of intolerance (January 2012) NICE TA241
  Dasatinib is **not** recommended for the treatment of chronic, accelerated or blast-crisis phase CML in adults with imatinib intolerance or whose CML is resistant to treatment with standard-dose imatinib.
  www.nice.org.uk/TA241

Scottish Medicines Consortium (SMC) Decisions
The *Scottish Medicines Consortium*) has advised (April 2007) that the use of dasatinib (*Sprycel* ®) in NHS Scotland is restricted to patients in the chronic phase of chronic myeloid leukaemia.

- MEDICINAL FORMS
  There can be variation in the licensing of different medicines containing the same drug.

Tablet
CAUTIONARY AND ADVISORY LABELS 25
- Sprycel (Bristol-Myers Squibb Pharmaceuticals Ltd)
  Dasatinib 20 mg Sprycel 20mg tablets | 60 tablet PoM £1,252.48
  Dasatinib 50 mg Sprycel 50mg tablets | 60 tablet PoM £2,504.96
  Dasatinib 80 mg Sprycel 80mg tablets | 30 tablet PoM £2,504.96
  Dasatinib 100 mg Sprycel 100mg tablets | 30 tablet PoM £2,504.96
  Dasatinib 140 mg Sprycel 140mg tablets | 30 tablet PoM £2,504.96

Erlotinib

18.4.2016

- DRUG ACTION Erlotinib is a tyrosine kinase inhibitor.

- INDICATIONS AND DOSE

Treatment of locally advanced or metastatic non-small cell lung cancer after failure of previous chemotherapy | Monotherapy for maintenance treatment of locally advanced or metastatic non-small cell lung cancer with stable disease after four cycles of platinum-based chemotherapy
- BY MOUTH
- Adult: 150 mg once daily

Treatment of metastatic pancreatic cancer (in combination with gemcitabine)
- BY MOUTH
- Adult: 100 mg once daily

IMPORTANT SAFETY INFORMATION

EPIDERMAL GROWTH FACTOR RECEPTOR (EGFR) INHIBITORS: SERIOUS CASES OF KERATITIS AND ULCERATIVE KERATITIS (MAY 2012)
Keratitis and ulcerative keratitis have been reported following treatment with epidermal growth factor receptor (EGFR) inhibitors for cancer (cetuximab, erlotinib, gefitinib and panitumumab). In rare cases, this has resulted in corneal perforation and blindness. Patients undergoing treatment with EGFR inhibitors who present with acute or worsening signs and symptoms suggestive of keratitis should be referred promptly to an opthalmology specialist. Treatment should be interupted or discontinued if ulcerative keratitis is diagnosed.

RISKS OF INCORRECT DOSING OF ORAL ANTI-CANCER MEDICINES See Cytotoxic drugs p. 787.

- CAUTIONS
  CAUTIONS, FURTHER INFORMATION
- Smoking Dose adjustment may be necessary if smoking started or stopped during treatment.
- INTERACTIONS → Appendix 1 (erlotinib).
  Caution with concomitant use with hepatotoxic drugs—monitor liver function.
- SIDE-EFFECTS
- **Common or very common** Abdominal pain · anorexia · conjunctivitis · depression · diarrhoea · dry skin · dyspepsia · fatigue · flatulence · headache · neuropathy · pruritus · rigor
- **Uncommon** Eyelash changes · gastro-intestinal perforation · interstitial lung disease—discontinue if unexplained symptoms such as dyspnoea, cough or fever occur
- **Rare** Hepatic failure
- **Very rare** Corneal perforation · corneal ulceration · Stevens-Johnson syndrome · toxic epidermal necrolysis
- **Frequency not known** Alopecia · bone-marrow suppression · hyperuricaemia · nausea · oral mucositis · thromboembolism · tumour lysis syndrome · vomiting
- CONCEPTION AND CONTRACEPTION Effective contraception required during and for at least 2 weeks after treatment.
- PREGNANCY Manufacturer advises avoid—toxicity in *animal* studies. See also *Pregnancy and reproductive function* in Cytotoxic drugs p. 787.
- BREAST FEEDING Manufacturer advises avoid- no information available.
- HEPATIC IMPAIRMENT Manufacturer advises caution in mild to moderate impairment. Avoid in severe impairment. Monitor liver function in pre-existing liver disease.

- RENAL IMPAIRMENT Manufacturer advises avoid in severe impairment.
- NATIONAL FUNDING/ACCESS DECISIONS

  NICE technology appraisals (TAs)

  ▶ Erlotinib monotherapy for maintenance treatment of non-small-cell lung cancer (June 2011) NICE TA227

  Erlotinib monotherapy is **not** recommended for maintenance treatment in patients with locally advanced or metastatic non-small-cell lung cancer who have stable disease after platinum-based first-line chemotherapy.

  www.nice.org.uk/TA227

  ▶ Erlotinib for the first-line treatment of locally advanced or metastatic EGFR-TK mutation-positive non-small-cell lung cancer (June 2012) NICE TA258

  Erlotinib is recommended as an option in patients for the first-line treatment of locally advanced or metastatic non-small-cell lung cancer if:
  - they test positive for the epidermal growth factor tyrosine kinase (EGFR-TK) mutation **and**
  - the manufacturer provides erlotinib at the discounted price agreed under the patient access scheme (as revised in 2012).

  www.nice.org.uk/TA258

  ▶ Erlotinib and gefitinib for treating non-small-cell lung cancer that has progressed after prior chemotherapy (December 2015) NICE TA374

  Erlotinib is recommended as an option for treating locally advanced or metastatic non-small-cell lung cancer that has progressed after non-targeted chemotherapy in patients with tumours of unknown epidermal growth factor receptor tyrosine kinase (EGFR-TK) mutation status, only if all of the following criteria are met:
  - the result of an EGFR-TK mutation diagnostic test is unobtainable because of an inadequate tissue sample or poor-quality DNA,
  - the treating clinician considers that the tumour is very likely to be EGFR-TK mutation-positive,
  - the patient's condition responds to the first 2 cycles of treatment with erlotinib, **and**,
  - the manufacturer provides erlotinib with the discount agreed in the patient access scheme.

  Erlotinib is **not** recommended for treating locally advanced or metastatic non-small-cell lung cancer that has progressed after non-targeted chemotherapy in patients with tumours that are EGFR-TK mutation-negative.

  Patients who are already receiving erlotinib should continue treatment until they and their clinician consider it appropriate to stop.

  www.nice.org.uk/TA374

- MEDICINAL FORMS

  There can be variation in the licensing of different medicines containing the same drug.

  Tablet

  CAUTIONARY AND ADVISORY LABELS 23

  ▶ Tarceva (Roche Products Ltd)

  Erlotinib (as Erlotinib hydrochloride) 25 mg Tarceva 25mg tablets | 30 tablet PoM £378.33

  Erlotinib (as Erlotinib hydrochloride) 100 mg Tarceva 100mg tablets | 30 tablet PoM £1,324.14

  Erlotinib (as Erlotinib hydrochloride) 150 mg Tarceva 150mg tablets | 30 tablet PoM £1,631.53

Everolimus

- DRUG ACTION Everolimus is a protein kinase inhibitor.

- INDICATIONS AND DOSE

  AFINITOR®

  Treatment of advanced renal cell carcinoma when the disease has progressed despite treatment with vascular endothelial growth factor-targeted therapy | Treatment of unresectable or metastatic, well- or moderately-differentiated neuroendocrine tumours of pancreatic origin | Treatment of hormone-receptor-positive, human epidermal growth factor-2 (HER-2) negative advanced breast cancer, in combination with exemestane, in postmenopausal women without symptomatic visceral disease after recurrence or progression following a non-steroidal aromatase inhibitor

  ▶ BY MOUTH
  ▸ Adult: 10 mg once daily

  CERTICAN®

  Liver transplantation

  ▶ BY MOUTH
  ▸ Adult: Initially 1 mg twice daily, to be started approximately 4 weeks after transplantation; maintenance, dose adjusted according to response and whole blood everolimus concentration; dose adjustments can be made every 4–5 days

  Renal transplantation | Heart transplantation

  ▶ BY MOUTH
  ▸ Adult: Initially 750 micrograms twice daily, to be started as soon as possible after transplantation; maintenance, dose adjusted according to response and whole blood everolimus concentration; dose adjustments can be made every 4–5 days

  VOTUBIA®

  Subependymal giant cell astrocytoma associated with tuberous sclerosis complex

  ▶ BY MOUTH
  ▸ Adult: (consult product literature)

  Renal angiomyolipoma associated with tuberous sclerosis complex

  ▶ BY MOUTH
  ▸ Adult: (consult product literature)

  IMPORTANT SAFETY INFORMATION

  RISKS OF INCORRECT DOSING OF ORAL ANTI-CANCER MEDICINES See Cytotoxic drugs p. 787.

- CAUTIONS History of bleeding disorders
- INTERACTIONS → Appendix 1 (everolimus). Caution with concomitant use of drugs that increase risk of bleeding.
- SIDE-EFFECTS

  ▶ **Common or very common** Abdominal pain · anorexia · arthralgia · asthenia · chest pain · convulsions · dehydration · diarrhoea · dry mouth · dysphagia · electrolyte disturbance · epistaxis · eyelid oedema · fatigue · hand-foot syndrome · headache · hypercholesterolaemia · hyperglycaemia · hyperlipidaemia · hypertension · hypoglycaemia · increased susceptibility to aspergillosis · increased susceptibility to candidiasis · increased susceptibility to infections · increased susceptibility to pneumonia · insomnia · interstitial lung disease · irritability · nail disorders · peripheral oedema · pneumonitis · renal failure · skin disorders · taste disturbance

  ▶ **Uncommon** Aggression · agitation · congestive heart failure · flushing · impaired wound healing · rhabdomyolysis

  ▶ **Frequency not known** Alopecia · bone-marrow suppression · haemorrhage · hepatitis B reactivation · hyperuricaemia ·

nausea · oral mucositis · thromboembolism · tumour lysis syndrome · vomiting

SIDE-EFFECTS, FURTHER INFORMATION

Reduce dose or discontinue if severe side-effects occur—consult product literature.

● CONCEPTION AND CONTRACEPTION Effective contraception must be used during and for up to 8 weeks after treatment.

● PREGNANCY Manufacturer advises avoid (toxicity in *animal* studies). See also *Pregnancy and reproductive function* in Cytotoxic drugs p. 787.

● BREAST FEEDING Manufacturer advises avoid.

● HEPATIC IMPAIRMENT Consult product literature.

● MONITORING REQUIREMENTS

▸ For *Certican*®: manufacturer advises pre-dose ('trough') whole blood everolimus concentration should be 3–8 nanograms/mL; monitoring should be performed every 4–5 days (using **chromatographic** assay) after initiation or dose adjustment until 2 consecutive stable concentrations; monitor patients with hepatic impairment taking concomitant strong CYP3A4 inducers and inhibitors when switching formulation, and/or if concomitant ciclosporin dose is reduced.

▸ Monitor blood-glucose concentration, serum-triglycerides and serum-cholesterol before treatment and periodically thereafter.

▸ Monitor renal function before treatment and periodically thereafter.

● DIRECTIONS FOR ADMINISTRATION

VOTUBIA® Tablets may be dispersed in approximately 30 mL of water by gently stirring, immediately before drinking. After solution has been swallowed, any residue must be re-dispersed in the same volume of water and swallowed.

● PATIENT AND CARER ADVICE

Pneumonitis Non-infectious pneumonitis reported. Patients should be advised to seek urgent medical advice if new or worsening respiratory symptoms occur.

● NATIONAL FUNDING/ACCESS DECISIONS

NICE technology appraisals (TAs)

▸ Everolimus for the second-line treatment of advanced renal cell carcinoma (April 2011) NICE TA219

Everolimus is **not** recommended for the second-line treatment of advanced renal cell carcinoma.
www.nice.org.uk/TA219

▸ Everolimus in combination with exemestane for treating advanced HER2-negative hormone-receptor-positive breast cancer after endocrine therapy (August 2013) NICE TA295

Everolimus, in combination with exemestane, is **not** recommended within its marketing authorisation for treating postmenopausal women with advanced human epidermal growth factor receptor 2 (HER2) negative hormone-receptor-positive breast cancer that has recurred or progressed following treatment with a non-steroidal aromatase inhibitor.
www.nice.org.uk/TA295

AFINITOR®

Scottish Medicines Consortium (SMC) Decisions

The *Scottish Medicines Consortium* has advised (April 2012) that everolimus (*Afinitor*®) is accepted for restricted use within NHS Scotland for the treatment of unresectable or metastatic, well- or moderately-differentiated neuroendocrine tumours of pancreatic origin (pNET) in adults with progressive disease.

CERTICAN®

NICE technology appraisals (TAs)

▸ Everolimus for preventing organ rejection in liver transplantation (July 2015) NICE TA348

Everolimus (*Certican*®) is **not** recommended within its marketing authorisation for preventing organ rejection in patients who have undergone a liver transplant. Patients currently receiving everolimus for this indication should have the option to continue treatment until they and their clinician consider it appropriate to stop.
www.nice.org.uk/TA348

● MEDICINAL FORMS

There can be variation in the licensing of different medicines containing the same drug.

Tablet

CAUTIONARY AND ADVISORY LABELS 25

▸ Afinitor (Novartis Pharmaceuticals UK Ltd)
Everolimus 2.5 mg Afinitor 2.5mg tablets | 30 tablet PoM £1,200.00
Everolimus 5 mg Afinitor 5mg tablets | 30 tablet PoM £2,250.00
Everolimus 10 mg Afinitor 10mg tablets | 30 tablet PoM £2,673.00

▸ Certican (Novartis Pharmaceuticals UK Ltd)
Everolimus 250 microgram Certican 0.25mg tablets | 60 tablet PoM £148.50
Everolimus 500 microgram Certican 0.5mg tablets | 60 tablet PoM £297.00
Everolimus 750 microgram Certican 0.75mg tablets | 60 tablet PoM £445.50

▸ Votubia (Novartis Pharmaceuticals UK Ltd)
Everolimus 2.5 mg Votubia 2.5mg tablets | 30 tablet PoM £1,200.00
Everolimus 5 mg Votubia 5mg tablets | 30 tablet PoM £2,250.00
Everolimus 10 mg Votubia 10mg tablets | 30 tablet PoM £2,970.00

Gefitinib

27.5.2016

● DRUG ACTION Gefitinib is a tyrosine kinase inhibitor.

● INDICATIONS AND DOSE

Treatment of locally advanced or metastatic non-small cell lung cancer with activating mutations of epidermal growth factor receptor

▸ BY MOUTH

▸ Adult: 250 mg once daily

IMPORTANT SAFETY INFORMATION

MHRA/CHM ADVICE: EPIDERMAL GROWTH FACTOR RECEPTOR (EGFR) INHIBITORS: SERIOUS CASES OF KERATITIS AND ULCERATIVE KERATITIS (MAY 2012)

Keratitis and ulcerative keratitis have been reported following treatment with epidermal growth factor receptor (EGFR) inhibitors for cancer (cetuximab, erlotinib, gefitinib and panitumumab). In rare cases, this has resulted in corneal perforation and blindness. Patients undergoing treatment with EGFR inhibitors who present with acute or worsening signs and symptoms suggestive of keratitis should be referred promptly to an opthalmology specialist. Treatment should be interupted or discontinued if ulcerative keratitis is diagnosed.

RISKS OF INCORRECT DOSING OF ORAL ANTI-CANCER MEDICINES
See Cytotoxic drugs p. 787.

● INTERACTIONS → Appendix 1 (gefitinib).

● SIDE-EFFECTS

▸ **Common or very common** Acne · anorexia · asthenia · blepharitis · conjunctivitis · diarrhoea · dry eye · dry mouth · dry skin · epistaxis · haematuria · interstitial lung disease—discontinue if confirmed · nail disorder · proteinuria · pruritus · pyrexia · rash · skin reactions

▸ **Uncommon** Corneal erosion · pancreatitis

▸ **Rare** Hepatitis · toxic epidermal necrolysis

▸ **Frequency not known** Alopecia · bone-marrow suppression · hyperuricaemia · nausea · oral mucositis · thromboembolism · tumour lysis syndrome · vomiting

● CONCEPTION AND CONTRACEPTION Contraceptive advice required, see *Pregnancy and reproductive function* in Cytotoxic drugs p. 787.

● PREGNANCY Manufacturer advises avoid unless essential—toxicity in *animal* studies. See also *Pregnancy and reproductive function* in Cytotoxic drugs p. 787.

● BREAST FEEDING Discontinue breast-feeding.

● HEPATIC IMPAIRMENT Manufacturer advises caution in moderate to severe impairment due to cirrhosis.

● RENAL IMPAIRMENT Manufacturer advises caution if creatinine clearance less than 20 mL/minute.

● MONITORING REQUIREMENTS
▸ Monitor for worsening of dyspnoea, cough and fever— discontinue if interstitial lung disease confirmed.
▸ Monitor liver function—consider discontinuing if severe changes in liver function occur.

● NATIONAL FUNDING/ACCESS DECISIONS

NICE technology appraisals (TAs)
▸ **Gefitinib for the first-line treatment of locally advanced or metastatic non-small-cell lung cancer (July 2010)** NICE TA192
Gefitinib is recommended as an option for the first-line treatment of locally advanced or metastatic non-small-cell lung cancer if the patient tests positive for the epidermal growth factor tyrosine kinase (EGFR-TK) mutation and the manufacturer provides gefitinib at the fixed price agreed under the patient access scheme.
www.nice.org.uk/TA192
▸ **Erlotinib and gefitinib for treating non-small-cell lung cancer that has progressed after prior chemotherapy (December 2015)** NICE TA374
Gefitinib is **not** recommended for treating locally advanced or metastatic non-small-cell lung cancer that has progressed after non-targeted chemotherapy in patients with tumours that are EGFR-TK mutation-positive.
   Patients who are already receiving gefitinib should continue treatment until they and their clinician consider it appropriate to stop.
www.nice.org.uk/TA374

Scottish Medicines Consortium (SMC) Decisions
The *Scottish Medicines Consortium* has advised (December 2015) that gefitinib (*Iressa* ®) is accepted for restricted use within NHS Scotland for the treatment of adult patients with previously untreated locally advanced or metastatic non-small cell lung cancer (NSCLC) with activating mutations of epidermal growth factor receptor tyrosine kinase (EGFR-TK).

● MEDICINAL FORMS
There can be variation in the licensing of different medicines containing the same drug.

Tablet
▸ Iressa (AstraZeneca UK Ltd)
   Gefitinib 250 mg Iressa 250mg tablets | 30 tablet PoM £2,167.71

Ibrutinib

● DRUG ACTION Ibrutinib is a tyrosine kinase inhibitor.

● INDICATIONS AND DOSE
Treatment of relapsed or refractory mantle cell lymphoma
▸ BY MOUTH
▸ Adult: 560 mg once daily, for dose adjustments due to side effects consult product literature

Treatment of chronic lymphocytic leukaemia, in patients who have received at least one prior therapy, or as first-line treatment in patients with 17p deletion or TP53 mutation who are unsuitable for chemo-immunotherapy | Treatment of Waldenstr m's macroglobulinaemia, in patients who have received at least one prior therapy, or as first-line treatment in patients who are unsuitable for chemo-immunotherapy
▸ BY MOUTH
▸ Adult: 420 mg once daily, for dose adjustments due to side effects consult product literature

Treatment of relapsed or refractory mantle cell lymphoma (reduced dose for patients taking concomitant moderate or potent CYP3A4 inhibitors) | Treatment of chronic lymphocytic leukaemia, in patients who have received at least one prior therapy, or as first-line treatment in patients with 17p deletion or TP53 mutation who are unsuitable for chemo-immunotherapy (reduced dose for patients taking concomitant moderate or potent CYP3A4 inhibitors) | Treatment of Waldenstr m's macroglobulinaemia, in patients who have received at least one prior therapy, or as first-line treatment in patients who are unsuitable for chemo-immunotherapy (reduced dose for patients taking concomitant moderate or potent CYP3A4 inhibitors)
▸ BY MOUTH
▸ Adult: 140 mg once daily, for dose adjustments due to side effects consult product literature

DOSE ADJUSTMENTS DUE TO INTERACTIONS
Reduce dose in patients taking concomitant potent CYP3A4 inhibitors (such as cobicistat, clarithromycin, darunavir boosted with ritonavir, indinavir, itraconazole, ketoconazole, ritonavir, saquinavir, telithromycin, and voriconazole) or moderate CYP3A4 inhibitors (such as amiodarone, aprepitant, atazanavir, ciprofloxacin, crizotinib, diltiazem, dronedarone, erythromycin, fluconazole, fosamprenavir, imatinib, and verapamil); alternatively temporarily stop ibrutinib if the potent CYP3A4 inhibitor is only required for 7 days or less. Avoid concomitant use with these drugs unless unavoidable.

IMPORTANT SAFETY INFORMATION
RISKS OF INCORRECT DOSING OF ORAL ANTI-CANCER MEDICINES
See Cytotoxic drugs p. 787.

● CAUTIONS Family history of congenital short QT syndrome · increased lymphocytes—increased risk of leukostasis, consider withholding treatment temporarily and monitor closely · patients at risk from further shortening of QTc interval · personal history of congenital short QT syndrome · risk of haemorrhagic events—withhold ibrutinib treatment for at least 3 to 7 days before and after surgery depending on risk of bleeding

● INTERACTIONS → Appendix 1 (ibrutinib).
Avoid concomitant use of drugs that increase risk of bleeding.

● SIDE-EFFECTS
▸ **Common or very common** Arthralgia · atrial fibrillation · blurred vision · bruising · constipation · dehydration · diarrhoea · dizziness · dry mouth · epistaxis · haemorrhage · headache · musculoskeletal pain · peripheral oedema · petechiae · pyrexia · rash · respiratory tract infection · sepsis · sinusitis · skin infection · subdural haematoma · urinary tract infection
▸ **Uncommon** Leukostasis
▸ **Frequency not known** Alopecia · bone-marrow suppression · hyperuricaemia · nausea · oral mucositis · thromboembolism · tumour lysis syndrome · vomiting

8

Immune system and malignant disease

- CONCEPTION AND CONTRACEPTION Highly effective contraception (must include a non-hormonal method) required during and for 3 months after stopping treatment.
- PREGNANCY Manufacturer advises avoid—toxicity in *animal* studies. See also *Pregnancy and reproductive function* in Cytotoxic drugs p. 787.
- BREAST FEEDING Manufacturer advises discontinue breastfeeding—no information available.
- HEPATIC IMPAIRMENT Reduce dose to 280 mg daily in mild impairment and reduce dose to 140 mg daily in moderate impairment—monitor for toxicity and adjust dose if necessary (consult product literature). Avoid in severe impairment.
- RENAL IMPAIRMENT Use in severe impairment only if benefit outweighs risk and with close monitoring for toxicity. Maintain hydration and monitor serum creatinine periodically in mild to moderate renal impairment.
- MONITORING REQUIREMENTS
- ▶ Monitor full blood count once a month.
- ▶ Monitor for atrial fibrillation (increased risk in cardiac risk factors, acute infections and history of atrial fibrillation), monitor all patients periodically and complete ECG if arrhythmic symptoms or dyspnoea develop—consult product literature for treatment options.
- MEDICINAL FORMS
There can be variation in the licensing of different medicines containing the same drug.

Capsule
CAUTIONARY AND ADVISORY LABELS 25
▶ Imbruvica (Janssen-Cilag Ltd) ▼
Ibrutinib 140 mg Imbruvica 140mg capsules | 90 capsule (PoM) £4,599.00 | 120 capsule (PoM) £6,132.00

Idelalisib

- DRUG ACTION Idelalisib is a protein kinase inhibitor.

- INDICATIONS AND DOSE
Treatment of chronic lymphocytic leukaemia in patients who have received at least one previous therapy, or as first-line treatment in the presence of 17p deletion or TP53 mutation in patients unsuitable for chemo-immunotherapy (in combination with rituximab) | Treatment of follicular lymphoma refractory to two lines of treatment (monotherapy)
- ▶ BY MOUTH
- ▶ Adult: 150 mg twice daily, for dose adjustment due to side effects, consult product literature

IMPORTANT SAFETY INFORMATION
RISKS OF INCORRECT DOSING OF ORAL ANTI-CANCER MEDICINES
See Cytotoxic drugs p. 787.

- CAUTIONS Active hepatitis · diarrhoea—symptomatic management recommended (consult product literature) · pneumonitis—withhold treatment (consult product literature)
- INTERACTIONS → Appendix 1 (idelalisib).
- SIDE-EFFECTS Alopecia · bone-marrow suppression · diarrhoea · hyperuricaemia · infections · nausea · neutropenia · oral mucositis · pneumonitis · pyrexia · rash · thromboembolism · tumour lysis syndrome · vomiting
- CONCEPTION AND CONTRACEPTION Highly effective contraception (in addition to barrier method) required during and for one month after treatment.
- PREGNANCY Manufacturer advises avoid (toxicity in *animal* studies). See also *Pregnancy and reproductive function* in Cytotoxic drugs p. 787.

- BREAST FEEDING Manufacturer advises avoid—no information available.
- HEPATIC IMPAIRMENT Manufacturer advises caution in hepatic impairment.
- MONITORING REQUIREMENTS Monitor liver function—consult product literature.
- NATIONAL FUNDING/ACCESS DECISIONS
NICE technology appraisals (TAs)
▶ Idelalisib for treating chronic lymphocytic leukaemia (October 2015) NICE TA359
Idelalisib, in combination with rituximab, is recommended as an option for treatment in adults:
  - who have untreated chronic lymphocytic leukaemia **or**
  - who have chronic lymphocytic leukaemia when the disease has been treated but has relapsed within 24 months **and**
  - if the manufacturer provides idelalisib with the discount agreed in the simple discount agreement.
Patients who are already receiving idelalisib should continue treatment until they and their clinician consider it appropriate to stop.
www.nice.org.uk/guidance/TA359

Scottish Medicines Consortium (SMC) Decisions
The *Scottish Medicines Consortium* has advised (March 2015) that idelalisib (*Zydelig*®) is accepted for restricted use within NHS Scotland, in combination with rituximab, for the treatment of relapsed chronic lymphocytic leukaemia in patients who are unsuitable for chemotherapy and treatment naïve patients with 17p depletion or TP53 mutation who are unsuitable for chemo-immunotherapy, only whilst idelalisib is available at the price agreed in the patient access scheme.

- MEDICINAL FORMS
There can be variation in the licensing of different medicines containing the same drug.

Tablet
CAUTIONARY AND ADVISORY LABELS 25
▶ Zydelig (Gilead Sciences International Ltd) ▼
Idelalisib 100 mg Zydelig 100mg tablets | 60 tablet (PoM) £3,114.75 (Hospital only)
Idelalisib 150 mg Zydelig 150mg tablets | 60 tablet (PoM) £3,114.75 (Hospital only)

Imatinib

- DRUG ACTION Imatinib is a tyrosine kinase inhibitor.

- INDICATIONS AND DOSE
Treatment of chronic myeloid leukaemia in chronic phase after failure with interferon alfa
- ▶ BY MOUTH
- ▶ Adult: 400 mg once daily, increased if necessary up to 800 mg daily in 2 divided doses

Treatment of chronic myeloid leukaemia in accelerated phase, or in blast crisis
- ▶ BY MOUTH
- ▶ Adult: 600 mg once daily, then increased if necessary up to 800 mg daily in 2 divided doses

Treatment of newly diagnosed acute lymphoblastic leukaemia (in combination with other chemotherapy) | Monotherapy for relapsed or refractory acute lymphoblastic leukaemia
- ▶ BY MOUTH
- ▶ Adult: 600 mg once daily

Treatment of c-kit (CD117)-positive unresectable or metastatic malignant gastro-intestinal stromal tumours (GIST) | Adjuvant treatment following resection of c-kit (CD117)-positive GIST, in patients at significant risk of relapse | Treatment of myelodysplastic/myeloproliferative diseases associated with platelet-derived growth factor receptor gene rearrangement
▶ BY MOUTH
 ▶ Adult: 400 mg once daily

Treatment of unresectable dermatofibrosarcoma protuberans | Recurrent or metastatic dermatofibrosarcoma protuberans, in patients who cannot have surgery
▶ BY MOUTH
 ▶ Adult: 800 mg daily in 2 divided doses

Treatment of advanced hypereosinophilic syndrome and chronic eosinophilic leukaemia
▶ BY MOUTH
 ▶ Adult: 100–400 mg once daily

● **IMPORTANT SAFETY INFORMATION**
RISKS OF INCORRECT DOSING OF ORAL ANTI-CANCER MEDICINES
See Cytotoxic drugs p. 787.

● **CAUTIONS** Cardiac disease · history of renal failure · risk factors for heart failure
● **INTERACTIONS** → Appendix 1 (imatinib).
● **SIDE-EFFECTS**
▶ **Common or very common** Abdominal pain · appetite changes · arthralgia · ascites · conjunctivitis · constipation · cough · cramps · diarrhoea · dizziness · dry eyes · dry mouth · dry skin · dyspnoea · epistaxis · fatigue · flatulence · flushing · gastro-oesophageal reflux · haemorrhage · headache · hypoaesthesia · increased lacrimation · influenza-like symptoms · insomnia · oedema · paraesthesia · photosensitivity · pleural effusion · pruritus · pulmonary oedema · rash · sweating · taste disturbance · visual disturbances · weight changes
▶ **Uncommon** Acute respiratory failure · anxiety · cold extremities · cough · depression · drowsiness · dysphagia · electrolyte disturbances · gastric ulceration · gout · gynaecomastia · haematoma · hearing loss · heart failure · hepatic dysfunction · hypertension · hypotension · impaired memory · irregular menstruation · menorrhagia · migraine · palpitation · pancreatitis · peripheral neuropathy · renal failure · sexual dysfunction · skin hyperpigmentation · syncope · tachycardia · tinnitus · tremor · urinary frequency · vertigo
▶ **Rare** Angina · angioedema · arrhythmia · aseptic necrosis of bone · atrial fibrillation · cataract · confusion · convulsions · exfoliative dermatitis · gastro-intestinal perforation · glaucoma · haemolytic anaemia · hepatic failure · hepatic necrosis · increased intracranial pressure · inflammatory bowel disease · intestinal obstruction · myocardial infarction · myopathy · pulmonary fibrosis · pulmonary hypertension · rhabdomyolysis · Stevens-Johnson syndrome
▶ **Frequency not known** Alopecia · bone-marrow suppression · drug rash with eosinophilia and systemic symptoms (DRESS) · growth retardation in children · hyperuricaemia · nausea · oral mucositis · thromboembolism · tumour lysis syndrome · vomiting
● **CONCEPTION AND CONTRACEPTION** Effective contraception required during treatment.
● **PREGNANCY** Manufacturer advises avoid unless potential benefit outweighs risk. See also *Pregnancy and reproductive function* in Cytotoxic drugs p. 787.
● **BREAST FEEDING** Discontinue breast-feeding.

● **HEPATIC IMPAIRMENT** Max. 400 mg daily; reduce dose further if not tolerated.
● **RENAL IMPAIRMENT** Maximum starting dose 400 mg daily if creatinine clearance less than 60 mL/minute; reduce dose further if not tolerated.
● **MONITORING REQUIREMENTS**
▶ Monitor for gastrointestinal haemorrhage.
▶ Monitor complete blood counts regularly.
▶ Monitor for fluid retention.
▶ Monitor liver function.
● **DIRECTIONS FOR ADMINISTRATION** Tablets may be dispersed in water or apple juice.
● **PATIENT AND CARER ADVICE** Patients or carers should be given advice on how to administer imatinib tablets.
● **NATIONAL FUNDING/ACCESS DECISIONS**
 NICE technology appraisals (TAs)
▶ Imatinib for the adjuvant treatment of gastro-intestinal stromal tumours (November 2014) NICE TA326
Imatinib is recommended as an option for adjuvant treatment of adult patients who are at high risk of relapse after surgery for KIT (CD117)-positive gastro-intestinal stromal tumours, as defined by the Miettinen 2006 criteria (based on tumour size, location, and mitotic rate), for up to 3 years.
  Patients currently receiving treatment initiated within the NHS with imatinib that is not recommended for them by NICE in this guidance should be able to continue treatment until they and their NHS clinician consider it appropriate to stop.
www.nice.org.uk/TA326
▶ Dasatinib, nilotinib and standard-dose imatinib for the first-line treatment of chronic myeloid leukaemia (April 2012) NICE TA251
Standard-dose imatinib is recommended as an option for the first-line treatment of adults with chronic phase Philadelphia-chromosome-positive chronic myeloid leukaemia (CML).
www.nice.org.uk/TA251
▶ Imatinib for chronic myeloid leukaemia (October 2003) NICE TA70
Imatinib is recommended as first-line treatment for Philadelphia-chromosome-positive chronic myeloid leukaemia in the chronic phase and as an option for patients presenting in the accelerated phase or with blast crisis, provided that imatinib has not been used previously.
www.nice.org.uk/TA70
▶ Dasatinib, high-dose imatinib and nilotinib for the treatment of imatinib-resistant chronic myeloid leukaemia (CML), and dasatinib and nilotinib for people with CML for whom treatment with imatinib has failed because of intolerance (January 2012) NICE TA241
High-dose imatinib is **not** recommended for the treatment of chronic, accelerated or blast-crisis phase Philadelphia-chromosome-positive CML that is resistant to standard-dose imatinib.
www.nice.org.uk/TA241
▶ Imatinib for the treatment of unresectable and/or metastatic gastro-intestinal stromal tumours (October 2004) NICE TA86
Imatinib 400 mg daily is recommended as first-line management of KIT (CD117)-positive unresectable or metastatic, or both, gastro-intestinal stromal tumours. Continued therapy is recommended only if a response to initial treatment [as defined by Southwest Oncology Group criteria available at www.nice.org.uk/TA86] is achieved within 12 weeks. Patients who have responded should be assessed at 12-week intervals. Discontinue if tumour ceases to respond.
www.nice.org.uk/TA86

▸ **Imatinib for the treatment of unresectable and/or metastatic gastro-intestinal stromal tumours (November 2010)** NICE TA209

Imatinib 600 mg daily or 800 mg daily is **not** recommended for unresectable or metastatic, or both, gastro-intestinal stromal tumours whose disease has progressed after treatment with imatinib 400 mg daily.

www.nice.org.uk/TA209

Scottish Medicines Consortium (SMC) Decisions

The *Scottish Medicines Consortium* has advised (March 2002) that imatinib (*Glivec*®) should be used for chronic myeloid leukaemia only under specialist supervision in accordance with British Society of Haematology guidelines (November 2001).

The *Scottish Medicines Consortium* has also advised (February 2012) that imatinib (*Glivec*®) is accepted for restricted use within NHS Scotland for the treatment of adult patients who are at significant risk of relapse following resection of a KIT (CD117) positive gastrointestinal stromal tumour (GIST) and who are at high risk of recurrence following complete resection (according to the Armed Forces Institute of Pathology (AFIP) risk criteria).

● **MEDICINAL FORMS**
There can be variation in the licensing of different medicines containing the same drug.

Tablet
CAUTIONARY AND ADVISORY LABELS 21, 27
▸ Glivec (Novartis Pharmaceuticals UK Ltd) ▼
Imatinib (as Imatinib mesilate) 100 mg Glivec 100mg tablets | 60 tablet PoM £973.32
Imatinib (as Imatinib mesilate) 400 mg Glivec 400mg tablets | 30 tablet PoM £1,946.67

Lapatinib

● DRUG ACTION Lapatinib is a tyrosine kinase inhibitor.

● **INDICATIONS AND DOSE**

Treatment of advanced or metastatic breast cancer in patients with tumours that overexpress human epidermal growth factor receptor-2 (HER2) with hormone-receptor-negative disease who have had previous treatment with trastuzumab in combination with chemotherapy (in combination with trastuzumab)
▸ BY MOUTH
▸ Adult: 1 g once daily

Treatment of advanced or metastatic breast cancer in patients with tumours that overexpress human epidermal growth factor receptor-2 (HER2), for patients who have had previous treatment with an anthracycline, a taxane, and trastuzumab (in combination with capecitabine)
▸ BY MOUTH
▸ Adult: 1.25 g once daily

Treatment of advanced or metastatic breast cancer with tumours that overexpress human epidermal growth factor receptor-2 (HER2), for postmenopausal women with hormone-receptor-positive disease (in combination with an aromatase inhibitor)
▸ BY MOUTH
▸ Adult: 1.5 g once daily

IMPORTANT SAFETY INFORMATION
RISKS OF INCORRECT DOSING OF ORAL ANTI-CANCER MEDICINES
See Cytotoxic drugs p. 787.

● CAUTIONS Diarrhoea—withhold treatment if severe (consult product literature) · low gastric pH (reduced absorption) · susceptibility to QT-interval prolongation (including electrolyte disturbances)

● INTERACTIONS → Appendix 1 (lapatinib).
Caution with concomitant use of drugs that prolong QT-interval.

● SIDE-EFFECTS
▸ **Common or very common** Anorexia · cardiac failure (fatal cases reported) · decreased left ventricular ejection fraction · diarrhoea (treat promptly) · hepatotoxicity (discontinue permanently if severe) · hyperbilirubinaemia · malaise · nail disorders · rash
▸ **Uncommon** Interstitial lung disease
▸ **Frequency not known** Alopecia · bone-marrow suppression · hyperuricaemia · nausea · oral mucositis · respiratory failure (including fatal cases) · thromboembolism · tumour lysis syndrome · vomiting

● CONCEPTION AND CONTRACEPTION Contraceptive advice required, see *Pregnancy and reproductive function* in Cytotoxic drugs p. 787.

● PREGNANCY Avoid unless potential benefit outweighs risk—toxicity in *animal* studies. See also Pregnancy and reproductive function in Cytotoxic drugs p. 787.

● BREAST FEEDING Discontinue breast-feeding.

● HEPATIC IMPAIRMENT Caution in moderate to severe impairment—metabolism reduced.

● RENAL IMPAIRMENT Caution in severe impairment—no information available.

● MONITORING REQUIREMENTS
▸ Monitor left ventricular function.
▸ Monitor for pulmonary toxicity.
▸ Monitor liver function before treatment and at monthly intervals.

● DIRECTIONS FOR ADMINISTRATION Always take at the same time in relation to food: either one hour before or one hour after food.

● PATIENT AND CARER ADVICE Counselling advised (administration). Patients should be advised to report any unexpected changes in bowel habit.

● NATIONAL FUNDING/ACCESS DECISIONS
NICE technology appraisals (TAs)
▸ **Lapatinib or trastuzumab in combination with an aromatase inhibitor for the first-line treatment of metastatic hormone-receptor-positive breast cancer that overexpresses HER2 (June 2012)** NICE TA257

Lapatinib or trastuzumab in combination with an aromatase inhibitor is **not** recommended for first-line treatment in postmenopausal women of metastatic hormone-receptor-positive breast cancer that overexpresses human epidermal growth factor receptor 2 (HER2).

Postmenopausal women currently receiving lapatinib or trastuzumab in combination with an aromatase inhibitor for this indication should have the option to continue treatment until they and their clinician consider it appropriate to stop.

www.nice.org.uk/TA257

● MEDICINAL FORMS
There can be variation in the licensing of different medicines containing the same drug.

Tablet
▸ Tyverb (Novartis Pharmaceuticals UK Ltd)
Lapatinib ditosylate monohydrate 250 mg Tyverb 250mg tablets | 84 tablet PoM £965.16 | 105 tablet PoM £1,206.45

Nilotinib

- **DRUG ACTION** Nilotinib is a tyrosine kinase inhibitor.

- ● **INDICATIONS AND DOSE**

Treatment of newly diagnosed chronic myeloid leukaemia in the chronic phase
- ▶ BY MOUTH
  - ▸ Adult: 300 mg twice daily

Treatment of chronic and accelerated phase chronic myeloid leukaemia in patients who have resistance to or intolerance of previous therapy, including imatinib
- ▶ BY MOUTH
  - ▸ Adult: 400 mg twice daily

IMPORTANT SAFETY INFORMATION
RISKS OF INCORRECT DOSING OF ORAL ANTI-CANCER MEDICINES
See Cytotoxic drugs p. 787.

- ● **CAUTIONS** History of pancreatitis · susceptibility to QT-interval prolongation (including electrolyte disturbances)
- ● **INTERACTIONS** → Appendix 1 (nilotinib).
  Caution with concomitant use of drugs that prolong QT interval.
- ● **SIDE-EFFECTS**
- ▶ **Common or very common** Abdominal pain · anorexia · arthralgia · asthenia · blood glucose changes · bone pain · constipation · cough · diarrhoea · dizziness · dry skin · dyspepsia · dysphonia · dyspnoea · erythema · fatigue · flatulence · flushing · headache · hyperhidrosis · hyperkalaemia · hypertension · hypomagnesaemia · insomnia · muscle spasm · oedema · palpitation · paraesthesia · pruritus · QT-interval prolongation · rash · urticaria · vertigo · weight changes
- ▶ **Uncommon** Anxiety · arrhythmias · bradycardia · breast pain · cardiac failure · cardiac murmur · cardiomegaly · chest pain · conjunctivitis · coronary artery disease · decreased visual acuity · dehydration · depression · dry eyes · dry mouth · dysuria · ecchymosis · epistaxis · erectile dysfunction · gynaecomastia · haematoma · haemorrhage · hepatitis · hyperaesthesia · hypertensive crisis · hyperthyroidism · hypoaesthesia · hypocalcaemia · hypokalaemia · hyponatraemia · hypophosphataemia · influenza-like symptoms · interstitial lung disease · melaena · migraine · pancreatitis · pericardial effusion · pleural effusion · tremor · urinary frequency
- ▶ **Frequency not known** Alopecia · bone-marrow suppression · hyperuricaemia · nausea · oral mucositis · thromboembolism · tumour lysis syndrome · vomiting
- ● **CONCEPTION AND CONTRACEPTION** Effective contraception required during treatment.
- ● **PREGNANCY** Manufacturer advises avoid unless potential benefit outweighs risk—toxicity in *animal* studies. See also *Pregnancy and reproductive function* in Cytotoxic drugs p. 787.
- ● **BREAST FEEDING** Manufacturer advises avoid—present in milk in *animal* studies.
- ● **HEPATIC IMPAIRMENT** Manufacturer advises caution.
- ● **NATIONAL FUNDING/ACCESS DECISIONS**

NICE technology appraisals (TAs)
- ▶ **Dasatinib, nilotinib and standard-dose imatinib for the first-line treatment of chronic myeloid leukaemia (April 2012)** NICE TA251
Nilotinib is recommended as an option for the first-line treatment of adults with chronic phase Philadelphia-chromosome-positive CML if the manufacturer makes nilotinib available with the discount agreed as part of the patient access scheme.
www.nice.org.uk/TA251

- ▶ **Dasatinib, high-dose imatinib and nilotinib for the treatment of imatinib-resistant chronic myeloid leukaemia (CML), and dasatinib and nilotinib for people with CML for whom treatment with imatinib has failed because of intolerance (January 2012)** NICE TA241
Nilotinib is recommended for the treatment of chronic or accelerated phase Philadelphia-chromosome-positive chronic myeloid leukaemia (CML) in adults:
  - ● whose CML is resistant to treatment with standard dose imatinib, **or**
  - ● who have imatinib intolerance, **and**
  - ● if the manufacturer makes nilotinib available with the discount agreed as part of the patient access scheme.
www.nice.org.uk/TA241

Scottish Medicines Consortium (SMC) Decisions
The *Scottish Medicines Consortium* has advised (February 2008) that nilotinib (*Tasigna*®) is accepted for restricted use within NHS Scotland for the treatment of chronic-phase chronic myeloid leukaemia in adults resistant to or intolerant of at least one previous therapy, including imatinib, and (July 2011) for the treatment of adults with newly diagnosed chronic myeloid leukaemia in the chronic phase.

- ● **MEDICINAL FORMS**
There can be variation in the licensing of different medicines containing the same drug.
Capsule
CAUTIONARY AND ADVISORY LABELS 23, 25, 27
- ▸ Tasigna (Novartis Pharmaceuticals UK Ltd)
  Nilotinib (as Nilotinib hydrochloride monohydrate)
  150 mg Tasigna 150mg capsules | 112 capsule [PoM] £2,432.85
  Nilotinib (as Nilotinib hydrochloride monohydrate)
  200 mg Tasigna 200mg capsules | 112 capsule [PoM] £2,432.85

Pazopanib

- **DRUG ACTION** Pazopanib is a tyrosine kinase inhibitor.

- ● **INDICATIONS AND DOSE**

First-line treatment of advanced renal cell carcinoma | Treatment of advanced renal cell carcinoma in patients who have had previous treatment with cytokine therapy
- ▶ BY MOUTH
  - ▸ Adult: 800 mg daily, adjust dose in steps of 200 mg according to tolerability; maximum 800 mg per day

Treatment of selective subtypes of advanced soft-tissue sarcoma
- ▶ BY MOUTH
  - ▸ Adult: (consult product literature)

IMPORTANT SAFETY INFORMATION
RISKS OF INCORRECT DOSING OF ORAL ANTI-CANCER MEDICINES
See Cytotoxic drugs p. 787.

- ● **CONTRA-INDICATIONS** Cerebral haemorrhage · clinically significant gastro-intestinal haemorrhage · haemoptysis in the past 6 months
- ● **CAUTIONS** Cardiac disease · increased risk of gastro-intestinal fistulas · increased risk of gastro-intestinal perforation · increased risk of haemorrhage · increased risk of thrombotic microangiopathy—permanently discontinue if symptoms develop · ischaemic stroke · myocardial infarction · risk of thrombotic events · susceptibility to QT-interval prolongation (including electrolyte disturbances) · transient ischaemic attack

CAUTIONS, FURTHER INFORMATION
- ▸ Elective surgery Discontinue treatment 7 days before

elective surgery and restart only if adequate wound healing.

▸ Blood pressure Blood pressure must be controlled before initiating treatment.

● INTERACTIONS → Appendix 1 (pazopanib).
Caution with concomitant use of drugs that prolong QT-interval.

● SIDE-EFFECTS

▸ Common or very common Abdominal distension · abdominal pain · anorexia · blood disorders · blurred vision · chest pain · cough · dehydration · diarrhoea · dizziness · dry mouth · dry skin · dyspepsia · dyspnoea · epistaxis · flatulence · flushing · hair discolouration · headache · hepatic dysfunction · hiccups · hyperalbuminaemia · hyperbilirubinaemia · hypertension · hypothyroidism · increased amylase · insomnia · malaise · muscle spasm · myalgia · nail disorders · oedema · paraesthesia · pneumothorax · proteinuria (discontinue if grade 4) · skin discolouration · skin reactions · sweating · taste disturbance · thrombocytopenia · venous thromboembolic events · voice changes · weight loss

▸ Uncommon Arthralgia · bradycardia · cardiac dysfunction · fistula · gastro-intestinal perforation · haemorrhage · hepatic failure · hypertensive crisis · hypomagnesaemia · menstrual disturbances · myocardial infarction · myocardial ischaemia · oropharyngeal pain · pancreatitis · peripheral neuropathy · peritonitis · photosensitivity reactions · pulmonary embolism · QT-interval prolongation · stroke · transient ischaemic attack

▸ Rare Thrombotic microangiopathy

▸ Frequency not known Alopecia · bone-marrow suppression · hyperuricaemia · nausea · oral mucositis · thromboembolism · tumour lysis syndrome · vomiting

● CONCEPTION AND CONTRACEPTION Effective contraception advised during treatment.

● PREGNANCY Avoid unless potential benefit outweighs risk—toxicity in *animal* studies. See also *Pregnancy and reproductive function* in Cytotoxic drugs p. 787.

● BREAST FEEDING Discontinue breast-feeding.

● HEPATIC IMPAIRMENT Reduce dose to 200 mg once daily in moderate impairment. Use with caution in mild to moderate impairment. Avoid in severe impairment.

● RENAL IMPAIRMENT Use with caution if creatinine clearance less than 30 mL/minute—no information available.

● MONITORING REQUIREMENTS

▸ Monitor liver function before treatment and at weeks 3, 5, 7, and 9, then at months 3 and 4, and periodically thereafter as clinically indicated—consult product literature if elevated liver enzymes observed.

▸ Monitor blood pressure within 1 week of treatment initiation, then frequently throughout treatment (consider dose reduction or interruption if hypertension uncontrolled despite anti-hypertensive therapy; discontinue if blood pressure persistently elevated despite anti-hypertensive therapy and pazopanib dose reduction—consult product literature).

▸ Monitor for signs or symptoms of congestive heart failure—monitor left ventricular ejection fraction in patients at risk of heart failure before and during treatment.

▸ Monitor for proteinuria.

▸ Monitor thyroid function.

▸ Monitor for signs and symptoms of posterior reversible encephalopathy syndrome (including headache, hypertension, seizure, lethargy, confusion, visual and neurological disturbances)—permanently discontinue treatment if symptoms occur.

● PATIENT AND CARER ADVICE Patients should be advised not to take antacids for at least 1 hour before or 2 hours after pazopanib.

● NATIONAL FUNDING/ACCESS DECISIONS

NICE technology appraisals (TAs)

▸ Pazopanib for the first-line treatment of advanced renal cell carcinoma (updated August 2013) NICE TA215
Pazopanib is recommended as a first-line treatment option for people with advanced renal cell carcinoma:
● who have not received prior cytokine therapy and have an Eastern Cooperative Oncology Group performance status of 0 or 1 **and**
● if the manufacturer provides pazopanib at the discounted price agreed under the patient access scheme.
www.nice.org.uk/TA215

Scottish Medicines Consortium (SMC) Decisions
The *Scottish Medicines Consortium* has advised (February 2011) that pazopanib (*Votrient*®) is accepted for restricted use within NHS Scotland for the first-line treatment of advanced renal cell carcinoma and (December 2012) is **not** recommended for use within NHS Scotland for the treatment of selective subtypes of advanced soft tissue sarcoma in patients who have received prior chemotherapy for metastatic disease, or who have progressed within 12 months after neoadjuvant therapy.

● MEDICINAL FORMS
There can be variation in the licensing of different medicines containing the same drug.

Tablet
CAUTIONARY AND ADVISORY LABELS 23, 25
▸ Votrient (Novartis Pharmaceuticals UK Ltd)
Pazopanib (as Pazopanib hydrochloride) 200 mg Votrient 200mg tablets | 30 tablet [PoM] £560.50
Pazopanib (as Pazopanib hydrochloride) 400 mg Votrient 400mg tablets | 30 tablet [PoM] £1,121.00

Ponatinib

● INDICATIONS AND DOSE

Treatment of chronic, accelerated, or blast phase chronic myeloid leukaemia in patients who have the T315I mutation or who have resistance to or intolerance of dasatinib or nilotinib, and for whom subsequent treatment with imatinib is not clinically appropriate | Treatment of Philadelphia chromosome-positive acute lymphoblastic leukaemia in patients who have the T315I mutation or who have resistance to or intolerance of dasatinib, and for whom subsequent treatment with imatinib is not clinically appropriate

▸ BY MOUTH

▸ Adult: 45 mg once daily, for dose adjustment due to side effects—consult product literature

DOSE ADJUSTMENTS DUE TO INTERACTIONS
Consider reducing the initial dose to 30 mg once daily with concomitant use of potent inhibitors of cytochrome P450 enzyme CYP3A4 (e.g. clarithromycin, indinavir, itraconazole, ritonavir, saquinavir, telithromycin or voriconazole).

IMPORTANT SAFETY INFORMATION
MHRA/CHM ADVICE: PONATINIB: RISK OF VASCULAR OCCLUSIVE EVENTS (NOVEMBER 2014)
The benefits and risks of ponatinib have been reviewed by the European Medicines Agency's Committee on Medicinal Products for Human Use, which has recommended that strengthened warnings should be added to the product information aimed at minimising the risk of blood clots and blockages in the arteries. The review concluded that available evidence shows that the

risk of blood vessel blockage with ponatinib is likely to be dose-dependent. However, the data is insufficient to recommend reducing the dose of ponatinib, and there is a risk that a lower dose might not be as effective as the current dose in all patients and in long-term treatment. Therefore, no change has been made to the recommended starting dose.

Prescribers may wish to consider reducing the dose in patients with chronic phase chronic myeloid leukaemia who are responding well to treatment, and who might be at high risk of blood vessel blockage. Stop ponatinib if a complete response has not occurred within 3 months of treatment, and monitor patients for high blood pressure or signs of heart problems.

RISKS OF INCORRECT DOSING OF ORAL ANTI-CANCER MEDICINES
See Cytotoxic drugs p. 787.

● CAUTIONS Alcohol abuse—increased risk of pancreatitis · current severe hypertriglyceridaemia—increased risk of pancreatitis · discontinue treatment if a complete haematologic response has not occurred within 3 months · history of myocardial infarction—do not use unless potential benefit outweighs potential risk · history of pancreatitis · history of stroke—do not use unless potential benefit outweighs potential risk · hypertension—medically control during treatment and interrupt treatment if uncontrolled

CAUTIONS, FURTHER INFORMATION
▸ Cardiovascular status Assess cardiovascular status before treatment—manage cardiovascular risk factors before and during treatment.

● INTERACTIONS → Appendix 1 (ponatinib).
● SIDE-EFFECTS
▸ **Common or very common** Abdominal discomfort · altered sensations · arthralgia · atrial fibrillation · biochemistry disturbances · blurred vision · bruising · cardiac disorders · cardiac events · cerebrovascular events · constipation · cough · decreased appetite · dehydration · diarrhoea · dizziness · dry eyes · dry mouth · dry skin · dyspepsia · dysphonia · dyspnoea · electrolyte disturbances · epistaxis · erectile dysfunction · exfoliative dermatitis · flushing · gastro-oesophageal reflux disease · headache · hyperhidrosis · hypertension · infection · insomnia · intermittent claudication · malaise · muscle spasms · musculoskeletal pain · oedema · pancreatitis · pericardial effusion · peripheral neuropathy · pleural effusion · pruritus · pyrexia · rash · thromboembolic events · vascular occlusion · weight loss
▸ **Uncommon** Atrial flutter · cerebral artery stenosis · cerebral infarction · gastric haemorrhage · hepatotoxicity · jaundice · retinal vein occlusion · retinal vein thrombosis · visual impairment
▸ **Frequency not known** Alopecia · bone-marrow suppression · hyperuricaemia · nausea · oral mucositis · thromboembolism · tumour lysis syndrome · vomiting

● CONCEPTION AND CONTRACEPTION Ensure effective contraception during treatment in men and women; effectiveness of hormonal contraception unknown—alternative or additional methods of contraception should be used.
● PREGNANCY Avoid—toxicity in *animal* studies. See also *Pregnancy and reproductive function* in Cytotoxic drugs p. 787.
● BREAST FEEDING Manufacturer advises discontinue breastfeeding—no information available.
● HEPATIC IMPAIRMENT Manufacturer advises caution in severe impairment.
● RENAL IMPAIRMENT No information available—manufacturer advises caution if creatinine clearance less than 50 mL/minute.

● MONITORING REQUIREMENTS
▸ Monitor serum lipase every 2 weeks for the first 2 months and periodically thereafter for all patients—withhold treatment if lipase elevated and abdominal symptoms occur.
▸ Monitor full blood count every 2 weeks for the first 3 months and then monthly thereafter or as clinically indicated.
▸ Monitor liver function periodically.
▸ Monitor for vascular occlusion or thromboembolism—interrupt treatment immediately if this occurs.

● MEDICINAL FORMS
There can be variation in the licensing of different medicines containing the same drug.
Tablet
CAUTIONARY AND ADVISORY LABELS 3, 25
▸ Iclusig (Ariad Pharma (UK) Ltd) ▼
  Ponatinib (as Ponatinib hydrochloride) 15 mg Iclusig 15mg tablets
  | 60 tablet [PoM] £5,050.00
  Ponatinib (as Ponatinib hydrochloride) 45 mg Iclusig 45mg tablets | 30 tablet [PoM] £5,050.00

Regorafenib

● DRUG ACTION Regorafenib is an inhibitor of several protein kinases.

● INDICATIONS AND DOSE
Treatment of metastatic colorectal cancer in patients who have previously been treated with, or who are unsuitable for standard treatment including fluoropyrimidine-based chemotherapy, a vascular endothelial growth factor inhibitor, and an epidermal growth factor receptor inhibitor | Treatment of unresectable or metastatic gastrointestinal stromal tumours in patients who progressed on or are intolerant to previous treatment with imatinib and sunitinib.
▸ BY MOUTH
▸ Adult: 160 mg once daily for 21 consecutive days of repeated 28-day cycles, for dose adjustment due to side effects—consult product literature

IMPORTANT SAFETY INFORMATION
RISKS OF INCORRECT DOSING OF ORAL ANTI-CANCER MEDICINES
See Cytotoxic drugs p. 787.

● CAUTIONS Ensure measures to prevent hand-foot skin reaction · Gilbert's syndrome—risk of hyperbilirubinaemia · history of ischaemic heart disease—monitor for signs and symptoms of myocardial ischaemia and interrupt treatment if signs of ischaemia or infarction develop · hypertension—control blood pressure before treatment initiation and monitor as clinically indicated during treatment (review dose and consider treatment interruption if severe or persistent hypertension develops; discontinue treatment if hypertensive crisis occurs) · may impair wound healing— withhold treatment for major surgical procedures · predisposition to bleeding
● INTERACTIONS → Appendix 1 (regorafenib).
Caution in concomitant treatment with drugs that may increase the risk of bleeding (increased risk of haemorrhagic events).
● SIDE-EFFECTS
▸ **Common or very common** Abnormal international normalised ratio · biochemical disturbances · decreased appetite · diarrhoea · dry mouth · dry skin · dysphonia · electrolyte disturbances · gastro-enteritis · gastro-oesophageal reflux · haemorrhage (including fatal) · hand-foot skin reaction · headache · hypertension · hypothyroidism · infection · malaise · mucosal

8

inflammation · musculoskeletal stiffness · nail disorder · pain · pyrexia · rash · taste disorders · tremor · weight loss
▸ **Uncommon** Gastro-intestinal perforation (including fatal cases) and fistula—discontinue treatment · hypertensive crisis · myocardial infarction · myocardial ischaemia · severe (including fatal) liver injury
▸ **Rare** Keratoacanthoma · posterior reversible encephalopathy syndrome · squamous cell carcinoma of the skin · Stevens-Johnson syndrome · toxic epidermal necrolysis
▸ **Frequency not known** Alopecia · bone-marrow suppression · hyperuricaemia · nausea · oral mucositis · thromboembolism · tumour lysis syndrome · vomiting
SIDE-EFFECTS, FURTHER INFORMATION
▸ **Hand-foot skin reaction** Consult product literature if signs or symptoms develop.
● **CONCEPTION AND CONTRACEPTION** Women of childbearing potential and men must use effective contraception during treatment and up to 8 weeks after last dose.
● **PREGNANCY** Manufacturer advises avoid unless potential benefit outweighs risk—toxicity in *animal* studies. See also *Pregnancy and reproductive function* in Cytotoxic drugs p. 787.
● **BREAST FEEDING** Avoid—present in milk in *animal* studies.
● **HEPATIC IMPAIRMENT** Manufacturer advises caution in moderate impairment. Avoid in severe impairment.
● **RENAL IMPAIRMENT** Caution in severe impairment—no information available.
● **MONITORING REQUIREMENTS**
▸ Monitor blood count and coagulation parameters and consider permanent discontinuation in event of severe bleeding.
▸ Monitor hepatic function before treatment, then at least every two weeks for the first 2 months, then at least monthly thereafter and as clinically indicated—consult product literature if changes in liver function observed.
▸ Monitor for signs and symptoms of posterior reversible encephalopathy syndrome (including seizure, headache, altered mental status, visual disturbances or cortical blindness, with or without hypertension)—discontinue treatment if symptoms occur.
▸ Monitor biochemical, electrolyte and metabolic parameters during treatment; ensure measures to prevent hand-foot skin reaction—consult product literature if signs or symptoms develop.
● **DIRECTIONS FOR ADMINISTRATION** Tablets should be taken at the same time each day, swallowed whole with water after a light meal that contains less than 30% fat.
● **PATIENT AND CARER ADVICE** Counselling advised (administration).

● **MEDICINAL FORMS**
There can be variation in the licensing of different medicines containing the same drug.
Tablet
CAUTIONARY AND ADVISORY LABELS 21
ELECTROLYTES: May contain Sodium
▸ Stivarga (Bayer Plc) ▼
Regorafenib 40 mg Stivarga 40mg tablets | 84 tablet [PoM] £3,744.00 (Hospital only)

Ruxolitinib
2.6.2016

● **DRUG ACTION** Ruxolitinib is a selective inhibitor of the Janus-associated tyrosine kinases JAK1 and JAK2.

● **INDICATIONS AND DOSE**

Treatment of disease-related splenomegaly or symptoms in patients with primary myelofibrosis, post-polycythaemia vera myelofibrosis, or post-essential thrombocythaemia myelofibrosis
▸ BY MOUTH
▸ **Adult:** (consult product literature or local protocols)

IMPORTANT SAFETY INFORMATION
RISKS OF INCORRECT DOSING OF ORAL ANTI-CANCER MEDICINES
See Cytotoxic drugs p. 787.

● **CAUTIONS** Assess risk of developing infection before treatment—do not initiate until active serious infections are resolved
CAUTIONS, FURTHER INFORMATION
▸ **Tuberculosis** Patients should be evaluated for latent and active tuberculosis before starting treatment and monitored for signs and symptoms of tuberculosis during treatment.
● **INTERACTIONS** → Appendix 1 (ruxolitinib).
● **SIDE-EFFECTS**
▸ **Common or very common** Dizziness · flatulence · headache · hypercholesterolaemia · weight gain
▸ **Uncommon** Tuberculosis
▸ **Frequency not known** Alopecia · bone-marrow suppression · hyperuricaemia · nausea · oral mucositis · progressive multifocal leucoencephalopathy · thromboembolism · tumour lysis syndrome · vomiting
● **CONCEPTION AND CONTRACEPTION** Contraceptive advice required, see *Pregnancy and reproductive function* in Cytotoxic drugs p. 787.
● **PREGNANCY** Avoid—toxicity in *animal* studies.
● **BREAST FEEDING** Avoid—present in milk in *animal* studies.
● **HEPATIC IMPAIRMENT** Reduce dose (consult product literature).
● **RENAL IMPAIRMENT** Reduce dose in severe impairment (consult product literature).
● **MONITORING REQUIREMENTS**
▸ Monitor full blood count (including differential white cell count) before treatment, then every 2–4 weeks until dose stabilised, then as clinically indicated.
▸ Monitor for infection during treatment.
▸ Monitor for symptoms of progressive multifocal leucoencephalopathy (presenting as new or worsening neurological, cognitive or psychiatric signs or symptoms)—withhold treatment if suspected.
● **NATIONAL FUNDING/ACCESS DECISIONS**
NICE technology appraisals (TAs)
▸ **Ruxolitinib for treating disease-related splenomegaly or symptoms in adults with myelofibrosis (March 2016)**
NICE TA386
Ruxolitinib is recommended as an option for treating disease-related splenomegaly or symptoms in patients with primary myelofibrosis (also known as chronic idiopathic myelofibrosis), post polycythaemia vera myelofibrosis or post essential thrombocythaemia myelofibrosis, only if the patient has intermediate-2 or high-risk disease, **and** if the manufacturer provides ruxolitinib with the discount agreed in the patient access scheme.
    Patients currently receiving ruxolitinib whose disease does not meet the above criteria should have the option to continue their treatment until they and their clinician consider it appropriate to stop.
www.nice.org.uk/TA386

- MEDICINAL FORMS
There can be variation in the licensing of different medicines containing the same drug.
Tablet
▸ Jakavi (Novartis Pharmaceuticals UK Ltd) ▼
  Ruxolitinib (as Ruxolitinib phosphate) 5 mg Jakavi 5mg tablets | 56 tablet [PoM] £1,428.00
  Ruxolitinib (as Ruxolitinib phosphate) 10 mg Jakavi 10mg tablets | 56 tablet [PoM] £2,856.00
  Ruxolitinib (as Ruxolitinib phosphate) 15 mg Jakavi 15mg tablets | 56 tablet [PoM] £2,856.00
  Ruxolitinib (as Ruxolitinib phosphate) 20 mg Jakavi 20mg tablets | 56 tablet [PoM] £2,856.00

Sorafenib

27.5.2016

- DRUG ACTION Sorafenib is an inhibitor of multiple kinases.

  - INDICATIONS AND DOSE

  Treatment of advanced renal cell carcinoma when treatment with interferon alfa or interleukin-2 has failed or is unsuitable | Treatment of progressive, locally advanced, or metastatic, differentiated thyroid carcinoma that is refractory to radioactive iodine | Treatment of hepatocellular carcinoma
  ▸ BY MOUTH
  ▸ Adult: 400 mg twice daily, for dose adjustments due to side effects, consult product literature

  IMPORTANT SAFETY INFORMATION
  RISKS OF INCORRECT DOSING OF ORAL ANTI-CANCER MEDICINES
  See Cytotoxic drugs p. 787.

- CAUTIONS Cardiac ischaemia · major surgical procedures · potential risk of bleeding—treat tracheal, bronchial, or oesophageal infiltration with localised therapy before initiating sorafenib in patients with differentiated thyroid carcinoma (DTC) and consider permanent withdrawal of sorafenib in any patient that requires medical intervention for bleeding · susceptibility to QT-interval prolongation
- INTERACTIONS → Appendix 1 (sorafenib).
- SIDE-EFFECTS
▸ **Common or very common** Acne · anorexia · arthralgia · asthenia · congestive heart failure · constipation · depression · dermatitis · desquamation · diarrhoea · dry skin · dysgeusia · dyspepsia · dysphagia · dysphonia · electrolyte disturbances · erectile dysfunction · erythema · fatigue · fever · flushing · gastro-oesophageal reflux disease · haemorrhage · hand-foot skin reaction · hoarseness · hyperkeratosis · hypertension · hypophosphataemia · hypophosphataemia · keratoacanthoma · malaise · muscle spasms · myalgia · myocardial infarction · myocardial ischaemia · peripheral neuropathy · proteinuria · pruritus · rash · renal failure · rhinorrhoea · thyroid dysfunction · tinnitus
▸ **Uncommon** Altered INR · altered prothrombin time · cholangitis · cholecystitis · dehydration · eczema · erythema multiforme · gastritis · gastro-intestinal perforations · gynaecomastia · hypertensive crisis · interstitial lung disease-like events · pancreatitis · posterior reversible encephalopathy syndrome
▸ **Rare** Hepatitis · leucocytoclastic vasculitis · nephrotic syndrome · QT-interval prolongation · rhabdomyolysis · Stevens-Johnson syndrome · toxic epidermal necrolysis
▸ **Frequency not known** Alopecia · bone-marrow suppression · hyperuricaemia · nausea · oral mucositis · thromboembolism · tumour lysis syndrome · vomiting
- CONCEPTION AND CONTRACEPTION Contraceptive advice required, see *Pregnancy and reproductive function* in Cytotoxic drugs p. 787.

- PREGNANCY Manufacturer advises avoid unless essential—toxicity in *animal* studies. See also *Pregnancy and reproductive function* in Cytotoxic drugs p. 787.
- BREAST FEEDING Discontinue breast-feeding.
- HEPATIC IMPAIRMENT Manufacturer advises caution in severe impairment—no information available.
- MONITORING REQUIREMENTS
▸ Consider periodic monitoring of ECG and electrolytes in patients susceptible to QT-interval prolongation.
▸ Monitor blood pressure regularly and consider permanent discontinuation of sorafenib if resistant to antihypertensive therapy.
▸ Monitor plasma-calcium concentration (increased risk of hypocalcaemia if history of hypoparathyroidism).
▸ Monitor thyroid stimulating hormone in patients with differentiated thyroid carcinoma.
- NATIONAL FUNDING/ACCESS DECISIONS

  NICE technology appraisals (TAs)
  ▸ Sorafenib for the treatment of advanced hepatocellular carcinoma (May 2010) NICE TA189
  Sorafenib is **not** recommended for the treatment of advanced hepatocellular carcinoma in patients for whom surgical or locoregional therapies have failed or are unsuitable.
  www.nice.org.uk/TA189
  ▸ Bevacizumab (first-line), sorafenib (first- and second-line), sunitinib (second-line) and temsirolimus (first-line) for the treatment of advanced or metastatic renal cell carcinoma (August 2009) NICE TA178
  Bevacizumab, sorafenib, and temsirolimus are **not** recommended as first-line treatments for people with advanced or metastatic renal cell carcinoma.
  Sorafenib and sunitinib are not recommended as second-line treatments for people with advanced or metastatic renal cell carcinoma.
  www.nice.org.uk/TA178

  Scottish Medicines Consortium (SMC) Decisions
  The *Scottish Medicines Consortium* has advised (January 2016) that sorafenib (*Nexavar*®) is accepted for restricted use within NHS Scotland for the treatment of advanced hepatocellular carcinoma in patients where surgical or loco-regional therapies have failed or are unsuitable.

- MEDICINAL FORMS
There can be variation in the licensing of different medicines containing the same drug.
Tablet
CAUTIONARY AND ADVISORY LABELS 23
▸ Nexavar (Bayer Plc)
  Sorafenib (as Sorafenib tosylate) 200 mg Nexavar 200mg tablets | 112 tablet [PoM] £3,576.56

Sunitinib

- DRUG ACTION Sunitinib is a tyrosine kinase inhibitor.

  - INDICATIONS AND DOSE

  Treatment of unresectable or metastatic malignant gastro-intestinal stromal tumours, after failure of imatinib | Treatment of advanced or metastatic renal cell carcinoma
  ▸ BY MOUTH
  ▸ Adult: 50 mg once daily for 4 weeks, followed by a 2-week treatment-free period to complete 6-week cycle, adjusted in steps of 12.5 mg, doses adjusted according to tolerability; usual dose 25–75 mg daily
  continued →

8

Immune system and malignant disease

Treatment of unresectable or metastatic pancreatic neuroendocrine tumours

▸ BY MOUTH

▸ Adult: 37.5 mg once daily without treatment-free period; adjusted in steps of 12.5 mg, doses adjusted according to tolerability; maximum 50 mg per day

---

IMPORTANT SAFETY INFORMATION

RISK OF OSTEONECROSIS OF THE JAW (JANUARY 2011)

Treatment with sunitinib may be a risk factor for the development of osteonecrosis of the jaw.

Patients treated with sunitinib, who have previously received bisphosphonates, or are treated concurrently with bisphosphonates, may be particularly at risk.

Dental examination and appropriate preventive dentistry should be considered before treatment with sunitinib.

If possible, invasive dental procedures should be avoided in patients treated with sunitinib who have previously received, or who are currently receiving, intravenous bisphosphonates.

RISKS OF INCORRECT DOSING OF ORAL ANTI-CANCER MEDICINES

See Cytotoxic drugs p. 787.

● CAUTIONS Cardiovascular disease—discontinue if congestive heart failure develops · hypertension · increased risk of bleeding · susceptibility to QT-interval prolongation

● INTERACTIONS → Appendix 1 (sunitinib).

● SIDE-EFFECTS

▸ **Rare** Nephrotic syndrome

▸ **Frequency not known** Abdominal pain · alopecia · anorexia · arthralgia · bone-marrow suppression · constipation · cough · dehydration · diarrhoea · dizziness · dry skin · dyspnoea · epistaxis · fatigue · fistula formation (interrupt treatment if occurs) · gastro-intestinal perforation · hair discoloration · hand-foot syndrome · headache · hepatic failure · hypertension · hyperuricaemia · hypothyroidism · increased lacrimation · insomnia · myalgia · nausea · oedema · oral mucositis · osteonecrosis of the jaw · pancreatitis · paraesthesia · peripheral neuropathy · proteinuria · rash · seizures · skin discoloration · taste disturbance · thromboembolism · tumour lysis syndrome · urine discoloration · vomiting

● CONCEPTION AND CONTRACEPTION Effective contraception required during treatment.

● PREGNANCY Manufacturer advises avoid unless potential benefit outweighs risk—toxicity in *animal* studies. See also *Pregnancy and reproductive function* in Cytotoxic drugs p. 787.

● BREAST FEEDING Discontinue breast-feeding.

● MONITORING REQUIREMENTS Monitor for thyroid dysfunction.

● NATIONAL FUNDING/ACCESS DECISIONS

NICE technology appraisals (TAs)

▸ **Sunitinib for advanced or metastatic renal cell carcinoma (March 2009)** NICE TA169

Sunitinib is recommended as first-line treatment for advanced or metastatic renal cell carcinoma in patients who are suitable for immunotherapy and have an Eastern Cooperative Oncology Group performance status of 0 or 1.
www.nice.org.uk/TA169

▸ **Sunitinib for the treatment of gastrointestinal stromal tumours (September 2009)** NICE TA179

Sunitinib is recommended as an option for treatment in patients with unresectable or metastatic gastrointestinal tumours if imatinib treatment has failed because of resistance or intolerance, and the cost of sunitinib for the first treatment cycle is met by the manufacturer.
www.nice.org.uk/TA179

▸ Bevacizumab (first-line), sorafenib (first- and second-line), sunitinib (second-line) and temsirolimus (first-line) for the treatment of advanced or metastatic renal cell carcinoma (August 2009) NICE TA178

Sorafenib and sunitinib are not recommended as second-line treatments for people with advanced or metastatic renal cell carcinoma.
www.nice.org.uk/TA178

Scottish Medicines Consortium (SMC) Decisions

The *Scottish Medicines Consortium* has advised (October 2009 and April 2011) that sunitinib (*Sutent ®*) is accepted for restricted use within NHS Scotland for the treatment of unresectable or metastatic malignant gastro-intestinal stromal tumours after failure of imatinib and for unresectable or metastatic pancreatic neuroendocrine tumours.

● MEDICINAL FORMS
There can be variation in the licensing of different medicines containing the same drug.

Capsule

CAUTIONARY AND ADVISORY LABELS 14

▸ Sutent (Pfizer Ltd)

Sunitinib (as Sunitinib malate) 12.5 mg Sutent 12.5mg capsules | 28 capsule [PoM] £784.70

Sunitinib (as Sunitinib malate) 25 mg Sutent 25mg capsules | 28 capsule [PoM] £1,569.40

Sunitinib (as Sunitinib malate) 50 mg Sutent 50mg capsules | 28 capsule [PoM] £3,138.80

Temsirolimus

● DRUG ACTION Temsirolimus is a protein kinase inhibitor.

● INDICATIONS AND DOSE

First-line treatment of advanced renal cell carcinoma | Treatment of relapsed or refractory mantle cell lymphoma

▸ BY INTRAVENOUS INFUSION

▸ Adult: (consult product literature or local protocols)

● INTERACTIONS → Appendix 1 (temsirolimus).
The main active metabolite of temsirolimus is sirolimus—*see also* interactions of sirolimus and consult product literature.

● SIDE-EFFECTS

▸ **Common or very common** Abdominal pain · acne · anorexia · anxiety · arthralgia · asthenia · bowel perforation · chest pain · cough · depression · diarrhoea · dizziness · drowsiness · dysphagia · dyspnoea · epistaxis · eye disorders · folliculitis · gastro-intestinal haemorrhage · hypercholesterolaemia · hyperglycaemia · hyperlipidaemia · hypersensitivity reactions · hypertension · hypokalaemia · hypophosphataemia · impaired wound healing · increased susceptibility to infection · increased susceptibility to pneumonia · increased susceptibility to urinary-tract infection · insomnia · interstitial lung disease · myalgia · oedema · paraesthesia · pyrexia · rash · renal failure · rhinitis · skin disorders · taste disturbance · thrombophlebitis · thrombosis

▸ **Uncommon** Intracerebral bleeding

▸ **Frequency not known** Alopecia · bone-marrow suppression · extravasation · hyperuricaemia · nausea · oral mucositis · thromboembolism · tumour lysis syndrome · vomiting

SIDE-EFFECTS, FURTHER INFORMATION

▸ Hypersensitivity reactions Hypersensitivity reactions, including some life-threatening and rare fatal reactions, are associated with temsirolimus therapy, usually during administration of the first dose. Symptoms include flushing, chest pain, dyspnoea, apnoea, hypotension, loss of consciousness, and anaphylaxis. Where possible, patients should receive an intravenous dose of antihistamine 30 minutes before starting the temsirolimus infusion. The infusion may have to be stopped temporarily for the treatment of infusion-related effects—consult product literature for appropriate management. If adverse reactions are not managed with dose delays, a dose reduction should be considered—consult product literature.

- CONCEPTION AND CONTRACEPTION Ensure effective contraception during treatment in men and women.
- PREGNANCY Manufacturer advises avoid (toxicity in *animal* studies). See also *Pregnancy and reproductive function* in Cytotoxic drugs p. 787.
- BREAST-FEEDING Manufacturer advises discontinue breast-feeding.
- HEPATIC IMPAIRMENT In renal cell carcinoma, reduce dose in severe impairment (consult product literature). Use with caution.
  In mantle cell lymphoma, avoid in moderate or severe impairment.
- RENAL IMPAIRMENT Manufacturer advises caution in severe impairment—no information available.
- MONITORING REQUIREMENTS
- ▶ Monitor respiratory function.
- ▶ Monitor blood lipids.
- NATIONAL FUNDING/ACCESS DECISIONS
  NICE technology appraisals (TAs)
- ▶ **Bevacizumab (first-line), sorafenib (first- and second-line), sunitinib (second-line) and temsirolimus (first-line) for the treatment of advanced or metastatic renal cell carcinoma (August 2009)** NICE TA178
  Bevacizumab, sorafenib, and temsirolimus are **not** recommended as first-line treatments for people with advanced or metastatic renal cell carcinoma.
  www.nice.org.uk/TA178

- MEDICINAL FORMS
  There can be variation in the licensing of different medicines containing the same drug.
  Solution for infusion
  EXCIPIENTS: May contain Ethanol, propylene glycol
  ▶ Torisel (Pfizer Ltd)
    Temsirolimus 25 mg per 1 ml Torisel 30mg/1.2ml concentrate for solution for infusion vials and diluent | 1 vial [PoM] £620.00 (Hospital only)

Vandetanib

- DRUG ACTION Vandetanib is a tyrosine kinase inhibitor.

● INDICATIONS AND DOSE

Treatment of aggressive and symptomatic medullary thyroid cancer in patients with unresectable locally advanced or metastatic disease
- ▶ BY MOUTH
- ▶ Adult: 300 mg once daily, for dose adjustment due to side effects—consult product literature

IMPORTANT SAFETY INFORMATION
RISKS OF INCORRECT DOSING OF ORAL ANTI-CANCER MEDICINES
See Cytotoxic drugs p. 787.

- CONTRA-INDICATIONS Congenital long QT syndrome · QT interval greater than 480 milliseconds
- CAUTIONS Brain metastases (intracranial haemorrhage reported) · electrolyte disturbances · history of torsades de pointes · hypertension · phototoxicity reactions reported (wear protective clothing and/or sunscreen) · susceptibility to QT-prolongation
- INTERACTIONS → Appendix 1 (vandetanib).
  Caution with concomitant use of drugs that prolong QT interval.

- ▷ SIDE-EFFECTS
- ▶ **Common or very common** Abdominal pain · alopecia · anxiety · asthenia · balance disorders · blurred vision · cholelithiasis · colitis · conjunctivitis · constipation · corneal changes (including opacity) · corneal deposits · decreased appetite · dehydration · depression · diarrhoea · dizziness · dry eye · dry mouth · dysaesthesia · dyspepsia · dysphagia · dysuria · electrolyte disturbances · epistaxis · gastritis · gastrointestinal haemorrhage · glaucoma · haematuria · haemoptysis · halo vision · hand-foot syndrome · headache · hyperglycaemia · hypertension · hypothyroidism · insomnia · ischaemic cerebrovascular conditions · keratopathy · lethargy · loss of consciousness · micturition urgency · nephrolithiasis · oedema · pain · paraesthesia · photopsia · photosensitivivity reactions · pneumonitis · pollakiuria · proteinuria · pyrexia · QT-interval prolongation · taste disturbance · tremor
- ▶ **Uncommon** Accommodation disorders · anuria · aspiration pneumonia · brain oedema · bullous dermatitis · cardiac arrest · cardiac conduction disorders · cardiac rate disorders · cardiac rhythm disorders · cataract · chromaturia · clonus · convulsions · erythema multiforme · faecal incontinence · heart failure · ileus · impaired healing · increased haemoglobin · interstitial lung disease (sometimes fatal) · intestinal perforation · pancreatitis · peritonitis · posterior reversible encephalopathy syndrome · respiratory failure · Stevens-Johnson syndrome · ventricular arrhythmia
- ▶ **Frequency not known** Alopecia · bone-marrow suppression · hyperuricaemia · nausea · oral mucositis · thromboembolism · tumour lysis syndrome · vomiting
- CONCEPTION AND CONTRACEPTION Effective contraception required during and for at least 4 months after treatment.
- PREGNANCY Manufacturer advises avoid unless potential benefit outweighs risk. Most cytotoxic drugs are teratogenic and should not be administered during pregnancy, especially during the first trimester. Considerable caution is necessary if a pregnant woman presents with cancer requiring chemotherapy, and specialist advice should always be sought.
- BREAST-FEEDING Avoid—no information available.
- HEPATIC IMPAIRMENT Manufacturer advises avoid in severe impairment (serum bilirubin greater than 1.5 times the upper limit of normal).
- RENAL IMPAIRMENT Reduce dose to 200 mg if creatinine clearance 30–49 mL/minute. Avoid if creatinine clearance less than 30 mL/minute.
- MONITORING REQUIREMENTS Monitor ECG, serum potassium, calcium, magnesium and thyroid stimulating hormone before treatment, then 1, 3, 6 and 12 weeks after starting treatment and following dose adjustment or interruption, then every 3 months for at least 1 year.
- DIRECTIONS FOR ADMINISTRATION Tablets may be dispersed in half a glass of water by stirring until dispersed (approximately 10 minutes), immediately before drinking (do not crush). After solution has been swallowed, any residue must be re-dispersed in the same volume of water and swallowed. The solution can also be administered via nasogastric or gastrostomy tubes.
- PATIENT AND CARER ADVICE Alert card should be provided. Patients or carers should be given advice on how to administer vandetanib tablets.
  Phototoxicity reactions Patients should be advised to wear protective clothing and/or sunscreen.

8

Immune system and malignant disease

● MEDICINAL FORMS
There can be variation in the licensing of different medicines containing the same drug.

Tablet
▸ Caprelsa (AstraZeneca UK Ltd) ▼
Vandetanib 100 mg Caprelsa 100mg tablets | 30 tablet PoM £2,500.00
Vandetanib 300 mg Caprelsa 300mg tablets | 30 tablet PoM £5,000.00

Vemurafenib

● DRUG ACTION Vemurafenib is a BRAF kinase inhibitor.

● INDICATIONS AND DOSE

Monotherapy for the treatment of BRAF V600 mutation-positive unresectable or metastatic melanoma
▸ BY MOUTH
▸ Adult: 960 mg twice daily, for dose adjustment due to side effects—consult product literature

IMPORTANT SAFETY INFORMATION
DRUG RASH WITH EOSINOPHILIA AND SYSTEMIC SYMPTOMS (DRESS SYNDROME)
DRESS syndrome has been reported in patients taking vemurafenib. DRESS syndrome starts with rash, fever, swollen glands, and increased white cell count, and it can affect the liver, kidneys and lungs; DRESS can also be fatal.
Patients should be advised to stop taking vemurafenib and consult their doctor immediately if skin rash develops. Treatment with vemurafenib should not be restarted.

MHRA/CHM ADVICE (NOVEMBER 2015): RISK OF POTENTIATION OF RADIATION TOXICITY
Potentiation of radiation toxicity has been reported in patients treated with vemurafenib before, during, or after radiotherapy— use with caution.

RISKS OF INCORRECT DOSING OF ORAL ANTI-CANCER MEDICINES
See Cytotoxic drugs p. 787.

● CONTRA-INDICATIONS Wild-type BRAF malignant melanoma

● CAUTIONS Electrolyte disturbances · prior or concurrent cancer associated with RAS mutation—increased risk of tumour progression · susceptibility to QT-prolongation

● INTERACTIONS → Appendix 1 (vemurafenib). Caution with concomitant use of drugs that prolong QT interval.

● SIDE-EFFECTS
▸ **Common or very common** Actinic keratosis · alopecia · arthralgia · arthritis · asthenia · basal cell carcinoma · Bell's palsy · constipation · cough · cutaneous squamous cell carcinoma · decreased appetite · diarrhoea · dizziness · dry skin · erythema · erythema nodosum · fatigue · folliculitis · hand-foot syndrome · headache · hyperkeratosis · keratosis pilaris · musculoskeletal pain · myalgia · new primary melanoma · pain in extremities · peripheral oedema · photosensitivity reactions · pyrexia · QT-interval prolongation · seborrhoeic keratosis · skin papilloma · taste disturbance · uveitis
▸ **Uncommon** Non-cutaneous squamous cell carcinoma · peripheral neuropathy · retinal vein occlusion · Stevens-Johnson syndrome · toxic epidermal necrolysis · vasculitis
▸ **Rare** Progression of pre-existing NRAS mutated chronic myelomonocytic leukaemia
▸ **Frequency not known** Alopecia · bone-marrow suppression · hypersensitivity reactions · hyperuricaemia · nausea · oral mucositis · thromboembolism · tumour lysis syndrome · vomiting

● CONCEPTION AND CONTRACEPTION Effective contraception required during for at least 6 months after treatment.

● PREGNANCY Manufacturer advises avoid unless potential benefit outweighs risk. See also *Pregnancy and reproductive function* in Cytotoxic drugs p. 787.

● BREAST FEEDING Avoid—no information available.

● HEPATIC IMPAIRMENT Manufacturer advises more frequent monitoring in moderate to severe hepatic impairment (including monthly ECG monitoring during first 3 months of treatment).

● RENAL IMPAIRMENT Manufacturer advises caution in severe impairment.

● MONITORING REQUIREMENTS
▸ Monitor ECG and electrolytes before treatment, after one month and following dose adjustment (treatment not recommended if QT interval greater than 500 milliseconds at baseline).
▸ Monitor liver function before treatment and periodically thereafter.
▸ Monitor for uveitis, iritis and retinal vein occlusion.
▸ Monitor for cutaneous and non-cutaneous squamous cell carcinoma and new primary melanoma before, during and for up to 6 months after treatment—consult product literature.

● DIRECTIONS FOR ADMINISTRATION Food may affect absorption (take at the same time with respect to food).

● PATIENT AND CARER ADVICE Counselling advised (administration).
Drug rash with eosinophilia and systemic symptoms (DRESS syndrome) Patients should be advised to stop taking vemurafenib and consult their doctor immediately if skin rash develops.

● NATIONAL FUNDING/ACCESS DECISIONS

NICE technology appraisals (TAs)
▸ **Vemurafenib for treating locally advanced or metastatic BRAF V600 mutation-positive malignant melanoma (December 2012)** NICE TA269
Vemurafenib is recommended as an option for the treatment of BRAF V600 mutation-positive unresectable or metastatic melanoma only if the manufacturer provides vemurafenib with the discount agreed in the patient access scheme.
www.nice.org.uk/TA269

Scottish Medicines Consortium (SMC) Decisions
The *Scottish Medicines Consortium* has advised (November 2013) that vemurafenib (*Zelboraf®*) is accepted for restricted use within NHS Scotland as monotherapy for the first-line treatment of BRAF V600 mutation-positive unresectable or metastatic melanoma.

● MEDICINAL FORMS
There can be variation in the licensing of different medicines containing the same drug.

Tablet
CAUTIONARY AND ADVISORY LABELS 25
▸ Zelboraf (Roche Products Ltd) ▼
Vemurafenib 240 mg Zelboraf 240mg tablets | 56 tablet PoM £1,750.00 (Hospital only)

ANTINEOPLASTIC DRUGS > PROTEIN KINASE
INHIBITORS > ANTIFIBROTICS

Nintedanib
23.2.2016

● DRUG ACTION Nintedanib is a tyrosine protein kinase
inhibitor.

● **INDICATIONS AND DOSE**

OFEV ®

Treatment of idiopathic pulmonary fibrosis
▶ BY MOUTH
  ▶ Adult: 150 mg twice daily, reduced if not tolerated to
    100 mg twice daily, for dose adjustments due to side-
    effects, consult product literature

VARGATEF ®

**Treatment of locally advanced, metastatic or locally
recurrent non-small cell lung cancer of adenocarcinoma
histology after first-line chemotherapy (in combination
with docetaxel) (initiated under specialist supervision)**
▶ BY MOUTH
  ▶ Adult: 200 mg twice daily on days 2–21 of a standard
    21 day docetaxel cycle, for treatment following
    discontinuation of docetaxel and for dose adjustments
    due to side-effects, consult product literature

IMPORTANT SAFETY INFORMATION

FOR *VARGATEF*®–RISKS OF INCORRECT DOSING OF ORAL ANTI-
CANCER MEDICINES
See Cytotoxic drugs p. 787.

● CAUTIONS History of organ perforation · history or risk
factors for QT prolongation · impaired wound healing ·
increased risk of bleeding · patients at high risk of
cardiovascular disease · previous abdominal surgery ·
theoretical increased risk of gastrointestinal perforation ·
theoretical increased risk of venous thromboembolism
● INTERACTIONS → Appendix 1 (nintedanib).
● SIDE-EFFECTS
▶ **Common or very common** Abdominal pain · decreased
appetite · diarrhoea · hyperbilirubinaemia · hypertension ·
nausea · raised hepatic enzymes · vomiting
  OFEV ® ▶ **Common or very common** Epistaxis · weight loss
  VARGATEF ® ▶ **Common or very common** Abscesses ·
  bleeding · dehydration · electrolyte imbalance · mucositis ·
  neutropenia · peripheral neuropathy · venous
  thromboembolism
▶ **Uncommon** Gastrointestinal perforation
● ALLERGY AND CROSS-SENSITIVITY Contra-indicated in
patients with peanut or soya hypersensitivity.
● CONCEPTION AND CONTRACEPTION Manufacturer advises
exclude pregnancy before treatment and ensure effective
contraception (in addition to barrier method) during
treatment and for at least 3 months after last dose.
● PREGNANCY Manufacturer advises avoid—toxicity in
animal studies.
  VARGATEF ® See also *Pregnancy and reproductive function*
  in Cytotoxic drugs p. 787.
● BREAST FEEDING Manufacturer advises avoid—present in
milk in *animal* studies.
● HEPATIC IMPAIRMENT Consult product literature for dose
adjustment in worsening liver function. Manufacturer
advises avoid in moderate to severe impairment—no
information available.
● RENAL IMPAIRMENT Manufacturer advises caution in
severe impairment—no information available.

● MONITORING REQUIREMENTS For *Vargatef*®, monitor full
blood count and hepatic function before each treatment
cycle and regularly thereafter, monitor prothrombin time
and INR if used concomitantly with anticoagulants and
monitor for signs and symptoms of cerebral bleeding.
● PRESCRIBING AND DISPENSING INFORMATION
VARGATEF ® Not to be taken on the same day as docetaxel
therapy.
● NATIONAL FUNDING/ACCESS DECISIONS
NICE technology appraisals (TAs)
▶ **Nintedanib for previously treated locally advanced,
metastatic, or locally recurrent non-small cell lung cancer
(July 2015)** NICE TA347
Nintedanib (*Vargatef*®), in combination with docetaxel is
recommended as an option for the treatment of patients
with locally advanced, metastatic, or locally recurrent non-
small cell lung cancer of adenocarcinoma histology, that
has progressed after first-line chemotherapy, only if the
manufacturer provides nintedanib with the discount
agreed in the patient access scheme.
www.nice.org.uk/TA347
▶ **Nintedanib for treating idiopathic pulmonary fibrosis
(January 2016)** NICE TA379
Nintedanib is recommended as an option for treating
idiopathic pulmonary fibrosis, only if:
  ● the patient has a forced vital capacity (FVC) between
    50% and 80% of predicted,
  ● the manufacturer provides nintedanib with the discount
    agreed in the patient access scheme, **and**,
  ● treatment is stopped if disease progresses (a confirmed
    decline in percent predicted FVC of 10% or more) in any
    12-month period.
www.nice.org.uk/TA379
Scottish Medicines Consortium (SMC) Decisions
The *Scottish Medicines Consortium* has advised (September
2015) that nintedanib (*Ofev*®) is accepted for restricted use
within NHS Scotland for the treatment of idiopathic
pulmonary fibrosis in patients with a predicted forced vital
capacity less than or equal to 80%.

● MEDICINAL FORMS
There can be variation in the licensing of different medicines
containing the same drug.
Capsule
CAUTIONARY AND ADVISORY LABELS 25
EXCIPIENTS: May contain Lecithin
  ▶ Ofev (Boehringer Ingelheim Ltd) ▼
    Nintedanib (as Nintedanib esilate) 100 mg Ofev 100mg capsules |
    60 capsule PoM £2,151.10 (Hospital only)
    Nintedanib (as Nintedanib esilate) 150 mg Ofev 150mg capsules |
    60 capsule PoM £2,151.10 (Hospital only)
  ▶ Vargatef (Boehringer Ingelheim Ltd) ▼
    Nintedanib (as Nintedanib esilate) 100 mg Vargatef 100mg
    capsules | 120 capsule PoM £2,151.10 (Hospital only)
    Nintedanib (as Nintedanib esilate) 150 mg Vargatef 150mg
    capsules | 60 capsule PoM £2,151.10 (Hospital only)

8

Immune system and malignant disease

ANTINEOPLASTIC DRUGS > OTHER

Bortezomib

14.4.2016

● DRUG ACTION Bortezomib is a proteasome inhibitor.

● INDICATIONS AND DOSE

Treatment of multiple myeloma that has progressed despite the use of at least one therapy, and where the patient has already had, or is unable to have, haematopoietic stem cell transplantation (either as monotherapy, or in combination with pegylated liposomal doxorubicin or dexamethasone) | Treatment of previously untreated multiple myeloma in patients who are not eligible for high-dose chemotherapy with haematopoietic stem cell transplantation (in combination with melphalan and prednisolone) | Induction treatment of previously untreated multiple myeloma in patients who are eligible for high-dose chemotherapy with haematopoietic stem cell transplantation (in combination with dexamethasone, or with dexamethasone and thalidomide)

▶ BY INTRAVENOUS INJECTION, OR BY SUBCUTANEOUS INJECTION

▶ Adult: (consult local protocol)

IMPORTANT SAFETY INFORMATION
Bortezomib injection is for **intravenous or subcutaneous administration** only. Inadvertent intrathecal administration with fatal outcome has been reported.

● CONTRA-INDICATIONS Acute diffuse infiltrative pulmonary disease · pericardial disease

● CAUTIONS Amyloidosis · cardiovascular disease · consider antiviral prophylaxis for herpes zoster infection · dehydration · history of syncope · pulmonary disease (discontinue if interstitial lung disease develops) · risk factors for seizures · risk of neuropathy—consult product literature

● INTERACTIONS → Appendix 1 (bortezomib).
Caution with concurrent use of medication which may cause hypotension.

● SIDE-EFFECTS
▶ **Common or very common** Constipation (cases of ileus reported) · decreased appetite · diarrhoea · dyspnoea · fatigue · headache · herpes zoster · hypotension · myalgia · paraesthesia · peripheral neuropathy · pyrexia · rash · reactivation of herpes zoster · sensory neuropathy
▶ **Uncommon** Acute diffuse infiltrative pulmonary disorders · heart failure · posterior reversible encephalopathy syndrome (discontinue treatment) · pulmonary hypertension · seizures
▶ **Rare** Autonomic neuropathy
▶ **Very rare** Progressive multifocal leucoencephalopathy
▶ **Frequency not known** Alopecia · bone-marrow suppression · extravasation · hyperuricaemia · nausea · oral mucositis · thromboembolism · tumour lysis syndrome · vomiting
SIDE-EFFECTS, FURTHER INFORMATION
For further information on side-effects, consult product literature.

● CONCEPTION AND CONTRACEPTION Manufacturer advises effective contraception during and for 3 months after treatment in men or women.

● PREGNANCY Toxicity in *animal* studies. See also *Pregnancy and reproductive function* in Cytotoxic drugs p. 787.

● BREAST FEEDING Discontinue breast-feeding.

● HEPATIC IMPAIRMENT Reduce dose in moderate to severe impairment—consult product literature.

● RENAL IMPAIRMENT No information available for creatinine clearance less than 20 mL/minute/1.73 m^2.

● MONITORING REQUIREMENTS
▶ Monitor blood-glucose concentration in patients on oral antidiabetics.
▶ Monitor for symptoms of progressive multifocal leucoencephalopathy (presenting as new or worsening neurological signs or symptoms)—discontinue treatment if diagnosed.
▶ Chest x-ray recommended before treatment to monitor for pulmonary disease—discontinue if interstitial lung disease develops.

● NATIONAL FUNDING/ACCESS DECISIONS
NICE technology appraisals (TAs)
▶ **Bortezomib for previously untreated mantle cell lymphoma (December 2015)** NICE TA370
Bortezomib is recommended as an option for the treatment of previously untreated mantle cell lymphoma in adults for whom haematopoietic stem cell transplantation is unsuitable.
www.nice.org.uk/TA370
▶ **Bortezomib for induction therapy in multiple myeloma before high-dose chemotherapy and autologous stem cell transplantation (April 2014)** NICE TA311
Bortezomib is recommended as an option within its marketing authorisation, in combination with dexamethasone, or with dexamethasone and thalidomide, for the induction treatment of adults with previously untreated multiple myeloma, who are eligible for high-dose chemotherapy with haematopoietic stem cell transplantation.
www.nice.org.uk/TA311
▶ **Bortezomib and thalidomide for the first-line treatment of multiple myeloma (July 2011)** NICE TA228
Bortezomib in combination with an alkylating drug and a corticosteroid is recommended as an option for the first-line treatment of multiple myeloma if:
● high-dose chemotherapy with stem cell transplantation is considered inappropriate **and**
● the person is unable to tolerate or has contra-indications to thalidomide.
www.nice.org.uk/TA228
▶ **Bortezomib monotherapy for relapsed multiple myeloma (October 2007)** NICE TA129
Bortezomib monotherapy is an option for the treatment of progressive multiple myeloma in patients who are at first relapse having received one prior therapy and who have undergone, or are unsuitable for, bone-marrow transplantation, under the following circumstances:
● the response to bortezomib is measured using serum M protein after a maximum of four cycles of treatment, and treatment is continued only in patients who have a reduction in serum M protein of 50% or more (where serum M protein is not measurable, an appropriate alternative biochemical measure of response should be used) **and**
● the manufacturer rebates the full cost of bortezomib if there is an inadequate response (as defined above) after four cycles of treatment.
www.nice.org.uk/TA129
Scottish Medicines Consortium (SMC) Decisions
The *Scottish Medicines Consortium*, has advised (December 2013) that bortezomib (*Velcade* ®) is accepted for restricted use within NHS Scotland in combination with dexamethasone and thalidomide for the induction treatment of adults with previously untreated multiple myeloma who are eligible for high-dose chemotherapy with haematopoietic stem cell transplantation.

- MEDICINAL FORMS
There can be variation in the licensing of different medicines containing the same drug.
Powder for solution for injection
▸ Velcade (Janssen-Cilag Ltd)
  Bortezomib 3.5 mg Velcade 3.5mg powder for solution for injection vials | 1 vial [PoM] £762.38 (Hospital only)

Olaparib

29.3.2016

- DRUG ACTION Olaparib is a PARP inhibitor. PARP are enzymes that repair damaged DNA in cancer cells and, in the absence of functional BRCA, inhibition of PARP results in an inability of cancer cells to repair. Therefore inhibition of PARP results in an antineoplastic effect.

- INDICATIONS AND DOSE
Monotherapy for the maintenance treatment of patients with platinum-senstive relapsed BRCA-mutated (germline and/or somatic) high grade serous epithelial ovarian, fallopian tube, or primary peritoneal cancer who are in response (complete response or partial response) to platinum-based chemotherapy (initiated under specialist supervision)
▸ BY MOUTH
▸ Adult: 400 mg twice daily; reduced if not tolerated to 200 mg twice daily, then reduced if not tolerated to 100 mg twice daily, take at least 1 hour after food and avoid food for 2 hours after taking, patients should start treatment within 8 weeks of receiving the final dose of their platinum-containing chemotherapy regimen

PHARMACOKINETICS
Peak plasma concentrations are typically achieved 1 to 3 hours after dosing; steady-state is achieved within 3 to 4 days.

- INTERACTIONS → Appendix 1 (olaparib).
- SIDE-EFFECTS
▸ **Common or very common** Anaemia · decreased appetite · diarrhoea · dizziness · dysgeusia · dyspepsia · fatigue · headache · lymphopaemia · nausea · neutropenia · stomatitis · thrombocytopaenia · upper abdominal pain · vomiting
▸ **Frequency not known** Pneumonitis (occasionally fatal)
SIDE-EFFECTS, FURTHER INFORMATION
▸ Haematological toxicity Withhold treatment if severe haematological toxicity develops; further analysis recommended if toxicity still present 4 weeks after treatment withdrawal.
▸ Pneumonitis If dyspnoea, cough and fever, or radiological abnormalities develop, withhold treatment and investigate; if pneumonitis confirmed, discontinue.
- CONCEPTION AND CONTRACEPTION Manufacturer advises effective contraception during treatment and for 1 month after receiving the last dose. Consider an additional non-hormonal method of contraception.
- PREGNANCY Manufacturer advises avoid—toxicity in *animal* studies.
- BREAST FEEDING Manufacturer advises avoid during treatment and for 1 month after last dose—no information available.
- HEPATIC IMPAIRMENT Manufacturer advises avoid—no information available.
- RENAL IMPAIRMENT Manufacturer advises avoid if creatinine clearance less than 50 mL/minute/1.73m^2 unless benefit outweighs potential risk—limited information available.
- MONITORING REQUIREMENTS Manufacturer advises monitor full blood count every month for the first 12 months of treatment and periodically thereafter.

- PATIENT AND CARER ADVICE
Missed doses
If a dose is missed, the missed dose should not be taken and the next dose should be taken at the usual time.
Driving and skilled tasks
Malaise and dizziness may affect performance of skilled tasks e.g. driving or operating machinery.
- NATIONAL FUNDING/ACCESS DECISIONS
NICE technology appraisals (TAs)
▸ Olaparib for maintenance treatment of relapsed, platinum-sensitive, BRCA mutation-positive ovarian, fallopian tube and peritoneal cancer after response to second-line or subsequent platinum-based chemotherapy (January 2016) NICE TA381
Olaparib is recommended as an option for treating adults with relapsed, platinum sensitive ovarian, fallopian tube or peritoneal cancer who have BRCA1 or BRCA2 mutations and whose disease has responded to platinum based chemotherapy only if:
  • they have had 3 or more courses of platinum-based chemotherapy and;
  • the drug cost of olaparib for people who remain on treatment after 15 months will be met by the company.
www.nice.org.uk/guidance/ta381
Scottish Medicines Consortium (SMC) Decisions
The *Scottish Medicines Consortium* has advised (June 2015) that olaparib (*Lynparza*®) is **not** recommended for use within NHS Scotland as monotherapy for the maintenance treatment of patients with platinum-sensitive relapsed BRCA-mutated (germline and/or somatic) high grade serous epithelial ovarian, fallopian tube, or primary peritoneal cancer who are in response (complete response or partial response) to platinum-based chemotherapy.

- MEDICINAL FORMS
There can be variation in the licensing of different medicines containing the same drug.
Capsule
▸ Lynparza (AstraZeneca UK Ltd) ▼
  Olaparib 50 mg Lynparza 50mg capsules | 448 capsule [PoM] £3,550.00

Vismodegib

- DRUG ACTION Vismodegib is a hedgehog pathway inhibitor.

- INDICATIONS AND DOSE
Symptomatic metastatic basal cell carcinoma | Locally advanced basal cell carcinoma not appropriate for surgery or radiotherapy
▸ BY MOUTH
▸ Adult: 150 mg once daily

IMPORTANT SAFETY INFORMATION
RISKS OF INCORRECT DOSING OF ORAL ANTI-CANCER MEDICINES
See Cytotoxic drugs p. 787.

- INTERACTIONS → Appendix 1 (vismodegib).
- SIDE-EFFECTS
▸ **Common or very common** Abdominal pain · abnormal hair growth · alopecia · amenorrhoea · arthralgia · constipation · decreased appetite · dehydration · diarrhoea · dyspepsia · hyponatraemia · malaise · muscle spasms · musculoskeletal pain · nausea · pruritus · rash · taste disturbances · vomiting · weight loss
- CONCEPTION AND CONTRACEPTION For women of child-bearing potential, pregnancy must be excluded before initiation of treatment, and monthly during treatment. Women must use two contraceptive methods (including one highly effective method and one barrier method) during treatment and for 24 months after the final dose of

8

Immune system and malignant disease

vismodegib. Men must use a condom during treatment and for 2 months after the final dose.

- ● PREGNANCY **Important: teratogenic risk**—may cause severe birth defects and embryo-foetal death.
- ● BREAST FEEDING Avoid during treatment and for 24 months after final dose.
- ● HEPATIC IMPAIRMENT No information available— manufacturer advises caution in moderate to severe impairment.
- ● RENAL IMPAIRMENT No information available— manufacturer advises caution in severe impairment.
- ● PRESCRIBING AND DISPENSING INFORMATION Prescribers and pharmacists must comply with prescribing and dispensing restrictions as specified in the manufacturer's Pregnancy Prevention Programme, and ensure that the patient fully acknowledges the programme's pregnancy prevention measures—consult product literature for further information.
- ● PATIENT AND CARER ADVICE

  Patient advice required around conception and contraception Counselling on pregnancy and contraception advised. Patients must comply with the manufacturer's pregnancy prevention programme.

- ● MEDICINAL FORMS
  There can be variation in the licensing of different medicines containing the same drug.
  Capsule
  CAUTIONARY AND ADVISORY LABELS 25
  ▸ Erivedge (Roche Products Ltd) ▼
     Vismodegib 150 mg Erivedge 150mg capsules | 28 capsule PoM £6,285.00 (Hospital only)

ANTINEOVASCULARISATION DRUGS ›
VASCULAR ENDOTHELIAL GROWTH FACTOR INHIBITORS

Aflibercept

- ● DRUG ACTION Aflibercept is a recombinant fusion protein that acts as a soluble decoy receptor and binds to vascular endothelial growth factors A and B (VEGF-A, VEGF-B) and placental growth factor (PlGF). Aflibercept inhibits the activation of VEGF receptors and the proliferation of endothelial cells, thereby inhibiting the growth of new vessels that supply tumours with oxygen and nutrients.

- ● INDICATIONS AND DOSE

  In combination with irinotecan, fluorouracil and folinic acid (FOLFIRI) chemotherapy, in metastatic colorectal cancer that is resistant to, or has progressed after, an oxaliplatin-containing regimen
  ▸ BY INTRAVENOUS INFUSION
  ▸ Adult: (consult local protocol)

- ● CONTRA-INDICATIONS Moderate or severe congestive heart failure · uncontrolled hypertension
- ● CAUTIONS Febrile neutropenia · history of cardiovascular disease (may be exacerbated by hypertension) · increased risk of haemorrhage (including fatal events) · increased risk of hypertension · increased risk of thromboembolic events (consult product literature if event occurs) · may impair wound healing—withhold treatment for at least 4 weeks before elective surgery and for at least 4 weeks after major surgery, or until wound fully healed · neutropenic infection · risk of fistula formation (discontinue if fistula develops) · risk of neutropenia · risk of thrombocytopenia

- ● SIDE-EFFECTS
  ▸ **Common or very common** Abdominal pain · aphthous stomatitis · decreased appetite · dehydration · diarrhoea ·

dysphonia · dyspnoea · fistula · haemorrhage (including nasal, rectal and gastro-intestinal) · haemorrhoids · hand-foot syndrome · headache · hypertension · infection · leucopenia · malaise · nasopharyngitis · neutropenia (including febrile neutropenia) · oropharyngeal pain · proctalgia · proteinuria · rhinorrhoea · sepsis · skin hyperpigmentation · stomatitis · thrombocytopenia · thromboembolic events (arterial and venous) · toothache · urinary tract infection · weight loss
▸ **Uncommon** Gastro-intestinal perforation · impaired wound healing · nephrotic syndrome · posterior reversible encephalopathy syndrome · thrombotic microangiopathy

- ● CONCEPTION AND CONTRACEPTION Exclude pregnancy before treatment. Effective contraception required during and for at least 6 months after treatment in men and women. Contraceptive advice should be given to men and women before therapy begins (and should cover the duration of contraception required after therapy has ended).
- ● PREGNANCY Manufacturer advises avoid—toxicity in *animal* studies. Considerable caution is necessary if a pregnant woman presents with cancer requiring chemotherapy, and specialist advice should always be sought.
- ● BREAST FEEDING Manufacturer advises avoid—no information available.
- ● HEPATIC IMPAIRMENT Caution in severe impairment—no information available.
- ● RENAL IMPAIRMENT Caution in severe impairment— no information available.
- ● MONITORING REQUIREMENTS Monitor blood pressure at initiation and at least fortnightly during treatment (do not initiate treatment if pre-existing hypertension is uncontrolled)—consult product literature if hypertension develops during treatment. Monitor for signs of gastro-intestinal perforation (discontinue if perforation develops). Monitor full blood count, including differential count and platelets at baseline and before each treatment cycle. Monitor for proteinuria before each treatment administration (consult product literature if symptoms develop). Monitor for signs and symptoms of diarrhoea and dehydration, particularly in elderly—consult product literature if severe diarrhoea occurs. Monitor for posterior reversible encephalopathy syndrome (presenting as seizures, altered mental status, nausea, vomiting, headache, or visual disturbance).

- ● NATIONAL FUNDING/ACCESS DECISIONS

  NICE technology appraisals (TAs)
  ▸ Aflibercept in combination with irinotecan and fluorouracil-based therapy for treating metastatic colorectal cancer that has progressed following prior oxaliplatin-based chemotherapy (March 2014) NICE TA307
  Aflibercept in combination with irinotecan and fluorouracil-based therapy is **not** recommended within its marketing authorisation for treating metastatic colorectal cancer that is resistant to or has progressed after an oxaliplatin-containing regimen.
  www.nice.org.uk/TA307

- ● MEDICINAL FORMS
  There can be variation in the licensing of different medicines containing the same drug.
  Solution for infusion
  ▸ Zaltrap (Sanofi) ▼
     Aflibercept 25 mg per 1 ml Zaltrap 200mg/8ml concentrate for solution for infusion vials | 1 vial PoM £591.30 (Hospital only)
     Zaltrap 100mg/4ml concentrate for solution for infusion vials | 1 vial PoM £295.65 (Hospital only)

Chapter 9
Blood and nutrition

CONTENTS

Blood and blood-forming organs

1   Anaemias

Anaemias

Initiation of treatment

Before initiating treatment for anaemia it is essential to determine which type is present. Iron salts may be harmful and result in iron overload if given alone to patients with anaemias other than those due to iron deficiency.

Sickle-cell anaemia

Sickle-cell disease is caused by a structural abnormality of haemoglobin resulting in deformed, less flexible red blood cells. Acute complications in the more severe forms include sickle-cell crisis, where infarction of the microvasculature and blood supply to organs results in severe pain. Sickle-cell crisis requires hospitalisation, intravenous fluids, analgesia and treatment of any concurrent infection. Chronic complications include skin ulceration, renal failure, and increased susceptibility to infection. Pneumococcal vaccine, haemophilus influenzae type b vaccine, an annual influenza vaccine and prophylactic penicillin reduce the risk of

infection. Hepatitis B vaccine should be considered if the patient is not immune.

In most forms of sickle-cell disease, varying degrees of haemolytic anaemia are present accompanied by increased erythropoiesis; this may increase folate requirements and folate supplementation may be necessary.

Hydroxycarbamide p. 823 can reduce the frequency of crises and the need for blood transfusions in sickle-cell disease. The beneficial effects of hydroxycarbamide may not become evident for several months.

G6PD deficiency

Glucose 6-phosphate dehydrogenase (G6PD) deficiency is highly prevalent in individuals originating from most parts of Africa, from most parts of Asia, from Oceania, and from Southern Europe; it can also occur, rarely, in any other individuals. G6PD deficiency is more common in males than it is in females.

Individuals with G6PD deficiency are susceptible to developing acute haemolytic anaemia when they take a number of common drugs. They are also susceptible to developing acute haemolytic anaemia when they eat fava beans (broad beans, *Vicia faba*); this is termed *favism* and can be more severe in children or when the fresh fava beans are eaten raw.

When prescribing drugs for patients with G6PD deficiency, the following three points should be kept in mind:

- G6PD deficiency is genetically heterogeneous; susceptibility to the haemolytic risk from drugs varies;

thus, a drug found to be safe in some G6PD-deficient individuals may not be equally safe in others;

- manufacturers do not routinely test drugs for their effects in G6PD-deficient individuals;
- the risk and severity of haemolysis is almost always dose-related.

The lists below should be read with these points in mind. Ideally, information about G6PD deficiency should be available before prescribing a drug listed below. However, in the absence of this information, the possibility of haemolysis should be considered, especially if the patient belongs to a group in which G6PD deficiency is common.

A very few G6PD-deficient individuals with chronic non-spherocytic haemolytic anaemia have haemolysis even in the absence of an exogenous trigger. These patients must be regarded as being at high risk of severe exacerbation of haemolysis following administration of any of the drugs listed below.

Drugs with definite risk of haemolysis in most G6PD-deficient individuals

- Dapsone and other sulfones (higher doses for dermatitis herpetiformis more likely to cause problems)
- Methylthioninium chloride
- Niridazole [not on UK market]
- Nitrofurantoin
- Pamaquin [not on UK market]
- Primaquine (30 mg weekly for 8 weeks has been found to be without undue harmful effects in African and Asian people)
- Quinolones (including ciprofloxacin, moxifloxacin, nalidixic acid, norfloxacin, and ofloxacin)
- Rasburicase
- Sulfonamides (including co-trimoxazole; some sulfonamides, e.g. sulfadiazine, have been tested and found not to be haemolytic in many G6PD-deficient individuals)

Drugs with possible risk of haemolysis in some G6PD-deficient individuals

- Aspirin (acceptable up to a dose of at least 1 g daily in most G6PD-deficient individuals)
- Chloroquine (acceptable in acute malaria and malaria chemoprophylaxis)
- Menadione, water-soluble derivatives (e.g. menadiol sodium phosphate)
- Quinidine (acceptable in acute malaria) [not on UK market]
- Quinine (acceptable in acute malaria)
- Sulfonylureas

Naphthalene in mothballs also causes haemolysis in individuals with Gana6PD deficiency.

Drugs used in hypoplastic, haemolytic, and renal anaemias

Anabolic steroids, pyridoxine hydrochloride p. 937, antilymphocyte immunoglobulin, and various corticosteroids are used in hypoplastic and haemolytic anaemias.

Antilymphocyte immunoglobulin given intravenously through a central line over 12–18 hours each day for 5 days produces a response in about 50% of cases of acquired *aplastic anaemia*; the response rate may be increased when ciclosporin p. 758 is given as well. Severe reactions are common in the first 2 days and profound immunosuppression can occur; antilymphocyte immunoglobulin should be given under specialist supervision with appropriate resuscitation facilities. Alternatively, oxymetholone tablets (available from 'special order' manufacturers or specialist importing companies) can be used in aplastic anaemia for 3 to 6 months.

It is unlikely that dietary deprivation of pyridoxine hydrochloride produces clinically relevant haematological effects. However, certain forms of *sideroblastic anaemia*

respond to pharmacological doses, possibly reflecting its role as a co-enzyme during haemoglobin synthesis. Pyridoxine hydrochloride is indicated in both *idiopathic acquired* and *hereditary sideroblastic anaemias*. Although complete cures have not been reported, some increase in haemoglobin can occur; the dose required is usually high. *Reversible sideroblastic anaemias* respond to treatment of the underlying cause but in pregnancy, haemolytic anaemias, and alcohol dependence, or during isoniazid p. 532 treatment, pyridoxine hydrochloride is also indicated.

Corticosteroids have an important place in the management of haematological disorders. They include conditions with an *autoimmune haemolytic anaemia*, *immune thrombocytopenias* and *neutropenias*, and *major transfusion reactions*. They are also used in chemotherapy schedules for many types of *lymphoma*, *lymphoid leukaemias*, and *paraproteinaemias*, including *multiple myeloma*.

Erythropoietins

Epoetins (recombinant human erythropoietins) are used to treat the anaemia associated with erythropoietin deficiency in chronic renal failure, to increase the yield of autologous blood in normal individuals and to shorten the period of symptomatic anaemia in patients receiving cytotoxic chemotherapy.

Epoetin beta p. 876 is also used for the prevention of anaemia in preterm neonates of low birth-weight; only unpreserved formulations should be used in neonates because other preparations may contain benzyl alcohol.

Darbepoetin alfa p. 873 is a hyperglycosylated derivative of epoetin; it has a longer half life and can be administered less frequently than epoetin.

Methoxy polyethylene glycol-epoetin beta p. 878 is a continuous erythropoietin receptor activator that is licensed for the treatment of symptomatic anaemia associated with chronic kidney disease. It has a longer duration of action than epoetin.

1.1 Hypoplastic, haemolytic, and renal anaemias

ANABOLIC STEROIDS > ANDROSTAN DERIVATIVES

Oxymetholone

- **INDICATIONS AND DOSE**
Aplastic anaemia
▶ BY MOUTH
▸ Adult: 1–5 mg/kg daily for 3 to 6 months

- **MEDICINAL FORMS**
There can be variation in the licensing of different medicines containing the same drug. Forms available from special-order manufacturers include: oral suspension
Capsule
▸ Oxymetholone (Non-proprietary)
  Oxymetholone 50 mg Oxymetholone 50mg capsules | 50 capsule [PoM] £475.00 [CD4-2]

EPOETINS

Epoetins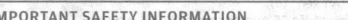

● CONTRA-INDICATIONS   Patients unable to receive thromboprophylaxis · pure red cell aplasia following erythropoietin therapy · uncontrolled hypertension

● CAUTIONS   Aluminium toxicity (can impair the response to erythropoietin) · concurrent infection (can impair the response to erythropoietin) · correct factors that contribute to the anaemia of chronic renal failure, such as iron or folate deficiency, before treatment. · during dialysis (increase in unfractionated or low molecular weight heparin dose may be needed) · epilepsy · inadequately treated or poorly controlled blood pressure—interrupt treatment if blood pressure uncontrolled · ischaemic vascular disease · malignant disease · other inflammatory disease (can impair the response to erythropoietin) · risk of thrombosis may be increased when used for anaemia before orthopaedic surgery—avoid in cardiovascular disease including recent myocardial infarction or cerebrovascular accident · risk of thrombosis may be increased when used for anaemia in adults receiving cancer chemotherapy · sickle-cell disease (lower target haemoglobin concentration may be appropriate) · sudden stabbing migraine-like pain (warning of a hypertensive crisis) · thrombocytosis (monitor platelet count for first 8 weeks)

● SIDE-EFFECTS

▶ **Common or very common**   Aggravation of hypertension (dose-dependent) · cardiovascular events · diarrhoea · dose-dependent increase in platelet count regressing during treatment (but thrombocytosis rare) · headache · hypertensive crisis (in isolated patients with normal or low blood pressure) · increase in blood pressure (dose-dependent) · influenza-like symptoms (may be reduced if intravenous injection given over 5 minutes) · nausea · shunt thrombosis especially if tendency to hypotension or arteriovenous shunt complications · vomiting

▶ **Very rare**   Sudden loss of efficacy because of pure red cell aplasia, particularly following subcutaneous administration in patients with chronic renal failure

▶ **Frequency not known**   Anaphylaxis · angioedema · hyperkalaemia · hypersensitivity reactions · injection-site reactions · peripheral oedema · skin reactions

SIDE-EFFECTS, FURTHER INFORMATION

▶ Hypertensive crisis   In isolated patients with normal or low blood pressure, hypertensive crisis with encephalopathy-like symptoms and generalised tonic-clonic seizures requiring immediate medical attention has occured with epoetin.

▶ Pure red cell aplasia   There have been very rare reports of pure red cell aplasia in patients treated with erythropoietins. In patients who develop a lack of efficacy with erythropoietin therapy and with a diagnosis of pure red cell aplasia, treatment with erythropoietins must be discontinued and testing for erythropoietin antibodies considered. Patients who develop pure red cell aplasia should **not** be switched to another form of erythropoietin.

● MONITORING REQUIREMENTS

▶ Monitor closely blood pressure, reticulocyte counts, haemoglobin, and electrolytes—interrupt treatment if blood pressure uncontrolled.

▶ Other factors, such as iron or folate deficiency, that contribute to the anaemia of chronic renal failure should be corrected before treatment and monitored during therapy. Supplemental iron may improve the response in resistant patients.

↰ above

Darbepoetin alfa

● INDICATIONS AND DOSE

Symptomatic anaemia associated with chronic renal failure in patients on dialysis

▶ BY SUBCUTANEOUS INJECTION, OR BY INTRAVENOUS INJECTION

▶ Adult: Initially 450 nanograms/kg once weekly, dose to be adjusted according to response by approximately 25% at intervals of at least 4 weeks, maintenance dose to be given once weekly or once every 2 weeks, reduce dose by approximately 25% if rise in haemoglobin concentration exceeds 2 g/100 mL over 4 weeks or if haemoglobin concentration exceeds 12 g/100 mL; if haemoglobin concentration continues to rise, despite dose reduction, suspend treatment until haemoglobin concentration decreases and then restart at a dose approximately 25% lower than the previous dose, when changing route give same dose then adjust according to weekly or fortnightly haemoglobin measurements, adjust doses not more frequently than every 2 weeks during maintenance treatment

Symptomatic anaemia associated with chronic renal failure in patients not on dialysis

▶ BY SUBCUTANEOUS INJECTION

▶ Adult: Initially 450 nanograms/kg once weekly, alternatively initially 750 nanograms/kg every 2 weeks, dose to be adjusted according to response by approximately 25% at intervals of at least continued →

9

Blood and nutrition

9

Blood and nutrition

4 weeks, maintenance dose can be given once weekly, every 2 weeks, or once a month, subcutaneous route preferred in patients not on haemodialysis, reduce dose by approximately 25% if rise in haemoglobin concentration exceeds 2 g/100 mL over 4 weeks or if haemoglobin concentration exceeds 12 g/100 mL; if haemoglobin concentration continues to rise, despite dose reduction, suspend treatment until haemoglobin concentration decreases and then restart at a dose approximately 25% lower than the previous dose, when changing route give same dose then adjust according to weekly or fortnightly haemoglobin measurements, adjust doses not more frequently than every 2 weeks during maintenance treatment

Symptomatic anaemia associated with chronic renal failure in patients not on dialysis

▸ BY INTRAVENOUS INJECTION

▸ Adult: Initially 450 nanograms/kg once weekly, dose to be adjusted according to response by approximately 25% at intervals of at least 4 weeks, maintenance dose given once weekly, subcutaneous route preferred in patients not on haemodialysis, reduce dose by approximately 25% if rise in haemoglobin concentration exceeds 2 g/100 mL over 4 weeks or if haemoglobin concentration exceeds 12 g/100 mL; if haemoglobin concentration continues to rise, despite dose reduction, suspend treatment until haemoglobin concentration decreases and then restart at a dose approximately 25% lower than the previous dose, when changing route give same dose then adjust according to weekly or fortnightly haemoglobin measurements, adjust doses not more frequently than every 2 weeks during maintenance treatment

Symptomatic anaemia in adults with non-myeloid malignancies receiving chemotherapy

▸ BY SUBCUTANEOUS INJECTION

▸ Adult: Initially 6.75 micrograms/kg every 3 weeks, alternatively initially 2.25 micrograms/kg once weekly, if response inadequate after 9 weeks further treatment may not be effective; if adequate response obtained then reduce dose by 25–50%, reduce dose by approximately 25–50% if rise in haemoglobin concentration exceeds 2 g/100 mL over 4 weeks or if haemoglobin concentration exceeds 12 g/100 mL; if haemoglobin concentration continues to rise, despite dose reduction, suspend treatment until haemoglobin concentration decreases and restart at a dose approximately 25% lower than the previous dose. Discontinue approximately 4 weeks after ending chemotherapy

● SIDE-EFFECTS Injection-site pain · oedema

● PREGNANCY No evidence of harm in *animal* studies—manufacturer advises caution.

● BREAST FEEDING Manufacturer advises avoid—no information available.

● HEPATIC IMPAIRMENT Manufacturer advises caution.

● NATIONAL FUNDING/ACCESS DECISIONS

NICE technology appraisals (TAs)

▸ Erythropoiesis-stimulating agents (epoetin and darbepoetin) for treating anaemia in people with cancer having chemotherapy (November 2014) NICE TA323
Erythropoiesis-stimulating agents (epoetin alfa, beta, theta and zeta, and darbepoetin alfa) are recommended, within their marketing authorisations, as options for treating anaemia in people with cancer who are having chemotherapy.

If different erythropoiesis-stimulating agents are equally suitable, the product with the lowest acquisition cost for the course of treatment should be used.
www.nice.org.uk/TA323

● MEDICINAL FORMS
There can be variation in the licensing of different medicines containing the same drug.

Solution for injection

▸ Aranesp (Amgen Ltd)

Darbepoetin alfa 25 microgram per 1 ml Aranesp
10micrograms/0.4ml solution for injection pre-filled syringes | 4 pre-filled disposable injection [PoM] £58.72

Darbepoetin alfa 40 microgram per 1 ml Aranesp
20micrograms/0.5ml solution for injection pre-filled syringes | 4 pre-filled disposable injection [PoM] £117.45

Darbepoetin alfa 100 microgram per 1 ml Aranesp
50micrograms/0.5ml solution for injection pre-filled syringes | 4 pre-filled disposable injection [PoM] £293.62
Aranesp 40micrograms/0.4ml solution for injection pre-filled syringes | 4 pre-filled disposable injection [PoM] £234.90
Aranesp 30micrograms/0.3ml solution for injection pre-filled syringes | 4 pre-filled disposable injection [PoM] £176.17

Darbepoetin alfa 200 microgram per 1 ml Aranesp
130micrograms/0.65ml solution for injection pre-filled syringes | 4 pre-filled disposable injection [PoM] £763.42
Aranesp 100micrograms/0.5ml solution for injection pre-filled syringes | 4 pre-filled disposable injection [PoM] £587.24
Aranesp 80micrograms/0.4ml solution for injection pre-filled syringes | 4 pre-filled disposable injection [PoM] £469.79
Aranesp 60micrograms/0.3ml solution for injection pre-filled syringes | 4 pre-filled disposable injection [PoM] £352.35

Darbepoetin alfa 500 microgram per 1 ml Aranesp
300micrograms/0.6ml solution for injection pre-filled syringes | 1 pre-filled disposable injection [PoM] £440.43
Aranesp 500micrograms/1ml solution for injection pre-filled syringes | 1 pre-filled disposable injection [PoM] £734.05
Aranesp 150micrograms/0.3ml solution for injection pre-filled syringes | 4 pre-filled disposable injection [PoM] £880.86

▸ Aranesp SureClick (Amgen Ltd)

Darbepoetin alfa 40 microgram per 1 ml Aranesp SureClick
20micrograms/0.5ml solution for injection pre-filled disposable devices | 1 pre-filled disposable injection [PoM] £29.36

Darbepoetin alfa 100 microgram per 1 ml Aranesp SureClick
40micrograms/0.4ml solution for injection pre-filled disposable devices | 1 pre-filled disposable injection [PoM] £58.72
Aranesp SureClick 80micrograms/0.4ml solution for injection pre-filled disposable devices | 1 pre-filled disposable injection [PoM] £117.45

Darbepoetin alfa 200 microgram per 1 ml Aranesp SureClick
60micrograms/0.3ml solution for injection pre-filled disposable devices | 1 pre-filled disposable injection [PoM] £88.09
Aranesp SureClick 100micrograms/0.5ml solution for injection pre-filled disposable devices | 1 pre-filled disposable injection [PoM] £146.81

Darbepoetin alfa 500 microgram per 1 ml Aranesp SureClick
150micrograms/0.3ml solution for injection pre-filled disposable devices | 1 pre-filled disposable injection [PoM] £220.22
Aranesp SureClick 300micrograms/0.6ml solution for injection pre-filled disposable devices | 1 pre-filled disposable injection [PoM] £440.43
Aranesp SureClick 500micrograms/1ml solution for injection pre-filled disposable devices | 1 pre-filled disposable injection [PoM] £734.05

F 873

Epoetin alfa

● INDICATIONS AND DOSE

BINOCRIT® PRE-FILLED SYRINGES

Symptomatic anaemia associated with chronic renal failure in patients on haemodialysis

▸ BY INTRAVENOUS INJECTION

▸ Adult: Initially 50 units/kg 3 times a week, adjusted in steps of 25 units/kg 3 times a week, dose adjusted according to response at intervals of at least 4 weeks; maintenance 25–100 units/kg 3 times a week, intravenous injection to be given over 1–5 minutes, reduce dose by approximately 25% if rise in haemoglobin concentration exceeds 2 g/100 mL over 4 weeks or if haemoglobin concentration exceeds 12 g/100 mL; if haemoglobin concentration continues to rise, despite dose reduction, suspend treatment until haemoglobin concentration decreases and then restart at a dose approximately 25% lower than the previous dose

Symptomatic anaemia associated with chronic renal failure in adults on peritoneal dialysis

▶ BY INTRAVENOUS INJECTION

▶ Adult: Initially 50 units/kg twice weekly; maintenance 25–50 units/kg twice weekly, intravenous injection to be given over 1–5 minutes, reduce dose by approximately 25% if rise in haemoglobin concentration exceeds 2 g/100 mL over 4 weeks or if haemoglobin concentration exceeds 12 g/100 mL; if haemoglobin concentration continues to rise, despite dose reduction, suspend treatment until haemoglobin concentration decreases and then restart at a dose approximately 25% lower than the previous dose

Severe symptomatic anaemia of renal origin in adults with renal insufficiency not yet on dialysis

▶ BY INTRAVENOUS INJECTION

▶ Adult: Initially 50 units/kg 3 times a week, increased in steps of 25 units/kg 3 times a week, adjusted according to response, dose to be increased at intervals of at least 4 weeks; maintenance 17–33 units/kg 3 times a week (max. per dose 200 units/kg 3 times a week), intravenous injection to be given over 1–5 minutes, reduce dose by approximately 25% if rise in haemoglobin concentration exceeds 2 g/100 mL over 4 weeks or if haemoglobin concentration exceeds 12 g/100 mL; if haemoglobin concentration continues to rise, despite dose reduction, suspend treatment until haemoglobin concentration decreases and then restart at a dose approximately 25% lower than the previous dose

Symptomatic anaemia in adults receiving cancer chemotherapy

▶ BY SUBCUTANEOUS INJECTION

▶ Adult: Initially 150 units/kg 3 times a week, alternatively initially 450 units/kg once weekly, increased to 300 units/kg 3 times a week, increased if appropriate rise in haemoglobin (or reticulocyte count) not achieved after 4 weeks; discontinue if inadequate response after 4 weeks at higher dose, subcutaneous injection maximum 1 mL per injection site, reduce dose by approximately 25–50% if rise in haemoglobin concentration exceeds 2 g/100 mL over 4 weeks or if haemoglobin concentration exceeds 12 g/100 mL; if haemoglobin concentration continues to rise, despite dose reduction, suspend treatment until haemoglobin concentration decreases and then restart at a dose approximately 25% lower than the previous dose. Discontinue approximately 4 weeks after ending chemotherapy

To increase yield of autologous blood (to avoid homologous blood) in predonation programme in moderate anaemia either when large volume of blood required or when sufficient blood cannot be saved for elective major surgery

▶ BY INTRAVENOUS INJECTION

▶ Adult: 600 units/kg twice weekly for 3 weeks before surgery, consult product literature for details and advice on ensuring high iron stores, intravenous injection to be given over 1–5 minutes

Moderate anaemia (haemoglobin concentration 10–13 g/100 mL) before elective orthopaedic surgery in adults with expected moderate blood loss to reduce exposure to allogeneic blood transfusion or if autologous transfusion unavailable

▶ BY SUBCUTANEOUS INJECTION

▶ Adult: 600 units/kg once weekly for 3 weeks before surgery and on day of surgery, alternatively 300 units/kg daily for 15 days starting 10 days before surgery, consult product literature for details, subcutaneous injection maximum 1 mL per injection site

EPREX® PRE-FILLED SYRINGES

Symptomatic anaemia associated with chronic renal failure in patients on haemodialysis

▶ BY INTRAVENOUS INJECTION, OR BY SUBCUTANEOUS INJECTION

▶ Adult: Initially 50 units/kg 3 times a week, adjusted in steps of 25 units/kg 3 times a week, dose adjusted according to response at intervals of at least 4 weeks; maintenance 75–300 units/kg once weekly, intravenous route preferred, intravenous injection to be given over 1–5 minutes, subcutaneous injection, maximum 1 mL per injection site, maintenance dose can be given as a single dose or in divided doses, reduce dose by approximately 25% if rise in haemoglobin concentration exceeds 2 g/100 mL over 4 weeks or if haemoglobin concentration exceeds 12 g/100 mL; if haemoglobin concentration continues to rise, despite dose reduction, suspend treatment until haemoglobin concentration decreases and then restart at a dose approximately 25% lower than the previous dose

Symptomatic anaemia associated with chronic renal failure in adults on peritoneal dialysis

▶ BY INTRAVENOUS INJECTION, OR BY SUBCUTANEOUS INJECTION

▶ Adult: Initially 50 units/kg twice weekly; maintenance 25–50 units/kg twice weekly, intravenous route preferred, intravenous injection to be given over 1–5 minutes, subcutaneous injection, maximum 1 mL per injection site, reduce dose by approximately 25% if rise in haemoglobin concentration exceeds 2 g/100 mL over 4 weeks or if haemoglobin concentration exceeds 12 g/100 mL; if haemoglobin concentration continues to rise, despite dose reduction, suspend treatment until haemoglobin concentration decreases and then restart at a dose approximately 25% lower than the previous dose

Severe symptomatic anaemia of renal origin in adults with renal insufficiency not yet on dialysis

▶ BY INTRAVENOUS INJECTION, OR BY SUBCUTANEOUS INJECTION

▶ Adult: Initially 50 units/kg 3 times a week, increased in steps of 25 units/kg 3 times a week, adjusted according to response, dose to be increased at intervals of at least 4 weeks; maintenance 17–33 units/kg 3 times a week (max. per dose 200 units/kg 3 times a week), intravenous route preferred, intravenous injection to be given over 1–5 minutes, subcutaneous injection, maximum 1 mL per injection site, reduce dose by approximately 25% if rise in haemoglobin concentration exceeds 2 g/100 mL over 4 weeks or if haemoglobin concentration exceeds 12 g/100 mL; if haemoglobin concentration continues to rise, despite dose reduction, suspend treatment until haemoglobin concentration decreases and then restart at a dose approximately 25% lower than the previous dose

Symptomatic anaemia in adults receiving cancer chemotherapy

▶ BY SUBCUTANEOUS INJECTION

▶ Adult: Initially 150 units/kg 3 times a week, alternatively initially 450 units/kg once weekly, increased to 300 units/kg 3 times a week, increased if appropriate rise in haemoglobin (or reticulocyte count) not achieved after 4 weeks; discontinue if inadequate response after 4 weeks at higher dose, subcutaneous injection maximum 1 mL per injection site, reduce dose by approximately 25–50% if rise in haemoglobin concentration exceeds 2 g/100 mL over 4 weeks or if haemoglobin concentration exceeds 12 g/100 mL; if haemoglobin concentration continues to rise, despite dose reduction, suspend treatment until haemoglobin concentration decreases and then restart at a dose approximately 25% lower than the previous dose. Discontinue approximately 4 weeks after ending chemotherapy continued →

To increase yield of autologous blood (to avoid homologous blood) in predonation programme in moderate anaemia either when large volume of blood required or when sufficient blood cannot be saved for elective major surgery

▸ BY INTRAVENOUS INJECTION

▸ Adult: 600 units/kg twice weekly for 3 weeks before surgery, consult product literature for details and advice on ensuring high iron stores, intravenous injection to be given over 1–5 minutes

Moderate anaemia (haemoglobin concentration 10–13 g/100 mL) before elective orthopaedic surgery in adults with expected moderate blood loss to reduce exposure to allogeneic blood transfusion or if autologous transfusion unavailable

▸ BY SUBCUTANEOUS INJECTION

▸ Adult: 600 units/kg once weekly for 3 weeks before surgery and on day of surgery, alternatively 300 units/kg daily for 15 days starting 10 days before surgery, consult product literature for details, subcutaneous injection maximum 1 mL per injection site

● PREGNANCY No evidence of harm. Benefits probably outweigh risk of anaemia and of blood transfusion in pregnancy.

● BREAST FEEDING Unlikely to be present in milk. Minimal effect on infant.

● HEPATIC IMPAIRMENT Manufacturers advise caution in chronic hepatic failure.

● PRESCRIBING AND DISPENSING INFORMATION Products containing epoetin alfa are not identical and although there should be no important differences in terms of safety and efficacy, when prescribing biological products it is good practice to use the brand name, see *Biosimilar medicines*, under Guidance on prescribing p. 1.

● NATIONAL FUNDING/ACCESS DECISIONS

NICE technology appraisals (TAs)

▸ Erythropoiesis-stimulating agents (epoetin and darbepoetin) for treating anaemia in people with cancer having chemotherapy (November 2014) NICE TA323
Erythropoiesis-stimulating agents (epoetin alfa, beta, theta and zeta, and darbepoetin alfa) are recommended, within their marketing authorisations, as options for treating anaemia in people with cancer who are having chemotherapy.

   If different erythropoiesis-stimulating agents are equally suitable, the product with the lowest acquisition cost for the course of treatment should be used.
www.nice.org.uk/TA323

● MEDICINAL FORMS
There can be variation in the licensing of different medicines containing the same drug.

Solution for injection

▸ Eprex (Janssen-Cilag Ltd)

Epoetin alfa 2000 unit per 1 ml Eprex 1,000units/0.5ml solution for injection pre-filled syringes | 6 pre-filled disposable injection [PoM] £33.18

Epoetin alfa 4000 unit per 1 ml Eprex 2,000units/0.5ml solution for injection pre-filled syringes | 6 pre-filled disposable injection [PoM] £66.37

Epoetin alfa 10000 unit per 1 ml Eprex 6,000units/0.6ml solution for injection pre-filled syringes | 6 pre-filled disposable injection [PoM] £199.11
Eprex 4,000units/0.4ml solution for injection pre-filled syringes | 6 pre-filled disposable injection [PoM] £132.74
Eprex 5,000units/0.5ml solution for injection pre-filled syringes | 6 pre-filled disposable injection [PoM] £165.92
Eprex 3,000units/0.3ml solution for injection pre-filled syringes | 6 pre-filled disposable injection [PoM] £99.55
Eprex 10,000units/1ml solution for injection pre-filled syringes | 6 pre-filled disposable injection [PoM] £331.85

Eprex 8,000units/0.8ml solution for injection pre-filled syringes | 6 pre-filled disposable injection [PoM] £265.48
Epoetin alfa 40000 unit per 1 ml Eprex 20,000units/0.5ml solution for injection pre-filled syringes | 1 pre-filled disposable injection [PoM] £110.62
Eprex 30,000units/0.75ml solution for injection pre-filled syringes | 1 pre-filled disposable injection [PoM] £199.11
Eprex 40,000units/1ml solution for injection pre-filled syringes | 1 pre-filled disposable injection [PoM] £265.48

☞ 873

Epoetin beta

● INDICATIONS AND DOSE

Symptomatic anaemia associated with chronic renal failure

▸ BY SUBCUTANEOUS INJECTION

▸ Adult: Initially 20 units/kg 3 times a week for 4 weeks, increased in steps of 20 units/kg 3 times a week, according to response at intervals of 4 weeks, total weekly dose may be divided into daily doses; maintenance dose, initially reduce dose by half then adjust according to response at intervals of 1–2 weeks, total weekly maintenance dose may be given as a single dose or in 3 or 7 divided doses. Subcutaneous route preferred in patients not on haemodialysis. Reduce dose by approximately 25% if rise in haemoglobin concentration exceeds 2 g/100 mL over 4 weeks or if haemoglobin concentration approaches or exceeds 12 g/100 mL; if haemoglobin concentration continues to rise, despite dose reduction, suspend treatment until haemoglobin concentration decreases and then restart at a dose approximately 25% lower than the previous dose; maximum 720 units/kg per week

▸ BY INTRAVENOUS INJECTION

▸ Adult: Initially 40 units/kg 3 times a week for 4 weeks, then increased to 80 units/kg 3 times a week, then increased in steps of 20 units/kg 3 times a week if required, at intervals of 4 weeks; maintenance dose, initially reduce dose by half then adjust according to response at intervals of 1–2 weeks. Intravenous injection to be administered over 2 minutes. Subcutaneous route preferred in patients not on haemodialysis. Reduce dose by approximately 25% if rise in haemoglobin concentration exceeds 2 g/100 mL over 4 weeks or if haemoglobin concentration approaches or exceeds 12 g/100 mL; if haemoglobin concentration continues to rise, despite dose reduction, suspend treatment until haemoglobin concentration decreases and then restart at a dose approximately 25% lower than the previous dose; maximum 720 units/kg per week

Symptomatic anaemia in adults with non-myeloid malignancies receiving chemotherapy

▸ BY SUBCUTANEOUS INJECTION

▸ Adult: Initially 450 units/kg once weekly for 4 weeks, dose to be given weekly as a single dose or in 3–7 divided doses, increase dose after 4 weeks (if a rise in haemoglobin of at least 1 g/100 mL not achieved), increased to 900 units/kg once weekly, dose to be given weekly as a single dose or in 3–7 divided doses, if adequate response obtained reduce dose by 25–50%, discontinue treatment if haemoglobin concentration does not increase by at least 1 g/100 mL after 8 weeks of therapy (response unlikely). Reduce dose by approximately 25–50% if rise in haemoglobin concentration exceeds 2 g/100 mL over 4 weeks or if haemoglobin concentration exceeds 12 g/100 mL; if haemoglobin concentration continues to rise, despite dose reduction, suspend treatment until haemoglobin concentration decreases and then restart at a dose approximately 25% lower than the previous dose. Discontinue approximately 4 weeks after ending chemotherapy; maximum 60 000 units per week

To increase yield of autologous blood (to avoid homologous blood) in predonation programme in moderate anaemia when blood-conserving procedures are insufficient or unavailable
▸ BY INTRAVENOUS INJECTION, OR BY SUBCUTANEOUS INJECTION
  ▸ Adult: (consult product literature)

● PREGNANCY No evidence of harm. Benefits probably outweigh risk of anaemia and of blood transfusion in pregnancy.

● BREAST FEEDING Unlikely to be present in milk. Minimal effect on infant.

● HEPATIC IMPAIRMENT Manufacturers advise caution in chronic hepatic failure.

● NATIONAL FUNDING/ACCESS DECISIONS
  NICE technology appraisals (TAs)
▸ Erythropoiesis-stimulating agents (epoetin and darbepoetin) for treating anaemia in people with cancer having chemotherapy (November 2014) NICE TA323
  Erythropoiesis-stimulating agents (epoetin alfa, beta, theta and zeta, and darbepoetin alfa) are recommended, within their marketing authorisations, as options for treating anaemia in people with cancer who are having chemotherapy.
  If different erythropoiesis-stimulating agents are equally suitable, the product with the lowest acquisition cost for the course of treatment should be used.
  www.nice.org.uk/TA323

● MEDICINAL FORMS
  There can be variation in the licensing of different medicines containing the same drug.
  Solution for injection
  EXCIPIENTS: May contain Phenylalanine
  ▸ NeoRecormon (Roche Products Ltd)
    Epoetin beta 1667 unit per 1 ml NeoRecormon 500units/0.3ml solution for injection pre-filled syringes | 6 pre-filled disposable injection PoM £21.05
    Epoetin beta 6667 unit per 1 ml NeoRecormon 2,000units/0.3ml solution for injection pre-filled syringes | 6 pre-filled disposable injection PoM £84.17
    Epoetin beta 10000 unit per 1 ml NeoRecormon 3,000units/0.3ml solution for injection pre-filled syringes | 6 pre-filled disposable injection PoM £126.25
    Epoetin beta 13333 unit per 1 ml NeoRecormon 4,000units/0.3ml solution for injection pre-filled syringes | 6 pre-filled disposable injection PoM £168.34
    Epoetin beta 16667 unit per 1 ml NeoRecormon 10,000units/0.6ml solution for injection pre-filled syringes | 6 pre-filled disposable injection PoM £420.85
    NeoRecormon 5,000units/0.3ml solution for injection pre-filled syringes | 6 pre-filled disposable injection PoM £210.42
    Epoetin beta 20000 unit per 1 ml NeoRecormon 6,000units/0.3ml solution for injection pre-filled syringes | 6 pre-filled disposable injection PoM £252.50
    Epoetin beta 33333 unit per 1 ml NeoRecormon 20,000units/0.6ml solution for injection pre-filled syringes | 6 pre-filled disposable injection PoM £841.71
    Epoetin beta 50000 unit per 1 ml NeoRecormon 30,000units/0.6ml solution for injection pre-filled syringes | 4 pre-filled disposable injection PoM £841.71

Epoetin zeta   ◀ 873

● INDICATIONS AND DOSE
  Symptomatic anaemia associated with chronic renal failure in patients on haemodialysis
▸ BY INTRAVENOUS INJECTION, OR BY SUBCUTANEOUS INJECTION
  ▸ Adult: Initially 50 units/kg 3 times a week, adjusted according to response, adjusted in steps of 25 units/kg 3 times a week, dose to be adjusted at intervals of at least 4 weeks; maintenance 25–100 units/kg 3 times a week, intravenous injection to be given over 1–5 minutes, if given by subcutaneous injection, a maximum of 1 mL can be given per injection site, avoid increasing haemoglobin concentration at a rate exceeding 2 g/100 mL over 4 weeks

  Symptomatic anaemia associated with chronic renal failure in adults on peritoneal dialysis
▸ BY INTRAVENOUS INJECTION, OR BY SUBCUTANEOUS INJECTION
  ▸ Adult: Initially 50 units/kg twice weekly; maintenance 25–50 units/kg twice weekly, intravenous injection to be given over 1–5 minutes, if given by subcutaneous injection, a maximum of 1 mL can be given per injection site, avoid increasing haemoglobin concentration at a rate exceeding 2 g/100 mL over 4 weeks

  Severe symptomatic anaemia of renal origin in adults with renal insufficiency not yet on dialysis
▸ BY INTRAVENOUS INJECTION, OR BY SUBCUTANEOUS INJECTION
  ▸ Adult: Initially 50 units/kg 3 times a week, adjusted according to response, adjusted in steps of 25 units/kg 3 times a week, dose to be increased at intervals of at least 4 weeks; maintenance 17–33 units/kg 3 times a week (max. per dose 200 units/kg 3 times a week), intravenous injection to be given over 1–5 minutes, if given by subcutaneous injection, a maximum of 1 mL can be given per injection site, avoid increasing haemoglobin concentration at a rate exceeding 2 g/100 mL over 4 weeks

  Symptomatic anaemia in adults receiving cancer chemotherapy
▸ BY SUBCUTANEOUS INJECTION
  ▸ Adult: Initially 150 units/kg 3 times a week, alternatively initially 450 units/kg once weekly, increased to 300 units/kg 3 times a week, only increase dose if appropriate rise in haemoglobin (or reticulocyte count) not achieved after 4 weeks; discontinue if inadequate response after 4 weeks at higher dose, maximum 1 mL per injection site, reduce dose by approximately 25–50% if rise in haemoglobin concentration exceeds 2 g/100 mL over 4 weeks or if haemoglobin concentration exceeds 12 g/100 mL; if haemoglobin concentration continues to rise, despite dose reduction, suspend treatment until haemoglobin concentration decreases and then restart at a dose approximately 25% lower than the previous dose. Discontinue approximately 4 weeks after ending chemotherapy

  To increase yield of autologous blood (to avoid homologous blood) in predonation programme in moderate anaemia either when large volume of blood required or when sufficient blood cannot be saved for elective major surgery
▸ BY INTRAVENOUS INJECTION
  ▸ Adult: 600 units/kg twice weekly for 3 weeks before surgery, intravenous injection to be given over 1–5 minutes, consult product literature for details and advice on ensuring high iron stores   continued →

Moderate anaemia (haemoglobin concentration 10–13 g/100 mL) before elective orthopaedic surgery in adults with expected moderate blood loss to reduce exposure to allogeneic blood transfusion or if autologous transfusion unavailable

▸ BY SUBCUTANEOUS INJECTION
▹ Adult: 600 units/kg every 1 week for 3 weeks before surgery and on day of surgery, alternatively 300 units/kg daily for 15 days starting 10 days before surgery, maximum 1 mL per injection site, consult product literature for details

● PREGNANCY No evidence of harm. Benefits probably outweigh risk of anaemia and of blood transfusion in pregnancy.

● BREAST FEEDING Unlikely to be present in milk. Minimal effect on infant.

● HEPATIC IMPAIRMENT Manufacturers advise caution in chronic hepatic failure.

● PRESCRIBING AND DISPENSING INFORMATION Products containing epoetin zeta are not identical and although there should be no important differences in terms of safety and efficacy, when prescribing biological products it is good practice to use the brand name, see *Biosimilar medicines*, under Guidance on prescribing p. 1.

● NATIONAL FUNDING/ACCESS DECISIONS

NICE technology appraisals (TAs)
▸ **Erythropoiesis-stimulating agents (epoetin and darbepoetin) for treating anaemia in people with cancer having chemotherapy (November 2014)** NICE TA323
Erythropoiesis-stimulating agents (epoetin alfa, beta, theta and zeta, and darbepoetin alfa) are recommended, within their marketing authorisations, as options for treating anaemia in people with cancer who are having chemotherapy.
  If different erythropoiesis-stimulating agents are equally suitable, the product with the lowest acquisition cost for the course of treatment should be used.
www.nice.org.uk/TA323

● MEDICINAL FORMS
There can be variation in the licensing of different medicines containing the same drug.
Solution for injection
EXCIPIENTS: May contain Phenylalanine
▸ Retacrit (Hospira UK Ltd)
  Epoetin zeta 3333 unit per 1 ml Retacrit 2,000units/0.6ml solution for injection pre-filled syringes | 6 pre-filled disposable injection PoM £67.88 (Hospital only)
  Retacrit 3,000units/0.9ml solution for injection pre-filled syringes | 6 pre-filled disposable injection PoM £101.82 (Hospital only)
  Retacrit 1,000units/0.3ml solution for injection pre-filled syringes | 6 pre-filled disposable injection PoM £33.94 (Hospital only)
  Epoetin zeta 10000 unit per 1 ml Retacrit 6,000units/0.6ml solution for injection pre-filled syringes | 6 pre-filled disposable injection PoM £203.63 (Hospital only)
  Retacrit 10,000units/1ml solution for injection pre-filled syringes | 6 pre-filled disposable injection PoM £339.39 (Hospital only)
  Retacrit 8,000units/0.8ml solution for injection pre-filled syringes | 6 pre-filled disposable injection PoM £271.52 (Hospital only)
  Retacrit 4,000units/0.4ml solution for injection pre-filled syringes | 6 pre-filled disposable injection PoM £135.76 (Hospital only)
  Retacrit 5,000units/0.5ml solution for injection pre-filled syringes | 6 pre-filled disposable injection PoM £169.70 (Hospital only)
  Epoetin zeta 40000 unit per 1 ml Retacrit 20,000units/0.5ml solution for injection pre-filled syringes | 1 pre-filled disposable injection PoM £96.16 (Hospital only)
  Retacrit 40,000units/1ml solution for injection pre-filled syringes | 1 pre-filled disposable injection PoM £226.26 (Hospital only)
  Retacrit 30,000units/0.75ml solution for injection pre-filled syringes | 1 pre-filled disposable injection PoM £169.70 (Hospital only)

Methoxy polyethylene glycol-epoetin beta

● INDICATIONS AND DOSE

Symptomatic anaemia associated with chronic kidney disease in patients on dialysis and not currently treated with erythropoietins

▸ BY SUBCUTANEOUS INJECTION, OR BY INTRAVENOUS INJECTION
▹ Adult: Initially 600 nanograms/kg every 2 weeks, dose to be adjusted according to response at intervals of at least 4 weeks, maintenance dose may be given every 4 weeks, reduce dose by approximately 25% if rise in haemoglobin concentration exceeds 2 g/100 mL over 4 weeks; or if haemoglobin concentration approaches or exceeds 12 g/100 mL; if haemoglobin concentration continues to rise, despite dose reduction, suspend treatment until haemoglobin concentration decreases and then restart at a dose approximately 25% lower than the previous dose

Symptomatic anaemia associated with chronic kidney disease in patients not on dialysis and not currently treated with erythropoietins

▸ INITIALLY BY SUBCUTANEOUS INJECTION
▹ Adult: Initially 1.2 micrograms/kg every 4 weeks, alternatively (by subcutaneous injection or by intravenous injection) initially 600 nanograms/kg every 2 weeks, dose to be adjusted according to response at intervals of at least 4 weeks, patients treated once every 2 weeks may be given a maintenance dose of double the previous fortnightly dose every 4 weeks, subcutaneous route preferred in patients not on haemodialysis. Reduce dose by approximately 25% if rise in haemoglobin concentration exceeds 2 g/100 mL over 4 weeks; or if haemoglobin concentration approaches or exceeds 12 g/100 mL; if haemoglobin concentration continues to rise, despite dose reduction, suspend treatment until haemoglobin concentration decreases and then restart at a dose approximately 25% lower than the previous dose

Symptomatic anaemia associated with chronic kidney disease in patients currently treated with erythropoietins

▸ BY SUBCUTANEOUS INJECTION, OR BY INTRAVENOUS INJECTION
▹ Adult: (consult product literature)

● SIDE-EFFECTS Hot flushes

● PREGNANCY No evidence of harm in *animal* studies—manufacturer advises caution.

● BREAST FEEDING Manufacturer advises use only if potential benefit outweighs risk—present in milk in *animal* studies.

● MEDICINAL FORMS
There can be variation in the licensing of different medicines containing the same drug.
Solution for injection
▸ Mircera (Roche Products Ltd)
  Methoxy polyethylene glycol-epoetin beta 100 microgram per 1 ml Mircera 30micrograms/0.3ml solution for injection pre-filled syringes | 1 pre-filled disposable injection PoM £44.05
  Methoxy polyethylene glycol-epoetin beta 166.667 microgram per 1 ml Mircera 50micrograms/0.3ml solution for injection pre-filled syringes | 1 pre-filled disposable injection PoM £73.41
  Methoxy polyethylene glycol-epoetin beta 250 microgram per 1 ml Mircera 75micrograms/0.3ml solution for injection pre-filled syringes | 1 pre-filled disposable injection PoM £110.11
  Methoxy polyethylene glycol-epoetin beta 333.333 microgram per 1 ml Mircera 100micrograms/0.3ml solution for injection pre-filled syringes | 1 pre-filled disposable injection PoM £146.81

9

Blood and nutrition

Methoxy polyethylene glycol-epoetin beta 400 microgram per 1 ml Mircera 120micrograms/0.3ml solution for injection pre-filled syringes | 1 pre-filled disposable injection PoM £176.18

Methoxy polyethylene glycol-epoetin beta 500 microgram per 1 ml Mircera 150micrograms/0.3ml solution for injection pre-filled syringes | 1 pre-filled disposable injection PoM £220.22

Methoxy polyethylene glycol-epoetin beta 600 microgram per 1 ml Mircera 360micrograms/0.6ml solution for injection pre-filled syringes | 1 pre-filled disposable injection PoM £528.56

Methoxy polyethylene glycol-epoetin beta 666.667 microgram per 1 ml Mircera 200micrograms/0.3ml solution for injection pre-filled syringes | 1 pre-filled disposable injection PoM £293.62

Methoxy polyethylene glycol-epoetin beta 833.333 microgram per 1 ml Mircera 250micrograms/0.3ml solution for injection pre-filled syringes | 1 pre-filled disposable injection PoM £367.03

1.1a Atypical haemolytic uraemic syndrome and paroxysmal nocturnal haemoglobinuria

IMMUNOSUPPRESSANTS > MONOCLONAL ANTIBODIES

Eculizumab

- **DRUG ACTION** Eculizumab a recombinant monoclonal antibody, inhibits terminal complement activation at the C5 protein and thereby reduces haemolysis and thrombotic microangiopathy.

- **INDICATIONS AND DOSE**

  Reduce haemolysis in paroxysmal nocturnal haemoglobinuria (PNH), in those with a history of blood transfusions (under expert supervision)
  ▸ BY INTRAVENOUS INFUSION
  ▸ Adult: Initially 600 mg once weekly for 4 weeks, then increased to 900 mg once weekly for 1 week; maintenance 900 mg every 12–16 days

  Reduce thrombotic microangiopathy in atypical haemolytic uraemic syndrome (aHUS) (specialist use only)
  ▸ BY INTRAVENOUS INFUSION
  ▸ Adult: Initially 900 mg once weekly for 4 weeks, then increased to 1.2 g once weekly for 1 week; maintenance 1.2 g every 12–16 days

- **CONTRA-INDICATIONS** Patients unvaccinated against *Neisseria meningitidis* · unresolved *Neisseria meningitidis* infection

- **CAUTIONS** Active systemic infection
  CAUTIONS, FURTHER INFORMATION
  ▸ Meningococcal infection Vaccinate against *Neisseria meningitidis* at least 2 weeks before treatment (tetravalent vaccine against serotypes A, C, W135 and Y recommended); revaccinate according to current medical guidelines. Patients receiving eculizumab less than 2 weeks after receiving meningococcal vaccine must be given prophylactic antibiotics until 2 weeks after vaccination. Advise patient to report promptly any signs of meningococcal infection. Other immunisations should also be up to date.

- **SIDE-EFFECTS**
  ▸ **Common or very common** Alopecia · arthralgia · blood disorders · cough · dizziness · dysgeusia · dysuria · fatigue · gastro-intestinal disturbances · headache · infection (including meningococcal infection) · influenza-like symptoms · infusion-related reactions · leucopenia · myalgia · nasopharyngitis · oedema · paraesthesia · pruritus · rash · spontaneous erection · thrombocytopenia · vertigo

- ▸ **Uncommon** Anorexia · anxiety · chest pain · depression · epistaxis · gingival pain · Graves' disease · haematoma · hot flushing · hyperhidrosis · hypotension · jaundice · malignant melanoma · menstrual disorders · mood changes · muscle spasms · myelodysplastic syndrome · palpitation · petechiae · renal impairment · skin depigmentation · sleep disturbances · syncope · tinnitus · tremor · visual disturbances

- **CONCEPTION AND CONTRACEPTION** Manufacturer advises effective contraception during and for 5 months after treatment.

- **PREGNANCY** No information available—use only if potential benefit outweighs risk. Human IgG antibodies known to cross placenta.

- **BREAST FEEDING** No information available—manufacturer advises avoid breast-feeding during and for 5 months after treatment.

- **MONITORING REQUIREMENTS**
  ▸ Monitor for 1 hour after infusion.
  ▸ For *paroxysmal nocturnal haemoglobinuria*, monitor for intravascular haemolysis (including serum-lactate dehydrogenase concentration) during treatment and for at least 8 weeks after discontinuation.
  ▸ For *atypical haemolytic uraemic syndrome*, monitor for thrombotic microangiopathy (measure platelet count, serum-lactate dehydrogenase concentration, and serum creatinine) during treatment and for at least 12 weeks after discontinuation.

- **DIRECTIONS FOR ADMINISTRATION**
  ▸ With intravenous use For *intravenous infusion* (*Soliris*®), give intermittently *in* Glucose 5% *or* Sodium chloride 0.9%. Dilute requisite dose to a concentration of 5 mg/mL and mix gently; give over 25–45 minutes (infusion time may be increased to 2 hours if infusion-related reactions occur).

- **PRESCRIBING AND DISPENSING INFORMATION** Consult product literature for details of supplemental doses with concomitant plasmapheresis, plasma exchange, or plasma infusion.

- **PATIENT AND CARER ADVICE** A patient information card should be provided.
  Patient or carers should be advised to report promptly any signs of meningococcal infection.

- **MEDICINAL FORMS**
  There can be variation in the licensing of different medicines containing the same drug.
  Solution for infusion
  ELECTROLYTES: May contain Sodium
  ▸ Soliris (Alexion Pharma UK Ltd)
  Eculizumab 10 mg per 1 ml Soliris 300mg/30ml concentrate for solution for infusion vials | 1 vial PoM £3,150.00 (Hospital only)

1.2 Iron deficiency anaemia

Anaemia, iron deficiency

Treatment and prophylaxis

Treatment with an iron preparation is justified only in the presence of a demonstrable iron-deficiency state. Before starting treatment, it is important to exclude any serious underlying cause of the anaemia (e.g. gastric erosion, gastro-intestinal cancer).

Prophylaxis with an iron preparation may be appropriate in malabsorption, menorrhagia, pregnancy, after subtotal or total gastrectomy, in haemodialysis patients, and in the management of low birth-weight infants such as preterm neonates.

9

Blood and nutrition

Oral iron

Iron salts should be given by mouth unless there are good reasons for using another route.

Ferrous salts show only marginal differences between one another in efficiency of absorption of iron. Haemoglobin regeneration rate is little affected by the type of salt used provided sufficient iron is given, and in most patients the speed of response is not critical. Choice of preparation is thus usually decided by the incidence of side-effects and cost.

The oral dose of elemental iron for iron-deficiency anaemia should be 100 to 200 mg daily. It is customary to give this as dried ferrous sulfate; for prophylaxis of iron-deficiency anaemia, ferrous sulfate may be effective.

Iron content of different iron salts

Iron salt/amount		Content of ferrous iron
ferrous fumarate	200 mg	65 mg
ferrous gluconate	300 mg	35 mg
ferrous sulfate	300 mg	60 mg
ferrous sulfate, dried	200 mg	65 mg

Compound preparations

Preparations containing iron and folic acid p. 886 are used during pregnancy in women who are at high risk of developing iron and folic acid deficiency; they should be distinguished from those used for the prevention of neural tube defects in women planning a pregnancy.

It is important to note that the small doses of folic acid contained in these preparations are inadequate for the treatment of megaloblastic anaemias.

Some oral preparations contain ascorbic acid p. 939 to aid absorption of the iron but the therapeutic advantage of such preparations is minimal and cost may be increased.

There is no justification for the inclusion of other ingredients, such as the **B group of vitamins** (except folic acid for pregnant women).

Modified-release preparations

Modified-release preparations of iron are licensed for once-daily dosage, but have no therapeutic advantage and should not be used. These preparations are formulated to release iron gradually; the low incidence of side-effects may reflect the small amounts of iron available for absorption as the iron is carried past the first part of the duodenum into an area of the gut where absorption may be poor.

Parenteral iron

Iron can be administered parenterally as iron dextran p. 881, iron sucrose p. 882, ferric carboxymaltose below, or iron isomaltoside 1000 p. 881. Parenteral iron is generally reserved for use when oral therapy is unsuccessful because the patient cannot tolerate oral iron, or does not take it reliably, or if there is continuing blood loss, or in malabsorption. Parenteral iron may also have a role in the management of chemotherapy-induced anaemia, when given with erythropoietins, in specific patient groups (see NICE guidance).

Many patients with chronic renal failure who are receiving haemodialysis (and some who are receiving peritoneal dialysis) also require iron by the intravenous route on a regular basis.

With the exception of patients with severe renal failure receiving haemodialysis, parenteral iron does not produce a faster haemoglobin response than oral iron provided that the oral iron preparation is taken reliably and is absorbed adequately. If parenteral iron is necessary, the dose should be calculated according to the patient's body-weight and total iron deficit. Depending on the preparation used, parenteral iron is given as a total dose or in divided doses.

Further treatment should be guided by monitoring haemoglobin and serum iron concentrations.

MINERALS AND TRACE ELEMENTS › IRON, INJECTABLE

Iron (injectable)

IMPORTANT SAFETY INFORMATION

MHRA/CHM ADVICE: SERIOUS HYPERSENSITIVITY REACTIONS WITH INTRAVENOUS IRON (AUGUST 2013)

Serious hypersensitivity reactions, including life-threatening and fatal anaphylactic reactions, have been reported in patients receiving intravenous iron. These reactions can occur even when a previous administration has been tolerated (including a negative test dose). Test doses are no longer recommended and caution is needed with every dose of intravenous iron.

Intravenous iron products should only be administered when appropriately trained staff and resuscitation facilities are immediately available; patients should be closely monitored for signs of hypersensitivity during and for at least 30 minutes after every administration. In the event of a hypersensitivity reaction, treatment should be stopped immediately and appropriate management initiated.

The risk of hypersensitivity is increased in patients with known allergies, immune or inflammatory conditions, or those with a history of severe asthma, eczema, or other atopic allergy; in these patients, intravenous iron should only be used if the benefits outweigh the risks.

Intravenous iron should be avoided in the first trimester of pregnancy and used in the second or third trimesters only if the benefit outweighs the potential risks for both mother and fetus.

● SIDE-EFFECTS Hypersensitivity reactions

SIDE-EFFECTS, FURTHER INFORMATION

➤ **Anaphylactic reactions** Anaphylactic reactions can occur with parenteral administration of iron complexes and facilities for cardiopulmonary resuscitation must be available.

Overdose

For details on the management of poisoning, see Iron salts, under Emergency treatment of poisoning p. 1194.

⚑ above

Ferric carboxymaltose

● **INDICATIONS AND DOSE**

Iron-deficiency anaemia

▸ BY SLOW INTRAVENOUS INJECTION, OR BY INTRAVENOUS INFUSION

▸ Adult: Dose calculated according to body-weight and iron deficit (consult product literature)

● CAUTIONS Allergic disorders · asthma · eczema · hypersensitivity can occur with parenteral iron and facilities for cardiopulmonary resuscitation must be available · infection (discontinue if ongoing bacteraemia) · oral iron should not be given until 5 days after last injection

● SIDE-EFFECTS

▸ **Common or very common** Dizziness · gastro-intestinal disturbances · headache · injection-site reactions · rash

▸ **Uncommon** Anaphylaxis · arthralgia · back pain · chest pain · fatigue · flushing · hypertension · hypotension · malaise · myalgia · paraesthesia · peripheral oedema · pruritus · pyrexia · rigors · urticaria

▸ **Rare** Dyspnoea

- PREGNANCY Avoid in first trimester; crosses the placenta in *animal* studies. May influence skeletal development.
- HEPATIC IMPAIRMENT Use with caution. Avoid in conditions where iron overload increases risk of impairment.
- DIRECTIONS FOR ADMINISTRATION
▸ With intravenous use For *intravenous infusion (Ferinject®)*, give intermittently in Sodium chloride 0.9%, dilute 200–500 mg in up to 100 mL infusion fluid and give over at least 6 minutes; dilute 0.5–1 g in up to 250 mL infusion fluid and give over at least 15 minutes.
- PRESCRIBING AND DISPENSING INFORMATION A ferric carboxymaltose complex containing 5% (50 mg/mL) of iron.

- MEDICINAL FORMS
There can be variation in the licensing of different medicines containing the same drug.
Solution for injection
ELECTROLYTES: May contain Sodium
▸ Ferinject (Vifor Pharma UK Ltd) ▼
  Iron (as Ferric carboxymaltose) 50 mg per 1 ml Ferinject 1000mg/20ml solution for injection vials | 1 vial PoM £154.23
Ferinject 100mg/2ml solution for injection vials | 5 vial PoM £81.18
Ferinject 500mg/10ml solution for injection vials | 5 vial PoM £405.88

☞ 880

Iron dextran

- INDICATIONS AND DOSE
Iron-deficiency anaemia
▸ BY DEEP INTRAMUSCULAR INJECTION
▸ Adult: Intramuscular injection to be administered into the gluteal muscle, doses calculated according to body-weight and iron deficit (consult product literature)
▸ BY SLOW INTRAVENOUS INJECTION, OR BY INTRAVENOUS INFUSION
▸ Adult: Doses calculated according to body-weight and iron deficit (consult product literature)

- CONTRA-INDICATIONS Active rheumatoid arthritis · asthma · eczema · history of allergic disorders · infection
- CAUTIONS Hypersensitivity can occur with parenteral iron and facilities for cardiopulmonary resuscitation must be available · oral iron should not be given until 5 days after last injection
- SIDE-EFFECTS
▸ **Uncommon** Abdominal pain · anaphylaxis · blurred vision · cramps · dyspnoea · flushing · nausea · numbness · pruritus · rash · vomiting
▸ **Rare** Angioedema · arrhythmias · arthralgia · chest pain · diarrhoea · dizziness · fatigue · hypotension · impaired consciousness · injection-site reactions · myalgia · restlessness · seizures · sweating · tachycardia · tremor
▸ **Very rare** Haemolysis · headache · hypertension · palpitation · paraesthesia · transient deafness
- PREGNANCY Avoid in first trimester.
- HEPATIC IMPAIRMENT Avoid in severe impairment.
- RENAL IMPAIRMENT Avoid in acute renal failure.
- DIRECTIONS FOR ADMINISTRATION
▸ With intravenous use For *intravenous infusion (Cosmofer®)*, give intermittently in Glucose 5% *or* Sodium chloride 0.9%, dilute 100–200 mg in 100 mL infusion fluid; give 25mg over 15 minutes initially, then give at a rate not exceeding 6.67 mg/minute; *total dose infusion* diluted in 500 mL infusion fluid and given over 4–6 hours (initial dose 25 mg over 15 minutes).
- PRESCRIBING AND DISPENSING INFORMATION A complex of ferric hydroxide with dextran containing 5% (50 mg/mL) of iron.

- MEDICINAL FORMS
There can be variation in the licensing of different medicines containing the same drug.
Solution for injection
▸ CosmoFer (Pharmacosmos UK Ltd) ▼
  Iron (as Iron dextran) 50 mg per 1 ml CosmoFer 500mg/10ml solution for injection ampoules | 2 ampoule PoM £79.70
CosmoFer 100mg/2ml solution for injection ampoules | 5 ampoule PoM £39.85

☞ 880

Iron isomaltoside 1000

- INDICATIONS AND DOSE
Iron-deficiency anaemia
▸ BY SLOW INTRAVENOUS INJECTION, OR BY INTRAVENOUS INFUSION
▸ Adult: Doses calculated according to body-weight and iron deficit (consult product literature)

- CONTRA-INDICATIONS Active rheumatoid arthritis · asthma · eczema · history of allergic disorders
- CAUTIONS Hypersensitivity can occur with parenteral iron and facilities for cardiopulmonary resuscitation must be available · infection (discontinue if ongoing bacteraemia) · oral iron should not be given until 5 days after last injection
- SIDE-EFFECTS
▸ **Uncommon** Abdominal pain · anaphylaxis · blurred vision · constipation · cramps · dysphonia · dyspnoea · fever · flushing · injection-site reactions · nausea · numbness · pruritus · rash · vomiting
▸ **Rare** Altered mental status · angioedema · arrhythmias · arthralgia · chest pain · diarrhoea · dizziness · hypotension · loss of consciousness · malaise · myalgia · restlessness · seizures · sweating · tachycardia · tremor
▸ **Very rare** Foetal bradycardia · haemolysis · headache · hypertension · palpitation · paraesthesia · transient deafness
- PREGNANCY Avoid in first trimester.
- HEPATIC IMPAIRMENT Avoid in decompensated liver disease and hepatitis.
- DIRECTIONS FOR ADMINISTRATION
▸ With intravenous use For *intravenous infusion (Monofer®)*, give intermittently *in* Sodium chloride 0.9%. For details consult product literature.
- PRESCRIBING AND DISPENSING INFORMATION A complex of ferric iron and isomaltosides containing 10% (100 mg/mL) of iron.

- MEDICINAL FORMS
There can be variation in the licensing of different medicines containing the same drug.
Solution for injection
▸ Diafer (Pharmacosmos UK Ltd) ▼
  Iron isomaltoside 1000 50 mg per 1 ml Diafer 100mg/2ml solution for injection ampoules | 25 ampoule PoM no price available
▸ Monofer (Pharmacosmos UK Ltd) ▼
  Iron isomaltoside 1000 100 mg per 1 ml Monofer 500mg/5ml solution for injection vials | 5 vial PoM no price available
Monofer 100mg/1ml solution for injection vials | 5 vial PoM no price available
Monofer 1g/10ml solution for injection vials | 2 vial PoM no price available

9

Blood and nutrition

Iron sucrose

F 880

- **INDICATIONS AND DOSE**

Iron-deficiency anaemia

▶ BY SLOW INTRAVENOUS INJECTION, OR BY INTRAVENOUS INFUSION

- Adult: Doses calculated according to body-weight and iron deficit (consult product literature)

- CONTRA-INDICATIONS Anaphylaxis · asthma · eczema · history of allergic disorders
- CAUTIONS Hypersensitivity reactions can occur with parenteral iron and facilities for cardiopulmonary resuscitation must be available · infection (discontinue if ongoing bacteraemia · oral iron should not be given until 5 days after last injection
- SIDE-EFFECTS
▶ **Common or very common** Taste disturbances
▶ **Uncommon** Abdominal pain · bronchospasm · chest pain · diarrhoea · dizziness · dyspnoea · fever · flushing · headache · hypotension · injection-site reactions · myalgia · nausea · palpitation · pruritus · rash · tachycardia · vomiting
▶ **Rare** Anaphylaxis · asthenia · fatigue · hypertension · paraesthesia · peripheral oedema
▶ **Frequency not known** Arthralgia · bradycardia · confusion · increased sweating
- PREGNANCY Avoid in first trimester.
- HEPATIC IMPAIRMENT Use with caution. Avoid in conditions where iron overload increases risk of impairment.
- DIRECTIONS FOR ADMINISTRATION
▶ With intravenous use For *intravenous infusion* (*Venofer*®), give intermittently in Sodium chloride 0.9%, dilute 100 mg in up to 100 mL infusion fluid; give 25 mg over 15 minutes initially, then give at a rate not exceeding 3.33 mg/minute.
- PRESCRIBING AND DISPENSING INFORMATION A complex of ferric hydroxide with sucrose containing 2% (20 mg/mL) of iron.

- MEDICINAL FORMS
There can be variation in the licensing of different medicines containing the same drug.
Solution for injection
▶ Venofer (Vifor Pharma UK Ltd, Imported (United States)) ▼
Iron (as Iron sucrose) 20 mg per 1 ml Venofer 100mg/5ml solution for injection vials | 5 vial [PoM] £43.52
Venofer 50mg/2.5ml solution for injection vials | 5 vial [PoM] no price available

MINERALS AND TRACE ELEMENTS > IRON, ORAL

Iron (oral)

- SIDE-EFFECTS Constipation · diarrhoea · epigastric pain (dose related) · faecal impaction · gastro-intestinal irritation · nausea (dose related)
  SIDE-EFFECTS, FURTHER INFORMATION
▶ Managing side-effects If side-effects occur, the dose may be reduced; alternatively, another iron salt may be used, but an improvement in tolerance may simply be a result of a lower content of elemental iron. The incidence of side-effects due to ferrous sulfate is no greater than with other iron salts when compared on the basis of equivalent amounts of elemental iron.
▶ Altered bowel habit Iron preparations taken orally can be constipating and occasionally lead to faecal impaction.
  Oral iron, particularly modified-release preparations, can exacerbate diarrhoea in patients with inflammatory bowel disease; care is also needed in patients with intestinal strictures and diverticular disease.

The relationship between dose and altered bowel habit (constipation or diarrhoea) is less clear than for nausea and epigastric pain.

Overdose
For details on the management of poisoning, see Iron salts, under Emergency treatment of poisoning p. 1194.
▶ In children Iron preparations are an important cause of accidental overdose in children and as little as 20 mg/kg of elemental iron can lead to symptoms of toxicity.

- MONITORING REQUIREMENTS
▶ Therapeutic response The haemoglobin concentration should rise by about 100–200 mg/100 mL (1–2 g/litre) per day *or* 2 g/100 mL (20 g/litre) over 3–4 weeks. When the haemoglobin is in the normal range, treatment should be continued for a further 3 months to replenish the iron stores. Epithelial tissue changes such as atrophic glossitis and koilonychia are usually improved, but the response is often slow.

- PRESCRIBING AND DISPENSING INFORMATION
▶ In children Express the dose in terms of elemental iron and iron salt and select the most appropriate preparation; specify both the iron salt and formulation on the prescription. The iron content of artificial formula feeds should also be considered.
▶ In children The most common reason for lack of response in children is poor compliance; poor absorption is rare in children.

- PATIENT AND CARER ADVICE Although iron preparations are best absorbed on an empty stomach they can be taken after food to reduce gastro-intestinal side-effects. May discolour stools.

F above

Ferrous fumarate

- **INDICATIONS AND DOSE**

Iron-deficiency anaemia (prophylactic)
▶ BY MOUTH USING TABLETS
- Child 12–17 years: 210 mg 1–2 times a day
- Adult: 210 mg 1–2 times a day
▶ BY MOUTH USING SYRUP
- Child 12–17 years: 140 mg twice daily
- Adult: 140 mg twice daily

Iron-deficiency anaemia (therapeutic)
▶ BY MOUTH USING TABLETS
- Child 12–17 years: 210 mg 2–3 times a day
- Adult: 210 mg 2–3 times a day
▶ BY MOUTH USING SYRUP
- Child 12–17 years: 280 mg twice daily
- Adult: 280 mg twice daily

FERSADAY®

Iron-deficiency anaemia (prophylactic)
▶ BY MOUTH
- Adult: 322 mg daily

Iron-deficiency anaemia (therapeutic)
▶ BY MOUTH
- Adult: 322 mg twice daily

GALFER® CAPSULES

Iron-deficiency anaemia (prophylactic)
▶ BY MOUTH
- Child 12–17 years: 305 mg daily
- Adult: 305 mg daily

Iron-deficiency anaemia (therapeutic)
▶ BY MOUTH
- Child 12–17 years: 305 mg twice daily
- Adult: 305 mg twice daily

9

Blood and nutrition

GALFER® SYRUP

Iron-deficiency anaemia (prophylaxis)
▸ BY MOUTH
▸ Child 1 month–11 years: 0.25 mL/kilogram twice daily, the total daily dose may alternatively be given in 3 divided doses, prophylactic iron supplementation may be required in babies of low birth-weight who are solely breast-fed; supplementation is started 4–6 weeks after birth and continued until mixed feeding is established; maximum 20 mL per day
▸ Child 12–17 years: 10 mL once daily
▸ Adult: 10 mL once daily

Iron-deficiency anaemia (therapeutic)
▸ BY MOUTH
▸ Child 1 month–11 years: 0.25 mL/kilogram twice daily, the total daily dose may alternatively be given in 3 divided doses; maximum 20 mL per day
▸ Child 12–17 years: 10 mL 1–2 times a day
▸ Adult: 10 mL 1–2 times a day

● INTERACTIONS → Appendix 1 (iron salts).

● PRESCRIBING AND DISPENSING INFORMATION Non-proprietary ferrous fumarate tablets may contain 210 mg (68 mg iron), syrup may contain approx. 140 mg (45 mg iron)/5 mL; *Galfer®* capsules contain ferrous fumarate 305 mg (100 mg iron); *Fersaday®* tablets contain ferrous fumarate 322 mg (100 mg iron).

● PATIENT AND CARER ADVICE
Medicines for Children leaflet: Ferrous fumarate for iron-deficiency anaemia www.medicinesforchildren.org.uk/ferrous-fumarate-for-iron-deficiency-anaemia

● MEDICINAL FORMS
There can be variation in the licensing of different medicines containing the same drug.
Tablet
▸ Ferrous fumarate (Non-proprietary)
   Ferrous fumarate 210 mg Ferrous fumarate 210mg tablets | 84 tablet no price available DT price = £2.75 | 84 tablet P £2.75 DT price = £2.75
   Ferrous fumarate 322 mg Ferrous fumarate 322mg tablets | 28 tablet no price available DT price = £0.95 | 28 tablet P £0.95–£1.00 DT price = £0.95
▸ Fersaday (AMCo)
   Ferrous fumarate 322 mg Fersaday 322mg tablets | 28 tablet P £0.95 DT price = £0.95
Capsule
▸ Galfer (Thornton & Ross Ltd)
   Ferrous fumarate 305 mg Galfer 305mg capsules | 100 capsule P £2.33 DT price = £2.33 | 250 capsule P £5.00
Oral solution
▸ Ferrous fumarate (Non-proprietary)
   Ferrous fumarate 28 mg per 1 ml Ferrous fumarate 140mg/5ml oral solution | 200 ml P £3.73 DT price = £3.73
▸ Galfer (Thornton & Ross Ltd)
   Ferrous fumarate 28 mg per 1 ml Galfer 140mg/5ml syrup sugar-free | 300 ml P £5.33 DT price = £5.33

Ferrous fumarate with folic acid

The properties listed below are those particular to the combination only. For the properties of the components please consider, ferrous fumarate p. 882, folic acid p. 886.

● INDICATIONS AND DOSE
Iron-deficiency anaemia
▸ BY MOUTH USING CAPSULES
▸ Adult: 1 capsule daily, to be taken before food
▸ BY MOUTH USING TABLETS
▸ Adult: 1 tablet daily

● PRESCRIBING AND DISPENSING INFORMATION *Pregaday®* contains ferrous fumarate 322 mg (100 mg iron),

folic acid 350 micrograms; *Galfer FA®* contains ferrous fumarate 305 mg (100 mg iron), folic acid 350 micrograms.

● MEDICINAL FORMS
There can be variation in the licensing of different medicines containing the same drug.
Tablet
▸ Pregaday (Focus Pharmaceuticals Ltd)
   Folic acid 350 microgram, Ferrous fumarate 322 mg Pregaday 322mg/350microgram tablets | 28 tablet P £1.25 DT price = £1.25
Capsule
▸ Galfer FA (Thornton & Ross Ltd)
   Folic acid 350 microgram, Ferrous fumarate 305 mg Galfer FA capsules | 100 capsule P £3.25 DT price = £3.25

◀ 882

Ferrous gluconate

● INDICATIONS AND DOSE
Prophylaxis of iron-deficiency anaemia
▸ BY MOUTH USING TABLETS
▸ Child 6–11 years: 300–900 mg daily
▸ Child 12–17 years: 600 mg daily
▸ Adult: 600 mg daily

Treatment of iron-deficiency anaemia
▸ BY MOUTH USING TABLETS
▸ Child 6–11 years: 300–900 mg daily
▸ Child 12–17 years: 1.2–1.8 g daily in divided doses
▸ Adult: 1.2–1.8 g daily in divided doses

● INTERACTIONS → Appendix 1 (iron salts).

● PRESCRIBING AND DISPENSING INFORMATION Ferrous gluconate 300 mg contains 35 mg iron.

● PATIENT AND CARER ADVICE
Medicines for Children leaflet: Ferrous gluconate for iron-deficiency anaemia www.medicinesforchildren.org.uk/ferrous-gluconate-for-iron-deficiency-anaemia

● MEDICINAL FORMS
There can be variation in the licensing of different medicines containing the same drug.
Tablet
▸ Ferrous gluconate (Non-proprietary)
   Ferrous gluconate 300 mg Ferrous gluconate 300mg tablets | 28 tablet P £3.35 DT price = £1.95 | 1000 tablet P £119.64

◀ 882

Ferrous sulfate

● INDICATIONS AND DOSE
Iron-deficiency anaemia (prophylactic)
▸ BY MOUTH USING TABLETS
▸ Child 6–17 years: 200 mg daily
▸ Adult: 200 mg daily

Iron-deficiency anaemia (therapeutic)
▸ BY MOUTH USING TABLETS
▸ Child 6–17 years: 200 mg 2–3 times a day
▸ Adult: 200 mg 2–3 times a day

FEOSPAN®

Iron-deficiency anaemia
▸ BY MOUTH
▸ Child 1–17 years: 1 capsule daily, capsule can be opened and sprinkled on food
▸ Adult: 1–2 capsules daily, capsule can be opened and sprinkled on food

FERROGRAD®

Iron-deficiency anaemia (prophylactic and therapeutic)
▸ BY MOUTH
▸ Child 12–17 years: 1 tablet daily
▸ Adult: 1 tablet daily

continued →

IRONORM® DROPS

Iron-deficiency anaemia (prophylactic)
▸ BY MOUTH
▸ Adult: 2.4–4.8 mL daily

Iron-deficiency anaemia (therapeutic)
▸ BY MOUTH
▸ Adult: 4 mL 1–2 times a day

● INTERACTIONS → Appendix 1 (iron salts).

● PRESCRIBING AND DISPENSING INFORMATION
Iron content Ferrous sulfate 200 mg is equivalent to 65 mg iron; *Ironorm*® drops contain ferrous sulfate 125 mg (equivalent to 25 mg iron)/mL; *Feospan*® spansules contains ferrous sulfate 150 mg (47 mg iron) (spansule (= capsules m/r)); *Ferrograd*® tablets contain ferrous sulfate 325 mg (105 mg iron).
▸ With oral use in adults Modified-release preparations of iron are licensed for once-daily dosage, but have no therapeutic advantage and should not be used. These preparations are formulated to release iron gradually; the low incidence of side-effects may reflect the small amounts of iron available for absorption as the iron is carried past the first part of the duodenum into an area of the gut where absorption may be poor.

● PATIENT AND CARER ADVICE
Medicines for Children leaflet: Ferrous sulfate for iron-deficiency anaemia www.medicinesforchildren.org.uk/ferrous-sulfate-iron-deficiency-anaemia

● NATIONAL FUNDING/ACCESS DECISIONS *Feospan*® and *Ferrograd*® are not prescribable under the National Health Service.

● LESS SUITABLE FOR PRESCRIBING *Feospan*® is less suitable for prescribing. *Ferrograd*® is less suitable for prescribing.

● MEDICINAL FORMS
There can be variation in the licensing of different medicines containing the same drug.
Tablet
▸ Ferrous sulfate (Non-proprietary)
Ferrous sulfate dried 200 mg Ferrous sulfate 200mg tablets | 28 tablet P £8.15 DT price = £2.75 | 60 tablet P £1.78 | 100 tablet P £14.96 | 1000 tablet P £108.93
Modified-release tablet
CAUTIONARY AND ADVISORY LABELS 25
▸ Ferrograd (Teofarma)
Ferrous sulfate dried 325 mg Ferrograd 325mg modified-release tablets | 30 tablet P £2.58 DT price = £2.58
Modified-release capsule
CAUTIONARY AND ADVISORY LABELS 25
▸ Feospan Spansules (Intrapharm Laboratories Ltd)
Ferrous sulfate dried 150 mg Feospan 150mg Spansules | 30 capsule P £3.95
Oral drops
▸ Ironorm (Wallace Manufacturing Chemists Ltd)
Ferrous sulfate 125 mg per 1 ml Ironorm 125mg/ml oral drops sugar-free | 15 ml P £30.00

Ferrous sulfate with ascorbic acid

The properties listed below are those particular to the combination only. For the properties of the components please consider, ferrous sulfate p. 883, ascorbic acid p. 939.

● INDICATIONS AND DOSE
Iron-deficiency anaemia
▸ BY MOUTH USING MODIFIED-RELEASE TABLETS
▸ Adult: 1 tablet daily, dose to be taken before food

● NATIONAL FUNDING/ACCESS DECISIONS
Ferrograd C® is not prescribable on the National Health Service.

● LESS SUITABLE FOR PRESCRIBING *Ferrograd C*® is less suitable for prescribing.

● MEDICINAL FORMS
There can be variation in the licensing of different medicines containing the same drug.
Modified-release tablet
CAUTIONARY AND ADVISORY LABELS 25
▸ Ferrograd C (Teofarma)
Ferrous sulfate dried 325 mg, Ascorbic acid (as Sodium ascorbate) 500 mg Ferrograd C modified-release tablets | 30 tablet P £3.20

Ferrous sulfate with folic acid

The properties listed below are those particular to the combination only. For the properties of the components please consider, ferrous sulfate p. 883, folic acid p. 886.

● INDICATIONS AND DOSE
Iron-deficiency anaemia
▸ BY MOUTH USING MODIFIED-RELEASE CAPSULES
▸ Adult: 1 capsule daily
▸ BY MOUTH USING MODIFIED-RELEASE TABLETS
▸ Child 12–17 years: 1 tablet daily, to be taken before food
▸ Adult: 1 tablet daily, to be taken before food

● NATIONAL FUNDING/ACCESS DECISIONS *Fefol*® is not prescribable under the National Health Service.

● LESS SUITABLE FOR PRESCRIBING *Fefol*® is less suitable for prescribing. *Ferrograd Folic*® is less suitable for prescribing.

● MEDICINAL FORMS
There can be variation in the licensing of different medicines containing the same drug.
Modified-release tablet
CAUTIONARY AND ADVISORY LABELS 25
▸ Ferrograd Folic (Teofarma)
Folic acid 350 microgram, Ferrous sulfate dried 325 mg Ferrograd Folic 325mg/350microgram modified-release tablets | 30 tablet P £2.64 DT price = £2.64
Modified-release capsule
CAUTIONARY AND ADVISORY LABELS 25
▸ Fefol Spansules (Intrapharm Laboratories Ltd)
Folic acid 500 microgram, Ferrous sulfate dried 150 mg Fefol Spansules | 30 capsule P £4.25

Polysaccharide-iron complex

● INDICATIONS AND DOSE
Iron-deficiency anaemia (prophylactic)
▸ BY MOUTH
▸ Child 1 month-1 year: 1 drop (approximately 500 micrograms iron) per 450 g body-weight to be to be given 3 times a daily, dose to be administered from dropper bottle, prophylactic iron supplementation may be required in babies of low birth-weight who are solely breast-fed; supplementation is started 4–6 weeks after birth and continued until mixed feeding is established
▸ Child 12–17 years: 2.5 mL daily
▸ Adult: 2.5 mL daily

Iron-deficiency anaemia (therapeutic)
▸ BY MOUTH
▸ Child 2–5 years: 2.5 mL daily
▸ Child 6–11 years: 5 mL daily
▸ Child 12–17 years: 5 mL 1–2 times a day
▸ Adult: 5 mL 1–2 times a day

Iron-deficiency anaemia (therapeutic) if required during second and third trimester of pregnancy
▸ BY MOUTH
▸ Child 12–17 years: 5 mL once daily
▸ Adult: 5 mL once daily

● INTERACTIONS → Appendix 1 (iron salts).

● PATIENT AND CARER ADVICE Counselling on the use of the dropper advised.

● NATIONAL FUNDING/ACCESS DECISIONS
Niferex® is not available on prescription under NHS, except 30-mL paediatric dropper bottle for prophylaxis and treatment of iron deficiency in infants born prematurely; endorse prescription 'SLS'.Service.

● MEDICINAL FORMS
There can be variation in the licensing of different medicines containing the same drug.
Oral solution
▸ Niferex (Tillomed Laboratories Ltd)
Iron (as Polysaccharide-iron complex) 100 mg Niferex 100mg/5ml elixir sugar-free | 30 ml P £2.16 sugar-free | 240 ml P £6.06

🔖 882

Sodium feredetate

(Sodium ironedetate)

● INDICATIONS AND DOSE
Iron-deficiency anaemia (therapeutic)
▸ BY MOUTH USING ORAL SOLUTION
▸ Child 1–11 months: Up to 2.5 mL twice daily, smaller doses to be used initially
▸ Child 1–4 years: 2.5 mL 3 times a day
▸ Child 5–11 years: 5 mL 3 times a day
▸ Child 12–17 years: 5 mL 3 times a day, increased to 10 mL 3 times a day, dose to be increased gradually
▸ Adult: 5 mL 3 times a day, increased to 10 mL 3 times a day, dose to be increased gradually

● UNLICENSED USE
▸ In children Not licensed for prophylaxis of iron deficiency.

● INTERACTIONS → Appendix 1 (iron salts).

● PRESCRIBING AND DISPENSING INFORMATION *Sytron*® contains 190 mg sodium feredetate, which is equivalent to 27.5 mg of iron/5 mL.

● PATIENT AND CARER ADVICE
Medicines for Children leaflet: Sytron (sodium feredetate) for the prevention of anaemia www.medicinesforchildren.org.uk/sytron-sodium-feredetate-for-prevention-of-anaemia
Medicines for Children leaflet: Sytron (sodium feredetate) for the treatment of anaemia www.medicinesforchildren.org.uk/sytron-sodium-feredetate-for-treatment-of-anaemia

● MEDICINAL FORMS
There can be variation in the licensing of different medicines containing the same drug.
Oral solution
▸ Sodium feredetate (Non-proprietary)
Sodium feredetate 38 mg per 1 ml Sodium feredetate 190mg/5ml oral solution sugar free sugar-free | 500 ml PoM £14.95–£17.94 DT price = £14.95
▸ Sytron (Forum Health Products Ltd)
Sodium feredetate 38 mg per 1 ml Sytron oral solution sugar-free | 500 ml P £14.95 DT price = £14.95

1.3 Megaloblastic anaemia

Anaemia, megaloblastic

Overview
Most megaloblastic anaemias result from a lack of either vitamin B_{12} or folate, and it is essential to establish in every case which deficiency is present and the underlying cause. In emergencies, when delay might be dangerous, it is sometimes necessary to administer both substances after the bone marrow test while plasma assay results are awaited. Normally, however, appropriate treatment should not be instituted until the results of tests are available.

One cause of megaloblastic anaemia in the UK is *pernicious anaemia* in which lack of gastric intrinsic factor resulting from an autoimmune gastritis causes malabsorption of vitamin B_{12}.

Vitamin B_{12} is also needed in the treatment of megaloblastosis caused by *prolonged nitrous oxide anaesthesia*, which inactivates the vitamin, and in the rare syndrome of *congenital transcobalamin II deficiency*.

Vitamin B_{12} should be given prophylactically after *total gastrectomy* or *total ileal resection* (or after *partial gastrectomy* if a vitamin B_{12} absorption test shows vitamin B_{12} malabsorption).

Apart from dietary deficiency, all other causes of vitamin B_{12} deficiency are attributable to malabsorption. There is little place for the use of low-dose vitamin B_{12} orally and none for vitamin B_{12} intrinsic factor complexes given by mouth. Vitamin B_{12} in larger oral doses [unlicensed] may be effective.

Hydroxocobalamin p. 887 has completely replaced cyanocobalamin p. 886 as the form of vitamin B_{12} of choice for therapy; it is retained in the body longer than cyanocobalamin and thus for maintenance therapy can be given at intervals of up to 3 months. Treatment is generally initiated with frequent administration of intramuscular injections to replenish the depleted body stores. Thereafter, maintenance treatment, which is usually for life, can be instituted. There is no evidence that doses larger than those recommended provide any additional benefit in vitamin B_{12} neuropathy.

Folic acid p. 886 has few indications for long-term therapy since most causes of folate deficiency are self-limiting or will yield to a short course of treatment. It should not be used in undiagnosed megaloblastic anaemia unless vitamin B_{12} is administered concurrently otherwise neuropathy may be precipitated.

In *folate-deficient megaloblastic anaemia* (e.g. because of poor nutrition, pregnancy, or antiepileptic drugs), daily folic acid supplementation for 4 months brings about haematological remission and replenishes body stores.

For prophylaxis in *chronic haemolytic states*, *malabsorption*, or *in renal dialysis*, folic acid is given daily or sometimes weekly, depending on the diet and the rate of haemolysis.

Folic acid is also used for the prevention of methotrexate-induced side-effects in severe Crohn's disease, rheumatic disease, and severe psoriasis.

Folinic acid p. 827 is also effective in the treatment of folate deficient megaloblastic anaemia but it is generally used in association with cytotoxic drugs; it is given as calcium folinate.

There is **no** justification for prescribing multiple ingredient vitamin preparations containing vitamin B_{12} or folic acid.

For the use of folic acid before and during pregnancy, see Neural tube defects (prevention in pregnancy) p. 946.

9

Blood and nutrition

VITAMINS AND TRACE ELEMENTS > FOLATES

Folic acid

9.6.2016

- INDICATIONS AND DOSE

Folate-deficient megaloblastic anaemia
▸ BY MOUTH
- Child 1-11 months: Initially 500 micrograms/kg once daily (max. per dose 5 mg) for up to 4 months, doses up to 10 mg daily may be required in malabsorption states
- Child 1-17 years: 5 mg daily for 4 months (until term in pregnant women), doses up to 15 mg daily may be required in malabsorption states
- Adult: 5 mg daily for 4 months (until term in pregnant women), doses up to 15 mg daily may be required in malabsorption states

Prevention of neural tube defects (in those at a low risk of conceiving a child with a neural tube defect see p. 946)
▸ BY MOUTH
- Females of childbearing potential: 400 micrograms daily, to be taken before conception and until week 12 of pregnancy

Prevention of neural tube defects (in those in the high-risk group who wish to become pregnant or who are at risk of becoming pregnant see p. 946)
▸ BY MOUTH
- Females of childbearing potential: 5 mg daily, to be taken before conception and until week 12 of pregnancy

Prevention of neural tube defects (in those with sickle-cell disease)
▸ BY MOUTH
- Females of childbearing potential: 5 mg daily, patient should continue taking their normal dose of folic acid 5 mg daily (or increase the dose to 5 mg daily) before conception and continue this throughout pregnancy

Prevention of methotrexate-induced side-effects in rheumatic disease
▸ BY MOUTH
- Adult: 5 mg once weekly, dose to be taken on a different day to methotrexate dose

Prevention of methotrexate side-effects in severe Crohn's disease | Prevention of methotrexate side-effects in severe psoriasis
▸ BY MOUTH
- Adult: 5 mg once weekly, dose to be taken on a different day to methotrexate dose

Prophylaxis in chronic haemolytic states
▸ BY MOUTH
- Adult: 5 mg every 1–7 days, frequency dependent on underlying disease

Prophylaxis of folate deficiency in dialysis
▸ BY MOUTH
- Child 1 month–11 years: 250 micrograms/kg once daily (max. per dose 10 mg)
- Child 12–17 years: 5–10 mg once daily
- Adult: 5 mg every 1–7 days

Prophylaxis of folate deficiency in patients receiving parenteral nutrition
▸ BY INTRAVENOUS INFUSION
- Adult: 15 mg 1–2 times a week, usually given by *intravenous infusion* in the parenteral nutrition solution

- UNLICENSED USE Not licensed for prevention of methotrexate-induced side-effects in severe Crohn's disease. Not licensed for prevention of methotrexate-induced side-effects in rheumatic disease. Not licensed for prevention of methotrexate-induced side-effects in severe psoriasis.

- CAUTIONS Should never be given alone for pernicious anaemia (may precipitate subacute combined degeneration of the spinal cord)
- INTERACTIONS → Appendix 1 (folates).
- SIDE-EFFECTS
- Rare Gastro-intestinal disturbances
- PATIENT AND CARER ADVICE
  Medicines for Children leaflet: Folic acid for megaloblastic anaemia caused by folate deficiency and haemolytic anaemia
  www.medicinesforchildren.org.uk/
  folic-acid-megaloblastic-anaemia-caused-folate-deficiency-and-haemolytic-anaemia
- EXCEPTIONS TO LEGAL CATEGORY
- With oral use Can be sold to the public provided daily doses do not exceed 500 micrograms.
- MEDICINAL FORMS
  There can be variation in the licensing of different medicines containing the same drug. Forms available from special-order manufacturers include: capsule, oral suspension, oral solution, solution for injection

Tablet
- Folic acid (Non-proprietary)
  Folic acid 400 microgram Folic acid 400microgram tablets | 90 tablet [PoM] no price available DT price = £2.71 | 90 tablet £2.71 DT price = £2.71
  Folic acid 5 mg Folic acid 5mg tablets | 28 tablet [PoM] £2.00 DT price = £0.83 | 1000 tablet [PoM] £41.75

Oral solution
- Folic acid (Non-proprietary)
  Folic acid 500 microgram per 1 ml Folic acid 2.5mg/5ml oral solution sugar free sugar-free | 150 ml £9.16 DT price = £9.16 sugar-free | 150 ml [PoM] £9.16 DT price = £9.16
- Lexpec (Rosemont Pharmaceuticals Ltd)
  Folic acid 500 microgram per 1 ml Lexpec Folic Acid 2.5mg/5ml oral solution sugar-free | 150 ml [PoM] £9.16 DT price = £9.16

VITAMINS AND TRACE ELEMENTS > VITAMIN B GROUP

Cyanocobalamin

- INDICATIONS AND DOSE

Vitamin B$_{12}$ deficiency of dietary origin
▸ BY MOUTH
- Adult: 50–150 micrograms daily, dose to be taken between meals
▸ BY INTRAMUSCULAR INJECTION
- Adult: Initially 1 mg every 2–3 days for 11 doses; maintenance 1 mg every 1 month

- PRESCRIBING AND DISPENSING INFORMATION The BP directs that when vitamin B$_{12}$ injection is prescribed or demanded hydroxocobalamin injection shall be dispensed or supplied.
  Currently available brands of the tablet may not be suitable for vegans.
- NATIONAL FUNDING/ACCESS DECISIONS Cyanocobalamin liquid, *Cytacon*® tablets, and *Cytamen*® injection are not available on prescription under the NHS.
- LESS SUITABLE FOR PRESCRIBING Cyanocobalamin is less suitable for prescribing.

- MEDICINAL FORMS
  There can be variation in the licensing of different medicines containing the same drug. Forms available from special-order manufacturers include: tablet

Tablet
- Cyanocobalamin (Non-proprietary)
  Cyanocobalamin 50 microgram Cyanocobalamin 50microgram tablets | 50 tablet [P] £6.24 DT price = £8.99 | 50 tablet £8.99 DT price = £8.99 | 100 tablet no price available
  Cyanocobalamin 1 mg Behepan 1mg tablets | 100 tablet [PoM] no price available

▸ Cytacon (AMCo)
Cyanocobalamin 50 microgram Cytacon 50microgram tablets |
50 tablet P £8.99 DT price = £8.99

Oral solution

▸ Cyanocobalamin (Non-proprietary)
Cyanocobalamin 7 microgram per 1 ml Cyanocobalamin
35micrograms/5ml oral solution | 200 ml P £8.75

Solution for injection

▸ Cytamen (Focus Pharmaceuticals Ltd)
Cyanocobalamin 1 mg per 1 ml Cytamen 1000micrograms/1ml
solution for injection ampoules | 5 ampoule PoM £14.50 DT price =
£14.50

Hydroxocobalamin

● **INDICATIONS AND DOSE**

**Prophylaxis of macrocytic anaemias associated with
vitamin B₁₂ deficiency**

▸ BY INTRAMUSCULAR INJECTION

▸ Adult: 1 mg every 2–3 months

**Pernicious anaemia and other macrocytic anaemias
without neurological involvement**

▸ BY INTRAMUSCULAR INJECTION

▸ Adult: Initially 1 mg 3 times a week for 2 weeks, then
1 mg every 3 months

**Pernicious anaemia and other macrocytic anaemias with
neurological involvement**

▸ BY INTRAMUSCULAR INJECTION

▸ Adult: Initially 1 mg once daily on alternate days until
no further improvement, then 1 mg every 2 months

Tobacco amblyopia

▸ BY INTRAMUSCULAR INJECTION

▸ Adult: Initially 1 mg daily for 2 weeks, then 1 mg twice
weekly until no further improvement, then 1 mg every
1–3 months

Leber's optic atrophy

▸ BY INTRAMUSCULAR INJECTION

▸ Adult: Initially 1 mg daily for 2 weeks, then 1 mg twice
weekly until no further improvement, then 1 mg every
1–3 months

CYANOKIT®

Poisoning with cyanides

▸ BY INTRAVENOUS INFUSION

▸ Child (body-weight 5 kg and above): Initially 70 mg/kg
(max. per dose 5 g), to be given over 15 minutes, then
70 mg/kg (max. per dose 5 g) if required, this second
dose can be given over 15 minutes–2 hours depending
on severity of poisoning and patient stability

▸ Adult: Initially 5 g, to be given over 15 minutes, then
5 g if required, this second dose can be given over
15 minutes–2 hours depending on severity of
poisoning and patient stability

● CAUTIONS

▸ With intramuscular use Should not be given before diagnosis
fully established

● INTERACTIONS → Appendix 1 (hydroxocobalamin).

● SIDE-EFFECTS

GENERAL SIDE-EFFECTS
Dizziness · headache · pruritus

SPECIFIC SIDE-EFFECTS

▸ With intramuscular use Chromaturia · fever · hypersensitivity
reactions · hypokalaemia (during initial treatment) ·
injection-site reactions · nausea · rash · thrombocytosis
(during initial treatment)

▸ With intravenous use Dyspnoea · eye disorders · gastro-
intestinal disturbances · hot flush · lymphocytopenia ·
memory impairment · peripheral oedema · pustular rashes ·
red coloration of urine · restlessness · reversible red

coloration of skin and mucous membranes · throat
disorders · transient hypertension

● BREAST FEEDING Present in milk but not known to be
harmful.

● EFFECT ON LABORATORY TESTS

▸ With intravenous use Deep red colour of hydroxocobalamin
may interfere with laboratory tests.

● DIRECTIONS FOR ADMINISTRATION For *intravenous infusion
(Cyanokit)®*, given intermittently in Sodium chloride 0.9%,
reconstitute 5 g vial with 200 mL Sodium Chloride 0.9%;
gently invert vial for at least 1 minute to mix (do not
shake).

● PRESCRIBING AND DISPENSING INFORMATION

▸ With intramuscular use The BP directs that when vitamin B₁₂
injection is prescribed or demanded, hydroxocobalamin
injection shall be dispensed or supplied.
Poisoning by cyanides

▸ With intravenous use *Cyanokit®* is the only preparation of
hydroxocobalamin that is suitable for use in victims of
smoke inhalation who show signs of significant cyanide
poisoning.

● NATIONAL FUNDING/ACCESS DECISIONS
Cobalin-H® is not prescribable under the National Health
Service (NHS). *Neo-Cytamen®* is not prescribable under the
National Health Service (NHS).

● MEDICINAL FORMS
There can be variation in the licensing of different medicines
containing the same drug.

Solution for injection

▸ Hydroxocobalamin (Non-proprietary)
Hydroxocobalamin 1 mg per 1 ml Hydroxocobalamin 1mg/1ml
solution for injection ampoules | 5 ampoule PoM £12.49 DT price =
£7.18
Hydroxocobalamin 2.5 mg per 1 ml Hepavit 5mg/2ml solution for
injection ampoules | 2 ampoule PoM no price available
Hydroxocobalamin 5 mg per 1 ml Megamilbedoce 10mg/2ml
solution for injection ampoules | 10 ampoule PoM no price available

▸ Cobalin (AMCo)
Hydroxocobalamin 1 mg per 1 ml Cobalin-H 1mg/1ml solution for
injection ampoules | 5 ampoule PoM £9.50 DT price = £7.18

▸ Neo-Cytamen (Focus Pharmaceuticals Ltd)
Hydroxocobalamin 1 mg per 1 ml Neo-Cytamen
1000micrograms/1ml solution for injection ampoules |
5 ampoule PoM £12.49 DT price = £7.18

Powder for solution for infusion

▸ Cyanokit (Swedish Orphan Biovitrum Ltd)
Hydroxocobalamin 5 gram Cyanokit 5g powder for solution for
infusion vials | 1 vial PoM no price available

---

2   Iron overload

Iron overload

Overview

Severe tissue iron overload can occur in aplastic and other
refractory anaemias, mainly as the result of repeated blood
transfusions. It is a particular problem in refractory
anaemias with hyperplastic bone marrow, especially
thalassaemia major, where excessive iron absorption from
the gut and inappropriate iron therapy can add to the tissue
siderosis.

Iron overload associated with haemochromatosis can be
treated with repeated venesection. Venesection may also be
used for patients who have received multiple transfusions
and whose bone marrow has recovered. Where venesection is
contra-indicated, the long-term administration of the iron
chelating compound desferrioxamine mesilate p. 889 is
useful. Desferrioxamine mesilate (up to 2 g per unit of blood)
may also be given at the time of blood transfusion, provided

that the desferrioxamine mesilate is **not** added to the blood and is **not** given through the same line as the blood (but the two may be given through the same cannula).

Iron excretion induced by desferrioxamine mesilate is enhanced by administration of ascorbic acid p. 939 (vitamin C) daily by mouth; it should be given separately from food since it also enhances iron absorption. Ascorbic acid should not be given to patients with cardiac dysfunction; in patients with normal cardiac function ascorbic acid should be introduced 1 month after starting desferrioxamine mesilate.

Desferrioxamine mesilate infusion can be used to treat *aluminium overload* in dialysis patients; theoretically 100 mg of desferrioxamine binds with 4.1 mg of aluminium.

ANTIDOTES AND CHELATORS › IRON CHELATORS

Deferasirox

● DRUG ACTION Deferasirox is an oral iron chelator.

● INDICATIONS AND DOSE

Transfusion-related chronic iron overload when desferrioxamine is contra-indicated or inadequate in patients with thalassaemia major who receive infrequent blood transfusions (less than 7 mL/kg/month of packed red blood cells) | Transfusion-related chronic iron overload when desferrioxamine is contra-indicated or inadequate in patients with other anaemias | Treatment of chronic iron overload in patients with thalassaemia major who receive frequent blood transfusions (more than 7 mL/kg/month of packed red blood cells)

▸ BY MOUTH

▸ Adult: Initially 10–30 mg/kg once daily, dose adjusted according to serum-ferritin concentration and amount of transfused blood—consult product literature; adjusted in steps of 5–10 mg/kg every 3–6 months, maintenance dose adjusted according to serum-ferritin concentration; maximum 40 mg/kg per day; Usual maximum 30 micrograms/kg

Treatment of chronic iron overload when desferrioxamine is contra-indicated or inadequate (with non-transfusion-dependent thalassaemia syndromes)

▸ BY MOUTH

▸ Adult: Initially 10 mg/kg once daily; adjusted in steps of 5–10 mg/kg every 3–6 months, maintenance dose adjusted according to serum-ferritin concentration and liver-iron concentration (consult product literature); maximum 20 mg/kg per day

● CAUTIONS Elderly (increased risk of side-effects) · history of liver cirrhosis · not recommended in conditions which may reduce life expectancy (e.g. high-risk myelodysplastic syndromes) · platelet count less than 50×10^9/litre · risk of gastro-intestinal ulceration and haemorrhage · unexplained cytopenia—consider treatment interruption

● INTERACTIONS → Appendix 1 (deferasirox).

● SIDE-EFFECTS

▸ **Common or very common** Fatal gastro-intestinal haemorrhage · gastro-intestinal disturbances · gastro-intestinal ulceration · headache · proteinuria · pruritus · rash

▸ **Uncommon** Anxiety · cholelithiasis · disturbances of hearing and vision · dizziness · fatigue · glucosuria · hepatitis · lens opacity · maculopathy · oedema · pharyngitis · pyrexia · renal tubulopathy · skin pigmentation · sleep disorder

▸ **Frequency not known** Acute renal failure · agranulocytosis · alopecia · anaemia · anaphylaxis · angioedema · blood disorders · hepatic failure · hypersensitivity reactions · neutropenia · pancytopenia · thrombocytopenia · tubulointerstitial nephritis

● PREGNANCY Manufacturer advises avoid unless essential— toxicity in *animal* studies.

● BREAST FEEDING Manufacturer advises avoid—present in milk in *animal* studies.

● HEPATIC IMPAIRMENT Use with caution in moderate impairment, reduce dose considerably then gradually increase to max. 50% of normal dose. Avoid in severe impairment.

● RENAL IMPAIRMENT Reduce dose by 10 mg/kg if eGFR 60–90 mL/minute/1.73 m^2 and if serum creatinine increased by more than 33% of baseline measurement on 2 consecutive occasions—interrupt treatment if deterioration in renal function persists after dose reduction. Avoid if eGFR less than 60 mL/minute/1.73 m^2.

● MONITORING REQUIREMENTS

▸ Eye and ear examinations required before treatment and annually during treatment.

▸ Monitor serum-ferritin concentration monthly.

▸ Test liver function before treatment, then every 2 weeks during the first month, and then monthly.

▸ Measure baseline serum creatinine and monitor renal function weekly during the first month of treatment and monthly thereafter.

▸ Test for proteinuria monthly.

● DIRECTIONS FOR ADMINISTRATION Tablets should be dispersed in water, orange juice, or apple juice; if necessary resuspend residue.

● PATIENT AND CARER ADVICE Patient or carers should be given advice on how to administer deferasirox dispersible tablets.

● NATIONAL FUNDING/ACCESS DECISIONS

Scottish Medicines Consortium (SMC) Decisions
The *Scottish Medicines Consortium* has advised (January 2007) that deferasirox is accepted for restricted use within NHS Scotland for the treatment of chronic iron overload associated with the treatment of rare acquired or inherited anaemias requiring recurrent blood transfusions. It is not recommended for patients with myelodysplastic syndromes.

● MEDICINAL FORMS
There can be variation in the licensing of different medicines containing the same drug.
Dispersible tablet
CAUTIONARY AND ADVISORY LABELS 13, 22
▸ Exjade (Novartis Pharmaceuticals UK Ltd) ▼
Deferasirox 125 mg Exjade 125mg dispersible tablets sugar-free | 28 tablet PoM £117.60
Deferasirox 250 mg Exjade 250mg dispersible tablets sugar-free | 28 tablet PoM £235.20
Deferasirox 500 mg Exjade 500mg dispersible tablets sugar-free | 28 tablet PoM £470.40

Deferiprone

● DRUG ACTION Deferiprone is an oral iron chelator.

● INDICATIONS AND DOSE

Treatment of iron overload in patients with thalassaemia major in whom desferrioxamine is contra-indicated or is inadequate

▸ BY MOUTH

▸ Adult: 25 mg/kg 3 times a day; maximum 100 mg/kg per day

● CONTRA-INDICATIONS History of agranulocytosis or recurrent neutropenia

● INTERACTIONS → Appendix 1 (deferiprone).

● SIDE-EFFECTS Agranulocytosis · arthropathy · blood dyscrasias · gastro-intestinal disturbances (reducing dose and increasing gradually may improve tolerance) ·

headache · increased appetite · neutropenia · red-brown urine discoloration · zinc deficiency

- CONCEPTION AND CONTRACEPTION Manufacturer advises avoid before intended conception—teratogenic and embryotoxic in *animal* studies. Contraception advised in females of child-bearing potential.
- PREGNANCY Manufacturer advises avoid during pregnancy—teratogenic and embryotoxic in *animal* studies.
- BREAST FEEDING Manufacturer advises avoid—no information available.
- HEPATIC IMPAIRMENT Manufacturer advises monitor liver function—interrupt treatment if persistent elevation in serum alanine aminotransferase.
- RENAL IMPAIRMENT Manufacturer advises caution—no information available.
- MONITORING REQUIREMENTS
  ▶ Monitor neutrophil count weekly and discontinue treatment if neutropenia develops.
  ▶ Monitor plasma-zinc concentration.
- PATIENT AND CARER ADVICE
  Blood disorders Patients or their carers should be told how to recognise signs of neutropenia and advised to seek immediate medical attention if symptoms such as fever or sore throat develop.

- MEDICINAL FORMS
  There can be variation in the licensing of different medicines containing the same drug. Forms available from special-order manufacturers include: capsule, oral suspension, oral solution

Tablet
CAUTIONARY AND ADVISORY LABELS 14
  ▶ Ferriprox (Swedish Orphan Biovitrum Ltd)
    Deferiprone 500 mg Ferriprox 500mg tablets | 100 tablet PoM £152.39
    Deferiprone 1 gram Ferriprox 1000mg tablets | 50 tablet PoM £175.25

Oral solution
CAUTIONARY AND ADVISORY LABELS 14
  ▶ Ferriprox (Swedish Orphan Biovitrum Ltd)
    Deferiprone 100 mg per 1 ml Ferriprox 100mg/ml oral solution sugar-free | 500 ml PoM £152.39

Desferrioxamine mesilate

(Deferoxamine Mesilate)

- **INDICATIONS AND DOSE**

Iron poisoning
  ▶ BY CONTINUOUS INTRAVENOUS INFUSION
  ▶ Adult: Initially up to 15 mg/kg/hour, max. 80 mg/kg in 24 hours, dose to be reduced after 4–6 hours, in severe cases, higher doses may be given on advice from the National Poisons Information Service

Aluminium overload in dialysis patients
  ▶ BY INTRAVENOUS INFUSION
  ▶ Adult: (consult product literature or local protocols)

Chronic iron overload (low iron overload)
  ▶ BY SUBCUTANEOUS INFUSION
  ▶ Adult: The dose should reflect the degree of iron overload

Chronic iron overload (established overload)
  ▶ BY SUBCUTANEOUS INFUSION
  ▶ Adult: 20–50 mg/kg daily

- CAUTIONS Aluminium-related encephalopathy (may exacerbate neurological dysfunction)
- INTERACTIONS → Appendix 1 (desferrioxamine).
- SIDE-EFFECTS
  ▶ **Common or very common** Abdominal pain · arthralgia · bone disorders · growth retardation · headache · hearing

disturbances · injection-site reactions · myalgia · nausea · pyrexia · vomiting
  ▶ **Rare** Anaphylaxis · blood dyscrasias · bone pain · diarrhoea · hepatic impairment · hypotension (especially when given too rapidly by intravenous injection) · leg cramps · lens opacity · leucopenia · rash · retinopathy · thrombocytopenia · visual disturbances · Yersinia and mucormycosis infections
  ▶ **Very rare** Acute respiratory distress · convulsions · dizziness · neurological disturbances · neuropathy · paraesthesia · renal impairment
  ▶ **Frequency not known** Muscle spasms

- PREGNANCY Teratogenic in *animal* studies. Manufacturer advises use only if potential benefit outweighs risk.
- BREAST FEEDING Manufacturer advises use only if potential benefit outweighs risk—no information available.
- RENAL IMPAIRMENT Use with caution.
- MONITORING REQUIREMENTS Eye and ear examinations before treatment and at 3-month intervals during treatment.
- DIRECTIONS FOR ADMINISTRATION For full details and warnings relating to administration, consult product literature.
  For *intravenous infusion* (Desferal®), give continuously or intermittently in Glucose 5% or Sodium chloride 0.9%. Reconstitute with water for injections to a concentration of 100 mg/mL; dilute with infusion fluid.

- MEDICINAL FORMS
  There can be variation in the licensing of different medicines containing the same drug.

Powder for solution for injection
  ▶ Desferrioxamine mesilate (Non-proprietary)
    Desferrioxamine mesilate 500 mg Desferrioxamine 500mg powder for solution for injection vials | 10 vial PoM £39.90–£50.00
    Desferrioxamine mesilate 2 gram Desferrioxamine 2g powder for solution for injection vials | 1 vial PoM £17.95–£20.00
  ▶ Desferal (Novartis Pharmaceuticals UK Ltd)
    Desferrioxamine mesilate 500 mg Desferal 500mg powder for solution for injection vials | 10 vial PoM £46.63
    Desferrioxamine mesilate 2 gram Desferal 2g powder for solution for injection vials | 1 vial PoM £18.66

3 Neutropenia and stem cell mobilisation

3.1 Neutropenia

Neutropenia

Management

Recombinant human granulocyte-colony stimulating factor (rhG-CSF) stimulates the production of neutrophils and may reduce the duration of chemotherapy-induced neutropenia and thereby reduce the incidence of associated sepsis; there is as yet no evidence that it improves overall survival. Filgrastim p. 890 (unglycosylated rhG-CSF) and lenograstim p. 891 (glycosylated rhG-CSF) have similar effects; both have been used in a variety of clinical settings, but they do not have any clear-cut routine indications. In congenital neutropenia filgrastim usually increases the neutrophil count with an appropriate clinical response. Pegfilgrastim p. 892 is a polyethylene glycol-conjugated ('pegylated') derivative of filgrastim; pegylation increases the duration of filgrastim activity. Lipegfilgrastim p. 891 is a polyethylene glycol-conjugated via a glycine linker derivative of filgrastim.

Granulocyte-colony stimulating factors should only be prescribed by those experienced in their use.

9 Blood and nutrition

Granulocyte-colony stimulating factors

- DRUG ACTION Recombinant human granulocyte-colony stimulating factor (rhG-CSF) stimulates the production of neutrophils.
- CAUTIONS Malignant myeloid conditions · pre-malignant myeloid conditions · risk of splenomegaly and rupture—spleen size should be monitored · sickle-cell disease

  CAUTIONS, FURTHER INFORMATION
- Acute respiratory distress syndrome There have been reports of pulmonary infiltrates leading to acute respiratory distress syndrome—patients with a recent history of pulmonary infiltrates or pneumonia may be at higher risk.
- SIDE-EFFECTS
- Common or very common Alopecia · anorexia · asthenia · bone pain · chest pain · fever · gastro-intestinal disturbances · headache · injection-site reactions · leucocytosis · musculoskeletal pain · rash · thrombocytopenia
- Rare Acute febrile neutrophilic dermatosis · cutaneous vasculitis · pulmonary side-effects (particularly interstitial pneumonia)

  SIDE-EFFECTS, FURTHER INFORMATION
- Pulmonary infiltration Treatment should be withdrawn in patients who develop signs of pulmonary infiltration.
- PREGNANCY There have been reports of toxicity in *animal* studies and manufacturers advise not to use granulocyte-colony stimulating factors during pregnancy unless the potential benefit outweighs the risk.
- BREAST FEEDING There is no evidence for the use of granulocyte-colony stimulating factors during breast-feeding and manufacturers advise avoiding their use.
- MONITORING REQUIREMENTS
- Full blood counts including differential white cell and platelet counts should be monitored.
- Spleen size should be monitored during treatment—risk of splenomegaly and rupture.

◤ above

Filgrastim

(Recombinant human granulocyte-colony stimulating factor; G-CSF)

- INDICATIONS AND DOSE

Reduction in duration of neutropenia and incidence of febrile neutropenia in cytotoxic chemotherapy for malignancy (except chronic myeloid leukaemia and myelodysplastic syndromes) (specialist use only)
- ▸ BY SUBCUTANEOUS INJECTION, OR BY INTRAVENOUS INFUSION
- ▸ Adult: 5 micrograms/kg daily until neutrophil count in normal range, usually for up to 14 days (up to 38 days in acute myeloid leukaemia), to be started at least 24 hours after cytotoxic chemotherapy. Preferably given by subcutaneous injection; if given by intravenous infusion, administer over 30 minutes

Reduction in duration of neutropenia (and associated sequelae) in myeloablative therapy followed by bone-marrow transplantation (specialist use only)
- ▸ BY SUBCUTANEOUS INFUSION, OR BY INTRAVENOUS INFUSION
- ▸ Adult: 10 micrograms/kg daily, to be started at least 24 hours following cytotoxic chemotherapy and within 24 hours of bone-marrow infusion, then adjusted according to neutrophil count— consult product literature, doses administered over 30 minutes or

24 hours via intravenous route and over 24 hours via subcutaneous route

Mobilisation of peripheral blood progenitor cells for autologous infusion, used alone (specialist use only)
- ▸ BY SUBCUTANEOUS INFUSION, OR BY SUBCUTANEOUS INJECTION
- ▸ Adult: 10 micrograms/kg daily for 5–7 days, to be administered over 24 hours if given by subcutaneous infusion

Mobilisation of peripheral blood progenitor cells for autologous infusion, used following adjunctive myelosuppressive chemotherapy—to improve yield (specialist use only)
- ▸ BY SUBCUTANEOUS INJECTION
- ▸ Adult: 5 micrograms/kg daily until neutrophil count in normal range, to be started the day after completing chemotherapy, for timing of leucopheresis, consult product literature

Mobilisation of peripheral blood progenitor cells in normal donors for allogeneic infusion (specialist use only)
- ▸ BY SUBCUTANEOUS INJECTION
- ▸ Adult 18–59 years: 10 micrograms/kg daily for 4–5 days, for timing of leucopheresis, consult product literature

Severe congenital neutropenia and history of severe or recurrent infections (distinguish carefully from other haematological disorders) (specialist use only)
- ▸ BY SUBCUTANEOUS INJECTION
- ▸ Adult: Initially 12 micrograms/kg daily, adjusted according to response, can be given in single or divided doses, consult product literature and local protocol

Severe cyclic neutropenia, or idiopathic neutropenia and history of severe or recurrent infections (distinguish carefully from other haematological disorders) (specialist use only)
- ▸ BY SUBCUTANEOUS INJECTION
- ▸ Adult: Initially 5 micrograms/kg daily, adjusted according to response, can be given in single or divided doses, consult product literature and local protocol

Persistent neutropenia in HIV infection (specialist use only)
- ▸ BY SUBCUTANEOUS INJECTION
- ▸ Adult: Initially 1 microgram/kg daily, subsequent doses increased as necessary until neutrophil count in normal range, then adjusted to maintain neutrophil count in normal range—consult product literature; maximum 4 micrograms/kg per day

- CONTRA-INDICATIONS Severe congenital neutropenia (Kostmann's syndrome) with abnormal cytogenetics
- CAUTIONS Osteoporotic bone disease (monitor bone density if given for more than 6 months) · secondary acute myeloid leukaemia
- INTERACTIONS → Appendix 1 (filgrastim).
- SIDE-EFFECTS
- Common or very common Anaemia · dysuria · epistaxis · exacerbation of rheumatoid arthritis · haematuria · hepatomegaly · mucositis · osteoporosis · proteinuria · pseudogout · raised uric acid · splenic enlargement · transient decrease in blood glucose · transient hypotension · urinary abnormalities
- Uncommon Capillary leak syndrome (including fatal cases)
- Rare Splenic rupture
- MONITORING REQUIREMENTS Regular morphological and cytogenetic bone-marrow examinations recommended in severe congenital neutropenia (possible risk of myelodysplastic syndromes or leukaemia).
- DIRECTIONS FOR ADMINISTRATION
- With intravenous use For *intravenous infusion* (Neupogen®); (Nivestim®); (Ratiograstim®); (Zarzio®) give continuously

or intermittently *in* Glucose 5%; for a filgrastim concentration of less than 1 500 000 units/mL (15 micrograms/mL) albumin solution (human albumin solution) is added to produce a final albumin concentration of 2 mg/mL; should not be diluted to a filgrastim concentration of less than 200 000 units/mL (2 micrograms/mL) and should not be diluted with sodium chloride solution.

- PRESCRIBING AND DISPENSING INFORMATION Products containing filgrastim are not identical and although theoretically there should be no important differences in terms of safety and efficacy, when prescribing biological products it is good practice to use the brand name, see *Biosimilar medicines*, under Guidance on prescribing p. 1.
  1 million units of filgrastim solution for injection contains 10 micrograms filgrastim.

- MEDICINAL FORMS
  There can be variation in the licensing of different medicines containing the same drug.
  Solution for injection
  ▸ Accofil (Accord Healthcare Ltd) ▼
    Filgrastim 60 mega u per 1 ml Accofil 30million units/0.5ml solution for injection pre-filled syringes | 5 pre-filled disposable injection PoM £284.20
    Filgrastim 96 mega u per 1 ml Accofil 48million units/0.5ml solution for injection pre-filled syringes | 5 pre-filled disposable injection PoM £455.70
  ▸ Neupogen (Amgen Ltd)
    Filgrastim 30 mega u per 1 ml Neupogen 30million units/1ml solution for injection vials | 5 vial PoM £263.52
  ▸ Neupogen Singleject (Amgen Ltd)
    Filgrastim 60 mega u per 1 ml Neupogen Singleject 30million units/0.5ml solution for injection pre-filled syringes | 1 pre-filled disposable injection PoM £52.70 | 5 pre-filled disposable injection PoM £263.52
    Filgrastim 96 mega u per 1 ml Neupogen Singleject 48million units/0.5ml solution for injection pre-filled syringes | 1 pre-filled disposable injection PoM £84.06 | 5 pre-filled disposable injection PoM £420.29
  ▸ Nivestim (Hospira UK Ltd)
    Filgrastim 60 mega u per 1 ml Nivestim 30million units/0.5ml solution for injection pre-filled syringes | 5 pre-filled disposable injection PoM £290.00 (Hospital only)
    Nivestim 12million units/0.2ml solution for injection pre-filled syringes | 5 pre-filled disposable injection PoM £180.00 (Hospital only)
    Filgrastim 96 mega u per 1 ml Nivestim 48million units/0.5ml solution for injection pre-filled syringes | 5 pre-filled disposable injection PoM £465.00 (Hospital only)
  ▸ Zarzio (Sandoz Ltd)
    Filgrastim 60 mega u per 1 ml Zarzio 30million units/0.5ml solution for injection pre-filled syringes | 5 pre-filled disposable injection PoM £250.75
    Filgrastim 96 mega u per 1 ml Zarzio 48million units/0.5ml solution for injection pre-filled syringes | 5 pre-filled disposable injection PoM £399.50

◀ 890

Lenograstim

(Recombinant human granulocyte-colony stimulating factor; rHuG-CSF)

- INDICATIONS AND DOSE

Reduction in the duration of neutropenia and associated complications following bone-marrow transplantation for non-myeloid malignancy (specialist use only) | **Reduction in the duration of neutropenia and associated complications following peripheral stem cells transplantation for non-myeloid malignancy (specialist use only)**
  ▸ BY INTRAVENOUS INFUSION, OR BY SUBCUTANEOUS INJECTION
  ▸ Adult: 150 micrograms/m^2 daily until neutrophil count stable in acceptable range (max. 28 days), to be started the day after transplantation. Intravenous infusion to be given over 30 minutes

Reduction in the duration of neutropenia and associated complications following treatment with cytotoxic chemotherapy associated with a significant incidence of febrile neutropenia (specialist use only)
  ▸ BY SUBCUTANEOUS INJECTION
  ▸ Adult: 150 micrograms/m^2 daily until neutrophil count stable in acceptable range (max. 28 days), to be started on the day after completion of chemotherapy

Mobilisation of peripheral blood progenitor cells for harvesting and subsequent infusion, used alone (specialist use only)
  ▸ BY SUBCUTANEOUS INJECTION
  ▸ Adult: 10 micrograms/kg daily for 4–6 days (5–6 days in healthy donors)

Mobilisation of peripheral blood progenitor cells, used following adjunctive myelosuppressive chemotherapy (to improve yield) (specialist use only)
  ▸ BY SUBCUTANEOUS INJECTION
  ▸ Adult: 150 micrograms/m^2 daily until neutrophil count stable in acceptable range, to be started 1–5 days after completion of chemotherapy, for timing of leucopheresis, consult product literature

- SIDE-EFFECTS Mucositis · splenic rupture · toxic epidermal necrolysis

- DIRECTIONS FOR ADMINISTRATION
  ▸ With intravenous use For *intravenous infusion*(Granocyte$^®$), give intermittently *in* Sodium chloride 0.9%; initially reconstitute with 1 mL water for injection provided (do not shake vigorously) then dilute with up to 50 mL infusion fluid for each vial of *Granocyte*-13 or up to 100 mL infusion fluid for *Granocyte*-34; give over 30 minutes.

- PRESCRIBING AND DISPENSING INFORMATION *Granocyte$^®$* solution for injection contains 105 micrograms of lenograstim per 13.4 mega unit vial and 263 micrograms lenograstim per 33.6 mega unit vial.

- MEDICINAL FORMS
  There can be variation in the licensing of different medicines containing the same drug.
  Powder and solvent for solution for injection
  EXCIPIENTS: May contain Phenylalanine
  ▸ Granocyte (Chugai Pharma UK Ltd)
    Lenograstim 13.4 mega u Granocyte-13 powder and solvent for solution for injection vials | 1 vial PoM £40.11 | 5 vial PoM £200.55
    Lenograstim 33.6 mega u Granocyte-34 powder and solvent for solution for injection vials | 1 vial PoM £62.54 | 5 vial PoM £312.69

◀ 890

Lipegfilgrastim

(Glycopegylated recombinant methionyl human granulocyte-colony stimulating factor)

- INDICATIONS AND DOSE

Reduction in duration of neutropenia and incidence of febrile neutropenia in cytotoxic chemotherapy for malignancy (except chronic myeloid leukaemia and myelodysplastic syndromes)
  ▸ BY SUBCUTANEOUS INJECTION
  ▸ Adult (specialist use only): 6 mg, for each chemotherapy cycle, given approximately 24 hours after chemotherapy, dose expressed as filgrastim

- CAUTIONS Myelosuppressive chemotherapy
- INTERACTIONS → Appendix 1 (lipegfilgrastim).
- SIDE-EFFECTS Hypokalaemia

● **MEDICINAL FORMS**
There can be variation in the licensing of different medicines containing the same drug.
Solution for injection
▸ Lonquex (Teva UK Ltd) ▼
Lipegfilgrastim 10 mg per 1 ml Lonquex 6mg/0.6ml solution for injection pre-filled syringes | 1 pre-filled disposable injection PoM £652.06

F 890

Pegfilgrastim

(Pegylated recombinant methionyl human granulocyte-colony stimulating factor)

● **INDICATIONS AND DOSE**
Reduction in duration of neutropenia and incidence of febrile neutropenia in cytotoxic chemotherapy for malignancy (except chronic myeloid leukaemia and myelodysplastic syndromes) (specialist use only)
▸ BY SUBCUTANEOUS INJECTION
▸ Adult: 6 mg for each chemotherapy cycle, to be given at least 24 hours after chemotherapy, dose is expressed as filgrastim

● **CAUTIONS** Acute leukaemia · myelosuppressive chemotherapy
● **INTERACTIONS** → Appendix 1 (pegfilgrastim).
● **SIDE-EFFECTS**
▸ **Rare** Capillary leak syndrome (including fatal cases)
▸ **Very rare** Splenic rupture
● **MEDICINAL FORMS**
There can be variation in the licensing of different medicines containing the same drug.
Solution for injection
▸ Neulasta (Amgen Ltd)
Filgrastim (as Pegfilgrastim) 10 mg per 1 ml Neulasta 6mg/0.6ml solution for injection pre-filled syringes | 1 pre-filled disposable injection PoM £686.38

3.2 Stem cell mobilisation

IMMUNOSTIMULANTS › CHEMOKINE RECEPTOR ANTAGONISTS

Plerixafor

● **DRUG ACTION** Plerixafor is a chemokine receptor antagonist.

● **INDICATIONS AND DOSE**
Mobilise haematopoietic stem cells to peripheral blood for collection and subsequent autologous transplantation in patients with lymphoma or multiple myeloma (specialist use only)
▸ BY SUBCUTANEOUS INJECTION
▸ Adult: 240 micrograms/kg daily usually for 2–4 days (max 7 days), to be administered 6–11 hours before initiation of apheresis, dose to be given following 4 days treatment with a granulocyte-colony stimulating factor

● **SIDE-EFFECTS**
▸ **Common or very common** Arthralgia · dizziness · dry mouth · erythema · fatigue · gastro-intestinal disturbances · headache · injection-site reactions · insomnia · musculoskeletal pain · oral hypoaesthesia · sweating
▸ **Uncommon** Dyspnoea · hypersensitivity reactions · periorbital swelling

● **CONCEPTION AND CONTRACEPTION** Use effective contraception during treatment— teratogenic in *animal* studies.
● **PREGNANCY** Manufacturer advises avoid unless essential— teratogenic in *animal* studies.
● **BREAST FEEDING** Manufacturer advises avoid—no information available.
● **RENAL IMPAIRMENT** Reduce dose to 160 micrograms/kg daily if creatinine clearance 20–50 mL/minute. No information available if creatinine clearance less than 20 mL/minute.
● **MONITORING REQUIREMENTS** Monitor platelets and white blood cell count.
● **MEDICINAL FORMS**
There can be variation in the licensing of different medicines containing the same drug.
Solution for injection
▸ Mozobil (Sanofi)
Plerixafor 20 mg per 1 ml Mozobil 24mg/1.2ml solution for injection vials | 1 vial PoM £4,882.77

4 Platelet disorders

Platelet disorders

Idiopathic thrombocytopenic purpura

Acute idiopathic thrombocytopenic purpura is usually self-limiting in children. In adults, idiopathic thrombocytopenic purpura can be treated with a **corticosteroid**, e.g. prednisolone p. 614, gradually reducing the dose over several weeks. Splenectomy is considered if a satisfactory platelet count is not achieved or if there is a relapse on reducing the dose of corticosteroid or withdrawing it.

Immunoglobulin preparations, are also used in idiopathic thrombocytopenic purpura or where a temporary rapid rise in platelets is needed, as in pregnancy or pre-operatively; they are also used for children often in preference to a corticosteroid. anti-d (Rh0) immunoglobulin p. 1130 is effective in raising the platelet count in about 80% of unsplenectomised rhesus-positive individuals; its effects may last longer than normal immunoglobulin p. 1131 for intravenous use, but further doses are usually required.

Other therapy that has been tried in refractory idiopathic thrombocytopenic purpura includes azathioprine p. 757, cyclophosphamide p. 793, vincristine sulfate p. 820, ciclosporin p. 758, and danazol p. 670. Rituximab p. 783 may also be effective and in some cases induces prolonged remission. For patients with chronic severe thrombocytopenia refractory to other therapy, tranexamic acid p. 99 may be given to reduce the severity of haemorrhage.

Eltrombopag p. 893 and romiplostim p. 894 are thrombopoietin receptor agonists licensed for the treatment of chronic idiopathic thrombocytopenic purpura in splenectomised patients refractory to other treatments, such as corticosteroids or immunoglobulins, or as a second-line treatment in non-splenectomised patients when surgery is contra-indicated (see also NICE guidance). Eltrombopag is an oral preparation and romiplostim is an injection which is made biosynthetically by recombinant DNA technology; they should both be used under the supervision of a specialist.

Essential thrombocythaemia

Anagrelide p. 893 inhibits platelet formation. It is licensed for essential thrombocythaemia in patients at risk of thrombo-haemorrhagic events who have not responded adequately to other drugs or who cannot tolerate other drugs. An at risk patient is defined by one or more of the following features: over 60 years of age, or a platelet count greater than 1000 x 10⁹ /L or history of thrombo-haemorrhagic events. Anagrelide should be initiated under specialist supervision.

4.1 Essential thrombocythaemia

ANTITHROMBOTIC DRUGS > CYCLIC AMP PHOSPHODIESTERASE III INHIBITORS

Anagrelide

● **INDICATIONS AND DOSE**

Essential thrombocythaemia in patients at risk of thrombo-haemorrhagic events who have not responded adequately to other drugs or who cannot tolerate other drugs (initiated under specialist supervision)

▸ BY MOUTH
▸ Adult: Initially 500 micrograms twice daily, dose to be adjusted at weekly intervals according to response, increased in steps of 500 micrograms daily; usual dose 1–3 mg daily in divided doses (max. per dose 2.5 mg); maximum 10 mg per day

● CAUTIONS Cardiovascular disease—assess cardiac function before and regularly during treatment · concomitant use of drugs that prolong QT-interval—assess cardiac function before and regularly during treatment · risk factors for QT-interval prolongation—assess cardiac function before and regularly during treatment

● INTERACTIONS Caution with concomitant aspirin in patients at risk of haemorrhage.
Appendix 1 (anagrelide).

● SIDE-EFFECTS
▸ **Common or very common** Anaemia · dizziness · fatigue · fluid retention · gastro-intestinal disturbances · headache · palpitation · rash · tachycardia
▸ **Uncommon** Alopecia · amnesia · anorexia · arrhythmias · arthralgia · back pain · blood disorders · chest pain · confusion · congestive heart failure · depression · dry mouth · dyspnoea · ecchymosis · epistaxis · fever · gastro-intestinal haemorrhage · haemorrhage · hypertension · hypoaesthesia · impotence · malaise · myalgia · nervousness · oedema · pancreatitis · paraesthesia · pneumonia pleural effusion · pruritus · skin discoloration · sleep disturbances · syncope · weight changes
▸ **Rare** Angina · asthenia · cardiomegaly · cardiomyopathy · colitis · dry skin · dysarthria · gastritis · gingival bleeding · impaired coordination · migraine · myocardial infarction · nocturia · pericardial effusion · postural hypotension · pulmonary hypertension · pulmonary infiltrates · renal failure · somnolence · tinnitus · vasodilatation · visual disturbances
▸ **Frequency not known** Hepatitis · interstitial lung disease · Torsade de pointes · tubulointerstitial nephritis

● CONCEPTION AND CONTRACEPTION Effective contraception required during treatment.

● PREGNANCY Manufacturer advises avoid (toxicity in *animal* studies).

● BREAST FEEDING Manufacturer advises avoid—present in milk in *animal* studies.

● HEPATIC IMPAIRMENT Manufacturer advises caution in mild impairment. Avoid in moderate to severe impairment.

● RENAL IMPAIRMENT Manufacturer advises avoid if eGFR less than 50 mL/minute/1.73 m².

● MONITORING REQUIREMENTS
▸ Monitor full blood count (monitor platelet count every 2 days for 1 week, then weekly until maintenance dose established).
▸ Monitor liver function.
▸ Monitor serum creatinine.
▸ Monitor urea.
▸ Monitor electrolytes (including potassium, magnesium and calcium) before and during treatment.

● PATIENT AND CARER ADVICE
Driving and skilled tasks
Dizziness may affect performance of skilled tasks (e.g. cycling, driving).

● MEDICINAL FORMS
There can be variation in the licensing of different medicines containing the same drug.
Capsule
▸ Xagrid (Shire Pharmaceuticals Ltd) ▼
Anagrelide (as Anagrelide hydrochloride) 500 microgram Xagrid 500microgram capsules | 100 capsule PoM £404.57

4.2 Idiopathic thrombocytopenic purpura

ANTIHAEMORRHAGICS > THROMBOPOIETIN RECEPTOR AGONISTS

Eltrombopag

● **INDICATIONS AND DOSE**

Treatment of chronic idiopathic thrombocytopenic purpura in splenectomised patients refractory to other treatments (such as corticosteroids or immunoglobulins) (under expert supervision) | Second-line treatment of chronic idiopathic thrombocytopenic purpura in non-splenectomised patients when surgery is contra-indicated (under expert supervision)

▸ BY MOUTH
▸ Adult: Initially 50 mg once daily, dose to be adjusted to achieve a platelet count of 50x10⁹/litre or more—consult product literature for dose adjustments, discontinue if inadequate response after 4 weeks treatment at maximum dose; maximum 75 mg per day
▸ Adult (patients of East Asian origin): Initially 25 mg once daily, dose to be adjusted to achieve a platelet count of 50x10⁹/litre or more—consult product literature for dose adjustments, discontinue if inadequate response after 4 weeks treatment at maximum dose; maximum 75 mg per day.

Treatment of thrombocytopenia associated with chronic hepatitis C infection, where the degree of thrombocytopenia is the main factor preventing the initiation or limiting the ability to maintain optimal interferon-based therapy (under expert supervision)

▸ BY MOUTH
▸ Adult: Initially 25 mg once daily, dose to be adjusted to achieve a platelet count sufficient to initiate antiviral therapy then a platelet count of 50–75x10⁹/litre during antiviral therapy—consult product literature for dose adjustments, discontinue if inadequate response after 2 weeks treatment at maximum dose; maximum 100 mg per day

● CAUTIONS Patients of East Asian origin · risk factors for thromboembolism

● INTERACTIONS → Appendix 1 (eltrombopag).

- SIDE-EFFECTS
  ► **Common or very common** Abdominal pain · alopecia · arthralgia · bone pain · cataract · constipation · diarrhoea · dry eye · fatigue · gastro-intestinal disturbances · headache · insomnia · myalgia · nausea · paraesthesia · peripheral oedema · pruritus · rash
  ► **Uncommon** Acute myocardial infarction · anaemia · anorexia · anxiety · blood disorders · changes in appetite · cholestasis · cough · deep vein thrombosis · depression · dizziness · dry mouth · ecchymosis · eosinophilia · epistaxis · eye disorders · flushing · gingival bleeding · gout · haemolysis · haemorrhoids · hemiparesis · hepatitis · hypertension · migraine · mood changes · myelocytosis · nocturia · palpitation · peripheral neuropathy · pulmonary embolism · QT-interval prolongation · rectosigmoid cancer · renal failure · respiratory infections · skin reactions · sleep disorders · sweating · tachycardia · taste disturbances · thromboembolic events · tremor · urinary tract infections · vertigo · weight gain

- CONCEPTION AND CONTRACEPTION Ensure effective contraception during treatment.
- PREGNANCY Avoid—toxicity in *animal* studies.
- BREAST FEEDING Manufacturer advises avoid.
- HEPATIC IMPAIRMENT For *idiopathic thrombocytopenic purpura*, avoid unless potential benefit outweighs risk—reduce initial dose to 25 mg once daily. For *thrombocytopenia associated with chronic hepatitis C infection*, in severe hepatic impairment use only if potential benefit outweighs risk and monitor closely—increased risk of hepatic decompensation and thromboembolic events.
- RENAL IMPAIRMENT Use with caution.
- MONITORING REQUIREMENTS
  ► Monitor liver function before treatment, every two weeks when adjusting the dose, and monthly thereafter.
  ► Regular ophthalmological examinations for cataract formation recommended.
  ► For *idiopathic thrombocytopenic purpura*, monitor full blood count including platelet count and peripheral blood smears every week during treatment until a stable platelet count is reached (50x10⁹/litre or more for at least 4 weeks), then monthly thereafter.
  ► For *thrombocytopenia associated with chronic hepatitis C infection*, monitor platelet count every week before and during antiviral treatment until a stable platelet count is reached (50–75x10⁹/litre), then monitor full blood count including platelet count and peripheral blood smears monthly thereafter.
- DIRECTIONS FOR ADMINISTRATION Each dose should be taken at least 4 hours before or after any dairy products (or foods containing calcium), indigestion remedies, or medicines containing aluminium, calcium, iron, magnesium, zinc, or selenium to reduce possible interference with absorption.
- PATIENT AND CARER ADVICE Patient counselling is advised on how to administer eltrombopag tablets.
- NATIONAL FUNDING/ACCESS DECISIONS

  NICE technology appraisals (TAs)
  ► **Eltrombopag for treating chronic immune (idiopathic) thrombocytopenic purpura (July 2013)** NICE TA293
  Eltrombopag is recommended for the treatment of chronic immune (idiopathic) thrombocytopenic purpura in splenectomised adults refractory to other treatments, or as a second-line treatment in non-splenectomised adults when surgery is contra-indicated, only if:
  - the manufacturer provides eltrombopag at the agreed discount as part of the patient access scheme *and*
  - their condition is refractory to standard active treatments and rescue therapies *or*

  - they have severe disease and a high risk of bleeding that needs frequent courses of rescue therapies.
  Patients currently receiving eltrombopag whose disease does not meet these criteria should have the option to continue treatment until they and their clinician consider it appropriate to stop.
  www.nice.org.uk/TA293

  Scottish Medicines Consortium (SMC) Decisions
  The *Scottish Medicines Consortium* has advised (July 2010) that eltrombopag (*Revolade* ®) is accepted for restricted use within NHS Scotland for the treatment of both splenectomised and non-splenectomised patients with severe symptomatic immune (idiopathic) thrombocytopenic purpura or a high risk of bleeding.

- MEDICINAL FORMS
  There can be variation in the licensing of different medicines containing the same drug.
  Tablet
  ► Eltrombopag (Non-proprietary)
  Eltrombopag (as Eltrombopag olamine) 12.5 mg Promacta 12.5mg tablets | 30 tablet [PoM] no price available
  Eltrombopag olamine 75 mg Promacta 75mg tablets | 30 tablet [PoM] no price available
  ► Revolade (Novartis Pharmaceuticals UK Ltd)
  Eltrombopag (as Eltrombopag olamine) 25 mg Revolade 25mg tablets | 28 tablet [PoM] £770.00
  Eltrombopag (as Eltrombopag olamine) 50 mg Revolade 50mg tablets | 28 tablet [PoM] £1,540.00

Romiplostim

- INDICATIONS AND DOSE
  Treatment of chronic idiopathic thrombocytopenic purpura in splenectomised patients refractory to other treatments (such as corticosteroids or immunoglobulins) (under expert supervision) | Second-line treatment of chronic idiopathic thrombocytopenic purpura in non-splenectomised patients when surgery is contra-indicated (under expert supervision)
  ► BY SUBCUTANEOUS INJECTION
  ► Adult: Initially 1 microgram/kg once weekly, adjusted in steps of 1 microgram/kg once weekly (max. per dose 10 micrograms/kg once weekly) until a stable platelet count of 50x10⁹/litre or more is reached, discontinue treatment if inadequate response after 4 weeks at maximum dose, consult product literature for dose adjustments

- SIDE-EFFECTS Arthralgia · asthenia · bone pain · dizziness · ecchymosis · fatigue · flushing · gastro-intestinal disturbances · increased bone marrow reticulin · influenza-like symptoms · injection site reactions · insomnia · migraine · muscle spasm · myalgia · oedema · paraesthesia · rash
- PREGNANCY Manufacturer advises use only if essential—toxicity in *animal* studies.
- BREAST FEEDING Manufacturer advises avoid—no information available.
- HEPATIC IMPAIRMENT Avoid in moderate or severe impairment unless potential benefit outweighs risk (e.g. of portal vein thrombosis).
- RENAL IMPAIRMENT Manufacturer advises caution—no information available.
- MONITORING REQUIREMENTS
  ► Monitor full blood count and peripheral blood smears for morphological abnormalities before and during treatment.
  ► Monitor platelet count weekly until platelet count reaches 50x10⁹/litre or more for at least 4 weeks without dose adjustment, then monthly thereafter.

- PATIENT AND CARER ADVICE

Driving and skilled tasks
Dizziness may affect performance of skilled tasks (e.g. driving).

- NATIONAL FUNDING/ACCESS DECISIONS

NICE technology appraisals (TAs)

▸ **Romiplostim for the treatment of chronic immune (idiopathic) thrombocytopenic purpura (April 2011)** NICE TA221
Romiplostim is recommended for the treatment of chronic immune (idiopathic) thrombocytopenic purpura in adults:
- if the manufacturer provides romiplostin at the agreed discount as part of the patient access scheme *and*
- whose condition is refractory to standard active treatments and rescue therapies *or*
- who have severe disease and a high risk of bleeding that needs frequent courses of rescue therapies.

www.nice.org.uk/TA221

Scottish Medicines Consortium (SMC) Decisions
The *Scottish Medicines Consortium* has advised (September 2009) that romiplostim (*Nplate®*) is accepted for restricted use within NHS Scotland for patients with severe symptomatic idiopathic thrombocytopenic purpura or those at high risk of bleeding.

- MEDICINAL FORMS
There can be variation in the licensing of different medicines containing the same drug.

Powder and solvent for solution for injection
▸ Nplate (Amgen Ltd)
Romiplostim 250 microgram Nplate 250microgram powder and solvent for solution for injection pre-filled disposable devices | 1 pre-filled disposable injection PoM £482.00

Nutrition and metabolic disorders

1 Fluid and electrolyte imbalances

Fluids and electrolytes

Electrolyte replacement therapy

The electrolyte concentrations (intravenous fluid) table and the electrolyte content (gastro-intestinal secretions) table may be helpful in planning replacement electrolyte therapy; faeces, vomit, or aspiration should be saved and analysed where possible if abnormal losses are suspected.

Oral preparations for fluid and electrolyte imbalance

Sodium and potassium salts, may be given by mouth to prevent deficiencies or to treat established deficiencies of mild or moderate degree.

Oral potassium
Compensation for potassium loss is especially necessary:
- in those taking digoxin or anti-arrhythmic drugs, where potassium depletion may induce arrhythmias;
- in patients in whom secondary hyperaldosteronism occurs, e.g. renal artery stenosis, cirrhosis of the liver, the nephrotic syndrome, and severe heart failure;
- in patients with excessive losses of potassium in the faeces, e.g. chronic diarrhoea associated with intestinal malabsorption or laxative abuse.

Measures to compensate for potassium loss may also be required in the elderly since they frequently take inadequate amounts of potassium in the diet (but see **warning** on **renal insufficiency**). Measures may also be required during long-term administration of drugs known to induce potassium loss (e.g. corticosteroids). Potassium supplements are **seldom required** with the small doses of diuretics given to treat hypertension; **potassium-sparing diuretics** (rather than potassium supplements) are recommended for prevention of hypokalaemia due to diuretics such as furosemide p. 210 or the thiazides when these are given to eliminate oedema.

If potassium salts are used for the prevention of hypokalaemia, then doses of potassium chloride daily (in divided doses) by mouth are suitable in patients taking a normal diet. *Smaller doses* must be used if there is *renal insufficiency (common in the elderly)* to reduce the **risk** of **hyperkalaemia**.

Potassium salts cause nausea and vomiting and poor compliance is a major limitation to their effectiveness; when appropriate, potassium-sparing diuretics are preferable.

When there is *established potassium depletion* larger doses may be necessary, the quantity depending on the severity of any continuing potassium loss (monitoring of plasma-potassium concentration and specialist advice would be required). Potassium depletion is frequently associated with chloride depletion and with metabolic alkalosis, and these disorders require correction.

Management of hyperkalaemia
Acute severe hyperkalaemia (plasma-potassium concentration above 6.5 mmol/litre or in the presence of ECG changes) calls for urgent treatment with calcium gluconate 10% p. 907 by slow intravenous injection, titrated and adjusted to ECG improvement, to temporarily protect against myocardial excitability. An intravenous injection of soluble insulin (5–10 units) with 50 mL glucose 50% p. 903 given over 5-15 minutes, reduces serum-potassium concentration; this is repeated if necessary or a continuous infusion instituted. Salbutamol p. 233 [unlicensed indication], by nebulisation or slow intravenous injection may also reduce plasma-potassium concentration; it should be used with caution in patients with cardiovascular disease. The correction of causal or compounding acidosis with sodium bicarbonate infusion p. 898 should be considered (**important**: preparations of sodium bicarbonate and calcium salts should not be administered in the same line—risk of precipitation). Drugs exacerbating hyperkalaemia should be reviewed and stopped as appropriate; occasionally haemodialysis is needed.

Ion-exchange resins may be used to remove excess potassium in *mild hyperkalaemia* or in *moderate hyperkalaemia* when there are no ECG changes.

Oral sodium and water
Sodium chloride p. 901 is indicated in states of sodium depletion and usually needs to be given intravenously. In chronic conditions associated with mild or moderate degrees of sodium depletion, e.g. in salt-losing bowel or renal disease, oral supplements of sodium chloride or sodium bicarbonate, according to the acid-base status of the patient, may be sufficient.

Oral rehydration therapy (ORT)
As a worldwide problem *diarrhoea* is by far the most important indication for fluid and electrolyte replacement. Intestinal absorption of sodium and water is enhanced by glucose (and other carbohydrates). Replacement of fluid and electrolytes lost through diarrhoea can therefore be achieved by giving solutions containing sodium, potassium, and glucose or another carbohydrate such as rice starch.

Oral rehydration solutions should:
- enhance the absorption of water and electrolytes;
- replace the electrolyte deficit adequately and safely;
- contain an alkalinising agent to counter acidosis;

9

Blood and nutrition

- be slightly hypo-osmolar (about 250 mmol/litre) to prevent the possible induction of osmotic diarrhoea;
- be simple to use in hospital and at home;
- be palatable and acceptable, especially to children;
- be readily available.

It is the policy of the World Health Organization (WHO) to promote a single oral rehydration solution but to use it flexibly (e.g. by giving extra water between drinks of oral rehydration solution to moderately dehydrated infants).

The WHO oral rehydration salts formulation contains sodium chloride 2.6 g, potassium chloride 1.5 g, sodium citrate 2.9 g, anhydrous glucose 13.5 g. It is dissolved in sufficient water to produce 1 litre (providing Na^+ 75 mmol, K^+ 20 mmol, Cl^- 65 mmol, citrate 10 mmol, glucose 75 mmol/litre). This formulation is recommended by the WHO and the United Nations Children's fund, but it is not commonly used in the UK.

Oral rehydration solutions used in the UK are lower in sodium (50–60 mmol/litre) than the WHO formulation since, in general, patients suffer less severe sodium loss.

Rehydration should be rapid over 3 to 4 hours (except in hypernatraemic dehydration in which case rehydration should occur more slowly over 12 hours). The patient should be reassessed after initial rehydration and if still dehydrated rapid fluid replacement should continue.

Once rehydration is complete further dehydration is prevented by encouraging the patient to drink normal volumes of an appropriate fluid and by replacing continuing losses with an oral rehydration solution; in infants, breast-feeding or formula feeds should be offered between oral rehydration drinks.

Oral bicarbonate

Sodium bicarbonate is given by mouth for *chronic acidotic states* such as uraemic acidosis or renal tubular acidosis. The dose for correction of metabolic acidosis is not predictable and the response must be assessed. For severe *metabolic acidosis*, sodium bicarbonate can be given intravenously.

Sodium bicarbonate may also be used to increase the pH of the urine; it is also used in dyspepsia.

Sodium supplements may increase blood pressure or cause fluid retention and pulmonary oedema in those at risk; hypokalaemia may be exacerbated.

Where *hyperchloraemic acidosis* is associated with potassium deficiency, as in some renal tubular and gastrointestinal disorders it may be appropriate to give oral **potassium bicarbonate**, although acute or severe deficiency should be managed by intravenous therapy.

Parenteral preparations for fluid and electrolyte imbalance

Electrolytes and water

Solutions of electrolytes are given intravenously, to meet normal fluid and electrolyte requirements or to replenish substantial deficits or continuing losses, when the patient is nauseated or vomiting and is unable to take adequate amounts by mouth. When intravenous administration is not possible, fluid (as sodium chloride 0.9% p. 901 or glucose 5% p. 903) can also be given by subcutaneous infusion (hypodermoclysis).

The nature and severity of the electrolyte imbalance must be assessed from the history and clinical and biochemical investigations. Sodium, potassium, chloride, magnesium, phosphate, and water depletion can occur singly and in combination with or without disturbances of acid-base balance.

Isotonic solutions may be infused safely into a peripheral vein. Solutions more concentrated than plasma, e.g. 20% glucose, are best given through an indwelling catheter positioned in a large vein.

Intravenous sodium

Sodium chloride in isotonic solution provides the most important extracellular ions in near physiological concentrations and is indicated in *sodium depletion,* which can arise from such conditions as gastro-enteritis, diabetic ketoacidosis, ileus, and ascites. In a severe deficit of 4 to 8 litres, 2 to 3 litres of isotonic sodium chloride may be given over 2 to 3 hours; thereafter the infusion can usually be at a slower rate.

Chronic hyponatraemia arising from inappropriate secretion of antidiuretic hormone should ideally be corrected by fluid restriction. However, if sodium chloride is required for acute or chronic hyponatraemia, regardless of the cause, the deficit should be corrected slowly to avoid the risk of osmotic demyelination syndrome and the rise in plasma-sodium concentration should not exceed 10 mmol/litre in 24 hours. In severe hyponatraemia, sodium chloride 1.8% may be used cautiously.

Compound sodium lactate (Hartmann's solution) can be used instead of isotonic sodium chloride solution during or after surgery, or in the initial management of the injured or wounded; it may reduce the risk of hyperchloraemic acidosis.

Sodium chloride with glucose solutions p. 902 are indicated when there is combined *water and sodium depletion.* A 1:1 mixture of isotonic sodium chloride and 5% glucose allows some of the water (free of sodium) to enter body cells which suffer most from dehydration while the sodium salt with a volume of water determined by the normal plasma Na^+ remains extracellular.

Combined sodium, potassium, chloride, and water depletion may occur, for example, with severe diarrhoea or persistent vomiting; replacement is carried out with sodium chloride intravenous infusion 0.9% and glucose intravenous infusion 5% with potassium as appropriate.

Intravenous glucose

Glucose solutions (5%) are used mainly to replace water deficit. Average water requirements in a healthy adult are 1.5 to 2.5 litres daily and this is needed to balance unavoidable losses of water through the skin and lungs and to provide sufficient for urinary excretion. Water depletion (dehydration) tends to occur when these losses are not matched by a comparable intake, as may occur in coma or dysphagia or in the elderly or apathetic who may not drink enough water on their own initiative.

Excessive loss of water without loss of electrolytes is uncommon, occurring in fevers, hyperthyroidism, and in uncommon water-losing renal states such as diabetes insipidus or hypercalcaemia. The volume of glucose solution needed to replace deficits varies with the severity of the disorder, but usually lies within the range of 2 to 6 litres.

Glucose solutions are also used to correct and prevent hypoglycaemia and to provide a source of energy in those too ill to be fed adequately by mouth; glucose solutions are a key component of parenteral nutrition.

Glucose solutions are given in regimens with calcium and insulin for the emergency management of *hyperkalaemia.* They are also given, after correction of hyperglycaemia, during treatment of diabetic ketoacidosis, when they must be accompanied by continuing insulin infusion.

Intravenous potassium

Potassium chloride with sodium chloride intravenous infusion p. 900 is the initial treatment for the correction of *severe hypokalaemia* and when sufficient potassium cannot be taken by mouth.

Repeated measurement of plasma-potassium concentration is necessary to determine whether further infusions are required and to avoid the development of hyperkalaemia, which is especially likely in renal impairment.

Initial potassium replacement therapy should **not** involve glucose infusions, because glucose may cause a further decrease in the plasma-potassium concentration.

Fluids and electrolytes

Electrolyte concentrations—intravenous fluids

Intravenous infusion	Millimoles per litre				
	Na$^+$	K$^+$	HCO$_3^-$	Cl$^-$	Ca^{2+}
Normal plasma values	**142**	**4.5**	**26**	**103**	**2.5**
Sodium Chloride 0.9%	150	-	-	150	-
Compound Sodium Lactate (Hartmann's)	131	5	29	111	2
Sodium Chloride 0.18% and Glucose 4% (Adults only)	30	-	-	30	-
Sodium Chloride 0.45% and Glucose 5% (Children only)	75	-	-	75	-
Potassium Chloride 0.15% and Glucose 5% (Children only)	-	20	-	20	-
Potassium Chloride 0.15% and Sodium Chloride 0.9% (Children only)	150	20	-	170	-
Potassium Chloride 0.3% and Glucose 5%	-	40	-	40	-
Potassium Chloride 0.3% and Sodium Chloride 0.9%	150	40	-	190	-
To correct metabolic acidosis					
Sodium Bicarbonate 1.26%	150	-	150	-	-
Sodium Bicarbonate 8.4% for cardiac arrest	1000	-	1000	-	-
Sodium Lactate (m/6)	167	-	167	-	-

Electrolyte content—gastro-intestinal secretions

Type of fluid	Millimoles per litre				
	H$^+$	Na$^+$	K$^+$	HCO$_3^-$	Cl$^-$
Gastric	40-60	20-80	5-20	-	100-150
Biliary	-	120-140	5-15	30-50	80-120
Pancreatic	-	120-140	5-15	70-110	40-80
Small bowel	-	120-140	5-15	20-40	90-130

Bicarbonate and lactate

Sodium bicarbonate p. 898 is used to control severe *metabolic acidosis* (pH<7.1) particularly that caused by loss of bicarbonate (as in renal tubular acidosis or from excessive gastro-intestinal losses). Mild metabolic acidosis associated with volume depletion should first be managed by appropriate fluid replacement because acidosis usually resolves as tissue and renal perfusion are restored. In more severe metabolic acidosis or when the acidosis remains unresponsive to correction of anoxia or hypovolaemia, sodium bicarbonate (1.26%) can be infused over 3–4 hours with plasma-pH and electrolyte monitoring. In severe shock, for example in cardiac arrest, metabolic acidosis can develop without sodium or volume depletion; in these circumstances sodium bicarbonate is best given as a small volume of hypertonic solution, such as 50 mL of 8.4% solution intravenously.

Sodium lactate intravenous infusion is no longer used in metabolic acidosis because of the risk of producing lactic acidosis, particularly in seriously ill patients with poor tissue perfusion or impaired hepatic function.

For *chronic acidotic states*, sodium bicarbonate can be given by mouth.

Plasma and plasma substitutes

Plasma and plasma substitutes ('colloids') contain large molecules that do not readily leave the intravascular space where they exert osmotic pressure to maintain circulatory volume. Compared to fluids containing electrolytes such as sodium chloride and glucose ('crystalloids'), a smaller volume of colloid is required to produce the same expansion of blood volume, thereby shifting salt and water from the extravascular space. If resuscitation requires a volume of fluid that exceeds the maximum dose of the colloid then crystalloids can be given; packed red cells may also be required.

Albumin solution p. 908, prepared from whole blood, contain soluble proteins and electrolytes but no clotting factors, blood group antibodies, or plasma cholinesterases; they may be given without regard to the recipient's blood group.

Albumin is usually used after the acute phase of illness, to correct a plasma-volume deficit; hypoalbuminaemia itself is not an appropriate indication. The use of albumin solution in acute plasma or blood loss may be wasteful; plasma substitutes are more appropriate. Concentrated albumin solution (20%) can be used under specialist supervision in patients with an intravascular fluid deficit and oedema because of interstitial fluid overload, to restore intravascular plasma volume with less exacerbation of the salt and water overload than isotonic solutions. Concentrated albumin solution p. 908 may also be used to obtain a diuresis in hypoalbuminaemic patients (e.g. in hepatic cirrhosis).

Recent evidence does not support the previous view that the use of albumin increases mortality.

Plasma substitutes

Dextran, gelatin p. 909, and the hydroxyethyl starch, tetrastarch, are macromolecular substances which are metabolised slowly. **Dextran** and gelatin may be used at the outset to expand and maintain blood volume in shock arising from conditions such as burns or septicaemia; they may also be used as an immediate short-term measure to treat haemorrhage until blood is available. **Dextran** and gelatin are rarely needed when shock is due to sodium and water depletion because, in these circumstances, the shock responds to water and electrolyte repletion.

Hydroxyethyl starches should only be used for the treatment of hypovolaemia due to acute blood loss when crystalloids alone are not sufficient; they should be used at the lowest effective dose for the first 24 hours of fluid resuscitation.

Plasma substitutes should **not** be used to maintain plasma volume in conditions such as burns or peritonitis where there is loss of plasma protein, water, and electrolytes over periods of several days or weeks. In these situations, plasma or plasma protein fractions containing large amounts of albumin should be given.

Large volumes of *some* plasma substitutes can increase the risk of bleeding through depletion of coagulation factors.

BICARBONATE

Sodium bicarbonate

● INDICATIONS AND DOSE

Alkalinisation of urine | Relief of discomfort in mild urinary-tract infections
▶ BY MOUTH
▶ Adult: 3 g every 2 hours until urinary pH exceeds 7, to be dissolved in water

Maintenance of alkaline urine
▶ BY MOUTH
▶ Adult: 5–10 g daily, to be dissolved in water

Chronic acidotic states such as uraemic acidosis or renal tubular acidosis
▶ BY MOUTH
▶ Adult: 4.8 g daily, (57 mmol each of Na^+ and HCO_3^-), higher doses may be required and should be adjusted according to response

Severe metabolic acidosis
▶ BY SLOW INTRAVENOUS INJECTION, OR BY INTRAVENOUS INFUSION
▶ Adult: Administer an amount appropriate to the body base deficit, to be given by slow intravenous injection of a strong solution (up to 8.4%), or by continuous intravenous infusion of a weaker solution (usually 1.26%)

● CONTRA-INDICATIONS
▶ With oral use Salt restricted diet

● CAUTIONS
▶ With systemic use Avoid prolonged use in urinary conditions · cardiac disease · elderly · patients on sodium-restricted diet · respiratory acidosis

● INTERACTIONS → Appendix 1 (antacids).

● SIDE-EFFECTS
▶ When used for alkalinisation of urine With oral use for alkalinisation of urine alkalosis on prolonged use · eructation
▶ When used for chronic acidotic states such as uraemic acidosis or renal tubular acidosis With oral use for chronic acidotic states such as uraemic acidosis or renal tubular acidosis fluid retention (in those at risk) · hypokalaemia may be exacerbated · increase blood pressure · pulmonary oedema (in those at risk)
▶ When used for maintenance of alkaline urine With oral use for maintenance of alkaline urine fluid retention (in those at risk) · hypokalaemia may be exacerbated · increase blood pressure · pulmonary oedema (in those at risk)
▶ When used for relief of discomfort in mild urinary-tract infections With oral use for relief of discomfort in mild urinary-tract infections alkalosis on prolonged use · eructation

● PREGNANCY
▶ With oral use Use with caution in urinary conditions.

● HEPATIC IMPAIRMENT
▶ With intravenous use or oral use In patients with fluid retention, avoid large amounts of sodium.

● RENAL IMPAIRMENT
▶ With oral use Avoid (except for specialised role in some forms of renal disease).

● MONITORING REQUIREMENTS
▶ With intravenous use Plasma-pH and electrolytes should be monitored.

● DIRECTIONS FOR ADMINISTRATION
▶ With intravenous use For *slow intravenous injection* use a small volume of hypertonic solution (such as 50 mL of 8.4%). For *continuous intravenous infusion* a weaker solution of 1.26% solution can be infused over 3–4 hours.
▶ With oral use Sodium bicarbonate may affect the stability or absorption of other drugs if administered at the same time. If possible, allow 1–2 hours before administering other drugs orally.

● PRESCRIBING AND DISPENSING INFORMATION
▶ With oral use Sodium bicarbonate 500*mg* capsules contain approximately 6 mmol each of Na^+ and HCO_3^-; *Sodium bicarbonate* 600*mg* capsules contain approximately 7 mmol each of Na^+ and HCO_3^-. Oral solutions of sodium bicarbonate are required occasionally; these are available from 'special-order' manufacturers or specialist importing companies; the strength of sodium bicarbonate should be stated on the prescription.
▶ With intravenous use Usual strength Sodium bicarbonate 1.26% (12.6 g, 150 mmol each of Na^+ and HCO_3^-/litre), various other strengths available.

● PATIENT AND CARER ADVICE
▶ With oral use Patients or carers should be given advice on the administration of sodium bicarbonate oral medicines.

● MEDICINAL FORMS
There can be variation in the licensing of different medicines containing the same drug. Forms available from special-order manufacturers include: capsule, oral suspension, oral solution, solution for injection, liquid

Tablet
▶ Sodium bicarbonate (Non-proprietary)
Sodium bicarbonate 600 mg Sodium bicarbonate 600mg tablets | 100 tablet £125.50 | 100 tablet GSL £29.75
S-Bicarb 600mg tablets | 100 tablet £125.50

Capsule
▶ Sodium bicarbonate (Non-proprietary)
Sodium bicarbonate 500 mg Sodium bicarbonate 500mg capsules | 56 capsule P £17.56 DT price = £2.23 | 100 capsule PoM no price available

Oral solution
▶ Sodium bicarbonate (Non-proprietary)
Sodium bicarbonate 84 mg per 1 ml S-Bicarb SF 420mg/5ml (1mmol/ml) oral solution sugar-free | 100 ml £26.25 DT price = £39.80
S-Bicarb 420mg/5ml (1mmol/ml) oral solution | 100 ml no price available
SodiBic 420mg/5ml (1mmol/ml) oral solution sugar-free | 100 ml £17.71 DT price = £39.80
▶ Thamicarb (Thame Laboratories Ltd)
Sodium bicarbonate 84 mg per 1 ml Thamicarb 84mg/1ml (1mmol/ml) oral solution sugar-free | 100 ml P £39.80 DT price = £39.80 sugar-free | 500 ml P £199.20 DT price = £199.20

Solution for injection
▶ Sodium bicarbonate (Non-proprietary)
Sodium bicarbonate 84 mg per 1 ml Sodium bicarbonate 8.4% (1mmol/ml) solution for injection 10ml ampoules | 10 ampoule PoM £77.40
Sodium bicarbonate 8.4% solution for injection 10ml Minijet pre-filled syringes | 1 pre-filled disposable injection PoM £9.71
Sodium bicarbonate 8.4% (1mmol/ml) solution for injection 250ml bottles | 10 bottle PoM £65.34
Sodium bicarbonate 8.4% (1mmol/ml) solution for injection 100ml bottles | 10 bottle PoM £62.04

Infusion

▶ Sodium bicarbonate (Non-proprietary)

Sodium bicarbonate 12.6 mg per 1 ml Polyfusor BC sodium bicarbonate 1.26% infusion 500ml bottles | 1 bottle PoM £9.86 | 12 bottle PoM no price available

Sodium bicarbonate 14 mg per 1 ml Polyfusor BD sodium bicarbonate 1.4% infusion 500ml bottles | 1 bottle PoM £9.86 | 12 bottle PoM no price available

Sodium bicarbonate 27.4 mg per 1 ml Polyfusor V sodium bicarbonate 2.74% infusion 500ml bottles | 1 bottle PoM £9.86 | 12 bottle PoM no price available

Sodium bicarbonate 42 mg per 1 ml Polyfusor BE sodium bicarbonate 4.2% infusion 500ml bottles | 1 bottle PoM £9.86 | 12 bottle PoM no price available

Sodium bicarbonate 84 mg per 1 ml Polyfusor B sodium bicarbonate 8.4% infusion 200ml bottles | 1 bottle PoM £9.86 | 12 bottle PoM no price available

ELECTROLYTES AND MINERALS > POTASSIUM

Potassium chloride with calcium chloride and sodium chloride and sodium lactate

(Sodium Lactate Intravenous Infusion, Compound; Compound, Hartmann's Solution for Injection; Ringer-Lactate Solution for Injection)

The properties listed below are those particular to the combination only. For the properties of the components please consider, potassium chloride p. 917, sodium chloride p. 901, calcium chloride p. 907.

● **INDICATIONS AND DOSE**

For prophylaxis, and replacement therapy, requiring the use of sodium chloride and lactate, with minimal amounts of calcium and potassium

▶ BY INTRAVENOUS INFUSION

▶ Adult: (consult product literature)

● PRESCRIBING AND DISPENSING INFORMATION Compound sodium lactate intravenous infusion contains Na^+ 131 mmol, K^+ 5 mmol, Ca^{2+} 2 mmol, HCO_3^- (as lactate) 29 mmol, Cl^- 111 mmol/litre.

● MEDICINAL FORMS
There can be variation in the licensing of different medicines containing the same drug.

Infusion

▶ Potassium chloride with calcium chloride and sodium chloride and sodium lactate (Non-proprietary)

Calcium chloride 270 microgram per 1 ml, Potassium chloride 400 microgram per 1 ml, Sodium lactate 3.17 mg per 1 ml, Sodium chloride 6 mg per 1 ml Sodium lactate compound infusion 1litre Macoflex N bags | 1 bag PoM no price available | 10 bag PoM no price available
Sodium lactate compound infusion 1litre Viaflex bags | 1 bag PoM no price available | 10 bag PoM no price available
Sodium lactate compound infusion 1litre Macoflex bags | 1 bag PoM no price available | 12 bag PoM no price available
Sodium lactate compound infusion 1litre Viaflo bags | 1 bag PoM no price available | 10 bag PoM no price available
Ringer lactate infusion 1litre Viaflo bags | 1 bag PoM no price available | 10 bag PoM no price available

Potassium chloride with calcium chloride dihydrate and sodium chloride

(Ringer's solution)

The properties listed below are those particular to the combination only. For the properties of the components please consider, potassium chloride p. 917, sodium chloride p. 901.

● **INDICATIONS AND DOSE**

Electrolyte imbalance

▶ BY INTRAVENOUS INFUSION

▶ Adult: Dosed according to the deficit or daily maintenance requirements (consult product literature)

● PRESCRIBING AND DISPENSING INFORMATION Ringer's solution for injection provides the following ions (in mmol/litre). Ca^{2+} 2.2, K^+ 4, Na^+ 147, Cl^- 156.

● MEDICINAL FORMS
There can be variation in the licensing of different medicines containing the same drug.

Infusion

▶ Potassium chloride with calcium chloride dihydrate and sodium chloride (Non-proprietary)

Potassium chloride 300 microgram per 1 ml, Calcium chloride 320 microgram per 1 ml, Sodium chloride 8.6 mg per 1 ml Polyfusor C ringers infusion 500ml bottles | 1 bottle PoM £2.95 | 12 bottle PoM no price available
Steriflex No.9 ringers infusion 1litre bags | 1 bag PoM £2.22 | 10 bag PoM no price available
Steriflex No.9 ringers infusion 500ml bags | 1 bag PoM £1.96 | 15 bag PoM no price available

Potassium chloride with glucose

The properties listed below are those particular to the combination only. For the properties of the components please consider, potassium chloride p. 917, glucose p. 903.

● **INDICATIONS AND DOSE**

Electrolyte imbalance

▶ BY INTRAVENOUS INFUSION

▶ Adult: Dosed according to the deficit or daily maintenance requirements

● PRESCRIBING AND DISPENSING INFORMATION Potassium chloride 0.3% contains 40 mmol each of K^+ and Cl^-/litre or 0.15% contains 20 mmol each of K^+ and Cl^-/litre with 5% of anhydrous glucose.

● MEDICINAL FORMS
There can be variation in the licensing of different medicines containing the same drug. Forms available from special-order manufacturers include: infusion, solution for infusion

Infusion

▶ Potassium chloride with glucose (Non-proprietary)

Potassium chloride 3 mg per 1 ml, Glucose anhydrous 50 mg per 1 ml Potassium chloride 0.3% (potassium 40mmol/1litre) / Glucose 5% infusion 1litre Macoflex bags | 1 bag PoM no price available | 12 bag PoM no price available
Steriflex No.16 potassium chloride 0.3% (potassium 20mmol/500ml) / glucose 5% infusion 500ml bags | 1 bag PoM £1.67 | 15 bag PoM no price available
Potassium chloride 0.3% (potassium 20mmol/500ml) / Glucose 5% infusion 500ml Macoflex bags | 1 bag PoM no price available | 20 bag PoM no price available
Potassium chloride 0.3% (potassium 40mmol/1litre) / Glucose 5% infusion 1litre bags | 1 bag PoM £1.79
Steriflex No.16 potassium chloride 0.3% (potassium 40mmol/1litre) / glucose 5% infusion 1litre bags | 1 bag PoM £2.20 | 10 bag PoM no price available

9

Blood and nutrition

Potassium chloride 0.3% (potassium 20mmol/500ml) / Glucose 5% infusion 500ml Viaflo bags | 1 bag [PoM] no price available | 20 bag [PoM] no price available
Potassium chloride 0.3% (potassium 40mmol/1litre) / Glucose 5% infusion 1litre Viaflo bags | 1 bag [PoM] no price available | 10 bag [PoM] no price available
Potassium chloride 2 mg per 1 ml, Glucose anhydrous 50 mg per 1 ml Steriflex No.29 potassium chloride 0.2% (potassium 27mmol/1litre) / glucose 5% infusion 1litre bags | 1 bag [PoM] £2.20 | 10 bag [PoM] no price available
Steriflex No.29 potassium chloride 0.2% (potassium 13.3mmol/500ml) / glucose 5% infusion 500ml bags | 1 bag [PoM] £1.67 | 15 bag [PoM] no price available
Potassium chloride 1.5 mg per 1 ml, Glucose anhydrous 50 mg per 1 ml Steriflex No.13 potassium chloride 0.15% (potassium 10mmol/500ml) / glucose 5% infusion 500ml bags | 1 bag [PoM] £1.67 | 15 bag [PoM] no price available
Steriflex No.13 potassium chloride 0.15% (potassium 20mmol/1litre) / glucose 5% infusion 1litre bags | 1 bag [PoM] £2.20 | 10 bag [PoM] no price available
Potassium chloride 0.15% (potassium 20mmol/1litre) / Glucose 5% infusion 1litre Macoflex bags | 1 bag [PoM] no price available | 12 bag [PoM] no price available
Potassium chloride 0.15% (potassium 10mmol/500ml) / Glucose 5% infusion 500ml Macoflex bags | 1 bag [PoM] no price available | 20 bag [PoM] no price available
Potassium chloride 0.15% (potassium 20mmol/1litre) / Glucose 5% infusion 1litre Viaflo bags | 1 bag [PoM] no price available
Potassium chloride 0.15% (potassium 20mmol/1litre) / Glucose 5% infusion 1litre Viaflex bags | 1 bag [PoM] no price available | 10 bag [PoM] no price available

Potassium chloride with glucose and sodium chloride

The properties listed below are those particular to the combination only. For the properties of the components please consider, potassium chloride p. 917, glucose p. 903, sodium chloride p. 901.

- INDICATIONS AND DOSE

Electrolyte imbalance
▶ BY INTRAVENOUS INFUSION
▶ Adult: Dosed according to the deficit or daily maintenance requirements

- PRESCRIBING AND DISPENSING INFORMATION
Concentration of potassium chloride to be specified by the prescriber (usually K⁺ 10–40 mmol/litre).

- MEDICINAL FORMS
There can be variation in the licensing of different medicines containing the same drug. Forms available from special-order manufacturers include: infusion, solution for infusion
Infusion
▶ Potassium chloride with glucose and sodium chloride (Non-proprietary)
Sodium chloride 1.8 mg per 1 ml, Potassium chloride 3 mg per 1 ml, Glucose anhydrous 40 mg per 1 ml Steriflex No.17 potassium chloride 0.3% (potassium 40mmol/1litre) / glucose 4% / sodium chloride 0.18% infusion 1litre bags | 1 bag [PoM] £2.20 | 10 bag [PoM] no price available
Steriflex No.17 potassium chloride 0.3% (potassium 20mmol/500ml) / glucose 4% / sodium chloride 0.18% infusion 500ml bags | 1 bag [PoM] £1.67 | 15 bag [PoM] no price available
Potassium chloride 0.3% (potassium 20mmol/500ml) / Glucose 4% / Sodium chloride 0.18% infusion 500ml Macoflex bags | 1 bag [PoM] no price available | 20 bag [PoM] no price available
Potassium chloride 0.3% (potassium 40mmol/1litre) / Glucose 4% / Sodium chloride 0.18% infusion 1litre Macoflex bags | 1 bag [PoM] no price available | 12 bag [PoM] no price available
Potassium chloride 0.3% (potassium 40mmol/1litre) / Glucose 4% / Sodium chloride 0.18% infusion 1litre Viaflo bags | 1 bag [PoM] no price available | 10 bag [PoM] no price available
Potassium chloride 1.5 mg per 1 ml, Sodium chloride 1.8 mg per 1 ml, Glucose anhydrous 40 mg per 1 ml Potassium chloride 0.15% (potassium 20mmol/1litre) / Glucose 4% / Sodium chloride 0.18% infusion 1litre Viaflo bags | 1 bag [PoM] no price available | 10 bag [PoM] no price available

Steriflex No.14 potassium chloride 0.15% (potassium 20mmol/1litre) / glucose 4% / sodium chloride 0.18% infusion 1litre bags | 1 bag [PoM] £2.20 | 10 bag [PoM] no price available
Potassium chloride 0.15% (potassium 20mmol/1litre) / Glucose 4% / Sodium chloride 0.18% infusion 1litre Macoflex bags | 1 bag [PoM] no price available | 12 bag [PoM] no price available
Potassium chloride 0.15% (potassium 10mmol/500ml) / Glucose 4% / Sodium chloride 0.18% infusion 500ml Macoflex bags | 1 bag [PoM] no price available | 20 bag [PoM] no price available
Steriflex No.14 potassium chloride 0.15% (potassium 10mmol/500ml) / glucose 4% / sodium chloride 0.18% infusion 500ml bags | 1 bag [PoM] £1.67 | 15 bag [PoM] no price available
Sodium chloride 1.8 mg per 1 ml, Potassium chloride 2 mg per 1 ml, Glucose anhydrous 40 mg per 1 ml Steriflex No.30 potassium chloride 0.2% (potassium 13.3mmol/500ml) / glucose 4% / sodium chloride 0.18% infusion 500ml bags | 1 bag [PoM] £1.67 | 15 bag [PoM] no price available
Steriflex No.30 potassium chloride 0.2% (potassium 27mmol/1litre) / glucose 4% / sodium chloride 0.18% infusion 1litre bags | 1 bag [PoM] £2.20 | 10 bag [PoM] no price available
Potassium chloride 1.5 mg per 1 ml, Sodium chloride 4.5 mg per 1 ml, Glucose anhydrous 50 mg per 1 ml Intraven potassium chloride 0.15% (potassium 10mmol/500ml) / glucose 5% / sodium chloride 0.45% infusion 500ml bags | 1 bag [PoM] £3.12

Potassium chloride with potassium bicarbonate

The properties listed below are those particular to the combination only. For the properties of the components please consider, potassium chloride p. 917.

- INDICATIONS AND DOSE

Potassium depletion
▶ BY MOUTH
▶ Adult: Dosed according to the deficit or daily maintenance requirements (consult product literature)

- PRESCRIBING AND DISPENSING INFORMATION Each *Sando-K*® tablet contains potassium 470 mg (12 mmol of K⁺) and chloride 285mg (8 mmol of Cl⁻).

- MEDICINAL FORMS
There can be variation in the licensing of different medicines containing the same drug.
Effervescent tablet
CAUTIONARY AND ADVISORY LABELS 13, 21
▶ Sando-K (HK Pharma Ltd)
Potassium bicarbonate 400 mg, Potassium chloride 600 mg Sando-K effervescent tablets | 100 tablet [P] £7.65 DT price = £7.65

Potassium chloride with sodium chloride

The properties listed below are those particular to the combination only. For the properties of the components please consider, potassium chloride p. 917, sodium chloride p. 901.

- INDICATIONS AND DOSE

Electrolyte imbalance
▶ BY INTRAVENOUS INFUSION
▶ Adult: Depending on the deficit or the daily maintenance requirements (consult product literature)

- PRESCRIBING AND DISPENSING INFORMATION Potassium chloride 0.15% with sodium chloride 0.9% contains K⁺ 20 mmol, Na⁺ 150 mmol, and Cl⁻ 170 mmol/litre or potassium chloride 0.3% with sodium chloride 0.9% contains K⁺ 40 mmol, Na⁺ 150 mmol, and Cl⁻ 190 mmol/litre.

● MEDICINAL FORMS

There can be variation in the licensing of different medicines containing the same drug. Forms available from special-order manufacturers include: infusion, solution for infusion

Infusion

▸ Potassium chloride with sodium chloride (Non-proprietary)

Potassium chloride 3 mg per 1 ml, Sodium chloride 9 mg per 1 ml Steriflex No.15 potassium chloride 0.3% (potassium 20mmol/500ml) / sodium chloride 0.9% infusion 500ml bags | 1 bag [PoM] £1.67 | 15 bag [PoM] no price available
Potassium chloride 0.3% (potassium 20mmol/500ml) / Sodium chloride 0.9% infusion 500ml Macoflex bags | 1 bag [PoM] no price available | 20 bag [PoM] no price available
Potassium chloride 0.3% (potassium 20mmol/500ml) / Sodium chloride 0.9% infusion 500ml bags | 1 bag [PoM] £1.42
Potassium chloride 0.3% (potassium 20mmol/500ml) / Sodium chloride 0.9% infusion 500ml Viaflo bags | 1 bag [PoM] no price available | 20 bag [PoM] no price available
Potassium chloride 0.3% (potassium 40mmol/1litre) / Sodium chloride 0.9% infusion 1litre Macoflex bags | 1 bag [PoM] no price available | 12 bag [PoM] no price available
Potassium chloride 0.3% (potassium 40mmol/1litre) / Sodium chloride 0.9% infusion 1litre Viaflo bags | 1 bag [PoM] no price available | 10 bag [PoM] no price available
Steriflex No.15 potassium chloride 0.3% (potassium 40mmol/1litre) / sodium chloride 0.9% infusion 1litre bags | 1 bag [PoM] £2.20 | 10 bag [PoM] no price available

Potassium chloride 1.5 mg per 1 ml, Sodium chloride 9 mg per 1 ml Steriflex No.12 potassium chloride 0.15% (potassium 20mmol/1litre) / sodium chloride 0.9% infusion 1litre bags | 1 bag [PoM] £2.20 | 10 bag [PoM] no price available
Steriflex No.12 potassium chloride 0.15% (potassium 10mmol/500ml) / sodium chloride 0.9% infusion 500ml bags | 1 bag [PoM] £1.67 | 15 bag [PoM] no price available
Potassium chloride 0.15% (potassium 10mmol/500ml) / Sodium chloride 0.9% infusion 500ml Viaflo bags | 1 bag [PoM] no price available | 20 bag [PoM] no price available
Potassium chloride 0.15% (potassium 20mmol/1litre) / Sodium chloride 0.9% infusion 1litre Viaflex bags | 1 bag [PoM] no price available | 10 bag [PoM] no price available
Potassium chloride 0.15% (potassium 10mmol/500ml) / Sodium chloride 0.9% infusion 500ml Viaflex bags | 1 bag [PoM] no price available | 20 bag [PoM] no price available
Potassium chloride 0.15% (potassium 10mmol/500ml) / Sodium chloride 0.9% infusion 500ml Macoflex bags | 1 bag [PoM] no price available | 20 bag [PoM] no price available
Potassium chloride 0.15% (potassium 20mmol/1litre) / Sodium chloride 0.9% infusion 1litre Viaflo bags | 1 bag [PoM] no price available | 10 bag [PoM] no price available
Potassium chloride 0.15% (potassium 20mmol/1litre) / Sodium chloride 0.9% infusion 1litre Macoflex bags | 1 bag [PoM] no price available | 12 bag [PoM] no price available

Potassium chloride 2 mg per 1 ml, Sodium chloride 9 mg per 1 ml Steriflex No.28 potassium chloride 0.2% (potassium 13.3mmol/500ml) / sodium chloride 0.9% infusion 500ml bags | 1 bag [PoM] £1.67 | 15 bag [PoM] no price available
Steriflex No.28 potassium chloride 0.2% (potassium 27mmol/1litre) / sodium chloride 0.9% infusion 1litre bags | 1 bag [PoM] £2.20 | 10 bag [PoM] no price available

ELECTROLYTES AND MINERALS › SODIUM CHLORIDE

Sodium chloride

● INDICATIONS AND DOSE

Prophylaxis of sodium chloride deficiency

▸ BY MOUTH

▸ Adult: 4–8 tablets daily, to be taken with water, up to maximum 20 tablets daily in severe depletion

Chronic renal salt wasting

▸ BY MOUTH

▸ Adult: Up to 20 tablets daily, to be taken with appropriate fluid intake

Management of diabetic ketoacidosis (to restore circulating volume if systolic blood pressure is below 90 mmHg and adjusted for age, sex, and medication as appropriate)

▸ BY INTRAVENOUS INFUSION

▸ Adult: 500 mL, sodium chloride 0.9% to be given over 10–15 minutes, repeat if blood pressure remains below 90 mmHg and seek senior medical advice, when blood pressure is over 90 mmHg, sodium chloride 0.9% should be given by intravenous infusion at a rate that replaces deficit and provides maintenance, management regimen also includes administration of potassium chloride, soluble insulin, long acting insulin analogues and glucose 10% solution

Diluent for instillation of drugs to the bladder

▸ BY INTRAVESICAL INSTILLATION

▸ Adult: (consult product literature)

● CAUTIONS

▸ With intravenous use Avoid excessive administration · cardiac failure · dilutional hyponatraemia especially in the elderly · hypertension · peripheral oedema · pulmonary oedema · restrict intake in impaired renal function · toxaemia of pregnancy

● SIDE-EFFECTS

▸ With intravenous use Administration of large doses may give rise to sodium accumulation · hyperchloraemic acidosis · oedema

● MONITORING REQUIREMENTS

▸ With intravenous use The jugular venous pressure should be assessed, the bases of the lungs should be examined for crepitations, and in elderly or seriously ill patients it is often helpful to monitor the right atrial (central) venous pressure.

● PRESCRIBING AND DISPENSING INFORMATION

▸ With intravenous use Sodium chloride 0.9% intravenous infusion contains Na^+ and Cl^- each 150 mmol/litre. The term 'normal saline' should not be used to describe sodium chloride intravenous infusion 0.9%; the term 'physiological saline' is acceptable but it is preferable to give the composition (i.e. sodium chloride intravenous infusion 0.9%).

▸ With oral use Each *Slow Sodium* ® tablet contains approximately 10 mmol each of Na^+ and Cl^-; tablets can be crushed before administration.

● MEDICINAL FORMS

There can be variation in the licensing of different medicines containing the same drug. Forms available from special-order manufacturers include: capsule, solution for injection, infusion, solution for infusion, irrigation

Modified-release tablet

CAUTIONARY AND ADVISORY LABELS 25

▸ Slow Sodium (HK Pharma Ltd)

Sodium chloride 600 mg Slow Sodium 600mg tablets | 100 tablet [GSL] £6.05 DT price = £6.05

Solution for injection

▸ Sodium chloride (Non-proprietary)

Sodium chloride 9 mg per 1 ml Sodium chloride 0.9% solution for injection 5ml Sure-Amp ampoules | 20 ampoule [PoM] £7.15
Sodium chloride 0.9% solution for injection 50ml vials | 1 vial [PoM] £3.41 DT price = £3.41 | 25 vial [PoM] £75.00–£85.00
Sodium chloride 0.9% solution for injection 10ml ampoules | 10 ampoule [PoM] £2.30–£2.96 DT price = £2.96 | 50 ampoule [PoM] £14.75
Sodium chloride 0.9% solution for injection 20ml Mini-Plasco ampoules | 20 ampoule [PoM] £18.93
Sodium chloride 0.9% solution for injection 5ml Mini-Plasco ampoules | 20 ampoule [PoM] £8.96
Sodium chloride 0.9% solution for injection 2ml Sure-Amp ampoules | 20 ampoule [PoM] £7.15
Sodium chloride 0.9% solution for injection 20ml ampoules | 20 ampoule [PoM] £15.75
Sodium chloride 0.9% solution for injection 2ml ampoules | 10 ampoule [PoM] £1.80–£2.57 DT price = £2.07

Sodium chloride 0.9% solution for injection 5ml ampoules | 10 ampoule [PoM] £2.00–£2.11 DT price = £2.11 | 50 ampoule [PoM] £10.50

Sodium chloride 0.9% solution for injection 10ml Sure-Amp ampoules | 20 ampoule [PoM] £8.15

Sodium chloride 0.9% solution for injection 10ml Mini-Plasco ampoules | 20 ampoule [PoM] £10.21

Sodium chloride 300 mg per 1 ml Sodium chloride 30% solution for injection 10ml ampoules | 10 ampoule [PoM] £67.46

Sodium chloride 30% solution for injection 50ml vials | 1 vial [PoM] £12.09

▸ Drytec saline (GE Healthcare Biosciences)

Sodium chloride 9 mg per 1 ml Drytec saline eluent 5ml vials | 20 vial [PoM] no price available (Hospital only) | 100 vial [PoM] no price available (Hospital only)

Drytec saline eluent 10ml vials | 20 vial [PoM] no price available (Hospital only) | 100 vial [PoM] no price available (Hospital only)

Drytec saline eluent 20ml vials | 20 vial [PoM] no price available (Hospital only) | 100 vial [PoM] no price available (Hospital only)

Infusion

▸ Sodium chloride (Non-proprietary)

Sodium chloride 1.8 mg per 1 ml Polyfusor O sodium chloride 0.18% infusion 500ml bottles | 1 bottle [PoM] £3.44 | 12 bottle [PoM] no price available

Sodium chloride 4.5 mg per 1 ml Sodium chloride 0.45% infusion 500ml Viaflo bags | 1 bag [PoM] no price available | 20 bag [PoM] no price available

Polyfusor SB sodium chloride 0.45% infusion 500ml bottles | 1 bottle [PoM] £3.44 | 12 bottle [PoM] no price available

Sodium chloride 0.45% infusion 500ml Viaflex bags | 1 bag [PoM] no price available | 20 bag [PoM] no price available

Steriflex No.2 sodium chloride 0.45% infusion 500ml bags | 1 bag [PoM] £1.38 | 15 bag [PoM] no price available

Sodium chloride 9 mg per 1 ml Sodium chloride 0.9% infusion 100ml bags | 1 bag [PoM] £1.27

Sodium chloride 0.9% infusion 250ml Macoflex N bags | 1 bag [PoM] no price available | 30 bag [PoM] no price available

Sodium chloride 0.9% infusion 1litre Macoflex N bags | 1 bag [PoM] no price available | 10 bag [PoM] no price available

Sodium chloride 0.9% infusion 100ml Viaflo bags | 1 bag [PoM] no price available | 50 bag [PoM] no price available

Sodium chloride 0.9% infusion 500ml Viaflo bags | 1 bag [PoM] no price available | 20 bag [PoM] no price available

Sodium chloride 0.9% infusion 50ml Viaflo bags | 1 bag [PoM] no price available | 50 bag [PoM] no price available

Intraven sodium chloride 0.9% infusion 2litre bags | 1 bag [PoM] £3.01

Sodium chloride 0.9% infusion 500ml Macoflex N bags | 1 bag [PoM] no price available | 18 bag [PoM] no price available

Sodium chloride 0.9% infusion 50ml Easyflex N bags | 1 bag [PoM] no price available | 70 bag [PoM] no price available

Sodium chloride 0.9% infusion 250ml Viaflo bags | 1 bag [PoM] no price available | 30 bag [PoM] no price available

Sodium chloride 0.9% infusion 1litre Easyflex N bags | 1 bag [PoM] no price available | 10 bag [PoM] no price available

Sodium chloride 0.9% infusion 100ml polyethylene bottles | 1 bottle [PoM] £0.55 | 20 bottle [PoM] £11.00

Sodium chloride 0.9% infusion 100ml Macoflex N bags | 1 bag [PoM] no price available | 60 bag [PoM] no price available

Sodium chloride 0.9% infusion 250ml bags | 1 bag [PoM] £1.33

Sodium chloride 0.9% infusion 250ml Viaflex bags | 1 bag [PoM] no price available | 30 bag [PoM] no price available

Intraven sodium chloride 0.9% infusion 500ml bags | 1 bag [PoM] £1.61

Sodium chloride 0.9% infusion 500ml Easyflex N bags | 1 bag [PoM] no price available | 18 bag [PoM] no price available

Sodium chloride 0.9% infusion 50ml Mini-Bag Plus Viaflex bags | 1 bag [PoM] no price available | 30 bag [PoM] no price available

Sodium chloride 0.9% infusion 250ml Macoflex bags | 1 bag [PoM] no price available | 30 bag [PoM] no price available

Sodium chloride 0.9% infusion 500ml Viaflex bags | 1 bag [PoM] no price available | 20 bag [PoM] no price available

Sodium chloride 0.9% infusion 100ml Mini-Bag Plus Viaflex bags | 1 bag [PoM] no price available | 30 bag [PoM] no price available

Sodium chloride 0.9% infusion 500ml Macoflex bags | 1 bag [PoM] no price available | 20 bag [PoM] no price available

Sodium chloride 0.9% infusion 50ml Macoflex N bags | 1 bag [PoM] no price available | 70 bag [PoM] no price available

Sodium chloride 0.9% infusion 1litre Macoflex bags | 1 bag [PoM] no price available | 12 bag [PoM] no price available

Sodium chloride 0.9% infusion 50ml Viaflo bags | 1 bag [PoM] no price available | 50 bag [PoM] no price available

Sodium chloride 0.9% infusion 1litre Viaflo bags | 1 bag [PoM] no price available | 10 bag [PoM] no price available

Intraven sodium chloride 0.9% infusion 50ml bags | 1 bag [PoM] £1.49

Sodium chloride 0.9% infusion 50ml Macoflex bags | 1 bag [PoM] no price available | 70 bag [PoM] no price available

Intraven sodium chloride 0.9% infusion 250ml bags | 1 bag [PoM] £1.61

Sodium chloride 0.9% infusion 1litre Viaflex bags | 1 bag [PoM] no price available | 10 bag [PoM] no price available

Intraven sodium chloride 0.9% infusion 100ml bags | 1 bag [PoM] £1.49

Polyfusor S sodium chloride 0.9% infusion 500ml bottles | 1 bottle [PoM] £2.33 | 12 bottle [PoM] no price available

Sodium chloride 0.9% infusion 100ml Easyflex N bags | 1 bag [PoM] no price available | 60 bag [PoM] no price available

Sodium chloride 0.9% infusion 250ml Easyflex N bags | 1 bag [PoM] no price available | 30 bag [PoM] no price available

Intraven sodium chloride 0.9% infusion 1litre bags | 1 bag [PoM] £2.33

Polyfusor S sodium chloride 0.9% infusion 1litre bottles | 1 bottle [PoM] £3.10 | 6 bottle [PoM] no price available

Sodium chloride 0.9% infusion 100ml Macoflex bags | 1 bag [PoM] no price available | 60 bag [PoM] no price available

Sodium chloride 18 mg per 1 ml Polyfusor SC sodium chloride 1.8% infusion 500ml bottles | 1 bottle [PoM] £3.44 | 12 bottle [PoM] no price available

Sodium chloride 27 mg per 1 ml Polyfusor SD sodium chloride 2.7% infusion 500ml bottles | 1 bottle [PoM] £3.44 | 12 bottle [PoM] no price available

Sodium chloride 50 mg per 1 ml Polyfusor SE sodium chloride 5% infusion 500ml bottles | 1 bottle [PoM] £3.44 | 12 bottle [PoM] no price available

Solution for infusion

▸ Sodium chloride (Non-proprietary)

Sodium chloride 300 mg per 1 ml Sodium chloride 30% concentrate for solution for infusion 100ml vials | 10 vial [PoM] £44.20

Sodium chloride 30% concentrate for solution for infusion 50ml vials | 10 vial [PoM] £27.70

Sodium chloride 30% concentrate for solution for infusion 10ml ampoules | 10 ampoule [PoM] £16.40

Intravesical solution

▸ Sodium chloride (Non-proprietary)

Sodium chloride 9 mg per 1 ml Sodium chloride 0.9% intravesical solution 50ml bags | 1 bag [P] £5.00

Combinations available: *Potassium chloride with calcium chloride and sodium chloride and sodium lactate*, p. 899 · *Potassium chloride with calcium chloride dihydrate and sodium chloride*, p. 899 · *Potassium chloride with glucose and sodium chloride*, p. 900 · *Potassium chloride with sodium chloride*, p. 900

Sodium chloride with glucose

The properties listed below are those particular to the combination only. For the properties of the components please consider, sodium chloride p. 901, glucose p. 903.

● INDICATIONS AND DOSE

Combined water and sodium depletion

▸ BY INTRAVENOUS INFUSION

▸ Adult: (consult product literature)

● CAUTIONS

CAUTIONS, FURTHER INFORMATION

▸ With intravenous use in children Sodium Chloride 0.18% and Glucose 4% intravenous infusion fluid should not be used for fluid replacement in children aged 16 years or less because of the risk of hyponatraemia; availability of this infusion should be restricted to high dependency and intensive care units, and specialist wards, such as renal, liver, and cardiac units. Local guidelines on intravenous fluids should be consulted.

● MONITORING REQUIREMENTS Maintenance fluid should accurately reflect daily requirements and close monitoring is required to avoid fluid and electrolyte imbalance.

● MEDICINAL FORMS
There can be variation in the licensing of different medicines containing the same drug. Forms available from special-order manufacturers include: solution for infusion

Infusion

▸ Sodium chloride with glucose (Non-proprietary)
Sodium chloride 4.5 mg per 1 ml, Glucose anhydrous 25 mg per 1 ml Sodium chloride 0.45% / Glucose 2.5% infusion 500ml Viaflex bags | 1 bag [PoM] no price available | 20 bag [PoM] no price available
Sodium chloride 0.45% / Glucose 2.5% infusion 500ml Viaflo bags | 1 bag [PoM] no price available | 20 bag [PoM] no price available
Sodium chloride 1.8 mg per 1 ml, Glucose anhydrous 40 mg per 1 ml Polyfusor T glucose 4% / sodium chloride 0.18% infusion 500ml bottles | 1 bottle [PoM] £2.40 | 12 bottle [PoM] no price available
Sodium chloride 0.18% / Glucose 4% infusion 500ml Macoflex bags | 1 bag [PoM] no price available | 20 bag [PoM] no price available
Sodium chloride 0.18% / Glucose 4% infusion 500ml Viaflo bags | 1 bag [PoM] no price available | 20 bag [PoM] no price available
Sodium chloride 0.18% / Glucose 4% infusion 1litre Macoflex bags | 1 bag [PoM] no price available | 12 bag [PoM] no price available
Sodium chloride 0.18% / Glucose 4% infusion 500ml Viaflex bags | 1 bag [PoM] no price available | 20 bag [PoM] no price available
Sodium chloride 0.18% / Glucose 4% infusion 1litre Viaflo bags | 1 bag [PoM] no price available | 10 bag [PoM] no price available
Sodium chloride 9 mg per 1 ml, Glucose 50 mg per 1 ml Steriflex No.3 glucose 5% / sodium chloride 0.9% infusion 500ml bags | 1 bag [PoM] £1.47 | 15 bag [PoM] no price available
Sodium chloride 0.9% / Glucose 5% infusion 500ml bags | 1 bag [PoM] £1.27
Sodium chloride 0.9% / Glucose 5% infusion 500ml Viaflex bags | 1 bag [PoM] no price available | 20 bag [PoM] no price available
Steriflex No.3 glucose 5% / sodium chloride 0.9% infusion 1litre bags | 1 bag [PoM] £2.10 | 10 bag [PoM] no price available
Sodium chloride 4.5 mg per 1 ml, Glucose anhydrous 50 mg per 1 ml Sodium chloride 0.45% / Glucose 5% infusion 500ml Viaflex bags | 1 bag [PoM] no price available | 20 bag [PoM] no price available
Steriflex No.45 glucose 5% / sodium chloride 0.45% infusion 500ml bags | 1 bag [PoM] £2.02 | 15 bag [PoM] no price available
Sodium chloride 1.8 mg per 1 ml, Glucose anhydrous 100 mg per 1 ml Steriflex No.19 glucose 10% / sodium chloride 0.18% infusion 500ml bags | 1 bag [PoM] £2.02 | 15 bag [PoM] no price available

NUTRIENTS ⟩ SUGARS

Glucose

(Dextrose Monohydrate)

● INDICATIONS AND DOSE

Establish presence of gestational diabetes
▸ BY MOUTH
▸ Adult: Test dose 75 g, anhydrous glucose to be given to the fasting patient and blood-glucose concentrations measured at intervals, to be given with 200–300 mL fluid

Oral glucose tolerance test
▸ BY MOUTH
▸ Adult: Test dose 75 g, anhydrous glucose to be given to the fasting patient and blood-glucose concentrations measured at intervals, to be given with 200–300 mL fluid

Hypoglycaemia
▸ BY INTRAVENOUS INFUSION
▸ Child: 500 mg/kg, to be administered as Glucose 10% intravenous infusion into a large vein through a large-gauge needle; care is required since this concentration is irritant especially if extravasation occurs
▸ Adult: 10 g, to be administered as Glucose 20% intravenous infusion into a large vein through a large-gauge needle; care is required since this concentration is irritant especially if extravasation occurs

Energy source
▸ BY INTRAVENOUS INFUSION
▸ Adult: 1–3 litres daily, solution concentration of 20–50% to be administered

Water replacement
▸ BY INTRAVENOUS INFUSION
▸ Adult: The volume of glucose solution needed to replace deficits may vary (consult product literature)

Persistent cyanosis (in combination with propranolol) when blood glucose less than 3 mmol/litre (followed by morphine)
▸ BY INTRAVENOUS INFUSION
▸ Child: 200 mg/kg, to be administered as Glucose 10% intravenous infusion over 10 minutes

Management of diabetic ketoacidosis
▸ BY INTRAVENOUS INFUSION
▸ Child: Glucose 5% or 10% should be added to replacement fluid once blood-glucose concentration falls below 14 mmol/litre
▸ Adult: Glucose 10% should be given once blood-glucose concentration falls below 14 mmol/litre, to be administered into a large vein through a large-gauge needle at a rate of 125 mL/hour, in addition to the sodium chloride 0.9% infusion

DOSE EQUIVALENCE AND CONVERSION
75 g anhydrous glucose is equivalent to Glucose BP 82.5 g.

● CAUTIONS Do not give alone except when there is no significant loss of electrolytes · prolonged administration of glucose solutions without electrolytes can lead to hyponatreamia and other electrolyte disturbances

● SIDE-EFFECTS Glucose injections especially if hypertonic may have a low pH and may cause venous irritation and thrombophlebitis

● DIRECTIONS FOR ADMINISTRATION
▸ With intravenous use in children Injections containing more than 10% glucose can be irritant and should be given into a central venous line; however, solutions containing up to 12.5% can be administered for a short period into a peripheral line.

● PRESCRIBING AND DISPENSING INFORMATION Glucose BP is the monohydrate but Glucose Intravenous Infusion BP is a sterile solution of anhydrous glucose or glucose monohydrate, potency being expressed in terms of anhydrous glucose.

● EXCEPTIONS TO LEGAL CATEGORY
▸ With intravenous use Prescription only medicine restriction does not apply to 50% solution where administration is for saving life in emergency.

● MEDICINAL FORMS
There can be variation in the licensing of different medicines containing the same drug. Forms available from special-order manufacturers include: solution for injection, solution for infusion

Oral solution
▸ Rapilose OGTT (Aspire Pharma Ltd)
Glucose 250 mg per 1 ml Rapilose OGTT solution | 300 ml £3.48

Oral gel
▸ Dextrogel (Neoceuticals Ltd)
Glucose 400 mg per 1 gram Dextrogel 40% gel | 75 gram £7.16 DT price = £7.16 | 80 gram £6.84
▸ GlucoBoost (Ennogen Healthcare Ltd)
Glucose 400 mg per 1 gram GlucoBoost 40% gel | 75 gram £7.16 DT price = £7.16 | 80 gram £6.84
▸ GlucoGel (BBI Healthcare Ltd)
Glucose 400 mg per 1 gram GlucoGel 40% gel original | 75 gram [GSL] £7.16 DT price = £7.16 | 80 gram [GSL] £6.84
▸ Rapilose (Galen Ltd)
Glucose 400 mg per 1 gram Rapilose 40% gel | 75 gram £5.49 DT price = £7.16

Infusion
▸ Glucose (Non-proprietary)
Glucose anhydrous 50 mg per 1 ml Glucose 5% infusion 1litre Macoflex bags | 1 bag [PoM] no price available | 12 bag [PoM] no price available

9

Blood and nutrition

Glucose 5% infusion 500ml bags | 1 bag [PoM] £1.27
Glucose 5% infusion 500ml Macoflex N bags | 1 bag [PoM] no price available | 18 bag [PoM] no price available
Glucose 5% infusion 100ml bags | 1 bag [PoM] £1.27
Glucose 5% infusion 1litre Easyflex N bags | 1 bag [PoM] no price available | 10 bag [PoM] no price available
Glucose 5% infusion 100ml Easyflex N bags | 1 bag [PoM] no price available | 60 bag [PoM] no price available
Glucose 5% infusion 500ml Viaflo bags | 1 bag [PoM] no price available | 20 bag [PoM] no price available
Glucose 5% infusion 100ml Macoflex N bags | 1 bag [PoM] no price available | 60 bag [PoM] no price available
Glucose 5% infusion 500ml Viaflex bags | 1 bag [PoM] no price available | 20 bag [PoM] no price available
Glucose 5% infusion 250ml Macoflex N bags | 1 bag [PoM] no price available | 30 bag [PoM] no price available
Glucose 5% infusion 500ml Macoflex bags | 1 bag [PoM] no price available | 20 bag [PoM] no price available
Polyfusor D glucose 5% infusion 1litre bottles | 1 bottle [PoM] £3.02 | 6 bottle [PoM] no price available
Glucose 5% infusion 500ml Easyflex N bags | 1 bag [PoM] no price available | 18 bag [PoM] no price available
Glucose 5% infusion 1litre Viaflo bags | 1 bag [PoM] no price available | 10 bag [PoM] no price available
Glucose 5% infusion 50ml Viaflo bags | 1 bag [PoM] no price available | 50 bag [PoM] no price available
Glucose 5% infusion 250ml Easyflex N bags | 1 bag [PoM] no price available | 30 bag [PoM] no price available
Glucose 5% infusion 100ml Macoflex bags | 1 bag [PoM] no price available | 60 bag [PoM] no price available
Glucose 5% infusion 50ml Easyflex N bags | 1 bag [PoM] no price available | 70 bag [PoM] no price available
Glucose 5% infusion 50ml Macoflex N bags | 1 bag [PoM] no price available | 70 bag [PoM] no price available
Glucose 5% infusion 250ml Viaflex bags | 1 bag [PoM] no price available | 30 bag [PoM] no price available
Polyfusor D glucose 5% infusion 500ml bottles | 1 bottle [PoM] £2.25 | 12 bottle [PoM] no price available
Glucose 5% infusion 50ml Viaflex bags | 1 bag [PoM] no price available | 50 bag [PoM] no price available
Glucose 5% infusion 100ml Viaflex bags | 1 bag [PoM] no price available | 50 bag [PoM] no price available
Glucose 5% infusion 100ml Viaflo bags | 1 bag [PoM] no price available | 50 bag [PoM] no price available
Glucose 5% infusion 1litre Macoflex N bags | 1 bag [PoM] no price available | 10 bag [PoM] no price available
Glucose 5% infusion 250ml Macoflex bags | 1 bag [PoM] no price available | 30 bag [PoM] no price available
Glucose 5% infusion 50ml Macoflex bags | 1 bag [PoM] no price available | 70 bag [PoM] no price available
Glucose 5% infusion 250ml Viaflo bags | 1 bag [PoM] no price available | 30 bag [PoM] no price available
Glucose anhydrous 100 mg per 1 ml Steriflex No.7 glucose 10% infusion 1litre bags | 1 bag [PoM] £2.54 | 10 bag [PoM] no price available
Glucose 10% infusion 1litre Viaflo bags | 1 bag [PoM] no price available | 10 bag [PoM] no price available
Glucose 10% infusion 500ml Macoflex bags | 1 bag [PoM] no price available | 20 bag [PoM] no price available
Glucose 10% infusion 500ml Viaflo bags | 1 bag [PoM] no price available | 20 bag [PoM] no price available
Glucose 10% infusion 1litre Macoflex bags | 1 bag [PoM] no price available | 12 bag [PoM] no price available
Steriflex No.7 glucose 10% infusion 500ml bags | 1 bag [PoM] £1.85 | 15 bag [PoM] no price available
Glucose anhydrous 200 mg per 1 ml Steriflex No.31 glucose 20% infusion 500ml bags | 1 bag [PoM] £2.64 | 15 bag [PoM] no price available
Glucose 20% infusion 500ml bags | 1 bag [PoM] £2.31
Glucose (as Glucose monohydrate) 300 mg per 1 ml Glucose 30% infusion 500ml polyethylene bottles | 10 bottle [PoM] no price available
Glucose anhydrous 400 mg per 1 ml Steriflex No.33 glucose 40% infusion 500ml bags | 1 bag [PoM] £2.81 | 15 bag [PoM] no price available
Glucose anhydrous 500 mg per 1 ml Steriflex No.34 glucose 50% infusion 500ml bags | 1 bag [PoM] £3.11 | 15 bag [PoM] no price available
Glucose 50% infusion 500ml polyethylene bottles | 1 bottle [PoM] £2.94
Glucose anhydrous 700 mg per 1 ml Glucose 70% concentrate for solution for infusion 500ml Viaflex bags | 1 bag [PoM] no price available

Solution for infusion

‣ Glucose (Non-proprietary)

Glucose anhydrous 200 mg per 1 ml Glucose 20% solution for infusion 100ml vials | 1 vial [PoM] £3.50
Glucose anhydrous 500 mg per 1 ml Glucose 50% solution for infusion 20ml ampoules | 10 ampoule [PoM] £10.00–£12.50
Glucose 50% solution for infusion 50ml vials | 1 vial [PoM] £2.01 DT price = £2.01 | 25 vial [PoM] £45.00–£50.00

Combinations available: *Potassium chloride with glucose,* p. 899 · *Potassium chloride with glucose and sodium chloride,* p. 900 · *Sodium chloride with glucose,* p. 902

ORAL REHYDRATION SALTS

Disodium hydrogen citrate with glucose, potassium chloride and sodium chloride

(Formulated as oral rehydration salts)

● **INDICATIONS AND DOSE**

Fluid and electrolyte loss in diarrhoea

▶ BY MOUTH

▸ **Child 1–11 months:** 1–1½ times usual feed volume to be given
▸ **Child 1–11 years:** 200 mL, to be given after every loose motion
▸ **Child 12–17 years:** 200–400 mL, to be given after every loose motion, dose according to fluid loss
▸ **Adult:** 200–400 mL, to be given after every loose motion, dose according to fluid loss

● **DIRECTIONS FOR ADMINISTRATION** Reconstitute 1 sachet with 200mL of water (freshly boiled and cooled for infants); 5 sachets reconstituted with 1 litre of water provide Na^+ 60 mmol, K^+ 20 mmol, Cl^- 60 mmol, citrate 10 mmol, and glucose 90 mmol.

● **PRESCRIBING AND DISPENSING INFORMATION** Flavours of oral powder formulations may include black currant, citrus, or natural.

● **PATIENT AND CARER ADVICE**

Medicines for Children leaflet: Oral rehydration salts
www.medicinesforchildren.org.uk/oral-rehydration-salts

After reconstitution any unused solution should be discarded no later than 1 hour after preparation unless stored in a refrigerator when it may be kept for up to 24 hours.

● **MEDICINAL FORMS**
There can be variation in the licensing of different medicines containing the same drug.

Powder

▶ Dioralyte (Sanofi)
Potassium chloride 300 mg, Sodium chloride 470 mg, Disodium hydrogen citrate 530 mg, Glucose 3.56 gram Dioralyte oral powder sachets citrus | 20 sachet [P] £6.72
Dioralyte oral powder sachets plain | 20 sachet [P] £6.72
Dioralyte oral powder sachets blackcurrant | 20 sachet [P] £6.72

Glucose with potassium chloride, sodium bicarbonate and sodium chloride

(Formulated as oral rehydration salts)

● **INDICATIONS AND DOSE**

Fluid and electrolyte loss in diarrhoea

▶ BY MOUTH

▸ **Adult:** 200–400 mL, to be given after every loose motion, dose according to fluid loss

- DIRECTIONS FOR ADMINISTRATION Reconstitute 1 sachet with 200 mL of water (freshly boiled and cooled for infants); 5 sachets when reconstituted with 1 litre of water provide Na$^+$ 50 mmol, K$^+$ 20 mmol, Cl$^-$ 40 mmol, HCO$_3^-$ 30 mmol, and glucose 111 mmol.
- PRESCRIBING AND DISPENSING INFORMATION Flavours of oral powder formulations may include banana, orange, black current, lemon and lime, plain, or multiflavoured.
- PATIENT AND CARER ADVICE Patients and carers should be advised how to reconstitute *Electrolade®* oral powder. After reconstitution any unused solution should be discarded no later than 1 hour after preparation unless stored in a refrigerator when it may be kept for up to 24 hours.

- MEDICINAL FORMS
There can be variation in the licensing of different medicines containing the same drug.
No licensed medicines listed.

Potassium chloride with rice powder, sodium chloride and sodium citrate

(Formulated as oral rehydration salts)

- INDICATIONS AND DOSE
Fluid and electrolyte loss in diarrhoea
  ▸ BY MOUTH
  ▸ Adult: 200–400 mL, to be given after every loose motion, dose according to fluid loss

- DIRECTIONS FOR ADMINISTRATION Reconstitute 1 sachet with 200 mL of water (freshly boiled and cooled for infants); 5 sachets when reconstituted with 1 litre of water provide Na$^+$ 60 mmol, K$^+$ 20 mmol, Cl$^-$ 50 mmol and citrate 10 mmol.
- PRESCRIBING AND DISPENSING INFORMATION Flavours of oral powder formulations may include apricot, black currant, or raspberry.
- PATIENT AND CARER ADVICE Patients and carers should be advised how to reconstitute *Dioralyte®* Relief oral powder. After reconstitution any unused solution should be discarded no later than 1 hour after preparation unless stored in a refrigerator when it may be kept for up to 24 hours.

- MEDICINAL FORMS
There can be variation in the licensing of different medicines containing the same drug.
Powder
EXCIPIENTS: May contain Aspartame
  ▸ Dioralyte Relief (Sanofi)
  Potassium chloride 300 mg, Sodium chloride 350 mg, Sodium citrate 580 mg, Rice powder pre-cooked 6 gram Dioralyte Relief oral powder sachets raspberry sugar-free | 6 sachet GSL £2.50
  Dioralyte Relief oral powder sachets blackcurrant sugar-free | 20 sachet P £7.13

1.1 Calcium imbalance

Calcium

Calcium supplements
Calcium supplements are usually only required where dietary calcium intake is deficient. This dietary requirement varies with age and is relatively greater in childhood, pregnancy, and lactation, due to an increased demand, and in old age, due to impaired absorption. In osteoporosis, a calcium intake which is double the recommended amount reduces the rate of bone loss. If the actual dietary intake is less than

the recommended amount, a supplement of as much as 40 mmol is appropriate.

In severe acute hypocalcaemia or hypocalcaemic tetany, an initial slow intravenous injection of calcium gluconate injection 10% p. 907 should be given, with plasma-calcium and ECG monitoring (risk of arrhythmias if given too rapidly), and either repeated as required or, if only temporary improvement, followed by a continuous intravenous infusion to prevent recurrence. Calcium chloride injection p. 907 is also available, but is more irritant; care should be taken to prevent extravasation. Oral supplements of calcium and vitamin D may also be required in persistent hypocalcaemia. Concurrent hypomagnesaemia should be corrected with magnesium sulfate p. 911.

See the role of calcium gluconate in temporarily reducing the toxic effects of hyperkalaemia.

Severe hypercalcaemia
Severe hypercalcaemia calls for urgent treatment before detailed investigation of the cause. Dehydration should be corrected first with intravenous infusion of sodium chloride **0.9%** p. 901. Drugs (such as thiazides and vitamin D compounds) which promote hypercalcaemia, should be discontinued and dietary calcium should be restricted.

If *severe hypercalcaemia persists* drugs which inhibit mobilisation of calcium from the skeleton may be required. The **bisphosphonates** are useful and pamidronate disodium p. 657 is probably the most effective.

Corticosteroids are widely given, but may only be useful where hypercalcaemia is due to sarcoidosis or vitamin D intoxication; they often take several days to achieve the desired effect.

Calcitonin (salmon) p. 660 can be used for the treatment of hypercalcaemia associated with malignancy; it is rarely effective where bisphosphonates have failed to reduce serum calcium adequately.

After treatment of severe hypercalcaemia the underlying cause must be established. *Further treatment* is governed by the same principles as for initial therapy. Salt and water depletion and drugs promoting hypercalcaemia should be avoided; oral administration of a bisphosphonate may be useful.

Hyperparathyroidism
Paricalcitol p. 944 is licensed for the prevention and treatment of secondary hyperparathyroidism associated with chronic renal failure.

Parathyroidectomy may be indicated for hyperparathyroidism.

Hypercalciuria
Hypercalciuria should be investigated for an underlying cause, which should be treated. Where a cause is not identified (idiopathic hypercalciuria), the condition is managed by increasing fluid intake and giving bendroflumethiazide p. 152. Reducing dietary calcium intake may be beneficial but severe restriction of calcium intake has not proved beneficial and may even be harmful.

9

Blood and nutrition

1.1a Hypercalcaemia and hypercalciuria

CALCIUM REGULATING DRUGS > BONE RESORPTION INHIBITORS

Cinacalcet

- **DRUG ACTION** Cinacalcet reduces parathyroid hormone which leads to a decrease in serum calcium concentrations.

- **INDICATIONS AND DOSE**

Secondary hyperparathyroidism in patients with end-stage renal disease on dialysis
- ▸ BY MOUTH
- ▸ Adult: Initially 30 mg once daily, dose to be adjusted every 2–4 weeks; maximum 180 mg per day

Treatment of hypercalcaemia in parathyroid carcinoma | Primary hyperparathyroidism in patients where parathyroidectomy is inappropriate
- ▸ BY MOUTH
- ▸ Adult: Initially 30 mg twice daily (max. per dose 90 mg 4 times a day), dose to be adjusted every 2–4 weeks according to response

DOSE ADJUSTMENTS DUE TO INTERACTIONS
Dose adjustment may be necessary if smoking started or stopped during treatment.

- **CAUTIONS** Treatment should not be initiated in patients with hypocalcaemia
- **INTERACTIONS** → Appendix 1 (cinacalcet).
- **SIDE-EFFECTS**
- ▸ **Common or very common** Anorexia · asthenia · dizziness · myalgia · nausea · paraesthesia · rash · reduced testosterone concentrations · vomiting
- ▸ **Uncommon** Diarrhoea · dyspepsia · seizures
- ▸ **Frequency not known** Allergic reactions · angioedema · heart failure · hypotension
- **PREGNANCY** Manufacturer advises use only if potential benefit outweighs risk—no information available.
- **BREAST FEEDING** Manufacturer advises avoid—present in milk in *animal* studies.
- **HEPATIC IMPAIRMENT** Manufacturer advises caution in moderate to severe impairment. Monitor closely in hepatic impairment especially when increasing dose.
- **MONITORING REQUIREMENTS**
- ▸ Measure serum-calcium concentration before initiation of treatment and within 1 week after starting treatment or adjusting dose, then monthly for secondary hyperparathyroidism, and every 2–3 months for primary hyperparathyroidism and parathyroid carcinoma.
- ▸ In secondary hyperparathyroidism measure parathyroid hormone concentration 1–4 weeks after starting treatment or adjusting dose, then every 1–3 months.
- **NATIONAL FUNDING/ACCESS DECISIONS**

NICE technology appraisals (TAs)
- ▸ **Cinacalcet for the treatment of secondary hyperparathyroidism in patients with end-stage renal disease on maintenance dialysis therapy** (January 2007) NICE TA117 Cinacalcet is not recommended for the routine treatment of secondary hyperparathyroidism in patients with end-stage renal disease on maintenance dialysis therapy.

  Cinacalcet is recommended for the treatment of refractory secondary hyperparathyroidism in patients with end-stage renal disease (including those with calciphylaxis) **only** in those:
  - who have 'very uncontrolled' plasma concentration of

intact parathyroid hormone (defined as greater than 85 picomol/litre) refractory to standard therapy, and a normal or high adjusted serum calcium concentration, **and**
- in whom surgical parathyroidectomy is contra-indicated, in that the risks of surgery outweigh the benefits.
Response to treatment should be monitored regularly and treatment should be continued only if a reduction in the plasma concentration of intact parathyroid hormone of 30% or greater is seen within 4 months of treatment.
www.nice.org.uk/TA117

- **MEDICINAL FORMS**
There can be variation in the licensing of different medicines containing the same drug.
Tablet
CAUTIONARY AND ADVISORY LABELS 21
- ▸ Mimpara (Amgen Ltd)
  Cinacalcet (as Cinacalcet hydrochloride) 30 mg Mimpara 30mg tablets | 28 tablet [PoM] £125.75 DT price = £125.75
  Cinacalcet (as Cinacalcet hydrochloride) 60 mg Mimpara 60mg tablets | 28 tablet [PoM] £231.97
  Cinacalcet (as Cinacalcet hydrochloride) 90 mg Mimpara 90mg tablets | 28 tablet [PoM] £347.96

1.1b Hypocalcaemia

ELECTROLYTES AND MINERALS > CALCIUM

Calcium salts

- **CONTRA-INDICATIONS** Conditions associated with hypercalcaemia (e.g. some forms of malignant disease) · conditions associated with hypercalciuria (e.g. some forms of malignant disease)
- **CAUTIONS** History of nephrolithiasis · sarcoidosis
- **INTERACTIONS** → Appendix 1 (antacids, calcium salts).
- **SIDE-EFFECTS**
GENERAL SIDE-EFFECTS
- ▸ **Rare** Gastro-intestinal disturbances
- ▸ **Frequency not known** Hypercalcaemia
SPECIFIC SIDE-EFFECTS
- ▸ With intravenous use Arrhythmias · bradycardia · fall in blood pressure · injection-site reactions · peripheral vasodilatation · severe tissue damage with extravasation · sweating
- **RENAL IMPAIRMENT** Use with caution.

↑ above

Calcium carbonate

- **INDICATIONS AND DOSE**

Phosphate binding in renal failure and hyper-phosphataemia
- ▸ BY MOUTH
- ▸ Adult: (consult product literature)

Calcium deficiency
- ▸ BY MOUTH
- ▸ Adult: (consult product literature)

- **PRESCRIBING AND DISPENSING INFORMATION** *Adcal*® contains calcium carbonate 1.5 g (calcium 600 mg or Ca²⁺ 15 mmol); *Calcichew*® contains calcium carbonate 1.25 g (calcium 500 mg or Ca²⁺ 12.5 mmol); *Calcichew Forte*® contains calcium carbonate 2.5 g (calcium 1 g or Ca²⁺ 25 mmol); *Cacit*® contains calcium carbonate 1.25 g, providing calcium citrate when dispersed in water (calcium 500 mg or Ca²⁺ 12.5 mmol); consult product literature for details of other available products.

  Flavours of chewable tablet formulations may include orange or fruit flavour.

- MEDICINAL FORMS
  There can be variation in the licensing of different medicines containing the same drug. Forms available from special-order manufacturers include: tablet, capsule, oral suspension
  Tablet
  CAUTIONARY AND ADVISORY LABELS 25
  ▸ Calcium carbonate (Non-proprietary)
  Calcium carbonate 1.25 gram Calcium carbonate 1.25g tablets | 100 tablet no price available
  Chewable tablet
  CAUTIONARY AND ADVISORY LABELS 24
  EXCIPIENTS: May contain Aspartame
  ▸ Calcium carbonate (Non-proprietary)
  Calcium carbonate 1.25 gram Calcium carbonate 1.25g chewable tablets sugar free sugar-free | 100 tablet £12.50 DT price = £9.33
  ▸ Adcal (ProStrakan Ltd)
  Calcium carbonate 1.5 gram Adcal 1500mg chewable tablets sugar-free | 100 tablet P £8.70 DT price = £8.70
  ▸ Calcichew (Forum Health Products Ltd)
  Calcium carbonate 1.25 gram Calcichew 500mg chewable tablets sugar-free | 100 tablet P £9.33 DT price = £9.33
  Calcium carbonate 2.5 gram Calcichew Forte chewable tablets sugar-free | 60 tablet P £13.16 DT price = £13.16
  Effervescent tablet
  CAUTIONARY AND ADVISORY LABELS 13
  ▸ Cacit (Warner Chilcott UK Ltd)
  Calcium carbonate 1.25 gram Cacit 500mg effervescent tablets sugar-free | 76 tablet P £11.81 DT price = £11.81

Calcium carbonate with calcium lactate gluconate

The properties listed below are those particular to the combination only. For the properties of the components please consider, calcium carbonate p. 906.

- INDICATIONS AND DOSE
  Calcium deficiency
  ▸ BY MOUTH
  ▸ Adult: Dose according to requirements

- PRESCRIBING AND DISPENSING INFORMATION Each *Sandocal®* tablet contains 1 g calcium (Ca^{2+} 25 mmol); flavours of soluble tablet formulations may include orange.

- MEDICINAL FORMS
  There can be variation in the licensing of different medicines containing the same drug.
  Effervescent tablet
  CAUTIONARY AND ADVISORY LABELS 13
  EXCIPIENTS: May contain Aspartame
  ▸ Sandocal (Novartis Consumer Health UK Ltd)
  Calcium carbonate 1.75 gram, Calcium lactate gluconate 2.263 gram Sandocal 1000 effervescent tablets sugar-free | 30 tablet P £7.95 DT price = £7.95

⊏ 906

Calcium chloride

- INDICATIONS AND DOSE
  Severe acute hypocalcaemia or hypocalcaemic tetany
  ▸ BY INTRAVENOUS INJECTION
  ▸ Adult: Dose according to requirements

- CAUTIONS Avoid in respiratory acidosis · avoid in respiratory failure

- DIRECTIONS FOR ADMINISTRATION Care should be taken to avoid extravasation.

- PRESCRIBING AND DISPENSING INFORMATION Non-proprietary *Calcium chloride dihydrate 7.35%* (calcium 20 mg or Ca^{2+} 500 micromol/mL); *Calcium chloride dihydrate 10%* (calcium 27.3 mg or Ca^{2+} 680 micromol/mL);

Calcium chloride dihydrate 14.7% (calcium 40.1 mg or Ca^{2+} 1000 micromol/mL).

- MEDICINAL FORMS
  There can be variation in the licensing of different medicines containing the same drug. Forms available from special-order manufacturers include: solution for infusion
  Solution for injection
  ▸ Calcium chloride (Non-proprietary)
  Calcium chloride dihydrate 73.5 mg per 1 ml Calcium chloride 7.35% solution for injection 10ml ampoules | 10 ampoule PoM £66.38
  Calcium chloride dihydrate 100 mg per 1 ml Calcium chloride 10% solution for injection 10ml pre-filled syringes | 1 pre-filled disposable injection PoM £9.42
  Calcium chloride dihydrate 147 mg per 1 ml Calcium chloride 14.7% solution for injection 5ml ampoules | 10 ampoule PoM £95.22 Calcium chloride 14.7% solution for injection 10ml ampoules | 10 ampoule PoM £64.69–£66.38

⊏ 906

Calcium gluconate

- INDICATIONS AND DOSE
  Severe acute hypocalcaemia or hypocalcaemic tetany
  ▸ INITIALLY BY SLOW INTRAVENOUS INJECTION
  ▸ Adult: Initially 10–20 mL, calcium gluconate injection 10% (providing approximately 2.25–4.5 mmol of calcium) should be administered with plasma-calcium and ECG monitoring, and either repeated as required or, if only temporary improvement, followed by a continuous intravenous infusion to prevent recurrence, alternatively (by continuous intravenous infusion), initially 50 mL/hour, adjusted according to response, infusion to be administered using 100 mL of calcium gluconate 10% diluted in 1 litre of glucose 5% or sodium chloride 0.9%

  Acute severe hyperkalaemia (plasma-potassium concentration above 6.5 mmol/litre or in the presence of ECG changes)
  ▸ BY SLOW INTRAVENOUS INJECTION
  ▸ Adult: 10–20 mL, calcium gluconate 10% should be administered, dose titrated and adjusted to ECG improvement

  Calcium deficiency | Mild asymptomatic hypocalcaemia
  ▸ BY MOUTH
  ▸ Adult: Dose according to requirements
  DOSE EQUIVALENCE AND CONVERSION
  0.11 mmol/kg is equivalent to 0.5 mL/kg of calcium gluconate 10%.

  IMPORTANT SAFETY INFORMATION
  The MHRA has advised that repeated or prolonged administration of calcium gluconate injection packaged in 10 mL glass containers is contra-indicated in children under 18 years and in patients with renal impairment owing to the risk of aluminium accumulation; in these patients the use of calcium gluconate injection packaged in plastic containers is recommended.

- MONITORING REQUIREMENTS
  ▸ With intravenous use Plasma-calcium and ECG monitoring required for administration by slow intravenous injection (risk of arrhythmias if given too rapidly).

- DIRECTIONS FOR ADMINISTRATION
  ▸ With intravenous use For continuous intravenous infusion, dilute 100 mL of calcium gluconate 10% in 1 litre of glucose 5% or sodium chloride 0.9% and give at an initial rate of 50 mL/hour adjusted according to response. Avoid bicarbonates, phosphates, or sulfates.

- PRESCRIBING AND DISPENSING INFORMATION Calcium gluconate 1 g contains calcium 89 mg or Ca^{2+} 2.23 mmol.

● MEDICINAL FORMS

There can be variation in the licensing of different medicines containing the same drug. Forms available from special-order manufacturers include: tablet, capsule, oral suspension, oral solution, solution for infusion

Effervescent tablet

CAUTIONARY AND ADVISORY LABELS 13

ELECTROLYTES: May contain Sodium

▸ Calcium gluconate (Non-proprietary)

Calcium gluconate 1 gram Calcium gluconate 1g effervescent tablets | 28 tablet GSL £15.68 DT price = £15.68

Solution for injection

▸ Calcium gluconate (Non-proprietary)

Calcium gluconate 100 mg per 1 ml Calcium gluconate 10% solution for injection 10ml ampoules | 10 ampoule PoM £6.50–£7.50

↑ 906

Calcium lactate

● INDICATIONS AND DOSE

Calcium deficiency

▸ BY MOUTH

▸ Adult: Dose according to requirements

● MEDICINAL FORMS

There can be variation in the licensing of different medicines containing the same drug.

Tablet

▸ Calcium lactate (Non-proprietary)

Calcium lactate 300 mg Calcium lactate 300mg tablets | 84 tablet no price available DT price = £4.57 | 84 tablet GSL £4.57 DT price = £4.57

↑ 906

Calcium phosphate

● INDICATIONS AND DOSE

Indications listed in combination monographs (available in the UK only in combination with other drugs)

▸ BY MOUTH

▸ Adult: Doses listed in combination monographs

● MEDICINAL FORMS

There can be variation in the licensing of different medicines containing the same drug.

No licensed medicines listed.

1.2   Low blood volume

BLOOD AND RELATED PRODUCTS › PLASMA PRODUCTS

Albumin solution

(Human Albumin Solution)

● INDICATIONS AND DOSE

Acute or sub-acute loss of plasma volume e.g. in burns, pancreatitis, trauma, and complications of surgery (with isotonic solutions)|Plasma exchange (with isotonic solutions)|Severe hypoalbuminaemia associated with low plasma volume and generalised oedema where salt and water restriction with plasma volume expansion are required (with concentrated solutions 20%)| Paracentesis of large volume ascites associated with portal hypertension (with concentrated solutions 20%)

▸ BY INTRAVENOUS INFUSION

▸ Adult: (consult product literature)

● CONTRA-INDICATIONS Cardiac failure · severe anaemia

● CAUTIONS Correct dehydration when administering concentrated solution · history of cardiac disease

(administer slowly to avoid rapid rise in blood pressure and cardiac failure, and monitor cardiovascular and respiratory function) · history of circulatory disease (administer slowly to avoid rapid rise in blood pressure and cardiac failure, and monitor cardiovascular and respiratory function) · increased capillary permeability

● SIDE-EFFECTS Anaphylaxis · chills · fever · hypersensitivity reactions · hypotension · increased salivation · nausea · tachycardia · vomiting

● MONITORING REQUIREMENTS Plasma and plasma substitutes are often used in very ill patients whose condition is unstable. Therefore, close monitoring is required and fluid and electrolyte therapy should be adjusted according to the patient's condition at all times.

● PRESCRIBING AND DISPENSING INFORMATION A solution containing protein derived from plasma, serum, or normal placentas; at least 95% of the protein is albumin. The solution may be isotonic (containing 3.5–5% protein) or concentrated (containing 15–25% protein).

● MEDICINAL FORMS

There can be variation in the licensing of different medicines containing the same drug.

Infusion

▸ Flexbumin (Baxalta UK Ltd)

Albumin solution human 200 gram per 1 litre Flexbumin 20% infusion 100ml bags | 1 bag PoM no price available | 12 bag PoM no price available

Flexbumin 20% infusion 50ml bags | 1 bag PoM no price available | 24 bag PoM no price available

Solution for infusion

▸ Albunorm (Octapharma Ltd)

Albumin solution human 50 mg per 1 ml Albunorm 5% solution for infusion 250ml bottles | 1 bottle PoM £25.50

Albunorm 5% solution for infusion 100ml bottles | 1 bottle PoM £10.20

Albunorm 5% solution for infusion 500ml bottles | 1 bottle PoM £51.00

Albumin solution human 200 mg per 1 ml Albunorm 20% solution for infusion 100ml bottles | 1 bottle PoM £40.80

▸ Alburex (CSL Behring UK Ltd)

Albumin solution human 50 mg per 1 ml Alburex 5% solution for infusion 500ml vials | 1 vial PoM £42.50

Albumin solution human 200 mg per 1 ml Alburex 20% solution for infusion 100ml vials | 1 vial PoM £34.00

▸ Albutein (Grifols UK Ltd)

Albumin solution human 50 mg per 1 ml Albutein 5% solution for infusion 500ml vials | 1 vial PoM no price available

Albutein 5% solution for infusion 250ml vials | 1 vial PoM no price available

Albumin solution human 200 mg per 1 ml Albutein 20% solution for infusion 100ml vials | 1 vial PoM no price available

Albutein 20% solution for infusion 50ml vials | 1 vial PoM no price available

Albumin solution human 250 mg per 1 ml Albutein 25% solution for infusion 100ml vials | 1 vial PoM no price available

Albutein 25% solution for infusion 20ml vials | 1 vial PoM no price available

Albutein 25% solution for infusion 50ml vials | 1 vial PoM no price available

▸ Biotest (Biotest (UK) Ltd)

Albumin solution human 50 mg per 1 ml Human Albumin Biotest 5% solution for infusion 250ml vials | 1 vial PoM £29.75

Albumin solution human 200 mg per 1 ml Human Albumin Biotest 20% solution for infusion 50ml vials | 1 vial PoM £23.80

Human Albumin Biotest 20% solution for infusion 100ml vials | 1 vial PoM £47.60

▸ Grifols (Grifols UK Ltd)

Albumin solution human 50 mg per 1 ml Human albumin Grifols 5% solution for infusion 500ml bottles | 1 bottle PoM £49.50 | 6 bottle PoM no price available

Human albumin Grifols 5% solution for infusion 250ml bottles | 1 bottle PoM £24.75 | 10 bottle PoM no price available

Human albumin Grifols 5% solution for infusion 100ml bottles | 1 bottle PoM £9.90 | 10 bottle PoM no price available

▸ Zenalb (Bio Products Laboratory Ltd)
Albumin solution human 45 mg per 1 ml Zenalb 4.5% solution for infusion 250ml bottles | 1 bottle [PoM] £26.31 | 10 bottle [PoM] no price available
Zenalb 4.5% solution for infusion 100ml bottles | 1 bottle [PoM] £11.15
Zenalb 4.5% solution for infusion 500ml bottles | 1 bottle [PoM] £52.61 | 20 bottle [PoM] no price available
Albumin solution human 200 mg per 1 ml Zenalb 20% solution for infusion 100ml bottles | 1 bottle [PoM] £50.07 | 20 bottle [PoM] no price available
Zenalb 20% solution for infusion 50ml bottles | 1 bottle [PoM] £24.72 | 20 bottle [PoM] no price available

PLASMA SUBSTITUTES

Dextran 70 with sodium chloride

● **INDICATIONS AND DOSE**

Initial treatment of hypovolaemia with hypotension induced by traumatic injury
▸ BY INTRAVENOUS INFUSION
▸ Adult: 250 mL, to be given over 2–5 minutes using *RescueFlow*®, followed immediately by administration of isotonic fluids.

● CAUTIONS Cardiac disease · hyperosmolality · severe hypoglycaemia · severe liver disease
● SIDE-EFFECTS
▸ **Rare** Severe anaphylactic reactions
▸ **Frequency not known** Hypersensitivity reactions · transient increase in bleeding time
● PREGNANCY Avoid—reports of anaphylaxis in mother causing fetal anoxia, neurological damage and death.
● HEPATIC IMPAIRMENT Use with caution in severe impairment.
● RENAL IMPAIRMENT Use with caution.
● MONITORING REQUIREMENTS
▸ Where possible, monitor central venous pressure.
▸ Urine output should be monitored. Care should be taken to avoid haematocrit concentration from falling below 25–30% and the patient should be monitored for hypersensitivity reactions.
▸ Plasma and plasma substitutes are often used in very ill patients whose condition is unstable. Therefore, close monitoring is required and fluid and electrolyte therapy should be adjusted according to the patient's condition at all times.
● EFFECT ON LABORATORY TESTS Can interfere with some laboratory tests—dextran may interfere with blood group cross-matching or biochemical measurements, and these should be carried out before infusion is begun.
● PRESCRIBING AND DISPENSING INFORMATION Dextran 70 is dextran with an average molecular weight of about '70 000'.
● MEDICINAL FORMS
There can be variation in the licensing of different medicines containing the same drug.
Infusion
▸ RescueFlow (Pharmacosmos UK Ltd)
Dextran 70 60 mg per 1 ml, Sodium chloride 75 mg per 1 ml RescueFlow 6% infusion 250ml bags | 1 bag [PoM] no price available (Hospital only)

Gelatin

● **INDICATIONS AND DOSE**

Low blood volume in hypovolaemic shock, burns and cardiopulmonary bypass
▸ BY INTRAVENOUS INFUSION
▸ Adult: Initially 500–1000 mL, use 3.5–4% solution

● CAUTIONS Cardiac disease · severe liver disease
● SIDE-EFFECTS
▸ **Rare** Severe anaphylactic reactions
▸ **Frequency not known** Hypersensitivity reactions · transient increase in bleeding time
● PREGNANCY Manufacturer of *Geloplasma*® advises avoid at the end of pregnancy.
● HEPATIC IMPAIRMENT Use with caution in severe impairment.
● RENAL IMPAIRMENT Use with caution in renal impairment.
● MONITORING REQUIREMENTS
▸ Urine output should be monitored. Care should be taken to avoid haematocrit concentration from falling below 25–30% and the patient should be monitored for hypersensitivity reactions.
▸ Plasma and plasma substitutes are often used in very ill patients whose condition is unstable. Therefore, close monitoring is required and fluid and electrolyte therapy should be adjusted according to the patient's condition at all times.
● PRESCRIBING AND DISPENSING INFORMATION The gelatin is partially degraded.
Gelaspan® contains succinylated gelatin (modified fluid gelatin, average molecular weight 26 500) 40 g, Na^+ 151 mmol, K^+ 4 mmol, Mg^{2+} 1 mmol, Cl^- 103 mmol, Ca^{2+} 1 mmol, acetate 24 mmol/litre; *Gelofusine*® contains succinylated gelatin (modified fluid gelatin, average molecular weight 30 000) 40 g (4%), Na^+ 154 mmol, Cl^- 124 mmol/litre; *Geloplasma*® contains partially hydrolysed and succinylated gelatin (modified liquid gelatin) (as anhydrous gelatin) 30 g (3%), Na^+ 150 mmol, K^+ 5 mmol, Mg^{2+} 1.5mmol, Cl^- 100 mmol, lactate 30 mmol/litre; *Isoplex*® contains succinylated gelatin (modified fluid gelatin, average molecular weight 30 000) 40g (4%), Na^+ 145 mmol, K^+ 4 mmol, Mg^{2+} 0.9 mmol, Cl^- 105 mmol, lactate 25mmol/litre; *Volplex*® contains succinylated gelatin (modified fluid gelatin, average molecular weight 30 000) 40 g (4%), Na^+ 154 mmol, Cl^- 125 mmol/litre.

● MEDICINAL FORMS
There can be variation in the licensing of different medicines containing the same drug.
Infusion
▸ Gelaspan (B.Braun Medical Ltd)
Gelatin 40 mg per 1 ml Gelaspan 4% infusion 500ml Ecobags | 1 bag [PoM] £5.78 (Hospital only) | 20 bag [PoM] no price available (Hospital only)
▸ Gelofusine (B.Braun Medical Ltd)
Gelatin 40 mg per 1 ml Gelofusine 4% infusion 1litre Ecobags | 1 bag [PoM] £9.04 | 10 bag [PoM] no price available
Gelofusine 4% infusion 500ml Ecobags | 1 bag [PoM] £4.83 | 20 bag [PoM] no price available
▸ Geloplasma (Fresenius Kabi Ltd)
Gelatin 30 mg per 1 ml Geloplasma 3% infusion 500ml Freeflex bags | 15 bag [PoM] no price available (Hospital only)
▸ Isoplex (Beacon Pharmaceuticals Ltd)
Gelatin 40 mg per 1 ml Isoplex 4% infusion 500ml bags | 10 bag [PoM] £75.30 (Hospital only)
▸ Volplex (Beacon Pharmaceuticals Ltd)
Gelatin 40 mg per 1 ml Volplex 4% infusion 500ml bags | 10 bag [PoM] £47.00 (Hospital only)
Volplex 4% infusion 1litre bags | 6 bag [PoM] £54.54 (Hospital only)

9

Blood and nutrition

Tetrastarch

- **INDICATIONS AND DOSE**

VOLULYTE® INFUSION

Treatment of hypovolaemia due to acute blood loss when crystalloids alone are not sufficient
- ▶ BY INTRAVENOUS INFUSION
- ▶ Adult: Initially 10–20 mL, then increased to up to 30 mL/kilogram daily for a maximum duration of treatment of 24 hours, the initial dose must be given slowly and with careful monitoring of the patient to allow any anaphylactic reaction to be detected as early as possible

VOLUVEN® INFUSION

Treatment of hypovolaemia due to acute blood loss when crystalloids alone are not sufficient
- ▶ BY INTRAVENOUS INFUSION
- ▶ Adult: Initially 10–20 mL, then increased to up to 30 mL/kilogram daily for maximum duration of treatment of 24 hours, the initial dose must be given slowly and with careful monitoring of the patient to allow any anaphylactic reaction to be detected as early as possible

- **CONTRA-INDICATIONS** Burns · cerebral haemorrhage · critically ill patients · dehydration · hyperhydration · intracranial haemorrhage · pulmonary oedema · sepsis · severe coagulopathy
- **CAUTIONS** Cardiac disease · care should be taken to avoid haematocrit concentration from falling below 25–30% · renal impairment · severe liver disease · surgery · trauma
- **SIDE-EFFECTS**
- ▶ **Rare** Severe anaphylactic reactions
- ▶ **Frequency not known** Hypersensitivity reactions · pruritus · raised serum amylase · transient increase in bleeding time
- **HEPATIC IMPAIRMENT** Avoid in severe impairment.
- **RENAL IMPAIRMENT** Avoid.
- **MONITORING REQUIREMENTS**
- ▶ Plasma and plasma substitutes are often used in very ill patients whose condition is unstable. Therefore, close monitoring is required and fluid and electrolyte therapy should be adjusted according to the patient's condition at all times. Treatment with hydroxyethyl starches should be guided by continuous haemodynamic monitoring so that the infusion is stopped as soon as appropriate haemodynamic goals have been achieved.
- ▶ Monitor renal function.
- ▶ Monitor for hypersensitivity reactions.
- ▶ Urine output should be monitored.
- **PRESCRIBING AND DISPENSING INFORMATION** Hydroxyethyl starch is composed of more than 90% of amylopectin that has been etherified with hydroxyethyl groups; the term tetrastarch reflects the degree of etherification. Hydroxyethyl starches should only be used for the treatment of hypovolaemia due to acute blood loss when crystalloids alone are not sufficient; they should be used at the lowest effective dose for the first 24 hours of fluid resuscitation.

Volulyte® contains hydroxyethyl starch 6% (average molecular weight 130 000) in sodium chloride intravenous infusion 0.6%, containing Na^+ 137 mmol, K^+ 4 mmol, Mg^{2+} 1.5 mmol, Cl^- 110 mmol, acetate 34 mmol/litre.

- **MEDICINAL FORMS**
There can be variation in the licensing of different medicines containing the same drug.

Infusion
- ▶ Volulyte (Fresenius Kabi Ltd) ▼
Magnesium chloride hexahydrate 300 mg per 1 litre, Potassium chloride 300 mg per 1 litre, Sodium acetate trihydrate 4.63 gram per 1 litre, Sodium chloride 6.02 gram per 1 litre, Tetrastarch 60 gram per 1 litre Volulyte 6% infusion 500ml Freeflex bags | 15 bag [PoM] £229.60
- ▶ Voluven (Fresenius Kabi Ltd) ▼
Tetrastarch 100 mg per 1 ml Voluven 10% infusion 500ml Freeflex bags | 1 bag [PoM] no price available
Tetrastarch 60 mg per 1 gram Voluven 6% infusion 500ml Freeflex bags | 1 bag [PoM] £10.63 | 15 bag [PoM] no price available

1.3 Magnesium imbalance

Magnesium

Magnesium is an essential constituent of many enzyme systems, particularly those involved in energy generation; the largest stores are in the skeleton.

Magnesium salts are not well absorbed from the gastrointestinal tract, which explains the use of magnesium sulfate as an osmotic laxative.

Magnesium is excreted mainly by the kidneys and is therefore retained in renal failure, but significant *hypermagnesaemia* (causing muscle weakness and arrhythmias) is rare.

Hypomagnesaemia
Since magnesium is secreted in large amounts in the gastro-intestinal fluid, excessive losses in diarrhoea, stoma or fistula are the most common causes of *hypomagnesaemia*; deficiency may also occur in alcoholism or as a result of treatment with certain drugs. Hypomagnesaemia often causes secondary hypocalcaemia, and also hypokalaemia and hyponatraemia.

Symptomatic *hypomagnesaemia* is associated with a deficit of 0.5–1 mmol/kg; up to 160 mmol Mg^{2+} over up to 5 days may be required to replace the deficit (allowing for urinary losses). Magnesium is given initially by intravenous infusion or by intramuscular injection of magnesium sulfate; the intramuscular injection is painful. Plasma magnesium concentration should be measured to determine the rate and duration of infusion and the dose should be reduced in renal impairment. To prevent *recurrence of the deficit*, magnesium may be given by mouth, but there is limited evidence of benefit. Magnesium aspartate powder for oral solution p. 911 is available as a licensed preparation and, magnesium glycerophosphate tablets and liquid p. 911 [unlicensed] are available from 'special-order' manufacturers or specialist importing companies.

Arrhythmias
Magnesium sulfate injection has also been recommended for the emergency treatment of *serious arrhythmias*, especially in the presence of hypokalaemia (when hypomagnesaemia may also be present) and when salvos of rapid ventricular tachycardia show the characteristic twisting wave front known as *torsade de pointes*.

Myocardial infarction
Limited evidence that magnesium sulfate prevents arrhythmias and reperfusion injury in patients with suspected myocardial infarction has not been confirmed by large studies. Routine use of magnesium sulfate for this purpose is not recommended.

Eclampsia and pre-eclampsia
Magnesium sulfate injection is the drug of choice for the treatment of seizures and the prevention of recurrent seizures in women with *eclampsia*. Regimens may vary

between hospitals. Calcium gluconate injection is used for the management of magnesium toxicity.

Magnesium sulfate injection is also of benefit in women with *pre-eclampsia* in whom there is concern about developing eclampsia. The patient should be monitored carefully.

1.3a Hypomagnesaemia

ELECTROLYTES AND MINERALS > MAGNESIUM

Magnesium aspartate

● **INDICATIONS AND DOSE**

Treatment and prevention of magnesium deficiency
▸ BY MOUTH
▸ Adult: 10–20 mmol daily, taken as 1–2 sachets of *Magnaspartate*® powder.

● CONTRA-INDICATIONS Disorders of cardiac conduction
● INTERACTIONS → Appendix 1 (magnesium salts, oral).
● SIDE-EFFECTS
▸ **Uncommon** Diarrhoea
▸ **Rare** Hypermagnesaemia
▸ **Frequency not known** Dental caries (on long term use) · gastrointestinal irritation

SIDE-EFFECTS, FURTHER INFORMATION
Side-effects generally occur at higher doses; if side-effects (such as diarrhoea) occur, consider interrupting treatment and restarting at a reduced dose.

Overdose
Symptoms of hypermagnesaemia may include nausea, vomiting, flushing of the skin, thirst, hypotension due to peripheral vasodilatation, drowsiness, confusion, loss of tendon reflexes and respiratory depression due to neuromuscular blockade, slurred speech, double vision, muscle weakness, bradycardia, cardiac arrhythmias, coma, and cardiac arrest.

● RENAL IMPAIRMENT Avoid in severe impairment (eGFR less than 30 mL/minute/1.73^2).
● DIRECTIONS FOR ADMINISTRATION Dissolve sachet contents in 50–200 mL water, tea or orange juice and take immediately.
● PRESCRIBING AND DISPENSING INFORMATION *Magnaspartate*® contains magnesium aspartate 6.5 g (10 mmol Mg^{2+})/sachet.
● PATIENT AND CARER ADVICE Patients and carers should be given advice on how to administer magnesium aspartate powder.

● MEDICINAL FORMS
There can be variation in the licensing of different medicines containing the same drug.
Powder
EXCIPIENTS: May contain Sucrose
▸ Magnesium aspartate (Non-proprietary)
Magnesium (as Magnesium aspartate) 243 mg Magnaspartate 243mg (magnesium 10mmol) oral powder sachets | 10 sachet PoM £8.95

Magnesium glycerophosphate

● **INDICATIONS AND DOSE**

Prevent recurrence of magnesium deficit
▸ BY MOUTH
▸ Adult: 6 g daily in divided doses
DOSE EQUIVALENCE AND CONVERSION
Magnesium glycerophosphate 1 g is equivalent to approximately magnesium 97 mg or Mg^{2+} 4 mmol.

● UNLICENSED USE Not licensed.
● INTERACTIONS → Appendix 1 (magnesium salts, oral).
● SIDE-EFFECTS Arrhythmias · colic · coma · confusion · diarrhoea · drowsiness · flushing of skin · hypermagnesaemia associated side-effects · hypotension · loss of tendon reflexes · muscle weakness · nausea · respiratory depression · thirst · vomiting
● RENAL IMPAIRMENT Avoid or reduce dose. Increased risk of toxicity.
● MONITORING REQUIREMENTS Monitor blood pressure, respiratory rate, urinary output and for signs of overdosage (loss of patellar reflexes, weakness, nausea, sensation of warmth, flushing, drowsiness, double vision, and slurred speech).
● DIRECTIONS FOR ADMINISTRATION Tablets may be dispersed in water.

● MEDICINAL FORMS
There can be variation in the licensing of different medicines containing the same drug. Forms available from special-order manufacturers include: tablet, chewable tablet, capsule, oral suspension, oral solution, powder
Tablet
▸ Magnesium glycerophosphate (Non-proprietary)
Magnesium (as Magnesium glycerophosphate) 97.2 mg Mag-4 (magnesium 97.2mg (4mmol)) tablets | 30 tablet £84.50
Chewable tablet
▸ Magnesium glycerophosphate (Non-proprietary)
Magnesium (as Magnesium glycerophosphate) 97.2 mg YourMAG (magnesium 97.2mg (4mmol)) chewable tablets | 50 tablet £20.00
Mag-4 (magnesium 97.2mg (4mmol)) chewable tablets sugar-free | 30 tablet £84.50
Neomag (magnesium 97mg (4mmol)) chewable tablets sugar-free | 50 tablet £20.00
▸ MagnaPhate (Arjun Products Ltd)
Magnesium (as Magnesium glycerophosphate) 97.2 mg MagnaPhate (magnesium 97.2mg (4mmol)) chewable tablets sugar-free | 50 tablet £22.64
Capsule
▸ Magnesium glycerophosphate (Non-proprietary)
Magnesium (as Magnesium glycerophosphate) 48.6 mg Mag-4 (magnesium 48.6mg (2mmol)) capsules | 30 capsule £85.70
Magnesium (as Magnesium glycerophosphate) 97.2 mg Mag-4 (magnesium 97.2mg (4mmol)) capsules | 30 capsule £89.30
Oral solution
▸ LiquaMag GP (Fontus Health Ltd)
Magnesium (as Magnesium glycerophosphate) 24.25 mg per 1 ml LiquaMag GP (magnesium 121.25mg/5ml (5mmol/5ml)) oral solution sugar-free | 250 ml £55.00

Magnesium sulfate

● **INDICATIONS AND DOSE**

Severe acute asthma | Continuing respiratory deterioration in anaphylaxis
▸ BY INTRAVENOUS INFUSION
▸ Child 2-17 years: 40 mg/kg (max. per dose 2 g), to be given over 20 minutes
▸ Adult: 1.2–2 g, to be given over 20 minutes continued →

9

Blood and nutrition

Prevention of seizures in pre-eclampsia
▸ INITIALLY BY INTRAVENOUS INJECTION
▸ **Adult:** Initially 4 g, to be given over 5–15 minutes, followed by (by intravenous infusion) 1 gram/hour for 24 hours, if seizure occurs, additional dose of 2 g by intravenous injection to be administered

Treatment of seizures and prevention of seizure recurrence in eclampsia
▸ INITIALLY BY INTRAVENOUS INJECTION
▸ **Adult:** Initially 4 g, to be given over 5–15 minutes, followed by (by intravenous infusion) 1 gram/hour for 24 hours after seizure or delivery (whichever is later), if seizure recurs, increase the infusion rate to 1.5–2 g/hour or give an additional dose of 2 g by intravenous injection

Hypomagnesaemia
▸ BY INTRAVENOUS INFUSION, OR BY INTRAMUSCULAR INJECTION
▸ **Adult:** Up to 40 g, given over a period of up to 5 days, dose given depends on the amount required to replace the deficit (allowing for urinary losses)

Hypomagnesaemia maintenance (e.g. in intravenous nutrition)
▸ BY INTRAVENOUS INFUSION, OR BY INTRAMUSCULAR INJECTION
▸ **Adult:** 2.5–5 g daily, usual dose 3 g daily

Emergency treatment of serious arrhythmias
▸ BY INTRAVENOUS INJECTION
▸ **Adult:** 2 g, to be given over 10-15 minutes, dose may be repeated once if necessary

Rapid bowel evacuation (acts in 2-4 hours)
▸ BY MOUTH
▸ **Adult:** 5–10 g, dose to be mixed in a glass of water, taken preferably before breakfast

DOSE EQUIVALENCE AND CONVERSION
Magnesium sulfate heptahydrate 1 g equivalent to Mg^{2+} approx. 4 mmol.

● UNLICENSED USE
▸ With intravenous use Unlicensed indication in severe acute asthma. Continuing respiratory deterioration in anaphylaxis.

● CONTRA-INDICATIONS
▸ With oral use In rapid bowel evacuation—acute gastro-intestinal conditions

● CAUTIONS
▸ With oral use In rapid bowel evacuation—elderly and debilitated patients

● INTERACTIONS → Appendix 1 (magnesium, parenteral).

● SIDE-EFFECTS
GENERAL SIDE-EFFECTS
Arrhythmias · coma · confusion · drowsiness · flushing of skin · hypermagnesaemia associated side-effects · hypotension · loss of tendon reflexes · muscle weakness · nausea · respiratory depression · thirst · vomiting
SPECIFIC SIDE-EFFECTS
▸ With oral use Colic · diarrhoea

● PREGNANCY
▸ When used for Hypomagnesaemia or Arrhythmias or Prevention of seizures in pre-eclampsia or Treatment of seizures and prevention of seizure recurrence in eclampsia or Severe acute asthma or Continuing respiratory deterioration in anaphylaxis Not known to be harmful for short-term intravenous administration in eclampsia, but sufficient amount may cross the placenta in mothers treated with high doses e.g. in pre-eclampsia, causing hypotonia and respiratory depression in newborns.

● HEPATIC IMPAIRMENT Avoid in hepatic coma if risk of renal failure.

● RENAL IMPAIRMENT Avoid or reduce dose. Increased risk of toxicity.

● MONITORING REQUIREMENTS Monitor blood pressure, respiratory rate, urinary output and for signs of overdosage (loss of patellar reflexes, weakness, nausea, sensation of warmth, flushing, drowsiness, double vision, and slurred speech).

● DIRECTIONS FOR ADMINISTRATION
▸ With intravenous use In severe hypomagnesaemia administer initially via controlled infusion device (preferably syringe pump).
▸ With intravenous use in adults For *intravenous injection*, in arrhythmias, hypomagnesaemia, eclampsia, and pre-eclampsia, give continuously in Glucose 5% or Sodium chloride 0.9%. Concentration of magnesium sulfate heptahydrate should not exceed 20% (200 mg/mL or 0.8 mmol/mL Mg^{2+}); dilute 1 part of magnesium sulfate injection 50% with at least 1.5 parts of water for injections. Max. rate 150 mg/minute (0.6 mmol/minute Mg^{2+}).

● PRESCRIBING AND DISPENSING INFORMATION
▸ With intramuscular use or intravenous use The BP directs that the label states the strength as the % w/v of magnesium sulfate heptahydrate and as the approximate concentration of magnesium ions (Mg^{2+}) in mmol/mL. Magnesium Sulfate Injection BP is a sterile solution of Magnesium Sulfate Heptahydrate.

● EXCEPTIONS TO LEGAL CATEGORY
▸ With oral use in adults Magnesium sulfate is on sale to the public as Epsom Salts.

● MEDICINAL FORMS
There can be variation in the licensing of different medicines containing the same drug. Forms available from special-order manufacturers include: capsule, solution for injection, infusion, solution for infusion

Solution for injection
▸ Magnesium sulfate (Non-proprietary)
  Magnesium sulfate heptahydrate 500 mg per 1 ml Magnesium sulfate 50% (magnesium 2mmol/ml) solution for injection 10ml ampoules | 10 ampoule [PoM] £11.85–£35.25
  Magnesium sulfate 50% (magnesium 2mmol/ml) solution for injection 20ml vials | 10 vial [PoM] £46.40
  Magnesium sulfate 50% (magnesium 2mmol/ml) solution for injection 5ml ampoules | 10 ampoule [PoM] £21.80–£58.34
  Magnesium sulfate 50% (magnesium 2mmol/ml) solution for injection 2ml ampoules | 10 ampoule [PoM] £11.72–£17.90 DT price = £11.85

Solution for infusion
▸ Magnesium sulfate (Non-proprietary)
  Magnesium sulfate heptahydrate 100 mg per 1 ml Magnesium sulfate 10% (magnesium 0.4mmol/ml) solution for injection 10ml ampoules | 10 ampoule [PoM] £57.12–£58.80
  Magnesium sulfate heptahydrate 500 mg per 1 ml Magnesium sulfate 50% (magnesium 2mmol/ml) solution for infusion 50ml vials | 10 vial [PoM] £63.70

Powder
▸ Magnesium sulfate (Non-proprietary)
  Magnesium sulfate dried 1 mg per 1 mg Numark Magnesium sulfate powder | 300 gram [GSL] £1.91–£2.02 | 500 gram [GSL] £3.20 DT price = £3.20 | 2000 gram [GSL] £5.60 | 5000 gram [GSL] £11.49
▸ Brands may include Epsom salts

1.4 Phosphate imbalance

Phosphorus

Phosphate supplements
Oral phosphate supplements p. 915 may be required in addition to vitamin D in a small minority of patients with hypophosphataemic vitamin D-resistant rickets.

Phosphate infusion is occasionally needed in alcohol dependence or in phosphate deficiency arising from use of parenteral nutrition deficient in phosphate supplements; phosphate depletion also occurs in severe diabetic ketoacidosis.

For phosphate requirements in total parenteral nutrition regimens, see Intravenous nutrition p. 928.

Phosphate-binding agents

Calcium-containing preparations are used as phosphate-binding agents in the management of hyperphosphataemia complicating renal failure. Aluminium-containing preparations are rarely used as phosphate binding agents and can cause aluminium accumulation.

Sevelamer p. 914 is licensed for the treatment of hyperphosphataemia in patients on haemodialysis or peritoneal dialysis. Sevelamer carbonate is also licensed for the treatment of patients with chronic kidney disease not on dialysis who have a serum-phosphate concentration of 1.78 mmol/litre or more.

Lanthanum p. 914 is licensed for the control of hyperphosphataemia in patients with chronic renal failure on haemodialysis or continuous ambulatory peritoneal dialysis (CAPD), and in patients with chronic kidney disease not on dialysis who have a serum-phosphate concentration of 1.78 mmol/litre or more that cannot be controlled by a low-phosphate diet.

Sucroferric oxyhydroxide p. 915 is licensed for the control of hyperphosphataemia in patients with chronic kidney disease on haemodialysis or peritoneal dialysis. It is used as part of a multiple therapeutic approach to control the development of renal bone disease; this could include the concomitant use of a calcium supplement, a vitamin D analogue or calcimimetics.

1.4a Hyperphosphataemia

ELECTROLYTES AND MINERALS > ALUMINIUM

▌Aluminium hydroxide

● **INDICATIONS AND DOSE**

Hyperphosphataemia in renal failure
▶ BY MOUTH USING CAPSULES
▶ Adult: 4–20 capsules daily in divided doses, to be taken with meals

Antacid
▶ BY MOUTH USING CAPSULES
▶ Adult: 475 mg 5 times a day, last dose to be taken at bedtime

● **CONTRA-INDICATIONS** Hypophosphataemia

● **INTERACTIONS** → Appendix 1 (antacids).
Antacids should preferably not be taken at the same time as other drugs since they may impair absorption. Antacids may damage enteric coatings designed to prevent dissolution in the stomach.

● **SIDE-EFFECTS** Constipation · hyperaluminaemia

● **HEPATIC IMPAIRMENT** Avoid; can cause constipation which can precipitate coma.

● **RENAL IMPAIRMENT** There is a risk of accumulation and aluminium toxicity with antacids containing aluminium salts. Absorption of aluminium from aluminium salts is increased by citrates, which are contained in many effervescent preparations (such as effervescent analgesics).

● **MEDICINAL FORMS**
There can be variation in the licensing of different medicines containing the same drug.
Capsule
▶ Alu-Cap (Meda Pharmaceuticals Ltd)
Aluminium hydroxide 475 mg Alu-Cap 475mg capsules | 120 capsule [P] £13.71 DT price = £13.71

ELECTROLYTES AND MINERALS >
CALCIUM

▐**☞ 906**

▌Calcium acetate

● **INDICATIONS AND DOSE**
PHOSEX® TABLETS

Hyperphosphataemia
▶ BY MOUTH
▶ Adult: Initially 1 tablet 3 times a day, to be taken with meals, dose to be adjusted according to serum-phosphate concentration, usual dose 4–6 tablets daily in divided doses, (1 or 2 tablets with each meal); maximum 12 tablets per day

RENACET® TABLETS

Hyperphosphataemia
▶ BY MOUTH
▶ Adult: 475–950 mg, to be taken with breakfast and with snacks, 0.95–2.85 g, to be taken with main meals and 0.95–1.9 g, to be taken with supper, dose to be adjusted according to serum-phosphate concentration; maximum 6.65 g per day

● **DIRECTIONS FOR ADMINISTRATION**

PHOSEX® TABLETS *Phosex®* tablets are taken with meals. Tablets can be broken to aid swallowing, but not chewed (bitter taste).

RENACET® TABLETS Manufacturer advises that other drugs should be taken 1 to 2 hours before or after *Renacet®* to reduce the possible interference with absorption of other drugs. *Renacet®* tablets are taken with meals.

● **PRESCRIBING AND DISPENSING INFORMATION** *Renacet®* tablets contain calcium acetate 475 mg (equivalent to calcium 120.25 mg or Ca^{2+} 3 mmol); *Phosex®* tablets contain calcium acetate 1 g (equivalent to calcium 250 mg or Ca^{2+} 6.2 mmol).

● **PATIENT AND CARER ADVICE**

PHOSEX® TABLETS Patients or carers should be given advice on how to administer *Phosex®* tablets.

RENACET® TABLETS Patients or carers should be given advice on how to administer *Renacet®* tablets.

● **MEDICINAL FORMS**
There can be variation in the licensing of different medicines containing the same drug. Forms available from special-order manufacturers include: tablet
Tablet
CAUTIONARY AND ADVISORY LABELS 25
▶ Phosex (Pharmacosmos UK Ltd)
Calcium acetate 1 gram Phosex 1g tablets | 180 tablet [PoM] £19.79 DT price = £19.79
▶ Renacet (Stanningley Pharma Ltd)
Calcium acetate 475 mg Renacet 475mg tablets | 200 tablet [PoM] £9.71 DT price = £9.71
Calcium acetate 950 mg Renacet 950mg tablets | 200 tablet [PoM] £18.45 DT price = £18.45

Combinations available: *Calcium acetate with magnesium carbonate*, p. 914

9

Blood and nutrition

PHOSPHATE BINDERS

Calcium acetate with magnesium carbonate

The properties listed below are those particular to the combination only. For the properties of the components please consider, calcium acetate p. 913, magnesium carbonate p. 63.

- **INDICATIONS AND DOSE**

Hyperphosphataemia
▶ BY MOUTH
▶ Adult: Initially 1 tablet 3 times a day, adjusted according to serum-phosphate concentration, to be taken with food; usual dose 3–10 tablets daily; maximum 12 tablets per day

- **CONTRA-INDICATIONS** Hypercalcaemia · hypermagnesaemia · myasthenia gravis · third-degree AV block
- **DIRECTIONS FOR ADMINISTRATION** Manufacturer advises that other drugs should be taken at least 2 hours before or 3 hours after calcium acetate with magnesium carbonate to reduce possible interference with absorption of other drugs.
- **PATIENT AND CARER ADVICE** Patients or carers should be given advice on how to administer calcium acetate with magnesium carbonate tablets.
- **MEDICINAL FORMS** There can be variation in the licensing of different medicines containing the same drug.

Tablet
CAUTIONARY AND ADVISORY LABELS 25
▶ Rephoren (Vifor Fresenius Medical Care Renal Pharma UK Ltd)
Magnesium carbonate heavy 235 mg, Calcium acetate 435 mg Osvaren 435mg/235mg tablets | 180 tablet [PoM] £24.00

Lanthanum

- **INDICATIONS AND DOSE**

Hyperphosphataemia in patients with chronic renal failure on haemodialysis or continuous ambulatory peritoneal dialysis (CAPD) | Hyperphosphataemia in patients with chronic kidney disease not on dialysis who have a serum-phosphate concentration of 1.78 mmol/litre or more that cannot be controlled by a low-phosphate diet
▶ BY MOUTH
▶ Adult: 1.5–3 g daily in divided doses, dose to be adjusted according to serum-phosphate concentration every 2–3 weeks, to be taken with or immediately after meals

- **CAUTIONS** Acute peptic ulcer · bowel obstruction · Crohn's disease · ulcerative colitis
- **INTERACTIONS** → Appendix 1 (lanthanum).
- **SIDE-EFFECTS**
▶ **Common or very common** Gastro-intestinal disturbances · headache · hypocalcaemia
▶ **Uncommon** Alopecia · anorexia · arthralgia · asthenia · chest pain · dizziness · dry mouth · eosinophilia · hypercalcaemia · hyperglycaemia · hyperparathyroidism · hypophosphataemia · increased appetite · malaise · myalgia · osteoporosis · peripheral oedema · stomatitis · sweating · taste disturbances · thirst · vertigo
▶ **Frequency not known** Accumulation of lanthanum in bone · transient changes in QT interval
- **PREGNANCY** Manufacturer advises avoid—toxicity in *animal* studies.

- **BREAST-FEEDING** Manufacturer advises caution—no information available.
- **HEPATIC IMPAIRMENT** Lanthanum excreted in bile—possible accumulation in obstructive jaundice.
- **DIRECTIONS FOR ADMINISTRATION** Tablets are to be chewed. Each sachet of powder to be mixed with soft food and consumed within 15 minutes.
- **PATIENT AND CARER ADVICE** Patient and carers should be given advice on how to administer lanthanum tablets and powder.
- **NATIONAL FUNDING/ACCESS DECISIONS**

Scottish Medicines Consortium (SMC) Decisions
The *Scottish Medicines Consortium* has advised (March 2007) that lanthanum (*Fosrenol®*) is accepted for restricted use within NHS Scotland for the control of hyperphosphataemia in patients with chronic renal failure on haemodialysis or continuous ambulatory peritoneal dialysis, as a second-line agent, where a non-aluminium, non-calcium phosphate binder is required.

- **MEDICINAL FORMS** There can be variation in the licensing of different medicines containing the same drug.

Chewable tablet
CAUTIONARY AND ADVISORY LABELS 21
▶ Fosrenol (Shire Pharmaceuticals Ltd)
Lanthanum (as Lanthanum carbonate) 500 mg Fosrenol 500mg chewable tablets sugar-free | 90 tablet [PoM] £124.06 DT price = £124.06
Lanthanum (as Lanthanum carbonate) 750 mg Fosrenol 750mg chewable tablets sugar-free | 90 tablet [PoM] £182.60 DT price = £182.60
Lanthanum (as Lanthanum carbonate) 1 gram Fosrenol 1000mg chewable tablets sugar-free | 90 tablet [PoM] £193.59 DT price = £193.59

Powder
CAUTIONARY AND ADVISORY LABELS 21
▶ Fosrenol (Shire Pharmaceuticals Ltd)
Lanthanum (as Lanthanum carbonate) 750 mg Fosrenol 750mg oral powder sachets | 90 sachet [PoM] £182.60 DT price = £182.60
Lanthanum (as Lanthanum carbonate) 1 gram Fosrenol 1000mg oral powder sachets | 90 sachet [PoM] £193.59 DT price = £193.59

Sevelamer

- **INDICATIONS AND DOSE**

RENAGEL®

Hyperphosphataemia in patients on haemodialysis or peritoneal dialysis
▶ BY MOUTH
▶ Adult: Initially 2.4–4.8 g daily in 3 divided doses, dose to be given with meals and adjusted according to serum-phosphate concentration; usual dose 2.4–12 g daily in 3 divided doses

RENVELA® 800MG TABLETS (SANOFI)

Hyperphosphataemia in patients on haemodialysis or peritoneal dialysis | Hyperphosphataemia in patients with chronic kidney disease not on dialysis who have a serum-phosphate concentration of 1.78 mmol/litre or more
▶ BY MOUTH
▶ Adult: Initially 2.4–4.8 g daily in 3 divided doses, dose to be taken with meals and adjusted according to serum-phosphate concentration every 2–4 weeks; usual dose 6 g daily in 3 divided doses

- **CONTRA-INDICATIONS** Bowel obstruction
- **CAUTIONS** Gastro-intestinal disorders
- **INTERACTIONS** → Appendix 1 (sevelamer).

- SIDE-EFFECTS
▶ **Common or very common** Abdominal pain · constipation · diarrhoea · dyspepsia · flatulence · nausea · vomiting
▶ **Frequency not known** Ileus · intestinal obstruction (higher incidence with sevelamer hydrochloride salt) · intestinal perforation · pruritus · rash
  RENAGEL® Diverticulitis

- PREGNANCY Manufacturer advises use only if potential benefit outweighs risk.

- BREAST FEEDING
  RENVELA® 800MG TABLETS (SANOFI) Unlikely to be present in milk (however, manufacturer advises avoid).
  RENAGEL® Manufacturer advises use only if potential benefit outweighs risk.

- DIRECTIONS FOR ADMINISTRATION
  RENVELA® 800MG TABLETS (SANOFI) For powder for oral suspension, each sachet to be dispersed in 60 mL water.

- MEDICINAL FORMS
  There can be variation in the licensing of different medicines containing the same drug.
  Tablet
  CAUTIONARY AND ADVISORY LABELS 25
  EXCIPIENTS: May contain Propylene glycol
  ▶ Renagel (Sanofi)
    Sevelamer 800 mg Renagel 800mg tablets | 180 tablet [PoM] £167.04 DT price = £87.00
  ▶ Renvela (Sanofi)
    Sevelamer 800 mg Renvela 800mg tablets | 180 tablet [PoM] £167.04 DT price = £87.00

Sucroferric oxyhydroxide

16.2.2016

- INDICATIONS AND DOSE
  Hyperphosphataemia in patients with chronic kidney disease on haemodialysis or peritoneal dialysis
  ▶ BY MOUTH
  ▶ Adult: Initially 1.5 g daily in 3 divided doses, dose to be taken with meals, then adjusted in steps of 500 mg every 2–4 weeks, dose adjusted according to serum-phosphate concentration; maintenance 1.5–2 g daily in divided doses; maximum 3 g per day

- CONTRA-INDICATIONS Haemochromatosis · iron accumulation disorders

- CAUTIONS Gastric disorders · hepatic disorders · major gastrointestinal surgery · peritonitis in the last 3 months

- INTERACTIONS → Appendix 1 (iron salts).

- SIDE-EFFECTS
▶ **Common or very common** Abdominal pain · constipation · diarrhoea · discoloured faeces · dyspepsia · flatulence · nausea · taste disturbance · tooth discolouration · vomiting
▶ **Uncommon** Abdominal discomfort · abdominal distension · dysphagia · dyspnoea · fatigue · gastritis · gastro-oesophageal reflux disease · headache · hypercalcaemia · hypocalcaemia · rash · tongue discolouration
  SIDE-EFFECTS, FURTHER INFORMATION
▶ Discoloured faeces Discoloured faeces may mask the visual signs of gastrointestinal bleeding.

- PREGNANCY Manufacturer advises use only if potential benefit outweighs risk—no information available.

- BREAST FEEDING Manufacturer advises avoid—no information available.

- DIRECTIONS FOR ADMINISTRATION *Velphoro*® tablets must be chewed or crushed, not swallowed whole.

- PATIENT AND CARER ADVICE Patients or carers should be counselled on administration of sucroferric oxyhydroxide tablets and advised that this medication can cause discoloured black stools.

- MEDICINAL FORMS
  There can be variation in the licensing of different medicines containing the same drug.
  Chewable tablet
  ▶ Velphoro (Vifor Fresenius Medical Care Renal Pharma UK Ltd) ▼
    Iron (as Sucroferric oxyhydroxide) 500 mg Velphoro 500mg chewable tablets | 90 tablet [PoM] £179.00

1.4b Hypophosphataemia

ELECTROLYTES AND MINERALS > PHOSPHATES

Phosphate

- INDICATIONS AND DOSE
  Treatment of moderate to severe hypophosphatemia
  ▶ BY INTRAVENOUS INFUSION
  ▶ Adult: (consult product literature)
  For established hypophosphataemia (with monobasic potassium phosphate)
  ▶ BY INTRAVENOUS INFUSION
  ▶ Adult: 9 mmol every 12 hours, increased if necessary up to 0.5 mmol/kg (max. per dose 50 mmol), dose only increased in critically ill patients; dose in critically ill patients is approximately equivalent to 30 mmol in adults, dose to be infused over 6–12 hours, according to severity
  Vitamin D-resistant hypophosphataemic osteomalacia
  ▶ BY MOUTH USING EFFERVESCENT TABLETS
  ▶ Adult: 4–6 tablets daily, using *Phosphate Sandoz*®.

- SIDE-EFFECTS
▶ **Common or very common** Diarrhoea
▶ **Frequency not known** Acute renal failure · hypocalcaemia · hypotension · metastatic calcification · nausea · oedema · phlebitis · tissue necrosis on extravasation
  SIDE-EFFECTS, FURTHER INFORMATION
  Diarrhoea is a common side-effect and should prompt a reduction in dosage.

- RENAL IMPAIRMENT Reduce dose. Monitor closely in renal impairment.

- MONITORING REQUIREMENTS It is essential to monitor closely plasma concentrations of calcium, phosphate, potassium, and other electrolytes—excessive doses of phosphates may cause hypocalcaemia and metastatic calcification.

- PRESCRIBING AND DISPENSING INFORMATION *Phosphate Sandoz*® contains sodium dihydrogen phosphate anhydrous (anhydrous sodium acid phosphate) 1.936 g, sodium bicarbonate 350 mg, potassium bicarbonate 315 mg, equivalent to phosphorus 500 mg (phosphate 16.1 mmol), sodium 468.8 mg (Na^+ 20.4 mmol), potassium 123 mg (K^+ 3.1 mmol); *Polyfusor NA*® contains Na^+ 162 mmol/litre, K^+ 19 mmol/litre, PO_4^{3-} 100 mmol/litre; non-proprietary *potassium dihydrogen phosphate injection* (potassium acid phosphate)13.6% may contain 1 mmol/mL phosphate, 1 mmol/mL potassium.

- MEDICINAL FORMS
  There can be variation in the licensing of different medicines containing the same drug. Forms available from special-order manufacturers include: infusion, solution for infusion
  Effervescent tablet
  CAUTIONARY AND ADVISORY LABELS 13
  ▶ Phosphate Sandoz (HK Pharma Ltd)
    Sodium dihydrogen phosphate anhydrous 1.936 gram Phosphate Sandoz effervescent tablets | 100 tablet [P] £16.43

9

Blood and nutrition

Infusion

▸ Phosphate (Non-proprietary)

Potassium dihydrogen phosphate 1.295 gram per 1 litre, Disodium hydrogen phosphate anhydrous 5.75 gram per 1 litre Polyfusor NA phosphates infusion 500ml bottles | 1 bottle PoM £5.15

Solution for infusion

▸ Phosphate (Non-proprietary)

Potassium dihydrogen phosphate 136 mg per 1 ml Potassium dihydrogen phosphate 13.6% (potassium 10mmol/10ml) solution for infusion 10ml ampoules | 10 ampoule PoM £72.95–£80.25

1.5 Potassium imbalance

1.5a Hyperkalaemia

> **Drugs used for Hyperkalaemia not listed below** Calcium gluconate, p. 907 · Insulin, p. 644

ANTIDOTES AND CHELATORS > CATION EXCHANGE RESINS

Calcium polystyrene sulfonate

● **INDICATIONS AND DOSE**

Hyperkalaemia associated with anuria or severe oliguria, and in dialysis patients

▸ BY MOUTH

▸ Adult: 15 g 3–4 times a day

▸ BY RECTUM

▸ Adult: 30 g, retained for 9 hours followed by irrigation to remove resin from colon

SORBISTERIT® POWDER

Hyperkalaemia associated with anuria or severe oliguria, and in dialysis patients

▸ BY MOUTH

▸ Adult: 20 g 1–3 times a day

▸ BY RECTUM

▸ Adult: 40 g 1–3 times a day, retained for 6 hours followed by irrigation to remove resin from colon

● **CONTRA-INDICATIONS** Hyperparathyroidism · metastatic carcinoma · multiple myeloma · obstructive bowel disease · sarcoidosis

● **INTERACTIONS** → Appendix 1 (polystyrene sulfonate resins).

● **SIDE-EFFECTS**

GENERAL SIDE-EFFECTS

Anorexia · constipation (discontinue treatment—avoid magnesium-containing laxatives) · diarrhoea · gastric irritation · gastro-intestinal obstruction · hypercalcaemia (including in dialysed patients and occasionally in those with renal impairment) · hypomagnesaemia · intestinal necrosis (reported with concomitant sorbitol) · ischaemic colitis · nausea · necrosis · ulceration · vomiting

SPECIFIC SIDE-EFFECTS

▸ With oral use Gastro-intestinal concretions

▸ With rectal use Faecal impaction

● **PREGNANCY** Manufacturers advise use only if potential benefit outweighs risk—no information available.

● **BREAST FEEDING** Manufacturers advise use only if potential benefit outweighs risk—no information available.

● **MONITORING REQUIREMENTS** Monitor for electrolyte disturbances (stop if plasma-potassium concentration below 5 mmol/litre).

● **DIRECTIONS FOR ADMINISTRATION**

▸ With rectal use Mix each 30 g of resin with 150 mL of water or 10% glucose.

SORBISTERIT® POWDER *By mouth*, administer in a small amount of water or soft drink—do not give with fruit juice or squash, which have a high potassium content.

By rectum, mix each 40 g of resin with 150 mL of 5% glucose.

● **MEDICINAL FORMS**

There can be variation in the licensing of different medicines containing the same drug. Forms available from special-order manufacturers include: enema

Powder

CAUTIONARY AND ADVISORY LABELS 13, 21 (Sorbisterit® powder only)

EXCIPIENTS: May contain Sucrose

▸ Calcium Resonium (Sanofi)

Calcium polystyrene sulfonate 999.34 mg per 1 gram Calcium Resonium powder sugar-free | 300 gram P £82.16

Sodium polystyrene sulfonate

● **INDICATIONS AND DOSE**

Hyperkalaemia associated with anuria or severe oliguria, and in dialysis patients

▸ BY MOUTH

▸ Adult: 15 g 3–4 times a day

▸ BY RECTUM

▸ Adult: 30 g, retain for 9 hours followed by irrigation to remove resin from colon

● **CONTRA-INDICATIONS** Obstructive bowel disease

● **CAUTIONS** Congestive heart failure · hypertension · oedema

● **INTERACTIONS** → Appendix 1 (polystyrene sulfonate resins).

● **SIDE-EFFECTS**

GENERAL SIDE-EFFECTS

Anorexia · constipation (discontinue treatment—avoid magnesium-containing laxatives) · diarrhoea · gastric irritation · gastro-intestinal obstruction · hypocalcaemia · hypomagnesaemia · intestinal necrosis (reported with concomitant use of sorbitol) · ischaemic colitis · nausea · necrosis · sodium retention · ulceration · vomiting

SPECIFIC SIDE-EFFECTS

▸ With oral use Gastro-intestinal concretions

▸ With rectal use Faecal impaction

● **PREGNANCY** Manufacturers advise use only if potential benefit outweighs risk—no information available.

● **BREAST FEEDING** Manufacturers advise use only if potential benefit outweighs risk—no information available.

● **RENAL IMPAIRMENT** Use with caution.

● **MONITORING REQUIREMENTS** Monitor for electrolyte disturbances (stop if plasma-potassium concentration below 5 mmol/litre).

● **DIRECTIONS FOR ADMINISTRATION**

▸ With rectal use Mix each 30 g of resin with 150 mL of water or 10% glucose.

▸ With oral use Administer dose (powder) in a small amount of water or honey—do not give with fruit juice or squash, which have a high potassium content.

● **MEDICINAL FORMS**
There can be variation in the licensing of different medicines containing the same drug. Forms available from special-order manufacturers include: oral suspension

Powder
CAUTIONARY AND ADVISORY LABELS 13
▸ Resonium A (Sanofi)
Sodium polystyrene sulfonate 999.34 mg per 1 gram Resonium A powder sugar-free | 454 gram Ⓟ £81.11

1.5b Hypokalaemia

ELECTROLYTES AND MINERALS ⟩ POTASSIUM

Potassium bicarbonate with potassium acid tartrate

● **INDICATIONS AND DOSE**

Hyperchloraemic acidosis associated with potassium deficiency (as in some renal tubular and gastro-intestinal disorders)
▸ BY MOUTH
▸ Adult: (consult product literature)

● CONTRA-INDICATIONS Hypochloraemia · plasma-potassium concentration above 5 mmol/litre
● CAUTIONS Cardiac disease · elderly
● INTERACTIONS → Appendix 1 (potassium salts).
● SIDE-EFFECTS Abdominal pain · diarrhoea · flatulence · nausea · vomiting
● RENAL IMPAIRMENT Avoid in severe impairment. Close monitoring required in renal impairment—high risk of hyperkalaemia.
● DIRECTIONS FOR ADMINISTRATION To be dissolved in water before administration.
● PRESCRIBING AND DISPENSING INFORMATION These tablets do not contain chloride.

● **MEDICINAL FORMS**
There can be variation in the licensing of different medicines containing the same drug.
Effervescent tablet
CAUTIONARY AND ADVISORY LABELS 13, 21
▸ Potassium bicarbonate with potassium acid tartrate (Non-proprietary)
Potassium acid tartrate 300 mg, Potassium bicarbonate 500 mg Potassium (potassium 6.5mmol) effervescent tablets BPC 1968 | 56 tablet GSL £77.77–£99.15 DT price = £92.02

Potassium chloride

● **INDICATIONS AND DOSE**

Prevention of hypokalaemia (patients with normal diet)
▸ BY MOUTH
▸ Adult: 2–4 g daily in divided doses
Electrolyte imbalance
▸ BY INTRAVENOUS INFUSION
▸ Adult: Dose dependent on deficit or the daily maintenance requirements

IMPORTANT SAFETY INFORMATION
SAFE PRACTICE
Potassium overdose can be fatal. Ready-mixed infusion solutions containing potassium should be used. Exceptionally, if potassium chloride concentrate is used for preparing an infusion, the infusion solution should be **thoroughly mixed**. Local policies on avoiding

inadvertent use of potassium chloride concentrate should be followed.

● CONTRA-INDICATIONS Plasma-potassium concentration above 5 mmol/litre
● CAUTIONS
▸ With intravenous use Seek specialist advice in very severe potassium depletion or difficult cases
▸ With oral use Cardiac disease · elderly · hiatus hernia (*with modified-release preparations*) · history of peptic ulcer (*with modified-release preparations*) · intestinal stricture (*with modified-release preparations*)
● INTERACTIONS → Appendix 1 (potassium salts).
● SIDE-EFFECTS
▸ **Common or very common**
▸ With oral use Abdominal pain · diarrhoea · flatulence · nausea · vomiting
▸ **Frequency not known**
▸ With intravenous use Heart toxicity (with rapid infusion)
▸ With oral use Bleeding (*with modified-release preparations*) · gastro-intestinal obstruction (*with modified-release preparations*) · ulceration (*with modified-release preparations*)
● RENAL IMPAIRMENT Smaller doses must be used in the prevention of hypokalaemia, to reduce the risk of hyperkalaemia. Avoid in severe impairment. Close monitoring required in renal impairment—high risk of hyperkalaemia.
● MONITORING REQUIREMENTS
▸ Regular monitoring of plasma-potassium concentration is essential in those taking potassium supplements.
▸ With intravenous use ECG monitoring should be performed in difficult cases.
● DIRECTIONS FOR ADMINISTRATION
▸ With oral use Potassium salts are preferably given as a liquid (or effervescent) preparation, rather than modified-release tablets; they should be given as the chloride (the use of effervescent potassium tablets BPC 1968 should be restricted to *hyperchloraemic* states).
▸ With intravenous use Potassium chloride concentrate must be diluted not **less** than 50 times its volume of sodium chloride intravenous infusion 0.9% or other suitable diluent and **mixed well**.
▸ With intravenous use Ready-mixed infusion solutions should be used where possible; alternatively, potassium chloride concentrate as ampoules containing 1.5 g (K⁺ 20 mmol) in 10 mL, is **thoroughly mixed** with 500 mL of sodium chloride 0.9% intravenous infusion and given slowly over 2 to 3 hours with specialist advice and ECG monitoring in difficult cases. For *peripheral intravenous infusion*, the concentration of potassium should not usually exceed 40 mmol/L. Higher concentrations of potassium chloride may be given in very severe depletion, but require specialist advice.
● PRESCRIBING AND DISPENSING INFORMATION Kay-Cee-L® contains 1 mmol/mL each of K⁺ and Cl⁻.
Potassium Tablets
▸ With oral use Do not confuse Effervescent Potassium Tablets BPC 1968 with effervescent potassium chloride tablets. Effervescent Potassium Tablets BPC 1968 do not contain chloride ions and their use should be restricted to hyperchloraemic states.
● PATIENT AND CARER ADVICE
Patient or carers should be given advice on how to administer potassium chloride modified-release tablets.
Salt substitutes A number of salt substitutes which contain significant amounts of potassium chloride are readily available as health food products (e.g. *LoSalt®* and *Ruthmol®*). These should not be used by patients with renal failure as potassium intoxication may result.

9

Blood and nutrition

- LESS SUITABLE FOR PRESCRIBING Modified-release tablets are less suitable for prescribing. Modified-release preparations should be avoided unless effervescent tablets or liquid preparations inappropriate.

- MEDICINAL FORMS
There can be variation in the licensing of different medicines containing the same drug. Forms available from special-order manufacturers include: modified-release tablet, modified-release capsule, oral solution, solution for injection, infusion, solution for infusion

Modified-release tablet
CAUTIONARY AND ADVISORY LABELS 25, 27
▸ Potassium chloride (Non-proprietary)
  Potassium chloride 600 mg Kaleorid LP 600mg tablets | 30 tablet PoM no price available
  Duro-K 600mg tablets | 100 tablet PoM no price available

Oral solution
CAUTIONARY AND ADVISORY LABELS 21
▸ Kay-Cee-L (Geistlich Sons Ltd)
  Potassium chloride 75 mg per 1 ml Kay-Cee-L syrup sugar-free | 500 ml P £7.57

Solution for infusion
▸ Potassium chloride (Non-proprietary)
  Potassium chloride 150 mg per 1 ml Potassium chloride 15% (potassium 20mmol/10ml) solution for infusion 10ml ampoules | 10 ampoule PoM £6.50 | 20 ampoule PoM £6.50
  Potassium chloride 15% (potassium 20mmol/10ml) solution for infusion 10ml Mini-Plasco ampoules | 20 ampoule PoM £10.70
  Potassium chloride 200 mg per 1 ml Potassium chloride 20% (potassium 13.3mmol/5ml) solution for infusion 5ml ampoules | 10 ampoule PoM £3.84-£4.00
  Potassium chloride 20% (potassium 27mmol/10ml) solution for infusion 10ml ampoules | 10 ampoule PoM £115.48

2 Metabolic disorders
2.1 Acute porphyrias

Acute porphyrias

Overview

The acute porphyrias (acute intermittent porphyria, variegate porphyria, hereditary coproporphyria, and 5-aminolaevulinic acid dehydratase deficiency porphyria) are hereditary disorders of haem biosynthesis; they have a prevalence of about 1 in 10 000 of the population.

Great care must be taken when prescribing for patients with acute porphyria, since certain drugs can induce acute porphyric crises. Since acute porphyrias are hereditary, relatives of affected individuals should be screened and advised about the potential danger of certain drugs.

Treatment of serious or life-threatening conditions should not be withheld from patients with acute porphyria. When there is no safe alternative, treatment should be started and urinary porphobilinogen excretion should be measured regularly; if it increases or symptoms occur, the drug can be withdrawn and the acute attack treated. If an acute attack of porphyria occurs during pregnancy, contact an expert porphyria service for further advice.

Haem arginate p. 919 is administered by short intravenous infusion as haem replacement in moderate, severe, or unremitting acute porphyria crises.

In the United Kingdom the National Acute Porphyria Service (NAPS) provides clinical support and treatment with haem arginate from three centres (University Hospital of Wales, Addenbrooke's Hospital, and King's College Hospital). To access the service telephone (029) 2074 7747 and ask for the Acute Porphyria Service.

Drugs unsafe for use in acute porphyrias

The following list contains drugs on the UK market that have been classified as 'unsafe' in porphyria because they have been shown to be porphyrinogenic in animals or in vitro, or have been associated with acute attacks in patients. Absence of a drug from the following lists does not necessarily imply that the drug is safe. For many drugs no information about porphyria is available.

An up-to-date list of drugs considered **safe** in acute porphyrias is available at
www.wmic.wales.nhs.uk/porphyria_info.php.
Further information may be obtained from:
www.porphyria-europe.org and also from:
Welsh Medicines Information Centre
University Hospital of Wales
CF14 4XW
Cardiff
(029) 2074 2979/3877
Quite modest changes in chemical structure can lead to changes in porphyrinogenicity but where possible general statements have been made about groups of drugs; these should be checked first.

Unsafe Drug Groups (check first)

- Alkylating drugs (contact Welsh Medicines Information Centre for further advice)
- Anabolic steroids
- Antidepressants (includes tricyclic (and related) antidepressants and MAOIs; fluoxetine, duloxetine, venlafaxine, and trazodone thought to be safe)
- Antihistamines (alimemazine, chlorphenamine, desloratadine, fexofenadine, ketotifen, loratadine, and promethazine thought to be safe)
- Barbiturates (includes primidone and thiopental)
- Calcium channel blockers (amlodipine, felodipine, and nifedipine thought to be safe)
- Contraceptives, hormonal (progestogens are more porphyrinogenic than oestrogens; oestrogens may be safe at least in replacement doses. Progestogens should be avoided whenever possible by all women susceptible to acute porphyria; however, when non-hormonal contraception is inappropriate, progestogens may be used with extreme caution if the potential benefit outweighs risk. The risk of an acute attack is greatest in women who have had a previous attack or are aged under 30 years. Long-acting progestogen preparations should **never** be used in those at risk of acute porphyria.)
- Ergot derivatives (includes ergometrine (oxytocin probably safe) and pergolide)
- Hormone replacement therapy (progestogens are more porphyrinogenic than oestrogens; oestrogens may be safe at least in replacement doses. Progestogens should be avoided whenever possible by all women susceptible to acute porphyria; however, when non-hormonal contraception is inappropriate, progestogens may be used with extreme caution if the potential benefit outweighs risk. The risk of an acute attack is greatest in women who have had a previous attack or are aged under 30 years. Long-acting progestogen preparations should **never** be used in those at risk of acute porphyria.)
- Imidazole antifungals (applies to oral and intravenous use; topical antifungals are thought to be safe due to low systemic exposure)
- Non-nucleoside reverse transcriptase inhibitors (contact Welsh Medicines Information Centre for further advice)
- Progestogens (progestogens are more porphyrinogenic than oestrogens; oestrogens may be safe at least in replacement doses. Progestogens should be avoided whenever possible by all women susceptible to acute porphyria; however, when non-hormonal contraception is inappropriate, progestogens may be used with extreme caution if the potential benefit outweighs risk. The risk of

an acute attack is greatest in women who have had a previous attack or are aged under 30 years. Long-acting progestogen preparations should **never** be used in those at risk of acute porphyria.)

- Protease inhibitors (contact Welsh Medicines Information Centre for further advice)
- Sulfonamides (includes co-trimoxazole and sulfasalazine)
- Sulfonylureas (glipizide and glimepiride are thought to be safe)
- Taxanes (contact Welsh Medicines Information Centre for further advice)
- Thiazolidinediones (contact Welsh Medicines Information Centre for further advice)
- Triazole antifungals (applies to oral and intravenous use; topical antifungals are thought to be safe due to low systemic exposure)

Unsafe Drugs (check groups above first)

- Aceclofenac
- Alcohol
- Amiodarone
- Aprepitant (contact Welsh Medicines Information Centre for further advice)
- Artemether with lumefantrine
- Bexarotene
- Bosentan
- Bromocriptine
- Buspirone
- Cabergoline
- Carbamazepine
- Chloral hydrate (although evidence of hazard is uncertain, manufacturer advises avoid)
- Chloramphenicol
- Chloroform (small amounts in medicines probably safe)
- Clindamycin
- Cocaine
- Colistimethate sodium
- Danazol
- Dapsone
- Dexfenfluramine
- Disopyramide
- Disulfiram
- Erythromycin
- Etamsylate
- Ethosuximide
- Etomidate
- Fenfluramine
- Flupentixol
- Flutamide
- Fosaprepitant (contact Welsh Medicines Information Centre for further advice)
- Fosphenytoin
- Griseofulvin
- Hydralazine
- Indapamide
- Isometheptene mucate
- Isoniazid (safety uncertain, contact Welsh Medicines Information Centre for further advice)
- Ketamine
- Mefenamic acid (may be used with caution if safer alternative not available)
- Meprobamate
- Methyldopa
- Metolazone
- Metyrapone
- Mifepristone
- Minoxidil (may be used with caution if safer alternative not available)
- Mitotane
- Nalidixic acid
- Nitrazepam
- Nitrofurantoin

- Orphenadrine
- Oxcarbazepine
- Oxybutynin
- Pentazocine (buprenorphine, codeine, diamorphine, dihydrocodeine, fentanyl, methadone, morphine, oxycodone, pethidine, and tramadol are thought to be safe)
- Pentoxifylline
- Phenoxybenzamine
- Phenytoin
- Pivmecillinam
- Porfimer
- Raloxifene
- Rifabutin (safety uncertain, contact Welsh Medicines Information Centre for further advice)
- Rifampicin
- Riluzole
- Risperidone
- Selegiline
- Spironolactone
- Sulfinpyrazone
- Tamoxifen
- Telithromycin
- Temoporfin
- Tiagabine
- Tibolone
- Tinidazole
- Topiramate
- Toremifene
- Trimethoprim
- Valproate
- Xipamide
- Zidovudine (contact Welsh Medicines Information Centre for further advice)
- Zuclopenthixol

BLOOD AND RELATED PRODUCTS > HAEM DERIVATIVES

| Haem arginate

(Human hemin)

- **● INDICATIONS AND DOSE**

Acute porphyrias | Acute intermittent porphyria | Porphyria variegata | Hereditary coproporphyria

▸ **BY INTRAVENOUS INFUSION**

▸ **Adult:** Initially 3 mg/kg once daily for 4 days, if response inadequate, repeat 4-day course with close biochemical monitoring; maximum 250 mg per day

- **● SIDE-EFFECTS**
- ▸ **Common or very common** Pain at injection site · thrombophlebitis at injection site
- ▸ **Rare** Fever · hypersensitivity reactions
- ▸ **Frequency not known** Headache
- **● PREGNANCY** Manufacturer advises avoid unless essential.
- **● BREAST FEEDING** Manufacturer advises avoid unless essential—no information available.
- **● DIRECTIONS FOR ADMINISTRATION**
- ▸ With intravenous use For *intravenous infusion* (*Normosang*®), give intermittently in Sodium chloride 0.9%; dilute requisite dose in 100 mL infusion fluid in glass bottle and give over at least 30 minutes through a filter *via* large antebrachial or central vein; administer within 1 hour after dilution.

9

Blood and nutrition

● MEDICINAL FORMS
There can be variation in the licensing of different medicines
containing the same drug.
Solution for infusion
▸ Normosang (Orphan Europe (UK) Ltd)
Haem arginate 25 mg per 1 ml Normosang 250mg/10ml solution for
infusion ampoules | 4 ampoule PoM £1,737.00

▸ Carnitor (Sigma-Tau Pharma Ltd)
L-Carnitine 100 mg per 1 ml Carnitor oral single dose 1g solution
sugar-free | 10 unit dose PoM £35.00
Solution for injection
▸ Carnitor (Sigma-Tau Pharma Ltd)
L-Carnitine 200 mg per 1 ml Carnitor 1g/5ml solution for injection
ampoules | 5 ampoule PoM £59.50

2.2 Carnitine deficiency

AMINO ACIDS AND DERIVATIVES

| Levocarnitine

(Carnitine)

● INDICATIONS AND DOSE

**Primary carnitine deficiency due to inborn errors of
metabolism**
▸ BY MOUTH
▸ Adult: Up to 200 mg/kg daily in 2–4 divided doses;
maximum 3 g per day
▸ BY SLOW INTRAVENOUS INJECTION
▸ Adult: Up to 100 mg/kg daily in 2–4 divided doses, to be
administered over 2–3 minutes
Secondary carnitine deficiency in haemodialysis patients
▸ INITIALLY BY SLOW INTRAVENOUS INJECTION
▸ Adult: 20 mg/kg, to be administered over 2–3 minutes,
after each dialysis session, dosage adjusted according
to plasma-carnitine concentration, then (by mouth)
maintenance 1 g daily, administered if benefit is gained
from first intravenous course

● CAUTIONS Diabetes mellitus
● SIDE-EFFECTS Abdominal pain · body odour · diarrhoea ·
nausea · vomiting
SIDE-EFFECTS, FURTHER INFORMATION
Side-effects may be dose-related—monitor tolerance
during first week and after any dose increase.
● PREGNANCY Appropriate to use; no evidence of
teratogenicity in *animal* studies.
● RENAL IMPAIRMENT Accumulation of metabolites may
occur with chronic oral administration in severe
impairment.
● MONITORING REQUIREMENTS
▸ Monitoring of free and acyl carnitine in blood and urine
recommended.
● MEDICINAL FORMS
There can be variation in the licensing of different medicines
containing the same drug. Forms available from special-order
manufacturers include: capsule
Tablet
▸ Carnitor (Sigma-Tau Pharma Ltd)
L-Carnitine 330 mg Carnitor 330mg tablets | 90 tablet PoM
£103.95
Chewable tablet
▸ Carnitor (Sigma-Tau Pharma Ltd)
L-Carnitine 1 gram Carnitor 1g chewable tablets | 10 tablet PoM
£35.00
Capsule
▸ Levocarnitine (Non-proprietary)
L-Carnitine 250 mg Bio-Carnitine 250mg capsules | 125 capsule
£11.06
L-Carnitine 500 mg Lamberts L-Carnitine 500mg capsules |
60 capsule £11.67
Oral solution
▸ Levocarnitine (Non-proprietary)
L-Carnitine 300 mg per 1 ml Levocarnitine 1.5g/5ml (30%) oral
solution paediatric | 20 ml PoM £71.40 DT price = £71.40

2.3 Fabry's disease

ENZYMES

| Agalsidase alfa

● DRUG ACTION Agalsidase alfa, an enzyme produced by
recombinant DNA technology are licensed for long-term
enzyme replacement therapy in Fabry's disease (a
lysosomal storage disorder caused by deficiency of alpha-
galactosidase A).

● INDICATIONS AND DOSE

Fabry's disease (specialist use only)
▸ BY INTRAVENOUS INFUSION
▸ Adult: 200 micrograms/kg every 2 weeks

● INTERACTIONS → Appendix 1 (agalsidase alfa and beta).
● SIDE-EFFECTS
▸ **Common or very common** Acne · angioedema · arthralgia ·
asthenia · bradycardia · chest pain · cough · dizziness ·
dyspnoea · eye irritation · fatigue · flushing · gastro-
intestinal disturbances · headache · hypersensitivity
reactions · hypertension · hypotension · influenza- like
symptoms · muscle spasms · myalgia · nasopharyngitis ·
neuropathic pain · oedema · palpitation · paraesthesia ·
pruritus · rash · rhinorrhoea · sleep disturbances · syncope ·
tachycardia · taste disturbances · tinnitus · tremor ·
urticaria
▸ **Uncommon** Cold extremities · ear pain · ear swelling ·
injection-site reactions · parosmia · skin discoloration
SIDE-EFFECTS, FURTHER INFORMATION
▸ Infusion-related reactions Infusion-related reactions very
common; manage by slowing the infusion rate or
interrupting the infusion, or minimise by pre-treatment
with an antihistamine, antipyretic, or corticosteroid—
consult product literature.
● PREGNANCY Use with caution.
● BREAST FEEDING Use with caution—no information
available.
● DIRECTIONS FOR ADMINISTRATION Administration for
intravenous infusion, give intermittently *in* sodium chloride
0.9%; dilute requisite dose with 100 mL infusion fluid and
give over 40 minutes using an in-line filter; use within
3 hours of dilution.
● MEDICINAL FORMS
There can be variation in the licensing of different medicines
containing the same drug.
Solution for infusion
▸ Replagal (Shire Pharmaceuticals Ltd)
Agalsidase alfa 1 mg per 1 ml Replagal 3.5mg/3.5ml solution for
infusion vials | 1 vial PoM £1,068.64

Agalsidase beta

- DRUG ACTION Agalsidase beta, an enzyme produced by recombinant DNA technology are licensed for long-term enzyme replacement therapy in Fabry's disease (a lysosomal storage disorder caused by deficiency of alpha-galactosidase A).

- INDICATIONS AND DOSE

Fabry's disease (specialist use only)
▸ BY INTRAVENOUS INFUSION
  ▸ Adult: 1 mg/kg every 2 weeks

- INTERACTIONS → Appendix 1 (agalsidase alfa and beta).

- SIDE-EFFECTS
▸ **Common or very common** Acne · angioedema · arthralgia · asthenia · bradycardia · chest pain · cough · dizziness · dyspnoea · eye irritation · fatigue · flushing · gastro-intestinal disturbances · headache · hypersensitivity reactions · hypertension · hypotension · influenza- like symptoms · muscle spasms · myalgia · nasopharyngitis · neuropathic pain · oedema · palpitation · paraesthesia · pruritus · rash · rhinorrhoea · sleep disturbances · syncope · tachycardia · taste disturbances · tinnitus · tremor · urticaria
▸ **Uncommon** Cold extremities · ear pain · ear swelling · injection-site reactions · parosmia · skin discoloration
  SIDE-EFFECTS, FURTHER INFORMATION
▸ Infusion-related reactions Infusion-related reactions very common; manage by slowing the infusion rate or interrupting the infusion, or minimise by pre-treatment with an antihistamine, antipyretic, or corticosteroid—consult product literature.

- PREGNANCY Use with caution.

- BREAST FEEDING Use with caution—no information available.

- DIRECTIONS FOR ADMINISTRATION For *intravenous infusion*, given intermittently in Sodium chloride 0.9%, reconstitute initially with Water for Injections (5 mg in 1.1 mL, 35 mg in 7.2 mL) to produce a solution containing 5 mg/mL. Dilute with Sodium Chloride 0.9% (for doses less than 35 mg dilute with at least 50 mL; doses 35–70 mg dilute with at least 100 mL; doses 70–100 mg dilute with at least 250 mL; doses greater than 100 mg dilute with 500 mL) and give through an in-line low protein-binding 0.2 micron filter at an initial rate of no more than 15 mg/hour; for subsequent infusions, infusion rate may be increased gradually once tolerance has been established.

- MEDICINAL FORMS
There can be variation in the licensing of different medicines containing the same drug.
Powder for solution for infusion
  ▸ Fabrazyme (Genzyme Therapeutics Ltd)
    Agalsidase beta 5 mg Fabrazyme 5mg powder for solution for infusion vials | 1 vial [PoM] £315.08
    Agalsidase beta 35 mg Fabrazyme 35mg powder for solution for infusion vials | 1 vial [PoM] £2,196.59

2.4 Gaucher's disease

Drugs used for Gaucher's disease not listed below;
Miglustat, p. 924

ENZYMES

Imiglucerase

- DRUG ACTION Imiglucerase is an enzyme produced by recombinant DNA technology that is administered as enzyme replacement therapy for non-neurological manifestations of type I or type III Gaucher's disease, a familial disorder affecting principally the liver, spleen, bone marrow, and lymph nodes.

- INDICATIONS AND DOSE

Non-neurological manifestations of type I Gaucher's disease (specialist use only) | Non-neurological manifestations of type III Gaucher's disease (specialist use only)
▸ BY INTRAVENOUS INFUSION
  ▸ Adult: Initially 60 units/kg every 2 weeks; maintenance, adjusted according to response, doses as low as 15 units/kg once every 2 weeks may improve haematological parameters and organomegaly

- SIDE-EFFECTS
▸ **Common or very common** Angioedema · backache · cyanosis · flushing · hypersensitivity reactions · hypotension · paraesthesia · tachycardia · urticaria
▸ **Uncommon** Abdominal cramps · arthralgia · diarrhoea · dizziness · fatigue · fever · headache · injection-site reactions · nausea · vomiting

- PREGNANCY Manufacturer advises use with caution—limited information available.

- BREAST FEEDING No information available.

- MONITORING REQUIREMENTS
▸ Monitor for immunoglobulin G (IgG) antibodies to imiglucerase.
▸ When stabilised, monitor all parameters and response to treatment at intervals of 6–12 months.

- DIRECTIONS FOR ADMINISTRATION For *intravenous infusion* (*Cerezyme*®), give intermittently in Sodium chloride 0.9%; initially reconstitute with water for injections (200 units in 5.1 mL, 400 units in 10.2 mL) to give 40 units/mL solution; dilute requisite dose with infusion fluid to a final volume of 100–200 mL and give initial dose at a rate not exceeding 0.5 units/kg/minute, subsequent doses to be given at a rate not exceeding 1 unit/kg/minute; administer within 3 hours after reconstitution.

- MEDICINAL FORMS
There can be variation in the licensing of different medicines containing the same drug.
Powder for solution for infusion
ELECTROLYTES: May contain Sodium
  ▸ Cerezyme (Genzyme Therapeutics Ltd)
    Imiglucerase 400 unit Cerezyme 400unit powder for solution for infusion vials | 1 vial [PoM] £1,071.29

9

Blood and nutrition

Velaglucerase alfa

- **DRUG ACTION** Velaglucerase alfa is an enzyme produced by recombinant DNA technology that is administered as enzyme replacement therapy for the treatment of type I Gaucher's disease.

- **INDICATIONS AND DOSE**

  Type I Gaucher's disease (specialist use only)
  ▸ BY INTRAVENOUS INFUSION
  ▸ Adult: Initially 60 units/kg every 2 weeks; adjusted according to response to 15–60 units/kg every 2 weeks

- **SIDE-EFFECTS** Abdominal pain · arthralgia · back pain · bone pain · dizziness · flushing · headache · hypersensitivity reactions · hypertension · hypotension · malaise · nausea · pyrexia · rash · tachycardia · urticaria

  SIDE-EFFECTS, FURTHER INFORMATION
  ▸ Infusion-related reactions Infusion-related reactions very common; manage by slowing the infusion rate, or interrupting the infusion, or minimise by pre-treatment with an antihistamine, antipyretic, or corticosteroid—consult product literature.

- **PREGNANCY** Manufacturer advises use with caution—limited information available.

- **BREAST FEEDING** Manufacturer advises use with caution—no information available.

- **MONITORING REQUIREMENTS** Monitor immunoglobulin G (IgG) antibody concentration in severe infusion-related reactions or if there is a lack or loss of effect with velaglucerase alfa.

- **DIRECTIONS FOR ADMINISTRATION** For *intravenous infusion* (*VPRIV*®), give intermittently *in* Sodium chloride 0.9%; reconstitute each 400-unit vial with 4.3 mL water for injections to produce a 100 units/mL solution; dilute requisite dose in 100 mL infusion fluid; give over 60 minutes through a 0.22 micron filter; start infusion within 24 hours of reconstitution.

- **MEDICINAL FORMS** There can be variation in the licensing of different medicines containing the same drug.
  Powder for solution for infusion
  ELECTROLYTES: May contain Sodium
  ▸ VPRIV (Shire Pharmaceuticals Ltd)
  Velaglucerase alfa 400 unit VPRIV 400units powder for solution for infusion vials | 1 vial [PoM] £1,410.20

2.5 Homocystinuria

METHYL DONORS

Betaine

- **INDICATIONS AND DOSE**

  Adjunctive treatment of homocystinuria involving deficiencies or defects in cystathionine beta-synthase, 5,10-methylene-tetrahydrofolate reductase, or cobalamin cofactor metabolism (specialist use only)
  ▸ BY MOUTH
  ▸ Adult: 3 g twice daily (max. per dose 10 g), adjusted according to response; maximum 20 g per day

- **SIDE-EFFECTS**
  ▸ **Uncommon** Agitation · alopecia · anorexia · depression · gastro-intestinal disorders · personality disorder · reversible cerebral oedema · sleep disturbances · urinary incontinence · urticaria

- **PREGNANCY** Manufacturer advises avoid unless essential—limited information available.

- **BREAST FEEDING** Manufacturer advises caution—no information available.

- **MONITORING REQUIREMENTS** Monitor plasma-methionine concentration before and during treatment—interrupt treatment if symptoms of cerebral oedema occur.

- **DIRECTIONS FOR ADMINISTRATION** Powder should be mixed with water, juice, milk, formula, or food until completely dissolved and taken immediately; measuring spoons are provided to measure 1 g, 150 mg, and 100 mg of *Cystadane*® powder.

- **PRESCRIBING AND DISPENSING INFORMATION** Betaine should be used in conjunction with dietary restrictions and may be given with supplements of Vitamin B_{12}, pyridoxine, and folate under specialist advice.

- **NATIONAL FUNDING/ACCESS DECISIONS**
  Scottish Medicines Consortium (SMC) Decisions
  The *Scottish Medicines Consortium* has advised (July 2010) that betaine anhydrous (Cystadane®) is accepted for restricted use within NHS Scotland for the adjunctive treatment of homocystinuria involving deficiencies or defects in cystathionine beta-synthase, 5,10-methylene-tetrahydrofolate reductase, or cobalamin cofactor metabolism in patients who are not responsive to pyridoxine treatment.

- **MEDICINAL FORMS** There can be variation in the licensing of different medicines containing the same drug. Forms available from special-order manufacturers include: tablet, oral solution
  Powder
  ▸ Cystadane (Orphan Europe (UK) Ltd)
  Betaine 1 gram per 1 gram Cystadane oral powder | 180 gram [PoM] £347.00

2.6 Mucopolysaccharidosis

ENZYMES

Galsulfase

- **DRUG ACTION** Galsulfase is a recombinant form of human N-acetylgalactosamine-4-sulfatase.

- **INDICATIONS AND DOSE**

  Mucopolysaccharidosis VI (specialist use only)
  ▸ BY INTRAVENOUS INFUSION
  ▸ Adult: 1 mg/kg once weekly

- **CAUTIONS** Acute febrile illness (consider delaying treatment) · acute respiratory illness (consider delaying treatment) · infusion-related reactions can occur · respiratory disease

- **SIDE-EFFECTS** Abdominal pain · apnoea · areflexia · chest pain · conjunctivitis · corneal opacity · dyspnoea · ear pain · facial oedema · gastroenteritis · hypertension · infusion-related reactions · malaise · nasal congestion · pharyngitis · rigors · umbilical hernia

  SIDE-EFFECTS, FURTHER INFORMATION
  ▸ Infusion-related reactions Infusion-related reactions often occur, they can be managed by slowing the infusion rate or interrupting the infusion, and can be minimised by pre-treatment with an antihistamine and an antipyretic. Recurrent infusion-related reactions may require pre-treatment with a corticosteroid—consult product literature for details.

- **PREGNANCY** Manufacturer advises avoid unless essential.

- **BREAST FEEDING** Manufacturer advises avoid—no information available.

- **DIRECTIONS FOR ADMINISTRATION** For *intravenous infusion* (*Naglazyme*®), give intermittently *in* Sodium chloride 0.9%;

dilute requisite dose with infusion fluid to final volume of 250 mL and mix gently; infuse through a 0.2 micron in-line filter; give approx. 2.5% of the total volume over 1 hour, then infuse remaining volume over next 3 hours; if body-weight under 20 kg and at risk of fluid overload, dilute requisite dose in 100 mL infusion fluid and give over at least 4 hours.

● MEDICINAL FORMS
There can be variation in the licensing of different medicines containing the same drug.
Solution for infusion
▸ Naglazyme (BioMarin Europe Ltd) ▼
   Galsulfase 1 mg per 1 ml Naglazyme 5mg/5ml solution for infusion vials | 1 vial PoM £982.00

Idursulfase

● DRUG ACTION Idursulfase is an enzyme produced by recombinant DNA technology licensed for long-term replacement therapy in mucopolysaccharidosis II (Hunter syndrome), a lysosomal storage disorder caused by deficiency of iduronate-2-sulfatase.

● INDICATIONS AND DOSE
Mucopolysaccharidosis II (specialist use only)
▸ BY INTRAVENOUS INFUSION
▸ Adult: 500 micrograms/kg once weekly

● CAUTIONS Acute febrile respiratory illness (consider delaying treatment) · infusion-related reactions can occur · severe respiratory disease
● SIDE-EFFECTS
▸ **Common or very common** Arrhythmia · arthralgia · bronchospasm · chest pain · cough · cyanosis · dizziness · dyspnoea · erythema · facial oedema · flushing · gastro-intestinal disturbances · headache · hypertension · hypotension · hypoxia · infusion-site swelling · peripheral oedema · pruritus · pyrexia · rash · swollen tongue · tachycardia · tachypnoea · tremor · urticaria · wheezing
▸ **Frequency not known** Anaphylaxis · infusion-related reactions · pulmonary embolism
  SIDE-EFFECTS, FURTHER INFORMATION
▸ Infusion-related reactions Infusion-related reactions often occur, they can be managed by slowing the infusion rate or interrupting the infusion, and can be minimised by pre-treatment with an antihistamine and an antipyretic. Recurrent infusion-related reactions may require pre-treatment with a corticosteroid—consult product literature for details.
● CONCEPTION AND CONTRACEPTION Contra-indicated in women of child-bearing potential.
● PREGNANCY Manufacturer advises avoid.
● BREAST FEEDING Manufacturer advises avoid—present in milk in *animal* studies.
● DIRECTIONS FOR ADMINISTRATION For *intravenous infusion* (*Elaprase®*), give intermittently *in* Sodium chloride 0.9%; dilute requisite dose in 100 mL infusion fluid and mix gently (do not shake); give over 3 hours (gradually reduced to 1 hour if no infusion-related reactions).

● MEDICINAL FORMS
There can be variation in the licensing of different medicines containing the same drug.
Solution for infusion
▸ Elaprase (Shire Pharmaceuticals Ltd) ▼
   Idursulfase 2 mg per 1 ml Elaprase 6mg/3ml concentrate for solution for infusion vials | 1 vial PoM £1,985.00

Laronidase

● DRUG ACTION Laronidase is an enzyme produced by recombinant DNA technology licensed for long-term replacement therapy in the treatment of non-neurological manifestations of mucopolysaccharidosis I, a lysosomal storage disorder caused by deficiency of alpha-L-iduronidase.

● INDICATIONS AND DOSE
Non-neurological manifestations of mucopolysaccharidosis I (specialist use only)
▸ BY INTRAVENOUS INFUSION
▸ Adult: 100 units/kg once weekly

● CAUTIONS Infusion-related reactions can occur
● INTERACTIONS → Appendix 1 (laronidase).
● SIDE-EFFECTS
▸ **Common or very common** Abdominal pain · alopecia · anaphylaxis · angioedema · blood pressure changes · cold extremities · cough · diarrhoea · dizziness · dyspnoea · fatigue · flushing · headache · influenza-like symptoms · infusion-site reactions · musculoskeletal pain · nausea · pain in extremities · pallor · paraesthesia · pruritus · rash · restlessness · tachycardia · urticaria · vomiting
▸ **Frequency not known** Bronchospasm · infusion-related reactions · respiratory arrest
  SIDE-EFFECTS, FURTHER INFORMATION
▸ Infusion-related reactions Infusion-related reactions often occur, they can be managed by slowing the infusion rate or interrupting the infusion, and can be minimised by pre-treatment with an antihistamine and an antipyretic. Recurrent infusion-related reactions may require pre-treatment with a corticosteroid—consult product literature for details.
● PREGNANCY Manufacturer advises avoid unless essential—no information available.
● BREAST FEEDING Manufacturer advises avoid—no information available.
● MONITORING REQUIREMENTS Monitor immunoglobulin G (IgG) antibody concentration.
● DIRECTIONS FOR ADMINISTRATION For *intravenous infusion* (*Aldurazyme®*), give intermittently in Sodium chloride 0.9%; body-weight under 20 kg, use 100 mL infusion fluid; body-weight over 20 kg use 250 mL infusion fluid; withdraw volume of infusion fluid equivalent to volume of laronidase concentrate being added; give through in-line filter (0.22 micron) initially at a rate of 2 units/kg/hour then increase gradually every 15 minutes to max. 43 units/kg/hour.

● MEDICINAL FORMS
There can be variation in the licensing of different medicines containing the same drug.
Solution for infusion
ELECTROLYTES: May contain Sodium
▸ Aldurazyme (Genzyme Therapeutics Ltd)
   Laronidase 100 unit per 1 ml Aldurazyme 500units/5ml solution for infusion vials | 1 vial PoM £444.70

9

Blood and nutrition

2.7 Nephropathic cystinosis

AMINO ACIDS AND DERIVATIVES

Mercaptamine

(Cysteamine)

● INDICATIONS AND DOSE

Nephropathic cystinosis (specialist use only)
▸ BY MOUTH
▸ Adult (body-weight 50 kg and above): Initially one-sixth
  to one-quarter of the expected maintenance dose,
  increased gradually over 4–6 weeks to avoid
  intolerance, maintenance 2 g daily in 4 divided doses
DOSE EQUIVALENCE AND CONVERSION
1.3 g/m^2 is approximately equivalent to 50 mg/kg.

IMPORTANT SAFETY INFORMATION
SAFE PRACTICE
Mercaptamine has been confused with mercaptopurine;
care must be taken to ensure the correct drug is
prescribed and dispensed.

● CAUTIONS Dose of phosphate supplement may need to be
adjusted if transferring from phosphocysteamine to
mercaptamine
● SIDE-EFFECTS
▸ **Common or very common** Abdominal pain · anorexia ·
breath and body odour · diarrhoea · dyspepsia ·
encephalopathy · fever · gastroenteritis · headache ·
malaise · nausea · rash · vomiting
▸ **Uncommon** Drowsiness · gastro-intestinal ulcer ·
hallucinations · leucopenia · nephrotic syndrome ·
nervousness · seizures
● ALLERGY AND CROSS-SENSITIVITY Contra-indicated if
history of hypersensitivity to penicillamine.
● PREGNANCY Avoid—teratogenic and toxic in *animal*
studies.
● BREAST FEEDING Avoid.
● MONITORING REQUIREMENTS Leucocyte-cystine
concentration and haematological monitoring required—
consult product literature.
● PRESCRIBING AND DISPENSING INFORMATION
Mercaptamine has a very unpleasant taste and smell,
which can affect compliance.

● MEDICINAL FORMS
There can be variation in the licensing of different medicines
containing the same drug.
Capsule
CAUTIONARY AND ADVISORY LABELS 21
▸ Cystagon (Orphan Europe (UK) Ltd)
  Mercaptamine (as Mercaptamine bitartrate) 50 mg Cystagon
  50mg capsules | 100 capsule [PoM] £70.00
  Mercaptamine (as Mercaptamine bitartrate) 150 mg Cystagon
  150mg capsules | 100 capsule [PoM] £190.00
Gastro-resistant capsule
▸ Procysbi (Raptor Pharmaceuticals)
  Mercaptamine (as Mercaptamine bitartrate) 25 mg Procysbi
  25mg gastro-resistant capsules | 60 capsule [PoM] £335.97
  Mercaptamine (as Mercaptamine bitartrate) 75 mg Procysbi
  75mg gastro-resistant capsules | 250 capsule [PoM] £4,199.65

2.8 Niemann-pick type C disease

ENZYME INHIBITORS > GLUCOSYLCERAMIDE SYNTHASE INHIBITORS

Miglustat

● DRUG ACTION Miglustat is an inhibitor of
glucosylceramide synthase.

● INDICATIONS AND DOSE

**Mild to moderate type I Gaucher's disease for whom
enzyme replacement therapy is unsuitable (under expert
supervision)**
▸ BY MOUTH
▸ Adult: 100 mg 3 times a day, reduced if not tolerated to
  100 mg 1–2 times a day
**Treatment of progressive neurological manifestations of
Niemann-Pick type C disease (under expert supervision)**
▸ BY MOUTH
▸ Adult: 200 mg 3 times a day

● SIDE-EFFECTS Abdominal pain · amnesia · anorexia · ataxia
· chills · constipation · decreased libido · depression ·
diarrhoea · dizziness · dyspepsia · flatulence · headache ·
hypoaesthesia · insomnia · malaise · muscle spasm · muscle
weakness · nausea · paraesthesia · peripheral neuropathy ·
thrombocytopenia · tremor · vomiting · weight changes
● CONCEPTION AND CONTRACEPTION Effective
contraception must be used during treatment. Men should
avoid fathering a child during and for 3 months after
treatment.
● PREGNANCY Manufacturer advises avoid—toxicity in
animal studies.
● BREAST FEEDING Manufacturer advises avoid—no
information available.
● HEPATIC IMPAIRMENT No information available—
manufacturer advises caution.
● RENAL IMPAIRMENT For Gaucher's disease initially 100 mg
twice daily if eGFR 50–70 mL/minute/1.73 m^2. Initially
100 mg once daily if eGFR 30–50 mL/minute/1.73 m^2. For
Niemann-Pick type C disease, initially 200 mg twice daily if
eGFR 50–70 mL/minute/1.73 m^2. Initially 100 mg twice
daily if eGFR 30–50 mL/minute/1.73 m^2 Avoid if eGFR less
than 30 mL/minute/1.73 m^2.
● MONITORING REQUIREMENTS
▸ Monitor cognitive and neurological function.
▸ Monitor growth and platelet count in Niemann-Pick type C
  disease.

● MEDICINAL FORMS
There can be variation in the licensing of different medicines
containing the same drug.
Capsule
▸ Zavesca (Actelion Pharmaceuticals UK Ltd)
  Miglustat 100 mg Zavesca 100mg capsules | 84 capsule [PoM]
  £3,934.17 (Hospital only)

2.9 Pompe disease

ENZYMES

Alglucosidase alfa

- DRUG ACTION Alglucosidase alfa is an enzyme produced by recombinant DNA technology licensed for long-term replacement therapy in Pompe disease, a lysosomal storage disorder caused by deficiency of acid alpha-glucosidase.

- INDICATIONS AND DOSE

Pompe disease (specialist use only)
▶ BY INTRAVENOUS INFUSION
▶ Adult: 20 mg/kg every 2 weeks

- CAUTIONS Cardiac dysfunction · infusion-related reactions—consult product literature · respiratory dysfunction

- SIDE-EFFECTS
▶ **Common or very common** Agitation · anaphylaxis · antibody formation · blood pressure changes · bronchospasm · chest discomfort · cold extremities · cough · cyanosis · diarrhoea · dizziness · facial oedema · fatigue · flushing · headache · hypersensitivity reactions · injection-site reactions · irritability · muscle spasm · myalgia · nausea · paraesthesia · pruritus · pyrexia · rash · restlessness · sweating · tachycardia · tachypnoea · tremor · urticaria · vomiting
▶ **Frequency not known** Infusion-related reactions · necrotising skin lesions · severe skin reactions · ulcerative skin lesions

SIDE-EFFECTS, FURTHER INFORMATION
▶ **Infusion-related reactions** Infusion-related reactions very common, calling for use of antihistamine, antipyretic, or corticosteroid; consult product literature for details.

- PREGNANCY Toxicity in *animal* studies, but treatment should not be withheld.

- BREAST FEEDING Manufacturer advises avoid—no information available.

- MONITORING REQUIREMENTS
▶ Monitor closely if cardiac dysfunction.
▶ Monitor closely if respiratory dysfunction.
▶ Monitor immunoglobulin G (IgG) antibody concentration.

- DIRECTIONS FOR ADMINISTRATION For *intravenous infusion* (*Myozyme®*), give intermittently *in* Sodium chloride 0.9%; reconstitute 50 mg with 10.3 mL water for injections to produce 5 mg/mL solution; gently rotate vial without shaking; dilute requisite dose with infusion fluid to give a final concentration of 0.5–4 mg/mL; give through a low protein-binding in-line filter (0.2 micron) at an initial rate of 1 mg/kg/hour increased by 2 mg/kg/hour every 30 minutes to max. 7 mg/kg/hour.

- MEDICINAL FORMS
There can be variation in the licensing of different medicines containing the same drug.
Powder for solution for infusion
▶ Myozyme (Genzyme Therapeutics Ltd)
Alglucosidase alfa 50 mg Myozyme 50mg powder for concentrate for solution for infusion vials | 1 vial [PoM] £356.06 (Hospital only)

2.10 Tyrosinaemia type I

ENZYME INHIBITORS ＞ 4-HYDROXYPHENYLPYRUVATE DIOXYGENASE INHIBITORS

Nitisinone

(NTBC)

- INDICATIONS AND DOSE

Hereditary tyrosinaemia type I (in combination with dietary restriction of tyrosine and phenylalanine) (specialist use only)
▶ BY MOUTH
▶ Adult: Initially 500 micrograms/kg twice daily, adjusted according to response; maximum 2 mg/kg per day

- SIDE-EFFECTS
▶ **Common or very common** Conjunctivitis · corneal opacity · eye pain · granulocytopenia · keratitis · leucopenia · photophobia · thrombocytopenia
▶ **Uncommon** Blepharitis · erythematous rash · exfoliative dermatitis · leucocytosis · pruritus

- PREGNANCY Manufacturer advises avoid unless potential benefit outweighs risk—toxicity in *animal* studies.

- BREAST FEEDING Manufacturer advises avoid—adverse effects in *animal* studies.

- PRE-TREATMENT SCREENING Slit-lamp examination of eyes recommended before treatment.

- MONITORING REQUIREMENTS
▶ Monitor liver function regularly.
▶ Monitor platelet and white blood cell count every 6 months.

- DIRECTIONS FOR ADMINISTRATION Capsules can be opened and the contents suspended in a small amount of water or formula diet and taken immediately.

- MEDICINAL FORMS
There can be variation in the licensing of different medicines containing the same drug.
Capsule
▶ Orfadin (Swedish Orphan Biovitrum Ltd)
Nitisinone 2 mg Orfadin 2mg capsules | 60 capsule [PoM] £564.00
Nitisinone 5 mg Orfadin 5mg capsules | 60 capsule [PoM] £1,127.00
Nitisinone 10 mg Orfadin 10mg capsules | 60 capsule [PoM] £2,062.00
Nitisinone 20 mg Orfadin 20mg capsules | 60 capsule [PoM] £4,512.00
Oral suspension
▶ Orfadin (Swedish Orphan Biovitrum Ltd)
Nitisinone 4 mg per 1 ml Orfadin 4mg/1ml oral suspension sugar-free | 90 ml [PoM] £1,692.00

2.11 Urea cycle disorders

AMINO ACIDS AND DERIVATIVES

Carglumic acid

- INDICATIONS AND DOSE

Hyperammonaemia due to N-acetylglutamate synthase deficiency (under expert supervision)
▶ BY MOUTH
▶ Adult: Initially 50–125 mg/kg twice daily, to be taken immediately before food, dose adjusted according to plasma–ammonia concentration; maintenance 5–50 mg/kg twice daily, the total daily dose may alternatively be given in 3–4 divided doses   continued →

Hyperammonaemia due to organic acidaemia (under expert supervision)

▶ BY MOUTH

▶ Adult: Initially 50–125 mg/kg twice daily, to be taken immediately before food, dose adjusted according to plasma-ammonia concentration, the total daily dose may alternatively be given in 3–4 divided doses

> **IMPORTANT SAFETY INFORMATION**
> EMERGENCY MANAGEMENT OF UREA CYCLE DISORDERS
> For further information on the emergency management of urea cycle disorders consult the British Inherited Metabolic Disease Group (BIMDG) website at www.bimdg.org.uk.

● SIDE-EFFECTS
▶ **Common or very common** Sweating
▶ **Uncommon** Bradycardia · diarrhoea · pyrexia · vomiting

● PREGNANCY Manufacturer advises avoid unless essential—no information available.

● BREAST FEEDING Manufacturer advises avoid—present in milk in *animal* studies.

● DIRECTIONS FOR ADMINISTRATION
▶ With oral use Dispersible tablets must be dispersed in at least 5–10 mL of water and taken orally immediately, or administered via a nasogastric tube.

● MEDICINAL FORMS
There can be variation in the licensing of different medicines containing the same drug.
Dispersible tablet
CAUTIONARY AND ADVISORY LABELS 13
▶ Carbaglu (Orphan Europe (UK) Ltd)
Carglumic acid 200 mg Carbaglu 200mg dispersible tablets sugar-free | 5 tablet [PoM] £299.00 sugar-free | 60 tablet [PoM] £3,499.00

DRUGS FOR METABOLIC DISORDERS >
AMMONIA LOWERING DRUGS

Sodium phenylbutyrate

● INDICATIONS AND DOSE

Long-term treatment of urea cycle disorders (as adjunctive therapy in all patients with neonatal-onset disease and in those with late-onset disease who have a history of hyperammonaemic encephalopathy) (under expert supervision)

▶ BY MOUTH

▶ Adult: 9.9–13 g/m^2 daily in divided doses, with meals; maximum 20 g per day

> **IMPORTANT SAFETY INFORMATION**
> EMERGENCY MANAGEMENT OF UREA CYCLE DISORDERS
> For further information on the emergency management of urea cycle disorders consult the British Inherited Metabolic Disease Group (BIMDG) website at www.bimdg.org.uk.

● CAUTIONS Congestive heart failure (preparations contain significant amounts of sodium)

● INTERACTIONS → Appendix 1 (sodium phenylbutyrate).

● SIDE-EFFECTS
▶ **Common or very common** Alkalosis · blood disorders · body odour · decreased appetite · depression · gastro-intestinal disturbances · headache · irritability · menstrual disorders · metabolic acidosis · oedema · rash · renal tubular acidosis · syncope · taste disturbance · weight gain
▶ **Uncommon** Arrhythmias · pancreatitis · peptic ulcer · rectal bleeding

SIDE-EFFECTS, FURTHER INFORMATION
Gastro-intestinal side-effects may be reduced by giving smaller doses more frequently.

● CONCEPTION AND CONTRACEPTION Manufacturer advises adequate contraception during administration in women of child-bearing potential.

● PREGNANCY Avoid—toxicity in *animal* studies.

● BREAST FEEDING Manufacturer advises avoid—no information available.

● HEPATIC IMPAIRMENT Manufacturer advises use with caution.

● RENAL IMPAIRMENT Manufacturer advises use with caution (preparations contain significant amounts of sodium).

● DIRECTIONS FOR ADMINISTRATION Granules should be mixed with food before taking. *Pheburane*® granules must not be administered by nasogastric or gastrostromy tubes.

● MEDICINAL FORMS
There can be variation in the licensing of different medicines containing the same drug. Forms available from special-order manufacturers include: capsule, oral suspension, oral solution
Tablet
▶ Ammonaps (Swedish Orphan Biovitrum Ltd)
Sodium phenylbutyrate 500 mg Ammonaps 500mg tablets | 250 tablet [PoM] £493.00
Granules
▶ Ammonaps (Swedish Orphan Biovitrum Ltd)
Sodium phenylbutyrate 940 mg per 1 gram Ammonaps 940mg/g granules sugar-free | 266 gram [PoM] £860.00
▶ Pheburane (Lucane Pharma Ltd)
Sodium phenylbutyrate 483 mg per 1 gram Pheburane 483mg/g granules | 174 gram [PoM] £331.00

2.12 Wilson's disease

> Drugs used for Wilson's disease not listed below;
> Penicillamine, p. 952

ANTIDOTES AND CHELATORS > COPPER ABSORPTION INHIBITORS

Zinc acetate

● DRUG ACTION Zinc prevents the absorption of copper in Wilson's disease.

● INDICATIONS AND DOSE

Wilson's disease (initiated under specialist supervision)

▶ BY MOUTH

▶ Adult: 50 mg 3 times a day (max. per dose 50 mg 5 times a day), adjusted according to response

DOSE EQUIVALENCE AND CONVERSION
Doses expressed as elemental zinc.

PHARMACOKINETICS
Symptomatic Wilson's disease patients should be treated initially with a chelating agent because zinc has a slow onset of action. When transferring from chelating treatment to zinc maintenance therapy, chelating treatment should be co-administered for 2–3 weeks until zinc produces its maximal effect.

● CAUTIONS Portal hypertension (risk of hepatic decompensation when switching from chelating agent)

● INTERACTIONS → Appendix 1 (zinc).

● SIDE-EFFECTS
▶ **Common or very common** Gastric irritation (usually transient)
▶ **Uncommon** Leucopenia · sideroblastic anaemia

SIDE-EFFECTS, FURTHER INFORMATION
Transient gastric irritation may be reduced if first dose is taken mid-morning or with a little protein.

● PREGNANCY Reduce dose to 25 mg 3 times daily adjusted according to plasma-copper concentration and urinary copper excretion.

● BREAST FEEDING Manufacturer advises avoid; present in milk—may cause zinc-induced copper deficiency in infant.

● MONITORING REQUIREMENTS Monitor full blood count and serum cholesterol.

● MEDICINAL FORMS
There can be variation in the licensing of different medicines containing the same drug.
Capsule
CAUTIONARY AND ADVISORY LABELS 23
▸ Wilzin (Orphan Europe (UK) Ltd)
Zinc (as Zinc acetate) 25 mg Wilzin 25mg capsules | 250 capsule [PoM] £132.00
Zinc (as Zinc acetate) 50 mg Wilzin 50mg capsules | 250 capsule [PoM] £242.00

ANTIDOTES AND CHELATORS ⟩ COPPER CHELATORS

Trientine dihydrochloride

● INDICATIONS AND DOSE
Wilson's disease in patients intolerant of penicillamine
▸ BY MOUTH
▸ Adult: 1.2–2.4 g daily in 2–4 divided doses, adjusted according to response, to be taken before food

● INTERACTIONS → Appendix 1 (trientine).

● SIDE-EFFECTS
▸ **Common or very common** Nausea · rash
▸ **Very rare** Anaemia
▸ **Frequency not known** Colitis · duodenitis

● PREGNANCY Teratogenic in *animal* studies—use only if benefit outweighs risk. Monitor maternal and neonatal serum-copper concentrations.

● PRESCRIBING AND DISPENSING INFORMATION Trientine is **not** an alternative to penicillamine for rheumatoid arthritis or cystinuria. Penicillamine-induced systemic lupus erythematosus may not resolve on transfer to trientine.

● MEDICINAL FORMS
There can be variation in the licensing of different medicines containing the same drug.
Capsule
CAUTIONARY AND ADVISORY LABELS 6, 22
▸ Trientine dihydrochloride (Non-proprietary)
Trientine dihydrochloride 300 mg Trientine dihydrochloride 300mg capsules | 100 capsule [PoM] no price available

3 Mineral and trace elements deficiencies

3.1 Selenium deficiency

Selenium

Selenium deficiency can occur as a result of inadequate diet or prolonged parenteral nutrition. A selenium supplement should not be given unless there is good evidence of deficiency.

VITAMINS AND TRACE ELEMENTS

Selenium

● INDICATIONS AND DOSE
Selenium deficiency
▸ BY MOUTH, OR BY INTRAMUSCULAR INJECTION, OR BY INTRAVENOUS INJECTION
▸ Adult: 100–500 micrograms daily

● INTERACTIONS → Appendix 1 (selenium).

● MEDICINAL FORMS
There can be variation in the licensing of different medicines containing the same drug.
Tablet
▸ Selenium (Non-proprietary)
Selenium (as L-Selenomethionine) 100 microgram Solgar Selenium 100microgram tablets | 100 tablet no price available
L-Selenomethionine 200 microgram EN-Selenium 200microgram tablets | 30 tablet £88.60
Solgar Selenium 200microgram tablets | 50 tablet no price available | 250 tablet no price available
HealthAid Selenium 200microgram tablets | 60 tablet £3.90
Lamberts Selenium 200microgram tablets | 60 tablet £4.08
▸ SelenoPrecise (Pharma Nord (UK) Ltd)
Selenium (as L-Selenomethionine) 100 microgram SelenoPrecise 100microgram tablets | 60 tablet £6.75
L-Selenomethionine 200 microgram SelenoPrecise 200microgram tablets | 60 tablet £4.02
Capsule
▸ Selenium (Non-proprietary)
L-Selenomethionine 200 microgram Selenium 200microgram capsules | 30 capsule £3.20 | 60 capsule £5.79
Oral solution
▸ Selenase (Baxter Healthcare Ltd)
Selenium (as Sodium selenite) 50 microgram per 1 ml Selenase 100micrograms/2ml oral solution 2ml unit dose ampoules | 20 unit dose [P] no price available
Selenase 500micrograms/10ml oral solution unit dose vials | 10 unit dose [P] no price available
Solution for injection
▸ Selenase (Baxter Healthcare Ltd)
Selenium (as Sodium selenite) 50 microgram per 1 ml Selenase 100micrograms/2ml solution for injection ampoules | 10 ampoule [PoM] no price available
Selenase 500micrograms/10ml solution for injection vials | 10 vial [PoM] no price available

3.2 Zinc deficiency

Zinc

Zinc supplements should not be given unless there is good evidence of deficiency (hypoproteinaemia spuriously lowers plasma-zinc concentration) or in zinc-losing conditions. Zinc deficiency can occur as a result of inadequate diet or malabsorption; excessive loss of zinc can occur in trauma, burns, and protein-losing conditions. A zinc supplement is given until clinical improvement occurs, but it may need to be continued in severe malabsorption, metabolic disorders, or in zinc-losing states.

Zinc is used in the treatment of Wilson's disease and acrodermatitis enteropathica, a rare inherited abnormality of zinc absorption.

Parenteral nutrition regimens usually include trace amounts of zinc. If necessary, further zinc can be added to intravenous feeding regimens.

9

Blood and nutrition

ELECTROLYTES AND MINERALS > ZINC

Zinc sulfate

● INDICATIONS AND DOSE

Zinc deficiency or supplementation in zinc-losing conditions

▸ BY MOUTH USING EFFERVESCENT TABLETS

▸ Child (body-weight up to 10 kg): 22.5 mg daily, dose to be adjusted as necessary, to be dissolved in water and taken after food, dose expressed as elemental zinc

▸ Child (body-weight 10–30 kg): 22.5 mg 1–3 times a day, dose to be adjusted as necessary, to be dissolved in water and taken after food, dose expressed as elemental zinc

▸ Child (body-weight 30 kg and above): 45 mg 1–3 times a day, dose to be adjusted as necessary, to be dissolved in water and taken after food, dose expressed as elemental zinc

▸ Adult (body-weight 30 kg and above): 45 mg 1–3 times a day, dose to be adjusted as necessary, to be dissolved in water and taken after food, dose expressed as elemental zinc

Additional elemental zinc for intravenous nutrition

▸ BY INTRAVENOUS INJECTION

▸ Adult: 6.5 mg daily (Zn^{2+} 100 micromol)

● UNLICENSED USE *Solvazinc*® is not licensed for use in acrodermatitis enteropathica.

● INTERACTIONS → Appendix 1 (zinc).

● SIDE-EFFECTS Abdominal pain · diarrhoea · dyspepsia · gastric irritation · gastritis · headache · irritability · lethargy · nausea · vomiting

● PREGNANCY Crosses placenta; risk theoretically minimal, but no information available.

● BREAST FEEDING Present in milk; risk theoretically minimal, but no information available.

● RENAL IMPAIRMENT Accumulation may occur in acute renal failure.

● PRESCRIBING AND DISPENSING INFORMATION Each *Solvazinc*® tablet contains zinc sulfate monohydrate 125 mg (45 mg zinc).

● MEDICINAL FORMS
There can be variation in the licensing of different medicines containing the same drug. Forms available from special-order manufacturers include: solution for injection

Effervescent tablet
CAUTIONARY AND ADVISORY LABELS 13, 21
▸ Solvazinc (Galen Ltd)
Zinc sulfate monohydrate 125 mg Solvazinc 125mg effervescent tablets sugar-free | 90 tablet P £14.95 DT price = £14.95

4   Nutrition (intravenous)

Intravenous nutrition

Overview

When adequate feeding through the alimentary tract is not possible, nutrients may be given by intravenous infusion. This may be in addition to ordinary oral or tube feeding—**supplemental parenteral nutrition**, or may be the sole source of nutrition—**total parenteral nutrition** (TPN). Indications for this method include preparation of undernourished patients for surgery, chemotherapy, or radiation therapy; severe or prolonged disorders of the gastro-intestinal tract; major surgery, trauma, or burns; prolonged coma or refusal to eat; and some patients with renal or hepatic failure. The composition of proprietary

preparations available is given under Proprietary Infusion Fluids for Parenteral Feeding p. 929.

Parenteral nutrition requires the use of a solution containing amino acids, glucose, fat, electrolytes, trace elements, and vitamins. This is now commonly provided by the pharmacy in the form of a 3-litre bag. A single dose of vitamin B_{12}, as hydroxocobalamin p. 887, is given by intramuscular injection; regular vitamin B_{12} injections are not usually required unless total parenteral nutrition continues for many months. Folic acid p. 886 is given in a dose of 15 mg once or twice each week, usually in the nutrition solution. Other vitamins are usually given daily; they are generally introduced in the parenteral nutrition solution. Alternatively, if the patient is able to take small amounts by mouth, vitamins may be given orally.

The nutrition solution is infused through a central venous catheter inserted under full surgical precautions. Alternatively, infusion through a peripheral vein may be used for supplementary as well as total parenteral nutrition for periods of up to a month, depending on the availability of peripheral veins; factors prolonging cannula life and preventing thrombophlebitis include the use of soft polyurethane paediatric cannulas and use of feeds of low osmolality and neutral pH. Only nutritional fluids should be given by the dedicated intravenous line.

Before starting, the patient should be well oxygenated with a near normal circulating blood volume and attention should be given to renal function and acid-base status. Appropriate biochemical tests should have been carried out beforehand and serious deficits corrected. Nutritional and electrolyte status must be monitored throughout treatment.

Complications of long-term parenteral nutrition include gall bladder sludging, gall stones, cholestasis and abnormal liver function tests. For details of the prevention and management of parenteral nutrition complications, specialist literature should be consulted.

Protein is given as mixtures of essential and non-essential synthetic L-amino acids. Ideally, all essential amino acids should be included with a wide variety of nonessential ones to provide sufficient nitrogen together with electrolytes. Solutions vary in their composition of amino acids; they often contain an energy source (usually glucose p. 903) and electrolytes.

Energy is provided in a ratio of 0.6 to 1.1 megajoules (150–250 kcals) per gram of protein nitrogen. Energy requirements must be met if amino acids are to be utilised for tissue maintenance. A mixture of carbohydrate and fat energy sources (usually 30–50% as fat) gives better utilisation of amino acids than glucose alone.

Glucose is the preferred source of carbohydrate, but if more than 180 g is given per day frequent monitoring of blood glucose is required, and insulin may be necessary. Glucose in various strengths from 10 to 50% must be infused through a central venous catheter to avoid thrombosis.

In parenteral nutrition regimens, it is necessary to provide adequate **phosphate** in order to allow phosphorylation of glucose and to prevent hypophosphataemia; between 20 and 30 mmol of phosphate is required daily.

Fructose and sorbitol have been used in an attempt to avoid the problem of hyperosmolar hyperglycaemic non-ketotic acidosis but other metabolic problems may occur, as with xylitol and ethanol which are now rarely used.

Fat emulsions have the advantages of a high energy to fluid volume ratio, neutral pH, and iso-osmolarity with plasma, and provide essential fatty acids. Several days of adaptation may be required to attain maximal utilisation. Reactions include occasional febrile episodes (usually only with 20% emulsions) and rare anaphylactic responses. Interference with biochemical measurements such as those for blood gases and calcium may occur if samples are taken before fat has been cleared. Daily checks are necessary to ensure complete clearance from the plasma in conditions

Proprietary Infusion Fluids for Parenteral Feeding

Preparation	Nitrogen g/litre	[1,2]Energy kJ/litre	K$^+$	Mg^{2+}	Na$^+$	Acet$^-$	Cl$^-$	Other components/litre
			Electrolytes mmol/litre					
Aminoven 25 (Fresenius Kabi Ltd) Net price 500 ml = £19.72	25.7	–	–	–	–	–	–	
Clinimix N9G20E (Baxter Healthcare Ltd) Net price (dual compartment bag of amino acids with electrolytes 1000 mL and glucose 20% with calcium 1000 mL) 2 litre: no price available	4.6	1680	30.0	2.5	35.0	50.0	40.0	Ca^{2+} 2.3 mmol, phosphate 15 mmol, anhydrous glucose 100 g
Clinimix N14G30E (Baxter Healthcare Ltd) Net price (dual compartment bag of amino acids with electrolytes 1000 mL and glucose 30% with calcium 1000 mL) 2 litre: no price available	7.0	2520	30.0	2.5	35.0	70.0	40.0	Ca^{2+} 2.3 mmol, phosphate 15 mmol, anhydrous glucose 150 g
ClinOleic 20% (Baxter Healthcare Ltd) Net price 100 ml: no price available; Net price 250 ml: no price available; Net price 500 ml: no price available	–	8360	–	–	–	–	–	purified olive and soya oil 200 g, glycerol 22.5 g, egg phosphatides 12 g
Hyperamine 30 (B.Braun Medical Ltd) Net price 500 ml: no price available	30.0	–	–	–	5.0	–	–	
Intralipid 10% (Fresenius Kabi Ltd) Net price 100 ml = £4.12; Net price 500 ml = £9.01	–	4600	–	–	–	–	–	soya oil 100 g, glycerol 22 g, purified egg phospholipids 12 g, phosphate 15 mmol
Intralipid 20% (Fresenius Kabi Ltd) Net price 100 ml = £6.21; Net price 250 ml = £10.16; Net price 500 ml = £13.52	–	8400	–	–	–	–	–	soya oil 200 g, glycerol 22 g, purified egg phospholipids 12 g, phosphate 15 mmol
Intralipid 30% (Fresenius Kabi Ltd) Net price 333 ml = £17.80	–	12600	–	–	–	–	–	soya oil 300 g, glycerol 16.7 g, purified egg phospholipids 12 g, phosphate 15 mmol
Kabiven (Fresenius Kabi Ltd) Net price (triple compartment bag of amino acids and electrolytes 300 mL, 450 mL, 600 mL, or 750 mL; glucose 526 mL, 790 mL, 1053 mL, or 1316 mL; lipid emulsion 200 mL, 300 mL, 400 mL, or 500 mL) 1.026 litre: no price available; Net price 1.54 litre = £44.09; Net price 2.053 litre = £57.42; Net price 2.566 litre = £59.92	5.3	3275	23.0	4.0	31.0	38.0	45.0	Ca^{2+} 2 mmol, phosphate 9.7 mmol, anhydrous glucose 97 g, soya oil 39 g
Kabiven peripheral (Fresenius Kabi Ltd) Net price (triple compartment bag of amino acids and electrolytes 300 mL, 400 mL, or 500 mL; glucose 885 mL, 1180 mL, or 1475 mL; lipid emulsion 255 mL, 340 mL, or 425 mL) 1.44 litre = £30.77; Net price 1.92 litre = £44.09; Net price 2.4 litre = £55.72	3.75	2625	17.0	2.8	22.0	27.0	33.0	Ca^{2+} 1.4 mmol, phosphate 7.5 mmol, anhydrous glucose 67.5 g, soya oil 35.4 g
Lipidem (B.Braun Medical Ltd) Net price 100 ml = £19.11; Net price 250 ml = £31.85; Net price 500 ml = £40.34	–	7900	–	–	–	–	–	omega-3-acid triglycerides 20 g, soya oil 80 g, medium chain triglycerides 100 g
Lipofundin MCT/LCT 10% (B.Braun Medical Ltd) Net price 100 ml: no price available; Net price 500 ml = £13.70	–	4430	–	–	–	–	–	soya oil 50 g, medium-chain triglycerides 50 g
Lipofundin MCT/LCT 20% (B.Braun Medical Ltd) Net price 100 ml = £13.28; Net price 250 ml: no price available; Net price 500 ml = £20.36	–	8000	–	–	–	–	–	soya oil 100 g, medium-chain triglycerides 100 g

1 1000 kcal = 4200kJ; 1000 kJ = 238.8 kcal. All entries are Prescription-only medicines.

2 Excludes protein- or amino acid-derived energy

9

Blood and nutrition

Preparation	Nitrogen g/litre	[1,2]Energy kJ/litre	Electrolytes mmol/litre					Other components/litre
			K$^+$	Mg^{2+}	Na$^+$	Acet$^-$	Cl$^-$	
Nutriflex basal (B.Braun Medical Ltd) Net price (dual compartment bag of amino acids 400 mL or 800 mL; glucose 600 mL or 1200 mL) 1 litre: no price available; Net price 2 litre = £29.20	4.6	2095	30.0	5.7	49.9	35.0	50.0	Ca^{2+} 3.6 mmol, acid phosphate 12.8 mmol, anhydrous glucose 125 g
Nutriflex peri (B.Braun Medical Ltd) Net price (dual compartment bag of amino acids 400 mL or 800 mL; glucose 600 mL or 1200 mL) 1 litre: no price available; Net price 2 litre = £30.47	5.7	1340	15.0	4.0	27.0	19.5	31.6	Ca^{2+} 2.5 mmol, acid phosphate 5.7 mmol, anhydrous glucose 80 g
Nutriflex plus (B.Braun Medical Ltd) Net price (dual compartment bag of amino acids 400 mL or 800 mL; glucose 600 mL or 1200 mL) 1 litre: no price available; Net price 2 litre = £33.02	6.8	2510	25.0	5.7	37.2	22.9	35.5	Ca^{2+} 3.6 mmol, acid phosphate 20 mmol, anhydrous glucose 150 g
Nutriflex special (B.Braun Medical Ltd) Net price (dual compartment bag of amino acids 500 mL or 750 mL; glucose 500 mL or 750 mL) 1 litre: no price available; Net price 1.5 litre = £27.60	10.0	4020	25.7	5.0	40.5	22.0	49.5	Ca^{2+} 4.1 mmol, acid phosphate 14.7 mmol, anhydrous glucose 240 g
NuTRIflex Lipid peri (B.Braun Medical Ltd) Net price (triple compartment bag of amino acids 500 mL, 750 mL or 1000 mL; glucose 500 mL, 750 mL or 1000 mL; lipid emulsion 20% 250 mL, 375 mL or 500 mL) 1.25 litre = £42.83; Net price 1.875 litre = £54.37; Net price 2.5 litre = £64.22	4.56	2664	24.0	2.4	40.0	32.0	38.4	Ca^{2+} 2.4 mmol, Zn^{2+} 24 micromol, phosphate 6 mmol, anhydrous glucose 64 g, soya oil 20 g, medium-chain triglycerides 20 g
NuTRIflex Lipid plus (B.Braun Medical Ltd) Net price (triple compartment bag of amino acids 500 mL, 750 mL or 1000 mL; glucose 500 mL, 750 mL or 1000 mL; lipid emulsion 20% 250 mL, 375 mL or 500 mL) 1.25 litre = £46.56; Net price 1.875 litre = £59.46; Net price 2.5 litre = £68.39	5.44	3600	28.0	3.2	40.0	36.0	36.0	Ca^{2+} 3.2 mmol, Zn^{2+} 24 micromol, phosphate 12 mmol, anhydrous glucose 120 g, soya oil 20 g, medium-chain triglycerides 20 g
NuTRIflex Lipid plus without Electrolytes (B.Braun Medical Ltd) Net price (triple compartment bag of amino acids 500 mL, 750 mL or 1000 mL; glucose 500 mL, 750 mL or 1000 mL; lipid emulsion 20% 250 mL, 375 mL or 500 mL) 1.25 litre = £46.56; Net price 1.875 litre = £59.45; Net price 2.5 litre = £68.39	5.44	3600	–	–	–	–	–	anhydrous glucose 120 g, soya oil 20 g, medium-chain triglycerides 20 g
NuTRIflex Lipid special (B.Braun Medical Ltd) Net price (triple compartment bag of amino acids 500 mL, 750 mL or 1000 mL; glucose 500 mL, 750 mL or 1000 mL; lipid emulsion 20% 250 mL, 375 mL or 500 mL) 1.25 litre = £56.96; Net price 1.875 litre = £74.62; Net price 2.5 litre: no price available	8.0	4004	37.6	4.24	53.6	48.0	48.0	Ca^{2+} 4.24 mmol, Zn^{2+} 32 micromol, phosphate 16 mmol, anhydrous glucose 144 g, soya oil 20 g, medium-chain triglycerides 20 g
NuTRIflex Lipid special without Electrolytes (B.Braun Medical Ltd) Net price (triple compartment bag of amino acids 500 mL, 750 mL or 1000 mL; glucose 500 mL, 750 mL or 1000 mL; lipid emulsion 20% 250 mL, 375 mL or 500 mL) 1.25 litre = £56.96; Net price 1.875 litre = £74.62	8.0	4004	–	–	–	–	–	anhydrous glucose 144 g, soya oil 20 g, medium-chain triglycerides 20 g

1 1000 kcal = 4200kJ; 1000 kJ = 238.8 kcal. All entries are Prescription-only medicines.
2 Excludes protein- or amino acid-derived energy

Preparation	Nitrogen g/litre	[1,2]Energy kJ/litre	Electrolytes mmol/litre					Other components/litre
			K$^+$	Mg^{2+}	Na$^+$	Acet$^-$	Cl$^-$	
NuTRIflex Omega plus (B.Braun Medical Ltd) Net price (triple compartment bag of amino acids 500 mL, 750 mL or 1000 mL; glucose 500 mL, 750 mL or 1000 mL; lipid emulsion 250 mL, 375 mL or 500 mL) 1.25 litre = £47.43; Net price 1.875 litre = £60.57; Net price 2.5 litre = £69.66	5.4	3600	28.0	3.2	40.0	36.0	36.0	Ca^{2+} 3.2 mmol, Zn^{2+} 24 micromol, phosphate 12 mmol, anhydrous glucose 120 g, refined soya oil 16 g, medium-chain triglycerides 20 g, omega-3-acid triglycerides 4 g
NuTRIflex Omega special (B.Braun Medical Ltd) Net price (triple compartment bag of amino acids 250 mL, 500 mL, 750 mL or 1000 mL; glucose 250 mL, 500 mL, 750 mL or 1000 mL; lipid emulsion 125 mL, 250 mL, 375 mL or 500 mL) 625 ml = £43.62; Net price 1.25 litre = £58.01; Net price 1.875 litre = £76.01; Net price 2.5 litre = £89.71	8.0	4004	37.6	4.24	53.6	48.0	48.0	Ca^{2+} 4.24 mmol, Zn^{2+} 30 micromol, phosphate 16 mmol, anhydrous glucose 144 g, refined soya oil 16 g, medium-chain triglycerides 20 g, omega-3-acid triglycerides 4 g
OliClinomel N4-550E (Baxter Healthcare Ltd) Net price (triple compartment bag of amino acids with electrolytes 1000 mL; glucose 20% 1000 mL; lipid emulsion 10% 500 mL) 2.5 litre: no price available	3.6	2184	16.0	2.2	21.0	30.0	33.0	Ca^{2+} 2 mmol, phosphate 8.5 mmol, refined olive and soya oil 20 g, anhydrous glucose 80 g
OliClinomel N4-720E (Baxter Healthcare Ltd) Net price (triple compartment bag of amino acids with electrolytes 1000 mL; glucose 20% 1000 mL; lipid emulsion 20% 500 mL) 2.5 litre: no price available	3.64	3024	24.0	2.0	28.0	40.0	40.0	Ca^{2+} 1.8 mmol, phosphate 8 mmol, refined olive and soya oil 40 g, anhydrous glucose 80 g
OliClinomel N5-800E (Baxter Healthcare Ltd) Net price (triple compartment bag of amino acids with electrolytes 800 mL or 1000 mL; glucose 25% 800 mL or 1000 mL; lipid emulsion 20% 400 mL or 500 mL) 2 litre: no price available; Net price 2.5 litre: no price available	4.6	3360	24.0	2.2	32.0	49.0	44.0	Ca^{2+} 2 mmol, phosphate 10 mmol, refined olive and soya oil 40 g, anhydrous glucose 100 g
OliClinomel N6-900E (Baxter Healthcare Ltd) Net price (triple compartment bag of amino acids with electrolytes 800 mL or 1000 mL; glucose 30% 800 mL or 1000 mL; lipid emulsion 20% 400 mL or 500 mL) 2 litre: no price available; Net price 2.5 litre: no price available	5.6	3696	24.0	2.2	32.0	53.0	46.0	Ca^{2+} 2 mmol, phosphate 10 mmol, refined olive and soya oil 40 g, anhydrous glucose 120 g
OliClinomel N7-1000 (Baxter Healthcare Ltd) Net price (triple compartment bag of amino acids 600 mL; glucose 40% 600 mL; lipid emulsion 20% 300 mL) 1.5 litre: no price available	6.6	4368	–	–	–	37.0	16.0	phosphate 3 mmol, refined olive and soya oil 40 g, anhydrous glucose 160 g
OliClinomel N7-1000E (Baxter Healthcare Ltd) Net price (triple compartment bag of amino acids with electrolytes 800 mL; glucose 40% 800 mL; lipid emulsion 20% 400 mL) 2 litre: no price available	6.6	4368	24.0	2.2	32.0	57.0	48.0	Ca^{2+} 2 mmol, phosphate 10 mmol, refined olive and soya oil 40 g, anhydrous glucose 160 g
OliClinomel N8-800 (Baxter Healthcare Ltd) Net price (triple compartment bag of amino acids 800 mL; glucose 31.25% 800 mL; lipid emulsion 15% 400 mL) 2 litre: no price available	8.25	3360	–	–	–	42.5	20.0	phosphate 2.25 mmol, refined olive and soya oil 30 g, anhydrous glucose 125 g

1　1000 kcal = 4200kJ; 1000 kJ = 238.8 kcal. All entries are Prescription-only medicines.
2　Excludes protein- or amino acid-derived energy

Preparation	Nitrogen g/litre	[1,2]Energy kJ/litre	Electrolytes mmol/litre					Other components/litre
			K⁺	Mg²⁺	Na⁺	Acet⁻	Cl⁻	
Omegaven (Fresenius Kabi Ltd) Net price 100 ml: no price available	–	4700	–	–	–	–	–	highly refined fish oil 100 g, glycerol 25 g, egg phosphatide 12 g
Plasma-Lyte 148 (water) (Baxter Healthcare Ltd) Net price 1 litre: no price available	–		5.0	1.5	140.0	27.0	98.0	gluconate 23 mmol
Plasma-Lyte 148 (dextrose 5%) (Baxter Healthcare Ltd) Net price 1 litre: no price available	–	840	5.0	1.5	140.0	27.0	98.0	gluconate 23 mmol, anhydrous glucose 50 g
Plasma-Lyte M (dextrose 5%) (Baxter Healthcare Ltd) Net price 1 litre: no price available	–	840	16.0	1.5	40.0	12.0	40.0	Ca^{2+} 2.5 mmol, lactate 12 mmol, anhydrous glucose 50 g
Primene 10% (Baxter Healthcare Ltd) Net price 100 ml: no price available; Net price 250 ml: no price available	15.0	–	–	–	–	–	19.0	
SMOFlipid (Fresenius Kabi Ltd) Net price 500 ml = £174.30	–	8400	–	–	–	–	–	fish oil 30 g, olive oil 50 g, soya oil 60 g, medium-chain triglycerides 60 g
Synthamin 9 (Baxter Healthcare Ltd) Net price 500 ml: no price available; Net price 1 litre: no price available	9.1	–	60.0	5.0	70.0	100.0	70.0	acid phosphate 30 mmol
Synthamin 9 EF (electrolyte-free) (Baxter Healthcare Ltd) Net price 500 ml: no price available; Net price 1 litre: no price available	9.1	–	–	–	–	44.0	22.0	
Synthamin 14 (Baxter Healthcare Ltd) Net price 500 ml: no price available; Net price 1 litre: no price available; Net price 3 litre: no price available	14.0	–	60.0	5.0	70.0	140.0	70.0	acid phosphate 30 mmol
Synthamin 14 EF (electrolyte-free) (Baxter Healthcare Ltd) Net price 500 ml: no price available; Net price 1 litre: no price available	14.0	–	–	–	–	68.0	34.0	
Synthamin 17 (Baxter Healthcare Ltd) Net price 500 ml: no price available; Net price 1 litre: no price available	16.5	–	60.0	5.0	70.0	150.0	70.0	acid phosphate 30 mmol
Synthamin 17 EF (electrolyte-free) (Baxter Healthcare Ltd) Net price 500 ml: no price available; Net price 3 litre: no price available	16.5	–	–	–	–	82.0	40.0	
Vamin 9 Glucose (Fresenius Kabi Ltd) Net price 100 ml = £3.90; Net price 500 ml = £7.95; Net price 1 litre = £13.80	9.4	1700	20.0	1.5	50.0	–	50.0	CA^{2+} 2.5 mmol, anhydrous glucose 100 g
Vamin 14 (Fresenius Kabi Ltd) Net price 500 ml = £9.48; Net price 1 litre = £16.02	13.5	–	50.0	8.0	100.0	135.0	100.0	CA^{2+} 5 mmol, SO_4^{2-} 8 mmol
Vamin 14 (electrolyte-free) (Fresenius Kabi Ltd) Net price 500 ml = £9.48; Net price 1 litre = £16.02	13.5	–	–	–	–	90.0	–	
Vamin 18 (electrolyte-free) (Fresenius Kabi Ltd) Net price 500 ml = £11.99; Net price 1 litre = £23.38	18.0	–	–	–	–	110.0	–	
Vaminolact (Fresenius Kabi Ltd) Net price 100 ml = £3.70; Net price 500 ml = £8.50	9.3	–						

1 1000 kcal = 4200kJ; 1000 kJ = 238.8 kcal. All entries are Prescription-only medicines.
2 Excludes protein- or amino acid-derived energy

where fat metabolism may be disturbed. **Additives should not be mixed with fat emulsions unless compatibility is known.**

Administration
Because of the complex requirements relating to parenteral nutrition full details relating to administration have been omitted. In all cases *product literature and other specialist literature should be consulted.*

NUTRIENTS > PARENTERAL NUTRITION

Parenteral nutrition supplements

● INDICATIONS AND DOSE

DIPEPTIVEN 20G/100ML CONCENTRATE FOR SOLUTION FOR INFUSION BOTTLES

Amino acid supplement for hypercatabolic or hypermetabolic states

▶ BY INTRAVENOUS INFUSION

▶ Adult: 300–400 mg/kg daily, dose not to exceed 20% of total amino acid intake

● CAUTIONS

PEDITRACE SOLUTION FOR INFUSION 10ML VIALS Reduced biliary excretion · reduced biliary excretion in cholestatic liver disease · reduced biliary excretion in markedly reduced urinary excretion (careful biochemical monitoring required) · total parenteral nutrition exceeding one month

CAUTIONS, FURTHER INFORMATION

▶ Total parenteral nutrition exceeding one month Measure serum manganese concentration and check liver function before commencing treatment and regularly during treatment— discontinue if manganese concentration raised or if cholestasis develops.

● DIRECTIONS FOR ADMINISTRATION Because of the complex requirements relating to parenteral nutrition, full details relating to administration have been omitted. In all cases *specialist pharmacy advice, product literature, and other specialist literature should be consulted.* Compatibility with the infusion solution must be ascertained before adding supplementary preparations. **Additives should not be mixed with fat emulsions unless compatibility is known.**

CERNEVIT SOLUTION FOR INJECTION VIALS AND DILUENT Dissolve in 5 mL water for injections.

PEDITRACE SOLUTION FOR INFUSION 10ML VIALS For addition to *Vaminolact* ®, *Vamin* ® 14 *Electrolyte-Free* solutions, and glucose intravenous infusions.

TRACUTIL® AMPOULES For addition to infusion solutions.

DECAN CONCENTRATE FOR SOLUTION FOR INFUSION 40ML BOTTLES For addition to infusion solutions.

ADDIPHOS® VIALS For addition to *Vamin* ® solutions and glucose intravenous infusions.

DIPEPTIVEN 20G/100ML CONCENTRATE FOR SOLUTION FOR INFUSION BOTTLES For addition to infusion solutions containing amino acids.

ADDITRACE SOLUTION FOR INFUSION 10ML AMPOULES For adddition to *Vamin* ® solutions and glucose intravenous infusions.

GLYCOPHOS® VIALS For addition to *Vamin* ® and *Vaminolact* ® solutions, and glucose intravenous infusions.

SOLIVITO N POWDER FOR SOLUTION FOR INFUSION VIALS Dissolve in water for injections or glucose intravenous infusion for adding to glucose intravenous infusion or *Intralipid* ®; dissolve in *Vitlipid N* ® or *Intralipid* ® for adding to *Intralipid* ® only.

VITLIPID N INFANT EMULSION FOR INJECTION 10ML AMPOULES For addition to *Intralipid* ®.

VITLIPID N ADULT EMULSION FOR INJECTION 10ML AMPOULES For addition to *Intralipid* ®.

● PRESCRIBING AND DISPENSING INFORMATION

CERNEVIT SOLUTION FOR INJECTION VIALS AND DILUENT *Cernevit* ® solution contains *dl*-alpha tocopherol 11.2 units, ascorbic acid 125 mg, biotin 69 micrograms, colecalciferol 220 units, cyanocobalamin 6 micrograms, folic acid 414 micrograms, glycine 250 mg, nicotinamide 46 mg, pantothenic acid (as dexpanthenol) 17.25 mg, pyridoxine hydrochloride 5.5 mg, retinol (as palmitate) 3500 units, riboflavin (as dihydrated sodium phosphate) 4.14 mg, thiamine (as cocarboxylase tetrahydrate) 3.51 mg.

PEDITRACE SOLUTION FOR INFUSION 10ML VIALS *Peditrace* ® solution contains traces of Zn^{2+}, Cu^{2+}, Mn^{2+}, Se^{4+}, F^-, I^-.

TRACUTIL® AMPOULES *Tracutil* ® solution contains trace elements Fe^{2+}, Zn^{2+}, Mn^{2+}, Cu^{2+}, Cr^{3+}, Se^{4+}, Mo^{6+}, I^-, F^-.

DECAN CONCENTRATE FOR SOLUTION FOR INFUSION 40ML BOTTLES For patients over 40 kg. *Decan* ® solution contains trace elements Fe^{2+}, Zn^{2+}, Cu^{2+}, Mn^{2+}, F^-, Co^{2+}, I^-, Se^{4+}, Mo^{6+}, Cr^{3+}.

ADDIPHOS® VIALS *Addiphos* ® sterile solution contains phosphate 40 mmol, K^+ 30 mmol, Na^+ 30 mmol/20 mL.

DIPEPTIVEN 20G/100ML CONCENTRATE FOR SOLUTION FOR INFUSION BOTTLES *Dipeptiven* ® solution contains N(2)-L-alanyl-L-glutamine 200 mg/mL (providing L-alanine 82 mg, L-glutamine 134.6 mg).

ADDITRACE SOLUTION FOR INFUSION 10ML AMPOULES For patients over 40 kg. *Additrace* ® solution contains traces of Fe^{3+}, Zn^{2+}, Mn^{2+}, Cu^{2+}, Cr^{3+}, Se^{4+}, Mo^{6+}, F^-, I^-.

GLYCOPHOS® VIALS *Glycophos* ® Sterile Concentrate solution contains phosphate 20 mmol, Na^+ 40 mmol/20 mL.

SOLIVITO N POWDER FOR SOLUTION FOR INFUSION VIALS *Solivito N* ® powder for reconstitution contains biotin 60 micrograms, cyanocobalamin 5 micrograms, folic acid 400 micrograms, glycine 300 mg, nicotinamide 40 mg, pyridoxine hydrochloride 4.9 mg, riboflavin sodium phosphate 4.9 mg, sodium ascorbate 113 mg, sodium pantothenate 16.5 mg, thiamine mononitrate 3.1 mg.

VITLIPID N INFANT EMULSION FOR INJECTION 10ML AMPOULES *Vitlipid N* ® infant emulsion contains vitamin A 230 units, ergocalciferol 40 units, *dl*-alpha tocopherol 0.7 unit, phytomenadione 20 micrograms/mL.

VITLIPID N ADULT EMULSION FOR INJECTION 10ML AMPOULES *Vitlipid N* ® adult emulsion contains vitamin A 330 units, ergocalciferol 20 units, *dl*-alpha tocopherol 1 unit, phytomenadione 15 micrograms/mL. For adults and children over 11 years.

● MEDICINAL FORMS
There can be variation in the licensing of different medicines containing the same drug. Forms available from special-order manufacturers include: solution for infusion

Solution for injection
▶ Cernevit (Baxter Healthcare Ltd)
Alpha tocopherol 11.2 unit, Cyanocobalamin 6 microgram, Biotin 69 microgram, Folic acid 414 microgram, Thiamine 3.51 mg, Riboflavin (as Riboflavin sodium phosphate) 4.14 mg, Pyridoxine (as Pyridoxine hydrochloride) 4.53 mg, Ascorbic acid 125 mg, Colecalciferol 220 unit, Pantothenic acid (as Dexpanthenol) 17.25 mg, Nicotinamide 46 mg, Retinol 3500 unit Cernevit solution for injection vials and diluent | 10 vial PoM no price available

9

Blood and nutrition

9

Blood and nutrition

Emulsion for injection

▸ Vitlipid N Adult (Fresenius Kabi Ltd)
Alpha tocopherol 910 microgram per 1 ml, Ergocalciferol
500 nanogram per 1 ml, Phytomenadione 15 microgram per 1 ml,
Retinol palmitate 99 microgram per 1 ml Vitlipid N Adult emulsion
for injection 10ml ampoules | 1 ampoule [PoM] £1.97 |
10 ampoule [PoM] no price available

▸ Vitlipid N Infant (Fresenius Kabi Ltd)
Ergocalciferol 1 microgram per 1 ml, Phytomenadione
20 microgram per 1 ml, Retinol palmitate 69 microgram per 1 ml,
Alpha tocopherol 640 microgram per 1 ml Vitlipid N Infant
emulsion for injection 10ml ampoules | 1 ampoule [PoM] £1.97 |
10 ampoule [PoM] no price available

Solution for infusion

▸ Parenteral nutrition supplements (Non-proprietary)
Sodium glycerophosphate 216 mg per 1 ml Sodium
glycerophosphate 4.32g/20ml concentrate for solution for infusion
vials | 1 vial [PoM] £4.83 | 10 vial [PoM] no price available

▸ Additrace (Fresenius Kabi Ltd)
Sodium molybdate 4.85 microgram per 1 ml, Chromic chloride
5.33 microgram per 1 ml, Sodium selenite 10.5 microgram per
1 ml, Potassium iodide 16.6 microgram per 1 ml, Manganese
chloride 99 microgram per 1 ml, Sodium fluoride 210 microgram
per 1 ml, Copper chloride 340 microgram per 1 ml, Ferric chloride
544 microgram per 1 ml, Zinc chloride 1.36 mg per 1 ml Additrace
solution for infusion 10ml ampoules | 1 ampoule [PoM] £1.96 |
20 ampoule [PoM] no price available

▸ Dipeptiven (Fresenius Kabi Ltd)
N(2)-L-alanyl-L-glutamine 200 mg per 1 ml Dipeptiven 20g/100ml
concentrate for solution for infusion bottles | 1 bottle [PoM] £25.93 |
10 bottle [PoM] no price available
Dipeptiven 10g/50ml concentrate for solution for infusion bottles |
1 bottle [PoM] £13.94 | 10 bottle [PoM] no price available

▸ Peditrace (Fresenius Kabi Ltd)
Manganese (as Manganese chloride) 1 microgram per 1 ml, Iodine
(as Potassium iodide) 1 microgram per 1 ml, Selenium (as Sodium
selenite) 2 microgram per 1 ml, Copper (as Copper chloride)
20 microgram per 1 ml, Fluoride (as Sodium fluoride)
57 microgram per 1 ml, Zinc (as Zinc chloride) 250 microgram per
1 ml Peditrace solution for infusion 10ml vials | 1 vial [PoM] £3.55 |
10 vial [PoM] no price available

▸ Tracutil (B.Braun Medical Ltd)
Sodium molybdate dihydrate 2.42 microgram per 1 ml, Chromic
chloride 5.3 microgram per 1 ml, Sodium selenite pentahydrate
7.89 microgram per 1 ml, Potassium iodide 16.6 microgram per
1 ml, Sodium fluoride 126 microgram per 1 ml, Manganese
chloride 197.9 microgram per 1 ml, Copper chloride
204.6 microgram per 1 ml, Zinc chloride 681.5 microgram per
1 ml, Ferrous chloride 695.8 microgram per 1 ml Tracutil
concentrate for solution for infusion 10ml ampoules |
5 ampoule [PoM] £7.96

Powder for solution for infusion

▸ Solivito N (Fresenius Kabi Ltd)
Cyanocobalamin 5 microgram, Biotin 60 microgram, Folic acid
400 microgram, Thiamine nitrate 3.1 mg, Pyridoxine
hydrochloride 4.9 mg, Riboflavin sodium phosphate 4.9 mg,
Sodium pantothenate 16.5 mg, Nicotinamide 40 mg, Sodium
ascorbate 113 mg Solivito N powder for solution for infusion vials |
1 vial [PoM] £1.97 | 10 vial [PoM] no price available

5   Nutrition (oral)

Enteral nutrition

Overview

The body's reserves of protein rapidly become exhausted in
severely ill patients, especially during chronic illness or in
those with severe burns, extensive trauma, pancreatitis, or
intestinal fistula. Much can be achieved by frequent meals
and by persuading the patient to take supplementary snacks
of ordinary food between the meals.

However, extra calories, protein, other nutrients, and
vitamins are often best given by supplementing ordinary
meals with enteral sip or tube feeds.

When patients cannot feed normally, for example, patients
with severe facial injury, oesophageal obstruction, or coma, a
nutritionally complete diet of enteral feeds must be given.
The advice of a dietitian should be sought to determine the
protein and total energy requirement of the patient and the
form and relative contribution of carbohydrate and fat to the
energy requirements.

Most enteral feeds contain protein derived from cows' milk
or soya. Elemental feeds containing protein hydrolysates or
free amino acids can be used for patients who have
diminished ability to break down protein, for example in
inflammatory bowel disease or pancreatic insufficiency.

Even when nutritionally complete feeds are given, water
and electrolyte balance should be monitored.
Haematological and biochemical parameters should also be
monitored, particularly in clinically unstable patients. Extra
minerals (e.g. magnesium and zinc) may be needed in
patients where gastro-intestinal secretions are being lost.
Additional vitamins may also be needed.

Enteral nutrition in children

Children have special requirements and in most situations
liquid feeds prepared for adults are totally unsuitable—the
advice of a paediatric dietitian should be sought.

5.1   Special diets

Nutrition in special diets

Overview

These are preparations that have been modified to eliminate
a particular constituent from a food or that are nutrient
mixtures formulated as food substitutes for patients who
either cannot tolerate or cannot metabolise certain common
constituents of food. In certain clinical conditions, some
food preparations are regarded as drugs and can be
prescribed within the NHS if they have been approved by the
Advisory Committee on Borderline Substances (ACBS).

Phenylketonuria

Phenylketonuria (hyperphenylalaninaemia, PKU), which
results from the inability to metabolise **phenylalanine**, is
managed by restricting dietary intake of **phenylalanine** to a
small amount sufficient for tissue building and repair.

Sapropterin dihydrochloride p. 935, a synthetic form of
tetrahydrobiopterin, is licensed as an adjunct to dietary
restriction of **phenylalanine** in the management of patients
with *phenylketonuria* and *tetrahydrobiopterin deficiency*.

Aspartame (used as a sweetener in some foods and
medicines) contributes to the **phenylalanine** intake and
may affect control of *phenylketonuria*. Where the presence of
aspartame is specified in the product literature this is
indicated in the BNF against the preparation; the patient
should be informed of this.

Coeliac disease

Intolerance to **gluten** in *coeliac disease* is managed by
completely eliminating **gluten** from the diet. A range of
gluten-free products is available for prescription.

5.1a Phenylketonuria

DRUGS FOR METABOLIC DISORDERS ›
TETRAHYDROBIOPTERIN AND DERIVATIVES

Sapropterin dihydrochloride

● **INDICATIONS AND DOSE**

Phenylketonuria (adjunct to dietary restriction of phenylalanine) (specialist use only)
▸ BY MOUTH
▸ Adult: Initially 10 mg/kg once daily, adjusted according to response; usual dose 5–20 mg/kg once daily, dose to be taken preferably in the morning

Tetrahydrobiopterin deficiency (adjunct to dietary restriction of phenylalanine) (specialist use only)
▸ BY MOUTH
▸ Adult: Initially 2–5 mg/kg once daily, adjusted according to response, dose to be taken preferably in the morning, the total daily dose may alternatively be given in 2–3 divided doses; maximum 20 mg/kg per day

● CAUTIONS History of convulsions
● SIDE-EFFECTS
▸ **Common or very common** Abdominal pain · cough · diarrhoea · headache · nasal congestion · pharyngolaryngeal pain · vomiting
▸ **Frequency not known** Hypersensitivity reactions
● PREGNANCY Manufacturer advises caution—consider only if strict dietary management inadequate.
● BREAST FEEDING Manufacturer advises avoid—no information available.
● HEPATIC IMPAIRMENT Manufacturer advises caution—no information available.
● RENAL IMPAIRMENT Manufacturer advises caution—no information available.
● MONITORING REQUIREMENTS
▸ Monitor blood-phenylalanine concentration before and after first week of treatment—if unsatisfactory response increase dose at weekly intervals to max. dose and monitor blood-phenylalanine concentration weekly; discontinue treatment if unsatisfactory response after 1 month.
▸ Monitor blood-phenylalanine and tyrosine concentrations 1–2 weeks after dose adjustment and during treatment.
● DIRECTIONS FOR ADMINISTRATION Tablets should be dissolved in water and taken within 20 minutes.
● PRESCRIBING AND DISPENSING INFORMATION Sapropterin is a synthetic form of tetrahydrobiopterin.
● PATIENT AND CARER ADVICE Patient or carers should be given advice on how to administer sapropterin dihydrochloride dispersible tablets.

● MEDICINAL FORMS
There can be variation in the licensing of different medicines containing the same drug.
Tablet
▸ Sapropterin dihydrochloride (Non-proprietary)
Sapropterin dihydrochloride 10 mg Tetrahydrobiopterin 10mg tablets | 100 tablet [PoM] no price available
Soluble tablet
CAUTIONARY AND ADVISORY LABELS 13, 21
▸ Kuvan (BioMarin Europe Ltd)
Sapropterin dihydrochloride 100 mg Kuvan 100mg soluble tablets sugar-free | 30 tablet [PoM] £597.22

6 Vitamin deficiency

Vitamins

Overview

Vitamins are used for the prevention and treatment of specific deficiency states or where the diet is known to be inadequate; they may be prescribed in the NHS to prevent or treat deficiency but not as dietary supplements.

Their use as general 'pick-me-ups' is of unproven value and, in the case of preparations containing vitamin A or D, may actually be harmful if patients take more than the prescribed dose. The 'fad' for mega-vitamin therapy with water-soluble vitamins, such as ascorbic acid p. 939 and pyridoxine hydrochloride p. 937, is unscientific and can be harmful.

Dietary reference values for vitamins are available in the Department of Health publication:

Dietary Reference Values for Food Energy and Nutrients for the United Kingdom: Report of the Panel on Dietary Reference Values of the Committee on Medical Aspects of Food Policy. *Report on Health and Social Subjects* 41. London: HMSO, 1991.

Dental patients

It is unjustifiable to treat stomatitis or glossitis with mixtures of vitamin preparations; this delays diagnosis and correct treatment.

Most patients who develop a nutritional deficiency despite an adequate intake of vitamins have malabsorption and if this is suspected the patient should be referred to a medical practitioner.

Vitamin A

Deficiency of vitamin A (retinol) p. 937 is associated with ocular defects (particularly xerophthalmia) and an increased susceptibility to infections, but deficiency is rare in the UK (even in disorders of fat absorption).

Vitamin B group

Deficiency of the B vitamins, other than vitamin B_{12}, is rare in the UK and is usually treated by preparations containing thiamine (B_1), riboflavin (B_2), and nicotinamide, which is used in preference to nicotinic acid, as it does not cause vasodilatation see p. 938. Other members (or substances traditionally classified as members) of the vitamin B complex such as aminobenzoic acid, biotin, choline, inositol nicotinate, and pantothenic acid or panthenol may be included in vitamin B preparations but there is no evidence of their value.

The severe deficiency states Wernicke's encephalopathy and Korsakoff's psychosis, especially as seen in chronic alcoholism, are best treated initially by the parenteral administration of B vitamins (*Pabrinex*®), followed by oral administration of thiamine in the longer term. Anaphylaxis has been reported with parenteral B vitamins.

As with other vitamins of the B group, pyridoxine hydrochloride (B_6) deficiency is rare, but it may occur during isoniazid p. 532 therapy or penicillamine p. 952 treatment in Wilson's disease and is characterised by peripheral neuritis. High doses of pyridoxine hydrochloride are given in some metabolic disorders, such as hyperoxaluria, and it is also used in sideroblastic anaemia. There is evidence to suggest that pyridoxine hydrochloride may provide some benefit in premenstrual syndrome. It has been tried for a wide variety of other disorders, but there is little sound evidence to support the claims of efficacy.

Nicotinic acid inhibits the synthesis of cholesterol and triglyceride. Folic acid p. 886 and vitamin B_{12} are used in the treatment of megaloblastic anaemia. Folinic acid p. 827

(available as calcium folinate) is used in association with cytotoxic therapy.

Vitamin C

Vitamin C (ascorbic acid) therapy is essential in scurvy, but less florid manifestations of vitamin C deficiency are commonly found, especially in the elderly.

Severe scurvy causes gingival swelling and bleeding margins as well as petechiae on the skin. This is, however, exceedingly rare and a patient with these signs is more likely to have leukaemia. Investigation should not be delayed by a trial period of vitamin treatment.

Claims that vitamin C ameliorates colds or promotes wound healing have not been proven.

Vitamin D

The term Vitamin D is used for a range of compounds which possess the property of preventing or curing rickets. They include ergocalciferol (calciferol, vitamin D$_2$) p. 943, colecalciferol (vitamin D$_3$) p. 941, dihydrotachysterol p. 943, alfacalcidol (1α-hydroxycholecalciferol) p. 940, and calcitriol (1,25-dihydroxycholecalciferol) p. 941.

Simple vitamin D deficiency can be prevented by taking an oral supplement of ergocalciferol (calciferol, vitamin D$_2$) or colecalciferol (vitamin D$_3$) daily. Vitamin D deficiency can occur in people whose exposure to sunlight is limited and in those whose diet is deficient in vitamin D. In these individuals, ergocalciferol or colecalciferol daily by mouth may be given to treat vitamin D deficiency; higher doses may be necessary for *severe* deficiency. Patients who do not respond should be referred to a specialist.

Preparations containing colecalciferol with calcium carbonate p. 942 are available for the management of combined calcium and vitamin D deficiency, or for those at high risk of deficiency.

Vitamin D deficiency caused by *intestinal malabsorption* or *chronic liver disease* usually requires vitamin D in pharmacological doses.

Vitamin D requires hydroxylation by the kidney to its active form, therefore the hydroxylated derivatives alfacalcidol or calcitriol should be prescribed if patients with *severe renal impairment* require vitamin D therapy. Calcitriol is also licensed for the management of postmenopausal osteoporosis.

Paricalcitol p. 944, a synthetic vitamin D analogue, is licensed for the prevention and treatment of secondary hyperparathyroidism associated with chronic renal failure.

Vitamin E

The daily requirement of vitamin E (tocopherol) has not been well defined but is probably 3 to 15 mg daily. There is little evidence that oral supplements of vitamin E are essential in adults, even where there is fat malabsorption secondary to cholestasis. In young children with congenital cholestasis, abnormally low vitamin E concentrations may be found in association with neuromuscular abnormalities, which usually respond only to the parenteral administration of vitamin E.

Vitamin E has been tried for various other conditions but there is little scientific evidence of its value.

Vitamin K

Vitamin K is necessary for the production of blood clotting factors and proteins necessary for the normal calcification of bone.

Because vitamin K is fat soluble, patients with fat malabsorption, especially in biliary obstruction or hepatic disease, may become deficient. Menadiol sodium phosphate p. 945 is a water-soluble synthetic vitamin K derivative that can be given orally to prevent vitamin K deficiency in malabsorption syndromes.

Oral coumarin anticoagulants act by interfering with vitamin K metabolism in the hepatic cells and their effects can be antagonised by giving vitamin K.

Other compounds

Potassium aminobenzoate p. 937 has been used in the treatment of various disorders associated with excessive fibrosis such as scleroderma and Peyronie's disease. In Peyronie's disease there is some evidence to support efficacy in reducing progression when given early in the disease; however, there is no evidence for reversal of the condition. The therapeutic value of potassium aminobenzoate p. 937 in scleroderma is doubtful.

VITAMINS AND TRACE ELEMENTS ›
MULTIVITAMINS

Vitamins A and D

- ● INDICATIONS AND DOSE

Prevention of vitamin A and D deficiency
▸ BY MOUTH
- ▸ Child: 1 capsule daily, 1 capsule contains 4000 units vitamin A and 400 units (10 micrograms) vitamin D
- ▸ Adult: (consult product literature)

- ● UNLICENSED USE
- ▸ In children Not licensed in children under 6 months of age.
- ● INTERACTIONS → Appendix 1 (vitamins).
- ● SIDE-EFFECTS

Overdose
Excessive ingestion Prolonged excessive ingestion of vitamins A and D can lead to hypervitaminosis.

- ● PRESCRIBING AND DISPENSING INFORMATION This drug contains vitamin D; consult individual vitamin D monographs.

- ● MEDICINAL FORMS
There can be variation in the licensing of different medicines containing the same drug.
Capsule
- ▸ Vitamins A and D (Non-proprietary)
Vitamin D 400 unit, Vitamin A 4000 unit Vitamins A and D capsules BPC 1973 | 28 capsule £2.81 | 28 capsule GSL £2.81 | 84 capsule £8.42 DT price = £8.42

Vitamins A, C and D

The properties listed below are those particular to the combination only. For the properties of the components please consider, vitamin A p. 937, ascorbic acid p. 939.

- ● INDICATIONS AND DOSE

Prevention of vitamin deficiency
▸ BY MOUTH
- ▸ Child 1 month-4 years: 5 drops daily, 5 drops contain vitamin A approx. 700 units, vitamin D approx. 300 units (7.5 micrograms), ascorbic acid approx. 20 mg

- ● PRESCRIBING AND DISPENSING INFORMATION This drug contains vitamin D; consult individual vitamin D monographs.
Available free of charge to children under 4 years in families on the Healthy Start Scheme, or alternatively may be available direct to the public—further information for healthcare professionals can be accessed at www.healthystart.nhs.uk. Beneficiaries can contact their midwife or health visitor for further information on where to obtain supplies.
Healthy Start Vitamins for women (containing ascorbic acid, vitamin D, and folic acid) are also available free of charge to women on the Healthy Start Scheme during

pregnancy and until their baby is one year old, or alternatively may be available direct to the public—further information for healthcare professionals can be accessed at www.healthystart.nhs.uk. Beneficiaries can contact their midwife or health visitor for further information on where to obtain supplies.

● MEDICINAL FORMS
There can be variation in the licensing of different medicines containing the same drug.
Oral drops
▶ Healthy Start Children's Vitamin (Secretary of State for Health)
Vitamin A and D3 concentrate.55 mg per 1 ml, Sodium ascorbate 18.58 mg per 1 ml, Ascorbic acid 150 mg per 1 ml, Vitamin D 2000 iu per 1 ml, Vitamin A 5000 iu per 1 ml Healthy Start Children's Vitamin drops | 10 ml no price available

VITAMINS AND TRACE ELEMENTS ⟩ VITAMIN A

Vitamin A

(Retinol)

● INDICATIONS AND DOSE
Vitamin A deficiency
▶ BY MOUTH
▶ Child 1–11 months: 5000 units daily, to be taken with or after food, higher doses may be used initially for treatment of severe deficiency
▶ Child 1–17 years: 10 000 units daily, to be taken with or after food, higher doses may be used initially for treatment of severe deficiency

● UNLICENSED USE Preparations containing only vitamin A are not licensed.
● INTERACTIONS → Appendix 1 (vitamins).
● SIDE-EFFECTS
Overdose
Massive overdose can cause rough skin, dry hair, an enlarged liver, and a raised erythrocyte sedimentation rate and raised serum calcium and serum alkaline phosphatase concentrations.
● PREGNANCY Excessive doses may be teratogenic. In view of evidence suggesting that high levels of vitamin A may cause birth defects, women who are (or may become) pregnant are advised not to take vitamin A supplements (including tablets and fish liver oil drops), except on the advice of a doctor or an antenatal clinic; nor should they eat liver or products such as liver paté or liver sausage.
● BREAST FEEDING Theoretical risk of toxicity in infants of mothers taking large doses.
● MONITORING REQUIREMENTS Treatment is sometimes initiated with very high doses of vitamin A and the child should be monitored closely; very high doses are associated with acute toxicity.

● MEDICINAL FORMS
There can be variation in the licensing of different medicines containing the same drug. Forms available from special-order manufacturers include: drops
Drops
▶ Vitamin A (Non-proprietary)
Vitamin A 150000 unit per 1 ml Arovit 150,000units/ml drops | 7.5 ml PoM no price available

Combinations available: *Vitamins A, C and D,* p. 936

VITAMINS AND TRACE ELEMENTS ⟩ VITAMIN B GROUP

Potassium aminobenzoate

● INDICATIONS AND DOSE
Peyronie's disease | Scleroderma
▶ BY MOUTH
▶ Adult: 12 g daily in divided doses, to be taken after food

● INTERACTIONS → Appendix 1 (potassium aminobenzoate).

● MEDICINAL FORMS
There can be variation in the licensing of different medicines containing the same drug.
Capsule
CAUTIONARY AND ADVISORY LABELS 21
▶ Potaba (Cheplapharm Arzneimittel GmbH)
Potassium aminobenzoate 500 mg Potaba 500mg capsules | 240 capsule P £44.75
Powder
CAUTIONARY AND ADVISORY LABELS 13, 21
▶ Potaba (Cheplapharm Arzneimittel GmbH)
Potassium aminobenzoate 3 gram Potaba 3g sachets | 40 sachet P £34.31

Pyridoxine hydrochloride

(Vitamin B$_6$)

● INDICATIONS AND DOSE
Deficiency states
▶ BY MOUTH
▶ Adult: 20–50 mg 1–3 times a day
Isoniazid-induced neuropathy (prophylaxis)
▶ BY MOUTH
▶ Adult: 10–20 mg daily
Isoniazid-induced neuropathy (treatment)
▶ BY MOUTH
▶ Adult: 50 mg 3 times a day
Idiopathic sideroblastic anaemia
▶ BY MOUTH
▶ Adult: 100–400 mg daily in divided doses
Prevention of penicillamine-induced neuropathy in Wilson's disease
▶ BY MOUTH
▶ Adult: 20 mg daily
Premenstrual syndrome
▶ BY MOUTH
▶ Adult: 50–100 mg daily

● UNLICENSED USE Not licensed for prophylaxis of penicillamine-induced neuropathy in Wilson's disease. Not licensed for treatment of premenstrual syndrome.

> IMPORTANT SAFETY INFORMATION
> Prolonged use of pyridoxine in a dose of 10 mg daily is considered safe but the long-term use of pyridoxine in a dose of 200 mg or more daily has been associated with neuropathy. The safety of long-term pyridoxine supplementation with doses above 10 mg daily has not been established.

● INTERACTIONS → Appendix 1 (vitamins).
● SIDE-EFFECTS Sensory neuropathy (with high doses when given for extended periods)
Overdose
Overdosage induces toxic effects.

9

Blood and nutrition

● MEDICINAL FORMS
There can be variation in the licensing of different medicines containing the same drug. Forms available from special-order manufacturers include: capsule, oral suspension, oral solution

Tablet
▸ Pyridoxine hydrochloride (Non-proprietary)
Pyridoxine hydrochloride 10 mg Pyridoxine 10mg tablets | 28 tablet £12.95–£14.50 | 28 tablet GSL no price available | 30 tablet GSL no price available | 60 tablet GSL no price available | 60 tablet no price available | 500 tablet £8.48 | 500 tablet GSL no price available
Pyridoxine (as Pyridoxine hydrochloride) 20 mg Pyridoxine 20mg tablets | 500 tablet GSL no price available | 500 tablet no price available
Pyridoxine hydrochloride 50 mg Pyridoxine 50mg tablets | 28 tablet P no price available DT price = £5.95 | 28 tablet GSL £6.62 DT price = £5.95 | 500 tablet P no price available

Capsule
▸ Pyridoxine hydrochloride (Non-proprietary)
Pyridoxine (as Pyridoxine hydrochloride) 100 mg capsules | 100 capsule no price available

Solution for injection
▸ Pyridoxine hydrochloride (Non-proprietary)
Pyridoxine hydrochloride 50 mg per 1 ml Vitamin B6 Streuli 100mg/2ml solution for injection ampoules | 10 ampoule PoM no price available

Thiamine

(Vitamin B₁)

● INDICATIONS AND DOSE
Mild deficiency
▸ BY MOUTH
▸ Adult: 25–100 mg daily
Severe deficiency
▸ BY MOUTH
▸ Adult: 200–300 mg daily in divided doses

IMPORTANT SAFETY INFORMATION
MHRA/CHM ADVICE (SEPTEMBER 2007)
Although potentially serious allergic adverse reactions may rarely occur during, or shortly after, parenteral administration, the CHM has recommended that:
• This should not preclude the use of parenteral thiamine in patients where this route of administration is required, particularly in patients at risk of Wernicke-Korsakoff syndrome where treatment with thiamine is essential;
• Intravenous administration should be by infusion over 30 minutes;
• Facilities for treating anaphylaxis (including resuscitation facilities) should be available when parenteral thiamine is administered.

● CAUTIONS Anaphylaxis may occasionally follow injection
● BREAST FEEDING Severely thiamine-deficient mothers should avoid breast-feeding as toxic methyl-glyoxal present in milk.
● PRESCRIBING AND DISPENSING INFORMATION
▸ With intramuscular use or intravenous use Some preparations may contain phenol as a preservative.

● MEDICINAL FORMS
There can be variation in the licensing of different medicines containing the same drug. Forms available from special-order manufacturers include: oral suspension, oral solution

Tablet
▸ Thiamine (Non-proprietary)
Thiamine hydrochloride 50 mg Thiamine 50mg tablets | 28 tablet P £1.80–£2.00 | 100 tablet P £7.13 DT price = £7.13 | 100 tablet no price available DT price = £7.13

Thiamine hydrochloride 100 mg Thiamine 100mg tablets | 28 tablet P £2.50–£2.82 | 100 tablet no price available DT price = £9.99 | 100 tablet P £10.08 DT price = £9.99
▸ Tyvera (Auden McKenzie (Pharma Division) Ltd, Almus Pharmaceuticals Ltd, Teva UK Ltd)
Thiamine hydrochloride 50 mg Tyvera 50mg tablets | 100 tablet P £4.99–£7.13 DT price = £7.13
Thiamine hydrochloride 100 mg Tyvera 100mg tablets | 100 tablet P £6.99–£10.13 DT price = £9.99

Modified-release tablet
▸ Thiamine (Non-proprietary)
Thiamine hydrochloride 100 mg HealthAid Vitamin B1 100mg modified-release tablets | 90 tablet £4.18

Vitamin B complex

● INDICATIONS AND DOSE
Treatment of deficiency
▸ BY MOUTH USING TABLETS
▸ Adult: 1–2 tablets 3 times a day, this dose is for vitamin B compound **strong** tablets
Prophylaxis of deficiency
▸ BY MOUTH USING TABLETS
▸ Adult: 1–2 tablets daily, this dose is for vitamin B compound tablets

● NATIONAL FUNDING/ACCESS DECISIONS
Vigranon® syrup is not prescribable under the National Health Service (NHS).
● LESS SUITABLE FOR PRESCRIBING Vitamin B compound tablets and vitamin B compound strong tablets are less suitable for prescribing.

● MEDICINAL FORMS
There can be variation in the licensing of different medicines containing the same drug.
Tablet
▸ Vitamin B complex (Non-proprietary)
Riboflavin 1 mg, Thiamine hydrochloride 1 mg, Nicotinamide 15 mg Vitamin B compound tablets | 28 tablet P no price available DT price = £26.63 | 28 tablet GSL £26.63 DT price = £26.63 | 100 tablet GSL £95.11 | 1000 tablet £10.50
Pyridoxine hydrochloride 2 mg, Riboflavin 2 mg, Thiamine hydrochloride 5 mg, Nicotinamide 20 mg Vitamin B compound strong tablets | 28 tablet GSL £1.71–£6.95 DT price = £1.55 | 28 tablet P no price available DT price = £1.55 | 1000 tablet no price available | 1000 tablet P no price available

Vitamin B substances with ascorbic acid

The properties listed below are those particular to the combination only. For the properties of the components please consider, thiamine above, ascorbic acid p. 939.

● INDICATIONS AND DOSE
Parenteral vitamins B and C for rapid correction of severe depletion or malabsorption (e.g. in alcoholism, after acute infections, postoperatively, or in psychiatric states) | Maintenance of vitamins B and C in chronic intermittent haemodialysis
▸ BY INTRAVENOUS INFUSION
▸ Adult: See MHRA/CHM advice in thiamine monograph (consult product literature).
Treatment of Wernicke's encephalopathy
▸ INITIALLY BY INTRAVENOUS INFUSION
▸ Adult: 2–3 pairs 3 times a day for 2 days, discontinue if no response, continue treatment if symptoms respond after 2 days; (by intravenous infusion or by deep intramuscular injection) 1 pair once daily for 5 days or for as long as improvement continues, give deep intramuscular injection into the gluteal muscle

Prophylaxis of Wernicke's encephalopathy in alcohol dependence
▸ BY INTRAVENOUS INFUSION, OR BY DEEP INTRAMUSCULAR INJECTION
▸ Adult: 1 pair once daily for at least 3–5 days, give deep intramuscular injection into the gluteal muscle

Psychosis following narcosis or electroconvulsive therapy | Toxicity from acute infections
▸ BY INTRAVENOUS INFUSION, OR BY DEEP INTRAMUSCULAR INJECTION
▸ Adult: 1 pair twice daily for up to 7 days, give deep intramuscular injection into the gluteal muscle

Haemodialysis
▸ BY INTRAVENOUS INFUSION
▸ Adult: 1 pair every 2 weeks

● UNLICENSED USE *Pabrinex*® doses in BNF may differ from those in product literature.

● DIRECTIONS FOR ADMINISTRATION Give (*Pabrinex*® *I/V High Potency*) intermittently *or via* drip tubing *in* Glucose 5% *or* Sodium chloride 0.9%. Ampoules contents should be mixed, diluted, and administered without delay; give over 30 minutes.

● PRESCRIBING AND DISPENSING INFORMATION Some formulations of *Pabrinex*® may contain benzyl alcohol. *Pabrinex*® I/M High Potency injection is for intramuscular use only. *Pabrinex*® I/V High Potency injection is for intravenous use only.

● MEDICINAL FORMS
There can be variation in the licensing of different medicines containing the same drug.
Solution for injection
EXCIPIENTS: May contain Benzyl alcohol
▸ Pabrinex Intramuscular High Potency (ProStrakan Ltd)
Pabrinex Intramuscular High Potency solution for injection 5ml and 2ml ampoules | 20 ampoule [PoM] £22.53 DT price = £22.53
▸ Pabrinex Intravenous High Potency (ProStrakan Ltd)
Pabrinex Intravenous High Potency solution for injection 5ml and 5ml ampoules | 20 ampoule [PoM] £22.53 DT price = £22.53

Vitamins with minerals and trace elements

● INDICATIONS AND DOSE
FORCEVAL® CAPSULES

Vitamin and mineral deficiency and as adjunct in synthetic diets
▸ BY MOUTH
▸ Adult: 1 capsule daily, one hour after a meal

KETOVITE® LIQUID

Prevention of vitamin deficiency in disorders of carbohydrate or amino-acid metabolism | Adjunct in restricted, specialised, or synthetic diets
▸ BY MOUTH
▸ Adult: 5 mL daily, use with *Ketovite*® *Tablets* for complete vitamin supplementation.

KETOVITE® TABLETS

Prevention of vitamin deficiency in disorders of carbohydrate or amino-acid metabolism | Adjunct in restricted, specialised, or synthetic diets
▸ BY MOUTH
▸ Adult: 1 tablet 3 times a day, use with *Ketovite*® *Liquid* for complete vitamin supplementation.

● PRESCRIBING AND DISPENSING INFORMATION To avoid potential toxicity, the content of all vitamin preparations, particularly vitamin A, should be considered when used together with other supplements.

● PATIENT AND CARER ADVICE
KETOVITE® LIQUID *Ketovite*® liquid may be mixed with milk, cereal, or fruit juice.
KETOVITE® TABLETS Tablets may be crushed immediately before use.

● MEDICINAL FORMS
There can be variation in the licensing of different medicines containing the same drug.
Tablet
▸ Ketovite (Essential Pharmaceuticals Ltd)
Biotin 170 microgram, Folic acid 250 microgram, Pyridoxine hydrochloride 330 microgram, Acetomenaphthone 500 microgram, Riboflavin 1 mg, Thiamine hydrochloride 1 mg, Calcium pantothenate 1.16 mg, Nicotinamide 3.3 mg, Alpha tocopheryl acetate 5 mg, Ascorbic acid 16.6 mg, Inositol 50 mg Ketovite tablets | 100 tablet [PoM] £9.21
Capsule
▸ Forceval (Alliance Pharmaceuticals Ltd)
Cyanocobalamin 3 microgram, Selenium 50 microgram, Biotin 100 microgram, Iodine 140 microgram, Chromium 200 microgram, Molybdenum 250 microgram, Folic acid 400 microgram, Thiamine 1.2 mg, Riboflavin 1.6 mg, Copper 2 mg, Pyridoxine 2 mg, Manganese 3 mg, Pantothenic acid 4 mg, Potassium 4 mg, Tocopheryl acetate 10 mg, Iron 12 mg, Zinc 15 mg, Nicotinamide 18 mg, Magnesium 30 mg, Ascorbic acid 60 mg, Phosphorus 77 mg, Calcium 100 mg, Ergocalciferol 400 unit, Vitamin A 2500 unit Forceval capsules | 15 capsule [P] £4.42 | 30 capsule [P] £7.71 | 90 capsule [P] £18.62
Oral emulsion
▸ Ketovite (Non-proprietary)
Cyanocobalamin 2.5 microgram per 1 ml, Choline chloride 30 mg per 1 ml, Ergocalciferol 80 unit per 1 ml, Vitamin A 500 unit per 1 ml Ketovite liquid sugar-free | 150 ml [P] £19.10

VITAMINS AND TRACE ELEMENTS › VITAMIN C

Ascorbic acid
(Vitamin C)

● INDICATIONS AND DOSE
Prevention of scurvy
▸ BY MOUTH
▸ Adult: 25–75 mg daily
Treatment of scurvy
▸ BY MOUTH
▸ Adult: Not less than 250 mg daily in divided doses

● CAUTIONS
CAUTIONS, FURTHER INFORMATION
▸ Iron overload Ascorbic acid should not be given to patients with cardiac dysfunction.
In patients with normal cardiac function ascorbic acid should be introduced 1 month after starting desferrioxamine.

● INTERACTIONS → Appendix 1 (vitamins).

● PRESCRIBING AND DISPENSING INFORMATION It is rarely necessary to prescribe more than 100 mg daily except early in the treatment of scurvy.

● MEDICINAL FORMS
There can be variation in the licensing of different medicines containing the same drug. Forms available from special-order manufacturers include: oral suspension, oral solution
Tablet
EXCIPIENTS: May contain Aspartame
▸ Ascorbic acid (Non-proprietary)
Ascorbic acid 50 mg Ascorbic acid 50mg tablets | 28 tablet [GSL] £15.10 DT price = £15.01 | 28 tablet no price available DT price = £15.01 | 500 tablet [GSL] no price available
Ascorbic acid 100 mg Ascorbic acid 100mg tablets | 28 tablet no price available DT price = £14.30 | 28 tablet [GSL] £14.30 DT price = £14.30

9

Blood and nutrition

Ascorbic acid 200 mg Ascorbic acid 200mg tablets | 28 tablet no price available DT price = £19.89 | 28 tablet GSL £19.77 DT price = £19.89 | 100 tablet GSL no price available

Ascorbic acid 250 mg Ascorbic acid 250mg tablets | 1000 tablet PoM no price available

Ascorbic acid 500 mg Ascorbic acid 500mg tablets | 28 tablet GSL £26.87 DT price = £26.87 | 28 tablet no price available DT price = £26.87 | 100 tablet GSL no price available

Chewable tablet

CAUTIONARY AND ADVISORY LABELS 24
EXCIPIENTS: May contain Aspartame

▸ Ascorbic acid (Non-proprietary)

Ascorbic acid 60 mg chewable tablets | 60 tablet no price available | 180 tablet no price available

Ascorbic acid 500 mg chewable tablets

Ascorbic acid 1 gram chewable tablets | 30 tablet £2.30 | 60 tablet £4.20

▸ Ascur (Ennogen Healthcare Ltd)

Ascorbic acid 100 mg Ascur 100mg chewable tablets | 30 tablet £3.95

Ascorbic acid (as Sodium ascorbate) 500 mg Ascur 500mg chewable tablets sugar-free | 30 tablet £2.99

Capsule

▸ Ascorbic acid (Non-proprietary)

Ascorbic acid 500 mg capsules | 100 capsule no price available

Ascorbic acid 1 gram capsules | 100 capsule no price available | 250 capsule no price available

Combinations available: *Vitamin B substances with ascorbic acid*, p. 938 · *Vitamins A, C and D*, p. 936

VITAMINS AND TRACE ELEMENTS > VITAMIN D AND ANALOGUES

Vitamin D and analogues (systemic)

● CONTRA-INDICATIONS Hypercalcaemia · metastatic calcification

● INTERACTIONS → Appendix 1 (vitamins).

● SIDE-EFFECTS

Overdose

Symptoms of overdosage include anorexia, lassitude, nausea and vomiting, diarrhoea, constipation, weight loss, polyuria, sweating, headache, thirst, vertigo, and raised concentrations of calcium and phosphate in plasma and urine.

● PREGNANCY High doses teratogenic in *animals* but therapeutic doses unlikely to be harmful.

● BREAST FEEDING Caution with high doses; may cause hypercalcaemia in infant—monitor serum-calcium concentration.

● MONITORING REQUIREMENTS **Important:** All patients receiving pharmacological doses of vitamin D should have their plasma-calcium concentration checked at intervals (initially once or twice weekly) and whenever nausea or vomiting occur.

☞ above

Alfacalcidol

(1α-Hydroxycholecalciferol)

● INDICATIONS AND DOSE

Patients with severe renal impairment requiring vitamin D therapy

▸ BY MOUTH, OR BY INTRAVENOUS INJECTION

▸ **Adult:** Initially 1 microgram daily, dose to be adjusted to avoid hypercalcaemia; maintenance 0.25–1 microgram daily

▸ **Elderly:** Initially 500 nanograms daily, dose adjusted to avoid hypercalcaemia; maintenance 0.25–1 microgram daily

Hypophosphataemic rickets | Persistent hypocalcaemia due to hypoparathyroidism or pseudohypoparathyroidism

▸ BY MOUTH, OR BY INTRAVENOUS INJECTION

▸ **Child 1 month–11 years:** 25–50 nanograms/kg once daily, dose to be adjusted as necessary; maximum 1 microgram per day

▸ **Child 12–17 years:** 1 microgram once daily, dose to be adjusted as necessary

Prevention of vitamin D deficiency in renal or cholestatic liver disease

▸ BY MOUTH, OR BY INTRAVENOUS INJECTION

▸ **Child 1 month–11 years (body-weight up to 20 kg):** 15–30 nanograms/kg once daily (max. per dose 500 nanograms)

▸ **Child 1 month–11 years (body-weight 20 kg and above):** 250–500 nanograms once daily, dose to be adjusted as necessary

▸ **Child 12–17 years:** 250–500 nanograms once daily, dose to be adjusted as necessary

DOSE EQUIVALENCE AND CONVERSION

One drop of alfacalcidol 2 microgram/mL oral drops contains approximately 100 nanograms alfacalcidol.

● CAUTIONS Nephrolithiasis · take care to ensure correct dose in infants

● SIDE-EFFECTS

▸ **Rare** Nephrocalcinosis · pruritus · rash · urticaria

● RENAL IMPAIRMENT

Monitoring

Monitor plasma-calcium concentration in renal impairment.

● MONITORING REQUIREMENTS Monitor plasma-calcium concentration in patients receiving high doses.

● DIRECTIONS FOR ADMINISTRATION

▸ With intravenous use For injection, shake ampoule for at least 5 seconds before use, and give over 30 seconds.

● MEDICINAL FORMS

There can be variation in the licensing of different medicines containing the same drug. Forms available from special-order manufacturers include: oral suspension, oral solution

Capsule

EXCIPIENTS: May contain Sesame oil

▸ Alfacalcidol (Non-proprietary)

Alfacalcidol 250 nanogram Alfacalcidol 250nanogram capsules | 30 capsule PoM £6.33 DT price = £1.82

Alfacalcidol 500 nanogram Alfacalcidol 500nanogram capsules | 30 capsule PoM £10.00 DT price = £3.96

Alfacalcidol 1 microgram Alfacalcidol 1microgram capsules | 30 capsule no price available DT price = £4.19 | 30 capsule PoM £14.03 DT price = £4.19

▸ One-Alpha (LEO Pharma)

Alfacalcidol 250 nanogram One-Alpha 250nanogram capsules | 30 capsule PoM £3.37 DT price = £1.82

Alfacalcidol 500 nanogram One-Alpha 0.5microgram capsules | 30 capsule PoM £6.27 DT price = £3.96

Alfacalcidol 1 microgram One-Alpha 1microgram capsules | 30 capsule PoM £8.75 DT price = £4.19

Oral drops

EXCIPIENTS: May contain Alcohol

▸ One-Alpha (LEO Pharma)

Alfacalcidol 2 microgram per 1 ml One-Alpha 2micrograms/ml oral drops sugar-free | 10 ml PoM £21.30 DT price = £21.30

Solution for injection

EXCIPIENTS: May contain Alcohol, propylene glycol

▸ One-Alpha (LEO Pharma)

Alfacalcidol 2 microgram per 1 ml One-Alpha 2micrograms/1ml solution for injection ampoules | 10 ampoule PoM £41.13 One-Alpha 1micrograms/0.5ml solution for injection ampoules | 10 ampoule PoM £21.57

9

Blood and nutrition

⌐ 940

Calcitriol

(1,25-Dihydroxycholecalciferol)

● INDICATIONS AND DOSE

Renal osteodystrophy

▸ BY MOUTH

▸ Adult: Initially 250 nanograms daily, adjusted in steps of 250 nanograms every 2–4 weeks if required; usual dose 0.5–1 microgram daily

Renal osteodystrophy (in patients with normal or only slightly reduced plasma-calcium concentration)

▸ BY MOUTH

▸ Adult: Initially 250 nanograms once daily on alternate days, adjusted in steps of 250 nanograms every 2–4 weeks if required; usual dose 0.5–1 microgram daily

Established postmenopausal osteoporosis

▸ BY MOUTH

▸ Adult: 250 nanograms twice daily, plasma-calcium concentration and creatinine to be monitored (consult product literature)

● HEPATIC IMPAIRMENT Manufacturer advises avoid—no information available.

● RENAL IMPAIRMENT Manufacturer advises avoid—no information available. Monitor plasma-calcium concentration in renal impairment.

● MONITORING REQUIREMENTS Monitor plasma calcium, phosphate, and creatinine during dosage titration. Monitor plasma-calcium concentration in patients receiving high doses.

● DIRECTIONS FOR ADMINISTRATION Contents of capsule may be administered by oral syringe.

● MEDICINAL FORMS
There can be variation in the licensing of different medicines containing the same drug. Forms available from special-order manufacturers include: oral suspension, oral solution

Capsule

▸ Calcitriol (Non-proprietary)
Calcitriol 250 nanogram Calcitriol 250nanogram capsules | 30 capsule PoM £18.04 | 100 capsule PoM no price available DT price = £18.04
Calcitriol 500 nanogram Calcitriol 500nanogram capsules | 30 capsule PoM £32.25 | 100 capsule PoM no price available DT price = £32.25

▸ Rocaltrol (Roche Products Ltd)
Calcitriol 250 nanogram Rocaltrol 250nanogram capsules | 100 capsule PoM £18.04 DT price = £18.04
Calcitriol 500 nanogram Rocaltrol 500nanogram capsules | 100 capsule PoM £32.25 DT price = £32.25

Oral solution

▸ Calcitriol (Non-proprietary)
Calcitriol 1 microgram per 1 ml Rocaltrol 1micrograms/ml oral solution sugar-free | 10 ml PoM no price available

⌐ 940

Colecalciferol

(Cholecalciferol; Vitamin D_3)

● INDICATIONS AND DOSE

Prevention of vitamin D deficiency

▸ BY MOUTH

▸ Adult: 400 units daily

Treatment of vitamin D deficiency

▸ BY MOUTH

▸ Adult: 800 units daily, higher doses may be necessary for severe deficiency

● RENAL IMPAIRMENT

Monitoring
Monitor plasma-calcium concentration in renal impairment.

● MONITORING REQUIREMENTS Monitor plasma-calcium concentration in patients receiving high doses.

● DIRECTIONS FOR ADMINISTRATION

INVITA D3® 25,000UNITS/1ML ORAL SOLUTION (CONSILIENT HEALTH LTD) May be mixed with a small amount of cold or lukewarm food immediately before administration.

● MEDICINAL FORMS
There can be variation in the licensing of different medicines containing the same drug. Forms available from special-order manufacturers include: tablet, capsule, oral suspension, oral solution, oral drops

Tablet

▸ Colecalciferol (Non-proprietary)
Colecalciferol 400 unit Colecalciferol 400unit tablets | 30 tablet no price available | 60 tablet £15.50
Colecalciferol 1000 unit Colecalciferol 1,000unit tablets | 28 tablet £20.95-£22.95 | 30 tablet no price available | 90 tablet £34.50 | 180 tablet no price available
Colecalciferol 5000 unit tablets | 100 tablet £3.50
Colecalciferol 10000 unit Colecalciferol 10,000unit tablets | 30 tablet £36.00
Colecalciferol 20000 unit Colecalciferol 20,000unit tablets | 20 tablet £36.00 | 30 tablet no price available

▸ Desunin (Meda Pharmaceuticals Ltd)
Colecalciferol 800 unit Desunin 800unit tablets | 30 tablet PoM £3.60 DT price = £3.60 | 90 tablet PoM £10.17
Colecalciferol 4000 unit Desunin 4,000unit tablets | 70 tablet PoM £15.90

▸ Stexerol-D3 (ProStrakan Ltd)
Colecalciferol 1000 unit Stexerol-D3 1,000unit tablets | 28 tablet PoM £2.95
Colecalciferol 25000 unit Stexerol-D3 25,000unit tablets | 12 tablet PoM £17.00

Chewable tablet

▸ Colecalciferol (Non-proprietary)
Colecalciferol 280 unit chewable tablets | 180 tablet £5.00
Colecalciferol 1000 unit chewable tablets | 100 tablet no price available

Orodispersible tablet

▸ Colecalciferol (Non-proprietary)
Colecalciferol 2000 unit tablets sugar-free | 120 tablet £4.88

Capsule
CAUTIONARY AND ADVISORY LABELS 25

▸ Colecalciferol (Non-proprietary)
Colecalciferol 400 unit Colecalciferol 400unit capsules | 30 capsule no price available
Colecalciferol 500 unit Vitamin D3 500IU capsules | 90 capsule GSL no price available
Colecalciferol 600 unit Colecalciferol 600unit capsules | 30 capsule no price available
Colecalciferol 800 unit Colecalciferol 800unit capsules | 30 capsule £3.60 DT price = £3.60
Colecalciferol 1000 unit Colecalciferol 1,000unit capsules | 28 capsule £36.50 | 30 capsule £29.50
Colecalciferol 2200 unit Colecalciferol 2,200unit capsules | 30 capsule no price available
Colecalciferol 2500 unit Colecalciferol 2,500unit capsules | 30 capsule no price available
Colecalciferol 3000 unit Colecalciferol 3,000unit capsules | 30 capsule no price available
Colecalciferol 4000 unit capsules | 60 capsule no price available | 120 capsule no price available
Colecalciferol 5000 unit Colecalciferol 5,000unit capsules | 30 capsule no price available | 40 capsule no price available | 100 capsule PoM no price available
Colecalciferol 10000 unit Colecalciferol 10,000unit capsules | 30 capsule no price available
Colecalciferol 20000 unit Colecalciferol 20,000unit capsules | 20 capsule £37.99 | 30 capsule £35.99 DT price = £29.00 | 30 capsule PoM £29.00 DT price = £29.00
Colecalciferol 30000 unit Colecalciferol 30,000unit capsules | 10 capsule no price available

9

Blood and nutrition

Colecalciferol **50000 unit** Colecalciferol 50,000unit capsules | 10 capsule £36.00 | 100 capsule [PoM] no price available
‣ Aviticol (Colonis Pharma Ltd)
Colecalciferol **800 unit** Aviticol 800unit capsules | 30 capsule [PoM] £3.60 DT price = £3.60
Colecalciferol **1000 unit** Aviticol 1,000unit capsules | 30 capsule [PoM] £3.16
Colecalciferol **20000 unit** Aviticol 20,000unit capsules | 30 capsule [PoM] £29.00 DT price = £29.00
‣ Fultium-D3 (Internis Pharmaceuticals Ltd)
Colecalciferol **800 unit** Fultium-D3 800unit capsules | 30 capsule [PoM] £3.60 DT price = £3.60 | 90 capsule [PoM] £8.85
Colecalciferol **3200 unit** Fultium-D3 3,200unit capsules | 30 capsule [PoM] £13.32 DT price = £13.32 | 90 capsule [PoM] £39.96
Colecalciferol **20000 unit** Fultium-D3 20,000unit capsules | 15 capsule [PoM] £17.04 DT price = £17.04 | 30 capsule [PoM] £29.00 DT price = £29.00
‣ Plenachol (Auden McKenzie (Pharma Division) Ltd)
Colecalciferol **20000 unit** Plenachol 20,000unit capsules | 10 capsule [PoM] £9.00
Colecalciferol **40000 unit** Plenachol 40,000unit capsules | 10 capsule [PoM] £15.00 DT price = £15.00
‣ Strivit-D3 (Strides Arcolab International Ltd)
Colecalciferol **800 unit** Strivit-D3 800unit capsules | 30 capsule [PoM] £2.34 DT price = £3.60

Oral solution
CAUTIONARY AND ADVISORY LABELS 21
‣ Colecalciferol (Non-proprietary)
Colecalciferol **3000 unit per 1 ml** Colecalciferol 3,000units/ml oral solution | 100 ml [PoM] £119.70–£144.00 DT price = £144.00
Colecalciferol **10000 unit per 1 ml** Colecalciferol 10,000units/ml oral solution | 10 ml no price available
‣ InVita D3 (Consilient Health Ltd)
Colecalciferol **25000 unit per 1 ml** InVita D3 25,000units/1ml oral solution sugar-free | 3 ampoule [PoM] £4.45 DT price = £4.45
Colecalciferol **50000 unit per 1 ml** InVita D3 50,000units/1ml oral solution sugar-free | 3 ampoule [PoM] £6.25 DT price = £6.25
‣ Thorens (Galen Ltd)
Colecalciferol **10000 unit per 1 ml** Thorens 25,000units/2.5ml oral solution sugar-free | 2.5 ml [PoM] £1.55 DT price = £1.55 sugar-free | 10 ml [PoM] £5.85 DT price = £5.85

Oral drops
‣ Colecalciferol (Non-proprietary)
Colecalciferol **20000 unit per 1 ml** Vigantol 20,000units/ml oral drops | 10 ml no price available
Colecalciferol **200 unit per 1 drop** Natures Aid Vitamin D3 200units/drop for infants and children oral drops sugar-free | 50 ml £3.86
Healthaid Vitamin D3 200units/drop oral drops sugar-free | 15 ml £4.46
‣ Fultium-D3 (Internis Pharmaceuticals Ltd)
Colecalciferol **2740 unit per 1 ml** Fultium-D3 2,740units/ml oral drops sugar-free | 25 ml [PoM] £10.70
‣ InVita D3 (Consilient Health Ltd)
Colecalciferol **2400 unit per 1 ml** InVita D3 2,400units/ml oral drops sugar-free | 10 ml [PoM] £3.60
‣ Thorens (Galen Ltd)
Colecalciferol **10000 unit per 1 ml** Thorens 10,000units/ml oral drops sugar-free | 10 ml [PoM] £5.85 DT price = £5.85

| Colecalciferol with calcium carbonate

The properties listed below are those particular to the combination only. For the properties of the components please consider, colecalciferol p. 941, calcium carbonate p. 906.

● INDICATIONS AND DOSE

Prevention and treatment of vitamin D and calcium deficiency
▸ BY MOUTH
▸ Adult: Dosed according to the deficit or daily maintenance requirements (consult product literature)

● PRESCRIBING AND DISPENSING INFORMATION *Accrete D3*®
contains calcium carbonate 1.5 g (calcium 600 mg or Ca^{2+} 15 mmol), colecalciferol 10 micrograms (400 units); *Adcal-*

D3® tablets contain calcium carbonate 1.5 g (calcium 600 mg or Ca^{2+} 15 mmol), colecalciferol 10 micrograms (400 units); *Cacit*® *D3* contains calcium carbonate 1.25 g (calcium 500 mg or Ca^{2+} 12.5 mmol), colecalciferol 11 micrograms (440 units)/sachet; *Calceos*® contains calcium carbonate 1.25 g (calcium 500 mg or Ca^{2+} 12.5 mmol), colecalciferol 10 micrograms (400 units); *Calcichew-D3*® tablets contain calcium carbonate 1.25 g (calcium 500 mg or Ca^{2+} 12.5 mmol), colecalciferol 5 micrograms (200 units); *Calcichew-D3*® *Forte* tablets contain calcium carbonate 1.25 g (calcium 500 mg or Ca^{2+} 12.5 mmol), colecalciferol 10 micrograms (400 units); *Calcichew-D3*® 500 mg/400 unit caplets contain calcium carbonate (calcium 500 mg or Ca^{2+} 12.5 mmol), colecalciferol 10 micrograms (400 units); *Kalcipos-D*® contains calcium carbonate (calcium 500 mg or Ca^{2+} 12.5 mmol), colecalciferol 20 micrograms (800 units); *Natecal D3*® contains calcium carbonate 1.5 g (calcium 600 mg or Ca^{2+} 15 mmol), colecalciferol 10 micrograms (400 units); consult product literature for details of other available products.

Flavours of chewable and soluble forms may include orange, lemon, aniseed, peppermint, molasses, or tutti-frutti.

● MEDICINAL FORMS
There can be variation in the licensing of different medicines containing the same drug.

Tablet
EXCIPIENTS: May contain Propylene glycol
‣ Colecalciferol with calcium carbonate (Non-proprietary)
Calcium carbonate 400 mg, Colecalciferol 100 unit tablets | 30 tablet no price available | 60 tablet no price available
Valupak Calcium & Vitamin D tablets | 30 tablet £0.59
‣ Accrete D3 (Internis Pharmaceuticals Ltd)
Calcium carbonate 1.5 gram, Colecalciferol 400 unit Accrete D3 tablets | 60 tablet [P] £2.95 DT price = £2.95
‣ Adcal-D3 (ProStrakan Ltd)
Calcium carbonate 750 mg, Colecalciferol 200 unit Adcal-D3 750mg/200unit caplets | 112 tablet [P] £2.95 DT price = £2.95
‣ Calcichew D3 (Forum Health Products Ltd)
Calcium carbonate 1.25 gram, Colecalciferol 400 unit Calcichew D3 500mg/400unit caplets | 100 tablet [P] £7.43 DT price = £7.43
‣ Kalcipos-D (Meda Pharmaceuticals Ltd)
Calcium carbonate 1.25 gram, Colecalciferol 800 unit Kalcipos-D 500mg/800unit tablets | 30 tablet [PoM] £4.21 DT price = £4.21

Chewable tablet
CAUTIONARY AND ADVISORY LABELS 24
EXCIPIENTS: May contain Aspartame
‣ Colecalciferol with calcium carbonate (Non-proprietary)
Calcium carbonate 1.25 gram, Colecalciferol 400 unit Colecalciferol 400unit / Calcium carbonate 1.25g chewable tablets | 100 tablet £14.75
Calcium carbonate 1.5 gram, Colecalciferol 400 unit Colecalciferol 400unit / Calcium carbonate 1.5g chewable tablets | 60 tablet [P] £4.38
‣ Adcal-D3 (ProStrakan Ltd)
Calcium carbonate 1.5 gram, Colecalciferol 400 unit Adcal-D3 Lemon chewable tablets | 56 tablet [P] £3.65 DT price = £3.65 | 112 tablet [P] £7.49
Adcal-D3 chewable tablets tutti frutti | 56 tablet [P] £3.65 DT price = £3.65 | 112 tablet [P] £7.49
‣ Calceos (Galen Ltd)
Calcium carbonate 1.25 gram, Colecalciferol 400 unit Calceos 500mg/400unit chewable tablets | 60 tablet [P] £3.58 DT price = £4.24
‣ Calci-D (Consilient Health Ltd)
Calcium carbonate 2.5 gram, Colecalciferol 1000 iu Calci-D 1000mg/1,000unit chewable tablets | 28 tablet [PoM] £2.25
‣ Calcichew D3 (Forum Health Products Ltd)
Calcium carbonate 2.5 gram, Colecalciferol 800 iu Calcichew D3 1000mg/800unit Once Daily chewable tablets | 30 tablet [P] £6.75 DT price = £6.75
Calcium carbonate 1.25 gram, Colecalciferol 200 unit Calcichew D3 chewable tablets | 100 tablet [P] £7.68 DT price = £7.68

- Calcichew D3 Forte (Forum Health Products Ltd)
  Calcium carbonate 1.25 gram, Colecalciferol 400 unit Calcichew D3 Forte chewable tablets | 60 tablet P £4.24 DT price = £4.24 | 100 tablet P £7.08
- Evacal D3 (Teva UK Ltd)
  Calcium carbonate 1.5 gram, Colecalciferol 400 unit Evacal D3 1500mg/400unit chewable tablets | 56 tablet P £2.75 DT price = £3.65 | 112 tablet P £5.50
- Kalcipos-D (Meda Pharmaceuticals Ltd)
  Calcium carbonate 1.25 gram, Colecalciferol 800 unit Kalcipos-D 500mg/800unit chewable tablets | 30 tablet PoM £4.21 DT price = £4.21
- Natecal (Chiesi Ltd)
  Calcium carbonate 1.5 gram, Colecalciferol 400 unit Natecal D3 600mg/400unit chewable tablets | 60 tablet P £3.63
- TheiCal-D3 (Stirling Anglian Pharmaceuticals Ltd)
  Calcium carbonate 2.5 gram, Colecalciferol 880 unit TheiCal-D3 1000mg/880unit chewable tablets | 30 tablet P £2.95 DT price = £2.95

Effervescent tablet

CAUTIONARY AND ADVISORY LABELS 13

- Adcal-D3 (ProStrakan Ltd)
  Calcium carbonate 1.5 gram, Colecalciferol 400 unit Adcal-D3 Dissolve 1500mg/400unit effervescent tablets | 56 tablet P £5.99 DT price = £5.99

Effervescent granules

CAUTIONARY AND ADVISORY LABELS 13

- Colecalciferol with calcium carbonate (Non-proprietary)
  Calcium carbonate 2.5 gram, Colecalciferol 880 unit Colecalciferol 880unit / Calcium carbonate 2.5g effervescent granules sachets | 24 sachet PoM no price available
- Cacit D3 (Warner Chilcott UK Ltd)
  Calcium carbonate 1.25 gram, Colecalciferol 440 unit Cacit D3 effervescent granules sachets | 30 sachet P £4.06 DT price = £4.06

Colecalciferol with calcium phosphate

The properties listed below are those particular to the combination only. For the properties of the components please consider, colecalciferol p. 941, calcium phosphate p. 908.

- **INDICATIONS AND DOSE**

Calcium and vitamin D deficiency
- BY MOUTH
- Adult: (consult product literature)

- MEDICINAL FORMS
There can be variation in the licensing of different medicines containing the same drug.

Powder

CAUTIONARY AND ADVISORY LABELS 13, 21

- Calfovit D3 (A. Menarini Farmaceutica Internazionale SRL)
  Calcium phosphate 3.1 gram, Colecalciferol 800 unit Calfovit D3 oral powder sachets | 30 sachet P £4.32 DT price = £4.32

F 940

Dihydrotachysterol

- **INDICATIONS AND DOSE**

Acute, chronic, and latent forms of hypocalcaemic tetany due to hypoparathyroidism
- BY MOUTH
- Adult: (consult product literature)

- RENAL IMPAIRMENT

Monitoring
Monitor plasma-calcium concentration in renal impairment.

- MONITORING REQUIREMENTS Monitor plasma-calcium concentration in patients receiving high doses.

- MEDICINAL FORMS
There can be variation in the licensing of different medicines containing the same drug.

Oral solution

EXCIPIENTS: May contain Arachis (peanut) oil

- AT10 (Intrapharm Laboratories Ltd)
  Dihydrotachysterol 250 microgram per 1 ml AT10 250micrograms/ml oral solution sugar-free | 15 ml P £22.87

F 940

Ergocalciferol

(Calciferol; Vitamin D$_2$)

- **INDICATIONS AND DOSE**

Vitamin D deficiency caused by intestinal malabsorption or chronic liver disease
- BY MOUTH
- Adult: Up to 40 000 units daily

Hypocalcaemia of hypoparathyroidism to achieve normocalcaemia
- BY MOUTH
- Adult: Up to 100 000 units daily

Prevention of vitamin D deficiency
- BY MOUTH
- Adult: 400 units daily

Treatment of vitamin D deficiency
- BY MOUTH
- Adult: 800 units daily, higher doses may be necessary for severe deficiency

- RENAL IMPAIRMENT

Monitoring
Monitor plasma-calcium concentration in renal impairment.

- MONITORING REQUIREMENTS Monitor plasma-calcium concentration in patients receiving high doses.

- PRESCRIBING AND DISPENSING INFORMATION The BP directs that when calciferol is prescribed or demanded, colecalciferol or ergocalciferol should be dispensed or supplied.
  When the strength of the tablets ordered or prescribed is not clear, the intention of the prescriber with respect to the strength (expressed in micrograms or milligrams per tablet) should be ascertained.

- MEDICINAL FORMS
There can be variation in the licensing of different medicines containing the same drug. Forms available from special-order manufacturers include: tablet, oral suspension, oral solution

Tablet

- Ergocalciferol (Non-proprietary)
  Ergocalciferol 12.5 microgram Ergocalciferol 12.5microgram tablets | 30 tablet no price available
- Ergoral (Cubic Pharmaceuticals Ltd)
  Ergocalciferol 125 microgram Ergoral D2 5,000unit tablets | 30 tablet £19.95
  Ergocalciferol 250 microgram Ergoral D2 10,000unit tablets | 30 tablet £23.95

Capsule

- Ergocalciferol (Non-proprietary)
  Ergocalciferol 1.25 mg Ergocalciferol 1.25mg capsules | 30 capsule PoM no price available | 50 capsule PoM £230.00
- Eciferol (Rhodes Pharma Ltd)
  Ergocalciferol 1.25 mg Eciferol D2 50,000unit capsules | 10 capsule £29.99
- Ergoral (Cubic Pharmaceuticals Ltd)
  Ergocalciferol 1.25 mg Ergoral D2 50,000unit capsules | 10 capsule £19.95

Oral solution

- Ergocalciferol (Non-proprietary)
  Ergocalciferol 1500 unit per 1 ml Uvesterol D 1,500units/ml oral solution sugar-free | 20 ml PoM no price available

9

Blood and nutrition

Ergocalciferol 20000 unit per 1 ml Sterogyl 100,000units/5ml oral solution | 20 ml [PoM] no price available DT price = £181.96
  ▸ Eciferol (Rhodes Pharma Ltd)
Ergocalciferol 3000 unit per 1 ml Eciferol D2 3,000units/ml liquid | 60 ml £55.00 DT price = £111.25

Ergocalciferol with calcium lactate and calcium phosphate

(Calcium and vitamin D)

The properties listed below are those particular to the combination only. For the properties of the components please consider, ergocalciferol p. 943, calcium lactate p. 908.

● INDICATIONS AND DOSE

Prevention of calcium and vitamin D deficiency | Treatment of calcium and vitamin D deficiency
  ▸ BY MOUTH
  ▸ Adult: (consult product literature)

● DIRECTIONS FOR ADMINISTRATION Tablets may be crushed before administration, or may be chewed.

● PRESCRIBING AND DISPENSING INFORMATION Each tablet contains calcium lactate 300 mg, calcium phosphate 150 mg (calcium 97 mg or Ca^{2+} 2.4 mmol), ergocalciferol 10 micrograms (400 units).

● PATIENT AND CARER ADVICE Patient or carers should be given advice on how to administer calcium and ergocalciferol tablets.

● MEDICINAL FORMS
There can be variation in the licensing of different medicines containing the same drug.
Tablet
  ▸ Ergocalciferol with calcium lactate and calcium phosphate (Non-proprietary)
Ergocalciferol 10 microgram, Calcium phosphate 150 mg, Calcium lactate 300 mg Calcium and Ergocalciferol tablets | 28 tablet no price available DT price = £15.43 | 28 tablet [P] £15.39 DT price = £15.43 | 500 tablet [P] no price available

◤ 940

Paricalcitol

● INDICATIONS AND DOSE

For prevention and treatment of secondary hyperparathyroidism associated with chronic renal failure
  ▸ BY MOUTH
  ▸ Adult: (consult product literature)

For prevention and treatment of secondary hyperparathyroidism associated with chronic renal failure in patients on haemodialysis
  ▸ Adult: To be administered via haemodialysis access (consult product literature)

● SIDE-EFFECTS Acne · breast tenderness · dyspepsia · pruritus · rash · taste disturbance

● PREGNANCY Toxicity in *animal* studies—manufacturer advises avoid unless potential benefit outweighs risk.

● BREAST FEEDING Manufacturer advises caution—no information available.

● MONITORING REQUIREMENTS
  ▸ Monitor plasma calcium and phosphate during dose titration and at least monthly when stabilised.
  ▸ Monitor parathyroid hormone concentration.

● MEDICINAL FORMS
There can be variation in the licensing of different medicines containing the same drug.
Capsule
  ▸ Zemplar (AbbVie Ltd)
Paricalcitol 1 microgram Zemplar 1microgram capsules | 28 capsule [PoM] £69.44
Paricalcitol 2 microgram Zemplar 2microgram capsules | 28 capsule [PoM] £138.88
Solution for injection
EXCIPIENTS: May contain Propylene glycol
  ▸ Zemplar (AbbVie Ltd)
Paricalcitol 5 microgram per 1 ml Zemplar 5micrograms/1ml solution for injection ampoules | 5 ampoule [PoM] £62.00 (Hospital only)
Zemplar 5micrograms/1ml solution for injection vials | 5 vial [PoM] £62.00 (Hospital only)

VITAMINS AND TRACE ELEMENTS ⟩ VITAMIN E

Alpha tocopherol

(Tocopherol)

● INDICATIONS AND DOSE

Vitamin E deficiency because of malabsorption in congenital or hereditary chronic cholestasis
  ▸ BY MOUTH USING ORAL SOLUTION
  ▸ Child: 17 mg/kg daily, dose to be adjusted as necessary

● CAUTIONS Predisposition to thrombosis

● INTERACTIONS → Appendix 1 (Vitamin E).

● SIDE-EFFECTS
  ▸ **Common or very common** Diarrhoea
  ▸ **Uncommon** Alopecia · asthenia · disturbances in serum-potassium concentration · disturbances in serum-sodium concentration · headache · pruritus · rash

● PREGNANCY Manufacturer advises caution, no evidence of harm in *animal* studies.

● BREAST FEEDING Manufacturer advises use only if potential benefit outweighs risk—no information available.

● HEPATIC IMPAIRMENT Manufacturer advises caution—no information available. Manufacturer advises monitor closely in hepatic impairment.

● RENAL IMPAIRMENT Manufacturer advises caution. Risk of renal toxicity due to polyethylene glycol content. Manufacturer advises monitor closely in renal impairment.

● PRESCRIBING AND DISPENSING INFORMATION Tocofersolan is a water-soluble form of D-alpha tocopherol.

● MEDICINAL FORMS
There can be variation in the licensing of different medicines containing the same drug.
Oral solution
  ▸ Vedrop (Orphan Europe (UK) Ltd) ▼
D-alpha tocopherol (as Tocofersolan) 50 mg per 1 ml Vedrop 50mg/ml oral solution sugar-free | 20 ml [PoM] £54.55 sugar-free | 60 ml [PoM] £163.65

Alpha tocopheryl acetate

(Tocopherol)

● INDICATIONS AND DOSE

Vitamin E deficiency
  ▸ BY MOUTH
  ▸ Child: 2–10 mg/kg daily, increased if necessary up to 20 mg/kg daily

Malabsorption in cystic fibrosis
▶ BY MOUTH
▶ Child 1–11 months: 50 mg once daily, dose to be adjusted as necessary, to be taken with food and pancreatic enzymes
▶ Child 1–11 years: 100 mg once daily, dose to be adjusted as necessary, to be taken with food and pancreatic enzymes
▶ Child 12–17 years: 100–200 mg once daily, dose to be adjusted as necessary, to be taken with food and pancreatic enzymes
▶ Adult: 100–200 mg once daily, dose to be adjusted as necessary, to be taken with food and pancreatic enzymes

Vitamin E deficiency in cholestasis and severe liver disease
▶ BY MOUTH
▶ Child 1 month–11 years: Initially 100 mg daily, adjusted according to response, increased if necessary up to 200 mg/kg daily
▶ Child 12–17 years: Initially 200 mg daily, adjusted according to response, increased if necessary up to 200 mg/kg daily

Malabsorption in abetalipoproteinaemia
▶ BY MOUTH
▶ Adult: 50–100 mg/kg once daily

● INTERACTIONS → Appendix 1 (Vitamins).
● SIDE-EFFECTS Abdominal pain (particularly with high doses) · diarrhoea (particularly with high doses)
● PREGNANCY No evidence of safety of high doses.
● BREAST FEEDING Excreted in milk; minimal risk, although caution with large doses.
● MONITORING REQUIREMENTS Increased bleeding tendency in vitamin-K deficient patients or those taking anticoagulants (prothrombin time and INR should be monitored).

● MEDICINAL FORMS
There can be variation in the licensing of different medicines containing the same drug. Forms available from special-order manufacturers include: chewable tablet
Chewable tablet
▶ Alpha tocopheryl acetate (Non-proprietary)
Alpha tocopheryl acetate 100 mg Alpha tocopheryl acetate 100mg chewable tablets | 30 tablet no price available
▶ E-Tabs (Ennogen Healthcare Ltd)
Alpha tocopheryl acetate 100 mg E-Tabs 100mg chewable tablets | 30 tablet £87.30
Capsule
▶ Alpha tocopheryl acetate (Non-proprietary)
Alpha tocopherol 100 unit capsules | 30 capsule £0.59
Alpha tocopherol 200 unit capsules | 100 capsule £6.60
Alpha tocopherol 250 unit capsules | 100 capsule £6.11
Alpha tocopherol 400 unit capsules | 30 capsule £6.69 | 60 capsule £11.72
Alpha tocopherol 500 unit capsules | 60 capsule £7.75
Alpha tocopherol 600 unit capsules | 30 capsule no price available
HealthAid Natural Vitamin E 600unit capsules | 30 capsule £8.37 | 60 capsule £13.95
Alpha tocopherol 1000 unit 1,000unit capsules | 30 capsule £6.64
▶ E-Caps (Ennogen Healthcare Ltd)
Alpha tocopherol 75 unit E-Caps 75unit capsules | 100 capsule £109.50
Alpha tocopherol 100 unit E-Caps 100unit capsules | 30 capsule £84.40
Alpha tocopherol 200 unit E-Caps 200unit capsules | 30 capsule £89.50
Alpha tocopherol 400 unit E-Caps 400unit capsules | 30 capsule £128.50
Alpha tocopherol 1000 unit E-Caps 1,000unit capsules | 30 capsule £130.20

▶ Vita-E (Typharm Ltd)
Alpha tocopherol 75 unit Vita-E 75unit capsules | 100 capsule £3.69
Alpha tocopherol 200 unit Vita-E 200unit capsules | 30 capsule £2.84 | 100 capsule £8.76
Alpha tocopherol 400 unit Vita-E 400unit capsules | 30 capsule £4.27 | 100 capsule £13.93
Oral suspension
EXCIPIENTS: May contain Sucrose
▶ Alpha tocopheryl acetate (Non-proprietary)
Alpha tocopheryl acetate 100 mg per 1 ml Alpha tocopheryl acetate 500mg/5ml oral suspension | 100 ml GSL £53.50 DT price = £53.50

VITAMINS AND TRACE ELEMENTS > VITAMIN K

Menadiol sodium phosphate

● INDICATIONS AND DOSE
Prevention of Vitamin K deficiency in malabsorption syndromes
▶ BY MOUTH
▶ Adult: 10–40 mg daily, dose to be adjusted as necessary

● CAUTIONS G6PD deficiency (risk of haemolysis) · vitamin E deficiency (risk of haemolysis)
● INTERACTIONS → Appendix 1 (Vitamins).
● PREGNANCY Avoid in late pregnancy and labour unless benefit outweighs risk of neonatal haemolytic anaemia, hyperbilirubinaemia, and kernicterus in neonate.

● MEDICINAL FORMS
There can be variation in the licensing of different medicines containing the same drug. Forms available from special-order manufacturers include: oral suspension, oral solution
Tablet
▶ Menadiol sodium phosphate (Non-proprietary)
Menadiol phosphate (as Menadiol sodium phosphate) 10 mg Menadiol 10mg tablets | 100 tablet P £169.00 DT price = £169.00

Phytomenadione

(Vitamin K₁)

● INDICATIONS AND DOSE
Major bleeding in patients on warfarin (in combination with dried prothrombin complex or fresh frozen plasma)
▶ BY SLOW INTRAVENOUS INJECTION
▶ Adult: 5 mg for 1 dose, stop warfarin treatment

INR > 8.0 with minor bleeding in patients on warfarin
▶ BY SLOW INTRAVENOUS INJECTION
▶ Adult: 1–3 mg, stop warfarin treatment, dose may be repeated if INR still too high after 24 hours, restart warfarin treatment when INR <5

INR > 8.0 with no bleeding in patients on warfarin
▶ BY MOUTH
▶ Adult: 1–5 mg, intravenous preparation to be used orally, stop warfarin treatment, repeat dose if INR still too high after 24 hours, restart warfarin treatment when INR <5

INR 5.0–8.0 with minor bleeding in patients on warfarin
▶ BY SLOW INTRAVENOUS INJECTION
▶ Adult: 1–3 mg, stop warfarin treatment, restart warfarin treatment when INR <5

Reversal of anticoagulation prior to elective surgery (after warfarin stopped)
▶ BY MOUTH
▶ Adult: 1–5 mg, intravenous preparation to be used orally, dose to be given the day before surgery if INR ≥1.5

continued →

Reversal of anticoagulation prior to emergency surgery (when surgery can be delayed 6–12 hours)
► BY INTRAVENOUS INJECTION
► Adult: 5 mg as a single dose, if surgery cannot be delayed, dried prothrombin complex can be given in addition to phytomenadione and the INR checked before surgery

● UNLICENSED USE Oral use of intravenous preparations is unlicensed.
● CAUTIONS Intravenous injections should be given very slowly—risk of vascular collapse
KONAKION® MM
► With intravenous use Reduce dose in elderly
● INTERACTIONS → Appendix 1 (Vitamins).
● SIDE-EFFECTS
KONAKION® MM Anaphylactoid reactions
● PREGNANCY Use if potential benefit outweighs risk.
● BREAST FEEDING Present in milk.
● HEPATIC IMPAIRMENT
KONAKION® MM Caution—glycocholic acid may displace bilirubin.
● DIRECTIONS FOR ADMINISTRATION
KONAKION® MM PAEDIATRIC *Konakion® MM Paediatric* may be administered *by mouth* or *by intravenous injection*.
For *intravenous injection*, may be diluted with Glucose 5% if necessary.
KONAKION® MM *Konakion® MM* may be administered by slow intravenous injection or by intravenous infusion in glucose 5%; **not** for intramuscular injection.
► With intravenous use For *intravenous infusion (Konakion® MM)*, give intermittently in Glucose 5%; dilute with 55 mL; may be injected into lower part of infusion apparatus.

● MEDICINAL FORMS
There can be variation in the licensing of different medicines containing the same drug.
Solution for injection
EXCIPIENTS: May contain Glycocholic acid, lecithin
► Konakion MM (Roche Products Ltd)
Phytomenadione 10 mg per 1 ml Konakion MM Paediatric 2mg/0.2ml solution for injection ampoules | 5 ampoule PoM £4.71
Konakion MM 10mg/1ml solution for injection ampoules | 10 ampoule PoM £3.78 DT price = £3.78

6.1 Neural tube defects (prevention in pregnancy)

Neural tube defects (prevention in pregnancy)

Prevention in pregnancy
Folic acid supplements p. 886 taken before and during pregnancy can reduce the occurrence of neural tube defects. The risk of a neural tube defect occurring in a child should be assessed and folic acid given as follows:
● Women at a low risk of conceiving a child with a neural tube defect should be advised to take folic acid as a medicinal or food supplement daily (at low-risk group dose) before conception and until week 12 of pregnancy. Women who have not been taking folic acid and who suspect they are pregnant should start at once and continue until week 12 of pregnancy.
● Couples are at a high risk of conceiving a child with a neural tube defect if either partner has a neural tube defect (or either partner has a family history of neural tube defects), if they have had a previous pregnancy affected by a neural tube defect, or if the woman has *coeliac disease* (or other malabsorption state), diabetes mellitus, sickle-cell anaemia, or is taking **antiepileptic medicines**.
● Women in the high-risk group who wish to become pregnant (or who are at risk of becoming pregnant) should be advised to take folic acid daily (at high-risk group dose) and continue until week 12 of pregnancy (women with sickle-cell disease should continue taking their normal dose of folic acid (or to increase the dose to high-risk group daily dose) and continue this throughout pregnancy).

There is no justification for prescribing multiple-ingredient vitamin preparations containing vitamin B_{12} or folic acid.

Chapter 10
Musculoskeletal system

CONTENTS

1 Arthritis

Arthritis

Rheumatoid arthritis and other inflammatory disorders

A non-steroidal anti-inflammatory drug (NSAID) is indicated for pain and stiffness resulting from inflammatory rheumatic disease; analgesics such as paracetamol p. 406 or codeine phosphate p. 413 can also be used.

Drugs are also used to influence the rheumatic disease process itself. For *rheumatoid arthritis* these disease-modifying antirheumatic drugs (DMARDs) include methotrexate p. 807, cytokine modulators, azathioprine p. 757, ciclosporin p. 758, cyclophosphamide p. 793, leflunomide p. 951, penicillamine p. 952, gold, antimalarials (chloroquine p. 560 and hydroxychloroquine sulfate p. 950), and sulfasalazine p. 38. Corticosteroids also have a significant role in the management of rheumatoid arthritis.

Drugs which may affect the disease process in *psoriatic arthritis* include sulfasalazine, gold, azathioprine, methotrexate, leflunomide, and cytokine modulators.

Osteoarthritis and soft-tissue disorders

For pain relief in osteoarthritis and soft-tissue disorders, paracetamol should be used first and may need to be taken regularly. A topical NSAID or topical capsaicin 0.025% p. 438 should also be considered, particularly in knee or hand osteoarthritis. An oral NSAID can be substituted for, or used in addition to, paracetamol. If further pain relief is required in osteoarthritis, then the addition of an opioid analgesic may be considered, but with a substantial risk of adverse effects; however, an opioid analgesic should be considered before a NSAID in patients taking low-dose aspirin.

Intra-articular corticosteroid injections may produce temporary benefit in osteoarthritis, especially if associated with soft-tissue inflammation.

Non-drug measures, such as weight reduction and exercise, should also be encouraged.

Glucosamine p. 949 and rubefacients are not recommended for the treatment of osteoarthritis.

Hyaluronic acid and its derivatives are available for osteoarthritis of the knee, but are not recommended. Sodium hyaluronate (*Durolane* ®, *Euflexxa* ®, *Fermathron* ®, *Hyalgan* ®, *Orthovisc* ®, *Ostenil* ®, *Ostenil Plus* ®, *RenehaVis* ®, *Suplasyn* ®, *Synocrom* ®, *Synopsis* ®) or hylan G-F 20 (*Synvisc* ®) is injected intra-articularly to supplement natural hyaluronic acid in the synovial fluid. These injections may reduce pain over 1–6 months, but are associated with a short-term increase in knee inflammation. Sodium hyaluronate (*SportVis* ®) is also licensed for the relief of pain and optimisation of recovery following ankle sprain, and for the relief of chronic pain and disability associated with tennis elbow.

Rheumatic disease, suppressing drugs

Overview

Certain drugs such as those affecting the immune response can suppress the disease process in *rheumatoid arthritis* and *psoriatic arthritis*; gold, penicillamine p. 952, hydroxychloroquine sulfate p. 950, chloroquine p. 560, and sulfasalazine p. 38 can also suppress the disease process in *rheumatoid arthritis* while sulfasalazine and possibly gold can suppress the disease process in *psoriatic arthritis*. Unlike NSAIDs, which are used only for symptom control, disease-modifying anti-rheumatic drugs (DMARDs) can affect the progression of disease but may require 2–6 months of treatment for a full therapeutic response. Response to DMARDs may allow the NSAID dose to be reduced or withdrawn. All patients with suspected inflammatory joint disease should be referred to a specialist as soon as possible to confirm diagnosis and evaluate disease activity; early initiation of DMARDs is recommended to control the signs and symptoms, and to limit joint damage.

Choice

The choice of a disease-modifying antirheumatic drug should take into account co-morbidity and patient preference. Methotrexate p. 807, sulfasalazine, intramuscular gold, and penicillamine are similar in efficacy. However, methotrexate or sulfasalazine may be better tolerated.

A combination of **DMARDs** (including methotrexate and at least one other DMARD) and a short-term **corticosteroid**, should be given to patients with newly diagnosed active rheumatoid arthritis, ideally within 3 months of the onset of persistent symptoms. If the use of particular DMARDs is contra-indicated and combination therapy is not possible, monotherapy with a suitable DMARD should be given and the dose rapidly increased until clinically effective. In patients with established and stable rheumatoid arthritis, cautiously reduce drug doses to the lowest that are clinically effective. Response to drug treatment often produces a reduction in requirements of both corticosteroids and other drugs.

Gold and penicillamine are effective in *palindromic rheumatism. Systemic* and *discoid lupus erythematosus* are sometimes treated with chloroquine or hydroxychloroquine sulfate.

If a disease-modifying anti-rheumatic drug does not lead to an objective benefit within 6 months, it should be replaced by a different one.

Gold

Gold can be given as sodium aurothiomalate p. 953 for active progressive rheumatoid arthritis; it must be given by deep intramuscular injection and the area gently massaged. A test dose must be given followed by doses at weekly intervals until there is definite evidence of remission. In patients who do respond, the interval between injections is then gradually increased to 4 weeks and treatment is continued for up to 5 years after complete remission. If relapse occurs the dosage frequency may be immediately increased and only once control has been obtained again should the dosage frequency be decreased; if no response is seen within 2 months, alternative treatment should be sought. It is important to avoid complete relapse since second courses of gold are not usually effective.

Penicillamine

Penicillamine has a similar action to gold. More patients are able to continue treatment than with gold but side-effects are common.

Patients should be warned not to expect improvement for at least 6 to 12 weeks after treatment is initiated. Penicillamine should be discontinued if there is no improvement within 1 year.

Sulfasalazine

Sulfasalazine has a beneficial effect in suppressing the inflammatory activity of rheumatoid arthritis. Sulfasalazine may also be used by specialists, in the management of psoriatic arthritis affecting peripheral joints [unlicensed indication]. Haematological abnormalities occur usually in the first 3 to 6 months of treatment and are reversible on cessation of treatment.

Antimalarials

The antimalarial hydroxychloroquine sulfate is used to treat rheumatoid arthritis of moderate inflammatory activity; chloroquine is also licensed for treating inflammatory disorders but is used much less frequently and is generally reserved for use if other drugs have failed.

Chloroquine and hydroxychloroquine sulfate are effective for mild systemic lupus erythematosus, particularly involving the skin and joints. These drugs should not be used for psoriatic arthritis. Chloroquine and hydroxychloroquine sulfate are better tolerated than gold or penicillamine. Retinopathy rarely occurs provided that the recommended doses are not exceeded; in the elderly it is difficult to distinguish drug-induced retinopathy from changes of ageing.

Mepacrine hydrochloride is sometimes used in discoid lupus erythematosus [unlicensed].

Drugs affecting the immune response

Methotrexate is a disease-modifying antirheumatic drug suitable for moderate to severe rheumatoid arthritis. Azathioprine p. 757, ciclosporin p. 758, cyclophosphamide p. 793, leflunomide p. 951, and the **cytokine modulators** are considered more toxic and they are used in cases that have not responded to other disease-modifying drugs.

Methotrexate is usually given by mouth once a week, adjusted according to response. In patients who experience mucosal or gastro-intestinal side-effects with methotrexate, folic acid p. 886 given every week [unlicensed indication], on a different day from the methotrexate, may help to reduce the frequency of such side-effects.

Leflunomide acts on the immune system as a disease-modifying antirheumatic drug. Its therapeutic effect starts after 4–6 weeks and improvement may continue for a further 4–6 weeks. Leflunomide, which is similar in efficacy to sulfasalazine and methotrexate, may be chosen when these drugs cannot be used.

Ciclosporin is licensed for severe active rheumatoid arthritis when conventional second-line therapy is inappropriate or ineffective. There is some evidence that ciclosporin may retard the rate of erosive progression and improve symptom control in those who respond only partially to methotrexate.

Cyclophosphamide may be used for rheumatoid arthritis with severe systemic manifestations [unlicensed indication]; it is toxic and regular blood counts (including platelet counts) should be carried out. Cyclophosphamide can also be given for *severe systemic rheumatoid arthritis* and for other connective tissue diseases (especially with active vasculitis).

Drugs that affect the immune response are also used in the management of severe cases of *systemic lupus erythematosus* and other connective tissue disorders. They are often given in conjunction with corticosteroids for patients with severe or progressive renal disease. They may be used in cases of *polymyositis* that are resistant to corticosteroids. They are used for their corticosteroid-sparing effect in patients whose corticosteroid requirements are excessive. Azathioprine is usually used.

In the specialist management of psoriatic arthritis affecting peripheral joints, leflunomide, methotrexate, or azathioprine [unlicensed indication] may be used.

Juvenile idiopathic arthritis

Many children with *juvenile idiopathic arthritis* (juvenile chronic arthritis) do not require disease-modifying antirheumatic drugs. Methotrexate is effective; sulfasalazine is an alternative [unlicensed indication] but it should be avoided in *systemic-onset juvenile idiopathic arthritis*. Gold and penicillamine are no longer used. Cytokine modulators have a role in *juvenile idiopathic arthritis*.

Cytokine modulators

Cytokine modulators should be used under specialist supervision.

Adalimumab p. 957, certolizumab pegol p. 959, etanercept p. 961, golimumab p. 962, and infliximab p. 964 inhibit the activity of tumour necrosis factor alpha (TNF-α).

Adalimumab is licensed for moderate to severe active *rheumatoid arthritis* when response to other disease modifying antirheumatic drugs (including methotrexate p. 807) has been inadequate; it is also licensed for severe, active, and progressive disease in adults not previously treated with methotrexate. In the treatment of rheumatoid arthritis, adalimumab should be used in combination with methotrexate, but it can be given alone if methotrexate is inappropriate. Adalimumab is also licensed for the treatment of active and progressive *psoriatic arthritis* and severe active *ankylosing spondylitis* that have not responded adequately to other disease-modifying antirheumatic drugs. It is also licensed for the treatment of severe axial spondyloarthritis without radiographic evidence of ankylosing spondylitis but with objective signs of inflammation, in patients who have had an inadequate response to, or are intolerant of NSAIDs. Adalimumab also has a role in inflammatory bowel disease and plaque psoriasis.

Certolizumab pegol is licensed for use in patients with moderate to severe active *rheumatoid arthritis* when response to disease-modifying antirheumatic drugs (including methotrexate) has been inadequate. Certolizumab pegol can be used in combination with methotrexate, or as a monotherapy if methotrexate is not tolerated or is contra-indicated. Certolizumab pegol is also licensed for the treatment of severe active *ankylosing spondylitis* in patients who have had an inadequate response to, or are intolerant of NSAIDs. It is also licensed for the treatment of severe active *axial spondyloarthritis*, without radiographic evidence of ankylosing spondylitis but with objective signs of inflammation, in patients who have had an inadequate response to, or are intolerant of NSAIDs.

Etanercept is licensed for the treatment of moderate to severe active *rheumatoid arthritis* either alone or in combination with methotrexate when the response to other disease-modifying antirheumatic drugs is inadequate and in severe, active and progressive *rheumatoid arthritis* in patients not previously treated with methotrexate. It is also licensed for the treatment of active and progressive *psoriatic arthritis* inadequately responsive to other disease-modifying antirheumatic drugs, and for severe *ankylosing spondylitis* inadequately responsive to conventional therapy. Etanercept also has a role in plaque psoriasis.

Golimumab is licensed in combination with methotrexate for the treatment of moderate to severe active *rheumatoid arthritis* when response to disease-modifying antirheumatic drug (DMARD) therapy (including methotrexate has been inadequate; it is also licensed in combination with methotrexate for patients with severe, active, and progressive rheumatoid arthritis not previously treated with methotrexate. Golimumab is also licensed for the treatment of active and progressive *psoriatic arthritis*, as monotherapy or in combination with methotrexate, when response to DMARD therapy has been inadequate; it is also licensed for the treatment of severe active *ankylosing spondylitis* when there is an inadequate response to conventional treatment.

Infliximab is licensed for the treatment of active *rheumatoid arthritis* in combination with methotrexate when the response to other disease-modifying antirheumatic drugs, including methotrexate, is inadequate; it is also licensed in combination with methotrexate for patients not previously treated with methotrexate or other DMARDs who have severe, active, and progressive rheumatoid arthritis. Infliximab is also licensed for the treatment of *ankylosing spondylitis*, in patients with severe axial symptoms who have not responded adequately to conventional therapy, and in combination with methotrexate (or alone if methotrexate is not tolerated or is contra-indicated) for the treatment of active and progressive *psoriatic arthritis* which has not responded adequately to disease-modifying antirheumatic drugs.

Rituximab p. 783 is licensed in combination with methotrexate for the treatment of severe active *rheumatoid arthritis* in patients whose condition has not responded adequately to other disease-modifying antirheumatic drugs (including one or more tumour necrosis factor inhibitors) or who are intolerant of them. Rituximab has a role in malignant disease.

Abatacept p. 956 prevents the full activation of T-lymphocytes. It is licensed for moderate to severe active *rheumatoid arthritis* in combination with methotrexate, in patients unresponsive to other disease-modifying antirheumatic drugs (including methotrexate or a tumour necrosis factor (TNF) inhibitor. Abatacept is not recommended for use in combination with TNF inhibitors.

Anakinra p. 953 inhibits the activity of interleukin-1. Anakinra (in combination with methotrexate) is licensed for the treatment of *rheumatoid arthritis* which has not responded to methotrexate alone. Anakinra is not recommended for the treatment of rheumatoid arthritis except when used in a controlled long-term clinical study. Patients who are already receiving anakinra for rheumatoid arthritis should continue treatment until they and their specialist consider it appropriate to stop.

Belimumab p. 765 inhibits the activity of B-lymphocyte stimulator. Belimumab is licensed as adjunctive therapy in patients with active, autoantibody-positive systemic lupus

erythematosus with a high degree of disease activity despite standard therapy.

Secukinumab p. 954 inhibits the activity of interleukin-17A. Secukinumab is licensed for the treatment of active *psoriatic arthritis*, in combination with methotrexate or alone, which has not responded adequately to disease-modifying antirheumatic drugs; it is also licensed for the treatment of *ankylosing spondylitis*, in patients who have not responded adequately to conventional therapy. Secukinumab also has a role in plaque psoriasis.

Tocilizumab p. 954 antagonises the actions of interleukin-6. Tocilizumab is licensed for use in patients with moderate to severe active *rheumatoid arthritis* when response to at least one disease-modifying antirheumatic drug or tumour necrosis factor inhibitor has been inadequate, or in those who are intolerant of these drugs. Tocilizumab can be used in combination with methotrexate, or as monotherapy if methotrexate is not tolerated or is contra-indicated.

Ustekinumab p. 955 inhibits the activity of interleukins 12 and 23. It is licensed for the treatment of active *psoriatic arthritis* (in combination with methotrexate or alone) in patients who have had an inadequate response to one or more disease-modifying antirheumatic drugs.

> **Drugs used for Arthritis not listed below** Aceclofenac, p. 976 · Acemetacin, p. 977 · Celecoxib, p. 977 · Dexibuprofen, p. 978 · Diclofenac potassium, p. 980 · Diclofenac sodium, p. 980 · Etodolac, p. 983 · Etoricoxib, p. 984 · Fenoprofen, p. 985 · Flurbiprofen, p. 986 · Ibuprofen, p. 987 · Indometacin, p. 989 · Ketoprofen, p. 991 · Mefenamic acid, p. 992 · Meloxicam, p. 993 · Nabumetone, p. 994 · Naproxen, p. 995 · Piroxicam, p. 996 · Prednisone, p. 615 · Sulindac, p. 997 · Tenoxicam, p. 998 · Tiaprofenic acid, p. 998

CHONDROPROTECTIVE DRUGS

Glucosamine

- **DRUG ACTION** Glucosamine is a natural substance found in mucopolysaccharides, mucoproteins, and chitin.

- **INDICATIONS AND DOSE**

ALATERIS®

Symptomatic relief of mild to moderate osteoarthritis of the knee
- ▸ BY MOUTH
- ▸ Adult: 1250 mg once daily, review treatment if no benefit after 2–3 months

DOLENIO®

Symptomatic relief of mild to moderate osteoarthritis of the knee
- ▸ BY MOUTH
- ▸ Adult: 1500 mg once daily, review treatment if no benefit after 2–3 months

GLUSARTEL®

Symptomatic relief of mild to moderate osteoarthritis of the knee
- ▸ BY MOUTH
- ▸ Adult: 1500 mg once daily, dose to be dissolved in at least 250 mL of water, review treatment if no benefit after 2–3 months

- **CAUTIONS** Asthma · impaired glucose tolerance · predisposition to cardiovascular disease

- **INTERACTIONS** → Appendix 1 (glucosamine).

- **SIDE-EFFECTS**
- ▸ **Common or very common** Abdominal pain · constipation · diarrhoea · drowsiness · dyspepsia · fatigue · flatulence · headache · nausea
- ▸ **Uncommon** Flushing · pruritus · rash
- ▸ **Frequency not known** Hair loss · visual disturbances

- ALLERGY AND CROSS-SENSITIVITY Contra-indicated if patient has a shellfish allergy.
- PREGNANCY Manufacturers advise avoid—no information available.
- BREAST FEEDING Manufacturers advise avoid—no information available.
- MONITORING REQUIREMENTS
  ▶ Monitor blood-glucose concentration before treatment and periodically thereafter in patients with impaired glucose tolerance.
  ▶ Monitor cholesterol in patients with predisposition to cardiovascular disease.
- NATIONAL FUNDING/ACCESS DECISIONS
  Scottish Medicines Consortium (SMC) Decisions
  The *Scottish Medicines Consortium* has advised (May 2008) that glucosamine (*Alateris* ®) and (July 2011) glucosamine (*Glusartel* ®) are **not** recommended for use within NHS Scotland for the symptomatic relief of mild to moderate osteoarthritis of the knee.
- LESS SUITABLE FOR PRESCRIBING Less suitable for prescribing—the mechanism of action is not understood and there is limited evidence to show it is effective.

- MEDICINAL FORMS
  There can be variation in the licensing of different medicines containing the same drug.
  Tablet
  ELECTROLYTES: May contain Sodium
  ▶ Alateris (MWK Healthcare Ltd)
    Glucosamine (as Glucosamine hydrochloride) 625 mg Alateris 625mg tablets | 60 tablet [PoM] £18.40 DT price = £18.40
  ▶ Dolenio (Alissa Healthcare Research Ltd)
    Dolenio 1500mg tablets | 30 tablet [PoM] £18.20 DT price = £18.20
  Powder
  CAUTIONARY AND ADVISORY LABELS 13
  EXCIPIENTS: May contain Aspartame
  ELECTROLYTES: May contain Sodium
  ▶ Glusartel (HFA Healthcare Ltd)
    Glusartel 1500mg oral powder sachets sugar-free | 30 sachet [PoM] £18.40

DISEASE-MODIFYING ANTI-RHEUMATIC DRUGS

Hydroxychloroquine sulfate

- INDICATIONS AND DOSE
  Active rheumatoid arthritis (administered on expert advice) | Systemic and discoid lupus erythematosus (administered on expert advice) | Dermatological conditions caused or aggravated by sunlight (administered on expert advice)
  ▶ BY MOUTH
  ▶ Adult: 200–400 mg daily, daily maximum dose to be based on ideal body-weight; maximum 6.5 mg/kg per day

- CAUTIONS Acute porphyrias p. 918 · elderly · G6PD deficiency · may aggravate myasthenia gravis · may exacerbate psoriasis · neurological disorders (especially in those with a history of epilepsy) · severe gastro-intestinal disorders

  CAUTIONS, FURTHER INFORMATION
  ▶ Screening for ocular toxicity A review group convened by the Royal College of Ophthalmologists has updated guidelines for screening to prevent ocular toxicity on long-term treatment with chloroquine and hydroxychloroquine (*Hydroxychloroquine and Ocular Toxicity: Recommendations on Screening* 2009). The following recommendations relate to hydroxychloroquine, which is only rarely associated with toxicity.
    Before treatment:
    ● Assess renal and liver function (adjust dose if impaired)

- Ask patient about visual impairment (not corrected by glasses). If impairment or eye disease present, assessment by an optometrist is advised and any abnormality should be referred to an ophthalmologist
- Record near visual acuity of each eye (with glasses where appropriate) using a standard reading chart
- Initiate hydroxychloroquine treatment if no abnormality detected (at a dose not exceeding hydroxychloroquine sulfate 6.5 mg/kg daily)
  During treatment:
- Ask patient about visual symptoms and monitor visual acuity annually using the standard reading chart
- Refer to ophthalmologist if visual acuity changes or if vision blurred and warn patient to seek prescribing doctor's advice about stopping treatment
- If long-term treatment is required (more than 5 years), individual arrangement should be agreed with the local ophthalmologist

- INTERACTIONS → Appendix 1 (hydroxychloroquine). Concurrent use of hepatotoxic drugs should be avoided.

- SIDE-EFFECTS
  ▶ **Common or very common** Gastro-intestinal disturbances · headache · pruritus · rashes · skin reactions
  ▶ **Uncommon** Convulsions · discoloration of skin, nails, and mucous membranes · ECG changes · hair depigmentation · hair loss · keratopathy · ototoxicity · retinal damage · visual changes
  ▶ **Rare** Acute generalised exanthematous pustulosis · agranulocytosis · angioedema · aplastic anaemia · blood disorders · cardiomyopathy · emotional disturbances · exfoliative dermatitis · hepatic damage · mental changes · myopathy · neuromyopathy · photosensitivity · psychosis · Stevens-Johnson syndrome · thrombocytopenia
  ▶ **Frequency not known** Bronchospasm · diffuse parenchymal lung disease · drug rash with eosinophilia and systemic symptoms

  Overdose
  Hydroxychloroquine is very toxic in overdosage; overdosage is extremely hazardous and difficult to treat. Urgent advice from the National Poisons Information Service is essential. Life-threatening features include arrhythmias (which can have a very rapid onset) and convulsions (which can be intractable).

- PREGNANCY It is not necessary to withdraw an antimalarial drug during pregnancy if the rheumatic disease is well controlled; however, the manufacturer of hydroxychloroquine advises avoiding use.

- BREAST FEEDING Avoid—risk of toxicity in infant.

- HEPATIC IMPAIRMENT Caution in moderate to severe hepatic impairment.

- RENAL IMPAIRMENT Manufacturer advises caution. Monitor plasma-hydroxychloroquine concentration in severe renal impairment.

- MONITORING REQUIREMENTS Manufacturers recommend regular ophthalmological examination but the evidence of practical value is unsatisfactory (see advice of the Royal College of Ophthalmologists).

- PRESCRIBING AND DISPENSING INFORMATION To avoid excessive dosage in obese patients, the dose of hydroxychloroquine should be calculated on the basis of ideal body-weight.

- PATIENT AND CARER ADVICE Do not take antacids for at least 4 hours before or after hydroxychloroquine to reduce possible interference with hydroxychloroquine absorption.

● MEDICINAL FORMS
There can be variation in the licensing of different medicines containing the same drug. Forms available from special-order manufacturers include: oral suspension, oral solution

Tablet
CAUTIONARY AND ADVISORY LABELS 21
▸ Hydroxychloroquine sulfate (Non-proprietary)
Hydroxychloroquine sulfate 200 mg Hydroxychloroquine 200mg tablets | 60 tablet [PoM] £5.15 DT price = £3.83
▸ Plaquenil (Sanofi)
Hydroxychloroquine sulfate 200 mg Plaquenil 200mg tablets | 60 tablet [PoM] £5.15 DT price = £3.83
▸ Quinoric (Bristol Laboratories Ltd)
Hydroxychloroquine sulfate 200 mg Quinoric 200mg tablets | 60 tablet [PoM] £5.10 DT price = £3.83

Leflunomide

● INDICATIONS AND DOSE
Moderate to severe active rheumatoid arthritis (specialist use only)
▸ BY MOUTH
▸ Adult: Initially 100 mg once daily for 3 days, then reduced to 10–20 mg once daily

Active psoriatic arthritis (specialist use only)
▸ BY MOUTH
▸ Adult: Initially 100 mg once daily for 3 days, then reduced to 20 mg once daily

● CONTRA-INDICATIONS Serious infection · severe hypoproteinaemia · severe immunodeficiency
● CAUTIONS Anaemia (avoid if significant and due to causes other than rheumatoid arthritis) · history of tuberculosis · impaired bone-marrow function (avoid if significant and due to causes other than rheumatoid arthritis) · leucopenia (avoid if significant and due to causes other than rheumatoid arthritis) · thrombocytopenia (avoid if significant and due to causes other than rheumatoid arthritis)
● INTERACTIONS → Appendix 1 (leflunomide).
Increased risk of toxicity with other haematotoxic and hepatotoxic drugs.
Caution if recent treatment with other hepatotoxic disease-modifying anti-rheumatic drugs.
Caution if recent treatment with other myelotoxic disease-modifying anti-rheumatic drugs.
Caution—washout procedures recommended before switching to other disease-modifying antirheumatic drugs (consult product literature).
● SIDE-EFFECTS
▸ **Common or very common** Abdominal pain · alopecia · anorexia · asthenia · diarrhoea · dizziness · dry skin · headache · increased blood pressure · leucopenia · nausea · oral mucosal disorders · paraesthesia · pruritus · rash · tenosynovitis · vomiting
▸ **Uncommon** Anaemia · anxiety · hyperlipidaemia · hypokalaemia · hypophosphataemia · taste disturbance · tendon rupture · thrombocytopenia
▸ **Rare** Hepatitis · eosinophilia · interstitial lung disease · jaundice · pancytopenia · severe infection
▸ **Very rare** Hepatic failure · pancreatitis · peripheral neuropathy · progressive multifocal leucoencephalopathy · Stevens-Johnson syndrome · toxic epidermal necrolysis · vasculitis
▸ **Frequency not known** Bone-marrow toxicity · hypouricaemia · malignancy · reduced sperm count · renal failure

SIDE-EFFECTS, FURTHER INFORMATION
Discontinue treatment and institute washout procedure in case of serious side-effect (consult product literature).

▸ Hepatotoxicity Potentially life-threatening hepatotoxicity reported usually in the first 6 months. Discontinue treatment (and institute washout procedure—consult product literature) or reduce dose according to liver-function abnormality; if liver-function abnormality persists after dose reduction, discontinue treatment and institute washout procedure.

● CONCEPTION AND CONTRACEPTION Effective contraception **essential** during treatment and for at least 2 years after treatment in women and at least 3 months after treatment in men (plasma concentration monitoring required; waiting time before conception may be reduced with washout procedure—consult product literature). The concentration of the active metabolite after washout should be less than 20 micrograms/litre (measured on 2 occasions 14 days apart) in men or women before conception—consult product literature.
● PREGNANCY Avoid—active metabolite teratogenic in *animal* studies.
● BREAST FEEDING Present in milk in *animal* studies—manufacturer advises avoid.
● HEPATIC IMPAIRMENT Avoid—active metabolite may accumulate.
● RENAL IMPAIRMENT Manufacturer advises avoid in moderate or severe impairment—no information available.
● PRE-TREATMENT SCREENING Exclude pregnancy before treatment.
● MONITORING REQUIREMENTS
▸ Monitor full blood count (including differential white cell count and platelet count) before treatment and every 2 weeks for 6 months then every 8 weeks.
▸ Monitor liver function before treatment and every 2 weeks for first 6 months then every 8 weeks.
▸ Monitor blood pressure.
● TREATMENT CESSATION
Washout Procedure The active metabolite persists for a long period; to aid drug elimination in case of serious adverse effect, or before starting another disease-modifying antirheumatic drug, or before conception, stop treatment and give *either* colestyramine p. 180 *or* charcoal, activated p. 1201. Procedure may be repeated as necessary.

● MEDICINAL FORMS
There can be variation in the licensing of different medicines containing the same drug.
Tablet
CAUTIONARY AND ADVISORY LABELS 4
▸ Leflunomide (Non-proprietary)
Leflunomide 10 mg Leflunomide 10mg tablets | 30 tablet [PoM] £46.00 DT price = £6.73
Leflunomide 15 mg Leflunomide 15mg tablets | 30 tablet [PoM] £46.00
Leflunomide 20 mg Leflunomide 20mg tablets | 30 tablet [PoM] £61.36 DT price = £4.96
▸ Arava (Sanofi)
Leflunomide 10 mg Arava 10mg tablets | 30 tablet [PoM] £51.13 DT price = £6.73
Leflunomide 20 mg Arava 20mg tablets | 30 tablet [PoM] £61.36 DT price = £4.96
Leflunomide 100 mg Arava 100mg tablets | 3 tablet [PoM] £30.67

Penicillamine

- **DRUG ACTION** Penicillamine aids the elimination of copper ions in Wilson's disease (hepatolenticular degeneration).

- **INDICATIONS AND DOSE**

Severe active rheumatoid arthritis (administered on expert advice)
▸ BY MOUTH
- Adult: Initially 125–250 mg daily for 1 month, then increased in steps of 125–250 mg, at intervals of not less than 4 weeks; maintenance 500–750 mg daily in divided doses, then reduced in steps of 125–250 mg every 12 weeks, dose reduction attempted only if remission sustained for 6 months; maximum 1.5 g per day
- Elderly: Initially up to 125 mg daily for 1 month, then increased in steps of up to 125 mg, at intervals of at least 4 weeks; maximum 1 g per day

Wilson's disease
▸ BY MOUTH
- Adult: 1.5–2 g daily in divided doses, adjusted according to response, to be taken before food; maintenance 0.75–1 g daily, a dose of 2 g daily should not be continued for more than one year; maximum 2 g per day
- Elderly: 20 mg/kg daily in divided doses, adjusted according to response

Autoimmune hepatitis (used rarely; after disease controlled with corticosteroids)
▸ BY MOUTH
- Adult: Initially 500 mg daily in divided doses, to be increased slowly over 3 months; maintenance 1.25 g daily

Cystinuria, therapeutic
▸ BY MOUTH
- Adult: 1–3 g daily in divided doses, to be adjusted to maintain urinary cystine below 200 mg/litre, to be taken before food

Cystinuria, prophylactic
▸ BY MOUTH
- Adult: 0.5–1 g daily, maintain urinary cystine below 300 mg/litre and adequate fluid intake (at least 3 litres daily), to be taken at bedtime
- Elderly: Minimum dose to maintain urinary cystine below 200 mg/litre is recommended

- **CONTRA-INDICATIONS** Lupus erythematosus
- **CAUTIONS** Neurological involvement in Wilson's disease
- **INTERACTIONS** → Appendix 1 (penicillamine). Caution with concomitant nephrotoxic drugs (increased risk of toxicity). Caution with gold treatment (avoid concomitant use if adverse reactions to gold).
- **SIDE-EFFECTS**
▸ **Common or very common** Anorexia · fever · nausea · proteinuria · rash · thrombocytopenia
▸ **Rare** Alopecia · breast enlargement (male and female) · elastosis perforans · haematuria (withdraw immediately if cause unknown) · mouth ulceration · pseudoxanthoma elasticum · skin laxity · stomatitis
▸ **Frequency not known** Agranulocytosis · aplastic anaemia · blood disorders · bronchiolitis · cholestatic jaundice · dermatomyositis · glomerulonephritis · Goodpasture's syndrome · haemolytic anaemia · haemolytic leucopenia · late rashes (consider dose reduction) · lupus erythematosus · myasthenia gravis · nephrotic syndrome · neuropathy (especially if neurological involvement in Wilson's disease—prophylactic pyridoxine recommended) · neutropenia · pancreatitis · pemphigus · pneumonitis · polymyositis · pulmonary haemorrhage · rheumatoid

arthritis · septic arthritis (in patients with rheumatoid arthritis) · Stevens-Johnson syndrome · taste loss (mineral supplements not recommended) · urticaria · vomiting

SIDE-EFFECTS, FURTHER INFORMATION
▸ Proteinuria Proteinuria, associated with immune complex nephritis, occurs in up to 30% of patients, but may resolve despite continuation of treatment; treatment may be continued provided that renal function tests remain normal, oedema is absent, and the 24-hour urinary excretion of protein does not exceed 2 g.
▸ Rash Rashes are a common side-effect. Those that occur in the first few months of treatment disappear when the drug is stopped and treatment may then be re-introduced at a lower dose level and gradually increased.
▸ Taste loss Loss of taste can occur about 6 weeks after treatment is started but usually returns 6 weeks later irrespective of whether treatment is discontinued.
▸ Nausea Nausea may occur but is not usually a problem provided that penicillamine is taken before food or on retiring and that low initial doses are used and only gradually increased.

- **ALLERGY AND CROSS-SENSITIVITY** Patients who are hypersensitive to penicillin may react rarely to penicillamine.
- **PREGNANCY** Fetal abnormalities reported rarely; avoid if possible.
- **BREAST FEEDING** Manufacturer advises avoid unless potential benefit outweighs risk—no information available.
- **RENAL IMPAIRMENT** Reduce dose and monitor renal function or avoid (consult product literature).
- **MONITORING REQUIREMENTS**
▸ Consider withdrawal if platelet count falls below 120 000/mm^3 or white blood cells below 2500/mm^3 or if 3 successive falls within reference range (can restart at reduced dose when counts return to within reference range but permanent withdrawal necessary if recurrence of leucopenia or thrombocytopenia).
▸ Blood counts, including platelets, and urine examinations should be carried out before starting treatment and then every 1 or 2 weeks for the first 2 months then every 4 weeks to detect blood disorders and proteinuria (they should also be carried out in the week after any dose increase).
▸ A reduction in platelet count calls for discontinuation with subsequent re-introduction at a lower dosage and then, if possible, gradual increase.
▸ Longer intervals may be adequate in cystinuria and Wilson's disease.
- **PATIENT AND CARER ADVICE** Counselling on the symptoms of blood disorders is advised. Warn patient and carers to tell doctor immediately if sore throat, fever, infection, non-specific illness, unexplained bleeding and bruising, purpura, mouth ulcers, or rashes develop.

- **MEDICINAL FORMS**
There can be variation in the licensing of different medicines containing the same drug. Forms available from special-order manufacturers include: oral solution

Tablet
CAUTIONARY AND ADVISORY LABELS 6, 22
▸ Penicillamine (Non-proprietary)
Penicillamine 125 mg Penicillamine 125mg tablets | 56 tablet [PoM] £45.00 DT price = £44.03
Penicillamine 250 mg Penicillamine 250mg tablets | 56 tablet [PoM] £90.00 DT price = £86.25
▸ Distamine (Alliance Pharmaceuticals Ltd)
Penicillamine 125 mg Distamine 125mg tablets | 100 tablet [PoM] £10.34
Penicillamine 250 mg Distamine 250mg tablets | 100 tablet [PoM] £17.78

Sodium aurothiomalate

- **INDICATIONS AND DOSE**

Active progressive rheumatoid arthritis (administered on expert advice)
▸ BY DEEP INTRAMUSCULAR INJECTION
▸ Adult: Test dose 10 mg, followed by 50 mg once weekly until there is definite evidence of remission, then reduced to 50 mg every 4 weeks continued for up to 5 years after complete remission, dose to be reduced gradually. Benefit is not expected until 300–500 mg has been given; it should be discontinued if there is no remission after 1 g has been given

Relapse in patients who have previously received sodium aurothiomalate therapy for active progressive rheumatoid arthritis (administered on expert advice)
▸ BY DEEP INTRAMUSCULAR INJECTION
▸ Adult: 50 mg once weekly until control has been obtained again, then reduced to 50 mg every 4 weeks continued for up to 5 years after complete remission, if no response is seen within 2 months, alternative treatment should be sought

- **CONTRA-INDICATIONS** Exfoliative dermatitis · history of blood disorders · history of bone marrow aplasia · necrotising enterocolitis · pulmonary fibrosis · systemic lupus erythematosus
- **CAUTIONS** Colitis · eczema · elderly · history of urticaria
  CAUTIONS, FURTHER INFORMATION
  Sodium aurothiomalate should be discontinued in the presence of blood disorders, gastro-intestinal bleeding (associated with ulcerative enterocolitis), or unexplained proteinuria (associated with immune complex nephritis) which is repeatedly above 300 mg/litre.
- **INTERACTIONS** → Appendix 1 (sodium aurothiomalate).
- **SIDE-EFFECTS** Alopecia · blood disorders (sometimes sudden and fatal) · colitis · gold deposits in eye · hepatotoxicity with cholestatic jaundice · irreversible pigmentation in sun-exposed areas (on prolonged parenteral treatment) · mouth ulcers · nephrotic syndrome · peripheral neuropathy · proteinuria · pulmonary fibrosis · severe anaphylactic reactions · skin reactions · stomatitis · taste disturbances
  SIDE-EFFECTS, FURTHER INFORMATION
  Rashes with pruritus often occur after 2 to 6 months of treatment and may necessitate discontinuation.
- **PREGNANCY** Consider reducing dose and frequency. Manufacturer advises avoid but limited data suggests usually not necessary to withdraw if condition well controlled.
- **BREAST FEEDING** Manufacturer advises avoid—present in milk; theoretical possibility of rashes and idiosyncratic reactions.
- **HEPATIC IMPAIRMENT** Caution in mild to moderate impairment. Avoid in severe impairment.
- **RENAL IMPAIRMENT** Caution in mild to moderate impairment. Avoid in severe impairment.
- **MONITORING REQUIREMENTS**
▸ Urine tests and full blood counts (including total and differential white cell and platelet counts) must be performed before starting treatment and before each intramuscular injection.
▸ Monitor for pulmonary fibrosis with annual chest X-ray.
- **PATIENT AND CARER ADVICE** Patients should be advised to seek prompt medical attention if diarrhoea, sore throat, fever, infection, non-specific illness, unexplained bleeding and bruising, purpura, mouth ulcers, metallic taste, rash, breathlessness, or cough develop.

- **MEDICINAL FORMS**
There can be variation in the licensing of different medicines containing the same drug.
Solution for injection
CAUTIONARY AND ADVISORY LABELS 11
▸ Myocrisin (Sanofi)
  Sodium aurothiomalate 20 mg per 1 ml Myocrisin 10mg/0.5ml solution for injection ampoules | 10 ampoule [PoM] £45.55
  Sodium aurothiomalate 100 mg per 1 ml Myocrisin 50mg/0.5ml solution for injection ampoules | 10 ampoule [PoM] £134.80

IMMUNOSUPPRESSANTS > INTERLEUKIN INHIBITORS

Anakinra

- **INDICATIONS AND DOSE**

Treatment of rheumatoid arthritis (in combination with methotrexate) which has not responded to methotrexate alone
▸ BY SUBCUTANEOUS INJECTION
▸ Adult: 100 mg once daily

- **CONTRA-INDICATIONS** Neutropenia
- **CAUTIONS** History of asthma (risk of serious infection) · predisposition to infection
- **INTERACTIONS** → Appendix 1 (anakinra).
- **SIDE-EFFECTS**
▸ **Common or very common** Neutropenia
▸ **Frequency not known** Antibody formation · headache · infections · injection-site reactions · malignancy
  SIDE-EFFECTS, FURTHER INFORMATION
▸ Blood disorders Neutropenia reported commonly—discontinue if neutropenia develops.
- **CONCEPTION AND CONTRACEPTION** Effective contraception must be used during treatment.
- **PREGNANCY** Manufacturer advises avoid.
- **BREAST FEEDING** Manufacturer advises avoid—no information available.
- **RENAL IMPAIRMENT** Caution if eGFR 30–50 mL/minute/1.73 m^2. Avoid if eGFR less than 30 mL/minute/1.73 m^2.
- **MONITORING REQUIREMENTS** Monitor neutrophil count before treatment, then every month for 6 months, then every 3 months.
- **PATIENT AND CARER ADVICE**
Blood disorders Patients should be instructed to seek medical advice if symptoms suggestive of neutropenia (such as fever, sore throat, bruising or, bleeding) develop.
- **NATIONAL FUNDING/ACCESS DECISIONS**
Scottish Medicines Consortium (SMC) Decisions
The *Scottish Medicines Consortium* has advised (July 2002) that anakinra is **not** recommended for the treatment of rheumatoid arthritis within NHS Scotland.

- **MEDICINAL FORMS**
There can be variation in the licensing of different medicines containing the same drug.
Solution for injection
▸ Kineret (Swedish Orphan Biovitrum Ltd)
  Anakinra 150 mg per 1 ml Kineret 100mg/0.67ml solution for injection pre-filled syringes | 28 pre-filled disposable injection [PoM] £734.44

10

Musculoskeletal system

Secukinumab
16.3.2016

- **DRUG ACTION** Secukinumab is a recombinant human monoclonal antibody that selectively binds to cytokine interleukin-17A (IL-17A) and inhibits the release of proinflammatory cytokines and chemokines.

- **INDICATIONS AND DOSE**

Psoriatic arthritis | Ankylosing spondylitis
▶ BY SUBCUTANEOUS INJECTION
▶ Adult: 150 mg every 1 week for 5 doses, then maintenance 150 mg every 1 month, review treatment if no response within 16 weeks of initial dose

Psoriatic arthritis with concomitant moderate to severe plaque psoriasis or if inadequate response to anti-TNFα treatment | Plaque psoriasis
▶ BY SUBCUTANEOUS INJECTION
▶ Adult: 300 mg every 1 week for 5 doses, then maintenance 300 mg every 1 month, review treatment if no response within 16 weeks of initial dose

- **CONTRA-INDICATIONS** Severe active infection
- **CAUTIONS** Chronic infection · Crohn's disease (monitor for exacerbations) · history of recurrent infection · predisposition to infection (discontinue if new serious infection develops)
  CAUTIONS, FURTHER INFORMATION
▶ Tuberculosis Manufacturer advises that patients with latent tuberculosis should complete anti-tuberculosis therapy before starting secukinumab.
- **INTERACTIONS** → Appendix 1 (secukinumab).
- **SIDE-EFFECTS**
▶ **Common or very common** Diarrhoea · oral herpes · rhinorrhoea · upper respiratory tract infections
▶ **Uncommon** Conjunctivitis · neutropenia (usually mild and reversible) · oral candidiasis · otitis externa · tinea pedis
▶ **Rare** Anaphylactic reactions
- **CONCEPTION AND CONTRACEPTION** Manufacturer advises that women of childbearing potential should use effective contraception during treatment and for at least 20 weeks after stopping treatment.
- **PREGNANCY** Manufacturer advises avoid—no information available.
- **BREAST FEEDING** Manufacturer advises avoid during treatment and for up to 20 weeks after discontinuing treatment—no information available.
- **DIRECTIONS FOR ADMINISTRATION** Manufacturer advises to take the syringe or pen out of the refrigerator 20 minutes before administration and to avoid injecting into areas of the skin that show psoriasis. Patients may self-administer *Cosentyx®* pre-filled pen.
- **PATIENT AND CARER ADVICE**
  Self-administration Patients and their carers should be given training in subcutaneous injection technique.
  Infection Patients and their carers should be advised to seek immediate medical attention if symptoms of infection develop during treatment with secukinumab.
- **NATIONAL FUNDING/ACCESS DECISIONS**
  NICE technology appraisals (TAs)
▶ Secukinumab for treating moderate to severe plaque psoriasis (July 2015) NICE TA350
  Secukinumab is recommended as an option for the treatment of moderate to severe plaque psoriasis in adults if:
  - the disease has failed to respond to standard systemic treatments (including ciclosporin, methotreaxate, and PUVA), or when standard treatments are contra-indicated or not tolerated; *and*
  - the manufacturer provides secukinumab with the discount agreed in the patient access scheme

Secukinumab should be withdrawn in patients whose psoriasis has not responded adequately within 12 weeks of initial dose; further treatment cycles are not recommended.
  Patients whose treatment with secukinumab was started before this guidance was published, but does not meet these criteria, should have the option to continue treatment until they and their clinician consider it appropriate to stop.
www.nice.org.uk/TA350

Scottish Medicines Consortium (SMC) Decisions
The *Scottish Medicines Consortium* has advised (May 2015) that secukinumab *(Cosentyx®)* is accepted for restricted use within NHS Scotland for the treatment of moderate to severe plaque psoriasis in adults who have failed to respond to standard systemic therapies (including ciclosporin, methotrexate and phototherapy), or when standard treatments cannot be used because of intolerance or contra-indications.

- **MEDICINAL FORMS**
  There can be variation in the licensing of different medicines containing the same drug.
  Solution for injection
▶ Cosentyx (Novartis Pharmaceuticals UK Ltd) ▼
  Secukinumab 150 mg per 1 ml Cosentyx 150mg/1ml solution for injection pre-filled pens | 2 pre-filled disposable injection [PoM] no price available
  Cosentyx 150mg/1ml solution for injection pre-filled syringes | 2 pre-filled disposable injection [PoM] no price available

Tocilizumab
31.5.2016

- **INDICATIONS AND DOSE**

Moderate to severe active rheumatoid arthritis (in combination with methotrexate or alone if methotrexate inappropriate) when response to at least one disease-modifying antirheumatic drug or tumour necrosis factor inhibitor has been inadequate, or in those who are intolerant of these drugs
▶ BY INTRAVENOUS INFUSION
▶ Adult: 8 mg/kg every 4 weeks (max. per dose 800 mg), for dose adjustments in patients with liver enzyme abnormalities, or low absolute neutrophil or platelet count, consult product literature

- **CONTRA-INDICATIONS** Do not initiate if absolute neutrophil count less than 2×10^9/litre · severe active infection
- **CAUTIONS** History of diverticulitis · history of intestinal ulceration · history of recurrent or chronic infection (interrupt treatment if serious infection occurs) · low absolute neutrophil count · low platelet count · predisposition to infection (interrupt treatment if serious infection occurs)
  CAUTIONS, FURTHER INFORMATION
▶ Tuberculosis Patients with latent tuberculosis should be treated with standard therapy before starting tocilizumab.
- **INTERACTIONS** → Appendix 1 (tocilizumab).
- **SIDE-EFFECTS**
▶ **Common or very common** Abdominal pain · antibody formation · dizziness · gastritis · headache · hypercholesterolaemia · hypersensitivity · hypertension · infection · leucopenia · mouth ulceration · neutropenia · peripheral oedema · pruritus · raised hepatic transaminases · rash · upper respiratory-tract infection
▶ **Uncommon** Anaphylaxis · gastric ulcer · gastro-intestinal perforation · hypertriglyceridaemia · hypothyroidism · infusion related reactions · nephrolithiasis
▶ **Frequency not known** Thrombocytopenia

SIDE-EFFECTS, FURTHER INFORMATION
▸ Neutrophil and platelet counts Discontinue if absolute neutrophil count less than 0.5×10^9/litre or platelet count less than 50×10^3/microlitre).

● CONCEPTION AND CONTRACEPTION Effective contraception required during and for 3 months after treatment.

● PREGNANCY Manufacturer advises avoid unless essential—toxicity in *animal* studies.

● BREAST FEEDING Manufacturer advises use only if potential benefit outweighs risk—no information available.

● HEPATIC IMPAIRMENT Manufacturer advises caution—consult product literature.

● RENAL IMPAIRMENT Manufacturer advises monitor renal function closely in moderate or severe impairment.

● PRE-TREATMENT SCREENING
Tuberculosis Patients should be evaluated for tuberculosis before treatment.

● MONITORING REQUIREMENTS
▸ Monitor lipid profile 4–8 weeks after starting treatment and then as indicated.
▸ Monitor for demyelinating disorders.
▸ Monitor hepatic transaminases every 4–8 weeks for first 6 months, then every 12 weeks.
▸ Monitor neutrophil and platelet counts 4–8 weeks after starting treatment and then as indicated.

● DIRECTIONS FOR ADMINISTRATION For *intravenous infusion* (*RoActemra*®), give intermittently in Sodium chloride 0.9%; dilute requisite dose to a volume of 100 mL with infusion fluid and give over 1 hour.

● PATIENT AND CARER ADVICE An alert card should be provided.

Patients and their carers should be advised to seek immediate medical attention if symptoms of infection occur, or if symptoms of diverticular perforation such as abdominal pain, haemorrhage, or fever accompanying change in bowel habits occur.

● NATIONAL FUNDING/ACCESS DECISIONS

NICE technology appraisals (TAs)
▸ Adalimumab, etanercept, infliximab, certolizumab pegol, golimumab, tocilizumab and abatacept for rheumatoid arthritis not previously treated with DMARDs or after conventional DMARDs only have failed (January 2016) NICE TA375

Tocilizumab, in combination with methotrexate, is recommended as an option for treating rheumatoid arthritis, only if **all** the following criteria are met:
● disease is severe, that is, a disease activity score (DAS28) greater than 5.1,
● disease has not responded to intensive therapy with a combination of conventional disease-modifying antirheumatic drugs (DMARDs),
● the manufacturers provides tocilizumab as agreed in the patient access schemes.

Tocilizumab can be used as monotherapy in patients who cannot take methotrexate because it is contra-indicated or because of intolerance, when the criteria above are met.

Continue treatment only if there is a moderate response measured using European League Against Rheumatism (EULAR) criteria at 6 months after starting therapy. After initial response within 6 months, withdraw treatment if a moderate EULAR response is not maintained.

Patients currently receiving tocilizumab whose disease does not meet the above criteria should have the option to continue their treatment until they and their clinician consider it appropriate to stop.
www.nice.org.uk/TA375

▸ Tocilizumab for the treatment of rheumatoid arthritis (February 2012—updated February 2016) NICE TA247
Tocilizumab, in combination with methotrexate, is recommended as an option for the treatment of rheumatoid arthritis in adults if:
● the disease has responded inadequately to DMARDs and a TNF inhibitor and the patient cannot receive rituximab because of contra-indications or intolerance, **and** tocilizumab is used as described for TNF inhibitor treatments (specifically the recommendations on disease activity) in the NICE guidance (August 2010) Adalimumab, etanercept, infliximab, rituximab and abatacept for the treatment of rheumatoid arthritis after the failure of a TNF inhibitor, *or*
● the disease has responded inadequately to one or more TNF inhibitor treatments and to rituximab
● **and** the manufacturer provides tocilizumab with the discount agreed as part of the patient access scheme.

Patients currently receiving tocilizumab for the treatment of rheumatoid arthritis who do not meet these criteria should have the option to continue treatment until they and their clinicians consider it appropriate to stop.
www.nice.org.uk/TA247

● MEDICINAL FORMS
There can be variation in the licensing of different medicines containing the same drug.

Solution for infusion
▸ RoActemra (Roche Products Ltd)
Tocilizumab 20 mg per 1 ml RoActemra 400mg/20ml concentrate for solution for infusion vials | 1 vial [PoM] £512.00 (Hospital only)
RoActemra 200mg/10ml concentrate for solution for infusion vials | 1 vial [PoM] £256.00 (Hospital only)
RoActemra 80mg/4ml concentrate for solution for infusion vials | 1 vial [PoM] £102.40 (Hospital only)

Ustekinumab

● INDICATIONS AND DOSE

Severe plaque psoriasis that has not responded to at least 2 standard systemic treatments and photochemotherapy, or when these treatments cannot be used because of intolerance or contra-indications
▸ BY SUBCUTANEOUS INJECTION
▸ Adult (body-weight up to 100 kg): Initially 45 mg, then 45 mg after 4 weeks, then 45 mg every 12 weeks, discontinue if no response within 16 weeks
▸ Adult (body-weight 100 kg and above): Initially 45–90 mg, then 45–90 mg after 4 weeks, then 45–90 mg every 12 weeks, discontinue if no response within 16 weeks

Active psoriatic arthritis (in combination with methotrexate or alone) in patients who have had an inadequate response to one or more disease-modifying antirheumatic drugs
▸ BY SUBCUTANEOUS INJECTION
▸ Adult (body-weight up to 100 kg): Initially 45 mg, then 45 mg after 4 weeks, then 45 mg every 12 weeks, review treatment if no response within 28 weeks
▸ Adult (body-weight 100 kg and above): Initially 45–90 mg, then 45–90 mg after 4 weeks, then 45–90 mg every 12 weeks, review treatment if no response within 28 weeks

● CONTRA-INDICATIONS Active infection
● CAUTIONS Development of malignancy · elderly · history of malignancy · predisposition to infection · start appropriate treatment if widespread erythema and skin exfoliation develop, and stop ustekinumab treatment if exfoliative dermatitis suspected

Musculoskeletal system

10

CAUTIONS, FURTHER INFORMATION

▶ Tuberculosis Active tuberculosis should be treated with standard treatment for at least 2 months before starting ustekinumab. Patients who have previously received adequate treatment for tuberculosis can start ustekinumab but should be monitored every 3 months for possible recurrence. In patients without active tuberculosis but who were previously not treated adequately, chemoprophylaxis should ideally be completed before starting ustekinumab. In patients at high risk of tuberculosis who cannot be assessed by tuberculin skin test, chemoprophylaxis can be given concurrently with ustekinumab.

● INTERACTIONS → Appendix 1 (ustekinumab).

● SIDE-EFFECTS

▶ **Common or very common** Arthralgia · diarrhoea · dizziness · headache · infections (sometimes severe) · injection-site reactions · malaise · myalgia · nausea · oropharyngeal pain · pruritus

▶ **Uncommon** Depression · facial palsy · hypersensitivity reactions (possibly delayed onset) · nasal congestion · pustular psoriasis

▶ **Rare** Exfoliative dermatitis

● CONCEPTION AND CONTRACEPTION Manufacturer advises effective contraception during treatment and for 15 weeks after stopping treatment.

● PREGNANCY Avoid.

● BREAST FEEDING Manufacturer advises avoid—present in milk in *animal* studies.

● PRE-TREATMENT SCREENING
Tuberculosis Patients should be evaluated for tuberculosis before treatment.

● MONITORING REQUIREMENTS

▶ Monitor for non-melanoma skin cancer, especially in patients with a history of PUVA treatment or prolonged immunosuppressant therapy, or those over 60 years of age.

▶ Monitor for signs and symptoms of exfoliative dermatitis or erythrodermic psoriasis.

● PATIENT AND CARER ADVICE
Exfoliative dermatitis Patients should be advised to seek prompt medical attention if symptoms suggestive of exfoliative dermatitis or erythrodermic psoriasis (such as increased redness and shedding of skin over a larger area of the body) develop.
Tuberculosis Patients should be advised to seek medical attention if symptoms suggestive of tuberculosis (e.g. persistent cough, weight loss, and fever) develop.

● NATIONAL FUNDING/ACCESS DECISIONS

NICE technology appraisals (TAs)

▶ **Ustekinumab for plaque psoriasis in adults (September 2009)** NICE TA180
Ustekinumab is recommended for the treatment of severe plaque psoriasis which has failed to respond to standard systemic treatments (including ciclosporin and methotrexate) and to photochemotherapy, or when standard treatments cannot be used because of intolerance or contra-indications. Ustekinumab should be withdrawn if the response is not adequate after 16 weeks. For patients weighing over 100 kg, the manufacturer should provide the 90-mg dose of ustekinumab at the same price as the 45-mg dose.
www.nice.org.uk/TA180

▶ **Ustekinumab for treating active psoriatic arthritis (June 2015)** NICE TA340
Ustekinumab is an option, alone or in combination with methotrexate, for the treatment of active psoriatic arthritis in adults only when:
● treatment with tumour necrosis factor (TNF) alpha inhibitors is contra-indicated but would otherwise be considered (as described in the NICE guidance on

etanercept, infliximab and adalimumab for the treatment of psoriatic arthritis (August 2010) and golimumab for the treatment of psoriatic arthritis (April 2011) **or**
● the patient has had treatment with 1 or more TNF-alpha inhibitors.
Ustekinumab is recommended only if the manufacturer provides the 90 mg dose of ustekinumab for patients who weigh more than 100 kg at the same cost as the 45 mg dose, as agreed in the patient access scheme.
Ustekinumab treatment should be stopped if the patient's psoriatic arthritis has not shown an adequate response using the Psoriatic Arthritis Response Criteria (PsARC) at 24 weeks.
Patients currently receiving ustekinumab whose disease does not meet the above criteria should have the option to continue treatment until they and their clinician consider it appropriate to stop.
www.nice.org.uk/TA340

Scottish Medicines Consortium (SMC) Decisions
The *Scottish Medicines Consortium* has advised (February 2014) that ustekinumab (*Stelara*®) is accepted for restricted use within NHS Scotland either alone or in combination with methotrexate, for the treatment of active psoriatic arthritis in adults who have responded inadequately to previous therapy with a non-biological disease-modifying anti-rheumatic drug, and failed on, or are unsuitable for, treatment with a TNF inhibitor.

● MEDICINAL FORMS
There can be variation in the licensing of different medicines containing the same drug.
Solution for injection
CAUTIONARY AND ADVISORY LABELS 10
▶ Stelara (Janssen-Cilag Ltd)
Ustekinumab 90 mg per 1 ml Stelara 90mg/1ml solution for injection pre-filled syringes | 1 pre-filled disposable injection [PoM] £2,147.00
Stelara 45mg/0.5ml solution for injection vials | 1 vial [PoM] £2,147.00
Stelara 45mg/0.5ml solution for injection pre-filled syringes | 1 pre-filled disposable injection [PoM] £2,147.00

IMMUNOSUPPRESSANTS 〉T-CELL ACTIVATION INHIBITORS

| Abatacept | 31.5.2016 |

● INDICATIONS AND DOSE

Moderate to severe active rheumatoid arthritis (in combination with methotrexate) in patients unresponsive to other disease-modifying antirheumatic drugs (including methotrexate or a tumour necrosis factor (TNF) inhibitor)

▶ INITIALLY BY INTRAVENOUS INFUSION

▶ Adult (body-weight up to 60 kg): 500 mg every 2 weeks for 3 doses (loading dose), then (by intravenous infusion) 500 mg every 4 weeks, alternatively (by subcutaneous injection) 125 mg once weekly, first subcutaneous dose to be given within 1 day of the intravenous loading dose; patients who are unable to receive an infusion may initiate subcutaneous abatacept without receiving an intravenous loading dose

▶ Adult (body-weight 60-100 kg): 750 mg every 2 weeks for 3 doses (loading dose), then (by intravenous infusion) 750 mg every 4 weeks, alternatively (by subcutaneous injection) 125 mg once weekly, first subcutaneous dose to be given within 1 day of the intravenous loading dose; patients who are unable to receive an infusion may initiate subcutaneous abatacept without receiving an intravenous loading dose

▸ Adult (body-weight 101 kg and above): 1 g every 2 weeks for 3 doses (loading dose), then (by intravenous infusion) 1 g every 4 weeks, alternatively (by subcutaneous injection) 125 mg once weekly, first subcutaneous dose to be given within 1 day of the intravenous loading dose; patients who are unable to receive an infusion may initiate subcutaneous abatacept without receiving an intravenous loading dose

● CONTRA-INDICATIONS Severe infection

● CAUTIONS Do not initiate until active infections are controlled · elderly (increased risk of side-effects) · predisposition to infection (screen for latent tuberculosis and viral hepatitis) · progressive multifocal leucoencephalopathy (discontinue treatment if neurological symptoms present)

● INTERACTIONS → Appendix 1 (abatacept).

● SIDE-EFFECTS

▸ **Common or very common** Abdominal pain · conjunctivitis · cough · diarrhoea · dizziness · dyspepsia · fatigue · flushing · headache · hypertension · infection · leucopenia · nausea · pain in extremities · paraesthesia · stomatitis · vomiting

▸ **Uncommon** Psoriasis · alopecia · anxiety · arthralgia · basal and squamous cell carcinoma · bradycardia · bronchospasm · bruising · depression · dry eye · dry skin · dyspnoea · gastritis · hyperhidrosis · hypotension · menstrual disturbances · palpitation · skin papilloma · sleep disorder · tachycardia · thrombocytopenia · visual disturbance · weight gain

▸ **Frequency not known** Lung cancer · lymphoma

● CONCEPTION AND CONTRACEPTION Effective contraception required during treatment and for 14 weeks after last dose.

● PREGNANCY Manufacturer advises avoid unless essential.

● BREAST FEEDING Present in milk in *animal* studies— manufacturer advises avoid breast-feeding during treatment and for 14 weeks after last dose.

● DIRECTIONS FOR ADMINISTRATION For *intravenous infusion*, given intermittently *in* Sodium chloride 0.9%; reconstitute each vial with 10 mL water for injections using the silicone-free syringe provided; dilute requisite dose in Sodium Chloride 0.9% to 100 mL (using the same silicone-free syringe); give over 30 minutes through a low protein-binding filter (pore size 0.2–1.2 micron).

● NATIONAL FUNDING/ACCESS DECISIONS

NICE technology appraisals (TAs)

▸ **Adalimumab, etanercept, infliximab, rituximab, and abatacept for the treatment of rheumatoid arthritis after the failure of a TNF inhibitor (August 2010)** NICE TA195 Abatacept, in combination with methotrexate, is an option for the treatment of severe active rheumatoid arthritis in adults who have had an inadequate response to, or have an intolerance of, other disease-modifying antirheumatic drugs (DMARDs) including at least 1 tumour necrosis factor (TNF) inhibitor, and who cannot use rituximab because of contra-indications or intolerance. Treatment should be continued only if there is adequate response. Patients should be monitored at least every 6 months. www.nice.org.uk/TA195

▸ **Adalimumab, etanercept, infliximab, certolizumab pegol, golimumab, tocilizumab and abatacept for rheumatoid arthritis not previously treated with DMARDs or after conventional DMARDs only have failed (January 2016)** NICE TA375 Abatacept, in combination with methotrexate, is recommended as an option for treating rheumatoid arthritis, only if **all** the following criteria are met:
  ● disease is severe, that is, a disease activity score (DAS28) greater than 5.1,

● disease has not responded to intensive therapy with a combination of conventional disease-modifying antirheumatic drugs (DMARDs),
● the manufacturers provides abatacept as agreed in the patient access schemes.

Continue treatment only if there is a moderate response measured using European League Against Rheumatism (EULAR) criteria at 6 months after starting therapy. After initial response within 6 months, withdraw treatment if a moderate EULAR response is not maintained.

Patients currently receiving abatacept whose disease does not meet the above criteria should have the option to continue their treatment until they and their clinician consider it appropriate to stop. www.nice.org.uk/TA375

● MEDICINAL FORMS
There can be variation in the licensing of different medicines containing the same drug.

Powder for solution for infusion
ELECTROLYTES: May contain Sodium

▸ Orencia (Bristol-Myers Squibb Pharmaceuticals Ltd)
Abatacept 250 mg Orencia 250mg powder for concentrate for solution for infusion vials | 1 vial [PoM] £302.40 (Hospital only)

IMMUNOSUPPRESSANTS > TUMOR NECROSIS FACTOR ALPHA (TNF-α) INHIBITORS

Adalimumab
31.5.2016

● INDICATIONS AND DOSE

Severe plaque psoriasis either refractory to at least 2 standard systemic treatments or photochemotherapy, or when standard treatments cannot be used because of intolerance or contra-indications

▸ BY SUBCUTANEOUS INJECTION

▸ Adult: Initially 80 mg, then 40 mg every 2 weeks, to be started 1 week after initial dose, discontinue treatment if no response within 16 weeks

Moderate to severe active rheumatoid arthritis (in combination with methotrexate or alone if methotrexate inappropriate) when response to other disease-modifying drugs (including methotrexate) has been inadequate | Severe, active, and progressive rheumatoid arthritis (in combination with methotrexate or alone if methotrexate inappropriate) not previously treated with methotrexate

▸ BY SUBCUTANEOUS INJECTION

▸ Adult: 40 mg every 2 weeks, then increased if necessary to 40 mg once weekly, dose to be increased only in patients receiving adalimumab alone, review treatment if no response within 12 weeks

Active and progressive psoriatic arthritis that has not responded adequately to other disease-modifying antirheumatic drugs | Severe active ankylosing spondylitis that has not responded adequately to other disease-modifying antirheumatic drugs | Severe axial spondyloarthritis without radiographic evidence of ankylosing spondylitis but with objective signs of inflammation, in patients who have had an inadequate response to, or are intolerant of, NSAIDs

▸ BY SUBCUTANEOUS INJECTION

▸ Adult: 40 mg every 2 weeks, discontinue treatment if no response within 12 weeks

Severe active Crohn's disease

▸ BY SUBCUTANEOUS INJECTION

▸ Adult: Initially 80 mg, then 40 mg after 2 weeks; maintenance 40 mg every 2 weeks, increased if necessary to 40 mg once weekly, maximum 40 mg administered at a single site, review treatment if no response within 12 weeks of initial dose continued →

Severe active Crohn's disease (accelerated regimen)
▸ BY SUBCUTANEOUS INJECTION
▸ **Adult:** Initially 160 mg, dose can alternatively be given as divided injections over 2 days, then 80 mg after 2 weeks; maintenance 40 mg every 2 weeks, increased if necessary to 40 mg once weekly, maximum 40 mg administered at a single site, review treatment if no response within 12 weeks of initial dose

Severe active ulcerative colitis
▸ BY SUBCUTANEOUS INJECTION
▸ **Adult:** Initially 160 mg, dose can alternatively be given as divided injections over 2 days, then 80 mg after 2 weeks; maintenance 40 mg every 2 weeks, increased if necessary to 40 mg once weekly, maximum 40 mg administered at a single site, review treatment if no response within 8 weeks of initial dose

Active moderate to severe hidradenitis suppurativa (acne inversa) in patients with an inadequate response to conventional systemic therapy
▸ BY SUBCUTANEOUS INJECTION
▸ **Adult:** Initially 160 mg, given as either four 40 mg injections in one day or as two 40 mg injections per day for 2 consecutive days, followed by 80 mg after 2 weeks, given as two 40 mg injections in one day, then 40 mg after 2 weeks; maintenance 40 mg once weekly, review treatment if no response within 12 weeks; if treatment interrupted—consult product literature

● CONTRA-INDICATIONS Moderate or severe heart failure · severe infection
● CAUTIONS Demyelinating disorders (risk of exacerbation) · development of malignancy · do not initiate until active infections are controlled (discontinue if new serious infection develops) · hepatitis B virus—monitor for active infection · history of malignancy · mild heart failure (discontinue if symptoms develop or worsen) · predisposition to infection
   CAUTIONS, FURTHER INFORMATION
▸ Tuberculosis Active tuberculosis should be treated with standard treatment for at least 2 months before starting adalimumab. Patients who have previously received adequate treatment for tuberculosis can start adalimumab but should be monitored every 3 months for possible recurrence. In patients without active tuberculosis but who were previously not treated adequately, chemoprophylaxis should ideally be completed before starting adalimumab. In patients at high risk of tuberculosis who cannot be assessed by tuberculin skin test, chemoprophylaxis can be given concurrently with adalimumab.
● INTERACTIONS → Appendix 1 (adalimumab).
● SIDE-EFFECTS
▸ **Common or very common** Anxiety · benign tumours · chest pain · cough · dehydration · dermatitis · dizziness · dyspepsia · dyspnoea · electrolyte disturbances · eye disorders · flushing · gastrointestinal haemorrhage · haematuria · hyperlipidaemia · hypertension · hyperuricaemia · impaired healing · mood changes · musculoskeletal pain · oedema · onycholysis · paraesthesia · rash · renal impairment · skin cancer · sleep disturbances · tachycardia · vomiting
▸ **Uncommon** Aortic aneurysm · arrhythmias · cholecystitis · cholelithiasis · dysphagia · erectile dysfunction · hearing loss · hepatic steatosis · interstitial lung disease · leukaemia · lymphoma · malignancy · neuropathy · nocturia · pancreatitis · pneumonitis · rhabdomyolysis · solid tumours · tinnitus · tremor · vascular occlusion
▸ **Rare** Autoimmune hepatitis · demyelinating disorders · myocardial infarction
▸ **Frequency not known** Abdominal pain · anaemia · antibody formation · aplastic anaemia · blood disorders · cutaneous

vasculitis · depression · fever · headache · hypersensitivity reactions · injection-site reactions · leucopenia · lupus erythematosus-like syndrome · nausea · new onset psoriasis · pancytopenia · pleural effusion · pruritus · pulmonary embolism · sarcoidosis · Stevens-Johnson syndrome · thrombocytopenia · worsening heart failure · worsening of symptoms of dermatomyositis · worsening psoriasis

SIDE-EFFECTS, FURTHER INFORMATION
Associated with infections, sometimes severe, including tuberculosis, septicaemia, and hepatitis B reactivation.
● CONCEPTION AND CONTRACEPTION Manufacturer advises effective contraception required during treatment and for at least 5 months after last dose.
● PREGNANCY Avoid.
● BREAST FEEDING Avoid; manufacturer advises avoid for at least 5 months after last dose.
● PRE-TREATMENT SCREENING
   Tuberculosis Patients should be evaluated for tuberculosis before treatment.
● MONITORING REQUIREMENTS
▸ Monitor for infection before, during, and for 4 months after treatment.
▸ Monitor for non-melanoma skin cancer before and during treatment, especially in patients with a history of PUVA treatment for psoriasis or extensive immunosuppressant therapy.
● PATIENT AND CARER ADVICE An alert card should be provided.
   Tuberculosis Patients and their carers should be advised to seek medical attention if symptoms suggestive of tuberculosis (e.g. persistent cough, weight loss, and fever) develop.
   Blood disorders Patients and their carers should be advised to seek medical attention if symptoms suggestive of blood disorders (such as fever, sore throat, bruising, or bleeding) develop.
▸ When used for Hidradenitis suppurativa Patients and their carers should be advised to use a daily topical antiseptic wash on lesions during treatment with adalimumab.
● NATIONAL FUNDING/ACCESS DECISIONS

NICE technology appraisals (TAs)
▸ **Adalimumab for plaque psoriasis in adults (June 2008)** NICE TA146
   Adalimumab is recommended for the treatment of severe plaque psoriasis which has failed to respond to standard systemic treatments (including ciclosporin and methotrexate) and photochemotherapy, or when standard treatments cannot be used because of intolerance or contra-indications. Adalimumab should be withdrawn if the response is not adequate after 16 weeks.
   www.nice.org.uk/TA146
▸ **Infliximab and adalimumab for Crohn's disease (May 2010)** NICE TA187
   Adalimumab is recommended for the treatment of severe active Crohn's disease that has not responded to conventional therapy (including corticosteroids and other drugs affecting the immune response) or when conventional therapy cannot be used because of intolerance or contra-indications.

   Adalimumab should be given as a planned course of treatment for 12 months or until treatment failure, whichever is shorter. Treatment should be continued beyond 12 months only if there is evidence of active disease—in these cases the need for treatment should be reviewed at least annually. If the disease relapses after stopping treatment, adalimumab can be restarted.
   www.nice.org.uk/TA187

▶ **Infliximab, adalimumab and golimumab for treating moderately to severely active ulcerative colitis after the failure of conventional therapy (February 2015)** NICE TA329
Adalimumab is an option for treating moderately to severely active ulcerative colitis in adults whose disease has responded inadequately to conventional therapy including corticosteroids and mercaptopurine or azathioprine, or in adults who are intolerant to or have contra-indications for conventional therapies.

The choice of treatment should be made on an individual basis and if more than one treatment is suitable, the least expensive should be chosen.

Adalimumab should be given as a planned course of treatment until treatment fails (including the need for surgery) or until 12 months after starting treatment, whichever is shorter. Treatment should be continued only if there is clear evidence of a response. Patients who continue treatment should be reassessed at least every 12 months to determine whether ongoing treatment is still clinically appropriate.
www.nice.org.uk/TA329

▶ **Etanercept, infliximab, and adalimumab for the treatment of psoriatic arthritis (August 2010)** NICE TA199
Adalimumab is recommended for the treatment of active and progressive psoriatic arthritis in adults who have peripheral arthritis with at least 3 tender joints and at least 3 swollen joints, and who have not responded adequately to at least 2 standard disease-modifying antirheumatic drugs (used alone or in combination).

Adalimumab should be discontinued if there is an inadequate response at 12 weeks.
www.nice.org.uk/TA199

▶ **Adalimumab, etanercept, infliximab, rituximab, and abatacept for the treatment of rheumatoid arthritis after the failure of a TNF inhibitor (August 2010)** NICE TA195
Adalimumab, in combination with methotrexate, is an option for the treatment of severe active rheumatoid arthritis in adults who have had an inadequate response to, or have an intolerance of, other DMARDs including at least 1 TNF inhibitor, and who cannot use rituximab because of contra-indications or intolerance. In patients who cannot use methotrexate because of intolerance or contra-indications, adalimumab can be given as monotherapy. Treatment should be continued only if there is adequate response. Patients should be monitored at least every 6 months.
www.nice.org.uk/TA195

▶ **Adalimumab, etanercept, infliximab, certolizumab pegol, golimumab, tocilizumab and abatacept for rheumatoid arthritis not previously treated with DMARDs or after conventional DMARDs only have failed (January 2016)** NICE TA375
Adalimumab, in combination with methotrexate, is recommended as an option for treating rheumatoid arthritis, only if the following criteria are met:
• disease is severe, that is, a disease activity score (DAS28) greater than 5.1, **and**,
• disease has not responded to intensive therapy with a combination of conventional disease-modifying antirheumatic drugs (DMARDs).
Adalimumab can be used as monotherapy in patients who cannot take methotrexate because it is contra-indicated or because of intolerance, when the criteria above are met.

Continue treatment only if there is a moderate response measured using European League Against Rheumatism (EULAR) criteria at 6 months after starting therapy. After initial response within 6 months, withdraw treatment if a moderate EULAR response is not maintained.

Patients currently receiving adalimumab whose disease does not meet the above criteria should have the option to continue their treatment until they and their clinician consider it appropriate to stop.
www.nice.org.uk/TA375

▶ **TNF-alpha inhibitors for ankylosing spondylitis and non-radiographic axial spondyloarthritis (February 2016)** NICE TA383
Adalimumab, certolizumab pegol, etanercept, golimumab and infliximab are recommended as options for treating severe active ankylosing spondylitis in patients whose disease has responded inadequately to, or who are intolerant of, non-steroidal anti-inflammatory drugs (NSAIDs).

Adalimumab, certolizumab pegol and etanercept are also recommended as options for treating severe non-radiographic axial spondyloarthritis in patients whose disease has responded inadequately to, or who are intolerant of, NSAIDs.

The response to treatment should be assessed 12 weeks after the start of treatment and should only be continued if there is clear evidence of response.

Treatment with another tumour necrosis factor (TNF)-alpha inhibitor is recommended in those who cannot tolerate, or whose disease has not responded to, treatment with the first TNF-alpha inhibitor, or in those whose disease has stopped responding after an initial response.
www.nice.org.uk/TA383

Scottish Medicines Consortium (SMC) Decisions
The *Scottish Medicines Consortium* issued similar advice for plaque psoriasis to NICE TA146 in May 2008.

● MEDICINAL FORMS
There can be variation in the licensing of different medicines containing the same drug.
Solution for injection
CAUTIONARY AND ADVISORY LABELS 10
▶ Humira (AbbVie Ltd)
Adalimumab 50 mg per 1 ml Humira 40mg/0.8ml solution for injection pre-filled syringes | 2 pre-filled disposable injection [PoM] £704.28
Humira 40mg/0.8ml solution for injection vials | 2 vial [PoM] £704.28
Humira 40mg/0.8ml solution for injection pre-filled pen | 2 pre-filled disposable injection [PoM] £704.28

Certolizumab pegol
31.5.2016

● INDICATIONS AND DOSE
Moderate to severe active rheumatoid arthritis when response to disease-modifying antirheumatic drugs (including methotrexate) has been inadequate (as monotherapy or in combination with methotrexate) | Severe, active and progressive rheumatoid arthritis in patients not previously treated with methotrexate or other disease-modifying antirheumatic drugs (in combination with methotrexate) | Active psoriatic arthritis when response to disease-modifying antirheumatic drugs has been inadequate (as monotherapy or in combination with methotrexate)
▶ BY SUBCUTANEOUS INJECTION
▶ Adult: Loading dose 400 mg every 2 weeks for 3 doses, then maintenance 200 mg every 2 weeks, once clinical response is confirmed, an alternative maintenance dosing of 400 mg every 4 weeks can be considered, review treatment if no response within 12 weeks

Treatment of severe active ankylosing spondylitis in patients who have had an inadequate response to, or are intolerant of NSAIDs | Treatment of severe active axial spondyloarthritis, without radiographic evidence of ankylosing spondylitis but with objective signs of inflammation, in patients who have had an inadequate response to, or are intolerant of NSAIDs
▶ BY SUBCUTANEOUS INJECTION
▶ Adult: Loading dose 400 mg every 2 weeks for 3 doses, then maintenance 200 mg every 2 weeks, alternatively maintenance 400 mg every 4 weeks, review treatment if no response within 12 weeks

● CONTRA-INDICATIONS Moderate to severe heart failure · severe active infection

● CAUTIONS Demyelinating CNS disorders (risk of exacerbation) · do not initiate until active infections are controlled (discontinue if new serious infection develops and until infection controlled) · hepatitis B virus (monitor for active infection) · history or development of malignancy · mild heart failure (discontinue if symptoms develop or worsen) · predisposition to infection

CAUTIONS, FURTHER INFORMATION

▸ Tuberculosis Active tuberculosis should be treated with standard treatment for at least 2 months before starting certolizumab pegol. Patients who have previously received adequate treatment for tuberculosis can start certolizumab pegol but should be monitored every 3 months for possible recurrence. In patients without active tuberculosis but who were previously not treated adequately, chemoprophylaxis should ideally be completed before starting certolizumab pegol. In patients at high risk of tuberculosis who cannot be assessed by tuberculin skin test, chemoprophylaxis can be given concurrently with certolizumab pegol.

● INTERACTIONS → Appendix 1 (certolizumab pegol).

● SIDE-EFFECTS

▸ Common or very common Hypertension · rash · sensory abnormalities

▸ Uncommon Acne · alopecia · anxiety · appetite disorders · arrhythmias · ascites · asthma · benign tumours · cardiomyopathies · cholestasis · cough · dermatitis · dizziness · dyslipidaemia · ecchymosis · electrolyte disorders · gastro-intestinal disorders · gastro-intestinal perforation · gastro-intestinal ulcer · haematuria · haemorrhage · heart failure · hepatic disorders · impaired healing · influenza-like illness · ischaemic coronary artery disorders · leukaemia · lymphoma · malignancy · menstrual disorders · mood disorders · muscle disorders · nail disorders · new onset or worsening psoriasis · ocular inflammation · oedema · peripheral neuropathy · photosensitivity · pleural effusion · renal impairment · skin cancer · skin discoloration · solid tumours · syncope · tinnitus · tremor · visual disturbance

▸ Rare Atrioventricular block · cerebrovascular accident · cholelithiasis · impaired coordination · interstitial lung disease · nephropathy · Raynaud's phenomenon · seizures · sexual dysfunction · splenomegaly · thyroid disorders · trigeminal neuralgia

▸ Frequency not known Abdominal pain · anaemia · antibody formation · aplastic anaemia · blood disorders · depression · fever · headache · hypersensitivity reactions · infections · injection-site reactions · leucopenia · lupus erythematosus-like syndrome · multiple sclerosis · nausea · pancytopenia · pruritus · thrombocytopenia · worsening heart failure

SIDE-EFFECTS, FURTHER INFORMATION

▸ Infection Associated with infections, sometimes severe, including tuberculosis, septicaemia, and hepatitis B reactivation.

● CONCEPTION AND CONTRACEPTION Manufacturer advises adequate contraception during treatment and for at least 5 months after last dose.

● PREGNANCY Avoid.

● BREAST FEEDING Manufacturer advises use only if potential benefit outweighs risk—no information available.

● PRE-TREATMENT SCREENING

Tuberculosis Patients should be evaluated for tuberculosis before treatment.

● MONITORING REQUIREMENTS Monitor for infection before, during, and for 5 months after treatment.

● PATIENT AND CARER ADVICE An alert card should be provided.

Blood disorders Patients should be advised to seek medical attention if symptoms suggestive of blood disorders (such as fever, sore throat, bruising, or bleeding) develop.

Tuberculosis Patients should be advised to seek medical attention if symptoms suggestive of tuberculosis (e.g persistent cough, weight loss and fever) develop.

● NATIONAL FUNDING/ACCESS DECISIONS

NICE technology appraisals (TAs)

▸ **Adalimumab, etanercept, infliximab, certolizumab pegol, golimumab, tocilizumab and abatacept for rheumatoid arthritis not previously treated with DMARDs or after conventional DMARDs only have failed (January 2016)**

NICE TA375

Certolizumab pegol, in combination with methotrexate, is recommended as an option for treating rheumatoid arthritis, only if all the following criteria are met:

● disease is severe, that is, a disease activity score (DAS28) greater than 5.1,

● disease has not responded to intensive therapy with a combination of conventional disease-modifying antirheumatic drugs (DMARDs),

● the manufacturers provide certolizumab pegol as agreed in the patient access schemes.

Certolizumab pegol can be used as monotherapy in patients who cannot take methotrexate because it is contra-indicated or because of intolerance, when the criteria above are met.

Continue treatment only if there is a moderate response measured using European League Against Rheumatism (EULAR) criteria at 6 months after starting therapy. After initial response within 6 months, withdraw treatment if a moderate EULAR response is not maintained.

Patients currently receiving certolizumab pegol whose disease does not meet the above criteria should have the option to continue their treatment until they and their clinician consider it appropriate to stop.

www.nice.org.uk/TA375

▸ **TNF-alpha inhibitors for ankylosing spondylitis and non-radiographic axial spondyloarthritis (February 2016)**

NICE TA383

Adalimumab, certolizumab pegol, etanercept, golimumab and infliximab are recommended as options for treating severe active ankylosing spondylitis in adults patients whose disease has responded inadequately to, or who are intolerant of, non-steroidal anti-inflammatory drugs.

Adalimumab, certolizumab pegol and etanercept are also recommended as options for treating severe non-radiographic axial spondyloarthritis in patients whose disease has responded inadequately to, or who are intolerant of, non-steroidal anti-inflammatory drugs (NSAIDs).

The response to treatment should be assessed 12 weeks after the start of treatment. Treatment should only be continued if there is clear evidence of response.

Treatment with another tumour necrosis factor (TNF)-alpha inhibitor is recommended in those who cannot tolerate, or whose disease has not responded to, treatment with the first TNF-alpha inhibitor, or in those whose disease has stopped responding after an initial response.

www.nice.org.uk/TA383

Scottish Medicines Consortium (SMC) Decisions

The *Scottish Medicines Consortium* has advised (July 2014) that certolizumab pegol is accepted for restricted use within NHS Scotland, in combination with methotrexate, for the treatment of active psoriatic arthritis in patients whose disease has not responded to adequate trials of at least two standard disease-modifying antirheumatic drugs (DMARDs), administered either individually or in combination.

- MEDICINAL FORMS
There can be variation in the licensing of different medicines
containing the same drug.
Solution for injection
CAUTIONARY AND ADVISORY LABELS 10
▸ Cimzia (UCB Pharma Ltd)
Certolizumab pegol 200 mg per 1 ml Cimzia 200mg/1ml solution
for injection pre-filled syringes | 2 syringe [PoM] £715.00

Etanercept
4.5.2016

- INDICATIONS AND DOSE

**Moderate to severe active rheumatoid arthritis (alone or
in combination with methotrexate) when the response to
other disease-modifying antirheumatic drugs is
inadequate | Severe, active, and progressive rheumatoid
arthritis not previously treated with methotrexate |
Active and progressive psoriatic arthritis inadequately
responsive to other disease-modifying antirheumatic
drugs | Severe ankylosing spondylitis inadequately
responsive to conventional therapy**
▸ BY SUBCUTANEOUS INJECTION
▸ Adult: 25 mg twice weekly, alternatively 50 mg once
weekly

**Severe plaque psoriasis either refractory to at least 2
standard systemic treatments and photochemotherapy,
or when standard treatments cannot be used because of
intolerance or contra-indications**
▸ BY SUBCUTANEOUS INJECTION
▸ Adult: 25 mg twice weekly for up to 24 weeks,
alternatively 50 mg once weekly for up to 24 weeks,
discontinue if no response after 12 weeks

- CONTRA-INDICATIONS Active infection
- CAUTIONS Development of malignancy · diabetes mellitus
· heart failure (risk of exacerbation) · hepatitis B virus—
monitor for active infection · hepatitis C infection
(monitor for worsening infection) · history of blood
disorders · history of malignancy · history or increased risk
of demyelinating disorders · predisposition to infection
(avoid if predisposition to septicaemia) · significant
exposure to herpes zoster virus—interrupt treatment and
consider varicella–zoster immunoglobulin

CAUTIONS, FURTHER INFORMATION
▸ Tuberculosis Active tuberculosis should be treated with
standard treatment for at least 2 months before starting
etanercept. Patients who have previously received
adequate treatment for tuberculosis can start etanercept
but should be monitored every 3 months for possible
recurrence. In patients without active tuberculosis but
who were previously not treated adequately,
chemoprophylaxis should ideally be completed before
starting etanercept. In patients at high risk of tuberculosis
who cannot be assessed by tuberculin skin test,
chemoprophylaxis can be given concurrently with
etanercept.

- INTERACTIONS → Appendix 1 (etanercept).
- SIDE-EFFECTS
▸ **Uncommon** Interstitial lung disease · new onset or
worsening psoriasis · rash · skin cancer · uveitis
▸ **Rare** Demyelinating disorders · lymphoma · seizures ·
Stevens-Johnson syndrome · vasculitis
▸ **Very rare** Toxic epidermal necrolysis
▸ **Frequency not known** Abdominal pain · anaemia · antibody
formation · aplastic anaemia · appendicitis · blood
disorders · cutaneous ulcer · depression · diabetes mellitus ·
fever · gastritis · headache · hypersensitivity reactions ·
inflammatory bowel disease · injection-site reactions ·
leucopenia · leukaemia · lupus erythematosus-like
syndrome · macrophage activation syndrome · malignancy
· nausea · oesophagitis · pancytopenia · pruritus · solid

tumours · thrombocytopenia · vomiting · worsening heart
failure
SIDE-EFFECTS, FURTHER INFORMATION
Associated with infections, sometimes severe, including
tuberculosis, septicaemia, and hepatitis B reactivation.

- CONCEPTION AND CONTRACEPTION Manufacturer advises
effective contraception required during treatment and for
3 weeks after last dose.
- PREGNANCY Avoid—limited information available.
- BREAST FEEDING Manufacturer advises avoid—present in
milk in *animal* studies.
- HEPATIC IMPAIRMENT Use with caution in moderate to
severe alcoholic hepatitis.
- PRE-TREATMENT SCREENING
Tuberculosis Patients should be evaluated for tuberculosis
before treatment.
- MONITORING REQUIREMENTS Monitor for skin cancer
before and during treatment, particularly in those at risk
(including patients with psoriasis or a history of PUVA
treatment).
- PRESCRIBING AND DISPENSING INFORMATION Products
containing etanercept are not identical and although there
should be no important differences in terms of safety and
efficacy, when prescribing biological products it is good
practice to use the brand name, see *Biosimilar medicines*,
under Guidance on prescribing p. 1.
- PATIENT AND CARER ADVICE An alert card should be
provided.
Blood disorders Patients and their carers should be advised
to seek medical attention if symptoms suggestive of blood
disorders (such as fever, sore throat, bruising, or bleeding)
develop.
Tuberculosis Patients and their carers should be advised to
seek medical attention if symptoms suggestive of
tuberculosis (e.g. persistent cough, weight loss, and fever)
develop.
- NATIONAL FUNDING/ACCESS DECISIONS
NICE technology appraisals (TAs)
▸ **Etanercept and efalizumab for plaque psoriasis (July 2006)**
NICE TA103
Etanercept is recommended for severe plaque psoriasis
which has failed to respond to standard systemic
treatments (including ciclosporin and methotrexate) and
to photochemotherapy, or when standard treatments
cannot be used because of intolerance or contra-
indications. Etanercept should be withdrawn if the
response is not adequate after 12 weeks.
www.nice.org.uk/TA103
▸ **Adalimumab, etanercept, infliximab, rituximab, and
abatacept for the treatment of rheumatoid arthritis after the
failure of a TNF inhibitor (August 2010)** NICE TA195
Etanercept, in combination with methotrexate, is an
option for the treatment of severe active rheumatoid
arthritis in adults who have had an inadequate response
to, or have an intolerance of, other DMARDs including at
least 1 TNF inhibitor, and who cannot use rituximab
because of contra-indications or intolerance. In patients
who cannot use methotrexate because of intolerance or
contra-indications, etanercept can be given as
monotherapy. Treatment should be continued only if there
is adequate response. Patients should be monitored at
least every 6 months.
www.nice.org.uk/TA195
▸ **Etanercept, infliximab, and adalimumab for the treatment of
psoriatic arthritis (August 2010)** NICE TA199
Etanercept is recommended for the treatment of active
and progressive psoriatic arthritis in adults who have
peripheral arthritis with at least 3 tender joints and at least
3 swollen joints, and who have not responded adequately

to at least 2 standard disease-modifying antirheumatic drugs (used alone or in combination).

Etanercept should be discontinued if there is an inadequate response at 12 weeks.
www.nice.org.uk/TA199

▶ **Adalimumab, etanercept, infliximab, certolizumab pegol, golimumab, tocilizumab and abatacept for rheumatoid arthritis not previously treated with DMARDs or after conventional DMARDs only have failed (January 2016)** NICE TA375

Etanercept, in combination with methotrexate, is recommended as an option for treating rheumatoid arthritis, only if the following criteria are met:
- disease is severe, that is, a disease activity score (DAS28) greater than 5.1, **and**
- disease has not responded to intensive therapy with a combination of conventional disease-modifying antirheumatic drugs (DMARDs)

Etanercept can be used as monotherapy in patients who cannot take methotrexate because it is contra-indicated or because of intolerance, when the criteria above are met.

Continue treatment only if there is a moderate response measured using European League Against Rheumatism (EULAR) criteria at 6 months after starting therapy. After initial response within 6 months, withdraw treatment if a moderate EULAR response is not maintained.

Patients currently receiving etanercept whose disease does not meet the above criteria should have the option to continue their treatment until they and their clinician consider it appropriate to stop.
www.nice.org.uk/TA375

▶ **TNF-alpha inhibitors for ankylosing spondylitis and non-radiographic axial spondyloarthritis (February 2016)** NICE TA383

Adalimumab, certolizumab pegol, etanercept, golimumab and infliximab are recommended as options for treating severe active ankylosing spondylitis in patients whose disease has responded inadequately to, or who are intolerant of, non-steroidal anti-inflammatory drugs (NSAIDs).

Adalimumab, certolizumab pegol and etanercept are also recommended as options for treating severe non-radiographic axial spondyloarthritis in patients whose disease has responded inadequately to, or who are intolerant of, NSAIDs.

The response to treatment should be assessed 12 weeks after the start of treatment and should only be continued if there is clear evidence of response.

Treatment with another tumour necrosis factor (TNF) -alpha inhibitor is recommended in those who cannot tolerate, or whose disease has not responded to, treatment with the first TNF-alpha inhibitor, or in those whose disease has stopped responding after an initial response.
www.nice.org.uk/TA383

Scottish Medicines Consortium (SMC) Decisions
The *Scottish Medicines Consortium* issued similar advice to NICE TA103 on the use of etanercept for severe plaque psoriasis in adults (August 2009) and children over 6 years old (April 2012).

● MEDICINAL FORMS
There can be variation in the licensing of different medicines containing the same drug.
Solution for injection
CAUTIONARY AND ADVISORY LABELS 10
▶ Benepali (Biogen Idec Ltd) ▼
Etanercept 50 mg per 1 ml Benepali 50mg/1ml solution for injection pre-filled syringes | 4 pre-filled disposable injection [PoM] £656.00
Benepali 50mg/1ml solution for injection pre-filled pen | 4 pre-filled disposable injection [PoM] £656.00
▶ Enbrel (Pfizer Ltd)
Etanercept 50 mg per 1 ml Enbrel 50mg/1ml solution for injection pre-filled syringes | 4 pre-filled disposable injection [PoM] £715.00

Enbrel 25mg/0.5ml solution for injection pre-filled syringes | 4 pre-filled disposable injection [PoM] £357.50
▶ Enbrel MyClic (Pfizer Ltd)
Etanercept 50 mg per 1 ml Enbrel 50mg/1ml solution for injection pre-filled MyClic pen | 4 pre-filled disposable injection [PoM] £715.00
Powder and solvent for solution for injection
CAUTIONARY AND ADVISORY LABELS 10
EXCIPIENTS: May contain Benzyl alcohol
▶ Enbrel (Pfizer Ltd)
Etanercept 10 mg Enbrel Paediatric 10mg powder and solvent for solution for injection vials | 4 vial [PoM] £143.00
Etanercept 25 mg Enbrel 25mg powder and solvent for solution for injection vials | 4 vial [PoM] £357.50

Golimumab

31.5.2016

● INDICATIONS AND DOSE

Treatment of severe ulcerative colitis in patients whose condition has not responded adequately to conventional therapy, or who are intolerant of it
▶ BY SUBCUTANEOUS INJECTION
▶ Adult (body-weight up to 80 kg): Initially 200 mg, then 100 mg after 2 weeks; maintenance 50 mg every 4 weeks, review treatment if no response after 4 doses
▶ Adult (body-weight 80 kg and above): Initially 200 mg, then 100 mg after 2 weeks; maintenance 100 mg every 4 weeks, review treatment if no response after 4 doses

Treatment of moderate to severe active rheumatoid arthritis (in combination with methotrexate) when response to disease-modifying antirheumatic drug (DMARD) therapy (including methotrexate) has been inadequate | Treatment of severe, active, and progressive rheumatoid arthritis (in combination with methotrexate) in patients not previously treated with methotrexate | Treatment of active and progressive psoriatic arthritis as monotherapy or in combination with methotrexate when response to DMARD therapy has been inadequate | Treatment of severe active ankylosing spondylitis when there is inadequate reponse to conventional treatment
▶ BY SUBCUTANEOUS INJECTION
▶ Adult (body-weight up to 100 kg): 50 mg once a month, on the same date each month, review treatment if no response after 3–4 doses
▶ Adult (body-weight 100 kg and above): Initially 50 mg once a month for 3–4 doses, on the same date each month, dose may be increased if inadequate response, increased to 100 mg once a month, review treatment if inadequate response to this higher dose after 3–4 doses

● CONTRA-INDICATIONS Moderate or severe heart failure · severe active infection

● CAUTIONS Active infection (do not initiate until active infections are controlled; discontinue if new serious infection develops until infection controlled) · demyelinating disorders (risk of exacerbation) · hepatitis B virus—monitor for active infection · history or development of malignancy · mild heart failure (discontinue if symptoms develop or worsen) · predisposition to infection · risk factors for dysplasia or carcinoma of the colon—screen for dysplasia regularly

CAUTIONS, FURTHER INFORMATION
▶ Tuberculosis Active tuberculosis should be treated with standard treatment for at least 2 months before starting golimumab. Patients who have previously received adequate treatment for tuberculosis can start golimumab but should be monitored every 3 months for possible recurrence. In patients without active tuberculosis but who were previously not treated adequately, chemoprophylaxis should ideally be completed before starting golimumab. In patients at high risk of tuberculosis

who cannot be assessed by tuberculin skin test, chemoprophylaxis can be given concurrently with golimumab. Patients who have tested negative for latent tuberculosis, and those who are receiving or who have completed treatment for latent tuberculosis, should be monitored closely for symptoms of active infection.

● INTERACTIONS → Appendix 1 (golimumab).

● SIDE-EFFECTS
▶ **Common or very common** Asthenia · dizziness · dyspepsia · hypertension
▶ **Uncommon** Alopecia · arrhythmia · bone fractures · bronchospasm · cholelithiasis · colitis · constipation · demyelinating disorders · dermatitis · eye irritation · flushing · gastritis · gastro-oesophageal reflux disease · heart failure · hepatic disorders · hyperglycaemia · hyperlipidaemia · insomnia · interstitial lung disease · ischaemic coronary artery disorders · lymphoma · malignancy · melanoma · menstrual disorders · new onset or worsening psoriasis · paraesthesia · Raynaud's syndrome · stomatitis · taste disturbance · thrombosis · thyroid disorders · visual disturbance
▶ **Rare** Impaired wound healing
▶ **Frequency not known** Abdominal pain · anaemia · antibody formation · aplastic anaemia · blood disorders · depression · fever · headache · hypersensitivity reactions · injection-site reactions · leucopenia · lupus erythematosus-like syndrome · nausea · pancytopenia · pruritus · thrombocytopenia · worsening heart failure

SIDE-EFFECTS, FURTHER INFORMATION
Associated with infections, sometimes severe, including tuberculosis, septicaemia, and hepatitis B reactivation.

● CONCEPTION AND CONTRACEPTION Manufacturer advises adequate contraception during treatment and for at least 6 months after last dose.

● PREGNANCY Use only if essential.

● BREAST-FEEDING Manufacturer advises avoid during and for at least 6 months after treatment—present in milk in *animal* studies.

● HEPATIC IMPAIRMENT Manufacturer advises caution—no information available.

● PRE-TREATMENT SCREENING
Tuberculosis Patients should be evaluated for tuberculosis before treatment.

● MONITORING REQUIREMENTS Monitor for infection before, during, and for 5 months after treatment.

● DIRECTIONS FOR ADMINISTRATION For doses requiring multiple injections, each injection should be administered at a different site.
Missed dose If dose administered more than 2 weeks late, subsequent doses should be administered on the new monthly due date.

● PATIENT AND CARER ADVICE An alert card should be provided.
Tuberculosis All patients and their carers should be advised to seek medical attention if symptoms suggestive of tuberculosis (e.g. persistent cough, weight loss, and fever) develop.
Blood disorders Patients and their carers should be advised to seek medical attention if symptoms suggestive of blood disorders (such as fever, sore throat, bruising, or bleeding) develop.

● NATIONAL FUNDING/ACCESS DECISIONS

NICE technology appraisals (TAs)
▶ **Golimumab for the treatment of psoriatic arthritis (April 2011)** NICE TA220
Golimumab is an option for the treatment of active and progressive psoriatic arthritis in adults only if:
● golimumab is used as described in the NICE guidance (August 2010) for other tumour necrosis factor (TNF) inhibitors, *and*

● the manufacturer provides the 100-mg dose of golimumab at the same price as the 50-mg dose.
www.nice.org.uk/TA220

▶ **Infliximab, adalimumab and golimumab for treating moderately to severely active ulcerative colitis after the failure of conventional therapy (February 2015)** NICE TA329
Golimumab is an option for treating moderately to severely active ulcerative colitis in adults whose disease has responded inadequately to conventional therapy including corticosteroids and mercaptopurine or azathioprine, or in adults who are intolerant to or have contra-indications for conventional therapies.

Golimumab is recommended only if the manufacturer provides the 100 mg dose of golimumab at the same cost as the 50 mg dose, as agreed in the patient access scheme.

The choice of treatment should be made on an individual basis and if more than one treatment is suitable, the least expensive should be chosen.

Golimumab should be given as a planned course of treatment until treatment fails (including the need for surgery) or until 12 months after starting treatment, whichever is shorter. Treatment should be continued only if there is clear evidence of a response. Patients who continue treatment should be reassessed at least every 12 months to determine whether ongoing treatment is still clinically appropriate.
www.nice.org.uk/TA329

▶ **Adalimumab, etanercept, infliximab, certolizumab pegol, golimumab, tocilizumab and abatacept for rheumatoid arthritis not previously treated with DMARDs or after conventional DMARDs only have failed (January 2016)** NICE TA375
Golimumab, in combination with methotrexate, is recommended as an option for treating rheumatoid arthritis, only if **all** the following criteria are met:
● disease is severe, that is, a disease activity score (DAS28) greater than 5.1,
● disease has not responded to intensive therapy with a combination of conventional disease-modifying antirheumatic drugs (DMARDs),
● the manufacturers provides golimumab as agreed in the patient access schemes.
Continue treatment only if there is a moderate response measured using European League Against Rheumatism (EULAR) criteria at 6 months after starting therapy. After initial response within 6 months, withdraw treatment if a moderate EULAR response is not maintained.

Patients currently receiving treatment with golimumab whose disease does not meet the above criteria should have the option to continue their treatment until they and their clinician consider it appropriate to stop.
www.nice.org.uk/TA375

▶ **TNF-alpha inhibitors for ankylosing spondylitis and non-radiographic axial spondyloarthritis (February 2016)** NICE TA383
Adalimumab, certolizumab pegol, etanercept, golimumab and infliximab are recommended as options for treating severe active ankylosing spondylitis in patients whose disease has responded inadequately to, or who are intolerant of, non-steroidal anti-inflammatory drugs (NSAIDs).

The response to treatment should be assessed 12 weeks after the start of treatment. Treatment should only be continued if there is clear evidence of response.

Treatment with another tumour necrosis factor (TNF)-alpha inhibitor is recommended in those who cannot tolerate, or whose disease has not responded to, treatment with the first TNF-alpha inhibitor, or in those whose disease has stopped responding after an initial response.
www.nice.org.uk/TA383

10

Musculoskeletal system

▸ **Golimumab for the treatment of rheumatoid arthritis after the failure of previous disease-modifying antirheumatic drugs (June 2011—updated February 2016)** NICE TA225
Golimumab, in combination with methotrexate, is an option for the treatment of rheumatoid arthritis in patients who have had an inadequate response to DMARDs, including a TNF inhibitor, if golimumab is used as described in the NICE technology appraisal guidance 195 (August 2010) for other TNF inhibitors, **and** the manufacturer provides the 100-mg dose of golimumab at the same price as the 50-mg dose.
www.nice.org.uk/TA225

Scottish Medicines Consortium (SMC) Decisions
The *Scottish Medicines Consortium* has advised (June 2012) that golimumab (*Simponi*®) is accepted for restricted use within NHS Scotland at a dose of 50 mg, alone or in combination with methotrexate, for the treatment of active and progressive psoriatic arthritis in adults whose disease has not responded to adequate trials of at least two standard DMARDs, administered either individually or in combination.

● MEDICINAL FORMS
There can be variation in the licensing of different medicines containing the same drug.
Solution for injection
CAUTIONARY AND ADVISORY LABELS 10
▸ Simponi (Merck Sharp & Dohme Ltd)
 Golimumab 100 mg per 1 ml Simponi 50mg/0.5ml solution for injection pre-filled disposable devices | 1 pre-filled disposable injection PoM £762.97
 Simponi 100mg/1ml solution for injection pre-filled pen | 1 pre-filled disposable injection PoM £1,525.94
 Simponi 50mg/0.5ml solution for injection pre-filled syringes | 1 pre-filled disposable injection PoM £762.97

Infliximab
31.5.2016

● INDICATIONS AND DOSE
Severe active Crohn's disease
▸ BY INTRAVENOUS INFUSION
▸ **Adult:** Initially 5 mg/kg, then 5 mg/kg after 2 weeks, then 5 mg/kg after 4 weeks, if condition has responded, then maintenance 5 mg/kg every 8 weeks

Fistulating Crohn's disease
▸ BY INTRAVENOUS INFUSION
▸ **Adult:** Initially 5 mg/kg, then 5 mg/kg after 2 weeks, followed by 5 mg/kg after 4 weeks, if condition has responded consult product literature for guidance on further doses

Severe active ulcerative colitis
▸ BY INTRAVENOUS INFUSION
▸ **Adult:** Initially 5 mg/kg, then 5 mg/kg after 2 weeks, followed by 5 mg/kg after 4 weeks, then 5 mg/kg every 8 weeks, discontinue if no response 14 weeks after initial dose

Rheumatoid arthritis (in combination with methotrexate)
▸ BY INTRAVENOUS INFUSION
▸ **Adult:** Initially 3 mg/kg, then 3 mg/kg after 2 weeks, followed by 3 mg/kg after 4 weeks, then 3 mg/kg every 8 weeks, dose to be increased only if response is inadequate after 12 weeks of initial treatment; increased in steps of 1.5 mg/kg every 8 weeks, increased if necessary up to 7.5 mg/kg every 8 weeks, alternatively increased if necessary to 3 mg/kg every 4 weeks, discontinue if no response by 12 weeks of initial infusion or after dose adjustment

Ankylosing spondylitis
▸ BY INTRAVENOUS INFUSION
▸ **Adult:** 5 mg/kg, then 5 mg/kg after 2 weeks, followed by 5 mg/kg after 4 weeks, then 5 mg/kg every 6–8 weeks,

discontinue if no response by 6 weeks of initial infusion

Psoriatic arthritis (in combination with methotrexate)
▸ BY INTRAVENOUS INFUSION
▸ **Adult:** 5 mg/kg, then 5 mg/kg after 2 weeks, followed by 5 mg/kg after 4 weeks, followed by 5 mg/kg every 8 weeks

Plaque psoriasis
▸ BY INTRAVENOUS INFUSION
▸ **Adult:** 5 mg/kg, then 5 mg/kg after 2 weeks, followed by 5 mg/kg after 4 weeks, then 5 mg/kg every 8 weeks, discontinue if no response within 14 weeks of initial infusion

> IMPORTANT SAFETY INFORMATION
> Adequate resuscitation facilities must be available when infliximab is used.

● CONTRA-INDICATIONS Moderate or severe heart failure · severe infections

● CAUTIONS Demyelinating disorders (risk of exacerbation) · dermatomyositis · development of malignancy · hepatitis B virus—monitor for active infection · history of colon carcinoma (in inflammatory bowel disease) · history of dysplasia (in inflammatory bowel disease) · history of malignancy · history of prolonged immunosuppressant or PUVA treatment in patients with psoriasis · mild heart failure (discontinue if symptoms develop or worsen) · predisposition to infection (discontinue if new serious infection develops) · risk of delayed hypersensitivity reactions if drug-free interval exceeds 16 weeks (re-administration after interval exceeding 16 weeks not recommended)

CAUTIONS, FURTHER INFORMATION
▸ Tuberculosis Manufacturer advises to evaluate patients for active and latent tuberculosis before treatment. Active tuberculosis should be treated with standard treatment for at least 2 months before starting infliximab. If latent tuberculosis is diagnosed, treatment should be started before commencing treatment with infliximab. Patients who have previously received adequate treatment for tuberculosis can start infliximab but should be monitored every 3 months for possible recurrence. In patients without active tuberculosis but who were previously not treated adequately, chemoprophylaxis should ideally be completed before starting infliximab. In patients at high risk of tuberculosis who cannot be assessed by tuberculin skin test, chemoprophylaxis can be given concurrently with infliximab. Patients should be advised to seek medical attention if symptoms suggestive of tuberculosis develop (e.g. persistent cough, weight loss and fever).
▸ Hypersensitivity reactions Hypersensitivity reactions (including fever, chest pain, hypotension, hypertension, dyspnoea, transient visual loss, pruritus, urticaria, serum sickness-like reactions, angioedema, anaphylaxis) reported during or within 1–2 hours after infusion (risk greatest during first or second infusion or in patients who discontinue other immunosuppressants). Manufacturer advises prophylactic antipyretics, antihistamines, or hydrocortisone may be administered.

● INTERACTIONS → Appendix 1 (infliximab).
● SIDE-EFFECTS
▸ **Common or very common** Alopecia · arthralgia · constipation · diarrhoea · dizziness · dry skin · dyspepsia · ecchymosis · epistaxis · flushing · gastro-intestinal haemorrhage · gastro-oesophageal reflux · hyperhydrosis · hypertension · hypoaesthesia · hypotension · myalgia · new onset or worsening psoriasis · palpitation · paraesthesia · rash · sleep disturbances · tachycardia
▸ **Uncommon** Abnormal skin pigmentation · agitation · amnesia · arrhythmia · bradycardia · bullous eruption ·

cheilitis · cholecystitis · confusion · eye disorders · heart failure · hepatitis · hyperkeratosis · impaired healing · intestinal perforation · nervousness · neuropathy · pancreatitis · peripheral ischaemia · pleurisy · pulmonary oedema · rosacea · seborrhoea · seizures · syncope · vaginitis
▸ **Rare** Demyelinating disorders · interstitial lung disease · leukaemia · lymphoma · melanoma · pericardial effusion · Stevens-Johnson syndrome · toxic epidermal necrolysis · vasospasm
▸ **Frequency not known** Abdominal pain · anaemia · antibody formation · aplastic anaemia · blood disorders · depression · fever · headache · hepatic failure · hepatosplenic T-cell lymphoma (more likely in inflammatory bowel disease) · hypersensitivity reactions · injection-site reactions · leucopenia · lupus erythematosus-like syndrome · Merkel cell carcinoma · nausea · pancytopenia · pruritus · thrombocytopenia · worsening heart failure · worsening symptoms of dermatomyositis

SIDE-EFFECTS, FURTHER INFORMATION
Associated with infections, sometimes severe, including tuberculosis, septicaemia, and hepatitis B reactivation.
● CONCEPTION AND CONTRACEPTION Manufacturer advises adequate contraception during and for at least 6 months after last dose.
● PREGNANCY Use only if essential.
● BREAST FEEDING Amount probably too small to be harmful.
● PRE-TREATMENT SCREENING
Tuberculosis Patients should be evaluated for tuberculosis before treatment.
● MONITORING REQUIREMENTS
▸ Monitor for infection before, during, and for 6 months after treatment.
▸ All patients should be observed carefully for 1–2 hours after infusion and resuscitation equipment should be available for immediate use (risk of hypersensitivity reactions).
▸ Monitor for symptoms of delayed hypersensitivity if re-administered after a prolonged period.
▸ Manufacturer advises periodic skin examination for non-melanoma skin cancer, particularly in patients with risk factors.
● DIRECTIONS FOR ADMINISTRATION For *intravenous infusion* (*Remicade*®), give intermittently *in* Sodium chloride 0.9%; reconstitute each 100-mg vial with 10 mL water for injections using a 21-gauge or smaller needle; gently swirl vial without shaking to dissolve; allow to stand for 5 minutes; dilute requisite dose with infusion fluid to a final volume of 250 mL and give through a low protein-binding filter (1.2 micron or less) over at least 2 hours (adults over 18 years who have tolerated 3 initial 2-hour infusions may be given subsequent infusions of up to 6 mg/kg over at least 1 hour); start infusion within 3 hours of reconstitution.
● PRESCRIBING AND DISPENSING INFORMATION Products containing infliximab are not identical and although there should be no important differences in terms of safety and efficacy, when prescribing biological products it is good practice to use the brand name, see *Biosimilar medicines*, under Guidance on prescribing p. 1.
● PATIENT AND CARER ADVICE An alert card should be provided.
Tuberculosis Patients and carers should be advised to seek medical attention if symptoms suggestive of tuberculosis (e.g. persistent cough, weight loss, and fever) develop.
Blood disorders Patients and carers should be advised to seek medical attention if symptoms suggestive of blood

disorders (such as fever, sore throat, bruising, or bleeding) develop.
Hypersensitivity reactions Patients and carers should be advised to keep Alert card with them at all times and seek medical advice if symptoms of delayed hypersensitivity develop.
● NATIONAL FUNDING/ACCESS DECISIONS
NICE technology appraisals (TAs)
▸ **Infliximab for plaque psoriasis in adults (January 2008)** NICE TA134
Infliximab is recommended for the treatment of very severe plaque psoriasis which has failed to respond to standard systemic treatments (including ciclosporin and methotrexate) or to photochemotherapy, or when standard treatments cannot be used because of intolerance or contra-indications. Infliximab should be withdrawn if the response is not adequate after 10 weeks.
www.nice.org.uk/TA134
▸ **Infliximab for acute exacerbations of ulcerative colitis (December 2008)** NICE TA163
Infliximab is recommended as an option for the treatment of acute exacerbations of severe ulcerative colitis when treatment with ciclosporin is contra-indicated or inappropriate.
www.nice.org.uk/TA163
▸ **Infliximab and adalimumab for Crohn's disease (May 2010)** NICE TA187
Infliximab is recommended for the treatment of severe active Crohn's disease that has not responded to conventional therapy (including corticosteroids and other drugs affecting the immune response) or when conventional therapy cannot be used because of intolerance or contra-indications; infliximab can also be used in a similar way in children over 6 years of age. In adults over 18 years of age, infliximab is recommended for the treatment of fistulating Crohn's disease that has not responded to conventional therapy (including antibacterials, drainage, and other drugs affecting the immune response) or when conventional therapy cannot be used because of intolerance or contra-indications.
    Infliximab should be given as a planned course of treatment for 12 months or until treatment failure, whichever is shorter. Treatment should be continued beyond 12 months only if there is evidence of active disease—in these cases the need for treatment should be reviewed at least annually. If the disease relapses after stopping treatment, infliximab can be restarted.
www.nice.org.uk/TA187
▸ **Adalimumab, etanercept, infliximab, rituximab, and abatacept for the treatment of rheumatoid arthritis after the failure of a TNF inhibitor (August 2010)** NICE TA195
Infliximab, in combination with methotrexate, is an option for the treatment of severe active rheumatoid arthritis in adults who have had an inadequate response to, or have an intolerance of, other DMARDs including at least 1 TNF inhibitor, and who cannot use rituximab because of contra-indications or intolerance. Treatment should be continued only if there is adequate response. Patients should be monitored at least every 6 months.
www.nice.org.uk/TA195
▸ **Etanercept, infliximab, and adalimumab for the treatment of psoriatic arthritis (August 2010)** NICE TA199
Infliximab is recommended for the treatment of active and progressive psoriatic arthritis in adults who have peripheral arthritis with at least 3 tender joints and at least 3 swollen joints, and who have not responded adequately to at least 2 standard disease-modifying antirheumatic drugs (used alone or in combination).
    Infliximab should be discontinued if there is an inadequate response at 12 weeks.
www.nice.org.uk/TA199

10 Musculoskeletal system

▶ **Infliximab, adalimumab and golimumab for treating moderately to severely active ulcerative colitis after the failure of conventional therapy (February 2015)** NICE TA329
Infliximab is an option for treating moderately to severely active ulcerative colitis in adults whose disease has responded inadequately to conventional therapy including corticosteroids and mercaptopurine or azathioprine, or in adults who are intolerant to or have contra-indications for conventional therapies.

The choice of treatment should be made on an individual basis and if more than one treatment is suitable, the least expensive should be chosen.

Infliximab should be given as a planned course of treatment until treatment fails (including the need for surgery) or until 12 months after starting treatment, whichever is shorter. Treatment should be continued only if there is clear evidence of a response. Patients who continue treatment should be reassessed at least every 12 months to determine whether ongoing treatment is still clinically appropriate.
www.nice.org.uk/TA329

▶ **Adalimumab, etanercept, infliximab, certolizumab pegol, golimumab, tocilizumab and abatacept for rheumatoid arthritis not previously treated with DMARDs or after conventional DMARDs only have failed (January 2016)** NICE TA375
Infliximab, in combination with methotrexate, is recommended as an option for treating rheumatoid arthritis, only if the following criteria are met:
• disease is severe, that is, a disease activity score (DAS28) greater than 5.1, **and**,
• disease has not responded to intensive therapy with a combination of conventional disease-modifying antirheumatic drugs (DMARDs).
Continue treatment only if there is a moderate response measured using European League Against Rheumatism (EULAR) criteria at 6 months after starting therapy. After initial response within 6 months, withdraw treatment if a moderate EULAR response is not maintained.

Patients currently receiving infliximab whose disease does not meet the above criteria should have the option to continue their treatment until they and their clinician consider it appropriate to stop.
www.nice.org.uk/TA375

▶ **TNF-alpha inhibitors for ankylosing spondylitis and non-radiographic axial spondyloarthritis (February 2016)** NICE TA383
Adalimumab, certolizumab pegol, etanercept, golimumab and infliximab are recommended as options for treating severe active ankylosing spondylitis in patients whose disease has responded inadequately to, or who are intolerant of, non-steroidal anti-inflammatory drugs (NSAIDs). Infliximab is recommended only if treatment is started with the least expensive infliximab product. Patients currently receiving infliximab should continue treatment with the same infliximab product until they and their clinician considers it appropriate to stop.

The response to treatment should be assessed 12 weeks after the start of treatment and should only be continued if there is clear evidence of response.

Treatment with another tumour necrosis factor (TNF) -alpha inhibitor is recommended in those who cannot tolerate, or whose disease has not responded to, treatment with the first TNF-alpha inhibitor, or in those whose disease has stopped responding after an initial response.
www.nice.org.uk/TA383

● MEDICINAL FORMS
There can be variation in the licensing of different medicines containing the same drug.
Powder for solution for infusion
CAUTIONARY AND ADVISORY LABELS 10
▶ Inflectra (Hospira UK Ltd) ▼
Infliximab 100 mg Inflectra 100mg powder for concentrate for solution for infusion vials | 1 vial PoM £377.66 (Hospital only)
▶ Remicade (Merck Sharp & Dohme Ltd)
Infliximab 100 mg Remicade 100mg powder for concentrate for solution for infusion vials | 1 vial PoM £419.62 (Hospital only)
▶ Remsima (Napp Pharmaceuticals Ltd) ▼
Infliximab 100 mg Remsima 100mg powder for concentrate for solution for infusion vials | 1 vial PoM £377.66 (Hospital only)

PHOSPHODIESTERASE TYPE-4 INHIBITORS

Apremilast

● DRUG ACTION Apremilast inhibits the activity of phosphodiesterase type-4 (PDE4) which results in suppression of pro-inflammatory mediator synthesis and promotes anti-inflammatory mediators.

● INDICATIONS AND DOSE
Active psoriatic arthritis (in combination with disease-modifying antirheumatic drugs or alone) in patients who have had an inadequate response or who have been intolerant to a prior disease-modifying antirheumatic drug therapy | Moderate to severe chronic plaque psoriasis that has not responded to standard systemic treatments or photochemotherapy, or when these treatments cannot be used because of intolerance or contra-indications
  ▶ BY MOUTH
   ▶ Adult: Initially 10 mg daily on day 1, then 10 mg twice daily on day 2, then 10 mg in the morning and 20 mg in the evening on day 3, then 20 mg twice daily on day 4, then 20 mg in the morning and 30 mg in the evening on day 5, then maintenance 30 mg twice daily, doses should be taken approximately 12 hours apart; review treatment if no response within 24 weeks of initiation

● CAUTIONS Low body-weight—consider discontinuation if weight loss is unexplained or clinically significant

● INTERACTIONS → Appendix 1 (apremilast).

● SIDE-EFFECTS
▶ **Common or very common** Back pain · bronchitis · cough · decreased appetite · diarrhoea · dyspepsia · fatigue · gastroesophageal reflux disease · headache · insomnia · migraine · nasopharyngitis · nausea · tension headache · upper abdominal pain · upper respiratory tract infections · vomiting
▶ **Uncommon** Rash · weight loss

● CONCEPTION AND CONTRACEPTION Exclude pregnancy before treatment and ensure effective contraception during treatment.

● PREGNANCY Avoid—teratogenic in *animal* studies.

● BREAST FEEDING Manufacturer advises avoid—present in milk in *animal* studies.

● RENAL IMPAIRMENT Reduce dose if eGFR less than 30 mL/minute/1.73 m^2; consult product literature for initial dose titration.

● MONITORING REQUIREMENTS Monitor body-weight regularly.

● NATIONAL FUNDING/ACCESS DECISIONS
NICE technology appraisals (TAs)
▶ **Apremilast for treating moderate to severe plaque psoriasis (November 2015)** NICE TA368
Apremilast is not recommended for the treatment of moderate to severe chronic plaque psoriasis in patients who have had an inadequate response to or intolerant of

systemic therapy, or when systemic therapy is contra-indicated.

www.nice.org.uk/TA368

▸ **Apremilast for treating active psoriatic arthritis (December 2015)** NICE TA372

Apremilast, alone or in combination with disease-modifying antirheumatic drugs (DMARDs), is not recommended for the treatment of active psoriatic arthritis that has not responded to prior DMARD therapy, or when DMARD therapy is not tolerated.

www.nice.org.uk/TA372

Scottish Medicines Consortium (SMC) Decisions

The *Scottish Medicines Consortium* has advised (June 2015) that apremilast (*Otezla*®) is accepted for restricted use within NHS Scotland for the treatment of active psoriatic arthritis in patients who have had an inadequate response with at least two prior Disease Modifying Antirheumatic Drug (DMARD) therapies or who are intolerant to such therapies.

● MEDICINAL FORMS
There can be variation in the licensing of different medicines containing the same drug.

Tablet

CAUTIONARY AND ADVISORY LABELS 25
▸ Otezla (Celgene Ltd) ▼
  Apremilast 10 mg Otezla 10mg tablets | 4 tablet PoM no price available
  Apremilast 20 mg Otezla 20mg tablets | 4 tablet PoM no price available
  Apremilast 30 mg Otezla 30mg tablets | 19 tablet PoM no price available | 56 tablet PoM £550.00

2 Hyperuricaemia and gout

Gout

Overview

It is important to distinguish drugs used for the treatment of acute attacks of gout from those used in the long-term control of the disease. The latter exacerbate and prolong the acute manifestations if started during an attack. The management of gout in adolescents requires specialist supervision.

Acute attacks of gout

Acute attacks of gout are usually treated with high doses of NSAIDs such as diclofenac sodium p. 980, diclofenac potassium p. 980, etoricoxib p. 984, indometacin p. 989, ketoprofen p. 991, naproxen p. 995 or sulindac p. 997. Colchicine below is an alternative in patients in whom NSAIDs are contra-indicated. Aspirin p. 109 is *not* indicated in gout. Allopurinol p. 968, febuxostat p. 969, and uricosurics are not effective in treating an acute attack and may prolong it indefinitely if started during the acute episode.

The use of colchicine is limited by the development of toxicity at higher doses, but it is of value in patients with heart failure since, unlike NSAIDs, it does not induce fluid retention; moreover, it can be given to patients receiving anticoagulants.

Oral or parenteral corticosteroids are an effective alternative in those who cannot tolerate NSAIDs or who are resistant to other treatments. Intra-articular injection of a corticosteroid can be used in acute monoarticular gout [unlicensed indication]. A corticosteroid by intramuscular injection can be effective in podagra.

Canakinumab p. 764, a recombinant monoclonal antibody, can be used for the symptomatic treatment of frequent gouty arthritis attacks (at least 3 in the previous 12 months). It is licensed for use in patients whose condition has not responded adequately to treatment with NSAIDs or colchicine, or who are intolerant of them.

Long-term control of gout

Frequent recurrence of acute attacks of gout, the presence of tophi, or signs of chronic gouty arthritis may call for the initiation of long-term ('interval') treatment. For long-term control of gout the formation of uric acid from purines may be reduced with the xanthine-oxidase inhibitors allopurinol or febuxostat alternatively the uricosuric drug sulfinpyrazone p. 968 may be used to increase the excretion of uric acid in the urine. Treatment should be continued indefinitely to prevent further attacks of gout by correcting the hyperuricaemia. These drugs should never be started during an acute attack; they are usually started 1–2 weeks after the attack has settled. The initiation of treatment may precipitate an acute attack, and therefore an anti-inflammatory analgesic or colchicine should be used as a prophylactic and continued for at least one month after the hyperuricaemia has been corrected. However, if an acute attack develops during treatment, then the treatment should continue at the same dosage and the acute attack treated in its own right.

Allopurinol is widely used and is especially useful in patients with renal impairment or urate stones when uricosuric drugs cannot be used; it is *not* indicated for the treatment of asymptomatic hyperuricaemia. It can cause rashes.

Febuxostat is licensed for the treatment of chronic hyperuricaemia where urate deposition has already occurred; it is *not* indicated for patients in whom the rate of urate formation is greatly increased, such as in malignant disease or in Lesch-Nyhan syndrome.

Sulfinpyrazone can be used instead of allopurinol or in conjunction with it in cases that are resistant to treatment.

Benzbromarone (available from 'special-order' manufacturers or specialist importing companies) is a uricosuric drug that can be used in patients with mild renal impairment.

Crystallisation of urate in the urine can occur with the uricosuric drugs and it is important to ensure an adequate urine output especially in the first few weeks of treatment. As an additional precaution the urine may be rendered alkaline.

Aspirin and other salicylates antagonise the uricosuric drugs; they do not antagonise allopurinol but are nevertheless *not* indicated in gout.

Drugs used for Hyperuricaemia and gout not listed below
Ketoprofen with omeprazole, p. 992 · Naproxen with esomeprazole, p. 995 · Naproxen with misoprostol, p. 996

ALKALOIDS ⟩ PLANT ALKALOIDS

▌Colchicine

● INDICATIONS AND DOSE

Acute gout
▸ BY MOUTH
  ▸ Adult: 500 micrograms 2–4 times a day until symptoms relieved, maximum 6 mg per course, do not repeat course within 3 days

Short-term prophylaxis during initial therapy with allopurinol and uricosuric drugs
▸ BY MOUTH
  ▸ Adult: 500 micrograms twice daily

Prophylaxis of familial Mediterranean fever (recurrent polyserositis)
▸ BY MOUTH
  ▸ Adult: 0.5–2 mg once daily

Musculoskeletal system

10

- UNLICENSED USE BNF doses may differ from those in the product literature. Use of colchicine for prophylaxis of familial Mediterranean fever (recurrent polyserositis) is an unlicensed indication.
- CONTRA-INDICATIONS Blood disorders
- CAUTIONS Cardiac disease · elderly · gastro-intestinal disease
- INTERACTIONS → Appendix 1 (colchicine).
- SIDE-EFFECTS
- ▶ **Common or very common** Abdominal pain · nausea · vomiting
- ▶ **Rare** Alopecia · blood disorders with prolonged treatment · inhibition of spermatogenesis · myopathy · peripheral neuritis
- ▶ **Frequency not known** Excessive doses may cause profuse diarrhoea · gastrointestinal haemorrhage · hepatic damage · rash · renal damage
- PREGNANCY Avoid—teratogenicity in *animal* studies.
- BREAST FEEDING Present in milk but no adverse effects reported. Manufacturers advise caution.
- HEPATIC IMPAIRMENT Use with caution.
- RENAL IMPAIRMENT Reduce dose or increase dosage interval if eGFR 10–50 mL/minute/1.73 m^2. Avoid if eGFR less than 10 mL/minute/1.73 m^2.

- MEDICINAL FORMS
There can be variation in the licensing of different medicines containing the same drug. Forms available from special-order manufacturers include: oral solution

Tablet
- ▶ Colchicine (Non-proprietary)
Colchicine 500 microgram Colchicine 500microgram tablets | 100 tablet [PoM] £72.75 DT price = £22.42

URICOSURICS

Sulfinpyrazone

(Sulphinpyrazone)

- INDICATIONS AND DOSE
Gout prophylaxis | Hyperuricaemia
- ▶ BY MOUTH
- ▶ Adult: Initially 100–200 mg daily, dose to be taken with food (or milk); increased to 600–800 mg daily over 2–3 weeks, 800 mg daily is rarely given; continue until serum uric acid concentration normal then reduce dose for maintenance (maintenance dose may be as low as 200 mg daily)

- CONTRA-INDICATIONS Acute gout attack · Acute porphyrias p. 918 · history of blood disorders · peptic ulceration
- CAUTIONS Cardiac disease (may cause salt and water retention) · ensure adequate fluid intake (about 2–3 litres daily) and render urine alkaline during initial treatment
- INTERACTIONS → Appendix 1 (sulfinpyrazone).
- SIDE-EFFECTS
- ▶ **Rare** Acute renal failure · blood disorders · gastro-intestinal bleeding · gastro-intestinal ulceration · hepatitis · jaundice · raised liver enzymes
- ▶ **Frequency not known** Allergic skin reactions · gastro-intestinal disturbances · salt retention · water retention
- ALLERGY AND CROSS-SENSITIVITY Avoid in hypersensitivity to aspirin, salicylates, NSAIDs.
- PREGNANCY Manufacturer advises caution—no information available.
- BREAST FEEDING No information available.
- HEPATIC IMPAIRMENT Avoid in severe impairment.

- RENAL IMPAIRMENT Reduce dose. Avoid in severe impairment.
- MONITORING REQUIREMENTS Regular blood counts before treatment and at regular intervals during treatment.

- MEDICINAL FORMS
There can be variation in the licensing of different medicines containing the same drug.
No licensed medicines listed.

XANTHINE OXIDASE INHIBITORS

Allopurinol

- INDICATIONS AND DOSE
Prophylaxis of gout and of uric acid and calcium oxalate renal stones | Prophylaxis of hyperuricaemia associated with cancer chemotherapy
- ▶ BY MOUTH
- ▶ Adult: Initially 100 mg daily, for maintenance adjust dose according to plasma or urinary uric acid concentration, dose to be taken preferably after food

Prophylaxis of gout and of uric acid and calcium oxalate renal stones (usual maintenance in mild conditions) | Prophylaxis of hyperuricaemia associated with cancer chemotherapy (usual maintenance in mild conditions)
- ▶ BY MOUTH
- ▶ Adult: 100–200 mg daily, dose to be taken preferably after food

Prophylaxis of gout and of uric acid and calcium oxalate renal stones (usual maintenance in moderately severe conditions) | Prophylaxis of hyperuricaemia associated with cancer chemotherapy (usual maintenance in moderately severe conditions)
- ▶ BY MOUTH
- ▶ Adult: 300–600 mg daily in divided doses (max. per dose 300 mg), dose to be taken preferably after food

Prophylaxis of gout and of uric acid and calcium oxalate renal stones (usual maintenance in severe conditions) | Prophylaxis of hyperuricaemia associated with cancer chemotherapy (usual maintenance in severe conditions)
- ▶ BY MOUTH
- ▶ Adult: 700–900 mg daily in divided doses (max. per dose 300 mg), dose to be taken preferably after food

- CONTRA-INDICATIONS Not a treatment for acute gout but continue if attack develops when already receiving allopurinol, and treat attack separately
- CAUTIONS Ensure adequate fluid intake (2–3 litres/day) · for hyperuricaemia associated with cancer therapy, allopurinol treatment should be started before cancer therapy
CAUTIONS, FURTHER INFORMATION
Administer prophylactic NSAID (*not* aspirin or salicylates) or colchicine until at least 1 month after hyperuricaemia corrected (usually for first 3 months) to avoid precipitating an acute attack.
- INTERACTIONS → Appendix 1 (allopurinol).
- SIDE-EFFECTS
- ▶ **Common or very common** Gastro-intestinal disorders · rashes (**withdraw** therapy; if rash mild re-introduce cautiously but **discontinue** promptly if recurrence)
- ▶ **Rare** Alopecia · aplastic anaemia · arthralgia · blood disorders · drowsiness · eosinophilia resembling Stevens-Johnson syndrome · eosinophilia resembling toxic epidermal necrolysis · exfoliation · fever · gynaecomastia · haemolytic anaemia · headache · hepatitis · hepatotoxicity · hypersensitivity reactions · hypertension · leucopenia · lymphadenopathy · malaise · neuropathy · paraesthesia · renal impairment · taste disturbances · thrombocytopenia · vasculitis · vertigo · visual disturbances
- ▶ **Very rare** Seizures

- PREGNANCY Toxicity not reported. Manufacturer advises use only if no safer alternative and disease carries risk for mother or child.
- BREAST FEEDING Present in milk—not known to be harmful.
- HEPATIC IMPAIRMENT Reduce dose.
- RENAL IMPAIRMENT Max. 100 mg daily, increased only if response inadequate; in severe impairment, reduce daily dose below 100 mg, or increase dose interval; if facilities available, adjust dose to maintain plasma-oxipurinol concentration below 100 micromol/litre.

- MEDICINAL FORMS
  There can be variation in the licensing of different medicines containing the same drug. Forms available from special-order manufacturers include: oral suspension, oral solution, mouthwash

  Tablet
  CAUTIONARY AND ADVISORY LABELS 8, 21, 27
  ▸ Allopurinol (Non-proprietary)
    Allopurinol 100 mg Allopurinol 100mg tablets | 28 tablet [PoM] £1.64 DT price = £0.80
    Allopurinol 300 mg Allopurinol 300mg tablets | 28 tablet [PoM] £1.72 DT price = £0.90
  ▸ Uricto (Ennogen Pharma Ltd)
    Allopurinol 100 mg Uricto 100mg tablets | 28 tablet [PoM] £1.25 DT price = £0.80
    Allopurinol 300 mg Uricto 300mg tablets | 28 tablet [PoM] £0.94 DT price = £0.90
  ▸ Zyloric (Aspen Pharma Trading Ltd)
    Allopurinol 100 mg Zyloric 100mg tablets | 100 tablet [PoM] £10.19
    Allopurinol 300 mg Zyloric 300mg tablets | 28 tablet [PoM] £7.31 DT price = £0.90

Febuxostat

- INDICATIONS AND DOSE

Treatment of chronic hyperuricaemia in gout
▸ BY MOUTH
▸ **Adult:** Initially 80 mg once daily, if after 2–4 weeks of initial dose, serum uric acid greater than 6 mg/100 mL then increase dose; increased if necessary to 120 mg once daily

IMPORTANT SAFETY INFORMATION
MHRA/CHM ADVICE: SERIOUS HYPERSENSITIVITY REACTIONS (JUNE 2012)
There have been rare but serious reports of hypersensitivity reactions, including Stevens-Johnson syndrome and acute anaphylactic shock with febuxostat. Patients should be advised of the signs and symptoms of severe hypersensitivity; febuxostat must be stopped immediately if these occur (early withdrawal is associated with a better prognosis), and must not be restarted in patients who have ever developed a hypersensitivity reaction to febuxostat. Most cases occur during the first month of treatment; a prior history of hypersensitivity to allopurinol and/or renal disease may indicate potential hypersensitivity to febuxostat.

- CONTRA-INDICATIONS Not a treatment for acute gout but continue if attack develops when already receiving febuxostat, and treat attack separately
- CAUTIONS Congestive heart failure · ischaemic heart disease · thyroid disorders · transplant recipients
  CAUTIONS, FURTHER INFORMATION
  Administer prophylactic NSAID (*not* aspirin or salicylates) or colchicine for at least 6 months after starting febuxostat to avoid precipitating an acute attack.
- INTERACTIONS → Appendix 1 (febuxostat).

- SIDE-EFFECTS
▸ **Common or very common** Abnormal liver function tests · gastro-intestinal disturbances · headache · oedema · rash
▸ **Uncommon** Renal failure · appetite change · arthralgia · arthritis · atrial fibrillation · bronchitis · bursitis · chest pain · cholelithiasis · cough · decreased libido · dermatitis · diabetes mellitus · dizziness · drowsiness · dyspnoea · ECG abnormalities · erectile dysfunction · flushing · haematuria · hemiparesis · hyperlipidaemia · hypertension · hypoaesthesia · increased thyroid stimulating hormone · increased urinary frequency · insomnia · muscle spasm · muscle weakness · myalgia · nephrolithiasis · palpitation · paraesthesia · proteinuria · smell disturbances · taste disturbances · upper respiratory tract infection · weight change
▸ **Rare** Asthenia · blurred vision · hepatitis · jaundice · mouth ulceration · nervousness · pancreatitis · pancytopenia · rhabdomyolysis · thirst · thrombocytopenia · tinnitus · tubulointerstitial nephritis
- PREGNANCY Manufacturer advises avoid—limited information available.
- BREAST FEEDING Manufacturer advises avoid—present in milk in *animal* studies.
- HEPATIC IMPAIRMENT Max. 80 mg daily in mild impairment. No dose information available in moderate or severe impairment.
- RENAL IMPAIRMENT Use with caution if eGFR less than 30 mL/minute/1.73 m^2—no information available.
- PRE-TREATMENT SCREENING Monitor liver function tests before treatment as indicated.
- MONITORING REQUIREMENTS Monitor liver function tests periodically during treatment as indicated.
- NATIONAL FUNDING/ACCESS DECISIONS

NICE technology appraisals (TAs)
▸ Febuxostat for the management of hyperuricaemia in patients with gout (December 2008) NICE TA164
Febuxostat is recommended as an option for the management of chronic hyperuricaemia in gout only for patients who are intolerant of allopurinol or for whom allopurinol is contra-indicated.
   For the purposes of this guidance, intolerance of allopurinol is defined as adverse effects that are sufficiently severe to warrant discontinuation, or to prevent full dose escalation for optimal effectiveness.
www.nice.org.uk/TA164

Scottish Medicines Consortium (SMC) Decisions
The *Scottish Medicines Consortium* issued similar advice to NICE guidance: Febuxostat for the management of hyperuricaemia in patients with gout (December 2008), in August 2010.

- MEDICINAL FORMS
  There can be variation in the licensing of different medicines containing the same drug.

  Tablet
  ▸ Febuxostat (Non-proprietary)
    Febuxostat 80 mg Febuxostat 80mg tablets | 28 tablet [PoM] no price available DT price = £24.36
    Febuxostat 120 mg Febuxostat 120mg tablets | 28 tablet [PoM] no price available DT price = £24.36
  ▸ Adenuric (A. Menarini Farmaceutica Internazionale SRL)
    Febuxostat 80 mg Adenuric 80mg tablets | 28 tablet [PoM] £24.36 DT price = £24.36
    Febuxostat 120 mg Adenuric 120mg tablets | 28 tablet [PoM] £24.36 DT price = £24.36

10

Musculoskeletal system

3 Neuromuscular disorders

Neuromuscular disorders

Drugs that enhance neuromuscular transmission

Anticholinesterases are used as first-line treatment in *ocular myasthenia gravis* and as an adjunct to immunosuppressant therapy for *generalised myasthenia gravis*.

Corticosteroids are used when anticholinesterases do not control symptoms completely. A second-line immunosuppressant such as azathioprine p. 757 is frequently used to reduce the dose of corticosteroid.

Plasmapheresis or infusion of intravenous immunoglobulin [unlicensed indication] may induce temporary remission in severe relapses, particularly where bulbar or respiratory function is compromised or before thymectomy.

Anticholinesterases

Anticholinesterase drugs enhance neuromuscular transmission in voluntary and involuntary muscle in myasthenia gravis. Excessive dosage of these drugs can impair neuromuscular transmission and precipitate cholinergic crises by causing a depolarising block. This may be difficult to distinguish from a worsening myasthenic state.

Muscarinic side-effects of anticholinesterases include increased sweating, increased salivary and gastric secretions, increased gastro-intestinal and uterine motility, and bradycardia. These parasympathomimetic effects are antagonised by atropine sulfate p. 1169.

Neostigmine p. 971 produces a therapeutic effect for up to 4 hours. Its pronounced muscarinic action is a disadvantage, and simultaneous administration of an antimuscarinic drug such as atropine sulfate or propantheline bromide p. 78 may be required to prevent colic, excessive salivation, or diarrhoea. In severe disease neostigmine can be given every 2 hours. The maximum that most patients can tolerate is 180 mg daily.

Pyridostigmine bromide p. 972 is less powerful and slower in action than neostigmine but it has a longer duration of action. It is preferable to neostigmine because of its smoother action and the need for less frequent dosage. It is particularly preferred in patients whose muscles are weak on waking. It has a comparatively mild gastrointestinal effect but an antimuscarinic drug may still be required.

Neostigmine is also used to reverse the actions of the non-depolarising neuromuscular blocking drugs.

Immunosuppressant therapy

Corticosteroids are established as treatment for myasthenia gravis; although they are commonly given on alternate days there is little evidence of benefit over daily administration. Corticosteroid treatment is usually initiated under in-patient supervision and all patients should receive osteoporosis prophylaxis.

In *generalised myasthenia gravis* prednisolone p. 614 is given. About 10% of patients experience a transient but very serious worsening of symptoms in the first 2–3 weeks, especially if the corticosteroid is started at a high dose. Smaller doses of corticosteroid are usually required in *ocular myasthenia*. Once clinical remission has occurred (usually after 2–6 months), the dose of prednisolone should be reduced slowly to the minimum effective dose.

In generalised myasthenia gravis azathioprine is usually started at the same time as the corticosteroid and it allows a lower maintenance dose of the corticosteroid to be used. Ciclosporin p. 758, methotrexate p. 807, or mycophenolate mofetil p. 765 can be used in patients unresponsive or intolerant to other treatments [unlicensed indications].

Acetylcholine-release enhancers

Amifampridine p. 972 is licensed for the symptomatic treatment of Lambert-Eaton myasthenic syndrome (LEMS), a rare disorder of neuromuscular transmission.

Fampridine p. 767 is licensed for the improvement of walking in patients with multiple sclerosis who have a walking disability.

Skeletal muscle relaxants

The drugs described are used for the relief of chronic muscle spasm or spasticity associated with multiple sclerosis or other neurological damage; they are not indicated for spasm associated with minor injuries. Baclofen, diazepam, and tizanidine act principally on the central nervous system. Dantrolene has a peripheral site of action; cannabis extract has both a central and a peripheral action. Skeletal muscle relaxants differ in action from the muscle relaxants used in anaesthesia, which block transmission at the neuromuscular junction.

The underlying cause of spasticity should be treated and any aggravating factors (e.g. pressure sores, infection) remedied. Skeletal muscle relaxants are effective in most forms of spasticity except the rare alpha variety. The major disadvantage of treatment with these drugs is that reduction in muscle tone can cause a loss of splinting action of the spastic leg and trunk muscles and sometimes lead to an increase in disability.

Baclofen p. 973 inhibits transmission at spinal level and also depresses the central nervous system. The dose should be increased slowly to avoid the major side-effects of sedation and muscular hypotonia (other adverse events are uncommon).

A cannabis extract p. 972 containing dronabinol (delta-9-tetrahydrocannabinol) and cannabidiol is licensed as an adjunct treatment for moderate to severe spasticity associated with multiple sclerosis in patients who have not responded adequately to other skeletal muscle relaxants. The dose should be titrated over 2 weeks; response to treatment should be reviewed after 4 weeks and treatment stopped if an adequate response is not achieved.

Dantrolene sodium p. 1181 acts directly on skeletal muscle and produces fewer central adverse effects making it a drug of choice. The dose should be increased slowly.

Diazepam p. 313 can also be used. Sedation and occasionally extensor hypotonus are disadvantages. Other benzodiazepines also have muscle-relaxant properties. Muscle-relaxant doses of benzodiazepines are similar to anxiolytic doses.

Tizanidine p. 974 is an alpha$_2$-adrenoceptor agonist indicated for spasticity associated with multiple sclerosis or spinal cord injury.

Other muscle relaxants

The clinical efficacy of methocarbamol p. 974 and meprobamate p. 316 as muscle relaxants is **not** well established, although they have been included in compound analgesic preparations.

NEUROPROTECTIVE DRUGS

| Riluzole

- **INDICATIONS AND DOSE**

To extend life in patients with amyotrophic lateral sclerosis, initiated by specialist experienced in the management of motor neurone disease

▸ BY MOUTH

▸ Adult: 50 mg twice daily

- CONTRA-INDICATIONS Acute porphyria
- CAUTIONS History of abnormal hepatic function (consult product literature for details) · interstitial lung disease

CAUTIONS, FURTHER INFORMATION
▸ Interstitial lung disease Perform chest radiography if symptoms such as dry cough or dyspnoea develop; discontinue if interstitial lung disease is diagnosed.

● **SIDE-EFFECTS**
▸ **Common or very common** Abdominal pain · asthenia · diarrhoea · dizziness · drowsiness · headache · nausea · oral paraesthesia · tachycardia · vomiting
▸ **Uncommon** Anaemia · angioedema · interstitial lung disease · pancreatitis
▸ **Rare** Neutropenia
▸ **Very rare** Hepatitis

SIDE-EFFECTS, FURTHER INFORMATION
▸ Neutropenia White blood cell counts should be determined in febrile illness; neutropenia requires discontinuation of riluzole.

● **PREGNANCY** Avoid—no information available.

● **BREAST FEEDING** Avoid—no information available.

● **HEPATIC IMPAIRMENT** Avoid.

● **RENAL IMPAIRMENT** Avoid—no information available.

● **PATIENT AND CARER ADVICE**
Blood disorders Patients or their carers should be told how to recognise signs of neutropenia and advised to seek immediate medical attention if symptoms such as fever occur.

Driving and skilled tasks
Dizziness or vertigo may affect performance of skilled tasks (e.g. driving).

● **NATIONAL FUNDING/ACCESS DECISIONS**
NICE technology appraisals (TAs)
▸ **Riluzole for motor neurone disease (January 2001)** NICE TA20
Riluzole is recommended for treating the amyotrophic lateral sclerosis (ALS) form of motor neurone disease (MND). Treatment should be initiated by a specialist in MND but it can then be supervised under a shared-care arrangement involving the general practitioner.
www.nice.org.uk/TA20

● **MEDICINAL FORMS**
There can be variation in the licensing of different medicines containing the same drug. Forms available from special-order manufacturers include: oral suspension, oral solution, powder
Tablet
▸ Riluzole (Non-proprietary)
  Riluzole 50 mg Riluzole 50mg tablets | 56 tablet [PoM] £320.00 DT price = £19.10
▸ Rilutek (Sanofi)
  Riluzole 50 mg Rilutek 50mg tablets | 56 tablet [PoM] £320.33 DT price = £19.10
Oral suspension
▸ Teglutik (Martindale Pharmaceuticals Ltd)
  Riluzole 5 mg per 1 ml Teglutik 5mg/1ml oral suspension sugar-free | 300 ml [PoM] £100.00 DT price = £100.00

3.1 Myasthenia gravis and Lambert-Eaton myasthenic syndrome

ANTICHOLINESTERASES

Anticholinesterases

● **DRUG ACTION** They prolong the action of acetylcholine by inhibiting the action of the enzyme acetylcholinesterase.

● **CONTRA-INDICATIONS** Intestinal obstruction · urinary obstruction

● **CAUTIONS** Arrhythmias · asthma (extreme caution) · atropine or other antidote to muscarinic effects may be

necessary (particularly when neostigmine is given by injection) but not given routinely because it may mask signs of overdosage · bradycardia · epilepsy · hyperthyroidism · hypotension · parkinsonism · peptic ulceration · recent myocardial infarction · vagotonia

● **INTERACTIONS** → Appendix 1 (parasympathomimetics).

● **SIDE-EFFECTS** Abdominal cramps (more marked with higher doses) · diarrhoea · increased salivation · nausea · vomiting

Overdose
Signs of overdosage include bronchoconstriction, increased bronchial secretions, lacrimation, excessive sweating, involuntary defaecation, involuntary micturition, miosis, nystagmus, bradycardia, heart block, arrhythmias, hypotension, agitation, excessive dreaming, and weakness eventually leading to fasciculation and paralysis.

● **PREGNANCY** Manufacturer advises use only if potential benefit outweighs risk.

● **BREAST FEEDING** Amount probably too small to be harmful.

◤ above

Neostigmine
(Neostigmine methylsulfate)

● **INDICATIONS AND DOSE**
Treatment of myasthenia gravis
▸ BY MOUTH
▸ Adult: Initially 15–30 mg, dose repeated at suitable intervals throughout the day, total daily dose 75–300 mg, the maximum that most patients can tolerate is 180 mg daily
▸ BY SUBCUTANEOUS INJECTION, OR BY INTRAMUSCULAR INJECTION
▸ Adult: 1–2.5 mg, dose repeated at suitable intervals throughout the day (usual total daily dose 5–20 mg)

Reversal of non-depolarising (competitive) neuromuscular blockade
▸ BY INTRAVENOUS INJECTION
▸ Adult: 2.5 mg (max. per dose 5 mg), repeated if necessary after or with glycopyrronium or atropine, to be given over 1 minute

● **CAUTIONS**
▸ With intravenous use Glycopyrronium or atropine should also be given when reversing neuromuscular blockade

● **INTERACTIONS** → Appendix 1 (parasympathomimetics).

● **RENAL IMPAIRMENT** May need dose reduction.

● **MEDICINAL FORMS**
There can be variation in the licensing of different medicines containing the same drug. Forms available from special-order manufacturers include: oral solution
Tablet
▸ Neostigmine (Non-proprietary)
  Neostigmine bromide 15 mg Prostigmin 15mg tablets | 100 tablet [PoM] no price available
  Neostigmine 15mg tablets | 140 tablet [PoM] £99.60
Solution for injection
▸ Neostigmine (Non-proprietary)
  Neostigmine metilsulfate 2.5 mg per 1 ml Neostigmine 2.5mg/1ml solution for injection ampoules | 10 ampoule [PoM] £4.95–£5.06

⌐ 971

Pyridostigmine bromide

- **DRUG ACTION** Pyridostigmine bromide has weaker muscarinic action than neostigmine.

- **INDICATIONS AND DOSE**

Myasthenia gravis

▶ INITIALLY BY MOUTH
▶ Adult: 30–120 mg, doses to be given at suitable intervals throughout day; (by mouth) usual dose 0.3–1.2 g daily in divided doses, it is inadvisable to exceed a total daily dose of 450 mg in order to avoid acetylcholine receptor down-regulation; patients requiring doses exceeding 450 mg daily will usually require input from a specialised neuromuscular service. Immunosuppressant therapy is usually considered if the dose of pyridostigmine exceeds 360 mg daily

- **RENAL IMPAIRMENT** Reduce dose; excreted by kidney.

- **MEDICINAL FORMS**
There can be variation in the licensing of different medicines containing the same drug. Forms available from special-order manufacturers include: oral suspension, oral solution
Tablet
▶ Pyridostigmine bromide (Non-proprietary)
Pyridostigmine bromide 60 mg Pyridostigmine bromide 60mg tablets | 200 tablet [PoM] £45.58 DT price = £45.58
▶ Mestinon (Meda Pharmaceuticals Ltd)
Pyridostigmine bromide 60 mg Mestinon 60mg tablets | 200 tablet [PoM] £45.57 DT price = £45.58

CHOLINERGIC RECEPTOR STIMULATING DRUGS

Amifampridine

- **INDICATIONS AND DOSE**

Symptomatic treatment of Lambert-Eaton myasthenic syndrome (specialist use only)

▶ BY MOUTH
▶ Adult: Initially 15 mg daily in 3 divided doses, then increased in steps of 5 mg every 4–5 days, increased to up to 60 mg daily in 3–4 divided doses (max. per dose 20 mg); maximum 60 mg per day

- **CONTRA-INDICATIONS** Congenital QT syndromes · epilepsy · uncontrolled asthma

- **CAUTIONS** Non-paraneoplastic form of Lambert-Eaton myasthenic syndrome

- **INTERACTIONS** Caution if concomitant use of drugs that lower convulsive threshold.
Avoid concomitant use of drugs that prolong QT interval.
Avoid concomitant use of drugs with a narrow therapeutic index.

- **SIDE-EFFECTS** Anxiety · arrhythmias · blurred vision · bronchial hypersecretion · chorea · convulsions · cough · dizziness · drowsiness · exacerbation or precipitation of asthma · gastro-intestinal disorders · headache · myoclonia · palpitations · paraesthesia · Raynaud's syndrome · sleep disturbances · weakness

- **CONCEPTION AND CONTRACEPTION** Ensure effective contraception during treatment in men and women.

- **PREGNANCY** Manufacturer advises avoid.

- **BREAST FEEDING** Manufacturer advises avoid—no information available.

- **HEPATIC IMPAIRMENT** In mild impairment reduce initial dose to 10 mg daily in divided doses, increased in steps of 5 mg every 7 days. In moderate or severe impairment reduce initial dose to 5 mg daily in divided doses, increased in steps of 5 mg every 7 days. Use with caution.

- **RENAL IMPAIRMENT** In mild impairment reduce initial dose to 10 mg daily in divided doses, increased in steps of 5 mg every 7 days. In moderate or severe impairment reduce initial dose to 5 mg daily in divided doses, increased in steps of 5 mg every 7 days. Use with caution.

- **MONITORING REQUIREMENTS** Clinical and ECG monitoring required at treatment initiation and yearly thereafter.

- **NATIONAL FUNDING/ACCESS DECISIONS**

Scottish Medicines Consortium (SMC) Decisions
The *Scottish Medicines Consortium* has advised (July 2012) that amifampridine phosphate (*Firdapse*®) is not recommended for use within NHS Scotland for the symptomatic treatment of Lambert-Eaton myasthenic syndrome (LEMS).

- **MEDICINAL FORMS**
There can be variation in the licensing of different medicines containing the same drug. Forms available from special-order manufacturers include: tablet
Tablet
CAUTIONARY AND ADVISORY LABELS 3, 21
▶ Firdapse (BioMarin Europe Ltd) ▼
Amifampridine (as Amifampridine phosphate) 10 mg Firdapse 10mg tablets | 100 tablet [PoM] £1,815.00

3.2 Nocturnal leg cramps

Nocturnal leg cramps

Quinine salts

Quinine salts p. 564, such as quinine sulfate are effective in reducing the frequency of nocturnal leg cramps by about 25% in ambulatory patients; however, because of potential toxicity, quinine is not recommended for routine treatment and should not be used unless cramps cause regular disruption to sleep. Quinine should only be considered when cramps are very painful or frequent; when other treatable causes of cramp have been excluded; and when non-pharmacological treatments have not worked (e.g. passive stretching exercises). It may take up to 4 weeks for improvement to become apparent; if there is benefit, quinine treatment can be continued. Treatment should be interrupted at intervals of approximately 3 months to assess the need for further quinine treatment. In patients taking quinine long term, a trial discontinuation may be considered. Quinine is toxic in overdosage and accidental fatalities have occurred.

3.3 Spasticity

Drugs used for spasticity not listed below Dantrolene sodium, p. 1181 · Diazepam, p. 313

CANNIBINOIDS

Cannabis extract

- **INDICATIONS AND DOSE**

Adjunct in moderate to severe spasticity in multiple sclerosis (specialist use only)

▶ BY BUCCAL ADMINISTRATION
▶ Adult: (consult product literature)

- **CONTRA-INDICATIONS** Family history of psychosis · history of other severe psychiatric disorder · personal history of psychosis

- CAUTIONS History of epilepsy · significant cardiovascular disease
- INTERACTIONS → Appendix 1 (cannabis extract).
- SIDE-EFFECTS
▸ **Common or very common** Amnesia · blurred vision · constipation · depression · diarrhoea · disorientation · dissociation · dizziness · drowsiness · dry mouth · dysarthria · impaired attention · increased or decreased appetite · malaise · mood disturbance · mouth ulcers · nausea · oral pain · taste disturbance · vertigo · vomiting
▸ **Uncommon** Abdominal pain · delusions · hallucinations · hypertension · oromucosal discolouration · palpitation · paranoia · pharyngitis · stomatitis · suicidal thoughts · syncope · tachycardia · tooth discolouration
▸ **Frequency not known** Anxiety · seizures
- CONCEPTION AND CONTRACEPTION Manufacturer recommends effective contraception during and for 3 months after treatment in men and women.
- PREGNANCY Manufacturer advises use only if potential benefit outweighs risks.
- BREAST FEEDING Avoid—present in milk.
- HEPATIC IMPAIRMENT Manufacturer advises more frequent monitoring in significant hepatic impairment—possible risk of prolonged or enhanced effect.
- RENAL IMPAIRMENT Manufacturer advises more frequent monitoring in significant renal impairment—possible risk of prolonged or enhanced effect.
- MONITORING REQUIREMENTS Monitor oral mucosa—interrupt treatment if lesions or persistent soreness.
- PATIENT AND CARER ADVICE
  Driving and skilled tasks
  For information on 2015 legislation regarding driving whilst taking certain controlled drugs, including cannabis, see Drugs and driving under Guidance on prescribing p. 1.

- MEDICINAL FORMS
  There can be variation in the licensing of different medicines containing the same drug.
  Spray
  EXCIPIENTS: May contain Propylene glycol
  ▸ Sativex (Bayer Plc)
  Cannabidiol 2.5 mg per 1 dose, Dronabinol 2.7 mg per 1 dose Sativex oromucosal spray | 270 dose [PoM] £375.00 [CD4-1]

MUSCLE RELAXANTS > CENTRALLY ACTING

Baclofen

- INDICATIONS AND DOSE
Pain of muscle spasm in palliative care
▸ BY MOUTH
  ▸ Adult: 5–10 mg 3 times a day
Hiccup due to gastric distension (in palliative care)
▸ BY MOUTH
  ▸ Adult: 5 mg twice daily
Chronic severe spasticity resulting from disorders such as multiple sclerosis or traumatic partial section of spinal cord
▸ BY MOUTH
  ▸ Adult: Initially 5 mg 3 times a day, gradually increased; maintenance up to 60 mg daily in divided doses, review treatment if no benefit within 6 weeks of achieving maximum dose; maximum 100 mg per day
Severe chronic spasticity unresponsive to oral antispastic drugs (or where side-effects of oral therapy unacceptable) or as alternative to ablative neurosurgical procedures (specialist use only)
▸ BY INTRATHECAL INJECTION
  ▸ Adult: Test dose 25–50 micrograms, to be given over at least 1 minute via catheter or lumbar puncture, then

increased in steps of 25 micrograms (max. per dose 100 micrograms), not given more often than every 24 hours to determine appropriate dose, then *dose-titration phase*, most often using infusion pump (implanted into chest wall or abdominal wall tissues) to establish maintenance dose (ranging from 12 micrograms to 2 mg daily for spasticity of spinal origin or 22 micrograms to 1.4 mg daily for spasticity of cerebral origin) retaining some spasticity to avoid sensation of paralysis

> **IMPORTANT SAFETY INFORMATION**
> Consult product literature for details on test dose and titration—important to monitor patients closely in appropriately equipped and staffed environment during screening and immediately after pump implantation. Resuscitation equipment must be available for immediate use. Treatment with continuous pump-administered intrathecal baclofen should be initiated within 3 months of a satisfactory response to intrathecal baclofen testing.

- CONTRA-INDICATIONS
▸ **With intrathecal use** Local infection · systemic infection
▸ **With oral use** Avoid oral route in active peptic ulceration
- CAUTIONS
  GENERAL CAUTIONS
  Cerebrovascular disease · diabetes · elderly · epilepsy · history of peptic ulcer · hypertonic bladder sphincter · Parkinson's disease · psychiatric illness · respiratory impairment
  SPECIFIC CAUTIONS
▸ **With intrathecal use** Coagulation disorders · malnutrition (increased risk of post-surgical complications) · previous spinal fusion procedure
- INTERACTIONS → Appendix 1 (muscle relaxants).
- SIDE-EFFECTS
▸ **Common or very common** Agitation · anxiety · ataxia · cardiovascular depression · confusion · depression · dizziness · drowsiness · dry mouth · euphoria · gastro-intestinal disturbances · hallucinations · headache · hyperhidrosis · hypotension · insomnia · myalgia · nightmares · rash · respiratory depression · sedation · seizure · tremor · urinary disturbances · visual disorders
▸ **Rare** Abdominal pain · changes in hepatic function · dysarthria · erectile dysfunction · paraesthesia · taste disturbances
▸ **Very rare** Hypothermia
- PREGNANCY Manufacturer advises use only if potential benefit outweighs risk (toxicity in *animal* studies).
- BREAST FEEDING Present in milk—amount probably too small to be harmful.
- HEPATIC IMPAIRMENT
▸ **With oral use** Manufacturer advises use with caution.
- RENAL IMPAIRMENT
▸ **With oral use** Risk of toxicity—use smaller doses (e.g. 5 mg daily by mouth) and if necessary increase dosage interval; if eGFR less than 15 mL/minute/1.73 m^2 manufacturer advises use by mouth only if potential benefit outweighs risk. Excreted by the kidney.
- TREATMENT CESSATION Avoid abrupt withdrawal (risk of hyperactive state, may exacerbate spasticity, and precipitate autonomic dysfunction including hyperthermia, psychiatric reactions and convulsions; to minimise risk, discontinue by gradual dose reduction over at least 1–2 weeks (longer if symptoms occur)).
- PRESCRIBING AND DISPENSING INFORMATION Flavours of oral liquid formulations may include raspberry.

10

Musculoskeletal system

- **PATIENT AND CARER ADVICE**
  Driving and skilled tasks
  Drowsiness may affect performance of skilled tasks (e.g. driving); effects of alcohol enhanced.

- **MEDICINAL FORMS**
  There can be variation in the licensing of different medicines containing the same drug. Forms available from special-order manufacturers include: oral suspension, oral solution

  Tablet
  CAUTIONARY AND ADVISORY LABELS 2, 8, 21
  EXCIPIENTS: May contain Gluten
  ▸ Baclofen (Non-proprietary)
    Baclofen 10 mg Baclofen 10mg tablets | 84 tablet [PoM] £9.99 DT price = £2.69
  ▸ Lioresal (Novartis Pharmaceuticals UK Ltd)
    Baclofen 10 mg Lioresal 10mg tablets | 100 tablet [PoM] £14.86

  Oral solution
  CAUTIONARY AND ADVISORY LABELS 2, 8, 21
  ▸ Baclofen (Non-proprietary)
    Baclofen 1 mg per 1 ml Baclofen 5mg/5ml oral solution sugar free sugar-free | 300 ml [PoM] £22.45 DT price = £3.43
  ▸ Lioresal (Novartis Pharmaceuticals UK Ltd)
    Baclofen 1 mg per 1 ml Lioresal 5mg/5ml liquid sugar-free | 300 ml [PoM] £10.31 DT price = £3.43
  ▸ Lyflex (Chemidex Pharma Ltd)
    Baclofen 1 mg per 1 ml Lyflex 5mg/5ml oral solution sugar-free | 300 ml [PoM] £7.95 DT price = £3.43

  Solution for injection
  ▸ Baclofen (Non-proprietary)
    Baclofen 50 microgram per 1 ml Baclofen 50micrograms/1ml solution for injection ampoules | 5 ampoule [PoM] £10.95 | 10 ampoule [PoM] £25.00-£27.60
  ▸ Lioresal (Novartis Pharmaceuticals UK Ltd)
    Baclofen 50 microgram per 1 ml Lioresal Intrathecal 50micrograms/1ml solution for injection ampoules | 1 ampoule [PoM] £3.16

  Solution for infusion
  ▸ Baclofen (Non-proprietary)
    Baclofen 500 microgram per 1 ml Baclofen 10mg/20ml solution for infusion ampoules | 1 ampoule [PoM] £48.62-£57.00
    Baclofen 2 mg per 1 ml Baclofen 40mg/20ml solution for infusion ampoules | 1 ampoule [PoM] £228.00-£250.00
    Baclofen 10mg/5ml solution for infusion ampoules | 5 ampoule [PoM] £243.10 | 10 ampoule [PoM] £500.00-£570.00
  ▸ Lioresal (Novartis Pharmaceuticals UK Ltd)
    Baclofen 500 microgram per 1 ml Lioresal Intrathecal 10mg/20ml solution for infusion ampoules | 1 ampoule [PoM] £70.01
    Baclofen 2 mg per 1 ml Lioresal Intrathecal 10mg/5ml solution for infusion ampoules | 1 ampoule [PoM] £70.01

Methocarbamol

- **INDICATIONS AND DOSE**
  Short-term symptomatic relief of muscle spasm
  ▸ BY MOUTH
  ▸ Adult: 1.5 g 4 times a day; reduced to 750 mg 3 times a day if required
  ▸ Elderly: Up to 750 mg 4 times a day, dose may be sufficient

- **CONTRA-INDICATIONS** Brain damage · coma · epilepsy · myasthenia gravis · pre-coma
- **INTERACTIONS** → Appendix 1 (muscle relaxants).
- **SIDE-EFFECTS** Amnesia · anaphylaxis · angioedema · anxiety · blurred vision · bradycardia · cholestatic jaundice · confusion · dizziness · drowsiness · dyspepsia · fever · headache · hypersensitivity reactions · hypotension · leucopenia · nasal congestion · nausea · pruritus · rash · restlessness · seizures · tremor · urticaria · vomiting
- **PREGNANCY** Manufacturer advises avoid unless potential benefit outweighs risk.
- **BREAST FEEDING** Present in milk in *animal studies*—manufacturer advises caution.

- **HEPATIC IMPAIRMENT** Manufacturer advises caution; half-life may be prolonged.
- **RENAL IMPAIRMENT** Manufacturer advises caution.
- **PATIENT AND CARER ADVICE**
  Driving and skilled tasks
  Drowsiness may affect performance of skilled tasks (e.g. driving); effects of alcohol enhanced.
- **LESS SUITABLE FOR PRESCRIBING** Less suitable for prescribing.

- **MEDICINAL FORMS**
  There can be variation in the licensing of different medicines containing the same drug. Forms available from special-order manufacturers include: oral suspension

  Tablet
  CAUTIONARY AND ADVISORY LABELS 2
  ▸ Methocarbamol (Non-proprietary)
    Methocarbamol 750 mg Methocarbamol 750mg tablets | 100 tablet [PoM] £47.13 DT price = £43.57
  ▸ Robaxin (Almirall Ltd)
    Methocarbamol 750 mg Robaxin 750 tablets | 100 tablet [PoM] £12.65 DT price = £43.57

Tizanidine

- **INDICATIONS AND DOSE**
  Spasticity associated with multiple sclerosis or spinal cord injury or disease
  ▸ BY MOUTH
  ▸ Adult: Initially 2 mg daily, then increased in steps of 2 mg daily in divided doses, increased at intervals of at least 3–4 days and adjust according to response; usual dose up to 24 mg daily in 3–4 divided doses; maximum 36 mg per day

- **CAUTIONS** Elderly
- **INTERACTIONS** → Appendix 1 (muscle relaxants). Caution with concomitant administration of drugs that prolong QT interval.
- **SIDE-EFFECTS**
  ▸ **Common or very common** Altered liver enzymes (discontinue if persistently raised—consult product literature) · dizziness · drowsiness · dry mouth · fatigue · gastro-intestinal disturbance · hypotension · nausea
  ▸ **Uncommon** Bradycardia
  ▸ **Frequency not known** Asthenia · blurred vision · confusion · convulsions · hallucinations · hepatitis · insomnia · liver failure · syncope
- **PREGNANCY** Avoid (toxicity in *animal* studies).
- **BREAST FEEDING** Avoid (present in milk in *animal* studies).
- **HEPATIC IMPAIRMENT** Avoid in severe impairment; use in moderate impairment only if potential benefit outweighs risk.
- **RENAL IMPAIRMENT** Manufacturer advises caution.
- **MONITORING REQUIREMENTS** Monitor liver function monthly for first 4 months and in those who develop unexplained nausea, anorexia or fatigue.
- **TREATMENT CESSATION** Avoid abrupt withdrawal (risk of rebound hypertension and tachycardia); to minimise risk, discontinue gradually and monitor blood pressure.
- **PATIENT AND CARER ADVICE**
  Driving and skilled tasks
  Drowsiness may affect performance of skilled tasks (e.g. driving); effects of alcohol enhanced.

● MEDICINAL FORMS
There can be variation in the licensing of different medicines containing the same drug. Forms available from special-order manufacturers include: oral suspension, oral solution

Tablet
CAUTIONARY AND ADVISORY LABELS 2, 8
▶ Tizanidine (Non-proprietary)
Tizanidine (as Tizanidine hydrochloride) 2 mg Tizanidine 2mg tablets | 120 tablet PoM £28.89 DT price = £3.33
Tizanidine (as Tizanidine hydrochloride) 4 mg Tizanidine 4mg tablets | 120 tablet PoM £40.07 DT price = £25.09
▶ Zanaflex (Teva UK Ltd)
Tizanidine (as Tizanidine hydrochloride) 2 mg Zanaflex 2mg tablets | 120 tablet PoM £30.41 DT price = £3.33
Tizanidine (as Tizanidine hydrochloride) 4 mg Zanaflex 4mg tablets | 120 tablet PoM £42.18 DT price = £25.09

4   Pain and inflammation in musculoskeletal disorders

Non-steroidal anti-inflammatory drugs

Therapeutic effects

In *single doses* non-steroidal anti-inflammatory drugs (NSAIDs) have analgesic activity comparable to that of paracetamol p. 406, but paracetamol is preferred, particularly in the elderly.

In regular *full dosage* NSAIDs have both a lasting analgesic and an anti-inflammatory effect which makes them particularly useful for the treatment of continuous or regular pain associated with inflammation. Therefore, although paracetamol often gives adequate pain control in osteoarthritis, NSAIDs are more appropriate than paracetamol or the opioid analgesics in the *inflammatory arthritides* (e.g. rheumatoid arthritis) and in some cases of *advanced osteoarthritis*. NSAIDs can also be of benefit in the less well defined conditions of *back pain* and *soft-tissue disorders*.

Choice

Differences in anti-inflammatory activity between NSAIDs are small, but there is considerable variation in individual response and tolerance to these drugs. About 60% of patients will respond to any NSAID; of the others, those who do not respond to one may well respond to another. Pain relief starts soon after taking the first dose and a full analgesic effect should normally be obtained within a week, whereas an anti-inflammatory effect may not be achieved (or may not be clinically assessable) for up to 3 weeks. If appropriate responses are not obtained within these times, another NSAID should be tried.

NSAIDs reduce the production of prostaglandins by inhibiting the enzyme cyclo-oxygenase. They vary in their selectivity for inhibiting different types of cyclo-oxygenase; selective inhibition of cyclo-oxygenase-2 is associated with less gastro-intestinal intolerance. Several other factors also influence susceptibility to gastrointestinal effects, and a NSAID should be chosen on the basis of the incidence of gastro-intestinal and other side-effects.

Ibuprofen p. 987 is a propionic acid derivative with anti-inflammatory, analgesic, and antipyretic properties. It has fewer side-effects than other non-selective NSAIDs but its anti-inflammatory properties are weaker. It is unsuitable for conditions where inflammation is prominent, such as acute gout. Dexibuprofen p. 978 is the active enantiomer of ibuprofen. It has similar properties to ibuprofen and is licensed for the relief of mild to moderate pain and inflammation.

Other propionic acid derivatives:
Naproxen p. 995 is one of the first choices because it combines good efficacy with a low incidence of side-effects (but more than ibuprofen).
Fenoprofen p. 985 is as effective as naproxen, and flurbiprofen p. 986 may be slightly more effective. Both are associated with slightly more gastro-intestinal side-effects than ibuprofen.
Ketoprofen p. 991 has anti-inflammatory properties similar to ibuprofen and has more side-effects.
Dexketoprofen p. 979, an isomer of ketoprofen, has been introduced for the short-term relief of mild to moderate pain.
Tiaprofenic acid p. 998 is as effective as naproxen; it has more side-effects than ibuprofen.
Drugs with properties similar to those of propionic acid derivatives:
Diclofenac sodium p. 980 and aceclofenac p. 976 are similar in efficacy to naproxen.
Etodolac p. 983 is comparable in efficacy to naproxen; it is licensed for symptomatic relief of osteoarthritis and rheumatoid arthritis.
Indometacin p. 989 has an action equal to or superior to that of naproxen, but with a high incidence of side-effects including headache, dizziness, and gastro-intestinal disturbances.
Mefenamic acid p. 992 has minor anti-inflammatory properties. It has occasionally been associated with diarrhoea and haemolytic anaemia which require discontinuation of treatment.
Meloxicam p. 993 is licensed for the short-term relief of pain in osteoarthritis and for long-term treatment of rheumatoid arthritis and ankylosing spondylitis.
Nabumetone p. 994 is comparable in effect to naproxen.
Phenylbutazone is licensed for ankylosing spondylitis, but is not recommended because it is associated with serious side-effects, in particular haematological reactions; it should be used only by a specialist in severe cases where other treatments have been found unsuitable.
Piroxicam p. 996 is as effective as naproxen and has a long duration of action which permits once-daily administration. However, it has more gastro-intestinal side-effects than most other NSAIDs, and is associated with more frequent serious skin reactions.
Sulindac p. 997 is similar in tolerance to naproxen.
Tenoxicam p. 998 is similar in activity and tolerance to naproxen. Its long duration of action allows once-daily administration.
Tolfenamic acid p. 432 is licensed for the treatment of migraine.
Ketorolac trometamol p. 1176 and the selective inhibitor of cyclo-oxygenase-2, parecoxib p. 1177, are licensed for the short-term management of postoperative pain.
The selective inhibitors of cyclo-oxygenase-2, etoricoxib p. 984 and celecoxib p. 977, are as effective as non-selective NSAIDs such as diclofenac sodium and naproxen. Although selective inhibitors can cause serious gastro-intestinal events, available evidence appears to indicate that the risk of serious upper gastro-intestinal events is lower with selective inhibitors compared to non-selective NSAIDs; this advantage may be lost in patients who require concomitant low-dose aspirin.
Celecoxib and etoricoxib are licensed for the relief of pain in osteoarthritis, rheumatoid arthritis, and ankylosing spondylitis; etoricoxib is also licensed for the relief of pain from acute gout.
Aspirin p. 109 has been used in high doses to treat rheumatoid arthritis, but other NSAIDs are now preferred.

Dental and orofacial pain
Most mild to moderate dental pain and inflammation is effectively relieved by NSAIDs. Those used for dental pain

include ibuprofen, diclofenac sodium, and diclofenac potassium p. 980.

Asthma

Any degree of worsening of asthma may be related to the ingestion of NSAIDs, either prescribed or (in the case of ibuprofen **and** others) purchased over the counter.

NSAIDs and cardiovascular events

All NSAID use (including cyclo-oxygenase-2 selective inhibitors) can, to varying degrees, be associated with a small increased risk of thrombotic events (e.g. myocardial infarction and stroke) independent of baseline cardiovascular risk factors or duration of NSAID use; however, the greatest risk may be in those receiving high doses long term.

Cyclo-oxygenase-2 selective inhibitors, diclofenac (150 mg daily) and ibuprofen (2.4 g daily) are associated with an increased risk of thrombotic events. Although there are limited data regarding the thrombotic effects of aceclofenac, treatment advice has been updated in line with diclofenac, based on aceclofenac's structural similarity to diclofenac and its metabolism to diclofenac. The increased risk for diclofenac is similar to that of licensed doses of etoricoxib. Naproxen (1 g daily) is associated with a lower thrombotic risk, and low doses of ibuprofen (1.2 g daily or less) have not been associated with an increased risk of myocardial infarction.

The lowest effective dose of NSAID should be prescribed for the shortest period of time to control symptoms and the need for long-term treatment should be reviewed periodically.

NSAIDs and gastro-intestinal events

All NSAIDs are associated with serious gastro-intestinal toxicity; the risk is higher in the elderly. Evidence on the relative safety of non-selective NSAIDs indicates differences in the risks of serious upper gastro-intestinal side-effects—piroxicam p. 996, ketoprofen p. 991, and ketorolac trometamol p. 1176 are associated with the highest risk; indometacin p. 989, diclofenac, and naproxen p. 995 are associated with intermediate risk, and ibuprofen p. 987 with the lowest risk (although high doses of ibuprofen have been associated with intermediate risk). Selective inhibitors of cyclo-oxygenase-2 are associated with a *lower risk* of serious upper gastro-intestinal side-effects than non-selective NSAIDs.

Recommendations are that NSAIDs associated with a low risk e.g. ibuprofen are *generally preferred*, to start at the *lowest recommended dose* **and** not to use more than one oral NSAID at a time.

The combination of a NSAID **and** low-dose aspirin can increase the risk of gastro-intestinal side-effects; this combination should be used only if absolutely necessary **and** the patient should be monitored closely.

While it is preferable to avoid NSAIDs in patients with active or previous gastro-intestinal ulceration or bleeding, and to withdraw them if gastro-intestinal lesions develop, nevertheless patients with serious rheumatic diseases (e.g. rheumatoid arthritis) are usually dependent on NSAIDs for effective relief of pain and stiffness.

Patients at risk of gastro-intestinal ulceration (including the elderly), who need NSAID treatment should receive gastroprotective treatment.

Systemic as well as local effects of NSAIDs contribute to gastro-intestinal damage; taking oral formulations with milk or food, or using enteric-coated formulations, or changing the route of administration may only partially reduce symptoms such as dyspepsia.

Aceclofenac

● **INDICATIONS AND DOSE**

Pain and inflammation in rheumatoid arthritis, osteoarthritis and ankylosing spondylitis
▶ BY MOUTH
 ▶ Adult: 100 mg twice daily

● CONTRA-INDICATIONS Active gastro-intestinal bleeding · active gastro-intestinal ulceration · cerebrovascular disease · history of gastro-intestinal bleeding related to previous NSAID therapy · history of gastro-intestinal perforation related to previous NSAID therapy · history of recurrent gastro-intestinal haemorrhage (two or more distinct episodes) · history of recurrent gastro-intestinal ulceration (two or more distinct episodes) · ischaemic heart disease · mild heart failure · peripheral arterial disease · severe heart failure

● CAUTIONS Allergic disorders · avoid in Acute porphyrias p. 918 · cardiac impairment (NSAIDs may impair renal function) · coagulation defects · connective-tissue disorders · Crohn's disease (may be exacerbated) · elderly (risk of serious side-effects and fatalities) · history of cardiac failure · hypertension · left ventricular dysfunction · oedema · risk factors for cardiovascular events · ulcerative colitis (may be exacerbated)

● INTERACTIONS → Appendix 1 (NSAIDs).

● SIDE-EFFECTS
▶ **Rare** Alveolitis · aseptic meningitis (patients with connective-tissue disorders such as systemic lupus erythematosus may be especially susceptible) · hepatic damage · interstitial fibrosis associated with NSAIDs can lead to renal failure · pancreatitis · papillary necrosis associated with NSAIDs can lead to renal failure · pulmonary eosinophilia · Stevens-Johnson syndrome · toxic epidermal necrolysis · visual disturbances
▶ **Frequency not known** Angioedema · blood disorders · bronchospasm · colitis (induction of or exacerbation of) · Crohn's disease (induction of or exacerbation of) · depression · diarrhoea · dizziness · drowsiness · fluid retention (rarely precipitating congestive heart failure) · gastro-intestinal bleeding · gastro-intestinal discomfort · gastro-intestinal disturbances · gastro-intestinal ulceration · haematuria · headache · hearing disturbances · hypersensitivity reactions · insomnia · nausea · nervousness · photosensitivity · raised blood pressure · rashes · renal failure (especially in patients with pre-existing renal impairment) · tinnitus · vertigo

SIDE-EFFECTS, FURTHER INFORMATION
▶ **Serious side-effects** For information about cardiovascular and gastro-intestinal side-effects, and a possible exacerbation of symptoms in asthma, see Non-steroidal anti-inflammatory drugs p. 975.

● ALLERGY AND CROSS-SENSITIVITY Contra-indicated in patients with a history of hypersensitivity to aspirin or any other NSAID—which includes those in whom attacks of asthma, angioedema, urticaria or rhinitis have been precipitated by aspirin or any other NSAID.

● CONCEPTION AND CONTRACEPTION Caution—long-term use of some NSAIDs is associated with reduced female fertility, which is reversible on stopping treatment.

● PREGNANCY Most manufacturers advise avoiding the use of NSAIDs during pregnancy or avoiding them unless the potential benefit outweighs the risk. NSAIDs should be avoided during the third trimester because use is associated with a risk of closure of fetal ductus arteriosus *in utero* and possibly persistent pulmonary hypertension of the newborn. In addition, the onset of labour may be delayed and its duration may be increased.

- **BREAST FEEDING** Use with caution during breast-feeding. Manufacturer advises avoid.
- **HEPATIC IMPAIRMENT** Initially 100 mg daily. Use with caution; there is an increased risk of gastro-intestinal bleeding and fluid retention. Avoid in severe liver disease.
- **RENAL IMPAIRMENT** The lowest effective dose should be used for the shortest possible duration. Avoid if possible or use with caution; avoid in moderate to severe impairment. In renal impairment monitor renal function; sodium and water retention may occur and renal function may deteriorate, possibly leading to renal failure.

- **MEDICINAL FORMS**
There can be variation in the licensing of different medicines containing the same drug.
Tablet
CAUTIONARY AND ADVISORY LABELS 21
  ▸ Aceclofenac (Non-proprietary)
    Aceclofenac 100 mg Aceclofenac 100mg tablets | 60 tablet PoM
    £10.78 DT price = £9.63
  ▸ Preservex (Almirall Ltd)
    Aceclofenac 100 mg Preservex 100mg tablets | 60 tablet PoM
    £9.63 DT price = £9.63

Acemetacin

- **DRUG ACTION** Glycolic acid ester of indometacin.

- **INDICATIONS AND DOSE**

Pain and inflammation in rheumatic disease | Pain and inflammation in other musculoskeletal disorders | Postoperative analgesia
  ▸ BY MOUTH
  ▸ Adult: 120 mg daily in divided doses, then increased if necessary to 180 mg daily in divided doses, dose to be taken with food

- **CONTRA-INDICATIONS** Active gastro-intestinal bleeding · active gastro-intestinal ulceration · history of gastro-intestinal bleeding related to previous NSAID therapy · history of gastro-intestinal perforation related to previous NSAID therapy · history of recurrent gastro-intestinal haemorrhage (two or more distinct episodes) · history of recurrent gastro-intestinal ulceration (two or more distinct episodes) · severe heart failure

- **CAUTIONS** Allergic disorders · cardiac impairment (NSAIDs may impair renal function) · cerebrovascular disease · coagulation defects · connective-tissue disorders · Crohn's disease (may be exacerbated) · elderly (risk of serious side-effects and fatalities) · epilepsy · heart failure · ischaemic heart disease · parkinsonism · peripheral arterial disease · psychiatric disturbances · risk factors for cardiovascular events · ulcerative colitis (may be exacerbated) · uncontrolled hypertension

- **INTERACTIONS** → Appendix 1 (NSAIDs).

- **SIDE-EFFECTS**
  ▸ **Rare** Alveolitis · aseptic meningitis (patients with connective-tissue disorders such as systemic lupus erythematosus may be especially susceptible) · blood disorders · confusion · convulsions · hepatic damage · hyperglycaemia · interstitial fibrosis associated with NSAIDs can lead to renal failure · intestinal strictures · pancreatitis · papillary necrosis associated with NSAIDs can lead to renal failure · peripheral neuropathy · psychiatric disturbances · pulmonary eosinophilia · Stevens-Johnson syndrome · syncope · thrombocytopenia · toxic epidermal necrolysis · visual disturbances
  ▸ **Frequency not known** Angioedema · blood disorders · bronchospasm · colitis (induction of or exacerbation of) · Crohn's disease (induction of or exacerbation of) ·

depression · diarrhoea · dizziness · drowsiness · fluid retention (rarely precipitating congestive heart failure) · gastro-intestinal bleeding · gastro-intestinal discomfort · gastro-intestinal disturbances · gastro-intestinal ulceration · haematuria · headache · hearing disturbances · hyperkalaemia · hypersensitivity reactions · insomnia · nausea · nervousness · photosensitivity · raised blood pressure · rashes · renal failure (especially in patients with pre-existing renal impairment) · tinnitus · vertigo

SIDE-EFFECTS, FURTHER INFORMATION
  ▸ Serious side-effects For information about cardiovascular and gastro-intestinal side-effects, and a possible exacerbation of symptoms in asthma, see Non-steroidal anti-inflammatory drugs p. 975.

- **ALLERGY AND CROSS-SENSITIVITY** Contra-indicated in patients with a history of hypersensitivity to aspirin or any other NSAID—which includes those in whom attacks of asthma, angioedema, urticaria or rhinitis have been precipitated by aspirin or any other NSAID.

- **CONCEPTION AND CONTRACEPTION** Caution—long-term use of some NSAIDs is associated with reduced female fertility, which is reversible on stopping treatment.

- **PREGNANCY** Most manufacturers advise avoiding the use of NSAIDs during pregnancy or avoiding them unless the potential benefit outweighs the risk. NSAIDs should be avoided during the third trimester because use is associated with a risk of closure of fetal ductus arteriosus *in utero* and possibly persistent pulmonary hypertension of the newborn. In addition, the onset of labour may be delayed and its duration may be increased.

- **BREAST FEEDING** Use with caution during breast-feeding. Manufacturer advises avoid.

- **HEPATIC IMPAIRMENT** Use with caution; there is an increased risk of gastro-intestinal bleeding and fluid retention. Avoid in severe liver disease.

- **RENAL IMPAIRMENT** The lowest effective dose should be used for the shortest possible duration. Avoid if possible or use with caution. In renal impairment monitor renal function; sodium and water retention may occur and renal function may deteriorate, possibly leading to renal failure.

- **MONITORING REQUIREMENTS** During prolonged therapy ophthalmic and blood examinations particularly advisable.

- **PATIENT AND CARER ADVICE**
Driving and skilled tasks
Dizziness may affect performance of skilled tasks (e.g. driving).

- **MEDICINAL FORMS**
There can be variation in the licensing of different medicines containing the same drug.
Capsule
CAUTIONARY AND ADVISORY LABELS 21
  ▸ Emflex (Merck Serono Ltd)
    Acemetacin 60 mg Emflex 60mg capsules | 90 capsule PoM
    £28.20 DT price = £28.20

Celecoxib

- **INDICATIONS AND DOSE**

Pain and inflammation in osteoarthritis
  ▸ BY MOUTH
  ▸ Adult: 200 mg daily in 1–2 divided doses, then increased if necessary up to 200 mg twice daily, discontinue if no improvement after 2 weeks on maximum dose continued →

Musculoskeletal system

Pain and inflammation in rheumatoid arthritis

▶ BY MOUTH
▶ Adult: 100 mg twice daily, then increased if necessary to 200 mg twice daily, discontinue if no improvement after 2 weeks on maximum dose

Ankylosing spondylitis

▶ BY MOUTH
▶ Adult: 200 mg daily in 1–2 divided doses, then increased if necessary up to 400 mg daily in 1–2 divided doses, discontinue if no improvement after 2 weeks on maximum dose

● CONTRA-INDICATIONS Active gastro-intestinal bleeding · active gastro-intestinal ulceration · cerebrovascular disease · inflammatory bowel disease · ischaemic heart disease · mild to severe heart failure · peripheral arterial disease

● CAUTIONS Allergic disorders · cardiac impairment (NSAIDs may impair renal function) · coagulation defects · connective-tissue disorders · Crohn's disease (may be exacerbated) · elderly (risk of serious side-effects and fatalities) · history of cardiac failure · hypertension · left ventricular dysfunction · oedema · risk factors for cardiovascular events · ulcerative colitis (may be exacerbated)

● INTERACTIONS → Appendix 1 (NSAIDs).

● SIDE-EFFECTS
▶ **Common or very common** Dyspnoea · influenza-like symptoms
▶ **Uncommon** Cerebral infarction · fatigue · muscle cramps · palpitation · paraesthesia · stomatitis
▶ **Rare** Alopecia · alveolitis · aseptic meningitis (patients with connective-tissue disorders such as systemic lupus erythematosus may be especially susceptible) · hepatic damage · interstitial fibrosis associated with NSAIDs can lead to renal failure · pancreatitis · papillary necrosis associated with NSAIDs can lead to renal failure · pulmonary eosinophilia · Stevens-Johnson syndrome · taste disturbance · toxic epidermal necrolysis · visual disturbances
▶ **Very rare** Seizures
▶ **Frequency not known** Angioedema · blood disorders · bronchospasm · chest pain · colitis (induction of or exacerbation of) · Crohn's disease (induction of or exacerbation of) · depression · diarrhoea · dizziness · drowsiness · fluid retention (rarely precipitating congestive heart failure) · gastro-intestinal bleeding · gastro-intestinal discomfort · gastro-intestinal disturbances · gastro-intestinal ulceration · haematuria · headache · hearing disturbances · hypersensitivity reactions · insomnia · nausea · nervousness · photosensitivity · raised blood pressure · rashes · renal failure (especially in patients with pre-existing renal impairment) · tinnitus · vertigo

SIDE-EFFECTS, FURTHER INFORMATION
▶ Serious side-effects For information about cardiovascular and gastro-intestinal side-effects, and a possible exacerbation of symptoms in asthma, see Non-steroidal anti-inflammatory drugs p. 975.

● ALLERGY AND CROSS-SENSITIVITY Contra-indicated in patients with a history of hypersensitivity to aspirin or any other NSAID—which includes those in whom attacks of asthma, angioedema, urticaria or rhinitis have been precipitated by aspirin or any other NSAID.
Contra-indicated in patients with sulfonamide sensitivity.

● CONCEPTION AND CONTRACEPTION Caution—long-term use of some NSAIDs is associated with reduced female fertility, which is reversible on stopping treatment.

● PREGNANCY Avoid (teratogenic in *animal* studies).

● BREAST FEEDING Avoid—present in milk in *animal* studies.

● HEPATIC IMPAIRMENT Halve initial dose in moderate impairment. Use with caution; there is an increased risk of gastro-intestinal bleeding and fluid retention. Avoid in severe liver disease.

● RENAL IMPAIRMENT The lowest effective dose should be used for the shortest possible duration. Avoid if possible or use with caution. Avoid if eGFR less than 30 mL/minute/1.73 m². In renal impairment monitor renal function; sodium and water retention may occur and renal function may deteriorate, possibly leading to renal failure.

● MONITORING REQUIREMENTS Monitor blood pressure before and during treatment.

● MEDICINAL FORMS
There can be variation in the licensing of different medicines containing the same drug.

Capsule
▶ Celecoxib (Non-proprietary)
Celecoxib 100 mg Celecoxib 100mg capsules | 60 capsule [PoM]
£21.55 DT price = £1.96
Celecoxib 200 mg Celecoxib 200mg capsules | 30 capsule [PoM]
£21.55 DT price = £1.76
▶ Celebrex (Pfizer Ltd)
Celecoxib 100 mg Celebrex 100mg capsules | 60 capsule [PoM]
£21.55 DT price = £1.96
Celecoxib 200 mg Celebrex 200mg capsules | 30 capsule [PoM]
£21.55 DT price = £1.76

Dexibuprofen

● INDICATIONS AND DOSE

Pain and inflammation associated with osteoarthritis and other musculoskeletal disorders | Mild to moderate pain and inflammation including dental pain

▶ BY MOUTH
▶ Adult: 600–900 mg daily in up to 3 divided doses; increased if necessary up to 1.2 g daily (max. per dose 400 mg)

Mild to moderate pain and inflammation in dysmenorrhoea

▶ BY MOUTH
▶ Adult: 600–900 mg daily in up to 3 divided doses (max. per dose 300 mg); maximum 900 mg per day

● CONTRA-INDICATIONS Active gastro-intestinal bleeding · active gastro-intestinal ulceration · history of gastro-intestinal bleeding related to previous NSAID therapy · history of gastro-intestinal perforation related to previous NSAID therapy · history of recurrent gastro-intestinal haemorrhage (two or more distinct episodes) · history of recurrent gastro-intestinal ulceration (two or more distinct episodes) · severe heart failure

● CAUTIONS Allergic disorders · cardiac impairment (NSAIDs may impair renal function) · cerebrovascular disease · coagulation defects · connective-tissue disorders · Crohn's disease (may be exacerbated) · elderly (risk of serious side-effects and fatalities) · heart failure · ischaemic heart disease · peripheral arterial disease · risk factors for cardiovascular events · ulcerative colitis (may be exacerbated) · uncontrolled hypertension

CAUTIONS, FURTHER INFORMATION
▶ High-dose dexibuprofen A small increase in cardiovascular risk, similar to the risk associated with cyclo-oxygenase-2 inhibitors and diclofenac, has been reported with high-dose dexibuprofen (≥ 1.2 g daily); use should be avoided in patients with established ischaemic heart disease, peripheral arterial disease, cerebrovascular disease, congestive heart failure (New York Heart Association classification II-III), and uncontrolled hypertension.

● INTERACTIONS → Appendix 1 (NSAIDs).

- SIDE-EFFECTS
▶ **Rare** Alveolitis · aseptic meningitis (patients with connective-tissue disorders such as systemic lupus erythematosus may be especially susceptible) · hepatic damage · interstitial fibrosis associated with NSAIDs can lead to renal failure · pancreatitis · papillary necrosis associated with NSAIDs can lead to renal failure · pulmonary eosinophilia · Stevens-Johnson syndrome · toxic epidermal necrolysis · visual disturbances
▶ **Frequency not known** Angioedema · blood disorders · bronchospasm · colitis (induction of or exacerbation of) · Crohn's disease (induction of or exacerbation of) · depression · diarrhoea · dizziness · drowsiness · fluid retention (rarely precipitating congestive heart failure) · gastro-intestinal bleeding · gastro-intestinal discomfort · gastro-intestinal disturbances · gastro-intestinal ulceration · haematuria · headache · hearing disturbances · hypersensitivity reactions · insomnia · nausea · nervousness · photosensitivity · raised blood pressure · rashes · renal failure (especially in patients with pre-existing renal impairment) · tinnitus · vertigo

SIDE-EFFECTS, FURTHER INFORMATION
▶ Serious side-effects For information about cardiovascular and gastro-intestinal side-effects, and a possible exacerbation of symptoms in asthma, see Non-steroidal anti-inflammatory drugs p. 975.

- ALLERGY AND CROSS-SENSITIVITY Contra-indicated in patients with a history of hypersensitivity to aspirin or any other NSAID—which includes those in whom attacks of asthma, angioedema, urticaria or rhinitis have been precipitated by aspirin or any other NSAID.

- CONCEPTION AND CONTRACEPTION Caution—long-term use of some NSAIDs is associated with reduced female fertility, which is reversible on stopping treatment.

- PREGNANCY Avoid unless the potential benefit outweighs the risk. Avoid during the third trimester (risk of closure of fetal ductus arteriosus *in utero* and possibly persistent pulmonary hypertension of the newborn); onset of labour may be delayed and duration may be increased.

- BREAST FEEDING Use with caution during breast-feeding. Present in milk—but risk to infant minimal.

- HEPATIC IMPAIRMENT Use with caution; there is an increased risk of gastro-intestinal bleeding and fluid retention. Avoid in severe liver disease.

- RENAL IMPAIRMENT Reduce initial dose. The lowest effective dose should be used for the shortest possible duration. Avoid if possible or use with caution. Avoid if eGFR less than 30 mL/minute/1.73 m^2. In renal impairment monitor renal function; sodium and water retention may occur and renal function may deteriorate, possibly leading to renal failure.

- MEDICINAL FORMS
There can be variation in the licensing of different medicines containing the same drug.
Tablet
CAUTIONARY AND ADVISORY LABELS 21
▶ Seractil (Thornton & Ross Ltd)
  Dexibuprofen 400 mg Seractil 400mg tablets | 60 tablet [PoM]
  £8.47 DT price = £9.97

Dexketoprofen

- INDICATIONS AND DOSE
Short-term treatment of mild to moderate pain including dysmenorrhoea
▶ BY MOUTH
▶ Adult: 12.5 mg every 4–6 hours, alternatively 25 mg every 8 hours; maximum 75 mg per day

▶ Elderly: 12.5 mg every 4–6 hours, alternatively 25 mg every 8 hours, initial max. 50 mg; maximum 75 mg daily

- CONTRA-INDICATIONS Active gastro-intestinal bleeding · active gastro-intestinal ulceration · history of gastro-intestinal bleeding related to previous NSAID therapy · history of gastro-intestinal perforation related to previous NSAID therapy · history of recurrent gastro-intestinal haemorrhage (two or more distinct episodes) · history of recurrent gastro-intestinal ulceration (two or more distinct episodes) · severe heart failure

- CAUTIONS Allergic disorders · cardiac impairment (NSAIDs may impair renal function) · cerebrovascular disease · coagulation defects · connective-tissue disorders · Crohn's disease (may be exacerbated) · elderly (risk of serious side-effects and fatalities) · heart failure · ischaemic heart disease · peripheral arterial disease · risk factors for cardiovascular events · ulcerative colitis (may be exacerbated) · uncontrolled hypertension

- INTERACTIONS → Appendix 1 (NSAIDs).

- SIDE-EFFECTS
▶ **Rare** Alveolitis · aseptic meningitis (patients with connective-tissue disorders such as systemic lupus erythematosus may be especially susceptible) · hepatic damage · interstitial fibrosis associated with NSAIDs can lead to renal failure · pancreatitis · papillary necrosis associated with NSAIDs can lead to renal failure · pulmonary eosinophilia · Stevens-Johnson syndrome · toxic epidermal necrolysis · visual disturbances
▶ **Frequency not known** Angioedema · blood disorders · bronchospasm · colitis (induction of or exacerbation of) · Crohn's disease (induction of or exacerbation of) · depression · diarrhoea · dizziness · drowsiness · fluid retention (rarely precipitating congestive heart failure) · gastro-intestinal bleeding · gastro-intestinal discomfort · gastro-intestinal disturbances · gastro-intestinal ulceration · haematuria · headache · hearing disturbances · hypersensitivity reactions · insomnia · nausea · nervousness · photosensitivity · raised blood pressure · rashes · renal failure (especially in patients with pre-existing renal impairment) · tinnitus · vertigo

SIDE-EFFECTS, FURTHER INFORMATION
▶ Serious side-effects For information about cardiovascular and gastro-intestinal side-effects, and a possible exacerbation of symptoms in asthma, see Non-steroidal anti-inflammatory drugs p. 975.

- ALLERGY AND CROSS-SENSITIVITY Contra-indicated in patients with a history of hypersensitivity to aspirin or any other NSAID—which includes those in whom attacks of asthma, angioedema, urticaria or rhinitis have been precipitated by aspirin or any other NSAID.

- CONCEPTION AND CONTRACEPTION Caution—long-term use of some NSAIDs is associated with reduced female fertility, which is reversible on stopping treatment.

- PREGNANCY Avoid unless the potential benefit outweighs the risk. Avoid during the third trimester (risk of closure of fetal ductus arteriosus *in utero* and possibly persistent pulmonary hypertension of the newborn); onset of labour may be delayed and duration may be increased.

- BREAST FEEDING Use with caution during breast-feeding. Manufacturer advises avoid—no information available.

- HEPATIC IMPAIRMENT Reduce initial dose to max. 50 mg daily in mild to moderate impairment. Use with caution; there is an increased risk of gastro-intestinal bleeding and fluid retention. Avoid in severe liver disease.

- RENAL IMPAIRMENT Reduce initial dose to 50 mg daily. The lowest effective dose should be used for the shortest possible duration. Avoid if possible or use with caution. Avoid in moderate to severe impairment. In renal

10

Musculoskeletal system

impairment monitor renal function; sodium and water retention may occur and renal function may deteriorate, possibly leading to renal failure.

- MEDICINAL FORMS
There can be variation in the licensing of different medicines containing the same drug.

Tablet

CAUTIONARY AND ADVISORY LABELS 22
- Keral (A. Menarini Farmaceutica Internazionale SRL)
  Dexketoprofen (as Dexketoprofen trometamol) 25 mg Keral 25mg tablets | 20 tablet [PoM] £3.67 | 50 tablet [PoM] £9.18 DT price = £9.18

Diclofenac potassium

- INDICATIONS AND DOSE

Pain and inflammation in rheumatic disease and other musculoskeletal disorders
- BY MOUTH
- Child 14-17 years: 75–100 mg daily in 2–3 divided doses
- Adult: 75–150 mg daily in 2–3 divided doses

Acute gout
- BY MOUTH
- Adult: 75–150 mg daily in 2–3 divided doses

Postoperative pain
- BY MOUTH
- Child 9-13 years (body-weight 35 kg and above): Up to 2 mg/kg daily in 3 divided doses; maximum 100 mg per day
- Child 14-17 years: 75–100 mg daily in 2–3 divided doses
- Adult: 75–150 mg daily in 2–3 divided doses

Migraine
- BY MOUTH
- Adult: 50 mg, to be given at onset of migraine, then 50 mg after 2 hours if required, then 50 mg after 4–6 hours; maximum 200 mg per day

Fever in ear, nose, or throat infection
- BY MOUTH
- Child 9-17 years (body-weight 35 kg and above): Up to 2 mg/kg daily in 3 divided doses; maximum 100 mg per day

- UNLICENSED USE *Voltarol® Rapid* not licensed for use in children under 14 years or in fever.
- CONTRA-INDICATIONS Active gastro-intestinal bleeding · active gastro-intestinal ulceration · cerebrovascular disease · history of gastro-intestinal bleeding related to previous NSAID therapy · history of gastro-intestinal perforation related to previous NSAID therapy · history of recurrent gastro-intestinal haemorrhage (two or more distinct episodes) · history of recurrent gastro-intestinal ulceration (two or more distinct episodes) · ischaemic heart disease · mild to severe heart failure · peripheral arterial disease
- CAUTIONS Allergic disorders · cardiac impairment (NSAIDs may impair renal function) · coagulation defects · connective-tissue disorders · Crohn's disease (may be exacerbated) · elderly (risk of serious side-effects and fatalities) · history of cardiac failure · hypertension · left ventricular dysfunction · oedema · risk factors for cardiovascular events · ulcerative colitis (may be exacerbated)
- INTERACTIONS → Appendix 1 (NSAIDs).
- SIDE-EFFECTS
- **Rare** Alveolitis · aseptic meningitis (patients with connective-tissue disorders such as systemic lupus erythematosus may be especially susceptible) · hepatic damage · interstitial fibrosis associated with NSAIDs can lead to renal failure · pancreatitis · papillary necrosis associated with NSAIDs can lead to renal failure ·

pulmonary eosinophilia · Stevens-Johnson syndrome · toxic epidermal necrolysis · visual disturbances
- **Frequency not known** Angioedema · blood disorders · bronchospasm · colitis (induction of or exacerbation of) · Crohn's disease (induction of or exacerbation of) · depression · diarrhoea · dizziness · drowsiness · fluid retention (rarely precipitating congestive heart failure) · gastro-intestinal bleeding · gastro-intestinal discomfort · gastro-intestinal disturbances · gastro-intestinal ulceration · haematuria · headache · hearing disturbances · hypersensitivity reactions · insomnia · nausea · nervousness · photosensitivity · raised blood pressure · rashes · renal failure (especially in patients with pre-existing renal impairment) · tinnitus · vertigo
- ALLERGY AND CROSS-SENSITIVITY Contra-indicated in patients with a history of hypersensitivity to aspirin or any other NSAID—which includes those in whom attacks of asthma, angioedema, urticaria or rhinitis have been precipitated by aspirin or any other NSAID.
- CONCEPTION AND CONTRACEPTION Caution—long-term use of some NSAIDs is associated with reduced female fertility, which is reversible on stopping treatment.
- PREGNANCY Avoid unless the potential benefit outweighs the risk. Avoid during the third trimester (risk of closure of fetal ductus arteriosus *in utero* and possibly persistent pulmonary hypertension of the newborn); onset of labour may be delayed and duration may be increased.
- BREAST FEEDING Use with caution during breast-feeding. Amount in milk too small to be harmful.
- HEPATIC IMPAIRMENT Use with caution; there is an increased risk of gastro-intestinal bleeding and fluid retention. Avoid in severe liver disease.
- RENAL IMPAIRMENT The lowest effective dose should be used for the shortest possible duration. Avoid if possible or use with caution. Avoid in severe impairment. In renal impairment monitor renal function; sodium and water retention may occur and renal function may deteriorate, possibly leading to renal failure.
- PATIENT AND CARER ADVICE
Medicines for Children leaflet: Diclofenac for pain and inflammation www.medicinesforchildren.org.uk/diclofenac-for-pain-and-inflammation
- MEDICINAL FORMS
There can be variation in the licensing of different medicines containing the same drug.

Tablet

CAUTIONARY AND ADVISORY LABELS 21
- Diclofenac potassium (Non-proprietary)
  Diclofenac potassium 25 mg Diclofenac potassium 25mg tablets | 28 tablet [PoM] £3.87
  Diclofenac potassium 50 mg Diclofenac potassium 50mg tablets | 28 tablet [PoM] £7.41
- Voltarol Rapid (Novartis Pharmaceuticals UK Ltd)
  Diclofenac potassium 25 mg Voltarol Rapid 25mg tablets | 30 tablet [PoM] £4.15 DT price = £4.15
  Diclofenac potassium 50 mg Voltarol Rapid 50mg tablets | 30 tablet [PoM] £7.94 DT price = £7.94

Diclofenac sodium

- INDICATIONS AND DOSE

Pain and inflammation in musculoskeletal disorders | Acute gout
- BY MOUTH USING IMMEDIATE-RELEASE MEDICINES
- Adult: 75–150 mg daily in 2–3 divided doses
- BY RECTUM
- Adult: 75–150 mg daily in divided doses

Pain and inflammation in rheumatic disease including juvenile idiopathic arthritis
▸ BY MOUTH USING IMMEDIATE-RELEASE MEDICINES
▸ Adult: 75–150 mg daily in 2–3 divided doses
▸ BY RECTUM
▸ Adult: 75–150 mg daily in divided doses

Postoperative pain
▸ BY MOUTH USING IMMEDIATE-RELEASE MEDICINES
▸ Adult: 75–150 mg daily in 2–3 divided doses
▸ BY RECTUM
▸ Adult: 75–150 mg daily in divided doses

DICLOMAX RETARD®

Pain and inflammation in rheumatic disease (including juvenile idiopathic arthritis) and other musculoskeletal disorders | Acute gout | Postoperative pain
▸ BY MOUTH
▸ Adult: 1 capsule once daily

DICLOMAX SR®

Pain and inflammation in rheumatic disease (including juvenile idiopathic arthritis) and other musculoskeletal disorders | Acute gout | Postoperative pain
▸ BY MOUTH
▸ Adult: 1 capsule 1–2 times a day, alternatively 2 capsules once daily

DYLOJECT®

Acute exacerbations of pain and postoperative pain
▸ BY DEEP INTRAMUSCULAR INJECTION
▸ Adult: 75 mg once daily for maximum 2 days, to be administered into the gluteal muscle

Acute exacerbations of pain and postoperative pain (severe cases)
▸ BY DEEP INTRAMUSCULAR INJECTION
▸ Adult: 75 mg twice daily for maximum 2 days, to be administered into the gluteal muscle

Ureteric colic
▸ BY DEEP INTRAMUSCULAR INJECTION
▸ Adult: 75 mg, then 75 mg after 30 minutes if required

Acute postoperative pain (in supervised settings)
▸ BY INTRAVENOUS INJECTION
▸ Adult: 75 mg every 4–6 hours if required for maximum 2 days; maximum 150 mg per day

Prevention of postoperative pain
▸ BY INTRAVENOUS INJECTION
▸ Adult: 25–50 mg, to be given after surgery; further doses given after 4–6 hours if necessary; maximum 150 mg in 24 hours for 2 days

MOTIFENE®

Pain and inflammation in rheumatic disease (including juvenile idiopathic arthritis) and other musculoskeletal disorders | Acute gout | Postoperative pain
▸ BY MOUTH
▸ Adult: 1 capsule 1–2 times a day

VOLTAROL® 75MG SR TABLETS

Pain and inflammation in rheumatic disease (including juvenile idiopathic arthritis) and other musculoskeletal disorders | Acute gout | Postoperative pain
▸ BY MOUTH
▸ Adult: 1 tablet 1–2 times a day

VOLTAROL® EMULGEL

Relief of pain in musculoskeletal conditions | Adjunctive treatment in knee or hand osteoarthritis
▸ TO THE SKIN
▸ Adult: Apply 3–4 times a day, therapy should be reviewed after 14 days (or after 28 days for osteoarthritis)

VOLTAROL® RETARD

Pain and inflammation in rheumatic disease (including juvenile idiopathic arthritis) and other musculoskeletal disorders | Acute gout | Postoperative pain
▸ BY MOUTH
▸ Adult: 1 tablet once daily

VOLTAROL® SOLUTION FOR INJECTION

Postoperative pain
▸ BY DEEP INTRAMUSCULAR INJECTION
▸ Adult: 75 mg 1–2 times a day for maximum 2 days, twice daily administration in severe cases, to be injected into the gluteal muscle

Acute exacerbations of pain
▸ BY DEEP INTRAMUSCULAR INJECTION
▸ Adult: 75 mg 1–2 times a day for maximum 2 days, twice daily administration in severe cases, to be injected into the gluteal muscle

Ureteric colic
▸ BY DEEP INTRAMUSCULAR INJECTION
▸ Adult: 75 mg, then 75 mg after 30 minutes if required

Acute postoperative pain (in hospital setting)
▸ BY INTRAVENOUS INFUSION
▸ Adult: 75 mg, then 75 mg after 4–6 hours if required for maximum 2 days; maximum 150 mg per day

Prevention of postoperative pain (in hospital setting)
▸ BY INTRAVENOUS INFUSION
▸ Adult: Initially 25–50 mg, to be given after surgery over 15–60 minutes, then 5 mg/hour for maximum 2 days; maximum 150 mg per day

● CONTRA-INDICATIONS
▸ With intravenous use Dehydration · history of asthma · history of confirmed or suspected cerebrovascular bleeding · history of haemorrhagic diathesis · hypovolaemia · operations with high risk of haemorrhage
▸ With systemic use Active gastro-intestinal bleeding · active gastro-intestinal ulceration · avoid suppositories in proctitis · cerebrovascular disease · history of gastro-intestinal bleeding related to previous NSAID therapy · history of gastro-intestinal perforation related to previous NSAID therapy · history of recurrent gastro-intestinal haemorrhage (two or more distinct episodes) · history of recurrent gastro-intestinal ulceration (two or more distinct episodes) · ischaemic heart disease · mild to severe heart failure · peripheral arterial disease

● CAUTIONS
▸ With systemic use Allergic disorders · cardiac impairment (NSAIDs may impair renal function) · coagulation defects · connective-tissue disorders · Crohn's disease (may be exacerbated) · elderly (risk of serious side-effects and fatalities) · history of cardiac failure · hypertension · left ventricular dysfunction · oedema · risk factors for cardiovascular events · ulcerative colitis (may be exacerbated)
▸ With topical use Avoid contact with eyes · avoid contact with inflamed or broken skin · avoid contact with mucous membranes · not for use with occlusive dressings · topical application of large amounts can result in systemic effects, including hypersensitivity and asthma (renal disease has also been reported)

● INTERACTIONS → Appendix 1 (NSAIDs).
▸ With intravenous use Contra-indicated in concomitant NSAID use. Contra-indicated in concomitant anticoagulant use (including low-dose heparins).
▸ With topical use Interactions do not generally apply to topical NSAIDs.

● SIDE-EFFECTS
▸ Rare
▸ With systemic use Alveolitis · aseptic meningitis (patients with connective-tissue disorders such as systemic lupus

10

Musculoskeletal system

erythematosus may be especially susceptible) · hepatic damage · interstitial fibrosis associated with NSAIDs can lead to renal failure · pancreatitis · papillary necrosis associated with NSAIDs can lead to renal failure · pulmonary eosinophilia · Stevens-Johnson syndrome · toxic epidermal necrolysis · visual disturbances

▸ **Frequency not known**
▸ With intramuscular use Injection site reactions
▸ With intravenous use Injection site reactions
▸ With rectal use Suppositories may cause rectal irritation
▸ With systemic use Angioedema · blood disorders · bronchospasm · colitis (induction of or exacerbation of) · Crohn's disease (induction of or exacerbation of) · depression · diarrhoea · dizziness · drowsiness · fluid retention (rarely precipitating congestive heart failure) · gastro-intestinal bleeding · gastro-intestinal discomfort · gastro-intestinal disturbances · gastro-intestinal ulceration · haematuria · headache · hearing disturbances · hypersensitivity reactions · insomnia · nausea · nervousness · photosensitivity · raised blood pressure · rashes · renal failure (especially in patients with pre-existing renal impairment) · tinnitus · vertigo
▸ With topical use Paraesthesia · photosensitivity · rash (discontinue use if develops)

SIDE-EFFECTS, FURTHER INFORMATION
▸ Serious side-effects For information about cardiovascular and gastro-intestinal side-effects, and a possible exacerbation of symptoms in asthma, see Non-steroidal anti-inflammatory drugs p. 975.
▸ With topical use Topical application of large amounts can result in systemic effects, including hypersensitivity and asthma (renal disease has also been reported).

● ALLERGY AND CROSS-SENSITIVITY Contra-indicated in patients with a history of hypersensitivity to aspirin or any other NSAID—which includes those in whom attacks of asthma, angioedema, urticaria or rhinitis have been precipitated by aspirin or any other NSAID.

● CONCEPTION AND CONTRACEPTION
▸ With systemic use Caution—long-term use of some NSAIDs is associated with reduced female fertility, which is reversible on stopping treatment.

● PREGNANCY
▸ With systemic use Avoid unless the potential benefit outweighs the risk. Avoid during the third trimester (risk of closure of fetal ductus arteriosus *in utero* and possibly persistent pulmonary hypertension of the newborn); onset of labour may be delayed and duration may be increased.
▸ With topical use Patient packs for topical preparations carry a warning to avoid during pregnancy.

● BREAST FEEDING
▸ With systemic use Use with caution during breast-feeding. Amount in milk too small to be harmful.
▸ With topical use Patient packs for topical preparations carry a warning to avoid during breast-feeding.

● HEPATIC IMPAIRMENT
▸ With systemic use Use with caution; there is an increased risk of gastro-intestinal bleeding and fluid retention. Avoid in severe liver disease.

● RENAL IMPAIRMENT
▸ With systemic use Avoid if possible or use with caution. Avoid in severe impairment. The lowest effective dose should be used for the shortest possible duration. In renal impairment monitor renal function; sodium and water retention may occur and renal function may deteriorate, possibly leading to renal failure.
▸ With intravenous use Avoid intravenous use if serum creatinine greater than 160 micromol/litre. Contra-indicated in moderate or severe renal impairment.

● DIRECTIONS FOR ADMINISTRATION
▸ With intravenous use For *intravenous infusion* (*Voltarol*®), give continuously or intermittently in Glucose 5% or

Sodium chloride 0.9%. Dilute 75 mg with 100–500 mL infusion fluid (previously buffered with 0.5 mL sodium bicarbonate 8.4% solution *or* with 1 mL sodium bicarbonate 4.2% solution). For intermittent infusion give 25–50 mg over 15–60 minutes or 75 mg over 30–120 minutes. For continuous infusion give at a rate of 5 mg/hour.
▸ With topical use For topical preparations, apply with gentle massage only.

● PRESCRIBING AND DISPENSING INFORMATION
▸ With oral use *Voltarol*® dispersible tablets are more suitable for **short-term** use in acute conditions for which treatment required for no more than 3 months (no information on use beyond 3 months).
▸ With topical use Caution—topical preparations not generally suitable for children.

● PATIENT AND CARER ADVICE
▸ With topical use For topical preparations, patients and their carers should be advised to wash hands immediately after use.
Photosensitivity
▸ With topical use Patients should be advised against excessive exposure to sunlight of area treated in order to avoid possibility of photosensitivity.

● EXCEPTIONS TO LEGAL CATEGORY
▸ With topical use Various pack sizes of gel preparations may be available on sale to the public.

● PROFESSION SPECIFIC INFORMATION
Dental practitioners' formulary
▸ With oral use Diclofenac Sodium Tablets may be prescribed.

● NATIONAL FUNDING/ACCESS DECISIONS
DYLOJECT®
Scottish Medicines Consortium (SMC) Decisions
▸ With intravenous use The *Scottish Medicines Consortium* has advised (February 2008) that *Dyloject*® is accepted for restricted use within NHS Scotland for the treatment or prevention of postoperative pain by intravenous injection in supervised healthcare settings.

● MEDICINAL FORMS
There can be variation in the licensing of different medicines containing the same drug. Forms available from special-order manufacturers include: dispersible tablet, oral suspension, oral solution

Dispersible tablet
CAUTIONARY AND ADVISORY LABELS 13, 21
▸ Voltarol (Novartis Pharmaceuticals UK Ltd)
  Diclofenac sodium 50 mg Voltarol 50mg dispersible tablets sugar-free | 21 tablet [PoM] £7.43 DT price = £7.43

Modified-release tablet
CAUTIONARY AND ADVISORY LABELS 21, 25
▸ Voltarol Retard (Novartis Pharmaceuticals UK Ltd)
  Diclofenac sodium 100 mg Voltarol Retard 100mg tablets | 28 tablet [PoM] £11.36 DT price = £11.36
▸ Voltarol SR (Novartis Pharmaceuticals UK Ltd)
  Diclofenac sodium 75 mg Voltarol 75mg SR tablets | 28 tablet [PoM] £7.75 | 56 tablet [PoM] £15.50 DT price = £15.50

Gastro-resistant tablet
CAUTIONARY AND ADVISORY LABELS 5, 25
▸ Diclofenac sodium (Non-proprietary)
  Diclofenac sodium 25 mg Diclofenac sodium 25mg gastro-resistant tablets | 28 tablet [PoM] £2.25–£8.99 DT price = £2.45 | 84 tablet [PoM] £8.16
  Diclofenac sodium 50 mg Diclofenac sodium 50mg gastro-resistant tablets | 28 tablet [PoM] £4.97 DT price = £3.29 | 84 tablet [PoM] £15.00 | 100 tablet [PoM] no price available
▸ Dicloflex (Dexcel-Pharma Ltd, Almus Pharmaceuticals Ltd)
  Diclofenac sodium 25 mg Dicloflex 25mg gastro-resistant tablets | 84 tablet [PoM] £4.42
  Diclofenac sodium 50 mg Dicloflex 50mg gastro-resistant tablets | 28 tablet [PoM] £2.75 DT price = £3.29 (Hospital only) | 84 tablet [PoM] £8.05–£8.85

▶ Fenactol (Discovery Pharmaceuticals)
Diclofenac sodium 50 mg Fenactol 50mg gastro-resistant tablets |
100 tablet PoM £3.70
▶ Voltarol (Novartis Pharmaceuticals UK Ltd)
Diclofenac sodium 25 mg Voltarol 25mg gastro-resistant tablets |
84 tablet PoM £2.94
Diclofenac sodium 50 mg Voltarol 50mg gastro-resistant tablets |
10 tablet PoM £0.91 (Hospital only) | 14 tablet PoM no price
available (Hospital only) | 84 tablet PoM £4.57 | 90 tablet PoM
£5.88

Modified-release capsule
CAUTIONARY AND ADVISORY LABELS 21 (does not apply to
Motifene® 75 mg), 25
EXCIPIENTS: May contain Propylene glycol
▶ Diclomax Retard (Galen Ltd)
Diclofenac sodium 100 mg Diclomax Retard 100mg capsules |
28 capsule PoM £6.97 DT price = £6.97
▶ Diclomax SR (Galen Ltd)
Diclofenac sodium 75 mg Diclomax SR 75mg capsules |
56 capsule PoM £9.69 DT price = £9.69
▶ Motifene (Daiichi Sankyo UK Ltd)
Diclofenac sodium 75 mg Motifene 75mg modified-release capsules
| 56 capsule PoM £8.00 DT price = £8.00

Solution for injection
EXCIPIENTS: May contain Benzyl alcohol, propylene glycol
▶ Dyloject (Therabel Pharma UK Ltd)
Diclofenac sodium 37.5 mg per 1 ml Dyloject 75mg/2ml solution for
injection vials | 10 vial PoM no price available
▶ Voltarol (Novartis Pharmaceuticals UK Ltd)
Diclofenac sodium 25 mg per 1 ml Voltarol 75mg/3ml solution for
injection ampoules | 10 ampoule PoM £9.91 DT price = £9.91

Gel
▶ Voltarol (Novartis Consumer Health UK Ltd)
Diclofenac diethylammonium 11.6 mg per 1 gram Voltarol 1.16%
Emulgel P | 30 gram P £3.23 | 50 gram P £4.71 | 100 gram P
£7.71 DT price = £5.63
Voltarol 1.16% Emulgel | 100 gram PoM £5.63 DT price = £5.63

Suppository
▶ Diclofenac sodium (Non-proprietary)
Diclofenac sodium 100 mg Diclofenac 100mg suppositories |
10 suppository PoM £7.75 DT price = £3.64
▶ Econac (AMCo)
Diclofenac sodium 100 mg Econac 100mg suppositories |
10 suppository PoM £3.04 DT price = £3.64
▶ Voltarol (Novartis Pharmaceuticals UK Ltd)
Diclofenac sodium 12.5 mg Voltarol 12.5mg suppositories |
10 suppository PoM £0.70 DT price = £0.70
Diclofenac sodium 25 mg Voltarol 25mg suppositories |
10 suppository PoM £1.24 DT price = £1.24
Diclofenac sodium 50 mg Voltarol 50mg suppositories |
10 suppository PoM £2.04 DT price = £2.04
Diclofenac sodium 100 mg Voltarol 100mg suppositories |
10 suppository PoM £3.64 DT price = £3.64

Diclofenac sodium with misoprostol

The properties listed below are those particular to the
combination only. For the properties of the components
please consider, diclofenac sodium p. 980, misoprostol p. 70.

● INDICATIONS AND DOSE
ARTHROTEC® 50/200
**Prophylaxis against NSAID-induced gastroduodenal
ulceration in patients requiring diclofenac for
rheumatoid arthritis or osteoarthritis**
▶ BY MOUTH
▶ Adult: 1 tablet 2–3 times a day, take with food
ARTHROTEC® 75/200
**Prophylaxis against NSAID-induced gastroduodenal
ulceration in patients requiring diclofenac for
rheumatoid arthritis or osteoarthritis**
▶ BY MOUTH
▶ Adult: 1 tablet twice daily, take with food

MISOFEN® 50/200
**Prophylaxis against NSAID-induced gastroduodenal
ulceration in patients requiring diclofenac for
rheumatoid arthritis or osteoarthritis**
▶ BY MOUTH
▶ Adult: 1 tablet 2–3 times a day, take with food
MISOFEN® 75/200
**Prophylaxis against NSAID-induced gastroduodenal
ulceration in patients requiring diclofenac for
rheumatoid arthritis or osteoarthritis**
▶ BY MOUTH
▶ Adult: 1 tablet twice daily, take with food

● UNLICENSED USE The BNF recommends a higher starting
dose of misoprostol for prophylaxis against NSAID-
induced gastroduodenal ulceration than that provided by
the combination preparations of diclofenac and
misoprostol.

● MEDICINAL FORMS
There can be variation in the licensing of different medicines
containing the same drug.
Gastro-resistant tablet
CAUTIONARY AND ADVISORY LABELS 21, 25
▶ Arthrotec (Pfizer Ltd)
Misoprostol 200 microgram, Diclofenac sodium 50 mg Arthrotec
50 gastro-resistant tablets | 60 tablet PoM £11.98 DT price = £11.98
Misoprostol 200 microgram, Diclofenac sodium 75 mg Arthrotec
75 gastro-resistant tablets | 60 tablet PoM £15.83 DT price = £15.83
▶ Misofen (Morningside Healthcare Ltd)
Misoprostol 200 microgram, Diclofenac sodium 50 mg Misofen
50mg/200microgram gastro-resistant tablets | 60 tablet PoM £11.98
DT price = £11.98
Misoprostol 200 microgram, Diclofenac sodium 75 mg Misofen
75mg/200microgram gastro-resistant tablets | 60 tablet PoM £15.83
DT price = £15.83

Etodolac

● INDICATIONS AND DOSE
**Pain and inflammation in rheumatoid arthritis and
osteoarthritis**
▶ BY MOUTH USING IMMEDIATE-RELEASE MEDICINES
▶ Adult: 300–600 mg daily in 1–2 divided doses
▶ BY MOUTH USING MODIFIED-RELEASE MEDICINES
▶ Adult: 600 mg daily

● CONTRA-INDICATIONS Active gastro-intestinal bleeding ·
active gastro-intestinal ulceration · history of gastro-
intestinal bleeding related to previous NSAID therapy ·
history of gastro-intestinal perforation related to previous
NSAID therapy · history of recurrent gastro-intestinal
haemorrhage (two or more distinct episodes) · history of
recurrent gastro-intestinal ulceration (two or more
distinct episodes) · severe heart failure

● CAUTIONS Allergic disorders · cardiac impairment (NSAIDs
may impair renal function) · cerebrovascular disease ·
coagulation defects · connective-tissue disorders · Crohn's
disease (may be exacerbated) · elderly (risk of serious side-
effects and fatalities) · heart failure · ischaemic heart
disease · peripheral arterial disease · risk factors for
cardiovascular events · ulcerative colitis (may be
exacerbated) · uncontrolled hypertension

● INTERACTIONS → Appendix 1 (NSAIDs).

● SIDE-EFFECTS
▶ **Rare** Alveolitis · aseptic meningitis (patients with
connective-tissue disorders such as systemic lupus
erythematosus may be especially susceptible) · hepatic
damage · interstitial fibrosis associated with NSAIDs can
lead to renal failure · pancreatitis · papillary necrosis
associated with NSAIDs can lead to renal failure ·

pulmonary eosinophilia · Stevens-Johnson syndrome · toxic epidermal necrolysis · visual disturbances

▶ **Frequency not known** Angioedema · blood disorders · bronchospasm · colitis (induction of or exacerbation of) · confusion · Crohn's disease (induction of or exacerbation of) · depression · diarrhoea · dizziness · drowsiness · dyspnoea · dysuria · fatigue · fluid retention (rarely precipitating congestive heart failure) · gastro-intestinal bleeding · gastro-intestinal discomfort · gastro-intestinal disturbances · gastro-intestinal ulceration · haematuria · headache · hearing disturbances · hypersensitivity reactions · insomnia · nausea · nervousness · palpitation · paraesthesia · photosensitivity · pruritus · pyrexia · raised blood pressure · rashes · renal failure (especially in patients with pre-existing renal impairment) · stomatitis · tinnitus · tremor · urinary frequency · vasculitis · vertigo

SIDE-EFFECTS, FURTHER INFORMATION

▶ Serious side-effects For information about cardiovascular and gastro-intestinal side-effects, and a possible exacerbation of symptoms in asthma, see Non-steroidal anti-inflammatory drugs p. 975.

● ALLERGY AND CROSS-SENSITIVITY Contra-indicated in patients with a history of hypersensitivity to aspirin or any other NSAID—which includes those in whom attacks of asthma, angioedema, urticaria or rhinitis have been precipitated by aspirin or any other NSAID.

● CONCEPTION AND CONTRACEPTION Caution—long-term use of some NSAIDs is associated with reduced female fertility, which is reversible on stopping treatment.

● PREGNANCY Avoid unless the potential benefit outweighs the risk. Avoid during the third trimester (risk of closure of fetal ductus arteriosus *in utero* and possibly persistent pulmonary hypertension of the newborn); onset of labour may be delayed and duration may be increased.

● BREAST FEEDING Use with caution during breast-feeding. Manufacturer advises avoid.

● HEPATIC IMPAIRMENT Use with caution; there is an increased risk of gastro-intestinal bleeding and fluid retention. Avoid in severe liver disease.

● RENAL IMPAIRMENT The lowest effective dose should be used for the shortest possible duration. Avoid if possible or use with caution. Avoid in severe impairment. In renal impairment monitor renal function; sodium and water retention may occur and renal function may deteriorate, possibly leading to renal failure.

● MEDICINAL FORMS
There can be variation in the licensing of different medicines containing the same drug.
Modified-release tablet
CAUTIONARY AND ADVISORY LABELS 25
▶ Etodolac (Non-proprietary)
Etodolac 600 mg Etodolac 600mg modified-release tablets | 30 tablet [PoM] £21.40 DT price = £15.50
▶ Etopan XL (Taro Pharmaceuticals (UK) Ltd)
Etodolac 600 mg Etopan XL 600mg tablets | 30 tablet [PoM] £14.60 DT price = £15.50
▶ Lodine SR (Almirall Ltd)
Etodolac 600 mg Lodine SR 600mg tablets | 30 tablet [PoM] £15.50 DT price = £15.50
Capsule
▶ Eccoxolac (Meda Pharmaceuticals Ltd)
Etodolac 300 mg Eccoxolac 300mg capsules | 60 capsule [PoM] £8.14 DT price = £8.14

Etoricoxib

● INDICATIONS AND DOSE

Pain and inflammation in osteoarthritis
▶ BY MOUTH
▶ Child 16-17 years: 30 mg once daily, then increased if necessary to 60 mg once daily
▶ Adult: 30 mg once daily, then increased if necessary to 60 mg once daily

Pain and inflammation in rheumatoid arthritis | Ankylosing spondylitis
▶ BY MOUTH
▶ Child 16-17 years: 90 mg once daily
▶ Adult: 90 mg once daily

Acute gout
▶ BY MOUTH
▶ Child 16-17 years: 120 mg once daily for maximum 8 days
▶ Adult: 120 mg once daily for maximum 8 days

● CONTRA-INDICATIONS Active gastro-intestinal bleeding · active gastro-intestinal ulceration · cerebrovascular disease · inflammatory bowel disease · ischaemic heart disease · mild to severe heart failure · peripheral arterial disease · uncontrolled hypertension (persistently above 140/90 mmHg)

● CAUTIONS Allergic disorders · cardiac impairment (NSAIDs may impair renal function) · coagulation defects · connective-tissue disorders · Crohn's disease (may be exacerbated) · dehydration · elderly (risk of serious side-effects and fatalities) · history of cardiac failure · hypertension · left ventricular dysfunction · oedema · risk factors for cardiovascular events · ulcerative colitis (may be exacerbated)

● INTERACTIONS → Appendix 1 (NSAIDs).

● SIDE-EFFECTS

▶ **Common or very common** Ecchymosis · fatigue · influenza-like symptoms · palpitation

▶ **Uncommon** Anxiety · appetite change · arthralgia · atrial fibrillation · chest pain · cough · dry mouth · dyspnoea · electrolyte disturbance · epistaxis · flushing · mental acuity impaired · mouth ulcer · myalgia · paraesthesia · taste disturbance · transient ischaemic attack · weight change

▶ **Rare** Alveolitis · aseptic meningitis (patients with connective-tissue disorders such as systemic lupus erythematosus may be especially susceptible) · hepatic damage · interstitial fibrosis associated with NSAIDs can lead to renal failure · pancreatitis · papillary necrosis associated with NSAIDs can lead to renal failure · pulmonary eosinophilia · Stevens-Johnson syndrome · toxic epidermal necrolysis · visual disturbances

▶ **Very rare** Confusion · hallucinations

▶ **Frequency not known** Angioedema · blood disorders · bronchospasm · colitis (induction of or exacerbation of) · Crohn's disease (induction of or exacerbation of) · depression · diarrhoea · dizziness · drowsiness · fluid retention (rarely precipitating congestive heart failure) · gastro-intestinal bleeding · gastro-intestinal discomfort · gastro-intestinal disturbances · gastro-intestinal ulceration · haematuria · headache · hearing disturbances · hypersensitivity reactions · insomnia · nausea · nervousness · photosensitivity · raised blood pressure · rashes · renal failure (especially in patients with pre-existing renal impairment) · tinnitus · vertigo

SIDE-EFFECTS, FURTHER INFORMATION

▶ Serious side-effects For information about cardiovascular and gastro-intestinal side-effects, and a possible exacerbation of symptoms in asthma, see Non-steroidal anti-inflammatory drugs p. 975.

● ALLERGY AND CROSS-SENSITIVITY Contra-indicated in patients with a history of hypersensitivity to aspirin or any other NSAID—which includes those in whom attacks of asthma, angioedema, urticaria or rhinitis have been precipitated by aspirin or any other NSAID.

- CONCEPTION AND CONTRACEPTION Caution—long-term use of some NSAIDs is associated with reduced female fertility, which is reversible on stopping treatment.
- PREGNANCY Manufacturer advises avoid (teratogenic in *animal* studies). Avoid during the third trimester (risk of closure of fetal ductus arteriosus *in utero* and possibly persistent pulmonary hypertension of the newborn); onset of labour may be delayed and duration may be increased.
- BREAST FEEDING Use with caution during breast-feeding. Manufacturer advises avoid—present in milk in *animal* studies.
- HEPATIC IMPAIRMENT Max. 60 mg daily in mild impairment. Max. 60 mg on alternate days or 30 mg once daily in moderate impairment. Use with caution; there is an increased risk of gastro-intestinal bleeding and fluid retention. Avoid in severe liver disease.
- RENAL IMPAIRMENT The lowest effective dose should be used for the shortest possible duration. Avoid if possible or use with caution.

  In renal impairment monitor renal function; sodium and water retention may occur and renal function may deteriorate, possibly leading to renal failure.
  ‣ With systemic use in adults Avoid if eGFR less than 30 mL/minute/1.73 m².
  ‣ With systemic use in children Avoid if estimated glomerular filtration rate less than 30 mL/minute/1.73 m².
- MONITORING REQUIREMENTS Monitor blood pressure before treatment, 2 weeks after initiation and periodically during treatment.

- MEDICINAL FORMS
  There can be variation in the licensing of different medicines containing the same drug.
  Tablet
  ‣ Arcoxia (Grunenthal Ltd)
  Etoricoxib 30 mg Arcoxia 30mg tablets | 28 tablet PoM £13.99 DT price = £13.99
  Etoricoxib 60 mg Arcoxia 60mg tablets | 28 tablet PoM £20.11 DT price = £20.11
  Etoricoxib 90 mg Arcoxia 90mg tablets | 5 tablet PoM £4.10 | 28 tablet PoM £22.96 DT price = £22.96
  Etoricoxib 120 mg Arcoxia 120mg tablets | 7 tablet PoM £6.03 | 28 tablet PoM £24.11 DT price = £24.11

Felbinac

- DRUG ACTION Felbinac is an active metabolite of the NSAID fenbufen.

- INDICATIONS AND DOSE
  Relief of pain in musculoskeletal conditions | Treatment in knee or hand osteoarthritis (adjunct)
  ‣ TO THE SKIN
  ‣ Adult: Apply 2–4 times a day, therapy should be reviewed after 14 days; maximum 25 g per day

- CAUTIONS Avoid contact with eyes · avoid contact with inflamed or broken skin · avoid contact with mucous membranes · not for use with occlusive dressings · topical application of large amounts can result in systemic effects, including hypersensitivity and asthma (renal disease has also been reported)
- INTERACTIONS → Appendix 1 (NSAIDs).
  Interactions do not generally apply to topical NSAIDs.
- SIDE-EFFECTS Photosensitivity · rash (discontinue use if develops)

  SIDE-EFFECTS, FURTHER INFORMATION
  ‣ Serious side-effects For information about cardiovascular and gastro-intestinal side-effects, and a possible

exacerbation of symptoms in asthma, see Non-steroidal anti-inflammatory drugs p. 975.

Topical application of large amounts can result in systemic effects, including hypersensitivity and asthma (renal disease has also been reported).

- ALLERGY AND CROSS-SENSITIVITY Contra-indicated in patients with a history of hypersensitivity to aspirin or any other NSAID—which includes those in whom attacks of asthma, angioedema, urticaria or rhinitis have been precipitated by aspirin or any other NSAID.
- PREGNANCY Patient packs for topical preparations carry a warning to avoid during pregnancy.
- BREAST FEEDING Patient packs for topical preparations carry a warning to avoid during breast-feeding.
- RENAL IMPAIRMENT Deterioration in renal function has also been reported after topical use.
- DIRECTIONS FOR ADMINISTRATION For topical preparations, apply with gentle massage only.
- PATIENT AND CARER ADVICE For topical preparations patients and carers should be advised to wash hands immediately after use.
  Photosensitivity Patients should be advised against excessive exposure to sunlight of area treated in order to avoid possibility of photosensitivity.

- MEDICINAL FORMS
  There can be variation in the licensing of different medicines containing the same drug.
  Foam
  CAUTIONARY AND ADVISORY LABELS 15
  EXCIPIENTS: May contain Cetostearyl alcohol (including cetyl and stearyl alcohol)
  ‣ Traxam (AMCo)
  Felbinac 31.7 mg per 1 gram Traxam 3.17% foam | 100 gram PoM £8.41 DT price = £8.41
  Gel
  ‣ Traxam (AMCo)
  Felbinac 30 mg per 1 gram Traxam 3% gel | 100 gram PoM £8.03 DT price = £8.03
  Traxam Pain Relief 3% gel | 7.5 gram P £1.24 | 30 gram P £2.26 DT price = £2.26

Fenoprofen

- INDICATIONS AND DOSE
  Pain and inflammation in rheumatic disease and other musculoskeletal disease | Mild to moderate pain
  ‣ BY MOUTH
  ‣ Adult: 300–600 mg 3–4 times a day; maximum 3 g per day

- CONTRA-INDICATIONS Active gastro-intestinal bleeding · active gastro-intestinal ulceration · history of gastro-intestinal bleeding related to previous NSAID therapy · history of gastro-intestinal perforation related to previous NSAID therapy · history of recurrent gastro-intestinal haemorrhage (two or more distinct episodes) · history of recurrent gastro-intestinal ulceration (two or more distinct episodes) · severe heart failure
- CAUTIONS Allergic disorders · cardiac impairment (NSAIDs may impair renal function) · cerebrovascular disease · coagulation defects · connective-tissue disorders · Crohn's disease (may be exacerbated) · elderly (risk of serious side-effects and fatalities) · heart failure · ischaemic heart disease · peripheral arterial disease · risk factors for cardiovascular events · ulcerative colitis (may be exacerbated) · uncontrolled hypertension
- INTERACTIONS → Appendix 1 (NSAIDs).
- SIDE-EFFECTS
  ‣ Rare Alveolitis · aseptic meningitis (patients with connective-tissue disorders such as systemic lupus

10

Musculoskeletal system

erythematosus may be especially susceptible) · hepatic damage · interstitial fibrosis associated with NSAIDs can lead to renal failure · pancreatitis · papillary necrosis associated with NSAIDs can lead to renal failure · pulmonary eosinophilia · Stevens-Johnson syndrome · toxic epidermal necrolysis · visual disturbances

▸ **Frequency not known** Angioedema · blood disorders · bronchospasm · colitis (induction of or exacerbation of) · Crohn's disease (induction of or exacerbation of) · cystitis · depression · diarrhoea · dizziness · drowsiness · fluid retention (rarely precipitating congestive heart failure) · gastro-intestinal bleeding · gastro-intestinal discomfort · gastro-intestinal disturbances · gastro-intestinal ulceration · haematuria · headache · hearing disturbances · hypersensitivity reactions · insomnia · nasopharyngitis · nausea · nervousness · photosensitivity · raised blood pressure · rashes · renal failure (especially in patients with pre-existing renal impairment) · tinnitus · upper respiratory-tract infection · vertigo

SIDE-EFFECTS, FURTHER INFORMATION

▸ Serious side-effects For information about cardiovascular and gastro-intestinal side-effects, and a possible exacerbation of symptoms in asthma, see Non-steroidal anti-inflammatory drugs p. 975.

● ALLERGY AND CROSS-SENSITIVITY Contra-indicated in patients with a history of hypersensitivity to aspirin or any other NSAID—which includes those in whom attacks of asthma, angioedema, urticaria or rhinitis have been precipitated by aspirin or any other NSAID.

● CONCEPTION AND CONTRACEPTION Caution—long-term use of some NSAIDs is associated with reduced female fertility, which is reversible on stopping treatment.

● PREGNANCY Avoid unless the potential benefit outweighs the risk. Avoid during the third trimester (risk of closure of fetal ductus arteriosus *in utero* and possibly persistent pulmonary hypertension of the newborn); onset of labour may be delayed and duration may be increased.

● BREAST FEEDING Use with caution during breast-feeding. Amount too small to be harmful.

● HEPATIC IMPAIRMENT Use with caution; there is an increased risk of gastro-intestinal bleeding and fluid retention. Avoid in severe liver disease.

● RENAL IMPAIRMENT The lowest effective dose should be used for the shortest possible duration. Avoid if possible or use with caution. In renal impairment monitor renal function; sodium and water retention may occur and renal function may deteriorate, possibly leading to renal failure.

● MEDICINAL FORMS
There can be variation in the licensing of different medicines containing the same drug.
Tablet
CAUTIONARY AND ADVISORY LABELS 21
▸ Fenopron (Typharm Ltd)
Fenoprofen (as Fenoprofen calcium) 300 mg Fenopron 300 tablets | 100 tablet PoM £9.45

Flurbiprofen

● **INDICATIONS AND DOSE**

Pain and inflammation in rheumatic disease and other musculoskeletal disorders | Migraine | Postoperative analgesia | Mild to moderate pain

▸ BY MOUTH
▸ Child 12-17 years: 150–200 mg daily in 2–4 divided doses, then increased to 300 mg daily, dose to be increased only in acute conditions
▸ Adult: 150–200 mg daily in 2–4 divided doses, then increased to 300 mg daily, dose to be increased only in acute conditions

Dysmenorrhoea

▸ BY MOUTH
▸ Child 12-17 years: Initially 100 mg, then 50–100 mg every 4–6 hours; maximum 300 mg per day
▸ Adult: Initially 100 mg, then 50–100 mg every 4–6 hours; maximum 300 mg per day

● CONTRA-INDICATIONS Active gastro-intestinal bleeding · active gastro-intestinal ulceration · history of gastro-intestinal bleeding related to previous NSAID therapy · history of gastro-intestinal perforation related to previous NSAID therapy · history of recurrent gastro-intestinal haemorrhage (two or more distinct episodes) · history of recurrent gastro-intestinal ulceration (two or more distinct episodes) · severe heart failure

● CAUTIONS Allergic disorders · cardiac impairment (NSAIDs may impair renal function) · cerebrovascular disease · coagulation defects · connective-tissue disorders · Crohn's disease (may be exacerbated) · elderly (risk of serious side-effects and fatalities) (in adults) · heart failure · ischaemic heart disease · peripheral arterial disease · risk factors for cardiovascular events · ulcerative colitis (may be exacerbated) · uncontrolled hypertension

● INTERACTIONS → Appendix 1 (NSAIDs).

● SIDE-EFFECTS
▸ **Common or very common** Stomatitis
▸ **Uncommon** Confusion · fatigue · hallucinations · paraesthesia
▸ **Rare** Alveolitis · aseptic meningitis (patients with connective-tissue disorders such as systemic lupus erythematosus may be especially susceptible) · hepatic damage · interstitial fibrosis associated with NSAIDs can lead to renal failure · pancreatitis · papillary necrosis associated with NSAIDs can lead to renal failure · pulmonary eosinophilia · Stevens-Johnson syndrome · toxic epidermal necrolysis · visual disturbances
▸ **Frequency not known** Angioedema · blood disorders · bronchospasm · colitis (induction of or exacerbation of) · Crohn's disease (induction of or exacerbation of) · depression · diarrhoea · dizziness · drowsiness · fluid retention (rarely precipitating congestive heart failure) · gastro-intestinal bleeding · gastro-intestinal discomfort · gastro-intestinal disturbances · gastro-intestinal ulceration · haematuria · headache · hearing disturbances · hypersensitivity reactions · insomnia · nausea · nervousness · photosensitivity · raised blood pressure · rashes · renal failure (especially in patients with pre-existing renal impairment) · tinnitus · vertigo

SIDE-EFFECTS, FURTHER INFORMATION

▸ Serious side-effects For information about cardiovascular and gastro-intestinal side-effects, and a possible exacerbation of symptoms in asthma, see Non-steroidal anti-inflammatory drugs p. 975.

● ALLERGY AND CROSS-SENSITIVITY Contra-indicated in patients with a history of hypersensitivity to aspirin or any other NSAID—which includes those in whom attacks of asthma, angioedema, urticaria or rhinitis have been precipitated by aspirin or any other NSAID.

● CONCEPTION AND CONTRACEPTION Caution—long-term use of some NSAIDs is associated with reduced female fertility, which is reversible on stopping treatment.

● PREGNANCY Avoid unless the potential benefit outweighs the risk. Avoid during the third trimester (risk of closure of fetal ductus arteriosus *in utero* and possibly persistent pulmonary hypertension of the newborn); onset of labour may be delayed and duration may be increased.

● BREAST FEEDING Use with caution during breast-feeding. Small amount present in milk—manufacturer advises avoid.

• HEPATIC IMPAIRMENT Use with caution; there is an increased risk of gastro-intestinal bleeding and fluid retention. Avoid in severe liver disease.

• RENAL IMPAIRMENT Avoid if possible or use with caution. Avoid in severe impairment. The lowest effective dose should be used for the shortest possible duration. In renal impairment monitor renal function; sodium and water retention may occur and renal function may deteriorate, possibly leading to renal failure.

• MEDICINAL FORMS
There can be variation in the licensing of different medicines containing the same drug.

Tablet
CAUTIONARY AND ADVISORY LABELS 21
▸ Flurbiprofen (Non-proprietary)
  Flurbiprofen 50 mg Flurbiprofen 50mg tablets | 100 tablet PoM
  £21.30–£35.97 DT price = £30.29
  Flurbiprofen 100 mg Flurbiprofen 100mg tablets | 100 tablet PoM
  £64.34 DT price = £54.18

Ibuprofen

• INDICATIONS AND DOSE

Pain and inflammation in rheumatic disease and other musculoskeletal disorders | Mild to moderate pain including dysmenorrhoea | Postoperative analgesia | Migraine | Dental pain
▸ BY MOUTH USING IMMEDIATE-RELEASE MEDICINES
▸ Adult: Initially 300–400 mg 3–4 times a day; increased if necessary up to 600 mg 4 times a day; maintenance 200–400 mg 3 times a day, may be adequate
▸ BY MOUTH USING MODIFIED-RELEASE MEDICINES
▸ Adult: 1.6 g once daily, dose to be taken in the early evening, increased if necessary to 2.4 g daily in 2 divided doses, dose to be increased only in severe cases

Mild to moderate pain | Pain and inflammation of soft-tissue injuries | Pyrexia with discomfort
▸ BY MOUTH USING IMMEDIATE-RELEASE MEDICINES
▸ Child 3–5 months: 50 mg 3 times a day, maximum daily dose to be given in 3–4 divided doses; maximum 30 mg/kg per day
▸ Child 6–11 months: 50 mg 3–4 times a day, maximum daily dose to be given in 3–4 divided doses; maximum 30 mg/kg per day
▸ Child 1–3 years: 100 mg 3 times a day, maximum daily dose to be given in 3–4 divided doses; maximum 30 mg/kg per day
▸ Child 4–6 years: 150 mg 3 times a day, maximum daily dose to be given in 3–4 divided doses; maximum 30 mg/kg per day
▸ Child 7–9 years: 200 mg 3 times a day, maximum daily dose to be given in 3–4 divided doses; maximum 30 mg/kg per day; maximum 2.4 g per day
▸ Child 10–11 years: 300 mg 3 times a day, maximum daily dose to be given in 3–4 divided doses; maximum 30 mg/kg per day; maximum 2.4 g per day
▸ Child 12–17 years: Initially 300–400 mg 3–4 times a day; increased if necessary up to 600 mg 4 times a day; maintenance 200–400 mg 3 times a day, may be adequate

Pain and inflammation
▸ BY MOUTH USING MODIFIED-RELEASE MEDICINES
▸ Child 12–17 years: 1.6 g once daily, dose preferably taken in the early evening, increased to 2.4 g daily in 2 divided doses, dose to be increased only in severe cases

Pain and inflammation in rheumatic disease including juvenile idiopathic arthritis
▸ BY MOUTH USING IMMEDIATE-RELEASE MEDICINES
▸ Child 3 months–17 years: 30–40 mg/kg daily in 3–4 divided doses; maximum 2.4 g per day

Pain and inflammation in systemic juvenile idiopathic arthritis
▸ BY MOUTH USING IMMEDIATE-RELEASE MEDICINES
▸ Child 3 months–17 years: Up to 60 mg/kg daily in 4–6 divided doses; maximum 2.4 g per day

Post-immunisation pyrexia in infants (on doctor's advice only)
▸ BY MOUTH USING IMMEDIATE-RELEASE MEDICINES
▸ Child 2–3 months: 50 mg for 1 dose, followed by 50 mg after 6 hours if required

Pain relief in musculoskeletal conditions | Treatment in knee or hand osteoarthritis (adjunct)
▸ TO THE SKIN
▸ Adult: Apply up to 3 times a day, ibuprofen gel 5% gel to be administered

FENBID® FORTE

Pain relief in musculoskeletal conditions | Treatment in knee or hand osteoarthritis (adjunct)
▸ TO THE SKIN
▸ Adult: Apply up to 4 times a day, therapy should be reviewed after 14 days

IBUGEL® FORTE

Pain relief in musculoskeletal conditions | Treatment in knee or hand osteoarthritis (adjunct)
▸ TO THE SKIN
▸ Adult: Apply up to 3 times a day

• UNLICENSED USE Not licensed for use in children under 3 months or body-weight under 5 kg. Maximum dose for systemic juvenile idiopathic arthritis is unlicensed.

• CONTRA-INDICATIONS
▸ With systemic use Active gastro-intestinal bleeding · active gastro-intestinal ulceration · history of gastro-intestinal bleeding related to previous NSAID therapy · history of gastro-intestinal perforation related to previous NSAID therapy · history of recurrent gastro-intestinal haemorrhage (two or more distinct episodes) · history of recurrent gastro-intestinal ulceration (two or more distinct episodes) · severe heart failure

• CAUTIONS
▸ With systemic use Allergic disorders (in adults) · cardiac impairment (NSAIDs may impair renal function) · cerebrovascular disease · coagulation defects · connective-tissue disorders · Crohn's disease (may be exacerbated) · elderly (risk of serious side-effects and fatalities) · heart failure · ischaemic heart disease · peripheral arterial disease · risk factors for cardiovascular events · risk factors for cardiovascular events · ulcerative colitis (may be exacerbated) · uncontrolled hypertension
▸ With topical use Avoid contact with eyes · avoid contact with inflamed or broken skin · avoid contact with mucous membranes · not for use with occlusive dressings · topical application of large amounts can result in systemic effects, including hypersensitivity and asthma (renal disease has also been reported)

CAUTIONS, FURTHER INFORMATION
▸ High-dose ibuprofen A small increase in cardiovascular risk, similar to the risk associated with cyclo-oxygenase-2 inhibitors and diclofenac, has been reported with high-dose ibuprofen ($\geq$ 2.4 g daily); use should be avoided in patients with established ischaemic heart disease, peripheral arterial disease, cerebrovascular disease, congestive heart failure (New York Heart Association classification II–III), and uncontrolled hypertension.

10

Musculoskeletal system

- INTERACTIONS → Appendix 1 (NSAIDs).
▸ With topical use Interactions do not generally apply to topical NSAIDs.
- SIDE-EFFECTS
▸ **Rare**
▸ With systemic use Alveolitis · aseptic meningitis (patients with connective-tissue disorders such as systemic lupus erythematosus may be especially susceptible) · hepatic damage · interstitial fibrosis associated with NSAIDs can lead to renal failure · pancreatitis · papillary necrosis associated with NSAIDs can lead to renal failure · pulmonary eosinophilia · Stevens-Johnson syndrome · toxic epidermal necrolysis · visual disturbances
▸ **Frequency not known**
▸ With systemic use Angioedema · blood disorders · bronchospasm · colitis (induction of or exacerbation of) · Crohn's disease (induction of or exacerbation of) · depression · diarrhoea · dizziness · drowsiness · fluid retention (rarely precipitating congestive heart failure) · gastro-intestinal bleeding · gastro-intestinal discomfort · gastro-intestinal disturbances · gastro-intestinal ulceration · haematuria · headache · hearing disturbances · hypersensitivity reactions · insomnia · nausea · nervousness · photosensitivity · raised blood pressure · rashes · renal failure (especially in patients with pre-existing renal impairment) · tinnitus · vertigo
▸ With topical use Photosensitivity · rash (discontinue use if develops)

SIDE-EFFECTS, FURTHER INFORMATION
▸ Serious side-effects For information about cardiovascular and gastro-intestinal side-effects, and a possible exacerbation of symptoms in asthma, see Non-steroidal anti-inflammatory drugs p. 975.
▸ With topical use Topical application of large amounts can result in systemic effects, including hypersensitivity and asthma (renal disease has also been reported).

Overdose
Overdosage with ibuprofen may cause nausea, vomiting, epigastric pain, and tinnitus, but more serious toxicity is very uncommon. Charcoal, activated p. 1201 followed by symptomatic measures are indicated if more than 100 mg/kg has been ingested within the preceding hour.
    For details on the management of poisoning, see Emergency treatment of poisoning p. 1194.

- ALLERGY AND CROSS-SENSITIVITY Contra-indicated in patients with a history of hypersensitivity to aspirin or any other NSAID—which includes those in whom attacks of asthma, angioedema, urticaria or rhinitis have been precipitated by aspirin or any other NSAID.
- CONCEPTION AND CONTRACEPTION
▸ With systemic use Caution—long-term use of some NSAIDs is associated with reduced female fertility, which is reversible on stopping treatment.
- PREGNANCY
▸ With systemic use Avoid unless the potential benefit outweighs the risk. Avoid during the third trimester (risk of closure of fetal ductus arteriosus *in utero* and possibly persistent pulmonary hypertension of the newborn); onset of labour may be delayed and duration may be increased.
▸ With topical use Patient packs for topical preparations carry a warning to avoid during pregnancy.
- BREAST FEEDING
▸ With systemic use Use with caution during breast-feeding. Amount too small to be harmful but some manufacturers advise avoid.
▸ With topical use Patient packs for topical preparations carry a warning to avoid during breast-feeding.
- HEPATIC IMPAIRMENT
▸ With systemic use Use with caution; there is an increased risk of gastro-intestinal bleeding and fluid retention. Avoid in severe liver disease.

- RENAL IMPAIRMENT
▸ With systemic use Avoid if possible or use with caution. Avoid in severe impairment. The lowest effective dose should be used for the shortest possible duration. In renal impairment monitor renal function; sodium and water retention may occur and renal function may deteriorate, possibly leading to renal failure.
▸ With topical use Deterioration in renal function has also been reported after topical use.
- DIRECTIONS FOR ADMINISTRATION For topical preparations, apply with gentle massage only.
- PRESCRIBING AND DISPENSING INFORMATION Flavours of syrup may include orange.
- PATIENT AND CARER ADVICE
Medicines for Children leaflet: Ibuprofen for pain and inflammation www.medicinesforchildren.org.uk/ibuprofen-for-pain-and-inflammation
▸ With topical use For topical preparations, patients and their carers should be advised to wash hands immediately after use.
Photosensitivity
▸ With topical use For topical preparations, patients or their carers should be advised against excessive exposure to sunlight of area treated in order to avoid possibility of photosensitivity.
- PROFESSION SPECIFIC INFORMATION
Dental practitioners' formulary
Ibuprofen Oral Suspension Sugar-free may be prescribed.
Ibuprofen Tablets may be prescribed.
- EXCEPTIONS TO LEGAL CATEGORY
▸ With topical use Smaller pack sizes of gel preparations may be available on sale to the public.
▸ With oral use Oral preparations can be sold to the public in certain circumstances.

- MEDICINAL FORMS
There can be variation in the licensing of different medicines containing the same drug. Forms available from special-order manufacturers include: oral suspension
Tablet
CAUTIONARY AND ADVISORY LABELS 21
▸ Ibuprofen (Non-proprietary)
Ibuprofen 200 mg Ibuprofen 200mg tablets | 16 tablet Ⓟ £0.20 | 24 tablet Ⓟ £1.13 DT price = £0.82 | 48 tablet Ⓟ £1.93 | 84 tablet Ⓟ £3.57 DT price = £2.87 | 96 tablet Ⓟ £1.69
Ibuprofen 200mg tablets sugar coated | 84 tablet Ⓟ £3.92 DT price = £2.87
Ibuprofen 200mg tablets film coated | 84 tablet Ⓟ £1.38 DT price = £2.87
Ibuprofen 200mg caplets | 16 tablet Ⓟ £0.20 | 24 tablet Ⓟ no price available DT price = £0.82 | 48 tablet Ⓟ no price available | 96 tablet Ⓟ no price available | 100 tablet Ⓟ no price available
Ibuprofen 400 mg Ibuprofen 400mg tablets film coated | 24 tablet Ⓟ £1.02 DT price = £0.93 | 84 tablet Ⓟ £1.52 DT price = £3.26
Ibuprofen 400mg tablets | 24 tablet Ⓟ £1.39 DT price = £0.93 | 48 tablet Ⓟ £2.56 | 84 tablet Ⓟ £6.84 DT price = £3.26 | 96 tablet Ⓟ £2.46 | 250 tablet PoM £10.74
Ibuprofen 400mg caplets | 12 tablet Ⓟ no price available | 24 tablet Ⓟ no price available DT price = £0.93 | 48 tablet Ⓟ no price available | 96 tablet Ⓟ no price available
Ibuprofen 400mg tablets sugar coated | 24 tablet Ⓟ £1.50 DT price = £0.93 | 48 tablet Ⓟ £2.40
Ibuprofen 600 mg Ibuprofen 600mg tablets | 84 tablet PoM £6.95 DT price = £4.32
Ibuprofen 600mg tablets film coated | 84 tablet PoM £4.79 DT price = £4.32
▸ Brufen (BGP Products Ltd)
Ibuprofen 400 mg Brufen 400mg tablets | 60 tablet PoM £4.90
Ibuprofen 600 mg Brufen 600mg tablets | 60 tablet PoM £7.34
▸ Cuprofen (SSL International Plc)
Ibuprofen 400 mg Cuprofen Maximum Strength 400mg tablets | 12 tablet Ⓟ £1.03 | 24 tablet Ⓟ £1.61 DT price = £0.93 | 48 tablet Ⓟ £2.91 | 96 tablet Ⓟ £5.04

▸ Ibucalm (Aspar Pharmaceuticals Ltd)
Ibuprofen 200 mg Ibucalm 200mg tablets | 24 tablet P £0.77 DT price = £0.82 | 48 tablet P £1.43 | 96 tablet P £2.43
Ibuprofen 400 mg Ibucalm 400mg tablets | 16 tablet P £0.88 | 24 tablet P £1.36 DT price = £0.93 | 48 tablet P £2.44 | 96 tablet P £4.19

▸ Nurofen (Reckitt Benckiser Healthcare (UK) Ltd)
Ibuprofen 200 mg Nurofen 200mg caplets | 24 tablet P £2.48 DT price = £0.82
Nurofen 200mg tablets | 24 tablet P £2.37 DT price = £0.82 | 48 tablet P £4.36 | 96 tablet P £7.20
Ibuprofen (as Ibuprofen lysine) 400 mg Nurofen Maximum Strength Migraine Pain 684mg caplets | 12 tablet P £3.49

Modified-release tablet
CAUTIONARY AND ADVISORY LABELS 25, 27
▸ Brufen Retard (BGP Products Ltd)
Ibuprofen 800 mg Brufen Retard 800mg tablets | 56 tablet PoM £7.74 DT price = £7.74

Capsule
▸ Ibuprofen (Non-proprietary)
Ibuprofen 200 mg Ibuprofen 200mg capsules | 24 capsule P £4.05 | 30 capsule P no price available DT price = £4.40 | 32 capsule P £0.79
Ibuprofen 400 mg Ibuprofen 400mg capsules | 10 capsule P no price available | 20 capsule P no price available

Chewable capsule
▸ Nurofen (Reckitt Benckiser Healthcare (UK) Ltd)
Ibuprofen 100 mg Nurofen for Children 100mg chewable capsules | 12 capsule P £3.23

Effervescent granules
CAUTIONARY AND ADVISORY LABELS 13, 21
ELECTROLYTES: May contain Sodium
▸ Brufen (BGP Products Ltd)
Ibuprofen 600 mg Brufen 600mg effervescent granules sachets | 20 sachet PoM £6.80 DT price = £6.80

Oral suspension
CAUTIONARY AND ADVISORY LABELS 21
▸ Ibuprofen (Non-proprietary)
Ibuprofen 20 mg per 1 ml Ibuprofen 100mg/5ml oral suspension sugar free sugar-free | 100 ml P £1.38 DT price = £1.25 sugar-free | 150 ml P no price available sugar-free | 500 ml PoM £7.55 sugar-free | 500 ml P no price available
▸ Brufen (BGP Products Ltd)
Ibuprofen 20 mg per 1 ml Brufen 100mg/5ml syrup | 500 ml PoM £8.88 DT price = £8.88
▸ Calprofen (McNeil Products Ltd)
Ibuprofen 20 mg per 1 ml Calprofen 100mg/5ml oral suspension sugar-free | 200 ml P £3.42
▸ Mandafen (M & A Pharmachem Ltd)
Ibuprofen 20 mg per 1 ml Mandafen for Children 100mg/5ml oral suspension sugar free sugar-free | 100 ml P £0.69 DT price = £1.25
▸ Nurofen (Reckitt Benckiser Healthcare (UK) Ltd)
Ibuprofen 20 mg per 1 ml Nurofen for Children 100mg/5ml oral suspension orange sugar-free | 200 ml P £4.20
Nurofen for Children 100mg/5ml oral suspension strawberry sugar-free | 200 ml P £4.20
▸ Orbifen (Orbis Consumer Products Ltd)
Ibuprofen 20 mg per 1 ml Orbifen For Children 100mg/5ml oral suspension sugar-free | 100 ml P £1.67 DT price = £1.25 sugar-free | 150 ml P £2.71

Gel
EXCIPIENTS: May contain Benzyl alcohol
▸ Ibuprofen (Non-proprietary)
Ibuprofen 50 mg per 1 gram Ibuprofen 5% gel | 30 gram P £1.39 | 50 gram P £2.31 DT price = £2.31 | 50 gram GSL £2.54 DT price = £2.31 | 100 gram P £5.33 DT price = £4.62 | 100 gram GSL £4.28 DT price = £4.62
▸ Fenbid (AMCo)
Ibuprofen 50 mg per 1 gram Fenbid 5% gel | 100 gram P £1.50 DT price = £4.62
Ibuprofen 100 mg per 1 gram Fenbid Forte 10% gel | 100 gram PoM £4.00 DT price = £4.92
▸ Ibugel (Dermal Laboratories Ltd)
Ibuprofen 50 mg per 1 gram Ibugel 5% gel | 100 gram P £4.87 DT price = £4.62
Ibuprofen 100 mg per 1 gram Ibugel Forte 10% gel | 100 gram P £4.92 DT price = £4.92

▸ Ibuleve (Dendron Ltd)
Ibuprofen 50 mg per 1 gram Ibuleve 5% gel | 30 gram P £2.64 | 50 gram P £3.70 DT price = £2.31 | 100 gram P £6.80 DT price = £4.62
▸ Phorpain (AMCo)
Ibuprofen 50 mg per 1 gram Phorpain 5% gel | 100 gram P £1.50 DT price = £4.62

Indometacin
(Indomethacin)

● INDICATIONS AND DOSE

Pain and moderate to severe inflammation in rheumatic disease and other musculoskeletal disorders
▸ BY MOUTH USING IMMEDIATE-RELEASE MEDICINES
▸ Adult: 50–200 mg daily in divided doses
▸ BY RECTUM
▸ Adult: 100 mg twice daily if required, dose to be administered at night and in the morning, combined oral and rectal treatment, maximum total daily dose 150–200 mg
▸ BY MOUTH USING MODIFIED-RELEASE MEDICINES
▸ Adult: 75 mg 1–2 times a day

Acute gout
▸ BY MOUTH USING IMMEDIATE-RELEASE MEDICINES
▸ Adult: 150–200 mg daily in divided doses
▸ BY RECTUM
▸ Adult: 100 mg twice daily if required, dose to be administered at night and in the morning, combined oral and rectal treatment, maximum total daily dose 150–200 mg
▸ BY MOUTH USING MODIFIED-RELEASE MEDICINES
▸ Adult: 75 mg 1–2 times a day

Dysmenorrhoea
▸ BY MOUTH USING IMMEDIATE-RELEASE MEDICINES
▸ Adult: Up to 75 mg daily
▸ BY RECTUM
▸ Adult: 100 mg twice daily if required, dose to be administered at night and in the morning, combined oral and rectal treatment, maximum total daily dose 150–200 mg
▸ BY MOUTH USING MODIFIED-RELEASE MEDICINES
▸ Adult: 75 mg daily

● CONTRA-INDICATIONS
▸ With oral use Active gastro-intestinal bleeding · active gastro-intestinal ulceration · history of gastro-intestinal bleeding related to previous NSAID therapy · history of gastro-intestinal perforation related to previous NSAID therapy · history of recurrent gastro-intestinal haemorrhage (two or more distinct episodes) · history of recurrent gastro-intestinal ulceration (two or more distinct episodes) · severe heart failure
▸ With rectal use Active gastro-intestinal bleeding · active gastro-intestinal ulceration · history of gastro-intestinal bleeding related to previous NSAID therapy · history of gastro-intestinal perforation related to previous NSAID therapy · history of recurrent gastro-intestinal haemorrhage (two or more distinct episodes) · history of recurrent gastro-intestinal ulceration (two or more distinct episodes) · severe heart failure

● CAUTIONS
GENERAL CAUTIONS
Elderly (risk of serious side-effects and fatalities · heart failure · parkinsonism
SPECIFIC CAUTIONS
▸ With oral use Allergic disorders · cardiac impairment (NSAIDs may impair renal function) · cerebrovascular disease · coagulation defects · connective-tissue disorders · Crohn's disease (may be exacerbated) · epilepsy · ischaemic

10

Musculoskeletal system

heart disease · peripheral arterial disease · psychiatric disturbances · risk factors for cardiovascular events · ulcerative colitis (may be exacerbated) · uncontrolled hypertension

▸ With rectal use Allergic disorders · avoid rectal administration in haemorrhoids · avoid rectal administration in proctitis · cardiac impairment (NSAIDs may impair renal function) · cerebrovascular disease · coagulation defects · connective-tissue disorders · Crohn's disease (may be exacerbated) · epilepsy · ischaemic heart disease · peripheral arterial disease · psychiatric disturbances · risk factors for cardiovascular events · ulcerative colitis (may be exacerbated) · uncontrolled hypertension

● INTERACTIONS → Appendix 1 (NSAIDs).

● SIDE-EFFECTS

▸ **Rare**

▸ With oral use Alveolitis · aseptic meningitis (patients with connective-tissue disorders such as systemic lupus erythematosus may be especially susceptible) · blood disorders · confusion · convulsions · hepatic damage · hyperglycaemia · interstitial fibrosis associated with NSAIDs can lead to renal failure · intestinal strictures · pancreatitis · papillary necrosis associated with NSAIDs can lead to renal failure · peripheral neuropathy · psychiatric disturbances · pulmonary eosinophilia · Stevens-Johnson syndrome · syncope · thrombocytopenia · toxic epidermal necrolysis · visual disturbances

▸ With rectal use Alveolitis · aseptic meningitis (patients with connective-tissue disorders such as systemic lupus erythematosus may be especially susceptible) · blood disorders · confusion · convulsions · hepatic damage · hyperglycaemia · interstitial fibrosis associated with NSAIDs can lead to renal failure · intestinal strictures · pancreatitis · papillary necrosis associated with NSAIDs can lead to renal failure · peripheral neuropathy · psychiatric disturbances · pulmonary eosinophilia · Stevens-Johnson syndrome · syncope · thrombocytopenia · toxic epidermal necrolysis · visual disturbances

▸ **Frequency not known**

▸ With oral use Angioedema · blood disorders · bronchospasm · colitis (induction of or exacerbation of) · Crohn's disease (induction of or exacerbation of) · depression · diarrhoea · dizziness · drowsiness · fluid retention (rarely precipitating congestive heart failure) · gastro-intestinal bleeding · gastro-intestinal discomfort · gastro-intestinal disturbances · gastro-intestinal ulceration · haematuria · headache · hearing disturbances · hyperkalaemia · hypersensitivity reactions · insomnia · nausea · nervousness · photosensitivity · raised blood pressure · rashes · renal failure (especially in patients with pre-existing renal impairment) · tinnitus · vertigo

▸ With rectal use Angioedema · blood disorders · bronchospasm · colitis (induction of or exacerbation of) · Crohn's disease (induction of or exacerbation of) · depression · diarrhoea · dizziness · drowsiness · fluid retention (rarely precipitating congestive heart failure) · gastro-intestinal bleeding · gastro-intestinal discomfort · gastro-intestinal disturbances · gastro-intestinal ulceration · haematuria · headache · hearing disturbances · hyperkalaemia · hypersensitivity reactions · insomnia · nervousness · photosensitivity · raised blood pressure · rashes · renal failure (especially in patients with pre-existing renal impairment) · suppositories may cause occasional bleeding · suppositories may cause rectal irritation · tinnitus · vertigo

SIDE-EFFECTS, FURTHER INFORMATION

▸ Serious side-effects For information about cardiovascular and gastro-intestinal side-effects, and a possible exacerbation of symptoms in asthma, see Non-steroidal anti-inflammatory drugs p. 975.

● ALLERGY AND CROSS-SENSITIVITY Contra-indicated in patients with a history of hypersensitivity to aspirin or any other NSAID—which includes those in whom attacks of asthma, angioedema, urticaria or rhinitis have been precipitated by aspirin or any other NSAID.

● CONCEPTION AND CONTRACEPTION Caution—long-term use of some NSAIDs is associated with reduced female fertility, which is reversible on stopping treatment.

● PREGNANCY

▸ With oral use or rectal use Avoid unless the potential benefit outweighs the risk. Avoid during the third trimester (risk of closure of fetal ductus arteriosus *in utero* and possibly persistent pulmonary hypertension of the newborn); onset of labour may be delayed and duration may be increased.

● BREAST FEEDING

▸ With oral use or rectal use Amount probably too small to be harmful—manufacturers advise avoid. Use with caution during breast-feeding.

● HEPATIC IMPAIRMENT

▸ With oral use or rectal use Use with caution; there is an increased risk of gastro-intestinal bleeding and fluid retention. Avoid in severe liver disease.

● RENAL IMPAIRMENT

▸ With oral use or rectal use The lowest effective dose should be used for the shortest possible duration.

▸ With oral use or rectal use Avoid if possible or use with caution. Avoid in severe impairment. In renal impairment monitor renal function; sodium and water retention may occur and renal function may deteriorate, possibly leading to renal failure.

● MONITORING REQUIREMENTS

▸ With oral use or rectal use During prolonged therapy ophthalmic and blood examinations particularly advisable.

● PATIENT AND CARER ADVICE

Driving and skilled tasks

▸ With oral use or rectal use Dizziness may affect performance of skilled tasks (e.g. driving).

● MEDICINAL FORMS

There can be variation in the licensing of different medicines containing the same drug. Forms available from special-order manufacturers include: oral suspension, oral solution

Capsule

CAUTIONARY AND ADVISORY LABELS 21

▸ Indometacin (Non-proprietary)

Indometacin 25 mg Indometacin 25mg capsules | 28 capsule PoM £5.00 DT price = £0.98

Indometacin 50 mg Indometacin 50mg capsules | 28 capsule PoM £7.50 DT price = £1.39

Modified-release capsule

CAUTIONARY AND ADVISORY LABELS 21, 25

▸ Indometacin (Non-proprietary)

Indometacin 75 mg Indometacin 75mg modified-release capsules | 100 capsule PoM £8.09 DT price = £8.65

▸ Berlind Retard (Tillomed Laboratories Ltd)

Indometacin 75 mg Berlind 75 Retard capsules | 100 capsule PoM £8.65 DT price = £8.65

Suppository

▸ Indometacin (Non-proprietary)

Indometacin 100 mg Indometacin 100mg suppositories | 10 suppository PoM £19.25 DT price = £17.61

▸ Indocid (Aspen Pharma Trading Ltd)

Indometacin 100 mg Indocid 100mg suppositories | 10 suppository PoM £17.61 DT price = £17.61

Ketoprofen

- **INDICATIONS AND DOSE**

Pain and mild inflammation in rheumatic disease
▸ BY MOUTH USING IMMEDIATE-RELEASE MEDICINES
▸ Adult: 100–200 mg daily in 2–4 divided doses
▸ BY MOUTH USING MODIFIED-RELEASE MEDICINES
▸ Adult: 100–200 mg once daily, dose to be taken with food
▸ BY RECTUM
▸ Adult: 100 mg once daily, to be administered at bedtime, combined oral and rectal treatment, maximum total daily dose 200 mg

Pain in musculoskeletal disorders | Pain after orthopaedic surgery | Dysmenorrhoea | Acute gout
▸ BY MOUTH USING IMMEDIATE-RELEASE MEDICINES
▸ Adult: 50 mg up to 3 times a day
▸ BY MOUTH USING MODIFIED-RELEASE MEDICINES
▸ Adult: 100–200 mg once daily, dose to be taken with food

Relief of pain in musculoskeletal disorders | Treatment in knee or hand osteoarthritis (adjunct)
▸ TO THE SKIN
▸ Adult: Apply 2–4 times a day for up to 7 days, ketoprofen 2.5% gel to be administered; maximum 15 g per day

POWERGEL®
Relief of pain in musculoskeletal conditions | Adjunctive treatment in knee or hand osteoarthritis
▸ TO THE SKIN
▸ Adult: Apply 2–3 times a day for up to max. 10 days

- **CONTRA-INDICATIONS**
▸ With systemic use Active gastro-intestinal bleeding · active gastro-intestinal ulceration · history of gastro-intestinal bleeding · history of gastro-intestinal perforation · history of gastro-intestinal ulceration · severe heart failure

- **CAUTIONS**
▸ With systemic use Allergic disorders · cardiac impairment (NSAIDs may impair renal function) · cerebrovascular disease · coagulation defects · connective-tissue disorders · Crohn's disease (may be exacerbated) · elderly (risk of serious side-effects and fatalities) · heart failure · ischaemic heart disease · peripheral arterial disease · risk factors for cardiovascular events · ulcerative colitis (may be exacerbated) · uncontrolled hypertension
▸ With topical use Avoid contact with eyes · avoid contact with inflamed or broken skin · avoid contact with mucous membranes · not for use with occlusive dressings · topical application of large amounts can result in systemic effects, including hypersensitivity and asthma (renal disease has also been reported)

- **INTERACTIONS** → Appendix 1 (NSAIDs).
▸ With topical use Interactions do not generally apply to topical NSAIDs.

- **SIDE-EFFECTS**
GENERAL SIDE-EFFECTS
Photosensitivity
SPECIFIC SIDE-EFFECTS
▸ **Rare**
▸ With systemic use Alveolitis · aseptic meningitis (patients with connective-tissue disorders such as systemic lupus erythematosus may be especially susceptible) · hepatic damage · interstitial fibrosis associated with NSAIDs can lead to renal failure · pancreatitis · papillary necrosis associated with NSAIDs can lead to renal failure · pulmonary eosinophilia · Stevens-Johnson syndrome · toxic epidermal necrolysis · visual disturbances
▸ **Frequency not known**
▸ With rectal use Suppositories may cause rectal irritation

▸ With systemic use Angioedema · blood disorders · bronchospasm · colitis (induction of or exacerbation of) · Crohn's disease (induction of or exacerbation of) · depression · diarrhoea · dizziness · drowsiness · fluid retention (rarely precipitating congestive heart failure) · gastro-intestinal bleeding · gastro-intestinal discomfort · gastro-intestinal disturbances · gastro-intestinal ulceration · haematuria · headache · hearing disturbances · hypersensitivity reactions · insomnia · nausea · nervousness · raised blood pressure · rashes · renal failure (especially in patients with pre-existing renal impairment) · tinnitus · vertigo
▸ With topical use Rash (discontinue use if develops)

SIDE-EFFECTS, FURTHER INFORMATION
▸ Serious side-effects For information about cardiovascular and gastro-intestinal side-effects, and a possible exacerbation of symptoms in asthma, see Non-steroidal anti-inflammatory drugs p. 975.
▸ With topical use Topical application of large amounts can result in systemic effects, including hypersensitivity and asthma (renal disease has also been reported).

- **ALLERGY AND CROSS-SENSITIVITY** Contra-indicated in patients with a history of hypersensitivity to aspirin or any other NSAID—which includes those in whom attacks of asthma, angioedema, urticaria or rhinitis have been precipitated by aspirin or any other NSAID.

- **CONCEPTION AND CONTRACEPTION**
▸ With systemic use Caution—long-term use of some NSAIDs is associated with reduced female fertility, which is reversible on stopping treatment.

- **PREGNANCY**
▸ With systemic use Avoid unless the potential benefit outweighs the risk. Avoid during the third trimester (risk of closure of fetal ductus arteriosus *in utero* and possibly persistent pulmonary hypertension of the newborn); onset of labour may be delayed and duration may be increased.
▸ With topical use Patient packs for topical preparations carry a warning to avoid during pregnancy.

- **BREAST FEEDING**
▸ With systemic use Use with caution during breast-feeding. Amount probably too small to be harmful but manufacturers advise avoid.
▸ With topical use Patient packs for topical preparations carry a warning to avoid during breast-feeding.

- **HEPATIC IMPAIRMENT**
▸ With systemic use Use with caution; there is an increased risk of gastro-intestinal bleeding and fluid retention. Should be avoided in severe liver disease.

- **RENAL IMPAIRMENT**
▸ With systemic use Avoid if possible or use with caution. Avoid in severe impairment. The lowest effective dose should be given for the shortest possible duration. Monitor renal function; sodium and water retention may occur and renal function may deteriorate, possibly leading to renal failure.
▸ With topical use Deterioration in renal function has also been reported after topical use.

- **DIRECTIONS FOR ADMINISTRATION**
▸ With topical use For topical preparations apply with gentle massage only.

- **PRESCRIBING AND DISPENSING INFORMATION**
▸ With topical use Caution—topical preparations not generally suitable for children.
▸ With oral use Flavours of oral liquid formulations may include strawberry.

- **PATIENT AND CARER ADVICE**
▸ With topical use For topical preparations, patients and their carers should be advised to wash hands immediately after use.
Photosensitivity For topical preparations, patients should be advised against excessive exposure to sunlight of area

10

Musculoskeletal system

treated in order to avoid possibility of photosensitivity. Patients should be advised not to expose area treated to sunbeds or sunlight (even on a bright but cloudy day) during, and for two weeks after stopping treatment; treated areas should be protected with clothing.

● EXCEPTIONS TO LEGAL CATEGORY
▸ With topical use Smaller pack sizes of gel preparations may be available on sale to the public.

● MEDICINAL FORMS
There can be variation in the licensing of different medicines containing the same drug.
Capsule
CAUTIONARY AND ADVISORY LABELS 21
▸ Tiloket (Tillomed Laboratories Ltd)
  Ketoprofen 50 mg Tiloket 50mg capsules | 28 capsule [PoM] £3.99 | 112 capsule [PoM] £17.20 DT price = £17.20
Modified-release capsule
CAUTIONARY AND ADVISORY LABELS 21, 25
▸ Ketoprofen (Non-proprietary)
  Ketoprofen 200 mg Ketoprofen 200mg modified-release capsules | 28 capsule [PoM] £23.85 DT price = £23.85
▸ Larafen CR (Ennogen Pharma Ltd)
  Ketoprofen 200 mg Larafen CR 200mg capsules | 28 capsule [PoM] £19.08 DT price = £23.85
▸ Oruvail (Sanofi)
  Ketoprofen 100 mg Oruvail 100 modified-release capsules | 56 capsule [PoM] £23.93 DT price = £23.93
  Ketoprofen 200 mg Oruvail 200 modified-release capsules | 28 capsule [PoM] £23.85 DT price = £23.85
▸ Tiloket CR (Tillomed Laboratories Ltd)
  Ketoprofen 100 mg Tiloket CR 100mg capsules | 56 capsule [PoM] £10.70 DT price = £23.93
  Ketoprofen 200 mg Tiloket CR 200mg capsules | 28 capsule [PoM] £10.70 DT price = £23.85
▸ Valket Retard (Tillomed Laboratories Ltd)
  Ketoprofen 200 mg Valket 200 Retard capsules | 28 capsule [PoM] £10.70 DT price = £23.85
Gel
EXCIPIENTS: May contain Fragrances
▸ Ketoprofen (Non-proprietary)
  Ketoprofen 25 mg per 1 gram Ketoprofen 2.5% gel | 50 gram [PoM] £2.03 DT price = £1.64 | 100 gram [PoM] £3.62 DT price = £3.28
▸ Oruvail (Sanofi)
  Ketoprofen 25 mg per 1 gram Oruvail 2.5% gel | 100 gram [PoM] £6.84 DT price = £3.28
▸ Powergel (A. Menarini Farmaceutica Internazionale SRL)
  Ketoprofen 25 mg per 1 gram Powergel 2.5% gel | 50 gram [PoM] £3.06 DT price = £1.64 | 100 gram [PoM] £5.89 DT price = £3.28
▸ Tiloket (Tillomed Laboratories Ltd)
  Ketoprofen 25 mg per 1 gram Tiloket 2.5% gel | 50 gram [PoM] £3.00 DT price = £1.64 | 100 gram [PoM] £6.00 DT price = £3.28

Ketoprofen with omeprazole

The properties listed below are those particular to the combination only. For the properties of the components please consider, ketoprofen p. 991, omeprazole p. 73.

● INDICATIONS AND DOSE
Patients requiring ketoprofen for osteoarthritis, rheumatoid arthritis, and ankylosing spondylitis, who are at risk of NSAID associated duodenal or gastric ulcer or gastroduodenal erosions
  ▸ BY MOUTH USING MODIFIED-RELEASE MEDICINES
  ▸ Adult: Initially 100/20 mg daily, increased if necessary to 200/20 mg daily, depending on severity of symptoms, dose expressed as x/y mg ketoprofen/omeprazole

● PRESCRIBING AND DISPENSING INFORMATION Capsules enclose microgranules containing modified-release ketoprofen and gastro-resistant omperazole.

● MEDICINAL FORMS
There can be variation in the licensing of different medicines containing the same drug.
Modified-release capsule
CAUTIONARY AND ADVISORY LABELS 21, 25
EXCIPIENTS: May contain Propylene glycol
▸ Axorid (Meda Pharmaceuticals Ltd)
  Omeprazole 20 mg, Ketoprofen 100 mg Axorid 100mg/20mg modified-release capsules | 30 capsule [PoM] £13.80
  Omeprazole 20 mg, Ketoprofen 200 mg Axorid 200mg/20mg modified-release capsules | 30 capsule [PoM] £13.80

Mefenamic acid

● INDICATIONS AND DOSE
Pain and inflammation in rheumatoid arthritis and osteoarthritis | Postoperative pain | Mild to moderate pain
  ▸ BY MOUTH
  ▸ Adult: 500 mg 3 times a day

Acute pain including dysmenorrhoea | Menorrhagia
  ▸ BY MOUTH
  ▸ Child 12–17 years: 500 mg 3 times a day
  ▸ Adult: 500 mg 3 times a day

● CONTRA-INDICATIONS Active gastro-intestinal bleeding · active gastro-intestinal ulceration · history of gastro-intestinal bleeding related to previous NSAID therapy · history of gastro-intestinal perforation related to previous NSAID therapy · history of recurrent gastro-intestinal haemorrhage (two or more distinct episodes) · history of recurrent gastro-intestinal ulceration (two or more distinct episodes) · inflammatory bowel disease · severe heart failure

● CAUTIONS Acute porphyrias p. 918 · allergic disorders · cardiac impairment (NSAIDs may impair renal function) · cerebrovascular disease · coagulation defects · connective-tissue disorders · Crohn's disease (may be exacerbated) · elderly (risk of serious side-effects and fatalities) (in adults) · epilepsy · heart failure · ischaemic heart disease · peripheral arterial disease · risk factors for cardiovascular events · ulcerative colitis (may be exacerbated) · uncontrolled hypertension

● INTERACTIONS → Appendix 1 (NSAIDs).

● SIDE-EFFECTS
▸ **Common or very common** Diarrhoea (withdraw treatment) · rashes (withdraw treatment) · stomatitis
▸ **Uncommon** Fatigue · paraesthesia
▸ **Rare** Alveolitis · aplastic anaemia · aseptic meningitis (patients with connective-tissue disorders such as systemic lupus erythematosus may be especially susceptible) · glucose intolerance · haemolytic anaemia (positive Coombs' test) · hepatic damage · hypotension · interstitial fibrosis associated with NSAIDs can lead to renal failure · palpitation · pancreatitis · papillary necrosis associated with NSAIDs can lead to renal failure · pulmonary eosinophilia · Stevens-Johnson syndrome · thrombocytopenia · toxic epidermal necrolysis · visual disturbances
▸ **Frequency not known** Angioedema · blood disorders · bronchospasm · colitis (induction of or exacerbation of) · Crohn's disease (induction of or exacerbation of) · depression · dizziness · drowsiness · fluid retention (rarely precipitating congestive heart failure) · gastro-intestinal bleeding · gastro-intestinal discomfort · gastro-intestinal disturbances · gastro-intestinal ulceration · haematuria · headache · hearing disturbances · hypersensitivity reactions · insomnia · nausea · nervousness · photosensitivity · raised blood pressure · renal failure (especially in patients with pre-existing renal impairment) · tinnitus · vertigo

SIDE-EFFECTS, FURTHER INFORMATION
▸ Serious side-effects For information about cardiovascular and gastro-intestinal side-effects, and a possible exacerbation of symptoms in asthma, see Non-steroidal anti-inflammatory drugs p. 975.

Overdose
Mefenamic acid has important consequences in overdosage because it can cause convulsions, which if prolonged or recurrent, require treatment.
   For details on the management of poisoning, see Emergency treatment of poisoning p. 1194, in particular, Convulsions.

● ALLERGY AND CROSS-SENSITIVITY Contra-indicated in patients with a history of hypersensitivity to aspirin or any other NSAID—which includes those in whom attacks of asthma, angioedema, urticaria or rhinitis have been precipitated by aspirin or any other NSAID.

● CONCEPTION AND CONTRACEPTION Caution—long-term use of some NSAIDs is associated with reduced female fertility, which is reversible on stopping treatment.

● PREGNANCY Avoid unless the potential benefit outweighs the risk. Avoid during the third trimester (risk of closure of fetal ductus arteriosus *in utero* and possibly persistent pulmonary hypertension of the newborn); onset of labour may be delayed and duration may be increased.

● BREAST FEEDING Use with caution during breast-feeding. Amount too small to be harmful but manufacturer advises avoid.

● HEPATIC IMPAIRMENT Use with caution; there is an increased risk of gastro-intestinal bleeding and fluid retention. Avoid in severe liver disease.

● RENAL IMPAIRMENT The lowest effective dose should be used for the shortest possible duration. Avoid if possible or use with caution. Avoid in severe impairment. In renal impairment monitor renal function; sodium and water retention may occur and renal function may deteriorate, possibly leading to renal failure.

● MEDICINAL FORMS
There can be variation in the licensing of different medicines containing the same drug. Forms available from special-order manufacturers include: oral suspension

Tablet
CAUTIONARY AND ADVISORY LABELS 21
▸ Mefenamic acid (Non-proprietary)
   Mefenamic acid 500 mg Mefenamic acid 500mg tablets | 28 tablet [PoM] £18.00 DT price = £7.43 | 84 tablet [PoM] £44.99
▸ Ponstan (Chemidex Pharma Ltd)
   Mefenamic acid 500 mg Ponstan Forte 500mg tablets | 100 tablet [PoM] £15.72

Capsule
CAUTIONARY AND ADVISORY LABELS 21
▸ Mefenamic acid (Non-proprietary)
   Mefenamic acid 250 mg Mefenamic acid 250mg capsules | 100 capsule [PoM] £15.00 DT price = £12.04
▸ Ponstan (Chemidex Pharma Ltd)
   Mefenamic acid 250 mg Ponstan 250mg capsules | 100 capsule [PoM] £8.17 DT price = £12.04

Oral suspension
CAUTIONARY AND ADVISORY LABELS 21
EXCIPIENTS: May contain Ethanol
▸ Mefenamic acid (Non-proprietary)
   Mefenamic acid 10 mg per 1 ml Mefenamic acid 50mg/5ml oral suspension | 125 ml [PoM] £79.98 DT price = £79.98

Meloxicam

● INDICATIONS AND DOSE
Exacerbation of osteoarthritis (short-term)
▸ BY MOUTH
▸ Child 16-17 years: 7.5 mg once daily, then increased if necessary up to 15 mg once daily
▸ Adult: 7.5 mg once daily, then increased if necessary up to 15 mg once daily

Pain and inflammation in rheumatic disease | Ankylosing spondylitis
▸ BY MOUTH
▸ Child 16-17 years: 15 mg once daily, then reduced to 7.5 mg once daily if required
▸ Adult: 15 mg once daily, then reduced to 7.5 mg once daily if required
▸ Elderly: 7.5 mg once daily

Relief of pain and inflammation in juvenile idiopathic arthritis and other musculoskeletal disorders in children intolerant to other NSAIDs
▸ BY MOUTH
▸ Child 12-17 years (body-weight up to 50 kg): 7.5 mg once daily
▸ Child 12-17 years (body-weight 50 kg and above): 15 mg once daily

● UNLICENSED USE Not licensed for use in children under 16 years.

● CONTRA-INDICATIONS Active gastro-intestinal bleeding · active gastro-intestinal ulceration · history of gastro-intestinal bleeding related to previous NSAID therapy · history of gastro-intestinal perforation related to previous NSAID therapy · history of recurrent gastro-intestinal haemorrhage (two or more distinct episodes) · history of recurrent gastro-intestinal ulceration (two or more distinct episodes) · severe heart failure

● CAUTIONS Allergic disorders · cardiac impairment (NSAIDs may impair renal function) · cerebrovascular disease · coagulation defects · connective-tissue disorders · Crohn's disease (may be exacerbated) · elderly (risk of serious side-effects and fatalities) (in adults) · heart failure · ischaemic heart disease · peripheral arterial disease · risk factors for cardiovascular events · ulcerative colitis (may be exacerbated) · uncontrolled hypertension

● INTERACTIONS → Appendix 1 (NSAIDs).

● SIDE-EFFECTS
▸ **Rare** Alveolitis · aseptic meningitis (patients with connective-tissue disorders such as systemic lupus erythematosus may be especially susceptible) · hepatic damage · interstitial fibrosis associated with NSAIDs can lead to renal failure · pancreatitis · papillary necrosis associated with NSAIDs can lead to renal failure · pulmonary eosinophilia · Stevens-Johnson syndrome · toxic epidermal necrolysis · visual disturbances
▸ **Frequency not known** Angioedema · blood disorders · bronchospasm · colitis (induction of or exacerbation of) · Crohn's disease (induction of or exacerbation of) · depression · diarrhoea · dizziness · drowsiness · fluid retention (rarely precipitating congestive heart failure) · gastro-intestinal bleeding · gastro-intestinal discomfort · gastro-intestinal disturbances · gastro-intestinal ulceration · haematuria · headache · hearing disturbances · hypersensitivity reactions · insomnia · nausea · nervousness · photosensitivity · raised blood pressure · rashes · renal failure (especially in patients with pre-existing renal impairment) · tinnitus · vertigo
SIDE-EFFECTS, FURTHER INFORMATION
▸ Serious side-effects For information about cardiovascular and gastro-intestinal side-effects, and a possible exacerbation of symptoms in asthma, see Non-steroidal anti-inflammatory drugs p. 975.

10

Musculoskeletal system

- **ALLERGY AND CROSS-SENSITIVITY** Contra-indicated in patients with a history of hypersensitivity to aspirin or any other NSAID—which includes those in whom attacks of asthma, angioedema, urticaria or rhinitis have been precipitated by aspirin or any other NSAID.
- **CONCEPTION AND CONTRACEPTION** Caution—long-term use of some NSAIDs is associated with reduced female fertility, which is reversible on stopping treatment.
- **PREGNANCY** Avoid unless the potential benefit outweighs the risk. Avoid during the third trimester (risk of closure of fetal ductus arteriosus *in utero* and possibly persistent pulmonary hypertension of the newborn); onset of labour may be delayed and duration may be increased.
- **BREAST FEEDING** Use with caution during breast-feeding. Present in milk in *animal* studies—manufacturer advises avoid.
- **HEPATIC IMPAIRMENT** Use with caution; there is an increased risk of gastro-intestinal bleeding and fluid retention. Avoid in severe liver disease.
- **RENAL IMPAIRMENT** The lowest effective dose should be used for the shortest possible duration. Avoid if possible or use with caution.

   In renal impairment monitor renal function; sodium and water retention may occur and renal function may deteriorate, possibly leading to renal failure.
  ▸ In adults Avoid if eGFR less than 25 mL/minute/1.73 m².
  ▸ In children Avoid if estimated glomerular filtration rate less than 25 mL/minute/1.73 m².

- **MEDICINAL FORMS**
  There can be variation in the licensing of different medicines containing the same drug. Forms available from special-order manufacturers include: oral suspension
  Tablet
  CAUTIONARY AND ADVISORY LABELS 21
  ▸ Meloxicam (Non-proprietary)
  Meloxicam 7.5 mg Meloxicam 7.5mg tablets | 30 tablet [PoM] £8.20
  DT price = £0.92
  Meloxicam 15 mg Meloxicam 15mg tablets | 30 tablet [PoM] £4.00
  DT price = £0.99
  Orodispersible tablet
  ▸ Meloxicam (Non-proprietary)
  Meloxicam 7.5 mg Meloxicam 7.5mg orodispersible tablets sugar free sugar-free | 30 tablet [PoM] £15.50
  Meloxicam 15 mg Meloxicam 15mg orodispersible tablets sugar free sugar-free | 30 tablet [PoM] £15.50

Nabumetone

- **INDICATIONS AND DOSE**

Pain and inflammation in osteoarthritis and rheumatoid arthritis
  ▸ BY MOUTH
  ▸ Adult: 1 g once daily, dose to be taken at night
  ▸ Elderly: 0.5–1 g daily

Pain and inflammation in osteoarthritis and rheumatoid arthritis (severe and persistent symptoms)
  ▸ BY MOUTH
  ▸ Adult: 0.5–1 g, dose to be taken in the morning and 1 g, dose to be taken at night
  ▸ Elderly: 0.5–1 g daily

- **CONTRA-INDICATIONS** Active gastro-intestinal bleeding · active gastro-intestinal ulceration · history of gastro-intestinal bleeding related to previous NSAID therapy · history of gastro-intestinal perforation related to previous NSAID therapy · history of recurrent gastro-intestinal haemorrhage (two or more distinct episodes) · history of recurrent gastro-intestinal ulceration (two or more distinct episodes) · severe heart failure
- **CAUTIONS** Allergic disorders · cardiac impairment (NSAIDs may impair renal function) · cerebrovascular disease ·

coagulation defects · connective-tissue disorders · Crohn's disease (may be exacerbated) · elderly (risk of serious side-effects and fatalities) · heart failure · ischaemic heart disease · peripheral arterial disease · risk factors for cardiovascular events · ulcerative colitis (may be exacerbated) · uncontrolled hypertension

- **INTERACTIONS** → Appendix 1 (NSAIDs).
- **SIDE-EFFECTS**
  ▸ **Rare** Alveolitis · aseptic meningitis (patients with connective-tissue disorders such as systemic lupus erythematosus may be especially susceptible) · hepatic damage · interstitial fibrosis associated with NSAIDs can lead to renal failure · pancreatitis · papillary necrosis associated with NSAIDs can lead to renal failure · pulmonary eosinophilia · Stevens-Johnson syndrome · toxic epidermal necrolysis · visual disturbances
  ▸ **Frequency not known** Angioedema · blood disorders · bronchospasm · colitis (induction of or exacerbation of) · Crohn's disease (induction of or exacerbation of) · depression · diarrhoea · dizziness · drowsiness · fluid retention (rarely precipitating congestive heart failure) · gastro-intestinal bleeding · gastro-intestinal discomfort · gastro-intestinal disturbances · gastro-intestinal ulceration · haematuria · headache · hearing disturbances · hypersensitivity reactions · insomnia · nausea · nervousness · photosensitivity · raised blood pressure · rashes · renal failure (especially in patients with pre-existing renal impairment) · tinnitus · vertigo

  SIDE-EFFECTS, FURTHER INFORMATION
  ▸ **Serious side-effects** For information about cardiovascular and gastro-intestinal side-effects, and a possible exacerbation of symptoms in asthma, see Non-steroidal anti-inflammatory drugs p. 975.

- **ALLERGY AND CROSS-SENSITIVITY** Contra-indicated in patients with a history of hypersensitivity to aspirin or any other NSAID—which includes those in whom attacks of asthma, angioedema, urticaria or rhinitis have been precipitated by aspirin or any other NSAID.
- **CONCEPTION AND CONTRACEPTION** Caution—long-term use of some NSAIDs is associated with reduced female fertility, which is reversible on stopping treatment.
- **PREGNANCY** Avoid unless the potential benefit outweighs the risk. Avoid during the third trimester (risk of closure of fetal ductus arteriosus *in utero* and possibly persistent pulmonary hypertension of the newborn); onset of labour may be delayed and duration may be increased.
- **BREAST FEEDING** Use with caution during breast-feeding. Manufacturer advises avoid.
- **HEPATIC IMPAIRMENT** Use with caution; there is an increased risk of gastro-intestinal bleeding and fluid retention. Avoid in severe liver disease.
- **RENAL IMPAIRMENT** The lowest effective dose should be used for the shortest possible duration. Avoided if possible or use with caution. Avoid in severe impairment. In renal impairment monitor renal function; sodium and water retention may occur and renal function may deteriorate, possibly leading to renal failure.

- **MEDICINAL FORMS**
  There can be variation in the licensing of different medicines containing the same drug. Forms available from special-order manufacturers include: oral suspension
  Tablet
  CAUTIONARY AND ADVISORY LABELS 21
  ▸ Nabumetone (Non-proprietary)
  Nabumetone 500 mg Nabumetone 500mg tablets | 56 tablet [PoM] £20.00 DT price = £7.14
  ▸ Relifex (Meda Pharmaceuticals Ltd)
  Nabumetone 500 mg Relifex 500mg tablets | 56 tablet [PoM] £6.18 DT price = £7.14

Naproxen

- **INDICATIONS AND DOSE**

Pain and inflammation in rheumatic disease
▶ BY MOUTH
  ▸ Adult: 0.5–1 g daily in 1–2 divided doses

Pain and inflammation in musculoskeletal disorders | Dysmenorrhoea
▶ BY MOUTH
  ▸ Adult: Initially 500 mg, then 250 mg every 6–8 hours as required, maximum dose after the first day 1.25 g daily

Acute gout
▶ BY MOUTH
  ▸ Adult: Initially 750 mg, then 250 mg every 8 hours until attack has passed

- **CONTRA-INDICATIONS** Active gastro-intestinal bleeding · active gastro-intestinal ulceration · history of gastro-intestinal bleeding related to previous NSAID therapy · history of gastro-intestinal perforation related to previous NSAID therapy · history of recurrent gastro-intestinal haemorrhage (two or more distinct episodes) · history of recurrent gastro-intestinal ulceration (two or more distinct episodes) · severe heart failure

- **CAUTIONS** Allergic disorders · cardiac impairment (NSAIDs may impair renal function) · cerebrovascular disease · coagulation defects · connective-tissue disorders · Crohn's disease (may be exacerbated) · elderly (risk of serious side-effects and fatalities) · heart failure · ischaemic heart disease · peripheral arterial disease · risk factors for cardiovascular events · ulcerative colitis (may be exacerbated) · uncontrolled hypertension

- **INTERACTIONS** → Appendix 1 (NSAIDs).

- **SIDE-EFFECTS**
▶ **Rare** Alveolitis · aseptic meningitis (patients with connective-tissue disorders such as systemic lupus erythematosus may be especially susceptible) · hepatic damage · interstitial fibrosis associated with NSAIDs can lead to renal failure · pancreatitis · papillary necrosis associated with NSAIDs can lead to renal failure · pulmonary eosinophilia · Stevens-Johnson syndrome · toxic epidermal necrolysis · visual disturbances
▶ **Frequency not known** Angioedema · blood disorders · bronchospasm · colitis (induction of or exacerbation of) · Crohn's disease (induction of or exacerbation of) · depression · diarrhoea · dizziness · drowsiness · fluid retention (rarely precipitating congestive heart failure) · gastro-intestinal bleeding · gastro-intestinal discomfort · gastro-intestinal disturbances · gastro-intestinal ulceration · haematuria · headache · hearing disturbances · hypersensitivity reactions · insomnia · nausea · nervousness · photosensitivity · raised blood pressure · rashes · renal failure (especially in patients with pre-existing renal impairment) · tinnitus · vertigo

  SIDE-EFFECTS, FURTHER INFORMATION
▶ **Serious side-effects** For information about cardiovascular and gastro-intestinal side-effects, and a possible exacerbation of symptoms in asthma, see Non-steroidal anti-inflammatory drugs p. 975.

- **ALLERGY AND CROSS-SENSITIVITY** Contra-indicated in patients with a history of hypersensitivity to aspirin or any other NSAID—which includes those in whom attacks of asthma, angioedema, urticaria or rhinitis have been precipitated by aspirin or any other NSAID.

- **CONCEPTION AND CONTRACEPTION** Caution—long-term use of some NSAIDs is associated with reduced female fertility, which is reversible on stopping treatment.

- **PREGNANCY** Avoid unless the potential benefit outweighs the risk. Avoid during the third trimester (risk of closure of fetal ductus arteriosus *in utero* and possibly persistent

pulmonary hypertension of the newborn); onset of labour may be delayed and duration may be increased.

- **BREAST FEEDING** Use with caution during breast-feeding. Amount too small to be harmful but manufacturer advises avoid.

- **HEPATIC IMPAIRMENT** Use with caution; there is an increased risk of gastro-intestinal bleeding and fluid retention. Avoid in severe liver disease.

- **RENAL IMPAIRMENT** The lowest effective dose should be used for the shortest possible duration. Avoid if possible or use with caution.
  Avoid if eGFR less than 30 mL/minute/1.73 m^2. In renal impairment monitor renal function; sodium and water retention may occur and renal function may deteriorate, possibly leading to renal failure.

- **EXCEPTIONS TO LEGAL CATEGORY** Can be sold to the public for the treatment of primary dysmenorrhoea in women aged 15–50 years subject to max. single dose of 500 mg, max. daily dose of 750 mg for max. 3 days, and a max. pack size of 9 × 250 mg tablets.

- **MEDICINAL FORMS**
There can be variation in the licensing of different medicines containing the same drug. Forms available from special-order manufacturers include: oral suspension

Tablet
CAUTIONARY AND ADVISORY LABELS 21
▶ Naproxen (Non-proprietary)
  Naproxen 250 mg Naproxen 250mg tablets | 28 tablet [PoM] £6.98 DT price = £0.91 | 56 tablet [PoM] £2.33
  Naproxen 500 mg Naproxen 500mg tablets | 28 tablet [PoM] £8.76 DT price = £1.22 | 56 tablet [PoM] £3.99

Effervescent tablet
▶ Stirlescent (Stirling Anglian Pharmaceuticals Ltd)
  Naproxen 250 mg Stirlescent 250mg effervescent tablets sugar-free | 20 tablet [PoM] £7.90

Gastro-resistant tablet
CAUTIONARY AND ADVISORY LABELS 5, 25
▶ Naproxen (Non-proprietary)
  Naproxen 250 mg Naproxen 250mg gastro-resistant tablets | 56 tablet [PoM] £12.90 DT price = £3.27
  Naproxen 375 mg Naproxen 375mg gastro-resistant tablets | 56 tablet [PoM] £26.82 DT price = £26.82
  Naproxen 500 mg Naproxen 500mg gastro-resistant tablets | 56 tablet [PoM] £16.90 DT price = £7.91

Oral suspension
▶ Naproxen (Non-proprietary)
  Naproxen 25 mg per 1 ml Naproxen 25mg/ml oral suspension sugar free sugar-free | 100 ml [PoM] £110.00
  Naproxen 125mg/5ml oral suspension sugar free sugar-free | 100 ml [PoM] £110.00

Naproxen with esomeprazole

The properties listed below are those particular to the combination only. For the properties of the components please consider, naproxen above, esomeprazole p. 71.

- **INDICATIONS AND DOSE**

Patients requiring naproxen for osteoarthritis, rheumatoid arthritis, or ankylosing spondylitis, who are at risk of NSAID-associated duodenal or gastric ulcer and when treatment with lower doses of naproxen or other NSAIDs ineffective
▶ BY MOUTH
  ▸ Adult: 500/20 mg twice daily, dose expressed as *x*/*y* mg naproxen/esomeprazole

- **PRESCRIBING AND DISPENSING INFORMATION** Naproxen component is gastro-resistant.

10

Musculoskeletal system

● MEDICINAL FORMS
There can be variation in the licensing of different medicines containing the same drug.
Modified-release tablet
CAUTIONARY AND ADVISORY LABELS 22, 25
▸ Naproxen with esomeprazole (Non-proprietary)
Esomeprazole (as Esomeprazole magnesium trihydrate) 20 mg, Naproxen 500 mg Naproxen 500mg / Esomeprazole 20mg modified-release tablets | 60 tablet [PoM] no price available DT price = £14.95
▸ Vimovo (AstraZeneca UK Ltd)
Esomeprazole (as Esomeprazole magnesium trihydrate) 20 mg, Naproxen 500 mg Vimovo 500mg/20mg modified-release tablets | 60 tablet [PoM] £14.95 DT price = £14.95

Naproxen with misoprostol

The properties listed below are those particular to the combination only. For the properties of the components please consider, naproxen p. 995, misoprostol p. 70.

● INDICATIONS AND DOSE
Patients requiring naproxen for rheumatoid arthritis, osteoarthritis, or ankylosing spondylitis, with prophylaxis against NSAID-induced gastroduodenal ulceration
▸ BY MOUTH
▸ Adult: 500 mg twice daily, naproxen and 200 micrograms twice daily, misoprostol, taken together with food

● PRESCRIBING AND DISPENSING INFORMATION The BNF recommends a higher starting dose of misoprostol for prophylaxis against NSAID-induced gastroduodenal ulceration than that provided by the misoprostol with naproxen combination pack.

● MEDICINAL FORMS
There can be variation in the licensing of different medicines containing the same drug.
Tablet
▸ Napratec (Pfizer Ltd)
Napratec OP tablets | 112 tablet [PoM] £23.76 DT price = £23.76

Piroxicam

● INDICATIONS AND DOSE
Rheumatoid arthritis (initiated by a specialist) | Osteoarthritis (initiated by a specialist) | Ankylosing spondylitis (initiated by a specialist)
▸ BY MOUTH
▸ Adult: Up to 20 mg once daily

Pain relief in musculoskeletal conditions | Treatment in knee or hand osteoarthritis (adjunct)
▸ TO THE SKIN
▸ Adult: Apply 3–4 times a day, 0.5% gel to be applied; review treatment after 4 weeks

IMPORTANT SAFETY INFORMATION
CHMP ADVICE–PIROXICAM (JUNE 2007)
▸ With systemic use
The CHMP has recommended restrictions on the use of piroxicam because of the increased risk of gastro-intestinal side effects and serious skin reactions. The CHMP has advised that:
● piroxicam should be initiated only by physicians experienced in treating inflammatory or degenerative rheumatic diseases
● piroxicam should not be used as first-line treatment
● in adults, use of piroxicam should be limited to the symptomatic relief of osteoarthritis, rheumatoid arthritis, and ankylosing spondylitis
● piroxicam dose should not exceed 20 mg daily

● piroxicam should no longer be used for the treatment of acute painful and inflammatory conditions
● treatment should be reviewed 2 weeks after initiating piroxicam, and periodically thereafter
● concomitant administration of a gastro-protective agent should be considered.
Topical preparations containing piroxicam are not affected by these restrictions.

● CONTRA-INDICATIONS
▸ With systemic use Active gastro-intestinal bleeding · active gastro-intestinal ulceration · history of gastro-intestinal bleeding · history of gastro-intestinal perforation · history of gastro-intestinal ulceration · inflammatory bowel disease · severe heart failure

● CAUTIONS
▸ With systemic use Allergic disorders · cardiac impairment (NSAIDs may impair renal function) · cerebrovascular disease · coagulation defects · connective-tissue disorders · Crohn's disease (may be exacerbated) · elderly (risk of serious side-effects and fatalities) · heart failure · ischaemic heart disease · peripheral arterial disease · risk factors for cardiovascular events · ulcerative colitis (may be exacerbated) · uncontrolled hypertension
▸ With topical use Avoid contact with eyes · avoid contact with inflamed or broken skin · avoid contact with mucous membranes · not for use with occlusive dressings · topical application of large amounts can result in systemic effects, including hypersensitivity and asthma (renal disease has also been reported)

● INTERACTIONS → Appendix 1 (NSAIDs).
▸ With topical use Interactions do not generally apply to topical NSAIDs.

● SIDE-EFFECTS
▸ **Rare**
▸ With systemic use Alveolitis · aseptic meningitis (patients with connective-tissue disorders such as systemic lupus erythematosus may be especially susceptible) · hepatic damage · interstitial fibrosis associated with NSAIDs can lead to renal failure · pancreatitis · papillary necrosis associated with NSAIDs can lead to renal failure · pulmonary eosinophilia · Stevens-Johnson syndrome · toxic epidermal necrolysis · visual disturbances
▸ **Frequency not known**
▸ With systemic use Angioedema · blood disorders · bronchospasm · colitis (induction of or exacerbation of) · Crohn's disease (induction of or exacerbation of) · depression · diarrhoea · dizziness · drowsiness · fluid retention (rarely precipitating congestive heart failure) · gastro-intestinal bleeding · gastro-intestinal discomfort · gastro-intestinal disturbances · gastro-intestinal ulceration · haematuria · headache · hearing disturbances · hypersensitivity reactions · insomnia · nausea · nervousness · photosensitivity · raised blood pressure · rashes · renal failure (especially in patients with pre-existing renal impairment) · tinnitus · vertigo
▸ With topical use Photosensitivity · rash (discontinue use if develops)

SIDE-EFFECTS, FURTHER INFORMATION
▸ Serious side-effects For information about cardiovascular and gastro-intestinal side-effects, and a possible exacerbation of symptoms in asthma, see Non-steroidal anti-inflammatory drugs p. 975.
▸ With topical use Topical application of large amounts can result in systemic effects, including hypersensitivity and asthma (renal disease has also been reported).

● ALLERGY AND CROSS-SENSITIVITY Contra-indicated in patients with a history of hypersensitivity to aspirin or any other NSAID—which includes those in whom attacks of asthma, angioedema, urticaria or rhinitis have been precipitated by aspirin or any other NSAID.

- CONCEPTION AND CONTRACEPTION
▶ With systemic use Caution—long-term use of some NSAIDs is associated with reduced female fertility, which is reversible on stopping treatment.

- PREGNANCY
▶ With systemic use Avoid unless the potential benefit outweighs the risk. Avoid during the third trimester (risk of closure of fetal ductus arteriosus *in utero* and possibly persistent pulmonary hypertension of the newborn); onset of labour may be delayed and duration may be increased.
▶ With topical use Patient packs for topical preparations carry a warning to avoid during pregnancy.

- BREAST FEEDING
▶ With systemic use Use with caution during breast-feeding. Amount too small to be harmful.
▶ With topical use Patient packs for topical preparations carry a warning to avoid during breast-feeding.

- HEPATIC IMPAIRMENT
▶ With systemic use Use with caution; there is an increased risk of gastro-intestinal bleeding and fluid retention. Avoid in severe liver disease.

- RENAL IMPAIRMENT
▶ With systemic use Avoid if possible or use with caution. The lowest effective dose should be given for the shortest possible duration. Monitor renal function; sodium and water retention may occur and renal function may deteriorate, possibly leading to renal failure.
▶ With topical use Deterioration in renal function has also been reported after topical use.

- DIRECTIONS FOR ADMINISTRATION For topical preparations apply with gentle massage only.
    Piroxicam orodispersible tablets can be taken by placing on the tongue and allowing to dissolve or by swallowing.

- PATIENT AND CARER ADVICE
▶ With topical use For topical preparations, patients and their carers should be advised to wash hands immediately after use.
Photosensitivity For topical preparations, patients should be advised against excessive exposure to sunlight of area treated in order to avoid possibility of photosensitivity.

- LESS SUITABLE FOR PRESCRIBING
▶ With oral use Piroxicam is less suitable for prescribing.

- MEDICINAL FORMS
There can be variation in the licensing of different medicines containing the same drug.

Orodispersible tablet
CAUTIONARY AND ADVISORY LABELS 10, 21
EXCIPIENTS: May contain Aspartame
▶ Feldene Melt (Pfizer Ltd)
    Piroxicam 20 mg Feldene Melt 20mg tablets sugar-free | 30 tablet [PoM] £10.53 DT price = £10.53

Capsule
CAUTIONARY AND ADVISORY LABELS 21
▶ Piroxicam (Non-proprietary)
    Piroxicam 10 mg Piroxicam 10mg capsules | 56 capsule [PoM] £16.82 DT price = £3.73
    Piroxicam 20 mg Piroxicam 20mg capsules | 28 capsule [PoM] £17.60 DT price = £3.13
▶ Feldene (Pfizer Ltd)
    Piroxicam 10 mg Feldene 10mg capsules | 30 capsule [PoM] £3.86
    Piroxicam 20 mg Feldene 20 capsules | 30 capsule [PoM] £7.71

Gel
EXCIPIENTS: May contain Benzyl alcohol, propylene glycol
▶ Piroxicam (Non-proprietary)
    Piroxicam 5 mg per 1 gram Piroxicam 0.5% gel | 60 gram [PoM] £3.50 DT price = £2.94 | 112 gram [PoM] £8.47 DT price = £5.49
▶ Feldene (Pfizer Ltd)
    Piroxicam 5 mg per 1 gram Feldene 0.5% gel | 60 gram [PoM] £6.00 DT price = £2.94 | 112 gram [PoM] £9.41 DT price = £5.49

Sulindac

- INDICATIONS AND DOSE

Pain and inflammation in rheumatic disease and other musculoskeletal disorders | Acute gout
▶ BY MOUTH
▶ Adult: 200 mg twice daily for maximum duration 7–10 days in peri-articular disorders, dose may be reduced according to response; acute gout should respond within 7 days; maximum 400 mg per day

- CONTRA-INDICATIONS Active gastro-intestinal bleeding · active gastro-intestinal ulceration · history of gastro-intestinal bleeding related to previous NSAID therapy · history of gastro-intestinal perforation related to previous NSAID therapy · history of recurrent gastro-intestinal haemorrhage (two or more distinct episodes) · history of recurrent gastro-intestinal ulceration (two or more distinct episodes) · severe heart failure

- CAUTIONS Allergic disorders · cardiac impairment (NSAIDs may impair renal function) · cerebrovascular disease · coagulation defects · connective-tissue disorders · Crohn's disease (may be exacerbated) · elderly (risk of serious side-effects and fatalities) · ensure adequate hydration · heart failure · history of renal stones · ischaemic heart disease · peripheral arterial disease · risk factors for cardiovascular events · ulcerative colitis (may be exacerbated) · uncontrolled hypertension

- INTERACTIONS → Appendix 1 (NSAIDs).

- SIDE-EFFECTS
▶ Rare Alveolitis · aseptic meningitis (patients with connective-tissue disorders such as systemic lupus erythematosus may be especially susceptible) · hepatic damage · interstitial fibrosis associated with NSAIDs can lead to renal failure · pancreatitis · papillary necrosis associated with NSAIDs can lead to renal failure · pulmonary eosinophilia · Stevens-Johnson syndrome · toxic epidermal necrolysis · visual disturbances
▶ Frequency not known Angioedema · blood disorders · bronchospasm · cholestasis · colitis (induction of or exacerbation of) · Crohn's disease (induction of or exacerbation of) · depression · diarrhoea · dizziness · drowsiness · fluid retention (rarely precipitating congestive heart failure) · gastro-intestinal bleeding · gastro-intestinal discomfort · gastro-intestinal disturbances · gastro-intestinal ulceration · haematuria · headache · hearing disturbances · hepatic failure · hepatitis · hypersensitivity reactions · insomnia · jaundice with fever · nausea · nervousness · photosensitivity · raised blood pressure · rashes · renal failure (especially in patients with pre-existing renal impairment) · tinnitus · urine discolouration · vertigo

SIDE-EFFECTS, FURTHER INFORMATION
▶ Serious side-effects For information about cardiovascular and gastro-intestinal side-effects, and a possible exacerbation of symptoms in asthma, see Non-steroidal anti-inflammatory drugs p. 975.

- ALLERGY AND CROSS-SENSITIVITY Contra-indicated in patients with a history of hypersensitivity to aspirin or any other NSAID—which includes those in whom attacks of asthma, angioedema, urticaria or rhinitis have been precipitated by aspirin or any other NSAID.

- CONCEPTION AND CONTRACEPTION Caution—long-term use of some NSAIDs is associated with reduced female fertility, which is reversible on stopping treatment.

- PREGNANCY Avoid unless the potential benefit outweighs the risk. Avoid during the third trimester (risk of closure of fetal ductus arteriosus *in utero* and possibly persistent pulmonary hypertension of the newborn); onset of labour may be delayed and duration may be increased.

10

Musculoskeletal system

Musculoskeletal system

10

- BREAST FEEDING Use with caution during breast-feeding.
- HEPATIC IMPAIRMENT Use with caution; there is an increased risk of gastro-intestinal bleeding and fluid retention. Avoid in severe liver disease.
- RENAL IMPAIRMENT The lowest effective dose should be used for the shortest possible duration. Avoid if possible or use with caution. Avoid in severe impairment. In renal impairment monitor renal function; sodium and water retention may occur and renal function may deteriorate, possibly leading to renal failure.

- MEDICINAL FORMS
There can be variation in the licensing of different medicines containing the same drug.
Tablet
CAUTIONARY AND ADVISORY LABELS 21
▸ Sulindac (Non-proprietary)
Sulindac 100 mg Sulindac 100mg tablets | 56 tablet PoM £43.75
DT price = £29.78
Sulindac 200 mg Sulindac 200mg tablets | 56 tablet PoM £56.25
DT price = £38.29

Tenoxicam

- INDICATIONS AND DOSE
Pain and inflammation in rheumatic disease
▸ BY MOUTH
▸ Adult: 20 mg once daily
▸ BY INTRAVENOUS INJECTION, OR BY INTRAMUSCULAR INJECTION
▸ Adult: 20 mg once daily as initial treatment for 1–2 days if oral administration not possible
Pain and inflammation in acute musculoskeletal disorders
▸ BY MOUTH
▸ Adult: 20 mg once daily for 7 days; maximum duration of treatment 14 days (including treatment by intravenous or intramuscular injection)
▸ BY INTRAVENOUS INJECTION, OR BY INTRAMUSCULAR INJECTION
▸ Adult: 20 mg once daily as initial treatment for 1–2 days if oral administration not possible

- CONTRA-INDICATIONS Active gastro-intestinal bleeding · active gastro-intestinal ulceration · history of gastro-intestinal bleeding related to previous NSAID therapy · history of gastro-intestinal perforation related to previous NSAID therapy · history of recurrent gastro-intestinal haemorrhage (two or more distinct episodes) · history of recurrent gastro-intestinal ulceration (two or more distinct episodes) · severe heart failure
- CAUTIONS Allergic disorders · cardiac impairment (NSAIDs may impair renal function) · cerebrovascular disease · coagulation defects · connective-tissue disorders · Crohn's disease (may be exacerbated) · elderly (risk of serious side-effects and fatalities) · heart failure · ischaemic heart disease · peripheral arterial disease · risk factors for cardiovascular events · ulcerative colitis (may be exacerbated) · uncontrolled hypertension
- INTERACTIONS → Appendix 1 (NSAIDs).
- SIDE-EFFECTS
▸ Rare Alveolitis · aseptic meningitis (patients with connective-tissue disorders such as systemic lupus erythematosus may be especially susceptible) · hepatic damage · interstitial fibrosis associated with NSAIDs can lead to renal failure · pancreatitis · papillary necrosis associated with NSAIDs can lead to renal failure · pulmonary eosinophilia · Stevens-Johnson syndrome · toxic epidermal necrolysis · visual disturbances
▸ Frequency not known Angioedema · blood disorders · bronchospasm · colitis (induction of or exacerbation of) · Crohn's disease (induction of or exacerbation of) ·

depression · diarrhoea · dizziness · drowsiness · fluid retention (rarely precipitating congestive heart failure) · gastro-intestinal bleeding · gastro-intestinal discomfort · gastro-intestinal disturbances · gastro-intestinal ulceration · haematuria · headache · hearing disturbances · hypersensitivity reactions · insomnia · nausea · nervousness · photosensitivity · raised blood pressure · rashes · renal failure (especially in patients with pre-existing renal impairment) · tinnitus · vertigo
SIDE-EFFECTS, FURTHER INFORMATION
▸ Serious side-effects For information about cardiovascular and gastro-intestinal side-effects, and a possible exacerbation of symptoms in asthma, see Non-steroidal anti-inflammatory drugs p. 975.
- ALLERGY AND CROSS-SENSITIVITY Contra-indicated in patients with a history of hypersensitivity to aspirin or any other NSAID—which includes those in whom attacks of asthma, angioedema, urticaria or rhinitis have been precipitated by aspirin or any other NSAID.
- CONCEPTION AND CONTRACEPTION Caution—long-term use of some NSAIDs is associated with reduced female fertility, which is reversible on stopping treatment.
- PREGNANCY Avoid unless the potential benefit outweighs the risk. Avoid during the third trimester (risk of closure of fetal ductus arteriosus *in utero* and possibly persistent pulmonary hypertension of the newborn); onset of labour may be delayed and duration may be increased.
- BREAST FEEDING Use with caution during breast-feeding. Present in milk in *animal* studies.
- HEPATIC IMPAIRMENT Use with caution; there is an increased risk of gastro-intestinal bleeding and fluid retention. Avoid in severe liver disease.
- RENAL IMPAIRMENT The lowest effective dose should be used for the shortest possible duration. Avoid if possible or use with caution. Avoid in severe impairment. In renal impairment monitor renal function; sodium and water retention may occur and renal function may deteriorate, possibly leading to renal failure.

- MEDICINAL FORMS
There can be variation in the licensing of different medicines containing the same drug.
Tablet
CAUTIONARY AND ADVISORY LABELS 21
▸ Tenoxicam (Non-proprietary)
Tenoxicam 20 mg Tenoxicam 20mg tablets | 28 tablet PoM £16.16
DT price = £16.16
▸ Mobiflex (Meda Pharmaceuticals Ltd)
Tenoxicam 20 mg Mobiflex 20mg tablets | 30 tablet PoM £13.42
Powder and solvent for solution for injection
▸ Tenoxicam (Non-proprietary)
Tenoxicam 20 mg Tenoxicam 20mg powder and solvent for solution for injection vials | 1 vial PoM £3.98

Tiaprofenic acid

- INDICATIONS AND DOSE
Pain and inflammation in rheumatic disease and other musculoskeletal disorders
▸ BY MOUTH
▸ Adult: 300 mg twice daily

IMPORTANT SAFETY INFORMATION
CSM ADVICE
Following reports of **severe cystitis** the CSM has recommended that tiaprofenic acid should not be given to patients with urinary-tract disorders and should be stopped if urinary symptoms develop.
Patients should be advised to stop taking tiaprofenic acid and to report to their doctor promptly if they

develop urinary-tract symptoms (such as increased frequency, nocturia, urgency, pain on urinating, or blood in urine).

- CONTRA-INDICATIONS Active bladder disease (or symptoms) · active gastro-intestinal bleeding · active gastro-intestinal ulceration · active prostate disease (or symptoms) · history of gastro-intestinal bleeding related to previous NSAID therapy · history of gastro-intestinal perforation related to previous NSAID therapy · history of recurrent gastro-intestinal haemorrhage (two or more distinct episodes) · history of recurrent gastro-intestinal ulceration (two or more distinct episodes) · history of recurrent urinary-tract disorders (if urinary symptoms develop discontinue immediately and perform urine tests and culture) · severe heart failure
- CAUTIONS Allergic disorders · cardiac impairment (NSAIDs may impair renal function) · cerebrovascular disease · coagulation defects · connective-tissue disorders · Crohn's disease (may be exacerbated) · elderly (risk of serious side-effects and fatalities) · heart failure · ischaemic heart disease · peripheral arterial disease · risk factors for cardiovascular events · ulcerative colitis (may be exacerbated) · uncontrolled hypertension
- INTERACTIONS → Appendix 1 (NSAIDs).
- SIDE-EFFECTS
  ▸ Rare Alveolitis · aseptic meningitis (patients with connective-tissue disorders such as systemic lupus erythematosus may be especially susceptible) · hepatic damage · interstitial fibrosis associated with NSAIDs can lead to renal failure · pancreatitis · papillary necrosis associated with NSAIDs can lead to renal failure · pulmonary eosinophilia · Stevens-Johnson syndrome · toxic epidermal necrolysis · visual disturbances
  ▸ Frequency not known Angioedema · blood disorders · bronchospasm · colitis (induction of or exacerbation of) · Crohn's disease (induction of or exacerbation of) · depression · diarrhoea · dizziness · drowsiness · fluid retention (rarely precipitating congestive heart failure) · gastro-intestinal bleeding · gastro-intestinal discomfort · gastro-intestinal disturbances · gastro-intestinal ulceration · haematuria · headache · hearing disturbances · hypersensitivity reactions · insomnia · nausea · nervousness · photosensitivity · raised blood pressure · rashes · renal failure (especially in patients with pre-existing renal impairment) · tinnitus · vertigo
  SIDE-EFFECTS, FURTHER INFORMATION
  ▸ Serious side-effects For information about cardiovascular and gastro-intestinal side-effects, and a possible exacerbation of symptoms in asthma, see Non-steroidal anti-inflammatory drugs p. 975.
- ALLERGY AND CROSS-SENSITIVITY Contra-indicated in patients with a history of hypersensitivity to aspirin or any other NSAID—which includes those in whom attacks of asthma, angioedema, urticaria or rhinitis have been precipitated by aspirin or any other NSAID.
- CONCEPTION AND CONTRACEPTION Caution—long-term use of some NSAIDs is associated with reduced female fertility, which is reversible on stopping treatment.
- PREGNANCY Avoid unless the potential benefit outweighs the risk. Avoid during the third trimester (risk of closure of fetal ductus arteriosus *in utero* and possibly persistent pulmonary hypertension of the newborn); onset of labour may be delayed and duration may be increased.
- BREAST FEEDING Use with caution during breast-feeding. Amount too small to be harmful.
- HEPATIC IMPAIRMENT Reduce dose in mild or moderate impairment. Use with caution; there is an increased risk of gastro-intestinal bleeding and fluid retention. Avoid in severe liver disease.

- RENAL IMPAIRMENT Reduce dose in mild or moderate impairment. The lowest effective dose should be used for the shortest possible duration. Avoid if possible or use with caution. Avoid in severe impairment. In renal impairment monitor renal function; sodium and water retention may occur and renal function may deteriorate, possibly leading to renal failure.

- MEDICINAL FORMS
  There can be variation in the licensing of different medicines containing the same drug.
  Tablet
  CAUTIONARY AND ADVISORY LABELS 21
  ▸ Surgam (Sanofi)
  Tiaprofenic acid 300 mg Surgam 300mg tablets | 56 tablet [PoM]
  £14.95 DT price = £14.95

5   Soft tissue and joint disorders

5.1 Local inflammation of joints and soft tissue

> Drugs used for Local inflammation of joints and soft tissue not listed below Betamethasone, p. 610

CORTICOSTEROIDS

Corticosteroids, inflammatory disorders

Systemic corticosteroids

Short-term treatment with corticosteroids can help to rapidly improve symptoms of rheumatoid arthritis. Long-term treatment in rheumatoid arthritis should be considered only after evaluating the risks and all other treatment options have been considered. Corticosteroids can induce osteoporosis, and prophylaxis should be considered on long-term treatment.

In severe, possibly life-threatening, situations a high initial dose of corticosteroid is given to induce remission and the dose is then reduced gradually and discontinued altogether. Relapse may occur as the dose of corticosteroid is reduced, particularly if the reduction is too rapid. The tendency is therefore to increase the maintenance dose and consequently the patient becomes dependent on corticosteroids. For this reason pulse doses of corticosteroids (e.g. methylprednisolone p. 613 up to 1 g intravenously on 3 consecutive days) are used to suppress highly active inflammatory disease while longer-term treatment with a disease-modifying drug is commenced.

Prednisolone p. 1001 may reduce the rate of joint destruction in moderate to severe *rheumatoid arthritis* of less than 2 years' duration. The reduction in joint destruction must be distinguished from mere symptomatic improvement (which lasts only 6 to 12 months at this dose) and care should be taken to avoid increasing the dose above 7.5 mg daily. Evidence supports maintenance of this anti-erosive dose for 2–4 years only after which treatment should be tapered off to reduce long-term adverse effects.

A modified-release preparation of prednisone p. 615 is also available for the treatment of moderate to severe rheumatoid arthritis.

Polymyalgia rheumatica and *giant cell (temporal) arteritis* are always treated with corticosteroids. Relapse is common if therapy is stopped prematurely. Many patients require treatment for at least 2 years and in some patients it may be necessary to continue long-term low-dose corticosteroid treatment.

Polyarteritis nodosa and *polymyositis* are usually treated with corticosteroids.

Systemic lupus erythematosus is treated with corticosteroids when necessary using a similar dosage regimen to that for polyarteritis nodosa and polymyositis. Patients with pleurisy, pericarditis, or other systemic manifestations will respond to corticosteroids. It may then be possible to reduce the dosage; alternate-day treatment is sometimes adequate, and the drug may be gradually withdrawn. In some mild cases corticosteroid treatment may be stopped after a few months. Many mild cases of systemic lupus erythematosus do not require corticosteroid treatment. Alternative treatment with anti-inflammatory analgesics, and possibly chloroquine p. 560 or hydroxychloroquine sulfate p. 950, should be considered.

Ankylosing spondylitis should not be treated with long-term corticosteroids; rarely, pulse doses may be needed and may be useful in extremely active disease that does not respond to conventional treatment.

Local corticosteroid injections

Corticosteroids are injected locally for an anti-inflammatory effect. In inflammatory conditions of the joints, particularly in rheumatoid arthritis, they are given by *intra-articular injection* to relieve pain, increase mobility, and reduce deformity in one or a few joints; they can also provide symptomatic relief while waiting for DMARDs to take effect. Full aseptic precautions are essential; infected areas should be avoided. Occasionally an acute inflammatory reaction develops after an intra-articular or soft-tissue injection of a corticosteroid. This may be a reaction to the microcrystalline suspension of the corticosteroid used, but must be distinguished from sepsis introduced into the injection site.

Smaller amounts of corticosteroids may also be injected directly into soft tissues for the relief of inflammation in conditions such as *tennis* or *golfer's elbow* or *compression neuropathies*. In *tendinitis*, injections should be made into the tendon sheath and not directly into the tendon (due to the absence of a true tendon sheath and a high risk of rupture, the Achilles tendon should not be injected).

Hydrocortisone below acetate or one of the synthetic analogues is generally used for local injection. Intra-articular corticosteroid injections can cause flushing and may affect the hyaline cartilage. Each joint should not usually be treated more than 4 times in one year.

Corticosteroid injections are also injected into soft tissues for the treatment of skin lesions.

F 608

Dexamethasone

6.6.2016

● INDICATIONS AND DOSE

Local inflammation of joints
▸ BY INTRA-ARTICULAR INJECTION
▸ Adult: 0.3–3.3 mg, where appropriate, dose may be repeated at intervals of 3–21 days according to response, dose given according to size—consult product literature

Local inflammation of soft tissues
▸ BY LOCAL INFILTRATION
▸ Adult: 1.7–5 mg, dose given according to size—consult product literature., where appropriate may be repeated at intervals of 3–21 days, use the 3.3 mg/mL injection preparation for this dose

● PREGNANCY Dexamethasone readily crosses the placenta.

● PRESCRIBING AND DISPENSING INFORMATION
Dexamethasone 3.8mg/mL Injection has replaced Dexamethasone 4mg/mL Injection. All dosage

recommendations for intra-articular use or local infiltration are given in units of dexamethasone base.

● MEDICINAL FORMS
There can be variation in the licensing of different medicines containing the same drug.
Solution for injection
CAUTIONARY AND ADVISORY LABELS 10
▸ Dexamethasone (Non-proprietary)
Dexamethasone (as Dexamethasone sodium phosphate) 3.3 mg per 1 ml Dexamethasone 6.6mg/2ml solution for injection vials | 5 vial PoM £24.00
Dexamethasone 6.6mg/2ml solution for injection ampoules | 5 ampoule PoM £11.00
Dexamethasone 3.3mg/1ml solution for injection ampoules | 5 ampoule PoM £12.00 | 10 ampoule PoM £12.00
Dexamethasone (as Dexamethasone sodium phosphate) 3.8 mg per 1 ml Dexamethasone 3.8mg/1ml solution for injection vials | 10 vial PoM £19.99 DT price = £19.99

F 608

Hydrocortisone

● INDICATIONS AND DOSE
HYDROCORTISTAB®

Local inflammation of joints and soft-tissues
▸ BY INTRA-ARTICULAR INJECTION
▸ Adult: 5–50 mg, select dose according to size of patient and joint; where appropriate dose may be repeated at intervals of 21 days. Not more than 3 joints should be treated on any one day, for details consult product literature

● MEDICINAL FORMS
There can be variation in the licensing of different medicines containing the same drug.
Suspension for injection
▸ Hydrocortistab (AMCo)
Hydrocortisone acetate 25 mg per 1 ml Hydrocortistab 25mg/1ml suspension for injection ampoules | 10 ampoule PoM £68.72 DT price = £68.72

F 608

Methylprednisolone

● INDICATIONS AND DOSE
DEPO-MEDRONE®

Local inflammation of joints and soft tissues
▸ BY INTRA-ARTICULAR INJECTION
▸ Adult: 4–80 mg, select dose according to size; where appropriate dose may be repeated at intervals of 7–35 days, for details consult product literature

● PATIENT AND CARER ADVICE Patient counselling is advised for methylprednisolone tablets and injections (steroid card).

● MEDICINAL FORMS
There can be variation in the licensing of different medicines containing the same drug.
Suspension for injection
CAUTIONARY AND ADVISORY LABELS 10
▸ Depo-Medrone (Pfizer Ltd)
Methylprednisolone acetate 40 mg per 1 ml Depo-Medrone 40mg/1ml suspension for injection vials | 1 vial PoM £3.44 DT price = £3.44 | 10 vial PoM £34.04
Depo-Medrone 80mg/2ml suspension for injection vials | 1 vial PoM £6.18 DT price = £6.18 | 10 vial PoM £61.39
Depo-Medrone 120mg/3ml suspension for injection vials | 1 vial PoM £8.96 DT price = £8.96 | 10 vial PoM £88.81

Methylprednisolone with lidocaine

The properties listed below are those particular to the combination only. For the properties of the components please consider, methylprednisolone p. 1000, lidocaine hydrochloride p. 1187.

- **INDICATIONS AND DOSE**

Local inflammation of joints

▸ BY INTRA-ARTICULAR INJECTION

▸ Adult: 4–80 mg, dose adjusted according to size; where appropriate may be repeated at intervals of 7–35 days, for details consult product literature

- **MEDICINAL FORMS**

There can be variation in the licensing of different medicines containing the same drug.

Suspension for injection

▸ Depo-Medrone with Lidocaine (Pfizer Ltd)

Lidocaine hydrochloride 10 mg per 1 ml, Methylprednisolone acetate 40 mg per 1 ml Depo-Medrone with Lidocaine suspension for injection 2ml vials | 1 vial PoM £7.06 DT price = £7.06 | 10 vial PoM £70.13

Depo-Medrone with Lidocaine suspension for injection 1ml vials | 1 vial PoM £3.94 DT price = £3.94 | 10 vial PoM £38.88

F 608

Prednisolone

- **INDICATIONS AND DOSE**

DELTASTAB®

Local inflammation of joints

▸ BY INTRA-ARTICULAR INJECTION

▸ Adult: 5–25 mg, dose according to size; not more than 3 joints should be treated on any one day; where appropriate may be repeated when relapse occurs, for details consult product literature

- **PREGNANCY** As it crosses the placenta 88% of prednisolone is inactivated.

- **BREAST FEEDING** Prednisolone appears in small amounts in breast milk but maternal doses of up to 40 mg daily are unlikely to cause systemic effects in the infant.

- **MEDICINAL FORMS**

There can be variation in the licensing of different medicines containing the same drug.

Suspension for injection

▸ Deltastab (AMCo)

Prednisolone acetate 25 mg per 1 ml Deltastab 25mg/1ml suspension for injection ampoules | 10 ampoule PoM £68.72

F 608

Triamcinolone acetonide

- **INDICATIONS AND DOSE**

ADCORTYL® INTRA-ARTICULAR/INTRADERMAL

Local inflammation of joints and soft tissues

▸ BY INTRA-ARTICULAR INJECTION

▸ Adult: 2.5–15 mg, adjusted according to size (for larger doses use Kenalog®). Where appropriate dose may be repeated when relapse occurs, for details consult product literature.

▸ BY INTRADERMAL INJECTION

▸ Adult: 2–3 mg, max. 5 mg at any one site (total max. 30 mg). Where appropriate may be repeated at intervals of 1–2 weeks, for details consult product literature

KENALOG® VIALS

Local inflammation of joints and soft tissues

▸ BY INTRA-ARTICULAR INJECTION

▸ Adult: 5–40 mg (max. per dose 80 mg), for further details consult product literature, select dose according

to size. For doses below 5 mg use Adcortyl® Intra-articular/Intradermal injection, where appropriate dose may be repeated when relapse occurs.

- **MEDICINAL FORMS**

There can be variation in the licensing of different medicines containing the same drug.

Suspension for injection

CAUTIONARY AND ADVISORY LABELS 10

EXCIPIENTS: May contain Benzyl alcohol

▸ Adcortyl Intra-articular / Intradermal (Bristol-Myers Squibb Pharmaceuticals Ltd)

Triamcinolone acetonide 10 mg per 1 ml Adcortyl Intra-articular / Intradermal 50mg/5ml suspension for injection vials | 1 vial PoM £3.63

Adcortyl Intra-articular / Intradermal 10mg/1ml suspension for injection ampoules | 5 ampoule PoM £4.47 DT price = £4.47

▸ Kenalog (Bristol-Myers Squibb Pharmaceuticals Ltd)

Triamcinolone acetonide 40 mg per 1 ml Kenalog Intra-articular / Intramuscular 40mg/1ml suspension for injection vials | 5 vial PoM £7.45 DT price = £7.45

F 608

Triamcinolone hexacetonide

- **INDICATIONS AND DOSE**

Local inflammation of joints and soft-tissues (for details, consult product literature)

▸ BY INTRA-ARTICULAR INJECTION

▸ Adult: 2–20 mg, adjusted according to size of joint, no more than 2 joints should be treated on any one day, where appropriate, may be repeated at intervals of 3–4 weeks

▸ BY PERI-ARTICULAR INJECTION

▸ Adult: 10–20 mg, adjusted according to size of joint, no more than 2 joints should be treated on any one day

- **CONTRA-INDICATIONS** Consult product literature
- **CAUTIONS** Consult product literature
- **SIDE-EFFECTS** Consult product literature
- **PRESCRIBING AND DISPENSING INFORMATION** Various strengths available from 'special order' manufacturers or specialist importing companies.

- **MEDICINAL FORMS**

There can be variation in the licensing of different medicines containing the same drug.

Suspension for injection

EXCIPIENTS: May contain Benzyl alcohol

▸ Triamcinolone hexacetonide (Non-proprietary)

Triamcinolone hexacetonide 20 mg per 1 ml Triamcinolone hexacetonide 20mg/1ml suspension for injection ampoules | 10 ampoule PoM £120.00

5.2 Soft tissue disorders

Soft-tissue disorders

Extravasation

Local guidelines for the management of extravasation should be followed where they exist or specialist advice sought.

Extravasation injury follows leakage of drugs or intravenous fluids from the veins or inadvertent administration into the subcutaneous or subdermal tissue. It must be dealt with **promptly** to prevent tissue necrosis.

Acidic or alkaline preparations and those with an osmolarity greater than that of plasma can cause extravasation injury; excipients including alcohol and polyethylene glycol have also been implicated. Cytotoxic drugs commonly cause extravasation injury. In addition, certain patients such as the very young and the elderly are at increased risk. Those receiving anticoagulants are more likely to lose blood into surrounding tissues if extravasation occurs, while those receiving sedatives or analgesics may not notice the early signs or symptoms of extravasation.

Prevention of extravasation
Precautions should be taken to avoid extravasation; ideally, drugs likely to cause extravasation injury should be given through a central line and patients receiving repeated doses of hazardous drugs peripherally should have the cannula resited at regular intervals. Attention should be paid to the manufacturers' recommendations for administration. Placing a glyceryl trinitrate patch p. 201 distal to the cannula may improve the patency of the vessel in patients with small veins or in those whose veins are prone to collapse.

Patients should be asked to report any pain or burning at the site of injection immediately.

Management of extravasation
If extravasation is suspected the infusion should be stopped immediately but the cannula should not be removed until after an attempt has been made to aspirate the area (through the cannula) in order to remove as much of the drug as possible. Aspiration is sometimes possible if the extravasation presents with a raised bleb or blister at the injection site and is surrounded by hardened tissue, but it is often unsuccessful if the tissue is soft or soggy.
Corticosteroids are usually given to treat inflammation, although there is little evidence to support their use in extravasation. Hydrocortisone p. 1000 or dexamethasone p. 1000 can be given either locally by subcutaneous injection or intravenously at a site distant from the injury.
Antihistamines and **analgesics** may be required for symptom relief.

The management of extravasation beyond these measures is not well standardised and calls for specialist advice. Treatment depends on the nature of the offending substance; one approach is to localise and neutralise the substance whereas another is to spread and dilute it.

The first method may be appropriate following extravasation of vesicant drugs and involves administration of an antidote (if available) and the application of cold compresses 3–4 times a day (consult specialist literature for details of specific antidotes). Spreading and diluting the offending substance involves infiltrating the area with physiological saline, applying warm compresses, elevating the affected limb, and administering hyaluronidase p. 1003. A saline flush-out technique (involving flushing the subcutaneous tissue with physiological saline) may be effective but requires specialist advice. Hyaluronidase should not be administered following extravasation of vesicant drugs (unless it is either specifically indicated or used in the saline flush-out technique). Dexrazoxane p. 826 is licensed for the treatment of anthracycline-induced extravasation.

Enzymes
Collagenase
Collagenase below are proteolytic enzymes that are derived from the fermentation of *Clostridium histolyticum* and have the ability to break down collagen. A preparation containing a mixture of two collagenases is licensed for the treatment of Dupuytren's contracture; the preparation should be injected into a palpable cord with a contracture of a metacarpophalangeal joint or proximal interphalangeal joint.

Hyaluronidase
Hyaluronidase is used to render the tissues more readily permeable to injected fluids, e.g. for introduction of fluids by subcutaneous infusion (termed hypodermoclysis).

Rubefacients, topical NSAIDs, capsaicin, and poultices
Rubefacients act by counter-irritation. Pain, whether superficial or deep-seated, is relieved by any method that itself produces irritation of the skin. Topical rubefacient preparations may contain nicotinate and salicylate compounds, essential oils, capsicum, and camphor. The evidence available does not support the use of topical rubefacients in acute or chronic musculoskeletal pain.

Topical NSAIDs
The use of a NSAID by mouth is effective for relieving musculoskeletal pain. **Topical NSAIDs** (e.g. felbinac p. 985, ibuprofen p. 987, ketoprofen p. 991, and piroxicam p. 996 may provide some relief of pain in musculoskeletal conditions; they can be considered as an adjunctive treatment in knee or hand osteoarthritis.

Capsaicin
A preparation containing capsaicin 0.025% p. 438 can be considered as an adjunct in hand or knee osteoarthritis.It may need to be used for 1–2 weeks before pain is relieved.

A capsaicin 0.075% cream is licensed for the symptomatic relief of postherpetic neuralgia after lesions have healed, and for the relief of painful diabetic neuropathy.

A self-adhesive patch containing capsaicin 8% is licensed for the treatment of peripheral neuropathic pain in non-diabetic patients.

ENZYMES

Collagenase

- **INDICATIONS AND DOSE**

Dupuytren's contracture in patients with a palpable cord
▶ BY INTRALESIONAL INJECTION
▶ Adult: 580 micrograms, then 580 micrograms every 4 weeks if required, inject into palpable cord, maximum 3 injections per cord, maximum 8 injections in total and only one cord may be treated at a time

- CONTRA-INDICATIONS Avoid injecting into other structures containing collagen (e.g. tendons, nerves, and blood vessels)—risk of tendon rupture or ligament damage
- CAUTIONS Coagulation disorders · use of anticoagulants
- SIDE-EFFECTS
▶ **Common or very common** Arthralgia · burning sensation · ecchymosis · hyperhidrosis · hypoaesthesia · injection site reactions · joint swelling · lymphadenopathy · myalgia · paraesthesia
▶ **Uncommon** Complex regional pain syndrome · crepitus · ligament injury · monoplegia · muscle spasm · muscle weakness · tendon rupture · tremor · wound dehiscence
- PREGNANCY Manufacturer advises avoid.
- BREAST FEEDING Systemic absorption by mother negligible.
- DIRECTIONS FOR ADMINISTRATION Reconstitution and injected volumes vary with site of injection—consult product literature.
- NATIONAL FUNDING/ACCESS DECISIONS

Scottish Medicines Consortium (SMC) Decisions
The *Scottish Medicines Consortium* has advised (April 2012) that collagenase *Clostridium histolyticum* (*Xiapex*®) is accepted for restricted use within NHS Scotland as an alternative to limited fasciectomy, for the treatment of Dupuytren's contracture of moderate severity (as defined by the British Society for Surgery of the Hand) in patients with a palpable cord and up to two affected joints per hand, who are suitable for limited fasciectomy, but for whom percutaneous needle fasciectomy is not considered a suitable treatment option.

● MEDICINAL FORMS
There can be variation in the licensing of different medicines
containing the same drug.
Powder and solvent for solution for injection
▸ Xiapex (Swedish Orphan Biovitrum Ltd)
  Collagenase clostridium histolyticum 900 microgram Xiapex
  0.9mg powder and solvent for solution for injection vials | 1 vial [PoM]
  £650.00

Hyaluronidase

● INDICATIONS AND DOSE
**Enhance permeation of subcutaneous or intramuscular
injections**
▸ BY SUBCUTANEOUS INJECTION, OR BY INTRAMUSCULAR
  INJECTION
▸ Adult: 1500 units, to be dissolved directly into the
  solution to be injected (ensure compatibility)
Enhance permeation of local anaesthetics
▸ BY LOCAL INFILTRATION
▸ Adult: 1500 units, to be mixed with the local
  anaesthetic solution
Enhance permeation of ophthalmic local anaesthetic
▸ TO THE EYE
▸ Adult: 15 units/mL, to be mixed with the local
  anaesthetic solution
Hypodermoclysis
▸ BY SUBCUTANEOUS INJECTION
▸ Adult: 1500 units, to be dissolved in 1 mL water for
  injections or 0.9% sodium chloride injection,
  administered before start of 500–1000 mL infusion
  fluid
Extravasation
▸ BY LOCAL INFILTRATION
▸ Adult: 1500 units, to be dissolved in 1 mL water for
  injections or 0.9% sodium chloride and infiltrated into
  affected area as soon as possible after extravasation
Haematoma
▸ BY LOCAL INFILTRATION
▸ Adult: 1500 units, to be dissolved in 1 mL water for
  injections or 0.9% sodium chloride and infiltrated into
  affected area

● CONTRA-INDICATIONS Avoid sites where infection is
present · avoid sites where malignancy is present · do not
apply direct to cornea · not for anaesthesia in unexplained
premature labour · not for intravenous administration · not
to be used to enhance the absorption and dispersion of
dopamine and/or alpha-adrenoceptor agonists · not to be
used to reduce swelling of bites · not to be used to reduce
swelling of stings
● CAUTIONS Elderly (control speed and total volume and
avoid overhydration especially in renal impairment)
● SIDE-EFFECTS
▸ **Common or very common** Oedema
▸ **Rare** Bleeding · bruising · infection · local irritation
▸ **Frequency not known** Anaphylaxis · severe allergy

● MEDICINAL FORMS
There can be variation in the licensing of different medicines
containing the same drug.
Powder for solution for injection
▸ Hyaluronidase (Non-proprietary)
  Hyaluronidase 1500 unit Hyaluronidase 1,500unit powder for
  solution for injection ampoules | 10 ampoule [PoM] £104.24

Chapter 11
Eye

CONTENTS

Eye

Administration of drugs to the eye

Drugs are most commonly administered to the eye by topical application as eye drops or eye ointments. When a higher drug concentration is required within the eye, a local injection may be necessary.

Eye-drop dispenser devices are available to aid the instillation of eye drops from plastic bottles and some are prescribable on the NHS (consult Drug Tariff—see Appliances and Reagents). Product-specific devices may be supplied by manufacturers—consult individual manufacturers for information. They are particularly useful for the elderly, visually impaired, arthritic, or otherwise physically limited patients.

Eye drops and eye ointments

Eye drops are generally instilled into the pocket formed by gently pulling down the lower eyelid and keeping the eye closed for as long as possible after application; one drop is all that is needed. Instillation of more than one drop should be discouraged because it may increase systemic side-effects. A small amount of eye ointment is applied similarly; the ointment melts rapidly and blinking helps to spread it.

When two different eye-drop preparations are used at the same time of day, dilution and overflow may occur when one immediately follows the other. The patient should therefore leave an interval of at least 5 minutes between the two; the interval should be extended when eye drops with a prolonged contact time, such as gels and suspensions, are used. Eye ointment should be applied after drops.

Systemic effects may arise from absorption of drugs into the general circulation from conjunctival vessels or from the nasal mucosa after the excess preparation has drained down through the tear ducts. The extent of systemic absorption following ocular administration is highly variable; nasal drainage of drugs is associated with eye drops much more often than with eye ointments. Pressure on the lacrimal punctum for at least a minute after applying eye drops reduces nasolacrimal drainage and therefore decreases systemic absorption from the nasal mucosa.

After using eye drops or eye ointments, patients should be warned not to drive or perform other skilled tasks until vision is clear.

Also see warnings relating to eye drops and contact lenses.

Eye lotions

These are solutions for the irrigation of the conjunctival sac. They act mechanically to flush out irritants or foreign bodies as a first-aid treatment. Sterile sodium chloride 0.9% p. 1014 solution is usually used. Clean water will suffice in an emergency.

Other preparations administered to the eye

Subconjunctival injection may be used to administer anti-infective drugs, mydriatics, or corticosteroids for conditions not responding to topical therapy; intracameral and intravitreal routes can also be used to administer certain drugs, for example antibacterials. These injections should only be used under specialist supervision.

Drugs such as antimicrobials and corticosteroids may be administered systemically to treat susceptible eye conditions.

Ophthalmic Specials

Certain eye drops, e.g. amphotericin, ceftazidime, cefuroxime, colistimethate sodium, desferrioxamine mesilate, dexamethasone, gentamicin, and vancomycin can be prepared aseptically from material supplied for injection.

The Royal College of Ophthalmologists and the UK Ophthalmic Pharmacy Group have produced the Ophthalmic Specials Guidance to help prescribers and pharmacists manage and restrict the use of unlicensed eye preparations. 'Specials' should only be prescribed in situations where a licensed product is not suitable for a patient's needs. The Ophthalmic Specials Guidance can be accessed on the Royal College of Ophthalmologists website (www.rcophth.ac.uk). The guidance will be reviewed every six months to ensure the most accurate and up-to-date information is available.

Preservatives and sensitisers

Information on preservatives and substances identified as skin sensitisers is provided under Excipients statements in preparation entries. Very rarely, cases of corneal calcification have been reported with the use of phosphate-containing eye drops in patients with significantly damaged corneas—consult product literature for further information.

Control of microbial contamination

Preparations for the eye should be sterile when issued. Care should be taken to avoid contamination of the contents during use.

Eye drops in multiple-application containers for *domiciliary use* should not be used for more than 4 weeks after first opening (unless otherwise stated by the manufacturer).

Multiple application eye drops for use in *hospital wards* are normally discarded 1 week after first opening—local practice may vary. Individual containers should be provided for each patient. A separate container should be supplied for each eye only if there are special concerns about contamination. Containers used before an eye operation should be discarded at the time of the operation and fresh containers supplied postoperatively. A fresh supply should also be provided upon discharge from hospital; in specialist ophthalmology units, it may be acceptable to issue containers that have been dispensed to the patient on the day of discharge.

In *out-patient departments* single-application containers should be used; if multiple-application containers are used, they should be discarded after single patient use within one clinical session.

In *eye surgery* single-application containers should be used if possible; if a multiple-application container is used, it should be discarded after single use. Preparations used during intra-ocular procedures and others that may penetrate into the anterior chamber must be isotonic and without preservatives and buffered if necessary to a neutral pH. Specially formulated fluids should be used for intra-ocular surgery; intravenous infusion preparations are not usually suitable for this purpose (Hartmann's solution may be used in some ocular surgery). For all surgical procedures, a previously unopened container is used for each patient.

Contact lenses

For cosmetic reasons many people prefer to wear contact lenses rather than spectacles; contact lenses are also sometimes required for medical indications. Visual defects are corrected by either rigid ('hard' or gas permeable) lenses or soft (hydrogel or silicone hydrogel—in adults only) lenses; soft lenses are the most popular type, because they are initially the most comfortable, but they may not give the best vision. Lenses should usually be worn for a specified number of hours each day and removed for sleeping. The risk of infectious and non-infectious keratitis is increased by extended continuous contact lens wear, which is not recommended, except when medically indicated.

Contact lenses require meticulous care. Poor compliance with directions for use, and with daily cleaning and disinfection, can result in complications including ulcerative keratitis or conjunctivitis. One-day disposable lenses, which are worn only once and therefore require no disinfection or cleaning, are becoming increasingly popular.

Acanthamoeba keratitis, a painful and sight-threatening condition, is associated with ineffective lens cleaning and disinfection, the use of contaminated lens cases, or tap water coming into contact with the lenses. The condition is especially associated with the use of soft lenses (including frequently replaced lenses) and should be treated by specialists.

Contact lenses and drug treatment

Special care is required in prescribing eye preparations for contact lens users. Some drugs and preservatives in eye preparations can accumulate in hydrogel lenses and may induce toxic and adverse reactions. Therefore, unless medically indicated, the lenses should be removed before instillation of the eye preparation and not worn during the period of treatment. Alternatively, unpreserved drops can be used. Eye drops may, however, be instilled while patients are wearing rigid corneal contact lenses. Ointment preparations should never be used in conjunction with contact lens wear; oily eye drops should also be avoided.

Many drugs given systemically can also have adverse effects on contact lens wear. These include oral contraceptives (particularly those with a higher oestrogen content), drugs which reduce blink rate (e.g. anxiolytics, hypnotics, antihistamines, and muscle relaxants), drugs which reduce lacrimation (e.g. antihistamines, antimuscarinics, phenothiazines and related drugs, some beta-blockers, diuretics, and tricyclic antidepressants), and drugs which increase lacrimation (including ephedrine

hydrochloride p. 248 and hydralazine hydrochloride p. 166). Other drugs that may affect contact lens wear are isotretinoin p. 1114 (can cause conjunctival inflammation), aspirin p. 109 (salicylic acid appears in tears and can be absorbed by contact lenses—leading to irritation), and rifampicin p. 527 and sulfasalazine p. 38 (can discolour lenses).

1 Allergic and inflammatory eye conditions

Eye, allergy and inflammation

Corticosteroids

Corticosteroids administered locally to the eye or given by mouth are effective for treating anterior segment inflammation, including that which results from surgery.

Topical corticosteroids are applied frequently for the first 24–48 hours; once inflammation is controlled, the frequency of application is reduced. They should normally only be used under expert supervision; three main dangers are associated with their use:

- a 'red eye', when the diagnosis is unconfirmed, may be due to herpes simplex virus, and a corticosteroid may aggravate the condition, leading to corneal ulceration, with possible damage to vision and even loss of the eye. Bacterial, fungal, and amoebic infections pose a similar hazard;
- 'steroid glaucoma' can follow the use of corticosteroid eye preparations in susceptible individuals;
- a 'steroid cataract' can follow prolonged use.

Combination products containing a corticosteroid with an anti-infective drug are sometimes used after ocular surgery to reduce inflammation and prevent infection; use of combination products is otherwise rarely justified.

Systemic corticosteroids may be useful for ocular conditions. The risk of producing a 'steroid cataract' increases with the dose and duration of corticosteroid use.

Intravitreal corticosteroids

An intravitreal implant containing dexamethasone p. 1008 (*Ozurdex*®) is licensed for the treatment of adults with macular oedema following either branch retinal vein occlusion or central retinal vein occlusion; it is also licensed for the treatment of adult patients with inflammation of the posterior segment of the eye presenting as non-infectious uveitis.

An intravitreal implant containing fluocinolone acetonide p. 1037 (*Iluvien*®) is licensed for the treatment of visual impairment associated with chronic diabetic macular oedema which is insufficiently responsive to available therapies. It should be administered by specialists experienced in the use of intravitreal injections.

Other anti-inflammatory preparations

Other preparations used for the topical treatment of inflammation and allergic conjunctivitis include antihistamines, lodoxamide p. 1007, and sodium cromoglicate p. 1007.

Eye drops containing antihistamines, such as **antazoline** (with xylometazoline hydrochloride p. 1046 as *Otrivine-Antistin*®), azelastine hydrochloride p. 1006, epinastine hydrochloride p. 1006, ketotifen p. 1006, and olopatadine p. 1007, can be used for allergic conjunctivitis.

Sodium cromoglicate (sodium cromoglycate) and nedocromil sodium p. 1007 eye drops can be useful for vernal keratoconjunctivitis and other allergic forms of conjunctivitis.

11

Eye

Lodoxamide eye drops are used for allergic conjunctival conditions including seasonal allergic conjunctivitis.

Diclofenac sodium eye drops p. 1023 and emedastine eye drops below are also licensed for seasonal allergic conjunctivitis.

Non-steroidal anti-inflammatory eye drops are used for the prophylaxis and treatment of inflammation of the eye following surgery or laser treatment.

1.1 Allergic conjunctivitis

ANTIHISTAMINES

Antazoline with xylometazoline

- ● **INDICATIONS AND DOSE**

Allergic conjunctivitis
▸ TO THE EYE
- ▸ Child 12–17 years: Apply 2–3 times a day for maximum 7 days
- ▸ Adult: Apply 2–3 times a day for maximum 7 days

- ● CAUTIONS Angle-closure glaucoma · cardiovascular disease · diabetes mellitus · hypertension · hyperthyroidism · phaeochromocytoma · urinary retention
- ● INTERACTIONS → Appendix 1 (antihistamines and sympathomimetics).
Absorption of antazoline and xylometazoline may result in the possibility of interaction with other drugs.
- ● SIDE-EFFECTS
- ▸ **Common or very common** Transient stinging
- ▸ **Frequency not known** Blurred vision · eye irritation · mydriasis
SIDE-EFFECTS, FURTHER INFORMATION
Absorption of antazoline and xylometazoline may result in systemic side-effects.

- ● MEDICINAL FORMS
There can be variation in the licensing of different medicines containing the same drug.
Eye drops
EXCIPIENTS: May contain Benzalkonium chloride, disodium edetate
▸ Otrivine Antistin (Thea Pharmaceuticals Ltd)
Xylometazoline hydrochloride 500 microgram per 1 ml, Antazoline sulfate 5 mg per 1 ml Otrivine Antistin 0.5%/0.05% eye drops | 10 ml ℗ £2.35 DT price = £2.35

Azelastine hydrochloride

- ● **INDICATIONS AND DOSE**

Seasonal allergic conjunctivitis
▸ TO THE EYE
- ▸ Child 4–17 years: Apply twice daily, increased if necessary to 4 times a day
- ▸ Adult: Apply twice daily, increased if necessary to 4 times a day

Perennial conjunctivitis
▸ TO THE EYE
- ▸ Child 12–17 years: Apply twice daily; increased if necessary to 4 times a day, maximum duration of treatment 6 weeks
- ▸ Adult: Apply twice daily; increased if necessary to 4 times a day, maximum duration of treatment 6 weeks

- ● SIDE-EFFECTS
- ▸ **Frequency not known** Bitter taste · mild transient irritation

- ● MEDICINAL FORMS
There can be variation in the licensing of different medicines containing the same drug.
Eye drops
EXCIPIENTS: May contain Benzalkonium chloride, disodium edetate
▸ Optilast (Meda Pharmaceuticals Ltd)
Azelastine hydrochloride 500 microgram per 1 ml Optilast 0.05% eye drops | 8 ml PoM £6.40 DT price = £6.40

Emedastine

- ● **INDICATIONS AND DOSE**

Seasonal allergic conjunctivitis
▸ TO THE EYE
- ▸ Child 3–17 years: Apply twice daily
- ▸ Adult: Apply twice daily

- ● SIDE-EFFECTS Blurred vision · corneal infiltrates (discontinue) · corneal staining · dry eye · headache · irritation · keratitis · lacrimation · local oedema · photophobia · rhinitis · transient burning · transient stinging

- ● MEDICINAL FORMS
There can be variation in the licensing of different medicines containing the same drug.
Eye drops
EXCIPIENTS: May contain Benzalkonium chloride
▸ Emadine (Alcon Laboratories (UK) Ltd)
Emedastine (as Emedastine difumarate) 500 microgram per 1 ml Emadine 0.5mg/ml eye drops | 5 ml PoM £7.31 DT price = £7.31

Epinastine hydrochloride

- ● **INDICATIONS AND DOSE**

Seasonal allergic conjunctivitis
▸ TO THE EYE
- ▸ Child 12–17 years: Apply twice daily for maximum 8 weeks
- ▸ Adult: Apply twice daily for maximum 8 weeks

- ● SIDE-EFFECTS
- ▸ **Common or very common** Burning
- ▸ **Uncommon** Conjunctival hyperaemia · dry eye · eye pain · eye pruritus · headache · increased lacrimation · nasal irritation · rhinitis · taste disturbance · visual disturbance

- ● MEDICINAL FORMS
There can be variation in the licensing of different medicines containing the same drug.
Eye drops
EXCIPIENTS: May contain Benzalkonium chloride, disodium edetate
▸ Relestat (Allergan Ltd)
Epinastine hydrochloride 500 microgram per 1 ml Relestat 500micrograms/ml eye drops | 5 ml PoM £9.90 DT price = £9.90

Ketotifen

- ● **INDICATIONS AND DOSE**

Seasonal allergic conjunctivitis
▸ TO THE EYE
- ▸ Child 3–17 years: Apply twice daily
- ▸ Adult: Apply twice daily

- ● INTERACTIONS Interactions do not generally apply to antihistamines used for topical action.
- ● SIDE-EFFECTS
- ▸ **Common or very common** Punctate corneal epithelial erosion · transient burning · transient stinging
- ▸ **Uncommon** Dry eye · photophobia · subconjunctival haemorrhage

▶ **Frequency not known** Drowsiness · dry mouth · headache · skin reactions

● MEDICINAL FORMS
There can be variation in the licensing of different medicines containing the same drug.
Eye drops
EXCIPIENTS: May contain Benzalkonium chloride
▶ Zaditen (Thea Pharmaceuticals Ltd)
Ketotifen (as Ketotifen fumarate) 250 microgram per 1 ml Zaditen 250micrograms/ml eye drops | 5 ml [PoM] £7.80 DT price = £7.80

Olopatadine

● INDICATIONS AND DOSE
Seasonal allergic conjunctivitis
▶ TO THE EYE
▶ **Child 3-17 years:** Apply twice daily for maximum 4 months
▶ **Adult:** Apply twice daily for maximum 4 months

● SIDE-EFFECTS
▶ **Common or very common** Local irritation
▶ **Uncommon** Asthenia · dizziness · dry eye · headache · keratitis · local oedema · photophobia
▶ **Frequency not known** Dry nose

● MEDICINAL FORMS
There can be variation in the licensing of different medicines containing the same drug.
Eye drops
EXCIPIENTS: May contain Benzalkonium chloride
▶ Opatanol (Alcon Laboratories (UK) Ltd)
Olopatadine (as Olopatadine hydrochloride) 1 mg per 1 ml Opatanol 1mg/ml eye drops | 5 ml [PoM] £4.68 DT price = £4.68

MAST-CELL STABILISERS

Lodoxamide

● INDICATIONS AND DOSE
Allergic conjunctivitis
▶ TO THE EYE
▶ **Child 4-17 years:** Apply 4 times a day, improvement of symptoms may sometimes require treatment for up to 4 weeks
▶ **Adult:** Apply 4 times a day, improvement of symptoms may sometimes require treatment for up to 4 weeks

● SIDE-EFFECTS
▶ **Common or very common** Blurred vision · burning · itching · ocular discomfort · stinging · tear production disturbance
▶ **Uncommon** Blepharitis · dizziness · drowsiness · flushing · headache · keratitis · nasal dryness
● EXCEPTIONS TO LEGAL CATEGORY Lodoxamide 0.1% eye drops can be sold to the public for treatment of allergic conjunctivitis in adults and children over 4 years.

● MEDICINAL FORMS
There can be variation in the licensing of different medicines containing the same drug.
Eye drops
EXCIPIENTS: May contain Benzalkonium chloride, disodium edetate
▶ Alomide (Alcon Laboratories (UK) Ltd)
Lodoxamide (as Lodoxamide trometamol) 1 mg per 1 ml Alomide 0.1% eye drops | 10 ml [PoM] £5.21 DT price = £5.21
Alomide Allergy 0.1% eye drops | 5 ml [P] £3.12

Nedocromil sodium

● INDICATIONS AND DOSE
Seasonal and perennial conjunctivitis
▶ TO THE EYE
▶ **Child 6-17 years:** Apply twice daily, increased if necessary to 4 times a day, max.12 weeks duration of treatment for seasonal allergic conjunctivitis
▶ **Adult:** Apply twice daily, increased if necessary to 4 times a day, max.12 weeks duration of treatment for seasonal allergic conjunctivitis
Seasonal keratoconjunctivitis
▶ TO THE EYE
▶ **Child 6-17 years:** Apply 4 times a day
▶ **Adult:** Apply 4 times a day

● SIDE-EFFECTS Distinctive taste · transient burning · transient stinging

● MEDICINAL FORMS
There can be variation in the licensing of different medicines containing the same drug.
Eye drops
EXCIPIENTS: May contain Benzalkonium chloride, disodium edetate
▶ Rapitil (Sanofi)
Nedocromil sodium 20 mg per 1 ml Rapitil 2% eye drops | 5 ml [PoM] £2.86 DT price = £2.86

Sodium cromoglicate

(Sodium cromoglycate)

● INDICATIONS AND DOSE
Allergic conjunctivitis | Seasonal keratoconjunctivitis
▶ TO THE EYE
▶ **Child:** Apply 4 times a day
▶ **Adult:** Apply 4 times a day

● SIDE-EFFECTS Transient burning · transient stinging

● EXCEPTIONS TO LEGAL CATEGORY Sodium cromoglicate 2% eye drops can be sold to the public (in max. pack size of 10 mL) for treatment of acute seasonal and perennial allergic conjunctivitis.

● MEDICINAL FORMS
There can be variation in the licensing of different medicines containing the same drug. Forms available from special-order manufacturers include: eye drops
Eye drops
▶ Sodium cromoglicate (Non-proprietary)
Sodium cromoglicate 20 mg per 1 ml Sodium cromoglicate 2% eye drops | 13.5 ml [PoM] £3.85 DT price = £2.06
▶ Catacrom (Moorfields Pharmaceuticals)
Sodium cromoglicate 20 mg per 1 ml Catacrom 2% eye drops 0.3ml unit dose | 30 unit dose [P] £8.99 DT price = £8.99
▶ Cromolux (Tubilux Pharma Ltd)
Sodium cromoglicate 20 mg per 1 ml Cromolux 2% eye drops | 13.5 ml [PoM] £3.20 DT price = £2.06
▶ Opticrom (Sanofi)
Sodium cromoglicate 20 mg per 1 ml Opticrom Allergy 2% eye drops | 5 ml [P] £2.74 | 10 ml [P] £3.35
Opticrom Aqueous 2% eye drops | 13.5 ml [PoM] £8.03 DT price = £2.06
▶ Optrex Allergy (Reckitt Benckiser Healthcare (UK) Ltd)
Sodium cromoglicate 20 mg per 1 ml Optrex Allergy 2% eye drops | 10 ml [P] £3.88
▶ Pollenase (sodium cromoglicate) (E M Pharma)
Sodium cromoglicate 20 mg per 1 ml Pollenase Allergy 2% eye drops | 10 ml [P] £2.08
▶ Vividrin (Bausch & Lomb UK Ltd)
Sodium cromoglicate 20 mg per 1 ml Vividrin 2% eye drops | 13.5 ml [PoM] £10.95 DT price = £2.06

11

Eye

1.2 Inflammatory eye conditions

ANALGESICS > NON-STEROIDAL ANTI-INFLAMMATORY DRUGS

Nepafenac

- **INDICATIONS AND DOSE**

Prophylaxis and treatment of postoperative pain and inflammation associated with cataract surgery | Reduction in the risk of postoperative macular oedema associated with cataract surgery in diabetic patients

- ▸ TO THE EYE
- ▸ Adult: (consult product literature)

- CAUTIONS Avoid sunlight · corneal epithelial breakdown (if evidence of, then discontinue immediately)

- SIDE-EFFECTS
- ▸ **Common or very common** Punctate keratitis
- ▸ **Uncommon** Allergic conjunctivitis · blurred vision · choroidal effusion · conjunctival hyperaemia · corneal deposits · corneal epithelium defect · dry eye · eye pruritus · headache · increased lacrimation · iritis · keratitis · nausea · ocular discomfort · photophobia
- ▸ **Frequency not known** Corneal opacity · dermatochalasis · dizziness · eye swelling · impaired corneal healing · reduced visual acuity

- MEDICINAL FORMS
There can be variation in the licensing of different medicines containing the same drug.
Eye drops
EXCIPIENTS: May contain Benzalkonium chloride, disodium edetate
- ▹ Nevanac (Alcon Laboratories (UK) Ltd)
  Nepafenac 1 mg per 1 ml Nevanac 1mg/ml eye drops | 5 ml PoM £14.92

CORTICOSTEROIDS

Betamethasone

- **INDICATIONS AND DOSE**

Local treatment of inflammation (short term)

- ▸ TO THE EYE USING EYE DROP
- ▸ Child: Apply every 1–2 hours until controlled then reduce frequency
- ▸ Adult: Apply every 1–2 hours until controlled then reduce frequency
- ▸ TO THE EYE USING EYE OINTMENT
- ▸ Child: Apply 2–4 times a day, alternatively apply at night when used in combination with eye drops
- ▸ Adult: Apply 2–4 times a day, alternatively apply at night when used in combination with eye drops

- SIDE-EFFECTS Corneal thinning · scleral thinning

- MEDICINAL FORMS
There can be variation in the licensing of different medicines containing the same drug.
Ear/eye/nose drops solution
EXCIPIENTS: May contain Benzalkonium chloride, disodium edetate
- ▹ Betamethasone (Non-proprietary)
  Betamethasone sodium phosphate 1 mg per 1 ml Betamethasone 0.1% ear/eye/nose drops | 5 ml PoM no price available
- ▹ Betnesol (Focus Pharmaceuticals Ltd)
  Betamethasone sodium phosphate 1 mg per 1 ml Betnesol 0.1% eye/ear/nose drops | 10 ml PoM £2.32 DT price = £2.32
- ▹ Vistamethasone (Martindale Pharmaceuticals Ltd)
  Betamethasone sodium phosphate 1 mg per 1 ml Vistamethasone 0.1% ear/eye/nose drops | 5 ml PoM £0.87 | 10 ml PoM £0.99 DT price = £2.32

Eye ointment
- ▸ Betnesol (Focus Pharmaceuticals Ltd)
  Betamethasone sodium phosphate 1 mg per 1 gram Betnesol 0.1% eye ointment | 3 gram PoM £1.41 DT price = £1.41

Combinations available: *Betamethasone with neomycin,* p. 1010

Dexamethasone

- **INDICATIONS AND DOSE**

Local treatment of inflammation (short-term)

- ▸ TO THE EYE USING EYE DROP
- ▸ Child: Apply 4–6 times a day
- ▸ Adult: Apply every 30–60 minutes until controlled, then reduced to 4–6 times a day

Short term local treatment of inflammation (severe conditions)

- ▸ TO THE EYE USING EYE DROP
- ▸ Child: Apply every 30–60 minutes until controlled, reduce frequency when control achieved

Macular oedema following either branch retinal vein occlusion or central retinal vein occlusion (specialist use only) | Visual impairment due to diabetic macular oedema in adults who are pseudophakic, or who are insufficiently responsive to, or unsuitable for non-corticosteroid therapy (specialist use only) | For the treatment of inflammation of the posterior segment of the eye presenting as non-infectious uveitis (specialist use only)

- ▸ BY INTRAVITREAL INJECTION
- ▸ Adult: 700 micrograms, to be administered into the affected eye, concurrent administration to both eyes not recommended. For further information on pre-treatment, administration and repeat dosing, consult product literature

- UNLICENSED USE *Maxidex*® not licensed for use in children under 2 years. *Dropodex*® not licensed for use in children.

- CONTRA-INDICATIONS
- ▸ With intravitreal use Active ocular herpes simplex · active or suspected ocular infection · active or suspected periocular infection · rupture of the posterior lens capsule in patients with aphakia, iris or transscleral fixated intra-ocular lens or anterior chamber intra-ocular lens · uncontrolled advanced glaucoma

- CAUTIONS
- ▸ With intravitreal use History of ocular viral infection (including herpes simplex) · posterior capsule tear or iris defect (risk of implant migration into the anterior chamber which may cause corneal oedema and, in persistent severe cases, the need for corneal transplantation) · retinal vein occlusion with significant retinal ischaemia

- INTERACTIONS
- ▸ With intravitreal use in adults Caution with concomitant administration of anticoagulant or antiplatelet drugs—increased risk of haemorrhagic events.

- SIDE-EFFECTS
- ▸ **Uncommon**
- ▸ With intravitreal use Eyelid pruritus · glaucoma · migraine · necrotising retinitis
- ▸ **Frequency not known**
- ▸ When used by eye Corneal thinning · scleral thinning
- ▸ With intravitreal use Blepharitis · cataract · headache · ocular hypertension · raised intra-ocular pressure · secondary ocular infection · visual disturbance

- PREGNANCY
- ▸ With intravitreal use Manufacturer advises avoid unless potential benefit outweighs risk—no information available.

- BREAST FEEDING
▸ With intravitreal use Manufacturer advises avoid unless potential benefit outweighs risk—no information available.
- MONITORING REQUIREMENTS
▸ With intravitreal use Monitor intra-ocular pressure and for signs of ocular infection. In patients with posterior capsule tear or iris defect monitor for implant migration to allow for; early diagnosis and management.
- PRESCRIBING AND DISPENSING INFORMATION Although multi-dose Dexamethasone eye drops commonly contain preservatives, preservative-free unit dose vials may be available.
- NATIONAL FUNDING/ACCESS DECISIONS

NICE technology appraisals (TAs)
▸ Dexamethasone intravitreal implant for the treatment of macular oedema secondary to retinal vein occlusion (July 2011) NICE TA229
▸ With intravitreal use Dexamethasone intravitreal implant is recommended as an option for the treatment of macular oedema following central retinal vein occlusion. Dexamethasone intravitreal implant is also recommended as an option for the treatment of macular oedema following branch retinal vein occlusion when:
  - treatment with laser photocoagulation has not been beneficial, or
  - treatment with laser photocoagulation is not considered suitable because of the extent of macular haemorrhage.
  www.nice.org.uk/TA229
▸ Dexamethasone intravitreal implant for treating diabetic macular oedema (July 2015) NICE TA349
▸ With intravitreal use Dexamethasone intravitreal implant is recommended as an option for treating diabetic macular oedema only if:
  - the implant is to be used in an eye with an intraocular (pseudophakic) lens and
  - the diabetic macular oedema does not respond to non-corticosteroid treatment, or such treatment is unsuitable.
  www.nice.org.uk/TA349

Scottish Medicines Consortium (SMC) Decisions
▸ With intravitreal use The *Scottish Medicines Consortium* has advised (May 2012) that dexamethasone intravitreal implant (*Ozurdex* ®) is accepted for restricted use within NHS Scotland for the treatment of adults with macular oedema (i) following central retinal vein occlusion, and (ii) with branch retinal vein occlusion who are not clinically suitable for laser treatment, including patients with dense macular haemorrhage, or patients who have received and failed on previous laser treatment.

- MEDICINAL FORMS
There can be variation in the licensing of different medicines containing the same drug. Forms available from special-order manufacturers include: eye drops
Eye drops
EXCIPIENTS: May contain Benzalkonium chloride, disodium edetate, polysorbates
▸ Dexamethasone (Non-proprietary)
  Dexamethasone sodium phosphate 1 mg per 1 ml Dexamethasone 0.1% eye drops 0.4ml unit dose preservative free | 20 unit dose [PoM] £9.75 DT price = £9.75
  Minims dexamethasone 0.1% eye drops 0.5ml unit dose | 20 unit dose [PoM] £11.46 DT price = £11.46
▸ Dexafree (Thea Pharmaceuticals Ltd)
  Dexamethasone sodium phosphate 1 mg per 1 ml Dexafree 1mg/1ml eye drops 0.4ml unit dose | 30 unit dose [PoM] £9.70
▸ Dropodex (Moorfields Pharmaceuticals)
  Dexamethasone sodium phosphate 1 mg per 1 ml Dropodex 0.1% eye drops 0.4ml unit dose | 20 unit dose [PoM] £9.75 DT price = £9.75
▸ Maxidex (Alcon Laboratories (UK) Ltd)
  Dexamethasone 1 mg per 1 ml Maxidex 0.1% eye drops | 5 ml [PoM] £1.42 DT price = £1.42 | 10 ml [PoM] £2.80 DT price = £2.80

Implant
▸ Ozurdex (Allergan Ltd)
  Dexamethasone 700 microgram Ozurdex 700microgram intravitreal implant in applicator | 1 device [PoM] £870.00 (Hospital only)

Combinations available: *Dexamethasone with framycetin sulfate and gramicidin*, p. 1010 · *Dexamethasone with hypromellose, neomycin and polymyxin B sulfate*, p. 1010 · *Dexamethasone with tobramycin*, p. 1011

Fluorometholone

- INDICATIONS AND DOSE
Local treatment of inflammation (short term)
▸ TO THE EYE
▸ Child 2-17 years: Apply every 1 hour for 24–48 hours, then reduced to 2–4 times a day
▸ Adult: Apply every 1 hour for 24–48 hours, then reduced to 2–4 times a day

- UNLICENSED USE Not licensed for use in children under 2 years.
- SIDE-EFFECTS Corneal thinning · scleral thinning

- MEDICINAL FORMS
There can be variation in the licensing of different medicines containing the same drug.
Eye drops
EXCIPIENTS: May contain Benzalkonium chloride, disodium edetate, polysorbates
▸ FML Liquifilm (Allergan Ltd)
  Fluorometholone 1 mg per 1 ml FML Liquifilm 0.1% ophthalmic suspension | 5 ml [PoM] £1.71 DT price = £1.71 | 10 ml [PoM] £2.95 DT price = £2.95

Prednisolone

- INDICATIONS AND DOSE
Local treatment of inflammation (short-term)
▸ TO THE EYE
▸ Child: Apply every 1–2 hours until controlled then reduce frequency
▸ Adult: Apply every 1–2 hours until controlled then reduce frequency

- UNLICENSED USE *Pred Forte* ® not licensed for use in children (age range not specified by manufacturer).
- SIDE-EFFECTS Corneal thinning · scleral thinning
- PRESCRIBING AND DISPENSING INFORMATION Although multi-dose prednisolone eye drops commonly contain preservatives, preservative-free unit dose vials may be available.

- MEDICINAL FORMS
There can be variation in the licensing of different medicines containing the same drug. Forms available from special-order manufacturers include: eye drops
Ear/eye drops solution
EXCIPIENTS: May contain Benzalkonium chloride, disodium edetate
▸ Predsol (Focus Pharmaceuticals Ltd)
  Prednisolone sodium phosphate 5 mg per 1 ml Predsol 0.5% ear/eye drops | 10 ml [PoM] £2.00 DT price = £2.00
Eye drops
EXCIPIENTS: May contain Benzalkonium chloride, disodium edetate, polysorbates
▸ Prednisolone (Non-proprietary)
  Prednisolone sodium phosphate 300 microgram per 1 ml Prednisolone sodium phosphate 0.03% eye drops preservative free | 10 ml [PoM] £34.24 DT price = £34.24
  Prednisolone sodium phosphate 1 mg per 1 ml Prednisolone sodium phosphate 0.1% eye drops preservative free | 10 ml [PoM] £27.10 DT price = £27.10

11

Eye

Prednisolone sodium phosphate 3 mg per 1 ml Prednisolone
sodium phosphate 0.3% eye drops preservative free | 10 ml PoM
£22.53 DT price = £22.53

Prednisolone sodium phosphate 5 mg per 1 ml Minims
prednisolone sodium phosphate 0.5% eye drops 0.5ml unit dose |
20 unit dose PoM £11.78 DT price = £11.78

▸ Pred Forte (Allergan Ltd)

Prednisolone acetate 10 mg per 1 ml Pred Forte 1% eye drops |
5 ml PoM £1.82 DT price = £1.82 | 10 ml PoM £3.66 DT price =
£3.66

Rimexolone

- **INDICATIONS AND DOSE**

**Local treatment of postoperative inflammation (short
term use)**

▸ TO THE EYE

▸ Adult: Apply 4 times a day for 2 weeks, treatment to
begin 24 hours after surgery

**Local treatment of steroid-responsive inflammation
(short term use)**

▸ TO THE EYE

▸ Adult: Apply in at least 4 times a day divided doses for
up to 4 weeks

Uveitis (short term use)

▸ TO THE EYE

▸ Adult: Apply every 1 hour during the day time for week
1, then apply every 2 hours for week 2, then apply
4 times a day for week 3, then apply twice daily for the
first 4 days of week 4, then apply once daily for the
remaining 3 days of week 4

- **SIDE-EFFECTS** Corneal thinning · scleral thinning

- **MEDICINAL FORMS**
There can be variation in the licensing of different medicines
containing the same drug.
No licensed medicines listed.

CORTICOSTEROIDS > CORTICOSTEROID
COMBINATIONS WITH ANTI-INFECTIVES

Betamethasone with neomycin

The properties listed below are those particular to the
combination only. For the properties of the components
please consider, betamethasone p. 1008.

- **INDICATIONS AND DOSE**

**Local treatment of eye inflammation and bacterial
infection (short-term)**

▸ TO THE EYE USING EYE DROP

▸ Adult: Apply up to 6 times a day

- **LESS SUITABLE FOR PRESCRIBING** Betamethasone with
neomycin eye-drops are less suitable for prescribing.

- **MEDICINAL FORMS**
There can be variation in the licensing of different medicines
containing the same drug.
Ear/eye/nose drops solution
EXCIPIENTS: May contain Benzalkonium chloride, disodium edetate
▸ Betnesol-N (Focus Pharmaceuticals Ltd)
**Betamethasone (as Betamethasone sodium phosphate) 1 mg per
1 ml, Neomycin sulfate 5 mg per 1 ml** Betnesol-N ear/eye/nose
drops | 10 ml PoM £2.39 DT price = £2.39

Dexamethasone with framycetin sulfate and gramicidin

The properties listed below are those particular to the
combination only. For the properties of the components
please consider, dexamethasone p. 1008.

- **INDICATIONS AND DOSE**

Local treatment of inflammation (short-term)

▸ TO THE EYE

▸ Child: Apply 4–6 times a day, may be administered
every 30–60 minutes in severe conditions until
controlled, then reduce frequency

▸ Adult: Apply 4–6 times a day, may be administered
every 30–60 minutes in severe conditions until
controlled, then reduce frequency

- **LESS SUITABLE FOR PRESCRIBING** *Sofradex*® is less
suitable for prescribing.

- **MEDICINAL FORMS**
There can be variation in the licensing of different medicines
containing the same drug.
Ear/eye drops solution
EXCIPIENTS: May contain Polysorbates
▸ Sofradex (Sanofi)
**Gramicidin 50 microgram per 1 ml, Dexamethasone (as
Dexamethasone sodium metasulfobenzoate) 500 microgram per
1 ml, Framycetin sulfate 5 mg per 1 ml** Sofradex ear/eye drops |
10 ml PoM £7.50

Dexamethasone with hypromellose, neomycin and polymyxin B sulfate

The properties listed below are those particular to the
combination only. For the properties of the components
please consider, dexamethasone p. 1008.

- **INDICATIONS AND DOSE**

Local treatment of inflammation (short-term)

▸ TO THE EYE USING EYE DROP

▸ Adult: Apply every 30–60 minutes until controlled,
then reduced to 4–6 times a day

Local treatment of inflammation (short-term)

▸ TO THE EYE USING EYE OINTMENT

▸ Adult: Apply 3–4 times a day, alternatively, apply at
night when used with eye drops

- **LESS SUITABLE FOR PRESCRIBING** Dexamethasone with
neomycin and polymixin B sulfate is less suitable for
prescribing.

- **MEDICINAL FORMS**
There can be variation in the licensing of different medicines
containing the same drug.
Eye drops
EXCIPIENTS: May contain Benzalkonium chloride, polysorbates
▸ Maxitrol (Alcon Laboratories (UK) Ltd)
**Dexamethasone 1 mg per 1 ml, Neomycin (as Neomycin sulfate)
3.5 mg per 1 ml, Hypromellose 5 mg per 1 ml, Polymyxin B sulfate
6000 unit per 1 ml** Maxitrol eye drops | 5 ml PoM £1.68
Eye ointment
EXCIPIENTS: May contain Hydroxybenzoates (parabens), wool fat and
related substances including lanolin
▸ Maxitrol (Alcon Laboratories (UK) Ltd)
**Dexamethasone 1 mg per 1 gram, Neomycin (as Neomycin
sulfate) 3500 unit per 1 gram, Polymyxin B sulfate 6000 unit per
1 gram** Maxitrol eye ointment | 3.5 gram PoM £1.44

Dexamethasone with tobramycin

The properties listed below are those particular to the combination only. For the properties of the components please consider, dexamethasone p. 1008.

● **INDICATIONS AND DOSE**

Local treatment of inflammation (short-term)
▶ TO THE EYE
▶ Adult: (consult product literature)

● **LESS SUITABLE FOR PRESCRIBING** Dexamethasone with tobramycin eye-drops are less suitable for prescribing.

● **MEDICINAL FORMS**
There can be variation in the licensing of different medicines containing the same drug.
Eye drops
EXCIPIENTS: May contain Benzalkonium chloride, disodium edetate
▶ Tobradex (Alcon Laboratories (UK) Ltd)
   Dexamethasone 1 mg per 1 ml, Tobramycin 3 mg per 1 ml Tobradex 3mg/ml / 1mg/ml eye drops | 5 ml [PoM] £5.37 DT price = £5.37

1.2a Anterior uveitis

ANTIMUSCARINICS

Antimuscarinics (eye) 🔲

● CAUTIONS Children under 3 months owing to the possible association between cycloplegia and the development of amblyopia (in children) · darkly pigmented iris is more resistant to pupillary dilatation and caution should be exercised to avoid overdosage · mydriasis can precipitate acute angle-closure glaucoma (usually in those aged over 60 years and hypermetropic (long-sighted), who are predisposed to the condition because of a shallow anterior chamber) (in adults) · mydriasis can precipitate acute angle-closure glaucoma (usually in those who are predisposed to the condition because of a shallow anterior chamber) (in children)

● SIDE-EFFECTS Conjunctivitis (on prolonged administration) · contact dermatitis · eye oedema (on prolonged administration) · hyperaemia (on prolonged administration) · local irritation (on prolonged administration) · raised intraocular pressure · transient stinging

● PATIENT AND CARER ADVICE Patients may not be able to undertake skilled tasks until vision clears after mydriasis.

◄ above

Atropine sulfate

● **INDICATIONS AND DOSE**

Cycloplegia
▶ TO THE EYE USING EYE DROP
▶ Adult: (consult product literature)

Anterior uveitis
▶ TO THE EYE USING EYE DROP
▶ Adult: (consult product literature)

● SIDE-EFFECTS Systemic side-effects can occur, particularly in children and the elderly.

● PRESCRIBING AND DISPENSING INFORMATION Although multi-dose atropine sulfate eye drops commonly contain preservatives, preservative-free unit dose vials may be available.

● MEDICINAL FORMS
There can be variation in the licensing of different medicines containing the same drug. Forms available from special-order manufacturers include: eye drops
Eye drops
▶ Atropine sulfate (Non-proprietary)
   Atropine sulfate 10 mg per 1 ml Atropine 1% eye drops | 10 ml [PoM] £41.99 DT price = £35.15
▶ Atropine sulfate (Bausch & Lomb UK Ltd)
   Atropine sulfate 10 mg per 1 ml Minims atropine sulfate 1% eye drops 0.5ml unit dose | 20 unit dose [PoM] £15.10 DT price = £15.10

◄ above

Cyclopentolate hydrochloride

● **INDICATIONS AND DOSE**

Cycloplegia
▶ TO THE EYE
▶ Child 3 months-11 years: Apply 1 drop, 30–60 minutes before examination, using 1% eye drops
▶ Child 12-17 years: Apply 1 drop, 30–60 minutes before examination, using 0.5% eye drops

Uveitis
▶ TO THE EYE
▶ Child 3 months-17 years: Apply 1 drop 2–4 times a day, using 0.5% eye drops (1% for deeply pigmented eyes)

Anterior uveitis | Cycloplegia
▶ TO THE EYE
▶ Adult: (consult product literature)

● SIDE-EFFECTS

SIDE-EFFECTS, FURTHER INFORMATION
Toxic systemic reactions can occur in neonates and children. Systemic side-effects can occur, particularly in children and the elderly.

● PRESCRIBING AND DISPENSING INFORMATION Although multi-dose cyclopentolate eye drops commonly contain preservatives, preservative-free unit dose vials may be available.

● MEDICINAL FORMS
There can be variation in the licensing of different medicines containing the same drug.
Eye drops
EXCIPIENTS: May contain Benzalkonium chloride
▶ Cyclopentolate hydrochloride (Bausch & Lomb UK Ltd)
   Cyclopentolate hydrochloride 5 mg per 1 ml Minims cyclopentolate hydrochloride 0.5% eye drops 0.5ml unit dose | 20 unit dose [PoM] £10.97 DT price = £10.97
   Cyclopentolate hydrochloride 10 mg per 1 ml Minims cyclopentolate hydrochloride 1% eye drops 0.5ml unit dose | 20 unit dose [PoM] £11.23 DT price = £11.23
▶ Mydrilate (Intrapharm Laboratories Ltd)
   Cyclopentolate hydrochloride 5 mg per 1 ml Mydrilate 0.5% solution | 5 ml [PoM] £6.73 DT price = £6.73
   Cyclopentolate hydrochloride 10 mg per 1 ml Mydrilate 1% solution | 5 ml [PoM] £6.73 DT price = £6.73

◄ above

Homatropine hydrobromide

● **INDICATIONS AND DOSE**

Anterior uveitis
▶ TO THE EYE
▶ Adult: (consult product literature)

● MEDICINAL FORMS
There can be variation in the licensing of different medicines containing the same drug. Forms available from special-order manufacturers include: eye drops

11

Eye

2 Dry eye conditions

Dry eye

Tear deficiency, ocular lubricants, and astringents

Chronic soreness of the eyes associated with reduced or abnormal tear secretion (e.g. in Sjögren's syndrome) often responds to tear replacement therapy or pilocarpine p. 1051 given by mouth in adults. The severity of the condition and patient preference will often guide the choice of preparation.

Hypromellose p. 1013 is the traditional choice of treatment for tear deficiency. It may need to be instilled frequently (e.g. hourly) for adequate relief. Ocular surface mucin is often abnormal in tear deficiency and the combination of hypromellose with a mucolytic such as acetylcysteine below can be helpful.

The ability of **carbomers** to cling to the eye surface may help reduce frequency of application to 4 times daily.

Polyvinyl alcohol p. 1014 increases the persistence of the tear film and is useful when the ocular surface mucin is reduced.

Sodium hyaluronate eye drops p. 1015 are also used in the management of tear deficiency.

Sodium chloride 0.9% drops p. 1014 are sometimes useful in tear deficiency, and can be used as 'comfort drops' by contact lens wearers, and to facilitate lens removal. They are also used to irrigate the eye. Special presentations of sodium chloride 0.9% and other irrigation solutions are used routinely for intra-ocular surgery. Sodium chloride 5% eye drops are used for the short-term treatment of corneal oedema in adults.

Eye ointments containing a paraffin can be used to lubricate the eye surface, especially in cases of recurrent corneal epithelial erosion. They may cause temporary visual disturbance and are best suited for application before sleep. Ointments should not be used during contact lens wear.

OCULAR LUBRICANTS

Acetylcysteine

● INDICATIONS AND DOSE

Tear deficiency | Impaired or abnormal mucus production
▸ TO THE EYE
▸ Adult: Apply 3–4 times a day

● MEDICINAL FORMS
There can be variation in the licensing of different medicines containing the same drug. Forms available from special-order manufacturers include: eye drops

Eye drops
EXCIPIENTS: May contain Benzalkonium chloride, disodium edetate
▸ Ilube (Moorfields Pharmaceuticals)
Acetylcysteine 50 mg per 1 ml Ilube 5% eye drops | 10 ml [PoM]
£14.93 DT price = £14.93

Carbomers

(Polyacrylic acid)

● INDICATIONS AND DOSE

Dry eyes including keratoconjunctivitis sicca, unstable tear film
▸ TO THE EYE
▸ Child: Apply 3–4 times a day or when required
▸ Adult: Apply 3–4 times a day or when required

● UNLICENSED USE Some preparations not licensed for use in children.

● PRESCRIBING AND DISPENSING INFORMATION Synthetic high molecular weight polymers of acrylic acid cross-linked with either allyl ethers of sucrose or allyl ethers of pentaerithrityl.

● MEDICINAL FORMS
There can be variation in the licensing of different medicines containing the same drug.
Eye drops
▸ Carbomers (Non-proprietary)
Carbomer 980 2 mg per 1 gram Carbomer '980' 0.2% eye drops | 10 gram [P] £2.80 DT price = £2.80
Carbomer 0.2% eye gel | 10 gram £2.80 DT price = £2.80
▸ Artelac Nighttime (Bausch & Lomb UK Ltd)
Carbomer 980 2 mg per 1 gram Artelac Nighttime 0.2% eye gel | 10 gram £2.96 DT price = £2.80
▸ Clinitas Carbomer (Altacor Ltd)
Carbomer 980 2 mg per 1 gram Clinitas Carbomer 0.2% eye gel | 10 gram £1.49 DT price = £2.80
▸ GelTears (Bausch & Lomb UK Ltd)
Carbomer 980 2 mg per 1 gram GelTears 0.2% gel | 10 gram [P] £2.80 DT price = £2.80
▸ Lumecare Long Lasting (Medicom Healthcare Ltd)
Carbomer 980 2 mg per 1 gram Lumecare Carbomer 0.2% eye gel | 10 gram £1.51 DT price = £2.80
▸ Viscotears (Alcon Laboratories (UK) Ltd)
Carbomer 980 2 mg per 1 gram Viscotears 2mg/g liquid gel | 10 gram [P] £1.59 DT price = £2.80
Viscotears 2mg/g eye gel 0.6ml unit dose | 30 unit dose [P] £5.42
▸ Xailin (Nicox Pharma)
Carbomer 980 2 mg per 1 gram Xailin 0.2% eye gel | 10 gram £3.25 DT price = £2.80
Eye gel
EXCIPIENTS: May contain Benzalkonium chloride, cetrimide, disodium edetate
▸ Blephagel (Thea Pharmaceuticals Ltd)
Carbomer 3.5 mg per 1 gram Blephagel 0.35% eye gel | 40 gram £6.66
Carbomer 3.6 mg per 1 gram Blephagel 0.36% eye gel preservative free | 30 gram £7.53
▸ Liquivisc (Thea Pharmaceuticals Ltd)
Carbomer 974P 2.5 mg per 1 gram Liquivisc 0.25% eye gel | 10 gram [P] £4.50 DT price = £4.50

Carmellose sodium

● INDICATIONS AND DOSE

Dry eye conditions
▸ TO THE EYE
▸ Child: Apply as required
▸ Adult: Apply as required

● PRESCRIBING AND DISPENSING INFORMATION Some preparations are contained units which are resealable and may be used for up to 12 hours.

● MEDICINAL FORMS
There can be variation in the licensing of different medicines containing the same drug.
Eye drops
▸ Carmellose sodium (Non-proprietary)
Carmellose sodium 5 mg per 1 ml Carmellose 0.5% eye drops 0.4ml unit dose preservative free | 30 unit dose [P] no price available DT price = £4.80 | 30 unit dose £5.75 DT price = £4.80 | 90 unit dose [P] no price available
Carmellose 0.5% eye drops | 10 ml £7.49
Carmellose 1% eye drops 0.4ml unit dose preservative free | 30 unit dose [PoM] no price available DT price = £3.00 | 30 unit dose £3.00 DT price = £3.00 | 30 unit dose [P] no price available DT price = £3.00 | 60 unit dose [P] no price available
▸ Carmeleze (Martindale Pharmaceuticals Ltd)
Carmellose sodium 5 mg per 1 ml Melophthal 0.5% eye drops 0.4ml unit dose | 30 unit dose £5.75 DT price = £4.80
Melophthal 1% eye drops 0.4ml unit dose | 30 unit dose £3.00 DT price = £3.00

11

Eye

Carmellose sodium 5 mg per 1 ml Carmize 0.5% eye drops 0.4ml unit dose preservative free | 30 unit dose £5.75 DT price = £4.80 | 90 unit dose £15.53
▸ Carmize (Aspire Pharma Ltd)
Carmellose sodium 5 mg per 1 ml Carmize 0.5% eye drops 0.4ml unit dose preservative free | 30 unit dose £5.75 DT price = £4.80 | 90 unit dose £15.53
Carmize 1% eye drops | 10 ml £8.49
Carmize 1% eye drops 0.4ml unit dose preservative free | 30 unit dose £3.00 DT price = £3.00 | 60 unit dose £6.00
Carmize 0.5% eye drops | 10 ml £7.49
▸ Cellusan (Farmigea S.p.A.)
Carmellose sodium 5 mg per 1 ml Cellusan Light 0.5% eye drops 0.4ml unit dose preservative free | 30 unit dose £5.75 DT price = £4.80
Cellusan 1% eye drops preservative free | 10 ml £4.80
Cellusan Light 0.5% eye drops preservative free | 10 ml £4.80
Cellusan 1% eye drops 0.4ml unit dose preservative free | 30 unit dose £3.00 DT price = £3.00
▸ Celluvisc (Allergan Ltd)
Carmellose sodium 5 mg per 1 ml Celluvisc 0.5% eye drops 0.4ml unit dose | 30 unit dose P £4.80 DT price = £4.80 | 90 unit dose P £15.53
Celluvisc 1% eye drops 0.4ml unit dose | 30 unit dose P £3.00 DT price = £3.00 | 60 unit dose P £10.99
▸ Lumecare (Carmellose) (Medicom Healthcare Ltd)
Carmellose sodium 5 mg per 1 ml Lumecare Singles Carmellose 0.5% eye drops 0.4ml unit dose | 30 unit dose £4.60 DT price = £4.80
Lumecare Advance Carmellose 0.5% eye drops | 10 ml £5.99
▸ Optive (Allergan Ltd)
Optive 0.5% eye drops | 10 ml £7.49
▸ Optive Plus (Allergan Ltd)
Optive Plus 0.5% eye drops | 10 ml £7.49
▸ Xailin Fresh (Nicox Pharma)
Carmellose sodium 5 mg per 1 ml Xailin Fresh 0.5% eye drops 0.4ml unit dose | 30 unit dose £3.84 DT price = £4.80

Hydroxyethylcellulose

● **INDICATIONS AND DOSE**

Tear deficiency
▸ TO THE EYE
▸ Child: Apply as required
▸ Adult: Apply as required

● PRESCRIBING AND DISPENSING INFORMATION Although multi-dose hydroxyethylcellulose eye drops commonly contain preservatives, preservative-free unit dose vials may be available.

● MEDICINAL FORMS
There can be variation in the licensing of different medicines containing the same drug.
Eye drops
▸ Artificial tears (Bausch & Lomb UK Ltd)
Hydroxyethylcellulose 4.4 mg per 1 ml Minims artificial tears 0.44% eye drops 0.5ml unit dose | 20 unit dose P £8.97

Hydroxypropyl guar with polyethylene glycol and propylene glycol

(Formulated as an ocular lubricant)

● **INDICATIONS AND DOSE**

Dry eye conditions
▸ TO THE EYE
▸ Child: Apply as required
▸ Adult: Apply as required

● MEDICINAL FORMS
There can be variation in the licensing of different medicines containing the same drug.
Eye drops
▸ Systane (Alcon Laboratories (UK) Ltd)
Systane Gel eye drops | 10 ml £7.49

Hypromellose

● **INDICATIONS AND DOSE**

Tear deficiency
▸ TO THE EYE
▸ Child: Apply as required
▸ Adult: Apply as required

● PRESCRIBING AND DISPENSING INFORMATION The Royal Pharmaceutical Society has stated that where it is not possible to ascertain the strength of hypromellose prescribed, the prescriber should be contacted to clarify the strength intended.
    Although multi-dose hypromellose eye drops commonly contain preservatives, preservative-free unit dose vials may be available.

● MEDICINAL FORMS
There can be variation in the licensing of different medicines containing the same drug. Forms available from special-order manufacturers include: eye drops
Eye drops
EXCIPIENTS: May contain Benzalkonium chloride, cetrimide, disodium edetate
▸ Hypromellose (Non-proprietary)
Hypromellose 2.5 mg per 1 ml Hypromellose 0.25% eye drops preservative free | 10 ml PoM £14.24 DT price = £14.24
Hypromellose 3 mg per 1 ml Hypromellose 0.3% eye drops preservative free | 10 ml £5.75
▸ Artelac (Bausch & Lomb UK Ltd)
Hypromellose 3.2 mg per 1 ml Artelac Single Dose Unit 0.32% eye drops 0.5ml unit dose | 30 unit dose P £16.95 | 60 unit dose P £32.85
Artelac 0.32% eye drops | 10 ml P £4.99
▸ Brolene Cool (Sanofi)
Hypromellose 3 mg per 1 ml Brolene Cool Eyes 0.3% eye drops | 10 ml GSL £2.38 DT price = £0.99
▸ Hydromoor (Moorfields Pharmaceuticals)
Hydromoor 0.3% eye drops 0.4ml unit dose preservative free | 30 unit dose £5.75
▸ Hypromellose (Moorfields Pharmaceuticals)
Hypromellose 3 mg per 1 ml PF Drops Hypromellose 0.3% eye drops preservative free | 10 ml £5.75
▸ Hypromol (Ennogen Healthcare Ltd)
Hypromellose 3 mg per 1 ml Hypromol 0.3% eye drops preservative free | 10 ml £4.55
▸ Isopto Alkaline (Alcon Laboratories (UK) Ltd)
Hypromellose 10 mg per 1 ml Isopto Alkaline 1% eye drops | 10 ml P £0.94 DT price = £0.94
▸ Isopto Plain (Alcon Laboratories (UK) Ltd)
Hypromellose 5 mg per 1 ml Isopto Plain 0.5% eye drops | 10 ml P £0.81 DT price = £0.81
▸ Lumecare (Hypromellose) (Medicom Healthcare Ltd)
Hypromellose 3 mg per 1 ml Lumecare Hypromellose 0.3% eye drops | 10 ml £1.67 DT price = £0.99
▸ Lumecare Tear Drops (Medicom Healthcare Ltd)
Hypromellose 3 mg per 1 ml Lumecare Tear Drops 0.3% eye drops | 10 ml £0.95 DT price = £0.99
▸ Mandanol (Hydroxypropyl methylcellulose) (M & A Pharmachem Ltd)
Hypromellose 3 mg per 1 ml Mandanol eye drops | 10 ml £1.33 DT price = £0.99
▸ Ocu-Lube (Sai-Meds Ltd)
Hypromellose 3 mg per 1 ml Ocu-Lube 0.3% eye drops preservative free | 10 ml £5.75
▸ SoftDrops (Farmigea S.p.A.)
Hypromellose 3 mg per 1 ml SoftDrops 0.3% eye drops | 10 ml £1.67 DT price = £0.99
▸ Tear-Lac (Scope Ophthalmics Ltd)
Hypromellose 3 mg per 1 ml Tear-Lac Hypromellose 0.3% eye drops preservative free | 10 ml £5.75
▸ Xailin Hydrate (Nicox Pharma)
Hypromellose 3 mg per 1 ml Xailin Hydrate 0.3% eye drops preservative free | 10 ml £4.60

11

Eye

Hypromellose with dextran 70

The properties listed below are those particular to the combination only. For the properties of the components please consider, hypromellose p. 1013.

● INDICATIONS AND DOSE

Tear deficiency
▸ TO THE EYE
▸ Adult: Apply as required

● MEDICINAL FORMS
There can be variation in the licensing of different medicines containing the same drug.
Eye drops
EXCIPIENTS: May contain Benzalkonium chloride, disodium edetate
▸ Tears Naturale (Alcon Laboratories (UK) Ltd)
Dextran 70 1 mg per 1 ml, Hypromellose 3 mg per 1 ml Tears Naturale eye drops | 15 ml P £1.89
Tears Naturale eye drops 0.4ml unit dose | 28 unit dose P £13.26

Liquid paraffin with white soft paraffin and wool alcohols

● INDICATIONS AND DOSE

Dry eye conditions
▸ TO THE EYE
▸ Child: Apply as required, best suited for application before sleep
▸ Adult: Apply as required, best suited for application before sleep

● PATIENT AND CARER ADVICE May cause temporary visual disturbance. Should not be used during contact lens wear.

● MEDICINAL FORMS
There can be variation in the licensing of different medicines containing the same drug.
Eye ointment
▸ Lacri-Lube (Allergan Ltd)
Wool alcohols 2 mg per 1 gram, Liquid paraffin 425 mg per 1 gram, White soft paraffin 573 mg per 1 gram Lacri-lube eye ointment | 3.5 gram P £2.94 | 5 gram P £3.88

Paraffin, yellow, soft

● INDICATIONS AND DOSE

Eye surface lubrication
▸ TO THE EYE
▸ Child: Apply every 2 hours as required
▸ Adult: Apply every 2 hours as required

● PATIENT AND CARER ADVICE Ophthalmic preparations may cause temporary visual disturbance. Should not be used during contact lens wear.

● MEDICINAL FORMS
There can be variation in the licensing of different medicines containing the same drug.
Eye ointment
▸ Paraffin, yellow, soft (Non-proprietary)
Liquid paraffin 100 mg per 1 gram, Wool fat 100 mg per 1 gram, Yellow soft paraffin 800 mg per 1 gram Simple eye ointment | 4 gram P £6.98 DT price = £5.82

Polyvinyl alcohol

● INDICATIONS AND DOSE

Tear deficiency
▸ TO THE EYE
▸ Child: Apply as required
▸ Adult: Apply as required

● PRESCRIBING AND DISPENSING INFORMATION Although multi-dose polyvinyl alcohol eye drops commonly contain preservatives, preservative-free unit dose vials may be available.

● MEDICINAL FORMS
There can be variation in the licensing of different medicines containing the same drug. Forms available from special-order manufacturers include: eye drops
Eye drops
EXCIPIENTS: May contain Benzalkonium chloride, disodium edetate
▸ Polyvinyl alcohol (Non-proprietary)
Polyvinyl alcohol 14 mg per 1 ml Polyvinyl alcohol 1.4% eye drops 0.4ml unit dose preservative free | 30 unit dose P no price available
Polyvinyl alcohol 1.4% eye drops | 10 ml P no price available | 15 ml P no price available
▸ Liquifilm Tears (Allergan Ltd)
Polyvinyl alcohol 14 mg per 1 ml Liquifilm Tears 1.4% eye drops | 15 ml P £1.93
Liquifilm Tears 1.4% eye drops 0.4ml unit dose preservative free | 30 unit dose P £5.35
▸ PVA (Tubilux Pharma Ltd)
Polyvinyl alcohol 14 mg per 1 ml PVA 1.4% eye drops | 15 ml £1.63
▸ Refresh Ophthalmic (Allergan Ltd)
Polyvinyl alcohol 14 mg per 1 ml Refresh Ophthalmic 1.4% eye drops 0.4ml unit dose | 30 unit dose P £2.25
▸ Sno Tears (Bausch & Lomb UK Ltd)
Polyvinyl alcohol 14 mg per 1 ml Sno Tears 1.4% eye drops | 10 ml P £1.06

Retinol palmitate with white soft paraffin and light liquid paraffin and liquid paraffin and wool fat

(Formulated as an ocular lubricant)

● INDICATIONS AND DOSE

Dry eye conditions
▸ TO THE EYE
▸ Adult: (consult product literature)

● MEDICINAL FORMS
There can be variation in the licensing of different medicines containing the same drug.
Eye ointment
▸ VitA-POS (Scope Ophthalmics Ltd)
VitA-POS eye ointment preservative free | 5 gram £2.75

Sodium chloride

● INDICATIONS AND DOSE

Tear deficiency | Ocular lubricants and astringents | Irrigation, including first-aid removal of harmful substances | Intra-ocular or topical irrigation during surgical procedures
▸ TO THE EYE USING 0.9% SOLUTION
▸ Child: Apply as required
▸ Adult: Apply as required

Corneal oedema
▸ TO THE EYE USING 5% EYE DROPS OR EYE OINTMENT
▸ Child: Consult product literature
▸ Adult: Consult product literature

- **PRESCRIBING AND DISPENSING INFORMATION** Although multi-dose sodium chloride eye drops commonly contain preservatives, preservative-free unit dose vials may be available.

- **MEDICINAL FORMS**
There can be variation in the licensing of different medicines containing the same drug. Forms available from special-order manufacturers include: eye drops, eye ointment

Eye drops
- Sodium chloride (Non-proprietary)
Sodium chloride 50 mg per 1 ml Sodium chloride 5% eye drops | 10 ml £25.25
- Hypersal (Ennogen Healthcare Ltd)
Sodium chloride 50 mg per 1 ml Hypersal 5% eye drops | 10 ml £25.25
- ODM5 (Kestrel Ophthalmics Ltd)
Sodium chloride 50 mg per 1 ml ODM5 5% eye drops preservative free | 10 ml £24.00 DT price = £0.00
- Saline (Bausch & Lomb UK Ltd)
Sodium chloride 9 mg per 1 ml Minims saline 0.9% eye drops 0.5ml unit dose | 20 unit dose P £7.14 DT price = £7.14
- Sodium chloride (Essential Pharmaceuticals Ltd, Moorfields Pharmaceuticals)
Sodium chloride 50 mg per 1 ml NaCl 5% eye drops 0.45ml unit dose preservative free | 20 unit dose £19.70
PF Drops Sodium Chloride 5% eye drops preservative free | 10 ml £25.20 DT price = £0.00

Eye ointment
- Sodium chloride (Non-proprietary)
Sodium chloride 50 mg per 1 ml Sodium chloride 5% eye ointment preservative free | 5 gram £22.50
Sodium chloride 50 mg per 1 gram Muro 128 5% eye ointment | 3.5 gram PoM no price available

Sodium hyaluronate

- **INDICATIONS AND DOSE**
Dry eye conditions
- TO THE EYE
- Adult: Apply as required

- **PRESCRIBING AND DISPENSING INFORMATION** Some preparations are contained in units which are resealable and may be used for up to 12 hours.
Although multi-dose sodium hyaluronate eye drops commonly contain preservatives, preservative-free unit dose vials may be available.

- **MEDICINAL FORMS**
There can be variation in the licensing of different medicines containing the same drug.

Eye drops
- Sodium hyaluronate (Non-proprietary)
Vislube 0.18% eye drops 0.3ml unit dose preservative free | 20 unit dose no price available
- Artelac Rebalance (Bausch & Lomb UK Ltd)
Artelac Rebalance 0.15% eye drops | 10 ml £4.00
- Artelac Splash (Bausch & Lomb UK Ltd)
Artelac Splash 0.2% eye drops 0.5ml unit dose | 30 unit dose £7.00 | 60 unit dose £11.20
- Blink Intensive (AMO UK Ltd)
Blink Intensive Tears 0.2% eye drops 0.4ml unit dose | 20 unit dose £2.97
Blink Intensive Tears 0.2% eye drops | 10 ml £2.97
- Clinitas (Altacor Ltd)
Clinitas Multi 0.4% eye drops preservative free | 10 ml £6.99
Clinitas 0.4% eye drops 0.5ml unit dose | 30 unit dose £5.70
- Evolve HA (Medicom Healthcare Ltd)
Evolve HA 0.2% eye drops preservative free | 10 ml £5.99
- Hy-Opti (Alissa Healthcare Research Ltd)
Hy-Opti 0.1% eye drops preservative free | 10 ml £8.50
Hy-Opti 0.2% eye drops preservative free | 10 ml £9.50
- Hyabak (Thea Pharmaceuticals Ltd)
Hyabak UD 0.15% eye drops 0.4ml unit dose preservative free | 30 unit dose £4.99
Hyabak 0.15% eye drops | 10 ml £7.99

- Hycosan (Scope Ophthalmics Ltd)
Hycosan Extra 0.2% eye drops | 7.5 ml no price available
Hycosan 0.1% eye drops | 7.5 ml no price available
- HydraMed (Farmigea S.p.A.)
HydraMed 0.2% eye drops preservative free | 10 ml £5.60
HydraMed 0.2% eye drops 0.5ml unit dose preservative free | 30 unit dose £5.60
- Hylo-Comod (Scope Ophthalmics Ltd)
Hylo-Tear 0.1% eye drops preservative free | 10 ml £8.50
Hylo-Forte 0.2% eye drops preservative free | 10 ml £9.50
- Hylo-fresh (Scope Ophthalmics Ltd)
Hylo-Fresh 0.03% eye drops preservative free | 10 ml £4.95
- Lubristil (Moorfields Pharmaceuticals)
Lubristil 0.15% eye drops 0.3ml unit dose preservative free | 20 unit dose £4.99
- Ocusan (Agepha Pharma s.r.o.)
Ocusan 0.2% eye drops 0.5ml unit dose | 20 unit dose £5.31
- Optive Fusion (Allergan Ltd)
Optive Fusion 0.1% eye drops | 10 ml £7.49
- Oxyal (Bausch & Lomb UK Ltd)
Oxyal 0.15% eye drops | 10 ml £4.15
- Vismed (TRB Chemidica (UK) Ltd)
Vismed Gel Multi 0.3% eye drops preservative free | 10 ml £7.95
Vismed Multi 0.18% eye drops preservative free | 10 ml £6.81
Vismed 0.18% eye drops 0.3ml unit dose preservative free | 20 unit dose £5.10
- Xailin HA (Nicox Pharma)
Xailin HA 0.2% eye drops preservative free | 10 ml £7.13

Eye gel
- Lubristil (Moorfields Pharmaceuticals)
Lubristil 0.15% eye gel 0.4ml unit dose preservative free | 20 unit dose £6.49
- Vismed (TRB Chemidica (UK) Ltd)
Vismed 0.3% eye gel 0.45ml unit dose preservative free | 20 unit dose £5.98

Soybean oil

- **INDICATIONS AND DOSE**
Dry eye conditions
- TO THE EYE
- Child: Apply up to 4 times a day
- Adult: Apply up to 4 times a day

- **MEDICINAL FORMS**
There can be variation in the licensing of different medicines containing the same drug.

Eye drops
- Emustil (Moorfields Pharmaceuticals)
Emustil eye drops 0.3ml unit dose preservative free | 20 unit dose £6.22

3   Eye infections

Eye, infections of

Eye infections

Most acute superficial eye infections can be treated topically. Blepharitis and conjunctivitis are often caused by staphylococci; keratitis and endophthalmitis may be bacterial, viral, or fungal.

Bacterial *blepharitis* is treated by application of an antibacterial eye ointment to the conjunctival sac or to the lid margins. Systemic treatment may occasionally be required and is usually undertaken after culturing organisms from the lid margin and determining their antimicrobial sensitivity; antibiotics such as the tetracyclines given for 3 months or longer may be appropriate.

Most cases of acute bacterial conjunctivitis are self limiting; where treatment is appropriate, antibacterial eye drops or an eye ointment are used. A poor response might indicate viral or allergic conjunctivitis.

11
Eye

Corneal ulcer and *keratitis* require specialist treatment and may call for hospital admission for intensive therapy.

Endophthalmitis is a medical emergency which also calls for specialist management and requires intravitreal administration of antimicrobials; concomitant systemic treatment is required in some cases. Surgical intervention, such as vitrectomy, is sometimes indicated.

Antibacterials

Bacterial eye infections are generally treated topically with eye drops and eye ointments. Systemic administration is sometimes appropriate in blepharitis.

Chloramphenicol p. 1018 has a broad spectrum of activity and is the drug of choice for *superficial eye infections*. Chloramphenicol eye drops are well tolerated and the recommendation that chloramphenicol eye drops should be avoided because of an increased risk of aplastic anaemia is not well founded.

Other antibacterials with a broad spectrum of activity include the quinolones, ciprofloxacin p. 1017, levofloxacin p. 1018, moxifloxacin p. 1018, and ofloxacin p. 1018; the aminoglycosides, gentamicin below and tobramycin below are also active against a wide variety of bacteria. Gentamicin, tobramycin, quinolones (except moxifloxacin), and **polymyxin B** are effective for infections caused by *Pseudomonas aeruginosa*.

Ciprofloxacin eye drops are licensed for corneal ulcers; intensive application (especially in the first 2 days) is required throughout the day and night.

Azithromycin eye drops p. 1017 are licensed for trachomatous conjunctivitis caused by *Chlamydia trachomatis* and for purulent bacterial conjunctivitis. *Trachoma* which results from chronic infection with *Chlamydia trachomatis* can be treated with azithromycin by mouth [unlicensed indication].

Fusidic acid is useful for staphylococcal infections.

Propamidine isetionate p. 1019 is of little value in bacterial infections but is used by specialists to treat the rare, but potentially sight-threatening, condition of *acanthamoeba keratitis* [unlicensed indication].

Cefuroxime p. 1017 can be administered by intracameral injection for the prophylaxis of endophthalmitis following cataract surgery.

With corticosteroids

Many antibacterial preparations also incorporate a corticosteroid but such mixtures should **not** be used unless a patient is under close specialist supervision. In particular they should not be prescribed for undiagnosed 'red eye' which is sometimes caused by the herpes simplex virus and may be difficult to diagnose.

Administration

Frequency of application depends on the severity of the infection and the potential for irreversible ocular damage; antibacterial eye preparations are usually administered as follows:

- *Eye drops*, apply 1 drop at least every 2 hours then reduce frequency as infection is controlled and continue for 48 hours after healing.
- *Eye ointment*, apply *either* at night (if eye drops used during the day) *or* 3–4 times daily (if eye ointment used alone).

Antifungals

Fungal infections of the cornea are rare but can occur after agricultural injuries, especially in hot and humid climates. Orbital mycosis is rarer, and when it occurs it is usually because of direct spread of infection from the paranasal sinuses. Increasing age, debility, or immunosuppression can encourage fungal proliferation. The spread of infection through blood occasionally produces metastatic endophthalmitis.

Many different fungi are capable of producing ocular infection; they can be identified by appropriate laboratory procedures.

Antifungal preparations for the eye are not generally available. Treatment will normally be carried out at specialist centres, but requests for information about supplies of preparations not available commercially should be addressed to the Strategic Health Authority (or equivalent), or to the nearest hospital ophthalmology unit, or to Moorfields Eye Hospital, 162 City Road, London EC1V 2PD (tel. (020) 7253 3411) or www.moorfields.nhs.uk.

Antivirals

Herpes simplex infections producing, for example, dendritic corneal ulcers can be treated with aciclovir p. 1019 or ganciclovir p. 1020. Aciclovir eye ointment is used in combination with systemic treatment for ophthalmic zoster.

Slow-release ocular implants containing ganciclovir (available on a named-patient basis from specialist importing companies) may be inserted surgically to treat immediate sight-threatening CMV retinitis. Local treatments do not protect against systemic infection or infection in the other eye. See systemic treatment of CMV retinitis.

3.1 Bacterial eye infection

ANTIBACTERIALS › AMINOGLYCOSIDES

Gentamicin

- **INDICATIONS AND DOSE**

Bacterial eye infections
▶ TO THE EYE
▶ Child: Apply 1 drop at least every 2 hours in severe infection, reduce frequency as infection is controlled and continue for 48 hours after healing, frequency of eye drops depends on the severity of the infection and the potential for irreversible ocular damage; for less severe infection 3–4 times daily is generally sufficient
▶ Adult: Apply 1 drop at least every 2 hours, reduce frequency as infection is controlled and continue for 48 hours after healing, frequency of eye drops depends on the severity of the infection and the potential for irreversible ocular damage; for less severe infection 3–4 times daily is generally sufficient

- **PRESCRIBING AND DISPENSING INFORMATION** Eye drops may be sourced as a manufactured special or from specialist importing companies.

- **MEDICINAL FORMS**
There can be variation in the licensing of different medicines containing the same drug. Forms available from special-order manufacturers include: eye drops
Ear/eye drops solution
EXCIPIENTS: May contain Benzalkonium chloride
▶ Gentamicin (Non-proprietary)
Gentamicin (as Gentamicin sulfate) 3 mg per 1 ml Gentamicin 0.3% ear/eye drops | 10 ml PoM £2.55 DT price = £2.13
Gentamicin 0.3% eye/ear drops | 10 ml PoM £2.13 DT price = £2.13

Tobramycin

- **INDICATIONS AND DOSE**

Local treatment of infections
▶ TO THE EYE
▶ Child 1-17 years: Apply twice daily for 6–8 days
▶ Adult: Apply twice daily for 6–8 days

Local treatment of infections (severe infection)
▸ TO THE EYE
  ▸ Child 1-17 years: Apply 4 times a day for first day, then apply twice daily for 5-7 days
  ▸ Adult: Apply 4 times a day for first day, then apply twice daily for 5-7 days

● MEDICINAL FORMS
There can be variation in the licensing of different medicines containing the same drug.
Eye drops
EXCIPIENTS: May contain Benzododecinium bromide
  ▸ Tobravisc (Alcon Laboratories (UK) Ltd)
    Tobramycin 3 mg per 1 ml Tobravisc 3mg/ml eye drops | 5 ml PoM £4.74

ANTIBACTERIALS › CEPHALOSPORINS, SECOND-GENERATION

Cefuroxime

● INDICATIONS AND DOSE
APROKAM® INTRACAMERAL INJECTION
Prophylaxis of endophthalmitis after cataract surgery
▸ BY INTRACAMERAL INJECTION
  ▸ Adult: 1 mg, dose to be injected into the anterior chamber of the eye at the end of cataract surgery

● CAUTIONS Combined operations with cataract surgery · complicated cataracts · reduced corneal endothelial cells (less than 2000) · severe risk of infection · severe thyroid disease

● PREGNANCY Not known to be harmful.

● BREAST FEEDING Present in milk in low concentration, but appropriate to use.

● MEDICINAL FORMS
There can be variation in the licensing of different medicines containing the same drug.
Powder for solution for injection
  ▸ Aprokam (Thea Pharmaceuticals Ltd)
    Cefuroxime (as Cefuroxime sodium) 50 mg Aprokam 50mg powder for solution for injection vials | 10 vial PoM £79.50

ANTIBACTERIALS › MACROLIDES

Azithromycin

● INDICATIONS AND DOSE
Trachomatous conjunctivitis caused by *Chlamydia trachomatis* | Purulent bacterial conjunctivitis
▸ TO THE EYE
  ▸ Child: Apply twice daily for 3 days, review if no improvement after 3 days of treatment
  ▸ Adult: Apply twice daily for 3 days, review if no improvement after 3 days of treatment

● SIDE-EFFECTS
▸ **Common or very common** Blurred vision · ocular burning · ocular discomfort · ocular pruritus
▸ **Uncommon** Conjunctival hyperaemia · eyelid eczema · eyelid erythema · eyelid oedema · keratitis

● MEDICINAL FORMS
There can be variation in the licensing of different medicines containing the same drug.
Eye drops
  ▸ Azyter (Thea Pharmaceuticals Ltd)
    Azithromycin dihydrate 15 mg per 1 gram Azyter 15mg/g eye drops 0.25g unit dose | 6 unit dose PoM £6.99 DT price = £6.99

ANTIBACTERIALS › QUINOLONES

Ciprofloxacin

● INDICATIONS AND DOSE
Superficial bacterial eye infection
▸ TO THE EYE USING EYE DROP
  ▸ Child: Apply 4 times a day for maximum duration of treatment 21 days
  ▸ Adult: Apply 4 times a day for maximum duration of treatment 21 days
▸ TO THE EYE USING EYE OINTMENT
  ▸ Child 1-17 years: Apply 1.25 centimetres 3 times a day for 2 days, then apply 1.25 centimetres twice daily for 5 days
  ▸ Adult: Apply 1.25 centimetres 3 times a day for 2 days, then apply 1.25 centimetres twice daily for 5 days
Superficial bacterial eye infection (severe infection)
▸ TO THE EYE USING EYE DROP
  ▸ Child: Apply every 2 hours during waking hours for 2 days, then apply 4 times a day for maximum duration of treatment 21 days
  ▸ Adult: Apply every 2 hours during waking hours for 2 days, then apply 4 times a day for maximum duration of treatment 21 days
Corneal ulcer
▸ TO THE EYE USING EYE DROP
  ▸ Child: Apply every 15 minutes for 6 hours, then apply every 30 minutes for the remainder of day 1, then apply every 1 hour on day 2, then apply every 4 hours on days 3-14, maximum duration of treatment 21 days, to be administered throughout the day and night
  ▸ Adult: Apply every 15 minutes for 6 hours, then apply every 30 minutes for the remainder of day 1, then apply every 1 hour on day 2, then apply every 4 hours on days 3-14, maximum duration of treatment 21 days, to be administered throughout the day and night
▸ TO THE EYE USING EYE OINTMENT
  ▸ Child 1-17 years: Apply 1.25 centimetres every 1-2 hours for 2 days, then apply 1.25 centimetres every 4 hours for the next 12 days, to be administered throughout the day and night
  ▸ Adult: Apply 1.25 centimetres every 1-2 hours for 2 days, then apply 1.25 centimetres every 4 hours for the next 12 days, to be administered throughout the day and night

● UNLICENSED USE Eye ointment not licensed for use in children under 1 year.

● SIDE-EFFECTS
▸ **Common or very common** Corneal deposits (reversible after completion of treatment) · ocular discomfort · ocular hyperaemia · taste disturbance
▸ **Uncommon** Increased lacrimation · blurred vision · conjunctival hyperaemia · corneal infiltrates · corneal staining · eye dryness · eye irritation · eye pain · eye pruritus · eye swelling · eyelid disorders · eyelid erythema · eyelid exfoliation · eyelid oedema · headache · keratopathy · nausea · photophobia
▸ **Rare** Abdominal pain · asthenopia · corneal disorders · corneal epithelium defect · dermatitis · diarrhoea · diplopia · dizziness · ear pain · eye hypoaesthesia · keratitis · paranasal sinus hypersecretion · rhinitis

● PREGNANCY Manufacturer advises use only if potential benefit outweighs risk.

● BREAST FEEDING Manufacturer advises caution.

11

Eye

- MEDICINAL FORMS
There can be variation in the licensing of different medicines containing the same drug. Forms available from special-order manufacturers include: eye drops

Eye drops
EXCIPIENTS: May contain Benzalkonium chloride
▸ Ciloxan (Alcon Laboratories (UK) Ltd)
Ciprofloxacin (as Ciprofloxacin hydrochloride) 3 mg per 1 ml Ciloxan 0.3% eye drops | 5 ml [PoM] £4.70 DT price = £4.70

Eye ointment
▸ Ciloxan (Alcon Laboratories (UK) Ltd)
Ciprofloxacin (as Ciprofloxacin hydrochloride) 3 mg per 1 gram Ciloxan 3mg/g eye ointment | 3.5 gram [PoM] £5.22

Levofloxacin

- INDICATIONS AND DOSE

Local treatment of eye infections
▸ TO THE EYE
▸ Child 1-17 years: Apply every 2 hours for first 2 days, to be applied maximum 8 times a day, then apply 4 times a day for 3 days
▸ Adult: Apply every 2 hours for first 2 days, to be applied maximum 8 times a day, then apply 4 times a day for 3 days

- SIDE-EFFECTS
▸ **Common or very common** Ocular burning · visual disturbances
▸ **Uncommon** Conjunctival follicles · headache · lid erythema · lid oedema · ocular discomfort · ocular dryness · ocular itching · ocular pain · photophobia · rhinitis
- PREGNANCY Manufacturer advises use only if potential benefit outweighs risk.
- BREAST FEEDING Manufacturer advises use only if potential benefit outweighs risk.
- PRESCRIBING AND DISPENSING INFORMATION Although multi-dose levofloxacin eye drops commonly contain preservatives, preservative-free unit dose vials may be available.

- MEDICINAL FORMS
There can be variation in the licensing of different medicines containing the same drug.

Eye drops
EXCIPIENTS: May contain Benzalkonium chloride
▸ Oftaquix (Santen UK Ltd)
Levofloxacin (as Levofloxacin hemihydrate) 5 mg per 1 ml Oftaquix 5mg/ml eye drops 0.5ml unit dose | 30 unit dose [PoM] £17.95
Oftaquix 5mg/ml eye drops | 5 ml [PoM] £6.95

Moxifloxacin

- INDICATIONS AND DOSE

Local treatment of infections
▸ TO THE EYE
▸ Child: Apply 3 times a day continue treatment for 2–3 days after infection improves; review if no improvement within 5 days
▸ Adult: Apply 3 times a day continue treatment for 2–3 days after infection improves; review if no improvement within 5 days

- SIDE-EFFECTS
▸ **Common or very common** Hyperaemia · ocular discomfort · ocular dryness · ocular irritation · ocular pain · taste disturbances
▸ **Uncommon** Conjunctival haemorrhage · corneal disorders · corneal erosion · corneal keratitis · corneal staining · eyelid erythema · headache · nasal discomfort ·

paraesthesia · pharyngolaryngeal pain · visual disturbances · vomiting
▸ **Frequency not known** Dizziness · dyspnoea · nausea · palpitation · photophobia · pruritus · raised intra-ocular pressure · rash

- MEDICINAL FORMS
There can be variation in the licensing of different medicines containing the same drug.

Eye drops
▸ Moxivig (Alcon Laboratories (UK) Ltd)
Moxifloxacin (as Moxifloxacin hydrochloride) 5 mg per 1 ml Moxivig 0.5% eye drops | 5 ml [PoM] £9.80

Ofloxacin

- INDICATIONS AND DOSE

Local treatment of infections
▸ TO THE EYE
▸ Child 1-17 years: Apply every 2–4 hours for the first 2 days, then reduced to 4 times a day for maximum 10 days treatment
▸ Adult: Apply every 2–4 hours for the first 2 days, then reduced to 4 times a day for maximum 10 days treatment

- CAUTIONS Corneal ulcer (risk of corneal perforation) · epithelial defect (risk of corneal perforation)
- SIDE-EFFECTS
▸ **Common or very common** Eye irritation · ocular discomfort
▸ **Frequency not known** Dry eyes · facial oedema · increased lacrimation · keratitis · ocular hyperaemia · ocular oedema · photophobia · visual disturbances
- PREGNANCY Manufacturer advises use only if benefit outweighs risk (systemic quinolones have caused arthropathy in *animal* studies).
- BREAST FEEDING Manufacturer advises avoid.

- MEDICINAL FORMS
There can be variation in the licensing of different medicines containing the same drug.

Eye drops
EXCIPIENTS: May contain Benzalkonium chloride
▸ Exocin (Allergan Ltd)
Ofloxacin 3 mg per 1 ml Exocin 0.3% eye drops | 5 ml [PoM] £2.17 DT price = £2.17

ANTIBACTERIALS 〉 OTHER

Chloramphenicol

- DRUG ACTION Chloramphenicol is a potent broad-spectrum antibiotic.

- INDICATIONS AND DOSE

Superficial eye infections
▸ TO THE EYE USING EYE DROP
▸ Child: Apply 1 drop every 2 hours then reduce frequency as infection is controlled and continue for 48 hours after healing, frequency dependent on the severity of the infection. For less severe infection 3–4 times daily is generally sufficient
▸ Adult: Apply 1 drop every 2 hours then reduce frequency as infection is controlled and continue for 48 hours after healing, frequency dependent on the severity of the infection. For less severe infection 3–4 times daily is generally sufficient
▸ TO THE EYE USING EYE OINTMENT
▸ Child: Apply daily, to be applied at night (if eye drops used during the day), alternatively apply 3–4 times a day, if ointment used alone

‣ **Adult:** Apply daily, to be applied at night (if eye drops used during the day), alternatively apply 3–4 times a day, if ointment used alone

- SIDE-EFFECTS Transient stinging
- PREGNANCY Avoid unless essential—no information on *topical* use but risk of 'neonatal grey-baby syndrome' with *oral* use in third trimester.
- BREAST FEEDING Avoid unless essential—*theoretical* risk of bone-marrow toxicity.
- PRESCRIBING AND DISPENSING INFORMATION Although multi-dose chloramphenicol eye drops commonly contain preservatives, preservative-free unit dose vials may be available.
- PATIENT AND CARER ADVICE
  Medicines for Children leaflet: Chloramphenicol for eye infections www.medicinesforchildren.org.uk/chloramphenicol-eye-infections-0
- EXCEPTIONS TO LEGAL CATEGORY Chloramphenicol 0.5% eye drops (in max. pack size 10 mL) and 1% eye ointment (in max. pack size 4 g) can be sold to the public for treatment of acute bacterial conjunctivitis in adults and children over 2 years; max. duration of treatment 5 days.

- MEDICINAL FORMS
  There can be variation in the licensing of different medicines containing the same drug. Forms available from special-order manufacturers include: eye drops

Eye drops
EXCIPIENTS: May contain Phenylmercuric acetate
‣ Chloramphenicol (Non-proprietary)
   Chloramphenicol 5 mg per 1 ml Minims chloramphenicol 0.5% eye drops 0.5ml unit dose | 20 unit dose [PoM] £10.99 DT price = £10.99
   Chloramphenicol 0.5% eye drops | 10 ml [PoM] £2.20 DT price = £1.12
‣ Brochlor (Sanofi)
   Chloramphenicol 5 mg per 1 ml Brochlor 0.5% eye drops | 10 ml [P] £2.83 DT price = £1.12
‣ Brolene Antibiotic (Sanofi)
   Chloramphenicol 5 mg per 1 ml Brolene Antibiotic 0.5% eye drops | 10 ml [P] £3.00 DT price = £1.12
‣ Chloromycetin (AMCo)
   Chloramphenicol 5 mg per 1 ml Chloromycetin Redidrops 0.5% | 10 ml [PoM] £0.90 DT price = £1.12
‣ Optrex Infected Eyes (Reckitt Benckiser Healthcare (UK) Ltd)
   Chloramphenicol 5 mg per 1 ml Optrex Infected Eyes 0.5% eye drops | 10 ml [P] £3.88 DT price = £1.12

Eye ointment
‣ Chloramphenicol (Non-proprietary)
   Chloramphenicol 10 mg per 1 gram Chloramphenicol 1% eye ointment | 4 gram [PoM] £4.25 DT price = £1.63
‣ Brochlor (Sanofi)
   Chloramphenicol 10 mg per 1 gram Brochlor 1% eye ointment | 4 gram [P] £2.95 DT price = £1.63
‣ Chloromycetin (AMCo)
   Chloramphenicol 10 mg per 1 gram Chloromycetin 1% eye ointment | 4 gram [P] £1.08 DT price = £1.63
‣ Klorafect (Blumont Pharma Ltd)
   Chloramphenicol 10 mg per 1 gram Klorafect 1% eye ointment | 4 gram [PoM] £1.81 DT price = £1.63
‣ Optrex Infected Eyes (Reckitt Benckiser Healthcare (UK) Ltd)
   Chloramphenicol 10 mg per 1 gram Optrex Infected Eyes 1% eye ointment | 4 gram [P] £3.88 DT price = £1.63

Fusidic acid

- DRUG ACTION Fusidic acid and its salts are narrow-spectrum antibiotics used for staphylococcal infections.

- INDICATIONS AND DOSE

Staphylococcal eye infections
▸ TO THE EYE
‣ **Child:** Apply twice daily
‣ **Adult:** Apply twice daily

- MEDICINAL FORMS
  There can be variation in the licensing of different medicines containing the same drug.
Modified-release drops
EXCIPIENTS: May contain Benzalkonium chloride, disodium edetate
‣ Fusidic acid (Non-proprietary)
   Fusidic acid 10 mg per 1 gram Fusidic acid 1% modified-release eye drops | 5 gram [PoM] £29.06 DT price = £29.06

ANTIPROTOZOALS

Propamidine isetionate

- INDICATIONS AND DOSE

***Acanthamoeba keratitis* infections (specialist use only) | Local treatment of eye infections**
▸ TO THE EYE USING EYE OINTMENT
‣ **Adult:** Apply 1–2 times a day
▸ TO THE EYE USING EYE DROP
‣ **Adult:** Apply up to 4 times a day

- UNLICENSED USE Not licensed for *acanthamoeba keratitis* infections.
- SIDE-EFFECTS Eye irritation · eye pain
- PREGNANCY Manufacturer advises avoid unless essential—no information available.
- BREAST FEEDING Manufacturer advises avoid unless essential—no information available.

- MEDICINAL FORMS
  There can be variation in the licensing of different medicines containing the same drug.
Eye drops
EXCIPIENTS: May contain Benzalkonium chloride
‣ Brolene (Propamidine) (Sanofi)
   Propamidine isetionate 1 mg per 1 ml Brolene 0.1% eye drops | 10 ml [P] £2.80
‣ Golden eye (Cambridge Healthcare Supplies Ltd)
   Propamidine isetionate 1 mg per 1 ml Golden Eye 0.1% drops | 10 ml [P] £3.26

Eye ointment
‣ Brolene (Dibrompropamidine) (Sanofi)
   Dibrompropamidine isetionate 1.5 mg per 1 gram Brolene 0.15% eye ointment | 5 gram [P] £2.92 DT price = £3.49
‣ Golden eye (Cambridge Healthcare Supplies Ltd)
   Dibrompropamidine isetionate 1.5 mg per 1 gram Golden Eye 0.15% ointment | 5 gram [P] £3.49 DT price = £3.49

3.2 Viral eye infection
3.2a Ophthalmic herpes simplex

ANTIVIRALS › NUCLEOSIDE ANALOGUES

Aciclovir

(Acyclovir)

- INDICATIONS AND DOSE

Herpes simplex infection (local treatment)
▸ TO THE EYE USING EYE OINTMENT
‣ **Child:** Apply 1 centimetre 5 times a day continue for at least 3 days after complete healing
‣ **Adult:** Apply 1 centimetre 5 times a day continue for at least 3 days after complete healing

- SIDE-EFFECTS
- **Common or very common** Local inflammation · local irritation · superficial punctate keratopathy
- **Rare** Blepharitis
- **Very rare** Angioedema · hypersensitivity reactions

11

Eye

- PATIENT AND CARER ADVICE
Medicines for Children leaflet: Aciclovir eye ointment for herpes simplex infections www.medicinesforchildren.org.uk/aciclovir-eye-ointment-for-herpes-simplex-infection

- MEDICINAL FORMS
There can be variation in the licensing of different medicines containing the same drug.
Eye ointment
▸ Zovirax (GlaxoSmithKline UK Ltd)
   Aciclovir 30 mg per 1 gram Zovirax 3% ophthalmic ointment | 4.5 gram [PoM] £9.34 DT price = £9.34

Ganciclovir

- INDICATIONS AND DOSE
Local treatment of herpes simplex infections
▸ TO THE EYE
▸ Adult: Apply 5 times a day until healing complete, then apply 3 times a day for a further 7 days

- SIDE-EFFECTS Burning sensation · superficial punctate keratitis · tingling

- ALLERGY AND CROSS-SENSITIVITY Contra-indicated in patients hypersensitive to valganciclovir, aciclovir, or valaciclovir.

- MEDICINAL FORMS
There can be variation in the licensing of different medicines containing the same drug.
Eye gel
EXCIPIENTS: May contain Benzalkonium chloride
▸ Virgan (Thea Pharmaceuticals Ltd)
   Ganciclovir 1.5 mg per 1 gram Virgan 0.15% eye gel | 5 gram [PoM] £19.99 DT price = £19.99

4   Eye procedures

Mydriatics and cycloplegics

Overview

Antimuscarinics dilate the pupil and paralyse the ciliary muscle; they vary in potency and duration of action.

Short-acting, relatively weak mydriatics, such as tropicamide 0.5% below (action lasts for 4–6 hours), facilitate the examination of the fundus of the eye. Longer-acting options include cyclopentolate hydrochloride 1% p. 1011 (action up to 24 hours) or atropine sulfate p. 1011 (action up to 7 days).

Phenylephrine hydrochloride p. 1021 is used for mydriasis in diagnostic or therapeutic procedures; mydriasis occurs within 60–90 minutes and lasts up to 5–7 hours.

Mydriatics and cycloplegics are used in the treatment of anterior uveitis, usually as an adjunct to corticosteroids. Atropine sulfate is used in anterior uveitis mainly to prevent posterior synechiae and to relieve ciliary spasm; cyclopentolate hydrochloride or homatropine hydrobromide p. 1011 (action up to 3 days) can also be used and may be preferred because they have a shorter duration of action.

Drugs used for Eye procedures not listed below Lidocaine hydrochloride, p. 1187

ANTIMUSCARINICS

☞ 1011

Tropicamide

- INDICATIONS AND DOSE
Funduscopy
▸ TO THE EYE
▸ Child: 0.5% eye drops to be applied 20 minutes before examination
▸ Adult: (consult product literature)

- PRESCRIBING AND DISPENSING INFORMATION Although multi-dose tropicamide eye drops commonly contain preservatives, preservative-free unit dose vials may be available.

- MEDICINAL FORMS
There can be variation in the licensing of different medicines containing the same drug.
Eye drops
EXCIPIENTS: May contain Benzalkonium chloride, edetic acid (edta)
▸ Mydriacyl (Alcon Laboratories (UK) Ltd)
   Tropicamide 5 mg per 1 ml Mydriacyl 0.5% eye drops | 5 ml [PoM] £1.29
   Tropicamide 10 mg per 1 ml Mydriacyl 1% eye drops | 5 ml [PoM] £1.60
▸ Tropicamide (Bausch & Lomb UK Ltd)
   Tropicamide 5 mg per 1 ml Minims tropicamide 0.5% eye drops 0.5ml unit dose | 20 unit dose [PoM] £10.75
   Tropicamide 10 mg per 1 ml Minims tropicamide 1% eye drops 0.5ml unit dose | 20 unit dose [PoM] £10.77

Combinations available: *Phenylephrine with tropicamide*, p. 1022

ANTISEPTICS AND DISINFECTANTS > IODINE PRODUCTS

Povidone-iodine

- INDICATIONS AND DOSE
Cutaneous peri-ocular and conjunctival antisepsis before ocular surgery
▸ TO THE EYE
▸ Adult: Apply, leave for 2 minutes, then irrigate thoroughly with sodium chloride 0.9%

- CONTRA-INDICATIONS Concomitant use of ocular antimicrobial drugs · concomitant use of ocular formulations containing mercury-based preservatives

- SIDE-EFFECTS
▸ **Rare** Conjunctival hyperaemia · superficial punctuate keratitis
▸ **Frequency not known** Cytotoxicity on deep tissue · cytotoxicity on mucous membranes · residual yellow coloration of the conjunctiva

- PRESCRIBING AND DISPENSING INFORMATION Although multi-dose povidone iodine eye drops commonly contain preservatives, preservative-free unit dose vials may be available.

- MEDICINAL FORMS
There can be variation in the licensing of different medicines containing the same drug. Forms available from special-order manufacturers include: eye drops, eye lotion
Eye drops
▸ Povidone iodine (Bausch & Lomb UK Ltd)
   Povidone-Iodine 50 mg per 1 ml Minims povidone iodine 5% eye drops 0.4ml unit dose | 20 unit dose [PoM] £16.00

DIAGNOSTIC AGENTS > DYES

Fluorescein sodium

- **INDICATIONS AND DOSE**

Detection of lesions and foreign bodies
▶ TO THE EYE USING EYE DROP
▷ Adult: Use sufficient amount to stain damaged areas

- PRESCRIBING AND DISPENSING INFORMATION Although multi-dose fluorescein eye drops commonly contain preservatives, preservative-free unit dose vials may be available.

- MEDICINAL FORMS
There can be variation in the licensing of different medicines containing the same drug.
Eye drops
▶ Fluorescein sodium (Bausch & Lomb UK Ltd)
Fluorescein sodium 10 mg per 1 ml Minims fluorescein sodium 1% eye drops 0.5ml unit dose | 20 unit dose P £8.89
Fluorescein sodium 20 mg per 1 ml Minims fluorescein sodium 2% eye drops 0.5ml unit dose | 20 unit dose P £8.89

Fluorescein with lidocaine

- **INDICATIONS AND DOSE**

Local anaesthesia
▶ TO THE EYE
▷ Adult: Apply as required

- PRESCRIBING AND DISPENSING INFORMATION Although multi-dose lidocaine and fluorescein eye drops commonly contain preservatives, preservative-free unit dose vials may be available.

- MEDICINAL FORMS
There can be variation in the licensing of different medicines containing the same drug.
Eye drops
▶ Lidocaine and Fluorescein (Bausch & Lomb UK Ltd)
Fluorescein sodium 2.5 mg per 1 ml, Lidocaine hydrochloride 40 mg per 1 ml Minims lidocaine and fluorescein eye drops 0.5ml unit dose | 20 unit dose PoM £11.24

MIOTICS > PARASYMPATHOMIMETICS

Acetylcholine chloride

- **INDICATIONS AND DOSE**

Cataract surgery | Penetrating keratoplasty | Iridectomy | Anterior segment surgery requiring rapid complete miosis
▶ TO THE EYE
▷ Adult: (consult product literature)

- CAUTIONS Asthma · gastro-intestinal spasm · heart failure · hyperthyroidism · parkinsonism · peptic ulcer · urinary-tract obstruction
- SIDE-EFFECTS
▶ Rare Bradycardia · breathing difficulty · flushing · hypotension · sweating
- PREGNANCY Avoid unless potential benefit outweighs risk—no information available.
- BREAST FEEDING Avoid unless potential benefit outweighs risk—no information available.

- MEDICINAL FORMS
There can be variation in the licensing of different medicines containing the same drug.
Irrigation
▶ Miochol-E (Bausch & Lomb UK Ltd)
Acetylcholine chloride 20 mg Miochol-E 20mg powder and solvent for solution for intraocular irrigation vials | 1 vial PoM £7.28
▶ Miphtel (Alan Pharmaceuticals)
Acetylcholine chloride 20 mg Miphtel 20mg powder and solvent for solution for intraocular irrigation ampoules | 6 ampoule PoM £43.68 (Hospital only)

SYMPATHOMIMETICS > VASOCONSTRICTOR

Phenylephrine hydrochloride

- **INDICATIONS AND DOSE**

Mydriasis
▶ TO THE EYE
▷ Child: Apply 1 drop, to be administered before procedure, a drop of proxymetacaine topical anaesthetic may be applied to the eye a few minutes before using phenylephrine to prevent stinging
▷ Adult: Apply 1 drop, to be administered before procedure, then apply 1 drop after 60 minutes if required, a drop of topical anaesthetic may be applied to the eye a few minutes before using phenylephrine to prevent stinging

- CONTRA-INDICATIONS 10% strength eye drops in children and the elderly · aneurysms · cardiovascular disease · hypertension · thyrotoxicosis
- CAUTIONS Asthma · cerebral arteriosclerosis (in adults) · corneal epithelial damage · darkly pigmented iris is more resistant to pupillary dilatation and caution should be exercised to avoid overdosage. · diabetes (avoid eye drops in long standing diabetes) · mydriasis can precipitate acute angle-closure glaucoma in a few patients, usually over 60 years and hypermetropic (long-sighted), who are pre-disposed to the condition because of a shallow anterior chamber · ocular hyperaemia · susceptibility to angle-closure glaucoma
- INTERACTIONS → Appendix 1 (sympathomimetics). Phenylephrine may interact with systemically administered monoamine-oxidase inhibitors.
- SIDE-EFFECTS Arrhythmias · blurred vision · conjunctivitis on prolonged administration · coronary artery spasm · extrasystoles · hyperaemia on prolonged administration · hypertension · local irritation on prolonged administration · myocardial infarction (usually after use of 10% strength in patients with pre-existing cardiovascular disease) · oedema on prolonged administration · palpitation · photophobia · raised intraocular pressure · tachycardia · transient stinging
- PREGNANCY Use only if potential benefit outweighs risk.
- BREAST FEEDING Use only if potential benefit outweighs risk—no information available.
- PRESCRIBING AND DISPENSING INFORMATION Although multi-dose phenylephrine eye drops commonly contain preservatives, preservative-free unit dose vials may be available.
- PATIENT AND CARER ADVICE
Driving and skilled tasks
Patients should be warned not to undertake skilled tasks (e.g. driving) until vision clears after mydriasis.

- **MEDICINAL FORMS**
There can be variation in the licensing of different medicines containing the same drug. Forms available from special-order manufacturers include: eye drops
Eye drops
EXCIPIENTS: May contain Disodium edetate, sodium metabisulfite
- ▸ Phenylephrine hydrochloride (Bausch & Lomb UK Ltd)
Phenylephrine hydrochloride 25 mg per 1 ml Minims phenylephrine hydrochloride 2.5% eye drops 0.5ml unit dose | 20 unit dose P £11.41
Phenylephrine hydrochloride 100 mg per 1 ml Minims phenylephrine hydrochloride 10% eye drops 0.5ml unit dose | 20 unit dose P £11.41

Phenylephrine with tropicamide

The properties listed below are those particular to the combination only. For the properties of the components please consider, phenylephrine hydrochloride p. 1021, tropicamide p. 1020.

- **INDICATIONS AND DOSE**

Pre-operative mydriasis | Diagnostic procedures when monotherapy insufficient
- ▸ TO THE EYE
- ▸ Adult: One insert to be applied into the lower conjunctival sac up to max. 2 hours before procedure; remove insert within 30 minutes of satisfactory mydriasis, and within 2 hours of application

- **DIRECTIONS FOR ADMINISTRATION** Patients with severe dry eyes may require a drop of saline to improve insert tolerance.

- **MEDICINAL FORMS**
There can be variation in the licensing of different medicines containing the same drug.
Ophthalmic insert
- ▸ Mydriasert (Thea Pharmaceuticals Ltd)
Tropicamide.28 mg, Phenylephrine hydrochloride 5.4 mg Mydriasert 5.4mg / 0.28mg ophthalmic inserts | 20 insert PoM £84.00

4.1 Post-operative pain and inflammation

Eye, surgical and peri-operative drug use

Ocular peri-operative drugs

Drugs used to prepare the eye for surgery, drugs that are injected into the anterior chamber at the time of surgery, and those used after eye surgery, are included here.

Cefuroxime p. 1017, administered by intra-ocular injection into the anterior chamber of the eye (intracameral use), is used for the prophylaxis of endophthalmitis after cataract surgery.

Non-steroidal anti-inflammatory eye drops such as diclofenac sodium p. 1023, flurbiprofen p. 1023, ketorolac trometamol p. 1023, and nepafenac p. 1008, are used for the prophylaxis and treatment of inflammation, pain, and other symptoms associated with ocular surgery or laser treatment of the eye. Bromfenac p. 1023 is used for the treatment of postoperative inflammation following cataract surgery. Diclofenac sodium and flurbiprofen are also used to prevent miosis during ocular surgery.

Apraclonidine p. 1032, an alpha$_2$-adrenoreceptor agonist, reduces intra-ocular pressure possibly by reducing the production of aqueous humour. It is used to control increases in intra-ocular pressure associated with ocular

surgery and as short-term treatment to reduce intraocular pressure prior to surgery.

Acetylcholine chloride p. 1021, administered into the anterior chamber of the eye during surgery, rapidly produces miosis which lasts approximately 20 minutes. If prolonged miosis is required, it can be applied again.

Intra-ocular sodium hyaluronate p. 1015 and balanced salt solution are used during surgical procedures on the eye.

Povidone-iodine p. 1020 is used for peri-ocular and conjunctival antisepsis before ocular surgery to support postoperative infection control.

Local anaesthetics

Oxybuprocaine hydrochloride below and tetracaine p. 1023 are widely used topical local anaesthetics. Proxymetacaine hydrochloride below causes less initial stinging and is useful for children. Oxyprocaine hydrochloride or a combined preparation of lidocaine hydrochloride p. 1187 and fluorescein sodium p. 1021 is used for tonometry. Tetracaine produces a more profound anaesthesia and is suitable for use before minor surgical procedures, such as the removal of corneal sutures. It has a temporary disruptive effect on the corneal epithelium. Lidocaine hydrochloride, with or without adrenaline/epinephrine p. 205, is injected into the eyelids for minor surgery. Local anaesthetics should never be used for the management of ocular symptoms.

ANAESTHETICS, LOCAL

Oxybuprocaine hydrochloride

(Benoxinate hydrochloride)

- **INDICATIONS AND DOSE**
Local anaesthetic
- ▸ TO THE EYE
- ▸ Adult: Apply as required

- **PRESCRIBING AND DISPENSING INFORMATION** Although multi-dose oxybuprocaine eye drops commonly contain preservatives, preservative-free unit dose vials may be available.

- **MEDICINAL FORMS**
There can be variation in the licensing of different medicines containing the same drug.
Eye drops
- ▸ Oxybuprocaine hydrochloride (Bausch & Lomb UK Ltd)
Oxybuprocaine hydrochloride 4 mg per 1 ml Minims oxybuprocaine hydrochloride 0.4% eye drops 0.5ml unit dose | 20 unit dose PoM £10.15

Proxymetacaine hydrochloride

- **INDICATIONS AND DOSE**
Local anaesthetic
- ▸ TO THE EYE
- ▸ Adult: Apply as required

- **PRESCRIBING AND DISPENSING INFORMATION** Although multi-dose proxymetacaine eye drops commonly contain preservatives, preservative-free unit dose vials may be available.

- **MEDICINAL FORMS**
There can be variation in the licensing of different medicines containing the same drug.
Eye drops
- ▸ Proxymetacaine (Bausch & Lomb UK Ltd)
Proxymetacaine hydrochloride 5 mg per 1 ml Minims proxymetacaine hydrochloride 0.5% eye drops 0.5ml unit dose | 20 unit dose PoM £11.54

Tetracaine

(Amethocaine)

- INDICATIONS AND DOSE

Local anaesthetic
- ▶ TO THE EYE
- ▶ Adult: Apply as required

- SIDE-EFFECTS Local skin reactions
- PRESCRIBING AND DISPENSING INFORMATION Although multi-dose tetracaine eye drops commonly contain preservatives, preservative-free unit dose vials may be available.

- MEDICINAL FORMS
There can be variation in the licensing of different medicines containing the same drug.
Eye drops
- ▶ Tetracaine (Non-proprietary)
  Tetracaine hydrochloride 5 mg per 1 ml Minims tetracaine hydrochloride 0.5% eye drops 0.5ml unit dose | 20 unit dose PoM £10.16
  Tetracaine hydrochloride 10 mg per 1 ml Minims tetracaine hydrochloride 1% eye drops 0.5ml unit dose | 20 unit dose PoM £10.16

ANALGESICS > NON-STEROIDAL ANTI-INFLAMMATORY DRUGS

Bromfenac

- INDICATIONS AND DOSE

Postoperative inflammation following cataract surgery
- ▶ TO THE EYE
- ▶ Adult: (consult product literature)

- MEDICINAL FORMS
There can be variation in the licensing of different medicines containing the same drug.
Eye drops
EXCIPIENTS: May contain Benzalkonium chloride, disodium edetate, sulfites
- ▶ Bromfenac (Non-proprietary)
  Bromfenac (as Bromfenac sodium sesquihydrate)
  900 microgram per 1 ml Bromfenac 900micrograms/ml eye drops | 5 ml PoM no price available
- ▶ Yellox (Bausch & Lomb UK Ltd)
  Bromfenac (as Bromfenac sodium sesquihydrate)
  900 microgram per 1 ml Yellox 900micrograms/ml eye drops | 5 ml PoM £8.50

Diclofenac sodium

- INDICATIONS AND DOSE

Inhibition of intra-operative miosis during cataract surgery (but does not possess intrinsic mydriatic properties) | Postoperative inflammation in cataract surgery, strabismus surgery or argon laser trabeculoplasty | Pain in corneal epithelial defects after photorefractive keratectomy, radial keratotomy or accidental trauma | Seasonal allergic conjunctivitis
- ▶ TO THE EYE
- ▶ Adult: (consult product literature)

- ALLERGY AND CROSS-SENSITIVITY Contra-indicated in patients with a history of hypersensitivity to aspirin or any other NSAID—which includes those in whom attacks of asthma, angioedema, urticaria or rhinitis have been precipitated by aspirin or any other NSAID.

- PRESCRIBING AND DISPENSING INFORMATION Although multi-dose diclofenac sodium eye drops commonly contain preservatives, preservative-free unit dose vials may be available.

- MEDICINAL FORMS
There can be variation in the licensing of different medicines containing the same drug.
Eye drops
EXCIPIENTS: May contain Benzalkonium chloride, disodium edetate, propylene glycol
- ▶ Voltarol Ophtha (Thea Pharmaceuticals Ltd)
  Diclofenac sodium 1 mg per 1 ml Voltarol Ophtha 0.1% eye drops 0.3ml unit dose | 5 unit dose PoM £4.00 | 40 unit dose PoM £32.00
- ▶ Voltarol Ophtha Multidose (Thea Pharmaceuticals Ltd)
  Diclofenac sodium 1 mg per 1 ml Voltarol Ophtha Multidose 0.1% eye drops | 5 ml PoM £6.68

Flurbiprofen

- INDICATIONS AND DOSE

Inhibition of intra-operative miosis (but does not possess intrinsic mydriatic properties) | Control of anterior segment inflammation following postoperative and post-laser trabeculoplasty when corticosteroids contra-indicated
- ▶ TO THE EYE
- ▶ Adult: (consult product literature)

- ALLERGY AND CROSS-SENSITIVITY Contra-indicated in patients with a history of hypersensitivity to aspirin or any other NSAID—which includes those in whom attacks of asthma, angioedema, urticaria or rhinitis have been precipitated by aspirin or any other NSAID.

- MEDICINAL FORMS
There can be variation in the licensing of different medicines containing the same drug.
Eye drops
- ▶ Ocufen (Allergan Ltd)
  Flurbiprofen sodium 300 microgram per 1 ml Ocufen 0.03% eye drops 0.4ml unit dose | 40 unit dose PoM £37.15

Ketorolac trometamol

- INDICATIONS AND DOSE

Prophylaxis and reduction of inflammation and associated symptoms following ocular surgery
- ▶ TO THE EYE
- ▶ Adult: (consult product literature)

- ALLERGY AND CROSS-SENSITIVITY Contra-indicated in patients with a history of hypersensitivity to aspirin or any other NSAID—which includes those in whom attacks of asthma, angioedema, urticaria or rhinitis have been precipitated by aspirin or any other NSAID.

- MEDICINAL FORMS
There can be variation in the licensing of different medicines containing the same drug.
Eye drops
EXCIPIENTS: May contain Benzalkonium chloride, disodium edetate
- ▶ Acular (Allergan Ltd)
  Ketorolac trometamol 5 mg per 1 ml Acular 0.5% eye drops | 5 ml PoM £3.00 DT price = £3.00

11

Eye

CORTICOSTEROIDS

▌Loteprednol etabonate

- ● **INDICATIONS AND DOSE**

Treatment of post-operative inflammation following ocular surgery

▸ TO THE EYE

▸ **Adult:** Apply 4 times a day for maximum duration of treatment of 14 days, to be started 24 hours after surgery

- ● **SIDE-EFFECTS** Corneal thinning · scleral thinning

- ● **MEDICINAL FORMS**
There can be variation in the licensing of different medicines containing the same drug.

Eye drops
EXCIPIENTS: May contain Benzalkonium chloride, disodium edetate

▸ Lotemax (Bausch & Lomb UK Ltd)
Loteprednol etabonate 5 mg per 1 ml Lotemax 0.5% eye drops | 5 ml [PoM] £5.50 DT price = £5.50

---

5 Glaucoma and ocular hypertension

Glaucoma

Overview

Glaucoma describes a group of disorders characterised by a loss of visual field associated with cupping of the optic disc and optic nerve damage. While glaucoma is generally associated with raised intra-ocular pressure, it can occur when the intra-ocular pressure is within the normal range.

The most common form of glaucoma is primary open-angle glaucoma (chronic open-angle glaucoma), where drainage of the aqueous humour through the trabecular meshwork is restricted. The condition is often asymptomatic, but the patient may present with significant loss of visual-field. Patients with ocular hypertension are at high risk of developing primary open-angle glaucoma.

Drugs that reduce intra-ocular pressure by different mechanisms are available for managing ocular hypertension and glaucoma. A topical beta-blocker or a prostaglandin analogue is usually the drug of first choice for the treatment of ocular hypertension. A prostaglandin analogue should be used to manage patients with early or moderate primary open-angle glaucoma. After checking compliance and eye drop instillation technique, it may be necessary to combine these drugs or add others, such as sympathomimetics, carbonic anhydrase inhibitors, or miotics to control intra-ocular pressure.

Acute angle-closure glaucoma

Acute angle-closure glaucoma occurs when the outflow of aqueous humour from the eye is obstructed by bowing of the iris against the trabecular meshwork; it is a medical emergency that requires urgent reduction of intra-ocular pressure to prevent loss of vision. Patients with acute angle-closure glaucoma should be referred immediately for specialist ophthalmology assessment and treatment.

Standard antiglaucoma therapy is used if supplementary treatment is required after iridotomy, iridectomy, laser treatment, or drainage surgery in either primary open-angle or acute angle-closure glaucoma.

Beta-blockers

Topical application of a beta-blocker to the eye reduces intra-ocular pressure effectively in *primary open-angle*

glaucoma, probably by reducing the rate of production of aqueous humour. Administration by mouth also reduces intra-ocular pressure but this route is not used since side-effects may be troublesome.

Beta-blockers used as eye drops include betaxolol p. 1025, carteolol hydrochloride p. 1025, levobunolol hydrochloride p. 1025, and timolol maleate p. 1025.

Prostaglandin analogues and prostamides

The prostaglandin analogues latanoprost p. 1030, tafluprost and travoprost p. 1030, and the synthetic prostamide, bimatoprost, increase uveoscleral outflow and subsequently reduce intra-ocular pressure. They are used to reduce intra-ocular pressure in ocular hypertension or open-angle glaucoma.

Sympathomimetics

Brimonidine tartrate, a selective alpha$_2$-adrenoceptor agonist, is thought to lower intra-ocular pressure by reducing aqueous humour formation and increasing uveoscleral outflow. It is licensed for the reduction of intra-ocular pressure in open-angle glaucoma or ocular hypertension in patients for whom beta-blockers are inappropriate; it may also be used as adjunctive therapy when intra-ocular pressure is inadequately controlled by other anti-glaucoma therapy.

Apraclonidine p. 1021 is another alpha$_2$- adrenoceptor agonist that lowers intra-ocular pressure by reducing aqueous humour formation. Eye drops containing apraclonidine 0.5% are used short-term to delay laser treatment or surgery in patients with glaucoma not adequately controlled by another drug; eye drops containing 1% are used for control of intra-ocular pressure after anterior segment laser surgery. Apraclonidine may not provide additional benefit in patients already using two drugs that suppress the production of aqueous humour.

Carbonic anhydrase inhibitors and systemic drugs

The **carbonic anhydrase inhibitors**, acetazolamide p. 1026, brinzolamide p. 1027, and dorzolamide p. 1027, reduce intra-ocular pressure by reducing aqueous humour production. Systemic use of acetazolamide also produces weak diuresis.

Acetazolamide is given by mouth or by intravenous injection (intramuscular injections are painful because of the alkaline pH of the solution). It is used as an adjunct to other treatment for reducing intra-ocular pressure. Acetazolamide is not generally recommended for long-term use.

Dorzolamide and brinzolamide are topical carbonic anhydrase inhibitors. They are licensed for use in patients resistant to beta-blockers or those in whom beta-blockers are contra-indicated. They are used alone or as an adjunct to a topical beta-blocker. Brinzolamide can also be used as an adjunct to a prostaglandin analogue. Systemic absorption can rarely cause sulfonamide-like side-effects and may require discontinuation if severe.

The **osmotic diuretics**, intravenous hypertonic mannitol p. 211 or glycerol p. 54 by mouth are useful short-term ocular hypotensive drugs.

Miotics

Miotics act by opening the inefficient drainage channels in the trabecular meshwork.

Pilocarpine p. 1028, a miotic, is not commonly used for the treatment of primary open-angle glaucoma because side-effects are poorly tolerated. It is used mainly in the treatment of primary angle-closure glaucoma and in some secondary glaucomas.

BETA-ADRENOCEPTOR BLOCKERS

Betaxolol

- **INDICATIONS AND DOSE**

Primary open-angle glaucoma
- ▶ TO THE EYE
- ▶ Adult: Apply twice daily

- CONTRA-INDICATIONS Also consider contra-indications listed for systemically administered beta blockers · bradycardia · heart block

- CAUTIONS Patients with corneal disease
  CAUTIONS, FURTHER INFORMATION
  Systemic absorption can follow topical application to the eyes; consider cautions listed for systemically administered beta blockers.

- INTERACTIONS → Appendix 1 (beta-blockers).
  Since systemic absorption may follow topical application the possibility of interactions, in particular, with drugs such as verapamil should be borne in mind.

- SIDE-EFFECTS Anaphylaxis · blepharoconjunctivitis · burning · corneal disorders · dry eyes · erythema · itching · ocular stinging · pain
  SIDE-EFFECTS, FURTHER INFORMATION
  Systemic absorption can follow topical application to the eyes; consider side effects listed for systemically administered beta blockers.

- PRESCRIBING AND DISPENSING INFORMATION Although multi-dose bextaxolol eye drops commonly contain preservatives, preservative-free unit dose vials may be available.

- MEDICINAL FORMS
  There can be variation in the licensing of different medicines containing the same drug.
  Eye drops
  EXCIPIENTS: May contain Benzalkonium chloride, disodium edetate
  ▶ Betaxolol (Non-proprietary)
  Betaxolol (as Betaxolol hydrochloride) 2.5 mg per 1 ml Betaxolol 0.25% eye drops 0.25ml unit dose preservative free | 50 unit dose [PoM] no price available
  Betaxolol (as Betaxolol hydrochloride) 5 mg per 1 ml Betaxolol 0.5% eye drops | 5 ml [PoM] £1.90 DT price = £1.90
  ▶ Betoptic (Alcon Laboratories (UK) Ltd)
  Betaxolol (as Betaxolol hydrochloride) 2.5 mg per 1 ml Betoptic 0.25% suspension eye drops | 5 ml [PoM] £2.66 DT price = £2.66
  Betoptic 0.25% eye drops suspension 0.25ml unit dose | 50 unit dose [PoM] £13.77
  Betaxolol (as Betaxolol hydrochloride) 5 mg per 1 ml Betoptic 0.5% eye drops | 5 ml [PoM] £1.90 DT price = £1.90

Carteolol hydrochloride

- **INDICATIONS AND DOSE**

Primary open-angle glaucoma
- ▶ TO THE EYE
- ▶ Adult: Apply twice daily

- CONTRA-INDICATIONS Also consider contra-indications listed for systemically administered beta blockers · bradycardia · heart block

- CAUTIONS Patients with corneal disease
  CAUTIONS, FURTHER INFORMATION
  Systemic absorption can follow topical application to the eyes; consider cautions listed for systemically administered beta blockers.

- INTERACTIONS → Appendix 1 (beta-blockers).
  Since systemic absorption may follow topical application the possibility of interactions, in particular, with drugs such as verapamil should be borne in mind.

- SIDE-EFFECTS Anaphylaxis · blepharoconjunctivitis · burning · corneal disorders · dry eyes · erythema · itching · ocular stinging · pain
  SIDE-EFFECTS, FURTHER INFORMATION
  Systemic absorption can follow topical application to the eyes; consider side effects listed for systemically administered beta blockers.

- MEDICINAL FORMS
  There can be variation in the licensing of different medicines containing the same drug.
  Eye drops
  EXCIPIENTS: May contain Benzalkonium chloride
  ▶ Teoptic (Thea Pharmaceuticals Ltd)
  Carteolol hydrochloride 10 mg per 1 ml Teoptic 1% eye drops | 5 ml [PoM] £7.60 DT price = £7.60
  Carteolol hydrochloride 20 mg per 1 ml Teoptic 2% eye drops | 5 ml [PoM] £8.40 DT price = £8.40

Levobunolol hydrochloride

- **INDICATIONS AND DOSE**

Primary open-angle glaucoma
- ▶ TO THE EYE
- ▶ Adult: Apply 1–2 times a day

- CONTRA-INDICATIONS Also consider contra-indications listed for systemically administered beta blockers · bradycardia · heart block

- CAUTIONS Patients with corneal disease
  CAUTIONS, FURTHER INFORMATION
  Systemic absorption can follow topical application to the eyes; consider cautions listed for systemically administered beta blockers.

- INTERACTIONS → Appendix 1 (beta-blockers).
  Since systemic absorption may follow topical application the possibility of interactions, in particular, with drugs such as verapamil should be borne in mind.

- SIDE-EFFECTS Anaphylaxis · anterior uveitis · blepharoconjunctivitis · burning · corneal disorders · dry eyes · erythema · itching · ocular stinging · pain
  SIDE-EFFECTS, FURTHER INFORMATION
  Systemic absorption can follow topical application to the eyes; consider side effects listed for systemically administered beta blockers.

- PRESCRIBING AND DISPENSING INFORMATION Although multi-dose (Levobunolol) eye drops commonly contain preservatives, preservative-free unit dose vials may be available.

- MEDICINAL FORMS
  There can be variation in the licensing of different medicines containing the same drug.
  Eye drops
  EXCIPIENTS: May contain Benzalkonium chloride, disodium edetate, sodium metabisulfite
  ▶ Betagan (Allergan Ltd)
  Levobunolol hydrochloride 5 mg per 1 ml Betagan 0.5% eye drops | 5 ml [PoM] £1.85 DT price = £1.85
  Betagan Unit Dose 0.5% eye drops 0.4ml unit dose | 30 unit dose [PoM] £9.98

Timolol maleate

- **INDICATIONS AND DOSE**

Reduction of intra-ocular pressure in primary open-angle glaucoma
- ▶ TO THE EYE
- ▶ Adult: Apply twice daily

continued →

Eye

TIMOPTOL-LA®

Reduction of intra-ocular pressure in primary open-angle glaucoma

▸ TO THE EYE
▸ Adult: Apply once daily

TIOPEX®

Reduction of intra-ocular pressure in primary open-angle glaucoma

▸ TO THE EYE
▸ Adult: Apply once daily, to be applied in the morning

- CONTRA-INDICATIONS Also consider contra-indications listed for systemically administered beta blockers · bradycardia · heart block
- CAUTIONS Consider also cautions listed for systemically administered beta blockers · patients with corneal disease
- INTERACTIONS Since systemic absorption may follow topical application the possibility of interactions, in particular, with drugs such as verapamil should be borne in mind.
- SIDE-EFFECTS Anaphylaxis · blepharoconjunctivitis · burning · corneal disorders · dry eyes · erythema · itching · ocular stinging · pain

SIDE-EFFECTS, FURTHER INFORMATION
Systemic absorption can follow topical application to the eyes; consider side effects listed for systemically administered beta blockers.

- BREAST FEEDING Manufacturer advises avoidance.
- PRESCRIBING AND DISPENSING INFORMATION Although multi-dose timolol eye drops commonly contain preservatives, preservative-free unit dose vials may be available.
- NATIONAL FUNDING/ACCESS DECISIONS
TIOPEX®

Scottish Medicines Consortium (SMC) Decisions
The *Scottish Medicines Consortium* has advised (February 2014) that timolol gel eye drops (*Tiopex*®) are accepted for restricted use within NHS Scotland for the reduction of elevated intraocular pressure in patients with ocular hypertension or chronic open angle glaucoma who have proven sensitivity to preservatives.

- MEDICINAL FORMS
There can be variation in the licensing of different medicines containing the same drug. Forms available from special-order manufacturers include: eye drops

Eye drops
EXCIPIENTS: May contain Benzalkonium chloride
▸ Timolol maleate (Non-proprietary)
  Timolol (as Timolol maleate) 2.5 mg per 1 ml Timolol 0.25% eye drops | 5 ml [PoM] £1.80 DT price = £1.02
  Timolol (as Timolol maleate) 5 mg per 1 ml Timolol 0.5% eye drops | 5 ml [PoM] £1.95 DT price = £1.04
▸ Timoptol (Santen UK Ltd)
  Timolol (as Timolol maleate) 2.5 mg per 1 ml Timoptol 0.25% eye drops | 5 ml [PoM] £3.12 DT price = £1.02
  Timoptol Unit Dose 0.25% ophthalmic solution 0.2ml unit dose | 30 unit dose [PoM] £8.45
  Timolol (as Timolol maleate) 5 mg per 1 ml Timoptol 0.5% eye drops | 5 ml [PoM] £3.12 DT price = £1.04
  Timoptol Unit Dose 0.5% ophthalmic solution 0.2ml unit dose | 30 unit dose [PoM] £9.65 DT price = £9.65
▸ Tiopex (Thea Pharmaceuticals Ltd)
  Timolol (as Timolol maleate) 1 mg per 1 gram Tiopex 1mg/g eye gel 0.4g unit dose | 30 unit dose [PoM] £7.49 DT price = £7.49

Eye gel
EXCIPIENTS: May contain Benzododecinium bromide
▸ Timoptol-LA (Santen UK Ltd)
  Timolol (as Timolol maleate) 2.5 mg per 1 ml Timoptol-LA 0.25% ophthalmic gel-forming solution | 2.5 ml [PoM] £3.12 DT price = £3.12

Timolol (as Timolol maleate) 5 mg per 1 ml Timoptol-LA 0.5% ophthalmic gel-forming solution | 2.5 ml [PoM] £3.12 DT price = £3.12

Combinations available: *Bimatoprost with timolol,* p. 1029 · *Brimonidine with timolol,* p. 1033 · *Brinzolamide with timolol,* p. 1027 · *Dorzolamide with timolol,* p. 1028 · *Latanoprost with timolol,* p. 1030 · *Tafluprost with timolol,* p. 1031 · *Travoprost with timolol,* p. 1032

CARBONIC ANHYDRASE INHIBITORS

Acetazolamide

- INDICATIONS AND DOSE

Reduction of intra-ocular pressure in open-angle glaucoma | Reduction of intra-ocular pressure in secondary glaucoma | Reduction of intra-ocular pressure perioperatively in angle-closure glaucoma

▸ BY MOUTH USING IMMEDIATE-RELEASE MEDICINES, OR BY INTRAVENOUS INJECTION, OR BY INTRAMUSCULAR INJECTION
▸ Adult: 0.25–1 g daily in divided doses, intramuscular injection preferably avoided because of alkalinity

Glaucoma
▸ BY MOUTH USING MODIFIED-RELEASE MEDICINES
▸ Adult: 250–500 mg daily

Epilepsy
▸ BY MOUTH USING IMMEDIATE-RELEASE MEDICINES, OR BY INTRAVENOUS INJECTION, OR BY INTRAMUSCULAR INJECTION
▸ Adult: 0.25–1 g daily in divided doses, intramuscular injection preferably avoided because of alkalinity

- CONTRA-INDICATIONS Adrenocortical insufficiency · hyperchloraemic acidosis · hypokalaemia · hyponatraemia · long-term administration in chronic angle-closure glaucoma
- CAUTIONS Avoid extravasation at injection site (risk of necrosis) · diabetes mellitus · elderly · impaired alveolar ventilation (risk of acidosis) · not generally recommended for long-term use · pulmonary obstruction (risk of acidosis) · renal calculi
- INTERACTIONS → Appendix 1 (diuretics)
- SIDE-EFFECTS
▸ **Common or very common** Ataxia · depression · diarrhoea · dizziness · excitement · fatigue · flushing · headache · irritability · loss of appetite · nausea · paraesthesia · polyuria · reduced libido · taste disturbance · thirst · vomiting
▸ **Uncommon** Blood disorders · bone marrow suppression · confusion · crystalluria · drowsiness · electrolyte disturbances on long-term therapy · fever · glycosuria · haematuria · hearing disturbances · melaena · metabolic acidosis · rash · renal calculi · renal colic · renal failure · renal lesions · Stevens-Johnson syndrome · toxic epidermal necrosis · ureteric colic
▸ **Rare** Cholestatic jaundice · convulsions · flaccid paralysis · fulminant hepatic necrosis · hepatitis · photosensitivity
▸ **Frequency not known** Transient myopia

SIDE-EFFECTS, FURTHER INFORMATION
Acetazolamide is a sulfonamide derivative; blood disorders, rashes, and other sulfonamide-related side-effects occur occasionally—patients should be told to report any unusual skin rash.
  If electrolyte disturbances and metabolic acidosis occur, these can be corrected by administering potassium bicarbonate (as effervescent potassium tablets).

- ALLERGY AND CROSS-SENSITIVITY Contra-indicated if history of sulfonamide hypersensitivity.
- PREGNANCY Manufacturer advises avoid, especially in first trimester (toxicity in *animal* studies).
- BREAST FEEDING Amount too small to be harmful.
- HEPATIC IMPAIRMENT Manufacturer advises avoid.

- RENAL IMPAIRMENT Avoid—risk of metabolic acidosis.
- MONITORING REQUIREMENTS Monitor blood count and plasma electrolyte concentrations with prolonged use.

- MEDICINAL FORMS
There can be variation in the licensing of different medicines containing the same drug. Forms available from special-order manufacturers include: oral suspension, oral solution

Tablet
CAUTIONARY AND ADVISORY LABELS 3
▸ Acetazolamide (Non-proprietary)
Acetazolamide 250 mg Acetazolamide 250mg tablets | 100 tablet PoM no price available | 112 tablet PoM £75.36 DT price = £64.00

Modified-release capsule
CAUTIONARY AND ADVISORY LABELS 3, 25
▸ Diamox SR (AMCo)
Acetazolamide 250 mg Diamox SR 250mg capsules | 30 capsule PoM £16.66 DT price = £16.66
▸ Eytazox (Auden McKenzie (Pharma Division) Ltd)
Acetazolamide 250 mg Eytazox 250mg modified-release capsules | 30 capsule PoM £16.60 DT price = £16.66

Powder for solution for injection
▸ Diamox (AMCo)
Acetazolamide 500 mg Diamox Sodium Parenteral 500mg powder for solution for injection vials | 1 vial PoM £14.76

Brinzolamide

- INDICATIONS AND DOSE

Reduction of intra-ocular pressure in ocular hypertension and open-angle glaucoma either as adjunct to beta-blockers or prostaglandin analogues or used alone in patients unresponsive to beta-blockers or if beta-blockers contra-indicated
▸ TO THE EYE
▸ Adult: Apply twice daily, then increased if necessary up to 3 times a day

- CONTRA-INDICATIONS Hyperchloraemic acidosis
- CAUTIONS Renal tubular immaturity or abnormality · systemic absorption follows topical application
- INTERACTIONS → Appendix 1 (brinzolamide).
Since systemic absorption may follow topical application of brinzolamide to the eye, the possibility of interactions should be borne in mind.
- SIDE-EFFECTS
▸ Common or very common Corneal erosion · corneal oedema · dry mouth · headache · ocular disturbances · photophobia · reduced visual acuity · taste disturbances
▸ Uncommon Alopecia · amnesia · bradycardia · chest pain · cough · decreased libido · depression · diarrhoea · dizziness · drowsiness · dyspepsia · dyspnoea · epistaxis · erectile dysfunction · flatulence · malaise · nasal dryness · nausea · nervousness · oesophagitis · oral hypoaesthesia and paraesthesia · palpitation · paraesthesia · pharyngitis · renal pain · sinusitis · sleep disturbances · throat irritation · tinnitus · upper respiratory tract congestion · vomiting
▸ Frequency not known Arrhythmia · asthma · dermatitis · erythema · hypertension · peripheral oedema · rhinitis · tachycardia · tremor · vertigo
SIDE-EFFECTS, FURTHER INFORMATION
Systemic absorption can rarely cause sulfonamide-like side-effects and may require discontinuation if severe.
- ALLERGY AND CROSS-SENSITIVITY Contra-indicated if history of sulfonamide hypersensitivity.
- PREGNANCY Avoid—toxicity in *animal* studies.
- BREAST FEEDING Use only if benefit outweighs risk.
- HEPATIC IMPAIRMENT Manufacturer advises avoid.
- RENAL IMPAIRMENT Avoid if eGFR less than 30 mL/minute/1.73 m².

- MEDICINAL FORMS
There can be variation in the licensing of different medicines containing the same drug.
Eye drops
EXCIPIENTS: May contain Benzalkonium chloride, disodium edetate
▸ Brinzolamide (Non-proprietary)
Brinzolamide 10 mg per 1 ml Brinzolamide 10mg/ml eye drops | 5 ml PoM £6.92 DT price = £3.36
▸ Azopt (Alcon Laboratories (UK) Ltd)
Brinzolamide 10 mg per 1 ml Azopt 10mg/ml eye drops | 5 ml PoM £6.92 DT price = £3.36

Brinzolamide with timolol

The properties listed below are those particular to the combination only. For the properties of the components please consider, brinzolamide above, timolol maleate p. 1025.

- INDICATIONS AND DOSE

Raised intra-ocular pressure in open-angle glaucoma or ocular hypertension when beta-blocker alone not adequate
▸ TO THE EYE
▸ Adult: Apply twice daily

- MEDICINAL FORMS
There can be variation in the licensing of different medicines containing the same drug.
Eye drops
EXCIPIENTS: May contain Benzalkonium chloride, disodium edetate
▸ Azarga (Alcon Laboratories (UK) Ltd)
Timolol (as Timolol maleate) 5 mg per 1 ml, Brinzolamide 10 mg per 1 ml Azarga 10mg/ml / 5mg/ml eye drops | 5 ml PoM £11.05 DT price = £11.05

Dorzolamide

- INDICATIONS AND DOSE

Raised intra-ocular pressure in ocular hypertension used alone in patients unresponsive to beta-blockers or if beta-blockers contra-indicated | Open-angle glaucoma used alone in patients unresponsive to beta-blockers or if beta-blockers contra-indicated | Pseudo-exfoliative glaucoma used alone in patients unresponsive to beta-blockers or if beta-blockers contra-indicated
▸ TO THE EYE
▸ Adult: Apply 3 times a day

Raised intra-ocular pressure in ocular hypertension as adjunct to beta-blocker | Open-angle glaucoma as adjunct to beta-blocker | Pseudo-exfoliative glaucoma as adjunct to beta-blocker
▸ TO THE EYE
▸ Adult: Apply twice daily

- CONTRA-INDICATIONS Hyperchloraemic acidosis
- CAUTIONS Chronic corneal defects · history of intra-ocular surgery · history of renal calculi · low endothelial cell count · systemic absorption follows topical application
- INTERACTIONS → Appendix 1 (dorzolamide).
Since systemic absorption may follow topical application of dorzolamide to the eye, the possibility of interactions should be borne in mind.
- SIDE-EFFECTS
▸ Common or very common Asthenia · bitter taste · blurred vision · conjunctivitis · eyelid inflammation · headache · lacrimation · nausea · ocular irritation · superficial punctate keratitis
▸ Uncommon Iridocyclitis
▸ Rare Contact dermatitis · corneal oedema · dizziness · dry mouth · epistaxis · eyelid crusting · paraesthesia · Stevens-

11

Eye

Johnson syndrome · throat irritation · toxic epidermal necrolysis · transient myopia · urolithiasis

SIDE-EFFECTS, FURTHER INFORMATION
Systemic absorption can rarely cause sulfonamide-like side-effects and may require discontinuation if severe.

● ALLERGY AND CROSS-SENSITIVITY Contra-indicated if history of sulfonamide hypersensitivity.

● PREGNANCY Manufacturer advises avoid—toxicity in *animal* studies.

● BREAST FEEDING Manufacturer advises avoid—no information available.

● HEPATIC IMPAIRMENT Manufacturer advises caution— no information available.

● RENAL IMPAIRMENT Avoid if eGFR less than 30 mL/minute/1.73 m^2.

● PRESCRIBING AND DISPENSING INFORMATION Although multi-dose dorzolamide eye drops commonly contain preservatives, preservative-free unit dose vials may be available.

● MEDICINAL FORMS
There can be variation in the licensing of different medicines containing the same drug.

Eye drops
EXCIPIENTS: May contain Benzalkonium chloride
▸ Dorzolamide (Non-proprietary)
Dorzolamide (as Dorzolamide hydrochloride) 20 mg per 1 ml Dorzolamide 2% eye drops | 5 ml [PoM] £6.33 DT price = £1.92
▸ Trusopt (Santen UK Ltd)
Dorzolamide (as Dorzolamide hydrochloride) 20 mg per 1 ml Trusopt 2% eye drops | 5 ml [PoM] £6.33 DT price = £1.92
Trusopt 2% eye drops 0.2ml unit dose preservative free | 60 unit dose [PoM] £24.18 DT price = £24.18

Dorzolamide with timolol

The properties listed below are those particular to the combination only. For the properties of the components please consider, dorzolamide p. 1027, timolol maleate p. 1025.

● INDICATIONS AND DOSE
Raised intra-ocular pressure in ocular hypertension when beta-blockers alone not adequate | Raised intra-ocular pressure in open-angle glaucoma when beta-blockers alone not adequate | Raised intra-ocular pressure in pseudo-exfoliative glaucoma when beta-blockers alone not adequate
▸ TO THE EYE
▸ Adult: Apply twice daily

● PRESCRIBING AND DISPENSING INFORMATION Although multi-dose dorzolamide with timolol eye drops commonly contain preservatives, preservative-free unit dose vials may be available.

● MEDICINAL FORMS
There can be variation in the licensing of different medicines containing the same drug.

Eye drops
EXCIPIENTS: May contain Benzalkonium chloride
▸ Dorzolamide with timolol (Non-proprietary)
Timolol (as Timolol maleate) 5 mg per 1 ml, Dorzolamide (as Dorzolamide hydrochloride) 20 mg per 1 ml Dorzolamide 2% / Timolol 0.5% eye drops | 5 ml [PoM] £27.16 DT price = £2.20
Dorzolamide 2% / Timolol 0.5% eye drops 0.2ml unit dose preservative free | 60 unit dose [PoM] £27.16 DT price = £28.59
▸ Cosopt (Santen UK Ltd)
Timolol (as Timolol maleate) 5 mg per 1 ml, Dorzolamide (as Dorzolamide hydrochloride) 20 mg per 1 ml Cosopt eye drops 0.2ml unit dose preservative free | 60 unit dose [PoM] £28.59 DT price = £28.59
Cosopt eye drops | 5 ml [PoM] £10.05 DT price = £2.20

MIOTICS ⟩ PARASYMPATHOMIMETICS

Pilocarpine

● DRUG ACTION Pilocarpine acts by opening the inefficient drainage channels in the trabecular meshwork.

● INDICATIONS AND DOSE
Primary angle-closure glaucoma | Some secondary glaucomas
▸ TO THE EYE
▸ Adult: Apply up to 4 times a day

● CONTRA-INDICATIONS Acute inflammatory disease of the anterior segment · acute iritis · anterior uveitis · conditions where pupillary constriction is undesirable · some forms of secondary glaucoma (where pupillary constriction is undesirable)

● CAUTIONS A darkly pigmented iris may require a higher concentration of the miotic or more frequent administration and care should be taken to avoid overdosage · asthma · cardiac disease · care in conjunctival damage · care in corneal damage · epilepsy · gastro-intestinal spasm · hypertension · hyperthyroidism · hypotension · marked vasomotor instability · Parkinson's disease · peptic ulceration · retinal detachment has occurred in susceptible individuals and those with retinal disease · urinary-tract obstruction

● INTERACTIONS → Appendix 1 (parasympathomimetics). Systemic effects rare following application to the eye.

● SIDE-EFFECTS
▸ **Rare** Parasympathomimetics systemic side effects
▸ **Frequency not known** Blurred vision · ciliary spasm (leads to headache and browache which may be more severe in the initial 2–4 weeks of treatment—a particular disadvantage in patients under 40 years of age) · conjunctival vascular congestion · lens changes (with chronic use) · myopia · ocular burning · ocular itching · pupillary block · smarting · vitreous haemorrhage

● PREGNANCY Avoid unless the potential benefit outweighs risk—limited information available.

● BREAST FEEDING Avoid unless the potential benefit outweighs risk—no information available.

● PRE-TREATMENT SCREENING Fundus examination is advised before starting treatment with a miotic (retinal detachment has occurred).

● MONITORING REQUIREMENTS Intra-ocular pressure and visual fields should be monitored in those with chronic simple glaucoma and those receiving long-term treatment with a miotic.

● PRESCRIBING AND DISPENSING INFORMATION Although multi-dose pilocarpine eye drops commonly contain preservatives, preservative-free unit dose vials may be available.

● PATIENT AND CARER ADVICE
Driving and skilled tasks
Blurred vision may affect performance of skilled tasks (e.g. driving) particularly at night or in reduced lighting.

● MEDICINAL FORMS
There can be variation in the licensing of different medicines containing the same drug. Forms available from special-order manufacturers include: eye drops

Eye drops
EXCIPIENTS: May contain Benzalkonium chloride
▸ Pilocarpine (Non-proprietary)
Pilocarpine hydrochloride 10 mg per 1 ml Pilocarpine hydrochloride 1% eye drops | 10 ml [PoM] £6.30 DT price = £5.33
Pilocarpine hydrochloride 20 mg per 1 ml Pilocarpine hydrochloride 2% eye drops | 10 ml [PoM] £7.74 DT price = £6.51
Pilocarpine hydrochloride 40 mg per 1 ml Pilocarpine hydrochloride 4% eye drops | 10 ml [PoM] £8.70 DT price = £7.32

▸ **Pilocarpine nitrate** (Bausch & Lomb UK Ltd)
Pilocarpine nitrate 20 mg per 1 ml Minims pilocarpine nitrate 2%
eye drops 0.5ml unit dose | 20 unit dose [PoM] £11.99

PROSTAGLANDIN ANALOGUES AND PROSTAMIDES

Bimatoprost

- **INDICATIONS AND DOSE**

Raised intra-ocular pressure in open-angle glaucoma | Ocular hypertension
▸ TO THE EYE
▸ Adult: Apply once daily, to be administered preferably in the evening

- CAUTIONS Angle-closure glaucoma (no experience of use) · aphakia · asthma · chronic obstructive pulmonary disease · compromised respiratory function · congenital glaucoma (no experience of use) · contact lens wearers · history of significant ocular viral infections · inflammatory ocular conditions (no experience of use) · narrow-angle glaucoma (no experience of use) · neovascular glaucoma (no experience of use) · predisposition to bradycardia · predisposition to hypotension · pseudophakia with torn posterior lens capsule or anterior chamber lenses · risk factors for cystoid macular oedema · risk factors for iritis · risk factors for uveitis

- SIDE-EFFECTS
▸ **Common or very common** Blepharitis · blood pressure changes · brown pigmentation particularly in those with mixed-colour irides · conjunctival disorders · corneal erosion · darkening, thickening and lengthening of eye lashes · eyelash and vellus hair changes · headache · ocular discomfort · photophobia · pigmentation of periocular skin · punctate keratitis · reduced visual acuity · transient punctate epithelial erosion
▸ **Uncommon** Asthenopia · dizziness · skin rash
▸ **Rare** Arthralgia · darkening of palpebral skin · facial oedema · iritis · macular oedema · myalgia · uveitis
▸ **Very rare** Chest pain · exacerbation of angina · palpitation · periorbital changes resulting in deepening of the eyelid sulcus
▸ **Frequency not known** Asthma · blepharospasm · bradycardia · dyspnoea · exacerbation of asthma · exacerbation of COPD · eyelid retraction · malaise · nausea · ocular infection · reactivation of previous corneal infiltrates · retinal haemorrhage

- PREGNANCY Manufacturer advises use only if potential benefit outweighs risk.

- BREAST FEEDING Manufacturer advises avoid—present in milk in *animal* studies.

- HEPATIC IMPAIRMENT Use with caution in moderate to severe impairment—no information available.

- RENAL IMPAIRMENT Use with caution—no information available.

- PRESCRIBING AND DISPENSING INFORMATION Although multi-dose bimatoprost eye drops commonly contain preservatives, preservative-free unit dose vials may be available.

- PATIENT AND CARER ADVICE
Changes to eye colour Before initiating treatment, patients should be warned of a possible change in eye colour as an increase in the brown pigment in the iris can occur, which may be permanent; particular care is required in those with mixed coloured irides and those receiving treatment to one eye only. Changes in eyelashes and vellus hair can also occur, and patients should also be advised to avoid repeated contact of the eye drop solution with skin as this can lead to hair growth or skin pigmentation.

- NATIONAL FUNDING/ACCESS DECISIONS
LUMIGAN®

Scottish Medicines Consortium (SMC) Decisions
The *Scottish Medicines Consortium* has advised (March 2013) that bimatoprost 300 micrograms/mL preservative-free eye drops (*Lumigan®* single-dose eye drops) are accepted for restricted use within NHS Scotland for the reduction of elevated intra-ocular pressure in chronic open-angle glaucoma and ocular hypertension (as monotherapy or as adjunctive therapy to beta-blockers) in adults who have proven sensitivity to benzalkonium chloride.

- MEDICINAL FORMS
There can be variation in the licensing of different medicines containing the same drug.
Eye drops
EXCIPIENTS: May contain Benzalkonium chloride
▸ Lumigan (Allergan Ltd)
Bimatoprost 100 microgram per 1 ml Lumigan 100micrograms/ml eye drops | 3 ml [PoM] £11.71 DT price = £11.71 | 9 ml [PoM] £35.13
Bimatoprost 300 microgram per 1 ml Lumigan 300micrograms/ml eye drops 0.4ml unit dose | 30 unit dose [PoM] £13.75 DT price = £13.75

Bimatoprost with timolol

The properties listed below are those particular to the combination only. For the properties of the components please consider, bimatoprost above, timolol maleate p. 1025.

- **INDICATIONS AND DOSE**

Raised intra-ocular pressure in patients with open-angle glaucoma or ocular hypertension when beta-blocker or prostaglandin analogue alone not adequate
▸ TO THE EYE
▸ Adult: Apply once daily

- NATIONAL FUNDING/ACCESS DECISIONS
GANFORT® SINGLE USE

Scottish Medicines Consortium (SMC) Decisions
The Scottish Medicines Consortium has advised (October 2013) that *Ganfort®* unit dose eye drops are accepted for restricted use within NHS Scotland for the reduction of intra-ocular pressure in patients with open-angle glaucoma or ocular hypertension insufficiently responsive to topical beta-blockers or prostaglandin analogues who have proven sensitivity to preservatives.

- MEDICINAL FORMS
There can be variation in the licensing of different medicines containing the same drug.
Eye drops
EXCIPIENTS: May contain Benzalkonium chloride
▸ Ganfort (Allergan Ltd)
Bimatoprost 300 microgram per 1 ml, Timolol (as Timolol maleate) 5 mg per 1 ml Ganfort 0.3mg/ml / 5mg/ml eye drops | 3 ml [PoM] £13.95 DT price = £13.95 | 9 ml [PoM] £37.59
Ganfort 0.3mg/ml / 5mg/ml eye drops 0.4ml unit dose | 30 unit dose [PoM] £17.50

11

Eye

Latanoprost

- **INDICATIONS AND DOSE**

Raised intra-ocular pressure in open-angle glaucoma | Ocular hypertension
- ▶ TO THE EYE
- ▶ **Adult:** Apply once daily, to be administered preferably in the evening

---

IMPORTANT SAFETY INFORMATION

MHRA/CHM ADVICE: LATANOPROST (*XALATAN*®): INCREASED REPORTING OF EYE IRRITATION SINCE REFORMULATION (JULY 2015)

Following reformulation of *Xalatan*®, to allow for long-term storage at room temperature, there has been an increase in the number of reports of eye irritation from across the EU. Patients should be advised to tell their health professional promptly (within a week) if they experience eye irritation (e.g. excessive watering) severe enough to make them consider stopping treatment. Review treatment and prescribe a different formulation if necessary.

- **CONTRA-INDICATIONS** Active herpes simplex keratitis · history of recurrent herpetic keratitis associated with prostaglandin analogues
- **CAUTIONS** Angle-closure glaucoma (no experience of use) · aphakia · asthma · chronic obstructive pulmonary disease · compromised respiratory function · congenital glaucoma (no experience of use) · contact lens wearers · do not use within 5 minutes of thiomersal-containing preparations · history of significant ocular viral infections · inflammatory ocular conditions (no experience of use) · narrow-angle glaucoma (no experience of use) · neovascular glaucoma (no experience of use) · peri-operative period of cataract surgery · pseudophakia with torn posterior lens capsule or anterior chamber lenses · risk factors for cystoid macular oedema · risk factors for iritis · risk factors for uveitis
- **SIDE-EFFECTS**
- ▶ **Common or very common** Blepharitis · blood pressure changes · brown pigmentation particularly in those with mixed-colour irides · conjunctival disorders · corneal erosion · darkening, thickening and lengthening of eye lashes · eyelash and vellus hair changes · headache · ocular discomfort · photophobia · pigmentation of periocular skin · punctate keratitis · reduced visual acuity · transient punctate epithelial erosion
- ▶ **Uncommon** Asthenopia · dizziness · skin rash
- ▶ **Rare** Arthralgia · darkening of palpebral skin · facial oedema · iritis · macular oedema · myalgia · uveitis
- ▶ **Very rare** Chest pain · exacerbation of angina · palpitation · periorbital changes resulting in deepening of the eyelid sulcus
- ▶ **Frequency not known** Asthma · dyspnoea · exacerbation of asthma · exacerbation of COPD · iris cyst · nasopharyngitis · pyrexia
- **PREGNANCY** Manufacturer advises avoid.
- **BREAST FEEDING** May be present in milk—manufacturer advises avoid.
- **PRESCRIBING AND DISPENSING INFORMATION** Although multi-dose latanoprost eye drops commonly contain preservatives, preservative-free unit dose vials may be available.
- **PATIENT AND CARER ADVICE**
Changes in eye colour Before initiating treatment, patients should be warned of a possible change in eye colour as an increase in the brown pigment in the iris can occur, which may be permanent; particular care is required in those with mixed coloured irides and those receiving treatment to one eye only. Changes in eyelashes and vellus hair can

also occur, and patients should also be advised to avoid repeated contact of the eye drop solution with skin as this can lead to hair growth or skin pigmentation.

- **NATIONAL FUNDING/ACCESS DECISIONS**
MONOPOST®

Scottish Medicines Consortium (SMC) Decisions
The *Scottish Medicines Consortium* has advised (June 2013) that *Monopost*® is accepted for restricted use within NHS Scotland for the reduction of elevated intra-ocular pressure in patients with open-angle glaucoma and ocular hypertension who have proven sensitivity to benzalkonium chloride.

- **MEDICINAL FORMS**
There can be variation in the licensing of different medicines containing the same drug.

Eye drops
EXCIPIENTS: May contain Benzalkonium chloride
- ▶ Latanoprost (Non-proprietary)
  Latanoprost 50 microgram per 1 ml Latanoprost 50micrograms/ml eye drops | 2.5 ml [PoM] £12.48 DT price = £1.56
- ▶ Monopost (Thea Pharmaceuticals Ltd)
  Latanoprost 50 microgram per 1 ml Monopost 50micrograms/ml eye drops 0.2ml unit dose | 30 unit dose [PoM] £8.49 DT price = £8.49 | 90 unit dose [PoM] £25.47 DT price = £25.47
- ▶ Xalatan (Pfizer Ltd)
  Latanoprost 50 microgram per 1 ml Xalatan 50micrograms/ml eye drops | 2.5 ml [PoM] £12.48 DT price = £1.56

Latanoprost with timolol

The properties listed below are those particular to the combination only. For the properties of the components please consider, latanoprost above, timolol maleate p. 1025.

- **INDICATIONS AND DOSE**

Raised intra-ocular pressure in patients with open-angle glaucoma and ocular hypertension when beta-blocker or prostaglandin analogue alone not adequate
- ▶ TO THE EYE
- ▶ **Adult:** Apply once daily

- **MEDICINAL FORMS**
There can be variation in the licensing of different medicines containing the same drug.

Eye drops
EXCIPIENTS: May contain Benzalkonium chloride
- ▶ Latanoprost with timolol (Non-proprietary)
  Latanoprost 50 microgram per 1 ml, Timolol (as Timolol maleate) 5 mg per 1 ml Latanoprost 50micrograms/ml / Timolol 5mg/ml eye drops | 2.5 ml [PoM] £14.32 DT price = £2.02
- ▶ Xalacom (Pfizer Ltd)
  Latanoprost 50 microgram per 1 ml, Timolol (as Timolol maleate) 5 mg per 1 ml Xalacom eye drops | 2.5 ml [PoM] £14.32 DT price = £2.02

Tafluprost

- **INDICATIONS AND DOSE**

Raised intra-ocular pressure in open-angle glaucoma | Ocular hypertension
- ▶ TO THE EYE
- ▶ **Adult:** Apply once daily, to be administered preferably in the evening

- **CAUTIONS** Angle-closure glaucoma (no experience of use) · aphakia · asthma · chronic obstructive pulmonary disease · compromised respiratory function · congenital glaucoma (no experience of use) · contact lens wearers · history of significant ocular viral infections · inflammatory ocular conditions (no experience of use) · narrow-angle glaucoma (no experience of use) · neovascular glaucoma (no experience of use) · pseudophakia with torn posterior lens capsule or anterior chamber lenses · risk factors for cystoid macular oedema · risk factors for iritis · risk factors for uveitis

- **SIDE-EFFECTS**
- ▶ **Common or very common** Blepharitis · blood pressure changes · brown pigmentation particularly in those with mixed-colour irides · conjunctival disorders · corneal erosion · darkening, thickening and lengthening of eye lashes · eyelash and vellus hair changes · headache · ocular discomfort · photophobia · pigmentation of periocular skin · punctuate keratitis · reduced visual acuity · transient punctate epithelial erosion
- ▶ **Uncommon** Asthenopia · dizziness · skin rash
- ▶ **Rare** Arthralgia · darkening of palpebral skin · facial oedema · iritis · macular oedema · myalgia · uveitis
- ▶ **Very rare** Chest pain · exacerbation of angina · palpitation · periorbital changes resulting in deepening of the eyelid sulcus
- ▶ **Frequency not known** Asthma · dyspnoea · exacerbation of asthma · exacerbation of COPD
- **PREGNANCY** Manufacturer advises avoid unless potential benefit outweighs risk—toxicity in *animal* studies.
- **BREAST FEEDING** Manufacturer advises avoid—present in milk in *animal* studies.
- **HEPATIC IMPAIRMENT** Use with caution—no information available.
- **RENAL IMPAIRMENT** Use with caution—no information available.
- **PRESCRIBING AND DISPENSING INFORMATION** Although multi-dose tafluprost eye drops commonly contain preservatives, preservative-free unit dose vials may be available.
- **PATIENT AND CARER ADVICE**
  Changes to eye colour Before initiating treatment, patients should be warned of a possible change in eye colour as an increase in the brown pigment in the iris can occur, which may be permanent; particular care is required in those with mixed coloured irides and those receiving treatment to one eye only. Changes in eyelashes and vellus hair can also occur, and patients should also be advised to avoid repeated contact of the eye drop solution with skin as this can lead to hair growth or skin pigmentation.

- **MEDICINAL FORMS**
  There can be variation in the licensing of different medicines containing the same drug.

  Eye drops
  EXCIPIENTS: May contain Disodium edetate
  ▶ Tafluprost (Non-proprietary)
      Tafluprost 15 microgram per 1 ml Taflotan 15micrograms/ml eye drops | 2.5 ml PoM no price available
  ▶ Saflutan (Santen UK Ltd)
      Tafluprost 15 microgram per 1 ml Saflutan 15micrograms/ml eye drops 0.3ml unit dose | 30 unit dose PoM £12.20 DT price = £12.20

Tafluprost with timolol
30.3.2016

The properties listed below are those particular to the combination only. For the properties of the components please consider, tafluprost p. 1030, timolol maleate p. 1025.

- **INDICATIONS AND DOSE**

Raised intra-ocular pressure in open-angle glaucoma and ocular hypertension when beta-blocker or prostaglandin analogue alone not adequate
- ▶ TO THE EYE
- ▶ Adult: Apply 1 drop once daily

- **SIDE-EFFECTS**
- ▶ **Common or very common** Blurred vision · ocular hyperaemia

- ▶ **Uncommon** Anterior chamber inflammation · conjunctivitis
- **PATIENT AND CARER ADVICE**
  Driving and skilled tasks
  Blurred vision may affect performance of skilled tasks (e.g. driving or operating machinery).
- **NATIONAL FUNDING/ACCESS DECISIONS**
  Scottish Medicines Consortium (SMC) Decisions
  The *Scottish Medicines Consortium* has advised (September 2015) that *Taptiqom* ® (tafluprost with timolol) is accepted for restricted use within NHS Scotland, within the licensed indications, in patients who have proven sensitivity to preservatives.

- **MEDICINAL FORMS**
  There can be variation in the licensing of different medicines containing the same drug.

  Eye drops
  EXCIPIENTS: May contain Disodium edetate
  ▶ Taptiqom (Santen UK Ltd)
      Tafluprost 15 microgram per 1 ml, Timolol (as Timolol maleate) 5 mg per 1 ml Taptiqom 15micrograms/ml / 5mg/ml eye drops | 30 unit dose PoM £14.50

Travoprost

- **INDICATIONS AND DOSE**

Raised intra-ocular pressure in open-angle glaucoma | Ocular hypertension
- ▶ TO THE EYE
- ▶ Adult: Apply once daily, to be administered preferably in the evening

- **CAUTIONS** History of significant ocular viral infections · angle-closure glaucoma (no experience of use) · aphakia · asthma · chronic obstructive pulmonary disease · compromised respiratory function · congenital glaucoma (no experience of use) · contact lens wearers · inflammatory ocular conditions (no experience of use) · narrow-angle glaucoma (no experience of use) · neovascular glaucoma (no experience of use) · pseudophakia with torn posterior lens capsule or anterior chamber lenses · risk factors for cystoid macular oedema · risk factors for iritis · risk factors for uveitis
- **SIDE-EFFECTS**
- ▶ **Common or very common** Blepharitis · blood pressure changes · brown pigmentation particularly in those with mixed-colour irides · conjunctival disorders · corneal erosion · darkening, thickening and lengthening of eye lashes · eyelash and vellus hair changes · headache · ocular discomfort · photophobia · pigmentation of periocular skin · punctuate keratitis · reduced visual acuity · transient punctate epithelial erosion
- ▶ **Uncommon** Asthenopia · dizziness · skin rash
- ▶ **Rare** Arthralgia · darkening of palpebral skin · facial oedema · iritis · macular oedema · myalgia · uveitis
- ▶ **Very rare** Chest pain · exacerbation of angina · palpitation · periorbital changes resulting in deepening of the eyelid sulcus
- ▶ **Frequency not known** Asthma · bradycardia · cataract · constipation · cough · dry mouth · dysgeusia · dysphonia · dyspnoea · exacerbation of asthma · exacerbation of COPD · gastro-intestinal disorders · herpes simplex · malaise · mydriasis · nasal congestion · oropharyngeal pain · peptic ulcer reactivation · photopsia · throat irritation · tinnitus · vertigo
- **PREGNANCY** Manufacturer advises avoid unless potential benefit outweighs risk—toxicity in *animal* studies.
- **BREAST FEEDING** Present in milk in *animal* studies; manufacturer advises avoid.

● PATIENT AND CARER ADVICE
Changes to eye colour Before initiating treatment, patients should be warned of a possible change in eye colour as an increase in the brown pigment in the iris can occur, which may be permanent; particular care is required in those with mixed coloured irides and those receiving treatment to one eye only. Changes in eyelashes and vellus hair can also occur, and patients should also be advised to avoid repeated contact of the eye drop solution with skin as this can lead to hair growth or skin pigmentation.

● MEDICINAL FORMS
There can be variation in the licensing of different medicines containing the same drug.
Eye drops
EXCIPIENTS: May contain Propylene glycol
▸ Travatan (Alcon Laboratories (UK) Ltd)
Travoprost 40 microgram per 1 ml Travatan 40micrograms/ml eye drops | 2.5 ml [PoM] £10.95 DT price = £10.95

Travoprost with timolol

The properties listed below are those particular to the combination only. For the properties of the components please consider, travoprost p. 1031, timolol maleate p. 1025.

● INDICATIONS AND DOSE
Raised intra-ocular pressure in patients with open-angle glaucoma or ocular hypertension when beta-blocker or prostaglandin analogue alone not adequate
▸ TO THE EYE
▸ Adult: Apply once daily

● MEDICINAL FORMS
There can be variation in the licensing of different medicines containing the same drug.
Eye drops
EXCIPIENTS: May contain Propylene glycol
▸ DuoTrav (Alcon Laboratories (UK) Ltd)
Travoprost 40 microgram per 1 ml, Timolol (as Timolol maleate) 5 mg per 1 ml DuoTrav 40micrograms/ml / 5mg/ml eye drops | 2.5 ml [PoM] £13.95 DT price = £13.95 | 7.5 ml [PoM] £39.68

SYMPATHOMIMETICS › ALPHA₂-ADRENOCEPTOR
AGONISTS

Apraclonidine

● DRUG ACTION Apraclonidine is an alpha₂-adrenoceptor agonist that lowers intra-ocular pressure by reducing aqueous humour formation. It is a derivative of clonidine.

● INDICATIONS AND DOSE
Control or prevention of postoperative elevation of intra-ocular pressure after anterior segment laser surgery
▸ TO THE EYE
▸ Adult: Apply 1 drop, 1 hour before laser procedure, then 1 drop, immediately after completion of procedure, 1% eye drops to be administered
Short-term adjunctive treatment of chronic glaucoma in patients not adequately controlled by another drug
▸ TO THE EYE
▸ Adult: Apply 1 drop 3 times a day usually for maximum 1 month, 0.5% eye drops to be administered, may not provide additional benefit if patient already using two drugs that suppress the production of aqueous humour

● CONTRA-INDICATIONS History of severe or unstable and uncontrolled cardiovascular disease
● CAUTIONS Cerebrovascular disease · depression · heart failure · history of angina · hypertension · loss of effect may occur over time · Parkinson's syndrome · Raynaud's syndrome · recent myocardial infarction · reduction in

vision in end-stage glaucoma (suspend treatment) · severe coronary insufficiency · thromboangiitis obliterans · vasovagal attack

● INTERACTIONS → Appendix 1 (apraclonidine).

● SIDE-EFFECTS
▸ **Common or very common** Conjunctivitis · dry eye · ocular intolerance · rhinitis · taste disturbance
▸ **Uncommon** Asthma · blepharitis · blepharospasm · chest pain · conjunctival vascular disorders · corneal erosion and infiltrates · dyspnoea · eyelid ptosis or retraction · impaired co-ordination · irritability · keratitis · keratopathy · myalgia · mydriasis · nervousness · parosmia · photophobia · rhinorrhoea · throat irritation · visual impairment

SIDE-EFFECTS, FURTHER INFORMATION
▸ **Ocular intolerance** Withdraw if eye pruritus, ocular hyperaemia, increased lacrimation, or oedema of the eyelids and conjunctiva occur.
▸ **Systemic effects** Since absorption may follow topical application, see clonidine hydrochloride p. 131.

● PREGNANCY Manufacturer advises avoid—no information available.
● BREAST FEEDING Manufacturer advises avoid—no information available.
● HEPATIC IMPAIRMENT Manufacturer advises caution.
● RENAL IMPAIRMENT Use with caution in chronic renal failure.
● MONITORING REQUIREMENTS
▸ Monitor intra-ocular pressure and visual fields.
▸ Monitor for excessive reduction in intra-ocular pressure following peri-operative use.
● PATIENT AND CARER ADVICE
Driving and skilled tasks
Drowsiness may affect performance of skilled tasks (e.g. driving).

● MEDICINAL FORMS
There can be variation in the licensing of different medicines containing the same drug.
Eye drops
EXCIPIENTS: May contain Benzalkonium chloride
▸ Iopidine (Alcon Laboratories (UK) Ltd)
Apraclonidine (as Apraclonidine hydrochloride) 5 mg per 1 ml Iopidine 5mg/ml eye drops | 5 ml [PoM] £10.88 DT price = £10.88
Apraclonidine (as Apraclonidine hydrochloride) 10 mg per 1 ml Iopidine 1% eye drops 0.25ml unit dose | 24 unit dose [PoM] £77.85 DT price = £77.85

Brimonidine tartrate

● DRUG ACTION Brimonidine, an alpha₂-adrenoceptor agonist, is thought to lower intra-ocular pressure by reducing aqueous humour formation and increasing uveoscleral outflow.

● INDICATIONS AND DOSE
Raised intra-ocular pressure in open-angle glaucoma in patients for whom beta-blockers are inappropriate | Ocular hypertension in patients for whom beta-blockers are inappropriate | Adjunctive therapy when intra-ocular pressure is inadequately controlled by other antiglaucoma therapy
▸ TO THE EYE
▸ Adult: Apply twice daily

● CAUTIONS Cerebral insufficiency · coronary insufficiency · depression · postural hypotension · Raynaud's syndrome · severe cardiovascular disease · thromboangiitis obliterans
● INTERACTIONS → Appendix 1 (brimonidine).

- SIDE-EFFECTS
► **Common or very common** Burning sensation at application · conjunctival blanching · conjunctival disturbances · conjunctival follicles · conjunctival infection · corneal erosion · corneal staining · dizziness · drowsiness · dry mouth · eyelid inflammation · gastro-intestinal disturbances · headache · malaise · ocular disturbances · ocular dryness · ocular hyperaemia · ocular pain · ocular pruritus · photophobia · stinging at application site · taste disturbances · upper respiratory symptoms · visual disturbances
► **Uncommon** Arrhythmia · bradycardia · depression · nasal dryness · palpitation · tachycardia
► **Rare** Dyspnoea
► **Very rare** Hypertension · hypotension · insomnia · iritis · miosis · syncope

- PREGNANCY Limited information available; manufacturer advises use only if benefit outweighs risk.

- BREAST FEEDING Manufacturer advises avoid—no information available.

- HEPATIC IMPAIRMENT Manufacturer advises use with caution.

- RENAL IMPAIRMENT Manufacturer advises use with caution.

- PATIENT AND CARER ADVICE
Driving and skilled tasks
Drowsiness may affect performance of skilled tasks (e.g. driving).

- MEDICINAL FORMS
There can be variation in the licensing of different medicines containing the same drug.
Eye drops
EXCIPIENTS: May contain Benzalkonium chloride
► Brimonidine tartrate (Non-proprietary)
Brimonidine tartrate 2 mg per 1 ml Brimonidine 0.2% eye drops | 5 ml [PoM] £6.85 DT price = £1.80
► Alphagan (Allergan Ltd)
Brimonidine tartrate 2 mg per 1 ml Alphagan 0.2% eye drops | 5 ml [PoM] £6.85 DT price = £1.80
► Brymont (Blumont Pharma Ltd)
Brimonidine tartrate 2 mg per 1 ml Brymont 2mg/ml eye drops | 5 ml [PoM] £2.27 DT price = £1.80

Brimonidine with timolol

The properties listed below are those particular to the combination only. For the properties of the components please consider, brimonidine tartrate p. 1032, timolol maleate p. 1025.

- INDICATIONS AND DOSE
Raised intra-ocular pressure in open-angle glaucoma and for ocular hypertension when beta-blocker alone not adequate
► TO THE EYE
► Adult: Apply twice daily

- MEDICINAL FORMS
There can be variation in the licensing of different medicines containing the same drug.
Eye drops
EXCIPIENTS: May contain Benzalkonium chloride
► Combigan (Allergan Ltd)
Brimonidine tartrate 2 mg per 1 ml, Timolol (as Timolol maleate) 5 mg per 1 ml Combigan eye drops | 5 ml [PoM] £10.00 DT price = £10.00 | 15 ml [PoM] £27.00

6 Retinal disorders
6.1 Macular degeneration

Subfoveal choroidal neovascularisation

Treatment
Aflibercept below, pegaptanib sodium p. 1034 and ranibizumab p. 1035 are vascular endothelial growth factor inhibitors licensed for the treatment of neovascular (wet) age-related macular degeneration. Aflibercept is also licensed for the treatment of macular oedema secondary to central retinal vein occlusion, and diabetic macular oedema; ranibizumab is also licensed for the treatment of visual impairment due to diabetic macular oedema, macular oedema secondary to branch or central retinal vein occlusion, and choroidal neovascularisation secondary to pathologic myopia. Ranibizumab can be administered concomitantly with laser photocoagulation for the treatment of diabetic macular oedema and for macular oedema secondary to branch retinal vein occlusion.

ANTINEOVASCULARISATION DRUGS >
VASCULAR ENDOTHELIAL GROWTH FACTOR INHIBITORS

Aflibercept

- DRUG ACTION Aflibercept is a recombinant fusion protein that acts as a soluble decoy receptor and binds to vascular endothelial growth factors A and B (VEGF-A, VEGF-B) and placental growth factor (PlGF). Aflibercept inhibits the activation of VEGF receptors and the proliferation of endothelial cells, thereby inhibiting the growth of new vessels that supply tumours with oxygen and nutrients.

- INDICATIONS AND DOSE
Neovascular (wet) age-related macular degeneration (specialist use only)
► BY INTRAVITREAL INJECTION
► Adult: Initially 2 mg once a month for 3 months, to be injected into the affected eye, then 2 mg every 2 months, review treatment frequency after 12 months
Macular oedema secondary to central retinal vein occlusion (specialist use only)
► BY INTRAVITREAL INJECTION
► Adult: Initially 2 mg once a month, to be injected into the affected eye, monitor visual and anatomic outcomes monthly; continue treatment until visual and anatomic outcomes are stable for 3 monthly assessments (discontinue treatment if no improvement in visual and anatomic outcomes after initial 3 injections); if necessary subsequent doses may be given at least 1 month apart
Diabetic macular oedema (specialist use only)
► BY INTRAVITREAL INJECTION
► Adult: Initially 2 mg once a month for 5 months, then maintenance 2 mg every 2 months, to be injected into the affected eye, review treatment frequency after 12 months (discontinue treatment if no improvement in visual and anatomic outcomes)

- CONTRA-INDICATIONS Clinical signs of irreversible ischaemic visual function loss · ocular or periocular infection · severe intra-ocular inflammation

- CAUTIONS Active systemic infection · diabetic patients with uncontrolled hypertension · discontinue treatment if

11

Eye

stage 3 or 4 macular holes develop—consult product literature for full details · discontinue treatment in the event of a retinal break—consult product literature for full details · discontinue treatment in the event of rhegmatogenous retinal detachment—consult product literature for full details · patients at risk of retinal pigment epithelial tear · poorly controlled glaucoma · recent history of myocardial infarction · recent history of stroke · recent history of transient ischaemic attack

CAUTIONS, FURTHER INFORMATION
Aflibercept is given by intravitreal injection by specialists experienced in the management of this condition. There is a potential risk of arterial thromboembolic events and non-ocular haemorrhage following the intravitreal injection of vascular endothelial growth factor inhibitors. Endophthalmitis can occur after intravitreal injections—patients should be advised to report any signs of infection immediately.

● SIDE-EFFECTS
▶ **Common or very common** Blurred vision · cataract formation · conjunctival haemorrhage · conjunctival hyperaemia · corneal abrasion or oedema · corneal erosion · eye pain · eyelid oedema · foreign body sensation in eye · increased lacrimation · injection-site haemorrhage · injection-site pain · ocular hyperaemia · punctate keratitis · raised intra-ocular pressure · reduced visual acuity · retinal degeneration · retinal pigment epithelium detachment · retinal pigment epithelium tear · vitreous detachment · vitreous floaters · vitreous haemorrhage
▶ **Uncommon** Anterior chamber flare · blindness · corneal epithelium defect · eyelid irritation · iridocyclitis · iritis · lenticular opacities · retinal detachment · retinal tear · uveitis
▶ **Rare** Hypopyon · vitritis

● CONCEPTION AND CONTRACEPTION Manufacturer recommends women use effective contraception during and for at least 3 months after treatment.

● PREGNANCY Manufacturer advises avoid unless potential benefit outweighs risk.

● BREAST FEEDING Manufacturer advises avoid—no information available.

● MONITORING REQUIREMENTS Monitor intra-ocular pressure following injection.

● DIRECTIONS FOR ADMINISTRATION For further information on administration, consult product literature.

● NATIONAL FUNDING/ACCESS DECISIONS
NICE technology appraisals (TAs)
▶ **Aflibercept solution for injection for treating wet age-related macular degeneration (July 2013)** NICE TA294
Aflibercept solution for injection is recommended as an option for treating wet age-related macular degeneration only if:
● it is used in accordance with the recommendations for ranibizumab in NICE TA 155 **and**
● the manufacturer provides aflibercept solution for injection with the discount agreed in the patient access scheme
www.nice.org.uk/TA294
▶ **Aflibercept for treating visual impairment caused by macular oedema secondary to central retinal vein occlusion (February 2014)** NICE TA305
Aflibercept solution for injection is recommended as an option for treating visual impairment caused by macular oedema secondary to central retinal vein occlusion only if the manufacturer provides aflibercept solution for injection with the discount agreed in the patient access scheme.
www.nice.org.uk/TA305

▶ **Aflibercept for treating diabetic macular oedema (July 2015)** NICE TA346
Aflibercept solution for injection is recommended as an option for treating visual impairment caused by diabetic macular oedema only if:
● the eye has a central retinal thickness of 400 micrometres or more at the start of treatment and
● the company provides aflibercept with the discount agreed in the patient access scheme.
www.nice.org.uk/TA346

● MEDICINAL FORMS
There can be variation in the licensing of different medicines containing the same drug.
Solution for injection
▶ Eylea (Bayer Plc) ▼
Aflibercept 40 mg per 1 ml Eylea 2mg/50microlitres solution for injection vials | 1 vial [PoM] £816.00

Pegaptanib sodium

● INDICATIONS AND DOSE
Treatment of neovascular (wet) age-related macular degeneration (specialist use only)
▶ BY INTRAVITREAL INJECTION
▶ Adult: 300 micrograms every 6 weeks, to be administered into the affected eye, review treatment if no benefit after 2 consecutive injections

● CONTRA-INDICATIONS Ocular or periocular infection
● CAUTIONS
CAUTIONS, FURTHER INFORMATION
Pegaptanib is given by intravitreal injection by specialists. There is a potential risk of arterial thromboembolic events and non-ocular haemorrhage following the intravitreal injection of vascular endothelial growth factor inhibitors. Endophthalmitis can occur after intravitreal injections—patients should be advised to report any signs of infection immediately.

● SIDE-EFFECTS
▶ **Common or very common** Anterior chamber inflammation · cataract · conjunctival haemorrhage · conjunctivitis · corneal dystrophy · dry eye · eye discharge · eye irritation · eye pain · flashing lights · headache · local oedema · macular degeneration · mydriasis · periorbital haematoma · photophobia · punctate keratitis · raised intra-ocular pressure · retinal haemorrhage · rhinorrhoea · vitreous disorders · vitreous floaters
▶ **Uncommon** Aortic aneurysm · asthenopia · back pain · blepharitis · chalazion · changes in hair colour · chest pain · corneal deposits · deafness · decreased intra-ocular pressure · depression · dyspepsia · ectropion · eczema · eye movement disorder · eyelid ptosis · hypertension · influenza-like symptoms · injection-site reactions · iritis · nasopharyngitis · night sweats · nightmares · occlusion of retinal blood vessels · optic nerve cupping · palpitation · pruritus · pupillary disorder · rash · retinal detachment · retinal exudates · vertigo · vitreous haemorrhage · vomiting

● PREGNANCY Manufacturer advises avoid unless potential benefit outweighs risk.

● BREAST FEEDING Manufacturer advises avoid—no information available.

● MONITORING REQUIREMENTS
▶ Monitor intra-ocular pressure (transient increase may occur following injection, and small, sustained increases reported after repeated dosing).
▶ Monitor for vitreous haemorrhage and for signs of ocular infection for 2 weeks following injection.

● DIRECTIONS FOR ADMINISTRATION For further information on administration, consult product literature.

● NATIONAL FUNDING/ACCESS DECISIONS

NICE technology appraisals (TAs)

▶ Ranibizumab and pegaptanib for the treatment of age-related macular degeneration (updated May 2012) NICE TA155
Pegaptanib is not recommended for the treatment of wet age-related macular degeneration; patients currently receiving pegaptanib for any lesion type can continue therapy until they and their specialist consider it appropriate to stop.
www.nice.org.uk/TA155

● MEDICINAL FORMS
There can be variation in the licensing of different medicines containing the same drug.
No licensed medicines listed.

Ranibizumab

● INDICATIONS AND DOSE

Neovascular (wet) age-related macular degeneration (specialist use only)
▶ BY INTRAVITREAL INJECTION
▶ Adult: 500 micrograms once a month, to be administered into the affected eye, monitor visual acuity monthly, continue treatment until visual acuity is stable for 3 consecutive months, thereafter monitor visual acuity monthly, if necessary subsequent doses may be given at least 1 month apart

Diabetic macular oedema | Macular oedema secondary to retinal vein occlusion (specialist use only)
▶ BY INTRAVITREAL INJECTION
▶ Adult: Initially 500 micrograms once a month, to be administered into the affected eye, monitor visual acuity monthly, continue treatment until visual acuity is stable for 3 consecutive months (discontinue treatment if no improvement in visual acuity after initial 3 injections), thereafter monitor visual acuity monthly, if necessary subsequent doses may be given at least 1 month apart

Choroidal neovascularisation secondary to pathologic myopia (specialist use only)
▶ BY INTRAVITREAL INJECTION
▶ Adult: Initially 500 micrograms, to be administered as a single injection into the affected eye, monitor for disease activity monthly for first 2 months, then at least every 3 months thereafter during the first year, then as required, if necessary subsequent doses may be given at least 1 month apart

Concomitant treatment of diabetic macular oedema, or macular oedema secondary to branch retinal vein occlusion, with laser photocoagulation (specialist use only)
▶ BY INTRAVITREAL INJECTION
▶ Adult: 500 micrograms, to be administered at least 30 minutes after laser photocoagulation

● CONTRA-INDICATIONS Ocular or periocular infection · severe intra-ocular inflammation · signs of irreversible ischaemic visual function loss in patients with retinal vein occlusion

● CAUTIONS Active systemic infection · diabetic macular oedema due to type 1 diabetes (limited information available) · diabetic patients with HbA_{1c} over 12% · history of stroke · history of transient ischaemic attack · patients at risk of retinal pigment epithelial tear · previous intravitreal injections · proliferative diabetic retinopathy · retinal detachment or macular hole (discontinue treatment if rhegmatogenous retinal detachment or stage 3 or 4 macular holes develop) · uncontrolled hypertension

CAUTIONS, FURTHER INFORMATION
Ranibizumab is given by intravitreal injection by specialists. There is a potential risk of arterial thromboembolic events and non-ocular haemorrhage following the intravitreal injection of vascular endothelial growth factor inhibitors. Endophthalmitis can occur after intravitreal injections—patients should be advised to report any signs of infection immediately.

● SIDE-EFFECTS
▶ **Common or very common** Allergic skin reactions · anaemia · anterior chamber flare · anxiety · arthralgia · blepharitis · cataract · conjunctival disorders · conjunctivitis · cough · eye haemorrhage · eyelid oedema · headache · iridocyclitis · iritis · nasopharyngitis · nausea · ocular discomfort · photophobia · photopsia · posterior capsule opacification · punctuate keratitis · raised intra-ocular pressure · retinal disorders · urinary tract infection · uveitis · visual disturbance · vitreous disorders
▶ **Uncommon** Blindness · corneal disorders · hyphaema · hypopyon · iris adhesion · keratopathy

● CONCEPTION AND CONTRACEPTION Manufacturer recommends women use effective contraception during and for at least 3 months after treatment.

● PREGNANCY Manufacturer advises avoid unless potential benefit outweighs risk.

● BREAST FEEDING Manufacturer advises avoid—no information available.

● MONITORING REQUIREMENTS
▶ Monitor intra-ocular pressure, perfusion of the optic nerve head, and for signs of ocular infection following injection.
▶ Monitor visual acuity, see individual indications and dose for frequency.

● DIRECTIONS FOR ADMINISTRATION For further information on administration, consult product literature.

● NATIONAL FUNDING/ACCESS DECISIONS

NICE technology appraisals (TAs)
▶ **Ranibizumab for treating choroidal neovascularisation associated with pathological myopia (November 2013)** NICE TA298
Ranibizumab is recommended as an option for treating visual impairment due to choroidal neovascularisation secondary to pathological myopia when the manufacturer provides ranibizumab with the discount agreed in the patient access scheme.
www.nice.org.uk/TA298
▶ **Ranibizumab for the treatment of visual impairment caused by macular oedema secondary to retinal vein occlusion (May 2013)** NICE TA283
Ranibizumab is recommended as an option for treating visual impairment caused by macular oedema:
● following central retinal vein occlusion **or**
● following branch retinal vein occlusion only if treatment with laser photocoagulation has not been beneficial, or when laser photocoagulation is not suitable because of the extent of macular haemorrhage **and**
● only if the manufacturer provides ranibizumab with the discount agreed in the patient access scheme revised in the context of NICE technology appraisal guidance 274.
www.nice.org.uk/TA283
▶ **Ranibizumab for the treatment of diabetic macular oedema (February 2013)** NICE TA274
Ranibizumab is recommended as an option for the treatment of visual impairment due to diabetic macular oedema only if:
● the eye has a central retinal thickness of 400 micrometres or more at the start of treatment **and**
● the manufacturer provides ranibizumab with the discount agreed in the patient access scheme (as revised in 2012).
Patients currently receiving ranibizumab for treating visual impairment due to diabetic macular oedema whose

11

Eye

disease does not meet the criteria should be able to continue treatment until they and their clinician consider it appropriate to stop.
www.nice.org.uk/TA274

▶ **Ranibizumab and pegaptanib for the treatment of age-related macular degeneration (updated May 2012)** NICE TA155
Ranibizumab is recommended for the treatment of wet age-related macular degeneration if all of the following apply:

• the best corrected visual acuity is between 6/12 and 6/96;
• there is no permanent structural damage to the central fovea;
• the lesion size is less than or equal to 12 disc areas in greatest linear dimension;
• there is evidence of recent disease progression;
• the manufacturer provides ranibizumab with the discount agreed in the patient access scheme (as revised in 2012).

Ranibizumab should only be continued in patients who maintain adequate response to therapy.
www.nice.org.uk/TA155

Scottish Medicines Consortium (SMC) Decisions
The *Scottish Medicines Consortium* has advised (May 2007) that ranibizumab (*Lucentis ®*) is accepted for use within NHS Scotland for the treatment of neovascular (wet) age-related macular degeneration.

The *Scottish Medicines Consortium* has advised (October 2011 and April 2013) that ranibizumab (*Lucentis ®*) is accepted for use within NHS Scotland for the treatment of macular oedema secondary to branch or central retinal vein occlusion, and (November 2012) for restricted use for the treatment of visual impairment due to diabetic macular oedema in adults with best corrected visual acuity 75 Early Treatment Diabetic Retinopathy Study letters or less at baseline, and (October 2013) for the treatment of visual impairment due to choroidal neovascularisation secondary to pathologic myopia in adults; SMC advice is contingent upon the continuing availability of ranibizumab at the price agreed in the patient access scheme.

● MEDICINAL FORMS
There can be variation in the licensing of different medicines containing the same drug.
Solution for injection
▶ Lucentis (Novartis Pharmaceuticals UK Ltd)
  Ranibizumab 10 mg per 1 ml Lucentis 2.3mg/0.23ml solution for injection vials | 1 vial [PoM] £742.00 (Hospital only)
  Lucentis 1.65mg/0.165ml solution for injection pre-filled syringes | 1 pre-filled disposable injection [PoM] £742.00

PHOTOSENSITISERS

Verteporfin

● DRUG ACTION Following intravenous infusion, verteporfin is activated by local irradiation using non-thermal red light to produce cytotoxic derivatives.

● INDICATIONS AND DOSE
Photodynamic treatment of age-related macular degeneration associated with predominantly classic subfoveal choroidal neovascularisation or with pathological myopia (specialist use only)
▶ BY INTRAVENOUS INFUSION
▶ Adult: 6 mg/m^2, dose to be given over 10 minutes

● CONTRA-INDICATIONS Acute porphyria
● CAUTIONS Avoid extravasation · biliary obstruction · photosensitivity
● INTERACTIONS Caution on concomitant use with other photosensitising drugs.

● SIDE-EFFECTS
▶ **Common or very common** Back pain · flashing lights · hypercholesterolaemia · malaise · nausea · photosensitivity · reduced visual acuity · visual disturbances · visual-field defects
▶ **Uncommon** Hyperaesthesia · hypertension · pyrexia · retinal detachment · subretinal, retinal or vitreous haemorrhage
▶ **Rare** Retinal or choroidal vessel non-perfusion
▶ **Frequency not known** Chest pain · macular oedema · myocardial infarction · retinal oedema · vasovagal reactions

● PREGNANCY Manufacturer advises use only if potential benefit outweighs risk (teratogenic in *animal* studies).

● BREAST FEEDING No information available—manufacturer advises avoid breast-feeding for 48 hours after administration.

● HEPATIC IMPAIRMENT Use with caution in moderate hepatic impairment. Avoid in severe hepatic impairment.

● DIRECTIONS FOR ADMINISTRATION For information on administration and light activation, consult product literature.
    For *intravenous infusion* (*Visudyne ®*), give intermittently in Glucose 5%; reconstitute each 15 mg with 7 ml water for injections to produce a 2 mg/ml solution then dilute requisite dose with infusion fluid to a final volume of 30 mL and give over 10 minutes; protect infusion from light and administer within 4 hours of reconstitution. Incompatible with sodium chloride infusion.

● PATIENT AND CARER ADVICE Photosensitivity—avoid exposure of unprotected skin and eyes to bright light during infusion and for 48 hours afterwards.

● NATIONAL FUNDING/ACCESS DECISIONS
NICE technology appraisals (TAs)
▶ **Verteporfin photodynamic therapy for wet age-related macular degeneration (September 2003)** NICE TA68
Photodynamic therapy is recommended for wet age-related macular degeneration with a confirmed diagnosis of classic (no occult) subfoveal choroidal neovascularisation and best-corrected visual acuity of 6/60 or better.
    Photodynamic therapy is **not** recommended for wet age-related macular degeneration with predominantly classic but partly occult subfoveal choroidal neovascularisation *except* in clinical studies.
www.nice.org.uk/TA68

● MEDICINAL FORMS
There can be variation in the licensing of different medicines containing the same drug.
Powder for solution for infusion
EXCIPIENTS: May contain Butylated hydroxytoluene
▶ Visudyne (Novartis Pharmaceuticals UK Ltd)
  Verteporfin 15 mg Visudyne 15mg powder for solution for infusion vials | 1 vial [PoM] £850.00 (Hospital only)

6.2 Macular oedema

> **Drugs used for Macular oedema not listed below**
> Aflibercept, p. 1033 · Dexamethasone p. 1008 · Ranibizumab, p. 1035

Fluocinolone acetonide

- ● **INDICATIONS AND DOSE**
  Treatment of visual impairment associated with chronic diabetic macular oedema which is insufficiently responsive to available therapies (specialist use only)
  ▶ BY INTRAVITREAL INJECTION
  ▶ Adult: 190 micrograms, to be administered into the affected eye

- ● CONTRA-INDICATIONS Active or suspected ocular infection · active or suspected peri-ocular infection · pre-existing glaucoma
- ● CAUTIONS Raised baseline intra-ocular pressure
- ● INTERACTIONS Caution with concomitant administration of anticoagulant or antiplatelet drugs (higher incidence of conjunctival haemorrhage).
- ● SIDE-EFFECTS
  ▶ **Common or very common** Blurred vision · cataract · conjunctival haemorrhage · glaucoma · ocular discomfort · raised intra-ocular pressure · reduced visual acuity · vitreous floaters · vitreous haemorrhage
  ▶ **Uncommon** Conjunctival ulcer · endophthalmitis · eye discharge · eye pruritus · headache · iris adhesions · iris neovascularisation · maculopathy · ocular hyperaemia · optic atrophy · optic nerve disorder · posterior capsule opacification · retinal exudates · retinal vascular occlusion · sclera thinning · vitreous degeneration · vitreous detachment
- ● PREGNANCY Manufacturer advises avoid unless potential benefit outweighs risk—no information available.
- ● BREAST FEEDING Manufacturer advises avoid unless essential.
- ● MONITORING REQUIREMENTS Monitor for raised intra-ocular pressure (particularly if raised at baseline), retinal detachment, endophthalmitis, vitreous haemorrhage or detachment within 2–7 days following the procedure. Monitor intra-ocular pressure at least every 3 months thereafter (for approximately 36 months).
- ● DIRECTIONS FOR ADMINISTRATION Concurrent administration to both eyes not recommended. For further information on administration and repeat dosing, consult product literature.
- ● NATIONAL FUNDING/ACCESS DECISIONS
  NICE technology appraisals (TAs)
  ▶ **Fluocinolone acetonide intravitreal implant for treating chronic diabetic macular oedema after an inadequate response to prior therapy (November 2013)** NICE TA301
  Fluocinolone acetonide intravitreal implant is recommended as an option for treating chronic diabetic macular oedema that is insufficiently responsive to available therapies only if:
  - the implant is to be used in an eye with an intra-ocular (pseudophakic lens) **and**
  - the manufacturer provides fluocinolone acetonide intravitreal implant with the discount agreed in the patient access scheme.
  www.nice.org.uk/TA301

  Scottish Medicines Consortium (SMC) Decisions
  The *Scottish Medicines Consortium* has advised (February 2014) that fluocinolone acetonide intravitreal implant

(*Iluvien* ®) is recommended for restricted use within NHS Scotland for the treatment of vision impairment associated with chronic diabetic macular oedema, considered insufficiently responsive to available therapies, only in patients in whom the affected eye is pseudophakic (has an artificial lens after cataract surgery), **and** retreatment would take place only if the patient had previously responded to treatment with fluocinolone acetonide and subsequently best corrected visual acuity had deteriorated to less than 20/32.

- ● MEDICINAL FORMS
  There can be variation in the licensing of different medicines containing the same drug.
  Implant
  ▶ Iluvien (Alimera Sciences Ltd)
  Fluocinolone acetonide 190 microgram ILUVIEN 190microgram intravitreal implant in applicator | 1 device PoM £5,500.00

6.3 Vitreomacular traction

RECOMBINANT PROTEOLYTIC ENZYMES

Ocriplasmin

- ● **INDICATIONS AND DOSE**
  Treatment of vitreomacular traction, including when associated with a macular hole of diameter less than or equal to 400 microns (specialist use only)
  ▶ BY INTRAVITREAL INJECTION
  ▶ Adult: 125 micrograms for 1 dose, to be administered into the affected eye, concurrent administration to both eyes is not recommended

- ● CONTRA-INDICATIONS Active or suspected ocular or periocular infection · aphakia · exudative age-related macular degeneration · high myopia · history of rhegmatogenous retinal detachment · ischaemic retinopathies · large diameter macular hole (> 400 microns) · lens zonule instability · proliferative diabetic retinopathy · recent intra-ocular injection (including laser therapy) · recent ocular surgery · retinal vein occlusions · vitreous haemorrhage
- ● CAUTIONS History of uveitis (including severe active inflammation) · non-proliferative diabetic retinopathy · significant eye trauma
- ● SIDE-EFFECTS
  ▶ **Common or very common** Abnormal retinograph · anterior chamber cell or flare · chromatopsia · conjunctival disorders · eyelid oedema · iritis · macular degeneration · macular hole · macular oedema · metamorphopsia · ocular discomfort · ocular hyperaemia · photophobia · photopsia · raised intra-ocular pressure · reduced visual acuity · retinal disorders · retinal pigment epitheliopathy · vitreous disorders
  ▶ **Uncommon** Anterior chamber inflammation · corneal abrasion · diplopia · eye inflammation · hyphaema · lens subluxation · miosis · scotoma · transient blindness · unequal pupils · visual field defect
- ● PREGNANCY Manufacturer advises use only if potential benefit outweighs risk—no information available.
- ● BREAST FEEDING Manufacturer advises use only if potential benefit outweighs risk—no information available.
- ● MONITORING REQUIREMENTS Monitor intra-ocular pressure, visual acuity, and for signs of intra-ocular inflammation or infection following injection.
- ● DIRECTIONS FOR ADMINISTRATION For further information on administration, consult product literature.

● NATIONAL FUNDING/ACCESS DECISIONS

NICE technology appraisals (TAs)

▶ Ocriplasmin for treating vitreomacular traction (October 2013) NICE TA297

Ocriplasmin is recommended as an option for treating vitreomacular traction in adults, only if:
- an epiretinal membrane is not present **and**
- they have a stage II full-thickness macular hole with a diameter of 400 microns or less **and/or**
- they have severe symptoms.

www.nice.org.uk/TA297

Scottish Medicines Consortium (SMC) Decisions

The *Scottish Medicines Consortium* has advised (July 2014) that ocriplasmin (*Jetrea*®) is accepted for restricted use within NHS Scotland for the treatment of patients with vitreomacular traction plus macular hole, regardless of whether they have epiretinal membrane formation, and in patients with vitreomacular traction alone (no epiretinal membrane and no macular hole).

● MEDICINAL FORMS

There can be variation in the licensing of different medicines containing the same drug.

Solution for injection

▶ Jetrea (Alcon Laboratories (UK) Ltd) ▼
  Ocriplasmin 2.5 mg per 1 ml Jetrea 0.5mg/0.2ml concentrate for solution for injection vials | 1 vial PoM £2,500.00

Chapter 12
Ear, nose and oropharynx

CONTENTS

12

Ear, nose and oropharynx

Ear

Ear

Otitis externa

Otitis externa is an inflammatory reaction of the meatal skin. It is important to exclude an underlying chronic otitis media before treatment is commenced. Many cases recover after thorough cleansing of the external ear canal by suction or dry mopping. A frequent problem in resistant cases is the difficulty in applying lotions and ointments satisfactorily to the relatively inaccessible affected skin. The most effective method is to introduce a ribbon gauze dressing or sponge wick soaked with **corticosteroid** ear drops or with an astringent such as aluminium acetate solution p. 1043. When this is not practical, the ear should be gently cleansed with a probe covered in cotton wool and the patient encouraged to lie with the affected ear uppermost for ten minutes after the canal has been filled with a liberal quantity of the appropriate solution.

If infection is present, a topical anti-infective which is not used systemically (such as neomycin sulfate p. 1041 or **clioquinol**) may be used, but for only about a week as excessive use may result in fungal infections; these may be difficult to treat and require expert advice. Sensitivity to the anti-infective or solvent may occur and resistance to antibacterials is a possibility with prolonged use. Aluminium acetate ear drops are also effective against bacterial infection and inflammation of the ear. Chloramphenicol p. 1041 may be used but the ear drops contain propylene glycol and cause hypersensitivity reactions in about 10% of patients. Solutions containing an anti-infective and a corticosteroid are used for treating cases where infection is present with inflammation and eczema.

In view of reports of ototoxicity, manufacturers contra-indicate treatment with topical **aminoglycosides** or **polymyxins** in patients with a perforated tympanic membrane (eardrum) or patent grommet. However, some specialists do use these drops cautiously in the presence of a perforation or patent grommet in patients with chronic suppurative otitis media and when other measures have failed for otitis externa; treatment should be considered only **by specialists** in the following circumstances:

• drops should only be used in the presence of obvious infection;
• treatment should be for no longer than 2 weeks;

• patients should be counselled on the risk of ototoxicity and given justification for the use of these topical antibiotics;
• baseline audiometry should be performed, if possible, before treatment is commenced.

Clinical expertise and judgement should be used to assess the risk of treatment versus the benefit to the patient in such circumstances.

A solution of **acetic acid** 2% acts as an antifungal and antibacterial in the external ear canal. It may be used to treat mild otitis externa but in severe cases an antiinflammatory preparation with or without an anti-infective drug is required. A proprietary preparation containing acetic acid 2% (*EarCalm®* spray) is on sale to the public.

For severe pain associated with otitis externa, a simple analgesic, such as paracetamol p. 406 or ibuprofen p. 987, can be used. A systemic antibacterial can be used if there is spreading cellulitis or if the patient is systemically unwell. When a resistant staphylococcal infection (a boil) is present in the external auditory meatus, flucloxacillin p. 503 is the drug of choice; ciprofloxacin p. 506 (or an aminoglycoside) may be needed in pseudomonal infections which may occur if the patient has diabetes or is immunocompromised.

The skin of the pinna adjacent to the ear canal is often affected by eczema. A topical corticosteroid cream or ointment is then required, but prolonged use should be avoided.

Otitis media

Acute otitis media

Acute otitis media is the commonest cause of severe aural pain in small children. Many infections, especially those accompanying coryza, are caused by viruses. Most uncomplicated cases resolve without antibacterial treatment and a **simple analgesic**, such as paracetamol, may be sufficient. In children without systemic features, a **systemic antibacterial** may be started after 72 hours if there is no improvement, or earlier if there is deterioration, if the patient is systemically unwell, if the patient is at high risk of serious complications (e.g. in immunosuppression, cystic fibrosis), if mastoiditis is present, or in children under 2 years of age with bilateral otitis media. Perforation of the tympanic membrane in patients with *acute otitis media* usually heals spontaneously without treatment; if there is no improvement, e.g. pain or discharge persists, a systemic antibacterial can be given. Topical treatment of acute otitis media is ineffective and there is no place for drops containing a local anaesthetic.

Otitis media with effusion

Otitis media with effusion (glue ear) occurs in about 10% of children and in 90% of children with cleft palates. Systemic antibacterials are not usually required. If glue ear persists for more than a month or two, the child should be referred for assessment and follow up because of the risk of long-term hearing impairment which can delay language development. Untreated or resistant glue ear may be responsible for some types of *chronic otitis media.*

Chronic otitis media

Opportunistic organisms are often present in the debris, keratin, and necrotic bone of the middle ear and mastoid in patients with chronic otitis media. The mainstay of treatment is thorough cleansing with aural microsuction which may completely resolve long-standing infection. Local cleansing of the meatal and middle ear may be followed by treatment with a sponge wick or ribbon gauze dressing soaked with corticosteroid ear drops or with an astringent such as aluminium acetate solution; this is particularly beneficial for discharging ears or infections of the mastoid cavity. An antibacterial ear ointment may also be used. Acute exacerbations of chronic infection may also require systemic treatment with amoxicillin p. 498 (or erythromycin p. 488 if penicillin-allergic); treatment is adjusted according to the results of sensitivity testing.

In view of reports of ototoxicity, manufacturers contraindicate topical treatment with ototoxic antibacterials in the presence of a tympanic perforation or patent grommet. Ciprofloxacin or ofloxacin eye drops p. 510 used in the ear [unlicensed use] or ear drops [both unlicensed; available from 'special-order' manufacturers or specialist importing companies] are an effective alternative to such ototoxic ear drops for chronic otitis media in patients with perforation of the tympanic membrane.

However, some specialists do use ear drops containing **aminoglycosides** or **polymyxins** [unlicensed indications] cautiously in patients with chronic suppurative otitis media and a perforation of the tympanic membrane, if the otitis media has failed to settle with systemic antibacterials; treatment should be considered only **by specialists** in the following circumstances:

- drops should only be used in the presence of obvious infection;
- treatment should be for no longer than 2 weeks;
- patients should be counselled on the risk of ototoxicity and given justification for the use of these topical antibiotics;
- baseline audiometry should be performed, if possible, before treatment is commenced.

Clinical expertise and judgement should be used to assess the risk of treatment versus the benefit to the patient in such circumstances. It is considered that the pus in the middle ear associated with otitis media also carries a risk of ototoxicity.

Removal of ear wax

Ear wax (cerumen) is a normal bodily secretion which provides a protective film on the meatal skin and need only be removed if it causes hearing loss or interferes with a proper view of the ear drum.

Ear wax can be softened using simple remedies such as **olive oil** ear drops or **almond oil** ear drops; sodium bicarbonate ear drops p. 1043 are also effective, but may cause dryness of the ear canal. If the wax is hard and impacted, the drops can be used twice daily for several days and this may reduce the need for mechanical removal of the wax. The patient should lie with the affected ear uppermost for 5 to 10 minutes after a generous amount of the softening remedy has been introduced into the ear. Some proprietary preparations containing organic solvents can irritate the meatal skin, and in most cases the simple remedies indicated above are just as effective and less likely to cause irritation. Docusate sodium p. 1043 or urea hydrogen peroxide p. 1044

are ingredients in a number of proprietary preparations for softening ear wax.

If necessary, wax may be removed by irrigation with water (warmed to body temperature). Ear irrigation is generally best avoided in young children, in patients unable to co-operate with the procedure, in those with otitis media in the last six weeks, in otitis externa, in patients with cleft palate, a history of ear drum perforation, or previous ear surgery. A person who has hearing in one ear only should not have that ear irrigated because even a very slight risk of damage is unacceptable in this situation.

1 Otitis externa

Drugs used for Otitis externa not listed below
Hydrocortisone with miconazole, p. 1097

ANTIBACTERIALS > AMINOGLYCOSIDES

Framycetin sulfate

- **INDICATIONS AND DOSE**

Bacterial infection in otitis externa
- TO THE EAR
- Adult: (consult product literature)

- **CONTRA-INDICATIONS** Perforated tympanic membrane
- **CAUTIONS** Avoid prolonged use
- **SIDE-EFFECTS** Local sensitivity

- **MEDICINAL FORMS**
There can be variation in the licensing of different medicines containing the same drug.
No licensed medicines listed.

Combinations available: *Dexamethasone with framycetin sulfate and gramicidin*, p. 1042

Gentamicin

- **INDICATIONS AND DOSE**

Bacterial infection in otitis externa
- TO THE EAR
- Child: Apply 2–3 drops 4–5 times a day, (including a dose at bedtime)
- Adult: Apply 2–3 drops 4–5 times a day, (including a dose at bedtime)

- **CONTRA-INDICATIONS** Patent grommet (although may be used by specialists (see Ear p. 1039) · perforated tympanic membrane (although may be used by specialists (see Ear p. 1039)
- **CAUTIONS** Avoid prolonged use
- **SIDE-EFFECTS** Local sensitivity

- **MEDICINAL FORMS**
There can be variation in the licensing of different medicines containing the same drug.
Ear/eye drops solution
EXCIPIENTS: May contain Benzalkonium chloride
- Gentamicin (Non-proprietary)
Gentamicin (as Gentamicin sulfate) 3 mg per 1 ml Gentamicin 0.3% ear/eye drops | 10 ml PoM £2.55 DT price = £2.13
Gentamicin 0.3% eye/ear drops | 10 ml PoM £2.13 DT price = £2.13

Gentamicin with hydrocortisone

- **INDICATIONS AND DOSE**

Eczematous inflammation in otitis externa
▸ TO THE EAR
- Child: Apply 2–4 drops 4–5 times a day, (including a dose at bedtime)
- Adult: Apply 2–4 drops 4–5 times a day, (including a dose at bedtime)

- **CONTRA-INDICATIONS** Patent grommet (although may be used by specialists, see Ear p. 1039) · perforated tympanic membrane (although may be used by specialists, see Ear p. 1039)
- **CAUTIONS** Avoid prolonged use
- **SIDE-EFFECTS** Local sensitivity reactions
- **PATIENT AND CARER ADVICE**
Medicines for Children leaflet: Gentamicin and hydrocortisone ear drops for inflammatory ear infections www. medicinesforchildren.org.uk/gentamicin-and-hydrocortisone-ear-drops-inflammatory-ear-infections

- **MEDICINAL FORMS**
There can be variation in the licensing of different medicines containing the same drug.
Ear drops
EXCIPIENTS: May contain Benzalkonium chloride, disodium edetate
▸ Gentamicin with hydrocortisone (Non-proprietary)
Gentamicin (as Gentamicin sulfate) 3 mg per 1 ml, Hydrocortisone acetate 10 mg per 1 ml Gentamicin 0.3% / Hydrocortisone acetate 1% ear drops | 10 ml [PoM] £23.92 DT price = £23.92

Neomycin sulfate

- **INDICATIONS AND DOSE**

Bacterial infection in otitis externa
▸ TO THE EAR
- Child: (consult product literature)
- Adult: (consult product literature)

- **CONTRA-INDICATIONS** Patent grommet (although may be used by specialists, see Ear p. 1039) · perforated tympanic membrane (although may be used by specialists, see Ear p. 1039)
- **CAUTIONS** Avoid prolonged use (in adults)
- **SIDE-EFFECTS** Local sensitivity

- **MEDICINAL FORMS**
There can be variation in the licensing of different medicines containing the same drug.

Combinations available: *Betamethasone with neomycin*, p. 1042 · *Dexamethasone with glacial acetic acid and neomycin sulfate*, p. 1042

ANTIBACTERIALS > OTHER

Chloramphenicol

- **DRUG ACTION** Chloramphenicol is a potent broad-spectrum antibiotic.

- **INDICATIONS AND DOSE**

Bacterial infection in otitis externa
▸ TO THE EAR
- Child: Apply 2–3 drops 2–3 times a day
- Adult: Apply 2–3 drops 2–3 times a day

- **CAUTIONS** Avoid prolonged use
- **SIDE-EFFECTS**
- **Common or very common** High incidence of sensitivity reactions to vehicle

- **PATIENT AND CARER ADVICE**
Medicines for Children leaflet: Chloramphenicol ear drops for ear infections (otitis externa) www.medicinesforchildren.org.uk/chloramphenicol-ear-drops-ear-infections-otitis-externa-0
- **LESS SUITABLE FOR PRESCRIBING** Chloramphenicol ear drops are less suitable for prescribing.

- **MEDICINAL FORMS**
There can be variation in the licensing of different medicines containing the same drug.
Ear drops
EXCIPIENTS: May contain Propylene glycol
▸ Chloramphenicol (Non-proprietary)
Chloramphenicol 50 mg per 1 ml Chloramphenicol 5% ear drops | 10 ml [PoM] £75.99 DT price = £57.90
Chloramphenicol 100 mg per 1 ml Chloramphenicol 10% ear drops | 10 ml [PoM] £42.18

ANTIFUNGALS > IMIDAZOLE ANTIFUNGALS

Clotrimazole

- **INDICATIONS AND DOSE**

Fungal infection in otitis externa
▸ TO THE EAR
- Child: Apply 2–3 times a day continue for at least 14 days after disappearance of infection
- Adult: Apply 2–3 times a day continue for at least 14 days after disappearance of infection

- **SIDE-EFFECTS** Local irritation · local sensitivity

- **MEDICINAL FORMS**
There can be variation in the licensing of different medicines containing the same drug.
Liquid
▸ Canesten (clotrimazole) (Bayer Plc)
Clotrimazole 10 mg per 1 ml Canesten 1% solution | 20 ml [P] £2.30 DT price = £2.30

CORTICOSTEROIDS

Betamethasone

- **INDICATIONS AND DOSE**
BETNESOL®
Eczematous inflammation in otitis externa
▸ TO THE EAR
- Adult: Apply 2–3 drops every 2–3 hours, reduce frequency when relief obtained
VISTAMETHASONE®
Eczematous inflammation in otitis externa
▸ TO THE EAR
- Adult: Apply 2–3 drops every 3–4 hours, reduce frequency when relief obtained

- **CONTRA-INDICATIONS** Avoid alone in the presence of untreated infection (combine with suitable anti-infective)
- **CAUTIONS** Avoid prolonged use
- **SIDE-EFFECTS** Local sensitivity reactions

- **MEDICINAL FORMS**
There can be variation in the licensing of different medicines containing the same drug.
Ear/eye/nose drops solution
EXCIPIENTS: May contain Benzalkonium chloride, disodium edetate
▸ Betnesol (Focus Pharmaceuticals Ltd)
Betamethasone sodium phosphate 1 mg per 1 ml Betnesol 0.1% eye/ear/nose drops | 10 ml [PoM] £2.32 DT price = £2.32
▸ Vistamethasone (Martindale Pharmaceuticals Ltd)
Betamethasone sodium phosphate 1 mg per 1 ml Vistamethasone 0.1% ear/eye/nose drops | 5 ml [PoM] £0.87 | 10 ml [PoM] £0.99 DT price = £2.32

Combinations available: *Betamethasone with neomycin*, p. 1042

12

Ear, nose and oropharynx

Clioquinol with flumetasone pivalate

- **INDICATIONS AND DOSE**

Eczematous inflammation in otitis externa | Mild bacterial or fungal infections in otitis externa
- ▶ TO THE EAR
- ▶ Child 2-17 years: 2–3 drops twice daily for 7–10 days, to be instilled into the ear
- ▶ Adult: 2–3 drops twice daily for 7–10 days, to be instilled into the ear

- **CONTRA-INDICATIONS** Iodine sensitivity
- **CAUTIONS** Avoid prolonged use · manufacturer advises avoid in perforated tympanic membrane (but used by specialists for short periods)
- **SIDE-EFFECTS** Local sensitivity
- **PATIENT AND CARER ADVICE** Clioquinol stains skin and clothing

- **MEDICINAL FORMS**
There can be variation in the licensing of different medicines containing the same drug.
Ear drops
- ▶ Clioquinol with flumetasone pivalate (Non-proprietary)
Flumetasone pivalate 200 microgram per 1 ml, Clioquinol 10 mg per 1 ml Flumetasone 0.02% / Clioquinol 1% ear drops | 7.5 ml [PoM] £10.37 DT price = £10.37 | 10 ml [PoM] £13.82 DT price = £13.82

Prednisolone

- **INDICATIONS AND DOSE**

Eczematous inflammation in otitis externa
- ▶ TO THE EAR
- ▶ Child: Apply 2–3 drops every 2–3 hours, frequency to be reduced when relief obtained
- ▶ Adult: Apply 2–3 drops every 2–3 hours, frequency to be reduced when relief obtained

- **CONTRA-INDICATIONS** Avoid alone in the presence of untreated infection (combine with suitable anti-infective)
- **CAUTIONS** Avoid prolonged use
- **SIDE-EFFECTS** Local sensitivity reactions

- **MEDICINAL FORMS**
There can be variation in the licensing of different medicines containing the same drug. Forms available from special-order manufacturers include: ear drops
Ear/eye drops solution
EXCIPIENTS: May contain Benzalkonium chloride, disodium edetate
- ▶ Predsol (Focus Pharmaceuticals Ltd)
Prednisolone sodium phosphate 5 mg per 1 ml Predsol 0.5% ear/eye drops | 10 ml [PoM] £2.00 DT price = £2.00

CORTICOSTEROIDS > CORTICOSTEROID COMBINATIONS WITH ANTI-INFECTIVES

Betamethasone with neomycin

The properties listed below are those particular to the combination only. For the properties of the components please consider, betamethasone p. 1041, neomycin sulfate p. 1041.

- **INDICATIONS AND DOSE**

Eczematous inflammation in otitis externa
- ▶ TO THE EAR USING EAR DROPS
- ▶ Child: Apply 2–3 drops 3–4 times a day
- ▶ Adult: Apply 2–3 drops 3–4 times a day

- **CONTRA-INDICATIONS** Patent grommet (although may be used by specialists, see Ear p. 1039) · perforated tympanic

membrane (although may be used by specialists, see Ear p. 1039)
- **CAUTIONS** Avoid prolonged use
- **SIDE-EFFECTS** Local sensitivity

- **MEDICINAL FORMS**
There can be variation in the licensing of different medicines containing the same drug.
Ear/eye/nose drops solution
EXCIPIENTS: May contain Benzalkonium chloride, disodium edetate
- ▶ Betnesol-N (Focus Pharmaceuticals Ltd)
Betamethasone (as Betamethasone sodium phosphate) 1 mg per 1 ml, Neomycin sulfate 5 mg per 1 ml Betnesol-N ear/eye/nose drops | 10 ml [PoM] £2.39 DT price = £2.39

Dexamethasone with framycetin sulfate and gramicidin

The properties listed below are those particular to the combination only. For the properties of the components please consider, framycetin sulfate p. 1040.

- **INDICATIONS AND DOSE**

Eczematous inflammation in otitis externa
- ▶ TO THE EAR
- ▶ Child: 2–3 drops 3–4 times a day
- ▶ Adult: 2–3 drops 3–4 times a day

- **LESS SUITABLE FOR PRESCRIBING** Sofradex® is less suitable for prescribing.

- **MEDICINAL FORMS**
There can be variation in the licensing of different medicines containing the same drug.
Ear/eye drops solution
EXCIPIENTS: May contain Polysorbates
- ▶ Sofradex (Sanofi)
Gramicidin 50 microgram per 1 ml, Dexamethasone (as Dexamethasone sodium metasulfobenzoate) 500 microgram per 1 ml, Framycetin sulfate 5 mg per 1 ml Sofradex ear/eye drops | 10 ml [PoM] £7.50

Dexamethasone with glacial acetic acid and neomycin sulfate

- **INDICATIONS AND DOSE**

Eczematous inflammation in otitis externa
- ▶ TO THE EAR
- ▶ Child 2-17 years: Apply 1 spray 3 times a day
- ▶ Adult: Apply 1 spray 3 times a day

- **CONTRA-INDICATIONS** Patent grommet (although may be used by specialists, see Ear p. 1039) · perforated tympanic membrane (although may be used by specialists, see Ear p. 1039)
- **CAUTIONS** Avoid prolonged use
- **SIDE-EFFECTS** Local sensitivity

- **MEDICINAL FORMS**
There can be variation in the licensing of different medicines containing the same drug.
Spray
EXCIPIENTS: May contain Hydroxybenzoates (parabens)
- ▶ Otomize (Forest Laboratories UK Ltd)
Dexamethasone 1 mg per 1 gram, Neomycin sulfate 5 mg per 1 gram, Acetic acid glacial 20 mg per 1 gram Otomize ear spray | 5 ml [PoM] £3.27

Aluminium acetate

- **INDICATIONS AND DOSE**
Inflammation in otitis externa
▸ TO THE EAR
▸ Adult: To be inserted into meatus or apply on a ribbon gauze dressing or sponge wick which should be kept saturated with the ear drops

- **DIRECTIONS FOR ADMINISTRATION** For ear drops 8%— dilute 8 parts aluminium acetate ear drops (13%) with 5 parts purified water. Must be freshly prepared.

- **MEDICINAL FORMS** There can be variation in the licensing of different medicines containing the same drug. Forms available from special-order manufacturers include: ear drops

2   Removal of earwax

BICARBONATE

Sodium bicarbonate

- **INDICATIONS AND DOSE**
Removal of earwax (with 5% ear drop solution)
▸ TO THE EAR
▸ Child: (consult product literature)
▸ Adult: (consult product literature)

- **SIDE-EFFECTS** Dryness of the ear canal

- **MEDICINAL FORMS** There can be variation in the licensing of different medicines containing the same drug.
Ear drops
▸ Sodium bicarbonate (Non-proprietary)
Sodium bicarbonate 50 mg per 1 ml Sodium bicarbonate 5% ear drops | 10 ml £1.23-£1.25

SOFTENING DRUGS

Almond oil

- **INDICATIONS AND DOSE**
Removal of earwax
▸ TO THE EAR
▸ Child: Allow drops to warm to room temperature before use (consult product literature)
▸ Adult: Allow drops to warm to room temperature before use (consult product literature)

- **DIRECTIONS FOR ADMINISTRATION** The patient should lie with the affected ear uppermost for 5 to 10 minutes after a generous amount of the softening remedy has been introduced into the ear.

- **MEDICINAL FORMS** There can be variation in the licensing of different medicines containing the same drug.
Liquid
▸ Almond oil (Non-proprietary)
Almond oil 1 ml per 1 ml Almond oil liquid | 50 ml £0.85 DT price = £0.85 | 70 ml £0.73 | 200 ml £2.01-£2.37 | 500 ml £11.67

Arachis oil with chlorobutanol

- **INDICATIONS AND DOSE**
Removal of earwax
▸ TO THE EAR
▸ Adult: (consult product literature)

- **LESS SUITABLE FOR PRESCRIBING** Arachis (peanut) oil with chlorobutanol ear drops are less suitable for prescribing.

- **MEDICINAL FORMS** There can be variation in the licensing of different medicines containing the same drug.
Ear drops
▸ Cerumol (Thornton & Ross Ltd)
Chlorobutanol 50 mg per 1 ml, Arachis oil 573 mg per 1 ml Cerumol ear drops | 11 ml Ⓟ £2.05

Docusate sodium
(Dioctyl sodium sulphosuccinate)

- **INDICATIONS AND DOSE**
Removal of ear wax
▸ TO THE EAR
▸ Adult: (consult product literature)

- **LESS SUITABLE FOR PRESCRIBING** Ear drops less suitable for prescribing.

- **MEDICINAL FORMS** There can be variation in the licensing of different medicines containing the same drug.
Ear drops
EXCIPIENTS: May contain Propylene glycol
▸ Molcer (Wallace Manufacturing Chemists Ltd)
Docusate sodium 50 mg per 1 ml Molcer ear drops | 15 ml Ⓟ £8.08
▸ Waxsol (Meda Pharmaceuticals Ltd)
Docusate sodium 5 mg per 1 ml Waxsol ear drops | 10 ml Ⓟ £1.95 DT price = £1.95

Olive oil

- **INDICATIONS AND DOSE**
Removal of earwax
▸ TO THE EAR
▸ Child: Apply twice daily for several days (if wax is hard and impacted)
▸ Adult: Apply twice daily for several days (if wax is hard and impacted)

- **DIRECTIONS FOR ADMINISTRATION** The patient should lie with the affected ear uppermost for 5 to 10 minutes after a generous amount of the softening remedy has been introduced into the ear. Allow ear drops to warm to room temperature before use.

- **MEDICINAL FORMS** There can be variation in the licensing of different medicines containing the same drug.
Ear drops
▸ Olive oil (Non-proprietary)
Olive oil ear drops | 10 ml £1.42 | 20 ml £2.70
▸ Arjun (Arjun Products Ltd)
Arjun ear drops | 10 ml £1.25
▸ Cerumol (olive oil) (Thornton & Ross Ltd)
Cerumol olive oil ear drops | 10 ml no price available
▸ Oleax (JR Biomedical Ltd)
Oleax ear drops | 15 ml £1.40
▸ Olive oil (Thornton & Ross Ltd)
Care olive oil ear drops | 10 ml £1.42
Spray
▸ Earol (HL Healthcare Ltd)
Earol olive oil ear spray | 10 ml no price available

Urea hydrogen peroxide

● INDICATIONS AND DOSE
Softening and removal of earwax
▸ TO THE EAR
▸ **Adult:** (consult product literature)

● PATIENT AND CARER ADVICE The patient should lie with the affected ear uppermost for 5 to 10 minutes after a generous amount of the softening remedy has been introduced into the ear.

● LESS SUITABLE FOR PRESCRIBING Urea-hydrogen peroxide ear drops are less suitable for prescribing.

● MEDICINAL FORMS
There can be variation in the licensing of different medicines containing the same drug.
Ear drops
▸ Exterol (Dermal Laboratories Ltd)
Urea hydrogen peroxide 50 mg per 1 gram Exterol 5% ear drops | 8 ml P £1.75 DT price = £2.89
▸ Otex (Dendron Ltd)
Urea hydrogen peroxide 50 mg per 1 gram Otex 5% ear drops | 8 ml P £2.89 DT price = £2.89

Nose

Nose

Rhinitis and bacterial sinusitis

Rhinitis is often self-limiting but bacterial sinusitis may require treatment with antibacterials. There are few indications for nasal sprays and drops except in allergic rhinitis and perennial rhinitis. Many nasal preparations contain sympathomimetic drugs which may damage the nasal cilia. Sodium chloride 0.9% solution p. 901 may be used as a douche or 'sniff' following endonasal surgery.

Drugs used in nasal allergy

Mild allergic rhinitis is controlled by **antihistamines** (see under Antihistamines, allergen immunotherapy and allergic emergencies p. 253) or topical **nasal corticosteroids**; systemic nasal decongestants are of doubtful value. Topical nasal decongestants can be used for a short period to relieve congestion and allow penetration of a topical nasal corticosteroid.

More persistent symptoms and nasal congestion can be relieved by topical nasal **corticosteroids**; sodium cromoglicate p. 1050 is an alternative, but may be less effective. The topical antihistamine azelastine hydrochloride is useful for controlling breakthrough symptoms in allergic rhinitis. Topical antihistamines are considered less effective than topical corticosteroids but probably more effective than cromoglicate. In seasonal allergic rhinitis (e.g. hay fever), treatment should begin 2 to 3 weeks before the season commences and may have to be continued for several months; continuous treatment may be required for years in perennial rhinitis.

Montelukast p. 245 is less effective than topical nasal corticosteroids; montelukast can be used in patients with seasonal allergic rhinitis and concomitant asthma.

Sometimes allergic rhinitis is accompanied by vasomotor rhinitis. In this situation, the addition of topical nasal ipratropium bromide can reduce watery rhinorrhoea.

Very occasionally symptoms occasionally justify the use of **systemic corticosteroids** for short periods, for example, in students taking important examinations. They may also be used at the beginning of a course of treatment with a corticosteroid spray to relieve severe mucosal oedema and allow the spray to penetrate the nasal cavity.

Corticosteroids

Corticosteroid nasal preparations should be avoided in the presence of untreated nasal infections, after nasal surgery (until healing has occurred), and in pulmonary tuberculosis. Patients transferred from systemic corticosteroids may experience exacerbation of some symptoms. Systemic absorption may follow nasal administration particularly if high doses are used or if treatment is prolonged; for cautions and side-effects of systemic corticosteroids. The risk of systemic effects may be greater with nasal drops than with nasal sprays; drops are administered incorrectly more often than sprays. The height of children receiving prolonged treatment with nasal corticosteroids should be monitored; if growth is slowed, referral to a paediatrician should be considered.

Nasal polyps

Short-term use of corticosteroid nasal drops helps to shrink nasal polyps; to be effective, the drops must be administered with the patient in the 'head down' position. A short course of a systemic corticosteroid may be required initially to shrink large polyps. A corticosteroid nasal spray can be used to maintain the reduction in swelling and also for the initial treatment of small polyps.

Pregnancy

If a pregnant woman cannot tolerate the symptoms of allergic rhinitis, treatment with nasal beclometasone dipropionate p. 1048, budesonide p. 1048, fluticasone p. 1049, or sodium cromoglicate may be considered.

Topical nasal decongestants

The nasal mucosa is sensitive to changes in atmospheric temperature and humidity and these alone may cause slight nasal congestion. The nose and nasal sinuses produce a litre of mucus in 24 hours and much of this finds its way silently into the stomach via the nasopharynx. Slight changes in the nasal airway, accompanied by an awareness of mucus passing along the nasopharynx causes some patients to be inaccurately diagnosed as suffering from chronic sinusitis. These symptoms are particularly noticeable in the later stages of the common cold. Sodium chloride 0.9% given as nasal drops or spray may relieve nasal congestion by helping to liquefy mucous secretions.

Inhalation of **warm moist air** is useful in the treatment of symptoms of acute infective conditions. The addition of volatile substances such as menthol and eucalyptus may encourage the use of warm moist air (see under Aromatic inhalations, cough preparations and systemic nasal decongestants p. 270).

Symptoms of nasal congestion associated with vasomotor rhinitis and the common cold can be relieved by the short-term use (usually not longer than 7 days) of decongestant nasal drops and sprays. These all contain sympathomimetic drugs which exert their effect by vasoconstriction of the mucosal blood vessels which in turn reduces oedema of the nasal mucosa. They are of limited value because they can give rise to a rebound congestion (rhinitis medicamentosa) on withdrawal, due to a secondary vasodilatation with a subsequent temporary increase in nasal congestion. This in turn tempts the further use of the decongestant, leading to a vicious cycle of events. Ephedrine hydrochloride nasal drops p. 1045 are the safest sympathomimetic preparation and can give relief for several hours. The more potent sympathomimetic drugs oxymetazoline and xylometazoline hydrochloride p. 1046 are more likely to cause a rebound effect.

Non-allergic watery rhinorrhoea often responds well to treatment with the antimuscarinic ipratropium bromide p. 1047.

Sinusitis and oral pain

Sinusitis affecting the maxillary antrum can cause pain in the upper jaw. Where this is associated with blockage of the opening from the sinus into the nasal cavity, it may be helpful to relieve the congestion with inhalation of warm moist air or with ephedrine hydrochloride nasal drops.

Systemic antibacterials may sometimes be required for sinusitis (see under Nose infections, bacterial p. 467).

Nasal preparations for infection

There is **no** evidence that topical anti-infective nasal preparations have any therapeutic value in rhinitis or sinusitis; see elimination of nasal staphylococci.

Nasal staphylococci

Elimination of organisms such as staphylococci from the nasal vestibule can be achieved by the use of a cream containing **chlorhexidine** and **neomycin** (*Naseptin*®), but re-colonisation frequently occurs. Coagulase-positive staphylococci are present in the noses of 40% of the population.

A nasal ointment containing mupirocin p. 1047 is also available; it should probably be held in reserve for resistant infections. In hospitals or in care establishments, mupirocin nasal ointment should be reserved for the eradication (in both patients and staff) of nasal carriage of meticillin-resistant *Staphylococcus aureus* (MRSA). A sample should be taken 2 days after treatment to confirm eradication. The course may be repeated if the sample is positive (and the throat is not colonised). To avoid the development of resistance, the treatment course should not exceed 7 days and the course should not be repeated on more than one occasion. If the MRSA strain is mupirocin-resistant or does not respond after 2 courses, consider alternative products such as chlorhexidine and neomycin cream.

1 Nasal congestion

SYMPATHOMIMETICS > VASOCONSTRICTOR

Ephedrine hydrochloride

● **INDICATIONS AND DOSE**

Nasal congestion | Sinusitis affecting the maxillary antrum
▸ BY INTRANASAL ADMINISTRATION
▹ Child 12-17 years: Apply 1–2 drops up to 4 times a day as required for a maximum of 7 days, to be instilled into each nostril, administer ephedrine 0.5% nasal drops
▹ Adult: Apply 1–2 drops up to 4 times a day as required for a maximum of 7 days, to be instilled into each nostril

---

IMPORTANT SAFETY INFORMATION
CHM/MHRA ADVICE
▸ With intranasal use in children
The CHM/MHRA has stated that non-prescription cough and cold medicines containing ephedrine can be considered for up to 5 days' treatment in children aged 6–12 years after basic principles of best care have been tried; these medicines should not be used in children under 6 years of age.

● CAUTIONS Avoid excessive or prolonged use · cardiovascular disease (in children) · diabetes mellitus · elderly · hypertension · hyperthyroidism · ischaemic heart disease (in adults) · prostatic hypertrophy (risk of acute urinary retention)
● INTERACTIONS → Appendix 1 (sympathomimetics).
● SIDE-EFFECTS
▸ **Common or very common** Headache · nausea
▸ **Frequency not known** After excessive use tolerance with diminished effect · cardiovascular effect · local irritation · rebound congestion

● PREGNANCY Manufacturer advises avoid.
● BREAST FEEDING Present in milk; manufacturer advises avoid—irritability and disturbed sleep reported.
● PRESCRIBING AND DISPENSING INFORMATION For nasal drops, the BP directs that if no strength is specified 0.5% drops should be supplied.
● PROFESSION SPECIFIC INFORMATION
Dental practitioners' formulary
Ephedrine nasal drops may be prescribed.
● EXCEPTIONS TO LEGAL CATEGORY Ephedrine nasal drops can be sold to the public provided no more than 180 mg of ephedrine base (or salts) are supplied at one time, and pseudoephedrine salts are not supplied at the same time; for conditions that apply to supplies made at the request of a patient, see *Medicines, Ethics and Practice*, London, Pharmaceutical Press (always consult latest edition).

● MEDICINAL FORMS
There can be variation in the licensing of different medicines containing the same drug. Forms available from special-order manufacturers include: nasal drops
Nasal drops
▸ Ephedrine hydrochloride (Non-proprietary)
  Ephedrine hydrochloride 5 mg per 1 ml Ephedrine 0.5% nasal drops | 10 ml ℗ £1.73–£1.75 DT price = £1.74
  Ephedrine hydrochloride 10 mg per 1 ml Ephedrine 1% nasal drops | 10 ml ℗ £1.79–£1.81 DT price = £1.80

Pseudoephedrine hydrochloride

● **INDICATIONS AND DOSE**

Congestion of mucous membranes of upper respiratory tract
▸ BY MOUTH
▹ Child 6-11 years: 30 mg 3–4 times a day
▹ Child 12-17 years: 60 mg 3–4 times a day
▹ Adult: 60 mg 3–4 times a day

IMPORTANT SAFETY INFORMATION
MHRA/CHM ADVICE (MARCH 2008 AND FEBRUARY 2009): OVER-THE-COUNTER COUGH AND COLD MEDICINES FOR CHILDREN
Children under 6 years should not be given over-the-counter cough and cold medicines containing pseudoephedrine.

● CAUTIONS Diabetes · heart disease · hypertension · hyperthyroidism · ischaemic heart disease (in adults) · prostatic hypertrophy (in adults) · raised intra-ocular pressure (in children) · susceptibility to angle-closure glaucoma
● INTERACTIONS → Appendix 1 (sympathomimetics). Contra-indicated in patients taking monoamine oxidase inhibitors within the previous 2 weeks.
● SIDE-EFFECTS
▸ **Common or very common** Anxiety · headache · hypertension · insomnia · nausea · restlessness · tachycardia · vomiting
▸ **Rare** Hallucinations · rash
▸ **Very rare** Angle-closure glaucoma
▸ **Frequency not known** Urinary retention
● PREGNANCY Defective closure of the abdominal wall (gastroschisis) reported very rarely in newborns after first trimester exposure.
● BREAST FEEDING May suppress lactation; avoid if lactation not well established or if milk production insufficient.
● HEPATIC IMPAIRMENT Manufacturer advises use with caution in severe impairment.
● RENAL IMPAIRMENT Use with caution in mild to moderate renal impairment. Manufacturer advises avoid in severe renal impairment.

Ear, nose and oropharynx

12

- LESS SUITABLE FOR PRESCRIBING Pseudoephedrine hydrochloride is less suitable for prescribing.
- EXCEPTIONS TO LEGAL CATEGORY *Galpseud®* and *Sudafed®* can be sold to the public provided no more than 720 mg of pseudoephedrine salts are supplied, and ephedrine base (or salts) are not supplied at the same time; for details see *Medicines, Ethics and Practice*, London, Pharmaceutical Press (always consult latest edition).

- MEDICINAL FORMS
  There can be variation in the licensing of different medicines containing the same drug.

Tablet
▸ Pseudoephedrine hydrochloride (Non-proprietary)
  Pseudoephedrine hydrochloride 60 mg | 12 tablet P no price available
▸ Galpseud (Thornton & Ross Ltd)
  Pseudoephedrine hydrochloride 60 mg Galpseud 60mg tablets | 24 tablet PoM £2.25 | 100 tablet PoM £5.42 DT price = £5.42
▸ Sudafed Non-Drowsy Decongestant (pseudoephedrine) (McNeil Products Ltd)
  Pseudoephedrine hydrochloride 60 mg Sudafed Decongestant 60mg tablets | 12 tablet P £2.04

Oral solution
EXCIPIENTS: May contain Alcohol
▸ Pseudoephedrine hydrochloride (Non-proprietary)
  Pseudoephedrine hydrochloride 6 mg per 1 ml Decongestant 30mg/5ml oral liquid sugar-free | 100 ml P £1.57 DT price = £1.57
▸ Galpseud (Thornton & Ross Ltd)
  Pseudoephedrine hydrochloride 6 mg per 1 ml Galpseud 30mg/5ml linctus sugar-free | 2000 ml PoM £14.00
▸ Sudafed Non-Drowsy Decongestant (pseudoephedrine) (McNeil Products Ltd)
  Pseudoephedrine hydrochloride 6 mg per 1 ml Sudafed Decongestant 30mg/5ml liquid | 100 ml P £1.92

Xylometazoline hydrochloride

- DRUG ACTION Xylometazoline is a sympathomimetic.

- INDICATIONS AND DOSE
Nasal congestion
▸ BY INTRANASAL ADMINISTRATION USING NASAL DROPS
▸ Child 6–11 years: 1–2 drops 1–2 times a day as required for maximum duration of 5 days, 0.05% solution to be administered into each nostril
▸ Child 12–17 years: 2–3 drops 2–3 times a day as required for maximum duration of 7 days, 0.1% solution to be administered into each nostril
▸ Adult: 2–3 drops 2–3 times a day as required for maximum duration of 7 days, 0.1% solution to be administered into each nostril
▸ BY INTRANASAL ADMINISTRATION USING NASAL SPRAY
▸ Child 12–17 years: 1 spray 1–3 times a day as required for maximum duration of 7 days, to be administered into each nostril
▸ Adult: 1 spray 1–3 times a day as required for maximum duration of 7 days, to be administered into each nostril

IMPORTANT SAFETY INFORMATION
The CHM/MHRA has stated that non-prescription cough and cold medicines containing oxymetazoline or xylometazoline can be considered for up to 5 days' treatment in children aged 6–12 years after basic principles of best care have been tried; these medicines should not be used in children under 6 years of age.

- CAUTIONS Angle-closure glaucoma · avoid excessive or prolonged use · cardiovascular disease (in children) · diabetes mellitus · elderly (in adults) · hypertension · hyperthyroidism · ischaemic heart disease (in adults) · prostatic hypertrophy (risk of acute retention) (in adults) · rebound congestion

CAUTIONS, FURTHER INFORMATION
▸ Rebound congestion Sympathomimetic drugs are of limited value in the treatment of nasal congestion because they can, following prolonged use (more than 7 days), give rise to a rebound congestion (rhinitis medicamentosa) on withdrawal, due to a secondary vasodilatation with a subsequent temporary increase in nasal congestion. This in turn tempts the further use of the decongestant, leading to a vicious cycle of events.

- SIDE-EFFECTS Cardiovascular effects · hallucinations in small children · headache · local irritation · nausea · rebound congestion · restlessness in small children · sleep disturbances in small children · tolerance with diminished effect (after excessive use) · transient visual disturbances
SIDE-EFFECTS, FURTHER INFORMATION
▸ Hallucinations (in small children) Discontinue treatment if the hallucinations occur.

- PREGNANCY Manufacturer advises avoid.
- BREAST FEEDING Manufacturer advises caution—no information available.

- MEDICINAL FORMS
  There can be variation in the licensing of different medicines containing the same drug.

Spray
▸ Otrivine (Novartis Consumer Health UK Ltd)
  Xylometazoline hydrochloride 1 mg per 1 ml Otrivine Congestion Relief 0.1% nasal spray | 10 ml GSL £3.05 DT price = £2.18
  Otrivine Adult Measured Dose Sinusitis spray | 10 ml GSL £2.62 DT price = £2.18
  Otrivine Allergy Relief 0.1% nasal spray | 10 ml GSL £2.62 DT price = £2.18
  Otrivine Adult nasal spray | 10 ml GSL £2.18 DT price = £2.18
  Otrivine Adult Metered Dose 0.1% nasal spray | 10 ml GSL £2.62 DT price = £2.18
▸ Sudafed Congestion Relief (McNeil Products Ltd)
  Xylometazoline hydrochloride 1 mg per 1 ml Sudafed Congestion Relief 0.1% nasal spray | 10 ml GSL £3.25 DT price = £2.18
▸ Sudafed Mucus Relief (McNeil Products Ltd)
  Xylometazoline hydrochloride 1 mg per 1 ml Sudafed Mucus Relief 0.1% nasal spray | 15 ml GSL £2.37
▸ Sudafed Non-Drowsy Decongestant (xylometazoline) (McNeil Products Ltd)
  Xylometazoline hydrochloride 1 mg per 1 ml Sudafed Blocked Nose 0.1% spray | 15 ml GSL £2.38

Nasal drops
▸ Otrivine (Novartis Consumer Health UK Ltd)
  Xylometazoline hydrochloride 500 microgram per 1 ml Otrivine Child nasal drops | 10 ml P £1.91 DT price = £1.91
  Xylometazoline hydrochloride 1 mg per 1 ml Otrivine Adult 0.1% nasal drops | 10 ml GSL £2.18 DT price = £2.18

2   Nasal infection

ANTIBACTERIALS > AMINOGLYCOSIDES

Chlorhexidine with neomycin

- INDICATIONS AND DOSE
Eradication of nasal carriage of staphylococci
▸ BY INTRANASAL ADMINISTRATION
▸ Child: Apply 4 times a day for 10 days
▸ Adult: Apply 4 times a day for 10 days
Preventing nasal carriage of staphylococci
▸ BY INTRANASAL ADMINISTRATION
▸ Child: Apply twice daily
▸ Adult: Apply twice daily

- MEDICINAL FORMS
  There can be variation in the licensing of different medicines containing the same drug.
  Cream
  EXCIPIENTS: May contain Arachis (peanut) oil, cetostearyl alcohol (including cetyl and stearyl alcohol)
  ▸ Naseptin (Alliance Pharmaceuticals Ltd)
  Chlorhexidine hydrochloride 1 mg per 1 gram, Neomycin sulfate 5 mg per 1 gram Naseptin nasal cream | 15 gram PoM £2.24 DT price = £2.24

ANTIBACTERIALS > OTHER

Mupirocin

- INDICATIONS AND DOSE
  BACTROBAN NASAL®
  For eradication of nasal carriage of staphylococci, including meticillin-resistant *Staphylococcus aureus* (MRSA)
  ▸ BY INTRANASAL ADMINISTRATION
  ▸ Child: Apply 2–3 times a day for 5 days; a sample should be taken 2 days after treatment to confirm eradication. Course may be repeated once if sample positive (and throat not colonised), dose to be applied to the inner surface of each nostril
  ▸ Adult: Apply 2–3 times a day for 5 days; a sample should be taken 2 days after treatment to confirm eradication. Course may be repeated once if sample positive (and throat not colonised), dose to be applied to the inner surface of each nostril

- PREGNANCY Manufacturer advises avoid unless potential benefit outweighs risk—no information available.
- BREAST FEEDING No information available.

- MEDICINAL FORMS
  There can be variation in the licensing of different medicines containing the same drug.
  Nasal ointment
  ▸ Bactroban (GlaxoSmithKline UK Ltd)
  Mupirocin (as Mupirocin calcium) 20 mg per 1 gram Bactroban 2% nasal ointment | 3 gram PoM £3.89 DT price = £3.89

CORTICOSTEROIDS > CORTICOSTEROID COMBINATIONS WITH ANTI-INFECTIVES

Betamethasone with neomycin

The properties listed below are those particular to the combination only. For the properties of the components please consider, betamethasone p. 1048.

- INDICATIONS AND DOSE
  Nasal infection
  ▸ BY INTRANASAL ADMINISTRATION USING NASAL DROPS
  ▸ Child: Apply 2–3 drops 2–3 times a day, to be applied into each nostril
  ▸ Adult: Apply 2–3 drops 2–3 times a day, to be applied into each nostril

- LESS SUITABLE FOR PRESCRIBING Betamethasone with neomycin nasal-drops are less suitable for prescribing; there is no evidence that topical anti-infective nasal preparations have any therapeutic value in rhinitis or sinusitis.

- MEDICINAL FORMS
  There can be variation in the licensing of different medicines containing the same drug.
  Ear/eye/nose drops solution
  EXCIPIENTS: May contain Benzalkonium chloride, disodium edetate
  ▸ Betnesol-N (Focus Pharmaceuticals Ltd)
  Betamethasone (as Betamethasone sodium phosphate) 1 mg per 1 ml, Neomycin sulfate 5 mg per 1 ml Betnesol-N ear/eye/nose drops | 10 ml PoM £2.39 DT price = £2.39

3 Nasal inflammation, nasal polyps and rhinitis

> **Drugs used for Nasal inflammation, nasal polyps and rhinitis not listed below** Desloratadine, p. 256 · Fexofenadine hydrochloride, p. 257 · Ketotifen, p. 263

ANTIMUSCARINICS

Ipratropium bromide   24.2.2016

- INDICATIONS AND DOSE
  Rhinorrhoea associated with allergic and non-allergic rhinitis
  ▸ BY INTRANASAL ADMINISTRATION
  ▸ Child 12–17 years: 2 sprays 2–3 times a day, dose to be sprayed into each nostril
  ▸ Adult: 2 sprays 2–3 times a day, dose to be sprayed into each nostril
  DOSE EQUIVALENCE AND CONVERSION
  1 metered spray of nasal spray = 21 micrograms.

- CAUTIONS Avoid spraying near eyes · bladder outflow obstruction · cystic fibrosis · prostatic hyperplasia (in adults) · susceptibility to angle-closure glaucoma
- SIDE-EFFECTS
  ▸ Common or very common Epistaxis · nasal dryness · nasal irritation
  ▸ Uncommon Headache · nausea
  ▸ Very rare Gastro-intestinal motility disturbances · palpitations · urinary retention
- PREGNANCY Manufacturer advises only use if potential benefit outweighs the risk.
- BREAST FEEDING No information available—manufacturer advises only use if potential benefit outweighs risk.

- MEDICINAL FORMS
  There can be variation in the licensing of different medicines containing the same drug.
  Spray
  EXCIPIENTS: May contain Benzalkonium chloride, disodium edetate
  ▸ Rinatec (Boehringer Ingelheim Ltd)
  Ipratropium bromide 21 microgram per 1 dose Rinatec 21micrograms/dose nasal spray | 180 dose PoM £6.54 DT price = £6.54

CORTICOSTEROIDS

Corticosteroids (intranasal)

- CAUTIONS Avoid after nasal surgery (until healing has occurred) · avoid in pulmonary tuberculosis · avoid in the presence of untreated nasal infections · patients transferred from systemic corticosteroids may experience exacerbation of some symptoms

  CAUTIONS, FURTHER INFORMATION
  ▸ Systemic absorption Systemic absorption may follow nasal administration particularly if high doses are used or if treatment is prolonged; therefore also consider the

cautions and side-effects of systemic corticosteroids. The risk of systemic effects may be greater with nasal drops than with nasal sprays; drops are administered incorrectly more often than sprays.

- SIDE-EFFECTS
- ▶ **Rare** Glaucoma · raised intra-ocular pressure
- ▶ **Very rare** Nasal septal perforation (usually following nasal surgery)
- ▶ **Frequency not known** Aggression (particularly in children) · anxiety (particularly in children) · bronchospasm · depression (particularly in children) · dryness · epistaxis · headache · hyperactivity (particularly in children) · hypersensitivity reactions · nasal irritation · nasal ulceration · sleep disturbances (particularly in children) · smell disturbances · taste disturbances · throat irritation

SIDE-EFFECTS, FURTHER INFORMATION
- ▶ Systemic absorption Systemic absorption may follow nasal administration particularly if high doses are used or if treatment is prolonged. Therefore also consider the side-effects of systemic corticosteroids. The risk of systemic effects may be greater with nasal drops than with nasal sprays; drops are administered incorrectly more often than sprays.

- MONITORING REQUIREMENTS
- ▶ In children The height of children receiving prolonged treatment with nasal corticosteroids should be monitored; if growth is slowed, referral to a paediatrician should be considered.

🔖 1047

Beclometasone dipropionate

(Beclomethasone dipropionate)

- INDICATIONS AND DOSE

Prophylaxis and treatment of allergic and vasomotor rhinitis
- ▶ BY INTRANASAL ADMINISTRATION
- ▶ Child 6–17 years: 100 micrograms twice daily, dose to be administered into each nostril, reduced to 50 micrograms twice daily, dose to be administered into each nostril, dose to be reduced when symptoms controlled; maximum 400 micrograms per day
- ▶ Adult: 100 micrograms twice daily, dose to be administered into each nostril, reduced to 50 micrograms twice daily, dose to be administered into each nostril, dose to be reduced when symptoms controlled; maximum 400 micrograms per day

- EXCEPTIONS TO LEGAL CATEGORY
- ▶ In adults Preparations of beclometasone dipropionate can be sold to the public for nasal administration as a nasal spray if supplied for the prevention and treatment of allergic rhinitis in adults over 18 years subject to max. single dose of 100 micrograms per nostril, max. daily dose of 200 micrograms per nostril for max. 3 months, and a pack size of 20 mg.

- MEDICINAL FORMS
There can be variation in the licensing of different medicines containing the same drug.
Spray
EXCIPIENTS: May contain Benzalkonium chloride, polysorbates
- ▶ Beclometasone dipropionate (Non-proprietary)
Beclometasone dipropionate 50 microgram per 1 dose Beclometasone 50micrograms/dose nasal spray | 200 dose [PoM] no price available DT price = £2.02 | 200 dose [P] £5.70 DT price = £2.02
- ▶ Beconase (GlaxoSmithKline UK Ltd, Omega Pharma Ltd)
Beclometasone dipropionate 50 microgram per 1 dose Beconase Aqueous 50micrograms/dose nasal spray | 200 dose [PoM] £2.19 DT price = £2.02
Beconase Hayfever 50micrograms/dose nasal spray | 180 dose [P] £6.46

- ▶ Nasobec (Teva UK Ltd)
Beclometasone dipropionate 50 microgram per 1 dose Nasobec Aqueous 50micrograms/dose nasal spray | 200 dose [PoM] £3.06 DT price = £2.02
Nasobec Hayfever 50micrograms/dose nasal spray | 180 dose [P] £5.78
- ▶ Pollenase (beclometasone) (E M Pharma)
Beclometasone dipropionate 50 microgram per 1 dose Pollenase Hayfever 50micrograms/dose nasal spray | 200 dose [P] £3.36 DT price = £2.02

🔖 1047

Betamethasone

- INDICATIONS AND DOSE

BETNESOL®

Non-infected inflammatory conditions of nose
- ▶ BY INTRANASAL ADMINISTRATION
- ▶ Adult: Apply 2–3 drops 2–3 times a day, dose to be applied into each nostril

VISTAMETHASONE®

Non-infected inflammatory conditions of nose
- ▶ BY INTRANASAL ADMINISTRATION
- ▶ Adult: Apply 2–3 drops twice daily, dose to be applied into each nostril

- MEDICINAL FORMS
There can be variation in the licensing of different medicines containing the same drug.
Ear/eye/nose drops solution
EXCIPIENTS: May contain Benzalkonium chloride, disodium edetate
- ▶ Betnesol (Focus Pharmaceuticals Ltd)
Betamethasone sodium phosphate 1 mg per 1 ml Betnesol 0.1% eye/ear/nose drops | 10 ml [PoM] £2.32 DT price = £2.32
- ▶ Vistamethasone (Martindale Pharmaceuticals Ltd)
Betamethasone sodium phosphate 1 mg per 1 ml Vistamethasone 0.1% ear/eye/nose drops | 5 ml [PoM] £0.87 | 10 ml [PoM] £0.99 DT price = £2.32

🔖 1047

Budesonide

- INDICATIONS AND DOSE

Prophylaxis and treatment of allergic and vasomotor rhinitis
- ▶ BY INTRANASAL ADMINISTRATION
- ▶ Child 12–17 years: Initially 200 micrograms once daily, dose to be administered into each nostril in the morning, alternatively initially 100 micrograms twice daily, dose to be administered to each nostril; reduced to 100 micrograms once daily, dose to be administered into each nostril, dose can be reduced when control achieved
- ▶ Adult: Initially 200 micrograms once daily, dose to be administered into each nostril in the morning, alternatively initially 100 micrograms twice daily, dose to be administered to each nostril; reduced to 100 micrograms once daily, dose to be administered into each nostril, dose can be reduced when control achieved

Nasal polyps
- ▶ BY INTRANASAL ADMINISTRATION
- ▶ Child 12–17 years: 100 micrograms twice daily for up to 3 months, dose to be administered into each nostril
- ▶ Adult: 100 micrograms twice daily for up to 3 months, dose to be administered into each nostril

RHINOCORT AQUA®

Rhinitis
- ▶ BY INTRANASAL ADMINISTRATION
- ▶ Adult: 128 micrograms once daily, dose to be administered into each nostril in the morning, alternatively 64 micrograms twice daily, dose to be

administered into each nostril; reduced to
64 micrograms once daily when control achieved. Use
for maximum 3 months, doses to be administered into
each nostril

Nasal polyps
▶ BY INTRANASAL ADMINISTRATION
▶ Adult: 64 micrograms twice daily for up to 3 months,
dose to be administered into each nostril

● EXCEPTIONS TO LEGAL CATEGORY
▶ In adults Preparations of budesonide can be sold to the
public for nasal administration as a nasal spray if supplied
for the prevention and treatment of seasonal allergic
rhinitis in adults over 18 years subject to max. single dose
of 200 micrograms per nostril, max. daily dose of
200 micrograms per nostril for max. period of 3 months,
and a pack size of 10 mg.

● MEDICINAL FORMS
There can be variation in the licensing of different medicines
containing the same drug.
Spray
EXCIPIENTS: May contain Disodium edetate, polysorbates, potassium
sorbate
▶ Budesonide (Non-proprietary)
Budesonide 100 microgram per 1 dose Budeflam Aquanase
100micrograms/dose nasal spray | 150 dose [PoM] no price available
Aircort 100micrograms/dose nasal spray | 200 dose [PoM] no price
available
▶ Rhinocort (AstraZeneca UK Ltd)
Budesonide 64 microgram per 1 dose Rhinocort Aqua 64 nasal
spray | 120 dose [PoM] £3.49 DT price = £4.77

⚑ 1047

Fluticasone
4.1.2016

● INDICATIONS AND DOSE
**Prophylaxis and treatment of allergic rhinitis and
perennial rhinitis**
▶ BY INTRANASAL ADMINISTRATION USING NASAL SPRAY
▶ Child 4–11 years: 50 micrograms once daily, to be
administered into each nostril preferably in the
morning, increased if necessary to 50 micrograms twice
daily
▶ Child 12–17 years: 100 micrograms once daily, to be
administered into each nostril preferably in the
morning, increased if necessary to 100 micrograms
twice daily; reduced to 50 micrograms once daily, dose
to be administered into each nostril, dose to be reduced
when control achieved
▶ Adult: 100 micrograms once daily, to be administered
into each nostril preferably in the morning, increased if
necessary to 100 micrograms twice daily; reduced to
50 micrograms once daily, dose to be administered into
each nostril, dose to be reduced when control achieved

Nasal polyps
▶ BY INTRANASAL ADMINISTRATION USING NASAL DROPS
▶ Child 16–17 years: 200 micrograms 1–2 times a day, to
be administered into each nostril, alternative
treatment should be considered if no improvement
after 4–6 weeks, (200 micrograms is equivalent to
approximately 6 drops)
▶ Adult: 200 micrograms 1–2 times a day, to be
administered into each nostril, alternative treatment
should be considered if no improvement after
4–6 weeks, (200 micrograms is equivalent to
approximately 6 drops)

AVAMYS® SPRAY
Prophylaxis and treatment of allergic rhinitis
▶ BY INTRANASAL ADMINISTRATION
▶ Child 6–11 years: 27.5 micrograms once daily, dose to be
sprayed into each nostril, increased if necessary to

55 micrograms once daily if required, reduced to
27.5 micrograms once daily, dose to be reduced once
control achieved; use minimum effective dose
▶ Child 12–17 years: 55 micrograms once daily, dose to be
sprayed into each nostril, reduced to 27.5 micrograms
once daily, to be sprayed into each nostril, dose to be
reduced once control achieved; use minimum effective
dose
▶ Adult: 55 micrograms once daily, dose to be sprayed
into each nostril, reduced to 27.5 micrograms once
daily, to be sprayed into each nostril, dose to be
reduced once control achieved; use minimum effective
dose

DOSE EQUIVALENCE AND CONVERSION
For *Avamys*® spray: 1 spray equivalent to
27.5 micrograms.

● SIDE-EFFECTS
SIDE-EFFECTS, FURTHER INFORMATION
Nasal ulceration occurs commonly with nasal preparations
containing fluticasone furoate.

● EXCEPTIONS TO LEGAL CATEGORY
▶ In adults Preparations of fluticasone propionate can be sold
to the public for nasal administration (other than by
pressurised nasal spray) if supplied for the prevention and
treatment of allergic rhinitis in adults over 18 years,
subject to max. single dose of 100 micrograms per nostril,
max. daily dose of 200 micrograms per nostril for max.
3 months, and a pack size of 3 mg.

● MEDICINAL FORMS
There can be variation in the licensing of different medicines
containing the same drug.
Spray
EXCIPIENTS: May contain Benzalkonium chloride, disodium edetate,
polysorbates
▶ Fluticasone (Non-proprietary)
Fluticasone propionate 50 microgram per 1 dose Fluticasone
propionate 50micrograms/dose nasal spray | 60 dose [PoM] no price
available | 150 dose [PoM] £29.50 DT price = £11.01
▶ Avamys (GlaxoSmithKline UK Ltd)
Fluticasone furoate 27.5 microgram per 1 dose Avamys
27.5micrograms/dose nasal spray | 120 dose [PoM] £6.44 DT price =
£6.44
▶ Flixonase (GlaxoSmithKline UK Ltd)
Fluticasone propionate 50 microgram per 1 dose Flixonase
50micrograms/dose aqueous nasal spray | 150 dose [PoM] £11.01 DT
price = £11.01
▶ Nasofan (Teva UK Ltd)
Fluticasone propionate 50 microgram per 1 dose Nasofan Allergy
50micrograms/dose nasal spray | 60 dose [P] £4.68
Nasofan 50micrograms/dose aqueous nasal spray | 150 dose [PoM]
£8.04 DT price = £11.01
▶ Pirinase Hayfever (GlaxoSmithKline Consumer Healthcare)
Fluticasone propionate 50 microgram per 1 dose Pirinase
Hayfever 0.05% nasal spray | 60 dose [P] £4.59
Pirinase Hayfever Relief for Adults 0.05% nasal spray | 60 dose [GSL]
£4.59

Nasal drops
EXCIPIENTS: May contain Polysorbates
▶ Flixonase (GlaxoSmithKline UK Ltd)
Fluticasone propionate 400 microgram Flixonase Nasule
400microgram/unit dose nasal drops | 28 unit dose [PoM] £12.99 DT
price = £12.99

12

Ear, nose and oropharynx

Fluticasone with azelastine

The properties listed below are those particular to the combination only. For the properties of the components please consider, fluticasone p. 1049, azelastine hydrochloride p. 1006.

● **INDICATIONS AND DOSE**

Moderate to severe seasonal and perennial allergic rhinitis, if monotherapy with antihistamine or corticosteroid is inadequate

▸ BY INTRANASAL ADMINISTRATION
▸ Child 12-17 years: 1 spray twice daily, dose to be administered into each nostril
▸ Adult: 1 spray twice daily, dose to be administered into each nostril

● MEDICINAL FORMS
There can be variation in the licensing of different medicines containing the same drug.
Spray
EXCIPIENTS: May contain Benzalkonium chloride, polysorbates
▸ Fluticasone with azelastine (Non-proprietary)
Fluticasone propionate 50 microgram per 1 actuation, Azelastine hydrochloride 137 microgram per 1 actuation Fluticasone propionate 50micrograms/dose / Azelastine 137micrograms/dose nasal spray | 120 dose [PoM] no price available
▸ Dymista (Meda Pharmaceuticals Ltd)
Fluticasone propionate 50 microgram per 1 actuation, Azelastine hydrochloride 137 microgram per 1 actuation Dymista 137micrograms/dose / 50micrograms/dose nasal spray | 120 dose [PoM] £14.80

▼ 1047

Mometasone furoate

● **INDICATIONS AND DOSE**

Prophylaxis and treatment of allergic rhinitis
▸ BY INTRANASAL ADMINISTRATION
▸ Child 6-11 years: 50 micrograms daily, dose to be sprayed into each nostril
▸ Child 12-17 years: 100 micrograms daily, increased if necessary up to 200 micrograms daily, dose to be sprayed into each nostril; reduced to 50 micrograms daily, dose to be reduced when control achieved, dose to be sprayed into each nostril
▸ Adult: 100 micrograms daily, increased if necessary up to 200 micrograms daily, dose to be sprayed into each nostril; reduced to 50 micrograms daily, dose to be reduced when control achieved, dose to be sprayed into each nostril

Nasal polyps
▸ BY INTRANASAL ADMINISTRATION
▸ Adult: Initially 100 micrograms daily for 5–6 weeks, dose to be sprayed into each nostril, then increased if necessary to 100 micrograms twice daily, dose to be sprayed into each nostril, consider alternative treatment if no improvement after further 5–6 weeks, reduce to the lowest effective dose when control achieved

● **SIDE-EFFECTS**
SIDE-EFFECTS, FURTHER INFORMATION
Nasal ulceration occurs commonly with preparations containing mometasone furoate.

● MEDICINAL FORMS
There can be variation in the licensing of different medicines containing the same drug.
Spray
EXCIPIENTS: May contain Benzalkonium chloride, polysorbates
▸ Mometasone furoate (Non-proprietary)
Mometasone furoate 50 microgram per 1 dose Mometasone 50micrograms/dose nasal spray | 140 dose [PoM] £7.30 DT price = £2.01
▸ Nasonex (Merck Sharp & Dohme Ltd)
Mometasone furoate 50 microgram per 1 dose Nasonex 50micrograms/dose nasal spray | 140 dose [PoM] £7.68 DT price = £2.01

▼ 1047

Triamcinolone acetonide

● **INDICATIONS AND DOSE**

Prophylaxis and treatment of allergic rhinitis
▸ BY INTRANASAL ADMINISTRATION
▸ Child 6-11 years: 55 micrograms once daily, dose to be sprayed into each nostril, increased if necessary to 110 micrograms once daily, dose to be sprayed into each nostril; reduced to 55 micrograms once daily, dose to be sprayed into each nostril, reduce dose when control achieved; maximum duration of treatment 3 months
▸ Child 12-17 years: 110 micrograms once daily, dose to be sprayed into each nostril, reduced to 55 micrograms once daily, dose to be sprayed into each nostril, reduce dose when control achieved
▸ Adult: 110 micrograms once daily, dose to be sprayed into each nostril, reduced to 55 micrograms once daily, dose to be sprayed into each nostril, reduce dose when control achieved

● UNLICENSED USE Not licensed for use in children under 6 years.

● EXCEPTIONS TO LEGAL CATEGORY
▸ In adults Preparations of triamcinolone acetonide can be sold to the public for nasal administration as a non-pressurised nasal spray if supplied for the symptomatic treatment of seasonal allergic rhinitis in adults over 18 years, subject to maximum daily dose of 110 micrograms per nostril for maximum 3 months, and a pack size of 3.575 mg.

● MEDICINAL FORMS
There can be variation in the licensing of different medicines containing the same drug.
Spray
EXCIPIENTS: May contain Benzalkonium chloride, disodium edetate, polysorbates
▸ Nasacort (Sanofi)
Triamcinolone acetonide 55 microgram per 1 dose Nasacort Allergy 55micrograms/dose nasal spray | 30 dose [P] £3.01 Nasacort 55micrograms/dose nasal spray | 120 dose [PoM] £7.39 DT price = £7.39

MAST-CELL STABILISERS

Sodium cromoglicate

(Sodium cromoglycate)

● **INDICATIONS AND DOSE**

Prophylaxis of allergic rhinitis
▸ BY INTRANASAL ADMINISTRATION
▸ Child: 1 spray 2–4 times a day, to be administered into each nostril
▸ Adult: 1 spray 2–4 times a day, to be administered into each nostril

● UNLICENSED USE Licensed for use in children (age range not specified by manufacturers).

- SIDE-EFFECTS
▶ **Rare** Transient bronchospasm
▶ **Frequency not known** Local irritation

- MEDICINAL FORMS
There can be variation in the licensing of different medicines
containing the same drug.
No licensed medicines listed.

Oropharynx

1 Dry mouth

Treatment of dry mouth

Overview

Dry mouth (xerostomia) may be caused by drugs with
antimuscarinic (anticholinergic) side-effects (e.g.
antispasmodics, tricyclic antidepressants, and some
antipsychotics), by diuretics, by irradiation of the head and
neck region or by damage to or disease of the salivary glands.
Patients with a persistently dry mouth may develop a
burning or scalded sensation and have poor oral hygiene;
they may develop increased dental caries, periodontal
disease, intolerance of dentures, and oral infections
(particularly candidiasis). Dry mouth may be relieved in
many patients by simple measures such as frequent sips of
cool drinks or sucking pieces of ice or sugar-free fruit
pastilles. Sugar-free chewing gum stimulates salivation in
patients with residual salivary function.

    Artificial saliva can provide useful relief of dry mouth. A
properly balanced artificial saliva should be of a neutral pH
and contain electrolytes (including fluoride) to correspond
approximately to the composition of saliva. The acidic pH of
some artificial saliva products may be inappropriate. Of the
proprietary preparations, *Aquoral ®*, *Biotène Oralbalance ®* gel
or *Xerotin ®* can be used for any condition giving rise to a dry
mouth. *BioXtra ®*, *Glandosane ®*, *Saliva Orthana ®*, and
Saliveze ®, have ACBS approval for dry mouth associated only
with radiotherapy or sicca syndrome. *Salivix ®* pastilles,
which act locally as salivary stimulants, are also available for
any condition leading to a dry mouth and SST tablets may be
prescribed for dry mouth in patients with salivary gland
impairment (and patent salivary ducts).

    Pilocarpine tablets, below, are licensed for the treatment
of xerostomia following irradiation for head and neck cancer
and for dry mouth and dry eyes (xerophthalmia) in Sjögren's
syndrome. They are effective only in patients who have some
residual salivary gland function, and therefore should be
withdrawn if there is no response.

PARASYMPATHOMIMETICS

▌ Pilocarpine

- INDICATIONS AND DOSE
Xerostomia following irradiation for head and neck cancer
▶ BY MOUTH
▶ Adult: 5 mg 3 times a day for 4 weeks, then increased if
tolerated to up to 30 mg daily in divided doses if
required, dose to be taken with or immediately after
meals (last dose always with evening meal), maximum
therapeutic effect normally within 4–8 weeks;
discontinue if no improvement after 2–3 months
Dry mouth and dry eyes in Sjögren's syndrome
▶ BY MOUTH
▶ Adult: 5 mg 4 times a day; increased if tolerated to up
to 30 mg daily in divided doses if required, dose to be

taken with meals and at bedtime, discontinue if no
improvement after 2–3 months

- CONTRA-INDICATIONS Acute iritis · chronic obstructive
pulmonary disease (increased bronchial secretions and
increased airways resistance) · uncontrolled asthma
(increased bronchial secretions and increased airways
resistance) · uncontrolled cardiorenal disease

- CAUTIONS Asthma (avoid if uncontrolled) · biliary-tract
disease · cardiovascular disease (avoid if uncontrolled) ·
cholelithiasis · chronic obstructive pulmonary disease
(avoid if uncontrolled) · cognitive disturbances · maintain
adequate fluid intake to avoid dehydration associated with
excessive sweating · peptic ulceration · psychiatric
disturbances · risk of increased renal colic · risk of
increased urethral smooth muscle tone · susceptibility to
angle-closure glaucoma

- INTERACTIONS → Appendix 1 (parasympathomimetics).

- SIDE-EFFECTS
▶ **Common or very common** Influenza-like symptoms ·
abdominal pain · asthenia · conjunctivitis · constipation ·
diarrhoea · dizziness · dyspepsia · flushing · headache ·
hypertension · increased urinary frequency · lacrimation ·
nausea · ocular pain · palpitation · pruritus · rash · rhinitis ·
sweating · visual disturbances · vomiting
▶ **Uncommon** Flatulence · urinary urgency

- PREGNANCY Avoid—smooth muscle stimulant; toxicity in
animal studies.

- BREAST FEEDING Manufacturer advises avoid—present in
milk in *animal* studies.

- HEPATIC IMPAIRMENT Reduce initial oral dose in moderate
or severe cirrhosis.

- RENAL IMPAIRMENT Manufacturer advises caution with
tablets.

- PATIENT AND CARER ADVICE

Driving and skilled tasks
Blurred vision may affect performance of skilled tasks (e.g.
driving) particularly at night or in reduced lighting.

- MEDICINAL FORMS
There can be variation in the licensing of different medicines
containing the same drug. Forms available from special-order
manufacturers include: oral solution
Tablet
CAUTIONARY AND ADVISORY LABELS 21, 27
▶ Salagen (Merus Labs Luxco S.a R.L.)
    Pilocarpine hydrochloride 5 mg Salagen 5mg tablets |
    84 tablet [PoM] £41.14 DT price = £41.14

LUBRICANTS

▌ Artificial saliva products

- ARTIFICIAL SALIVA PRODUCTS
AS SALIVA ORTHANA® LOZENGES
Mucin 65 mg, xylitol 59 mg, in a sorbitol basis, pH neutral

- INDICATIONS AND DOSE
**Dry mouth as a result of having (or having undergone)
radiotherapy | Sicca syndrome**
▶ BY MOUTH
▶ Adult: 1 lozenge as required, allow to dissolve slowly in
the mouth

- PRESCRIBING AND DISPENSING INFORMATION *AS Saliva
Orthana ®* lozenges do not contain fluoride.

    AS Saliva Orthana lozenges (A S Pharma Ltd)
    30 lozenge(ACBS) · NHS indicative price = £3.50

12

Ear, nose and oropharynx

12

Ear, nose and oropharynx

AS SALIVA ORTHANA® SPRAY

Gastric mucin (porcine) 3.5%, xylitol 2%, sodium fluoride 4.2 mg/litre, with preservatives and flavouring agents, pH neutral.

● INDICATIONS AND DOSE

Symptomatic treatment of dry mouth
▸ BY MOUTH
▸ Adult: Apply 2–3 sprays as required, spray onto oral and pharyngeal mucosa

● PROFESSION SPECIFIC INFORMATION

Dental practitioners' formulary
AS Saliva Orthana ® Oral Spray may be prescribed.

BIOXTRA® GEL

Lactoperoxidase, lactoferrin, lysozyme, whey colostrum, xylitol and other ingredients.

● INDICATIONS AND DOSE

Dry mouth as a result of having (or having undergone) radiotherapy (ACBS) | Dry mouth as a result of sicca syndrome (ACBS)
▸ BY MOUTH
▸ Adult: Apply as required, apply to oral mucosa

● PROFESSION SPECIFIC INFORMATION

Dental practitioners' formulary
BioXtra ® Gel may be prescribed.

BioXtra moisturising gel for dry mouths (R.I.S. Products Ltd)
40 ml · NHS indicative price = £3.94

BIOTENE ORALBALANCE®

Lactoperoxidase, lactoferrin, lysozyme, glucose oxidase, xylitol in a gel basis

● INDICATIONS AND DOSE

Symptomatic treatment of dry mouth
▸ BY MOUTH
▸ Adult: Apply as required, apply to gums and tongue

● PATIENT AND CARER ADVICE Avoid use with toothpastes containing detergents (including foaming agents).

● PROFESSION SPECIFIC INFORMATION

Dental practitioners' formulary
Biotene Oralbalance ® Saliva Replacement Gel may be prescribed as Artificial Saliva Gel.

Biotene Oralbalance dry mouth saliva replacement gel
(GlaxoSmithKline Consumer Healthcare)
  Glucose oxidase 12000 unit, Lactoferrin 12 mg, Lactoperoxidase 12000 unit, Muramidase 12 mg 50 gram · NHS indicative price = £4.46 · Drug Tariff (Part IXa)

GLANDOSANE®

Carmellose sodium 500 mg, sorbitol 1.5 g, potassium chloride 60 mg, sodium chloride 42.2 mg, magnesium chloride 2.6 mg, calcium chloride 7.3 mg, and dipotassium hydrogen phosphate 17.1 mg/50 g, pH 5.75.

● INDICATIONS AND DOSE

Dry mouth as a result of having (or having undergone) radiotherapy (ACBS) | Dry mouth as a result of sicca syndrome (ACBS)
▸ BY MOUTH
▸ Adult: Apply as required, spray onto oral and pharyngeal mucosa

● PROFESSION SPECIFIC INFORMATION

Dental practitioners' formulary
Glandosane ® Aerosol Spray may be prescribed.

Glandosane synthetic saliva spray lemon (Fresenius Kabi Ltd)
50 ml(ACBS) · NHS indicative price = £5.58

Glandosane synthetic saliva spray natural (Fresenius Kabi Ltd)
50 ml(ACBS) · NHS indicative price = £5.58

Glandosane synthetic saliva spray peppermint (Fresenius Kabi Ltd)
50 ml(ACBS) · NHS indicative price = £5.58

ORALIEVE GEL

● INDICATIONS AND DOSE

Symptomatic treatment of dry mouth
▸ BY MOUTH
▸ Adult: Apply as required, particularly at night, to oral mucosa

● PRESCRIBING AND DISPENSING INFORMATION Contains traces of milk protein and egg white protein.

SST®

Sugar-free, citric acid, malic acid and other ingredients in a sorbitol base.

● INDICATIONS AND DOSE

Symptomatic treatment of dry mouth in patients with impaired salivary gland function and patent salivary ducts
▸ BY MOUTH
▸ Adult: 1 tablet as required, allow tablet to dissolve slowly in the mouth

● PROFESSION SPECIFIC INFORMATION

Dental practitioners' formulary
May be prescribed as Saliva Stimulating Tablets.

SST saliva stimulating tablets (Sinclair IS Pharma Plc)
100 tablet · NHS indicative price = £4.86 · Drug Tariff (Part IXa)

SALIVEZE®

Carmellose sodium (sodium carboxymethylcellulose), calcium chloride, magnesium chloride, potassium chloride, sodium chloride, and dibasic sodium phosphate, pH neutral

● INDICATIONS AND DOSE

Dry mouth as a result of having (or having undergone) radiotherapy (ACBS) | Dry mouth as a result of sicca syndrome (ACBS)
▸ BY MOUTH
▸ Adult: Apply 1 spray as required, spray onto oral mucosa

● PROFESSION SPECIFIC INFORMATION

Dental practitioners' formulary
Saliveze ® Oral Spray may be prescribed.

Saliveze mouth spray (Wyvern Medical Ltd)
50 ml(ACBS) · NHS indicative price = £3.50

SALIVIX®

Sugar-free, reddish-amber, acacia, malic acid and other ingredients.

● INDICATIONS AND DOSE

Symptomatic treatment of dry mouth
▸ BY MOUTH USING PASTILLES
▸ Adult: 1 unit as required, suck pastille

● PROFESSION SPECIFIC INFORMATION

Dental practitioners' formulary
Salivix ® Pastilles may be prescribed as Artificial Saliva Pastilles.

Salivix pastilles (Galen Ltd)
50 pastille · NHS indicative price = £3.55 · Drug Tariff (Part IXa)

XEROTIN®
Sugar-free, water, sorbitol, carmellose
(carboxymethylcellulose), potassium chloride, sodium
chloride, potassium phosphate, magnesium chloride,
calcium chloride and other ingredients, pH neutral.

● **INDICATIONS AND DOSE**

Symptomatic treatment of dry mouth
▸ BY MOUTH
▸ Adult: 1 spray as required

● PROFESSION SPECIFIC INFORMATION

Dental practitioners' formulary
Xerotin® Oral Spray may be prescribed as Artificial Saliva
Oral Spray.

Xerotin spray (SpePharm UK Ltd)
100 ml · NHS indicative price = £6.86 · Drug Tariff (Part IXa)

2   Oral hygiene

Mouthwashes and other preparations for oropharyngeal use

Lozenges and sprays

There is no convincing evidence that antiseptic lozenges and
sprays have a beneficial action and they sometimes irritate
and cause sore tongue and sore lips. Some of these
preparations also contain local anaesthetics which relieve
pain but may cause sensitisation.

Mouthwashes, gargles, and dentifrices

Superficial infections of the mouth are often helped by warm
mouthwashes which have a mechanical cleansing effect and
cause some local hyperaemia. However, to be effective, they
must be used frequently and vigorously. A warm saline
mouthwash is ideal and can be prepared either by dissolving
half a teaspoonful of salt in a glassful of warm water or by
diluting compound sodium chloride mouthwash p. 1055 with
an equal volume of warm water.

Mouthwashes containing an oxidising agent, such as
hydrogen peroxide p. 1054, may be useful in the treatment of
acute ulcerative gingivitis (Vincent's infection) since the
organisms involved are anaerobes. It also has a mechanical
cleansing effect arising from frothing when in contact with
oral debris.

Chlorhexidine below is an effective antiseptic which has
the advantage of inhibiting plaque formation on the teeth. It
does not, however, completely control plaque deposition and
is not a substitute for effective toothbrushing. Moreover,
chlorhexidine preparations do not penetrate significantly
into stagnation areas and are therefore of little value in the
control of dental caries or of periodontal disease once
pocketing has developed.

Chlorhexidine mouthwash is used in the treatment of
denture stomatitis. It is also used in the prevention of oral
candidiasis in immunocompromised patients. Chlorhexidine
mouthwash reduces the incidence of alveolar osteitis
following tooth extraction. Chlorhexidine mouthwash
should not be used for the prevention of endocarditis in
patients undergoing dental procedures.

Chlorhexidine can be used as a mouthwash, spray or gel
for secondary infection in mucosal ulceration and for
controlling gingivitis, as an adjunct to other oral hygiene
measures. These preparations may also be used instead of
toothbrushing where there is a painful periodontal condition
(e.g. primary herpetic stomatitis) or if the patient has a
haemorrhagic disorder, or is disabled.

Chlorhexidine preparations are of little value in the control
of acute necrotising ulcerative gingivitis. With prolonged
use, chlorhexidine causes reversible brown staining of teeth
and tongue. Chlorhexidine may be incompatible with some
ingredients in toothpaste, causing an unpleasant taste in the
mouth; rinse the mouth thoroughly with water between
using toothpaste and chlorhexidine-containing products.

There is no convincing evidence that gargles are effective
in adults.

ANTISEPTICS AND DISINFECTANTS ⟩ OTHER

Chlorhexidine

● **INDICATIONS AND DOSE**

**Oral hygiene and plaque inhibition | Oral candidiasis |
Gingivitis | Management of aphthous ulcers**
▸ BY MOUTH USING MOUTHWASH
▸ Child: Rinse or gargle 10 mL twice daily (rinse or gargle
for about 1 minute)
▸ Adult: Rinse or gargle 10 mL twice daily (rinse or gargle
for about 1 minute)

Denture stomatitis
▸ MOUTHWASH
▸ Adult: Cleanse and soak dentures in mouthwash
solution for 15 minutes twice daily

Oral hygiene and plaque inhibition and gingivitis
▸ BY MOUTH USING DENTAL GEL
▸ Child: Apply 1–2 times a day, to be brushed on the
teeth
▸ Adult: Apply 1–2 times a day, to be brushed on the
teeth

Oral candidiasis | Management of aphthous ulcers
▸ BY MOUTH USING DENTAL GEL
▸ Child: Apply 1–2 times a day, to affected areas
▸ Adult: Apply 1–2 times a day, to affected areas

**Oral hygiene and plaque inhibition | Oral candidiasis |
Gingivitis | Management of aphthous ulcers**
▸ BY MOUTH USING OROMUCOSAL SPRAY
▸ Child: Apply up to 12 sprays twice daily as required, to
be applied tooth, gingival, or ulcer surfaces
▸ Adult: Apply up to 12 sprays twice daily as required, to
be applied tooth, gingival, or ulcer surfaces

Bladder irrigation and catheter patency solutions
▸ BY INTRAVESICAL INSTILLATION
▸ Adult: (consult product literature)

● UNLICENSED USE *Corsodyl*® not licensed for use in
children under 12 years (unless on the advice of a
healthcare professional).

● SIDE-EFFECTS Anaphylaxis · hypersensitivity · mucosal
irritation · parotid gland swelling · reversible brown
staining of composite restorations · reversible brown
staining of silicate compositions · reversible brown
staining of teeth · taste disturbance · tongue discolouration

SIDE-EFFECTS, FURTHER INFORMATION
If desquamation occurs with mucosal irritation,
discontinue treatment or dilute mouthwash with an equal
volume of water.

● PATIENT AND CARER ADVICE Chlorhexidine gluconate may
be incompatible with some ingredients in toothpaste;
rinse the mouth thoroughly with water between using
toothpaste and chlorhexidine-containing product.

● PROFESSION SPECIFIC INFORMATION

Dental practitioners' formulary
Corsodyl® dental gel may be prescribed as Chlorhexidine
Gluconate Gel; *Corsodyl*® mouthwash may be prescribed as
Chlorhexidine Mouthwash; *Corsodyl*® oral spray may be
prescribed as Chlorhexidine Oral Spray.

12

Ear, nose and oropharynx

● MEDICINAL FORMS
There can be variation in the licensing of different medicines containing the same drug.
Dental gel
▸ Corsodyl (GlaxoSmithKline Consumer Healthcare)
Chlorhexidine gluconate 10 mg per 1 gram Corsodyl 1% dental gel sugar-free | 50 gram P £1.26 DT price = £1.26
Mouthwash
▸ Chlorhexidine (Non-proprietary)
Chlorhexidine gluconate 2 mg per 1 ml Chlorhexidine gluconate 0.2% mouthwash natural | 300 ml GSL £3.65 DT price = £3.48
Chlorhexidine gluconate 0.2% mouthwash | 300 ml GSL £1.99–£2.09 DT price = £3.48
Chlorhexidine gluconate 0.2% mouthwash plain | 300 ml GSL £3.48 DT price = £3.48
Chlorhexidine gluconate 0.2% mouthwash peppermint | 300 ml GSL £3.65 DT price = £3.48
Chlorhexidine gluconate 0.2% mouthwash original | 300 ml GSL £3.65 DT price = £3.48
Chlorhexidine gluconate 0.2% mouthwash alcohol free | 300 ml GSL no price available DT price = £3.48 | 500 ml GSL no price available
▸ Corsodyl (GlaxoSmithKline Consumer Healthcare)
Chlorhexidine gluconate 2 mg per 1 ml Corsodyl 0.2% mouthwash aniseed | 300 ml GSL £2.44 DT price = £3.48
Corsodyl Mint 0.2% mouthwash | 300 ml GSL £2.44 DT price = £3.48 | 600 ml GSL £4.76
Corsodyl 0.2% mouthwash alcohol free | 300 ml GSL £3.06 DT price = £3.48
▸ Curasept (Curaprox (UK) Ltd)
Chlorhexidine gluconate 2 mg per 1 ml Curasept 0.2% oral rinse | 200 ml no price available
Irrigation
▸ Chlorhexidine (Non-proprietary)
Chlorhexidine acetate 200 microgram per 1 ml Chlorhexidine acetate 0.02% catheter maintenance solution | 100 ml P no price available
▸ Uro-Tainer (chlorhexidine) (B.Braun Medical Ltd)
Chlorhexidine acetate 200 microgram per 1 ml Uro-Tainer chlorhexidine 1:5000 catheter maintenance solution | 100 ml P £2.70

Chlorhexidine with chlorobutanol

The properties listed below are those particular to the combination only. For the properties of the components please consider, chlorhexidine p. 1053.

● INDICATIONS AND DOSE
Oral hygiene and plaque inhibition
▸ BY MOUTH USING MOUTHWASH
▸ **Child 6–17 years:** Rinse or gargle 10–15 mL 2–3 times a day, to be diluted with lukewarm water in measuring cup provided
▸ **Adult:** Rinse or gargle 10–15 mL 2–3 times a day, to be diluted with lukewarm water in measuring cup provided

Denture disinfection
▸ **Adult:** Soak previously cleansed dentures in mouthwash (diluted with 2 volumes of water) for 60 minutes

● PRESCRIBING AND DISPENSING INFORMATION Flavours of mouthwash may include mint.

● MEDICINAL FORMS
There can be variation in the licensing of different medicines containing the same drug.
No licensed medicines listed.

Hexetidine

● INDICATIONS AND DOSE
Oral hygiene
▸ BY MOUTH USING MOUTHWASH
▸ **Child 6–17 years:** Rinse or gargle 15 mL 2–3 times a day, to be used undiluted
▸ **Adult:** Rinse or gargle 15 mL 2–3 times a day, to be used undiluted

● SIDE-EFFECTS
▸ **Very rare** Taste disturbance · transient anaesthesia
▸ **Frequency not known** Local irritation

● MEDICINAL FORMS
There can be variation in the licensing of different medicines containing the same drug.
Mouthwash
▸ Oraldene (McNeil Products Ltd)
Hexetidine 1 mg per 1 ml Oraldene Icemint 0.1% mouthwash sugar-free | 200 ml GSL £2.21 DT price = £2.21
Oraldene 0.1% mouthwash peppermint sugar-free | 100 ml GSL £1.43 sugar-free | 200 ml GSL £2.21 DT price = £2.21

Hydrogen peroxide

● DRUG ACTION Hydrogen peroxide is an oxidising agent.

● INDICATIONS AND DOSE
Oral hygiene (with hydrogen peroxide 6%)
▸ BY MOUTH USING MOUTHWASH
▸ **Child:** Rinse or gargle 15 mL 2–3 times a day for 2–3 minutes, to be diluted in half a tumblerful of warm water
▸ **Adult:** Rinse or gargle 15 mL 2–3 times a day for 2–3 minutes, to be diluted in half a tumblerful of warm water

PEROXYL®
Oral hygiene
▸ BY MOUTH USING MOUTHWASH
▸ **Child 6–17 years:** Rinse or gargle 10 mL 3 times a day for about 1 minute, for maximum 7 days, to be used after meals and at bedtime
▸ **Adult:** Rinse or gargle 10 mL up to 4 times a day for about 1 minute, to be used after meals and at bedtime

● SIDE-EFFECTS Hypertrophy of papillae of tongue with prolonged use

● PRESCRIBING AND DISPENSING INFORMATION When prepared extemporaneously, the BP states Hydrogen Peroxide Mouthwash, BP consists of hydrogen peroxide 6% solution (= approx. 20 volume) BP.

● HANDLING AND STORAGE Hydrogen peroxide bleaches fabric.

● PROFESSION SPECIFIC INFORMATION
Dental practitioners' formulary
Hydrogen Peroxide Mouthwash may be prescribed.

● MEDICINAL FORMS
There can be variation in the licensing of different medicines containing the same drug.
Mouthwash
▸ Peroxyl (Colgate-Palmolive (UK) Ltd)
Hydrogen peroxide 15 mg per 1 ml Peroxyl 1.5% mouthwash sugar-free | 300 ml GSL £2.94

Sodium bicarbonate with sodium chloride

● **INDICATIONS AND DOSE**

Oral hygiene

▸ BY MOUTH USING MOUTHWASH
▸ Adult: (consult product literature)

● DIRECTIONS FOR ADMINISTRATION For mouthwash, extemporaneous preparations should be prepared according to the following formula: sodium chloride 1.5 g, sodium bicarbonate 1 g, concentrated peppermint emulsion 2.5 mL, double-strength chloroform water 50 mL, water to 100 mL. To be diluted with an equal volume of warm water prior to administration.

● PRESCRIBING AND DISPENSING INFORMATION Flavours of mouthwash may include peppermint.

● PROFESSION SPECIFIC INFORMATION

Dental practitioners' formulary
Compound sodium chloride mouthwash may be prescribed.

● MEDICINAL FORMS
There can be variation in the licensing of different medicines containing the same drug. Forms available from special-order manufacturers include: mouthwash

Sodium chloride

● **INDICATIONS AND DOSE**

Oral hygiene

▸ BY MOUTH USING MOUTHWASH
▸ Child: Rinse or gargle as required
▸ Adult: Rinse or gargle as required

● DIRECTIONS FOR ADMINISTRATION Extemporaneous mouthwash preparations should be prepared according to the following formula: sodium chloride 1.5 g, sodium bicarbonate 1 g, concentrated peppermint emulsion 2.5 mL, double-strength chloroform water 50 mL, water to 100 mL. To be diluted with an equal volume of warm water.

● PRESCRIBING AND DISPENSING INFORMATION No mouthwash preparations available—when prepared extemporaneously, the BP states Sodium Chloride Mouthwash, Compound, BP consists of sodium bicarbonate 1%, sodium chloride 1.5% in a suitable vehicle with peppermint flavour.

● PROFESSION SPECIFIC INFORMATION

Dental practitioners' formulary
Compound Sodium Chloride Mouthwash may be prescribed.

● MEDICINAL FORMS
There can be variation in the licensing of different medicines containing the same drug.
No licensed medicines listed.

2.1 Dental caries

Fluoride

Availability of adequate fluoride confers significant resistance to dental caries. It is now considered that the topical action of fluoride on enamel and plaque is more important than the systemic effect.

When the fluoride content of drinking water is less than 700 micrograms per litre (0.7 parts per million), daily administration of fluoride tablets or drops provides suitable supplementation. Systemic fluoride supplements should not

be prescribed without reference to the fluoride content of the local water supply. Infants need not receive fluoride supplements until the age of 6 months.

Dentifrices which incorporate sodium fluoride or monofluorophosphate are also a convenient source of fluoride.

Individuals who are either particularly caries prone or medically compromised may be given additional protection by use of fluoride rinses or by application of fluoride gels. Rinses may be used daily or weekly; daily use of a less concentrated rinse is more effective than weekly use of a more concentrated one. High-strength gels must be applied regularly under professional supervision; extreme caution is necessary to prevent children from swallowing any excess. Less concentrated gels are available for home use. Varnishes are also available and are particularly valuable for young or disabled children since they adhere to the teeth and set in the presence of moisture.

VITAMINS AND TRACE ELEMENTS

Sodium fluoride

● **INDICATIONS AND DOSE**

Prophylaxis of dental caries for water content less than 300micrograms/litre (0.3 parts per million) of fluoride ion

▸ BY MOUTH USING TABLETS
▸ Child 6 months-2 years: 250 micrograms daily, doses expressed as fluoride ion (F^-)
▸ Child 3-5 years: 500 micrograms daily, doses expressed as fluoride ion (F^-)
▸ Child 6-17 years: 1 mg daily, doses expressed as fluoride ion (F^-)
▸ Adult: 1 mg daily, doses expressed as fluoride ion (F^-)

Prophylaxis of dental caries for water content between 300 and 700micrograms/litre (0.3-0.7 parts per million) of fluoride ion

▸ BY MOUTH USING TABLETS
▸ Child 3-5 years: 250 micrograms daily, doses expressed as fluoride ion (F^-)
▸ Child 6-17 years: 500 micrograms daily, doses expressed as fluoride ion (F^-)
▸ Adult: 500 micrograms daily, doses expressed as fluoride ion (F^-)

Prophylaxis of dental caries for water content above 700micrograms/litre (0.7 parts per million) of fluoride ion

▸ Child 6 months-17 years: Supplements not advised
▸ Adult: Supplements not advised

Prophylaxis of dental caries for individuals who are caries prone or medically compromised

▸ BY MOUTH USING MOUTHWASH
▸ Adult: Rinse or gargle 10 mL daily

COLGATE DURAPHAT® 2800PPM FLUORIDE TOOTHPASTE

Prophylaxis of dental caries

▸ BY MOUTH USING PASTE
▸ Child 10-17 years: Apply 1 centimetre twice daily, to be applied using a toothbrush
▸ Adult: Apply 1 centimetre twice daily, to be applied using a toothbrush

COLGATE DURAPHAT® 5000PPM FLUORIDE TOOTHPASTE

Prophylaxis of dental caries

▸ BY MOUTH USING PASTE
▸ Child 16-17 years: Apply 2 centimetres 3 times a day, to be applied after meals using a toothbrush
▸ Adult: Apply 2 centimetres 3 times a day, to be applied after meals using a toothbrush   continued →

EN-DE-KAY® FLUORINSE

Prophylaxis of dental carries for individuals who are caries prone or medically compromised
▸ BY MOUTH USING MOUTHWASH
▸ Adult: 5 drops daily, dilute 5 drops to 10 mL of water, alternatively 20 drops once weekly, dilute 20 drops to 10 mL

DOSE EQUIVALENCE AND CONVERSION
Sodium fluoride 2.2 mg provides approx. 1 mg fluoride ion.
These doses reflect the recommendations of the British Dental Association, the British Society of Paediatric Dentistry and the British Association for the Study of Community Dentistry (*Br Dent J* 1997; **182**: 6–7).

● CONTRA-INDICATIONS Not for areas where drinking water is fluoridated
● SIDE-EFFECTS
▸ **Uncommon** Occasional white flecks on teeth with recommended doses
▸ **Rare** Yellowish-brown discoloration if recommended doses are exceeded
● DIRECTIONS FOR ADMINISTRATION
▸ With oral use Tablets should be sucked or dissolved in the mouth and taken preferably in the evening.
▸ With oral (topical) use For mouthwash, rinse mouth for 1 minute and then spit out.
COLGATE DURAPHAT® 2800PPM FLUORIDE TOOTHPASTE Brush teeth for 1 minute before spitting out.
COLGATE DURAPHAT® 5000PPM FLUORIDE TOOTHPASTE Brush teeth for 3 minutes before spitting out.
● PRESCRIBING AND DISPENSING INFORMATION Flavours of oral tablet formulations may include orange.
● PATIENT AND CARER ADVICE
Mouthwash
▸ With oral (topical) use Avoid eating, drinking, or rinsing mouth for 15 minutes after use.
COLGATE DURAPHAT® 2800PPM FLUORIDE TOOTHPASTE Patients or carers should be given advice on how to administer sodium fluoride toothpaste. Avoid drinking or rinsing mouth for 30 minutes after use.
COLGATE DURAPHAT® 5000PPM FLUORIDE TOOTHPASTE Patients or carers should be given advice on how to administer Sodium fluoride toothpaste.
● PROFESSION SPECIFIC INFORMATION

Dental practitioners' formulary
Tablets may be prescribed as Sodium Fluoride Tablets. Oral drops may be prescribed as Sodium Fluoride Oral Drops. Mouthwashes may be prescribed as Sodium Fluoride Mouthwash 0.05% or Sodium Fluoride Mouthwash 2%.
COLGATE DURAPHAT® 2800PPM FLUORIDE TOOTHPASTE May be prescribed as Sodium Fluoride Toothpaste 0.619%.
COLGATE DURAPHAT® 5000PPM FLUORIDE TOOTHPASTE May be prescribed as Sodium Fluoride Toothpaste 1.1%.

Dental information
Fluoride mouthwash, oral drops, tablets and toothpaste are prescribable on form FP10D (GP14 in Scotland, WP10D in Wales).
There are also arrangements for health authorities to supply fluoride tablets in the course of pre-school dental schemes, and they may also be supplied in school dental schemes.
Fluoride gels are not prescribable on form FP10D (GP14 in Scotland, WP10D in Wales).

● MEDICINAL FORMS
There can be variation in the licensing of different medicines containing the same drug.
Tablet
▸ Endekay (Manx Healthcare Ltd)
Sodium fluoride 1.1 mg Endekay Fluotabs 3-6 Years 1.1mg tablets | 200 tablet Ⓟ £2.38 DT price = £2.38
Sodium fluoride 2.2 mg Endekay Fluotabs 6+ Years 2.2mg tablets | 200 tablet Ⓟ £2.38 DT price = £2.38
Chewable tablet
▸ Fluor-a-day (Dental Health Products Ltd)
Sodium fluoride 1.1 mg Fluor-a-day 1.1mg chewable tablets sugar-free | 200 tablet Ⓟ £2.79 DT price = £2.79
Sodium fluoride 2.2 mg Fluor-a-day 2.2mg chewable tablets sugar-free | 200 tablet Ⓟ £2.79 DT price = £2.79
Oral drops
▸ Endekay (Manx Healthcare Ltd)
Sodium fluoride 3.7 mg per 1 ml Endekay Fluodrops 0.37% drops paediatric sugar-free | 60 ml Ⓟ £2.38 DT price = £2.38
Paste
▸ Colgate Duraphat (Colgate-Palmolive (UK) Ltd)
Fluoride (as Sodium fluoride) 2.8 mg per 1 gram Colgate Duraphat 2800ppm fluoride toothpaste sugar-free | 75 ml ⒫oM £3.26 DT price = £3.26
Fluoride (as Sodium fluoride) 5 mg per 1 gram Colgate Duraphat 5000ppm fluoride toothpaste sugar-free | 51 gram ⒫oM £6.50 DT price = £6.50
Mouthwash
▸ Sodium fluoride (Non-proprietary)
Sodium fluoride 500 microgram per 1 ml Sodium fluoride 0.05% mouthwash sugar free sugar-free | 250 ml Ⓖsl no price available sugar-free | 400 ml Ⓖsl no price available sugar-free | 500 ml Ⓖsl no price available
▸ Colgate FluoriGard (Colgate-Palmolive (UK) Ltd)
Sodium fluoride 500 microgram per 1 ml Colgate FluoriGard 0.05% daily dental rinse alcohol free sugar-free | 400 ml £2.99 Colgate FluoriGard 0.05% daily dental rinse sugar-free | 400 ml Ⓖsl £2.99
▸ Endekay (Manx Healthcare Ltd)
Sodium fluoride 500 microgram per 1 ml Endekay 0.05% daily fluoride mouthrinse sugar-free | 250 ml Ⓖsl £1.50 sugar-free | 500 ml Ⓖsl £2.43
Sodium fluoride 20 mg per 1 ml Endekay Fluorinse 2% mouthwash sugar-free | 100 ml ⒫oM £4.97

3 Oral ulceration and inflammation

Oral ulceration and inflammation

Ulceration and inflammation

Ulceration of the oral mucosa may be caused by trauma (physical or chemical), recurrent aphthae, infections, carcinoma, dermatological disorders, nutritional deficiencies, gastro-intestinal disease, haematopoietic disorders, and drug therapy (see also *Chemotherapy induced mucositis and myelosuppression* under Cytotoxic drugs p. 787). It is important to establish the diagnosis in each case as the majority of these lesions require specific management in addition to local treatment. Local treatment aims to protect the ulcerated area, to relieve pain, to reduce inflammation, or to control secondary infection. Patients with an unexplained mouth ulcer of more than 3 weeks' duration require urgent referral to hospital to exclude oral cancer.

Simple mouthwashes

A **saline** mouthwash may relieve the pain of traumatic ulceration. The mouthwash is made up with warm water and used at frequent intervals until the discomfort and swelling subsides.

Antiseptic mouthwashes

Secondary bacterial infection may be a feature of any mucosal ulceration; it can increase discomfort and delay healing. Use of a chlorhexidine mouthwash p. 1053 is often beneficial and may accelerate healing of recurrent aphthae.

Corticosteroids

Topical corticosteroid therapy may be used for some forms of oral ulceration. In the case of aphthous ulcers it is most effective if applied in the 'prodromal' phase.

Thrush or other types of candidiasis are recognised complications of corticosteroid treatment.

Hydrocortisone **oromucosal tablets** p. 1059 are allowed to dissolve next to an ulcer and are useful in recurrent aphthae and erosive lichenoid lesions.

Beclometasone dipropionate inhaler p. 1048 sprayed on the oral mucosa is used to manage oral ulceration [unlicensed indication]. Alternatively, betamethasone soluble tablets p. 1059 dissolved in water can be used as a mouthwash to treat oral ulceration [unlicensed indication].

Systemic corticosteroid therapy (see under Corticosteroids, inflammatory disorders p. 999), is reserved for severe conditions such as pemphigus vulgaris.

Local analgesics

Local analgesics have a limited role in the management of oral ulceration. When applied topically their action is of a relatively short duration so that analgesia cannot be maintained continuously throughout the day. The main indication for a topical local analgesic is to relieve the pain of otherwise intractable oral ulceration particularly when it is due to major aphthae. For this purpose lidocaine hydrochloride 5% ointment or lozenges below containing a local anaesthetic are applied to the ulcer. Lidocaine hydrochloride 10% solution as spray can be applied thinly to the ulcer [unlicensed indication] using a cotton bud. When local anaesthetics are used in the mouth care must be taken not to produce anaesthesia of the pharynx before meals as this might lead to choking.

Preparations on sale to the public: many mouth ulcer preparations, throat lozenges, and throat sprays on sale to the public contain a local anaesthetic. To identify the active ingredients in such preparations, consult the product literature of the manufacturer— the correct proprietary name should be ascertained as many products have very similar names but different active ingredients.

Benzydamine hydrochloride p. 1058 and flurbiprofen p. 1058 are non-steroidal anti-inflammatory drugs (NSAIDs). Benzydamine hydrochloride mouthwash or spray may be useful in reducing the discomfort associated with a variety of ulcerative conditions. It has also been found to be effective in reducing the discomfort of tonsillectomy and post-irradiation mucositis. Some patients find the full-strength mouthwash causes some stinging and, for them, it should be diluted with an equal volume of water. Flurbiprofen lozenges are licensed for the relief of sore throat.

Choline salicylate p. 1059 is a derivative of salicylic acid and has some analgesic action. The dental gel may provide relief for recurrent aphthae, but excessive application or confinement under a denture irritates the mucosa and can itself cause ulceration.

Other preparations

Doxycycline p. 1060 rinsed in the mouth may be of value for recurrent aphthous ulceration.

Periodontitis

Low-dose doxycycline (*Periostat®*) is licensed as an adjunct to scaling and root planing for the treatment of periodontitis; a low dose of doxycycline reduces collagenase activity without inhibiting bacteria associated with periodontitis.

For anti-infectives used in the treatment of destructive (refractory) forms of periodontal disease, see under Oropharyngeal bacterial infections p. 1060. See also

Mouthwashes and other preparations for oropharyngeal use p. 1053 for mouthwashes used for oral hygiene and plaque inhibition.

ANAESTHETICS, LOCAL

Lidocaine hydrochloride

(Lignocaine hydrochloride)

● **INDICATIONS AND DOSE**

Dental practice
▸ BY BUCCAL ADMINISTRATION USING OINTMENT
▸ Adult: Rub gently into dry gum

Relief of pain in oral lesions
▸ TO THE LESION USING OINTMENT
▸ Adult: Apply as required, rub sparingly and gently on affected areas

LARYNGOJET®

Anaesthesia of mucous membranes of oropharynx, trachea, or respiratory tract
▸ TO MUCOUS MEMBRANES
▸ Adult: 40–200 mg, to be given as a single dose sprayed, instilled (if a cavity), or applied with a swab (reduce dose according to size, age and condition of patient); usual dose 160 mg

XYLOCAINE®

Bronchoscopy | Laryngoscopy | Oesophagoscopy | Endotracheal intubation
▸ TO MUCOUS MEMBRANES
▸ Adult: Up to 20 doses

Dental practice
▸ TO MUCOUS MEMBRANES
▸ Adult: 1–5 doses

Maxillary sinus puncture
▸ TO MUCOUS MEMBRANES
▸ Adult: 3 doses

Relief of pain in oral lesions
▸ TO THE LESION
▸ Adult: Apply thinly to the ulcer using a cotton bud

● UNLICENSED USE Spray not licensed for the relief of pain in oral lesions.

● CAUTIONS Avoid anaesthesia of the pharynx before meals—risk of choking (in adults) · can damage plastic cuffs of endotracheal tubes

● INTERACTIONS → Appendix 1 (lidocaine). Interactions less likely when lidocaine used topically.

● SIDE-EFFECTS

SIDE-EFFECTS, FURTHER INFORMATION
▸ Topical application A single application of a topical lidocaine preparation does not generally cause systemic side-effects.

● ALLERGY AND CROSS-SENSITIVITY
▸ Hypersensitivity and cross-sensitivity Hypersensitivity reactions occur mainly with the ester-type local anaesthetics, such as tetracaine and chloroprocaine; reactions are less frequent with the amide types, such as articaine, bupivacaine, levobupivacaine, lidocaine, mepivacaine, prilocaine, and ropivacaine. Cross-sensitivity reactions may be avoided by using the alternative chemical type.

● PREGNANCY Crosses the placenta but not known to be harmful in *animal* studies—use if benefit outweighs risk. When used as a local anaesthetic, large doses can cause fetal bradycardia; if given during delivery can also cause neonatal respiratory depression, hypotonia, or bradycardia after paracervical or epidural block.

● BREAST FEEDING Present in milk but amount too small to be harmful.

12

Ear, nose and oropharynx

- HEPATIC IMPAIRMENT Caution—increased risk of side-effects.
- RENAL IMPAIRMENT Possible accumulation of lidocaine and active metabolite; caution in severe impairment.
- PROFESSION SPECIFIC INFORMATION

Dental practitioners' formulary
Lidocaine ointment 5% may be prescribed. Spray may be prescribed as Lidocaine Spray 10%.
XYLOCAINE® May be prescribed as lidocaine spray 10%.

- MEDICINAL FORMS
There can be variation in the licensing of different medicines containing the same drug.
Ointment
▸ Lidocaine hydrochloride (Non-proprietary)
Lidocaine hydrochloride 50 mg per 1 gram Lidocaine 5% ointment | 15 gram P £6.50 DT price = £6.18
Spray
▸ Xylocaine (AstraZeneca UK Ltd)
Lidocaine 10 mg per 1 actuation Xylocaine 10mg/dose spray sugar-free | 50 ml P £6.29
Liquid
▸ Laryngojet (UCB Pharma Ltd)
Lidocaine hydrochloride 40 mg per 1 mL Lidocaine 4% oromucosal solution | 1 pre-filled disposable injection PoM £5.10

ANALGESICS > NON-STEROIDAL ANTI-INFLAMMATORY DRUGS

Benzydamine hydrochloride

- INDICATIONS AND DOSE

Painful inflammatory conditions of oropharynx
▸ TO THE LESION USING MOUTHWASH
▸ Child 13-17 years: Rinse or gargle 15 mL every 1.5–3 hours as required usually for not more than 7 days, dilute with an equal volume of water if stinging occurs
▸ Adult: Rinse or gargle 15 mL every 1.5–3 hours as required usually for not more than 7 days, dilute with an equal volume of water if stinging occurs
▸ TO THE LESION USING OROMUCOSAL SPRAY
▸ Child 1 month–5 years (body-weight 4-7 kg): 1 spray every 1.5–3 hours, to be administered onto the affected area
▸ Child 1 month–5 years (body-weight 8-11 kg): 2 sprays every 1.5–3 hours, to be administered onto the affected area
▸ Child 1 month–5 years (body-weight 12-15 kg): 3 sprays every 1.5–3 hours, to be administered onto the affected area
▸ Child 1 month–5 years (body-weight 16 kg and above): 4 sprays every 1.5–3 hours, to be administered onto the affected area
▸ Child 6-11 years: 4 sprays every 1.5–3 hours, to be administered onto affected area
▸ Child 12-17 years: 4–8 sprays every 1.5–3 hours, to be administered onto affected area
▸ Adult: 4–8 sprays every 1.5–3 hours, to be administered onto affected area

- SIDE-EFFECTS
▸ Rare Hypersensitivity reactions
▸ **Frequency not known** Occasional numbness or stinging
- PROFESSION SPECIFIC INFORMATION

Dental practitioners' formulary
Benzydamine Oromucosal Spray 0.15% may be prescribed.
Benzydamine mouthwash may be prescribed as Benzydamine Mouthwash 0.15%.

- MEDICINAL FORMS
There can be variation in the licensing of different medicines containing the same drug.
Spray
▸ Benzydamine hydrochloride (Non-proprietary)
Benzydamine hydrochloride 1.5 mg per 1 ml Benzydamine 0.15% oromucosal spray sugar free sugar-free | 30 ml P £4.64 DT price = £4.49
▸ Difflam (Meda Pharmaceuticals Ltd)
Benzydamine hydrochloride 1.5 mg per 1 ml Difflam 0.15% spray sugar-free | 30 ml P £4.24 DT price = £4.49
Mouthwash
▸ Benzydamine hydrochloride (Non-proprietary)
Benzydamine hydrochloride 1.5 mg per 1 ml Benzydamine 0.15% mouthwash sugar free sugar-free | 300 ml P £7.14 DT price = £6.01
▸ Difflam (Meda Pharmaceuticals Ltd)
Benzydamine hydrochloride 1.5 mg per 1 ml Difflam Oral Rinse 0.15% solution sugar-free | 300 ml P £6.50 DT price = £6.01
Difflam 0.15% Sore Throat Rinse sugar-free | 200 ml P £4.64

Flurbiprofen

- INDICATIONS AND DOSE

Relief of sore throat
▸ BY MOUTH USING LOZENGES
▸ Child 12-17 years: 1 lozenge every 3–6 hours for maximum 3 days, allow lozenge to dissolve slowly in the mouth; maximum 5 lozenges per day
▸ Adult: 1 lozenge every 3–6 hours for maximum 3 days, allow lozenge to dissolve slowly in the mouth; maximum 5 lozenges per day

- INTERACTIONS → Appendix 1 (NSAIDs).
- SIDE-EFFECTS Mouth ulcers (move lozenge around mouth) · taste disturbance
- ALLERGY AND CROSS-SENSITIVITY Contra-indicated in patients with a history of hypersensitivity to aspirin or any other NSAID—which includes those in whom attacks of asthma, angioedema, urticaria or rhinitis have been precipitated by aspirin or any other NSAID.

- MEDICINAL FORMS
There can be variation in the licensing of different medicines containing the same drug.
Lozenge
▸ Strefen (Reckitt Benckiser Healthcare (UK) Ltd)
Flurbiprofen 8.75 mg Strefen 8.75mg lozenges | 16 lozenge P £2.58 DT price = £2.58

CORTICOSTEROIDS

Beclometasone dipropionate

(Beclomethasone dipropionate)

- INDICATIONS AND DOSE

Management of oral ulceration
▸ BY BUCCAL ADMINISTRATION
▸ Adult: 50–100 micrograms twice daily, use inhaler device to spray dose on to the oral mucosa

- UNLICENSED USE Use of inhaler unlicensed in oral ulceration.
- MEDICINAL FORMS
For preparations see inhaled beclometasone p. 238

Betamethasone

- **INDICATIONS AND DOSE**

Oral ulceration

▸ BY MOUTH USING SOLUBLE TABLETS

- ▸ Child 12-17 years: 500 micrograms 4 times a day, to be dissolved in 20 mL water and rinsed around the mouth; not to be swallowed
- ▸ Adult: 500 micrograms 4 times a day, to be dissolved in 20 mL water and rinsed around the mouth; not to be swallowed

- **UNLICENSED USE**
▸ In children Betamethasone soluble tablets not licensed for use as mouthwash or in oral ulceration.
- **CONTRA-INDICATIONS** Untreated local infection
- **SIDE-EFFECTS** Candidal infection · exacerbation of local infection
- **PATIENT AND CARER ADVICE** Patient counselling is advised for betamethasone soluble tablets (administration).
- **PROFESSION SPECIFIC INFORMATION**

Dental practitioners' formulary
Betamethasone Soluble Tablets 500 micrograms may be prescribed for oral ulceration.

- **MEDICINAL FORMS**
There can be variation in the licensing of different medicines containing the same drug.
Soluble tablet
CAUTIONARY AND ADVISORY LABELS 10, 13, 21 (not for use as mouthwash for oral ulceration)
▸ Betamethasone (Non-proprietary)
Betamethasone (as Betamethasone sodium phosphate)
500 microgram Betamethasone 500microgram soluble tablets sugar free sugar-free | 100 tablet PoM £42.60 DT price = £42.04

Hydrocortisone

- **INDICATIONS AND DOSE**

Oral and perioral lesions

▸ TO THE LESION USING BUCCAL TABLET

- ▸ Child 1 month–11 years: Only on medical advice
- ▸ Child 12-17 years: 1 lozenge 4 times a day, allowed to dissolve slowly in the mouth in contact with the ulcer
- ▸ Adult: 1 lozenge 4 times a day, allowed to dissolve slowly in the mouth in contact with the ulcer

- **UNLICENSED USE** *Hydrocortisone mucoadhesive buccal tablets* licensed for use in children (under 12 years—on medical advice only).
- **CONTRA-INDICATIONS** Untreated local infection
- **SIDE-EFFECTS** Candidal infection · exacerbation of local infection
- **PROFESSION SPECIFIC INFORMATION**

Dental practitioners' formulary
Mucoadhesive buccal tablets may be prescribed as Hydrocortisone Oromucosal Tablets.

- **MEDICINAL FORMS**
There can be variation in the licensing of different medicines containing the same drug.
Muco-adhesive buccal tablet
▸ Hydrocortisone (Non-proprietary)
Hydrocortisone (as Hydrocortisone sodium succinate)
2.5 mg Hydrocortisone 2.5mg muco-adhesive buccal tablets sugar free sugar-free | 20 tablet P £5.81 DT price = £5.05

SALICYLIC ACID AND DERIVATIVES

Choline salicylate

- **INDICATIONS AND DOSE**

Mild oral and perioral lesions

▸ TO THE LESION

- ▸ Child 16-17 years: Apply 0.5 inch, apply with gentle massage, not more often than every 3 hours
- ▸ Adult: Apply 0.5 inch, apply with gentle massage, not more often than every 3 hours

- **CONTRA-INDICATIONS** Children under 16 years
CONTRA-INDICATIONS, FURTHER INFORMATION
▸ Reye's syndrome The CHM has advised that topical oral pain relief products containing salicylate salts should not be used in children under 16 years, as a cautionary measure due to the theoretical risk of Reye's syndrome.
- **CAUTIONS**
Frequent application, especially in children, may give rise to salicylate poisoning · Not to be applied to dentures—leave at least 30 minutes before re-insertion of dentures (in adults)
- **SIDE-EFFECTS** Transient local burning sensation
- **PRESCRIBING AND DISPENSING INFORMATION** When prepared extemporaneously, the BP states Choline Salicylate Dental Gel, BP consists of choline salicylate 8.7% in a flavoured gel basis.
- **PROFESSION SPECIFIC INFORMATION**

Dental practitioners' formulary
Choline Salicylate Dental Gel may be prescribed.

- **MEDICINAL FORMS**
There can be variation in the licensing of different medicines containing the same drug.
Oromucosal gel
▸ Bonjela (Reckitt Benckiser Healthcare (UK) Ltd)
Choline salicylate 87 mg per 1 gram Bonjela Cool Mint gel sugar-free | 15 gram GSL £3.07 DT price = £2.58
Bonjela Original gel sugar-free | 15 gram GSL £2.58 DT price = £2.58

Salicylic acid with rhubarb extract

- **INDICATIONS AND DOSE**

Mild oral and perioral lesions

▸ TO THE LESION

- ▸ Child 16-17 years: Apply 3–4 times a day maximum duration 7 days
- ▸ Adult: Apply 3–4 times a day maximum duration 7 days

- **CONTRA-INDICATIONS** Children under 16 years
CONTRA-INDICATIONS, FURTHER INFORMATION
▸ Reye's syndrome The CHM has advised that topical oral pain relief products containing salicylate salts should not be used in children under 16 years, as a cautionary measure due to the theoretical risk of Reye's syndrome.
- **CAUTIONS**
Frequent application, especially in children, may give rise to salicylate poisoning · Not to be applied to dentures—leave at least 30 minutes before re-insertion of dentures (in adults)
- **SIDE-EFFECTS** Temporary discolouration of oral mucosa · temporary discolouration of teeth · transient local burning sensation
- **PATIENT AND CARER ADVICE** May cause temporary discolouration of teeth and oral mucosa

12

Ear, nose and oropharynx

- MEDICINAL FORMS
There can be variation in the licensing of different medicines containing the same drug.
Paint
EXCIPIENTS: May contain Ethanol
▸ Pyralvex (Meda Pharmaceuticals Ltd)
Salicylic acid 10 mg per 1 ml, Rhubarb extract 50 mg per 1 ml Pyralvex solution | 10 ml P £3.25

4 Oropharyngeal bacterial infections

Oropharyngeal bacterial infections

Antibacterial therapy for pericoronitis

Antibacterial required only in presence of systemic features of infection, or of trismus, or persistent swelling despite local treatment.

- Metronidazole p. 492, or *alternatively*, amoxicillin p. 498
▸ *Suggested duration of treatment* 3 days or until symptoms resolve.

Antibacterial therapy for gingivitis: acute necrotising ulcerative

Antibacterial required only if systemic features of infection.

- Metronidazole, or *alternatively*, amoxicillin
▸ *Suggested duration of treatment* 3 days or until symptoms resolve.

Antibacterial therapy for periapical or periodontal abscess

Antibacterial required only in severe disease with cellulitis or if systemic features of infection.

- Amoxicillin, or *alternatively*, metronidazole
▸ *Suggested duration of treatment* 5 days.

Antibacterial therapy for periodontitis

Antibacterial used as an adjunct to debridement in severe disease or disease unresponsive to local treatment alone.

- Metronidazole, or *alternatively in adults and children over 12 years*, doxycycline below

Antibacterial therapy for throat infections

Most throat infections are caused by viruses and many do not require antibacterial therapy. Consider antibacterial, if history of valvular heart disease, if marked systemic upset, if peritonsillar cellulitis or abscess, or if at increased risk from acute infection (e.g. in immunosuppression, cystic fibrosis); prescribe antibacterial for beta-haemolytic streptococcal pharyngitis.

- Phenoxymethylpenicillin p. 497
▸ In severe infection, initial parenteral therapy with benzylpenicillin sodium p. 496, then oral therapy with phenoxymethylpenicillin *or* amoxicillin (*or* ampicillin p. 499). **Avoid** amoxicillin if possibility of glandular fever.
▸ *Suggested duration of treatment* 10 days.
▸ *If penicillin-allergic*, clarithromycin p. 487 (*or* azithromycin p. 486 *or* erythromycin p. 488)
▸ *Suggested duration of treatment* 10 days

⫶ 513

Doxycycline

- INDICATIONS AND DOSE

Treatment of recurrent aphthous ulceration
▸ BY MOUTH USING SOLUBLE TABLETS
▸ Child 12-17 years: 100 mg 4 times a day usually for 3 days, dispersible tablet can be stirred into a small amount of water then rinsed around the mouth for 2–3 minutes, it should preferably not be swallowed
▸ Adult: 100 mg 4 times a day usually for 3 days, dispersible tablet can be stirred into a small amount of water then rinsed around the mouth for 2–3 minutes, it should preferably not be swallowed

- UNLICENSED USE Not licensed for use in children under 12 years.
Not licensed for severe recurrent aphthous ulceration.
- CAUTIONS Alcohol dependence
- INTERACTIONS The metabolism of doxycycline may be influenced by antiepileptics.
- SIDE-EFFECTS Anorexia · anxiety · dry mouth · flushing · tinnitus
- RENAL IMPAIRMENT Use with caution (avoid excessive doses).
- PATIENT AND CARER ADVICE Counselling on administration advised.
Photosensitivity Patients should be advised to avoid exposure to sunlight or sun lamps.
- PROFESSION SPECIFIC INFORMATION

Dental practitioners' formulary
Dispersible tablets may be prescribed as Dispersible Doxycycline Tablets.

- MEDICINAL FORMS
There can be variation in the licensing of different medicines containing the same drug.
Dispersible tablet
CAUTIONARY AND ADVISORY LABELS 6, 9, 11, 13
▸ Vibramycin-D (Pfizer Ltd)
Doxycycline (as Doxycycline monohydrate) 100 mg Vibramycin-D 100mg dispersible tablets sugar-free | 8 tablet PoM £4.91 DT price = £4.91

5 Oropharyngeal fungal infections

Oropharyngeal fungal infections

Overview

Fungal infections of the mouth are usually caused by *Candida* spp. (candidiasis or candidosis). Different types of oropharyngeal candidiasis are managed as follows:

Thrush

Acute pseudomembranous candidiasis (thrush), is usually an acute infection but it may persist for months in patients receiving inhaled corticosteroids, cytotoxics or broad-spectrum antibacterials. Thrush also occurs in patients with serious systemic disease associated with reduced immunity such as leukaemia, other malignancies, and HIV infection. Any predisposing condition should be managed appropriately. When thrush is associated with corticosteroid inhalers, rinsing the mouth with water (or cleaning a child's teeth) immediately after using the inhaler may avoid the problem. Treatment with nystatin p. 1062 or miconazole, below, may be needed. Fluconazole p. 540 is effective for unresponsive infections or if a topical antifungal drug cannot be used or if the patient has dry mouth. Topical therapy may not be adequate in immunocompromised patients and an oral triazole antifungal is preferred.

Acute erythematous candidiasis
Acute erythematous (atrophic) candidiasis is a relatively uncommon condition associated with corticosteroid and broad-spectrum antibacterial use and with HIV disease. It is usually treated with fluconazole.

Denture stomatitis
Patients with denture stomatitis (chronic atrophic candidiasis), should cleanse their dentures thoroughly and leave them out as often as possible during the treatment period. To prevent recurrence of the problem, dentures should not normally be worn at night. New dentures may be required if these measures fail despite good compliance.

Miconazole oral gel can be applied to the fitting surface of the denture before insertion (for short periods only). Denture stomatitis is not always associated with candidiasis and other factors such as mechanical or chemical irritation, bacterial infection, or rarely allergy to the dental base material, may be the cause.

Chronic hyperplastic candidiasis
Chronic hyperplastic candidiasis (candidal leucoplakia) carries an increased risk of malignancy; biopsy is essential—this type of candidiasis may be associated with varying degrees of dysplasia, with oral cancer present in a high proportion of cases. Chronic hyperplastic candidiasis is treated with a systemic antifungal such as fluconazole to eliminate candidal overlay. Patients should avoid the use of tobacco.

Angular cheilitis
Angular cheilitis (angular stomatitis) is characterised by soreness, erythema and fissuring at the angles of the mouth. It is commonly associated with denture stomatitis but may represent a nutritional deficiency or it may be related to orofacial granulomatosis or HIV infection. Both yeasts (*Candida* spp.) and bacteria (*Staphylococcus aureus* and beta-haemolytic streptococci) are commonly involved as interacting, infective factors. A reduction in facial height related to ageing and tooth loss with maceration in the deep occlusive folds that may subsequently arise, predisposes to such infection. While the underlying cause is being identified and treated, it is often helpful to apply miconazole cream or fusidic acid ointment p. 519; if the angular cheilitis is unresponsive to treatment, hydrocortisone with miconazole cream or ointment p. 1097 can be used.

Immunocompromised patients
See advice on prevention of fungal infections in *Immunocompromised patients* under Antifungals, systemic use p. 536.

Drugs used in oropharyngeal candidiasis
Nystatin is not absorbed from the gastro-intestinal tract and is applied locally (as a suspension) to the mouth for treating local fungal infections. Miconazole is applied locally (as an oral gel) in the mouth but it is absorbed to the extent that potential interactions need to be considered. Miconazole also has some activity against Gram-positive bacteria including streptococci and staphylococci. Fluconazole is given by mouth for infections that do not respond to topical therapy or when topical therapy cannot be used. It is reliably absorbed and effective. Itraconazole p. 542 can be used for fluconazole-resistant infections.

If candidal infection fails to respond to 1 to 2 weeks of treatment with antifungal drugs the patient should be sent for investigation to eliminate the possibility of underlying disease. Persistent infection may also be caused by reinfection from the genito-urinary or gastro-intestinal tract. Infection can be eliminated from these sources by appropriate anticandidal therapy; the patient's partner may also require treatment to prevent reinfection.

Antiseptic mouthwashes are used in the prevention of oral candidiasis in immunocompromised patients and in the treatment of denture stomatitis.

ANTIFUNGALS > IMIDAZOLE ANTIFUNGALS

Miconazole

● **INDICATIONS AND DOSE**

Prevention and treatment of oral candidiasis
▸ BY MOUTH USING ORAL GEL
▸ Child 2–17 years: 2.5 mL 4 times a day treatment should be continued for at least 7 days after lesions have healed or symptoms have cleared, to be administered after meals, retain near oral lesions before swallowing (dental prostheses and orthodontic appliances should be removed at night and brushed with gel)
▸ Adult: 2.5 mL 4 times a day treatment should be continued for at least 7 days after lesions have healed or symptoms have cleared, to be administered after meals, retain near oral lesions before swallowing (dental prostheses and orthodontic appliances should be removed at night and brushed with gel)

Prevention and treatment of intestinal candidiasis
▸ BY MOUTH USING ORAL GEL
▸ Child 4 months–17 years: 5 mg/kg 4 times a day (max. per dose 250 mg 4 times a day) treatment should be continued for at least 7 days after lesions have healed or symptoms have cleared
▸ Adult: 5 mg/kg 4 times a day (max. per dose 250 mg 4 times a day) treatment should be continued for at least 7 days after lesions have healed or symptoms have cleared

● **UNLICENSED USE** Not licensed for use in children under 4 months of age or during first 5–6 months of life of an infant born pre-term.

● **CONTRA-INDICATIONS** Infants with impaired swallowing reflex

● **CAUTIONS** Avoid in Acute porphyrias p. 918

● **INTERACTIONS** → Appendix 1 (antifungals, imidazole).

● **SIDE-EFFECTS**
▸ **Common or very common** Nausea · rash · vomiting
▸ **Very rare** Diarrhoea (usually on long term treatment) · hepatitis · rash (in children) · Stevens-Johnson syndrome · toxic epidermal necrolysis

● **PREGNANCY** Manufacturer advises avoid if possible—toxicity at high doses in *animal* studies.

● **BREAST FEEDING** Manufacturer advises caution—no information available.

● **HEPATIC IMPAIRMENT** Avoid.

● **DIRECTIONS FOR ADMINISTRATION** Oral gel should be held in mouth, after food.

● **PRESCRIBING AND DISPENSING INFORMATION** Flavours of oral gel may include orange.

● **PATIENT AND CARER ADVICE** Patients or carers should be given advice on how to administer miconazole oromucosal gel.

● **PROFESSION SPECIFIC INFORMATION**

Dental practitioners' formulary
Miconazole Oromucosal Gel may be prescribed.

● **EXCEPTIONS TO LEGAL CATEGORY** 15-g tube of oral gel can be sold to the public.

● MEDICINAL FORMS
There can be variation in the licensing of different medicines containing the same drug.

Oromucosal gel
CAUTIONARY AND ADVISORY LABELS 9
▸ Daktarin (McNeil Products Ltd, Janssen-Cilag Ltd)
Miconazole 20 mg per 1 gram Daktarin 20mg/g oromucosal gel sugar-free | 15 gram [P] £3.23 DT price = £3.23 sugar-free | 80 gram [PoM] £4.38 DT price = £4.38

ANTIFUNGALS › POLYENE ANTIFUNGALS

Nystatin

6.6.2016

● INDICATIONS AND DOSE
Oral and perioral fungal infections
▸ BY MOUTH
▸ Child 1 month-1 year: 200 000 units 4 times a day usually for 7 days, and continued for 48 hours after lesions have resolved, divide administration of the dose between both sides of the mouth
▸ Child 2-17 years: 400 000-600 000 units 4 times a day usually for 7 days, and continued for 48 hours after lesions have resolved, divide administration of the dose between both sides of the mouth
▸ Adult: 400 000-600 000 units 4 times a day usually for 7 days, and continued for 48 hours after lesions have resolved, divide administration of the dose between both sides of the mouth

● SIDE-EFFECTS Local irritation · local sensitisation · nausea
● PATIENT AND CARER ADVICE
Medicines for Children leaflet: Nystatin for Candida infection
www.medicinesforchildren.org.uk/nystatin-for-candida-infection
Counselling advised with oral suspension (use of pipette, hold in mouth, after food).

● PROFESSION SPECIFIC INFORMATION
Dental practitioners' formulary
Nystatin Oral Suspension may be prescribed.

● MEDICINAL FORMS
There can be variation in the licensing of different medicines containing the same drug. Forms available from special-order manufacturers include: oral suspension

Oral suspension
CAUTIONARY AND ADVISORY LABELS 9
EXCIPIENTS: May contain Ethanol
▸ Nystatin (Non-proprietary)
Nystatin 100000 unit per 1 ml Nystatin 100,000units/ml oral suspension | 30 ml [PoM] £22.44 DT price = £2.73
▸ Nystan (Bristol-Myers Squibb Pharmaceuticals Ltd)
Nystatin 100000 unit per 1 ml Nystan 100,000units/ml oral suspension (ready mixed) | 30 ml [PoM] £1.80 DT price = £2.73

6   Oropharyngeal viral infections

Oropharyngeal viral infections

Management
Viral infections are the most common cause of a sore throat. They do not benefit from anti-infective treatment.
The management of primary herpetic gingivostomatitis is a soft diet, adequate fluid intake, and analgesics as required, including local use of benzydamine hydrochloride p. 1058. The use of chlorhexidine mouthwash p. 1053 will control plaque accumulation if toothbrushing is painful and will also help to control secondary infection in general.

In the case of severe herpetic stomatitis, a systemic antiviral such as aciclovir p. 576 is required. Valaciclovir p. 579 and famciclovir p. 578 are suitable alternatives for oral lesions associated with herpes zoster. Aciclovir and valaciclovir are also used for the prevention of frequently recurring herpes simplex lesions of the mouth, particularly when implicated in the initiation of erythema multiforme.

Chapter 13
Skin

CONTENTS

Skin conditions, management

Vehicles

The British Association of Dermatologists list of preferred unlicensed dermatological preparations (specials) is available at www.bad.org.uk/specials.

Both vehicle and active ingredients are important in the treatment of skin conditions; the vehicle alone may have more than a mere placebo effect. The vehicle affects the degree of hydration of the skin, has a mild anti-inflammatory effect, and aids the penetration of active drug.

Applications are usually viscous solutions, emulsions, or suspensions for application to the skin (including the scalp) or nails.

Collodions are painted on the skin and allowed to dry to leave a flexible film over the site of application.

Creams are emulsions of oil and water and are generally well absorbed into the skin. They may contain an antimicrobial preservative unless the active ingredient or basis is intrinsically bactericidal and fungicidal. Generally, creams are cosmetically more acceptable than ointments because they are less greasy and easier to apply.

Gels consist of active ingredients in suitable hydrophilic or hydrophobic bases; they generally have a high water content. Gels are particularly suitable for application to the face and scalp.

Lotions have a cooling effect and may be preferred to ointments or creams for application over a hairy area. Lotions in alcoholic basis can sting if used on broken skin. *Shake lotions* (such as calamine lotion) contain insoluble powders which leave a deposit on the skin surface.

Ointments are greasy preparations which are normally anhydrous and insoluble in water, and are more occlusive than creams. They are particularly suitable for chronic, dry lesions. The most commonly used ointment bases consist of soft paraffin or a combination of soft, liquid, and hard paraffin. Some ointment bases have both *hydrophilic and lipophilic* properties; they may have occlusive properties on the skin surface, encourage hydration, and also be miscible with water; they often have a mild anti-inflammatory effect. *Water-soluble ointments* contain macrogols which are freely soluble in water and are therefore readily washed off; they

have a limited but useful role where ready removal is desirable.

Pastes are stiff preparations containing a high proportion of finely powdered solids such as zinc oxide and starch suspended in an ointment. They are used for circumscribed lesions such as those which occur in lichen simplex, chronic eczema, or psoriasis. They are less occlusive than ointments and can be used to protect inflamed, lichenified, or excoriated skin.

Dusting powders are used only rarely. They reduce friction between opposing skin surfaces. Dusting powders should not be applied to moist areas because they can cake and abrade the skin. Talc is a lubricant but it does not absorb moisture; it can cause respiratory irritation. Starch is less lubricant but absorbs water.

Dilution

The BP directs that creams and ointments should **not** normally be diluted but that should dilution be necessary care should be taken, in particular, to prevent microbial contamination. The appropriate diluent should be used and heating should be avoided during mixing; excessive dilution may affect the stability of some creams. Diluted creams should normally be used within 2 weeks of preparation.

Suitable quantities for prescribing

Suitable quantities of dermatological preparations to be prescribed for specific areas of the body		
Area of body	**Creams and Ointments**	**Lotions**
Face	15–30 g	100 ml
Both hands	25–50 g	200 ml
Scalp	50–100 g	200 ml
Both arms or both legs	100–200 g	200 ml
Trunk	400 g	500 ml
Groins and genitalia	15–25 g	100 ml
These amounts are usually suitable for an adult for twice daily application for 1 week. The recommendations **do not apply** to corticosteroid preparations. For suitable quantities of corticosteroid preparations, see relevant table.		

13

Skin

Excipients and sensitisation

Excipients in topical products rarely cause problems. If a patch test indicates allergy to an excipient, products containing the substance should be avoided. The following excipients in topical preparations are associated, rarely, with sensitisation; the presence of these excipients is indicated in the entries for topical products.

- Beeswax
- Benzyl alcohol
- Butylated hydroxyanisole
- Butylated hydroxytoluene
- Cetostearyl alcohol (including cetyl and stearyl alcohol)
- Chlorocresol
- Edetic acid (EDTA)
- Ethylenediamine
- Fragrances
- Hydroxybenzoates (parabens)
- Imidurea
- Isopropyl palmitate
- N-(3-Chloroallyl)hexaminium chloride (quaternium 15)
- Polysorbates
- Propylene glycol
- Sodium metabisulfite
- Sorbic acid
- Wool fat and related substances including lanolin (purified versions of wool fat have reduced the problem)

1 Dry and scaling skin disorders

Emollient and barrier preparations

Borderline substances

The preparations marked 'ACBS' are regarded as drugs when prescribed in accordance with the advice of the Advisory Committee on Borderline Substances for the clinical conditions listed. Prescriptions issued in accordance with this advice and endorsed 'ACBS' will normally not be investigated.

Emollients

Emollients soothe, smooth and hydrate the skin and are indicated for all dry or scaling disorders. Their effects are short lived and they should be applied frequently even after improvement occurs. They are useful in dry and eczematous disorders, and to a lesser extent in psoriasis. The choice of an appropriate emollient will depend on the severity of the condition, patient preference, and the site of application. Some ingredients rarely cause sensitisation and this should be suspected if an eczematous reaction occurs. The use of aqueous cream as a leave-on emollient may increase the risk of skin reactions, particularly in eczema.

Preparations such as **aqueous cream** and **emulsifying ointment** can be used as soap substitutes for hand washing and in the bath; the preparation is rubbed on the skin before rinsing off completely. The addition of a bath oil may also be helpful.

Urea is occasionally used with other topical agents such as corticosteroids to enhance penetration of the skin.

Emollient bath and shower preparations

Emollient bath additives should be added to bath water; hydration can be improved by soaking in the bath for 10–20 minutes. Some bath emollients can be applied to wet skin undiluted and rinsed off. In dry skin conditions soap should be avoided.

The quantities of bath additives recommended for adults are suitable for an adult-size bath. Proportionately less should be used for a child-size bath or a washbasin; recommended bath additive quantities for children reflect this.

Barrier preparations

Barrier preparations often contain water-repellent substances such as dimeticone or other silicones. They are used on the skin around stomas, bedsores, and pressure areas in the elderly where the skin is intact. Where the skin has broken down, barrier preparations have a limited role in protecting adjacent skin. Barrier preparations are not a substitute for adequate nursing care.

Nappy rash

The first line of treatment is to ensure that nappies are changed frequently and that tightly fitting water-proof pants are avoided. The rash may clear when left exposed to the air and a barrier preparation, applied with each nappy change, can be helpful. A mild corticosteroid such as hydrocortisone 0.5% or 1% p. 1092 can be used if inflammation is causing discomfort, but it should be avoided in neonates. The barrier preparation should be applied after the corticosteroid preparation to prevent further damage. Preparations containing hydrocortisone should be applied for no more than a week; the hydrocortisone should be discontinued as soon as the inflammation subsides. The occlusive effect of nappies and waterproof pants may increase absorption of corticosteroids. If the rash is associated with candidal infection, a topical antifungal such as clotrimazole cream p. 750 can be used. Topical antibacterial preparations can be used if bacterial infection is present; treatment with an oral antibacterial may occasionally be required in severe or recurrent infection. Hydrocortisone may be used in combination with antimicrobial preparations if there is considerable inflammation, erosion, and infection.

DERMATOLOGICAL DRUGS > BARRIER PREPARATIONS

Barrier creams and ointments

- **INDICATIONS AND DOSE**

For use as a barrier preparation
▶ TO THE SKIN
▶ Child: (consult product literature)
▶ Adult: (consult product literature)

- **MEDICINAL FORMS**
There can be variation in the licensing of different medicines containing the same drug.

Cream
EXCIPIENTS: May contain Beeswax, butylated hydroxyanisole, butylated hydroxytoluene, cetostearyl alcohol (including cetyl and stearyl alcohol), chlorocresol, fragrances, hydroxybenzoates (parabens), propylene glycol, wool fat and related substances including lanolin

▶ Conotrane (Astellas Pharma Ltd)
Benzalkonium chloride 1 mg per 1 gram, Dimeticone 220 mg per 1 gram Conotrane cream | 100 gram (GSL) £0.88 DT price = £0.88 | 500 gram (GSL) £3.51

▶ Drapolene (Omega Pharma Ltd)
Benzalkonium chloride 100 microgram per 1 gram, Cetrimide 2 mg per 1 gram Drapolene cream | 100 gram (GSL) £1.76 | 200 gram (GSL) £2.86 | 350 gram (GSL) £4.28

▶ Siopel (Derma UK Ltd)
Cetrimide 3 mg per 1 gram, Dimeticone 1000 100 mg per 1 gram Siopel cream | 50 gram (GSL) £2.15

▶ Sudocrem (Forest Laboratories UK Ltd)
Benzyl cinnamate 1.5 mg per 1 gram, Benzyl alcohol 3.9 mg per 1 gram, Benzyl benzoate 10.1 mg per 1 gram, Wool fat hydrous 40 mg per 1 gram, Zinc oxide 152.5 mg per 1 gram Sudocrem antiseptic healing cream | 60 gram (GSL) £1.45 | 125 gram (GSL) £2.15 | 250 gram (GSL) £3.67 | 400 gram (GSL) £5.25

Ointment

EXCIPIENTS: May contain Wool fat and related substances including lanolin

▸ Barrier creams and ointments (Non-proprietary)
   Cetostearyl alcohol 20 mg per 1 gram, Zinc oxide 75 mg per 1 gram, Beeswax white 100 mg per 1 gram, Arachis oil 305 mg per 1 gram, Castor oil 500 mg per 1 gram Zinc and Castor oil ointment | 15 gram GSL £1.08 | 50 gram GSL £2.01 | 100 gram GSL £1.41 | 500 gram GSL £4.99–£5.34 DT price = £5.34 Zinc and Castor oil cream | 100 gram GSL £1.41
▸ Brands may include Metanium

Spray

CAUTIONARY AND ADVISORY LABELS 15
EXCIPIENTS: May contain Cetostearyl alcohol (including cetyl and stearyl alcohol), hydroxybenzoates (parabens), wool fat and related substances including lanolin

▸ Sprilon (J M Loveridge Ltd)
   Dimeticone 10.4 mg per 1 gram, Zinc oxide 125 mg per 1 gram Sprilon aerosol spray | 115 gram GSL £8.90 DT price = £8.90

DERMATOLOGICAL DRUGS > EMOLLIENTS

Emollient bath and shower products, antimicrobial-containing

● INDICATIONS AND DOSE

DERMOL® 200 SHOWER EMOLLIENT

Dry and pruritic skin conditions including eczema and dermatitis

▸ TO THE SKIN
▸ Child: To be applied to the skin or used as a soap substitute
▸ Adult: To be applied to the skin or used as a soap substitute

DERMOL® 600® BATH EMOLLIENT

Dry and pruritic skin conditions including eczema and dermatitis

▸ TO THE SKIN
▸ Child 1–23 months: 5–15 mL/bath, not to be used undiluted
▸ Child 2–17 years: 15–30 mL/bath, not to be used undiluted
▸ Adult: Up to 30 mL/bath, not to be used undiluted

DERMOL® WASH EMULSION

Dry and pruritic skin conditions including eczema and dermatitis

▸ TO THE SKIN
▸ Child: To be applied to the skin or used as a soap substitute
▸ Adult: To be applied to the skin or used as a soap substitute

EMULSIDERM®

Dry skin conditions including eczema and ichthyosis

▸ TO THE SKIN
▸ Child 1–23 months: 5–10 mL/bath, alternatively, to be rubbed into dry skin until absorbed
▸ Child 2–17 years: 7–30 mL/bath, alternatively, to be rubbed into dry skin until absorbed
▸ Adult: 7–30 mL/bath, alternatively, to be rubbed into dry skin until absorbed

OILATUM® PLUS

Topical treatment of eczema, including eczema at risk from infection

▸ TO THE SKIN
▸ Child 6–11 months: 1 mL/bath, not to be used undiluted
▸ Child 1–17 years: 1–2 capfuls/bath, not to be used undiluted
▸ Adult: 1–2 capfuls/bath, not to be used undiluted

IMPORTANT SAFETY INFORMATION

FIRE HAZARD WITH PARAFFIN-BASED EMOLLIENTS

Emulsifying ointment or 50% Liquid Paraffin and 50% White Soft Paraffin Ointment in contact with dressings and clothing is easily ignited by a naked flame. The risk is greater when these preparations are applied to large areas of the body, and clothing or dressings become soaked with the ointment. Patients should be told to keep away from fire or flames, and not to smoke when using these preparations. The risk of fire should be considered when using large quantities of any paraffin-based emollient.

These preparations make skin and surfaces slippery—particular care is needed when bathing.

● DIRECTIONS FOR ADMINISTRATION Emollient bath additives should be added to bath water; hydration can be improved by soaking in the bath for 10–20 minutes. Some bath emollients can be applied to wet skin undiluted and rinsed off. Emollient preparations contained in tubs should be removed with a clean spoon or spatula to reduce bacterial contamination of the emollient. Emollients should be applied in the direction of hair growth to reduce the risk of folliculitis.

● PRESCRIBING AND DISPENSING INFORMATION Preparations containing an antibacterial should be avoided unless infection is present or is a frequent complication.

● MEDICINAL FORMS There can be variation in the licensing of different medicines containing the same drug.

Liquid

EXCIPIENTS: May contain Cetostearyl alcohol (including cetyl and stearyl alcohol)

▸ Dermol 200 (Dermal Laboratories Ltd)
   Benzalkonium chloride 1 mg per 1 gram, Chlorhexidine hydrochloride 1 mg per 1 gram, Isopropyl myristate 25 mg per 1 gram, Liquid paraffin 25 mg per 1 gram Dermol 200 shower emollient | 200 ml P £3.55
▸ Dermol Wash (Dermal Laboratories Ltd)
   Benzalkonium chloride 1 mg per 1 gram, Chlorhexidine hydrochloride 1 mg per 1 gram, Isopropyl myristate 25 mg per 1 gram, Liquid paraffin 25 mg per 1 gram Dermol Wash cutaneous emulsion | 200 ml P £3.55

Bath additive

EXCIPIENTS: May contain Acetylated lanolin alcohols, isopropyl palmitate, polysorbates

▸ Dermol 600 (Dermal Laboratories Ltd)
   Benzalkonium chloride 5 mg per 1 gram, Isopropyl myristate 250 mg per 1 gram, Liquid paraffin 250 mg per 1 gram Dermol 600 bath emollient | 600 ml P £7.55
▸ Emulsiderm (Dermal Laboratories Ltd)
   Benzalkonium chloride 5 mg per 1 gram, Isopropyl myristate 250 mg per 1 gram, Liquid paraffin 250 mg per 1 gram Emulsiderm emollient | 300 ml P £3.85 | 1000 ml P £12.00
▸ Oilatum Plus (GlaxoSmithKline Consumer Healthcare)
   Triclosan 20 mg per 1 gram, Benzalkonium chloride 60 mg per 1 gram, Liquid paraffin light 525 mg per 1 gram Oilatum Plus bath additive | 500 ml GSL £6.98

13

Skin

Emollient bath and shower products, colloidal oatmeal-containing

● **INDICATIONS AND DOSE**

Endogenous and exogenous eczema | Xeroderma | Ichthyosis

▸ TO THE SKIN
▸ Child 2-17 years: 20–30 mL/bath, alternatively apply to wet skin and rinse
▸ Adult: 20–30 mL/bath, alternatively apply to wet skin and rinse

Pruritus of the elderly associated with dry skin

▸ TO THE SKIN
▸ Elderly: 20–30 mL/bath, alternatively apply to wet skin and rinse

> **IMPORTANT SAFETY INFORMATION**
> These preparations make skin and surfaces slippery—particular care is needed when bathing.

● **DIRECTIONS FOR ADMINISTRATION** Emollient bath additives should be added to bath water; hydration can be improved by soaking in the bath for 10–20 minutes. Some bath emollients can be applied to wet skin undiluted and rinsed off. Emollient preparations contained in tubs should be removed with a clean spoon or spatula to reduce bacterial contamination of the emollient. Emollients should be applied in the direction of hair growth to reduce the risk of folliculitis.

● **MEDICINAL FORMS**
There can be variation in the licensing of different medicines containing the same drug.

Bath additive
EXCIPIENTS: May contain Beeswax, fragrances
▸ Aveeno (Johnson & Johnson Ltd)
Aveeno bath oil | 250 ml (ACBS) £4.49

Emollient bath and shower products, paraffin-containing

● **INDICATIONS AND DOSE**

AQUAMAX® WASH

Dry skin conditions

▸ TO THE SKIN
▸ Child: To be applied to wet or dry skin and rinse
▸ Adult: To be applied to wet or dry skin and rinse

CETRABEN® BATH

Dry skin conditions, including eczema

▸ TO THE SKIN
▸ Child 1 month-11 years: 0.5–1 capful/bath, alternatively, to be applied to wet skin and rinse
▸ Child 12-17 years: 1–2 capfuls/bath, alternatively, to be applied to wet skin and rinse
▸ Adult: 1–2 capfuls/bath, alternatively, to be applied to wet skin and rinse

DERMALO®

Dermatitis | Dry skin conditions, including ichthyosis

▸ TO THE SKIN
▸ Child 1 month-11 years: 5–10 mL/bath, alternatively, to be applied to wet skin and rinse
▸ Child 12-17 years: 15–20 mL/bath, alternatively, to be applied to wet skin and rinse
▸ Adult: 15–20 mL/bath, alternatively, to be applied to wet skin and rinse

Pruritus of the elderly

▸ TO THE SKIN
▸ Elderly: 15–20 mL/bath, alternatively, to be applied to wet skin and rinse

DOUBLEBASE® EMOLLIENT BATH ADDITIVE

Dry skin conditions including dermatitis and ichthyosis

▸ TO THE SKIN
▸ Child 1 month-11 years: 5–10 mL/bath
▸ Child 12-17 years: 15–20 mL/bath
▸ Adult: 15–20 mL/bath

Pruritus of the elderly

▸ TO THE SKIN
▸ Elderly: 15–20 mL/bath

DOUBLEBASE® EMOLLIENT SHOWER GEL

Dry, chapped, or itchy skin conditions

▸ TO THE SKIN
▸ Child: To be applied to wet or dry skin and rinse, or apply to dry skin after showering
▸ Adult: To be applied to wet or dry skin and rinse, or apply to dry skin after showering

E45® BATH OIL

Endogenous and exogenous eczema, xeroderma, and ichthyosis

▸ TO THE SKIN
▸ Child 1 month-11 years: 5–10 mL/bath, alternatively, to be applied to wet skin and rinse
▸ Child 12-17 years: 15 mL/bath, alternatively, to be applied to wet skin and rinse
▸ Adult: 15 mL/bath, alternatively, to be applied to wet skin and rinse

Pruritus of the elderly associated with dry skin

▸ TO THE SKIN
▸ Elderly: 15 mL/bath, alternatively, to be applied to wet skin and rinse

E45® WASH CREAM

Endogenous and exogenous eczema, xeroderma, and ichthyosis

▸ TO THE SKIN
▸ Child: To be used as a soap substitute
▸ Adult: To be used as a soap substitute

Pruritus of the elderly associated with dry skin

▸ TO THE SKIN
▸ Elderly: To be used as a soap substitute

HYDROMOL® BATH AND SHOWER EMOLLIENT

Dry skin conditions | Eczema | Ichthyosis

▸ TO THE SKIN
▸ Child 1 month-11 years: 0.5–2 capfuls/bath, alternatively apply to wet skin and rinse
▸ Child 12-17 years: 1–3 capfuls/bath, alternatively apply to wet skin and rinse
▸ Adult: 1–3 capfuls/bath, alternatively apply to wet skin and rinse

Pruritus of the elderly

▸ TO THE SKIN
▸ Elderly: 1–3 capfuls/bath, alternatively apply to wet skin and rinse

LPL 63.4®

Dry skin conditions

▸ TO THE SKIN
▸ Child 1 month-11 years: 0.5–2 capfuls/bath, alternatively, to be applied to wet skin and rinse
▸ Child 12-17 years: 1–3 capfuls/bath, alternatively, to be applied to wet skin and rinse
▸ Adult: 1–3 capfuls/bath, alternatively, to be applied to wet skin and rinse

13

Skin

OILATUM® EMOLLIENT BATH ADDITIVE

Dry skin conditions including dermatitis and ichthyosis

▶ TO THE SKIN

- Child 1 month-11 years: Apply 0.5–2 capfuls/bath, alternatively, to be applied to wet skin and rinse
- Child 12-17 years: 1–3 capfuls/bath, alternatively, to be applied to wet skin and rinse
- Adult: 1–3 capfuls/bath, alternatively, to be applied to wet skin and rinse

Pruritus of the elderly

▶ TO THE SKIN

- Elderly: 1–3 capfuls/bath, alternatively, to be applied to wet skin and rinse

OILATUM® JUNIOR BATH ADDITIVE

Dry skin conditions including dermatitis and ichthyosis

▶ TO THE SKIN

- Child 1 month-11 years: 0.5–2 capfuls/bath, alternatively, apply to wet skin and rinse
- Child 12-17 years: 1–3 capfuls/bath, alternatively, apply to wet skin and rinse
- Adult: 1–3 capfuls/bath, alternatively, apply to wet skin and rinse

Pruritus of the elderly

▶ TO THE SKIN

- Elderly: 1–3 capfuls/bath, alternatively, apply to wet skin and rinse

QV® BATH OIL

Dry skin conditions including eczema, psoriasis, ichthyosis, and pruritus

▶ TO THE SKIN

- Child 1-11 months: 5 mL/bath, alternatively, to be applied to wet skin and rinse
- Child 1-17 years: 10 mL/bath, alternatively, to be applied to wet skin and rinse
- Adult: 10 mL/bath, alternatively, to be applied to wet skin and rinse

QV® GENTLE WASH

Dry skin conditions including eczema, psoriasis, ichthyosis, and pruritus

▶ TO THE SKIN

- Child: To be used as a soap substitute
- Adult: To be used as a soap substitute

ZEROLATUM®

Dry skin conditions | Dermatitis | Ichthyosis

▶ TO THE SKIN

- Child 1 month-11 years: 5–10 mL/bath
- Child 12-17 years: 15–20 mL/bath
- Adult: 15–20 mL/bath

Pruritus of the elderly

▶ TO THE SKIN

- Elderly: 15–20 mL/bath

IMPORTANT SAFETY INFORMATION

FIRE HAZARD WITH PARAFFIN-BASED EMOLLIENTS

Emulsifying ointment or 50% Liquid Paraffin and 50% White Soft Paraffin Ointment in contact with dressings and clothing is easily ignited by a naked flame. The risk is greater when these preparations are applied to large areas of the body, and when clothing or dressings become soaked with the ointment. Patients should be told to keep away from fire or flames, and not to smoke when using these preparations. The risk of fire should be considered when using large quantities of any paraffin-based emollient.

These preparations make the skin and surfaces slippery—particular care is needed when bathing.

● DIRECTIONS FOR ADMINISTRATION Emollient bath additives should be added to bath water; hydration can be improved by soaking in the bath for 10–20 minutes. Some bath emollients can be applied to wet skin undiluted and rinsed off. Emollient preparations contained in tubs should be removed with a clean spoon or spatula to reduce bacterial contamination of the emollient. Emollients should be applied in the direction of hair growth to reduce the risk of folliculitis.

● MEDICINAL FORMS
There can be variation in the licensing of different medicines containing the same drug.

Cream
EXCIPIENTS: May contain Cetostearyl alcohol (including cetyl and stearyl alcohol)

▶ Emollient bath and shower products, paraffin-containing (Non-proprietary)
Phenoxyethanol 10 mg per 1 gram, Liquid paraffin 60 mg per 1 gram, Emulsifying wax 90 mg per 1 gram, White soft paraffin 150 mg per 1 gram, Purified water 690 mg per 1 gram Aqueous cream | 30 gram GSL £1.35 | 100 gram GSL £2.15 DT price = £0.86 | 500 gram GSL £6.35 DT price = £4.30

Gel
EXCIPIENTS: May contain Cetostearyl alcohol (including cetyl and stearyl alcohol)

▶ Doublebase (Dermal Laboratories Ltd)
Isopropyl myristate 150 mg per 1 gram, Liquid paraffin 150 mg per 1 gram Doublebase Dayleve gel | 100 gram P £2.65 DT price = £2.65 | 500 gram P £6.29 DT price = £5.83
Doublebase gel | 100 gram P £2.65 DT price = £2.65 | 500 gram P £5.83 DT price = £5.83
Doublebase emollient wash gel | 200 gram P £5.21
Doublebase emollient shower gel | 200 gram P £5.21

Bath additive
EXCIPIENTS: May contain Acetylated lanolin alcohols, cetostearyl alcohol (including cetyl and stearyl alcohol), fragrances, isopropyl palmitate

▶ Emollient bath and shower products, paraffin-containing (Non-proprietary)
Liquid paraffin light 634 mg per 1 ml Liquid paraffin light 63.4% bath additive | 150 ml GSL no price available DT price = £2.84 | 250 ml GSL no price available DT price = £2.75 | 300 ml GSL no price available DT price = £4.88 | 500 ml GSL no price available DT price = £4.57

▶ Cetraben (Genus Pharmaceuticals Ltd)
Liquid paraffin light 828 mg per 1 gram Cetraben emollient 82.8% bath additive | 500 ml GSL £5.75

▶ Dermalo (Dermal Laboratories Ltd)
Acetylated wool alcohols 50 mg per 1 gram, Liquid paraffin 650 mg per 1 gram Dermalo bath emollient | 500 ml GSL £3.44

▶ Doublebase emollient bath (Dermal Laboratories Ltd)
Liquid paraffin 650 mg per 1 gram Doublebase emollient bath additive | 500 ml GSL £5.45

▶ E45 emollient bath (Forum Health Products Ltd)
E45 emollient bath oil | 250 ml (ACBS) £3.43 | 500 ml (ACBS) £5.32

▶ Hydromol (Alliance Pharmaceuticals Ltd)
Isopropyl myristate 130 mg per 1 ml, Liquid paraffin light 378 mg per 1 ml Hydromol Bath & Shower emollient | 350 ml GSL £3.88 | 500 ml GSL £4.42 | 1000 ml GSL £8.80

▶ LPL (Huxley Europe Ltd)
Liquid paraffin light 634 mg per 1 ml LPL 63.4 bath additive and emollient | 500 ml £3.10 DT price = £4.57

▶ Oilatum (GlaxoSmithKline Consumer Healthcare)
Liquid paraffin light 634 mg per 1 ml Oilatum Bath Formula | 150 ml GSL £2.84 DT price = £2.84 | 300 ml GSL £4.88 DT price = £4.88
Oilatum Emollient | 250 ml GSL £2.75 DT price = £2.75 | 500 ml GSL £4.57 DT price = £4.57

▶ Oilatum junior (GlaxoSmithKline Consumer Healthcare)
Liquid paraffin light 634 mg per 1 ml Oilatum Junior bath additive | 150 ml GSL £2.84 DT price = £2.84 | 250 ml GSL £4.05 DT price = £2.75 | 500 ml GSL £4.88 DT price = £4.88 | 600 ml GSL £5.89 DT price = £5.89

▶ QV (Crawford Healthcare Ltd)
Liquid paraffin light 850.9 mg per 1 gram QV 85.09% bath oil | 250 ml £2.91 | 500 ml £4.76

▶ Zerolatum (Thornton & Ross Ltd)
Acetylated wool alcohols 50 mg per 1 gram, Liquid paraffin 650 mg per 1 gram Zerolatum Emollient bath additive | 500 ml £4.79

13

Skin

13
Skin

Wash

EXCIPIENTS: May contain Cetostearyl alcohol (including cetyl and stearyl alcohol), polysorbates

▸ Aquamax (Intrapharm Laboratories Ltd)
Aquamax wash | 250 gram £2.99

▸ E45 emollient wash (Forum Health Products Ltd)
E45 emollient wash cream | 250 ml (ACBS) £3.43

EXCIPIENTS: May contain Hydroxybenzoates (parabens)

▸ QV Gentle (Crawford Healthcare Ltd)
QV Gentle wash | 250 ml £3.17 | 500 ml £5.29

Emollient bath and shower products, soya-bean oil-containing

● **INDICATIONS AND DOSE**

BALNEUM® BATH OIL

Dry skin conditions including those associated with dermatitis and eczema

▸ TO THE SKIN

▸ Child 1-23 months: 5–15 mL/bath, not to be used undiluted

▸ Child 2-17 years: 20–60 mL/bath, not to be used undiluted

▸ Adult: 20–60 mL/bath, not to be used undiluted

BALNEUM® PLUS BATH OIL

Dry skin conditions including those associated with dermatitis and eczema where pruritus also experienced

▸ TO THE SKIN

▸ Child 1-23 months: 5 mL/bath, alternatively, to be applied to wet skin and rinse

▸ Child 2-17 years: 10–20 mL/bath, alternatively, to be applied to wet skin and rinse

▸ Adult: 20 mL/bath, alternatively, to be applied to wet skin and rinse

ZERONEUM®

Dry skin conditions including eczema

▸ TO THE SKIN

▸ Child 1 month-11 years: 5 mL/bath

▸ Child 12-17 years: 20 mL/bath

▸ Adult: 20 mL/bath

IMPORTANT SAFETY INFORMATION

These preparations make skin and surfaces slippery—particular care is needed when bathing.

● DIRECTIONS FOR ADMINISTRATION Emollient bath additives should be added to bath water; hydration can be improved by soaking in the bath for 10–20 minutes. Some bath emollients can be applied to wet skin undiluted and rinsed off. Emollient preparations contained in tubs should be removed with a clean spoon or spatula to reduce bacterial contamination of the emollient. Emollients should be applied in the direction of hair growth to reduce the risk of folliculitis.

● MEDICINAL FORMS
There can be variation in the licensing of different medicines containing the same drug.

Bath additive

EXCIPIENTS: May contain Butylated hydroxytoluene, fragrances, propylene glycol

▸ Emollient bath and shower products, soya-bean oil-containing (Non-proprietary)
Lauromacrogols 150 mg per 1 gram, Soya oil 829.5 mg per 1 gram Soya oil 82.95% / Lauromacrogols 15% bath oil | 500 ml (GSL) no price available
Soya oil 847.5 mg per 1 gram Soya oil 84.75% bath oil | 500 ml (GSL) no price available

▸ Balneum (Almirall Ltd)
Lauromacrogols 150 mg per 1 gram, Soya oil 829.5 mg per 1 gram Balneum Plus bath oil | 500 ml (GSL) £6.66
Soya oil 847.5 mg per 1 gram Balneum 84.75% bath oil | 200 ml (GSL) £2.48 | 500 ml (GSL) £5.38 | 1000 ml (GSL) £10.39

▸ Zeroneum (Thornton & Ross Ltd)
Soya oil 833.5 mg per 1 gram Zeroneum 83.35% bath additive | 500 ml £4.48

Emollient bath and shower products, tar-containing

● **INDICATIONS AND DOSE**

POLYTAR EMOLLIENT®

Psoriasis, eczema, atopic and pruritic dermatoses

▸ TO THE SKIN

▸ Adult: 2–4 capfuls/bath, add 15–30 mL to an adult-size bath; soak for 20 minutes

PSORIDERM® EMULSION

Psoriasis

▸ TO THE SKIN

▸ Adult: Up to 30 mL/bath, use 30mL in adult-size bath, soak for 5 minutes

---

IMPORTANT SAFETY INFORMATION

FIRE HAZARD WITH PARAFFIN-BASED EMOLLIENTS

Emulsifying ointment or 50% Liquid Paraffin and 50% White Soft Paraffin Ointment in contact with dressings and clothing is easily ignited by a naked flame. The risk is greater when these preparations are applied to large areas of the body, and clothing or dressings become soaked with the ointment. Patients should be told to keep away from fire or flames, and not to smoke when using these preparations. The risk of fire should be considered when using large quantities of any paraffin-based emollient.

These preparations make skin and surfaces slippery—particular care is needed when bathing.

● DIRECTIONS FOR ADMINISTRATION Emollient bath additives should be added to bath water; hydration can be improved by soaking in the bath for 10–20 minutes. Some bath emollients can be applied to wet skin undiluted and rinsed off. Emollient preparations contained in tubs should be removed with a clean spoon or spatula to reduce bacterial contamination of the emollient. Emollients should be applied in the direction of hair growth to reduce the risk of folliculitis.

● MEDICINAL FORMS
There can be variation in the licensing of different medicines containing the same drug.

Bath additive

EXCIPIENTS: May contain Isopropyl palmitate, polysorbates

▸ Psoriderm (Dermal Laboratories Ltd)
Coal tar distilled 400 mg per 1 ml Psoriderm Emulsion 40% bath additive | 200 ml (P) £2.74

Emollient creams and ointments, antimicrobial-containing

● INDICATIONS AND DOSE

Dry and pruritic skin conditions including eczema and dermatitis
▸ TO THE SKIN
▸ Child: To be applied to the skin or used as a soap substitute
▸ Adult: To be applied to the skin or used as a soap substitute

---

IMPORTANT SAFETY INFORMATION

FIRE HAZARD WITH PARAFFIN-BASED EMOLLIENTS

Emulsifying ointment *or* 50% Liquid Paraffin and 50% White Soft Paraffin Ointment in contact with dressings and clothing is easily ignited by a naked flame. The risk is greater when these preparations are applied to large areas of the body, and clothing or dressings become soaked with the ointment. Patients should be told to keep away from fire or flames, and not to smoke when using these preparations. The risk of fire should be considered when using large quantities of any paraffin-based emollient.

These preparations make skin and surfaces slippery—particular care is needed when bathing.

● DIRECTIONS FOR ADMINISTRATION Emollients should be applied immediately after washing or bathing to maximise the effect of skin hydration. Emollient preparations contained in tubs should be removed with a clean spoon or spatula to reduce bacterial contamination of the emollient. Emollients should be applied in the direction of hair growth to reduce the risk of folliculitis.

● PRESCRIBING AND DISPENSING INFORMATION Preparations containing an antibacterial should be avoided unless infection is present or is a frequent complication.

● MEDICINAL FORMS There can be variation in the licensing of different medicines containing the same drug.

Liquid
EXCIPIENTS: May contain Cetostearyl alcohol (including cetyl and stearyl alcohol)
▸ Dermol 500 (Dermal Laboratories Ltd)
Benzalkonium chloride 1 mg per 1 gram, Chlorhexidine hydrochloride 1 mg per 1 gram, Isopropyl myristate 25 mg per 1 gram, Liquid paraffin 25 mg per 1 gram Dermol 500 lotion | 500 ml P £6.04

Cream
EXCIPIENTS: May contain Cetostearyl alcohol (including cetyl and stearyl alcohol)
▸ Dermol (Dermal Laboratories Ltd)
Benzalkonium chloride 1 mg per 1 gram, Chlorhexidine hydrochloride 1 mg per 1 gram, Isopropyl myristate 100 mg per 1 gram, Liquid paraffin 100 mg per 1 gram Dermol cream | 100 gram P £2.86 | 500 gram P £6.63
▸ Eczmol (Genus Pharmaceuticals Ltd)
Chlorhexidine gluconate 10 mg per 1 gram Eczmol 1% cream | 250 ml GSL £3.70

Emollient creams and ointments, colloidal oatmeal-containing

● INDICATIONS AND DOSE

Endogenous and exogenous eczema | Xeroderma | Ichthyosis
▸ TO THE SKIN
▸ Child: (consult product literature)
▸ Adult: (consult product literature)

Senile pruritus (pruritus of the elderly) associated with dry skin
▸ TO THE SKIN
▸ Elderly: (consult product literature)

● DIRECTIONS FOR ADMINISTRATION Emollients should be applied immediately after washing or bathing to maximise the effect of skin hydration. Emollient preparations contained in tubs should be removed with a clean spoon or spatula to reduce bacterial contamination of the emollient. Emollients should be applied in the direction of hair growth to reduce the risk of folliculitis.

● MEDICINAL FORMS There can be variation in the licensing of different medicines containing the same drug.

Cream and lotion
EXCIPIENTS: May contain Benzyl alcohol, cetostearyl alcohol (including cetyl and stearyl alcohol), isopropyl palmitate
▸ Aveeno (Johnson & Johnson Ltd)
Aveeno lotion | 500 ml (ACBS) £6.66
Aveeno cream | 100 ml (ACBS) £3.97 | 300 ml (ACBS) £6.80 | 500 ml (ACBS) £7.19

Emollient creams and ointments, paraffin-containing

● INDICATIONS AND DOSE

Dry skin conditions | Eczema | Psoriasis | Ichthyosis | Pruritus
▸ TO THE SKIN
▸ Adult: (consult product literature)

IMPORTANT SAFETY INFORMATION

FIRE HAZARD WITH PARAFFIN-BASED EMOLLIENTS

Emulsifying ointment *or* 50% Liquid Paraffin and 50% White Soft Paraffin Ointment in contact with dressings and clothing is easily ignited by a naked flame. The risk is greater when these preparations are applied to large areas of the body, and clothing or dressings become soaked with the ointment. Patients should be told to keep away from fire or flames, and not to smoke when using these preparations. The risk of fire should be considered when using large quantities of any paraffin-based emollient.

● DIRECTIONS FOR ADMINISTRATION Emollients should be applied immediately after washing or bathing to maximise the effect of skin hydration. Emollient preparations contained in tubs should be removed with a clean spoon or spatula to reduce bacterial contamination of the emollient. Emollients should be applied in the direction of hair growth to reduce the risk of folliculitis.

● MEDICINAL FORMS There can be variation in the licensing of different medicines containing the same drug.

Liquid
EXCIPIENTS: May contain Benzyl alcohol, cetostearyl alcohol (including cetyl and stearyl alcohol), hydroxybenzoates (parabens), isopropyl palmitate
▸ Cetraben
Cetraben lotion | 200 ml £4.00 | 500 ml £5.64
▸ E45 (Forum Health Products Ltd)
E45 lotion | 200 ml £2.40 | 500 ml £4.50
▸ QV (Crawford Healthcare Ltd)
White soft paraffin 50 mg per 1 gram QV 5% skin lotion | 250 ml £3.17 | 500 ml £5.29

13

Skin

Cream

EXCIPIENTS: May contain Benzyl alcohol, cetostearyl alcohol (including cetyl and stearyl alcohol), chlorocresol, disodium edetate, fragrances, hydroxybenzoates (parabens), polysorbates, propylene glycol, sorbic acid, lanolin

▸ Emollient creams and ointments, paraffin-containing (Non-proprietary)

Liquid paraffin light 60 mg per 1 gram, White soft paraffin 150 mg per 1 gram White soft paraffin 15% / Liquid paraffin light 6% cream | 150 gram GSL no price available DT price = £3.06 | 500 ml GSL no price available DT price = £5.28 | 1050 ml GSL no price available DT price = £9.98

▸ Aquamax (Intrapharm Laboratories Ltd)
Aquamax cream | 100 gram £1.89 | 500 gram £3.99

▸ Aquamol (Thornton & Ross Ltd)
Aquamol cream | 50 gram £1.22 | 500 gram £6.40

▸ Cetraben (Thornton & Ross Ltd)
Liquid paraffin light 105 mg per 1 gram, White soft paraffin 132 mg per 1 gram Cetraben cream | 50 gram £1.40 | 150 gram £3.98 | 500 gram £5.99 | 1050 gram £11.62

▸ Diprobase (Bayer Plc)
Diprobase cream | 50 gram GSL £1.28 | 500 gram GSL £6.32

▸ E45 (Forum Health Products Ltd)
Wool fat 10 mg per 1 gram, Liquid paraffin light 126 mg per 1 gram, White soft paraffin 145 mg per 1 gram E45 cream | 50 gram GSL £1.61 | 125 gram GSL £2.90 | 350 gram GSL £5.17 | 500 gram GSL £5.62

▸ Enopen (Ennogen Healthcare Ltd)
Liquid paraffin light 105 mg per 1 gram, White soft paraffin 132 mg per 1 gram Enopen cream | 500 gram £5.99

▸ Epaderm (Molnlycke Health Care Ltd)
Epaderm cream | 50 gram £1.70 | 500 gram £6.95

▸ Hydromol (Alliance Pharmaceuticals Ltd)
Sodium lactate 10 mg per 1 gram, Sodium pidolate 25 mg per 1 gram, Isopropyl myristate 50 mg per 1 gram, Liquid paraffin 100 mg per 1 gram Hydromol 2.5% cream | 50 gram GSL £2.19 | 100 gram GSL £4.09 | 500 gram GSL £11.92

▸ Lipobase (Astellas Pharma Ltd)
Lipobase cream | 50 gram P £1.46

▸ Oilatum (GlaxoSmithKline Consumer Healthcare)
Liquid paraffin light 60 mg per 1 gram, White soft paraffin 150 mg per 1 gram Oilatum cream | 50 gram GSL £1.67 DT price = £1.67 | 150 gram GSL £3.06 DT price = £3.06 | 500 ml GSL £5.28 DT price = £5.28 | 1050 ml GSL £9.98 DT price = £9.98

▸ Oilatum junior (GlaxoSmithKline Consumer Healthcare)
Liquid paraffin light 60 mg per 1 gram, White soft paraffin 150 mg per 1 gram Oilatum Junior cream | 150 gram GSL £3.06 DT price = £3.06 | 350 ml GSL £4.65 DT price = £4.65 | 500 ml GSL £5.28 DT price = £5.28 | 1050 ml GSL £9.98 DT price = £9.98

▸ QV (Crawford Healthcare Ltd)
White soft paraffin 50 mg per 1 gram, Glycerol 100 mg per 1 gram, Liquid paraffin light 100 mg per 1 gram QV cream | 100 gram £2.06 | 500 gram £5.92 | 1050 gram £12.05

▸ Soffen (Vitame Ltd)
Liquid paraffin light 105 mg per 1 gram, White soft paraffin 132 mg per 1 gram Soffen cream | 500 gram £4.79

▸ Unguentum M (Almirall Ltd)
Unguentum M cream | 50 gram GSL £1.41 | 60 gram GSL no price available | 100 gram GSL £2.78 | 200 ml GSL £5.50 | 500 gram GSL £8.48

▸ ZeroAQS (Thornton & Ross Ltd)
ZeroAQS emollient cream | 500 gram £3.29

▸ Zerobase (Thornton & Ross Ltd)
Liquid paraffin 110 mg per 1 gram Zerobase 11% cream | 50 gram £1.04 | 500 gram £5.26

▸ Zerocream (Thornton & Ross Ltd)
Liquid paraffin 126 mg per 1 gram, White soft paraffin 145 mg per 1 gram Zerocream | 50 gram £1.17 | 500 gram £4.08

▸ Zeroguent (Thornton & Ross Ltd)
White soft paraffin 40 mg per 1 gram, Soya oil 50 mg per 1 gram, Liquid paraffin light 80 mg per 1 gram Zeroguent cream | 100 gram £2.33 | 500 gram £6.99

Ointment

EXCIPIENTS: May contain Cetostearyl alcohol (including cetyl and stearyl alcohol), polysorbates

▸ Emollient creams and ointments, paraffin-containing (Non-proprietary)

Cetraben ointment | 125 gram £3.49 | 450 gram £5.39

Liquid paraffin 200 mg per 1 gram, Emulsifying wax 300 mg per 1 gram, White soft paraffin 500 mg per 1 gram Emulsifying ointment | 100 gram GSL £2.82 | 500 gram GSL £3.26 DT price = £1.84 | 500 gram PoM no price available DT price = £1.84

White soft paraffin 1 mg per 1 mg White soft paraffin solid | 500 gram GSL £4.18 DT price = £3.23 | 4500 gram GSL £18.62-£29.07

Liquid paraffin 500 mg per 1 gram, White soft paraffin 500 mg per 1 gram Pure Health Liquid Paraffin 50% in White Soft Paraffin ointment | 500 gram £3.66 DT price = £4.57

Bell's Emollient 50 ointment | 250 gram £1.99 | 500 gram £3.17 DT price = £4.57

The 50:50 Ointment | 500 gram P £4.57 DT price = £4.57

White soft paraffin 50% / Liquid paraffin 50% ointment | 250 gram £1.87 | 500 gram £6.80 DT price = £4.57 | 500 gram P £4.57 DT price = £4.57

Magnesium sulfate dried 5 mg per 1 gram, Phenoxyethanol 10 mg per 1 gram, Wool alcohols ointment 500 mg per 1 gram Hydrous ointment | 500 gram GSL £4.89 DT price = £4.89

Yellow soft paraffin 1 mg per 1 mg Yellow soft paraffin solid | 15 gram GSL £1.16 | 500 gram GSL £13.02 DT price = £13.27 | 4500 gram GSL £18.29

▸ Diprobase (Bayer Plc)
Liquid paraffin 50 mg per 1 gram, White soft paraffin 950 mg per 1 gram Diprobase ointment | 50 gram GSL £1.28 DT price = £1.28 | 500 gram GSL £5.99 DT price = £5.99

▸ Emelpin (Vitame Ltd)
Emulsifying wax 300 mg per 1 gram, Yellow soft paraffin 300 mg per 1 gram Emelpin ointment | 125 gram £3.08 | 500 gram £5.22

▸ Epaderm (Molnlycke Health Care Ltd)
Emulsifying wax 300 mg per 1 gram, Yellow soft paraffin 300 mg per 1 gram Epaderm ointment | 125 gram £3.85 | 500 gram £6.53 | 1000 gram £12.02

▸ Fifty:50 (Ennogen Healthcare Ltd)
Liquid paraffin 500 mg per 1 gram, White soft paraffin 500 mg per 1 gram Fifty:50 ointment | 250 gram £1.83 | 500 gram £3.66 DT price = £4.57

▸ Hydromol (Alliance Pharmaceuticals Ltd)
Emulsifying wax 300 mg per 1 gram, Yellow soft paraffin 300 mg per 1 gram Hydromol ointment | 125 gram £2.88 | 500 gram £4.89 | 1000 gram £9.09

▸ QV intensive (Crawford Healthcare Ltd)
QV Intensive ointment | 450 gram £5.71

▸ Thirty:30 (Ennogen Healthcare Ltd)
Emulsifying wax 300 mg per 1 gram, Yellow soft paraffin 300 mg per 1 gram Thirty:30 ointment | 125 gram £3.81 | 250 gram £4.29 | 500 gram £6.47

▸ Vaseline (Unilever UK Home & Personal Care)
White soft paraffin 1 mg per 1 mg Vaseline Pure Petroleum jelly | 50 ml GSL no price available | 100 ml GSL no price available | 250 ml GSL no price available

Spray

CAUTIONARY AND ADVISORY LABELS 15

▸ Dermamist (Alliance Pharmaceuticals Ltd)
White soft paraffin 100 mg per 1 gram Dermamist 10% spray | 250 ml P £5.97

▸ Emollin (C D Medical Ltd)
Emollin aerosol spray | 150 ml £4.00 | 240 ml £6.39

Emollients, urea-containing

● DRUG ACTION Urea is a keratin softener and hydrating agent used in the treatment of dry, scaling conditions (including ichthyosis) and may be useful in elderly patients.

● INDICATIONS AND DOSE

AQUADRATE®

Dry, scaling, and itching skin
▸ TO THE SKIN
▸ Child: Apply twice daily, to be applied thinly
▸ Adult: Apply twice daily, to be applied thinly

13

Skin

BALNEUM® CREAM

Dry skin conditions
▸ TO THE SKIN
▸ Child: Apply twice daily
▸ Adult: Apply twice daily

BALNEUM® PLUS CREAM

Dry, scaling, and itching skin
▸ TO THE SKIN
▸ Child: Apply twice daily
▸ Adult: Apply twice daily

CALMURID®

Dry, scaling, and itching skin
▸ TO THE SKIN
▸ Child: Apply twice daily, apply a thick layer for 3–5 minutes, massage into area, and remove excess. Can be diluted with aqueous cream (life of diluted cream is 14 days). Half-strength cream can be used for 1 week if stinging occurs
▸ Adult: Apply twice daily, apply a thick layer for 3–5 minutes, massage into area, and remove excess. Can be diluted with aqueous cream (life of diluted cream is 14 days). Half-strength cream can be used for 1 week if stinging occurs

DERMATONICS ONCE HEEL BALM®

Dry skin on soles of feet
▸ TO THE SKIN
▸ Child 12–17 years: Apply once daily
▸ Adult: Apply once daily

E45® ITCH RELIEF CREAM

Dry, scaling, and itching skin
▸ TO THE SKIN
▸ Child: Apply twice daily
▸ Adult: Apply twice daily

EUCERIN® INTENSIVE CREAM

Dry skin conditions including eczema, ichthyosis, xeroderma, and hyperkeratosis
▸ TO THE SKIN
▸ Child: Apply twice daily, to be applied thinly and rubbed into area
▸ Adult: Apply twice daily, to be applied thinly and rubbed into area

EUCERIN® INTENSIVE LOTION

Dry skin conditions including eczema, ichthyosis, xeroderma, and hyperkeratosis
▸ TO THE SKIN
▸ Child: Apply twice daily, to be applied sparingly and rubbed into area
▸ Adult: Apply twice daily, to be applied sparingly and rubbed into area

FLEXITOL®

Dry skin on soles of feet and heels
▸ TO THE SKIN
▸ Child 12–17 years: Apply 1–2 times a day
▸ Adult: Apply 1–2 times a day

HYDROMOL® INTENSIVE

Dry, scaling, and itching skin
▸ TO THE SKIN
▸ Child: Apply twice daily, to be applied thinly
▸ Adult: Apply twice daily, to be applied thinly

IMUDERM® EMOLLIENT

Dry skin conditions including eczema, psoriasis or dermatitis
▸ TO THE SKIN
▸ Adult: Apply to skin or use as a soap substitute

NUTRAPLUS®

Dry, scaling, and itching skin
▸ TO THE SKIN
▸ Child: Apply 2–3 times a day
▸ Adult: Apply 2–3 times a day

● DIRECTIONS FOR ADMINISTRATION Emollients should be applied immediately after washing or bathing to maximise the effect of skin hydration. Emollient preparations contained in tubs should be removed with a clean spoon or spatula to reduce bacterial contamination of the emollient. Emollients should be applied in the direction of hair growth to reduce the risk of folliculitis.

● MEDICINAL FORMS
There can be variation in the licensing of different medicines containing the same drug.

Liquid
EXCIPIENTS: May contain Benzyl alcohol, isopropyl palmitate
▸ Eucerin (Beiersdorf UK Ltd)
 Urea 100 mg per 1 gram Eucerin Intensive 10% lotion | 250 ml [GSL] £7.93

Cream
EXCIPIENTS: May contain Benzyl alcohol, cetostearyl alcohol (including cetyl and stearyl alcohol), hydroxybenzoates (parabens), isopropyl palmitate, polysorbates, propylene glycol, wool fat and related substances including lanolin
▸ Emollients, urea-containing (Non-proprietary)
 Lauromacrogols 30 mg per 1 gram, Urea 50 mg per 1 gram Urea 5% / Lauromacrogols 3% cream | 500 gram [GSL] no price available
 Urea 100 mg per 1 gram Urea 10% cream | 100 gram [P] no price available
▸ Aquadrate (Alliance Pharmaceuticals Ltd)
 Urea 100 mg per 1 gram Aquadrate 10% cream | 100 gram [P] £4.37
▸ Balneum (Almirall Ltd)
 Balneum cream | 50 gram £2.85 | 500 gram £9.97
▸ Balneum Plus (Almirall Ltd)
 Lauromacrogols 30 mg per 1 gram, Urea 50 mg per 1 gram Balneum Plus cream | 100 gram [GSL] £3.29 | 500 gram [GSL] £14.99
▸ Calmurid (Galderma (UK) Ltd)
 Lactic acid 50 mg per 1 gram, Urea 100 mg per 1 gram Calmurid cream | 100 gram [P] £5.75 DT price = £5.75 | 500 gram [P] £33.40 DT price = £33.40
▸ E45 Itch Relief (Forum Health Products Ltd)
 Lauromacrogols 30 mg per 1 gram, Urea 50 mg per 1 gram E45 Itch Relief cream | 50 gram [GSL] £2.81 | 100 gram [GSL] £3.74 | 500 gram [GSL] £14.99
▸ Eucerin (Beiersdorf UK Ltd)
 Urea 100 mg per 1 gram Eucerin Intensive 10% cream | 100 ml [GSL] £7.59
▸ Hydromol Intensive (Alliance Pharmaceuticals Ltd)
 Urea 100 mg per 1 gram Hydromol Intensive 10% cream | 30 gram [P] £1.64 | 100 gram [P] £4.37
▸ Nutraplus (Galderma (UK) Ltd)
 Urea 100 mg per 1 gram Nutraplus 10% cream | 100 gram [P] £4.37

Balms
EXCIPIENTS: May contain Beeswax, benzyl alcohol, cetostearyl alcohol (including cetyl and stearyl alcohol), fragrances, lanolin
▸ Emollients, urea-containing (Non-proprietary)
 imuDERM emollient | 500 gram £6.50
▸ Dermatonics once (Dermatonics Ltd)
 Dermatonics Once Heel Balm | 75 ml £3.60 | 200 ml £8.50
▸ Flexitol (Thornton & Ross Ltd)
 Flexitol Heel Balm | 40 gram £2.75 | 56 gram no price available | 75 gram £3.80 | 112 gram no price available | 200 gram £9.40 | 500 gram £14.75

13

Skin

2 Infections of the skin

Skin infections

Antibacterial preparations

Cellulitis, a rapidly spreading deeply seated inflammation of the skin and subcutaneous tissue, requires systemic antibacterial treatment. Lower leg infections or infections spreading around wounds are almost always cellulitis. *Erysipelas*, a superficial infection with clearly defined edges (and often affecting the face), is also treated with a systemic antibacterial.

In the community, acute *impetigo* on small areas of the skin may be treated by short-term topical application of fusidic acid p. 519; mupirocin p. 1076 should be used only to treat meticillin-resistant *Staphylococcus aureus*. If the impetigo is extensive or longstanding, an oral antibacterial such as flucloxacillin p. 503 (or clarithromycin p. 487 in penicillin allergy) should be used. Mild antiseptics can be used to soften crusts.

Although many antibacterial drugs are available in topical preparations, some are potentially hazardous and frequently their use is not necessary if adequate hygienic measures can be taken. Moreover, not all skin conditions that are oozing, crusted, or characterised by pustules are actually infected. Topical antibacterials should be **avoided** on *leg ulcers* unless used in short courses for defined infections; treatment of bacterial colonisation is generally inappropriate.

To minimise the development of resistant organisms it is advisable to limit the choice of antibacterials applied topically to those not used systemically. Unfortunately some of these, for example neomycin sulfate p. 1074, may cause sensitisation, and there is cross-sensitivity with other aminoglycoside antibiotics, such as gentamicin p. 471. If *large areas of skin* are being treated, ototoxicity may also be a hazard with aminoglycoside antibiotics (and also with polymyxins p. 1075), particularly in children, in the elderly, and in those with renal impairment. *Resistant organisms* are more common in hospitals, and whenever possible swabs should be taken for bacteriological examination before beginning treatment.

Mupirocin is not related to any other antibacterial in use; it is effective for skin infections, particularly those due to Gram-positive organisms but it is not indicated for pseudomonal infection. Although *Staphylococcus aureus* strains with low-level resistance to mupirocin are emerging, it is generally useful in infections resistant to other antibacterials. To avoid the development of resistance, mupirocin or fusidic acid should not be used for longer than 10 days and local microbiology advice should be sought before using it in hospital. In the presence of mupirocin-resistant MRSA infection, a topical antiseptic such as povidone-iodine p. 1119, chlorhexidine p. 1120, or alcohol can be used; their use should be discussed with the local microbiologist.

Retapamulin p. 1076 can be used for impetigo and other superficial bacterial skin infections caused by *Staphylococcus aureus* and *Streptococcus pyogenes* that are resistant to first-line topical antibacterials. However, it is not effective against MRSA.

Silver sulfadiazine p. 1075 is used in the treatment of infected burns.

Antibacterial preparations also used systemically

Fusidic acid is a narrow-spectrum antibacterial used for staphylococcal infections. Fusidic acid has a role in the treatment of impetigo.

An ointment containing fusidic acid is used in the fissures of angular cheilitis when associated with staphylococcal

infection. See Oropharyngeal fungal infections p. 1060 for further information on angular cheilitis.

Metronidazole p. 1074 is used topically for rosacea and to reduce the odour associated with anaerobic infections; oral metronidazole is used to treat wounds infected with anaerobic bacteria.

Antifungal preparations

Most localised fungal infections are treated with topical preparations. To prevent relapse, local antifungal treatment should be continued for 1–2 weeks after the disappearance of all signs of infection. Systemic therapy is necessary for scalp infection or if the skin infection is widespread, disseminated, or intractable; although topical therapy may be used to treat some nail infections, systemic therapy is more effective. Skin scrapings should be examined if systemic therapy is being considered or where there is doubt about the diagnosis.

Dermatophytoses

Ringworm infection can affect the scalp (tinea capitis), body (tinea corporis), groin (tinea cruris), hand (tinea manuum), foot (tinea pedis, athlete's foot), or nail (tinea unguium). Scalp infection requires systemic treatment; additional application of a topical antifungal, during the early stages of treatment, may reduce the risk of transmission. A topical antifungal can also be used to treat asymptomatic carriers of scalp ringworm. Most other local ringworm infections can be treated adequately with topical antifungal preparations (including shampoos). The imidazole antifungals clotrimazole p. 1076, econazole nitrate p. 1076, ketoconazole p. 1077, and miconazole p. 1077 are all effective. Terbinafine cream p. 1079 is also effective but it is more expensive. Other topical antifungals include griseofulvin p. 1078 and the **undecenoates**. **Compound benzoic acid ointment** (Whitfield's ointment) has been used for ringworm infections but it is cosmetically less acceptable than proprietary preparations. Topical preparations for athlete's foot containing **tolnaftate** are on sale to the public.

Antifungal dusting powders are of little therapeutic value in the treatment of fungal skin infections and may cause skin irritation; they may have some role in preventing re-infection.

Antifungal treatment may not be necessary in asymptomatic patients with tinea infection of the nails. If treatment is necessary, a systemic antifungal is more effective than topical therapy. However, topical application of amorolfine p. 1078 or tioconazole p. 1078 may be useful for treating early onychomycosis when involvement is limited to mild distal disease, or for superficial white onychomycosis, or where there are contra-indications to systemic therapy.

Pityriasis versicolor

Pityriasis (tinea) versicolor can be treated with ketoconazole shampoo. Alternatively, **selenium sulfide** shampoo [unlicensed indication] can be used as a lotion (diluting with a small amount of water can reduce irritation) and left on the affected area for 10 minutes before rinsing off; it should be applied once daily for 7 days, and the course repeated if necessary.

Topical imidazole antifungals such as clotrimazole, econazole nitrate, ketoconazole, and miconazole, or topical terbinafine are alternatives, but large quantities may be required.

If topical therapy fails, or if the infection is widespread, pityriasis versicolor is treated systemically with a triazole antifungal. Relapse is common, especially in the immunocompromised.

Candidiasis

Candidal skin infections can be treated with a topical imidazole antifungal, such as clotrimazole, econazole nitrate, ketoconazole, or miconazole; topical terbinafine is an alternative. Topical application of nystatin p. 1062 is also effective for candidiasis but it is ineffective against dermatophytosis. Refractory candidiasis requires systemic treatment generally with a triazole such as fluconazole p. 540; systemic treatment with terbinafine is **not appropriate** for refractory candidiasis.

Angular cheilitis

Miconazole cream is used in the fissures of angular cheilitis when associated with *Candida*.

Compound topical preparations

Combination of an imidazole and a mild corticosteroid (such as hydrocortisone 1%) p. 1092 may be of value in the treatment of eczematous intertrigo and, in the first few days only, of a severely inflamed patch of ringworm.

Combination of a mild corticosteroid with either an imidazole or nystatin p. 1062 may be of use in the treatment of intertrigo associated with candida.

Antiviral preparations

Aciclovir p. 1082 cream is licensed for the treatment of initial and recurrent labial and genital *herpes simplex infections*; treatment should begin as early as possible. Systemic treatment is necessary for buccal or vaginal infections and for *herpes zoster* (shingles).

Herpes labialis

Aciclovir cream can be used for the treatment of initial and recurrent labial herpes simplex infections (cold sores). It is best applied at the earliest possible stage, usually when prodromal changes of sensation are felt in the lip and before vesicles appear.

Penciclovir cream is also licensed for the treatment of herpes labialis; it needs to be applied more frequently than aciclovir cream.

Systemic treatment is necessary if cold sores recur frequently or for infections in the mouth.

Parasiticidal preparations

Suitable quantities of parasiticidal preparations

Area of body	Skin creams	Lotions	Cream rinses
Scalp (head lice)		50–100 mL	50–100 mL
Body (scabies)	30–60 g	100 mL	
Body (crab lice)	30–60 g	100 mL	

These amounts are usually suitable for an adult for single application.

Scabies

Permethrin p. 1082 is used for the treatment of *scabies* (*Sarcoptes scabiei*); malathion p. 1081 can be used if permethrin is inappropriate.

Benzyl benzoate p. 1081 is an irritant and should be avoided in children; it is less effective than malathion and permethrin.

Ivermectin p. 549 (available on a named patient basis from 'special-order' manufacturers or specialist importing companies) by mouth has been used, in combination with topical drugs, for the treatment of hyperkeratotic (crusted or 'Norwegian') scabies that does not respond to topical treatment alone; further doses may be required.

Application

Although acaricides have traditionally been applied after a hot bath, this is **not** necessary and there is even evidence that a hot bath may increase absorption into the blood, removing them from their site of action on the skin.

All members of the affected household should be treated simultaneously. Treatment should be applied to the whole body including the scalp, neck, face, and ears. Particular

attention should be paid to the webs of the fingers and toes and lotion brushed under the ends of nails. It is now recommended that malathion and permethrin should be applied twice, one week apart; in the case of benzyl benzoate in adults, up to 3 applications on consecutive days may be needed. It is important to warn users to reapply treatment to the hands if they are washed. Patients with hyperkeratotic scabies may require 2 or 3 applications of acaricide on consecutive days to ensure that enough penetrates the skin crusts to kill all the mites.

Itching

The *itch* and *eczema* of scabies persists for some weeks after the infestation has been eliminated and treatment for pruritus and eczema may be required. Application of crotamiton p. 1109 can be used to control itching after treatment with more effective acaricides. A topical corticosteroid may help to reduce itch and inflammation after scabies has been treated successfully; however, persistent symptoms suggest that scabies eradication was not successful. Oral administration of a **sedating antihistamine** at night may also be useful.

Head lice

Dimeticone p. 1081 is effective against head lice (*Pediculus humanus capitis*). It coats head lice and interferes with water balance in lice by preventing the excretion of water; it is less active against eggs and treatment should be repeated after 7 days. Malathion, an organophosphorus insecticide, is an alternative, but resistance has been reported. Benzyl benzoate is licensed for the treatment of head lice but it is less effective than other drugs and not recommended for use in children. Permethrin is active against head lice but the formulation and licensed methods of application of the current products make them unsuitable for the treatment of head lice.

Head lice infestation (pediculosis) should be treated using lotion or liquid formulations only if live lice are present. Shampoos are diluted too much in use to be effective. A contact time of 8–12 hours or overnight treatment is recommended for lotions and liquids; a 2-hour treatment is not sufficient to kill eggs.

In general, a course of treatment for head lice should be 2 applications of product 7 days apart to kill lice emerging from any eggs that survive the first application. All affected household members should be treated simultaneously.

Wet combing methods

Head lice can be mechanically removed by combing wet hair meticulously with a plastic detection comb (probably for at least 30 minutes each time) over the whole scalp at 4-day intervals for a minimum of 2 weeks, and continued until no lice are found on 3 consecutive sessions; hair conditioner or vegetable oil can be used to facilitate the process.

Several devices for the removal of head lice such as combs and topical solutions, are available and some are prescribable on the NHS.

The Drug Tariffs can be accessed online at:

- National Health Service Drug Tariff for England and Wales: www.ppa.org.uk/ppa/edt_intro.htm
- Health and Personal Social Services for Northern Ireland Drug Tariff: www.dhsspsni.gov.uk/pas-tariff
- Scottish Drug Tariff: www.isdscotland.org/Health-topics/ Prescribing-and-Medicines/Scottish-Drug-Tariff/

Crab lice

Permethrin and malathion are used to eliminate *crab lice* (*Pthirus pubis*). An aqueous preparation should be applied, allowed to dry naturally and washed off after 12 hours; a second treatment is needed after 7 days to kill lice emerging from surviving eggs. All surfaces of the body should be treated, including the scalp, neck, and face (paying particular attention to the eyebrows and other facial hair). A different insecticide should be used if a course of treatment fails.

13

Skin

2.1 Bacterial skin infections

ANTIBACTERIALS > AMINOGLYCOSIDES

Neomycin sulfate

- **INDICATIONS AND DOSE**

Bacterial skin infections

‣ TO THE SKIN

‣ Child: Apply up to 3 times a day, for short-term use only

‣ Adult: Apply up to 3 times a day, for short-term use only

- **UNLICENSED USE**
‣ With topical use in children *Neomycin Cream BPC*—no information available.
- **CONTRA-INDICATIONS**
‣ With topical use Neonates
- **CAUTIONS**

CAUTIONS, FURTHER INFORMATION

If large areas of skin are being treated ototoxicity may be a hazard, particularly in children, the elderly, and in those with renal impairment.

- **INTERACTIONS** → Appendix 1 (aminoglycosides).
- **SIDE-EFFECTS** Sensitisation (cross sensitivity with other aminoglycosides may occur)
- **RENAL IMPAIRMENT** Ototoxicity may be a hazard if large areas of skin are treated.
- **LESS SUITABLE FOR PRESCRIBING** Neomycin sulfate cream is less suitable for prescribing.
- **MEDICINAL FORMS**
There can be variation in the licensing of different medicines containing the same drug. Forms available from special-order manufacturers include: cream

ANTIBACTERIALS > NITROIMIDAZOLE DERIVATIVES

Metronidazole

- **DRUG ACTION** Metronidazole is an antimicrobial drug with high activity against anaerobic bacteria and protozoa.

- **INDICATIONS AND DOSE**

ACEA®

Acute inflammatory exacerbation of rosacea

‣ TO THE SKIN

‣ Adult: Apply twice daily for 8 weeks, to be applied thinly

ANABACT®

Malodorous fungating tumours and malodorous gravitational and decubitus ulcers

‣ TO THE SKIN

‣ Adult: Apply 1–2 times a day, to be applied to clean wound and covered with non-adherent dressing

METROGEL®

Acute inflammatory exacerbation of rosacea

‣ TO THE SKIN

‣ Adult: Apply twice daily for 8–9 weeks, to be applied thinly

Malodorous fungating tumours

‣ TO THE SKIN

‣ Adult: Apply 1–2 times a day, to be applied to clean wound and covered with non-adherent dressing

METROSA®

Acute exacerbation of rosacea

‣ TO THE SKIN

‣ Adult: Apply twice daily for up to 8 weeks, to be applied thinly

ROSICED®

Inflammatory papules and pustules of rosacea

‣ TO THE SKIN

‣ Adult: Apply twice daily for 6 weeks (longer if necessary)

ROZEX® CREAM

Inflammatory papules, pustules and erythema of rosacea

‣ TO THE SKIN

‣ Adult: Apply twice daily for 3–4 months

ROZEX® GEL

Inflammatory papules, pustules and erythema of rosacea

‣ TO THE SKIN

‣ Adult: Apply twice daily for 3–4 months

ZYOMET®

Acute inflammatory exacerbation of rosacea

‣ TO THE SKIN

‣ Adult: Apply twice daily for 8–9 weeks, to be applied thinly

- **CAUTIONS** Avoid exposure to strong sunlight or UV light
- **SIDE-EFFECTS** Skin irritation

- **MEDICINAL FORMS**
There can be variation in the licensing of different medicines containing the same drug. Forms available from special-order manufacturers include: cream, gel

Cream

EXCIPIENTS: May contain Benzyl alcohol, isopropyl palmitate, propylene glycol

‣ Rosiced (Pierre Fabre Dermo-Cosmetique)
Metronidazole 7.5 mg per 1 gram Rosiced 0.75% cream | 30 gram [PoM] £7.50 DT price = £6.60

‣ Rozex (Galderma (UK) Ltd)
Metronidazole 7.5 mg per 1 gram Rozex 0.75% cream | 30 gram [PoM] £6.60 DT price = £6.60 | 40 gram [PoM] £9.88 DT price = £9.88

Gel

EXCIPIENTS: May contain Benzyl alcohol, disodium edetate, hydroxybenzoates (parabens), propylene glycol

‣ Acea (Ferndale Pharmaceuticals Ltd)
Metronidazole 7.5 mg per 1 gram Acea 0.75% gel | 40 gram [PoM] £9.95

‣ Anabact (Cambridge Healthcare Supplies Ltd)
Metronidazole 7.5 mg per 1 gram Anabact 0.75% gel | 15 gram [PoM] £4.47 | 30 gram [PoM] £7.89

‣ Metrogel (Galderma (UK) Ltd)
Metronidazole 7.5 mg per 1 gram Metrogel 0.75% gel | 40 gram [PoM] £22.63

‣ Metrosa (M & A Pharmachem Ltd)
Metronidazole 7.5 mg per 1 gram Metrosa 0.75% gel | 30 gram [PoM] £12.00 | 40 gram [PoM] £19.90

‣ Rozex (Galderma (UK) Ltd)
Metronidazole 7.5 mg per 1 gram Rozex 0.75% gel | 30 gram [PoM] £6.60 | 40 gram [PoM] £9.88

‣ Zyomet (AMCo)
Metronidazole 7.5 mg per 1 gram Zyomet 0.75% gel | 30 gram [PoM] £12.00

ANTIBACTERIALS > POLYMYXINS

Polymyxins

- **INDICATIONS AND DOSE**

Bacterial skin infections
▸ TO THE SKIN
▸ Adult: Apply twice daily, may be applied more
  frequently if required

- **CAUTIONS**

CAUTIONS, FURTHER INFORMATION
▸ Large areas If large areas of skin are being treated
  nephrotoxicity and neurotoxicity may be a hazard,
  particularly in children, in the elderly, and in those with
  renal impairment.

- **SIDE-EFFECTS** Sensitisation

- **MEDICINAL FORMS**
  There can be variation in the licensing of different medicines
  containing the same drug.
  No licensed medicines listed.

ANTIBACTERIALS > SULFONAMIDES

Silver sulfadiazine

- **INDICATIONS AND DOSE**

Prophylaxis and treatment of infection in burn wounds
▸ TO THE SKIN
▸ Child: Apply daily, may be applied more frequently if
  very exudative
▸ Adult: Apply daily, may be applied more frequently if
  very exudative

For conservative management of finger-tip injuries
▸ TO THE SKIN
▸ Child: Apply every 2–3 days, consult product literature
  for details
▸ Adult: Apply every 2–3 days, consult product literature
  for details

**Adjunct to prophylaxis of infection in skin graft donor
sites and extensive abrasions**
▸ TO THE SKIN
▸ Adult: (consult product literature)

**Adjunct to short-term treatment of infection in pressure
sores**
▸ TO THE SKIN
▸ Adult: Apply once daily or on alternate days

**As an adjunct to short-term treatment of infection in leg
ulcers**
▸ TO THE SKIN
▸ Adult: Apply once daily or on alternate days, not
  recommended if ulcer is very exudative

- **UNLICENSED USE**
▸ With topical use in children No age range specified by
  manufacturer.
- **CONTRA-INDICATIONS** Not recommended for neonates
- **CAUTIONS** G6PD deficiency
  CAUTIONS, FURTHER INFORMATION
  Plasma-sulfadiazine concentrations may approach
  therapeutic levels with *side-effects* and *interactions* as for
  sulfonamides if large areas of skin are treated.
- **INTERACTIONS** → Appendix 1 (sulfonamides)—if large
  amounts given.
  May inactivate enzymatic debriding agents—concomitant
  use may be inappropriate.
- **SIDE-EFFECTS** Allergic reactions · argyria (following
  treatment of large areas of skin or prolonged use) · burning
  · itching · leucopenia · rashes

SIDE-EFFECTS, FURTHER INFORMATION
▸ Severe blood and skin disorders Owing to the association of
  sulfonamides with severe blood and skin disorders,
  treatment should be stopped immediately if blood
  disorders or rashes develop.
      Leucopenia developing 2–3 days after starting treatment
  of burns patients is reported usually to be self-limiting and
  silver sulfadiazine need not usually be discontinued
  provided blood counts are monitored carefully to ensure
  return to normality within a few days.

- **ALLERGY AND CROSS-SENSITIVITY** Contra-indicated in
  patients with sensitivity to sulfonamides.
- **PREGNANCY** Risk of neonatal haemolysis and
  methaemoglobinaemia in third trimester.
- **BREAST FEEDING** Small risk of kernicterus in jaundiced
  infants and of haemolysis in G6PD-deficient infants.
- **HEPATIC IMPAIRMENT** Manufacturer advises caution if
  significant impairment.
- **RENAL IMPAIRMENT** Manufacturer advises caution if
  significant impairment.
- **MONITORING REQUIREMENTS** Monitor for leucopenia.
- **DIRECTIONS FOR ADMINISTRATION** Apply with sterile
  applicator.
- **MEDICINAL FORMS**
  There can be variation in the licensing of different medicines
  containing the same drug.
  Cream
  EXCIPIENTS: May contain Cetostearyl alcohol (including cetyl and
  stearyl alcohol), polysorbates, propylene glycol
  ▸ Flamazine (Smith & Nephew Healthcare Ltd)
    Sulfadiazine silver 10 mg per 1 gram Flamazine 1% cream |
    20 gram [PoM] £2.91 | 50 gram [PoM] £3.85 DT price = £3.85 |
    250 gram [PoM] £10.32 DT price = £10.32 | 500 gram [PoM] £18.27 DT
    price = £18.27

ANTIBACTERIALS > OTHER

Bacitracin with polymyxin B

- **INDICATIONS AND DOSE**

Bacterial skin infections
▸ TO THE SKIN
▸ Child: Apply twice daily, can be applied more
  frequently if required
▸ Adult: Apply twice daily, can be applied more
  frequently if required

- **UNLICENSED USE**
▸ With topical use in children Licensed for use in children (age
  range not specified by manufacturer).
- **CAUTIONS** Nephrotoxicity · neurotoxicity
  CAUTIONS, FURTHER INFORMATION
  If large areas of skin are being treated nephrotoxicity and
  neurotoxicity may be a hazard, particularly in children
  with renal impairment.
- **SIDE-EFFECTS** Contact sensitisation
- **RENAL IMPAIRMENT** Renal impairment increases the risk
  of nephrotoxicity and neurotoxicity.

- **MEDICINAL FORMS**
  There can be variation in the licensing of different medicines
  containing the same drug.
  Ointment
  ▸ Polyfax (Teva UK Ltd)
    **Bacitracin zinc 500 unit per 1 gram, Polymyxin B sulfate
    10000 unit per 1 gram** Polyfax ointment | 4 gram [PoM] £3.26 |
    20 gram [PoM] £4.62 DT price = £4.62

Mupirocin

- **INDICATIONS AND DOSE**

Bacterial skin infections, particularly those caused by Gram-positive organisms (except pseudomonal infection)
- ▶ TO THE SKIN
- ▶ Child: Apply up to 3 times a day for up to 10 days
- ▶ Adult: Apply up to 3 times a day for up to 10 days

- **UNLICENSED USE**
- ▶ With topical use in children Mupirocin ointment is licensed for use in children (age range not specified by manufacturer). *Bactroban* ® cream not recommended for use in children under 1 year.
- **SIDE-EFFECTS** Burning sensation · local reactions · pruritus · rash · urticaria
- **PREGNANCY** Manufacturer advises avoid unless potential benefit outweighs risk—no information available.
- **BREAST FEEDING** No information available.
- **RENAL IMPAIRMENT** Manufacturer advises caution when mupirocin ointment used in moderate or severe impairment because it contains macrogols (polyethylene glycol).

- **MEDICINAL FORMS**
There can be variation in the licensing of different medicines containing the same drug.
Cream
EXCIPIENTS: May contain Benzyl alcohol, cetostearyl alcohol (including cetyl and stearyl alcohol)
- ▶ Bactroban (GlaxoSmithKline UK Ltd)
  Mupirocin (as Mupirocin calcium) 20 mg per 1 gram Bactroban 2% cream | 15 gram PoM £5.26 DT price = £5.26
Ointment
- ▶ Mupirocin (Non-proprietary)
  Mupirocin 20 mg per 1 gram Mupirocin 2% ointment | 15 gram PoM £9.50 DT price = £4.38
- ▶ Bactroban (GlaxoSmithKline UK Ltd)
  Mupirocin 20 mg per 1 gram Bactroban 2% ointment | 15 gram PoM £4.38 DT price = £4.38

Retapamulin

- **INDICATIONS AND DOSE**

Superficial bacterial skin infection caused by *Staphylococcus aureus* and *Streptococcus pyogenes* (if resistant to first line topical antibacterials)
- ▶ TO THE SKIN
- ▶ Child 9 months-17 years: Apply twice daily for 5 days, to be applied thinly, maximum area of skin treated 2% of body surface area, review treatment if no response within 2–3 days
- ▶ Adult: Apply twice daily for 5 days, to be applied thinly, maximum area of skin treated 100 cm^2 or lesion length 10 cm, review treatment if no response within 2–3 days

- **CONTRA-INDICATIONS** Contact with eyes · contact with mucous membranes
- **SIDE-EFFECTS** Contact dermatitis · localised erythema · localised irritation · localised pain · pruritus
- **NATIONAL FUNDING/ACCESS DECISIONS**

Scottish Medicines Consortium (SMC) Decisions
The *Scottish Medicines Consortium* has advised (March 2008) that retapamulin (*Altargo* ®) is **not** recommended for use within NHS Scotland for the treatment of superficial skin infections.

- **MEDICINAL FORMS**
There can be variation in the licensing of different medicines containing the same drug.
Ointment
CAUTIONARY AND ADVISORY LABELS 28
EXCIPIENTS: May contain Butylated hydroxytoluene
- ▶ Altargo (GlaxoSmithKline UK Ltd)
  Retapamulin 10 mg per 1 gram Altargo 10mg/g ointment | 5 gram PoM £7.89

2.2 Fungal skin infections

ANTIFUNGALS 〉 IMIDAZOLE ANTIFUNGALS

Clotrimazole

- **INDICATIONS AND DOSE**

Fungal skin infections
- ▶ TO THE SKIN
- ▶ Child: Apply 2–3 times a day
- ▶ Adult: Apply 2–3 times a day

- **CAUTIONS** Contact with eyes and mucous membranes should be avoided
- **SIDE-EFFECTS** Local irritation · erythema · hypersensitivity reactions · itching · mild burning sensation
  SIDE-EFFECTS, FURTHER INFORMATION
  Treatment should be discontinued if side-effects are severe.
- **PREGNANCY** Minimal absorption from skin; not known to be harmful.
- **PRESCRIBING AND DISPENSING INFORMATION** Spray may be useful for application of clotrimazole to large or hairy areas of the skin.

- **MEDICINAL FORMS**
There can be variation in the licensing of different medicines containing the same drug. Forms available from special-order manufacturers include: powder
Liquid
- ▶ Canesten (clotrimazole) (Bayer Plc)
  Clotrimazole 10 mg per 1 ml Canesten 1% solution | 20 ml P £2.30 DT price = £2.30
Cream
EXCIPIENTS: May contain Benzyl alcohol, cetostearyl alcohol (including cetyl and stearyl alcohol), polysorbates
- ▶ Clotrimazole (Non-proprietary)
  Clotrimazole 10 mg per 1 gram Clotrimazole 1% cream | 20 gram P £2.79 DT price = £1.04 | 50 gram P £5.45 DT price = £2.60
- ▶ Canesten (clotrimazole) (Bayer Plc)
  Clotrimazole 10 mg per 1 gram Canesten 1% cream | 20 gram P £2.14 DT price = £1.04 | 50 gram P £3.50 DT price = £2.60
  Canesten Antifungal 1% cream | 20 gram P £1.85 DT price = £1.04

Combinations available: *Hydrocortisone with clotrimazole*, p. 1097

Econazole nitrate

- **INDICATIONS AND DOSE**
Fungal skin infections
- ▶ TO THE SKIN
- ▶ Child: Apply twice daily
- ▶ Adult: Apply twice daily
Fungal nail infections
- ▶ BY TRANSUNGUAL APPLICATION
- ▶ Child: Apply once daily, applied under occlusive dressing
- ▶ Adult: Apply once daily, applied under occlusive dressing

- CAUTIONS Avoid contact with eyes and mucous membranes
- SIDE-EFFECTS Burning sensation · erythema · hypersensitivity reactions · itching · occasional local irritation

SIDE-EFFECTS, FURTHER INFORMATION
Treatment should be discontinued if side-effects are severe.

- PREGNANCY Minimal absorption from skin; not known to be harmful.

- MEDICINAL FORMS
There can be variation in the licensing of different medicines containing the same drug.
Cream
EXCIPIENTS: May contain Butylated hydroxyanisole, fragrances
▸ Pevaryl (Janssen-Cilag Ltd)
   Econazole nitrate 10 mg per 1 gram Pevaryl 1% cream | 30 gram P £3.71

Ketoconazole

- INDICATIONS AND DOSE
Tinea pedis
▸ TO THE SKIN USING CREAM
▸ Adult: Apply twice daily
Fungal skin infection (not Tinea pedis)
▸ TO THE SKIN USING CREAM
▸ Adult: Apply 1–2 times a day
Treatment of seborrhoeic dermatitis and dandruff
▸ TO THE SKIN USING SHAMPOO
▸ Child 12-17 years: Apply twice weekly for 2–4 weeks, leave preparation on for 3–5 minutes before rinsing
▸ Adult: Apply twice weekly for 2–4 weeks, leave preparation on for 3–5 minutes before rinsing
Prophylaxis of seborrhoeic dermatitis and dandruff
▸ TO THE SKIN USING SHAMPOO
▸ Child 12-17 years: Apply every 1–2 weeks, leave preparation on for 3–5 minutes before rinsing
▸ Adult: Apply every 1–2 weeks, leave preparation on for 3–5 minutes before rinsing
Treatment of pityriasis versicolor
▸ TO THE SKIN USING SHAMPOO
▸ Child 12-17 years: Apply once daily for maximum 5 days, leave preparation on for 3–5 minutes before rinsing
▸ Adult: Apply once daily for maximum 5 days, leave preparation on for 3–5 minutes before rinsing
Prophylaxis of pityriasis versicolor
▸ TO THE SKIN USING SHAMPOO
▸ Child 12-17 years: Apply once daily for up to 3 days before sun exposure, leave preparation on for 3–5 minutes before rinsing
▸ Adult: Apply once daily for up to 3 days before sun exposure, leave preparation on for 3–5 minutes before rinsing

- CAUTIONS Avoid contact with eyes · avoid contact with mucous membranes
- INTERACTIONS → Appendix 1 (antifungals, imidazole).
- SIDE-EFFECTS Erythema · hypersensitivity reactions · itching · mild burning sensation · occasional local irritation
SIDE-EFFECTS, FURTHER INFORMATION
Treatment should be discontinued if side-effects are severe.
- NATIONAL FUNDING/ACCESS DECISIONS
NHS restrictions Ketoconazole cream is not prescribable on the NHS except for seborrhoeic dermatitis and pityriasis versicolor and endorsed 'SLS'.

- EXCEPTIONS TO LEGAL CATEGORY
▸ With topical use for Fungal skin infections in adults A 15-g tube is available for sale to the public for the treatment of tinea pedis, tinea cruris, and candidal intertrigo.
▸ With topical use for Seborrhoeic dermatitis and dandruff Can be sold to the public for the prevention and treatment of dandruff and seborrhoeic dermatitis of the scalp as a shampoo formulation containing ketoconazole maximum 2%, in a pack containing maximum 120 mL and labelled to show a maximum frequency of application of once every 3 days.

- MEDICINAL FORMS
There can be variation in the licensing of different medicines containing the same drug.
Cream
EXCIPIENTS: May contain Cetostearyl alcohol (including cetyl and stearyl alcohol), polysorbates, propylene glycol
▸ Daktarin Gold (McNeil Products Ltd)
   Ketoconazole 20 mg per 1 gram Daktarin Gold 2% cream | 15 gram P £3.16
▸ Daktarin Intensiv (McNeil Products Ltd)
   Ketoconazole 20 mg per 1 gram Daktarin Intensiv 2% cream | 15 gram GSL £3.16
▸ Nizoral (Janssen-Cilag Ltd)
   Ketoconazole 20 mg per 1 gram Nizoral 2% cream | 30 gram PoM £4.24 DT price = £4.24
Shampoo
EXCIPIENTS: May contain Imidurea
▸ Ketoconazole (Non-proprietary)
   Ketoconazole 20 mg per 1 gram Ketoconazole 2% shampoo | 120 ml PoM £3.00 DT price = £2.71
▸ Dandrazol (Transdermal Ltd)
   Ketoconazole 20 mg per 1 gram Dandrazol Anti-dandruff 2% shampoo | 60 ml GSL £3.42 | 100 ml GSL £5.28
   Dandrazol 2% shampoo | 120 ml PoM £5.20 DT price = £2.71
▸ Nizoral (Janssen-Cilag Ltd, McNeil Products Ltd)
   Ketoconazole 20 mg per 1 gram Nizoral 2% shampoo | 120 ml PoM £3.59 DT price = £2.71
   Nizoral anti-dandruff 2% shampoo | 60 ml GSL £3.78
   Nizoral Dandruff 2% shampoo | 100 ml P £5.68

Miconazole

- INDICATIONS AND DOSE
Fungal skin infections
▸ TO THE SKIN
▸ Child: Apply twice daily continuing for 10 days after lesions have healed
▸ Adult: Apply twice daily continuing for 10 days after lesions have healed
Fungal nail infections
▸ TO THE SKIN
▸ Child: Apply 1–2 times a day
▸ Adult: Apply 1–2 times a day

- UNLICENSED USE
▸ With topical use in children Licensed for use in children (age range not specified by manufacturer).
- CAUTIONS Avoid in Acute porphyrias p. 918 · contact with eyes and mucous membranes should be avoided
- INTERACTIONS → Appendix 1 (antifungals, imidazole).
- SIDE-EFFECTS
SPECIFIC SIDE-EFFECTS
Burning sensation · erythema · hypersensitivity reactions · itching · occasional local irritation · rash
SIDE-EFFECTS, FURTHER INFORMATION
Treatment should be discontinued if side effects are severe.
- PREGNANCY Absorbed from the skin in small amounts; manufacturer advises caution.
- BREAST FEEDING Manufacturer advises caution—no information available.

13

Skin

- PROFESSION SPECIFIC INFORMATION
Dental practitioners' formulary
Miconazole cream may be prescribed.

- MEDICINAL FORMS
There can be variation in the licensing of different medicines containing the same drug.
Cream
EXCIPIENTS: May contain Butylated hydroxyanisole
▸ Daktarin (McNeil Products Ltd, Janssen-Cilag Ltd)
Miconazole nitrate 20 mg per 1 gram Daktarin 2% cream | 15 gram P £2.14 | 30 gram P £1.82 DT price = £1.82
Daktarin Aktiv 2% cream | 15 gram GSL £2.16 | 30 gram GSL £3.22 DT price = £1.82
Powder
▸ Daktarin (McNeil Products Ltd)
Miconazole nitrate 20 mg per 1 gram Daktarin 2% powder | 20 gram P £2.58 DT price = £2.58

Tioconazole

- INDICATIONS AND DOSE
Fungal nail infection
▸ BY TRANSUNGUAL APPLICATION
▸ Child: Apply twice daily usually for up to 6 months (may be extended to 12 months), apply to nails and surrounding skin
▸ Adult: Apply twice daily usually for up to 6 months (may be extended to 12 months), apply to nails and surrounding skin

- UNLICENSED USE
▸ With topical use in children Licensed for use in children (age range not specified by manufacturer).

- CAUTIONS Contact with eyes and mucous membranes should be avoided · use with caution if child likely to suck affected digits (in children)

- SIDE-EFFECTS Burning sensation · dry skin · erythema · exfoliation · hypersensitivity reactions · itching · local oedema · nail discoloration · nail pain · occasional local irritation · periungual inflammation · rash

SIDE-EFFECTS, FURTHER INFORMATION
Treatment should be discontinued if side-effects are severe.

- PREGNANCY Manufacturer advises avoid.

- MEDICINAL FORMS
There can be variation in the licensing of different medicines containing the same drug.
Paint
▸ Tioconazole (Non-proprietary)
Tioconazole 283 mg per 1 ml Tioconazole 283mg/ml medicated nail lacquer | 12 ml PoM £27.38-£28.74 DT price = £28.06
▸ Trosyl (Pfizer Ltd)
Tioconazole 283 mg per 1 ml Trosyl 283mg/ml nail solution | 12 ml PoM £27.38 DT price = £28.06

ANTIFUNGALS > OTHER

Amorolfine

- INDICATIONS AND DOSE
Fungal nail infections
▸ BY TRANSUNGUAL APPLICATION
▸ Child 12–17 years: Apply 1–2 times a week for 6 months to treat finger nails and for toe nails 9–12 months (review at intervals of 3 months), apply to infected nails after filing and cleansing, allow to dry for approximately 3 minutes
▸ Adult: Apply 1–2 times a week for 6 months to treat finger nails and for toe nails 9–12 months (review at intervals of 3 months), apply to infected nails after

filing and cleansing, allow to dry for approximately 3 minutes

- UNLICENSED USE Not licensed for use in children under 12 years.

- CAUTIONS Avoid contact with ears · avoid contact with eyes and mucous membranes · use with caution in child likely to suck affected digits

- SIDE-EFFECTS Burning sensation · erythema · hypersensitivity reactions · itching · occasional local irritation

SIDE-EFFECTS, FURTHER INFORMATION
Treatment should be discontinued if side-effects are severe.

- PATIENT AND CARER ADVICE Avoid nail varnish or artificial nails during treatment.

- EXCEPTIONS TO LEGAL CATEGORY
▸ In adults Amorolfine nail lacquer can be sold to the public if supplied for the treatment of mild cases of distal and lateral subungual onychomycoses caused by dermatophytes, yeasts and moulds; subject to treatment of max. 2 nails, max. strength of nail lacquer amorolfine 5% and a pack size of 3 mL.

- MEDICINAL FORMS
There can be variation in the licensing of different medicines containing the same drug.
Medicated nail lacquer
CAUTIONARY AND ADVISORY LABELS 10
▸ Amorolfine (Non-proprietary)
Amorolfine (as Amorolfine hydrochloride) 50 mg per 1 ml Amorolfine 5% medicated nail lacquer | 3 ml PoM no price available | 5 ml PoM £16.21 DT price = £7.45
▸ Loceryl (Galderma (UK) Ltd)
Amorolfine (as Amorolfine hydrochloride) 50 mg per 1 ml Loceryl Curanail 5% medicated nail lacquer | 3 ml P £12.31
Loceryl 5% medicated nail lacquer | 2.5 ml PoM £7.26 | 5 ml PoM £9.08 DT price = £7.45
▸ Omicur (Morningside Healthcare Ltd)
Amorolfine (as Amorolfine hydrochloride) 50 mg per 1 ml Omicur 5% medicated nail lacquer | 2.5 ml PoM £9.09 | 5 ml PoM £9.09 DT price = £7.45

Griseofulvin

- INDICATIONS AND DOSE
Tinea pedis
▸ TO THE SKIN
▸ Adult: Apply 400 micrograms once daily, apply to an area approximately 13 cm^2; increased if necessary to 1.2 mg once daily for maximum treatment duration of 4 weeks, allow each spray to dry between application

- CAUTIONS Avoid contact with eyes and mucous membranes

- INTERACTIONS → Appendix 1 (griseofulvin).

- SIDE-EFFECTS Burning sensation · erythema · hypersensitivity reactions · itching · occasional local irritation

SIDE-EFFECTS, FURTHER INFORMATION
Treatment should be discontinued if side-effects are severe.

- PREGNANCY Manufacturer advises avoid unless potential benefit outweighs risk.

- BREAST FEEDING Manufacturer advises avoid unless potential benefit outweighs risk.

● MEDICINAL FORMS
There can be variation in the licensing of different medicines containing the same drug.

Spray

CAUTIONARY AND ADVISORY LABELS 15
EXCIPIENTS: May contain Benzyl alcohol

‣ Grisol AF (Transdermal Ltd)
  Griseofulvin 10 mg per 1 gram Grisol AF 1% spray | 20 ml P £3.35

Terbinafine

● **INDICATIONS AND DOSE**

Tinea pedis

‣ TO THE SKIN USING CREAM
‣ Adult: Apply 1–2 times a day for up to 1 week, to be applied thinly
‣ BY MOUTH USING TABLETS
‣ Adult: 250 mg once daily for 2-6 weeks

Tinea corporis

‣ TO THE SKIN USING CREAM
‣ Adult: Apply 1–2 times a day for up to 1–2 weeks, to be applied thinly, review treatment after 2 weeks
‣ BY MOUTH USING TABLETS
‣ Adult: 250 mg once daily for 4 weeks

Tinea cruris

‣ TO THE SKIN USING CREAM
‣ Adult: Apply 1–2 times a day for up to 1–2 weeks, to be applied thinly, review treatment after 2 weeks
‣ BY MOUTH USING TABLETS
‣ Adult: 250 mg once daily for 2-4 weeks

Dermatophyte infections of the nails

‣ BY MOUTH USING TABLETS
‣ Adult: 250 mg once daily for 6 weeks-3 months (occasionally longer in toenail infections)

Cutaneous candidiasis | Pityriasis versicolor

‣ TO THE SKIN USING CREAM
‣ Adult: Apply 1–2 times a day for 2 weeks, to be applied thinly, review treatment after 2 weeks

● CAUTIONS
‣ With oral use Autoimmune disease (risk of lupus-erythematosus-like effect) · psoriasis (risk of exacerbation)
‣ With topical use Contact with eyes and mucous membranes should be avoided

● INTERACTIONS
‣ With oral use Appendix 1 (terbinafine).

● SIDE-EFFECTS
‣ **Common or very common**
‣ With oral use Abdominal discomfort · anorexia · arthralgia · diarrhoea · dyspepsia · headache · myalgia · nausea · rash · urticaria
‣ **Uncommon**
‣ With oral use Taste disturbance
‣ **Rare**
‣ With oral use Cholestasis · dizziness · hepatitis · hypoaesthesia · jaundice · liver toxicity · malaise · paraesthesia
‣ **Very rare**
‣ With oral use Alopecia · blood disorders · lupus erythematosus-like effect · neutropenia · photosensitivity · serious skin reactions · Stevens-Johnson syndrome · thrombocytopenia · toxic epidermal necrolysis
‣ **Frequency not known**
‣ With oral use Disturbances in smell · exacerbation of psoriasis · hearing disturbances · influenza-like symptoms · pancreatitis · rhabdomyolysis · vasculitis
‣ With topical use Erythema · hypersensitivity reactions · itching · mild burning sensation · occasional local irritation

SIDE-EFFECTS, FURTHER INFORMATION
‣ Liver toxicity
‣ With oral use Discontinue treatment if liver toxicity develops (including jaundice, cholestasis and hepatitis).
‣ Serious skin reactions
‣ With oral use Discontinue treatment in progressive skin rash (including Stevens-Johnson syndrome and toxic epidermal necrolysis).
‣ Topical application
‣ With topical use Treatment should be discontinued if side effects are severe.

● PREGNANCY
‣ With topical use Manufacturer advises use only if potential benefit outweighs risk—*animal* studies suggest no adverse effects.
‣ With oral use Manufacturer advises use only if potential benefit outweighs risk—no information available.

● BREAST FEEDING
‣ With topical use Manufacturer advises avoid—present in milk. Less than 5% of the dose is absorbed after topical application of terbinafine; avoid application to mother's chest.
‣ With oral use Avoid—present in milk.

● HEPATIC IMPAIRMENT
‣ With oral use Manufacturer advises avoid—elimination reduced.

● RENAL IMPAIRMENT
‣ With oral use Use half normal dose if eGFR less than 50 mL/minute/1.73 m^2 and no suitable alternative available.

● MONITORING REQUIREMENTS
‣ With oral use Monitor hepatic function before treatment and then every 4–6 weeks during treatment—discontinue if abnormalities in liver function tests.

● EXCEPTIONS TO LEGAL CATEGORY
‣ With topical use Preparations of terbinafine hydrochloride (maximum 1%) can be sold to the public for use in those over 16 years for external use for the treatment of tinea pedis as a cream in a pack containing maximum 15 g, or for the treatment of tinea pedis and cruris as a cream in a pack containing maximum 15 g, or for the treatment of tinea pedis, cruris, and corporis as a spray in a pack containing maximum 30 mL spray or as a gel in a pack containing maximum 30 g gel.

● MEDICINAL FORMS
There can be variation in the licensing of different medicines containing the same drug.

Tablet

CAUTIONARY AND ADVISORY LABELS 9

‣ Terbinafine (Non-proprietary)
  Terbinafine (as Terbinafine hydrochloride) 250 mg Terbinafine 250mg tablets | 14 tablet PoM £18.11 DT price = £1.22 | 28 tablet PoM £34.93
‣ Lamisil (Novartis Pharmaceuticals UK Ltd)
  Terbinafine (as Terbinafine hydrochloride) 250 mg Lamisil 250mg tablets | 14 tablet PoM £21.30 DT price = £1.22 | 28 tablet PoM £41.09

Cream

EXCIPIENTS: May contain Benzyl alcohol, cetostearyl alcohol (including cetyl and stearyl alcohol), polysorbates

‣ Terbinafine (Non-proprietary)
  Terbinafine hydrochloride 10 mg per 1 gram Terbinafine 1% cream | 7.5 gram GSL £5.50 | 7.5 gram PoM £1.06 | 15 gram GSL £4.59 DT price = £1.31 | 15 gram PoM £4.86 DT price = £1.31 | 30 gram PoM £8.76 DT price = £2.62
‣ Lamisil (Novartis Consumer Health UK Ltd)
  Terbinafine hydrochloride 10 mg per 1 gram Lamisil 1% cream | 30 gram PoM £7.45 DT price = £2.62
  Lamisil AT 1% cream | 7.5 gram GSL £2.39 | 15 gram GSL £3.60 DT price = £1.31

13

Skin

ANTISEPTICS AND DISINFECTANTS >
UNDECENOATES

Undecenoic acid with zinc undecenoate

- **INDICATIONS AND DOSE**

Treatment of athletes foot
▶ TO THE SKIN
▶ Child: Apply twice daily, continue use for 7 days after lesions have healed
▶ Adult: Apply twice daily, continue use for 7 days after lesions have healed

Prevention of athletes foot
▶ TO THE SKIN
▶ Child: Apply once daily
▶ Adult: Apply once daily

- **UNLICENSED USE**
▶ In children *Mycota*® licensed for use in children (age range not specified by manufacturer).

- **CAUTIONS** Avoid broken skin · contact with eyes should be avoided · contact with mucous membranes should be avoided

- **SIDE-EFFECTS** Erythema · hypersensitivity reactions · itching · local irritation · mild burning sensation
SIDE-EFFECTS, FURTHER INFORMATION
Treatment should be discontinued if side effects are severe.

- **MEDICINAL FORMS**
There can be variation in the licensing of different medicines containing the same drug.
Cream
EXCIPIENTS: May contain Cetostearyl alcohol (including cetyl and stearyl alcohol), fragrances
▶ Undecenoic acid with zinc undecenoate (Non-proprietary)
Undecenoic acid 50 mg per 1 gram, Zinc undecenoate 200 mg per 1 gram Mycota cream | 25 gram GSL £2.01
Powder
EXCIPIENTS: May contain Fragrances
▶ Undecenoic acid with zinc undecenoate (Non-proprietary)
Undecenoic acid 20 mg per 1 gram, Zinc undecenoate 200 mg per 1 gram Mycota powder | 70 gram GSL £2.71

ANTISEPTICS AND DISINFECTANTS > OTHER

Chlorhexidine with nystatin

- **INDICATIONS AND DOSE**

Skin infections due to Candida spp.
▶ TO THE SKIN
▶ Child: Apply 2–3 times a day, continuing for 7 days after lesions have healed
▶ Adult: Apply 2–3 times a day, continuing for 7 days after lesions have healed

- **UNLICENSED USE**
▶ With topical use in children Licensed for use in children (age range not specified by manufacturer).

- **CAUTIONS** Avoid contact with eyes and mucous membranes

- **SIDE-EFFECTS** Burning sensation · erythema · hypersensitivity reactions · itching · occasional local irritation
SIDE-EFFECTS, FURTHER INFORMATION
Treatment should be discontinued if side-effects are severe.

- **MEDICINAL FORMS**
There can be variation in the licensing of different medicines containing the same drug.
Cream
EXCIPIENTS: May contain Benzyl alcohol, cetostearyl alcohol (including cetyl and stearyl alcohol), polysorbates
▶ Nystaform (Typharm Ltd)
Chlorhexidine hydrochloride 10 mg per 1 gram, Nystatin 100000 unit per 1 gram Nystaform cream | 30 gram PoM £2.62 DT price = £2.62

BENZOATES

Benzoic acid with salicylic acid

- **INDICATIONS AND DOSE**

Ringworm (tinea)
▶ TO THE SKIN
▶ Child: Apply twice daily
▶ Adult: Apply twice daily

- **UNLICENSED USE**
▶ In children Licensed for use in children (age range not specified by manufacturer).

- **CAUTIONS** Avoid broken or inflamed skin · avoid contact with eyes · avoid contact with mucous membranes
CAUTIONS, FURTHER INFORMATION
▶ Salicylate toxicity Salicylate toxicity may occur particularly if applied on large areas of skin.

- **SIDE-EFFECTS** Erythema · hypersensitivity reactions · itching · mild burning sensation · occasional local irritation
SIDE-EFFECTS, FURTHER INFORMATION
Treatment should be discontinued if side effects are severe.

- **PRESCRIBING AND DISPENSING INFORMATION** Benzoic Acid Ointment, Compound, BP has also been referred to as Whitfield's ointment.

- **MEDICINAL FORMS**
There can be variation in the licensing of different medicines containing the same drug. Forms available from special-order manufacturers include: cream, ointment

SALICYLIC ACID AND DERIVATIVES

Boric acid with salicylic acid and tannic acid

- **INDICATIONS AND DOSE**

Fungal nail infection, particularly tinea
▶ BY TRANSUNGUAL APPLICATION
▶ Child 5-17 years: Apply twice daily, and after washing
▶ Adult: Apply twice daily, and after washing

- **CAUTIONS** Avoid broken or inflamed skin · contact with eyes and mucous membranes should be avoided · use with caution in children likely to suck affected digits
CAUTIONS, FURTHER INFORMATION
▶ Salicylate toxicity Salicylate toxicity can occur particularly if applied on large areas of skin.

- **SIDE-EFFECTS** Burning sensation · erythema · hypersensitivity reactions · itching · occasional local irritation
SIDE-EFFECTS, FURTHER INFORMATION
Treatment should be discontinued if side-effects are severe.

- **PREGNANCY** Avoid.

- **LESS SUITABLE FOR PRESCRIBING** *Phytex*® is less suitable for prescribing.

- **MEDICINAL FORMS**
There can be variation in the licensing of different medicines containing the same drug.
No licensed medicines listed.

2.3 Parasitic skin infections

PARASITICIDES

Benzyl benzoate

- **INDICATIONS AND DOSE**

Scabies
▸ TO THE SKIN
▸ Adult: Apply over the whole body; repeat without bathing on the following day and wash off 24 hours later; a third application may be required in some cases

- **CAUTIONS** Avoid contact with eyes and mucous membranes · children (not recommended) · do not use on broken or secondarily infected skin
- **SIDE-EFFECTS** Burning sensation (especially on genitalia and excoriations) · rashes · skin irritation
- **BREAST FEEDING** Suspend feeding until product has been washed off.
- **PRESCRIBING AND DISPENSING INFORMATION** When prepared extemporaneously, the BP states Benzyl Benzoate Application, BP consists of benzyl benzoate 25% in an emulsion basis.
    Some manufacturers recommend application to the body but to exclude the head and neck. However, application should be extended to the scalp, neck, face, and ears. Note—dilution to reduce irritant effect also reduces efficacy.
- **LESS SUITABLE FOR PRESCRIBING** Benzyl benzoate is less suitable for prescribing.

- **MEDICINAL FORMS**
There can be variation in the licensing of different medicines containing the same drug. Forms available from special-order manufacturers include: liquid

Dimeticone

- **INDICATIONS AND DOSE**

Head lice
▸ TO THE SKIN
▸ Child: Apply once weekly for 2 doses, rub into dry hair and scalp, allow to dry naturally, shampoo after minimum 8 hours (or overnight)
▸ Adult: Apply once weekly for 2 doses, rub into dry hair and scalp, allow to dry naturally, shampoo after minimum 8 hours (or overnight)

- **UNLICENSED USE**
▸ With topical use in children Not licensed for use in children under 6 months except under medical supervision.
- **CAUTIONS** Avoid contact with eyes · children under 6 months, medical supervision required
- **SIDE-EFFECTS** Skin irritation
- **PATIENT AND CARER ADVICE** Patients should be told to keep hair away from fire and flames during treatment.

- **MEDICINAL FORMS**
There can be variation in the licensing of different medicines containing the same drug.
Liquid
▸ Hedrin (Thornton & Ross Ltd)
Dimeticone 40 mg per 1 gram Hedrin 4% lotion | 50 ml Ⓟ £2.98 DT price = £2.98 | 150 ml Ⓟ £6.92 DT price = £6.92
Cutaneous spray solution
▸ Hedrin (Thornton & Ross Ltd)
Dimeticone 40 mg per 1 gram Hedrin 4% spray | 120 ml ⃞GSL £7.13

Gel
▸ Hedrin Once (Thornton & Ross Ltd)
Hedrin Once spray gel | 60 ml £4.16 | 100 ml £6.83
Hedrin Once liquid gel | 100 ml £5.95 | 250 ml £10.40

Malathion

- **INDICATIONS AND DOSE**

Head lice
▸ TO THE SKIN
▸ Child: Apply once weekly for 2 doses, rub preparation into dry hair and scalp, allow to dry naturally, remove by washing after 12 hours
▸ Adult: Apply once weekly for 2 doses, rub preparation into dry hair and scalp, allow to dry naturally, remove by washing after 12 hours

Crab lice
▸ TO THE SKIN
▸ Child: Apply once weekly for 2 doses, apply preparation over whole body, allow to dry naturally, wash off after 12 hours or overnight
▸ Adult: Apply once weekly for 2 doses, apply preparation over whole body, allow to dry naturally, wash off after 12 hours or overnight

Scabies
▸ TO THE SKIN
▸ Child: Apply once weekly for 2 doses, apply preparation over whole body, and wash off after 24 hours, if hands are washed with soap within 24 hours, they should be retreated
▸ Adult: Apply once weekly for 2 doses, apply preparation over whole body, and wash off after 24 hours, if hands are washed with soap within 24 hours, they should be retreated

- **UNLICENSED USE**
▸ With topical use in children Not licensed for use in children under 6 months except under medical supervision.
- **CAUTIONS** Alcoholic lotions **not** recommended for head lice in children with severe eczema or asthma, or for scabies or crab lice · avoid contact with eyes · children under 6 months, medical supervision required · do not use lotion more than once a week for 3 consecutive weeks · do not use on broken or secondarily infected skin
- **SIDE-EFFECTS** Chemical burns · hypersensitivity reactions · skin irritation
- **PRESCRIBING AND DISPENSING INFORMATION** For scabies, manufacturer recommends application to the body but not necessarily to the head and neck. However, application should be extended to the scalp, neck, face, and ears.

- **MEDICINAL FORMS**
There can be variation in the licensing of different medicines containing the same drug.
Liquid
EXCIPIENTS: May contain Cetostearyl alcohol (including cetyl and stearyl alcohol), fragrances, hydroxybenzoates (parabens)
▸ Derbac-M (G.R. Lane Health Products Ltd)
Malathion 5 mg per 1 gram Derbac-M 0.5% liquid | 50 ml Ⓟ £3.57 DT price = £3.57 | 200 ml Ⓟ £8.44 DT price = £8.44

13

Skin

Permethrin

- **INDICATIONS AND DOSE**

Scabies
▶ TO THE SKIN
▷ **Child:** Apply once weekly for 2 doses, apply 5% preparation over whole body including face, neck, scalp and ears then wash off after 8–12 hours. If hands are washed with soap within 8 hours of application, they should be treated again with cream
▷ **Adult:** Apply once weekly for 2 doses, apply 5% preparation over whole body including face, neck, scalp and ears then wash off after 8–12 hours. If hands are washed with soap within 8 hours of application, they should be treated again with cream

Crab lice
▶ TO THE SKIN
▷ **Adult:** Apply once weekly for 2 doses, apply 5% cream over whole body, allow to dry naturally and wash off after 12 hours or after leaving on overnight

Head lice
▶ TO THE SKIN
▷ **Adult:** Not recommended; no information given

- **UNLICENSED USE**
▶ With topical use in children *Dermal Cream* (scabies), not licensed for use in children under 2 months; not licensed for treatment of crab lice in children under 18 years. *Creme Rinse* (head lice) not licensed for use in children under 6 months except under medical supervision.
- **CAUTIONS** Avoid contact with eyes · children aged 2 months–2 years, medical supervision required for dermal cream (scabies) · children under 6 months, medical supervision required for cream rinse (head lice) · do not use on broken or secondarily infected skin
- **SIDE-EFFECTS**
▶ **Rare** Oedema · rashes
▶ **Frequency not known** Erythema · pruritus · stinging
- **PRESCRIBING AND DISPENSING INFORMATION** Manufacturer recommends application to the body but to exclude head and neck. However, application should be extended to the scalp, neck, face, and ears.
    Larger patients may require up to two 30-g packs for adequate treatment.
- **LESS SUITABLE FOR PRESCRIBING** Lyclear® Creme Rinse is less suitable for prescribing.

- **MEDICINAL FORMS** There can be variation in the licensing of different medicines containing the same drug.

Liquid
EXCIPIENTS: May contain Cetostearyl alcohol (including cetyl and stearyl alcohol)
▶ Lyclear (Omega Pharma Ltd)
    Permethrin 10 mg per 1 gram Lyclear 1% creme rinse | 59 ml P £3.55 DT price = £3.55 | 118 ml P £6.46 DT price = £6.46

Cream
CAUTIONARY AND ADVISORY LABELS 10 (Dermal cream only)
EXCIPIENTS: May contain Butylated hydroxytoluene, wool fat and related substances including lanolin
▶ Permethrin (Non-proprietary)
    Permethrin 50 mg per 1 gram Permethrin 5% cream | 30 gram P £7.46 DT price = £7.46
▶ Lyclear (Omega Pharma Ltd)
    Permethrin 50 mg per 1 gram Lyclear 5% dermal cream | 30 gram P £5.71 DT price = £7.46

2.4 Viral skin infections

ANTIVIRALS › NUCLEOSIDE ANALOGUES

Aciclovir

(Acyclovir)

- **INDICATIONS AND DOSE**

Herpes simplex infection (local treatment)
▶ TO THE SKIN
▷ **Child:** Apply 5 times a day for 5–10 days, to be applied to lesions approximately every 4 hours, starting at first sign of attack
▷ **Adult:** Apply 5 times a day for 5–10 days, to be applied to lesions approximately every 4 hours, starting at first sign of attack

- **UNLICENSED USE**
▶ With topical use in children Cream licensed for use in children (age range not specified by manufacturer).
- **CAUTIONS** Avoid cream coming in to contact with eyes and mucous membranes
- **SIDE-EFFECTS** Drying of the skin · erythema · itching of the skin · transient burning · transient stinging
- **PREGNANCY** Limited absorption from topical aciclovir preparations.
- **PATIENT AND CARER ADVICE** Medicines for Children leaflet: Aciclovir cream for herpes www.medicinesforchildren.org.uk/aciclovir-cream-for-herpes
- **PROFESSION SPECIFIC INFORMATION**

Dental practitioners' formulary
Aciclovir Cream may be prescribed.
- **EXCEPTIONS TO LEGAL CATEGORY** A 2-g tube and a pump pack are on sale to the public for the treatment of cold sores.

- **MEDICINAL FORMS** There can be variation in the licensing of different medicines containing the same drug.

Cream
EXCIPIENTS: May contain Cetostearyl alcohol (including cetyl and stearyl alcohol), propylene glycol
▶ Aciclovir (Non-proprietary)
    Aciclovir 50 mg per 1 gram Aciclovir 5% cream | 2 gram GSL £0.83 DT price = £1.05 | 2 gram PoM £4.17 DT price = £1.05 | 10 gram PoM £12.56 DT price = £5.25
▶ Zovirax (GlaxoSmithKline Consumer Healthcare, GlaxoSmithKline UK Ltd)
    Aciclovir 50 mg per 1 gram Zovirax Cold Sore 5% cream | 2 gram GSL £3.96–£4.28 DT price = £1.05
    Zovirax 5% cream | 2 gram PoM £4.63 DT price = £1.05 | 10 gram PoM £13.96 DT price = £5.25

3 Inflammatory skin conditions

3.1 Eczema and psoriasis

Eczema

Types and management

Eczema (dermatitis) has several causes, which may influence treatment. The main types of eczema are irritant, allergic contact, atopic, venous and discoid; different types may co-exist. Lichenification, due to scratching and rubbing, may complicate any chronic eczema. *Atopic eczema* is the most common type and it usually involves dry skin as well as infection and lichenification.

Management of eczema involves the removal or treatment of contributory factors including occupational and domestic irritants. Known or suspected contact allergens should be avoided. Rarely, ingredients in topical medicinal products may sensitise the skin; the BNF lists active ingredients together with excipients that have been associated with skin sensitisation.

Skin dryness and the consequent irritant eczema requires **emollients** applied regularly (at least twice daily) and liberally to the affected area; this can be supplemented with bath and shower emollients. The use of emollients should continue even if the eczema improves or if other treatment is being used.

Topical corticosteroids are also required in the management of eczema; the potency of the corticosteroid should be appropriate to the severity and site of the condition. Mild corticosteroids are generally used on the face and on flexures; potent corticosteroids are generally required for use on adults with discoid or lichenified eczema or with eczema on the scalp, limbs, and trunk. Treatment should be reviewed regularly, especially if a potent corticosteroid is required. In patients with frequent flares (2–3 per month), a topical corticosteroid can be applied on 2 consecutive days each week to prevent further flares.

Bandages (including those containing ichthammol with zinc oxide p. 1098) are sometimes applied over topical corticosteroids or emollients to treat eczema of the limbs. Dry-wrap dressings can be used to provide a physical barrier to help prevent scratching and improve retention of emollients. See *Wound management products and elasticated garments* for details of elasticated viscose stockinette tubular bandages and garments, and silk clothing.

See Eczema and psoriasis, drugs affecting the immune response below for the role of topical pimecrolimus p. 1101 and tacrolimus p. 1102 in atopic eczema.

Infection

Bacterial infection (commonly with *Staphylococcus aureus* and occasionally with *Streptococcus pyogenes*) can exacerbate eczema and requires treatment with topical or systemic **antibacterial drugs**. Antibacterial drugs should be used in short courses (typically 1 week) to reduce the risk of drug resistance or skin sensitisation. Associated eczema is treated simultaneously with a topical corticosteroid which can be combined with a topical antimicrobial.

Eczema involving widespread or recurrent infection requires the use of a systemic antibacterial that is active against the infecting organism. Products that combine an antiseptic with an emollient application and with a bath emollient can also be used; antiseptic shampoos can be used on the scalp.

Intertriginous eczema commonly involves candida and bacteria; it is best treated with a mild or moderately potent topical corticosteroid and a suitable antimicrobial drug.

Widespread herpes simplex infection may complicate atopic eczema and treatment with a systemic antiviral drug is indicated.

Management of other features of eczema

Lichenification, which results from repeated scratching is treated initially with a potent corticosteroid. Bandages containing ichthammol **paste** p. 1098 (to reduce pruritus) and other substances such as **zinc oxide** can be applied over the corticosteroid or emollient. **Coal tar** and ichthammol can be useful in some cases of *chronic eczema*.

A *non-sedating* **antihistamine** may be of some value in relieving severe itching or urticaria associated with eczema. A *sedating* antihistamine can be used if itching causes sleep disturbance.

Exudative ('weeping') eczema requires a potent corticosteroid initially; infection may also be present and require specific treatment. Potassium permanganate

solution (1 in 10,000) p. 1119 can be used in exudating eczema for its antiseptic and astringent effects; treatment should be stopped when exudation stops.

Severe refractory eczema

Severe refractory eczema is best managed under specialist supervision; it may require phototherapy or drugs that act on the immune system. Alitretinoin p. 1103 is licensed for the treatment of severe chronic hand eczema refractory to potent topical corticosteroids; patients with hyperkeratotic features are more likely to respond to alitretinoin than those with pompholyx.

Seborrhoeic dermatitis

Seborrhoeic dermatitis (seborrhoeic eczema) is associated with species of the yeast *Malassezia* and affects the scalp, paranasal areas, and eyebrows. Shampoos active against the yeast (including those containing ketoconazole p. 1077 and coal tar) and combinations of mild corticosteroids with suitable antimicrobials are used.

Eczema and psoriasis, drugs affecting the immune response

Overview

Drugs affecting the immune response are used for eczema or psoriasis. Systemic drugs acting on the immune system are used under specialist supervision.

Pimecrolimus p. 1101 by topical application is licensed for *mild to moderate atopic eczema*. Tacrolimus p. 1102 is licensed for topical use in *moderate to severe atopic eczema*. Both are drugs whose long-term safety is still being evaluated and they should not usually be considered first-line treatments unless there is a specific reason to avoid or reduce the use of topical corticosteroids. Treatment of atopic eczema with topical pimecrolimus or topical tacrolimus should be initiated only by prescribers experienced in managing the condition. Topical tacrolimus and pimecrolimus have a role in the treatment of psoriasis.

A short course of a systemic corticosteroid can be given for eczema flares that have not improved despite appropriate topical treatment.

Ciclosporin p. 758 by mouth can be used for *severe psoriasis* and for *severe eczema*. Azathioprine p. 757 or mycophenolate mofetil p. 765 are used for severe refractory eczema [unlicensed indication].

Methotrexate p. 807 can be used for *severe psoriasis*, the dose being adjusted according to severity of the condition and haematological and biochemical measurements. Folic acid p. 886 should be given to reduce the possibility of side-effects associated with methotrexate. Folic acid can be given once weekly [unlicensed indication], on a different day from the methotrexate; alternative regimens of folic acid may be used in some settings.

Etanercept p. 961, adalimumab p. 957, and infliximab p. 964 inhibit the activity of tumour necrosis factor (TNFα). They are used for *severe plaque psoriasis* either refractory to at least 2 standard systemic treatments and photochemotherapy, or when standard treatments cannot be used because of intolerance or contra-indications; while either etanercept or adalimumab is considered to be the first choice in stable disease, infliximab or adalimumab may be useful when rapid disease control is required. Secukinumab p. 954 inhibits the activity of interleukin-17A. It is used for *moderate to severe plaque psoriasis* in patients who are candidates for systemic therapy. Secukinumab is also licensed for psoriatic arthritis and ankylosing spondylitis. Ustekinumab p. 955 (a monoclonal antibody that inhibits interleukins 12 and 23) can be used for *severe plaque psoriasis* that has not responded to at least 2 standard systemic treatments and photochemotherapy, or when these

13

Skin

treatments cannot be used because of intolerance or contra-indications. Adalimumab is also licensed for the treatment of active moderate to severe hidradenitis suppurativa (acne inversa) in patients who have had inadequate response to conventional systemic therapy. Adalimumab, etanercept, infliximab and ustekinumab are also licensed for psoriatic arthritis.

Psoriasis

Management

Psoriasis is characterised by epidermal thickening and scaling. It commonly affects extensor surfaces and the scalp.

Occasionally, psoriasis is provoked or exacerbated by drugs such as lithium, chloroquine and hydroxychloroquine, beta-blockers, non-steroidal anti-inflammatory drugs, and ACE inhibitors. Psoriasis may not be seen until the drug has been taken for weeks or months.

Emollients, in addition to their effects on dryness, scaling and cracking, may have an anti-proliferative effect in psoriasis, and may be the only treatment necessary for mild psoriasis. They are particularly useful in *inflammatory psoriasis* and in *plaque psoriasis of palms and soles*, in which irritant factors can perpetuate the condition. Emollients are useful adjuncts to other more specific treatment.

More specific topical treatment for *chronic stable plaque psoriasis* on extensor surfaces of trunk and limbs involves the use of **vitamin D analogues**, coal tar p. 1099, dithranol p. 1098, and the retinoid tazarotene p. 1104. However, they can irritate the skin and they are not suitable for the more inflammatory forms of psoriasis; their use should be suspended during an inflammatory phase of psoriasis. The efficacy and the irritancy of each substance varies between patients. If a substance irritates significantly, it should be stopped or the concentration reduced; if it is tolerated, its effects should be assessed after 4 to 6 weeks and treatment continued if it is effective.

Scalp psoriasis is usually scaly, and the scale may be thick and adherent; this will require softening with an emollient cream, ointment, or oil. A tar-based shampoo is first-line treatment for scalp psoriasis; a keratolytic, such as salicylic acid, should also be used if there is significant scaling, to allow other treatments to work.

Some preparations prescribed for psoriasis affecting the scalp, combine salicylic acid with coal tar or sulfur. The product should be applied generously, and an adequate quantity should be prescribed. It should be left on for at least an hour, often more conveniently overnight, before washing off. The use of scalp preparations containing a potent corticosteroid or a vitamin D analogue, either alone or in combination, can also be helpful.

Facial, flexural and genital psoriasis can be managed with short-term use of a mild or moderate potency topical corticosteroid (a mild potency topical corticosteroid is preferred for the initial treatment of facial psoriasis). Calcitriol p. 1105 or calcitriol p. 1105 can be used for longer-term treatment, or if the response to mild or moderate potency topical corticosteroids is inadequate; calcipotriol p. 1105 is more likely to cause irritation. Low strength tar preparations can also be used. Pimecrolimus p. 1101 or tacrolimus p. 1102 by topical application [unlicensed indication] can be used short-term, under specialist supervision, in patients whose condition has not responded adequately to other treatments, or who are intolerant of them.

Widespread *unstable psoriasis* of erythrodermic or generalised pustular type requires urgent specialist assessment. Initial topical treatment should be limited to using emollients frequently and generously; emollients should be prescribed in quantities of 1 kg or more. More localised acute or subacute *inflammatory psoriasis* with hot,

spreading or itchy lesions, should be treated topically with emollients or with a corticosteroid of moderate potency.

Calcipotriol and tacalcitol are analogues of vitamin D that affect cell division and differentiation. Calcitriol is an active form of vitamin D. Vitamin D and its analogues are used first-line for the long-term treatment of plaque psoriasis; they do not smell or stain and they may be more acceptable than tar or dithranol products. Of the vitamin D analogues, tacalcitol and calcitriol are less likely to irritate.

Coal tar has anti-inflammatory properties that are useful in chronic plaque psoriasis; it also has antiscaling properties. Crude coal tar (coal tar, BP) is the most effective form, typically in a concentration of 1 to 10% in a soft paraffin base, but few outpatients tolerate the smell and mess. Cleaner extracts of coal tar included in proprietary preparations, are more practicable for home use but they are less effective and improvement takes longer. Contact of coal tar products with normal skin is not normally harmful and they can be used for widespread small lesions; however, irritation, contact allergy, and sterile folliculitis can occur. The milder tar extracts can be used on the face and flexures. Tar baths and tar shampoos are also helpful.

Dithranol is effective for chronic plaque psoriasis. Its major disadvantages are irritation (for which individual susceptibility varies) and staining of skin and of clothing. Dithranol is not generally suitable for widespread small lesions nor should it be used in the flexures or on the face. Proprietary preparations are more suitable for home use; they are usually washed off after 5 to 60 minutes ('short contact'). Specialist nurses may apply intensive treatment with dithranol paste which is covered by stockinette dressings and usually retained overnight. Dithranol should be discontinued if even a low concentration causes acute inflammation; continued use can result in the psoriasis becoming unstable.

Tazarotene, a retinoid, has a similar efficacy to vitamin D and its analogues, but is associated with a greater incidence of irritation. Although irritation is common, it is minimised by applying tazarotene sparingly to the plaques and avoiding normal skin; application to the face and in flexures should also be avoided. Tazarotene does not stain and is odourless.

A topical **corticosteroid** is not generally suitable for long-term use or as the sole treatment of extensive chronic plaque psoriasis; any early improvement is not usually maintained and there is a risk of the condition deteriorating or of precipitating an unstable form of psoriasis (e.g. erythrodermic psoriasis or generalised pustular psoriasis) on withdrawal. Topical use of potent corticosteroids on widespread psoriasis can also lead to systemic as well as local side-effects. However, topical corticosteroids used short-term may be appropriate to treat psoriasis in specific sites such as the face or flexures (with a mild or moderate corticosteroid), and psoriasis of the scalp, palms, and soles (with a potent corticosteroid). Very potent corticosteroids should only be used under specialist supervision.

Combining the use of a corticosteroid with another specific topical treatment may be beneficial in chronic plaque psoriasis; the drugs may be used separately at different times of the day or used together in a single formulation. *Eczema* co-existing with psoriasis may be treated with a corticosteroid, or coal tar, or both.

Phototherapy

Phototherapy is available in specialist centres under the supervision of a dermatologist. **Ultraviolet B** (UVB) radiation is usually effective for *chronic stable psoriasis* and for *guttate psoriasis*. It may be considered for patients with moderately severe psoriasis in whom topical treatment has failed, but it may irritate inflammatory psoriasis.

Photochemotherapy combining long-wave ultraviolet A radiation with a psoralen (PUVA) is available in specialist centres under the supervision of a dermatologist. The psoralen, which enhances the effect of irradiation, is administered either by mouth or topically. PUVA is effective in most forms of psoriasis, including *localised palmoplantar pustular psoriasis*. Early adverse effects include phototoxicity and pruritus. Higher cumulative doses exaggerate skin ageing, increase the risk of dysplastic and neoplastic skin lesions, especially squamous cancer, and pose a theoretical risk of cataracts.

Phototherapy combined with coal tar, dithranol, tazarotene, topical vitamin D or vitamin D analogues, or oral acitretin, allows reduction of the cumulative dose of phototherapy required to treat psoriasis.

Systemic treatment
Systemic treatment is required for severe, resistant, unstable or complicated forms of psoriasis, and it should be initiated only under specialist supervision. Systemic drugs for psoriasis include acitretin and drugs that affect the immune response (such as ciclosporin p. 758 and methotrexate p. 807).

Systemic corticosteroids should be used only rarely in psoriasis because rebound deterioration may occur on reducing the dose.

Acitretin p. 1102, a metabolite of etretinate, is a retinoid (vitamin A derivative); it is prescribed by specialists. The main indication for acitretin is *psoriasis*, but it is also used in disorders of keratinisation such as severe *Darier's disease* (keratosis follicularis), and some forms of *ichthyosis*. Although a minority of cases of psoriasis respond well to acitretin alone, it is only moderately effective in many cases and it is combined with other treatments. A therapeutic effect occurs after 2 to 4 weeks and the maximum benefit after 4 months. Consideration should be given to stopping acitretin if the response is inadequate after 4 months at the optimum dose. The manufacturers of acitretin do not recommend continuous treatment for longer than 6 months. However, some patients may benefit from longer treatment, provided that the lowest effective dose is used, patients are monitored carefully for adverse effects, and the need for treatment is reviewed regularly.

Apart from teratogenicity, which remains a risk for 3 years after stopping, acitretin is the least toxic systemic treatment for psoriasis; in women with a potential for child-bearing, the possibility of pregnancy must be excluded before treatment and effective contraception must be used during treatment and for at least 3 years afterwards (oral progestogen-only contraceptives not considered effective).

Topical treatment
The vitamin D and analogues, calcipotriol p. 1105, calcitriol p. 1105, and tacalcitol p. 1105 are used for the management of plaque psoriasis. They should be avoided by those with calcium metabolism disorders, and used with caution in generalised pustular or erythrodermic exfoliative psoriasis (enhanced risk of hypercalcaemia).

> **Drugs used for Eczema and psoriasis not listed below**
> Apremilast, p. 966

CORTICOSTEROIDS

Topical corticosteroids

Overview
Topical corticosteroids are used for the treatment of inflammatory conditions of the skin (other than those arising from an infection), in particular eczema, contact dermatitis, insect stings, and eczema of scabies. Corticosteroids suppress the inflammatory reaction during use; they are not curative and on discontinuation a rebound exacerbation of the condition may occur. They are generally used to relieve symptoms and suppress signs of the disorder when other measures such as emollients are ineffective.

Topical corticosteroids are not recommended in the routine treatment of urticaria; treatment should only be initiated and supervised by a specialist. They should not be used indiscriminately in pruritus (where they will only benefit if inflammation is causing the itch) and are **not** recommended for acne vulgaris.

Systemic or very potent topical corticosteroids should be avoided or given only under specialist supervision in *psoriasis* because, although they may suppress the psoriasis in the short term, relapse or vigorous rebound occurs on withdrawal (sometimes precipitating severe pustular psoriasis). See the role of topical corticosteroids in the treatment of psoriasis.

In general, the most potent topical corticosteroids should be reserved for recalcitrant dermatoses such as *chronic discoid lupus erythematosus, lichen simplex chronicus, hypertrophic lichen planus,* and *palmoplantar pustulosis*. Potent corticosteroids should generally be avoided on the face and skin flexures, but specialists occasionally prescribe them for use on these areas in certain circumstances.

When topical treatment has failed, intralesional corticosteroid injections may be used. These are more effective than the very potent topical corticosteroid preparations and should be reserved for severe cases where there are localised lesions such as *keloid scars, hypertrophic lichen planus,* or *localised alopecia areata*.

Perioral lesions
Hydrocortisone cream 1% p. 1092 can be used for up to 7 days to treat uninfected inflammatory lesions on the lips. Hydrocortisone with miconazole cream or ointment p. 1097 is useful where infection by susceptible organisms and inflammation co-exist, particularly for initial treatment (up to 7 days) e.g. in angular cheilitis. Organisms susceptible to miconazole include *Candida* spp. and many Gram-positive bacteria including streptococci and staphylococci.

Choice of formulation
Water-miscible corticosteroid *creams* are suitable for moist or weeping lesions whereas *ointments* are generally chosen for dry, lichenified or scaly lesions or where a more occlusive effect is required. *Lotions* may be useful when minimal application to a large or hair-bearing area is required or for the treatment of exudative lesions. *Occlusive polythene* or *hydrocolloid dressings* increase absorption, but also increase the risk of side effects; they are therefore used only under supervision on a short-term basis for areas of very thick skin (such as the palms and soles). The inclusion of urea or salicylic acid also increases the penetration of the corticosteroid.

In the BNF publications topical corticosteroids for the skin are categorised as 'mild', 'moderately potent', 'potent' or 'very potent'; the **least potent** preparation which is effective should be chosen but dilution should be avoided whenever possible.

Absorption through the skin
Mild and *moderately potent* topical corticosteroids are associated with few side-effects but care is required in the use of *potent* and *very potent* corticosteroids. Absorption through the skin can rarely cause adrenal suppression and even Cushing's syndrome, depending on the area of the body being treated and the duration of treatment. Absorption is greatest where the skin is thin or raw, and from intertriginous areas; it is increased by occlusion.

13

Skin

Suitable quantities of corticosteroid preparations to be prescribed for specific areas of the body

Area of body	Creams and Ointments
Face and neck	15 to 30 g
Both hands	15 to 30 g
Scalp	15 to 30 g
Both arms	30 to 60g
Both legs	100 g
Trunk	100 g
Groins and genitalia	15 to 30 g

These amounts are usually suitable for an adult for a single daily application for 2 weeks

Compound preparations

The advantages of including other substances (such as antibacterials or antifungals) with corticosteroids in topical preparations are uncertain, but such combinations may have a place where inflammatory skin conditions are associated with bacterial or fungal infection, such as infected eczema. In these cases the antimicrobial drug should be chosen according to the sensitivity of the infecting organism and used regularly for a short period (typically twice daily for 1 week). Longer use increases the likelihood of resistance and of sensitisation.

The keratolytic effect of salicylic acid facilitates the absorption of topical corticosteroids; however, excessive and prolonged use of topical preparations containing salicylic acid may cause salicylism.

Topical corticosteroid preparation potencies

Potency of a topical corticosteroid preparation is a result of the formulation as well as the corticosteroid. Therefore, proprietary names are shown.

Mild
- Hydrocortisone 0.1–2.5%
- Dioderm
- Mildison
- Synalar 1 in 10 dilution

Mild with antimicrobials
- Canesten HC
- Daktacort
- Econacort
- Fucidin H
- Nystaform-HC
- Terra-Cortril
- Timodine

Moderate
- Betnovate-RD
- Eumovate
- Haelan
- Modrasone
- Synalar 1 in 4 Dilution
- Ultralanum Plain

Moderate with antimicrobials
- Trimovate

Moderate with urea:
- Alphaderm

Potent
- Beclometasone dipropionate 0.025%
- Betamethasone valerate 0.1%
- Betacap
- Betesil
- Bettamousse
- Betnovate
- Cutivate
- Diprosone
- Elocon
- Hydrocortisone butyrate
- Locoid
- Locoid Crelo
- Metosyn
- Mometasone furoate 0.1%
- Nerisone
- Synalar

Potent with antimicrobials
- Aureocort
- Betamethasone and clioquinol
- Betamethasone and neomycin
- Fucibet
- Lotriderm
- Synalar C
- Synalar N

Potent with salicylic acid
- Diprosalic

Very potent
- Clarelux
- Dermovate
- Etrivex
- Nerisone Forte

Very potent with antimicrobials
- Clobetasol with neomycin and nystatin

Use in children

Children, especially infants, are particularly susceptible to side-effects. However, concern about the safety of topical corticosteroids in children should not result in the child being undertreated. The aim is to control the condition as well as possible; inadequate treatment will perpetuate the condition. A mild corticosteroid such as hydrocortisone 0.5% or 1% is useful for treating nappy rash and hydrocortisone1% for atopic eczema in childhood. A moderately potent or potent corticosteroid may be appropriate for severe atopic eczema on the limbs, for 1–2 weeks only, switching to a less potent preparation as the condition improves. In an acute flare-up of atopic eczema, it may be appropriate to use more potent formulations of topical corticosteroids for a short period to regain control of the condition. A very potent corticosteroid should be initiated under the supervision of a specialist. Carers of young children should be advised that treatment should **not** necessarily be reserved to 'treat only the worst areas' and they may need to be advised that patient information leaflets may contain inappropriate advice for the patient's condition.

Corticosteroids (topical)

- CONTRA-INDICATIONS Acne · perioral dermatitis · potent corticosteroids in widespread plaque psoriasis · rosacea (in adults) · untreated bacterial, fungal or viral skin lesions
- CAUTIONS Avoid prolonged use (particularly on the face) · cautions applicable to systemic corticosteroids may also apply if absorption occurs following topical and local use · dermatoses of infancy, including nappy rash (extreme caution required—treatment should be limited to 5–7 days) (in children) · infection · keep away from eyes · use potent or very potent topical corticosteroids under specialist supervision (in children) · use potent or very potent topical corticosteroids under specialist supervision in psoriasis (can result in rebound relapse, development of generalised pustular psoriasis, and local and systemic toxicity) (in adults)
- SIDE-EFFECTS
- ▶ Rare Adrenal suppression · Cushing's syndrome

▸ **Frequency not known** Acne · contact dermatitis · hypertrichosis · irreversible striae atrophicae · irreversible telangiectasia · mild depigmentation (may be reversible) · perioral dermatitis · side-effects applicable to systemic corticosteroids may also apply if absorption occurs following topical and local use · spread and worsening of untreated infection · thinning of the skin (may be restored over a period after stopping treatment but the original structure may never return) · worsening of acne · worsening of rosacea

SIDE-EFFECTS, FURTHER INFORMATION
In order to minimise the side-effects of a topical corticosteroid, it is important to apply it **thinly** to affected areas **only**, no more frequently than **twice daily**, and to use the least potent formulation which is fully effective.

● DIRECTIONS FOR ADMINISTRATION Topical corticosteroid preparations should be applied no more frequently than twice daily; once daily is often sufficient. Topical corticosteroids should be spread thinly on the skin but in sufficient quantity to cover the affected areas. The length of cream or ointment expelled from a tube may be used to specify the quantity to be applied to a given area of skin. This length can be measured in terms of a *fingertip unit* (the distance from the tip of the adult index finger to the first crease). One fingertip unit (approximately 500 mg from a tube with a standard 5 mm diameter nozzle) is sufficient to cover an area that is twice that of the flat adult handprint (palm and fingers). Mixing topical preparations on the skin should be avoided where possible; several minutes should elapse between application of different preparations.

▸ In children 'Wet-wrap bandaging' increases absorption into the skin, but should be initiated only by a dermatologist and application supervised by a healthcare professional trained in the technique.

● PRESCRIBING AND DISPENSING INFORMATION The potency of each topical corticosteroid should be included on the label with the directions for use. The label should be attached to the container (for example, the tube) rather than the outer packaging.

● PATIENT AND CARER ADVICE Patients or carers should be given advice on how to administer corticosteroid creams and ointments. If a patient is using topical corticosteroids of different potencies, the patient should be told when to use each corticosteroid. Patients and their carers should be reassured that side effects such as skin thinning and systemic effects rarely occur when topical corticosteroids are used appropriately.

⟲ 1086

Alclometasone dipropionate

● INDICATIONS AND DOSE

Inflammatory skin disorders such as eczemas
▸ TO THE SKIN
▸ Child: Apply 1–2 times a day, to be applied thinly
▸ Adult: Apply 1–2 times a day, to be applied thinly
POTENCY
Alclometasone dipropionate cream 0.05%: moderate

● UNLICENSED USE
▸ With topical use in children Licensed for use in children (age range not specified by manufacturer).

● PATIENT AND CARER ADVICE Patients or carers should be counselled on the application of alclometasone dipropionate cream.

● MEDICINAL FORMS
There can be variation in the licensing of different medicines containing the same drug.
Cream
CAUTIONARY AND ADVISORY LABELS 28
EXCIPIENTS: May contain Cetostearyl alcohol (including cetyl and stearyl alcohol), chlorocresol, propylene glycol
▸ Alclometasone dipropionate (Non-proprietary)
Alclometasone dipropionate 500 microgram per 1 gram Boots Derma Care Eczema & Dermatitis Flare-Up 0.05% cream ǀ 15 gram Ⓟ no price available
▸ Modrasone (Teva UK Ltd)
Alclometasone dipropionate 500 microgram per 1 gram Modrasone 0.05% cream ǀ 50 gram PoM £2.68 DT price = £2.68

⟲ 1086

Beclometasone dipropionate
(Beclomethasone dipropionate)

● INDICATIONS AND DOSE

Severe inflammatory skin disorders such as eczemas unresponsive to less potent corticosteroids ǀ Psoriasis
▸ TO THE SKIN
▸ Child: Apply 1–2 times a day, thin layer to be applied
▸ Adult: Apply 1–2 times a day, thin layer to be applied
POTENCY
Beclometasone dipropionate cream and ointment 0.025%: potent.

● UNLICENSED USE
▸ With topical use in children Not licensed for use in children under 1 year.

● MEDICINAL FORMS
There can be variation in the licensing of different medicines containing the same drug. Forms available from special-order manufacturers include: cream, ointment
Cream
CAUTIONARY AND ADVISORY LABELS 28
▸ Beclometasone dipropionate (Non-proprietary)
Beclometasone dipropionate 250 microgram per 1 gram Beclometasone 0.025% cream ǀ 30 gram PoM £68.00 DT price = £68.00
Ointment
CAUTIONARY AND ADVISORY LABELS 28
▸ Beclometasone dipropionate (Non-proprietary)
Beclometasone dipropionate 250 microgram per 1 gram Beclometasone 0.025% ointment ǀ 30 gram PoM £68.00 DT price = £68.00

⟲ 1086

Betamethasone

● INDICATIONS AND DOSE

Severe inflammatory skin disorders such as eczemas unresponsive to less potent corticosteroids ǀ Psoriasis
▸ TO THE SKIN
▸ Child: Apply 1–2 times a day, to be applied thinly
▸ Adult: Apply 1–2 times a day, to be applied thinly
POTENCY
Betamethasone valerate 0.025% cream and ointment: moderate.
Betamethasone valerate 0.1% cream, lotion, ointment, and scalp application: potent.
Betamethasone valerate 0.12% foam: potent.
Betamethasone dipropionate 0.05% cream, lotion, and ointment: potent.

● UNLICENSED USE
▸ With topical use in children *Betacap*®, *Betnovate*® and *Betnovate-RD*® are not licensed for use in children under 1 year. *Bettamousse*® is not licensed for use in children under 6 years.

13

Skin

- CAUTIONS Use of more than 100 g per week of 0.1% preparation likely to cause adrenal suppression
- PATIENT AND CARER ADVICE Patient counselling is advised for betamethasone cream, ointment, scalp application and foam (application).

● MEDICINAL FORMS
There can be variation in the licensing of different medicines containing the same drug. Forms available from special-order manufacturers include: cream, ointment

Foam
CAUTIONARY AND ADVISORY LABELS 28, 15
EXCIPIENTS: May contain Cetostearyl alcohol (including cetyl and stearyl alcohol), polysorbates, propylene glycol
▸ Bettamousse (Focus Pharmaceuticals Ltd)
Betamethasone (as Betamethasone valerate) 1 mg per 1 gram Bettamousse 0.1% cutaneous foam | 100 gram PoM £9.75 DT price = £9.75

Liquid
CAUTIONARY AND ADVISORY LABELS 15 (scalp lotion only), 28
EXCIPIENTS: May contain Cetostearyl alcohol (including cetyl and stearyl alcohol), hydroxybenzoates (parabens)
▸ Betacap (Dermal Laboratories Ltd)
Betamethasone (as Betamethasone valerate) 1 mg per 1 gram Betacap 0.1% scalp application | 100 ml PoM £3.19 DT price = £3.19
▸ Betnovate (GlaxoSmithKline UK Ltd)
Betamethasone (as Betamethasone valerate) 1 mg per 1 gram Betnovate 0.1% scalp application | 100 ml PoM £4.99 DT price = £3.19
Betnovate 0.1% lotion | 100 ml PoM £4.58 DT price = £4.58
▸ Diprosone (Merck Sharp & Dohme Ltd)
Betamethasone (as Betamethasone dipropionate) 500 microgram per 1 ml Diprosone 0.05% lotion | 30 ml PoM £2.73 DT price = £2.73 | 100 ml PoM £7.80 DT price = £7.80

Cream
CAUTIONARY AND ADVISORY LABELS 28
EXCIPIENTS: May contain Cetostearyl alcohol (including cetyl and stearyl alcohol), chlorocresol
▸ Betamethasone (Non-proprietary)
Betamethasone (as Betamethasone valerate) 1 mg per 1 gram Betamethasone valerate 0.1% cream | 30 gram PoM £5.99 DT price = £3.31 | 100 gram PoM £12.23 DT price = £11.03
▸ Audavate (Auden McKenzie (Pharma Division) Ltd)
Betamethasone (as Betamethasone valerate) 250 microgram per 1 gram Audavate RD 0.025% cream | 100 gram PoM £2.52 DT price = £3.15
▸ Betnovate (GlaxoSmithKline UK Ltd)
Betamethasone (as Betamethasone valerate) 250 microgram per 1 gram Betnovate RD 0.025% cream | 100 gram PoM £3.15 DT price = £3.15
Betamethasone (as Betamethasone valerate) 1 mg per 1 gram Betnovate 0.1% cream | 30 gram PoM £1.43 DT price = £3.31 | 100 gram PoM £4.05 DT price = £11.03
▸ Diprosone (Merck Sharp & Dohme Ltd)
Betamethasone (as Betamethasone dipropionate) 500 microgram per 1 gram Diprosone 0.05% cream | 30 gram PoM £2.16 DT price = £2.16 | 100 gram PoM £6.12 DT price = £6.12

Ointment
CAUTIONARY AND ADVISORY LABELS 28
▸ Betamethasone (Non-proprietary)
Betamethasone (as Betamethasone valerate) 1 mg per 1 gram Betamethasone 0.1% ointment | 30 gram PoM £5.55 DT price = £2.65 | 100 gram PoM £14.99 DT price = £8.83
▸ Audavate (Auden McKenzie (Pharma Division) Ltd)
Betamethasone (as Betamethasone valerate) 250 microgram per 1 gram Audavate RD 0.025% ointment | 100 gram PoM £2.52 DT price = £3.15
Betamethasone (as Betamethasone valerate) 1 mg per 1 gram Audavate 0.1% ointment | 30 gram PoM £1.14 DT price = £2.65 | 100 gram PoM £3.24 DT price = £8.83
▸ Betnovate (GlaxoSmithKline UK Ltd)
Betamethasone (as Betamethasone valerate) 250 microgram per 1 gram Betnovate RD 0.025% ointment | 100 gram PoM £3.15 DT price = £3.15

Betamethasone (as Betamethasone valerate) 1 mg per 1 gram Betnovate 0.1% ointment | 30 gram PoM £1.43 DT price = £2.65 | 100 gram PoM £4.05 DT price = £8.83
▸ Diprosone (Merck Sharp & Dohme Ltd)
Betamethasone (as Betamethasone dipropionate) 500 microgram per 1 gram Diprosone 0.05% ointment | 30 gram PoM £2.16 DT price = £2.16 | 100 gram PoM £6.12 DT price = £6.12

Combinations available: *Betamethasone with clioquinol,* p. 1093 · *Betamethasone with clotrimazole,* p. 1094 · *Betamethasone with fusidic acid,* p. 1094 · *Betamethasone with neomycin,* p. 1094 · *Betamethasone with salicylic acid,* p. 1094

Calcipotriol with betamethasone

The properties listed below are those particular to the combination only. For the properties of the components please consider, calcipotriol p. 1105, betamethasone p. 1087.

● INDICATIONS AND DOSE

DOVOBET® GEL

Scalp psoriasis
▸ TO THE SKIN
▸ Adult: Apply 1–4 g once daily usual duration of therapy 4 weeks; if necessary, treatment may be continued beyond 4 weeks or repeated, on the advice of a specialist, shampoo off after leaving on scalp overnight or during day, when different preparations containing calcipotriol used together, maximum total calcipotriol 5 mg in any one week

Mild to moderate plaque psoriasis
▸ TO THE SKIN
▸ Adult: Apply once daily for 8 weeks; if necessary, treatment may be continued beyond 8 weeks or repeated, on the advice of a specialist, apply to maximum 30% of body surface, when different preparations containing calcipotriol used together, max. total calcipotriol 5 mg in any one week; maximum 15 g per day

DOVOBET® OINTMENT

Stable plaque psoriasis
▸ TO THE SKIN
▸ Adult: Apply once daily for 4 weeks; if necessary, treatment may be continued beyond 4 weeks or repeated, on the advice of a specialist, apply to a maximum 30% of body surface, when different preparations containing calcipotriol used together, max. total calcipotriol 5 mg in any one week; maximum 15 g per day

● MEDICINAL FORMS
There can be variation in the licensing of different medicines containing the same drug.

Ointment
CAUTIONARY AND ADVISORY LABELS 28
EXCIPIENTS: May contain Butylated hydroxytoluene
▸ Dovobet (LEO Pharma)
Calcipotriol (as Calcipotriol hydrate) 50 microgram per 1 gram, Betamethasone (as Betamethasone dipropionate) 500 microgram per 1 gram Dovobet ointment | 30 gram PoM £19.84 DT price = £19.84 | 60 gram PoM £39.68 | 120 gram PoM £73.86

Gel
CAUTIONARY AND ADVISORY LABELS 28
EXCIPIENTS: May contain Butylated hydroxytoluene
▸ Dovobet (LEO Pharma)
Calcipotriol (as Calcipotriol monohydrate) 50 microgram per 1 gram, Betamethasone (as Betamethasone dipropionate) 500 microgram per 1 gram Dovobet gel Applicator | 60 gram PoM £37.21 DT price = £37.21
Dovobet gel | 60 gram PoM £37.21 DT price = £37.21 | 120 gram PoM £69.11

Clobetasol propionate

☞ 1086

● **INDICATIONS AND DOSE**

Short-term treatment only of severe resistant inflammatory skin disorders such as recalcitrant eczemas unresponsive to less potent corticosteroids | Psoriasis

▸ TO THE SKIN

▸ Child: Apply 1–2 times a day for up to 4 weeks, to be applied thinly

▸ Adult: Apply 1–2 times a day for up to 4 weeks, to be applied thinly, maximum 50 g of 0.05% preparation per week

ETRIVEX®

Moderate scalp psoriasis

▸ TO THE SKIN

▸ Adult: Apply once daily maximum duration of treatment 4 weeks, to be applied thinly then rinsed off after 15 minutes; frequency of application should be reduced after clinical improvement

POTENCY

Clobetasol propionate 0.05% cream, foam, ointment, scalp application, and shampoo: very potent.

● UNLICENSED USE

▸ With topical use in children *Dermovate*® not licensed for use in children under 1 year.

● PATIENT AND CARER ADVICE Patients or carers should be given advice on how to administer clobetasol propionate foam, liquid (scalp application), cream, ointment and shampoo.

Scalp application Patients or carers should be advised to apply foam directly to scalp lesions (foam begins to subside immediately on contact with skin).

● MEDICINAL FORMS

There can be variation in the licensing of different medicines containing the same drug. Forms available from special-order manufacturers include: cream, ointment, paste

Foam

CAUTIONARY AND ADVISORY LABELS 15, 28

EXCIPIENTS: May contain Cetostearyl alcohol (including cetyl and stearyl alcohol), polysorbates, propylene glycol

▸ Clarelux (Pierre Fabre Dermo-Cosmetique)

Clobetasol propionate 500 microgram per 1 gram Clarelux 500micrograms/g foam | 100 gram [PoM] £11.06

Liquid

CAUTIONARY AND ADVISORY LABELS 15, 28

▸ Dermovate (GlaxoSmithKline UK Ltd)

Clobetasol propionate 500 microgram per 1 gram Dermovate 0.05% scalp application | 30 ml [PoM] £3.07 DT price = £3.07 | 100 ml [PoM] £10.42 DT price = £10.42

Cream

CAUTIONARY AND ADVISORY LABELS 28

EXCIPIENTS: May contain Beeswax, cetostearyl alcohol (including cetyl and stearyl alcohol), chlorocresol, propylene glycol

▸ Clobetasol propionate (Non-proprietary)

Clobetasol propionate 500 microgram per 1 gram Clobetasol 0.05% cream | 30 gram [PoM] no price available DT price = £2.69 | 100 gram [PoM] no price available DT price = £7.90

▸ ClobaDerm (Auden McKenzie (Pharma Division) Ltd)

Clobetasol propionate 500 microgram per 1 gram ClobaDerm 0.05% cream | 30 gram [PoM] £2.15 DT price = £2.69 | 100 gram [PoM] £6.32 DT price = £7.90

▸ Dermovate (GlaxoSmithKline UK Ltd)

Clobetasol propionate 500 microgram per 1 gram Dermovate 0.05% cream | 30 gram [PoM] £2.69 DT price = £2.69 | 100 gram [PoM] £7.90 DT price = £7.90

Ointment

CAUTIONARY AND ADVISORY LABELS 28

EXCIPIENTS: May contain Propylene glycol

▸ Clobetasol propionate (Non-proprietary)

Clobetasol propionate 500 microgram per 1 gram Clobetasol 0.05% ointment | 30 gram [PoM] no price available DT price = £2.69 | 100 gram [PoM] no price available DT price = £7.90

▸ ClobaDerm (Auden McKenzie (Pharma Division) Ltd)

Clobetasol propionate 500 microgram per 1 gram ClobaDerm 0.05% ointment | 30 gram [PoM] £2.15 DT price = £2.69 | 100 gram [PoM] £6.32 DT price = £7.90

▸ Dermovate (GlaxoSmithKline UK Ltd)

Clobetasol propionate 500 microgram per 1 gram Dermovate 0.05% ointment | 30 gram [PoM] £2.69 DT price = £2.69 | 100 gram [PoM] £7.90 DT price = £7.90

Shampoo

CAUTIONARY AND ADVISORY LABELS 28

▸ Etrivex (Galderma (UK) Ltd)

Clobetasol propionate 500 microgram per 1 gram Etrivex 500micrograms/g shampoo | 125 ml [PoM] £10.29 DT price = £10.29

Combinations available: *Clobetasol propionate with neomycin sulfate and nystatin,* p. 1095

☞ 1086

Clobetasone butyrate

● **INDICATIONS AND DOSE**

Eczemas and dermatitis of all types | Maintenance between courses of more potent corticosteroids

▸ TO THE SKIN

▸ Child: Apply 1–2 times a day, to be applied thinly

▸ Adult: Apply 1–2 times a day, to be applied thinly

POTENCY

Clobetasone butyrate 0.05% cream and ointment: moderate.

● UNLICENSED USE

▸ With topical use in children Licensed for use in children (age range not specified by manufacturer).

● PATIENT AND CARER ADVICE

▸ With topical use Patients or carers should be advised on the application of clobetasone butyrate containing preparations.

● EXCEPTIONS TO LEGAL CATEGORY

▸ With topical use Cream can be sold to the public for short-term symptomatic treatment and control of patches of eczema and dermatitis (but not seborrhoeic dermatitis) in adults and children over 12 years provided pack does not contain more than 15 g.

● MEDICINAL FORMS

There can be variation in the licensing of different medicines containing the same drug. Forms available from special-order manufacturers include: cream, ointment

Cream

CAUTIONARY AND ADVISORY LABELS 28

EXCIPIENTS: May contain Cetostearyl alcohol (including cetyl and stearyl alcohol), chlorocresol

▸ Eumovate (GlaxoSmithKline Consumer Healthcare, GlaxoSmithKline UK Ltd)

Clobetasone butyrate 500 microgram per 1 gram Eumovate Eczema and Dermatitis 0.05% cream | 15 gram [P] £3.57 DT price = £3.57

Eumovate 0.05% cream | 30 gram [PoM] £1.86 DT price = £1.86 | 100 gram [PoM] £5.44 DT price = £5.44

Ointment

CAUTIONARY AND ADVISORY LABELS 28

▸ Clobavate (Auden McKenzie (Pharma Division) Ltd)

Clobetasone butyrate 500 microgram per 1 gram Clobavate 0.05% ointment | 30 gram [PoM] £1.49 DT price = £1.86 | 100 gram [PoM] £4.35 DT price = £5.44

13

Skin

> Eumovate (GlaxoSmithKline UK Ltd)
Clobetasone butyrate 500 microgram per 1 gram Eumovate 0.05% ointment | 30 gram [PoM] £1.86 DT price = £1.86 | 100 gram [PoM] £5.44 DT price = £5.44

Combinations available: *Clobetasone butyrate with nystatin and oxytetracycline,* p. 1095

Diflucortolone valerate ⚑ 1086

● INDICATIONS AND DOSE

Severe inflammatory skin disorders such as eczemas unresponsive to less potent corticosteroids (using 0.3% diflucortolone valerate) | Short-term treatment of severe exacerbations (using 0.3% diflucortolone valerate) | Psoriasis (using 0.3% diflucortolone valerate)

▶ TO THE SKIN

▶ Child 4–17 years: Apply 1–2 times a day for up to 2 weeks, reducing strength as condition responds, to be applied thinly; maximum 60 g per week

▶ Adult: Apply 1–2 times a day for up to 2 weeks, reducing strength as condition responds, to be applied thinly; maximum 60 g per week

Severe inflammatory skin disorders such as eczemas unresponsive to less potent corticosteroids (using 0.1% diflucortolone valerate) | Psoriasis (using 0.1% diflucortolone valerate)

▶ TO THE SKIN

▶ Child: Apply 1–2 times a day for up to 4 weeks, to be applied thinly

▶ Adult: Apply 1–2 times a day for up to 4 weeks, to be applied thinly

POTENCY

Diflucortolone valerate 0.1% cream and ointment: potent.
Diflucortolone valerate 0.3% cream and ointment: very potent.

● UNLICENSED USE

▶ With topical use in children *Nerisone*® licensed for use in children (age range not specified by manufacturer); *Nerisone Forte*® not licensed for use in children under 4 years.

● PRESCRIBING AND DISPENSING INFORMATION Patients or carers should be advised on application of diflucortolone valerate containing preparations.

● MEDICINAL FORMS
There can be variation in the licensing of different medicines containing the same drug.
Cream
CAUTIONARY AND ADVISORY LABELS 28
EXCIPIENTS: May contain Beeswax, cetostearyl alcohol (including cetyl and stearyl alcohol), disodium edetate, hydroxybenzoates (parabens)
▶ Nerisone (Meadow Laboratories Ltd)
Diflucortolone valerate 1 mg per 1 gram Nerisone 0.1% cream | 30 gram [PoM] £3.98
Nerisone 0.1% oily cream | 30 gram [PoM] £4.95 DT price = £4.95
Diflucortolone valerate 3 mg per 1 gram Nerisone Forte 0.3% oily cream | 15 gram [PoM] £4.70 DT price = £4.70
Ointment
CAUTIONARY AND ADVISORY LABELS 28
▶ Nerisone (Meadow Laboratories Ltd)
Diflucortolone valerate 1 mg per 1 gram Nerisone 0.1% ointment | 30 gram [PoM] £3.98
Diflucortolone valerate 3 mg per 1 gram Nerisone Forte 0.3% ointment | 15 gram [PoM] £4.70

Fludroxycortide ⚑ 1086

(Flurandrenolone)

● INDICATIONS AND DOSE

Inflammatory skin disorders such as eczemas

▶ TO THE SKIN

▶ Child: Apply 1–2 times a day, to be applied thinly

▶ Adult: Apply 1–2 times a day, to be applied thinly

HAELAN® TAPE

Chronic localised recalcitrant dermatoses (but not acute or weeping)

▶ TO THE SKIN

▶ Child: Cut tape to fit lesion, apply to clean, dry skin shorn of hair, usually for 12 hours daily

▶ Adult: Cut tape to fit lesion, apply to clean, dry skin shorn of hair, usually for 12 hours daily

POTENCY

Fludroxycortide 0.0125% cream and ointment: moderate.

● UNLICENSED USE

▶ With topical use in children Licensed for use in children (age range not specified by manufacturer).

● PATIENT AND CARER ADVICE Patients or carers should be counselled on application of fludroxycortide cream and ointment.

● MEDICINAL FORMS
There can be variation in the licensing of different medicines containing the same drug.
Cream
CAUTIONARY AND ADVISORY LABELS 28
EXCIPIENTS: May contain Cetostearyl alcohol (including cetyl and stearyl alcohol), propylene glycol
▶ Fludroxycortide (Non-proprietary)
Fludroxycortide 125 microgram per 1 gram Fludroxycortide 0.0125% cream | 60 gram [PoM] no price available
▶ Haelan (Typharm Ltd)
Fludroxycortide 125 microgram per 1 gram Haelan 0.0125% cream | 60 gram [PoM] £3.26
Ointment
CAUTIONARY AND ADVISORY LABELS 28
EXCIPIENTS: May contain Beeswax, cetostearyl alcohol (including cetyl and stearyl alcohol), polysorbates
▶ Fludroxycortide (Non-proprietary)
Fludroxycortide 125 microgram per 1 gram Fludroxycortide 0.0125% ointment | 60 gram [PoM] no price available
▶ Haelan (Typharm Ltd)
Fludroxycortide 125 microgram per 1 gram Haelan 0.0125% ointment | 60 gram [PoM] £3.26
Impregnated dressing
▶ Haelan (Typharm Ltd)
Fludroxycortide 4 microgram per 1 square cm Haelan 4micrograms/square cm tape 7.5cm | 20 cm [PoM] £8.19 | 50 cm [PoM] £9.27 DT price = £9.27

Fluocinolone acetonide ⚑ 1086

● INDICATIONS AND DOSE

Severe inflammatory skin disorders such as eczemas | Psoriasis

▶ TO THE SKIN

▶ Child 1–17 years: Apply 1–2 times a day, to be applied thinly, reduce strength as condition responds

▶ Adult: Apply 1–2 times a day, to be applied thinly, reduce strength as condition responds

POTENCY

Fluocinolone acetonide 0.025% cream, gel, and ointment: potent.
Fluocinolone acetonide 0.00625% cream and ointment: moderate.
Fluocinolone acetonide 0.0025% cream: mild.

- **UNLICENSED USE**
▸ With topical use in children Not licensed for use in children under 1 year.
- **PRESCRIBING AND DISPENSING INFORMATION** Gel is useful for application to the scalp and other hairy areas.
- **PATIENT AND CARER ADVICE** Patient counselling is advised for fluocinolone acetonide cream, gel and ointment (application).

- **MEDICINAL FORMS**
There can be variation in the licensing of different medicines containing the same drug.
Cream
CAUTIONARY AND ADVISORY LABELS 28
EXCIPIENTS: May contain Benzyl alcohol, cetostearyl alcohol (including cetyl and stearyl alcohol), polysorbates, propylene glycol
▸ Synalar (Derma UK Ltd)
Fluocinolone acetonide 25 microgram per 1 gram Synalar 1 in 10 Dilution 0.0025% cream | 50 gram PoM £4.58 DT price = £4.58
Fluocinolone acetonide 62.5 microgram per 1 gram Synalar 1 in 4 Dilution 0.00625% cream | 50 gram PoM £4.84 DT price = £4.84
Fluocinolone acetonide 250 microgram per 1 gram Synalar 0.025% cream | 30 gram PoM £4.14 DT price = £4.14 | 100 gram PoM £11.75 DT price = £11.75
Ointment
CAUTIONARY AND ADVISORY LABELS 28
EXCIPIENTS: May contain Propylene glycol, wool fat and related substances including lanolin
▸ Synalar (Derma UK Ltd)
Fluocinolone acetonide 62.5 microgram per 1 gram Synalar 1 in 4 Dilution 0.00625% ointment | 50 gram PoM £4.84 DT price = £4.84
Fluocinolone acetonide 250 microgram per 1 gram Synalar 0.025% ointment | 30 gram PoM £4.14 DT price = £4.14 | 100 gram PoM £11.75 DT price = £11.75
Gel
CAUTIONARY AND ADVISORY LABELS 28
EXCIPIENTS: May contain Hydroxybenzoates (parabens), propylene glycol
▸ Synalar (Derma UK Ltd)
Fluocinolone acetonide 250 microgram per 1 gram Synalar 0.025% gel | 30 gram PoM £5.56 DT price = £5.56 | 60 gram PoM £10.02 DT price = £10.02

Combinations available: *Fluocinolone acetonide with clioquinol*, p. 1096 · *Fluocinolone acetonide with neomycin*, p. 1096

F 1086

Fluocinonide

- **INDICATIONS AND DOSE**
Severe inflammatory skin disorders such as eczemas unresponsive to less potent corticosteroids | Psoriasis
▸ TO THE SKIN
▸ Child: Apply 1–2 times a day, to be applied thinly
▸ Adult: Apply 1–2 times a day, to be applied thinly
POTENCY
Fluocinonide 0.05% cream and ointment: potent.

- **UNLICENSED USE**
▸ With topical use in children Not licensed for use in children under 1 year.
- **PATIENT AND CARER ADVICE** Patients or carers should be advised on the application of fluocinonide preparations.

- **MEDICINAL FORMS**
There can be variation in the licensing of different medicines containing the same drug.
Cream
CAUTIONARY AND ADVISORY LABELS 28
EXCIPIENTS: May contain Propylene glycol
▸ Metosyn FAPG (Derma UK Ltd)
Fluocinonide 500 microgram per 1 gram Metosyn FAPG 0.05% cream | 25 gram PoM £3.96 DT price = £3.96 | 100 gram PoM £13.34 DT price = £13.34

Ointment
CAUTIONARY AND ADVISORY LABELS 28
EXCIPIENTS: May contain Propylene glycol, wool fat and related substances including lanolin
▸ Metosyn (Derma UK Ltd)
Fluocinonide 500 microgram per 1 gram Metosyn 0.05% ointment | 25 gram PoM £3.50 DT price = £3.50 | 100 gram PoM £13.15 DT price = £13.15

F 1086

Fluocortolone

- **INDICATIONS AND DOSE**
Severe inflammatory skin disorders such as eczemas unresponsive to less potent corticosteroids | Psoriasis
▸ TO THE SKIN
▸ Adult: Apply 1–2 times a day, to be applied thinly, reducing strength as condition responds
POTENCY
Fluocortolone hexanoate 0.25% cream and ointment; fluocortolone pivalate 0.25% cream and fluocortolone 0.25% ointment: moderate.

- **PRESCRIBING AND DISPENSING INFORMATION** Patients or carers should be counselled on the application of fluocortolone preparations.

- **MEDICINAL FORMS**
There can be variation in the licensing of different medicines containing the same drug.
Cream
CAUTIONARY AND ADVISORY LABELS 28
EXCIPIENTS: May contain Cetostearyl alcohol (including cetyl and stearyl alcohol), disodium edetate, fragrances, hydroxybenzoates (parabens)
▸ Ultralanum Plain (Fluocortolone hexanoate / Fluocortolone pivalate) (Meadow Laboratories Ltd)
Fluocortolone hexanoate 2.5 mg per 1 gram, Fluocortolone pivalate 2.5 mg per 1 gram Ultralanum Plain cream | 50 gram PoM £2.95
Ointment
CAUTIONARY AND ADVISORY LABELS 28
EXCIPIENTS: May contain Fragrances, wool fat and related substances including lanolin
▸ Ultralanum Plain (Fluocortolone / Fluocortolone hexanoate) (Meadow Laboratories Ltd)
Fluocortolone 2.5 mg per 1 gram, Fluocortolone hexanoate 2.5 mg per 1 gram Ultralanum Plain ointment | 50 gram PoM £2.95

F 1086

Fluticasone

4.1.2016

- **INDICATIONS AND DOSE**
Severe inflammatory skin disorders such as dermatitis and eczemas unresponsive to less potent corticosteroids | Psoriasis
▸ TO THE SKIN
▸ Child 3 months-17 years: Apply 1–2 times a day, to be applied thinly
▸ Adult: Apply 1–2 times a day, to be applied thinly
POTENCY
Fluticasone cream 0.05%: potent.
Fluticasone ointment 0.005%: potent.

- **UNLICENSED USE**
▸ With topical use in children Not licensed for use in children under 3 months.
- **PATIENT AND CARER ADVICE** Patients or carers should be given advice on application of fluticasone creams and ointments.

13

Skin

13

Skin

● MEDICINAL FORMS
There can be variation in the licensing of different medicines containing the same drug.

Cream

CAUTIONARY AND ADVISORY LABELS 28
EXCIPIENTS: May contain Cetostearyl alcohol (including cetyl and stearyl alcohol), imidurea, propylene glycol
▸ Cutivate (GlaxoSmithKline UK Ltd)
    Fluticasone propionate 500 microgram per 1 gram Cutivate 0.05% cream | 15 gram [PoM] £2.27 DT price = £2.27 | 30 gram [PoM] £4.24 DT price = £4.24

Ointment

CAUTIONARY AND ADVISORY LABELS 28
EXCIPIENTS: May contain Propylene glycol
▸ Cutivate (GlaxoSmithKline UK Ltd)
    Fluticasone propionate 50 microgram per 1 gram Cutivate 0.005% ointment | 15 gram [PoM] £2.27 DT price = £2.27 | 30 gram [PoM] £4.24 DT price = £4.24

[F 1086]

Hydrocortisone

● INDICATIONS AND DOSE

Mild inflammatory skin disorders such as eczemas
▸ TO THE SKIN
▸ Child: Apply 1–2 times a day, to be applied thinly
▸ Adult: Apply 1–2 times a day, to be applied thinly

Nappy rash
▸ TO THE SKIN
▸ Child: Apply as required for no more than 1 week, discontinue as soon as the inflammation subsides

POTENCY
Hydrocortisone cream and ointment 0.5 to 2.5%: mild

● PRESCRIBING AND DISPENSING INFORMATION When hydrocortisone cream or ointment is prescribed and no strength is stated, the 1% strength should be supplied. Although *Dioderm*® contains only 0.1% hydrocortisone, the formulation is designed to provide a clinical activity comparable to that of Hydrocortisone Cream 1% BP.

● PATIENT AND CARER ADVICE Patient counselling is advised for hydrocortisone cream and ointment (application).

● PROFESSION SPECIFIC INFORMATION

Dental practitioners' formulary
Hydrocortisone Cream 1% 15 g may be prescribed.

● EXCEPTIONS TO LEGAL CATEGORY
Over-the-counter hydrocortisone preparations Skin creams and ointments containing hydrocortisone (alone or with other ingredients) can be sold to the public for the treatment of allergic contact dermatitis, irritant dermatitis, insect bite reactions and mild to moderate eczema in patients over 10 years, to be applied sparingly over the affected area 1–2 times daily for max. 1 week. Over-the-counter hydrocortisone preparations should not be sold without medical advice for children under 10 years or for pregnant women; they should **not** be sold for application to the face, anogenital region, broken or infected skin (including cold sores, acne, and athlete's foot).

● MEDICINAL FORMS
There can be variation in the licensing of different medicines containing the same drug. Forms available from special-order manufacturers include: cream, ointment

Cream

CAUTIONARY AND ADVISORY LABELS 28
EXCIPIENTS: May contain Benzyl alcohol, cetostearyl alcohol (including cetyl and stearyl alcohol), hydroxybenzoates (parabens), propylene glycol
▸ Hydrocortisone (Non-proprietary)
    Hydrocortisone 5 mg per 1 gram Hydrocortisone 0.5% cream | 15 gram [PoM] £4.80 DT price = £1.12 | 30 gram [PoM] £2.84–£4.90
    Hydrocortisone 10 mg per 1 gram Hydrocortisone 1% cream | 15 gram [P] £1.64 DT price = £0.94 | 15 gram [PoM] £11.41 DT price = £0.94 | 30 gram [PoM] £14.30 DT price = £1.88 | 50 gram [PoM] £27.75 DT price = £3.13

    Hydrocortisone acetate 10 mg per 1 gram **Hydrocortisone 25 mg per 1 gram** Hydrocortisone 2.5% cream | 15 gram [PoM] £25.00 DT price = £4.88 | 30 gram [PoM] £44.00
▸ Derma Care Hydrocortisone (The Boots Company Plc)
    Hydrocortisone 10 mg per 1 gram Derma Care Hydrocortisone 1% cream | 15 gram [P] no price available DT price = £0.94
▸ Dermacort (Marlborough Pharmaceuticals Ltd)
    Hydrocortisone 1 mg per 1 gram Dermacort hydrocortisone 0.1% cream | 15 gram [P] £2.83 DT price = £2.83
▸ Dioderm (Dermal Laboratories Ltd)
    Hydrocortisone 1 mg per 1 gram Dioderm 0.1% cream | 30 gram [P] £2.03 DT price = £2.03
▸ Hc45 (Reckitt Benckiser Healthcare (UK) Ltd)
    Hydrocortisone acetate 10 mg per 1 gram Hc45 Hydrocortisone 1% cream | 15 gram [P] £2.58
▸ Mildison Lipocream (Astellas Pharma Ltd)
    Hydrocortisone 10 mg per 1 gram Mildison Lipocream 1% cream | 30 gram [PoM] £1.71 DT price = £1.88
▸ Zenoxone (Teva UK Ltd)
    Hydrocortisone 10 mg per 1 gram Zenoxone 1% cream | 15 gram [P] £1.25 DT price = £0.94

Ointment

CAUTIONARY AND ADVISORY LABELS 28
▸ Hydrocortisone (Non-proprietary)
    Hydrocortisone 5 mg per 1 gram Hydrocortisone 0.5% ointment | 15 gram [PoM] £5.55 DT price = £5.55 | 30 gram [PoM] £11.10–£12.00
    Hydrocortisone 10 mg per 1 gram Hydrocortisone 1% ointment | 15 gram [PoM] £11.41 DT price = £1.05 | 30 gram [PoM] £14.30 DT price = £2.10 | 30 gram [P] £3.31 DT price = £2.10 | 50 gram [PoM] £27.75 DT price = £3.50
    Hydrocortisone 25 mg per 1 gram Hydrocortisone 2.5% ointment | 15 gram [PoM] £25.37 DT price = £24.43 | 30 gram [PoM] £48.86

Combinations available: *Hydrocortisone with benzalkonium chloride, dimeticone, and nystatin*, p. 1096 · *Hydrocortisone with chlorhexidine hydrochloride and nystatin*, p. 1096 · *Hydrocortisone with fusidic acid*, p. 1097 · *Hydrocortisone with miconazole*, p. 1097 · *Hydrocortisone with oxytetracycline*, p. 1098

[F 1086]

Hydrocortisone butyrate

● INDICATIONS AND DOSE

Severe inflammatory skin disorders such as eczemas unresponsive to less potent corticosteroids | Psoriasis
▸ TO THE SKIN
▸ Child 1-17 years: Apply 1–2 times a day, to be applied thinly
▸ Adult: Apply 1–2 times a day, to be applied thinly

POTENCY
Hydrocortisone butyrate 0.1% cream, liquid, and ointment: potent

● PATIENT AND CARER ADVICE
Medicines for Children leaflet: Hydrocortisone (topical) for eczema www.medicinesforchildren.org.uk/hydrocortisone-topical-for-eczema

Patients or carers should be given advice on how to administer hydrocortisone butyrate lotion, cream, ointment and scalp lotion.

● MEDICINAL FORMS
There can be variation in the licensing of different medicines containing the same drug. Forms available from special-order manufacturers include: ointment

Liquid

CAUTIONARY AND ADVISORY LABELS 15 (excluding Locoid Crelo topical emulsion), 28
EXCIPIENTS: May contain Butylated hydroxytoluene, cetostearyl alcohol (including cetyl and stearyl alcohol), hydroxybenzoates (parabens), propylene glycol
▸ Locoid (Astellas Pharma Ltd)
    Hydrocortisone butyrate 1 mg per 1 ml Locoid 0.1% scalp lotion | 100 ml [PoM] £6.83 DT price = £6.83

▸ Locoid Crelo (Astellas Pharma Ltd)
Hydrocortisone butyrate 1 mg per 1 gram Locoid Crelo 0.1%
topical emulsion | 100 gram [PoM] £5.91

Cream
CAUTIONARY AND ADVISORY LABELS 28
EXCIPIENTS: May contain Benzyl alcohol, cetostearyl alcohol (including cetyl and stearyl alcohol), hydroxybenzoates (parabens)
▸ Locoid (Astellas Pharma Ltd)
Hydrocortisone butyrate 1 mg per 1 gram Locoid 0.1% cream |
30 gram [PoM] £1.60 DT price = £1.60 | 100 gram [PoM] £4.93 DT
price = £4.93
▸ Locoid Lipocream (Astellas Pharma Ltd)
Hydrocortisone butyrate 1 mg per 1 gram Locoid 0.1% Lipocream
| 30 gram [PoM] £1.69 DT price = £1.60 | 100 gram [PoM] £5.17 DT
price = £4.93

Ointment
CAUTIONARY AND ADVISORY LABELS 28
▸ Locoid (Astellas Pharma Ltd)
Hydrocortisone butyrate 1 mg per 1 gram Locoid 0.1% ointment |
30 gram [PoM] £1.60 DT price = £1.60 | 100 gram [PoM] £4.93 DT
price = £4.93

Hydrocortisone with urea

The properties listed below are those particular to the
combination only. For the properties of the components
please consider, hydrocortisone p. 1092.

● **INDICATIONS AND DOSE**

Mild inflammatory skin disorders such as eczemas
▸ TO THE SKIN
▸ Child: To be applied thinly (consult product literature)
▸ Adult: To be applied thinly (consult product literature)
POTENCY
Hydrocortisone 1% with urea cream: moderate

● **PATIENT AND CARER ADVICE** Patients or carers should be
advised on application of hydrocortisone with urea cream.

● **MEDICINAL FORMS**
There can be variation in the licensing of different medicines
containing the same drug.
Cream
CAUTIONARY AND ADVISORY LABELS 28
▸ Alphaderm (Alliance Pharmaceuticals Ltd)
**Hydrocortisone 10 mg per 1 gram, Urea 100 mg per
1 gram** Alphaderm 1%/10% cream | 30 gram [PoM] £2.38 DT price =
£2.38 | 100 gram [PoM] £7.03 DT price = £7.03

⌐ 1086

Mometasone furoate

● **INDICATIONS AND DOSE**

**Severe inflammatory skin disorders such as eczemas
unresponsive to less potent corticosteroids | Psoriasis**
▸ TO THE SKIN
▸ Child 2–17 years: Apply once daily, to be applied thinly
(to scalp in case of lotion)
▸ Adult: Apply once daily, to be applied thinly (to scalp in
case of lotion)
POTENCY
Mometasone furoate 0.1% cream, ointment, and scalp
lotion: potent.

● **UNLICENSED USE**
▸ With topical use in children Not licensed for use in children
under 2 years.

● **PATIENT AND CARER ADVICE**
Patients and carers should be advised on the application of
topical mometasone.

● **MEDICINAL FORMS**
There can be variation in the licensing of different medicines
containing the same drug. Forms available from special-order
manufacturers include: ointment
Liquid
CAUTIONARY AND ADVISORY LABELS 28
EXCIPIENTS: May contain Propylene glycol
▸ Elocon (Merck Sharp & Dohme Ltd)
Mometasone furoate 1 mg per 1 gram Elocon 0.1% scalp lotion |
30 ml [PoM] £4.36 DT price = £4.36
Cream
CAUTIONARY AND ADVISORY LABELS 28
EXCIPIENTS: May contain Beeswax
▸ Mometasone furoate (Non-proprietary)
Mometasone furoate 1 mg per 1 gram Mometasone 0.1% cream |
30 gram [PoM] £4.36 DT price = £2.07 | 100 gram [PoM] £12.58 DT
price = £6.90
▸ Elocon (Merck Sharp & Dohme Ltd)
Mometasone furoate 1 mg per 1 gram Elocon 0.1% cream |
30 gram [PoM] £4.80 DT price = £2.07 | 100 gram [PoM] £15.10 DT
price = £6.90
Ointment
CAUTIONARY AND ADVISORY LABELS 28
EXCIPIENTS: May contain Beeswax, propylene glycol
▸ Mometasone furoate (Non-proprietary)
Mometasone furoate 1 mg per 1 gram Mometasone 0.1% ointment
| 15 gram [PoM] £4.32 | 30 gram [PoM] £4.45 DT price = £2.18 |
50 gram [PoM] £12.44 | 100 gram [PoM] £12.82 DT price = £7.27
▸ Elocon (Merck Sharp & Dohme Ltd)
Mometasone furoate 1 mg per 1 gram Elocon 0.1% ointment |
30 gram [PoM] £4.32 DT price = £2.18 | 100 gram [PoM] £12.44 DT
price = £7.27

CORTICOSTEROIDS › CORTICOSTEROID
COMBINATIONS WITH ANTI-INFECTIVES

Betamethasone with clioquinol

The properties listed below are those particular to the
combination only. For the properties of the components
please consider, betamethasone p. 1087.

● **INDICATIONS AND DOSE**

**Severe inflammatory skin disorders such as eczemas
unresponsive to less potent corticosteroids | Psoriasis**
▸ TO THE SKIN
▸ Child: (consult product literature)
▸ Adult: (consult product literature)
POTENCY
Betamethasone (as valerate) 0.1% with clioquinol cream
and ointment: potent.

● **UNLICENSED USE**
▸ With topical use in children Betamethasone and clioquinol
preparations is not licensed for use in children under
1 year.

● **PATIENT AND CARER ADVICE** Stains clothing. Patients or
carers should be counselled on application of
betamethasone with clioquinol preparations.

● **MEDICINAL FORMS**
There can be variation in the licensing of different medicines
containing the same drug.
Cream
CAUTIONARY AND ADVISORY LABELS 28
EXCIPIENTS: May contain Cetostearyl alcohol (including cetyl and
stearyl alcohol), chlorocresol
▸ Betamethasone with clioquinol (Non-proprietary)
**Betamethasone (as Betamethasone valerate) 1 mg per 1 gram,
Clioquinol 30 mg per 1 gram** Betamethasone valerate 0.1% /
Clioquinol 3% cream | 30 gram [PoM] £28.88 DT price = £28.88

13

Skin

Ointment

CAUTIONARY AND ADVISORY LABELS 28
▶ Betamethasone with clioquinol (Non-proprietary)
   Betamethasone (as Betamethasone valerate) 1 mg per 1 gram, Clioquinol 30 mg per 1 gram Betamethasone valerate 0.1% / Clioquinol 3% ointment | 30 gram [PoM] £28.88 DT price = £28.88

Betamethasone with clotrimazole

The properties listed below are those particular to the combination only. For the properties of the components please consider, betamethasone p. 1087, clotrimazole p. 1076.

● **INDICATIONS AND DOSE**

Severe inflammatory skin disorders such as eczemas unresponsive to less potent corticosteroids | Psoriasis
▶ TO THE SKIN
▶ Child: (consult product literature)
▶ Adult: (consult product literature)
POTENCY
Betamethasone dipropionate 0.064% (=betamethasone 0.5%) with clotrimazole cream: potent.

● **UNLICENSED USE**
▶ With topical use in children *Lotriderm* ® not licensed for use in children under 12 years.

● **PATIENT AND CARER ADVICE** Patients or carers should be given advice on how to administer betamethasone with clotrimazole cream.

● **MEDICINAL FORMS**
There can be variation in the licensing of different medicines containing the same drug.
Cream
CAUTIONARY AND ADVISORY LABELS 28
EXCIPIENTS: May contain Benzyl alcohol, cetostearyl alcohol (including cetyl and stearyl alcohol), propylene glycol
▶ Lotriderm (Merck Sharp & Dohme Ltd)
   Betamethasone dipropionate 640 microgram per 1 gram, Clotrimazole 10 mg per 1 gram Lotriderm cream | 30 gram [PoM] £6.34 DT price = £6.34

Betamethasone with fusidic acid

The properties listed below are those particular to the combination only. For the properties of the components please consider, betamethasone p. 1087, fusidic acid p. 519.

● **INDICATIONS AND DOSE**

Severe inflammatory skin disorders such as eczemas unresponsive to less potent corticosteroids | Psoriasis
▶ TO THE SKIN
▶ Child: (consult product literature)
▶ Adult: (consult product literature)
POTENCY
Betamethasone (as valerate) 0.1% with fusidic acid cream: potent.

● **UNLICENSED USE**
▶ With topical use in children *Fucibet* ® *Lipid Cream* is not licensed for use in children under 6 years.

● **PATIENT AND CARER ADVICE** Patients or carers should be counselled on application of betamethasone with fusidic acid preparations.

● **MEDICINAL FORMS**
There can be variation in the licensing of different medicines containing the same drug.
Cream
CAUTIONARY AND ADVISORY LABELS 28
EXCIPIENTS: May contain Cetostearyl alcohol (including cetyl and stearyl alcohol), chlorocresol, hydroxybenzoates (parabens)

▶ Fucibet (LEO Pharma)
   Betamethasone (as Betamethasone valerate) 1 mg per 1 gram, Fusidic acid 20 mg per 1 gram Fucibet cream | 30 gram [PoM] £6.38 DT price = £6.38 | 60 gram [PoM] £12.76 DT price = £12.76
   Fucibet Lipid cream | 30 gram [PoM] £6.74 DT price = £6.38
▶ Xemacort (Mylan Ltd)
   Betamethasone (as Betamethasone valerate) 1 mg per 1 gram, Fusidic acid 20 mg per 1 gram Xemacort cream | 30 gram [PoM] £6.05 DT price = £6.38 | 60 gram [PoM] £12.45 DT price = £12.76

Betamethasone with neomycin

The properties listed below are those particular to the combination only. For the properties of the components please consider, betamethasone p. 1087, neomycin sulfate p. 1074.

● **INDICATIONS AND DOSE**

Severe inflammatory skin disorders such as eczemas unresponsive to less potent corticosteroids | Psoriasis
▶ TO THE SKIN USING OINTMENT, OR TO THE SKIN USING CREAM
▶ Child 2–17 years: Apply 1–2 times a day, to be applied thinly
▶ Adult: Apply 1–2 times a day, to be applied thinly
POTENCY
Betamethasone (as valerate) 0.1% with neomycin cream and ointment: potent.

● **UNLICENSED USE**
▶ With topical use in children Betamethasone and neomycin preparations not licensed for use in children under 2 years.

● **PATIENT AND CARER ADVICE**
Patient counselling is advised for betamethasone with neomycin cream and ointment (application).

● **MEDICINAL FORMS**
There can be variation in the licensing of different medicines containing the same drug.
Cream
CAUTIONARY AND ADVISORY LABELS 28
EXCIPIENTS: May contain Cetostearyl alcohol (including cetyl and stearyl alcohol), chlorocresol
▶ Betamethasone with neomycin (Non-proprietary)
   Betamethasone (as Betamethasone valerate) 1 mg per 1 gram, Neomycin sulfate 5 mg per 1 gram Betamethasone valerate 0.1% / Neomycin 0.5% cream | 30 gram [PoM] £28.88 DT price = £17.74 | 100 gram [PoM] £48.00 DT price = £59.14
Ointment
CAUTIONARY AND ADVISORY LABELS 28
▶ Betamethasone with neomycin (Non-proprietary)
   Betamethasone (as Betamethasone valerate) 1 mg per 1 gram, Neomycin sulfate 5 mg per 1 gram Betamethasone valerate 0.1% / Neomycin 0.5% ointment | 30 gram [PoM] £28.88 DT price = £17.74 | 100 gram [PoM] £48.00 DT price = £59.14

Betamethasone with salicylic acid

The properties listed below are those particular to the combination only. For the properties of the components please consider, betamethasone p. 1087, salicylic acid p. 1126.

● **INDICATIONS AND DOSE**

DIPROSALIC® OINTMENT

Severe inflammatory skin disorders such as eczemas unresponsive to less potent corticosteroids | Psoriasis
▶ TO THE SKIN
▶ Child: Apply 1–2 times a day, max. 60 g per week
▶ Adult: Apply 1–2 times a day, max. 60 g per week
POTENCY
For *Diprosalic* ® ointment: Betamethasone (as dipropionate) 0.05% with salicylic acid 3%: potent.

DIPROSALIC® SCALP APPLICATION

Severe inflammatory skin disorders such as eczemas unresponsive to less potent corticosteroids | Psoriasis
▸ TO THE SKIN
▸ Child: Apply 1–2 times a day, apply a few drops
▸ Adult: Apply 1–2 times a day, apply a few drops
POTENCY
For *Diprosalic®* scalp application: Betamethasone (as dipropionate) 0.05% with salicylic acid 2%: potent.

● PATIENT AND CARER ADVICE
DIPROSALIC® OINTMENT Patients or carers should be counselled on application of betamethasone and salicylic acid preparations.
DIPROSALIC® SCALP APPLICATION Patients or carers should be counselled on application of betamethasone and salicylic acid scalp application.

● MEDICINAL FORMS
There can be variation in the licensing of different medicines containing the same drug.
Liquid
CAUTIONARY AND ADVISORY LABELS 28
EXCIPIENTS: May contain Disodium edetate
▸ Diprosalic (Merck Sharp & Dohme Ltd)
　Betamethasone (as Betamethasone dipropionate) 500 microgram per 1 ml, Salicylic acid 20 mg per 1 ml Diprosalic 0.05%/2% scalp application | 100 ml [PoM] £10.10 DT price = £10.10
Ointment
CAUTIONARY AND ADVISORY LABELS 28
▸ Diprosalic (Merck Sharp & Dohme Ltd)
　Betamethasone (as Betamethasone dipropionate) 500 microgram per 1 gram, Salicylic acid 30 mg per 1 gram Diprosalic 0.05%/3% ointment | 30 gram [PoM] £3.18 DT price = £3.18 | 100 gram [PoM] £9.14 DT price = £9.14

Chlortetracycline with triamcinolone

● INDICATIONS AND DOSE
Severe inflammatory skin disorders such as eczemas unresponsive to less potent corticosteroids (associated with infection) | Psoriasis (associated with infection)
▸ TO THE SKIN
▸ Adult: To be applied thinly (consult product literature)
POTENCY
Triamcinolone acetonide 0.1%, chlortetracycline hydrochloride 3% ointment: potent.

● PATIENT AND CARER ADVICE Stains clothing. Patients or carers should be counselled on the application of chlortetracycline with triamcinolone products.

● MEDICINAL FORMS
There can be variation in the licensing of different medicines containing the same drug.
Ointment
CAUTIONARY AND ADVISORY LABELS 28
EXCIPIENTS: May contain Wool fat and related substances including lanolin
▸ Aureocort (AMCo)
　Triamcinolone acetonide 1 mg per 1 gram, Chlortetracycline hydrochloride 30.9 mg per 1 gram Aureocort ointment | 15 gram [PoM] £3.51

Clobetasol propionate with neomycin sulfate and nystatin

The properties listed below are those particular to the combination only. For the properties of the components please consider, clobetasol propionate p. 1089, neomycin sulfate p. 1074.

● INDICATIONS AND DOSE
Short-term treatment only of severe resistant inflammatory skin disorders such as recalcitrant eczemas associated with infection and unresponsive to less potent corticosteroids | Psoriasis associated with infection
▸ TO THE SKIN
▸ Adult: (consult product literature)
POTENCY
Clobetasol propionate 0.05% with neomycin sulfate and nystatin cream and ointment: very potent.

● PATIENT AND CARER ADVICE Patients or carers should be advised on application of clobetasol propionate, neomycin sulfate and nystatin containing preparations.

● MEDICINAL FORMS
There can be variation in the licensing of different medicines containing the same drug.
Cream
CAUTIONARY AND ADVISORY LABELS 28
▸ Clobetasol propionate with neomycin sulfate and nystatin (Non-proprietary)
　Clobetasol propionate 500 microgram per 1 gram, Neomycin sulfate 5 mg per 1 gram, Nystatin 100000 unit per 1 gram Clobetasol 500microgram / Neomycin 5mg / Nystatin 100,000units/g cream | 30 gram [PoM] £64.00 DT price = £64.00
Ointment
CAUTIONARY AND ADVISORY LABELS 28
▸ Clobetasol propionate with neomycin sulfate and nystatin (Non-proprietary)
　Clobetasol propionate 500 microgram per 1 gram, Neomycin sulfate 5 mg per 1 gram, Nystatin 100000 unit per 1 gram Clobetasol 500microgram / Neomycin 5mg / Nystatin 100,000units/g ointment | 30 gram [PoM] £64.00 DT price = £64.00

Clobetasone butyrate with nystatin and oxytetracycline

The properties listed below are those particular to the combination only. For the properties of the components please consider, clobetasone butyrate p. 1089, oxytetracycline p. 515.

● INDICATIONS AND DOSE
Steroid-responsive dermatoses where candidal or bacterial infection is present
▸ TO THE SKIN
▸ Adult: (consult product literature)
POTENCY
Clobetasone butyrate 0.05% with nystatin and oxytetracyline cream: moderate.

● PATIENT AND CARER ADVICE Stains clothing.

● MEDICINAL FORMS
There can be variation in the licensing of different medicines containing the same drug.
Cream
CAUTIONARY AND ADVISORY LABELS 28
EXCIPIENTS: May contain Cetostearyl alcohol (including cetyl and stearyl alcohol), chlorocresol, sodium metabisulfite
▸ Trimovate (GlaxoSmithKline UK Ltd)
　Clobetasone butyrate 500 microgram per 1 gram, Nystatin 100000 unit per 1 gram, Oxytetracycline (as Oxytetracycline calcium) 30 mg per 1 gram Trimovate cream | 30 gram [PoM] £3.29

13

Skin

Fluocinolone acetonide with clioquinol

The properties listed below are those particular to the combination only. For the properties of the components please consider, fluocinolone acetonide p. 1090.

● **INDICATIONS AND DOSE**

Inflammatory skin disorders such as eczemas associated with infection | Psoriasis associated with infection

▸ TO THE SKIN

▸ Adult: Apply 1–2 times a day, to be applied thinly, reducing strength as condition responds

POTENCY

Clioquinol 3% with fluocinolone acetonide 0.025% cream and ointment: potent

● **PATIENT AND CARER ADVICE** Patient counselling is advised for clioquinol with fluocinolone acetonide cream and ointment (application). Ointment stains clothing.

● **MEDICINAL FORMS**
There can be variation in the licensing of different medicines containing the same drug.

Cream
CAUTIONARY AND ADVISORY LABELS 28
EXCIPIENTS: May contain Cetostearyl alcohol (including cetyl and stearyl alcohol), disodium edetate, hydroxybenzoates (parabens), polysorbates, propylene glycol
▸ Synalar C (Derma UK Ltd)
Fluocinolone acetonide 250 microgram per 1 gram, Clioquinol 30 mg per 1 gram Synalar C cream | 15 gram [PoM] £2.66

Ointment
CAUTIONARY AND ADVISORY LABELS 28
EXCIPIENTS: May contain Propylene glycol, wool fat and related substances including lanolin
▸ Synalar C (Derma UK Ltd)
Fluocinolone acetonide 250 microgram per 1 gram, Clioquinol 30 mg per 1 gram Synalar C ointment | 15 gram [PoM] £2.66

Fluocinolone acetonide with neomycin

The properties listed below are those particular to the combination only. For the properties of the components please consider, fluocinolone acetonide p. 1090, neomycin sulfate p. 1074.

● **INDICATIONS AND DOSE**

Inflammatory skin disorders such as eczemas associated with infection | Psoriasis associated with infection

▸ TO THE SKIN

▸ Child 1-17 years: Apply 1–2 times a day, to be applied thinly, reducing strength as condition responds

▸ Adult: Apply 1–2 times a day, to be applied thinly, reducing strength as condition responds

POTENCY

Fluocinolone acetonide 0.025% with neomycin 0.5% cream and ointment: potent

● **PATIENT AND CARER ADVICE** Patients or carers should be counselled on the application of fluocinolone acetonide with neomycin preparations.

● **MEDICINAL FORMS**
There can be variation in the licensing of different medicines containing the same drug.

Cream
CAUTIONARY AND ADVISORY LABELS 28
EXCIPIENTS: May contain Cetostearyl alcohol (including cetyl and stearyl alcohol), hydroxybenzoates (parabens), polysorbates, propylene glycol
▸ Synalar N (Derma UK Ltd)
Fluocinolone acetonide 250 microgram per 1 gram, Neomycin sulfate 5 mg per 1 gram Synalar N cream | 30 gram [PoM] £4.36

Ointment
CAUTIONARY AND ADVISORY LABELS 28
EXCIPIENTS: May contain Propylene glycol, wool fat and related substances including lanolin
▸ Synalar N (Derma UK Ltd)
Fluocinolone acetonide 250 microgram per 1 gram, Neomycin sulfate 5 mg per 1 gram Synalar N ointment | 30 gram [PoM] £4.36

Hydrocortisone with benzalkonium chloride, dimeticone and nystatin

15.3.2016

The properties listed below are those particular to the combination only. For the properties of the components please consider, hydrocortisone p. 1092.

● **INDICATIONS AND DOSE**

Mild inflammatory skin disorders such as eczemas associated with infection

▸ TO THE SKIN

▸ Child: Apply 3 times a day until lesion has healed, to be applied thinly

▸ Adult: Apply 3 times a day until lesion has healed, to be applied thinly

POTENCY

Benzalkonium with dimeticone, hydrocortisone acetate 0.5%, and nystatin cream: mild.

● **PATIENT AND CARER ADVICE** Patients or carers should be advised on application of benzalkonium with dimeticone and hydrocortisone and nystatin preparations.

● **MEDICINAL FORMS**
There can be variation in the licensing of different medicines containing the same drug.

Cream
CAUTIONARY AND ADVISORY LABELS 28
EXCIPIENTS: May contain Butylated hydroxyanisole, cetostearyl alcohol (including cetyl and stearyl alcohol), hydroxybenzoates (parabens), sodium metabisulfite, sorbic acid
▸ Timodine (Alliance Pharmaceuticals Ltd)
Benzalkonium chloride 1 mg per 1 gram, Hydrocortisone 5 mg per 1 gram, Dimeticone 350 100 mg per 1 gram, Nystatin 100000 unit per 1 gram Timodine cream | 30 gram [PoM] £3.37

Hydrocortisone with chlorhexidine hydrochloride and nystatin

The properties listed below are those particular to the combination only. For the properties of the components please consider, hydrocortisone p. 1092, chlorhexidine p. 1120.

● **INDICATIONS AND DOSE**

Mild inflammatory skin disorders such as eczemas

▸ TO THE SKIN

▸ Child: To be applied thinly (consult product literature)

▸ Adult: To be applied thinly (consult product literature)

POTENCY

Hydrocortisone 0.5% with chlorhexidine hydrochloride 1% and nystatin cream: mild
Hydrocortisone 1% with chlorhexidine hydrochloride 1% and nystatin ointment: mild

● **PATIENT AND CARER ADVICE** Patients or carers should be given advice on application of chlorhexidine hydrochloride with hydrocortisone and nystatin preparations.

- MEDICINAL FORMS
There can be variation in the licensing of different medicines containing the same drug.

Cream
CAUTIONARY AND ADVISORY LABELS 28
EXCIPIENTS: May contain Benzyl alcohol, cetostearyl alcohol (including cetyl and stearyl alcohol), polysorbates
▸ Nystaform HC (Typharm Ltd)
  Hydrocortisone 5 mg per 1 gram, Chlorhexidine hydrochloride 10 mg per 1 gram, Nystatin 100000 iu per 1 gram Nystaform HC cream ⎮ 30 gram PoM £2.66

Ointment
CAUTIONARY AND ADVISORY LABELS 28
▸ Nystaform HC (Typharm Ltd)
  Chlorhexidine acetate 10 mg per 1 gram, Hydrocortisone 10 mg per 1 gram, Nystatin 100000 unit per 1 gram Nystaform HC ointment ⎮ 30 gram PoM £2.66

Hydrocortisone with clotrimazole

The properties listed below are those particular to the combination only. For the properties of the components please consider, hydrocortisone p. 1092, clotrimazole p. 1076.

- INDICATIONS AND DOSE
Mild inflammatory skin disorders such as eczemas (associated with fungal infection)
▸ TO THE SKIN
▸ Child: (consult product literature)
▸ Adult: (consult product literature)
POTENCY
Clotrimazole with hydrocortisone 1% cream: mild

- PATIENT AND CARER ADVICE Patients or carers should be given advice on how to administer clotrimazole with hydrocortisone cream.
- EXCEPTIONS TO LEGAL CATEGORY A 15-g tube is on sale to the public for the treatment of athlete's foot and fungal infection of skin folds with associated inflammation in patients 10 years and over.

- MEDICINAL FORMS
There can be variation in the licensing of different medicines containing the same drug.

Cream
CAUTIONARY AND ADVISORY LABELS 28
EXCIPIENTS: May contain Benzyl alcohol, cetostearyl alcohol (including cetyl and stearyl alcohol)
▸ Canesten HC (Bayer Plc)
  Clotrimazole 10 mg per 1 gram, Hydrocortisone 10 mg per 1 gram Canesten HC cream ⎮ 30 gram PoM £2.42 DT price = £2.42
▸ Canesten Hydrocortisone (Bayer Plc)
  Clotrimazole 10 mg per 1 gram, Hydrocortisone 10 mg per 1 gram Canesten Hydrocortisone cream ⎮ 15 gram P £3.11 DT price = £3.11

Hydrocortisone with fusidic acid

The properties listed below are those particular to the combination only. For the properties of the components please consider, hydrocortisone p. 1092, fusidic acid p. 519.

- INDICATIONS AND DOSE
Mild inflammatory skin disorders such as eczemas
▸ TO THE SKIN
▸ Child: To be applied thinly (consult product literature)
▸ Adult: To be applied thinly (consult product literature)
POTENCY
Hydrocortisone with fusidic acid cream: mild

- PATIENT AND CARER ADVICE Patients or carers should be advised on application of hydrocortisone with fusidic acid preparations.

- MEDICINAL FORMS
There can be variation in the licensing of different medicines containing the same drug.

Cream
CAUTIONARY AND ADVISORY LABELS 28
EXCIPIENTS: May contain Butylated hydroxyanisole, cetostearyl alcohol (including cetyl and stearyl alcohol), polysorbates, potassium sorbate
▸ Fucidin H (Fusidic acid / Hydrocortisone) (LEO Pharma)
  Hydrocortisone acetate 10 mg per 1 gram, Fusidic acid 20 mg per 1 gram Fucidin H cream ⎮ 30 gram PoM £6.02 DT price = £6.02 ⎮ 60 gram PoM £12.05 DT price = £12.05

Hydrocortisone with miconazole

The properties listed below are those particular to the combination only. For the properties of the components please consider, hydrocortisone p. 1092, miconazole p. 1077.

- INDICATIONS AND DOSE
Mild inflammatory skin disorders such as eczemas associated with infections
▸ TO THE SKIN
▸ Adult: (consult product literature)
POTENCY
Hydrocortisone 1% with miconazole cream and ointment: mild

- INTERACTIONS → Appendix 1 (antifungals, imidazole).
- PATIENT AND CARER ADVICE Patients or carers should be advised on application of hydrocortisone with miconazole preparations.
- PROFESSION SPECIFIC INFORMATION
Dental practitioners' formulary
May be prescribed as Miconazole and Hydrocortisone Cream or Ointment for max. 7 days.
- EXCEPTIONS TO LEGAL CATEGORY A 15-g tube of hydrocortisone with miconazole cream is on sale to the public for the treatment of athlete's foot and candidal intertrigo.

- MEDICINAL FORMS
There can be variation in the licensing of different medicines containing the same drug.

Cream
CAUTIONARY AND ADVISORY LABELS 28
EXCIPIENTS: May contain Butylated hydroxyanisole, disodium edetate
▸ Daktacort (McNeil Products Ltd, Janssen-Cilag Ltd)
  Hydrocortisone 10 mg per 1 gram, Miconazole nitrate 20 mg per 1 gram Daktacort Hydrocortisone cream ⎮ 15 gram P £3.17 DT price = £3.17
  Daktacort 2%/1% cream ⎮ 30 gram PoM £2.49 DT price = £2.49

Ointment
CAUTIONARY AND ADVISORY LABELS 28
▸ Daktacort (Janssen-Cilag Ltd)
  Hydrocortisone 10 mg per 1 gram, Miconazole nitrate 20 mg per 1 gram Daktacort ointment ⎮ 30 gram PoM £2.50 DT price = £2.50

13

Skin

Hydrocortisone with oxytetracycline

The properties listed below are those particular to the combination only. For the properties of the components please consider, hydrocortisone p. 1092, oxytetracycline p. 515.

- **INDICATIONS AND DOSE**

Mild inflammatory skin disorders such as eczemas
- ▸ TO THE SKIN
- ▸ Child 12–17 years: (consult product literature)
- ▸ Adult: (consult product literature)
POTENCY
Hydrocortisone 1% with oxytetracycline ointment: mild.

- **CONTRA-INDICATIONS** Children under 12 years
- **PREGNANCY** Tetracyclines should not be given to pregnant women. Effects on skeletal development have been documented when tetracyclines have been used in the first trimester in animal studies. Administration during the second or third trimester may cause discoloration of the child's teeth.
- **BREAST FEEDING** Tetracyclines should not be given to women who are breast-feeding (although absorption and therefore discoloration of teeth in the infant is probably usually prevented by chelation with calcium in milk).
- **PATIENT AND CARER ADVICE** Patients should be given advice on the application of hydrocortisone with oxytetracycline ointment.

- **MEDICINAL FORMS**
There can be variation in the licensing of different medicines containing the same drug.
Ointment
CAUTIONARY AND ADVISORY LABELS 28
- ▸ Terra-Cortril (Intrapharm Laboratories Ltd)
Hydrocortisone 10 mg per 1 gram, Oxytetracycline (as Oxytetracycline hydrochloride) 30 mg per 1 gram Terra-Cortril ointment | 30 gram [PoM] £5.01 DT price = £5.01

DERMATOLOGICAL DRUGS > ANTI-INFECTIVES

Ichthammol

- **INDICATIONS AND DOSE**

Chronic lichenified eczema
- ▸ TO THE SKIN
- ▸ Child 1–17 years: Apply 1–3 times a day
- ▸ Adult: Apply 1–3 times a day

- **UNLICENSED USE**
- ▸ In children No information available.
- **SIDE-EFFECTS** Skin irritation

- **MEDICINAL FORMS**
There can be variation in the licensing of different medicines containing the same drug. Forms available from special-order manufacturers include: ointment, paste
Liquid
- ▸ Ichthammol (Non-proprietary)
Ichthammol 1 mg per 1 mg Ichthammol liquid | 100 gram [GSL] £11.42 DT price = £11.42 | 500 gram [GSL] £34.27

Ichthammol with zinc oxide

The properties listed below are those particular to the combination only. For the properties of the components please consider, ichthammol above.

- **INDICATIONS AND DOSE**

Chronic lichenified eczema
- ▸ TO THE SKIN
- ▸ Adult: (consult product literature)

- **MEDICINAL FORMS**
There can be variation in the licensing of different medicines containing the same drug. Forms available from special-order manufacturers include: cream, ointment
Impregnated dressing
- ▸ Ichthopaste (Smith & Nephew Healthcare Ltd)
Ichthopaste bandage 7.5cm × 6m | 1 bandage £3.68

DERMATOLOGICAL DRUGS > ANTRACEN DERIVATIVES

Dithranol

(Anthralin)

- **INDICATIONS AND DOSE**

Subacute and chronic psoriasis
- ▸ TO THE SKIN
- ▸ Adult: (consult product literature)
DITHROCREAM®

Subacute and chronic psoriasis
- ▸ TO THE SKIN
- ▸ Adult: For application to skin or scalp, 0.1–0.5% cream suitable for overnight treatment, 1–2% cream for maximum 1 hour (consult product literature)
MICANOL®

Subacute and chronic psoriasis
- ▸ TO THE SKIN
- ▸ Adult: Apply once daily, for application to skin or scalp, to be applied for up to 30 minutes, apply 1% cream, if necessary 3% cream can be used under medical supervision

- **CONTRA-INDICATIONS** Acute and pustular psoriasis · hypersensitivity
- **CAUTIONS** Avoid sensitive areas of skin · avoid use near eyes
- **SIDE-EFFECTS** Local burning sensation · local irritation · stains hair · stains skin
- **PREGNANCY** No adverse effects reported.
- **BREAST FEEDING** No adverse effects reported.
- **DIRECTIONS FOR ADMINISTRATION** When applying dithranol, hands should be protected by gloves or they should be washed thoroughly afterwards. Dithranol should be applied to chronic extensor plaques only, carefully avoiding normal skin.
MICANOL® At the end of contact time, use plenty of lukewarm (not hot) water to rinse off cream; soap may be used after the cream has been rinsed off; use shampoo before applying cream to scalp and if necessary after cream has been rinsed off.
- **PRESCRIBING AND DISPENSING INFORMATION** Treatment should be started with a low concentration such as dithranol 0.1%, and the strength increased gradually every few days up to 3%, according to tolerance.
- **PATIENT AND CARER ADVICE** Dithranol can stain the skin, hair and fabrics.
- **EXCEPTIONS TO LEGAL CATEGORY** Prescription only medicine if dithranol content more than 1%, otherwise may be sold to the public.

- **MEDICINAL FORMS**
There can be variation in the licensing of different medicines containing the same drug. Forms available from special-order manufacturers include: ointment
Cream
CAUTIONARY AND ADVISORY LABELS 28
EXCIPIENTS: May contain Cetostearyl alcohol (including cetyl and stearyl alcohol), chlorocresol

- Dithrocream (Dermal Laboratories Ltd)
  - **Dithranol 1 mg per 1 gram** Dithrocream 0.1% cream | 50 gram P £3.77
  - **Dithranol 2.5 mg per 1 gram** Dithrocream 0.25% cream | 50 gram P £4.04
  - **Dithranol 5 mg per 1 gram** Dithrocream 0.5% cream | 50 gram P £4.66
  - **Dithranol 10 mg per 1 gram** Dithrocream HP 1% cream | 50 gram P £5.42
  - **Dithranol 20 mg per 1 gram** Dithrocream 2% cream | 50 gram PoM £5.77
- Micanol (Derma UK Ltd)
  - **Dithranol 10 mg per 1 gram** Micanol 1% cream | 50 gram P £16.18
  - **Dithranol 30 mg per 1 gram** Micanol 3% cream | 50 gram PoM £20.15

Combinations available: *Coal tar with dithranol and salicylic acid,* p. 1100

Dithranol with salicylic acid and zinc oxide

The properties listed below are those particular to the combination only. For the properties of the components please consider, dithranol p. 1098, salicylic acid p. 1126.

- ● **INDICATIONS AND DOSE**
  Subacute and chronic psoriasis
  - ▸ TO THE SKIN
  - ▸ Adult: (consult local protocol)

- ● **MEDICINAL FORMS**
  There can be variation in the licensing of different medicines containing the same drug. Forms available from special-order manufacturers include: ointment, paste

DERMATOLOGICAL DRUGS > TARS

Coal tar

- ● **INDICATIONS AND DOSE**
  Psoriasis | Chronic atopic eczema
  - ▸ TO THE SKIN USING PASTE
  - ▸ Child: Apply 1–3 times a day, start application with low-strength preparations
  - ▸ Adult: Apply 1–3 times a day, start application with low-strength preparations
  - ▸ TO THE SKIN
  - ▸ Child: 100 mL/bath, to be added to an adult sized bath; add proportionally less for a child's bath. Use Coal Tar Solution BP
  - ▸ Adult: 100 mL/bath, to be added to an adult sized bath. Use Coal Tar Solution BP

  ALPHOSYL 2 IN 1® SHAMPOO
  Psoriasis | Seborrhoeic dermatitis | Scaling | Itching
  - ▸ TO THE SKIN
  - ▸ Adult: Apply every 2–3 days

  Dandruff
  - ▸ TO THE SKIN
  - ▸ Adult: Apply 1–2 times a week as required

  EXOREX® LOTION
  Psoriasis
  - ▸ TO THE SKIN
  - ▸ Adult: Apply 2–3 times a day, to be applied to skin or scalp; in elderly, lotion can be diluted with a few drops of water before applying

- ● **CONTRA-INDICATIONS** Avoid broken or inflamed skin · avoid eye area · avoid genital area · avoid mucosal areas · avoid rectal area · infection · sore, acute, or pustular psoriasis

- ● **CAUTIONS** Application to face · application to skin flexures

- ● **SIDE-EFFECTS** Acne-like eruptions · photosensitivity · skin irritation

- ● **PRESCRIBING AND DISPENSING INFORMATION** Coal Tar Solution BP contains coal tar 20%, Strong Coal Tar Solution BP contains coal tar 40%.

- ● **HANDLING AND STORAGE** Use suitable chemical protection gloves for extemporaneous preparation. May stain skin, hair and fabric.

- ● **PATIENT AND CARER ADVICE** May stain skin, hair and fabric.

- ● **MEDICINAL FORMS**
  There can be variation in the licensing of different medicines containing the same drug. Forms available from special-order manufacturers include: cream, ointment, paste
  Bath additive
  - ▸ Psoriderm (Dermal Laboratories Ltd)
    - **Coal tar distilled 400 mg per 1 ml** Psoriderm Emulsion 40% bath additive | 200 ml P £2.74

  Shampoo
  EXCIPIENTS: May contain Fragrances, hydroxybenzoates (parabens)
  - ▸ Coal tar (Non-proprietary)
    - **Coal tar extract 20 mg per 1 gram** Coal tar extract 2% shampoo | 125 ml GSL no price available DT price = £3.61 | 250 ml GSL no price available DT price = £5.38
  - ▸ Brands may include Alphosyl 2 in 1, Neutrogena T/Gel Therapeutic, Polytar Scalp

  Cutaneous emulsion
  EXCIPIENTS: May contain Hydroxybenzoates (parabens)
  - ▸ Exorex (Forest Laboratories UK Ltd)
    - **Coal tar solution 50 mg per 1 gram** Exorex lotion | 100 ml GSL £8.11 DT price = £8.11 | 250 ml GSL £16.24 DT price = £16.24

Coal tar with arachis oil extract of coal tar, cade oil, light liquid paraffin and tar

The properties listed below are those particular to the combination only. For the properties of the components please consider, coal tar above.

- ● **INDICATIONS AND DOSE**
  Psoriasis | Eczema | Atopic dermatoses | Pruritic dermatoses
  - ▸ TO THE SKIN
  - ▸ Child: 2–4 capfuls/bath, alternatively 15–30 mL, to be added in an adult-size bath and soak for 20 minutes (proportionally less for a child's bath)
  - ▸ Adult: 2–4 capfuls/bath, alternatively 15–30 mL, to be added in an adult-size bath and soak for 20 minutes

- ● **MEDICINAL FORMS**
  There can be variation in the licensing of different medicines containing the same drug.
  No licensed medicines listed.

Coal tar with calamine

The properties listed below are those particular to the combination only. For the properties of the components please consider, coal tar above.

- ● **INDICATIONS AND DOSE**
  Psoriasis | Chronic atopic eczema (occasionally)
  - ▸ TO THE SKIN
  - ▸ Adult: Apply 1–2 times a day

- ● **PRESCRIBING AND DISPENSING INFORMATION** When prepared extemporaneously, the BP states Calamine and Coal Tar Ointment BP, consists of calamine 12.5 g, strong coal tar solution 2.5 g, zinc oxide 12.5 g, hydrous wool fat 25 g, white soft paraffin 47.5 g.

13

Skin

● MEDICINAL FORMS
There can be variation in the licensing of different medicines containing the same drug. Forms available from special-order manufacturers include: ointment

Coal tar with coconut oil and salicylic acid

The properties listed below are those particular to the combination only. For the properties of the components please consider, coal tar p. 1099, salicylic acid p. 1126.

● INDICATIONS AND DOSE

Scaly scalp disorders | Psoriasis | Seborrhoeic dermatitis | Dandruff | Cradle cap
▸ TO THE SKIN USING SHAMPOO
▸ Child: Apply daily as required
▸ Adult: Apply daily as required

● MEDICINAL FORMS
There can be variation in the licensing of different medicines containing the same drug.
Shampoo
▸ Capasal (Dermal Laboratories Ltd)
Salicylic acid 5 mg per 1 gram, Coal tar distilled 10 mg per 1 gram, Coconut oil 10 mg per 1 gram Capasal Therapeutic shampoo | 250 ml Ⓟ £4.69

Coal tar with dithranol and salicylic acid

The properties listed below are those particular to the combination only. For the properties of the components please consider, coal tar p. 1099, dithranol p. 1098, salicylic acid p. 1126.

● INDICATIONS AND DOSE

Subacute and chronic psoriasis
▸ TO THE SKIN
▸ Child: Apply up to twice daily
▸ Adult: Apply up to twice daily

● UNLICENSED USE
▸ In children Psorin ® is licensed for use in children (age range not specified by manufacturer).

● MEDICINAL FORMS
There can be variation in the licensing of different medicines containing the same drug. Forms available from special-order manufacturers include: ointment

Coal tar with lecithin

The properties listed below are those particular to the combination only. For the properties of the components please consider, coal tar p. 1099.

● INDICATIONS AND DOSE

PSORIDERM® CREAM

Psoriasis
▸ TO THE SKIN
▸ Child: Apply 1–2 times a day, cream to be applied to the skin or scalp
▸ Adult: Apply 1–2 times a day, cream to be applied to the skin or scalp

PSORIDERM® SCALP LOTION

Scalp psoriasis
▸ TO THE SKIN
▸ Child: Apply as required
▸ Adult: Apply as required

● MEDICINAL FORMS
There can be variation in the licensing of different medicines containing the same drug.
Cream
EXCIPIENTS: May contain Isopropyl palmitate, propylene glycol
▸ Psoriderm (Dermal Laboratories Ltd)
Lecithin 4 mg per 1 gram, Coal tar distilled 60 mg per 1 gram Psoriderm cream | 225 ml Ⓟ £9.42
Shampoo
EXCIPIENTS: May contain Disodium edetate
▸ Psoriderm (Dermal Laboratories Ltd)
Lecithin 3 mg per 1 ml, Coal tar distilled 25 mg per 1 ml Psoriderm scalp lotion | 250 ml Ⓟ £4.74

Coal tar with salicylic acid

The properties listed below are those particular to the combination only. For the properties of the components please consider, coal tar p. 1099, salicylic acid p. 1126.

● INDICATIONS AND DOSE

Psoriasis | Chronic atopic eczema
▸ TO THE SKIN USING OINTMENT
▸ Adult: Apply 1–2 times a day

● PRESCRIBING AND DISPENSING INFORMATION When prepared extemporaneously, the BP states Coal Tar and Salicylic Acid Ointment, BP consists of coal tar 2 g, salicylic acid 2 g, emulsifying wax 11.4 g, white soft paraffin 19 g, coconut oil 54 g, polysorbate '80' 4 g, liquid paraffin 7.6 g.

● MEDICINAL FORMS
There can be variation in the licensing of different medicines containing the same drug. Forms available from special-order manufacturers include: cream, ointment

Coal tar with salicylic acid and precipitated sulfur

The properties listed below are those particular to the combination only. For the properties of the components please consider, coal tar p. 1099, salicylic acid p. 1126.

● INDICATIONS AND DOSE

COCOIS® OINTMENT

Scaly scalp disorders including psoriasis, eczema, seborrhoeic dermatitis and dandruff
▸ INITIALLY TO THE SKIN USING SCALP OINTMENT
▸ Child 6–11 years: Medical supervision required
▸ Child 12–17 years: Apply once weekly as required, alternatively (to the skin) apply daily for the first 3–7 days (if severe), shampoo off after 1 hour
▸ Adult: Apply once weekly as required, alternatively (to the skin) apply daily for the first 3–7 days (if severe), shampoo off after 1 hour

SEBCO® OINTMENT

Scaly scalp disorders including psoriasis, eczema, seborrhoeic dermatitis and dandruff
▸ TO THE SKIN USING SCALP OINTMENT
▸ Child 6–11 years: Medical supervision required
▸ Child 12–17 years: Apply as required, alternatively apply daily for the first 3–7 days (if severe), shampoo off after 1 hour
▸ Adult: Apply as required, alternatively apply daily for the first 3–7 days (if severe), shampoo off after 1 hour

- MEDICINAL FORMS
There can be variation in the licensing of different medicines containing the same drug.

Ointment
EXCIPIENTS: May contain Cetostearyl alcohol (including cetyl and stearyl alcohol)

▸ Cocois (Focus Pharmaceuticals Ltd)
Salicylic acid 20 mg per 1 gram, Sulfur precipitated 40 mg per 1 gram, Coal tar solution 120 mg per 1 gram Cocois ointment | 40 gram GSL £6.22 | 100 gram GSL £11.69

▸ Sebco (Derma UK Ltd)
Salicylic acid 20 mg per 1 gram, Sulfur precipitated 40 mg per 1 gram, Coal tar solution 120 mg per 1 gram Sebco ointment | 40 gram GSL £5.91 | 100 gram GSL £11.11

Coal tar with zinc oxide

The properties listed below are those particular to the combination only. For the properties of the components please consider, coal tar p. 1099.

- INDICATIONS AND DOSE
Psoriasis | Chronic atopic eczema
▸ TO THE SKIN
▸ Child: Apply 1–2 times a day
▸ Adult: Apply 1–2 times a day

- PRESCRIBING AND DISPENSING INFORMATION No preparations available—when prepared extemporaneously, the BP states Zinc and Coal Tar Paste, BP consists of zinc oxide 6%, coal tar 6%, emulsifying wax 5%, starch 38%, yellow soft paraffin 45%.

- MEDICINAL FORMS
There can be variation in the licensing of different medicines containing the same drug. Forms available from special-order manufacturers include: ointment, paste

Extract of coal tar with arachis oil

The properties listed below are those particular to the combination only. For the properties of the components please consider, coal tar p. 1099.

- INDICATIONS AND DOSE
Scalp disorders | Psoriasis | Seborrhoea | Eczema | Pruritus | Dandruff
▸ TO THE SKIN
▸ Child: Apply 1–2 times a week, to the scalp
▸ Adult: Apply 1–2 times a week, to the scalp

- MEDICINAL FORMS
There can be variation in the licensing of different medicines containing the same drug.
No licensed medicines listed.

IMMUNOSUPPRESSANTS > CALCINEURIN INHIBITORS AND RELATED DRUGS

Pimecrolimus

- INDICATIONS AND DOSE
Short-term treatment of mild to moderate atopic eczema (including flares) when topical corticosteroids cannot be used (initiated by a specialist)
▸ TO THE SKIN
▸ Adult: Apply twice daily until symptoms resolve (stop treatment if eczema worsens or no response after 6 weeks)

Short-term treatment of facial, flexural, or genital psoriasis in patients unresponsive to, or intolerant of other topical therapy (initiated by a specialist)
▸ TO THE SKIN
▸ Adult: Apply twice daily until symptoms resolve (maximum duration of treatment 4 weeks)

- UNLICENSED USE Pimecrolimus is not licensed for short-term treatment of facial, flexural, or genital psoriasis in patients unresponsive to, or intolerant of other topical therapy.

- CONTRA-INDICATIONS Application to malignant or potentially malignant skin lesions · application under occlusion · congenital epidermal barrier defects · contact with eyes · contact with mucous membranes · generalised erythroderma · immunodeficiency · infection at treatment site

- CAUTIONS Alcohol consumption (risk of facial flushing and skin irritation) · avoid other topical treatments except emollients at treatment site · UV light (avoid excessive exposure to sunlight and sunlamps)

- INTERACTIONS Concomitant use with drugs that cause immunosuppression is contra-indicated (may be prescribed in exceptional circumstances by specialists).

- SIDE-EFFECTS
▸ **Common or very common** Burning sensation · erythema · folliculitis · pruritus · skin infections
▸ **Uncommon** Herpes simplex · herpes zoster · impetigo · molluscum contagiosum
▸ **Rare** Dryness · local reactions including pain · oedema · papilloma · paraesthesia · peeling · skin discoloration · worsening of eczema
▸ **Frequency not known** Skin malignancy

- PREGNANCY Manufacturer advises avoid; toxicity in *animal* studies following systemic administration.

- BREAST FEEDING Manufacturer advises caution; ensure infant does not come in contact with treated areas.

- NATIONAL FUNDING/ACCESS DECISIONS

NICE technology appraisals (TAs)
▸ Tacrolimus and pimecrolimus for atopic eczema (August 2004) NICE TA82
Topical pimecrolimus is an option for atopic eczema not controlled by maximal topical corticosteroid treatment or if there is a risk of important corticosteroid side-effects (particularly skin atrophy).
  Pimecrolimus should be used within its licensed indications.
www.nice.org.uk/TA82

- MEDICINAL FORMS
There can be variation in the licensing of different medicines containing the same drug.

Cream
CAUTIONARY AND ADVISORY LABELS 4, 11, 28
EXCIPIENTS: May contain Benzyl alcohol, cetostearyl alcohol (including cetyl and stearyl alcohol), propylene glycol

▸ Elidel (Meda Pharmaceuticals Ltd)
Pimecrolimus 10 mg per 1 gram Elidel 1% cream | 30 gram PoM £19.69 DT price = £19.69 | 60 gram PoM £37.41 DT price = £37.41 | 100 gram PoM £59.07 DT price = £59.07

13

Skin

Tacrolimus

- **DRUG ACTION** Tacrolimus is a calcineurin inhibitor.

- **INDICATIONS AND DOSE**

  Short-term treatment of moderate to severe atopic eczema (including flares) in patients unresponsive to, or intolerant of conventional therapy (initiated by a specialist)
  ▶ TO THE SKIN
  ▶ Adult: Apply twice daily until lesion clears (consider other treatment if eczema worsens or no improvement after 2 weeks), initially 0.1% ointment to be applied thinly, reduce frequency to once daily or strength of ointment to 0.03% if condition allows

  Prevention of flares in patients with moderate to severe atopic eczema and 4 or more flares a year who have responded to initial treatment with topical tacrolimus (initiated by a specialist)
  ▶ TO THE SKIN
  ▶ Adult: Apply twice weekly, 0.1% ointment to be applied thinly, with an interval of 2–3 days between applications, use short-term treatment regimen during an acute flare; review need for preventative therapy after 1 year

  Short-term treatment of facial, flexural, or genital psoriasis in patients unresponsive to, or intolerant of other topical therapy (initiated under specialist supervision)
  ▶ TO THE SKIN
  ▶ Adult: Apply twice daily until symptoms resolve, 0.1% ointment to be applied thinly, reduce to once daily or switch to 0.03% ointment if condition allows, maximum duration of treatment 4 weeks

- **UNLICENSED USE** Short-term treatment of facial, flexural, or genital psoriasis is unlicensed.

- **CONTRA-INDICATIONS** Application to malignant or potentially malignant skin lesions · application under occlusion · avoid contact with eyes · avoid contact with mucous membranes · congenital epidermal barrier defects · generalised erythroderma · immunodeficiency · infection at treatment site

- **CAUTIONS** UV light (avoid excessive exposure to sunlight and sunlamps)

- **INTERACTIONS** Interactions do not generally apply to tacrolimus used topically. Concomitant use with drugs that cause immunosuppression (may be prescribed in exceptional circumstances by specialists). Risk of facial flushing and skin irritation with alcohol consumption (does not apply to tacrolimus taken systemically).

- **SIDE-EFFECTS**
  ▶ **Common or very common** Application-site infections · application-site reactions · herpes simplex infection · irritation (at application-site) · Kaposi's varicelliform eruption · pain at application-site · rash
  ▶ **Uncommon** Acne
  ▶ **Frequency not known** Cutaneous lymphoma · malignancies · other types of lymphomas · rosacea · skin malignancy

- **ALLERGY AND CROSS-SENSITIVITY** Contra-indicated if history of hypersensitivity to macrolides.

- **PREGNANCY** Manufacturer advises avoid unless essential; toxicity in *animal* studies following systemic administration.

- **BREAST FEEDING** Avoid—present in breast milk (following systemic administration).

- **PATIENT AND CARER ADVICE** Avoid excessive exposure to UV light including sunlight.

- **NATIONAL FUNDING/ACCESS DECISIONS**

  NICE technology appraisals (TAs)
  ▶ **Tacrolimus and pimecrolimus for atopic eczema (August 2004) NICE TA82**
  Topical tacrolimus is an option for atopic eczema not controlled by maximal topical corticosteroid treatment or if there is a risk of important corticosteroid side-effects (particularly skin atrophy). Topical tacrolimus is recommended for moderate to severe atopic eczema in adults and children over 2 years. Tacrolimus should be used within its licensed indications.
  www.nice.org.uk/TA82

  Scottish Medicines Consortium (SMC) Decisions
  The *Scottish Medicines Consortium* has advised (March 2010) that tacrolimus ointment (*Protopic*®) is accepted for restricted use within NHS Scotland for the prevention of flares in patients aged over 2 years with moderate to severe atopic eczema in accordance with the licensed indications; initiation of treatment is restricted to doctors (including general practitioners) with a specialist interest and experience in treating atopic eczema with immunomodulatory therapy.

- **MEDICINAL FORMS**
  There can be variation in the licensing of different medicines containing the same drug.
  Ointment
  CAUTIONARY AND ADVISORY LABELS 4, 11, 28
  EXCIPIENTS: May contain Beeswax
  ▶ Protopic (Astellas Pharma Ltd)
    Tacrolimus (as Tacrolimus monohydrate) 300 microgram per 1 gram Protopic 0.03% ointment | 30 gram [PoM] £19.44 DT price = £19.44 | 60 gram [PoM] £35.46 DT price = £35.46
    Tacrolimus (as Tacrolimus monohydrate) 1 mg per 1 gram Protopic 0.1% ointment | 30 gram [PoM] £21.60 DT price = £21.60 | 60 gram [PoM] £39.40 DT price = £39.40

RETINOID AND RELATED DRUGS

Acitretin

- **DRUG ACTION** Acitretin is a metabolite of etretinate.

- **INDICATIONS AND DOSE**

  Severe extensive psoriasis resistant to other forms of therapy (under expert supervision) | Palmoplantar pustular psoriasis (under expert supervision) | Severe congenital ichthyosis (under expert supervision)
  ▶ BY MOUTH
  ▶ Adult: Initially 25–30 mg daily for 2–4 weeks, then adjusted according to response to 25–50 mg daily, increased to up to 75 mg daily, dose only increased to 75 mg daily for short periods in psoriasis

  Severe Darier's disease (keratosis follicularis) (under expert supervision)
  ▶ BY MOUTH
  ▶ Adult: Initially 10 mg daily for 2–4 weeks, then adjusted according to response to 25–50 mg daily

- **CONTRA-INDICATIONS** Hyperlipidaemia

- **CAUTIONS** Avoid excessive exposure to sunlight and unsupervised use of sunlamps · diabetes (can alter glucose tolerance—initial frequent blood glucose checks) · do not donate blood during and for 2 years after stopping therapy (teratogenic risk) · investigate atypical musculoskeletal symptoms

- **INTERACTIONS** → Appendix 1 (retinoids). Avoid concomitant use of keratolytics.

- **SIDE-EFFECTS**
  ▶ **Common or very common** Abdominal pain · abnormal hair texture · alopecia (reversible on withdrawal) · arthralgia · brittle nails · dermatitis · diarrhoea · dryness and inflammation of mucous membranes · dryness of

conjunctiva (causing conjunctivitis and decreased tolerance to contact lenses) · epidermal fragility · erythema · headache · myalgia · nausea · paronychia · peripheral oedema · pruritus · reversible increase in serum-cholesterol (with high doses) · reversible increase in serum-triglyceride concentrations (with high doses) · skin exfoliation · sticky skin · vomiting
▶ **Uncommon** Dizziness · hepatitis · photosensitivity · visual disturbances
▶ **Rare** Peripheral neuropathy
▶ **Very rare** Benign intracranial hypertension · bone pain · exostosis · night blindness · ulcerative keratitis
▶ **Frequency not known** Drowsiness · dry skin · flushing · granulomatous lesions · impaired hearing · initial worsening of psoriasis · malaise · rectal haemorrhage · sweating · taste disturbance · tinnitus

SIDE-EFFECTS, FURTHER INFORMATION
▶ **Exostosis** Skeletal hyperostosis and extra-osseous calcification reported following long-term treatment with etretinate (of which Acitretin is a metabolite).
▶ **Benign intracranial hypertension** Discontinue if severe headache, nausea, vomiting, or visual disturbances occur.

● **CONCEPTION AND CONTRACEPTION** Effective contraception must be used.
Pregnancy prevention In females of child-bearing potential (including those with a history of infertility), exclude pregnancy up to 3 days before treatment, every month during treatment, and every 1–3 months for 3 years after stopping treatment. Treatment should be started on day 2 or 3 of menstrual cycle. Females of child-bearing age must practise effective contraception for at least 1 month before starting treatment, during treatment, and for at least 3 years after stopping treatment. Females should be advised to use at least 1 method of contraception, but ideally they should use 2 methods of contraception. Oral progestogen-only contraceptives are not considered effective. Barrier methods should not be used alone but can be used in conjunction with other contraceptive methods. Females should be advised to seek medical attention immediately if they become pregnant during treatment or within 3 years of stopping treatment. They should also be advised to avoid alcohol during treatment and for 2 months after stopping treatment.

● **PREGNANCY** Avoid—teratogenic.
● **BREAST FEEDING** Avoid.
● **HEPATIC IMPAIRMENT** Avoid in severe impairment—risk of further impairment.
● **RENAL IMPAIRMENT** Avoid in severe impairment; increased risk of toxicity.
● **MONITORING REQUIREMENTS**
▶ Monitor serum-triglyceride and serum-cholesterol concentrations before treatment, 1 month after starting, then every 3 months.
▶ Check liver function at start, then every 2–4 weeks for first 2 months and then every 3 months.
● **PRESCRIBING AND DISPENSING INFORMATION**
Prescribing for women of child-bearing potential Each prescription for acitretin should be limited to a supply of up to 30 days' treatment and dispensed within 7 days of the date stated on the prescription.
● **PATIENT AND CARER ADVICE** A patient information leaflet should be provided.
Patient advice required around conception and contraception Females of child-bearing potential must be advised on pregnancy prevention.

● **MEDICINAL FORMS**
There can be variation in the licensing of different medicines containing the same drug. Forms available from special-order manufacturers include: oral suspension, oral solution

Capsule
CAUTIONARY AND ADVISORY LABELS 10, 11, 21
▶ Acitretin (Non-proprietary)
  Acitretin 10 mg Acitretin 10mg capsules | 60 capsule [PoM] £23.80 DT price = £23.80
  Acitretin 25 mg Acitretin 25mg capsules | 60 capsule [PoM] £55.24 DT price = £55.24
▶ Neotigason (Actavis UK Ltd)
  Acitretin 10 mg Neotigason 10mg capsules | 60 capsule [PoM] £17.30 DT price = £23.80 (Hospital only)
  Acitretin 25 mg Neotigason 25mg capsules | 60 capsule [PoM] £43.00 DT price = £55.24 (Hospital only)

Alitretinoin

● **INDICATIONS AND DOSE**
Severe chronic hand eczema refractory to potent topical corticosteroids
▶ BY MOUTH
▶ Adult (prescribed by or under supervision of a consultant dermatologist): 30 mg once daily; reduced if not tolerated to 10 mg once daily for 12–24 weeks total duration of treatment, discontinue if no response after 12 weeks, course may be repeated in those who relapse

Severe chronic hand eczema refractory to potent topical corticosteroids in patients with diabetes, history of hyperlipidaemia, or risk factors for cardiovascular disease
▶ BY MOUTH
▶ Adult (prescribed by or under supervision of a consultant dermatologist): Initially 10 mg once daily, increased if necessary up to 30 mg once daily for 12–24 weeks total duration of treatment, discontinue if no response after 12 weeks, course may be repeated in those who relapse

● **CONTRA-INDICATIONS** Hypervitaminosis A · uncontrolled hyperlipidaemia · uncontrolled hypothyroidism
● **CAUTIONS** Avoid blood donation during treatment and for at least 1 month after stopping treatment · dry eye syndrome · history of depression
● **INTERACTIONS** → Appendix 1 (retinoids).
● **SIDE-EFFECTS**
▶ **Common or very common** Alopecia · anaemia · arthralgia · changes in thyroid function tests · cheilitis · conjunctivitis · dry eyes · dryness of lips · dryness of skin · erythema · eye irritation · flushing · headache · myalgia · raised creatine kinase · raised serum concentration of triglycerides and of cholesterol (risk of pancreatitis if triglycerides above 9 mmol/litre)
▶ **Uncommon** Ankylosing spondylitis · asteototic eczema · blurred vision · cataracts · epistaxis · hyperostosis · pruritus
▶ **Rare** Benign intracranial hypertension · vasculitis
▶ **Frequency not known** Decreased tolerance to contact lenses · depression · impaired night vision · keratitis · mood changes · suicidal ideation

SIDE-EFFECTS, FURTHER INFORMATION
▶ **Dry eyes** Dry eyes may respond to lubricating eye ointment or tear replacement therapy.
▶ **Benign intracranial hypertension** Discontinue treatment if severe headache, nausea, vomiting, papilloedema, or visual disturbances occur.
● **CONCEPTION AND CONTRACEPTION** Effective contraception must be used.
Pregnancy prevention In women of child-bearing potential, exclude pregnancy 1 month before treatment, up to 3 days before treatment, every month during treatment (unless there are compelling reasons to indicate that there is no

risk of pregnancy), and 5 weeks after stopping treatment—perform pregnancy test in the first 3 days of the menstrual cycle.

Women must practise effective contraception for at least 1 month before starting treatment, during treatment, and for at least 1 month after stopping treatment. Women should be advised to use at least 1 method of contraception but ideally they should use 2 methods of contraception. Oral progestogen-only contraceptives are not considered effective. Barrier methods should not be used alone but can be used in conjunction with other contraceptive methods.

Women should be advised to discontinue treatment and to seek prompt medical attention if they become pregnant during treatment or within 1 month of stopping treatment.

- PREGNANCY Avoid—teratogenic.
- BREAST FEEDING Manufacturer advises avoid.
- HEPATIC IMPAIRMENT Manufacturer advises avoid—no information available.
- RENAL IMPAIRMENT Manufacturer advises avoid in severe impairment—no information available.
- MONITORING REQUIREMENTS Monitor serum lipids (more frequently in those with diabetes, history of hyperlipidaemia, or risk factors for cardiovascular disease)—discontinue if uncontrolled hyperlipidaemia.
- PRESCRIBING AND DISPENSING INFORMATION Prescribing for women of child-bearing potential Each prescription for alitretinoin should be limited to a supply of up to 30 days' treatment and dispensed within 7 days of the date stated on the prescription.

Alitretinoin is **teratogenic** and must **not** be given to women of child-bearing potential unless they practise effective contraception and then only after detailed assessment and explanation by the physician.

- PATIENT AND CARER ADVICE A patient information leaflet should be provided.
Patient advice required around conception and contraception Women of child-bearing potential must be counselled on pregnancy prevention.
- NATIONAL FUNDING/ACCESS DECISIONS

NICE technology appraisals (TAs)
▸ **Alitretinoin for the treatment of severe chronic hand eczema in adults (August 2009)** NICE TA177
Alitretinoin is recommended for the treatment of severe chronic hand eczema that has not responded to potent topical corticosteroids. Treatment should be stopped as soon as an adequate response has been achieved (hands clear or almost clear), or if the eczema remains severe after 12 weeks, or if an adequate response has not been achieved by 24 weeks.
www.nice.org.uk/TA177

- MEDICINAL FORMS
There can be variation in the licensing of different medicines containing the same drug.
Capsule
CAUTIONARY AND ADVISORY LABELS 10, 11, 21
▸ Toctino (Stiefel Laboratories (UK) Ltd)
Alitretinoin 10 mg Toctino 10mg capsules | 30 capsule [PoM] £411.43
Alitretinoin 30 mg Toctino 30mg capsules | 30 capsule [PoM] £411.43

Tazarotene

- INDICATIONS AND DOSE
Mild to moderate plaque psoriasis affecting up to 10% of skin area
▸ TO THE SKIN
▸ Adult: Apply once daily usually for up to 12 weeks, apply in the evening

- CAUTIONS Avoid contact with eczematous skin · avoid contact with eyes · avoid contact with face · avoid contact with hair-covered scalp · avoid contact with inflamed skin · avoid contact with intertriginous areas
- SIDE-EFFECTS
▸ **Rare** Dry or painful skin · stinging and inflamed skin
▸ **Frequency not known** Burning · contact dermatitis · desquamation · erythema · local irritation · non-specific rash · pruritus · worsening of psoriasis
SIDE-EFFECTS, FURTHER INFORMATION
▸ Local irritation Local irritation is more common with higher concentration and may require discontinuation.
- CONCEPTION AND CONTRACEPTION Effective contraception required (oral progestogen-only contraceptives not considered effective).
- PREGNANCY Avoid.
- BREAST FEEDING Manufacturer advises avoid—present in milk in *animal* studies.
- PATIENT AND CARER ADVICE Avoid excessive exposure to UV light (including sunlight, solariums, PUVA or UVB treatment). Do not apply emollients or cosmetics within 1 hour of application. Wash hands immediately after use.

- MEDICINAL FORMS
There can be variation in the licensing of different medicines containing the same drug.
Gel
EXCIPIENTS: May contain Benzyl alcohol, butylated hydroxyanisole, butylated hydroxytoluene, disodium edetate, polysorbates
▸ Zorac (Allergan Ltd)
Tazarotene 500 microgram per 1 gram Zorac 0.05% gel | 30 gram [PoM] £14.09
Tazarotene 1 mg per 1 gram Zorac 0.1% gel | 30 gram [PoM] £14.80

SALICYLIC ACID AND DERIVATIVES

Salicylic acid with zinc oxide

- INDICATIONS AND DOSE
Hyperkeratotic skin disorders
▸ TO THE SKIN
▸ Adult: Apply twice daily

- CAUTIONS Avoid broken skin · avoid inflamed skin
CAUTIONS, FURTHER INFORMATION
▸ Salicylate toxicity Salicylate toxicity may occur particularly if applied on large areas of skin or neonatal skin.
- SIDE-EFFECTS Excessive drying · irritation · sensitivity · systemic effects (after widespread use)
- PRESCRIBING AND DISPENSING INFORMATION Zinc and Salicylic Acid Paste BP is also referred to as Lassar's Paste. When prepared extemporaneously, the BP states Zinc and Salicylic Acid Paste, BP (Lassar's Paste) consists of zinc oxide 24%, salicylic acid 2%, starch 24%, white soft paraffin 50%.

- MEDICINAL FORMS
There can be variation in the licensing of different medicines containing the same drug. Forms available from special-order manufacturers include: paste

VITAMINS AND TRACE ELEMENTS > VITAMIN D AND ANALOGUES

Calcipotriol

● **INDICATIONS AND DOSE**

Plaque psoriasis

▸ TO THE SKIN USING OINTMENT

▸ Adult: Apply 1–2 times a day, when preparations are used together maximum total calcipotriol 5 mg in any one week (e.g. scalp solution 60 mL with ointment 30 g or scalp solution 30 mL with ointment 60 g); maximum 100 g per week

Scalp psoriasis

▸ TO THE SKIN USING SCALP LOTION

▸ Adult: Apply twice daily, when preparations are used together maximum total calcipotriol 5 mg in any one week (e.g. scalp solution 60 mL with ointment 30 g or scalp solution 30 mL with ointment 60 g); maximum 60 mL per week

● CONTRA-INDICATIONS Calcium metabolism disorders

● CAUTIONS Avoid excessive exposure to sunlight and sunlamps · avoid use on face · erythrodermic exfoliative psoriasis (enhanced risk of hypercalcaemia) · generalised pustular psoriasis (enhanced risk of hypercalcaemia)

● SIDE-EFFECTS

▸ **Common or very common** Burning · dermatitis · erythema · itching · local skin reactions · paraesthesia

▸ **Rare** Facial dermatitis · perioral dermatitis

▸ **Frequency not known** Aggravation of psoriasis · dry skin · photosensitivity

● PREGNANCY Manufacturers advise avoid unless essential.

● BREAST FEEDING No information available.

● PATIENT AND CARER ADVICE
Advice on application Patient information leaflet for *Dovonex*® ointment advises liberal application. However, patients should be advised of maximum recommended weekly dose.

    Hands should be washed thoroughly after application to avoid inadvertent transfer to other body areas.

● MEDICINAL FORMS
There can be variation in the licensing of different medicines containing the same drug. Forms available from special-order manufacturers include: ointment

Liquid

▸ Calcipotriol (Non-proprietary)
Calcipotriol (as Calcipotriol hydrate) 50 microgram per 1 ml Calcipotriol 50micrograms/ml scalp solution | 60 ml PoM £56.94 DT price = £56.94 | 120 ml PoM £113.88 DT price = £113.88

Ointment
EXCIPIENTS: May contain Disodium edetate, propylene glycol

▸ Calcipotriol (Non-proprietary)
Calcipotriol 50 microgram per 1 gram Calcipotriol 50micrograms/g ointment | 30 gram PoM £7.37 DT price = £5.78 | 60 gram PoM £11.56–£13.86 | 120 gram PoM £23.12–£27.72

▸ Dovonex (LEO Pharma)
Calcipotriol 50 microgram per 1 gram Dovonex 50micrograms/g ointment | 30 gram PoM £5.78 DT price = £5.78 | 60 gram PoM £11.56

Combinations available: *Calcipotriol with betamethasone,* p. 1088

Calcitriol

(1,25-Dihydroxycholecalciferol)

● **INDICATIONS AND DOSE**

Mild to moderate plaque psoriasis

▸ TO THE SKIN

▸ Adult: Apply twice daily, not more than 35% of body surface to be treated daily; maximum 30 g per day

● CONTRA-INDICATIONS Do not apply under occlusion · patients with calcium metabolism disorders

● CAUTIONS Erythrodermic exfoliative psoriasis (enhanced risk of hypercalcaemia) · generalised pustular psoriasis (enhanced risk of hypercalcaemia)

● SIDE-EFFECTS

▸ **Common or very common** Burning · dermatitis · erythema · itching · local skin reactions · paraesthesia

▸ **Frequency not known** Aggravation of psoriasis

● PREGNANCY Manufacturer advises use in restricted amounts only if clearly necessary.

    Monitor urine- and serum-calcium concentration in pregnancy.

● BREAST FEEDING Manufacturer advises avoid.

● HEPATIC IMPAIRMENT Manufacturer advises avoid—no information available.

● RENAL IMPAIRMENT Manufacturer advises avoid—no information available.

● HANDLING AND STORAGE Hands should be washed thoroughly after application to avoid inadvertent transfer to other body areas.

● MEDICINAL FORMS
There can be variation in the licensing of different medicines containing the same drug. Forms available from special-order manufacturers include: oral suspension, oral solution

Ointment

▸ Silkis (Galderma (UK) Ltd)
Calcitriol 3 microgram per 1 gram Silkis ointment | 100 gram PoM £18.06 DT price = £18.06

Tacalcitol

● **INDICATIONS AND DOSE**

Plaque psoriasis

▸ TO THE SKIN

▸ Adult: Apply once daily, preferably at bedtime, maximum 10 g ointment or 10 mL lotion daily, when lotion and ointment used together, maximum total tacalcitol 280 micrograms in any one week (e.g. lotion 30 mL with ointment 40 g)

● CONTRA-INDICATIONS Calcium metabolism disorders

● CAUTIONS Avoid eyes · erythrodermic exfoliative psoriasis (enhanced risk of hypercalcaemia) · generalised pustular psoriasis (enhanced risk of hypercalcaemia) · if used in conjunction with UV treatment

CAUTIONS, FURTHER INFORMATION

▸ UV treatment If tacalcitol is used in conjunction with UV treatment, UV radiation should be given in the morning and tacalcitol applied at bedtime.

● SIDE-EFFECTS

▸ **Common or very common** Burning · dermatitis · erythema · itching · local skin reactions · paraesthesia

▸ **Frequency not known** Aggravation of psoriasis

● PREGNANCY Manufacturer advises avoid unless no safer alternative—no information available.

● BREAST FEEDING Manufacturer advises avoid application to breast area; no information available on presence in milk.

13

Skin

- MONITORING REQUIREMENTS Monitor serum calcium if risk of hypercalcaemia.
- PATIENT AND CARER ADVICE Hands should be washed thoroughly after application to avoid inadvertent transfer to other body areas.

- MEDICINAL FORMS
There can be variation in the licensing of different medicines containing the same drug.
Liquid
EXCIPIENTS: May contain Disodium edetate, propylene glycol
 ‣ Curatoderm (Almirall Ltd)
   Tacalcitol (as Tacalcitol monohydrate) 4 microgram per 1 gram Curatoderm 4micrograms/g lotion | 30 ml PoM £12.73
Ointment
 ‣ Curatoderm (Almirall Ltd)
   Tacalcitol (as Tacalcitol monohydrate) 4 microgram per 1 gram Curatoderm 4micrograms/g ointment | 30 gram PoM £13.40 DT price = £13.40 | 60 gram PoM £23.14 DT price = £23.14 | 100 gram PoM £30.86 DT price = £30.86

4 Perspiration

Antiperspirants

Overview

Aluminium chloride hexahydrate below is a potent antiperspirant used in the treatment of hyperhidrosis. Aluminium salts are also incorporated in preparations used for minor fungal skin infections associated with hyperhidrosis.

In more severe cases specialists use glycopyrronium bromide below as a 0.05% solution in the iontophoretic treatment of hyperhidrosis of plantar and palmar areas. *Botox*® contains botulinum toxin type A **complex** p. 372 and is licensed for use intradermally for severe hyperhidrosis of the axillae unresponsive to topical antiperspirant or other antihidrotic treatment.

4.1 Hyperhidrosis

ANTIMUSCARINICS

Glycopyrronium bromide

(Glycopyrrolate)

- INDICATIONS AND DOSE
Iontophoretic treatment of hyperhidrosis
 ‣ TO THE SKIN
 ‣ Adult: Only 1 site to be treated at a time, maximum 2 sites treated in any 24 hours, treatment not to be repeated within 7 days (consult product literature)

- CONTRA-INDICATIONS Infections affecting the treatment site
CONTRA-INDICATIONS, FURTHER INFORMATION
Contra-indications applicable to systemic use should be considered; however, glycopyrronium is poorly absorbed and systemic effects unlikely with topical use.
- CAUTIONS Cautions applicable to systemic use should be considered; however, glycopyrronium is poorly absorbed and systemic effects unlikely with topical use.
- SIDE-EFFECTS Tingling at administration site
SIDE-EFFECTS, FURTHER INFORMATION
The possibility of systemic side-effects should be considered; however; glycopyrrhonium is poorly absorbed and systemic effects unlikely with topical use.

- MEDICINAL FORMS
There can be variation in the licensing of different medicines containing the same drug.
Powder for solution for iontophoresis
 ‣ Glycopyrronium bromide (Non-proprietary)
   Glycopyrronium bromide 1 mg per 1 mg Glycopyrronium bromide powder for solution for iontophoresis | 3 gram PoM £313.92

DERMATOLOGICAL DRUGS > ASTRINGENTS

Aluminium chloride hexahydrate

- INDICATIONS AND DOSE
Hyperhidrosis affecting axillae, hands or feet
 ‣ TO THE SKIN
 ‣ Adult: Apply once daily, apply liquid formulation at night to dry skin, wash off the following morning, reduce frequency as condition improves—do not bathe immediately before use

Hyperhidrosis | Bromidrosis | Intertrigo | Prevention of tinea pedis and related conditions
 ‣ TO THE SKIN
 ‣ Adult: Apply powder to dry skin

- CAUTIONS Avoid contact with eyes · avoid contact with mucous membranes · avoid use on broken or irritated skin · do not shave axillae or use depilatories within 12 hours of application
- SIDE-EFFECTS Skin irritation
- PATIENT AND CARER ADVICE Avoid contact with clothing.
- EXCEPTIONS TO LEGAL CATEGORY A 30 mL pack of aluminium chloride hexahydrate 20% is on sale to the public.

- MEDICINAL FORMS
There can be variation in the licensing of different medicines containing the same drug.
Liquid
CAUTIONARY AND ADVISORY LABELS 15
 ‣ Aluminium chloride hexahydrate (Non-proprietary)
   Aluminium chloride 200 mg per 1 ml Aluminium chloride 20% solution | 60 ml P no price available DT price = £2.51
 ‣ Anhydrol (Dermal Laboratories Ltd)
   Aluminium chloride 200 mg per 1 ml Anhydrol Forte 20% solution | 60 ml P £2.51 DT price = £2.51
 ‣ Driclor (GlaxoSmithKline Consumer Healthcare)
   Aluminium chloride 200 mg per 1 ml Driclor 20% solution | 75 ml P £3.01 DT price = £3.01

5 Photodamage

Photodamage

Patients should be advised to use a high-SPF sunscreen and to minimise exposure of the skin to direct sunlight or sun lamps.

Topical treatments can be used for actinic keratosis. An emollient may be sufficient for mild lesions. Diclofenac sodium gel p. 1107 is suitable for the treatment of superficial lesions in mild disease. Fluorouracil cream p. 1107 is effective against most types of non-hypertrophic actinic keratosis; a solution containing fluorouracil with salicylic acid p. 1107 is available for the treatment of low or moderately thick hyperkeratotic actinic keratosis. Imiquimod p. 1126 is used for lesions on the face and scalp when cryotherapy or other topical treatments cannot be used. Fluorouracil and imiquimod produce a more marked inflammatory reaction than diclofenac sodium but lesions resolve faster. A short course of ingenol mebutate p. 1108 is licensed for the treatment of non-hypertrophic actinic

13

Skin

keratosis; response to treatment can usually be assessed 8 weeks after the course. Photodynamic therapy in combination with methyl-5-aminolevulinate cream (Metvix®, available from Galderma) or 5-aminolaevulinic acid gel (Ameluz®, available from Spirit Healthcare) is used in specialist centres for treating superficial and confluent, non-hypertrophic actinic keratosis when other treatments are inadequate or unsuitable; it is particularly suitable for multiple lesions, for periorbital lesions, or for lesions located at sites of poor healing.

Imiquimod or topical fluorouracil is used for treating superficial basal cell carcinomas. Photodynamic therapy in combination with methyl-5-aminolevulinate cream is used in specialist centres for treating superficial, nodular basal cell carcinomas when other treatments are unsuitable.

ANALGESICS > NON-STEROIDAL ANTI-INFLAMMATORY DRUGS

Diclofenac sodium

- **INDICATIONS AND DOSE**

SOLARAZE®

Actinic keratosis
▶ TO THE SKIN
▶ Adult: Apply twice daily for 60–90 days, to be applied thinly; maximum 8 g per day

- **CAUTIONS** Avoid contact with eyes · avoid contact with inflamed or broken skin · avoid contact with mucous membranes · not for use with occlusive dressings · topical application of large amounts can result in systemic effects, including hypersensitivity and asthma (renal disease has also been reported)
- **INTERACTIONS** → Appendix 1 (NSAIDs).
▶ With topical use Interactions do not generally apply to topical NSAIDs.
- **SIDE-EFFECTS** Paraesthesia · photosensitivity · rash (discontinue use if develops)
  SIDE-EFFECTS, FURTHER INFORMATION
  Topical application of large amounts can result in systemic effects, including hypersensitivity and asthma (renal disease has also been reported).
- **ALLERGY AND CROSS-SENSITIVITY** Contra-indicated in patients with a history of hypersensitivity to aspirin or any other NSAID—which includes those in whom attacks of asthma, angioedema, urticaria or rhinitis have been precipitated by aspirin or any other NSAID.
- **PREGNANCY** Patient packs for topical preparations carry a warning to avoid during pregnancy.
- **BREAST FEEDING** Patient packs for topical preparations carry a warning to avoid during breast-feeding.
- **DIRECTIONS FOR ADMINISTRATION** Apply with gentle massage only.
- **PATIENT AND CARER ADVICE** For topical preparations, patients and their carers should be advised to wash hands immediately after use.
  Photosensitivity Patients should be advised against excessive exposure to sunlight of area treated in order to avoid possibility of photosensitivity.
- **MEDICINAL FORMS**
  There can be variation in the licensing of different medicines containing the same drug.
  Gel
  EXCIPIENTS: May contain Benzyl alcohol, fragrances, propylene glycol
  ▶ Solaraze (Almirall Ltd)
    Diclofenac sodium 30 mg per 1 gram Solaraze 3% gel | 50 gram [PoM] £38.30 DT price = £38.30 | 100 gram [PoM] £76.60

ANTINEOPLASTIC DRUGS > ANTIMETABOLITES

Fluorouracil

- **INDICATIONS AND DOSE**

Superficial malignant and pre-malignant skin lesions
▶ TO THE SKIN USING CREAM
▶ Adult: Apply 1–2 times a day for 3–4 weeks (usual duration of initial therapy), apply thinly to the affected area, maximum area of skin 500 cm^2 (e.g. 23 cm × 23 cm) treated at one time, alternative regimens may be used in some settings

- **CAUTIONS** Avoid contact with eyes and mucous membranes · do not apply to bleeding lesions
- **SIDE-EFFECTS** Erythema multiforme · local irritation (use a topical corticosteroid for severe discomfort associated with inflammatory reactions) · photosensitivity
- **CONCEPTION AND CONTRACEPTION** Contraceptive advice required, see *Pregnancy and reproductive function* in Cytotoxic drugs p. 787.
- **PREGNANCY** Manufacturers advise avoid (teratogenic).
- **BREAST FEEDING** Manufacturers advise avoid.
- **HANDLING AND STORAGE** Caution in handling—irritant to tissues.
- **MEDICINAL FORMS**
  There can be variation in the licensing of different medicines containing the same drug.
  Cream
  EXCIPIENTS: May contain Cetostearyl alcohol (including cetyl and stearyl alcohol), hydroxybenzoates (parabens), polysorbates, propylene glycol
  ▶ Efudix (Meda Pharmaceuticals Ltd)
    Fluorouracil 50 mg per 1 gram Efudix 5% cream | 40 gram [PoM] £32.90 DT price = £32.90

Fluorouracil with salicylic acid

The properties listed below are those particular to the combination only. For the properties of the components please consider, fluorouracil above, salicylic acid p. 1126.

- **INDICATIONS AND DOSE**

Low or moderately thick hyperkeratotic actinic keratosis
▶ TO THE SKIN
▶ Adult: Apply once daily for up to 12 weeks, reduced to 3 times a week if severe side effects occur and until side-effects improve, to be applied to the affected area, if treating area with thin epidermis, reduce frequency of application and monitor response more often; maximum area of skin treated at one time, 25 cm^2 (e.g. 5 cm × 5 cm)

- **MEDICINAL FORMS**
  There can be variation in the licensing of different medicines containing the same drug.
  Cutaneous solution
  CAUTIONARY AND ADVISORY LABELS 15
  ▶ Actikerall (Almirall Ltd)
    Fluorouracil 5 mg/g, Salicylic acid 100 mg/g Actikerall 5mg/g / 100mg/g cutaneous solution | 25 ml [PoM] £38.30

PROTEIN KINASE C ACTIVATORS

Ingenol mebutate

- ● **INDICATIONS AND DOSE**

Actinic keratosis on face and scalp
- ▶ TO THE SKIN
- ▶ Adult: Apply once daily for 3 days, use the 150 microgram/g gel

Actinic keratosis on trunk and extremities
- ▶ TO THE SKIN
- ▶ Adult: Apply once daily for 2 days, use the 500 microgram/g gel

- ● CAUTIONS Avoid contact with broken skin · avoid contact with eyes · avoid contact with inside of ears · avoid contact with inside of nostrils · avoid contact with lips · avoid occlusive dressings on treated area

- ● SIDE-EFFECTS
- ▶ **Common or very common** Blistering · crusting · erosion · erythema · exfoliation · headache · infection · local reactions · oedema · pain · pruritus
- ▶ **Uncommon** Local ulceration · paraesthesia

- ● PREGNANCY Not absorbed from skin, but manufacturer advises avoid.

- ● BREAST FEEDING Not absorbed from skin; ensure infant does not come in contact with treated area for 6 hours after application.

- ● DIRECTIONS FOR ADMINISTRATION One tube covers skin area of 25 cm². Allow gel to dry on treatment area for 15 minutes. Avoid washing or touching the treated area for 6 hours after application; after this time, area may be washed with mild soap and water. Avoid use immediately after shower or less than 2 hours before bedtime.

- ● MEDICINAL FORMS
There can be variation in the licensing of different medicines containing the same drug.

Gel
CAUTIONARY AND ADVISORY LABELS 15
EXCIPIENTS: May contain Benzyl alcohol
- ▶ Picato (LEO Pharma) ▼
  Ingenol mebutate 150 microgram per 1 gram Picato 150micrograms/g gel | 1.41 gram PoM £65.00
  Ingenol mebutate 500 microgram per 1 gram Picato 500micrograms/g gel | .94 gram PoM £65.00

6   Pruritus

Topical local antipruritics

Overview

Pruritus may be caused by systemic disease (such as obstructive jaundice, endocrine disease, chronic renal disease, iron deficiency, and certain malignant diseases), skin disease (e.g. psoriasis, eczema, urticaria, and scabies), drug hypersensitivity, or as a side-effect of opioid analgesics. Where possible, the underlying causes should be treated. An **emollient** may be of value where the pruritus is associated with dry skin. Pruritus that occurs in otherwise healthy elderly people can also be treated with an emollient. Levomenthol **cream** p. 1109 can be used to relieve pruritus; it exerts a cooling effect on the skin. Local antipruritics have a role in the treatment of pruritus in palliative care.

Preparations containing crotamiton p. 1109 are sometimes used but are of uncertain value. Preparations containing calamine are often ineffective.

A topical preparation containing doxepin 5% p. 1109 is licensed for the relief of pruritus in eczema; it can cause drowsiness and there may be a risk of sensitisation.

Pruritus is common in biliary obstruction, especially in primary biliary cirrhosis and drug-induced cholestasis. Oral administration of colestyramine p. 180 is the treatment of choice.

Topical antihistamines and local anaesthetics are only marginally effective and occasionally cause hypersensitivity. For *insect stings* and *insect bites*, a short course of a topical corticosteroid is appropriate. Short-term treatment with a **sedating antihistamine** may help in insect stings and in intractable pruritus where sedation is desirable. Calamine preparations are of little value for the treatment of insect stings or bites.

Topical local anaesthetics are indicated for the relief of local pain. Preparations may be absorbed, especially through mucosal surfaces, therefore excessive application should be avoided and they should preferably not be used for more than 3 days; not generally suitable for young children and are less suitable for prescribing.

Topical antihistamines should be avoided in eczema and are not recommended for longer than 3 days. They are less suitable for prescribing.

> **Drugs used for Pruritus not listed below** Alimemazine tartrate, p. 259 · Cetirizine hydrochloride, p. 256 · Chlorphenamine maleate, p. 260 · Hydroxyzine hydrochloride, p. 262 · Levocetirizine hydrochloride, p. 257

ANTIPRURITICS

Calamine with zinc oxide

- ● **INDICATIONS AND DOSE**

Pruritus
- ▶ TO THE SKIN
- ▶ Child: (consult product literature)
- ▶ Adult: (consult product literature)

- ● CONTRA-INDICATIONS Avoid application of preparations containing zinc oxide prior to x-ray (zinc oxide may affect outcome of x-ray)

- ● LESS SUITABLE FOR PRESCRIBING Less suitable for prescribing.

- ● MEDICINAL FORMS
There can be variation in the licensing of different medicines containing the same drug.

Liquid
- ▶ Calamine with zinc oxide (Non-proprietary)
  Phenol liquefied 5 mg per 1 ml, Sodium citrate 5 mg per 1 ml, Bentonite 30 mg per 1 ml, Glycerol 50 mg per 1 ml, Zinc oxide 50 mg per 1 ml, Calamine 150 mg per 1 ml Calamine lotion | 200 ml GSL £0.81–£0.96 DT price = £0.96
- ▶ Cala Soothe (Ennogen Healthcare Ltd)
  Phenol liquefied 5 mg per 1 ml, Sodium citrate 5 mg per 1 ml, Bentonite 30 mg per 1 ml, Glycerol 50 mg per 1 ml, Zinc oxide 50 mg per 1 ml, Calamine 150 mg per 1 ml Cala Soothe lotion | 200 ml £19.50 DT price = £0.96

Cream
- ▶ Calamine with zinc oxide (Non-proprietary)
  Phenoxyethanol 5 mg per 1 gram, Zinc oxide 30 mg per 1 gram, Calamine 40 mg per 1 gram, Cetomacrogol emulsifying wax 50 mg per 1 gram, Self-emulsifying glyceryl monostearate 50 mg per 1 gram, Liquid paraffin 200 mg per 1 gram Aqueous calamine cream | 100 gram GSL £1.29 DT price = £1.29
- ▶ Cala Soothe (Ennogen Healthcare Ltd)
  Phenoxyethanol 5 mg per 1 gram, Zinc oxide 30 mg per 1 gram, Calamine 40 mg per 1 gram, Cetomacrogol emulsifying wax 50 mg per 1 gram, Self-emulsifying glyceryl monostearate 50 mg per 1 gram, Liquid paraffin 200 mg per 1 gram Cala Soothe cream | 100 ml £18.80

13

Skin

Crotamiton

- **INDICATIONS AND DOSE**

Pruritus (including pruritus after scabies)
▸ TO THE SKIN
- Child 1 month-2 years (on doctor's advice only): Apply once daily
- Child 3-17 years: Apply 2–3 times a day
- Adult: Apply 2–3 times a day

- **CONTRA-INDICATIONS** Acute exudative dermatoses
- **CAUTIONS** Avoid use in buccal mucosa · avoid use near eyes · avoid use on broken skin · avoid use on very inflamed skin · use on doctor's advice for children under 3 years
- **PREGNANCY** Manufacturer advises avoid, especially during the first trimester—no information available.
- **BREAST FEEDING** No information available; avoid application to nipple area.
- **MEDICINAL FORMS**
There can be variation in the licensing of different medicines containing the same drug.

Cream
EXCIPIENTS: May contain Beeswax, cetostearyl alcohol (including cetyl and stearyl alcohol), fragrances, hydroxybenzoates (parabens)
▸ Crotamiton (Non-proprietary)
Crotamiton 100 mg per 1 gram Boots Derma Care Itch Relief cream | 30 gram GSL no price available DT price = £2.50
▸ Brands may include Eurax

Doxepin

- **INDICATIONS AND DOSE**

Pruritus in eczema
▸ TO THE SKIN
- Child 12-17 years: Apply up to 3 g 3–4 times a day, apply thinly; coverage should be less than 10% of body surface area; maximum 12 g per day
- Adult: Apply up to 3 g 3–4 times a day, apply thinly; coverage should be less than 10% of body surface area; maximum 12 g per day

- **CAUTIONS** Avoid application to large areas · cardiac arrhythmias · mania · severe heart disease · susceptibility to angle-closure glaucoma · urinary retention
- **INTERACTIONS** → Appendix 1 (antidepressants, tricyclic).
- **SIDE-EFFECTS**
▸ **Common or very common** Dizziness · drowsiness
▸ **Frequency not known** Antimuscarinic effects · fever · gastro-intestinal disturbances · headache · irritation · local burning · rash · stinging · tingling
- **PREGNANCY** Manufacturer advises use only if potential benefit outweighs risk.
- **BREAST FEEDING** Manufacturer advises use only if potential benefit outweighs risk.
- **HEPATIC IMPAIRMENT** Manufacturer advises caution in severe liver disease.
- **PATIENT AND CARER ADVICE**
A patient information leaflet should be provided.
Driving and skilled tasks
Drowsiness may affect performance of skilled tasks (e.g. driving). Effects of alcohol enhanced.

- **MEDICINAL FORMS**
There can be variation in the licensing of different medicines containing the same drug.

Cream
CAUTIONARY AND ADVISORY LABELS 2, 10
EXCIPIENTS: May contain Benzyl alcohol
▸ Xepin (Cambridge Healthcare Supplies Ltd)
Doxepin hydrochloride 50 mg per 1 gram Xepin 5% cream | 30 gram PoM £11.70

MENTHOL AND DERIVATIVES

Levomenthol

- **INDICATIONS AND DOSE**

Pruritus
▸ TO THE SKIN
- Adult: Apply 1–2 times a day

- **MEDICINAL FORMS**
There can be variation in the licensing of different medicines containing the same drug. Forms available from special-order manufacturers include: cream, ointment

Cream
▸ Aqua-cool (Pinewood Healthcare)
Menthol 5 mg per 1 gram Aqua-cool 0.5% cream | 500 gram £15.30 DT price = £16.07
Menthol 10 mg per 1 gram Aqua-cool 1% cream | 100 gram £3.25 DT price = £3.97 | 500 gram £15.30 DT price = £16.59
Menthol 20 mg per 1 gram Aqua-cool 2% cream | 500 gram £15.30 DT price = £16.97
▸ AquaSoothe (Ennogen Healthcare Ltd)
Menthol 10 mg per 1 gram AquaSoothe 1% cream | 100 gram £3.70 DT price = £3.97 | 500 gram £15.43 DT price = £16.59
Menthol 20 mg per 1 gram AquaSoothe 2% cream | 50 gram £1.86 | 500 gram £15.43 DT price = £16.97
▸ Arjun (Arjun Products Ltd)
Menthol 5 mg per 1 gram Arjun 0.5% cream | 500 gram £15.30 DT price = £16.07
Menthol 10 mg per 1 gram Arjun 1% cream | 100 gram £3.25 DT price = £3.97 | 500 gram £15.30 DT price = £16.59
Menthol 20 mg per 1 gram Arjun 2% cream | 500 gram £15.30 DT price = £16.97
▸ Dermacool (Pern Consumer Products Ltd)
Menthol 5 mg per 1 gram Dermacool 0.5% cream | 100 gram £3.85 | 500 gram £16.07 DT price = £16.07
Menthol 10 mg per 1 gram Dermacool 1% cream | 100 gram £3.97 DT price = £3.97 | 500 gram £16.59 DT price = £16.59
Menthol 20 mg per 1 gram Dermacool 2% cream | 100 gram £4.07 | 500 gram £16.97 DT price = £16.97
Menthol 50 mg per 1 gram Dermacool 5% cream | 100 gram £4.69 | 500 gram £17.48

7 Rosacea and acne

Rosacea and Acne

Acne

Treatment of acne should be commenced early to prevent scarring. Patients should be counselled that an improvement may not be seen for at least a couple of months. The choice of treatment depends on whether the acne is predominantly inflammatory or comedonal and its severity.

Mild to moderate acne is generally treated with topical preparations. Systemic treatment with oral antibacterials is generally used for *moderate to severe acne* or where topical preparations are not tolerated or are ineffective or where application to the site is difficult. Another oral preparation used for acne is the hormone treatment co-cyprindiol (cyproterone acetate with ethinylestradiol) p. 1111; it is for women only.

13

Skin

Severe acne, acne unresponsive to prolonged courses of oral antibacterials, scarring, or acne associated with psychological problems calls for early referral to a consultant dermatologist who may prescribe isotretinoin p. 1114 for administration by mouth.

Topical preparations for acne

In mild to moderate acne, comedones and inflamed lesions respond well to benzoyl peroxide p. 1112 or to a topical retinoid. Alternatively, topical application of an antibacterial such as erythromycin or clindamycin p. 1111 may be effective for inflammatory acne. If topical preparations prove inadequate, oral preparations may be needed.

Benzoyl peroxide and azelaic acid

Benzoyl peroxide is effective in mild to moderate acne. Both comedones and inflamed lesions respond well to benzoyl peroxide. The lower concentrations seem to be as effective as higher concentrations in reducing inflammation. It is usual to start with a lower strength and to increase the concentration of benzoyl peroxide gradually. Adverse effects include local skin irritation, particularly when therapy is initiated, but the scaling and redness often subside with treatment continued at a reduced frequency of application. If the acne does not respond after 2 months then use of a topical antibacterial should be considered.

Azelaic acid p. 1113 has antimicrobial and anticomedonal properties. It may be an alternative to benzoyl peroxide or to a topical retinoid for treating mild to moderate comedonal acne, particularly of the face. Some patients prefer azelaic acid because it is less likely to cause local irritation than benzoyl peroxide.

Topical antibacterials for acne

For many patients with mild to moderate inflammatory acne, topical antibacterials may be no more effective than topical benzoyl peroxide or tretinoin. Topical antibacterials are probably best reserved for patients who wish to avoid oral antibacterials or who cannot tolerate them. Topical preparations of erythromycin and clindamycin are effective for inflammatory acne. Topical antibacterials can produce mild irritation of the skin, and on rare occasions cause sensitisation; gastro-intestinal disturbances have been reported with topical clindamycin.

Antibacterial resistance of *Propionibacterium acnes* is increasing; there is cross-resistance between erythromycin and clindamycin. To avoid development of resistance:

- when possible use non-antibiotic antimicrobials (such as benzoyl peroxide or azelaic acid);
- avoid concomitant treatment with different oral and topical antibacterials;
- if a particular antibacterial is effective, use it for repeat courses if needed (short intervening courses of benzoyl peroxide or azelaic acid may eliminate any resistant propionibacteria);
- do not continue treatment for longer than necessary (however, treatment with a topical preparation should be continued for at least 6 months).

Some manufacturers of topical antibacterial preparations for acne advise that preparations containing alcohol are not suitable for use with benzoyl peroxide.

Topical retinoids and related preparations for acne

Topical tretinoin, its isomer isotretinoin, and adapalene p. 1113 (a retinoid-like drug), are useful for treating comedones and inflammatory lesions in mild to moderate acne. Several months of treatment may be needed to achieve an optimal response and the treatment should be continued until no new lesions develop. Isotretinoin is given by mouth in severe acne.

Other topical preparations for acne

Preparations containing aluminium oxide p. 1112 are not considered beneficial in acne.

A topical preparation of nicotinamide p. 1116 is available for inflammatory acne.

Oral preparations for acne

Systemic antibacterial treatment is useful for inflammatory acne if topical treatment is not adequately effective or if it is inappropriate. Anticomedonal treatment (e.g. with topical benzoyl peroxide) may also be required.

Either oxytetracycline p. 515 or tetracycline p. 515 is usually given for acne. If there is no improvement after the first 3 months another oral antibacterial should be used. Maximum improvement usually occurs after 4 to 6 months but in more severe cases treatment may need to be continued for 2 years or longer.

Doxycycline p. 513 and lymecycline p. 514 are alternatives to tetracycline.

Although minocycline p. 515 is as effective as other tetracyclines for acne, it is associated with a greater risk of lupus erythematosus-like syndrome. Minocycline sometimes causes irreversible pigmentation; it is given in a once or twice daily dose.

Erythromycin in a twice daily dose is an alternative for the management of acne but *propionibacteria* strains resistant to erythromycin are becoming widespread and this may explain poor response.

Trimethoprim p. 521 may be used for acne resistant to other antibacterials [unlicensed indication]. Prolonged treatment with trimethoprim may depress haematopoiesis; it should generally be initiated by specialists.

Concomitant use of different topical and systemic antibacterials is undesirable owing to the increased likelihood of the development of bacterial resistance.

Hormone treatment for acne

Co-cyprindiol (cyproterone acetate with ethinylestradiol) contains an anti-androgen. It is licensed for use in women with moderate to severe acne that has not responded to topical therapy or oral antibacterials, and for moderately severe hirsutism. Although it is an effective hormonal contraceptive, it should not be used solely for contraception.

Improvement of acne with co-cyprindiol probably occurs because of decreased sebum secretion which is under androgen control. Some women with moderately severe hirsutism may also benefit because hair growth is also androgen-dependent.

Oral retinoid for acne

The retinoid isotretinoin reduces sebum secretion. It is used for the systemic treatment of nodulo-cystic and conglobate acne, severe acne, scarring, acne which has not responded to an adequate course of a systemic antibacterial, or acne which is associated with psychological problems. It is also useful in women who develop acne in the third or fourth decades of life, since late onset acne is frequently unresponsive to antibacterials.

Isotretinoin is a toxic drug that should be prescribed **only** by, or under the supervision of, a consultant dermatologist. It is given for at least 16 weeks; repeat courses are not normally required.

Side-effects of isotretinoin include severe dryness of the skin and mucous membranes, nose bleeds, and joint pains. The drug is **teratogenic** and must **not** be given to women of child-bearing age unless they practise effective contraception (oral progestogen-only contraceptives not considered effective) and then only after detailed assessment and explanation by the physician. Women must also be registered with a pregnancy prevention programme.

Although a causal link between isotretinoin p. 1114 use and psychiatric changes (including suicidal ideation) has not been established, the possibility should be considered before initiating treatment; if psychiatric changes occur during treatment, isotretinoin should be stopped, the prescriber informed, and specialist psychiatric advice should be sought.

Rosacea

Rosacea is not comedonal (but may exist with acne which may be comedonal). Brimonidine tartrate p. 1116 is licensed for the treatment of facial erythema in rosacea. The pustules and papules of rosacea respond to topical azelaic acid p. 1113, topical ivermectin or to topical metronidazole p. 1074. Alternatively oral administration of oxytetracycline p. 515 or tetracycline p. 515, or erythromycin p. 488, can be used; courses usually last 6–12 weeks and are repeated intermittently. Doxycycline p. 513 can be used [unlicensed indication] if oxytetracycline or tetracycline is inappropriate (e.g. in renal impairment). A modified-release preparation of doxycycline is licensed in low daily doses for the treatment of facial rosacea. Isotretinoin is occasionally given in refractory cases [unlicensed indication]. Camouflagers may be required for the redness.

7.1 Acne

ANTI-ANDROGENS

Co-cyprindiol

- ● INDICATIONS AND DOSE

Moderate to severe acne in females of child-bearing age refractory to topical therapy or oral antibacterials | Moderately severe hirsutism
- ▸ BY MOUTH
- ▸ Females of childbearing potential: 1 tablet daily for 21 days, to be started on day 1 of menstrual cycle; subsequent courses repeated after a 7-day interval (during which withdrawal bleeding occurs), time to symptom remission, at least 3 months; review need for treatment regularly

- ● CONTRA-INDICATIONS Acute porphyria · gallstones · heart disease associated with pulmonary hypertension or risk of embolus · history during pregnancy of cholestatic jaundice · history during pregnancy of chorea · history during pregnancy of pemphigoid gestationis · history during pregnancy of pruritus · history of breast cancer but can be used after 5 years if no evidence of disease and non-hormonal methods unacceptable · history of haemolytic uraemic syndrome · migraine with aura · personal history of venous or arterial thrombosis · sclerosing treatment for varicose veins · severe or multiple risk factors for arterial disease or for venous thromboembolism · systemic lupus erythematosus with (or unknown) antiphospholipid antibodies · transient cerebral ischaemic attacks without headaches · undiagnosed vaginal bleeding
- ● CAUTIONS Active trophoblastic disease (until return to normal of urine- and plasma-gonadotrophin concentration)—seek specialist advice · arterial disease · gene mutations associated with breast cancer (e.g. BRCA 1) · history of severe depression especially if induced by hormonal contraceptive—seek specialist advice · hyperprolactinaemia—seek specialist advice · inflammatory bowel disease including Crohn's disease · migraine · personal or family history of hypertriglyceridaemia (increased risk of pancreatitis) · risk factors for venous thromboembolism · sickle-cell disease · undiagnosed breast mass

CAUTIONS, FURTHER INFORMATION
- ▸ Venous thromboembolism There is an increased risk of venous thromboembolism in women taking co-cyprindiol, particularly during the first year of use. The incidence of venous thromboembolism is 1.5–2 times higher in women using co-cyprindiol than in women using combined oral contraceptives containing levonorgestrel, but the risk may be similar to that associated with use of combined oral contraceptives containing third generation progestogens (desogestrel and gestodene) or drospirenone. Women

requiring co-cyprindiol may have an inherently increased risk of cardiovascular disease.
- ● INTERACTIONS → Appendix 1 (oestrogens).
- ● SIDE-EFFECTS
- ▸ **Rare** Rarely gallstones · systemic lupus erythematosus
- ▸ **Very rare** Photosensitivity
- ▸ **Frequency not known** Abdominal cramps · absence of withdrawal bleeding · amenorrhoea after discontinuation · breast enlargement · breast secretion · breast tenderness · cervical erosion · changes in libido · changes in lipid metabolism · changes in vaginal discharge · chloasma · chorea · contact lenses may irritate · depression · fluid retention · headache · hepatic tumours · hypertension · irritability · leg cramps · liver impairment · nausea · nervousness · reduced menstrual loss · skin reactions · thrombosis (more common when factor V Leiden present or in blood groups A, B, and AB · visual disturbances · vomiting · 'spotting' in early cycles
- ● PREGNANCY Avoid—risk of feminisation of male fetus with cyproterone.
- ● BREAST FEEDING Manufacturer advises avoid; possibility of anti-androgen effects in neonate with cyproterone.
- ● HEPATIC IMPAIRMENT Avoid in active liver disease including disorders of hepatic excretion (e.g. Dubin-Johnson or Rotor syndromes), infective hepatitis (until liver function returns to normal), and liver tumours.
- ● PRESCRIBING AND DISPENSING INFORMATION A mixture of cyproterone acetate and ethinylestradiol in the mass proportions 2000 parts to 35 parts, respectively.

- ● MEDICINAL FORMS
There can be variation in the licensing of different medicines containing the same drug.

Tablet
- ▸ Co-cyprindiol (Non-proprietary)
  Ethinylestradiol 35 microgram, Cyproterone acetate 2 mg Co-cyprindiol 2000microgram/35microgram tablets | 63 tablet [PoM] £5.70 DT price = £5.56
- ▸ Clairette (Stragen UK Ltd) ▼
  Ethinylestradiol 35 microgram, Cyproterone acetate 2 mg Clairette 2000/35 tablets | 63 tablet [PoM] £5.90 DT price = £5.56
- ▸ Dianette (Bayer Plc, Mylan Ltd) ▼
  Ethinylestradiol 35 microgram, Cyproterone acetate 2 mg Dianette tablets | 63 tablet [PoM] £7.71–£11.10 DT price = £5.56
- ▸ Teragezza (Morningside Healthcare Ltd)
  Ethinylestradiol 35 microgram, Cyproterone acetate 2 mg Teragezza 2000microgram/35microgram tablets | 63 tablet [PoM] £11.10 DT price = £5.56

ANTIBACTERIALS ❭ LINCOSAMIDES

Clindamycin

- ● INDICATIONS AND DOSE
DALACIN T ® LOTION
Acne vulgaris
- ▸ TO THE SKIN
- ▸ Child: Apply twice daily, to be applied thinly
- ▸ Adult: Apply twice daily, to be applied thinly
DALACIN T ® SOLUTION
Acne vulgaris
- ▸ TO THE SKIN
- ▸ Child: Apply twice daily, to be applied thinly
- ▸ Adult: Apply twice daily, to be applied thinly
ZINDACLIN ® GEL
Acne vulgaris
- ▸ TO THE SKIN
- ▸ Child 12–17 years: Apply once daily, to be applied thinly
- ▸ Adult: Apply once daily, to be applied thinly

13

Skin

- **MEDICINAL FORMS**
There can be variation in the licensing of different medicines containing the same drug.
Liquid
EXCIPIENTS: May contain Cetostearyl alcohol (including cetyl and stearyl alcohol), hydroxybenzoates (parabens), propylene glycol
  - Dalacin T (Pfizer Ltd)
  Clindamycin (as Clindamycin phosphate) 10 mg per 1 ml Dalacin T 1% topical lotion | 30 ml [PoM] £5.08 DT price = £5.08 | 60 ml [PoM] £10.16
  Dalacin T 1% topical solution | 30 ml [PoM] £4.34 DT price = £4.34 | 50 ml [PoM] £7.23
Gel
EXCIPIENTS: May contain Propylene glycol
  - Zindaclin (Crawford Healthcare Ltd)
  Clindamycin (as Clindamycin phosphate) 10 mg per 1 gram Zindaclin 1% gel | 30 gram [PoM] £8.66 DT price = £8.66

Combinations available: *Benzoyl peroxide with clindamycin,* below · *Tretinoin with clindamycin,* p. 1115

ANTIBACTERIALS > MACROLIDES

Erythromycin with zinc acetate

- **INDICATIONS AND DOSE**

Acne vulgaris
▸ TO THE SKIN
  - Child: Apply twice daily
  - Adult: Apply twice daily

- **CAUTIONS** Some manufacturers advise preparations containing alcohol are not suitable for use with benzoyl peroxide

- **MEDICINAL FORMS**
There can be variation in the licensing of different medicines containing the same drug.
Liquid
  - Zineryt (Astellas Pharma Ltd)
  Zinc acetate 12 mg per 1 ml, Erythromycin 40 mg per 1 ml Zineryt lotion | 30 ml [PoM] £7.71 DT price = £7.71 | 90 ml [PoM] £16.68 DT price = £16.68

ANTISEPTICS AND DISINFECTANTS > PEROXIDES

Benzoyl peroxide

- **INDICATIONS AND DOSE**

Acne vulgaris
▸ TO THE SKIN
  - Child 12-17 years: Apply 1-2 times a day, preferably apply after washing with soap and water, start treatment with lower-strength preparations
  - Adult: Apply 1-2 times a day, preferably apply after washing with soap and water, start treatment with lower-strength preparations

- **CAUTIONS** Avoid contact with broken skin · avoid contact with eyes · avoid contact with mouth · avoid contact with mucous membranes · avoid excessive exposure to sunlight
- **SIDE-EFFECTS** Skin irritation
SIDE-EFFECTS, FURTHER INFORMATION
▸ Skin irritation Reduce frequency or suspend use until irritation subsides and re-introduce at reduced frequency.
- **PATIENT AND CARER ADVICE** May bleach fabrics and hair.

- **MEDICINAL FORMS**
There can be variation in the licensing of different medicines containing the same drug.
Cream
EXCIPIENTS: May contain Cetostearyl alcohol (including cetyl and stearyl alcohol), fragrances, isopropyl palmitate, propylene glycol
  - Brevoxyl (GlaxoSmithKline Consumer Healthcare)
  Benzoyl peroxide 40 mg per 1 gram Brevoxyl 4% cream | 50 gram [P] £4.13 DT price = £4.13

  - PanOxyl (GlaxoSmithKline Consumer Healthcare)
  Benzoyl peroxide 50 mg per 1 gram PanOxyl 5 cream | 40 gram [P] £1.89 DT price = £1.89
Gel
EXCIPIENTS: May contain Fragrances, propylene glycol
  - Acnecide (Galderma (UK) Ltd)
  Benzoyl peroxide 50 mg per 1 gram Acnecide 5% gel | 30 gram [P] £5.44 DT price = £5.44 | 60 gram [P] £10.68
  Acnecide Wash 5% gel | 50 gram [P] £5.44
  - PanOxyl Aquagel (GlaxoSmithKline Consumer Healthcare)
  Benzoyl peroxide 25 mg per 1 gram PanOxyl 2.5 Aquagel | 40 gram [P] £1.76 DT price = £1.76
  Benzoyl peroxide 50 mg per 1 gram PanOxyl 5 Aquagel | 40 gram [P] £1.92 DT price = £1.92
  Benzoyl peroxide 100 mg per 1 gram PanOxyl 10 Aquagel | 40 gram [P] £2.13 DT price = £2.13
  - Panoxyl Acnegel (GlaxoSmithKline Consumer Healthcare)
  Benzoyl peroxide 100 mg per 1 gram PanOxyl 10 Acnegel | 40 gram [P] £1.99 DT price = £2.13

Combinations available: *Adapalene with benzoyl peroxide,* p. 1113

Benzoyl peroxide with clindamycin

The properties listed below are those particular to the combination only. For the properties of the components please consider, benzoyl peroxide above, clindamycin p. 1111.

- **INDICATIONS AND DOSE**

Acne vulgaris
▸ TO THE SKIN
  - Child 12-17 years: Apply once daily, dose to be applied in the evening
  - Adult: Apply once daily, dose to be applied in the evening

- **MEDICINAL FORMS**
There can be variation in the licensing of different medicines containing the same drug.
Gel
EXCIPIENTS: May contain Disodium edetate
  - Duac (Stiefel Laboratories (UK) Ltd)
  Clindamycin (as Clindamycin phosphate) 10 mg per 1 gram, Benzoyl peroxide 30 mg per 1 gram Duac Once Daily gel (3% and 1%) | 30 gram [PoM] £13.14 DT price = £13.14 | 60 gram [PoM] £26.28
  Clindamycin (as Clindamycin phosphate) 10 mg per 1 gram, Benzoyl peroxide 50 mg per 1 gram Duac Once Daily gel (5% and 1%) | 30 gram [PoM] £13.14 DT price = £13.14 | 60 gram [PoM] £26.28 DT price = £26.28

DERMATOLOGICAL DRUGS > ABRASIVE AGENTS

Aluminium oxide

- **INDICATIONS AND DOSE**

Acne vulgaris
▸ TO THE SKIN
  - Adult: Apply 1-3 times a day, to be used instead of soap

- **CONTRA-INDICATIONS** Superficial venules · telangiectasia
- **CAUTIONS** Avoid contact with eyes
- **SIDE-EFFECTS** Skin irritation (discontinue use temporarily)
- **PATIENT AND CARER ADVICE** Patients should discontinue use temporarily if skin becomes irritated.
- **LESS SUITABLE FOR PRESCRIBING** Less suitable for prescribing (not considered beneficial).

13

Skin

- MEDICINAL FORMS
There can be variation in the licensing of different medicines containing the same drug.

Paste

EXCIPIENTS: May contain Fragrances, n-(3-chloroallyl)hexaminium chloride (quaternium 15)

▸ Brasivol (GlaxoSmithKline Consumer Healthcare)
Aluminium oxide 380 mg per 1 gram Brasivol Fine No.1 38% paste | 75 gram GSL £2.76

DERMATOLOGICAL DRUGS > ANTICOMEDONALS

Azelaic acid

- INDICATIONS AND DOSE
FINACEA®

Facial acne vulgaris
▸ TO THE SKIN
▸ Child 12-17 years: Apply twice daily, discontinue if no improvement after 1 month
▸ Adult: Apply twice daily, discontinue if no improvement after 1 month

Papulopustular rosacea
▸ TO THE SKIN
▸ Adult: Apply twice daily, discontinue if no improvement after 2 months

SKINOREN®

Acne vulgaris
▸ TO THE SKIN
▸ Child 12-17 years: Apply twice daily
▸ Adult: Apply twice daily

Acne vulgaris in patients with sensitive skin
▸ TO THE SKIN
▸ Child 12-17 years: Apply once daily for 1 week, then apply twice daily
▸ Adult: Apply once daily for 1 week, then apply twice daily

- CAUTIONS Avoid contact with eyes · avoid contact with mouth · avoid contact with mucous membranes
- SIDE-EFFECTS
▸ Common or very common Local irritation (reduce frequency or discontinue temporarily)
▸ Uncommon Skin discoloration
▸ Frequency not known Worsening of asthma

- MEDICINAL FORMS
There can be variation in the licensing of different medicines containing the same drug.

Cream
EXCIPIENTS: May contain Propylene glycol
▸ Skinoren (Bayer Plc)
Azelaic acid 200 mg per 1 gram Skinoren 20% cream | 30 gram PoM £3.74 DT price = £3.74

Gel
EXCIPIENTS: May contain Disodium edetate, polysorbates, propylene glycol
▸ Finacea (Bayer Plc)
Azelaic acid 150 mg per 1 gram Finacea 15% gel | 30 gram PoM £7.48 DT price = £7.48

RETINOID AND RELATED DRUGS

Adapalene

- INDICATIONS AND DOSE
Mild to moderate acne vulgaris
▸ TO THE SKIN
▸ Child 12-17 years: Apply once daily, apply thinly in the evening
▸ Adult: Apply once daily, apply thinly in the evening

- CAUTIONS Avoid accumulation in angles of the nose · avoid contact with eyes, nostrils, mouth and mucous membranes, eczematous, broken or sunburned skin · avoid exposure to UV light (including sunlight, solariums) · avoid in severe acne involving large areas · caution in sensitive areas such as the neck
- CONCEPTION AND CONTRACEPTION Females of child-bearing age must use effective contraception (oral progestogen-only contraceptives not considered effective).
- PREGNANCY Avoid.
- BREAST FEEDING Amount of drug in milk probably too small to be harmful; ensure infant does not come in contact with treated areas.
- PATIENT AND CARER ADVICE If sun exposure is unavoidable, an appropriate sunscreen or protective clothing should be used.

- MEDICINAL FORMS
There can be variation in the licensing of different medicines containing the same drug.

Cream
CAUTIONARY AND ADVISORY LABELS 11
EXCIPIENTS: May contain Disodium edetate, hydroxybenzoates (parabens)
▸ Adapalene (Non-proprietary)
Adapalene 1 mg per 1 gram Adapalene 0.1% cream | 45 gram PoM £19.73 DT price = £16.43
▸ Differin (Galderma (UK) Ltd)
Adapalene 1 mg per 1 gram Differin 0.1% cream | 45 gram PoM £16.43 DT price = £16.43

Gel
CAUTIONARY AND ADVISORY LABELS 11
EXCIPIENTS: May contain Disodium edetate, hydroxybenzoates (parabens), propylene glycol
▸ Adapalene (Non-proprietary)
Adapalene 1 mg per 1 gram Adapalene 0.1% gel | 45 gram PoM £19.73 DT price = £16.43
▸ Differin (Galderma (UK) Ltd)
Adapalene 1 mg per 1 gram Differin 0.1% gel | 45 gram PoM £16.43 DT price = £16.43

Adapalene with benzoyl peroxide

The properties listed below are those particular to the combination only. For the properties of the components please consider, adapalene above, benzoyl peroxide p. 1112.

- INDICATIONS AND DOSE
Acne vulgaris
▸ TO THE SKIN
▸ Child 9-17 years: Apply once daily, to be applied thinly in the evening
▸ Adult: Apply once daily, to be applied thinly in the evening

- CONCEPTION AND CONTRACEPTION Females of child-bearing age must use effective contraception (oral progestogen-only contraceptives not considered effective).
- PATIENT AND CARER ADVICE Gel may bleach clothing and hair.
- NATIONAL FUNDING/ACCESS DECISIONS
Scottish Medicines Consortium (SMC) Decisions
The *Scottish Medicines Consortium* has advised (March 2014) that *Epiduo®* should be restricted for use in mild to moderate facial acne when monotherapy with benzoyl peroxide or adapalene is inappropriate.

13

Skin

- **MEDICINAL FORMS**
There can be variation in the licensing of different medicines containing the same drug.

Gel

CAUTIONARY AND ADVISORY LABELS 11

EXCIPIENTS: May contain Disodium edetate, polysorbates, propylene glycol

- Adapalene with benzoyl peroxide (Non-proprietary)
Adapalene 1 mg per 1 gram, Benzoyl peroxide 25 mg per 1 gram Adapalene 0.1% / Benzoyl peroxide 2.5% gel | 45 gram [PoM] no price available DT price = £19.05

- Epiduo (Galderma (UK) Ltd)
Adapalene 1 mg per 1 gram, Benzoyl peroxide 25 mg per 1 gram Epiduo 0.1%/2.5% gel | 45 gram [PoM] £19.05 DT price = £19.05

Isotretinoin

- **INDICATIONS AND DOSE**

Topical treatment of mild to moderate acne
- TO THE SKIN
- Adult: Apply 1–2 times a day, to be applied thinly

Severe acne (under expert supervision) | Acne which is associated with psychological problems (under expert supervision) | Acne which has not responded to an adequate course of a systemic antibacterial (under expert supervision) | Acne with scarring (under expert supervision) | Systemic treatment of nodulo-cystic and conglobate acne (under expert supervision)
- BY MOUTH
- Adult: Initially 500 micrograms/kg daily in 1–2 divided doses, increased if necessary to 1 mg/kg daily for 16–24 weeks, repeat treatment course after a period of at least 8 weeks if relapse after first course; maximum 150 mg/kg per course

- **CONTRA-INDICATIONS**
- With oral use Hyperlipidaemia · hypervitaminosis A
- With topical use Perioral dermatitis · rosacea

- **CAUTIONS**
- With oral use Avoid blood donation during treatment and for at least 1 month after treatment · diabetes · dry eye syndrome (associated with risk of keratitis) · history of depression · monitor for depression
- With topical use Allow peeling (resulting from other irritant treatments) to subside before using a topical retinoid · alternating a preparation that causes peeling with a topical retinoid may give rise to contact dermatitis (reduce frequency of retinoid application) · avoid accumulation in angles of the nose · avoid contact with eyes, nostrils, mouth and mucous membranes, eczematous, broken or sunburned skin · avoid exposure to UV light (including sunlight, solariums) · avoid in severe acne involving large areas · avoid use of topical retinoids with abrasive cleaners, comedogenic or astringent cosmetics · caution in sensitive areas such as the neck · personal or familial history of non-melanoma skin cancer

- **INTERACTIONS**
- With oral use Appendix 1 (retinoids). Avoid keratolytics.

- **SIDE-EFFECTS**
- **Common or very common**
- With oral use Anaemia · arthralgia · dryness of eyes (with blepharitis and conjunctivitis) · dryness of lips (sometimes cheilitis) · dryness of nasal mucosa (with epistaxis) · dryness of pharyngeal mucosa (with hoarseness) · dryness of skin (with dermatitis, scaling, thinning, erythema, pruritus) · epidermal fragility (trauma may cause blistering) · haematuria · headache · myalgia · neutropenia · proteinuria · raised blood-glucose concentration · raised plasma-triglyceride concentration · raised serum-cholesterol concentration (with reduced high-density lipoprotein concentration) · raised serum-transaminase concentration · thrombocytopenia · thrombocytosis
- **Rare**
- With oral use Aggressive behaviour · alopecia · anxiety · depression · mood changes · skin reactions
- **Very rare**
- With oral use Acne fulminans · allergic vasculitis · arthritis · benign intracranial hypertension · blurred vision · bone changes following long-term administration · calcification of tendons and ligaments following long-term administration · cataracts · colour blindness · convulsions · corneal opacities · decreased night vision · decreased tolerance to contact lenses · diabetes mellitus · dizziness · drowsiness · early epiphyseal closure following long-term administration · exacerbation of acne · gastrointestinal haemorrhage · glomerulonephritis · Gram-positive infections of skin and mucous membranes · granulomatous lesions · haemorrhagic diarrhoea · hepatitis · hirsutism · hyperuricaemia · impaired hearing · increased sweating · inflammatory bowel disease · keratitis · lymphadenopathy · malaise · nail dystrophy · nausea · papilloedema · paronychia · photophobia · photosensitivity · psychosis · raised serum-creatine kinase concentration · reduced bone density following long-term administration · skeletal hyperostosis following long-term administration · skin hyperpigmentation · suicidal ideation · tendinitis · visual disturbances
- **Frequency not known**
- With oral use Stevens-Johnson syndrome · toxic epidermal necrolysis
- With topical use Blistering of skin · burning · crusting of skin · dry or peeling skin · erythema · eye irritation · increased sensitivity to UVB light or sunlight · oedema · pruritus · stinging

SIDE-EFFECTS, FURTHER INFORMATION
- Management of side-effects Risk of pancreatitis if triglycerides above 9 mmol/litre—discontinue if uncontrolled hypertriglyceridaemia or pancreatitis.
  Psychiatric side-effects require expert referral.
  Discontinue treatment if skin peeling severe or haemorrhagic diarrhoea develops.
  Visual disturbances require expert referral and possible withdrawal.

- **CONCEPTION AND CONTRACEPTION**
Pregnancy prevention
- With oral use Effective contraception must be used. In women of child-bearing potential, exclude pregnancy up to 3 days before treatment (start treatment on day 2 or 3 of menstrual cycle), every month during treatment (unless there are compelling reasons to indicate that there is no risk of pregnancy), and 5 weeks after stopping treatment—perform pregnancy test in the first 3 days of the menstrual cycle. Women must practise effective contraception for at least 1 month before starting treatment, during treatment, and for at least 1 month after stopping treatment. Women should be advised to use at least 1 method of contraception, but ideally they should use 2 methods of contraception. Oral progestogen-only contraceptives are not considered effective. Barrier methods should not be used alone, but can be used in conjunction with other contraceptive methods. Each prescription for isotretinoin should be limited to a supply of up to 30 days' treatment and dispensed within 7 days of the date stated on the prescription; repeat prescriptions or faxed prescriptions are not acceptable. Women should be advised to discontinue treatment and to seek prompt medical attention if they become pregnant during treatment or within 1 month of stopping treatment.
- With topical use Females of child-bearing age must use effective contraception (oral progestogen-only contraceptives not considered effective).

- **PREGNANCY** Contra-indicated in pregnancy (teratogenic).

● BREAST FEEDING Avoid.

● HEPATIC IMPAIRMENT

▸ With oral use Avoid—further impairment may occur.

● RENAL IMPAIRMENT

▸ With oral use In severe impairment, reduce initial dose (e.g. 10 mg daily) and increase gradually up to 1 mg/kg daily as tolerated.

● MONITORING REQUIREMENTS

▸ With oral use Measure hepatic function and serum lipids before treatment, 1 month after starting and then every 3 months (reduce dose or discontinue if transaminase or serum lipids persistently raised).

● PRESCRIBING AND DISPENSING INFORMATION Isotretinoin is an isomer of tretinoin.

● PATIENT AND CARER ADVICE

▸ With oral use Warn patient to avoid wax epilation (risk of epidermal stripping), dermabrasion, and laser skin treatments (risk of scarring) during treatment and for at least 6 months after stopping; patient should avoid exposure to UV light (including sunlight) and use sunscreen and emollient (including lip balm) preparations from the start of treatment.

▸ With oral use Patients and carers should be told how to recognise signs and symptoms of psychiatric disorders such as depression, anxiety, and rarely suicidal thoughts.

▸ With topical use Patients should be warned that some redness and skin peeling can occur initially but settles with time. If undue irritation occurs, the frequency of application should be reduced or treatment suspended until the reaction subsides; if irritation persists, discontinue treatment. Several months of treatment may be needed to achieve an optimal response and the treatment should be continued until no new lesions develop. If sun exposure is unavoidable, an appropriate sunscreen or protective clothing should be used.

● MEDICINAL FORMS
There can be variation in the licensing of different medicines containing the same drug.

Capsule

CAUTIONARY AND ADVISORY LABELS 10, 11, 21
 ▸ Isotretinoin (Non-proprietary)

  Isotretinoin 5 mg Isotretinoin 5mg capsules | 30 capsule PoM £10.15 | 56 capsule PoM £14.78
  Isotretinoin 10 mg Isotretinoin 10mg capsules | 30 capsule PoM £15.00 DT price = £14.54
  Isotretinoin 20 mg Isotretinoin 20mg capsules | 30 capsule PoM £20.00 DT price = £17.08 | 56 capsule PoM £37.85
  Isotretinoin 40 mg Isotretinoin 40mg capsules | 30 capsule PoM £38.98 DT price = £38.98
 ▸ Roaccutane (Roche Products Ltd)
  Roaccutane 10 mg Roaccutane 10mg capsules | 30 capsule PoM £14.54 DT price = £14.54
  Roaccutane 20 mg Roaccutane 20mg capsules | 30 capsule PoM £20.02 DT price = £17.08

Gel

CAUTIONARY AND ADVISORY LABELS 11
EXCIPIENTS: May contain Butylated hydroxytoluene
 ▸ Isotrex (Stiefel Laboratories (UK) Ltd)
  Isotretinoin 500 microgram per 1 gram Isotrex 0.05% gel | 30 gram PoM £5.94 DT price = £5.94

Isotretinoin with erythromycin

The properties listed below are those particular to the combination only. For the properties of the components please consider, isotretinoin p. 1114.

● INDICATIONS AND DOSE

Topical treatment of mild to moderate acne
 ▸ TO THE SKIN
 ▸ Adult: (consult product literature)

● MEDICINAL FORMS
There can be variation in the licensing of different medicines containing the same drug.

Gel

CAUTIONARY AND ADVISORY LABELS 11
EXCIPIENTS: May contain Butylated hydroxytoluene
 ▸ Isotrexin (Stiefel Laboratories (UK) Ltd)
  Isotretinoin 500 microgram per 1 gram, Erythromycin 20 mg per 1 gram Isotrexin gel | 30 gram PoM £7.47 DT price = £7.47

Tretinoin with clindamycin

The properties listed below are those particular to the combination only. For the properties of the components please consider, clindamycin p. 1111.

● INDICATIONS AND DOSE

Facial acne
 ▸ TO THE SKIN
 ▸ Child 12–17 years: Apply daily, (to be applied thinly at bedtime)
 ▸ Adult: Apply daily, (to be applied thinly at bedtime)

● CONTRA-INDICATIONS Perioral dermatitis · personal or familial history of non-melanoma skin cancer · rosacea

● CAUTIONS Allow peeling (resulting from other irritant treatments) to subside before using a topical retinoid · alternating a preparation that causes peeling with a topical retinoid may give rise to contact dermatitis (reduce frequency of retinoid application) · avoid accumulation in angles of the nose · avoid contact with eyes, nostrils, mouth and mucous membranes, eczematous, broken or sunburned skin · avoid exposure to UV light (including sunlight, solariums) · avoid in severe acne involving large areas · avoid use of topical retinoids with abrasive cleaners, comedogenic or astringent cosmetics · caution in sensitive areas such as the neck

● SIDE-EFFECTS Blistering of skin · burning · crusting of skin · dry or peeling skin (discontinue if severe) · erythema · eye irritation · increased sensitivity to UVB light or sunlight · oedema · pruritus · stinging · temporary changes of skin pigmentation

● CONCEPTION AND CONTRACEPTION Females of child-bearing age must use effective contraception (oral progestogen-only contraceptives not considered effective).

● PREGNANCY Contra-indicated in pregnancy.

● BREAST FEEDING Amount of drug in milk after topical application probably too small to be harmful; ensure infant does not come in contact with treated areas.

● PATIENT AND CARER ADVICE If sun exposure is unavoidable, an appropriate sunscreen or protective clothing should be used.

Patients and carers should be warned that some redness and skin peeling can occur initially but settles with time. If undue irritation occurs, the frequency of application should be reduced or treatment suspended until the reaction subsides; if irritation persists, discontinue treatment. Several months of treatment may be needed to achieve an optimal response and the treatment should be continued until no new lesions develop.

● MEDICINAL FORMS
There can be variation in the licensing of different medicines containing the same drug.

Gel

CAUTIONARY AND ADVISORY LABELS 11
EXCIPIENTS: May contain Butylated hydroxytoluene, hydroxybenzoates (parabens), polysorbates
 ▸ Treclin (Meda Pharmaceuticals Ltd)
  Tretinoin 250 microgram per 1 gram, Clindamycin (as Clindamycin phosphate) 10 mg per 1 gram Treclin 1%/0.025% gel | 30 gram PoM £11.94

13

Skin

Tretinoin with erythromycin

- **INDICATIONS AND DOSE**

Acne
▶ TO THE SKIN
  ▶ Child: Apply 1–2 times a day, apply thinly
  ▶ Adult: Apply 1–2 times a day, apply thinly

- **CONTRA-INDICATIONS** Perioral dermatitis · personal or familial history of non-melanoma skin cancer · rosacea
- **CAUTIONS** Allow peeling (resulting from other irritant treatments) to subside before using a topical retinoid · alternating a preparation that causes peeling with a topical retinoid may give rise to contact dermatitis (reduce frequency of retinoid application) · avoid accumulation in angles of the nose · avoid contact with eyes, nostrils, mouth and mucous membranes, eczematous, broken or sunburned skin · avoid exposure to UV light (including sunlight, solariums) · avoid in severe acne involving large areas · avoid use of topical retinoids with abrasive cleaners, comedogenic or astringent cosmetics · caution in sensitive areas such as the neck
- **SIDE-EFFECTS** Blistering of skin · burning · crusting of skin · dry or peeling skin (discontinue if severe) · erythema · eye irritation · increased sensitivity to UVB light or sunlight · oedema · pruritus · stinging · temporary changes of skin pigmentation
- **CONCEPTION AND CONTRACEPTION** Females of child-bearing age must use effective contraception (oral progestogen-only contraceptives not considered effective).
- **PREGNANCY** Contra-indicated in pregnancy.
- **BREAST FEEDING** Amount of drug in milk after topical application probably too small to be harmful; ensure infant does not come in contact with treated areas.
- **PATIENT AND CARER ADVICE** Patients and carers should be warned that some redness and skin peeling can occur initially but settles with time. If undue irritation occurs, the frequency of application should be reduced or treatment suspended until the reaction subsides; if irritation persists, discontinue treatment. Several months of treatment may be needed to achieve an optimal response and the treatment should be continued until no new lesions develop. If sun exposure is unavoidable, an appropriate sunscreen or protective clothing should be used.
- **MEDICINAL FORMS** There can be variation in the licensing of different medicines containing the same drug.
Liquid
CAUTIONARY AND ADVISORY LABELS 11
  ▶ Aknemycin Plus (Almirall Ltd)
    Tretinoin 250 microgram per 1 gram, Erythromycin 40 mg per 1 gram Aknemycin Plus solution | 25 ml PoM £7.05 DT price = £7.05

VITAMINS AND TRACE ELEMENTS > VITAMIN B GROUP

Nicotinamide

- **INDICATIONS AND DOSE**

Inflammatory acne vulgaris
▶ TO THE SKIN
  ▶ Adult: Apply twice daily, reduced to once daily or on alternate days, dose reduced if irritation occurs

- **CAUTIONS** Avoid contact with eyes · avoid contact with mucous membranes (including nose and mouth) · reduce frequency of application if excessive dryness, irritation or peeling

- **SIDE-EFFECTS** Burning · dry skin · erythema · irritation · pruritus

- **MEDICINAL FORMS** There can be variation in the licensing of different medicines containing the same drug.
Gel
  ▶ Freederm (Dendron Ltd)
    Nicotinamide 40 mg per 1 gram Freederm 4% gel | 25 gram P £5.56
  ▶ Nicam (Dermal Laboratories Ltd)
    Nicotinamide 40 mg per 1 gram Nicam 4% gel | 60 gram P £7.10

7.2 Rosacea

SYMPATHOMIMETICS > ALPHA₂-ADRENOCEPTOR AGONISTS

Brimonidine tartrate

- **DRUG ACTION Brimonidine**, an alpha₂-adrenoceptor agonist, is used to reduce erythema in rosacea by cutaneous vasoconstriction.

- **INDICATIONS AND DOSE**

Facial erythema in rosacea
▶ TO THE SKIN
  ▶ Adult: Apply once daily until erythema subsides, apply thinly, divide dose over forehead, chin, nose, and cheeks; maximum 5 mg per day

- **CAUTIONS** Cerebral insufficiency · coronary insufficiency · depression · postural hypotension · Raynaud's syndrome · severe cardiovascular disease · thromboangitis obliterans
- **INTERACTIONS** → Appendix 1 (brimonidine).
- **SIDE-EFFECTS**
  ▶ **Common or very common** Burning sensation at application site · stinging at application site
  ▶ **Uncommon** Dry mouth · dry skin · headache · paraesthesia · skin irritation
- **PREGNANCY** Limited information available; manufacturer advises avoid (gel).
- **BREAST FEEDING** Manufacturer advises avoid—no information available.
- **HEPATIC IMPAIRMENT** Manufacturer advises use with caution.
- **RENAL IMPAIRMENT** Manufacturer advises use with caution.
- **DIRECTIONS FOR ADMINISTRATION** Avoid contact with eyes, mouth, and mucous membranes; avoid use on irritated skin or open wounds; apply other topical preparations (including cosmetics) only after brimonidine gel has dried on skin.
- **PATIENT AND CARER ADVICE** Patients should be advised on administration of gel.
Driving and skilled tasks
Drowsiness may affect performance of skilled tasks (e.g. driving).
- **NATIONAL FUNDING/ACCESS DECISIONS**
Scottish Medicines Consortium (SMC) Decisions
The *Scottish Medicines Consortium* has advised (December 2014) that brimonidine (*Mirvaso®*) is accepted for restricted use within NHS Scotland for the symptomatic treatment of moderate to severe persistent facial erythema associated with rosacea in adult patients.

● MEDICINAL FORMS

There can be variation in the licensing of different medicines containing the same drug.

Gel

CAUTIONARY AND ADVISORY LABELS 28

EXCIPIENTS: May contain Hydroxybenzoates (parabens), propylene glycol

▸ Mirvaso (Galderma (UK) Ltd)

　Brimonidine (as Brimonidine tartrate) 3 mg per 1 gram Mirvaso 3mg/g gel | 30 gram PoM £33.69

8　Scalp and hair conditions

Scalp and hair conditions

Overview

Dandruff is considered to be a mild form of seborrhoeic dermatitis. Shampoos containing antimicrobial agents such as **pyrithione zinc** (which are widely available) and selenium below may have beneficial effects. Shampoos containing **tar** extracts may be useful and they are also used in *psoriasis*. Ketoconazole shampoo p. 1077 should be considered for more persistent or severe dandruff or for seborrhoeic dermatitis of the scalp.

Corticosteroid gels and lotions can be used. Shampoos containing coal tar with salicylic acid p. 1100 may also be useful. A cream or an ointment containing coal tar with salicylic acid is very helpful in Psoriasis p. 1084 that affects the scalp. Patients who do not respond to these treatments may need to be referred to exclude the possibility of other skin conditions.

Cradle cap in infants may be treated with **coconut oil** or **olive oil** applications followed by shampooing.

Hirsutism

Hirsutism may result from hormonal disorders or as a side-effect of drugs such as minoxidil p. 1118, corticosteroids, anabolic steroids, androgens, danazol p. 670, and progestogens.

Weight loss can reduce hirsutism in obese women.

Women should be advised about local methods of hair removal, and in the mildest cases this may be all that is required.

Eflornithine p. 1118 an antiprotozoal drug, inhibits the enzyme ornithine decarboxylase in hair follicles. Topical eflornithine can be used as an adjunct to laser therapy for facial hirsutism in women.

Co-cyprindiol p. 1111 may be effective for moderately severe hirsutism. Metformin hydrochloride p. 624 is an alternative in women with polycystic ovary syndrome [unlicensed indication]. Systemic treatment is required for 6–12 months before benefit is seen.

Androgenetic alopecia

Finasteride p. 712 is licensed for the treatment of androgenetic alopecia in men. Continuous use for 3–6 months is required before benefit is seen, and effects are reversed 6–12 months after treatment is discontinued.

Topical application of minoxidil may stimulate limited hair growth in a small proportion of adults but only for as long as it is used.

Drugs used for Scalp and hair conditions not listed below

Coal tar, p. 1099 · Coal tar with lecithin, p. 1100 · Coal tar with salicylic acid and precipitated sulfur, p. 1100

ANTISEPTICS AND DISINFECTANTS ❯
UNDECENOATES

Cetrimide with undecenoic acid

● INDICATIONS AND DOSE

Scalp psoriasis | Seborrhoeic dermatitis | Dandruff

▸ TO THE SKIN

▸ Child: Apply 3 times a week for 1 week, then apply twice weekly

▸ Adult: Apply 3 times a week for 1 week, then apply twice weekly

● MEDICINAL FORMS

There can be variation in the licensing of different medicines containing the same drug.

Shampoo

▸ Ceanel (Alliance Pharmaceuticals Ltd)

　Undecenoic acid 10 mg per 1 ml, Phenylethyl alcohol 75 mg per 1 ml, Cetrimide 100 mg per 1 ml Ceanel Concentrate shampoo | 150 ml P £3.40 | 500 ml P £9.80

ANTISEPTICS AND DISINFECTANTS ❯ OTHER

Benzalkonium chloride

● INDICATIONS AND DOSE

Seborrhoeic scalp conditions associated with dandruff and scaling

▸ TO THE SKIN

▸ Child: Apply as required

▸ Adult: Apply as required

● MEDICINAL FORMS

There can be variation in the licensing of different medicines containing the same drug.

Shampoo

▸ Dermax (Dermal Laboratories Ltd)

　Benzalkonium chloride 5 mg per 1 ml Dermax Therapeutic 0.5% shampoo | 250 ml P £5.69

VITAMINS AND TRACE ELEMENTS

Selenium

● INDICATIONS AND DOSE

Seborrhoeic dermatitis | Dandruff

▸ TO THE SKIN USING SHAMPOO

▸ Child 5–17 years: Apply twice weekly for 2 weeks, then apply once weekly for 2 weeks, then apply as required

▸ Adult: Apply twice weekly for 2 weeks, then apply once weekly for 2 weeks, then apply as required

Pityriasis versicolor

▸ TO THE SKIN USING SHAMPOO

▸ Adult: Apply once daily for 7 days, apply to the affected area and leave on for 10 minutes before rinsing off. The course may be repeated if necessary. Diluting with a small amount of water prior to application can reduce irritation

● UNLICENSED USE The use of selenium sulfide shampoo as a lotion for the treatment of pityriasis (tinea) versicolor is an unlicensed indication.

● PATIENT AND CARER ADVICE Avoid using 48 hours before or after applying hair colouring, straightening or waving preparations.

13

Skin

● MEDICINAL FORMS
There can be variation in the licensing of different medicines containing the same drug.

Shampoo

EXCIPIENTS: May contain Fragrances

▸ Selsun (Chattem (U.K.) Ltd)
Selenium sulfide 25 mg per 1 ml Selsun 2.5% shampoo | 50 ml [P]
£1.61 DT price = £1.61 | 100 ml [P] £2.15 DT price = £2.15 |
150 ml [P] £3.06 DT price = £3.06

8.1 Alopecia

VASODILATORS

| Minoxidil

● INDICATIONS AND DOSE

REGAINE® FOR MEN EXTRA STRENGTH FOAM

Androgenetic alopecia
▸ TO THE SKIN
▸ Adult: Apply 0.5 capful twice daily, to be applied to the affected areas of scalp; discontinue if no improvement after 16 weeks

REGAINE® FOR MEN EXTRA STRENGTH SOLUTION

Androgenetic alopecia
▸ TO THE SKIN
▸ Adult: Apply 1 mL twice daily, to be applied to the affected areas of scalp; discontinue if no improvement after 1 year

REGAINE® FOR WOMEN REGULAR STRENGTH

Androgenetic alopecia
▸ TO THE SKIN
▸ Adult: Apply 1 mL twice daily, to be applied to the affected areas of scalp; discontinue if no improvement after 1 year

● CONTRA-INDICATIONS Phaeochromocytoma

● CAUTIONS Avoid contact with broken, infected, shaved, or inflamed skin · avoid contact with eyes · avoid contact with mouth · avoid contact with mucous membranes · avoid inhalation of spray mist · avoid occlusive dressings

CAUTIONS, FURTHER INFORMATION
When used topically systemic effects unlikely; only about 1–2% absorbed (greater absorption may occur with use on inflamed skin).

● INTERACTIONS Caution—avoid topical drugs which enhance absorption.

● SIDE-EFFECTS
▸ Common or very common Headache · local irritation
▸ Uncommon Changes in hair colour or texture (discontinue if increased hair loss persists for more than 2 weeks) · hypotension

SIDE-EFFECTS, FURTHER INFORMATION
When used topically systemic effects unlikely; only about 1–2% absorbed (greater absorption may occur with use on inflamed skin).

● PREGNANCY Avoid—possible toxicity including reduced placental perfusion. Neonatal hirsutism reported.

● BREAST FEEDING Present in milk but not known to be harmful.

● PATIENT AND CARER ADVICE Ensure hair and scalp dry before application. Patients and their carers should be advised to wash hands after application of liquid or foam.

● MEDICINAL FORMS
There can be variation in the licensing of different medicines containing the same drug.

Foam

CAUTIONARY AND ADVISORY LABELS 15
EXCIPIENTS: May contain Butylated hydroxytoluene, cetostearyl alcohol (including cetyl and stearyl alcohol), polysorbates

▸ Regaine (McNeil Products Ltd)
Minoxidil 50 mg per 1 gram Regaine for Men Extra Strength 5% scalp foam | 180 gram [P] £46.83

Liquid

CAUTIONARY AND ADVISORY LABELS 15
EXCIPIENTS: May contain Propylene glycol

▸ Regaine (McNeil Products Ltd)
Minoxidil 20 mg per 1 ml Regaine for Women Regular Strength 2% solution | 60 ml [GSL] £14.16
Minoxidil 50 mg per 1 ml Regaine for Men Extra Strength 5% solution | 180 ml [P] £39.71

8.2 Hirsutism

ANTIPROTOZOALS

| Eflornithine

● DRUG ACTION An antiprotozoal drug that inhibits the enzyme ornithine decarboxylase in hair follicles.

● INDICATIONS AND DOSE

Adjunct to laser therapy for facial hirsutism in women
▸ TO THE SKIN
▸ Adult: Apply twice daily, to be applied thinly, discontinue use if no improvement after 4 months of treatment

● SIDE-EFFECTS
▸ Common or very common Acne · burning at application site · rash · stinging at application site
▸ Uncommon Abnormal hair growth · abnormal hair texture

● PREGNANCY Toxicity in *animal* studies—manufacturer advises avoid.

● BREAST FEEDING Manufacturer advises avoid—no information available.

● PATIENT AND CARER ADVICE Medicines must be rubbed in thoroughly. Cosmetics may be applied over treated area 5 minutes after eflornithine, do not wash treated area for 4 hours after application.

● NATIONAL FUNDING/ACCESS DECISIONS

Scottish Medicines Consortium (SMC) Decisions
The *Scottish Medicines Consortium* has advised (September 2005) that eflornithine for facial hirsutism be restricted for use in women in whom alternative drug treatment cannot be used.

● MEDICINAL FORMS
There can be variation in the licensing of different medicines containing the same drug.

Cream

EXCIPIENTS: May contain Cetostearyl alcohol (including cetyl and stearyl alcohol), hydroxybenzoates (parabens)

▸ Vaniqa (Almirall Ltd)
Eflornithine (as Eflornithine monohydrate chloride) 115 mg per 1 gram Vaniqa 11.5% cream | 60 gram [PoM] £56.87 DT price = £56.87

9 Skin cleansers, antiseptics and desloughing agents

Skin cleansers, antiseptics and desloughing agents

Skin cleansers and antiseptics

Soap or detergent is used with water to cleanse intact skin; emollient preparations such as aqueous cream or emulsifying ointment can be used in place of soap or detergent for cleansing dry skin.

An antiseptic is used for skin that is infected or that is susceptible to recurrent infection. Detergent preparations containing chlorhexidine p. 1120 or povidone-iodine below, which should be thoroughly rinsed off, are used. Emollients may also contain antiseptics.

Antiseptics such as chlorhexidine or povidone-iodine are used on intact skin before surgical procedures; their antiseptic effect is enhanced by an alcoholic solvent. Antiseptic solutions containing cetrimide can be used if a detergent effect is also required.

Hydrogen peroxide p. 1122, an oxidising agent, can be used in solutions of up to 6% for skin disinfection, such as cleansing and deodorising wounds and ulcers. Hydrogen peroxide is also available as a cream for superficial bacterial skin infections.

For irrigating ulcers or wounds, lukewarm sterile sodium chloride 0.9% solution is used, but tap water is often appropriate.

Potassium permanganate below solution 1 in 10000, a mild antiseptic with astringent properties, can be used for exudative eczematous areas; treatment should be stopped when the skin becomes dry.

Desloughing agents

Alginate, hydrogel and hydrocolloid dressings are effective at wound debridement. Sterile larvae (maggots) (available from BioMonde) are also used for managing sloughing wounds and are prescribable on the NHS.

Desloughing solutions and creams are of little clinical value. Substances applied to an open area are easily absorbed and perilesional skin is easily sensitised. Gravitational dermatitis may be complicated by superimposed contact sensitivity to substances such as neomycin sulfate p. 1074 or lanolin.

ANTISEPTICS AND DISINFECTANTS

Potassium permanganate

- **INDICATIONS AND DOSE**

Cleansing and deodorising suppurating eczematous reactions and wounds
▶ TO THE SKIN
▶ Adult: For wet dressings or baths, use approximately 0.01% (1 in 10 000) solution

- **CAUTIONS** Irritant to mucous membranes
- **DIRECTIONS FOR ADMINISTRATION** Potassium permanganate 0.1% solution to be diluted 1 in 10 to provide a 0.01% (1 in 10 000) solution. With potassium permanganate tablets for solution, 1 tablet dissolved in 4 litres of water provides a 0.01% (1 in 10 000) solution.
- **PATIENT AND CARER ADVICE** Can stain clothing, skin and nails (especially with prolonged use).

- **MEDICINAL FORMS**
There can be variation in the licensing of different medicines containing the same drug. Forms available from special-order manufacturers include: liquid
Tablet for cutaneous solution
▶ Potassium permanganate (Non-proprietary)
  Potassium permanganate 400 mg Potassium permanganate 400mg tablets for cutaneous solution | 30 tablet no price available DT price = £17.50
  EN-Potab 400mg tablets for cutaneous solution | 30 tablet no price available DT price = £17.50
▶ Permitabs (Alliance Pharmaceuticals Ltd)
  Potassium permanganate 400 mg Permitabs 400mg tablets for cutaneous solution | 30 tablet £17.50 DT price = £17.50

ANTISEPTICS AND DISINFECTANTS > ALCOHOL DISINFECTANTS

Alcohol

(Industrial methylated spirit)

- **INDICATIONS AND DOSE**

Skin preparation before injection
▶ TO THE SKIN
▶ Child: Apply as required
▶ Adult: Apply as required

- **CONTRA-INDICATIONS** Neonates
- **CAUTIONS** Avoid broken skin · flammable · patients have suffered severe burns when diathermy has been preceded by application of alcoholic skin disinfectants
- **INTERACTIONS** For the interactions following the *ingestion* of alcohol, see Appendix 1 (alcohol).
- **SIDE-EFFECTS**

Overdose
Features of acute alcohol intoxication include ataxia, dysarthria, nystagmus, and drowsiness, which may progress to coma, with hypotension and acidosis.

For details on the management of poisoning, see Alcohol, under Emergency treatment of poisoning p. 1194.

- **PRESCRIBING AND DISPENSING INFORMATION** Industrial methylated spirits defined by the BP as a mixture of 19 volumes of ethyl alcohol of an appropriate strength with 1 volume of approved wood naphtha.

- **MEDICINAL FORMS**
There can be variation in the licensing of different medicines containing the same drug.
Liquid
▶ Alcohol (Non-proprietary)
  Wood naphtha 50 ml per 1 litre, Ethanol 950 ml per 1 litre Industrial methylated spirit 95% | 600 ml £5.04 | 1000 ml £4.42–£6.02
  Industrial methylated spirit 70% | 600 ml £6.00

ANTISEPTICS AND DISINFECTANTS > IODINE PRODUCTS

Povidone-iodine

- **INDICATIONS AND DOSE**

Skin disinfection
▶ TO THE SKIN
▶ Child: (consult product literature)
▶ Adult: (consult product literature)

BETADINE® DRY POWDER SPRAY

Skin disinfection, particularly minor wounds and infections
▶ TO THE SKIN
▶ Adult: Not for use in serous cavities (consult product literature)

continued →

Skin
13

SAVLON® DRY

Skin disinfection of minor wounds

▶ TO THE SKIN
▶ Adult: (consult product literature)

VIDENE® SOLUTION

Skin disinfection

▶ TO THE SKIN
▶ Child: Apply undiluted in pre-operative skin disinfection and general antisepsis
▶ Adult: Apply undiluted in pre-operative skin disinfection and general antisepsis

VIDENE® SURGICAL SCRUB®

Skin disinfection

▶ TO THE SKIN
▶ Child: Use as a pre-operative scrub for hand and skin disinfection
▶ Adult: Use as a pre-operative scrub for hand and skin disinfection

VIDENE® TINCTURE

Skin disinfection

▶ TO THE SKIN
▶ Adult: Apply undiluted in pre-operative skin disinfection

● CONTRA-INDICATIONS Avoid regular use in patients with thyroid disorders (in adults) · concomitant use of lithium · corrected gestational age under 32 weeks (in children) · infants body-weight under 1.5 kg (in children) · regular use in neonates (in children)

● CAUTIONS Broken skin · large open wounds

CAUTIONS, FURTHER INFORMATION

▶ Large open wounds The application of povidone–iodine to large wounds or severe burns may produce systemic adverse effects such as metabolic acidosis, hypernatraemia and impairment of renal function.

VIDENE® TINCTURE Procedures involving hot wire cautery and diathermy

● SIDE-EFFECTS
▶ Rare Sensitivity

● PREGNANCY Sufficient iodine may be absorbed to affect the fetal thyroid in the second and third trimester.

● BREAST FEEDING Avoid regular or excessive use.

● RENAL IMPAIRMENT Avoid regular application to inflamed or broken skin or mucosa.

● EFFECT ON LABORATORY TESTS May interfere with thyroid function tests.

● MEDICINAL FORMS
There can be variation in the licensing of different medicines containing the same drug. Forms available from special-order manufacturers include: liquid

Liquid

CAUTIONARY AND ADVISORY LABELS 15 (Only for use with alcoholic solutions)

▶ Videne (Ecolab Healthcare Division)
Povidone-Iodine 75 mg per 1 ml Videne 7.5% surgical scrub solution | 500 ml [P] £7.30
Povidone-Iodine 100 mg per 1 ml Videne 10% antiseptic solution | 500 ml [GSL] £7.30

Spray

▶ Betadine (J M Loveridge Ltd)
Povidone-Iodine 25 mg per 1 gram Betadine 2.5% dry powder spray | 100 ml [GSL] £9.95 DT price = £9.95
▶ Savlon Dry (Novartis Consumer Health UK Ltd)
Povidone-Iodine 11.4 mg per 1 gram Savlon Dry 1.14% spray | 50 ml [GSL] £2.51 DT price = £2.51

Impregnated dressing

▶ Povidone-iodine (Non-proprietary)
Povidone-Iodine 100 mg per 1 gram Povitulle dressing 9.5cm × 9.5cm | 1 dressing £0.42 | 10 dressing no price available
Povitulle dressing 5cm × 5cm | 1 dressing £0.28 | 25 dressing no price available
▶ Inadine (Systagenix Wound Management Ltd)
Povidone-Iodine 100 mg per 1 gram Inadine dressing 5cm × 5cm | 1 dressing £0.33 | 25 dressing no price available
Inadine dressing 9.5cm × 9.5cm | 1 dressing £0.49 | 10 dressing no price available

ANTISEPTICS AND DISINFECTANTS > OTHER

Chlorhexidine

● INDICATIONS AND DOSE

CX ANTISEPTIC DUSTING POWDER

For skin disinfection

▶ TO THE SKIN
▶ Adult: (consult product literature)

CEPTON® LOTION

For skin disinfection in acne

▶ TO THE SKIN
▶ Child: (consult product literature)
▶ Adult: (consult product literature)

CEPTON® SKIN WASH

For use as skin wash in acne

▶ TO THE SKIN
▶ Child: (consult product literature)
▶ Adult: (consult product literature)

HIBITANE® PLUS 5% CONCENTRATE SOLUTION

General and pre-operative skin disinfection

▶ TO THE SKIN
▶ Child: (consult product literature)

HIBISCRUB®

Pre-operative hand and skin disinfection | General hand and skin disinfection

▶ TO THE SKIN
▶ Child: Use as alternative to soap (consult product literature)
▶ Adult: Use as alternative to soap (consult product literature)

HIBITANE OBSTETRIC®

For use in obstetrics and gynaecology as an antiseptic and lubricant

▶ TO THE SKIN
▶ Adult: To be applied to skin around vulva and perineum and to hands of midwife or doctor

HIBI® LIQUID HAND RUB+

Hand and skin disinfection

▶ TO THE SKIN
▶ Child: To be used undiluted (consult product literature)
▶ Adult: To be used undiluted (consult product literature)

HYDREX® SOLUTION

For pre-operative skin disinfection

▶ TO THE SKIN
▶ Child: (consult product literature)
▶ Adult: (consult product literature)

HYDREX® SURGICAL SCRUB

For pre-operative hand and skin disinfection | General hand disinfection

▶ TO THE SKIN
▶ Child: (consult product literature)
▶ Adult: (consult product literature)

UNISEPT®

For cleansing and disinfecting wounds and burns and swabbing in obstetrics
▶ TO THE SKIN
▶ Child: (consult product literature)
▶ Adult: (consult product literature)

IMPORTANT SAFETY INFORMATION
In preterm neonates, use sparingly, monitor for skin reactions, and do not allow solution to pool—risk of severe chemical burns.

● CONTRA-INDICATIONS Alcoholic solutions not suitable before diathermy · alcoholic solutions not suitable for use on neonatal skin · not for use in body cavities
● CAUTIONS Avoid contact with brain · avoid contact with eyes · avoid contact with meninges · avoid contact with middle ear
● SIDE-EFFECTS Chemical burns in preterm neonates · sensitivity
● DIRECTIONS FOR ADMINISTRATION

HIBITANE® PLUS 5% CONCENTRATE SOLUTION For pre-operative skin preparation, dilute 1 in 10 (0.5%) with alcohol 70%. For general skin disinfection, dilute 1 in 100 (0.05%) with water. Alcoholic solutions not suitable for use before diathermy or on neonatal skin.

● MEDICINAL FORMS
There can be variation in the licensing of different medicines containing the same drug.
Liquid
CAUTIONARY AND ADVISORY LABELS 15 (For ethanolic solutions (e.g. ChloraPrep® and Hydrex® only)
EXCIPIENTS: May contain Fragrances
▶ Cepton (Boston Healthcare Ltd)
Chlorhexidine gluconate 10 mg per 1 ml Cepton 1% medicated skin wash | 150 ml GSL £6.78
▶ HiBiTane Plus (Molnlycke Health Care Ltd)
Chlorhexidine gluconate 50 mg per 1 ml HiBiTane Plus 5% concentrate solution | 5000 ml GSL £14.50
▶ Hibi (Molnlycke Health Care Ltd)
Chlorhexidine gluconate 5 mg per 1 ml HiBi Liquid Hand Rub+ 0.5% solution | 500 ml GSL £5.25
▶ Hibiscrub (Molnlycke Health Care Ltd)
Chlorhexidine gluconate 40 mg per 1 ml Hibiscrub 4% solution | 250 ml GSL £4.25 | 500 ml GSL £5.25 | 5000 ml GSL £24.00
▶ Hydrex (Ecolab Healthcare Division)
Chlorhexidine gluconate 5 mg per 1 ml Hydrex pink chlorhexidine gluconate 0.5% solution | 600 ml GSL £4.50
Hydrex clear chlorhexidine gluconate 0.5% solution | 600 ml GSL £4.50
Chlorhexidine gluconate 40 mg per 1 ml Hydrex 4% Surgical Scrub | 250 ml GSL £4.09 | 500 ml GSL £4.34 | 5000 ml GSL £38.22
▶ Sterets Unisept (Molnlycke Health Care Ltd)
Chlorhexidine gluconate 500 microgram per 1 ml Sterets Unisept 0.05% solution 25ml sachets | 25 sachet P £5.54
Sterets Unisept 0.05% solution 100ml sachets | 10 sachet P £6.83
Cream
EXCIPIENTS: May contain Cetostearyl alcohol (including cetyl and stearyl alcohol)
▶ Hibitane (Derma UK Ltd)
Chlorhexidine gluconate 10 mg per 1 gram Hibitane Obstetric 1% cream | 250 ml GSL £12.00
Powder
▶ CX - brand name (Ecolab Healthcare Division)
Chlorhexidine acetate 10 mg per 1 gram CX 1% powder | 15 gram GSL £4.76

Chlorhexidine gluconate with isopropyl alcohol

The properties listed below are those particular to the combination only. For the properties of the components please consider, chlorhexidine p. 1120.

● INDICATIONS AND DOSE
Skin disinfection before invasive procedures
▶ TO THE SKIN
▶ Child 2 months-17 years: (consult product literature)
▶ Adult: (consult product literature)

● MEDICINAL FORMS
There can be variation in the licensing of different medicines containing the same drug.
Liquid
CAUTIONARY AND ADVISORY LABELS 15
▶ ChloraPrep (CareFusion U.K. Ltd)
Chlorhexidine gluconate 20 mg per 1 ml, Isopropyl alcohol 700 ml per 1 litre ChloraPrep with Tint solution 10.5ml applicators | 25 applicator GSL £76.65
ChloraPrep with Tint solution 26ml applicators | 25 applicator GSL £170.75
ChloraPrep solution 3ml applicators | 25 applicator GSL £21.25
ChloraPrep solution 1.5ml applicators | 20 applicator GSL £11.00
ChloraPrep with Tint solution 3ml applicators | 25 applicator GSL £22.31
ChloraPrep solution 0.67ml applicators | 200 applicator GSL £60.00
ChloraPrep solution 10.5ml applicators | 25 applicator GSL £73.00
ChloraPrep solution 26ml applicators | 25 applicator GSL £162.50

Chlorhexidine with cetrimide

The properties listed below are those particular to the combination only. For the properties of the components please consider, chlorhexidine p. 1120.

● INDICATIONS AND DOSE
Skin disinfection such as wound cleansing and obstetrics
▶ TO THE SKIN
▶ Child: To be used undiluted
▶ Adult: To be used undiluted

● MEDICINAL FORMS
There can be variation in the licensing of different medicines containing the same drug.
Liquid
▶ Savlon disinfectant (Novartis Consumer Health UK Ltd)
Chlorhexidine gluconate 3 mg per 1 ml, Cetrimide 30 mg per 1 ml Savlon disinfectant liquid | 500 ml £1.32
▶ Sterets Tisept (Molnlycke Health Care Ltd)
Chlorhexidine gluconate 150 microgram per 1 ml, Cetrimide 1.5 mg per 1 ml Sterets Tisept solution 25ml sachets | 25 sachet P £5.33
Sterets Tisept solution 100ml sachets | 10 sachet P £6.85
Cream
▶ Chlorhexidine with cetrimide (Non-proprietary)
Chlorhexidine gluconate 1 mg per 1 gram, Cetrimide 5 mg per 1 gram Savlon antiseptic cream | 15 gram GSL £0.86 | 30 gram GSL £1.14 | 60 gram GSL £1.82 | 100 gram GSL £2.65
Irrigation solution
▶ Chlorhexidine with cetrimide (Non-proprietary)
Chlorhexidine acetate 150 microgram per 1 ml, Cetrimide 1.5 mg per 1 ml Chlorhexidine acetate 0.015% / Cetrimide 0.15% irrigation solution 1litre bottles | 1 bottle P no price available

13

Skin

Diethyl phthalate with methyl salicylate

● INDICATIONS AND DOSE

Skin preparation before injection

▸ TO THE SKIN

▸ Adult: Apply to the area to be disinfected

● MEDICINAL FORMS
There can be variation in the licensing of different medicines containing the same drug.
Liquid
CAUTIONARY AND ADVISORY LABELS 15
▸ Diethyl phthalate with methyl salicylate (Non-proprietary)
Methyl salicylate 5 ml per 1 litre, Diethyl phthalate 20 ml per 1 litre, Castor oil 25 ml per 1 litre, Industrial methylated spirit 950 ml per 1 litre Surgical spirit | 200 ml [GSL] £1.06–£1.11 DT price = £1.11 | 500 ml [GSL] £1.95 | 1000 ml [GSL] £3.29

Hydrogen peroxide

● DRUG ACTION Hydrogen peroxide is an oxidising agent.

● INDICATIONS AND DOSE

For skin disinfection, particularly cleansing and deodorising wounds and ulcers

▸ TO THE SKIN

▸ Adult: Use 3% and 6% solutions (consult product literature)

CRYSTACIDE®

Superficial bacterial skin infection

▸ TO THE SKIN

▸ Child: Apply 2–3 times a day for up to 3 weeks

▸ Adult: Apply 2–3 times a day for up to 3 weeks

● UNLICENSED USE
▸ With topical use in children Licensed for use in children (age range not specified by manufacturer).

● CONTRA-INDICATIONS Closed body cavities (in adults) · deep wounds (in adults) · large wounds (in adults) · use as disinfection agent for surgical instruments (in adults) · use as enema (in adults) · use during surgery (in adults)

● CAUTIONS Avoid on eyes · avoid on healthy skin · incompatible with products containing iodine or potassium permanganate

● PRESCRIBING AND DISPENSING INFORMATION The BP directs that when hydrogen peroxide is prescribed, hydrogen peroxide solution 6% (20 vols) should be dispensed. Strong solutions of hydrogen peroxide which contain 27% (90 vols) and 30% (100 vols) are only for the preparation of weaker solutions.

● HANDLING AND STORAGE Hydrogen peroxide bleaches fabric.

● MEDICINAL FORMS
There can be variation in the licensing of different medicines containing the same drug. Forms available from special-order manufacturers include: liquid
Liquid
▸ Hydrogen peroxide (Non-proprietary)
Hydrogen peroxide 60 mg per 1 ml Hydrogen peroxide 6% solution | 200 ml [GSL] £0.61 | 500 ml [GSL] £2.54 | 2000 ml [GSL] £7.74
Hydrogen peroxide 90 mg per 1 ml Hydrogen peroxide 9% solution | 200 ml [GSL] £0.65
Hydrogen peroxide 30 ml per 1 litre Hydrogen peroxide 3% solution | 200 ml [GSL] £0.58
Cream
EXCIPIENTS: May contain Edetic acid (edta), propylene glycol
▸ Crystacide (Derma UK Ltd)
Hydrogen peroxide 10 mg per 1 gram Crystacide 1% cream | 25 gram [P] £8.07 DT price = £8.07 | 40 gram [P] £11.62

Proflavine

● INDICATIONS AND DOSE

Infected wounds | Infected burns

▸ TO THE SKIN

▸ Adult: (consult product literature)

● PATIENT AND CARER ADVICE Stains clothing.

● MEDICINAL FORMS
There can be variation in the licensing of different medicines containing the same drug. Forms available from special-order manufacturers include: liquid

Irrigation solutions

● IRRIGATION SOLUTIONS

Flowfusor sodium chloride 0.9% irrigation solution 120ml bottles (Fresenius Kabi Ltd)
Sodium chloride 9 mg per 1 ml | 1 bottle · NHS indicative price = £1.53 · Drug Tariff (Part IXa)

Irriclens sodium chloride 0.9% irrigation solution aerosol spray (ConvaTec Ltd)
Sodium chloride 9 mg per 1 ml | 240 ml · NHS indicative price = £3.50 · Drug Tariff (Part IXa)

Normasol sodium chloride 0.9% irrigation solution 100ml sachets (Molnlycke Health Care Ltd)
Sodium chloride 9 mg per 1 ml | 10 unit dose · NHS indicative price = £7.83 · Drug Tariff (Part IXa)

Normasol sodium chloride 0.9% irrigation solution 25ml sachets (Molnlycke Health Care Ltd)
Sodium chloride 9 mg per 1 ml | 25 unit dose · NHS indicative price = £6.42 · Drug Tariff (Part IXa)

Sodium chloride 0.9% irrigation solution 20ml Clinipod unit dose (Mayors Healthcare Ltd)
Sodium chloride 9 mg per 1 ml | 25 unit dose · NHS indicative price = £4.80 · Drug Tariff (Part IXa)

Sodium chloride 0.9% irrigation solution 20ml ISO-POD unit dose (St Georges Medical Ltd)
Sodium chloride 9 mg per 1 ml | 25 unit dose · NHS indicative price = £4.95 · Drug Tariff (Part IXa)

Sodium chloride 0.9% irrigation solution 20ml Irripod unit dose (C D Medical Ltd)
Sodium chloride 9 mg per 1 ml | 25 unit dose · NHS indicative price = £5.84 · Drug Tariff (Part IXa)

Sodium chloride 0.9% irrigation solution 20ml Sal-e Pods unit dose (Ennogen Healthcare Ltd)
Sodium chloride 9 mg per 1 ml | 25 unit dose · NHS indicative price = £4.80 · Drug Tariff (Part IXa)

Sodium chloride 0.9% irrigation solution 20ml Steripod unit dose (Molnlycke Health Care Ltd)
Sodium chloride 9 mg per 1 ml | 25 unit dose · NHS indicative price = £7.90 · Drug Tariff (Part IXa)

Sodium chloride 0.9% irrigation solution 20ml Sterowash unit dose (Steroplast Healthcare Ltd)
Sodium chloride 9 mg per 1 ml | 25 unit dose · NHS indicative price = £5.40 · Drug Tariff (Part IXa)

Sodium chloride 0.9% irrigation solution 20ml unit dose (Alissa Healthcare Research Ltd)
Sodium chloride 9 mg per 1 ml | 25 unit dose · NHS indicative price = £7.36 · Drug Tariff (Part IXa)

Sodium chloride 0.9% irrigation solution 20ml unit dose (Crest Medical Ltd)
Sodium chloride 9 mg per 1 ml | 25 unit dose · NHS indicative price = £4.99 · Drug Tariff (Part IXa)

Sodium chloride 0.9% irrigation solution 20ml unit dose (Mylan Ltd)
Sodium chloride 9 mg per 1 ml | 25 unit dose · NHS indicative price = £5.50 · Drug Tariff (Part IXa)

Stericlens sodium chloride 0.9% irrigation solution aerosol spray (C D Medical Ltd)
> Sodium chloride 9 mg per 1 ml | 100 ml · NHS indicative price = £2.07 · Drug Tariff (Part IXa) | 240 ml · NHS indicative price = £3.15 · Drug Tariff (Part IXa)

9.1   Minor cuts and abrasions

Minor cuts and abrasions

Management
Many preparations traditionally used to manage minor burns, and abrasions have fallen out of favour. Preparations containing camphor and sulfonamides should be avoided. Preparations such as magnesium sulfate paste are now rarely used to treat carbuncles and boils as these are best treated with antibiotics.

Cetrimide is used to treat minor cuts and abrasions and proflavine p. 1122 may be used to treat infected wounds or burns, but its use has now been largely superseded by other antiseptics or suitable antibacterials. The effervescent effect of hydrogen peroxide p. 1122 is used to clean minor cuts and abrasions.

Flexible colloidon (see castor oil with collodion and colophony below) may be used to seal minor cuts and wounds that have partially healed; skin tissue adhesives are used similarly, and also for additional suture support.

ANTISEPTICS AND DISINFECTANTS

Glycerol with magnesium sulfate and phenol

- **INDICATIONS AND DOSE**
Treat carbuncles and boils
▸ TO THE SKIN
▸ Adult: To be applied under dressing

- **DIRECTIONS FOR ADMINISTRATION** Paste should be stirred before use.

- **MEDICINAL FORMS**
There can be variation in the licensing of different medicines containing the same drug.
Paste
▸ Glycerol with magnesium sulfate and phenol (Non-proprietary)
Phenol 5 mg per 1 gram, Magnesium sulfate dried 450 mg per 1 gram, Glycerol 550 mg per 1 gram   Magnesium sulfate paste | 25 gram GSL £1.29 | 50 gram GSL £2.57 DT price = £2.40

DERMATOLOGICAL DRUGS > COLLODIONS

Castor oil with collodion and colophony

- **INDICATIONS AND DOSE**
Used to seal minor cuts and wounds that have partially healed
▸ TO THE SKIN
▸ Child: (consult product literature)
▸ Adult: (consult product literature)

- **ALLERGY AND CROSS-SENSITIVITY** Contra-indicated if patient has an allergy to colophony in elastic adhesive plasters and tape.

- **MEDICINAL FORMS**
There can be variation in the licensing of different medicines containing the same drug.
Liquid
▸ Castor oil with collodion and colophony (Non-proprietary)
Castor oil 25 mg per 1 ml, Collodion methylated 950 microlitre per 1 ml, Colophony 25 mg per 1 ml   Flexible collodion methylated | 100 ml £13.54 | 500 ml £27.52

Skin adhesives

- **SKIN ADHESIVES**
Derma+Flex skin adhesive (Chemence Ltd)
.5 ml · NHS indicative price = £5.36 · Drug Tariff (Part IXa)

Dermabond ProPen skin adhesive (Ethicon Ltd)
.5 ml · NHS indicative price = £19.26 · Drug Tariff (Part IXa)

Histoacryl L skin adhesive (B.Braun Medical Ltd)
.2 gram · NHS indicative price = £6.20 · Drug Tariff (Part IXa).5 gram · NHS indicative price = £6.72 · Drug Tariff (Part IXa)

Histoacryl skin adhesive (B.Braun Medical Ltd)
.2 gram · NHS indicative price = £6.41 · Drug Tariff (Part IXa).5 gram · NHS indicative price = £6.50 · Drug Tariff (Part IXa)

Indermil skin adhesive (Covidien (UK) Commercial Ltd)
.5 gram · NHS indicative price = £6.50 · Drug Tariff (Part IXa)

LiquiBand flow control tissue adhesive (MedLogic Global Ltd)
.5 gram · NHS indicative price = £5.50 · Drug Tariff (Part IXa)

LiquiBand tissue adhesive (MedLogic Global Ltd)
.5 gram · NHS indicative price = £5.50 · Drug Tariff (Part IXa)

10   Skin disfigurement

Camouflagers

Overview
Disfigurement of the skin can be very distressing to patients and may have a marked psychological effect. In skilled hands, or with experience, camouflage cosmetics can be very effective in concealing scars and birthmarks. The depigmented patches in vitiligo are also very disfiguring and camouflage creams are of great cosmetic value.

Opaque cover foundation or cream is used to mask skin pigment abnormalities; careful application using a combination of dark- and light-coloured cover creams set with powder helps to minimise the appearance of skin deformities.

Borderline substances
The preparations marked 'ACBS' can be prescribed on the NHS for postoperative scars and other deformities and as adjunctive therapy in the relief of emotional disturbances due to disfiguring skin disease, such as vitiligo.

Camouflages

- **CAMOUFLAGES**
Covermark classic foundation (Derma UK Ltd)
15 ml(ACBS) · NHS indicative price = £11.86

Covermark finishing powder (Derma UK Ltd)
25 gram(ACBS) · NHS indicative price = £11.86

Dermacolor camouflage creme (Charles H Fox Ltd)
25 ml(ACBS) · NHS indicative price = £10.52

Dermacolor fixing powder (Charles H Fox Ltd)
60 gram(ACBS) · NHS indicative price = £9.05

Keromask finishing powder (Bellava Ltd)
20 gram(ACBS) · NHS indicative price = £5.80

Keromask masking cream (Bellava Ltd)
15 ml(ACBS) · NHS indicative price = £5.80

13

Skin

Veil cover cream (Thomas Blake Cosmetic Creams Ltd)
19 gram(ACBS) · NHS indicative price = £22.42 44 gram(ACBS) · NHS
indicative price = £33.35 70 gram(ACBS) · NHS indicative price = £42.10

Veil finishing powder (Thomas Blake Cosmetic Creams Ltd)
35 gram(ACBS) · NHS indicative price = £24.58

11 Superficial soft-tissue injuries and superficial thrombophlebitis

Topical circulatory preparations

Overview

These preparations are used to improve circulation in
conditions such as bruising, superficial thrombophlebitis,
chilblains and varicose veins but are of little value. Chilblains
are best managed by avoidance of exposure to cold; neither
systemic nor topical vasodilator therapy is established as
being effective.

HEPARINOIDS

Heparinoid

- ● INDICATIONS AND DOSE

Superficial thrombophlebitis | Bruising | Haematoma
▸ TO THE SKIN
 ▸ Adult: Apply up to 4 times a day

- ● CONTRA-INDICATIONS Should not be used on large areas of
skin, broken or sensitive skin, or mucous membranes
- ● LESS SUITABLE FOR PRESCRIBING Hirudoid® is less
suitable for prescribing.

- ● MEDICINAL FORMS
There can be variation in the licensing of different medicines
containing the same drug.
Cream
EXCIPIENTS: May contain Cetostearyl alcohol (including cetyl and
stearyl alcohol), hydroxybenzoates (parabens)
 ▸ Hirudoid (Genus Pharmaceuticals Ltd)
 Heparinoid 3 mg per 1 gram Hirudoid 0.3% cream | 50 gram P
 £3.99 DT price = £3.99
Gel
EXCIPIENTS: May contain Fragrances, propylene glycol
 ▸ Hirudoid (Genus Pharmaceuticals Ltd)
 Heparinoid 3 mg per 1 gram Hirudoid 0.3% gel | 50 gram P £3.99
 DT price = £3.99

12 Warts and calluses

Warts and calluses

Overview

Warts (verrucas) are caused by a human papillomavirus,
which most frequently affects the hands, feet (plantar warts),
and the anogenital region; treatment usually relies on local
tissue destruction. Warts may regress on their own and
treatment is required only if the warts are painful, unsightly,
persistent, or cause distress.

Preparations of salicylic acid p. 1126, formaldehyde
p. 1125, glutaraldehyde p. 1125 or silver nitrate p. 1125 are
available for purchase by the public; they are suitable for the
removal of warts on hands and feet. Salicylic acid is a useful
keratolytic which may be considered first-line; it is also
suitable for the removal of *corns and calluses*. Preparations of

salicylic acid in a collodion basis are available but some
patients may develop an allergy to colophony in the
formulation; collodion should be avoided in children allergic
to elastic adhesive plaster. Cryotherapy causes pain,
swelling, and blistering, and may be no more effective than
topical salicylic acid in the treatment of warts.

Anogenital warts

The treatment of anogenital warts (condylomata acuminata)
should be accompanied by screening for other sexually
transmitted infections. Podophyllotoxin p. 1124 (the major
active ingredient of podophyllum) may be used for *soft, non-
keratinised* external anogenital warts. Patients with a limited
number of external warts or *keratinised* lesions may be better
treated with cryotherapy or other forms of physical ablation.

Imiquimod p. 1126 cream is licensed for the treatment of
external anogenital warts; it may be used for both
keratinised and non-keratinised lesions. It is also licensed
for the treatment of superficial basal cell carcinoma and
actinic keratosis.

Inosine pranobex p. 576 is licensed for adjunctive
treatment of genital warts but it has been superseded by
more effective drugs.

ANTINEOPLASTIC DRUGS › PLANT ALKALOIDS

Podophyllotoxin

- ● INDICATIONS AND DOSE

CONDYLINE®

**Condylomata acuminata affecting the penis or the female
external genitalia**
▸ TO THE LESION
 ▸ Adult: Apply twice daily for 3 consecutive days,
 treatment may be repeated at weekly intervals if
 necessary for a total of five 3-day treatment courses,
 direct medical supervision for lesions in the female and
 for lesions greater than 4 cm² in the male, maximum 50
 single applications ('loops') per session (consult
 product literature)

WARTICON® CREAM

**Condylomata acuminata affecting the penis or the female
external genitalia**
▸ TO THE LESION
 ▸ Adult: Apply twice daily for 3 consecutive days,
 treatment may be repeated at weekly intervals if
 necessary for a total of four 3-day treatment courses,
 direct medical supervision for lesions greater than
 4 cm²

WARTICON® LIQUID

**Condylomata acuminata affecting the penis or the female
external genitalia**
▸ TO THE LESION
 ▸ Adult: Apply twice daily for 3 consecutive days,
 treatment may be repeated at weekly intervals if
 necessary for a total of four 3-day treatment courses,
 direct medical supervision for lesions greater than
 4 cm², maximum 50 single applications ('loops') per
 session (consult product literature)

- ● CAUTIONS Avoid normal skin · avoid open wounds · keep
away from face · very irritant to eyes
- ● SIDE-EFFECTS Local irritation
- ● PREGNANCY Avoid.
- ● BREAST FEEDING Avoid.

- MEDICINAL FORMS
There can be variation in the licensing of different medicines containing the same drug.

Liquid

CAUTIONARY AND ADVISORY LABELS 15

▸ Condyline (Takeda UK Ltd)
Podophyllotoxin 5 mg per 1 ml Condyline 0.5% solution | 3.5 ml [PoM] £14.49

▸ Warticon (Stiefel Laboratories (UK) Ltd)
Podophyllotoxin 5 mg per 1 ml Warticon 0.5% solution | 3 ml [PoM] £14.86

Cream

EXCIPIENTS: May contain Butylated hydroxyanisole, cetostearyl alcohol (including cetyl and stearyl alcohol), hydroxybenzoates (parabens), sorbic acid

▸ Warticon (Stiefel Laboratories (UK) Ltd)
Podophyllotoxin 1.5 mg per 1 gram Warticon 0.15% cream | 5 gram [PoM] £17.83 DT price = £17.83

ANTISEPTICS AND DISINFECTANTS ›
ALDEHYDES AND DERIVATIVES

Formaldehyde

- INDICATIONS AND DOSE

Warts, particularly plantar warts

▸ TO THE LESION

▸ Child: Apply twice daily

▸ Adult: Apply twice daily

- UNLICENSED USE
▸ In children Licensed for use in children (age range not specified by manufacturer).

- CAUTIONS Impaired peripheral circulation · not suitable for application to anogenital region · not suitable for application to face · not suitable for application to large areas · patients with diabetes at risk of neuropathic ulcers · protect surrounding skin and avoid broken skin · significant peripheral neuropathy

- SIDE-EFFECTS Skin irritation · skin ulceration (with high concentrations)

- MEDICINAL FORMS
There can be variation in the licensing of different medicines containing the same drug. Forms available from special-order manufacturers include: liquid

Liquid

▸ Formaldehyde (Non-proprietary)
Formaldehyde 40 mg per 1 ml Formaldehyde (Buffered) 4% solution | 1000 ml £3.90

Gel

▸ Veracur (Typharm Ltd)
Formaldehyde 7.5 mg per 1 gram Veracur 0.75% gel | 15 gram [GSL] £2.41

Form unstated

▸ Formaldehyde (Non-proprietary)
Formaldehyde 350 mg per 1 gram Formaldehyde solution | 500 ml £5.84 DT price = £5.84 | 2000 ml £9.22–£16.77

Glutaraldehyde

- INDICATIONS AND DOSE

Warts, particularly plantar warts

▸ TO THE LESION

▸ Child: Apply twice daily

▸ Adult: Apply twice daily

- UNLICENSED USE
▸ In children Licensed for use in children (age range not specified by manufacturer).

- CAUTIONS Not for application to anogenital areas · not for application to face · not for application to mucosa · protect surrounding skin

- SIDE-EFFECTS Rashes · skin irritation (discontinue if severe) · stains skin brown

- MEDICINAL FORMS
There can be variation in the licensing of different medicines containing the same drug.

Paint

▸ Glutarol (Dermal Laboratories Ltd)
Glutaraldehyde 100 mg per 1 ml Glutarol 10% cutaneous solution | 10 ml [P] £2.07 DT price = £2.07

ANTISEPTICS AND DISINFECTANTS › OTHER

Silver nitrate

- INDICATIONS AND DOSE

Common warts

▸ TO THE LESION

▸ Child: Apply every 24 hours for up to 3 applications, apply moistened caustic pencil tip for 1–2 minutes. Instructions in proprietary packs generally incorporate advice to remove dead skin before use by gentle filing and to cover with adhesive dressing after application

▸ Adult: Apply every 24 hours for up to 3 applications, apply moistened caustic pencil tip for 1–2 minutes. Instructions in proprietary packs generally incorporate advice to remove dead skin before use by gentle filing and to cover with adhesive dressing after application

Verrucas

▸ TO THE LESION

▸ Child: Apply every 24 hours for up to 6 applications, apply moistened caustic pencil tip for 1–2 minutes. Instructions in proprietary packs generally incorporate advice to remove dead skin before use by gentle filing and to cover with adhesive dressing after application

▸ Adult: Apply every 24 hours for up to 6 applications, apply moistened caustic pencil tip for 1–2 minutes. Instructions in proprietary packs generally incorporate advice to remove dead skin before use by gentle filing and to cover with adhesive dressing after application

Umbilical granulomas

▸ TO THE SKIN

▸ Child: Apply moistened caustic pencil tip (usually containing silver nitrate 40%) for 1–2 minutes, protect surrounding skin with soft paraffin

▸ Adult: Apply moistened caustic pencil tip (usually containing silver nitrate 40%) for 1–2 minutes, protect surrounding skin with soft paraffin

- UNLICENSED USE
▸ In children No age range specified by manufacturer.

- CAUTIONS Avoid broken skin · not suitable for application to ano-genital region · not suitable for application to face · not suitable for application to large areas · protect surrounding skin

- SIDE-EFFECTS Chemical burns on surrounding skin · stains skin

- PATIENT AND CARER ADVICE Patients should be advised that silver nitrate may stain fabric.

- MEDICINAL FORMS
There can be variation in the licensing of different medicines containing the same drug.

Stick

▸ Silver nitrate (Non-proprietary)
Silver nitrate 400 mg per 1 gram Silver nitrate 40% caustic pencils | 1 applicator [P] no price available

▸ Avoca (Bray Group Ltd)
Silver nitrate 400 mg per 1 gram Avoca 40% silver nitrate pencils | 1 applicator [P] £1.03
Silver nitrate 750 mg per 1 gram Avoca 75% silver nitrate applicators | 100 applicator [P] £44.48

13

Skin

Avoca 75% silver nitrate applicators with thick handles |
50 applicator [P] £43.41
Silver nitrate 950 mg per 1 gram Avoca 95% silver nitrate
applicators | 100 applicator [P] £44.52
Avoca 95% silver nitrate pencils | 1 applicator [P] £1.99 DT price =
£2.44

Imiquimod

● **INDICATIONS AND DOSE**

ALDARA®

Warts (external genital and perianal)
▸ TO THE LESION
▸ Adult: Apply 3 times a week until lesions resolve
(maximum 16 weeks), to be applied thinly at night

Superficial basal cell carcinoma
▸ TO THE LESION
▸ Adult: Apply daily for 5 nights of each week for
6 weeks, to be applied to lesion and 1 cm beyond it,
assess response 12 weeks after completing treatment

Actinic keratosis
▸ TO THE LESION
▸ Adult: Apply 3 times a week for 4 weeks, to be applied
to lesion at night, assess response after a 4 week
treatment-free interval; repeat 4-week course if lesions
persist, maximum 2 courses

ZYCLARA®

Actinic keratosis
▸ TO THE SKIN
▸ Adult: Apply once daily for 2 weeks, to be applied at
bedtime to lesion on face or balding scalp, repeat
course after a 2-week treatment-free interval, assess
response 8 weeks after second course; maximum
2 sachets per day

● CAUTIONS Autoimmune disease · avoid broken skin · avoid
contact with eyes · avoid contact with lips · avoid contact
with nostrils · avoid open wounds · immunosuppressed
patients · not suitable for internal genital warts ·
uncircumcised males (risk of phimosis or stricture of
foreskin)

● SIDE-EFFECTS
▸ **Common or very common** Burning sensation · erosion ·
erythema · excoriation · headache · influenza-like
symptoms · itching · local reactions · myalgia · oedema ·
scabbing
▸ **Uncommon** Alopecia · local ulceration
▸ **Rare** Cutaneous lupus erythematosus-like effect · Stevens-
Johnson syndrome
▸ **Very rare** Dysuria
▸ **Frequency not known** Permanent hyperpigmentation ·
permanent hypopigmentation

● CONCEPTION AND CONTRACEPTION May damage latex
condoms and diaphragms.

● PREGNANCY No evidence of teratogenicity or toxicity in
animal studies; manufacturer advises caution.

● BREAST FEEDING No information available.

● DIRECTIONS FOR ADMINISTRATION
ZYCLARA® ▸ **Important** Should be rubbed in and allowed
to stay on the treated area for 8 hours, then washed off
with mild soap and water.
ALDARA® ▸ **Important** Should be rubbed in and allowed
to stay on the treated area for 6–10 hours for warts or for
8 hours for basal cell carcinoma and actinic keratosis, then
washed off with mild soap and water (uncircumcised males
treating warts under foreskin should wash the area daily).
The cream should be washed off before sexual contact.

● PATIENT AND CARER ADVICE A patient information leaflet
should be provided.

● MEDICINAL FORMS
There can be variation in the licensing of different medicines
containing the same drug.
Cream
CAUTIONARY AND ADVISORY LABELS 10
EXCIPIENTS: May contain Benzyl alcohol, cetostearyl alcohol (including
cetyl and stearyl alcohol), hydroxybenzoates (parabens), polysorbates
▸ Aldara (Meda Pharmaceuticals Ltd)
Imiquimod 50 mg per 1 gram Aldara 5% cream 250mg sachets |
12 sachet [PoM] £48.60 DT price = £48.60
▸ Zyclara (Meda Pharmaceuticals Ltd)
Imiquimod 37.5 mg per 1 gram Zyclara 3.75% cream 250mg sachets
| 28 sachet [PoM] £113.00

SALICYLIC ACID AND DERIVATIVES

Salicylic acid

● **INDICATIONS AND DOSE**

OCCLUSAL®

Common and plantar warts
▸ TO THE LESION
▸ Child: Apply daily, treatment may need to be continued
for up to 3 months
▸ Adult: Apply daily, treatment may need to be
continued for up to 3 months

VERRUGON®

For plantar warts
▸ TO THE LESION
▸ Child: Apply daily, treatment may need to be continued
for up to 3 months
▸ Adult: Apply daily, treatment may need to be
continued for up to 3 months

● UNLICENSED USE
▸ In children Not licensed for use in children under 2 years.

● CAUTIONS Avoid broken skin · impaired peripheral
circulation · not suitable for application to anogenital
region · not suitable for application to face · not suitable
for application to large areas · patients with diabetes at risk
of neuropathic ulcers · significant peripheral neuropathy

● SIDE-EFFECTS Skin irritation · skin ulceration (with high
concentrations)

● PATIENT AND CARER ADVICE Advise patient to apply
carefully to wart and to protect surrounding skin (e.g. with
soft paraffin or specially designed plaster); rub wart
surface gently with file or pumice stone once weekly.

● MEDICINAL FORMS
There can be variation in the licensing of different medicines
containing the same drug.
Liquid
CAUTIONARY AND ADVISORY LABELS 15
▸ Occlusal - brand name (Alliance Pharmaceuticals Ltd)
Salicylic acid 260 mg per 1 ml Occlusal 26% solution | 10 ml [P]
£3.56 DT price = £3.56
Ointment
▸ Verrugon (Optima Consumer Health Ltd)
Salicylic acid 500 mg per 1 gram Verrugon complete 50% ointment
| 6 gram [P] £3.12

Salicylic acid with lactic acid

The properties listed below are those particular to the combination only. For the properties of the components please consider, salicylic acid p. 1126.

● **INDICATIONS AND DOSE**

CUPLEX®

Plantar and mosaic warts | Corns | Calluses
▸ TO THE LESION
▸ Adult: Apply daily, treatment may need to be continued for up to 3 months

DUOFILM®

Plantar and mosaic warts
▸ TO THE LESION
▸ Adult: Apply daily, treatment may need to be continued for up to 3 months

SALACTOL®

Warts, particularly plantar warts | Verrucas | Corns | Calluses
▸ TO THE LESION
▸ Adult: Apply daily, treatment may need to be continued for up to 3 months

SALATAC®

Warts | Verrucas | Corns | Calluses
▸ TO THE LESION
▸ Adult: Apply daily, treatment may need to be continued for up to 3 months

● **PRESCRIBING AND DISPENSING INFORMATION**
Preparations of salicylic acid in a collodion basis (Cuplex® and Salactol®) are available but some patients may develop an allergy to colophony in the formulation.

● **MEDICINAL FORMS**
There can be variation in the licensing of different medicines containing the same drug.

Gel
CAUTIONARY AND ADVISORY LABELS 15
▸ Cuplex (Crawford Healthcare Ltd)
  Lactic acid 40 mg per 1 gram, Salicylic acid 110 mg per 1 gram Cuplex Verruca gel | 5 gram GSL £2.88 DT price = £2.88
▸ Salatac (Dermal Laboratories Ltd)
  Lactic acid 40 mg per 1 gram, Salicylic acid 120 mg per 1 gram Salatac gel | 8 gram P £2.98 DT price = £2.98

Paint
CAUTIONARY AND ADVISORY LABELS 15
▸ Duofilm (GlaxoSmithKline UK Ltd)
  Lactic acid 150 mg per 1 gram, Salicylic acid 167 mg per 1 gram Duofilm paint | 15 ml P £2.25
▸ Salactol (Dermal Laboratories Ltd)
  Lactic acid 167 mg per 1 gram, Salicylic acid 167 mg per 1 gram Salactol paint | 10 ml P £1.71 DT price = £1.71

Chapter 14
Vaccines

CONTENTS

1   Immunoglobulin therapy

IMMUNE SERA AND IMMUNOGLOBULINS >
IMMUNOGLOBULINS

Immunoglobulins

Passive immunity

Immunity with immediate protection against certain infective organisms can be obtained by injecting preparations made from the plasma of immune individuals with adequate levels of antibody to the disease for which protection is sought. The duration of this passive immunity varies according to the dose and the type of immunoglobulin. Passive immunity may last only a few weeks; when necessary, passive immunisation can be repeated. Antibodies of human origin are usually termed immunoglobulins. The term antiserum is applied to material prepared in animals. Because of serum sickness and other allergic-type reactions that may follow injections of antisera, this therapy has been replaced wherever possible by the use of immunoglobulins. Reactions are theoretically possible after injection of human immunoglobulins but reports of such reactions are very rare.

Two types of human immunoglobulin preparation are available, normal immunoglobulin p. 1131 and **disease-specific immunoglobulins**.

Human immunoglobulin is a sterile preparation of concentrated antibodies (immune globulins) recovered from pooled human plasma or serum obtained from outside the UK, tested and found non-reactive for hepatitis B surface antigen and for antibodies against hepatitis C virus and human immunodeficiency virus (types 1 and 2). A global shortage of human immunoglobulin and the rapidly increasing range of clinical indications for treatment with immunoglobulins has resulted in the need for a Demand Management programme in the UK, for further information consult www.ivig.nhs.uk and *Clinical Guidelines for Immunoglobulin Use*, www.gov.uk/dh.

Further information on the use of immunoglobulins is included in Public Health England's *Immunoglobulin Handbook* www.gov.uk/phe, and in the Department of Health's publication, *Immunisation against Infectious Disease*, www.gov.uk/dh.

Availability

Normal immunoglobulin for intramuscular administration is available from some regional Public Health laboratories for protection of contacts and the control of outbreaks of hepatitis A, measles, and rubella only. For other indications, subcutaneous or intravenous normal immunoglobulin should be purchased from the manufacturer.

Disease-specific immunoglobulins are available from some regional Public Health laboratories, with the exception of tetanus immunoglobulin p. 1133 which is available from

BPL, hospital pharmacies, or blood transfusion departments. Rabies immunoglobulin p. 1133 is available from the Specialist and Reference Microbiology Division, Public Health England, Colindale. Hepatitis B immunoglobulin p. 1131 required by transplant centres should be obtained commercially.

In Scotland all immunoglobulins are available from the *Scottish National Blood Transfusion Service* (SNBTS).

In Wales all immunoglobulins are available from the *Welsh Blood Service* (WBS).

In Northern Ireland all immunoglobulins are available from the *Northern Ireland Blood Transfusion Service* (NIBTS).

Normal immunoglobulin

Human normal immunoglobulin ('HNIG') is prepared from pools of at least 1000 donations of human plasma; it contains immunoglobulin G (IgG) and antibodies to hepatitis A, measles, mumps, rubella, varicella, and other viruses that are currently prevalent in the general population.

Uses

Normal immunoglobulin (containing 10%–18% protein) is administered by *intramuscular injection* for the protection of susceptible contacts against **hepatitis A** virus (infectious hepatitis), **measles** and, to a lesser extent, **rubella**. Injection of immunoglobulin produces immediate protection lasting several weeks.

Normal immunoglobulin (containing 3%–12% protein) for *intravenous administration* is used as *replacement therapy* for patients with congenital agammaglobulinaemia and hypogammaglobulinaemia, and for the short-term treatment of idiopathic thrombocytopenic purpura and Kawasaki disease; it is also used for the prophylaxis of infection following bone-marrow transplantation and in children with symptomatic HIV infection who have recurrent bacterial infections. Normal immunoglobulin for replacement therapy may also be given intramuscularly or subcutaneously, but intravenous formulations are normally preferred. Intravenous immunoglobulin is also used in the treatment of Guillain-Barré syndrome as an alternative to plasma exchange.

For guidance on the use of intravenous normal immunoglobulin and alternative therapies for certain conditions, consult *Clinical Guidelines for Immunoglobulin Use* (www.gov.uk/dh).

Hepatitis A

Hepatitis A vaccine p. 1154 is preferred for individuals at risk of infection including those visiting areas where the disease is highly endemic (all countries excluding Northern and Western Europe,North America, Japan, Australia, and New Zealand). In unimmunised individuals, transmission of hepatitis A is reduced by good hygiene. Intramuscular normal immunoglobulin is no longer recommended for routine prophylaxis in travellers, but it may be indicated for immunocompromised patients if their antibody response to the vaccine is unlikely to be adequate.

Intramuscular normal immunoglobulin is recommended for prevention of infection in close contacts (of confirmed cases of hepatitis A) who have chronic liver disease or HIV infection, or who are immunosuppressed or over 50 years of age; normal immunoglobulin should be given as soon as possible, preferably within 14 days of exposure to the primary case. However, normal immunoglobulin can still be given to contacts at risk of severe disease up to 28 days after exposure to the primary case. Hepatitis A vaccine can be given at the same time, but it should be given at a separate injection site.

Measles

Intravenous or subcutaneous normal immunoglobulin may be given to prevent or attenuate an attack of measles in individuals who do not have adequate immunity. Patients with compromised immunity who have come into contact with measles should receive intravenous or subcutaneous normal immunoglobulin as soon as possible after exposure. It is most effective if given within 72 hours but can be effective if given within 6 days.

Subcutaneous or intramuscular normal immunoglobulin should also be considered for the following individuals if they have been in contact with a confirmed case of measles or with a person associated with a local outbreak:

- non-immune pregnant women
- infants under 9 months

Further advice should be sought from the Centre for Infections, Public Health England (tel. (020) 8200 6868).

Individuals with normal immunity who are not in the above categories and who have not been fully immunised against measles, can be given measles, mumps and rubella vaccine, live p. 1159 for prophylaxis following exposure to measles.

Rubella

Intramuscular immunoglobulin after exposure to rubella does **not** prevent infection in non-immune contacts and is **not** recommended for protection of pregnant women exposed to rubella. It may, however, reduce the likelihood of a clinical attack which may possibly reduce the risk to the fetus. Risk of intra-uterine transmission is greatest in the first 11 weeks of pregnancy, between 16 and 20 weeks there is minimal risk of deafness only, after 20 weeks there is no increased risk. Intramuscular normal immunoglobulin should be used only if termination of pregnancy would be unacceptable to the pregnant woman—it should be given as soon as possible after exposure. Serological follow-up of recipients is essential to determine if the woman has become infected despite receiving immunoglobulin.

For routine prophylaxis against Rubella, see measles, mumps and rubella vaccine, live p. 1159.

Disease-specific immunoglobulins

Specific immunoglobulins are prepared by pooling the plasma of selected human donors with high levels of the specific antibody required. For further information, see *Immunoglobulin Handbook* (www.gov.uk/phe).

There are no specific immunoglobulins for hepatitis A, measles, or rubella—normal immunoglobulin p. 1131 is used in certain circumstances. There is no specific immunoglobulin for mumps; neither normal immunoglobulin nor measles, mumps and rubella vaccine, live is effective as post-exposure prophylaxis.

Hepatitis B immunoglobulin

Disease-specific hepatitis B immunoglobulin ('HBIG') p. 1131 is available for use in association with hepatitis B vaccine p. 1155 for the prevention of infection in laboratory and other personnel who have been accidentally inoculated with hepatitis B virus, and in infants born to mothers who have become infected with this virus in pregnancy or who are high-risk carriers. Hepatitis B immunoglobulin will not inhibit the antibody response when given at the same time as hepatitis B vaccine but should be given at different sites.

An intravenous and subcutaneous preparation of hepatitis B immunoglobulin is licensed for the prevention of hepatitis B recurrence in HBV-DNA negative patients who have undergone liver transplantation for liver failure caused by the virus.

Rabies immunoglobulin

Following exposure of an unimmunised individual to an animal in or from a country where the risk of rabies is high the site of the bite should be washed with soapy water and specific rabies immunoglobulin p. 1133 of human origin administered. All of the dose should be injected around the site of the wound; if this is difficult or the wound has completely healed it can be given in the anterolateral thigh (remote from the site used for vaccination).

Rabies vaccine p. 1160 should also be given intramuscularly at a different site (for details see rabies vaccine). If there is delay in giving the rabies immunoglobulin, it should be given within 7 days of starting the course of rabies vaccine.

Tetanus immunoglobulin

For the management of tetanus-prone wounds, tetanus immunoglobulin p. 1133 should be used in addition to wound cleansing and, where appropriate, antibacterial prophylaxis and a tetanus-containing vaccine. Tetanus immunoglobulin, together with metronidazole p. 492 and wound cleansing, should also be used for the treatment of established cases of tetanus.

Varicella–zoster immunoglobulin

Varicella-zoster immunoglobulin (VZIG) p. 1134 is recommended for individuals who are at increased risk of severe varicella *and* who have no antibodies to varicella–zoster virus *and* who have significant exposure to chickenpox or herpes zoster. Those at increased risk include:

- neonates whose mothers develop chickenpox in the period 7 days before to 7 days after delivery;
- susceptible neonates exposed in the first 7 days of life;
- susceptible neonates or infants exposed whilst requiring intensive or prolonged special care nursing;
- susceptible women exposed at any stage of pregnancy (but when supplies of VZIG are short, may only be issued to those exposed in the first 20 weeks' gestation or to those near term) providing VZIG is given within 10 days of contact;
- immunocompromised individuals including those who have received corticosteroids in the previous 3 months at the following dose equivalents of prednisolone: *children* 2 mg/kg daily for at least 1 week or 1 mg/kg daily for 1 month; *adults* about 40 mg daily for more than 1 week.

Important: for full details consult *Immunisation against Infectious Disease*. Varicella-zoster vaccine p. 1161 is available.

Anti-D (Rh$_0$) immunoglobulin

Anti-D (Rh$_0$) immunoglobulin p. 1130 is prepared from plasma taken from rhesus-negative donors who have been immunised against the anti-D-antigen. Anti-D (Rh$_0$) immunoglobulin is used to prevent a rhesus-negative mother from forming antibodies to fetal rhesus-positive cells which may pass into the maternal circulation. The objective is to protect any subsequent child from the hazard of haemolytic disease of the newborn.

Anti-D (Rh$_0$) immunoglobulin should be administered to the mother following any sensitising episode (e.g. abortion, miscarriage and birth); it should be injected within 72 hours of the episode but even if a longer period has elapsed it may still give protection and should be administered. Anti-D (Rh$_0$) immunoglobulin is also given when significant feto-maternal haemorrhage occurs in rhesus-negative women during delivery. The dose of anti-D (Rh$_0$) immunoglobulin is

14

Vaccines

determined according to the level of exposure to rhesus-positive blood.

Use of routine *antenatal* anti-D prophylaxis should be given irrespective of previous anti-D prophylaxis for a sensitising event early in the same pregnancy. Similarly, *postpartum* anti-D prophylaxis should be given irrespective of previous routine antenatal anti-D prophylaxis or antenatal anti-D prophylaxis for a sensitising event in the same pregnancy.

Anti-D (Rh_0) immunoglobulin is also given to women of child-bearing potential after the inadvertent transfusion of rhesus-incompatible blood components and is used for the treatment of idiopathic thrombocytopenia purpura.

MMR vaccine
Measles, mumps and rubella vaccine, live may be given in the postpartum period with anti-D (Rh_0) immunoglobulin injection provided that separate syringes are used and the products are administered into different limbs. If blood is transfused, the antibody response to the vaccine may be inhibited—measure rubella antibodies after 6–8 weeks and revaccinate if necessary.

Anti-D (Rh_0) immunoglobulin

- ● INDICATIONS AND DOSE
To rhesus-negative woman for prevention of Rh_0(D) sensitisation, following birth of rhesus-positive infant
▸ BY DEEP INTRAMUSCULAR INJECTION
▹ Females of childbearing potential: 500 units, dose to be administered immediately or within 72 hours; for transplacental bleed of over 4 mL fetal red cells, extra 100–125 units per mL fetal red cells, subcutaneous route used for patients with bleeding disorders

To rhesus-negative woman for prevention of Rh_0(D) sensitisation, following any potentially sensitising episode (e.g. stillbirth, abortion, amniocentesis) up to 20 weeks' gestation
▸ BY DEEP INTRAMUSCULAR INJECTION
▹ Females of childbearing potential: 250 units per episode, dose to be administered immediately or within 72 hours, subcutaneous route used for patients with bleeding disorders

To rhesus-negative woman for prevention of Rh_0(D) sensitisation, following any potentially sensitising episode (e.g. stillbirth, abortion, amniocentesis) after 20 weeks' gestation
▸ BY DEEP INTRAMUSCULAR INJECTION
▹ Females of childbearing potential: 500 units per episode, dose to be administered immediately or within 72 hours, subcutaneous route used for patients with bleeding disorders

To rhesus-negative woman for prevention of Rh_0(D) sensitisation, antenatal prophylaxis
▸ BY DEEP INTRAMUSCULAR INJECTION
▹ Females of childbearing potential: 500 units, dose to be given at weeks 28 and 34 of pregnancy, if infant rhesus-positive, a further dose is still needed immediately or within 72 hours of delivery, subcutaneous route used for patients with bleeding disorders

To rhesus-negative woman for prevention of Rh_0(D) sensitisation, antenatal prophylaxis (alternative NICE recommendation)
▸ BY DEEP INTRAMUSCULAR INJECTION
▹ Females of childbearing potential: 1000–1650 units, dose to be given at weeks 28 and 34 of pregnancy, alternatively 1500 units for 1 dose, dose to be given between 28 and 30 weeks gestation

To rhesus-negative woman for prevention of Rh_0(D) sensitisation, following Rh_0(D) incompatible blood transfusion
▸ BY DEEP INTRAMUSCULAR INJECTION
▹ Females of childbearing potential: 100–125 units per mL of transfused rhesus-positive red cells, subcutaneous route used for patients with bleeding disorders

RHOPHYLAC®
To rhesus-negative woman for prevention of Rh_0(D) sensitisation, following birth of rhesus-positive infant
▸ BY INTRAMUSCULAR INJECTION, OR BY INTRAVENOUS INJECTION
▹ Females of childbearing potential: 1000–1500 units, dose to administered immediately or within 72 hours; for large transplacental bleed, extra 100 units per mL fetal red cells (preferably by intravenous injection), intravenous route recommended for patients with bleeding disorders

To rhesus-negative woman for prevention of Rh_0(D) sensitisation, following any potentially sensitising episode (e.g. abortion, amniocentesis, chorionic villous sampling) up to 12 weeks' gestation
▸ BY INTRAMUSCULAR INJECTION, OR BY INTRAVENOUS INJECTION
▹ Females of childbearing potential: 1000 units per episode, dose to be administered immediately or within 72 hours, intravenous route recommended for patients with bleeding disorders, higher doses may be required after 12 weeks gestation

To rhesus-negative woman for prevention of Rh_0(D) sensitisation, antenatal prophylaxis
▸ BY INTRAMUSCULAR INJECTION, OR BY INTRAVENOUS INJECTION
▹ Females of childbearing potential: 1500 units, dose to be given between weeks 28–30 of pregnancy; if infant rhesus-positive, a further dose is still needed immediately or within 72 hours of delivery, intravenous route recommended for patients with bleeding disorders

To rhesus-negative woman for prevention of Rh_0(D) sensitisation, following Rh_0(D) incompatible blood transfusion
▸ BY INTRAVENOUS INJECTION
▹ Females of childbearing potential: 50 units per mL of transfused rhesus-positive blood, alternatively 100 units per of mL of erythrocyte concentrate, intravenous route recommended for patients with bleeding disorders

- ● CONTRA-INDICATIONS Treatment of idiopathic thrombocytopenia purpura in rhesus negative patients · treatment of idiopathic thrombocytopenia purpura in splenectomised patients
- ● CAUTIONS Immunoglobulin A deficiency · possible interference with live virus vaccines
CAUTIONS, FURTHER INFORMATION
MMR vaccine may be given in the postpartum period with anti-D (Rh_0) immunoglobulin injection provided that separate syringes are used and the products are administered into different limbs. If blood is transfused, the antibody response to the vaccine may be inhibited—measure rubella antibodies after 6–8 weeks and revaccinate if necessary.
- ● INTERACTIONS → Appendix 1 (immunoglobulins).
- ● SIDE-EFFECTS
GENERAL SIDE-EFFECTS
▸ Rare Anaphylaxis · dyspnoea · hypotension · tachycardia · urticaria
▸ Frequency not known Abdominal pain · arthralgia · asthenia · back pain · diarrhoea · dizziness · drowsiness · fever ·

14

Vaccines

headache · hypertension · hypotension · injection site pain · malaise · myalgia · nausea · pruritus · rash · sweating · vomiting

SPECIFIC SIDE-EFFECTS
▸ With intravenous use Abdominal distension · blood pressure fluctuations · deep vein thrombosis · haemolytic anaemia · injection site reactions · myocardial infarction · pulmonary embolism · stroke · thromboembolic events

● HANDLING AND STORAGE Care must be taken to store all immunological products under the conditions recommended in the product literature, otherwise the preparation may become ineffective. **Refrigerated storage** is usually necessary; many immunoglobulins need to be stored at 2–8°C and not allowed to freeze. Immunoglobulins should be protected from light. Opened multidose vials must be used within the period recommended in the product literature.

● NATIONAL FUNDING/ACCESS DECISIONS
NICE technology appraisals (TAs)
▸ Routine antenatal anti-D prophylaxis for rhesus-negative women (August 2008) NICE TA156
Routine antenatal anti-D prophylaxis should be offered to all non-sensitised pregnant women who are rhesus negative.
www.nice.org.uk/TA156

● MEDICINAL FORMS
There can be variation in the licensing of different medicines containing the same drug.
Solution for injection
▸ D-Gam (Bio Products Laboratory Ltd)
Anti-D (RHO) immunoglobulin 250 unit D-Gam Anti-D immunoglobulin 250unit solution for injection vials | 1 vial [PoM] £23.75
Anti-D (RHO) immunoglobulin 500 unit D-Gam Anti-D immunoglobulin 500unit solution for injection vials | 1 vial [PoM] £33.75
Anti-D (RHO) immunoglobulin 1500 unit D-Gam Anti-D immunoglobulin 1,500unit solution for injection vials | 1 vial [PoM] £58.00
▸ Rhophylac (CSL Behring UK Ltd)
Anti-D (RHO) immunoglobulin 750 unit per 1 ml Rhophylac 1,500units/2ml solution for injection pre-filled syringes | 1 pre-filled disposable injection [PoM] £39.52

Hepatitis B immunoglobulin

● INDICATIONS AND DOSE
Prophylaxis against hepatitis B infection
▸ BY INTRAMUSCULAR INJECTION
▸ Adult: 500 units, dose to be administered as soon as possible after exposure; ideally within 12–48 hours, but no later than 7 days after exposure

Prophylaxis against hepatitis B infection, after exposure to hepatitis B virus-contaminated material
▸ BY INTRAVENOUS INFUSION
▸ Adult: Dose to be administered as soon as possible after exposure, but no later than 72 hours (consult product literature)

Prevention of hepatitis B in haemodialysed patients
▸ BY INTRAVENOUS INFUSION
▸ Adult: (consult product literature)

Prophylaxis against re-infection of transplanted liver
▸ BY INTRAVENOUS INFUSION
▸ Adult: (consult product literature)

Prevention of hepatitis B re-infection more than 6 months after liver transplantation in stable HBV-DNA negative patients
▸ BY SUBCUTANEOUS INJECTION
▸ Adult (body-weight up to 75 kg): 500 units once weekly, increased if necessary up to 1000 units once weekly,

dose to be started 2–3 weeks after last dose of intravenous hepatitis B immunoglobulin
▸ Adult (body-weight 75 kg and above): 1000 units once weekly, dose to be started 2–3 weeks after last dose of intravenous hepatitis B immunoglobulin

● CAUTIONS IgA deficiency · interference with live virus vaccines

● SIDE-EFFECTS
GENERAL SIDE-EFFECTS
▸ **Common or very common** Injection site reactions
▸ **Uncommon** Abdominal pain · anaphylaxis · arthralgia · buccal ulceration · chest pain · dizziness · dyspnoea · glossitis · headache · tremor

SPECIFIC SIDE-EFFECTS
▸ With intravenous use Abdominal distension · blood pressure fluctuations · deep vein thrombosis · haemolytic anaemia · injection site reactions · myocardial infarction · pulmonary embolism · stroke · thromboembolic events

● PRESCRIBING AND DISPENSING INFORMATION Vials containing 200 units or 500 units (for intramuscular injection), available from selected Public Health England and NHS laboratories (except for Transplant Centres), also available from BPL.

● HANDLING AND STORAGE Care must be taken to store all immunological products under the conditions recommended in the product literature, otherwise the preparation may become ineffective. **Refrigerated storage** is usually necessary; many immunoglobulins need to be stored at 2–8°C and not allowed to freeze. Immunoglobulins should be protected from light. Opened multidose vials must be used within the period recommended in the product literature.

● MEDICINAL FORMS
There can be variation in the licensing of different medicines containing the same drug.
Solution for injection
▸ Hepatitis B immunoglobulin (Non-proprietary)
Hepatitis B immunoglobulin human 200 unit Hepatitis B immunoglobulin human 200unit solution for injection vials | 1 vial [PoM] £122.44
Hepatitis B immunoglobulin human 500 unit Hepatitis B immunoglobulin human 500unit solution for injection vials | 1 vial [PoM] £266.33
▸ Zutectra (Biotest (UK) Ltd)
Zutectra 500units/1ml solution for injection pre-filled syringes | 5 syringe [PoM] £1,275.00
Solution for infusion
▸ Hepatect CP (Biotest (UK) Ltd)
Hepatitis B immunoglobulin human 50 unit per 1 ml Hepatect CP 100units/2ml solution for infusion vials | 1 vial [PoM] £51.00
Hepatect CP 2000units/40ml solution for infusion vials | 1 vial [PoM] £935.00
Hepatect CP 500units/10ml solution for infusion vials | 1 vial [PoM] £255.00
Hepatect CP 5000units/100ml solution for infusion vials | 1 vial [PoM] £2,550.00
▸ Omri-Hep-B (Imported (Israel))
Hepatitis B immunoglobulin human 50 unit per 1 ml Omri-Hep-B 5000units/100ml solution for infusion vials | 1 vial [PoM] no price available

Normal immunoglobulin

● INDICATIONS AND DOSE
To control outbreaks of hepatitis A
▸ BY DEEP INTRAMUSCULAR INJECTION
▸ Adult: 500 mg

Rubella in pregnancy, prevention of clinical attack
▸ BY DEEP INTRAMUSCULAR INJECTION
▸ Females of childbearing potential: 750 mg   continued →

14

Vaccines

Antibody deficiency syndromes
▸ BY SUBCUTANEOUS INFUSION
▸ Adult: (consult product literature)
SUBGAM®

Hepatitis A prophylaxis in outbreaks
▸ BY INTRAMUSCULAR INJECTION
▸ Adult: 750 mg

● UNLICENSED USE
SUBGAM® *Subgam®* is not licensed for prophylactic use, but due to difficulty in obtaining suitable immunoglobulin products, Public Health England recommends intramuscular use for prophylaxis against Hepatitis A or rubella.

● CONTRA-INDICATIONS Patients with selective IgA deficiency who have known antibody against IgA
PRIVIGEN® Hyperprolinaemia (contains -proline)
GAMMAPLEX® Hereditary fructose intolerance (contains sorbitol)
HIZENTRA® Hyperprolinaemia (contains -proline)
FLEBOGAMMA® DIF Hereditary fructose intolerance (contains sorbitol)

● CAUTIONS Agammaglobulinaemia with or without IgA deficiency · hypogammaglobulinaemia with or without IgA deficiency · interference with live virus vaccines
CAUTIONS, FURTHER INFORMATION
▸ Interference with live virus vaccines Normal immunoglobulin may **interfere with the immune response to live virus vaccines** which should therefore only be given **at least 3 weeks before or 3 months after** an injection of normal immunoglobulin (this does not apply to yellow fever vaccine since normal immunoglobulin does not contain antibody to this virus).
OCTAGAM® Falsely elevated results with blood glucose testing systems (contains maltose)

● INTERACTIONS → Appendix 1 (immunoglobulins).

● SIDE-EFFECTS
▸ Rare Acute renal failure · anaphylaxis · aseptic meningitis · cutaneous skin reactions · hypotension
▸ Frequency not known Arthralgia · chills · diarrhoea · dizziness · fever · headache · low back pain · muscle spasms · myalgia · nausea
SIDE-EFFECTS, FURTHER INFORMATION
Adverse reactions are more likely to occur in patients receiving normal immunoglobulin for the first time, or following a prolonged period between treatments, or when a different brand of normal immunoglobulin is administered.

● MONITORING REQUIREMENTS Monitor for acute renal failure; consider discontinuation if renal function deteriorates. Intravenous preparations with added sucrose have been associated with cases of renal dysfunction and acute renal failure.

● DIRECTIONS FOR ADMINISTRATION
Preparations for subcutaneous use May be administered by intramuscular injection if subcutaneous route not possible; intramuscular route **not** for patients with thrombocytopenia or other bleeding disorders.
GAMUNEX® Use Glucose 5% intravenous infusion if dilution prior to infusion is required.
KIOVIG® Use Glucose 5% intravenous infusion if dilution prior to infusion is required.

● PRESCRIBING AND DISPENSING INFORMATION Antibody titres can vary widely between normal immunoglobulin preparations from different manufacturers—formulations are **not interchangeable**; patients should be maintained on the same formulation throughout long-term treatment to avoid adverse effects.

▸ With intramuscular use Available from the Centre for Infections and other regional Public Health England offices (for contacts and control of outbreaks only).

● HANDLING AND STORAGE Care must be taken to store all immunological products under the conditions recommended in the product literature, otherwise the preparation may become ineffective. **Refrigerated storage** is usually necessary; many immunoglobulins need to be stored at 2–8°C and not allowed to freeze. Immunoglobulins should be protected from light. Opened multidose vials must be used within the period recommended in the product literature.

● MEDICINAL FORMS
There can be variation in the licensing of different medicines containing the same drug.

Solution for injection
ELECTROLYTES: May contain Sodium
▸ Gammanorm (Octapharma Ltd)
Normal immunoglobulin human 165 mg per 1 ml Gammanorm 8g/48ml solution for injection vials | 1 vial [PoM] £469.20
Gammanorm 2g/12ml solution for injection vials | 1 vial [PoM] £117.30
Gammanorm 4g/24ml solution for injection vials | 1 vial [PoM] £234.60
Gammanorm 1.65g/10ml solution for injection vials | 1 vial [PoM] £96.77 | 10 vial [PoM] no price available (Hospital only)
Gammanorm 3.3g/20ml solution for injection vials | 1 vial [PoM] £193.55 | 10 vial [PoM] no price available (Hospital only)
Gammanorm 1g/6ml solution for injection vials | 1 vial [PoM] £58.65
▸ Subcuvia (Baxalta UK Ltd)
Normal immunoglobulin human 160 mg per 1 ml Subcuvia 800mg/5ml solution for injection vials | 1 vial [PoM] no price available
Subcuvia 1.6g/10ml solution for injection vials | 1 vial [PoM] no price available
▸ Subgam (Bio Products Laboratory Ltd)
Normal immunoglobulin human 150 mg per 1 ml Subgam 750mg/5ml solution for injection vials | 1 vial [PoM] £34.20
Subgam 1.5g/10ml solution for injection vials | 1 vial [PoM] £68.40

Powder and solvent for solution for injection
▸ Gammagard S/D (Baxalta UK Ltd)
Normal immunoglobulin human 500 mg Gammagard S/D 500mg powder and solvent for solution for injection bottles | 1 bottle [PoM] no price available
Normal immunoglobulin human 2.5 gram Gammagard S/D 2.5g powder and solvent for solution for injection bottles | 1 bottle [PoM] no price available
Normal immunoglobulin human 5 gram Gammagard S/D 5g powder and solvent for solution for injection bottles | 1 bottle [PoM] no price available
Normal immunoglobulin human 10 gram Gammagard S/D 10g powder and solvent for solution for injection bottles | 1 bottle [PoM] no price available

Solution for infusion
EXCIPIENTS: May contain Glucose, maltose, sorbitol, sucrose
▸ Normal immunoglobulin (Non-proprietary)
Normal immunoglobulin human 100 mg per 1 ml Normal immunoglobulin human 5g/50ml solution for infusion vials | 1 vial [PoM] no price available
Normal immunoglobulin human 2.5g/25ml solution for infusion vials | 1 vial [PoM] no price available
Normal immunoglobulin human 20g/200ml solution for infusion vials | 1 vial [PoM] no price available
Normal immunoglobulin human 10g/100ml solution for infusion vials | 1 vial [PoM] no price available
Normal immunoglobulin human 30g/300ml solution for infusion vials | 1 vial [PoM] no price available
▸ Aragam (Oxbridge Pharma Ltd)
Normal immunoglobulin human 50 mg per 1 ml Aragam 5g/100ml solution for infusion vials | 1 vial [PoM] no price available
Aragam 2.5g/50ml solution for infusion vials | 1 vial [PoM] no price available
▸ Flebogammadif (Grifols UK Ltd)
Normal immunoglobulin human 50 mg per 1 ml Flebogamma DIF 10g/200ml solution for infusion vials | 1 vial [PoM] £510.00
Flebogamma DIF 2.5g/50ml solution for infusion vials | 1 vial [PoM] £127.50

Flebogamma DIF 5g/100ml solution for infusion vials | 1 vial [PoM]
£255.00
Flebogamma DIF 500mg/10ml solution for infusion vials | 1 vial [PoM]
£30.00
Flebogamma DIF 20g/400ml solution for infusion vials | 1 vial [PoM]
£1,020.00
Normal immunoglobulin human 100 mg per 1 ml Flebogamma DIF
10g/100ml solution for infusion vials | 1 vial [PoM] £510.00
Flebogamma DIF 20g/200ml solution for infusion vials | 1 vial [PoM]
£1,020.00
Flebogamma DIF 5g/50ml solution for infusion vials | 1 vial [PoM]
£255.00

▸ Gammaplex (Bio Products Laboratory Ltd)
Normal immunoglobulin human 50 mg per 1 ml Gammaplex
10g/200ml solution for infusion vials | 1 vial [PoM] £418.00 (Hospital
only)
Gammaplex 5g/100ml solution for infusion vials | 1 vial [PoM]
£209.00 (Hospital only)
Gammaplex 20g/400ml solution for infusion vials | 1 vial [PoM]
£660.00 (Hospital only)
Gammaplex 2.5g/50ml solution for infusion vials | 1 vial [PoM]
£104.50 (Hospital only)

▸ Gamunex (Grifols UK Ltd)
Normal immunoglobulin human 100 mg per 1 ml Gamunex 10%
1g/10ml solution for infusion vials | 1 vial [PoM] £42.50
Gamunex 10% 10g/100ml solution for infusion vials | 1 vial [PoM]
£425.00
Gamunex 10% 20g/200ml solution for infusion vials | 1 vial [PoM]
£850.00
Gamunex 10% 5g/50ml solution for infusion vials | 1 vial [PoM]
£212.50

▸ Hizentra (CSL Behring UK Ltd)
Normal immunoglobulin human 200 mg per 1 ml Hizentra
2g/10ml solution for infusion vials | 1 vial [PoM] £91.80
Hizentra 1g/5ml solution for infusion vials | 1 vial [PoM] £45.90
Hizentra 4g/20ml solution for infusion vials | 1 vial [PoM] £183.60

▸ Intratect (Biotest (UK) Ltd)
Normal immunoglobulin human 50 mg per 1 ml Intratect
5g/100ml solution for infusion vials | 1 vial [PoM] £191.25
Intratect 1g/20ml solution for infusion vials | 1 vial [PoM] £38.25
Intratect 2.5g/50ml solution for infusion vials | 1 vial [PoM] £95.63
Intratect 10g/200ml solution for infusion vials | 1 vial [PoM] £382.50
Normal immunoglobulin human 100 mg per 1 ml Intratect
10g/100ml solution for infusion vials | 1 vial [PoM] £382.50
Intratect 20g/200ml solution for infusion vials | 1 vial [PoM] £765.00
Intratect 5g/50ml solution for infusion vials | 1 vial [PoM] £191.25
Intratect 1g/10ml solution for infusion vials | 1 vial [PoM] £38.25

▸ Kiovig (Baxalta UK Ltd)
Normal immunoglobulin human 100 mg per 1 ml Kiovig 5g/50ml
solution for infusion vials | 1 vial [PoM] no price available
Kiovig 20g/200ml solution for infusion vials | 1 vial [PoM] no price
available
Kiovig 10g/100ml solution for infusion vials | 1 vial [PoM] no price
available
Kiovig 2.5g/25ml solution for infusion vials | 1 vial [PoM] no price
available
Kiovig 1g/10ml solution for infusion vials | 1 vial [PoM] no price
available

▸ Octagam (Octapharma Ltd)
Normal immunoglobulin human 50 mg per 1 ml Octagam 5%
10g/200ml solution for infusion bottles | 1 bottle [PoM] £408.00
(Hospital only)
Octagam 5% 5g/200ml solution for infusion bottles | 1 bottle [PoM]
£204.00 (Hospital only)
Octagam 5% 2.5g/50ml solution for infusion bottles | 1 bottle [PoM]
£102.00 (Hospital only)
Normal immunoglobulin human 100 mg per 1 ml Octagam 10%
20g/200ml solution for infusion bottles | 1 bottle [PoM] £1,173.00
(Hospital only)
Octagam 10% 5g/50ml solution for infusion bottles | 1 bottle [PoM]
£293.25 (Hospital only)
Octagam 10% 10g/100ml solution for infusion bottles | 1 bottle [PoM]
£586.50 (Hospital only)
Octagam 10% 2g/20ml solution for infusion bottles | 1 bottle [PoM]
£117.30 (Hospital only)

▸ Privigen (CSL Behring UK Ltd)
Normal immunoglobulin human 100 mg per 1 ml Privigen
5g/50ml solution for infusion vials | 1 vial [PoM] £229.50
Privigen 10g/100ml solution for infusion vials | 1 vial [PoM] £459.00
Privigen 20g/200ml solution for infusion vials | 1 vial [PoM] £918.00
Privigen 2.5g/25ml solution for infusion vials | 1 vial [PoM] £114.75

▸ Vigam (Bio Products Laboratory Ltd)
Normal immunoglobulin human 50 mg per 1 ml Vigam Liquid
5g/100ml solution for infusion vials | 1 vial [PoM] £209.00
Vigam Liquid 10g/200ml solution for infusion vials | 1 vial [PoM]
£418.00

Rabies immunoglobulin

● INDICATIONS AND DOSE

Post-exposure prophylaxis against rabies infection

▸ BY LOCAL INFILTRATION, OR BY INTRAMUSCULAR INJECTION

▸ Child: 20 units/kg, dose administered by infiltration in
and around the cleansed wound; if the wound not
visible or healed or if infiltration of whole volume not
possible, give remainder by intramuscular injection
into anterolateral thigh (remote from vaccination site)

▸ Adult: 20 units/kg, dose administered by infiltration in
and around the cleansed wound; if the wound not
visible or healed or if infiltration of whole volume not
possible, give remainder by intramuscular injection
into anterolateral thigh (remote from vaccination site)

● CAUTIONS IgA deficiency · interference with live virus
vaccines

● SIDE-EFFECTS

▸ Rare Anaphylaxis · arthralgia · buccal ulceration · chest
tightness · dizziness · dyspnoea · glossitis · tremor

▸ Frequency not known Facial oedema · injection site pain ·
injection site swelling

● PRESCRIBING AND DISPENSING INFORMATION The potency
of individual batches of rabies immunoglobulin from the
manufacturer may vary; potency may also be described
differently by different manufacturers. It is therefore
critical to know the potency of the batch to be used and
the weight of the patient in order to calculate the specific
volume required to provide the necessary dose.
Available from Specialist and Reference Microbiology
Division, Public Health England (also from BPL).

● HANDLING AND STORAGE Care must be taken to store all
immunological products under the conditions
recommended in the product literature, otherwise the
preparation may become ineffective. **Refrigerated
storage** is usually necessary; many immunoglobulins need
to be stored at 2–8°C and not allowed to freeze.
Immunoglobulins should be protected from light. Opened
multidose vials must be used within the period
recommended in the product literature.

● MEDICINAL FORMS
There can be variation in the licensing of different medicines
containing the same drug.
Solution for injection
▸ Rabies immunoglobulin (Non-proprietary)
Rabies immunoglobulin human 500 unit Rabies immunoglobulin
human 500unit solution for injection vials | 1 vial [PoM] £412.13

Tetanus immunoglobulin

● INDICATIONS AND DOSE

Post-exposure prophylaxis

▸ BY INTRAMUSCULAR INJECTION

▸ Child: Initially 250 units, then increased to 500 units,
dose is only increased if more than 24 hours have
elapsed or there is risk of heavy contamination or
following burns

▸ Adult: Initially 250 units, then increased to 500 units,
dose is only increased if more than 24 hours have
elapsed or there is risk of heavy contamination or
following burns

continued →

14

Vaccines

Treatment of tetanus infection

▶ BY INTRAMUSCULAR INJECTION

▸ **Child:** 150 units/kg, dose may be given over multiple sites

▸ **Adult:** 150 units/kg, dose may be given over multiple sites

● CAUTIONS IgA deficiency · interference with live virus vaccines

● SIDE-EFFECTS

▶ **Rare** Anaphylaxis · arthralgia (in children) · buccal ulceration (in children) · chest tightness (in children) · dizziness (in children) · dyspnoea (in children) · glossitis (in children) · tremor (in children)

▶ **Frequency not known** Facial oedema (in children) · injection site swelling · pain at injection site

● HANDLING AND STORAGE Care must be taken to store all immunological products under the conditions recommended in the product literature, otherwise the preparation may become ineffective. **Refrigerated storage** is usually necessary; many immunoglobulins need to be stored at 2–8°C and not allowed to freeze. Immunoglobulins should be protected from light. Opened multidose vials must be used within the period recommended in the product literature.

● MEDICINAL FORMS
There can be variation in the licensing of different medicines containing the same drug.
Solution for injection
▸ Tetanus immunoglobulin (Non-proprietary)
   Tetanus immunoglobulin human 250 unit Tetanus immunoglobulin human 250unit solution for injection vials | 1 vial [PoM] £45.00

Varicella-zoster immunoglobulin

(Antivaricella-zoster Immunoglobulin)

● INDICATIONS AND DOSE

Prophylaxis against varicella infection

▶ BY DEEP INTRAMUSCULAR INJECTION

▸ **Adult:** 1 g, to be administered as soon as possible—not later than 10 days after exposure, second dose to be given if further exposure occurs more than 3 weeks after first dose, no evidence that effective in severe disease

● CAUTIONS IgA deficiency · interference with live virus vaccines

● SIDE-EFFECTS

▶ **Rare** Anaphylaxis

▶ **Frequency not known** Injection site pain · injection site swelling

● DIRECTIONS FOR ADMINISTRATION Normal immunoglobulin for intravenous use may be used in those unable to receive intramuscular injections.

● PRESCRIBING AND DISPENSING INFORMATION Available from selected Public Health England and NHS laboratories (also from BPL).

● HANDLING AND STORAGE Care must be taken to store all immunological products under the conditions recommended in the product literature, otherwise the preparation may become ineffective. **Refrigerated storage** is usually necessary; many immunoglobulins need to be stored at 2–8°C and not allowed to freeze. Immunoglobulins should be protected from light. Opened multidose vials must be used within the period recommended in the product literature.

● MEDICINAL FORMS
There can be variation in the licensing of different medicines containing the same drug.
Solution for injection
▸ Varicella-Zoster (Bio Products Laboratory Ltd)
   Varicella-Zoster immunoglobulin human 250 mg Varicella-Zoster immunoglobulin human 250mg solution for injection vials | 1 vial [PoM] £350.00

2 Post-exposure prophylaxis

IMMUNE SERA AND IMMUNOGLOBULINS ⟩ ANTITOXINS

Botulism antitoxin

● DRUG ACTION A preparation containing the specific antitoxic globulins that have the power of neutralising the toxins formed by types A, B, and E of *Clostridium botulinum*.

● INDICATIONS AND DOSE

Post exposure prophylaxis of botulism

▶ BY INTRAMUSCULAR INJECTION

▸ **Adult:** (consult product literature)

● SIDE-EFFECTS Hypersensitivity reactions

SIDE-EFFECTS, FURTHER INFORMATION

▸ Hypersensitivity reactions It is essential to read the contra-indications, warnings, and details of sensitivity tests on the package insert. Prior to treatment checks should be made regarding previous administration of any antitoxin and history of any allergic condition, e.g. asthma, hay fever, etc.

● PRE-TREATMENT SCREENING All patients should be tested for sensitivity (diluting the antitoxin if history of allergy).

● PRESCRIBING AND DISPENSING INFORMATION Available from local designated centres, for details see TOXBASE (requires registration) www.toxbase.org. For supplies outside working hours apply to other designated centres or to the Public Health England Colindale duty doctor (Tel (020) 8200 6868). For major incidents, obtain supplies from the local blood bank.

   The BP title Botulinum Antitoxin is not used because the preparation currently in use may have a different specification.

● MEDICINAL FORMS
There can be variation in the licensing of different medicines containing the same drug.
Solution for infusion
▸ Botulism-antitoxin (Novartis Vaccines and Diagnostics Ltd)
   Botulinum antitoxin type E 50 unit per 1 ml, Botulinum antitoxin type B 500 unit per 1 ml, Botulinum antitoxin type A 750 unit per 1 ml Botulism-Antitoxin Behring 25g/250ml solution for infusion bottles | 1 bottle [PoM] no price available

Diphtheria antitoxin

(Dip/Ser)

● INDICATIONS AND DOSE

Passive immunisation in suspected cases of diphtheria

▶ BY INTRAVENOUS INFUSION

▸ **Adult:** Dose should be given without waiting for bacteriological confirmation (consult product literature)

- CAUTIONS
  CAUTIONS, FURTHER INFORMATION
  ▸ Hypersensitivity Hypersensitivity is common after administration; resuscitation facilities should be available.
    Diphtheria antitoxin is no longer used for prophylaxis because of the risk of hypersensitivity; unimmunised contacts should be promptly investigated and given antibacterial prophylaxis and vaccine.
- SIDE-EFFECTS
  ▸ **Common or very common** Hypersensitivity reactions
- PRE-TREATMENT SCREENING Diphtheria antitoxin is derived from horse serum and reactions are common; tests for hypersensitivity should be carried out before use.
- PRESCRIBING AND DISPENSING INFORMATION Available from Centre for Infections (Tel (020) 8200 6868) or in Northern Ireland from Public Health Laboratory, Belfast City Hospital (Tel (028) 9032 9241).

- MEDICINAL FORMS
  There can be variation in the licensing of different medicines containing the same drug.
  Solution for injection
  ▸ Diphtheria antitoxin (Non-proprietary)
    Diphtheria antitoxin 1000 unit per 1 ml Antidiphtheria serum 10,000units/10ml solution for injection ampoules | 1 ampoule PoM no price available

3 Tuberculosis diagnostic test

DIAGNOSTIC AGENTS ⟩ OTHER

Tuberculin purified protein derivative
(Tuberculin PPD)

- INDICATIONS AND DOSE
Mantoux test
  ▸ BY INTRADERMAL INJECTION
  ▸ Child: 2 units for one dose
  ▸ Adult: 2 units for one dose

Mantoux test (if first test is negative and a further test is considered appropriate)
  ▸ BY INTRADERMAL INJECTION
  ▸ Child: 10 units for 1 dose
  ▸ Adult: 10 units for 1 dose

DOSE EQUIVALENCE AND CONVERSION
2 units is equivalent to 0.1 mL of 20 units/mL strength.
10 units is equivalent to 0.1 mL of 100 units/mL strength.

- CAUTIONS
  CAUTIONS, FURTHER INFORMATION
  ▸ Mantoux test Response to tuberculin may be suppressed by viral infection, sarcoidosis, corticosteroid therapy, or immunosuppression due to disease or treatment and the MMR vaccine. If a tuberculin skin test has already been initiated, then the MMR should be delayed until the skin test has been read unless protection against measles is required urgently. If a child has had a recent MMR, and requires a tuberculin test, then a 4 week interval should be observed. Apart from tuberculin and MMR, all other live vaccines can be administered at any time before or after tuberculin.
- PRESCRIBING AND DISPENSING INFORMATION Available from ImmForm (SSI brand).
    The strength of tuberculin PPD in currently available products may be different to the strengths of products used previously for the Mantoux test; care is required to select the correct strength.

- MEDICINAL FORMS
  There can be variation in the licensing of different medicines containing the same medicine. Forms available from special-order manufacturers include: solution for injection
  Solution for injection
  ▸ Tuberculin purified protein derivative (Non-proprietary)
    Tuberculin purified protein derivative 20 tuberculin unit per 1 ml Tuberculin PPD RT 23 SSI 20 tuberculin units/ml solution for injection 1.5ml vials | 1 vial no price available
    Tuberculin purified protein derivative 100 tuberculin unit per 1 ml Tuberculin PPD RT 23 SSI 100 tuberculin units/ml solution for injection 1.5ml vials | 1 vial no price available

4 Vaccination

Vaccines

Active immunity

Active immunity can be acquired by natural disease or by vaccination. **Vaccines** stimulate production of antibodies and other components of the immune mechanism; they consist of either:

- a *live attenuated* form of a virus (e.g. measles, mumps and rubella vaccine) or bacteria (e.g. BCG vaccine), or
- *inactivated* preparations of the virus (e.g. influenza vaccine) or bacteria, or
- *detoxified exotoxins* produced by a micro-organism (e.g. tetanus vaccine), or
- *extracts of* a micro-organism, which may be derived from the organism (e.g. pneumococcal vaccine) or produced by recombinant DNA technology (e.g. hepatitis B vaccine).

Live attenuated vaccines usually produce a durable immunity, but not always as long-lasting as that resulting from natural infection.

Inactivated vaccines may require a primary series of injections of vaccine to produce an adequate antibody response, and in most cases booster (reinforcing) injections are required; the duration of immunity varies from months to many years. Some inactivated vaccines are adsorbed onto an adjuvant (such as aluminium hydroxide) to enhance the antibody response.

Advice reflects that in the handbook *Immunisation against Infectious Disease* (2013), which in turn reflects the guidance of the Joint Committee on Vaccination and Immunisation (JCVI).

Chapters from the handbook are available at www.immunisation.dh.gov.uk

The advice also incorporates changes announced by the Chief Medical Officer and Health Department Updates.

Immunisation schedule

Vaccines for the childhood immunisation schedule should be obtained from **local health organisations** or from **ImmForm** (www.immform.dh.gov.uk)—not to be prescribed on FP10 (HS21 in Northern Ireland; GP10 in Scotland; WP10 in Wales).

For the most up to date immunisation schedule consult 'The complete routine immunisation schedule', available at www.gov.uk.

Preterm birth

Babies born preterm should receive all routine immunisations based on their actual date of birth. The risk of apnoea following vaccination is increased in preterm babies, particularly in those born at or before 28 weeks gestational age. If babies at risk of apnoea are in hospital at the time of their first immunisation, they should be monitored for 48 hours after immunisation. If a baby develops apnoea, bradycardia, or desaturation after the first immunisation, the second immunisation should also be given in hospital with

Routine immunisation schedule

When to immunise	Vaccine given and dose schedule (for details of dose, see under individual vaccines)
Neonates at risk only	‣ Bacillus Calmette-Guérin vaccine p. 1149 ‣ Hepatitis B vaccine p. 1155
2 months	‣ Diphtheria with haemophilus influenzae type b vaccine, pertussis, poliomyelitis and tetanus p. 1147 First dose ‣ Meningococcal group B vaccine (rDNA, component, adsorbed) p. 1150 First dose ‣ Pneumococcal polysaccharide conjugate vaccine (adsorbed) p. 1152 First dose ‣ Rotavirus vaccine p. 1160 First dose
3 months	‣ Diphtheria with haemophilus influenzae type b vaccine, pertussis, poliomyelitis and tetanus p. 1147 Second dose ‣ Meningococcal group C vaccine p. 1151 First dose ‣ Rotavirus vaccine p. 1160 Second dose
4 months	‣ Diphtheria with haemophilus influenzae type b vaccine, pertussis, poliomyelitis and tetanus p. 1147 Third dose ‣ Meningococcal group B vaccine (rDNA, component, adsorbed) p. 1150 Second dose ‣ Pneumococcal polysaccharide conjugate vaccine (adsorbed) p. 1152 Second dose
12–13 months	‣ Measles, mumps and rubella vaccine, live p. 1159 First dose ‣ Meningococcal group B vaccine (rDNA, component, adsorbed) p. 1150 Single booster dose ‣ Pneumococcal polysaccharide conjugate vaccine (adsorbed) p. 1152 Single booster dose ‣ Haemophilus influenzae type B with meningococcal group C vaccine p. 1150 Single booster dose
2–6 years (including children in school years 1 and 2)	‣ Influenza vaccine p. 1157 Each year from September **Note:** Flu nasal spray is recommended (*Fluenz Tetra*®). If contra-indicated and child is in clinical risk group, use inactivated flu vaccine
Between 3 years and 4 months, and 5 years	‣ Diphtheria with pertussis, poliomyelitis vaccine and tetanus p. 1148 Single booster dose. **Note:** Preferably allow interval of at least 3 years after completing primary course. ‣ Measles, mumps and rubella vaccine, live p. 1159 Second dose
11–14 years (females only). First dose of HPV vaccine will be offered to females aged 12–13 years of age in England, Wales, and Northern Ireland, and 11–14 years of age in Scotland.	‣ Human papillomavirus vaccines p. 1157 2 doses; second dose 12 months after first dose. If a 3-dose course of HPV vaccine has been started under the 2013/2014 programme, where possible, the course should be completed. The two human papillomavirus vaccines are not interchangeable and, ideally, one vaccine product should be used for the entire course. However, for those females who started the schedule with *Cervarix*® under the national immunisation programme, but did not complete the vaccination course, the course can be completed with *Gardasil*®.
13–15 years	‣ Meningococcal groups A with C and W135 and Y vaccine p. 1151 Single booster dose
13–18 years	‣ Diphtheria with poliomyelitis and tetanus vaccine p. 1148 Single booster dose. **Note:** Can be given at the same time as the dose of meningococcal group A with C and W135 and Y vaccine at 13–15 years of age.
During adult life, women of child-bearing age susceptible to rubella	‣ Measles, mumps and rubella vaccine, live p. 1159 Women of child-bearing age who have not received 2 doses of a rubella-containing vaccine or who do not have a positive antibody test for rubella should be offered rubella immunisation (using the MMR vaccine)—exclude pregnancy before immunisation.
During adult life, those entering or being at university who are at risk of meningococcal group C disease	‣ Meningococcal group C vaccine p. 1151 Single dose. **Note:** Should be offered to those of any age entering or being at university who have never been vaccinated against meningococcal group C disease, or those born after September 1995 who are entering university and only received meningococcal group C vaccine under the age of 10 years
During adult life, if not previously immunised	‣ Diphtheria with poliomyelitis and tetanus vaccine p. 1148
70 years	‣ Varicella-zoster vaccine p. 1161 Single dose

similar monitoring. Seroconversion may be unreliable in babies born earlier than 28 weeks' gestation or in babies treated with corticosteroids for chronic lung disease; consideration should be given to testing for antibodies against *Haemophilus influenzae* type b, meningococcal C, and hepatitis B after primary immunisation.

Vaccines and HIV infection
HIV-positive individuals with or without symptoms can receive the following live vaccines:
- MMR (but avoid if immunity significantly impaired; use of normal immunoglobulin should be considered after exposure to measles), varicella-zoster vaccine against chickenpox (but avoid if immunity significantly impaired—consult product literature; varicella–zoster

immunoglobulin should be considered after exposure to chickenpox or herpes zoster), rotavirus;

and the following inactivated vaccines:
- anthrax, cholera (oral), diphtheria, haemophilus influenzae type b, hepatitis A, hepatitis B, human papillomavirus, influenza (injection), meningococcal, pertussis, pneumococcal, poliomyelitis, rabies, tetanus, tick-borne encephalitis, typhoid (injection).

HIV-positive individuals should **not** receive:
- BCG, influenza nasal spray (unless stable HIV infection and receiving antiretroviral therapy), typhoid (oral), yellow fever (if yellow fever risk is unavoidable, specialist advice should be sought)

The above advice differs from that for other immunocompromised patients; *Immunisation Guidelines for*

HIV-infected Adults issued by *British HIV Association* (BHIVA) are available at www.bhiva.org and, *Immunisation of HIV-infected Children* issued by *Children's HIV Association* (CHIVA) are available at www.chiva.org.uk

Vaccines and asplenia

The following vaccines are recommended for asplenic patients, those with splenic dysfunction or complement disorders, depending on the age at which their condition is diagnosed:

- Haemophilus influenzae type B with meningococcal group C vaccine;
- Influenza vaccine;
- Meningococcal groups A with C and W135 and Y vaccine;
- pneumococcal polysaccharide vaccine.

Children first diagnosed under 2 *years of age* should be vaccinated according to the Immunisation Schedule, including the 12 month boosters. If meningococcal group C vaccine p. 1151 has not yet been given as part of routine schedule, give one dose of meningococcal groups A with C and W135 and Y vaccine p. 1151 followed by a second dose at least one month apart. If meningococcal group C vaccine has already been given as part of routine schedule, then give one additional dose of meningococcal groups A with C and W135 and Y vaccine at least one month later. Following routine 12 month booster vaccines, give a dose of meningococcal groups A with C and W135 and Y vaccine and an additional dose of 13-valent pneumococcal polysaccharide vaccine 2 months later. An additional dose of haemophilus influenzae type B with meningococcal group C vaccine p. 1150 and 23-valent pneumococcal polysaccharide vaccine should be given after the second birthday. The influenza vaccine should be administered annually in children aged 6 months or older.

Children first diagnosed over 2 *years of age* should be vaccinated according to the Immunisation schedule, including the 12 month boosters. The child should receive one additional booster dose of haemophilus influenzae type B with meningococcal group C vaccine along with the 23-valent pneumococcal polysaccharide vaccine, followed by one dose of meningococcal groups A with C and W135 and Y vaccine after 2 months. The influenza vaccine should be administered annually.

Vaccines and antisera availability

Anthrax vaccine p. 1149 and yellow fever vaccine, live p. 1162, botulism antitoxin p. 1134, diphtheria antitoxin p. 1134, and snake and spider venom antitoxins are available from local designated holding centres.

For antivenom, see Emergency treatment of poisoning p. 1194.

Enquiries for vaccines not available commercially can also be made to:

Vaccines and Countermeasures Response Department
Public Health England
Wellington House
133–155 Waterloo Road
London
SE1 8UG
vaccinesupply@phe.gov.uk

In Scotland information about availability of vaccines can be obtained from a Specialist in Pharmaceutical Public Health.

In Wales enquiries for vaccines not available commercially should be directed to:

Welsh Medicines Information Centre
University Hospital of Wales
Cardiff
CF14 4XW
(029) 2074 2979

In Northern Ireland:

Pharmacy and Medicines Management Centre
Northern Health and Social Care Trust
Beech House
Antrim Hospital Site
Bush Road
Antrim
BT41 2RL
rphps.admin@northerntrust.hscni.net

For further details of availability, see under individual vaccines.

Anthrax vaccine

Anthrax vaccine is made from antigens from *B. anthracis*. Anthrax immunisation is indicated for individuals who handle infected animals, for those exposed to imported infected animal products, and for laboratory staff who work with *B. anthracis*. A 4-dose regimen is used for primary immunisation; booster doses should be given annually to workers at continued risk of exposure to anthrax.

In the event of possible contact with *B. anthracis*, post-exposure immunisation may be indicated, in addition to antimicrobial prophylaxis. Advice on the use of anthrax vaccine for post-exposure prophylaxis must be obtained from Public Health England Colindale (Tel. 020 8200 4400).

BCG vaccine

Bacillus Calmette-Guérin vaccine p. 1149 should be given intradermally by operators skilled in the technique.

The expected reaction to successful Bacillus Calmette-Guérin vaccine is induration at the site of injection followed by a local lesion which starts as a papule 2 or more weeks after vaccination; the lesion may ulcerate then subside over several weeks or months, leaving a small, flat scar. A dry dressing may be used if the ulcer discharges, but air should **not** be excluded.

BCG is recommended for the following groups if BCG immunisation has not previously been carried out and they are negative for tuberculoprotein hypersensitivity:

- neonates with a family history of tuberculosis in the last 5 years;
- all neonates and infants (0–12 months) born in areas where the incidence of tuberculosis is greater than 40 per 100 000;
- neonates, infants, and children under 16 years with a parent or grandparent born in a country with an incidence of tuberculosis greater than 40 per 100 000;
- new immigrants aged under 16 years who were born in, or lived for more than 3 months in a country with an incidence of tuberculosis greater than 40 per 100 000;
- new immigrants aged 16–35 years from Sub-Saharan Africa or a country with an incidence of tuberculosis greater than 500 per 100 000;
- contacts aged under 36 years of those with active respiratory tuberculosis (for healthcare or laboratory workers who have had contact with clinical materials or patients with tuberculosis, age limit does not apply);
- healthcare workers and laboratory staff (irrespective of age) who are likely to have contact with patients, clinical materials, or derived isolates; other individuals under 35 years (there is inadequate evidence of protection by BCG vaccine in adults aged over 35 years; however, vaccination is recommended for healthcare workers irrespective of age because of the increased risk to them or their patients) at occupational risk including veterinary and other staff who handle animal species susceptible to tuberculosis, and staff working directly with prisoners, in care homes for the elderly, or in hostels or facilities for the homeless or refugees;
- individuals under 16 years intending to live with local people for more than 3 months in a country with an

incidence of tuberculosis greater than 40 per 100 000.

List of countries or primary care trusts where the incidence of tuberculosis is greater than 40 cases per 100 000 is available at www.gov.uk/phe.

Bladder instillations of BCG are licensed for the management of bladder carcinoma.

See also Tuberculosis p. 525 for advice on chemoprophylaxis; for the treatment of infection following vaccination, seek expert advice.

Tuberculosis Diagnostic Agents

The *Mantoux test* is recommended for tuberculin skin testing, but no licensed preparation is currently available. Guidance for healthcare professionals is available at www.dh.gov.uk/immunisation.

In the Mantoux test, the diagnostic dose is administered by intradermal injection of tuberculin purified protein derivative p. 1135 (PPD).

The *Heaf test* (involving the use of multiple-puncture apparatus) is no longer available.

Two interferon gamma release assay (IGRA) tests are also available as an aid in the diagnosis of tuberculosis infection: *QuantiFERON® TB Gold* and *T-SPOT®.TB*. Both tests measure T-cell mediated immune response to synthetic antigens. For further information on the use of interferon gamma release assay tests for tuberculosis, see www.gov.uk/phe.

Botulism antitoxin

A polyvalent botulism antitoxin is available for the post-exposure prophylaxis of botulism and for the treatment of persons thought to be suffering from botulism. It specifically neutralises the toxins produced by *Clostridium botulinum* types A, B, and E. It is not effective against infantile botulism as the toxin (type A) is seldom, if ever, found in the blood in this type of infection.

Cholera vaccine

Cholera vaccine p. 1149 (oral) contains inactivated Inaba (including El-Tor biotype) and Ogawa strains of *Vibrio cholerae*, serotype O1 together with recombinant B-subunit of the cholera toxin produced in Inaba strains of *V.cholerae*, serotype O1.

Oral cholera vaccine p. 1149 is licensed for travellers to endemic or epidemic areas on the basis of current recommendations. Immunisation should be completed at least 1 week before potential exposure. However, there is no requirement for cholera vaccination for international travel.

Injectable cholera vaccine provides unreliable protection and is no longer available in the UK.

Diphtheria vaccine

Diphtheria-containing vaccines are prepared from the toxin of *Corynebacterium diphtheriae* and adsorption on aluminium hydroxide or aluminium phosphate improves antigenicity. The vaccine stimulates the production of the protective antibody. The quantity of diphtheria toxoid in a preparation determines whether the vaccine is defined as 'high dose' or 'low dose'. Vaccines containing the higher dose of diphtheria toxoid are used for primary immunisation of children under 10 years of age. Vaccines containing the lower dose of diphtheria toxoid are used for primary immunisation in adults and children over 10 years. Single-antigen diphtheria vaccine is not available and adsorbed diphtheria vaccine is given as a combination product containing other vaccines.

For primary immunisation *of children aged between 2 months and 10 years* vaccination is recommended usually in the form of 3 doses (separated by 1-month intervals) of **diphtheria, tetanus, pertussis (acellular, component), poliomyelitis (inactivated) and haemophilus type b conjugate vaccine (adsorbed)** (see Immunisation schedule). In unimmunised individuals aged *over* 10 *years* the primary course comprises of 3 doses of **adsorbed diphtheria**

[low dose], **tetanus and poliomyelitis (inactivated) vaccine**.

A booster dose should be given 3 years after the primary course (this interval can be reduced to a minimum of 1 year if the primary course was delayed). Children *under* 10 *years* should receive *either* **adsorbed diphtheria, tetanus, pertussis (acellular, component) and poliomyelitis (inactivated) vaccine** *or* **adsorbed diphtheria** [low dose], **tetanus, pertussis (acellular, component) and poliomyelitis (inactivated) vaccine**. Individuals aged *over* 10 *years* should receive **adsorbed diphtheria** [low dose], **tetanus, and poliomyelitis (inactivated) vaccine**.

A second booster dose, of adsorbed diphtheria [low dose], tetanus and poliomyelitis (inactivated) vaccine, should be given 10 years after the previous booster dose (this interval can be reduced to a minimum of 5 years if previous doses were delayed).

Diphtheria-containing vaccines for children over 10 years and adults

A **low dose** of diphtheria toxoid is sufficient to recall immunity in individuals previously immunised against diphtheria but whose immunity may have diminished with time; it is insufficient to cause serious reactions in an individual who is already immune. Preparations containing low dose diphtheria should be used for adults and children *over* 10 *years*, for both primary immunisation and booster doses.

Travel

Those intending to travel to areas with a risk of diphtheria infection should be fully immunised according to the UK schedule. If more than 10 years have lapsed since completion of the UK schedule, a dose of **adsorbed diphtheria** [low dose], **tetanus and poliomyelitis (inactivated) vaccine** should be administered.

Contacts

Staff in contact with diphtheria patients or with potentially pathogenic clinical specimens or working directly with *C. diphtheriae* or *C. ulcerans* should receive a booster dose if fully immunised (with 5 doses of diphtheria-containing vaccine given at appropriate intervals); further doses should be given at 10-year intervals if risk persists. Individuals at risk who are not fully immunised should complete the primary course; a booster dose should be given after 5 years and then at 10-year intervals. **Adsorbed diphtheria** [low dose], **tetanus and poliomyelitis (inactivated) vaccine** is used for this purpose; immunity should be checked by antibody testing at least 3 months after completion of immunisation.

Advice on the management of cases, carriers, contacts and outbreaks must be sought from health protection units. The immunisation history of infected individuals and their contacts should be determined; those who have been incompletely immunised should complete their immunisation and fully immunised individuals should receive a reinforcing dose. See advice on antibacterial treatment to prevent a secondary case of diphtheria in a non-immune individual.

Haemophilus influenzae type B conjugate vaccine

Haemophilus influenzae type b (Hib) vaccine is made from capsular polysaccharide; it is conjugated with a protein such as tetanus toxoid to increase immunogenicity, especially in young children. Haemophilus influenzae type b vaccine immunisation is given in combination with diphtheria, tetanus, pertussis (acellular, component) and poliomyelitis (inactivated) vaccine, as a component of the primary course of childhood immunisation (see Immunisation schedule). For infants under 1 year, the course consists of 3 doses of a vaccine containing *Haemophilus influenzae* type b component with an interval of 1 month between doses. A booster dose of haemophilus influenzae type b vaccine (combined with meningococcal group C conjugate vaccine) should be given at 12–13 months of age.

Children 1–10 years who have not been immunised against *Haemophilus influenzae* type b need to receive only 1 dose of Haemophilus influenzae type b vaccine (combined with meningococcal group C conjugate vaccine). However, if a primary course of immunisation has not been completed, these children should be given 3 doses of diphtheria with haemophilus influenzae type b vaccine, pertussis, poliomyelitis and tetanus p. 1147. The risk of infection falls sharply in older children and the vaccine is not normally required for children over 10 years.

Haemophilus influenzae type b vaccine may be given to those over 10 years who are considered to be at increased risk of invasive *H. influenzae* type b disease (such as those with sickle-cell disease or complement deficiency, or those receiving treatment for malignancy).

Invasive *Haemophilus influenzae* type b disease

After recovery from infection, unimmunised and partially immunised index cases under 10 years of age should complete their age-specific course of immunisation. Previously vaccinated cases under 10 years of age should be given an additional dose of haemophilus influenzae type b vaccine (combined with meningococcal group C conjugate vaccine) if Hib antibody concentrations are low or if it is not possible to measure antibody concentrations. Index cases of any age with asplenia or splenic dysfunction should complete their immunisation according to the recommendations below; fully vaccinated cases with asplenia or splenic dysfunction should be given an additional dose of haemophilus influenzae type b vaccine (combined with meningococcal group C conjugate vaccine) if they received their previous dose over 1 year ago.

See also use of rifampicin p. 527 in the prevention of secondary cases of *Haemophilus influenzae* type b disease.

Hepatitis A vaccine

Hepatitis A vaccine p. 1154 is prepared from formaldehyde-inactivated hepatitis A virus grown in human diploid cells.

Immunisation is recommended for:

- laboratory staff who work directly with the virus;
- staff and residents of homes for those with severe learning difficulties;
- workers at risk of exposure to untreated sewage;
- individuals who work with primates;
- patients with haemophilia or other conditions treated with plasma-derived clotting factors;
- patients with severe liver disease;
- travellers to high-risk areas;
- individuals who are at risk due to their sexual behaviour;
- parenteral drug abusers.

  Immunisation should be considered for:

- patients with chronic liver disease including chronic hepatitis B or chronic hepatitis C;
- prevention of secondary cases in close contacts of confirmed cases of hepatitis A, within 14 days of exposure to the primary case (within 8 weeks of exposure to the primary case where there is more than 1 contact in the household).

A booster dose is usually given 6–12 months after the initial dose. A second booster dose can be given 20 years after the previous booster dose to those who continue to be at risk. Specialist advice should be sought on re-immunisation of immunocompromised individuals.

For rapid protection against hepatitis A after exposure or during an outbreak, in adults a single dose of a monovalent vaccine is recommended; for children under 16 years, a single dose of the combined vaccine Ambirix® can also be used.

Intramuscular normal immunoglobulin p. 1131 is recommended for use in addition to hepatitis A vaccine for close contacts (of confirmed cases of hepatitis A) who have chronic liver disease or HIV infection, or who are immunosuppressed or over 50 years of age.

Post-exposure prophylaxis is not required for healthy children under 1 year of age, so long as all those involved in nappy changing are vaccinated against hepatitis A. However, children 2–12 months of age can be given a dose of hepatitis A vaccine if it is not possible to vaccinate their carers, or if the child becomes a source of infection to others [unlicensed use]; in these cases, if the child goes on to require long-term protection against hepatitis A after the first birthday, the full course of 2 doses should be given.

Hepatitis B vaccine

Hepatitis B vaccine p. 1155 contains inactivated hepatitis B virus surface antigen (HBsAg) adsorbed onto aluminium hydroxide adjuvant. It is made biosynthetically using recombinant DNA technology. The vaccine is used in individuals at high risk of contracting hepatitis B.

In the UK, groups at high-risk of hepatitis B include:

- parenteral drug misusers, their sexual partners, and household contacts; other drug misusers who are likely to 'progress' to injecting;
- individuals who change sexual partners frequently;
- close family contacts of a case or individual with chronic hepatitis B infection;
- babies whose mothers have had acute hepatitis B during pregnancy *or* are positive for hepatitis B surface antigen (regardless of e-antigen markers); hepatitis B vaccination is started immediately on delivery and *hepatitis B immunoglobulin* given at the same time (but preferably at a different site). Babies whose mothers are positive for hepatitis B surface antigen and for e-antigen antibody should receive the vaccine only (but babies weighing 1.5 kg or less should also receive the immunoglobulin regardless of the mother's e-antigen antibody status);
- individuals with haemophilia, those receiving regular blood transfusions or blood products, and carers responsible for the administration of such products;
- patients with chronic renal failure including those on haemodialysis. Haemodialysis patients should be monitored for antibodies annually and re-immunised if necessary. Home carers (of dialysis patients) should be vaccinated;
- individuals with chronic liver disease;
- healthcare personnel (including trainees) who have direct contact with blood or blood-stained body fluids or with patients' tissues;
- laboratory staff who handle material that may contain the virus;
- other occupational risk groups such as morticians and embalmers;
- staff and patients of day-care or residential accommodation for those with severe learning difficulties;
- staff and inmates of custodial institutions;
- those travelling to areas of high or intermediate prevalence who are at increased risk or who plan to remain there for lengthy periods;
- families adopting children from countries with a high or intermediate prevalence of hepatitis B;
- foster carers and their families.

Different immunisation schedules for hepatitis B vaccine are recommended for specific circumstances. Generally, three or four doses are required for primary immunisation; an 'accelerated schedule' is recommended for pre-exposure prophylaxis in high-risk groups where rapid protection is required, and for post-exposure prophylaxis.

Immunisation may take up to 6 months to confer adequate protection; the duration of immunity is not known precisely, but a single booster 5 years after the primary course may be sufficient to maintain immunity for those who continue to be at risk.

14

Vaccines

Immunisation does not eliminate the need for commonsense precautions for avoiding the risk of infection from known carriers by the routes of infection which have been clearly established, consult *Guidance for Clinical Health Care Workers: Protection against Infection with Blood-borne Viruses* (available at www.dh.gov.uk). Accidental inoculation of hepatitis B virus-infected blood into a wound, incision, needle-prick, or abrasion may lead to infection, whereas it is unlikely that indirect exposure to a carrier will do so.

Following significant exposure to hepatitis B, an accelerated schedule, with the second dose given 1 month, and the third dose 2 months after the first dose, is recommended. For those at continued risk, a fourth dose should be given 12 months after the first dose. More detailed guidance is given in the handbook *Immunisation against Infectious Disease*. Specific hepatitis B immunoglobulin ('HBIG') p. 1131 is available for use with the vaccine in those accidentally inoculated and in neonates at special risk of infection.

A combined hepatitis A and B vaccine p. 1153 is also available.

Human papillomavirus vaccine

Human papillomavirus vaccine is available as a bivalent vaccine (*Cervarix*®) or a quadrivalent vaccine (*Gardasil* ®). *Cervarix*® is licensed for use in females for the prevention of cervical cancer and other pre-cancerous lesions caused by human papillomavirus types 16 and 18. *Gardasil* is licensed for use in females for the prevention of cervical and anal cancers, genital warts and pre-cancerous genital (cervical, vulvar, and vaginal) and anal lesions caused by human papillomavirus types 6, 11, 16, and 18. The vaccines may also provide limited protection against disease caused by other types of human papillomavirus. The two vaccines are not interchangeable and one vaccine product should be used for an entire course.

Human papillomavirus vaccine will be most effective if given before sexual activity starts. From September 2014, a 2-dose schedule is recommended, as long as the first dose is received before the age of 15 years. The first dose is given to females aged 11 to 14 years, and the second dose is given 6–24 months after the first dose (for the purposes of planning the national immunisation programme, it is appropriate to give the second dose 12 months after the first (see Immunisation schedule). If the course is interrupted, it should be resumed (using the same vaccine) but not repeated, even if more than 24 months have elapsed since the first dose or if the girl is then aged 15 years or more. Females receiving their first dose aged 15 years or older require a 3-dose schedule (see *Cervarix*® and *Gardasil*®), with the second and third doses given 1 and 4–6 months after the first dose; all 3 doses should be given within a 12-month period. If the course is interrupted, it should be resumed (using the same vaccine) but not repeated, allowing the appropriate interval between the remaining doses. If a 3-dose course of vaccination has been started before September 2014, then where possible this should be completed; if the course is interrupted, it should be resumed (using the same vaccine) but not repeated, allowing the appropriate interval between the remaining doses. Under the national programme in England, females remain eligible to receive the human papillomavirus vaccine up to the age of 18 years if they did not receive the vaccine when scheduled. Where appropriate, immunisation with human papillomavirus vaccine should be offered to females coming into the UK as they may not have been offered protection in their country of origin. The duration of protection has not been established, but current studies suggest that protection is maintained for at least 6 years after completion of the primary course.

As the vaccines do not protect against all strains of human papillomavirus, routine cervical screening should continue.

Influenza vaccine

While most viruses are antigenically stable, the influenza viruses A and B (especially A) are constantly altering their antigenic structure as indicated by changes in the haemagglutinins (H) and neuraminidases (N) on the surface of the viruses. It is essential that influenza vaccine p. 1157 in use contain the H and N components of the prevalent strain or strains as recommended each year by the World Health Organization.

Immunisation is recommended *for persons at high risk*, and to reduce transmission of infection. Annual immunisation is strongly recommended for individuals aged over 6 months with the following conditions:

- chronic respiratory disease (includes asthma treated with continuous or repeated use of inhaled or systemic corticosteroids or asthma with previous exacerbations requiring hospital admission);
- chronic heart disease;
- chronic liver disease;
- chronic renal disease;
- chronic neurological disease;
- complement disorders;
- diabetes mellitus;
- immunosuppression because of disease (including asplenia or splenic dysfunction) or treatment (including prolonged systemic corticosteroid treatment [for over 1 month at dose equivalents of prednisolone: *adult and child over 20 kg*, 20 mg or more daily; *child under 20 kg*, 1 mg/kg or more daily] and chemotherapy);
- HIV infection (regardless of immune status).

Seasonal influenza vaccine is also recommended for all pregnant women, for all persons aged over 65 years, for residents of nursing or residential homes for the elderly and other long-stay facilities, and for carers of persons whose welfare may be at risk if the carer falls ill. Influenza immunisation should also be considered for household contacts of immunocompromised individuals.

As part of winter planning, NHS employers should offer vaccination to healthcare workers who are directly involved in patient care. Employers of social care workers should consider similar action.

Unless contra-indicated, the live influenza vaccine, *Fluenz Tetra*®, is preferred in children aged 2–18 years because it provides a higher level of protection than inactivated influenza vaccine. From September 2015, seasonal influenza vaccine will also be offered to all children aged 2–6 years (including those in school years 1 and 2).

Information on pandemic influenza, avian influenza and swine influenza may be found at www.dh.gov.uk/pandemicflu and at www.gov.uk/phe.

Japanese encephalitis vaccine

Japanese encephalitis vaccine p. 1158 is indicated for travellers to areas in Asia and the Far East where infection is endemic and for laboratory staff at risk of exposure to the virus. The primary immunisation course of 2 doses should be completed at least one week before potential exposure to Japanese encephalitis virus.

Up-to-date information on the risk of Japanese encephalitis in specific countries can be obtained from the National Travel Health Network and Centre (www.nathnac.org).

Measles, Mumps and Rubella vaccine

Measles vaccine has been replaced by a combined live measles, mumps and rubella vaccine, live (MMR vaccine) p. 1159.

Measles, mumps and rubella vaccine, live aims to eliminate measles, mumps, and rubella (German measles) and congenital rubella syndrome. Every child should receive two doses of measles, mumps and rubella vaccine, live by entry to primary school, unless there is a valid contra-indication. Measles, mumps and rubella vaccine, live should be given irrespective of previous measles, mumps, or rubella infection or vaccination.

The first dose of measles, mumps and rubella vaccine, live is given to children aged 12–13 months. A second dose is given before starting school at 3 years and 4 months–5 years of age (see Immunisation Schedule).

Children presenting for pre-school booster who have not received the first dose of measles, mumps and rubella vaccine, live should be given a dose of measles, mumps and rubella vaccine, live followed 3 months later by a second dose.

At school-leaving age or at entry into further education, measles, mumps and rubella vaccine, live immunisation should be offered to individuals of both sexes who have not received 2 doses during childhood. In those who have received only a single dose of measles, mumps and rubella vaccine, live in childhood, a second dose is recommended to achieve full protection. If 2 doses of measles, mumps and rubella vaccine, live are required, the second dose should be given one month after the initial dose. The decision on whether to vaccinate adults should take into consideration their vaccination history, the likelihood of the individual remaining susceptible, and the future risk of exposure and disease.

Measles, mumps and rubella vaccine, live should be used to protect against rubella in *seronegative women of child-bearing age* (see Immunisation Schedule); unimmunised healthcare workers who might put pregnant women and other vulnerable groups at risk of rubella or measles should be vaccinated. Measles, mumps and rubella vaccine, live may also be offered to previously *unimmunised and seronegative post-partum women* (see measles, mumps and rubella vaccine, live p. 1159)—vaccination a few days after delivery is important because about 60% of congenital abnormalities from rubella infection occur in babies of women who have borne more than one child. Immigrants arriving after the age of school immunisation are particularly likely to require immunisation.

Contacts

Measles, mumps and rubella vaccine, live may also be used in the control of outbreaks of measles and should be offered to susceptible children aged over 6 months who are contacts of a case, within 3 days of exposure to infection. Children immunised before 12 months of age should still receive two doses of measles, mumps and rubella vaccine, live at the recommended ages. If one dose of measles, mumps and rubella vaccine, live has already been given to a child, then the second dose may be brought forward to at least one month after the first, to ensure complete protection. If the child is under 18 months of age and the second dose is given within 3 months of the first, then the routine dose before starting school at 3 years and 4 months–5 years should still be given. Children aged under 9 months for whom avoidance of measles infection is particularly important (such as those with history of recent severe illness) can be given normal immunoglobulin after exposure to measles; routine measles, mumps and rubella vaccine, live immunisation should then be given after at least 3 months at the appropriate age.

Measles, mumps and rubella vaccine, live is **not suitable** for prophylaxis following exposure to mumps or rubella since the antibody response to the mumps and rubella components is too slow for effective prophylaxis.

Children and adults with impaired immune response should not receive live vaccines (see advice on HIV). If they have been exposed to measles infection they should be given normal immunoglobulin.

Travel

Unimmunised travellers, including children over 6 months, to areas where measles is endemic or epidemic should receive measles, mumps and rubella vaccine, live. Children

immunised before 12 months of age should still receive two doses of measles, mumps and rubella vaccine, live at the recommended ages. If one dose of measles, mumps and rubella vaccine, live has already been given to a child, then the second dose should be brought forward to at least one month after the first, to ensure complete protection. If the child is under 18 months of age and the second dose is given within 3 months of the first, then the routine dose before starting school at 3 years and 4 months–5 years should still be given.

Meningococcal vaccines

Almost all childhood meningococcal disease in the UK is caused by *Neisseria meningitidis* serogroups B and C. **Meningococcal group C conjugate vaccine** protects only against infection by serogroup C and **Meningococcal group B vaccine** protects only against infection by serogroup B. The risk of meningococcal disease declines with age—immunisation is not generally recommended after the age of 25 years.

Tetravalent meningococcal vaccines that cover serogroups A, C, W135, and Y are available. Although the duration of protection has not been established, the **meningococcal groups A, C, W135, and Y conjugate vaccine** is likely to provide longer-lasting protection than the unconjugated meningococcal polysaccharide vaccine. The antibody response to serogroup C in unconjugated meningococcal polysaccharide vaccines in young children may be suboptimal [not currently available in the UK].

A **meningococcal group B vaccine**, *Bexsero®*, is licensed in the UK against infection caused by *Neisseria meningitidis* serogroup B and is recommended in the Immunisation Schedule. *Bexsero®* contains 3 recombinant *Neisseria meningitidis* serogroup B proteins and the outer membrane vesicles from the NZ 98/254 strain, in order to achieve broad protection against *Neisseria meningitidis* serogroup B; the proteins are adsorbed onto an aluminium compound to stimulate an enhanced immune response.

Childhood immunisation

Meningococcal group C conjugate vaccine provides long-term protection against infection by serogroup C of *Neisseria meningitidis*. Immunisation consists of 1 dose given at 3 months of age; 2 booster doses are recommended, the first is given at 12–13 months of age (combined with haemophilus influenzae type b vaccine), and the second is given at 13–15 years of age (combined with meningococcal A, W135 and Y vaccine) (see Immunisation Schedule).

Meningococcal group B vaccine provides protection against infection by serogroup B of *Neisseria meningitidis*. Immunisation consists of 1 dose given at 2 months of age, a second dose at 4 months of age, and a booster dose at 12 months of age (see Immunisation Schedule).

Unimmunised children aged under 12 months should be given 1 dose of meningococcal group B and group C conjugate vaccines, followed by a second dose of meningococcal group B vaccine (rDNA, component, adsorbed) p. 1150 two months later. They should then be vaccinated according to the Immunisation Schedule. Unimmunised children aged 12–23 months should be given a single dose of the meningococcal group C vaccine p. 1151 and 2 doses of meningococcal group B vaccine (rDNA, component, adsorbed) separated by an interval of two months. Children aged 2–9 years who have not received the meningococcal group C vaccine since 12-13 months should be given a single dose of meningococcal group C vaccine only, followed by a booster dose of meningococcal groups A with C and W135 and Y vaccine p. 1151 at 13–15 years of age.

From 2015, unimmunised individuals aged 10–25 years, including those aged under 25 years who are attending university for the first time, should be given a single dose of meningococcal groups A with C and W135 and Y vaccine; a booster dose is not required. All students attending

14

Vaccines

university for the first time who are unvaccinated against meningococcal group C, irrespective of age, should be offered a single dose of meningococcal group C vaccine.

Patients under 25 years of age with confirmed serogroup C disease, who have previously been immunised with meningococcal group C vaccine, should be offered meningococcal group C conjugate vaccine before discharge from hospital.

Travel

Individuals travelling to countries of risk should be immunised with meningococcal groups A, C, W135, and Y conjugate vaccine, even if they have previously received meningococcal group C conjugate vaccine. If an individual has recently received meningococcal group C conjugate vaccine, an interval of at least 4 weeks should be allowed before administration of the tetravalent (meningococcal groups A, C, and Y) vaccine.

Vaccination is particularly important for those living or working with local people or visiting an area of risk during outbreaks.

Immunisation recommendations and requirements for visa entry for individual countries should be checked before travelling, particularly to countries in Sub-Saharan Africa, Asia, and the Indian sub-continent where epidemics of meningococcal outbreaks and infection are reported. Country-by-country information is available from the National Travel Health Network and Centre (www.nathnac.org).

Proof of vaccination with the tetravalent meningococcal groups A with C and W135 and Y vaccine is required for those travelling to Saudi Arabia during the Hajj and Umrah pilgrimages (where outbreaks of the W135 strain have occurred).

Contacts

For advice on the immunisation of *laboratory workers and close contacts* of cases of meningococcal disease in the UK and on the role of the vaccine in the control of *local outbreaks*, consult Guidance for Public Health Management of Meningococcal Disease in the UK at www.gov.uk/phe. Also see for antibacterial prophylaxis for prevention of secondary cases of meningococcal meningitis.

The need for immunisation of laboratory staff who work directly with *Neisseria meningitidis* should be considered.

Pertussis vaccine

Pertussis vaccine is given as a combination preparation containing other vaccines. Acellular vaccines are derived from highly purified components of *Bordetella pertussis*. Primary immunisation against pertussis (whooping cough) requires 3 doses of an acellular pertussis-containing vaccine (see Immunisation schedule), given at intervals of 1 month from the age of 2 months.

All children up to the age of 10 years should receive primary immunisation with diphtheria, tetanus, pertussis (acellular, component), poliomyelitis (inactivated) and haemophilus type b conjugate vaccine (adsorbed).

A booster dose of an acellular pertussis-containing vaccine should ideally be given 3 years after the primary course, although, the interval can be reduced to 1 year if the primary course was delayed. Children aged 1–10 years who have not received a *pertussis-containing* vaccine as part of their primary immunisation should be offered 1 dose of a suitable pertussis-containing vaccine; after an interval of at least 1 year, a booster dose of a suitable pertussis-containing vaccine should be given. Immunisation against pertussis is not routinely recommended in individuals over 10 years of age.

Vaccination of pregnant women against pertussis

In response to the pertussis outbreak, the UK health departments introduced a temporary programme (October 2012) to vaccinate pregnant women against pertussis, and

this programme will continue until further notice. The aim of the programme is to boost the levels of pertussis–specific antibodies that are transferred through the placenta, from the mother to the fetus, so that the newborn is protected before routine immunisation begins at 2 months of age.

Pregnant women should be offered a single dose of acellular pertussis-containing vaccine (as adsorbed diphtheria [low dose], tetanus, pertussis (acellular, component) and poliomyelitis (inactivated) vaccine; *Boostrix-IPV®*) between 28 to 38 weeks of pregnancy; the optimal time for vaccination is between 28–32 weeks of pregnancy. Pregnant women should be offered a single dose of acellular pertussis-containing vaccine up to the onset of labour if they missed the opportunity for vaccination at 28–38 weeks of pregnancy. A single dose of acellular pertussis-containing vaccine may also be offered to new mothers, who have never previously been vaccinated against pertussis, until the child receives the first vaccination.

While this programme is in place, women who become pregnant again should be offered vaccination during each pregnancy to maximise transplacental transfer of antibody.

Contacts

Vaccination against pertussis should be considered for close contacts of cases with pertussis who have been offered antibacterial prophylaxis. Unimmunised or partially immunised contacts under 10 years of age should complete their vaccination against pertussis. A booster dose of an acellular pertussis-containing vaccine is recommended for contacts aged over 10 years who have not received a pertussis-containing vaccine in the last 5 years and who have not received adsorbed diphtheria [low dose], tetanus, and poliomyelitis (inactivated) vaccine in the last month.

Side-effects

Local reactions do not contra-indicate further doses.

The vaccine should not be withheld from children with a history to a preceding dose of:

- fever, irrespective of severity;
- persistent crying or screaming for more than 3 hours;
- severe local reaction, irrespective of extent.

Pneumococcal vaccine

Pneumococcal polysaccharide conjugate vaccine (adsorbed) p. 1152 protects against infection with *Streptococcus pneumoniae* (pneumococcus); the vaccines contain polysaccharide from capsular pneumococci. **Pneumococcal polysaccharide vaccine** contains purified polysaccharide from 23 capsular types of pneumococci, whereas **pneumococcal polysaccharide conjugate vaccine (adsorbed)** contains polysaccharide from either 10 capsular types (*Synflorix®*) or 13 capsular types (*Prevenar* 13®) and the polysaccharide is conjugated to protein.

The 13-valent conjugate vaccine (*Prevenar* 13®) is used in the childhood immunisation schedule. The recommended schedule consists of 3 doses, the first at 2 months of age, the second at 4 months, and the third at 12–13 months (see Immunisation Schedule).

Pneumococcal polysaccharide conjugate vaccine (adsorbed) is recommended for individuals at increased risk of pneumococcal infection as follows:

- age over 65 years;
- asplenia or splenic dysfunction (including homozygous sickle cell disease and coeliac disease which could lead to splenic dysfunction);
- chronic respiratory disease (includes asthma treated with continuous or frequent use of a systemic corticosteroid);
- chronic heart disease;
- chronic renal disease;
- chronic liver disease;
- chronic neurological conditions;
- complement disorders;

- diabetes mellitus requiring insulin or oral hypoglycaemic drugs;
- immune deficiency because of disease (e.g. HIV infection) or treatment (including prolonged systemic corticosteroid treatment for over 1 month at dose equivalents of prednisolone: *adult and child over* 20 *kg*, 20 mg or more daily; *child under* 20 *kg*, 1 mg/kg or more daily);
- presence of cochlear implant;
- conditions where leakage of cerebrospinal fluid may occur;
- child under 5 years with a history of invasive pneumococcal disease;
- at risk of occupational exposure to metal fume (e.g. welders).

Where possible, the vaccine should be given at least 2 weeks before splenectomy, cochlear implant surgery, chemotherapy, or radiotherapy; patients should be given advice about increased risk of pneumococcal infection. If it is not practical to vaccinate at least 2 weeks before splenectomy, chemotherapy, or radiotherapy, the vaccine should be given at least 2 weeks after the splenectomy or, where possible, at least 3 months after completion of chemotherapy or radiotherapy. Prophylactic antibacterial therapy against pneumococcal infection should not be stopped after immunisation. A patient card and information leaflet for patients with asplenia are available from the Department of Health or in Scotland from the Scottish Government, Health Protection Division (Tel (0131) 244 2879).

Choice of vaccine
Children under 2 years at increased risk of pneumococcal infection (see list) should receive the 13-valent pneumococcal polysaccharide conjugate vaccine (adsorbed) at the recommended ages, followed by a single dose of the 23-valent pneumococcal polysaccharide vaccine after their second birthday. Children at increased risk of pneumococcal infection presenting late for vaccination should receive 2 doses (separated by at least 1 month) of the 13-valent pneumococcal polysaccharide conjugate vaccine (adsorbed) before the age of 12 months, and a third dose at 12–13 months. Children over 12 months and under 5 years (who have not been vaccinated or not completed the primary course) should receive a single dose of the 13-valent pneumococcal polysaccharide conjugate vaccine (adsorbed) (2 doses separated by an interval of 2 months in the immunocompromised or those with asplenia or splenic dysfunction). All children under 5 years at increased risk of pneumococcal infection should receive a single dose of the 23-valent pneumococcal polysaccharide vaccine after their second birthday and at least 2 months after the final dose of the 13-valent pneumococcal polysaccharide conjugate vaccine (adsorbed).

Children over 5 years and adults who are at increased risk of pneumococcal disease should receive a single dose of the 23-valent unconjugated pneumococcal polysaccharide vaccine.

Revaccination
In individuals with higher concentrations of antibodies to pneumococcal polysaccharides, revaccination with the 23-valent pneumococcal polysaccharide vaccine more commonly produces adverse reactions. Revaccination is therefore not recommended, except every 5 years in individuals in whom the antibody concentration is likely to decline rapidly (e.g. asplenia, splenic dysfunction and nephrotic syndrome). If there is doubt, the need for revaccination should be discussed with a haematologist, immunologist, or microbiologist.

Poliomyelitis vaccine
Two types of poliomyelitis vaccines (containing strains of poliovirus types 1, 2, and 3) are available, inactivated poliomyelitis vaccine (for injection) and live (oral) poliomyelitis vaccine. **Inactivated** poliomyelitis vaccines, only available in combined preparation, is recommended for routine immunisation.

A course of primary immunisation consists of 3 doses of a combined preparation containing inactivated poliomyelitis vaccines, starting at 2 months of age with intervals of 1 month between doses (see Immunisation schedule). A course of 3 doses should also be given to all unimmunised adults; no adult should remain unimmunised against poliomyelitis.

Two booster doses of a preparation containing inactivated poliomyelitis vaccines are recommended, the first before school entry and the second before leaving school (see Immunisation schedule). Further booster doses are only necessary for adults at special risk, such as travellers to endemic areas, or laboratory staff likely to be exposed to the viruses, or healthcare workers in possible contact with cases; booster doses should be given to such individuals every 10 years.

Live (oral) poliomyelitis vaccine is no longer available for routine use; its use may be considered during large outbreaks, but advice should be sought from Public Health England. The live (oral) vaccine poses a very rare risk of vaccine-associated paralytic polio because the attenuated strain of the virus can revert to a virulent form. For this reason the live (oral) vaccine must **not** be used for immunosuppressed individuals or their household contacts. The use of inactivated poliomyelitis vaccines removes the risk of vaccine-associated paralytic polio altogether.

Travel
Unimmunised travellers to areas with a high incidence of poliomyelitis should receive a full 3-dose course of a preparation containing inactivated poliomyelitis vaccines. Those who have not been vaccinated in the last 10 years should receive a booster dose of **adsorbed diphtheria [low dose], tetanus and poliomyelitis (inactivated) vaccine**. Information about countries with a high incidence of poliomyelitis can be obtained from www.travax.nhs.uk or from the National Travel Health Network and Centre (www.nathnac.org).

Rabies vaccine
Rabies vaccine p. 1160 contains inactivated rabies virus cultivated in either human diploid cells or purified chick embryo cells; vaccines are used for pre- and post-exposure prophylaxis.

Pre-exposure prophylaxis
Immunisation should be offered to those at high risk of exposure to rabies— laboratory staff who handle the rabies virus, those working in quarantine stations, animal handlers, veterinary surgeons and field workers who are likely to be bitten by infected wild animals, certain port officials, and bat handlers. Transmission of rabies by humans has not been recorded but it is advised that those caring for patients with the disease should be vaccinated.

Immunisation against rabies is also recommended where there is limited access to prompt medical care for those living in areas where rabies is enzootic, for those travelling to such areas for longer than 1 month, and for those on shorter visits who may be exposed to unusual risk.

Immunisation against rabies is indicated during pregnancy if there is substantial risk of exposure to rabies and rapid access to post-exposure prophylaxis is likely to be limited.

Up-to-date country-by-country information on the incidence of rabies can be obtained from the National Travel Health Network and Centre (www.nathnac.org) and, in Scotland, from Health Protection Scotland (www.hps.scot.nhs.uk).

Immunisation against rabies requires 3 doses of rabies vaccine, with further booster doses for those who remain at frequent risk. To ensure continued protection in persons at high risk (e.g. laboratory workers), the concentration of antirabies antibodies in plasma is used to determine the intervals between doses.

Post-exposure management

Following potential exposure to rabies, the wound or site of exposure (e.g. mucous membrane) should be cleansed under running water and washed for several minutes with soapy water as soon as possible after exposure. Disinfectant and a simple dressing can be applied, but suturing should be delayed because it may increase the risk of introducing rabies virus into the nerves.

Post-exposure prophylaxis against rabies depends on the level of risk in the country, the nature of exposure, and the individual's immunity. In each case, expert risk assessment and advice on appropriate management should be obtained from the local Public Health England Centre or Public Health England's Virus Reference Department, Colindale (tel. (020) 8200 4400) or the PHE Colindale Duty Doctor (tel. (020) 8200 6868), in Wales from the Public Health Wales local Health Protection Team or Public Health Wales Virus Reference Laboratory (tel. (029) 2074 7747), in Scotland from the local on-call infectious diseases consultant, and in Northern Ireland from the Public Health Agency Duty Room (tel (028) 9055 3997/(028) 9063 2662) or the Regional Virology Service (tel. (028) 9024 0503).

There are no specific contra-indications to the use of rabies vaccine for post-exposure prophylaxis and its use should be considered whenever a patient has been attacked by an animal in a country where rabies is enzootic, even if there is no direct evidence of rabies in the attacking animal. Because of the potential consequences of untreated rabies exposure and because rabies vaccination has not been associated with fetal abnormalities, pregnancy is not considered a contra-indication to post-exposure prophylaxis.

For post-exposure prophylaxis of *fully immunised* individuals (who have previously received pre-exposure or post-exposure prophylaxis with cell-derived rabies vaccine), 2 doses of cell-derived vaccine are likely to be sufficient; the first dose is given on day 0 and the second dose is given between day 3–7. Rabies immunoglobulin p. 1133 is not necessary in such cases.

Post-exposure treatment for *unimmunised individuals* (or those whose prophylaxis is possibly incomplete) comprises 5 doses of rabies vaccine given over 1 month (on days 0, 3, 7, 14, and the fifth dose is given between day 28–30); also, depending on the level of risk (determined by factors such as the nature of the bite and the country where it was sustained), rabies immunoglobulin p. 1133 is given to unimmunised individuals on day 0 or within 7 days of starting the course of rabies vaccine p. 1160. The immunisation course can be discontinued if it is proved that the individual was not at risk.

Rotavirus vaccine

Rotavirus vaccine p. 1160 is a live, oral vaccine that protects young children against gastro-enteritis caused by rotavirus infection. The recommended schedule consists of 2 doses, the first at 2 months of age, and the second at 3 months of age (see Immunisation schedule). The first dose of rotavirus vaccine must be given between 6–15 weeks of age and the second dose should be given after an interval of at least 4 weeks; the vaccine should not be started in children 15 weeks of age or older. Ideally, the full course should be completed before 16 weeks of age to provide protection before the main burden of disease, and to avoid a temporal association between vaccination and intussusception; the course must be completed before 24 weeks of age.

The rotavirus vaccine virus is excreted in the stool and may be transmitted to close contacts; however, vaccination of those with *immunosuppressed* close contacts may protect the contacts from wild-type rotavirus disease and outweigh any risk from transmission of vaccine virus. Carers of a

recently vaccinated baby should be advised of the need to wash their hands after changing the baby's nappies.

Smallpox vaccine

Limited supplies of **smallpox vaccine** are held at the Specialist and Reference Microbiology Division, Public Health England Colindale (Tel. (020) 8200 4400) for the exclusive use of workers in laboratories where pox viruses (such as vaccinia) are handled.

If a wider use of the vaccine is being considered, *Guidelines for smallpox response and management in the post-eradication era* should be consulted at www.gov.uk/phe.

Tetanus vaccine

Tetanus vaccine contains a cell-free purified toxin of *Clostridium tetani* adsorbed on aluminium hydroxide or aluminium phosphate to improve antigenicity.

Primary immunisation for children under 10 years consists of 3 doses of a combined preparation containing adsorbed tetanus vaccine, with an interval of 1 month between doses. Following routine childhood vaccination, 2 booster doses of a preparation containing adsorbed tetanus vaccine are recommended, the first before school entry and the second before leaving school (see Immunisation schedule).

The recommended schedule of tetanus vaccination not only gives protection against tetanus in childhood but also gives the basic immunity for subsequent booster doses. In most circumstances, a total of 5 doses of tetanus vaccine is considered sufficient for long term protection.

For primary immunisation of adults and children over 10 years previously unimmunised against tetanus, 3 doses of **adsorbed diphtheria [low dose], tetanus and poliomyelitis (inactivated) vaccine** are given with an interval of 1 month between doses (see Diphtheria-containing Vaccines).

When an individual presents for a booster dose but has been vaccinated following a tetanus-prone wound, the vaccine preparation administered at the time of injury should be determined. If this is not possible, the booster should still be given to ensure adequate protection against all antigens in the booster vaccine.

Very rarely, tetanus has developed after abdominal surgery; patients awaiting elective surgery should be asked about tetanus immunisation and immunised if necessary.

Parenteral drug abuse is also associated with tetanus; those abusing drugs by injection should be vaccinated if unimmunised—booster doses should be given if there is any doubt about their immunisation status.

All laboratory staff should be offered a primary course if unimmunised.

Wounds

Wounds are considered to be tetanus-prone if they are sustained more than 6 hours before surgical treatment or at any interval after injury and are puncture-type (particularly if contaminated with soil or manure) *or* show much devitalised tissue *or* are septic *or* are compound fractures *or* contain foreign bodies. All wounds should receive thorough cleansing.

- For *clean wounds*: fully immunised individuals (those who have received a total of 5 doses of a tetanus-containing vaccine at appropriate intervals) and those whose primary immunisation is complete (with boosters up to date), do not require tetanus vaccine; individuals whose primary immunisation is incomplete or whose boosters are not up to date require a reinforcing dose of a tetanus-containing vaccine (followed by further doses as required to complete the schedule); non-immunised individuals (or those whose immunisation status is not known or who have been fully immunised but are now immunocompromised) should be given a dose of the appropriate tetanus-containing vaccine immediately (followed by completion of the full course of the vaccine if records confirm the need)
- For *tetanus-prone wounds*: management is as for clean

wounds with the addition of a dose of tetanus immunoglobulin given at a different site; in fully immunised individuals and those whose primary immunisation is complete (with boosters up to date) the immunoglobulin is needed only if the risk of infection is especially high (e.g. contamination with manure). Antibacterial prophylaxis (with benzylpenicillin, co-amoxiclav, or metronidazole) may also be required for tetanus-prone wounds.

Tick-borne encephalitis vaccine

Tick-borne encephalitis vaccine, inactivated p. 1161 contains inactivated tick-borne encephalitis virus cultivated in chick embryo cells. It is recommended for immunisation of those working in, or visiting, high-risk areas (see International Travel). Those working, walking or camping in warm forested areas of Central and Eastern Europe, Scandinavia, Northern and Eastern China, and some parts of Japan, particularly from April to November when ticks are most prevalent, are at greatest risk of tick-borne encephalitis. For full protection, 3 doses of the vaccine are required; booster doses are required every 3–5 years for those still at risk. Ideally, immunisation should be completed at least one month before travel.

Typhoid vaccine

Typhoid vaccine p. 1152 is available as Vi capsular polysaccharide (from *Salmonella typhi*) vaccine for injection and as live attenuated *Salmonella typhi* for oral use.
    Typhoid immunisation is advised for:
* travellers to areas where typhoid is endemic, especially if staying in or visiting local people;
* travellers to endemic areas where frequent or prolonged exposure to poor sanitation and poor food hygiene is likely
* laboratory personnel who, in the course of their work, may be exposed to *Salmonella typhi*.

Typhoid vaccination is not a substitute for scrupulous personal hygiene.
    Capsular **polysaccharide** typhoid vaccine is usually given by *intramuscular injection*. Children under 2 years may respond suboptimally to the vaccine, but children aged between 1–2 years should be immunised if the risk of typhoid fever is considered high (immunisation is not recommended for infants under 12 months). Revaccination is needed every 3 years on continued exposure.
    Oral typhoid vaccine p. 1152 is a **live attenuated** vaccine contained in an enteric-coated capsule. One capsule taken on alternate days for a total of 3 doses, provides protection 7–10 days after the last dose. Protection may persist for up to 3 years in those constantly (or repeatedly) exposed to *Salmonella typhi*, but those who only occasionally travel to endemic areas require further courses at intervals of 1 year.

Varicella-zoster vaccine

The live varicella-zoster vaccine, *Varilrix*® and *Varivax*®, p. 1161 are licensed for immunisation against varicella (chickenpox) in seronegative individuals. They are not recommended for routine use in children, but can be given to seronegative healthy children over 1 year who come into close contact with individuals at high risk of severe varicella infections. The Department of Health recommends these vaccines for seronegative healthcare workers who come into direct contact with patients. Those with a history of chickenpox or shingles can be considered immune, but healthcare workers with a negative or uncertain history should be tested.
    Rarely, the varicella-zoster vaccine virus has been transmitted from the vaccinated individual to close contacts. Therefore, contact with the following should be avoided if a vaccine-related cutaneous rash develops within 4–6 weeks of the first or second dose:

* varicella-susceptible pregnant women;
* individuals at high risk of severe varicella, including those with immunodeficiency or those receiving immunosuppressive therapy;

Healthcare workers who develop a generalised papular or vesicular rash on vaccination should avoid contact with patients until the lesions have crusted. Those who develop a localised rash after vaccination should cover the lesions and be allowed to continue working unless in contact with patients at high risk of severe varicella.
    The high potency, live varicella-zoster vaccine, *Zostavax*®, is recommended for the prevention of *herpes zoster* (shingles) in adults who are, or were, 70 years of age on 1 September 2014. The 2014-15, catch-up programme with *Zostavax*® will be offered to all who are, or were, 78 or 79 years of age on 1 September 2014. A single dose of *Zostavax*® is likely to give protection for at least 7 years, but the need for, or timing of, a booster dose has not been established. Although *Zostavax*® is not recommended for the treatment of shingles or post-herpetic neuralgia, it can be given to those with a previous history of shingles; ideally the vaccine should be delayed until systemic antiviral therapy has been completed.
    Varicella-zoster immunoglobulin p. 1134 is used to protect susceptible individuals at increased risk of varicella infection.

Yellow fever vaccine

Yellow fever vaccine, live p. 1162 is indicated for those travelling or living in areas where infection is endemic and for laboratory staff who handle the virus or who handle clinical material from suspected cases. Infants under 6 months of age should not be vaccinated because there is a small risk of encephalitis; infants aged 6–9 months should be vaccinated only if the risk of yellow fever is high and unavoidable (seek expert advice). The immunity which probably lasts for life is officially accepted for 10 years starting from 10 days after primary immunisation and for a further 10 years immediately after revaccination.

Vaccines for travel

Immunisation

See advice on Malaria, treatment p. 557.
    No special immunisation is required for travellers to the United States, Europe, Australia, or New Zealand, although all travellers should have immunity to tetanus and poliomyelitis (and childhood immunisations should be up to date); Tick-borne encephalitis vaccine is recommended for immunisation of those working in, or visiting, high-risk areas. Certain special precautions are required in non-European areas surrounding the Mediterranean, in Africa, the Middle East, Asia, and South America.
    Travellers to areas that have a high incidence of **poliomyelitis** or **tuberculosis** should be immunised with the appropriate vaccine; in the case of poliomyelitis previously immunised travellers may be given a booster dose of a preparation containing inactivated poliomyelitis vaccine. BCG immunisation is recommended for travellers aged under 16 years proposing to stay for longer than 3 months (or in close contact with the local population) in countries with an incidence of tuberculosis greater than 40 per 100 000 (list of countries where the incidence of tuberculosis is greater than 40 cases per 100 000 is available from www.gov.uk/phe); it should preferably be given 3 months or more before departure.
    Yellow fever immunisation is recommended for travel to the endemic zones of Africa and South America. Many countries require an International Certificate of Vaccination from individuals arriving from, or who have been travelling

14

Vaccines

through, endemic areas; other countries require a certificate from all entering travellers (consult the Department of Health handbook, *Health Information for Overseas Travel*, www.dh.gov.uk).

Immunisation against **meningococcal meningitis** is recommended for a number of areas of the world.

Protection against **hepatitis A** is recommended for travellers to high-risk areas outside Northern and Western Europe, North America, Japan, Australia and New Zealand. Hepatitis A vaccine is preferred and it is likely to be effective even if given shortly before departure; normal immunoglobulin is no longer given routinely but may be indicated in the immunocompromised. Special care must also be taken with food hygiene.

Hepatitis B vaccine is recommended for those travelling to areas of high or intermediate prevalence who intend to seek employment as healthcare workers or who plan to remain there for lengthy periods and who may therefore be at increased risk of acquiring infection as the result of medical or dental procedures carried out in those countries. Short-term tourists or business travellers are not generally at increased risk of infection but may put themselves at risk by their sexual behaviour when abroad.

Prophylactic immunisation against **rabies** is recommended for travellers to enzootic areas on long journeys or to areas out of reach of immediate medical attention.

Travellers who have not had a **tetanus** booster in the last 10 years and are visiting areas where medical attention may not be accessible should receive a booster dose of adsorbed diphtheria [low dose], tetanus and poliomyelitis (inactivated) vaccine, even if they have received 5 doses of a tetanus-containing vaccine previously.

Typhoid vaccine is indicated for travellers to countries where typhoid is endemic, but the vaccine is no substitute for personal precautions.

There is no requirement for cholera vaccination as a condition for entry into any country, but **oral cholera vaccine** should be considered for backpackers and those travelling to situations where the risk is greatest (e.g. refugee camps). Regardless of vaccination, travellers to areas where cholera is endemic should take special care with food hygiene.

Advice on **diphtheria**, on **Japanese encephalitis**, and on **tick-borne encephalitis** is included in *Health Information for Overseas Travel*.

Food hygiene

In areas where sanitation is poor, good food hygiene is important to help prevent hepatitis A, typhoid, cholera, and other diarrhoeal diseases (including travellers' diarrhoea). Food should be freshly prepared and hot, and uncooked vegetables (including green salads) should be avoided; only fruits which can be peeled should be eaten. Only suitable bottled water, or tap water that has been boiled or treated with sterilising tablets, should be used for drinking.

Information on health advice for travellers

Health professionals and travellers can find the latest information on immunisation requirements and precautions for avoiding disease while travelling from: www.nathnac.org.

The handbook, *Health Information for Overseas Travel* (2010), which draws together essential information *for healthcare professionals* regarding health advice for travellers, can also be obtained from this website.

Immunisation requirements change from time to time, and information on the current requirements for any particular country may be obtained from the embassy or legation of the appropriate country or from:

National Travel Health Network and Centre
UCLH NHS Foundation Trust
3rd Floor Central,
250 Euston Road,
London, NW1 2PG
Tel: 0845 602 6712
(8:30–11:45 a.m, 1–3:15 p.m. weekdays for healthcare professionals **only**)
www.nathnac.org

Travel Medicine Team
Health Protection Scotland
Meridian Court,
5 Cadogan Street,
Glasgow, G2 6QE
Tel: (0141) 300 1130
(2–4 p.m. Monday to Wednesday, 9:30–11:30 a.m. Friday; for registered TRAVAX users **only**)
www.travax.nhs.uk

(free for NHS Scotland users, registration required; subscription fee may be payable for users outside NHS Scotland)

Welsh Assembly Government
Tel (029) 2082 5397
(9 a.m.–5:30 p.m. weekdays)

Department of Health, Social Services and Public Safety
Castle Buildings,
Stormont,
Belfast, BT4 3SQ
Tel: (028) 9052 2118
(9 a.m.–5. p.m. weekdays)
www.dhsspsni.gov.uk

VACCINES

Vaccines

> **IMPORTANT SAFETY INFORMATION**
> MHRA/CHM ADVICE (APRIL 2016)
> Following reports of death in neonates who received a live attenuated vaccine after exposure to a tumor necrosis factor alpha (TNF-a) inhibitor in utero, the MHRA has issued the following advice:
> - any infant who has been exposed to immunosuppressive treatment from the mother either in utero during pregnancy or via breastfeeding should have any live attenuated vaccination deferred for as long as a postnatal influence on the immune status of the infant remains possible;
> - in the case of infants who have been exposed to TNF-a inhibitors and other biological medicines in utero, any live attenuated vaccination should be deferred until the infant is age 6 months, after which time vaccination should be considered.

● CONTRA-INDICATIONS

CONTRA-INDICATIONS, FURTHER INFORMATION

▸ Impaired immune response Severely immunosuppressed patients should not be given live vaccines (including those with severe primary immunodeficiency).

● CAUTIONS Acute illness · minor illnesses

CAUTIONS, FURTHER INFORMATION

Vaccination may be postponed if the individual is suffering from an acute illness; however, it is not necessary to postpone immunisation in patients with minor illnesses without fever or systemic upset.

▸ Impaired immune response and drugs affecting immune response Immune response to vaccines may be reduced in immunosuppressed patients and there is also a risk of generalised infection with live vaccines.

Specialist advice should be sought for those being treated with high doses of corticosteroids (dose equivalents of prednisolone: **adults**, at least 40 mg daily for more than 1 week; **children**, 2 mg/kg (or more than 40 mg) daily for at least 1 week or 1 mg/kg daily for 1 month), or other immunosuppressive drugs, and those being treated for malignant conditions with chemotherapy or generalised radiotherapy. Live vaccines should be postponed until at least 3 months after stopping high-dose systemic corticosteroids and at least 6 months after stopping other immunosuppressive drugs or generalised radiotherapy (at least 12 months after discontinuing immunosuppressants following bone-marrow transplantation).

The Royal College of Paediatrics and Child Health has produced a statement, *Immunisation of the Immunocompromised Child* (2002) (available at www.rcpch.ac.uk).

▹ Predisposition to neurological problems When there is a personal or family history of *febrile* convulsions, there is an increased risk of these occurring during fever from any cause including immunisation, but this is not a contra-indication to immunisation. In children who have had a seizure associated with fever without neurological deterioration, immunisation is *recommended*; advice on the *management of fever* (see Post-immunisation Pyrexia in Infants) should be given before immunisation. When a child has had a convulsion not associated with fever, and the neurological condition is not deteriorating, immunisation is *recommended*.

Children with stable neurological disorders (e.g. spina bifida, congenital brain abnormality, and peri-natal hypoxic-ischaemic encephalopathy) should be immunised according to the recommended schedule.

When there is a *still evolving neurological problem*, including poorly controlled epilepsy, immunisation should be deferred and the child referred to a specialist. Immunisation is recommended if a cause for the neurological disorder is identified. If a cause is not identified, immunisation should be deferred until the condition is stable.

● INTERACTIONS → Appendix 1 (vaccines).

● SIDE-EFFECTS

SIDE-EFFECTS

GENERAL SIDE-EFFECTS

▹ **Common or very common** Fatigue · fever · gastro-intestinal disturbances · headache · irritability · loss of appetite · lymphangitis · malaise · myalgia

▹ **Very rare** Anaphylaxis (can be fatal) · angioedema (can be fatal) · bronchospasm (can be fatal) · hypersensitivity reactions (can be fatal) · urticaria (can be fatal)

▹ **Frequency not known** Arthralgia · asthenia · dizziness · drowsiness · influenza-like symptoms · lymphadenopathy · paraesthesia · rash

SPECIFIC SIDE-EFFECTS

▹ **Common or very common**

▹ **With intradermal or intramuscular or subcutaneous use** Induration may develop at the injection site · inflammation · local reactions · pain · redness · sterile abscess may develop at the injection site

SIDE-EFFECTS, FURTHER INFORMATION

Occasionally serious adverse reactions can occur—these should always be reported to the CHM.

▹ Post-immunisation pyrexia in infants The parent should be advised that if pyrexia develops after childhood immunisation, and the infant seems distressed, paracetamol can be given. Ibuprofen can be used if paracetamol is unsuitable. The parent should be warned to seek medical advice if the pyrexia persists.

● ALLERGY AND CROSS-SENSITIVITY Contra-indicated in patients with a confirmed anaphylactic reaction to a preceding dose of a vaccine containing the same antigens or vaccine component (such as antibacterials in viral vaccines).

● PREGNANCY Live vaccines should not be administered routinely to pregnant women because of the theoretical risk of fetal infection but where there is a significant risk of exposure to disease, the need for vaccination usually outweighs any possible risk to the fetus. Termination of pregnancy following inadvertent immunisation is not recommended. There is no evidence of risk from vaccinating pregnant women with inactivated viral or bacterial vaccines or toxoids.

● BREAST FEEDING Although there is a theoretical risk of live vaccine being present in breast milk, vaccination is not contra-indicated for women who are breast-feeding when there is significant risk of exposure to disease. There is no evidence of risk from vaccinating women who are breast-feeding, with inactivated viral or bacterial vaccines or toxoids.

● DIRECTIONS FOR ADMINISTRATION If alcohol or disinfectant is used for cleansing the skin it should be allowed to evaporate before vaccination to prevent possible inactivation of live vaccines.

When 2 or more live vaccines are required (and are not available as a combined preparation), they can be administered at any time before or after each other at different sites, preferably in a different limb; if more than one injection is to be given in the same limb, they should be administered at least 2.5 cm apart. See also Bacillus Calmette-Guérin vaccine p. 1149.

Vaccines should not be given intravenously. Most vaccines are given by the intramuscular route, although some are given by either the intradermal, deep subcutaneous, or oral route. The intramuscular route should not be used in patients with **bleeding disorders** such as haemophilia or thrombocytopenia, vaccines usually given by the intramuscular route should be given by deep subcutaneous injection instead.

The Department of Health has advised *against the use of jet guns* for vaccination owing to the risk of transmitting blood borne infections, such as HIV.

Particular attention must be paid to instructions on the use of diluents. Vaccines which are liquid suspensions or are reconstituted before use should be adequately mixed to ensure uniformity of the material to be injected.

● HANDLING AND STORAGE Care must be taken to store all vaccines under the conditions recommended in the product literature, otherwise the preparation may become ineffective. **Refrigerated storage** is usually necessary; many vaccines need to be stored at 2–8°C and not allowed to freeze. Vaccines should be protected from light. Reconstituted vaccines and opened multidose vials must be used within the period recommended in the product literature. Unused vaccines should be disposed of by incineration at a registered disposal contractor.

VACCINES › BACTERIAL AND VIRAL VACCINES, COMBINED

F 1146

Diphtheria with haemophilus influenzae type b vaccine, pertussis, poliomyelitis and tetanus

● INDICATIONS AND DOSE

Primary immunisation

▸ BY INTRAMUSCULAR INJECTION

▹ Child 2 months-10 years: 0.5 mL every 1 month for 3 doses

● UNLICENSED USE *Infanrix-IPV + Hib* ® not licensed for use in children over 36 months; *Pediacel* ® not licensed in

14

Vaccines

children over 4 years. However, the Department of Health recommends that these be used for children up to 10 years.

- SIDE-EFFECTS Atopic dermatitis · hypotonia · restlessness · sleep disturbances · unusual crying in infants

  SIDE-EFFECTS, FURTHER INFORMATION
  ► Side effects of vaccines containing pertussis The incidence of local and systemic effects is generally lower with vaccines containing acellular pertussis components than with the whole-cell pertussis vaccine used previously. However, compared with primary vaccination, booster doses with vaccines containing acellular pertussis are reported to increase the risk of injection-site reactions (some of which affect the entire limb); local reactions do not contra-indicate further doses.

  The vaccine should not be withheld from children with a history to a preceding dose of:
  - fever, irrespective of severity;
  - persistent crying or screaming for more than 3 hours;
  - severe local reaction, irrespective of extent.

- PRESCRIBING AND DISPENSING INFORMATION Available as part of childhood schedule from health organisations or ImmForm.

- MEDICINAL FORMS
  There can be variation in the licensing of different medicines containing the same drug.
  Suspension for injection
  EXCIPIENTS: May contain Neomycin, polymyxin b, streptomycin
  ► Pediacel (sanofi pasteur MSD Ltd)
  Pediacel vaccine suspension for injection 0.5ml vials | 1 vial [PoM] £32.00
  Powder and suspension for suspension for injection
  ► Infanrix-IPV + Hib (GlaxoSmithKline UK Ltd)
  Infanrix-IPV + Hib vaccine powder and suspension for suspension for injection 0.5ml pre-filled syringes | 1 pre-filled disposable injection [PoM] £27.86

F 1146

Diphtheria with pertussis, poliomyelitis vaccine and tetanus

- INDICATIONS AND DOSE
  First booster dose
  ► BY INTRAMUSCULAR INJECTION
  ► Child 3–9 years: 0.5 mL, to be given 3 years after primary immunisation
  Vaccination of pregnant women against pertussis (using low dose vaccines)
  ► BY INTRAMUSCULAR INJECTION
  ► Females of childbearing potential: 0.5 mL for 1 dose

- SIDE-EFFECTS Restlessness · sleep disturbances · unusual crying in infants

  SIDE-EFFECTS, FURTHER INFORMATION
  ► Side effects of vaccines containing pertussis The incidence of local and systemic effects is generally lower with vaccines containing acellular pertussis components than with the whole-cell pertussis vaccine used previously. However, compared with primary vaccination, booster doses with vaccines containing acellular pertussis are reported to increase the risk of injection-site reactions (some of which affect the entire limb); local reactions do not contra-indicate further doses.

  The vaccine should not be withheld from children with a history to a preceding dose of:
  - fever, irrespective of severity;
  - persistent crying or screaming for more than 3 hours;
  - severe local reaction, irrespective of extent.

- PREGNANCY Contra-indicated in pregnant women with a history of encephalopathy of unknown origin within 7 days of previous immunisation with a pertussis-containing vaccine. Contra-indicated in pregnant women with a

history of transient thrombocytopenia or neurological complications following previous immunisation against diphtheria or tetanus.

- PRESCRIBING AND DISPENSING INFORMATION Pregnant women should be vaccinated using low dose vaccines (brands may include *Boostrix-IPV*® or *Repevax*®).

  Available as part of childhood immunisation schedule from health organisations or ImmForm.

  Available for vaccination of pregnant women from ImmForm.

- MEDICINAL FORMS
  There can be variation in the licensing of different medicines containing the same drug.
  Suspension for injection
  EXCIPIENTS: May contain Neomycin, polymyxin b, streptomycin
  ► Boostrix-IPV (GlaxoSmithKline UK Ltd)
  Boostrix-IPV suspension for injection 0.5ml pre-filled syringes | 1 pre-filled disposable injection [PoM] £22.74
  ► Infanrix-IPV (GlaxoSmithKline UK Ltd)
  Infanrix-IPV vaccine suspension for injection 0.5ml pre-filled syringes | 1 pre-filled disposable injection [PoM] £17.56
  ► Repevax (sanofi pasteur MSD Ltd)
  Repevax vaccine suspension for injection 0.5ml pre-filled syringes | 1 pre-filled disposable injection [PoM] £20.00

F 1146

Diphtheria with poliomyelitis and tetanus vaccine

- INDICATIONS AND DOSE
  Primary immunisation
  ► BY INTRAMUSCULAR INJECTION
  ► Child 10–17 years: 0.5 mL every 1 month for 3 doses
  ► Adult: 0.5 mL every 1 month for 3 doses
  Booster doses
  ► BY INTRAMUSCULAR INJECTION
  ► Child 10–17 years: 0.5 mL for 1 dose, first booster dose—should be given 3 years after primary course (this interval can be reduced to a minimum of 1 year if the primary course was delayed), then 0.5 mL for 1 dose, second booster dose—should be given 10 years after first booster dose (this interval can be reduced to a minimum of 5 years if previous doses were delayed), second booster dose may also be used as first booster dose in those over 10 years who have received only 3 previous doses of a diphtheria-containing vaccine
  ► Adult: 0.5 mL for 1 dose, first booster dose—should be given 3 years after primary course (this interval can be reduced to a minimum of 1 year if the primary course was delayed), then 0.5 mL for 1 dose, second booster dose—should be given 10 years after first booster dose (this interval can be reduced to a minimum of 5 years if previous doses were delayed), second booster dose may also be used as first booster dose in those over 10 years who have received only 3 previous doses of a diphtheria-containing vaccine

- SIDE-EFFECTS Restlessness · sleep disturbances · unusual crying in infants

- PRESCRIBING AND DISPENSING INFORMATION Available as part of childhood schedule from health organisations or ImmForm.

- MEDICINAL FORMS
  There can be variation in the licensing of different medicines containing the same drug.
  Suspension for injection
  EXCIPIENTS: May contain Neomycin, polymyxin b, streptomycin
  ► Revaxis (sanofi pasteur MSD Ltd)
  Revaxis vaccine suspension for injection 0.5ml pre-filled syringes | 1 pre-filled disposable injection [PoM] £6.50

VACCINES > BACTERIAL VACCINES

☞ 1146

Anthrax vaccine

● **INDICATIONS AND DOSE**

Pre-exposure immunisation against anthrax | Post-exposure immunisation

▸ BY INTRAMUSCULAR INJECTION

▸ Adult: Initially 1 dose every 3 weeks for 3 doses, followed by 1 dose after 6 months, to be administered in the deltoid region, 1 dose is equivalent to 0.5 mL

Booster

▸ BY INTRAMUSCULAR INJECTION

▸ Adult: 1 dose every 12 months, to be administered in deltoid region, 1 dose is equivalent to 0.5 mL

● PRESCRIBING AND DISPENSING INFORMATION Available from Public Health England's Centre for Emergency Preparedness and Response (Porton Down).

● MEDICINAL FORMS
There can be variation in the licensing of different medicines containing the same drug.
Suspension for injection
EXCIPIENTS: May contain Thiomersal
▸ Anthrax vaccine (Non-proprietary)
Anthrax vaccine (alum precipitated sterile filtrate) suspension for injection 0.5ml ampoules | 5 ampoule [PoM] no price available

☞ 1146

Bacillus Calmette-Guérin vaccine

(BCG Vaccine)

● DRUG ACTION BCG (Bacillus Calmette-Guérin) is a live attenuated strain derived from *Mycobacterium bovis* which stimulates the development of immunity to *M. tuberculosis*.

● **INDICATIONS AND DOSE**

Immunisation against tuberculosis

▸ BY INTRADERMAL INJECTION

▸ Child 1–11 months: 0.05 mL, to be injected at insertion of deltoid muscle onto humerus (keloid formation more likely with sites higher on arm); tip of shoulder should be **avoided**

▸ Child 1–17 years: 0.1 mL, to be injected at insertion of deltoid muscle onto humerus (keloid formation more likely with sites higher on arm); tip of shoulder should be **avoided**

▸ Adult: 0.1 mL, to be injected at insertion of deltoid muscle onto humerus (keloid formation more likely with sites higher on arm); tip of shoulder should be **avoided**

● CONTRA-INDICATIONS Generalised septic skin conditions · neonate in household contact with known or suspected case of active tuberculosis

CONTRA-INDICATIONS, FURTHER INFORMATION
A lesion-free site should be used to administer BCG vaccine to patients with eczema.

● CAUTIONS

CAUTIONS, FURTHER INFORMATION
BCG vaccine can be given simultaneously with another live vaccine, but if they are not given at the same time an interval of 4 weeks should normally be allowed. When BCG is given to infants, there is no need to delay routine primary immunisations. No further vaccination should be given in the arm used for BCG vaccination for at least 3 months because of the risk of regional lymphadenitis.

● SIDE-EFFECTS
▸ **Rare** Disseminated complications · osteitis · osteomyelitis
▸ **Frequency not known** Prolonged ulceration at the injection site · subcutaneous abscess at the injection site

● PRE-TREATMENT SCREENING Apart from children under 6 years, any person being considered for BCG immunisation must first be given a skin test for hypersensitivity to tuberculoprotein (see tuberculin purified protein derivative p. 1135). A skin test is not necessary for a child under 6 years provided that the child has not stayed for longer than 3 months in a country with an incidence of tuberculosis greater than 40 per 100 000, the child has not had contact with a person with tuberculosis, and there is no family history of tuberculosis within the last 5 years.

● DIRECTIONS FOR ADMINISTRATION
Intradermal injection technique Skin is stretched between thumb and forefinger and needle (size 25G or 26G) inserted (bevel upwards) for about 3 mm into superficial layers of dermis (almost parallel with surface). Needle should be short with short bevel (can usually be seen through epidermis during insertion). Tense raised blanched bleb showing tips of hair follicles is sign of correct injection; 7 mm bleb ≡ 0.1 mL injection, 3 mm bleb ≡ 0.05 mL injection; if considerable resistance not felt, needle too deep and should be removed and reinserted before giving more vaccine.

● PRESCRIBING AND DISPENSING INFORMATION Available from health organisations or direct from ImmForm www.immform.dh.gov.uk (SSI brand, multidose vial with diluent).

● MEDICINAL FORMS
There can be variation in the licensing of different medicines containing the same drug.
Powder and solvent for suspension for injection
▸ Bacillus calmette-guérin vaccine (Non-proprietary)
Bacillus Calmette-Guerin vaccine powder and solvent for suspension for injection vials | 10 vial [PoM] no price available

☞ 1146

Cholera vaccine

● **INDICATIONS AND DOSE**

Immunisation against cholera (for travellers to endemic or epidemic areas on the basis of current recommendations)

▸ BY MOUTH

▸ Child 2–5 years: 1 dose every 1–6 weeks for 3 doses, if more than 6 weeks have elapsed between doses, the primary course should be restarted, immunisation should be completed at least one week before potential exposure

▸ Child 6–17 years: 1 dose every 1–6 weeks for 2 doses, if more than 6 weeks have elapsed between doses, the primary course should be restarted, immunisation should be completed at least one week before potential exposure

▸ Adult: 1 dose every 1–6 weeks for 2 doses, if more than 6 weeks have elapsed between doses, the primary course should be restarted, immunisation should be completed at least one week before potential exposure

Booster

▸ BY MOUTH

▸ Child 2–5 years: A single booster dose can be given within 6 months after primary course, if more than 6 months have elapsed since the last vaccination, the primary course should be repeated

▸ Child 6–17 years: A single booster dose can be given within 2 years after primary course, if more than 2 years have elapsed since the last vaccination, the primary course should be repeated continued →

14

Vaccines

▸ **Adult:** A single booster dose can be given within 2 years after primary course, if more than 2 years have elapsed since the last vaccination, the primary course should be repeated

● CONTRA-INDICATIONS Acute gastro-intestinal illness
● SIDE-EFFECTS
▸ **Rare** Cough · respiratory symptoms · rhinitis
▸ **Very rare** Insomnia · sore throat
▸ **Frequency not known** Abdominal pain and cramps · diarrhoea · nausea · vomiting
● DIRECTIONS FOR ADMINISTRATION
▸ In children Dissolve effervescent sodium bicarbonate granules in a glassful of water *or* chlorinated water (approximately 150 mL). For children over 6 years, add vaccine suspension to make one dose. For child 2–5 years, discard half (approximately 75 mL) of the solution, then add vaccine suspension to make one dose. Drink within 2 hours. Food, drink, and other oral medicines should be avoided for 1 hour before and after vaccination.
▸ In adults Dissolve effervescent sodium bicarbonate granules in a glassful of water *or* chlorinated water (approximately 150 mL). Add vaccine suspension to make one dose. Drink within 2 hours. Food, drink, and other oral medicines should be avoided for 1 hour before and after vaccination.
● PATIENT AND CARER ADVICE Counselling on administration advised. Immunisation with cholera vaccine does not provide complete protection and all travellers to a country where cholera exists should be warned that scrupulous attention to food, water, and personal hygiene is **essential**.

● MEDICINAL FORMS
There can be variation in the licensing of different medicines containing the same drug.
Oral suspension
▸ Dukoral (Valneva UK Ltd)
Dukoral cholera vaccine oral suspension | 2 dose PoM £23.42

⌐ 1146

Haemophilus influenzae type B with meningococcal group C vaccine

● INDICATIONS AND DOSE
Booster dose (for infants who have received primary immunisation with a vaccine containing *Haemophilus influenzae* type b component)
▸ BY INTRAMUSCULAR INJECTION
▸ Child 12–13 months: 0.5 mL for 1 dose
Booster dose (for children who have not been immunised against *Haemophilus influenza* type b) | Booster dose after recovery from *Haemophilus influenzae* type b disease (for index cases previously vaccinated, with low Hib antibody concentration or if it is not possible to measure antibody concentration)
▸ BY INTRAMUSCULAR INJECTION
▸ Child 1–9 years: 0.5 mL for 1 dose
Booster dose after recovery from *Haemophilus influenzae* type b disease (for fully vaccinated index cases with asplenia or splenic dysfunction, if previous dose received over 1 year ago)
▸ BY INTRAMUSCULAR INJECTION
▸ Child 1–17 years: 0.5 mL for 1 dose
▸ Adult: 0.5 mL for 1 dose

Booster dose (for patients diagnosed with asplenia, splenic dysfunction or complement deficiency at under 2 years of age)
▸ BY INTRAMUSCULAR INJECTION
▸ Child 12–13 months: 0.5 mL for 1 dose, this booster dose should be followed 1 month later by one dose of meningococcal A, C, W135, and Y conjugate vaccine, followed by 0.5 mL for 1 dose, the second dose should be given after the second birthday
Booster dose (for patients diagnosed with asplenia, splenic dysfunction or complement deficiency at over 2 years of age)
▸ BY INTRAMUSCULAR INJECTION
▸ Child 2–17 years: 0.5 mL for 1 dose, this booster dose should be followed 1 month later by one dose of meningococcal A, C, W135, and Y conjugate vaccine
▸ Adult: 0.5 mL for 1 dose, this booster dose should be followed 1 month later by one dose of meningococcal A, C, W135, and Y conjugate vaccine

● UNLICENSED USE Not licensed for use in patients over 2 years.
● SIDE-EFFECTS
▸ **Rare** Symptoms of meningitis reported (but no evidence that the vaccine causes meningococcal C meningitis)
▸ **Frequency not known** Atopic dermatitis · hypotonia
● PRESCRIBING AND DISPENSING INFORMATION Available as part of the childhood immunisation schedule from ImmForm.

● MEDICINAL FORMS
There can be variation in the licensing of different medicines containing the same drug.
Powder and solvent for solution for injection
▸ Menitorix (GlaxoSmithKline UK Ltd)
Menitorix vaccine powder and solvent for solution for injection 0.5ml vials | 1 vial PoM £37.76

⌐ 1146

Meningococcal group B vaccine (rDNA, component, adsorbed)

● INDICATIONS AND DOSE
Immunisation against *Neisseria meningitidis*, primary immunisation
▸ BY DEEP INTRAMUSCULAR INJECTION
▸ Child 2 months: 0.5 mL for 1 dose, injected preferably into deltoid region (or anterolateral thigh in infants). Three doses of 60 mg prophylactic paracetamol should be given post primary meningococcal B immunisation, at 2 months and 4 months of age. Further information can be found at www.gov.uk.
▸ Child 4 months: 0.5 mL for 1 dose, injected preferably into deltoid region (or anterolateral thigh in infants). Three doses of 60 mg prophylactic paracetamol should be given post primary meningococcal B immunisation, at 2 months and 4 months of age. Further information can be found at www.gov.uk.
Immunisation against *Neisseria meningitidis*, primary immunisation booster dose
▸ BY DEEP INTRAMUSCULAR INJECTION
▸ Child 12–23 months: 0.5 mL for 1 dose, injected preferably into deltoid region (or anterolateral thigh in infants)
Immunisation against *Neisseria meningitidis*, primary immunisation (in unimmunised patients)
▸ BY DEEP INTRAMUSCULAR INJECTION
▸ Child 6–11 months: 0.5 mL for 2 doses, separated by an interval of at least 2 months; booster dose of 0.5 mL given between 1–2 years of age and at least 2 months after completion of primary immunisation, injected

preferably into deltoid region (or anterolateral thigh in infants)
- Child 12-23 months: 0.5 mL for 2 doses, separated by an interval of at least 2 months; booster dose of 0.5 mL given 12–24 months after completion of primary immunisation, injected preferably into deltoid region (or anterolateral thigh in infants)
- Child 2-10 years: 0.5 mL for 2 doses, separated by an interval of at least 2 months. Injected preferably into deltoid region (or anterolateral thigh in infants)
- Child 11-17 years: 0.5 mL for 2 doses, separated by an interval of at least 1 month. Injected preferably into deltoid region
- Adult: 0.5 mL for 2 doses, separated by an interval of at least 1 month. Injected preferably into deltoid region

● SIDE-EFFECTS
▶ **Rare** Kawasaki disease (in children) · symptoms of meningitis reported (but no evidence that the vaccine causes meningococcal C meningitis)
▶ **Frequency not known** Unusual crying (in children)

● MEDICINAL FORMS
There can be variation in the licensing of different medicines containing the same drug.
Suspension for injection
EXCIPIENTS: May contain Kanamycin
▶ Bexsero (GlaxoSmithKline UK Ltd) ▼
Bexsero vaccine suspension for injection 0.5ml pre-filled syringes | 1 pre-filled disposable injection [PoM] £75.00

◤ 1146

Meningococcal group C vaccine

● INDICATIONS AND DOSE
Primary immunisation against *Neisseria meningitidis*
▶ BY INTRAMUSCULAR INJECTION
- Child 3 months: 0.5 mL for 1 dose, the primary immunisation dose is followed by a booster dose of meningococcal group C conjugate vaccine combined with haemophilus influenzae type b vaccine at 12–13 months of age

Second booster dose for immunisation against *Neisseria meningitidis*
▶ BY INTRAMUSCULAR INJECTION
- Child 13-15 years: 0.5 mL for 1 dose

Immunisation against *Neisseria meningitidis* in an unimmunised patient
▶ BY INTRAMUSCULAR INJECTION
- Child 4-11 months: 0.5 mL for 1 dose, the primary immunisation dose is followed by a booster dose of meningococcal group C conjugate vaccine combined with haemophilus influenzae type b vaccine at 12–13 months of age, then 0.5 mL for 1 dose, this second booster dose to be given at 13–15 years of age
- Child 1-9 years: 0.5 mL for 1 dose, then 0.5 mL for 1 dose, this booster dose to be given at 13–15 years of age
- Child 10-17 years: 0.5 mL for 1 dose, booster dose is not required
- Adult 18-24 years: 0.5 mL for 1 dose, booster dose is not required

Patients attending university for the first time (who did not receive second booster dose at 13–15 years)
▶ BY INTRAMUSCULAR INJECTION
- Adult 18-24 years: 0.5 mL for 1 dose

Patients with confirmed serogroup C disease (who have previously been immunised)
▶ BY INTRAMUSCULAR INJECTION
- Child 1-17 years: 0.5 mL for 1 dose, dose to be given before discharge from hospital
- Adult 18-24 years: 0.5 mL for 1 dose, dose to be given before discharge from hospital

● SIDE-EFFECTS
▶ **Rare** Symptoms of meningitis (but no evidence that vaccine causes meningococcal C meningitis)
● DIRECTIONS FOR ADMINISTRATION
▶ In children *Menjugate Kit* ® may be used via subcutaneous route in children with bleeding disorders.
● PRESCRIBING AND DISPENSING INFORMATION Available as part of childhood immunisation schedule from www.immform.dh.gov.uk.

● MEDICINAL FORMS
There can be variation in the licensing of different medicines containing the same drug.
Powder and solvent for suspension for injection
▶ Menjugate (Novartis Vaccines and Diagnostics Ltd)
Menjugate vaccine powder and solvent for suspension for injection 0.5ml vials | 1 vial [PoM] no price available | 10 vial [PoM] no price available
Suspension for injection
▶ Meningitec (Nuron Biotech B.V.)
Meningitec vaccine suspension for injection 0.5ml pre-filled syringes | 1 pre-filled disposable injection [PoM] £4.33 | 10 pre-filled disposable injection [PoM] £43.30
▶ NeisVac-C (Pfizer Ltd)
NeisVac-C vaccine suspension for injection 0.5ml pre-filled syringes | 10 pre-filled disposable injection [PoM] £187.50

◤ 1146

Meningococcal groups A with C and W135 and Y vaccine

● INDICATIONS AND DOSE
MENVEO®
Primary immunisation against *Neisseria meningitidis*
▶ BY INTRAMUSCULAR INJECTION
- Child 13-15 years: 0.5 mL for 1 dose, dose preferably injected into deltoid region
Immunisation against *Neisseria meningitidis* in those at risk of exposure to prevent invasive disease
▶ BY INTRAMUSCULAR INJECTION
- Child 3-11 months: 0.5 mL every 1 month for 2 doses, dose preferably injected into deltoid region
- Child 1-17 years: 0.5 mL for 1 dose, dose preferably injected into deltoid region
- Adult: 0.5 mL for 1 dose, dose preferably injected into deltoid region

NIMENRIX®
Primary immunisation against *Neisseria meningitidis*
▶ BY INTRAMUSCULAR INJECTION
- Child 13-15 years: 0.5 mL for 1 dose, to be injected preferably into deltoid region
Immunisation against *Neisseria meningitidis* in those at risk of exposure
▶ BY INTRAMUSCULAR INJECTION
- Child 1-17 years: 0.5 mL for 1 dose, to be injected preferably into deltoid region (or anterolateral thigh in child 12–23 months), then 0.5 mL after 1 year if required for 1 dose, second dose should be considered in those who continue to be at risk of *Neisseria meningitidis* serogroup A infection
- Adult: 0.5 mL for 1 dose, to be injected preferably into deltoid region, then 0.5 mL after 1 year if required for 1 dose, second dose should be considered in those who continue to be at risk of *Neisseria meningitidis* serogroup A infection

● UNLICENSED USE
MENVEO® *Menveo* ® is not licensed for use in children under 2 years.

- SIDE-EFFECTS
- ▶ **Rare** Symptoms of meningitis reported (but no evidence that the vaccine causes meningococcal C meningitis)

- MEDICINAL FORMS
  There can be variation in the licensing of different medicines containing the same drug.
  Powder and solvent for solution for injection
  - ▶ Menveo (GlaxoSmithKline UK Ltd)
    Menveo vaccine powder and solvent for solution for injection 0.5ml vials | 1 vial [PoM] £30.00
  - ▶ Nimenrix (Pfizer Ltd) ▼
    Nimenrix vaccine powder and solvent for solution for injection 0.5ml pre-filled syringes | 1 pre-filled disposable injection [PoM] £30.00

F 1146

Pneumococcal polysaccharide conjugate vaccine (adsorbed)

- INDICATIONS AND DOSE
  PREVENAR 13®
  Primary immunisation against pneumococcal infection (first dose)
  - ▶ BY INTRAMUSCULAR INJECTION
  - ▶ Child 2 months: 0.5 mL for 1 dose, anterolateral thigh is preferred site of injection in infants
  Primary immunisation against pneumococcal infection (second dose)
  - ▶ BY INTRAMUSCULAR INJECTION
  - ▶ Child 4 months: 0.5 mL for 1 dose, anterolateral thigh is preferred site of injection in infants
  Primary immunisation against pneumococcal infection (booster dose)
  - ▶ BY INTRAMUSCULAR INJECTION
  - ▶ Child 12-13 months: 0.5 mL for 1 dose, anterolateral thigh is preferred site of injection in infants
  Immunisation against pneumococcal infection (in patients who have not been vaccinated or not completed the primary course)
  - ▶ BY INTRAMUSCULAR INJECTION
  - ▶ Child 12 months-4 years: 0.5 mL for 1 dose, deltoid muscle is preferred site of injection in young children; anterolateral thigh is preferred site in infants
  Immunisation against pneumococcal infection, in immunocompromised or asplenic patients or patients with splenic dysfunction (who have not been vaccinated or not completed the primary course)
  - ▶ BY INTRAMUSCULAR INJECTION
  - ▶ Child 12 months-4 years: 0.5 mL every 2 months for 2 doses, deltoid muscle is preferred site of injection in young children; anterolateral thigh is preferred site in infants
  SYNFLORIX®
  Immunisation against pneumococcal infection
  - ▶ BY INTRAMUSCULAR INJECTION
  - ▶ Child 6 weeks-4 years: Deltoid muscle is preferred site of injection in young children; anterolateral thigh is preferred site in infants (consult product literature)

- UNLICENSED USE
  PREVENAR 13® The dose in BNF publications may differ from that in product literature.
- CONTRA-INDICATIONS Concomitant use of high potency varicella-zoster vaccine (Zostavax®) with pneumococcal polysaccharide vaccine (in adults)
- PRESCRIBING AND DISPENSING INFORMATION
  PREVENAR 13® Available as part of childhood immunisation schedule from ImmForm
  www.immform.dh.gov.uk.

- MEDICINAL FORMS
  There can be variation in the licensing of different medicines containing the same drug.
  Suspension for injection
  - ▶ Prevenar (Pfizer Ltd)
    Prevenar 13 vaccine suspension for injection 0.5ml pre-filled syringes | 1 pre-filled disposable injection [PoM] £49.10 | 10 pre-filled disposable injection [PoM] £491.00
  - ▶ Synflorix (GlaxoSmithKline UK Ltd)
    Synflorix vaccine suspension for injection 0.5ml pre-filled syringes | 1 pre-filled disposable injection [PoM] £27.60

F 1146

Pneumococcal polysaccharide vaccine

- INDICATIONS AND DOSE
  Immunisation against pneumococcal infection
  - ▶ BY INTRAMUSCULAR INJECTION, OR BY SUBCUTANEOUS INJECTION
  - ▶ Child 2-17 years: 0.5 mL for 1 dose
  - ▶ Adult: 0.5 mL for 1 dose
  Immunisation in patients at increased risk of pneumococcal disease
  - ▶ BY INTRAMUSCULAR INJECTION, OR BY SUBCUTANEOUS INJECTION
  - ▶ Child 2-4 years: 0.5 mL for 1 dose, dose should be administered after the second birthday or at least 2 months after the final dose of the 13-valent pneumococcal polysaccharide conjugate vaccine (adsorbed)
  - ▶ Child 5-17 years: 0.5 mL for 1 dose
  - ▶ Adult: 0.5 mL for 1 dose

- MEDICINAL FORMS
  There can be variation in the licensing of different medicines containing the same drug.
  Solution for injection
  - ▶ Pneumococcal polysaccharide vaccine (Non-proprietary)
    Pneumococcal polysaccharide vaccine solution for injection 0.5ml vials | 1 vial [PoM] £8.32

F 1146

Typhoid vaccine

- INDICATIONS AND DOSE
  Immunisation against typhoid fever in children at high risk of typhoid fever
  - ▶ BY INTRAMUSCULAR INJECTION
  - ▶ Child 12-23 months: 0.5 mL for 1 dose, dose should be given at least 2 weeks before potential exposure to typhoid infection, response may be suboptimal
  Immunisation against typhoid fever
  - ▶ BY INTRAMUSCULAR INJECTION
  - ▶ Child 2-17 years: 0.5 mL for 1 dose, dose should be given at least 2 weeks before potential exposure to typhoid infection
  - ▶ Adult: 0.5 mL for 1 dose, dose should be given at least 2 weeks before potential exposure to typhoid infection
  - ▶ BY MOUTH
  - ▶ Child 6-17 years: 1 capsule every 2 days for 3 doses (on days 1, 3, and 5)
  - ▶ Adult: 1 capsule every 2 days for 3 doses (on days 1, 3, and 5)

- UNLICENSED USE
  - ▶ With intramuscular use in children Not licensed for use in children under 2 years.
- CONTRA-INDICATIONS
  - ▶ With oral use Acute gastro-intestinal illness

- INTERACTIONS → Appendix 1 (vaccines).
Oral typhoid vaccine is inactivated by concomitant administration of antibacterials or antimalarials:
  - antibacterials should be avoided for 3 days before and after oral typhoid vaccination;
  - *Mefloquine* should be avoided for at least 12 hours before or after oral typhoid;
  - For other antimalarials vaccination with oral typhoid vaccine should be completed at least 3 days before the first dose of the antimalarial (except proguanil hydrochloride with atovaquone, which may be given concomitantly).

- SIDE-EFFECTS
  - With oral use Abdominal cramps · abdominal pain · diarrhoea · nausea · vomiting

- DIRECTIONS FOR ADMINISTRATION Capsule should be taken one hour before a meal. Swallow as soon as possible after placing in mouth with a cold or lukewarm drink.

- HANDLING AND STORAGE
  - With oral use It is important to store capsules in a refrigerator.

- PATIENT AND CARER ADVICE
  - With oral use Patients or carers should be given advice on how to administer and store typhoid vaccine capsules.

- MEDICINAL FORMS
There can be variation in the licensing of different medicines containing the same drug.
Gastro-resistant capsule
CAUTIONARY AND ADVISORY LABELS 25
  - Vivotif (PaxVax Ltd)
Vivotif vaccine gastro-resistant capsules | 3 capsule PoM £14.77
Solution for injection
  - Typherix (GlaxoSmithKline UK Ltd)
Salmonella typhi Vi capsular polysaccharide 50 microgram per 1 ml Typherix 25micrograms/0.5ml vaccine solution for injection pre-filled syringes | 1 pre-filled disposable injection PoM £9.93 | 10 pre-filled disposable injection PoM £99.32
  - Typhim Vi (sanofi pasteur MSD Ltd)
Salmonella typhi Vi capsular polysaccharide 50 microgram per 1 ml Typhim Vi 25micrograms/0.5ml vaccine solution for injection pre-filled syringes | 1 pre-filled disposable injection PoM £9.30 | 10 pre-filled disposable injection PoM £93.00

Combinations available: *Hepatitis A with typhoid vaccine,* p. 1155.

VACCINES ⟩ VIRAL VACCINES

Hepatitis A and B vaccine

The properties listed below are those particular to the combination only. For the properties of the components please consider, hepatitis A vaccine p. 1154, hepatitis B vaccine p. 1155.

- INDICATIONS AND DOSE

AMBIRIX®
Immunisation against hepatitis A and hepatitis B infection (primary course)
▸ BY INTRAMUSCULAR INJECTION
  - Child 1–15 years: Initially 1 mL for 1 dose, then 1 mL after 6–12 months for 1 dose, the deltoid region is the preferred site of injection in older children; anterolateral thigh is the preferred site in infants; not to be injected into the buttock (vaccine efficacy reduced), subcutaneous route used for patients with bleeding disorders (but immune response may be reduced)

TWINRIX® ADULT
Immunisation against hepatitis A and hepatitis B infection (primary course)
▸ BY INTRAMUSCULAR INJECTION
  - Child 16–17 years: Initially 1 mL every 1 month for 2 doses, then 1 mL after 5 months for 1 dose, the deltoid region is the preferred site of injection; not to be injected into the buttock (vaccine efficacy reduced), subcutaneous route used for patients with bleeding disorders (but immune response may be reduced)
  - Adult: Initially 1 mL every 1 month for 2 doses, then 1 mL after 5 months for 1 dose, the deltoid region is the preferred site of injection; not to be injected into the buttock (vaccine efficacy reduced), subcutaneous route used for patients with bleeding disorders (but immune response may be reduced)

Immunisation against hepatitis A and hepatitis B infection—accelerated schedule for travellers departing within 1 month
▸ BY INTRAMUSCULAR INJECTION
  - Child 16–17 years: Initially 1 mL for 1 dose, then 1 mL after 7 days for 1 dose, then 1 mL after 14 days for 1 dose, then 1 mL for 1 dose given 12 months after the first dose, the deltoid region is the preferred site of injection; not to be injected into the buttock (vaccine efficacy reduced), subcutaneous route used for patients with bleeding disorders (but immune response may be reduced)
  - Adult: Initially 1 mL for 1 dose, then 1 mL after 7 days for 1 dose, then 1 mL after 14 days for 1 dose, then 1 mL for 1 dose given 12 months after the first dose, the deltoid region is the preferred site of injection; not to be injected into the buttock (vaccine efficacy reduced), subcutaneous route used for patients with bleeding disorders (but immune response may be reduced)

TWINRIX® PAEDIATRIC
Immunisation against hepatitis A and hepatitis B infection (primary course)
▸ BY INTRAMUSCULAR INJECTION
  - Child 1–15 years: Initially 0.5 mL every 1 month for 2 doses, then 0.5 mL after 5 months for 1 dose, the deltoid region is the preferred site of injection in older children; anterolateral thigh is the preferred site in infants; not to be injected into the buttock (vaccine efficacy reduced), subcutaneous route used for patients with bleeding disorders (but immune response may be reduced)

IMPORTANT SAFETY INFORMATION
Ambirix® and *Twinrix®* are not recommended for post-exposure prophylaxis following percutaneous (needle-stick), ocular, or mucous membrane exposure to hepatitis B virus.

- PRESCRIBING AND DISPENSING INFORMATION
TWINRIX® PAEDIATRIC Primary course should be completed with *Twinrix®* (single component vaccines given at appropriate intervals may be used for booster dose).
AMBIRIX® Primary course should be completed with *Ambirix®* (single component vaccines given at appropriate intervals may be used for booster dose).
TWINRIX® ADULT Primary course should be completed with *Twinrix®* (single component vaccines given at appropriate intervals may be used for booster dose).

14

Vaccines

● MEDICINAL FORMS
There can be variation in the licensing of different medicines containing the same drug.

Suspension for injection
EXCIPIENTS: May contain Neomycin
▸ Ambirix (GlaxoSmithKline UK Ltd)
Ambirix vaccine suspension for injection 1ml pre-filled syringes | 1 pre-filled disposable injection PoM £31.18
▸ Twinrix (GlaxoSmithKline UK Ltd)
Twinrix Paediatric vaccine suspension for injection 0.5ml pre-filled syringes | 1 pre-filled disposable injection PoM £20.79
Twinrix Adult vaccine suspension for injection 1ml pre-filled syringes | 1 pre-filled disposable injection PoM £33.31 | 10 pre-filled disposable injection PoM £333.13

📖 1146

Hepatitis A vaccine

● INDICATIONS AND DOSE
AVAXIM®
Immunisation against hepatitis A infection
▸ BY INTRAMUSCULAR INJECTION
▸ Child 16–17 years: Initially 0.5 mL for 1 dose, then 0.5 mL after 6–12 months, dose given as booster; booster dose may be delayed by up to 3 years if not given after recommended interval following primary dose, the deltoid region is the preferred site of injection. The subcutaneous route may be used for patients with bleeding disorders; not to be injected into the buttock (vaccine efficacy reduced)
▸ Adult: Initially 0.5 mL for 1 dose, then 0.5 mL after 6–12 months, dose given as booster; booster dose may be delayed by up to 3 years if not given after recommended interval following primary dose, the deltoid region is the preferred site of injection. The subcutaneous route may be used for patients with bleeding disorders; not to be injected into the buttock (vaccine efficacy reduced)

EPAXAL®
Immunisation against hepatitis A infection
▸ BY INTRAMUSCULAR INJECTION
▸ Child 1–17 years: Initially 0.5 mL for 1 dose, then 0.5 mL after 6–12 months, dose given as booster; booster dose may be delayed by up to 4 years if not given after recommended interval following primary dose. The deltoid region is the preferred site of injection. The subcutaneous route may be used for patients with bleeding disorders
▸ Adult: Initially 0.5 mL for 1 dose, then 0.5 mL after 6–12 months, dose given as booster; booster dose may be delayed by up to 4 years if not given after recommended interval following primary dose. The deltoid region is the preferred site of injection. The subcutaneous route may be used for patients with bleeding disorders

Immunisation against hepatitis A infection (splenectomised patients)
▸ BY INTRAMUSCULAR INJECTION
▸ Child 1–17 years: Initially 0.5 mL for 1 dose, then 0.5 mL after 1–6 months, dose given as booster; booster dose may be delayed by up to 4 years if not given after recommended interval following primary dose. The deltoid region is the preferred site of injection. The subcutaneous route may be used for patients with bleeding disorders
▸ Adult: Initially 0.5 mL for 1 dose, then 0.5 mL after 1–6 months, dose given as booster; booster dose may be delayed by up to 4 years if not given after recommended interval following primary dose. The deltoid region is the preferred site of injection. The subcutaneous route may be used for patients with bleeding disorders

HAVRIX MONODOSE®
Immunisation against hepatitis A infection
▸ BY INTRAMUSCULAR INJECTION
▸ Child 1–15 years: Initially 0.5 mL for 1 dose, then 0.5 mL after 6–12 months, dose given as booster; booster dose may be delayed by up to 3 years if not given after recommended interval following primary dose, the deltoid region is the preferred site of injection. The subcutaneous route may be used for patients with bleeding disorders
▸ Child 16–17 years: Initially 1 mL for 1 dose, then 1 mL after 6–12 months, dose given as booster; booster dose may be delayed by up to 3 years if not given after recommended interval following primary dose, the deltoid region is the preferred site of injection. The subcutaneous route may be used for patients with bleeding disorders
▸ Adult: Initially 1 mL for 1 dose, then 1 mL after 6–12 months, dose given as booster; booster dose may be delayed by up to 3 years if not given after recommended interval following primary dose, the deltoid region is the preferred site of injection. The subcutaneous route may be used for patients with bleeding disorders

VAQTA® ADULT
Immunisation against hepatitis A infection
▸ BY INTRAMUSCULAR INJECTION
▸ Adult: Initially 1 mL for 1 dose, then 1 mL after 6–18 months, dose given as booster, the deltoid region is the preferred site of injection. The subcutaneous route may be used for patients with bleeding disorders (but immune response may be delayed)

VAQTA® PAEDIATRIC
Immunisation against hepatitis A infection
▸ BY INTRAMUSCULAR INJECTION
▸ Child 1–17 years: Initially 0.5 mL for 1 dose, then 0.5 mL after 6–18 months, dose given as booster, the deltoid region is the preferred site of injection. The subcutaneous route may be used for patients with bleeding disorders (but immune response may be reduced)

● ALLERGY AND CROSS-SENSITIVITY *Epaxal*® contains influenza virus haemagglutinin grown in the allantoic cavity of chick embryos, therefore contra-indicated in those hypersensitive to eggs or chicken protein.

● MEDICINAL FORMS
There can be variation in the licensing of different medicines containing the same drug.
Suspension for injection
EXCIPIENTS: May contain Neomycin
▸ Avaxim (sanofi pasteur MSD Ltd)
Avaxim vaccine suspension for injection 0.5ml pre-filled syringes | 1 pre-filled disposable injection PoM £18.10 | 10 pre-filled disposable injection PoM £181.00
▸ Havrix (GlaxoSmithKline UK Ltd)
Havrix Monodose vaccine suspension for injection 1ml pre-filled syringes | 1 pre-filled disposable injection PoM £22.14 | 10 pre-filled disposable injection PoM £221.43
Havrix Junior Monodose vaccine suspension for injection 0.5ml pre-filled syringes | 1 pre-filled disposable injection PoM £16.77 | 10 pre-filled disposable injection PoM £167.68
Havrix Junior Monodose vaccine suspension for injection 0.5ml vials | 1 vial PoM £16.77
Havrix Monodose vaccine suspension for injection 1ml vials | 1 vial PoM £22.14
▸ VAQTA (sanofi pasteur MSD Ltd)
VAQTA Adult vaccine suspension for injection 1ml pre-filled syringes | 1 pre-filled disposable injection PoM £18.10
VAQTA Paediatric vaccine suspension for injection 0.5ml pre-filled syringes | 1 pre-filled disposable injection PoM £14.74

Emulsion for injection

▸ Epaxal (Janssen-Cilag Ltd)
Epaxal vaccine emulsion for injection 0.5ml pre-filled syringes | 1 pre-filled disposable injection [PoM] £23.81 | 10 pre-filled disposable injection [PoM] £238.10

Hepatitis A with typhoid vaccine

The properties listed below are those particular to the combination only. For the properties of the components please consider, hepatitis A vaccine p. 1154, typhoid vaccine p. 1152.

● INDICATIONS AND DOSE

HEPATYRIX®

Immunisation against hepatitis A and typhoid infection (primary course)

▸ BY INTRAMUSCULAR INJECTION

▸ Child 15-17 years: 1 mL for 1 dose, the deltoid region is the preferred site of injection; not to be injected into the buttock (vaccine efficacy reduced). The subcutaneous route may be used for patients with bleeding disorders, booster dose given using single component vaccines

▸ Adult: 1 mL for 1 dose, the deltoid region is the preferred site of injection; not to be injected into the buttock (vaccine efficacy reduced). The subcutaneous route may be used for patients with bleeding disorders, booster dose given using single component vaccines

VIATIM®

Immunisation against hepatitis A and typhoid infection (primary course)

▸ BY INTRAMUSCULAR INJECTION

▸ Child 16-17 years: 1 mL for 1 dose, the deltoid region is the preferred site of injection; not to be injected into the buttock (vaccine efficacy reduced). The subcutaneous route may be used for patients with bleeding disorders, booster dose given using single component vaccines

▸ Adult: 1 mL for 1 dose, the deltoid region is the preferred site of injection; not to be injected into the buttock (vaccine efficacy reduced). The subcutaneous route may be used for patients with bleeding disorders, booster dose given using single component vaccines

● MEDICINAL FORMS
There can be variation in the licensing of different medicines containing the same drug.

Suspension for injection
EXCIPIENTS: May contain Neomycin

▸ Hepatyrix (GlaxoSmithKline UK Ltd)
Hepatyrix vaccine suspension for injection 1ml pre-filled syringes | 1 pre-filled disposable injection [PoM] £37.21 | 10 pre-filled disposable injection [PoM] £372.10

▸ ViATIM (sanofi pasteur MSD Ltd)
ViATIM vaccine suspension for injection 1ml pre-filled syringes | 1 pre-filled disposable injection [PoM] £29.80

F 1146

Hepatitis B vaccine

● INDICATIONS AND DOSE

ENGERIX B®

Immunisation against hepatitis B infection

▸ BY INTRAMUSCULAR INJECTION

▸ Child 1 month-15 years: 10 micrograms for 1 dose, then 10 micrograms after 1 month for 1 dose, followed by 10 micrograms after 5 months for 1 dose, deltoid muscle is preferred site of injection in older children; anterolateral thigh is preferred site in infants and young children; not to be injected into the buttock (vaccine efficacy reduced)

▸ Child 16-17 years: 20 micrograms for 1 dose, then 20 micrograms after 1 month for 1 dose, followed by 20 micrograms after 5 months for 1 dose, deltoid muscle is preferred site of injection; not to be injected into the buttock (vaccine efficacy reduced)

▸ Adult: 20 micrograms for 1 dose, then 20 micrograms after 1 month for 1 dose, followed by 20 micrograms after 5 months for 1 dose, deltoid muscle is preferred site of injection; not to be injected into the buttock (vaccine efficacy reduced)

Immunisation against hepatitis B infection (accelerated schedule)

▸ BY INTRAMUSCULAR INJECTION

▸ Child 1 month-15 years: 10 micrograms every 1 month for 3 doses, followed by 10 micrograms after 10 months for 1 dose, deltoid muscle is preferred site of injection in older children; anterolateral thigh is preferred site in infants and young children; not to be injected into the buttock (vaccine efficacy reduced)

▸ Child 16-17 years: 20 micrograms every 1 month for 3 doses, followed by 20 micrograms after 10 months for 1 dose, deltoid muscle is preferred site of injection; not to be injected into the buttock (vaccine efficacy reduced)

▸ Adult: 20 micrograms every 1 month for 3 doses, followed by 20 micrograms after 10 months for 1 dose, deltoid muscle is preferred site of injection; not to be injected into the buttock (vaccine efficacy reduced)

Immunisation against hepatitis B infection, alternative accelerated schedule

▸ BY INTRAMUSCULAR INJECTION

▸ Child 11-15 years: 20 micrograms for 1 dose, followed by 20 micrograms after 6 months, this schedule is not suitable if high risk of infection between doses or if compliance with second dose uncertain, deltoid muscle is preferred site of injection; not to be injected into the buttock (vaccine efficacy reduced)

Immunisation against hepatitis B infection (accelerated schedule in exceptional cases, e.g. for travellers departing within 1 month)

▸ BY INTRAMUSCULAR INJECTION

▸ Adult: 20 micrograms for 1 dose, then 20 micrograms after 7 days for 1 dose, followed by 20 micrograms after 14 days for 1 dose, followed by 20 micrograms for 1 dose, to be given 12 months after the first dose, deltoid muscle is preferred site of injection; not to be injected into the buttock (vaccine efficacy reduced)

Immunisation against hepatitis B infection (in renal insufficiency, including haemodialysis patients)

▸ BY INTRAMUSCULAR INJECTION

▸ Child 1 month-15 years: 10 micrograms every 1 month for 2 doses, followed by 10 micrograms after 5 months for 1 dose, immunisation schedule and booster doses may need to be adjusted in those with low antibody concentration, deltoid muscle is preferred site of injection in older children; anterolateral thigh is preferred site in infants and young children; not to be injected into the buttock (vaccine efficacy reduced)

▸ Child 16-17 years: 40 micrograms every 1 month for 3 doses, followed by 40 micrograms after 4 months for 1 dose, immunisation schedule and booster doses may need to be adjusted in those with low antibody concentration, deltoid muscle is preferred site of injection; not to be injected into the buttock (vaccine efficacy reduced)

▸ Adult: 40 micrograms every 1 month for 3 doses, followed by 40 micrograms after 4 months for 1 dose, immunisation schedule and booster doses may need to be adjusted in those with low antibody concentration, deltoid muscle is preferred site of injection; not to be injected into the buttock (vaccine efficacy reduced)

continued →

Immunisation against hepatitis B infection (in renal insufficiency, including haemodialysis patients (accelerated schedule))
▸ BY INTRAMUSCULAR INJECTION
▸ Child 1 month–15 years: 10 micrograms every 1 month for 3 doses, followed by 10 micrograms after 10 months for 1 dose, immunisation schedule and booster doses may need to be adjusted in those with low antibody concentration, deltoid muscle is preferred site of injection in older children; anterolateral thigh is preferred site in infants and young children; not to be injected into the buttock (vaccine efficacy reduced)

Immunisation against hepatitis B infection in renal insufficiency (including pre-haemodialysis and haemodialysis patients)
▸ BY INTRAMUSCULAR INJECTION
▸ Child 15–17 years: 20 micrograms every 1 month for 3 doses, followed by 20 micrograms after 4 months for 1 dose, immunisation schedule and booster doses may need to be adjusted in those with low antibody concentration, deltoid muscle is preferred site of injection; not to be injected into the buttock (vaccine efficacy reduced)
▸ Adult: 20 micrograms every 1 month for 3 doses, followed by 20 micrograms after 4 months for 1 dose, immunisation schedule and booster doses may need to be adjusted in those with low antibody concentration, deltoid muscle is preferred site of injection; not to be injected into the buttock (vaccine efficacy reduced)

Immunisation against hepatitis B infection
▸ BY INTRAMUSCULAR INJECTION
▸ Neonate: 5 micrograms for 1 dose, followed by 5 micrograms after 1 month for 1 dose, then 5 micrograms after 5 months for 1 dose, booster doses may be required in immunocompromised patients with low antibody concentration, anterolateral thigh is preferred site in neonates; not to be injected into the buttock (vaccine efficacy reduced), dose not to be used for neonate born to hepatitis B surface antigen positive mother.
▸ Child 1 month–15 years: 5 micrograms for 1 dose, followed by 5 micrograms after 1 month for 1 dose, then 5 micrograms after 5 months for 1 dose, booster doses may be required in immunocompromised patients with low antibody concentration, deltoid muscle is preferred site of injection in adults and older children; anterolateral thigh is preferred site in infants; not to be injected into the buttock (vaccine efficacy reduced)
▸ Child 16–17 years: 10 micrograms for 1 dose, followed by 10 micrograms after 1 month for 1 dose, followed by 10 micrograms after 5 months for 1 dose, booster doses may be required in immunocompromised patients with low antibody concentration, deltoid muscle is preferred site of injection in adults and older children; not to be injected into the buttock (vaccine efficacy reduced)
▸ Adult: 10 micrograms for 1 dose, followed by 10 micrograms after 1 month for 1 dose, followed by 10 micrograms after 5 months for 1 dose, booster doses may be required in immunocompromised patients with low antibody concentration, deltoid muscle is preferred site of injection in adults and older children; not to be injected into the buttock (vaccine efficacy reduced)

Immunisation against hepatitis B infection (accelerated schedule)
▸ BY INTRAMUSCULAR INJECTION
▸ Neonate: 5 micrograms every 1 month for 3 doses, followed by 5 micrograms after 10 months for 1 dose, booster doses may be required in immunocompromised patients with low antibody concentration, anterolateral thigh is preferred site in neonates; not to be injected into the buttock (vaccine efficacy reduced), dose not to be used for neonate born to hepatitis B surface antigen positive mother.
▸ Child 1 month–15 years: 5 micrograms every 1 month for 3 doses, followed by 5 micrograms after 10 months for 1 dose, booster doses may be required in immunocompromised patients with low antibody concentration, deltoid muscle is preferred site of injection in adults and older children; anterolateral thigh is preferred site in infants; not to be injected into the buttock (vaccine efficacy reduced)
▸ Child 16–17 years: 10 micrograms every 1 month for 3 doses, followed by 10 micrograms after 10 months for 1 dose, booster doses may be required in immunocompromised patients with low antibody concentration, deltoid muscle is preferred site of injection in adults and older children; not to be injected into the buttock (vaccine efficacy reduced)
▸ Adult: 10 micrograms every 1 month for 3 doses, followed by 10 micrograms after 10 months for 1 dose, booster doses may be required in immunocompromised patients with low antibody concentration, deltoid muscle is preferred site of injection in adults and older children; not to be injected into the buttock (vaccine efficacy reduced)

Neonate born to hepatitis B surface antigen-positive mother
▸ BY INTRAMUSCULAR INJECTION
▸ Neonate: 5 micrograms every 1 month for 3 doses, first dose given at birth with hepatitis B immunoglobulin injection (separate site), followed by 5 micrograms after 10 months for 1 dose, anterolateral thigh is preferred site in neonates; not to be injected into the buttock (vaccine efficacy reduced).

Chronic haemodialysis patients
▸ BY INTRAMUSCULAR INJECTION
▸ Child 16–17 years: 40 micrograms every 1 month for 2 doses, followed by 40 micrograms after 5 months for 1 dose, booster doses may be required in those with low antibody concentration, deltoid muscle is preferred site of injection in adults and older children; not to be injected into the buttock (vaccine efficacy reduced)
▸ Adult: 40 micrograms every 1 month for 2 doses, followed by 40 micrograms after 5 months for 1 dose, booster doses may be required in those with low antibody concentration, deltoid muscle is preferred site of injection in adults and older children; not to be injected into the buttock (vaccine efficacy reduced)

● MEDICINAL FORMS
There can be variation in the licensing of different medicines containing the same drug.
Suspension for injection
EXCIPIENTS: May contain Thiomersal
▸ Engerix B (GlaxoSmithKline UK Ltd)
Hepatitis B virus surface antigen 20 microgram per 1 ml Engerix B 20micrograms/1ml vaccine suspension for injection vials | 1 vial [PoM] £12.34 | 10 vial [PoM] £123.41
Engerix B 10micrograms/0.5ml vaccine suspension for injection pre-filled syringes | 1 pre-filled disposable injection [PoM] £9.67
Engerix B 20micrograms/1ml vaccine suspension for injection pre-filled syringes | 1 pre-filled disposable injection [PoM] £12.99 | 10 pre-filled disposable injection [PoM] £129.92

▸ Fendrix (GlaxoSmithKline UK Ltd)
Hepatitis B virus surface antigen 40 microgram per 1 ml Fendrix
20micrograms/0.5ml vaccine suspension for injection pre-filled
syringes | 1 pre-filled disposable injection PoM £38.10
▸ HBVAXPRO (sanofi pasteur MSD Ltd)
**Hepatitis B virus surface antigen 10 microgram per
1 ml** HBVAXPRO 10micrograms/1ml vaccine suspension for injection
pre-filled syringes | 1 pre-filled disposable injection PoM £12.20
HBVAXPRO 5micrograms/0.5ml vaccine suspension for injection pre-
filled syringes | 1 pre-filled disposable injection PoM £8.95
**Hepatitis B virus surface antigen 40 microgram per
1 ml** HBvaxPRO 40micrograms/1ml vaccine suspension for injection
vials | 1 vial PoM £27.60

📖 1146

Human papillomavirus vaccines

● **INDICATIONS AND DOSE**
CERVARIX®
**Prevention of premalignant genital lesions and cervical
cancer**
▸ BY INTRAMUSCULAR INJECTION
▸ **Child 9-14 years (female):** 0.5 mL for 1 dose, followed by
0.5 mL after 5–7 months for 1 dose, if second dose
administered earlier than 5 months after the first, a
third dose should be administered, dose to be
administered into deltoid region, if the course is
interrupted, it should be resumed (using the same
vaccine) but not repeated, even if more than 24 months
have elapsed since the first dose or if the girl is then
aged 15 years or more.
▸ **Child 15-17 years (female):** 0.5 mL for 1 dose, followed by
0.5 mL after 1–2.5 months for 1 dose, then 0.5 mL after
5–12 months from the first dose for 1 dose, dose to be
administered into deltoid region, if the course is
interrupted, it should be resumed (using the same
vaccine) but not repeated, allowing the appropriate
interval between the remaining doses.
▸ **Adult (female):** 0.5 mL for 1 dose, followed by 0.5 mL
after 1–2.5 months for 1 dose, then 0.5 mL after
5–12 months from the first dose for 1 dose, dose to be
administered into deltoid region, if the course is
interrupted, it should be resumed (using the same
vaccine) but not repeated, allowing the appropriate
interval between the remaining doses.

GARDASIL®
**Prevention of premalignant genital (cervical, vulvar and
vaginal) and anal lesions, cervical and anal cancers, and
genital warts**
▸ BY INTRAMUSCULAR INJECTION
▸ **Child 9-17 years (female):** 0.5 mL for 1 dose, followed by
0.5 mL for 1 dose, second dose to be given at least
1 month after the first dose, then 0.5 mL for 1 dose,
third dose to be given at least 3 months after the
second dose, schedule should be completed within
12 months of the first dose, dose to be administered
preferably into deltoid region or higher anterolateral
thigh, if the course is interrupted, it should be resumed
(using the same vaccine) but not repeated, allowing the
appropriate interval between the remaining doses.
▸ **Adult (female):** 0.5 mL for 1 dose, followed by 0.5 mL for
1 dose, second dose to be given at least 1 month after
the first dose, then 0.5 mL for 1 dose, third dose to be
given at least 3 months after the second dose, schedule
should be completed within 12 months of the first
dose, dose to be administered preferably into deltoid
region or higher anterolateral thigh, if the course is
interrupted, it should be resumed (using the same
vaccine) but not repeated, allowing the appropriate
interval between the remaining doses.

**Prevention of premalignant genital (cervical, vulvar, and
vaginal) and anal lesions, cervical and anal cancers, and
genital warts (alternative schedule)**
▸ BY INTRAMUSCULAR INJECTION
▸ **Child 9-13 years (female):** 0.5 mL, for 1 dose, followed by
0.5 mL after 6 months for 1 dose, if the second dose is
administered earlier than 6 months after the first dose,
a third dose should be administered, dose to be
administered preferably into deltoid region or higher
anterolateral thigh, if the course is interrupted, it
should be resumed (using the same vaccine) but not
repeated, even if more than 24 months have elapsed
since the first dose or if the girl is then aged 15 years or
more.

● PREGNANCY Not known to be harmful, but vaccination
should be postponed until completion of pregnancy.

● PRESCRIBING AND DISPENSING INFORMATION To avoid
confusion, prescribers should specify the brand to be
dispensed.

● MEDICINAL FORMS
There can be variation in the licensing of different medicines
containing the same drug.
Suspension for injection
▸ Cervarix (GlaxoSmithKline UK Ltd)
Cervarix vaccine suspension for injection 0.5ml pre-filled syringes |
1 pre-filled disposable injection PoM £80.50
▸ Gardasil (sanofi pasteur MSD Ltd)
Gardasil vaccine suspension for injection 0.5ml pre-filled syringes |
1 pre-filled disposable injection PoM £86.50

📖 1146

Influenza vaccine

● **INDICATIONS AND DOSE**
**Annual immunisation against seasonal influenza (for
children who have not received seasonal influenza
vaccine previously)**
▸ BY INTRAMUSCULAR INJECTION
▸ **Child 6 months-9 years:** 0.5 mL for 1 dose, followed by
0.5 mL after at least 4 weeks for 1 dose
▸ BY INTRANASAL ADMINISTRATION
▸ **Child 2-9 years:** 0.1 mL for 1 dose, followed by 0.1 mL
after at least 4 weeks for 1 dose, 0.1 mL dose to be
administered into each nostril
Annual immunisation against seasonal influenza
▸ BY INTRAMUSCULAR INJECTION
▸ **Child 6 months-17 years:** 0.5 mL for 1 dose
▸ **Adult:** 0.5 mL for 1 dose
▸ BY INTRADERMAL INJECTION
▸ **Adult 18-59 years:** 9 micrograms for 1 dose, dose to be
injected into deltoid region
▸ **Adult 60 years and over:** 15 micrograms for 1 dose, dose
to be injected into deltoid region
▸ BY INTRANASAL ADMINISTRATION
▸ **Child 2-17 years:** 0.1 mL for 1 dose, dose to be
administered into each nostril

● UNLICENSED USE Some products containing inactivated
influenza vaccine (surface antigen) are not licensed for use
in children under 4 years—check product literature.
FLUVIRIN® Not licensed for use in children under 4 years.
FLUARIX TETRA® Not licensed for use in children under
3 years of age.
OPTAFLU® Not licensed for use in children and
adolescents under 18 years.

● CONTRA-INDICATIONS Preparations marketed by Pfizer, or
CSL Biotherapies in child under 5 years— increased risk of
febrile convulsions
FLUENZ TETRA® Active wheezing · concomitant use with

antiviral therapy for influenza · severe asthma

CONTRA-INDICATIONS, FURTHER INFORMATION

▸ Concomitant use with antivirals Avoid antivirals for at least 2 weeks after immunisation; avoid immunisation for at least 48 hours after stopping the antiviral.

ENZIRA® Child under 5 years—increased risk of febrile convulsions

● CAUTIONS Increased risk of fever in child 5–9 years with preparations marketed by Pfizer or CSL Biotherapies—use alternative influenza vaccine if available

ENZIRA® Child 5–9 years (increased risk of fever)—use alternative influenza vaccine if available

● SIDE-EFFECTS

GENERAL SIDE-EFFECTS

▸ **Uncommon** Epistaxis

▸ **Frequency not known** Febrile convulsions · transient thrombocytopenia · vasculitis (in adults)

SPECIFIC SIDE-EFFECTS

● With intranasal use Rhinorrhoea

● ALLERGY AND CROSS-SENSITIVITY Individuals with a history of egg allergy can be immunised with either an egg free influenza vaccine, if available, or an influenza vaccine with an ovalbumin content less than 120 nanograms/mL (facilities should be available to treat anaphylaxis). Vaccines with an ovalbumin content more than 120 nanograms/mL or where content is not stated should not be used in individuals with egg allergy. If an influenza vaccine containing ovalbumin is being considered in those with a history of anaphylaxis to egg or egg allergy with uncontrolled asthma, these individuals should be referred to a specialist in hospital.

● PREGNANCY Inactivated vaccines not known to be harmful.

FLUENZ TETRA® Avoid in pregnancy.

● BREAST FEEDING Inactivated vaccines not known to be harmful.

FLUENZ TETRA® Avoid in breast-feeding.

● PRESCRIBING AND DISPENSING INFORMATION

FLUARIX TETRA® Ovalbumin content less than 100 nanograms/mL.

● PATIENT AND CARER ADVICE

FLUENZ TETRA® Avoid close contact with severely immunocompromised patients for 1–2 weeks after vaccination.

● MEDICINAL FORMS
There can be variation in the licensing of different medicines containing the same drug.

Suspension for injection
EXCIPIENTS: May contain Gentamicin, kanamycin, neomycin penicillins, polymyxin b, thiomersal

▸ Influenza vaccine (Non-proprietary)
Influenza vaccine (split virion, inactivated) suspension for injection 0.5ml pre-filled syringes | 1 pre-filled disposable injection PoM £5.00–£6.59 | 10 pre-filled disposable injection PoM £65.90
Influenza vaccine (surface antigen, inactivated) suspension for injection 0.5ml pre-filled syringes | 10 pre-filled disposable injection PoM £41.50

▸ Agrippal (Novartis Vaccines and Diagnostics Ltd)
Agrippal vaccine suspension for injection 0.5ml pre-filled syringes | 10 pre-filled disposable injection PoM £58.50

▸ Enzira (Pfizer Ltd)
Enzira vaccine suspension for injection 0.5ml pre-filled syringes | 1 pre-filled disposable injection PoM £5.25 | 10 pre-filled disposable injection PoM £52.50

▸ Fluarix Tetra (GlaxoSmithKline UK Ltd) ▼
Fluarix Tetra vaccine suspension for injection 0.5ml pre-filled syringes | 1 pre-filled disposable injection PoM £9.94 | 10 pre-filled disposable injection PoM £99.40

▸ Imuvac (BGP Products Ltd)
Imuvac vaccine suspension for injection 0.5ml pre-filled syringes | 1 pre-filled disposable injection PoM £6.59 | 10 pre-filled disposable injection PoM £65.90

▸ Influvac Sub-unit (BGP Products Ltd)
Influvac Sub-unit vaccine suspension for injection 0.5ml pre-filled syringes | 1 pre-filled disposable injection PoM £5.22 | 10 pre-filled disposable injection PoM £52.20

▸ Intanza (sanofi pasteur MSD Ltd)
Intanza 15microgram strain vaccine suspension for injection 0.1ml pre-filled syringes | 1 pre-filled disposable injection PoM £9.05 | 10 pre-filled disposable injection PoM £90.50

▸ Optaflu (Novartis Vaccines and Diagnostics Ltd)
Optaflu vaccine suspension for injection 0.5ml pre-filled syringes | 1 pre-filled disposable injection PoM £6.59

Spray
EXCIPIENTS: May contain Gelatin, gentamicin

▸ FluMist Quadrivalent (AstraZeneca UK Ltd)
FluMist Quadrivalent vaccine nasal suspension 0.2ml unit dose | 10 unit dose PoM £180.00

▸ Fluenz Tetra (AstraZeneca UK Ltd) ▼
Fluenz Tetra vaccine nasal suspension 0.2ml unit dose | 10 unit dose PoM £180.00

F 1146

Japanese encephalitis vaccine

● INDICATIONS AND DOSE

Immunisation against Japanese encephalitis
▸ BY INTRAMUSCULAR INJECTION

▸ Child 2 months-2 years: 0.25 mL every 28 days for 2 doses, anterolateral thigh is preferred site of injection in infants, the subcutaneous route may be used for patients with bleeding disorders

▸ Child 3-17 years: 0.5 mL every 28 days for 2 doses, deltoid muscle is preferred site in older children; anterolateral thigh is preferred in infants, the subcutaneous route may be used for patients with bleeding disorders

▸ Adult: 0.5 mL every 28 days for 2 doses, deltoid muscle is preferred site of injection, the subcutaneous route may be used for patients with bleeding disorders

Booster dose
▸ BY INTRAMUSCULAR INJECTION

▸ Adult: 0.5 mL after 1–2 years, deltoid muscle is preferred site of injection, the subcutaneous route may be used for patients with bleeding disorders, for those at continued risk, the booster dose should be given 1 year after completing the primary course

● SIDE-EFFECTS

▸ **Uncommon** Cough (in children) · migraine (in adults) · vertigo (in adults)

▸ **Rare** Dyspnoea (in adults) · neuritis (in adults) · palpitation (in adults) · tachycardia (in adults) · thrombocytopenia (in adults)

● PREGNANCY Although manufacturer advises avoid because of limited information, miscarriage has been associated with Japanese encephalitis virus infection acquired during the first 2 trimesters of pregnancy.

● MEDICINAL FORMS
There can be variation in the licensing of different medicines containing the same drug.

Solution for injection
▸ Japanese encephalitis vaccine (Non-proprietary)
Japanese encephalitis GCVC vaccine solution for injection 1ml vials | 1 vial no price available
Japanese encephalitis GCVC vaccine solution for injection 20ml vials | 1 vial no price available
Japanese encephalitis GCVC vaccine solution for injection 10ml vials | 1 vial no price available

Suspension for injection
▸ Ixiaro (Valneva UK Ltd)
Ixiaro vaccine suspension for injection 0.5ml pre-filled syringes | 1 pre-filled disposable injection PoM £59.50

⟆ 1146

Measles, mumps and rubella vaccine, live

● **INDICATIONS AND DOSE**

Primary immunisation against measles, mumps, and rubella (first dose)

▸ BY INTRAMUSCULAR INJECTION, OR BY DEEP SUBCUTANEOUS INJECTION
▸ Child 12-13 months: 0.5 mL for 1 dose

Primary immunisation against measles, mumps, and rubella (second dose)

▸ BY INTRAMUSCULAR INJECTION, OR BY DEEP SUBCUTANEOUS INJECTION
▸ Child 40 months-5 years: 0.5 mL for 1 dose

Rubella immunisation (in seronegative women, susceptible to rubella and in unimmunised, seronegative women, post-partum)

▸ BY INTRAMUSCULAR INJECTION, OR BY DEEP SUBCUTANEOUS INJECTION
▸ Females of childbearing potential: (consult product literature or local protocols)

Children presenting for pre-school booster, who have not received the primary immunisation (first dose) | Immunisation for patients at school-leaving age or at entry into further education, who have not completed the primary immunisation course | Control of measles outbreak | Immunisation for patients travelling to areas where measles is endemic or epidemic, who have not completed the primary immunisation

▸ BY INTRAMUSCULAR INJECTION, OR BY DEEP SUBCUTANEOUS INJECTION
▸ Child 6 months-17 years: (consult product literature or local protocols)
▸ Adult: (consult product literature or local protocols)

● **UNLICENSED USE**

▸ In children Not licensed for use in children under 9 months.

> **IMPORTANT SAFETY INFORMATION**
> MMR VACCINATION AND BOWEL DISEASE OR AUTISM
> Reviews undertaken on behalf of the CSM, the Medical Research Council, and the Cochrane Collaboration, have not found any evidence of a link between MMR vaccination and bowel disease or autism. The Chief Medical Officers have advised that the MMR vaccine is the safest and best way to protect children against measles, mumps, and rubella. Information (including fact sheets and a list of references) may be obtained from   www.dh.gov.uk/immunisation.

● **CAUTIONS** Antibody response to measles component may be reduced after immunoglobulin administration or blood transfusion–leave an interval of at least 3 months before MMR immunisation

CAUTIONS, FURTHER INFORMATION
▸ Administration with other vaccines MMR vaccine should not be administered on the same day as yellow fever vaccine; there should be a 4-week minimum interval between the vaccines. When protection is rapidly required, the vaccines can be given at any interval and an additional dose of MMR may be considered.

MMR and varicella-zoster vaccine can be given on the same day or separated by a 4-week minimum interval. When protection is rapidly required, the vaccines can be given at any interval and an additional dose of MMR vaccine given second may be considered.

● **SIDE-EFFECTS**

▸ **Uncommon** Parotid swelling (usually in the third week) · sleep disturbances · unusual crying in infants

▸ **Rare** Arthropathy (2 to 3 weeks after immunisation) · idiopathic thrombocytopenic purpura
▸ **Frequency not known** Optic neuritis · peripheral neuritis

SIDE-EFFECTS, FURTHER INFORMATION
Malaise, fever, or a rash can occur after the first dose of MMR vaccine–most commonly about a week after vaccination and lasting about 2 to 3 days. Leaflets are available for parents on advice for reducing fever (including the use of paracetamol).

Febrile seizures–occur rarely 6 to 11 days after MMR vaccination (the incidence is lower than that following measles infection)

▸ Idiopathic thrombocytopenic purpura Idiopathic thrombocytopenic purpura has occurred rarely following MMR vaccination, usually within 6 weeks of the first dose. The risk of idiopathic thrombocytopenic purpura after MMR vaccine is much less than the risk after infection with wild measles or rubella virus. Children who develop idiopathic thrombocytopenic purpura within 6 weeks of the first dose of MMR should undergo serological testing before the second dose is due; if the results suggest incomplete immunity against measles, mumps or rubella then a second dose of MMR is recommended. The Specialist and Reference Microbiology Division, Health Protection Agency offers free serological testing for children who develop idiopathic thrombocytopenic purpura *within* 6 *weeks* of the first dose of MMR.

▸ Aseptic meningitis Post-vaccination aseptic meningitis was reported (rarely and with complete recovery) following vaccination with MMR vaccine containing Urabe mumps vaccine, which has now been discontinued; no cases have been confirmed in association with the currently used Jeryl Lynn mumps vaccine. Children with post-vaccination symptoms are not infectious.

▸ Frequency of side effects Adverse reactions are considerably less frequent after the second dose of MMR vaccine than after the first.

● **ALLERGY AND CROSS-SENSITIVITY** MMR vaccine can be given safely even when the child has had an anaphylactic reaction to food containing egg. Dislike of eggs, refusal to eat egg, or confirmed anaphylactic reactions to egg-containing food is not a contra-indication to MMR vaccination. Children with a confirmed anaphylactic reaction to the MMR vaccine should be assessed by a specialist.

● **CONCEPTION AND CONTRACEPTION** Exclude pregnancy before immunisation. Avoid pregnancy for at least 1 month after vaccination.

● **PRESCRIBING AND DISPENSING INFORMATION** Available as part of childhood immunisation schedule from health organisations or ImmForm www.immform.dh.gov.uk.

● **MEDICINAL FORMS**
There can be variation in the licensing of different medicines containing the same drug.

Powder and solvent for solution for injection
EXCIPIENTS: May contain Neomycin
▸ Priorix (GlaxoSmithKline UK Ltd)
  Priorix vaccine powder and solvent for solution for injection 0.5ml vials | 1 vial [PoM] £7.64

Powder and solvent for suspension for injection
EXCIPIENTS: May contain Gelatin, neomycin
▸ M-M-RVAXPRO (sanofi pasteur MSD Ltd)
  M-M-RVAXPRO vaccine powder and solvent for suspension for injection 0.5ml pre-filled syringes | 1 pre-filled disposable injection [PoM] £11.00

14

Vaccines

14

Vaccines

Rabies vaccine

↱ 1146

● INDICATIONS AND DOSE

Pre-exposure prophylaxis
▸ BY INTRAMUSCULAR INJECTION
▸ Child: 1 mL for 2 doses (on days 0 and 7), followed by 1 mL for 1 dose (on day 28), to be administered in deltoid region or anterolateral thigh in infants, for those at continuous risk, measure plasma-concentration of antirabies antibodies every 6 months and give a booster dose if the titre is less than 0.5 units/mL, final dose may be given from day 21, if insufficient time before travel
▸ Adult: 1 mL for 2 doses (on days 0 and 7), followed by 1 mL for 1 dose (on day 28), to be administered in deltoid region, for those at continuous risk, measure plasma-concentration of antirabies antibodies every 6 months and give a booster dose if the titre is less than 0.5 units/mL, final dose may be given from day 21, if insufficient time before travel

Pre-exposure prophylaxis booster dose (for patients at frequent risk of exposure)
▸ BY INTRAMUSCULAR INJECTION
▸ Child: 1 mL after 1 year for 1 dose, to be given 1 year after primary course is completed, then 1 mL every 3–5 years, to be administered in deltoid region or anterolateral thigh in infants, the frequency of booster doses may alternatively be determined according to plasma-concentration of antirabies antibodies
▸ Adult: 1 mL for 1 dose, to be given 1 year after primary course is completed, then 1 mL every 3–5 years, to be administered in deltoid region, the frequency of booster doses may alternatively be determined according to plasma-concentration of antirabies antibodies

Pre-exposure prophylaxis booster dose (for patients at infrequent risk of exposure)
▸ BY INTRAMUSCULAR INJECTION
▸ Child: 1 mL for 1 dose, to be given 10 years after primary course is completed, administered in deltoid region or anterolateral thigh in infants
▸ Adult: 1 mL for 1 dose, to be given 10 years after primary course is completed, administered in deltoid region

Post-exposure prophylaxis of fully immunised individuals (who have previously received pre-exposure or post-exposure prophylaxis with cell-derived rabies vaccine)
▸ BY INTRAMUSCULAR INJECTION
▸ Child (administered on expert advice): 1 mL for 1 dose, followed by 1 mL after 3–7 days for 1 dose, to be administered in deltoid region or anterolateral thigh in infants, rabies immunoglobulin is not necessary
▸ Adult (administered on expert advice): 1 mL for 1 dose, followed by 1 mL after 3–7 days for 1 dose, to be administered in deltoid region, rabies immunoglobulin is not necessary

Post-exposure treatment for unimmunised individuals (or those whose prophylaxis is possibly incomplete)
▸ BY INTRAMUSCULAR INJECTION
▸ Child (administered on expert advice): 1 mL 5 times a month for 1 month, doses should be given on days 0, 3, 7, 14, and the fifth dose is given between day 28–30, to be administered in deltoid region or anterolateral thigh in infants, depending on the level of risk (determined by factors such as the nature of the bite and the country where it was sustained), rabies immunoglobulin is given to unimmunised individuals on day 0 or within 7 days of starting the course of rabies vaccine, the immunisation course can be

discontinued if it is proved that the individual was not at risk
▸ Adult (administered on expert advice): 1 mL 5 times a month for 1 month, doses should be given on days 0, 3, 7, 14, and the fifth dose is given between day 28–30, to be administered in deltoid region, depending on the level of risk (determined by factors such as the nature of the bite and the country where it was sustained), rabies immunoglobulin is given to unimmunised individuals on day 0 or within 7 days of starting the course of rabies vaccine, the immunisation course can be discontinued if it is proved that the individual was not at risk

● SIDE-EFFECTS Paresis
● PREGNANCY Because of the potential consequences of untreated rabies exposure and because rabies vaccination has not been associated with fetal abnormalities, pregnancy is not considered a contra-indication to post-exposure prophylaxis. Immunisation against rabies is indicated during pregnancy if there is substantial risk of exposure to rabies and rapid access to post-exposure prophylaxis is likely to be limited.

● MEDICINAL FORMS
There can be variation in the licensing of different medicines containing the same drug.
Powder and solvent for solution for injection
EXCIPIENTS: May contain Neomycin
▸ Rabipur (GlaxoSmithKline UK Ltd)
Rabipur vaccine powder and solvent for solution for injection 1ml vials | 1 vial [PoM] £34.56
Powder and solvent for suspension for injection
EXCIPIENTS: May contain Neomycin
▸ Rabies vaccine (Non-proprietary)
Verorab powder and solvent for suspension for injection 0.5ml vials | 1 vial [PoM] no price available
Rabies vaccine powder and solvent for suspension for injection 1ml vials | 1 vial [PoM] £33.90

Rotavirus vaccine

↱ 1146

● DRUG ACTION Rotavirus vaccine is a live, oral vaccine that protects young children against gastro-enteritis caused by rotavirus infection.

● INDICATIONS AND DOSE

Immunisation against gastro-enteritis caused by rotavirus
▸ BY MOUTH
▸ Child 6–23 weeks: 1.5 mL for 2 doses separated by an interval of at least 4 weeks, first dose must be given between 6–14 weeks of age; course should be completed before 24 weeks of age (preferably before 16 weeks)

● CONTRA-INDICATIONS History of intussusception · predisposition to intussusception · severe combined immunosuppression
CONTRA-INDICATIONS, FURTHER INFORMATION
▸ Immunosuppresion With the exception of severe combined immunodeficiency, rotavirus vaccine is not contra-indicated in immunosuppressed patients—benefit from vaccination is likely to outweigh the risk, if there is any doubt, seek specialist advice.

● CAUTIONS Diarrhoea (postpone vaccination) · immunosuppressed close contacts · vomiting (postpone vaccination)
CAUTIONS, FURTHER INFORMATION
The rotavirus vaccine virus is excreted in the stool and may be transmitted to close contacts; however, vaccination of those with immunosuppressed close contacts may protect the contacts from wild-type rotavirus

disease and outweigh any risk from transmission of vaccine virus.

- SIDE-EFFECTS Abdominal cramps · abdominal pain · diarrhoea · nausea · vomiting
- PATIENT AND CARER ADVICE The rotavirus vaccine virus is excreted in the stool and may be transmitted to close contacts; carers of a recently vaccinated baby should be advised of the need to wash their hands after changing the baby's nappies.

- MEDICINAL FORMS
There can be variation in the licensing of different medicines containing the same drug.
Oral suspension
‣ Rotarix (GlaxoSmithKline UK Ltd)
  Rotarix vaccine live oral suspension 1.5ml pre-filled syringes | 1 unit dose PoM £34.76

🏳 1146

Tick-borne encephalitis vaccine, inactivated

- INDICATIONS AND DOSE
Initial immunisation against tick-borne encephalitis
‣ BY INTRAMUSCULAR INJECTION
‣ Child 1–15 years: 0.25 mL for 1 dose, followed by 0.25 mL after 1–3 months for 1 dose, then 0.25 mL after further 5–12 months for 1 dose, to achieve more rapid protection, second dose may be given 14 days after first dose, dose to be administered in deltoid region or anterolateral thigh in infants, in immunocompromised patients (including those receiving immunosuppressants), antibody concentration may be measured 4 weeks after second dose and dose repeated if protective levels not achieved
‣ Child 16–17 years: 0.5 mL for 1 dose, followed by 0.5 mL after 1–3 months for 1 dose, then 0.5 mL after further 5–12 months for 1 dose, to achieve more rapid protection, second dose may be given 14 days after first dose, dose to be administered in deltoid region, in immunocompromised patients (including those receiving immunosuppressants), antibody concentration may be measured 4 weeks after second dose and dose repeated if protective levels not achieved
‣ Adult: 0.5 mL for 1 dose, followed by 0.5 mL after 1–3 months for 1 dose, then 0.5 mL after further 5–12 months for 1 dose, to achieve more rapid protection, second dose may be given 14 days after first dose, dose to be administered in deltoid region, in immunocompromised patients (including those receiving immunosuppressants), antibody concentration may be measured 4 weeks after second dose and dose repeated if protective levels not achieved
‣ Elderly: 0.5 mL for 1 dose, followed by 0.5 mL after 1–3 months for 1 dose, then 0.5 mL after further 5–12 months for 1 dose, to achieve more rapid protection, second dose may be given 14 days after first dose, dose to be administered in deltoid region, antibody concentration may be measured 4 weeks after second dose and dose repeated if protective levels not achieved

Immunisation against tick-borne encephalitis, booster doses
‣ BY INTRAMUSCULAR INJECTION
‣ Child 1–17 years: First dose to be given within 3 years after initial course completed and then every 3–5 years, dose to be administered in deltoid region or anterolateral thigh in infants (consult product literature)

‣ Adult: First dose to be given within 3 years after initial course completed and then every 3–5 years, dose to be administered in deltoid region (consult product literature)

- ALLERGY AND CROSS-SENSITIVITY Individuals with evidence of previous anaphylactic reaction to egg should not be given tick-borne encephalitis vaccine.

- MEDICINAL FORMS
There can be variation in the licensing of different medicines containing the same drug.
Suspension for injection
EXCIPIENTS: May contain Gentamicin, neomycin
‣ TicoVac (Masta Ltd)
  TicoVac Junior vaccine suspension for injection 0.25ml pre-filled syringes | 1 pre-filled disposable injection PoM £28.00
  TicoVac vaccine suspension for injection 0.5ml pre-filled syringes | 1 pre-filled disposable injection PoM £32.00

🏳 1146

Varicella-zoster vaccine

- INDICATIONS AND DOSE
VARILRIX®
Prevention of varicella infection (chickenpox)
‣ BY SUBCUTANEOUS INJECTION
‣ Child 1–17 years: 0.5 mL every 4–6 weeks for 2 doses, to be administered preferably into the deltoid region
‣ Adult: 0.5 mL every 4–6 weeks for 2 doses, to be administered preferably into the deltoid region

VARIVAX®
Prevention of varicella infection (chickenpox)
‣ BY SUBCUTANEOUS INJECTION, OR BY INTRAMUSCULAR INJECTION
‣ Child 1–12 years: 0.5 mL for 2 doses, interval of at least 4 weeks between each dose, to be administered into the deltoid region (or higher anterolateral thigh in young children)
‣ Child 13–17 years: 0.5 mL every 4–8 weeks for 2 doses, to be administered preferably into the deltoid region
‣ Adult: 0.5 mL every 4–8 weeks for 2 doses, to be administered preferably into the deltoid region

Prevention of varicella infection (chickenpox) in children with asymptomatic HIV infection
‣ BY SUBCUTANEOUS INJECTION, OR BY INTRAMUSCULAR INJECTION
‣ Child 1–12 years: 0.5 mL every 12 weeks for 2 doses, to be administered into the deltoid region (or higher anterolateral thigh in young children)

ZOSTAVAX®
Prevention of herpes zoster (shingles)
‣ BY SUBCUTANEOUS INJECTION
‣ Adult 70–79 years: 0.65 mL for 1 dose, to be administered preferably into the deltoid region

- CAUTIONS Post-vaccination close contact with susceptible individuals
CAUTIONS, FURTHER INFORMATION
Rarely, the varicella–zoster vaccine virus has been transmitted from the vaccinated individual to close contacts. Therefore, contact with the following should be avoided if a vaccine-related cutaneous rash develops within 4–6 weeks of the first or second dose:
- varicella-susceptible pregnant women;
- individuals at high risk of severe varicella, including those with immunodeficiency or those receiving immunosuppressive therapy.

Healthcare workers who develop a generalised papular or vesicular rash on vaccination should avoid contact with patients until the lesions have crusted. Those who develop

14

Vaccines

a localised rash after vaccination should cover the lesions and be allowed to continue working unless in contact with patients at high risk of severe varicella.
▸ Administration with MMR vaccine Varicella–zoster and MMR vaccines can be given on the same day or separated by a 4-week minimum interval. When protection is rapidly required, the vaccines can be given at any interval and an additional dose of the vaccine given second may be considered.

● SIDE-EFFECTS
▸ **Rare** Thrombocytopenia
▸ **Frequency not known** Conjunctivitis · varicella-like rash

● CONCEPTION AND CONTRACEPTION Avoid pregnancy for 3 months after vaccination.

● PRESCRIBING AND DISPENSING INFORMATION
ZOSTAVAX® Advice in the BNF may differ from that in product literature.

● MEDICINAL FORMS
There can be variation in the licensing of different medicines containing the same drug.
Powder and solvent for solution for injection
EXCIPIENTS: May contain Neomycin
▸ Varilrix (GlaxoSmithKline UK Ltd)
Varilrix vaccine powder and solvent for solution for injection 0.5ml vials | 1 vial [PoM] £27.31
Powder and solvent for suspension for injection
EXCIPIENTS: May contain Gelatin, neomycin
▸ Varivax (sanofi pasteur MSD Ltd)
Varivax vaccine powder and solvent for suspension for injection 0.5ml vials | 1 vial [PoM] £30.28

⌐ 1146

Yellow fever vaccine, live

● **INDICATIONS AND DOSE**
Immunisation against yellow fever
▸ BY DEEP SUBCUTANEOUS INJECTION
▸ Child 6–8 months (administered on expert advice): Infants under 9 months should be vaccinated only if the risk of yellow fever is high and unavoidable (consult product literature or local protocols)
▸ Child 9 months–17 years: 0.5 mL for 1 dose
▸ Adult: 0.5 mL for 1 dose

● CONTRA-INDICATIONS Children under 6 months · history of thymus dysfunction
● CAUTIONS Individuals over 60 years—greater risk of vaccine-associated adverse effects (in adults)
CAUTIONS, FURTHER INFORMATION
▸ Administration with MMR vaccine Yellow fever and MMR vaccines should not be administered on the same day; there should be a 4-week minimum interval between the vaccines. When protection is rapidly required, the vaccines can be given at any interval and an additional dose of MMR may be considered.

● SIDE-EFFECTS Neurotropic disease · viscerotropic disease
SIDE-EFFECTS, FURTHER INFORMATION
▸ Vaccine-associated adverse effects *Very rare* adverse effects, such as viscerotropic disease (yellow-fever vaccine-associated viscerotropic disease, YEL-AVD), a syndrome which may include metabolic acidosis, muscle and liver cirrhosis, and multi-organ failure. Neurological disorders (yellow fever vaccine-associated neurotropic disease, YEL-AND) such as encephalitis have also been reported. These *very rare* adverse effects usually occur after the first dose of yellow fever vaccine in those with no previous immunity.
● ALLERGY AND CROSS-SENSITIVITY Yellow fever vaccine should only be considered under the guidance of a specialist in individuals with evidence of previous anaphylactic reaction to egg.

● PREGNANCY Live yellow fever vaccine should not be given during pregnancy because there is a theoretical risk of fetal infection. Pregnant women should be advised not to travel to areas at high risk of yellow fever. If exposure cannot be avoided during pregnancy, then the vaccine should be given if the risk from disease in the mother outweighs the risk to the fetus from vaccination.

● BREAST FEEDING Avoid; seek specialist advice if exposure to virus cannot be avoided.

● MEDICINAL FORMS
There can be variation in the licensing of different medicines containing the same drug.
Powder and solvent for suspension for injection
▸ Stamaril (sanofi pasteur MSD Ltd)
Stamaril vaccine powder and solvent for suspension for injection 0.5ml vials | 1 vial [PoM] £33.10

Chapter 15
Anaesthesia

CONTENTS

General anaesthesia

General anaesthesia

Overview

Several different types of drug are given together during general anaesthesia. Anaesthesia is induced with either a volatile drug given by inhalation or with an intravenously administered drug; anaesthesia is maintained with an intravenous or inhalational anaesthetic. Analgesics, usually short-acting opioids, are also used. The use of neuromuscular blocking drugs necessitates intermittent positive-pressure ventilation. Following surgery, anticholinesterases can be given to reverse the effects of neuromuscular blocking drugs; specific antagonists can be used to reverse central and respiratory depression caused by some drugs used in surgery. A local topical anaesthetic can be used to reduce pain at the injection site.

Individual requirements vary considerably and the recommended doses are only a guide. Smaller doses are indicated in ill, shocked, or debilitated patients and in significant hepatic impairment, while robust individuals may require larger doses. The required dose of induction agent may be less if the patient has been premedicated with a sedative agent or if an opioid analgesic has been used.

Intravenous anaesthetics

Intravenous anaesthetics may be used either to induce anaesthesia or for maintenance of anaesthesia throughout surgery. Intravenous anaesthetics nearly all produce their effect in one arm-brain circulation time. Extreme care is required in surgery of the mouth, pharynx, or larynx where the airway may be difficult to maintain (e.g. in the presence of a tumour in the pharynx or larynx).

To facilitate tracheal intubation, induction is usually followed by a neuromuscular blocking drug or a short-acting opioid.

The doses of all intravenous anaesthetic drugs should be titrated to effect (except when using 'rapid sequence induction'); lower doses may be required in premedicated patients.

Total intravenous anaesthesia

This is a technique in which major surgery is carried out with all drugs given intravenously. Respiration can be spontaneous, or controlled with oxygen-enriched air. Neuromuscular blocking drugs can be used to provide relaxation and prevent reflex muscle movements. The main problem to be overcome is the assessment of depth of anaesthesia. Target Controlled Infusion (TCI) systems can be used to titrate intravenous anaesthetic infusions to

predicted plasma-drug concentrations in ventilated adult patients.

Drugs used for intravenous anaesthesia

Propofol p. 1165, the most widely used intravenous anaesthetic, can be used for induction or maintenance of anaesthesia in adults and children, but it is not commonly used in neonates. Propofol is associated with rapid recovery and less hangover effect than other intravenous anaesthetics. Propofol can also be used for sedation during diagnostic procedures and sedation in adults in intensive care.

Thiopental sodium p. 308 is a barbiturate that is used for induction of anaesthesia, but has no analgesic properties. Induction is generally smooth and rapid, but dose-related cardiovascular and respiratory depression can occur. Awakening from a moderate dose of thiopental sodium is rapid because the drug redistributes into other tissues, particularly fat. However, metabolism is slow and sedative effects can persist for 24 hours. Repeated doses have a cumulative effect and recovery is much slower.

Etomidate p. 1165 is an intravenous agent associated with rapid recovery without a hangover effect. Etomidate causes less hypotension than thiopental sodium and propofol during induction. It produces a high incidence of extraneous muscle movements, which can be minimised by an opioid analgesic or a short-acting benzodiazepine given just before induction.

Ketamine p. 1179 is used rarely. Ketamine causes less hypotension than thiopental sodium and propofol during induction. It is used mainly for paediatric anaesthesia, particularly when repeated administration is required (such as for serial burns dressings); recovery is relatively slow and there is a high incidence of extraneous muscle movements. The main disadvantage of ketamine is the high incidence of hallucinations, nightmares, and other transient psychotic effects; these can be reduced by a benzodiazepine such as diazepam p. 313 or midazolam p. 310.

Inhalational anaesthetics

Inhalational anaesthetics include gases and volatile liquids. *Gaseous anaesthetics* require suitable equipment for storage and administration. *Volatile liquid anaesthetics* are administered using calibrated vaporisers, using air, oxygen, or nitrous oxide-oxygen mixtures as the carrier gas. To prevent hypoxia, the inspired gas mixture should contain a minimum of 25% oxygen at all times. Higher concentrations of oxygen (greater than 30%) are usually required during inhalational anaesthesia when nitrous oxide p. 1167 is being administered.

increase in sedation required), patients over 55 years or debilitated may require lower initial dose and rate of administration

Maintenance of sedation for surgical and diagnostic procedures using 1% injection
▸ INITIALLY BY INTRAVENOUS INFUSION
▸ Adult: Initially 1.5–4.5 mg/kg/hour, dose and rate of administration adjusted according to desired level of sedation and response, followed by (by slow intravenous injection) 10–20 mg, (if rapid increase in sedation required), patients over 55 years or debilitated may require lower initial dose and rate of administration

Maintenance of sedation for surgical and diagnostic procedures using 2% injection
▸ INITIALLY BY INTRAVENOUS INFUSION
▸ Adult: Initially 1.5–4.5 mg/kg/hour, dose and rate of administration adjusted according to desired level of sedation and response, followed by (by slow intravenous injection) 10–20 mg, using 0.5% or 1% injection (if rapid increase in sedation required), patients over 55 years or debilitated may require lower initial dose and rate of administration

> **IMPORTANT SAFETY INFORMATION**
> Propofol should only be administered by, or under the direct supervision of, personnel experienced in its use, with adequate training in anaesthesia and airway management, and when resuscitation equipment is available.

● CAUTIONS Acute circulatory failure (shock) · cardiac impairment · cardiovascular disease · elderly · epilepsy · fixed cardiac output · hypotension · hypovolaemia · raised intracranial pressure · respiratory impairment
● INTERACTIONS → Appendix 1 (anaesthetics, general).
● SIDE-EFFECTS
▸ **Common or very common** Headache · hypotension · tachycardia · transient apnoea
▸ **Uncommon** Phlebitis · thrombosis
▸ **Rare** Anaphylaxis · arrhythmia · convulsions (onset can be delayed) · delayed recovery from anaesthesia · euphoria
▸ **Very rare** Discoloration of urine · pancreatitis · pulmonary oedema · sexual disinhibition
▸ **Frequency not known** Bradycardia · pain on intravenous injection · propofol infusion syndrome · significant extraneous muscle movements
SIDE-EFFECTS, FURTHER INFORMATION
▸ Bradycardia Bradycardia may be profound and may be treated with intravenous administration of an antimuscarinic drug.
▸ Extraneous muscle movement Extraneous muscle movements can be minimised by an opioid analgesic or a short-acting benzodiazepine given just before induction.
▸ Pain on injection Can be reduced by intravenous lidocaine.
▸ Propofol infusion syndrome Prolonged infusion of propofol doses exceeding 4 mg/kg/hour may result in potentially fatal effects, including metabolic acidosis, arrhythmias, cardiac failure, rhabdomyolysis, hyperlipidaemia, hyperkalaemia, hepatomegaly, and renal failure.
● PREGNANCY Max. dose for maintenance of anaesthesia 6 mg/kg/hour. May depress neonatal respiration if used during delivery.
● BREAST FEEDING Breast-feeding can be resumed as soon as mother has recovered sufficiently from anaesthesia.
● HEPATIC IMPAIRMENT Use with caution.
● RENAL IMPAIRMENT Use with caution.
● MONITORING REQUIREMENTS Monitor blood-lipid concentration if risk of fat overload or if sedation longer than 3 days.

● DIRECTIONS FOR ADMINISTRATION Shake before use; microbiological filter not recommended; may be administered via a Y-piece close to injection site co-administered with Glucose 5% or Sodium chloride 0.9%. 0.5% **emulsion** for injection or intermittent infusion; may be administered undiluted, or diluted with Glucose 5% or Sodium chloride 0.9%; dilute to a concentration not less than 1 mg/mL. 1% **emulsion** for injection or infusion; may be administered undiluted, or diluted with Glucose 5% (*Diprivan®*) or (*Propofol-Lipuro®*) or Sodium chloride 0.9% (*Propofol-Lipuro®* only); dilute to a concentration not less than 2 mg/mL; use within 6 hours of preparation. 2% **emulsion** for infusion; do not dilute.
● PATIENT AND CARER ADVICE
Driving and skilled tasks
Patients given sedatives and analgesics during minor outpatient procedures should be very carefully warned about the risk of driving or undertaking skilled tasks afterwards. For a short general anaesthetic the risk extends to **at least 24 hours** after administration. Responsible persons should be available to take patients home. The dangers of taking **alcohol** should also be emphasised.

● MEDICINAL FORMS
There can be variation in the licensing of different medicines containing the same drug.
Emulsion for injection
▸ Diprivan (AstraZeneca UK Ltd)
Propofol 10 mg per 1 ml Diprivan 1% emulsion for injection 20ml ampoules | 5 ampoule [PoM] £15.36 (Hospital only)
▸ Propofol-Lipuro (B.Braun Medical Ltd)
Propofol 5 mg per 1 ml Propofol-Lipuro 0.5% emulsion for injection 20ml ampoules | 5 ampoule [PoM] £14.71
Emulsion for infusion
▸ Diprivan (AstraZeneca UK Ltd)
Propofol 10 mg per 1 ml Diprivan 1% emulsion for infusion 50ml pre-filled syringes | 1 pre-filled disposable injection [PoM] £10.68
Propofol 20 mg per 1 ml Diprivan 2% emulsion for infusion 50ml pre-filled syringes | 1 pre-filled disposable injection [PoM] £15.16

ANAESTHETICS, GENERAL ⟩ VOLATILE LIQUID ANAESTHETICS

Volatile halogenated anaesthetics

> **IMPORTANT SAFETY INFORMATION**
> Should only be administered by, or under the direct supervision of, personnel experienced in their use, with adequate training in anaesthesia and airway management, and when resuscitation equipment is available.

● CONTRA-INDICATIONS Susceptibility to malignant hyperthermia
● CAUTIONS Can trigger malignant hyperthermia · raised intracranial pressure (can increase cerebrospinal pressure)
● SIDE-EFFECTS
▸ **Common or very common** Arrhythmias · cardiorespiratory depression · hypotension
▸ **Frequency not known** Convulsions · mood changes (that can last several days)
● ALLERGY AND CROSS-SENSITIVITY Can cause hepatotoxicity in those sensitised to halogenated anaesthetics.
● DIRECTIONS FOR ADMINISTRATION Volatile liquid anaesthetics are administered using calibrated vaporisers, using air, oxygen, or nitrous oxide-oxygen mixtures as the carrier gas. To prevent hypoxia, the inspired gas mixture should contain a minimum of 25% oxygen at all times.

- PATIENT AND CARER ADVICE

Driving and skilled tasks

Patients given sedatives and analgesics during minor outpatient procedures should be very carefully warned about the risks of driving or undertaking skilled tasks afterwards. For a short general anaesthetic, the risk extends **to at least 24 hours** after administration. Responsible persons should be available to take patients home. The dangers of taking **alcohol** should also be emphasised.

ℱ 1166

Desflurane

- INDICATIONS AND DOSE

Induction of anaesthesia (but not recommended)

▸ BY INHALATION
▸ Adult: 4–11 %, to be inhaled through specifically calibrated vaporiser

Maintenance of anaesthesia (in nitrous oxide–oxygen)

▸ BY INHALATION
▸ Adult: 2–6 %, to be inhaled through a specifically calibrated vaporiser

Maintenance of anaesthesia (in oxygen or oxygen-enriched air)

▸ BY INHALATION
▸ Adult: 2.5–8.5 %, to be inhaled through a specifically calibrated vaporiser

- INTERACTIONS → Appendix 1 (anaesthetics, general).
- SIDE-EFFECTS Apnoea · breath-holding · cough · increased secretions · laryngospasm
- PREGNANCY May depress neonatal respiration if used during delivery.
- BREAST FEEDING Breast-feeding can be resumed as soon as mother has recovered sufficiently from anaesthesia.
- PATIENT AND CARER ADVICE

Driving and skilled tasks

Patients given sedatives and analgesics during minor outpatient procedures should be very carefully warned about the risk of driving or undertaking skilled tasks afterwards. For a short general anaesthetic the risk extends to **at least 24 hours** after administration. Responsible persons should be available to take patients home. The dangers of taking **alcohol** should also be emphasised.

- MEDICINAL FORMS

There can be variation in the licensing of different medicines containing the same drug.

Inhalation vapour

▸ Suprane (Baxter Healthcare Ltd)
Desflurane 1 ml per 1 ml Suprane volatile liquid | 240 ml [PoM] no price available (Hospital only)

ℱ 1166

Isoflurane

- INDICATIONS AND DOSE

Induction of anaesthesia (in oxygen or nitrous oxide-oxygen)

▸ BY INHALATION
▸ Adult: Initially 0.5 %, increased to 3 %, adjusted according to response, administered using specifically calibrated vaporiser

Maintenance of anaesthesia (in nitrous oxide–oxygen)

▸ BY INHALATION
▸ Adult: 1–2.5 %, to be administered using specifically calibrated vaporiser; an additional 0.5–1% may be required when given with oxygen alone

Maintenance of anaesthesia in caesarean section (in nitrous oxide–oxygen)

▸ BY INHALATION
▸ Adult: 0.5–0.75 %, to be administered using specifically calibrated vaporiser

- INTERACTIONS → Appendix 1 (anaesthetics, general).
- SIDE-EFFECTS Breath-holding · cough · irritate mucous membrane · laryngospasm
- PREGNANCY May depress neonatal respiration if used during delivery.
- BREAST FEEDING Breast-feeding can be resumed as soon as mother has recovered sufficiently from anaesthesia.
- PATIENT AND CARER ADVICE

Driving and skilled tasks

Patients given sedatives and analgesics during minor outpatient procedures should be very carefully warned about the risk of driving or undertaking skilled tasks afterwards. For a short general anaesthetic the risk extends to **at least 24 hours** after administration. Responsible persons should be available to take patients home. The dangers of taking **alcohol** should also be emphasised.

- MEDICINAL FORMS

There can be variation in the licensing of different medicines containing the same drug.

Inhalation vapour

▸ Isoflurane (Non-proprietary)
Isoflurane 1 ml per 1 ml Isoflurane inhalation vapour | 250 ml [PoM] £35.29 (Hospital only)
Isoflurane volatile liquid | 250 ml [P] £47.50 (Hospital only)
▸ AErrane (Baxter Healthcare Ltd)
Isoflurane 1 ml per 1 ml AErrane volatile liquid | 250 ml [P] no price available (Hospital only)

Nitrous oxide

- INDICATIONS AND DOSE

Maintenance of anaesthesia in conjunction with other anaesthetic agents

▸ BY INHALATION
▸ Adult: 50–66 %, to be administered using suitable anaesthetic apparatus in oxygen

Analgesia

▸ BY INHALATION
▸ Adult: Up to 50 %, to be administered using suitable anaesthetic apparatus in oxygen, adjusted according to the patient's needs

IMPORTANT SAFETY INFORMATION

Nitrous oxide should only be administered by, or under the direct supervision of, personnel experienced in its use, with adequate training in anaesthesia and airway management, and when resuscitation equipment is available.

- CAUTIONS Entrapped air following recent underwater dive · pneumothorax · presence of intracranial air after head injury · recent intra-ocular gas injection

CAUTIONS, FURTHER INFORMATION

Nitrous oxide may have a deleterious effect if used in patients with an air-containing closed space since nitrous oxide diffuses into such a space with a resulting increase in pressure. This effect may be dangerous in conditions such as pneumothorax, which may enlarge to compromise respiration, or in the presence of intracranial air after head injury, entrapped air following recent underwater dive, or recent intra-ocular gas injection.

- INTERACTIONS → Appendix 1 (anaesthetics, general).

- SIDE-EFFECTS Depression of white cell formation · hypoxia · megaloblastic anaemia · neurological toxic effects

  SIDE-EFFECTS, FURTHER INFORMATION

  ‣ Hypoxia Hypoxia can occur immediately following the administration of nitrous oxide; additional oxygen should always be given for several minutes after stopping the flow of nitrous oxide.

  ‣ Prolonged exposure Exposure of patients to nitrous oxide for prolonged periods, either by continuous or by intermittent administration, may result in megaloblastic anaemia owing to interference with the action of vitamin B_{12}; neurological toxic effects can occur without preceding overt haematological changes. Depression of white cell formation may also occur.

- PREGNANCY May depress neonatal respiration if used during delivery.

- BREAST FEEDING Breast-feeding can be resumed as soon as mother has recovered sufficiently from anaesthesia.

- MONITORING REQUIREMENTS

  ‣ Assessment of plasma-vitamin B_{12} concentration should be considered in those at risk of deficiency, including the elderly, those who have a poor, vegetarian, or vegan diet, and those with a history of anaemia.

  ‣ Nitrous oxide should **not** be given continuously for longer than 24 hours or more frequently than every 4 days without close supervision and haematological monitoring.

- DIRECTIONS FOR ADMINISTRATION For analgesia (without loss of consciousness), a mixture of nitrous oxide and oxygen containing 50% of each gas (Entonox®, Equanox®) is used.

- HANDLING AND STORAGE Exposure of theatre staff to nitrous oxide should be minimised (risk of serious side-effects).

- MEDICINAL FORMS

  There can be variation in the licensing of different medicines containing the same drug.

  Inhalation gas

  ‣ Nitrous oxide (Non-proprietary)

  Nitrous oxide 1 ml per 1 ml Nitrous oxide cylinders size E | 1800 litre P no price available

  Medical Nitrous Oxide cylinders size D | 900 litre P no price available

  Medical Nitrous Oxide cylinders size G | 9000 litre P no price available

  Nitrous oxide cylinders size F | 3600 litre P no price available

  Nitrous oxide cylinders size J | 18000 litre P no price available

  Nitrous oxide cylinders size G | 9000 litre P no price available

  Nitrous oxide cylinders size C | 450 litre P no price available

  Medical Nitrous Oxide cylinders size F | 3600 litre P no price available

  Nitrous oxide cylinders size D | 900 litre P no price available

  Medical Nitrous Oxide cylinders size E | 1800 litre P no price available

  F 1166

Sevoflurane

- INDICATIONS AND DOSE

  Induction of anaesthesia (in oxygen or nitrous oxide-oxygen)

  ‣ BY INHALATION

  ‣ Adult: Initially 0.5–1 %, then increased to up to 8 %, increased gradually, according to response, to be administered using specifically calibrated vaporiser

  Maintenance of anaesthesia (in oxygen or nitrous oxide-oxygen)

  ‣ BY INHALATION

  ‣ Adult: 0.5–3 %, adjusted according to response, to be administered using specifically calibrated vaporiser

- CAUTIONS Susceptibility to QT-interval prolongation

- INTERACTIONS → Appendix 1 (anaesthetics, general). Sevoflurane can interact with carbon dioxide absorbents to form compound A, a potentially nephrotoxic vinyl ether. However, in spite of extensive use, no cases of sevoflurane-induced permanent renal injury have been reported and the carbon dioxide absorbents used in the UK produce very low concentrations of compound A, even in low-flow anaesthetic systems.

- SIDE-EFFECTS Cardiac arrest · dystonia · leucopenia · torsade de pointes · urinary retention

- PREGNANCY May depress neonatal respiration if used during delivery.

- BREAST FEEDING Breast-feeding can be resumed as soon as mother has recovered sufficiently from anaesthesia.

- RENAL IMPAIRMENT Use with caution.

- PATIENT AND CARER ADVICE

  Driving and skilled tasks

  Patients given sedatives and analgesics during minor outpatient procedures should be very carefully warned about the risk of driving or undertaking skilled tasks afterwards. For a short general anaesthetic the risk extends to **at least 24 hours** after administration. Responsible persons should be available to take patients home. The dangers of taking **alcohol** should also be emphasised.

- MEDICINAL FORMS

  There can be variation in the licensing of different medicines containing the same drug.

  Inhalation vapour

  ‣ Sevoflurane (Non-proprietary)

  Sevoflurane 1 ml per 1 ml Sevoflurane volatile liquid | 250 ml PoM £123.00 (Hospital only)

1 Anaesthesia adjuvants

Pre-medication and peri-operative drugs

Drugs that affect gastric pH

Regurgitation and aspiration of gastric contents (Mendelson's syndrome) can be an important complication of general anaesthesia, particularly in obstetrics and during emergency surgery, and requires prophylaxis against acid aspiration. Prophylaxis is also needed in those with gastro-oesophageal reflux disease and in circumstances where gastric emptying may be delayed.

A **H_2-receptor antagonist** can be used before surgery to increase the pH and reduce the volume of gastric fluid. It does not affect the pH of fluid already in the stomach and this limits its value in emergency procedures; an oral H_2-receptor antagonist can be given 1–2 hours before the procedure. Antacids are frequently used to neutralise the acidity of the fluid already in the stomach; 'clear' (non-particulate) antacids such as sodium citrate p. 713 are preferred.

Antimuscarinic drugs

Antimuscarinic drugs are used (less commonly nowadays) as premedicants to dry bronchial and salivary secretions which are increased by intubation, upper airway surgery, or some inhalational anaesthetics. They are also used before or with neostigmine p. 971 to prevent bradycardia, excessive salivation, and other muscarinic actions of neostigmine. They also prevent bradycardia and hypotension associated with drugs such as propofol p. 1165 and suxamethonium chloride p. 1171.

Atropine sulfate p. 1169 is now rarely used for premedication but still has an emergency role in the treatment of vagotonic side-effects. Atropine sulfate may have a role in acute arrhythmias after myocardial infarction.

Hyoscine hydrobromide p. 401 reduces secretions and also provides a degree of amnesia, sedation, and anti-emesis. Unlike atropine sulfate it may produce bradycardia rather than tachycardia.

Glycopyrronium bromide p. 1170 reduces salivary secretions. When given intravenously it produces less tachycardia than atropine sulfate. It is widely used with neostigmine for reversal of non-depolarising neuromuscular blocking drugs.

Phenothiazines do not effectively reduce secretions when used alone.

Sedative drugs

Fear and anxiety before a procedure (including the night before) can be minimised by using a sedative drug, usually a **benzodiazepine**. Premedication may also augment the action of anaesthetics and provide some degree of pre-operative amnesia. The choice of drug depends on the individual, the nature of the procedure, the anaesthetic to be used, and other prevailing circumstances such as outpatients, obstetrics, and availability of recovery facilities. The choice also varies between elective and emergency procedures.

Premedicants can be given the night before major surgery; a further, smaller dose may be required before surgery. Alternatively, the first dose may be given on the day of the procedure.

Benzodiazepines

Benzodiazepines possess useful properties for premedication including relief of anxiety, sedation, and amnesia; short-acting benzodiazepines taken by mouth are the most common premedicants. Benzodiazepines are also used in intensive care units for sedation, particularly in those receiving assisted ventilation. Flumazenil p. 1203 is used to antagonise the effects of benzodiazepines.

Diazepam p. 313 is used to produce mild sedation with amnesia. It is a long-acting drug with active metabolites and a second period of drowsiness can occur several hours after its administration. Peri-operative use of diazepam in children is not recommended; its effect and timing of response are unreliable and paradoxical effects may occur.

Diazepam is relatively insoluble in water and preparations formulated in organic solvents are painful on intravenous injection and give rise to a high incidence of venous thrombosis (which may not be noticed for several days after the injection). Intramuscular injection of diazepam is painful and absorption is erratic. An emulsion formulated for intravenous injection is less irritant and reduces the risk of venous thrombosis; it is not suitable for intramuscular injection.

Temazepam p. 443 is given by mouth for premedication and has a shorter duration of action and a more rapid onset than oral diazepam; anxiolytic and sedative effects last about 90 minutes although there may be residual drowsiness.

Lorazepam p. 308 produces more prolonged sedation than temazepam and it has marked amnesic effects.

Midazolam p. 310 is a water-soluble benzodiazepine that is often used in preference to intravenous diazepam; recovery is faster than from diazepam, but may be significantly longer in the elderly, in patients with a low cardiac output, or after repeated dosing. Midazolam is associated with profound sedation when high doses are given intravenously or when it is used with certain other drugs.

Other drugs for sedation

Dexmedetomidine p. 1180 and clonidine hydrochloride p. 131 are alpha$_2$-adrenergic agonists with sedative properties. Dexmedetomidine is licensed for the sedation of patients receiving intensive care who need to remain responsive to verbal stimulation. Clonidine hydrochloride

[unlicensed indication] can be used by mouth or by intravenous injection as a sedative agent when adequate sedation cannot be achieved with standard treatment.

Antagonists for central and respiratory depression

Respiratory depression is a major concern with opioid analgesics and it may be treated by artificial ventilation or be reversed by naloxone hydrochloride p. 1204. Naloxone hydrochloride will immediately reverse opioid-induced respiratory depression but the dose may have to be repeated because of the short duration of action of naloxone hydrochloride; however, naloxone hydrochloride will also antagonise the analgesic effect.

Flumazenil is a benzodiazepine antagonist for the reversal of the central sedative effects of benzodiazepines after anaesthetic and similar procedures. Flumazenil has a shorter half-life and duration of action than diazepam or midazolam so patients may become resedated.

Doxapram hydrochloride p. 273 is a central and respiratory stimulant but is of limited value in anaesthesia.

ANTIMUSCARINICS

> ☞ 703

Atropine sulfate

● INDICATIONS AND DOSE

Bradycardia due to acute massive overdosage of beta-blockers
▶ BY INTRAVENOUS INJECTION
▹ Child: 40 micrograms/kg (max. per dose 3 mg)
▹ Adult: 3 mg

Treatment of poisoning by organophosphorus insecticide or nerve agent (in combination with pralidoxime chloride)
▶ BY INTRAVENOUS INJECTION
▹ Child: 20 micrograms/kg every 5–10 minutes (max. per dose 2 mg) until the skin becomes flushed and dry, the pupils dilate, and bradycardia is abolished, frequency of administration dependent on the severity of poisoning
▹ Adult: 2 mg every 5–10 minutes until the skin becomes flushed and dry, the pupils dilate, and bradycardia is abolished, frequency of administration dependent on the severity of poisoning

Symptomatic relief of gastro-intestinal disorders characterised by smooth muscle spasm
▶ BY MOUTH
▹ Adult: 0.6–1.2 mg daily, dose to be taken at night

Premedication
▶ BY INTRAVENOUS INJECTION
▹ Child 12-17 years: 300–600 micrograms, to be administered immediately before induction of anaesthesia
▹ Adult: 300–600 micrograms, to be administered immediately before induction of anaesthesia
▶ BY SUBCUTANEOUS INJECTION, OR BY INTRAMUSCULAR INJECTION
▹ Child 12-17 years: 300–600 micrograms, to be administered 30–60 minutes before induction of anaesthesia
▹ Adult: 300–600 micrograms, to be administered 30–60 minutes before induction of anaesthesia

Intra-operative bradycardia
▶ BY INTRAVENOUS INJECTION
▹ Child 12-17 years: 300–600 micrograms, larger doses may be used in emergencies
▹ Adult: 300–600 micrograms, larger doses may be used in emergencies　　　　continued →

Control of muscarinic side-effects of neostigmine in reversal of competitive neuromuscular block

▶ BY INTRAVENOUS INJECTION

▸ Child 12-17 years: 0.6–1.2 mg

▸ Adult: 0.6–1.2 mg

Excessive bradycardia associated with beta-blocker use

▶ BY INTRAVENOUS INJECTION

▸ Adult: 0.6–2.4 mg in divided doses (max. per dose 600 micrograms)

Bradycardia following myocardial infarction (particularly if complicated by hypotension)

▶ BY INTRAVENOUS INJECTION

▸ Adult: 500 micrograms every 3–5 minutes; maximum 3 mg per course

● UNLICENSED USE Not licensed for use in children under 12 years for intra-operative bradycardia or by intravenous route for premedication.

┌───┐
IMPORTANT SAFETY INFORMATION
Antimuscarinic drugs used for premedication to general anaesthesia should only be administered by, or under the direct supervision of, personnel experienced in their use.
└───┘

● PREGNANCY Not known to be harmful; manufacturer advises caution.

● BREAST FEEDING May suppress lactation; small amount present in milk—manufacturer advises caution.

● MONITORING REQUIREMENTS

● Control of muscarinic side-effects of neostigmine in reversal of competitive neuromuscular block Since atropine has a shorter duration of action than neostigmine, late unopposed bradycardia may result; close monitoring of the patient is necessary.

● LESS SUITABLE FOR PRESCRIBING Atropine tablets less suitable for prescribing. Any clinical benefit as a gastro-intestinal antispasmodic is outweighed by atropinic side-effects.

● EXCEPTIONS TO LEGAL CATEGORY

▶ With intramuscular use or intravenous use or subcutaneous use Prescription only medicine restriction does not apply where administration is for saving life in emergency.

● MEDICINAL FORMS
There can be variation in the licensing of different medicines containing the same drug. Forms available from special-order manufacturers include: oral suspension, oral solution, solution for injection, solution for infusion

Tablet

▸ Atropine sulfate (Non-proprietary)
Atropine sulfate 600 microgram Atropine 600microgram tablets | 28 tablet PoM £25.75 DT price = £25.75

Solution for injection

▸ Atropine sulfate (Non-proprietary)
Atropine sulfate 100 microgram per 1 ml Atropine 500micrograms/5ml solution for injection pre-filled syringes | 1 pre-filled disposable injection PoM £7.40–£13.00 | 10 pre-filled disposable injection PoM £69.00–£130.00
Atropine sulfate 200 microgram per 1 ml Atropine 1mg/5ml solution for injection pre-filled syringes | 1 pre-filled disposable injection PoM £7.08–£13.00 | 10 pre-filled disposable injection PoM £130.00
Atropine sulfate 300 microgram per 1 ml Atropine 3mg/10ml solution for injection pre-filled syringes | 1 pre-filled disposable injection PoM £7.08–£13.00 | 10 pre-filled disposable injection PoM £130.00
Atropine sulfate 400 microgram per 1 ml Atropine 400micrograms/1ml solution for injection ampoules | 10 ampoule PoM £67.78–£74.56 DT price = £71.17
Atropine sulfate 600 microgram per 1 ml Atropine 600micrograms/1ml solution for injection ampoules | 10 ampoule PoM £11.71 DT price = £11.70

Atropine 600micrograms/1ml solution for injection pre-filled syringes | 1 pre-filled disposable injection PoM £7.08
Atropine sulfate 1 mg per 1 ml Atropine 1mg/1ml solution for injection ampoules | 10 ampoule PoM £57.66–£63.43 DT price = £60.55

━ 703

Glycopyrronium bromide

(Glycopyrrolate)

● INDICATIONS AND DOSE

Premedication at induction

▶ BY INTRAMUSCULAR INJECTION, OR BY INTRAVENOUS INJECTION

▸ Adult: 200–400 micrograms, alternatively 4–5 micrograms/kg (max. per dose 400 micrograms)

Intra-operative bradycardia

▶ BY INTRAVENOUS INJECTION

▸ Adult: 200–400 micrograms, alternatively 4–5 micrograms/kg (max. per dose 400 micrograms), repeated if necessary

Control of muscarinic side-effects of neostigmine in reversal of non-depolarising neuromuscular block

▶ BY INTRAVENOUS INJECTION

▸ Adult: 10–15 micrograms/kg, alternatively, 200 micrograms per 1 mg of neostigmine to be administered

Bowel colic in palliative care | Excessive respiratory secretions in palliative care

▶ BY SUBCUTANEOUS INJECTION

▸ Adult: 200 micrograms every 4 hours and when required, hourly use is occasionally necessary, particularly in excessive respiratory secretions

▶ BY SUBCUTANEOUS INFUSION

▸ Adult: 0.6–1.2 mg/24 hours

┌───┐
IMPORTANT SAFETY INFORMATION
Antimuscarinic drugs used for premedication to general anaesthesia should only be administered by, or under the direct supervision of, personnel experienced in their use.
└───┘

● MEDICINAL FORMS
There can be variation in the licensing of different medicines containing the same drug.
Solution for injection

▸ Glycopyrronium bromide (Non-proprietary)
Glycopyrronium bromide 200 microgram per 1 ml Glycopyrronium bromide 200micrograms/1ml solution for injection ampoules | 10 ampoule PoM £14.00 DT price = £8.28
Glycopyrronium bromide 600micrograms/3ml solution for injection ampoules | 3 ampoule PoM £8.00–£8.56 | 10 ampoule PoM £11.50

Combinations available: *Neostigmine with glycopyrronium bromide*, p. 1174

1.1 Neuromuscular blockade

Neuromuscular blockade

Neuromuscular blocking drugs

Neuromuscular blocking drugs used in anaesthesia are also known as **muscle relaxants**. By specific blockade of the neuromuscular junction they enable light anaesthesia to be used with adequate relaxation of the muscles of the abdomen and diaphragm. They also relax the vocal cords and allow the passage of a tracheal tube. Their action differs from the muscle relaxants used in musculoskeletal disorders that act on the spinal cord or brain.

Patients who have received a neuromuscular blocking drug should **always** have their respiration assisted or controlled until the drug has been inactivated or antagonised. They should also receive sufficient concomitant inhalational or intravenous anaesthetic or sedative drugs to prevent awareness.

Non-depolarising neuromuscular blocking drugs

Non-depolarising neuromuscular blocking drugs (also known as competitive muscle relaxants) compete with acetylcholine for receptor sites at the neuromuscular junction and their action can be reversed with anticholinesterases such as neostigmine p. 971. Non-depolarising neuromuscular blocking drugs can be divided into the **aminosteroid** group, comprising pancuronium bromide p. 1173, rocuronium bromide p. 1173, and vecuronium bromide p. 1174, and the **benzylisoquinolinium** group, comprising atracurium besilate p. 1172, cisatracurium p. 1172, and mivacurium p. 1173.

Non-depolarising neuromuscular blocking drugs have a slower onset of action than suxamethonium chloride below. These drugs can be classified by their duration of action as short-acting (15–30 minutes), intermediate-acting (30–40 minutes), and long-acting (60–120 minutes), although duration of action is dose-dependent. Drugs with a shorter or intermediate duration of action, such as atracurium besilate and vecuronium bromide, are more widely used than those with a longer duration of action, such as pancuronium bromide.

Non-depolarising neuromuscular blocking drugs have no sedative or analgesic effects and are not considered to trigger malignant hyperthermia.

For patients receiving intensive care and who require tracheal intubation and mechanical ventilation, a non-depolarising neuromuscular blocking drug is chosen according to its onset of effect, duration of action, and side-effects. Rocuronium bromide, with a rapid onset of effect, may facilitate intubation. Atracurium besilate or cisatracurium may be suitable for long-term neuromuscular blockade since their duration of action is not dependent on elimination by the liver or the kidneys.

Atracurium besilate, a mixture of 10 isomers, is a benzylisoquinolinium neuromuscular blocking drug with an intermediate duration of action. It undergoes non-enzymatic metabolism which is independent of liver and kidney function, thus allowing its use in patients with hepatic or renal impairment. Cardiovascular effects are associated with significant histamine release; histamine release can be minimised by administering slowly or in divided doses over at least 1 minute.

Cisatracurium is a single isomer of atracurium besilate. It is more potent and has a slightly longer duration of action than atracurium besilate and provides greater cardiovascular stability because cisatracurium lacks histamine-releasing effects.

Mivacurium, a benzylisoquinolinium neuromuscular blocking drug, has a short duration of action. It is metabolised by plasma cholinesterase and muscle paralysis is prolonged in individuals deficient in this enzyme. It is not associated with vagolytic activity or ganglionic blockade although histamine release can occur, particularly with rapid injection.

Pancuronium bromide, an aminosteroid neuromuscular blocking drug, has a long duration of action and is often used in patients receiving long-term mechanical ventilation in intensive care units. It lacks a histamine-releasing effect, but vagolytic and sympathomimetic effects can cause tachycardia and hypertension.

Rocuronium bromide exerts an effect within 2 minutes and has the most rapid onset of any of the non-depolarising neuromuscular blocking drugs. It is an aminosteroid neuromuscular blocking drug with an intermediate duration

of action. It is reported to have minimal cardiovascular effects; high doses produce mild vagolytic activity.

Vecuronium bromide, an aminosteroid neuromuscular blocking drug, has an intermediate duration of action. It does not generally produce histamine release and lacks cardiovascular effects.

Depolarising neuromuscular blocking drugs

Suxamethonium chloride has the most rapid onset of action of any of the neuromuscular blocking drugs and is ideal if fast onset and brief duration of action are required, e.g. with tracheal intubation. Unlike the non-depolarising neuromuscular blocking drugs, its action cannot be reversed and recovery is spontaneous; anticholinesterases such as neostigmine potentiate the neuromuscular block.

Suxamethonium chloride should be given after anaesthetic induction because paralysis is usually preceded by painful muscle fasciculations. While tachycardia occurs with single use, bradycardia may occur with repeated doses in adults and with the first dose in children. Premedication with atropine reduces bradycardia as well as the excessive salivation associated with suxamethonium chloride use.

Prolonged paralysis may occur in **dual block**, which occurs with high or repeated doses of suxamethonium chloride and is caused by the development of a non-depolarising block following the initial depolarising block. Individuals with myasthenia gravis are resistant to suxamethonium chloride but can develop dual block resulting in delayed recovery. Prolonged paralysis may also occur in those with low or atypical plasma cholinesterase. Assisted ventilation should be continued until muscle function is restored.

NEUROMUSCULAR BLOCKING DRUGS ›
DEPOLARISING

▌Suxamethonium chloride

(Succinylcholine chloride)

- **DRUG ACTION** Suxamethonium acts by mimicking acetylcholine at the neuromuscular junction but hydrolysis is much slower than for acetylcholine; depolarisation is therefore prolonged, resulting in neuromuscular blockade.

- **INDICATIONS AND DOSE**

Neuromuscular blockade (short duration) during surgery and intubation

▸ BY INTRAVENOUS INJECTION
▸ Adult: 1–1.5 mg/kg

- **UNLICENSED USE** Doses of suxamethonium in BNF may differ from those in product literature.

> IMPORTANT SAFETY INFORMATION
> Should only be administered by, or under the direct supervision of, personnel experienced in its use.

- **CONTRA-INDICATIONS** Duchenne muscular dystrophy · family history of malignant hyperthermia · hyperkalaemia · low plasma-cholinesterase activity (including severe liver disease) · major trauma · neurological disease involving acute wasting of major muscle · personal or family history of congenital myotonic disease · prolonged immobilisation (risk of hyperkalaemia) · severe burns

- **CAUTIONS** Cardiac disease · neuromuscular disease · raised intra-ocular pressure (avoid in penetrating eye injury) · respiratory disease · severe sepsis (risk of hyperkalaemia)

- **INTERACTIONS** → Appendix 1 (muscle relaxants).

- **SIDE-EFFECTS**
▸ **Common or very common** Flushing · hyperkalaemia · increased gastric pressure · increased intra-ocular pressure · myoglobinaemia · myoglobinuria · postoperative muscle pain · rash

- ▸ **Rare** Apnoea · arrhythmias · bronchospasm · cardiac arrest · limited jaw mobility · prolonged respiratory depression
- ▸ **Very rare** Anaphylactic reactions · malignant hyperthermia
- ▸ **Frequency not known** Bradycardia (may occur with repeated doses) · hypertension · hypotension · rhabdomyolysis · tachycardia (occurs with single use)
  SIDE-EFFECTS, FURTHER INFORMATION
- ▸ Bradycardia Premedication with atropine reduces bradycardia as well as the excessive salivation associated with suxamethonium use.
- ● ALLERGY AND CROSS-SENSITIVITY Allergic cross-reactivity between neuromuscular blocking drugs has been reported; caution is advised in cases of hypersensitivity to these drugs.
- ● PREGNANCY Mildly prolonged maternal neuromuscular blockade may occur.
- ● BREAST FEEDING Unlikely to be present in breast milk in significant amounts (ionised at physiological pH). Breast-feeding may be resumed once the mother recovered from neuromuscular block.
- ● HEPATIC IMPAIRMENT Prolonged apnoea may occur in severe liver disease because of reduced hepatic synthesis of pseudocholinesterase.

- ● MEDICINAL FORMS
  There can be variation in the licensing of different medicines containing the same drug. Forms available from special-order manufacturers include: solution for injection
  Solution for injection
  - ▸ Suxamethonium chloride (Non-proprietary)
    Suxamethonium chloride 50 mg per 1 ml Suxamethonium chloride 100mg/2ml solution for injection ampoules | 10 ampoule [PoM] £28.80–£50.00
  - ▸ Anectine (GlaxoSmithKline UK Ltd)
    Suxamethonium chloride 50 mg per 1 ml Anectine 100mg/2ml solution for injection ampoules | 5 ampoule [PoM] £3.57

NEUROMUSCULAR BLOCKING DRUGS > NON-DEPOLARISING

Non-depolarising neuromuscular blocking drugs

> IMPORTANT SAFETY INFORMATION
> Non-depolarising neuromuscular blocking drugs should only be administered by, or under direct supervision of, personnel experienced in their use, with adequate training in anaesthesia and airway management.

- ● CAUTIONS Burns (resistance can develop, increased doses may be required) · cardiovascular disease (reduce rate of administration) · electrolyte disturbances (response unpredictable) · fluid disturbances (response unpredictable) · hypothermia (activity prolonged, lower doses required) · myasthenia gravis (activity prolonged, lower doses required) · neuromuscular disorders (response unpredictable)
- ● INTERACTIONS → Appendix 1 (muscle relaxants).
- ● ALLERGY AND CROSS-SENSITIVITY Allergic cross-reactivity between neuromuscular blocking drugs has been reported; caution is advised in cases of hypersensitivity to these drugs.
- ● PREGNANCY Non-depolarising neuromuscular blocking drugs are highly ionised at physiological pH and are therefore unlikely to cross the placenta in significant amounts.
- ● BREAST FEEDING Non-depolarising neuromuscular blocking drugs are ionised at physiological pH and are

unlikely to be present in milk in significant amounts. Breast-feeding may be resumed once the mother has recovered from neuromuscular block.

◀ above

Atracurium besilate

(Atracurium besylate)

- ● INDICATIONS AND DOSE
  Neuromuscular blockade (short to intermediate duration) for surgery and intubation
  - ▸ INITIALLY BY INTRAVENOUS INJECTION
  - ▸ Adult: Initially 300–600 micrograms/kg, then (by intravenous injection) 100–200 micrograms/kg as required, alternatively (by intravenous injection) initially 300–600 micrograms/kg, followed by (by intravenous infusion) 300–600 micrograms/kg/hour
  Neuromuscular blockade during intensive care
  - ▸ INITIALLY BY INTRAVENOUS INJECTION
  - ▸ Adult: Initially 300–600 micrograms/kg, initial dose is optional, then (by intravenous infusion) 270–1770 micrograms/kg/hour; (by intravenous infusion) usual dose 650–780 micrograms/kg/hour
  DOSES AT EXTREMES OF BODY-WEIGHT
  To avoid excessive dosage in obese patients, dose should be calculated on the basis of ideal body-weight.

- ● SIDE-EFFECTS
  - ▸ **Very rare** Anaphylactoid reactions
  - ▸ **Frequency not known** Acute myopathy (after prolonged use in intensive care) · bronchospasm · hypotension · seizures · skin flushing · tachycardia
    SIDE-EFFECTS, FURTHER INFORMATION
  - ▸ Cardiovascular effects Cardiovascular effects are associated with significant histamine release; histamine release can be minimised by administering slowly or in divided doses over at least 1 minute.
- ● DIRECTIONS FOR ADMINISTRATION For *intravenous infusion* (*Tracrium*®; Atracurium besilate injection, Hospira; Atracurium injection/infusion, Genus), give continuously in Glucose 5% or Sodium Chloride 0.9%; stability varies with diluent; dilute requisite dose with infusion fluid to a concentration of 0.5–5 mg/mL.

- ● MEDICINAL FORMS
  There can be variation in the licensing of different medicines containing the same drug.
  Solution for injection
  - ▸ Atracurium besilate (Non-proprietary)
    Atracurium besilate 10 mg per 1 ml Atracurium besilate 250mg/25ml solution for injection vials | 1 vial [PoM] £16.50
    Atracurium besilate 25mg/2.5ml solution for injection ampoules | 5 ampoule [PoM] £8.50–£9.25
    Atracurium besilate 50mg/5ml solution for injection ampoules | 5 ampoule [PoM] £15.00–£17.50 | 10 ampoule [PoM] £35.00
  - ▸ Tracrium (GlaxoSmithKline UK Ltd)
    Atracurium besilate 10 mg per 1 ml Tracrium 250mg/25ml solution for injection vials | 2 vial [PoM] £25.81
    Tracrium 25mg/2.5ml solution for injection ampoules | 5 ampoule [PoM] £8.28
    Tracrium 50mg/5ml solution for injection ampoules | 5 ampoule [PoM] £15.02

◀ above

Cisatracurium

- ● INDICATIONS AND DOSE
  Neuromuscular blockade (intermediate duration) during surgery and intubation
  - ▸ INITIALLY BY INTRAVENOUS INJECTION
  - ▸ Adult: Initially 150 micrograms/kg, then (by intravenous injection) maintenance 30 micrograms/kg every 20 minutes, alternatively (by intravenous

infusion) initially 180 micrograms/kg/hour, then (by intravenous infusion) maintenance 60–120 micrograms/kg/hour, maintenance dose administered after stabilisation

Neuromuscular blockade (intermediate duration) during intensive care

▶ INITIALLY BY INTRAVENOUS INJECTION
▶ Adult: Initially 150 micrograms/kg, initial dose is optional, then (by intravenous infusion) 180 micrograms/kg/hour, adjusted according to response; (by intravenous infusion) usual dose 30–600 micrograms/kg/hour

DOSES AT EXTREMES OF BODY-WEIGHT
To avoid excessive dosage in obese patients, dose should be calculated on the basis of ideal body-weight.

● SIDE-EFFECTS Acute myopathy (after prolonged use in intensive care) · bradycardia

● DIRECTIONS FOR ADMINISTRATION For *intravenous infusion* (Nimbex®, Nimbex Forte®), give continuously in Glucose 5% or Sodium Chloride 0.9%; solutions of 2 mg/mL and 5 mg/mL may be infused undiluted; alternatively dilute with infusion fluid to a concentration of 0.1–2 mg/mL.

● MEDICINAL FORMS
There can be variation in the licensing of different medicines containing the same drug.
Solution for injection
▶ Cisatracurium (Non-proprietary)
Cisatracurium (as Cisatracurium besilate) 2 mg per 1 ml Cisatracurium besilate 20mg/10ml solution for injection ampoules | 5 ampoule PoM £13.03
Cisatracurium besilate 20mg/10ml solution for injection vials | 5 vial PoM £37.75 (Hospital only) | 5 vial PoM £37.75
Cisatracurium (as Cisatracurium besilate) 5 mg per 1 ml Cisatracurium besilate 150mg/30ml solution for injection vials | 1 vial PoM £45.00 (Hospital only) | 1 vial PoM £18.66
▶ Nimbex (GlaxoSmithKline UK Ltd)
Cisatracurium (as Cisatracurium besilate) 2 mg per 1 ml Nimbex 20mg/10ml solution for injection ampoules | 5 ampoule PoM £37.75
Cisatracurium (as Cisatracurium besilate) 5 mg per 1 ml Nimbex Forte 150mg/30ml solution for injection vials | 1 vial PoM £31.09

◤ 1172

Mivacurium

● INDICATIONS AND DOSE

Neuromuscular blockade (short duration) during surgery and intubation

▶ INITIALLY BY INTRAVENOUS INJECTION
▶ Adult: 70–250 micrograms/kg; (by intravenous injection) maintenance 100 micrograms/kg every 15 minutes, alternatively (by intravenous infusion) maintenance 8–10 micrograms/kg/minute, (by intravenous infusion) adjusted in steps of 1 microgram/kg/minute every 3 minutes if required; (by intravenous infusion) usual dose 6–7 micrograms/kg/minute

DOSES AT EXTREMES OF BODY-WEIGHT
To avoid excessive dosage in obese patients, dose should be calculated on the basis of ideal bodyweight.

● CAUTIONS Burns (low plasma cholinesterase activity; dose titration required) · elderly

● SIDE-EFFECTS
▶ Very rare Anaphylactoid reactions
▶ Frequency not known Bronchospasm · hypotension · skin flushing · tachycardia

● HEPATIC IMPAIRMENT Reduce dose in severe impairment.

● RENAL IMPAIRMENT Clinical effect prolonged in renal failure—reduce dose according to response.

● DIRECTIONS FOR ADMINISTRATION For *intravenous infusion*, give continuously in Glucose 5% or Sodium

chloride 0.9%. Dilute to a concentration of 500 micrograms/mL; may also be given undiluted. Doses up to 150 micrograms/kg may be given over 5–15 seconds, higher doses should be given over 30 seconds. In asthma, cardiovascular disease or in those sensitive to reduced arterial blood pressure, give over 60 seconds.

● MEDICINAL FORMS
There can be variation in the licensing of different medicines containing the same drug.
Solution for injection
▶ Mivacron (GlaxoSmithKline UK Ltd)
Mivacurium (as Mivacurium chloride) 2 mg per 1 ml Mivacron 10mg/5ml solution for injection ampoules | 5 ampoule PoM £13.95
Mivacron 20mg/10ml solution for injection ampoules | 5 ampoule PoM £22.57

◤ 1172

Pancuronium bromide

● INDICATIONS AND DOSE

Neuromuscular blockade (long duration) during surgery and intubation

▶ BY INTRAVENOUS INJECTION
▶ Adult: Initially 100 micrograms/kg, then 20 micrograms/kg as required

Neuromuscular blockade (long duration) during intensive care

▶ BY INTRAVENOUS INJECTION
▶ Adult: Initially 100 micrograms/kg, initial dose is optional, then 60 micrograms/kg every 60–90 minutes

DOSES AT EXTREMES OF BODY-WEIGHT
To avoid excessive dosage in obese patients, dose should be calculated on the basis of ideal bodyweight.

● SIDE-EFFECTS Acute myopathy (after prolonged use in intensive care) · hypertension · tachycardia
SIDE-EFFECTS, FURTHER INFORMATION
Pancuronium lacks histamine-releasing effect, but vagolytic and sympathomimetic effects can cause tachycardia and hypertension.

● HEPATIC IMPAIRMENT Possibly slower onset, higher dose requirement, and prolonged recovery time.

● RENAL IMPAIRMENT Use with caution; prolonged duration of block.

● MEDICINAL FORMS
There can be variation in the licensing of different medicines containing the same drug.
Solution for injection
▶ Pancuronium bromide (Non-proprietary)
Pancuronium bromide 2 mg per 1 ml Pancuronium bromide 4mg/2ml solution for injection ampoules | 10 ampoule PoM £50.00

◤ 1172

Rocuronium bromide

● INDICATIONS AND DOSE

Neuromuscular blockade (intermediate duration) during surgery and intubation

▶ INITIALLY BY INTRAVENOUS INJECTION
▶ Adult: Initially 600 micrograms/kg; (by intravenous injection) maintenance 150 micrograms/kg, alternatively (by intravenous infusion) maintenance 300–600 micrograms/kg/hour, adjusted according to response
▶ Elderly: Initially 600 micrograms/kg; (by intravenous injection) maintenance 75–100 micrograms/kg, alternatively (by intravenous infusion) maintenance up to 400 micrograms/kg/hour, adjusted according to response

continued →

Neuromuscular blockade (intermediate duration) during intensive care
▶ INITIALLY BY INTRAVENOUS INJECTION
▶ Adult: Initially 600 micrograms/kg, initial dose is optional; (by intravenous infusion) maintenance 300–600 micrograms/kg/hour for first hour, then (by intravenous infusion), adjusted according to response

DOSES AT EXTREMES OF BODY-WEIGHT
To avoid excessive dosage in obese patients, dose should be calculated on the basis of ideal bodyweight.

● SIDE-EFFECTS
▶ **Very rare** Anaphylactoid reactions
▶ **Frequency not known** Acute myopathy (after prolonged use in intensive care) · bronchospasm · hypotension · skin flushing · tachycardia
● HEPATIC IMPAIRMENT Reduce dose.
● RENAL IMPAIRMENT Reduce maintenance dose; prolonged paralysis.
● DIRECTIONS FOR ADMINISTRATION For *continuous intravenous infusion* or via drip tubing, may be diluted with Glucose 5% or Sodium Chloride 0.9%.

● MEDICINAL FORMS
There can be variation in the licensing of different medicines containing the same drug.
Solution for injection
▶ Rocuronium bromide (Non-proprietary)
 Rocuronium bromide 10 mg per 1 ml Rocuronium bromide 50mg/5ml solution for injection vials | 10 vial [PoM] £28.00–£30.00
 Rocuronium bromide 100mg/10ml solution for injection vials | 10 vial [PoM] £57.00–£60.00
▶ Esmeron (Merck Sharp & Dohme Ltd)
 Rocuronium bromide 10 mg per 1 ml Esmeron 50mg/5ml solution for injection vials | 10 vial [PoM] £28.92 (Hospital only)
 Esmeron 100mg/10ml solution for injection vials | 10 vial [PoM] £57.85 (Hospital only)

▸ 1172

Vecuronium bromide

● INDICATIONS AND DOSE
Neuromuscular blockade (intermediate duration) during surgery and intubation
▶ INITIALLY BY INTRAVENOUS INJECTION
▶ Adult: 80–100 micrograms/kg; (by intravenous injection) maintenance 20–30 micrograms/kg, adjusted according to response, max. 100 micrograms/kg in caesarian section, alternatively (by intravenous infusion) maintenance 0.8–1.4 micrograms/kg/minute, adjusted according to response

DOSES AT EXTREMES OF BODY-WEIGHT
To avoid excessive dosage in obese patients, dose should be calculated on the basis of ideal bodyweight.

● SIDE-EFFECTS
▶ **Very rare** Anaphylactoid reactions
▶ **Frequency not known** Acute myopathy (after prolonged use in intensive care) · bronchospasm · hypotension · skin flushing · tachycardia
● HEPATIC IMPAIRMENT Use with caution in significant impairment.
● RENAL IMPAIRMENT Use with caution.
● DIRECTIONS FOR ADMINISTRATION Reconstitute each vial with 5 mL Water for Injections to give 2 mg/mL solution; *alternatively* reconstitute with up to 10 mL Glucose 5% *or* Sodium Chloride 0.9% *or* Water for Injections—unsuitable for further dilution if not reconstituted with Water for Injections. For *continuous intravenous infusion*, dilute reconstituted solution to a concentration up to 40 micrograms/mL with Glucose 5% or Sodium Chloride 0.9%; reconstituted solution can also be given via drip tubing.

● MEDICINAL FORMS
There can be variation in the licensing of different medicines containing the same drug.
Powder and solvent for solution for injection
▶ Norcuron (Merck Sharp & Dohme Ltd)
 Vecuronium bromide 10 mg Norcuron 10mg powder and solvent for solution for injection vials | 10 vial [PoM] £33.73 (Hospital only)

1.2 Neuromuscular blockade reversal

Neuromuscular blockade

Drugs for reversal of neuromuscular blockade
Anticholinesterases
Anticholinesterases reverse the effects of the non-depolarising (competitive) neuromuscular blocking drugs such as pancuronium bromide but they prolong the action of the depolarising neuromuscular blocking drug suxamethonium chloride.

Neostigmine is used specifically for reversal of non-depolarising (competitive) blockade. It acts within one minute of intravenous injection and its effects last for 20 to 30 minutes; a second dose may then be necessary. Glycopyrronium bromide p. 1170 or alternatively atropine sulfate p. 1169, given before or with neostigmine, prevent bradycardia, excessive salivation, and other muscarinic effects of neostigmine.

Other drugs for reversal of neuromuscular blockade
Sugammadex p. 1175 is a modified gamma cyclodextrin that can be used for rapid reversal of neuromuscular blockade induced by rocuronium bromide or vecuronium bromide. In practice, sugammadex is used mainly for rapid reversal of neuromuscular blockade in an emergency.

ANTICHOLINESTERASES

Neostigmine with glycopyrronium bromide

The properties listed below are those particular to the combination only. For the properties of the components please consider, neostigmine p. 971, glycopyrronium bromide p. 1170.

● INDICATIONS AND DOSE
Reversal of non-depolarising neuromuscular blockade
▶ BY INTRAVENOUS INJECTION
▶ Adult: 1–2 mL, repeated if necessary, alternatively 0.02 mL/kilogram, repeated if necessary; maximum 2 mL per course

● DIRECTIONS FOR ADMINISTRATION For *intravenous injection*, give over 10–30 seconds.

● MEDICINAL FORMS
There can be variation in the licensing of different medicines containing the same drug.
Solution for injection
▶ Neostigmine with glycopyrronium bromide (Non-proprietary)
 Glycopyrronium bromide 500 microgram per 1 ml, Neostigmine metilsulfate 2.5 mg per 1 ml Neostigmine 2.5mg/1ml / Glycopyrronium bromide 500micrograms/1ml solution for injection ampoules | 10 ampoule [PoM] £11.50

ANTIDOTES AND CHELATORS

Sugammadex

● INDICATIONS AND DOSE

Routine reversal of neuromuscular blockade induced by rocuronium or vecuronium
▶ BY INTRAVENOUS INJECTION
▶ Adult: Initially 2–4 mg/kg, then 4 mg/kg if required, administered if recurrence of neuromuscular blockade occurs; consult product literature for further details

Immediate reversal of neuromuscular blockade induced by rocuronium
▶ BY INTRAVENOUS INJECTION
▶ Adult: 16 mg/kg (consult product literature)

IMPORTANT SAFETY INFORMATION
Should only be administered by, or under the direct supervision of, personnel experienced in its use.

● CAUTIONS Cardiovascular disease (recovery may be delayed) · elderly (recovery may be delayed) · pre-existing coagulation disorders · recurrence of neuromuscular blockade— monitor respiratory function until fully recovered · use of anticoagulants (unrelated to surgery) · wait 24 hours before re-administering rocuronium · wait 24 hours before re-administering vecuronium
● INTERACTIONS → Appendix 1 (sugammadex).
● SIDE-EFFECTS Bradycardia · bronchospasm · cardiac arrest · hypersensitivity reactions
● PREGNANCY Use with caution—no information available.
● RENAL IMPAIRMENT Avoid if eGFR less than 30 mL/minute/1.73 m².
● NATIONAL FUNDING/ACCESS DECISIONS
Scottish Medicines Consortium (SMC) Decisions
The *Scottish Medicines Consortium,* has advised (February 2013) that sugammadex (*Bridion* ®) is accepted for restricted use within NHS Scotland for the routine reversal of neuromuscular blockade in high-risk patients only, or where prompt reversal of neuromuscular block is required.

● MEDICINAL FORMS
There can be variation in the licensing of different medicines containing the same drug.
Solution for injection
ELECTROLYTES: May contain Sodium
▶ Bridion (Merck Sharp & Dohme Ltd)
　Sugammadex (as Sugammadex sodium) 100 mg per 1 ml Bridion 500mg/5ml solution for injection vials | 10 vial [PoM] £1,491.00 (Hospital only)
　Bridion 200mg/2ml solution for injection vials | 10 vial [PoM] £596.40 (Hospital only)

1.3　Peri-operative analgesia

Peri-operative analgesia

Non-opioid analgesics

Since non-steroidal anti-inflammatory drugs (NSAIDs) do not depress respiration, do not impair gastro-intestinal motility, and do not cause dependence, they may be useful alternatives or adjuncts to opioids for the relief of postoperative pain. NSAIDs may be inadequate for the relief of severe pain. Acemetacin p. 977, diclofenac sodium p. 980, diclofenac potassium p. 980, flurbiprofen p. 986, ibuprofen p. 987, ketoprofen p. 991, paracetamol p. 406, parecoxib p. 1177, and ketorolac trometamol p. 1176 are licensed for postoperative use. Diclofenac and paracetamol can be given by injection as well as by mouth. Diclofenac sodium can be

given by intravenous infusion for the treatment or prevention of postoperative pain. Intramuscular injections of diclofenac sodium and ketoprofen are rarely used; they are given deep into the gluteal muscle to minimise pain and tissue damage. Ketorolac trometamol is less irritant on intramuscular injection but pain has been reported; it can also be given by intravenous injection.

Suppositories of diclofenac sodium and ketoprofen may be effective alternatives to the parenteral use of these drugs.

Opioid analgesics

Opioid analgesics are now rarely used as premedicants; they are more likely to be administered at induction. Pre-operative use of opioid analgesics is generally limited to those patients who require control of existing pain. See general notes on opioid analgesics and their use in postoperative pain.

See the management of opioid-induced respiratory depression in Pre-medication and peri-operative drugs p. 1168.

Intra-operative analgesia
Opioid analgesics given in small doses before or with induction reduce the dose requirement of some drugs used during anaesthesia.

Alfentanil p. 1177, fentanyl p. 416, and remifentanil p. 1178 are particularly useful because they act within 1–2 minutes and have short durations of action. The initial doses of alfentanil or fentanyl are followed either by successive intravenous injections or by an intravenous infusion; prolonged infusions increase the duration of effect. Repeated intra-operative doses of alfentanil or fentanyl should be given with care since the resulting respiratory depression can persist postoperatively and occasionally it may become apparent for the first time postoperatively when monitoring of the patient might be less intensive. Alfentanil, fentanyl, and remifentanil can cause muscle rigidity, particularly of the chest wall or jaw; this can be managed by the use of neuromuscular blocking drugs.

In contrast to other opioids which are metabolised in the liver, remifentanil undergoes rapid metabolism by nonspecific blood and tissue esterases; its short duration of action allows prolonged administration at high dosage, without accumulation, and with little risk of residual postoperative respiratory depression. Remifentanil should not be given by intravenous injection intraoperatively, but it is well suited to continuous infusion; a supplementary analgesic is given before stopping the infusion of remifentanil.

ANAESTHETICS, LOCAL

Bupivacaine with fentanyl

The properties listed below are those particular to the combination only. For the properties of the components please consider, bupivacaine hydrochloride p. 1183, fentanyl p. 416.

● INDICATIONS AND DOSE
During labour (once epidural block established)
▶ BY CONTINUOUS LUMBAR EPIDURAL INFUSION
▶ Adult: 10–18.75 mg/hour, dose of bupivacaine to be administered, maximum 400 mg bupivacaine in 24 hours and 16–30 micrograms/hour, dose of fentanyl to be administered, maximum 720 micrograms fentanyl in 24 hours　　　　　continued →

15　Anaesthesia

Postoperative pain (once epidural block established)

▶ BY CONTINUOUS EPIDURAL INFUSION

▶ Adult: 4–18.75 mg/hour, dose of bupivacaine to be administered, maximum 400 mg bupivacaine in 24 hours and 8–30 micrograms/hour, dose of fentanyl to be administered, maximum 720 micrograms fentanyl in 24 hours, to be administered by thoracic, upper abdominal or lower abdominal epidural infusion

● MEDICINAL FORMS

There can be variation in the licensing of different medicines containing the same drug. Forms available from special-order manufacturers include: infusion, solution for infusion

Solution for infusion

▶ Bufyl (AMCo)

Fentanyl 2 microgram per 1 ml, Bupivacaine hydrochloride 1 mg per 1 ml Bufyl 1mg/ml and 2micrograms/ml 250ml infusion bags | 20 bag [PoM] £170.00 (Hospital only) [CD2]

Bufyl 1mg/ml and 2micrograms/ml 500ml infusion bags | 10 bag [PoM] £92.00 (Hospital only) [CD2]

Fentanyl (as Fentanyl citrate) 2 microgram per 1 ml, Bupivacaine hydrochloride 1.25 mg per 1 ml Bufyl 1.25mg/ml and 2micrograms/ml 250ml infusion bags | 20 bag [PoM] £181.00 (Hospital only) [CD2]

Bufyl 1.25mg/ml and 2micrograms/ml 500ml infusion bags | 10 bag [PoM] £92.00 (Hospital only) [CD2]

ANALGESICS > NON-STEROIDAL ANTI-INFLAMMATORY DRUGS

Ketorolac trometamol

● INDICATIONS AND DOSE

Short-term management of moderate to severe acute postoperative pain only

▶ BY INTRAMUSCULAR INJECTION, OR BY INTRAVENOUS INJECTION

▶ Adult (body-weight up to 50 kg): Initially 10 mg, then 10–30 mg every 4–6 hours as required for maximum duration of treatment 2 days, frequency may be increased to up to every 2 hours during initial postoperative period; maximum 60 mg per day

▶ Adult (body-weight 50 kg and above): Initially 10 mg, then 10–30 mg every 4–6 hours as required for maximum duration of treatment 2 days, frequency may be increased to up to every 2 hours during initial postoperative period; maximum 90 mg per day

▶ Elderly: Initially 10 mg, then 10–30 mg every 4–6 hours as required for maximum duration of treatment 2 days, frequency may be increased to up to every 2 hours during initial postoperative period; maximum 60 mg per day

● CONTRA-INDICATIONS Active or history of gastro-intestinal bleeding · active or history of gastro-intestinal ulceration · coagulation disorders · complete or partial syndrome of nasal polyps · confirmed or suspected cerebrovascular bleeding · dehydration · following operations with high risk of haemorrhage or incomplete haemostasis · haemorrhagic diatheses · history of gastro-intestinal perforation · hypovolaemia · severe heart failure

● CAUTIONS Allergic disorders · cardiac impairment (NSAIDs may impair renal function) · cerebrovascular disease · coagulation defects · connective-tissue disorders · Crohn's disease (may be exacerbated) · elderly (risk of serious side-effects and fatalities) · heart failure · ischaemic heart disease · peripheral arterial disease · risk factors for cardiovascular events · ulcerative colitis (may be exacerbated) · uncontrolled hypertension

● INTERACTIONS → Appendix 1 (NSAIDs).

● SIDE-EFFECTS

▶ **Rare** Alveolitis · aseptic meningitis (patients with connective-tissue disorders such as systemic lupus erythematosus may be especially susceptible) · hepatic damage · interstitial fibrosis associated with NSAIDs can lead to renal failure · pancreatitis · papillary necrosis associated with NSAIDs can lead to renal failure · pulmonary eosinophilia · Stevens-Johnson syndrome · toxic epidermal necrolysis

▶ **Frequency not known** Abnormal dreams · angioedema · asthma · blood disorders · bradycardia · bronchospasm · chest pain · colitis (induction of or exacerbation of) · confusion · convulsions · Crohn's disease (induction of or exacerbation of) · depression · diarrhoea · dizziness · drowsiness · dry mouth · dyspnoea · euphoria · fluid retention (rarely precipitating congestive heart failure) · flushing · gastro-intestinal bleeding · gastro-intestinal discomfort · gastro-intestinal disturbances · gastro-intestinal ulceration · haematuria · hallucinations · headache · hearing disturbances · hyperkalaemia · hyperkinesia · hypersensitivity reactions · hypertension · hyponatraemia · insomnia · malaise · myalgia · nausea · nervousness · optic neuritis · pain at injection site · pallor · palpitation · paraesthesia · photosensitivity · psychosis · purpura · raised blood pressure · rashes · renal failure (especially in patients with pre-existing renal impairment) · sweating · taste disturbances · thirst · tinnitus · urinary frequency · vertigo · visual disturbances

SIDE-EFFECTS, FURTHER INFORMATION

▶ **Serious side-effects** For information about cardiovascular and gastro-intestinal side-effects, and a possible exacerbation of symptoms in asthma, see Non-steroidal anti-inflammatory drugs p. 975.

● ALLERGY AND CROSS-SENSITIVITY Contra-indicated in patients with a history of hypersensitivity to aspirin or any other NSAID—which includes those in whom attacks of asthma, angioedema, urticaria or rhinitis have been precipitated by aspirin or any other NSAID.

● CONCEPTION AND CONTRACEPTION Caution—long-term use of some NSAIDs is associated with reduced female fertility, which is reversible on stopping treatment.

● PREGNANCY Avoid unless the potential benefit outweighs the risk. Avoid during the third trimester (risk of closure of fetal ductus arteriosus *in utero* and possibly persistent pulmonary hypertension of the newborn); onset of labour may be delayed and duration may be increased.

● BREAST FEEDING Amount too small to be harmful.

● HEPATIC IMPAIRMENT Use with caution; there is an increased risk of gastro-intestinal bleeding and fluid retention. Avoid in severe liver disease.

● RENAL IMPAIRMENT Avoid if possible or use with caution. Avoid if serum creatinine greater than 160 micromol/litre. The lowest effective dose should be used for the shortest possible duration. Max. 60 mg daily by intramuscular injection or intravenous injection.

Monitor renal function; sodium and water retention may occur and renal function may deteriorate, possibly leading to renal failure.

● DIRECTIONS FOR ADMINISTRATION For *intravenous injection*, give over at least 15 seconds.

● MEDICINAL FORMS

There can be variation in the licensing of different medicines containing the same drug.

Solution for injection

▶ Ketorolac trometamol (Non-proprietary)

Ketorolac trometamol 30 mg per 1 ml Ketorolac 30mg/1ml solution for injection ampoules | 6 ampoule [PoM] £6.56

Parecoxib

- DRUG ACTION Parecoxib is a selective inhibitor of cyclo-oxygenase-2.

  ● INDICATIONS AND DOSE

  Short-term management of acute postoperative pain
  ▸ BY DEEP INTRAMUSCULAR INJECTION, OR BY INTRAVENOUS INJECTION
  ▸ Adult: Initially 40 mg, then 20–40 mg every 6–12 hours as required for up to 3 days; maximum 80 mg per day
  ▸ Elderly (body-weight up to 50 kg): Initially 20 mg; maximum 40 mg per day

- CONTRA-INDICATIONS Active gastro-intestinal bleeding · active gastro-intestinal ulceration · cerebrovascular disease · inflammatory bowel disease · ischaemic heart disease · mild to severe heart failure · peripheral arterial disease
- CAUTIONS Allergic disorders · cardiac impairment (NSAIDs may impair renal function) · coagulation defects · connective-tissue disorders · Crohn's disease (may be exacerbated) · dehydration · elderly (risk of serious side-effects and fatalities) · following coronary artery bypass graft surgery · history of cardiac failure · hypertension · left ventricular dysfunction · oedema · risk factors for cardiovascular events · ulcerative colitis (may be exacerbated)
- INTERACTIONS → Appendix 1 (NSAIDs).
- SIDE-EFFECTS
  ▸ **Common or very common** Alveolar osteitis · flatulence · hypoaesthesia · hypokalaemia · hypotension · postoperative anaemia · sweating
  ▸ **Uncommon** Anorexia · arthralgia · bradycardia · cardiovascular events · ecchymosis · hyperglycaemia · malaise · pulmonary embolism
  ▸ **Rare** Alveolitis · aseptic meningitis (patients with connective-tissue disorders such as systemic lupus erythematosus may be especially susceptible) · hepatic damage · interstitial fibrosis associated with NSAIDs can lead to renal failure · pancreatitis · papillary necrosis associated with NSAIDs can lead to renal failure · pulmonary eosinophilia · Stevens-Johnson syndrome · toxic epidermal necrolysis · visual disturbances
  ▸ **Frequency not known** Angioedema · blood disorders · blood pressure may be raised · bronchospasm · circulatory collapse · colitis (induction of or exacerbation of) · Crohn's disease (induction of or exacerbation of) · depression · diarrhoea · dizziness · drowsiness · fluid retention (rarely precipitating congestive heart failure) · gastro-intestinal bleeding · gastro-intestinal discomfort · gastro-intestinal disturbances · gastro-intestinal ulceration · haematuria · headache · hearing disturbances · hypersensitivity reactions · insomnia · nausea · nervousness · photosensitivity · rashes · renal failure (especially in patients with pre-existing renal impairment) · tachycardia · tinnitus · vertigo

  SIDE-EFFECTS, FURTHER INFORMATION
  ▸ **Serious side-effects** For information about cardiovascular and gastro-intestinal side-effects, and a possible exacerbation of symptoms in asthma, see Non-steroidal anti-inflammatory drugs p. 975.
- ALLERGY AND CROSS-SENSITIVITY Contra-indicated in patients with a history of hypersensitivity to aspirin or any other NSAID—which includes those in whom attacks of asthma, angioedema, urticaria or rhinitis have been precipitated by aspirin or any other NSAID. Contra-indicated in patients with a history of allergic drug reactions including sulfonamide hypersensitivity.

- CONCEPTION AND CONTRACEPTION Caution—long-term use of some NSAIDs is associated with reduced female fertility, which is reversible on stopping treatment.
- PREGNANCY Avoid unless the potential benefit outweighs the risk. Avoid during the third trimester (risk of closure of fetal ductus arteriosus *in utero* and possibly persistent pulmonary hypertension of the newborn); onset of labour may be delayed and duration may be increased.
- BREAST FEEDING Avoid—present in milk.
- HEPATIC IMPAIRMENT Halve dose in moderate impairment (max. 40 mg daily). Use with caution; there is an increased risk of gastro-intestinal bleeding and fluid retention. Avoid in severe liver disease.
- RENAL IMPAIRMENT The lowest effective dose should be used for the shortest possible duration. Avoid if possible or use with caution. In renal impairment monitor renal function; sodium and water retention may occur and renal function may deteriorate, possibly leading to renal failure.
- NATIONAL FUNDING/ACCESS DECISIONS

  Scottish Medicines Consortium (SMC) Decisions
  The *Scottish Medicines Consortium* has advised (January 2003) that parecoxib is **not** recommended for use within NHS Scotland.

- MEDICINAL FORMS
  There can be variation in the licensing of different medicines containing the same drug.

  Powder for solution for injection
  ▸ Dynastat (Pfizer Ltd)
    Parecoxib (as Parecoxib sodium) 40 mg Dynastat 40mg powder for solution for injection vials | 10 vial PoM £49.60

  Powder and solvent for solution for injection
  ▸ Dynastat (Pfizer Ltd)
    Parecoxib (as Parecoxib sodium) 40 mg Dynastat 40mg powder and solvent for solution for injection vials | 5 vial PoM £28.34

ANALGESICS > OPIOIDS

Papaveretum with hyoscine hydrobromide

The properties listed below are those particular to the combination only. For the properties of the components please consider, papaveretum p. 426, hyoscine hydrobromide p. 401.

● INDICATIONS AND DOSE

Premedication
▸ BY SUBCUTANEOUS INJECTION, OR BY INTRAMUSCULAR INJECTION
▸ Adult: 0.5–1 mL

- LESS SUITABLE FOR PRESCRIBING Hyoscine hydrobromide with papaveretum is less suitable for prescribing.
- MEDICINAL FORMS
  There can be variation in the licensing of different medicines containing the same drug.
  No licensed medicines listed.

Alfentanil

● INDICATIONS AND DOSE

Spontaneous respiration: analgesia and enhancement of anaesthesia for short procedures
▸ BY INTRAVENOUS INJECTION
▸ Adult: Initially up to 500 micrograms, dose to be administered over 30 seconds; supplemental doses 250 micrograms continued →

Assisted ventilation: analgesia and enhancement of anaesthesia for short procedures

▸ BY INTRAVENOUS INJECTION
▸ Adult: Initially 30–50 micrograms/kg, supplemental doses 15 micrograms/kg

Assisted ventilation: analgesia and enhancement of anaesthesia during maintenance of anaesthesia for longer procedures

▸ BY INTRAVENOUS INFUSION
▸ Adult: Initially 50–100 micrograms/kg, dose to be administered over 10 minutes or as a bolus, followed by maintenance 30–60 micrograms/kg/hour

Assisted ventilation: analgesia and suppression of respiratory activity during intensive care for up to 4 days

▸ BY INTRAVENOUS INFUSION
▸ Adult: Initially 2 mg/hour, adjusted according to response; usual dose 0.5–10 mg/hour, alternatively initially 5 mg in divided doses, to be administered over 10 minutes; dose used for more rapid initial control, reduce rate of administration if hypotension or bradycardia occur; additional doses of 0.5–1 mg may be given by intravenous injection during short painful procedures

DOSES AT EXTREMES OF BODY-WEIGHT
To avoid excessive dosage in obese patients, dose should be calculated on the basis of ideal body-weight.

● CAUTIONS
CAUTIONS, FURTHER INFORMATION
▸ Repeated intra-operative doses Repeated intra-operative doses of alfentanil should be given with care since the resulting respiratory depression can persist postoperatively and occasionally it may become apparent for the first time postoperatively when monitoring of the patient might be less intensive.

● SIDE-EFFECTS
▸ **Common or very common** Hypertension · myoclonic movements
▸ **Uncommon** Arrhythmias · hiccup · laryngospasm
▸ **Rare** Epistaxis
▸ **Frequency not known** Cardiac arrest · convulsions · cough · muscle rigidity · pyrexia

SIDE-EFFECTS, FURTHER INFORMATION
▸ Muscle rigidity Alfentanil can cause muscle rigidity, particularly of the chest wall or jaw; this can be managed by the use of neuromuscular blocking drugs.

● BREAST FEEDING Present in milk—withhold breast-feeding for 24 hours.

● RENAL IMPAIRMENT Avoid use or reduce dose; opioid effects increased and prolonged and increased cerebral sensitivity occurs.

● DIRECTIONS FOR ADMINISTRATION 5 mg/mL injection to be diluted before use. For *continuous or intermittent intravenous infusion* dilute in Glucose 5% *or* Sodium Chloride 0.9%.

● MEDICINAL FORMS
There can be variation in the licensing of different medicines containing the same drug. Forms available from special-order manufacturers include: solution for injection
Solution for injection
▸ Alfentanil (Non-proprietary)
  Alfentanil (as Alfentanil hydrochloride) 500 microgram per 1 ml Alfentanil 1mg/2ml solution for injection ampoules | 10 ampoule [PoM] £7.00 [CD2]
  Alfentanil 5mg/10ml solution for injection ampoules | 5 ampoule [PoM] £16.00 [CD2]
  Alfentanil (as Alfentanil hydrochloride) 5 mg per 1 ml Alfentanil 5mg/1ml solution for injection ampoules | 10 ampoule [PoM] £25.00 [CD2]

▸ Rapifen (Janssen-Cilag Ltd)
  Alfentanil (as Alfentanil hydrochloride) 500 microgram per 1 ml Rapifen 5mg/10ml solution for injection ampoules | 5 ampoule [PoM] £14.50 [CD2]
  Rapifen 1mg/2ml solution for injection ampoules | 10 ampoule [PoM] £6.34 [CD2]
  Alfentanil (as Alfentanil hydrochloride) 5 mg per 1 ml Rapifen Intensive Care 5mg/1ml solution for injection ampoules | 10 ampoule [PoM] £23.19 (Hospital only) [CD2]

☞ 408

Remifentanil

● INDICATIONS AND DOSE

Analgesia and enhancement of anaesthesia at induction (initial bolus injection)

▸ BY INTRAVENOUS INJECTION
▸ Adult: Initially 0.25–1 microgram/kg, dose to be administered over at least 30 seconds, if patient is to be intubated more than 8 minutes after start of intravenous infusion, initial bolus intravenous injection dose is not necessary

Analgesia and enhancement of anaesthesia at induction with or without initial bolus dose

▸ BY INTRAVENOUS INFUSION
▸ Adult: 30–60 micrograms/kg/hour, if patient is to be intubated more than 8 minutes after start of intravenous infusion, initial bolus intravenous injection dose is not necessary

Assisted ventilation: analgesia and enhancement of anaesthesia during maintenance of anaesthesia (initial bolus injection)

▸ BY INTRAVENOUS INJECTION
▸ Adult: Initially 0.25–1 microgram/kg, dose to be administered over at least 30 seconds

Assisted ventilation: analgesia and enhancement of anaesthesia during maintenance of anaesthesia with or without initial bolus dose

▸ BY INTRAVENOUS INFUSION
▸ Adult: 3–120 micrograms/kg/hour, dose to be administered according to anaesthetic technique and adjusted according to response, in light anaesthesia additional doses can be given *by intravenous injection* every 2–5 minutes during the intravenous infusion

Spontaneous respiration: analgesia and enhancement of anaesthesia during maintenance of anaesthesia

▸ BY INTRAVENOUS INFUSION
▸ Adult: Initially 2.4 micrograms/kg/hour, adjusted according to response; usual dose 1.5–6 micrograms/kg/hour

Assisted ventilation: analgesia and sedation in intensive-care patients (for max 3 days)

▸ BY INTRAVENOUS INFUSION
▸ Adult: Initially 6–9 micrograms/kg/hour, then adjusted in steps of 1.5 micrograms/kg/hour, allow at least 5 minutes between dose adjustments; usual dose 0.36–44.4 micrograms/kg/hour, if an infusion rate of 12 micrograms/kg/hour does not produce adequate sedation add another sedative (consult product literature for details)

Assisted ventilation: additional analgesia during stimulating or painful procedures in intensive-care patients

▸ BY INTRAVENOUS INFUSION
▸ Adult: Usual dose 15–45 micrograms/kg/hour, maintain infusion rate of at least 6 micrograms/kg/hour for at least 5 minutes before procedure and adjust every 2–5 minutes according to requirements

Cardiac surgery

▸ Adult: (consult product literature)

DOSES AT EXTREMES OF BODY-WEIGHT
To avoid excessive dosage in obese patients, dose should be calculated on the basis of ideal body-weight.

● UNLICENSED USE Remifentanil doses in BNF may differ from those in product literature.

● CONTRA-INDICATIONS Analgesia in conscious patients

● SIDE-EFFECTS

▸ **Common or very common** Hypertension

▸ **Uncommon** Hypoxia

▸ **Rare** Asystole

▸ **Frequency not known** AV block · convulsions

SIDE-EFFECTS, FURTHER INFORMATION

▸ Muscle rigidity Alfentanil can cause muscle rigidity, particularly of the chest wall or jaw; this can be managed by the use of neuromuscular blocking drugs.

▸ Respiratory depression In contrast to other opioids which are metabolised in the liver, remifentanil undergoes rapid metabolism by non-specific blood and tissue esterases; its short duration of action allows prolonged administration at high dosage, without accumulation, and with little risk of residual postoperative respiratory depression.

● PREGNANCY No information available.

● BREAST FEEDING Avoid breast-feeding for 24 hours after administration—present in milk in *animal* studies.

● RENAL IMPAIRMENT No dose adjustment necessary in renal impairment.

● DIRECTIONS FOR ADMINISTRATION For *intravenous infusion* (*Ultiva*®), give continuously in Glucose 5% or Sodium Chloride 0.9% or Water for Injections; reconstitute with infusion fluid to a concentration of 1 mg/mL then dilute further to a concentration of 20–250 micrograms/mL (50 micrograms/mL recommended for general anaesthesia, 20–50 micrograms/mL recommended when used with target controlled infusion (TCI) device).

● PRESCRIBING AND DISPENSING INFORMATION
Remifentanil should not be given by intravenous injection intra-operatively, but it is well suited to continuous infusion; a supplementary analgesic is given before stopping the infusion of remifentanil.

● MEDICINAL FORMS
There can be variation in the licensing of different medicines containing the same drug.

Powder for solution for injection

▸ Remifentanil (Non-proprietary)

Remifentanil (as Remifentanyl hydrochloride) 1 mg Remifentanil 1mg powder for concentrate for solution for injection vials | 5 vial PoM £25.58–£25.60 (Hospital only) CD2

Remifentanil (as Remifentanyl hydrochloride) 2 mg Remifentanil 2mg powder for concentrate for solution for injection vials | 5 vial PoM £51.13–£51.15 (Hospital only) CD2

Remifentanil (as Remifentanyl hydrochloride) 5 mg Remifentanil 5mg powder for concentrate for solution for injection vials | 5 vial PoM £127.00–£127.90 (Hospital only) CD2

▸ Ultiva (GlaxoSmithKline UK Ltd)

Remifentanil (as Remifentanyl hydrochloride) 1 mg Ultiva 1mg powder for solution for injection vials | 5 vial PoM £25.58 (Hospital only) CD2

Remifentanil (as Remifentanyl hydrochloride) 2 mg Ultiva 2mg powder for solution for injection vials | 5 vial PoM £51.15 (Hospital only) CD2

Remifentanil (as Remifentanyl hydrochloride) 5 mg Ultiva 5mg powder for solution for injection vials | 5 vial PoM £127.88 (Hospital only) CD2

1.4 Peri-operative sedation

Conscious sedation for clinical procedures

Overview

Sedation of patients during diagnostic and therapeutic procedures is used to reduce fear and anxiety, to control pain, and to minimise excessive movement. The choice of sedative drug will depend upon the intended procedure; some procedures are safer and more successful under anaesthesia. The patient should be *monitored carefully*; monitoring should begin as soon as the sedative is given or when the patient becomes drowsy, and should be continued until the patient wakes up.

ANAESTHETICS, GENERAL > NMDA RECEPTOR ANTAGONISTS

Ketamine

● INDICATIONS AND DOSE

Induction and maintenance of anaesthesia for short procedures

▸ BY INTRAMUSCULAR INJECTION

▸ Adult: Initially 6.5–13 mg/kg, adjusted according to response, a dose of 10 mg/kg usually produces 12–25 minutes of surgical anaesthesia

▸ BY INTRAVENOUS INJECTION

▸ Adult: Initially 1–4.5 mg/kg, adjusted according to response, to be administered over at least 60 seconds, a dose of 2 mg/kg usually produces 5–10 minutes of surgical anaesthesia

Diagnostic manoeuvres and procedures not involving intense pain

▸ BY INTRAMUSCULAR INJECTION

▸ Adult: Initially 4 mg/kg

Induction and maintenance of anaesthesia for long procedures

▸ BY INTRAVENOUS INFUSION

▸ Adult: Initially 0.5–2 mg/kg, using an infusion solution containing 1 mg/ml; maintenance 10–45 micrograms/kg/minute, adjusted according to response

IMPORTANT SAFETY INFORMATION
Ketamine should only be administered by, or under the direct supervision of, personnel experienced in its use, with adequate training in anaesthesia and airway management, and when resuscitation equipment is available.

● CONTRA-INDICATIONS Acute porphyrias p. 918 · eclampsia · head trauma · hypertension · pre-eclampsia · raised intracranial pressure · severe cardiac disease · stroke

● CAUTIONS Acute circulatory failure (shock) · cardiovascular disease · dehydration · elderly · fixed cardiac output · hallucinations · head injury · hypertension · hypovolaemia · increased cerebrospinal fluid pressure · intracranial mass lesions · nightmares · predisposition to seizures · psychotic disorders · raised intra-ocular pressure · respiratory tract infection · thyroid dysfunction

● INTERACTIONS → Appendix 1 (anaesthetics, general).

● SIDE-EFFECTS

▸ **Common or very common** Diplopia · hallucinations · hypertension · nausea · nightmares · nystagmus · rash · tachycardia · transient psychotic effects · vomiting

15

Anaesthesia

▶ **Uncommon** Arrhythmias · bradycardia · hypotension · laryngospasm · respiratory depression
▶ **Rare** Apnoea · cystitis · haemorrhagic cystitis · hypersalivation · insomnia
▶ **Frequency not known** Raised intra-ocular pressure

SIDE-EFFECTS, FURTHER INFORMATION
▶ Transient psychotic effects Incidence of hallucinations, nightmares, and other transient psychotic effects can be reduced by a benzodiazepine such as diazepam or midazolam.
● PREGNANCY May depress neonatal respiration if used during delivery.
● BREAST FEEDING Avoid for at least 12 hours after last dose.
● HEPATIC IMPAIRMENT Consider dose reduction.
● DIRECTIONS FOR ADMINISTRATION For *continuous intravenous infusion*, dilute to a concentration of 1 mg/mL with Glucose 5% *or* Sodium Chloride 0.9%; use microdrip infusion for maintenance of anaesthesia. For *intravenous injection*, dilute 100 mg/mL strength to a concentration of not more than 50 mg/mL with Glucose 5% *or* Sodium Chloride 0.9% *or* Water for Injections.
● PATIENT AND CARER ADVICE
Driving and skilled tasks
Patients given sedatives and analgesics during minor outpatient procedures should be very carefully warned about the risk of driving or undertaking skilled tasks afterwards. For a short general anaesthetic the risk extends to **at least 24 hours** after administration. Responsible persons should be available to take patients home. The dangers of taking **alcohol** should also be emphasised.
  For information on 2015 legislation regarding driving whilst taking certain controlled drugs, including ketamine, see *Drugs and driving* under Guidance on prescribing p. 1.

● MEDICINAL FORMS
There can be variation in the licensing of different medicines containing the same drug. Forms available from special-order manufacturers include: solution for injection
Solution for injection
▶ Ketamine (Non-proprietary)
  Ketamine (as Ketamine hydrochloride) 10 mg per 1 ml Ketamin 10 Curamed 50mg/5ml solution for injection ampoules | 10 ampoule [PoM] no price available [CD2]
  Ketamine (as Ketamine hydrochloride) 50 mg per 1 ml Ketamine 500mg/10ml solution for injection vials | 10 vial [PoM] £87.70 [CD2] Ketamin 100mg/2ml solution for injection ampoules | 10 ampoule [PoM] no price available [CD2]
▶ Ketalar (Pfizer Ltd)
  Ketamine (as Ketamine hydrochloride) 10 mg per 1 ml Ketalar 200mg/20ml solution for injection vials | 1 vial [PoM] £5.06 (Hospital only) [CD2]
  Ketamine (as Ketamine hydrochloride) 50 mg per 1 ml Ketalar 500mg/10ml solution for injection vials | 1 vial [PoM] £8.77 (Hospital only) [CD2]
  Ketamine (as Ketamine hydrochloride) 100 mg per 1 ml Ketalar 1g/10ml solution for injection vials | 1 vial [PoM] £16.10 (Hospital only) [CD2]

HYPNOTICS, SEDATIVES AND ANXIOLYTICS ›
NON-BENZODIAZEPINE HYPNOTICS AND SEDATIVES

Dexmedetomidine

● INDICATIONS AND DOSE
Maintenance of sedation during intensive care
▶ BY INTRAVENOUS INFUSION
▶ Adult: 0.7 microgram/kg/hour, adjusted according to response; usual dose 0.2–1.4 micrograms/kg/hour

> IMPORTANT SAFETY INFORMATION
> Dexmedetomidine should only be administered by, or under the direct supervision of, personnel experienced in its use, with adequate training in anaesthesia and airway management.

● CONTRA-INDICATIONS Acute cerebrovascular disorders · second- or third-degree AV block (unless pacemaker fitted) · uncontrolled hypotension
● CAUTIONS Abrupt withdrawal after prolonged use · bradycardia · ischaemic heart disease · malignant hyperthermia · severe cerebrovascular disease (especially at higher doses) · severe neurological disorders · spinal cord injury
● SIDE-EFFECTS
▶ **Common or very common** Agitation · blood pressure changes · bradycardia · changes in blood sugar · dry mouth · hyperthermia · myocardial infarction · myocardial ischaemia · nausea · tachycardia · vomiting
▶ **Uncommon** Abdominal distension · AV block · decreased cardiac output · dyspnoea · hallucination · hypoalbuminaemia · metabolic acidosis · thirst
● PREGNANCY Manufacturer advises avoid unless potential benefit outweighs risk—toxicity in *animal* studies.
● BREAST FEEDING Manufacturer advises avoid unless potential benefit outweighs risk—present in milk in *animal* studies.
● HEPATIC IMPAIRMENT Dose reduction may be required. Manufacturer advises caution.
● MONITORING REQUIREMENTS
▶ Monitor cardiac function.
▶ Monitor respiratory function in non-intubated patients.
● DIRECTIONS FOR ADMINISTRATION To be diluted before use. For *intravenous infusion* given continuously *in* Glucose 5% or Sodium chloride 0.9%, dilute to a concentration of 4 micrograms/mL.

● MEDICINAL FORMS
There can be variation in the licensing of different medicines containing the same drug.
Solution for infusion
▶ Dexdor (Orion Pharma (UK) Ltd)
  Dexmedetomidine (as Dexmedetomidine hydrochloride) 100 microgram per 1 ml Dexdor 1mg/10ml concentrate for solution for infusion vials | 4 vial [PoM] £313.20 (Hospital only)
  Dexdor 400micrograms/4ml concentrate for solution for infusion vials | 4 vial [PoM] £125.28 (Hospital only)
  Dexdor 200micrograms/2ml concentrate for solution for infusion ampoules | 5 ampoule [PoM] £78.30 (Hospital only) | 25 ampoule [PoM] £391.50 (Hospital only)

2   Malignant hyperthermia

MUSCLE RELAXANTS > MUSCLE RELAXANTS, DIRECTLY ACTING

Dantrolene sodium

- **DRUG ACTION** Acts on skeletal muscle cells by interfering with calcium efflux, thereby stopping the contractile process.

- **INDICATIONS AND DOSE**
  Malignant hyperthermia
  ▸ BY RAPID INTRAVENOUS INJECTION
  ▸ Adult: Initially 2–3 mg/kg, then 1 mg/kg, repeated if necessary; maximum 10 mg/kg per course
  Chronic severe spasticity of voluntary muscle
  ▸ BY MOUTH
  ▸ Adult: Initially 25 mg daily, then increased to up to 100 mg 4 times a day, dose increased at weekly intervals; usual dose 75 mg 3 times a day

  > IMPORTANT SAFETY INFORMATION
  > Should only be administered by, or under the direct supervision of, personnel experienced in the use of dantrolene when used for malignant hyperthermia.

- **CONTRA-INDICATIONS**
  ▸ With oral use Acute muscle spasm · avoid when spasticity is useful, for example, locomotion
- **CAUTIONS**
  ▸ With intravenous use Avoid extravasation (risk of tissue necrosis)
  ▸ With oral use Females (hepatotoxicity) · history of liver disorders (hepatotoxicity) · if doses greater than 400 mg daily (hepatotoxicity) · impaired cardiac function · impaired pulmonary function · patients over 30 years (hepatotoxicity) · therapeutic effect may take a few weeks to develop— discontinue if no response within 6–8 weeks
- **INTERACTIONS** → Appendix 1 (muscle relaxants).
  ▸ With oral use Caution if concomitant use of hepatotoxic drugs.
- **SIDE-EFFECTS**
  ▸ **Common or very common**
  ▸ With oral use Abdominal pain · anorexia · asthenia · chills · diarrhoea (withdraw if severe, discontinue treatment if recurs on re-introduction) · dizziness · drowsiness · fatigue · fever · headache · hepatotoxicity · nausea · pericarditis · pleural effusion · rash · respiratory depression · seizures · speech disturbances · visual disturbances · vomiting
  ▸ **Uncommon**
  ▸ With oral use Confusion · constipation · crystalluria · depression · dysphagia · dyspnoea · erratic blood pressure · exacerbation of cardiac insufficiency · haematuria · increased sweating · increased urinary frequency · insomnia · nervousness · tachycardia · urinary incontinence · urinary retention
  ▸ **Frequency not known**
  ▸ With intravenous use Dizziness · erythema · hepatotoxicity · injection-site reactions · pulmonary oedema · rash · swelling · thrombophlebitis · weakness
  SIDE-EFFECTS, FURTHER INFORMATION
  ▸ Hepatotoxicity Potentially life-threatening hepatotoxicity reported—discontinue if abnormal liver function tests or symptoms of liver disorder; re-introduce only if complete reversal of hepatotoxicity.

- **PREGNANCY**
  ▸ With intravenous use Use only if potential benefit outweighs risk.
  ▸ With oral use Avoid use in chronic spasticity—embryotoxic in *animal* studies.
- **BREAST FEEDING**
  ▸ With intravenous use Present in milk—use only if potential benefit outweighs risk.
  ▸ With oral use Present in milk—manufacturer advises avoid use in chronic spasticity.
- **HEPATIC IMPAIRMENT** Avoid—may cause severe liver damage (injection may be used in an emergency for malignant hyperthermia).
- **MONITORING REQUIREMENTS**
  ▸ With oral use Test liver function before and at intervals during therapy.
- **PATIENT AND CARER ADVICE**
  Driving and skilled tasks
  ▸ With oral use Drowsiness may affect performance of skilled tasks (e.g. driving); effects of alcohol enhanced.
  Hepatotoxicity
  ▸ With oral use Patients should be told how to recognise signs of liver disorder and advised to seek prompt medical attention if symptoms such as anorexia, nausea, vomiting, fatigue, abdominal pain, dark urine, or pruritus develop.

- **MEDICINAL FORMS**
  There can be variation in the licensing of different medicines containing the same drug. Forms available from special-order manufacturers include: oral suspension, oral solution
  Capsule
  CAUTIONARY AND ADVISORY LABELS 2
  ▸ Dantrium (Norgine Pharmaceuticals Ltd)
  Dantrolene sodium 25 mg Dantrium 25mg capsules | 100 capsule [PoM] £16.87 DT price = £16.87
  Dantrolene sodium 100 mg Dantrium 100mg capsules | 100 capsule [PoM] £43.07 DT price = £43.07
  Powder for solution for injection
  ▸ Dantrium (Norgine Pharmaceuticals Ltd)
  Dantrolene sodium 20 mg Dantrium Intravenous 20mg powder for solution for injection vials | 12 vial [PoM] £612.00 (Hospital only) | 36 vial [PoM] £1,836.00 (Hospital only)

Local anaesthesia

Local anaesthesia

Local anaesthetic drugs

The use of local anaesthetics by injection or by application to mucous membranes to produce local analgesia is discussed in this section.

Local anaesthetic drugs act by causing a reversible block to conduction along nerve fibres. They vary widely in their potency, toxicity, duration of action, stability, solubility in water, and ability to penetrate mucous membranes. These factors determine their application, e.g. topical (surface), infiltration, peripheral nerve block, intravenous regional anaesthesia (Bier's block), plexus, epidural (extradural), or spinal (intrathecal or subarachnoid) block. Local anaesthetics may also be used for postoperative pain relief, thereby reducing the need for analgesics such as opioids.

Bupivacaine hydrochloride p. 1183 has a longer duration of action than other local anaesthetics. It has a slow onset of action, taking up to 30 minutes for full effect. It is often used in lumbar epidural blockade and is particularly suitable for continuous epidural analgesia in labour, or for postoperative pain relief. It is the principal drug used for spinal anaesthesia. Hyperbaric solutions containing glucose may be used for spinal block.

Chloroprocaine hydrochloride p. 1185, a para-aminobenzoic acid ester, is used for spinal anaesthesia in adults where the planned procedure should not exceed 40 minutes.

Levobupivacaine p. 1186, an isomer of bupivacaine, has anaesthetic and analgesic properties similar to bupivacaine hydrochloride, but is thought to have fewer adverse effects.

Lidocaine hydrochloride p. 1187 is effectively absorbed from mucous membranes and is a useful surface anaesthetic in concentrations up to 10%. Except for surface anaesthesia and dental anaesthesia, solutions should **not** usually exceed 1% in strength. The duration of the block (with adrenaline/epinephrine p. 205) is about 90 minutes.

Prilocaine hydrochloride p. 1191 is a local anaesthetic of low toxicity which is similar to lidocaine hydrochloride. A hyperbaric solution of prilocaine hydrochloride (containing glucose) may be used for spinal anaesthesia.

Ropivacaine hydrochloride p. 1192 is an amide-type local anaesthetic agent similar to bupivacaine hydrochloride. It is less cardiotoxic than bupivacaine hydrochloride, but also less potent.

Tetracaine p. 1193, a para-aminobenzoic acid ester, is an effective local anaesthetic for topical application; a 4% gel is indicated for anaesthesia before venepuncture or venous cannulation. It is rapidly absorbed from mucous membranes and should **never** be applied to inflamed, traumatised, or highly vascular surfaces. It should never be used to provide anaesthesia for bronchoscopy or cystoscopy because lidocaine hydrochloride is a safer alternative.

Administration

The dose of local anaesthetic depends on the injection site and the procedure used. In determining the safe dosage, it is important to take account of the rate of absorption and excretion, and of the potency. The patient's age, weight, physique, and clinical condition, and the vascularity of the administration site and the duration of administration, must also be considered.

Uptake of local anaesthetics into the systemic circulation determines their duration of action and produces toxicity.

Great care must be taken to avoid accidental intravascular injection; local anaesthetic injections should be given slowly in order to detect inadvertent intravascular administration. When prolonged analgesia is required, a long-acting local anaesthetic is preferred to minimise the likelihood of cumulative systemic toxicity. Local anaesthesia around the oral cavity may impair swallowing and therefore increases the risk of aspiration.

Epidural anaesthesia is commonly used during surgery, often combined with general anaesthesia, because of its protective effect against the stress response of surgery. It is often used when good postoperative pain relief is essential.

Use of vasoconstrictors

Local anaesthetics cause dilatation of blood vessels. The addition of a vasoconstrictor such as adrenaline/epinephrine to the local anaesthetic preparation diminishes local blood flow, slowing the rate of absorption and thereby prolonging the anaesthetic effect. Great care should be taken to avoid inadvertent intravenous administration of a preparation containing adrenaline/epinephrine, and it is **not** advisable to give adrenaline/epinephrine with a local anaesthetic injection in digits or appendages because of the risk of ischaemic necrosis.

Adrenaline/epinephrine must be used in a low concentration when administered with a local anaesthetic. Care must also be taken to calculate a safe maximum dose of local anaesthetic when using combination products.

In patients with severe hypertension or unstable cardiac rhythm, the use of adrenaline/epinephrine with a local anaesthetic may be hazardous. For these patients an anaesthetic without adrenaline/epinephrine should be used.

Dental anaesthesia

Lidocaine hydrochloride is widely used in dental procedures; it is most often used in combination with adrenaline/epinephrine. Lidocaine hydrochloride 2% combined with adrenaline/epinephrine 1 in 80 000 (12.5 micrograms/mL) is a safe and effective preparation; there is no justification for using higher concentrations of adrenaline/epinephrine.

The amide-type local anaesthetics **articaine** and mepivacaine hydrochloride p. 1190 are also used in dentistry; they are available in cartridges suitable for dental use. Mepivacaine hydrochloride is available with or without adrenaline/epinephrine and articaine is available with adrenaline.

In patients with severe hypertension or unstable cardiac rhythm, mepivacaine hydrochloride without adrenaline/epinephrine may be used. Alternatively, prilocaine hydrochloride with or without felypressin can be used but there is no evidence that it is any safer. Felypressin can cause coronary vasoconstriction when used at high doses; limit dose in patients with coronary artery disease.

Toxicity

For management of toxicity see Severe local anaesthetic-induced cardiovascular toxicity below.

Severe local anaesthetic-induced cardiovascular toxicity

Overview

After injection of a bolus of local anaesthetic, toxicity may develop at any time in the following hour. In the event of signs of toxicity during injection, the administration of the local anaesthetic must be stopped immediately.

Cardiovascular status must be assessed and cardiopulmonary resuscitation procedures must be followed.

In the event of local anaesthetic-induced cardiac arrest, standard cardiopulmonary resuscitation should be initiated immediately. Lidocaine must not be used as anti-arrhythmic therapy.

If the patient does not respond rapidly to standard procedures, 20% lipid emulsion such as *Intralipid*® [unlicensed indication] should be given intravenously at an initial bolus dose of 1.5 mL/kg over 1 minute, followed by an infusion of 15 mL/kg/hour. After 5 minutes, if cardiovascular stability has not been restored or circulation deteriorates, give a maximum of two further bolus doses of 1.5 mL/kg over 1 minute, 5 minutes apart, and increase the infusion rate to 30 mL/kg/hour. Continue infusion until cardiovascular stability and adequate circulation are restored or maximum cumulative dose of 12 mL/kg is given.

Standard cardiopulmonary resuscitation must be maintained throughout lipid emulsion treatment.

Propofol is not a suitable alternative to lipid emulsion.

Further advice on ongoing treatment should be obtained from the National Poisons Information Service.

Detailed treatment algorithms and accompanying notes are available at www.toxbase.org *or* can be found in the Association of Anaesthetists of Great Britain and Ireland safety guideline, Management of Severe Local Anaesthetic Toxicity and Management of Severe Local Anaesthetic Toxicity – Accompanying notes.

ANAESTHETICS, LOCAL

Adrenaline with articaine hydrochloride

(Carticaine hydrochloride with epinephrine)

● **INDICATIONS AND DOSE**

Infiltration anaesthesia in dentistry
▸ BY REGIONAL ADMINISTRATION
▸ Adult: Consult expert dental sources
DOSES AT EXTREMES OF BODY-WEIGHT
To avoid excessive dosage in obese patients, dose should be calculated on the basis of ideal body-weight.

IMPORTANT SAFETY INFORMATION
Should only be administered by, or under the direct supervision of, personnel experienced in their use, with adequate training in anaesthesia and airway management, and should not be administered parenterally unless adequate resuscitation equipment is available.

Adrenaline/epinephrine must be used in a low concentration when administered with a local anaesthetic. The total dose of adrenaline should not exceed 500 micrograms and it is essential not to exceed a concentration of 1 in 200 000 (5 micrograms/mL) if more than 50 mL of the mixture is to be injected.

● CONTRA-INDICATIONS Application to damaged skin · application to the middle ear (may cause ototoxicity) · complete heart block · injection into infected tissues · injection into inflamed tissues · preparations containing preservatives should not be used for caudal, epidural, or spinal block, or for intravenous regional anaesthesia (Bier's block)

CONTRA-INDICATIONS, FURTHER INFORMATION
▸ Injection site Local anaesthetics should not be injected into inflamed or infected tissues nor should they be applied to damaged skin. Increased absorption into the blood increases the possibility of systemic side-effects, and the local anaesthetic effect may also be reduced by altered local pH.

● CAUTIONS Arrhythmias · arteriosclerosis · cardiovascular disease · cerebrovascular disease · cor pulmonale · debilitated patients (consider dose reduction) · diabetes mellitus · elderly (consider dose reduction) · epilepsy · hypercalcaemia · hyperreflexia · hypertension · hyperthyroidism · hypokalaemia · hypovolaemia · impaired cardiac conduction · impaired respiratory function · ischaemic heart disease · myasthenia gravis · obstructive cardiomyopathy · occlusive vascular disease · organic brain damage · phaeochromocytoma · prostate disorders · psychoneurosis · severe angina · shock · susceptibility to angle-closure glaucoma

CAUTIONS, FURTHER INFORMATION
▸ Use of vasoconstrictors In patients with severe hypertension or unstable cardiac rhythm, the use of adrenaline with a local anaesthetic may be hazardous. For these patients an anaesthetic without adrenaline should be used.

● INTERACTIONS → Appendix 1 (sympathomimetics).

● SIDE-EFFECTS Angina · angle-closure glaucoma · anorexia · anxiety · arrhythmias · blurred vision · cardiac arrest · cold extremities · confusion · convulsions · difficulty in micturition · dizziness · drowsiness · dry mouth · dyspnoea · feeling of inebriation · headache · hyperglycaemia · hypersalavation · hypertension (risk of cerebral haemorrhage) · hypokalaemia · insomnia · lightheadedness · metabolic acidosis · methaemoglobinaemia · muscle twitching · mydriasis · myocardial depression (resulting in hypotension and bradycardia) · myocardial infarction · nausea · numbness of the tongue and perioral region · pallor · palpitation · paraesthesia (including sensations of hot and cold) · peripheral vasodilatation (resulting in hypotension and bradycardia) · psychosis · pulmonary oedema (on excessive dosage or extreme sensitivity) · restlessness · sweating · tachycardia · tinnitus · tissue necrosis at injection site and of extremities, bowel, liver and kidneys · transient excitation (followed by depression with drowsiness, respiratory failure, unconsciousness, and coma) · tremor · urinary retention · vomiting · weakness

SIDE-EFFECTS, FURTHER INFORMATION
▸ Toxic effects Toxic effects after administration of local anaesthetics are a result of excessively high plasma concentrations; severe toxicity usually results from inadvertent intravascular injection or too rapid injection.

Following most regional anaesthetic procedures, maximum arterial plasma concentration of anaesthetic develops within about 10 to 25 minutes, so careful surveillance for toxic effects is necessary during the first 30 minutes after injection.

The systemic toxicity of local anaesthetics mainly involves the central nervous and cardiovascular systems.

● ALLERGY AND CROSS-SENSITIVITY
▸ Hypersensitivity and cross-sensitivity Hypersensitivity reactions occur mainly with the ester-type local anaesthetics, such as tetracaine and chloroprocaine; reactions are less frequent with the amide types, such as articaine, bupivacaine, levobupivacaine, lidocaine, mepivacaine, prilocaine, and ropivacaine. Cross-sensitivity reactions may be avoided by using the alternative chemical type.

● PREGNANCY Use only if potential benefit outweighs risk—no information available.

● BREAST FEEDING Avoid breast-feeding for 48 hours after administration.

● HEPATIC IMPAIRMENT Use with caution; increased risk of side-effects in severe impairment.

● RENAL IMPAIRMENT Manufacturers advise use with caution in severe impairment.

● MONITORING REQUIREMENTS Consider monitoring blood pressure and ECG (advised with systemic adrenaline/epinephrine).

● MEDICINAL FORMS
There can be variation in the licensing of different medicines containing the same drug.
Solution for injection
EXCIPIENTS: May contain Sulfites
▸ Septanest (Septodont Ltd)
Adrenaline (as Adrenaline acid tartrate) 10 microgram per 1 ml, Articaine hydrochloride 40 mg per 1 ml Septanest 1 in 100,000 solution for injection cartridges | 50 cartridge [PoM] no price available
Adrenaline (as Adrenaline acid tartrate) 5 microgram per 1 ml, Articaine hydrochloride 40 mg per 1 ml Septanest 1 in 200,000 solution for injection cartridges | 50 cartridge [PoM] no price available

Bupivacaine hydrochloride

● **INDICATIONS AND DOSE**

Surgical anaesthesia, lumbar epidural block
▸ BY REGIONAL ADMINISTRATION
▸ Adult: 75–150 mg, dose administered using a 5 mg/mL (0.5%) solution

Surgical anaesthesia, field block
▸ BY REGIONAL ADMINISTRATION
▸ Adult: Up to 150 mg, dose administered using a 2.5 mg/mL (0.25%) or 5 mg/mL (0.5%) solution

continued →

Surgical anaesthesia, thoracic epidural block
▸ BY THORACIC EPIDURAL
▸ Adult: 12.5–50 mg, dose administered using a
2.5 mg/mL (0.25%) or 5 mg/mL (0.5%) solution

Surgical anaesthesia, caudal epidural block
▸ BY REGIONAL ADMINISTRATION
▸ Adult: 50–150 mg, dose administered using a
2.5 mg/mL (0.25%) or 5 mg/mL (0.5%) solution

Surgical anaesthesia, major nerve block
▸ BY REGIONAL ADMINISTRATION
▸ Adult: 50–175 mg, dose administered using 5 mg/mL
(0.5%) solution

Acute pain, intra-articular block
▸ BY INTRA-ARTICULAR INJECTION
▸ Adult: Up to 100 mg, dose administered using a
2.5 mg/mL (0.25%) solution; when co-administered
with bupivacaine by another route, total max. 150 mg

Acute pain, thoracic epidural block
▸ BY CONTINUOUS EPIDURAL INFUSION
▸ Adult: 6.3–18.8 mg/hour, dose administered using a
1.25 mg/mL (0.125%) or 2.5 mg/mL (0.25%) solution;
maximum 400 mg per day

Acute pain, labour
▸ BY CONTINUOUS EPIDURAL INFUSION
▸ Adult: 6.25–12.5 mg/hour, dose administered using a
1.25 mg/mL (0.125%) solution; maximum 400 mg per
day

Acute pain, lumbar epidural block
▸ INITIALLY BY LUMBAR EPIDURAL
▸ Adult: 15–37.5 mg, then (by lumbar epidural)
15–37.5 mg, repeated when required at intervals of at
least 30 minutes, dose administered by intermittent
injection using a 2.5 mg/mL (0.25%) solution,
alternatively (by continuous epidural infusion)
12.5–18.8 mg/hour, dose administered using a
1.25 mg/mL (0.125%) or 2.5 mg/mL (0.25%) solution;
maximum 400 mg per day

Acute pain, field block
▸ BY REGIONAL ADMINISTRATION
▸ Adult: Up to 150 mg, dose administered using a
2.5 mg/mL (0.25%) solution

MARCAIN HEAVY®

Intrathecal anaesthesia for surgery
▸ BY INTRATHECAL INJECTION
▸ Adult: 10–20 mg

DOSES AT EXTREMES OF BODY-WEIGHT
To avoid excessive dosage in obese patients, dose should
be calculated on the basis of ideal body-weight.

IMPORTANT SAFETY INFORMATION
The licensed doses stated may not be appropriate in
some settings and expert advice should be sought.
Should only be administered by, or under the direct
supervision of, personnel experienced in their use, with
adequate training in anaesthesia and airway
management, and should not be administered
parenterally unless adequate resuscitation equipment is
available.

● CONTRA-INDICATIONS Application to the middle ear (can
cause ototoxicity) · avoid injection into infected tissues ·
avoid injection into inflamed tissues · complete heart block
· preparations containing preservatives should not be used
for caudal, epidural, or spinal block, or for intravenous
regional anaesthesia (Bier's block) · should not be applied
to damaged skin

CONTRA-INDICATIONS, FURTHER INFORMATION
▸ Injection site Local anaesthetics should not be injected into
inflamed or infected tissues nor should they be applied to

damaged skin. Increased absorption into the blood
increases the possibility of systemic side-effects, and the
local anaesthetic effect may also be reduced by altered
local pH.

● CAUTIONS Cardiovascular disease · cerebral atheroma ·
debilitated patients (consider dose reduction) · elderly
(consider dose reduction) · epilepsy · hypertension ·
hypotension · hypovolaemia · impaired cardiac conduction
· impaired respiratory function · myasthenia gravis ·
myocardial depression may be more severe and more
resistant to treatment · shock

● INTERACTIONS → Appendix 1 (bupivacaine).

● SIDE-EFFECTS Arrhythmias · blurred vision · cardiac arrest
· convulsions · dizziness · drowsiness · feeling of
inebriation · headache · lightheadedness · muscle twitching
· myocardial depression (resulting in hypotension and
bradycardia) · nausea · numbness of the tongue and
perioral region · paraesthesia (including sensations of hot
and cold) · peripheral vasodilatation (resulting in
hypotension and bradycardia) · restlessness · tinnitus ·
transient excitation (followed by depression with
drowsiness, respiratory failure, unconsciousness, and
coma) · tremors · vomiting

SIDE-EFFECTS, FURTHER INFORMATION
▸ Toxic effects Toxic effects after administration of local
anaesthetics are a result of excessively high plasma
concentrations; severe toxicity usually results from
inadvertent intravascular injection or too rapid injection.
Following most regional anaesthetic procedures,
maximum arterial plasma concentration of anaesthetic
develops within about 10 to 25 minutes, so careful
surveillance for toxic effects is necessary during the first
30 minutes after injection.
The systemic toxicity of local anaesthetics mainly
involves the central nervous and cardiovascular systems.

● ALLERGY AND CROSS-SENSITIVITY
▸ Hypersensitivity and cross-sensitivity Hypersensitivity
reactions occur mainly with the ester-type local
anaesthetics, such as tetracaine and chloroprocaine;
reactions are less frequent with the amide types, such as
articaine, bupivacaine, levobupivacaine, lidocaine,
mepivacaine, prilocaine, and ropivacaine. Cross-
sensitivity reactions may be avoided by using the
alternative chemical type.

● PREGNANCY Use lower doses for intrathecal use during
late pregnancy. Large doses during delivery can cause
neonatal respiratory depression, hypotonia, and
bradycardia after epidural block.

● BREAST FEEDING Amount too small to be harmful.

● HEPATIC IMPAIRMENT Use with caution in severe
impairment.

● RENAL IMPAIRMENT Use with caution in severe
impairment.

● MEDICINAL FORMS
There can be variation in the licensing of different medicines
containing the same drug. Forms available from special-order
manufacturers include: solution for injection, infusion,
solution for infusion

Solution for injection
▸ Bupivacaine hydrochloride (Non-proprietary)
Bupivacaine hydrochloride 2.5 mg per 1 ml Bupivacaine 0.25%
solution for injection 10ml Sure-Amp ampoules | 20 ampoule [PoM]
£17.50
Bupivacaine hydrochloride 5 mg per 1 ml Bupivacaine 0.5%
solution for injection 10ml Sure-Amp ampoules | 20 ampoule [PoM]
£18.30
Bupivacaine 50mg/10ml (0.5%) solution for injection ampoules |
10 ampoule [PoM] no price available
▸ Marcain (AstraZeneca UK Ltd)
Bupivacaine hydrochloride 2.5 mg per 1 ml Marcain 0.25% solution
for injection 10ml Polyamp Steripack ampoules | 5 ampoule [PoM]
£7.92

Bupivacaine hydrochloride 5 mg per 1 ml Marcain 0.5% solution for injection 10ml Polyamp Steripack ampoules | 5 ampoule [PoM] £9.25

Infusion

▶ Bupivacaine hydrochloride (Non-proprietary)
Bupivacaine hydrochloride 1 mg per 1 ml Bupivacaine 100mg/100ml (0.1%) infusion bags | 20 bag [PoM] no price available
Bupivacaine 250mg/250ml (0.1%) infusion bags | 20 bag [PoM] no price available
Bupivacaine hydrochloride 1.25 mg per 1 ml Bupivacaine 312.5mg/250ml (0.125%) infusion bags | 20 bag [PoM] no price available

Bupivacaine with adrenaline

The properties listed below are those particular to the combination only. For the properties of the components please consider, bupivacaine hydrochloride p. 1183, adrenaline/epinephrine p. 205.

● INDICATIONS AND DOSE

Surgical anaesthesia
▶ BY LUMBAR EPIDURAL, OR BY LOCAL INFILTRATION, OR BY CAUDAL EPIDURAL
▶ Adult: (consult product literature)

Acute pain management
▶ BY LUMBAR EPIDURAL, OR BY LOCAL INFILTRATION
▶ Adult: (consult product literature)

IMPORTANT SAFETY INFORMATION
Adrenaline/epinephrine must be used in a low concentration when administered with a local anaesthetic. The total dose of adrenaline should not exceed 500 micrograms and it is essential not to exceed a concentration of 1 in 200 000 (5 micrograms/mL) if more than 50 mL of the mixture is to be injected.

● CAUTIONS

CAUTIONS, FURTHER INFORMATION
In patients with severe hypertension or unstable cardiac rhythm, the use of adrenaline with a local anaesthetic may be hazardous. For these patients an anaesthetic without adrenaline should be used.

● MEDICINAL FORMS
There can be variation in the licensing of different medicines containing the same drug.

Solution for injection
▶ Bupivacaine with adrenaline (Non-proprietary)
Adrenaline (as Adrenaline acid tartrate) 5 microgram per 1 ml, Bupivacaine hydrochloride 2.5 mg per 1 ml Bupivacaine 25mg/10ml (0.25%) / Adrenaline (base) 50micrograms/10ml (1 in 200,000) solution for injection ampoules | 10 ampoule [PoM] £40.00
Adrenaline (as Adrenaline acid tartrate) 5 microgram per 1 ml, Bupivacaine hydrochloride anhydrous 2.5 mg per 1 ml Carbostesin-adrenaline 0.25% / 100micrograms/20ml (1 in 200,000) solution for injection ampoules | 1 ampoule [PoM] no price available
Carbostesin-adrenaline 0.25% / 25micrograms/5ml (1 in 200,000) solution for injection ampoules | 1 ampoule [PoM] no price available
Adrenaline (as Adrenaline acid tartrate) 5 microgram per 1 ml, Bupivacaine hydrochloride 5 mg per 1 ml Bupivacaine 50mg/10ml (0.5%) / Adrenaline (base) 50micrograms/10ml (1 in 200,000) solution for injection ampoules | 10 ampoule [PoM] £45.00
Adrenaline (as Adrenaline acid tartrate) 5 microgram per 1 ml, Bupivacaine hydrochloride anhydrous 5 mg per 1 ml Carbostesin-adrenaline 0.5% / 25micrograms/5ml (1 in 200,000) solution for injection ampoules | 1 ampoule [PoM] no price available
Carbostesin-adrenaline 0.5% / 100micrograms/20ml (1 in 200,000) solution for injection ampoules | 1 ampoule [PoM] no price available

Chloroprocaine hydrochloride

● INDICATIONS AND DOSE

Intrathecal anaesthesia for surgical procedures lasting up to 40 minutes
▶ BY SLOW INTRATHECAL INJECTION
▶ Adult: 40–50 mg, dose depends on desired length of block

DOSES AT EXTREMES OF BODY-WEIGHT
To avoid excessive dosage in obese patients, dose may need to be calculated on the basis of ideal body-weight.

IMPORTANT SAFETY INFORMATION
The licensed doses stated above may not be appropriate in some settings and expert advice should be sought.
Should only be administered by, or under the direct supervision of, personnel experienced in their use, with adequate training in anaesthesia and airway management, and should not be administered parenterally unless adequate resuscitation equipment is available.

● CONTRA-INDICATIONS Application to the middle ear (can cause ototoxicity) · avoid injection into infected tissues · avoid injection into inflamed tissues · complete heart block · preparations containing preservatives should not be used for caudal, epidural, or spinal block, or for intravenous regional anaesthesia (Bier's block) · severe anaemia · should not be applied to damaged skin

CONTRA-INDICATIONS, FURTHER INFORMATION
▶ Injection site Local anaesthetics should not be injected into inflamed or infected tissues nor should they be applied to damaged skin. Increased absorption into the blood increases the possibility of systemic side-effects, and the local anaesthetic effect may also be reduced by altered local pH.

● CAUTIONS Acute porphyrias p. 918 · cardiovascular disease · debilitated patients (consider dose reduction) · elderly (consider dose reduction) · epilepsy · hypovolaemia · impaired cardiac conduction · impaired respiratory function · myasthenia gravis · shock

● INTERACTIONS → Appendix 1 (chloroprocaine).

● SIDE-EFFECTS
▶ **Uncommon** Hypertension
▶ **Frequency not known** Arrhythmias · blurred vision · cardiac arrest · convulsions · dizziness · drowsiness · feeling of inebriation · headache · lightheadedness · muscle twitching · myocardial depression (resulting in hypotension and bradycardia) · nausea · numbness of the tongue and perioral region · paraesthesia (including sensations of hot and cold) · peripheral vasodilatation (resulting in hypotension and bradycardia) · restlessness · tinnitus · transient excitation (followed by depression with drowsiness, respiratory failure, unconsciousness, and coma) · tremors · vomiting

SIDE-EFFECTS, FURTHER INFORMATION
▶ Toxic effects Toxic effects after administration of local anaesthetics are a result of excessively high plasma concentrations; severe toxicity usually results from inadvertent intravascular injection or too rapid injection.
Following most regional anaesthetic procedures, maximum arterial plasma concentration of anaesthetic develops within about 10 to 25 minutes, so careful surveillance for toxic effects is necessary during the first 30 minutes after injection.
The systemic toxicity of local anaesthetics mainly involves the central nervous and cardiovascular systems.

● ALLERGY AND CROSS-SENSITIVITY
▶ Hypersensitivity and cross-sensitivity Hypersensitivity reactions occur mainly with the ester-type local

15

Anaesthesia

anaesthetics, such as tetracaine and chloroprocaine; reactions are less frequent with the amide types, such as articaine, bupivacaine, levobupivacaine, lidocaine, mepivacaine, prilocaine, and ropivacaine. Cross-sensitivity reactions may be avoided by using the alternative chemical type.

● PREGNANCY Avoid—no information available.

● BREAST FEEDING Avoid—no information available.

● HEPATIC IMPAIRMENT Use with caution in severe impairment.

● RENAL IMPAIRMENT Use with caution in severe impairment.

● MEDICINAL FORMS
There can be variation in the licensing of different medicines containing the same drug.
Solution for injection
 ▹ Ampres (AMCo)
  Chloroprocaine hydrochloride 10 mg per 1 ml Ampres 50mg/5ml solution for injection ampoules | 10 ampoule PoM £87.50

Levobupivacaine

● INDICATIONS AND DOSE
Acute postoperative pain
 ▹ BY CONTINUOUS EPIDURAL INFUSION
 ▹ Adult: 12.5–18.75 mg/hour, dose administered using a 1.25 mg/mL (0.125%) or 2.5 mg/mL (0.25%) solution; maximum 400 mg per day
Acute labour pain
 ▹ BY LUMBAR EPIDURAL
 ▹ Adult: 15–25 mg, repeated at intervals of at least 15 minutes, dose administered using a 2.5 mg/mL (0.25%) solution; maximum 400 mg per day
 ▹ BY CONTINUOUS EPIDURAL INFUSION
 ▹ Adult: 5–12.5 mg/hour, dose administered using a 1.25 mg/mL (0.125%) solution; maximum 400 mg per day
Surgical anaesthesia, peripheral nerve block
 ▹ BY REGIONAL ADMINISTRATION
 ▹ Adult: 2.5–150 mg, dose administered using a 2.5 mg/mL (0.25%) or 5 mg/mL (0.5%) solution
Surgical anaesthesia, peribulbular nerve block
 ▹ BY REGIONAL ADMINISTRATION
 ▹ Adult: 37.5–112.5 mg, dose administered using a 7.5 mg/mL (0.75%) solution
Surgical anaesthesia for caesarean section
 ▹ BY LUMBAR EPIDURAL
 ▹ Adult: 75–150 mg, to be given over 15 –20 minutes, dose administered using a 5 mg/mL (0.5%) solution
Surgical anaesthesia
 ▹ BY LUMBAR EPIDURAL
 ▹ Adult: 50–150 mg, to be given over 5 minutes, dose administered using a 5 mg/mL (0.5%) or 7.5 mg/mL (0.75%) solution
 ▹ BY INTRATHECAL INJECTION
 ▹ Adult: 15 mg, dose administered using a 5 mg/mL (0.5%) solution
 ▹ BY LOCAL INFILTRATION
 ▹ Adult: 2.5–150 mg, dose administered using a 2.5 mg/mL (0.25%) solution

DOSES AT EXTREMES OF BODY-WEIGHT
To avoid excessive dosage in obese patients, dose should be calculated on the basis of ideal body-weight.

IMPORTANT SAFETY INFORMATION
The licensed doses stated may not be appropriate in some settings and expert advice should be sought.

Should only be administered by, or under the direct supervision of, personnel experienced in their use, with adequate training in anaesthesia and airway management, and should not be administered parenterally unless adequate resuscitation equipment is available.

● CONTRA-INDICATIONS Application to the middle ear (can cause ototoxicity) · avoid injection into infected tissues · avoid injection into inflamed tissues · complete heart block · preparations containing preservatives should not be used for caudal, epidural, or spinal block, or for intravenous regional anaesthesia (Bier's block) · should not be applied to damaged skin

CONTRA-INDICATIONS, FURTHER INFORMATION
 ▹ Injection site Local anaesthetics should not be injected into inflamed or infected tissues nor should they be applied to damaged skin. Increased absorption into the blood increases the possibility of systemic side-effects, and the local anaesthetic effect may also be reduced by altered local pH.

● CAUTIONS Cardiovascular disease · debilitated patients (consider dose reduction) · elderly (consider dose reduction) · epilepsy · hypovolaemia · impaired cardiac conduction · impaired respiratory function · myasthenia gravis · shock

● INTERACTIONS → Appendix 1 (levobupivacaine).

● SIDE-EFFECTS Anaemia · arrhythmias · blurred vision · cardiac arrest · convulsions · dizziness · drowsiness · feeling of inebriation · headache · lightheadedness · muscle twitching · myocardial depression (resulting in hypotension and bradycardia) · nausea · numbness of the tongue and perioral region · paraesthesia (including sensations of hot and cold) · peripheral vasodilatation (resulting in hypotension and bradycardia) · pyrexia · restlessness · sweating · tinnitus · transient excitation (followed by depression with drowsiness, respiratory failure, unconsciousness, and coma) · tremors · vomiting

SIDE-EFFECTS, FURTHER INFORMATION
 ▹ Toxic effects Toxic effects after administration of local anaesthetics are a result of excessively high plasma concentrations; severe toxicity usually results from inadvertent intravascular injection or too rapid injection.
  Following most regional anaesthetic procedures, maximum arterial plasma concentration of anaesthetic develops within about 10 to 25 minutes, so careful surveillance for toxic effects is necessary during the first 30 minutes after injection.
  The systemic toxicity of local anaesthetics mainly involves the central nervous and cardiovascular systems.

● ALLERGY AND CROSS-SENSITIVITY
 ▹ Hypersensitivity and cross-sensitivity Hypersensitivity reactions occur mainly with the ester-type local anaesthetics, such as tetracaine and chloroprocaine; reactions are less frequent with the amide types, such as articaine, bupivacaine, levobupivacaine, lidocaine, mepivacaine, prilocaine, and ropivacaine. Cross-sensitivity reactions may be avoided by using the alternative chemical type.

● PREGNANCY Large doses during delivery can cause neonatal respiratory depression, hypotonia, and bradycardia after epidural block. Avoid if possible in the first trimester—toxicity in *animal* studies. May cause fetal distress syndrome. Do not use for paracervical block in obstetrics. Do not use 7.5 mg/mL strength in obstetrics.

● BREAST FEEDING Amount too small to be harmful.

● HEPATIC IMPAIRMENT Use with caution.

● DIRECTIONS FOR ADMINISTRATION For 1.25 mg/mL concentration dilute standard solutions with sodium chloride 0.9%.

● PRESCRIBING AND DISPENSING INFORMATION
Levobupivacaine is an isomer of bupivacaine.

● MEDICINAL FORMS
There can be variation in the licensing of different medicines
containing the same drug.

Solution for injection
▸ Chirocaine (AbbVie Ltd)
**Levobupivacaine (as Levobupivacaine hydrochloride) 2.5 mg per
1 ml** Chirocaine 25mg/10ml solution for injection ampoules |
10 ampoule PoM £14.11 (Hospital only)
**Levobupivacaine (as Levobupivacaine hydrochloride) 5 mg per
1 ml** Chirocaine 50mg/10ml solution for injection ampoules |
10 ampoule PoM £16.15 (Hospital only)
**Levobupivacaine (as Levobupivacaine hydrochloride) 7.5 mg per
1 ml** Chirocaine 75mg/10ml solution for injection ampoules |
10 ampoule PoM £24.23 (Hospital only)

Infusion
▸ Chirocaine (AbbVie Ltd)
**Levobupivacaine (as Levobupivacaine hydrochloride) 1.25 mg per
1 ml** Chirocaine 125mg/100ml infusion bags | 24 bag PoM £174.22
Chirocaine 250mg/200ml infusion bags | 12 bag PoM no price
available

Lidocaine hydrochloride

(Lignocaine hydrochloride)

● INDICATIONS AND DOSE

Infiltration anaesthesia
▸ BY LOCAL INFILTRATION
▸ Adult: Dose to be given according to patient's weight
and nature of procedure; max. 200 mg, maximum dose
500 mg if given in solutions containing adrenaline

DOSES AT EXTREMES OF BODY-WEIGHT
▸ When used by local infiltration To avoid excessive dosage in
obese patients, dose may need to be calculated on the
basis of ideal body-weight.

Intravenous regional anaesthesia and nerve block
▸ BY REGIONAL ADMINISTRATION
▸ Adult: Seek expert advice

**Pain relief (in anal fissures, haemorrhoids, pruritus ani,
pruritus vulvae, herpes zoster, or herpes labialis) |
Lubricant in cystoscopy | Lubricant in proctoscopy**
▸ TO THE SKIN USING OINTMENT
▸ Adult: Apply 1–2 mL as required, avoid long-term use

Sore nipples from breast-feeding
▸ TO THE SKIN USING OINTMENT
▸ Adult: Apply using gauze and wash off immediately
before next feed

LMX 4®

Anaesthesia before venous cannulation or venepuncture
▸ TO THE SKIN
▸ Child 1-2 months: Apply up to 1 g, apply thick layer to
small area (2.5 cm × 2.5 cm) of non-irritated skin at
least 30 minutes before procedure; may be applied
under an occlusive dressing; max. application time
60 minutes, remove cream with gauze and perform
procedure after approximately 5 minutes
▸ Child 3-11 months: Apply up to 1 g, apply thick layer to
small area (2.5 cm × 2.5 cm) of non-irritated skin at
least 30 minutes before procedure; may be applied
under an occlusive dressing; max. application time
4 hours, remove cream with gauze and perform
procedure after approximately 5 minutes
▸ Child 1-17 years: Apply 1–2.5 g, apply thick layer to
small area (2.5 cm × 2.5 cm) of non-irritated skin at
least 30 minutes before procedure; may be applied
under an occlusive dressing; max. application time
5 hours, remove cream with gauze and perform
procedure after approximately 5 minutes

▸ Adult: Apply 1–2.5 g, apply thick layer to small area
(2.5 cm × 2.5 cm) of non-irritated skin at least
30 minutes before procedure; may be applied under an
occlusive dressing; max. application time 5 hours,
remove cream with gauze and perform procedure after
approximately 5 minutes

VERSATIS®

Postherpetic neuralgia
▸ TO THE SKIN
▸ Adult: Apply once daily for up to 12 hours, followed by
a 12-hour plaster-free period; discontinue if no
response after 4 weeks, to be applied to intact, dry,
non-hairy, non-irritated skin, up to 3 plasters may be
used to cover large areas; plasters may be cut

XYLOCAINE®

During delivery in obstetrics
▸ TO THE SKIN
▸ Adult: Up to 20 doses

> IMPORTANT SAFETY INFORMATION
> ▸ When used by local infiltration
> The licensed doses stated may not be appropriate in
> some settings and expert advice should be sought.
> Should only be administered by, or under the direct
> supervision of, personnel experienced in their use, with
> adequate training in anaesthesia and airway
> management, and should not be administered
> parenterally unless adequate resuscitation equipment is
> available.

● CONTRA-INDICATIONS
▸ When used by regional administration All grades of
atrioventricular block · application to the middle ear (can
cause ototoxicity) · avoid injection into infected tissues ·
avoid injection into inflamed tissues · preparations
containing preservatives should not be used for caudal,
epidural, or spinal block, or for intravenous regional
anaesthesia (Bier's block) · severe myocardial depression ·
should not be applied to damaged skin · sino-atrial
disorders

CONTRA-INDICATIONS, FURTHER INFORMATION
▸ Injection site
▸ When used by regional administration Local anaesthetics
should not be injected into inflamed or infected tissues nor
should they be applied to damaged skin. Increased
absorption into the blood increases the possibility of
systemic side-effects, and the local anaesthetic effect may
also be reduced by altered local pH.

● CAUTIONS
▸ When used by regional administration Acute porphyria
(consider infusion with glucose for its anti-
porphyrinogenic effects) · congestive cardiac failure
(consider lower dose) · debilitated patients (consider dose
reduction) · elderly (consider dose reduction) · epilepsy ·
hypovolaemia · impaired cardiac conduction · impaired
respiratory function · myasthenia gravis · post cardiac
surgery (consider lower dose) · shock

● INTERACTIONS → Appendix 1 (lidocaine).
Interactions less likely when lidocaine used topically.

● SIDE-EFFECTS
▸ **Common or very common**
▸ When used by regional administration Bradycardia (may lead
to cardiac arrest) · confusion · convulsions · hypotension
(may lead to cardiac arrest) · respiratory depression
▸ **Rare**
▸ When used by regional administration Anaphylaxis
▸ **Frequency not known**
▸ When used by regional administration Transient excitation
(followed by depression with drowsiness, respiratory
failure, unconsciousness, and coma) · arrhythmias · blurred

vision · cardiac arrest · feeling of inebriation · headache · hypoglycaemia (following intrathecal or extradural administration) · methaemoglobinaemia · muscle twitching · myocardial depression (resulting in hypotension and bradycardia) · nausea · numbness of the tongue and perioral region · nystagmus · peripheral vasodilatation (resulting in hypotension and bradycardia) · rash · restlessness · tinnitus · tremors · vomiting

SIDE-EFFECTS, FURTHER INFORMATION

‣ Topical application A single application of a topical lidocaine preparation does not generally cause systemic side-effects.
‣ Toxic effects
‣ When used by regional administration Toxic effects after administration of local anaesthetics are a result of excessively high plasma concentrations; severe toxicity usually results from inadvertent intravascular injection or too rapid injection. Following most regional anaesthetic procedures, maximum arterial plasma concentration of anaesthetic develops within about 10 to 25 minutes, so careful surveillance for toxic effects is necessary during the first 30 minutes after injection. The systemic toxicity of local anaesthetics mainly involves the central nervous and cardiovascular systems.
‣ Methaemoglobinaemia
‣ When used by regional administration Methaemoglobinaemia can be treated with an intravenous injection of methylthioninium chloride.

● ALLERGY AND CROSS-SENSITIVITY
‣ Hypersensitivity and cross-sensitivity Hypersensitivity reactions occur mainly with the ester-type local anaesthetics, such as tetracaine and chloroprocaine; reactions are less frequent with the amide types, such as articaine, bupivacaine, levobupivacaine, lidocaine, mepivacaine, prilocaine, and ropivacaine. Cross-sensitivity reactions may be avoided by using the alternative chemical type.

● PREGNANCY Crosses the placenta but not known to be harmful in *animal* studies—use if benefit outweighs risk. When used as a local anaesthetic, large doses can cause fetal bradycardia; if given during delivery can also cause neonatal respiratory depression, hypotonia, or bradycardia after paracervical or epidural block.

● BREAST FEEDING Present in milk but amount too small to be harmful.

● HEPATIC IMPAIRMENT Caution—increased risk of side-effects.

● RENAL IMPAIRMENT Possible accumulation of lidocaine and active metabolite; caution in severe impairment.

● MONITORING REQUIREMENTS
‣ With systemic use Monitor ECG and have resuscitation facilities available.

● PROFESSION SPECIFIC INFORMATION

Dental practitioners' formulary
Lidocaine ointment 5% may be prescribed. Spray may be prescribed as Lidocaine Spray 10%

● NATIONAL FUNDING/ACCESS DECISIONS

Scottish Medicines Consortium (SMC) Decisions
The *Scottish Medicines Consortium* has advised (July 2008) that *Versatis*® is accepted for restricted use within NHS Scotland for the treatment of postherpetic neuralgia in patients who are intolerant of first-line systemic therapies or when they have been ineffective.

● MEDICINAL FORMS
There can be variation in the licensing of different medicines containing the same drug.

Solution for injection
‣ Lidocaine hydrochloride (Non-proprietary)
  Lidocaine hydrochloride 5 mg per 1 ml Lidocaine 50mg/10ml (0.5%) solution for injection ampoules | 10 ampoule [PoM] £7.00
  Lidocaine hydrochloride 10 mg per 1 ml Lidocaine 100mg/10ml (1%) solution for injection Mini-Plasco ampoules | 20 ampoule [PoM] £10.89
  Lidocaine 100mg/10ml (1%) solution for injection ampoules | 10 ampoule [PoM] £4.50 DT price = £4.01
  Lidocaine 100mg/10ml (1%) solution for injection Sure-Amp ampoules | 20 ampoule [PoM] £8.80
  Lidocaine 200mg/20ml (1%) solution for injection vials | 10 vial [PoM] £18.00–£19.00
  Lidocaine 200mg/20ml (1%) solution for injection ampoules | 10 ampoule [PoM] £7.00–£8.75 DT price = £8.75
  Lidocaine 50mg/5ml (1%) solution for injection ampoules | 10 ampoule [PoM] £2.35–£3.10 DT price = £2.36
  Lidocaine 20mg/2ml (1%) solution for injection ampoules | 10 ampoule [PoM] £3.50 DT price = £1.98
  Lidocaine 50mg/5ml (1%) solution for injection Sure-Amp ampoules | 20 ampoule [PoM] £6.00
  Lidocaine hydrochloride 20 mg per 1 ml Lidocaine 100mg/5ml (2%) solution for injection ampoules | 10 ampoule [PoM] £2.40–£3.80 DT price = £2.41
  Lidocaine 400mg/20ml (2%) solution for injection vials | 10 vial [PoM] £18.50–£19.50
  Lidocaine 200mg/10ml (2%) solution for injection Mini-Plasco ampoules | 20 ampoule [PoM] £14.52
  Lidocaine 40mg/2ml (2%) solution for injection ampoules | 10 ampoule [PoM] £4.00 DT price = £2.11
  Lidocaine 100mg/5ml (2%) solution for injection Sure-Amp ampoules | 20 ampoule [PoM] £6.00
  Lidocaine 400mg/20ml (2%) solution for injection ampoules | 10 ampoule [PoM] £8.00–£9.00 DT price = £9.00

Cream
EXCIPIENTS: May contain Benzyl alcohol, propylene glycol
‣ LMX 4 (Ferndale Pharmaceuticals Ltd)
  Lidocaine 40 mg per 1 gram LMX 4 cream | 5 gram [P] £2.98 DT price = £2.98 | 30 gram [P] £14.90

Ointment
‣ Lidocaine hydrochloride (Non-proprietary)
  Lidocaine hydrochloride 50 mg per 1 gram Lidocaine 5% ointment | 15 gram [P] £6.50 DT price = £6.18

Medicated plaster
EXCIPIENTS: May contain Hydroxybenzoates (parabens), propylene glycol
‣ Versatis (Grunenthal Ltd)
  Lidocaine 50 mg per 1 gram Versatis 5% medicated plasters | 30 plaster [PoM] £72.40 DT price = £72.40

Lidocaine with adrenaline

The properties listed below are those particular to the combination only. For the properties of the components please consider, lidocaine hydrochloride p. 1187, adrenaline/epinephrine p. 205.

● INDICATIONS AND DOSE

Local anaesthesia
▸ BY LOCAL INFILTRATION
▸ Adult: Dosed according to the type of nerve block required (consult product literature)

IMPORTANT SAFETY INFORMATION
Adrenaline/epinephrine must be used in a low concentration when administered with a local anaesthetic. The total dose of adrenaline should not exceed 500 micrograms and it is essential not to exceed a concentration of 1 in 200 000 (5 micrograms/mL) if more than 50 mL of the mixture is to be injected.

● PROFESSION SPECIFIC INFORMATION

Dental information
A variety of lidocaine injections with adrenaline is available in dental cartridges.
  Consult expert dental sources for specific advice in relation to dose of lidocaine for dental anaesthesia.

● MEDICINAL FORMS
There can be variation in the licensing of different medicines containing the same drug. Forms available from special-order manufacturers include: solution for injection
Solution for injection
EXCIPIENTS: May contain Sulfites
‣ Lignospan Special (Kent Pharmaceuticals Ltd)
  Adrenaline (as Adrenaline acid tartrate) 12.5 microgram per 1 ml, Lidocaine hydrochloride 20 mg per 1 ml Lignospan Special 2% injection 2.2ml cartridges | 50 cartridge PoM £18.11
‣ Rexocaine (Henry Schein Ltd)
  Adrenaline (as Adrenaline acid tartrate) 12.5 microgram per 1 ml, Lidocaine hydrochloride 20 mg per 1 ml Rexocaine 2% injection 2.2ml cartridges | 50 cartridge PoM no price available
‣ Xylocaine with Adrenaline (AstraZeneca UK Ltd)
  Adrenaline (as Adrenaline acid tartrate) 5 microgram per 1 ml, Lidocaine hydrochloride 10 mg per 1 ml Xylocaine 1% with Adrenaline 100micrograms/20ml (1 in 200,000) solution for injection vials | 5 vial PoM £9.66 DT price = £9.66
  Adrenaline (as Adrenaline acid tartrate) 5 microgram per 1 ml, Lidocaine hydrochloride 20 mg per 1 ml Xylocaine 2% with Adrenaline 100micrograms/20ml (1 in 200,000) solution for injection vials | 5 vial PoM £8.85 DT price = £8.85

Lidocaine with phenylephrine

The properties listed below are those particular to the combination only. For the properties of the components please consider, lidocaine hydrochloride p. 1187, phenylephrine hydrochloride p. 173.

● INDICATIONS AND DOSE

Anaesthesia before nasal surgery, endoscopy, laryngoscopy, or removal of foreign bodies from the nose
▸ BY INTRANASAL ADMINISTRATION
‣ Adult: Up to 8 sprays

● MEDICINAL FORMS
There can be variation in the licensing of different medicines containing the same drug.
Spray
▸ Lidocaine with phenylephrine (Non-proprietary)
  Phenylephrine hydrochloride 5 mg per 1 ml, Lidocaine hydrochloride 50 mg per 1 ml Lidocaine 5% / Phenylephrine 0.5% nasal spray | 2.5 ml PoM £11.48 DT price = £11.48

Lidocaine with prilocaine

The properties listed below are those particular to the combination only. For the properties of the components please consider, lidocaine hydrochloride p. 1187, prilocaine hydrochloride p. 1191.

● INDICATIONS AND DOSE

Anaesthesia before minor skin procedures including venepuncture
▸ TO THE SKIN
‣ Child 1-2 months: Apply up to 1 g for maximum 1 hour before procedure, to be applied under occlusive dressing, shorter application time of 15–30 minutes is recommended for children with atopic dermatitis (30 minutes before removal of mollusca); maximum 1 dose per day
‣ Child 3-11 months: Apply up to 2 g for maximum 4 hours before procedure, to be applied under occlusive dressing, shorter application time of 15–30 minutes is

recommended for children with atopic dermatitis (30 minutes before removal of mollusca); maximum 2 doses per day
‣ Child 1-11 years: Apply 1–5 hours before procedure (2–5 hours before procedures on large areas e.g. split skin grafting), a thick layer should be applied under occlusive dressing, shorter application time of 15–30 minutes is recommended for children with atopic dermatitis (30 minutes before removal of mollusca); maximum 2 doses per day
‣ Child 12-17 years: Apply 1–5 hours before procedure (2–5 hours before procedures on large areas e.g. split skin grafting), a thick layer should be applied under occlusive dressing, shorter application time of 15–30 minutes is recommended for children with atopic dermatitis (30 minutes before removal of mollusca)
‣ Adult: Apply 1–5 hours before procedure (2–5 hours before procedures on large areas e.g. split skin grafting), a thick layer should be applied under occlusive dressing

Anaesthesia on genital skin before injection of local anaesthetics
▸ TO THE SKIN
‣ Adult: Apply for 15 minutes (in adult men) and 60 minutes (in adult women), to be applied under occlusive dressing

Anaesthesia before surgical treatment of lesions on genital mucosa
▸ TO THE SKIN
‣ Adult: Apply up to 10 g, to be applied 5–10 minutes before procedure

Anaesthesia before cervical curettage
▸ TO THE SKIN
‣ Adult: Apply 10 g in lateral vaginal fornices for 10 minutes

Anaesthesia before mechanical cleansing or debridement of leg ulcer
▸ TO THE SKIN
‣ Adult: Apply up to 10 g for 30–60 minutes, to be applied under occlusive dressing

● CONTRA-INDICATIONS Use in child less than 37 weeks corrected gestational age

● PATIENT AND CARER ADVICE
Medicines for Children leaflet: EMLA cream for local anaesthesia www.medicinesforchildren.org.uk/emla-cream-for-local-anaesthesia

● MEDICINAL FORMS
There can be variation in the licensing of different medicines containing the same drug.
Cream
▸ Lidocaine with prilocaine (Non-proprietary)
  Lidocaine 25 mg per 1 gram, Prilocaine 25 mg per 1 gram Lidocaine 2.5% / Prilocaine 2.5% cream | 5 gram P no price available
▸ Denela (Auden McKenzie (Pharma Division) Ltd)
  Lidocaine 25 mg per 1 gram, Prilocaine 25 mg per 1 gram Denela 5% cream | 5 gram P £2.84-£3.29 | 25 gram P £12.99 | 30 gram P £14.75 DT price = £12.30
▸ Emla (AstraZeneca UK Ltd)
  Lidocaine 25 mg per 1 gram, Prilocaine 25 mg per 1 gram Emla 5% cream | 5 gram P £2.25-£2.99 | 25 gram P £11.70 | 30 gram P £12.30 DT price = £12.30

15

Anaesthesia

Lidocaine with tetracaine

The properties listed below are those particular to the combination only. For the properties of the components please consider, lidocaine hydrochloride p. 1187, tetracaine p. 1193.

● **INDICATIONS AND DOSE**

Anaesthesia before dermatological procedures and venepuncture
▸ TO THE SKIN
 ▸ Adult: Apply 1 mm layer using a spatula 30 minutes before procedure, then peel off immediately before procedure; max. application area 400 cm², application time of 60 minutes indicated for certain procedures, such as laser–assisted tattoo removal and laser leg vein ablation

● **MEDICINAL FORMS**
There can be variation in the licensing of different medicines containing the same drug.
Cream
 EXCIPIENTS: May contain Hydroxybenzoates (parabens)
 ▸ Pliaglis (Galderma (UK) Ltd)
  Lidocaine 70 mg, Tetracaine 70 mg Pliaglis 70mg/g / 70mg/g cream | 15 gram PoM £22.95

Mepivacaine hydrochloride

● **INDICATIONS AND DOSE**

Infiltration anaesthesia and nerve block in dentistry
 ▸ Child 3-17 years: Consult expert dental sources
 ▸ Adult: Consult expert dental sources
DOSES AT EXTREMES OF BODY-WEIGHT
To avoid excessive dosage in obese patients, dose should be calculated on the basis of ideal body-weight.

IMPORTANT SAFETY INFORMATION
Should only be administered by, or under the direct supervision of, personnel experienced in their use, with adequate training in anaesthesia and airway management, and should not be administered parenterally unless adequate resuscitation equipment is available.

● **CONTRA-INDICATIONS** Application to the middle ear (can cause ototoxicity) · avoid injection into infected tissues · avoid injection into inflamed tissues · complete heart block · preparations containing preservatives should not be used for caudal, epidural, or spinal block, or for intravenous regional anaesthesia (Bier's block) · should not be applied to damaged skin
 CONTRA-INDICATIONS, FURTHER INFORMATION
▸ Injection site Local anaesthetics should not be injected into inflamed or infected tissues nor should they be applied to damaged skin. Increased absorption into the blood increases the possibility of systemic side-effects, and the local anaesthetic effect may also be reduced by altered local pH.
● **CAUTIONS** Cardiovascular disease · children (consider dose reduction) (in children) · debilitated patients (consider dose reduction) · elderly (consider dose reduction) (in adults) · epilepsy · hypovolaemia · impaired cardiac conduction · impaired respiratory function · myasthenia gravis · shock
● **SIDE-EFFECTS** Arrhythmias · blurred vision · cardiac arrest · convulsions · dizziness · drowsiness · feeling of inebriation · headache · lightheadedness · muscle twitching · myocardial depression (resulting in hypotension and bradycardia) · nausea · numbness of the tongue and

perioral region · paraesthesia (including sensations of hot and cold) · peripheral vasodilatation (resulting in hypotension and bradycardia) · restlessness · tinnitus · transient excitation (followed by depression with drowsiness, respiratory failure, unconsciousness, and coma) · tremors · vomiting
 SIDE-EFFECTS, FURTHER INFORMATION
▸ Toxic effects Toxic effects after administration of local anaesthetics are a result of excessively high plasma concentrations; severe toxicity usually results from inadvertent intravascular injection or too rapid injection.
  Following most regional anaesthetic procedures, maximum arterial plasma concentration of anaesthetic develops within about 10 to 25 minutes, so careful surveillance for toxic effects is necessary during the first 30 minutes after injection.
  The systemic toxicity of local anaesthetics mainly involves the central nervous and cardiovascular systems.
● **ALLERGY AND CROSS-SENSITIVITY**
▸ Hypersensitivity and cross-sensitivity Hypersensitivity reactions occur mainly with the ester-type local anaesthetics, such as tetracaine and chloroprocaine; reactions are less frequent with the amide types, such as articaine, bupivacaine, levobupivacaine, lidocaine, mepivacaine, prilocaine, and ropivacaine. Cross-sensitivity reactions may be avoided by using the alternative chemical type.
● **PREGNANCY** Use with caution in early pregnancy.
● **BREAST FEEDING** Use with caution.
● **HEPATIC IMPAIRMENT** Use with caution; increased risk of side-effects in severe impairment.
● **RENAL IMPAIRMENT** Use with caution; increased risk of side-effects.

● **MEDICINAL FORMS**
There can be variation in the licensing of different medicines containing the same drug.
Solution for injection
 ▸ Scandonest plain (Deproco UK Ltd)
  Mepivacaine hydrochloride 30 mg per 1 ml Scandonest plain 3% solution for injection 2.2ml cartridges | 50 cartridge PoM no price available

Mepivacaine with adrenaline

The properties listed below are those particular to the combination only. For the properties of the components please consider, mepivacaine hydrochloride above, adrenaline/epinephrine p. 205.

● **INDICATIONS AND DOSE**

Infiltration anaesthesia and nerve block in dentistry
 ▸ BY LOCAL INFILTRATION
 ▸ Adult: (consult product literature)

IMPORTANT SAFETY INFORMATION
Adrenaline/epinephrine must be used in a low concentration when administered with a local anaesthetic. The total dose of adrenaline should not exceed 500 micrograms and it is essential not to exceed a concentration of 1 in 200 000 (5 micrograms/mL) if more than 50 mL of the mixture is to be injected.

● **MEDICINAL FORMS**
There can be variation in the licensing of different medicines containing the same drug.
Solution for injection
 EXCIPIENTS: May contain Sulfites
 ▸ Scandonest special (Deproco UK Ltd)
  Adrenaline 10 microgram per 1 ml, Mepivacaine hydrochloride 20 mg per 1 ml Scandonest special 2% solution for injection 2.2ml cartridges | 50 cartridge PoM no price available

Prilocaine hydrochloride

- **INDICATIONS AND DOSE**

CITANEST 1%®

Infiltration anaesthesia | Nerve block
- ▸ BY REGIONAL ADMINISTRATION
- ▸ Adult: 100–200 mg/minute, alternatively may be given in incremental doses; dose adjusted according to site of administration and response, and in elderly and debilitated patients (smaller doses may be required); maximum 400 mg per course

PRILOTEKAL®

Spinal anaesthesia
- ▸ BY INTRATHECAL INJECTION
- ▸ Adult: Usual dose 40–60 mg (max. per dose 80 mg), dose may need to be reduced in elderly or debilitated patients, or in late pregnancy

DOSES AT EXTREMES OF BODY-WEIGHT
To avoid excessive dosage in obese patients, dose should be calculated on the basis of ideal body-weight.

IMPORTANT SAFETY INFORMATION
Should only be administered by, or under the direct supervision of, personnel experienced in their use, with adequate training in anaesthesia and airway management, and should not be administered parenterally unless adequate resuscitation equipment is available.

- **CONTRA-INDICATIONS** Acquired methaemoglobinaemia · anaemia · application to the middle ear (can cause ototoxicity) · avoid injection into infected tissues · avoid injection into inflamed tissues · complete heart block · congenital methaemoglobinaemia · preparations containing preservatives should not be used for caudal, epidural, or spinal block, or for intravenous regional anaesthesia (Bier's block) · should not be applied to damaged skin

CONTRA-INDICATIONS, FURTHER INFORMATION
- ▸ Injection site Local anaesthetics should not be injected into inflamed or infected tissues nor should they be applied to damaged skin. Increased absorption into the blood increases the possibility of systemic side-effects, and the local anaesthetic effect may also be reduced by altered local pH.

- **CAUTIONS** Acute porphyrias p. 918 · cardiovascular disease · debilitated patients (consider dose reduction) · elderly (consider dose reduction) · epilepsy · hypovolaemia · impaired cardiac conduction · impaired respiratory function · myasthenia gravis · severe or untreated hypertension · shock

- **INTERACTIONS** → Appendix 1 (prilocaine). Caution with concomitant use of drugs that cause methaemoglobinaemia.

- **SIDE-EFFECTS** Arrhythmias · blurred vision · cardiac arrest · convulsions · dizziness · drowsiness · feeling of inebriation · headache · hypertension · lightheadedness · methaemoglobinaemia (with high doses) · muscle twitching · myocardial depression (resulting in hypotension and bradycardia) · nausea · numbness of the tongue and perioral region · paraesthesia (including sensations of hot and cold) · peripheral vasodilatation (resulting in hypotension and bradycardia) · restlessness · tinnitus · transient excitation (followed by depression with drowsiness, respiratory failure, unconsciousness, and coma) · tremors · vomiting

SIDE-EFFECTS, FURTHER INFORMATION
- ▸ Toxic effects Toxic effects after administration of local anaesthetics are a result of excessively high plasma concentrations; severe toxicity usually results from inadvertent intravascular injection or too rapid injection.
  Following most regional anaesthetic procedures, maximum arterial plasma concentration of anaesthetic develops within about 10 to 25 minutes, so careful surveillance for toxic effects is necessary during the first 30 minutes after injection.
  The systemic toxicity of local anaesthetics mainly involves the central nervous and cardiovascular systems.
- ▸ Methaemoglobinaemia Methaemoglobinaemia can be treated with an intravenous injection of **methylthioninium chloride**.

- **ALLERGY AND CROSS-SENSITIVITY**
- ▸ Hypersensitivity and cross-sensitivity Hypersensitivity reactions occur mainly with the ester-type local anaesthetics, such as tetracaine and chloroprocaine; reactions are less frequent with the amide types, such as articaine, bupivacaine, levobupivacaine, lidocaine, mepivacaine, prilocaine, and ropivacaine. Cross-sensitivity reactions may be avoided by using the alternative chemical type.

- **PREGNANCY** Use lower doses for intrathecal use during late pregnancy. Large doses during delivery can cause neonatal respiratory depression, hypotonia, and bradycardia after epidural block. Avoid paracervical or pudendal block in obstetrics (neonatal methaemoglobinaemia reported).

- **BREAST FEEDING** Present in milk but not known to be harmful.

- **HEPATIC IMPAIRMENT** Lower doses may be required for intrathecal anaesthesia. Use with caution.

- **RENAL IMPAIRMENT** Lower doses may be required for intrathecal anaesthesia. Use with caution.

- **NATIONAL FUNDING/ACCESS DECISIONS**

Scottish Medicines Consortium (SMC) Decisions
The *Scottish Medicines Consortium* has advised (December 2010) that prilocaine 2% hyperbaric solution for injection (*Prilotekal*®) is accepted for restricted use within NHS Scotland for use in spinal anaesthesia in ambulatory surgery settings.

- **MEDICINAL FORMS**
There can be variation in the licensing of different medicines containing the same drug.
Solution for injection
- ▸ Citanest (AstraZeneca UK Ltd)
  Prilocaine hydrochloride 10 mg per 1 ml Citanest 1% solution for injection 50ml vials | 1 vial PoM £5.06
- ▸ Prilotekal (AMCo)
  Prilocaine hydrochloride 20 mg per 1 ml Prilotekal 100mg/5ml hyperbaric solution for injection ampoules | 10 ampoule PoM £78.75

Prilocaine with felypressin

The properties listed below are those particular to the combination only. For the properties of the components please consider, prilocaine hydrochloride above.

- **INDICATIONS AND DOSE**

Dental anaesthesia
- ▸ BY REGIONAL ADMINISTRATION
- ▸ Adult: Consult expert dental sources for specific advice

15

Anaesthesia

- **MEDICINAL FORMS**
There can be variation in the licensing of different medicines containing the same drug.

Solution for injection
- Citanest with Octapressin (Dentsply Ltd)
Felypressin.03 unit per 1 ml, Prilocaine hydrochloride 30 mg per 1 ml Citanest 3% with Octapressin Dental 0.054units/1.8ml solution for injection self aspirating cartridges | 100 cartridge [PoM] no price available
Citanest 3% with Octapressin Dental 0.066units/2.2ml solution for injection self aspirating cartridges | 100 cartridge [PoM] no price available

DOSES AT EXTREMES OF BODY-WEIGHT
To avoid excessive dosage in obese patients, dose may need to be calculated on the basis of ideal bodyweight.

> **IMPORTANT SAFETY INFORMATION**
> Should only be administered by, or under the direct supervision of, personnel experienced in their use, with adequate training in anaesthesia and airway management, and should not be administered parenterally unless adequate resuscitation equipment is available.

Ropivacaine hydrochloride

- **INDICATIONS AND DOSE**

Acute pain, peripheral nerve block
▶ BY REGIONAL ADMINISTRATION
▶ Adult: 10–20 mg/hour, dose administered as a continuous infusion or by intermittent injection using a 2 mg/mL (0.2%) solution

Acute pain, field block
▶ BY REGIONAL ADMINISTRATION
▶ Adult: 2–200 mg, dose administered using a 2 mg/mL (0.2%) solution

Acute pain, lumbar epidural block
▶ BY LUMBAR EPIDURAL
▶ Adult: 20–40 mg, followed by 20–30 mg at least every 30 minutes, dose administered using a 2 mg/mL (0.2%) solution

Acute labour pain
▶ BY CONTINUOUS EPIDURAL INFUSION
▶ Adult: 12–20 mg/hour, dose administered using a 2 mg/mL (0.2%) solution

Acute postoperative pain
▶ BY CONTINUOUS EPIDURAL INFUSION
▶ Adult: Up to 28 mg/hour, dose administered using a 2 mg/mL (0.2%) solution

Postoperative pain, thoracic epidural block
▶ BY CONTINUOUS EPIDURAL INFUSION
▶ Adult: 12–28 mg/hour, dose administered using a 2 mg/mL (0.2%) solution

Surgical anaesthesia, field block
▶ BY REGIONAL ADMINISTRATION
▶ Adult: 7.5–225 mg, dose administered using a 7.5 mg/mL (0.75%) solution

Surgical anaesthesia, major nerve block (brachial plexus block)
▶ BY REGIONAL ADMINISTRATION
▶ Adult: 225–300 mg, dose administered using a 7.5 mg/mL (0.75%) solution

Surgical anaesthesia, thoracic epidural block (to establish block for postoperative pain)
▶ BY THORACIC EPIDURAL
▶ Adult: 38–113 mg, dose administered using a 7.5 mg/mL (0.75%) solution

Surgical anaesthesia for caesarean section
▶ BY LUMBAR EPIDURAL
▶ Adult: 113–150 mg, to be administered in incremental doses using a 7.5 mg/mL (0.75%) solution

Surgical anaesthesia, lumbar epidural block
▶ BY LUMBAR EPIDURAL
▶ Adult: 113–200 mg, dose administered using a 7.5 mg/mL (0.75%) or 10 mg/mL (1%) solution

- **CONTRA-INDICATIONS** Application to the middle ear (can cause ototoxicity) · avoid injection into infected tissues · avoid injection into inflamed tissues · complete heart block · preparations containing preservatives should not be used for caudal, epidural, or spinal block, or for intravenous regional anaesthesia (Bier's block) · should not be applied to damaged skin

CONTRA-INDICATIONS, FURTHER INFORMATION
▶ Injection site Local anaesthetics should not be injected into inflamed or infected tissues nor should they be applied to damaged skin. Increased absorption into the blood increases the possibility of systemic side-effects, and the local anaesthetic effect may also be reduced by altered local pH.

- **CAUTIONS** Acute porphyrias p. 918 · cardiovascular disease · debilitated patients (consider dose reduction) · elderly (consider dose reduction) · epilepsy · hypovolaemia · impaired cardiac conduction · impaired respiratory function · myasthenia gravis · shock

- **INTERACTIONS** → Appendix 1 (ropivacaine).

- **SIDE-EFFECTS**
▶ **Common or very common** Hypertension · pyrexia
▶ **Uncommon** Hypothermia · syncope
▶ **Frequency not known** Arrhythmias · blurred vision · cardiac arrest · convulsions · dizziness · drowsiness · feeling of inebriation · headache · lightheadedness · muscle twitching · myocardial depression (resulting in hypotension and bradycardia) · nausea · numbness of the tongue and perioral region · paraesthesia (including sensations of hot and cold) · peripheral vasodilatation (resulting in hypotension and bradycardia) · restlessness · tinnitus · transient excitation (followed by depression with drowsiness, respiratory failure, unconsciousness, and coma) · tremors · vomiting

SIDE-EFFECTS, FURTHER INFORMATION
▶ Toxic effects Toxic effects after administration of local anaesthetics are a result of excessively high plasma concentrations; severe toxicity usually results from inadvertent intravascular injection or too rapid injection.
Following most regional anaesthetic procedures, maximum arterial plasma concentration of anaesthetic develops within about 10 to 25 minutes, so careful surveillance for toxic effects is necessary during the first 30 minutes after injection.
The systemic toxicity of local anaesthetics mainly involves the central nervous and cardiovascular systems.

- **ALLERGY AND CROSS-SENSITIVITY**
▶ Hypersensitivity and cross-sensitivity Hypersensitivity reactions occur mainly with the ester-type local anaesthetics, such as tetracaine and chloroprocaine; reactions are less frequent with the amide types, such as articaine, bupivacaine, levobupivacaine, lidocaine, mepivacaine, prilocaine, and ropivacaine. Cross-sensitivity reactions may be avoided by using the alternative chemical type.

- **PREGNANCY** Not known to be harmful. Do not use for paracervical block in obstetrics.

- **BREAST FEEDING** Not known to be harmful.

- **HEPATIC IMPAIRMENT** Use with caution in severe impairment.
- **RENAL IMPAIRMENT** Caution in severe impairment. Increased risk of systemic toxicity in chronic renal failure.
- **MEDICINAL FORMS**
There can be variation in the licensing of different medicines containing the same drug.

Solution for injection
ELECTROLYTES: May contain Sodium
▸ Ropivacaine hydrochloride (Non-proprietary)
Ropivacaine hydrochloride 2 mg per 1 ml Ropivacaine 20mg/10ml solution for injection ampoules | 10 ampoule PoM £16.50 (Hospital only)
Ropivacaine hydrochloride 7.5 mg per 1 ml Ropivacaine 75mg/10ml solution for injection ampoules | 10 ampoule PoM £25.00 (Hospital only)
Ropivacaine hydrochloride 10 mg per 1 ml Ropivacaine 100mg/10ml solution for injection ampoules | 10 ampoule PoM £30.00 (Hospital only)
▸ Naropin (AstraZeneca UK Ltd)
Ropivacaine hydrochloride 2 mg per 1 ml Naropin 20mg/10ml solution for injection ampoules | 5 ampoule PoM £12.79
Ropivacaine hydrochloride 7.5 mg per 1 ml Naropin 75mg/10ml solution for injection ampoules | 5 ampoule PoM £15.90
Ropivacaine hydrochloride 10 mg per 1 ml Naropin 100mg/10ml solution for injection ampoules | 5 ampoule PoM £19.22

Infusion
ELECTROLYTES: May contain Sodium
▸ Ropivacaine hydrochloride (Non-proprietary)
Ropivacaine hydrochloride 2 mg per 1 ml Ropivacaine 400mg/200ml infusion bags | 5 bag PoM £72.25 | 10 bag PoM £137.00 (Hospital only)
▸ Naropin (AstraZeneca UK Ltd)
Ropivacaine hydrochloride 2 mg per 1 ml Naropin 400mg/200ml infusion Polybags | 5 bag PoM £86.70

Tetracaine
(Amethocaine)

- **INDICATIONS AND DOSE**

Anaesthesia before venepuncture or venous cannulation
▸ TO THE SKIN
▸ Child 1 month–4 years: Apply contents of up to 1 tube (applied at separate sites at a single time or appropriate proportion) to site of venepuncture or venous cannulation and cover with occlusive dressing; remove gel and dressing after 30 minutes for venepuncture and after 45 minutes for venous cannulation
▸ Child 5–17 years: Apply contents of up to 5 tubes (applied at separate sites at a single time or appropriate proportion) to site of venepuncture or venous cannulation and cover with occlusive dressing; remove gel and dressing after 30 minutes for venepuncture and after 45 minutes for venous cannulation
▸ Adult: Apply contents of up to 5 tubes (applied at separate sites at a single time or appropriate proportion) to site of venepuncture or venous cannulation and cover with occlusive dressing; remove gel and dressing after 30 minutes for venepuncture and after 45 minutes for venous cannulation

- **UNLICENSED USE** Not licensed for use in neonates.
- **CONTRA-INDICATIONS** Should not be applied to damaged skin
- **SIDE-EFFECTS** Local skin reactions
SIDE-EFFECTS, FURTHER INFORMATION
The systemic toxicity of local anaesthetics mainly involves the central nervous and cardiovascular systems; systemic side effects unlikely as minimal absorption following topical application.

- **ALLERGY AND CROSS-SENSITIVITY**
▸ Hypersensitivity and cross-sensitivity Hypersensitivity reactions occur mainly with the ester-type local anaesthetics, such as tetracaine and chloroprocaine; reactions are less frequent with the amide types, such as articaine, bupivacaine, levobupivacaine, lidocaine, mepivacaine, prilocaine, and ropivacaine. Cross-sensitivity reactions may be avoided by using the alternative chemical type.
- **BREAST FEEDING** Not known to be harmful.
- **PATIENT AND CARER ADVICE**
Medicines for Children leaflet: Tetracaine gel for local anaesthesia www.medicinesforchildren.org.uk/tetracaine-gel-for-local-anaesthesia
- **MEDICINAL FORMS**
There can be variation in the licensing of different medicines containing the same drug.
Gel
EXCIPIENTS: May contain Hydroxybenzoates (parabens)
▸ Ametop (Smith & Nephew Healthcare Ltd)
Tetracaine 40 mg per 1 gram Ametop 4% gel | 1.5 gram P £1.08 | 18 gram P no price available

15
Anaesthesia

Chapter 16
Emergency treatment of poisoning

CONTENTS

Emergency treatment of poisoning

Overview

These notes provide only an overview of the treatment of poisoning, and it is strongly recommended that either **TOXBASE** or the **UK National Poisons Information Service** be consulted when there is doubt about the degree of risk or about management.

Hospital admission

Patients who have features of poisoning should generally be admitted to hospital. Patients who have taken poisons with delayed action should also be admitted, even if they appear well. Delayed-action poisons include aspirin p. 109, iron, paracetamol p. 406, tricyclic antidepressants, and co-phenotrope (diphenoxylate with atropine, *Lomotil®*) p. 58; the effects of modified-release preparations are also delayed. A note of all relevant information, including what treatment has been given, should accompany the patient to hospital.

Further information

TOXBASE, the primary clinical toxicology database of the National Poisons Information Service, is available on the internet to registered users at www.toxbase.org (a backup site is available at www.toxbasebackup.org if the main site cannot be accessed). It provides information about routine diagnosis, treatment, and management of patients exposed to drugs, household products, and industrial and agricultural chemicals.

Specialist information and advice on the treatment of poisoning is available day and night from the **UK National Poisons Information Service** on the following number: Tel: 0344 892 0111.

Advice on laboratory analytical services can be obtained from TOXBASE or from the National Poisons Information Service. Help with identifying capsules or tablets may be available from a regional medicines information centre or from the National Poisons Information Service (out of hours).

General care

It is often impossible to establish with certainty the identity of the poison and the size of the dose. This is not usually important because only a few poisons (such as opioids, paracetamol, and iron) have specific antidotes; few patients require active removal of the poison. In most patients, treatment is directed at managing symptoms as they arise. Nevertheless, knowledge of the type and timing of poisoning can help in anticipating the course of events. All relevant information should be sought from the poisoned individual and from carers or parents. However, such information

should be interpreted with care because it may not be complete or entirely reliable. Sometimes symptoms arise from other illnesses and patients should be assessed carefully. Accidents may involve domestic and industrial products (the contents of which are not generally known). The **National Poisons Information Service** should be consulted when there is doubt about any aspect of suspected poisoning.

Respiration

Respiration is often impaired in unconscious patients. An obstructed airway requires immediate attention. In the absence of trauma, the airway should be opened with simple measures such as chin lift or jaw thrust. An oropharyngeal or nasopharyngeal airway may be useful in patients with reduced consciousness to prevent obstruction, provided ventilation is adequate. Intubation and ventilation should be considered in patients whose airway cannot be protected or who have respiratory acidosis because of inadequate ventilation; such patients should be monitored in a critical care area.

Most poisons that impair consciousness also depress respiration. Assisted ventilation (either mouth-to-mouth or using a bag-valve-mask device) may be needed. Oxygen is not a substitute for adequate ventilation, although it should be given in the highest concentration possible in poisoning with carbon monoxide and irritant gases.

Blood pressure

Hypotension is common in severe poisoning with central nervous system depressants. A systolic blood pressure of less than 70 mmHg may lead to irreversible brain damage or renal tubular necrosis. Hypotension should be corrected initially by raising the foot of the bed and administration of an infusion of either sodium chloride p. 901 or a colloid. Vasoconstrictor sympathomimetics are rarely required and their use may be discussed with the National Poisons Information Service.

Fluid depletion without hypotension is common after prolonged coma and after aspirin poisoning due to vomiting, sweating, and hyperpnoea.

Hypertension, often transient, occurs less frequently than hypotension in poisoning; it may be associated with sympathomimetic drugs such as amfetamines, phencyclidine, and cocaine.

Heart

Cardiac conduction defects and arrhythmias can occur in acute poisoning, notably with tricyclic antidepressants, some antipsychotics, and some antihistamines. Arrhythmias often respond to correction of underlying hypoxia, acidosis, or other biochemical abnormalities, but ventricular arrhythmias that cause serious hypotension require treatment. If the QT interval is prolonged, specialist advice should be sought because the use of some anti-arrhythmic drugs may be inappropriate. Supraventricular arrhythmias are seldom life-threatening and drug treatment is best withheld until the patient reaches hospital.

Body temperature

Hypothermia may develop in patients of any age who have been deeply unconscious for some hours, particularly following overdose with barbiturates or phenothiazines. It may be missed unless core temperature is measured using a low-reading rectal thermometer or by some other means. Hypothermia should be managed by prevention of further heat loss and appropriate re-warming as clinically indicated.

Hyperthermia can develop in patients taking CNS stimulants; children and the elderly are also at risk when taking therapeutic doses of drugs with antimuscarinic properties. Hyperthermia is initially managed by removing all unnecessary clothing and using a fan. Sponging with **tepid** water will promote evaporation. Advice should be sought from the National Poisons Information Service on the management of severe hyperthermia resulting from conditions such as the serotonin syndrome.

Both hypothermia and hyperthermia require **urgent** hospitalisation for assessment and supportive treatment.

Convulsions

Single short-lived convulsions (lasting less than 5 minutes) do not require treatment. If convulsions are protracted or recur frequently, lorazepam p. 308 or diazepam p. 313 (preferably as emulsion) should be given by slow intravenous injection into a large vein. Benzodiazepines should not be given by the intramuscular route for convulsions. If the intravenous route is not readily available, midazolam oromucosal solution p. 310 [unlicensed use in adults and children under 3 months] can be given by the buccal route or diazepam can be administered as a rectal solution.

Methaemoglobinaemia

Drug- or chemical-induced methaemoglobinaemia should be treated with methylthioninium chloride p. 1206 if the methaemoglobin concentration is 30% or higher, *or* if symptoms of tissue hypoxia are present despite oxygen therapy. Methylthioninium chloride reduces the ferric iron of methaemoglobin back to the ferrous iron of haemoglobin; in high doses, methylthioninium chloride can itself cause methaemoglobinaemia.

Removal and elimination

Prevention of absorption

Given by mouth, charcoal, activated p. 1201 can bind many poisons in the gastro-intestinal system, thereby reducing their absorption. The **sooner** it is given the **more effective** it is, but it may still be effective up to 1 hour after ingestion of the poison—longer in the case of modified-release preparations or of drugs with antimuscarinic (anticholinergic) properties. It is particularly useful for the prevention of absorption of poisons that are toxic in small amounts, such as antidepressants.

Active elimination techniques

Repeated doses of charcoal, activated p. 1201 by mouth *enhance the elimination* of some drugs after they have been absorbed; repeated doses are given after overdosage with:

- Carbamazepine
- Dapsone
- Phenobarbital
- Quinine
- Theophylline

If vomiting occurs after dosing it should be treated (e.g. with an antiemetic drug) since it may reduce the efficacy of charcoal treatment. In cases of intolerance, the dose may be reduced and the frequency increased but this may compromise efficacy.

Charcoal, activated should **not** be used for poisoning with petroleum distillates, corrosive substances, alcohols, malathion, cyanides and metal salts including iron and lithium salts.

Other techniques intended to enhance the elimination of poisons after absorption are only practicable in hospital and are only suitable for a small number of severely poisoned patients. Moreover, they only apply to a limited number of poisons. Examples include:

- haemodialysis for ethylene glycol, lithium, methanol, phenobarbital, salicylates, and sodium valproate;
- alkalinisation of the urine for salicylates.

Removal from the gastro-intestinal tract

Gastric lavage is rarely required; for substances that cannot be removed effectively by other means (e.g. iron), it should be considered only if a life-threatening amount has been ingested within the previous hour. It should be carried out only if the airway can be protected adequately. Gastric lavage is contra-indicated if a corrosive substance or a petroleum distillate has been ingested, but it may occasionally be considered in patients who have ingested drugs that are not adsorbed by charcoal, such as iron or lithium. Induction of *emesis* (e.g. with ipecacuanha) is **not** recommended because there is no evidence that it affects absorption and it may increase the risk of aspiration.

Whole bowel irrigation (by means of a bowel cleansing preparation) has been used in poisoning with certain modified-release or enteric-coated formulations, in severe poisoning with iron and lithium salts, and if illicit drugs are carried in the gastro-intestinal tract ('body-packing'). However, it is not clear that the procedure improves outcome and advice should be sought from the National Poisons Information Service.

Alcohol

Acute intoxication with alcohol (ethanol) is common in adults but also occurs in children. The features include ataxia, dysarthria, nystagmus, and drowsiness, which may progress to coma, with hypotension and acidosis. Aspiration of vomit is a special hazard and hypoglycaemia may occur in children and some adults. Patients are managed supportively, with particular attention to maintaining a clear airway and measures to reduce the risk of aspiration of gastric contents. The blood glucose is measured and glucose given if indicated.

Aspirin

The main features of salicylate poisoning are hyperventilation, tinnitus, deafness, vasodilatation, and sweating. Coma is uncommon but indicates very severe poisoning. The associated acid-base disturbances are complex.

Treatment must be in hospital, where plasma salicylate, pH, and electrolytes can be measured; absorption of aspirin may be slow and the plasma-salicylate concentration may continue to rise for several hours, requiring repeated measurement. Plasma-salicylate concentration may not correlate with clinical severity in the young and the elderly, and clinical and biochemical assessment is necessary. Generally, the clinical severity of poisoning is less below a plasma-salicylate concentration of 500 mg/litre (3.6 mmol/litre), unless there is evidence of metabolic acidosis. Activated charcoal can be given within 1 hour of ingesting more than 125 mg/kg of aspirin. Fluid losses should be replaced and intravenous sodium bicarbonate may be given (ensuring plasma-potassium concentration is within the reference range) to enhance urinary salicylate excretion (optimum urinary pH 7.5–8.5).

Paracetamol overdose treatment graph

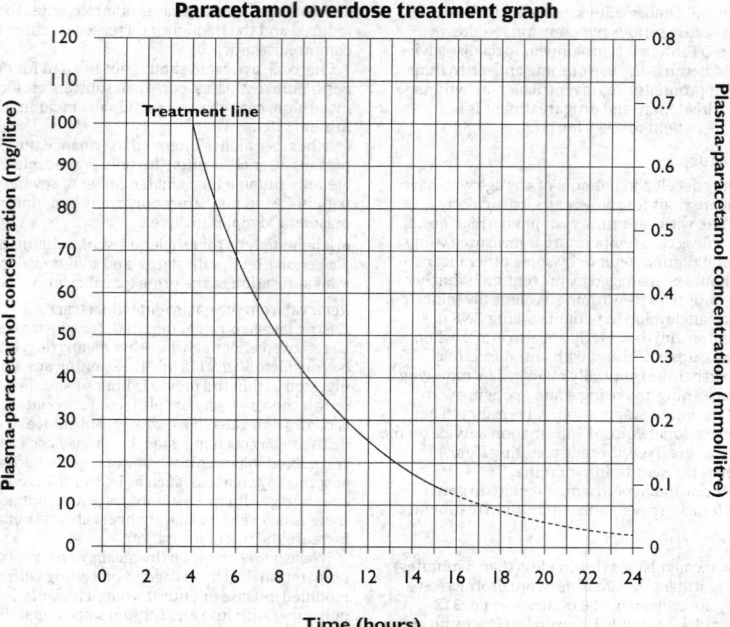

Patients whose plasma-paracetamol concentrations are on or above the **treatment line** should be treated with acetylcysteine by intravenous infusion.

The prognostic accuracy after 15 hours is uncertain, but a plasma-paracetamol concentration on or above the treatment line should be regarded as carrying a serious risk of liver damage.

Graph reproduced courtesy of Medicines and Healthcare products Regulatory Agency

Plasma-potassium concentration should be corrected before giving sodium bicarbonate as hypokalaemia may complicate alkalinisation of the urine.

Haemodialysis is the treatment of choice for severe salicylate poisoning and should be considered when the plasma-salicylate concentration exceeds 700 mg/litre (5.1 mmol/litre) or in the presence of severe metabolic acidosis.

Opioids

Opioids (narcotic analgesics) cause coma, respiratory depression, and pinpoint pupils. The specific antidote naloxone hydrochloride p. 1204 is indicated if there is coma or bradypnoea. Since naloxone has a shorter duration of action than many opioids, close monitoring and repeated injections are necessary according to the respiratory rate and depth of coma. When repeated administration of naloxone is required, it can be given by continuous intravenous infusion instead and the rate of infusion adjusted according to vital signs. The effects of some opioids, such as buprenorphine, are only partially reversed by naloxone.

Dextropropoxyphene and methadone have very long durations of action; patients may need to be monitored for long periods following large overdoses.

Naloxone reverses the opioid effects of dextropropoxyphene. The long duration of action of dextropropoxyphene calls for prolonged monitoring and further doses of naloxone may be required. Norpropoxyphene, a metabolite of dextropropoxyphene, also has cardiotoxic effects which may require treatment

with sodium bicarbonate p. 898 or magnesium sulfate p. 911, or both. Arrhythmias may occur for up to 12 hours.

Paracetamol

In cases of **intravenous paracetamol poisoning** contact the National Poisons Information Service for advice on risk assessment and management.

Toxic doses of paracetamol may cause severe hepatocellular necrosis and, much less frequently, renal tubular necrosis. Nausea and vomiting, the only early features of poisoning, usually settle within 24 hours. Persistence beyond this time, often associated with the onset of right subcostal pain and tenderness, usually indicates development of hepatic necrosis. Liver damage is maximal 3–4 days after paracetamol overdose and may lead to encephalopathy, haemorrhage, hypoglycaemia, cerebral oedema, and death. Therefore, despite a lack of significant early symptoms, patients who have taken an overdose of paracetamol should be transferred to hospital urgently.

To avoid underestimating the potentially toxic paracetamol dose ingested by obese patients who weigh more than 110 kg, use a body-weight of 110 kg (rather than their actual body-weight) when calculating the total dose of paracetamol ingested (in mg/kg).

Acetylcysteine p. 1205 protects the liver if infused up to, and possibly beyond, 24 hours of ingesting paracetamol. It is most effective if given within 8 hours of ingestion, after which effectiveness declines. Very rarely, giving acetylcysteine by mouth [unlicensed route] is an alternative if intravenous access is not possible—contact the National Poisons Information Service for advice.

Neonates less than 45 weeks corrected gestational age may be more susceptible to paracetamol-induced liver toxicity, therefore, treatment with acetylcysteine p. 1205 should be considered in all paracetamol overdoses, and advice should be sought from the National Poisons Information Service.

Acute overdose
Hepatotoxicity may occur after a single ingestion of more than 150 mg/kg paracetamol taken in less than 1 hour. Rarely, hepatotoxicity may develop with single ingestions as low as 75 mg/kg of paracetamol taken in less than 1 hour. Patients who have ingested 75 mg/kg or more of paracetamol in less than 1 hour should be referred to hospital. Administration of charcoal, activated p. 1201 should be considered if paracetamol in excess of 150 mg/kg is thought to have been ingested within the previous hour.

Patients at risk of liver damage and, therefore, requiring acetylcysteine, can be identified from a single measurement of the plasma-paracetamol concentration, related to the time from ingestion, provided this time interval is not less than 4 hours; earlier samples may be misleading. The concentration is plotted on a paracetamol treatment graph, with a reference line ('treatment line') joining plots of 100 mg/litre (0.66 mmol/litre) at 4 hours and 3.13 mg/litre (0.02 mmol/litre) at 24 hours. Acetylcysteine treatment should commence immediately in patients:

- whose plasma-paracetamol concentration falls on or above the *treatment line* on the paracetamol treatment graph;
- who present 8–24 hours after taking an acute overdose of more than 150 mg/kg of paracetamol, even if the plasma-paracetamol concentration is not yet available; acetylcysteine can be discontinued if the plasma-paracetamol concentration is later reported to be below the *treatment line* on the paracetamol treatment graph, provided that the patient is asymptomatic and liver function tests, serum creatinine and INR are normal.

The prognostic accuracy of a plasma-paracetamol concentration taken after 15 hours is uncertain, but a concentration on or above the *treatment line* on the paracetamol treatment graph should be regarded as carrying a serious risk of liver damage. If more than 15 hours have elapsed since ingestion, or there is doubt about appropriate management, advice should be sought from the National Poisons Information Service.

'Staggered' overdose, uncertain time of overdose, or therapeutic excess
A 'staggered' overdose involves ingestion of a potentially toxic dose of paracetamol over more than one hour, with the possible intention of causing self-harm. Therapeutic excess is the inadvertent ingestion of a potentially toxic dose of paracetamol during its clinical use. The paracetamol treatment graph is unreliable if a 'staggered' overdose is taken, if there is uncertainty about the time of the overdose, or if there is therapeutic excess. In these cases, patients who have taken more than 150 mg/kg of paracetamol in any 24-hour period are at risk of toxicity and should be commenced on acetylcysteine immediately, unless it is more than 24 hours since the last ingestion, the patient is asymptomatic, the plasma-paracetamol concentration is undetectable, and liver function tests, serum creatinine and INR are normal.

Rarely, toxicity can occur with paracetamol doses between 75–150 mg/kg in any 24-hour period; clinical judgement of the individual case is necessary to determine whether to treat those who have ingested this amount of paracetamol. For small adults, this may be within the licensed dose, but ingestion of a licensed dose of paracetamol is not considered an overdose.

Although there is some evidence suggesting that factors such as the use of liver enzyme-inducing drugs (e.g. carbamazepine p. 283, efavirenz p. 585, nevirapine p. 586, phenobarbital p. 304, phenytoin p. 294, primidone p. 305,

rifabutin p. 522, rifampicin p. 527, St John's wort), chronic alcoholism, and starvation may increase the risk of hepatotoxicity, the CHM has advised that these should no longer be used in the assessment of paracetamol toxicity.

Significant toxicity is unlikely if, 24 hours or longer after the last paracetamol ingestion, the patient is asymptomatic, the plasma-paracetamol concentration is undetectable, and liver function tests, serum creatinine and INR are normal. Patients with clinical features of hepatic injury such as jaundice or hepatic tenderness should be treated urgently with acetylcysteine. If there is uncertainty about a patient's risk of toxicity after paracetamol overdose, treatment with acetylcysteine should be commenced. Advice should be sought from the National Poisons Information Service whenever necessary.

Acetylcysteine dose and administration
For paracetamol overdosage, acetylcysteine is given in a total dose that is divided into 3 consecutive intravenous infusions over a total of 21 hours. The tables below include the dose of acetylcysteine, for adults and children of body-weight 40 kg and over, in terms of the volume of acetylcysteine Concentrate for Intravenous Infusion required for each of the 3 infusions. The requisite dose of acetylcysteine is added to glucose Intravenous Infusion 5%.

First infusion	
Body-weight	**Volume of Acetylcysteine Concentrate for Intravenous Infusion 200 mg/mL required to prepare first infusion**
40–49 kg	34 mL
50–59 kg	42 mL
60–69 kg	49 mL
70–79 kg	57 mL
80–89 kg	64 mL
90–99 kg	72 mL
100–109 kg	79 mL
≥110 kg	83 mL (max. dose)

First infusion (based on an acetylcysteine dose of approx. 150 mg/kg)—add requisite volume of Acetylcysteine Concentrate for Intravenous Infusion to 200 mL Glucose Intravenous Infusion 5%; infuse over 1 hour.

Second infusion	
Body-weight	**Volume of Acetylcysteine Concentrate for Intravenous Infusion 200 mg/mL required to prepare second infusion**
40–49 kg	12 mL
50–59 kg	14 mL
60–69 kg	17 mL
70–79 kg	19 mL
80–89 kg	22 mL
90–99 kg	24 mL
100–109 kg	27 mL
≥110 kg	28 mL (max. dose)

Second infusion (based on an acetylcysteine dose of approx. 50 mg/kg; start immediately after completion of first infusion)—add requisite volume of Acetylcysteine Concentrate for Intravenous Infusion to 500 mL Glucose Intravenous Infusion 5%; infuse over 4 hours.

Third infusion	
Body-weight	Volume of Acetylcysteine Concentrate for Intravenous Infusion 200 mg/mL required to prepare third infusion
40–49 kg	23 mL
50–59 kg	28 mL
60–69 kg	33 mL
70–79 kg	38 mL
80–89 kg	43 mL
90–99 kg	48 mL
100–109 kg	53 mL
≥110 kg	55 mL (max. dose)

Third infusion (based on an acetylcysteine dose of approx. 100 mg/kg; start immediately after completion of second infusion)—add requisite volume of Acetylcysteine Concentrate for Intravenous Infusion to 1 litre Glucose Intravenous Infusion 5%; infuse over 16 hours.

Antidepressants

Tricyclic and related antidepressants

Tricyclic and related antidepressants cause dry mouth, coma of varying degree, hypotension, hypothermia, hyperreflexia, extensor plantar responses, convulsions, respiratory failure, cardiac conduction defects, and arrhythmias. Dilated pupils and urinary retention also occur. Metabolic acidosis may complicate severe poisoning; delirium with confusion, agitation, and visual and auditory hallucinations are common during recovery.

Assessment in hospital is strongly advised in case of poisoning by tricyclic and related antidepressants but symptomatic treatment can be given before transfer. Supportive measures to ensure a clear airway and adequate ventilation during transfer are mandatory. Intravenous lorazepam or intravenous diazepam (preferably in emulsion form) may be required to treat convulsions. Activated charcoal given within 1 hour of the overdose reduces absorption of the drug. Although arrhythmias are worrying, some will respond to correction of hypoxia and acidosis. The use of anti-arrhythmic drugs is best avoided, but intravenous infusion of sodium bicarbonate can arrest arrhythmias or prevent them in those with an extended QRS duration. Diazepam given by mouth is usually adequate to sedate delirious patients but large doses may be required.

Selective serotonin re-uptake inhibitors (SSRIs)

Symptoms of poisoning by selective serotonin re-uptake inhibitors include nausea, vomiting, agitation, tremor, nystagmus, drowsiness, and sinus tachycardia; convulsions may occur. Rarely, severe poisoning results in the serotonin syndrome, with marked neuropsychiatric effects, neuromuscular hyperactivity, and autonomic instability; hyperthermia, rhabdomyolysis, renal failure, and coagulopathies may develop.

Management of SSRI poisoning is supportive. Activated charcoal given within 1 hour of the overdose reduces absorption of the drug. Convulsions can be treated with lorazepam, diazepam, or midazolam oromucosal solution [unlicensed use in adults and children under 3 months] (see *Convulsions*). Contact the National Poisons Information Service for the management of hyperthermia or the serotonin syndrome.

Antimalarials

Overdosage with quinine, chloroquine, or hydroxychloroquine is extremely hazardous and difficult to treat. Urgent advice from the National Poisons Information Service is essential. Life-threatening features include arrhythmias (which can have a very rapid onset) and convulsions (which can be intractable).

Antipsychotics

Phenothiazines and related drugs

Phenothiazines cause less depression of consciousness and respiration than other sedatives. Hypotension, hypothermia, sinus tachycardia, and arrhythmias may complicate poisoning. Dystonic reactions can occur with therapeutic doses (particularly with prochlorperazine and trifluoperazine), and convulsions may occur in severe cases. Arrhythmias may respond to correction of hypoxia, acidosis, and other biochemical abnormalities, but specialist advice should be sought if arrhythmias result from a prolonged QT interval; the use of some anti-arrhythmic drugs can worsen such arrhythmias. Dystonic reactions are rapidly abolished by injection of drugs such as procyclidine hydrochloride p. 376 or diazepam p. 313 (emulsion preferred).

Second-generation antipsychotic drugs

Features of poisoning by second-generation antipsychotic drugs include drowsiness, convulsions, extrapyramidal symptoms, hypotension, and ECG abnormalities (including prolongation of the QT interval). Management is supportive. Charcoal, activated p. 1201 can be given within 1 hour of ingesting a significant quantity of a second-generation antipsychotic drug.

Benzodiazepines

Benzodiazepines taken alone cause drowsiness, ataxia, dysarthria, nystagmus, and occasionally respiratory depression, and coma. Charcoal, activated can be given within 1 hour of ingesting a significant quantity of benzodiazepine, provided the patient is awake and the airway is protected. Benzodiazepines potentiate the effects of other central nervous system depressants taken concomitantly. Use of the benzodiazepine antagonist flumazenil p. 1203 [unlicensed indication] can be hazardous, particularly in mixed overdoses involving tricyclic antidepressants or in benzodiazepine-dependent patients. Flumazenil may prevent the need for ventilation, particularly in patients with severe respiratory disorders; it should be used on expert advice only and not as a diagnostic test in patients with a reduced level of consciousness.

Beta blockers

Therapeutic overdosages with beta-blockers may cause lightheadedness, dizziness, and possibly syncope as a result of bradycardia and hypotension; heart failure may be precipitated or exacerbated. These complications are most likely in patients with conduction system disorders or impaired myocardial function. Bradycardia is the most common arrhythmia caused by beta-blockers, but sotalol may induce ventricular tachyarrhythmias (sometimes of the torsade de pointes type). The effects of massive overdosage can vary from one beta-blocker to another; propranolol overdosage in particular may cause coma and convulsions.

Acute massive overdosage must be managed in hospital and expert advice should be obtained. Maintenance of a clear airway and adequate ventilation is mandatory. An intravenous injection of atropine sulfate p. 1169 is required to treat bradycardia. Cardiogenic shock unresponsive to atropine sulfate is probably best treated with an intravenous injection of glucagon p. 652 [unlicensed indication] in glucose 5% (with precautions to protect the airway in case of vomiting) followed by an intravenous infusion. If glucagon is not available, intravenous isoprenaline (available from 'special-order' manufacturers or specialist importing companies) is an alternative. A cardiac pacemaker can be used to increase the heart rate.

Calcium-channel blockers

Features of calcium-channel blocker poisoning include nausea, vomiting, dizziness, agitation, confusion, and coma in severe poisoning. Metabolic acidosis and hyperglycaemia may occur. Verapamil and diltiazem have a profound cardiac depressant effect causing hypotension and arrhythmias, including complete heart block and asystole. The dihydropyridine calcium-channel blockers cause severe hypotension secondary to profound peripheral vasodilatation.

Charcoal, activated should be considered if the patient presents within 1 hour of overdosage with a calcium-channel blocker; repeated doses of activated charcoal are considered if a modified-release preparation is involved. In patients with significant features of poisoning, calcium chloride p. 907 or calcium gluconate p. 907 is given by injection; atropine sulfate is given to correct symptomatic bradycardia. In severe cases, an insulin and glucose infusion may be required in the management of hypotension and myocardial failure. For the management of hypotension, the choice of inotropic sympathomimetic depends on whether hypotension is secondary to vasodilatation or to myocardial depression—advice should be sought from the National Poisons Information Service.

Iron salts

Iron poisoning in childhood is usually accidental. The symptoms are nausea, vomiting, abdominal pain, diarrhoea, haematemesis, and rectal bleeding. Hypotension and hepatocellular necrosis can occur later. Coma, shock, and metabolic acidosis indicate severe poisoning.

Advice should be sought from the National Poisons Information Service if a significant quantity of iron has been ingested within the previous hour.

Mortality is reduced by intensive and specific therapy with desferrioxamine mesilate p. 889, which chelates iron. The serum-iron concentration is measured as an emergency and intravenous desferrioxamine mesilate given to chelate absorbed iron in excess of the expected iron binding capacity. In severe toxicity intravenous desferrioxamine mesilate should be given immediately without waiting for the result of the serum-iron measurement.

Lithium

Most cases of lithium intoxication occur as a complication of long-term therapy and are caused by reduced excretion of the drug because of a variety of factors including dehydration, deterioration of renal function, infections, and co-administration of diuretics or NSAIDs (or other drugs that interact). Acute deliberate overdoses may also occur with delayed onset of symptoms (12 hours or more) owing to slow entry of lithium into the tissues and continuing absorption from modified-release formulations.

The early clinical features are non-specific and may include apathy and restlessness which could be confused with mental changes arising from the patient's depressive illness. Vomiting, diarrhoea, ataxia, weakness, dysarthria, muscle twitching, and tremor may follow. Severe poisoning is associated with convulsions, coma, renal failure, electrolyte imbalance, dehydration, and hypotension.

Therapeutic serum-lithium concentrations are within the range of 0.4–1 mmol/litre; concentrations in excess of 2 mmol/litre are usually associated with serious toxicity and such cases may need treatment with haemodialysis if neurological symptoms or renal failure are present. In acute overdosage much higher serum-lithium concentrations may be present without features of toxicity and all that is usually necessary is to take measures to increase urine output (e.g. by increasing fluid intake but avoiding diuretics). Otherwise, treatment is supportive with special regard to electrolyte balance, renal function, and control of convulsions. Gastric lavage may be considered if it can be performed within

1 hour of ingesting significant quantities of lithium. Whole-bowel irrigation should be considered for significant ingestion, but advice should be sought from the National Poisons Information Service.

Stimulants

Amfetamines cause wakefulness, excessive activity, paranoia, hallucinations, and hypertension followed by exhaustion, convulsions, hyperthermia, and coma. The early stages can be controlled by diazepam p. 313 or lorazepam p. 308; advice should be sought from the National Poisons Information Service on the management of hypertension. Later, tepid sponging, anticonvulsants, and artificial respiration may be needed.

Cocaine

Cocaine stimulates the central nervous system, causing agitation, dilated pupils, tachycardia, hypertension, hallucinations, hyperthermia, hypertonia, and hyperreflexia; cardiac effects include chest pain, myocardial infarction, and arrhythmias.

Initial treatment of cocaine poisoning involves intravenous administration of diazepam to control agitation and cooling measures for hyperthermia (see Body temperature); hypertension and cardiac effects require specific treatment and expert advice should be sought.

Ecstasy

Ecstasy (methylenedioxymethamfetamine, MDMA) may cause severe reactions, even at doses that were previously tolerated. The most serious effects are delirium, coma, convulsions, ventricular arrhythmias, hyperthermia, rhabdomyolysis, acute renal failure, acute hepatitis, disseminated intravascular coagulation, adult respiratory distress syndrome, hyperreflexia, hypotension and intracerebral haemorrhage; hyponatraemia has also been associated with ecstasy use.

Treatment of methylenedioxymethamfetamine poisoning is supportive, with diazepam to control severe agitation or persistent convulsions and close monitoring including ECG. Self-induced water intoxication should be considered in patients with ecstasy poisoning.

'Liquid ecstasy' is a term used for sodium oxybate (gamma-hydroxybutyrate, GHB), which is a sedative.

Theophylline

Theophylline and related drugs are often prescribed as modified-release formulations and toxicity can therefore be delayed. They cause vomiting (which may be severe and intractable), agitation, restlessness, dilated pupils, sinus tachycardia, and hyperglycaemia. More serious effects are haematemesis, convulsions, and supraventricular and ventricular arrhythmias. Severe hypokalaemia may develop rapidly.

Repeated doses of activated charcoal can be used to eliminate theophylline even if more than 1 hour has elapsed after ingestion and especially if a modified-release preparation has been taken (see also under Active Elimination Techniques). Ondansetron p. 397 may be effective for severe vomiting that is resistant to other antiemetics [unlicensed indication]. Hypokalaemia is corrected by intravenous infusion of potassium chloride p. 917 and may be so severe as to require 60 mmol/hour (high doses require ECG monitoring). Convulsions should be controlled by intravenous administration of lorazepam or diazepam (see Convulsions). Sedation with diazepam may be necessary in agitated patients.

Provided the patient does not suffer from asthma, a short-acting beta-blocker can be administered intravenously to reverse severe tachycardia, hypokalaemia, and hyperglycaemia.

16

Emergency treatment of poisoning

Other poisons

Consult either the National Poisons Information Service day and night or TOXBASE, see under the National Poisons Information Service.

Cyanides

Oxygen should be administered to patients with cyanide poisoning. The choice of antidote depends on the severity of poisoning, certainty of diagnosis, and the cause. Dicobalt edetate p. 1202 is the antidote of choice when there is a strong clinical suspicion of severe cyanide poisoning, but it should **not** be used as a precautionary measure. Dicobalt edetate itself is toxic, associated with anaphylactoid reactions, and is potentially fatal if administered in the absence of cyanide poisoning. A regimen of sodium nitrite p. 1202 followed by sodium thiosulfate p. 1202 is an alternative if dicobalt edetate is not available.

Hydroxocobalamin p. 887 (*Cyanokit*®—no other preparation of hydroxocobalamin is suitable) can be considered for use in victims of smoke inhalation who show signs of significant cyanide poisoning.

Ethylene glycol and methanol

Fomepizole (available from 'special-order' manufacturers or specialist importing companies) is the treatment of choice for ethylene glycol and methanol (methyl alcohol) poisoning. If necessary, **ethanol** (by mouth or by intravenous infusion) can be used, but with caution. Advice on the treatment of ethylene glycol and methanol poisoning should be obtained from the National Poisons Information Service. It is important to start antidote treatment promptly in cases of suspected poisoning with these agents.

Heavy metals

Heavy metal antidotes include succimer (DMSA) [unlicensed], unithiol (DMPS) [unlicensed], sodium calcium edetate [unlicensed], and dimercaprol. Dimercaprol in the management of heavy metal poisoning has been superseded by other chelating agents. In all cases of heavy metal poisoning, the advice of the National Poisons Information Service should be sought.

Noxious gases

Carbon monoxide

Carbon monoxide poisoning is usually due to inhalation of smoke, car exhaust, or fumes caused by blocked flues or incomplete combustion of fuel gases in confined spaces.

Immediate treatment of carbon monoxide poisoning is essential. The person should be moved to fresh air, the airway cleared, and high-flow **oxygen** 100% administered through a tight-fitting mask with an inflated face seal. Artificial respiration should be given as necessary and continued until adequate spontaneous breathing starts, or stopped only after persistent and efficient treatment of cardiac arrest has failed. The patient should be admitted to hospital because complications may arise after a delay of hours or days. Cerebral oedema may occur in severe poisoning and is treated with an intravenous infusion of mannitol p. 211. Referral for hyperbaric oxygen treatment should be discussed with the National Poisons Information Service if the patient is pregnant or in cases of severe poisoning, such as if the patient is or has been unconscious, or has psychiatric or neurological features other than a headache, or has myocardial ischaemia or an arrhythmia, or has a blood carboxyhaemoglobin concentration of more than 20%.

Sulfur dioxide, chlorine, phosgene, ammonia

All of these gases can cause upper respiratory tract and conjunctival irritation. Pulmonary oedema, with severe breathlessness and cyanosis may develop suddenly up to 36 hours after exposure. Death may occur. Patients are kept under observation and those who develop pulmonary oedema are given oxygen. Assisted ventilation may be necessary in the most serious cases.

CS Spray

CS spray, which is used for riot control, irritates the eyes (hence 'tear gas') and the respiratory tract; symptoms normally settle spontaneously within 15 minutes. If symptoms persist, the patient should be removed to a well-ventilated area, and the exposed skin washed with soap and water after removal of contaminated clothing. Contact lenses should be removed and rigid ones washed (soft ones should be discarded). Eye symptoms should be treated by irrigating the eyes with physiological saline (or water if saline is not available) and advice sought from an ophthalmologist. Patients with features of severe poisoning, particularly respiratory complications, should be admitted to hospital for symptomatic treatment.

Nerve agents

Treatment of nerve agent poisoning is similar to organophosphorus insecticide poisoning, but advice must be sought from the National Poisons Information Service. The risk of cross-contamination is significant; adequate decontamination and protective clothing for healthcare personnel are essential. In emergencies involving the release of nerve agents, kits ('NAAS pods') containing pralidoxime chloride p. 1202 can be obtained through the Ambulance Service from the National Blood Service (or the Welsh Blood Service in South Wales or designated hospital pharmacies in Northern Ireland and Scotland—see TOXBASE for list of designated centres).

Pesticides

Organophosphorus insecticides

Organophosphorus insecticides are usually supplied as powders or dissolved in organic solvents. All are absorbed through the bronchi and intact skin as well as through the gut and inhibit cholinesterase activity, thereby prolonging and intensifying the effects of acetylcholine. Toxicity between different compounds varies considerably, and onset may be delayed after skin exposure.

Anxiety, restlessness, dizziness, headache, miosis, nausea, hypersalivation, vomiting, abdominal colic, diarrhoea, bradycardia, and sweating are common features of organophosphorus poisoning. Muscle weakness and fasciculation may develop and progress to generalised flaccid paralysis, including the ocular and respiratory muscles. Convulsions, coma, pulmonary oedema with copious bronchial secretions, hypoxia, and arrhythmias occur in severe cases. Hyperglycaemia and glycosuria without ketonuria may also be present.

Further absorption of the organophosphorus insecticide should be prevented by moving the patient to fresh air, removing soiled clothing, and washing contaminated skin. In severe poisoning it is vital to ensure a clear airway, frequent removal of bronchial secretions, and adequate ventilation and oxygenation; gastric lavage may be considered provided that the airway is protected. Atropine sulfate p. 1169 will reverse the muscarinic effects of acetylcholine and is given by intravenous injection until the skin becomes flushed and dry, the pupils dilate, and bradycardia is abolished.

Pralidoxime chloride, a cholinesterase reactivator, is used as an adjunct to atropine sulfate in moderate or severe poisoning. It improves muscle tone within 30 minutes of administration. Pralidoxime chloride is continued until the patient has not required atropine sulfate for 12 hours. Pralidoxime chloride can be obtained from designated centres, the names of which are held by the National Poisons Information Service.

Snake bites and animal stings

Snake bites

Envenoming from snake bite is uncommon in the UK. Many exotic snakes are kept, some illegally, but the only indigenous venomous snake is the adder (*Vipera berus*). The bite may cause local and systemic effects. Local effects include pain, swelling, bruising, and tender enlargement of regional lymph nodes. Systemic effects include early anaphylactic symptoms (transient hypotension with syncope, angioedema, urticaria, abdominal colic, diarrhoea, and vomiting), with later persistent or recurrent hypotension, ECG abnormalities, spontaneous systemic bleeding, coagulopathy, adult respiratory distress syndrome, and acute renal failure. Fatal envenoming is rare but the potential for severe envenoming must not be underestimated.

Early anaphylactic symptoms should be treated with **adrenaline/epinephrine** p. 205. Indications for european viper snake venom antiserum treatment p. 1206 include *systemic envenoming*, especially hypotension, ECG abnormalities, vomiting, haemostatic abnormalities, and marked local envenoming such that after bites on the hand or foot, swelling extends beyond the wrist or ankle within 4 hours of the bite. For those patients who present with clinical features of *severe envenoming* (e.g. shock, ECG abnormalities, or local swelling that has advanced from the foot to above the knee or from the hand to above the elbow within 2 hours of the bite), a higher initial dose of the european viper snake venom antiserum is recommended; if symptoms of *systemic envenoming* persist contact the National Poisons Information Service.

Adrenaline/epinephrine injection must be immediately to hand for treatment of anaphylactic reactions to the european viper snake venom antiserum.

European viper snake venom antiserum is available for bites by certain foreign snakes and spiders, stings by scorpions and fish. For information on identification, management, and for supply in an emergency, telephone the National Poisons Information Service. Whenever possible the TOXBASE entry should be read, and relevant information collected, before telephoning the National Poisons Information Service.

Insect stings

Stings from ants, wasps, hornets, and bees cause local pain and swelling but seldom cause severe direct toxicity unless many stings are inflicted at the same time. If the sting is in the mouth or on the tongue local swelling may threaten the upper airway. The stings from these insects are usually treated by cleaning the area with a topical antiseptic. Bee stings should be removed as quickly as possible. Anaphylactic reactions require immediate treatment with intramuscular **adrenaline/epinephrine**; self-administered intramuscular adrenaline/epinephrine (e.g. *EpiPen*®) is the best first-aid treatment for patients with severe hypersensitivity. An inhaled bronchodilator should be used for asthmatic reactions, see also the management of anaphylaxis. A short course of an **oral antihistamine** or a **topical corticosteroid** may help to reduce inflammation and relieve itching. A vaccine containing extracts of bee and wasp venom can be used to reduce the risk of anaphylaxis and systemic reactions in patients with systemic hypersensitivity to bee or wasp stings.

Marine stings

The severe pain of weeverfish (*Trachinus vipera*) and Portuguese man-o'-war stings can be relieved by immersing the stung area immediately in uncomfortably hot, but not scalding, water (not more than 45° C). People stung by jellyfish and Portuguese man-o'-war around the UK coast should be removed from the sea as soon as possible. Adherent tentacles should be lifted off carefully (wearing gloves or using tweezers) or washed off with seawater.

Alcoholic solutions, including suntan lotions, should **not** be applied because they can cause further discharge of stinging hairs. Ice packs can be used to reduce pain.

Other poisons

Consult either the National Poisons Information Service day and night or TOXBASE.

The National Poisons Information Service (Tel: 0344 892 0111) will provide specialist advice on all aspects of poisoning day and night.

1   Active elimination from the gastro-intestinal tract

ANTIDOTES AND CHELATORS > INTESTINAL ADSORBENTS

Charcoal, activated

- **INDICATIONS AND DOSE**

Reduction of absorption of poisons in the gastro-intestinal system
▸ BY MOUTH
- Child 1 month–11 years: 1 g/kg (max. per dose 50 g)
- Child 12–17 years: 50 g
▸ Adult: 50 g

Active elimination of poisons
▸ BY MOUTH
- Child 1 month–11 years: 1 g/kg every 4 hours (max. per dose 50 g), dose may be reduced and the frequency increased if not tolerated, reduced dose may compromise efficacy
- Child 12–17 years: Initially 50 g, then 50 g every 4 hours, reduced if not tolerated to 25 g every 2 hours, alternatively 12.5 g every 1 hour, reduced dose may compromise efficacy
- Adult: Initially 50 g, then 50 g every 4 hours, reduced if not tolerated to 25 g every 2 hours, alternatively 12.5 g every 1 hour, reduced dose may compromise efficacy

Accelerated elimination of teriflunomide
▸ BY MOUTH USING GRANULES
- Adult: 50 g every 12 hours for 11 days

Accelerated elimination of leflunomide (washout procedure)
▸ BY MOUTH USING GRANULES
- Adult: 50 g 4 times a day for 11 days

- **UNLICENSED USE** Activated charcoal doses in BNF may differ from those in product literature.

- **CAUTIONS** Comatose patient (risk of aspiration—ensure airway is protected) · drowsy patient (risk of aspiration—ensure airway protected) · reduced gastrointestinal motility (risk of obstruction)

- **SIDE-EFFECTS** Black stools

- **DIRECTIONS FOR ADMINISTRATION** Suspension or reconstituted powder may be mixed with soft drinks (e.g. caffeine-free diet cola) or fruit juices to mask the taste.

- **MEDICINAL FORMS**
There can be variation in the licensing of different medicines containing the same drug.
Granules
▸ Carbomix (Beacon Pharmaceuticals Ltd)
   Activated charcoal 813 mg per 1 gram Carbomix 81.3% granules sugar-free | 50 gram Ⓟ £11.90
Oral suspension
▸ Actidose-Aqua Advance (Alliance Pharmaceuticals Ltd)
   Activated charcoal 208 mg per 1 ml Actidose-Aqua Advance 1.04g/5ml oral suspension | 240 ml Ⓟ £12.89

16

Emergency treatment of poisoning

▸ Charcodote (Teva UK Ltd)
Activated charcoal 200 mg per 1 ml Charcodote 200mg/ml oral
suspension sugar-free | 250 ml P £11.88

2 Chemical toxicity

2.1 Cyanide toxicity

ANTIDOTES AND CHELATORS

Dicobalt edetate

● **INDICATIONS AND DOSE**

Severe poisoning with cyanides
▸ **BY INTRAVENOUS INJECTION**
▸ Child: Consult the National Poisons Information
  Service
▸ Adult: 300 mg, to be given over 1 minute (or 5 minutes
  if condition less serious), dose to be followed
  immediately by 50 mL of glucose intravenous infusion
  50%; if response inadequate a second dose of both may
  be given, but risk of cobalt toxicity

● CAUTIONS Owing to toxicity to be used only for definite
cyanide poisoning when patient tending to lose, or has
lost, consciousness

● SIDE-EFFECTS Anaphylactoid reactions · cardiac
abnormalities · facial oedema · hypotension · laryngeal
oedema · tachycardia · vomiting

● EXCEPTIONS TO LEGAL CATEGORY Prescription only
medicine restriction does not apply where administration
is for saving life in emergency.

● MEDICINAL FORMS
There can be variation in the licensing of different medicines
containing the same drug.
Solution for injection
▸ Dicobalt edetate (Non-proprietary)
  Dicobalt edetate 15 mg per 1 ml Dicobalt edetate 300mg/20ml
  solution for injection ampoules | 6 ampoule PoM £117.20

Sodium nitrite

● **INDICATIONS AND DOSE**

**Poisoning with cyanides (used in conjunction with sodium
thiosulfate)**
▸ **BY INTRAVENOUS INJECTION**
▸ Child: 4–10 mg/kg (max. per dose 300 mg), to be given
  over 5–20 minutes followed by sodium thiosulphate
  injection
▸ Adult: 300 mg, to be given over 5–20 minutes (as
  sodium nitrite injection 30 mg/mL)

DOSE EQUIVALENCE AND CONVERSION
4–10 mg/kg equates to 0.13–0.33 mL/kg of a 3% solution.
Dose max. of 300 mg equates to 10 mL of a 3% solution.

● SIDE-EFFECTS Flushing (due to vasodilatation) · headache
(due to vasodilatation)

● EXCEPTIONS TO LEGAL CATEGORY Prescription only
medicine restriction does not apply where administration
is for saving life in emergency.

● MEDICINAL FORMS
There can be variation in the licensing of different medicines
containing the same drug. Forms available from special-order
manufacturers include: solution for injection

Sodium thiosulfate

● **INDICATIONS AND DOSE**

**Poisoning with cyanides (used in conjunction with sodium
nitrite)**
▸ **BY INTRAVENOUS INJECTION**
▸ Child: 400 mg/kg (max. per dose 12.5 g), to be given
  over 10 minutes, dose may be repeated in severe
  cyanide poisoning if dicobalt edetate not available
▸ Adult: 12.5 g, to be given over 10 minutes (as sodium
  thiosulfate injection 500 mg/mL), dose may be
  repeated in severe cyanide poisoning if dicobalt
  edetate not available

DOSE EQUIVALENCE AND CONVERSION
400 mg/kg equates to 0.8 mL/kg of a 50% solution.
12.5 g equates to 25 mL of a 50% solution.

● EXCEPTIONS TO LEGAL CATEGORY Prescription only
medicine restriction does not apply where administration
is for saving life in emergency.

● MEDICINAL FORMS
There can be variation in the licensing of different medicines
containing the same drug. Forms available from special-order
manufacturers include: solution for injection

2.2 Organophosphorus toxicity

**Drugs used for organophosphorus toxicity not listed
below** Atropine sulfate, p. 1169

ANTIDOTES AND CHELATORS

Pralidoxime chloride

● **INDICATIONS AND DOSE**

**Adjunct to atropine in the treatment of poisoning by
organophosphorus insecticide or nerve agent**
▸ **BY INTRAVENOUS INFUSION**
▸ Child: Initially 30 mg/kg, to be given over 20 minutes,
  followed by 8 mg/kg/hour; maximum 12 g per day
▸ Adult: Initially 30 mg/kg, to be given over 20 minutes,
  followed by 8 mg/kg/hour; maximum 12 g per day

● UNLICENSED USE Pralidoxime chloride doses may differ
from those in product literature. Licensed for use in
children (age range not specified by manufacturer).

● CONTRA-INDICATIONS Poisoning with carbamates ·
poisoning with organophosphorus compounds without
anticholinesterase activity

● CAUTIONS Myasthenia gravis

● SIDE-EFFECTS Disturbances of vision · dizziness ·
drowsiness · headache · hyperventilation · muscular
weakness · nausea · tachycardia

● RENAL IMPAIRMENT Use with caution.

● DIRECTIONS FOR ADMINISTRATION The loading dose may
be administered by intravenous injection (diluted to a
concentration of 50 mg/mL with water for injections) over
at least 5 minutes if pulmonary oedema is present or if it is
not practical to administer an intravenous infusion.
▸ With intravenous use in children For *intravenous infusion*,
reconstitute each vial with 20 mL Water for Injections,
then dilute to a concentration of 10–20 mg/mL with
Sodium Chloride 0.9%.

● PRESCRIBING AND DISPENSING INFORMATION Available
from designated centres for organophosphorus insecticide
poisoning or from the National Blood Service (or Welsh
Ambulance Services for Mid West and South East Wales)—
see TOXBASE for list of designated centres).

- EXCEPTIONS TO LEGAL CATEGORY Prescription only medicine restriction does not apply where administration is for saving life in emergency.

- MEDICINAL FORMS
  There can be variation in the licensing of different medicines containing the same drug.
  Powder for solution for injection
  ▸ Pralidoxime chloride (Non-proprietary)
    Pralidoxime chloride 1 gram Protopam Chloride 1g powder for solution for injection vials | 6 vial [PoM] no price available

3 Drug toxicity

3.1 Benzodiazepine toxicity

ANTIDOTES AND CHELATORS >
BENZODIAZEPINE ANTAGONISTS

Flumazenil

- INDICATIONS AND DOSE
  Reversal of sedative effects of benzodiazepines in anaesthesia and clinical procedures
  ▸ BY INTRAVENOUS INJECTION
  ▸ Adult: 200 micrograms, dose to be administered over 15 seconds, then 100 micrograms every 1 minute if required; usual dose 300–600 micrograms; maximum 1 mg per course
  Reversal of sedative effects of benzodiazepines in intensive care
  ▸ BY INTRAVENOUS INJECTION
  ▸ Adult: 300 micrograms, dose to be administered over 15 seconds, then 100 micrograms every 1 minute if required; maximum 2 mg per course
  Reversal of sedative effects of benzodiazepines in intensive care (if drowsiness recurs after injection)
  ▸ INITIALLY BY INTRAVENOUS INFUSION
  ▸ Adult: 100–400 micrograms/hour, adjusted according to response, alternatively (by intravenous injection) 300 micrograms, adjusted according to response

  IMPORTANT SAFETY INFORMATION
  Flumazenil should only be administered by, or under the direct supervision of, personnel experienced in its use.

- CONTRA-INDICATIONS Life-threatening condition (e.g. raised intracranial pressure, status epilepticus) controlled by benzodiazepines
- CAUTIONS Avoid rapid injection following major surgery · avoid rapid injection in high-risk or anxious patients · benzodiazepine dependence (may precipitate withdrawal symptoms) · elderly · ensure neuromuscular blockade cleared before giving · head injury (rapid reversal of benzodiazepine sedation may cause convulsions) · history of panic disorders (risk of recurrence) · prolonged benzodiazepine therapy for epilepsy (risk of convulsions) · short-acting (repeat doses may be necessary—benzodiazepine effects may persist for at least 24 hours)
- SIDE-EFFECTS
  ▸ **Common or very common** Nausea · vomiting
  ▸ **Uncommon** Anxiety · fear · palpitation
  ▸ **Frequency not known** Agitation · chills · convulsions (particularly in those with epilepsy) · dizziness · flushing · sensory disturbance · sweating · tachycardia · transient hypertension
- PREGNANCY Not known to be harmful.
- BREAST FEEDING Avoid breast-feeding for 24 hours.
- HEPATIC IMPAIRMENT Carefully titrate dose.

- DIRECTIONS FOR ADMINISTRATION For *continuous intravenous infusion*, dilute with Glucose 5% or Sodium Chloride 0.9%.

- MEDICINAL FORMS
  There can be variation in the licensing of different medicines containing the same drug.
  Solution for injection
  ▸ Flumazenil (Non-proprietary)
    Flumazenil 100 microgram per 1 ml Flumazenil 500micrograms/5ml solution for injection ampoules | 5 ampoule [PoM] £65.50–£72.46

3.2 Digoxin toxicity

ANTIDOTES AND CHELATORS > ANTIBODIES

Digoxin-specific antibody

- INDICATIONS AND DOSE
  Treatment of known or strongly suspected life-threatening digoxin toxicity associated with ventricular arrhythmias or bradyarrhythmias unresponsive to atropine and when measures beyond the withdrawal of digoxin and correction of any electrolyte abnormalities are considered necessary
  ▸ BY INTRAVENOUS INFUSION
  ▸ Child: Serious cases of digoxin toxicity should be discussed with the National Poisons Information Service (consult product literature)
  ▸ Adult: Serious cases of digoxin toxicity should be discussed with the National Poisons Information Service (consult product literature)

- DIRECTIONS FOR ADMINISTRATION
  ▸ In adults For *intravenous infusion (DigiFab®)*, given intermittently in Sodium chloride 0.9%. Reconstitute with water for injections (4 mL/vial), then dilute with infusion fluid and give over 30 minutes.

- MEDICINAL FORMS
  There can be variation in the licensing of different medicines containing the same drug.
  Powder for solution for infusion
  ▸ DigiFab (BTG International Ltd)
    Digoxin-specific antibody fragments 40 mg DigiFab 40mg powder for solution for infusion vials | 1 vial [PoM] £750.00 (Hospital only)

3.3 Heparin toxicity

ANTIDOTES AND CHELATORS

Protamine sulfate

- INDICATIONS AND DOSE
  Overdosage with intravenous injection of unfractionated heparin
  ▸ BY INTRAVENOUS INJECTION
  ▸ Adult: Dose to be administered at a rate not exceeding 5 mg/minute, 1 mg neutralises 80–100 units heparin when given within 15 minutes; if longer than 15 minute since heparin, less protamine required (consult product literature for details) as heparin rapidly excreted; maximum 50 mg
  Overdosage with intravenous infusion of unfractionated heparin
  ▸ BY INTRAVENOUS INJECTION
  ▸ Adult: 25–50 mg, to be administered once heparin infusion stopped at a rate not exceeding 5 mg/minute
  continued →

16

Emergency treatment of poisoning

Overdosage with subcutaneous injection of unfractionated heparin

▶ INITIALLY BY INTRAVENOUS INJECTION

▶ Adult: Initially 25–50 mg, to be administered at a rate not exceeding 5 mg/minute, 1 mg neutralises 100 units heparin, then (by intravenous infusion), any remaining dose to be administered over 8–16 hours; maximum 50 mg per course

Overdosage with subcutaneous injection of low molecular weight heparin

▶ BY INTRAVENOUS INJECTION, OR BY CONTINUOUS INTRAVENOUS INFUSION

▶ Adult: Dose to be administered by intermittent intravenous injection at a rate not exceeding 5 mg/minute, 1 mg neutralises approx. 100 units low molecular weight heparin (consult product literature of low molecular weight heparin for details); maximum 50 mg

● CAUTIONS Excessive doses can have an anticoagulant effect

● SIDE-EFFECTS Anaphylaxis · angioedema · back pain · bradycardia · dyspnoea · flushing · hypersensitivity reactions · hypertension · hypotension · lassitude · nausea · pulmonary oedema · rebound bleeding · vomiting

● ALLERGY AND CROSS-SENSITIVITY Caution if increased risk of allergic reaction to protamine (includes previous treatment with protamine or protamine insulin, allergy to fish, men who are infertile or who have had a vasectomy and who may have antibodies to protamine).

● MONITORING REQUIREMENTS Monitor activated partial thromboplastin time or other appropriate blood clotting parameters.

● PRESCRIBING AND DISPENSING INFORMATION The long half-life of low molecular weight heparins should be taken into consideration when determining the dose of protamine sulfate; the effects of low molecular weight heparins can persist for up to 24 hours after administration.

● MEDICINAL FORMS
There can be variation in the licensing of different medicines containing the same drug.
Solution for injection
▶ Protamine sulfate (Non-proprietary)
Protamine sulfate 10 mg per 1 ml Protamine sulfate 100mg/10ml solution for injection ampoules | 5 ampoule [PoM] no price available
Protamine sulfate 50mg/5ml solution for injection ampoules | 10 ampoule [PoM] £49.55

3.4 Opioid toxicity

OPIOID RECEPTOR ANTAGONISTS

Naloxone hydrochloride

● INDICATIONS AND DOSE
Overdosage with opioids
▶ BY INTRAVENOUS INJECTION, OR BY SUBCUTANEOUS INJECTION, OR BY INTRAMUSCULAR INJECTION
▶ Child 1 month–11 years: Initially 100 micrograms/kg, if no response, repeat at intervals of 1 minute to a total max. 2 mg, then review diagnosis; further doses may be required if respiratory function deteriorates
▶ Child 12–17 years: Initially 400 micrograms, then 800 micrograms for up to 2 doses at 1 minute intervals if no response to preceding dose, then increased to 2 mg for 1 dose if still no response (4 mg dose may be required in seriously poisoned patients), then review

diagnosis; further doses may be required if respiratory function deteriorates
▶ Adult: Initially 400 micrograms, then 800 micrograms for up to 2 doses at 1 minute intervals if no response to preceding dose, then increased to 2 mg for 1 dose if still no response (4 mg dose may be required in seriously poisoned patients), then review diagnosis; further doses may be required if respiratory function deteriorates
▶ BY CONTINUOUS INTRAVENOUS INFUSION
▶ Child: Using an infusion pump, adjust rate according to response (initially, rate may be set at 60% of the initial resuscitative intravenous injection dose per hour). The initial resuscitative *intravenous injection* dose is that which maintained satisfactory ventilation for at least 15 minutes
▶ Adult: Using an infusion pump, adjust rate according to response (initially, rate may be set at 60% of the initial resuscitative intravenous injection dose per hour). The initial resuscitative *intravenous injection* dose is that which maintained satisfactory ventilation for at least 15 minutes

Overdosage with opioids in a non-medical setting
▶ BY INTRAMUSCULAR INJECTION
▶ Adult: 400 micrograms every 2–3 minutes, each dose given in subsequent resuscitation cycles if patient not breathing normally, continue until consciousness regained, breathing normally, medical assistance available, or contents of syringe used up; to be injected into deltoid region or anterolateral thigh

Reversal of postoperative respiratory depression
▶ INITIALLY BY INTRAVENOUS INJECTION
▶ Child 1 month–11 years: 1 microgram/kg, repeated every 2–3 minutes if required
▶ Child 12–17 years: Initially 100–200 micrograms, alternatively (by intravenous injection) initially 1.5–3 micrograms/kg, if response inadequate, give subsequent doses, (by intravenous injection) 100 micrograms every 2 minutes, alternatively (by intramuscular injection) 100 micrograms every 1–2 hours
▶ Adult: Initially 100–200 micrograms, alternatively (by intravenous injection) initially 1.5–3 micrograms/kg, if response inadequate, give subsequent doses, (by intravenous injection) 100 micrograms every 2 minutes, alternatively (by intramuscular injection) 100 micrograms every 1–2 hours

PHARMACOKINETICS
Naloxone has a short duration of action; repeated doses or infusion may be necessary to reverse effects of opioids with longer duration of action.
Important: Only give by subcutaneous or intramuscular routes if intravenous route is not feasible; intravenous administration has more rapid onset of action.

● UNLICENSED USE Naloxone doses in BNF may differ from those in product literature.

IMPORTANT SAFETY INFORMATION
SAFE PRACTICE
Doses used in acute opioid overdosage may not be appropriate for the management of opioid-induced respiratory depression and sedation in those receiving palliative care and in chronic opioid use.

● CAUTIONS Cardiovascular disease or those receiving cardiotoxic drugs (serious adverse cardiovascular effects reported) · maternal physical dependence on opioids (may precipitate withdrawal in newborn) · pain · physical dependence on opioids (precipitates withdrawal)

CAUTIONS, FURTHER INFORMATION
‣ **Titration of dose** In postoperative use, the dose should be titrated for each patient in order to obtain sufficient respiratory response; however, naloxone antagonises analgesia.

● SIDE-EFFECTS
‣ **Common or very common** Cardiac arrest (in children) · dizziness · dyspnoea (in children) · headache · hypertension · hyperventilation (in children) · hypotension · nausea · pulmonary oedema (in children) · tachycardia · ventricular fibrillation (in children) · vomiting
‣ **Uncommon** Agitation (in children) · arrhythmia (in adults) · bradycardia (in adults) · diarrhoea · dry mouth · excitement (in children) · hypertension (in adults) · paraesthesia (in children) · sweating · tremor
‣ **Rare** Seizures (in adults)
‣ **Very rare** Anaphylaxis (in adults) · cardiac arrest (in adults) · erythema multiforme · hypersensitivity reactions (in adults) · pulmonary oedema (in adults) · seizures (in children) · ventricular fibrillation (in adults)
‣ **Frequency not known** Agitation (in adults)
● PREGNANCY Use only if potential benefit outweighs risk.
● BREAST FEEDING Not orally bioavailable.
● DIRECTIONS FOR ADMINISTRATION
‣ **With intravenous use in children** For *continuous intravenous infusion*, dilute to a concentration of up to 200 micrograms/mL with Glucose 5% or Sodium Chloride 0.9%.
‣ **With intravenous use in adults** For *intravenous infusion* (*Minijet*® Naloxone Hydrochloride), give continuously in Glucose 5% or Sodium Chloide 0.9%. Dilute to a concentration of up to 200 micrograms/mL and administer via an infusion pump.

● MEDICINAL FORMS
There can be variation in the licensing of different medicines containing the same drug.
Solution for injection
‣ Naloxone hydrochloride (Non-proprietary)
Naloxone hydrochloride 20 microgram per 1 ml Naloxone 40micrograms/2ml solution for injection ampoules | 10 ampoule PoM £55.00
Naloxone hydrochloride 400 microgram per 1 ml Naloxone 400micrograms/1ml solution for injection Minijet pre-filled syringes | 1 pre-filled disposable injection PoM £20.40
Naloxone 2mg/5ml solution for injection Minijet pre-filled syringes | 1 pre-filled disposable injection PoM £20.40
Naloxone 400micrograms/1ml solution for injection ampoules | 10 ampoule PoM £41.00–£53.70
Naloxone 800micrograms/2ml solution for injection Minijet pre-filled syringes | 1 pre-filled disposable injection PoM £20.40
Naloxone hydrochloride 1 mg per 1 ml Naloxone 2mg/2ml solution for injection pre-filled syringes | 1 pre-filled disposable injection PoM £16.80
‣ Prenoxad (Martindale Pharmaceuticals Ltd)
Naloxone hydrochloride 1 mg per 1 ml Prenoxad 2mg/2ml solution for injection pre-filled syringes | 1 pre-filled disposable injection PoM £15.30

3.5 Paracetamol toxicity

ANTIDOTES AND CHELATORS

| Acetylcysteine

● INDICATIONS AND DOSE
Paracetamol overdosage
‣ BY INTRAVENOUS INFUSION
‣ **Child (body-weight up to 20 kg):** Initially 150 mg/kg over 1 hour, dose to be administered in 3 mL/kg glucose 5%, followed by 50 mg/kg over 4 hours, dose to be

administered in 7 mL/kg glucose 5%, then 100 mg/kg over 16 hours, dose to be administered in 14 mL/kg glucose 5%
‣ **Child (body-weight 20–39 kg):** Initially 150 mg/kg over 1 hour, dose to be administered in 100 mL glucose 5%, followed by 50 mg/kg over 4 hours, dose to be administered in 250 mL glucose 5%, then 100 mg/kg over 16 hours, dose to be administered in 500 mL glucose 5%
‣ **Child (body-weight 40 kg and above):** 150 mg/kg over 1 hour, dose to be administered in 200 mL Glucose Intravenous Infusion 5%, then 50 mg/kg over 4 hours, to be started immediately after completion of first infusion, dose to be administered in 500 mL Glucose Intravenous Infusion 5%, then 100 mg/kg over 16 hours, to be started immediately after completion of second infusion, dose to be administered in 1 litre Glucose Intravenous Infusion 5%
‣ **Adult (body-weight 40 kg and above):** 150 mg/kg over 1 hour, dose to be administered in 200 mL Glucose Intravenous Infusion 5%, then 50 mg/kg over 4 hours, to be started immediately after completion of first infusion, dose to be administered in 500 mL Glucose Intravenous Infusion 5%, then 100 mg/kg over 16 hours, to be started immediately after completion of second infusion, dose to be administered in 1 litre Glucose Intravenous Infusion 5%

● CAUTIONS Asthma (see Side-effects for management of asthma but do not delay acetylcysteine treatment) · atopy · may slightly increase INR · may slightly increase prothrombin time
● SIDE-EFFECTS
Hypersensitivity-like reactions · rashes · slight increase in INR and prothrombin time
SIDE-EFFECTS, FURTHER INFORMATION
‣ **Hypersensitivity-like reactions** Hypersensitivity-like reactions managed by reducing infusion rate or suspending until reaction settled (rash also managed by giving antihistamine; acute asthma managed by giving nebulised short-acting beta₂ agonist)—contact the National Poisons Information Service if reaction severe.
● DIRECTIONS FOR ADMINISTRATION
‣ **With intravenous use in children** Glucose 5% is preferred fluid; Sodium Chloride 0.9% is an alternative if Glucose 5% unsuitable.
‣ **With intravenous use in adults** For *intravenous infusion* (*Parvolex*®), give continuously in Glucose 5% or Sodium chloride 0.9%. Glucose Intravenous Infusion 5% is the preferred fluid; Sodium Chloride Intravenous Infusion 0.9% is an alternative if Glucose Intravenous Infusion 5% is unsuitable.

● MEDICINAL FORMS
There can be variation in the licensing of different medicines containing the same drug.
Solution for infusion
ELECTROLYTES: May contain Sodium
‣ Acetylcysteine (Non-proprietary)
Acetylcysteine 200 mg per 1 ml Acetylcysteine 2g/10ml solution for infusion ampoules | 10 ampoule PoM £21.26–£24.99
‣ Parvolex (Phoenix Labs Ltd)
Acetylcysteine 200 mg per 1 ml Parvolex 2g/10ml concentrate for solution for infusion ampoules | 10 ampoule PoM £22.50

16

Emergency treatment of poisoning

4 Methaemoglobinaemia

ANTIDOTES AND CHELATORS

Methylthioninium chloride
(Methylene blue)

● **INDICATIONS AND DOSE**

Drug- or chemical-induced methaemoglobinaemia
▸ BY SLOW INTRAVENOUS INJECTION
▸ Child 3 months–17 years: Initially 1–2 mg/kg, then 1–2 mg/kg after 30–60 minutes if required, to be given over 5 minutes, seek advice from National Poisons Information Service if further repeat doses are required; maximum 7 mg/kg per course
▸ Adult: Initially 1–2 mg/kg, then 1–2 mg/kg after 30–60 minutes if required, to be given over 5 minutes, seek advice from National Poisons Information Service if further repeat doses are required; maximum 7 mg/kg per course

Aniline- or dapsone-induced methaemoglobinaemia
▸ BY SLOW INTRAVENOUS INJECTION
▸ Child 3 months–17 years: Initially 1–2 mg/kg, then 1–2 mg/kg after 30–60 minutes if required, to be given over 5 minutes, seek advice from National Poisons Information Service if further repeat doses are required; maximum 4 mg/kg per course
▸ Adult: Initially 1–2 mg/kg, then 1–2 mg/kg after 30–60 minutes if required, to be given over 5 minutes, seek advice from National Poisons Information Service if further repeat doses are required; maximum 4 mg/kg per course

● CAUTIONS Children under 3 months (more susceptible to methaemoglobinaemia from high doses of methylthioninium) · chlorate poisoning (reduces efficacy of methylthioninium) · G6PD deficiency (seek advice from National Poisons Information Service) · methaemoglobinaemia due to treatment of cyanide poisoning with sodium nitrite (seek advice from National Poisons Information Service) · pulse oximetry may give false estimation of oxygen saturation

● INTERACTIONS → Appendix 1 (methylthioninium).

● SIDE-EFFECTS Abdominal pain · agitation · anxiety · arrhythmia · blue-green discoloration of faeces · blue-green discoloration of skin · blue-green discoloration of urine · chest pain · confusion · dizziness · dyspnoea · fever · haemolytic anaemia · headache · hyperbilirubinaemia (in infants) · hypertension · hypotension · methaemoglobinaemia · mydriasis · nausea · sweating · tachypnoea · tremor · vomiting

● PREGNANCY No information available, but risk to fetus of untreated methaemoglobinaemia likely to be significantly higher than risk of treatment.

● BREAST FEEDING Manufacturer advises avoid breastfeeding for up to 6 days after administration—no information available.

● RENAL IMPAIRMENT Use with caution in severe impairment; dose reduction may be required.

● DIRECTIONS FOR ADMINISTRATION
▸ With intravenous use in children For *intravenous injection*, may be diluted with Glucose 5% to minimise injection-site pain; not compatible with Sodium Chloride 0.9%.

● MEDICINAL FORMS There can be variation in the licensing of different medicines containing the same drug. Forms available from special-order manufacturers include: solution for injection
Solution for injection
▸ Methylthioninium chloride (Non-proprietary)
  Methylthioninium chloride 5 mg per 1 ml Methylthioninium chloride Proveblue 50mg/10ml solution for injection ampoules | 5 ampoule [PoM] £167.36

5 Snake bites

IMMUNE SERA AND IMMUNOGLOBULINS ›
ANTITOXINS

European viper snake venom antiserum

● **INDICATIONS AND DOSE**

Systemic envenoming from snake bites | Marked local envenoming
▸ BY INTRAVENOUS INJECTION, OR BY INTRAVENOUS INFUSION
▸ Child: Initially 10 mL for 1 dose, then 10 mL after 1–2 hours if required, the second dose should only be given if symptoms of systemic envenoming persist after the first dose, if symptoms of systemic envenoming persist contact the National Poisons Information Service
▸ Adult: Initially 10 mL for 1 dose, then 10 mL after 1–2 hours if required, the second dose should only be given if symptoms of systemic envenoming persist after the first dose, if symptoms of systemic envenoming persist contact the National Poisons Information Service

Severe systemic envenoming from snake bites in patients presenting with clinical features
▸ BY INTRAVENOUS INJECTION, OR BY INTRAVENOUS INFUSION
▸ Child: Initially 20 mL for 1 dose, if symptoms of systemic envenoming persist contact the National Poisons Information Service
▸ Adult: Initially 20 mL for 1 dose, if symptoms of systemic envenoming persist contact the National Poisons Information Service

● DIRECTIONS FOR ADMINISTRATION By *intravenous injection* given over 10–15 minutes or by *intravenous infusion* over 30 minutes after diluting in sodium chloride 0.9% (use 5 mL diluent/kg body-weight).

● PRESCRIBING AND DISPENSING INFORMATION To order, email immform@dh.gsi.gov.uk.

● MEDICINAL FORMS There can be variation in the licensing of different medicines containing the same drug.
Solution for injection
▸ European viper snake venom antiserum (Non-proprietary)
  European viper snake venom antiserum 100 mg per 1 ml Viper venom antiserum, European (equine) 1g/10ml solution for injection vials | 1 vial [PoM] no price available

Appendix 1
Interactions

Two or more drugs given at the same time may exert their effects independently or may interact. The interaction may be potentiation or antagonism of one drug by another, or occasionally some other effect. Adverse drug interactions should be reported to the Medicines and Healthcare products Regulatory Agency (MHRA), through the Yellow Card Scheme (see Adverse Reactions to Drugs), as for other adverse drug reactions.

Drug interactions may be **pharmacodynamic** or **pharmacokinetic**.

Pharmacodynamic interactions

These are interactions between drugs which have similar or antagonistic pharmacological effects or side-effects. They may be due to competition at receptor sites, or occur between drugs acting on the same physiological system. They are usually predictable from a knowledge of the pharmacology of the interacting drugs; in general, those demonstrated with one drug are likely to occur with related drugs. They occur to a greater or lesser extent in most patients who receive the interacting drugs.

Pharmacokinetic interactions

These occur when one drug alters the absorption, distribution, metabolism, or excretion of another, thus increasing or reducing the amount of drug available to produce its pharmacological effects. They are not easily predicted and many of them affect only a small proportion of patients taking the combination of drugs. Pharmacokinetic interactions occurring with one drug cannot be assumed to occur with related drugs unless their pharmacokinetic properties are known to be similar.

Pharmacokinetic interactions are of several types:

Affecting absorption The rate of absorption or the total amount absorbed can both be altered by drug interactions. Delayed absorption is rarely of clinical importance unless high peak plasma concentrations are required (e.g. when giving an analgesic). Reduction in the total amount absorbed, however, may result in ineffective therapy.

Due to changes in protein binding To a variable extent most drugs are loosely bound to plasma proteins. Protein-binding sites are non-specific and one drug can displace another thereby increasing its proportion free to diffuse from plasma to its site of action. This only produces a detectable increase in effect if it is an extensively bound drug (more than 90%) that is not widely distributed throughout the body. Even so displacement rarely produces more than transient potentiation because this increased concentration of free drug results in an increased rate of elimination.

Displacement from protein binding plays a part in the potentiation of warfarin by sulfonamides and tolbutamide but the importance of these interactions is due mainly to the fact that warfarin metabolism is also inhibited.

Affecting metabolism Many drugs are metabolised in the liver. Induction of the hepatic microsomal enzyme system by one drug can gradually increase the rate of metabolism of another, resulting in lower plasma concentrations and a reduced effect. On withdrawal of the inducer plasma concentrations increase and toxicity may occur. Barbiturates, griseofulvin, many antiepileptics, and rifampicin are the most important enzyme inducers. Drugs affected include warfarin and the oral contraceptives.

Conversely when one drug inhibits the metabolism of another higher plasma concentrations are produced, rapidly resulting in an increased effect with risk of toxicity. Some drugs which potentiate warfarin and phenytoin do so by this mechanism.

Isoenzymes of the hepatic cytochrome P450 system interact with a wide range of drugs. Drugs may be substrates, inducers or inhibitors of the different isoenzymes. A great deal of *in-vitro* information is available on the effect of drugs on the isoenzymes; however, since drugs are eliminated by a number of different metabolic routes as well as renal excretion, the clinical effects of interactions cannot be predicted accurately from laboratory data on the cytochrome P450 isoenzymes. Except where a combination of drugs is specifically contra-indicated, the BNF presents only interactions that have been reported in clinical practice. In all cases the possibility of an interaction must be considered if toxic effects occur or if the activity of a drug diminishes.

Affecting renal excretion Drugs are eliminated through the kidney both by glomerular filtration and by active tubular secretion. Competition occurs between those which share active transport mechanisms in the proximal tubule. For example, salicylates and some other NSAIDs delay the excretion of methotrexate; serious methotrexate toxicity is possible.

Relative importance of interactions

Many drug interactions are harmless and many of those which are potentially harmful only occur in a small proportion of patients; moreover, the severity of an interaction varies from one patient to another. Drugs with a small therapeutic ratio (e.g. phenytoin) and those which require careful control of dosage (e.g. anticoagulants, antihypertensives, and antidiabetics) are most often involved.

Patients at increased risk from drug interactions include the elderly and those with impaired renal or liver function.

Serious interactions The symbol ● has been placed against interactions that are **potentially serious** and where concomitant administration of the drugs involved should be **avoided** (or only undertaken with caution and appropriate monitoring).

Interactions that have no symbol do not usually have serious consequences.

List of drug interactions

The following is an alphabetical list of drugs and their interactions; to avoid excessive cross-referencing each drug or group is listed twice: in the alphabetical list and also against the drug or group with which it interacts.

Abacavir
▸ Analgesics: abacavir possibly reduces plasma concentration of METHADONE
▸ Antibacterials: plasma concentration of abacavir possibly reduced by RIFAMPICIN
▸ Antiepileptics: plasma concentration of abacavir possibly reduced by FOSPHENYTOIN, PHENOBARBITAL, PHENYTOIN and PRIMIDONE
● Antivirals: abacavir possibly reduces effects of ● RIBAVIRIN; plasma concentration of abacavir reduced by ● TIPRANAVIR
● Orlistat: absorption of abacavir possibly reduced by ● ORLISTAT

Abatacept
● Cytotoxics: increased risk of side-effects when abatacept given with ADALIMUMAB; avoid concomitant use of abatacept with ● CERTOLIZUMAB PEGOL, ● GOLIMUMAB or ● INFLIXIMAB
● Etanercept: avoid concomitant use of abatacept with ● ETANERCEPT
● Vaccines: risk of generalised infections when abatacept given with live ● VACCINES—avoid concomitant use

Abiraterone
▸ Analgesics: abiraterone increases plasma concentration of DEXTROMETHORPHAN
● Antibacterials: plasma concentration of abiraterone possibly reduced by ● RIFABUTIN—manufacturer of abiraterone advises avoid concomitant use; plasma concentration of abiraterone reduced by ● RIFAMPICIN—manufacturer of abiraterone advises avoid concomitant use
● Antidepressants: plasma concentration of abiraterone possibly reduced by ● ST JOHN'S WORT—manufacturer of abiraterone advises avoid concomitant use
● Antiepileptics: plasma concentration of abiraterone possibly reduced by ● CARBAMAZEPINE, ● FOSPHENYTOIN, ● PHENOBARBITAL, ● PHENYTOIN and ● PRIMIDONE—manufacturer of abiraterone advises avoid concomitant use
▸ Diuretics: manufacturer of abiraterone advises avoid concomitant use with SPIRONOLACTONE

Acarbose see Antidiabetics

ACE Inhibitors
▸ Alcohol: enhanced hypotensive effect when ACE inhibitors given with ALCOHOL
▸ Aldesleukin: enhanced hypotensive effect when ACE inhibitors given with ALDESLEUKIN
● Aliskiren: increased risk of hyperkalaemia, hypotension, and impaired renal function when ACE inhibitors given with ● ALISKIREN—avoid concomitant use
● Allopurinol: manufacturers state possible increased risk of leucopenia and hypersensitivity reactions when ACE inhibitors given with ALLOPURINOL especially in renal impairment
▸ Alpha-blockers: enhanced hypotensive effect when ACE inhibitors given with ALPHA-BLOCKERS
▸ Anaesthetics, General: enhanced hypotensive effect when ACE inhibitors given with GENERAL ANAESTHETICS
▸ Analgesics: increased risk of renal impairment when ACE inhibitors given with NSAIDs, also hypotensive effect antagonised
● Angiotensin-II Receptor Antagonists: increased risk of hyperkalaemia, hypotension, and impaired renal function when ACE inhibitors given with ● ANGIOTENSIN-II RECEPTOR ANTAGONISTS—avoid concomitant use
▸ Antacids: absorption of ACE inhibitors possibly reduced by ANTACIDS; absorption of captopril, enalapril and fosinopril reduced by ANTACIDS
▸ Antibacterials: plasma concentration of active metabolite of imidapril reduced by RIFAMPICIN (reduced antihypertensive effect); quinapril tablets reduce absorption of TETRACYCLINES (quinapril tablets contain magnesium carbonate); possible increased risk of hyperkalaemia when ACE inhibitors given with TRIMETHOPRIM

ACE Inhibitors (continued)
▸ Anticoagulants: increased risk of hyperkalaemia when ACE inhibitors given with HEPARINS
▸ Antidepressants: hypotensive effect of ACE inhibitors possibly enhanced by MAOIs
▸ Antidiabetics: ACE inhibitors possibly enhance hypoglycaemic effect of INSULIN, METFORMIN and SULFONYLUREAS
▸ Antipsychotics: enhanced hypotensive effect when ACE inhibitors given with ANTIPSYCHOTICS
▸ Anxiolytics and Hypnotics: enhanced hypotensive effect when ACE inhibitors given with ANXIOLYTICS AND HYPNOTICS
▸ Avanafil: hypotensive effect of enalapril possibly enhanced by AVANAFIL
▸ Azathioprine: increased risk of anaemia or leucopenia when captopril given with AZATHIOPRINE especially in renal impairment; increased risk of anaemia when enalapril given with AZATHIOPRINE especially in renal impairment
● Bee Venom Extracts: possible severe anaphylactoid reaction when ACE inhibitors given with ● BEE VENOM EXTRACTS
▸ Beta-blockers: enhanced hypotensive effect when ACE inhibitors given with BETA-BLOCKERS
▸ Calcium-channel Blockers: enhanced hypotensive effect when ACE inhibitors given with CALCIUM-CHANNEL BLOCKERS
▸ Cardiac Glycosides: captopril possibly increases plasma concentration of DIGOXIN
● Ciclosporin: increased risk of hyperkalaemia when ACE inhibitors given with ● CICLOSPORIN
● Clonidine: enhanced hypotensive effect when ACE inhibitors given with CLONIDINE; antihypertensive effect of captopril possibly delayed by previous treatment with CLONIDINE
● Corticosteroids: hypotensive effect of ACE inhibitors antagonised by CORTICOSTEROIDS
● Cytotoxics: increased risk of angioedema when ACE inhibitors given with ● EVEROLIMUS
▸ Diazoxide: enhanced hypotensive effect when ACE inhibitors given with DIAZOXIDE
▸ Diuretics: enhanced hypotensive effect when ACE inhibitors given with ● DIURETICS; increased risk of severe hyperkalaemia when ACE inhibitors given with ● AMILORIDE, ● POTASSIUM CANRENOATE or ● TRIAMTERENE; increased risk of severe hyperkalaemia when ACE inhibitors given with ● EPLERENONE and ● SPIRONOLACTONE—avoid concurrent use or use lowest possible doses of both drugs
● Dopaminergics: enhanced hypotensive effect when ACE inhibitors given with CO-BENELDOPA, CO-CARELDOPA or LEVODOPA
● Lithium: ACE inhibitors reduce excretion of ● LITHIUM (increased plasma concentration)
▸ Methyldopa: enhanced hypotensive effect when ACE inhibitors given with METHYLDOPA
▸ Moxisylyte: enhanced hypotensive effect when ACE inhibitors given with MOXISYLYTE
▸ Moxonidine: enhanced hypotensive effect when ACE inhibitors given with MOXONIDINE
▸ Muscle Relaxants: enhanced hypotensive effect when ACE inhibitors given with BACLOFEN or TIZANIDINE
▸ Nitrates: enhanced hypotensive effect when ACE inhibitors given with NITRATES
▸ Oestrogens: hypotensive effect of ACE inhibitors antagonised by OESTROGENS
● Potassium Salts: increased risk of severe hyperkalaemia when ACE inhibitors given with ● POTASSIUM SALTS
▸ Prostaglandins: enhanced hypotensive effect when ACE inhibitors given with ALPROSTADIL
● Sacubitril: manufacturer of sacubitril advises avoid ACE inhibitors for 36 hours before or after ● SACUBITRIL
● Sodium Aurothiomalate: flushing and hypotension reported when ACE inhibitors given with ● SODIUM AUROTHIOMALATE
▸ Vasodilator Antihypertensives: enhanced hypotensive effect when ACE inhibitors given with HYDRALAZINE, MINOXIDIL or SODIUM NITROPRUSSIDE
● Wasp Venom Extracts: possible severe anaphylactoid reaction when ACE inhibitors given with ● WASP VENOM EXTRACTS

Acebutolol see Beta-blockers
Aceclofenac see NSAIDs
Acemetacin see NSAIDs

Acenocoumarol *see* Coumarins

Acetazolamide *see* Diuretics

Aciclovir

NOTE Interactions do not apply to topical aciclovir preparations

▸ Aminophylline: aciclovir possibly increases plasma concentration of AMINOPHYLLINE

▸ Ciclosporin: increased risk of nephrotoxicity when aciclovir given with CICLOSPORIN

▸ Mycophenolate: plasma concentration of aciclovir increased by MYCOPHENOLATE, also plasma concentration of inactive metabolite of mycophenolate increased

▸ Tacrolimus: possible increased risk of nephrotoxicity when aciclovir given with TACROLIMUS

▸ Theophylline: aciclovir possibly increases plasma concentration of THEOPHYLLINE

Acitretin *see* Retinoids

Aclidinium *see* Antimuscarinics

Acrivastine *see* Antihistamines

Adalimumab

▸ Abatacept: increased risk of side-effects when adalimumab given with ABATACEPT

● Anakinra: avoid concomitant use of adalimumab with ● ANAKINRA

● Antipsychotics: avoid concomitant use of cytotoxics with ● CLOZAPINE (increased risk of agranulocytosis)

● Vaccines: risk of generalised infections when monoclonal antibodies given with live ● VACCINES—avoid concomitant use

Adefovir

▸ Antivirals: avoidance of adefovir advised by manufacturer of TENOFOVIR

▸ Interferons: manufacturer of adefovir advises caution with PEGINTERFERON ALFA

Adenosine

NOTE Possibility of interaction with drugs tending to impair myocardial conduction

▸ Aminophylline: anti-arrhythmic effect of adenosine antagonised by AMINOPHYLLINE—manufacturer of adenosine advises avoid aminophylline for 24 hours before adenosine

▸ Anaesthetics, Local: increased myocardial depression when anti-arrhythmics given with BUPIVACAINE, LEVOBUPIVACAINE, PRILOCAINE or ROPIVACAINE

● Anti-arrhythmics: increased myocardial depression when anti-arrhythmics given with other ● ANTI-ARRHYTHMICS

● Antipsychotics: increased risk of ventricular arrhythmias when anti-arrhythmics that prolong the QT interval given with ● ANTIPSYCHOTICS that prolong the QT interval

▸ Beta-blockers: increased myocardial depression when anti-arrhythmics given with ● BETA-BLOCKERS

▸ Caffeine citrate: anti-arrhythmic effect of adenosine antagonised by CAFFEINE CITRATE—manufacturer of adenosine advises avoid caffeine citrate for at least 12 hours before adenosine

● Dipyridamole: effect of adenosine enhanced and extended by ● DIPYRIDAMOLE (important risk of toxicity)—reduce dose of adenosine, see p. 96

▸ Nicotine: effects of adenosine possibly enhanced by NICOTINE

▸ Theophylline: anti-arrhythmic effect of adenosine antagonised by THEOPHYLLINE—manufacturer of adenosine advises avoid theophylline for 24 hours before adenosine

Adrenaline (epinephrine) *see* Sympathomimetics

Adrenergic Neurone Blockers

▸ Alcohol: enhanced hypotensive effect when adrenergic neurone blockers given with ALCOHOL

▸ Alpha-blockers: enhanced hypotensive effect when adrenergic neurone blockers given with ALPHA-BLOCKERS

● Anaesthetics, General: enhanced hypotensive effect when adrenergic neurone blockers given with ● GENERAL ANAESTHETICS

▸ Analgesics: hypotensive effect of adrenergic neurone blockers antagonised by NSAIDs

▸ Angiotensin-II Receptor Antagonists: enhanced hypotensive effect when adrenergic neurone blockers given with ANGIOTENSIN-II RECEPTOR ANTAGONISTS

Adrenergic Neurone Blockers (continued)

▸ Antidepressants: enhanced hypotensive effect when adrenergic neurone blockers given with MAOIs; hypotensive effect of adrenergic neurone blockers antagonised by TRICYCLICS

▸ Antipsychotics: hypotensive effect of adrenergic neurone blockers antagonised by HALOPERIDOL; hypotensive effect of adrenergic neurone blockers antagonised by higher doses of CHLORPROMAZINE; enhanced hypotensive effect when adrenergic neurone blockers given with PHENOTHIAZINES

▸ Anxiolytics and Hypnotics: enhanced hypotensive effect when adrenergic neurone blockers given with ANXIOLYTICS AND HYPNOTICS

▸ Beta-blockers: enhanced hypotensive effect when adrenergic neurone blockers given with BETA-BLOCKERS

▸ Calcium-channel Blockers: enhanced hypotensive effect when adrenergic neurone blockers given with CALCIUM-CHANNEL BLOCKERS

▸ Clonidine: enhanced hypotensive effect when adrenergic neurone blockers given with CLONIDINE

▸ Corticosteroids: hypotensive effect of adrenergic neurone blockers antagonised by CORTICOSTEROIDS

▸ Diazoxide: enhanced hypotensive effect when adrenergic neurone blockers given with DIAZOXIDE

▸ Diuretics: enhanced hypotensive effect when adrenergic neurone blockers given with DIURETICS

▸ Dopaminergics: enhanced hypotensive effect when adrenergic neurone blockers given with CO-BENELDOPA, CO-CARELDOPA or LEVODOPA

▸ Methyldopa: enhanced hypotensive effect when adrenergic neurone blockers given with METHYLDOPA

▸ Moxisylyte: enhanced hypotensive effect when adrenergic neurone blockers given with MOXISYLYTE

▸ Moxonidine: enhanced hypotensive effect when adrenergic neurone blockers given with MOXONIDINE

▸ Muscle Relaxants: enhanced hypotensive effect when adrenergic neurone blockers given with BACLOFEN or TIZANIDINE

▸ Nitrates: enhanced hypotensive effect when adrenergic neurone blockers given with NITRATES

▸ Oestrogens: hypotensive effect of adrenergic neurone blockers antagonised by OESTROGENS

▸ Pizotifen: hypotensive effect of adrenergic neurone blockers antagonised by PIZOTIFEN

▸ Prostaglandins: enhanced hypotensive effect when adrenergic neurone blockers given with ALPROSTADIL

● Sympathomimetics: increased risk of hypertension when guanethidine given with ● ADRENALINE (EPINEPHRINE); hypotensive effect of guanethidine antagonised by ● DEXAMFETAMINE and ● LISDEXAMFETAMINE; hypotensive effect of adrenergic neurone blockers antagonised by ● EPHEDRINE, ● ISOMETHEPTENE, ● METARAMINOL, ● METHYLPHENIDATE, ● NORADRENALINE (NOREPINEPHRINE), ● OXYMETAZOLINE, ● PHENYLEPHRINE, ● PSEUDOEPHEDRINE and ● XYLOMETAZOLINE; avoidance of guanethidine advised by manufacturer of MIDODRINE

▸ Vasodilator Antihypertensives: enhanced hypotensive effect when adrenergic neurone blockers given with HYDRALAZINE, MINOXIDIL or SODIUM NITROPRUSSIDE

Adsorbents *see* Kaolin

Afatinib

▸ Anti-arrhythmics: plasma concentration of afatinib possibly increased by AMIODARONE—manufacturer of afatinib advises separating administration of amiodarone by 6 to 12 hours

▸ Antibacterials: plasma concentration of afatinib possibly increased by ERYTHROMYCIN—manufacturer of afatinib advises separating administration of erythromycin by 6 to 12 hours; plasma concentration of afatinib reduced by RIFAMPICIN

▸ Antifungals: plasma concentration of afatinib possibly increased by ITRACONAZOLE and KETOCONAZOLE—manufacturer of afatinib advises separating administration of itraconazole and ketoconazole by 6 to 12 hours

● Antipsychotics: avoid concomitant use of cytotoxics with ● CLOZAPINE (increased risk of agranulocytosis)

▸ Antivirals: plasma concentration of afatinib increased by RITONAVIR—manufacturer of afatinib advises separating administration of ritonavir by 6 to 12 hours; plasma

Afatinib

Antivirals (continued)
concentration of afatinib possibly increased by SAQUINAVIR—manufacturer of afatinib advises separating administration of saquinavir by 6 to 12 hours
▸ **Calcium-channel Blockers:** plasma concentration of afatinib possibly increased by VERAPAMIL—manufacturer of afatinib advises separating administration of verapamil by 6 to 12 hours
▸ **Ciclosporin:** plasma concentration of afatinib possibly increased by CICLOSPORIN—manufacturer of afatinib advises separating administration of ciclosporin by 6 to 12 hours
▸ **Tacrolimus:** plasma concentration of afatinib possibly increased by TACROLIMUS—manufacturer of afatinib advises separating administration of tacrolimus by 6 to 12 hours

Agalsidase Alfa and Beta
▸ **Anti-arrhythmics:** effects of agalsidase alfa and beta possibly inhibited by AMIODARONE (manufacturers of agalsidase alfa and beta advise avoid concomitant use)
▸ **Antibacterials:** effects of agalsidase alfa and beta possibly inhibited by GENTAMICIN (manufacturers of agalsidase alfa and beta advise avoid concomitant use)
▸ **Antimalarials:** effects of agalsidase alfa and beta possibly inhibited by CHLOROQUINE and HYDROXYCHLOROQUINE (manufacturers of agalsidase alfa and beta advise avoid concomitant use)

Agomelatine
● **Antibacterials:** manufacturer of agomelatine advises avoid concomitant use with ● CIPROFLOXACIN
● **Antidepressants:** metabolism of agomelatine inhibited by ● FLUVOXAMINE (increased plasma concentration)
● **Antimalarials:** avoidance of antidepressants advised by manufacturer of ● ARTEMETHER WITH LUMEFANTRINE and ● ARTENIMOL WITH PIPERAQUINE
▸ **Atomoxetine:** possible increased risk of convulsions when antidepressants given with ATOMOXETINE

Albendazole
▸ **Anthelmintics:** plasma concentration of both drugs possibly reduced when albendazole given with LEVAMISOLE
● **Antiepileptics:** plasma concentration of albendazole reduced by ● CARBAMAZEPINE, ● FOSPHENYTOIN, ● PHENOBARBITAL, ● PHENYTOIN and ● PRIMIDONE—consider increasing albendazole dose when given for systemic infections
● **Antivirals:** plasma concentration of active metabolite of albendazole reduced by ● RITONAVIR—consider increasing albendazole dose when given for systemic infections
▸ **Corticosteroids:** plasma concentration of active metabolite of albendazole increased by DEXAMETHASONE
▸ **Grapefruit Juice:** plasma concentration of active metabolite of albendazole increased by GRAPEFRUIT JUICE
▸ **Ulcer-healing Drugs:** effects of albendazole possibly enhanced by CIMETIDINE

Albiglutide see Antidiabetics

Alcohol
▸ **ACE Inhibitors:** enhanced hypotensive effect when alcohol given with ACE INHIBITORS
▸ **Adrenergic Neurone Blockers:** enhanced hypotensive effect when alcohol given with ADRENERGIC NEURONE BLOCKERS
▸ **Alpha-blockers:** increased sedative effect when alcohol given with INDORAMIN; enhanced hypotensive effect when alcohol given with ALPHA-BLOCKERS
▸ **Analgesics:** enhanced hypotensive and sedative effects when alcohol given with OPIOID ANALGESICS
▸ **Angiotensin-II Receptor Antagonists:** enhanced hypotensive effect when alcohol given with ANGIOTENSIN-II RECEPTOR ANTAGONISTS
▸ **Anthelmintics:** possibility of disulfiram-like reaction when alcohol given with LEVAMISOLE
● **Antibacterials:** disulfiram-like reaction when alcohol given with METRONIDAZOLE; possibility of disulfiram-like reaction when alcohol given with TINIDAZOLE; increased risk of convulsions when alcohol given with ● CYCLOSERINE
● **Anticoagulants:** major changes in consumption of alcohol may affect anticoagulant control with ● COUMARINS or ● PHENINDIONE

Alcohol (continued)
● **Antidepressants:** some beverages containing alcohol and some dealcoholised beverages contain tyramine which interacts with ● MAOIS (hypertensive crisis)—if no tyramine, enhanced hypotensive effect; sedative effects possibly increased when alcohol given with SSRIS; increased sedative effect when alcohol given with ● MIRTAZAPINE, ●TRICYCLIC-RELATED ANTIDEPRESSANTS or ● TRICYCLICS
▸ **Antidiabetics:** alcohol enhances hypoglycaemic effect of ANTIDIABETICS; increased risk of lactic acidosis when alcohol given with METFORMIN
▸ **Antiepileptics:** alcohol possibly increases CNS side-effects of CARBAMAZEPINE; chronic heavy consumption of alcohol possibly reduces plasma concentration of FOSPHENYTOIN and PHENYTOIN; increased sedative effect when alcohol given with PHENOBARBITAL or PRIMIDONE; increased risk of blurred vision when alcohol given with RETIGABINE
▸ **Antifungals:** possibility of disulfiram-like reaction when alcohol given with KETOCONAZOLE; effects of alcohol possibly enhanced by GRISEOFULVIN
▸ **Antihistamines:** increased sedative effect when alcohol given with ANTIHISTAMINES (possibly less effect with non-sedating antihistamines)
▸ **Antimuscarinics:** increased sedative effect when alcohol given with HYOSCINE
▸ **Antipsychotics:** increased sedative effect when alcohol given with ANTIPSYCHOTICS
▸ **Anxiolytics and Hypnotics:** increased sedative effect when alcohol given with ANXIOLYTICS AND HYPNOTICS
▸ **Avanafil:** possible enhanced hypotensive effect when alcohol given with AVANAFIL
▸ **Beta-blockers:** enhanced hypotensive effect when alcohol given with BETA-BLOCKERS
▸ **Calcium-channel Blockers:** enhanced hypotensive effect when alcohol given with CALCIUM-CHANNEL BLOCKERS; plasma concentration of alcohol possibly increased by VERAPAMIL
▸ **Clonidine:** enhanced hypotensive effect when alcohol given with CLONIDINE
● **Cytotoxics:** disulfiram-like reaction when alcohol given with PROCARBAZINE; avoidance of alcohol advised by manufacturer of ● TRABECTEDIN
● **Dapoxetine:** increased sedative effect when alcohol given with ● DAPOXETINE
▸ **Diazoxide:** enhanced hypotensive effect when alcohol given with DIAZOXIDE
▸ **Disulfiram:** disulfiram reaction when alcohol given with DISULFIRAM
▸ **Diuretics:** enhanced hypotensive effect when alcohol given with DIURETICS
▸ **Dopaminergics:** alcohol reduces tolerance to BROMOCRIPTINE
▸ **Guanfacine:** sedative effects possibly increased when alcohol given with GUANFACINE
▸ **Lipid-regulating Drugs:** avoidance of alcohol advised by manufacturer of LOMITAPIDE
▸ **Lofexidine:** increased sedative effect when alcohol given with LOFEXIDINE
▸ **Methyldopa:** enhanced hypotensive effect when alcohol given with METHYLDOPA
▸ **Metoclopramide:** absorption of alcohol possibly increased by METOCLOPRAMIDE
▸ **Moxonidine:** enhanced hypotensive effect when alcohol given with MOXONIDINE
▸ **Muscle Relaxants:** increased sedative effect when alcohol given with BACLOFEN, METHOCARBAMOL or TIZANIDINE
▸ **Nicorandil:** alcohol possibly enhances hypotensive effect of NICORANDIL
▸ **Nitrates:** enhanced hypotensive effect when alcohol given with NITRATES
● **Paraldehyde:** increased sedative effect when alcohol given with ● PARALDEHYDE
● **Retinoids:** presence of alcohol causes etretinate to be formed from ● ACITRETIN (increased risk of teratogenicity in women of child-bearing potential)
▸ **Sympathomimetics:** alcohol possibly enhances effects of METHYLPHENIDATE

Alcohol (continued)
▸ Vasodilator Antihypertensives: enhanced hypotensive effect when alcohol given with HYDRALAZINE, MINOXIDIL or SODIUM NITROPRUSSIDE

Aldesleukin
▸ ACE Inhibitors: enhanced hypotensive effect when aldesleukin given with ACE INHIBITORS
▸ Alpha-blockers: enhanced hypotensive effect when aldesleukin given with ALPHA-BLOCKERS
▸ Angiotensin-II Receptor Antagonists: enhanced hypotensive effect when aldesleukin given with ANGIOTENSIN-II RECEPTOR ANTAGONISTS
▸ Antivirals: aldesleukin possibly increases plasma concentration of INDINAVIR
▸ Beta-blockers: enhanced hypotensive effect when aldesleukin given with BETA-BLOCKERS
▸ Calcium-channel Blockers: enhanced hypotensive effect when aldesleukin given with CALCIUM-CHANNEL BLOCKERS
▸ Clonidine: enhanced hypotensive effect when aldesleukin given with CLONIDINE
● Corticosteroids: manufacturer of aldesleukin advises avoid concomitant use with ● CORTICOSTEROIDS
● Cytotoxics: manufacturer of aldesleukin advises avoid concomitant use with ● CISPLATIN, ● DACARBAZINE and ● VINBLASTINE
▸ Diazoxide: enhanced hypotensive effect when aldesleukin given with DIAZOXIDE
▸ Diuretics: enhanced hypotensive effect when aldesleukin given with DIURETICS
▸ Methyldopa: enhanced hypotensive effect when aldesleukin given with METHYLDOPA
▸ Moxonidine: enhanced hypotensive effect when aldesleukin given with MOXONIDINE
▸ Nitrates: enhanced hypotensive effect when aldesleukin given with NITRATES
▸ Vasodilator Antihypertensives: enhanced hypotensive effect when aldesleukin given with HYDRALAZINE, MINOXIDIL or SODIUM NITROPRUSSIDE

Alemtuzumab
● Antipsychotics: avoid concomitant use of cytotoxics with ● CLOZAPINE (increased risk of agranulocytosis)
● Vaccines: risk of generalised infections when monoclonal antibodies given with ● VACCINES—avoid concomitant use

Alendronic Acid see Bisphosphonates
Alfacalcidol see Vitamins
Alfentanil see Opioid Analgesics
Alfuzosin see Alpha-blockers
Alimemazine see Antihistamines
Aliskiren
● ACE Inhibitors: increased risk of hyperkalaemia, hypotension, and impaired renal function when aliskiren given with ● ACE INHIBITORS—avoid concomitant use
▸ Analgesics: hypotensive effect of aliskiren possibly antagonised by NSAIDs
● Angiotensin-II Receptor Antagonists: increased risk of hyperkalaemia, hypotension, and impaired renal function when aliskiren given with ● ANGIOTENSIN-II RECEPTOR ANTAGONISTS—avoid concomitant use; plasma concentration of aliskiren possibly reduced by IRBESARTAN
▸ Antibacterials: plasma concentration of aliskiren reduced by RIFAMPICIN
▸ Anticoagulants: increased risk of hyperkalaemia when aliskiren given with HEPARINS
● Antifungals: plasma concentration of aliskiren increased by KETOCONAZOLE; plasma concentration of aliskiren increased by ● ITRACONAZOLE—avoid concomitant use
▸ Calcium-channel Blockers: plasma concentration of aliskiren increased by VERAPAMIL
● Ciclosporin: plasma concentration of aliskiren increased by ● CICLOSPORIN—avoid concomitant use
▸ Diuretics: aliskiren reduces plasma concentration of FUROSEMIDE; increased risk of hyperkalaemia when aliskiren given with POTASSIUM-SPARING DIURETICS AND ALDOSTERONE ANTAGONISTS
● Grapefruit Juice: plasma concentration of aliskiren reduced by ● GRAPEFRUIT JUICE—avoid concomitant use

Aliskiren (continued)
▸ Potassium Salts: increased risk of hyperkalaemia when aliskiren given with POTASSIUM SALTS
Alitretinoin see Retinoids
Alkylating Drugs see Bendamustine, Busulfan, Carmustine, Cyclophosphamide, Estramustine, Ifosfamide, Lomustine, Melphalan, and Thiotepa
Allopurinol
▸ ACE Inhibitors: manufacturers state possible increased risk of leucopenia and hypersensitivity reactions when allopurinol given with ACE INHIBITORS especially in renal impairment
▸ Aminophylline: allopurinol possibly increases plasma concentration of AMINOPHYLLINE
▸ Antibacterials: increased risk of rash when allopurinol given with AMOXICILLIN, AMPICILLIN or CO-AMOXICLAV
▸ Anticoagulants: allopurinol possibly enhances anticoagulant effect of COUMARINS
● Antivirals: allopurinol increases plasma concentration of ● DIDANOSINE (risk of toxicity)—avoid concomitant use
● Azathioprine: allopurinol enhances effects and increases toxicity of ● AZATHIOPRINE (reduce dose of azathioprine to one quarter of usual dose)
▸ Ciclosporin: allopurinol possibly increases plasma concentration of CICLOSPORIN (risk of nephrotoxicity)
● Cytotoxics: avoidance of allopurinol advised by manufacturer of ● CAPECITABINE; allopurinol enhances effects and increases toxicity of ● MERCAPTOPURINE (reduce dose of mercaptopurine to one quarter of usual dose)
▸ Diuretics: increased risk of hypersensitivity when allopurinol given with THIAZIDES AND RELATED DIURETICS especially in renal impairment
▸ Theophylline: allopurinol possibly increases plasma concentration of THEOPHYLLINE
Almotriptan see 5HT$_1$-receptor Agonists (under HT)
Alogliptin see Antidiabetics
Alpha$_2$-adrenoceptor Stimulants see Apraclonidine, Brimonidine, Clonidine, and Methyldopa
Alpha-blockers
▸ ACE Inhibitors: enhanced hypotensive effect when alpha-blockers given with ACE INHIBITORS
▸ Adrenergic Neurone Blockers: enhanced hypotensive effect when alpha-blockers given with ADRENERGIC NEURONE BLOCKERS
▸ Alcohol: enhanced hypotensive effect when alpha-blockers given with ALCOHOL; increased sedative effect when indoramin given with ALCOHOL
▸ Aldesleukin: enhanced hypotensive effect when alpha-blockers given with ALDESLEUKIN
● Anaesthetics, General: enhanced hypotensive effect when alpha-blockers given with ● GENERAL ANAESTHETICS
▸ Analgesics: hypotensive effect of alpha-blockers antagonised by NSAIDs
▸ Angiotensin-II Receptor Antagonists: enhanced hypotensive effect when alpha-blockers given with ANGIOTENSIN-II RECEPTOR ANTAGONISTS
● Antidepressants: manufacturer of indoramin advises avoid concomitant use with ● MAOIs; enhanced hypotensive effect when alpha-blockers given with MAOIs
▸ Antifungals: plasma concentration of alfuzosin possibly increased by KETOCONAZOLE; plasma concentration of tamsulosin increased by KETOCONAZOLE
▸ Antipsychotics: enhanced hypotensive effect when alpha-blockers given with ANTIPSYCHOTICS
● Antivirals: plasma concentration of doxazosin and tamsulosin possibly increased by BOCEPREVIR—manufacturer of boceprevir advises avoid concomitant use; plasma concentration of alfuzosin possibly increased by ● RITONAVIR—avoid concomitant use; avoidance of alfuzosin advised by manufacturer of ● TELAPREVIR
▸ Anxiolytics and Hypnotics: enhanced hypotensive and sedative effects when alpha-blockers given with ANXIOLYTICS AND HYPNOTICS
● Avanafil: enhanced hypotensive effect when alpha-blockers given with ● AVANAFIL—when patient is stable on the alpha blocker initiate avanafil at the lowest possible dose

A1

Interactions | Appendix 1

Alpha-blockers (continued)
- Beta-blockers: enhanced hypotensive effect when alpha-blockers given with ● BETA-BLOCKERS, also increased risk of first-dose hypotension with post-synaptic alpha-blockers such as prazosin
- Calcium-channel Blockers: enhanced hypotensive effect when alpha-blockers given with ● CALCIUM-CHANNEL BLOCKERS, also increased risk of first-dose hypotension with post-synaptic alpha-blockers such as prazosin; plasma concentration of tamsulosin increased by VERAPAMIL
▹ Cardiac Glycosides: prazosin increases plasma concentration of DIGOXIN
▹ Clonidine: enhanced hypotensive effect when alpha-blockers given with CLONIDINE
● Cobicistat: plasma concentration of alfuzosin possibly increased by ● COBICISTAT—manufacturer of cobicistat advises avoid concomitant use
▹ Corticosteroids: hypotensive effect of alpha-blockers antagonised by CORTICOSTEROIDS
▹ Cytotoxics: avoidance of alfuzosin advised by manufacturer of IDELALISIB
▹ Diazoxide: enhanced hypotensive effect when alpha-blockers given with DIAZOXIDE
● Diuretics: enhanced hypotensive effect when alpha-blockers given with ● DIURETICS, also increased risk of first-dose hypotension with post-synaptic alpha-blockers such as prazosin
▹ Dopaminergics: enhanced hypotensive effect when alpha-blockers given with CO-BENELDOPA, CO-CARELDOPA or LEVODOPA
▹ Methyldopa: enhanced hypotensive effect when alpha-blockers given with METHYLDOPA
▹ Moxisylyte: possible severe postural hypotension when alpha-blockers given with ● MOXISYLYTE
▹ Moxonidine: enhanced hypotensive effect when alpha-blockers given with MOXONIDINE
▹ Muscle Relaxants: enhanced hypotensive effect when alpha-blockers given with BACLOFEN or TIZANIDINE
▹ Nitrates: enhanced hypotensive effect when alpha-blockers given with NITRATES
▹ Oestrogens: hypotensive effect of alpha-blockers antagonised by OESTROGENS
▹ Prostaglandins: enhanced hypotensive effect when alpha-blockers given with ALPROSTADIL
● Sildenafil: enhanced hypotensive effect when alpha-blockers given with ● SILDENAFIL (avoid alpha-blockers for 4 hours after sildenafil)—when patient is stable on the alpha blocker initiate sildenafil at the lowest possible dose
● Sympathomimetics: avoid concomitant use of tolazoline with ● ADRENALINE (EPINEPHRINE) or ● DOPAMINE; alpha-blockers possibly antagonise effects of MIDODRINE
● Tadalafil: enhanced hypotensive effect when alpha-blockers given with ● TADALAFIL—when patient is stable on the alpha blocker initiate tadalafil at the lowest possible dose; enhanced hypotensive effect when doxazosin given with ● TADALAFIL—manufacturer of tadalafil advises avoid concomitant use
▹ Ulcer-healing Drugs: effects of tolazoline antagonised by ● CIMETIDINE and ● RANITIDINE
● Vardenafil: enhanced hypotensive effect when alpha-blockers given with ● VARDENAFIL—when patient is stable on the alpha blocker initiate vardenafil at the lowest possible dose—separate doses by 6 hours (except with tamsulosin)
▹ Vasodilator Antihypertensives: enhanced hypotensive effect when alpha-blockers given with HYDRALAZINE, MINOXIDIL or SODIUM NITROPRUSSIDE

Alpha-blockers (post-synaptic) see Alpha-blockers
Alprazolam see Anxiolytics and Hypnotics
Alprostadil see Prostaglandins
Aluminium Hydroxide see Antacids
Amantadine
▹ Antimalarials: plasma concentration of amantadine possibly increased by QUININE
▹ Antipsychotics: increased risk of extrapyramidal side-effects when amantadine given with ANTIPSYCHOTICS
▹ Bupropion: increased risk of side-effects when amantadine given with BUPROPION

Amantadine (continued)
● Memantine: increased risk of CNS toxicity when amantadine given with ● MEMANTINE (manufacturer of memantine advises avoid concomitant use); effects of dopaminergics possibly enhanced by MEMANTINE
▹ Methyldopa: increased risk of extrapyramidal side-effects when amantadine given with METHYLDOPA; antiparkinsonian effect of dopaminergics antagonised by METHYLDOPA
▹ Tetrabenazine: increased risk of extrapyramidal side-effects when amantadine given with TETRABENAZINE
Ambrisentan
▹ Antibacterials: plasma concentration of ambrisentan possibly increased by RIFAMPICIN
● Ciclosporin: plasma concentration of ambrisentan increased by ● CICLOSPORIN (see under Ambrisentan, p. 169)
Amikacin see Aminoglycosides
Amiloride see Diuretics
Aminoglycosides
▹ Agalsidase Alfa and Beta: gentamicin possibly inhibits effects of AGALSIDASE ALFA AND BETA (manufacturers of agalsidase alfa and beta advise avoid concomitant use)
▹ Analgesics: plasma concentration of amikacin and gentamicin in neonates possibly increased by INDOMETACIN
▹ Antibacterials: neomycin reduces absorption of PHENOXYMETHYLPENICILLIN; increased risk of nephrotoxicity when aminoglycosides given with COLISTIMETHATE SODIUM or POLYMYXINS; increased risk of nephrotoxicity and ototoxicity when aminoglycosides given with CAPREOMYCIN or ● VANCOMYCIN; possible increased risk of nephrotoxicity when aminoglycosides given with CEPHALOSPORINS
● Anticoagulants: experience in anticoagulant clinics suggests that INR possibly altered when neomycin (given for local action on gut) is given with ● COUMARINS or ● PHENINDIONE
▹ Antidiabetics: neomycin possibly enhances hypoglycaemic effect of ACARBOSE, also severity of gastro-intestinal effects increased
▹ Antifungals: increased risk of nephrotoxicity when aminoglycosides given with AMPHOTERICIN
▹ Bisphosphonates: increased risk of hypocalcaemia when aminoglycosides given with BISPHOSPHONATES
▹ Cardiac Glycosides: gentamicin possibly increases plasma concentration of DIGOXIN; neomycin reduces absorption of DIGOXIN
● Ciclosporin: increased risk of nephrotoxicity when aminoglycosides given with ● CICLOSPORIN
● Cytotoxics: neomycin possibly reduces absorption of METHOTREXATE; neomycin reduces bioavailability of SORAFENIB; increased risk of nephrotoxicity and possibly of ototoxicity when aminoglycosides given with ● PLATINUM COMPOUNDS
● Diuretics: increased risk of ototoxicity when aminoglycosides given with ● LOOP DIURETICS
▹ Mannitol: manufacturer of tobramycin advises avoid concomitant use with MANNITOL
● Muscle Relaxants: aminoglycosides enhance effects of ● NON-DEPOLARISING MUSCLE RELAXANTS and ● SUXAMETHONIUM
● Parasympathomimetics: aminoglycosides antagonise effects of ● NEOSTIGMINE and ● PYRIDOSTIGMINE
● Tacrolimus: increased risk of nephrotoxicity when aminoglycosides given with ● TACROLIMUS
▹ Vaccines: antibacterials inactivate ORAL TYPHOID VACCINE—see under Typhoid Vaccine in BNF
▹ Vitamins: neomycin possibly reduces absorption of VITAMIN A
Aminophylline
▹ Allopurinol: plasma concentration of aminophylline possibly increased by ALLOPURINOL
▹ Anaesthetics, General: increased risk of convulsions when aminophylline given with KETAMINE
▹ Anti-arrhythmics: aminophylline antagonises anti-arrhythmic effect of ADENOSINE—manufacturer of adenosine advises avoid aminophylline for 24 hours before adenosine; plasma concentration of aminophylline increased by PROPAFENONE
● Antibacterials: plasma concentration of aminophylline possibly increased by CLARITHROMYCIN and ISONIAZID; plasma concentration of aminophylline increased by ● ERYTHROMYCIN (also aminophylline may reduce absorption of *oral*

Aminophylline

- **Antibacterials** (continued)
erythromycin); plasma concentration of aminophylline
increased by ● CIPROFLOXACIN and ● NORFLOXACIN; metabolism
of aminophylline accelerated by RIFAMPICIN (reduced plasma
concentration); possible increased risk of convulsions when
aminophylline given with ● QUINOLONES
- **Antidepressants:** plasma concentration of aminophylline
increased by ● FLUVOXAMINE (concomitant use should usually
be avoided, but where not possible halve aminophylline dose
and monitor plasma-aminophylline concentration); plasma
concentration of aminophylline possibly reduced by ST JOHN'S
WORT
- **Antiepileptics:** metabolism of aminophylline accelerated by
CARBAMAZEPINE, ● PHENOBARBITAL and ● PRIMIDONE (reduced
effect); plasma concentration of both drugs reduced when
aminophylline given with ● FOSPHENYTOIN and ● PHENYTOIN
- **Antifungals:** plasma concentration of aminophylline possibly
increased by ● FLUCONAZOLE and ● KETOCONAZOLE
- **Antivirals:** plasma concentration of aminophylline possibly
increased by ACICLOVIR and VALACICLOVIR; metabolism of
aminophylline accelerated by RITONAVIR (reduced plasma
concentration)
- **Anxiolytics and Hypnotics:** aminophylline possibly reduces
effects of BENZODIAZEPINES
- **Caffeine citrate:** avoidance of aminophylline advised by
manufacturer of CAFFEINE CITRATE
- **Calcium-channel Blockers:** plasma concentration of
aminophylline possibly increased by ● CALCIUM-CHANNEL
BLOCKERS (enhanced effect); plasma concentration of
aminophylline increased by DILTIAZEM; plasma concentration
of aminophylline increased by VERAPAMIL (enhanced effect)
- **Corticosteroids:** increased risk of hypokalaemia when
aminophylline given with CORTICOSTEROIDS
- **Cytotoxics:** plasma concentration of aminophylline possibly
increased by METHOTREXATE
- **Deferasirox:** plasma concentration of aminophylline increased
by ● DEFERASIROX (consider reducing dose of aminophylline)
- **Disulfiram:** metabolism of aminophylline inhibited by
DISULFIRAM (increased risk of toxicity)
- **Diuretics:** increased risk of hypokalaemia when aminophylline
given with ACETAZOLAMIDE, LOOP DIURETICS or THIAZIDES AND
RELATED DIURETICS
- **Doxapram:** increased CNS stimulation when aminophylline
given with DOXAPRAM
- **Interferons:** metabolism of aminophylline inhibited by
● INTERFERON ALFA and ● PEGINTERFERON ALFA (consider
reducing dose of aminophylline)
- **Leukotriene Receptor Antagonists:** plasma concentration of
aminophylline possibly increased by ZAFIRLUKAST, also plasma
concentration of zafirlukast reduced
- **Lithium:** aminophylline increases excretion of LITHIUM
(reduced plasma concentration)
- **Oestrogens:** plasma concentration of aminophylline increased
by OESTROGENS (consider reducing dose of aminophylline)
- **Pentoxifylline:** plasma concentration of aminophylline
increased by PENTOXIFYLLINE
- **Roflumilast:** avoidance of aminophylline advised by
manufacturer of ROFLUMILAST
- **Sulfinpyrazone:** plasma concentration of aminophylline
reduced by SULFINPYRAZONE
- **Sympathomimetics:** manufacturer of aminophylline advises
avoid concomitant use with EPHEDRINE in children
- **Sympathomimetics, Beta₂:** increased risk of hypokalaemia when
aminophylline given with high doses of BETA₂
SYMPATHOMIMETICS
- **Ulcer-healing Drugs:** metabolism of aminophylline inhibited by
● CIMETIDINE (increased plasma concentration); absorption of
aminophylline possibly reduced by SUCRALFATE (give at least
2 hours apart)
- **Vaccines:** plasma concentration of aminophylline possibly
increased by INFLUENZA VACCINE

Aminosalicylates see individual drugs

Amiodarone

NOTE Amiodarone has a long half-life; there is a potential for
drug interactions to occur for several weeks (or even months)
after treatment with it has been stopped
- **Agalsidase Alfa and Beta:** amiodarone possibly inhibits effects
of AGALSIDASE ALFA AND BETA (manufacturers of agalsidase alfa
and beta advise avoid concomitant use)
- **Anaesthetics, Local:** increased myocardial depression when
anti-arrhythmics given with BUPIVACAINE, LEVOBUPIVACAINE,
PRILOCAINE or ROPIVACAINE
- **Anti-arrhythmics:** increased myocardial depression when anti-
arrhythmics given with other ● ANTI-ARRHYTHMICS; increased
risk of ventricular arrhythmias when amiodarone given with
● DISOPYRAMIDE or ● DRONEDARONE—avoid concomitant use;
amiodarone increases plasma concentration of ● FLECAINIDE
(halve dose of flecainide)
- **Antibacterials:** increased risk of ventricular arrhythmias when
amiodarone given with *parenteral* ● ERYTHROMYCIN—avoid
concomitant use; increased risk of ventricular arrhythmias
when amiodarone given with ● LEVOFLOXACIN or
● MOXIFLOXACIN—avoid concomitant use; possible increased
risk of ventricular arrhythmias when amiodarone given with
SULFAMETHOXAZOLE and TRIMETHOPRIM (as co-trimoxazole)—
manufacturer of amiodarone advises avoid concomitant use
of co-trimoxazole; increased risk of ventricular arrhythmias
when amiodarone given with ● DELAMANID; avoidance of
amiodarone advised by manufacturer of FIDAXOMICIN; possible
increased risk of ventricular arrhythmias when amiodarone
given with ● TELITHROMYCIN
- **Anticoagulants:** amiodarone inhibits metabolism of
● COUMARINS and ● PHENINDIONE (enhanced anticoagulant
effect); amiodarone increases plasma concentration of
● DABIGATRAN (see under Dabigatran Etexilate, p. 123)
- **Antidepressants:** avoidance of amiodarone advised by
manufacturer of ● CITALOPRAM, ● ESCITALOPRAM and
● VENLAFAXINE (risk of ventricular arrhythmias); increased risk
of ventricular arrhythmias when amiodarone given with
● TRICYCLICS—avoid concomitant use
- **Antiepileptics:** amiodarone inhibits metabolism of
● FOSPHENYTOIN and ● PHENYTOIN (increased plasma
concentration)
- **Antihistamines:** increased risk of ventricular arrhythmias when
amiodarone given with ● MIZOLASTINE—avoid concomitant use
- **Antimalarials:** avoidance of amiodarone advised by
manufacturer of ● ARTEMETHER WITH LUMEFANTRINE (risk of
ventricular arrhythmias); avoidance of amiodarone advised by
manufacturer of ● ARTENIMOL WITH PIPERAQUINE (possible risk
of ventricular arrhythmias); increased risk of ventricular
arrhythmias when amiodarone given with ● CHLOROQUINE,
● HYDROXYCHLOROQUINE, ● MEFLOQUINE or ● QUININE—avoid
concomitant use
- **Antimuscarinics:** increased risk of ventricular arrhythmias when
amiodarone given with ● TOLTERODINE
- **Antipsychotics:** increased risk of ventricular arrhythmias when
anti-arrhythmics that prolong the QT interval given with
● ANTIPSYCHOTICS that prolong the QT interval; increased risk
of ventricular arrhythmias when amiodarone given with
● BENPERIDOL—manufacturer of benperidol advises avoid
concomitant use; increased risk of ventricular arrhythmias
when amiodarone given with ● AMISULPRIDE, ● DROPERIDOL,
● HALOPERIDOL, ● PHENOTHIAZINES, ● PIMOZIDE or
● ZUCLOPENTHIXOL—avoid concomitant use; increased risk of
ventricular arrhythmias when amiodarone given with
● SULPIRIDE
- **Antivirals:** plasma concentration of amiodarone possibly
increased by ● ATAZANAVIR; possible increased risk of
bradycardia when amiodarone given with ● DACLATASVIR,
● LEDIPASVIR and ● SIMEPREVIR (with sofosbuvir)—see under
Amiodarone, p. 94; plasma concentration of amiodarone
possibly increased by ● FOSAMPRENAVIR (increased risk of
ventricular arrhythmias—avoid concomitant use); plasma
concentration of amiodarone possibly increased by
● INDINAVIR—avoid concomitant use; plasma concentration of
amiodarone increased by ● RITONAVIR (increased risk of
ventricular arrhythmias—avoid concomitant use); increased
risk of ventricular arrhythmias when amiodarone given with

Amiodarone

- **Antivirals** (continued)
  - • SAQUINAVIR—avoid concomitant use; possible increased risk of bradycardia when amiodarone given with • SOFOSBUVIR—see under Amiodarone, p. 94; avoidance of amiodarone advised by manufacturer of • TELAPREVIR (risk of ventricular arrhythmias)
- • **Atomoxetine:** increased risk of ventricular arrhythmias when amiodarone given with • ATOMOXETINE
- • **Beta-blockers:** increased risk of bradycardia, AV block and myocardial depression when amiodarone given with • BETA-BLOCKERS; increased myocardial depression when anti-arrhythmics given with • BETA-BLOCKERS; increased risk of ventricular arrhythmias when amiodarone given with • SOTALOL—avoid concomitant use
- • **Calcium-channel Blockers:** increased risk of bradycardia, AV block and myocardial depression when amiodarone given with • DILTIAZEM or • VERAPAMIL
- • **Cardiac Glycosides:** amiodarone increases plasma concentration of • DIGOXIN (halve dose of digoxin)
- ▹ **Ciclosporin:** amiodarone possibly increases plasma concentration of CICLOSPORIN
- • **Cobicistat:** plasma concentration of amiodarone possibly increased by • COBICISTAT—manufacturer of cobicistat advises avoid concomitant use
- • **Colchicine:** amiodarone possibly increases risk of • COLCHICINE toxicity
- • **Cytotoxics:** amiodarone possibly increases the plasma concentration of AFATINIB—manufacturer of afatinib advises separating administration of amiodarone by 6 to 12 hours; possible increased risk of ventricular arrhythmias when amiodarone given with • BOSUTINIB; amiodarone possibly increases the plasma concentration of • IBRUTINIB—reduce dose of ibrutinib (see under Ibrutinib, p. 855); avoidance of amiodarone advised by manufacturer of • IDELALISIB; possible increased risk of ventricular arrhythmias when amiodarone given with • VANDETANIB—avoid concomitant use; increased risk of ventricular arrhythmias when amiodarone given with • ARSENIC TRIOXIDE
- ▹ **Diuretics:** increased cardiac toxicity with amiodarone if hypokalaemia occurs with ACETAZOLAMIDE, LOOP DIURETICS or THIAZIDES AND RELATED DIURETICS; amiodarone increases plasma concentration of EPLERENONE (reduce dose of eplerenone)
- • **Fingolimod:** possible increased risk of bradycardia when amiodarone given with • FINGOLIMOD
- ▹ **Grapefruit Juice:** plasma concentration of amiodarone increased by GRAPEFRUIT JUICE
- • **Ivabradine:** increased risk of ventricular arrhythmias when amiodarone given with • IVABRADINE
- • **Lipid-regulating Drugs:** increased risk of myopathy when amiodarone given with • SIMVASTATIN (see under Simvastatin, p. 188); separating administration from amiodarone by 12 hours advised by manufacturer of LOMITAPIDE
- • **Lithium:** manufacturer of amiodarone advises avoid concomitant use with • LITHIUM (risk of ventricular arrhythmias)
- ▹ **Orlistat:** plasma concentration of amiodarone possibly reduced by ORLISTAT
- • **Pentamidine Isetionate:** increased risk of ventricular arrhythmias when amiodarone given with • PENTAMIDINE ISETIONATE—avoid concomitant use
- ▹ **Tacrolimus:** amiodarone possibly increases plasma concentration of TACROLIMUS
- ▹ **Thyroid Hormones:** amiodarone can affect serum concentrations of THYROID HORMONES—monitor thyroid function closely
- ▹ **Ulcer-healing Drugs:** plasma concentration of amiodarone increased by CIMETIDINE

Amisulpride see Antipsychotics

Amitriptyline see Antidepressants, Tricyclic

Amlodipine see Calcium-channel Blockers

Amoxicillin see Penicillins

Amphotericin

NOTE Close monitoring required with concomitant administration of nephrotoxic drugs or cytotoxics

Amphotericin (continued)

- ▹ **Antibacterials:** increased risk of nephrotoxicity when amphotericin given with AMINOGLYCOSIDES or POLYMYXINS; possible increased risk of nephrotoxicity when amphotericin given with VANCOMYCIN
- ▹ **Antifungals:** amphotericin reduces renal excretion and increases cellular uptake of FLUCYTOSINE (toxicity possibly increased); effects of amphotericin possibly antagonised by IMIDAZOLES and TRIAZOLES; plasma concentration of amphotericin possibly increased by MICAFUNGIN
- • **Cardiac Glycosides:** hypokalaemia caused by amphotericin increases cardiac toxicity with • CARDIAC GLYCOSIDES
- • **Ciclosporin:** increased risk of nephrotoxicity when amphotericin given with • CICLOSPORIN
- • **Corticosteroids:** increased risk of hypokalaemia when amphotericin given with • CORTICOSTEROIDS—avoid concomitant use unless corticosteroids needed to control reactions
- • **Cytotoxics:** increased risk of ventricular arrhythmias when amphotericin given with • ARSENIC TRIOXIDE
- ▹ **Diuretics:** increased risk of hypokalaemia when amphotericin given with LOOP DIURETICS or THIAZIDES AND RELATED DIURETICS
- ▹ **Pentamidine Isetionate:** possible increased risk of nephrotoxicity when amphotericin given with PENTAMIDINE ISETIONATE
- • **Sodium Stibogluconate:** possible increased risk of arrhythmias when amphotericin given after • SODIUM STIBOGLUCONATE—manufacturer of sodium stibogluconate advises giving 14 days apart
- • **Tacrolimus:** increased risk of nephrotoxicity when amphotericin given with • TACROLIMUS

Ampicillin see Penicillins

Anabolic Steroids

- • **Anticoagulants:** anabolic steroids enhance anticoagulant effect of • COUMARINS and • PHENINDIONE
- • **Antidiabetics:** anabolic steroids possibly enhance hypoglycaemic effect of ANTIDIABETICS

Anaesthetics, General

NOTE See also Surgery and Long-term Medication, under General Anaesthesia in BNF

- ▹ **ACE Inhibitors:** enhanced hypotensive effect when general anaesthetics given with ACE INHIBITORS
- • **Adrenergic Neurone Blockers:** enhanced hypotensive effect when general anaesthetics given with • ADRENERGIC NEURONE BLOCKERS
- • **Alpha-blockers:** enhanced hypotensive effect when general anaesthetics given with • ALPHA-BLOCKERS
- ▹ **Aminophylline:** increased risk of convulsions when ketamine given with AMINOPHYLLINE
- ▹ **Analgesics:** metabolism of etomidate inhibited by FENTANYL (consider reducing dose of etomidate); effects of thiopental possibly enhanced by ASPIRIN; effects of intravenous general anaesthetics and volatile liquid general anaesthetics possibly enhanced by OPIOID ANALGESICS
- ▹ **Angiotensin-II Receptor Antagonists:** enhanced hypotensive effect when general anaesthetics given with ANGIOTENSIN-II RECEPTOR ANTAGONISTS
- ▹ **Antibacterials:** increased risk of hepatotoxicity when isoflurane given with ISONIAZID; effects of thiopental enhanced by SULFONAMIDES; hypersensitivity-like reactions can occur when general anaesthetics given with *intravenous* VANCOMYCIN
- ▹ **Antidepressants:** increased risk of arrhythmias and hypotension when general anaesthetics given with TRICYCLICS
- • **Antipsychotics:** enhanced hypotensive effect when general anaesthetics given with • ANTIPSYCHOTICS; effects of thiopental enhanced by DROPERIDOL
- ▹ **Anxiolytics and Hypnotics:** increased sedative effect when general anaesthetics given with ANXIOLYTICS AND HYPNOTICS
- ▹ **Beta-blockers:** enhanced hypotensive effect when general anaesthetics given with BETA-BLOCKERS
- • **Calcium-channel Blockers:** enhanced hypotensive effect when general anaesthetics or isoflurane given with CALCIUM-CHANNEL BLOCKERS; general anaesthetics enhance hypotensive effect of • VERAPAMIL (also AV delay)
- ▹ **Clonidine:** enhanced hypotensive effect when general anaesthetics given with CLONIDINE

Anaesthetics, General (continued)

- Cytotoxics: nitrous oxide increases antifolate effect of ● METHOTREXATE—avoid concomitant use
- ▸ Diazoxide: enhanced hypotensive effect when general anaesthetics given with DIAZOXIDE
- ▸ Diuretics: enhanced hypotensive effect when general anaesthetics given with DIURETICS
- Dopaminergics: increased risk of arrhythmias when volatile liquid general anaesthetics given with ● CO-BENELDOPA, ● CO-CARELDOPA or ● LEVODOPA
- Doxapram: increased risk of arrhythmias when volatile liquid general anaesthetics given with ● DOXAPRAM (avoid doxapram for at least 10 minutes after volatile liquid general anaesthetics)
- Memantine: increased risk of CNS toxicity when ketamine given with ● MEMANTINE (manufacturer of memantine advises avoid concomitant use)
- ▸ Methyldopa: enhanced hypotensive effect when general anaesthetics given with METHYLDOPA
- ▸ Metoclopramide: effects of thiopental enhanced by METOCLOPRAMIDE
- ▸ Moxonidine: enhanced hypotensive effect when general anaesthetics given with MOXONIDINE
- Muscle Relaxants: increased risk of myocardial depression and bradycardia when propofol given with ● SUXAMETHONIUM; volatile liquid general anaesthetics enhance effects of NON-DEPOLARISING MUSCLE RELAXANTS and SUXAMETHONIUM; ketamine enhances effects of ATRACURIUM
- ▸ Nitrates: enhanced hypotensive effect when general anaesthetics given with NITRATES
- ▸ Oxytocin: oxytocic effect possibly reduced, also enhanced hypotensive effect and risk of arrhythmias when volatile liquid general anaesthetics given with OXYTOCIN
- Sympathomimetics: manufacturer of isoflurane advises avoid concomitant use with ● SYMPATHOMIMETICS (risk of ventricular arrhythmias); increased risk of arrhythmias when volatile liquid general anaesthetics given with ● ADRENALINE (EPINEPHRINE) or ● NORADRENALINE (NOREPINEPHRINE); increased risk of hypertension when volatile liquid general anaesthetics given with ● METHYLPHENIDATE
- ▸ Theophylline: increased risk of convulsions when ketamine given with THEOPHYLLINE
- ▸ Vasodilator Antihypertensives: enhanced hypotensive effect when general anaesthetics given with HYDRALAZINE, MINOXIDIL or SODIUM NITROPRUSSIDE

Anaesthetics, General (intravenous) *see* Anaesthetics, General

Anaesthetics, General (volatile liquids) *see* Anaesthetics, General

Anaesthetics, Local *see* Bupivacaine, Chloroprocaine, Levobupivacaine, Lidocaine, Prilocaine, and Ropivacaine

Anagrelide

- Cilostazol: manufacturer of anagrelide advises avoid concomitant use with ● CILOSTAZOL
- Phosphodiesterase Type-3 Inhibitors: manufacturer of anagrelide advises avoid concomitant use with ● ENOXIMONE and ● MILRINONE

Anakinra

- Cytotoxics: avoid concomitant use of anakinra with ● ADALIMUMAB, ● CERTOLIZUMAB PEGOL, ● GOLIMUMAB or ● INFLIXIMAB
- Etanercept: avoid concomitant use of anakinra with ● ETANERCEPT
- Vaccines: risk of generalised infections when anakinra given with live ● VACCINES—avoid concomitant use

Analgesics *see* Aspirin, Nefopam, NSAIDs, Opioid Analgesics, and Paracetamol

Angiotensin-II Receptor Antagonists

- ACE Inhibitors: increased risk of hyperkalaemia, hypotension, and impaired renal function when angiotensin-II receptor antagonists given with ● ACE INHIBITORS—avoid concomitant use
- Adrenergic Neurone Blockers: enhanced hypotensive effect when angiotensin-II receptor antagonists given with ADRENERGIC NEURONE BLOCKERS
- Alcohol: enhanced hypotensive effect when angiotensin-II receptor antagonists given with ALCOHOL

Angiotensin-II Receptor Antagonists (continued)

- ▸ Aldesleukin: enhanced hypotensive effect when angiotensin-II receptor antagonists given with ALDESLEUKIN
- Aliskiren: increased risk of hyperkalaemia, hypotension, and impaired renal function when angiotensin-II receptor antagonists given with ● ALISKIREN—avoid concomitant use; irbesartan possibly reduces plasma concentration of ALISKIREN
- ▸ Alpha-blockers: enhanced hypotensive effect when angiotensin-II receptor antagonists given with ALPHA-BLOCKERS
- ▸ Anaesthetics, General: enhanced hypotensive effect when angiotensin-II receptor antagonists given with GENERAL ANAESTHETICS
- ▸ Analgesics: increased risk of renal impairment when angiotensin-II receptor antagonists given with NSAIDs, also hypotensive effect antagonised
- ▸ Antibacterials: plasma concentration of losartan and its active metabolite reduced by RIFAMPICIN; possible increased risk of hyperkalaemia when angiotensin-II receptor antagonists given with TRIMETHOPRIM
- ▸ Anticoagulants: increased risk of hyperkalaemia when angiotensin-II receptor antagonists given with HEPARINS
- ▸ Antidepressants: hypotensive effect of angiotensin-II receptor antagonists possibly enhanced by MAOIs
- ▸ Antipsychotics: enhanced hypotensive effect when angiotensin-II receptor antagonists given with ANTIPSYCHOTICS
- ▸ Antivirals: when given with valsartan manufacturer of PARITAPREVIR advises reduce dose of paritaprevir
- ▸ Anxiolytics and Hypnotics: enhanced hypotensive effect when angiotensin-II receptor antagonists given with ANXIOLYTICS AND HYPNOTICS
- ▸ Beta-blockers: enhanced hypotensive effect when angiotensin-II receptor antagonists given with BETA-BLOCKERS
- ▸ Calcium-channel Blockers: enhanced hypotensive effect when angiotensin-II receptor antagonists given with CALCIUM-CHANNEL BLOCKERS
- ▸ Ciclosporin: increased risk of hyperkalaemia when angiotensin-II receptor antagonists given with ● CICLOSPORIN
- ▸ Clonidine: enhanced hypotensive effect when angiotensin-II receptor antagonists given with CLONIDINE
- ▸ Corticosteroids: hypotensive effect of angiotensin-II receptor antagonists antagonised by CORTICOSTEROIDS
- ▸ Diazoxide: enhanced hypotensive effect when angiotensin-II receptor antagonists given with DIAZOXIDE
- ▸ Diuretics: enhanced hypotensive effect when angiotensin-II receptor antagonists given with ● DIURETICS; valsartan reduces plasma concentration of FUROSEMIDE; increased risk of severe hyperkalaemia when angiotensin-II receptor antagonists given with ● AMILORIDE, ● POTASSIUM CANRENOATE or ● TRIAMTERENE; increased risk of severe hyperkalaemia when angiotensin-II receptor antagonists given with ● EPLERENONE and ● SPIRONOLACTONE—avoid concurrent use or use lowest possible doses of both drugs
- ▸ Dopaminergics: enhanced hypotensive effect when angiotensin-II receptor antagonists given with CO-BENELDOPA, CO-CARELDOPA or LEVODOPA
- ▸ Lithium: angiotensin-II receptor antagonists reduce excretion of ● LITHIUM (increased plasma concentration)
- ▸ Methyldopa: enhanced hypotensive effect when angiotensin-II receptor antagonists given with METHYLDOPA
- ▸ Moxisylyte: enhanced hypotensive effect when angiotensin-II receptor antagonists given with MOXISYLYTE
- ▸ Moxonidine: enhanced hypotensive effect when angiotensin-II receptor antagonists given with MOXONIDINE
- ▸ Muscle Relaxants: enhanced hypotensive effect when angiotensin-II receptor antagonists given with BACLOFEN or TIZANIDINE
- ▸ Nitrates: enhanced hypotensive effect when angiotensin-II receptor antagonists given with NITRATES
- ▸ Oestrogens: hypotensive effect of angiotensin-II receptor antagonists antagonised by OESTROGENS
- Potassium Salts: increased risk of hyperkalaemia when angiotensin-II receptor antagonists given with ● POTASSIUM SALTS
- ▸ Prostaglandins: enhanced hypotensive effect when angiotensin-II receptor antagonists given with ALPROSTADIL

Angiotensin-II Receptor Antagonists (continued)
▸ Tacrolimus: increased risk of hyperkalaemia when angiotensin-II receptor antagonists given with TACROLIMUS
▸ Vasodilator Antihypertensives: enhanced hypotensive effect when angiotensin-II receptor antagonists given with HYDRALAZINE, MINOXIDIL or SODIUM NITROPRUSSIDE

Antacids
NOTE Antacids should preferably not be taken at the same time as other drugs since they may impair absorption
▸ ACE Inhibitors: antacids possibly reduce absorption of ACE INHIBITORS; antacids reduce absorption of CAPTOPRIL, ENALAPRIL and FOSINOPRIL
▸ Analgesics: antacids possibly reduce absorption of ACEMETACIN; alkaline urine due to some antacids increases excretion of ASPIRIN
▸ Anthelmintics: sodium bicarbonate reduces excretion of DIETHYLCARBAMAZINE
▸ Antibacterials: antacids reduce absorption of CEFACLOR, ISONIAZID, NORFLOXACIN and RIFAMPICIN; antacids reduce absorption of AZITHROMYCIN (give at least 2 hours before or 1 hour after antacids); antacids reduce absorption of CIPROFLOXACIN and LEVOFLOXACIN (give at least 2 hours before or 4 hours after ciprofloxacin and levofloxacin); antacids reduce absorption of MOXIFLOXACIN (give at least 6 hours apart); antacids reduce absorption of OFLOXACIN (give at least 2 hours apart); avoid concomitant use of antacids with METHENAMINE; oral magnesium salts (as magnesium trisilicate) reduce absorption of NITROFURANTOIN; antacids possibly reduce absorption of TETRACYCLINES (give at least 2 to 3 hours apart)
▸ Antiepileptics: antacids reduce absorption of FOSPHENYTOIN, GABAPENTIN and PHENYTOIN
▸ Antifungals: antacids reduce absorption of ITRACONAZOLE and KETOCONAZOLE
▸ Antihistamines: antacids reduce absorption of FEXOFENADINE
▸ Antimalarials: antacids reduce absorption of CHLOROQUINE and HYDROXYCHLOROQUINE; oral magnesium salts (as magnesium trisilicate) reduce absorption of PROGUANIL
▸ Antipsychotics: antacids reduce absorption of PHENOTHIAZINES and SULPIRIDE
▸ Antivirals: antacids reduce absorption of ATAZANAVIR (give at least 2 hours before or 1 hour after antacids); aluminium hydroxide reduces absorption of DOLUTEGRAVIR—manufacturer of dolutegravir advises give at least 2 hours before or 6 hours after aluminium hydroxide; oral magnesium salts reduce absorption of DOLUTEGRAVIR—manufacturer of dolutegravir advises give at least 2 hours before or 6 hours after oral magnesium salts; aluminium hydroxide reduces absorption of ELVITEGRAVIR (give at least 4 hours apart); oral magnesium salts reduce absorption of ELVITEGRAVIR (give at least 4 hours apart); separating administration from antacids by 4 hours advised by manufacturer of LEDIPASVIR; oral magnesium salts reduce plasma concentration of RALTEGRAVIR—manufacturer of raltegravir advises avoid concomitant use; aluminium hydroxide reduces plasma concentration of RALTEGRAVIR—manufacturer of raltegravir advises avoid concomitant use; manufacturer of rilpivirine advises give antacids 2 hours before or 4 hours after RILPIVIRINE; antacids reduce absorption of TIPRANAVIR (give at least 2 hours apart)
▸ Bile Acids: antacids possibly reduce absorption of BILE ACIDS; aluminium hydroxide probably reduces effects of CHOLIC ACID (manufacturer of cholic acid advises give at least 5 hours apart)
▸ Bisphosphonates: antacids reduce absorption of BISPHOSPHONATES
▸ Cardiac Glycosides: antacids possibly reduce absorption of DIGOXIN
▸ Corticosteroids: antacids reduce absorption of DEFLAZACORT
● Cytotoxics: aluminium hydroxide and oral magnesium salts possibly reduce absorption of ESTRAMUSTINE—manufacturer of estramustine advises avoid concomitant administration; separating administration with antacids by about 12 hours advised by manufacturer of BOSUTINIB; antacids possibly reduce plasma concentration of ● ERLOTINIB—give antacids at least 4 hours before or 2 hours after erlotinib

Antacids (continued)
▸ Deferasirox: antacids containing aluminium possibly reduce absorption of DEFERASIROX (manufacturer of deferasirox advises avoid concomitant use)
▸ Deferiprone: antacids containing aluminium possibly reduce absorption of DEFERIPRONE (manufacturer of deferiprone advises avoid concomitant use)
▸ Dipyridamole: antacids possibly reduce absorption of DIPYRIDAMOLE
▸ Eltrombopag: antacids reduce absorption of ELTROMBOPAG (give at least 4 hours apart)
▸ Folates: antacids possibly reduce absorption of FOLIC ACID (manufacturer of folic acid advises give at least 2 hours apart)
▸ Iron Salts: oral magnesium salts (as magnesium trisilicate) reduce absorption of *oral* IRON SALTS
▸ Lipid-regulating Drugs: antacids reduce absorption of ROSUVASTATIN
▸ Lithium: sodium bicarbonate increases excretion of LITHIUM (reduced plasma concentration)
▸ Misoprostol: antacids possibly reduce absorption of MISOPROSTOL
▸ Mycophenolate: antacids reduce absorption of MYCOPHENOLATE
▸ Penicillamine: antacids reduce absorption of PENICILLAMINE
▸ Polystyrene Sulfonate Resins: risk of intestinal obstruction when aluminium hydroxide given with POLYSTYRENE SULFONATE RESINS; risk of metabolic alkalosis when oral magnesium salts given with POLYSTYRENE SULFONATE RESINS
▸ Riociguat: antacids reduce absorption of RIOCIGUAT (give at least 2 hours before or 1 hour after riociguat)
▸ Sympathomimetics: aluminium hydroxide possibly increases absorption of PSEUDOEPHEDRINE
▸ Thyroid Hormones: antacids possibly reduce absorption of LEVOTHYROXINE
▸ Ulcer-healing Drugs: antacids possibly reduce absorption of LANSOPRAZOLE

Antazoline *see* Antihistamines
Anthelmintics *see* individual drugs
Anthrax Vaccine *see* Vaccines
Anti-D Immunoglobulins *see* Immunoglobulins
Anti-arrhythmics *see* Adenosine, Amiodarone, Disopyramide, Dronedarone, Flecainide, Lidocaine, and Propafenone
Antibacterials *see* individual drugs
Antibiotics (cytotoxic) *see* Bleomycin, Daunorubicin, Doxorubicin, Epirubicin, Idarubicin, Mitomycin, Mitoxantrone, and Pixantrone
Anticoagulants *see* Apixaban, Argatroban, Bivalirudin, Coumarins, Dabigatran, Danaparoid, Edoxaban, Fondaparinux, Heparins, Phenindione, and Rivaroxaban
Antidepressants *see* Agomelatine; Antidepressants, SSRI; Antidepressants, Tricyclic; Antidepressants, Tricyclic (related); MAOIs; Mirtazapine; Moclobemide; Reboxetine; St John's Wort; Venlafaxine; Vortioxetine
Antidepressants, Noradrenaline Re-uptake Inhibitors *see* Reboxetine
Antidepressants, SSRI
NOTE *see also* Dapoxetine
▸ Alcohol: sedative effects possibly increased when SSRIs given with ALCOHOL
● Aminophylline: fluvoxamine increases plasma concentration of ● AMINOPHYLLINE (concomitant use should usually be avoided, but where not possible halve aminophylline dose and monitor plasma-aminophylline concentration)
▸ Anaesthetics, Local: fluvoxamine inhibits metabolism of ROPIVACAINE—avoid prolonged administration of ropivacaine
▸ Analgesics: increased risk of bleeding when SSRIs given with ● NSAIDS or ● ASPIRIN; possible increased serotonergic effects when SSRIs given with FENTANYL; fluoxetine, fluvoxamine, paroxetine and sertraline increase plasma concentration of METHADONE; increased risk of CNS toxicity when SSRIs given with ● TRAMADOL
● Anti-arrhythmics: manufacturer of citalopram and escitalopram advises avoid concomitant use with ● AMIODARONE (risk of ventricular arrhythmias); manufacturer of citalopram and escitalopram advises avoid concomitant use with ● DISOPYRAMIDE (risk of ventricular arrhythmias); manufacturer of citalopram and escitalopram advises avoid

Antidepressants, SSRI
- **Anti-arrhythmics** (continued)
  concomitant use with ● DRONEDARONE (risk of ventricular arrhythmias); fluoxetine increases plasma concentration of FLECAINIDE; fluoxetine and paroxetine possibly inhibit metabolism of PROPAFENONE
- **Antibacterials:** manufacturer of citalopram and escitalopram advises avoid concomitant use with *intravenous* ● ERYTHROMYCIN (risk of ventricular arrhythmias); manufacturer of citalopram and escitalopram advises avoid concomitant use with ● MOXIFLOXACIN (risk of ventricular arrhythmias); possible increased risk of ventricular arrhythmias when citalopram given with ● TELITHROMYCIN
- **Anticoagulants:** SSRIs possibly enhance anticoagulant effect of ● COUMARINS; possible increased risk of bleeding when SSRIs given with ● DABIGATRAN
- **Antidepressants:** avoidance of fluvoxamine advised by manufacturer of ● REBOXETINE; possible increased serotonergic effects when SSRIs given with DULOXETINE; fluvoxamine inhibits metabolism of ● DULOXETINE—avoid concomitant use; citalopram, escitalopram, fluvoxamine, paroxetine or sertraline should not be started until 2 weeks after stopping ● MAOIS, also MAOIs should not be started until at least 1 week after stopping citalopram, escitalopram, fluvoxamine, paroxetine or sertraline; fluoxetine should not be started until 2 weeks after stopping ● MAOIS, also MAOIs should not be started until at least 5 weeks after stopping fluoxetine; CNS effects of SSRIs increased by ● MAOIS (risk of serious toxicity); increased risk of CNS toxicity when escitalopram given with ● MOCLOBEMIDE, preferably avoid concomitant use; after stopping citalopram, fluvoxamine, paroxetine or sertraline do not start ● MOCLOBEMIDE for at least 1 week; after stopping fluoxetine do not start ● MOCLOBEMIDE for 5 weeks; increased serotonergic effects when SSRIs given with ● ST JOHN'S WORT—avoid concomitant use; fluvoxamine inhibits metabolism of ● AGOMELATINE (increased plasma concentration); possible increased serotonergic effects when fluoxetine or fluvoxamine given with MIRTAZAPINE; SSRIs increase plasma concentration of some ● TRICYCLICS; manufacturer of citalopram and escitalopram advises avoid concomitant use with ● TRICYCLICS (risk of ventricular arrhythmias); possible increased risk of convulsions when SSRIs given with ● VORTIOXETINE; fluoxetine and paroxetine possibly increase plasma concentration of VORTIOXETINE (consider reducing dose of vortioxetine)
- **Antiepileptics:** SSRIs antagonise anticonvulsant effect of ● ANTIEPILEPTICS (convulsive threshold lowered); fluoxetine and fluvoxamine increase plasma concentration of ● CARBAMAZEPINE; fluoxetine and fluvoxamine increase plasma concentration of ● FOSPHENYTOIN; plasma concentration of sertraline possibly reduced by FOSPHENYTOIN and PHENYTOIN, also plasma concentration of fosphenytoin and phenytoin possibly increased; plasma concentration of paroxetine reduced by FOSPHENYTOIN, PHENOBARBITAL, PHENYTOIN and PRIMIDONE; fluoxetine and fluvoxamine increase plasma concentration of ● PHENYTOIN
- ▸ **Antifungals:** plasma concentration of paroxetine possibly increased by TERBINAFINE
- **Antihistamines:** manufacturer of citalopram and escitalopram advises avoid concomitant use with ● MIZOLASTINE (risk of ventricular arrhythmias); antidepressant effect of SSRIs possibly antagonised by CYPROHEPTADINE
- **Antimalarials:** avoidance of antidepressants advised by manufacturer of ● ARTEMETHER WITH LUMEFANTRINE and ● ARTENIMOL WITH PIPERAQUINE; possible increased risk of ventricular arrhythmias when citalopram or escitalopram given with ● ARTEMETHER WITH LUMEFANTRINE—avoid concomitant use; possible increased risk of ventricular arrhythmias when citalopram or escitalopram given with ● ARTENIMOL WITH PIPERAQUINE—avoid concomitant use; possible increased risk of ventricular arrhythmias when citalopram and escitalopram given with ● CHLOROQUINE; possible increased risk of ventricular arrhythmias when citalopram or escitalopram given with ● QUININE—avoid concomitant use

Antidepressants, SSRI (continued)
- ▸ **Antimuscarinics:** paroxetine increases plasma concentration of DARIFENACIN and PROCYCLIDINE
- **Antipsychotics:** avoidance of fluoxetine, fluvoxamine and sertraline advised by manufacturer of ● DROPERIDOL (risk of ventricular arrhythmias); manufacturer of citalopram and escitalopram advises avoid concomitant use with ● HALOPERIDOL (risk of ventricular arrhythmias); fluoxetine increases plasma concentration of ● CLOZAPINE, ● HALOPERIDOL and RISPERIDONE; fluvoxamine possibly increases plasma concentration of ASENAPINE and HALOPERIDOL; paroxetine inhibits metabolism of PERPHENAZINE (reduce dose of perphenazine); fluoxetine and paroxetine possibly increase plasma concentration of ● ARIPIPRAZOLE (reduce dose of aripiprazole—consult aripiprazole product literature); plasma concentration of paroxetine possibly increased by ASENAPINE; fluvoxamine, paroxetine and sertraline increase plasma concentration of ● CLOZAPINE; citalopram possibly increases plasma concentration of CLOZAPINE (increased risk of toxicity); fluvoxamine increases plasma concentration of OLANZAPINE; manufacturer of citalopram and escitalopram advises avoid concomitant use with ● PHENOTHIAZINES (risk of ventricular arrhythmias); manufacturer of citalopram and escitalopram advises avoid concomitant use with ● PIMOZIDE (risk of ventricular arrhythmias); SSRIs possibly increase plasma concentration of ● PIMOZIDE (increased risk of ventricular arrhythmias—avoid concomitant use); paroxetine possibly increases plasma concentration of RISPERIDONE (increased risk of toxicity)
- **Antivirals:** plasma concentration of paroxetine and sertraline possibly reduced by DARUNAVIR; plasma concentration of SSRIs possibly increased by RITONAVIR; plasma concentration of paroxetine possibly reduced by RITONAVIR
- **Anxiolytics and Hypnotics:** fluoxetine increases plasma concentration of ALPRAZOLAM; fluvoxamine increases plasma concentration of some BENZODIAZEPINES; fluvoxamine increases plasma concentration of ● MELATONIN—avoid concomitant use; sedative effects possibly increased when sertraline given with ZOLPIDEM
- ▸ **Atomoxetine:** possible increased risk of convulsions when antidepressants given with ATOMOXETINE; fluoxetine and paroxetine possibly inhibit metabolism of ATOMOXETINE
- **Beta-blockers:** citalopram and escitalopram increase plasma concentration of METOPROLOL; paroxetine possibly increases the plasma concentration of ● METOPROLOL—increased risk of AV block (manufacturer of paroxetine advises avoid concomitant use in cardiac insufficiency); fluvoxamine increases plasma concentration of PROPRANOLOL; increased risk of ventricular arrhythmias when citalopram given with ● SOTALOL—avoid concomitant use; manufacturer of escitalopram advises avoid concomitant use with ● SOTALOL (risk of ventricular arrhythmias)
- ▸ **Bupropion:** plasma concentration of citalopram possibly increased by BUPROPION
- ▸ **Calcium-channel Blockers:** fluoxetine possibly inhibits metabolism of NIFEDIPINE (increased plasma concentration)
- **Clopidogrel:** fluoxetine and fluvoxamine possibly reduce antiplatelet effect of ● CLOPIDOGREL
- **Dapoxetine:** possible increased risk of serotonergic effects when SSRIs given with ● DAPOXETINE (manufacturer of dapoxetine advises SSRIs should not be started until 1 week after stopping dapoxetine, avoid dapoxetine for 2 weeks after stopping SSRIs)
- **Dopaminergics:** increased risk of CNS toxicity when SSRIs given with ● RASAGILINE; fluvoxamine should not be started until 2 weeks after stopping ● RASAGILINE; fluoxetine should not be started until 2 weeks after stopping ● RASAGILINE, also rasagiline should not be started until at least 5 weeks after stopping fluoxetine; avoidance of citalopram and escitalopram advised by manufacturer of ● SELEGILINE; increased risk of hypertension and CNS excitation when fluvoxamine or sertraline given with ● SELEGILINE (selegiline should not be started until 1 week after stopping fluvoxamine or sertraline, avoid fluvoxamine or sertraline for 2 weeks after stopping selegiline); increased risk of hypertension and CNS excitation when paroxetine given with ● SELEGILINE (selegiline

Antidepressants, SSRI

- **Dopaminergics** (continued)
  should not be started until 2 weeks after stopping paroxetine, avoid paroxetine for 2 weeks after stopping selegiline; increased risk of hypertension and CNS excitation when fluoxetine given with • SELEGILINE (selegiline should not be started until 5 weeks after stopping fluoxetine, avoid fluoxetine for 2 weeks after stopping selegiline)
- ▸ **Grapefruit Juice**: plasma concentration of sertraline possibly increased by GRAPEFRUIT JUICE
- **Hormone Antagonists**: fluoxetine and paroxetine possibly inhibit metabolism of • TAMOXIFEN to active metabolite (avoid concomitant use)
- **5HT₁-receptor Agonists**: increased risk of CNS toxicity when citalopram given with • 5HT₁ AGONISTS (manufacturer of citalopram advises avoid concomitant use); fluvoxamine inhibits the metabolism of FROVATRIPTAN; possible increased serotonergic effects when SSRIs given with NARATRIPTAN; CNS toxicity reported when sertraline given with SUMATRIPTAN; increased risk of CNS toxicity when citalopram, escitalopram, fluoxetine, fluvoxamine or paroxetine given with • SUMATRIPTAN; fluvoxamine possibly inhibits metabolism of ZOLMITRIPTAN (reduce dose of zolmitriptan)
- ▸ **5HT₃-receptor Antagonists**: possible increased serotonergic effects when SSRIs given with 5HT₃ ANTAGONISTS
- ▸ **Lipid-regulating Drugs**: separating administration from fluoxetine and fluvoxamine by 12 hours advised by manufacturer of LOMITAPIDE
- **Lithium**: Increased risk of CNS effects when SSRIs given with • LITHIUM (lithium toxicity reported)
- **Methylthioninium**: risk of CNS toxicity when SSRIs given with • METHYLTHIONINIUM—avoid concomitant use (if avoidance not possible, use lowest possible dose of methylthioninium and observe patient for up to 4 hours after administration)
- ▸ **Metoclopramide**: CNS toxicity reported when SSRIs given with METOCLOPRAMIDE
- **Muscle Relaxants**: fluvoxamine increases plasma concentration of • TIZANIDINE (increased risk of toxicity)—avoid concomitant use
- ▸ **Parasympathomimetics**: paroxetine increases plasma concentration of GALANTAMINE
- **Pentamidine Isetionate**: manufacturer of citalopram and escitalopram advises avoid concomitant use with • PENTAMIDINE ISETIONATE (risk of ventricular arrhythmias)
- ▸ **Pirfenidone**: fluvoxamine increases plasma concentration of • PIRFENIDONE—manufacturer of pirfenidone advises avoid concomitant use
- ▸ **Pomalidomide**: fluvoxamine increases plasma concentration of • POMALIDOMIDE
- ▸ **Ranolazine**: paroxetine increases plasma concentration of RANOLAZINE
- ▸ **Roflumilast**: fluvoxamine inhibits the metabolism of ROFLUMILAST
- ▸ **Sympathomimetics**: metabolism of SSRIs possibly inhibited by METHYLPHENIDATE
- **Theophylline**: fluvoxamine increases plasma concentration of • THEOPHYLLINE (concomitant use should usually be avoided, but where not possible halve theophylline dose and monitor plasma-theophylline concentration)
- ▸ **Ticagrelor**: possible increased risk of bleeding when citalopram, paroxetine or sertraline given with TICAGRELOR
- ▸ **Ulcer-healing Drugs**: plasma concentration of citalopram, escitalopram and sertraline increased by CIMETIDINE; fluvoxamine possibly increases plasma concentration of LANSOPRAZOLE; plasma concentration of escitalopram increased by OMEPRAZOLE

Antidepressants, SSRI (related) *see* Duloxetine and Venlafaxine

Antidepressants, Tricyclic

- ▸ **Adrenergic Neurone Blockers**: tricyclics antagonise hypotensive effect of ADRENERGIC NEURONE BLOCKERS
- **Alcohol**: increased sedative effect when tricyclics given with • ALCOHOL
- ▸ **Alpha₂-adrenoceptor Stimulants**: avoidance of tricyclics advised by manufacturer of APRACLONIDINE and BRIMONIDINE
- ▸ **Anaesthetics, General**: increased risk of arrhythmias and hypotension when tricyclics given with GENERAL ANAESTHETICS

Antidepressants, Tricyclic (continued)

- **Analgesics**: increased risk of CNS toxicity when tricyclics given with • TRAMADOL; side-effects possibly increased when tricyclics given with NEFOPAM; sedative effects possibly increased when tricyclics given with OPIOID ANALGESICS
- **Anti-arrhythmics**: increased risk of ventricular arrhythmias when tricyclics given with • AMIODARONE—avoid concomitant use; increased risk of ventricular arrhythmias when tricyclics given with • DISOPYRAMIDE or • FLECAINIDE; avoidance of tricyclics advised by manufacturer of • DRONEDARONE (risk of ventricular arrhythmias); increased risk of arrhythmias when tricyclics given with • PROPAFENONE
- **Antibacterials**: increased risk of ventricular arrhythmias when tricyclics given with • MOXIFLOXACIN—avoid concomitant use; possible increased risk of ventricular arrhythmias when tricyclics that prolong the QT interval given with • DELAMANID; possible increased risk of ventricular arrhythmias when tricyclics given with • TELITHROMYCIN
- **Anticoagulants**: tricyclics may enhance or reduce anticoagulant effect of • COUMARINS
- **Antidepressants**: avoidance of tricyclics advised by manufacturer of • CITALOPRAM and • ESCITALOPRAM (risk of ventricular arrhythmias); possible increased serotonergic effects when amitriptyline or clomipramine given with DULOXETINE; increased risk of hypertension and CNS excitation when tricyclics given with • MAOIs, tricyclics should not be started until 2 weeks after stopping MAOIs (3 weeks if starting clomipramine or imipramine), also MAOIs should not be started for at least 1–2 weeks after stopping tricyclics (3 weeks in the case of clomipramine or imipramine); after stopping tricyclics do not start • MOCLOBEMIDE for at least 1 week; plasma concentration of some tricyclics increased by • SSRIs; plasma concentration of amitriptyline reduced by ST JOHN'S WORT; possible increased risk of convulsions when tricyclics given with • VORTIOXETINE
- **Antiepileptics**: tricyclics antagonise anticonvulsant effect of • ANTIEPILEPTICS (convulsive threshold lowered); metabolism of tricyclics accelerated by • CARBAMAZEPINE (reduced plasma concentration and reduced effect); plasma concentration of tricyclics possibly reduced by • FOSPHENYTOIN and • PHENYTOIN; metabolism of tricyclics possibly accelerated by • PHENOBARBITAL and • PRIMIDONE (reduced plasma concentration)
- ▸ **Antifungals**: plasma concentration of amitriptyline and nortriptyline possibly increased by FLUCONAZOLE; plasma concentration of tricyclics possibly increased by TERBINAFINE
- ▸ **Antihistamines**: increased antimuscarinic and sedative effects when tricyclics given with ANTIHISTAMINES
- **Antimalarials**: avoidance of antidepressants advised by manufacturer of • ARTEMETHER WITH LUMEFANTRINE and • ARTENIMOL WITH PIPERAQUINE
- ▸ **Antimuscarinics**: increased risk of antimuscarinic side-effects when tricyclics given with ANTIMUSCARINICS
- **Antipsychotics**: avoidance of tricyclics advised by manufacturer of • DROPERIDOL, • FLUPHENAZINE, • HALOPERIDOL, • SULPIRIDE and • ZUCLOPENTHIXOL (risk of ventricular arrhythmias); possible increased antimuscarinic side-effects when tricyclics given with CLOZAPINE; increased risk of antimuscarinic side-effects when tricyclics given with PHENOTHIAZINES; possible increased risk of ventricular arrhythmias when tricyclics given with • RISPERIDONE
- **Antivirals**: plasma concentration of tricyclics possibly increased by • RITONAVIR; increased risk of ventricular arrhythmias when tricyclics given with • SAQUINAVIR—avoid concomitant use
- ▸ **Anxiolytics and Hypnotics**: increased sedative effect when tricyclics given with ANXIOLYTICS AND HYPNOTICS
- **Atomoxetine**: increased risk of ventricular arrhythmias when tricyclics given with • ATOMOXETINE; possible increased risk of convulsions when antidepressants given with ATOMOXETINE
- **Beta-blockers**: plasma concentration of imipramine increased by LABETALOL and PROPRANOLOL; increased risk of ventricular arrhythmias when tricyclics given with • SOTALOL
- ▸ **Bupropion**: plasma concentration of tricyclics possibly increased by BUPROPION (possible increased risk of convulsions)

Antidepressants, Tricyclic (continued)

▸ Calcium-channel Blockers: plasma concentration of imipramine increased by DILTIAZEM and VERAPAMIL; plasma concentration of tricyclics possibly increased by DILTIAZEM and VERAPAMIL

▸ Cannabis Extract: possible increased risk of hypertension and tachycardia when tricyclics given with CANNABIS EXTRACT

● Clonidine: tricyclics antagonise hypotensive effect of ● CLONIDINE, also increased risk of hypertension on clonidine withdrawal

● Cytotoxics: increased risk of ventricular arrhythmias when amitriptyline or clomipramine given with ● ARSENIC TRIOXIDE

● Dapoxetine: possible increased risk of serotonergic effects when tricyclics given with ● DAPOXETINE (manufacturer of dapoxetine advises tricyclics should not be started until 1 week after stopping dapoxetine, avoid dapoxetine for 2 weeks after stopping tricyclics)

▸ Disulfiram: metabolism of tricyclics inhibited by DISULFIRAM (increased plasma concentration); concomitant amitriptyline reported to increase DISULFIRAM reaction with alcohol

▸ Diuretics: increased risk of postural hypotension when tricyclics given with DIURETICS

● Dopaminergics: caution with tricyclics advised by manufacturer of ENTACAPONE; increased risk of CNS toxicity when tricyclics given with ● RASAGILINE; CNS toxicity reported when tricyclics given with ● SELEGILINE

▸ Histamine: tricyclics theoretically antagonise effects of HISTAMINE—manufacturer of histamine advises avoid concomitant use

● Lithium: risk of toxicity when tricyclics given with LITHIUM

● Methylthioninium: risk of CNS toxicity when clomipramine given with ● METHYLTHIONINIUM—avoid concomitant use (if avoidance not possible, use lowest possible dose of methylthioninium and observe patient for up to 4 hours after administration)

▸ Moxonidine: tricyclics possibly antagonise hypotensive effect of MOXONIDINE (manufacturer of moxonidine advises avoid concomitant use)

▸ Muscle Relaxants: tricyclics enhance muscle relaxant effect of BACLOFEN

▸ Nicorandil: tricyclics possibly enhance hypotensive effect of NICORANDIL

▸ Nitrates: tricyclics reduce effects of sublingual tablets of NITRATES (failure to dissolve under tongue owing to dry mouth)

▸ Oestrogens: antidepressant effect of tricyclics antagonised by OESTROGENS (but side-effects of tricyclics possibly increased due to increased plasma concentration)

● Pentamidine Isetionate: increased risk of ventricular arrhythmias when tricyclics given with ● PENTAMIDINE ISETIONATE

▸ Sodium Oxybate: increased risk of side-effects when tricyclics given with SODIUM OXYBATE

● Sympathomimetics: increased risk of hypertension and arrhythmias when tricyclics given with ● ADRENALINE (EPINEPHRINE) (but local anaesthetics with adrenaline appear to be safe); metabolism of tricyclics possibly inhibited by METHYLPHENIDATE; avoidance of tricyclics advised by manufacturer of MIDODRINE; increased risk of hypertension and arrhythmias when tricyclics given with ● NORADRENALINE (NOREPINEPHRINE) or PHENYLEPHRINE

▸ Thyroid Hormones: effects of tricyclics possibly enhanced by THYROID HORMONES; effects of amitriptyline and imipramine enhanced by THYROID HORMONES

▸ Ulcer-healing Drugs: plasma concentration of tricyclics possibly increased by CIMETIDINE; metabolism of amitriptyline, doxepin, imipramine and nortriptyline inhibited by CIMETIDINE (increased plasma concentration)

Antidepressants, Tricyclic (related)

● Alcohol: increased sedative effect when tricyclic-related antidepressants given with ● ALCOHOL

▸ Alpha₂-adrenoceptor Stimulants: avoidance of tricyclic-related antidepressants advised by manufacturer of APRACLONIDINE and BRIMONIDINE

● Antibacterials: plasma concentration of trazodone possibly increased by CLARITHROMYCIN

Antidepressants, Tricyclic (related) (continued)

▸ Anticoagulants: trazodone may enhance or reduce anticoagulant effect of WARFARIN

● Antidepressants: tricyclic-related antidepressants should not be started until 2 weeks after stopping ● MAOIS, also MAOIs should not be started until at least 1–2 weeks after stopping tricyclic-related antidepressants; after stopping tricyclic-related antidepressants do not start ● MOCLOBEMIDE for at least 1 week

● Antiepileptics: tricyclic-related antidepressants possibly antagonise anticonvulsant effect of ● ANTIEPILEPTICS (convulsive threshold lowered); plasma concentration of mianserin and trazodone reduced by ● CARBAMAZEPINE; plasma concentration of mianserin reduced by ● FOSPHENYTOIN and ● PHENYTOIN; metabolism of mianserin accelerated by ● PHENOBARBITAL and ● PRIMIDONE (reduced plasma concentration)

▸ Antihistamines: possible increased antimuscarinic and sedative effects when tricyclic-related antidepressants given with ANTIHISTAMINES

● Antimalarials: avoidance of antidepressants advised by manufacturer of ● ARTEMETHER WITH LUMEFANTRINE and ● ARTENIMOL WITH PIPERAQUINE

▸ Antimuscarinics: possible increased antimuscarinic side-effects when tricyclic-related antidepressants given with ANTIMUSCARINICS

● Antivirals: plasma concentration of trazodone increased by ● RITONAVIR (increased risk of toxicity); increased risk of ventricular arrhythmias when trazodone given with ● SAQUINAVIR—avoid concomitant use; plasma concentration of trazodone possibly increased by TELAPREVIR

▸ Anxiolytics and Hypnotics: increased sedative effect when tricyclic-related antidepressants given with ANXIOLYTICS AND HYPNOTICS

▸ Atomoxetine: possible increased risk of convulsions when antidepressants given with ATOMOXETINE

▸ Diazoxide: enhanced hypotensive effect when tricyclic-related antidepressants given with DIAZOXIDE

▸ Nitrates: tricyclic-related antidepressants possibly reduce effects of sublingual tablets of NITRATES (failure to dissolve under tongue owing to dry mouth)

▸ Vasodilator Antihypertensives: enhanced hypotensive effect when tricyclic-related antidepressants given with HYDRALAZINE or SODIUM NITROPRUSSIDE

Antidiabetics

NOTE Other drugs administered orally may need to be taken at least 1 hour before or 4 hours after lixisenatide injection, or taken with a meal when lixisenatide is not administered, to minimise possible interference with absorption

NOTE Other drugs administered orally may need to be taken at least 1 hour before or 4 hours after exenatide injection, or taken with a meal when exenatide is not administered, to minimise possible interference with absorption

▸ ACE Inhibitors: hypoglycaemic effect of insulin, metformin and sulfonylureas possibly enhanced by ACE INHIBITORS

▸ Alcohol: hypoglycaemic effect of antidiabetics enhanced by ALCOHOL; increased risk of lactic acidosis when metformin given with ALCOHOL

▸ Anabolic Steroids: hypoglycaemic effect of antidiabetics possibly enhanced by ANABOLIC STEROIDS

● Analgesics: effects of sulfonylureas possibly enhanced by ● NSAIDS; lixisenatide possibly reduces the absorption of PARACETAMOL when given 1 to 4 hours before paracetamol

▸ Anti-arrhythmics: hypoglycaemic effect of gliclazide, insulin and metformin possibly enhanced by DISOPYRAMIDE

● Antibacterials: hypoglycaemic effect of acarbose possibly enhanced by NEOMYCIN, also severity of gastro-intestinal effects increased; effects of repaglinide enhanced by CLARITHROMYCIN; effects of glibenclamide possibly enhanced by NORFLOXACIN; plasma concentration of canagliflozin and nateglinide reduced by ● RIFAMPICIN; effects of linagliptin possibly reduced by RIFAMPICIN; hypoglycaemic effect of repaglinide possibly antagonised by RIFAMPICIN; effects of sulfonylureas enhanced by ● CHLORAMPHENICOL; metabolism of sulfonylureas possibly accelerated by ● RIFAMYCINS (reduced effect); metabolism of tolbutamide accelerated by

Antidiabetics

- **Antibacterials** (continued)
  - RIFAMYCINS (reduced effect); effects of sulfonylureas rarely enhanced by SULFONAMIDES and TRIMETHOPRIM; hypoglycaemic effect of sulfonylureas possibly enhanced by TETRACYCLINES; hypoglycaemic effect of repaglinide possibly enhanced by TRIMETHOPRIM—manufacturer advises avoid concomitant use
- **Anticoagulants:** exenatide possibly enhances anticoagulant effect of WARFARIN; hypoglycaemic effect of sulfonylureas possibly enhanced by • COUMARINS, also possible changes to anticoagulant effect
- **Antidepressants:** hypoglycaemic effect of antidiabetics possibly enhanced by MAOIs; hypoglycaemic effect of insulin, metformin and sulfonylureas enhanced by MAOIs
- **Antidiabetics:** manufacturer of dapagliflozin advises avoid concomitant use with PIOGLITAZONE; plasma concentration of dulaglutide increased by SITAGLIPTIN
- **Antiepileptics:** tolbutamide transiently increases plasma concentration of FOSPHENYTOIN and PHENYTOIN (possibility of toxicity); plasma concentration of glibenclamide possibly reduced by TOPIRAMATE; plasma concentration of metformin possibly increased by TOPIRAMATE
- **Antifungals:** plasma concentration of pioglitazone, saxagliptin and tolbutamide increased by KETOCONAZOLE; plasma concentration of sulfonylureas increased by • FLUCONAZOLE and • MICONAZOLE; hypoglycaemic effect of gliclazide and glipizide enhanced by MICONAZOLE—avoid concomitant use; hypoglycaemic effect of nateglinide possibly enhanced by FLUCONAZOLE; hypoglycaemic effect of repaglinide possibly enhanced by ITRACONAZOLE; hypoglycaemic effect of glipizide possibly enhanced by POSACONAZOLE; plasma concentration of sulfonylureas possibly increased by VORICONAZOLE
- **Antihistamines:** thrombocyte count depressed when metformin given with KETOTIFEN (manufacturer of ketotifen advises avoid concomitant use)
- **Antipsychotics:** hypoglycaemic effect of sulfonylureas possibly antagonised by PHENOTHIAZINES
- **Antivirals:** plasma concentration of metformin increased by DOLUTEGRAVIR—consider reducing dose of metformin; plasma concentration of tolbutamide possibly increased by RITONAVIR; plasma concentration of metformin increased by TELAPREVIR (consider reducing dose of metformin)
- **Aprepitant:** plasma concentration of tolbutamide reduced by APREPITANT
- **Beta-blockers:** warning signs of hypoglycaemia (such as tremor) with antidiabetics may be masked when given with BETA-BLOCKERS; hypoglycaemic effect of insulin enhanced by BETA-BLOCKERS
- **Bosentan:** increased risk of hepatotoxicity when glibenclamide given with • BOSENTAN—avoid concomitant use
- **Calcium-channel Blockers:** glucose tolerance occasionally impaired when insulin given with NIFEDIPINE
- **Cardiac Glycosides:** canagliflozin and sitagliptin increase plasma concentration of DIGOXIN; acarbose possibly reduces plasma concentration of DIGOXIN
- **Ciclosporin:** hypoglycaemic effect of repaglinide possibly enhanced by CICLOSPORIN
- **Corticosteroids:** hypoglycaemic effect of antidiabetics antagonised by CORTICOSTEROIDS
- **Cytotoxics:** avoidance of repaglinide advised by manufacturer of • LAPATINIB; plasma concentration of metformin possibly increased by VANDETANIB (consider reducing dose of metformin)
- **Deferasirox:** plasma concentration of repaglinide increased by DEFERASIROX
- **Diazoxide:** hypoglycaemic effect of antidiabetics antagonised by DIAZOXIDE
- **Diuretics:** canagliflozin possibly enhances diuretic effect of DIURETICS; hypoglycaemic effect of antidiabetics antagonised by LOOP DIURETICS and THIAZIDES AND RELATED DIURETICS; dapagliflozin possibly enhances diuretic effect of LOOP DIURETICS and THIAZIDES AND RELATED DIURETICS; manufacturer of canagliflozin advises avoid concomitant use with LOOP DIURETICS

Antidiabetics (continued)

- **Fosaprepitant:** plasma concentration of tolbutamide reduced by FOSAPREPITANT
- **Hormone Antagonists:** requirements for antidiabetics possibly reduced by LANREOTIDE, OCTREOTIDE and PASIREOTIDE
- **Leflunomide:** hypoglycaemic effect of tolbutamide possibly enhanced by LEFLUNOMIDE
- **Lipid-regulating Drugs:** absorption of glibenclamide and glipizide reduced by COLESEVELAM; absorption of glimepiride reduced by COLESEVELAM—manufacturer of glimepiride advises give at least 4 hours before colesevelam; hypoglycaemic effect of acarbose possibly enhanced by COLESTYRAMINE; hypoglycaemic effect of nateglinide possibly enhanced by GEMFIBROZIL; increased risk of severe hypoglycaemia when repaglinide given with • GEMFIBROZIL—avoid concomitant use; plasma concentration of glibenclamide possibly increased by FLUVASTATIN; manufacturer of canagliflozin advises give at least 1 hour before or 4–6 hours after BILE ACID SEQUESTRANTS; may be improved glucose tolerance and an additive effect when insulin or sulfonylureas given with FIBRATES; separating administration from linagliptin by 12 hours advised by manufacturer of LOMITAPIDE
- **Oestrogens:** hypoglycaemic effect of antidiabetics antagonised by OESTROGENS
- **Orlistat:** avoidance of acarbose advised by manufacturer of ORLISTAT
- **Pancreatin:** hypoglycaemic effect of acarbose antagonised by PANCREATIN
- **Progestogens:** hypoglycaemic effect of antidiabetics antagonised by PROGESTOGENS
- **Sulfinpyrazone:** effects of sulfonylureas enhanced by • SULFINPYRAZONE
- **Teriflunomide:** plasma concentration of repaglinide increased by TERIFLUNOMIDE
- **Testosterone:** hypoglycaemic effect of antidiabetics possibly enhanced by TESTOSTERONE
- **Ulcer-healing Drugs:** excretion of metformin reduced by CIMETIDINE (increased plasma concentration); hypoglycaemic effect of sulfonylureas enhanced by CIMETIDINE

Antiepileptics see Carbamazepine, Eslicarbazepine, Ethosuximide, Fosphenytoin, Gabapentin, Lacosamide, Lamotrigine, Levetiracetam, Oxcarbazepine, Perampanel, Phenobarbital, Phenytoin, Pregabalin, Primidone, Retigabine, Rufinamide, Sodium valproate, Stiripentol, Tiagabine, Topiramate, Valproic acid, Vigabatrin, and Zonisamide

Antifungals see Amphotericin; Antifungals, Imidazole; Antifungals, Triazole; Caspofungin; Flucytosine; Griseofulvin; Micafungin; Terbinafine

Antifungals, Imidazole

- **Alcohol:** possibility of disulfiram-like reaction when ketoconazole given with ALCOHOL
- **Aliskiren:** ketoconazole increases plasma concentration of ALISKIREN
- **Alpha-blockers:** ketoconazole possibly increases plasma concentration of ALFUZOSIN; ketoconazole increases plasma concentration of • TAMSULOSIN
- **Aminophylline:** ketoconazole possibly increases plasma concentration of • AMINOPHYLLINE
- **Analgesics:** ketoconazole inhibits metabolism of • BUPRENORPHINE (reduce dose of buprenorphine); possible increased risk of ventricular arrhythmias when ketoconazole given with • METHADONE—manufacturer of ketoconazole advises avoid concomitant use; ketoconazole increases plasma concentration of OXYCODONE; manufacturer of ketoconazole advises avoid concomitant use with PARACETAMOL
- **Antacids:** absorption of ketoconazole reduced by ANTACIDS
- **Anthelmintics:** ketoconazole increases plasma concentration of PRAZIQUANTEL
- **Anti-arrhythmics:** increased risk of ventricular arrhythmias when ketoconazole given with • DISOPYRAMIDE—avoid concomitant use; ketoconazole increases plasma concentration of • DRONEDARONE—avoid concomitant use
- **Antibacterials:** manufacturer of ketoconazole advises avoid concomitant • CLARITHROMYCIN in severe renal impairment;

Antifungals, Imidazole
- **Antibacterials** (continued)
  metabolism of ketoconazole accelerated by ● RIFAMPICIN (reduced plasma concentration), also plasma concentration of rifampicin may be reduced by ketoconazole; ketoconazole increases plasma concentration of BEDAQUILINE—avoid concomitant use if ketoconazole given for more than 14 days; avoidance of ketoconazole advised by manufacturer of FIDAXOMICIN; plasma concentration of ketoconazole possibly reduced by ISONIAZID; ketoconazole increases the plasma concentration of ● TELITHROMYCIN—avoid in severe renal and hepatic impairment
- **Anticoagulants:** ketoconazole increases plasma concentration of ● APIXABAN—manufacturer of apixaban advises avoid concomitant use; miconazole (including oral gel and possibly vaginal and topical formulations) greatly enhances the anticoagulant effect of ● COUMARINS—avoid concomitant use if possible; ketoconazole enhances anticoagulant effect of ● COUMARINS; ketoconazole increases plasma concentration of ● DABIGATRAN and ● RIVAROXABAN—avoid concomitant use; ketoconazole increases plasma concentration of ● EDOXABAN (reduce dose of edoxaban—see under Edoxaban, p. 113)
- **Antidepressants:** avoidance of imidazoles advised by manufacturer of ● REBOXETINE; ketoconazole increases plasma concentration of MIRTAZAPINE
- **Antidiabetics:** miconazole enhances hypoglycaemic effect of ● GLICLAZIDE and ● GLIPIZIDE—avoid concomitant use; ketoconazole increases plasma concentration of PIOGLITAZONE, SAXAGLIPTIN and TOLBUTAMIDE; miconazole increases plasma concentration of ● SULFONYLUREAS
- **Antiepileptics:** miconazole possibly increases plasma concentration of CARBAMAZEPINE; plasma concentration of ketoconazole possibly reduced by CARBAMAZEPINE, also plasma concentration of carbamazepine possibly increased; plasma concentration of ketoconazole reduced by ● FOSPHENYTOIN and ● PHENYTOIN; miconazole enhances anticonvulsant effect of ● FOSPHENYTOIN and ● PHENYTOIN (plasma concentration of fosphenytoin and phenytoin increased); ketoconazole increases plasma concentration of PERAMPANEL
- ▸ **Antifungals:** imidazoles possibly antagonise effects of AMPHOTERICIN
- **Antihistamines:** imidazoles possibly inhibit metabolism of ● MIZOLASTINE (avoid concomitant use)
- **Antimalarials:** avoidance of imidazoles advised by manufacturer of ● ARTEMETHER WITH LUMEFANTRINE; avoidance of imidazoles advised by manufacturer of ● ARTENIMOL WITH PIPERAQUINE (possible risk of ventricular arrhythmias); ketoconazole increases plasma concentration of MEFLOQUINE
- **Antimuscarinics:** absorption of ketoconazole reduced by ANTIMUSCARINICS; ketoconazole increases plasma concentration of DARIFENACIN—avoid concomitant use; manufacturer of fesoterodine advises dose reduction when ketoconazole given with FESOTERODINE—consult fesoterodine product literature; ketoconazole increases plasma concentration of ● OXYBUTYNIN; ketoconazole increases plasma concentration of ● SOLIFENACIN—see under Solifenacin, p. 705; avoidance of ketoconazole advised by manufacturer of ● TOLTERODINE
- **Antipsychotics:** ketoconazole inhibits metabolism of ● ARIPIPRAZOLE (reduce dose of aripiprazole); ketoconazole increases plasma concentration of ● LURASIDONE—avoid concomitant use; increased risk of ventricular arrhythmias when imidazoles given with ● PIMOZIDE—avoid concomitant use; imidazoles possibly increase plasma concentration of ● QUETIAPINE—manufacturer of quetiapine advises avoid concomitant use
- **Antivirals:** ketoconazole increases plasma concentration of ● BOCEPREVIR; ketoconazole increases the plasma concentration of ● DACLATASVIR—reduce dose of daclatasvir (see under Daclatasvir, p. 568); plasma concentration of both drugs increased when ketoconazole given with DARUNAVIR; plasma concentration of both drugs increased when ketoconazole given with ● DASABUVIR and ● PARITAPREVIR—avoid concomitant use; plasma concentration of ketoconazole reduced by ● EFAVIRENZ; plasma concentration of

Antifungals, Imidazole
- **Antivirals** (continued)
  ketoconazole increased by FOSAMPRENAVIR (also plasma concentration of fosamprenavir possibly increased); ketoconazole increases plasma concentration of ● INDINAVIR and ● MARAVIROC (consider reducing dose of indinavir and maraviroc); plasma concentration of ketoconazole reduced by ● NEVIRAPINE—avoid concomitant use; avoidance of ketoconazole advised by manufacturer of OMBITASVIR and ● SIMEPREVIR; plasma concentration of ketoconazole increased by ● RITONAVIR (reduce dose of ketoconazole); imidazoles possibly increase plasma concentration of SAQUINAVIR; ketoconazole increases plasma concentration of ● SAQUINAVIR—manufacturer of ketoconazole advises avoid concomitant use; plasma concentration of both drugs possibly increased when ketoconazole given with TELAPREVIR (increased risk of ventricular arrhythmias)—reduce dose of ketoconazole
- **Anxiolytics and Hypnotics:** ketoconazole increases plasma concentration of ● ALPRAZOLAM—manufacturer of ketoconazole advises avoid concomitant use; ketoconazole increases plasma concentration of ● MIDAZOLAM (risk of prolonged sedation—avoid concomitant use of *oral* midazolam); ketoconazole increases plasma concentration of ZOLPIDEM
- ▸ **Aprepitant:** ketoconazole increases plasma concentration of APREPITANT
- **Avanafil:** ketoconazole increases plasma concentration of ● AVANAFIL—avoid concomitant use
- ▸ **Beta-blockers:** ketoconazole possibly increases plasma concentration of NADOLOL
- ▸ **Bosentan:** ketoconazole increases plasma concentration of BOSENTAN
- **Calcium-channel Blockers:** ketoconazole inhibits metabolism of ● FELODIPINE (increased plasma concentration)—manufacturer of ketoconazole advises avoid concomitant use; avoidance of ketoconazole advised by manufacturer of LERCANIDIPINE; ketoconazole possibly inhibits metabolism of DIHYDROPYRIDINES (increased plasma concentration)
- ▸ **Cannabis Extract:** ketoconazole increases plasma concentration of CANNABIS EXTRACT
- **Ciclosporin:** ketoconazole inhibits metabolism of ● CICLOSPORIN (increased plasma concentration); miconazole possibly inhibits metabolism of ● CICLOSPORIN (increased plasma concentration)
- **Cilostazol:** ketoconazole increases plasma concentration of ● CILOSTAZOL (see under Cilostazol, p. 215)
- ▸ **Cinacalcet:** ketoconazole inhibits metabolism of CINACALCET (increased plasma concentration)
- **Clopidogrel:** ketoconazole possibly reduces antiplatelet effect of ● CLOPIDOGREL
- ▸ **Cobicistat:** plasma concentration of ketoconazole possibly increased by COBICISTAT—manufacturer of cobicistat advises reduce dose of ketoconazole
- **Colchicine:** ketoconazole possibly increases risk of ● COLCHICINE toxicity—suspend or reduce dose of colchicine (avoid concomitant use in hepatic or renal impairment)
- **Corticosteroids:** ketoconazole possibly inhibits metabolism of CORTICOSTEROIDS; ketoconazole increases the plasma concentration of *inhaled* and *oral* (and possibly also *intranasal* and *rectal*) ● BUDESONIDE; ketoconazole increases plasma concentration of active metabolite of ● CICLESONIDE; ketoconazole possibly increases plasma concentration of *inhaled* FLUTICASONE; ketoconazole inhibits the metabolism of METHYLPREDNISOLONE; ketoconazole increases plasma concentration of *inhaled* MOMETASONE
- **Cytotoxics:** ketoconazole inhibits the metabolism of IFOSFAMIDE; possible increased risk of neutropenia when ketoconazole given with ● BRENTUXIMAB VEDOTIN; ketoconazole possibly increases the plasma concentration of AFATINIB—manufacturer of afatinib advises separating administration of ketoconazole by 6 to 12 hours; ketoconazole increases plasma concentration of AXITINIB (reduce dose of axitinib—consult axitinib product literature); ketoconazole increases the plasma concentration of ● BOSUTINIB—manufacturer of bosutinib advises avoid or

Antifungals, Imidazole

- **Cytotoxics** (continued)
consider reducing dose of bosutinib; ketoconazole increases plasma concentration of BORTEZOMIB, CABOZANTINIB, DABRAFENIB, ETOPOSIDE, IDELALISIB, IMATINIB, ● NINTEDANIB and PONATINIB; ketoconazole increases plasma concentration of ● CRIZOTINIB, ● LAPATINIB, ● NILOTINIB and ● REGORAFENIB— avoid concomitant use; ketoconazole possibly increases plasma concentration of DASATINIB; ketoconazole inhibits metabolism of ERLOTINIB and SUNITINIB (increased plasma concentration); ketoconazole increases plasma concentration of ● EVEROLIMUS—manufacturer of ketoconazole advises avoid concomitant use; ketoconazole increases plasma concentration of ● IBRUTINIB—reduce dose of ibrutinib (see under Ibrutinib, p. 855); ketoconazole increases plasma concentration of ● PAZOPANIB (reduce dose of pazopanib); manufacturer of ruxolitinib advises dose reduction when ketoconazole given with ● RUXOLITINIB—consult ruxolitinib product literature; ketoconazole increases plasma concentration of active metabolite of ● TEMSIROLIMUS—avoid concomitant use; avoidance of ketoconazole advised by manufacturer of ● CABAZITAXEL; *in vitro* studies suggest a possible interaction between ketoconazole and DOCETAXEL (consult docetaxel product literature); ketoconazole reduces plasma concentration of ● IRINOTECAN (but concentration of active metabolite of irinotecan increased)—avoid concomitant use; ketoconazole increases plasma concentration of ● VINFLUNINE—manufacturer of vinflunine advises avoid concomitant use
- **Dapoxetine:** ketoconazole increases plasma concentration of ● DAPOXETINE—manufacturer of dapoxetine advises avoid concomitant use
- **Diuretics:** ketoconazole increases plasma concentration of ● EPLERENONE—avoid concomitant use
- **Domperidone:** manufacturer of ketoconazole advises avoid concomitant use with ● DOMPERIDONE (risk of ventricular arrhythmias)
- **Ergot Alkaloids:** manufacturer of ketoconazole advises avoid concomitant use with ● ERGOT ALKALOIDS; increased risk of ergotism when imidazoles given with ● ERGOTAMINE—avoid concomitant use
- **Fingolimod:** ketoconazole increases plasma concentration of ● FINGOLIMOD
▸ **Fosaprepitant:** ketoconazole increases plasma concentration of FOSAPREPITANT
- **Guanfacine:** ketoconazole increases plasma concentration of ● GUANFACINE (halve dose of guanfacine)
▸ **Hormone Antagonists:** manufacturer of ketoconazole advises avoid concomitant use with PASIREOTIDE
- **5HT₁-receptor Agonists:** ketoconazole increases plasma concentration of ALMOTRIPTAN (increased risk of toxicity); ketoconazole increases plasma concentration of ● ELETRIPTAN (risk of toxicity)—avoid concomitant use
- **Ivabradine:** ketoconazole increases plasma concentration of ● IVABRADINE—avoid concomitant use
- **Ivacaftor:** ketoconazole increases plasma concentration of ● IVACAFTOR (see under Ivacaftor, p. 269)
▸ **Lanthanum:** absorption of ketoconazole possibly reduced by LANTHANUM (give at least 2 hours apart)
- **Lenalidomide:** ketoconazole possibly increases plasma concentration of ● LENALIDOMIDE (increased risk of toxicity)
- **Lipid-regulating Drugs:** possible increased risk of myopathy when imidazoles given with ATORVASTATIN; possible increased risk of myopathy when ketoconazole given with ● ATORVASTATIN—manufacturer of ketoconazole advises avoid concomitant use; increased risk of myopathy when ketoconazole given with ● SIMVASTATIN (avoid concomitant use); possible increased risk of myopathy when miconazole given with ● SIMVASTATIN; ketoconazole increases plasma concentration of ● LOMITAPIDE—avoid concomitant use
▸ **Macitentan:** ketoconazole increases plasma concentration of MACITENTAN
▸ **Mirabegron:** when given with ketoconazole avoid or reduce dose of MIRABEGRON in hepatic or renal impairment—see Mirabegron, p. 707

Antifungals, Imidazole (continued)

▸ **Netupitant:** ketoconazole possibly increases plasma concentration of NETUPITANT
▸ **Oestrogens:** anecdotal reports of contraceptive failure when imidazoles given with OESTROGENS; ketoconazole increases plasma concentration of ETHINYLESTRADIOL
▸ **Parasympathomimetics:** ketoconazole increases plasma concentration of GALANTAMINE
▸ **Progestogens:** ketoconazole increases plasma concentration of DROSPIRENONE
- **Ranolazine:** ketoconazole increases plasma concentration of ● RANOLAZINE—avoid concomitant use
- **Retinoids:** ketoconazole increases plasma concentration of ALITRETINOIN; ketoconazole possibly increases risk of ● TRETINOIN toxicity
▸ **Riociguat:** avoidance of ketoconazole advised by manufacturer of RIOCIGUAT
- **Sildenafil:** ketoconazole increases plasma concentration of ● SILDENAFIL—reduce initial dose of sildenafil for erectile dysfunction and avoid concomitant use of sildenafil for pulmonary hypertension
- **Sirolimus:** ketoconazole increases plasma concentration of ● SIROLIMUS—avoid concomitant use; miconazole increases plasma concentration of ● SIROLIMUS
- **Sympathomimetics, Beta₂:** ketoconazole increases plasma concentration of ● OLODATEROL; ketoconazole inhibits metabolism of ● SALMETEROL (increased plasma concentration)
- **Tacrolimus:** ketoconazole increases plasma concentration of ● TACROLIMUS (consider reducing dose of tacrolimus); miconazole *oral gel* possibly increases plasma concentration of ● TACROLIMUS
- **Tadalafil:** ketoconazole increases plasma concentration of ● TADALAFIL—avoid concomitant use of tadalafil for pulmonary hypertension
- **Theophylline:** ketoconazole possibly increases plasma concentration of ● THEOPHYLLINE
- **Ticagrelor:** ketoconazole increases plasma concentration of ● TICAGRELOR—manufacturer of ticagrelor advises avoid concomitant use
- **Tolvaptan:** ketoconazole increases plasma concentration of TOLVAPTAN—manufacturer of ketoconazole advises avoid concomitant use
▸ **Ulcer-healing Drugs:** absorption of ketoconazole reduced by HISTAMINE H₂-ANTAGONISTS, PROTON PUMP INHIBITORS and SUCRALFATE
▸ **Ulipristal:** ketoconazole increases plasma concentration of *low-dose* ULIPRISTAL—manufacturer of *low-dose* ulipristal advises avoid concomitant use
- **Vardenafil:** ketoconazole increases plasma concentration of ● VARDENAFIL—avoid concomitant use
▸ **Vitamins:** miconazole possibly reduces effects of ALFACALCIDOL, CALCITRIOL, COLECALCIFEROL, DIHYDROTACHYSTEROL, ERGOCALCIFEROL, PARICALCITOL and VITAMIN D; ketoconazole possibly increases plasma concentration of PARICALCITOL

Antifungals, Polyene *see* Amphotericin

Antifungals, Triazole

NOTE In general, fluconazole interactions relate to multiple-dose treatment

- **Aliskiren:** itraconazole increases plasma concentration of ● ALISKIREN—avoid concomitant use
- **Aminophylline:** fluconazole possibly increases plasma concentration of ● AMINOPHYLLINE
- **Analgesics:** fluconazole increases plasma concentration of CELECOXIB (halve dose of celecoxib); voriconazole increases plasma concentration of DICLOFENAC, IBUPROFEN and ● OXYCODONE; fluconazole increases plasma concentration of FLURBIPROFEN, IBUPROFEN and METHADONE; fluconazole increases plasma concentration of PARECOXIB (reduce dose of parecoxib); voriconazole increases plasma concentration of ● ALFENTANIL and ● METHADONE (consider reducing dose of alfentanil and methadone); fluconazole inhibits metabolism of ALFENTANIL (risk of prolonged or delayed respiratory depression); itraconazole possibly inhibits metabolism of ALFENTANIL; triazoles possibly increase plasma concentration of ● FENTANYL; itraconazole possibly increases plasma

Antifungals, Triazole

- **Analgesics** (continued)
concentration of ● METHADONE (increased risk of ventricular arrhythmias); itraconazole increases plasma concentration of OXYCODONE
▸ **Antacids:** absorption of itraconazole reduced by ANTACIDS
- **Anti-arrhythmics:** manufacturer of itraconazole advises avoid concomitant use with ● DISOPYRAMIDE; avoidance of itraconazole, posaconazole and voriconazole advised by manufacturer of ● DRONEDARONE
- **Antibacterials:** plasma concentration of itraconazole increased by CLARITHROMYCIN; manufacturer of fluconazole advises avoid concomitant use with ERYTHROMYCIN; triazoles possibly increase plasma concentration of ● RIFABUTIN (increased risk of uveitis—reduce rifabutin dose); posaconazole increases plasma concentration of ● RIFABUTIN (also plasma concentration of posaconazole reduced); voriconazole increases plasma concentration of ● RIFABUTIN, also rifabutin reduces plasma concentration of voriconazole (increase dose of voriconazole and also monitor for rifabutin toxicity); fluconazole increases plasma concentration of ● RIFABUTIN (increased risk of uveitis—reduce rifabutin dose); plasma concentration of itraconazole reduced by ● RIFABUTIN and ● RIFAMPICIN—manufacturer of itraconazole advises avoid concomitant use; plasma concentration of posaconazole reduced by ● RIFAMPICIN; plasma concentration of voriconazole reduced by ● RIFAMPICIN—avoid concomitant use; metabolism of fluconazole accelerated by ● RIFAMPICIN (reduced plasma concentration); fluconazole possibly increases plasma concentration of BEDAQUILINE—avoid concomitant use if fluconazole given for more than 14 days
- **Anticoagulants:** avoidance of itraconazole, posaconazole and voriconazole advised by manufacturer of APIXABAN; fluconazole, itraconazole and voriconazole enhance anticoagulant effect of ● COUMARINS; avoidance of itraconazole advised by manufacturer of DABIGATRAN and RIVAROXABAN; avoidance of posaconazole and voriconazole advised by manufacturer of RIVAROXABAN
- **Antidepressants:** avoidance of triazoles advised by manufacturer of ● REBOXETINE; fluconazole possibly increases plasma concentration of AMITRIPTYLINE and NORTRIPTYLINE; plasma concentration of voriconazole reduced by ● ST JOHN'S WORT—avoid concomitant use
- **Antidiabetics:** posaconazole possibly enhances hypoglycaemic effect of GLIPIZIDE; fluconazole possibly enhances hypoglycaemic effect of NATEGLINIDE; itraconazole possibly enhances hypoglycaemic effect of REPAGLINIDE; voriconazole possibly increases plasma concentration of SULFONYLUREAS; fluconazole increases plasma concentration of ● SULFONYLUREAS
- **Antiepileptics:** plasma concentration of itraconazole and posaconazole possibly reduced by ● CARBAMAZEPINE; fluconazole possibly increases plasma concentration of CARBAMAZEPINE; plasma concentration of voriconazole possibly reduced by ● CARBAMAZEPINE, ● PHENOBARBITAL and ● PRIMIDONE—avoid concomitant use; plasma concentration of itraconazole reduced by ● FOSPHENYTOIN and ● PHENYTOIN—avoid concomitant use; fluconazole increases plasma concentration of ● FOSPHENYTOIN and ● PHENYTOIN (consider reducing dose of fosphenytoin and phenytoin); voriconazole increases plasma concentration of ● FOSPHENYTOIN and ● PHENYTOIN, also fosphenytoin and phenytoin reduces plasma concentration of voriconazole (increase dose of voriconazole and also monitor for fosphenytoin and phenytoin toxicity); plasma concentration of posaconazole reduced by ● FOSPHENYTOIN and ● PHENYTOIN; plasma concentration of itraconazole and posaconazole possibly reduced by ● PHENOBARBITAL; plasma concentration of itraconazole and posaconazole possibly reduced by ● PRIMIDONE
▸ **Antifungals:** triazoles possibly antagonise effects of AMPHOTERICIN; monitoring for increased voriconazole side effects advised by manufacturer of FLUCONAZOLE if voriconazole given after fluconazole; plasma concentration of itraconazole increased by MICAFUNGIN (consider reducing dose of itraconazole); plasma concentration of fluconazole increased by TERBINAFINE

Antifungals, Triazole (continued)

- **Antihistamines:** itraconazole inhibits metabolism of ● MIZOLASTINE—avoid concomitant use
- **Antimalarials:** avoidance of triazoles advised by manufacturer of ● ARTEMETHER WITH LUMEFANTRINE; avoidance of triazoles advised by manufacturer of ● ARTENIMOL WITH PIPERAQUINE (possible risk of ventricular arrhythmias)
- **Antimuscarinics:** avoidance of itraconazole advised by manufacturer of DARIFENACIN and TOLTERODINE; manufacturer of fesoterodine advises dose reduction when itraconazole given with FESOTERODINE—consult fesoterodine product literature; itraconazole possibly increases plasma concentration of ● SOLIFENACIN—see under Solifenacin, p. 705
- **Antipsychotics:** itraconazole possibly increases plasma concentration of HALOPERIDOL; itraconazole possibly increases plasma concentration of ● ARIPIPRAZOLE (reduce dose of aripiprazole—consult aripiprazole product literature); itraconazole, posaconazole and voriconazole possibly increase plasma concentration of ● LURASIDONE—avoid concomitant use; fluconazole possibly increases the plasma concentration of ● LURASIDONE (see under Lurasidone, p. 364); increased risk of ventricular arrhythmias when triazoles given with ● PIMOZIDE—avoid concomitant use; triazoles possibly increase plasma concentration of ● QUETIAPINE—manufacturer of quetiapine advises avoid concomitant use; itraconazole possibly increases side-effects of RISPERIDONE
- **Antivirals:** posaconazole increases plasma concentration of ● ATAZANAVIR; plasma concentration of voriconazole increased or decreased by ● ATAZANAVIR and plasma concentration of atazanavir also reduced; itraconazole, posaconazole and voriconazole possibly increase the plasma concentration of ● DACLATASVIR—reduce dose of daclatasvir (see under Daclatasvir, p. 568); plasma concentration of voriconazole possibly affected by DARUNAVIR; plasma concentration of both drugs possibly increased when itraconazole and posaconazole given with ● DASABUVIR—avoid concomitant use; plasma concentration of voriconazole reduced by ● EFAVIRENZ, also plasma concentration of efavirenz increased (increase voriconazole dose and reduce efavirenz dose); plasma concentration of itraconazole and posaconazole reduced by ● EFAVIRENZ; plasma concentration of both drugs may increase when itraconazole given with FOSAMPRENAVIR; plasma concentration of posaconazole possibly reduced by FOSAMPRENAVIR; itraconazole increases plasma concentration of ● INDINAVIR (consider reducing dose of indinavir); fluconazole increases plasma concentration of ● NEVIRAPINE, RITONAVIR and TIPRANAVIR; plasma concentration of itraconazole possibly reduced by NEVIRAPINE—consider increasing dose of itraconazole; plasma concentration of both drugs possibly increased when itraconazole and posaconazole given with ● PARITAPREVIR—avoid concomitant use; plasma concentration of voriconazole reduced by ● RITONAVIR—avoid concomitant use; combination of itraconazole with ● RITONAVIR may increase plasma concentration of either drug (or both); triazoles possibly increase plasma concentration of SAQUINAVIR; fluconazole, itraconazole, posaconazole and voriconazole possibly increase plasma concentration of ● SIMEPREVIR—manufacturer of simeprevir advises avoid concomitant use; plasma concentration of voriconazole possibly affected by ● TELAPREVIR (possible increased risk of ventricular arrhythmias); plasma concentration of posaconazole possibly increased by ● TELAPREVIR (increased risk of ventricular arrhythmias); plasma concentration of itraconazole possibly increased by TELAPREVIR; fluconazole increases plasma concentration of ● ZIDOVUDINE (increased risk of toxicity)
- **Anxiolytics and Hypnotics:** itraconazole increases plasma concentration of ALPRAZOLAM; fluconazole and voriconazole increase plasma concentration of ● DIAZEPAM (risk of prolonged sedation); fluconazole, itraconazole, posaconazole and voriconazole increase plasma concentration of ● MIDAZOLAM (risk of prolonged sedation); itraconazole increases plasma concentration of BUSPIRONE (reduce dose of buspirone)

A1

Antifungals, Triazole (continued)

- Avanafil: itraconazole and voriconazole possibly increase plasma concentration of • AVANAFIL—manufacturer of avanafil advises avoid concomitant use; fluconazole possibly increases plasma concentration of • AVANAFIL—see under Avanafil, p. 735
- Bosentan: fluconazole possibly increases plasma concentration of • BOSENTAN—avoid concomitant use; itraconazole possibly increases plasma concentration of BOSENTAN
- Calcium-channel Blockers: negative inotropic effect possibly increased when itraconazole given with CALCIUM-CHANNEL BLOCKERS; itraconazole inhibits metabolism of • FELODIPINE (increased plasma concentration); avoidance of itraconazole advised by manufacturer of LERCANIDIPINE; itraconazole possibly inhibits metabolism of DIHYDROPYRIDINES (increased plasma concentration)
- Cardiac Glycosides: itraconazole increases plasma concentration of • DIGOXIN
- Ciclosporin: fluconazole, itraconazole, posaconazole and voriconazole inhibit metabolism of • CICLOSPORIN (increased plasma concentration)
- Cilostazol: itraconazole possibly increases plasma concentration of • CILOSTAZOL (see under Cilostazol, p. 215)
- Clopidogrel: fluconazole, itraconazole and voriconazole possibly reduce antiplatelet effect of CLOPIDOGREL
- Cobicistat: plasma concentration of itraconazole possibly increased by COBICISTAT—manufacturer of cobicistat advises reduce dose of itraconazole
- Colchicine: itraconazole possibly increases risk of • COLCHICINE toxicity—suspend or reduce dose of colchicine (avoid concomitant use in hepatic or renal impairment)
- Corticosteroids: itraconazole possibly inhibits metabolism of CORTICOSTEROIDS and METHYLPREDNISOLONE; itraconazole increases the plasma concentration of *inhaled* and *oral* (and possibly also *intranasal* and *rectal*) • BUDESONIDE; itraconazole increases plasma concentration of *inhaled* FLUTICASONE
- Cytotoxics: itraconazole inhibits metabolism of BUSULFAN (increased risk of toxicity); fluconazole and itraconazole possibly increase side-effects of CYCLOPHOSPHAMIDE; itraconazole possibly increases the plasma concentration of AFATINIB—manufacturer of afatinib advises separating administration of itraconazole by 6 to 12 hours; itraconazole possibly increases plasma concentration of AXITINIB (reduce dose of axitinib—consult axitinib product literature); fluconazole, itraconazole, posaconazole and voriconazole possibly increase the plasma concentration of • BOSUTINIB— manufacturer of bosutinib advises avoid or consider reducing dose of bosutinib; itraconazole possibly increases plasma concentration of CABOZANTINIB; itraconazole and voriconazole possibly increase plasma concentration of • CRIZOTINIB— manufacturer of crizotinib advises avoid concomitant use; avoidance of itraconazole advised by manufacturer of DASATINIB and • TEMSIROLIMUS (plasma concentration of dasatinib and temsirolimus possibly increased); itraconazole, posaconazole and voriconazole possibly increase plasma concentration of • EVEROLIMUS—manufacturer of everolimus advises avoid concomitant use; itraconazole increases plasma concentration of GEFITINIB; fluconazole, itraconazole and voriconazole possibly increase the plasma concentration of • IBRUTINIB—reduce dose of ibrutinib (see under Ibrutinib, p. 855); avoidance of itraconazole, posaconazole and voriconazole advised by manufacturer of • LAPATINIB; avoidance of itraconazole and voriconazole advised by manufacturer of • NILOTINIB; itraconazole and voriconazole possibly increase plasma concentration of • PAZOPANIB (reduce dose of pazopanib); itraconazole and voriconazole possibly increase plasma concentration of • PONATINIB— consider reducing initial dose of ponatinib (see under Ponatinib, p. 860); manufacturer of ruxolitinib advises dose reduction when fluconazole, itraconazole, posaconazole and voriconazole given with • RUXOLITINIB—consult ruxolitinib product literature; itraconazole and voriconazole possibly increase the plasma concentration of • CABAZITAXEL— manufacturer of cabazitaxel advises avoid or consider reducing dose of cabazitaxel; itraconazole and voriconazole possibly increase plasma concentration of • DOCETAXEL—

Antifungals, Triazole

- Cytotoxics (continued)
  manufacturer of docetaxel advises avoid concomitant use or consider reducing docetaxel dose; increased risk of toxicity when itraconazole given with • IRINOTECAN—avoid concomitant use; avoidance of itraconazole advised by manufacturer of • OLAPARIB; posaconazole possibly inhibits metabolism of • VINBLASTINE and • VINCRISTINE (increased risk of neurotoxicity); itraconazole possibly increases risk of • VINBLASTINE, • VINDESINE, • VINFLUNINE and • VINORELBINE toxicity; itraconazole increases risk of • VINCRISTINE toxicity
- Dapoxetine: manufacturer of dapoxetine advises dose reduction when fluconazole given with DAPOXETINE (see under Dapoxetine, p. 742); avoidance of itraconazole advised by manufacturer of • DAPOXETINE (increased risk of toxicity)
- Diuretics: fluconazole increases plasma concentration of EPLERENONE (reduce dose of eplerenone); itraconazole increases plasma concentration of • EPLERENONE—avoid concomitant use; plasma concentration of fluconazole increased by HYDROCHLOROTHIAZIDE
- Domperidone: possible increased risk of ventricular arrhythmias when itraconazole or voriconazole given with • DOMPERIDONE—avoid concomitant use
- Ergot Alkaloids: increased risk of ergotism when voriconazole given with • ERGOMETRINE—avoid concomitant use; manufacturer of itraconazole advises avoid concomitant use with • ERGOMETRINE (increased risk of ergotism); increased risk of ergotism when triazoles given with • ERGOTAMINE— avoid concomitant use
- Guanfacine: fluconazole, itraconazole and posaconazole possibly increase the plasma concentration of • GUANFACINE (halve dose of guanfacine)
- 5HT$_1$-receptor Agonists: itraconazole increases plasma concentration of • ELETRIPTAN (risk of toxicity)—avoid concomitant use
- Ivabradine: fluconazole increases plasma concentration of IVABRADINE—reduce initial dose of ivabradine; itraconazole possibly increases plasma concentration of • IVABRADINE— avoid concomitant use
- Ivacaftor: itraconazole, posaconazole and voriconazole possibly increase plasma concentration of • IVACAFTOR (see under Ivacaftor, p. 269); fluconazole increases plasma concentration of • IVACAFTOR (see under Ivacaftor, p. 269)
- Lenalidomide: itraconazole possibly increases plasma concentration of • LENALIDOMIDE (increased risk of toxicity)
- Leukotriene Receptor Antagonists: fluconazole increases plasma concentration of ZAFIRLUKAST
- Lipid-regulating Drugs: increased risk of myopathy when itraconazole, posaconazole or voriconazole given with • ATORVASTATIN; possible increased risk of myopathy when fluconazole given with • ATORVASTATIN or • SIMVASTATIN; fluconazole increases plasma concentration of FLUVASTATIN— possible increased risk of myopathy; itraconazole increases plasma concentration of • ROSUVASTATIN—adjust dose of rosuvastatin (consult product literature); increased risk of myopathy when itraconazole or posaconazole given with • SIMVASTATIN (avoid concomitant use); increased risk of myopathy when voriconazole given with • SIMVASTATIN; avoidance of triazoles advised by manufacturer of • LOMITAPIDE (plasma concentration of lomitapide possibly increased)
- Mirabegron: when given with itraconazole avoid or reduce dose of MIRABEGRON in hepatic or renal impairment—see Mirabegron, p. 707
- Oestrogens: plasma concentration of voriconazole increased by OESTROGENS
- Progestogens: plasma concentration of voriconazole possibly increased by PROGESTOGENS
- Ranolazine: itraconazole, posaconazole and voriconazole possibly increase plasma concentration of • RANOLAZINE— manufacturer of ranolazine advises avoid concomitant use
- Retinoids: fluconazole and voriconazole possibly increase risk of • TRETINOIN toxicity
- Riociguat: avoidance of itraconazole and voriconazole advised by manufacturer of RIOCIGUAT

Antifungals, Triazole (continued)

▸ Sildenafil: itraconazole increases plasma concentration of SILDENAFIL—reduce initial dose of sildenafil
● Sirolimus: fluconazole and posaconazole possibly increase plasma concentration of SIROLIMUS; itraconazole and voriconazole increase plasma concentration of ● SIROLIMUS—avoid concomitant use
● Tacrolimus: fluconazole, itraconazole, posaconazole and voriconazole increase plasma concentration of ● TACROLIMUS (consider reducing dose of tacrolimus)
▸ Tadalafil: itraconazole possibly increases plasma concentration of TADALAFIL
● Theophylline: fluconazole possibly increases plasma concentration of ● THEOPHYLLINE
● Ulcer-healing Drugs: plasma concentration of posaconazole reduced by ● CIMETIDINE and ● ESOMEPRAZOLE—manufacturer of posaconazole *suspension* advises avoid concomitant use; plasma concentration of posaconazole possibly reduced by ● FAMOTIDINE, ● LANSOPRAZOLE, ● NIZATIDINE, ● OMEPRAZOLE, ● PANTOPRAZOLE, ● RABEPRAZOLE and ● RANITIDINE—manufacturer of posaconazole *suspension* advises avoid concomitant use; voriconazole possibly increases plasma concentration of ESOMEPRAZOLE; voriconazole increases plasma concentration of OMEPRAZOLE (consider reducing dose of omeprazole); absorption of itraconazole reduced by HISTAMINE H₂-ANTAGONISTS and PROTON PUMP INHIBITORS
▸ Ulipristal: avoidance of itraconazole advised by manufacturer of ULIPRISTAL
● Vardenafil: itraconazole possibly increases plasma concentration of ● VARDENAFIL—avoid concomitant use

Antihistamines

NOTE Sedative interactions apply to a lesser extent to the non-sedating antihistamines. Interactions do not generally apply to antihistamines used for topical action (including inhalation)

▸ Alcohol: increased sedative effect when antihistamines given with ALCOHOL (possibly less effect with non-sedating antihistamines)
● Analgesics: sedative effects possibly increased when sedating antihistamines given with ● OPIOID ANALGESICS
▸ Antacids: absorption of fexofenadine reduced by ANTACIDS
● Anti-arrhythmics: increased risk of ventricular arrhythmias when mizolastine given with ● AMIODARONE, ● DISOPYRAMIDE or ● FLECAINIDE—avoid concomitant use; manufacturer of mizolastine advises avoid concomitant use with PROPAFENONE (possible risk of ventricular arrhythmias)
● Antibacterials: manufacturer of loratadine advises plasma concentration possibly increased by ERYTHROMYCIN; metabolism of mizolastine inhibited by ● ERYTHROMYCIN—avoid concomitant use; increased risk of ventricular arrhythmias when mizolastine given with ● MOXIFLOXACIN—avoid concomitant use; effects of fexofenadine possibly reduced by RIFAMPICIN; metabolism of mizolastine possibly inhibited by ● MACROLIDES (avoid concomitant use)
● Antidepressants: avoidance of mizolastine advised by manufacturer of ● CITALOPRAM and ● ESCITALOPRAM (risk of ventricular arrhythmias); increased antimuscarinic and sedative effects when antihistamines given with MAOIs or TRICYCLICS; manufacturer of promethazine advises avoid for 2 weeks after stopping MAOIs; manufacturer of hydroxyzine advises avoid concomitant use with MAOIs; cyproheptadine possibly antagonises antidepressant effect of SSRIs; possible increased antimuscarinic and sedative effects when antihistamines given with TRICYCLIC-RELATED ANTIDEPRESSANTS
▸ Antidiabetics: thrombocyte count depressed when ketotifen given with METFORMIN (manufacturer of ketotifen advises avoid concomitant use)
● Antifungals: metabolism of mizolastine inhibited by ● ITRACONAZOLE—avoid concomitant use; metabolism of mizolastine possibly inhibited by ● IMIDAZOLES (avoid concomitant use)
● Antimalarials: avoidance of mizolastine advised by manufacturer of ● ARTENIMOL WITH PIPERAQUINE (possible risk of ventricular arrhythmias)
▸ Antimuscarinics: increased risk of antimuscarinic side-effects when antihistamines given with ANTIMUSCARINICS

Antihistamines (continued)

● Antivirals: plasma concentration of chlorphenamine possibly increased by LOPINAVIR; plasma concentration of non-sedating antihistamines possibly increased by RITONAVIR; increased risk of ventricular arrhythmias when mizolastine given with ● SAQUINAVIR—avoid concomitant use
▸ Anxiolytics and Hypnotics: increased sedative effect when antihistamines given with ANXIOLYTICS AND HYPNOTICS
● Beta-blockers: increased risk of ventricular arrhythmias when mizolastine given with ● SOTALOL—avoid concomitant use
▸ Betahistine: antihistamines theoretically antagonise effect of BETAHISTINE
● Cytotoxics: possible increased risk of ventricular arrhythmias when mizolastine given with ● VANDETANIB—avoid concomitant use
● Grapefruit Juice: plasma concentration of bilastine reduced by GRAPEFRUIT JUICE
▸ Histamine: antihistamines theoretically antagonise effects of HISTAMINE—manufacturer of histamine advises avoid concomitant use
▸ Sympathomimetics: avoidance of antihistamines advised by manufacturer of MIDODRINE
▸ Ulcer-healing Drugs: manufacturer of loratadine advises plasma concentration possibly increased by CIMETIDINE; plasma concentration of hydroxyzine increased by CIMETIDINE
▸ Ulipristal: manufacturer of ulipristal advises give fexofenadine at least 1.5 hours before or after ULIPRISTAL

Antihistamines, Non-sedating *see* Antihistamines
Antihistamines, Sedating *see* Antihistamines
Antimalarials *see* Artemether with Lumefantrine, Artenimol with Piperaquine, Chloroquine, Hydroxychloroquine, Mefloquine, Primaquine, Proguanil, Pyrimethamine, and Quinine
Antimetabolites *see* Capecitabine, Cladribine, Cytarabine, Decitabine, Fludarabine, Fluorouracil, Gemcitabine, Mercaptopurine, Methotrexate, Pemetrexed, Raltitrexed, Tegafur, and Tioguanine
Antimuscarinics

NOTE Many drugs have antimuscarinic effects; concomitant use of two or more such drugs can increase side-effects such as dry mouth, urine retention, and constipation; concomitant use can also lead to confusion in the elderly. Interactions do not generally apply to antimuscarinics used by inhalation

▸ Alcohol: increased sedative effect when hyoscine given with ALCOHOL
▸ Analgesics: possible increased risk of antimuscarinic side-effects when antimuscarinics given with CODEINE; increased risk of antimuscarinic side-effects when antimuscarinics given with NEFOPAM
● Anti-arrhythmics: increased risk of ventricular arrhythmias when tolterodine given with ● AMIODARONE, ● DISOPYRAMIDE or ● FLECAINIDE; increased risk of antimuscarinic side-effects when antimuscarinics given with DISOPYRAMIDE
● Antibacterials: manufacturer of fesoterodine advises dose reduction when fesoterodine given with CLARITHROMYCIN and TELITHROMYCIN—consult fesoterodine product literature; manufacturer of tolterodine advises avoid concomitant use with CLARITHROMYCIN and ERYTHROMYCIN; plasma concentration of darifenacin possibly increased by ERYTHROMYCIN; plasma concentration of active metabolite of fesoterodine reduced by ● RIFAMPICIN—avoid concomitant use
● Antidepressants: plasma concentration of darifenacin and procyclidine increased by PAROXETINE; increased risk of antimuscarinic side-effects when antimuscarinics given with MAOIs or TRICYCLICS; plasma concentration of active metabolite of fesoterodine possibly reduced by ● ST JOHN'S WORT—manufacturer of fesoterodine advises avoid concomitant use; possible increased antimuscarinic side-effects when antimuscarinics given with TRICYCLIC-RELATED ANTIDEPRESSANTS
● Antiepileptics: plasma concentration of active metabolite of fesoterodine possibly reduced by ● CARBAMAZEPINE, ● PHENOBARBITAL and ● PHENYTOIN—manufacturer of fesoterodine advises avoid concomitant use
● Antifungals: antimuscarinics reduce absorption of KETOCONAZOLE; manufacturer of fesoterodine advises dose

Antimuscarinics

- **Antifungals** (continued)
reduction when fesoterodine given with ITRACONAZOLE and KETOCONAZOLE—consult fesoterodine product literature; plasma concentration of darifenacin increased by KETOCONAZOLE—avoid concomitant use; plasma concentration of solifenacin increased by ● KETOCONAZOLE—see under Solifenacin, p. 705; plasma concentration of oxybutynin increased by KETOCONAZOLE; manufacturer of tolterodine advises avoid concomitant use with ITRACONAZOLE and ● KETOCONAZOLE; manufacturer of darifenacin advises avoid concomitant use with ITRACONAZOLE; plasma concentration of solifenacin possibly increased by ● ITRACONAZOLE—see under Solifenacin, p. 705
▸ **Antihistamines:** increased risk of antimuscarinic side-effects when antimuscarinics given with ANTIHISTAMINES
▸ **Antipsychotics:** antimuscarinics possibly reduce effects of HALOPERIDOL; increased risk of antimuscarinic side-effects when antimuscarinics given with CLOZAPINE; antimuscarinics reduce plasma concentration of PHENOTHIAZINES, but risk of antimuscarinic side-effects increased
- **Antivirals:** manufacturer of darifenacin advises avoid concomitant use with ATAZANAVIR, FOSAMPRENAVIR, INDINAVIR, LOPINAVIR, RITONAVIR, SAQUINAVIR and TIPRANAVIR; manufacturer of fesoterodine advises dose reduction when fesoterodine given with ATAZANAVIR, INDINAVIR, RITONAVIR and SAQUINAVIR—consult fesoterodine product literature; manufacturer of tolterodine advises avoid concomitant use with FOSAMPRENAVIR, INDINAVIR, LOPINAVIR, RITONAVIR and SAQUINAVIR; plasma concentration of solifenacin possibly increased by ● RITONAVIR—see under Solifenacin, p. 705
- **Beta-blockers:** increased risk of ventricular arrhythmias when tolterodine given with ● SOTALOL
▸ **Calcium-channel Blockers:** plasma concentration of solifenacin increased by VERAPAMIL; manufacturer of darifenacin advises avoid concomitant use with VERAPAMIL
▸ **Cardiac Glycosides:** darifenacin possibly increases plasma concentration of DIGOXIN
▸ **Ciclosporin:** manufacturer of darifenacin advises avoid concomitant use with CICLOSPORIN
▸ **Domperidone:** antimuscarinics antagonise effects of DOMPERIDONE on gastro-intestinal activity
▸ **Dopaminergics:** antimuscarinics possibly reduce absorption of CO-BENELDOPA, CO-CARELDOPA and LEVODOPA
▸ **Hormone Antagonists:** possible increased risk of bradycardia when ipratropium or oxybutynin given with PASIREOTIDE
▸ **Memantine:** effects of antimuscarinics possibly enhanced by MEMANTINE
▸ **Metoclopramide:** antimuscarinics antagonise effects of METOCLOPRAMIDE on gastro-intestinal activity
▸ **Nitrates:** antimuscarinics possibly reduce effects of sublingual tablets of NITRATES (failure to dissolve under tongue owing to dry mouth)
▸ **Parasympathomimetics:** antimuscarinics antagonise effects of PARASYMPATHOMIMETICS

Antipsychotics

NOTE Increased risk of toxicity with myelosuppressive drugs
NOTE Avoid concomitant use of clozapine with drugs that have a substantial potential for causing agranulocytosis
▸ **ACE Inhibitors:** enhanced hypotensive effect when antipsychotics given with ACE INHIBITORS
▸ **Adrenergic Neurone Blockers:** enhanced hypotensive effect when phenothiazines given with ADRENERGIC NEURONE BLOCKERS; higher doses of chlorpromazine antagonise hypotensive effect of ADRENERGIC NEURONE BLOCKERS; haloperidol antagonises hypotensive effect of ADRENERGIC NEURONE BLOCKERS
▸ **Adsorbents:** absorption of phenothiazines possibly reduced by KAOLIN
▸ **Alcohol:** increased sedative effect when antipsychotics given with ALCOHOL
▸ **Alpha-blockers:** enhanced hypotensive effect when antipsychotics given with ALPHA-BLOCKERS
- **Anaesthetics, General:** droperidol enhances effects of THIOPENTAL; enhanced hypotensive effect when antipsychotics given with ● GENERAL ANAESTHETICS

Antipsychotics (continued)

- **Analgesics:** possible severe drowsiness when haloperidol given with ACEMETACIN or INDOMETACIN; increased risk of ventricular arrhythmias when antipsychotics that prolong the QT interval given with ● METHADONE; increased risk of ventricular arrhythmias when amisulpride given with ● METHADONE—avoid concomitant use; increased risk of convulsions when antipsychotics given with TRAMADOL; enhanced hypotensive and sedative effects when antipsychotics given with OPIOID ANALGESICS
▸ **Angiotensin-II Receptor Antagonists:** enhanced hypotensive effect when antipsychotics given with ANGIOTENSIN-II RECEPTOR ANTAGONISTS
▸ **Antacids:** absorption of phenothiazines and sulpiride reduced by ANTACIDS
- **Anti-arrhythmics:** increased risk of ventricular arrhythmias when antipsychotics that prolong the QT interval given with ● ANTI-ARRHYTHMICS that prolong the QT interval; increased risk of ventricular arrhythmias when amisulpride, droperidol, haloperidol, phenothiazines, pimozide or zuclopenthixol given with ● AMIODARONE—avoid concomitant use; increased risk of ventricular arrhythmias when benperidol given with ● AMIODARONE—manufacturer of benperidol advises avoid concomitant use; increased risk of ventricular arrhythmias when sulpiride given with ● AMIODARONE or ● DISOPYRAMIDE; increased risk of ventricular arrhythmias when amisulpride, droperidol, pimozide or zuclopenthixol given with ● DISOPYRAMIDE—avoid concomitant use; possible increased risk of ventricular arrhythmias when haloperidol given with ● DISOPYRAMIDE—avoid concomitant use; increased risk of ventricular arrhythmias when phenothiazines given with ● DISOPYRAMIDE; avoidance of phenothiazines advised by manufacturer of ● DRONEDARONE (risk of ventricular arrhythmias); increased risk of arrhythmias when clozapine given with ● FLECAINIDE
- **Antibacterials:** plasma concentration of lurasidone possibly increased by ● CLARITHROMYCIN and ● TELITHROMYCIN—avoid concomitant use; increased risk of ventricular arrhythmias when pimozide given with ● CLARITHROMYCIN, ● MOXIFLOXACIN or ● TELITHROMYCIN—avoid concomitant use; plasma concentration of quetiapine possibly increased by ● CLARITHROMYCIN—manufacturer of quetiapine advises avoid concomitant use; plasma concentration of lurasidone possibly increased by ● ERYTHROMYCIN (see under Lurasidone, p. 364); increased risk of ventricular arrhythmias when amisulpride given with ● ERYTHROMYCIN—avoid concomitant use; plasma concentration of clozapine possibly increased by ● ERYTHROMYCIN (possible increased risk of convulsions); possible increased risk of ventricular arrhythmias when pimozide given with ● ERYTHROMYCIN—avoid concomitant use; plasma concentration of quetiapine increased by ● ERYTHROMYCIN—manufacturer of quetiapine advises avoid concomitant use; increased risk of ventricular arrhythmias when sulpiride given with *parenteral* ● ERYTHROMYCIN; increased risk of ventricular arrhythmias when zuclopenthixol given with *parenteral* ● ERYTHROMYCIN—avoid concomitant use; plasma concentration of clozapine increased by CIPROFLOXACIN; plasma concentration of olanzapine possibly increased by CIPROFLOXACIN; increased risk of ventricular arrhythmias when droperidol, haloperidol, phenothiazines or zuclopenthixol given with ● MOXIFLOXACIN—avoid concomitant use; increased risk of ventricular arrhythmias when benperidol given with ● MOXIFLOXACIN—manufacturer of benperidol advises avoid concomitant use; plasma concentration of aripiprazole possibly reduced by ● RIFABUTIN and ● RIFAMPICIN (avoid concomitant use or consider increasing the dose of aripiprazole—consult aripiprazole product literature); plasma concentration of lurasidone reduced by ● RIFAMPICIN—avoid concomitant use; plasma concentration of clozapine possibly reduced by RIFAMPICIN; metabolism of haloperidol accelerated by ● RIFAMPICIN (reduced plasma concentration); avoid concomitant use of clozapine with ● CHLORAMPHENICOL or ● SULFONAMIDES (increased risk of agranulocytosis); increased risk of ventricular arrhythmias when droperidol, haloperidol or pimozide given with ● DELAMANID; increased risk of

Antipsychotics

- **Antibacterials** (continued)
  ventricular arrhythmias when phenothiazines that prolong the QT interval given with • DELAMANID; manufacturer of droperidol advises avoid concomitant use with • MACROLIDES (risk of ventricular arrhythmias); possible increased risk of ventricular arrhythmias when chlorpromazine given with • TELITHROMYCIN; plasma concentration of quetiapine possibly increased by TELITHROMYCIN
- **Antidepressants:** plasma concentration of clozapine possibly increased by CITALOPRAM (increased risk of toxicity); avoidance of haloperidol, phenothiazines and pimozide advised by manufacturer of • CITALOPRAM (risk of ventricular arrhythmias); avoidance of haloperidol, phenothiazines and pimozide advised by manufacturer of • ESCITALOPRAM (risk of ventricular arrhythmias); plasma concentration of aripiprazole possibly increased by • FLUOXETINE and • PAROXETINE (reduce dose of aripiprazole—consult aripiprazole product literature); plasma concentration of clozapine, haloperidol and risperidone increased by • FLUOXETINE; manufacturer of droperidol advises avoid concomitant use with • FLUOXETINE, • FLUVOXAMINE, • SERTRALINE and • TRICYCLICS (risk of ventricular arrhythmias); plasma concentration of asenapine and haloperidol possibly increased by FLUVOXAMINE; plasma concentration of clozapine and olanzapine increased by • FLUVOXAMINE; asenapine possibly increases plasma concentration of PAROXETINE; plasma concentration of clozapine increased by • PAROXETINE and • SERTRALINE; plasma concentration of risperidone possibly increased by PAROXETINE (increased risk of toxicity); metabolism of perphenazine inhibited by PAROXETINE (reduce dose of perphenazine); plasma concentration of haloperidol increased by VENLAFAXINE; clozapine possibly increases CNS effects of • MAOIS; plasma concentration of pimozide possibly increased by • SSRIS (increased risk of ventricular arrhythmias—avoid concomitant use); plasma concentration of lurasidone possibly reduced by • ST JOHN'S WORT—avoid concomitant use; plasma concentration of aripiprazole possibly reduced by • ST JOHN'S WORT (avoid concomitant use or consider increasing the dose of aripiprazole—consult aripiprazole product literature); manufacturer of fluphenazine, haloperidol, sulpiride and zuclopenthixol advises avoid concomitant use with • TRICYCLICS (risk of ventricular arrhythmias); increased risk of antimuscarinic side-effects when phenothiazines given with TRICYCLICS; possible increased risk of ventricular arrhythmias when risperidone given with • TRICYCLICS; possible increased antimuscarinic side-effects when clozapine given with TRICYCLICS; possible increased risk of convulsions when butyrophenones, phenothiazines or thioxanthenes given with • VORTIOXETINE
- ‣ **Antidiabetics:** phenothiazines possibly antagonise hypoglycaemic effect of SULFONYLUREAS
- **Antiepileptics:** antipsychotics antagonise anticonvulsant effect of • ANTIEPILEPTICS (convulsive threshold lowered); metabolism of haloperidol, olanzapine, quetiapine and risperidone accelerated by CARBAMAZEPINE (reduced plasma concentration); metabolism of clozapine accelerated by • CARBAMAZEPINE (reduced plasma concentration), also avoid concomitant use of drugs with substantial potential for causing agranulocytosis; plasma concentration of aripiprazole reduced by CARBAMAZEPINE (avoid concomitant use or consider increasing the dose of aripiprazole —consult aripiprazole product literature); plasma concentration of paliperidone reduced by CARBAMAZEPINE; plasma concentration of lurasidone possibly reduced by • CARBAMAZEPINE, • FOSPHENYTOIN, • PHENOBARBITAL, • PHENYTOIN and • PRIMIDONE—avoid concomitant use; chlorpromazine possibly increases or decreases plasma concentration of FOSPHENYTOIN and PHENYTOIN; metabolism of clozapine and quetiapine accelerated by FOSPHENYTOIN (reduced plasma concentration); plasma concentration of aripiprazole possibly reduced by • FOSPHENYTOIN, • PHENOBARBITAL, • PHENYTOIN and • PRIMIDONE (avoid concomitant use or consider increasing the dose of

Antipsychotics

- **Antiepileptics** (continued)
  aripiprazole—consult aripiprazole product literature); plasma concentration of haloperidol reduced by FOSPHENYTOIN and PHENYTOIN; metabolism of haloperidol accelerated by PHENOBARBITAL and PRIMIDONE (reduced plasma concentration); plasma concentration of both drugs reduced when chlorpromazine given with PHENOBARBITAL and PRIMIDONE; plasma concentration of clozapine possibly reduced by PHENOBARBITAL and PRIMIDONE; metabolism of clozapine and quetiapine accelerated by PHENYTOIN (reduced plasma concentration); increased risk of side-effects including neutropenia when olanzapine given with • SODIUM VALPROATE and • VALPROIC ACID; plasma concentration of clozapine possibly increased or decreased by SODIUM VALPROATE and VALPROIC ACID
- **Antifungals:** plasma concentration of lurasidone increased by • KETOCONAZOLE—avoid concomitant use; metabolism of aripiprazole inhibited by • KETOCONAZOLE (reduce dose of aripiprazole); plasma concentration of lurasidone possibly increased by • FLUCONAZOLE (see under Lurasidone, p. 364); plasma concentration of lurasidone possibly increased by • ITRACONAZOLE, • POSACONAZOLE and • VORICONAZOLE—avoid concomitant use; plasma concentration of aripiprazole possibly increased by • ITRACONAZOLE (reduce dose of aripiprazole—consult aripiprazole product literature); side-effects of risperidone possibly increased by ITRACONAZOLE; plasma concentration of haloperidol possibly increased by ITRACONAZOLE; increased risk of ventricular arrhythmias when pimozide given with • IMIDAZOLES or • TRIAZOLES—avoid concomitant use; plasma concentration of quetiapine possibly increased by • IMIDAZOLES and • TRIAZOLES—manufacturer of quetiapine advises avoid concomitant use
- **Antimalarials:** avoidance of antipsychotics advised by manufacturer of • ARTEMETHER WITH LUMEFANTRINE; avoidance of droperidol, haloperidol, phenothiazines and pimozide advised by manufacturer of • ARTENIMOL WITH PIPERAQUINE (possible risk of ventricular arrhythmias); increased risk of ventricular arrhythmias when droperidol given with • CHLOROQUINE, • HYDROXYCHLOROQUINE or • QUININE—avoid concomitant use; possible increased risk of ventricular arrhythmias when haloperidol given with • MEFLOQUINE or • QUININE—avoid concomitant use; manufacturer of risperidone advises possible risk of ventricular arrhythmias when risperidone given with • MEFLOQUINE; increased risk of ventricular arrhythmias when pimozide given with • MEFLOQUINE or • QUININE—avoid concomitant use; manufacturer of amisulpride advises avoid concomitant use with MEFLOQUINE; possible increased risk of ventricular arrhythmias when risperidone given with • QUININE
- ‣ **Antimuscarinics:** increased risk of antimuscarinic side-effects when clozapine given with ANTIMUSCARINICS; plasma concentration of phenothiazines reduced by ANTIMUSCARINICS, but risk of antimuscarinic side-effects increased; effects of haloperidol possibly reduced by ANTIMUSCARINICS
- **Antipsychotics:** increased risk of ventricular arrhythmias when amisulpride, pimozide or sulpiride given with • DROPERIDOL—avoid concomitant use; increased risk of ventricular arrhythmias when phenothiazines that prolong the QT interval given with • DROPERIDOL—avoid concomitant use; avoid concomitant use of clozapine with depot formulation of • FLUPENTIXOL, • FLUPHENAZINE, • HALOPERIDOL, • RISPERIDONE or • ZUCLOPENTHIXOL as cannot be withdrawn quickly if neutropenia occurs; increased risk of ventricular arrhythmias when sulpiride given with • HALOPERIDOL; chlorpromazine possibly increases plasma concentration of HALOPERIDOL; increased risk of ventricular arrhythmias when droperidol given with • HALOPERIDOL—avoid concomitant use; increased risk of ventricular arrhythmias when pimozide given with • PHENOTHIAZINES—avoid concomitant use; lurasidone possibly increases plasma concentration of PIMOZIDE (increased risk of toxicity); possible increased risk of ventricular arrhythmias when antipsychotics that prolong the QT interval given with • RISPERIDONE; increased risk of ventricular arrhythmias when pimozide given with • SULPIRIDE

A1

Interactions | **Appendix 1**

Antipsychotics (continued)

- **Antivirals:** plasma concentration of aripiprazole possibly increased by ● ATAZANAVIR, ● DARUNAVIR, ● FOSAMPRENAVIR, ● INDINAVIR, ● LOPINAVIR, ● RITONAVIR, ● SAQUINAVIR and ● TIPRANAVIR (reduce dose of aripiprazole—consult aripiprazole product literature); plasma concentration of quetiapine possibly increased by ● ATAZANAVIR, ● BOCEPREVIR, ● DARUNAVIR, ● FOSAMPRENAVIR, ● INDINAVIR, ● LOPINAVIR, ● RITONAVIR, ● SAQUINAVIR, ● TELAPREVIR and ● TIPRANAVIR—manufacturer of quetiapine advises avoid concomitant use; plasma concentration of pimozide possibly increased by ● ATAZANAVIR—avoid concomitant use; avoidance of pimozide advised by manufacturer of ● BOCEPREVIR and ● TELAPREVIR; plasma concentration of lurasidone possibly increased by ● BOCEPREVIR, ● INDINAVIR, ● RITONAVIR, ● SAQUINAVIR and ● TELAPREVIR—avoid concomitant use; plasma concentration of aripiprazole possibly reduced by ● EFAVIRENZ and ● NEVIRAPINE (avoid concomitant use or consider increasing the dose of aripiprazole—consult aripiprazole product literature); plasma concentration of pimozide possibly increased by ● EFAVIRENZ, ● INDINAVIR and ● SAQUINAVIR (increased risk of ventricular arrhythmias—avoid concomitant use); plasma concentration of pimozide increased by ● FOSAMPRENAVIR and ● RITONAVIR (increased risk of ventricular arrhythmias—avoid concomitant use); plasma concentration of antipsychotics possibly increased by ● RITONAVIR; plasma concentration of olanzapine reduced by ● RITONAVIR—consider increasing dose of olanzapine; avoidance of clozapine advised by manufacturer of ● RITONAVIR (increased risk of toxicity); increased risk of ventricular arrhythmias when clozapine, haloperidol or phenothiazines given with ● SAQUINAVIR—avoid concomitant use
- **Anxiolytics and Hypnotics:** increased sedative effect when antipsychotics given with ANXIOLYTICS AND HYPNOTICS; plasma concentration of haloperidol possibly increased by ALPRAZOLAM; lurasidone increases plasma concentration of MIDAZOLAM; serious adverse events reported with concomitant use of clozapine and ● BENZODIAZEPINES (causality not established); increased risk of hypotension, bradycardia and respiratory depression when *intramuscular* olanzapine given with *parenteral* ● BENZODIAZEPINES; plasma concentration of haloperidol increased by BUSPIRONE
- **Aprepitant:** avoidance of pimozide advised by manufacturer of ● APREPITANT
- **Atomoxetine:** increased risk of ventricular arrhythmias when antipsychotics that prolong the QT interval given with ● ATOMOXETINE
- **Beta-blockers:** enhanced hypotensive effect when phenothiazines given with BETA-BLOCKERS; plasma concentration of both drugs may increase when chlorpromazine given with ● PROPRANOLOL; increased risk of ventricular arrhythmias when droperidol or zuclopenthixol given with ● SOTALOL—avoid concomitant use; increased risk of ventricular arrhythmias when amisulpride, phenothiazines, pimozide or sulpiride given with ● SOTALOL; possible increased risk of ventricular arrhythmias when risperidone given with ● SOTALOL; possible increased risk of ventricular arrhythmias when haloperidol given with ● SOTALOL—avoid concomitant use
- **Calcium-channel Blockers:** enhanced hypotensive effect when antipsychotics given with CALCIUM-CHANNEL BLOCKERS; plasma concentration of lurasidone increased by ● DILTIAZEM (see under Lurasidone, p. 364); plasma concentration of lurasidone possibly increased by ● VERAPAMIL (see under Lurasidone, p. 364)
- **Clonidine:** enhanced hypotensive effect when phenothiazines given with CLONIDINE
- **Cobicistat:** plasma concentration of lurasidone possibly increased by ● COBICISTAT—avoid concomitant use; plasma concentration of pimozide possibly increased by ● COBICISTAT—manufacturer of cobicistat advises avoid concomitant use
- **Cytotoxics:** avoid concomitant use of clozapine with ● CYTOTOXICS (increased risk of agranulocytosis); possible increased risk of ventricular arrhythmias when haloperidol given with ● BOSUTINIB; caution with pimozide advised by

Antipsychotics

- **Cytotoxics** (continued)
  manufacturer of ● CRIZOTINIB; avoidance of pimozide and quetiapine advised by manufacturer of IDELALISIB; avoidance of pimozide advised by manufacturer of ● LAPATINIB; possible increased risk of ventricular arrhythmias when amisulpride, chlorpromazine, haloperidol, pimozide, sulpiride or zuclopenthixol given with VANDETANIB—avoid concomitant use; increased risk of ventricular arrhythmias when antipsychotics that prolong the QT interval given with ● ARSENIC TRIOXIDE; increased risk of ventricular arrhythmias when haloperidol given with ● ARSENIC TRIOXIDE
- **Deferasirox:** avoidance of clozapine advised by manufacturer of DEFERASIROX
- **Desferrioxamine:** manufacturer of levomepromazine advises avoid concomitant use with DESFERRIOXAMINE; avoidance of prochlorperazine advised by manufacturer of DESFERRIOXAMINE
- **Diazoxide:** enhanced hypotensive effect when phenothiazines given with DIAZOXIDE
- **Diuretics:** risk of ventricular arrhythmias with amisulpride increased by hypokalaemia caused by ● DIURETICS; risk of ventricular arrhythmias with pimozide increased by hypokalaemia caused by ● DIURETICS (avoid concomitant use); enhanced hypotensive effect when phenothiazines given with DIURETICS
- **Dopaminergics:** increased risk of extrapyramidal side-effects when antipsychotics given with AMANTADINE; antipsychotics antagonise effects of APOMORPHINE, CO-BENELDOPA, CO-CARELDOPA, LEVODOPA and PERGOLIDE; antipsychotics antagonise hypoprolactinaemic and antiparkinsonian effects of BROMOCRIPTINE and CABERGOLINE; manufacturer of amisulpride advises avoid concomitant use of CO-BENELDOPA, CO-CARELDOPA and LEVODOPA (antagonism of effect); avoidance of antipsychotics advised by manufacturer of PRAMIPEXOLE, ROPINIROLE and ROTIGOTINE (antagonism of effect)
- **Ergot Alkaloids:** lurasidone possibly increases plasma concentration of ERGOT ALKALOIDS (increased risk of toxicity)
- **Fosaprepitant:** avoidance of pimozide advised by manufacturer of ● FOSAPREPITANT
- **Grapefruit Juice:** manufacturer of lurasidone and pimozide advises avoid concomitant use with GRAPEFRUIT JUICE; plasma concentration of quetiapine possibly increased by ● GRAPEFRUIT JUICE—manufacturer of quetiapine advises avoid concomitant use
- **Guanfacine:** sedative effects possibly increased when antipsychotics given with GUANFACINE
- **Histamine:** antipsychotics theoretically antagonise effects of HISTAMINE—manufacturer of histamine advises avoid concomitant use
- **Hormone Antagonists:** manufacturer of droperidol advises avoid concomitant use with ● TAMOXIFEN (risk of ventricular arrhythmias)
- **Ivabradine:** increased risk of ventricular arrhythmias when pimozide given with ● IVABRADINE
- **Lithium:** increased risk of extrapyramidal side-effects and possibly neurotoxicity when clozapine, flupentixol, haloperidol, phenothiazines, risperidone or zuclopenthixol given with ● LITHIUM; possible risk of toxicity when olanzapine given with LITHIUM; extrapyramidal side-effects of quetiapine possibly increased by LITHIUM; increased risk of extrapyramidal side-effects when sulpiride given with LITHIUM
- **Memantine:** effects of antipsychotics possibly reduced by MEMANTINE
- **Methyldopa:** enhanced hypotensive effect when antipsychotics given with METHYLDOPA (also increased risk of extrapyramidal effects)
- **Metoclopramide:** increased risk of extrapyramidal side-effects when antipsychotics given with METOCLOPRAMIDE
- **Moxonidine:** enhanced hypotensive effect when phenothiazines given with MOXONIDINE
- **Muscle Relaxants:** promazine possibly enhances effects of SUXAMETHONIUM
- **Nitrates:** enhanced hypotensive effect when phenothiazines given with NITRATES

Antipsychotics (continued)

- Penicillamine: increased risk of haematological toxicity when clozapine given with • PENICILLAMINE—manufacturer of penicillamine advises avoid concomitant use
- Pentamidine Isetionate: increased risk of ventricular arrhythmias when amisulpride or droperidol given with • PENTAMIDINE ISETIONATE—avoid concomitant use; increased risk of ventricular arrhythmias when phenothiazines given with • PENTAMIDINE ISETIONATE
▸ Sodium Benzoate: haloperidol possibly reduces effects of SODIUM BENZOATE
▸ Sodium Oxybate: antipsychotics possibly enhance effects of SODIUM OXYBATE
▸ Sodium Phenylbutyrate: haloperidol possibly reduces effects of SODIUM PHENYLBUTYRATE
▸ Sympathomimetics: antipsychotics antagonise hypertensive effect of SYMPATHOMIMETICS; antipsychotic effects of chlorpromazine possibly antagonised by DEXAMFETAMINE; chlorpromazine possibly reduces effects of LISDEXAMFETAMINE; side-effects of risperidone possibly increased by METHYLPHENIDATE
- Tacrolimus: manufacturer of droperidol advises avoid concomitant use with • TACROLIMUS (risk of ventricular arrhythmias)
- Tetrabenazine: increased risk of extrapyramidal side-effects when antipsychotics given with TETRABENAZINE
▸ Ulcer-healing Drugs: effects of antipsychotics, chlorpromazine and clozapine possibly enhanced by CIMETIDINE; plasma concentration of clozapine possibly reduced by OMEPRAZOLE; absorption of sulpiride reduced by SUCRALFATE
▸ Vasodilator Antihypertensives: enhanced hypotensive effect when phenothiazines given with HYDRALAZINE, MINOXIDIL or SODIUM NITROPRUSSIDE

Antivirals *see* individual drugs

Anxiolytics and Hypnotics

▸ ACE Inhibitors: enhanced hypotensive effect when anxiolytics and hypnotics given with ACE INHIBITORS
▸ Adrenergic Neurone Blockers: enhanced hypotensive effect when anxiolytics and hypnotics given with ADRENERGIC NEURONE BLOCKERS
- Alcohol: increased sedative effect when anxiolytics and hypnotics given with ALCOHOL
▸ Alpha-blockers: enhanced hypotensive and sedative effects when anxiolytics and hypnotics given with ALPHA-BLOCKERS
▸ Aminophylline: effects of benzodiazepines possibly reduced by AMINOPHYLLINE
▸ Anaesthetics, General: increased sedative effect when anxiolytics and hypnotics given with GENERAL ANAESTHETICS
▸ Analgesics: metabolism of midazolam possibly inhibited by FENTANYL; increased sedative effect when anxiolytics and hypnotics given with OPIOID ANALGESICS
▸ Angiotensin-II Receptor Antagonists: enhanced hypotensive effect when anxiolytics and hypnotics given with ANGIOTENSIN-II RECEPTOR ANTAGONISTS
- Antibacterials: metabolism of midazolam inhibited by • CLARITHROMYCIN, • ERYTHROMYCIN and • TELITHROMYCIN (increased plasma concentration with increased sedation); plasma concentration of buspirone increased by ERYTHROMYCIN (reduce dose of buspirone); metabolism of zopiclone inhibited by ERYTHROMYCIN; manufacturer of zolpidem advises avoid concomitant use with CIPROFLOXACIN; metabolism of benzodiazepines possibly accelerated by RIFAMPICIN (reduced plasma concentration); metabolism of diazepam and zaleplon accelerated by RIFAMPICIN (reduced plasma concentration); metabolism of buspirone possibly accelerated by RIFAMPICIN; metabolism of zolpidem accelerated by RIFAMPICIN (reduced plasma concentration and reduced effect); plasma concentration of zopiclone significantly reduced by RIFAMPICIN; metabolism of diazepam inhibited by ISONIAZID
▸ Anticoagulants: chloral may transiently enhance anticoagulant effect of COUMARINS
- Antidepressants: plasma concentration of alprazolam increased by FLUOXETINE; plasma concentration of melatonin increased by • FLUVOXAMINE—avoid concomitant use; plasma concentration of some benzodiazepines increased by

Anxiolytics and Hypnotics

- **Antidepressants** (continued)
FLUVOXAMINE; sedative effects possibly increased when zolpidem given with SERTRALINE; manufacturer of buspirone advises avoid concomitant use with MAOIs; avoidance of buspirone for 14 days after stopping • TRANYLCYPROMINE advised by manufacturer of tranylcypromine; plasma concentration of *oral* midazolam possibly reduced by ST JOHN'S WORT; increased sedative effect when anxiolytics and hypnotics given with MIRTAZAPINE, TRICYCLIC-RELATED ANTIDEPRESSANTS or TRICYCLICS
▸ Antiepileptics: plasma concentration of midazolam reduced by CARBAMAZEPINE and PERAMPANEL; plasma concentration of clonazepam often reduced by CARBAMAZEPINE, FOSPHENYTOIN, PHENOBARBITAL, PHENYTOIN and PRIMIDONE; benzodiazepines possibly increase or decrease plasma concentration of FOSPHENYTOIN and PHENYTOIN; diazepam increases or decreases plasma concentration of FOSPHENYTOIN and PHENYTOIN; increased sedative effect when anxiolytics and hypnotics given with PHENOBARBITAL or PRIMIDONE; increased risk of side-effects when clonazepam given with SODIUM VALPROATE or VALPROIC ACID; clobazam possibly increases plasma concentration of SODIUM VALPROATE and VALPROIC ACID; plasma concentration of diazepam and lorazepam possibly increased by SODIUM VALPROATE; plasma concentration of clobazam increased by STIRIPENTOL; plasma concentration of diazepam and lorazepam possibly increased by VALPROIC ACID
- Antifungals: plasma concentration of alprazolam increased by • KETOCONAZOLE—manufacturer of ketoconazole advises avoid concomitant use; plasma concentration of midazolam increased by • KETOCONAZOLE (risk of prolonged sedation—avoid concomitant use of *oral* midazolam); plasma concentration of zolpidem increased by KETOCONAZOLE; plasma concentration of diazepam and midazolam increased by • FLUCONAZOLE (risk of prolonged sedation); plasma concentration of alprazolam increased by ITRACONAZOLE; plasma concentration of midazolam increased by • ITRACONAZOLE, • POSACONAZOLE and • VORICONAZOLE (risk of prolonged sedation); plasma concentration of buspirone increased by ITRACONAZOLE (reduce dose of buspirone); plasma concentration of diazepam increased by • VORICONAZOLE (risk of prolonged sedation)
▸ Antihistamines: increased sedative effect when anxiolytics and hypnotics given with ANTIHISTAMINES
- Antipsychotics: increased sedative effect when anxiolytics and hypnotics given with ANTIPSYCHOTICS; alprazolam possibly increases plasma concentration of HALOPERIDOL; buspirone increases plasma concentration of HALOPERIDOL; serious adverse events reported with concomitant use of benzodiazepines and • CLOZAPINE (causality not established); plasma concentration of midazolam increased by LURASIDONE; increased risk of hypotension, bradycardia and respiratory depression when *parenteral* benzodiazepines given with *intramuscular* • OLANZAPINE
- Antivirals: plasma concentration of midazolam possibly increased by • ATAZANAVIR—avoid concomitant use of *oral* midazolam; plasma concentration of *oral* midazolam increased by • BOCEPREVIR—manufacturer of boceprevir advises avoid concomitant use; increased risk of prolonged sedation when midazolam given with • EFAVIRENZ—avoid concomitant use; plasma concentration of midazolam possibly increased by • FOSAMPRENAVIR, • INDINAVIR, • RITONAVIR and • TELAPREVIR (risk of prolonged sedation—avoid concomitant use of *oral* midazolam); increased risk of prolonged sedation when alprazolam given with • INDINAVIR—avoid concomitant use; plasma concentration of alprazolam, diazepam, flurazepam and zolpidem possibly increased by • RITONAVIR (risk of extreme sedation and respiratory depression—avoid concomitant use); plasma concentration of anxiolytics and hypnotics possibly increased by • RITONAVIR; plasma concentration of buspirone increased by RITONAVIR (increased risk of toxicity); plasma concentration of midazolam increased by • SAQUINAVIR (risk of prolonged sedation—avoid concomitant use of *oral* midazolam); plasma concentration of *oral* midazolam increased by SIMEPREVIR

Anxiolytics and Hypnotics (continued)

▸ Aprepitant: plasma concentration of midazolam increased by APREPITANT (risk of prolonged sedation)

▸ Beta-blockers: enhanced hypotensive effect when anxiolytics and hypnotics given with BETA-BLOCKERS

▸ Calcium-channel Blockers: enhanced hypotensive effect when anxiolytics and hypnotics given with CALCIUM-CHANNEL BLOCKERS; midazolam increases absorption of LERCANIDIPINE; metabolism of midazolam inhibited by DILTIAZEM and VERAPAMIL (increased plasma concentration with increased sedation); plasma concentration of buspirone increased by DILTIAZEM and VERAPAMIL (reduce dose of buspirone)

▸ Cardiac Glycosides: alprazolam increases plasma concentration of DIGOXIN (increased risk of toxicity)

▸ Clonidine: enhanced hypotensive effect when anxiolytics and hypnotics given with CLONIDINE

● Cobicistat: avoidance of *oral* midazolam advised by manufacturer of ● COBICISTAT

▸ Cytotoxics: plasma concentration of midazolam increased by ● CRIZOTINIB and NILOTINIB; avoidance of *oral* midazolam advised by manufacturer of IDELALISIB

▸ Deferasirox: plasma concentration of midazolam possibly reduced by DEFERASIROX

▸ Diazoxide: enhanced hypotensive effect when anxiolytics and hypnotics given with DIAZOXIDE

▸ Disulfiram: metabolism of benzodiazepines inhibited by DISULFIRAM (increased sedative effects); increased risk of temazepam toxicity when given with DISULFIRAM

▸ Diuretics: enhanced hypotensive effect when anxiolytics and hypnotics given with DIURETICS; administration of chloral with *parenteral* FUROSEMIDE may displace thyroid hormone from binding sites

▸ Dopaminergics: benzodiazepines possibly antagonise effects of CO-BENELDOPA, CO-CARELDOPA and LEVODOPA

▸ Fosaprepitant: plasma concentration of midazolam increased by FOSAPREPITANT (risk of prolonged sedation)

▸ Grapefruit Juice: plasma concentration of *oral* midazolam possibly increased by GRAPEFRUIT JUICE; plasma concentration of buspirone increased by GRAPEFRUIT JUICE

▸ Guanfacine: sedative effects possibly increased when anxiolytics and hypnotics given with GUANFACINE

● Hormone Antagonists: plasma concentration of midazolam reduced by ● ENZALUTAMIDE

▸ Ivacaftor: plasma concentration of midazolam increased by IVACAFTOR

▸ Lipid-regulating Drugs: plasma concentration of *intravenous* midazolam increased by ATORVASTATIN; separating administration from alprazolam by 12 hours advised by manufacturer of LOMITAPIDE

▸ Lithium: increased risk of neurotoxicity when clonazepam given with LITHIUM

▸ Lofexidine: increased sedative effect when anxiolytics and hypnotics given with LOFEXIDINE

▸ Methyldopa: enhanced hypotensive effect when anxiolytics and hypnotics given with METHYLDOPA

● Methylthioninium: possible risk of CNS toxicity when buspirone given with ● METHYLTHIONINIUM—avoid concomitant use (if avoidance not possible, use lowest possible dose of methylthioninium and observe patient for up to 4 hours after administration)

● Moxonidine: enhanced hypotensive effect when anxiolytics and hypnotics given with MOXONIDINE; sedative effects possibly increased when benzodiazepines given with MOXONIDINE

▸ Muscle Relaxants: increased sedative effect when anxiolytics and hypnotics given with BACLOFEN or TIZANIDINE

▸ Netupitant: plasma concentration of midazolam increased by NETUPITANT

▸ Nitrates: enhanced hypotensive effect when anxiolytics and hypnotics given with NITRATES

▸ Oestrogens: plasma concentration of melatonin increased by OESTROGENS; plasma concentration of chlordiazepoxide, diazepam and nitrazepam possibly increased by OESTROGENS; plasma concentration of lorazepam, oxazepam and temazepam possibly reduced by OESTROGENS

▸ Progestogens: plasma concentration of chlordiazepoxide, diazepam and nitrazepam possibly increased by

Anxiolytics and Hypnotics

Progestogens (continued)

PROGESTOGENS; plasma concentration of lorazepam, oxazepam and temazepam possibly reduced by PROGESTOGENS

● Sodium Oxybate: benzodiazepines enhance effects of ● SODIUM OXYBATE (avoid concomitant use)

▸ Theophylline: effects of benzodiazepines possibly reduced by THEOPHYLLINE

▸ Ulcer-healing Drugs: plasma concentration of melatonin increased by CIMETIDINE; metabolism of benzodiazepines, clomethiazole and zaleplon inhibited by CIMETIDINE (increased plasma concentration); metabolism of diazepam possibly inhibited by ESOMEPRAZOLE and OMEPRAZOLE (increased plasma concentration)

▸ Vasodilator Antihypertensives: enhanced hypotensive effect when anxiolytics and hypnotics given with HYDRALAZINE, MINOXIDIL or SODIUM NITROPRUSSIDE

Apixaban

● Analgesics: increased risk of haemorrhage when anticoagulants given with *intravenous* ● DICLOFENAC (avoid concomitant use, including low-dose heparins); increased risk of haemorrhage when anticoagulants given with ● KETOROLAC (avoid concomitant use, including low-dose heparins)

● Antibacterials: manufacturer of apixaban advises avoid concomitant use with CLARITHROMYCIN and TELITHROMYCIN; plasma concentration of apixaban possibly reduced by ● RIFAMPICIN—manufacturer of apixaban advises avoid concomitant use when given for treatment of deep-vein thrombosis or pulmonary embolism

● Anticoagulants: increased risk of haemorrhage when apixaban given with other ● ANTICOAGULANTS (avoid concomitant use except when switching with other anticoagulants or using heparin to maintain catheter patency); increased risk of haemorrhage when other anticoagulants given with ● DABIGATRAN, ● EDOXABAN and ● RIVAROXABAN (avoid concomitant use except when switching with other anticoagulants or using heparin to maintain catheter patency)

● Antidepressants: plasma concentration of apixaban possibly reduced by ● ST JOHN'S WORT—manufacturer of apixaban advises avoid concomitant use when given for treatment of deep-vein thrombosis or pulmonary embolism

● Antiepileptics: plasma concentration of apixaban possibly reduced by CARBAMAZEPINE—manufacturer of apixaban advises avoid concomitant use when given for treatment of deep-vein thrombosis or pulmonary embolism; plasma concentration of apixaban possibly reduced by ● FOSPHENYTOIN, ● PHENOBARBITAL, ● PHENYTOIN and ● PRIMIDONE

● Antifungals: plasma concentration of apixaban increased by ● KETOCONAZOLE—manufacturer of apixaban advises avoid concomitant use; manufacturer of apixaban advises avoid concomitant use with ITRACONAZOLE, POSACONAZOLE and VORICONAZOLE

▸ Antivirals: manufacturer of apixaban advises avoid concomitant use with ATAZANAVIR, BOCEPREVIR, DARUNAVIR, FOSAMPRENAVIR, INDINAVIR, LOPINAVIR, RITONAVIR, SAQUINAVIR, TELAPREVIR and TIPRANAVIR

▸ Cobicistat: manufacturer of apixaban advises avoid concomitant use with COBICISTAT

▸ Sulfinpyrazone: increased risk of bleeding when apixaban given with SULFINPYRAZONE

Apomorphine

▸ Antipsychotics: effects of apomorphine antagonised by ANTIPSYCHOTICS

● Domperidone: possible increased risk of ventricular arrhythmias when apomorphine given with ● DOMPERIDONE

▸ Dopaminergics: effects of apomorphine possibly enhanced by ENTACAPONE

● 5HT$_3$-receptor Antagonists: possible increased hypotensive effect when apomorphine given with ● ONDANSETRON—avoid concomitant use

▸ Memantine: effects of dopaminergics possibly enhanced by MEMANTINE

▸ Methyldopa: antiparkinsonian effect of dopaminergics antagonised by METHYLDOPA

Apraclonidine

▸ Antidepressants: manufacturer of apraclonidine advises avoid concomitant use with MAOIs, TRICYCLIC-RELATED ANTIDEPRESSANTS and TRICYCLICS
▸ Sympathomimetics: manufacturer of apraclonidine advises avoid concomitant use with SYMPATHOMIMETICS

Apremilast

● Antibacterials: plasma concentration of apremilast reduced by ● RIFAMPICIN—avoid concomitant use
● Antidepressants: plasma concentration of apremilast possibly reduced by ● ST JOHN'S WORT—avoid concomitant use
● Antiepileptics: plasma concentration of apremilast possibly reduced by ● CARBAMAZEPINE, ● PHENOBARBITAL and ● PHENYTOIN—avoid concomitant use

Aprepitant

▸ Antibacterials: plasma concentration of aprepitant possibly increased by CLARITHROMYCIN and TELITHROMYCIN; plasma concentration of aprepitant reduced by RIFAMPICIN
▸ Anticoagulants: aprepitant possibly reduces anticoagulant effect of WARFARIN
● Antidepressants: manufacturer of aprepitant advises avoid concomitant use with ● ST JOHN'S WORT
▸ Antidiabetics: aprepitant reduces plasma concentration of TOLBUTAMIDE
▸ Antiepileptics: plasma concentration of aprepitant possibly reduced by CARBAMAZEPINE, FOSPHENYTOIN, PHENOBARBITAL, PHENYTOIN and PRIMIDONE
▸ Antifungals: plasma concentration of aprepitant increased by KETOCONAZOLE
● Antipsychotics: manufacturer of aprepitant advises avoid concomitant use with ● PIMOZIDE
▸ Antivirals: plasma concentration of aprepitant possibly increased by RITONAVIR
▸ Anxiolytics and Hypnotics: aprepitant increases plasma concentration of MIDAZOLAM (risk of prolonged sedation)
● Avanafil: aprepitant possibly increases plasma concentration of ● AVANAFIL—see under Avanafil, p. 735
▸ Calcium-channel Blockers: plasma concentration of both drugs may increase when aprepitant given with DILTIAZEM
▸ Corticosteroids: aprepitant inhibits metabolism of DEXAMETHASONE and METHYLPREDNISOLONE (reduce dose of dexamethasone and methylprednisolone)
● Cytotoxics: aprepitant possibly increases the plasma concentration of ● BOSUTINIB—manufacturer of bosutinib advises avoid or consider reducing dose of bosutinib; aprepitant possibly increases the plasma concentration of ● IBRUTINIB—reduce dose of ibrutinib (see under Ibrutinib, p. 855)
▸ Dapoxetine: manufacturer of dapoxetine advises dose reduction when aprepitant given with DAPOXETINE (see under Dapoxetine, p. 742)
▸ Guanfacine: aprepitant possibly increases plasma concentration of GUANFACINE (halve dose of guanfacine)
● Oestrogens: aprepitant possibly causes contraceptive failure of hormonal contraceptives containing ● OESTROGENS (alternative contraception recommended)
● Progestogens: aprepitant possibly causes contraceptive failure of hormonal contraceptives containing ● PROGESTOGENS (alternative contraception recommended)

Argatroban

● Analgesics: increased risk of haemorrhage when anticoagulants given with *intravenous* ● DICLOFENAC (avoid concomitant use, including low-dose heparins); increased risk of haemorrhage when anticoagulants given with ● KETOROLAC (avoid concomitant use, including low-dose heparins)
● Anticoagulants: increased risk of haemorrhage when other anticoagulants given with ● APIXABAN, ● DABIGATRAN, ● EDOXABAN and ● RIVAROXABAN (avoid concomitant use except when switching with other anticoagulants or using heparin to maintain catheter patency)

Aripiprazole *see* Antipsychotics

Arsenic Trioxide

● Anti-arrhythmics: increased risk of ventricular arrhythmias when arsenic trioxide given with ● AMIODARONE or ● DISOPYRAMIDE

Arsenic Trioxide (continued)

● Antibacterials: increased risk of ventricular arrhythmias when arsenic trioxide given with ● DELAMANID, ● ERYTHROMYCIN, ● LEVOFLOXACIN or ● MOXIFLOXACIN
● Antidepressants: increased risk of ventricular arrhythmias when arsenic trioxide given with ● AMITRIPTYLINE or ● CLOMIPRAMINE
● Antifungals: increased risk of ventricular arrhythmias when arsenic trioxide given with ● AMPHOTERICIN
● Antimalarials: avoidance of arsenic trioxide advised by manufacturer of ● ARTENIMOL WITH PIPERAQUINE (possible risk of ventricular arrhythmias)
● Antipsychotics: increased risk of ventricular arrhythmias when arsenic trioxide given with ● ANTIPSYCHOTICS that prolong the QT interval; increased risk of ventricular arrhythmias when arsenic trioxide given with ● HALOPERIDOL; avoid concomitant use of cytotoxics with ● CLOZAPINE (increased risk of agranulocytosis)
● Beta-blockers: increased risk of ventricular arrhythmias when arsenic trioxide given with ● SOTALOL
● Cytotoxics: possible increased risk of ventricular arrhythmias when arsenic trioxide given with ● VANDETANIB—avoid concomitant use
● Diuretics: risk of ventricular arrhythmias with arsenic trioxide increased by hypokalaemia caused by ● ACETAZOLAMIDE, ● LOOP DIURETICS or ● THIAZIDES AND RELATED DIURETICS
● Lithium: increased risk of ventricular arrhythmias when arsenic trioxide given with ● LITHIUM

Artemether with Lumefantrine

● Anti-arrhythmics: manufacturer of artemether with lumefantrine advises avoid concomitant use with ● AMIODARONE, ● DISOPYRAMIDE and ● FLECAINIDE (risk of ventricular arrhythmias)
● Antibacterials: manufacturer of artemether with lumefantrine advises avoid concomitant use with ● MACROLIDES and ● QUINOLONES
● Antidepressants: possible increased risk of ventricular arrhythmias when artemether with lumefantrine given with ● CITALOPRAM or ● ESCITALOPRAM—avoid concomitant use; manufacturer of artemether with lumefantrine advises avoid concomitant use with ● ANTIDEPRESSANTS
● Antifungals: manufacturer of artemether with lumefantrine advises avoid concomitant use with ● IMIDAZOLES and ● TRIAZOLES
● Antimalarials: manufacturer of artemether with lumefantrine advises avoid concomitant use with ● ANTIMALARIALS; increased risk of ventricular arrhythmias when artemether with lumefantrine given with ● QUININE
● Antipsychotics: manufacturer of artemether with lumefantrine advises avoid concomitant use with ● ANTIPSYCHOTICS
● Antivirals: manufacturer of artemether with lumefantrine advises caution with ATAZANAVIR, FOSAMPRENAVIR, INDINAVIR, LOPINAVIR, RITONAVIR, SAQUINAVIR and TIPRANAVIR; avoidance of artemether with lumefantrine advised by manufacturer of ● BOCEPREVIR; plasma concentration of lumefantrine increased when artemether with lumefantrine given with DARUNAVIR; plasma concentration of artemether with lumefantrine reduced by ● EFAVIRENZ and ETRAVIRINE
● Beta-blockers: manufacturer of artemether with lumefantrine advises avoid concomitant use with ● METOPROLOL and ● SOTALOL
● Cytotoxics: possible increased risk of ventricular arrhythmias when artemether with lumefantrine given with ● VANDETANIB—avoid concomitant use
▸ Grapefruit Juice: plasma concentration of artemether with lumefantrine possibly increased by GRAPEFRUIT JUICE
▸ Histamine: avoidance of antimalarials advised by manufacturer of HISTAMINE
▸ Penicillamine: increased risk of haematological toxicity when antimalarials given with PENICILLAMINE—manufacturer of penicillamine advises avoid concomitant use
● Ulcer-healing Drugs: manufacturer of artemether with lumefantrine advises avoid concomitant use with ● CIMETIDINE
▸ Vaccines: antimalarials inactivate ORAL TYPHOID VACCINE—see under Typhoid Vaccine in BNF

A1

Interactions | **Appendix 1**

Artenimol with Piperaquine

NOTE Piperaquine has a long half-life; there is a potential for drug interactions to occur for up to 3 months after treatment has been stopped

- Analgesics: manufacturer of artenimol with piperaquine advises avoid concomitant use with ● METHADONE (possible risk of ventricular arrhythmias)
- Anti-arrhythmics: manufacturer of artenimol with piperaquine advises avoid concomitant use with ● AMIODARONE and ● DISOPYRAMIDE (possible risk of ventricular arrhythmias)
- Antibacterials: manufacturer of artenimol with piperaquine advises avoid concomitant use with ● MACROLIDES and ● MOXIFLOXACIN (possible risk of ventricular arrhythmias); manufacturer of artenimol with piperaquine advises avoid concomitant use with RIFAMPICIN
- Antidepressants: possible increased risk of ventricular arrhythmias when artenimol with piperaquine given with ● CITALOPRAM or ● ESCITALOPRAM—avoid concomitant use; manufacturer of artenimol with piperaquine advises avoid concomitant use with ● ANTIDEPRESSANTS
- Antiepileptics: manufacturer of artenimol with piperaquine advises avoid concomitant use with CARBAMAZEPINE, FOSPHENYTOIN, PHENOBARBITAL, PHENYTOIN and PRIMIDONE
- Antifungals: manufacturer of artenimol with piperaquine advises avoid concomitant use with ● IMIDAZOLES and ● TRIAZOLES (possible risk of ventricular arrhythmias)
- Antihistamines: manufacturer of artenimol with piperaquine advises avoid concomitant use with ● MIZOLASTINE (possible risk of ventricular arrhythmias)
- Antimalarials: avoidance of antimalarials advised by manufacturer of ● ARTEMETHER WITH LUMEFANTRINE
- Antipsychotics: manufacturer of artenimol with piperaquine advises avoid concomitant use with ● DROPERIDOL, ● HALOPERIDOL, ● PHENOTHIAZINES and ● PIMOZIDE (possible risk of ventricular arrhythmias)
- Antivirals: manufacturer of artenimol with piperaquine advises avoid concomitant use with ● SAQUINAVIR (possible risk of ventricular arrhythmias)
- Beta-blockers: manufacturer of artenimol with piperaquine advises avoid concomitant use with ● SOTALOL (possible risk of ventricular arrhythmias)
- Cytotoxics: manufacturer of artenimol with piperaquine advises avoid concomitant use with ● ARSENIC TRIOXIDE (possible risk of ventricular arrhythmias); manufacturer of artenimol with piperaquine advises avoid concomitant use with ● VINBLASTINE, ● VINCRISTINE, ● VINFLUNINE and ● VINORELBINE
- Domperidone: manufacturer of artenimol with piperaquine advises avoid concomitant use with ● DOMPERIDONE (possible risk of ventricular arrhythmias)
- Grapefruit Juice: manufacturer of artenimol with piperaquine advises avoid concomitant use with GRAPEFRUIT JUICE
- Histamine: avoidance of antimalarials advised by manufacturer of HISTAMINE
- Penicillamine: increased risk of haematological toxicity when antimalarials given with PENICILLAMINE—manufacturer of penicillamine advises avoid concomitant use
- Pentamidine Isetionate: manufacturer of artenimol with piperaquine advises avoid concomitant use with ● PENTAMIDINE ISETIONATE (possible risk of ventricular arrhythmias)
- Vaccines: antimalarials inactivate ORAL TYPHOID VACCINE—see under Typhoid Vaccine in BNF

Ascorbic acid see Vitamins

Asenapine see Antipsychotics

Aspirin

- Adsorbents: absorption of aspirin possibly reduced by KAOLIN
- Anaesthetics, General: aspirin possibly enhances effects of THIOPENTAL
- Analgesics: avoid concomitant use of aspirin with ● NSAIDS (increased side-effects); antiplatelet effect of aspirin possibly reduced by IBUPROFEN
- Antacids: excretion of aspirin increased by alkaline urine due to some ANTACIDS
- Anticoagulants: increased risk of bleeding when aspirin given with ● COUMARINS or ● PHENINDIONE (due to antiplatelet

Aspirin

- Anticoagulants (continued)
effect); increased risk of bleeding when high-dose aspirin given with ● EDOXABAN (avoid concomitant use); aspirin enhances anticoagulant effect of ● HEPARINS
- Antidepressants: increased risk of bleeding when aspirin given with ● SSRIs or ● VENLAFAXINE
- Antiepileptics: aspirin enhances effects of FOSPHENYTOIN, PHENYTOIN, SODIUM VALPROATE and VALPROIC ACID
- Clopidogrel: increased risk of bleeding when aspirin given with CLOPIDOGREL
- Corticosteroids: increased risk of gastro-intestinal bleeding and ulceration when aspirin given with CORTICOSTEROIDS, also corticosteroids reduce plasma concentration of salicylate
- Cytotoxics: aspirin reduces excretion of ● METHOTREXATE (increased risk of toxicity); aspirin possibly reduces renal excretion of PEMETREXED—consult product literature
- Diuretics: increased risk of toxicity when high-dose aspirin given with ● ACETAZOLAMIDE; aspirin antagonises diuretic effect of SPIRONOLACTONE; possible increased risk of toxicity when high-dose aspirin given with LOOP DIURETICS (also possible reduced effect of loop diuretics)
- Iloprost: increased risk of bleeding when aspirin given with ILOPROST
- Leukotriene Receptor Antagonists: aspirin increases plasma concentration of ZAFIRLUKAST
- Metoclopramide: rate of absorption of aspirin increased by METOCLOPRAMIDE (enhanced effect)
- Nicorandil: increased risk of gastro-intestinal bleeding and ulceration when aspirin given with NICORANDIL
- Sulfinpyrazone: aspirin antagonises effects of SULFINPYRAZONE

Atazanavir

- Analgesics: atazanavir increases plasma concentration of BUPRENORPHINE
- Antacids: absorption of atazanavir reduced by ANTACIDS (give at least 2 hours before or 1 hour after antacids)
- Anti-arrhythmics: atazanavir possibly increases plasma concentration of ● AMIODARONE and ● LIDOCAINE
- Antibacterials: plasma concentration of both drugs increased when atazanavir given with CLARITHROMYCIN; atazanavir increases plasma concentration of RIFABUTIN (reduce dose of rifabutin); plasma concentration of atazanavir reduced by ● RIFAMPICIN—avoid concomitant use; avoidance of concomitant atazanavir in severe renal and hepatic impairment advised by manufacturer of ● TELITHROMYCIN
- Anticoagulants: atazanavir may enhance or reduce anticoagulant effect of WARFARIN; avoidance of atazanavir advised by manufacturer of APIXABAN and RIVAROXABAN
- Antidepressants: plasma concentration of atazanavir reduced by ● ST JOHN'S WORT—avoid concomitant use
- Antifungals: plasma concentration of atazanavir increased by ● POSACONAZOLE; atazanavir increases or decreases the plasma concentration of ● VORICONAZOLE and plasma concentration of atazanavir also reduced
- Antimalarials: caution with atazanavir advised by manufacturer of ARTEMETHER WITH LUMEFANTRINE; atazanavir possibly increases plasma concentration of ● QUININE (increased risk of toxicity)
- Antimuscarinics: avoidance of atazanavir advised by manufacturer of DARIFENACIN; manufacturer of fesoterodine advises dose reduction when atazanavir given with FESOTERODINE—consult fesoterodine product literature
- Antipsychotics: atazanavir possibly increases plasma concentration of ● ARIPIPRAZOLE (reduce dose of aripiprazole—consult aripiprazole product literature); atazanavir possibly increases plasma concentration of ● PIMOZIDE—avoid concomitant use; atazanavir possibly increases plasma concentration of ● QUETIAPINE—manufacturer of quetiapine advises avoid concomitant use
- Antivirals: plasma concentration of atazanavir reduced by ● BOCEPREVIR; atazanavir increases the plasma concentration of ● DACLATASVIR—reduce dose of daclatasvir (see under Daclatasvir, p. 568); absorption of atazanavir reduced by DIDANOSINE *tablets* (give at least 2 hours before or 1 hour after didanosine *tablets*); manufacturer of atazanavir advises avoid concomitant use with ● EFAVIRENZ (plasma concentration of

Atazanavir

- **Antivirals** (continued)
atazanavir reduced); atazanavir boosted with ritonavir increases plasma concentration of ● ELVITEGRAVIR (reduce dose of elvitegravir); avoid concomitant use of atazanavir with ● INDINAVIR; atazanavir increases plasma concentration of ● MARAVIROC (consider reducing dose of maraviroc); plasma concentration of atazanavir possibly reduced by ● NEVIRAPINE—avoid concomitant use; atazanavir increases plasma concentration of ● PARITAPREVIR; increased risk of ventricular arrhythmias when atazanavir given with ● SAQUINAVIR—avoid concomitant use; atazanavir possibly reduces plasma concentration of TELAPREVIR, also plasma concentration of atazanavir possibly increased; plasma concentration of atazanavir reduced by TENOFOVIR, also plasma concentration of tenofovir possibly increased; atazanavir increases plasma concentration of TIPRANAVIR (also plasma concentration of atazanavir reduced)
- **Anxiolytics and Hypnotics:** atazanavir possibly increases plasma concentration of ● MIDAZOLAM—avoid concomitant use of *oral* midazolam
- **Calcium-channel Blockers:** atazanavir increases plasma concentration of ● DILTIAZEM (reduce dose of diltiazem); atazanavir possibly increases plasma concentration of VERAPAMIL
- **Ciclosporin:** atazanavir possibly increases plasma concentration of ● CICLOSPORIN
- **Colchicine:** atazanavir possibly increases risk of ● COLCHICINE toxicity—suspend or reduce dose of colchicine (avoid concomitant use in hepatic or renal impairment)
- **Cytotoxics:** atazanavir possibly increases plasma concentration of AXITINIB (reduce dose of axitinib—consult axitinib product literature); atazanavir possibly increases the plasma concentration of ● BOSUTINIB—manufacturer of bosutinib advises avoid or consider reducing dose of bosutinib; atazanavir possibly increases plasma concentration of ● CRIZOTINIB and ● EVEROLIMUS—manufacturer of crizotinib and everolimus advises avoid concomitant use; atazanavir possibly increases the plasma concentration of ● IBRUTINIB— reduce dose of ibrutinib (see under Ibrutinib, p. 855); atazanavir possibly increases plasma concentration of ● PAZOPANIB (reduce dose of pazopanib); avoidance of atazanavir advised by manufacturer of ● CABAZITAXEL; atazanavir possibly inhibits metabolism of ● IRINOTECAN (increased risk of toxicity)
- **Dapoxetine:** avoidance of atazanavir advised by manufacturer of ● DAPOXETINE (increased risk of toxicity)
- **Ergot Alkaloids:** atazanavir possibly increases plasma concentration of ● ERGOT ALKALOIDS—avoid concomitant use
▸ **Guanfacine:** atazanavir possibly increases plasma concentration of GUANFACINE (halve dose of guanfacine)
- **Lipid-regulating Drugs:** possible increased risk of myopathy when atazanavir given with ● ATORVASTATIN or PRAVASTATIN; atazanavir increases plasma concentration of ● ROSUVASTATIN—adjust dose of rosuvastatin (consult product literature); increased risk of myopathy when atazanavir given with ● SIMVASTATIN (avoid concomitant use)
▸ **Oestrogens:** atazanavir increases plasma concentration of ETHINYLESTRADIOL
- **Orlistat:** absorption of atazanavir possibly reduced by ● ORLISTAT
▸ **Progestogens:** atazanavir increases plasma concentration of NORETHISTERONE
- **Ranolazine:** atazanavir possibly increases plasma concentration of ● RANOLAZINE—manufacturer of ranolazine advises avoid concomitant use
- **Sirolimus:** atazanavir possibly increases plasma concentration of ● SIROLIMUS
▸ **Sympathomimetics, Beta₂:** atazanavir possibly increases plasma concentration of SALMETEROL—manufacturer of atazanavir advises avoid concomitant use
- **Tacrolimus:** atazanavir possibly increases plasma concentration of ● TACROLIMUS
- **Ticagrelor:** atazanavir possibly increases plasma concentration of ● TICAGRELOR—manufacturer of ticagrelor advises avoid concomitant use

Atazanavir (continued)
- **Ulcer-healing Drugs:** manufacturer of atazanavir advises adjust doses of both drugs when atazanavir given with CIMETIDINE and NIZATIDINE—consult atazanavir product literature; plasma concentration of atazanavir reduced by ● FAMOTIDINE and ● RANITIDINE (adjust doses of both drugs—consult atazanavir product literature); plasma concentration of atazanavir reduced by PROTON PUMP INHIBITORS—avoid or adjust dose of both drugs (consult product literature)

Atenolol *see* Beta-blockers

Atomoxetine
- **Analgesics:** increased risk of ventricular arrhythmias when atomoxetine given with ● METHADONE; possible increased risk of convulsions when atomoxetine given with TRAMADOL
- **Anti-arrhythmics:** increased risk of ventricular arrhythmias when atomoxetine given with ● AMIODARONE or ● DISOPYRAMIDE
- **Antibacterials:** increased risk of ventricular arrhythmias when atomoxetine given with *parenteral* ● ERYTHROMYCIN; increased risk of ventricular arrhythmias when atomoxetine given with ● MOXIFLOXACIN
- **Antidepressants:** metabolism of atomoxetine possibly inhibited by FLUOXETINE and PAROXETINE; possible increased risk of convulsions when atomoxetine given with ANTIDEPRESSANTS; atomoxetine should not be started until 2 weeks after stopping ● MAOIS, also MAOIs should not be started until at least 2 weeks after stopping atomoxetine; increased risk of ventricular arrhythmias when atomoxetine given with ● TRICYCLICS
- **Antimalarials:** increased risk of ventricular arrhythmias when atomoxetine given with ● MEFLOQUINE
- **Antipsychotics:** increased risk of ventricular arrhythmias when atomoxetine given with ● ANTIPSYCHOTICS that prolong the QT interval
- **Beta-blockers:** increased risk of ventricular arrhythmias when atomoxetine given with ● SOTALOL
▸ **Bupropion:** possible increased risk of convulsions when atomoxetine given with BUPROPION
- **Diuretics:** risk of ventricular arrhythmias with atomoxetine increased by hypokalaemia caused by ● DIURETICS
▸ **Sympathomimetics, Beta₂:** increased risk of cardiovascular side-effects when atomoxetine given with *parenteral* SALBUTAMOL

Atorvastatin *see* Statins

Atovaquone
- **Antibacterials:** manufacturer of atovaquone advises avoid concomitant use with RIFABUTIN (plasma concentration of both drugs reduced); plasma concentration of atovaquone reduced by RIFAMPICIN (and concentration of rifampicin increased)—avoid concomitant use; plasma concentration of atovaquone reduced by TETRACYCLINE
- **Antivirals:** plasma concentration of atovaquone reduced by ● EFAVIRENZ—avoid concomitant use; atovaquone possibly reduces plasma concentration of INDINAVIR; plasma concentration of atovaquone possibly reduced by RITONAVIR— manufacturer of atovaquone advises avoid concomitant use; atovaquone increases plasma concentration of ZIDOVUDINE (increased risk of toxicity)
▸ **Cytotoxics:** atovaquone possibly increases plasma concentration of ETOPOSIDE
▸ **Histamine:** avoidance of atovaquone advised by manufacturer of HISTAMINE
▸ **Metoclopramide:** plasma concentration of atovaquone reduced by METOCLOPRAMIDE—avoid concomitant use

Atracurium *see* Muscle Relaxants

Atropine *see* Antimuscarinics

Avanafil
▸ **ACE Inhibitors:** avanafil possibly enhances hypotensive effect of ENALAPRIL
▸ **Alcohol:** possible enhanced hypotensive effect when avanafil given with ALCOHOL
- **Alpha-blockers:** enhanced hypotensive effect when avanafil given with ● ALPHA-BLOCKERS—when patient is stable on the alpha blocker initiate avanafil at the lowest possible dose
- **Antibacterials:** plasma concentration of avanafil possibly increased by ● CLARITHROMYCIN and ● TELITHROMYCIN— manufacturer of avanafil advises avoid concomitant use;

Avanafil

- **Antibacterials** (continued)
  plasma concentration of avanafil increased by
  • ERYTHROMYCIN—see under Avanafil, p. 735; plasma
  concentration of avanafil possibly reduced by RIFAMPICIN—
  manufacturer of avanafil advises avoid concomitant use
- ▸ **Antiepileptics:** plasma concentration of avanafil possibly
  reduced by CARBAMAZEPINE, PHENOBARBITAL and PRIMIDONE—
  manufacturer of avanafil advises avoid concomitant use
- **Antifungals:** plasma concentration of avanafil increased by
  • KETOCONAZOLE—avoid concomitant use; plasma
  concentration of avanafil possibly increased by
  • FLUCONAZOLE—see under Avanafil, p. 735; plasma
  concentration of avanafil possibly increased by
  • ITRACONAZOLE and • VORICONAZOLE—manufacturer of
  avanafil advises avoid concomitant use
- **Antivirals:** plasma concentration of avanafil possibly reduced
  by EFAVIRENZ—manufacturer of avanafil advises avoid
  concomitant use; plasma concentration of avanafil possibly
  increased by • FOSAMPRENAVIR—see under Avanafil, p. 735;
  plasma concentration of avanafil possibly increased by
  • INDINAVIR and • SAQUINAVIR—manufacturer of avanafil
  advises avoid concomitant use; plasma concentration of
  avanafil significantly increased by • RITONAVIR—avoid
  concomitant use
- **Aprepitant:** plasma concentration of avanafil possibly
  increased by APREPITANT—see under Avanafil, p. 735
- ▸ **Bosentan:** plasma concentration of avanafil possibly reduced
  by BOSENTAN—manufacturer of avanafil advises avoid
  concomitant use
- **Calcium-channel Blockers:** plasma concentration of avanafil
  possibly increased by • DILTIAZEM and • VERAPAMIL—see under
  Avanafil, p. 735
- **Cobicistat:** plasma concentration of avanafil possibly increased
  by • COBICISTAT—avoid concomitant use
- ▸ **Fosaprepitant:** plasma concentration of avanafil possibly
  increased by FOSAPREPITANT
- ▸ **Grapefruit Juice:** plasma concentration of avanafil possibly
  increased by GRAPEFRUIT JUICE— manufacturer of avanafil
  advises avoid grapefruit juice for 24 hours before avanafil
- **Nicorandil:** avanafil significantly enhances hypotensive effect
  of • NICORANDIL (avoid concomitant use)
- **Nitrates:** avanafil significantly enhances hypotensive effect of
  • NITRATES (avoid concomitant use)
- **Riociguat:** possible enhanced hypotensive effect when avanafil
  given with • RIOCIGUAT—avoid concomitant use

Axitinib

- ▸ **Antibacterials:** plasma concentration of axitinib possibly
  increased by CLARITHROMYCIN, ERYTHROMYCIN and
  TELITHROMYCIN (reduce dose of axitinib—consult axitinib
  product literature); plasma concentration of axitinib possibly
  decreased by RIFABUTIN (increase dose of axitinib—consult
  axitinib product literature); plasma concentration of axitinib
  decreased by RIFAMPICIN (increase dose of axitinib—consult
  axitinib product literature)
- ▸ **Antidepressants:** plasma concentration of axitinib possibly
  reduced by ST JOHN'S WORT—consider increasing dose of
  axitinib
- ▸ **Antiepileptics:** plasma concentration of axitinib possibly
  decreased by CARBAMAZEPINE, FOSPHENYTOIN, PHENOBARBITAL,
  PHENYTOIN and PRIMIDONE (increase dose of axitinib—consult
  axitinib product literature)
- ▸ **Antifungals:** plasma concentration of axitinib increased by
  KETOCONAZOLE (reduce dose of axitinib—consult axitinib
  product literature); plasma concentration of axitinib possibly
  increased by ITRACONAZOLE (reduce dose of axitinib—consult
  axitinib product literature)
- **Antipsychotics:** avoid concomitant use of cytotoxics with
  • CLOZAPINE (increased risk of agranulocytosis)
- ▸ **Antivirals:** plasma concentration of axitinib possibly increased
  by ATAZANAVIR, INDINAVIR, RITONAVIR and SAQUINAVIR (reduce
  dose of axitinib—consult axitinib product literature)
- ▸ **Corticosteroids:** plasma concentration of axitinib possibly
  decreased by DEXAMETHASONE (increase dose of axitinib—
  consult axitinib product literature)

Axitinib (continued)

- ▸ **Grapefruit Juice:** plasma concentration of axitinib possibly
  increased by GRAPEFRUIT JUICE

Azathioprine

- ▸ **ACE Inhibitors:** increased risk of anaemia or leucopenia when
  azathioprine given with CAPTOPRIL especially in renal
  impairment; increased risk of anaemia when azathioprine
  given with ENALAPRIL especially in renal impairment
- **Allopurinol:** enhanced effects and increased toxicity of
  azathioprine when given with • ALLOPURINOL (reduce dose of
  azathioprine to one quarter of usual dose)
- ▸ **Analgesics:** manufacturer of azathioprine advises
  increased risk of myelosuppression when azathioprine given
  with INDOMETACIN
- **Antibacterials:** increased risk of haematological toxicity when
  azathioprine given with • SULFAMETHOXAZOLE (as co-
  trimoxazole); increased risk of haematological toxicity when
  azathioprine given with • TRIMETHOPRIM (also with co-
  trimoxazole)
- **Anticoagulants:** azathioprine possibly reduces anticoagulant
  effect of • ACENOCOUMAROL; azathioprine reduces
  anticoagulant effect of • WARFARIN
- **Antivirals:** myelosuppressive effects of azathioprine possibly
  enhanced by • RIBAVIRIN
- **Febuxostat:** avoidance of azathioprine advised by
  manufacturer of • FEBUXOSTAT
- ▸ **Ulcer-healing Drugs:** manufacturer of azathioprine advises
  possible increased risk of myelosuppression when
  azathioprine given with CIMETIDINE
- **Vaccines:** risk of generalised infections when azathioprine
  given with live • VACCINES—avoid concomitant use

Azelastine see Antihistamines

Azilsartan see Angiotensin-II Receptor Antagonists

Azithromycin see Macrolides

Aztreonam

- **Anticoagulants:** aztreonam possibly enhances anticoagulant
  effect of • COUMARINS
- **Vaccines:** antibacterials inactivate ORAL TYPHOID VACCINE—see
  under Typhoid Vaccine in BNF

Baclofen see Muscle Relaxants

Bambuterol see Sympathomimetics, Beta$_2$

Basiliximab

- **Antipsychotics:** avoid concomitant use of cytotoxics with
  • CLOZAPINE (increased risk of agranulocytosis)
- **Vaccines:** risk of generalised infections when monoclonal
  antibodies given with live • VACCINES—avoid concomitant use

BCG Vaccine see Vaccines

Beclometasone see Corticosteroids

Bedaquiline

- **Antibacterials:** plasma concentration of bedaquiline possibly
  increased by CIPROFLOXACIN, CLARITHROMYCIN and
  ERYTHROMYCIN—avoid concomitant use if ciprofloxacin,
  clarithromycin and erythromycin given for more than 14 days;
  manufacturer of bedaquiline advises avoid concomitant use
  with MOXIFLOXACIN; plasma concentration of bedaquiline
  possibly reduced by RIFABUTIN—manufacturer of bedaquiline
  advises avoid concomitant use; plasma concentration of
  bedaquiline reduced by • RIFAMPICIN—manufacturer of
  bedaquiline advises avoid concomitant use; possible
  increased risk of ventricular arrhythmias when bedaquiline
  given with • CLOFAZIMINE
- ▸ **Antidepressants:** plasma concentration of bedaquiline possibly
  reduced by ST JOHN'S WORT—manufacturer of bedaquiline
  advises avoid concomitant use
- **Antiepileptics:** plasma concentration of bedaquiline possibly
  reduced by • CARBAMAZEPINE, • FOSPHENYTOIN and
  • PHENYTOIN—manufacturer of bedaquiline advises avoid
  concomitant use
- ▸ **Antifungals:** plasma concentration of bedaquiline increased by
  KETOCONAZOLE—avoid concomitant use if ketoconazole given
  for more than 14 days; plasma concentration of bedaquiline
  possibly increased by FLUCONAZOLE—avoid concomitant use if
  fluconazole given for more than 14 days
- ▸ **Antivirals:** plasma concentration of bedaquiline possibly
  reduced by EFAVIRENZ and ETRAVIRINE—manufacturer of
  bedaquiline advises avoid concomitant use; plasma

Bedaquiline

Antivirals (continued)

concentration of bedaquiline possibly increased by RITONAVIR—manufacturer of ritonavir advises avoid concomitant use

▸ Vaccines: antibacterials inactivate ORAL TYPHOID VACCINE—see under Typhoid Vaccine in BNF

Bee Venom Extracts

• ACE Inhibitors: possible severe anaphylactoid reaction when bee venom extracts given with • ACE INHIBITORS

Belimumab

• Antipsychotics: avoid concomitant use of cytotoxics with • CLOZAPINE (increased risk of agranulocytosis)
• Vaccines: risk of generalised infections when monoclonal antibodies given with live • VACCINES—avoid concomitant use

Bendamustine

• Antipsychotics: avoid concomitant use of cytotoxics with • CLOZAPINE (increased risk of agranulocytosis)

Bendroflumethiazide see Diuretics

Benperidol see Antipsychotics

Benzodiazepines see Anxiolytics and Hypnotics

Benzthiazide see Diuretics

Benzylpenicillin see Penicillins

Beta-blockers

NOTE Since systemic absorption may follow topical application of beta-blockers to the eye the possibility of interactions, in particular, with drugs such as verapamil should be borne in mind

▸ ACE Inhibitors: enhanced hypotensive effect when beta-blockers given with ACE INHIBITORS
▸ Adrenergic Neurone Blockers: enhanced hypotensive effect when beta-blockers given with ADRENERGIC NEURONE BLOCKERS
▸ Alcohol: enhanced hypotensive effect when beta-blockers given with ALCOHOL
▸ Aldesleukin: enhanced hypotensive effect when beta-blockers given with ALDESLEUKIN
• Alpha-blockers: enhanced hypotensive effect when beta-blockers given with • ALPHA-BLOCKERS, also increased risk of first-dose hypotension with post-synaptic alpha-blockers such as prazosin
• Anaesthetics, General: enhanced hypotensive effect when beta-blockers given with GENERAL ANAESTHETICS
• Anaesthetics, Local: propranolol increases risk of • BUPIVACAINE toxicity
▸ Analgesics: hypotensive effect of beta-blockers antagonised by NSAIDs; plasma concentration of esmolol possibly increased by MORPHINE
▸ Angiotensin-II Receptor Antagonists: enhanced hypotensive effect when beta-blockers given with ANGIOTENSIN-II RECEPTOR ANTAGONISTS
• Anti-arrhythmics: increased myocardial depression when beta-blockers given with • ANTI-ARRHYTHMICS; increased risk of ventricular arrhythmias when sotalol given with • AMIODARONE, • DISOPYRAMIDE or • DRONEDARONE—avoid concomitant use; increased risk of bradycardia, AV block and myocardial depression when beta-blockers given with • AMIODARONE; plasma concentration of metoprolol and propranolol possibly increased by DRONEDARONE; increased risk of myocardial depression and bradycardia when beta-blockers given with • FLECAINIDE; nadolol possibly increases risk of LIDOCAINE toxicity; propranolol increases risk of • LIDOCAINE toxicity; plasma concentration of metoprolol and propranolol increased by PROPAFENONE
• Antibacterials: increased risk of ventricular arrhythmias when sotalol given with • MOXIFLOXACIN—avoid concomitant use; metabolism of bisoprolol and propranolol accelerated by RIFAMPICIN (plasma concentration significantly reduced); plasma concentration of carvedilol, celiprolol and metoprolol reduced by RIFAMPICIN; plasma concentration of *oral* timolol possibly reduced by RIFAMPICIN; increased risk of ventricular arrhythmias when sotalol given with • DELAMANID
• Antidepressants: plasma concentration of metoprolol increased by CITALOPRAM and ESCITALOPRAM; increased risk of ventricular arrhythmias when sotalol given with • CITALOPRAM—avoid concomitant use; avoidance of sotalol advised by manufacturer of • ESCITALOPRAM and • VENLAFAXINE (risk of

Beta-blockers

• Antidepressants (continued)

ventricular arrhythmias); plasma concentration of propranolol increased by FLUVOXAMINE; plasma concentration of metoprolol possibly increased by • PAROXETINE—increased risk of AV block (manufacturer of paroxetine advises avoid concomitant use in cardiac insufficiency); labetalol and propranolol increase plasma concentration of IMIPRAMINE; enhanced hypotensive effect when beta-blockers given with MAOIs; increased risk of ventricular arrhythmias when sotalol given with • TRICYCLICS

▸ Antidiabetics: beta-blockers may mask warning signs of hypoglycaemia (such as tremor) with ANTIDIABETICS; beta-blockers enhance hypoglycaemic effect of INSULIN
▸ Antiepileptics: plasma concentration of propranolol possibly reduced by PHENOBARBITAL and PRIMIDONE
▸ Antifungals: plasma concentration of nadolol possibly increased by KETOCONAZOLE
• Antihistamines: increased risk of ventricular arrhythmias when sotalol given with • MIZOLASTINE—avoid concomitant use
• Antimalarials: avoidance of metoprolol and sotalol advised by manufacturer of • ARTEMETHER WITH LUMEFANTRINE; avoidance of sotalol advised by manufacturer of • ARTENIMOL WITH PIPERAQUINE (possible risk of ventricular arrhythmias); increased risk of bradycardia when beta-blockers given with MEFLOQUINE
• Antimuscarinics: increased risk of ventricular arrhythmias when sotalol given with • TOLTERODINE
• Antipsychotics: increased risk of ventricular arrhythmias when sotalol given with • DROPERIDOL or • ZUCLOPENTHIXOL—avoid concomitant use; possible increased risk of ventricular arrhythmias when sotalol given with • HALOPERIDOL—avoid concomitant use; plasma concentration of both drugs may increase when propranolol given with • CHLORPROMAZINE; increased risk of ventricular arrhythmias when sotalol given with • AMISULPRIDE, • PHENOTHIAZINES, • PIMOZIDE or • SULPIRIDE; enhanced hypotensive effect when beta-blockers given with PHENOTHIAZINES; possible increased risk of ventricular arrhythmias when sotalol given with • RISPERIDONE
• Antivirals: increased risk of ventricular arrhythmias when sotalol given with • SAQUINAVIR—avoid concomitant use; avoidance of sotalol advised by manufacturer of • TELAPREVIR (risk of ventricular arrhythmias); avoidance of metoprolol for heart failure advised by manufacturer of • TIPRANAVIR
▸ Anxiolytics and Hypnotics: enhanced hypotensive effect when beta-blockers given with ANXIOLYTICS AND HYPNOTICS
• Atomoxetine: increased risk of ventricular arrhythmias when sotalol given with • ATOMOXETINE
• Calcium-channel Blockers: enhanced hypotensive effect when beta-blockers given with CALCIUM-CHANNEL BLOCKERS; possible severe hypotension and heart failure when beta-blockers given with • NIFEDIPINE; increased risk of AV block and bradycardia when beta-blockers given with • DILTIAZEM; asystole, severe hypotension and heart failure when beta-blockers given with • VERAPAMIL (see under Verapamil, p. 150)
• Cardiac Glycosides: increased risk of AV block and bradycardia when beta-blockers given with CARDIAC GLYCOSIDES
• Ciclosporin: carvedilol increases plasma concentration of • CICLOSPORIN
• Clonidine: increased risk of withdrawal hypertension when beta-blockers given with • CLONIDINE (withdraw beta-blockers several days before slowly withdrawing clonidine)
▸ Corticosteroids: hypotensive effect of beta-blockers antagonised by CORTICOSTEROIDS
• Cytotoxics: possible increased risk of ventricular arrhythmias when sotalol given with • BOSUTINIB; possible increased risk of bradycardia when beta-blockers given with CRIZOTINIB; possible increased risk of ventricular arrhythmias when sotalol given with • VANDETANIB—avoid concomitant use; increased risk of ventricular arrhythmias when sotalol given with • ARSENIC TRIOXIDE
▸ Diazoxide: enhanced hypotensive effect when beta-blockers given with DIAZOXIDE
• Diuretics: enhanced hypotensive effect when beta-blockers given with DIURETICS; risk of ventricular arrhythmias with

Beta-blockers

- Diuretics (continued)
sotalol increased by hypokalaemia caused by ● LOOP DIURETICS or ● THIAZIDES AND RELATED DIURETICS
- Dopaminergics: enhanced hypotensive effect when beta-blockers given with CO-BENELDOPA, CO-CARELDOPA or LEVODOPA
- Ergot Alkaloids: increased peripheral vasoconstriction when beta-blockers given with ERGOT ALKALOIDS
- Fingolimod: possible increased risk of bradycardia when beta-blockers given with ● FINGOLIMOD
- Hormone Antagonists: possible increased risk of bradycardia when carteolol, metoprolol, propranolol or sotalol given with PASIREOTIDE
▹ 5HT₁-receptor Agonists: propranolol increases plasma concentration of RIZATRIPTAN (manufacturer of rizatriptan advises halve dose and avoid within 2 hours of propranolol)
- Ivabradine: increased risk of ventricular arrhythmias when sotalol given with ● IVABRADINE
▹ Methyldopa: enhanced hypotensive effect when beta-blockers given with METHYLDOPA
▹ Mirabegron: plasma concentration of metoprolol increased by MIRABEGRON
- Moxisylyte: possible severe postural hypotension when beta-blockers given with ● MOXISYLYTE
- Moxonidine: enhanced hypotensive effect when beta-blockers given with MOXONIDINE
▹ Muscle Relaxants: propranolol enhances effects of MUSCLE RELAXANTS; enhanced hypotensive effect when beta-blockers given with BACLOFEN; possible enhanced hypotensive effect and bradycardia when beta-blockers given with TIZANIDINE
▹ Nitrates: enhanced hypotensive effect when beta-blockers given with NITRATES
- Oestrogens: hypotensive effect of beta-blockers antagonised by OESTROGENS
▹ Parasympathomimetics: propranolol antagonises effects of NEOSTIGMINE and PYRIDOSTIGMINE; increased risk of arrhythmias when beta-blockers given with PILOCARPINE
▹ Prostaglandins: enhanced hypotensive effect when beta-blockers given with ALPROSTADIL
- Ranolazine: avoidance of sotalol advised by manufacturer of ● RANOLAZINE
- Sympathomimetics: increased risk of severe hypertension and bradycardia when non-cardioselective beta-blockers given with ● ADRENALINE (EPINEPHRINE), also reponse to adrenaline (epinephrine) may be reduced; increased risk of severe hypertension and bradycardia when non-cardioselective beta-blockers given with ● DOBUTAMINE; possible increased risk of severe hypertension and bradycardia when non-cardioselective beta-blockers given with ● NORADRENALINE (NOREPINEPHRINE)
▹ Thyroid Hormones: metabolism of propranolol accelerated by LEVOTHYROXINE
▹ Ulcer-healing Drugs: plasma concentration of labetalol, metoprolol and propranolol increased by CIMETIDINE; plasma concentration of *oral* timolol possibly increased by CIMETIDINE
▹ Vasodilator Antihypertensives: enhanced hypotensive effect when beta-blockers given with HYDRALAZINE, MINOXIDIL or SODIUM NITROPRUSSIDE

Betahistine

▹ Antihistamines: effect of betahistine theoretically antagonised by ANTIHISTAMINES

Betamethasone see Corticosteroids

Betaxolol see Beta-blockers

Bethanechol see Parasympathomimetics

Bevacizumab

- Antipsychotics: avoid concomitant use of cytotoxics with ● CLOZAPINE (increased risk of agranulocytosis)
- Cytotoxics: avoidance of bevacizumab advised by manufacturer of ● PANITUMUMAB
- Vaccines: risk of generalised infections when monoclonal antibodies given with live ● VACCINES—avoid concomitant use

Bexarotene

- Antipsychotics: avoid concomitant use of cytotoxics with ● CLOZAPINE (increased risk of agranulocytosis)
- Lipid-regulating Drugs: plasma concentration of bexarotene increased by ● GEMFIBROZIL—avoid concomitant use

Bezafibrate see Fibrates

Bicalutamide

- Anticoagulants: bicalutamide possibly enhances anticoagulant effect of COUMARINS
▹ Lipid-regulating Drugs: separating administration from bicalutamide by 12 hours advised by manufacturer of LOMITAPIDE

Biguanides see Antidiabetics

Bilastine see Antihistamines

Bile Acid Sequestrants see Colesevelam, Colestipol, and Colestyramine

Bile Acids

▹ Antacids: absorption of bile acids possibly reduced by ANTACIDS; effects of cholic acid probably reduced by ALUMINIUM HYDROXIDE (manufacturer of cholic acid advises give at least 5 hours apart)
- Antiepileptics: manufacturer of cholic acid advises avoid concomitant use with ● PHENOBARBITAL
- Ciclosporin: manufacturer of cholic acid advises avoid concomitant use with CICLOSPORIN; ursodeoxycholic acid increases absorption of ● CICLOSPORIN
▹ Lipid-regulating Drugs: effects of cholic acid probably reduced by COLESEVELAM, COLESTIPOL and COLESTYRAMINE (manufacturer of cholic acid advises give at least 5 hours apart); absorption of bile acids possibly reduced by COLESTIPOL and COLESTYRAMINE

Bisoprolol see Beta-blockers

Bisphosphonates

▹ Antacids: absorption of bisphosphonates reduced by ANTACIDS
▹ Antibacterials: increased risk of hypocalcaemia when bisphosphonates given with AMINOGLYCOSIDES
▹ Calcium Salts: absorption of bisphosphonates reduced by CALCIUM SALTS
- Cytotoxics: sodium clodronate increases plasma concentration of ● ESTRAMUSTINE
▹ Iron Salts: absorption of bisphosphonates reduced by *oral* IRON SALTS

Bivalirudin

- Analgesics: increased risk of haemorrhage when anticoagulants given with *intravenous* ● DICLOFENAC (avoid concomitant use, including low-dose heparins); increased risk of haemorrhage when anticoagulants given with ● KETOROLAC (avoid concomitant use, including low-dose heparins)
- Anticoagulants: increased risk of haemorrhage when other anticoagulants given with ● APIXABAN, ● DABIGATRAN, ● EDOXABAN and ● RIVAROXABAN (avoid concomitant use except when switching with other anticoagulants or using heparin to maintain catheter patency)

Bleomycin

- Antipsychotics: avoid concomitant use of cytotoxics with ● CLOZAPINE (increased risk of agranulocytosis)
▹ Cardiac Glycosides: bleomycin possibly reduces absorption of DIGOXIN *tablets*
- Cytotoxics: increased risk of pulmonary toxicity when bleomycin given with ● BRENTUXIMAB VEDOTIN—avoid concomitant use; increased pulmonary toxicity when bleomycin given with ● CISPLATIN
- Vaccines: risk of generalised infections when cytotoxic antibiotics given with live ● VACCINES—avoid concomitant use

Boceprevir

▹ Alpha-blockers: boceprevir possibly increases plasma concentration of DOXAZOSIN and TAMSULOSIN—manufacturer of boceprevir advises avoid concomitant use
- Analgesics: possible increased risk of prolonged sedation and respiratory depression when boceprevir given with BUPRENORPHINE; boceprevir possibly affects plasma concentration of METHADONE
- Antibacterials: manufacturer of boceprevir advises avoid concomitant use with ● RIFAMPICIN (plasma concentration of boceprevir possibly reduced)
- Anticoagulants: avoidance of boceprevir advised by manufacturer of APIXABAN
- Antiepileptics: manufacturer of boceprevir advises avoid concomitant use with ● CARBAMAZEPINE, ● FOSPHENYTOIN, ● PHENOBARBITAL, ● PHENYTOIN and ● PRIMIDONE (plasma concentration of boceprevir possibly reduced)

Boceprevir (continued)

- Antifungals: plasma concentration of boceprevir increased by ● KETOCONAZOLE
- Antimalarials: manufacturer of boceprevir advises avoid concomitant use with ● ARTEMETHER WITH LUMEFANTRINE
- Antipsychotics: boceprevir possibly increases plasma concentration of ● LURASIDONE—avoid concomitant use; manufacturer of boceprevir advises avoid concomitant use with ● PIMOZIDE; boceprevir possibly increases plasma concentration of ● QUETIAPINE—manufacturer of quetiapine advises avoid concomitant use
- Antivirals: boceprevir reduces plasma concentration of ● ATAZANAVIR; boceprevir possibly increases the plasma concentration of ● DACLATASVIR—reduce dose of daclatasvir (see under Daclatasvir, p. 568); avoid concomitant use of boceprevir with ● DARUNAVIR; effects of both drugs possibly reduced when boceprevir given with ● ETRAVIRINE; avoidance of boceprevir advised by manufacturer of ● FOSAMPRENAVIR, NEVIRAPINE and TIPRANAVIR; manufacturers advise avoid concomitant use of boceprevir with ● LOPINAVIR; boceprevir increases plasma concentration of MARAVIROC (consider reducing dose of maraviroc); plasma concentration of both drugs reduced when boceprevir given with ● RITONAVIR
- Anxiolytics and Hypnotics: boceprevir increases plasma concentration of *oral* ● MIDAZOLAM—manufacturer of boceprevir advises avoid concomitant use
- Cardiac Glycosides: boceprevir possibly increases side-effects of DIGOXIN
- Ciclosporin: boceprevir increases plasma concentration of ● CICLOSPORIN
- Cilostazol: boceprevir possibly increases plasma concentration of ● CILOSTAZOL (see under Cilostazol, p. 215)
- Cobicistat: avoidance of boceprevir advised by manufacturer of COBICISTAT
- Cytotoxics: boceprevir possibly increases the plasma concentration of ● BOSUTINIB—manufacturer of bosutinib advises avoid or consider reducing dose of bosutinib; manufacturer of boceprevir advises avoid concomitant use with ● DASATINIB, ● ERLOTINIB, ● GEFITINIB, ● IMATINIB, ● LAPATINIB, ● NILOTINIB, ● PAZOPANIB, ● SORAFENIB and ● SUNITINIB; manufacturer of ruxolitinib advises dose reduction when boceprevir given with ● RUXOLITINIB—consult ruxolitinib product literature; avoidance of boceprevir advised by manufacturer of ● OLAPARIB
- Domperidone: possible increased risk of ventricular arrhythmias when boceprevir given with ● DOMPERIDONE—avoid concomitant use
- Ergot Alkaloids: manufacturer of boceprevir advises avoid concomitant use with ● ERGOT ALKALOIDS
- Guanfacine: boceprevir possibly increases plasma concentration of ● GUANFACINE (halve dose of guanfacine)
- Lipid-regulating Drugs: boceprevir increases plasma concentration of ATORVASTATIN (reduce dose of atorvastatin); boceprevir increases plasma concentration of PRAVASTATIN; manufacturers advise avoid concomitant use of boceprevir with ● SIMVASTATIN
- Progestogens: boceprevir increases plasma concentration of DROSPIRENONE (increased risk of toxicity)
- Sirolimus: boceprevir increases plasma concentration of ● SIROLIMUS (increased risk of toxicity—reduce sirolimus dose)
- Tacrolimus: boceprevir increases plasma concentration of ● TACROLIMUS (reduce dose of tacrolimus)

Bortezomib

- Antibacterials: plasma concentration of bortezomib reduced by ● RIFAMPICIN—manufacturer of bortezomib advises avoid concomitant use
- Antidepressants: plasma concentration of bortezomib possibly reduced by ST JOHN'S WORT—manufacturer of bortezomib advises avoid concomitant use
- Antiepileptics: plasma concentration of bortezomib possibly reduced by CARBAMAZEPINE, FOSPHENYTOIN, PHENOBARBITAL, PHENYTOIN and PRIMIDONE—manufacturer of bortezomib advises avoid concomitant use
- Antifungals: plasma concentration of bortezomib increased by KETOCONAZOLE

Bortezomib (continued)

- Antipsychotics: avoid concomitant use of cytotoxics with ● CLOZAPINE (increased risk of agranulocytosis)

Bosentan

- Antibacterials: plasma concentration of bosentan reduced by ● RIFAMPICIN—avoid concomitant use
- Anticoagulants: manufacturer of bosentan recommends monitoring anticoagulant effect of COUMARINS
- Antidiabetics: increased risk of hepatotoxicity when bosentan given with ● GLIBENCLAMIDE—avoid concomitant use
- Antifungals: plasma concentration of bosentan increased by KETOCONAZOLE; plasma concentration of bosentan possibly increased by ● FLUCONAZOLE—avoid concomitant use; plasma concentration of bosentan possibly increased by ITRACONAZOLE
- Antivirals: avoidance of bosentan advised by manufacturer of ELVITEGRAVIR and TIPRANAVIR; bosentan possibly reduces plasma concentration of INDINAVIR; plasma concentration of bosentan increased by ● LOPINAVIR and ● RITONAVIR (consider reducing dose of bosentan); bosentan possibly reduces plasma concentration of TELAPREVIR, also plasma concentration of bosentan possibly increased
- Avanafil: bosentan possibly reduces plasma concentration of AVANAFIL—manufacturer of avanafil advises avoid concomitant use
- Ciclosporin: plasma concentration of bosentan increased by ● CICLOSPORIN (also plasma concentration of ciclosporin reduced—avoid concomitant use)
- Cobicistat: avoidance of bosentan advised by manufacturer of COBICISTAT
- Cytotoxics: bosentan possibly reduces plasma concentration of ● BOSUTINIB—manufacturer of bosutinib advises avoid concomitant use
- Guanfacine: bosentan possibly reduces plasma concentration of ● GUANFACINE—increase dose of guanfacine
- Lipid-regulating Drugs: bosentan reduces plasma concentration of SIMVASTATIN
- Oestrogens: bosentan possibly causes contraceptive failure of hormonal contraceptives containing ● OESTROGENS (alternative contraception recommended)
- Progestogens: bosentan possibly causes contraceptive failure of hormonal contraceptives containing ● PROGESTOGENS (alternative contraception recommended)
- Riociguat: bosentan reduces plasma concentration of RIOCIGUAT
- Sildenafil: bosentan reduces plasma concentration of SILDENAFIL, also plasma concentration of bosentan increased
- Tadalafil: bosentan reduces plasma concentration of TADALAFIL

Bosutinib

- Analgesics: possible increased risk of ventricular arrhythmias when bosutinib given with ● METHADONE
- Antacids: manufacturer of bosutinib advises separating administration with ANTACIDS by about 12 hours
- Anti-arrhythmics: possible increased risk of ventricular arrhythmias when bosutinib given with ● AMIODARONE and ● DISOPYRAMIDE; plasma concentration of bosutinib possibly increased by ● DRONEDARONE—manufacturer of bosutinib advises avoid or consider reducing dose of bosutinib
- Antibacterials: plasma concentration of bosutinib possibly increased by ● CIPROFLOXACIN, ● CLARITHROMYCIN, ● ERYTHROMYCIN and ● TELITHROMYCIN—manufacturer of bosutinib advises avoid or consider reducing dose of bosutinib; possible increased risk of ventricular arrhythmias when bosutinib given with ● MOXIFLOXACIN; plasma concentration of bosutinib possibly reduced by ● RIFABUTIN—manufacturer of bosutinib advises avoid concomitant use; plasma concentration of bosutinib reduced by ● RIFAMPICIN—manufacturer of bosutinib advises avoid concomitant use
- Antidepressants: plasma concentration of bosutinib possibly reduced by ● ST JOHN'S WORT—manufacturer of bosutinib advises avoid concomitant use
- Antiepileptics: plasma concentration of bosutinib possibly reduced by ● CARBAMAZEPINE, ● FOSPHENYTOIN, ● PHENOBARBITAL, ● PHENYTOIN and ● PRIMIDONE—manufacturer of bosutinib advises avoid concomitant use
- Antifungals: plasma concentration of bosutinib increased by ● KETOCONAZOLE—manufacturer of bosutinib advises avoid or

Bosutinib

- **Antifungals** (continued)
consider reducing dose of bosutinib; plasma concentration of bosutinib possibly increased by ● FLUCONAZOLE, ● ITRACONAZOLE, ● POSACONAZOLE and ● VORICONAZOLE—manufacturer of bosutinib advises avoid or consider reducing dose of bosutinib
- **Antimalarials:** possible increased risk of ventricular arrhythmias when bosutinib given with ● CHLOROQUINE and ● HYDROXYCHLOROQUINE
- **Antipsychotics:** possible increased risk of ventricular arrhythmias when bosutinib given with ● HALOPERIDOL; avoid concomitant use of cytotoxics with ● CLOZAPINE (increased risk of agranulocytosis)
- **Antivirals:** plasma concentration of bosutinib possibly increased by ● ATAZANAVIR, ● BOCEPREVIR, ● DARUNAVIR, ● FOSAMPRENAVIR, ● INDINAVIR, ● RITONAVIR, ● SAQUINAVIR and ● TELAPREVIR—manufacturer of bosutinib advises avoid or consider reducing dose of bosutinib; plasma concentration of bosutinib possibly reduced by ● EFAVIRENZ and ● ETRAVIRINE—manufacturer of bosutinib advises avoid concomitant use
- **Aprepitant:** plasma concentration of bosutinib possibly increased by ● APREPITANT—manufacturer of bosutinib advises avoid or consider reducing dose of bosutinib
- **Beta-blockers:** possible increased risk of ventricular arrhythmias when bosutinib given with ● SOTALOL
- **Bosentan:** plasma concentration of bosutinib possibly reduced by ● BOSENTAN—manufacturer of bosutinib advises avoid concomitant use
- **Calcium-channel Blockers:** plasma concentration of bosutinib possibly increased by ● DILTIAZEM and ● VERAPAMIL—manufacturer of bosutinib advises avoid or consider reducing dose of bosutinib
- **Cytotoxics:** plasma concentration of bosutinib possibly increased by ● IMATINIB—manufacturer of bosutinib advises avoid or consider reducing dose of bosutinib
- **Domperidone:** manufacturer of bosutinib advises avoid concomitant use with ● DOMPERIDONE (risk of ventricular arrhythmias)
- **Fosaprepitant:** plasma concentration of bosutinib possibly increased by ● FOSAPREPITANT—manufacturer of bosutinib advises avoid or consider reducing dose of bosutinib
- **Grapefruit Juice:** plasma concentration of bosutinib possibly increased by ● GRAPEFRUIT JUICE—manufacturer of bosutinib advises avoid or consider reducing dose of bosutinib
- **Modafinil:** plasma concentration of bosutinib possibly reduced by ● MODAFINIL—manufacturer of bosutinib advises avoid concomitant use
▷ **Ulcer-healing Drugs:** plasma concentration of bosutinib reduced by LANSOPRAZOLE

Brentuximab vedotin

▷ **Antibacterials:** effects of brentuximab vedotin possibly reduced by RIFAMPICIN
- **Antifungals:** possible increased risk of neutropenia when brentuximab vedotin given with ● KETOCONAZOLE
- **Antipsychotics:** avoid concomitant use of cytotoxics with ● CLOZAPINE (increased risk of agranulocytosis)
- **Cytotoxics:** increased risk of pulmonary toxicity when brentuximab vedotin given with ● BLEOMYCIN—avoid concomitant use
- **Vaccines:** risk of generalised infections when monoclonal antibodies given with live ● VACCINES—avoid concomitant use

Brimonidine

▷ **Antidepressants:** manufacturer of brimonidine advises avoid concomitant use with MAOIs, TRICYCLIC-RELATED ANTIDEPRESSANTS and TRICYCLICS

Brinzolamide see Diuretics

Bromocriptine

▷ **Alcohol:** tolerance of bromocriptine reduced by ALCOHOL
▷ **Antibacterials:** plasma concentration of bromocriptine increased by ERYTHROMYCIN (increased risk of toxicity); plasma concentration of bromocriptine possibly increased by MACROLIDES (increased risk of toxicity)
▷ **Antipsychotics:** hypoprolactinaemic and antiparkinsonian effects of bromocriptine antagonised by ANTIPSYCHOTICS

Bromocriptine (continued)

▷ **Domperidone:** hypoprolactinaemic effect of bromocriptine possibly antagonised by DOMPERIDONE
▷ **Hormone Antagonists:** plasma concentration of bromocriptine increased by OCTREOTIDE
▷ **Memantine:** effects of dopaminergics possibly enhanced by MEMANTINE
▷ **Methyldopa:** antiparkinsonian effect of dopaminergics antagonised by METHYLDOPA
▷ **Metoclopramide:** hypoprolactinaemic effect of bromocriptine antagonised by METOCLOPRAMIDE
- **Sympathomimetics:** risk of toxicity when bromocriptine given with ● ISOMETHEPTENE

Buclizine see Antihistamines

Budesonide see Corticosteroids

Bumetanide see Diuretics

Bupivacaine

▷ **Anti-arrhythmics:** increased myocardial depression when bupivacaine given with ANTI-ARRHYTHMICS
- **Beta-blockers:** increased risk of bupivacaine toxicity when given with ● PROPRANOLOL

Buprenorphine see Opioid Analgesics

Bupropion

- **Antidepressants:** bupropion possibly increases plasma concentration of CITALOPRAM; manufacturer of bupropion advises avoid for 2 weeks after stopping ● MAOIs; manufacturer of bupropion advises avoid concomitant use with ● MOCLOBEMIDE; bupropion possibly increases plasma concentration of TRICYCLICS (possible increased risk of convulsions); bupropion increases plasma concentration of VORTIOXETINE (consider reducing dose of vortioxetine)
▷ **Antiepileptics:** plasma concentration of bupropion reduced by CARBAMAZEPINE, FOSPHENYTOIN and PHENYTOIN; metabolism of bupropion inhibited by SODIUM VALPROATE and VALPROIC ACID
▷ **Antivirals:** metabolism of bupropion accelerated by EFAVIRENZ (reduced plasma concentration); plasma concentration of bupropion reduced by RITONAVIR
▷ **Atomoxetine:** possible increased risk of convulsions when bupropion given with ATOMOXETINE
▷ **Dopaminergics:** increased risk of side-effects when bupropion given with AMANTADINE, CO-BENELDOPA, CO-CARELDOPA or LEVODOPA
- **Hormone Antagonists:** bupropion possibly inhibits metabolism of ● TAMOXIFEN to active metabolite (avoid concomitant use)
- **Methylthioninium:** possible risk of CNS toxicity when bupropion given with ● METHYLTHIONINIUM—avoid concomitant use (if avoidance not possible, use lowest possible dose of methylthioninium and observe patient for up to 4 hours after administration)

Buspirone see Anxiolytics and Hypnotics

Busulfan

▷ **Analgesics:** metabolism of *intravenous* busulfan possibly inhibited by PARACETAMOL (manufacturer of *intravenous* busulfan advises caution within 72 hours of paracetamol)
- **Antibacterials:** plasma concentration of busulfan increased by ● METRONIDAZOLE (increased risk of toxicity)
▷ **Antiepileptics:** plasma concentration of busulfan possibly reduced by FOSPHENYTOIN and PHENYTOIN
▷ **Antifungals:** metabolism of busulfan inhibited by ITRACONAZOLE (increased risk of toxicity)
- **Antipsychotics:** avoid concomitant use of cytotoxics with ● CLOZAPINE (increased risk of agranulocytosis)
▷ **Cytotoxics:** increased risk of hepatotoxicity when busulfan given with TIOGUANINE

Butyrophenones see Antipsychotics

Cabazitaxel

- **Antibacterials:** plasma concentration of cabazitaxel possibly increased by ● CLARITHROMYCIN and ● TELITHROMYCIN—manufacturer of cabazitaxel advises avoid or consider reducing dose of cabazitaxel; manufacturer of cabazitaxel advises avoid concomitant use with ● RIFABUTIN; plasma concentration of cabazitaxel reduced by ● RIFAMPICIN—manufacturer of cabazitaxel advises avoid concomitant use
- **Antidepressants:** manufacturer of cabazitaxel advises avoid concomitant use with ● ST JOHN'S WORT

Cabazitaxel (continued)
- Antiepileptics: manufacturer of cabazitaxel advises avoid concomitant use with ● CARBAMAZEPINE, ● FOSPHENYTOIN, ● PHENOBARBITAL, ● PHENYTOIN and ● PRIMIDONE
- Antifungals: manufacturer of cabazitaxel advises avoid concomitant use with ● KETOCONAZOLE; plasma concentration of cabazitaxel possibly increased by ● ITRACONAZOLE and ● VORICONAZOLE—manufacturer of cabazitaxel advises avoid or consider reducing dose of cabazitaxel
- Antipsychotics: avoid concomitant use of cytotoxics with ● CLOZAPINE (increased risk of agranulocytosis)
- Antivirals: manufacturer of cabazitaxel advises avoid concomitant use with ● ATAZANAVIR; plasma concentration of cabazitaxel possibly increased by ● INDINAVIR, ● RITONAVIR and ● SAQUINAVIR—manufacturer of cabazitaxel advises avoid or consider reducing dose of cabazitaxel

Cabergoline
▸ Antibacterials: plasma concentration of cabergoline increased by ERYTHROMYCIN (increased risk of toxicity); plasma concentration of cabergoline possibly increased by MACROLIDES (increased risk of toxicity)
▸ Antipsychotics: hypoprolactinaemic and antiparkinsonian effects of cabergoline antagonised by ANTIPSYCHOTICS
▸ Domperidone: hypoprolactinaemic effect of cabergoline possibly antagonised by DOMPERIDONE
▸ Memantine: effects of dopaminergics possibly enhanced by MEMANTINE
▸ Methyldopa: antiparkinsonian effect of dopaminergics antagonised by METHYLDOPA
▸ Metoclopramide: hypoprolactinaemic effect of cabergoline antagonised by METOCLOPRAMIDE

Cabozantinib
- Antibacterials: plasma concentration of cabozantinib possibly increased by CLARITHROMYCIN and ERYTHROMYCIN; plasma concentration of cabozantinib reduced by ● RIFAMPICIN—avoid concomitant use
▸ Antidepressants: plasma concentration of cabozantinib possibly reduced by ST JOHN'S WORT—manufacturer of cabozantinib advises avoid concomitant use
▸ Antiepileptics: plasma concentration of cabozantinib possibly reduced by ● CARBAMAZEPINE, ● FOSPHENYTOIN, ● PHENOBARBITAL, ● PHENYTOIN and ● PRIMIDONE—avoid concomitant use
▸ Antifungals: plasma concentration of cabozantinib increased by KETOCONAZOLE; plasma concentration of cabozantinib possibly increased by ITRACONAZOLE
- Antipsychotics: avoid concomitant use of cytotoxics with ● CLOZAPINE (increased risk of agranulocytosis)
▸ Antivirals: plasma concentration of cabozantinib possibly increased by RITONAVIR
▸ Corticosteroids: plasma concentration of cabozantinib possibly reduced by DEXAMETHASONE—manufacturer of cabozantinib advises avoid concomitant use
▸ Grapefruit Juice: plasma concentration of cabozantinib possibly increased by GRAPEFRUIT JUICE

Caffeine citrate
▸ Aminophylline: manufacturer of caffeine citrate advises avoid concomitant use with AMINOPHYLLINE
▸ Anti-arrhythmics: caffeine citrate antagonises anti-arrhythmic effect of ADENOSINE—manufacturer of adenosine advises avoid caffeine citrate for at least 12 hours before adenosine
▸ Antiepileptics: plasma concentration of caffeine citrate reduced by FOSPHENYTOIN and PHENYTOIN; caffeine citrate possibly antagonises effects of PHENOBARBITAL and PRIMIDONE
▸ Theophylline: manufacturer of caffeine citrate advises avoid concomitant use with THEOPHYLLINE
▸ Ulcer-healing Drugs: plasma concentration of caffeine citrate increased by CIMETIDINE

Calcitriol *see* Vitamins

Calcium Salts
NOTE *see also* Antacids
▸ Antibacterials: calcium salts reduce absorption of CIPROFLOXACIN (give at least 2 hours before or 4 hours after ciprofloxacin); calcium salts possibly reduce absorption of TETRACYCLINES (give at least 2 to 3 hours apart)

Calcium Salts (continued)
▸ Antivirals: calcium salts reduce absorption of DOLUTEGRAVIR—manufacturer of dolutegravir advises give at least 2 hours before or 6 hours after calcium salts; separating administration from calcium salts by 4 hours advised by manufacturer of LEDIPASVIR; manufacturer of rilpivirine advises give calcium salts 2 hours before or 4 hours after RILPIVIRINE
▸ Bisphosphonates: calcium salts reduce absorption of BISPHOSPHONATES
▸ Cardiac Glycosides: large *intravenous* doses of calcium salts can precipitate arrhythmias when given with CARDIAC GLYCOSIDES
▸ Corticosteroids: absorption of calcium salts reduced by CORTICOSTEROIDS
▸ Cytotoxics: calcium salts reduce absorption of ESTRAMUSTINE (manufacturer of estramustine advises avoid concomitant administration)
▸ Diuretics: increased risk of hypercalcaemia when calcium salts given with THIAZIDES AND RELATED DIURETICS
▸ Eltrombopag: calcium salts possibly reduce absorption of ELTROMBOPAG (give at least 4 hours apart)
▸ Fluorides: calcium salts reduce absorption of FLUORIDES
▸ Iron Salts: calcium salts reduce absorption of *oral* IRON SALTS
▸ Thyroid Hormones: calcium salts reduce absorption of LEVOTHYROXINE
▸ Zinc: calcium salts reduce absorption of ZINC

Calcium-channel Blockers
NOTE Dihydropyridine calcium-channel blockers include amlodipine, felodipine, isradipine, lacidipine, lercanidipine, nicardipine, nifedipine, and nimodipine
▸ ACE Inhibitors: enhanced hypotensive effect when calcium-channel blockers given with ACE INHIBITORS
▸ Adrenergic Neurone Blockers: enhanced hypotensive effect when calcium-channel blockers given with ADRENERGIC NEURONE BLOCKERS
▸ Alcohol: enhanced hypotensive effect when calcium-channel blockers given with ALCOHOL; verapamil possibly increases plasma concentration of ALCOHOL
▸ Aldesleukin: enhanced hypotensive effect when calcium-channel blockers given with ALDESLEUKIN
▸ Aliskiren: verapamil increases plasma concentration of ALISKIREN
▸ Alpha-blockers: verapamil increases plasma concentration of TAMSULOSIN; enhanced hypotensive effect when calcium-channel blockers given with ● ALPHA-BLOCKERS, also increased risk of first-dose hypotension with post-synaptic alpha-blockers such as prazosin
- Aminophylline: calcium-channel blockers possibly increase plasma concentration of ● AMINOPHYLLINE (enhanced effect); diltiazem increases plasma concentration of AMINOPHYLLINE; verapamil increases plasma concentration of ● AMINOPHYLLINE (enhanced effect)
- Anaesthetics, General: enhanced hypotensive effect when calcium-channel blockers given with GENERAL ANAESTHETICS or ISOFLURANE; hypotensive effect of verapamil enhanced by ● GENERAL ANAESTHETICS (also AV delay)
▸ Analgesics: hypotensive effect of calcium-channel blockers antagonised by NSAIDs; diltiazem inhibits metabolism of ALFENTANIL (risk of prolonged or delayed respiratory depression)
▸ Angiotensin-II Receptor Antagonists: enhanced hypotensive effect when calcium-channel blockers given with ANGIOTENSIN-II RECEPTOR ANTAGONISTS
- Anti-arrhythmics: increased risk of bradycardia, AV block and myocardial depression when diltiazem or verapamil given with ● AMIODARONE; increased risk of myocardial depression and asystole when verapamil given with ● DISOPYRAMIDE or ● FLECAINIDE; nifedipine increases plasma concentration of ● DRONEDARONE; increased risk of bradycardia and myocardial depression when diltiazem and verapamil given with ● DRONEDARONE
- Antibacterials: metabolism of calcium-channel blockers possibly inhibited by ● CLARITHROMYCIN, ● ERYTHROMYCIN and ● TELITHROMYCIN (increased risk of side-effects); manufacturer of lercanidipine advises avoid concomitant use with ERYTHROMYCIN; metabolism of diltiazem, nifedipine,

A1

Interactions | Appendix 1

Calcium-channel Blockers

- **Antibacterials** (continued)
  nimodipine and verapamil accelerated by • RIFAMPICIN (plasma concentration significantly reduced); metabolism of isradipine and nicardipine possibly accelerated by • RIFAMPICIN (possible significantly reduced plasma concentration); plasma concentration of felodipine possibly reduced by RIFAMPICIN; avoidance of verapamil advised by manufacturer of FIDAXOMICIN
- **Anticoagulants**: verapamil possibly increases plasma concentration of • DABIGATRAN (see under Dabigatran Etexilate, p. 123); verapamil increases plasma concentration of EDOXABAN
- **Antidepressants**: metabolism of nifedipine possibly inhibited by FLUOXETINE (increased plasma concentration); diltiazem and verapamil increase plasma concentration of IMIPRAMINE; enhanced hypotensive effect when calcium-channel blockers given with MAOIs; plasma concentration of amlodipine and felodipine possibly reduced by ST JOHN'S WORT; plasma concentration of verapamil significantly reduced by • ST JOHN'S WORT; plasma concentration of nifedipine reduced by ST JOHN'S WORT; diltiazem and verapamil possibly increase plasma concentration of TRICYCLICS
- **Antidiabetics**: glucose tolerance occasionally impaired when nifedipine given with INSULIN
- **Antiepileptics**: effects of felodipine and isradipine reduced by CARBAMAZEPINE; effects of dihydropyridines, nicardipine and nifedipine probably reduced by CARBAMAZEPINE; diltiazem and verapamil enhance effects of • CARBAMAZEPINE; manufacturer of nimodipine advises avoid concomitant use with CARBAMAZEPINE, FOSPHENYTOIN and PHENYTOIN (plasma concentration of nimodipine possibly reduced); effects of felodipine and verapamil reduced by FOSPHENYTOIN; diltiazem increases plasma concentration of • FOSPHENYTOIN and • PHENYTOIN but also effect of diltiazem reduced; manufacturer of isradipine advises avoid concomitant use with FOSPHENYTOIN, PHENOBARBITAL, PHENYTOIN and PRIMIDONE; effects of calcium-channel blockers probably reduced by • PHENOBARBITAL and • PRIMIDONE; manufacturer of nimodipine advises avoid concomitant use with • PHENOBARBITAL and • PRIMIDONE (plasma concentration of nimodipine reduced); effects of felodipine and verapamil reduced by PHENYTOIN
- **Antifungals**: metabolism of dihydropyridines possibly inhibited by ITRACONAZOLE and KETOCONAZOLE (increased plasma concentration); metabolism of felodipine is inhibited by • KETOCONAZOLE (increased plasma concentration)—manufacturer of ketoconazole advises avoid concomitant use; manufacturer of lercanidipine advises avoid concomitant use with ITRACONAZOLE and KETOCONAZOLE; negative inotropic effect possibly increased when calcium-channel blockers given with ITRACONAZOLE; metabolism of felodipine inhibited by • ITRACONAZOLE (increased plasma concentration); plasma concentration of nifedipine increased by MICAFUNGIN
- **Antimalarials**: possible increased risk of bradycardia when calcium-channel blockers given with MEFLOQUINE
- **Antimuscarinics**: avoidance of verapamil advised by manufacturer of DARIFENACIN; verapamil increases plasma concentration of SOLIFENACIN
- **Antipsychotics**: enhanced hypotensive effect when calcium-channel blockers given with ANTIPSYCHOTICS; verapamil possibly increases the plasma concentration of • LURASIDONE (see under Lurasidone, p. 364); diltiazem increases the plasma concentration of • LURASIDONE (see under Lurasidone, p. 364)
- **Antivirals**: plasma concentration of verapamil possibly increased by ATAZANAVIR; plasma concentration of diltiazem increased by • ATAZANAVIR (reduce dose of diltiazem); plasma concentration of diltiazem reduced by EFAVIRENZ; manufacturer of lercanidipine advises avoid concomitant use with RITONAVIR; plasma concentration of amlodipine increased by • RITONAVIR (reduce dose of amlodipine); plasma concentration of calcium-channel blockers possibly increased by • RITONAVIR; caution with diltiazem, felodipine, nicardipine, nifedipine and verapamil advised by manufacturer of TELAPREVIR; plasma concentration of

Calcium-channel Blockers

- **Antivirals** (continued)
  amlodipine increased by TELAPREVIR (consider reducing dose of amlodipine)
- **Anxiolytics and Hypnotics**: enhanced hypotensive effect when calcium-channel blockers given with ANXIOLYTICS AND HYPNOTICS; diltiazem and verapamil inhibit metabolism of MIDAZOLAM (increased plasma concentration with increased sedation); absorption of lercanidipine increased by MIDAZOLAM; diltiazem and verapamil increase plasma concentration of BUSPIRONE (reduce dose of buspirone)
- **Aprepitant**: plasma concentration of both drugs may increase when diltiazem given with APREPITANT
- **Avanafil**: diltiazem and verapamil possibly increase plasma concentration of • AVANAFIL—see under Avanafil, p. 735
- **Beta-blockers**: enhanced hypotensive effect when calcium-channel blockers given with BETA-BLOCKERS; increased risk of AV block and bradycardia when diltiazem given with • BETA-BLOCKERS; asystole, severe hypotension and heart failure when verapamil given with • BETA-BLOCKERS (see under Verapamil, p. 150); possible severe hypotension and heart failure when nifedipine given with • BETA-BLOCKERS
- **Calcium-channel Blockers**: plasma concentration of both drugs may increase when diltiazem given with NIFEDIPINE
- **Cardiac Glycosides**: verapamil increases plasma concentration of • DIGOXIN, also increased risk of AV block and bradycardia; diltiazem, lercanidipine and nicardipine increase plasma concentration of • DIGOXIN; nifedipine possibly increases plasma concentration of • DIGOXIN
- **Ciclosporin**: diltiazem, nicardipine and verapamil increase plasma concentration of • CICLOSPORIN; combination of lercanidipine with • CICLOSPORIN may increase plasma concentration of either drug (or both)—avoid concomitant use; plasma concentration of nifedipine possibly increased by CICLOSPORIN (increased risk of toxicity including gingival hyperplasia)
- **Cilostazol**: diltiazem increases plasma concentration of CILOSTAZOL (consider reducing dose of cilostazol)
- **Clonidine**: enhanced hypotensive effect when calcium-channel blockers given with CLONIDINE
- **Colchicine**: diltiazem and verapamil possibly increase risk of • COLCHICINE toxicity—suspend or reduce dose of colchicine (avoid concomitant use in hepatic or renal impairment)
- **Corticosteroids**: hypotensive effect of calcium-channel blockers antagonised by CORTICOSTEROIDS; diltiazem increases plasma concentration of METHYLPREDNISOLONE
- **Cytotoxics**: verapamil possibly increases plasma concentration of DOXORUBICIN; verapamil possibly increases the plasma concentration of AFATINIB—manufacturer of afatinib advises separating administration of verapamil by 6 to 12 hours; diltiazem and verapamil possibly increase the plasma concentration of • BOSUTINIB—manufacturer of bosutinib advises avoid or consider reducing dose of bosutinib; possible increased risk of bradycardia when diltiazem or verapamil given with CRIZOTINIB; plasma concentration of both drugs may increase when verapamil given with • EVEROLIMUS (consider reducing the dose of everolimus —consult everolimus product literature); diltiazem and verapamil possibly increase the plasma concentration of • IBRUTINIB—reduce dose of ibrutinib (see under Ibrutinib, p. 855); nifedipine possibly inhibits metabolism of VINCRISTINE
- **Dapoxetine**: manufacturer of dapoxetine advises dose reduction when diltiazem and verapamil given with DAPOXETINE (see under Dapoxetine, p. 742)
- **Diazoxide**: enhanced hypotensive effect when calcium-channel blockers given with DIAZOXIDE
- **Diuretics**: enhanced hypotensive effect when calcium-channel blockers given with DIURETICS; diltiazem and verapamil increase plasma concentration of EPLERENONE (reduce dose of eplerenone)
- **Dopaminergics**: enhanced hypotensive effect when calcium-channel blockers given with CO-BENELDOPA, CO-CARELDOPA or LEVODOPA
- **Fingolimod**: possible increased risk of bradycardia when diltiazem or verapamil given with • FINGOLIMOD

Calcium-channel Blockers (continued)

▸ Fosaprepitant: plasma concentration of both drugs may increase when diltiazem given with FOSAPREPITANT

▸ Grapefruit Juice: plasma concentration of felodipine, isradipine, lacidipine, lercanidipine, nicardipine, nifedipine, nimodipine and verapamil increased by GRAPEFRUIT JUICE; plasma concentration of amlodipine possibly increased by GRAPEFRUIT JUICE

● Guanfacine: diltiazem and verapamil possibly increase the plasma concentration of GUANFACINE (halve dose of guanfacine)

● Hormone Antagonists: diltiazem and verapamil increase plasma concentration of DUTASTERIDE; possible increased risk of bradycardia when diltiazem or verapamil given with PASIREOTIDE

● Ivabradine: diltiazem and verapamil increase plasma concentration of ● IVABRADINE—avoid concomitant use

● Lenalidomide: verapamil possibly increases plasma concentration of ● LENALIDOMIDE (increased risk of toxicity)

● Lipid-regulating Drugs: diltiazem increases plasma concentration of ATORVASTATIN—possible increased risk of myopathy; plasma concentration of verapamil increased by ● ATORVASTATIN, also possible increased risk of myopathy (consider reducing dose of atorvastatin); possible increased risk of myopathy when amlodipine and diltiazem given with ● SIMVASTATIN (see under Simvastatin, p. 188); increased risk of myopathy when verapamil given with ● SIMVASTATIN (see under Simvastatin, p. 188); separating administration from amlodipine and lacidipine by 12 hours advised by manufacturer of LOMITAPIDE; avoidance of diltiazem and verapamil advised by manufacturer of ● LOMITAPIDE (plasma concentration of lomitapide possibly increased)

▸ Lithium: neurotoxicity may occur when diltiazem or verapamil given with LITHIUM without increased plasma concentration of lithium

● Magnesium (parenteral): profound hypotension reported with concomitant use of nifedipine and ● PARENTERAL MAGNESIUM in pre-eclampsia

▸ Methyldopa: enhanced hypotensive effect when calcium-channel blockers given with METHYLDOPA

▸ Moxisylyte: enhanced hypotensive effect when calcium-channel blockers given with MOXISYLYTE

▸ Moxonidine: enhanced hypotensive effect when calcium-channel blockers given with MOXONIDINE

▸ Muscle Relaxants: verapamil enhances effects of NON-DEPOLARISING MUSCLE RELAXANTS and SUXAMETHONIUM; enhanced hypotensive effect when calcium-channel blockers given with BACLOFEN or TIZANIDINE; manufacturer of verapamil advises avoid concomitant use of *intravenous* DANTROLENE; possible increased risk of ventricular arrhythmias when diltiazem given with *intravenous* DANTROLENE—manufacturer of diltiazem advises avoid concomitant use; calcium-channel blockers possibly enhance effects of NON-DEPOLARISING MUSCLE RELAXANTS

▸ Nitrates: enhanced hypotensive effect when calcium-channel blockers given with NITRATES

▸ Oestrogens: hypotensive effect of calcium-channel blockers antagonised by OESTROGENS

▸ Prostaglandins: enhanced hypotensive effect when calcium-channel blockers given with ALPROSTADIL

▸ Ranolazine: diltiazem and verapamil increase plasma concentration of RANOLAZINE (consider reducing dose of ranolazine)

▸ Sildenafil: enhanced hypotensive effect when amlodipine given with SILDENAFIL

● Sirolimus: diltiazem increases plasma concentration of ● SIROLIMUS; plasma concentration of both drugs increased when verapamil given with ● SIROLIMUS; nicardipine possibly increases plasma concentration of SIROLIMUS

▸ Sulfinpyrazone: plasma concentration of verapamil reduced by SULFINPYRAZONE

● Tacrolimus: diltiazem, nicardipine and nifedipine increase plasma concentration of ● TACROLIMUS; felodipine and verapamil possibly increase plasma concentration of TACROLIMUS

Calcium-channel Blockers (continued)

● Theophylline: calcium-channel blockers possibly increase plasma concentration of ● THEOPHYLLINE (enhanced effect); diltiazem increases plasma concentration of THEOPHYLLINE; verapamil increases plasma concentration of ● THEOPHYLLINE (enhanced effect)

▸ Ticagrelor: diltiazem increases plasma concentration of TICAGRELOR

▸ Ulcer-healing Drugs: metabolism of calcium-channel blockers possibly inhibited by CIMETIDINE (increased plasma concentration); plasma concentration of isradipine increased by CIMETIDINE (halve dose of isradipine)

▸ Ulipristal: avoidance of verapamil advised by manufacturer of *low-dose* ULIPRISTAL

▸ Vardenafil: enhanced hypotensive effect when nifedipine given with VARDENAFIL

▸ Vasodilator Antihypertensives: enhanced hypotensive effect when calcium-channel blockers given with HYDRALAZINE, MINOXIDIL or SODIUM NITROPRUSSIDE

Calcium-channel Blockers (dihydropyridines) *see* Calcium-channel Blockers

Canagliflozin *see* Antidiabetics

Canakinumab

● Antipsychotics: avoid concomitant use of cytotoxics with ● CLOZAPINE (increased risk of agranulocytosis)

● Vaccines: risk of generalised infections when monoclonal antibodies given with live ● VACCINES—avoid concomitant use

Candesartan *see* Angiotensin-II Receptor Antagonists

Cannabis Extract

● Antibacterials: plasma concentration of cannabis extract reduced by ● RIFAMPICIN—manufacturer of cannabis extract advises avoid concomitant use

● Antidepressants: plasma concentration of cannabis extract possibly reduced by ● ST JOHN'S WORT—manufacturer of cannabis extract advises avoid concomitant use; possible increased risk of hypertension and tachycardia when cannabis extract given with TRICYCLICS

● Antiepileptics: plasma concentration of cannabis extract possibly reduced by ● CARBAMAZEPINE, ● FOSPHENYTOIN, ● PHENOBARBITAL, ● PHENYTOIN and ● PRIMIDONE—manufacturer of cannabis extract advises avoid concomitant use

▸ Antifungals: plasma concentration of cannabis extract increased by KETOCONAZOLE

Capecitabine

● Allopurinol: manufacturer of capecitabine advises avoid concomitant use with ● ALLOPURINOL

● Antibacterials: metabolism of capecitabine inhibited by METRONIDAZOLE (increased toxicity)

● Anticoagulants: capecitabine enhances anticoagulant effect of ● COUMARINS

▸ Antiepileptics: capecitabine possibly inhibits metabolism of FOSPHENYTOIN and PHENYTOIN (increased risk of toxicity)

● Antipsychotics: avoid concomitant use of cytotoxics with ● CLOZAPINE (increased risk of agranulocytosis)

▸ Cytotoxics: capecitabine possibly increases plasma concentration of ERLOTINIB

▸ Filgrastim: neutropenia possibly exacerbated when capecitabine given with FILGRASTIM

● Folates: toxicity of capecitabine increased by ● FOLIC ACID—avoid concomitant use

▸ Lipegfilgrastim: neutropenia possibly exacerbated when capecitabine given with LIPEGFILGRASTIM

▸ Pegfilgrastim: neutropenia possibly exacerbated when capecitabine given with PEGFILGRASTIM

▸ Ulcer-healing Drugs: metabolism of capecitabine inhibited by CIMETIDINE (increased plasma concentration)

Capreomycin

▸ Antibacterials: increased risk of nephrotoxicity when capreomycin given with COLISTIMETHATE SODIUM or POLYMYXINS; increased risk of nephrotoxicity and ototoxicity when capreomycin given with AMINOGLYCOSIDES or VANCOMYCIN

▸ Cytotoxics: increased risk of nephrotoxicity and ototoxicity when capreomycin given with PLATINUM COMPOUNDS

Capreomycin (continued)

▸ Vaccines: antibacterials inactivate ORAL TYPHOID VACCINE—see under Typhoid Vaccine in BNF

Captopril see ACE Inhibitors

Carbamazepine

▸ Alcohol: CNS side-effects of carbamazepine possibly increased by ALCOHOL

▸ Aminophylline: carbamazepine accelerates metabolism of AMINOPHYLLINE (reduced effect)

● Analgesics: effects of carbamazepine enhanced by ● DEXTROPROPOXYPHENE; carbamazepine possibly accelerates metabolism of FENTANYL (reduced effect); carbamazepine reduces plasma concentration of METHADONE; carbamazepine reduces effects of TRAMADOL; carbamazepine possibly accelerates metabolism of PARACETAMOL (also isolated reports of hepatotoxicity)

● Anthelmintics: carbamazepine reduces plasma concentration of ● ALBENDAZOLE and ● PRAZIQUANTEL—consider increasing albendazole and praziquantel dose when given for systemic infections

● Anti-arrhythmics: carbamazepine possibly reduces plasma concentration of ● DRONEDARONE—avoid concomitant use

● Antibacterials: plasma concentration of carbamazepine increased by ● CLARITHROMYCIN (consider reducing dose of carbamazepine); plasma concentration of carbamazepine increased by ● ERYTHROMYCIN; plasma concentration of carbamazepine reduced by RIFABUTIN; carbamazepine accelerates metabolism of DOXYCYCLINE (reduced effect); carbamazepine possibly reduces plasma concentration of ● BEDAQUILINE—manufacturer of bedaquiline advises avoid concomitant use; avoidance of carbamazepine advised by manufacturer of DELAMANID; plasma concentration of carbamazepine increased by ● ISONIAZID (also possibly increased isoniazid hepatotoxicity); carbamazepine reduces plasma concentration of ● TELITHROMYCIN (avoid during and for 2 weeks after carbamazepine)

● Anticoagulants: carbamazepine possibly reduces plasma concentration of ● APIXABAN—manufacturer of apixaban advises avoid concomitant use when given for treatment of deep-vein thrombosis or pulmonary embolism; carbamazepine accelerates metabolism of ● COUMARINS (reduced anticoagulant effect); carbamazepine possibly reduces plasma concentration of DABIGATRAN—manufacturer of dabigatran advises avoid concomitant use; carbamazepine possibly reduces plasma concentration of ● EDOXABAN; carbamazepine possibly reduces plasma concentration of ● RIVAROXABAN—manufacturer of rivaroxaban advises monitor for signs of thrombosis

● Antidepressants: carbamazepine possibly reduces plasma concentration of ● REBOXETINE; plasma concentration of carbamazepine increased by ● FLUOXETINE and ● FLUVOXAMINE; carbamazepine reduces plasma concentration of ● MIANSERIN, MIRTAZAPINE and TRAZODONE; anticonvulsant effect of antiepileptics possibly antagonised by MAOIs and ● TRICYCLIC-RELATED ANTIDEPRESSANTS (convulsive threshold lowered); manufacturer of antidepressants advises avoid for 2 weeks after stopping ● MAOIs, also antagonism of anticonvulsant effect; anticonvulsant effect of antiepileptics antagonised by ● SSRIs and ● TRICYCLICS (convulsive threshold lowered); plasma concentration of carbamazepine possibly reduced by ST JOHN'S WORT; carbamazepine accelerates metabolism of ● TRICYCLICS (reduced plasma concentration and reduced effect); carbamazepine possibly reduces plasma concentration of ● VORTIOXETINE—consider increasing dose of vortioxetine

● Antiepileptics: carbamazepine possibly reduces plasma concentration of ESLICARBAZEPINE but risk of side-effects increased; carbamazepine possibly reduces plasma concentration of ETHOSUXIMIDE and RETIGABINE; plasma concentration of both drugs often reduced when carbamazepine given with FOSPHENYTOIN or PHENYTOIN, also plasma concentration of fosphenytoin or phenytoin may be increased; carbamazepine often reduces plasma concentration of LAMOTRIGINE, also plasma concentration of an active metabolite of carbamazepine sometimes raised (but evidence is conflicting); possible increased risk of carbamazepine toxicity when given with LEVETIRACETAM;

Carbamazepine

● Antiepileptics (continued)

plasma concentration of carbamazepine sometimes reduced by OXCARBAZEPINE (but concentration of an active metabolite of carbamazepine may be increased), also plasma concentration of an active metabolite of oxcarbazepine often reduced; carbamazepine reduces plasma concentration of ● PERAMPANEL (see under Perampanel, p. 293); carbamazepine possibly increases plasma concentration of PHENOBARBITAL and PRIMIDONE; plasma concentration of both drugs possibly reduced when carbamazepine given with RUFINAMIDE; carbamazepine reduces plasma concentration of SODIUM VALPROATE and VALPROIC ACID, also plasma concentration of active metabolite of carbamazepine increased; plasma concentration of carbamazepine increased by ● STIRIPENTOL; carbamazepine reduces plasma concentration of TIAGABINE and ZONISAMIDE; carbamazepine often reduces plasma concentration of TOPIRAMATE

● Antifungals: plasma concentration of carbamazepine possibly increased by KETOCONAZOLE, also plasma concentration of ketoconazole possibly reduced; plasma concentration of carbamazepine possibly increased by FLUCONAZOLE and MICONAZOLE; carbamazepine possibly reduces plasma concentration of ITRACONAZOLE and ● POSACONAZOLE; carbamazepine possibly reduces plasma concentration of ● VORICONAZOLE—avoid concomitant use; carbamazepine possibly reduces plasma concentration of CASPOFUNGIN—consider increasing dose of caspofungin

● Antimalarials: avoidance of carbamazepine advised by manufacturer of ARTENIMOL WITH PIPERAQUINE; anticonvulsant effect of antiepileptics antagonised by MEFLOQUINE

● Antimuscarinics: carbamazepine possibly reduces plasma concentration of active metabolite of ● FESOTERODINE—manufacturer of fesoterodine advises avoid concomitant use

● Antipsychotics: anticonvulsant effect of antiepileptics antagonised by ● ANTIPSYCHOTICS (convulsive threshold lowered); carbamazepine accelerates metabolism of HALOPERIDOL, OLANZAPINE, QUETIAPINE and RISPERIDONE (reduced plasma concentration); carbamazepine reduces plasma concentration of ● ARIPIPRAZOLE (avoid concomitant use or consider increasing the dose of aripiprazole —consult aripiprazole product literature); carbamazepine accelerates metabolism of ● CLOZAPINE (reduced plasma concentration), also avoid concomitant use of drugs with substantial potential for causing agranulocytosis; carbamazepine possibly reduces plasma concentration of ● LURASIDONE—avoid concomitant use; carbamazepine reduces plasma concentration of PALIPERIDONE

● Antivirals: avoidance of carbamazepine advised by manufacturer of ● BOCEPREVIR and ● RILPIVIRINE (plasma concentration of boceprevir and rilpivirine possibly reduced); carbamazepine possibly reduces plasma concentration of ● DACLATASVIR and ● SIMEPREVIR—manufacturer of daclatasvir and simeprevir advises avoid concomitant use; carbamazepine possibly reduces plasma concentration of DARUNAVIR, FOSAMPRENAVIR, LOPINAVIR, SAQUINAVIR and TIPRANAVIR; carbamazepine reduces plasma concentration of ● DASABUVIR, ● OMBITASVIR and ● PARITAPREVIR—avoid concomitant use; carbamazepine reduces the plasma concentration of ● DOLUTEGRAVIR (see under Dolutegravir, p. 584); plasma concentration of both drugs reduced when carbamazepine given with EFAVIRENZ; avoidance of carbamazepine advised by manufacturer of ● ELVITEGRAVIR, ETRAVIRINE, LEDIPASVIR, SOFOSBUVIR and ● TELAPREVIR; carbamazepine possibly reduces plasma concentration of ● INDINAVIR, also plasma concentration of carbamazepine possibly increased; carbamazepine reduces plasma concentration of NEVIRAPINE; plasma concentration of carbamazepine possibly increased by ● RITONAVIR

▸ Anxiolytics and Hypnotics: carbamazepine often reduces plasma concentration of CLONAZEPAM; carbamazepine reduces plasma concentration of MIDAZOLAM

● Apremilast: carbamazepine possibly reduces plasma concentration of ● APREMILAST—avoid concomitant use

▸ Aprepitant: carbamazepine possibly reduces plasma concentration of APREPITANT

Carbamazepine (continued)

▸ Avanafil: carbamazepine possibly reduces plasma concentration of AVANAFIL—manufacturer of avanafil advises avoid concomitant use
▸ Bupropion: carbamazepine reduces plasma concentration of BUPROPION
● Calcium-channel Blockers: carbamazepine reduces effects of FELODIPINE and ISRADIPINE; carbamazepine probably reduces effects of DIHYDROPYRIDINES, NICARDIPINE and NIFEDIPINE; avoidance of carbamazepine advised by manufacturer of NIMODIPINE (plasma concentration of nimodipine possibly reduced); effects of carbamazepine enhanced by ● DILTIAZEM and ● VERAPAMIL
● Cannabis Extract: carbamazepine possibly reduces plasma concentration of ● CANNABIS EXTRACT—manufacturer of cannabis extract advises avoid concomitant use
● Ciclosporin: carbamazepine accelerates metabolism of ● CICLOSPORIN (reduced plasma concentration)
● Clopidogrel: carbamazepine possibly reduces antiplatelet effect of ● CLOPIDOGREL
● Cobicistat: carbamazepine possibly reduces plasma concentration of ● COBICISTAT—manufacturer of cobicistat advises avoid concomitant use
● Corticosteroids: carbamazepine accelerates metabolism of ● CORTICOSTEROIDS (reduced effect)
● Cytotoxics: carbamazepine possibly decreases plasma concentration of AXITINIB (increase dose of axitinib—consult axitinib product literature); carbamazepine possibly reduces plasma concentration of BORTEZOMIB, ● BOSUTINIB, CRIZOTINIB, ● IBRUTINIB, ● IDELALISIB and PONATINIB—manufacturer of bortezomib, bosutinib, crizotinib, ibrutinib, idelalisib and ponatinib advises avoid concomitant use; carbamazepine possibly reduces plasma concentration of ● CABOZANTINIB— avoid concomitant use; avoidance of carbamazepine advised by manufacturer of ● CABAZITAXEL, DABRAFENIB, GEFITINIB, ● OLAPARIB and VEMURAFENIB; avoidance of carbamazepine advised by manufacturer of DASATINIB, VANDETANIB and ● VISMODEGIB (plasma concentration of dasatinib, vandetanib and vismodegib possibly reduced); carbamazepine reduces plasma concentration of ● IMATINIB and ● LAPATINIB—avoid concomitant use; carbamazepine possibly reduces plasma concentration of ERIBULIN; carbamazepine reduces plasma concentration of IRINOTECAN and its active metabolite; manufacturer of procarbazine advises possible increased risk of hypersensitivity reactions when carbamazepine given with PROCARBAZINE
● Diuretics: increased risk of hyponatraemia when carbamazepine given with DIURETICS; plasma concentration of carbamazepine increased by ● ACETAZOLAMIDE; carbamazepine reduces plasma concentration of ● EPLERENONE—avoid concomitant use
▸ Fingolimod: carbamazepine reduces plasma concentration of FINGOLIMOD
▸ Fosaprepitant: carbamazepine possibly reduces plasma concentration of FOSAPREPITANT
● Guanfacine: carbamazepine possibly reduces plasma concentration of ● GUANFACINE—increase dose of guanfacine
● Hormone Antagonists: carbamazepine possibly reduces plasma concentration of ● ABIRATERONE—manufacturer of abiraterone advises avoid concomitant use; metabolism of carbamazepine inhibited by ● DANAZOL (increased risk of toxicity); carbamazepine possibly accelerates metabolism of TOREMIFENE (reduced plasma concentration)
▸ 5HT$_3$-receptor Antagonists: carbamazepine accelerates metabolism of ONDANSETRON (reduced effect)
● Ivacaftor: carbamazepine possibly reduces plasma concentration of ● IVACAFTOR—manufacturer of ivacaftor advises avoid concomitant use
● Lipid-regulating Drugs: carbamazepine reduces plasma concentration of SIMVASTATIN—consider increasing dose of simvastatin
▸ Lithium: neurotoxicity may occur when carbamazepine given with LITHIUM without increased plasma concentration of lithium
▸ Macitentan: avoidance of carbamazepine advised by manufacturer of MACITENTAN

Carbamazepine (continued)

▸ Muscle Relaxants: carbamazepine antagonises muscle relaxant effect of NON-DEPOLARISING MUSCLE RELAXANTS (accelerated recovery from neuromuscular blockade)
● Oestrogens: carbamazepine accelerates metabolism of ● OESTROGENS (reduced contraceptive effect with combined oral contraceptives, contraceptive patches, and vaginal rings—see Contraceptive Interactions in BNF)
● Orlistat: possible increased risk of convulsions when antiepileptics given with ● ORLISTAT
● Progestogens: carbamazepine accelerates metabolism of ● PROGESTOGENS (reduced contraceptive effect with combined oral contraceptives, progestogen-only oral contraceptives, contraceptive patches, vaginal rings, etonogestrel-releasing implant, and emergency hormonal contraception—see Contraceptive Interactions in BNF)
▸ Retinoids: plasma concentration of carbamazepine possibly reduced by ISOTRETINOIN
▸ Roflumilast: carbamazepine possibly inhibits effects of ROFLUMILAST (manufacturer of roflumilast advises avoid concomitant use)
▸ Theophylline: carbamazepine accelerates metabolism of THEOPHYLLINE (reduced effect)
▸ Thyroid Hormones: carbamazepine accelerates metabolism of THYROID HORMONES (may increase requirements for thyroid hormones in hypothyroidism)
▸ Tibolone: carbamazepine accelerates metabolism of TIBOLONE (reduced plasma concentration)
▸ Ticagrelor: carbamazepine possibly reduces plasma concentration of TICAGRELOR
● Ulcer-healing Drugs: metabolism of carbamazepine inhibited by ● CIMETIDINE (increased plasma concentration)
● Ulipristal: avoidance of carbamazepine advised by manufacturer of ● ULIPRISTAL (contraceptive effect of ulipristal possibly reduced)
▸ Vitamins: carbamazepine possibly increases requirements for ALFACALCIDOL, CALCITRIOL, COLECALCIFEROL, DIHYDROTACHYSTEROL, ERGOCALCIFEROL, PARICALCITOL or VITAMIN D

Carbapenems see Ertapenem, Imipenem with Cilastatin, and Meropenem

Carbimazole

▸ Anticoagulants: carbimazole possibly enhances anticoagulant effect of COUMARINS

Carbonic Anhydrase Inhibitors see Diuretics

Carboplatin see Platinum Compounds

Carboprost see Prostaglandins

Cardiac Glycosides

▸ ACE Inhibitors: plasma concentration of digoxin possibly increased by CAPTOPRIL
▸ Alpha-blockers: plasma concentration of digoxin increased by PRAZOSIN
▸ Aminosalicylates: absorption of digoxin possibly reduced by SULFASALAZINE
▸ Analgesics: plasma concentration of cardiac glycosides possibly increased by NSAIDs, also possible exacerbation of heart failure and reduction of renal function
▸ Antacids: absorption of digoxin possibly reduced by ANTACIDS
● Anti-arrhythmics: plasma concentration of digoxin increased by ● AMIODARONE, ● DRONEDARONE and ● PROPAFENONE (halve dose of digoxin)
▸ Antibacterials: plasma concentration of digoxin possibly increased by GENTAMICIN, TELITHROMYCIN and TRIMETHOPRIM; absorption of digoxin reduced by NEOMYCIN; plasma concentration of digoxin possibly reduced by RIFAMPICIN; plasma concentration of digoxin increased by MACROLIDES (increased risk of toxicity)
● Antidepressants: plasma concentration of digoxin reduced by ● ST JOHN'S WORT—avoid concomitant use
▸ Antidiabetics: plasma concentration of digoxin possibly reduced by ACARBOSE; plasma concentration of digoxin increased by CANAGLIFLOZIN and SITAGLIPTIN
▸ Antiepileptics: plasma concentration of digoxin possibly reduced by FOSPHENYTOIN and PHENYTOIN

A1

Interactions | Appendix 1

A1

Cardiac Glycosides (continued)

- Antifungals: increased cardiac toxicity with cardiac glycosides if hypokalaemia occurs with ● AMPHOTERICIN; plasma concentration of digoxin increased by ● ITRACONAZOLE
- Antimalarials: plasma concentration of digoxin possibly increased by ● CHLOROQUINE and HYDROXYCHLOROQUINE; possible increased risk of bradycardia when digoxin given with MEFLOQUINE; plasma concentration of digoxin increased by ● QUININE
▸ Antimuscarinics: plasma concentration of digoxin possibly increased by DARIFENACIN
- Antivirals: side-effects of digoxin possibly increased by BOCEPREVIR; plasma concentration of digoxin increased by ● DACLATASVIR, ETRAVIRINE, SIMEPREVIR and TELAPREVIR; plasma concentration of digoxin possibly increased by PARITAPREVIR (consider reducing dose of digoxin); plasma concentration of digoxin possibly increased by RITONAVIR
▸ Anxiolytics and Hypnotics: plasma concentration of digoxin increased by ALPRAZOLAM (increased risk of toxicity)
▸ Beta-blockers: increased risk of AV block and bradycardia when cardiac glycosides given with BETA-BLOCKERS
- Calcium Salts: arrhythmias can be precipitated when cardiac glycosides given with large *intravenous* doses of CALCIUM SALTS
- Calcium-channel Blockers: plasma concentration of digoxin increased by ● DILTIAZEM, ● LERCANIDIPINE and ● NICARDIPINE; plasma concentration of digoxin possibly increased by ● NIFEDIPINE; plasma concentration of digoxin increased by ● VERAPAMIL, also increased risk of AV block and bradycardia
- Ciclosporin: plasma concentration of digoxin increased by ● CICLOSPORIN (increased risk of toxicity)
▸ Cobicistat: plasma concentration of digoxin possibly increased by COBICISTAT—reduce initial dose of digoxin
- Colchicine: possible increased risk of myopathy when digoxin given with ● COLCHICINE
▸ Corticosteroids: increased risk of hypokalaemia when cardiac glycosides given with CORTICOSTEROIDS
▸ Cytotoxics: absorption of digoxin *tablets* possibly reduced by BLEOMYCIN; CARMUSTINE, CYCLOPHOSPHAMIDE, CYTARABINE, DOXORUBICIN, MELPHALAN, METHOTREXATE, PROCARBAZINE and VINCRISTINE; possible increased risk of bradycardia when digoxin given with CRIZOTINIB; manufacturer of digoxin advises give IBRUTINIB at least 6 hours before or after ibrutinib; plasma concentration of digoxin increased by VANDETANIB—possible increased risk of bradycardia
- Diuretics: increased cardiac toxicity with cardiac glycosides if hypokalaemia occurs with ● ACETAZOLAMIDE, ● LOOP DIURETICS or ● THIAZIDES AND RELATED DIURETICS; plasma concentration of digoxin possibly increased by POTASSIUM CANRENOATE; plasma concentration of digoxin increased by ● SPIRONOLACTONE
▸ Ivacaftor: plasma concentration of digoxin increased by IVACAFTOR
▸ Lenalidomide: plasma concentration of digoxin possibly increased by LENALIDOMIDE
▸ Lipid-regulating Drugs: absorption of cardiac glycosides possibly reduced by COLESTIPOL and COLESTYRAMINE; plasma concentration of digoxin possibly increased by ATORVASTATIN
▸ Mirabegron: plasma concentration of digoxin increased by MIRABEGRON—reduce initial dose of digoxin
- Muscle Relaxants: risk of ventricular arrhythmias when cardiac glycosides given with SUXAMETHONIUM; possible increased risk of bradycardia when cardiac glycosides given with TIZANIDINE
▸ Penicillamine: plasma concentration of digoxin possibly reduced by PENICILLAMINE
▸ Ranolazine: plasma concentration of digoxin increased by RANOLAZINE
▸ Sympathomimetics: avoidance of digoxin advised by manufacturer of MIDODRINE
▸ Sympathomimetics, Beta₂: plasma concentration of digoxin possibly reduced by SALBUTAMOL
- Ticagrelor: plasma concentration of digoxin increased by ● TICAGRELOR
▸ Tolvaptan: plasma concentration of digoxin increased by TOLVAPTAN (increased risk of toxicity)
▸ Ulcer-healing Drugs: plasma concentration of digoxin possibly slightly increased by PROTON PUMP INHIBITORS; absorption of cardiac glycosides possibly reduced by SUCRALFATE

Cardiac Glycosides (continued)

▸ Ulipristal: manufacturer of ulipristal advises give digoxin at least 1.5 hours before or after ULIPRISTAL

Carmustine

- Antipsychotics: avoid concomitant use of cytotoxics with ● CLOZAPINE (increased risk of agranulocytosis)
▸ Cardiac Glycosides: carmustine possibly reduces absorption of DIGOXIN *tablets*
▸ Ulcer-healing Drugs: myelosuppressive effects of carmustine possibly enhanced by CIMETIDINE

Carteolol *see* Beta-blockers

Carvedilol *see* Beta-blockers

Caspofungin

▸ Antibacterials: plasma concentration of caspofungin initially increased and then reduced by RIFAMPICIN (consider increasing dose of caspofungin)
▸ Antiepileptics: plasma concentration of caspofungin possibly reduced by CARBAMAZEPINE, FOSPHENYTOIN and PHENYTOIN—consider increasing dose of caspofungin
▸ Antivirals: plasma concentration of caspofungin possibly reduced by EFAVIRENZ and NEVIRAPINE—consider increasing dose of caspofungin
- Ciclosporin: plasma concentration of caspofungin increased by ● CICLOSPORIN (manufacturer of caspofungin recommends monitoring liver enzymes)
▸ Corticosteroids: plasma concentration of caspofungin possibly reduced by DEXAMETHASONE—consider increasing dose of caspofungin
- Tacrolimus: caspofungin reduces plasma concentration of ● TACROLIMUS

Catumaxomab

- Antipsychotics: avoid concomitant use of cytotoxics with ● CLOZAPINE (increased risk of agranulocytosis)
- Vaccines: risk of generalised infections when monoclonal antibodies given with live ● VACCINES—avoid concomitant use

Cefaclor *see* Cephalosporins
Cefadroxil *see* Cephalosporins
Cefalexin *see* Cephalosporins
Cefixime *see* Cephalosporins
Cefotaxime *see* Cephalosporins
Cefradine *see* Cephalosporins
Ceftaroline *see* Cephalosporins
Ceftazidime *see* Cephalosporins
Ceftobiprole *see* Cephalosporins
Ceftriaxone *see* Cephalosporins
Cefuroxime *see* Cephalosporins
Celecoxib *see* NSAIDs
Celiprolol *see* Beta-blockers

Cephalosporins

▸ Antacids: absorption of cefaclor reduced by ANTACIDS
▸ Antibacterials: possible increased risk of nephrotoxicity when cephalosporins given with AMINOGLYCOSIDES
- Anticoagulants: cephalosporins possibly enhance anticoagulant effect of ● COUMARINS
▸ Teriflunomide: plasma concentration of cefaclor increased by TERIFLUNOMIDE
▸ Vaccines: antibacterials inactivate ORAL TYPHOID VACCINE—see under Typhoid Vaccine in BNF

Certolizumab pegol

- Abatacept: avoid concomitant use of certolizumab pegol with ● ABATACEPT
- Anakinra: avoid concomitant use of certolizumab pegol with ● ANAKINRA
- Antipsychotics: avoid concomitant use of cytotoxics with ● CLOZAPINE (increased risk of agranulocytosis)
- Vaccines: risk of generalised infections when monoclonal antibodies given with live ● VACCINES—avoid concomitant use

Cetirizine *see* Antihistamines

Cetuximab

- Antipsychotics: avoid concomitant use of cytotoxics with ● CLOZAPINE (increased risk of agranulocytosis)
- Vaccines: risk of generalised infections when monoclonal antibodies given with live ● VACCINES—avoid concomitant use

Chenodeoxycholic Acid *see* Bile Acids
Chloral *see* Anxiolytics and Hypnotics

Chloramphenicol
- Antibacterials: metabolism of chloramphenicol accelerated by RIFAMPICIN (reduced plasma concentration)
- Anticoagulants: chloramphenicol enhances anticoagulant effect of ● COUMARINS
- Antidiabetics: chloramphenicol enhances effects of ● SULFONYLUREAS
- Antiepileptics: chloramphenicol increases plasma concentration of ● FOSPHENYTOIN and ● PHENYTOIN (increased risk of toxicity); metabolism of chloramphenicol possibly accelerated by ● PHENOBARBITAL and ● PRIMIDONE (reduced plasma concentration)
- Antipsychotics: avoid concomitant use of chloramphenicol with ● CLOZAPINE (increased risk of agranulocytosis)
- Ciclosporin: chloramphenicol possibly increases plasma concentration of ● CICLOSPORIN
- Clopidogrel: chloramphenicol possibly reduces antiplatelet effect of ● CLOPIDOGREL
- Guanfacine: when given with chloramphenicol manufacturer of GUANFACINE advises halve dose
- Hydroxocobalamin: chloramphenicol reduces response to HYDROXOCOBALAMIN
- Iron Salts: chloramphenicol possibly inhibits effects of IRON SALTS
- Tacrolimus: chloramphenicol possibly increases plasma concentration of ● TACROLIMUS
- Vaccines: antibacterials inactivate ORAL TYPHOID VACCINE—see under Typhoid Vaccine in BNF

Chlordiazepoxide see Anxiolytics and Hypnotics
Chloroprocaine
- Antibacterials: chloroprocaine possibly inhibits effects of ● SULFONAMIDES (manufacturer of chloroprocaine advises avoid concomitant use)
Chloroquine
- Adsorbents: absorption of chloroquine reduced by KAOLIN
- Agalsidase Alfa and Beta: chloroquine possibly inhibits effects of AGALSIDASE ALFA AND BETA (manufacturers of agalsidase alfa and beta advise avoid concomitant use)
- Antacids: absorption of chloroquine reduced by ANTACIDS
- Anthelmintics: chloroquine reduces plasma concentration of ● PRAZIQUANTEL—consider increasing praziquantel dose when given for systemic infections
- Anti-arrhythmics: increased risk of ventricular arrhythmias when chloroquine given with ● AMIODARONE—avoid concomitant use
- Antibacterials: increased risk of ventricular arrhythmias when chloroquine given with ● MOXIFLOXACIN—avoid concomitant use
- Antidepressants: possible increased risk of ventricular arrhythmias when chloroquine given with ● CITALOPRAM and ● ESCITALOPRAM
- Antimalarials: avoidance of antimalarials advised by manufacturer of ● ARTEMETHER WITH LUMEFANTRINE; increased risk of convulsions when chloroquine given with ● MEFLOQUINE
- Antipsychotics: increased risk of ventricular arrhythmias when chloroquine given with ● DROPERIDOL—avoid concomitant use
- Cardiac Glycosides: chloroquine possibly increases plasma concentration of ● DIGOXIN
- Ciclosporin: chloroquine increases plasma concentration of ● CICLOSPORIN (increased risk of toxicity)
- Cytotoxics: possible increased risk of ventricular arrhythmias when chloroquine given with ● BOSUTINIB
- Histamine: avoidance of antimalarials advised by manufacturer of HISTAMINE
- Lanthanum: absorption of chloroquine possibly reduced by LANTHANUM (give at least 2 hours apart)
- Laronidase: chloroquine possibly inhibits effects of LARONIDASE (manufacturer of laronidase advises avoid concomitant use)
- Parasympathomimetics: chloroquine has potential to increase symptoms of myasthenia gravis and thus diminish effect of NEOSTIGMINE and PYRIDOSTIGMINE
- Penicillamine: increased risk of haematological toxicity when antimalarials given with PENICILLAMINE—manufacturer of penicillamine advises avoid concomitant use
- Ulcer-healing Drugs: metabolism of chloroquine inhibited by CIMETIDINE (increased plasma concentration)

Chloroquine (continued)
- Vaccines: antimalarials inactivate ORAL TYPHOID VACCINE—see under Typhoid Vaccine in BNF
Chlorothiazide see Diuretics
Chlorphenamine see Antihistamines
Chlorpromazine see Antipsychotics
Chlortalidone see Diuretics
Cholera Vaccine see Vaccines
Cholic Acid see Bile Acids
Ciclesonide see Corticosteroids
Ciclosporin
- ACE Inhibitors: increased risk of hyperkalaemia when ciclosporin given with ● ACE INHIBITORS
- Aliskiren: ciclosporin increases plasma concentration of ● ALISKIREN—avoid concomitant use
- Allopurinol: plasma concentration of ciclosporin possibly increased by ALLOPURINOL (risk of nephrotoxicity)
- Ambrisentan: ciclosporin increases plasma concentration of ● AMBRISENTAN (see under Ambrisentan, p. 169)
- Analgesics: increased risk of nephrotoxicity when ciclosporin given with ● NSAIDS; ciclosporin increases plasma concentration of ● DICLOFENAC (halve dose of diclofenac)
- Angiotensin-II Receptor Antagonists: increased risk of hyperkalaemia when ciclosporin given with ● ANGIOTENSIN-II RECEPTOR ANTAGONISTS
- Anti-arrhythmics: plasma concentration of ciclosporin possibly increased by AMIODARONE and PROPAFENONE
- Antibacterials: plasma concentration of ciclosporin increased by ● AZITHROMYCIN; metabolism of ciclosporin inhibited by ● CLARITHROMYCIN and ● ERYTHROMYCIN (increased concentration); metabolism of ciclosporin accelerated by ● RIFAMPICIN (reduced plasma concentration); plasma concentration of ciclosporin possibly reduced by ● SULFADIAZINE; increased risk of nephrotoxicity when ciclosporin given with ● AMINOGLYCOSIDES, ● POLYMYXINS, ● QUINOLONES, ● SULFONAMIDES or ● VANCOMYCIN; plasma concentration of ciclosporin possibly increased by ● CHLORAMPHENICOL and ● TELITHROMYCIN; increased risk of myopathy when ciclosporin given with ● DAPTOMYCIN (preferably avoid concomitant use); avoidance of ciclosporin advised by manufacturer of FIDAXOMICIN; metabolism of ciclosporin possibly inhibited by ● MACROLIDES (increased plasma concentration); ciclosporin increases plasma concentration of ● RIFAXIMIN; increased risk of nephrotoxicity when ciclosporin given with ● TRIMETHOPRIM, also plasma concentration of ciclosporin reduced by intravenous trimethoprim
- Anticoagulants: ciclosporin possibly increases plasma concentration of ● DABIGATRAN—manufacturer of dabigatran advises avoid concomitant use; ciclosporin increases plasma concentration of ● EDOXABAN (reduce dose of edoxaban—see under Edoxaban, p. 113)
- Antidepressants: plasma concentration of ciclosporin reduced by ● ST JOHN'S WORT—avoid concomitant use
- Antidiabetics: ciclosporin possibly enhances hypoglycaemic effect of REPAGLINIDE
- Antiepileptics: metabolism of ciclosporin accelerated by ● CARBAMAZEPINE, ● FOSPHENYTOIN, ● PHENOBARBITAL, ● PHENYTOIN and ● PRIMIDONE (reduced plasma concentration); plasma concentration of ciclosporin possibly reduced by OXCARBAZEPINE
- Antifungals: metabolism of ciclosporin inhibited by ● FLUCONAZOLE, ● ITRACONAZOLE, ● KETOCONAZOLE, ● POSACONAZOLE and ● VORICONAZOLE (increased plasma concentration); metabolism of ciclosporin possibly inhibited by ● MICONAZOLE (increased plasma concentration); increased risk of nephrotoxicity when ciclosporin given with ● AMPHOTERICIN; ciclosporin increases plasma concentration of ● CASPOFUNGIN (manufacturer of caspofungin recommends monitoring liver enzymes); plasma concentration of ciclosporin possibly reduced by GRISEOFULVIN and TERBINAFINE; plasma concentration of ciclosporin possibly increased by MICAFUNGIN
- Antimalarials: plasma concentration of ciclosporin increased by ● CHLOROQUINE and ● HYDROXYCHLOROQUINE (increased risk of toxicity)

A1

Interactions | Appendix 1

Ciclosporin (continued)

▸ Antimuscarinics: avoidance of ciclosporin advised by manufacturer of DARIFENACIN
● Antivirals: increased risk of nephrotoxicity when ciclosporin given with ACICLOVIR or VALACICLOVIR; plasma concentration of ciclosporin possibly increased by ● ATAZANAVIR and ● RITONAVIR; plasma concentration of ciclosporin increased by ● BOCEPREVIR, ● FOSAMPRENAVIR and ● INDINAVIR; plasma concentration of ciclosporin possibly reduced by ● EFAVIRENZ; plasma concentration of both drugs increased when ciclosporin given with ● SAQUINAVIR; plasma concentration of both drugs increased when ciclosporin given with ● TELAPREVIR (reduce dose of ciclosporin)
● Beta-blockers: plasma concentration of ciclosporin increased by ● CARVEDILOL
● Bile Acids: avoidance of ciclosporin advised by manufacturer of CHOLIC ACID; absorption of ciclosporin increased by ● URSODEOXYCHOLIC ACID
● Bosentan: ciclosporin increases plasma concentration of ● BOSENTAN (also plasma concentration of ciclosporin reduced—avoid concomitant use)
● Calcium-channel Blockers: combination of ciclosporin with ● LERCANIDIPINE may increase plasma concentration of either drug (or both)—avoid concomitant use; plasma concentration of ciclosporin increased by ● DILTIAZEM, ● NICARDIPINE and ● VERAPAMIL; ciclosporin possibly increases plasma concentration of NIFEDIPINE (increased risk of toxicity including gingival hyperplasia)
● Cardiac Glycosides: ciclosporin increases plasma concentration of ● DIGOXIN (increased risk of toxicity)
● Colchicine: possible increased risk of nephrotoxicity and myotoxicity when ciclosporin given with ● COLCHICINE—suspend or reduce dose of colchicine (avoid concomitant use in hepatic or renal impairment)
● Corticosteroids: plasma concentration of ciclosporin increased by high-dose ● METHYLPREDNISOLONE (risk of convulsions); ciclosporin increases plasma concentration of PREDNISOLONE
● Cytotoxics: increased risk of nephrotoxicity when ciclosporin given with ● MELPHALAN; increased risk of neurotoxicity when ciclosporin given with ● DOXORUBICIN; ciclosporin increases plasma concentration of ● EPIRUBICIN and ● IDARUBICIN; ciclosporin reduces excretion of MITOXANTRONE (increased plasma concentration); risk of toxicity when ciclosporin given with ● METHOTREXATE; ciclosporin possibly increases the plasma concentration of AFATINIB—manufacturer of afatinib advises separating administration of ciclosporin by 6 to 12 hours; caution with ciclosporin advised by manufacturer of ● CRIZOTINIB; ciclosporin increases plasma concentration of ● EVEROLIMUS (consider reducing the dose of everolimus — consult everolimus product literature); plasma concentration of ciclosporin possibly increased by IMATINIB; *in vitro* studies suggest a possible interaction between ciclosporin and DOCETAXEL (consult docetaxel product literature); ciclosporin possibly increases plasma concentration of ETOPOSIDE (increased risk of toxicity)
▸ Dexrazoxane: increased risk of immunosupression with ciclosporin advised by manufacturer of DEXRAZOXANE
● Diuretics: plasma concentration of ciclosporin possibly increased by ● ACETAZOLAMIDE; increased risk of hyperkalaemia when ciclosporin given with ● POTASSIUM-SPARING DIURETICS AND ALDOSTERONE ANTAGONISTS; increased risk of nephrotoxicity and possibly hypermagnesaemia when ciclosporin given with THIAZIDES AND RELATED DIURETICS
● Grapefruit Juice: plasma concentration of ciclosporin increased by ● GRAPEFRUIT JUICE (increased risk of toxicity)
● Hormone Antagonists: metabolism of ciclosporin inhibited by ● DANAZOL (increased plasma concentration); plasma concentration of ciclosporin reduced by LANREOTIDE and ● OCTREOTIDE; plasma concentration of ciclosporin possibly reduced by ● PASIREOTIDE
● Lenalidomide: ciclosporin possibly increases plasma concentration of ● LENALIDOMIDE (increased risk of toxicity)
● Lipid-regulating Drugs: absorption of ciclosporin reduced by ● COLESEVELAM; increased risk of renal impairment when ciclosporin given with BEZAFIBRATE or FENOFIBRATE; increased risk of myopathy when ciclosporin given with

Ciclosporin
● Lipid-regulating Drugs (continued)
● ATORVASTATIN (see under Atorvastatin, p. 186); increased risk of myopathy when ciclosporin given with ● FLUVASTATIN or ● PRAVASTATIN; increased risk of myopathy when ciclosporin given with ● ROSUVASTATIN or ● SIMVASTATIN (avoid concomitant use); plasma concentration of both drugs may increase when ciclosporin given with ● EZETIMIBE; separating administration from ciclosporin by 12 hours advised by manufacturer of LOMITAPIDE
▸ Mannitol: possible increased risk of nephrotoxicity when ciclosporin given with MANNITOL
● Metoclopramide: plasma concentration of ciclosporin increased by ● METOCLOPRAMIDE
▸ Mifamurtide: avoidance of ciclosporin advised by manufacturer of MIFAMURTIDE
▸ Modafinil: plasma concentration of ciclosporin reduced by ● MODAFINIL
▸ Oestrogens: plasma concentration of ciclosporin possibly increased by OESTROGENS
● Orlistat: absorption of ciclosporin possibly reduced by ● ORLISTAT
● Potassium Salts: increased risk of hyperkalaemia when ciclosporin given with ● POTASSIUM SALTS
▸ Progestogens: plasma concentration of ciclosporin possibly increased by PROGESTOGENS
▸ Ranolazine: plasma concentration of both drugs may increase when ciclosporin given with RANOLAZINE
▸ Sevelamer: plasma concentration of ciclosporin possibly reduced by SEVELAMER
● Sirolimus: ciclosporin increases plasma concentration of SIROLIMUS
● Sulfinpyrazone: plasma concentration of ciclosporin reduced by ● SULFINPYRAZONE
▸ Tacrolimus: plasma concentration of ciclosporin increased by ● TACROLIMUS (increased risk of nephrotoxicity)—avoid concomitant use
▸ Ticagrelor: ciclosporin increases plasma concentration of TICAGRELOR
▸ Ulcer-healing Drugs: plasma concentration of ciclosporin possibly increased by ● CIMETIDINE; plasma concentration of ciclosporin possibly affected by OMEPRAZOLE
▸ Vitamins: plasma concentration of ciclosporin possibly affected by VITAMIN E

Cilostazol
● Anagrelide: avoidance of cilostazol advised by manufacturer of ● ANAGRELIDE
● Antibacterials: plasma concentration of cilostazol possibly increased by ● CLARITHROMYCIN (see under Cilostazol, p. 215); plasma concentration of cilostazol increased by ● ERYTHROMYCIN (see under Cilostazol, p. 215)
● Antifungals: plasma concentration of cilostazol increased by ● KETOCONAZOLE (see under Cilostazol, p. 215); plasma concentration of cilostazol possibly increased by ● ITRACONAZOLE (see under Cilostazol, p. 215)
● Antivirals: plasma concentration of cilostazol possibly increased by ● BOCEPREVIR, ● RITONAVIR and ● TELAPREVIR (see under Cilostazol, p. 215)
▸ Calcium-channel Blockers: plasma concentration of cilostazol increased by DILTIAZEM (consider reducing dose of cilostazol)
▸ Lipid-regulating Drugs: separating administration from cilostazol by 12 hours advised by manufacturer of LOMITAPIDE
▸ Ulcer-healing Drugs: plasma concentration of cilostazol increased by ● OMEPRAZOLE (see under Cilostazol, p. 215)

Cimetidine see Histamine H₂-antagonists

Cinacalcet
▸ Antifungals: metabolism of cinacalcet inhibited by KETOCONAZOLE (increased plasma concentration)
● Hormone Antagonists: cinacalcet possibly inhibits metabolism of ● TAMOXIFEN to active metabolite (avoid concomitant use)

Cinnarizine see Antihistamines
Ciprofibrate see Fibrates
Ciprofloxacin see Quinolones
Cisatracurium see Muscle Relaxants
Cisplatin see Platinum Compounds
Citalopram see Antidepressants, SSRI

Cladribine
- Antipsychotics: avoid concomitant use of cytotoxics with ● CLOZAPINE (increased risk of agranulocytosis)
- Antivirals: avoidance of cladribine advised by manufacturer of ● LAMIVUDINE

Clarithromycin see Macrolides
Clemastine see Antihistamines
Clindamycin
- Muscle Relaxants: clindamycin enhances effects of ● NON-DEPOLARISING MUSCLE RELAXANTS and ● SUXAMETHONIUM
▸ Parasympathomimetics: clindamycin antagonises effects of NEOSTIGMINE and PYRIDOSTIGMINE
▸ Vaccines: antibacterials inactivate ORAL TYPHOID VACCINE—see under Typhoid Vaccine in BNF

Clobazam see Anxiolytics and Hypnotics
Clofazimine
- Antibacterials: possible increased risk of ventricular arrhythmias when clofazimine given with ● BEDAQUILINE
▸ Vaccines: antibacterials inactivate ORAL TYPHOID VACCINE—see under Typhoid Vaccine in BNF

Clomethiazole see Anxiolytics and Hypnotics
Clomipramine see Antidepressants, Tricyclic
Clonazepam see Anxiolytics and Hypnotics
Clonidine
▸ ACE Inhibitors: enhanced hypotensive effect when clonidine given with ACE INHIBITORS; previous treatment with clonidine possibly delays antihypertensive effect of CAPTOPRIL
▸ Adrenergic Neurone Blockers: enhanced hypotensive effect when clonidine given with ADRENERGIC NEURONE BLOCKERS
▸ Alcohol: enhanced hypotensive effect when clonidine given with ALCOHOL
▸ Aldesleukin: enhanced hypotensive effect when clonidine given with ALDESLEUKIN
▸ Alpha-blockers: enhanced hypotensive effect when clonidine given with ALPHA-BLOCKERS
▸ Anaesthetics, General: enhanced hypotensive effect when clonidine given with GENERAL ANAESTHETICS
▸ Analgesics: hypotensive effect of clonidine antagonised by NSAIDs
▸ Angiotensin-II Receptor Antagonists: enhanced hypotensive effect when clonidine given with ANGIOTENSIN-II RECEPTOR ANTAGONISTS
- Antidepressants: enhanced hypotensive effect when clonidine given with MAOIs; hypotensive effect of clonidine possibly antagonised by MIRTAZAPINE; hypotensive effect of clonidine antagonised by ● TRICYCLICS, also increased risk of hypertension on clonidine withdrawal
- Antipsychotics: enhanced hypotensive effect when clonidine given with PHENOTHIAZINES
▸ Anxiolytics and Hypnotics: enhanced hypotensive effect when clonidine given with ANXIOLYTICS AND HYPNOTICS
- Beta-blockers: increased risk of withdrawal hypertension when clonidine given with ● BETA-BLOCKERS (withdraw beta-blockers several days before slowly withdrawing clonidine)
▸ Calcium-channel Blockers: enhanced hypotensive effect when clonidine given with CALCIUM-CHANNEL BLOCKERS
▸ Corticosteroids: hypotensive effect of clonidine antagonised by CORTICOSTEROIDS
▸ Cytotoxics: possible increased risk of bradycardia when clonidine given with CRIZOTINIB
▸ Diazoxide: enhanced hypotensive effect when clonidine given with DIAZOXIDE
▸ Diuretics: enhanced hypotensive effect when clonidine given with DIURETICS
▸ Dopaminergics: enhanced hypotensive effect when clonidine given with CO-BENELDOPA, CO-CARELDOPA or LEVODOPA
▸ Histamine: avoidance of clonidine advised by manufacturer of HISTAMINE
▸ Methyldopa: enhanced hypotensive effect when clonidine given with METHYLDOPA
▸ Moxisylyte: enhanced hypotensive effect when clonidine given with MOXISYLYTE
▸ Moxonidine: enhanced hypotensive effect when clonidine given with MOXONIDINE
▸ Muscle Relaxants: enhanced hypotensive effect when clonidine given with BACLOFEN or TIZANIDINE

Clonidine (continued)
▸ Nitrates: enhanced hypotensive effect when clonidine given with NITRATES
▸ Oestrogens: hypotensive effect of clonidine antagonised by OESTROGENS
▸ Prostaglandins: enhanced hypotensive effect when clonidine given with ALPROSTADIL
- Sympathomimetics: possible risk of hypertension when clonidine given with ADRENALINE (EPINEPHRINE) or NORADRENALINE (NOREPINEPHRINE); serious adverse events reported with concomitant use of clonidine and ● METHYLPHENIDATE (causality not established)
▸ Vasodilator Antihypertensives: enhanced hypotensive effect when clonidine given with HYDRALAZINE, MINOXIDIL or SODIUM NITROPRUSSIDE

Clopamide see Diuretics
Clopidogrel
▸ Analgesics: increased risk of bleeding when clopidogrel given with NSAIDs or ASPIRIN
- Antibacterials: antiplatelet effect of clopidogrel possibly reduced by ● CHLORAMPHENICOL, ● CIPROFLOXACIN and ● ERYTHROMYCIN
- Anticoagulants: manufacturer of clopidogrel advises avoid concomitant use with ● WARFARIN; antiplatelet action of clopidogrel enhances anticoagulant effect of ● COUMARINS and ● PHENINDIONE; increased risk of bleeding when clopidogrel given with HEPARINS
- Antidepressants: antiplatelet effect of clopidogrel possibly reduced by ● FLUOXETINE, ● FLUVOXAMINE and ● MOCLOBEMIDE
- Antiepileptics: antiplatelet effect of clopidogrel possibly reduced by ● CARBAMAZEPINE and ● OXCARBAZEPINE
- Antifungals: antiplatelet effect of clopidogrel possibly reduced by ● FLUCONAZOLE, ● ITRACONAZOLE, ● KETOCONAZOLE and ● VORICONAZOLE
- Antivirals: antiplatelet effect of clopidogrel possibly reduced by ● ETRAVIRINE
▸ Dipyridamole: increased risk of bleeding when clopidogrel given with DIPYRIDAMOLE
▸ Iloprost: increased risk of bleeding when clopidogrel given with ILOPROST
- Lipid-regulating Drugs: clopidogrel increases plasma concentration of ● ROSUVASTATIN—adjust dose of rosuvastatin (consult product literature)
▸ Prasugrel: possible increased risk of bleeding when clopidogrel given with PRASUGREL
- Ulcer-healing Drugs: antiplatelet effect of clopidogrel possibly reduced by ● CIMETIDINE, LANSOPRAZOLE, PANTOPRAZOLE and RABEPRAZOLE; antiplatelet effect of clopidogrel reduced by ● ESOMEPRAZOLE and ● OMEPRAZOLE

Clotrimazole see Antifungals, Imidazole
Clozapine see Antipsychotics
Co-amoxiclav see Penicillins
Co-beneldopa
▸ ACE Inhibitors: enhanced hypotensive effect when co-beneldopa given with ACE INHIBITORS
▸ Adrenergic Neurone Blockers: enhanced hypotensive effect when co-beneldopa given with ADRENERGIC NEURONE BLOCKERS
▸ Alpha-blockers: enhanced hypotensive effect when co-beneldopa given with ALPHA-BLOCKERS
- Anaesthetics, General: increased risk of arrhythmias when co-beneldopa given with ● VOLATILE LIQUID GENERAL ANAESTHETICS
▸ Angiotensin-II Receptor Antagonists: enhanced hypotensive effect when co-beneldopa given with ANGIOTENSIN-II RECEPTOR ANTAGONISTS
▸ Antibacterials: effects of co-beneldopa possibly reduced by ISONIAZID
- Antidepressants: risk of hypertensive crisis when co-beneldopa given with ● MAOIs, avoid co-beneldopa for at least 2 weeks after stopping MAOIs; increased risk of side-effects when co-beneldopa given with MOCLOBEMIDE
▸ Antiepileptics: effects of co-beneldopa possibly reduced by FOSPHENYTOIN and PHENYTOIN
▸ Antimuscarinics: absorption of co-beneldopa possibly reduced by ANTIMUSCARINICS

Co-beneldopa (continued)

▸ **Antipsychotics:** effects of co-beneldopa antagonised by ANTIPSYCHOTICS; avoidance of co-beneldopa advised by manufacturer of AMISULPRIDE (antagonism of effect)
▸ **Anxiolytics and Hypnotics:** effects of co-beneldopa possibly antagonised by BENZODIAZEPINES
▸ **Beta-blockers:** enhanced hypotensive effect when co-beneldopa given with BETA-BLOCKERS
▸ **Bupropion:** increased risk of side-effects when co-beneldopa given with BUPROPION
▸ **Calcium-channel Blockers:** enhanced hypotensive effect when co-beneldopa given with CALCIUM-CHANNEL BLOCKERS
▸ **Clonidine:** enhanced hypotensive effect when co-beneldopa given with CLONIDINE
▸ **Diazoxide:** enhanced hypotensive effect when co-beneldopa given with DIAZOXIDE
▸ **Diuretics:** enhanced hypotensive effect when co-beneldopa given with DIURETICS
▸ **Dopaminergics:** enhanced effects and increased toxicity of co-beneldopa when given with SELEGILINE (reduce dose of co-beneldopa)
▸ **Iron Salts:** absorption of co-beneldopa possibly reduced by *oral* IRON SALTS
▸ **Memantine:** effects of dopaminergics possibly enhanced by MEMANTINE
▸ **Methyldopa:** enhanced hypotensive effect when co-beneldopa given with METHYLDOPA; antiparkinsonian effect of dopaminergics antagonised by METHYLDOPA
▸ **Moxonidine:** enhanced hypotensive effect when co-beneldopa given with MOXONIDINE
▸ **Muscle Relaxants:** possible agitation, confusion and hallucinations when co-beneldopa given with BACLOFEN
▸ **Nitrates:** enhanced hypotensive effect when co-beneldopa given with NITRATES
▸ **Vasodilator Antihypertensives:** enhanced hypotensive effect when co-beneldopa given with HYDRALAZINE, MINOXIDIL or SODIUM NITROPRUSSIDE

Cobicistat

● **Alpha-blockers:** cobicistat possibly increases plasma concentration of ● ALFUZOSIN—manufacturer of cobicistat advises avoid concomitant use
● **Anti-arrhythmics:** cobicistat possibly increases plasma concentration of ● AMIODARONE—manufacturer of cobicistat advises avoid concomitant use
● **Antibacterials:** plasma concentration of cobicistat reduced by ● RIFABUTIN (adjust dose—consult product literature); plasma concentration of cobicistat possibly reduced by ● RIFAMPICIN—manufacturer of cobicistat advises avoid concomitant use
● **Anticoagulants:** avoidance of cobicistat advised by manufacturer of APIXABAN; cobicistat possibly enhances anticoagulant effect of ● RIVAROXABAN—avoid concomitant use
● **Antidepressants:** plasma concentration of cobicistat possibly reduced by ● ST JOHN'S WORT—manufacturer of cobicistat advises avoid concomitant use
● **Antiepileptics:** plasma concentration of cobicistat possibly reduced by ● CARBAMAZEPINE, ● FOSPHENYTOIN, ● PHENOBARBITAL, ● PHENYTOIN and ● PRIMIDONE—manufacturer of cobicistat advises avoid concomitant use
▸ **Antifungals:** cobicistat possibly increases plasma concentration of ITRACONAZOLE and KETOCONAZOLE—manufacturer of cobicistat advises reduce dose of itraconazole and ketoconazole
● **Antipsychotics:** cobicistat possibly increases plasma concentration of ● LURASIDONE—avoid concomitant use; cobicistat possibly increases plasma concentration of ● PIMOZIDE—manufacturer of cobicistat advises avoid concomitant use
● **Antivirals:** manufacturer of cobicistat advises avoid concomitant use with BOCEPREVIR and RITONAVIR; cobicistat possibly increases the plasma concentration of ● DACLATASVIR—reduce dose of daclatasvir (see under Daclatasvir, p. 568); avoidance of cobicistat advised by manufacturer of DASABUVIR, NEVIRAPINE, OMBITASVIR and PARITAPREVIR; cobicistat possibly increases plasma concentration of ● MARAVIROC (reduce dose of maraviroc);

Cobicistat

● **Antivirals** (continued)
cobicistat possibly increases plasma concentration of ● SIMEPREVIR—manufacturer of simeprevir advises avoid concomitant use; plasma concentration of both drugs reduced when cobicistat given with ● TIPRANAVIR (avoid concomitant use)
● **Anxiolytics and Hypnotics:** manufacturer of cobicistat advises avoid concomitant use with *oral* ● MIDAZOLAM
● **Avanafil:** cobicistat possibly increases plasma concentration of ● AVANAFIL—avoid concomitant use
▸ **Bosentan:** manufacturer of cobicistat advises avoid concomitant use with BOSENTAN
▸ **Cardiac Glycosides:** cobicistat possibly increases plasma concentration of DIGOXIN—reduce initial dose of digoxin
● **Cytotoxics:** cobicistat possibly increases the plasma concentration of ● IBRUTINIB—reduce dose of ibrutinib (see under Ibrutinib, p. 855)
● **Domperidone:** possible increased risk of ventricular arrhythmias when cobicistat given with ● DOMPERIDONE—avoid concomitant use
● **Ergot Alkaloids:** cobicistat possibly increases plasma concentration of ● ERGOT ALKALOIDS—manufacturer of cobicistat advises avoid concomitant use
● **Lipid-regulating Drugs:** cobicistat possibly increases plasma concentration of ● ATORVASTATIN—manufacturer of cobicistat advises reduce dose of atorvastatin; manufacturer of cobicistat advises avoid concomitant use with ● SIMVASTATIN
● **Oestrogens:** cobicistat accelerates metabolism of ● OESTROGENS (reduced contraceptive effect with combined oral contraceptives, contraceptive patches, and vaginal rings—see Contraceptive Interactions in BNF)
▸ **Progestogens:** cobicistat increases plasma concentration of NORGESTIMATE
● **Sildenafil:** cobicistat possibly increases plasma concentration of ● SILDENAFIL—manufacturer of cobicistat advises avoid concomitant use of sildenafil for pulmonary arterial hypertension or reduce dose of sildenafil for erectile dysfunction—consult cobicistat product literature
▸ **Sympathomimetics, Beta₂:** manufacturer of cobicistat advises avoid concomitant use with SALMETEROL
● **Tadalafil:** cobicistat possibly increases plasma concentration of ● TADALAFIL—manufacturer of cobicistat advises reduce dose of tadalafil (consult cobicistat product literature)
● **Vardenafil:** cobicistat possibly increases plasma concentration of ● VARDENAFIL—manufacturer of cobicistat advises reduce dose of vardenafil (consult cobicistat product literature)

Co-careldopa

▸ **ACE Inhibitors:** enhanced hypotensive effect when co-careldopa given with ACE INHIBITORS
▸ **Adrenergic Neurone Blockers:** enhanced hypotensive effect when co-careldopa given with ADRENERGIC NEURONE BLOCKERS
▸ **Alpha-blockers:** enhanced hypotensive effect when co-careldopa given with ALPHA-BLOCKERS
● **Anaesthetics, General:** increased risk of arrhythmias when co-careldopa given with ● VOLATILE LIQUID GENERAL ANAESTHETICS
▸ **Angiotensin-II Receptor Antagonists:** enhanced hypotensive effect when co-careldopa given with ANGIOTENSIN-II RECEPTOR ANTAGONISTS
▸ **Antibacterials:** effects of co-careldopa possibly reduced by ISONIAZID
● **Antidepressants:** risk of hypertensive crisis when co-careldopa given with ● MAOIs, avoid co-careldopa for at least 2 weeks after stopping MAOIs; increased risk of side-effects when co-careldopa given with MOCLOBEMIDE
▸ **Antiepileptics:** effects of co-careldopa possibly reduced by FOSPHENYTOIN and PHENYTOIN
▸ **Antimuscarinics:** absorption of co-careldopa possibly reduced by ANTIMUSCARINICS
▸ **Antipsychotics:** effects of co-careldopa antagonised by ANTIPSYCHOTICS; avoidance of co-careldopa advised by manufacturer of AMISULPRIDE (antagonism of effect)
▸ **Anxiolytics and Hypnotics:** effects of co-careldopa possibly antagonised by BENZODIAZEPINES
▸ **Beta-blockers:** enhanced hypotensive effect when co-careldopa given with BETA-BLOCKERS

Co-careldopa (continued)

▸ Bupropion: increased risk of side-effects when co-careldopa given with BUPROPION
▸ Calcium-channel Blockers: enhanced hypotensive effect when co-careldopa given with CALCIUM-CHANNEL BLOCKERS
▸ Clonidine: enhanced hypotensive effect when co-careldopa given with CLONIDINE
▸ Diazoxide: enhanced hypotensive effect when co-careldopa given with DIAZOXIDE
▸ Diuretics: enhanced hypotensive effect when co-careldopa given with DIURETICS
▸ Dopaminergics: enhanced effects and increased toxicity of co-careldopa when given with SELEGILINE (reduce dose of co-careldopa)
▸ Iron Salts: absorption of co-careldopa possibly reduced by *oral* IRON SALTS
▸ Memantine: effects of dopaminergics possibly enhanced by MEMANTINE
▸ Methyldopa: enhanced hypotensive effect when co-careldopa given with METHYLDOPA; antiparkinsonian effect of dopaminergics antagonised by METHYLDOPA
▸ Moxonidine: enhanced hypotensive effect when co-careldopa given with MOXONIDINE
▸ Muscle Relaxants: possible agitation, confusion and hallucinations when co-careldopa given with BACLOFEN
▸ Nitrates: enhanced hypotensive effect when co-careldopa given with NITRATES
▸ Vasodilator Antihypertensives: enhanced hypotensive effect when co-careldopa given with HYDRALAZINE, MINOXIDIL or SODIUM NITROPRUSSIDE

Codeine *see* Opioid Analgesics

Co-fluampicil *see* Penicillins

Colchicine

● Anti-arrhythmics: possible increased risk of colchicine toxicity when given with ● AMIODARONE
● Antibacterials: possible increased risk of colchicine toxicity when given with ● AZITHROMYCIN, ● CLARITHROMYCIN, ● ERYTHROMYCIN and ● TELITHROMYCIN—suspend or reduce dose of colchicine (avoid concomitant use in hepatic or renal impairment)
● Antifungals: possible increased risk of colchicine toxicity when given with ● ITRACONAZOLE and ● KETOCONAZOLE—suspend or reduce dose of colchicine (avoid concomitant use in hepatic or renal impairment)
● Antivirals: possible increased risk of colchicine toxicity when given with ● ATAZANAVIR, ● INDINAVIR, ● RITONAVIR and ● TELAPREVIR—suspend or reduce dose of colchicine (avoid concomitant use in hepatic or renal impairment)
● Calcium-channel Blockers: possible increased risk of colchicine toxicity when given with ● DILTIAZEM and ● VERAPAMIL—suspend or reduce dose of colchicine (avoid concomitant use in hepatic or renal impairment)
● Cardiac Glycosides: possible increased risk of myopathy when colchicine given with ● DIGOXIN
● Ciclosporin: possible increased risk of nephrotoxicity and myotoxicity when colchicine given with ● CICLOSPORIN—suspend or reduce dose of colchicine (avoid concomitant use in hepatic or renal impairment)
● Grapefruit Juice: possible increased risk of colchicine toxicity when given with ● GRAPEFRUIT JUICE
● Lipid-regulating Drugs: possible increased risk of myopathy when colchicine given with ● FIBRATES or ● STATINS
▸ Netupitant: caution with colchicine advised by manufacturer of NETUPITANT

Colecalciferol *see* Vitamins

Colesevelam

NOTE Other drugs should be taken at least 4 hours before or after colesevelam to reduce possible interference with absorption

▸ Antidiabetics: colesevelam reduces absorption of GLIBENCLAMIDE and GLIPIZIDE; colesevelam reduces absorption of GLIMEPIRIDE—manufacturer of glimepiride advises give at least 4 hours before colesevelam; manufacturer of canagliflozin advises give bile acid sequestrants at least 1 hour after or 4–6 before CANAGLIFLOZIN

Colesevelam (continued)

▸ Antiepileptics: colesevelam possibly reduces absorption of FOSPHENYTOIN and PHENYTOIN
▸ Bile Acids: colesevelam probably reduces effects of CHOLIC ACID (manufacturer of cholic acid advises give at least 5 hours apart)
● Ciclosporin: colesevelam reduces absorption of ● CICLOSPORIN
▸ Lipid-regulating Drugs: bile acid sequestrants possibly reduce absorption of LOMITAPIDE (give at least 4 hours apart)
▸ Oestrogens: colesevelam reduces absorption of ETHINYLESTRADIOL
▸ Thyroid Hormones: colesevelam reduces absorption of LEVOTHYROXINE

Colestipol

NOTE Other drugs should be taken at least 1 hour before or 4–6 hours after colestipol to reduce possible interference with absorption

▸ Antibacterials: colestipol possibly reduces absorption of TETRACYCLINE
▸ Antidiabetics: manufacturer of canagliflozin advises give bile acid sequestrants at least 1 hour after or 4–6 before CANAGLIFLOZIN
▸ Bile Acids: colestipol possibly reduces absorption of BILE ACIDS; colestipol probably reduces effects of CHOLIC ACID (manufacturer of cholic acid advises give at least 5 hours apart)
▸ Cardiac Glycosides: colestipol possibly reduces absorption of CARDIAC GLYCOSIDES
▸ Diuretics: colestipol reduces absorption of THIAZIDES AND RELATED DIURETICS (give at least 2 hours apart)
▸ Lipid-regulating Drugs: bile acid sequestrants possibly reduce absorption of LOMITAPIDE (give at least 4 hours apart)
▸ Thyroid Hormones: colestipol reduces absorption of THYROID HORMONES

Colestyramine

NOTE Other drugs should be taken at least 1 hour before or 4–6 hours after colestyramine to reduce possible interference with absorption

▸ Analgesics: colestyramine increases the excretion of MELOXICAM; colestyramine reduces absorption of PARACETAMOL
▸ Antibacterials: colestyramine possibly reduces absorption of TETRACYCLINE; colestyramine antagonises effects of *oral* VANCOMYCIN
● Anticoagulants: colestyramine may enhance or reduce anticoagulant effect of ● COUMARINS and ● PHENINDIONE
▸ Antidiabetics: colestyramine possibly enhances hypoglycaemic effect of ACARBOSE; manufacturer of canagliflozin advises give bile acid sequestrants at least 1 hour after or 4–6 before CANAGLIFLOZIN
▸ Antiepileptics: colestyramine possibly reduces absorption of SODIUM VALPROATE and VALPROIC ACID
▸ Bile Acids: colestyramine possibly reduces absorption of BILE ACIDS; colestyramine probably reduces effects of CHOLIC ACID (manufacturer of cholic acid advises give at least 5 hours apart)
▸ Cardiac Glycosides: colestyramine possibly reduces absorption of CARDIAC GLYCOSIDES
▸ Diuretics: colestyramine reduces absorption of THIAZIDES AND RELATED DIURETICS (give at least 2 hours apart)
▸ Leflunomide: colestyramine significantly decreases effect of LEFLUNOMIDE (enhanced elimination)—avoid unless drug elimination desired
▸ Lipid-regulating Drugs: bile acid sequestrants possibly reduce absorption of LOMITAPIDE (give at least 4 hours apart)
▸ Mycophenolate: colestyramine reduces absorption of MYCOPHENOLATE
▸ Raloxifene: colestyramine reduces absorption of RALOXIFENE (manufacturer of raloxifene advises avoid concomitant administration)
▸ Teriflunomide: colestyramine significantly decreases effect of TERIFLUNOMIDE (enhanced elimination)—avoid unless drug elimination desired
▸ Thyroid Hormones: colestyramine reduces absorption of THYROID HORMONES
▸ Vitamins: colestyramine possibly reduces absorption of CALCITRIOL (give at least 1 hour before or 4 to 6 hours after colestyramine)

A1

Interactions | Appendix 1

Colistimethate Sodium *see* Polymyxins

Contraceptives, oral *see* Oestrogens and Progestogens

Corticosteroids

NOTE Interactions do not generally apply to corticosteroids used for topical action (including inhalation) unless specified

▸ ACE Inhibitors: corticosteroids antagonise hypotensive effect of ACE INHIBITORS

▸ Adrenergic Neurone Blockers: corticosteroids antagonise hypotensive effect of ADRENERGIC NEURONE BLOCKERS

● Aldesleukin: avoidance of corticosteroids advised by manufacturer of ● ALDESLEUKIN

▸ Alpha-blockers: corticosteroids antagonise hypotensive effect of ALPHA-BLOCKERS

▸ Aminophylline: increased risk of hypokalaemia when corticosteroids given with AMINOPHYLLINE

▸ Analgesics: increased risk of gastro-intestinal bleeding and ulceration when corticosteroids given with NSAIDs; increased risk of gastro-intestinal bleeding and ulceration when corticosteroids given with ASPIRIN, also corticosteroids reduce plasma concentration of salicylate

▸ Angiotensin-II Receptor Antagonists: corticosteroids antagonise hypotensive effect of ANGIOTENSIN-II RECEPTOR ANTAGONISTS

▸ Antacids: absorption of deflazacort reduced by ANTACIDS

▸ Anthelmintics: dexamethasone increases plasma concentration of active metabolite of ALBENDAZOLE; continuous use of dexamethasone possibly reduces plasma concentration of PRAZIQUANTEL

● Antibacterials: plasma concentration of methylprednisolone possibly increased by CLARITHROMYCIN; metabolism of corticosteroids possibly inhibited by ERYTHROMYCIN; metabolism of methylprednisolone inhibited by ERYTHROMYCIN; corticosteroids possibly reduce plasma concentration of ISONIAZID; metabolism of corticosteroids accelerated by ● RIFAMYCINS (reduced effect)

● Anticoagulants: corticosteroids may enhance or reduce anticoagulant effect of ● COUMARINS (high-dose corticosteroids enhance anticoagulant effect); corticosteroids may enhance or reduce anticoagulant effect of PHENINDIONE

▸ Antidiabetics: corticosteroids antagonise hypoglycaemic effect of ANTIDIABETICS

● Antiepileptics: metabolism of corticosteroids accelerated by ● CARBAMAZEPINE, ● FOSPHENYTOIN, ● PHENOBARBITAL, ● PHENYTOIN and ● PRIMIDONE (reduced effect)

● Antifungals: metabolism of corticosteroids possibly inhibited by ITRACONAZOLE and KETOCONAZOLE; plasma concentration of active metabolite of ciclesonide increased by ● KETOCONAZOLE; plasma concentration of *inhaled* mometasone increased by KETOCONAZOLE; plasma concentration of *inhaled* and *oral* (and possibly also *intranasal* and *rectal*) budesonide increased by ● ITRACONAZOLE and ● KETOCONAZOLE; *inhaled* fluticasone plasma concentration is possibly increased by KETOCONAZOLE; metabolism of methylprednisolone inhibited by KETOCONAZOLE; increased risk of hypokalaemia when corticosteroids given with ● AMPHOTERICIN—avoid concomitant use unless corticosteroids needed to control reactions; plasma concentration of *inhaled* fluticasone increased by ITRACONAZOLE; metabolism of methylprednisolone possibly inhibited by ITRACONAZOLE; dexamethasone possibly reduces plasma concentration of CASPOFUNGIN—consider increasing dose of caspofungin

● Antivirals: dexamethasone possibly reduces plasma concentration of DACLATASVIR and SIMEPREVIR—manufacturer of daclatasvir and simeprevir advises avoid concomitant use; dexamethasone possibly reduces plasma concentration of INDINAVIR, LOPINAVIR, SAQUINAVIR and TELAPREVIR; avoidance of dexamethasone (except when given as a single dose) advised by manufacturer of ● RILPIVIRINE; plasma concentration of *inhaled* and *intranasal* fluticasone increased by ● RITONAVIR—increased risk of adrenal suppression; plasma concentration of budesonide (including *inhaled*, *intranasal*, and *rectal* budesonide) possibly increased by ● RITONAVIR—increased risk of adrenal suppresion; plasma concentration of corticosteroids possibly increased by ● RITONAVIR—increased risk of adrenal suppression; plasma concentration of triamcinolone *injection* increased by ● RITONAVIR—increased risk of adrenal suppression; plasma concentration of *inhaled*

Corticosteroids

● Antivirals (continued)

and *intranasal* budesonide and fluticasone possibly increased by TELAPREVIR

▸ Aprepitant: metabolism of dexamethasone and methylprednisolone inhibited by APREPITANT (reduce dose of dexamethasone and methylprednisolone)

▸ Beta-blockers: corticosteroids antagonise hypotensive effect of BETA-BLOCKERS

▸ Calcium Salts: corticosteroids reduce absorption of CALCIUM SALTS

▸ Calcium-channel Blockers: corticosteroids antagonise hypotensive effect of CALCIUM-CHANNEL BLOCKERS; plasma concentration of methylprednisolone increased by DILTIAZEM

▸ Cardiac Glycosides: increased risk of hypokalaemia when corticosteroids given with CARDIAC GLYCOSIDES

● Ciclosporin: high-dose methylprednisolone increases plasma concentration of ● CICLOSPORIN (risk of convulsions); plasma concentration of prednisolone increased by CICLOSPORIN

▸ Clonidine: corticosteroids antagonise hypotensive effect of CLONIDINE

▸ Cytotoxics: possible increased risk of hepatoxicity when dexamethasone given with *high-dose* METHOTREXATE; dexamethasone possibly decreases plasma concentration of AXITINIB (increase dose of axitinib—consult axitinib product literature); dexamethasone possibly reduces plasma concentration of CABOZANTINIB—manufacturer of cabozantinib advises avoid concomitant use

▸ Diazoxide: corticosteroids antagonise hypotensive effect of DIAZOXIDE

▸ Diuretics: corticosteroids antagonise diuretic effect of DIURETICS; increased risk of hypokalaemia when corticosteroids given with ACETAZOLAMIDE, LOOP DIURETICS or THIAZIDES AND RELATED DIURETICS

▸ Fosaprepitant: metabolism of dexamethasone and methylprednisolone inhibited by FOSAPREPITANT (reduce dose of dexamethasone and methylprednisolone)

● Grapefruit Juice: plasma concentration of *oral* budesonide increased by ● GRAPEFRUIT JUICE—avoid concurrent use or separate administration by as much as possible and consider reducing *oral* budesonide dose

▸ Histamine: avoidance of corticosteroids advised by manufacturer of HISTAMINE

▸ Methyldopa: corticosteroids antagonise hypotensive effect of METHYLDOPA

▸ Mifamurtide: avoidance of corticosteroids advised by manufacturer of MIFAMURTIDE

▸ Mifepristone: effect of corticosteroids (including *inhaled* corticosteroids) may be reduced for 3–4 days after MIFEPRISTONE

▸ Moxonidine: corticosteroids antagonise hypotensive effect of MOXONIDINE

▸ Muscle Relaxants: corticosteroids possibly antagonise effects of PANCURONIUM and VECURONIUM

▸ Netupitant: plasma concentration of dexamethasone increased by ● NETUPITANT (halve dose of dexamethasone)

▸ Nicorandil: increased risk of gastro-intestinal bleeding and ulceration when corticosteroids given with NICORANDIL

▸ Nitrates: corticosteroids antagonise hypotensive effect of NITRATES

▸ Oestrogens: plasma concentration of corticosteroids increased by oral contraceptives containing OESTROGENS

▸ Sodium Benzoate: corticosteroids possibly reduce effects of SODIUM BENZOATE

▸ Sodium Phenylbutyrate: corticosteroids possibly reduce effects of SODIUM PHENYLBUTYRATE

▸ Somatropin: corticosteroids may inhibit growth-promoting effect of SOMATROPIN

▸ Sympathomimetics: metabolism of dexamethasone accelerated by EPHEDRINE; possible risk of hypertension when corticosteroids given with MIDODRINE

▸ Sympathomimetics, Beta$_2$: increased risk of hypokalaemia when corticosteroids given with high doses of BETA$_2$ SYMPATHOMIMETICS

▸ Theophylline: increased risk of hypokalaemia when corticosteroids given with THEOPHYLLINE

Corticosteroids (continued)

- Vaccines: high doses of corticosteroids impair immune response to ● VACCINES—avoid concomitant use with live vaccines
▸ Vasodilator Antihypertensives: corticosteroids antagonise hypotensive effect of HYDRALAZINE, MINOXIDIL and SODIUM NITROPRUSSIDE

Co-trimoxazole see Trimethoprim and Sulfamethoxazole
Coumarins

NOTE Change in patient's clinical condition, particularly associated with liver disease, intercurrent illness, or drug administration, necessitates more frequent testing. Major changes in diet (especially involving salads and vegetables) and in alcohol consumption may also affect anticoagulant control

- Alcohol: anticoagulant control with coumarins may be affected by major changes in consumption of ● ALCOHOL
▸ Allopurinol: anticoagulant effect of coumarins possibly enhanced by ALLOPURINOL
- Anabolic Steroids: anticoagulant effect of coumarins enhanced by ● ANABOLIC STEROIDS
- Analgesics: anticoagulant effect of coumarins possibly enhanced by ● NSAIDS; increased risk of haemorrhage when anticoagulants given with *intravenous* ● DICLOFENAC (avoid concomitant use, including low-dose heparins); increased risk of haemorrhage when anticoagulants given with ● KETOROLAC (avoid concomitant use, including low-dose heparins); anticoagulant effect of coumarins enhanced by ● TRAMADOL; increased risk of bleeding when coumarins given with ● ASPIRIN (due to antiplatelet effect); anticoagulant effect of coumarins possibly enhanced by prolonged regular use of PARACETAMOL
- Anthelmintics: anticoagulant effect of coumarins possibly enhanced by IVERMECTIN; anticoagulant effect of warfarin possibly enhanced by ● LEVAMISOLE
- Anti-arrhythmics: metabolism of coumarins inhibited by ● AMIODARONE (enhanced anticoagulant effect); anticoagulant effect of warfarin may be enhanced or reduced by DISOPYRAMIDE; anticoagulant effect of coumarins possibly enhanced by ● DRONEDARONE; anticoagulant effect of coumarins enhanced by ● PROPAFENONE
- Antibacterials: experience in anticoagulant clinics suggests that INR possibly altered when coumarins are given with ● NEOMYCIN (given for local action on gut); anticoagulant effect of coumarins possibly enhanced by ● AZITHROMYCIN, ● AZTREONAM, ● CEPHALOSPORINS, CIPROFLOXACIN, LEVOFLOXACIN, ● TETRACYCLINES, TIGECYCLINE and TRIMETHOPRIM; anticoagulant effect of coumarins enhanced by ● CHLORAMPHENICOL, ● CLARITHROMYCIN, ● ERYTHROMYCIN, ● METRONIDAZOLE, ● NALIDIXIC ACID, ● NORFLOXACIN, ● OFLOXACIN and ● SULFONAMIDES; plasma concentration of warfarin possibly increased by ORITAVANCIN; an interaction between coumarins and broad-spectrum PENICILLINS has not been demonstrated in studies, but common experience in anticoagulant clinics is that INR can be altered; metabolism of coumarins accelerated by ● RIFAMYCINS (reduced anticoagulant effect); anticoagulant effect of warfarin possibly reduced by RIFAXIMIN
- Anticoagulants: increased risk of haemorrhage when other anticoagulants given with ● APIXABAN, ● DABIGATRAN, ● EDOXABAN and ● RIVAROXABAN (avoid concomitant use except when switching with other anticoagulants or using heparin to maintain catheter patency)
- Antidepressants: anticoagulant effect of warfarin possibly enhanced by ● VENLAFAXINE; anticoagulant effect of warfarin may be enhanced or reduced by TRAZODONE; anticoagulant effect of coumarins possibly enhanced by ● SSRIs; anticoagulant effect of coumarins reduced by ● ST JOHN'S WORT (avoid concomitant use); anticoagulant effect of warfarin enhanced by MIRTAZAPINE; anticoagulant effect of coumarins may be enhanced or reduced by ● TRICYCLICS
- Antidiabetics: anticoagulant effect of warfarin possibly enhanced by EXENATIDE; coumarins possibly enhance hypoglycaemic effect of ● SULFONYLUREAS, also possible changes to anticoagulant effect

Coumarins (continued)

- Antiepileptics: metabolism of coumarins accelerated by ● CARBAMAZEPINE, ● PHENOBARBITAL and ● PRIMIDONE (reduced anticoagulant effect); plasma concentration of warfarin reduced by ESLICARBAZEPINE; metabolism of coumarins accelerated by ● FOSPHENYTOIN and ● PHENYTOIN (possibility of reduced anticoagulant effect, but enhancement also reported); anticoagulant effect of coumarins possibly enhanced by SODIUM VALPROATE and VALPROIC ACID
- Antifungals: anticoagulant effect of coumarins enhanced by ● FLUCONAZOLE, ● ITRACONAZOLE, ● KETOCONAZOLE and ● VORICONAZOLE; anticoagulant effect of coumarins greatly enhanced by ● MICONAZOLE (including oral gel and possibly vaginal and topical formulations)—avoid concomitant use if possible; anticoagulant effect of coumarins reduced by ● GRISEOFULVIN
▸ Antimalarials: isolated reports that anticoagulant effect of warfarin may be enhanced by PROGUANIL; plasma concentration of both drugs increased when warfarin given with QUININE
- Antivirals: anticoagulant effect of warfarin may be enhanced or reduced by ATAZANAVIR, ● NEVIRAPINE and ● RITONAVIR; plasma concentration of coumarins possibly affected by ● EFAVIRENZ; anticoagulant effect of coumarins may be enhanced or reduced by FOSAMPRENAVIR; anticoagulant effect of coumarins possibly enhanced by ● RITONAVIR; anticoagulant effect of warfarin possibly enhanced by SAQUINAVIR; plasma concentration of warfarin possibly affected by ● TELAPREVIR
▸ Anxiolytics and Hypnotics: anticoagulant effect of coumarins may transiently be enhanced by CHLORAL
▸ Aprepitant: anticoagulant effect of warfarin possibly reduced by APREPITANT
- Azathioprine: anticoagulant effect of acenocoumarol possibly reduced by ● AZATHIOPRINE; anticoagulant effect of warfarin reduced by ● AZATHIOPRINE
▸ Bosentan: monitoring anticoagulant effect of coumarins recommended by manufacturer of BOSENTAN
▸ Carbimazole: anticoagulant effect of coumarins possibly enhanced by CARBIMAZOLE
- Clopidogrel: anticoagulant effect of coumarins enhanced due to antiplatelet action of ● CLOPIDOGREL; avoidance of warfarin advised by manufacturer of ● CLOPIDOGREL
- Corticosteroids: anticoagulant effect of coumarins may be enhanced or reduced by ● CORTICOSTEROIDS (high-dose corticosteroids enhance anticoagulant effect)
- Cranberry Juice: anticoagulant effect of coumarins possibly enhanced by ● CRANBERRY JUICE—avoid concomitant use
- Cytotoxics: anticoagulant effect of coumarins possibly enhanced by ● ETOPOSIDE, ● IFOSFAMIDE and ● SORAFENIB; anticoagulant effect of coumarins enhanced by ● CAPECITABINE, ● FLUOROURACIL and ● TEGAFUR; anticoagulant effect of warfarin possibly enhanced by ● GEFITINIB, GEMCITABINE and ● VEMURAFENIB; anticoagulant effect of coumarins possibly reduced by ● MERCAPTOPURINE and ● MITOTANE; plasma concentration of warfarin reduced by DABRAFENIB; increased risk of bleeding when coumarins given with ● ERLOTINIB; avoidance of coumarins advised by manufacturer of ● IBRUTINIB; replacement of warfarin with a heparin advised by manufacturer of IMATINIB (possibility of enhanced warfarin effect); increased risk of bleeding when warfarin given with ● REGORAFENIB
- Dipyridamole: anticoagulant effect of coumarins enhanced due to antiplatelet action of ● DIPYRIDAMOLE
- Disulfiram: anticoagulant effect of coumarins enhanced by ● DISULFIRAM
- Dopaminergics: anticoagulant effect of warfarin enhanced by ● ENTACAPONE
- Enteral Feeds: anticoagulant effect of coumarins antagonised by vitamin K (present in some ● ENTERAL FEEDS)
▸ Fosaprepitant: anticoagulant effect of warfarin possibly reduced by FOSAPREPITANT
- Glucosamine: anticoagulant effect of warfarin enhanced by ● GLUCOSAMINE (avoid concomitant use)
- Hormone Antagonists: anticoagulant effect of coumarins possibly enhanced by BICALUTAMIDE and ● TOREMIFENE; metabolism of coumarins inhibited by ● DANAZOL (enhanced

A1

Interactions | Appendix 1

Coumarins
- Hormone Antagonists (continued)
  anticoagulant effect); plasma concentration of coumarins possibly reduced by ● ENZALUTAMIDE; anticoagulant effect of coumarins enhanced by ● FLUTAMIDE and ● TAMOXIFEN
▹ Iloprost: anticoagulant effect of coumarins possibly enhanced by ILOPROST
▹ Lactulose: anticoagulant effect of coumarins possibly enhanced by LACTULOSE
▹ Leflunomide: anticoagulant effect of warfarin possibly enhanced by LEFLUNOMIDE
▹ Leukotriene Receptor Antagonists: anticoagulant effect of warfarin enhanced by ZAFIRLUKAST
▹ Levocarnitine: anticoagulant effect of coumarins possibly enhanced by LEVOCARNITINE
● Lipid-regulating Drugs: anticoagulant effect of coumarins may be enhanced or reduced by ● COLESTYRAMINE; anticoagulant effect of warfarin may be transiently reduced by ATORVASTATIN; anticoagulant effect of coumarins enhanced by ● FIBRATES and ● FLUVASTATIN; anticoagulant effect of coumarins possibly enhanced by EZETIMIBE and ● ROSUVASTATIN; anticoagulant effect of coumarins can be enhanced by SIMVASTATIN; anticoagulant effect of warfarin possibly enhanced by LOMITAPIDE
▹ Memantine: anticoagulant effect of warfarin possibly enhanced by MEMANTINE
▹ Oestrogens: anticoagulant effect of coumarins may be enhanced or reduced by OESTROGENS
▹ Orlistat: monitoring anticoagulant effect of coumarins recommended by manufacturer of ORLISTAT
▹ Prasugrel: possible increased risk of bleeding when coumarins given with PRASUGREL
▹ Progestogens: anticoagulant effect of coumarins may be enhanced or reduced by PROGESTOGENS
▹ Raloxifene: anticoagulant effect of coumarins antagonised by RALOXIFENE
▹ Retinoids: anticoagulant effect of coumarins possibly reduced by ● ACITRETIN
● Sulfinpyrazone: anticoagulant effect of coumarins enhanced by ● SULFINPYRAZONE
● Sympathomimetics: anticoagulant effect of coumarins possibly enhanced by METHYLPHENIDATE
● Testolactone: anticoagulant effect of coumarins enhanced by ● TESTOLACTONE
● Testosterone: anticoagulant effect of coumarins enhanced by ● TESTOSTERONE
● Thyroid Hormones: anticoagulant effect of coumarins enhanced by ● THYROID HORMONES
▹ Ubidecarenone: anticoagulant effect of warfarin may be enhanced or reduced by UBIDECARENONE
● Ulcer-healing Drugs: metabolism of coumarins inhibited by ● CIMETIDINE (enhanced anticoagulant effect); anticoagulant effect of coumarins possibly enhanced by ● ESOMEPRAZOLE and ● OMEPRAZOLE; anticoagulant effect of coumarins might be enhanced by PANTOPRAZOLE; absorption of coumarins possibly reduced by ● SUCRALFATE (reduced anticoagulant effect)
▹ Vaccines: anticoagulant effect of warfarin possibly enhanced by INFLUENZA VACCINE
● Vitamins: anticoagulant effect of coumarins possibly enhanced by ● VITAMIN E; anticoagulant effect of coumarins antagonised by ● VITAMIN K

Cranberry Juice
● Anticoagulants: cranberry juice possibly enhances anticoagulant effect of ● COUMARINS—avoid concomitant use

Crizotinib
● Analgesics: manufacturer of crizotinib advises caution with ● ALFENTANIL and ● FENTANYL
● Antibacterials: plasma concentration of crizotinib possibly increased by ● CLARITHROMYCIN and ● TELITHROMYCIN—manufacturer of crizotinib advises avoid concomitant use; plasma concentration of crizotinib possibly reduced by RIFABUTIN—manufacturer of crizotinib advises avoid concomitant use; plasma concentration of crizotinib reduced by ● RIFAMPICIN—manufacturer of crizotinib advises avoid concomitant use

Crizotinib (continued)
▹ Antidepressants: plasma concentration of crizotinib possibly reduced by ST JOHN'S WORT—manufacturer of crizotinib advises avoid concomitant use
▹ Antiepileptics: plasma concentration of crizotinib possibly reduced by CARBAMAZEPINE, FOSPHENYTOIN, PHENOBARBITAL, PHENYTOIN and PRIMIDONE—manufacturer of crizotinib advises avoid concomitant use
● Antifungals: plasma concentration of crizotinib increased by ● KETOCONAZOLE—avoid concomitant use; plasma concentration of crizotinib possibly increased by ● ITRACONAZOLE and ● VORICONAZOLE—manufacturer of crizotinib advises avoid concomitant use
● Antimalarials: possible increased risk of bradycardia when crizotinib given with MEFLOQUINE
● Antipsychotics: avoid concomitant use of cytotoxics with ● CLOZAPINE (increased risk of agranulocytosis); manufacturer of crizotinib advises caution with ● PIMOZIDE
● Antivirals: plasma concentration of crizotinib possibly increased by ● ATAZANAVIR, ● INDINAVIR, ● RITONAVIR and ● SAQUINAVIR—manufacturer of crizotinib advises avoid concomitant use
● Anxiolytics and Hypnotics: crizotinib increases plasma concentration of ● MIDAZOLAM
▹ Beta-blockers: possible increased risk of bradycardia when crizotinib given with BETA-BLOCKERS
▹ Calcium-channel Blockers: possible increased risk of bradycardia when crizotinib given with DILTIAZEM or VERAPAMIL
▹ Cardiac Glycosides: possible increased risk of bradycardia when crizotinib given with DIGOXIN
● Ciclosporin: manufacturer of crizotinib advises caution with ● CICLOSPORIN
▹ Clonidine: possible increased risk of bradycardia when crizotinib given with CLONIDINE
● Cytotoxics: crizotinib possibly increases the plasma concentration of ● IBRUTINIB—reduce dose of ibrutinib (see under Ibrutinib, p. 855)
● Ergot Alkaloids: manufacturer of crizotinib advises caution with ● ERGOT ALKALOIDS
▹ Grapefruit Juice: plasma concentration of crizotinib possibly increased by GRAPEFRUIT JUICE—manufacturer of crizotinib advises avoid concomitant use
▹ Guanfacine: crizotinib possibly increases plasma concentration of GUANFACINE (halve dose of guanfacine)
▹ Oestrogens: manufacturer of crizotinib advises contraceptive effect of ● OESTROGENS possibly reduced
▹ Parasympathomimetics: possible increased risk of bradycardia when crizotinib given with PILOCARPINE
▹ Progestogens: manufacturer of crizotinib advises contraceptive effect of ● PROGESTOGENS possibly reduced
● Sirolimus: manufacturer of crizotinib advises caution with ● SIROLIMUS
● Tacrolimus: manufacturer of crizotinib advises caution with ● TACROLIMUS

Cyclizine see Antihistamines
Cyclopenthiazide see Diuretics
Cyclopentolate see Antimuscarinics

Cyclophosphamide
▹ Antifungals: side-effects of cyclophosphamide possibly increased by FLUCONAZOLE and ITRACONAZOLE
● Antipsychotics: avoid concomitant use of cytotoxics with ● CLOZAPINE (increased risk of agranulocytosis)
▹ Cardiac Glycosides: cyclophosphamide possibly reduces absorption of DIGOXIN *tablets*
● Cytotoxics: increased toxicity when high-dose cyclophosphamide given with ● PENTOSTATIN—avoid concomitant use
▹ Muscle Relaxants: cyclophosphamide enhances effects of SUXAMETHONIUM

Cycloserine
● Alcohol: increased risk of convulsions when cycloserine given with ● ALCOHOL
▹ Antibacterials: increased risk of CNS toxicity when cycloserine given with ISONIAZID
▹ Vaccines: antibacterials inactivate ORAL TYPHOID VACCINE—see under Typhoid Vaccine in BNF

Cyproheptadine *see* Antihistamines

Cytarabine

▸ Antifungals: cytarabine possibly reduces plasma concentration of FLUCYTOSINE

● Antipsychotics: avoid concomitant use of cytotoxics with ● CLOZAPINE (increased risk of agranulocytosis)

▸ Cardiac Glycosides: cytarabine possibly reduces absorption of DIGOXIN *tablets*

▸ Cytotoxics: intracellular concentration of cytarabine increased by FLUDARABINE

Cytotoxics *see* individual drugs

Dabigatran

● Analgesics: possible increased risk of bleeding when dabigatran given with ● NSAIDS; increased risk of haemorrhage when anticoagulants given with *intravenous* ● DICLOFENAC (avoid concomitant use, including low-dose heparins); increased risk of haemorrhage when anticoagulants given with ● KETOROLAC (avoid concomitant use, including low-dose heparins)

● Anti-arrhythmics: plasma concentration of dabigatran increased by ● AMIODARONE (see under Dabigatran Etexilate, p. 123); plasma concentration of dabigatran increased by ● DRONEDARONE—avoid concomitant use

● Antibacterials: possible increased risk of bleeding when dabigatran given with CLARITHROMYCIN; plasma concentration of dabigatran reduced by ● RIFAMPICIN—manufacturer of dabigatran advises avoid concomitant use

● Anticoagulants: increased risk of haemorrhage when dabigatran given with other ● ANTICOAGULANTS (avoid concomitant use except when switching with other anticoagulants or using heparin to maintain catheter patency); increased risk of haemorrhage when other anticoagulants given with ● APIXABAN, ● EDOXABAN and ● RIVAROXABAN (avoid concomitant use except when switching with other anticoagulants or using heparin to maintain catheter patency)

● Antidepressants: possible increased risk of bleeding when dabigatran given with ● SSRI-RELATED ANTIDEPRESSANTS or ● SSRIS; plasma concentration of dabigatran possibly reduced by ST JOHN'S WORT—manufacturer of dabigatran advises avoid concomitant use

▸ Antiepileptics: plasma concentration of dabigatran possibly reduced by CARBAMAZEPINE, FOSPHENYTOIN and PHENYTOIN—manufacturer of dabigatran advises avoid concomitant use

● Antifungals: plasma concentration of dabigatran increased by ● KETOCONAZOLE—avoid concomitant use; manufacturer of dabigatran advises avoid concomitant use with ITRACONAZOLE

▸ Antivirals: manufacturers advise avoid concomitant use of dabigatran with DARUNAVIR; plasma concentration of dabigatran possibly increased by RILPIVIRINE and TELAPREVIR

● Calcium-channel Blockers: plasma concentration of dabigatran possibly increased by ● VERAPAMIL (see under Dabigatran Etexilate, p. 123)

● Ciclosporin: plasma concentration of dabigatran increased by ● CICLOSPORIN—manufacturer of dabigatran advises avoid concomitant use

▸ Netupitant: caution with dabigatran advised by manufacturer of NETUPITANT

● Sulfinpyrazone: possible increased risk of bleeding when dabigatran given with ● SULFINPYRAZONE

● Tacrolimus: plasma concentration of dabigatran possibly increased by ● TACROLIMUS—manufacturer of dabigatran advises avoid concomitant use

● Ticagrelor: plasma concentration of dabigatran increased by ● TICAGRELOR

▸ Ulipristal: manufacturer of ulipristal advises give dabigatran at least 1.5 hours before or after ULIPRISTAL

Dabrafenib

▸ Antibacterials: manufacturer of dabrafenib advises avoid concomitant use with RIFAMPICIN

▸ Anticoagulants: dabrafenib reduces plasma concentration of WARFARIN

▸ Antidepressants: manufacturer of dabrafenib advises avoid concomitant use with ST JOHN'S WORT

▸ Antiepileptics: manufacturer of dabrafenib advises avoid concomitant use with CARBAMAZEPINE, FOSPHENYTOIN, PHENOBARBITAL, PHENYTOIN and PRIMIDONE

Dabrafenib (continued)

▸ Antifungals: plasma concentration of dabrafenib increased by KETOCONAZOLE

● Antipsychotics: avoid concomitant use of cytotoxics with ● CLOZAPINE (increased risk of agranulocytosis)

▸ Lipid-regulating Drugs: plasma concentration of dabrafenib increased by GEMFIBROZIL

● Oestrogens: manufacturer of dabrafenib advises contraceptive effect of hormonal contraceptives containing ● OESTROGENS possibly reduced (alternative contraceptive recommended)

● Progestogens: manufacturer of dabrafenib advises contraceptive effect of hormonal contraceptives containing ● PROGESTOGENS possibly reduced (alternative contraceptive recommended)

▸ Ulcer-healing Drugs: manufacturer of dabrafenib advises avoid concomitant use with PROTON PUMP INHIBITORS (plasma concentration of dabrafenib possibly reduced)

Dacarbazine

● Aldesleukin: avoidance of dacarbazine advised by manufacturer of ● ALDESLEUKIN

● Antipsychotics: avoid concomitant use of cytotoxics with ● CLOZAPINE (increased risk of agranulocytosis)

Daclatasvir

● Anti-arrhythmics: possible increased risk of bradycardia when daclatasvir (with sofosbuvir) given with ● AMIODARONE—see under Amiodarone, p. 94

● Antibacterials: plasma concentration of daclatasvir possibly increased by ● CLARITHROMYCIN and ● TELITHROMYCIN—reduce dose of daclatasvir (see under Daclatasvir, p. 568); plasma concentration of daclatasvir possibly reduced by ● RIFABUTIN—manufacturer of daclatasvir advises avoid concomitant use; plasma concentration of daclatasvir reduced by ● RIFAMPICIN—avoid concomitant use

▸ Antidepressants: plasma concentration of daclatasvir possibly reduced by ST JOHN'S WORT—manufacturer of daclatasvir advises avoid concomitant use

● Antiepileptics: plasma concentration of daclatasvir possibly reduced by ● CARBAMAZEPINE, ● FOSPHENYTOIN, ● OXCARBAZEPINE, ● PHENOBARBITAL, ● PHENYTOIN and ● PRIMIDONE—manufacturer of daclatasvir advises avoid concomitant use

● Antifungals: plasma concentration of daclatasvir increased by ● KETOCONAZOLE—reduce dose of daclatasvir (see under Daclatasvir, p. 568); plasma concentration of daclatasvir possibly increased by ● ITRACONAZOLE, ● POSACONAZOLE and ● VORICONAZOLE—reduce dose of daclatasvir (see under Daclatasvir, p. 568)

● Antivirals: plasma concentration of daclatasvir increased by ● ATAZANAVIR and ● TELAPREVIR—reduce dose of daclatasvir (see under Daclatasvir, p. 568); plasma concentration of daclatasvir possibly increased by ● BOCEPREVIR—reduce dose of daclatasvir (see under Daclatasvir, p. 568); manufacturer of daclatasvir advises avoid concomitant use with DARUNAVIR (plasma concentration of daclatasvir possibly increased); plasma concentration of daclatasvir reduced by ● EFAVIRENZ—increase dose of daclatasvir (see under Daclatasvir, p. 568); manufacturer of daclatasvir advises avoid concomitant use with ETRAVIRINE and NEVIRAPINE (plasma concentration of daclatasvir possibly reduced)

● Cardiac Glycosides: daclatasvir increases plasma concentration of ● DIGOXIN

● Cobicistat: plasma concentration of daclatasvir possibly increased by ● COBICISTAT—reduce dose of daclatasvir (see under Daclatasvir, p. 568)

▸ Corticosteroids: plasma concentration of daclatasvir possibly reduced by DEXAMETHASONE—manufacturer of daclatasvir advises avoid concomitant use

▸ Lipid-regulating Drugs: daclatasvir increases plasma concentration of ROSUVASTATIN

Dactinomycin

● Antipsychotics: avoid concomitant use of cytotoxics with ● CLOZAPINE (increased risk of agranulocytosis)

● Cytotoxics: increased risk of hepatotoxicity when dactinomycin given with ● VINCRISTINE

● Vaccines: risk of generalised infections when cytotoxic antibiotics given with live ● VACCINES—avoid concomitant use

Dactinomycin (continued)

▸ **Vitamins:** dactinomycin possibly reduces effects of ALFACALCIDOL, CALCITRIOL, COLECALCIFEROL, DIHYDROTACHYSTEROL, ERGOCALCIFEROL, PARICALCITOL and VITAMIN D

Dairy Products

▸ **Antibacterials:** dairy products reduce absorption of CIPROFLOXACIN (give at least 2 hours apart); dairy products reduce absorption of NORFLOXACIN; dairy products reduce absorption of TETRACYCLINES (except doxycycline and minocycline)

▸ **Cytotoxics:** dairy products possibly reduce plasma concentration of MERCAPTOPURINE—manufacturer of mercaptopurine advises give at least 1 hour before or 3 hours after dairy products

▸ **Eltrombopag:** dairy products possibly reduce absorption of ELTROMBOPAG (give at least 4 hours apart)

Dalteparin *see* Heparins

Danaparoid

● **Analgesics:** increased risk of haemorrhage when anticoagulants given with *intravenous* ● DICLOFENAC (avoid concomitant use, including low-dose heparins); increased risk of haemorrhage when anticoagulants given with ● KETOROLAC (avoid concomitant use, including low-dose heparins)

● **Anticoagulants:** increased risk of haemorrhage when other anticoagulants given with ● APIXABAN, ● DABIGATRAN, ● EDOXABAN and ● RIVAROXABAN (avoid concomitant use except when switching with other anticoagulants or using heparin to maintain catheter patency)

Danazol

● **Anticoagulants:** danazol inhibits metabolism of ● COUMARINS (enhanced anticoagulant effect)

● **Antiepileptics:** danazol inhibits metabolism of ● CARBAMAZEPINE (increased risk of toxicity)

● **Ciclosporin:** danazol inhibits metabolism of ● CICLOSPORIN (increased plasma concentration)

● **Lipid-regulating Drugs:** possible increased risk of myopathy when danazol given with ● SIMVASTATIN—avoid concomitant use

▸ **Tacrolimus:** danazol possibly increases plasma concentration of TACROLIMUS

Dantrolene *see* Muscle Relaxants

Dapagliflozin *see* Antidiabetics

Dapoxetine

● **Alcohol:** increased sedative effect when dapoxetine given with ● ALCOHOL

● **Analgesics:** possible increased risk of serotonergic effects when dapoxetine given with ● TRAMADOL (manufacturer of dapoxetine advises tramadol should not be started until 1 week after stopping dapoxetine, avoid dapoxetine for 2 weeks after stopping tramadol)

● **Antibacterials:** manufacturer of dapoxetine advises dose reduction when dapoxetine given with CLARITHROMYCIN and ERYTHROMYCIN (see under Dapoxetine, p. 742); manufacturer of dapoxetine advises avoid concomitant use with ● TELITHROMYCIN (increased risk of toxicity)

● **Antidepressants:** possible increased risk of serotonergic effects when dapoxetine given with ● SSRIs, ● ST JOHN'S WORT, ● DULOXETINE, ● TRICYCLICS and ● VENLAFAXINE (manufacturer of dapoxetine advises SSRIs, St John's wort, duloxetine, tricyclics and venlafaxine should not be started until 1 week after stopping dapoxetine, avoid dapoxetine for 2 weeks after stopping SSRIs, St John's wort, duloxetine, tricyclics and venlafaxine); increased risk of serotonergic effects when dapoxetine given with ● MAOIS (MAOIs should not be started until 1 week after stopping dapoxetine, avoid dapoxetine for 2 weeks after stopping MAOIs)

● **Antifungals:** plasma concentration of dapoxetine increased by ● KETOCONAZOLE—manufacturer of dapoxetine advises avoid concomitant use; manufacturer of dapoxetine advises dose reduction when dapoxetine given with FLUCONAZOLE (see under Dapoxetine, p. 742); manufacturer of dapoxetine advises avoid concomitant use with ● ITRACONAZOLE (increased risk of toxicity)

● **Antivirals:** manufacturer of dapoxetine advises avoid concomitant use with ● ATAZANAVIR, ● RITONAVIR and

Dapoxetine

● **Antivirals** (continued)

● SAQUINAVIR (increased risk of toxicity); manufacturer of dapoxetine advises dose reduction when dapoxetine given with FOSAMPRENAVIR (see under Dapoxetine, p. 742)

▸ **Aprepitant:** manufacturer of dapoxetine advises dose reduction when dapoxetine given with APREPITANT (see under Dapoxetine, p. 742)

▸ **Calcium-channel Blockers:** manufacturer of dapoxetine advises dose reduction when dapoxetine given with DILTIAZEM and VERAPAMIL (see under Dapoxetine, p. 742)

● **5HT₁-receptor Agonists:** possible increased risk of serotonergic effects when dapoxetine given with ● 5HT₁ AGONISTS (manufacturer of dapoxetine advises 5HT₁ agonists should not be started until 1 week after stopping dapoxetine, avoid dapoxetine for 2 weeks after stopping 5HT₁ agonists)

● **Lithium:** possible increased risk of serotonergic effects when dapoxetine given with ● LITHIUM (manufacturer of dapoxetine advises lithium should not be started until 1 week after stopping dapoxetine, avoid dapoxetine for 2 weeks after stopping lithium)

▸ **Sildenafil:** manufacturer of dapoxetine advises avoid concomitant use with SILDENAFIL

▸ **Tadalafil:** manufacturer of dapoxetine advises avoid concomitant use with TADALAFIL

▸ **Vardenafil:** manufacturer of dapoxetine advises avoid concomitant use with VARDENAFIL

Dapsone

▸ **Antibacterials:** plasma concentration of dapsone reduced by RIFAMYCINS; plasma concentration of both drugs may increase when dapsone given with TRIMETHOPRIM

▸ **Antivirals:** increased risk of ventricular arrhythmias when dapsone given with SAQUINAVIR—avoid concomitant use

▸ **Vaccines:** antibacterials inactivate ORAL TYPHOID VACCINE—see under Typhoid Vaccine in BNF

Daptomycin

● **Ciclosporin:** increased risk of myopathy when daptomycin given with ● CICLOSPORIN (preferably avoid concomitant use)

● **Lipid-regulating Drugs:** increased risk of myopathy when daptomycin given with ● FIBRATES or ● STATINS (preferably avoid concomitant use)

▸ **Vaccines:** antibacterials inactivate ORAL TYPHOID VACCINE—see under Typhoid Vaccine in BNF

Darifenacin *see* Antimuscarinics

Darunavir

▸ **Anti-arrhythmics:** darunavir possibly increases plasma concentration of LIDOCAINE—avoid concomitant use

● **Antibacterials:** darunavir increases plasma concentration of ● RIFABUTIN (reduce dose of rifabutin); plasma concentration of darunavir significantly reduced by ● RIFAMPICIN—avoid concomitant use

▸ **Anticoagulants:** avoidance of darunavir advised by manufacturer of APIXABAN and RIVAROXABAN; manufacturers advise avoid concomitant use of darunavir with DABIGATRAN

● **Antidepressants:** darunavir possibly increases plasma concentration of PAROXETINE and SERTRALINE; plasma concentration of darunavir reduced by ● ST JOHN'S WORT—avoid concomitant use

● **Antiepileptics:** plasma concentration of darunavir possibly reduced by CARBAMAZEPINE, FOSPHENYTOIN, PHENOBARBITAL, PHENYTOIN and PRIMIDONE

● **Antifungals:** plasma concentration of both drugs increased when darunavir given with KETOCONAZOLE; darunavir possibly affects plasma concentration of VORICONAZOLE

● **Antimalarials:** plasma concentration of lumefantrine increased when darunavir given with ARTEMETHER WITH LUMEFANTRINE; darunavir possibly increases plasma concentration of ● QUININE (increased risk of toxicity)

● **Antipsychotics:** darunavir possibly increases plasma concentration of ● ARIPIPRAZOLE (reduce dose of aripiprazole—consult aripiprazole product literature); darunavir possibly increases plasma concentration of ● QUETIAPINE—manufacturer of quetiapine advises avoid concomitant use

● **Antivirals:** avoid concomitant use of darunavir with ● BOCEPREVIR or ● TELAPREVIR; avoidance of darunavir advised

Darunavir

- Antivirals (continued)

    by manufacturer of DACLATASVIR (plasma concentration of daclatasvir possibly increased); manufacturer of darunavir advises take DIDANOSINE 1 hour before or 2 hours after darunavir; plasma concentration of darunavir reduced by • EFAVIRENZ (adjust dose—consult product literature); plasma concentration of both drugs increased when darunavir given with INDINAVIR; plasma concentration of darunavir reduced by • LOPINAVIR and SAQUINAVIR—avoid concomitant use; darunavir increases plasma concentration of • MARAVIROC (consider reducing dose of maraviroc); darunavir increases plasma concentration of • PARITAPREVIR and plasma concentration of darunavir decreased; increased risk of rash when darunavir given with RALTEGRAVIR; plasma concentration of both drugs increased when darunavir given with • SIMEPREVIR—manufacturer of simeprevir advises avoid concomitant use

- Cytotoxics: darunavir possibly increases the plasma concentration of • BOSUTINIB—manufacturer of bosutinib advises avoid or consider reducing dose of bosutinib; darunavir possibly increases plasma concentration of • EVEROLIMUS—manufacturer of everolimus advises avoid concomitant use; darunavir possibly increases the plasma concentration of • IBRUTINIB—reduce dose of ibrutinib (see under Ibrutinib, p. 855)

- Ergot Alkaloids: increased risk of ergotism when darunavir given with • ERGOT ALKALOIDS—manufacturer of darunavir advises avoid concomitant use

- Lipid-regulating Drugs: possible increased risk of myopathy when darunavir given with ATORVASTATIN; darunavir possibly increases plasma concentration of PRAVASTATIN (use lowest possible dose of pravastatin); darunavir increases plasma concentration of • ROSUVASTATIN—adjust dose of rosuvastatin (consult product literature); avoidance of darunavir advised by manufacturer of • LOMITAPIDE (plasma concentration of lomitapide possibly increased)

- Orlistat: absorption of darunavir possibly reduced by • ORLISTAT

- Ranolazine: darunavir possibly increases plasma concentration of • RANOLAZINE—manufacturer of ranolazine advises avoid concomitant use

Dasabuvir

- Antibacterials: manufacturer of dasabuvir advises avoid concomitant use with CLARITHROMYCIN and TELITHROMYCIN; plasma concentration of dasabuvir possibly reduced by • RIFAMPICIN—avoid concomitant use

- Antidepressants: plasma concentration of dasabuvir possibly reduced by • ST JOHN'S WORT—manufacturer of dasabuvir advises avoid concomitant use

- Antiepileptics: plasma concentration of dasabuvir reduced by • CARBAMAZEPINE—avoid concomitant use; plasma concentration of dasabuvir possibly reduced by • FOSPHENYTOIN, • PHENOBARBITAL, • PHENYTOIN and • PRIMIDONE—avoid concomitant use

- Antifungals: plasma concentration of both drugs increased when dasabuvir given with • KETOCONAZOLE—avoid concomitant use; plasma concentration of both drugs possibly increased when dasabuvir given with • ITRACONAZOLE and • POSACONAZOLE—avoid concomitant use

▸ Antivirals: manufacturer of dasabuvir advises avoid concomitant use with EFAVIRENZ, ETRAVIRINE and NEVIRAPINE

▸ Cobicistat: manufacturer of dasabuvir advises avoid concomitant use with COBICISTAT

▸ Cytotoxics: manufacturer of dasabuvir advises avoid concomitant use with MITOTANE

- Diuretics: dasabuvir increases plasma concentration of • FUROSEMIDE (reduce dose of furosemide)

▸ Hormone Antagonists: manufacturer of dasabuvir advises avoid concomitant use with ENZALUTAMIDE

- Lipid-regulating Drugs: manufacturer of dasabuvir advises avoid concomitant use with • ATORVASTATIN, GEMFIBROZIL and • SIMVASTATIN; dasabuvir increases plasma concentration of • ROSUVASTATIN (reduce dose of rosuvastatin—see under Rosuvastatin, p. 188)

Dasabuvir (continued)

- Oestrogens: manufacturer of dasabuvir advises avoid concomitant use of • ETHINYLESTRADIOL—use alternative form of contraception

Dasatinib

- Antibacterials: manufacturer of dasatinib advises avoid concomitant use with CLARITHROMYCIN, ERYTHROMYCIN and TELITHROMYCIN (plasma concentration of dasatinib possibly increased); metabolism of dasatinib accelerated by • RIFAMPICIN (reduced plasma concentration—avoid concomitant use)

▸ Antiepileptics: manufacturer of dasatinib advises avoid concomitant use with CARBAMAZEPINE, FOSPHENYTOIN, PHENOBARBITAL, PHENYTOIN and PRIMIDONE (plasma concentration of dasatinib possibly reduced)

▸ Antifungals: plasma concentration of dasatinib possibly increased by KETOCONAZOLE; manufacturer of dasatinib advises avoid concomitant use with ITRACONAZOLE (plasma concentration of dasatinib possibly increased)

- Antipsychotics: avoid concomitant use of cytotoxics with • CLOZAPINE (increased risk of agranulocytosis)

- Antivirals: avoidance of dasatinib advised by manufacturer of • BOCEPREVIR; manufacturer of dasatinib advises avoid concomitant use with RITONAVIR (plasma concentration of dasatinib possibly increased)

▸ Grapefruit Juice: manufacturer of dasatinib advises avoid concomitant use with GRAPEFRUIT JUICE (plasma concentration of dasatinib possibly increased)

▸ Lipid-regulating Drugs: dasatinib possibly increases plasma concentration of SIMVASTATIN

▸ Ulcer-healing Drugs: plasma concentration of dasatinib possibly reduced by FAMOTIDINE

Daunorubicin

- Antipsychotics: avoid concomitant use of cytotoxics with • CLOZAPINE (increased risk of agranulocytosis)

- Cytotoxics: possible increased risk of cardiotoxicity when daunorubicin given with • TRASTUZUMAB—avoid concomitant use for up to 28 weeks after stopping trastuzumab

- Vaccines: risk of generalised infections when cytotoxic antibiotics given with live • VACCINES—avoid concomitant use

Decitabine

- Antipsychotics: avoid concomitant use of cytotoxics with • CLOZAPINE (increased risk of agranulocytosis)

Deferasirox

- Aminophylline: deferasirox increases plasma concentration of • AMINOPHYLLINE (consider reducing dose of aminophylline)

▸ Antacids: absorption of deferasirox possibly reduced by ANTACIDS containing aluminium (manufacturer of deferasirox advises avoid concomitant use)

▸ Antibacterials: plasma concentration of deferasirox reduced by RIFAMPICIN

▸ Antidiabetics: deferasirox increases plasma concentration of REPAGLINIDE

▸ Antipsychotics: manufacturer of deferasirox advises avoid concomitant use with CLOZAPINE

▸ Anxiolytics and Hypnotics: deferasirox possibly reduces plasma concentration of MIDAZOLAM

▸ Muscle Relaxants: manufacturer of deferasirox advises avoid concomitant use with TIZANIDINE

- Theophylline: deferasirox increases plasma concentration of • THEOPHYLLINE (consider reducing dose of theophylline)

Deferiprone

▸ Antacids: absorption of deferiprone possibly reduced by ANTACIDS containing aluminium (manufacturer of deferiprone advises avoid concomitant use)

Deflazacort see Corticosteroids

Delamanid

- Analgesics: increased risk of ventricular arrhythmias when delamanid given with • METHADONE

- Anti-arrhythmics: increased risk of ventricular arrhythmias when delamanid given with • AMIODARONE or • DISOPYRAMIDE

- Antibacterials: possible increased risk of ventricular arrhythmias when delamanid given with • CLARITHROMYCIN and • ERYTHROMYCIN; increased risk of ventricular arrhythmias when delamanid given with • MOXIFLOXACIN; plasma

Delamanid
- Antibacterials (continued)
  concentration of delamanid reduced by • RIFAMPICIN;
  delamanid increases plasma concentration of ETHAMBUTOL
- Antidepressants: possible increased risk of ventricular
  arrhythmias when delamanid given with • TRICYCLICS that
  prolong the QT interval
▸ Antiepileptics: manufacturer of delamanid advises avoid
  concomitant use with CARBAMAZEPINE
- Antipsychotics: increased risk of ventricular arrhythmias when
  delamanid given with • DROPERIDOL, • HALOPERIDOL or
  • PIMOZIDE; increased risk of ventricular arrhythmias when
  delamanid given with • PHENOTHIAZINES that prolong the QT
  interval
- Antivirals: plasma concentration of delamanid increased by
  LOPINAVIR and RITONAVIR; increased risk of ventricular
  arrhythmias when delamanid given with • SAQUINAVIR
- Beta-blockers: increased risk of ventricular arrhythmias when
  delamanid given with • SOTALOL
- Cytotoxics: increased risk of ventricular arrhythmias when
  delamanid given with • ARSENIC TRIOXIDE or • VINFLUNINE;
  possible increased risk of ventricular arrhythmias when
  delamanid given with • VINBLASTINE, • VINCRISTINE, • VINDESINE
  and • VINORELBINE
- Domperidone: possible increased risk of ventricular
  arrhythmias when delamanid given with • DOMPERIDONE
- Pentamidine Isetionate: increased risk of ventricular
  arrhythmias when delamanid given with • PENTAMIDINE
  ISETIONATE
▸ Vaccines: antibacterials inactivate ORAL TYPHOID VACCINE—see
  under Typhoid Vaccine in BNF

Demeclocycline see Tetracyclines

Desferrioxamine
▸ Antipsychotics: avoidance of desferrioxamine advised by
  manufacturer of LEVOMEPROMAZINE; manufacturer of
  desferrioxamine advises avoid concomitant use with
  PROCHLORPERAZINE

Desflurane see Anaesthetics, General

Desloratadine see Antihistamines

Desmopressin
▸ Analgesics: effects of desmopressin enhanced by INDOMETACIN
▸ Loperamide: plasma concentration of *oral* desmopressin
  increased by LOPERAMIDE

Desogestrel see Progestogens

Dexamethasone see Corticosteroids

Dexamfetamine see Sympathomimetics

Dexibuprofen see NSAIDs

Dexketoprofen see NSAIDs

Dexrazoxane
- Antiepileptics: dexrazoxane possibly reduces absorption of
  • FOSPHENYTOIN and • PHENYTOIN
▸ Ciclosporin: manufacturer of dexrazoxane advises increased
  risk of immunosuppression with CICLOSPORIN
▸ Tacrolimus: manufacturer of dexrazoxane advises increased
  risk of immunosuppression with TACROLIMUS
- Vaccines: risk of generalised infections when dexrazoxane
  given with live • VACCINES—avoid concomitant use

Dextromethorphan see Opioid Analgesics

Dextropropoxyphene see Opioid Analgesics

Diamorphine see Opioid Analgesics

Diazepam see Anxiolytics and Hypnotics

Diazoxide
▸ ACE Inhibitors: enhanced hypotensive effect when diazoxide
  given with ACE INHIBITORS
▸ Adrenergic Neurone Blockers: enhanced hypotensive effect
  when diazoxide given with ADRENERGIC NEURONE BLOCKERS
▸ Alcohol: enhanced hypotensive effect when diazoxide given
  with ALCOHOL
▸ Aldesleukin: enhanced hypotensive effect when diazoxide
  given with ALDESLEUKIN
▸ Alpha-blockers: enhanced hypotensive effect when diazoxide
  given with ALPHA-BLOCKERS
▸ Anaesthetics, General: enhanced hypotensive effect when
  diazoxide given with GENERAL ANAESTHETICS
▸ Analgesics: hypotensive effect of diazoxide antagonised by
  NSAIDs

Diazoxide (continued)
▸ Angiotensin-II Receptor Antagonists: enhanced hypotensive
  effect when diazoxide given with ANGIOTENSIN-II RECEPTOR
  ANTAGONISTS
▸ Antidepressants: enhanced hypotensive effect when diazoxide
  given with MAOIs or TRICYCLIC-RELATED ANTIDEPRESSANTS
▸ Antidiabetics: diazoxide antagonises hypoglycaemic effect of
  ANTIDIABETICS
▸ Antiepileptics: diazoxide reduces plasma concentration of
  FOSPHENYTOIN and PHENYTOIN, also effect of diazoxide may be
  reduced
▸ Antipsychotics: enhanced hypotensive effect when diazoxide
  given with PHENOTHIAZINES
▸ Anxiolytics and Hypnotics: enhanced hypotensive effect when
  diazoxide given with ANXIOLYTICS AND HYPNOTICS
▸ Beta-blockers: enhanced hypotensive effect when diazoxide
  given with BETA-BLOCKERS
▸ Calcium-channel Blockers: enhanced hypotensive effect when
  diazoxide given with CALCIUM-CHANNEL BLOCKERS
▸ Clonidine: enhanced hypotensive effect when diazoxide given
  with CLONIDINE
▸ Corticosteroids: hypotensive effect of diazoxide antagonised by
  CORTICOSTEROIDS
▸ Diuretics: enhanced hypotensive and hyperglycaemic effects
  when diazoxide given with DIURETICS
▸ Dopaminergics: enhanced hypotensive effect when diazoxide
  given with CO-BENELDOPA, CO-CARELDOPA or LEVODOPA
▸ Methyldopa: enhanced hypotensive effect when diazoxide
  given with METHYLDOPA
▸ Moxisylyte: enhanced hypotensive effect when diazoxide given
  with MOXISYLYTE
▸ Moxonidine: enhanced hypotensive effect when diazoxide
  given with MOXONIDINE
▸ Muscle Relaxants: enhanced hypotensive effect when diazoxide
  given with BACLOFEN or TIZANIDINE
▸ Nitrates: enhanced hypotensive effect when diazoxide given
  with NITRATES
▸ Prostaglandins: enhanced hypotensive effect when diazoxide
  given with ALPROSTADIL
▸ Vasodilator Antihypertensives: enhanced hypotensive effect
  when diazoxide given with HYDRALAZINE, MINOXIDIL or SODIUM
  NITROPRUSSIDE

Diclofenac see NSAIDs

Dicycloverine see Antimuscarinics

Didanosine
NOTE Antacids in tablet formulation might affect absorption of
other drugs—give at least 2 hours apart
- Allopurinol: plasma concentration of didanosine increased by
  • ALLOPURINOL (risk of toxicity)—avoid concomitant use
▸ Analgesics: plasma concentration of didanosine possibly
  reduced by METHADONE
▸ Antibacterials: didanosine *tablets* reduce absorption of
  CIPROFLOXACIN (give at least 2 hours before or 4 hours after
  ciprofloxacin); manufacturer of levofloxacin advises give
  didanosine *tablets* at least 2 hours before or after
  LEVOFLOXACIN; manufacturer of moxifloxacin advises give
  didanosine *tablets* at least 6 hours before or after
  MOXIFLOXACIN; manufacturer of norfloxacin advises give
  didanosine at least 2 hours before or after NORFLOXACIN
- Antivirals: didanosine *tablets* reduce absorption of ATAZANAVIR
  (give at least 2 hours before or 1 hour after didanosine
  tablets); manufacturer of darunavir advises take didanosine
  1 hour before or 2 hours after DARUNAVIR; plasma
  concentration of didanosine possibly increased by
  GANCICLOVIR and VALGANCICLOVIR; didanosine *tablets* reduce
  absorption of INDINAVIR (give at least 1 hour apart); increased
  risk of side-effects when didanosine given with • RIBAVIRIN—
  avoid concomitant use; manufacturer of rilpivirine advises
  give didanosine 2 hours before or 4 hours after RILPIVIRINE;
  manufacturer of ritonavir advises didanosine and RITONAVIR
  should be taken 2.5 hours apart; increased risk of side-effects
  when didanosine given with • STAVUDINE; plasma
  concentration of didanosine increased by • TENOFOVIR
  (increased risk of toxicity)—avoid concomitant use; plasma
  concentration of didanosine reduced by TIPRANAVIR—

Didanosine
- Antivirals (continued)
  manufacturer of tipranavir advises tipranavir and didanosine *capsules* should be taken at least 2 hours apart
- Cytotoxics: increased risk of toxicity when didanosine given with ● HYDROXYCARBAMIDE—avoid concomitant use
- Orlistat: absorption of didanosine possibly reduced by ● ORLISTAT

Dienogest *see* Progestogens

Diethylcarbamazine
▸ Antacids: excretion of diethylcarbamazine reduced by SODIUM BICARBONATE

Digoxin *see* Cardiac Glycosides

Dihydrocodeine *see* Opioid Analgesics

Dihydrotachysterol *see* Vitamins

Diltiazem *see* Calcium-channel Blockers

Dimethyl sulfoxide
- Analgesics: avoid concomitant use of dimethyl sulfoxide with ● SULINDAC

Dinoprostone *see* Prostaglandins

Diphenoxylate *see* Opioid Analgesics

Diphtheria Vaccines *see* Vaccines

Dipipanone *see* Opioid Analgesics

Dipyridamole
▸ Antacids: absorption of dipyridamole possibly reduced by ANTACIDS
- Anti-arrhythmics: dipyridamole enhances and extends effect of ● ADENOSINE (important risk of toxicity)—reduce dose of adenosine, see p. 96
- Anticoagulants: antiplatelet action of dipyridamole enhances anticoagulant effect of ● COUMARINS and ● PHENINDIONE; dipyridamole enhances anticoagulant effect of HEPARINS
▸ Clopidogrel: increased risk of bleeding when dipyridamole given with CLOPIDOGREL
▸ Cytotoxics: dipyridamole possibly reduces effects of ● FLUDARABINE

Disopyramide
▸ Anaesthetics, Local: increased myocardial depression when anti-arrhythmics given with BUPIVACAINE, LEVOBUPIVACAINE, PRILOCAINE or ROPIVACAINE
- Anti-arrhythmics: increased myocardial depression when anti-arrhythmics given with other ● ANTI-ARRHYTHMICS; increased risk of ventricular arrhythmias when disopyramide given with ● AMIODARONE or ● DRONEDARONE—avoid concomitant use
- Antibacterials: plasma concentration of disopyramide possibly increased by ● AZITHROMYCIN (increased risk of toxicity); plasma concentration of disopyramide possibly increased by ● CLARITHROMYCIN (increased risk of ventricular arrhythmias); plasma concentration of disopyramide increased by ● ERYTHROMYCIN (increased risk of toxicity); increased risk of ventricular arrhythmias when disopyramide given with ● MOXIFLOXACIN—avoid concomitant use; increased risk of ventricular arrhythmias when disopyramide given with ● DELAMANID; metabolism of disopyramide accelerated by ● RIFAMYCINS (reduced plasma concentration); possible increased risk of ventricular arrhythmias when disopyramide given with ● TELITHROMYCIN
▸ Anticoagulants: disopyramide may enhance or reduce anticoagulant effect of WARFARIN
- Antidepressants: avoidance of disopyramide advised by manufacturer of ● CITALOPRAM and ● ESCITALOPRAM (risk of ventricular arrhythmias); increased risk of ventricular arrhythmias when disopyramide given with ● TRICYCLICS
- Antidiabetics: disopyramide possibly enhances hypoglycaemic effect of GLICLAZIDE, INSULIN and METFORMIN
- Antiepileptics: plasma concentration of disopyramide reduced by FOSPHENYTOIN and PHENYTOIN; metabolism of disopyramide accelerated by PHENOBARBITAL and PRIMIDONE (reduced plasma concentration)
- Antifungals: increased risk of ventricular arrhythmias when disopyramide given with ● KETOCONAZOLE—avoid concomitant use; avoidance of disopyramide advised by manufacturer of ● ITRACONAZOLE
- Antihistamines: increased risk of ventricular arrhythmias when disopyramide given with ● MIZOLASTINE—avoid concomitant use

Disopyramide (continued)
- Antimalarials: avoidance of disopyramide advised by manufacturer of ● ARTEMETHER WITH LUMEFANTRINE (risk of ventricular arrhythmias); avoidance of disopyramide advised by manufacturer of ● ARTENIMOL WITH PIPERAQUINE (possible risk of ventricular arrhythmias)
- Antimuscarinics: increased risk of antimuscarinic side-effects when disopyramide given with ANTIMUSCARINICS; increased risk of ventricular arrhythmias when disopyramide given with ● TOLTERODINE
- Antipsychotics: increased risk of ventricular arrhythmias when anti-arrhythmics that prolong the QT interval given with ● ANTIPSYCHOTICS that prolong the QT interval; increased risk of ventricular arrhythmias when disopyramide given with ● AMISULPRIDE, ● DROPERIDOL, ● PIMOZIDE or ● ZUCLOPENTHIXOL—avoid concomitant use; possible increased risk of ventricular arrhythmias when disopyramide given with ● HALOPERIDOL—avoid concomitant use; increased risk of ventricular arrhythmias when disopyramide given with ● PHENOTHIAZINES or ● SULPIRIDE
- Antivirals: plasma concentration of disopyramide possibly increased by ● RITONAVIR (increased risk of toxicity); increased risk of ventricular arrhythmias when disopyramide given with ● SAQUINAVIR—avoid concomitant use; avoidance of disopyramide advised by manufacturer of ● TELAPREVIR (risk of ventricular arrhythmias)
- Atomoxetine: increased risk of ventricular arrhythmias when disopyramide given with ● ATOMOXETINE
- Beta-blockers: increased myocardial depression when anti-arrhythmics given with ● BETA-BLOCKERS; increased risk of ventricular arrhythmias when disopyramide given with ● SOTALOL—avoid concomitant use
- Calcium-channel Blockers: increased risk of myocardial depression and asystole when disopyramide given with ● VERAPAMIL
- Cytotoxics: possible increased risk of ventricular arrhythmias when disopyramide given with ● BOSUTINIB; possible increased risk of ventricular arrhythmias when disopyramide given with ● VANDETANIB—avoid concomitant use; increased risk of ventricular arrhythmias when disopyramide given with ● ARSENIC TRIOXIDE
- Diuretics: increased cardiac toxicity with disopyramide if hypokalaemia occurs with ● ACETAZOLAMIDE, ● LOOP DIURETICS or ● THIAZIDES and RELATED DIURETICS
- Fingolimod: possible increased risk of bradycardia when disopyramide given with ● FINGOLIMOD
- Ivabradine: increased risk of ventricular arrhythmias when disopyramide given with ● IVABRADINE
▸ Nitrates: disopyramide reduces effects of sublingual tablets of NITRATES (failure to dissolve under tongue owing to dry mouth)
- Pentamidine Isetionate: possible increased risk of ventricular arrhythmias when disopyramide given with ● PENTAMIDINE ISETIONATE
- Ranolazine: avoidance of disopyramide advised by manufacturer of ● RANOLAZINE
▸ Sildenafil: manufacturer of disopyramide advises avoid concomitant use with SILDENAFIL (risk of ventricular arrhythmias)
▸ Tadalafil: manufacturer of disopyramide advises avoid concomitant use with TADALAFIL (risk of ventricular arrhythmias)
▸ Vardenafil: manufacturer of disopyramide advises avoid concomitant use with VARDENAFIL (risk of ventricular arrhythmias)

Disulfiram
▸ Alcohol: disulfiram reaction when disulfiram given with ALCOHOL
▸ Aminophylline: disulfiram inhibits metabolism of AMINOPHYLLINE (increased risk of toxicity)
▸ Antibacterials: psychotic reaction reported when disulfiram given with METRONIDAZOLE; CNS effects of disulfiram possibly increased by ISONIAZID
- Anticoagulants: disulfiram enhances anticoagulant effect of ● COUMARINS

Disulfiram (continued)
▸ Antidepressants: increased disulfiram reaction with alcohol reported with concomitant AMITRIPTYLINE; disulfiram inhibits metabolism of TRICYCLICS (increased plasma concentration)
● Antiepileptics: disulfiram inhibits metabolism of
  ● FOSPHENYTOIN and ● PHENYTOIN (increased risk of toxicity)
▸ Anxiolytics and Hypnotics: disulfiram increases risk of TEMAZEPAM toxicity; disulfiram inhibits metabolism of BENZODIAZEPINES (increased sedative effects)
● Paraldehyde: risk of toxicity when disulfiram given with
  ● PARALDEHYDE
▸ Theophylline: disulfiram inhibits metabolism of THEOPHYLLINE (increased risk of toxicity)

Diuretics
NOTE Since systemic absorption may follow topical application of brinzolamide to the eye, the possibility of interactions should be borne in mind
NOTE Since systemic absorption may follow topical application of dorzolamide to the eye, the possibility of interactions should be borne in mind
● ACE Inhibitors: enhanced hypotensive effect when diuretics given with ● ACE INHIBITORS; increased risk of severe hyperkalaemia when amiloride, potassium canrenoate or triamterene given with ● ACE INHIBITORS; increased risk of severe hyperkalaemia when eplerenone and spironolactone given with ● ACE INHIBITORS—avoid concurrent use or use lowest possible doses of both drugs
▸ Adrenergic Neurone Blockers: enhanced hypotensive effect when diuretics given with ADRENERGIC NEURONE BLOCKERS
▸ Alcohol: enhanced hypotensive effect when diuretics given with ALCOHOL
▸ Aldesleukin: enhanced hypotensive effect when diuretics given with ALDESLEUKIN
▸ Aliskiren: plasma concentration of furosemide reduced by ALISKIREN; increased risk of hyperkalaemia when potassium-sparing diuretics and aldosterone antagonists given with ALISKIREN
▸ Allopurinol: increased risk of hypersensitivity when thiazides and related diuretics given with ALLOPURINOL especially in renal impairment
● Alpha-blockers: enhanced hypotensive effect when diuretics given with ● ALPHA-BLOCKERS, also increased risk of first-dose hypotension with post-synaptic alpha-blockers such as prazosin
▸ Aminophylline: increased risk of hypokalaemia when acetazolamide, loop diuretics or thiazides and related diuretics given with AMINOPHYLLINE
▸ Anaesthetics, General: enhanced hypotensive effect when diuretics given with GENERAL ANAESTHETICS
● Analgesics: diuretics increase risk of nephrotoxicity of NSAIDs, also antagonism of diuretic effect; diuretic effect of potassium canrenoate possibly antagonised by NSAIDs; possible increased risk of hyperkalaemia when potassium-sparing diuretics and aldosterone antagonists given with NSAIDs; furosemide possibly increases the excretion of ACEMETACIN; effects of diuretics antagonised by INDOMETACIN and KETOROLAC; increased risk of hyperkalaemia when potassium-sparing diuretics and aldosterone antagonists given with INDOMETACIN; occasional reports of reduced renal function when triamterene given with ● INDOMETACIN—avoid concomitant use; diuretic effect of spironolactone antagonised by ASPIRIN; possible increased risk of toxicity when loop diuretics given with high-dose ASPIRIN (also possible reduced effect of loop diuretics); increased risk of toxicity when acetazolamide given with high-dose ● ASPIRIN
● Angiotensin-II Receptor Antagonists: enhanced hypotensive effect when diuretics given with ● ANGIOTENSIN-II RECEPTOR ANTAGONISTS; increased risk of severe hyperkalaemia when amiloride, potassium canrenoate or triamterene given with ● ANGIOTENSIN-II RECEPTOR ANTAGONISTS; increased risk of severe hyperkalaemia when eplerenone and spironolactone given with ● ANGIOTENSIN-II RECEPTOR ANTAGONISTS—avoid concurrent use or use lowest possible doses of both drugs; plasma concentration of furosemide reduced by VALSARTAN
● Anti-arrhythmics: hypokalaemia caused by acetazolamide, loop diuretics or thiazides and related diuretics increases cardiac

Diuretics
● Anti-arrhythmics (continued)
toxicity with AMIODARONE; plasma concentration of eplerenone increased by AMIODARONE (reduce dose of eplerenone); hypokalaemia caused by acetazolamide, loop diuretics or thiazides and related diuretics increases cardiac toxicity with ● DISOPYRAMIDE; hypokalaemia caused by acetazolamide, loop diuretics or thiazides and related diuretics increases cardiac toxicity with ● FLECAINIDE; hypokalaemia caused by acetazolamide, loop diuretics or thiazides and related diuretics antagonises action of
  ● LIDOCAINE
● Antibacterials: plasma concentration of eplerenone increased by ● CLARITHROMYCIN and ● TELITHROMYCIN—avoid concomitant use; plasma concentration of eplerenone increased by ERYTHROMYCIN (reduce dose of eplerenone); plasma concentration of eplerenone reduced by
  ● RIFAMPICIN—avoid concomitant use; avoidance of diuretics advised by manufacturer of LYMECYCLINE; increased risk of otoxicity when loop diuretics given with ● AMINOGLYCOSIDES,
  ● POLYMYXINS or ● VANCOMYCIN; acetazolamide antagonises effects of ● METHENAMINE; increased risk of hyperkalaemia when eplerenone given with TRIMETHOPRIM; possible increased risk of hyperkalaemia when spironolactone given with TRIMETHOPRIM
● Antidepressants: possible increased risk of hypokalaemia when loop diuretics or thiazides and related diuretics given with REBOXETINE; enhanced hypotensive effect when diuretics given with MAOIs; plasma concentration of eplerenone reduced by ● ST JOHN'S WORT—avoid concomitant use; increased risk of postural hypotension when diuretics given with TRICYCLICS
▸ Antidiabetics: loop diuretics and thiazides and related diuretics antagonise hypoglycaemic effect of ANTIDIABETICS; diuretic effect of diuretics possibly enhanced by CANAGLIFLOZIN; avoidance of loop diuretics advised by manufacturer of CANAGLIFLOZIN; diuretic effect of loop diuretics and thiazides and related diuretics enhanced by DAPAGLIFLOZIN
● Antiepileptics: increased risk of hyponatraemia when diuretics given with CARBAMAZEPINE; acetazolamide increases plasma concentration of ● CARBAMAZEPINE; plasma concentration of eplerenone reduced by ● CARBAMAZEPINE, ● FOSPHENYTOIN,
  ● PHENOBARBITAL, ● PHENYTOIN and ● PRIMIDONE—avoid concomitant use; increased risk of osteomalacia when carbonic anhydrase inhibitors given with FOSPHENYTOIN, PHENOBARBITAL, PHENYTOIN or PRIMIDONE; effects of furosemide antagonised by FOSPHENYTOIN and PHENYTOIN; acetazolamide possibly increases plasma concentration of
  ● FOSPHENYTOIN and ● PHENYTOIN; hydrochlorothiazide possibly increases plasma concentration of TOPIRAMATE; avoidance of carbonic anhydrase inhibitors in children advised by manufacturer of ZONISAMIDE
● Antifungals: plasma concentration of eplerenone increased by
  ● ITRACONAZOLE and ● KETOCONAZOLE—avoid concomitant use; increased risk of hypokalaemia when loop diuretics or thiazides and related diuretics given with AMPHOTERICIN; hydrochlorothiazide increases plasma concentration of FLUCONAZOLE; plasma concentration of eplerenone increased by FLUCONAZOLE (reduce dose of eplerenone)
● Antipsychotics: hypokalaemia caused by diuretics increases risk of ventricular arrhythmias with ● AMISULPRIDE; enhanced hypotensive effect when diuretics given with PHENOTHIAZINES; hypokalaemia caused by diuretics increases risk of ventricular arrhythmias with ● PIMOZIDE (avoid concomitant use)
● Antivirals: plasma concentration of furosemide increased by
  ● DASABUVIR, ● OMBITASVIR and ● PARITAPREVIR (reduce dose of furosemide); plasma concentration of eplerenone increased by ● RITONAVIR—avoid concomitant use; plasma concentration of eplerenone increased by SAQUINAVIR (reduce dose of eplerenone)
▸ Anxiolytics and Hypnotics: enhanced hypotensive effect when diuretics given with ANXIOLYTICS AND HYPNOTICS; administration of *parenteral* furosemide given with CHLORAL may displace thyroid hormone from binding sites
● Atomoxetine: hypokalaemia caused by diuretics increases risk of ventricular arrhythmias with ● ATOMOXETINE

Diuretics (continued)

- Beta-blockers: enhanced hypotensive effect when diuretics given with BETA-BLOCKERS; hypokalaemia caused by loop diuretics or thiazides and related diuretics increases risk of ventricular arrhythmias with ● SOTALOL
▹ Calcium Salts: increased risk of hypercalcaemia when thiazides and related diuretics given with CALCIUM SALTS
▹ Calcium-channel Blockers: enhanced hypotensive effect when diuretics given with CALCIUM-CHANNEL BLOCKERS; plasma concentration of eplerenone increased by DILTIAZEM and VERAPAMIL (reduce dose of eplerenone)
- Cardiac Glycosides: hypokalaemia caused by acetazolamide, loop diuretics or thiazides and related diuretics increases cardiac toxicity with ● CARDIAC GLYCOSIDES; potassium cannrenoate possibly increases plasma concentration of DIGOXIN; spironolactone increases plasma concentration of ● DIGOXIN
- Ciclosporin: increased risk of nephrotoxicity and possibly hypermagnesaemia when thiazides and related diuretics given with CICLOSPORIN; increased risk of hyperkalaemia when potassium-sparing diuretics and aldosterone antagonists given with ● CICLOSPORIN; acetazolamide possibly increases plasma concentration of ● CICLOSPORIN
▹ Clonidine: enhanced hypotensive effect when diuretics given with CLONIDINE
▹ Corticosteroids: diuretic effect of diuretics antagonised by CORTICOSTEROIDS; increased risk of hypokalaemia when acetazolamide, loop diuretics or thiazides and related diuretics given with CORTICOSTEROIDS
- Cytotoxics: alkaline urine due to acetazolamide increases excretion of METHOTREXATE; hypokalaemia caused by acetazolamide, loop diuretics or thiazides and related diuretics increases risk of ventricular arrhythmias with ● ARSENIC TRIOXIDE; avoidance of spironolactone advised by manufacturer of MITOTANE (antagonism of effect); increased risk of nephrotoxicity and ototoxicity when diuretics given with PLATINUM COMPOUNDS
▹ Diazoxide: enhanced hypotensive and hyperglycaemic effects when diuretics given with DIAZOXIDE
▹ Diuretics: increased risk of hypokalaemia when loop diuretics or thiazides and related diuretics given with ACETAZOLAMIDE; profound diuresis possible when metolazone given with FUROSEMIDE; increased risk of hypokalaemia when thiazides and related diuretics given with LOOP DIURETICS
▹ Dopaminergics: enhanced hypotensive effect when diuretics given with CO-BENELDOPA, CO-CARELDOPA or LEVODOPA
▹ Hormone Antagonists: avoidance of spironolactone advised by manufacturer of ABIRATERONE; increased risk of hypercalcaemia when thiazides and related diuretics given with TOREMIFENE
▹ Lipid-regulating Drugs: absorption of thiazides and related diuretics reduced by COLESTIPOL and COLESTYRAMINE (give at least 2 hours apart)
- Lithium: loop diuretics and thiazides and related diuretics reduce excretion of ● LITHIUM (increased plasma concentration and risk of toxicity)—loop diuretics safer than thiazides; potassium-sparing diuretics and aldosterone antagonists reduce excretion of ● LITHIUM (increased plasma concentration and risk of toxicity); acetazolamide increases the excretion of ● LITHIUM
▹ Methyldopa: enhanced hypotensive effect when diuretics given with METHYLDOPA
▹ Moxisylyte: enhanced hypotensive effect when diuretics given with MOXISYLYTE
▹ Moxonidine: enhanced hypotensive effect when diuretics given with MOXONIDINE
▹ Muscle Relaxants: enhanced hypotensive effect when diuretics given with BACLOFEN or TIZANIDINE
▹ Nitrates: enhanced hypotensive effect when diuretics given with NITRATES
▹ Oestrogens: diuretic effect of diuretics antagonised by OESTROGENS
- Potassium Salts: increased risk of hyperkalaemia when potassium-sparing diuretics and aldosterone antagonists given with ● POTASSIUM SALTS

Diuretics (continued)

▹ Progestogens: risk of hyperkalaemia when potassium-sparing diuretics and aldosterone antagonists given with DROSPIRENONE (monitor serum potassium during first cycle)
▹ Prostaglandins: enhanced hypotensive effect when diuretics given with ALPROSTADIL
▹ Sacubitril: plasma concentration of furosemide reduced by SACUBITRIL
▹ Sympathomimetics, Beta₂: increased risk of hypokalaemia when acetazolamide, loop diuretics or thiazides and related diuretics given with high doses of BETA₂ SYMPATHOMIMETICS
▹ Tacrolimus: increased risk of hyperkalaemia when potassium-sparing diuretics and aldosterone antagonists given with ● TACROLIMUS
▹ Theophylline: increased risk of hypokalaemia when acetazolamide, loop diuretics or thiazides and related diuretics given with THEOPHYLLINE
▹ Vasodilator Antihypertensives: enhanced hypotensive effect when diuretics given with HYDRALAZINE, MINOXIDIL or SODIUM NITROPRUSSIDE
▹ Vitamins: increased risk of hypercalcaemia when thiazides and related diuretics given with ALFACALCIDOL, CALCITRIOL, COLECALCIFEROL, DIHYDROTACHYSTEROL, ERGOCALCIFEROL, PARICALCITOL or VITAMIN D

Diuretics, Loop see Diuretics
Diuretics, Potassium-sparing and Aldosterone Antagonists see Diuretics
Diuretics, Thiazide and related see Diuretics
Dobutamine see Sympathomimetics
Docetaxel

- Antibacterials: plasma concentration of docetaxel possibly increased by ● CLARITHROMYCIN and ● TELITHROMYCIN—manufacturer of docetaxel advises avoid concomitant use or consider reducing docetaxel dose
- Antifungals: in vitro studies suggest a possible interaction between docetaxel and KETOCONAZOLE (consult docetaxel product literature); plasma concentration of docetaxel possibly increased by ● ITRACONAZOLE and ● VORICONAZOLE—manufacturer of docetaxel advises avoid concomitant use or consider reducing docetaxel dose
- Antipsychotics: avoid concomitant use of cytotoxics with ● CLOZAPINE (increased risk of agranulocytosis)
- Antivirals: plasma concentration of docetaxel possibly increased by ● INDINAVIR, ● RITONAVIR and ● SAQUINAVIR—manufacturer of docetaxel advises avoid concomitant use or consider reducing docetaxel dose
- Ciclosporin: in vitro studies suggest a possible interaction between docetaxel and CICLOSPORIN (consult docetaxel product literature)
- Cytotoxics: possible increased risk of neutropenia when docetaxel given with LAPATINIB; plasma concentration of docetaxel increased by SORAFENIB
- Netupitant: plasma concentration of docetaxel increased by NETUPITANT

Dolutegravir

- Antacids: absorption of dolutegravir reduced by ALUMINIUM HYDROXIDE and ORAL MAGNESIUM SALTS—manufacturer of dolutegravir advises give at least 2 hours before or 6 hours after aluminium hydroxide and oral magnesium salts
- Antibacterials: plasma concentration of dolutegravir reduced by ● RIFAMPICIN (see under Dolutegravir, p. 584)
- Antidepressants: plasma concentration of dolutegravir possibly reduced by ● ST JOHN'S WORT (see under Dolutegravir, p. 584)
- Antidiabetics: dolutegravir increases the plasma concentration of METFORMIN—consider reducing dose of metformin
- Antiepileptics: plasma concentration of dolutegravir reduced by ● CARBAMAZEPINE (see under Dolutegravir, p. 584); plasma concentration of dolutegravir possibly reduced by ● FOSPHENYTOIN, ● OXCARBAZEPINE, ● PHENOBARBITAL, ● PHENYTOIN and ● PRIMIDONE (see under Dolutegravir, p. 584)
- Antivirals: plasma concentration of dolutegravir reduced by ● EFAVIRENZ, ● ETRAVIRINE and ● TIPRANAVIR (see under Dolutegravir, p. 584); plasma concentration of dolutegravir reduced by ● FOSAMPRENAVIR; plasma concentration of dolutegravir possibly reduced by ● NEVIRAPINE (see under Dolutegravir, p. 584)

A1

Interactions | Appendix 1

Dolutegravir (continued)

‣ Calcium Salts: absorption of dolutegravir reduced by CALCIUM SALTS—manufacturer of dolutegravir advises give at least 2 hours before or 6 hours after calcium salts
‣ Iron Salts: absorption of dolutegravir reduced by *oral* IRON SALTS—manufacturer of dolutegravir advises give at least 2 hours before or 6 hours after *oral* iron salts

Domperidone

‣ Analgesics: effects of domperidone on gastro-intestinal activity antagonised by OPIOID ANALGESICS
● Antibacterials: possible increased risk of ventricular arrhythmias when domperidone given with ● CLARITHROMYCIN or ● TELITHROMYCIN—avoid concomitant use; plasma concentration of domperidone increased by ● ERYTHROMYCIN (increased risk of ventricular arrhythmias—avoid concomitant use); possible increased risk of ventricular arrhythmias when domperidone given with ● DELAMANID
● Antifungals: avoidance of domperidone advised by manufacturer of ● KETOCONAZOLE (risk of ventricular arrhythmias); possible increased risk of ventricular arrhythmias when domperidone given with ● ITRACONAZOLE or ● VORICONAZOLE—avoid concomitant use
● Antimalarials: avoidance of domperidone advised by manufacturer of ● ARTENIMOL WITH PIPERAQUINE (possible risk of ventricular arrhythmias)
‣ Antimuscarinics: effects of domperidone on gastro-intestinal activity antagonised by ANTIMUSCARINICS
● Antivirals: possible increased risk of ventricular arrhythmias when domperidone given with ● BOCEPREVIR, ● RITONAVIR, ● SAQUINAVIR or ● TELAPREVIR—avoid concomitant use
● Cobicistat: possible increased risk of ventricular arrhythmias when domperidone given with ● COBICISTAT—avoid concomitant use
● Cytotoxics: avoidance of domperidone advised by manufacturer of ● BOSUTINIB (risk of ventricular arrhythmias)
● Dopaminergics: possible increased risk of ventricular arrhythmias when domperidone given with ● APOMORPHINE; domperidone possibly antagonises hypoprolactinaemic effects of BROMOCRIPTINE and CABERGOLINE

Donepezil *see* Parasympathomimetics
Dopamine *see* Sympathomimetics
Dopaminergics *see* Amantadine, Apomorphine, Bromocriptine, Cabergoline, Entacapone, Levodopa, Pergolide, Pramipexole, Quinagolide, Rasagiline, Ropinirole, Rotigotine, Selegiline, and Tolcapone
Dopexamine *see* Sympathomimetics
Dorzolamide *see* Diuretics
Dosulepin *see* Antidepressants, Tricyclic
Doxapram

‣ Aminophylline: increased CNS stimulation when doxapram given with AMINOPHYLLINE
● Anaesthetics, General: increased risk of arrhythmias when doxapram given with ● VOLATILE LIQUID GENERAL ANAESTHETICS (avoid doxapram for at least 10 minutes after volatile liquid general anaesthetics)
‣ Antidepressants: effects of doxapram enhanced by MAOIs
‣ Sympathomimetics: increased risk of hypertension when doxapram given with SYMPATHOMIMETICS
‣ Theophylline: increased CNS stimulation when doxapram given with THEOPHYLLINE

Doxazosin *see* Alpha-blockers
Doxepin *see* Antidepressants, Tricyclic
Doxorubicin

● Antipsychotics: avoid concomitant use of cytotoxics with ● CLOZAPINE (increased risk of agranulocytosis)
‣ Antivirals: doxorubicin possibly inhibits effects of STAVUDINE
‣ Calcium-channel Blockers: plasma concentration of doxorubicin possibly increased by VERAPAMIL
‣ Cardiac Glycosides: doxorubicin possibly reduces absorption of DIGOXIN *tablets*
● Ciclosporin: increased risk of neurotoxicity when doxorubicin given with ● CICLOSPORIN
● Cytotoxics: possible increased risk of cardiotoxicity when doxorubicin given with ● TRASTUZUMAB—avoid concomitant use for up to 28 weeks after stopping trastuzumab; plasma concentration of doxorubicin increased by SORAFENIB

Doxorubicin (continued)

‣ Ulcer-healing Drugs: plasma concentration of doxorubicin reduced by CIMETIDINE
● Vaccines: risk of generalised infections when cytotoxic antibiotics given with live ● VACCINES—avoid concomitant use

Doxycycline *see* Tetracyclines
Dronedarone

● Anaesthetics, Local: increased myocardial depression when anti-arrhythmics given with BUPIVACAINE, LEVOBUPIVACAINE, PRILOCAINE or ROPIVACAINE
● Anti-arrhythmics: increased myocardial depression when anti-arrhythmics given with other ● ANTI-ARRHYTHMICS; increased risk of ventricular arrhythmias when dronedarone given with ● AMIODARONE or ● DISOPYRAMIDE—avoid concomitant use
● Antibacterials: manufacturer of dronedarone advises avoid concomitant use with ● CLARITHROMYCIN (risk of ventricular arrhythmias); plasma concentration of dronedarone increased by ● ERYTHROMYCIN (increased risk of ventricular arrhythmias—avoid concomitant use); plasma concentration of dronedarone reduced by ● RIFAMPICIN—avoid concomitant use; avoidance of dronedarone advised by manufacturer of FIDAXOMICIN; increased risk of ventricular arrhythmias when dronedarone given with ● TELITHROMYCIN—avoid concomitant use
● Anticoagulants: dronedarone possibly enhances anticoagulant effect of ● COUMARINS and ● PHENINDIONE; dronedarone increases plasma concentration of ● DABIGATRAN—avoid concomitant use; dronedarone increases plasma concentration of ● EDOXABAN (reduce dose of edoxaban—see under Edoxaban, p. 113); avoidance of dronedarone advised by manufacturer of RIVAROXABAN
● Antidepressants: avoidance of dronedarone advised by manufacturer of ● CITALOPRAM and ● ESCITALOPRAM (risk of ventricular arrhythmias); plasma concentration of dronedarone possibly reduced by ● ST JOHN'S WORT—avoid concomitant use; manufacturer of dronedarone advises avoid concomitant use with ● TRICYCLICS (risk of ventricular arrhythmias)
● Antiepileptics: plasma concentration of dronedarone possibly reduced by ● CARBAMAZEPINE, ● FOSPHENYTOIN, ● PHENOBARBITAL, ● PHENYTOIN and ● PRIMIDONE—avoid concomitant use
● Antifungals: plasma concentration of dronedarone increased by ● KETOCONAZOLE—avoid concomitant use; manufacturer of dronedarone advises avoid concomitant use with ● ITRACONAZOLE, ● POSACONAZOLE and ● VORICONAZOLE
● Antipsychotics: increased risk of ventricular arrhythmias when anti-arrhythmics that prolong the QT interval given with ● ANTIPSYCHOTICS that prolong the QT interval; manufacturer of dronedarone advises avoid concomitant use with ● PHENOTHIAZINES (risk of ventricular arrhythmias)
● Antivirals: manufacturer of dronedarone advises avoid concomitant use with ● RITONAVIR; increased risk of ventricular arrhythmias when dronedarone given with ● SAQUINAVIR—avoid concomitant use
● Beta-blockers: increased myocardial depression when anti-arrhythmics given with ● BETA-BLOCKERS; dronedarone possibly increases plasma concentration of METOPROLOL and PROPRANOLOL; increased risk of ventricular arrhythmias when dronedarone given with ● SOTALOL—avoid concomitant use
● Calcium-channel Blockers: plasma concentration of dronedarone increased by ● NIFEDIPINE; increased risk of bradycardia and myocardial depression when dronedarone given with ● DILTIAZEM and ● VERAPAMIL
● Cardiac Glycosides: dronedarone increases plasma concentration of ● DIGOXIN (halve dose of digoxin)
● Cytotoxics: dronedarone possibly increases the plasma concentration of ● BOSUTINIB—manufacturer of bosutinib advises avoid or consider reducing dose of bosutinib; dronedarone possibly increases the plasma concentration of ● IBRUTINIB—reduce dose of ibrutinib (see under Ibrutinib, p. 855)
● Fingolimod: possible increased risk of bradycardia when dronedarone given with ● FINGOLIMOD
● Grapefruit Juice: plasma concentration of dronedarone increased by ● GRAPEFRUIT JUICE—avoid concomitant use

Dronedarone (continued)

- Lipid-regulating Drugs: dronedarone possibly increases plasma concentration of ATORVASTATIN; dronedarone increases plasma concentration of ● ROSUVASTATIN—adjust dose of rosuvastatin (consult product literature); increased risk of myopathy when dronedarone given with ● SIMVASTATIN; avoidance of dronedarone advised by manufacturer of ● LOMITAPIDE (plasma concentration of lomitapide possibly increased)
- ▸ Sirolimus: manufacturer of dronedarone advises caution with SIROLIMUS
- ▸ Tacrolimus: manufacturer of dronedarone advises caution with TACROLIMUS

Droperidol see Antipsychotics

Drospirenone see Progestogens

Dulaglutide see Antidiabetics

Duloxetine

- ▸ Analgesics: possible increased serotonergic effects when SSRI-related antidepressants given with ● FENTANYL; possible increased serotonergic effects when duloxetine given with PETHIDINE or TRAMADOL
- Antibacterials: metabolism of duloxetine inhibited by ● CIPROFLOXACIN—avoid concomitant use
- Anticoagulants: possible increased risk of bleeding when SSRI-related antidepressants given with ● DABIGATRAN
- Antidepressants: metabolism of duloxetine inhibited by ● FLUVOXAMINE—avoid concomitant use; possible increased serotonergic effects when duloxetine given with SSRIs, ST JOHN'S WORT, AMITRIPTYLINE, CLOMIPRAMINE, ● MOCLOBEMIDE or VENLAFAXINE; duloxetine should not be started until 2 weeks after stopping ● MAOIS, also MAOIs should not be started until at least 5 days after stopping duloxetine; after stopping SSRI-related antidepressants do not start ● MOCLOBEMIDE for at least 1 week; possible increased risk of convulsions when SSRI-related antidepressants given with ● VORTIOXETINE
- Antimalarials: avoidance of antidepressants advised by manufacturer of ● ARTEMETHER WITH LUMEFANTRINE and ● ARTENIMOL WITH PIPERAQUINE
- ▸ Atomoxetine: possible increased risk of convulsions when antidepressants given with ATOMOXETINE
- Dapoxetine: possible increased risk of serotonergic effects when duloxetine given with ● DAPOXETINE (manufacturer of dapoxetine advises duloxetine should not be started until 1 week after stopping dapoxetine, avoid dapoxetine for 2 weeks after stopping duloxetine)
- ▸ 5HT₁-receptor Agonists: possible increased serotonergic effects when duloxetine given with 5HT₁ AGONISTS
- ▸ 5HT₃-receptor Antagonists: possible increased serotonergic effects when SSRI-related antidepressants given with 5HT₃ ANTAGONISTS
- Methylthioninium: risk of CNS toxicity when SSRI-related antidepressants given with ● METHYLTHIONINIUM—avoid concomitant use (if inhibition not possible, use lowest possible dose of methylthioninium and observe patient for up to 4 hours after administration)

Dutasteride

- ▸ Calcium-channel Blockers: plasma concentration of dutasteride increased by DILTIAZEM and VERAPAMIL

Dydrogesterone see Progestogens

Edoxaban

- Analgesics: increased risk of bleeding when edoxaban given with ● NSAIDS (manufacturer of edoxaban advises avoid long-term NSAIDs); increased risk of haemorrhage when anticoagulants given with *intravenous* ● DICLOFENAC (avoid concomitant use, including low-dose heparins); increased risk of haemorrhage when anticoagulants given with ● KETOROLAC (avoid concomitant use, including low-dose heparins); increased risk of bleeding when edoxaban given with high-dose ● ASPIRIN (avoid concomitant use)
- Anti-arrhythmics: plasma concentration of edoxaban increased by ● DRONEDARONE (reduce dose of edoxaban—see under Edoxaban, p. 113)
- Antibacterials: plasma concentration of edoxaban increased by ● ERYTHROMYCIN (reduce dose of edoxaban—see under Edoxaban, p. 113); plasma concentration of edoxaban reduced by ● RIFAMPICIN

Edoxaban (continued)

- Anticoagulants: increased risk of haemorrhage when edoxaban given with other ● ANTICOAGULANTS (avoid concomitant use except when switching with other anticoagulants or using heparin to maintain catheter patency); increased risk of haemorrhage when other anticoagulants given with ● APIXABAN, ● DABIGATRAN and ● RIVAROXABAN (avoid concomitant use except when switching with other anticoagulants or using heparin to maintain catheter patency)
- Antidepressants: plasma concentration of edoxaban possibly reduced by ● ST JOHN'S WORT
- Antiepileptics: plasma concentration of edoxaban possibly reduced by ● CARBAMAZEPINE, ● FOSPHENYTOIN, ● PHENOBARBITAL, ● PHENYTOIN and ● PRIMIDONE
- Antifungals: plasma concentration of edoxaban increased by ● KETOCONAZOLE (reduce dose of edoxaban—see under Edoxaban, p. 113)
- ▸ Calcium-channel Blockers: plasma concentration of edoxaban increased by VERAPAMIL
- Ciclosporin: plasma concentration of edoxaban increased by ● CICLOSPORIN (reduce dose of edoxaban—see under Edoxaban, p. 113)

Efavirenz

- ▸ Analgesics: efavirenz reduces plasma concentration of METHADONE
- ▸ Antibacterials: efavirenz reduces plasma concentration of CLARITHROMYCIN, also plasma concentration of active metabolite of clarithromycin increased; efavirenz reduces plasma concentration of RIFABUTIN—increase dose of rifabutin; plasma concentration of efavirenz reduced by RIFAMPICIN—increase dose of efavirenz; efavirenz possibly reduces plasma concentration of BEDAQUILINE—manufacturer of bedaquiline advises avoid concomitant use
- Anticoagulants: efavirenz possibly affects plasma concentration of ● COUMARINS
- Antidepressants: plasma concentration of efavirenz reduced by ● ST JOHN'S WORT—avoid concomitant use
- ▸ Antiepileptics: plasma concentration of both drugs reduced when efavirenz given with CARBAMAZEPINE
- Antifungals: efavirenz reduces plasma concentration of ITRACONAZOLE, ● KETOCONAZOLE and ● POSACONAZOLE; efavirenz reduces plasma concentration of ● VORICONAZOLE, also plasma concentration of efavirenz increased (increase voriconazole dose and reduce efavirenz dose); efavirenz possibly reduces plasma concentration of CASPOFUNGIN—consider increasing dose of caspofungin
- Antimalarials: efavirenz reduces plasma concentration of ● ARTEMETHER WITH LUMEFANTRINE; efavirenz possibly affects plasma concentration of PROGUANIL
- Antipsychotics: efavirenz possibly reduces plasma concentration of ● ARIPIPRAZOLE (avoid concomitant use or consider increasing the dose of aripiprazole—consult aripiprazole product literature); efavirenz possibly increases plasma concentration of ● PIMOZIDE (increased risk of ventricular arrhythmias—avoid concomitant use)
- Antivirals: avoidance of efavirenz advised by manufacturer of ● ATAZANAVIR (plasma concentration of atazanavir reduced); efavirenz reduces the plasma concentration of ● DACLATASVIR—increase dose of daclatasvir (see under Daclatasvir, p. 568); efavirenz reduces plasma concentration of ● DARUNAVIR (adjust dose—consult product literature); avoidance of efavirenz advised by manufacturer of DASABUVIR, ELVITEGRAVIR, OMBITASVIR and PARITAPREVIR; efavirenz reduces the plasma concentration of ● DOLUTEGRAVIR (see under Dolutegravir, p. 584); efavirenz possibly reduces plasma concentration of ● ETRAVIRINE—avoid concomitant use; efavirenz reduces plasma concentration of INDINAVIR and SIMEPREVIR; efavirenz reduces plasma concentration of ● LOPINAVIR—consider increasing dose of lopinavir; efavirenz possibly reduces plasma concentration of ● MARAVIROC—consider increasing dose of maraviroc; plasma concentration of efavirenz reduced by ● NEVIRAPINE—avoid concomitant use; toxicity of efavirenz increased by ● RITONAVIR, monitor liver function tests —manufacturer of *Atripla*® advises avoid concomitant use with *high-dose* ritonavir; efavirenz significantly reduces plasma concentration of SAQUINAVIR;

Efavirenz
- **Antivirals** (continued)
  efavirenz reduces plasma concentration of • TELAPREVIR—increase dose of telaprevir
- **Anxiolytics and Hypnotics:** increased risk of prolonged sedation when efavirenz given with • MIDAZOLAM—avoid concomitant use
- **Atovaquone:** efavirenz reduces plasma concentration of • ATOVAQUONE—avoid concomitant use
- ▸ **Avanafil:** efavirenz possibly reduces plasma concentration of AVANAFIL—manufacturer of avanafil advises avoid concomitant use
- ▸ **Bupropion:** efavirenz accelerates metabolism of BUPROPION (reduced plasma concentration)
- ▸ **Calcium-channel Blockers:** efavirenz reduces plasma concentration of DILTIAZEM
- **Ciclosporin:** efavirenz possibly reduces plasma concentration of • CICLOSPORIN
- **Cytotoxics:** efavirenz possibly reduces plasma concentration of • BOSUTINIB—manufacturer of bosutinib advises avoid concomitant use
- **Ergot Alkaloids:** increased risk of ergotism when efavirenz given with • ERGOT ALKALOIDS—avoid concomitant use
- ▸ **Grapefruit Juice:** plasma concentration of efavirenz possibly increased by GRAPEFRUIT JUICE
- **Guanfacine:** efavirenz possibly reduces plasma concentration of • GUANFACINE—increase dose of guanfacine
- **Lipid-regulating Drugs:** efavirenz reduces plasma concentration of ATORVASTATIN, PRAVASTATIN and SIMVASTATIN
- **Orlistat:** absorption of efavirenz possibly reduced by • ORLISTAT
- **Progestogens:** efavirenz possibly reduces contraceptive effect of • PROGESTOGENS
- **Tacrolimus:** efavirenz possibly affects plasma concentration of • TACROLIMUS

Eletriptan see 5HT$_1$-receptor Agonists (under HT)

Eltrombopag
- ▸ **Antacids:** absorption of eltrombopag reduced by ANTACIDS (give at least 4 hours apart)
- ▸ **Antivirals:** plasma concentration of eltrombopag possibly reduced by LOPINAVIR
- ▸ **Calcium Salts:** absorption of eltrombopag possibly reduced by CALCIUM SALTS (give at least 4 hours apart)
- ▸ **Dairy Products:** absorption of eltrombopag possibly reduced by DAIRY PRODUCTS (give at least 4 hours apart)
- ▸ **Iron Salts:** absorption of eltrombopag possibly reduced by *oral* IRON SALTS (give at least 4 hours apart)
- **Lipid-regulating Drugs:** eltrombopag increases plasma concentration of • ROSUVASTATIN—adjust dose of rosuvastatin (consult product literature)
- ▸ **Selenium:** absorption of eltrombopag possibly reduced by SELENIUM (give at least 4 hours apart)
- ▸ **Zinc:** absorption of eltrombopag possibly reduced by ZINC (give at least 4 hours apart)

Elvitegravir
- ▸ **Antacids:** absorption of elvitegravir reduced by ALUMINIUM HYDROXIDE and ORAL MAGNESIUM SALTS (give at least 4 hours apart)
- **Antibacterials:** plasma concentration of elvitegravir reduced by • RIFABUTIN also plasma concentration of active metabolite of rifabutin increased—reduce dose of rifabutin; manufacturer of elvitegravir advises avoid concomitant use with • RIFAMPICIN
- **Antidepressants:** manufacturer of elvitegravir advises avoid concomitant use with • ST JOHN'S WORT
- **Antiepileptics:** manufacturer of elvitegravir advises avoid concomitant use with • CARBAMAZEPINE, • FOSPHENYTOIN, • PHENOBARBITAL, • PHENYTOIN and • PRIMIDONE
- **Antivirals:** plasma concentration of elvitegravir increased by • ATAZANAVIR and • LOPINAVIR boosted with ritonavir (reduce dose of elvitegravir); manufacturer of elvitegravir advises avoid concomitant use with EFAVIRENZ and NEVIRAPINE
- ▸ **Bosentan:** manufacturer of elvitegravir advises avoid concomitant use with BOSENTAN
- **Orlistat:** absorption of elvitegravir possibly reduced by • ORLISTAT
- ▸ **Progestogens:** elvitegravir increases plasma concentration of NORGESTIMATE

Empagliflozin see Antidiabetics

Emtricitabine
- ▸ **Antivirals:** manufacturer of emtricitabine advises avoid concomitant use with LAMIVUDINE
- **Orlistat:** absorption of emtricitabine possibly reduced by • ORLISTAT

Enalapril see ACE Inhibitors

Enfuvirtide
- **Orlistat:** absorption of enfuvirtide possibly reduced by • ORLISTAT

Enoxaparin see Heparins

Enoximone see Phosphodiesterase Inhibitors

Entacapone
- **Anticoagulants:** entacapone enhances anticoagulant effect of • WARFARIN
- **Antidepressants:** manufacturer of entacapone advises caution with MOCLOBEMIDE, TRICYCLICS and VENLAFAXINE; avoid concomitant use of entacapone with non-selective • MAOIS
- ▸ **Dopaminergics:** entacapone possibly enhances effects of APOMORPHINE; entacapone possibly reduces plasma concentration of RASAGILINE; manufacturer of entacapone advises max. dose of 10 mg SELEGILINE if used concomitantly
- ▸ **Iron Salts:** absorption of entacapone reduced by *oral* IRON SALTS
- ▸ **Memantine:** effects of dopaminergics possibly enhanced by MEMANTINE
- ▸ **Methyldopa:** entacapone possibly enhances effects of METHYLDOPA; antiparkinsonian effect of dopaminergics antagonised by METHYLDOPA
- ▸ **Sympathomimetics:** entacapone possibly enhances effects of ADRENALINE (EPINEPHRINE), DOBUTAMINE, DOPAMINE and NORADRENALINE (NOREPINEPHRINE)

Enteral Feeds
- **Anticoagulants:** the presence of vitamin K in some enteral feeds can antagonise the anticoagulant effect of • COUMARINS and • PHENINDIONE
- ▸ **Antiepileptics:** enteral feeds possibly reduce absorption of FOSPHENYTOIN and PHENYTOIN

Enzalutamide
- **Anticoagulants:** enzalutamide possibly reduces plasma concentration of • COUMARINS
- **Antivirals:** avoidance of enzalutamide advised by manufacturer of DASABUVIR, OMBITASVIR and PARITAPREVIR
- **Anxiolytics and Hypnotics:** enzalutamide reduces plasma concentration of • MIDAZOLAM
- **Lipid-regulating Drugs:** plasma concentration of enzalutamide increased by • GEMFIBROZIL—manufacturer of enzalutamide advises avoid concomitant use or halve dose of enzalutamide
- ▸ **Ulcer-healing Drugs:** enzalutamide reduces plasma concentration of OMEPRAZOLE

Ephedrine see Sympathomimetics

Epinephrine
  NOTE Epinephrine interactions as for adrenaline, see under sympathomimetics

Epirubicin
- **Antipsychotics:** avoid concomitant use of cytotoxics with • CLOZAPINE (increased risk of agranulocytosis)
- **Ciclosporin:** plasma concentration of epirubicin increased by • CICLOSPORIN
- **Cytotoxics:** possible increased risk of cardiotoxicity when epirubicin given with • TRASTUZUMAB—avoid concomitant use for up to 28 weeks after stopping trastuzumab
- **Ulcer-healing Drugs:** plasma concentration of epirubicin increased by • CIMETIDINE
- **Vaccines:** risk of generalised infections when cytotoxic antibiotics given with live • VACCINES—avoid concomitant use

Eplerenone see Diuretics

Eprosartan see Angiotensin-II Receptor Antagonists

Eptifibatide
- ▸ **Iloprost:** increased risk of bleeding when eptifibatide given with ILOPROST

Ergocalciferol see Vitamins

Ergometrine see Ergot Alkaloids

Ergot Alkaloids
- **Antibacterials:** increased risk of ergotism when ergot alkaloids given with • CLARITHROMYCIN, • ERYTHROMYCIN or

Ergot Alkaloids

- **Antibacterials** (continued)
  - ● TELITHROMYCIN—avoid concomitant use; increased risk of ergotism when ergotamine given with TETRACYCLINES
- ▸ **Antidepressants:** possible risk of hypertension when ergotamine given with REBOXETINE
- **Antifungals:** avoidance of ergot alkaloids advised by manufacturer of ● KETOCONAZOLE; avoidance of ergometrine advised by manufacturer of ● ITRACONAZOLE (increased risk of ergotism); increased risk of ergotism when ergometrine given with ● VORICONAZOLE—avoid concomitant use; increased risk of ergotism when ergotamine given with ● IMIDAZOLES or ● TRIAZOLES—avoid concomitant use
- ▸ **Antipsychotics:** plasma concentration of ergot alkaloids possibly increased by LURASIDONE (increased risk of toxicity)
- **Antivirals:** plasma concentration of ergot alkaloids possibly increased by ● ATAZANAVIR—avoid concomitant use; avoidance of ergot alkaloids advised by manufacturer of ● BOCEPREVIR and ● TELAPREVIR; increased risk of ergotism when ergot alkaloids given with ● DARUNAVIR—manufacturer of darunavir advises avoid concomitant use; increased risk of ergotism when ergot alkaloids given with ● EFAVIRENZ or ● RITONAVIR—avoid concomitant use; increased risk of ergotism when ergotamine given with ● FOSAMPRENAVIR, ● INDINAVIR or ● SAQUINAVIR—avoid concomitant use; increased risk of ergotism when ergometrine given with ● INDINAVIR—avoid concomitant use
- ▸ **Beta-blockers:** increased peripheral vasoconstriction when ergot alkaloids given with BETA-BLOCKERS
- **Cobicistat:** plasma concentration of ergot alkaloids possibly increased by ● COBICISTAT—manufacturer of cobicistat advises avoid concomitant use
- **Cytotoxics:** caution with ergot alkaloids advised by manufacturer of ● CRIZOTINIB; avoidance of ergotamine advised by manufacturer of ● IDELALISIB
- **5HT$_1$-receptor Agonists:** increased risk of vasospasm when ergotamine given with ● ALMOTRIPTAN, ● RIZATRIPTAN, ● SUMATRIPTAN or ● ZOLMITRIPTAN (avoid ergotamine for 6 hours after almotriptan, rizatriptan, sumatriptan or zolmitriptan; avoid almotriptan, rizatriptan, sumatriptan or zolmitriptan for 24 hours after ergotamine); increased risk of vasospasm when ergotamine given with ● ELETRIPTAN, ● FROVATRIPTAN or ● NARATRIPTAN (avoid ergotamine for 24 hours after eletriptan, frovatriptan or naratriptan, avoid eletriptan, frovatriptan or naratriptan for 24 hours after ergotamine)
- ▸ **Sympathomimetics:** increased risk of ergotism when ergot alkaloids given with SYMPATHOMIMETICS
- **Ticagrelor:** plasma concentration of ergot alkaloids possibly increased by ● TICAGRELOR
- **Ulcer-healing Drugs:** increased risk of ergotism when ergotamine given with ● CIMETIDINE—avoid concomitant use

Ergotamine *see* Ergot Alkaloids

Eribulin

- ▸ **Antibacterials:** plasma concentration of eribulin possibly reduced by RIFAMPICIN
- ▸ **Antidepressants:** plasma concentration of eribulin possibly reduced by ST JOHN'S WORT
- ▸ **Antiepileptics:** plasma concentration of eribulin possibly reduced by CARBAMAZEPINE, FOSPHENYTOIN and PHENYTOIN
- **Antipsychotics:** avoid concomitant use of cytotoxics with ● CLOZAPINE (increased risk of agranulocytosis)

Erlotinib

- **Analgesics:** increased risk of bleeding when erlotinib given with ● NSAIDS
- **Antacids:** plasma concentration of erlotinib possibly reduced by ● ANTACIDS—give antacids at least 4 hours before or 2 hours after erlotinib
- **Antibacterials:** plasma concentration of erlotinib increased by CIPROFLOXACIN; metabolism of erlotinib accelerated by RIFAMPICIN (reduced plasma concentration)
- **Anticoagulants:** increased risk of bleeding when erlotinib given with ● COUMARINS
- ▸ **Antifungals:** metabolism of erlotinib inhibited by KETOCONAZOLE (increased plasma concentration)

Erlotinib (continued)

- **Antipsychotics:** avoid concomitant use of cytotoxics with ● CLOZAPINE (increased risk of agranulocytosis)
- **Antivirals:** avoidance of erlotinib advised by manufacturer of ● BOCEPREVIR
- ▸ **Cytotoxics:** plasma concentration of erlotinib possibly increased by CAPECITABINE
- **Ulcer-healing Drugs:** manufacturer of erlotinib advises avoid concomitant use with ● CIMETIDINE, ● ESOMEPRAZOLE, ● FAMOTIDINE, ● LANSOPRAZOLE, ● NIZATIDINE, ● PANTOPRAZOLE and ● RABEPRAZOLE; plasma concentration of erlotinib reduced by ● RANITIDINE—manufacturer of erlotinib advises give at least 2 hours before or 10 hours after ranitidine; plasma concentration of erlotinib reduced by ● OMEPRAZOLE—manufacturer of erlotinib advises avoid concomitant use

Ertapenem

- **Antiepileptics:** carbapenems reduce plasma concentration of ● SODIUM VALPROATE and ● VALPROIC ACID—avoid concomitant use
- ▸ **Vaccines:** antibacterials inactivate ORAL TYPHOID VACCINE—see under Typhoid Vaccine in BNF

Erythromycin *see* Macrolides

Escitalopram *see* Antidepressants, SSRI

Eslicarbazepine

- ▸ **Anticoagulants:** eslicarbazepine reduces plasma concentration of WARFARIN
- **Antidepressants:** anticonvulsant effect of antiepileptics possibly antagonised by MAOIs and ● TRICYCLIC-RELATED ANTIDEPRESSANTS (convulsive threshold lowered); anticonvulsant effect of antiepileptics antagonised by ● SSRIS and ● TRICYCLICS (convulsive threshold lowered)
- ▸ **Antiepileptics:** plasma concentration of eslicarbazepine possibly reduced by CARBAMAZEPINE but risk of side-effects increased; plasma concentration of eslicarbazepine reduced by FOSPHENYTOIN and PHENYTOIN, also plasma concentration of fosphenytoin and phenytoin increased; manufacturer of eslicarbazepine advises avoid concomitant use with OXCARBAZEPINE
- **Antimalarials:** anticonvulsant effect of antiepileptics antagonised by ● MEFLOQUINE
- **Antipsychotics:** anticonvulsant effect of antiepileptics antagonised by ● ANTIPSYCHOTICS (convulsive threshold lowered)
- ▸ **Lipid-regulating Drugs:** eslicarbazepine reduces plasma concentration of ROSUVASTATIN; eslicarbazepine reduces plasma concentration of SIMVASTATIN—consider increasing dose of simvastatin
- **Oestrogens:** eslicarbazepine accelerates metabolism of ● OESTROGENS (reduced contraceptive effect with combined oral contraceptives, contraceptive patches, and vaginal rings—see Contraceptive Interactions in BNF)
- **Orlistat:** possible increased risk of convulsions when antiepileptics given with ● ORLISTAT
- **Progestogens:** eslicarbazepine accelerates metabolism of ● PROGESTOGENS (reduced contraceptive effect with combined oral contraceptives, progestogen-only oral contraceptives, contraceptive patches, vaginal rings, etonogestrel-releasing implant, and emergency hormonal contraception—see Contraceptive Interactions in BNF)

Esmolol *see* Beta-blockers

Esomeprazole *see* Proton Pump Inhibitors

Estradiol *see* Oestrogens

Estramustine

- ▸ **Antacids:** absorption of estramustine possibly reduced by ALUMINIUM HYDROXIDE and ORAL MAGNESIUM SALTS—manufacturer of estramustine advises avoid concomitant administration
- **Antipsychotics:** avoid concomitant use of cytotoxics with ● CLOZAPINE (increased risk of agranulocytosis)
- **Bisphosphonates:** plasma concentration of estramustine increased by ● SODIUM CLODRONATE
- ▸ **Calcium Salts:** absorption of estramustine reduced by CALCIUM SALTS (manufacturer of estramustine advises avoid concomitant administration)

Estriol *see* Oestrogens

Estrone *see* Oestrogens

Etanercept
- Abatacept: avoid concomitant use of etanercept with
  - ABATACEPT
- Anakinra: avoid concomitant use of etanercept with
  - ANAKINRA
- Vaccines: risk of generalised infections when etanercept given with live ● VACCINES—avoid concomitant use

Ethambutol
▸ Antibacterials: plasma concentration of ethambutol increased by DELAMANID
▸ Vaccines: antibacterials inactivate ORAL TYPHOID VACCINE—see under Typhoid Vaccine in BNF

Ethinylestradiol *see* Oestrogens

Ethosuximide
- Antibacterials: metabolism of ethosuximide inhibited by ● ISONIAZID (increased plasma concentration and risk of toxicity)
- Antidepressants: anticonvulsant effect of antiepileptics possibly antagonised by MAOIs and ● TRICYCLIC-RELATED ANTIDEPRESSANTS (convulsive threshold lowered); anticonvulsant effect of antiepileptics antagonised by ● SSRIs and ● TRICYCLICS (convulsive threshold lowered)
- Antiepileptics: plasma concentration of ethosuximide possibly reduced by CARBAMAZEPINE, PHENOBARBITAL and PRIMIDONE; plasma concentration of ethosuximide possibly reduced by ● FOSPHENYTOIN and ● PHENYTOIN, also plasma concentration of fosphenytoin and phenytoin possibly increased; plasma concentration of ethosuximide possibly increased by SODIUM VALPROATE and VALPROIC ACID
- Antimalarials: anticonvulsant effect of antiepileptics antagonised by ● MEFLOQUINE
- Antipsychotics: anticonvulsant effect of antiepileptics antagonised by ● ANTIPSYCHOTICS (convulsive threshold lowered)
- Orlistat: possible increased risk of convulsions when antiepileptics given with ● ORLISTAT

Etodolac *see* NSAIDs

Etomidate *see* Anaesthetics, General

Etonogestrel *see* Progestogens

Etoposide
- Anticoagulants: etoposide possibly enhances anticoagulant effect of ● COUMARINS
▸ Antiepileptics: plasma concentration of etoposide possibly reduced by FOSPHENYTOIN, PHENOBARBITAL, PHENYTOIN and PRIMIDONE
▸ Antifungals: plasma concentration of etoposide increased by KETOCONAZOLE
- Antipsychotics: avoid concomitant use of cytotoxics with ● CLOZAPINE (increased risk of agranulocytosis)
▸ Atovaquone: plasma concentration of etoposide possibly increased by ATOVAQUONE
▸ Ciclosporin: plasma concentration of etoposide possibly increased by CICLOSPORIN (increased risk of toxicity)
▸ Netupitant: plasma concentration of etoposide increased by NETUPITANT

Etoricoxib *see* NSAIDs

Etravirine
- Antibacterials: etravirine reduces plasma concentration of ● CLARITHROMYCIN (but concentration of an active metabolite increased), also plasma concentration of etravirine increased; plasma concentration of both drugs reduced when etravirine given with ● RIFABUTIN; manufacturer of etravirine advises avoid concomitant use with RIFAMPICIN; etravirine possibly reduces plasma concentration of ● BEDAQUILINE—manufacturer of bedaquiline advises avoid concomitant use
▸ Antidepressants: manufacturer of etravirine advises avoid concomitant use with ST JOHN'S WORT
▸ Antiepileptics: manufacturer of etravirine advises avoid concomitant use with CARBAMAZEPINE, FOSPHENYTOIN, PHENOBARBITAL, PHENYTOIN and PRIMIDONE
▸ Antimalarials: etravirine reduces plasma concentration of ARTEMETHER WITH LUMEFANTRINE
- Antivirals: effects of both drugs possibly reduced when etravirine given with BOCEPREVIR; avoidance of etravirine advised by manufacturer of DACLATASVIR (plasma concentration of daclatasvir possibly reduced); avoidance of

Etravirine
- Antivirals (continued)
  etravirine advised by manufacturer of DASABUVIR, OMBITASVIR, PARITAPREVIR and SIMEPREVIR; etravirine reduces the plasma concentration of ● DOLUTEGRAVIR (see under Dolutegravir, p. 584); plasma concentration of etravirine possibly reduced by ● EFAVIRENZ and ● NEVIRAPINE—avoid concomitant use; etravirine increases plasma concentration of ● FOSAMPRENAVIR (consider reducing dose of fosamprenavir); etravirine possibly reduces plasma concentration of ● INDINAVIR—avoid concomitant use; etravirine possibly reduces plasma concentration of MARAVIROC; plasma concentration of etravirine reduced by ● TIPRANAVIR, also plasma concentration of tipranavir increased (avoid concomitant use)
▸ Cardiac Glycosides: etravirine increases plasma concentration of DIGOXIN
- Clopidogrel: etravirine possibly reduces antiplatelet effect of ● CLOPIDOGREL
- Cytotoxics: etravirine possibly reduces plasma concentration of ● BOSUTINIB—manufacturer of bosutinib advises avoid concomitant use
- Guanfacine: etravirine possibly reduces plasma concentration of ● GUANFACINE—increase dose of guanfacine
▸ Lipid-regulating Drugs: etravirine possibly reduces plasma concentration of ATORVASTATIN
- Orlistat: absorption of etravirine possibly reduced by ● ORLISTAT
▸ Sildenafil: etravirine reduces plasma concentration of SILDENAFIL

Everolimus
- ACE Inhibitors: increased risk of angioedema when everolimus given with ● ACE INHIBITORS
- Antibacterials: plasma concentration of everolimus possibly increased by ● CLARITHROMYCIN and ● TELITHROMYCIN—manufacturer of everolimus advises avoid concomitant use; plasma concentration of everolimus increased by ● ERYTHROMYCIN (consider reducing the dose of everolimus — consult everolimus product literature); plasma concentration of everolimus reduced by ● RIFAMPICIN (avoid concomitant use or consider increasing the dose of everolimus —consult everolimus product literature)
▸ Antidepressants: plasma concentration of everolimus possibly reduced by ST JOHN'S WORT—manufacturer of everolimus advises avoid concomitant use
- Antifungals: plasma concentration of everolimus increased by ● KETOCONAZOLE—manufacturer of ketoconazole advises avoid concomitant use; plasma concentration of everolimus possibly increased by ● ITRACONAZOLE, ● POSACONAZOLE and ● VORICONAZOLE—manufacturer of everolimus advises avoid concomitant use
- Antipsychotics: avoid concomitant use of cytotoxics with ● CLOZAPINE (increased risk of agranulocytosis)
- Antivirals: plasma concentration of everolimus possibly increased by ● ATAZANAVIR, ● DARUNAVIR, ● INDINAVIR, ● RITONAVIR and ● SAQUINAVIR—manufacturer of everolimus advises avoid concomitant use
- Calcium-channel Blockers: plasma concentration of both drugs may increase when everolimus given with ● VERAPAMIL (consider reducing the dose of everolimus —consult everolimus product literature)
- Ciclosporin: plasma concentration of everolimus increased by ● CICLOSPORIN (consider reducing the dose of everolimus — consult everolimus product literature)
- Cytotoxics: plasma concentration of everolimus increased by ● IMATINIB (consider reducing the dose of everolimus —consult everolimus product literature)
▸ Grapefruit Juice: manufacturer of everolimus advises avoid concomitant use with GRAPEFRUIT JUICE

Exemestane
▸ Antibacterials: plasma concentration of exemestane possibly reduced by RIFAMPICIN

Exenatide *see* Antidiabetics

Ezetimibe
▸ Anticoagulants: ezetimibe possibly enhances anticoagulant effect of COUMARINS

Ezetimibe (continued)
- Ciclosporin: plasma concentration of both drugs may increase when ezetimibe given with ● CICLOSPORIN
- Lipid-regulating Drugs: ezetimibe increases plasma concentration of ● ROSUVASTATIN—adjust dose of rosuvastatin (consult product literature); increased risk of cholelithiasis and gallbladder disease when ezetimibe given with FIBRATES—discontinue if suspected

Famotidine see Histamine H_2-antagonists
Fampridine
- Ulcer-healing Drugs: manufacturer of fampridine advises avoid concomitant use with ● CIMETIDINE

Febuxostat
- Azathioprine: manufacturer of febuxostat advises avoid concomitant use with ● AZATHIOPRINE
- Cytotoxics: manufacturer of febuxostat advises avoid concomitant use with ● MERCAPTOPURINE

Felodipine see Calcium-channel Blockers
Fenofibrate see Fibrates
Fenoprofen see NSAIDs
Fentanyl see Opioid Analgesics
Ferrous Fumarate see Iron salts
Ferrous Gluconate see Iron salts
Ferrous Sulfate see Iron salts
Fesoterodine see Antimuscarinics
Fexofenadine see Antihistamines
Fibrates
- Antibacterials: increased risk of myopathy when fibrates given with ● DAPTOMYCIN (preferably avoid concomitant use)
- Anticoagulants: fibrates enhance anticoagulant effect of ● COUMARINS and ● PHENINDIONE
- Antidiabetics: fibrates may improve glucose tolerance and have an additive effect with INSULIN or SULFONYLUREAS; gemfibrozil possibly enhances hypoglycaemic effect of NATEGLINIDE; increased risk of severe hypoglycaemia when gemfibrozil given with ● REPAGLINIDE—avoid concomitant use
- Antivirals: avoidance of gemfibrozil advised by manufacturer of DASABUVIR; gemfibrozil increases plasma concentration of ● PARITAPREVIR—manufacturer of paritaprevir advises avoid concomitant use
- Ciclosporin: increased risk of renal impairment when bezafibrate or fenofibrate given with CICLOSPORIN
- Colchicine: possible increased risk of myopathy when fibrates given with ● COLCHICINE
- Cytotoxics: gemfibrozil increases plasma concentration of DABRAFENIB; gemfibrozil increases plasma concentration of ● BEXAROTENE—avoid concomitant use
- Hormone Antagonists: gemfibrozil increases plasma concentration of ● ENZALUTAMIDE—manufacturer of enzalutamide advises avoid concomitant use or halve dose of enzalutamide
- Leukotriene Receptor Antagonists: gemfibrozil increases plasma concentration of MONTELUKAST
- Lipid-regulating Drugs: increased risk of myopathy when gemfibrozil given with ● ATORVASTATIN, ● FLUVASTATIN or ● PRAVASTATIN (preferably avoid concomitant use); increased risk of myopathy when fibrates given with ● ROSUVASTATIN (see under Rosuvastatin, p. 188); possible increased risk of myopathy with bezafibrate given with ● SIMVASTATIN (see under Simvastatin, p. 188); possible increased risk of myopathy when ciprofibrate given with ● SIMVASTATIN (see under Simvastatin, p. 188); increased risk of myopathy when gemfibrozil given with ● SIMVASTATIN (avoid concomitant use); increased risk of cholelithiasis and gallbladder disease when fibrates given with EZETIMIBE—discontinue if suspected; increased risk of myopathy when fibrates given with ● STATINS; reduce maximum dose of fenofibrate when given with STATINS—see under Fenofibrate, p. 183

Fidaxomicin
- Anti-arrhythmics: manufacturer of fidaxomicin advises avoid concomitant use with AMIODARONE and DRONEDARONE
- Antibacterials: manufacturer of fidaxomicin advises avoid concomitant use with CLARITHROMYCIN and ERYTHROMYCIN
- Antifungals: manufacturer of fidaxomicin advises avoid concomitant use with KETOCONAZOLE

Fidaxomicin (continued)
- Calcium-channel Blockers: manufacturer of fidaxomicin advises avoid concomitant use with VERAPAMIL
- Ciclosporin: manufacturer of fidaxomicin advises avoid concomitant use with CICLOSPORIN
- Vaccines: antibacterials inactivate ORAL TYPHOID VACCINE—see under Typhoid Vaccine in BNF

Filgrastim
- Cytotoxics: neutropenia possibly exacerbated when filgrastim given with CAPECITABINE, FLUOROURACIL or TEGAFUR

Fingolimod
- Anti-arrhythmics: possible increased risk of bradycardia when fingolimod given with ● AMIODARONE, ● DISOPYRAMIDE or ● DRONEDARONE
- Antidepressants: plasma concentration of fingolimod possibly reduced by ST JOHN'S WORT—manufacturer of fingolimod advises avoid concomitant use
- Antiepileptics: plasma concentration of fingolimod reduced by CARBAMAZEPINE
- Antifungals: plasma concentration of fingolimod increased by ● KETOCONAZOLE
- Beta-blockers: possible increased risk of bradycardia when fingolimod given with ● BETA-BLOCKERS
- Calcium-channel Blockers: possible increased risk of bradycardia when fingolimod given with ● DILTIAZEM or ● VERAPAMIL

Flavoxate see Antimuscarinics
Flecainide
- Anaesthetics, Local: increased myocardial depression when anti-arrhythmics given with BUPIVACAINE, LEVOBUPIVACAINE, PRILOCAINE or ROPIVACAINE
- Anti-arrhythmics: increased myocardial depression when anti-arrhythmics given with other ● ANTI-ARRHYTHMICS; plasma concentration of flecainide increased by ● AMIODARONE (halve dose of flecainide)
- Antidepressants: plasma concentration of flecainide increased by FLUOXETINE; increased risk of ventricular arrhythmias when flecainide given with ● TRICYCLICS
- Antihistamines: increased risk of ventricular arrhythmias when flecainide given with ● MIZOLASTINE—avoid concomitant use
- Antimalarials: avoidance of flecainide advised by manufacturer of ● ARTEMETHER WITH LUMEFANTRINE (risk of ventricular arrhythmias); plasma concentration of flecainide increased by ● QUININE
- Antimuscarinics: increased risk of ventricular arrhythmias when flecainide given with ● TOLTERODINE
- Antipsychotics: increased risk of ventricular arrhythmias when anti-arrhythmics that prolong the QT interval given with ● ANTIPSYCHOTICS that prolong the QT interval; increased risk of arrhythmias when flecainide given with ● CLOZAPINE
- Antivirals: plasma concentration of flecainide possibly increased by ● FOSAMPRENAVIR, ● INDINAVIR, ● LOPINAVIR and ● RITONAVIR (increased risk of ventricular arrhythmias—avoid concomitant use); increased risk of ventricular arrhythmias when flecainide given with ● SAQUINAVIR—avoid concomitant use; caution with flecainide advised by manufacturer of ● TELAPREVIR (risk of ventricular arrhythmias)
- Beta-blockers: increased risk of myocardial depression and bradycardia when flecainide given with ● BETA-BLOCKERS; increased myocardial depression when anti-arrhythmics given with ● BETA-BLOCKERS
- Calcium-channel Blockers: increased risk of myocardial depression and asystole when flecainide given with ● VERAPAMIL
- Diuretics: increased cardiac toxicity with flecainide if hypokalaemia occurs with ● ACETAZOLAMIDE, ● LOOP DIURETICS or ● THIAZIDES AND RELATED DIURETICS
- Ulcer-healing Drugs: metabolism of flecainide inhibited by CIMETIDINE (increased plasma concentration)

Flucloxacillin see Penicillins
Fluconazole see Antifungals, Triazole
Flucytosine
- Antifungals: renal excretion of flucytosine decreased and cellular uptake increased by AMPHOTERICIN (toxicity possibly increased)
- Cytotoxics: plasma concentration of flucytosine possibly reduced by CYTARABINE

A1

Interactions | Appendix 1

Fludarabine

- Antipsychotics: avoid concomitant use of cytotoxics with ● CLOZAPINE (increased risk of agranulocytosis)
- Cytotoxics: fludarabine increases intracellular concentration of CYTARABINE; increased pulmonary toxicity when fludarabine given with ● PENTOSTATIN (unacceptably high incidence of fatalities)
- ▶ Dipyridamole: effects of fludarabine possibly reduced by DIPYRIDAMOLE

Fludrocortisone see Corticosteroids

Fluorides

- ▶ Calcium Salts: absorption of fluorides reduced by CALCIUM SALTS

Fluorouracil

- ▶ Antibacterials: metabolism of fluorouracil inhibited by METRONIDAZOLE (increased toxicity)
- Anticoagulants: fluorouracil enhances anticoagulant effect of ● COUMARINS
- Antiepileptics: fluorouracil possibly inhibits metabolism of FOSPHENYTOIN and PHENYTOIN (increased risk of toxicity)
- Antipsychotics: avoid concomitant use of cytotoxics with ● CLOZAPINE (increased risk of agranulocytosis)
- Cytotoxics: avoidance of fluorouracil advised by manufacturer of ● PANITUMUMAB
- Filgrastim: neutropenia possibly exacerbated when fluorouracil given with FILGRASTIM
- Folates: toxicity of fluorouracil increased by ● FOLIC ACID— avoid concomitant use
- Lipegfilgrastim: neutropenia possibly exacerbated when fluorouracil given with LIPEGFILGRASTIM
- Pegfilgrastim: neutropenia possibly exacerbated when fluorouracil given with PEGFILGRASTIM
- Temoporfin: increased skin photosensitivity when *topical* fluorouracil used with ● TEMOPORFIN
- ▶ Ulcer-healing Drugs: metabolism of fluorouracil inhibited by CIMETIDINE (increased plasma concentration)

Fluoxetine see Antidepressants, SSRI

Flupentixol see Antipsychotics

Fluphenazine see Antipsychotics

Flurazepam see Anxiolytics and Hypnotics

Flurbiprofen see NSAIDs

Flutamide

- Anticoagulants: flutamide enhances anticoagulant effect of ● COUMARINS

Fluticasone see Corticosteroids

Fluvastatin see Statins

Fluvoxamine see Antidepressants, SSRI

Folates

- ▶ Aminosalicylates: absorption of folic acid possibly reduced by SULFASALAZINE
- ▶ Antacids: absorption of folic acid possibly reduced by ANTACIDS (manufacturer of folic acid advises give at least 2 hours apart)
- ▶ Antiepileptics: folates possibly reduce plasma concentration of FOSPHENYTOIN, PHENOBARBITAL, PHENYTOIN and PRIMIDONE
- Cytotoxics: folic acid increases toxicity of ● CAPECITABINE, ● FLUOROURACIL and ● TEGAFUR—avoid concomitant use; avoidance of folates advised by manufacturer of ● RALTITREXED; avoidance of folinic acid advised by manufacturer of ● PANITUMUMAB

Folic Acid see Folates

Folinic Acid see Folates

Fondaparinux

- Analgesics: increased risk of haemorrhage when anticoagulants given with *intravenous* ● DICLOFENAC (avoid concomitant use, including low-dose heparins); increased risk of haemorrhage when anticoagulants given with ● KETOROLAC (avoid concomitant use, including low-dose heparins)
- Anticoagulants: increased risk of haemorrhage when other anticoagulants given with ● APIXABAN, ● DABIGATRAN, ● EDOXABAN and ● RIVAROXABAN (avoid concomitant use except when switching with other anticoagulants or using heparin to maintain catheter patency)

Formoterol see Sympathomimetics, Beta$_2$

Fosamprenavir

NOTE Fosamprenavir is a prodrug of amprenavir

- ▶ Analgesics: fosamprenavir reduces plasma concentration of METHADONE

Fosamprenavir (continued)

- Anti-arrhythmics: fosamprenavir possibly increases plasma concentration of ● AMIODARONE, ● FLECAINIDE and ● PROPAFENONE (increased risk of ventricular arrhythmias— avoid concomitant use); fosamprenavir possibly increases plasma concentration of ● LIDOCAINE—avoid concomitant use
- Antibacterials: fosamprenavir increases plasma concentration of ● RIFABUTIN (reduce dose of rifabutin); plasma concentration of fosamprenavir significantly reduced by ● RIFAMPICIN—avoid concomitant use; avoidance of concomitant fosamprenavir in severe renal and hepatic impairment advised by manufacturer of ● TELITHROMYCIN
- ▶ Anticoagulants: avoidance of fosamprenavir advised by manufacturer of APIXABAN and RIVAROXABAN; fosamprenavir may enhance or reduce anticoagulant effect of COUMARINS
- Antidepressants: plasma concentration of fosamprenavir reduced by ● ST JOHN'S WORT—avoid concomitant use
- ▶ Antiepileptics: plasma concentration of fosamprenavir possibly reduced by CARBAMAZEPINE, PHENOBARBITAL and PRIMIDONE
- Antifungals: fosamprenavir increases plasma concentration of KETOCONAZOLE (also plasma concentration of fosamprenavir possibly increased); plasma concentration of both drugs may increase when fosamprenavir given with ITRACONAZOLE; fosamprenavir possibly reduces plasma concentration of POSACONAZOLE
- Antimalarials: caution with fosamprenavir advised by manufacturer of ARTEMETHER WITH LUMEFANTRINE; fosamprenavir possibly increases plasma concentration of ● QUININE (increased risk of toxicity)
- ▶ Antimuscarinics: avoidance of fosamprenavir advised by manufacturer of DARIFENACIN and TOLTERODINE
- Antipsychotics: fosamprenavir possibly increases plasma concentration of ● ARIPIPRAZOLE (reduce dose of aripiprazole—consult aripiprazole product literature); fosamprenavir increases plasma concentration of ● PIMOZIDE (increased risk of ventricular arrhythmias—avoid concomitant use); fosamprenavir possibly increases plasma concentration of ● QUETIAPINE—manufacturer of quetiapine advises avoid concomitant use
- Antivirals: manufacturer of fosamprenavir advises avoid concomitant use with ● BOCEPREVIR and ● RALTEGRAVIR; fosamprenavir reduces plasma concentration of ● DOLUTEGRAVIR; plasma concentration of fosamprenavir increased by ● ETRAVIRINE (consider reducing dose of fosamprenavir); plasma concentration of fosamprenavir reduced by LOPINAVIR, effect on lopinavir plasma concentration not predictable—avoid concomitant use; plasma concentration of fosamprenavir reduced by ● MARAVIROC—avoid concomitant use; plasma concentration of fosamprenavir possibly reduced by NEVIRAPINE—avoid unboosted fosamprenavir; manufacturers advise avoid concomitant use of fosamprenavir with ● TELAPREVIR; plasma concentration of fosamprenavir reduced by ● TIPRANAVIR
- Anxiolytics and Hypnotics: fosamprenavir possibly increases plasma concentration of ● MIDAZOLAM (risk of prolonged sedation—avoid concomitant use of *oral* midazolam)
- Avanafil: fosamprenavir possibly increases plasma concentration of ● AVANAFIL—see under Avanafil, p. 735
- Ciclosporin: fosamprenavir increases plasma concentration of ● CICLOSPORIN
- Cytotoxics: fosamprenavir possibly increases the plasma concentration of ● BOSUTINIB—manufacturer of bosutinib advises avoid or consider reducing dose of bosutinib; fosamprenavir possibly increases the plasma concentration of ● IBRUTINIB—reduce dose of ibrutinib (see under Ibrutinib, p. 855)
- ▶ Dapoxetine: manufacturer of dapoxetine advises dose reduction when fosamprenavir given with DAPOXETINE (see under Dapoxetine, p. 742)
- Ergot Alkaloids: increased risk of ergotism when fosamprenavir given with ● ERGOTAMINE—avoid concomitant use
- ▶ Guanfacine: fosamprenavir possibly increases plasma concentration of GUANFACINE (halve dose of guanfacine)
- Lipid-regulating Drugs: possible increased risk of myopathy when fosamprenavir given with ATORVASTATIN; possible increased risk of myopathy when fosamprenavir given with

Fosamprenavir

- Lipid-regulating Drugs (continued)
  - ROSUVASTATIN—manufacturer of rosuvastatin advises avoid concomitant use; possible increased risk of myopathy when fosamprenavir given with • SIMVASTATIN—avoid concomitant use; avoidance of fosamprenavir advised by manufacturer of • LOMITAPIDE (plasma concentration of lomitapide possibly increased)
- Orlistat: absorption of fosamprenavir possibly reduced by • ORLISTAT
- Ranolazine: fosamprenavir possibly increases plasma concentration of • RANOLAZINE—manufacturer of ranolazine advises avoid concomitant use
- Sildenafil: fosamprenavir possibly increases plasma concentration of SILDENAFIL
- Tacrolimus: fosamprenavir increases plasma concentration of • TACROLIMUS
- Tadalafil: fosamprenavir possibly increases plasma concentration of TADALAFIL
- Vardenafil: fosamprenavir possibly increases plasma concentration of VARDENAFIL

Fosaprepitant

- Antibacterials: plasma concentration of fosaprepitant possibly increased by CLARITHROMYCIN and TELITHROMYCIN; plasma concentration of fosaprepitant reduced by RIFAMPICIN
- Anticoagulants: fosaprepitant possibly reduces anticoagulant effect of WARFARIN
- Antidepressants: manufacturer of fosaprepitant advises avoid concomitant use with • ST JOHN'S WORT
- Antidiabetics: fosaprepitant reduces plasma concentration of TOLBUTAMIDE
- Antiepileptics: plasma concentration of fosaprepitant possibly reduced by CARBAMAZEPINE, FOSPHENYTOIN, PHENOBARBITAL, PHENYTOIN and PRIMIDONE
- Antifungals: plasma concentration of fosaprepitant increased by KETOCONAZOLE
- Antipsychotics: manufacturer of fosaprepitant advises avoid concomitant use with • PIMOZIDE
- Antivirals: plasma concentration of fosaprepitant possibly increased by RITONAVIR
- Anxiolytics and Hypnotics: fosaprepitant increases plasma concentration of MIDAZOLAM (risk of prolonged sedation)
- Avanafil: fosaprepitant possibly increases plasma concentration of AVANAFIL
- Calcium-channel Blockers: plasma concentration of both drugs may increase when fosaprepitant given with DILTIAZEM
- Corticosteroids: fosaprepitant inhibits metabolism of DEXAMETHASONE and METHYLPREDNISOLONE (reduce dose of dexamethasone and methylprednisolone)
- Cytotoxics: fosaprepitant possibly increases the plasma concentration of • BOSUTINIB—manufacturer of bosutinib advises avoid or consider reducing dose of bosutinib; fosaprepitant possibly increases plasma concentration of IBRUTINIB
- Guanfacine: fosaprepitant possibly increases plasma concentration of GUANFACINE (halve dose of guanfacine)
- Lipid-regulating Drugs: separating administration from fosaprepitant by 12 hours advised by manufacturer of LOMITAPIDE
- Oestrogens: fosaprepitant possibly causes contraceptive failure of hormonal contraceptives containing • OESTROGENS (alternative contraception recommended)
- Progestogens: fosaprepitant possibly causes contraceptive failure of hormonal contraceptives containing • PROGESTOGENS (alternative contraception recommended)

Foscarnet

- Pentamidine Isetionate: increased risk of hypocalcaemia when foscarnet given with *parenteral* • PENTAMIDINE ISETIONATE

Fosfomycin

- Metoclopramide: plasma concentration of fosfomycin reduced by METOCLOPRAMIDE
- Vaccines: antibacterials inactivate ORAL TYPHOID VACCINE—see under Typhoid Vaccine in BNF

Fosinopril see ACE Inhibitors

Fosphenytoin

- Alcohol: plasma concentration of fosphenytoin possibly reduced by chronic heavy consumption of ALCOHOL
- Aminophylline: plasma concentration of both drugs reduced when fosphenytoin given with • AMINOPHYLLINE
- Analgesics: excretion of fosphenytoin possibly reduced by ACEMETACIN (increased risk of toxicity); fosphenytoin possibly accelerates metabolism of FENTANYL (reduced effect); fosphenytoin accelerates metabolism of METHADONE (reduced effect and risk of withdrawal effects); fosphenytoin possibly increases risk of • PETHIDINE toxicity; effects of fosphenytoin enhanced by ASPIRIN; fosphenytoin possibly accelerates metabolism of PARACETAMOL (also isolated reports of hepatotoxicity)
- Antacids: absorption of fosphenytoin reduced by ANTACIDS
- Anthelmintics: fosphenytoin reduces plasma concentration of • ALBENDAZOLE and • PRAZIQUANTEL—consider increasing albendazole and praziquantel dose when given for systemic infections; plasma concentration of fosphenytoin possibly increased by LEVAMISOLE
- Anti-arrhythmics: metabolism of fosphenytoin inhibited by • AMIODARONE (increased plasma concentration); fosphenytoin reduces plasma concentration of DISOPYRAMIDE; fosphenytoin possibly reduces plasma concentration of • DRONEDARONE—avoid concomitant use
- Antibacterials: metabolism of fosphenytoin inhibited by CLARITHROMYCIN (increased plasma concentration); metabolism of fosphenytoin possibly inhibited by METRONIDAZOLE (increased plasma concentration); plasma concentration of fosphenytoin increased or decreased by CIPROFLOXACIN; fosphenytoin accelerates metabolism of DOXYCYCLINE (reduced plasma concentration); fosphenytoin possibly reduces plasma concentration of • BEDAQUILINE—manufacturer of bedaquiline advises avoid concomitant use; plasma concentration of fosphenytoin increased by • CHLORAMPHENICOL (increased risk of toxicity); metabolism of fosphenytoin possibly inhibited by ISONIAZID (increased risk of toxicity); metabolism of fosphenytoin accelerated by • RIFAMYCINS (reduced plasma concentration); plasma concentration of fosphenytoin possibly increased by SULFONAMIDES; fosphenytoin reduces plasma concentration of • TELITHROMYCIN (avoid during and for 2 weeks after fosphenytoin); plasma concentration of fosphenytoin increased by • TRIMETHOPRIM (also increased antifolate effect)
- Anticoagulants: fosphenytoin possibly reduces plasma concentration of • APIXABAN and • EDOXABAN; fosphenytoin accelerates metabolism of COUMARINS (possibility of reduced anticoagulant effect, but enhancement also reported); fosphenytoin possibly reduces plasma concentration of DABIGATRAN—manufacturer of dabigatran advises avoid concomitant use; fosphenytoin possibly reduces plasma concentration of • RIVAROXABAN—manufacturer of rivaroxaban advises monitor for signs of thrombosis
- Antidepressants: plasma concentration of fosphenytoin increased by • FLUOXETINE and • FLUVOXAMINE; fosphenytoin reduces plasma concentration of • MIANSERIN, MIRTAZAPINE and PAROXETINE; plasma concentration of fosphenytoin possibly increased by SERTRALINE, also plasma concentration of sertraline possibly reduced; anticonvulsant effect of antiepileptics possibly antagonised by MAOIs and • TRICYCLIC-RELATED ANTIDEPRESSANTS (convulsive threshold lowered); anticonvulsant effect of antiepileptics antagonised by • SSRIS and • TRICYCLICS (convulsive threshold lowered); plasma concentration of fosphenytoin possibly reduced by • ST JOHN'S WORT—avoid concomitant use; fosphenytoin possibly reduces plasma concentration of • TRICYCLICS; fosphenytoin possibly reduces plasma concentration of • VORTIOXETINE—consider increasing dose of vortioxetine
- Antidiabetics: plasma concentration of fosphenytoin transiently increased by TOLBUTAMIDE (possibility of toxicity)
- Antiepileptics: plasma concentration of both drugs often reduced when fosphenytoin given with CARBAMAZEPINE, also plasma concentration of fosphenytoin may be increased; fosphenytoin reduces plasma concentration of ESLICARBAZEPINE, also plasma concentration of fosphenytoin increased; plasma concentration of fosphenytoin possibly

Fosphenytoin

- **Antiepileptics** (continued)
  increased by ● ETHOSUXIMIDE, also plasma concentration of ethosuximide possibly reduced; fosphenytoin reduces plasma concentration of LAMOTRIGINE, TIAGABINE and ZONISAMIDE; plasma concentration of fosphenytoin increased by OXCARBAZEPINE, also plasma concentration of an active metabolite of oxcarbazepine reduced; fosphenytoin reduces plasma concentration of ● PERAMPANEL (see under Perampanel, p. 293); fosphenytoin often increases plasma concentration of PHENOBARBITAL and PRIMIDONE, plasma concentration of fosphenytoin often reduced but may be increased; fosphenytoin possibly reduces plasma concentration of RETIGABINE; fosphenytoin possibly reduces plasma concentration of RUFINAMIDE, also plasma concentration of fosphenytoin possibly increased; plasma concentration of fosphenytoin increased or possibly reduced when given with SODIUM VALPROATE and VALPROIC ACID, also plasma concentration of sodium valproate and valproic acid reduced; plasma concentration of fosphenytoin increased by ● STIRIPENTOL; plasma concentration of fosphenytoin increased by ● TOPIRAMATE (also plasma concentration of topiramate reduced); plasma concentration of fosphenytoin reduced by VIGABATRIN
- **Antifungals:** fosphenytoin reduces plasma concentration of ● KETOCONAZOLE and ● POSACONAZOLE; anticonvulsant effect of fosphenytoin enhanced by ● MICONAZOLE (plasma concentration of fosphenytoin increased); plasma concentration of fosphenytoin increased by ● FLUCONAZOLE (consider reducing dose of fosphenytoin); fosphenytoin reduces plasma concentration of ● ITRACONAZOLE—avoid concomitant use; plasma concentration of fosphenytoin increased by ● VORICONAZOLE, also fosphenytoin reduces plasma concentration of voriconazole (increase dose of voriconazole and also monitor for fosphenytoin toxicity); fosphenytoin possibly reduces plasma concentration of CASPOFUNGIN—consider increasing dose of caspofungin
- **Antimalarials:** avoidance of fosphenytoin advised by manufacturer of ARTENIMOL WITH PIPERAQUINE; anticonvulsant effect of antiepileptics antagonised by ● MEFLOQUINE; anticonvulsant effect of fosphenytoin antagonised by ● PYRIMETHAMINE, also increased antifolate effect
- **Antipsychotics:** anticonvulsant effect of antiepileptics antagonised by ● ANTIPSYCHOTICS (convulsive threshold lowered); fosphenytoin reduces plasma concentration of HALOPERIDOL; plasma concentration of fosphenytoin possibly increased or decreased by CHLORPROMAZINE; fosphenytoin possibly reduces plasma concentration of ● ARIPIPRAZOLE (avoid concomitant use or consider increasing the dose of aripiprazole—consult aripiprazole product literature); fosphenytoin accelerates metabolism of CLOZAPINE and QUETIAPINE (reduced plasma concentration); fosphenytoin possibly reduces plasma concentration of ● LURASIDONE—avoid concomitant use
- **Antivirals:** fosphenytoin possibly reduces plasma concentration of ABACAVIR, DARUNAVIR, LOPINAVIR and SAQUINAVIR; avoidance of fosphenytoin advised by manufacturer of ● BOCEPREVIR and ● RILPIVIRINE (plasma concentration of boceprevir and rilpivirine possibly reduced); fosphenytoin possibly reduces plasma concentration of ● DACLATASVIR and ● SIMEPREVIR—manufacturer of daclatasvir and simeprevir advises avoid concomitant use; fosphenytoin possibly reduces plasma concentration of ● DASABUVIR, ● OMBITASVIR and ● PARITAPREVIR—avoid concomitant use; fosphenytoin possibly reduces plasma concentration of ● DOLUTEGRAVIR (see under Dolutegravir, p. 584); avoidance of fosphenytoin advised by manufacturer of ● ELVITEGRAVIR, ETRAVIRINE, LEDIPASVIR, SOFOSBUVIR and ● TELAPREVIR; fosphenytoin possibly reduces plasma concentration of ● INDINAVIR, also plasma concentration of fosphenytoin possibly increased; fosphenytoin possibly reduces plasma concentration of RITONAVIR, also plasma concentration of fosphenytoin possibly affected; plasma concentration of fosphenytoin increased or decreased by ZIDOVUDINE
- **Anxiolytics and Hypnotics:** fosphenytoin often reduces plasma concentration of CLONAZEPAM; plasma concentration of

Fosphenytoin

Anxiolytics and Hypnotics (continued)
fosphenytoin increased or decreased by DIAZEPAM; plasma concentration of fosphenytoin possibly increased or decreased by BENZODIAZEPINES
- **Aprepitant:** fosphenytoin possibly reduces plasma concentration of APREPITANT
- **Bupropion:** fosphenytoin reduces plasma concentration of BUPROPION
- **Caffeine citrate:** fosphenytoin reduces plasma concentration of CAFFEINE CITRATE
- **Calcium-channel Blockers:** fosphenytoin reduces effects of FELODIPINE and VERAPAMIL; avoidance of fosphenytoin advised by manufacturer of ISRADIPINE; avoidance of fosphenytoin advised by manufacturer of NIMODIPINE (plasma concentration of nimodipine possibly reduced); plasma concentration of fosphenytoin increased by ● DILTIAZEM but also effect of diltiazem reduced
- **Cannabis Extract:** fosphenytoin possibly reduces plasma concentration of ● CANNABIS EXTRACT—manufacturer of cannabis extract advises avoid concomitant use
- **Cardiac Glycosides:** fosphenytoin possibly reduces plasma concentration of DIGOXIN
- **Ciclosporin:** fosphenytoin accelerates metabolism of ● CICLOSPORIN (reduced plasma concentration)
- **Cobicistat:** fosphenytoin possibly reduces plasma concentration of ● COBICISTAT—manufacturer of cobicistat advises avoid concomitant use
- **Corticosteroids:** fosphenytoin accelerates metabolism of ● CORTICOSTEROIDS (reduced effect)
- **Cytotoxics:** fosphenytoin possibly reduces plasma concentration of BUSULFAN, ERIBULIN and ETOPOSIDE; metabolism of fosphenytoin possibly inhibited by CAPECITABINE, FLUOROURACIL and TEGAFUR (increased risk of toxicity); fosphenytoin increases antifolate effect of METHOTREXATE; plasma concentration of fosphenytoin possibly reduced by CISPLATIN; fosphenytoin possibly decreases plasma concentration of AXITINIB (increase dose of axitinib—consult axitinib product literature); fosphenytoin possibly reduces plasma concentration of BORTEZOMIB, ● BOSUTINIB, CRIZOTINIB, ● IBRUTINIB, ● IDELALISIB and PONATINIB—manufacturer of bortezomib, bosutinib, crizotinib, ibrutinib, idelalisib and ponatinib advises avoid concomitant use; fosphenytoin possibly reduces plasma concentration of ● CABOZANTINIB—avoid concomitant use; avoidance of fosphenytoin advised by manufacturer of ● CABAZITAXEL, DABRAFENIB, GEFITINIB, ● LAPATINIB and VEMURAFENIB; avoidance of fosphenytoin advised by manufacturer of ● DASATINIB and ● VISMODEGIB (plasma concentration of dasatinib and vismodegib possibly reduced); fosphenytoin reduces plasma concentration of ● IMATINIB—avoid concomitant use; fosphenytoin reduces plasma concentration of IRINOTECAN and its active metabolite; manufacturer of procarbazine advises possible increased risk of hypersensitivity reactions when fosphenytoin given with PROCARBAZINE
- **Dexrazoxane:** absorption of fosphenytoin possibly reduced by ● DEXRAZOXANE
- **Diazoxide:** plasma concentration of fosphenytoin reduced by DIAZOXIDE, also effect of diazoxide may be reduced
- **Disulfiram:** metabolism of fosphenytoin inhibited by ● DISULFIRAM (increased risk of toxicity)
- **Diuretics:** plasma concentration of fosphenytoin possibly increased by ● ACETAZOLAMIDE; fosphenytoin antagonises effects of FUROSEMIDE; fosphenytoin reduces plasma concentration of ● EPLERENONE—avoid concomitant use; increased risk of osteomalacia when fosphenytoin given with CARBONIC ANHYDRASE INHIBITORS
- **Dopaminergics:** fosphenytoin possibly reduces effects of CO-BENELDOPA, CO-CARELDOPA and LEVODOPA
- **Enteral Feeds:** absorption of fosphenytoin possibly reduced by ENTERAL FEEDS
- **Folates:** plasma concentration of fosphenytoin possibly reduced by FOLATES
- **Fosaprepitant:** fosphenytoin possibly reduces plasma concentration of FOSAPREPITANT

Fosphenytoin (continued)
- Hormone Antagonists: fosphenytoin possibly reduces plasma concentration of ● ABIRATERONE—manufacturer of abiraterone advises avoid concomitant use; fosphenytoin possibly accelerates metabolism of TOREMIFENE
▹ 5HT₃-receptor Antagonists: fosphenytoin accelerates metabolism of ONDANSETRON (reduced effect)
- Ivacaftor: fosphenytoin possibly reduces plasma concentration of ● IVACAFTOR—manufacturer of ivacaftor advises avoid concomitant use
▹ Leflunomide: plasma concentration of fosphenytoin possibly increased by LEFLUNOMIDE
▹ Lipid-regulating Drugs: absorption of fosphenytoin possibly reduced by COLESEVELAM; combination of fosphenytoin with FLUVASTATIN may increase plasma concentration of either drug (or both)
▹ Lithium: neurotoxicity may occur when fosphenytoin given with LITHIUM without increased plasma concentration of lithium
▹ Macitentan: avoidance of fosphenytoin advised by manufacturer of MACITENTAN
▹ Modafinil: plasma concentration of fosphenytoin possibly increased by MODAFINIL
- Muscle Relaxants: *long-term use* of fosphenytoin reduces effects of ● NON-DEPOLARISING MUSCLE RELAXANTS (but *acute use* of fosphenytoin might increase effects of non-depolarising muscle relaxants)
- Oestrogens: fosphenytoin accelerates metabolism of ● OESTROGENS (reduced contraceptive effect with combined oral contraceptives, contraceptive patches, and vaginal rings—see Contraceptive Interactions in BNF)
- Orlistat: possible increased risk of convulsions when antiepileptics given with ● ORLISTAT
- Progestogens: fosphenytoin accelerates metabolism of ● PROGESTOGENS (reduced contraceptive effect with combined oral contraceptives, progestogen-only oral contraceptives, contraceptive patches, vaginal rings, etonogestrel-releasing implant, and emergency hormonal contraception—see Contraceptive Interactions in BNF)
▹ Roflumilast: fosphenytoin possibly inhibits effects of ROFLUMILAST (manufacturer of roflumilast advises avoid concomitant use)
- Sulfinpyrazone: plasma concentration of fosphenytoin increased by ● SULFINPYRAZONE
▹ Sympathomimetics: plasma concentration of fosphenytoin increased by METHYLPHENIDATE
▹ Tacrolimus: fosphenytoin reduces plasma concentration of TACROLIMUS, also plasma concentration of fosphenytoin possibly increased
- Theophylline: plasma concentration of both drugs reduced when fosphenytoin given with ● THEOPHYLLINE
▹ Thyroid Hormones: fosphenytoin accelerates metabolism of THYROID HORMONES (may increase requirements in hypothyroidism), also plasma concentration of fosphenytoin possibly increased
▹ Tibolone: fosphenytoin accelerates metabolism of TIBOLONE
▹ Ticagrelor: fosphenytoin possibly reduces plasma concentration of TICAGRELOR
- Ulcer-healing Drugs: metabolism of fosphenytoin inhibited by CIMETIDINE (increased plasma concentration); effects of fosphenytoin enhanced by ● ESOMEPRAZOLE; effects of fosphenytoin possibly enhanced by OMEPRAZOLE; absorption of fosphenytoin reduced by ● SUCRALFATE
- Ulipristal: avoidance of fosphenytoin advised by manufacturer of ● ULIPRISTAL (contraceptive effect of ulipristal possibly reduced)
▹ Vaccines: effects of fosphenytoin enhanced by INFLUENZA VACCINE
▹ Vitamins: fosphenytoin possibly increases requirements for ALFACALCIDOL, CALCITRIOL, COLECALCIFEROL, DIHYDROTACHYSTEROL, ERGOCALCIFEROL, PARICALCITOL or VITAMIN D

Frovatriptan *see* 5HT₁-receptor Agonists (under HT)
Furosemide *see* Diuretics

Fusidic Acid
- Antivirals: plasma concentration of both drugs increased when fusidic acid given with ● RITONAVIR—avoid concomitant use; plasma concentration of both drugs may increase when fusidic acid given with SAQUINAVIR
- Lipid-regulating Drugs: risk of myopathy and rhabdomyolysis when fusidic acid given with ● STATINS—avoid concomitant use and for 7 days after last fusidic acid dose
▹ Sugammadex: fusidic acid possibly reduces response to SUGAMMADEX
▹ Vaccines: antibacterials inactivate ORAL TYPHOID VACCINE—see under Typhoid Vaccine in BNF

Gabapentin
▹ Analgesics: bioavailability of gabapentin increased by MORPHINE
▹ Antacids: absorption of gabapentin reduced by ANTACIDS
- Antidepressants: anticonvulsant effect of antiepileptics possibly antagonised by MAOIs & ● TRICYCLIC-RELATED ANTIDEPRESSANTS (convulsive threshold lowered); anticonvulsant effect of antiepileptics antagonised by ● SSRIs and ● TRICYCLICS (convulsive threshold lowered)
- Antimalarials: anticonvulsant effect of antiepileptics antagonised by ● MEFLOQUINE
- Antipsychotics: anticonvulsant effect of antiepileptics antagonised by ● ANTIPSYCHOTICS (convulsive threshold lowered)
- Orlistat: possible increased risk of convulsions when antiepileptics given with ● ORLISTAT

Galantamine *see* Parasympathomimetics
Ganciclovir
NOTE Increased risk of myelosuppression with other myelosuppressive drugs—consult product literature
- Antibacterials: increased risk of convulsions when ganciclovir given with ● IMIPENEM WITH CILASTATIN
- Antivirals: ganciclovir possibly increases plasma concentration of DIDANOSINE; profound myelosuppression when ganciclovir given with ● ZIDOVUDINE (if possible avoid concomitant administration, particularly during initial ganciclovir therapy)
▹ Mycophenolate: plasma concentration of ganciclovir possibly increased by MYCOPHENOLATE, also plasma concentration of inactive metabolite of mycophenolate possibly increased
▹ Tacrolimus: possible increased risk of nephrotoxicity when ganciclovir given with TACROLIMUS

Gefitinib
- Antibacterials: plasma concentration of gefitinib reduced by ● RIFAMPICIN—avoid concomitant use
- Anticoagulants: gefitinib possibly enhances anticoagulant effect of ● WARFARIN
- Antidepressants: manufacturer of gefitinib advises avoid concomitant use with ST JOHN'S WORT
▹ Antiepileptics: manufacturer of gefitinib advises avoid concomitant use with CARBAMAZEPINE, FOSPHENYTOIN, PHENOBARBITAL, PHENYTOIN and PRIMIDONE
▹ Antifungals: plasma concentration of gefitinib increased by ITRACONAZOLE
- Antipsychotics: avoid concomitant use of cytotoxics with ● CLOZAPINE (increased risk of agranulocytosis)
- Antivirals: avoidance of gefitinib advised by manufacturer of ● BOCEPREVIR
- Ulcer-healing Drugs: plasma concentration of gefitinib reduced by ● RANITIDINE

Gemcitabine
▹ Anticoagulants: gemcitabine possibly enhances anticoagulant effect of WARFARIN
- Antipsychotics: avoid concomitant use of cytotoxics with ● CLOZAPINE (increased risk of agranulocytosis)

Gemeprost *see* Prostaglandins
Gemfibrozil *see* Fibrates
Gentamicin *see* Aminoglycosides
Gestodene *see* Progestogens
Glibenclamide *see* Antidiabetics
Gliclazide *see* Antidiabetics
Glimepiride *see* Antidiabetics
Glipizide *see* Antidiabetics

A1

Interactions | Appendix 1

Glucosamine
- Anticoagulants: glucosamine enhances anticoagulant effect of
  - WARFARIN (avoid concomitant use)

Glyceryl Trinitrate *see* Nitrates

Glycopyrronium *see* Antimuscarinics

Gold

NOTE *see* Sodium Aurothiomalate

Golimumab
- Abatacept: avoid concomitant use of golimumab with
  - ABATACEPT
- Anakinra: avoid concomitant use of golimumab with
  - ANAKINRA
- Antipsychotics: avoid concomitant use of cytotoxics with
  - CLOZAPINE (increased risk of agranulocytosis)
- Vaccines: risk of generalised infections when monoclonal antibodies given with live ● VACCINES—avoid concomitant use

Granisetron *see* 5HT₃-receptor Antagonists (under HT)

Grapefruit Juice
- Aliskiren: grapefruit juice reduces plasma concentration of
  - ALISKIREN—avoid concomitant use
- Anthelmintics: grapefruit juice increases plasma concentration of active metabolite of ALBENDAZOLE; grapefruit juice increases plasma concentration of PRAZIQUANTEL
- Anti-arrhythmics: grapefruit juice increases plasma concentration of AMIODARONE; grapefruit juice increases plasma concentration of ● DRONEDARONE—avoid concomitant use
- Antidepressants: grapefruit juice possibly increases plasma concentration of SERTRALINE
- Antihistamines: grapefruit juice reduces plasma concentration of BILASTINE
- Antimalarials: grapefruit juice possibly increases plasma concentration of ARTEMETHER WITH LUMEFANTRINE; avoidance of grapefruit juice advised by manufacturer of ARTENIMOL WITH PIPERAQUINE
- Antipsychotics: avoidance of grapefruit juice advised by manufacturer of LURASIDONE and PIMOZIDE; grapefruit juice possibly increases plasma concentration of ● QUETIAPINE—manufacturer of quetiapine advises avoid concomitant use
- Antivirals: grapefruit juice possibly increases plasma concentration of EFAVIRENZ
- Anxiolytics and Hypnotics: grapefruit juice possibly increases plasma concentration of *oral* MIDAZOLAM; grapefruit juice increases plasma concentration of BUSPIRONE
- Avanafil: grapefruit juice possibly increases plasma concentration of AVANAFIL— manufacturer of avanafil advises avoid grapefruit juice for 24 hours before avanafil
- Calcium-channel Blockers: grapefruit juice possibly increases plasma concentration of AMLODIPINE; grapefruit juice increases plasma concentration of FELODIPINE, ISRADIPINE, LACIDIPINE, LERCANIDIPINE, NICARDIPINE, NIFEDIPINE, NIMODIPINE and VERAPAMIL
- Ciclosporin: grapefruit juice increases plasma concentration of ● CICLOSPORIN (increased risk of toxicity)
- Colchicine: grapefruit juice possibly increases risk of
  - COLCHICINE toxicity
- Corticosteroids: grapefruit juice increases plasma concentration of *oral* ● BUDESONIDE—avoid concurrent use or separate administration by as much as possible and consider reducing *oral* budesonide dose
- Cytotoxics: grapefruit juice increases plasma concentration of AXITINIB, CABOZANTINIB and PONATINIB; grapefruit juice possibly increases the plasma concentration of ● BOSUTINIB—manufacturer of bosutinib advises avoid or consider reducing dose of bosutinib; grapefruit juice possibly increases plasma concentration of ● CRIZOTINIB and VINFLUNINE—manufacturer of crizotinib and vinflunine advises avoid concomitant use; avoidance of grapefruit juice advised by manufacturer of DASATINIB (plasma concentration of dasatinib possibly increased); avoidance of grapefruit juice advised by manufacturer of EVEROLIMUS, IBRUTINIB, ● LAPATINIB, ● NILOTINIB and ● PAZOPANIB
- Guanfacine: avoidance of grapefruit juice advised by manufacturer of GUANFACINE
- Ivabradine: grapefruit juice increases plasma concentration of IVABRADINE

Grapefruit Juice (continued)
- Ivacaftor: grapefruit juice possibly increases plasma concentration of IVACAFTOR—manufacturer of ivacaftor advises avoid concomitant use
- Lipid-regulating Drugs: grapefruit juice possibly increases plasma concentration of ATORVASTATIN; grapefruit juice increases plasma concentration of ● SIMVASTATIN—avoid concomitant use; avoidance of grapefruit juice advised by manufacturer of LOMITAPIDE
- Pirfenidone: avoidance of grapefruit juice advised by manufacturer of PIRFENIDONE
- Ranolazine: grapefruit juice possibly increases plasma concentration of ● RANOLAZINE—manufacturer of ranolazine advises avoid concomitant use
- Sildenafil: grapefruit juice possibly increases plasma concentration of SILDENAFIL
- Sirolimus: grapefruit juice increases plasma concentration of
  - SIROLIMUS—avoid concomitant use
- Tacrolimus: grapefruit juice increases plasma concentration of
  - TACROLIMUS
- Tadalafil: grapefruit juice possibly increases plasma concentration of TADALAFIL
- Tolvaptan: grapefruit juice increases plasma concentration of
  - TOLVAPTAN—avoid concomitant use
- Ulipristal: avoidance of grapefruit juice advised by manufacturer of *low-dose* ULIPRISTAL
- Vardenafil: grapefruit juice possibly increases plasma concentration of ● VARDENAFIL—avoid concomitant use

Griseofulvin
- Alcohol: griseofulvin possibly enhances effects of ALCOHOL
- Anticoagulants: griseofulvin reduces anticoagulant effect of
  - COUMARINS
- Antiepileptics: absorption of griseofulvin reduced by PHENOBARBITAL and PRIMIDONE (reduced effect)
- Ciclosporin: griseofulvin possibly reduces plasma concentration of CICLOSPORIN
- Oestrogens: anecdotal reports of contraceptive failure and menstrual irregularities when griseofulvin given with OESTROGENS
- Progestogens: anecdotal reports of contraceptive failure and menstrual irregularities when griseofulvin given with PROGESTOGENS

Guanethidine *see* Adrenergic Neurone Blockers

Guanfacine
- Alcohol: sedative effects possibly increased when guanfacine given with ALCOHOL
- Antibacterials: plasma concentration of guanfacine possibly increased by ● CLARITHROMYCIN, ERYTHROMYCIN and ● TELITHROMYCIN (halve dose of guanfacine); plasma concentration of guanfacine possibly reduced by ● RIFABUTIN—increase dose of guanfacine; plasma concentration of guanfacine reduced by ● RIFAMPICIN—increase dose of guanfacine; manufacturer of guanfacine advises halve dose when given with CHLORAMPHENICOL
- Antidepressants: plasma concentration of guanfacine possibly reduced by ● ST JOHN'S WORT—increase dose of guanfacine
- Antiepileptics: plasma concentration of guanfacine possibly reduced by ● CARBAMAZEPINE, ● OXCARBAZEPINE, ● PHENOBARBITAL, ● PHENYTOIN and ● PRIMIDONE—increase dose of guanfacine; guanfacine increases plasma concentration of SODIUM VALPROATE and VALPROIC ACID
- Antifungals: plasma concentration of guanfacine increased by ● KETOCONAZOLE (halve dose of guanfacine); plasma concentration of guanfacine possibly increased by FLUCONAZOLE, ● ITRACONAZOLE and ● POSACONAZOLE (halve dose of guanfacine)
- Antipsychotics: sedative effects possibly increased when guanfacine given with ANTIPSYCHOTICS
- Antivirals: plasma concentration of guanfacine possibly increased by ATAZANAVIR, ● BOCEPREVIR, FOSAMPRENAVIR, ● INDINAVIR, ● RITONAVIR, ● SAQUINAVIR and ● TELAPREVIR (halve dose of guanfacine); plasma concentration of guanfacine possibly reduced by ● EFAVIRENZ, ● ETRAVIRINE and ● NEVIRAPINE—increase dose of guanfacine
- Anxiolytics and Hypnotics: sedative effects possibly increased when guanfacine given with ANXIOLYTICS AND HYPNOTICS

Guanfacine (continued)

▸ Aprepitant: plasma concentration of guanfacine possibly increased by APREPITANT (halve dose of guanfacine)
● Bosentan: plasma concentration of guanfacine possibly reduced by ● BOSENTAN—increase dose of guanfacine
– Calcium-channel Blockers: plasma concentration of guanfacine possibly increased by DILTIAZEM and VERAPAMIL (halve dose of guanfacine)
▸ Cytotoxics: plasma concentration of guanfacine possibly increased by CRIZOTINIB and IMATINIB (halve dose of guanfacine)
▸ Fosaprepitant: plasma concentration of guanfacine possibly increased by FOSAPREPITANT (halve dose of guanfacine)
▸ Grapefruit Juice: manufacturer of guanfacine advises avoid concomitant use with GRAPEFRUIT JUICE
● Modafinil: plasma concentration of guanfacine possibly reduced by ● MODAFINIL—increase dose of guanfacine

Haemophilus Vaccine see Vaccines
Haloperidol see Antipsychotics
Heparin see Heparins
Heparins

▸ ACE Inhibitors: increased risk of hyperkalaemia when heparins given with ACE INHIBITORS
▸ Aliskiren: increased risk of hyperkalaemia when heparins given with ALISKIREN
● Analgesics: possible increased risk of bleeding when heparins given with NSAIDs; increased risk of haemorrhage when anticoagulants given with *intravenous* ● DICLOFENAC (avoid concomitant use, including low-dose heparins); increased risk of haemorrhage when anticoagulants given with ● KETOROLAC (avoid concomitant use, including low-dose heparins); anticoagulant effect of heparins enhanced by ● ASPIRIN
▸ Angiotensin-II Receptor Antagonists: increased risk of hyperkalaemia when heparins given with ANGIOTENSIN-II RECEPTOR ANTAGONISTS
● Anticoagulants: increased risk of haemorrhage when other anticoagulants given with ● APIXABAN, ● DABIGATRAN, ● EDOXABAN and ● RIVAROXABAN (avoid concomitant use except when switching with other anticoagulants or using heparin to maintain catheter patency)
▸ Clopidogrel: increased risk of bleeding when heparins given with CLOPIDOGREL
▸ Dipyridamole: anticoagulant effect of heparins enhanced by DIPYRIDAMOLE
▸ Iloprost: anticoagulant effect of heparins possibly enhanced by ILOPROST
● Nitrates: anticoagulant effect of heparins reduced by *infusion* of ● GLYCERYL TRINITRATE

Hepatitis Vaccines see Vaccines
Histamine

▸ Antidepressants: manufacturer of histamine advises avoid concomitant use with MAOIs; effects of histamine theoretically antagonised by TRICYCLICS—manufacturer of histamine advises avoid concomitant use
▸ Antihistamines: effects of histamine theoretically antagonised by ANTIHISTAMINES—manufacturer of histamine advises avoid concomitant use
▸ Antimalarials: manufacturer of histamine advises avoid concomitant use with ANTIMALARIALS
▸ Antipsychotics: effects of histamine theoretically antagonised by ANTIPSYCHOTICS—manufacturer of histamine advises avoid concomitant use
▸ Atovaquone: manufacturer of histamine advises avoid concomitant use with ATOVAQUONE
▸ Clonidine: manufacturer of histamine advises avoid concomitant use with CLONIDINE
▸ Corticosteroids: manufacturer of histamine advises avoid concomitant use with CORTICOSTEROIDS
▸ Ulcer-healing Drugs: effects of histamine theoretically antagonised by HISTAMINE H$_2$-ANTAGONISTS—manufacturer of histamine advises avoid concomitant use

Histamine H$_2$-antagonists

● Alpha-blockers: cimetidine and ranitidine antagonise effects of ● TOLAZOLINE
● Aminophylline: cimetidine inhibits metabolism of ● AMINOPHYLLINE (increased plasma concentration)

Histamine H$_2$-antagonists (continued)

▸ Analgesics: cimetidine inhibits metabolism of OPIOID ANALGESICS (increased plasma concentration)
▸ Anthelmintics: cimetidine possibly enhances effects of ALBENDAZOLE; cimetidine possibly inhibits metabolism of MEBENDAZOLE (increased plasma concentration); cimetidine increases plasma concentration of PRAZIQUANTEL
● Anti-arrhythmics: cimetidine increases plasma concentration of AMIODARONE and ● PROPAFENONE; cimetidine inhibits metabolism of FLECAINIDE (increased plasma concentration); cimetidine increases plasma concentration of ● LIDOCAINE (increased risk of toxicity)
▸ Antibacterials: cimetidine increases plasma concentration of ERYTHROMYCIN (increased risk of toxicity, including deafness); cimetidine inhibits metabolism of METRONIDAZOLE (increased plasma concentration); metabolism of cimetidine accelerated by RIFAMPICIN (reduced plasma concentration)
● Anticoagulants: cimetidine inhibits metabolism of ● COUMARINS (enhanced anticoagulant effect)
▸ Antidepressants: cimetidine increases plasma concentration of CITALOPRAM, ESCITALOPRAM, MIRTAZAPINE and SERTRALINE; cimetidine inhibits metabolism of AMITRIPTYLINE, DOXEPIN, IMIPRAMINE and NORTRIPTYLINE (increased plasma concentration); cimetidine increases plasma concentration of MOCLOBEMIDE (halve dose of moclobemide); cimetidine possibly increases plasma concentration of TRICYCLICS
▸ Antidiabetics: cimetidine reduces excretion of METFORMIN (increased plasma concentration); cimetidine enhances hypoglycaemic effect of SULFONYLUREAS
● Antiepileptics: cimetidine inhibits metabolism of ● CARBAMAZEPINE, ● FOSPHENYTOIN, ● PHENYTOIN, ● SODIUM VALPROATE and ● VALPROIC ACID (increased plasma concentration)
● Antifungals: histamine H$_2$-antagonists reduce absorption of ITRACONAZOLE and KETOCONAZOLE; cimetidine reduces plasma concentration of ● POSACONAZOLE—manufacturer of posaconazole *suspension* advises avoid concomitant use; famotidine, nizatidine and ranitidine possibly reduce plasma concentration of ● POSACONAZOLE—manufacturer of posaconazole *suspension* advises avoid concomitant use; cimetidine increases plasma concentration of TERBINAFINE
▸ Antihistamines: manufacturer of loratadine advises cimetidine possibly increases plasma concentration of LORATADINE; cimetidine increases plasma concentration of HYDROXYZINE
● Antimalarials: avoidance of cimetidine advised by manufacturer of ● ARTEMETHER WITH LUMEFANTRINE; cimetidine inhibits metabolism of CHLOROQUINE, HYDROXYCHLOROQUINE and QUININE (increased plasma concentration)
▸ Antipsychotics: cimetidine possibly enhances effects of ANTIPSYCHOTICS, CHLORPROMAZINE and CLOZAPINE
● Antivirals: famotidine and ranitidine reduce the plasma concentration of ● ATAZANAVIR (adjust doses of both drugs—consult atazanavir product literature; manufacturer of atazanavir advises adjust doses of both drugs when cimetidine and nizatidine given with ATAZANAVIR—consult atazanavir product literature; famotidine reduces plasma concentration of LEDIPASVIR; famotidine increases plasma concentration of RALTEGRAVIR; avoidance of histamine H$_2$-antagonists for 12 hours before or 4 hours after RILPIVIRINE advised by manufacturer of rilpivirine—consult product literature; cimetidine possibly increases plasma concentration of SAQUINAVIR
▸ Anxiolytics and Hypnotics: cimetidine inhibits metabolism of BENZODIAZEPINES, CLOMETHIAZOLE and ZALEPLON (increased plasma concentration); cimetidine increases plasma concentration of MELATONIN
▸ Azathioprine: manufacturer of azathioprine advises possible increased risk of myelosuppression when cimetidine given with AZATHIOPRINE
▸ Beta-blockers: cimetidine increases plasma concentration of LABETALOL, METOPROLOL and PROPRANOLOL; cimetidine possibly increases plasma concentration of *oral* TIMOLOL
▸ Caffeine citrate: cimetidine increases plasma concentration of CAFFEINE CITRATE
▸ Calcium-channel Blockers: cimetidine possibly inhibits metabolism of CALCIUM-CHANNEL BLOCKERS (increased plasma

Histamine H$_2$-antagonists

Calcium-channel Blockers (continued)
concentration); cimetidine increases plasma concentration of
ISRADIPINE (halve dose of isradipine)

• Ciclosporin: cimetidine possibly increases plasma
concentration of • CICLOSPORIN

• Clopidogrel: cimetidine possibly reduces antiplatelet effect of
• CLOPIDOGREL

• Cytotoxics: cimetidine possibly enhances myelosuppressive
effects of CARMUSTINE and LOMUSTINE; cimetidine reduces
plasma concentration of DOXORUBICIN; cimetidine increases
plasma concentration of • EPIRUBICIN; cimetidine inhibits
metabolism of CAPECITABINE, FLUOROURACIL and TEGAFUR
(increased plasma concentration); famotidine possibly
reduces plasma concentration of DASATINIB; avoidance of
cimetidine, famotidine and nizatidine advised by
manufacturer of • ERLOTINIB; ranitidine reduces plasma
concentration of • ERLOTINIB—manufacturer of erlotinib
advises give at least 2 hours before or 10 hours after
ranitidine; ranitidine reduces plasma concentration of
• GEFITINIB; histamine H$_2$-antagonists possibly reduce
absorption of LAPATINIB; histamine H$_2$-antagonists possibly
reduce absorption of PAZOPANIB—manufacturer of pazopanib
advises give at least 2 hours before or 10 hours after histamine
H$_2$-antagonists

▸ Dopaminergics: cimetidine reduces excretion of PRAMIPEXOLE
(increased plasma concentration)

• Ergot Alkaloids: increased risk of ergotism when cimetidine
given with • ERGOTAMINE—avoid concomitant use

• Fampridine: avoidance of cimetidine advised by manufacturer
of • FAMPRIDINE

• Histamine: histamine H$_2$-antagonists theoretically antagonise
effects of HISTAMINE—manufacturer of histamine advises
avoid concomitant use

▸ Hormone Antagonists: absorption of cimetidine possibly
delayed by OCTREOTIDE

▸ 5HT$_1$-receptor Agonists: cimetidine inhibits metabolism of
ZOLMITRIPTAN (reduce dose of zolmitriptan)

▸ Lipid-regulating Drugs: separating administration from
cimetidine and ranitidine by 12 hours advised by
manufacturer of LOMITAPIDE

▸ Roflumilast: cimetidine inhibits the metabolism of
ROFLUMILAST

▸ Sildenafil: cimetidine increases plasma concentration of
SILDENAFIL—consider reducing dose of sildenafil for erectile
dysfunction

▸ Sympathomimetics: cimetidine possibly inhibits metabolism of
DOBUTAMINE

• Theophylline: cimetidine inhibits metabolism of
• THEOPHYLLINE (increased plasma concentration)

▸ Thyroid Hormones: cimetidine reduces absorption of
LEVOTHYROXINE

Homatropine *see* Antimuscarinics

Hormone Antagonists *see* Abiraterone, Bicalutamide, Danazol,
Dutasteride, Enzalutamide, Exemestane, Flutamide,
Lanreotide, Octreotide, Pasireotide, Tamoxifen, and
Toremifene

5HT$_1$-receptor Agonists

• Antibacterials: plasma concentration of eletriptan increased by
• CLARITHROMYCIN and • ERYTHROMYCIN (risk of toxicity)—avoid
concomitant use; metabolism of zolmitriptan possibly
inhibited by QUINOLONES (reduce dose of zolmitriptan)

• Antidepressants: increased risk of CNS toxicity when 5HT$_1$
agonists given with • CITALOPRAM (manufacturer of citalopram
advises avoid concomitant use); increased risk of CNS toxicity
when sumatriptan given with • CITALOPRAM, • ESCITALOPRAM,
• FLUOXETINE, • FLUVOXAMINE or • PAROXETINE; metabolism of
frovatriptan inhibited by FLUVOXAMINE; metabolism of
zolmitriptan possibly inhibited by FLUVOXAMINE (reduce dose
of zolmitriptan); CNS toxicity reported when sumatriptan
given with SERTRALINE; possible increased serotonergic effects
when 5HT$_1$ agonists given with • DULOXETINE, VENLAFAXINE or
VORTIOXETINE; risk of CNS toxicity when rizatriptan or
sumatriptan given with • MAOIS (avoid rizatriptan or
sumatriptan for 2 weeks after MAOIs); risk of CNS toxicity
when zolmitriptan given with • MAOIS or

5HT$_1$-receptor Agonists

• Antidepressants (continued)
• MOCLOBEMIDE (reduce dose of zolmitriptan); risk of CNS
toxicity when rizatriptan or sumatriptan given with
• MOCLOBEMIDE (avoid rizatriptan or sumatriptan for 2 weeks
after moclobemide); possible increased serotonergic effects
when naratriptan given with SSRIs; increased serotonergic
effects when 5HT$_1$ agonists given with • ST JOHN'S WORT—
avoid concomitant use

• Antifungals: plasma concentration of eletriptan increased by
• ITRACONAZOLE and • KETOCONAZOLE (risk of toxicity)—avoid
concomitant use; plasma concentration of almotriptan
increased by KETOCONAZOLE (increased risk of toxicity)

• Antivirals: plasma concentration of eletriptan increased by
• INDINAVIR and • RITONAVIR (risk of toxicity)—avoid
concomitant use

▸ Beta-blockers: plasma concentration of rizatriptan increased
by PROPRANOLOL (manufacturer of rizatriptan advises halve
dose and avoid within 2 hours of propranolol)

• Dapoxetine: possible increased risk of serotonergic effects
when 5HT$_1$ agonists given with • DAPOXETINE (manufacturer of
dapoxetine advises 5HT$_1$ agonists should not be started until
1 week after stopping dapoxetine, avoid dapoxetine for
2 weeks after stopping 5HT$_1$ agonists)

▸ Dopaminergics: avoidance of 5HT$_1$ agonists advised by
manufacturer of SELEGILINE

• Ergot Alkaloids: increased risk of vasospasm when eletriptan,
frovatriptan or naratriptan given with • ERGOTAMINE (avoid
ergotamine for 24 hours after eletriptan, frovatriptan or
naratriptan, avoid eletriptan, frovatriptan or naratriptan for
24 hours after ergotamine); increased risk of vasospasm when
almotriptan, rizatriptan, sumatriptan or zolmitriptan given
with • ERGOTAMINE (avoid ergotamine for 6 hours after
almotriptan, rizatriptan, sumatriptan or zolmitriptan, avoid
almotriptan, rizatriptan, sumatriptan or zolmitriptan for
24 hours after ergotamine)

▸ Lithium: possible risk of toxicity when sumatriptan given with
LITHIUM

▸ Ulcer-healing Drugs: metabolism of zolmitriptan inhibited by
CIMETIDINE (reduce dose of zolmitriptan)

5HT$_3$-receptor Antagonists

▸ Analgesics: ondansetron possibly antagonises effects of
TRAMADOL

▸ Antibacterials: metabolism of ondansetron accelerated by
RIFAMPICIN (reduced effect)

▸ Antidepressants: possible increased serotonergic effects when
5HT$_3$ antagonists given with SSRI-RELATED ANTIDEPRESSANTS or
SSRIs

▸ Antiepileptics: metabolism of ondansetron accelerated by
CARBAMAZEPINE, FOSPHENYTOIN and PHENYTOIN (reduced effect)

• Cytotoxics: increased risk of ventricular arrhythmias when
ondansetron given with • VANDETANIB—avoid concomitant use

• Dopaminergics: possible increased hypotensive effect when
ondansetron given with • APOMORPHINE—avoid concomitant
use

Human papillomavirus Vaccine *see* Vaccines

Hydralazine *see* Vasodilator Antihypertensives

Hydrochlorothiazide *see* Diuretics

Hydrocortisone *see* Corticosteroids

Hydroflumethiazide *see* Diuretics

Hydromorphone *see* Opioid Analgesics

Hydrotalcite *see* Antacids

Hydroxocobalamin

▸ Antibacterials: response to hydroxocobalamin reduced by
CHLORAMPHENICOL

Hydroxycarbamide

• Antipsychotics: avoid concomitant use of cytotoxics with
• CLOZAPINE (increased risk of agranulocytosis)

• Antivirals: increased risk of toxicity when hydroxycarbamide
given with • DIDANOSINE and • STAVUDINE—avoid concomitant
use

• Vaccines: risk of generalised infections when
hydroxycarbamide given with live • VACCINES—avoid
concomitant use

Hydroxychloroquine

▸ Adsorbents: absorption of hydroxychloroquine reduced by
KAOLIN

Hydroxychloroquine (continued)

‣ Agalsidase Alfa and Beta: hydroxychloroquine possibly inhibits effects of AGALSIDASE ALFA AND BETA (manufacturers of agalsidase alfa and beta advise avoid concomitant use)
‣ Antacids: absorption of hydroxychloroquine reduced by ANTACIDS
• Anti-arrhythmics: increased risk of ventricular arrhythmias when hydroxychloroquine given with • AMIODARONE—avoid concomitant use
• Antibacterials: increased risk of ventricular arrhythmias when hydroxychloroquine given with • MOXIFLOXACIN—avoid concomitant use
• Antimalarials: avoidance of antimalarials advised by manufacturer of • ARTEMETHER WITH LUMEFANTRINE; increased risk of convulsions when hydroxychloroquine given with • MEFLOQUINE
• Antipsychotics: increased risk of ventricular arrhythmias when hydroxychloroquine given with • DROPERIDOL—avoid concomitant use
• Cardiac Glycosides: hydroxychloroquine possibly increases plasma concentration of • DIGOXIN
• Ciclosporin: hydroxychloroquine increases plasma concentration of • CICLOSPORIN (increased risk of toxicity)
• Cytotoxics: possible increased risk of ventricular arrhythmias when hydroxychloroquine given with • BOSUTINIB
‣ Histamine: avoidance of antimalarials advised by manufacturer of HISTAMINE
‣ Lanthanum: absorption of hydroxychloroquine possibly reduced by LANTHANUM (give at least 2 hours apart)
‣ Laronidase: hydroxychloroquine possibly inhibits effects of LARONIDASE (manufacturer of laronidase advises avoid concomitant use)
‣ Parasympathomimetics: hydroxychloroquine has potential to increase symptoms of myasthenia gravis and thus diminish effect of NEOSTIGMINE and PYRIDOSTIGMINE
‣ Penicillamine: increased risk of haematological toxicity when antimalarials given with PENICILLAMINE—manufacturer of penicillamine advises avoid concomitant use
‣ Ulcer-healing Drugs: metabolism of hydroxychloroquine inhibited by CIMETIDINE (increased plasma concentration)
‣ Vaccines: antimalarials inactivate ORAL TYPHOID VACCINE—see under Typhoid Vaccine in BNF

Hydroxyzine see Antihistamines
Hyoscine see Antimuscarinics
Ibandronic Acid see Bisphosphonates
Ibrutinib
• Anti-arrhythmics: plasma concentration of ibrutinib possibly increased by • AMIODARONE and • DRONEDARONE—reduce dose of ibrutinib (see under Ibrutinib, p. 855)
• Antibacterials: plasma concentration of ibrutinib possibly increased by • CIPROFLOXACIN, • CLARITHROMYCIN, • ERYTHROMYCIN and • TELITHROMYCIN—reduce dose of ibrutinib (see under Ibrutinib, p. 855); plasma concentration of ibrutinib reduced by • RIFAMPICIN—avoid concomitant use
‣ Anticoagulants: manufacturer of ibrutinib advises avoid concomitant use with COUMARINS and PHENINDIONE
• Antidepressants: plasma concentration of ibrutinib possibly reduced by • ST JOHN'S WORT—manufacturer of ibrutinib advises avoid concomitant use
• Antiepileptics: plasma concentration of ibrutinib possibly reduced by • CARBAMAZEPINE, • FOSPHENYTOIN and • PHENYTOIN—manufacturer of ibrutinib advises avoid concomitant use
• Antifungals: plasma concentration of ibrutinib increased by • KETOCONAZOLE—reduce dose of ibrutinib (see under Ibrutinib, p. 855); plasma concentration of ibrutinib possibly increased by • FLUCONAZOLE, • ITRACONAZOLE and • VORICONAZOLE—reduce dose of ibrutinib (see under Ibrutinib, p. 855)
• Antipsychotics: avoid concomitant use of cytotoxics with • CLOZAPINE (increased risk of agranulocytosis)
• Antivirals: plasma concentration of ibrutinib possibly increased by • ATAZANAVIR, • DARUNAVIR, • FOSAMPRENAVIR, • INDINAVIR, • RITONAVIR and • SAQUINAVIR—reduce dose of ibrutinib (see under Ibrutinib, p. 855)

Ibrutinib (continued)
• Aprepitant: plasma concentration of ibrutinib possibly increased by • APREPITANT—reduce dose of ibrutinib (see under Ibrutinib, p. 855)
• Calcium-channel Blockers: plasma concentration of ibrutinib possibly increased by • DILTIAZEM and • VERAPAMIL—reduce dose of ibrutinib (see under Ibrutinib, p. 855)
‣ Cardiac Glycosides: manufacturer of ibrutinib advises give DIGOXIN at least 6 hours before or after ibrutinib
• Cobicistat: plasma concentration of ibrutinib possibly increased by • COBICISTAT—reduce dose of ibrutinib (see under Ibrutinib, p. 855)
• Cytotoxics: plasma concentration of ibrutinib possibly increased by • CRIZOTINIB and • IMATINIB—reduce dose of ibrutinib (see under Ibrutinib, p. 855)
‣ Fosaprepitant: plasma concentration of ibrutinib possibly increased by FOSAPREPITANT
‣ Grapefruit Juice: manufacturer of ibrutinib advises avoid concomitant use with GRAPEFRUIT JUICE
‣ Vitamins: manufacturer of ibrutinib advises avoid concomitant use with VITAMIN E

Ibuprofen see NSAIDs
Idarubicin
• Antipsychotics: avoid concomitant use of cytotoxics with • CLOZAPINE (increased risk of agranulocytosis)
• Ciclosporin: plasma concentration of idarubicin increased by • CICLOSPORIN
• Cytotoxics: possible increased risk of cardiotoxicity when idarubicin given with • TRASTUZUMAB—avoid concomitant use for up to 28 weeks after stopping trastuzumab
• Vaccines: risk of generalised infections when cytotoxic antibiotics given with live • VACCINES—avoid concomitant use

Idelalisib
‣ Alpha-blockers: manufacturer of idelalisib advises avoid concomitant use with ALFUZOSIN
‣ Anti-arrhythmics: manufacturer of idelalisib advises avoid concomitant use with AMIODARONE
• Antibacterials: plasma concentration of idelalisib reduced by • RIFAMPICIN—avoid concomitant use
• Antidepressants: plasma concentration of idelalisib possibly reduced by • ST JOHN'S WORT—manufacturer of idelalisib advises avoid concomitant use
• Antiepileptics: plasma concentration of idelalisib possibly reduced by • CARBAMAZEPINE, • FOSPHENYTOIN and • PHENYTOIN—manufacturer of idelalisib advises avoid concomitant use
‣ Antifungals: plasma concentration of idelalisib increased by KETOCONAZOLE
• Antipsychotics: avoid concomitant use of cytotoxics with • CLOZAPINE (increased risk of agranulocytosis); manufacturer of idelalisib advises avoid concomitant use with PIMOZIDE and QUETIAPINE
‣ Anxiolytics and Hypnotics: manufacturer of idelalisib advises avoid concomitant use of oral MIDAZOLAM
‣ Ergot Alkaloids: manufacturer of idelalisib advises avoid concomitant use with ERGOTAMINE
‣ Lipid-regulating Drugs: manufacturer of idelalisib advises avoid concomitant use with SIMVASTATIN
‣ Sildenafil: manufacturer of idelalisib advises avoid concomitant use of SILDENAFIL for pulmonary arterial hypertension
‣ Sympathomimetics, Beta$_2$: manufacturer of idelalisib advises avoid concomitant use with SALMETEROL

Ifosfamide
• Anticoagulants: ifosfamide possibly enhances anticoagulant effect of • COUMARINS
‣ Antifungals: metabolism of ifosfamide inhibited by KETOCONAZOLE
• Antipsychotics: avoid concomitant use of cytotoxics with • CLOZAPINE (increased risk of agranulocytosis)
‣ Cytotoxics: increased risk of otoxicity when ifosfamide given with CISPLATIN

Iloprost
‣ Analgesics: increased risk of bleeding when iloprost given with NSAIDs or ASPIRIN

Iloprost (continued)

▸ Anticoagulants: iloprost possibly enhances anticoagulant effect of COUMARINS and HEPARINS; increased risk of bleeding when iloprost given with PHENINDIONE

▸ Clopidogrel: increased risk of bleeding when iloprost given with CLOPIDOGREL

▸ Eptifibatide: increased risk of bleeding when iloprost given with EPTIFIBATIDE

▸ Tirofiban: increased risk of bleeding when iloprost given with TIROFIBAN

Imatinib

▸ Analgesics: manufacturer of imatinib advises caution with PARACETAMOL

● Antibacterials: plasma concentration of imatinib reduced by ● RIFAMPICIN—avoid concomitant use

● Anticoagulants: manufacturer of imatinib advises replacement of WARFARIN with a heparin (possibility of enhanced warfarin effect)

● Antidepressants: plasma concentration of imatinib reduced by ● ST JOHN'S WORT—avoid concomitant use

● Antiepileptics: plasma concentration of imatinib reduced by ● CARBAMAZEPINE, ● FOSPHENYTOIN, ● OXCARBAZEPINE and ● PHENYTOIN—avoid concomitant use

▸ Antifungals: plasma concentration of imatinib increased by KETOCONAZOLE

● Antipsychotics: avoid concomitant use of cytotoxics with ● CLOZAPINE (increased risk of agranulocytosis)

● Antivirals: avoidance of imatinib advised by manufacturer of ● BOCEPREVIR

● Ciclosporin: imatinib possibly increases plasma concentration of CICLOSPORIN

● Cytotoxics: imatinib possibly increases the plasma concentration of ● BOSUTINIB—manufacturer of bosutinib advises avoid or consider reducing dose of bosutinib; imatinib increases plasma concentration of ● EVEROLIMUS (consider reducing the dose of everolimus —consult everolimus product literature); imatinib possibly increases the plasma concentration of ● IBRUTINIB—reduce dose of ibrutinib (see under Ibrutinib, p. 855)

▸ Guanfacine: imatinib possibly increases plasma concentration of GUANFACINE (halve dose of guanfacine)

▸ Lipid-regulating Drugs: imatinib increases plasma concentration of SIMVASTATIN

▸ Tacrolimus: imatinib increases plasma concentration of TACROLIMUS

▸ Thyroid Hormones: imatinib possibly reduces plasma concentration of LEVOTHYROXINE

Imidapril *see* ACE Inhibitors

Imipenem with Cilastatin

● Antiepileptics: carbapenems reduce plasma concentration of ● SODIUM VALPROATE and ● VALPROIC ACID—avoid concomitant use

● Antivirals: increased risk of convulsions when imipenem with cilastatin given with ● GANCICLOVIR or ● VALGANCICLOVIR

▸ Vaccines: antibacterials inactivate ORAL TYPHOID VACCINE—see under Typhoid Vaccine in BNF

Imipramine *see* Antidepressants, Tricyclic

Immunoglobulins

● Vaccines: anti-d immunoglobulins and normal immunoglobulin might impair immune response to ● BCG VACCINE—give BCG vaccine at least 3 weeks before or 3 months after anti-d immunoglobulins and normal immunoglobulin; anti-d immunoglobulins and normal immunoglobulin might impair immune response to ● MMR VACCINE—give MMR vaccine at least 3 weeks before or 3 months after anti-d immunoglobulins and normal immunoglobulin; anti-d immunoglobulins and normal immunoglobulin might impair immune response to live ● INFLUENZA VACCINE—give live influenza vaccine at least 3 weeks before or 3 months after anti-d immunoglobulins and normal immunoglobulin; anti-d immunoglobulins and normal immunoglobulin might impair immune response to ● ORAL TYPHOID VACCINE—give oral typhoid vaccine at least 3 weeks before or 3 months after anti-d immunoglobulins and normal immunoglobulin; anti-d immunoglobulins and normal immunoglobulin might impair immune response to

Immunoglobulins

● Vaccines (continued)

oral ● POLIOMYELITIS VACCINE—give *oral* poliomyelitis vaccine at least 3 weeks before or 3 months after anti-d immunoglobulins and normal immunoglobulin; anti-d immunoglobulins and normal immunoglobulin might impair immune response to ● ROTAVIRUS VACCINE—give rotavirus vaccine at least 3 weeks before or 3 months after anti-d immunoglobulins and normal immunoglobulin; anti-d immunoglobulins and normal immunoglobulin might impair immune response to ● SMALLPOX VACCINE—give smallpox vaccine at least 3 weeks before or 3 months after anti-d immunoglobulins and normal immunoglobulin; anti-d immunoglobulins and normal immunoglobulin might impair immune response to ● VARICELLA-ZOSTER VACCINE—give varicella-zoster vaccine at least 3 weeks before or 3 months after anti-d immunoglobulins and normal immunoglobulin; anti-d immunoglobulins and normal immunoglobulin might impair immune response to ● YELLOW FEVER VACCINE—give yellow fever vaccine at least 3 weeks before or 3 months after anti-d immunoglobulins and normal immunoglobulin

Indacaterol *see* Sympathomimetics, Beta$_2$

Indapamide *see* Diuretics

Indinavir

▸ Aldesleukin: plasma concentration of indinavir possibly increased by ALDESLEUKIN

● Anti-arrhythmics: indinavir possibly increases plasma concentration of ● AMIODARONE—avoid concomitant use; indinavir possibly increases plasma concentration of ● FLECAINIDE (increased risk of ventricular arrhythmias—avoid concomitant use)

● Antibacterials: indinavir increases plasma concentration of ● RIFABUTIN, also plasma concentration of indinavir decreased (reduce dose of rifabutin and increase dose of indinavir); metabolism of indinavir accelerated by ● RIFAMPICIN (reduced plasma concentration—avoid concomitant use); avoidance of concomitant indinavir in severe renal and hepatic impairment advised by manufacturer of ● TELITHROMYCIN

▸ Anticoagulants: avoidance of indinavir advised by manufacturer of APIXABAN and RIVAROXABAN

● Antidepressants: plasma concentration of indinavir reduced by ● ST JOHN'S WORT—avoid concomitant use

● Antiepileptics: plasma concentration of indinavir possibly reduced by ● CARBAMAZEPINE, ● FOSPHENYTOIN and ● PHENYTOIN, also plasma concentration of carbamazepine, fosphenytoin and phenytoin possibly increased; plasma concentration of indinavir possibly reduced by ● PHENOBARBITAL and ● PRIMIDONE

● Antifungals: plasma concentration of indinavir increased by ● ITRACONAZOLE and ● KETOCONAZOLE (consider reducing dose of indinavir)

● Antimalarials: caution with indinavir advised by manufacturer of ARTEMETHER WITH LUMEFANTRINE; indinavir possibly increases plasma concentration of ● QUININE (increased risk of toxicity)

▸ Antimuscarinics: avoidance of indinavir advised by manufacturer of DARIFENACIN and TOLTERODINE; manufacturer of fesoterodine advises dose reduction when indinavir given with FESOTERODINE—consult fesoterodine product literature

● Antipsychotics: indinavir possibly increases plasma concentration of ● ARIPIPRAZOLE (reduce dose of aripiprazole—consult aripiprazole product literature); indinavir possibly increases plasma concentration of ● LURASIDONE—avoid concomitant use; indinavir possibly increases plasma concentration of ● PIMOZIDE (increased risk of ventricular arrhythmias—avoid concomitant use); indinavir possibly increases plasma concentration of ● QUETIAPINE—manufacturer of quetiapine advises avoid concomitant use

● Antivirals: avoid concomitant use of indinavir with ● ATAZANAVIR; plasma concentration of both drugs increased when indinavir given with DARUNAVIR; absorption of indinavir reduced by DIDANOSINE *tablets* (give at least 1 hour apart); plasma concentration of indinavir reduced by EFAVIRENZ and NEVIRAPINE; plasma concentration of indinavir possibly reduced by ● ETRAVIRINE—avoid concomitant use; indinavir increases plasma concentration of ● MARAVIROC (consider

Indinavir

- **Antivirals** (continued)
  reducing dose of maraviroc); avoidance of indinavir advised by manufacturer of PARITAPREVIR; plasma concentration of indinavir increased by RITONAVIR; indinavir increases plasma concentration of SAQUINAVIR
- **Anxiolytics and Hypnotics:** increased risk of prolonged sedation when indinavir given with ● ALPRAZOLAM—avoid concomitant use; indinavir possibly increases plasma concentration of ● MIDAZOLAM (risk of prolonged sedation—avoid concomitant use of *oral* midazolam)
- ▸ **Atovaquone:** plasma concentration of indinavir possibly reduced by ATOVAQUONE
- **Avanafil:** indinavir possibly increases plasma concentration of ● AVANAFIL—manufacturer of avanafil advises avoid concomitant use
- ▸ **Bosentan:** plasma concentration of indinavir possibly reduced by BOSENTAN
- **Ciclosporin:** indinavir increases plasma concentration of ● CICLOSPORIN
- **Colchicine:** indinavir possibly increases risk of ● COLCHICINE toxicity—suspend or reduce dose of colchicine (avoid concomitant use in hepatic or renal impairment)
- ▸ **Corticosteroids:** plasma concentration of indinavir possibly reduced by DEXAMETHASONE
- **Cytotoxics:** indinavir possibly increases plasma concentration of AXITINIB (reduce dose of axitinib—consult axitinib product literature); indinavir possibly increases the plasma concentration of ● BOSUTINIB and ● CABAZITAXEL—manufacturer of bosutinib and cabazitaxel advises avoid or consider reducing dose of bosutinib and cabazitaxel; indinavir possibly increases plasma concentration of ● CRIZOTINIB and ● EVEROLIMUS—manufacturer of crizotinib and everolimus advises avoid concomitant use; indinavir possibly increases the plasma concentration of ● IBRUTINIB—reduce dose of ibrutinib (see under Ibrutinib, p. 855); indinavir possibly increases plasma concentration of ● PAZOPANIB (reduce dose of pazopanib); indinavir possibly increases plasma concentration of PONATINIB—consider reducing initial dose of ponatinib (see under Ponatinib, p. 860); manufacturer of ruxolitinib advises dose reduction when indinavir given with ● RUXOLITINIB—consult ruxolitinib product literature; indinavir possibly increases plasma concentration of ● DOCETAXEL—manufacturer of docetaxel advises avoid concomitant use or consider reducing docetaxel dose; avoidance of indinavir advised by manufacturer of ● OLAPARIB
- **Ergot Alkaloids:** increased risk of ergotism when indinavir given with ● ERGOMETRINE or ● ERGOTAMINE—avoid concomitant use
- **Guanfacine:** indinavir possibly increases plasma concentration of ● GUANFACINE (halve dose of guanfacine)
- **5HT₁-receptor Agonists:** indinavir increases plasma concentration of ● ELETRIPTAN (risk of toxicity)—avoid concomitant use
- **Lipid-regulating Drugs:** possible increased risk of myopathy when indinavir given with ATORVASTATIN; possible increased risk of myopathy when indinavir given with ● ROSUVASTATIN—manufacturer of rosuvastatin advises avoid concomitant use; increased risk of myopathy when indinavir given with ● SIMVASTATIN (avoid concomitant use); avoidance of indinavir advised by manufacturer of ● LOMITAPIDE (plasma concentration of lomitapide possibly increased)
- **Orlistat:** absorption of indinavir possibly reduced by ● ORLISTAT
- **Ranolazine:** indinavir possibly increases plasma concentration of ● RANOLAZINE—manufacturer of ranolazine advises avoid concomitant use
- **Sildenafil:** indinavir increases plasma concentration of ● SILDENAFIL—reduce initial dose of sildenafil
- **Tadalafil:** indinavir possibly increases plasma concentration of TADALAFIL
- **Vardenafil:** indinavir increases plasma concentration of ● VARDENAFIL—avoid concomitant use

Indometacin *see* NSAIDs

Indoramin *see* Alpha-blockers

Infliximab

- **Abatacept:** avoid concomitant use of infliximab with ● ABATACEPT

Infliximab (continued)

- **Anakinra:** avoid concomitant use of infliximab with ● ANAKINRA
- **Antipsychotics:** avoid concomitant use of cytotoxics with ● CLOZAPINE (increased risk of agranulocytosis)
- **Vaccines:** risk of generalised infections when monoclonal antibodies given with live ● VACCINES—avoid concomitant use

Influenza Vaccine *see* Vaccines

Insulin *see* Antidiabetics

Interferon Alfa *see* Interferons

Interferon Gamma *see* Interferons

Interferons

- **Aminophylline:** interferon alfa and peginterferon alfa inhibit metabolism of ● AMINOPHYLLINE (consider reducing dose of aminophylline)
- **Antivirals:** caution with peginterferon alfa advised by manufacturer of ADEFOVIR; increased risk of peripheral neuropathy when interferon alfa and peginterferon alfa given with ● TELBIVUDINE
- **Theophylline:** interferon alfa and peginterferon alfa inhibit metabolism of ● THEOPHYLLINE (consider reducing dose of theophylline)
- ▸ **Vaccines:** manufacturer of interferon gamma advises avoid concomitant use with VACCINES

Ipilimumab

- ▸ **Antipsychotics:** avoid concomitant use of cytotoxics with ● CLOZAPINE (increased risk of agranulocytosis)
- ▸ **Cytotoxics:** manufacturer of ipilimumab advises avoid concomitant use with VEMURAFENIB
- **Vaccines:** risk of generalised infections when monoclonal antibodies given with live ● VACCINES—avoid concomitant use

Ipratropium *see* Antimuscarinics

Irbesartan *see* Angiotensin-II Receptor Antagonists

Irinotecan

- **Antidepressants:** metabolism of irinotecan accelerated by ● ST JOHN'S WORT (reduced plasma concentration—avoid concomitant use)
- ▸ **Antiepileptics:** plasma concentration of irinotecan and its active metabolite reduced by CARBAMAZEPINE, FOSPHENYTOIN, PHENOBARBITAL, PHENYTOIN and PRIMIDONE
- **Antifungals:** plasma concentration of irinotecan reduced by ● KETOCONAZOLE (but concentration of active metabolite of irinotecan increased)—avoid concomitant use; increased risk of toxicity when irinotecan given with ● ITRACONAZOLE—avoid concomitant use
- **Antipsychotics:** avoid concomitant use of cytotoxics with ● CLOZAPINE (increased risk of agranulocytosis)
- **Antivirals:** metabolism of irinotecan possibly inhibited by ● ATAZANAVIR (increased risk of toxicity)
- **Cytotoxics:** avoidance of irinotecan advised by manufacturer of ● PANITUMUMAB; plasma concentration of active metabolite of irinotecan increased by ● LAPATINIB—consider reducing dose of irinotecan; plasma concentration of irinotecan increased by REGORAFENIB; plasma concentration of irinotecan possibly increased by SORAFENIB

Iron Salts

- ▸ **Antacids:** absorption of *oral* iron salts reduced by ORAL MAGNESIUM SALTS (as magnesium trisilicate)
- ▸ **Antibacterials:** *oral* iron salts reduce absorption of CIPROFLOXACIN (give at least 2 hours before or 4 hours after ciprofloxacin); *oral* iron salts reduce absorption of LEVOFLOXACIN, NORFLOXACIN and OFLOXACIN (give at least 2 hours apart); *oral* iron salts reduce absorption of MOXIFLOXACIN (give at least 6 hours apart); effects of iron salts possibly inhibited by CHLORAMPHENICOL; *oral* iron salts reduce absorption of tetracyclines, also absorption of *oral* iron salts reduced by TETRACYCLINES (give at least 2 to 3 hours apart)
- ▸ **Antivirals:** *oral* iron salts reduce absorption of DOLUTEGRAVIR—manufacturer of dolutegravir advises give at least 2 hours before or 6 hours after *oral* iron salts
- ▸ **Bisphosphonates:** *oral* iron salts reduce absorption of BISPHOSPHONATES
- ▸ **Calcium Salts:** absorption of *oral* iron salts reduced by CALCIUM SALTS
- ▸ **Dopaminergics:** *oral* iron salts possibly reduce absorption of CO-BENELDOPA, CO-CARELDOPA and LEVODOPA; *oral* iron salts reduce absorption of ENTACAPONE

Iron Salts (continued)

▸ Eltrombopag: *oral* iron salts possibly reduce absorption of ELTROMBOPAG (give at least 4 hours apart)

▸ Methyldopa: *oral* iron salts antagonise hypotensive effect of METHYLDOPA

▸ Mycophenolate: *oral* iron salts reduce absorption of MYCOPHENOLATE

▸ Penicillamine: *oral* iron salts reduce absorption of PENICILLAMINE

▸ Thyroid Hormones: *oral* iron salts reduce absorption of LEVOTHYROXINE (give at least 2 hours apart)

▸ Trientine: absorption of *oral* iron salts reduced by TRIENTINE

▸ Zinc: *oral* iron salts reduce absorption of ZINC, also absorption of *oral* iron salts reduced by zinc

Isocarboxazid *see* MAOIs

Isoflurane *see* Anaesthetics, General

Isomethepteme *see* Sympathomimetics

Isoniazid

▸ Aminophylline: isoniazid possibly increases plasma concentration of AMINOPHYLLINE

▸ Anaesthetics, General: increased risk of hepatotoxicity when isoniazid given with ISOFLURANE

▸ Analgesics: avoidance of isoniazid advised by manufacturer of PETHIDINE

▸ Antacids: absorption of isoniazid reduced by ANTACIDS

▸ Antibacterials: increased risk of hepatotoxicity when isoniazid given with • RIFAMPICIN; increased risk of CNS toxicity when isoniazid given with CYCLOSERINE

▸ Antiepileptics: isoniazid increases plasma concentration of • CARBAMAZEPINE (also possibly increased isoniazid hepatotoxicity); isoniazid inhibits metabolism of • ETHOSUXIMIDE (increased plasma concentration and risk of toxicity); isoniazid possibly inhibits metabolism of FOSPHENYTOIN and PHENYTOIN (increased risk of toxicity)

▸ Antifungals: isoniazid possibly reduces plasma concentration of KETOCONAZOLE

▸ Anxiolytics and Hypnotics: isoniazid inhibits the metabolism of DIAZEPAM

▸ Corticosteroids: plasma concentration of isoniazid possibly reduced by CORTICOSTEROIDS

▸ Disulfiram: isoniazid possibly increases CNS effects of DISULFIRAM

▸ Dopaminergics: isoniazid possibly reduces effects of CO-BENELDOPA, CO-CARELDOPA and LEVODOPA

▸ Lipid-regulating Drugs: separating administration from isoniazid by 12 hours advised by manufacturer of LOMITAPIDE

▸ Theophylline: isoniazid possibly increases plasma concentration of THEOPHYLLINE

▸ Vaccines: antibacterials inactivate ORAL TYPHOID VACCINE—see under Typhoid Vaccine in BNF

Isosorbide Dinitrate *see* Nitrates

Isosorbide Mononitrate *see* Nitrates

Isotretinoin *see* Retinoids

Isradipine *see* Calcium-channel Blockers

Itraconazole *see* Antifungals, Triazole

Ivabradine

• Anti-arrhythmics: increased risk of ventricular arrhythmias when ivabradine given with • AMIODARONE or • DISOPYRAMIDE

• Antibacterials: plasma concentration of ivabradine possibly increased by • CLARITHROMYCIN and • TELITHROMYCIN—avoid concomitant use; increased risk of ventricular arrhythmias when ivabradine given with • ERYTHROMYCIN—avoid concomitant use

• Antidepressants: plasma concentration of ivabradine reduced by ST JOHN'S WORT—avoid concomitant use

• Antifungals: plasma concentration of ivabradine increased by • KETOCONAZOLE—avoid concomitant use; plasma concentration of ivabradine increased by FLUCONAZOLE—reduce initial dose of ivabradine; plasma concentration of ivabradine possibly increased by • ITRACONAZOLE—avoid concomitant use

• Antimalarials: increased risk of ventricular arrhythmias when ivabradine given with • MEFLOQUINE

• Antipsychotics: increased risk of ventricular arrhythmias when ivabradine given with • PIMOZIDE

Ivabradine (continued)

• Antivirals: plasma concentration of ivabradine possibly increased by • RITONAVIR—avoid concomitant use

• Beta-blockers: increased risk of ventricular arrhythmias when ivabradine given with • SOTALOL

• Calcium-channel Blockers: plasma concentration of ivabradine increased by • DILTIAZEM and • VERAPAMIL—avoid concomitant use

▸ Grapefruit Juice: plasma concentration of ivabradine increased by GRAPEFRUIT JUICE

• Pentamidine Isetionate: increased risk of ventricular arrhythmias when ivabradine given with • PENTAMIDINE ISETIONATE

Ivacaftor

• Antibacterials: plasma concentration of ivacaftor possibly increased by • CLARITHROMYCIN, • ERYTHROMYCIN and • TELITHROMYCIN (see under Ivacaftor, p. 269); plasma concentration of ivacaftor possibly reduced by • RIFABUTIN—manufacturer of ivacaftor advises avoid concomitant use; plasma concentration of ivacaftor reduced by • RIFAMPICIN—manufacturer of ivacaftor advises avoid concomitant use

• Antidepressants: plasma concentration of ivacaftor possibly reduced by • ST JOHN'S WORT—manufacturer of ivacaftor advises avoid concomitant use

• Antiepileptics: plasma concentration of ivacaftor possibly reduced by • CARBAMAZEPINE, • FOSPHENYTOIN, • PHENOBARBITAL, • PHENYTOIN and • PRIMIDONE—manufacturer of ivacaftor advises avoid concomitant use

• Antifungals: plasma concentration of ivacaftor increased by • FLUCONAZOLE and • KETOCONAZOLE (see under Ivacaftor, p. 269); plasma concentration of ivacaftor possibly increased by • ITRACONAZOLE, • POSACONAZOLE and • VORICONAZOLE (see under Ivacaftor, p. 269)

▸ Anxiolytics and Hypnotics: ivacaftor increases plasma concentration of MIDAZOLAM

▸ Cardiac Glycosides: ivacaftor increases plasma concentration of DIGOXIN

▸ Grapefruit Juice: plasma concentration of ivacaftor possibly increased by GRAPEFRUIT JUICE—manufacturer of ivacaftor advises avoid concomitant use

▸ Lipid-regulating Drugs: separating administration from ivacaftor by 12 hours advised by manufacturer of LOMITAPIDE

Ivermectin

▸ Anthelmintics: plasma concentration of ivermectin possibly increased by LEVAMISOLE

▸ Anticoagulants: ivermectin possibly enhances anticoagulant effect of COUMARINS

Japanese Encephalitis Vaccine *see* Vaccines

Kaolin

▸ Analgesics: kaolin possibly reduces absorption of ASPIRIN

▸ Antibacterials: kaolin possibly reduces absorption of TETRACYCLINES

▸ Antimalarials: kaolin reduces absorption of CHLOROQUINE and HYDROXYCHLOROQUINE

▸ Antipsychotics: kaolin possibly reduces absorption of PHENOTHIAZINES

Ketamine *see* Anaesthetics, General

Ketoconazole *see* Antifungals, Imidazole

Ketoprofen *see* NSAIDs

Ketorolac *see* NSAIDs

Ketotifen *see* Antihistamines

Labetalol *see* Beta-blockers

Lacidipine *see* Calcium-channel Blockers

Lacosamide

• Antidepressants: anticonvulsant effect of antiepileptics possibly antagonised by MAOIs and • TRICYCLIC-RELATED ANTIDEPRESSANTS (convulsive threshold lowered); anticonvulsant effect of antiepileptics antagonised by • SSRIS and • TRICYCLICS (convulsive threshold lowered)

• Antimalarials: anticonvulsant effect of antiepileptics antagonised by • MEFLOQUINE

• Antipsychotics: anticonvulsant effect of antiepileptics antagonised by • ANTIPSYCHOTICS (convulsive threshold lowered)

• Orlistat: possible increased risk of convulsions when antiepileptics given with • ORLISTAT

Lactulose
▸ Anticoagulants: lactulose possibly enhances anticoagulant effect of COUMARINS

Lamivudine
▸ Antibacterials: plasma concentration of lamivudine increased by TRIMETHOPRIM (as co-trimoxazole)—avoid concomitant use of high-dose co-trimoxazole
▸ Antivirals: avoidance of lamivudine advised by manufacturer of EMTRICITABINE
● Cytotoxics: manufacturer of lamivudine advises avoid concomitant use with ● CLADRIBINE
● Orlistat: absorption of lamivudine possibly reduced by ● ORLISTAT

Lamotrigine
● Antibacterials: plasma concentration of lamotrigine reduced by ● RIFAMPICIN
● Antidepressants: anticonvulsant effect of antiepileptics possibly antagonised by MAOIs and ● TRICYCLIC-RELATED ANTIDEPRESSANTS (convulsive threshold lowered); anticonvulsant effect of antiepileptics antagonised by ● SSRIs and ● TRICYCLICS (convulsive threshold lowered)
● Antiepileptics: plasma concentration of lamotrigine often reduced by CARBAMAZEPINE, also plasma concentration of an active metabolite of carbamazepine sometimes raised (but evidence is conflicting); plasma concentration of lamotrigine reduced by FOSPHENYTOIN, PHENOBARBITAL, PHENYTOIN and PRIMIDONE; plasma concentration of lamotrigine increased by ● SODIUM VALPROATE and ● VALPROIC ACID (increased risk of toxicity—reduce lamotrigine dose)
● Antimalarials: anticonvulsant effect of antiepileptics antagonised by ● MEFLOQUINE
● Antipsychotics: anticonvulsant effect of antiepileptics antagonised by ● ANTIPSYCHOTICS (convulsive threshold lowered)
▸ Antivirals: plasma concentration of lamotrigine possibly reduced by RITONAVIR
● Oestrogens: plasma concentration of lamotrigine reduced by ● OESTROGENS—consider increasing dose of lamotrigine
● Orlistat: possible increased risk of convulsions when antiepileptics given with ● ORLISTAT
▸ Progestogens: plasma concentration of lamotrigine possibly increased by DESOGESTREL

Lanreotide
▸ Antidiabetics: lanreotide possibly reduces requirements for ANTIDIABETICS
▸ Ciclosporin: lanreotide reduces plasma concentration of CICLOSPORIN

Lansoprazole see Proton Pump Inhibitors

Lanthanum
▸ Antibacterials: lanthanum possibly reduces absorption of QUINOLONES (give at least 2 hours before or 4 hours after lanthanum)
▸ Antifungals: lanthanum possibly reduces absorption of KETOCONAZOLE (give at least 2 hours apart)
▸ Antimalarials: lanthanum possibly reduces absorption of CHLOROQUINE and HYDROXYCHLOROQUINE (give at least 2 hours apart)
▸ Thyroid Hormones: lanthanum reduces absorption of LEVOTHYROXINE (give at least 2 hours apart)

Lapatinib
● Antibacterials: manufacturer of lapatinib advises avoid concomitant use with ● RIFABUTIN, ● RIFAMPICIN and ● TELITHROMYCIN
● Antidepressants: manufacturer of lapatinib advises avoid concomitant use with ● ST JOHN'S WORT
● Antidiabetics: manufacturer of lapatinib advises avoid concomitant use with ● REPAGLINIDE
● Antiepileptics: plasma concentration of lapatinib reduced by ● CARBAMAZEPINE—avoid concomitant use; manufacturer of lapatinib advises avoid concomitant use with ● FOSPHENYTOIN and ● PHENYTOIN
● Antifungals: plasma concentration of lapatinib increased by ● KETOCONAZOLE—avoid concomitant use; manufacturer of lapatinib advises avoid concomitant use with ● ITRACONAZOLE, ● POSACONAZOLE and ● VORICONAZOLE

Lapatinib (continued)
● Antipsychotics: avoid concomitant use of cytotoxics with ● CLOZAPINE (increased risk of agranulocytosis); manufacturer of lapatinib advises avoid concomitant use with ● PIMOZIDE
● Antivirals: avoidance of lapatinib advised by manufacturer of ● BOCEPREVIR; manufacturer of lapatinib advises avoid concomitant use with ● RITONAVIR and ● SAQUINAVIR
● Cytotoxics: lapatinib increases plasma concentration of PAZOPANIB; possible increased risk of neutropenia when lapatinib given with DOCETAXEL; increased risk of neutropenia when lapatinib given with ● PACLITAXEL; lapatinib increases plasma concentration of active metabolite of ● IRINOTECAN—consider reducing dose of irinotecan
● Grapefruit Juice: manufacturer of lapatinib advises avoid concomitant use with ● GRAPEFRUIT JUICE
● Lipid-regulating Drugs: separating administration from lapatinib by 12 hours advised by manufacturer of LOMITAPIDE
▸ Ulcer-healing Drugs: absorption of lapatinib possibly reduced by HISTAMINE H$_2$-ANTAGONISTS and PROTON PUMP INHIBITORS

Laronidase
▸ Antimalarials: effects of laronidase possibly inhibited by CHLOROQUINE and HYDROXYCHLOROQUINE (manufacturer of laronidase advises avoid concomitant use)

Ledipasvir
▸ Antacids: manufacturer of ledipasvir advises separating administration from ANTACIDS by 4 hours
▸ Anti-arrhythmics: possible increased risk of bradycardia when ledipasvir (with sofosbuvir) given with ● AMIODARONE—see under Amiodarone, p. 94
▸ Antibacterials: manufacturer of ledipasvir advises avoid concomitant use with RIFABUTIN and RIFAMPICIN
▸ Antidepressants: manufacturer of ledipasvir advises avoid concomitant use with ST JOHN'S WORT
▸ Antiepileptics: manufacturer of ledipasvir advises avoid concomitant use with CARBAMAZEPINE, FOSPHENYTOIN, OXCARBAZEPINE, PHENOBARBITAL, PHENYTOIN and PRIMIDONE
▸ Antivirals: plasma concentration of both drugs increased when ledipasvir given with SIMEPREVIR—manufacturer of ledipasvir advises avoid concomitant use
▸ Calcium Salts: manufacturer of ledipasvir advises separating administration from CALCIUM SALTS by 4 hours
● Lipid-regulating Drugs: possible increased risk of myopathy when ledipasvir given with ● ATORVASTATIN, ● FLUVASTATIN and ● SIMVASTATIN—manufacturer of ledipasvir advises consider reducing dose of atorvastatin, fluvastatin and simvastatin; manufacturer of ledipasvir advises avoid concomitant use with ● ROSUVASTATIN
▸ Ulcer-healing Drugs: plasma concentration of ledipasvir reduced by FAMOTIDINE and OMEPRAZOLE; manufacturer of ledipasvir advises do not take PROTON PUMP INHIBITORS before ledispavir

Leflunomide
NOTE Increased risk of toxicity with other haematotoxic and hepatotoxic drugs
▸ Antibacterials: plasma concentration of active metabolite of leflunomide possibly increased by RIFAMPICIN
▸ Anticoagulants: leflunomide possibly enhances anticoagulant effect of WARFARIN
▸ Antidiabetics: leflunomide possibly enhances hypoglycaemic effect of TOLBUTAMIDE
▸ Antiepileptics: leflunomide possibly increases plasma concentration of FOSPHENYTOIN and PHENYTOIN
● Cytotoxics: risk of toxicity when leflunomide given with ● METHOTREXATE
▸ Lipid-regulating Drugs: the effect of leflunomide is significantly decreased by COLESTYRAMINE (enhanced elimination)—avoid unless drug elimination desired
● Vaccines: risk of generalised infections when leflunomide given with live ● VACCINES—avoid concomitant use

Lenalidomide
● Antibacterials: plasma concentration of lenalidomide possibly increased by ● CLARITHROMYCIN (increased risk of toxicity)
● Antifungals: plasma concentration of lenalidomide possibly increased by ● ITRACONAZOLE and ● KETOCONAZOLE (increased risk of toxicity)

Lenalidomide (continued)

▸ Calcium-channel Blockers: plasma concentration of lenalidomide possibly increased by • VERAPAMIL (increased risk of toxicity)

▸ Cardiac Glycosides: lenalidomide possibly increases plasma concentration of DIGOXIN

▸ Ciclosporin: plasma concentration of lenalidomide possibly increased by • CICLOSPORIN (increased risk of toxicity)

Lercanidipine see Calcium-channel Blockers

Leukotriene Receptor Antagonists

▸ Aminophylline: zafirlukast possibly increases plasma concentration of AMINOPHYLLINE, also plasma concentration of zafirlukast reduced

▸ Analgesics: plasma concentration of zafirlukast increased by ASPIRIN

▸ Antibacterials: plasma concentration of zafirlukast reduced by ERYTHROMYCIN

▸ Anticoagulants: zafirlukast enhances anticoagulant effect of WARFARIN

▸ Antiepileptics: plasma concentration of montelukast reduced by PHENOBARBITAL and PRIMIDONE

▸ Antifungals: plasma concentration of zafirlukast increased by FLUCONAZOLE

▸ Lipid-regulating Drugs: plasma concentration of montelukast increased by GEMFIBROZIL

▸ Theophylline: zafirlukast possibly increases plasma concentration of THEOPHYLLINE, also plasma concentration of zafirlukast reduced

Levamisole

▸ Alcohol: possibility of disulfiram-like reaction when levamisole given with ALCOHOL

▸ Anthelmintics: plasma concentration of both drugs possibly reduced when levamisole given with ALBENDAZOLE; levamisole possibly increases plasma concentration of IVERMECTIN

• Anticoagulants: levamisole possibly enhances anticoagulant effect of • WARFARIN

▸ Antiepileptics: levamisole possibly increases plasma concentration of FOSPHENYTOIN and PHENYTOIN

Levetiracetam

• Antidepressants: anticonvulsant effect of antiepileptics possibly antagonised by MAOIs and • TRICYCLIC-RELATED ANTIDEPRESSANTS (convulsive threshold lowered); anticonvulsant effect of antiepileptics antagonised by • SSRIS and • TRICYCLICS (convulsive threshold lowered)

• Antiepileptics: levetiracetam possibly increases risk of CARBAMAZEPINE toxicity

• Antimalarials: anticonvulsant effect of antiepileptics antagonised by • MEFLOQUINE

• Antipsychotics: anticonvulsant effect of antiepileptics antagonised by • ANTIPSYCHOTICS (convulsive threshold lowered)

• Cytotoxics: levetiracetam possibly increases plasma concentration of • METHOTREXATE

• Orlistat: possible increased risk of convulsions when antiepileptics given with • ORLISTAT

Levobunolol see Beta-blockers

Levobupivacaine

▸ Anti-arrhythmics: increased myocardial depression when levobupivacaine given with ANTI-ARRHYTHMICS

Levocarnitine

• Anticoagulants: levocarnitine possibly enhances anticoagulant effect of COUMARINS

Levocetirizine see Antihistamines

Levodopa

• ACE Inhibitors: enhanced hypotensive effect when levodopa given with ACE INHIBITORS

▸ Adrenergic Neurone Blockers: enhanced hypotensive effect when levodopa given with ADRENERGIC NEURONE BLOCKERS

▸ Alpha-blockers: enhanced hypotensive effect when levodopa given with ALPHA-BLOCKERS

• Anaesthetics, General: increased risk of arrhythmias when levodopa given with • VOLATILE LIQUID GENERAL ANAESTHETICS

▸ Angiotensin-II Receptor Antagonists: enhanced hypotensive effect when levodopa given with ANGIOTENSIN-II RECEPTOR ANTAGONISTS

Levodopa (continued)

▸ Antibacterials: effects of levodopa possibly reduced by ISONIAZID

• Antidepressants: risk of hypertensive crisis when levodopa given with • MAOIS, avoid levodopa for at least 2 weeks after stopping MAOIs; increased risk of side-effects when levodopa given with MOCLOBEMIDE

▸ Antiepileptics: effects of levodopa possibly reduced by FOSPHENYTOIN and PHENYTOIN

▸ Antimuscarinics: absorption of levodopa possibly reduced by ANTIMUSCARINICS

▸ Antipsychotics: effects of levodopa antagonised by ANTIPSYCHOTICS; avoidance of levodopa advised by manufacturer of AMISULPRIDE (antagonism of effect)

▸ Anxiolytics and Hypnotics: effects of levodopa possibly antagonised by BENZODIAZEPINES

▸ Beta-blockers: enhanced hypotensive effect when levodopa given with BETA-BLOCKERS

▸ Bupropion: increased risk of side-effects when levodopa given with BUPROPION

▸ Calcium-channel Blockers: enhanced hypotensive effect when levodopa given with CALCIUM-CHANNEL BLOCKERS

▸ Clonidine: enhanced hypotensive effect when levodopa given with CLONIDINE

▸ Diazoxide: enhanced hypotensive effect when levodopa given with DIAZOXIDE

▸ Diuretics: enhanced hypotensive effect when levodopa given with DIURETICS

▸ Dopaminergics: enhanced effects and increased toxicity of levodopa when given with SELEGILINE (reduce dose of levodopa)

▸ Iron Salts: absorption of levodopa possibly reduced by *oral* IRON SALTS

▸ Memantine: effects of dopaminergics possibly enhanced by MEMANTINE

▸ Methyldopa: enhanced hypotensive effect when levodopa given with METHYLDOPA; antiparkinsonian effect of dopaminergics antagonised by METHYLDOPA

▸ Moxonidine: enhanced hypotensive effect when levodopa given with MOXONIDINE

▸ Muscle Relaxants: possible agitation, confusion and hallucinations when levodopa given with BACLOFEN

▸ Nitrates: enhanced hypotensive effect when levodopa given with NITRATES

▸ Vasodilator Antihypertensives: enhanced hypotensive effect when levodopa given with HYDRALAZINE, MINOXIDIL or SODIUM NITROPRUSSIDE

▸ Vitamins: effects of levodopa reduced by PYRIDOXINE when given without dopa-decarboxylase inhibitor

Levofloxacin see Quinolones

Levofolinic Acid see Folates

Levomepromazine see Antipsychotics

Levonorgestrel see Progestogens

Levosimendan

• Nitrates: possible severe postural hypotension when levosimendan given with • ISOSORBIDE MONONITRATE

Levothyroxine see Thyroid Hormones

Lidocaine

NOTE Interactions less likely when lidocaine used topically

▸ Anaesthetics, Local: increased myocardial depression when anti-arrhythmics given with BUPIVACAINE, LEVOBUPIVACAINE, PRILOCAINE or ROPIVACAINE

• Anti-arrhythmics: increased myocardial depression when anti-arrhythmics given with other • ANTI-ARRHYTHMICS

• Antipsychotics: increased risk of ventricular arrhythmias when anti-arrhythmics that prolong the QT interval given with • ANTIPSYCHOTICS that prolong the QT interval

• Antivirals: plasma concentration of lidocaine possibly increased by • ATAZANAVIR and LOPINAVIR; plasma concentration of lidocaine possibly increased by DARUNAVIR and • FOSAMPRENAVIR—avoid concomitant use; increased risk of ventricular arrhythmias when lidocaine given with • SAQUINAVIR—avoid concomitant use; caution with *intravenous* lidocaine advised by manufacturer of TELAPREVIR

• Beta-blockers: increased myocardial depression when anti-arrhythmics given with • BETA-BLOCKERS; possible increased

Lidocaine

- **Beta-blockers** (continued)
  risk of lidocaine toxicity when given with NADOLOL; increased risk of lidocaine toxicity when given with ● PROPRANOLOL
- **Diuretics:** action of lidocaine antagonised by hypokalaemia caused by ● ACETAZOLAMIDE, ● LOOP DIURETICS or ● THIAZIDES AND RELATED DIURETICS
- ▸ **Muscle Relaxants:** neuromuscular blockade enhanced and prolonged when lidocaine given with SUXAMETHONIUM
- **Ulcer-healing Drugs:** plasma concentration of lidocaine increased by ● CIMETIDINE (increased risk of toxicity)

Linagliptin *see* Antidiabetics

Linezolid *see* MAOIs

Liothyronine *see* Thyroid Hormones

Lipegfilgrastim

- ▸ **Cytotoxics:** neutropenia possibly exacerbated when lipegfilgrastim given with CAPECITABINE, FLUOROURACIL or TEGAFUR

Lipid-regulating Drugs *see* Colesevelam, Colestipol, Colestyramine, Ezetimibe, Fibrates, Lomitapide, Nicotinic Acid, and Statins

Liraglutide *see* Antidiabetics

Lisdexamfetamine *see* Sympathomimetics

Lisinopril *see* ACE Inhibitors

Lithium

- **ACE Inhibitors:** excretion of lithium reduced by ● ACE INHIBITORS (increased plasma concentration)
- ▸ **Aminophylline:** excretion of lithium increased by AMINOPHYLLINE (reduced plasma concentration)
- **Analgesics:** excretion of lithium reduced by ● NSAIDS (increased risk of toxicity); excretion of lithium reduced by ● KETOROLAC (increased risk of toxicity)—avoid concomitant use
- **Angiotensin-II Receptor Antagonists:** excretion of lithium reduced by ● ANGIOTENSIN-II RECEPTOR ANTAGONISTS (increased plasma concentration)
- ▸ **Antacids:** excretion of lithium increased by SODIUM BICARBONATE (reduced plasma concentration)
- **Anti-arrhythmics:** avoidance of lithium advised by manufacturer of ● AMIODARONE (risk of ventricular arrhythmias)
- ▸ **Antibacterials:** increased risk of lithium toxicity when given with METRONIDAZOLE
- **Antidepressants:** possible increased serotonergic effects when lithium given with VENLAFAXINE; increased risk of CNS effects when lithium given with ● SSRIS (lithium toxicity reported); risk of toxicity when lithium given with TRICYCLICS
- ▸ **Antiepileptics:** neurotoxicity may occur when lithium given with CARBAMAZEPINE, FOSPHENYTOIN or PHENYTOIN without increased plasma concentration of lithium; plasma concentration of lithium possibly affected by TOPIRAMATE
- **Antipsychotics:** increased risk of extrapyramidal side-effects and possibly neurotoxicity when lithium given with CLOZAPINE, FLUPENTIXOL, HALOPERIDOL, PHENOTHIAZINES, ● RISPERIDONE or ZUCLOPENTHIXOL; possible risk of toxicity when lithium given with OLANZAPINE; lithium possibly increases extrapyramidal side-effects of QUETIAPINE; increased risk of extrapyramidal side-effects when lithium given with SULPIRIDE
- ▸ **Anxiolytics and Hypnotics:** increased risk of neurotoxicity when lithium given with CLONAZEPAM
- ▸ **Calcium-channel Blockers:** neurotoxicity may occur when lithium given with DILTIAZEM or VERAPAMIL without increased plasma concentration of lithium
- **Cytotoxics:** increased risk of ventricular arrhythmias when lithium given with ● ARSENIC TRIOXIDE
- **Dapoxetine:** possible increased risk of serotonergic effects when lithium given with ● DAPOXETINE (manufacturer of dapoxetine advises lithium should not be started until 1 week after stopping dapoxetine, avoid dapoxetine for 2 weeks after stopping lithium)
- **Diuretics:** excretion of lithium increased by ● ACETAZOLAMIDE; excretion of lithium reduced by ● LOOP DIURETICS and ● THIAZIDES AND RELATED DIURETICS (increased plasma concentration and risk of toxicity)—loop diuretics safer than thiazides; excretion of lithium reduced by

Lithium

- **Diuretics** (continued)
  ● POTASSIUM-SPARING DIURETICS AND ALDOSTERONE ANTAGONISTS (increased plasma concentration and risk of toxicity)
- ▸ **5HT$_1$-receptor Agonists:** possible risk of toxicity when lithium given with SUMATRIPTAN
- **Methyldopa:** neurotoxicity may occur when lithium given with ● METHYLDOPA without increased plasma concentration of lithium
- ▸ **Muscle Relaxants:** lithium enhances effects of MUSCLE RELAXANTS; hyperkinesis caused by lithium possibly aggravated by BACLOFEN
- ▸ **Parasympathomimetics:** lithium antagonises effects of NEOSTIGMINE
- ▸ **Theophylline:** excretion of lithium increased by THEOPHYLLINE (reduced plasma concentration)

Lixisenatide *see* Antidiabetics

Lofepramine *see* Antidepressants, Tricyclic

Lofexidine

- ▸ **Alcohol:** increased sedative effect when lofexidine given with ALCOHOL
- ▸ **Anxiolytics and Hypnotics:** increased sedative effect when lofexidine given with ANXIOLYTICS AND HYPNOTICS

Lomitapide

- ▸ **Alcohol:** manufacturer of lomitapide advises avoid concomitant use with ALCOHOL
- **Anti-arrhythmics:** manufacturer of lomitapide advises separating administration from AMIODARONE by 12 hours; manufacturer of lomitapide advises avoid concomitant use with ● DRONEDARONE (plasma concentration possibly increased)
- **Antibacterials:** manufacturer of lomitapide advises separating administration from AZITHROMYCIN and ISONIAZID by 12 hours; manufacturer of lomitapide advises avoid concomitant use with ● CLARITHROMYCIN, ● ERYTHROMYCIN and ● TELITHROMYCIN (plasma concentration of lomitapide possibly increased)
- ▸ **Anticoagulants:** lomitapide possibly enhances anticoagulant effect of WARFARIN
- ▸ **Antidepressants:** manufacturer of lomitapide advises separating administration from FLUOXETINE and FLUVOXAMINE by 12 hours
- ▸ **Antidiabetics:** manufacturer of lomitapide advises separating administration from LINAGLIPTIN by 12 hours
- **Antifungals:** plasma concentration of lomitapide increased by ● KETOCONAZOLE—avoid concomitant use; manufacturer of lomitapide advises avoid concomitant use with ● TRIAZOLES (plasma concentration of lomitapide possibly increased)
- **Antivirals:** manufacturer of lomitapide advises avoid concomitant use with ● DARUNAVIR, ● FOSAMPRENAVIR, ● INDINAVIR, ● LOPINAVIR, ● RITONAVIR, ● SAQUINAVIR, ● TELAPREVIR and ● TIPRANAVIR (plasma concentration of lomitapide possibly increased)
- ▸ **Anxiolytics and Hypnotics:** manufacturer of lomitapide advises separating administration from ALPRAZOLAM by 12 hours
- **Calcium-channel Blockers:** manufacturer of lomitapide advises separating administration from AMLODIPINE and LACIDIPINE by 12 hours; manufacturer of lomitapide advises avoid concomitant use with ● DILTIAZEM and ● VERAPAMIL (plasma concentration of lomitapide possibly increased)
- ▸ **Ciclosporin:** manufacturer of lomitapide advises separating administration from CICLOSPORIN by 12 hours
- ▸ **Cilostazol:** manufacturer of lomitapide advises separating administration from CILOSTAZOL by 12 hours
- ▸ **Cytotoxics:** manufacturer of lomitapide advises separating administration from LAPATINIB, NILOTINIB and PAZOPANIB by 12 hours
- ▸ **Fosaprepitant:** manufacturer of lomitapide advises separating administration from FOSAPREPITANT by 12 hours
- ▸ **Grapefruit Juice:** manufacturer of lomitapide advises avoid concomitant use with GRAPEFRUIT JUICE
- ▸ **Hormone Antagonists:** manufacturer of lomitapide advises separating administration from BICALUTAMIDE by 12 hours
- ▸ **Ivacaftor:** manufacturer of lomitapide advises separating administration from IVACAFTOR by 12 hours
- **Lipid-regulating Drugs:** lomitapide increases plasma concentration of ATORVASTATIN—manufacturer of lomitapide

Lomitapide
- Lipid-regulating Drugs (continued)
  advises reduce dose of atorvastatin by half or separate administration by 12 hours; lomitapide increases plasma concentration of • SIMVASTATIN (see under Simvastatin, p. 188); absorption of lomitapide possibly reduced by BILE ACID SEQUESTRANTS (give at least 4 hours apart)
- ▸ Oestrogens: manufacturer of lomitapide advises separating administration from OESTROGENS by 12 hours
- ▸ Ranolazine: manufacturer of lomitapide advises separating administration from RANOLAZINE by 12 hours
- ▸ Tacrolimus: manufacturer of lomitapide advises separating administration from TACROLIMUS by 12 hours
- ▸ Ticagrelor: manufacturer of lomitapide advises separating administration from TICAGRELOR by 12 hours
- ▸ Tolvaptan: manufacturer of lomitapide advises separating administration from TOLVAPTAN by 12 hours
- ▸ Ulcer-healing Drugs: manufacturer of lomitapide advises separating administration from CIMETIDINE and RANITIDINE by 12 hours

Lomustine
- Antipsychotics: avoid concomitant use of cytotoxics with • CLOZAPINE (increased risk of agranulocytosis)
- ▸ Ulcer-healing Drugs: myelosuppressive effects of lomustine possibly enhanced by CIMETIDINE

Loperamide
- ▸ Desmopressin: loperamide increases plasma concentration of *oral* DESMOPRESSIN

Lopinavir
NOTE In combination with ritonavir as *Kaletra*® (ritonavir is present to inhibit lopinavir metabolism and increase plasma-lopinavir concentration)—see also Ritonavir
- Anti-arrhythmics: lopinavir possibly increases plasma concentration of • FLECAINIDE (increased risk of ventricular arrhythmias—avoid concomitant use); lopinavir possibly increases plasma concentration of LIDOCAINE
- ▸ Antibacterials: plasma concentration of lopinavir reduced by • RIFAMPICIN—avoid concomitant use; lopinavir increases plasma concentration of DELAMANID; avoidance of concomitant lopinavir in severe renal and hepatic impairment advised by manufacturer of • TELITHROMYCIN
- ▸ Anticoagulants: avoidance of lopinavir advised by manufacturer of APIXABAN; manufacturers advise avoid concomitant use of lopinavir with RIVAROXABAN
- Antidepressants: plasma concentration of lopinavir reduced by • ST JOHN'S WORT—avoid concomitant use
- Antiepileptics: plasma concentration of lopinavir possibly reduced by CARBAMAZEPINE, FOSPHENYTOIN, • PHENOBARBITAL, PHENYTOIN and • PRIMIDONE
- ▸ Antihistamines: lopinavir possibly increases plasma concentration of CHLORPHENAMINE
- ▸ Antimalarials: caution with lopinavir advised by manufacturer of ARTEMETHER WITH LUMEFANTRINE
- Antimuscarinics: avoidance of lopinavir advised by manufacturer of DARIFENACIN and TOLTERODINE
- Antipsychotics: lopinavir possibly increases plasma concentration of • ARIPIPRAZOLE (reduce dose of aripiprazole—consult aripiprazole product literature); lopinavir possibly increases plasma concentration of • QUETIAPINE—manufacturer of quetiapine advises avoid concomitant use
- Antivirals: manufacturers advise avoid concomitant use of lopinavir with • BOCEPREVIR and • TELAPREVIR; lopinavir reduces plasma concentration of • DARUNAVIR—avoid concomitant use; plasma concentration of lopinavir reduced by • EFAVIRENZ—consider increasing dose of lopinavir; lopinavir boosted with ritonavir increases plasma concentration of • ELVITEGRAVIR (reduce dose of elvitegravir); lopinavir reduces plasma concentration of FOSAMPRENAVIR, effect on lopinavir plasma concentration not predictable—avoid concomitant use; lopinavir increases plasma concentration of • MARAVIROC (consider reducing dose of maraviroc); plasma concentration of lopinavir possibly reduced by • NEVIRAPINE—consider increasing dose of lopinavir; lopinavir increases plasma concentration of • PARITAPREVIR—manufacturer of paritaprevir advises avoid

Lopinavir
- Antivirals (continued)
  concomitant use; increased risk of ventricular arrhythmias when lopinavir given with • SAQUINAVIR—avoid concomitant use; lopinavir increases plasma concentration of TENOFOVIR; plasma concentration of lopinavir reduced by • TIPRANAVIR
- Bosentan: lopinavir increases plasma concentration of • BOSENTAN (consider reducing dose of bosentan)
- ▸ Corticosteroids: plasma concentration of lopinavir possibly reduced by DEXAMETHASONE
- Cytotoxics: manufacturer of ruxolitinib advises dose reduction when lopinavir given with • RUXOLITINIB—consult ruxolitinib product literature
- ▸ Eltrombopag: lopinavir possibly reduces plasma concentration of ELTROMBOPAG
- Lipid-regulating Drugs: possible increased risk of myopathy when lopinavir given with ATORVASTATIN; lopinavir increases plasma concentration of • ROSUVASTATIN—adjust dose of rosuvastatin (consult product literature); possible increased risk of myopathy when lopinavir given with • SIMVASTATIN—avoid concomitant use; avoidance of lopinavir advised by manufacturer of • LOMITAPIDE (plasma concentration of lomitapide possibly increased)
- Orlistat: absorption of lopinavir possibly reduced by • ORLISTAT
- Ranolazine: lopinavir possibly increases plasma concentration of • RANOLAZINE—manufacturer of ranolazine advises avoid concomitant use
- ▸ Sirolimus: lopinavir possibly increases plasma concentration of SIROLIMUS
- ▸ Sympathomimetics, Beta₂: manufacturer of lopinavir advises avoid concomitant use with SALMETEROL

Loprazolam *see* Anxiolytics and Hypnotics
Loratadine *see* Antihistamines
Lorazepam *see* Anxiolytics and Hypnotics
Lormetazepam *see* Anxiolytics and Hypnotics
Losartan *see* Angiotensin-II Receptor Antagonists
Lurasidone *see* Antipsychotics
Lymecycline *see* Tetracyclines

Macitentan
- Antibacterials: plasma concentration of macitentan reduced by • RIFAMPICIN—avoid concomitant use
- ▸ Antidepressants: manufacturer of macitentan advises avoid concomitant use with ST JOHN'S WORT
- ▸ Antiepileptics: manufacturer of macitentan advises avoid concomitant use with CARBAMAZEPINE, FOSPHENYTOIN and PHENYTOIN
- ▸ Antifungals: plasma concentration of macitentan increased by KETOCONAZOLE

Macrogols
NOTE Some manufacturers suggest taking other oral medication 1 hour before or 1 hour after macrogols to reduce possible interference with absorption

Macrolides
NOTE *See also* Telithromycin
NOTE Interactions do not apply to small amounts of erythromycin used topically
- Aminophylline: clarithromycin possibly increases plasma concentration of AMINOPHYLLINE; erythromycin increases plasma concentration of • AMINOPHYLLINE (also aminophylline may reduce absorption of *oral* erythromycin)
- ▸ Analgesics: erythromycin increases plasma concentration of ALFENTANIL; clarithromycin possibly increases plasma concentration of FENTANYL
- ▸ Antacids: absorption of azithromycin reduced by ANTACIDS (give at least 2 hours before or 1 hour after antacids)
- Anti-arrhythmics: increased risk of ventricular arrhythmias when *parenteral* erythromycin given with • AMIODARONE—avoid concomitant use; erythromycin increases plasma concentration of • DISOPYRAMIDE (increased risk of toxicity); clarithromycin possibly increases plasma concentration of • DISOPYRAMIDE (increased risk of ventricular arrhythmias); azithromycin possibly increases plasma concentration of • DISOPYRAMIDE (increased risk of toxicity); avoidance of clarithromycin advised by manufacturer of • DRONEDARONE (risk of ventricular arrhythmias); erythromycin increases

Macrolides

- **Anti-arrhythmics** (continued)
plasma concentration of ● DRONEDARONE (increased risk of ventricular arrhythmias—avoid concomitant use)
- **Antibacterials:** increased risk of ventricular arrhythmias when *parenteral* erythromycin given with ● MOXIFLOXACIN—avoid concomitant use; increased risk of side-effects including neutropenia when azithromycin given with ● RIFABUTIN; clarithromycin increases plasma concentration of ● RIFABUTIN (increased risk of toxicity—reduce rifabutin dose); erythromycin possibly increases plasma concentration of ● RIFABUTIN (increased risk of toxicity—reduce rifabutin dose); clarithromycin and erythromycin possibly increase plasma concentration of BEDAQUILINE—avoid concomitant use if clarithromycin and erythromycin given for more than 14 days; possible increased risk of ventricular arrhythmias when clarithromycin and erythromycin given with ● DELAMANID; avoidance of clarithromycin and erythromycin advised by manufacturer of FIDAXOMICIN; plasma concentration of clarithromycin reduced by RIFAMYCINS
- **Anticoagulants:** avoidance of clarithromycin advised by manufacturer of APIXABAN; clarithromycin and erythromycin enhance anticoagulant effect of ● COUMARINS; azithromycin possibly enhances anticoagulant effect of ● COUMARINS; possible increased risk of bleeding when clarithromycin given with DABIGATRAN; erythromycin increases plasma concentration of ● EDOXABAN (reduce dose of edoxaban—see under Edoxaban, p. 113)
- **Antidepressants:** avoidance of macrolides advised by manufacturer of ● REBOXETINE; avoidance of *intravenous* erythromycin advised by manufacturer of ● CITALOPRAM and ● ESCITALOPRAM (risk of ventricular arrhythmias); avoidance of erythromycin advised by manufacturer of ● VENLAFAXINE (risk of ventricular arrhythmias); clarithromycin possibly increases plasma concentration of TRAZODONE
- **Antidiabetics:** clarithromycin enhances effects of REPAGLINIDE
- **Antiepileptics:** erythromycin increases plasma concentration of ● CARBAMAZEPINE; clarithromycin increases plasma concentration of ● CARBAMAZEPINE (consider reducing dose of carbamazepine); clarithromycin inhibits metabolism of FOSPHENYTOIN and PHENYTOIN (increased plasma concentration); erythromycin possibly inhibits metabolism of SODIUM VALPROATE and VALPROIC ACID (increased plasma concentration)
- **Antifungals:** avoidance of concomitant clarithromycin in severe renal imapirment advised by manufacturer of ● KETOCONAZOLE; avoidance of erythromycin advised by manufacturer of FLUCONAZOLE; clarithromycin increases plasma concentration of ITRACONAZOLE
- **Antihistamines:** manufacturer of loratadine advises erythromycin possibly increases plasma concentration of LORATADINE; macrolides possibly inhibit metabolism of ● MIZOLASTINE (avoid concomitant use); erythromycin inhibits metabolism of ● MIZOLASTINE—avoid concomitant use
- **Antimalarials:** avoidance of macrolides advised by manufacturer of ● ARTEMETHER WITH LUMEFANTRINE; avoidance of macrolides advised by manufacturer of ● ARTENIMOL WITH PIPERAQUINE (possible risk of ventricular arrhythmias)
- **Antimuscarinics:** erythromycin possibly increases plasma concentration of DARIFENACIN; manufacturer of fesoterodine advises dose reduction when clarithromycin given with FESOTERODINE—consult fesoterodine product literature; avoidance of clarithromycin and erythromycin advised by manufacturer of TOLTERODINE
- **Antipsychotics:** avoidance of macrolides advised by manufacturer of ● DROPERIDOL (risk of ventricular arrhythmias); increased risk of ventricular arrhythmias when *parenteral* erythromycin given with ● ZUCLOPENTHIXOL—avoid concomitant use; increased risk of ventricular arrhythmias when erythromycin given with ● AMISULPRIDE—avoid concomitant use; erythromycin possibly increases plasma concentration of ● CLOZAPINE (possible increased risk of convulsions); clarithromycin possibly increases plasma concentration of ● LURASIDONE—avoid concomitant use; erythromycin possibly increases the plasma concentration of ● LURASIDONE (see under Lurasidone, p. 364); increased risk of

Macrolides

- **Antipsychotics** (continued)
ventricular arrhythmias when clarithromycin given with ● PIMOZIDE—avoid concomitant use; possible increased risk of ventricular arrhythmias when erythromycin given with ● PIMOZIDE—avoid concomitant use; clarithromycin possibly increases plasma concentration of ● QUETIAPINE—manufacturer of quetiapine advises avoid concomitant use; erythromycin increases plasma concentration of ● QUETIAPINE—manufacturer of quetiapine advises avoid concomitant use; increased risk of ventricular arrhythmias when *parenteral* erythromycin given with ● SULPIRIDE
- **Antivirals:** plasma concentration of both drugs increased when clarithromycin given with ATAZANAVIR; clarithromycin possibly increases the plasma concentration of ● DACLATASVIR—reduce dose of daclatasvir (see under Daclatasvir, p. 568); avoidance of clarithromycin advised by manufacturer of DASABUVIR and PARITAPREVIR; plasma concentration of clarithromycin reduced by EFAVIRENZ, also plasma concentration of active metabolite of clarithromycin increased; plasma concentration of clarithromycin reduced by ● ETRAVIRINE and NEVIRAPINE (but concentration of an active metabolite increased), also plasma concentration of etravirine and nevirapine increased; clarithromycin possibly increases plasma concentration of ● MARAVIROC (consider reducing dose of maraviroc); avoidance of clarithromycin and erythromycin advised by manufacturer of ● RILPIVIRINE (plasma concentration of rilpivirine possibly increased); plasma concentration of clarithromycin increased by ● RITONAVIR (reduce dose of clarithromycin in renal impairment); plasma concentration of azithromycin and erythromycin possibly increased by RITONAVIR; increased risk of ventricular arrhythmias when erythromycin given with ● SAQUINAVIR—avoid concomitant use; plasma concentration of both drugs possibly increased when clarithromycin given with ● SAQUINAVIR and ● TELAPREVIR (increased risk of ventricular arrhythmias); plasma concentration of both drugs increased when erythromycin given with ● SIMEPREVIR—manufacturer of simeprevir advises avoid concomitant use; clarithromycin possibly increases plasma concentration of ● SIMEPREVIR—manufacturer of simeprevir advises avoid concomitant use; plasma concentration of both drugs possibly increased when erythromycin given with ● TELAPREVIR (increased risk of ventricular arrhythmias); plasma concentration of clarithromycin increased by ● TIPRANAVIR (reduce dose of clarithromycin in renal impairment), also clarithromycin increases plasma concentration of tipranavir; clarithromycin tablets reduce absorption of ZIDOVUDINE (give at least 2 hours apart)
- **Anxiolytics and Hypnotics:** clarithromycin and erythromycin inhibit metabolism of ● MIDAZOLAM (increased plasma concentration with increased sedation); erythromycin increases plasma concentration of BUSPIRONE (reduce dose of buspirone); erythromycin inhibits the metabolism of ZOPICLONE
- **Aprepitant:** clarithromycin possibly increases plasma concentration of APREPITANT
- **Atomoxetine:** increased risk of ventricular arrhythmias when *parenteral* erythromycin given with ● ATOMOXETINE
- **Avanafil:** clarithromycin possibly increases plasma concentration of ● AVANAFIL—manufacturer of avanafil advises avoid concomitant use; erythromycin increases plasma concentration of ● AVANAFIL—see under Avanafil, p. 735
- **Calcium-channel Blockers:** clarithromycin and erythromycin possibly inhibit metabolism of ● CALCIUM-CHANNEL BLOCKERS (increased risk of side-effects); avoidance of erythromycin advised by manufacturer of LERCANIDIPINE
- **Cardiac Glycosides:** macrolides increase plasma concentration of DIGOXIN (increased risk of toxicity)
- **Ciclosporin:** clarithromycin possibly inhibit metabolism of ● CICLOSPORIN (increased plasma concentration); azithromycin increases plasma concentration of ● CICLOSPORIN; clarithromycin and erythromycin inhibit metabolism of ● CICLOSPORIN (increased plasma concentration)
- **Cilostazol:** clarithromycin possibly increases plasma concentration of ● CILOSTAZOL (see under Cilostazol, p. 215);

Macrolides

- Cilostazol (continued)
  erythromycin increases plasma concentration of ● CILOSTAZOL
  (see under Cilostazol, p. 215)
- Clopidogrel: erythromycin possibly reduces antiplatelet effect
  of ● CLOPIDOGREL
- Colchicine: azithromycin, clarithromycin and erythromycin
  possibly increase risk of COLCHICINE toxicity—suspend or
  reduce dose of colchicine (avoid concomitant use in hepatic or
  renal impairment)
- Corticosteroids: erythromycin possibly inhibits metabolism of
  CORTICOSTEROIDS; erythromycin inhibits the metabolism of
  METHYLPREDNISOLONE; clarithromycin possibly increases
  plasma concentration of METHYLPREDNISOLONE
- Cytotoxics: erythromycin possibly increases the plasma
  concentration of ● AFATINIB—manufacturer of afatinib advises
  separating administration of erythromycin by 6 to 12 hours;
  clarithromycin and erythromycin possibly increase plasma
  concentration of ● AXITINIB (reduce dose of axitinib—consult
  axitinib product literature); clarithromycin and erythromycin
  possibly increase the plasma concentration of ● BOSUTINIB—
  manufacturer of bosutinib advises avoid or consider reducing
  dose of bosutinib; clarithromycin and erythromycin possibly
  increase plasma concentration of CABOZANTINIB;
  clarithromycin possibly increases plasma concentration of
  ● CRIZOTINIB and ● EVEROLIMUS—manufacturer of crizotinib
  and everolimus advises avoid concomitant use; avoidance of
  clarithromycin and erythromycin advised by manufacturer of
  DASATINIB (plasma concentration of dasatinib possibly
  increased); erythromycin increases plasma concentration of
  ● EVEROLIMUS (consider reducing the dose of everolimus —
  consult everolimus product literature); clarithromycin and
  erythromycin possibly increase the plasma concentration of
  ● IBRUTINIB—reduce dose of ibrutinib (see under Ibrutinib,
  p. 855); avoidance of clarithromycin advised by manufacturer
  of ● NILOTINIB and ● OLAPARIB; clarithromycin possibly
  increases plasma concentration of ● PAZOPANIB (reduce dose
  of pazopanib); clarithromycin possibly increases plasma
  concentration of PONATINIB—consider reducing initial dose of
  ponatinib (see under Ponatinib, p. 860); manufacturer of
  ruxolitinib advises dose reduction when clarithromycin given
  with ● RUXOLITINIB—consult ruxolitinib product literature;
  possible increased risk of ventricular arrhythmias when
  parenteral erythromycin given with ● VANDETANIB—avoid
  concomitant use; clarithromycin possibly increases the
  plasma concentration of ● CABAZITAXEL—manufacturer of
  cabazitaxel advises avoid or consider reducing dose of
  cabazitaxel; clarithromycin possibly increases plasma
  concentration of ● DOCETAXEL—manufacturer of docetaxel
  advises avoid concomitant use or consider reducing docetaxel
  dose; increased risk of ventricular arrhythmias when
  erythromycin given with ● ARSENIC TRIOXIDE; erythromycin
  increases toxicity of ● VINBLASTINE—avoid concomitant use;
  possible increased risk of neutropenia when clarithromycin
  given with ● VINORELBINE
- Dapoxetine: manufacturer of dapoxetine advises dose
  reduction when clarithromycin and erythromycin given with
  DAPOXETINE (see under Dapoxetine, p. 742)
- Diuretics: clarithromycin increases plasma concentration of
  ● EPLERENONE—avoid concomitant use; erythromycin
  increases plasma concentration of EPLERENONE (reduce dose
  of eplerenone)
- Domperidone: possible increased risk of ventricular
  arrhythmias when clarithromycin given with ● DOMPERIDONE—
  avoid concomitant use; erythromycin increases plasma
  concentration of ● DOMPERIDONE (increased risk of ventricular
  arrhythmias—avoid concomitant use)
- Dopaminergics: macrolides possibly increase plasma
  concentration of BROMOCRIPTINE and CABERGOLINE (increased
  risk of toxicity); erythromycin increases plasma concentration
  of BROMOCRIPTINE and CABERGOLINE (increased risk of toxicity)
- Ergot Alkaloids: increased risk of ergotism when clarithromycin
  or erythromycin given with ● ERGOT ALKALOIDS—avoid
  concomitant use
- Fosaprepitant: clarithromycin possibly increases plasma
  concentration of FOSAPREPITANT

Macrolides (continued)

- Guanfacine: clarithromycin and erythromycin possibly increase
  the plasma concentration of ● GUANFACINE (halve dose of
  guanfacine)
- 5HT₁-receptor Agonists: clarithromycin and erythromycin
  increase plasma concentration of ● ELETRIPTAN (risk of
  toxicity)—avoid concomitant use
- Ivabradine: clarithromycin possibly increases plasma
  concentration of ● IVABRADINE—avoid concomitant use;
  increased risk of ventricular arrhythmias when erythromycin
  given with ● IVABRADINE—avoid concomitant use
- Ivacaftor: clarithromycin and erythromycin possibly increase
  plasma concentration of ● IVACAFTOR (see under Ivacaftor,
  p. 269)
- Lenalidomide: clarithromycin possibly increases plasma
  concentration of ● LENALIDOMIDE (increased risk of toxicity)
- Leukotriene Receptor Antagonists: erythromycin reduces plasma
  concentration of ZAFIRLUKAST
- Lipid-regulating Drugs: possible increased risk of myopathy
  when azithromycin or erythromycin given with
  ● ATORVASTATIN; clarithromycin increases plasma
  concentration of ● ATORVASTATIN and PRAVASTATIN;
  erythromycin increases plasma concentration of PRAVASTATIN;
  erythromycin reduces plasma concentration of ROSUVASTATIN;
  possible increased risk of myopathy when azithromycin given
  with ● SIMVASTATIN; increased risk of myopathy when
  clarithromycin or erythromycin given with ● SIMVASTATIN
  (avoid concomitant use); avoidance of clarithromycin and
  erythromycin advised by manufacturer of ● LOMITAPIDE
  (plasma concentration of lomitapide possibly increased);
  separating administration from azithromycin by 12 hours
  advised by manufacturer of LOMITAPIDE
- Mirabegron: when given with clarithromycin avoid or reduce
  dose of MIRABEGRON in hepatic or renal impairment—see
  Mirabegron, p. 707
- Netupitant: plasma concentration of erythromycin increased
  by NETUPITANT
- Oestrogens: erythromycin increases plasma concentration of
  ESTRADIOL
- Parasympathomimetics: erythromycin increases plasma
  concentration of GALANTAMINE
- Pentamidine Isetionate: increased risk of ventricular
  arrhythmias when *parenteral* erythromycin given with
  ● PENTAMIDINE ISETIONATE
- Progestogens: erythromycin increases plasma concentration of
  DIENOGEST
- Ranolazine: clarithromycin possibly increases plasma
  concentration of ● RANOLAZINE—manufacturer of ranolazine
  advises avoid concomitant use
- Sildenafil: clarithromycin increases the plasma concentration
  of ● SILDENAFIL—consider reducing initial dose of sildenafil for
  erectile dysfunction or reduce sildenafil dose frequency to
  once daily for pulmonary hypertension; erythromycin
  increases plasma concentration of SILDENAFIL—reduce initial
  dose of sildenafil for erectile dysfunction or reduce sildenafil
  dose frequency to twice daily for pulmonary hypertension
- Sirolimus: clarithromycin increases plasma concentration of
  ● SIROLIMUS—avoid concomitant use; plasma concentration of
  both drugs increased when erythromycin given with
  ● SIROLIMUS
- Tacrolimus: clarithromycin and erythromycin increase plasma
  concentration of ● TACROLIMUS
- Tadalafil: clarithromycin and erythromycin possibly increase
  plasma concentration of TADALAFIL
- Theophylline: clarithromycin possibly increases plasma
  concentration of THEOPHYLLINE; erythromycin increases
  plasma concentration of THEOPHYLLINE (also theophylline
  may reduce absorption of *oral* erythromycin)
- Ticagrelor: clarithromycin possibly increases plasma
  concentration of ● TICAGRELOR—manufacturer of ticagrelor
  advises avoid concomitant use; erythromycin possibly
  increases plasma concentration of TICAGRELOR
- Ulcer-healing Drugs: plasma concentration of erythromycin
  increased by CIMETIDINE (increased risk of toxicity, including
  deafness); plasma concentration of both drugs increased
  when clarithromycin given with OMEPRAZOLE

Macrolides (continued)

▸ Ulipristal: avoidance of clarithromycin advised by manufacturer of *low-dose* ULIPRISTAL; erythromycin increases plasma concentration of *low-dose* ULIPRISTAL—manufacturer of *low-dose* ulipristal advises avoid concomitant use

▸ Vaccines: antibacterials inactivate ORAL TYPHOID VACCINE—see under Typhoid Vaccine in BNF

▸ Vardenafil: clarithromycin possibly increases plasma concentration of VARDENAFIL (consider reducing initial dose of vardenafil); erythromycin increases plasma concentration of VARDENAFIL (reduce dose of vardenafil)

Magnesium (parenteral)

● Calcium-channel Blockers: profound hypotension reported with concomitant use of parenteral magnesium and ● NIFEDIPINE in pre-eclampsia

▸ Muscle Relaxants: parenteral magnesium enhances effects of NON-DEPOLARISING MUSCLE RELAXANTS and SUXAMETHONIUM

Magnesium Salts (oral) *see* Antacids

Mannitol

▸ Antibacterials: avoidance of mannitol advised by manufacturer of TOBRAMYCIN

▸ Ciclosporin: possible increased risk of nephrotoxicity when mannitol given with CICLOSPORIN

MAOIs

NOTE For interactions of reversible MAO-A inhibitors (RIMAs) see Moclobemide, and for interactions of MAO-B inhibitors see Rasagiline and Selegiline

NOTE Linezolid is a reversible, non-selective MAO inhibitor and an antibacterial

▸ ACE Inhibitors: MAOIs possibly enhance hypotensive effect of ACE INHIBITORS

▸ Adrenergic Neurone Blockers: enhanced hypotensive effect when MAOIs given with ADRENERGIC NEURONE BLOCKERS

● Alcohol: MAOIs interact with tyramine found in some beverages containing ● ALCOHOL and some dealcoholised beverages (hypertensive crisis)—if no tyramine, enhanced hypotensive effect

▸ Alpha₂-adrenoceptor Stimulants: avoidance of MAOIs advised by manufacturer of APRACLONIDINE and BRIMONIDINE

● Alpha-blockers: avoidance of MAOIs advised by manufacturer of ● INDORAMIN; enhanced hypotensive effect when MAOIs given with ALPHA-BLOCKERS

● Analgesics: possible increased serotonergic effects when MAOIs given with FENTANYL; CNS excitation or depression (hypertension or hypotension) when MAOIs given with ● PETHIDINE—avoid concomitant use and for 2 weeks after stopping MAOIs; possible increased serotonergic effects and increased risk of convulsions when MAOIs given with ● TRAMADOL—some manufacturers advise avoid concomitant use and for 2 weeks after stopping MAOIs; avoidance of MAOIs advised by manufacturer of ● NEFOPAM; possible CNS excitation or depression (hypertension or hypotension) when MAOIs given with ● OPIOID ANALGESICS—some manufacturers advise avoid concomitant use and for 2 weeks after stopping MAOIs

▸ Angiotensin-II Receptor Antagonists: MAOIs possibly enhance hypotensive effect of ANGIOTENSIN-II RECEPTOR ANTAGONISTS

▸ Antibacterials: plasma concentration of linezolid reduced by RIFAMPICIN (possible therapeutic failure of linezolid)

● Antidepressants: increased risk of hypertension and CNS excitation when MAOIs given with ● REBOXETINE (MAOIs should not be started until 1 week after stopping reboxetine, avoid reboxetine for 2 weeks after stopping MAOIs); after stopping MAOIs do not start ● CITALOPRAM, ● ESCITALOPRAM, ● FLUVOXAMINE, ● PAROXETINE or ● SERTRALINE for 2 weeks, also MAOIs should not be started until at least 1 week after stopping citalopram, escitalopram, fluvoxamine, paroxetine or sertraline; after stopping MAOIs do not start ● FLUOXETINE for 2 weeks, also MAOIs should not be started until at least 5 weeks after stopping fluoxetine; after stopping MAOIs do not start ● DULOXETINE for 2 weeks, also MAOIs should not be started until at least 5 days after stopping duloxetine; enhanced CNS effects and toxicity when MAOIs given with ● VENLAFAXINE (venlafaxine should not be started until 2 weeks after stopping MAOIs, avoid MAOIs for 1 week after stopping venlafaxine); increased risk of hypertension and

MAOIs

● Antidepressants (continued)
CNS excitation when MAOIs given with other ● MAOIS (avoid for at least 2 weeks after stopping previous MAOIs and then start at a reduced dose); after stopping MAOIs do not start ● MOCLOBEMIDE for at least 1 week; MAOIs increase CNS effects of ● SSRIS (risk of serious toxicity); after stopping MAOIs do not start ● MIRTAZAPINE for 2 weeks, also MAOIs should not be started until at least 2 weeks after stopping mirtazapine; after stopping MAOIs do not start ● TRICYCLIC-RELATED ANTIDEPRESSANTS for 2 weeks, also MAOIs should not be started until at least 1–2 weeks after stopping tricyclic-related antidepressants; increased risk of hypertension and CNS excitation when MAOIs given with ● TRICYCLICS, tricyclics should not be started until 2 weeks after stopping MAOIs (3 weeks if starting clomipramine or imipramine), also MAOIs should not be started for at least 1–2 weeks after stopping tricyclics (3 weeks in the case of clomipramine or imipramine); increased risk of hypertension and CNS excitation when MAOIs given with ● VORTIOXETINE (vortioxetine should not be started until 2 weeks after stopping MAOIs, avoid MAOIs for 2 weeks after stopping vortioxetine); avoidance of linezolid advised by manufacturer of ● VORTIOXETINE

▸ Antidiabetics: MAOIs possibly enhance hypoglycaemic effect of ANTIDIABETICS; MAOIs enhance hypoglycaemic effect of INSULIN, METFORMIN and SULFONYLUREAS

● Antiepileptics: MAOIs possibly antagonise anticonvulsant effect of ANTIEPILEPTICS (convulsive threshold lowered); avoidance for 2 weeks after stopping MAOIs advised by manufacturer of ● CARBAMAZEPINE, also antagonism of anticonvulsant effect

▸ Antihistamines: avoidance of MAOIs advised by manufacturer of HYDROXYZINE; avoidance of promethazine for 2 weeks after stopping MAOIs advised by manufacturer of PROMETHAZINE; increased antimuscarinic and sedative effects when MAOIs given with ANTIHISTAMINES

● Antimalarials: avoidance of antidepressants advised by manufacturer of ● ARTEMETHER WITH LUMEFANTRINE and ● ARTENIMOL WITH PIPERAQUINE

● Antimuscarinics: increased risk of antimuscarinic side-effects when MAOIs given with ANTIMUSCARINICS

● Antipsychotics: CNS effects of MAOIs possibly increased by ● CLOZAPINE

● Anxiolytics and Hypnotics: manufacturer of tranylcypromine advises avoid ● BUSPIRONE for 14 days after stopping tranylcypromine; avoidance of MAOIs advised by manufacturer of BUSPIRONE

● Atomoxetine: after stopping MAOIs do not start ● ATOMOXETINE for 2 weeks, also MAOIs should not be started until at least 2 weeks after stopping atomoxetine; possible increased risk of convulsions when antidepressants given with ATOMOXETINE

▸ Beta-blockers: enhanced hypotensive effect when MAOIs given with BETA-BLOCKERS

● Bupropion: avoidance of bupropion for 2 weeks after stopping MAOIs advised by manufacturer of ● BUPROPION

▸ Calcium-channel Blockers: enhanced hypotensive effect when MAOIs given with CALCIUM-CHANNEL BLOCKERS

▸ Clonidine: enhanced hypotensive effect when MAOIs given with CLONIDINE

● Dapoxetine: increased risk of serotonergic effects when MAOIs given with ● DAPOXETINE (MAOIs should not be started until 1 week after stopping dapoxetine, avoid dapoxetine for 2 weeks after stopping MAOIs)

▸ Diazoxide: enhanced hypotensive effect when MAOIs given with DIAZOXIDE

▸ Diuretics: enhanced hypotensive effect when MAOIs given with DIURETICS

● Dopaminergics: risk of hypertensive crisis when MAOIs given with ● CO-BENELDOPA, ● CO-CARELDOPA or ● LEVODOPA, avoid co-beneldopa, co-careldopa or levodopa for at least 2 weeks after stopping MAOIs; avoid concomitant use of non-selective MAOIs with ● ENTACAPONE; risk of hypertensive crisis when MAOIs given with ● RASAGILINE, avoid MAOIs for at least 2 weeks after stopping rasagiline; enhanced hypotensive effect when MAOIs given with ● SELEGILINE—manufacturer of

MAOIs

- **Dopaminergics** (continued)
  selegiline advises avoid concomitant use; avoid concomitant use of MAOIs with TOLCAPONE
- **Doxapram:** MAOIs enhance effects of DOXAPRAM
▸ **Histamine:** avoidance of MAOIs advised by manufacturer of HISTAMINE
- **5HT₁-receptor Agonists:** risk of CNS toxicity when MAOIs given with ● RIZATRIPTAN or ● SUMATRIPTAN (avoid rizatriptan or sumatriptan for 2 weeks after MAOIs); risk of CNS toxicity when MAOIs given with ● ZOLMITRIPTAN (reduce dose of zolmitriptan)
- **Methyldopa:** avoidance of MAOIs advised by manufacturer of ● METHYLDOPA
- **Moxonidine:** enhanced hypotensive effect when MAOIs given with MOXONIDINE
▸ **Muscle Relaxants:** phenelzine enhances effects of SUXAMETHONIUM
▸ **Nicorandil:** enhanced hypotensive effect when MAOIs given with NICORANDIL
▸ **Nitrates:** enhanced hypotensive effect when MAOIs given with NITRATES
- **Pholcodine:** avoidance of pholcodine for 2 weeks after stopping MAOIs advised by manufacturer of PHOLCODINE
- **Sympathomimetics:** risk of hypertensive crisis when MAOIs given with ● ADRENALINE (EPINEPHRINE), ● DOBUTAMINE, ● DOPAMINE, ● NORADRENALINE (NOREPINEPHRINE) or ● XYLOMETAZOLINE; risk of hypertensive crisis when MAOIs given with ● DEXAMFETAMINE, ● EPHEDRINE, ● ISOMETHEPTENE, ● LISDEXAMFETAMINE, ● METARAMINOL, ● METHYLPHENIDATE, ● PHENYLEPHRINE or ● PSEUDOEPHEDRINE, avoid dexamfetamine, ephedrine, isometheptene, lisdexamfetamine, metaraminol, methylphenidate, phenylephrine or pseudoephedrine for at least 2 weeks after stopping MAOIs; avoidance of MIDODRINE advised by manufacturer of MIDODRINE; risk of hypertensive crisis when MAOIs given with ● OXYMETAZOLINE, some manufacturers advise avoid oxymetazoline for at least 2 weeks after stopping MAOIs
- **Tetrabenazine:** risk of CNS toxicity when MAOIs given with ● TETRABENAZINE (avoid tetrabenazine for 2 weeks after MAOIs)
▸ **Vaccines:** antibacterials including linezolid inactivate ORAL TYPHOID VACCINE—see under Typhoid Vaccine in BNF
▸ **Vasodilator Antihypertensives:** enhanced hypotensive effect when MAOIs given with HYDRALAZINE, MINOXIDIL or SODIUM NITROPRUSSIDE

MAOIs, reversible see Moclobemide

Maraviroc
- **Antibacterials:** plasma concentration of maraviroc possibly increased by ● CLARITHROMYCIN and ● TELITHROMYCIN (consider reducing dose of maraviroc); plasma concentration of maraviroc reduced by ● RIFAMPICIN—consider increasing dose of maraviroc
- **Antidepressants:** plasma concentration of maraviroc possibly reduced by ● ST JOHN'S WORT—avoid concomitant use
- **Antifungals:** plasma concentration of maraviroc increased by ● KETOCONAZOLE (consider reducing dose of maraviroc)
- **Antivirals:** plasma concentration of maraviroc increased by ● ATAZANAVIR, BOCEPREVIR, ● DARUNAVIR, ● INDINAVIR, ● LOPINAVIR, ● SAQUINAVIR and TELAPREVIR (consider reducing dose of maraviroc); plasma concentration of maraviroc possibly reduced by ● EFAVIRENZ—consider increasing dose of maraviroc; plasma concentration of maraviroc possibly reduced by ETRAVIRINE; maraviroc reduces plasma concentration of ● FOSAMPRENAVIR—avoid concomitant use; plasma concentration of maraviroc increased by RITONAVIR
- **Cobicistat:** plasma concentration of maraviroc possibly increased by ● COBICISTAT (reduce dose of maraviroc)
- **Orlistat:** absorption of maraviroc possibly reduced by ● ORLISTAT

Mebendazole
▸ **Ulcer-healing Drugs:** metabolism of mebendazole possibly inhibited by CIMETIDINE (increased plasma concentration)

Medroxyprogesterone see Progestogens

Mefenamic Acid see NSAIDs

Mefloquine
- **Anti-arrhythmics:** increased risk of ventricular arrhythmias when mefloquine given with ● AMIODARONE—avoid concomitant use
- **Antibacterials:** increased risk of ventricular arrhythmias when mefloquine given with ● MOXIFLOXACIN—avoid concomitant use; plasma concentration of mefloquine reduced by ● RIFAMPICIN—avoid concomitant use
- **Antidepressants:** possible increased risk of convulsions when mefloquine given with ● VORTIOXETINE
- **Antiepileptics:** mefloquine antagonises anticonvulsant effect of ● ANTIEPILEPTICS
▸ **Antifungals:** plasma concentration of mefloquine increased by KETOCONAZOLE
- **Antimalarials:** avoidance of antimalarials advised by manufacturer of ● ARTEMETHER WITH LUMEFANTRINE; increased risk of convulsions when mefloquine given with ● CHLOROQUINE or ● HYDROXYCHLOROQUINE; increased risk of convulsions when mefloquine given with ● QUININE (but should not prevent the use of *intravenous* quinine in severe cases)
- **Antipsychotics:** possible increased risk of ventricular arrhythmias when mefloquine given with ● HALOPERIDOL—avoid concomitant use; avoidance of mefloquine advised by manufacturer of AMISULPRIDE; increased risk of ventricular arrhythmias when mefloquine given with ● PIMOZIDE—avoid concomitant use; manufacturer of risperidone advises possible risk of ventricular arrhythmias when mefloquine given with ● RISPERIDONE
▸ **Antivirals:** mefloquine possibly reduces plasma concentration of RITONAVIR
- **Atomoxetine:** increased risk of ventricular arrhythmias when mefloquine given with ● ATOMOXETINE
▸ **Beta-blockers:** increased risk of bradycardia when mefloquine given with BETA-BLOCKERS
▸ **Calcium-channel Blockers:** possible increased risk of bradycardia when mefloquine given with CALCIUM-CHANNEL BLOCKERS
▸ **Cardiac Glycosides:** possible increased risk of bradycardia when mefloquine given with DIGOXIN
▸ **Cytotoxics:** possible increased risk of bradycardia when mefloquine given with CRIZOTINIB
▸ **Histamine:** avoidance of antimalarials advised by manufacturer of HISTAMINE
- **Ivabradine:** increased risk of ventricular arrhythmias when mefloquine given with ● IVABRADINE
- **Penicillamine:** increased risk of haematological toxicity when antimalarials given with PENICILLAMINE—manufacturer of penicillamine advises avoid concomitant use
▸ **Vaccines:** antimalarials inactivate ORAL TYPHOID VACCINE—see under Typhoid Vaccine in BNF

Megestrol see Progestogens

Melatonin see Anxiolytics and Hypnotics

Meloxicam see NSAIDs

Melphalan
▸ **Antibacterials:** increased risk of melphalan toxicity when given with NALIDIXIC ACID
- **Antipsychotics:** avoid concomitant use of cytotoxics with ● CLOZAPINE (increased risk of agranulocytosis)
- **Cardiac Glycosides:** melphalan possibly reduces absorption of DIGOXIN *tablets*
- **Ciclosporin:** increased risk of nephrotoxicity when melphalan given with ● CICLOSPORIN

Memantine
- **Anaesthetics, General:** increased risk of CNS toxicity when memantine given with ● KETAMINE (manufacturer of memantine advises avoid concomitant use)
- **Analgesics:** increased risk of CNS toxicity when memantine given with ● DEXTROMETHORPHAN (manufacturer of memantine advises avoid concomitant use)
▸ **Anticoagulants:** memantine possibly enhances anticoagulant effect of WARFARIN
▸ **Antimuscarinics:** memantine possibly enhances effects of ANTIMUSCARINICS
▸ **Antipsychotics:** memantine possibly reduces effects of ANTIPSYCHOTICS

Memantine (continued)
- Dopaminergics: memantine possibly enhances effects of DOPAMINERGICS and SELEGILINE; increased risk of CNS toxicity when memantine given with ● AMANTADINE (manufacturer of memantine advises avoid concomitant use)
▸ Muscle Relaxants: memantine possibly modifies effects of BACLOFEN and DANTROLENE

Meningococcal Vaccines see Vaccines

Mepacrine
▸ Antimalarials: mepacrine increases plasma concentration of PRIMAQUINE (increased risk of toxicity)

Meprobamate see Anxiolytics and Hypnotics

Meptazinol see Opioid Analgesics

Mercaptopurine
- Allopurinol: enhanced effects and increased toxicity of mercaptopurine when given with ● ALLOPURINOL (reduce dose of mercaptopurine to one quarter of usual dose)
- Antibacterials: increased risk of haematological toxicity when mercaptopurine given with ● SULFAMETHOXAZOLE (as co-trimoxazole); increased risk of haematological toxicity when mercaptopurine given with ● TRIMETHOPRIM (also with co-trimoxazole)
- Anticoagulants: mercaptopurine possibly reduces anticoagulant effect of ● COUMARINS
- Antipsychotics: avoid concomitant use of cytotoxics with ● CLOZAPINE (increased risk of agranulocytosis)
▸ Dairy Products: plasma concentration of mercaptopurine possibly reduced by DAIRY PRODUCTS—manufacturer of mercaptopurine advises give at least 1 hour before or 3 hours after dairy products
- Febuxostat: avoidance of mercaptopurine advised by manufacturer of ● FEBUXOSTAT

Meropenem
- Antiepileptics: carbapenems reduce plasma concentration of ● SODIUM VALPROATE and ● VALPROIC ACID—avoid concomitant use
▸ Vaccines: antibacterials inactivate ORAL TYPHOID VACCINE—see under Typhoid Vaccine in BNF

Mestranol see Oestrogens

Metaraminol see Sympathomimetics

Metformin see Antidiabetics

Methadone see Opioid Analgesics

Methenamine
▸ Antacids: avoid concomitant use of methenamine with ANTACIDS
- Antibacterials: increased risk of crystalluria when methenamine given with ● SULFONAMIDES
- Diuretics: effects of methenamine antagonised by ● ACETAZOLAMIDE
▸ Potassium Salts: avoid concomitant use of methenamine with POTASSIUM CITRATE
▸ Sodium Citrate: avoid concomitant use of methenamine with SODIUM CITRATE
▸ Vaccines: antibacterials inactivate ORAL TYPHOID VACCINE—see under Typhoid Vaccine in BNF

Methocarbamol see Muscle Relaxants

Methotrexate
▸ Aminophylline: methotrexate possibly increases plasma concentration of AMINOPHYLLINE
- Anaesthetics, General: antifolate effect of methotrexate increased by ● NITROUS OXIDE—avoid concomitant use
- Analgesics: excretion of methotrexate probably reduced by ● NSAIDS (increased risk of toxicity); excretion of methotrexate reduced by ● ASPIRIN, ● DICLOFENAC, ● IBUPROFEN, ● INDOMETACIN, ● KETOPROFEN, ● MELOXICAM and ● NAPROXEN (increased risk of toxicity)
- Antibacterials: absorption of methotrexate possibly reduced by NEOMYCIN; excretion of methotrexate possibly reduced by CIPROFLOXACIN (increased risk of toxicity); increased risk of severe bone marrow depression (fatalities reported) and other haematological toxicites when methotrexate given with ● SULFAMETHOXAZOLE (as co-trimoxazole); increased risk of methotrexate toxicity when given with DOXYCYCLINE, SULFONAMIDES or TETRACYCLINE; excretion of methotrexate reduced by PENICILLINS (increased risk of toxicity); increased risk of severe bone marrow depression (fatalities reported) and other haematological toxicites when

Methotrexate
- Antibacterials (continued)
  methotrexate given with ● TRIMETHOPRIM (also with co-trimoxazole)
- Antiepileptics: antifolate effect of methotrexate increased by FOSPHENYTOIN and PHENYTOIN; plasma concentration of methotrexate possibly increased by ● LEVETIRACETAM
- Antimalarials: antifolate effect of methotrexate increased by ● PYRIMETHAMINE
- Antipsychotics: avoid concomitant use of cytotoxics with ● CLOZAPINE (increased risk of agranulocytosis)
▸ Cardiac Glycosides: methotrexate possibly reduces absorption of DIGOXIN *tablets*
- Ciclosporin: risk of toxicity when methotrexate given with ● CICLOSPORIN
- Corticosteroids: possible increased risk of hepatoxicity when *high-dose* methotrexate given with DEXAMETHASONE
- Cytotoxics: increased pulmonary toxicity when methotrexate given with ● CISPLATIN
- Diuretics: excretion of methotrexate increased by alkaline urine due to ACETAZOLAMIDE
- Leflunomide: risk of toxicity when methotrexate given with ● LEFLUNOMIDE
- Retinoids: plasma concentration of methotrexate increased by ● ACITRETIN (also increased risk of hepatotoxicity)—avoid concomitant use
▸ Theophylline: methotrexate possibly increases plasma concentration of THEOPHYLLINE
▸ Ulcer-healing Drugs: excretion of methotrexate possibly reduced by PROTON PUMP INHIBITORS (increased risk of toxicity)

Methyldopa
▸ ACE Inhibitors: enhanced hypotensive effect when methyldopa given with ACE INHIBITORS
▸ Adrenergic Neurone Blockers: enhanced hypotensive effect when methyldopa given with ADRENERGIC NEURONE BLOCKERS
▸ Alcohol: enhanced hypotensive effect when methyldopa given with ALCOHOL
▸ Aldesleukin: enhanced hypotensive effect when methyldopa given with ALDESLEUKIN
▸ Alpha-blockers: enhanced hypotensive effect when methyldopa given with ALPHA-BLOCKERS
▸ Anaesthetics, General: enhanced hypotensive effect when methyldopa given with GENERAL ANAESTHETICS
▸ Analgesics: hypotensive effect of methyldopa antagonised by NSAIDS
▸ Angiotensin-II Receptor Antagonists: enhanced hypotensive effect when methyldopa given with ANGIOTENSIN-II RECEPTOR ANTAGONISTS
- Antidepressants: manufacturer of methyldopa advises avoid concomitant use with ● MAOIS
▸ Antipsychotics: enhanced hypotensive effect when methyldopa given with ANTIPSYCHOTICS (also increased risk of extrapyramidal effects)
▸ Anxiolytics and Hypnotics: enhanced hypotensive effect when methyldopa given with ANXIOLYTICS AND HYPNOTICS
▸ Beta-blockers: enhanced hypotensive effect when methyldopa given with BETA-BLOCKERS
▸ Calcium-channel Blockers: enhanced hypotensive effect when methyldopa given with CALCIUM-CHANNEL BLOCKERS
▸ Clonidine: enhanced hypotensive effect when methyldopa given with CLONIDINE
▸ Corticosteroids: hypotensive effect of methyldopa antagonised by CORTICOSTEROIDS
▸ Diazoxide: enhanced hypotensive effect when methyldopa given with DIAZOXIDE
▸ Diuretics: enhanced hypotensive effect when methyldopa given with DIURETICS
▸ Dopaminergics: methyldopa antagonises antiparkinsonian effect of DOPAMINERGICS; increased risk of extrapyramidal side-effects when methyldopa given with AMANTADINE; enhanced hypotensive effect when methyldopa given with CO-BENELDOPA, CO-CARELDOPA or LEVODOPA; effects of methyldopa possibly enhanced by ENTACAPONE
▸ Iron Salts: hypotensive effect of methyldopa antagonised by *oral* IRON SALTS
- Lithium: neurotoxicity may occur when methyldopa given with ● LITHIUM without increased plasma concentration of lithium

Methyldopa (continued)

▸ Moxisylyte: enhanced hypotensive effect when methyldopa given with MOXISYLYTE

▸ Moxonidine: enhanced hypotensive effect when methyldopa given with MOXONIDINE

▸ Muscle Relaxants: enhanced hypotensive effect when methyldopa given with BACLOFEN or TIZANIDINE

▸ Nitrates: enhanced hypotensive effect when methyldopa given with NITRATES

▸ Oestrogens: hypotensive effect of methyldopa antagonised by OESTROGENS

▸ Prostaglandins: enhanced hypotensive effect when methyldopa given with ALPROSTADIL

● Sympathomimetics, Beta₂: acute hypotension reported when methyldopa given with *infusion* of ● SALBUTAMOL

▸ Vasodilator Antihypertensives: enhanced hypotensive effect when methyldopa given with HYDRALAZINE, MINOXIDIL or SODIUM NITROPRUSSIDE

Methylphenidate *see* Sympathomimetics

Methylprednisolone *see* Corticosteroids

Methylthioninium

● Antidepressants: risk of CNS toxicity when methylthioninium given with ● SSRI-RELATED ANTIDEPRESSANTS, ● SSRIs and ● CLOMIPRAMINE—avoid concomitant use (if avoidance not possible, use lowest possible dose of methylthioninium and observe patient for up to 4 hours after administration); possible risk of CNS toxicity when methylthioninium given with ● MIRTAZAPINE—avoid concomitant use (if avoidance not possible, use lowest possible dose of methylthioninium and observe patient for up to 4 hours after administration)

● Anxiolytics and Hypnotics: possible risk of CNS toxicity when methylthioninium given with ● BUSPIRONE—avoid concomitant use (if avoidance not possible, use lowest possible dose of methylthioninium and observe patient for up to 4 hours after administration)

● Bupropion: possible risk of CNS toxicity when methylthioninium given with ● BUPROPION—avoid concomitant use (if avoidance not possible, use lowest possible dose of methylthioninium and observe patient for up to 4 hours after administration)

Metoclopramide

▸ Alcohol: metoclopramide possibly increases absorption of ALCOHOL

▸ Anaesthetics, General: metoclopramide enhances effects of THIOPENTAL

▸ Analgesics: metoclopramide increases rate of absorption of ASPIRIN (enhanced effect); effects of metoclopramide on gastro-intestinal activity antagonised by OPIOID ANALGESICS; metoclopramide increases rate of absorption of PARACETAMOL

▸ Antibacterials: metoclopramide reduces plasma concentration of FOSFOMYCIN

▸ Antidepressants: CNS toxicity reported when metoclopramide given with SSRIs

▸ Antimuscarinics: effects of metoclopramide on gastro-intestinal activity antagonised by ANTIMUSCARINICS

▸ Antipsychotics: increased risk of extrapyramidal side-effects when metoclopramide given with ANTIPSYCHOTICS

▸ Atovaquone: metoclopramide reduces plasma concentration of ATOVAQUONE—avoid concomitant use

● Ciclosporin: metoclopramide increases plasma concentration of ● CICLOSPORIN

▸ Dopaminergics: metoclopramide antagonises hypoprolactinaemic effects of BROMOCRIPTINE and CABERGOLINE; metoclopramide antagonises antiparkinsonian effect of PERGOLIDE; avoidance of metoclopramide advised by manufacturer of ROPINIROLE and ROTIGOTINE (antagonism of effect)

▸ Muscle Relaxants: metoclopramide enhances effects of SUXAMETHONIUM

▸ Tetrabenazine: increased risk of extrapyramidal side-effects when metoclopramide given with TETRABENAZINE

Metolazone *see* Diuretics

Metoprolol *see* Beta-blockers

Metronidazole

NOTE Interactions do not apply to topical metronidazole preparations

Metronidazole (continued)

▸ Alcohol: disulfiram-like reaction when metronidazole given with ALCOHOL

● Anticoagulants: metronidazole enhances anticoagulant effect of ● COUMARINS

▸ Antiepileptics: metronidazole possibly inhibits metabolism of FOSPHENYTOIN and PHENYTOIN (increased plasma concentration); metabolism of metronidazole accelerated by PHENOBARBITAL and PRIMIDONE (reduced effect)

▸ Cytotoxics: metronidazole increases plasma concentration of ● BUSULFAN (increased risk of toxicity); metronidazole inhibits metabolism of CAPECITABINE, FLUOROURACIL and TEGAFUR (increased toxicity)

▸ Disulfiram: psychotic reaction reported when metronidazole given with DISULFIRAM

▸ Lithium: metronidazole increases risk of LITHIUM toxicity

▸ Mycophenolate: metronidazole possibly reduces bioavailability of MYCOPHENOLATE

▸ Ulcer-healing Drugs: metabolism of metronidazole inhibited by CIMETIDINE (increased plasma concentration)

▸ Vaccines: antibacterials inactivate ORAL TYPHOID VACCINE—see under Typhoid Vaccine in BNF

Mianserin *see* Antidepressants, Tricyclic (related)

Micafungin

▸ Antifungals: micafungin possibly increases plasma concentration of AMPHOTERICIN; micafungin increases plasma concentration of ITRACONAZOLE (consider reducing dose of itraconazole)

▸ Calcium-channel Blockers: micafungin increases plasma concentration of NIFEDIPINE

▸ Ciclosporin: micafungin possibly increases plasma concentration of CICLOSPORIN

▸ Sirolimus: micafungin increases plasma concentration of SIROLIMUS

Miconazole *see* Antifungals, Imidazole

Midazolam *see* Anxiolytics and Hypnotics

Midodrine *see* Sympathomimetics

Mifamurtide

▸ Analgesics: manufacturer of mifamurtide advises avoid concomitant use with high doses of NSAIDs

▸ Ciclosporin: manufacturer of mifamurtide advises avoid concomitant use with CICLOSPORIN

▸ Corticosteroids: manufacturer of mifamurtide advises avoid concomitant use with CORTICOSTEROIDS

▸ Tacrolimus: manufacturer of mifamurtide advises avoid concomitant use with TACROLIMUS

Mifepristone

▸ Corticosteroids: mifepristone may reduce effect of CORTICOSTEROIDS (including *inhaled* corticosteroids) for 3–4 days

Milrinone *see* Phosphodiesterase Inhibitors

Minocycline *see* Tetracyclines

Minoxidil *see* Vasodilator Antihypertensives

Mirabegron

▸ Antibacterials: avoid or reduce dose of mirabegron in hepatic or renal impairment when given with CLARITHROMYCIN—see Mirabegron, p. 707

▸ Antifungals: avoid or reduce dose of mirabegron in hepatic or renal impairment when given with ITRACONAZOLE and KETOCONAZOLE—see Mirabegron, p. 707

▸ Antivirals: avoid or reduce dose of mirabegron in hepatic or renal impairment when given with RITONAVIR—see Mirabegron, p. 707

▸ Beta-blockers: mirabegron increases plasma concentration of METOPROLOL

▸ Cardiac Glycosides: mirabegron increases plasma concentration of DIGOXIN—reduce initial dose of digoxin

Mirtazapine

● Alcohol: increased sedative effect when mirtazapine given with ● ALCOHOL

▸ Analgesics: possible increased serotonergic effects when mirtazapine given with TRAMADOL

▸ Anticoagulants: mirtazapine enhances anticoagulant effect of WARFARIN

● Antidepressants: possible increased serotonergic effects when mirtazapine given with FLUOXETINE, FLUVOXAMINE or

Mirtazapine
- **Antidepressants** (continued)
  VENLAFAXINE; mirtazapine should not be started until 2 weeks after stopping ● MAOIS, also MAOIs should not be started until at least 2 weeks after stopping mirtazapine; after stopping mirtazapine do not start ● MOCLOBEMIDE for at least 1 week
- ▸ **Antiepileptics:** plasma concentration of mirtazapine reduced by CARBAMAZEPINE, FOSPHENYTOIN and PHENYTOIN
- **Antifungals:** plasma concentration of mirtazapine increased by KETOCONAZOLE
- **Antimalarials:** avoidance of antidepressants advised by manufacturer of ● ARTEMETHER WITH LUMEFANTRINE and ● ARTENIMOL WITH PIPERAQUINE
- ▸ **Anxiolytics and Hypnotics:** increased sedative effect when mirtazapine given with ANXIOLYTICS AND HYPNOTICS
- ▸ **Atomoxetine:** possible increased risk of convulsions when antidepressants given with ATOMOXETINE
- **Clonidine:** mirtazapine possibly antagonises hypotensive effect of CLONIDINE
- **Methylthioninium:** possible risk of CNS toxicity when mirtazapine given with ● METHYLTHIONINIUM—avoid concomitant use (if avoidance not possible, use lowest possible dose of methylthioninium and observe patient for up to 4 hours after administration)
- ▸ **Ulcer-healing Drugs:** plasma concentration of mirtazapine increased by CIMETIDINE

Misoprostol
- ▸ **Antacids:** absorption of misoprostol possibly reduced by ANTACIDS

Mitomycin
- **Antipsychotics:** avoid concomitant use of cytotoxics with ● CLOZAPINE (increased risk of agranulocytosis)
- **Vaccines:** risk of generalised infections when cytotoxic antibiotics given with live ● VACCINES—avoid concomitant use

Mitotane
- **Anticoagulants:** mitotane possibly reduces anticoagulant effect of ● COUMARINS
- **Antipsychotics:** avoid concomitant use of cytotoxics with ● CLOZAPINE (increased risk of agranulocytosis)
- ▸ **Antivirals:** avoidance of mitotane advised by manufacturer of DASABUVIR, OMBITASVIR and PARITAPREVIR
- ▸ **Diuretics:** manufacturer of mitotane advises avoid concomitant use of SPIRONOLACTONE (antagonism of effect)

Mitoxantrone
- **Antipsychotics:** avoid concomitant use of cytotoxics with ● CLOZAPINE (increased risk of agranulocytosis)
- ▸ **Ciclosporin:** excretion of mitoxantrone reduced by CICLOSPORIN (increased plasma concentration)
- **Vaccines:** risk of generalised infections when cytotoxic antibiotics given with live ● VACCINES—avoid concomitant use

Mivacurium see Muscle Relaxants
Mizolastine see Antihistamines
MMR Vaccine see Vaccines

Moclobemide
- **Analgesics:** possible CNS excitation or depression (hypertension or hypotension) when moclobemide given with ● DEXTROMETHORPHAN or ● PETHIDINE—avoid concomitant use; possible CNS excitation or depression (hypertension or hypotension) when moclobemide given with ● OPIOID ANALGESICS—manufacturer of moclobemide advises consider reducing dose of opioid analgesics
- **Antidepressants:** moclobemide should not be started for at least 1 week after stopping ● MAOIS, ● SSRI-RELATED ANTIDEPRESSANTS, ● CITALOPRAM, ● FLUVOXAMINE, ● MIRTAZAPINE, ● PAROXETINE, ● SERTRALINE, ● TRICYCLIC-RELATED ANTIDEPRESSANTS or ● TRICYCLICS; increased risk of CNS toxicity when moclobemide given with ● ESCITALOPRAM, preferably avoid concomitant use; moclobemide should not be started until 5 weeks after stopping ● FLUOXETINE; possible increased serotonergic effects when moclobemide given with ● DULOXETINE; avoidance of moclobemide advised by manufacturer of ● VORTIOXETINE
- **Antimalarials:** avoidance of antidepressants advised by manufacturer of ● ARTEMETHER WITH LUMEFANTRINE and ● ARTENIMOL WITH PIPERAQUINE

Moclobemide (continued)
- ▸ **Atomoxetine:** possible increased risk of convulsions when antidepressants given with ATOMOXETINE
- **Bupropion:** avoidance of moclobemide advised by manufacturer of ● BUPROPION
- **Clopidogrel:** moclobemide possibly reduces antiplatelet effect of ● CLOPIDOGREL
- **Dopaminergics:** increased risk of side-effects when moclobemide given with CO-BENELDOPA, CO-CARELDOPA or LEVODOPA; caution with moclobemide advised by manufacturer of ENTACAPONE; avoid concomitant use of moclobemide with ● SELEGILINE
- **5HT₁-receptor Agonists:** risk of CNS toxicity when moclobemide given with ● RIZATRIPTAN or ● SUMATRIPTAN (avoid rizatriptan or sumatriptan for 2 weeks after moclobemide); risk of CNS toxicity when moclobemide given with ● ZOLMITRIPTAN (reduce dose of zolmitriptan)
- **Sympathomimetics:** risk of hypertensive crisis when moclobemide given with ● SYMPATHOMIMETICS
- ▸ **Ulcer-healing Drugs:** plasma concentration of moclobemide increased by CIMETIDINE (halve dose of moclobemide)

Modafinil
- ▸ **Antiepileptics:** modafinil possibly increases plasma concentration of FOSPHENYTOIN and PHENYTOIN
- **Ciclosporin:** modafinil reduces plasma concentration of ● CICLOSPORIN
- **Cytotoxics:** modafinil possibly reduces plasma concentration of ● BOSUTINIB—manufacturer of bosutinib advises avoid concomitant use
- **Guanfacine:** modafinil possibly reduces plasma concentration of ● GUANFACINE—increase dose of guanfacine
- **Oestrogens:** modafinil accelerates metabolism of ● OESTROGENS (reduced contraceptive effect with combined oral contraceptives, contraceptive patches, and vaginal rings—see Contraceptive Interactions in BNF)

Moexipril see ACE Inhibitors
Mometasone see Corticosteroids
Monobactams see Aztreonam
Monoclonal antibodies see individual drugs
Montelukast see Leukotriene Receptor Antagonists
Morphine see Opioid Analgesics
Moxifloxacin see Quinolones

Moxisylyte
- ▸ **ACE Inhibitors:** enhanced hypotensive effect when moxisylyte given with ACE INHIBITORS
- ▸ **Adrenergic Neurone Blockers:** enhanced hypotensive effect when moxisylyte given with ADRENERGIC NEURONE BLOCKERS
- **Alpha-blockers:** possible severe postural hypotension when moxisylyte given with ● ALPHA-BLOCKERS
- ▸ **Angiotensin-II Receptor Antagonists:** enhanced hypotensive effect when moxisylyte given with ANGIOTENSIN-II RECEPTOR ANTAGONISTS
- **Beta-blockers:** possible severe postural hypotension when moxisylyte given with ● BETA-BLOCKERS
- ▸ **Calcium-channel Blockers:** enhanced hypotensive effect when moxisylyte given with CALCIUM-CHANNEL BLOCKERS
- ▸ **Clonidine:** enhanced hypotensive effect when moxisylyte given with CLONIDINE
- ▸ **Diazoxide:** enhanced hypotensive effect when moxisylyte given with DIAZOXIDE
- ▸ **Diuretics:** enhanced hypotensive effect when moxisylyte given with DIURETICS
- ▸ **Methyldopa:** enhanced hypotensive effect when moxisylyte given with METHYLDOPA
- ▸ **Moxonidine:** enhanced hypotensive effect when moxisylyte given with MOXONIDINE
- ▸ **Nitrates:** enhanced hypotensive effect when moxisylyte given with NITRATES
- ▸ **Vasodilator Antihypertensives:** enhanced hypotensive effect when moxisylyte given with HYDRALAZINE, MINOXIDIL or SODIUM NITROPRUSSIDE

Moxonidine
- ▸ **ACE Inhibitors:** enhanced hypotensive effect when moxonidine given with ACE INHIBITORS
- ▸ **Adrenergic Neurone Blockers:** enhanced hypotensive effect when moxonidine given with ADRENERGIC NEURONE BLOCKERS

Moxonidine (continued)

▸ Alcohol: enhanced hypotensive effect when moxonidine given with ALCOHOL
▸ Aldesleukin: enhanced hypotensive effect when moxonidine given with ALDESLEUKIN
▸ Alpha-blockers: enhanced hypotensive effect when moxonidine given with ALPHA-BLOCKERS
▸ Anaesthetics, General: enhanced hypotensive effect when moxonidine given with GENERAL ANAESTHETICS
▸ Analgesics: hypotensive effect of moxonidine antagonised by NSAIDS
▸ Angiotensin-II Receptor Antagonists: enhanced hypotensive effect when moxonidine given with ANGIOTENSIN-II RECEPTOR ANTAGONISTS
▸ Antidepressants: enhanced hypotensive effect when moxonidine given with MAOIs; hypotensive effect of moxonidine possibly antagonised by TRICYCLICS (manufacturer of moxonidine advises avoid concomitant use)
▸ Antipsychotics: enhanced hypotensive effect when moxonidine given with PHENOTHIAZINES
▸ Anxiolytics and Hypnotics: enhanced hypotensive effect when moxonidine given with ANXIOLYTICS AND HYPNOTICS; sedative effects possibly increased when moxonidine given with BENZODIAZEPINES
▸ Beta-blockers: enhanced hypotensive effect when moxonidine given with BETA-BLOCKERS
▸ Calcium-channel Blockers: enhanced hypotensive effect when moxonidine given with CALCIUM-CHANNEL BLOCKERS
▸ Clonidine: enhanced hypotensive effect when moxonidine given with CLONIDINE
▸ Corticosteroids: hypotensive effect of moxonidine antagonised by CORTICOSTEROIDS
▸ Diazoxide: enhanced hypotensive effect when moxonidine given with DIAZOXIDE
▸ Diuretics: enhanced hypotensive effect when moxonidine given with DIURETICS
▸ Dopaminergics: enhanced hypotensive effect when moxonidine given with CO-BENELDOPA, CO-CARELDOPA or LEVODOPA
▸ Methyldopa: enhanced hypotensive effect when moxonidine given with METHYLDOPA
▸ Moxisylyte: enhanced hypotensive effect when moxonidine given with MOXISYLYTE
▸ Muscle Relaxants: enhanced hypotensive effect when moxonidine given with BACLOFEN or TIZANIDINE
▸ Nitrates: enhanced hypotensive effect when moxonidine given with NITRATES
▸ Oestrogens: hypotensive effect of moxonidine antagonised by OESTROGENS
▸ Prostaglandins: enhanced hypotensive effect when moxonidine given with ALPROSTADIL
▸ Vasodilator Antihypertensives: enhanced hypotensive effect when moxonidine given with HYDRALAZINE, MINOXIDIL or SODIUM NITROPRUSSIDE

Muscle Relaxants

▸ ACE Inhibitors: enhanced hypotensive effect when baclofen or tizanidine given with ACE INHIBITORS
▸ Adrenergic Neurone Blockers: enhanced hypotensive effect when baclofen or tizanidine given with ADRENERGIC NEURONE BLOCKERS
▸ Alcohol: increased sedative effect when baclofen, methocarbamol or tizanidine given with ALCOHOL
▸ Alpha-blockers: enhanced hypotensive effect when baclofen or tizanidine given with ALPHA-BLOCKERS
• Anaesthetics, General: effects of atracurium enhanced by KETAMINE; increased risk of myocardial depression and bradycardia when suxamethonium given with ● PROPOFOL; effects of non-depolarising muscle relaxants and suxamethonium enhanced by VOLATILE LIQUID GENERAL ANAESTHETICS
▸ Analgesics: excretion of baclofen possibly reduced by NSAIDs (increased risk of toxicity); excretion of baclofen reduced by IBUPROFEN (increased risk of toxicity); increased sedative effect when baclofen given with FENTANYL or MORPHINE
▸ Angiotensin-II Receptor Antagonists: enhanced hypotensive effect when baclofen or tizanidine given with ANGIOTENSIN-II RECEPTOR ANTAGONISTS

Muscle Relaxants (continued)

▸ Anti-arrhythmics: neuromuscular blockade enhanced and prolonged when suxamethonium given with LIDOCAINE
• Antibacterials: effects of non-depolarising muscle relaxants and suxamethonium enhanced by PIPERACILLIN; plasma concentration of tizanidine increased by ● CIPROFLOXACIN (increased risk of toxicity)—avoid concomitant use; plasma concentration of tizanidine possibly increased by NORFLOXACIN (increased risk of toxicity); plasma concentration of tizanidine possibly reduced by RIFAMPICIN; effects of non-depolarising muscle relaxants and suxamethonium enhanced by ● AMINOGLYCOSIDES; effects of non-depolarising muscle relaxants and suxamethonium enhanced by ● CLINDAMYCIN; effects of non-depolarising muscle relaxants enhanced by ● POLYMYXINS; effects of suxamethonium enhanced by ● VANCOMYCIN
• Antidepressants: plasma concentration of tizanidine increased by ● FLUVOXAMINE (increased risk of toxicity)—avoid concomitant use; effects of suxamethonium enhanced by PHENELZINE; muscle relaxant effect of baclofen enhanced by TRICYCLICS
• Antiepileptics: muscle relaxant effect of non-depolarising muscle relaxants antagonised by CARBAMAZEPINE (accelerated recovery from neuromuscular blockade); effects of non-depolarising muscle relaxants reduced by long-term use of ● FOSPHENYTOIN and ● PHENYTOIN (but effects of non-depolarising muscle relaxants might be increased by acute use of fosphenytoin and phenytoin)
▸ Antimalarials: effects of suxamethonium possibly enhanced by QUININE
▸ Antipsychotics: effects of suxamethonium possibly enhanced by PROMAZINE
▸ Anxiolytics and Hypnotics: increased sedative effect when baclofen or tizanidine given with ANXIOLYTICS AND HYPNOTICS
▸ Beta-blockers: enhanced hypotensive effect when baclofen given with BETA-BLOCKERS; possible enhanced hypotensive effect and bradycardia when tizanidine given with BETA-BLOCKERS; effects of muscle relaxants enhanced by PROPRANOLOL
▸ Calcium-channel Blockers: enhanced hypotensive effect when baclofen or tizanidine given with CALCIUM-CHANNEL BLOCKERS; effects of non-depolarising muscle relaxants possibly enhanced by CALCIUM-CHANNEL BLOCKERS; possible increased risk of ventricular arrhythmias when intravenous dantrolene given with DILTIAZEM—manufacturer of diltiazem advises avoid concomitant use; effects of non-depolarising muscle relaxants and suxamethonium enhanced by VERAPAMIL; avoidance of intravenous dantrolene advised by manufacturer of VERAPAMIL
▸ Cardiac Glycosides: possible increased risk of bradycardia when tizanidine given with CARDIAC GLYCOSIDES; risk of ventricular arrhythmias when suxamethonium given with CARDIAC GLYCOSIDES
▸ Clonidine: enhanced hypotensive effect when baclofen or tizanidine given with CLONIDINE
▸ Corticosteroids: effects of pancuronium and vecuronium possibly antagonised by CORTICOSTEROIDS
▸ Cytotoxics: effects of suxamethonium enhanced by CYCLOPHOSPHAMIDE and THIOTEPA
▸ Deferasirox: avoidance of tizanidine advised by manufacturer of DEFERASIROX
▸ Diazoxide: enhanced hypotensive effect when baclofen or tizanidine given with DIAZOXIDE
▸ Diuretics: enhanced hypotensive effect when baclofen or tizanidine given with DIURETICS
▸ Dopaminergics: possible agitation, confusion and hallucinations when baclofen given with CO-BENELDOPA, CO-CARELDOPA or LEVODOPA
▸ Lithium: effects of muscle relaxants enhanced by LITHIUM; baclofen possibly aggravates hyperkinesis caused by LITHIUM
▸ Magnesium (parenteral): effects of non-depolarising muscle relaxants and suxamethonium enhanced by PARENTERAL MAGNESIUM
▸ Memantine: effects of baclofen and dantrolene possibly modified by MEMANTINE

Muscle Relaxants (continued)

▸ **Methyldopa:** enhanced hypotensive effect when baclofen or tizanidine given with METHYLDOPA
▸ **Metoclopramide:** effects of suxamethonium enhanced by METOCLOPRAMIDE
▸ **Moxonidine:** enhanced hypotensive effect when baclofen or tizanidine given with MOXONIDINE
▸ **Nitrates:** enhanced hypotensive effect when baclofen or tizanidine given with NITRATES
▸ **Oestrogens:** plasma concentration of tizanidine possibly increased by OESTROGENS (increased risk of toxicity)
▸ **Parasympathomimetics:** effects of non-depolarising muscle relaxants possibly antagonised by DONEPEZIL; effects of suxamethonium possibly enhanced by DONEPEZIL; effects of suxamethonium enhanced by GALANTAMINE, NEOSTIGMINE, PYRIDOSTIGMINE and RIVASTIGMINE; effects of non-depolarising muscle relaxants antagonised by NEOSTIGMINE, PYRIDOSTIGMINE and RIVASTIGMINE
▸ **Progestogens:** plasma concentration of tizanidine possibly increased by PROGESTOGENS (increased risk of toxicity)
▸ **Sympathomimetics, Beta$_2$:** effects of suxamethonium enhanced by BAMBUTEROL
▸ **Vasodilator Antihypertensives:** enhanced hypotensive effect when baclofen or tizanidine given with HYDRALAZINE; enhanced hypotensive effect when baclofen or tizanidine given with MINOXIDIL; enhanced hypotensive effect when baclofen or tizanidine given with SODIUM NITROPRUSSIDE

Muscle Relaxants, depolarising see Muscle Relaxants
Muscle Relaxants, non-depolarising see Muscle Relaxants
Mycophenolate

▸ **Antacids:** absorption of mycophenolate reduced by ANTACIDS
● **Antibacterials:** bioavailability of mycophenolate possibly reduced by METRONIDAZOLE and NORFLOXACIN; plasma concentration of mycophenolate possibly reduced by CO-AMOXICLAV; plasma concentration of active metabolite of mycophenolate reduced by ● RIFAMPICIN
▸ **Antivirals:** mycophenolate increases plasma concentration of ACICLOVIR and VALACICLOVIR, also plasma concentration of inactive metabolite of mycophenolate increased; mycophenolate possibly increases plasma concentration of GANCICLOVIR and VALGANCICLOVIR, also plasma concentration of inactive metabolite of mycophenolate possibly increased
▸ **Iron Salts:** absorption of mycophenolate reduced by *oral* IRON SALTS
▸ **Lipid-regulating Drugs:** absorption of mycophenolate reduced by COLESTYRAMINE
▸ **Sevelamer:** plasma concentration of mycophenolate possibly reduced by SEVELAMER

Nabumetone see NSAIDs
Nadolol see Beta-blockers
Nalidixic Acid see Quinolones
Nalmefene

● **Analgesics:** manufacturer of nalmefene advises avoid concomitant use with ● OPIOID ANALGESICS

Nandrolone see Anabolic Steroids
Naproxen see NSAIDs
Naratriptan see 5HT$_1$-receptor Agonists (under HT)
Natalizumab

● **Antipsychotics:** avoid concomitant use of cytotoxics with ● CLOZAPINE (increased risk of agranulocytosis)
● **Vaccines:** risk of generalised infections when monoclonal antibodies given with live ● VACCINES—avoid concomitant use

Nateglinide see Antidiabetics
Nebivolol see Beta-blockers
Nefopam

● **Antidepressants:** manufacturer of nefopam advises avoid concomitant use with ● MAOIS; side-effects possibly increased when nefopam given with TRICYCLICS
▸ **Antimuscarinics:** increased risk of antimuscarinic side-effects when nefopam given with ANTIMUSCARINICS

Neomycin see Aminoglycosides
Neostigmine see Parasympathomimetics
Netupitant

▸ **Analgesics:** manufacturer of netupitant advises caution with MORPHINE

Netupitant (continued)

● **Antibacterials:** netupitant increases plasma concentration of ERYTHROMYCIN; plasma concentration of netupitant reduced by ● RIFAMPICIN—avoid concomitant use
▸ **Anticoagulants:** manufacturer of netupitant advises caution with DABIGATRAN
▸ **Antiepileptics:** manufacturer of netupitant advises caution with VALPROIC ACID
▸ **Antifungals:** plasma concentration of netupitant possibly increased by KETOCONAZOLE
▸ **Antivirals:** manufacturer of netupitant advises caution with ZIDOVUDINE
▸ **Anxiolytics and Hypnotics:** netupitant increases plasma concentration of MIDAZOLAM
● **Colchicine:** manufacturer of netupitant advises caution with COLCHICINE
● **Corticosteroids:** netupitant increases plasma concentration of ● DEXAMETHASONE (halve dose of dexamethasone)
▸ **Cytotoxics:** netupitant increases plasma concentration of DOCETAXEL and ETOPOSIDE

Nevirapine

▸ **Analgesics:** nevirapine possibly reduces plasma concentration of METHADONE
● **Antibacterials:** nevirapine reduces plasma concentration of CLARITHROMYCIN (but concentration of an active metabolite increased), also plasma concentration of nevirapine increased; nevirapine possibly increases plasma concentration of RIFABUTIN; plasma concentration of nevirapine reduced by ● RIFAMPICIN—avoid concomitant use
● **Anticoagulants:** nevirapine may enhance or reduce anticoagulant effect of ● WARFARIN
● **Antidepressants:** plasma concentration of nevirapine reduced by ● ST JOHN'S WORT—avoid concomitant use
▸ **Antiepileptics:** plasma concentration of nevirapine reduced by CARBAMAZEPINE
● **Antifungals:** nevirapine reduces plasma concentration of ● KETOCONAZOLE—avoid concomitant use; plasma concentration of nevirapine increased by ● FLUCONAZOLE; nevirapine possibly reduces plasma concentration of CASPOFUNGIN and ITRACONAZOLE—consider increasing dose of caspofungin and itraconazole
● **Antipsychotics:** nevirapine possibly reduces plasma concentration of ● ARIPIPRAZOLE (avoid concomitant use or consider increasing the dose of aripiprazole—consult aripiprazole product literature)
● **Antivirals:** nevirapine possibly reduces plasma concentration of ● ATAZANAVIR and ● ETRAVIRINE—avoid concomitant use; manufacturer of nevirapine advises avoid concomitant use with BOCEPREVIR and RILPIVIRINE; avoidance of nevirapine advised by manufacturer of DACLATASVIR (plasma concentration of daclatasvir possibly reduced); avoidance of nevirapine advised by manufacturer of DASABUVIR, ELVITEGRAVIR, OMBITASVIR and PARITAPREVIR; nevirapine possibly reduces the plasma concentration of ● DOLUTEGRAVIR (see under Dolutegravir, p. 584); nevirapine reduces plasma concentration of ● EFAVIRENZ—avoid concomitant use; nevirapine possibly reduces plasma concentration of FOSAMPRENAVIR—avoid unboosted fosamprenavir; nevirapine reduces plasma concentration of INDINAVIR; nevirapine possibly reduces plasma concentration of ● LOPINAVIR and TELAPREVIR—consider increasing dose of lopinavir and telaprevir; nevirapine possibly reduces plasma concentration of ● SIMEPREVIR—manufacturer of simeprevir advises avoid concomitant use; increased risk of granulocytopenia when nevirapine given with ● ZIDOVUDINE
▸ **Cobicistat:** manufacturer of nevirapine advises avoid concomitant use with COBICISTAT
● **Cytotoxics:** avoidance of nevirapine advised by manufacturer of ● OLAPARIB
● **Guanfacine:** nevirapine possibly reduces plasma concentration of ● GUANFACINE—increase dose of guanfacine
● **Oestrogens:** nevirapine accelerates metabolism of ● OESTROGENS (reduced contraceptive effect with combined oral contraceptives, contraceptive patches, and vaginal rings—see Contraceptive Interactions in BNF)

A1

Interactions | **Appendix 1**

Nevirapine (continued)

- Orlistat: absorption of nevirapine possibly reduced by
  - ORLISTAT
- Progestogens: nevirapine accelerates metabolism of
  - PROGESTOGENS (reduced contraceptive effect with combined oral contraceptives, progestogen-only oral contraceptives, contraceptive patches, vaginal rings, etonogestrel-releasing implant, and emergency hormonal contraception—see Contraceptive Interactions in BNF)

Nicardipine see Calcium-channel Blockers

Nicorandil

- ▶ Alcohol: hypotensive effect of nicorandil possibly enhanced by ALCOHOL
- ▶ Analgesics: increased risk of gastro-intestinal bleeding and ulceration when nicorandil given with NSAIDs or ASPIRIN
- ▶ Antidepressants: enhanced hypotensive effect when nicorandil given with MAOIs; hypotensive effect of nicorandil possibly enhanced by TRICYCLICS
- Avanafil: hypotensive effect of nicorandil significantly enhanced by ● AVANAFIL (avoid concomitant use)
- ▶ Corticosteroids: increased risk of gastro-intestinal bleeding and ulceration when nicorandil given with CORTICOSTEROIDS
- Riociguat: possible enhanced hypotensive effect when nicorandil given with ● RIOCIGUAT—avoid concomitant use
- Sildenafil: hypotensive effect of nicorandil significantly enhanced by ● SILDENAFIL (avoid concomitant use)
- Tadalafil: hypotensive effect of nicorandil significantly enhanced by ● TADALAFIL (avoid concomitant use)
- Vardenafil: possible increased hypotensive effect when nicorandil given with ● VARDENAFIL—avoid concomitant use
- ▶ Vasodilator Antihypertensives: possible enhanced hypotensive effect when nicorandil given with HYDRALAZINE, MINOXIDIL or SODIUM NITROPRUSSIDE

Nicotine

- ▶ Anti-arrhythmics: nicotine possibly enhances effects of ADENOSINE

Nicotinic Acid

- Lipid-regulating Drugs: increased risk of myopathy when nicotinic acid given with ● STATINS (applies to lipid regulating doses of nicotinic acid)

Nifedipine see Calcium-channel Blockers

Nilotinib

- Antibacterials: manufacturer of nilotinib advises avoid concomitant use with ● CLARITHROMYCIN and ● TELITHROMYCIN; plasma concentration of nilotinib reduced by ● RIFAMPICIN— avoid concomitant use
- Antifungals: plasma concentration of nilotinib increased by ● KETOCONAZOLE—avoid concomitant use; manufacturer of nilotinib advises avoid concomitant use with ● ITRACONAZOLE and ● VORICONAZOLE
- Antipsychotics: avoid concomitant use of cytotoxics with ● CLOZAPINE (increased risk of agranulocytosis)
- Antivirals: avoidance of nilotinib advised by manufacturer of ● BOCEPREVIR; plasma concentration of nilotinib possibly increased by RITONAVIR—manufacturer of nilotinib advises avoid concomitant use
- ▶ Anxiolytics and Hypnotics: nilotinib increases plasma concentration of MIDAZOLAM
- Grapefruit Juice: manufacturer of nilotinib advises avoid concomitant use with ● GRAPEFRUIT JUICE
- ▶ Lipid-regulating Drugs: separating administration from nilotinib by 12 hours advised by manufacturer of LOMITAPIDE

Nimodipine see Calcium-channel Blockers

Nintedanib

- Antibacterials: plasma concentration of nintedanib reduced by ● RIFAMPICIN—avoid concomitant use
- Antifungals: plasma concentration of nintedanib increased by ● KETOCONAZOLE
- Antipsychotics: avoid concomitant use of cytotoxics with ● CLOZAPINE (increased risk of agranulocytosis)

Nitrates

- ▶ ACE Inhibitors: enhanced hypotensive effect when nitrates given with ACE INHIBITORS
- ▶ Adrenergic Neurone Blockers: enhanced hypotensive effect when nitrates given with ADRENERGIC NEURONE BLOCKERS

Nitrates (continued)

- ▶ Alcohol: enhanced hypotensive effect when nitrates given with ALCOHOL
- ▶ Aldesleukin: enhanced hypotensive effect when nitrates given with ALDESLEUKIN
- ▶ Alpha-blockers: enhanced hypotensive effect when nitrates given with ALPHA-BLOCKERS
- ▶ Anaesthetics, General: enhanced hypotensive effect when nitrates given with GENERAL ANAESTHETICS
- ▶ Analgesics: hypotensive effect of nitrates antagonised by NSAIDs
- ▶ Angiotensin-II Receptor Antagonists: enhanced hypotensive effect when nitrates given with ANGIOTENSIN-II RECEPTOR ANTAGONISTS
- ▶ Anti-arrhythmics: effects of sublingual tablets of nitrates reduced by DISOPYRAMIDE (failure to dissolve under tongue owing to dry mouth)
- Anticoagulants: *infusion* of glyceryl trinitrate reduces anticoagulant effect of ● HEPARINS
- ▶ Antidepressants: enhanced hypotensive effect when nitrates given with MAOIs; effects of sublingual tablets of nitrates possibly reduced by TRICYCLIC-RELATED ANTIDEPRESSANTS (failure to dissolve under tongue owing to dry mouth); effects of sublingual tablets of nitrates reduced by TRICYCLICS (failure to dissolve under tongue owing to dry mouth)
- ▶ Antimuscarinics: effects of sublingual tablets of nitrates possibly reduced by ANTIMUSCARINICS (failure to dissolve under tongue owing to dry mouth)
- ▶ Antipsychotics: enhanced hypotensive effect when nitrates given with PHENOTHIAZINES
- ▶ Anxiolytics and Hypnotics: enhanced hypotensive effect when nitrates given with ANXIOLYTICS AND HYPNOTICS
- Avanafil: hypotensive effect of nitrates significantly enhanced by ● AVANAFIL (avoid concomitant use)
- ▶ Beta-blockers: enhanced hypotensive effect when nitrates given with BETA-BLOCKERS
- ▶ Calcium-channel Blockers: enhanced hypotensive effect when nitrates given with CALCIUM-CHANNEL BLOCKERS
- ▶ Clonidine: enhanced hypotensive effect when nitrates given with CLONIDINE
- ▶ Corticosteroids: hypotensive effect of nitrates antagonised by CORTICOSTEROIDS
- ▶ Diazoxide: enhanced hypotensive effect when nitrates given with DIAZOXIDE
- ▶ Diuretics: enhanced hypotensive effect when nitrates given with DIURETICS
- ▶ Dopaminergics: enhanced hypotensive effect when nitrates given with CO-BENELDOPA, CO-CARELDOPA or LEVODOPA
- Levosimendan: possible severe postural hypotension when isosorbide mononitrate given with ● LEVOSIMENDAN
- ▶ Methyldopa: enhanced hypotensive effect when nitrates given with METHYLDOPA
- ▶ Moxisylyte: enhanced hypotensive effect when nitrates given with MOXISYLYTE
- ▶ Moxonidine: enhanced hypotensive effect when nitrates given with MOXONIDINE
- ▶ Muscle Relaxants: enhanced hypotensive effect when nitrates given with BACLOFEN or TIZANIDINE
- ▶ Oestrogens: hypotensive effect of nitrates antagonised by OESTROGENS
- ▶ Prostaglandins: enhanced hypotensive effect when nitrates given with ALPROSTADIL
- ▶ Riociguat: possible enhanced hypotensive effect when nitrates given with ● RIOCIGUAT—avoid concomitant use
- Sildenafil: hypotensive effect of nitrates significantly enhanced by ● SILDENAFIL (avoid concomitant use)
- Tadalafil: hypotensive effect of nitrates significantly enhanced by ● TADALAFIL (avoid concomitant use)
- Vardenafil: possible increased hypotensive effect when nitrates given with ● VARDENAFIL—avoid concomitant use
- ▶ Vasodilator Antihypertensives: enhanced hypotensive effect when nitrates given with HYDRALAZINE, MINOXIDIL or SODIUM NITROPRUSSIDE

Nitrazepam see Anxiolytics and Hypnotics

Nitrofurantoin

- ▶ Antacids: absorption of nitrofurantoin reduced by ORAL MAGNESIUM SALTS (as magnesium trisilicate)

Nitrofurantoin (continued)

▸ **Antibacterials:** nitrofurantoin possibly antagonises effects of NALIDIXIC ACID

▸ **Sulfinpyrazone:** excretion of nitrofurantoin reduced by SULFINPYRAZONE (increased risk of toxicity)

▸ **Vaccines:** antibacterials inactivate ORAL TYPHOID VACCINE—see under Typhoid Vaccine in BNF

Nitroimidazoles see Metronidazole and Tinidazole

Nitrous Oxide see Anaesthetics, General

Nizatidine see Histamine H$_2$-antagonists

Nomegestrol see Progestogens

Noradrenaline (norepinephrine) see Sympathomimetics

Norelgestromin see Progestogens

Norepinephrine

NOTE Norepinephrine interactions as for noradrenaline, see under sympathomimetics

Norethisterone see Progestogens

Norfloxacin see Quinolones

Norgestimate see Progestogens

Norgestrel see Progestogens

Normal Immunoglobulin see Immunoglobulins

Nortriptyline see Antidepressants, Tricyclic

NSAIDs

NOTE *See also* Aspirin. Interactions do not generally apply to topical NSAIDs

▸ **ACE Inhibitors:** increased risk of renal impairment when NSAIDs given with ACE INHIBITORS, also hypotensive effect antagonised

▸ **Adrenergic Neurone Blockers:** NSAIDs antagonise hypotensive effect of ADRENERGIC NEURONE BLOCKERS

▸ **Aliskiren:** NSAIDs possibly antagonise hypotensive effect of ALISKIREN

▸ **Alpha-blockers:** NSAIDs antagonise hypotensive effect of ALPHA-BLOCKERS

● **Analgesics:** avoid concomitant use of NSAIDs with ● NSAIDs or ● ASPIRIN (increased side-effects); avoid concomitant use of NSAIDs with ● KETOROLAC (increased side-effects and haemorrhage); ibuprofen possibly reduces antiplatelet effect of ASPIRIN

▸ **Angiotensin-II Receptor Antagonists:** increased risk of renal impairment when NSAIDs given with ANGIOTENSIN-II RECEPTOR ANTAGONISTS, also hypotensive effect antagonised

▸ **Antacids:** absorption of acemetacin possibly reduced by ANTACIDS

● **Antibacterials:** indometacin possibly increases plasma concentration of AMIKACIN and GENTAMICIN in neonates; plasma concentration of celecoxib, diclofenac and etoricoxib reduced by RIFAMPICIN; possible increased risk of convulsions when NSAIDs given with ● QUINOLONES

● **Anticoagulants:** increased risk of haemorrhage when *intravenous* diclofenac given with ● ANTICOAGULANTS (avoid concomitant use, including low-dose heparins); increased risk of haemorrhage when ketorolac given with ● ANTICOAGULANTS (avoid concomitant use, including low-dose heparins); NSAIDs possibly enhance anticoagulant effect of ● COUMARINS and ● PHENINDIONE; possible increased risk of bleeding when NSAIDs given with ● DABIGATRAN or HEPARINS; increased risk of bleeding when NSAIDs given with ● EDOXABAN (manufacturer of edoxaban advises avoid long-term NSAIDs)

● **Antidepressants:** increased risk of bleeding when NSAIDs given with ● SSRIs or ● VENLAFAXINE

● **Antidiabetics:** NSAIDs possibly enhance effects of ● SULFONYLUREAS

▸ **Antiepileptics:** acemetacin possibly reduces excretion of FOSPHENYTOIN and PHENYTOIN (increased risk of toxicity)

▸ **Antifungals:** plasma concentration of parecoxib increased by FLUCONAZOLE (reduce dose of parecoxib); plasma concentration of celecoxib increased by FLUCONAZOLE (halve dose of celecoxib); plasma concentration of flurbiprofen and ibuprofen increased by FLUCONAZOLE; plasma concentration of diclofenac and ibuprofen increased by VORICONAZOLE

▸ **Antipsychotics:** possible severe drowsiness when acemetacin or indometacin given with HALOPERIDOL

● **Antivirals:** plasma concentration of NSAIDs possibly increased by RITONAVIR; plasma concentration of piroxicam increased by ● RITONAVIR (risk of toxicity)—avoid concomitant use;

NSAIDs

● **Antivirals** (continued)
increased risk of haematological toxicity when NSAIDs given with ZIDOVUDINE

▸ **Azathioprine:** manufacturer of azathioprine advises possible increased risk of myelosuppression when indometacin given with AZATHIOPRINE

▸ **Beta-blockers:** NSAIDs antagonise hypotensive effect of BETA-BLOCKERS

▸ **Calcium-channel Blockers:** NSAIDs antagonise hypotensive effect of CALCIUM-CHANNEL BLOCKERS

▸ **Cardiac Glycosides:** NSAIDs possibly increase plasma concentration of CARDIAC GLYCOSIDES, also possible exacerbation of heart failure and reduction of renal function

● **Ciclosporin:** increased risk of nephrotoxicity when NSAIDs given with ● CICLOSPORIN; plasma concentration of diclofenac increased by ● CICLOSPORIN (halve dose of diclofenac)

▸ **Clonidine:** NSAIDs antagonise hypotensive effect of CLONIDINE

▸ **Clopidogrel:** increased risk of bleeding when NSAIDs given with CLOPIDOGREL

● **Corticosteroids:** increased risk of gastro-intestinal bleeding and ulceration when NSAIDs given with CORTICOSTEROIDS

● **Cytotoxics:** NSAIDs probably reduce excretion of ● METHOTREXATE (increased risk of toxicity); diclofenac, ibuprofen, indometacin, ketoprofen, meloxicam and naproxen reduce excretion of ● METHOTREXATE (increased risk of toxicity); NSAIDs possibly reduce renal excretion of PEMETREXED—consult product literature; increased risk of bleeding when NSAIDs given with ● ERLOTINIB; avoidance of mefenamic acid advised by manufacturer of REGORAFENIB

▸ **Desmopressin:** indometacin enhances effects of DESMOPRESSIN

▸ **Diazoxide:** NSAIDs antagonise hypotensive effect of DIAZOXIDE

● **Dimethyl sulfoxide:** avoid concomitant use of sulindac with ● DIMETHYL SULFOXIDE

▸ **Diuretics:** risk of nephrotoxicity of NSAIDs increased by DIURETICS, also antagonism of diuretic effect; indometacin and ketorolac antagonise effects of DIURETICS; excretion of acemetacin possibly increased by FUROSEMIDE; NSAIDs possibly antagonise diuretic effect of POTASSIUM CANRENOATE; occasional reports of reduced renal function when indometacin given with ● TRIAMTERENE—avoid concomitant use; increased risk of hyperkalaemia when indometacin given with POTASSIUM-SPARING DIURETICS AND ALDOSTERONE ANTAGONISTS; possible increased risk of hyperkalaemia when NSAIDs given with POTASSIUM-SPARING DIURETICS AND ALDOSTERONE ANTAGONISTS

▸ **Iloprost:** increased risk of bleeding when NSAIDs given with ILOPROST

▸ **Lipid-regulating Drugs:** excretion of meloxicam increased by COLESTYRAMINE

● **Lithium:** NSAIDs reduce excretion of ● LITHIUM (increased risk of toxicity); ketorolac reduces excretion of ● LITHIUM (increased risk of toxicity)—avoid concomitant use

▸ **Methyldopa:** NSAIDs antagonise hypotensive effect of METHYLDOPA

▸ **Mifamurtide:** avoidance of high doses of NSAIDs advised by manufacturer of MIFAMURTIDE

▸ **Moxonidine:** NSAIDs antagonise hypotensive effect of MOXONIDINE

▸ **Muscle Relaxants:** ibuprofen reduces excretion of BACLOFEN (increased risk of toxicity); NSAIDs possibly reduce excretion of BACLOFEN (increased risk of toxicity)

● **Nicorandil:** increased risk of gastro-intestinal bleeding and ulceration when NSAIDs given with NICORANDIL

▸ **Nitrates:** NSAIDs antagonise hypotensive effect of NITRATES

▸ **Oestrogens:** etoricoxib increases plasma concentration of ETHINYLESTRADIOL

● **Penicillamine:** possible increased risk of nephrotoxicity when NSAIDs given with PENICILLAMINE

● **Pentoxifylline:** possible increased risk of bleeding when NSAIDs given with PENTOXIFYLLINE; increased risk of bleeding when ketorolac given with ● PENTOXIFYLLINE (avoid concomitant use)

▸ **Prasugrel:** possible increased risk of bleeding when NSAIDs given with PRASUGREL

A1

Interactions | **Appendix 1**

NSAIDs (continued)
- Tacrolimus: possible increased risk of nephrotoxicity when NSAIDs given with TACROLIMUS; increased risk of nephrotoxicity when ibuprofen given with ● TACROLIMUS
▸ Vasodilator Antihypertensives: NSAIDs antagonise hypotensive effect of HYDRALAZINE, MINOXIDIL and SODIUM NITROPRUSSIDE

Obinutuzumab
- Antipsychotics: avoid concomitant use of cytotoxics with ● CLOZAPINE (increased risk of agranulocytosis)
- Vaccines: risk of generalised infections when monoclonal antibodies given with live ● VACCINES—avoid concomitant use

Octreotide
▸ Antidiabetics: octreotide possibly reduces requirements for ANTIDIABETICS
- Ciclosporin: octreotide reduces plasma concentration of ● CICLOSPORIN
▸ Dopaminergics: octreotide increases plasma concentration of BROMOCRIPTINE
▸ Ulcer-healing Drugs: octreotide possibly delays absorption of CIMETIDINE

Oestrogens
▸ ACE Inhibitors: oestrogens antagonise hypotensive effect of ACE INHIBITORS
▸ Adrenergic Neurone Blockers: oestrogens antagonise hypotensive effect of ADRENERGIC NEURONE BLOCKERS
▸ Alpha-blockers: oestrogens antagonise hypotensive effect of ALPHA-BLOCKERS
▸ Aminophylline: oestrogens increase plasma concentration of AMINOPHYLLINE (consider reducing dose of aminophylline)
▸ Analgesics: plasma concentration of ethinylestradiol increased by ETORICOXIB
▸ Angiotensin-II Receptor Antagonists: oestrogens antagonise hypotensive effect of ANGIOTENSIN-II RECEPTOR ANTAGONISTS
- Antibacterials: plasma concentration of estradiol increased by ERYTHROMYCIN; metabolism of oestrogens accelerated by ● RIFAMYCINS (reduced contraceptive effect with combined oral contraceptives, contraceptive patches, and vaginal rings—see Contraceptive Interactions in BNF)
- Anticoagulants: oestrogens may enhance or reduce anticoagulant effect of COUMARINS; oestrogens antagonise anticoagulant effect of ● PHENINDIONE
- Antidepressants: contraceptive effect of oestrogens reduced by ● ST JOHN'S WORT (avoid concomitant use); oestrogens antagonise antidepressant effect of TRICYCLICS (but side-effects of tricyclics possibly increased due to increased plasma concentration)
- Antidiabetics: oestrogens antagonise hypoglycaemic effect of ANTIDIABETICS
- Antiepileptics: metabolism of oestrogens accelerated by ● CARBAMAZEPINE, ● ESLICARBAZEPINE, ● FOSPHENYTOIN, ● OXCARBAZEPINE, ● PHENOBARBITAL, ● PHENYTOIN, ● PRIMIDONE, ● RUFINAMIDE and ● TOPIRAMATE (reduced contraceptive effect with combined oral contraceptives, contraceptive patches, and vaginal rings—see Contraceptive Interactions in BNF); oestrogens reduce plasma concentration of ● LAMOTRIGINE—consider increasing dose of lamotrigine; ethinylestradiol possibly reduces plasma concentration of SODIUM VALPROATE and VALPROIC ACID
▸ Antifungals: plasma concentration of ethinylestradiol increased by KETOCONAZOLE; oestrogens increase plasma concentration of VORICONAZOLE; anecdotal reports of contraceptive failure and menstrual irregularities when oestrogens given with GRISEOFULVIN; anecdotal reports of contraceptive failure when oestrogens given with IMIDAZOLES; occasional reports of breakthrough bleeding when oestrogens (used for contraception) given with TERBINAFINE
- Antivirals: plasma concentration of ethinylestradiol increased by ATAZANAVIR; avoidance of ethinylestradiol advised by manufacturer of ● DASABUVIR, ● OMBITASVIR and ● PARITAPREVIR—use alternative form of contraception; metabolism of oestrogens accelerated by ● NEVIRAPINE and ● RITONAVIR (reduced contraceptive effect with combined oral contraceptives, contraceptive patches, and vaginal rings—see Contraceptive Interactions in BNF); plasma concentration of ethinylestradiol possibly reduced by ● TELAPREVIR—

Oestrogens
- Antivirals (continued)
manufacturer of telaprevir advises additional contraceptive precautions
▸ Anxiolytics and Hypnotics: oestrogens possibly increase plasma concentration of CHLORDIAZEPOXIDE, DIAZEPAM and NITRAZEPAM; oestrogens possibly reduce plasma concentration of LORAZEPAM, OXAZEPAM and TEMAZEPAM; oestrogens increase plasma concentration of MELATONIN
- Aprepitant: possible contraceptive failure of hormonal contraceptives containing oestrogens when given with ● APREPITANT (alternative contraception recommended)
▸ Beta-blockers: oestrogens antagonise hypotensive effect of BETA-BLOCKERS
- Bosentan: possible contraceptive failure of hormonal contraceptives containing oestrogens when given with ● BOSENTAN (alternative contraception recommended)
▸ Calcium-channel Blockers: oestrogens antagonise hypotensive effect of CALCIUM-CHANNEL BLOCKERS
▸ Ciclosporin: oestrogens possibly increase plasma concentration of CICLOSPORIN
▸ Clonidine: oestrogens antagonise hypotensive effect of CLONIDINE
- Cobicistat: metabolism of oestrogens accelerated by ● COBICISTAT (reduced contraceptive effect with combined oral contraceptives, contraceptive patches, and vaginal rings—see Contraceptive Interactions in BNF)
▸ Corticosteroids: oral contraceptives containing oestrogens increase plasma concentration of CORTICOSTEROIDS
- Cytotoxics: possible reduction in contraceptive effect of oestrogens advised by manufacturer of ● CRIZOTINIB and ● VEMURAFENIB; possible reduced contraceptive effect of hormonal contraceptives containing oestrogens advised by manufacturer of ● DABRAFENIB (alternative contraception recommended)
▸ Diuretics: oestrogens antagonise diuretic effect of DIURETICS
- Dopaminergics: oestrogens increase plasma concentration of ROPINIROLE; oestrogens increase plasma concentration of ● SELEGILINE—manufacturer of selegiline advises avoid concomitant use
- Fosaprepitant: possible contraceptive failure of hormonal contraceptives containing oestrogens when given with ● FOSAPREPITANT (alternative contraception recommended)
▸ Lipid-regulating Drugs: absorption of ethinylestradiol reduced by COLESEVELAM; plasma concentration of ethinylestradiol increased by ATORVASTATIN and ROSUVASTATIN; separating administration from oestrogens by 12 hours advised by manufacturer of LOMITAPIDE
▸ Methyldopa: oestrogens antagonise hypotensive effect of METHYLDOPA
- Modafinil: metabolism of oestrogens accelerated by ● MODAFINIL (reduced contraceptive effect with combined oral contraceptives, contraceptive patches, and vaginal rings—see Contraceptive Interactions in BNF)
▸ Moxonidine: oestrogens antagonise hypotensive effect of MOXONIDINE
▸ Muscle Relaxants: oestrogens possibly increase plasma concentration of TIZANIDINE (increased risk of toxicity)
▸ Nitrates: oestrogens antagonise hypotensive effect of NITRATES
▸ Somatropin: oestrogens (when used as oral replacement therapy) may increase dose requirements of SOMATROPIN
▸ Tacrolimus: ethinylestradiol possibly increases plasma concentration of TACROLIMUS
▸ Teriflunomide: plasma concentration of ethinylestradiol increased by TERIFLUNOMIDE
▸ Theophylline: oestrogens increase plasma concentration of THEOPHYLLINE (consider reducing dose of theophylline)
▸ Thyroid Hormones: oestrogens may increase requirements for THYROID HORMONES in hypothyroidism
▸ Vasodilator Antihypertensives: oestrogens antagonise hypotensive effect of HYDRALAZINE, MINOXIDIL and SODIUM NITROPRUSSIDE

Oestrogens, conjugated see Oestrogens

Ofatumumab
- Antipsychotics: avoid concomitant use of cytotoxics with ● CLOZAPINE (increased risk of agranulocytosis)

Ofatumumab (continued)
- Vaccines: risk of generalised infections when monoclonal antibodies given with live • VACCINES—avoid concomitant use

Ofloxacin see Quinolones

Olanzapine see Antipsychotics

Olaparib
- Antibacterials: manufacturer of olaparib advises avoid concomitant use with • CLARITHROMYCIN, • RIFABUTIN, • RIFAMPICIN and • TELITHROMYCIN
- Antidepressants: manufacturer of olaparib advises avoid concomitant use with • ST JOHN'S WORT
- Antiepileptics: manufacturer of olaparib advises avoid concomitant use with • CARBAMAZEPINE, • PHENOBARBITAL and • PHENYTOIN
- Antifungals: manufacturer of olaparib advises avoid concomitant use with • ITRACONAZOLE
- Antipsychotics: avoid concomitant use of cytotoxics with • CLOZAPINE (increased risk of agranulocytosis)
- Antivirals: manufacturer of olaparib advises avoid concomitant use with • BOCEPREVIR, • INDINAVIR, • NEVIRAPINE, • SAQUINAVIR and • TELAPREVIR

Olmesartan see Angiotensin-II Receptor Antagonists

Olodaterol see Sympathomimetics, Beta$_2$

Ombitasvir
- Antibacterials: plasma concentration of ombitasvir possibly reduced by • RIFAMPICIN—avoid concomitant use
- Antidepressants: plasma concentration of ombitasvir possibly reduced by • ST JOHN'S WORT—manufacturer of ombitasvir advises avoid concomitant use
- Antiepileptics: plasma concentration of ombitasvir reduced by • CARBAMAZEPINE—avoid concomitant use; plasma concentration of ombitasvir possibly reduced by • FOSPHENYTOIN, • PHENOBARBITAL, • PHENYTOIN and • PRIMIDONE—avoid concomitant use
- Antifungals: manufacturer of ombitasvir advises avoid concomitant use with KETOCONAZOLE
- Antivirals: manufacturer of ombitasvir advises avoid concomitant use with EFAVIRENZ, ETRAVIRINE and NEVIRAPINE
- Cobicistat: manufacturer of ombitasvir advises avoid concomitant use with COBICISTAT
- Cytotoxics: manufacturer of ombitasvir advises avoid concomitant use with MITOTANE
- Diuretics: ombitasvir increases plasma concentration of • FUROSEMIDE (reduce dose of furosemide)
- Hormone Antagonists: manufacturer of ombitasvir advises avoid concomitant use with ENZALUTAMIDE
- Lipid-regulating Drugs: manufacturer of ombitasvir advises avoid concomitant use with • ATORVASTATIN and • SIMVASTATIN
- Oestrogens: manufacturer of ombitasvir advises avoid concomitant use of • ETHINYLESTRADIOL—use alternative form of contraception

Omeprazole see Proton Pump Inhibitors

Ondansetron see 5HT$_3$-receptor Antagonists (under HT)

Opioid Analgesics
- Alcohol: enhanced hypotensive and sedative effects when opioid analgesics given with ALCOHOL
- Anaesthetics, General: fentanyl inhibits metabolism of ETOMIDATE (consider reducing dose of etomidate); opioid analgesics possibly enhance effects of INTRAVENOUS GENERAL ANAESTHETICS and VOLATILE LIQUID GENERAL ANAESTHETICS
- Analgesics: possible opioid withdrawal when tapentadol given with • BUPRENORPHINE and • PENTAZOCINE; possible opioid withdrawal when buprenorphine given with • DIAMORPHINE, • DIPIPANONE, • HYDROMORPHONE, • METHADONE, • MORPHINE, • OXYCODONE, • PAPAVERETUM, • PETHIDINE and • TRAMADOL; avoidance of buprenorphine advised by manufacturer of FENTANYL; possible opioid withdrawal when diamorphine, dipipanone, hydromorphone, methadone, morphine, oxycodone and papaveretum given with • PENTAZOCINE; manufacturer of fentanyl advises avoid concomitant use with PENTAZOCINE; possible opioid withdrawal when pentazocine given with • PETHIDINE and • TRAMADOL
- Antibacterials: plasma concentration of fentanyl possibly increased by CLARITHROMYCIN; plasma concentration of alfentanil increased by ERYTHROMYCIN; metabolism of alfentanil, codeine, fentanyl, methadone and morphine

Opioid Analgesics
- Antibacterials (continued)
accelerated by RIFAMPICIN (reduced effect); metabolism of oxycodone possibly accelerated by RIFAMPICIN; increased risk of ventricular arrhythmias when methadone given with • DELAMANID; manufacturer of pethidine advises avoid concomitant use with ISONIAZID; metabolism of oxycodone inhibited by TELITHROMYCIN; possible increased risk of ventricular arrhythmias when methadone given with • TELITHROMYCIN
- Anticoagulants: tramadol enhances anticoagulant effect of • COUMARINS
- Antidepressants: plasma concentration of methadone possibly increased by FLUOXETINE, FLUVOXAMINE, PAROXETINE and SERTRALINE; possible increased serotonergic effects when pethidine or tramadol given with DULOXETINE; possible increased serotonergic effects when tramadol given with MIRTAZAPINE, VENLAFAXINE or VORTIOXETINE; possible increased serotonergic effects and increased risk of convulsions when tramadol given with • MAOIS—some manufacturers advise avoid concomitant use and for 2 weeks after stopping MAOIs; CNS excitation or depression (hypertension or hypotension) when pethidine given with • MAOIS—avoid concomitant use and for 2 weeks after stopping MAOIs; possible increased serotonergic effects when fentanyl given with MAOIs, SSRI-RELATED ANTIDEPRESSANTS or SSRIs; possible CNS excitation or depression (hypertension or hypotension) when opioid analgesics given with • MAOIS—some manufacturers advise avoid concomitant use and for 2 weeks after stopping MAOIs; possible CNS excitation or depression (hypertension or hypotension) when opioid analgesics given with • MOCLOBEMIDE—manufacturer of moclobemide advises consider reducing dose of opioid analgesics; possible CNS excitation or depression (hypertension or hypotension) when dextromethorphan or pethidine given with • MOCLOBEMIDE—avoid concomitant use; increased risk of CNS toxicity when tramadol given with • SSRIS or • TRICYCLICS; plasma concentration of methadone possibly reduced by ST JOHN'S WORT; sedative effects possibly increased when opioid analgesics given with TRICYCLICS
- Antiepileptics: metabolism of fentanyl possibly accelerated by CARBAMAZEPINE, FOSPHENYTOIN and PHENYTOIN (reduced effect); dextropropoxyphene enhances effects of • CARBAMAZEPINE; effects of tramadol reduced by CARBAMAZEPINE; plasma concentration of methadone reduced by CARBAMAZEPINE, PHENOBARBITAL and PRIMIDONE; possible increased risk of pethidine toxicity when given with • FOSPHENYTOIN and • PHENYTOIN; metabolism of methadone accelerated by FOSPHENYTOIN and PHENYTOIN (reduced effect and risk of withdrawal effects); morphine increases bioavailability of GABAPENTIN
- Antifungals: metabolism of buprenorphine inhibited by • KETOCONAZOLE (reduce dose of buprenorphine); possible increased risk of ventricular arrhythmias when methadone given with • KETOCONAZOLE—manufacturer of ketoconazole advises avoid concomitant use; plasma concentration of oxycodone increased by ITRACONAZOLE, KETOCONAZOLE and • VORICONAZOLE; metabolism of alfentanil inhibited by FLUCONAZOLE (risk of prolonged or delayed respiratory depression); plasma concentration of methadone increased by FLUCONAZOLE; metabolism of alfentanil possibly inhibited by ITRACONAZOLE; plasma concentration of methadone possibly increased by • ITRACONAZOLE (increased risk of ventricular arrhythmias); plasma concentration of alfentanil and methadone increased by • VORICONAZOLE (consider reducing dose of alfentanil and methadone); plasma concentration of fentanyl possibly increased by • TRIAZOLES
- Antihistamines: sedative effects possibly increased when opioid analgesics given with • SEDATING ANTIHISTAMINES
- Antimalarials: avoidance of methadone advised by manufacturer of • ARTENIMOL WITH PIPERAQUINE (possible risk of ventricular arrhythmias)
- Antimuscarinics: possible increased risk of antimuscarinic side-effects when codeine given with ANTIMUSCARINICS
- Antipsychotics: enhanced hypotensive and sedative effects when opioid analgesics given with ANTIPSYCHOTICS; increased

Opioid Analgesics

- Antipsychotics (continued)
  risk of ventricular arrhythmias when methadone given with
  ● ANTIPSYCHOTICS that prolong the QT interval; increased risk
  of convulsions when tramadol given with ANTIPSYCHOTICS;
  increased risk of ventricular arrhythmias when methadone
  given with ● AMISULPRIDE—avoid concomitant use
- Antivirals: plasma concentration of methadone possibly
  reduced by ABACAVIR, NEVIRAPINE and RILPIVIRINE; plasma
  concentration of buprenorphine increased by ATAZANAVIR;
  plasma concentration of methadone possibly affected by
  BOCEPREVIR; possible increased risk of prolonged sedation and
  respiratory depression when buprenorphine given with
  BOCEPREVIR; methadone possibly reduces plasma
  concentration of DIDANOSINE; plasma concentration of
  methadone reduced by EFAVIRENZ, FOSAMPRENAVIR and
  RITONAVIR; plasma concentration of alfentanil and fentanyl
  increased by ● RITONAVIR; plasma concentration of pethidine
  reduced by ● RITONAVIR, but plasma concentration of toxic
  pethidine metabolite increased (avoid concomitant use);
  plasma concentration of morphine possibly reduced by
  RITONAVIR; plasma concentration of dextropropoxyphene
  increased by ● RITONAVIR (risk of toxicity)—avoid concomitant
  use; plasma concentration of buprenorphine possibly
  increased by RITONAVIR; increased risk of ventricular
  arrhythmias when alfentanil, fentanyl or methadone given
  with ● SAQUINAVIR—avoid concomitant use; caution with
  methadone advised by manufacturer of ● TELAPREVIR (risk of
  ventricular arrhythmias); buprenorphine possibly reduces
  plasma concentration of TIPRANAVIR; methadone possibly
  increases plasma concentration of ZIDOVUDINE
- Anxiolytics and Hypnotics: increased sedative effect when opioid
  analgesics given with ANXIOLYTICS AND HYPNOTICS; fentanyl
  possibly inhibits metabolism of MIDAZOLAM
- Atomoxetine: increased risk of ventricular arrhythmias when
  methadone given with ● ATOMOXETINE; possible increased risk
  of convulsions when tramadol given with ATOMOXETINE
- Beta-blockers: morphine possibly increases plasma
  concentration of ESMOLOL
- Calcium-channel Blockers: metabolism of alfentanil inhibited by
  DILTIAZEM (risk of prolonged or delayed respiratory
  depression)
- Cytotoxics: possible increased risk of ventricular arrhythmias
  when methadone given with ● BOSUTINIB; caution with
  alfentanil and fentanyl advised by manufacturer of
  ● CRIZOTINIB; possible increased risk of ventricular
  arrhythmias when methadone given with ● VANDETANIB—
  avoid concomitant use
- Dapoxetine: possible increased risk of serotonergic effects
  when tramadol given with ● DAPOXETINE (manufacturer of
  dapoxetine advises tramadol should not be started until
  1 week after stopping dapoxetine, avoid dapoxetine for
  2 weeks after stopping tramadol)
- Domperidone: opioid analgesics antagonise effects of
  DOMPERIDONE on gastro-intestinal activity
- Dopaminergics: avoid concomitant use of dextromethorphan
  with ● RASAGILINE; risk of CNS toxicity when pethidine given
  with ● RASAGILINE (avoid pethidine for 2 weeks after
  rasagiline); avoidance of opioid analgesics advised by
  manufacturer of SELEGILINE; hyperpyrexia and CNS toxicity
  reported when pethidine given with ● SELEGILINE (avoid
  concomitant use)
- Hormone Antagonists: plasma concentration of
  dextromethorphan increased by ABIRATERONE
- 5HT$_3$-receptor Antagonists: effects of tramadol possibly
  antagonised by ONDANSETRON
- Memantine: increased risk of CNS toxicity when
  dextromethorphan given with ● MEMANTINE (manufacturer of
  memantine advises avoid concomitant use)
- Metoclopramide: opioid analgesics antagonise effects of
  METOCLOPRAMIDE on gastro-intestinal activity
- Muscle Relaxants: increased sedative effect when fentanyl or
  morphine given with BACLOFEN
- Nalmefene: avoidance of opioid analgesics advised by
  manufacturer of ● NALMEFENE

Opioid Analgesics (continued)

- Netupitant: caution with morphine advised by manufacturer of
  NETUPITANT
- Sodium Oxybate: opioid analgesics enhance effects of ● SODIUM
  OXYBATE (avoid concomitant use)
- Ulcer-healing Drugs: metabolism of opioid analgesics inhibited
  by CIMETIDINE (increased plasma concentration)

Oritavancin
- Anticoagulants: oritavancin possibly increases plasma
  concentration of WARFARIN
- Vaccines: antibacterials inactivate ORAL TYPHOID VACCINE—see
  under Typhoid Vaccine in BNF

Orlistat
- Anti-arrhythmics: orlistat possibly reduces plasma
  concentration of AMIODARONE
- Anticoagulants: manufacturer of orlistat recommends
  monitoring anticoagulant effect of COUMARINS
- Antidiabetics: manufacturer of orlistat advises avoid
  concomitant use with ACARBOSE
- Antiepileptics: possible increased risk of convulsions when
  orlistat given with ● ANTIEPILEPTICS
- Antivirals: orlistat possibly reduces absorption of ● ABACAVIR,
  ● ATAZANAVIR, ● DARUNAVIR, ● DIDANOSINE, ● EFAVIRENZ,
  ● ELVITEGRAVIR, ● EMTRICITABINE, ● ENFUVIRTIDE, ● ETRAVIRINE,
  ● FOSAMPRENAVIR, ● INDINAVIR, ● LAMIVUDINE, ● LOPINAVIR,
  ● MARAVIROC, ● NEVIRAPINE, ● RALTEGRAVIR, ● RILPIVIRINE,
  ● RITONAVIR, ● SAQUINAVIR, ● STAVUDINE, ● TENOFOVIR,
  ● TIPRANAVIR and ● ZIDOVUDINE
- Ciclosporin: orlistat possibly reduces absorption of
  ● CICLOSPORIN
- Thyroid Hormones: possible increased risk of hypothyroidism
  when orlistat given with LEVOTHYROXINE

Orphenadrine see Antimuscarinics
Oxaliplatin see Platinum Compounds
Oxandrolone see Anabolic Steroids
Oxazepam see Anxiolytics and Hypnotics
Oxcarbazepine
- Antidepressants: anticonvulsant effect of antiepileptics
  possibly antagonised by MAOIs and ● TRICYCLIC-RELATED
  ANTIDEPRESSANTS (convulsive threshold lowered);
  anticonvulsant effect of antiepileptics antagonised by SSRIs
  and ● TRICYCLICS (convulsive threshold lowered)
- Antiepileptics: oxcarbazepine sometimes reduces plasma
  concentration of CARBAMAZEPINE (but concentration of an
  active metabolite of carbamazepine may be increased), also
  plasma concentration of an active metabolite of
  oxcarbazepine often reduced; avoidance of oxcarbazepine
  advised by manufacturer of ESLICARBAZEPINE; oxcarbazepine
  increases plasma concentration of FOSPHENYTOIN,
  PHENOBARBITAL, PHENYTOIN and PRIMIDONE, also plasma
  concentration of an active metabolite of oxcarbazepine
  reduced; oxcarbazepine reduces plasma concentration of
  ● PERAMPANEL, also plasma concentration of oxcarbazepine
  increased (see under Perampanel, p. 293); plasma
  concentration of an active metabolite of oxcarbazepine
  sometimes reduced by SODIUM VALPROATE and VALPROIC ACID
- Antimalarials: anticonvulsant effect of antiepileptics
  antagonised by ● MEFLOQUINE
- Antipsychotics: anticonvulsant effect of antiepileptics
  antagonised by ANTIPSYCHOTICS (convulsive threshold
  lowered)
- Antivirals: oxcarbazepine possibly reduces plasma
  concentration of ● DACLATASVIR and ● SIMEPREVIR—
  manufacturer of daclatasvir and simeprevir advises avoid
  concomitant use; oxcarbazepine possibly reduces the plasma
  concentration of ● DOLUTEGRAVIR (see under Dolutegravir,
  p. 584); avoidance of oxcarbazepine advised by manufacturer
  of LEDIPASVIR and SOFOSBUVIR; avoidance of oxcarbazepine
  advised by manufacturer of ● RILPIVIRINE (plasma
  concentration of rilpivirine possibly reduced)
- Ciclosporin: oxcarbazepine possibly reduces plasma
  concentration of CICLOSPORIN
- Clopidogrel: oxcarbazepine possibly reduces antiplatelet effect
  of ● CLOPIDOGREL
- Cytotoxics: oxcarbazepine reduces plasma concentration of
  ● IMATINIB—avoid concomitant use

Oxcarbazepine (continued)

- Guanfacine: oxcarbazepine possibly reduces plasma concentration of ● GUANFACINE—increase dose of guanfacine
- Oestrogens: oxcarbazepine accelerates metabolism of ● OESTROGENS (reduced contraceptive effect with combined oral contraceptives, contraceptive patches, and vaginal rings—see Contraceptive Interactions in BNF)
- Orlistat: possible increased risk of convulsions when antiepileptics given with ● ORLISTAT
- Progestogens: oxcarbazepine accelerates metabolism of ● PROGESTOGENS (reduced contraceptive effect with combined oral contraceptives, progestogen-only oral contraceptives, contraceptive patches, vaginal rings, etonogestrel-releasing implant, and emergency hormonal contraception—see Contraceptive Interactions in BNF)

Oxprenolol see Beta-blockers

Oxybutynin see Antimuscarinics

Oxycodone see Opioid Analgesics

Oxymetazoline see Sympathomimetics

Oxytetracycline see Tetracyclines

Oxytocin

- Anaesthetics, General: oxytocic effect possibly reduced, also enhanced hypotensive effect and risk of arrhythmias when oxytocin given with VOLATILE LIQUID GENERAL ANAESTHETICS
- Prostaglandins: uterotonic effect of oxytocin potentiated by PROSTAGLANDINS
- Sympathomimetics: risk of hypertension when oxytocin given with vasoconstrictor SYMPATHOMIMETICS (due to enhanced vasopressor effect)

Paclitaxel

- Antipsychotics: avoid concomitant use of cytotoxics with ● CLOZAPINE (increased risk of agranulocytosis)
- Antivirals: plasma concentration of paclitaxel increased by RITONAVIR
- Cytotoxics: increased risk of neutropenia when paclitaxel given with ● LAPATINIB

Paliperidone see Antipsychotics

Palonosetron see 5HT₃-receptor Antagonists (under HT)

Pamidronate Disodium see Bisphosphonates

Pancreatin

- Antidiabetics: pancreatin antagonises hypoglycaemic effect of ACARBOSE

Pancuronium see Muscle Relaxants

Panitumumab

- Antipsychotics: avoid concomitant use of cytotoxics with ● CLOZAPINE (increased risk of agranulocytosis)
- Cytotoxics: manufacturer of panitumumab advises avoid concomitant use with ● BEVACIZUMAB, ● FLUOROURACIL, ● IRINOTECAN and ● OXALIPLATIN
- Folates: manufacturer of panitumumab advises avoid concomitant use with ● FOLINIC ACID
- Vaccines: risk of generalised infections when monoclonal antibodies given with live ● VACCINES—avoid concomitant use

Pantoprazole see Proton Pump Inhibitors

Papaveretum see Opioid Analgesics

Paracetamol

- Anticoagulants: prolonged regular use of paracetamol possibly enhances anticoagulant effect of COUMARINS
- Antidiabetics: absorption of paracetamol possibly reduced when given 1 to 4 hours after LIXISENATIDE
- Antiepileptics: metabolism of paracetamol possibly accelerated by CARBAMAZEPINE, FOSPHENYTOIN, PHENOBARBITAL, PHENYTOIN and PRIMIDONE (also isolated reports of hepatotoxicity)
- Antifungals: avoidance of paracetamol advised by manufacturer of KETOCONAZOLE
- Cytotoxics: paracetamol possibly inhibits metabolism of *intravenous* BUSULFAN (manufacturer of *intravenous* busulfan advises caution within 72 hours of paracetamol); caution with paracetamol advised by manufacturer of IMATINIB
- Lipid-regulating Drugs: absorption of paracetamol reduced by COLESTYRAMINE
- Metoclopramide: rate of absorption of paracetamol increased by METOCLOPRAMIDE

Paraldehyde

- Alcohol: increased sedative effect when paraldehyde given with ● ALCOHOL

Paraldehyde (continued)

- Disulfiram: risk of toxicity when paraldehyde given with ● DISULFIRAM

Parasympathomimetics

- Anti-arrhythmics: effects of neostigmine and pyridostigmine possibly antagonised by PROPAFENONE
- Antibacterials: plasma concentration of galantamine increased by ERYTHROMYCIN; effects of neostigmine and pyridostigmine antagonised by ● AMINOGLYCOSIDES; effects of neostigmine and pyridostigmine antagonised by CLINDAMYCIN; effects of neostigmine and pyridostigmine antagonised by ● POLYMYXINS
- Antidepressants: plasma concentration of galantamine increased by PAROXETINE
- Antifungals: plasma concentration of galantamine increased by KETOCONAZOLE
- Antimalarials: effects of neostigmine and pyridostigmine may be diminished because of potential for CHLOROQUINE to increase symptoms of myasthenia gravis; effects of neostigmine and pyridostigmine may be diminished because of potential for HYDROXYCHLOROQUINE to increase symptoms of myasthenia gravis
- Antimuscarinics: effects of parasympathomimetics antagonised by ANTIMUSCARINICS
- Beta-blockers: increased risk of arrhythmias when pilocarpine given with BETA-BLOCKERS; effects of neostigmine and pyridostigmine antagonised by PROPRANOLOL
- Cytotoxics: possible increased risk of bradycardia when pilocarpine given with CRIZOTINIB
- Lithium: effects of neostigmine antagonised by LITHIUM
- Muscle Relaxants: donepezil possibly enhances effects of SUXAMETHONIUM; galantamine, neostigmine, pyridostigmine and rivastigmine enhance effects of SUXAMETHONIUM; neostigmine, pyridostigmine and rivastigmine antagonise effects of NON-DEPOLARISING MUSCLE RELAXANTS; donepezil possibly antagonises effects of NON-DEPOLARISING MUSCLE RELAXANTS

Parecoxib see NSAIDs

Paricalcitol see Vitamins

Paritaprevir

- Angiotensin-II Receptor Antagonists: manufacturer of paritaprevir advises reduce dose when given with VALSARTAN
- Antibacterials: manufacturer of paritaprevir advises avoid concomitant use with CLARITHROMYCIN and TELITHROMYCIN; plasma concentration of paritaprevir possibly reduced by ● RIFAMPICIN—avoid concomitant use
- Antidepressants: plasma concentration of paritaprevir possibly reduced by ● ST JOHN'S WORT—manufacturer of paritaprevir advises avoid concomitant use
- Antiepileptics: plasma concentration of paritaprevir reduced by ● CARBAMAZEPINE—avoid concomitant use; plasma concentration of paritaprevir possibly reduced by ● FOSPHENYTOIN, ● PHENOBARBITAL, ● PHENYTOIN and ● PRIMIDONE—avoid concomitant use
- Antifungals: plasma concentration of both drugs increased when paritaprevir given with ● KETOCONAZOLE—avoid concomitant use; plasma concentration of both drugs possibly increased when paritaprevir given with ● ITRACONAZOLE and ● POSACONAZOLE—avoid concomitant use
- Antivirals: plasma concentration of paritaprevir increased by ● ATAZANAVIR; plasma concentration of paritaprevir increased by ● DARUNAVIR and plasma concentration of darunavir decreased; manufacturer of paritaprevir advises avoid concomitant use with EFAVIRENZ, ETRAVIRINE, INDINAVIR, NEVIRAPINE, SAQUINAVIR and TIPRANAVIR; plasma concentration of paritaprevir increased by ● LOPINAVIR—manufacturer of paritaprevir advises avoid concomitant use
- Cardiac Glycosides: paritaprevir possibly increases plasma concentration of DIGOXIN (consider reducing dose of digoxin)
- Cobicistat: manufacturer of paritaprevir advises avoid concomitant use with COBICISTAT
- Cytotoxics: manufacturer of paritaprevir advises avoid concomitant use with MITOTANE
- Diuretics: paritaprevir increases plasma concentration of ● FUROSEMIDE (reduce dose of furosemide)
- Hormone Antagonists: manufacturer of paritaprevir advises avoid concomitant use with ENZALUTAMIDE

Interactions | Appendix 1

A1

Paritaprevir (continued)

- Lipid-regulating Drugs: plasma concentration of paritaprevir increased by ● GEMFIBROZIL—manufacturer of paritaprevir advises avoid concomitant use; manufacturer of paritaprevir advises avoid concomitant use with ● ATORVASTATIN, FLUVASTATIN and ● SIMVASTATIN; paritaprevir increases plasma concentration of ● PRAVASTATIN (reduce dose of pravastatin); paritaprevir increases plasma concentration of ● ROSUVASTATIN (reduce dose of rosuvastatin—see under Rosuvastatin, p. 188)
- Oestrogens: manufacturer of paritaprevir advises avoid concomitant use of ● ETHINYLESTRADIOL—use alternative form of contraception

Paroxetine *see* Antidepressants, SSRI

Pasireotide
- ▷ Antidiabetics: pasireotide possibly reduces requirements for ANTIDIABETICS
- ▷ Antifungals: avoidance of pasireotide advised by manufacturer of KETOCONAZOLE
- ▷ Antimuscarinics: possible increased risk of bradycardia when pasireotide given with IPRATROPIUM or OXYBUTYNIN
- ▷ Beta-blockers: possible increased risk of bradycardia when pasireotide given with CARTEOLOL, METOPROLOL, PROPRANOLOL or SOTALOL
- ▷ Calcium-channel Blockers: possible increased risk of bradycardia when pasireotide given with DILTIAZEM or VERAPAMIL
- ● Ciclosporin: pasireotide possibly reduces plasma concentration of ● CICLOSPORIN

Pazopanib
- ● Antibacterials: plasma concentration of pazopanib possibly increased by ● CLARITHROMYCIN and ● TELITHROMYCIN (reduce dose of pazopanib); plasma concentration of pazopanib possibly reduced by ● RIFAMPICIN
- ● Antifungals: plasma concentration of pazopanib increased by ● KETOCONAZOLE (reduce dose of pazopanib); plasma concentration of pazopanib possibly increased by ● ITRACONAZOLE and ● VORICONAZOLE (reduce dose of pazopanib)
- ● Antipsychotics: avoid concomitant use of cytotoxics with ● CLOZAPINE (increased risk of agranulocytosis)
- ● Antivirals: plasma concentration of pazopanib possibly increased by ● ATAZANAVIR, ● INDINAVIR and ● RITONAVIR (reduce dose of pazopanib); avoidance of pazopanib advised by manufacturer of ● BOCEPREVIR; increased risk of ventricular arrhythmias when pazopanib given with ● SAQUINAVIR—avoid concomitant use
- ▷ Cytotoxics: plasma concentration of pazopanib increased by LAPATINIB
- ● Grapefruit Juice: manufacturer of pazopanib advises avoid concomitant use with ● GRAPEFRUIT JUICE
- ▷ Lipid-regulating Drugs: separating administration from pazopanib by 12 hours advised by manufacturer of LOMITAPIDE
- ▷ Ulcer-healing Drugs: absorption of pazopanib possibly reduced by HISTAMINE H₂-ANTAGONISTS—manufacturer of pazopanib advises give at least 2 hours before or 10 hours after histamine H₂-antagonists; absorption of pazopanib possibly reduced by PROTON PUMP INHIBITORS—manufacturer of pazopanib advises give at the same time as proton pump inhibitors

Pegfilgrastim
- ▷ Cytotoxics: neutropenia possibly exacerbated when pegfilgrastim given with CAPECITABINE, FLUOROURACIL or TEGAFUR

Peginterferon Alfa *see* Interferons

Pembrolizumab
- ● Antipsychotics: avoid concomitant use of cytotoxics with ● CLOZAPINE (increased risk of agranulocytosis)
- ● Vaccines: risk of generalised infections when monoclonal antibodies given with live ● VACCINES—avoid concomitant use

Pemetrexed
- ▷ Analgesics: renal excretion of pemetrexed possibly reduced by NSAIDs and ASPIRIN—consult product literature
- ● Antimalarials: antifolate effect of pemetrexed increased by ● PYRIMETHAMINE
- ● Antipsychotics: avoid concomitant use of cytotoxics with ● CLOZAPINE (increased risk of agranulocytosis)

Penicillamine
- ▷ Analgesics: possible increased risk of nephrotoxicity when penicillamine given with NSAIDs
- ▷ Antacids: absorption of penicillamine reduced by ANTACIDS
- ▷ Antimalarials: increased risk of haematological toxicity when penicillamine given with ANTIMALARIALS—manufacturer of penicillamine advises avoid concomitant use
- ● Antipsychotics: increased risk of haematological toxicity when penicillamine given with ● CLOZAPINE—manufacturer of penicillamine advises avoid concomitant use
- ▷ Cardiac Glycosides: penicillamine possibly reduces plasma concentration of DIGOXIN
- ▷ Iron Salts: absorption of penicillamine reduced by *oral* IRON SALTS
- ● Sodium Aurothiomalate: increased risk of haematological toxicity when penicillamine given with ● SODIUM AUROTHIOMALATE—see under Penicillamine, p. 952)
- ▷ Zinc: penicillamine reduces absorption of ZINC, also absorption of penicillamine reduced by zinc

Penicillins
- ▷ Allopurinol: increased risk of rash when amoxicillin, ampicillin or co-amoxiclav given with ALLOPURINOL
- ▷ Antibacterials: absorption of phenoxymethylpenicillin reduced by NEOMYCIN; effects of penicillins possibly antagonised by TETRACYCLINES
- ▷ Anticoagulants: an interaction between broad-spectrum penicillins and COUMARINS and PHENINDIONE has not been demonstrated in studies, but common experience in anticoagulant clinics is that INR can be altered
- ● Antiepileptics: manufacturer of pivmecillinam advises avoid concomitant use with ● SODIUM VALPROATE and ● VALPROIC ACID
- ▷ Cytotoxics: penicillins reduce excretion of METHOTREXATE (increased risk of toxicity)
- ▷ Muscle Relaxants: piperacillin enhances effects of NON-DEPOLARISING MUSCLE RELAXANTS and SUXAMETHONIUM
- ▷ Mycophenolate: co-amoxiclav possibly reduces plasma concentration of MYCOPHENOLATE
- ▷ Sulfinpyrazone: excretion of penicillins reduced by SULFINPYRAZONE
- ▷ Vaccines: antibacterials inactivate ORAL TYPHOID VACCINE—see under Typhoid Vaccine in BNF

Pentamidine Isetionate
- ● Anti-arrhythmics: increased risk of ventricular arrhythmias when pentamidine isetionate given with ● AMIODARONE—avoid concomitant use; possible increased risk of ventricular arrhythmias when pentamidine isetionate given with ● DISOPYRAMIDE
- ● Antibacterials: increased risk of ventricular arrhythmias when pentamidine isetionate given with *parenteral* ● ERYTHROMYCIN; increased risk of ventricular arrhythmias when pentamidine isetionate given with ● MOXIFLOXACIN—avoid concomitant use; increased risk of ventricular arrhythmias when pentamidine isetionate given with ● DELAMANID; possible increased risk of ventricular arrhythmias when *parenteral* pentamidine isetionate given with ● TELITHROMYCIN
- ● Antidepressants: avoidance of pentamidine isetionate advised by manufacturer of ● CITALOPRAM and ● ESCITALOPRAM (risk of ventricular arrhythmias); increased risk of ventricular arrhythmias when pentamidine isetionate given with ● TRICYCLICS
- ▷ Antifungals: possible increased risk of nephrotoxicity when pentamidine isetionate given with AMPHOTERICIN
- ● Antimalarials: avoidance of pentamidine isetionate advised by manufacturer of ● ARTENIMOL WITH PIPERAQUINE (possible risk of ventricular arrhythmias)
- ● Antipsychotics: increased risk of ventricular arrhythmias when pentamidine isetionate given with ● AMISULPRIDE or ● DROPERIDOL—avoid concomitant use; increased risk of ventricular arrhythmias when pentamidine isetionate given with ● PHENOTHIAZINES
- ● Antivirals: increased risk of hypocalcaemia when *parenteral* pentamidine isetionate given with ● FOSCARNET; increased risk of ventricular arrhythmias when pentamidine isetionate given with ● SAQUINAVIR—avoid concomitant use

Pentamidine Isetionate (continued)

- Cytotoxics: possible increased risk of ventricular arrhythmias when pentamidine isetionate given with • VANDETANIB—avoid concomitant use
- Ivabradine: increased risk of ventricular arrhythmias when pentamidine isetionate given with • IVABRADINE

Pentazocine *see* Opioid Analgesics

Pentostatin

- Antipsychotics: avoid concomitant use of cytotoxics with • CLOZAPINE (increased risk of agranulocytosis)
- Cytotoxics: increased toxicity when pentostatin given with high-dose • CYCLOPHOSPHAMIDE—avoid concomitant use; increased pulmonary toxicity when pentostatin given with • FLUDARABINE (unacceptably high incidence of fatalities)

Pentoxifylline

▸ Aminophylline: pentoxifylline increases plasma concentration of AMINOPHYLLINE
- Analgesics: possible increased risk of bleeding when pentoxifylline given with NSAIDs; increased risk of bleeding when pentoxifylline given with • KETOROLAC (avoid concomitant use)
▸ Theophylline: pentoxifylline increases plasma concentration of THEOPHYLLINE

Perampanel

- Antidepressants: anticonvulsant effect of antiepileptics possibly antagonised by MAOIs and • TRICYCLIC-RELATED ANTIDEPRESSANTS (convulsive threshold lowered); anticonvulsant effect of antiepileptics antagonised by • SSRIs and • TRICYCLICS (convulsive threshold lowered)
- Antiepileptics: plasma concentration of perampanel reduced by • CARBAMAZEPINE, • FOSPHENYTOIN and • PHENYTOIN (see under Perampanel, p. 293); plasma concentration of perampanel reduced by • OXCARBAZEPINE, also plasma concentration of oxcarbazepine increased (see under Perampanel, p. 293); plasma concentration of perampanel reduced by TOPIRAMATE
▸ Antifungals: plasma concentration of perampanel increased by KETOCONAZOLE
- Antimalarials: anticonvulsant effect of antiepileptics antagonised by • MEFLOQUINE
- Antipsychotics: anticonvulsant effect of antiepileptics antagonised by • ANTIPSYCHOTICS (convulsive threshold lowered)
▸ Anxiolytics and Hypnotics: perampanel reduces plasma concentration of MIDAZOLAM
- Orlistat: possible increased risk of convulsions when antiepileptics given with • ORLISTAT
- Progestogens: perampanel accelerates metabolism of • PROGESTOGENS (reduced contraceptive effect with combined oral contraceptives, progestogen-only oral contraceptives, contraceptive patches, vaginal rings, etonogestrel-releasing implant, and emergency hormonal contraception—see Contraceptive Interactions in BNF)

Pergolide

▸ Antipsychotics: effects of pergolide antagonised by ANTIPSYCHOTICS
▸ Memantine: effects of dopaminergics possibly enhanced by MEMANTINE
▸ Methyldopa: antiparkinsonian effect of dopaminergics antagonised by METHYLDOPA
▸ Metoclopramide: antiparkinsonian effect of pergolide antagonised by METOCLOPRAMIDE

Pericyazine *see* Antipsychotics
Perindopril *see* ACE Inhibitors
Perphenazine *see* Antipsychotics

Pertuzumab

- Antipsychotics: avoid concomitant use of cytotoxics with • CLOZAPINE (increased risk of agranulocytosis)
- Vaccines: risk of generalised infections when monoclonal antibodies given with live • VACCINES—avoid concomitant use

Pethidine *see* Opioid Analgesics
Phenelzine *see* MAOIs

Phenindione

NOTE Change in patient's clinical condition particularly associated with liver disease, intercurrent illness, or drug administration, necessitates more frequent testing. Major changes in diet (especially involving salads and vegetables)

Phenindione (continued)

and in alcohol consumption may also affect anticoagulant control

- Alcohol: anticoagulant control with phenindione may be affected by major changes in consumption of • ALCOHOL
- Anabolic Steroids: anticoagulant effect of phenindione enhanced by • ANABOLIC STEROIDS
- Analgesics: anticoagulant effect of phenindione possibly enhanced by • NSAIDs; increased risk of haemorrhage when anticoagulants given with *intravenous* • DICLOFENAC (avoid concomitant use, including low-dose heparins); increased risk of haemorrhage when anticoagulants given with • KETOROLAC (avoid concomitant use, including low-dose heparins); increased risk of bleeding when phenindione given with • ASPIRIN (due to antiplatelet effect)
- Anti-arrhythmics: metabolism of phenindione inhibited by • AMIODARONE (enhanced anticoagulant effect); anticoagulant effect of phenindione possibly enhanced by • DRONEDARONE
- Antibacterials: experience in anticoagulant clinics suggests that INR possibly altered when phenindione is given with • NEOMYCIN (given for local action on gut); anticoagulant effect of phenindione possibly enhanced by LEVOFLOXACIN and • TETRACYCLINES; an interaction between phenindione and broad-spectrum PENICILLINS has not been demonstrated in studies, but common experience in anticoagulant clinics is that INR can be altered; metabolism of phenindione possibly inhibited by SULFONAMIDES
- Anticoagulants: increased risk of haemorrhage when other anticoagulants given with • APIXABAN, • DABIGATRAN, • EDOXABAN and • RIVAROXABAN (avoid concomitant use except when switching with other anticoagulants or using heparin to maintain catheter patency)
- Antivirals: anticoagulant effect of phenindione possibly enhanced by • RITONAVIR
- Clopidogrel: anticoagulant effect of phenindione enhanced due to antiplatelet action of • CLOPIDOGREL
▸ Corticosteroids: anticoagulant effect of phenindione may be enhanced or reduced by CORTICOSTEROIDS
▸ Cytotoxics: avoidance of phenindione advised by manufacturer of IBRUTINIB
- Dipyridamole: anticoagulant effect of phenindione enhanced due to antiplatelet action of • DIPYRIDAMOLE
- Enteral Feeds: anticoagulant effect of phenindione antagonised by vitamin K (present in some • ENTERAL FEEDS)
▸ Iloprost: increased risk of bleeding when phenindione given with ILOPROST
- Lipid-regulating Drugs: anticoagulant effect of phenindione may be enhanced or reduced by • COLESTYRAMINE; anticoagulant effect of phenindione possibly enhanced by • ROSUVASTATIN; anticoagulant effect of phenindione enhanced by • FIBRATES
- Oestrogens: anticoagulant effect of phenindione antagonised by • OESTROGENS
▸ Prasugrel: possible increased risk of bleeding when phenindione given with PRASUGREL
- Progestogens: anticoagulant effect of phenindione antagonised by • PROGESTOGENS
- Testolactone: anticoagulant effect of phenindione enhanced by • TESTOLACTONE
- Testosterone: anticoagulant effect of phenindione enhanced by • TESTOSTERONE
- Thyroid Hormones: anticoagulant effect of phenindione enhanced by • THYROID HORMONES
- Vitamins: anticoagulant effect of phenindione antagonised by • VITAMIN K

Phenobarbital

▸ Alcohol: increased sedative effect when phenobarbital given with ALCOHOL
- Aminophylline: phenobarbital accelerates metabolism of • AMINOPHYLLINE (reduced effect)
▸ Analgesics: phenobarbital reduces plasma concentration of METHADONE; phenobarbital possibly accelerates metabolism of PARACETAMOL (also isolated reports of hepatotoxicity)
- Anthelmintics: phenobarbital reduces plasma concentration of • ALBENDAZOLE and • PRAZIQUANTEL—consider increasing

Phenobarbital

- **Anthelmintics** (continued)
albendazole and praziquantel dose when given for systemic infections
- **Anti-arrhythmics:** phenobarbital accelerates metabolism of DISOPYRAMIDE (reduced plasma concentration); phenobarbital possibly reduces plasma concentration of ● DRONEDARONE—avoid concomitant use; phenobarbital possibly accelerates metabolism of PROPAFENONE
- **Antibacterials:** phenobarbital accelerates metabolism of METRONIDAZOLE (reduced effect); phenobarbital possibly reduces plasma concentration of RIFAMPICIN; phenobarbital accelerates metabolism of DOXYCYCLINE (reduced plasma concentration); phenobarbital possibly accelerates metabolism of ● CHLORAMPHENICOL (reduced plasma concentration); phenobarbital reduces plasma concentration of ● TELITHROMYCIN (avoid during and for 2 weeks after phenobarbital)
- **Anticoagulants:** phenobarbital possibly reduces plasma concentration of ● APIXABAN and ● EDOXABAN; phenobarbital accelerates metabolism of ● COUMARINS (reduced anticoagulant effect); phenobarbital possibly reduces plasma concentration of ● RIVAROXABAN—manufacturer of rivaroxaban advises monitor for signs of thrombosis
- **Antidepressants:** phenobarbital possibly reduces plasma concentration of REBOXETINE; phenobarbital reduces plasma concentration of PAROXETINE; phenobarbital accelerates metabolism of MIANSERIN (reduced plasma concentration); anticonvulsant effect of antiepileptics possibly antagonised by MAOIs and ● TRICYCLIC-RELATED ANTIDEPRESSANTS (convulsive threshold lowered); anticonvulsant effect of antiepileptics antagonised by ● SSRIs and ● TRICYCLICS (convulsive threshold lowered); plasma concentration of phenobarbital possibly reduced by ● ST JOHN'S WORT—avoid concomitant use; phenobarbital possibly accelerates metabolism of ● TRICYCLICS (reduced plasma concentration)
- **Antiepileptics:** plasma concentration of phenobarbital possibly increased by CARBAMAZEPINE; phenobarbital possibly reduces plasma concentration of ETHOSUXIMIDE, RUFINAMIDE and TOPIRAMATE; plasma concentration of phenobarbital often increased by FOSPHENYTOIN and PHENYTOIN, plasma concentration of fosphenytoin and phenytoin often reduced but may be increased; phenobarbital reduces plasma concentration of LAMOTRIGINE, TIAGABINE and ZONISAMIDE; plasma concentration of phenobarbital increased by OXCARBAZEPINE, also plasma concentration of an active metabolite of oxcarbazepine reduced; plasma concentration of phenobarbital increased by SODIUM VALPROATE and VALPROIC ACID (also plasma concentration of sodium valproate and valproic acid reduced); plasma concentration of phenobarbital increased by STIRIPENTOL
- **Antifungals:** phenobarbital possibly reduces plasma concentration of ITRACONAZOLE and ● POSACONAZOLE; phenobarbital possibly reduces plasma concentration of ● VORICONAZOLE—avoid concomitant use; phenobarbital reduces absorption of GRISEOFULVIN (reduced effect)
- **Antimalarials:** avoidance of phenobarbital advised by manufacturer of ARTENIMOL WITH PIPERAQUINE; anticonvulsant effect of antiepileptics antagonised by ● MEFLOQUINE
- **Antimuscarinics:** phenobarbital possibly reduces plasma concentration of active metabolite of ● FESOTERODINE—manufacturer of fesoterodine advises avoid concomitant use
- **Antipsychotics:** anticonvulsant effect of antiepileptics antagonised by ● ANTIPSYCHOTICS (convulsive threshold lowered); phenobarbital accelerates metabolism of HALOPERIDOL (reduced plasma concentration); plasma concentration of both drugs reduced when phenobarbital given with CHLORPROMAZINE; phenobarbital possibly reduces plasma concentration of ● ARIPIPRAZOLE (avoid concomitant use or consider increasing the dose of aripiprazole—consult aripiprazole product literature); phenobarbital possibly reduces plasma concentration of CLOZAPINE; phenobarbital possibly reduces plasma concentration of ● LURASIDONE—avoid concomitant use
- **Antivirals:** phenobarbital possibly reduces plasma concentration of ABACAVIR, DARUNAVIR, FOSAMPRENAVIR,

Phenobarbital

- **Antivirals** (continued)
● INDINAVIR, ● LOPINAVIR and ● SAQUINAVIR; avoidance of phenobarbital advised by manufacturer of ● BOCEPREVIR and ● RILPIVIRINE (plasma concentration of boceprevir and rilpivirine possibly reduced); phenobarbital possibly reduces plasma concentration of ● DACLATASVIR and ● SIMEPREVIR—manufacturer of daclatasvir and simeprevir advises avoid concomitant use; phenobarbital possibly reduces plasma concentration of ● DASABUVIR, ● OMBITASVIR and ● PARITAPREVIR—avoid concomitant use; phenobarbital possibly reduces the plasma concentration of ● DOLUTEGRAVIR (see under Dolutegravir, p. 584); avoidance of phenobarbital advised by manufacturer of ● ELVITEGRAVIR, ETRAVIRINE, LEDIPASVIR, SOFOSBUVIR and ● TELAPREVIR
- **Anxiolytics and Hypnotics:** increased sedative effect when phenobarbital given with ANXIOLYTICS AND HYPNOTICS; phenobarbital often reduces plasma concentration of CLONAZEPAM
- **Apremilast:** phenobarbital possibly reduces plasma concentration of ● APREMILAST—avoid concomitant use
- **Aprepitant:** phenobarbital possibly reduces plasma concentration of APREPITANT
- **Avanafil:** phenobarbital possibly reduces plasma concentration of AVANAFIL—manufacturer of avanafil advises avoid concomitant use
- **Beta-blockers:** phenobarbital possibly reduces plasma concentration of PROPRANOLOL
- **Bile Acids:** avoidance of phenobarbital advised by manufacturer of ● CHOLIC ACID
- **Caffeine citrate:** effects of phenobarbital possibly antagonised by CAFFEINE CITRATE
- **Calcium-channel Blockers:** phenobarbital probably reduces effects of ● CALCIUM-CHANNEL BLOCKERS; avoidance of phenobarbital advised by manufacturer of ● ISRADIPINE; avoidance of phenobarbital advised by manufacturer of ● NIMODIPINE (plasma concentration of nimodipine reduced)
- **Cannabis Extract:** phenobarbital possibly reduces plasma concentration of ● CANNABIS EXTRACT—manufacturer of cannabis extract advises avoid concomitant use
- **Ciclosporin:** phenobarbital accelerates metabolism of ● CICLOSPORIN (reduced plasma concentration)
- **Cobicistat:** phenobarbital possibly reduces plasma concentration of ● COBICISTAT—manufacturer of cobicistat advises avoid concomitant use
- **Corticosteroids:** phenobarbital accelerates metabolism of ● CORTICOSTEROIDS (reduced effect)
- **Cytotoxics:** phenobarbital possibly decreases plasma concentration of AXITINIB (increase dose of axitinib—consult axitinib product literature); phenobarbital possibly reduces plasma concentration of BORTEZOMIB, ● BOSUTINIB, CRIZOTINIB and PONATINIB—manufacturer of bortezomib, bosutinib, crizotinib and ponatinib advises avoid concomitant use; phenobarbital possibly reduces plasma concentration of ● CABOZANTINIB—avoid concomitant use; avoidance of phenobarbital advised by manufacturer of ● CABAZITAXEL, DABRAFENIB, GEFITINIB and ● OLAPARIB; avoidance of phenobarbital advised by manufacturer of ● DASATINIB and VANDETANIB (plasma concentration of dasatinib and vandetanib possibly reduced); phenobarbital possibly reduces plasma concentration of ● ETOPOSIDE; phenobarbital reduces plasma concentration of IRINOTECAN and its active metabolite; manufacturer of procarbazine advises possible increased risk of hypersensitivity reactions when phenobarbital given with PROCARBAZINE
- **Diuretics:** phenobarbital reduces plasma concentration of ● EPLERENONE—avoid concomitant use; increased risk of osteomalacia when phenobarbital given with CARBONIC ANHYDRASE INHIBITORS
- **Folates:** plasma concentration of phenobarbital possibly reduced by FOLATES
- **Fosaprepitant:** phenobarbital possibly reduces plasma concentration of FOSAPREPITANT
- **Guanfacine:** phenobarbital possibly reduces plasma concentration of ● GUANFACINE—increase dose of guanfacine

Phenobarbital (continued)

- Hormone Antagonists: phenobarbital possibly reduces plasma concentration of ● ABIRATERONE—manufacturer of abiraterone advises avoid concomitant use; phenobarbital accelerates metabolism of TOREMIFENE (reduced plasma concentration)
- Ivacaftor: phenobarbital possibly reduces plasma concentration of ● IVACAFTOR—manufacturer of ivacaftor advises avoid concomitant use
- ▹ Leukotriene Receptor Antagonists: phenobarbital reduces plasma concentration of MONTELUKAST
- Oestrogens: phenobarbital accelerates metabolism of ● OESTROGENS (reduced contraceptive effect with combined oral contraceptives, contraceptive patches, and vaginal rings—see Contraceptive Interactions in BNF)
- Orlistat: possible increased risk of convulsions when antiepileptics given with ● ORLISTAT
- Progestogens: phenobarbital accelerates metabolism of ● PROGESTOGENS (reduced contraceptive effect with combined oral contraceptives, progestogen-only oral contraceptives, contraceptive patches, vaginal rings, etonogestrel-releasing implant, and emergency hormonal contraception—see Contraceptive Interactions in BNF)
- ▹ Roflumilast: phenobarbital possibly inhibits effects of ROFLUMILAST (manufacturer of roflumilast advises avoid concomitant use)
- ▹ Sodium Oxybate: avoidance of phenobarbital advised by manufacturer of SODIUM OXYBATE
- ▹ Sympathomimetics: plasma concentration of phenobarbital possibly increased by METHYLPHENIDATE
- Tacrolimus: phenobarbital reduces plasma concentration of ● TACROLIMUS
- Theophylline: phenobarbital accelerates metabolism of ● THEOPHYLLINE (reduced effect)
- ▹ Thyroid Hormones: phenobarbital accelerates metabolism of THYROID HORMONES (may increase requirements for thyroid hormones in hypothyroidism)
- ▹ Ticagrelor: phenobarbital possibly reduces plasma concentration of TICAGRELOR
- Ulipristal: avoidance of phenobarbital advised by manufacturer of ● ULIPRISTAL (contraceptive effect of ulipristal possibly reduced)
- ▹ Vitamins: phenobarbital possibly increases requirements for ALFACALCIDOL, CALCITRIOL, COLECALCIFEROL, DIHYDROTACHYSTEROL, ERGOCALCIFEROL, PARICALCITOL or VITAMIN D

Phenothiazines see Antipsychotics

Phenoxybenzamine see Alpha-blockers

Phenoxymethylpenicillin see Penicillins

Phentolamine see Alpha-blockers

Phenylephrine see Sympathomimetics

Phenytoin

- ▹ Alcohol: plasma concentration of phenytoin possibly reduced by chronic heavy consumption of ALCOHOL
- Aminophylline: plasma concentration of both drugs reduced when phenytoin given with ● AMINOPHYLLINE
- Analgesics: excretion of phenytoin possibly reduced by ACEMETACIN (increased risk of toxicity); phenytoin possibly accelerates metabolism of FENTANYL (reduced effect); phenytoin accelerates metabolism of METHADONE (reduced effect and risk of withdrawal effects); phenytoin possibly increases risk of ● PETHIDINE toxicity; effects of phenytoin enhanced by ASPIRIN; phenytoin possibly accelerates metabolism of PARACETAMOL (also isolated reports of hepatotoxicity)
- ▹ Antacids: absorption of phenytoin reduced by ANTACIDS
- Anthelmintics: phenytoin reduces plasma concentration of ● ALBENDAZOLE and ● PRAZIQUANTEL—consider increasing albendazole and praziquantel dose when given for systemic infections; plasma concentration of phenytoin possibly increased by LEVAMISOLE
- Anti-arrhythmics: metabolism of phenytoin inhibited by ● AMIODARONE (increased plasma concentration); phenytoin reduces plasma concentration of DISOPYRAMIDE; phenytoin possibly reduces plasma concentration of ● DRONEDARONE— avoid concomitant use

Phenytoin (continued)

- Antibacterials: metabolism of phenytoin inhibited by CLARITHROMYCIN (increased plasma concentration); metabolism of phenytoin possibly inhibited by METRONIDAZOLE (increased plasma concentration); plasma concentration of phenytoin increased or decreased by CIPROFLOXACIN; phenytoin accelerates metabolism of DOXYCYCLINE (reduced plasma concentration); phenytoin possibly reduces plasma concentration of ● BEDAQUILINE— manufacturer of bedaquiline advises avoid concomitant use; plasma concentration of phenytoin increased by ● CHLORAMPHENICOL (increased risk of toxicity); metabolism of phenytoin possibly inhibited by ISONIAZID (increased risk of toxicity); metabolism of phenytoin accelerated by ● RIFAMYCINS (reduced plasma concentration); plasma concentration of phenytoin possibly increased by SULFONAMIDES; phenytoin reduces plasma concentration of ● TELITHROMYCIN (avoid during and for 2 weeks after phenytoin); plasma concentration of phenytoin increased by ● TRIMETHOPRIM (also increased antifolate effect)
- Anticoagulants: phenytoin possibly reduces plasma concentration of ● APIXABAN and ● EDOXABAN; phenytoin accelerates metabolism of ● COUMARINS (possibility of reduced anticoagulant effect, but enhancement also reported); phenytoin possibly reduces plasma concentration of DABIGATRAN—manufacturer of dabigatran advises avoid concomitant use; phenytoin possibly reduces plasma concentration of ● RIVAROXABAN—manufacturer of rivaroxaban advises monitor for signs of thrombosis
- Antidepressants: plasma concentration of phenytoin increased by ● FLUOXETINE and ● FLUVOXAMINE; phenytoin reduces plasma concentration of ● MIANSERIN, MIRTAZAPINE and PAROXETINE; plasma concentration of phenytoin possibly increased by SERTRALINE, also plasma concentration of sertraline possibly reduced; anticonvulsant effect of antiepileptics possibly antagonised by MAOIs and ● TRICYCLIC-RELATED ANTIDEPRESSANTS (convulsive threshold lowered); anticonvulsant effect of antiepileptics antagonised by ● SSRIS and ● TRICYCLICS (convulsive threshold lowered); plasma concentration of phenytoin possibly reduced by ● ST JOHN'S WORT—avoid concomitant use; phenytoin possibly reduces plasma concentration of ● TRICYCLICS; phenytoin possibly reduces plasma concentration of ● VORTIOXETINE—consider increasing dose of vortioxetine
- ▹ Antidiabetics: plasma concentration of phenytoin transiently increased by TOLBUTAMIDE (possibility of toxicity)
- Antiepileptics: plasma concentration of both drugs often reduced when phenytoin given with CARBAMAZEPINE, also plasma concentration of phenytoin may be increased; phenytoin reduces plasma concentration of ESLICARBAZEPINE, also plasma concentration of phenytoin increased; plasma concentration of phenytoin possibly increased by ● ETHOSUXIMIDE, also plasma concentration of ethosuximide possibly reduced; phenytoin reduces plasma concentration of LAMOTRIGINE, TIAGABINE and ZONISAMIDE; plasma concentration of phenytoin increased by OXCARBAZEPINE, also plasma concentration of an active metabolite of oxcarbazepine reduced; phenytoin reduces plasma concentration of ● PERAMPANEL (see under Perampanel, p. 293); phenytoin often increases plasma concentration of PHENOBARBITAL and PRIMIDONE, plasma concentration of phenytoin often reduced but may be increased; phenytoin possibly reduces plasma concentration of RETIGABINE; phenytoin possibly reduces plasma concentration of RUFINAMIDE, also plasma concentration of phenytoin possibly increased; plasma concentration of phenytoin increased or possibly reduced when given with SODIUM VALPROATE and VALPROIC ACID, also plasma concentration of sodium valproate and valproic acid reduced; plasma concentration of phenytoin increased by ● STIRIPENTOL; plasma concentration of phenytoin increased by ● TOPIRAMATE (also plasma concentration of topiramate reduced); plasma concentration of phenytoin reduced by VIGABATRIN
- Antifungals: phenytoin reduces plasma concentration of ● KETOCONAZOLE and ● POSACONAZOLE; anticonvulsant effect of phenytoin enhanced by ● MICONAZOLE (plasma concentration

Phenytoin

- **Antifungals** (continued)
of phenytoin increased); plasma concentration of phenytoin
increased by ● FLUCONAZOLE (consider reducing dose of
phenytoin); phenytoin reduces plasma concentration of
● ITRACONAZOLE—avoid concomitant use; plasma
concentration of phenytoin increased by ● VORICONAZOLE, also
phenytoin reduces plasma concentration of voriconazole
(increase dose of voriconazole and also monitor for phenytoin
toxicity); phenytoin possibly reduces plasma concentration of
CASPOFUNGIN—consider increasing dose of caspofungin
- **Antimalarials**: avoidance of phenytoin advised by manufacturer
of ARTENIMOL WITH PIPERAQUINE; anticonvulsant effect of
antiepileptics antagonised by ● MEFLOQUINE; anticonvulsant
effect of phenytoin antagonised by ● PYRIMETHAMINE, also
increased antifolate effect
- **Antimuscarinics**: phenytoin possibly reduces plasma
concentration of active metabolite of ● FESOTERODINE—
manufacturer of fesoterodine advises avoid concomitant use
- **Antipsychotics**: anticonvulsant effect of antiepileptics
antagonised by ● ANTIPSYCHOTICS (convulsive threshold
lowered); phenytoin reduces plasma concentration of
HALOPERIDOL; plasma concentration of phenytoin possibly
increased or decreased by CHLORPROMAZINE; phenytoin
possibly reduces plasma concentration of ● ARIPIPRAZOLE
(avoid concomitant use or consider increasing the dose of
aripiprazole—consult aripiprazole product literature);
phenytoin accelerates metabolism of CLOZAPINE and
QUETIAPINE (reduced plasma concentration); phenytoin
possibly reduces plasma concentration of ● LURASIDONE—
avoid concomitant use
- **Antivirals**: phenytoin possibly reduces plasma concentration of
ABACAVIR, DARUNAVIR, LOPINAVIR and SAQUINAVIR; avoidance of
phenytoin advised by manufacturer of ● BOCEPREVIR and
● RILPIVIRINE (plasma concentration of boceprevir and
rilpivirine possibly reduced); phenytoin possibly reduces
plasma concentration of ● DACLATASVIR and ● SIMEPREVIR—
manufacturer of daclatasvir and simeprevir advises avoid
concomitant use; phenytoin possibly reduces plasma
concentration of ● DASABUVIR, ● OMBITASVIR and
● PARITAPREVIR—avoid concomitant use; phenytoin possibly
reduces the plasma concentration of ● DOLUTEGRAVIR (see
under Dolutegravir, p. 584); avoidance of phenytoin advised
by manufacturer of ● ELVITEGRAVIR, ETRAVIRINE, LEDIPASVIR,
SOFOSBUVIR and ● TELAPREVIR; phenytoin possibly reduces
plasma concentration of ● INDINAVIR, also plasma
concentration of phenytoin possibly increased; phenytoin
possibly reduces plasma concentration of RITONAVIR, also
plasma concentration of phenytoin possibly affected; plasma
concentration of phenytoin increased or decreased by
ZIDOVUDINE
▸ **Anxiolytics and Hypnotics**: phenytoin often reduces plasma
concentration of CLONAZEPAM; plasma concentration of
phenytoin increased or decreased by DIAZEPAM; plasma
concentration of phenytoin possibly increased or decreased
by BENZODIAZEPINES
- **Apremilast**: phenytoin possibly reduces plasma concentration
of ● APREMILAST—avoid concomitant use
▸ **Aprepitant**: phenytoin possibly reduces plasma concentration
of APREPITANT
▸ **Bupropion**: phenytoin reduces plasma concentration of
BUPROPION
▸ **Caffeine citrate**: phenytoin reduces plasma concentration of
CAFFEINE CITRATE
- **Calcium-channel Blockers**: phenytoin reduces effects of
FELODIPINE and VERAPAMIL; avoidance of phenytoin advised by
manufacturer of ISRADIPINE; avoidance of phenytoin advised
by manufacturer of NIMODIPINE (plasma concentration of
nimodipine possibly reduced); plasma concentration of
phenytoin increased by ● DILTIAZEM but also effect of diltiazem
reduced
- **Cannabis Extract**: phenytoin possibly reduces plasma
concentration of ● CANNABIS EXTRACT—manufacturer of
cannabis extract advises avoid concomitant use
▸ **Cardiac Glycosides**: phenytoin possibly reduces plasma
concentration of DIGOXIN

Phenytoin (continued)

- **Ciclosporin**: phenytoin accelerates metabolism of ● CICLOSPORIN
(reduced plasma concentration)
- **Cobicistat**: phenytoin possibly reduces plasma concentration of
● COBICISTAT—manufacturer of cobicistat advises avoid
concomitant use
- **Corticosteroids**: phenytoin accelerates metabolism of
● CORTICOSTEROIDS (reduced effect)
- **Cytotoxics**: phenytoin possibly reduces plasma concentration
of BUSULFAN, ERIBULIN and ETOPOSIDE; metabolism of
phenytoin possibly inhibited by CAPECITABINE, FLUOROURACIL
and TEGAFUR (increased risk of toxicity); phenytoin increases
antifolate effect of METHOTREXATE; plasma concentration of
phenytoin possibly reduced by CISPLATIN; phenytoin possibly
decreases plasma concentration of AXITINIB (increase dose of
axitinib—consult axitinib product literature); phenytoin
possibly reduces plasma concentration of BORTEZOMIB,
● BOSUTINIB, ● CRIZOTINIB, ● IBRUTINIB, ● IDELALISIB and
PONATINIB—manufacturer of bortezomib, bosutinib,
crizotinib, ibrutinib, idelalisib and ponatinib advises avoid
concomitant use; phenytoin possibly reduces plasma
concentration of ● CABOZANTINIB—avoid concomitant use;
avoidance of phenytoin advised by manufacturer of
● CABAZITAXEL, DABRAFENIB, GEFITINIB, ● LAPATINIB, ● OLAPARIB
and VEMURAFENIB; avoidance of phenytoin advised by
manufacturer of DASATINIB and ● VISMODEGIB (plasma
concentration of dasatinib and vismodegib possibly reduced);
phenytoin reduces plasma concentration of ● IMATINIB—avoid
concomitant use; phenytoin reduces plasma concentration of
IRINOTECAN and its active metabolite; manufacturer of
procarbazine advises possible increased risk of
hypersensitivity reactions when phenytoin given with
PROCARBAZINE
- **Dexrazoxane**: absorption of phenytoin possibly reduced by
● DEXRAZOXANE
▸ **Diazoxide**: plasma concentration of phenytoin reduced by
DIAZOXIDE, also effect of diazoxide may be reduced
- **Disulfiram**: metabolism of phenytoin inhibited by ● DISULFIRAM
(increased risk of toxicity)
- **Diuretics**: plasma concentration of phenytoin possibly
increased by ● ACETAZOLAMIDE; phenytoin antagonises effects
of FUROSEMIDE; phenytoin reduces plasma concentration of
● EPLERENONE—avoid concomitant use; increased risk of
osteomalacia when phenytoin given with CARBONIC
ANHYDRASE INHIBITORS
▸ **Dopaminergics**: phenytoin possibly reduces effects of CO-
BENELDOPA, CO-CARELDOPA and LEVODOPA
▸ **Enteral Feeds**: absorption of phenytoin possibly reduced by
ENTERAL FEEDS
▸ **Folates**: plasma concentration of phenytoin possibly reduced
by FOLATES
▸ **Fosaprepitant**: phenytoin possibly reduces plasma
concentration of FOSAPREPITANT
- **Guanfacine**: phenytoin possibly reduces plasma concentration
of ● GUANFACINE—increase dose of guanfacine
- **Hormone Antagonists**: phenytoin possibly reduces plasma
concentration of ● ABIRATERONE—manufacturer of abiraterone
advises avoid concomitant use; phenytoin possibly
accelerates metabolism of TOREMIFENE
▸ **5HT₃-receptor Antagonists**: phenytoin accelerates metabolism of
ONDANSETRON (reduced effect)
- **Ivacaftor**: phenytoin possibly reduces plasma concentration of
● IVACAFTOR—manufacturer of ivacaftor advises avoid
concomitant use
▸ **Leflunomide**: plasma concentration of phenytoin possibly
increased by LEFLUNOMIDE
▸ **Lipid-regulating Drugs**: absorption of phenytoin possibly
reduced by COLESEVELAM; combination of phenytoin with
FLUVASTATIN may increase plasma concentration of either drug
(or both)
- **Lithium**: neurotoxicity may occur when phenytoin given with
LITHIUM without increased plasma concentration of lithium
▸ **Macitentan**: avoidance of phenytoin advised by manufacturer
of MACITENTAN
▸ **Modafinil**: plasma concentration of phenytoin possibly
increased by MODAFINIL

Phenytoin (continued)

- Muscle Relaxants: *long-term use* of phenytoin reduces effects of ● NON-DEPOLARISING MUSCLE RELAXANTS (but *acute use* of phenytoin might increase effects of non-depolarising muscle relaxants)
- Oestrogens: phenytoin accelerates metabolism of ● OESTROGENS (reduced contraceptive effect with combined oral contraceptives, contraceptive patches, and vaginal rings—see Contraceptive Interactions in BNF)
- Orlistat: possible increased risk of convulsions when antiepileptics given with ● ORLISTAT
- Progestogens: phenytoin accelerates metabolism of ● PROGESTOGENS (reduced contraceptive effect with combined oral contraceptives, progestogen-only oral contraceptives, contraceptive patches, vaginal rings, etonogestrel-releasing implant, and emergency hormonal contraception—see Contraceptive Interactions in BNF)
- ▸ Roflumilast: phenytoin possibly inhibits effects of ROFLUMILAST (manufacturer of roflumilast advises avoid concomitant use)
- Sulfinpyrazone: plasma concentration of phenytoin increased by ● SULFINPYRAZONE
- ▸ Sympathomimetics: plasma concentration of phenytoin increased by METHYLPHENIDATE
- ▸ Tacrolimus: phenytoin reduces plasma concentration of TACROLIMUS, also plasma concentration of phenytoin possibly increased
- Theophylline: plasma concentration of both drugs reduced when phenytoin given with ● THEOPHYLLINE
- ▸ Thyroid Hormones: phenytoin accelerates metabolism of THYROID HORMONES (may increase requirements in hypothyroidism), also plasma concentration of phenytoin possibly increased
- ▸ Tibolone: phenytoin accelerates metabolism of TIBOLONE
- ▸ Ticagrelor: phenytoin possibly reduces plasma concentration of TICAGRELOR
- Ulcer-healing Drugs: metabolism of phenytoin inhibited by ● CIMETIDINE (increased plasma concentration); effects of phenytoin enhanced by ● ESOMEPRAZOLE; effects of phenytoin possibly enhanced by OMEPRAZOLE; absorption of phenytoin reduced by ● SUCRALFATE
- Ulipristal: avoidance of phenytoin advised by manufacturer of ● ULIPRISTAL (contraceptive effect of ulipristal possibly reduced)
- ▸ Vaccines: effects of phenytoin enhanced by INFLUENZA VACCINE
- ▸ Vitamins: phenytoin possibly increases requirements for ALFACALCIDOL, CALCITRIOL, COLECALCIFEROL, DIHYDROTACHYSTEROL, ERGOCALCIFEROL, PARICALCITOL or VITAMIN D

Pholcodine
- ▸ Antidepressants: manufacturer of pholcodine advises avoid for 2 weeks after stopping MAOIs

Phosphodiesterase Type-3 Inhibitors
- ● Anagrelide: avoidance of enoximone and milrinone advised by manufacturer of ● ANAGRELIDE

Pilocarpine see Parasympathomimetics

Pimozide see Antipsychotics

Pindolol see Beta-blockers

Pioglitazone see Antidiabetics

Piperacillin see Penicillins

Piperaquine see Artenimol with Piperaquine

Pirfenidone
- ● Antibacterials: plasma concentration of pirfenidone increased by ● CIPROFLOXACIN—see under Pirfenidone, p. 272
- ● Antidepressants: plasma concentration of pirfenidone increased by ● FLUVOXAMINE—manufacturer of pirfenidone advises avoid concomitant use
- ▸ Grapefruit Juice: manufacturer of pirfenidone advises avoid concomitant use with GRAPEFRUIT JUICE

Piroxicam see NSAIDs

Pivmecillinam see Penicillins

Pixantrone
- ● Antipsychotics: avoid concomitant use of cytotoxics with ● CLOZAPINE (increased risk of agranulocytosis)
- ● Vaccines: risk of generalised infections when cytotoxic antibiotics given with live ● VACCINES—avoid concomitant use

Pizotifen
- ▸ Adrenergic Neurone Blockers: pizotifen antagonises hypotensive effect of ADRENERGIC NEURONE BLOCKERS

Platinum Compounds
- ● Aldesleukin: avoidance of cisplatin advised by manufacturer of ● ALDESLEUKIN
- ● Antibacterials: increased risk of nephrotoxicity and possibly of ototoxicity when platinum compounds given with ● AMINOGLYCOSIDES or ● POLYMYXINS; increased risk of nephrotoxicity and ototoxicity when platinum compounds given with CAPREOMYCIN; increased risk of nephrotoxicity and possibly of ototoxicity when cisplatin given with VANCOMYCIN
- ▸ Antiepileptics: cisplatin possibly reduces plasma concentration of FOSPHENYTOIN and PHENYTOIN
- ● Antipsychotics: avoid concomitant use of cytotoxics with ● CLOZAPINE (increased risk of agranulocytosis)
- ● Cytotoxics: increased risk of otoxicity when cisplatin given with IFOSFAMIDE; increased pulmonary toxicity when cisplatin given with ● BLEOMYCIN and ● METHOTREXATE; avoidance of oxaliplatin advised by manufacturer of ● PANITUMUMAB
- ▸ Diuretics: increased risk of nephrotoxicity and ototoxicity when platinum compounds given with DIURETICS

Pneumococcal Vaccine see Vaccines

Poliomyelitis Vaccine see Vaccines

Polymyxins
- ▸ Antibacterials: increased risk of nephrotoxicity when colistimethate sodium or polymyxins given with AMINOGLYCOSIDES; increased risk of nephrotoxicity when colistimethate sodium or polymyxins given with CAPREOMYCIN; increased risk of nephrotoxicity when polymyxins given with VANCOMYCIN; increased risk of nephrotoxicity and ototoxicity when colistimethate sodium given with VANCOMYCIN
- ▸ Antifungals: increased risk of nephrotoxicity when polymyxins given with AMPHOTERICIN
- ● Ciclosporin: increased risk of nephrotoxicity when polymyxins given with ● CICLOSPORIN
- ● Cytotoxics: increased risk of nephrotoxicity and possibly of ototoxicity when polymyxins given with ● PLATINUM COMPOUNDS
- ▸ Diuretics: increased risk of ototoxicity when polymyxins given with ● LOOP DIURETICS
- ● Muscle Relaxants: polymyxins enhance effects of ● NON-DEPOLARISING MUSCLE RELAXANTS and ● SUXAMETHONIUM
- ● Parasympathomimetics: polymyxins antagonise effects of ● NEOSTIGMINE and ● PYRIDOSTIGMINE
- ▸ Vaccines: antibacterials inactivate ORAL TYPHOID VACCINE—see under Typhoid Vaccine in BNF

Polysaccharide-iron Complex see Iron salts

Polystyrene Sulfonate Resins
- ▸ Antacids: risk of intestinal obstruction when polystyrene sulfonate resins given with ALUMINIUM HYDROXIDE; risk of metabolic alkalosis when polystyrene sulfonate resins given with ORAL MAGNESIUM SALTS
- ▸ Thyroid Hormones: polystyrene sulfonate resins reduce absorption of LEVOTHYROXINE

Pomalidomide
- ● Antidepressants: plasma concentration of pomalidomide increased by ● FLUVOXAMINE

Ponatinib
- ● Antibacterials: plasma concentration of ponatinib possibly increased by CLARITHROMYCIN and TELITHROMYCIN—consider reducing initial dose of ponatinib (see under Ponatinib, p. 860); plasma concentration of ponatinib possibly reduced by RIFABUTIN—manufacturer of ponatinib advises avoid concomitant use; plasma concentration of ponatinib reduced by ● RIFAMPICIN—manufacturer of ponatinib advises avoid concomitant use
- ▸ Antidepressants: plasma concentration of ponatinib possibly reduced by ST JOHN'S WORT—manufacturer of ponatinib advises avoid concomitant use
- ▸ Antiepileptics: plasma concentration of ponatinib possibly reduced by CARBAMAZEPINE, FOSPHENYTOIN, PHENOBARBITAL, PHENYTOIN and PRIMIDONE—manufacturer of ponatinib advises avoid concomitant use

A1

Interactions | Appendix 1

Ponatinib (continued)

▸ Antifungals: plasma concentration of ponatinib increased by KETOCONAZOLE; plasma concentration of ponatinib possibly increased by ITRACONAZOLE and VORICONAZOLE—consider reducing initial dose of ponatinib (see under Ponatinib, p. 860)

● Antipsychotics: avoid concomitant use of cytotoxics with ● CLOZAPINE (increased risk of agranulocytosis)

▸ Antivirals: plasma concentration of ponatinib possibly increased by INDINAVIR, RITONAVIR and SAQUINAVIR—consider reducing initial dose of ponatinib (see under Ponatinib, p. 860)

▸ Grapefruit Juice: plasma concentration of ponatinib possibly increased by GRAPEFRUIT JUICE

Posaconazole see Antifungals, Triazole

Potassium Canrenoate see Diuretics

Potassium Aminobenzoate

▸ Antibacterials: potassium aminobenzoate inhibits effects of SULFONAMIDES

Potassium Bicarbonate see Potassium Salts

Potassium Chloride see Potassium Salts

Potassium Citrate see Potassium Salts

Potassium Salts

NOTE Includes salt substitutes

● ACE Inhibitors: increased risk of severe hyperkalaemia when potassium salts given with ● ACE INHIBITORS

● Aliskiren: increased risk of hyperkalaemia when potassium salts given with ALISKIREN

● Angiotensin-II Receptor Antagonists: increased risk of hyperkalaemia when potassium salts given with ● ANGIOTENSIN-II RECEPTOR ANTAGONISTS

▸ Antibacterials: avoid concomitant use of potassium citrate with METHENAMINE

● Ciclosporin: increased risk of hyperkalaemia when potassium salts given with ● CICLOSPORIN

● Diuretics: increased risk of hyperkalaemia when potassium salts given with ● POTASSIUM-SPARING DIURETICS AND ALDOSTERONE ANTAGONISTS

● Tacrolimus: increased risk of hyperkalaemia when potassium salts given with ● TACROLIMUS

▸ Ulcer-healing Drugs: avoidance of potassium citrate advised by manufacturer of SUCRALFATE

Pramipexole

▸ Antipsychotics: manufacturer of pramipexole advises avoid concomitant use of ANTIPSYCHOTICS (antagonism of effect)

▸ Memantine: effects of dopaminergics possibly enhanced by MEMANTINE

▸ Methyldopa: antiparkinsonian effect of dopaminergics antagonised by METHYLDOPA

▸ Ulcer-healing Drugs: excretion of pramipexole reduced by CIMETIDINE (increased plasma concentration)

Prasugrel

▸ Analgesics: possible increased risk of bleeding when prasugrel given with NSAIDs

▸ Anticoagulants: possible increased risk of bleeding when prasugrel given with COUMARINS or PHENINDIONE

▸ Clopidogrel: possible increased risk of bleeding when prasugrel given with CLOPIDOGREL

Pravastatin see Statins

Praziquantel

● Antibacterials: plasma concentration of praziquantel reduced by ● RIFAMPICIN—avoid concomitant use

● Antiepileptics: plasma concentration of praziquantel reduced by ● CARBAMAZEPINE, ● FOSPHENYTOIN, ● PHENOBARBITAL, ● PHENYTOIN and ● PRIMIDONE—consider increasing praziquantel dose when given for systemic infections

● Antifungals: plasma concentration of praziquantel increased by KETOCONAZOLE

● Antimalarials: plasma concentration of praziquantel reduced by ● CHLOROQUINE—consider increasing praziquantel dose when given for systemic infections

▸ Corticosteroids: plasma concentration of praziquantel possibly reduced by continuous use of DEXAMETHASONE

▸ Grapefruit Juice: plasma concentration of praziquantel increased by GRAPEFRUIT JUICE

Praziquantel (continued)

▸ Ulcer-healing Drugs: plasma concentration of praziquantel increased by CIMETIDINE

Prazosin see Alpha-blockers

Prednisolone see Corticosteroids

Prednisone see Corticosteroids

Pregabalin

● Antidepressants: anticonvulsant effect of antiepileptics possibly antagonised by MAOIs and ● TRICYCLIC-RELATED ANTIDEPRESSANTS (convulsive threshold lowered); anticonvulsant effect of antiepileptics antagonised by ● SSRIS and ● TRICYCLICS (convulsive threshold lowered)

● Antimalarials: anticonvulsant effect of antiepileptics antagonised by ● MEFLOQUINE

● Antipsychotics: anticonvulsant effect of antiepileptics antagonised by ● ANTIPSYCHOTICS (convulsive threshold lowered)

● Orlistat: possible increased risk of convulsions when antiepileptics given with ● ORLISTAT

Prilocaine

▸ Anti-arrhythmics: increased myocardial depression when prilocaine given with ANTI-ARRHYTHMICS

▸ Antibacterials: increased risk of methaemoglobinaemia when prilocaine given with SULFONAMIDES

Primaquine

● Antimalarials: avoidance of antimalarials advised by manufacturer of ● ARTEMETHER WITH LUMEFANTRINE

● Histamine: avoidance of antimalarials advised by manufacturer of HISTAMINE

▸ Mepacrine: plasma concentration of primaquine increased by MEPACRINE (increased risk of toxicity)

▸ Penicillamine: increased risk of haematological toxicity when antimalarials given with PENICILLAMINE—manufacturer of penicillamine advises avoid concomitant use

▸ Vaccines: antimalarials inactivate ORAL TYPHOID VACCINE—see under Typhoid Vaccine in BNF

Primidone

● Alcohol: increased sedative effect when primidone given with ALCOHOL

● Aminophylline: primidone accelerates metabolism of ● AMINOPHYLLINE (reduced effect)

● Analgesics: primidone reduces plasma concentration of METHADONE; primidone possibly accelerates metabolism of PARACETAMOL (also isolated reports of hepatotoxicity)

● Anthelmintics: primidone reduces plasma concentration of ● ALBENDAZOLE and ● PRAZIQUANTEL—consider increasing albendazole and praziquantel dose when given for systemic infections

● Anti-arrhythmics: primidone accelerates metabolism of DISOPYRAMIDE (reduced plasma concentration); primidone possibly reduces plasma concentration of ● DRONEDARONE—avoid concomitant use; primidone possibly accelerates metabolism of PROPAFENONE

● Antibacterials: primidone accelerates metabolism of METRONIDAZOLE (reduced effect); primidone possibly reduces plasma concentration of RIFAMPICIN; primidone accelerates metabolism of DOXYCYCLINE (reduced plasma concentration); primidone possibly accelerates metabolism of ● CHLORAMPHENICOL (reduced plasma concentration); primidone reduces plasma concentration of ● TELITHROMYCIN (avoid during and for 2 weeks after primidone)

● Anticoagulants: primidone possibly reduces plasma concentration of ● APIXABAN and ● EDOXABAN; primidone accelerates metabolism of ● COUMARINS (reduced anticoagulant effect); primidone possibly reduces plasma concentration of ● RIVAROXABAN—manufacturer of rivaroxaban advises monitor for signs of thrombosis

● Antidepressants: primidone possibly reduces plasma concentration of REBOXETINE; primidone reduces plasma concentration of PAROXETINE; primidone accelerates metabolism of ● MIANSERIN (reduced plasma concentration); anticonvulsant effect of antiepileptics possibly antagonised by MAOIs and ● TRICYCLIC-RELATED ANTIDEPRESSANTS (convulsive threshold lowered); anticonvulsant effect of antiepileptics antagonised by ● SSRIS and ● TRICYCLICS (convulsive threshold lowered); plasma concentration of

Primidone
- **Antidepressants** (continued)
  primidone possibly reduced by ● ST JOHN'S WORT—avoid concomitant use; primidone possibly accelerates metabolism of ● TRICYCLICS (reduced plasma concentration)
- **Antiepileptics:** plasma concentration of primidone possibly increased by CARBAMAZEPINE; primidone possibly reduces plasma concentration of ETHOSUXIMIDE, RUFINAMIDE and TOPIRAMATE; plasma concentration of primidone often increased by FOSPHENYTOIN and PHENYTOIN, plasma concentration of fosphenytoin and phenytoin often reduced but may be increased; primidone reduces plasma concentration of LAMOTRIGINE, TIAGABINE and ZONISAMIDE; plasma concentration of primidone increased by OXCARBAZEPINE, also plasma concentration of an active metabolite of oxcarbazepine reduced; plasma concentration of primidone increased by SODIUM VALPROATE and VALPROIC ACID (also plasma concentration of sodium valproate and valproic acid reduced); plasma concentration of primidone increased by ● STIRIPENTOL
- **Antifungals:** primidone possibly reduces plasma concentration of ITRACONAZOLE and ● POSACONAZOLE; primidone possibly reduces plasma concentration of ● VORICONAZOLE—avoid concomitant use; primidone reduces absorption of GRISEOFULVIN (reduced effect)
- **Antimalarials:** avoidance of primidone advised by manufacturer of ARTENIMOL WITH PIPERAQUINE; anticonvulsant effect of antiepileptics antagonised by ● MEFLOQUINE
- **Antipsychotics:** anticonvulsant effect of antiepileptics antagonised by ● ANTIPSYCHOTICS (convulsive threshold lowered); primidone accelerates metabolism of HALOPERIDOL (reduced plasma concentration); plasma concentration of both drugs reduced when primidone given with CHLORPROMAZINE; primidone possibly reduces plasma concentration of ● ARIPIPRAZOLE (avoid concomitant use or consider increasing the dose of aripiprazole—consult aripiprazole product literature); primidone possibly reduces plasma concentration of CLOZAPINE; primidone possibly reduces plasma concentration of ● LURASIDONE—avoid concomitant use
- **Antivirals:** primidone possibly reduces plasma concentration of ABACAVIR, DARUNAVIR, FOSAMPRENAVIR, ● INDINAVIR, ● LOPINAVIR and ● SAQUINAVIR; avoidance of primidone advised by manufacturer of ● BOCEPREVIR and ● RILPIVIRINE (plasma concentration of boceprevir and rilpivirine possibly reduced); primidone possibly reduces plasma concentration of ● DACLATASVIR and ● SIMEPREVIR—manufacturer of daclatasvir and simeprevir advises avoid concomitant use; primidone possibly reduces plasma concentration of ● DASABUVIR, ● OMBITASVIR and ● PARITAPREVIR—avoid concomitant use; primidone possibly reduces the plasma concentration of ● DOLUTEGRAVIR (see under Dolutegravir, p. 584); avoidance of primidone advised by manufacturer of ● ELVITEGRAVIR, ETRAVIRINE, LEDIPASVIR, SOFOSBUVIR and ● TELAPREVIR
- ▸ **Anxiolytics and Hypnotics:** increased sedative effect when primidone given with ANXIOLYTICS AND HYPNOTICS; primidone often reduces plasma concentration of CLONAZEPAM
- ▸ **Aprepitant:** primidone possibly reduces plasma concentration of APREPITANT
- ▸ **Avanafil:** primidone possibly reduces plasma concentration of AVANAFIL—manufacturer of avanafil advises avoid concomitant use
- ▸ **Beta-blockers:** primidone possibly reduces plasma concentration of PROPRANOLOL
- ▸ **Caffeine citrate:** effects of primidone possibly antagonised by CAFFEINE CITRATE
- **Calcium-channel Blockers:** primidone probably reduces effects of ● CALCIUM-CHANNEL BLOCKERS; avoidance of primidone advised by manufacturer of ISRADIPINE; avoidance of primidone advised by manufacturer of ● NIMODIPINE (plasma concentration of nimodipine reduced)
- **Cannabis Extract:** primidone possibly reduces plasma concentration of ● CANNABIS EXTRACT—manufacturer of cannabis extract advises avoid concomitant use
- **Ciclosporin:** primidone accelerates metabolism of ● CICLOSPORIN (reduced plasma concentration)

Primidone (continued)
- **Cobicistat:** primidone possibly reduces plasma concentration of ● COBICISTAT—manufacturer of cobicistat advises avoid concomitant use
- **Corticosteroids:** primidone accelerates metabolism of ● CORTICOSTEROIDS (reduced effect)
- **Cytotoxics:** primidone possibly decreases plasma concentration of AXITINIB (increase dose of axitinib—consult axitinib product literature); primidone possibly reduces plasma concentration of BORTEZOMIB, ● BOSUTINIB, CRIZOTINIB and PONATINIB—manufacturer of bortezomib, bosutinib, crizotinib and ponatinib advises avoid concomitant use; primidone possibly reduces plasma concentration of ● CABOZANTINIB—avoid concomitant use; avoidance of primidone advised by manufacturer of ● CABAZITAXEL, DABRAFENIB and GEFITINIB; avoidance of primidone advised by manufacturer of DASATINIB and VANDETANIB (plasma concentration of dasatinib and vandetanib possibly reduced); primidone possibly reduces plasma concentration of ETOPOSIDE; primidone reduces plasma concentration of IRINOTECAN and its active metabolite; manufacturer of procarbazine advises possible increased risk of hypersensitivity reactions when primidone given with PROCARBAZINE
- **Diuretics:** primidone reduces plasma concentration of ● EPLERENONE—avoid concomitant use; increased risk of osteomalacia when primidone given with CARBONIC ANHYDRASE INHIBITORS
- ▸ **Folates:** plasma concentration of primidone possibly reduced by FOLATES
- ▸ **Fosaprepitant:** primidone possibly reduces plasma concentration of FOSAPREPITANT
- ▸ **Guanfacine:** primidone possibly reduces plasma concentration of ● GUANFACINE—increase dose of guanfacine
- **Hormone Antagonists:** primidone possibly reduces plasma concentration of ● ABIRATERONE—manufacturer of abiraterone advises avoid concomitant use; primidone accelerates metabolism of TOREMIFENE (reduced plasma concentration)
- **Ivacaftor:** primidone possibly reduces plasma concentration of ● IVACAFTOR—manufacturer of ivacaftor advises avoid concomitant use
- ▸ **Leukotriene Receptor Antagonists:** primidone reduces plasma concentration of MONTELUKAST
- **Oestrogens:** primidone accelerates metabolism of ● OESTROGENS (reduced contraceptive effect with combined oral contraceptives, contraceptive patches, and vaginal rings—see Contraceptive Interactions in BNF)
- **Orlistat:** possible increased risk of convulsions when antiepileptics given with ● ORLISTAT
- **Progestogens:** primidone accelerates metabolism of ● PROGESTOGENS (reduced contraceptive effect with combined oral contraceptives, progestogen-only oral contraceptives, contraceptive patches, vaginal rings, etonogestrel-releasing implant, and emergency hormonal contraception—see Contraceptive Interactions in BNF)
- ▸ **Roflumilast:** primidone possibly inhibits effects of ROFLUMILAST (manufacturer of roflumilast advises avoid concomitant use)
- ▸ **Sodium Oxybate:** avoidance of primidone advised by manufacturer of SODIUM OXYBATE
- ▸ **Sympathomimetics:** plasma concentration of primidone possibly increased by METHYLPHENIDATE
- **Tacrolimus:** primidone reduces plasma concentration of ● TACROLIMUS
- **Theophylline:** primidone accelerates metabolism of ● THEOPHYLLINE (reduced effect)
- ▸ **Thyroid Hormones:** primidone accelerates metabolism of THYROID HORMONES (may increase requirements for thyroid hormones in hypothyroidism)
- ▸ **Ticagrelor:** primidone possibly reduces plasma concentration of TICAGRELOR
- **Ulipristal:** avoidance of primidone advised by manufacturer of ● ULIPRISTAL (contraceptive effect of ulipristal possibly reduced)
- **Vitamins:** primidone possibly increases requirements for ALFACALCIDOL, CALCITRIOL, COLECALCIFEROL, DIHYDROTACHYSTEROL, ERGOCALCIFEROL, PARICALCITOL or VITAMIN D

A1

Interactions | **Appendix 1**

Procarbazine

▸ Alcohol: disulfiram-like reaction when procarbazine given with ALCOHOL
▸ Antiepileptics: manufacturer of procarbazine advises possible increased risk of hypersensitivity reactions when given with CARBAMAZEPINE, FOSPHENYTOIN, PHENOBARBITAL, PHENYTOIN and PRIMIDONE
● Antipsychotics: avoid concomitant use of cytotoxics with ● CLOZAPINE (increased risk of agranulocytosis)
● Cardiac Glycosides: procarbazine possibly reduces absorption of DIGOXIN *tablets*

Prochlorperazine *see* Antipsychotics
Procyclidine *see* Antimuscarinics
Progesterone *see* Progestogens

Progestogens

● Antibacterials: plasma concentration of dienogest increased by ERYTHROMYCIN; metabolism of progestogens accelerated by ● RIFAMYCINS (reduced contraceptive effect with combined oral contraceptives, progestogen-only oral contraceptives, contraceptive patches, vaginal rings, etonogestrel-releasing implant, and emergency hormonal contraception—see Contraceptive Interactions in BNF)
● Anticoagulants: progestogens may enhance or reduce anticoagulant effect of COUMARINS; progestogens antagonise anticoagulant effect of ● PHENINDIONE
● Antidepressants: contraceptive effect of progestogens reduced by ● ST JOHN'S WORT (avoid concomitant use)
▸ Antidiabetics: progestogens antagonise hypoglycaemic effect of ANTIDIABETICS
● Antiepileptics: metabolism of progestogens accelerated by ● CARBAMAZEPINE, ● ESLICARBAZEPINE, ● FOSPHENYTOIN, ● OXCARBAZEPINE, ● PERAMPANEL, ● PHENOBARBITAL, ● PHENYTOIN, ● PRIMIDONE, ● RUFINAMIDE and ● TOPIRAMATE (reduced contraceptive effect with combined oral contraceptives, progestogen-only oral contraceptives, contraceptive patches, vaginal rings, etonogestrel-releasing implant, and emergency hormonal contraception—see Contraceptive Interactions in BNF); desogestrel possibly increases plasma concentration of LAMOTRIGINE
▸ Antifungals: plasma concentration of drospirenone increased by KETOCONAZOLE; progestogens possibly increase plasma concentration of VORICONAZOLE; anecdotal reports of contraceptive failure and menstrual irregularities when progestogens given with GRISEOFULVIN; occasional reports of breakthrough bleeding when progestogens (used for contraception) given with TERBINAFINE
● Antivirals: plasma concentration of norethisterone increased by ATAZANAVIR; plasma concentration of drospirenone increased by BOCEPREVIR (increased risk of toxicity); contraceptive effect of progestogens possibly reduced by ● EFAVIRENZ; plasma concentration of norgestimate increased by ELVITEGRAVIR; metabolism of progestogens accelerated by ● NEVIRAPINE (reduced contraceptive effect with combined oral contraceptives, progestogen-only oral contraceptives, contraceptive patches, vaginal rings, etonogestrel-releasing implant, and emergency hormonal contraception—see Contraceptive Interactions in BNF)
▸ Anxiolytics and Hypnotics: progestogens possibly increase plasma concentration of CHLORDIAZEPOXIDE, DIAZEPAM and NITRAZEPAM; progestogens possibly reduce plasma concentration of LORAZEPAM, OXAZEPAM and TEMAZEPAM
● Aprepitant: possible contraceptive failure of hormonal contraceptives containing progestogens when given with ● APREPITANT (alternative contraception recommended)
● Bosentan: possible contraceptive failure of hormonal contraceptives containing progestogens when given with ● BOSENTAN (alternative contraception recommended)
▸ Ciclosporin: progestogens possibly increase plasma concentration of CICLOSPORIN
▸ Cobicistat: plasma concentration of norgestimate increased by COBICISTAT
● Cytotoxics: possible reduction in contraceptive effect of progestogens advised by manufacturer of ● CRIZOTINIB and ● VEMURAFENIB; possible reduced contraceptive effect of hormonal contraceptives containing progestogens advised by

● Cytotoxics (continued)
manufacturer of ● DABRAFENIB (alternative contraception recommended)
▸ Diuretics: risk of hyperkalaemia when drospirenone given with POTASSIUM-SPARING DIURETICS AND ALDOSTERONE ANTAGONISTS (monitor serum potassium during first cycle)
● Dopaminergics: progestogens increase plasma concentration of ● SELEGILINE—manufacturer of selegiline advises avoid concomitant use
● Fosaprepitant: possible contraceptive failure of hormonal contraceptives containing progestogens when given with ● FOSAPREPITANT (alternative contraception recommended)
▸ Lipid-regulating Drugs: plasma concentration of norethisterone increased by ATORVASTATIN; plasma concentration of active metabolite of norgestimate increased by ROSUVASTATIN; plasma concentration of norgestrel increased by ROSUVASTATIN
● Muscle Relaxants: progestogens possibly increase plasma concentration of TIZANIDINE (increased risk of toxicity)
▸ Sugammadex: plasma concentration of progestogens possibly reduced by SUGAMMADEX—manufacturer of sugammadex advises additional contraceptive precautions
▸ Teriflunomide: plasma concentration of levonorgestrel increased by TERIFLUNOMIDE
● Ulipristal: contraceptive effect of progestogens possibly reduced by ● ULIPRISTAL

Proguanil

▸ Antacids: absorption of proguanil reduced by ORAL MAGNESIUM SALTS (as magnesium trisilicate)
▸ Anticoagulants: isolated reports that proguanil may enhance anticoagulant effect of WARFARIN
▸ Antimalarials: avoidance of antimalarials advised by manufacturer of ● ARTEMETHER WITH LUMEFANTRINE; increased antifolate effect when proguanil given with PYRIMETHAMINE
▸ Antivirals: plasma concentration of proguanil possibly affected by EFAVIRENZ
▸ Histamine: avoidance of antimalarials advised by manufacturer of HISTAMINE
▸ Penicillamine: increased risk of haematological toxicity when antimalarials given with PENICILLAMINE—manufacturer of penicillamine advises avoid concomitant use
▸ Vaccines: antimalarials inactivate ORAL TYPHOID VACCINE—see under Typhoid Vaccine in BNF

Promazine *see* Antipsychotics
Promethazine *see* Antihistamines

Propafenone

▸ Aminophylline: propafenone increases plasma concentration of AMINOPHYLLINE
▸ Anaesthetics, Local: increased myocardial depression when anti-arrhythmics given with BUPIVACAINE, LEVOBUPIVACAINE, PRILOCAINE or ROPIVACAINE
● Anti-arrhythmics: increased myocardial depression when anti-arrhythmics given with other ● ANTI-ARRHYTHMICS
● Antibacterials: metabolism of propafenone accelerated by ● RIFAMPICIN (reduced effect)
● Anticoagulants: propafenone enhances anticoagulant effect of ● COUMARINS
● Antidepressants: metabolism of propafenone possibly inhibited by FLUOXETINE and PAROXETINE; increased risk of arrhythmias when propafenone given with ● TRICYCLICS
▸ Antiepileptics: metabolism of propafenone possibly accelerated by PHENOBARBITAL and PRIMIDONE
▸ Antihistamines: avoidance of propafenone advised by manufacturer of MIZOLASTINE (possible risk of ventricular arrhythmias)
● Antipsychotics: increased risk of ventricular arrhythmias when anti-arrhythmics that prolong the QT interval given with ● ANTIPSYCHOTICS that prolong the QT interval
● Antivirals: plasma concentration of propafenone possibly increased by ● FOSAMPRENAVIR (increased risk of ventricular arrhythmias—avoid concomitant use); plasma concentration of propafenone increased by ● RITONAVIR (increased risk of ventricular arrhythmias—avoid concomitant use); increased risk of ventricular arrhythmias when propafenone given with ● SAQUINAVIR—avoid concomitant use; caution with

Propafenone
- Antivirals (continued)
  propafenone advised by manufacturer of • TELAPREVIR (risk of ventricular arrhythmias)
- Beta-blockers: increased myocardial depression when anti-arrhythmics given with • BETA-BLOCKERS; propafenone increases plasma concentration of METOPROLOL and PROPRANOLOL
- Cardiac Glycosides: propafenone increases plasma concentration of • DIGOXIN (halve dose of digoxin)
▸ Ciclosporin: propafenone possibly increases plasma concentration of CICLOSPORIN
▸ Parasympathomimetics: propafenone possibly antagonises effects of NEOSTIGMINE and PYRIDOSTIGMINE
▸ Theophylline: propafenone increases plasma concentration of THEOPHYLLINE
- Ulcer-healing Drugs: plasma concentration of propafenone increased by • CIMETIDINE

Propantheline see Antimuscarinics
Propiverine see Antimuscarinics
Propofol see Anaesthetics, General
Propranolol see Beta-blockers
Prostaglandins
▸ ACE Inhibitors: enhanced hypotensive effect when alprostadil given with ACE INHIBITORS
▸ Adrenergic Neurone Blockers: enhanced hypotensive effect when alprostadil given with ADRENERGIC NEURONE BLOCKERS
▸ Alpha-blockers: enhanced hypotensive effect when alprostadil given with ALPHA-BLOCKERS
▸ Angiotensin-II Receptor Antagonists: enhanced hypotensive effect when alprostadil given with ANGIOTENSIN-II RECEPTOR ANTAGONISTS
▸ Beta-blockers: enhanced hypotensive effect when alprostadil given with BETA-BLOCKERS
▸ Calcium-channel Blockers: enhanced hypotensive effect when alprostadil given with CALCIUM-CHANNEL BLOCKERS
▸ Clonidine: enhanced hypotensive effect when alprostadil given with CLONIDINE
▸ Diazoxide: enhanced hypotensive effect when alprostadil given with DIAZOXIDE
▸ Diuretics: enhanced hypotensive effect when alprostadil given with DIURETICS
▸ Methyldopa: enhanced hypotensive effect when alprostadil given with METHYLDOPA
▸ Moxonidine: enhanced hypotensive effect when alprostadil given with MOXONIDINE
▸ Nitrates: enhanced hypotensive effect when alprostadil given with NITRATES
▸ Oxytocin: prostaglandins potentiate uterotonic effect of OXYTOCIN
▸ Vasodilator Antihypertensives: enhanced hypotensive effect when alprostadil given with HYDRALAZINE, MINOXIDIL or SODIUM NITROPRUSSIDE

Protein Kinase Inhibitors see individual drugs
Proton Pump Inhibitors
▸ Antacids: absorption of lansoprazole possibly reduced by ANTACIDS
▸ Antibacterials: plasma concentration of both drugs increased when omeprazole given with CLARITHROMYCIN
- Anticoagulants: pantoprazole might enhance the anticoagulant effect of COUMARINS; esomeprazole and omeprazole possibly enhance anticoagulant effect of • COUMARINS
- Antidepressants: omeprazole increases plasma concentration of ESCITALOPRAM; plasma concentration of lansoprazole possibly increased by FLUVOXAMINE; plasma concentration of omeprazole possibly reduced by ST JOHN'S WORT
- Antiepileptics: esomeprazole enhances effects of • FOSPHENYTOIN and • PHENYTOIN; omeprazole possibly enhances effects of FOSPHENYTOIN and PHENYTOIN
- Antifungals: proton pump inhibitors reduce absorption of ITRACONAZOLE and KETOCONAZOLE; esomeprazole reduces plasma concentration of • POSACONAZOLE—manufacturer of posaconazole *suspension* advises avoid concomitant use; lansoprazole, omeprazole, pantoprazole and rabeprazole possibly reduce plasma concentration of • POSACONAZOLE—manufacturer of posaconazole *suspension* advises avoid

Proton Pump Inhibitors
- Antifungals (continued)
  concomitant use; plasma concentration of esomeprazole possibly increased by VORICONAZOLE; plasma concentration of omeprazole increased by VORICONAZOLE (consider reducing dose of omeprazole)
▸ Antipsychotics: omeprazole possibly reduces plasma concentration of CLOZAPINE
- Antivirals: proton pump inhibitors reduce plasma concentration of • ATAZANAVIR—avoid or adjust dose of both drugs (consult product literature); do not take proton pump inhibitors before LEDIPASVIR advised by manufacturer of ledipasvir; omeprazole reduces plasma concentration of LEDIPASVIR; omeprazole increases plasma concentration of RALTEGRAVIR; omeprazole reduces plasma concentration of • RILPIVIRINE—avoid concomitant use; avoidance of esomeprazole, lansoprazole, pantoprazole and rabeprazole advised by manufacturer of RILPIVIRINE (plasma concentration of rilpivirine possibly reduced); omeprazole increases plasma concentration of • SAQUINAVIR—manufacturer of saquinavir advises avoid concomitant use; esomeprazole, lansoprazole, pantoprazole and rabeprazole possibly increase plasma concentration of • SAQUINAVIR—manufacturer of saquinavir advises avoid concomitant use; plasma concentration of esomeprazole and omeprazole reduced by • TIPRANAVIR
▸ Anxiolytics and Hypnotics: esomeprazole and omeprazole possibly inhibit metabolism of DIAZEPAM (increased plasma concentration)
▸ Cardiac Glycosides: proton pump inhibitors possibly slightly increase plasma concentration of DIGOXIN
▸ Ciclosporin: omeprazole possibly affects plasma concentration of CICLOSPORIN
- Cilostazol: omeprazole increases plasma concentration of • CILOSTAZOL (see under Cilostazol, p. 215)
- Clopidogrel: esomeprazole and omeprazole reduce antiplatelet effect of • CLOPIDOGREL; lansoprazole, pantoprazole and rabeprazole possibly reduce antiplatelet effect of CLOPIDOGREL
- Cytotoxics: proton pump inhibitors possibly reduce excretion of METHOTREXATE (increased risk of toxicity); lansoprazole reduces plasma concentration of BOSUTINIB; avoidance of proton pump inhibitors advised by manufacturer of DABRAFENIB (plasma concentration of dabrafenib possibly reduced); avoidance of esomeprazole, lansoprazole, pantoprazole and rabeprazole advised by manufacturer of • ERLOTINIB; omeprazole reduces plasma concentration of • ERLOTINIB—manufacturer of erlotinib advises avoid concomitant use; proton pump inhibitors possibly reduce absorption of LAPATINIB; proton pump inhibitors possibly reduce absorption of PAZOPANIB—manufacturer of pazopanib advises give at the same time as proton pump inhibitors
▸ Hormone Antagonists: plasma concentration of omeprazole reduced by ENZALUTAMIDE
▸ Tacrolimus: omeprazole possibly increases plasma concentration of TACROLIMUS
▸ Ulcer-healing Drugs: absorption of lansoprazole possibly reduced by SUCRALFATE

Pseudoephedrine see Sympathomimetics
Pyrazinamide
▸ Sulfinpyrazone: pyrazinamide antagonises effects of SULFINPYRAZONE
▸ Vaccines: antibacterials inactivate ORAL TYPHOID VACCINE—see under Typhoid Vaccine in BNF
Pyridostigmine see Parasympathomimetics
Pyridoxine see Vitamins
Pyrimethamine
- Antibacterials: increased antifolate effect when pyrimethamine given with • SULFONAMIDES or • TRIMETHOPRIM
- Antiepileptics: pyrimethamine antagonises anticonvulsant effect of • FOSPHENYTOIN and • PHENYTOIN, also increased antifolate effect
- Antimalarials: avoidance of antimalarials advised by manufacturer of • ARTEMETHER WITH LUMEFANTRINE; increased antifolate effect when pyrimethamine given with PROGUANIL
▸ Antivirals: increased antifolate effect when pyrimethamine given with ZIDOVUDINE

A1

Interactions | Appendix 1

Pyrimethamine (continued)

- Cytotoxics: pyrimethamine increases antifolate effect of ● METHOTREXATE and ● PEMETREXED
‣ Histamine: avoidance of antimalarials advised by manufacturer of HISTAMINE
‣ Penicillamine: increased risk of haematological toxicity when antimalarials given with PENICILLAMINE—manufacturer of penicillamine advises avoid concomitant use
‣ Vaccines: antimalarials inactivate ORAL TYPHOID VACCINE—see under Typhoid Vaccine in BNF

Quetiapine *see* Antipsychotics

Quinagolide

‣ Memantine: effects of dopaminergics possibly enhanced by MEMANTINE
‣ Methyldopa: antiparkinsonian effect of dopaminergics antagonised by METHYLDOPA

Quinapril *see* ACE Inhibitors

Quinine

- Anti-arrhythmics: increased risk of ventricular arrhythmias when quinine given with ● AMIODARONE—avoid concomitant use; quinine increases plasma concentration of ● FLECAINIDE
- Antibacterials: increased risk of ventricular arrhythmias when quinine given with ● MOXIFLOXACIN—avoid concomitant use; plasma concentration of quinine reduced by ● RIFAMPICIN
‣ Anticoagulants: plasma concentration of both drugs increased when quinine given with WARFARIN
‣ Antidepressants: possible increased risk of ventricular arrhythmias when quinine given with ● CITALOPRAM or ● ESCITALOPRAM—avoid concomitant use
- Antimalarials: increased risk of ventricular arrhythmias when quinine given with ● ARTEMETHER WITH LUMEFANTRINE; avoidance of antimalarials advised by manufacturer of ● ARTEMETHER WITH LUMEFANTRINE; increased risk of convulsions when quinine given with ● MEFLOQUINE (but should not prevent the use of *intravenous* quinine in severe cases)
- Antipsychotics: increased risk of ventricular arrhythmias when quinine given with ● DROPERIDOL or ● PIMOZIDE—avoid concomitant use; possible increased risk of ventricular arrhythmias when quinine given with ● HALOPERIDOL—avoid concomitant use; possible increased risk of ventricular arrhythmias when quinine given with ● RISPERIDONE
- Antivirals: plasma concentration of quinine possibly increased by ● ATAZANAVIR, ● DARUNAVIR, ● FOSAMPRENAVIR, ● INDINAVIR and ● TIPRANAVIR (increased risk of toxicity); plasma concentration of quinine increased by ● RITONAVIR (increased risk of toxicity); increased risk of ventricular arrhythmias when quinine given with ● SAQUINAVIR—avoid concomitant use
- Cardiac Glycosides: quinine increases plasma concentration of ● DIGOXIN
‣ Dopaminergics: quinine possibly increases plasma concentration of AMANTADINE
‣ Histamine: avoidance of antimalarials advised by manufacturer of HISTAMINE
‣ Muscle Relaxants: quinine possibly enhances effects of SUXAMETHONIUM
‣ Penicillamine: increased risk of haematological toxicity when antimalarials given with PENICILLAMINE—manufacturer of penicillamine advises avoid concomitant use
‣ Ulcer-healing Drugs: metabolism of quinine inhibited by CIMETIDINE (increased plasma concentration)
‣ Vaccines: antimalarials inactivate ORAL TYPHOID VACCINE—see under Typhoid Vaccine in BNF

Quinolones

- Aminophylline: possible increased risk of convulsions when quinolones given with ● AMINOPHYLLINE; ciprofloxacin and norfloxacin increase plasma concentration of ● AMINOPHYLLINE
- Analgesics: possible increased risk of convulsions when quinolones given with ● NSAIDS
‣ Antacids: absorption of moxifloxacin reduced by ANTACIDS (give at least 6 hours apart); absorption of ciprofloxacin and levofloxacin reduced by ANTACIDS (give at least 2 hours before or 4 hours after ciprofloxacin and levofloxacin); absorption of norfloxacin reduced by ANTACIDS; absorption of ofloxacin reduced by ANTACIDS (give at least 2 hours apart)

Quinolones (continued)

- Anti-arrhythmics: increased risk of ventricular arrhythmias when levofloxacin or moxifloxacin given with ● AMIODARONE—avoid concomitant use; increased risk of ventricular arrhythmias when moxifloxacin given with ● DISOPYRAMIDE—avoid concomitant use
- Antibacterials: increased risk of ventricular arrhythmias when moxifloxacin given with *parenteral* ● ERYTHROMYCIN—avoid concomitant use; avoidance of moxifloxacin advised by manufacturer of BEDAQUILINE; ciprofloxacin possibly increases plasma concentration of BEDAQUILINE—avoid concomitant use if ciprofloxacin given for more than 14 days; increased risk of ventricular arrhythmias when moxifloxacin given with ● DELAMANID; effects of nalidixic acid possibly antagonised by NITROFURANTOIN; possible increased risk of ventricular arrhythmias when moxifloxacin given with ● TELITHROMYCIN
- Anticoagulants: ciprofloxacin and levofloxacin possibly enhance anticoagulant effect of COUMARINS; nalidixic acid, norfloxacin and ofloxacin enhance anticoagulant effect of ● COUMARINS; levofloxacin possibly enhances anticoagulant effect of PHENINDIONE
- Antidepressants: avoidance of moxifloxacin advised by manufacturer of ● CITALOPRAM, ● ESCITALOPRAM and ● VENLAFAXINE (risk of ventricular arrhythmias); ciprofloxacin inhibits metabolism of ● DULOXETINE—avoid concomitant use; avoidance of ciprofloxacin advised by manufacturer of ● AGOMELATINE; increased risk of ventricular arrhythmias when moxifloxacin given with ● TRICYCLICS—avoid concomitant use
‣ Antidiabetics: norfloxacin possibly enhances effects of GLIBENCLAMIDE
- Antiepileptics: ciprofloxacin increases or decreases plasma concentration of FOSPHENYTOIN and PHENYTOIN
- Antihistamines: increased risk of ventricular arrhythmias when moxifloxacin given with ● MIZOLASTINE—avoid concomitant use
- Antimalarials: avoidance of quinolones advised by manufacturer of ● ARTEMETHER WITH LUMEFANTRINE; avoidance of moxifloxacin advised by manufacturer of ● ARTENIMOL WITH PIPERAQUINE (possible risk of ventricular arrhythmias); increased risk of ventricular arrhythmias when moxifloxacin given with ● CHLOROQUINE, ● HYDROXYCHLOROQUINE, ● MEFLOQUINE or ● QUININE—avoid concomitant use
- Antipsychotics: increased risk of ventricular arrhythmias when moxifloxacin given with ● BENPERIDOL—manufacturer of benperidol advises avoid concomitant use; increased risk of ventricular arrhythmias when moxifloxacin given with ● DROPERIDOL, ● HALOPERIDOL, ● PHENOTHIAZINES, ● PIMOZIDE or ● ZUCLOPENTHIXOL—avoid concomitant use; ciprofloxacin increases plasma concentration of CLOZAPINE; ciprofloxacin possibly increases plasma concentration of OLANZAPINE
- Antivirals: manufacturer of levofloxacin advises give DIDANOSINE *tablets* at least 2 hours before or after levofloxacin; absorption of ciprofloxacin reduced by DIDANOSINE *tablets* (give at least 2 hours before or 4 hours after ciprofloxacin); manufacturer of moxifloxacin advises give DIDANOSINE *tablets* at least 6 hours before or after moxifloxacin; manufacturer of norfloxacin advises give DIDANOSINE at least 2 hours before or after norfloxacin; increased risk of ventricular arrhythmias when moxifloxacin given with ● SAQUINAVIR—avoid concomitant use
‣ Anxiolytics and Hypnotics: avoidance of ciprofloxacin advised by manufacturer of ZOLPIDEM
- Atomoxetine: increased risk of ventricular arrhythmias when moxifloxacin given with ● ATOMOXETINE
- Beta-blockers: increased risk of ventricular arrhythmias when moxifloxacin given with ● SOTALOL—avoid concomitant use
‣ Calcium Salts: absorption of ciprofloxacin reduced by CALCIUM SALTS (give at least 2 hours before or 4 hours after ciprofloxacin)
- Ciclosporin: increased risk of nephrotoxicity when quinolones given with ● CICLOSPORIN
- Clopidogrel: ciprofloxacin possibly reduces antiplatelet effect of ● CLOPIDOGREL
- Cytotoxics: nalidixic acid increases risk of MELPHALAN toxicity; ciprofloxacin possibly reduces excretion of METHOTREXATE (increased risk of toxicity); possible increased risk of

Quinolones

- Cytotoxics (continued)
  ventricular arrhythmias when moxifloxacin given with
  ● BOSUTINIB; ciprofloxacin possibly increases the plasma
  concentration of ● BOSUTINIB—manufacturer of bosutinib
  advises avoid or consider reducing dose of bosutinib;
  ciprofloxacin increases plasma concentration of ERLOTINIB;
  ciprofloxacin possibly increases the plasma concentration of
  ● IBRUTINIB—reduce dose of ibrutinib (see under Ibrutinib,
  p. 855); possible increased risk of ventricular arrhythmias
  when moxifloxacin given with ● VANDETANIB—avoid
  concomitant use; increased risk of ventricular arrhythmias
  when levofloxacin or moxifloxacin given with ● ARSENIC
  TRIOXIDE
- ▸ Dairy Products: absorption of ciprofloxacin reduced by DAIRY
  PRODUCTS (give at least 2 hours apart); absorption of
  norfloxacin reduced by DAIRY PRODUCTS
- ▸ Dopaminergics: ciprofloxacin increases plasma concentration
  of RASAGILINE; ciprofloxacin inhibits metabolism of
  ROPINIROLE (increased plasma concentration)
- ▸ 5HT₁-receptor Agonists: quinolones possibly inhibit metabolism
  of ZOLMITRIPTAN (reduce dose of zolmitriptan)
- ▸ Iron Salts: absorption of moxifloxacin reduced by IRON
  SALTS (give at least 6 hours apart); absorption of ciprofloxacin
  reduced by oral IRON SALTS (give at least 2 hours before or
  4 hours after ciprofloxacin); absorption of levofloxacin,
  norfloxacin and ofloxacin reduced by oral IRON SALTS (give at
  least 2 hours apart)
- ▸ Lanthanum: absorption of quinolones possibly reduced by
  LANTHANUM (give at least 2 hours before or 4 hours after
  lanthanum)
- Muscle Relaxants: ciprofloxacin increases plasma concentration
  of ● TIZANIDINE (increased risk of toxicity)—avoid concomitant
  use; norfloxacin possibly increases plasma concentration of
  TIZANIDINE (increased risk of toxicity)
- Mycophenolate: norfloxacin possibly reduces bioavailability of
  MYCOPHENOLATE
- Pentamidine Isetionate: increased risk of ventricular
  arrhythmias when moxifloxacin given with ● PENTAMIDINE
  ISETIONATE—avoid concomitant use
- Pirfenidone: ciprofloxacin increases plasma concentration of
  ● PIRFENIDONE—see under Pirfenidone, p. 272
- ▸ Sevelamer: absorption of ciprofloxacin reduced by SEVELAMER
  (give at least 2 hours before or 4 hours after ciprofloxacin)
- ▸ Strontium Ranelate: absorption of quinolones reduced by
  STRONTIUM RANELATE (manufacturer of strontium ranelate
  advises avoid concomitant use)
- Theophylline: possible increased risk of convulsions when
  quinolones given with ● THEOPHYLLINE; ciprofloxacin and
  norfloxacin increase plasma concentration of ● THEOPHYLLINE
- ▸ Ulcer-healing Drugs: absorption of moxifloxacin reduced by
  SUCRALFATE (give at least 6 hours apart); absorption of
  levofloxacin, norfloxacin and ofloxacin reduced by SUCRALFATE
  (give at least 2 hours apart); absorption of ciprofloxacin
  reduced by SUCRALFATE (give at least 2 hours before or 4 hours
  after ciprofloxacin)
- ▸ Vaccines: antibacterials inactivate ORAL TYPHOID VACCINE—see
  under Typhoid Vaccine in BNF
- ▸ Zinc: absorption of moxifloxacin reduced by ZINC (give at least
  6 hours apart); absorption of ciprofloxacin, levofloxacin,
  norfloxacin and ofloxacin reduced by ZINC (give at least
  2 hours apart)

Rabeprazole see Proton Pump Inhibitors

Rabies Vaccine see Vaccines

Raloxifene

- ▸ Anticoagulants: raloxifene antagonises anticoagulant effect of
  COUMARINS
- ▸ Lipid-regulating Drugs: absorption of raloxifene reduced by
  COLESTYRAMINE (manufacturer of raloxifene advises avoid
  concomitant administration)

Raltegravir

- ▸ Antacids: plasma concentration of raltegravir reduced by
  ALUMINIUM HYDROXIDE and ORAL MAGNESIUM SALTS—
  manufacturer of raltegravir advises avoid concomitant use
- Antibacterials: plasma concentration of raltegravir reduced by
  ● RIFAMPICIN—consider increasing dose of raltegravir

Raltegravir (continued)

- Antivirals: increased risk of rash when raltegravir given with
  DARUNAVIR; avoidance of raltegravir advised by manufacturer
  of ● FOSAMPRENAVIR
- Orlistat: absorption of raltegravir possibly reduced by
  ● ORLISTAT
- ▸ Ulcer-healing Drugs: plasma concentration of raltegravir
  increased by FAMOTIDINE and OMEPRAZOLE

Raltitrexed

- Antipsychotics: avoid concomitant use of cytotoxics with
  ● CLOZAPINE (increased risk of agranulocytosis)
- Folates: manufacturer of raltitrexed advises avoid concomitant
  use with ● FOLATES

Ramipril see ACE Inhibitors

Ramucirumab

- Antipsychotics: avoid concomitant use of cytotoxics with
  ● CLOZAPINE (increased risk of agranulocytosis)
- Vaccines: risk of generalised infections when monoclonal
  antibodies given with live ● VACCINES—avoid concomitant use

Ranitidine see Histamine H₂-antagonists

Ranolazine

- Anti-arrhythmics: manufacturer of ranolazine advises avoid
  concomitant use with ● DISOPYRAMIDE
- Antibacterials: plasma concentration of ranolazine possibly
  increased by ● CLARITHROMYCIN and ● TELITHROMYCIN—
  manufacturer of ranolazine advises avoid concomitant use;
  plasma concentration of ranolazine reduced by ● RIFAMPICIN—
  manufacturer of ranolazine advises avoid concomitant use
- ▸ Antidepressants: plasma concentration of ranolazine increased
  by PAROXETINE
- Antifungals: plasma concentration of ranolazine increased by
  KETOCONAZOLE—avoid concomitant use; plasma
  concentration of ranolazine possibly increased by
  ● ITRACONAZOLE, ● POSACONAZOLE and ● VORICONAZOLE—
  manufacturer of ranolazine advises avoid concomitant use
- Antivirals: plasma concentration of ranolazine possibly
  increased by ● ATAZANAVIR, ● DARUNAVIR, ● FOSAMPRENAVIR,
  ● INDINAVIR, ● LOPINAVIR, ● RITONAVIR, ● SAQUINAVIR and
  ● TIPRANAVIR—manufacturer of ranolazine advises avoid
  concomitant use
- Beta-blockers: manufacturer of ranolazine advises avoid
  concomitant use with ● SOTALOL
- ▸ Calcium-channel Blockers: plasma concentration of ranolazine
  increased by DILTIAZEM and VERAPAMIL (consider reducing dose
  of ranolazine)
- ▸ Cardiac Glycosides: ranolazine increases plasma concentration
  of DIGOXIN
- ▸ Ciclosporin: plasma concentration of both drugs may increase
  when ranolazine given with CICLOSPORIN
- Grapefruit Juice: plasma concentration of ranolazine possibly
  increased by ● GRAPEFRUIT JUICE—manufacturer of ranolazine
  advises avoid concomitant use
- Lipid-regulating Drugs: ranolazine increases plasma
  concentration of ● SIMVASTATIN (see under Simvastatin,
  p. 188); separating administration from ranolazine by
  12 hours advised by manufacturer of LOMITAPIDE
- Tacrolimus: ranolazine increases plasma concentration of
  ● TACROLIMUS

Rasagiline

NOTE Rasagiline is a MAO-B inhibitor

- Analgesics: avoid concomitant use of rasagiline with
  ● DEXTROMETHORPHAN; risk of CNS toxicity when rasagiline
  given with ● PETHIDINE (avoid pethidine for 2 weeks after
  rasagiline)
- ▸ Antibacterials: plasma concentration of rasagiline increased by
  CIPROFLOXACIN
- Antidepressants: after stopping rasagiline do not start
  ● FLUOXETINE for 2 weeks, also rasagiline should not be started
  until at least 5 weeks after stopping fluoxetine; after stopping
  rasagiline do not start ● FLUVOXAMINE for 2 weeks; risk of
  hypertensive crisis when rasagiline given with ● MAOIS, avoid
  MAOIs for at least 2 weeks after stopping rasagiline; increased
  risk of CNS toxicity when rasagiline given with ● SSRIS or
  ● TRICYCLICS; risk of CNS excitation and hypertension when
  rasagiline given with ● VORTIOXETINE

Rasagiline (continued)
- ▸ Dopaminergics: plasma concentration of rasagiline possibly reduced by ENTACAPONE
- ▸ Memantine: effects of dopaminergics possibly enhanced by MEMANTINE
- ▸ Methyldopa: antiparkinsonian effect of dopaminergics antagonised by METHYLDOPA
- • Sympathomimetics: avoid concomitant use of rasagiline with • SYMPATHOMIMETICS

Reboxetine
- • Antibacterials: manufacturer of reboxetine advises avoid concomitant use with • MACROLIDES
- • Antidepressants: manufacturer of reboxetine advises avoid concomitant use with • FLUVOXAMINE; increased risk of hypertension and CNS excitation when reboxetine given with • MAOIS (MAOIs should not be started until 1 week after stopping reboxetine, avoid reboxetine for 2 weeks after stopping MAOIs)
- ▸ Antiepileptics: plasma concentration of reboxetine possibly reduced by CARBAMAZEPINE, PHENOBARBITAL and PRIMIDONE
- • Antifungals: manufacturer of reboxetine advises avoid concomitant use with • IMIDAZOLES and • TRIAZOLES
- • Antimalarials: avoidance of antidepressants advised by manufacturer of • ARTEMETHER WITH LUMEFANTRINE and • ARTENIMOL WITH PIPERAQUINE
- ▸ Atomoxetine: possible increased risk of convulsions when antidepressants given with ATOMOXETINE
- ▸ Diuretics: possible increased risk of hypokalaemia when reboxetine given with LOOP DIURETICS or THIAZIDES AND RELATED DIURETICS
- ▸ Ergot Alkaloids: possible risk of hypertension when reboxetine given with ERGOTAMINE

Regorafenib
- ▸ Analgesics: manufacturer of regorafenib advises avoid concomitant use with MEFENAMIC ACID
- • Antibacterials: plasma concentration of regorafenib reduced by • RIFAMPICIN—manufacturer of regorafenib advises avoid concomitant use
- • Anticoagulants: increased risk of bleeding when regorafenib given with • WARFARIN
- • Antifungals: plasma concentration of regorafenib increased by • KETOCONAZOLE—avoid concomitant use
- • Antipsychotics: avoid concomitant use of cytotoxics with • CLOZAPINE (increased risk of agranulocytosis)
- ▸ Cytotoxics: regorafenib increases plasma concentration of IRINOTECAN

Remifentanil *see* Opioid Analgesics

Repaglinide *see* Antidiabetics

Retigabine
- • Alcohol: increased risk of blurred vision when retigabine given with ALCOHOL
- • Antidepressants: anticonvulsant effect of antiepileptics possibly antagonised by MAOIs and • TRICYCLIC-RELATED ANTIDEPRESSANTS (convulsive threshold lowered); anticonvulsant effect of antiepileptics antagonised by • SSRIS and • TRICYCLICS (convulsive threshold lowered)
- ▸ Antiepileptics: plasma concentration of retigabine possibly reduced by CARBAMAZEPINE, FOSPHENYTOIN and PHENYTOIN
- • Antimalarials: anticonvulsant effect of antiepileptics antagonised by • MEFLOQUINE
- • Antipsychotics: anticonvulsant effect of antiepileptics antagonised by • ANTIPSYCHOTICS (convulsive threshold lowered)
- • Orlistat: possible increased risk of convulsions when antiepileptics given with • ORLISTAT

Retinoids
- • Alcohol: etretinate formed from acitretin in presence of • ALCOHOL (increased risk of teratogenicity in women of child-bearing potential)
- • Antibacterials: possible increased risk of benign intracranial hypertension when retinoids given with • TETRACYCLINES (avoid concomitant use)
- • Anticoagulants: acitretin possibly reduces anticoagulant effect of • COUMARINS
- ▸ Antiepileptics: isotretinoin possibly reduces plasma concentration of CARBAMAZEPINE

Retinoids (continued)
- • Antifungals: plasma concentration of alitretinoin increased by KETOCONAZOLE; possible increased risk of tretinoin toxicity when given with • FLUCONAZOLE, • KETOCONAZOLE and • VORICONAZOLE
- • Cytotoxics: acitretin increases plasma concentration of • METHOTREXATE (also increased risk of hepatotoxicity)—avoid concomitant use
- ▸ Lipid-regulating Drugs: alitretinoin reduces plasma concentration of SIMVASTATIN
- • Vitamins: risk of hypervitaminosis A when retinoids given with • VITAMIN A—avoid concomitant use

Ribavirin
- • Antivirals: effects of ribavirin possibly reduced by • ABACAVIR; increased risk of side-effects when ribavirin given with • DIDANOSINE—avoid concomitant use; increased risk of toxicity when ribavirin given with • STAVUDINE; increased risk of anaemia when ribavirin given with • ZIDOVUDINE—avoid concomitant use
- • Azathioprine: ribavirin possibly enhances myelosuppressive effects of • AZATHIOPRINE

Rifabutin *see* Rifamycins

Rifampicin *see* Rifamycins

Rifamycins

NOTE Interactions do not apply to rifaximin
- ▸ ACE Inhibitors: rifampicin reduces plasma concentration of active metabolite of IMIDAPRIL (reduced antihypertensive effect)
- ▸ Aliskiren: rifampicin reduces plasma concentration of ALISKIREN
- ▸ Ambrisentan: rifampicin possibly increases plasma concentration of AMBRISENTAN
- ▸ Aminophylline: rifampicin accelerates metabolism of AMINOPHYLLINE (reduced plasma concentration)
- ▸ Analgesics: rifampicin reduces plasma concentration of CELECOXIB, DICLOFENAC and ETORICOXIB; rifampicin accelerates metabolism of ALFENTANIL, CODEINE, FENTANYL, METHADONE and MORPHINE (reduced effect); rifampicin possibly accelerates metabolism of OXYCODONE
- ▸ Angiotensin-II Receptor Antagonists: rifampicin reduces plasma concentration of LOSARTAN and its active metabolite
- ▸ Antacids: absorption of rifampicin reduced by ANTACIDS
- • Anthelmintics: rifampicin reduces plasma concentration of • PRAZIQUANTEL—avoid concomitant use
- • Anti-arrhythmics: rifamycins accelerate metabolism of • DISOPYRAMIDE (reduced plasma concentration); rifampicin reduces plasma concentration of • DRONEDARONE—avoid concomitant use; rifampicin accelerates metabolism of • PROPAFENONE (reduced effect)
- • Antibacterials: increased risk of side-effects including neutropenia when rifabutin given with • AZITHROMYCIN; rifamycins reduce plasma concentration of CLARITHROMYCIN and DAPSONE; plasma concentration of rifabutin increased by • CLARITHROMYCIN (increased risk of toxicity—reduce rifabutin dose); plasma concentration of rifabutin possibly increased by • ERYTHROMYCIN (increased risk of toxicity—reduce rifabutin dose); rifampicin possibly reduces plasma concentration of TINIDAZOLE and TRIMETHOPRIM; rifampicin reduces plasma concentration of DOXYCYCLINE—consider increasing dose of doxycycline; rifampicin reduces plasma concentration of • BEDAQUILINE—manufacturer of bedaquiline advises avoid concomitant use; rifabutin possibly reduces plasma concentration of BEDAQUILINE—manufacturer of bedaquiline advises avoid concomitant use; rifampicin accelerates metabolism of CHLORAMPHENICOL (reduced plasma concentration); rifampicin reduces plasma concentration of • DELAMANID; increased risk of hepatotoxicity when rifampicin given with • ISONIAZID; rifampicin reduces plasma concentration of • TELITHROMYCIN (avoid during and for 2 weeks after rifampicin)
- • Anticoagulants: rifampicin possibly reduces plasma concentration of • APIXABAN—manufacturer of apixaban advises avoid concomitant use when given for treatment of deep-vein thrombosis or pulmonary embolism; rifamycins accelerate metabolism of • COUMARINS (reduced anticoagulant effect); rifampicin reduces plasma concentration of

Rifamycins

- **Anticoagulants** (continued)
  - DABIGATRAN—manufacturer of dabigatran advises avoid concomitant use; rifampicin reduces plasma concentration of
  - EDOXABAN; rifampicin reduces plasma concentration of
  - RIVAROXABAN—manufacturer of rivaroxaban advises monitor for signs of thrombosis
- **Antidepressants:** rifampicin reduces plasma concentration of LINEZOLID (possible therapeutic failure of linezolid); rifampicin reduces plasma concentration of • VORTIOXETINE—consider increasing dose of vortioxetine
- **Antidiabetics:** rifampicins accelerate metabolism of
  - TOLBUTAMIDE (reduced effect); rifampicin reduces plasma concentration of • CANAGLIFLOZIN and NATEGLINIDE; rifampicin possibly reduces effects of LINAGLIPTIN; rifampicin possibly antagonises hypoglycaemic effect of REPAGLINIDE; rifampicins possibly accelerate metabolism of • SULFONYLUREAS (reduced effect)
- **Antiepileptics:** rifabutin reduces plasma concentration of
  - CARBAMAZEPINE; rifamycins accelerate metabolism of
  - FOSPHENYTOIN and • PHENYTOIN (reduced plasma concentration); rifampicin reduces plasma concentration of LAMOTRIGINE; plasma concentration of rifampicin possibly reduced by PHENOBARBITAL and PRIMIDONE
- **Antifungals:** rifampicin accelerates metabolism of
  - KETOCONAZOLE (reduced plasma concentration), also plasma concentration of rifampicin may be reduced by ketoconazole; plasma concentration of rifabutin increased by • FLUCONAZOLE (increased risk of uveitis—reduce rifabutin dose); rifampicin accelerates metabolism of • FLUCONAZOLE (reduced plasma concentration); rifabutin and rifampicin reduce plasma concentration of • ITRACONAZOLE—manufacturer of itraconazole advises avoid concomitant use; plasma concentration of rifabutin increased by • POSACONAZOLE (also plasma concentration of posaconazole reduced); rifampicin reduces plasma concentration of • POSACONAZOLE and
  - TERBINAFINE; plasma concentration of rifabutin increased by • VORICONAZOLE, also rifabutin reduces plasma concentration of voriconazole (increase dose of voriconazole and also monitor for rifabutin toxicity); rifampicin reduces plasma concentration of • VORICONAZOLE—avoid concomitant use; rifampicin initially increases and then reduces plasma concentration of CASPOFUNGIN (consider increasing dose of caspofungin); plasma concentration of rifabutin possibly increased by • TRIAZOLES (increased risk of uveitis—reduce rifabutin dose)
- ▸ **Antihistamines:** rifampicin possibly reduces effects of FEXOFENADINE
- **Antimalarials:** avoidance of rifampicin advised by manufacturer of ARTENIMOL WITH PIPERAQUINE; rifampicin reduces plasma concentration of • MEFLOQUINE—avoid concomitant use; rifampicin reduces plasma concentration of • QUININE
- **Antimuscarinics:** rifampicin reduces plasma concentration of active metabolite of • FESOTERODINE—avoid concomitant use
- **Antipsychotics:** rifampicin accelerates metabolism of
  - HALOPERIDOL (reduced plasma concentration); rifabutin and rifampicin possibly reduce plasma concentration of
  - ARIPIPRAZOLE (avoid concomitant use or consider increasing the dose of aripiprazole—consult aripiprazole product literature); rifampicin possibly reduces plasma concentration of CLOZAPINE; rifampicin reduces plasma concentration of
  - LURASIDONE—avoid concomitant use
- **Antivirals:** rifampicin possibly reduces plasma concentration of ABACAVIR; rifampicin reduces plasma concentration of
  - ATAZANAVIR, • DACLATASVIR, • LOPINAVIR, • NEVIRAPINE and
  - RILPIVIRINE—avoid concomitant use; plasma concentration of rifabutin increased by • ATAZANAVIR, • DARUNAVIR,
  - FOSAMPRENAVIR and • TIPRANAVIR (reduce dose of rifabutin); avoidance of rifampicin advised by manufacturer of
  - BOCEPREVIR (plasma concentration of boceprevir possibly reduced); rifampicin possibly reduces plasma concentration of
  - DACLATASVIR and SIMEPREVIR—manufacturer of daclatasvir and simeprevir advises avoid concomitant use; rifampicin significantly reduces plasma concentration of • DARUNAVIR,
  - FOSAMPRENAVIR and • TELAPREVIR—avoid concomitant use; rifampicin possibly reduces plasma concentration of

Rifamycins

- **Antivirals** (continued)
  - DASABUVIR, • OMBITASVIR, • PARITAPREVIR and • TIPRANAVIR—avoid concomitant use; rifampicin reduces the plasma concentration of • DOLUTEGRAVIR (see under Dolutegravir, p. 584); plasma concentration of rifabutin reduced by EFAVIRENZ—increase dose of rifabutin; rifampicin reduces plasma concentration of EFAVIRENZ—increase dose of efavirenz; rifampicin reduces plasma concentration of
  - ELVITEGRAVIR also plasma concentration of active metabolite of rifabutin increased—reduce dose of rifabutin; avoidance of rifampicin advised by manufacturer of • ELVITEGRAVIR, ETRAVIRINE, LEDIPASVIR, SOFOSBUVIR and ZIDOVUDINE; plasma concentration of both drugs reduced when rifabutin given with • ETRAVIRINE; rifampicin accelerates metabolism of
  - INDINAVIR (reduced plasma concentration—avoid concomitant use); plasma concentration of rifabutin increased by • INDINAVIR, also plasma concentration of indinavir decreased (reduce dose of rifabutin and increase dose of indinavir); avoidance of rifabutin advised by manufacturer of LEDIPASVIR, SOFOSBUVIR and • TELAPREVIR; rifampicin reduces plasma concentration of • MARAVIROC and
  - RALTEGRAVIR—consider increasing dose of maraviroc and raltegravir; plasma concentration of rifabutin increased by NEVIRAPINE; rifabutin decreases plasma concentration of • RILPIVIRINE (increase dose of rilpivirine—consult rilpivirine product literature); rifampicin reduces plasma concentration of RITONAVIR; plasma concentration of rifabutin increased by • RITONAVIR (increased risk of toxicity—reduce rifabutin dose); plasma concentration of rifabutin increased by • SAQUINAVIR (also plasma concentration of saquinavir reduced)—reduce rifabutin dose; rifampicin significantly reduces plasma concentration of • SAQUINAVIR, also risk of hepatotoxicity—avoid concomitant use; rifampicin reduces plasma concentration of • SIMEPREVIR—manufacturer of simeprevir advises avoid concomitant use
- ▸ **Anxiolytics and Hypnotics:** rifampicin accelerates metabolism of DIAZEPAM and ZALEPLON (reduced plasma concentration); rifampicin possibly accelerates metabolism of BENZODIAZEPINES (reduced plasma concentration); rifampicin possibly accelerates metabolism of BUSPIRONE; rifampicin accelerates metabolism of ZOLPIDEM (reduced plasma concentration and reduced effect); rifampicin significantly reduces plasma concentration of ZOPICLONE
- **Apremilast:** rifampicin reduces plasma concentration of
  - APREMILAST—avoid concomitant use
- **Aprepitant:** rifampicin reduces plasma concentration of APREPITANT
- **Atovaquone:** avoidance of concomitant rifabutin advised by manufacturer of ATOVAQUONE (plasma concentration of both drugs reduced); rifampicin reduces plasma concentration of
  - ATOVAQUONE (and concentration of rifampicin increased)—avoid concomitant use
- ▸ **Avanafil:** rifampicin possibly reduces plasma concentration of AVANAFIL—manufacturer of avanafil advises avoid concomitant use
- ▸ **Beta-blockers:** rifampicin accelerates metabolism of BISOPROLOL and PROPRANOLOL (plasma concentration significantly reduced); rifampicin reduces plasma concentration of CARVEDILOL, CELIPROLOL and METOPROLOL; rifampicin possibly reduces plasma concentration of *oral* TIMOLOL
- **Bosentan:** rifampicin reduces plasma concentration of
  - BOSENTAN—avoid concomitant use
- **Calcium-channel Blockers:** rifampicin possibly reduces plasma concentration of FELODIPINE; rifampicin possibly accelerates metabolism of • ISRADIPINE and • NICARDIPINE (possible significantly reduced plasma concentration); rifampicin accelerates metabolism of • DILTIAZEM, • NIFEDIPINE,
  - NIMODIPINE and • VERAPAMIL (plasma concentration significantly reduced)
- **Cannabis Extract:** rifampicin reduces plasma concentration of
  - CANNABIS EXTRACT—manufacturer of cannabis extract advises avoid concomitant use
- ▸ **Cardiac Glycosides:** rifampicin possibly reduces plasma concentration of DIGOXIN

Rifamycins (continued)

- Ciclosporin: rifampicin accelerates metabolism of • CICLOSPORIN (reduced plasma concentration)
- Cobicistat: rifabutin reduces plasma concentration of • COBICISTAT (adjust dose—consult product literature); rifampicin possibly reduces plasma concentration of • COBICISTAT—manufacturer of cobicistat advises avoid concomitant use
- Corticosteroids: rifamycins accelerate metabolism of • CORTICOSTEROIDS (reduced effect)
- Cytotoxics: rifampicin possibly reduces effects of BRENTUXIMAB VEDOTIN; rifampicin reduces plasma concentration of AFATINIB, RUXOLITINIB, SORAFENIB and • TRABECTEDIN; rifabutin possibly decreases plasma concentration of AXITINIB (increase dose of axitinib—consult axitinib product literature); rifampicin decreases plasma concentration of AXITINIB (increase dose of axitinib—consult axitinib product literature); rifabutin possibly reduces plasma concentration of • BOSUTINIB, CRIZOTINIB and PONATINIB—manufacturer of bosutinib, crizotinib and ponatinib advises avoid concomitant use; rifampicin reduces plasma concentration of • BORTEZOMIB, • BOSUTINIB, • CABAZITAXEL, • CRIZOTINIB, • PONATINIB, • REGORAFENIB and • VANDETANIB—manufacturer of bortezomib, bosutinib, cabazitaxel, crizotinib, ponatinib, regorafenib and vandetanib advises avoid concomitant use; rifampicin reduces plasma concentration of • CABOZANTINIB, • GEFITINIB, • IBRUTINIB, • IDELALISIB, • IMATINIB, • NILOTINIB and • NINTEDANIB—avoid concomitant use; avoidance of rifampicin advised by manufacturer of DABRAFENIB, • LAPATINIB, • OLAPARIB and VEMURAFENIB; rifampicin accelerates metabolism of • DASATINIB (reduced plasma concentration—avoid concomitant use); rifampicin accelerates metabolism of ERLOTINIB and SUNITINIB (reduced plasma concentration); rifampicin reduces plasma concentration of • EVEROLIMUS (avoid concomitant use or consider increasing the dose of everolimus—consult everolimus product literature); avoidance of rifabutin advised by manufacturer of • CABAZITAXEL, • LAPATINIB, • OLAPARIB and VEMURAFENIB; rifampicin possibly reduces plasma concentration of ERIBULIN and • PAZOPANIB; rifampicin reduces plasma concentration of active metabolite of • TEMSIROLIMUS—avoid concomitant use; rifampicin possibly reduces plasma concentration of • VINFLUNINE—manufacturer of vinflunine advises avoid concomitant use; avoidance of rifampicin advised by manufacturer of • VISMODEGIB (plasma concentration of vismodegib possibly reduced)
- Deferasirox: rifampicin reduces plasma concentration of DEFERASIROX
- Diuretics: rifampicin reduces plasma concentration of • EPLERENONE—avoid concomitant use
- Fosaprepitant: rifampicin reduces plasma concentration of FOSAPREPITANT
- Guanfacine: rifabutin possibly reduces plasma concentration of • GUANFACINE—increase dose of guanfacine; rifampicin reduces plasma concentration of • GUANFACINE—increase dose of guanfacine
- Hormone Antagonists: rifampicin reduces plasma concentration of • ABIRATERONE—manufacturer of abiraterone advises avoid concomitant use; rifabutin possibly reduces plasma concentration of • ABIRATERONE—manufacturer of abiraterone advises avoid concomitant use; rifampicin possibly reduces plasma concentration of EXEMESTANE; rifampicin accelerates metabolism of TAMOXIFEN (reduced plasma concentration)
- 5HT$_3$-receptor Antagonists: rifampicin accelerates metabolism of ONDANSETRON (reduced effect)
- Ivacaftor: rifabutin possibly reduces plasma concentration of • IVACAFTOR—manufacturer of ivacaftor advises avoid concomitant use; rifampicin reduces plasma concentration of • IVACAFTOR—manufacturer of ivacaftor advises avoid concomitant use
- Leflunomide: rifampicin possibly increases plasma concentration of active metabolite of LEFLUNOMIDE
- Lipid-regulating Drugs: rifampicin possibly reduces plasma concentration of ATORVASTATIN and SIMVASTATIN; rifampicin accelerates metabolism of FLUVASTATIN (reduced effect)

Rifamycins (continued)

- Macitentan: rifampicin reduces plasma concentration of • MACITENTAN—avoid concomitant use
- Muscle Relaxants: rifampicin possibly reduces plasma concentration of TIZANIDINE
- Mycophenolate: rifampicin reduces plasma concentration of active metabolite of • MYCOPHENOLATE
- Netupitant: rifampicin reduces plasma concentration of • NETUPITANT—avoid concomitant use
- Oestrogens: rifamycins accelerate metabolism of • OESTROGENS (reduced contraceptive effect with combined oral contraceptives, contraceptive patches, and vaginal rings—see Contraceptive Interactions in BNF)
- Progestogens: rifamycins accelerate metabolism of • PROGESTOGENS (reduced contraceptive effect with combined oral contraceptives, progestogen-only oral contraceptives, contraceptive patches, vaginal rings, etonogestrel-releasing implant, and emergency hormonal contraception—see Contraceptive Interactions in BNF)
- Ranolazine: rifampicin reduces plasma concentration of • RANOLAZINE—manufacturer of ranolazine advises avoid concomitant use
- Roflumilast: rifampicin inhibits effects of • ROFLUMILAST (manufacturer of roflumilast advises avoid concomitant use)
- Sirolimus: rifabutin and rifampicin reduce plasma concentration of • SIROLIMUS—avoid concomitant use
- Tacrolimus: rifabutin possibly reduces plasma concentration of TACROLIMUS; rifampicin reduces plasma concentration of • TACROLIMUS
- Tadalafil: rifampicin reduces plasma concentration of • TADALAFIL—manufacturer of tadalafil advises avoid concomitant use
- Teriflunomide: rifampicin reduces plasma concentration of TERIFLUNOMIDE
- Theophylline: rifampicin accelerates metabolism of THEOPHYLLINE (reduced plasma concentration)
- Thyroid Hormones: rifampicin accelerates metabolism of LEVOTHYROXINE (may increase requirements for levothyroxine in hypothyroidism)
- Tibolone: rifampicin accelerates metabolism of TIBOLONE (reduced plasma concentration)
- Ticagrelor: rifampicin reduces plasma concentration of • TICAGRELOR
- Tolvaptan: rifampicin reduces plasma concentration of TOLVAPTAN
- Ulcer-healing Drugs: rifampicin accelerates metabolism of CIMETIDINE (reduced plasma concentration)
- Ulipristal: avoidance of rifampicin advised by manufacturer of • ULIPRISTAL (contraceptive effect of ulipristal possibly reduced)
- Vaccines: antibacterials inactivate ORAL TYPHOID VACCINE—see under Typhoid Vaccine in BNF

Rifaximin

NOTE Rifamycins interactions do not apply to rifaximin

- Anticoagulants: rifaximin possibly reduces anticoagulant effect of WARFARIN
- Ciclosporin: plasma concentration of rifaximin increased by • CICLOSPORIN
- Vaccines: antibacterials inactivate ORAL TYPHOID VACCINE—see under Typhoid Vaccine in BNF

Rilpivirine

- Analgesics: rilpivirine possibly reduces plasma concentration of METHADONE
- Antacids: manufacturer of rilpivirine advises give ANTACIDS 2 hours before or 4 hours after rilpivirine
- Antibacterials: manufacturer of rilpivirine advises avoid concomitant use with • CLARITHROMYCIN and • ERYTHROMYCIN (plasma concentration of rilpivirine possibly increased); plasma concentration of rilpivirine decreased by • RIFABUTIN (increase dose of rilpivirine—consult rilpivirine product literature); plasma concentration of rilpivirine reduced by • RIFAMPICIN—avoid concomitant use
- Anticoagulants: rilpivirine possibly increases plasma concentration of DABIGATRAN

Rilpivirine (continued)

- Antidepressants: manufacturer of rilpivirine advises avoid concomitant use with • ST JOHN'S WORT (plasma concentration of rilpivirine possibly reduced)
- Antiepileptics: manufacturer of rilpivirine advises avoid concomitant use with • CARBAMAZEPINE, • FOSPHENYTOIN, • OXCARBAZEPINE, • PHENOBARBITAL, • PHENYTOIN and • PRIMIDONE (plasma concentration of rilpivirine possibly reduced)
- ▸ Antivirals: manufacturer of rilpivirine advises give DIDANOSINE 2 hours before or 4 hours after rilpivirine; avoidance of rilpivirine advised by manufacturer of NEVIRAPINE
- ▸ Calcium Salts: manufacturer of rilpivirine advises give CALCIUM SALTS 2 hours before or 4 hours after rilpivirine
- Corticosteroids: manufacturer of rilpivirine advises avoid concomitant use with • DEXAMETHASONE (except when given as a single dose)
- Orlistat: absorption of rilpivirine possibly reduced by • ORLISTAT
- Ulcer-healing Drugs: manufacturer of rilpivirine advises avoid concomitant use with ESOMEPRAZOLE, LANSOPRAZOLE, PANTOPRAZOLE and RABEPRAZOLE (plasma concentration of rilpivirine possibly reduced); plasma concentration of rilpivirine reduced by OMEPRAZOLE—avoid concomitant use; manufacturer of rilpivirine advises avoid HISTAMINE H₂-ANTAGONISTS for 12 hours before or 4 hours after rilpivirine—consult product literature

Riociguat

- ▸ Antacids: absorption of riociguat reduced by ANTACIDS (give at least 2 hours before or 1 hour after riociguat)
- ▸ Antifungals: manufacturer of riociguat advises avoid concomitant use with ITRACONAZOLE, KETOCONAZOLE and VORICONAZOLE
- ▸ Antivirals: manufacturer of riociguat advises avoid concomitant use with RITONAVIR
- Avanafil: possible enhanced hypotensive effect when riociguat given with • AVANAFIL—avoid concomitant use
- ▸ Bosentan: plasma concentration of riociguat reduced by BOSENTAN
- Nicorandil: possible enhanced hypotensive effect when riociguat given with • NICORANDIL—avoid concomitant use
- Nitrates: possible enhanced hypotensive effect when riociguat given with • NITRATES—avoid concomitant use
- Sildenafil: enhanced hypotensive effect when riociguat given with • SILDENAFIL—avoid concomitant use
- Tadalafil: possible enhanced hypotensive effect when riociguat given with • TADALAFIL—avoid concomitant use
- Vardenafil: possible enhanced hypotensive effect when riociguat given with • VARDENAFIL—avoid concomitant use

Risedronate Sodium *see* Bisphosphonates

Risperidone *see* Antipsychotics

Ritonavir

- Alpha-blockers: ritonavir possibly increases plasma concentration of • ALFUZOSIN—avoid concomitant use
- Aminophylline: ritonavir accelerates metabolism of • AMINOPHYLLINE (reduced plasma concentration)
- Analgesics: ritonavir possibly increases plasma concentration of NSAIDs and BUPRENORPHINE; ritonavir increases plasma concentration of • DEXTROPROPOXYPHENE and • PIROXICAM (risk of toxicity)—avoid concomitant use; ritonavir increases plasma concentration of • ALFENTANIL and • FENTANYL; ritonavir reduces plasma concentration of METHADONE; ritonavir possibly reduces plasma concentration of MORPHINE; ritonavir reduces plasma concentration of • PETHIDINE, but increases plasma concentration of toxic metabolite of pethidine (avoid concomitant use)
- Anthelmintics: ritonavir possibly reduces plasma concentration of active metabolite of • ALBENDAZOLE—consider increasing albendazole dose when given for systemic infections
- Anti-arrhythmics: ritonavir increases plasma concentration of • AMIODARONE and • PROPAFENONE (increased risk of ventricular arrhythmias—avoid concomitant use); ritonavir possibly increases plasma concentration of • DISOPYRAMIDE (increased risk of toxicity); avoidance of ritonavir advised by manufacturer of • DRONEDARONE; ritonavir possibly increases

Ritonavir

- Anti-arrhythmics (continued)
  plasma concentration of • FLECAINIDE (increased risk of ventricular arrhythmias—avoid concomitant use)
- Antibacterials: ritonavir possibly increases plasma concentration of AZITHROMYCIN and ERYTHROMYCIN; ritonavir increases plasma concentration of • CLARITHROMYCIN (reduce dose of clarithromycin in renal impairment); ritonavir increases plasma concentration of • RIFABUTIN (increased risk of toxicity—reduce rifabutin dose); plasma concentration of ritonavir reduced by RIFAMPICIN; ritonavir possibly increases plasma concentration of BEDAQUILINE—manufacturer of ritonavir advises avoid concomitant use; ritonavir increases plasma concentration of DELAMANID; plasma concentration of both drugs increased when ritonavir given with • FUSIDIC ACID—avoid concomitant use; avoidance of concomitant ritonavir in severe renal and hepatic impairment advised by manufacturer of • TELITHROMYCIN
- Anticoagulants: ritonavir may enhance or reduce anticoagulant effect of • WARFARIN; avoidance of ritonavir advised by manufacturer of APIXABAN; ritonavir possibly enhances anticoagulant effect of • COUMARINS and • PHENINDIONE; ritonavir increases plasma concentration of • RIVAROXABAN—avoid concomitant use
- Antidepressants: ritonavir possibly reduces plasma concentration of PAROXETINE; ritonavir increases plasma concentration of • TRAZODONE (increased risk of toxicity); ritonavir possibly increases plasma concentration of • SSRIs and • TRICYCLICS; plasma concentration of ritonavir reduced by • ST JOHN'S WORT—avoid concomitant use
- ▸ Antidiabetics: ritonavir possibly increases plasma concentration of TOLBUTAMIDE
- Antiepileptics: ritonavir possibly increases plasma concentration of • CARBAMAZEPINE; plasma concentration of ritonavir possibly reduced by FOSPHENYTOIN and PHENYTOIN, also plasma concentration of fosphenytoin and phenytoin possibly affected; ritonavir possibly reduces plasma concentration of LAMOTRIGINE, SODIUM VALPROATE and VALPROIC ACID
- Antifungals: ritonavir increases plasma concentration of • KETOCONAZOLE (reduce dose of ketoconazole); plasma concentration of ritonavir increased by FLUCONAZOLE; combination of ritonavir with • ITRACONAZOLE may increase plasma concentration of either drug (or both); ritonavir reduces plasma concentration of • VORICONAZOLE—avoid concomitant use
- ▸ Antihistamines: ritonavir possibly increases plasma concentration of NON-SEDATING ANTIHISTAMINES
- Antimalarials: caution with ritonavir advised by manufacturer of ARTEMETHER WITH LUMEFANTRINE; plasma concentration of ritonavir possibly reduced by MEFLOQUINE; ritonavir increases plasma concentration of • QUININE (increased risk of toxicity)
- Antimuscarinics: avoidance of ritonavir advised by manufacturer of DARIFENACIN and TOLTERODINE; manufacturer of fesoterodine advises dose reduction when ritonavir given with FESOTERODINE—consult fesoterodine product literature; ritonavir possibly increases plasma concentration of • SOLIFENACIN—see under Solifenacin, p. 705
- Antipsychotics: ritonavir possibly increases plasma concentration of • ANTIPSYCHOTICS; ritonavir possibly increases plasma concentration of • ARIPIPRAZOLE (reduce dose of aripiprazole—consult aripiprazole product literature); manufacturer of ritonavir advises avoid concomitant use with • CLOZAPINE (increased risk of toxicity); ritonavir possibly increases plasma concentration of • LURASIDONE—avoid concomitant use; ritonavir reduces plasma concentration of OLANZAPINE—consider increasing dose of olanzapine; ritonavir increases plasma concentration of • PIMOZIDE (increased risk of ventricular arrhythmias—avoid concomitant use); ritonavir possibly increases plasma concentration of • QUETIAPINE—manufacturer of quetiapine advises avoid concomitant use
- Antivirals: plasma concentration of both drugs reduced when ritonavir given with • BOCEPREVIR; manufacturer of ritonavir advises ritonavir and DIDANOSINE should be taken 2.5 hours apart; ritonavir increases the toxicity of • EFAVIRENZ, monitor

Interactions | **Appendix 1**

A1

Ritonavir

- **Antivirals** (continued)
  liver function tests —manufacturer of *Atripla*® advises avoid concomitant use with *high-dose* ritonavir; ritonavir increases plasma concentration of INDINAVIR, MARAVIROC and
  - SAQUINAVIR; ritonavir increases plasma concentration of
  - SIMEPREVIR—manufacturer of simeprevir advises avoid concomitant use; ritonavir possibly reduces plasma concentration of TELAPREVIR
- **Anxiolytics and Hypnotics:** ritonavir possibly increases plasma concentration of • ANXIOLYTICS AND HYPNOTICS; ritonavir possibly increases plasma concentration of • ALPRAZOLAM, • DIAZEPAM, • FLURAZEPAM and • ZOLPIDEM (risk of extreme sedation and respiratory depression—avoid concomitant use); ritonavir possibly increases plasma concentration of • MIDAZOLAM (risk of prolonged sedation—avoid concomitant use of *oral* midazolam); ritonavir increases plasma concentration of BUSPIRONE (increased risk of toxicity)
- **Aprepitant:** ritonavir possibly increases plasma concentration of APREPITANT
- **Atovaquone:** ritonavir possibly reduces plasma concentration of ATOVAQUONE—manufacturer of atovaquone advises avoid concomitant use
- **Avanafil:** ritonavir significantly increases plasma concentration of • AVANAFIL—avoid concomitant use
- **Bosentan:** ritonavir increases plasma concentration of • BOSENTAN (consider reducing dose of bosentan)
- **Bupropion:** ritonavir reduces plasma concentration of BUPROPION
- **Calcium-channel Blockers:** ritonavir possibly increases plasma concentration of • CALCIUM-CHANNEL BLOCKERS; ritonavir increases plasma concentration of • AMLODIPINE (reduce dose of amlodipine); avoidance of ritonavir advised by manufacturer of LERCANIDIPINE
- **Cardiac Glycosides:** ritonavir possibly increases plasma concentration of DIGOXIN
- **Ciclosporin:** ritonavir possibly increases plasma concentration of • CICLOSPORIN
- **Cilostazol:** ritonavir possibly increases plasma concentration of • CILOSTAZOL (see under Cilostazol, p. 215)
- **Cobicistat:** avoidance of ritonavir advised by manufacturer of COBICISTAT
- **Colchicine:** ritonavir possibly increases risk of • COLCHICINE toxicity—suspend or reduce dose of colchicine (avoid concomitant use in hepatic or renal impairment)
- **Corticosteroids:** ritonavir possibly increases plasma concentration of • CORTICOSTEROIDS—increased risk of adrenal supression; ritonavir possibly increases plasma concentration of • BUDESONIDE (including *inhaled*, *intranasal*, and *rectal* budesonide)—increased risk of adrenal suppresion; ritonavir increases plasma concentration of *inhaled* and *intranasal* • FLUTICASONE—increased risk of adrenal suppression; ritonavir increases plasma concentration of • TRIAMCINOLONE *injection*—increased risk of adrenal suppression
- **Cytotoxics:** ritonavir increases the plasma concentration of AFATINIB—manufacturer of afatinib advises separating administration of ritonavir by 6 to 12 hours; ritonavir possibly increases plasma concentration of AXITINIB (reduce dose of axitinib—consult axitinib product literature); ritonavir possibly increases the plasma concentration of • BOSUTINIB and • CABAZITAXEL—manufacturer of bosutinib and cabazitaxel advises avoid or consider reducing dose of bosutinib and cabazitaxel; ritonavir possibly increases plasma concentration of CABOZANTINIB and VINBLASTINE; ritonavir possibly increases plasma concentration of • CRIZOTINIB, • EVEROLIMUS, NILOTINIB and • VINFLUNINE—manufacturer of crizotinib, everolimus, nilotinib and vinflunine advises avoid concomitant use; avoidance of ritonavir advised by manufacturer of DASATINIB (plasma concentration of dasatinib possibly increased); ritonavir possibly increases the plasma concentration of • IBRUTINIB—reduce dose of ibrutinib (see under Ibrutinib, p. 855); avoidance of ritonavir advised by manufacturer of • LAPATINIB; ritonavir possibly increases plasma concentration of • PAZOPANIB (reduce dose of pazopanib); ritonavir possibly increases plasma concentration of PONATINIB—consider reducing initial dose of ponatinib (see

Ritonavir

- **Cytotoxics** (continued)
  under Ponatinib, p. 860); manufacturer of ruxolitinib advises dose reduction when ritonavir given with • RUXOLITINIB—consult ruxolitinib product literature; ritonavir possibly increases plasma concentration of • DOCETAXEL—manufacturer of docetaxel advises avoid concomitant use or consider reducing docetaxel dose; ritonavir increases plasma concentration of PACLITAXEL
- **Dapoxetine:** avoidance of ritonavir advised by manufacturer of • DAPOXETINE (increased risk of toxicity)
- **Diuretics:** ritonavir increases plasma concentration of • EPLERENONE—avoid concomitant use
- **Domperidone:** possible increased risk of ventricular arrhythmias when ritonavir given with • DOMPERIDONE—avoid concomitant use
- **Ergot Alkaloids:** increased risk of ergotism when ritonavir given with • ERGOT ALKALOIDS—avoid concomitant use
- **Fosaprepitant:** ritonavir possibly increases plasma concentration of FOSAPREPITANT
- **Guanfacine:** ritonavir possibly increases plasma concentration of • GUANFACINE (halve dose of guanfacine)
- **5HT₁-receptor Agonists:** ritonavir increases plasma concentration of • ELETRIPTAN (risk of toxicity)—avoid concomitant use
- **Ivabradine:** ritonavir possibly increases plasma concentration of • IVABRADINE—avoid concomitant use
- **Lipid-regulating Drugs:** ritonavir possibly increases plasma concentration of ATORVASTATIN (use lowest possible dose of atorvastatin); possible increased risk of myopathy when ritonavir given with • ROSUVASTATIN—manufacturer of rosuvastatin advises avoid concomitant use; increased risk of myopathy when ritonavir given with • SIMVASTATIN (avoid concomitant use); avoidance of ritonavir advised by manufacturer of • LOMITAPIDE (plasma concentration of lomitapide possibly increased)
- **Mirabegron:** when given with ritonavir avoid or reduce dose of MIRABEGRON in hepatic or renal impairment—see Mirabegron, p. 707
- **Oestrogens:** ritonavir accelerates metabolism of • OESTROGENS (reduced contraceptive effect with combined oral contraceptives, contraceptive patches, and vaginal rings—see Contraceptive Interactions in BNF)
- **Orlistat:** absorption of ritonavir possibly reduced by • ORLISTAT
- **Ranolazine:** ritonavir possibly increases plasma concentration of • RANOLAZINE—manufacturer of ranolazine advises avoid concomitant use
- **Riociguat:** avoidance of ritonavir advised by manufacturer of RIOCIGUAT
- **Sildenafil:** ritonavir significantly increases plasma concentration of • SILDENAFIL—avoid concomitant use of sildenafil for pulmonary arterial hypertension or reduce dose of sildenafil for erectile dysfunction (consult sildenafil product literature)
- **Sympathomimetics:** ritonavir possibly increases plasma concentration of DEXAMFETAMINE
- **Sympathomimetics, Beta₂:** manufacturer of ritonavir advises avoid concomitant use with SALMETEROL
- **Tacrolimus:** ritonavir possibly increases plasma concentration of • TACROLIMUS
- **Tadalafil:** ritonavir increases plasma concentration of • TADALAFIL—avoid concomitant use of tadalafil for pulmonary hypertension
- **Theophylline:** ritonavir accelerates metabolism of • THEOPHYLLINE (reduced plasma concentration)
- **Ticagrelor:** ritonavir possibly increases plasma concentration of • TICAGRELOR—manufacturer of ticagrelor advises avoid concomitant use
- **Ulipristal:** avoidance of ritonavir advised by manufacturer of • ULIPRISTAL (contraceptive effect of ulipristal possibly reduced)
- **Vardenafil:** ritonavir increases plasma concentration of • VARDENAFIL—avoid concomitant use

Rituximab

- **Antipsychotics:** avoid concomitant use of cytotoxics with • CLOZAPINE (increased risk of agranulocytosis)

Rituximab (continued)
- Vaccines: risk of generalised infections when monoclonal antibodies given with live ● VACCINES—avoid concomitant use

Rivaroxaban
- Analgesics: increased risk of haemorrhage when anticoagulants given with *intravenous* ● DICLOFENAC (avoid concomitant use, including low-dose heparins); increased risk of haemorrhage when anticoagulants given with ● KETOROLAC (avoid concomitant use, including low-dose heparins)
- ▷ Anti-arrhythmics: manufacturer of rivaroxaban advises avoid concomitant use with DRONEDARONE
- Antibacterials: plasma concentration of rivaroxaban reduced by ● RIFAMPICIN—manufacturer of rivaroxaban advises monitor for signs of thrombosis
- Anticoagulants: increased risk of haemorrhage when rivaroxaban given with other ● ANTICOAGULANTS (avoid concomitant use except when switching with other anticoagulants or using heparin to maintain catheter patency); increased risk of haemorrhage when other anticoagulants given with ● APIXABAN, ● DABIGATRAN and ● EDOXABAN (avoid concomitant use except when switching with other anticoagulants or using heparin to maintain catheter patency)
- Antidepressants: plasma concentration of rivaroxaban possibly reduced by ● ST JOHN'S WORT—manufacturer of rivaroxaban advises monitor for signs of thrombosis
- Antiepileptics: plasma concentration of rivaroxaban possibly reduced by ● CARBAMAZEPINE, ● FOSPHENYTOIN, ● PHENOBARBITAL, ● PHENYTOIN and ● PRIMIDONE—manufacturer of rivaroxaban advises monitor for signs of thrombosis
- Antifungals: plasma concentration of rivaroxaban increased by ● KETOCONAZOLE—avoid concomitant use; manufacturer of rivaroxaban advises avoid concomitant use with ITRACONAZOLE, POSACONAZOLE and VORICONAZOLE
- Antivirals: manufacturer of rivaroxaban advises avoid concomitant use with ATAZANAVIR, DARUNAVIR, FOSAMPRENAVIR, INDINAVIR, SAQUINAVIR and TIPRANAVIR; manufacturers advise avoid concomitant use of rivaroxaban with LOPINAVIR; plasma concentration of rivaroxaban increased by ● RITONAVIR—avoid concomitant use
- Cobicistat: anticoagulant effect of rivaroxaban possibly enhanced by ● COBICISTAT—avoid concomitant use

Rivastigmine *see* Parasympathomimetics

Rizatriptan *see* 5HT$_1$-receptor Agonists (under HT)

Rocuronium *see* Muscle Relaxants

Roflumilast
- ▷ Aminophylline: manufacturer of roflumilast advises avoid concomitant use with AMINOPHYLLINE
- Antibacterials: effects of roflumilast inhibited by ● RIFAMPICIN (manufacturer of roflumilast advises avoid concomitant use)
- ▷ Antidepressants: metabolism of roflumilast inhibited by FLUVOXAMINE
- ▷ Antiepileptics: effects of roflumilast possibly inhibited by CARBAMAZEPINE, FOSPHENYTOIN, PHENOBARBITAL, PHENYTOIN and PRIMIDONE (manufacturer of roflumilast advises avoid concomitant use)
- ▷ Theophylline: manufacturer of roflumilast advises avoid concomitant use with THEOPHYLLINE
- ▷ Ulcer-healing Drugs: metabolism of roflumilast inhibited by CIMETIDINE

Ropinirole
- ▷ Antibacterials: metabolism of ropinirole inhibited by CIPROFLOXACIN (increased plasma concentration)
- ▷ Antipsychotics: manufacturer of ropinirole advises avoid concomitant use of ANTIPSYCHOTICS (antagonism of effect)
- ▷ Memantine: effects of dopaminergics possibly enhanced by MEMANTINE
- ▷ Methyldopa: antiparkinsonian effect of dopaminergics antagonised by METHYLDOPA
- ▷ Metoclopramide: manufacturer of ropinirole advises avoid concomitant use of METOCLOPRAMIDE (antagonism of effect)
- ▷ Oestrogens: plasma concentration of ropinirole increased by OESTROGENS

Ropivacaine
- ▷ Anti-arrhythmics: increased myocardial depression when ropivacaine given with ANTI-ARRHYTHMICS
- ▷ Antidepressants: metabolism of ropivacaine inhibited by FLUVOXAMINE—avoid prolonged administration of ropivacaine

Rosuvastatin *see* Statins

Rotavirus Vaccine *see* Vaccines

Rotigotine
- ▷ Antipsychotics: manufacturer of rotigotine advises avoid concomitant use of ANTIPSYCHOTICS (antagonism of effect)
- ▷ Memantine: effects of dopaminergics possibly enhanced by MEMANTINE
- ▷ Methyldopa: antiparkinsonian effect of dopaminergics antagonised by METHYLDOPA
- ▷ Metoclopramide: manufacturer of rotigotine advises avoid concomitant use of METOCLOPRAMIDE (antagonism of effect)

Rufinamide
- Antidepressants: anticonvulsant effect of antiepileptics possibly antagonised by MAOIs and ● TRICYCLIC-RELATED ANTIDEPRESSANTS (convulsive threshold lowered); anticonvulsant effect of antiepileptics antagonised by ● SSRIS and ● TRICYCLICS (convulsive threshold lowered)
- ▷ Antiepileptics: plasma concentration of both drugs possibly reduced when rufinamide given with CARBAMAZEPINE; plasma concentration of rufinamide possibly reduced by FOSPHENYTOIN and PHENYTOIN, also plasma concentration of fosphenytoin and phenytoin possibly increased; plasma concentration of rufinamide possibly reduced by PHENOBARBITAL and PRIMIDONE; plasma concentration of rufinamide possibly increased by SODIUM VALPROATE and VALPROIC ACID (reduce dose of rufinamide)
- Antimalarials: anticonvulsant effect of antiepileptics antagonised by ● MEFLOQUINE
- Antipsychotics: anticonvulsant effect of antiepileptics antagonised by ● ANTIPSYCHOTICS (convulsive threshold lowered)
- Oestrogens: rufinamide accelerates metabolism of ● OESTROGENS (reduced contraceptive effect with combined oral contraceptives, contraceptive patches, and vaginal rings—see Contraceptive Interactions in BNF)
- Orlistat: possible increased risk of convulsions when antiepileptics given with ORLISTAT
- Progestogens: rufinamide accelerates metabolism of ● PROGESTOGENS (reduced contraceptive effect with combined oral contraceptives, progestogen-only oral contraceptives, contraceptive patches, vaginal rings, etonogestrel-releasing implant, and emergency hormonal contraception—see Contraceptive Interactions in BNF)

Ruxolitinib
- Antibacterials: manufacturer of ruxolitinib advises dose reduction when ruxolitinib given with ● CLARITHROMYCIN and ● TELITHROMYCIN—consult ruxolitinib product literature; plasma concentration of ruxolitinib reduced by RIFAMPICIN
- Antifungals: manufacturer of ruxolitinib advises dose reduction when ruxolitinib given with ● FLUCONAZOLE, ● ITRACONAZOLE, ● KETOCONAZOLE, ● POSACONAZOLE and ● VORICONAZOLE—consult ruxolitinib product literature
- Antipsychotics: avoid concomitant use of cytotoxics with ● CLOZAPINE (increased risk of agranulocytosis)
- Antivirals: manufacturer of ruxolitinib advises dose reduction when ruxolitinib given with ● BOCEPREVIR, ● INDINAVIR, ● LOPINAVIR, ● RITONAVIR, ● SAQUINAVIR and ● TELAPREVIR—consult ruxolitinib product literature

Sacubitril
- ACE Inhibitors: manufacturer of sacubitril advises avoid ● ACE INHIBITORS for 36 hours before or after sacubitril
- ▷ Diuretics: sacubitril reduces plasma concentration of FUROSEMIDE
- ▷ Lipid-regulating Drugs: sacubitril increases plasma concentration of ATORVASTATIN

St John's Wort
- ▷ Aminophylline: St John's wort possibly reduces plasma concentration of AMINOPHYLLINE
- ▷ Analgesics: St John's wort possibly reduces plasma concentration of METHADONE

St John's Wort (continued)

- Anti-arrhythmics: St John's wort possibly reduces plasma concentration of ● DRONEDARONE—avoid concomitant use
- Antibacterials: St John's wort possibly reduces plasma concentration of BEDAQUILINE—manufacturer of bedaquiline advises avoid concomitant use; St John's wort reduces plasma concentration of ● TELITHROMYCIN (avoid during and for 2 weeks after St John's wort)
- Anticoagulants: St John's wort reduces plasma concentration of ● APIXABAN—manufacturer of apixaban advises avoid concomitant use when given for treatment of deep-vein thrombosis or pulmonary embolism; St John's wort reduces anticoagulant effect of ● COUMARINS (avoid concomitant use); St John's wort reduces plasma concentration of DABIGATRAN—manufacturer of dabigatran advises avoid concomitant use; St John's wort possibly reduces plasma concentration of ● EDOXABAN; St John's wort possibly reduces plasma concentration of ● RIVAROXABAN— manufacturer of rivaroxaban advises monitor for signs of thrombosis
- Antidepressants: possible increased serotonergic effects when St John's wort given with DULOXETINE, VENLAFAXINE or VORTIOXETINE; St John's wort reduces plasma concentration of AMITRIPTYLINE; increased serotonergic effects when St John's wort given with ● SSRIS—avoid concomitant use
- Antiepileptics: St John's wort possibly reduces plasma concentration of CARBAMAZEPINE; St John's wort possibly reduces plasma concentration of ● FOSPHENYTOIN, ● PHENOBARBITAL, ● PHENYTOIN and ● PRIMIDONE—avoid concomitant use
- Antifungals: St John's wort reduces plasma concentration of ● VORICONAZOLE—avoid concomitant use
- Antimalarials: avoidance of antidepressants advised by manufacturer of ● ARTEMETHER WITH LUMEFANTRINE and ● ARTENIMOL WITH PIPERAQUINE
- Antimuscarinics: St John's wort possibly reduces plasma concentration of active metabolite of ● FESOTERODINE— manufacturer of fesoterodine advises avoid concomitant use
- Antipsychotics: St John's wort possibly reduces plasma concentration of ● ARIPIPRAZOLE (avoid concomitant use or consider increasing the dose of aripiprazole—consult aripiprazole product literature); St John's wort possibly reduces plasma concentration of LURASIDONE—avoid concomitant use
- Antivirals: St John's wort reduces plasma concentration of ● ATAZANAVIR, ● DARUNAVIR, ● EFAVIRENZ, ● FOSAMPRENAVIR, ● INDINAVIR, ● LOPINAVIR, ● NEVIRAPINE, ● RITONAVIR and ● SAQUINAVIR—avoid concomitant use; St John's wort possibly reduces plasma concentration of DACLATASVIR, ● DASABUVIR, ● OMBITASVIR, ● PARITAPREVIR and ● SIMEPREVIR—manufacturer of daclatasvir, dasabuvir, ombitasvir, paritaprevir and simeprevir advises avoid concomitant use; St John's wort possibly reduces the plasma concentration of ● DOLUTEGRAVIR (see under Dolutegravir, p. 584); avoidance of St John's wort advised by manufacturer of ● ELVITEGRAVIR, ETRAVIRINE, LEDIPASVIR, SOFOSBUVIR and ● TELAPREVIR; St John's wort possibly reduces plasma concentration of ● MARAVIROC and ● TIPRANAVIR—avoid concomitant use; avoidance of St John's wort advised by manufacturer of ● RILPIVIRINE (plasma concentration of rilpivirine possibly reduced)
▸ Anxiolytics and Hypnotics: St John's wort possibly reduces plasma concentration of *oral* MIDAZOLAM
- Apremilast: St John's wort possibly reduces plasma concentration of ● APREMILAST—avoid concomitant use
- Aprepitant: avoidance of St John's wort advised by manufacturer of ● APREPITANT
▸ Atomoxetine: possible increased risk of convulsions when antidepressants given with ATOMOXETINE
- Calcium-channel Blockers: St John's wort possibly reduces plasma concentration of AMLODIPINE and FELODIPINE; St John's wort reduces plasma concentration of NIFEDIPINE; St John's wort significantly reduces plasma concentration of ● VERAPAMIL
- Cannabis Extract: St John's wort possibly reduces plasma concentration of ● CANNABIS EXTRACT—manufacturer of cannabis extract advises avoid concomitant use

St John's Wort (continued)

- Cardiac Glycosides: St John's wort reduces plasma concentration of ● DIGOXIN—avoid concomitant use
- Ciclosporin: St John's wort reduces plasma concentration of ● CICLOSPORIN—avoid concomitant use
- Cobicistat: St John's wort possibly reduces plasma concentration of ● COBICISTAT—manufacturer of cobicistat advises avoid concomitant use
- Cytotoxics: St John's wort possibly reduces plasma concentration of AXITINIB—consider increasing dose of axitinib; St John's wort possibly reduces plasma concentration of BORTEZOMIB, ● BOSUTINIB, CABOZANTINIB, CRIZOTINIB, EVEROLIMUS, ● IBRUTINIB, ● IDELALISIB, PONATINIB and ● VINFLUNINE—manufacturer of bortezomib, bosutinib, cabozantinib, crizotinib, everolimus, ibrutinib, idelalisib, ponatinib and vinflunine advises avoid concomitant use; avoidance of St John's wort advised by manufacturer of ● CABAZITAXEL, DABRAFENIB, GEFITINIB, ● LAPATINIB, ● OLAPARIB and VEMURAFENIB; St John's wort reduces plasma concentration of ● IMATINIB—avoid concomitant use; avoidance of St John's wort advised by manufacturer of VANDETANIB and ● VISMODEGIB (plasma concentration of vandetanib and vismodegib possibly reduced); St John's wort possibly reduces plasma concentration of ● ERIBULIN; St John's wort accelerates metabolism of ● IRINOTECAN (reduced plasma concentration—avoid concomitant use)
- Dapoxetine: possible increased risk of serotonergic effects when St John's wort given with ● DAPOXETINE (manufacturer of dapoxetine advises St John's wort should not be started until 1 week after stopping dapoxetine, avoid dapoxetine for 2 weeks after stopping St John's wort)
- Diuretics: St John's wort reduces plasma concentration of ● EPLERENONE—avoid concomitant use
▸ Fingolimod: St John's wort possibly reduces plasma concentration of FINGOLIMOD—manufacturer of fingolimod advises avoid concomitant use
- Fosaprepitant: avoidance of St John's wort advised by manufacturer of ● FOSAPREPITANT
- Guanfacine: St John's wort possibly reduces plasma concentration of ● GUANFACINE—increase dose of guanfacine
- Hormone Antagonists: St John's wort possibly reduces plasma concentration of ● ABIRATERONE—manufacturer of abiraterone advises avoid concomitant use
- 5HT$_1$-receptor Agonists: increased serotonergic effects when St John's wort given with ● 5HT$_1$ AGONISTS—avoid concomitant use
- Ivabradine: St John's wort reduces plasma concentration of IVABRADINE—avoid concomitant use
- Ivacaftor: St John's wort possibly reduces plasma concentration of ● IVACAFTOR—manufacturer of ivacaftor advises avoid concomitant use
▸ Lipid-regulating Drugs: St John's wort reduces plasma concentration of SIMVASTATIN
▸ Macitentan: avoidance of St John's wort advised by manufacturer of MACITENTAN
- Oestrogens: St John's wort reduces contraceptive effect of ● OESTROGENS (avoid concomitant use)
- Progestogens: St John's wort reduces contraceptive effect of ● PROGESTOGENS (avoid concomitant use)
- Tacrolimus: St John's wort reduces plasma concentration of ● TACROLIMUS—avoid concomitant use
▸ Theophylline: St John's wort possibly reduces plasma concentration of THEOPHYLLINE
▸ Ulcer-healing Drugs: St John's wort possibly reduces plasma concentration of OMEPRAZOLE
- Ulipristal: avoidance of St John's wort advised by manufacturer of ● ULIPRISTAL (contraceptive effect of ulipristal possibly reduced)

Salbutamol see Sympathomimetics, Beta$_2$
Salmeterol see Sympathomimetics, Beta$_2$
Saquinavir

- Analgesics: increased risk of ventricular arrhythmias when saquinavir given with ● ALFENTANIL, ● FENTANYL or ● METHADONE—avoid concomitant use
- Anti-arrhythmics: increased risk of ventricular arrhythmias when saquinavir given with ● AMIODARONE, ● DISOPYRAMIDE,

Saquinavir

- **Anti-arrhythmics** (continued)
  - DRONEDARONE, ● FLECAINIDE, ● LIDOCAINE or ● PROPAFENONE—avoid concomitant use
- **Antibacterials:** plasma concentration of both drugs possibly increased when saquinavir given with ● CLARITHROMYCIN (increased risk of ventricular arrhythmias); increased risk of ventricular arrhythmias when saquinavir given with ● DAPSONE, ● ERYTHROMYCIN or ● MOXIFLOXACIN—avoid concomitant use; saquinavir increases plasma concentration of ● RIFABUTIN (also plasma concentration of saquinavir reduced)—reduce rifabutin dose; plasma concentration of saquinavir significantly reduced by ● RIFAMPICIN, also risk of hepatotoxicity—avoid concomitant use; increased risk of ventricular arrhythmias when saquinavir given with ● DELAMANID; plasma concentration of both drugs may increase when saquinavir given with FUSIDIC ACID; avoidance of saquinavir advised by manufacturer of ● TELITHROMYCIN (risk of ventricular arrhythmias)
- ▸ **Anticoagulants:** saquinavir possibly enhances anticoagulant effect of WARFARIN; avoidance of saquinavir advised by manufacturer of APIXABAN and RIVAROXABAN
- **Antidepressants:** increased risk of ventricular arrhythmias when saquinavir given with ● TRAZODONE or ● TRICYCLICS—avoid concomitant use; plasma concentration of saquinavir reduced by ● ST JOHN'S WORT—avoid concomitant use
- **Antiepileptics:** plasma concentration of saquinavir possibly reduced by CARBAMAZEPINE, FOSPHENYTOIN, ● PHENOBARBITAL, PHENYTOIN and ● PRIMIDONE
- **Antifungals:** plasma concentration of saquinavir increased by ● KETOCONAZOLE—manufacturer of ketoconazole advises avoid concomitant use; plasma concentration of saquinavir possibly increased by IMIDAZOLES and TRIAZOLES
- **Antihistamines:** increased risk of ventricular arrhythmias when saquinavir given with ● MIZOLASTINE—avoid concomitant use
- **Antimalarials:** caution with saquinavir advised by manufacturer of ARTEMETHER WITH LUMEFANTRINE; avoidance of saquinavir advised by manufacturer of ● ARTENIMOL WITH PIPERAQUINE (possible risk of ventricular arrhythmias); increased risk of ventricular arrhythmias when saquinavir given with ● QUININE—avoid concomitant use
- ▸ **Antimuscarinics:** avoidance of saquinavir advised by manufacturer of DARIFENACIN and TOLTERODINE; manufacturer of fesoterodine advises dose reduction when saquinavir given with FESOTERODINE—consult fesoterodine product literature
- **Antipsychotics:** increased risk of ventricular arrhythmias when saquinavir given with ● CLOZAPINE, ● HALOPERIDOL or ● PHENOTHIAZINES—avoid concomitant use; saquinavir possibly increases plasma concentration of ● ARIPIPRAZOLE (reduce dose of aripiprazole—consult aripiprazole product literature); saquinavir possibly increases plasma concentration of ● LURASIDONE—avoid concomitant use; saquinavir possibly increases plasma concentration of ● PIMOZIDE (increased risk of ventricular arrhythmias—avoid concomitant use); saquinavir possibly increases plasma concentration of ● QUETIAPINE—manufacturer of quetiapine advises avoid concomitant use
- **Antivirals:** increased risk of ventricular arrhythmias when saquinavir given with ● ATAZANAVIR or ● LOPINAVIR—avoid concomitant use; saquinavir reduces plasma concentration of DARUNAVIR—avoid concomitant use; plasma concentration of saquinavir significantly reduced by EFAVIRENZ; plasma concentration of saquinavir increased by INDINAVIR and ● RITONAVIR; saquinavir increases plasma concentration of ● MARAVIROC (consider reducing dose of maraviroc); avoidance of saquinavir advised by manufacturer of PARITAPREVIR; plasma concentration of saquinavir reduced by TIPRANAVIR
- **Anxiolytics and Hypnotics:** saquinavir increases plasma concentration of ● MIDAZOLAM (risk of prolonged sedation—avoid concomitant use of *oral* midazolam)
- **Avanafil:** saquinavir possibly increases plasma concentration of ● AVANAFIL—manufacturer of avanafil advises avoid concomitant use
- **Beta-blockers:** increased risk of ventricular arrhythmias when saquinavir given with ● SOTALOL—avoid concomitant use

Saquinavir (continued)

- **Ciclosporin:** plasma concentration of both drugs increased when saquinavir given with ● CICLOSPORIN
- ▸ **Corticosteroids:** plasma concentration of saquinavir possibly reduced by DEXAMETHASONE
- **Cytotoxics:** saquinavir possibly increases the plasma concentration of AFATINIB—manufacturer of afatinib advises separating administration of saquinavir by 6 to 12 hours; saquinavir possibly increases plasma concentration of AXITINIB (reduce dose of axitinib—consult axitinib product literature); saquinavir possibly increases the plasma concentration of ● BOSUTINIB and ● CABAZITAXEL—manufacturer of bosutinib and cabazitaxel advises avoid or consider reducing dose of bosutinib and cabazitaxel; saquinavir possibly increases plasma concentration of ● CRIZOTINIB and ● EVEROLIMUS—manufacturer of crizotinib and everolimus advises avoid concomitant use; saquinavir possibly increases the plasma concentration of ● IBRUTINIB—reduce dose of ibrutinib (see under Ibrutinib, p. 855); avoidance of saquinavir advised by manufacturer of ● LAPATINIB and ● OLAPARIB; increased risk of ventricular arrhythmias when saquinavir given with ● PAZOPANIB—avoid concomitant use; saquinavir possibly increases plasma concentration of ● PONATINIB—consider reducing initial dose of ponatinib (see under Ponatinib, p. 860); manufacturer of ruxolitinib advises dose reduction when saquinavir given with ● RUXOLITINIB—consult ruxolitinib product literature; saquinavir possibly increases plasma concentration of ● DOCETAXEL—manufacturer of docetaxel advises avoid concomitant use or consider reducing docetaxel dose
- **Dapoxetine:** avoidance of saquinavir advised by manufacturer of ● DAPOXETINE (increased risk of toxicity)
- ▸ **Diuretics:** saquinavir increases plasma concentration of EPLERENONE (reduce dose of eplerenone)
- **Domperidone:** possible increased risk of ventricular arrhythmias when saquinavir given with ● DOMPERIDONE—avoid concomitant use
- **Ergot Alkaloids:** increased risk of ergotism when saquinavir given with ● ERGOTAMINE—avoid concomitant use
- **Guanfacine:** saquinavir possibly increases plasma concentration of ● GUANFACINE (halve dose of guanfacine)
- **Lipid-regulating Drugs:** possible increased risk of myopathy when saquinavir given with ATORVASTATIN; possible increased risk of myopathy when saquinavir given with ● ROSUVASTATIN—manufacturer of rosuvastatin advises avoid concomitant use; increased risk of myopathy when saquinavir given with ● SIMVASTATIN (avoid concomitant use); avoidance of saquinavir advised by manufacturer of ● LOMITAPIDE (plasma concentration of lomitapide possibly increased)
- **Orlistat:** absorption of saquinavir possibly reduced by ● ORLISTAT
- **Pentamidine Isetionate:** increased risk of ventricular arrhythmias when saquinavir given with ● PENTAMIDINE ISETIONATE—avoid concomitant use
- **Ranolazine:** saquinavir possibly increases plasma concentration of ● RANOLAZINE—manufacturer of ranolazine advises avoid concomitant use
- **Sildenafil:** increased risk of ventricular arrhythmias when saquinavir given with ● SILDENAFIL—avoid concomitant use
- **Tacrolimus:** saquinavir increases plasma concentration of ● TACROLIMUS (consider reducing dose of tacrolimus)
- **Tadalafil:** increased risk of ventricular arrhythmias when saquinavir given with ● TADALAFIL—avoid concomitant use
- **Ulcer-healing Drugs:** plasma concentration of saquinavir possibly increased by CIMETIDINE; plasma concentration of saquinavir possibly increased by ● ESOMEPRAZOLE, ● LANSOPRAZOLE, ● PANTOPRAZOLE and ● RABEPRAZOLE—manufacturer of saquinavir advises avoid concomitant use; plasma concentration of saquinavir increased by ● OMEPRAZOLE—manufacturer of saquinavir advises avoid concomitant use
- **Vardenafil:** increased risk of ventricular arrhythmias when saquinavir given with ● VARDENAFIL—avoid concomitant use

Saxagliptin see Antidiabetics

A1

Interactions | Appendix 1

Secukinumab
- Antipsychotics: avoid concomitant use of cytotoxics with
  - CLOZAPINE (increased risk of agranulocytosis)
- Vaccines: risk of generalised infections when monoclonal antibodies given with live • VACCINES—avoid concomitant use

Selegiline

NOTE Selegiline is a MAO-B inhibitor

- Analgesics: hyperpyrexia and CNS toxicity reported when selegiline given with • PETHIDINE (avoid concomitant use); manufacturer of selegiline advises avoid concomitant use with OPIOID ANALGESICS
- Antidepressants: manufacturer of selegiline advises avoid concomitant use with CITALOPRAM and ESCITALOPRAM; increased risk of hypertension and CNS excitation when selegiline given with • FLUOXETINE (selegiline should not be started until 5 weeks after stopping fluoxetine, avoid fluoxetine for 2 weeks after stopping selegiline); increased risk of hypertension and CNS excitation when selegiline given with • FLUVOXAMINE, • SERTRALINE or • VENLAFAXINE (selegiline should not be started until 1 week after stopping fluvoxamine, sertraline or venlafaxine, avoid fluvoxamine, sertraline or venlafaxine for 2 weeks after stopping selegiline); increased risk of hypertension and CNS excitation when selegiline given with • PAROXETINE (selegiline should not be started until 2 weeks after stopping paroxetine, avoid paroxetine for 2 weeks after stopping selegiline); enhanced hypotensive effect when selegiline given with • MAOIS—manufacturer of selegiline advises avoid concomitant use; avoid concomitant use of selegiline with • MOCLOBEMIDE; CNS toxicity reported when selegiline given with • TRICYCLICS; risk of CNS excitation and hypertension when selegiline given with • VORTIOXETINE
- Dopaminergics: selegiline enhances effects and increases toxicity of CO-BENELDOPA, CO-CARELDOPA or LEVODOPA (reduce dose of co-beneldopa, co-careldopa or levodopa); max. dose of 10 mg selegiline advised by manufacturer of ENTACAPONE if used concomitantly
- 5HT$_1$-receptor Agonists: manufacturer of selegiline advises avoid concomitant use with 5HT$_1$ AGONISTS
- Memantine: effects of dopaminergics and selegiline possibly enhanced by MEMANTINE
- Methyldopa: antiparkinsonian effect of dopaminergics antagonised by METHYLDOPA
- Oestrogens: plasma concentration of selegiline increased by • OESTROGENS—manufacturer of selegiline advises avoid concomitant use
- Progestogens: plasma concentration of selegiline increased by • PROGESTOGENS—manufacturer of selegiline advises avoid concomitant use
- Sympathomimetics: manufacturer of selegiline advises avoid concomitant use with SYMPATHOMIMETICS; risk of hypertensive crisis when selegiline given with • DOPAMINE

Selenium
- Eltrombopag: selenium possibly reduces absorption of ELTROMBOPAG (give at least 4 hours apart)
- Vitamins: absorption of selenium possibly reduced by ASCORBIC ACID (give at least 4 hours apart)

Sertraline see Antidepressants, SSRI

Sevelamer
- Antibacterials: sevelamer reduces absorption of CIPROFLOXACIN (give at least 2 hours before or 4 hours after ciprofloxacin)
- Ciclosporin: sevelamer possibly reduces plasma concentration of CICLOSPORIN
- Mycophenolate: sevelamer possibly reduces plasma concentration of MYCOPHENOLATE
- Tacrolimus: sevelamer possibly reduces plasma concentration of TACROLIMUS
- Thyroid Hormones: sevelamer possibly reduces absorption of LEVOTHYROXINE
- Vitamins: sevelamer reduces absorption of CALCITRIOL (give at least 1 hour before or 3 hours after sevelamer)

Sevoflurane see Anaesthetics, General

Sildenafil
- Alpha-blockers: enhanced hypotensive effect when sildenafil given with • ALPHA-BLOCKERS (avoid alpha-blockers for 4 hours after sildenafil)—when patient is stable on the alpha blocker initiate sildenafil at the lowest possible dose

Sildenafil (continued)
- Anti-arrhythmics: avoidance of sildenafil advised by manufacturer of DISOPYRAMIDE (risk of ventricular arrhythmias)
- Antibacterials: plasma concentration of sildenafil increased by • CLARITHROMYCIN—consider reducing initial dose of sildenafil for erectile dysfunction or reduce sildenafil dose frequency to once daily for pulmonary hypertension; plasma concentration of sildenafil increased by ERYTHROMYCIN—reduce initial dose of sildenafil for erectile dysfunction or reduce sildenafil dose frequency to twice daily for pulmonary hypertension; plasma concentration of sildenafil possibly increased by • TELITHROMYCIN—consider reducing initial dose of sildenafil for erectile dysfunction or reduce sildenafil dose frequency to once daily for pulmonary hypertension
- Antifungals: plasma concentration of sildenafil increased by • KETOCONAZOLE—reduce initial dose of sildenafil for erectile dysfunction and avoid concomitant use of sildenafil for pulmonary hypertension; plasma concentration of sildenafil increased by ITRACONAZOLE—reduce initial dose of sildenafil
- Antivirals: plasma concentration of sildenafil reduced by ETRAVIRINE; plasma concentration of sildenafil possibly increased by FOSAMPRENAVIR; plasma concentration of sildenafil increased by • INDINAVIR—reduce initial dose of sildenafil; plasma concentration of sildenafil significantly increased by • RITONAVIR—avoid concomitant use of sildenafil for pulmonary arterial hypertension or reduce dose of sildenafil for erectile dysfunction (consult sildenafil product literature); increased risk of ventricular arrhythmias when sildenafil given with • SAQUINAVIR—avoid concomitant use; avoidance of sildenafil advised by manufacturer of • TELAPREVIR; avoidance of sildenafil for pulmonary arterial hypertension advised by manufacturer of TIPRANAVIR
- Bosentan: plasma concentration of sildenafil reduced by BOSENTAN, also plasma concentration of bosentan increased
- Calcium-channel Blockers: enhanced hypotensive effect when sildenafil given with AMLODIPINE
- Cobicistat: plasma concentration of sildenafil possibly increased by • COBICISTAT—manufacturer of cobicistat advises avoid concomitant use of sildenafil for pulmonary arterial hypertension or reduce dose of sildenafil for erectile dysfunction—consult cobicistat product literature
- Cytotoxics: avoidance of sildenafil for pulmonary arterial hypertension advised by manufacturer of IDELALISIB
- Dapoxetine: avoidance of sildenafil advised by manufacturer of DAPOXETINE
- Grapefruit Juice: plasma concentration of sildenafil possibly increased by GRAPEFRUIT JUICE
- Nicorandil: sildenafil significantly enhances hypotensive effect of • NICORANDIL (avoid concomitant use)
- Nitrates: sildenafil significantly enhances hypotensive effect of • NITRATES (avoid concomitant use)
- Riociguat: enhanced hypotensive effect when sildenafil given with • RIOCIGUAT—avoid concomitant use
- Ulcer-healing Drugs: plasma concentration of sildenafil increased by CIMETIDINE—consider reducing dose of sildenafil for erectile dysfunction

Siltuximab
- Antipsychotics: avoid concomitant use of cytotoxics with • CLOZAPINE (increased risk of agranulocytosis)
- Vaccines: risk of generalised infections when monoclonal antibodies given with live • VACCINES—avoid concomitant use

Simeprevir
- Anti-arrhythmics: possible increased risk of bradycardia when simeprevir (with sofosbuvir) given with • AMIODARONE—see under Amiodarone, p. 94
- Antibacterials: plasma concentration of simeprevir possibly increased by • CLARITHROMYCIN and • TELITHROMYCIN— manufacturer of simeprevir advises avoid concomitant use; plasma concentration of both drugs increased when simeprevir given with • ERYTHROMYCIN—manufacturer of simeprevir advises avoid concomitant use; plasma concentration of simeprevir possibly reduced by RIFABUTIN— manufacturer of simeprevir advises avoid concomitant use; plasma concentration of simeprevir reduced by • RIFAMPICIN— manufacturer of simeprevir advises avoid concomitant use

Simeprevir (continued)
- Antidepressants: plasma concentration of simeprevir possibly reduced by • ST JOHN'S WORT—manufacturer of simeprevir advises avoid concomitant use
- Antiepileptics: plasma concentration of simeprevir possibly reduced by • CARBAMAZEPINE, • FOSPHENYTOIN, • OXCARBAZEPINE, • PHENOBARBITAL, • PHENYTOIN and • PRIMIDONE—manufacturer of simeprevir advises avoid concomitant use
- Antifungals: manufacturer of simeprevir advises avoid concomitant use with • KETOCONAZOLE; plasma concentration of simeprevir possibly increased by • FLUCONAZOLE, • ITRACONAZOLE, • POSACONAZOLE and • VORICONAZOLE—manufacturer of simeprevir advises avoid concomitant use
- Antivirals: plasma concentration of both drugs increased when simeprevir given with • DARUNAVIR—manufacturer of simeprevir advises avoid concomitant use; plasma concentration of simeprevir reduced by EFAVIRENZ; manufacturer of simeprevir advises avoid concomitant use with ETRAVIRINE; plasma concentration of both drugs increased when simeprevir given with LEDIPASVIR—manufacturer of ledipasvir advises avoid concomitant use; plasma concentration of simeprevir possibly reduced by • NEVIRAPINE—manufacturer of simeprevir advises avoid concomitant use; plasma concentration of simeprevir increased by • RITONAVIR—manufacturer of simeprevir advises avoid concomitant use
▸ Anxiolytics and Hypnotics: simeprevir increases plasma concentration of *oral* MIDAZOLAM
- Cardiac Glycosides: simeprevir increases plasma concentration of DIGOXIN
- Cobicistat: plasma concentration of simeprevir possibly increased by • COBICISTAT—manufacturer of simeprevir advises avoid concomitant use
▸ Corticosteroids: plasma concentration of simeprevir possibly reduced by DEXAMETHASONE—manufacturer of simeprevir advises avoid concomitant use
▸ Lipid-regulating Drugs: simeprevir increases plasma concentration of ATORVASTATIN, ROSUVASTATIN and SIMVASTATIN (consider reducing dose of atorvastatin, rosuvastatin and simvastatin)

Simvastatin *see* Statins
Sirolimus
▸ Anti-arrhythmics: caution with sirolimus advised by manufacturer of DRONEDARONE
- Antibacterials: plasma concentration of sirolimus increased by • CLARITHROMYCIN and • TELITHROMYCIN—avoid concomitant use; plasma concentration of both drugs increased when sirolimus given with • ERYTHROMYCIN; plasma concentration of sirolimus reduced by • RIFABUTIN and • RIFAMPICIN—avoid concomitant use
- Antifungals: plasma concentration of sirolimus increased by • ITRACONAZOLE, • KETOCONAZOLE and • VORICONAZOLE—avoid concomitant use; plasma concentration of sirolimus increased by MICAFUNGIN and • MICONAZOLE; plasma concentration of sirolimus possibly increased by FLUCONAZOLE and POSACONAZOLE
- Antivirals: plasma concentration of sirolimus possibly increased by • ATAZANAVIR and LOPINAVIR; plasma concentration of sirolimus increased by • BOCEPREVIR (increased risk of toxicity—reduce sirolimus dose); plasma concentration of both drugs increased when sirolimus given with • TELAPREVIR (reduce dose of sirolimus)
- Calcium-channel Blockers: plasma concentration of sirolimus possibly increased by NICARDIPINE; plasma concentration of sirolimus increased by • DILTIAZEM; plasma concentration of both drugs increased when sirolimus given with • VERAPAMIL
- Ciclosporin: plasma concentration of sirolimus increased by CICLOSPORIN
- Cytotoxics: caution with sirolimus advised by manufacturer of • CRIZOTINIB
- Grapefruit Juice: plasma concentration of sirolimus increased by • GRAPEFRUIT JUICE—avoid concomitant use

Sitagliptin *see* Antidiabetics
Smallpox Vaccine *see* Vaccines

Sodium Aurothiomalate
- ACE Inhibitors: flushing and hypotension reported when sodium aurothiomalate given with • ACE INHIBITORS
- Penicillamine: increased risk of haematological toxicity when sodium aurothiomalate given with • PENICILLAMINE—see under Penicillamine, p. 952)

Sodium Benzoate
▸ Antiepileptics: effects of sodium benzoate possibly reduced by SODIUM VALPROATE and VALPROIC ACID
▸ Antipsychotics: effects of sodium benzoate possibly reduced by HALOPERIDOL
▸ Corticosteroids: effects of sodium benzoate possibly reduced by CORTICOSTEROIDS

Sodium Bicarbonate *see* Antacids
Sodium Citrate
▸ Antibacterials: avoid concomitant use of sodium citrate with METHENAMINE
▸ Ulcer-healing Drugs: avoidance of sodium citrate advised by manufacturer of SUCRALFATE

Sodium Clodronate *see* Bisphosphonates
Sodium Feredetate *see* Iron salts
Sodium Nitroprusside *see* Vasodilator Antihypertensives
Sodium Oxybate
- Analgesics: effects of sodium oxybate enhanced by • OPIOID ANALGESICS (avoid concomitant use)
▸ Antidepressants: increased risk of side-effects when sodium oxybate given with TRICYCLICS
- Antiepileptics: manufacturer of sodium oxybate advises avoid concomitant use with PHENOBARBITAL and PRIMIDONE; plasma concentration of sodium oxybate increased by • SODIUM VALPROATE and • VALPROIC ACID (see under Sodium Oxybate, p. 447)
▸ Antipsychotics: effects of sodium oxybate possibly enhanced by ANTIPSYCHOTICS
- Anxiolytics and Hypnotics: effects of sodium oxybate enhanced by • BENZODIAZEPINES (avoid concomitant use)

Sodium Phenylbutyrate
▸ Antiepileptics: effects of sodium phenylbutyrate possibly reduced by SODIUM VALPROATE and VALPROIC ACID
▸ Antipsychotics: effects of sodium phenylbutyrate possibly reduced by HALOPERIDOL
▸ Corticosteroids: effects of sodium phenylbutyrate possibly reduced by CORTICOSTEROIDS

Sodium Stibogluconate
- Antifungals: possible increased risk of arrhythmias when sodium stibogluconate given before • AMPHOTERICIN—manufacturer of sodium stibogluconate advises giving 14 days apart

Sodium Valproate
▸ Analgesics: effects of sodium valproate enhanced by ASPIRIN
- Antibacterials: metabolism of sodium valproate possibly inhibited by ERYTHROMYCIN (increased plasma concentration); avoidance of sodium valproate advised by manufacturer of • PIVMECILLINAM; plasma concentration of sodium valproate reduced by • CARBAPENEMS—avoid concomitant use
▸ Anticoagulants: sodium valproate possibly enhances anticoagulant effect of COUMARINS
- Antidepressants: anticonvulsant effect of antiepileptics possibly antagonised by MAOIs and • TRICYCLIC-RELATED ANTIDEPRESSANTS (convulsive threshold lowered); anticonvulsant effect of antiepileptics antagonised by • SSRIS and • TRICYCLICS (convulsive threshold lowered)
- Antiepileptics: plasma concentration of sodium valproate reduced by CARBAMAZEPINE, also plasma concentration of active metabolite of carbamazepine increased; sodium valproate possibly increases plasma concentration of ETHOSUXIMIDE; sodium valproate increases or possibly decreases plasma concentration of FOSPHENYTOIN and PHENYTOIN, also plasma concentration of sodium valproate reduced; sodium valproate increases plasma concentration of • LAMOTRIGINE (increased risk of toxicity—reduce lamotrigine dose); sodium valproate sometimes reduces plasma concentration of an active metabolite of OXCARBAZEPINE; sodium valproate increases plasma concentration of PHENOBARBITAL and PRIMIDONE (also plasma concentration of sodium valproate reduced); sodium valproate possibly

Sodium Valproate

- Antiepileptics (continued)
  increases plasma concentration of RUFINAMIDE (reduce dose of rufinamide); hyperammonaemia and CNS toxicity reported when sodium valproate given with ● TOPIRAMATE
- Antimalarials: anticonvulsant effect of antiepileptics antagonised by ● MEFLOQUINE
- Antipsychotics: anticonvulsant effect of antiepileptics antagonised by ● ANTIPSYCHOTICS (convulsive threshold lowered); sodium valproate possibly increases or decreases plasma concentration of CLOZAPINE; increased risk of side-effects including neutropenia when sodium valproate given with ● OLANZAPINE
- Antivirals: plasma concentration of sodium valproate possibly reduced by RITONAVIR; sodium valproate possibly increases plasma concentration of ZIDOVUDINE (increased risk of toxicity)
- Anxiolytics and Hypnotics: plasma concentration of sodium valproate possibly increased by CLOBAZAM; increased risk of side-effects when sodium valproate given with CLONAZEPAM; sodium valproate possibly increases plasma concentration of DIAZEPAM and LORAZEPAM
- Bupropion: sodium valproate inhibits the metabolism of BUPROPION
- Cytotoxics: sodium valproate increases plasma concentration of TEMOZOLOMIDE
- Guanfacine: plasma concentration of sodium valproate increased by GUANFACINE
- Lipid-regulating Drugs: absorption of sodium valproate possibly reduced by COLESTYRAMINE
- Oestrogens: plasma concentration of sodium valproate possibly reduced by ETHINYLESTRADIOL
- Orlistat: possible increased risk of convulsions when antiepileptics given with ● ORLISTAT
- Sodium Benzoate: sodium valproate possibly reduces effects of SODIUM BENZOATE
- Sodium Oxybate: sodium valproate increases the plasma concentration of ● SODIUM OXYBATE (see under Sodium Oxybate, p. 447)
- Sodium Phenylbutyrate: sodium valproate possibly reduces effects of SODIUM PHENYLBUTYRATE
- Ulcer-healing Drugs: metabolism of sodium valproate inhibited by ● CIMETIDINE (increased plasma concentration)

Sofosbuvir

- Anti-arrhythmics: possible increased risk of bradycardia when sofosbuvir given with ● AMIODARONE—see under Amiodarone, p. 94
- Antibacterials: manufacturer of sofosbuvir advises avoid concomitant use with RIFABUTIN and RIFAMPICIN
- Antidepressants: manufacturer of sofosbuvir advises avoid concomitant use with ST JOHN'S WORT
- Antiepileptics: manufacturer of sofosbuvir advises avoid concomitant use with CARBAMAZEPINE, FOSPHENYTOIN, OXCARBAZEPINE, PHENOBARBITAL, PHENYTOIN and PRIMIDONE

Solifenacin see Antimuscarinics

Somatropin

- Corticosteroids: growth-promoting effect of somatropin may be inhibited by CORTICOSTEROIDS
- Oestrogens: increased doses of somatropin may be needed when given with OESTROGENS (when used as oral replacement therapy)

Sorafenib

- Antibacterials: bioavailability of sorafenib reduced by NEOMYCIN; plasma concentration of sorafenib reduced by RIFAMPICIN
- Anticoagulants: sorafenib possibly enhances anticoagulant effect of ● COUMARINS
- Antipsychotics: avoid concomitant use of cytotoxics with ● CLOZAPINE (increased risk of agranulocytosis)
- Antivirals: avoidance of sorafenib advised by manufacturer of ● BOCEPREVIR
- Cytotoxics: sorafenib increases plasma concentration of DOCETAXEL and DOXORUBICIN; sorafenib possibly increases plasma concentration of IRINOTECAN

Sotalol see Beta-blockers

Spironolactone see Diuretics

Statins

- Antacids: absorption of rosuvastatin reduced by ANTACIDS
- Anti-arrhythmics: increased risk of myopathy when simvastatin given with ● AMIODARONE (see under Simvastatin, p. 188); plasma concentration of rosuvastatin increased by ● DRONEDARONE—adjust dose of rosuvastatin (consult product literature); increased risk of myopathy when simvastatin given with ● DRONEDARONE; plasma concentration of atorvastatin possibly increased by DRONEDARONE
- Antibacterials: possible increased risk of myopathy when atorvastatin or simvastatin given with ● AZITHROMYCIN; plasma concentration of atorvastatin and pravastatin increased by ● CLARITHROMYCIN; increased risk of myopathy when simvastatin given with ● CLARITHROMYCIN, ● ERYTHROMYCIN or ● TELITHROMYCIN (avoid concomitant use); plasma concentration of rosuvastatin reduced by ERYTHROMYCIN; possible increased risk of myopathy when atorvastatin given with ERYTHROMYCIN; plasma concentration of pravastatin increased by ERYTHROMYCIN; plasma concentration of atorvastatin and simvastatin possibly reduced by RIFAMPICIN; metabolism of fluvastatin accelerated by RIFAMPICIN (reduced effect); increased risk of myopathy when statins given with ● DAPTOMYCIN (preferably avoid concomitant use); risk of myopathy and rhabdomyolysis when statins given with ● FUSIDIC ACID—avoid concomitant use and for 7 days after last fusidic acid dose; possible increased risk of myopathy when pravastatin given with TELITHROMYCIN; increased risk of myopathy when atorvastatin given with ● TELITHROMYCIN (avoid concomitant use)
- Anticoagulants: atorvastatin may transiently reduce anticoagulant effect of WARFARIN; rosuvastatin possibly enhances anticoagulant effect of ● COUMARINS and ● PHENINDIONE; simvastatin can enhance the anticoagulant effect of COUMARINS; fluvastatin enhances anticoagulant effect of ● COUMARINS
- Antidepressants: plasma concentration of simvastatin reduced by ST JOHN'S WORT
- Antidiabetics: fluvastatin possibly increases plasma concentration of GLIBENCLAMIDE
- Antiepileptics: plasma concentration of simvastatin reduced by ● CARBAMAZEPINE and ESLICARBAZEPINE—consider increasing dose of simvastatin; plasma concentration of rosuvastatin reduced by ESLICARBAZEPINE; combination of fluvastatin with FOSPHENYTOIN or PHENYTOIN may increase plasma concentration of either drug (or both)
- Antifungals: possible increased risk of myopathy when atorvastatin given with ● KETOCONAZOLE—manufacturer of ketoconazole advises avoid concomitant use; increased risk of myopathy when simvastatin given with ● ITRACONAZOLE, ● KETOCONAZOLE or ● POSACONAZOLE (avoid concomitant use); possible increased risk of myopathy when simvastatin given with ● FLUCONAZOLE or ● MICONAZOLE; possible increased risk of myopathy when atorvastatin given with ● FLUCONAZOLE or IMIDAZOLES; plasma concentration of fluvastatin increased by FLUCONAZOLE—possible increased risk of myopathy; plasma concentration of rosuvastatin increased by ● ITRACONAZOLE—adjust dose of rosuvastatin (consult product literature); increased risk of myopathy when atorvastatin given with ● ITRACONAZOLE, ● POSACONAZOLE or ● VORICONAZOLE; increased risk of myopathy when simvastatin given with ● VORICONAZOLE
- Antivirals: increased risk of myopathy when simvastatin given with ● ATAZANAVIR, ● INDINAVIR, ● RITONAVIR or ● SAQUINAVIR (avoid concomitant use); possible increased risk of myopathy when atorvastatin or pravastatin given with ● ATAZANAVIR; plasma concentration of rosuvastatin increased by ● ATAZANAVIR, ● DARUNAVIR, ● LOPINAVIR and ● TIPRANAVIR—adjust dose of rosuvastatin (consult product literature); plasma concentration of pravastatin increased by BOCEPREVIR; plasma concentration of atorvastatin increased by BOCEPREVIR (reduce dose of atorvastatin); manufacturers advise avoid concomitant use of simvastatin with ● BOCEPREVIR and ● TELAPREVIR; plasma concentration of rosuvastatin increased by DACLATASVIR; plasma concentration of pravastatin possibly increased by DARUNAVIR (use lowest possible dose of pravastatin); possible increased risk of myopathy when atorvastatin given with DARUNAVIR, FOSAMPRENAVIR,

Statins

- **Antivirals** (continued)

  INDINAVIR, LOPINAVIR or SAQUINAVIR; plasma concentration of rosuvastatin increased by ● DASABUVIR and ● PARITAPREVIR (reduce dose of rosuvastatin—see under Rosuvastatin, p. 188); avoidance of atorvastatin advised by manufacturer of ● DASABUVIR; plasma concentration of atorvastatin, pravastatin and simvastatin reduced by EFAVIRENZ; plasma concentration of atorvastatin possibly reduced by ETRAVIRINE; possible increased risk of myopathy when rosuvastatin given with ● FOSAMPRENAVIR, ● INDINAVIR, ● RITONAVIR and ● SAQUINAVIR—manufacturer of rosuvastatin advises avoid concomitant use; possible increased risk of myopathy when simvastatin given with ● FOSAMPRENAVIR or ● LOPINAVIR—avoid concomitant use; possible increased risk of myopathy when atorvastatin, fluvastatin and simvastatin given with ● LEDIPASVIR—manufacturer of ledipasvir advises consider reducing dose of atorvastatin, fluvastatin and simvastatin; avoidance of rosuvastatin advised by manufacturer of ● LEDIPASVIR; avoidance of atorvastatin and simvastatin advised by manufacturer of ● OMBITASVIR; plasma concentration of pravastatin increased by ● PARITAPREVIR (reduce dose of pravastatin); avoidance of atorvastatin, fluvastatin and simvastatin advised by manufacturer of ● PARITAPREVIR; plasma concentration of atorvastatin possibly increased by RITONAVIR (use lowest possible dose of atorvastatin); plasma concentration of atorvastatin, rosuvastatin and simvastatin increased by SIMEPREVIR (consider reducing dose of atorvastatin, rosuvastatin and simvastatin); avoidance of atorvastatin advised by manufacturer of ● TELAPREVIR; increased risk of myopathy when atorvastatin given with ● TIPRANAVIR (see under Atorvastatin, p. 186); plasma concentration of simvastatin possibly increased by ● TIPRANAVIR—avoid concomitant use

- **Anxiolytics and Hypnotics:** atorvastatin increases plasma concentration of *intravenous* MIDAZOLAM

- **Bosentan:** plasma concentration of simvastatin reduced by BOSENTAN

- **Calcium-channel Blockers:** possible increased risk of myopathy when simvastatin given with ● AMLODIPINE and ● DILTIAZEM (see under Simvastatin, p. 188); plasma concentration of atorvastatin increased by DILTIAZEM—possible increased risk of myopathy; atorvastatin increases plasma concentration of ● VERAPAMIL, also possible increased risk of myopathy (consider reducing dose of atorvastatin); increased risk of myopathy when simvastatin given with ● VERAPAMIL (see under Simvastatin, p. 188)

- **Cardiac Glycosides:** atorvastatin possibly increases plasma concentration of DIGOXIN

- **Ciclosporin:** increased risk of myopathy when rosuvastatin or simvastatin given with ● CICLOSPORIN (avoid concomitant use); increased risk of myopathy when atorvastatin given with ● CICLOSPORIN (see under Atorvastatin, p. 186); increased risk of myopathy when fluvastatin or pravastatin given with ● CICLOSPORIN

- **Clopidogrel:** plasma concentration of rosuvastatin increased by ● CLOPIDOGREL—adjust dose of rosuvastatin (consult product literature)

- **Cobicistat:** plasma concentration of atorvastatin possibly increased by COBICISTAT—manufacturer of cobicistat advises reduce dose of atorvastatin; avoidance of simvastatin advised by manufacturer of ● COBICISTAT

- **Colchicine:** possible increased risk of myopathy when statins given with ● COLCHICINE

- **Cytotoxics:** plasma concentration of simvastatin possibly increased by DASATINIB; avoidance of simvastatin advised by manufacturer of IDELALISIB; plasma concentration of simvastatin increased by IMATINIB

- **Eltrombopag:** plasma concentration of rosuvastatin increased by ● ELTROMBOPAG—adjust dose of rosuvastatin (consult product literature)

- **Grapefruit Juice:** plasma concentration of atorvastatin possibly increased by GRAPEFRUIT JUICE; plasma concentration of simvastatin increased by GRAPEFRUIT JUICE—avoid concomitant use

Statins (continued)

- **Hormone Antagonists:** possible increased risk of myopathy when simvastatin given with ● DANAZOL—avoid concomitant use

- **Lipid-regulating Drugs:** possible increased risk of myopathy when simvastatin given with ● BEZAFIBRATE (see under Simvastatin, p. 188); possible increased risk of myopathy when simvastatin given with ● CIPROFIBRATE (see under Simvastatin, p. 188); when given with statins reduce maximum dose of FENOFIBRATE—see under Fenofibrate, p. 183; increased risk of myopathy when atorvastatin, fluvastatin or pravastatin given with ● GEMFIBROZIL (preferably avoid concomitant use); increased risk of myopathy when simvastatin given with ● GEMFIBROZIL (avoid concomitant use); plasma concentration of rosuvastatin increased by ● EZETIMIBE—adjust dose of rosuvastatin (consult product literature); increased risk of myopathy when statins given with ● FIBRATES; increased risk of myopathy when rosuvastatin given with ● FIBRATES (see under Rosuvastatin, p. 188); plasma concentration of simvastatin increased by ● LOMITAPIDE (see under Simvastatin, p. 188); plasma concentration of atorvastatin increased by LOMITAPIDE—manufacturer of lomitapide advises reduce dose of atorvastatin by half or separate administration by 12 hours; increased risk of myopathy when statins given with ● NICOTINIC ACID (applies to lipid regulating doses of nicotinic acid)

- **Oestrogens:** atorvastatin and rosuvastatin increase plasma concentration of ETHINYLESTRADIOL

- **Progestogens:** atorvastatin increases plasma concentration of NORETHISTERONE; rosuvastatin increases plasma concentration of active metabolite of NORGESTIMATE; rosuvastatin increases plasma concentration of NORGESTREL

- **Ranolazine:** plasma concentration of simvastatin increased by ● RANOLAZINE (see under Simvastatin, p. 188)

- **Retinoids:** plasma concentration of simvastatin reduced by ALITRETINOIN

- **Sacubitril:** plasma concentration of atorvastatin increased by SACUBITRIL

- **Teriflunomide:** plasma concentration of rosuvastatin increased by ● TERIFLUNOMIDE (consider reducing dose of rosuvastatin)

- **Ticagrelor:** plasma concentration of simvastatin increased by ● TICAGRELOR (increased risk of toxicity)

Stavudine

- **Antivirals:** increased risk of side-effects when stavudine given with ● DIDANOSINE; increased risk of toxicity when stavudine given with ● RIBAVIRIN; effects of stavudine possibly inhibited by ● ZIDOVUDINE (manufacturers advise avoid concomitant use)

- **Cytotoxics:** effects of stavudine possibly inhibited by DOXORUBICIN; increased risk of toxicity when stavudine given with ● HYDROXYCARBAMIDE—avoid concomitant use

- **Orlistat:** absorption of stavudine possibly reduced by ● ORLISTAT

Stiripentol

- **Antidepressants:** anticonvulsant effect of antiepileptics possibly antagonised by MAOIs and ● TRICYCLIC-RELATED ANTIDEPRESSANTS (convulsive threshold lowered); anticonvulsant effect of antiepileptics antagonised by ● SSRIS and ● TRICYCLICS (convulsive threshold lowered)

- **Antiepileptics:** stiripentol increases plasma concentration of ● CARBAMAZEPINE, ● FOSPHENYTOIN, ● PHENOBARBITAL, ● PHENYTOIN and ● PRIMIDONE

- **Antimalarials:** anticonvulsant effect of antiepileptics antagonised by ● MEFLOQUINE

- **Antipsychotics:** anticonvulsant effect of antiepileptics antagonised by ● ANTIPSYCHOTICS (convulsive threshold lowered)

- **Anxiolytics and Hypnotics:** stiripentol increases plasma concentration of CLOBAZAM

- **Orlistat:** possible increased risk of convulsions when antiepileptics given with ● ORLISTAT

Streptomycin see Aminoglycosides

Strontium Ranelate
▸ Antibacterials: strontium ranelate reduces absorption of QUINOLONES and TETRACYCLINES (manufacturer of strontium ranelate advises avoid concomitant use)

Sucralfate
▸ Aminophylline: sucralfate possibly reduces absorption of AMINOPHYLLINE (give at least 2 hours apart)
▸ Antibacterials: sucralfate reduces absorption of CIPROFLOXACIN (give at least 2 hours before or 4 hours after ciprofloxacin); sucralfate reduces absorption of LEVOFLOXACIN, NORFLOXACIN and OFLOXACIN (give at least 2 hours apart); sucralfate reduces absorption of MOXIFLOXACIN (give at least 6 hours apart); sucralfate reduces absorption of TETRACYCLINES
● Anticoagulants: sucralfate possibly reduces absorption of ● COUMARINS (reduced anticoagulant effect)
● Antiepileptics: sucralfate reduces absorption of ● FOSPHENYTOIN and ● PHENYTOIN
▸ Antifungals: sucralfate reduces absorption of KETOCONAZOLE
▸ Antipsychotics: sucralfate reduces absorption of SULPIRIDE
▸ Cardiac Glycosides: sucralfate possibly reduces absorption of CARDIAC GLYCOSIDES
▸ Potassium Salts: manufacturer of sucralfate advises avoid concomitant use with POTASSIUM CITRATE
▸ Sodium Citrate: manufacturer of sucralfate advises avoid concomitant use with SODIUM CITRATE
▸ Theophylline: sucralfate possibly reduces absorption of THEOPHYLLINE (give at least 2 hours apart)
▸ Thyroid Hormones: sucralfate reduces absorption of LEVOTHYROXINE
▸ Ulcer-healing Drugs: sucralfate possibly reduces absorption of LANSOPRAZOLE

Sucroferric Oxyhydroxide see Iron Salts

Sugammadex
▸ Antibacterials: response to sugammadex possibly reduced by FUSIDIC ACID
▸ Progestogens: sugammadex possibly reduces plasma concentration of PROGESTOGENS—manufacturer of sugammadex advises additional contraceptive precautions

Sulfadiazine see Sulfonamides

Sulfadoxine see Sulfonamides

Sulfamethoxazole see Sulfonamides

Sulfasalazine
▸ Cardiac Glycosides: sulfasalazine possibly reduces absorption of DIGOXIN
▸ Folates: sulfasalazine possibly reduces absorption of FOLIC ACID

Sulfinpyrazone
▸ Aminophylline: sulfinpyrazone reduces plasma concentration of AMINOPHYLLINE
▸ Analgesics: effects of sulfinpyrazone antagonised by ASPIRIN
▸ Antibacterials: sulfinpyrazone reduces excretion of NITROFURANTOIN (increased risk of toxicity); sulfinpyrazone reduces excretion of PENICILLINS; effects of sulfinpyrazone antagonised by PYRAZINAMIDE
● Anticoagulants: increased risk of bleeding when sulfinpyrazone given with APIXABAN; sulfinpyrazone enhances anticoagulant effect of ● COUMARINS; possible increased risk of bleeding when sulfinpyrazone given with ● DABIGATRAN
● Antidiabetics: sulfinpyrazone enhances effects of ● SULFONYLUREAS
● Antiepileptics: sulfinpyrazone increases plasma concentration of ● FOSPHENYTOIN and ● PHENYTOIN
▸ Calcium-channel Blockers: sulfinpyrazone reduces plasma concentration of VERAPAMIL
▸ Ciclosporin: sulfinpyrazone reduces plasma concentration of ● CICLOSPORIN
▸ Theophylline: sulfinpyrazone reduces plasma concentration of THEOPHYLLINE

Sulfonamides
▸ Anaesthetics, General: sulfonamides enhance effects of THIOPENTAL
● Anaesthetics, Local: effects of sulfonamides possibly inhibited by ● CHLOROPROCAINE (manufacturer of chloroprocaine advises avoid concomitant use); increased risk of methaemoglobinaemia when sulfonamides given with PRILOCAINE

Sulfonamides (continued)
▸ Anti-arrhythmics: possible increased risk of ventricular arrhythmias when sulfamethoxazole (as co-trimoxazole) given with AMIODARONE—manufacturer of amiodarone advises avoid concomitant use of co-trimoxazole
● Antibacterials: increased risk of crystalluria when sulfonamides given with ● METHENAMINE
● Anticoagulants: sulfonamides enhance anticoagulant effect of ● COUMARINS; sulfonamides possibly inhibit metabolism of PHENINDIONE
▸ Antidiabetics: sulfonamides rarely enhance the effects of SULFONYLUREAS
▸ Antiepileptics: sulfonamides possibly increase plasma concentration of FOSPHENYTOIN and PHENYTOIN
● Antimalarials: increased antifolate effect when sulfonamides given with ● PYRIMETHAMINE
● Antipsychotics: avoid concomitant use of sulfonamides with ● CLOZAPINE (increased risk of agranulocytosis)
● Azathioprine: increased risk of haematological toxicity when sulfamethoxazole (as co-trimoxazole) given with ● AZATHIOPRINE
● Ciclosporin: increased risk of nephrotoxicity when sulfonamides given with ● CICLOSPORIN; sulfadiazine possibly reduces plasma concentration of ● CICLOSPORIN
● Cytotoxics: increased risk of haematological toxicity when sulfamethoxazole (as co-trimoxazole) given with ● MERCAPTOPURINE; sulfonamides increase risk of METHOTREXATE toxicity; increased risk of severe bone marrow depression (fatalities reported) and other haematological toxicites when sulfamethoxazole (as co-trimoxazole) given with ● METHOTREXATE
▸ Potassium Aminobenzoate: effects of sulfonamides inhibited by POTASSIUM AMINOBENZOATE
● Tacrolimus: possible increased risk of nephrotoxicity when sulfamethoxazole given with ● TACROLIMUS
▸ Vaccines: antibacterials inactivate ORAL TYPHOID VACCINE—see under Typhoid Vaccine in BNF

Sulfonylureas see Antidiabetics

Sulindac see NSAIDs

Sulpiride see Antipsychotics

Sumatriptan see 5HT$_1$-receptor Agonists (under HT)

Sunitinib
▸ Antibacterials: metabolism of sunitinib accelerated by RIFAMPICIN (reduced plasma concentration)
▸ Antifungals: metabolism of sunitinib inhibited by KETOCONAZOLE (increased plasma concentration)
● Antipsychotics: avoid concomitant use of cytotoxics with ● CLOZAPINE (increased risk of agranulocytosis)
● Antivirals: avoidance of sunitinib advised by manufacturer of ● BOCEPREVIR

Suxamethonium see Muscle Relaxants

Sympathomimetics
● Adrenergic Neurone Blockers: ephedrine, isometheptene, metaraminol, methylphenidate, noradrenaline (norepinephrine), oxymetazoline, phenylephrine, pseudoephedrine and xylometazoline antagonise hypotensive effect of ● ADRENERGIC NEURONE BLOCKERS; manufacturer of midodrine advises avoid concomitant use with GUANETHIDINE; dexamfetamine and lisdexamfetamine antagonise hypotensive effect of ● GUANETHIDINE; increased risk of hypertension when adrenaline (epinephrine) given with ● GUANETHIDINE
▸ Alcohol: effects of methylphenidate possibly enhanced by ALCOHOL
▸ Alpha$_2$-adrenoceptor Stimulants: avoidance of sympathomimetics advised by manufacturer of APRACLONIDINE
● Alpha-blockers: effects of midodrine possibly antagonised by ALPHA-BLOCKERS; avoid concomitant use of adrenaline (epinephrine) or dopamine with ● TOLAZOLINE
▸ Aminophylline: avoidance of ephedrine in children advised by manufacturer of AMINOPHYLLINE
● Anaesthetics, General: avoidance of sympathomimetics advised by manufacturer of ● ISOFLURANE (risk of ventricular arrhythmias); increased risk of hypertension when methylphenidate given with ● VOLATILE LIQUID GENERAL ANAESTHETICS; increased risk of arrhythmias when adrenaline

Sympathomimetics

- Anaesthetics, General (continued)
  (epinephrine) or noradrenaline (norepinephrine) given with
  ● VOLATILE LIQUID GENERAL ANAESTHETICS
- Antacids: absorption of pseudoephedrine possibly increased by
  ALUMINIUM HYDROXIDE
- Anticoagulants: methylphenidate possibly enhances
  anticoagulant effect of ● COUMARINS
- Antidepressants: risk of hypertensive crisis when
  dexamfetamine, ephedrine, isometheptene,
  lisdexamfetamine, metaraminol, methylphenidate,
  phenylephrine or pseudoephedrine given with ● MAOIs, avoid
  dexamfetamine, ephedrine, isometheptene,
  lisdexamfetamine, metaraminol, methylphenidate,
  phenylephrine or pseudoephedrine for at least 2 weeks after
  stopping MAOIs; manufacturer of midodrine advises avoid
  concomitant use with MAOIs and TRICYCLICS; risk of
  hypertensive crisis when adrenaline (epinephrine),
  dobutamine, dopamine, noradrenaline (norepinephrine) or
  xylometazoline given with ● MAOIs; risk of hypertensive crisis
  when oxymetazoline given with ● MAOIs, some manufacturers
  advise avoid oxymetazoline for at least 2 weeks after stopping
  MAOIs; risk of hypertensive crisis when sympathomimetics
  given with ● MOCLOBEMIDE; methylphenidate possibly inhibits
  metabolism of SSRIs and TRICYCLICS; increased risk of
  hypertension and arrhythmias when noradrenaline
  (norepinephrine) or phenylephrine given with ● TRICYCLICS;
  increased risk of hypertension and arrhythmias when
  adrenaline (epinephrine) given with ● TRICYCLICS (but local
  anaesthetics with adrenaline appear to be safe)
- Antiepileptics: methylphenidate increases plasma
  concentration of FOSPHENYTOIN and PHENYTOIN;
  methylphenidate possibly increases plasma concentration of
  PHENOBARBITAL and PRIMIDONE
- Antihistamines: manufacturer of midodrine advises avoid
  concomitant use with ANTIHISTAMINES
- Antipsychotics: hypertensive effect of sympathomimetics
  antagonised by ANTIPSYCHOTICS; effects of lisdexamfetamine
  possibly reduced by CHLORPROMAZINE; dexamfetamine
  possibly antagonises antipsychotic effects of
  CHLORPROMAZINE; methylphenidate possibly increases side-
  effects of RISPERIDONE
- Antivirals: plasma concentration of dexamfetamine possibly
  increased by RITONAVIR
- Beta-blockers: increased risk of severe hypertension and
  bradycardia when adrenaline (epinephrine) given with non-
  cardioselective ● BETA-BLOCKERS, also response to adrenaline
  (epinephrine) may be reduced; increased risk of severe
  hypertension and bradycardia when dobutamine given with
  non-cardioselective ● BETA-BLOCKERS; possible increased risk
  of severe hypertension and bradycardia when noradrenaline
  (norepinephrine) given with non-cardioselective ● BETA-
  BLOCKERS
- Cardiac Glycosides: manufacturer of midodrine advises avoid
  concomitant use with DIGOXIN
- Clonidine: possible risk of hypertension when adrenaline
  (epinephrine) or noradrenaline (norepinephrine) given with
  CLONIDINE; serious adverse events reported with concomitant
  use of methylphenidate and ● CLONIDINE (causality not
  established)
- Corticosteroids: possible risk of hypertension when midodrine
  given with CORTICOSTEROIDS; ephedrine accelerates
  metabolism of DEXAMETHASONE
- Dopaminergics: risk of toxicity when isometheptene given with
  ● BROMOCRIPTINE; effects of adrenaline (epinephrine),
  dobutamine, dopamine and noradrenaline (norepinephrine)
  possibly enhanced by ENTACAPONE; avoid concomitant use of
  sympathomimetics with ● RASAGILINE; risk of hypertensive
  crisis when dopamine given with ● SELEGILINE; avoidance of
  sympathomimetics advised by manufacturer of SELEGILINE
- Doxapram: increased risk of hypertension when
  sympathomimetics given with DOXAPRAM
- Ergot Alkaloids: increased risk of ergotism when
  sympathomimetics given with ERGOT ALKALOIDS

- Oxytocin: risk of hypertension when vasoconstrictor
  sympathomimetics given with OXYTOCIN (due to enhanced
  vasopressor effect)
- Sympathomimetics: effects of adrenaline (epinephrine) possibly
  enhanced by ● DOPEXAMINE; dopexamine possibly enhances
  effects of ● NORADRENALINE (NOREPINEPHRINE)
- Theophylline: avoidance of ephedrine in children advised by
  manufacturer of THEOPHYLLINE
- Thyroid Hormones: manufacturer of midodrine advises avoid
  concomitant use with THYROID HORMONES
- Ulcer-healing Drugs: metabolism of dobutamine possibly
  inhibited by CIMETIDINE

Sympathomimetics, Beta$_2$

- Aminophylline: increased risk of hypokalaemia when high
  doses of beta$_2$ sympathomimetics given with AMINOPHYLLINE
- Antifungals: plasma concentration of olodaterol increased by
  KETOCONAZOLE; metabolism of salmeterol inhibited by
  ● KETOCONAZOLE (increased plasma concentration)
- Antivirals: plasma concentration of salmeterol possibly
  increased by ATAZANAVIR—manufacturer of atazanavir advises
  avoid concomitant use; avoidance of salmeterol advised by
  manufacturer of LOPINAVIR, RITONAVIR and TIPRANAVIR;
  avoidance of salmeterol advised by manufacturer of
  ● TELAPREVIR (risk of ventricular arrhythmias)
- Atomoxetine: increased risk of cardiovascular side-effects when
  parenteral salbutamol given with ATOMOXETINE
- Cardiac Glycosides: salbutamol possibly reduces plasma
  concentration of DIGOXIN
- Cobicistat: avoidance of salmeterol advised by manufacturer of
  COBICISTAT
- Corticosteroids: increased risk of hypokalaemia when high
  doses of beta$_2$ sympathomimetics given with CORTICOSTEROIDS
- Cytotoxics: avoidance of salmeterol advised by manufacturer of
  IDELALISIB
- Diuretics: increased risk of hypokalaemia when high doses of
  beta$_2$ sympathomimetics given with ACETAZOLAMIDE, LOOP
  DIURETICS or THIAZIDES AND RELATED DIURETICS
- Methyldopa: acute hypotension reported when *infusion* of
  salbutamol given with ● METHYLDOPA
- Muscle Relaxants: bambuterol enhances effects of
  SUXAMETHONIUM
- Theophylline: increased risk of hypokalaemia when high doses
  of beta$_2$ sympathomimetics given with THEOPHYLLINE

Tacrolimus

NOTE Interactions do not generally apply to tacrolimus used
topically; risk of facial flushing and skin irritation with topical
tacrolimus on consumption of alcohol

- Analgesics: possible increased risk of nephrotoxicity when
  tacrolimus given with NSAIDs; increased risk of nephrotoxicity
  when tacrolimus given with ● IBUPROFEN
- Angiotensin-II Receptor Antagonists: increased risk of
  hyperkalaemia when tacrolimus given with ANGIOTENSIN-II
  RECEPTOR ANTAGONISTS
- Anti-arrhythmics: plasma concentration of tacrolimus possibly
  increased by AMIODARONE; caution with tacrolimus advised by
  manufacturer of DRONEDARONE
- Antibacterials: plasma concentration of tacrolimus increased
  by ● CLARITHROMYCIN and ● ERYTHROMYCIN; plasma
  concentration of tacrolimus possibly reduced by RIFABUTIN;
  plasma concentration of tacrolimus reduced by ● RIFAMPICIN;
  possible increased risk of nephrotoxicity when tacrolimus
  given with ● SULFAMETHOXAZOLE, ● TRIMETHOPRIM or
  VANCOMYCIN; increased risk of nephrotoxicity when tacrolimus
  given with ● AMINOGLYCOSIDES; plasma concentration of
  tacrolimus possibly increased by ● CHLORAMPHENICOL and
  ● TELITHROMYCIN
- Anticoagulants: tacrolimus possibly increases plasma
  concentration of ● DABIGATRAN—manufacturer of dabigatran
  advises avoid concomitant use
- Antidepressants: plasma concentration of tacrolimus reduced
  by ● ST JOHN'S WORT—avoid concomitant use
- Antiepileptics: plasma concentration of tacrolimus reduced by
  FOSPHENYTOIN and PHENYTOIN, also plasma concentration of
  fosphenytoin and phenytoin possibly increased; plasma

Tacrolimus

- **Antiepileptics** (continued)
  concentration of tacrolimus reduced by • PHENOBARBITAL and
  • PRIMIDONE
- **Antifungals:** plasma concentration of tacrolimus increased by
  • FLUCONAZOLE, • ITRACONAZOLE, • KETOCONAZOLE,
  • POSACONAZOLE and • VORICONAZOLE (consider reducing dose
  of tacrolimus); plasma concentration of tacrolimus possibly
  increased by • MICONAZOLE *oral gel*; increased risk of
  nephrotoxicity when tacrolimus given with • AMPHOTERICIN;
  plasma concentration of tacrolimus reduced by • CASPOFUNGIN
- **Antipsychotics:** avoidance of tacrolimus advised by
  manufacturer of • DROPERIDOL (risk of ventricular
  arrhythmias)
- **Antivirals:** possible increased risk of nephrotoxicity when
  tacrolimus given with ACICLOVIR, GANCICLOVIR, VALACICLOVIR or
  VALGANCICLOVIR; plasma concentration of tacrolimus possibly
  increased by • ATAZANAVIR and • RITONAVIR; plasma
  concentration of tacrolimus increased by • BOCEPREVIR
  (reduce dose of tacrolimus); plasma concentration of
  tacrolimus possibly affected by • EFAVIRENZ; plasma
  concentration of tacrolimus increased by • FOSAMPRENAVIR;
  plasma concentration of tacrolimus increased by • SAQUINAVIR
  (consider reducing dose of tacrolimus); plasma concentration
  of both drugs increased when tacrolimus given with
  • TELAPREVIR (reduce dose of tacrolimus)
- **Calcium-channel Blockers:** plasma concentration of tacrolimus
  possibly increased by FELODIPINE and VERAPAMIL; plasma
  concentration of tacrolimus increased by • DILTIAZEM,
  NICARDIPINE and • NIFEDIPINE
- **Ciclosporin:** tacrolimus increases plasma concentration of
  • CICLOSPORIN (increased risk of nephrotoxicity)—avoid
  concomitant use
- **Cytotoxics:** tacrolimus possibly increases the plasma
  concentration of AFATINIB—manufacturer of afatinib advises
  separating administration of tacrolimus by 6 to 12 hours;
  caution with tacrolimus advised by manufacturer of
  • CRIZOTINIB; plasma concentration of tacrolimus increased by
  IMATINIB
- Dexrazoxane: increased risk of immunosupression with
  tacrolimus advised by manufacturer of DEXRAZOXANE
- **Diuretics:** increased risk of hyperkalaemia when tacrolimus
  given with • POTASSIUM-SPARING DIURETICS AND ALDOSTERONE
  ANTAGONISTS
- **Grapefruit Juice:** plasma concentration of tacrolimus increased
  by • GRAPEFRUIT JUICE
- Hormone Antagonists: plasma concentration of tacrolimus
  possibly increased by DANAZOL
- Lipid-regulating Drugs: separating administration from
  tacrolimus by 12 hours advised by manufacturer of LOMITAPIDE
- Mifamurtide: avoidance of tacrolimus advised by manufacturer
  of MIFAMURTIDE
- Oestrogens: plasma concentration of tacrolimus possibly
  increased by ETHINYLESTRADIOL
- Potassium Salts: increased risk of hyperkalaemia when
  tacrolimus given with • POTASSIUM SALTS
- Ranolazine: plasma concentration of tacrolimus increased by
  • RANOLAZINE
- Sevelamer: plasma concentration of tacrolimus possibly
  reduced by SEVELAMER
- Ulcer-healing Drugs: plasma concentration of tacrolimus
  possibly increased by OMEPRAZOLE

Tadalafil

- **Alpha-blockers:** enhanced hypotensive effect when tadalafil
  given with • DOXAZOSIN—manufacturer of tadalafil advises
  avoid concomitant use; enhanced hypotensive effect when
  tadalafil given with • ALPHA-BLOCKERS—when patient is stable
  on the alpha blocker initiate tadalafil at the lowest possible
  dose
- Anti-arrhythmics: avoidance of tadalafil advised by
  manufacturer of DISOPYRAMIDE (risk of ventricular
  arrhythmias)
- **Antibacterials:** plasma concentration of tadalafil possibly
  increased by CLARITHROMYCIN and ERYTHROMYCIN; plasma
  concentration of tadalafil reduced by • RIFAMPICIN—
  manufacturer of tadalafil advises avoid concomitant use

Tadalafil (continued)

- **Antifungals:** tadalafil concentration is increased by
  • KETOCONAZOLE—avoid concomitant use of tadalafil for
  pulmonary hypertension; plasma concentration of tadalafil
  possibly increased by ITRACONAZOLE
- **Antivirals:** plasma concentration of tadalafil possibly increased
  by FOSAMPRENAVIR and INDINAVIR; plasma concentration of
  tadalafil increased by • RITONAVIR—avoid concomitant use of
  tadalafil for pulmonary hypertension; increased risk of
  ventricular arrhythmias when tadalafil given with
  • SAQUINAVIR—avoid concomitant use; avoidance of high
  doses of tadalafil advised by manufacturer of • TELAPREVIR—
  consult product literature
- Bosentan: plasma concentration of tadalafil reduced by
  BOSENTAN
- **Cobicistat:** plasma concentration of tadalafil possibly increased
  by • COBICISTAT—manufacturer of cobicistat advises reduce
  dose of tadalafil (consult cobicistat product literature)
- Dapoxetine: avoidance of tadalafil advised by manufacturer of
  DAPOXETINE
- Grapefruit Juice: plasma concentration of tadalafil possibly
  increased by GRAPEFRUIT JUICE
- **Nicorandil:** tadalafil significantly enhances hypotensive effect
  of • NICORANDIL (avoid concomitant use)
- **Nitrates:** tadalafil significantly enhances hypotensive effect of
  • NITRATES (avoid concomitant use)
- **Riociguat:** possible enhanced hypotensive effect when tadalafil
  given with • RIOCIGUAT—avoid concomitant use

Tamoxifen

- Antibacterials: metabolism of tamoxifen accelerated by
  RIFAMPICIN (reduced plasma concentration)
- **Anticoagulants:** tamoxifen enhances anticoagulant effect of
  • COUMARINS
- **Antidepressants:** metabolism of tamoxifen to active metabolite
  possibly inhibited by • FLUOXETINE and • PAROXETINE (avoid
  concomitant use)
- **Antipsychotics:** avoidance of tamoxifen advised by
  manufacturer of • DROPERIDOL (risk of ventricular
  arrhythmias)
- **Bupropion:** metabolism of tamoxifen to active metabolite
  possibly inhibited by • BUPROPION (avoid concomitant use)
- **Cinacalcet:** metabolism of tamoxifen to active metabolite
  possibly inhibited by • CINACALCET (avoid concomitant use)

Tamsulosin see Alpha-blockers

Tapentadol see Opioid Analgesics

Taxanes see Cabazitaxel, Docetaxel, and Paclitaxel

Tegafur

- Antibacterials: metabolism of tegafur inhibited by
  METRONIDAZOLE (increased toxicity)
- **Anticoagulants:** tegafur enhances anticoagulant effect of
  • COUMARINS
- **Antiepileptics:** tegafur possibly inhibits metabolism of
  FOSPHENYTOIN and PHENYTOIN (increased risk of toxicity)
- **Antipsychotics:** avoid concomitant use of cytotoxics with
  • CLOZAPINE (increased risk of agranulocytosis)
- Filgrastim: neutropenia possibly exacerbated when tegafur
  given with FILGRASTIM
- **Folates:** toxicity of tegafur increased by • FOLIC ACID—avoid
  concomitant use
- Lipegfilgrastim: neutropenia possibly exacerbated when
  tegafur given with LIPEGFILGRASTIM
- Pegfilgrastim: neutropenia possibly exacerbated when tegafur
  given with PEGFILGRASTIM
- Ulcer-healing Drugs: metabolism of tegafur inhibited by
  CIMETIDINE (increased plasma concentration)

Teicoplanin

- Vaccines: antibacterials inactivate ORAL TYPHOID VACCINE—see
  under Typhoid Vaccine in BNF

Telaprevir

- **Alpha-blockers:** manufacturer of telaprevir advises avoid
  concomitant use with • ALFUZOSIN
- **Analgesics:** manufacturer of telaprevir advises caution with
  • METHADONE (risk of ventricular arrhythmias)
- **Anti-arrhythmics:** manufacturer of telaprevir advises avoid
  concomitant use with • AMIODARONE and • DISOPYRAMIDE (risk
  of ventricular arrhythmias); manufacturer of telaprevir

Telaprevir
- **Anti-arrhythmics** (continued)
advises caution with ● FLECAINIDE and ● PROPAFENONE (risk of ventricular arrhythmias); manufacturer of teleprevir advises caution with *intravenous* LIDOCAINE
- **Antibacterials:** plasma concentration of both drugs possibly increased when teleprevir given with ● CLARITHROMYCIN, ● ERYTHROMYCIN and ● TELITHROMYCIN (increased risk of ventricular arrhythmias); manufacturer of teleprevir advises avoid concomitant use with ● RIFABUTIN; plasma concentration of teleprevir significantly reduced by ● RIFAMPICIN—avoid concomitant use
- **Anticoagulants:** teleprevir possibly affects plasma concentration of ● WARFARIN; avoidance of teleprevir advised by manufacturer of APIXABAN; teleprevir possibly increases plasma concentration of DABIGATRAN
- **Antidepressants:** teleprevir possibly increases plasma concentration of TRAZODONE; manufacturer of teleprevir advises avoid concomitant use with ● ST JOHN'S WORT
▸ **Antidiabetics:** teleprevir increases plasma concentration of METFORMIN (consider reducing dose of metformin)
- **Antiepileptics:** manufacturer of teleprevir advises avoid concomitant use with ● CARBAMAZEPINE, ● FOSPHENYTOIN, ● PHENOBARBITAL, ● PHENYTOIN and ● PRIMIDONE
- **Antifungals:** plasma concentration of both drugs possibly increased when teleprevir given with KETOCONAZOLE (increased risk of ventricular arrhythmias)—reduce dose of ketoconazole; teleprevir possibly increases plasma concentration of ITRACONAZOLE; teleprevir possibly increases plasma concentration of ● POSACONAZOLE (increased risk of ventricular arrhythmias); teleprevir possibly affects plasma concentration of ● VORICONAZOLE (possible increased risk of ventricular arrhythmias)
- **Antipsychotics:** teleprevir possibly increases plasma concentration of ● LURASIDONE—avoid concomitant use; manufacturer of teleprevir advises avoid concomitant use with ● PIMOZIDE; teleprevir possibly increases plasma concentration of ● QUETIAPINE—manufacturer of quetiapine advises avoid concomitant use
- **Antivirals:** plasma concentration of teleprevir possibly reduced by ATAZANAVIR, also plasma concentration of atazanavir possibly increased; teleprevir increases the plasma concentration of ● DACLATASVIR—reduce dose of daclatasvir (see under Daclatasvir, p. 568); avoid concomitant use of teleprevir with ● DARUNAVIR; plasma concentration of teleprevir reduced by EFAVIRENZ—increase dose of teleprevir; manufacturers advise avoid concomitant use of teleprevir with ● FOSAMPRENAVIR and ● LOPINAVIR; teleprevir increases plasma concentration of MARAVIROC (consider reducing dose of maraviroc); plasma concentration of teleprevir possibly reduced by NEVIRAPINE—consider increasing dose of teleprevir; plasma concentration of teleprevir possibly reduced by RITONAVIR; teleprevir increases plasma concentration of TENOFOVIR; avoidance of teleprevir advised by manufacturer of TIPRANAVIR
- **Anxiolytics and Hypnotics:** teleprevir possibly increases plasma concentration of ● MIDAZOLAM (risk of prolonged sedation—avoid concomitant use of *oral* midazolam)
- **Beta-blockers:** manufacturer of teleprevir advises avoid concomitant use with ● SOTALOL (risk of ventricular arrhythmias)
▸ **Bosentan:** plasma concentration of teleprevir possibly reduced by BOSENTAN, also plasma concentration of bosentan possibly increased
▸ **Calcium-channel Blockers:** teleprevir increases plasma concentration of AMLODIPINE (consider reducing dose of amlodipine); manufacturer of teleprevir advises caution with DILTIAZEM, FELODIPINE, NICARDIPINE, NIFEDIPINE and VERAPAMIL
▸ **Cardiac Glycosides:** teleprevir increases plasma concentration of DIGOXIN
- **Ciclosporin:** plasma concentration of both drugs increased when teleprevir given with ● CICLOSPORIN (reduce dose of ciclosporin)
- **Cilostazol:** teleprevir possibly increases plasma concentration of ● CILOSTAZOL (see under Cilostazol, p. 215)

Teleprevir (continued)
- **Colchicine:** teleprevir possibly increases risk of ● COLCHICINE toxicity—suspend or reduce dose of colchicine (avoid concomitant use in hepatic or renal impairment)
▸ **Corticosteroids:** teleprevir possibly increases plasma concentration of *inhaled* and *intranasal* BUDESONIDE and FLUTICASONE; plasma concentration of teleprevir possibly reduced by DEXAMETHASONE
- **Cytotoxics:** teleprevir possibly increases the plasma concentration of ● BOSUTINIB—manufacturer of bosutinib advises avoid or consider reducing dose of bosutinib; manufacturer of ruxolitinib advises dose reduction when teleprevir given with ● RUXOLITINIB—consult ruxolitinib product literature; avoidance of teleprevir advised by manufacturer of ● OLAPARIB
- **Domperidone:** possible increased risk of ventricular arrhythmias when teleprevir given with ● DOMPERIDONE—avoid concomitant use
- **Ergot Alkaloids:** manufacturer of teleprevir advises avoid concomitant use with ● ERGOT ALKALOIDS
- **Guanfacine:** teleprevir possibly increases plasma concentration of ● GUANFACINE (halve dose of guanfacine)
- **Lipid-regulating Drugs:** manufacturer of teleprevir advises avoid concomitant use with ● ATORVASTATIN; manufacturers advise avoid concomitant use of teleprevir with ● SIMVASTATIN; avoidance of teleprevir advised by manufacturer of ● LOMITAPIDE (plasma concentration of lomitapide possibly increased)
- **Oestrogens:** teleprevir possibly reduces plasma concentration of ● ETHINYLESTRADIOL—manufacturer of teleprevir advises additional contraceptive precautions
- **Sildenafil:** manufacturer of teleprevir advises avoid concomitant use with ● SILDENAFIL
- **Sirolimus:** plasma concentration of both drugs increased when teleprevir given with ● SIROLIMUS (reduce dose of sirolimus)
- **Sympathomimetics, Beta₂:** manufacturer of teleprevir advises avoid concomitant use with ● SALMETEROL (risk of ventricular arrhythmias)
- **Tacrolimus:** plasma concentration of both drugs increased when teleprevir given with ● TACROLIMUS (reduce dose of tacrolimus)
- **Tadalafil:** manufacturer of teleprevir advises avoid concomitant use with high doses of ● TADALAFIL—consult product literature
- **Vardenafil:** manufacturer of teleprevir advises avoid concomitant use with ● VARDENAFIL

Telavancin
▸ **Vaccines:** antibacterials inactivate ORAL TYPHOID VACCINE—see under Typhoid Vaccine in BNF

Telbivudine
- **Interferons:** increased risk of peripheral neuropathy when telbivudine given with ● INTERFERON ALFA and ● PEGINTERFERON ALFA

Telithromycin
- **Analgesics:** possible increased risk of ventricular arrhythmias when telithromycin given with ● METHADONE; telithromycin inhibits the metabolism of OXYCODONE
- **Anti-arrhythmics:** possible increased risk of ventricular arrhythmias when telithromycin given with ● AMIODARONE and ● DISOPYRAMIDE; increased risk of ventricular arrhythmias when telithromycin given with ● DRONEDARONE—avoid concomitant use
- **Antibacterials:** possible increased risk of ventricular arrhythmias when telithromycin given with ● MOXIFLOXACIN; plasma concentration of telithromycin reduced by ● RIFAMPICIN (avoid during and for 2 weeks after rifampicin)
▸ **Anticoagulants:** avoidance of telithromycin advised by manufacturer of APIXABAN
- **Antidepressants:** possible increased risk of ventricular arrhythmias when telithromycin given with ● CITALOPRAM and ● TRICYCLICS; plasma concentration of telithromycin reduced by ● ST JOHN'S WORT (avoid during and for 2 weeks after St John's wort)
- **Antiepileptics:** plasma concentration of telithromycin reduced by ● CARBAMAZEPINE, ● FOSPHENYTOIN, ● PHENOBARBITAL, ● PHENYTOIN and ● PRIMIDONE (avoid during and for 2 weeks

A1

Interactions | **Appendix 1**

Telithromycin

- **Antiepileptics** (continued)
after carbamazepine, fosphenytoin, phenobarbital, phenytoin and primidone)
- **Antifungals:** plasma concentration of telithromycin increased by ● KETOCONAZOLE—avoid in severe renal and hepatic impairment
▸ **Antimuscarinics:** manufacturer of fesoterodine advises dose reduction when telithromycin given with FESOTERODINE—consult fesoterodine product literature
- **Antipsychotics:** possible increased risk of ventricular arrhythmias when telithromycin given with ● CHLORPROMAZINE; telithromycin possibly increases plasma concentration of ● LURASIDONE—avoid concomitant use; increased risk of ventricular arrhythmias when telithromycin given with ● PIMOZIDE—avoid concomitant use; telithromycin possibly increases plasma concentration of QUETIAPINE
- **Antivirals:** manufacturer of telithromycin advises avoid concomitant use with ● ATAZANAVIR, ● FOSAMPRENAVIR, ● INDINAVIR, ● LOPINAVIR, ● RITONAVIR and ● TIPRANAVIR in severe renal and hepatic impairment; telithromycin possibly increases the plasma concentration of ● DACLATASVIR—reduce dose of daclatasvir (see under Daclatasvir, p. 568); avoidance of telithromycin advised by manufacturer of DASABUVIR and PARITAPREVIR; telithromycin possibly increases plasma concentration of ● MARAVIROC (consider reducing dose of maraviroc); manufacturer of telithromycin advises avoid concomitant use with ● SAQUINAVIR (risk of ventricular arrhythmias); telithromycin possibly increases plasma concentration of ● SIMEPREVIR—manufacturer of simeprevir advises avoid concomitant use; plasma concentration of both drugs possibly increased when telithromycin given with ● TELAPREVIR (increased risk of ventricular arrhythmias)
- **Anxiolytics and Hypnotics:** telithromycin inhibits metabolism of ● MIDAZOLAM (increased plasma concentration with increased sedation)
▸ **Aprepitant:** telithromycin possibly increases plasma concentration of APREPITANT
- **Avanafil:** telithromycin possibly increases plasma concentration of ● AVANAFIL—manufacturer of avanafil advises avoid concomitant use
- **Calcium-channel Blockers:** telithromycin possibly inhibits metabolism of ● CALCIUM-CHANNEL BLOCKERS (increased risk of side-effects)
▸ **Cardiac Glycosides:** telithromycin possibly increases plasma concentration of DIGOXIN
- **Ciclosporin:** telithromycin possibly increases plasma concentration of ● CICLOSPORIN
- **Colchicine:** telithromycin possibly increases risk of ● COLCHICINE toxicity—suspend or reduce dose of colchicine (avoid concomitant use in hepatic or renal impairment)
- **Cytotoxics:** telithromycin possibly increases plasma concentration of AXITINIB (reduce dose of axitinib—consult axitinib product literature); telithromycin possibly increases the plasma concentration of ● BOSUTINIB and ● CABAZITAXEL—manufacturer of bosutinib and cabazitaxel advises avoid or consider reducing dose of bosutinib and cabazitaxel; telithromycin possibly increases plasma concentration of ● CRIZOTINIB and ● EVEROLIMUS—manufacturer of crizotinib and everolimus advises avoid concomitant use; avoidance of telithromycin advised by manufacturer of DASATINIB (plasma concentration of dasatinib possibly increased); telithromycin possibly increases the plasma concentration of ● IBRUTINIB—reduce dose of ibrutinib (see under Ibrutinib, p. 855); avoidance of telithromycin advised by manufacturer of ● LAPATINIB, ● NILOTINIB and ● OLAPARIB; telithromycin possibly increases plasma concentration of ● PAZOPANIB (reduce dose of pazopanib); telithromycin possibly increases plasma concentration of PONATINIB—consider reducing initial dose of ponatinib (see under Ponatinib, p. 860); manufacturer of ruxolitinib advises dose reduction when telithromycin given with ● RUXOLITINIB—consult ruxolitinib product literature; telithromycin possibly increases plasma concentration of ● DOCETAXEL—manufacturer of docetaxel advises avoid concomitant use or consider reducing docetaxel dose

Telithromycin (continued)

- **Dapoxetine:** avoidance of telithromycin advised by manufacturer of ● DAPOXETINE (increased risk of toxicity)
- **Diuretics:** telithromycin increases plasma concentration of ● EPLERENONE—avoid concomitant use
- **Domperidone:** possible increased risk of ventricular arrhythmias when telithromycin given with ● DOMPERIDONE—avoid concomitant use
- **Ergot Alkaloids:** increased risk of ergotism when telithromycin given with ● ERGOT ALKALOIDS—avoid concomitant use
▸ **Fosaprepitant:** telithromycin possibly increases plasma concentration of FOSAPREPITANT
- **Guanfacine:** telithromycin possibly increases plasma concentration of ● GUANFACINE (halve dose of guanfacine)
- **Ivabradine:** telithromycin possibly increases plasma concentration of ● IVABRADINE—avoid concomitant use
- **Ivacaftor:** telithromycin possibly increases plasma concentration of ● IVACAFTOR (see under Ivacaftor, p. 269)
- **Lipid-regulating Drugs:** increased risk of myopathy when telithromycin given with ● ATORVASTATIN or ● SIMVASTATIN (avoid concomitant use); possible increased risk of myopathy when telithromycin given with PRAVASTATIN; avoidance of telithromycin advised by manufacturer of ● LOMITAPIDE (plasma concentration of lomitapide possibly increased)
- **Pentamidine Isetionate:** possible increased risk of ventricular arrhythmias when telithromycin given with *parenteral* ● PENTAMIDINE ISETIONATE
- **Ranolazine:** telithromycin possibly increases plasma concentration of ● RANOLAZINE—manufacturer of ranolazine advises avoid concomitant use
- **Sildenafil:** telithromycin possibly increases plasma concentration of ● SILDENAFIL—consider reducing initial dose of sildenafil for erectile dysfunction or reduce sildenafil dose frequency to once daily for pulmonary hypertension
- **Sirolimus:** telithromycin increases plasma concentration of ● SIROLIMUS—avoid concomitant use
- **Tacrolimus:** telithromycin possibly increases plasma concentration of ● TACROLIMUS
- **Ulipristal:** avoidance of telithromycin advised by manufacturer of *low-dose* ULIPRISTAL
▸ **Vaccines:** antibacterials inactivate ORAL TYPHOID VACCINE—see under Typhoid Vaccine in BNF

Telmisartan *see* Angiotensin-II Receptor Antagonists

Temazepam *see* Anxiolytics and Hypnotics

Temocillin *see* Penicillins

Temoporfin

- **Cytotoxics:** increased skin photosensitivity when temoporfin given with *topical* ● FLUOROURACIL

Temozolomide

▸ **Antiepileptics:** plasma concentration of temozolomide increased by SODIUM VALPROATE and VALPROIC ACID
- **Antipsychotics:** avoid concomitant use of cytotoxics with ● CLOZAPINE (increased risk of agranulocytosis)

Temsirolimus

NOTE The main active metabolite of temsirolimus is sirolimus—*see also* interactions of sirolimus and consult product literature

- **Antibacterials:** plasma concentration of active metabolite of temsirolimus reduced by ● RIFAMPICIN—avoid concomitant use
- **Antifungals:** plasma concentration of active metabolite of temsirolimus increased by ● KETOCONAZOLE—avoid concomitant use; manufacturer of temsirolimus advises avoid concomitant use with ● ITRACONAZOLE (plasma concentration of temsirolimus possibly increased)
- **Antipsychotics:** avoid concomitant use of cytotoxics with ● CLOZAPINE (increased risk of agranulocytosis)

Tenofovir

- **Antivirals:** manufacturer of tenofovir advises avoid concomitant use with ADEFOVIR; tenofovir reduces plasma concentration of ATAZANAVIR, also plasma concentration of tenofovir possibly increased; tenofovir increases plasma concentration of ● DIDANOSINE (increased risk of toxicity)—avoid concomitant use; plasma concentration of tenofovir increased by LOPINAVIR and TELAPREVIR
- **Orlistat:** absorption of tenofovir possibly reduced by ● ORLISTAT

Tenoxicam *see* NSAIDs

Terazosin *see* Alpha-blockers

Terbinafine
- Antibacterials: plasma concentration of terbinafine reduced by ● RIFAMPICIN
- Antidepressants: terbinafine possibly increases plasma concentration of PAROXETINE and TRICYCLICS
- Antifungals: terbinafine increases plasma concentration of FLUCONAZOLE
- Ciclosporin: terbinafine possibly reduces plasma concentration of CICLOSPORIN
- Oestrogens: occasional reports of breakthrough bleeding when terbinafine given with OESTROGENS (when used for contraception)
- Progestogens: occasional reports of breakthrough bleeding when terbinafine given with PROGESTOGENS (when used for contraception)
- Ulcer-healing Drugs: plasma concentration of terbinafine increased by CIMETIDINE

Terbutaline *see* Sympathomimetics, Beta$_2$

Teriflunomide
- Antibacterials: teriflunomide increases plasma concentration of CEFACLOR; plasma concentration of teriflunomide reduced by RIFAMPICIN
- Antidiabetics: teriflunomide increases plasma concentration of REPAGLINIDE
- Lipid-regulating Drugs: the effect of teriflunomide is significantly decreased by COLESTYRAMINE (enhanced elimination)—avoid unless drug elimination desired; teriflunomide increases plasma concentration of ● ROSUVASTATIN (consider reducing dose of rosuvastatin)
- Oestrogens: teriflunomide increases plasma concentration of ETHINYLESTRADIOL
- Progestogens: teriflunomide increases plasma concentration of LEVONORGESTREL
- Vaccines: risk of generalised infections when teriflunomide given with live ● VACCINES—avoid concomitant use

Testolactone
- Anticoagulants: testolactone enhances anticoagulant effect of ● COUMARINS and ● PHENINDIONE

Testosterone
- Anticoagulants: testosterone enhances anticoagulant effect of ● COUMARINS and ● PHENINDIONE
- Antidiabetics: testosterone possibly enhances hypoglycaemic effect of ANTIDIABETICS

Tetrabenazine
- Antidepressants: risk of CNS toxicity when tetrabenazine given with ● MAOIS (avoid tetrabenazine for 2 weeks after MAOIs)
- Antipsychotics: increased risk of extrapyramidal side-effects when tetrabenazine given with ANTIPSYCHOTICS
- Dopaminergics: increased risk of extrapyramidal side-effects when tetrabenazine given with AMANTADINE
- Metoclopramide: increased risk of extrapyramidal side-effects when tetrabenazine given with METOCLOPRAMIDE

Tetracosactide *see* Corticosteroids

Tetracycline *see* Tetracyclines

Tetracyclines
- ACE Inhibitors: absorption of tetracyclines reduced by QUINAPRIL tablets (quinapril tablets contain magnesium carbonate)
- Adsorbents: absorption of tetracyclines possibly reduced by KAOLIN
- Antacids: absorption of tetracyclines possibly reduced by ANTACIDS (give at least 2 to 3 hours apart)
- Antibacterials: plasma concentration of doxycycline reduced by RIFAMPICIN—consider increasing dose of doxycycline; tetracyclines possibly antagonise effects of PENICILLINS
- Anticoagulants: tetracyclines possibly enhance anticoagulant effect of ● COUMARINS and ● PHENINDIONE
- Antidiabetics: tetracyclines possibly enhance hypoglycaemic effect of SULFONYLUREAS
- Antiepileptics: metabolism of doxycycline accelerated by CARBAMAZEPINE (reduced effect); metabolism of doxycycline accelerated by FOSPHENYTOIN, PHENOBARBITAL, PHENYTOIN and PRIMIDONE (reduced plasma concentration)
- Atovaquone: tetracycline reduces plasma concentration of ATOVAQUONE

Tetracyclines (continued)
- Calcium Salts: absorption of tetracyclines possibly reduced by CALCIUM SALTS (give at least 2 to 3 hours apart)
- Cytotoxics: doxycycline or tetracycline increase risk of METHOTREXATE toxicity
- Dairy Products: absorption of tetracyclines (except doxycycline and minocycline) reduced by DAIRY PRODUCTS
- Diuretics: manufacturer of lymecycline advises avoid concomitant use with DIURETICS
- Ergot Alkaloids: increased risk of ergotism when tetracyclines given with ERGOTAMINE
- Iron Salts: absorption of tetracyclines reduced by *oral* IRON SALTS, also absorption of *oral* iron salts reduced by tetracyclines (give at least 2 to 3 hours apart)
- Lipid-regulating Drugs: absorption of tetracycline possibly reduced by COLESTIPOL and COLESTYRAMINE
- Retinoids: possible increased risk of benign intracranial hypertension when tetracyclines given with ● RETINOIDS (avoid concomitant use)
- Strontium Ranelate: absorption of tetracyclines reduced by STRONTIUM RANELATE (manufacturer of strontium ranelate advises avoid concomitant use)
- Ulcer-healing Drugs: absorption of tetracyclines reduced by SUCRALFATE and TRIPOTASSIUM DICITRATOBISMUTHATE
- Vaccines: antibacterials inactivate ORAL TYPHOID VACCINE—see under Typhoid Vaccine in BNF
- Zinc: absorption of tetracyclines possibly reduced by ZINC (give at least 2 to 3 hours apart)

Theophylline
- Allopurinol: plasma concentration of theophylline possibly increased by ALLOPURINOL
- Anaesthetics, General: increased risk of convulsions when theophylline given with KETAMINE
- Anti-arrhythmics: theophylline antagonises anti-arrhythmic effect of ADENOSINE—manufacturer of adenosine advises avoid theophylline for 24 hours before adenosine; plasma concentration of theophylline increased by PROPAFENONE
- Antibacterials: plasma concentration of theophylline possibly increased by CLARITHROMYCIN and ISONIAZID; plasma concentration of theophylline increased by ● ERYTHROMYCIN (also theophylline may reduce absorption of *oral* erythromycin); plasma concentration of theophylline increased by ● CIPROFLOXACIN and NORFLOXACIN; metabolism of theophylline accelerated by RIFAMPICIN (reduced plasma concentration); possible increased risk of convulsions when theophylline given with ● QUINOLONES
- Antidepressants: plasma concentration of theophylline increased by ● FLUVOXAMINE (concomitant use should usually be avoided, but where not possible halve theophylline dose and monitor plasma-theophylline concentration); plasma concentration of theophylline possibly reduced by ST JOHN'S WORT
- Antiepileptics: metabolism of theophylline accelerated by CARBAMAZEPINE, ● PHENOBARBITAL and ● PRIMIDONE (reduced effect); plasma concentration of both drugs reduced when theophylline given with ● FOSPHENYTOIN and ● PHENYTOIN
- Antifungals: plasma concentration of theophylline possibly increased by ● FLUCONAZOLE and ● KETOCONAZOLE
- Antivirals: plasma concentration of theophylline possibly increased by ACICLOVIR and VALACICLOVIR; metabolism of theophylline accelerated by ● RITONAVIR (reduced plasma concentration)
- Anxiolytics and Hypnotics: theophylline possibly reduces effects of BENZODIAZEPINES
- Caffeine citrate: avoidance of theophylline advised by manufacturer of CAFFEINE CITRATE
- Calcium-channel Blockers: plasma concentration of theophylline possibly increased by ● CALCIUM-CHANNEL BLOCKERS (enhanced effect); plasma concentration of theophylline increased by DILTIAZEM; plasma concentration of theophylline increased by ● VERAPAMIL (enhanced effect)
- Corticosteroids: increased risk of hypokalaemia when theophylline given with CORTICOSTEROIDS
- Cytotoxics: plasma concentration of theophylline possibly increased by METHOTREXATE

Theophylline (continued)

- Deferasirox: plasma concentration of theophylline increased by ●DEFERASIROX (consider reducing dose of theophylline)
- ▹ Disulfiram: metabolism of theophylline inhibited by DISULFIRAM (increased risk of toxicity)
- Diuretics: increased risk of hypokalaemia when theophylline given with ACETAZOLAMIDE, LOOP DIURETICS or THIAZIDES AND RELATED DIURETICS
- Doxapram: increased CNS stimulation when theophylline given with DOXAPRAM
- Interferons: metabolism of theophylline inhibited by ●INTERFERON ALFA and ●PEGINTERFERON ALFA (consider reducing dose of theophylline)
- Leukotriene Receptor Antagonists: plasma concentration of theophylline possibly increased by ZAFIRLUKAST, also plasma concentration of zafirlukast reduced
- Lithium: theophylline increases excretion of LITHIUM (reduced plasma concentration)
- Oestrogens: plasma concentration of theophylline increased by OESTROGENS (consider reducing dose of theophylline)
- Pentoxifylline: plasma concentration of theophylline increased by PENTOXIFYLLINE
- Roflumilast: avoidance of theophylline advised by manufacturer of ROFLUMILAST
- Sulfinpyrazone: plasma concentration of theophylline reduced by SULFINPYRAZONE
- ▹ Sympathomimetics: manufacturer of theophylline advises avoid concomitant use with EPHEDRINE in children
- Sympathomimetics, Beta₂: increased risk of hypokalaemia when theophylline given with high doses of BETA₂ SYMPATHOMIMETICS
- Ulcer-healing Drugs: metabolism of theophylline inhibited by ●CIMETIDINE (increased plasma concentration); absorption of theophylline possibly reduced by SUCRALFATE (give at least 2 hours apart)
- ▹ Vaccines: plasma concentration of theophylline possibly increased by INFLUENZA VACCINE

Thiazolidinediones see Antidiabetics
Thiopental see Anaesthetics, General
Thiotepa
- Antipsychotics: avoid concomitant use of cytotoxics with ●CLOZAPINE (increased risk of agranulocytosis)
- Muscle Relaxants: thiotepa enhances effects of SUXAMETHONIUM

Thioxanthenes see Antipsychotics
Thyroid Hormones
- ▹ Antacids: absorption of levothyroxine possibly reduced by ANTACIDS
- ▹ Anti-arrhythmics: serum concentrations of thyroid hormones can be affected by AMIODARONE —monitor thyroid function closely
- ▹ Antibacterials: metabolism of levothyroxine accelerated by RIFAMPICIN (may increase requirements for levothyroxine in hypothyroidism)
- Anticoagulants: thyroid hormones enhance anticoagulant effect of ●COUMARINS and ●PHENINDIONE
- Antidepressants: thyroid hormones enhance effects of AMITRIPTYLINE and IMIPRAMINE ; thyroid hormones possibly enhance effects of TRICYCLICS
- Antiepileptics: metabolism of thyroid hormones accelerated by CARBAMAZEPINE, PHENOBARBITAL and PRIMIDONE (may increase requirements for thyroid hormones in hypothyroidism); metabolism of thyroid hormones accelerated by FOSPHENYTOIN and PHENYTOIN (may increase requirements in hypothyroidism), also plasma concentration of fosphenytoin and phenytoin possibly increased
- ▹ Beta-blockers: levothyroxine accelerates metabolism of PROPRANOLOL
- Calcium Salts: absorption of levothyroxine reduced by CALCIUM SALTS
- ▹ Cytotoxics: plasma concentration of levothyroxine possibly reduced by IMATINIB
- ▹ Iron Salts: absorption of levothyroxine reduced by oral IRON SALTS (give at least 2 hours apart)
- ▹ Lanthanum: absorption of levothyroxine reduced by LANTHANUM (give at least 2 hours apart)

Thyroid Hormones (continued)
- ▹ Lipid-regulating Drugs: absorption of levothyroxine reduced by COLESEVELAM ; absorption of thyroid hormones reduced by COLESTIPOL and COLESTYRAMINE
- ▹ Oestrogens: requirements for thyroid hormones in hypothyroidism may be increased by OESTROGENS
- ▹ Orlistat: possible increased risk of hypothyroidism when levothyroxine given with ORLISTAT
- ▹ Polystyrene Sulfonate Resins: absorption of levothyroxine reduced by POLYSTYRENE SULFONATE RESINS
- ▹ Sevelamer: absorption of levothyroxine possibly reduced by SEVELAMER
- ▹ Sympathomimetics: avoidance of thyroid hormones advised by manufacturer of MIDODRINE
- ▹ Ulcer-healing Drugs: absorption of levothyroxine reduced by CIMETIDINE and SUCRALFATE

Tiagabine
- Antidepressants: anticonvulsant effect of antiepileptics possibly antagonised by MAOIs and ●TRICYCLIC-RELATED ANTIDEPRESSANTS (convulsive threshold lowered); anticonvulsant effect of antiepileptics antagonised by ●SSRIs and ●TRICYCLICS (convulsive threshold lowered)
- ▹ Antiepileptics: plasma concentration of tiagabine reduced by CARBAMAZEPINE, FOSPHENYTOIN, PHENOBARBITAL, PHENYTOIN and PRIMIDONE
- Antimalarials: anticonvulsant effect of antiepileptics antagonised by ●MEFLOQUINE
- Antipsychotics: anticonvulsant effect of antiepileptics antagonised by ●ANTIPSYCHOTICS (convulsive threshold lowered)
- Orlistat: possible increased risk of convulsions when antiepileptics given with ●ORLISTAT

Tiaprofenic Acid see NSAIDs
Tibolone
- ▹ Antibacterials: metabolism of tibolone accelerated by RIFAMPICIN (reduced plasma concentration)
- ▹ Antiepileptics: metabolism of tibolone accelerated by CARBAMAZEPINE (reduced plasma concentration); metabolism of tibolone accelerated by FOSPHENYTOIN and PHENYTOIN

Ticagrelor
- Antibacterials: plasma concentration of ticagrelor possibly increased by ●CLARITHROMYCIN —manufacturer of ticagrelor advises avoid concomitant use; plasma concentration of ticagrelor possibly increased by ERYTHROMYCIN ; plasma concentration of ticagrelor reduced by ●RIFAMPICIN
- Anticoagulants: ticagrelor increases plasma concentration of ●DABIGATRAN
- ▹ Antidepressants: possible increased risk of bleeding when ticagrelor given with CITALOPRAM, PAROXETINE or SERTRALINE
- ▹ Antiepileptics: plasma concentration of ticagrelor possibly reduced by CARBAMAZEPINE, FOSPHENYTOIN, PHENOBARBITAL, PHENYTOIN and PRIMIDONE
- Antifungals: plasma concentration of ticagrelor increased by ●KETOCONAZOLE —manufacturer of ticagrelor advises avoid concomitant use
- Antivirals: plasma concentration of ticagrelor possibly increased by ●ATAZANAVIR and ●RITONAVIR —manufacturer of ticagrelor advises avoid concomitant use
- Calcium-channel Blockers: plasma concentration of ticagrelor increased by DILTIAZEM
- Cardiac Glycosides: ticagrelor increases plasma concentration of ●DIGOXIN
- ▹ Ciclosporin: plasma concentration of ticagrelor increased by CICLOSPORIN
- Ergot Alkaloids: ticagrelor possibly increases plasma concentration of ●ERGOT ALKALOIDS
- Lipid-regulating Drugs: ticagrelor increases plasma concentration of ●SIMVASTATIN (increased risk of toxicity); separating administration from ticagrelor by 12 hours advised by manufacturer of LOMITAPIDE

Ticarcillin see Penicillins
Tick-borne Encephalitis Vaccine see Vaccines
Tigecycline
- ▹ Anticoagulants: tigecycline possibly enhances anticoagulant effect of COUMARINS

Tigecycline (continued)

▸ Vaccines: antibacterials inactivate ORAL TYPHOID VACCINE—see under Typhoid Vaccine in BNF

Timolol *see* Beta-blockers

Tinidazole

▸ Alcohol: possibility of disulfiram-like reaction when tinidazole given with ALCOHOL

▸ Antibacterials: plasma concentration of tinidazole possibly reduced by RIFAMPICIN

▸ Vaccines: antibacterials inactivate ORAL TYPHOID VACCINE—see under Typhoid Vaccine in BNF

Tinzaparin *see* Heparins

Tioguanine

● Antipsychotics: avoid concomitant use of cytotoxics with ● CLOZAPINE (increased risk of agranulocytosis)

● Cytotoxics: increased risk of hepatotoxicity when tioguanine given with BUSULFAN

Tiotropium *see* Antimuscarinics

Tipranavir

▸ Analgesics: plasma concentration of tipranavir possibly reduced by BUPRENORPHINE

▸ Antacids: absorption of tipranavir reduced by ANTACIDS (give at least 2 hours apart)

● Antibacterials: tipranavir increases plasma concentration of ● CLARITHROMYCIN (reduce dose of clarithromycin in renal impairment), also plasma concentration of tipranavir increased by clarithromycin; tipranavir increases plasma concentration of ● RIFABUTIN (reduce dose of rifabutin); plasma concentration of tipranavir possibly reduced by ● RIFAMPICIN—avoid concomitant use; avoidance of concomitant tipranavir in severe renal and hepatic impairment advised by manufacturer of ● TELITHROMYCIN

▸ Anticoagulants: avoidance of tipranavir advised by manufacturer of APIXABAN and RIVAROXABAN

● Antidepressants: plasma concentration of tipranavir possibly reduced by ● ST JOHN'S WORT—avoid concomitant use

▸ Antiepileptics: plasma concentration of tipranavir possibly reduced by CARBAMAZEPINE

▸ Antifungals: plasma concentration of tipranavir increased by FLUCONAZOLE

● Antimalarials: caution with tipranavir advised by manufacturer of ARTEMETHER WITH LUMEFANTRINE; tipranavir possibly increases plasma concentration of ● QUININE (increased risk of toxicity)

▸ Antimuscarinics: avoidance of tipranavir advised by manufacturer of DARIFENACIN

● Antipsychotics: tipranavir possibly increases plasma concentration of ● ARIPIPRAZOLE (reduce dose of aripiprazole—consult aripiprazole product literature); tipranavir possibly increases plasma concentration of ● QUETIAPINE—manufacturer of quetiapine advises avoid concomitant use

● Antivirals: tipranavir reduces plasma concentration of ● ABACAVIR, ● FOSAMPRENAVIR, ● LOPINAVIR, ● SAQUINAVIR and ● ZIDOVUDINE; plasma concentration of tipranavir increased by ATAZANAVIR (also plasma concentration of atazanavir reduced); manufacturer of tipranavir advises avoid concomitant use with BOCEPREVIR and TELAPREVIR; tipranavir reduces plasma concentration of DIDANOSINE—manufacturer of tipranavir advises tipranavir and didanosine *capsules* should be taken at least 2 hours apart; tipranavir reduces plasma concentration of ● DOLUTEGRAVIR (see under Dolutegravir, p. 584); tipranavir reduces plasma concentration of ● ETRAVIRINE, also plasma concentration of tipranavir increased (avoid concomitant use); avoidance of tipranavir advised by manufacturer of PARITAPREVIR

● Beta-blockers: manufacturer of tipranavir advises avoid concomitant use with ● METOPROLOL for heart failure

▸ Bosentan: manufacturer of tipranavir advises avoid concomitant use with BOSENTAN

● Cobicistat: plasma concentration of both drugs reduced when tipranavir given with ● COBICISTAT (avoid concomitant use)

● Lipid-regulating Drugs: increased risk of myopathy when tipranavir given with ● ATORVASTATIN (see under Atorvastatin, p. 186); tipranavir increases plasma concentration of ● ROSUVASTATIN—adjust dose of rosuvastatin (consult product

Tipranavir

● Lipid-regulating Drugs (continued)
literature); tipranavir possibly increases plasma concentration of ● SIMVASTATIN—avoid concomitant use; avoidance of tipranavir advised by manufacturer of ● LOMITAPIDE (plasma concentration of lomitapide possibly increased)

● Orlistat: absorption of tipranavir possibly reduced by ● ORLISTAT

● Ranolazine: tipranavir possibly increases plasma concentration of ● RANOLAZINE—manufacturer of ranolazine advises avoid concomitant use

▸ Sildenafil: manufacturer of tipranavir advises avoid concomitant use of SILDENAFIL for pulmonary arterial hypertension

▸ Sympathomimetics, Beta$_2$: manufacturer of tipranavir advises avoid concomitant use with SALMETEROL

● Ulcer-healing Drugs: tipranavir reduces plasma concentration of ● ESOMEPRAZOLE and ● OMEPRAZOLE

▸ Vardenafil: manufacturer of tipranavir advises caution with VARDENAFIL

▸ Vitamins: increased risk of bleeding when tipranavir given with high doses of VITAMIN E

Tirofiban

▸ Iloprost: increased risk of bleeding when tirofiban given with ILOPROST

Tizanidine *see* Muscle Relaxants

Tobramycin *see* Aminoglycosides

Tocilizumab

● Antipsychotics: avoid concomitant use of cytotoxics with ● CLOZAPINE (increased risk of agranulocytosis)

● Vaccines: risk of generalised infections when monoclonal antibodies given with live ● VACCINES—avoid concomitant use

Tolazoline *see* Alpha-blockers

Tolbutamide *see* Antidiabetics

Tolcapone

▸ Antidepressants: avoid concomitant use of tolcapone with MAOIS

▸ Memantine: effects of dopaminergics possibly enhanced by MEMANTINE

▸ Methyldopa: antiparkinsonian effect of dopaminergics antagonised by METHYLDOPA

Tolfenamic Acid *see* NSAIDs

Tolterodine *see* Antimuscarinics

Tolvaptan

▸ Antibacterials: plasma concentration of tolvaptan reduced by RIFAMPICIN

▸ Antifungals: plasma concentration of tolvaptan increased by KETOCONAZOLE—manufacturer of ketoconazole advises avoid concomitant use

● Cardiac Glycosides: tolvaptan increases plasma concentration of DIGOXIN (increased risk of toxicity)

● Grapefruit Juice: plasma concentration of tolvaptan increased by ● GRAPEFRUIT JUICE—avoid concomitant use

▸ Lipid-regulating Drugs: separating administration from tolvaptan by 12 hours advised by manufacturer of LOMITAPIDE

Topiramate

● Antidepressants: anticonvulsant effect of antiepileptics possibly antagonised by MAOIS and ● TRICYCLIC-RELATED ANTIDEPRESSANTS (convulsive threshold lowered); anticonvulsant effect of antiepileptics antagonised by ● SSRIS and ● TRICYCLICS (convulsive threshold lowered)

▸ Antidiabetics: topiramate possibly increases plasma concentration of METFORMIN; topiramate possibly reduces plasma concentration of GLIBENCLAMIDE

● Antiepileptics: plasma concentration of topiramate often reduced by CARBAMAZEPINE; topiramate increases plasma concentration of ● FOSPHENYTOIN and ● PHENYTOIN (also plasma concentration of topiramate reduced); topiramate reduces plasma concentration of PERAMPANEL; plasma concentration of topiramate possibly reduced by PHENOBARBITAL and PRIMIDONE; hyperammonaemia and CNS toxicity reported when topiramate given with SODIUM VALPROATE and VALPROIC ACID

● Antimalarials: anticonvulsant effect of antiepileptics antagonised by ● MEFLOQUINE

A1

Interactions | Appendix 1

Topiramate (continued)

- Antipsychotics: anticonvulsant effect of antiepileptics antagonised by ● ANTIPSYCHOTICS (convulsive threshold lowered)
- Diuretics: plasma concentration of topiramate possibly increased by HYDROCHLOROTHIAZIDE
- Lithium: topiramate possibly affects plasma concentration of LITHIUM
- Oestrogens: topiramate accelerates metabolism of ● OESTROGENS (reduced contraceptive effect with combined oral contraceptives, contraceptive patches, and vaginal rings—see Contraceptive Interactions in BNF)
- Orlistat: possible increased risk of convulsions when antiepileptics given with ● ORLISTAT
- Progestogens: topiramate accelerates metabolism of ● PROGESTOGENS (reduced contraceptive effect with combined oral contraceptives, progestogen-only oral contraceptives, contraceptive patches, vaginal rings, etonogestrel-releasing implant, and emergency hormonal contraception—see Contraceptive Interactions in BNF)

Torasemide see Diuretics

Toremifene

- Anticoagulants: toremifene possibly enhances anticoagulant effect of ● COUMARINS
- Antiepileptics: metabolism of toremifene possibly accelerated by CARBAMAZEPINE (reduced plasma concentration); metabolism of toremifene possibly accelerated by FOSPHENYTOIN and PHENYTOIN; metabolism of toremifene accelerated by PHENOBARBITAL and PRIMIDONE (reduced plasma concentration)
- Cytotoxics: possible increased risk of ventricular arrhythmias when toremifene given with ● VANDETANIB—avoid concomitant use
- Diuretics: increased risk of hypercalcaemia when toremifene given with THIAZIDES AND RELATED DIURETICS

Trabectedin

- Alcohol: manufacturer of trabectedin advises avoid concomitant use with ● ALCOHOL
- Antibacterials: plasma concentration of trabectedin reduced by ● RIFAMPICIN
- Antipsychotics: avoid concomitant use of cytotoxics with ● CLOZAPINE (increased risk of agranulocytosis)
- Vaccines: risk of generalised infections when trabectedin given with live ● VACCINES—avoid concomitant use

Tramadol see Opioid Analgesics

Trandolapril see ACE Inhibitors

Tranylcypromine see MAOIs

Trastuzumab

- Antipsychotics: avoid concomitant use of cytotoxics with ● CLOZAPINE (increased risk of agranulocytosis)
- Cytotoxics: possible increased risk of cardiotoxicity when trastuzumab given with ● DAUNORUBICIN, ● DOXORUBICIN, ● EPIRUBICIN and ● IDARUBICIN—avoid concomitant use for up to 28 weeks after stopping trastuzumab
- Vaccines: risk of generalised infections when monoclonal antibodies given with live ● VACCINES—avoid concomitant use

Trazodone see Antidepressants, Tricyclic (related)

Tretinoin see Retinoids

Triamcinolone see Corticosteroids

Triamterene see Diuretics

Trientine

- Iron Salts: trientine reduces absorption of *oral* IRON SALTS
- Zinc: trientine reduces absorption of ZINC, also absorption of trientine reduced by zinc

Trifluoperazine see Antipsychotics

Trihexyphenidyl see Antimuscarinics

Trimethoprim

- ACE Inhibitors: possible increased risk of hyperkalaemia when trimethoprim given with ACE INHIBITORS
- Angiotensin-II Receptor Antagonists: possible increased risk of hyperkalaemia when trimethoprim given with ANGIOTENSIN-II RECEPTOR ANTAGONISTS
- Anti-arrhythmics: possible increased risk of ventricular arrhythmias when trimethoprim (as co-trimoxazole) given with AMIODARONE—manufacturer of amiodarone advises avoid concomitant use of co-trimoxazole

Trimethoprim (continued)

- Antibacterials: plasma concentration of trimethoprim possibly reduced by RIFAMPICIN; plasma concentration of both drugs may increase when trimethoprim given with DAPSONE
- Anticoagulants: trimethoprim possibly enhances anticoagulant effect of COUMARINS
- Antidiabetics: trimethoprim possibly enhances hypoglycaemic effect of REPAGLINIDE—manufacturer advises avoid concomitant use; trimethoprim rarely enhances the effects of SULFONYLUREAS
- Antiepileptics: trimethoprim increases plasma concentration of ● FOSPHENYTOIN and ● PHENYTOIN (also increased antifolate effect)
- Antimalarials: increased antifolate effect when trimethoprim given with ● PYRIMETHAMINE
- Antivirals: trimethoprim (as co-trimoxazole) increases plasma concentration of LAMIVUDINE—avoid concomitant use of high-dose co-trimoxazole
- Azathioprine: increased risk of haematological toxicity when trimethoprim (also with co-trimoxazole) given with ● AZATHIOPRINE
- Cardiac Glycosides: trimethoprim possibly increases plasma concentration of DIGOXIN
- Ciclosporin: increased risk of nephrotoxicity when trimethoprim given with ● CICLOSPORIN, also plasma concentration of ciclosporin reduced by *intravenous* trimethoprim
- Cytotoxics: increased risk of haematological toxicity when trimethoprim (also with co-trimoxazole) given with ● MERCAPTOPURINE; increased risk of severe bone marrow depression (fatalities reported) and other haematological toxicites when trimethoprim (also with co-trimoxazole) given with ● METHOTREXATE
- Diuretics: increased risk of hyperkalaemia when trimethoprim given with EPLERENONE; possible increased risk of hyperkalaemia when trimethoprim given with SPIRONOLACTONE
- Tacrolimus: possible increased risk of nephrotoxicity when trimethoprim given with ● TACROLIMUS
- Vaccines: antibacterials inactivate ORAL TYPHOID VACCINE—see under Typhoid Vaccine in BNF

Trimipramine see Antidepressants, Tricyclic

Tripotassium Dicitratobismuthate

- Antibacterials: tripotassium dicitratobismuthate reduces absorption of TETRACYCLINES

Tropicamide see Antimuscarinics

Trospium see Antimuscarinics

Typhoid Vaccine (oral) see Vaccines

Typhoid Vaccine (parenteral) see Vaccines

Ubidecarenone

- Anticoagulants: ubidecarenone may enhance or reduce anticoagulant effect of WARFARIN

Ulcer-healing Drugs see Histamine H$_2$-antagonists, Proton Pump Inhibitors, Sucralfate, and Tripotassium Dicitratobismuthate

Ulipristal

- Antibacterials: manufacturer of *low-dose* ulipristal advises avoid concomitant use with CLARITHROMYCIN and TELITHROMYCIN; plasma concentration of *low-dose* ulipristal increased by ERYTHROMYCIN—manufacturer of *low-dose* ulipristal advises avoid concomitant use; manufacturer of ulipristal advises avoid concomitant use with RIFAMPICIN (contraceptive effect of ulipristal possibly reduced)
- Anticoagulants: manufacturer of ulipristal advises give DABIGATRAN at least 1.5 hours before or after ulipristal
- Antidepressants: manufacturer of ulipristal advises avoid concomitant use with ● ST JOHN'S WORT (contraceptive effect of ulipristal possibly reduced)
- Antiepileptics: manufacturer of ulipristal advises avoid concomitant use with ● CARBAMAZEPINE, ● FOSPHENYTOIN, ● PHENOBARBITAL, ● PHENYTOIN and ● PRIMIDONE (contraceptive effect of ulipristal possibly reduced)
- Antifungals: plasma concentration of *low-dose* ulipristal increased by KETOCONAZOLE—manufacturer of *low-dose* ulipristal advises avoid concomitant use; manufacturer of ulipristal advises avoid concomitant use with ITRACONAZOLE

Ulipristal (continued)

▸ Antihistamines: manufacturer of ulipristal advises give FEXOFENADINE at least 1.5 hours before or after ulipristal

• Antivirals: manufacturer of ulipristal advises avoid concomitant use with ● RITONAVIR (contraceptive effect of ulipristal possibly reduced)

• Calcium-channel Blockers: manufacturer of *low-dose* ulipristal advises avoid concomitant use with VERAPAMIL

▸ Cardiac Glycosides: manufacturer of ulipristal advises give DIGOXIN at least 1.5 hours before or after ulipristal

▸ Grapefruit Juice: manufacturer of *low-dose* ulipristal advises avoid concomitant use with GRAPEFRUIT JUICE

• Progestogens: ulipristal possibly reduces contraceptive effect of ● PROGESTOGENS

Umeclidinium *see* Antimuscarinics

Ursodeoxycholic Acid *see* Bile Acids

Ustekinumab

• Antipsychotics: avoid concomitant use of cytotoxics with ● CLOZAPINE (increased risk of agranulocytosis)

• Vaccines: risk of generalised infections when monoclonal antibodies given with live ● VACCINES—avoid concomitant use

Vaccines

• Abatacept: risk of generalised infections when live vaccines given with ● ABATACEPT—avoid concomitant use

▸ Aminophylline: influenza vaccine possibly increases plasma concentration of AMINOPHYLLINE

• Anakinra: risk of generalised infections when live vaccines given with ● ANAKINRA—avoid concomitant use

▸ Antibacterials: oral typhoid vaccine inactivated by ANTIBACTERIALS—see under Typhoid Vaccine in BNF

▸ Anticoagulants: influenza vaccine possibly enhances anticoagulant effect of WARFARIN

▸ Antidepressants: oral typhoid vaccine inactivated by antibacterials including LINEZOLID—see under Typhoid Vaccine in BNF

▸ Antiepileptics: influenza vaccine enhances effects of FOSPHENYTOIN and PHENYTOIN

▸ Antimalarials: oral typhoid vaccine inactivated by ANTIMALARIALS—see under Typhoid Vaccine in BNF

• Azathioprine: risk of generalised infections when live vaccines given with ● AZATHIOPRINE—avoid concomitant use

• Corticosteroids: immune response to vaccines impaired by high doses of ● CORTICOSTEROIDS—avoid concomitant use with live vaccines

• Cytotoxics: risk of generalised infections when live vaccines given with ● CYTOTOXIC ANTIBIOTICS, ● HYDROXYCARBAMIDE, ● MONOCLONAL ANTIBODIES or ● TRABECTEDIN—avoid concomitant use

• Dexrazoxane: risk of generalised infections when live vaccines given with ● DEXRAZOXANE—avoid concomitant use

• Etanercept: risk of generalised infections when live vaccines given with ● ETANERCEPT—avoid concomitant use

• Immunoglobulins: impaired immune response to *oral* poliomyelitis vaccine might occur with ● ANTI-D IMMUNOGLOBULINS and ● NORMAL IMMUNOGLOBULIN—give *oral* poliomyelitis vaccine at least 3 weeks before or 3 months after anti-d immunoglobulins and normal immunoglobulin; impaired immune response to BCG vaccine, MMR vaccine, oral typhoid vaccine, rotavirus vaccine, smallpox vaccine, varicella-zoster vaccine and yellow fever vaccine might occur with ● ANTI-D IMMUNOGLOBULINS—give BCG vaccine, MMR vaccine, oral typhoid vaccine, rotavirus vaccine, smallpox vaccine, varicella-zoster vaccine and yellow fever vaccine at least 3 weeks before or 3 months after anti-d immunoglobulins; impaired immune response to live influenza vaccine might occur with ● ANTI-D IMMUNOGLOBULINS and ● NORMAL IMMUNOGLOBULIN—give live influenza vaccine at least 3 weeks before or 3 months after anti-d immunoglobulins and normal immunoglobulin; impaired immune response to BCG vaccine, MMR vaccine, oral typhoid vaccine, rotavirus vaccine, smallpox vaccine, varicella-zoster vaccine and yellow fever vaccine might occur with ● NORMAL IMMUNOGLOBULIN—give BCG vaccine, MMR vaccine, oral typhoid vaccine, rotavirus vaccine, smallpox vaccine, varicella-zoster vaccine and yellow fever vaccine at least 3 weeks before or 3 months after normal immunoglobulin

Vaccines (continued)

▸ Interferons: avoidance of vaccines advised by manufacturer of INTERFERON GAMMA

• Leflunomide: risk of generalised infections when live vaccines given with ● LEFLUNOMIDE—avoid concomitant use

• Teriflunomide: risk of generalised infections when live vaccines given with ● TERIFLUNOMIDE—avoid concomitant use

▸ Theophylline: influenza vaccine possibly increases plasma concentration of THEOPHYLLINE

Valaciclovir

▸ Aminophylline: valaciclovir possibly increases plasma concentration of AMINOPHYLLINE

▸ Ciclosporin: increased risk of nephrotoxicity when valaciclovir given with CICLOSPORIN

▸ Mycophenolate: plasma concentration of valaciclovir increased by MYCOPHENOLATE, also plasma concentration of inactive metabolite of mycophenolate increased

▸ Tacrolimus: possible increased risk of nephrotoxicity when valaciclovir given with TACROLIMUS

▸ Theophylline: valaciclovir possibly increases plasma concentration of THEOPHYLLINE

Valganciclovir

• Antibacterials: increased risk of convulsions when valganciclovir given with ● IMIPENEM WITH CILASTATIN

• Antivirals: valganciclovir possibly increases plasma concentration of DIDANOSINE; profound myelosuppression when valganciclovir given with ● ZIDOVUDINE (if possible avoid concomitant administration, particularly during initial valganciclovir therapy)

▸ Mycophenolate: plasma concentration of valganciclovir possibly increased by MYCOPHENOLATE, also plasma concentration of inactive metabolite of mycophenolate possibly increased

▸ Tacrolimus: possible increased risk of nephrotoxicity when valganciclovir given with TACROLIMUS

Valproic Acid

▸ Analgesics: effects of valproic acid enhanced by ASPIRIN

▸ Antibacterials: metabolism of valproic acid possibly inhibited by ERYTHROMYCIN (increased plasma concentration); avoidance of valproic acid advised by manufacturer of ● PIVMECILLINAM; plasma concentration of valproic acid reduced by ● CARBAPENEMS—avoid concomitant use

• Anticoagulants: valproic acid possibly enhances anticoagulant effect of COUMARINS

• Antidepressants: anticonvulsant effect of antiepileptics possibly antagonised by MAOIs and ● TRICYCLIC-RELATED ANTIDEPRESSANTS (convulsive threshold lowered); anticonvulsant effect of antiepileptics antagonised by ● SSRIs and ● TRICYCLICS (convulsive threshold lowered)

• Antiepileptics: plasma concentration of valproic acid reduced by CARBAMAZEPINE, also plasma concentration of active metabolite of carbamazepine increased; valproic acid possibly increases plasma concentration of ETHOSUXIMIDE; valproic acid increases or possibly decreases plasma concentration of FOSPHENYTOIN and PHENYTOIN, also plasma concentration of valproic acid reduced; valproic acid increases plasma concentration of ● LAMOTRIGINE (increased risk of toxicity—reduce lamotrigine dose); valproic acid sometimes reduces plasma concentration of an active metabolite of OXCARBAZEPINE; valproic acid increases plasma concentration of PHENOBARBITAL and PRIMIDONE (also plasma concentration of valproic acid reduced); valproic acid possibly increases plasma concentration of RUFINAMIDE (reduce dose of rufinamide); hyperammonaemia and CNS toxicity reported when valproic acid given with TOPIRAMATE

• Antimalarials: anticonvulsant effect of antiepileptics antagonised by ● MEFLOQUINE

• Antipsychotics: anticonvulsant effect of antiepileptics antagonised by ● ANTIPSYCHOTICS (convulsive threshold lowered); valproic acid possibly increases or decreases plasma concentration of CLOZAPINE; increased risk of side-effects including neutropenia when valproic acid given with ● OLANZAPINE

▸ Antivirals: plasma concentration of valproic acid possibly reduced by RITONAVIR; valproic acid possibly increases plasma concentration of ZIDOVUDINE (increased risk of toxicity)

Valproic Acid (continued)

▸ **Anxiolytics and Hypnotics:** plasma concentration of valproic acid possibly increased by CLOBAZAM; increased risk of side-effects when valproic acid given with CLONAZEPAM; valproic acid possibly increases plasma concentration of DIAZEPAM and LORAZEPAM

▸ **Bupropion:** valproic acid inhibits the metabolism of BUPROPION

▸ **Cytotoxics:** valproic acid increases plasma concentration of TEMOZOLOMIDE

▸ **Guanfacine:** plasma concentration of valproic acid increased by GUANFACINE

▸ **Lipid-regulating Drugs:** absorption of valproic acid possibly reduced by COLESTYRAMINE

▸ **Netupitant:** caution with valproic acid advised by manufacturer of NETUPITANT

▸ **Oestrogens:** plasma concentration of valproic acid possibly reduced by ETHINYLESTRADIOL

● **Orlistat:** possible increased risk of convulsions when antiepileptics given with ● ORLISTAT

● **Sodium Benzoate:** valproic acid possibly reduces effects of SODIUM BENZOATE

● **Sodium Oxybate:** valproic acid increases the plasma concentration of ● SODIUM OXYBATE (see under Sodium Oxybate, p. 447)

▸ **Sodium Phenylbutyrate:** valproic acid possibly reduces effects of SODIUM PHENYLBUTYRATE

● **Ulcer-healing Drugs:** metabolism of valproic acid inhibited by ● CIMETIDINE (increased plasma concentration)

Valsartan see Angiotensin-II Receptor Antagonists

Vancomycin

▸ **Anaesthetics, General:** hypersensitivity-like reactions can occur when *intravenous* vancomycin given with GENERAL ANAESTHETICS

● **Antibacterials:** increased risk of nephrotoxicity and ototoxicity when vancomycin given with ● AMINOGLYCOSIDES, CAPREOMYCIN or COLISTIMETHATE SODIUM; increased risk of nephrotoxicity when vancomycin given with POLYMYXINS

▸ **Antifungals:** possible increased risk of nephrotoxicity when vancomycin given with AMPHOTERICIN

● **Ciclosporin:** increased risk of nephrotoxicity when vancomycin given with ● CICLOSPORIN

▸ **Cytotoxics:** increased risk of nephrotoxicity and possibly of ototoxicity when vancomycin given with CISPLATIN

● **Diuretics:** increased risk of otoxicity when vancomycin given with ● LOOP DIURETICS

▸ **Lipid-regulating Drugs:** effects of *oral* vancomycin antagonised by COLESTYRAMINE

● **Muscle Relaxants:** vancomycin enhances effects of ● SUXAMETHONIUM

▸ **Tacrolimus:** possible increased risk of nephrotoxicity when vancomycin given with TACROLIMUS

▸ **Vaccines:** antibacterials inactivate ORAL TYPHOID VACCINE—see under Typhoid Vaccine in BNF

Vandetanib

● **Analgesics:** possible increased risk of ventricular arrhythmias when vandetanib given with ● METHADONE—avoid concomitant use

● **Anti-arrhythmics:** possible increased risk of ventricular arrhythmias when vandetanib given with ● AMIODARONE or ● DISOPYRAMIDE—avoid concomitant use

● **Antibacterials:** possible increased risk of ventricular arrhythmias when vandetanib given with *parenteral* ● ERYTHROMYCIN—avoid concomitant use; possible increased risk of ventricular arrhythmias when vandetanib given with ● MOXIFLOXACIN—avoid concomitant use; plasma concentration of vandetanib reduced by ● RIFAMPICIN—manufacturer of vandetanib advises avoid concomitant use

▸ **Antidepressants:** manufacturer of vandetanib advises avoid concomitant use with ST JOHN'S WORT (plasma concentration of vandetanib possibly reduced)

▸ **Antidiabetics:** vandetanib possibly increases plasma concentration of METFORMIN (consider reducing dose of metformin)

▸ **Antiepileptics:** manufacturer of vandetanib advises avoid concomitant use with CARBAMAZEPINE, PHENOBARBITAL and

Vandetanib

Antiepileptics (continued)

PRIMIDONE (plasma concentration of vandetanib possibly reduced)

● **Antihistamines:** possible increased risk of ventricular arrhythmias when vandetanib given with ● MIZOLASTINE—avoid concomitant use

● **Antimalarials:** possible increased risk of ventricular arrhythmias when vandetanib given with ● ARTEMETHER WITH LUMEFANTRINE—avoid concomitant use

● **Antipsychotics:** possible increased risk of ventricular arrhythmias when vandetanib given with ● AMISULPRIDE, ● CHLORPROMAZINE, ● HALOPERIDOL, ● PIMOZIDE, ● SULPIRIDE or ● ZUCLOPENTHIXOL—avoid concomitant use; avoid concomitant use of cytotoxics with ● CLOZAPINE (increased risk of agranulocytosis)

● **Beta-blockers:** possible increased risk of ventricular arrhythmias when vandetanib given with ● SOTALOL—avoid concomitant use

▸ **Cardiac Glycosides:** vandetanib increases plasma concentration of DIGOXIN—possible increased risk of bradycardia

● **Cytotoxics:** possible increased risk of ventricular arrhythmias when vandetanib given with ● ARSENIC TRIOXIDE—avoid concomitant use

● **Hormone Antagonists:** possible increased risk of ventricular arrhythmias when vandetanib given with ● TOREMIFENE—avoid concomitant use

● **5HT₃-receptor Antagonists:** increased risk of ventricular arrhythmias when vandetanib given with ● ONDANSETRON—avoid concomitant use

● **Pentamidine Isetionate:** possible increased risk of ventricular arrhythmias when vandetanib given with ● PENTAMIDINE ISETIONATE—avoid concomitant use

Vardenafil

● **Alpha-blockers:** enhanced hypotensive effect when vardenafil given with ● ALPHA-BLOCKERS—when patient is stable on the alpha blocker initiate vardenafil at the lowest possible dose—separate doses by 6 hours (except with tamsulosin)

▸ **Anti-arrhythmics:** avoidance of vardenafil advised by manufacturer of DISOPYRAMIDE (risk of ventricular arrhythmias)

▸ **Antibacterials:** plasma concentration of vardenafil possibly increased by CLARITHROMYCIN (consider reducing initial dose of vardenafil); plasma concentration of vardenafil increased by ERYTHROMYCIN (reduce dose of vardenafil)

● **Antifungals:** plasma concentration of vardenafil increased by ● KETOCONAZOLE—avoid concomitant use; plasma concentration of vardenafil possibly increased by ● ITRACONAZOLE—avoid concomitant use

● **Antivirals:** plasma concentration of vardenafil possibly increased by FOSAMPRENAVIR; plasma concentration of vardenafil increased by ● INDINAVIR and ● RITONAVIR—avoid concomitant use; increased risk of ventricular arrhythmias when vardenafil given with ● SAQUINAVIR—avoid concomitant use; avoidance of vardenafil advised by manufacturer of ● TELAPREVIR; caution with vardenafil advised by manufacturer of TIPRANAVIR

▸ **Calcium-channel Blockers:** enhanced hypotensive effect when vardenafil given with NIFEDIPINE

● **Cobicistat:** plasma concentration of vardenafil possibly increased by ● COBICISTAT—manufacturer of cobicistat advises reduce dose of vardenafil (consult cobicistat product literature)

▸ **Dapoxetine:** avoidance of vardenafil advised by manufacturer of DAPOXETINE

● **Grapefruit Juice:** plasma concentration of vardenafil possibly increased by ● GRAPEFRUIT JUICE—avoid concomitant use

● **Nicorandil:** possible increased hypotensive effect when vardenafil given with ● NICORANDIL—avoid concomitant use

● **Nitrates:** possible increased hypotensive effect when vardenafil given with ● NITRATES—avoid concomitant use

● **Riociguat:** possible enhanced hypotensive effect when vardenafil given with ● RIOCIGUAT—avoid concomitant use

Varicella-zoster Vaccine see Vaccines

Vasodilator Antihypertensives

▸ **ACE Inhibitors:** enhanced hypotensive effect when hydralazine, minoxidil or sodium nitroprusside given with ACE INHIBITORS
▸ **Adrenergic Neurone Blockers:** enhanced hypotensive effect when hydralazine, minoxidil or sodium nitroprusside given with ADRENERGIC NEURONE BLOCKERS
▸ **Alcohol:** enhanced hypotensive effect when hydralazine, minoxidil or sodium nitroprusside given with ALCOHOL
▸ **Aldesleukin:** enhanced hypotensive effect when hydralazine, minoxidil or sodium nitroprusside given with ALDESLEUKIN
▸ **Alpha-blockers:** enhanced hypotensive effect when hydralazine, minoxidil or sodium nitroprusside given with ALPHA-BLOCKERS
▸ **Anaesthetics, General:** enhanced hypotensive effect when hydralazine, minoxidil or sodium nitroprusside given with GENERAL ANAESTHETICS
▸ **Analgesics:** hypotensive effect of hydralazine, minoxidil and sodium nitroprusside antagonised by NSAIDs
▸ **Angiotensin-II Receptor Antagonists:** enhanced hypotensive effect when hydralazine, minoxidil or sodium nitroprusside given with ANGIOTENSIN-II RECEPTOR ANTAGONISTS
▸ **Antidepressants:** enhanced hypotensive effect when hydralazine, minoxidil or sodium nitroprusside given with MAOIs; enhanced hypotensive effect when hydralazine or sodium nitroprusside given with TRICYCLIC-RELATED ANTIDEPRESSANTS
▸ **Antipsychotics:** enhanced hypotensive effect when hydralazine, minoxidil or sodium nitroprusside given with PHENOTHIAZINES
▸ **Anxiolytics and Hypnotics:** enhanced hypotensive effect when hydralazine, minoxidil or sodium nitroprusside given with ANXIOLYTICS AND HYPNOTICS
▸ **Beta-blockers:** enhanced hypotensive effect when hydralazine, minoxidil or sodium nitroprusside given with BETA-BLOCKERS
▸ **Calcium-channel Blockers:** enhanced hypotensive effect when hydralazine, minoxidil or sodium nitroprusside given with CALCIUM-CHANNEL BLOCKERS
▸ **Clonidine:** enhanced hypotensive effect when hydralazine, minoxidil or sodium nitroprusside given with CLONIDINE
▸ **Corticosteroids:** hypotensive effect of hydralazine, minoxidil and sodium nitroprusside antagonised by CORTICOSTEROIDS
▸ **Diazoxide:** enhanced hypotensive effect when hydralazine, minoxidil or sodium nitroprusside given with DIAZOXIDE
▸ **Diuretics:** enhanced hypotensive effect when hydralazine, minoxidil or sodium nitroprusside given with DIURETICS
▸ **Dopaminergics:** enhanced hypotensive effect when hydralazine, minoxidil or sodium nitroprusside given with CO-BENELDOPA; enhanced hypotensive effect when hydralazine, minoxidil or sodium nitroprusside given with CO-CARELDOPA; enhanced hypotensive effect when hydralazine, minoxidil or sodium nitroprusside given with LEVODOPA
▸ **Methyldopa:** enhanced hypotensive effect when hydralazine, minoxidil or sodium nitroprusside given with METHYLDOPA
▸ **Moxisylyte:** enhanced hypotensive effect when hydralazine, minoxidil or sodium nitroprusside given with MOXISYLYTE
▸ **Moxonidine:** enhanced hypotensive effect when hydralazine, minoxidil or sodium nitroprusside given with MOXONIDINE
▸ **Muscle Relaxants:** enhanced hypotensive effect when hydralazine, minoxidil or sodium nitroprusside given with BACLOFEN; enhanced hypotensive effect when hydralazine, minoxidil or sodium nitroprusside given with TIZANIDINE
▸ **Nicorandil:** possible enhanced hypotensive effect when hydralazine, minoxidil or sodium nitroprusside given with NICORANDIL
▸ **Nitrates:** enhanced hypotensive effect when hydralazine, minoxidil or sodium nitroprusside given with NITRATES
▸ **Oestrogens:** hypotensive effect of hydralazine, minoxidil and sodium nitroprusside antagonised by OESTROGENS
▸ **Prostaglandins:** enhanced hypotensive effect when hydralazine, minoxidil or sodium nitroprusside given with ALPROSTADIL
▸ **Vasodilator Antihypertensives:** enhanced hypotensive effect when hydralazine given with MINOXIDIL or SODIUM NITROPRUSSIDE; enhanced hypotensive effect when minoxidil given with SODIUM NITROPRUSSIDE

Vecuronium *see* Muscle Relaxants

Vedolizumab

• **Antipsychotics:** avoid concomitant use of cytotoxics with ● CLOZAPINE (increased risk of agranulocytosis)
• **Vaccines:** risk of generalised infections when monoclonal antibodies given with live ● VACCINES—avoid concomitant use

Vemurafenib

▸ **Antibacterials:** manufacturer of vemurafenib advises avoid concomitant use with RIFABUTIN and RIFAMPICIN
▸ **Anticoagulants:** vemurafenib possibly enhances anticoagulant effect of ● WARFARIN
▸ **Antidepressants:** manufacturer of vemurafenib advises avoid concomitant use with ST JOHN'S WORT
▸ **Antiepileptics:** manufacturer of vemurafenib advises avoid concomitant use with CARBAMAZEPINE, FOSPHENYTOIN and PHENYTOIN
• **Antipsychotics:** avoid concomitant use of cytotoxics with ● CLOZAPINE (increased risk of agranulocytosis)
▸ **Cytotoxics:** avoidance of vemurafenib advised by manufacturer of IPILIMUMAB
• **Oestrogens:** manufacturer of vemurafenib advises contraceptive effect of ● OESTROGENS possibly reduced
• **Progestogens:** manufacturer of vemurafenib advises contraceptive effect of ● PROGESTOGENS possibly reduced

Venlafaxine

▸ **Analgesics:** increased risk of bleeding when venlafaxine given with ● NSAIDs or ● ASPIRIN; possible increased serotonergic effects when SSRI-related antidepressants given with FENTANYL; possible increased serotonergic effects when venlafaxine given with TRAMADOL
• **Anti-arrhythmics:** manufacturer of venlafaxine advises avoid concomitant use with ● AMIODARONE (risk of ventricular arrhythmias)
• **Antibacterials:** manufacturer of venlafaxine advises avoid concomitant use with ● ERYTHROMYCIN and ● MOXIFLOXACIN (risk of ventricular arrhythmias)
• **Anticoagulants:** venlafaxine possibly enhances anticoagulant effect of ● WARFARIN; possible increased risk of bleeding when SSRI-related antidepressants given with ● DABIGATRAN
• **Antidepressants:** possible increased serotonergic effects when venlafaxine given with ST JOHN'S WORT, DULOXETINE or MIRTAZAPINE; enhanced CNS effects and toxicity when venlafaxine given with ● MAOIS (venlafaxine should not be started until 2 weeks after stopping MAOIs, avoid MAOIs for 1 week after stopping venlafaxine); after stopping SSRI-related antidepressants do not start ● MOCLOBEMIDE for at least 1 week; possible increased risk of convulsions when SSRI-related antidepressants given with ● VORTIOXETINE
• **Antimalarials:** avoidance of antidepressants advised by manufacturer of ● ARTEMETHER WITH LUMEFANTRINE and ● ARTENIMOL WITH PIPERAQUINE
▸ **Antipsychotics:** venlafaxine increases plasma concentration of HALOPERIDOL
• **Atomoxetine:** possible increased risk of convulsions when antidepressants given with ATOMOXETINE
• **Beta-blockers:** manufacturer of venlafaxine advises avoid concomitant use with ● SOTALOL (risk of ventricular arrhythmias)
• **Dapoxetine:** possible increased risk of serotonergic effects when venlafaxine given with ● DAPOXETINE (manufacturer of dapoxetine advises venlafaxine should not be started until 1 week after stopping dapoxetine, avoid dapoxetine for 2 weeks after stopping venlafaxine)
• **Dopaminergics:** caution with venlafaxine advised by manufacturer of ENTACAPONE; increased risk of hypertension and CNS excitation when venlafaxine given with ● SELEGILINE (selegiline should not be started until 1 week after stopping venlafaxine, avoid venlafaxine for 2 weeks after stopping selegiline)
▸ **5HT₁-receptor Agonists:** possible increased serotonergic effects when venlafaxine given with 5HT₁ AGONISTS
▸ **5HT₃-receptor Antagonists:** possible increased serotonergic effects when SSRI-related antidepressants given with 5HT₃ ANTAGONISTS
▸ **Lithium:** possible increased serotonergic effects when venlafaxine given with LITHIUM

Venlafaxine (continued)

- Methylthioninium: risk of CNS toxicity when SSRI-related antidepressants given with ● METHYLTHIONINIUM—avoid concomitant use (if avoidance not possible, use lowest possible dose of methylthioninium and observe patient for up to 4 hours after administration)

Verapamil see Calcium-channel Blockers

Vigabatrin

- Antidepressants: anticonvulsant effect of antiepileptics possibly antagonised by MAOIs and ● TRICYCLIC-RELATED ANTIDEPRESSANTS (convulsive threshold lowered); anticonvulsant effect of antiepileptics antagonised by ● SSRIS and ● TRICYCLICS (convulsive threshold lowered)
- ▸ Antiepileptics: vigabatrin reduces plasma concentration of FOSPHENYTOIN and PHENYTOIN
- Antimalarials: anticonvulsant effect of antiepileptics antagonised by ● MEFLOQUINE
- Antipsychotics: anticonvulsant effect of antiepileptics antagonised by ● ANTIPSYCHOTICS (convulsive threshold lowered)
- Orlistat: possible increased risk of convulsions when antiepileptics given with ● ORLISTAT

Vilanterol see Sympathomimetics, Beta$_2$

Vildagliptin see Antidiabetics

Vinblastine

- Aldesleukin: avoidance of vinblastine advised by manufacturer of ● ALDESLEUKIN
- Antibacterials: toxicity of vinblastine increased by ● ERYTHROMYCIN—avoid concomitant use; possible increased risk of ventricular arrhythmias when vinblastine given with ● DELAMANID
- Antifungals: possible increased risk of vinblastine toxicity when given with ● ITRACONAZOLE; metabolism of vinblastine possibly inhibited by ● POSACONAZOLE (increased risk of neurotoxicity)
- Antimalarials: avoidance of vinblastine advised by manufacturer of ● ARTENIMOL WITH PIPERAQUINE
- Antipsychotics: avoid concomitant use of cytotoxics with ● CLOZAPINE (increased risk of agranulocytosis)
- ▸ Antivirals: plasma concentration of vinblastine possibly increased by RITONAVIR

Vincristine

- Antibacterials: possible increased risk of ventricular arrhythmias when vincristine given with ● DELAMANID
- Antifungals: increased risk of vincristine toxicity when given with ● ITRACONAZOLE; metabolism of vincristine possibly inhibited by ● POSACONAZOLE (increased risk of neurotoxicity)
- Antimalarials: avoidance of vincristine advised by manufacturer of ● ARTENIMOL WITH PIPERAQUINE
- Antipsychotics: avoid concomitant use of cytotoxics with ● CLOZAPINE (increased risk of agranulocytosis)
- ▸ Calcium-channel Blockers: metabolism of vincristine possibly inhibited by NIFEDIPINE
- ▸ Cardiac Glycosides: vincristine possibly reduces absorption of DIGOXIN *tablets*
- Cytotoxics: increased risk of hepatotoxicity when vincristine given with ● DACTINOMYCIN

Vindesine

- Antibacterials: possible increased risk of ventricular arrhythmias when vindesine given with ● DELAMANID
- Antifungals: possible increased risk of vindesine toxicity when given with ● ITRACONAZOLE
- Antipsychotics: avoid concomitant use of cytotoxics with ● CLOZAPINE (increased risk of agranulocytosis)

Vinflunine

- Antibacterials: plasma concentration of vinflunine possibly reduced by RIFAMPICIN—manufacturer of vinflunine advises avoid concomitant use; increased risk of ventricular arrhythmias when vinflunine given with ● DELAMANID
- Antidepressants: plasma concentration of vinflunine possibly reduced by ● ST JOHN'S WORT—manufacturer of vinflunine advises avoid concomitant use
- Antifungals: plasma concentration of vinflunine increased by ● KETOCONAZOLE—manufacturer of vinflunine advises avoid concomitant use; possible increased risk of vinflunine toxicity when given with ● ITRACONAZOLE

Vinflunine (continued)

- Antimalarials: avoidance of vinflunine advised by manufacturer of ● ARTENIMOL WITH PIPERAQUINE
- Antipsychotics: avoid concomitant use of cytotoxics with ● CLOZAPINE (increased risk of agranulocytosis)
- Antivirals: plasma concentration of vinflunine possibly increased by ● RITONAVIR—manufacturer of vinflunine advises avoid concomitant use
- ▸ Grapefruit Juice: plasma concentration of vinflunine possibly increased by GRAPEFRUIT JUICE—manufacturer of vinflunine advises avoid concomitant use

Vinorelbine

- Antibacterials: possible increased risk of neutropenia when vinorelbine given with ● CLARITHROMYCIN; possible increased risk of ventricular arrhythmias when vinorelbine given with ● DELAMANID
- Antifungals: possible increased risk of vinorelbine toxicity when given with ● ITRACONAZOLE
- Antimalarials: avoidance of vinorelbine advised by manufacturer of ● ARTENIMOL WITH PIPERAQUINE
- Antipsychotics: avoid concomitant use of cytotoxics with ● CLOZAPINE (increased risk of agranulocytosis)

Vismodegib

- Antibacterials: manufacturer of vismodegib advises avoid concomitant use with ● RIFAMPICIN (plasma concentration of vismodegib possibly reduced)
- Antidepressants: manufacturer of vismodegib advises avoid concomitant use with ● ST JOHN'S WORT (plasma concentration of vismodegib possibly reduced)
- Antiepileptics: manufacturer of vismodegib advises avoid concomitant use with ● CARBAMAZEPINE, ● FOSPHENYTOIN and ● PHENYTOIN (plasma concentration of vismodegib possibly reduced)
- Antipsychotics: avoid concomitant use of cytotoxics with ● CLOZAPINE (increased risk of agranulocytosis)

Vitamin A see Vitamins

Vitamin D see Vitamins

Vitamin E see Vitamins

Vitamin K (Phytomenadione) see Vitamins

Vitamins

- ▸ Antibacterials: absorption of vitamin A possibly reduced by NEOMYCIN
- Anticoagulants: vitamin E possibly enhances anticoagulant effect of ● COUMARINS; vitamin K antagonises anticoagulant effect of ● COUMARINS and ● PHENINDIONE
- ▸ Antiepileptics: alfacalcidol, calcitriol, colecalciferol, dihydrotachysterol, ergocalciferol, paricalcitol or vitamin D requirements possibly increased when given with CARBAMAZEPINE; alfacalcidol, calcitriol, colecalciferol, dihydrotachysterol, ergocalciferol, paricalcitol or vitamin D requirements possibly increased when given with FOSPHENYTOIN; alfacalcidol, calcitriol, colecalciferol, dihydrotachysterol, ergocalciferol, paricalcitol or vitamin D requirements possibly increased when given with PHENOBARBITAL; alfacalcidol, calcitriol, colecalciferol, dihydrotachysterol, ergocalciferol, paricalcitol or vitamin D requirements possibly increased when given with PHENYTOIN; alfacalcidol, calcitriol, colecalciferol, dihydrotachysterol, ergocalciferol, paricalcitol or vitamin D requirements possibly increased when given with PRIMIDONE
- ▸ Antifungals: plasma concentration of paricalcitol possibly increased by KETOCONAZOLE; effects of alfacalcidol, calcitriol, colecalciferol, dihydrotachysterol, ergocalciferol, paricalcitol and vitamin D possibly reduced by MICONAZOLE
- ▸ Antivirals: increased risk of bleeding when high doses of vitamin E given with TIPRANAVIR
- ▸ Ciclosporin: vitamin E possibly affects plasma concentration of CICLOSPORIN
- ▸ Cytotoxics: effects of alfacalcidol, calcitriol, colecalciferol, dihydrotachysterol, ergocalciferol, paricalcitol and vitamin D possibly reduced by DACTINOMYCIN; avoidance of vitamin E advised by manufacturer of IBRUTINIB
- ▸ Diuretics: increased risk of hypercalcaemia when alfacalcidol, calcitriol, colecalciferol, dihydrotachysterol, ergocalciferol, paricalcitol or vitamin D given with THIAZIDES AND RELATED DIURETICS

Vitamins (continued)

▸ **Dopaminergics:** pyridoxine reduces effects of LEVODOPA when given without dopa-decarboxylase inhibitor

▸ **Lipid-regulating Drugs:** absorption of calcitriol possibly reduced by COLESTYRAMINE (give at least 1 hour before or 4 to 6 hours after colestyramine)

● **Retinoids:** risk of hypervitaminosis A when vitamin A given with ● RETINOIDS—avoid concomitant use

● **Selenium:** ascorbic acid possibly reduces absorption of SELENIUM (give at least 4 hours apart)

▸ **Sevelamer:** absorption of calcitriol reduced by SEVELAMER (give at least 1 hour before or 3 hours after sevelamer)

Voriconazole see Antifungals, Triazole

Vortioxetine

▸ **Analgesics:** possible increased serotonergic effects when vortioxetine given with TRAMADOL

● **Antibacterials:** plasma concentration of vortioxetine reduced by ● RIFAMPICIN—consider increasing dose of vortioxetine

● **Antidepressants:** plasma concentration of vortioxetine possibly increased by FLUOXETINE and PAROXETINE (consider reducing dose of vortioxetine); increased risk of hypertension and CNS excitation when vortioxetine given with ● MAOIS (vortioxetine should not be started until 2 weeks after stopping MAOIs, avoid MAOIs for 2 weeks after stopping vortioxetine); manufacturer of vortioxetine advises avoid concomitant use with ● LINEZOLID and ● MOCLOBEMIDE; possible increased risk of convulsions when vortioxetine given with ● SSRI-RELATED ANTIDEPRESSANTS, ● SSRIS or ● TRICYCLICS; possible increased serotonergic effects when vortioxetine given with ST JOHN'S WORT

● **Antiepileptics:** plasma concentration of vortioxetine possibly reduced by ● CARBAMAZEPINE, ● FOSPHENYTOIN and ● PHENYTOIN—consider increasing dose of vortioxetine

● **Antimalarials:** avoidance of antidepressants advised by manufacturer of ● ARTEMETHER WITH LUMEFANTRINE and ● ARTENIMOL WITH PIPERAQUINE; possible increased risk of convulsions when vortioxetine given with ● MEFLOQUINE

● **Antipsychotics:** possible increased risk of convulsions when vortioxetine given with ● BUTYROPHENONES, ● PHENOTHIAZINES or ● THIOXANTHENES

▸ **Atomoxetine:** possible increased risk of convulsions when antidepressants given with ATOMOXETINE

▸ **Bupropion:** plasma concentration of vortioxetine increased by BUPROPION (consider reducing dose of vortioxetine)

● **Dopaminergics:** risk of CNS excitation and hypertension when vortioxetine given with ● RASAGILINE or ● SELEGILINE

▸ **5HT$_1$-receptor Agonists:** possible increased serotonergic effects when vortioxetine given with 5HT$_1$ AGONISTS

Warfarin see Coumarins

Wasp Venom Extracts

● **ACE Inhibitors:** possible severe anaphylactoid reaction when wasp venom extracts given with ● ACE INHIBITORS

Xipamide see Diuretics

Xylometazoline see Sympathomimetics

Yellow Fever Vaccine see Vaccines

Zafirlukast see Leukotriene Receptor Antagonists

Zaleplon see Anxiolytics and Hypnotics

Zidovudine

NOTE Increased risk of toxicity with nephrotoxic and myelosuppressive drugs—for further details consult product literature

▸ **Analgesics:** increased risk of haematological toxicity when zidovudine given with NSAIDs; plasma concentration of zidovudine possibly increased by METHADONE

▸ **Antibacterials:** absorption of zidovudine reduced by CLARITHROMYCIN tablets (give at least 2 hours apart); manufacturer of zidovudine advises avoid concomitant use with RIFAMPICIN

▸ **Antiepileptics:** zidovudine increases or decreases plasma concentration of FOSPHENYTOIN and PHENYTOIN; plasma concentration of zidovudine possibly increased by SODIUM VALPROATE and VALPROIC ACID (increased risk of toxicity)

● **Antifungals:** plasma concentration of zidovudine increased by ● FLUCONAZOLE (increased risk of toxicity)

▸ **Antimalarials:** increased antifolate effect when zidovudine given with PYRIMETHAMINE

Zidovudine (continued)

● **Antivirals:** profound myelosuppression when zidovudine given with ● GANCICLOVIR or ● VALGANCICLOVIR (if possible avoid concomitant administration, particularly during initial ganciclovir or valganciclovir therapy); increased risk of granulocytopenia when zidovudine given with ● NEVIRAPINE; increased risk of anaemia when zidovudine given with ● RIBAVIRIN—avoid concomitant use; zidovudine possibly inhibits effects of ● STAVUDINE (manufacturers advise avoid concomitant use); plasma concentration of zidovudine reduced by ● TIPRANAVIR

▸ **Atovaquone:** plasma concentration of zidovudine increased by ATOVAQUONE (increased risk of toxicity)

▸ **Netupitant:** caution with zidovudine advised by manufacturer of NETUPITANT

▸ **Orlistat:** absorption of zidovudine possibly reduced by ● ORLISTAT

Zinc

▸ **Antibacterials:** zinc reduces absorption of CIPROFLOXACIN, LEVOFLOXACIN, NORFLOXACIN and OFLOXACIN (give at least 2 hours apart); zinc reduces absorption of MOXIFLOXACIN (give at least 6 hours apart); zinc possibly reduces absorption of TETRACYCLINES (give at least 2 to 3 hours apart)

▸ **Calcium Salts:** absorption of zinc reduced by CALCIUM SALTS

▸ **Eltrombopag:** zinc possibly reduces absorption of ELTROMBOPAG (give at least 4 hours apart)

▸ **Iron Salts:** absorption of zinc reduced by *oral* IRON SALTS, also absorption of *oral* iron salts reduced by zinc

▸ **Penicillamine:** absorption of zinc reduced by PENICILLAMINE, also absorption of penicillamine reduced by zinc

▸ **Trientine:** absorption of zinc reduced by TRIENTINE, also absorption of trientine reduced by zinc

Zoledronic Acid see Bisphosphonates

Zolmitriptan see 5HT$_1$-receptor Agonists (under HT)

Zolpidem see Anxiolytics and Hypnotics

Zonisamide

● **Antidepressants:** anticonvulsant effect of antiepileptics possibly antagonised by MAOIS and ● TRICYCLIC-RELATED ANTIDEPRESSANTS (convulsive threshold lowered); anticonvulsant effect of antiepileptics antagonised by ● SSRIS and ● TRICYCLICS (convulsive threshold lowered)

▸ **Antiepileptics:** plasma concentration of zonisamide reduced by CARBAMAZEPINE, FOSPHENYTOIN, PHENOBARBITAL, PHENYTOIN and PRIMIDONE

● **Antimalarials:** anticonvulsant effect of antiepileptics antagonised by ● MEFLOQUINE

● **Antipsychotics:** anticonvulsant effect of antiepileptics antagonised by ● ANTIPSYCHOTICS (convulsive threshold lowered)

▸ **Diuretics:** manufacturer of zonisamide advises avoid concomitant use with CARBONIC ANHYDRASE INHIBITORS in children

● **Orlistat:** possible increased risk of convulsions when antiepileptics given with ● ORLISTAT

Zopiclone see Anxiolytics and Hypnotics

Zuclopenthixol see Antipsychotics

A1

Interactions | **Appendix 1**

Appendix 2
Borderline substances

CONTENTS

In certain conditions some foods (and toilet preparations) have characteristics of drugs and the Advisory Committee on Borderline Substances (ACBS) advises as to the circumstances in which such substances may be regarded as drugs. Prescriptions issued in accordance with the Committee's advice and endorsed 'ACBS' will normally not be investigated.

Information

General Practitioners are reminded that the ACBS recommends products on the basis that they may be regarded as drugs for the management of specified conditions. Doctors should satisfy themselves that the products can safely be prescribed, that patients are adequately monitored and that, where necessary, expert hospital supervision is available.

Foods which may be prescribed on FP10, GP10 (Scotland), or WP10 (Wales)

All the food products listed in this appendix have ACBS approval. The clinical condition for which the product has been approved is included with each entry.
Note Foods included in this appendix may contain cariogenic sugars and patients should be advised to take appropriate oral hygiene measures.

Enteral feeds and supplements

For most enteral feeds and nutritional supplements, the main source of **carbohydrate** is either maltodextrin or glucose syrup; other carbohydrate sources are listed in the relevant table, below. Feeds containing residual lactose (less than 1 g lactose/100 mL formula) are described as 'clinically lactose-free' or 'lactose-free' by some manufacturers. The presence of lactose (including residual lactose) in feeds is indicated in the relevant table, below. The primary sources of **protein** or **amino acids** are included with each product entry. The **fat** or **oil** content is derived from a variety of sources such as vegetables, soya bean, corn, palm nuts, and seeds; where the fat content is derived from animal or fish sources, this information is included in the relevant table,

below. The presence of medium chain triglycerides (MCT) is also noted where the quantity exceeds 30% of the fat content.
Enteral feeds and nutritional supplements can contain varying amounts of **vitamins, minerals,** and **trace elements**—the manufacturer's product literature should be consulted for more detailed information. Feeds containing vitamin K may affect the INR in patients receiving warfarin. The suitability of food products for patients requiring a vegan, kosher, halal, or other compliant diet should be confirmed with individual manufacturers.
Note Feeds containing more than 6 g/100 mL protein or 2 g/100 mL fibre should be avoided in children unless recommended by an appropriate specialist or dietician.

Nutritional values

Nutritional values of products vary with flavour and pack size—consult product literature.

Other conditions for which ACBS products can be prescribed

This is a list of clinical conditions for which the ACBS has approved toilet preparations.
Birthmarks
Dermatitis
Eczema and Pruritus
Aveeno® Bath Oil; *Aveeno*® Cream; *Aveeno*® Lotion; *E45*® Emollient Bath Oil; *E45*® Emollient Wash Cream; *E45*® Lotion
Disfiguring skin lesions (birthmarks, mutilating lesions, scars, vitiligo)
Covermark® classic foundation and finishing powder; *Dermablend*® *Ultra* corrective foundation; *Dermacolor*® Camouflage cream and fixing powder; *Keromask*® masking cream and finishing powder; *Veil*® Cover cream and Finishing Powder. (Cleansing Creams, Cleansing Milks, and Cleansing Lotions are excluded).
Disinfectants (antiseptics)
May be prescribed on an FP10 only when ordered in such quantities and with such directions as are appropriate for

the treatment of patients, but not for general hygenic purposes.

Dry mouth (xerostomia)

For patients suffering from dry mouth as a result of having (or having undergone) radiotherapy, or sicca syndrome. *AS Saliva Orthana*®; *Biotène Oralbalance*®; *BioXtra*®; *Glandosane*®; *Saliveze*®

Photodermatoses (skin protection in)

Anthelios® XL SPF 50+ Melt-in cream; *Sunsense*® Ultra; *Uvistat*® Lipscreen SPF 50, *Uvistat*® Suncream SPF 30 and 50

Standard ACBS Indications

Disease-related malnutrition, intractable malabsorption, pre-operative preparation of malnourished patients, dysphagia, proven inflammatory bowel disease, following total gastrectomy, short-bowel syndrome, bowel fistula.

Borderline substances | Appendix 2

A2

Table 1 Enteral feeds (non-disease specific)
Less than 5 g protein/100 mL

Enteral feeds: 1 kcal/mL and less than 5 g protein/100 mL
Not suitable for use in child under 1 year unless otherwise stated; not recommended for child 1-6 years

Product	Formulation	Energy	Protein	Carbohydrate	Fat	Fibre	Special Characteristics	ACBS Indications	Presentation & Flavour
Fresubin® 1500 Complete (Fresenius Kabi Ltd)	Liquid (tube feed) per 100 mL	420 kJ (100 kcal)	3.8 g cows' milk soya	13 g (sugars 0.9 g)	3.4 g	1.5 g	Gluten-free Residual lactose Contains fish oil	Standard, p. 1335 except bowel fistula and pre-operative preparation of malnourished patients. Not suitable for child under 2 years	Fresubin 1500 Complete liquid: 1.5 litre = £13.28
Fresubin® Original (Fresenius Kabi Ltd)	Liquid (sip or tube feed) per 100 mL	420 kJ (100 kcal)	3.8 g cows' milk soya	13.8 g (sugars 3.5 g)	3.4 g	Nil	Gluten-free Residual lactose Contains fish gelatin Feed in flexible pack contains fish oil and fish gelatin	Standard, p. 1335	Fresubin Original liquid: blackcurrant, chocolate, nut, peach, vanilla 200 ml = £2.14; unflavoured 500 ml = £4.17; 1000 ml = £8.26; 1500 ml = £12.39
Fresubin® Original Fibre (Fresenius Kabi Ltd)	Liquid (tube feed) per 100 mL	420 kJ (100 kcal)	3.8 g cows' milk soya	13 g (sugars 0.9 g)	3.4 g	1.5 g	Gluten-free Residual lactose Contains fish oil	Standard, p. 1335 except bowel fistula and pre-operative preparation of malnourished patients. Not suitable for child under 2 years	Fresubin Original Fibre liquid: 500 ml = £4.72; 1000 ml = £9.42
Jevity® (Abbott Laboratories Ltd)	Liquid (tube feed) per 100 mL	449 kJ (107 kcal)	4 g caseinates	14.1 g (sugars 470 mg)	3.47 g	1.76 g	Gluten-free Residual lactose	Standard, p. 1335 except bowel fistula. Not suitable for child under 2 years	Jevity liquid: 500 ml = £5.20; 1000 ml = £9.46; 1500 ml = £14.14
Nutrison® (Nutricia Ltd)	Liquid (tube feed) per 100 mL	420 kJ (100 kcal)	4 g cows' milk	12.3 g (sugars 1 g)	3.9 g	Nil	Gluten-free Residual lactose	Standard, p. 1335	Nutrison liquid: 500 ml = £4.43; 500 ml = £4.92; 1000 ml = £8.63; 1500 ml = £12.93
Nutrison® Multi Fibre (Nutricia Ltd)	Liquid (tube feed) per 100 mL	420 kJ (100 kcal)	4 g cows' milk	12.3 g (sugars 1 g)	3.9 g	1.5 g	Gluten-free Residual lactose	Standard, p. 1335 except bowel fistula	Nutrison Multi Fibre liquid: 500 ml = £5.31; 500 ml = £5.31; 1000 ml = £9.99; 1500 ml = £14.97
Osmolite® (Abbott Laboratories Ltd)	Liquid (tube feed) per 100 mL	424 kJ (100 kcal)	4 g caseinates soy isolate	13.6 g (sugars 630 mg)	3.4 g	Nil	Gluten-free Residual lactose	Standard, p. 1335	Osmolite liquid: 500 ml = £4.65; 1000 ml = £8.46; 1500 ml = £12.65
SOYA PROTEIN FORMULA									
Fresubin® Soya Fibre (Fresenius Kabi Ltd)	Liquid (tube feed) per 100 mL	420 kJ (100 kcal)	3.8 g soya protein	13.3 g (sugars 4.1 g)	3.6 g	2 g	Gluten-free Lactose-free Contains fish oil	Standard, p. 1335; also cows' milk protein intolerance, lactose intolerance	Fresubin Soya Fibre liquid: 500 ml = £4.88
Nutrison® Soya (Nutricia Ltd)	Liquid (tube feed) per 100 mL	420 kJ (100 kcal)	4 g soy isolate	12.3 g (sugars 1 g)	3.9 g	Nil	Gluten-free Residual lactose Milk protein-free	Standard, p. 1335; also cows' milk protein and lactose intolerance	Nutrison Soya liquid: 500 ml = £5.30; 1000 ml = £10.62
Nutrison® Soya Multi Fibre (Nutricia Ltd)	Liquid (tube feed) per 100 mL	420 kJ (100 kcal)	4 g soy isolate	12.3 g (sugars 700 mg)	3.9 g	1.5 g	Gluten-free Residual lactose Milk protein-free	Standard, p. 1335 except bowel fistula; also cows' milk protein and lactose intolerance	Nutrison Soya Multi Fibre liquid: 1.5 litre = £17.66

PEPTIDE-BASED FORMULA

Product	Formulation	Energy	Protein	Carbohydrate	Fat	Fibre	Special Characteristics	ACBS Indications	Presentation & Flavour
Nutrison Peptisorb® (Nutricia Ltd)	Liquid (tube feed) per 100 mL	425 kJ (100 kcal)	4 g whey protein hydrolysate	17.6 g (sugars 1.7 g)	1.7 g (MCT 47 %)	Nil	Gluten-free Residual lactose	Short bowel syndrome, intractable malabsorption, proven inflammatory bowel disease, bowel fistula	Nutrison Peptisorb liquid: 500 ml = £7.04; 500 ml = £7.73; 1000 ml = £13.94
Peptamen® (Nestle Health Science)	Liquid (sip or tube feed) per 100 mL	420 kJ (100 kcal)	4 g whey peptides	12.7 g (sugars 480 mg)	3.7 g (MCT 70 %)	Nil	Gluten-free Residual lactose	Short bowel syndrome, intractable malabsorption, proven inflammatory bowel disease, bowel fistula	Peptamen liquid: vanilla 800 ml = £12.14; unflavoured 500 ml = £6.82; 1000 ml = £12.80
Survimel® OPD (Fresenius Kabi Ltd)	Liquid (tube feed) per 100 mL	420 kJ (100 kcal)	4.5 g whey protein hydrolysate	14.3 g (sugars 1.1 g)	2.8 g (MCT 51 %)	0.1 g	Gluten-free Residual lactose Contains fish oil	Standard, p. 1335; also growth failure	Survimed OPD: liquid 500 ml = £6.96 800 ml = £12.84 1000 ml = £13.92 HN liquid 500 ml = £6.70

Enteral feeds: Less than 1 kcal/mL and less than 5 g protein/100 mL

AMINO ACID FORMULA (ESSENTIAL AND NON-ESSENTIAL AMINO ACIDS)

Not suitable for use in child under 1 year unless otherwise stated; not recommended for child 1-6 years

Product	Formulation	Energy	Protein	Carbohydrate	Fat	Fibre	Special Characteristics	ACBS Indications	Presentation & Flavour
Elemental 028® Extra (Nutricia Ltd)	Liquid (sip feed) per 100 mL	360 kJ (86 kcal)	2.5 g (protein equivalent)	11 g (sugars 4.7 g)	3.5 g (MCT 35 %)	Nil		Short bowel syndrome, intractable malabsorption, proven inflammatory bowel disease, bowel fistula	Elemental 028 Extra liquid summer fruits: 250 ml = £3.68
	Standard dilution (20 %) of powder (sip or tube feed) per 100 mL	374 kJ (89 kcal)	2.5 g (protein equivalent)	11.8 g (sugars 1.1 g)	3.5 g (MCT 35 %)	Nil		Short bowel syndrome, intractable malabsorption, proven inflammatory bowel disease, bowel fistula.	Elemental 028 Extra powder: plain, orange, banana 100 gram = £7.14

Powder provides protein equivalent 12.5 g, carbohydrate 59 g, fat 17.45 g, energy 1871 kJ (443 kcal)/100 g

Enteral feeds (non-disease specific): 5 g (or more) protein/100 mL

Not suitable for use in child under 1 year unless otherwise stated; not recommended for child 1-6 years

Enteral feeds: 1.5 kcal/mL and 5 g (or more) protein/100 mL

Not suitable for use in child under 1 year unless otherwise stated; not recommended for child 1-6 years

Product	Formulation	Energy	Protein	Carbohydrate	Fat	Fibre	Special Characteristics	ACBS Indications	Presentation & Flavour
Fresubin® 2250 Complete (Fresenius Kabi Ltd)	Liquid (tube feed) per 100 mL	630 kJ (150 kcal)	5.6 g cows' milk	18.8 g (sugars 1.5 g)	5.8 g	2 g	Gluten-free Residual lactose Contains fish oil and fish gelatin	Standard, p. 1335	Fresubin 2250 Complete liquid: 1.5 litre = £14.82
Fresubin® Energy (Fresenius Kabi Ltd)	Liquid (sip feed) per 100 mL	630 kJ (150 kcal)	5.6 g cows' milk	18.8 g (sugar content varies with flavour)	5.8 g	Nil	Gluten-free Residual lactose Contains fish gelatin Strawberry flavour may contain traces of wheat starch and egg.	Standard, p. 1335	liquid: 200 ml Fresubin Energy liquid: banana, blackcurrant, cappuccino, chocolate, lemon, strawberry, tropical fruits, vanilla 200 ml = £1.40 unflavoured 200 ml = £1.40
	Liquid (tube feed) per 100 mL	630 kJ (150 kcal)	5.6 g cows' milk	18.8 g (sugars 1.4 g)	5.8 g	Nil	Gluten-free Residual lactose Contains fish oil and fish gelatin	Standard, p. 1335	liquid: 1000 ml = £10.03 1500 ml = £13.45

Borderline substances | **Appendix 2**

A2

Enteral feeds: 1.5 kcal/mL and 5 g (or more) protein/100 mL (product list continued)

Not suitable for use in child under 1 year unless otherwise stated; not recommended for child 1-6 years

Product	Formulation	Energy	Protein	Carbohydrate	Fat	Fibre	Special Characteristics	ACBS Indications	Presentation & Flavour
Fresubin® Energy Fibre (Fresenius Kabi Ltd)	Liquid (sip feed) per 100 mL	630 kJ (150 kcal)	5.6 g cows' milk	18.8 g (sugar content varies with flavour)	5.8 g	2 g	Gluten-free Residual lactose Contains fish gelatin	Standard, p. 1335	Banana, caramel, cherry, chocolate, strawberry 200 ml = £2.05
	Liquid (tube feed) per 100 mL	630 kJ (150 kcal)	5.6 g cows' milk	18.8 g (sugars 1.5 g)	5.8 g	2 g	Gluten-free Residual lactose Contains fish oil and fish gelatin	Standard, p. 1335	Fresubin Energy Fibre liquid: unflavoured 500 ml = £5.60 1000 ml = £10.68
Fresubin® HP Energy (Fresenius Kabi Ltd)	Liquid (tube feed) per 100 mL	630 kJ (150 kcal)	7.5 g cows' milk	17 g (sugars 1 g)	5.8 g (MCT 57 %)	Nil	Gluten-free Residual lactose Contains fish oil and fish gelatin	Standard, p. 1335; also CAPD and haemodialysis	Fresubin HP Energy liquid: 500 ml = £5.20; 1000 ml = £10.40
Jevity® 1.5 kcal (Abbott Laboratories Ltd)	Liquid (tube feed) per 100 mL	649 kJ (154 kcal)	6.38 g caseinates and soy protein isolate	20.1 g (sugars 1.47 g)	4.9 g	2.2 g	Gluten-free Residual lactose	Standard, p. 1335 Not suitable for child under 2 years; not recommended for child 2-10 years	Jevity 1.5kcal liquid: 500 ml = £6.24; 1000 ml = £11.36; 1500 ml = £16.97
Nutrison® Energy (Nutricia Ltd)	Liquid (tube feed) per 100 mL	630 kJ (150 kcal)	6 g cows' milk	18.5 g (sugars 1.5 g)	5.8 g	Nil	Gluten-free Residual lactose	Standard, p. 1335	Nutrison Energy liquid: 500 ml = £5.72; 500 ml = £5.35; 1000 ml = £10.77; 1500 ml = £16.10
Nutrison® Energy Multi Fibre (Nutricia Ltd)	Liquid (tube feed) per 100 mL	630 kJ (150 kcal)	6 g cows' milk	18.5 g (sugars 1.5 g)	5.8 g	1.5 g	Gluten-free Residual lactose	Standard, p. 1335	Nutrison Energy Multi Fibre liquid: 500 ml = £5.99; 500 ml = £6.35; 1000 ml = £11.95; 1500 ml = £18.45
Osmolite® 1.5 kcal (Abbott Laboratories Ltd)	Liquid (tube feed) per 100 mL	632 kJ (150 kcal)	6.25 g cows' milk soya protein isolate	20 g (sugars 4.9 g)	5 g	Nil	Gluten-free Residual lactose	Standard, p. 1335	Osmolite 1.5kcal tube feed liquid: 500 ml = £5.60; 1000 ml = £10.19; 1500 ml = £15.23
Resource® Energy (Nestle Health Science)	Liquid (sip feed) per 100 mL	630 kJ (150 kcal)	5.6 g cows' milk	21 g (sugars 5.2 g)	5 g	less than 0.5 g	Gluten-free Residual lactose	Standard, p. 1335 Not suitable for use in child under 3 years	Resource Energy liquid: apricot, banana, chocolate, coffee, strawberry & raspberry, vanilla 800 ml = £7.67
Vital 1.5 kcal (Abbott Laboratories Ltd)	Liquid (sip or tube feed) per 100 mL	631 kJ (150 kcal)	6.75 g caseinate whey protein hydrolysate	18.4 g (sugars 3.6 g)	5.5 g (MCT 64%)	Nil	Gluten-free Residual lactose	Standard, p. 1335; except proven inflammatory bowel disease and following total gastrectomy; not recommended for use in children	Vital 1.5kcal liquid: 200 ml = £2.98; 1000 ml = £15.20

Enteral feeds: Less than 1.5 kcal/mL and 5 g (or more) protein/100 mL

Not suitable for use in child under 1 year unless otherwise stated; not recommended for child 1-6 years

Product	Formulation	Energy	Protein	Carbohydrate	Fat	Fibre	Special Characteristics	ACBS Indications	Presentation & Flavour
Fresubin® 1000 Complete (Fresenius Kabi Ltd)	Liquid (tube feed) per 100 mL	420 kJ (100 kcal)	5.5 g cows' milk	12.5 g (sugars 1.1 g)	3.1 g	2 g	Gluten-free Residual lactose Contains fish oil	Standard, p. 1335	Fresubin 1000 Complete liquid: 1 litre = £10.68
Fresubin® 1200 Complete (Fresenius Kabi Ltd)	Liquid (tube feed) per 100 mL	500 kJ (120 kcal)	6 g cows' milk	15 g (sugars 1.22 g)	4.1 g	2 g	Gluten-free Residual lactose Contains fish oil	Standard, p. 1335	Fresubin 1200 Complete liquid: 1 litre = £13.60

Product	Formulation	Energy per 100 mL	Protein	Carbohydrate	Fat	Fibre	Special characteristics	Notes	Presentation
Fresubin® 1800 Complete (Fresenius Kabi Ltd)	Liquid (tube feed) per 100 mL	500 kJ (120 kcal)	6 g cows' milk	15 g (sugars 1.22 g)	4.1 g	2 g	Gluten-free, Residual lactose, Contains fish oil	Standard, p. 1335	Fresubin 1800 Complete liquid: 1.5 litre = £13.60
Jevity® Plus (Abbott Laboratories Ltd)	Liquid (tube feed) per 100 mL	514 kJ (122 kcal)	5.5 g caseinates soy isolates	15.1 g (sugars 890 mg)	3.93 g	2.2 g	Gluten-free, Residual lactose	Standard, p. 1335. Not suitable for child under 2 years; not recommended for child 2-10 years	Jevity Plus liquid: 500 ml = £6.20; 1000 ml = £11.28; 1500 ml = £16.86
Jevity® Plus HP (Abbott Laboratories Ltd)	Liquid (tube feed) per 100 mL	551 kJ (131 kcal)	8.13 g cows' milk soy isolates	14.2 g (sugars 950 mg)	4.33 g	1.5 g	Gluten-free, Residual lactose	Standard, p. 1335; also CAPD, haemodialysis. Not suitable for child under 2 years; not recommended for child 2-10 years	Jevity Plus HP gluten free liquid: 500 ml = £6.20
Jevity® Promote (Abbott Laboratories Ltd)	Liquid (tube feed) per 100 mL	434 kJ (103 kcal)	5.55 g caseinates soy isolates	12 g (sugars 670 mg)	3.32 g	1.7 g	Gluten-free, Residual lactose	Standard, p. 1335. Not suitable for child under 2 years; not recommended for child 2-10 years	Jevity Promote liquid: 1 litre = £10.80
Nutrison® 800 Complete Multi Fibre (Nutricia Ltd)	Liquid (tube feed) per 100 mL	345 kJ (83 kcal)	5.5 g cows' milk pea protein soya protein	8.8 g (sugars 600 mg)	2.5 g	1.5 g	Gluten-free, Residual lactose, Contains fish oil	Standard, p. 1335 except bowel fistula. Not suitable for child under 6 years; not recommended for child 6-12 years	Nutrison 800 Complete Multi Fibre liquid: 1 litre = £10.45
Nutrison® 1000 Complete Multi Fibre (Nutricia Ltd)	Liquid (tube feed) per 100 mL	420 kJ (100 kcal)	5.5 g cows' milk	11.3 g (sugars 700 mg)	3.7 g	2 g	Gluten-free, Residual lactose	Disease related malnutrition in patients with low energy and/or low fluid requirements	Nutrison 1000 Complete Multi Fibre liquid: 1 litre = £11.08
Nutrison® 1200 Complete Multi Fibre (Nutricia Ltd)	Liquid (tube feed) per 100 mL	505 kJ (120 kcal)	5.5 g cows' milk	15 g (sugars 1.2 g)	4.3 g	2 g	Gluten-free, Residual lactose	Standard, p. 1335 except bowel fistula	Nutrison 1200 Complete Multi Fibre liquid: 1000 ml = £11.73; 1500 ml = £17.61
Nutrison® MCT (Nutricia Ltd)	Liquid (tube feed) per 100 mL	420 kJ (100 kcal)	5 g cows' milk	12.6 g (sugars 1 g)	3.3 g (MCT 61%)	Nil	Gluten-free, Residual lactose	Standard, p. 1335	Nutrison MCT liquid: 1000 ml = £9.98
Nutrison® Protein Plus (Nutricia Ltd)	Liquid (tube feed) per 100 mL	525 kJ (125 kcal)	6.3 g cows' milk	14.2 g (sugars 1.1 g)	4.9 g	Nil	Gluten-free, Residual lactose	Standard, p. 1335	Nutrison Protein Plus liquid: 1 litre = £10.25
Nutrison® Protein Plus Multi Fibre (Nutricia Ltd)	Liquid (tube feed) per 100 mL	525 kJ (125 kcal)	6.3 g cows' milk	14.1 g (sugars 1.1 g)	4.9 g	1.5 g	Gluten-free, Residual lactose	Disease related malnutrition	Nutrison Protein Plus Multifibre liquid: 1 litre = £11.42
Osmolite® Plus (Abbott Laboratories Ltd)	Liquid (tube feed) per 100 mL	508 kJ (121 kcal)	5.55 g caseinates	15.8 g (sugars 730 mg)	3.93 g	Nil	Gluten-free, Residual lactose	Standard, p. 1335. Not suitable for child under 10 years	Osmolite Plus liquid: 500 ml = £5.20; 1000 ml = £9.46; 1500 ml = £14.15
Peptamen® HN (Nestle Health Science)	Liquid (tube feed) per 100 mL	556 kJ (133 kcal)	6.6 g whey protein hydrolysates	15.6 g (sugars 1.4 g)	4.9 g (MCT 70%)	Nil	Gluten-free, Residual lactose, Hydrolysed with pork trypsin	Short bowel syndrome, intractable malabsorption, proven inflammatory bowel disease, bowel fistula. Not suitable for child under 3 years	Peptamen HN liquid: 500 ml = £7.34
Perative® (Abbott Laboratories Ltd)	Liquid (sip or tube feed) per 100 mL	552 kJ (131 kcal)	6.7 g caseinate whey protein hydrolysates	17.7 g (sugars 660 mg)	3.7 g (MCT 42%)	Nil	Gluten-free, Residual lactose	Standard, p. 1335. Not suitable for child under 5 years	Perative liquid: 500 ml = £7.50; 1000 ml = £13.66

A2

Borderline substances | **Appendix 2**

Borderline substances | Appendix 2

A2

Enteral feeds: More than 1.5 kcal/mL and 5 g (or more) protein/100 mL

Not suitable for use in child under 1 year unless otherwise stated; not recommended for child 1-6 years

Product	Formulation	Energy	Protein	Carbohydrate	Fat	Fibre	Special Characteristics	ACBS Indications	Presentation & Flavour
Ensure® Twocal (Abbott Laboratories Ltd)	Liquid (sip or tube feed) per 100 mL	838 kJ (200 kcal)	8.4 g cows' milk	21 g (sugars 4.5 g)	8.9 g	1 g	Gluten-free Residual lactose	Standard, p. 1335; also haemodialysis and CAPD	Ensure TwoCal liquid: banana, neutral, strawberry, vanilla 200 ml = £2.22
TwoCal® (Abbott Laboratories Ltd)	Liquid (tube feed) per 100 mL	837 kJ (200 kcal)	8.4 g cows' milk caseinates	21 g (sugars 4.5 g)	8.9 g	1 g	Gluten-free Residual lactose	Adults with or at risk of disease-related malnutrition, catabolic or fluid-restricted patients, and other patients requiring a 2 kcal/mL feed	TwoCal liquid: 1 litre = £14.80

Enteral feeds (non-disease specific): Child under 12 years see *BNF for Children*

Table 2 Nutritional supplements (non-disease specific)

Nutritional supplements: less than 5 g protein/100 mL.

Nutritional supplements: 1 kcal/mL and less than 5 g protein/100 mL

Not suitable for use in child under 1 year; use with caution in child 1-5 years unless otherwise stated

Product	Formulation	Energy	Protein	Carbohydrate	Fat	Fibre	Special Characteristics	ACBS Indications	Presentation & Flavour
Ensure® (Abbott Laboratories Ltd)	Liquid (sip or tube feed) per 100 mL	423 kJ (100 kcal)	4 g caseinates soy isolate	13.6 g (sugars 3.93 g)	3.36 g	Nil	Gluten-free Residual lactose	Standard, p. 1335	Ensure liquid: vanilla, chocolate, coffee 250 ml = £2.26

Nutritional supplements: More than 1 kcal/mL and less than 5 g protein/100 mL

Not suitable for use in child under 1 year; use with caution in child 1-5 years unless otherwise stated

Product	Formulation	Energy	Protein	Carbohydrate	Fat	Fibre	Special Characteristics	ACBS Indications	Presentation & Flavour
AYMES® Shake (Aymes International Ltd)	Standard dilution of powder (57 g in 200 mL water) (sip feed) per 100 mL	530.5 kJ (126 kcal)	4.5 g cows' milk	17.5 g (sugars 8.4 g)	4.2 g	Nil	Gluten-free Contains lactose	Standard, p. 1335 Use with caution in child 1-6 years.	Aymes Shake Sample Pack powder: 285 gram = £4.78 Aymes Shake powder: banana, chocolate, neutral, strawberry, vanilla 57 gram 399 gram = £4.90

Powder 57 g reconstituted with 200 mL whole milk provides: protein 15.8 g, carbohydrate 44.1 g, fat 16.4 g, energy 1625 kJ (388 kcal)

Product	Formulation	Energy	Protein	Carbohydrate	Fat	Fibre	Special Characteristics	ACBS Indications	Presentation & Flavour
Ensure® Plus Juce (Abbott Laboratories Ltd)	Liquid (sip feed) per 100 mL	638 kJ (150 kcal)	4.8 g whey protein isolate	32.7 g (sugars 9.4 g)	Nil	Nil	Gluten-free Residual lactose Non-milk taste	Standard, p. 1335	Ensure Plus Juce liquid: assorted 880 ml apple, fruit punch, lemon & lime, orange, peach 220 ml = £1.97
Fortijuce® (Nutricia Ltd)	Liquid (sip feed) per 100 mL	640 kJ (150 kcal)	4.0 g cows' milk	33.5 g (sugars 13.1 g)	Nil	Nil	Gluten-free Residual lactose Non-milk taste	Standard, p. 1335 Not suitable for child under 3 years	Fortijuce Starter Pack liquid: 800 ml = £8.08 Fortijuce liquid: apple, blackcurrant, forest fruits, lemon, orange, strawberry, tropical 200 ml = £2.02 assorted 800 ml
Fresubin® Jucy Drink (Fresenius Kabi Ltd)	Liquid (sip feed) per 100 mL	630 kJ (150 kcal)	4 g whey protein	33.5 g (sugars 8 g)	Nil	Nil	Gluten-free Residual lactose	Standard, p. 1335; also CAPD, haemodialysis	Fresubin Jucy drink: apple, blackcurrant, cherry, orange, pineapple 800 ml = £7.80

Product	Formulation	Energy	Protein	Carbohydrate	Fat	Fibre	Special Characteristics	ACBS Indications	Presentation & Flavour
Resource® Dessert Energy (Nestle Health Science)	Semi-solid per 100 g	671 kJ (160 kcal)	4.8 g cows' milk	21.2 g (sugars 9.9 g)	6.2 g	Nil	Gluten-free, Contains lactose	Standard, p. 1335; also CAPD, haemodialysis.	Resource Dessert Energy semi-solid food: caramel, chocolate, vanilla 125 gram = £1.63
Resource® Fruit (Nestle Health Science)	Liquid (sip feed) per 100 mL	520 kJ (125 kcal)	4 g whey protein hydrolysate	27 g (sugars 9.5 g)	less than 0.2 g	less than 0.2 g	Gluten-free, Residual lactose, Non-milk taste	Standard, p. 1335 Not suitable for child under 3 years.	Resource Fruit liquid: apple, orange, pear & cherry, raspberry & blackcurrant 800 ml = £7.35

Nutritional supplements: 5 g (or more) protein/100 mL

Not suitable for use in child under 1 year: use with caution in child 1-5 years unless otherwise stated

Nutritional supplements: 1.5 kcal/mL and 5 g (or more) protein/100 mL

Product	Formulation	Energy	Protein	Carbohydrate	Fat	Fibre	Special Characteristics	ACBS Indications	Presentation & Flavour
Altraplen® Protein (Nualtra Ltd)	Liquid (sip feed) per 100 mL	632 kJ (150 kcal)	10 g cows' milk soya protein	15 g (sugars 4.6 g)	5.6 g	Nil	Gluten-free, Residual lactose	Standard, p. 1335 Not suitable for child under 3 years; use with caution in child 3-6 years	Altraplen Protein liquid: strawberry, vanilla 800 ml = £8.00
Ensure® Plus Advance (Abbott Laboratories Ltd)	Liquid (sip or tube feed) per 100 mL	631 kJ (150 kcal)	9.1 g cows' milk soya protein isolate whey protein concentrate	16.8 g (sugars 6.8 g)	4.8 g	0.75 g	Gluten-free, Residual lactose	Frail elderly people (this is defined as older than 65 years with BMI less than or equal to 23 kg/m² where clinical assessment and nutritional screening show the individual to be at risk of undernutrition). Not suitable as the sole source of nutrition.	Ensure Plus Fibre liquid: banana, chocolate, coffee, strawberry, vanilla 200 ml = £2.02
Ensure® Plus Commence (Abbott Laboratories Ltd)	Starter pack (5-10 day's supply), contains: Ensure® Plus Milkshake Style (various flavours), 1 pack (10 x 200 mL) = £14.00								
Ensure® Plus Fibre (Abbott Laboratories Ltd)	Liquid (sip or tube feed) per 100 mL	652 kJ (155 kcal)	6.25 g cows' milk soya protein isolate	20.2 g (sugars 5.5 g)	4.92 g	2.5 g	Gluten-free, Residual lactose	Standard, p. 1335; also CAPD, haemodialysis.	Ensure Plus Fibre liquid: banana, chocolate, raspberry, strawberry, vanilla 200 ml = £2.02
Ensure® Plus Milkshake style (Abbott Laboratories Ltd)	Liquid (sip or tube feed) per 100 mL	632 kJ (150 kcal)	6.25 g cows' milk soya protein isolate	20.2 g (sugars 6.89 g)	4.92 g	Nil	Gluten-free, Residual lactose	Standard, p. 1335; also CAPD, haemodialysis	Ensure Plus milkshake style liquid: banana, chocolate, coffee, fruits of the forest, neutral, orange, peach, raspberry, strawberry, vanilla 220 ml = £1.40
Ensure® Plus Savoury (Abbott Laboratories Ltd)	Liquid (sip or tube feed) per 100 mL	632 kJ (150 kcal)	6.25 g cows' milk soy protein isolate	20.2 g (sugars 1.13 g)	4.92 g	Nil	Gluten-free, Residual lactose	Standard, p. 1335; also CAPD, haemodialysis.	Ensure Plus savoury liquid: chicken, mushroom 220 ml = £1.40
Ensure® Plus Yoghurt style (Abbott Laboratories Ltd)	Liquid (sip feed) per 100 mL	632 kJ (150 kcal)	6.25 g cows' milk	20.2 g (sugars 11.7 g)	4.92 g	Nil	Gluten-free, Residual lactose	Standard, p. 1335; also CAPD, haemodialysis	Ensure Plus yoghurt style liquid: orchard peach, strawberry swirl 220 ml = £1.40

Borderline substances | **Appendix 2**

A2

Nutritional supplements: 1.5 kcal/mL and 5 g (or more) protein/100 mL (product list continued)
Not suitable for use in child under 1 year; use with caution in child 1-5 years unless otherwise stated

Product	Formulation	Energy	Protein	Carbohydrate	Fat	Fibre	Special Characteristics	ACBS Indications	Presentation & Flavour
Fortisip® Bottle (Nutricia Ltd)	Liquid (sip feed) per 100 mL	630 kJ (150 kcal)	6 g cows' milk	18.4 g	5.8 g	Nil	Gluten-free; Residual lactose	Standard, p. 1335. Not suitable for child under 3 years; use with caution in child 3-5 years.	Fortisip Bottle: banana, caramel, chocolate, neutral, orange, strawberry, tropical fruit, vanilla 200 ml = £1.40 assorted 800 ml
Fortisip® Yoghurt Style (Nutricia Ltd)	Liquid (sip feed) per 100 mL	630 kJ (150 kcal)	6 g cows' milk	18.7 g (sugars 10.8 g)	5.8 g	0.2 g	Gluten-free; Contains lactose	Standard, p. 1335. Not suitable for child under 3 years	Fortisip Yogurt Style liquid vanilla & lemon: 200 ml = £2.02
Fortisip® Range (Nutricia Ltd)	Starter pack contains 4 x Fortisip® Bottle, 4 x Fortijuce®, 2 x Fortisip® Yoghurt Stye, 1 pack (10 x 200 mL) = £20.20								
Fresubin® Protein Energy Drink (Fresenius Kabi Ltd)	Liquid (sip feed) per 100 mL	630 kJ (150 kcal)	10 g cows' milk	12.4 g (sugars 6.4 g)	6.7 g	Nil	Gluten-free; Residual lactose; Contains fish gelatin	Standard, p. 1335; also CAPD, haemodialysis.	Fresubin Protein Energy drink: cappuccino, chocolate, tropical fruits, vanilla, wild strawberry 200 ml = £2.04
Fresubin® thickened (Fresenius Kabi Ltd)	Liquid (sip feed) per 100 mL	630 kJ (150 kcal)	10 g cows' milk	12.2 g (sugars 7.1 g)	6.7 g	0.48 g	Gluten-free; Residual lactose	Dysphagia or disease-related malnutrition. Not suitable for child under 3 years; use with caution in child 3-4 years.	Fresubin Thickened Stage 1 syrup: vanilla, wild strawberry 800 ml = £9.12 Fresubin Thickened Stage 2 custard: vanilla, wild strawberry 800 ml = £9.24
Fresubin® YOcrème (Fresenius Kabi Ltd)	Semi-solid per 100 g	630 kJ (150 kcal)	7.5 g whey protein	19.5 g (sugars 16.8 g)	4.7 g	Nil	Gluten-free; Contains lactose	Dysphagia, or presence or risk of malnutrition. Not suitable for child under 3 years	Fresubin YOcreme dessert: apricot-peach, biscuit, lemon, raspberry 500 gram = £8.00

Nutritional supplements: Less than 1.5 kcal/mL and 5 g (or more) protein/100 mL
Not suitable for use in child under 1 year; use with caution in child 1-5 years unless otherwise stated

Product	Formulation	Energy	Protein	Carbohydrate	Fat	Fibre	Special Characteristics	ACBS Indications	Presentation & Flavour
Ensure® Plus Crème (Abbott Laboratories Ltd)	Semi-solid per 100 g	574 kJ (137 kcal)	5.68 g cow's milk soy protein isolates	18.4 g (sugars 12.4 g)	4.47 g	Nil	Gluten-free; Residual lactose; Contains soya	Standard, p. 1335; also CAPD, haemodialysis. Not suitable for child under 3 years; use with caution in child 3-5 years.	Ensure Plus Crème: chocolate, neutral, vanilla 500 gram = £7.51
Nutilis® Fruit Stage 3 (Nutricia Ltd)	Semi-Solid per 100 g	560 kJ (133 kcal)	7 g whey isolate	16.7 g (sugars 11.3 g)	4 g	2.6 g	Gluten-free; Residual lactose	Standard, p. 1335 except bowel fistula; also CAPD, haemodialysis. Not suitable for child under 3 years; use with caution in child 3-5 years.	Nutilis Fruit Stage 3: apple, strawberry 450 gram = £7.08
Oral Impact® (Nestle Health Science)	Standard dilution of powder (74 g in 250 mL water) (sip feed) per 100 mL	425 kJ (101 kcal)	5.6 g cows' milk	13.4 g (sugars 7.4 g)	2.8 g	1 g	Residual lactose; Contains fish oil	Pre-operative nutritional supplement for malnourished patients or patients at risk of malnourishment. Not suitable for child under 3 years; use with caution in child 3-5 years.	Oral Impact oral powder 74g sachets: citrus, coffee, tropical 5 sachet = £16.93

Nutritional supplements: More than 1.5 kcal/mL and 5 g (or more) protein/100 mL
Not suitable for use in child under 1 year: use with caution in child 1-5 years unless otherwise stated

Product	Formulation	Energy	Protein	Carbohydrate	Fat	Fibre	Special Characteristics	ACBS Indications	Presentation & Flavour
Altraplen Compact® (Nualtra Ltd)	Liquid (sip feed) per 100 mL	1008 kJ (240 kcal)	9.6 g cows' milk	28.8 g (sugars 11.6 g)	9.6 g	Nil	Gluten-free Residual lactose	Standard, p. 1335 Not suitable for child under 3 years; use with caution in child 3-6 years.	Altraplen liquid: strawberry, vanilla 500 ml = £5.80
Complan® Shake (Nutricia Ltd)	Powder per 57 g	1057 kJ (251 kcal)	8.8 g cows' milk soya protein	35.2 g (sugars 22.7 g)	8.4 g	Trace	Gluten-free Contains lactose	Standard, p. 1335	Complan Shake Starter Pack sachets: 5 sachet = £4.79 Complan Shake oral powder 57 g sachets: banana, chocolate, milk, strawberry, vanilla 4 sachet = £3.12
Powder 57 g reconstituted with 200 mL whole milk provides: protein 15.6 g, carbohydrate 44.5 g, fat 16.4 g, energy 1621 kJ (387 kcal)									
Ensure® Compact (Abbott Laboratories Ltd)	Liquid (sip or tube feed) per 100 mL	1008 kJ (240 kcal)	10.2 g cows' milk	28.8 g (sugars 6.2 g)	9.35 g	Nil	Gluten-free Residual lactose	As a sole source of nutrition or as a nutritional supplement for the dietary management of patient with, or at risk of developing, disease-related malnutrition.	Ensure Compact liquid: banana, strawberry, vanilla 125 ml = £1.45
Ensure® Shake (Abbott Laboratories Ltd)	Powder per 100 g	1852 kJ (443 kcal)	17.8 g cows' milk whey protein concentrate	59 g (sugars 33.7 g)	15.1 g	Nil	Gluten-free Residual lactose	Standard, p. 1335	Ensure Shake oral powder 57 g sachets: banana, chocolate, strawberry, vanilla 7 sachet = £5.46
Powder 57 g reconstituted with 200 mL whole milk provides: protein 17 g, carbohydrate 43.2 g, fat 16.6 g, energy 1626 kJ (389 kcal)									
Foodlink® Complete (Nualtra Ltd)	Powder per 100 g	1826 kJ (434 kcal)	21.3 g cows' milk	56.7 g	13.5 g	Nil	Contains lactose	Standard, p. 1335	Foodlink Complete powder: banana, chocolate, natural, strawberry 399 gram = £4.27
Recommended serving = 4 heaped dessertspoonfuls in 200 mL full cream milk provides: protein 18.9 g, carbohydrate 41.8 g, fat 15.7 g, energy 1605 kJ (383 kcal)									
Foodlink® Complete with Fibre (Nualtra Ltd)	Powder per 100 g	1683 kJ (400 kcal)	19.4 g cows' milk	52.7 g (sugars 27.3 g)	12.4 g	7.2 g	Contains lactose	Standard, p. 1335	Foodlink Complete powder with fibre vanilla: 441 gram = £4.69
Recommended serving = 4 heaped dessertspoonfuls (or the contents of a 63 g sachet) in 200 mL full cream milk provides: protein 19.0 g, carbohydrate 42.7 g fat 15.8 g, fibre 4.5 g, energy 1624 kJ (388 kcal)									
Forticreme® Complete (Nutricia Ltd)	Semi-solid per 100 g	675 kJ (160 kcal)	9.5 g cows' milk	19.2 g (sugars 10.6 g)	5 g	0.1 g	Gluten-free Residual lactose	Standard, p. 1335; also CAPD, haemodialysis. Not suitable for child under 3 years; use with caution in child 3-5 years.	Forticreme Complete dessert: banana, chocolate, forest fruits, vanilla 500 gram = £7.84
Fortisip® Compact (Nutricia Ltd)	Liquid (sip feed) per 100 mL	1010 kJ (240 kcal)	9.6 g cows' milk	29.7 g (sugars 15 g)	9.3 g	Nil	Residual lactose	Standard, p. 1335 Not suitable for child under 3 years; use with caution in child 3-5 years.	Fortisip Compact liquid: apricot, banana, forest fruit, mocha, strawberry, vanilla 500 ml = £5.80 chocolate 500 ml = £5.80
Fortisip® Compact Fibre (Nutricia Ltd)	Liquid (sip feed) per 100 mL	1000 kJ (240 kcal)	9.4 g cows' milk	25.2 g (sugars 13.9 g)	10.4 g	3.6 g	Gluten-free Residual lactose	Standard, p. 1335 Not suitable for child under 3 years; use with caution in child 3-5 years.	Fortisip Compact Fibre Starter Pack liquid: 500 ml = £8.36 Fortisip Compact Fibre liquid: mocha, strawberry, vanilla 500 ml = £8.36

A2

Borderline substances | **Appendix 2**

Nutritional supplements: More than 1.5 kcal/mL and 5 g (or more) protein/100 mL (product list continued)

Not suitable for use in child under 1 year; use with caution in child 1–5 years unless otherwise stated

Product	Formulation	Energy	Protein	Carbohydrate	Fat	Fibre	Special Characteristics	ACBS Indications	Presentation & Flavour
Fortisip® Compact Protein (Nutricia Ltd)	Liquid (sip feed) per 100 mL	1010 kJ (240 kcal)	14.4 g cows' milk	24.4 g (sugars 13.3 g)	9.4 g	Nil	Gluten-free Residual lactose	Standard, p. 1335 Not suitable for child under 3 years; use with caution in child 3–5 years.	Fortisip Compact Protein Starter Pack liquid: 500 ml = £8.00 Fortisip Compact Protein liquid: banana, mocha, strawberry, vanilla 500 ml = £8.00
Fortisip® Extra (Nutricia Ltd)	Liquid (sip feed) per 100 mL	675 kJ (160 kcal)	10 g cows' milk	18.1 g (sugars 9 g)	5.3 g	Nil	Gluten-free Contains lactose	Standard, p. 1335 Not suitable for child under 3 years; use with caution in child 3–5 years.	Fortisip Extra Starter Pack liquid: 800 ml = £8.72 Fortisip Extra liquid: chocolate, forest fruits, mocha, strawberry, vanilla 200 ml = £2.18
Fresubin® 2 kcal Drink (Fresenius Kabi Ltd)	Liquid (sip feed) per 100 mL	840 kJ (200 kcal)	10 g cows' milk	22.5 g (sugars 5.8 g)	7.8 g	Nil	Gluten-free Residual lactose	Standard, p. 1335; also CAPD, haemodialysis.	Fresubin 2kcal drink: apricot-peach, cappuccino, fruits of the forest, neutral, toffee, vanilla 200 ml = £1.98
Fresubin® 2 kcal Fibre Drink (Fresenius Kabi Ltd)	Liquid (sip feed) per 100 mL	840 kJ (200 kcal)	10 g cows' milk	22.5 g (sugars 5.8 g)	7.8 g	1.6 g	Gluten-free Residual lactose	Standard, p. 1335; also CAPD, haemodialysis.	Fresubin 2kcal Fibre drink: apricot-peach, cappuccino, chocolate, lemon, neutral 200 ml = £1.98
Fresubin® Powder Extra (Fresenius Kabi Ltd)	Powder per 100 g	1764 kJ (420 kcal)	17.5 g cows' milk whey protein	63 g (sugars 24.7 g)	10.9 g	Nil	Gluten-free Contains lactose	Standard, p. 1335	Fresubin Powder Extra oral powder 62g sachets: chocolate, neutral, strawberry, vanilla 7 sachet = £5.32
Powder 62 g reconstituted with 200 mL whole milk provides: protein 17.7 g, carbohydrate 48.5 g, fat 14.8 g, energy 1658 kJ (397 kcal)									
Nutilis® Complete Stage 1 (Nutricia Ltd)	Liquid (pre-thickened) per 100 mL	1010 kJ (240 kcal)	9.6 g cows' milk	29.1 g (sugars 5.4 g)	9.3 g	3.2 g	Residual lactose	Standard, p. 1335 Not suitable for child under 3 years.	Nutilis Complete Stage 1 liquid: strawberry, vanilla 500 ml = £8.84
Nutilis® Complete Stage 2 (Nutricia Ltd)	Semi-solid per 100 g	1030 kJ (245 kcal)	9.6 g cows' milk	29.1 g (sugars 11.8 g)	9.4 g	3.2 g	Gluten-free Residual lactose	Standard, p. 1335 Not suitable for child under 3 years; use with caution in child 3–6 years.	Nutilis Complete Stage 2 custard: chocolate, strawberry, vanilla 500 gram = £8.84
Nutricrem® (Nualtra Ltd)	Semi-solid per 100 g	756 kJ (180 kcal)	10 g cows' milk soya protein	18.8 g (sugars 9.7 g)	7.2 g	Nil	Gluten-free Residual lactose	Standard, p. 1335 Not suitable for child under 3 years; use with caution in child 3–6 years.	Nutricrem dessert: strawberry, vanilla 500 gram = £5.60
Renilon® 7.5 (Nutricia Ltd)	Liquid (sip feed) per 100 mL	840 kJ (200 kcal)	7.5 g cows' milk	20 g (sugars 4.8 g)	10 g	Nil	Gluten-free Residual lactose	Standard, p. 1335 Not suitable for child under 3 years; use with caution in child 3–5 years.	Renilon 7.5 liquid: apricot, caramel 500 ml = £8.64
Resource® 2.0 Fibre (Nestle Health Science)	Liquid (sip feed) per 100 mL	836 kJ (200 kcal)	9 g cows' milk	21.4 g (sugars 5.5 g)	8.7 g	2.5 g	Gluten-free Residual lactose	Standard, p. 1335 Not suitable for child under 6 years; use with caution in child 6–10 years.	Resource Fibre 2.0 liquid: apricot, coffee, neutral, strawberry, summer fruit, vanilla 200 ml = £1.88

Table 3 Specialised formulas

Specialised formulas: Infant and child see *BNF for Children*

Specialised formulas for specific clinical conditions

Product	Formulation	Energy	Protein	Carbohydrate	Fat	Fibre	Special Characteristics	ACBS Indications	Presentation & Flavour
Alicalm® (Nutricia Ltd)	Standard dilution (30%) of powder per 100 mL	567 kJ (135 kcal)	4.5 g caseinate whey	17.4 g (sugars 3.2 g)	5.3 g	Nil	Residual lactose	Crohn's disease Not suitable for child under 1 year; use as nutritional supplement only in children 1–6 years.	Alicalm oral powder: 400 gram = £21.49
Powder provides: protein 15 g, carbohydrate 58 g, fat 17.5 g, energy 1889 kJ (450 kcal)/100 g									
Forticare® (Nutricia Ltd)	Liquid (sip feed) per 100 mL	675 kJ (160 kcal)	9 g cows' milk	19.1 g (sugars 13.6 g)	5.3 g	2.1 g	Gluten-free Residual lactose Contains fish oil	Nutritional supplement in patients with lung cancer undergoing chemotherapy, or with pancreatic cancer Not suitable in child under 3 years	Forticare liquid: cappuccino, orange & lemon, peach & ginger 500 ml = £8.92
Heparon® Junior (Nutricia Ltd)	Standard dilution (18%) of powder per 100 mL	363 kJ (86 kcal)	2 g cows' milk	11.6 g (sugars 2.9 g)	3.6 g	Nil	Contains lactose Electrolytes/100 mL: Na⁺ 0.56 mmol K⁺ 1.9 mmol Ca²⁺ 2.3 mmol P⁺ 1.6 mmol	Enteral feed or nutritional supplement for children with acute or chronic liver failure	Heparon Junior powder: 400 gram = £21.65
Powder provides: protein 11.1 g, carbohydrate 64.2 g, fat 19.9 g, energy 2016 kJ (480 kcal)/100 g									
KetoCal® (Nutricia Ltd)	Standard dilution (20 %) of powder per 100 mL	602 kJ (146 kcal)	3.1 g cows' milk with additional amino acids	600 mg (sugars 120 mg)	14.6 g (LCT 100 %)	Nil	Electrolytes/100 mL: Na⁺ 4.3 mmol K⁺ 4.1 mmol Ca²⁺ 2.15 mmol P⁺ 2.77 mmol	Enteral feed or nutritional supplement as part of ketogenic diet in management of epilepsy resistant to drug therapy, in children over 1 year, only on the advice of secondary care physician with experience of ketogenic diet.	KetoCal 4:1 powder: unflavoured, vanilla 300 gram = £30.48
Powder provides: protein 15.25 g, carbohydrate 3 g, fat 73 g, energy 3011 kJ (730 kcal)/100 g									
KetoCal® 3:1 (Nutricia Ltd)	Standard dilution (9.5%) of powder per 100 mL	276 kJ (66 kcal)	1.5 g	680 mg (sugars 570 mg)	6.4 g	Nil	Electrolytes/100 mL: Na⁺ 1.3 mmol K⁺ 2.4 mmol Ca²⁺ 2 mmol P⁺ 1.7 mmol	Enteral feed or nutritional supplement as part of ketogenic diet in management of drug resistant epilepsy or other conditions for which a ketogenic diet is indicated in children from birth to 6 years; as a nutritional supplement in children over 6 years.	KetoCal 3:1 powder: 300 gram = £29.50
Powder provides: protein 15.3 g, carbohydrate 7.2 g, fat 67.7 g, energy 2927 kJ (699 kcal)/100 g									
KetoCal® 4:1 LQ (Nutricia Ltd)	Liquid (sip or tube feed) per 100 mL	620 kJ (150 kcal)	3.09 g casein and whey with additional amino acids	610 mg (sugars 230 mg)	14.8 g (LCT 100 %)	1.12 g	Residual lactose Electrolytes/100 mL: Na⁺ 4.9 mmol K⁺ 4.7 mmol Ca²⁺ 2.4 mmol P⁺ 3.1 mmol	Enteral feed or nutritional supplement as part of ketogenic diet in management of drug resistant epilepsy or other conditions for which a ketogenic diet is indicated in children 1–10 years; as a nutritional supplement in children over 10 years.	KetoCal 4:1 LQ liquid: unflavoured, vanilla 200 ml = £4.35

A2

Borderline substances | **Appendix 2**

A2

Specialised formulas for specific clinical conditions (product list continued)

Product	Formulation	Energy	Protein	Carbohydrate	Fat	Fibre	Special Characteristics	ACBS Indications	Presentation & Flavour
Kindergen® (Nutricia Ltd)	Standard dilution (20 %) of powder per 100 mL	421 kJ (101 kcal)	1.5 g whey protein	11.8 g (sugars 1.2 g)	5.3 g (LCT 93 %)	Nil	Electrolytes/100 mL: Na^+ 2 mmol K^+ 0.6 mmol Ca^{2+} 2.8 mmol P 3 mmol Low Vitamin A	Enteral feed or nutritional supplement for children with chronic renal failure receiving peritoneal rapid overnight dialysis.	Kindergen powder: 400 gram = £29.06
Powder provides: protein 7.5 g, carbohydrate 59 g, fat 26.3 g, energy 2104 kJ (504 kcal)/100 g									
Modulen IBD® (Nestle Health Science)	Standard dilution (20%) of powder (sip or tube feed) per 100 mL	420 kJ (100 kcal)	3.6 g casein	11 g (sugars 3.98 g)	4.7 g	Nil	Gluten-free Residual lactose	Crohn's disease active phase, and in remission if malnourished	Modulen IBD powder: 400 gram = £15.06
Powder provides: protein 18 g, carbohydrate 54 g, fat 23 g, energy 2070 kJ (500 kcal)/100 g									
Nepro® (Abbott Laboratories Ltd)	Liquid (sip or tube feed) per 100 mL	838 kJ (200 kcal)	7 g cows' milk	20.6 g (sugars 3.26 g)	9.6 g	1.56 g	Gluten-free Residual lactose Electrolytes/100 mL: Na^+ 3.67 mmol K^+ 2.72 mmol Ca^{2+} 3.43 mmol P 2.23 mmol	Enteral feed or nutritional supplement in patients with chronic renal failure who are on haemodialysis or CAPD, or with cirrhosis, or other conditions requiring a high energy, low fluid, low electrolyte diet. Not suitable for child under 1 year; use with caution in child 1-5 years.	Nepro HP liquid: strawberry 220 ml = £2.98 vanilla 220 ml = £2.98, 500 ml = £6.80
ProSure® (Abbott Laboratories Ltd)	Liquid (sip or tube feed) per 100 mL	536 kJ (127 kcal)	6.65 g cows' milk	18.3 g (sugars 2.95 g)	2.56 g	2.07 g	Gluten-free Residual lactose Contains fish oil	Nutritional supplement for patients with pancreatic cancer. Not suitable for child under 1 year; use with caution in child 1-4 years.	ProSure liquid: 240 ml = £3.34
Renamil® (Stanningley Pharma Ltd)	Powder (sip or tube feed when reconstituted) per 100 g	2003 kJ (477 kcal)	4.6 g cows' milk	70.8 g	19.3 g	Nil	Contains lactose Gluten-free Electrolytes/100 g: Na^+ 1.04 mmol K^+ 0.13 mmol Ca^{2+} 10.22 mmol P 1.06 mmol Contains no vitamin A or vitamin D	Enteral feed or nutritional supplement for adults and children over 1 year with chronic renal failure.	Renamil powder: 10 x 100 gram = £25.40
Renapro® (Stanningley Pharma Ltd)	Powder per 100 g	1580 kJ (372 kcal)	90 g whey protein	800 mg	1 g	Nil	Gluten-free Residual lactose Electrolytes/100 g: Na^+ 23 mmol K^+ 2 mmol Ca^{2+} 4.99 mmol P 4.84 mmol	Nutritional supplement for biochemically proven hypoproteinaemia and patients undergoing dialysis. Not suitable for child under 1 year.	Renapro powder: 600 gram = £69.60

Powder provides: protein 18 g, energy 316 kJ (74 kcal)/20 g sachet

Product	Formulation	Energy	Protein	Carbohydrate	Fat	Fibre	Special Characteristics	ACBS Indications	Presentation & Flavour
Renastart® (Vitaflo International Ltd)	Standard dilution (20%) of powder per 100 mL	414 kJ (99 kcal)	1.5 g cows' milk soya	12.5 g (sugars 1.3 g)	4.8 g	Nil	Contains lactose Electrolytes/100 mL: Na⁺ 2.1 mmol K⁺ 0.6 mmol Ca²⁺ 0.6 mmol P⁺ 0.6 mmol	Dietary management of renal failure in child from birth to 10 years.	Renastart powder: 400 gram = £26.37

Powder provides: protein 7.5 g, carbohydrate 62.5 g, fat 23.8 g, energy 2071 kJ (494 kcal)/100 g

Product	Formulation	Energy	Protein	Carbohydrate	Fat	Fibre	Special Characteristics	ACBS Indications	Presentation & Flavour
Respifor® (Nutricia Ltd)	Liquid (sip feed) per 100 mL	633 kJ (150 kcal)	7.5 g cows' milk	22.5 g (sugars 6.4 g)	3.3 g	Nil	Contains lactose	Nutritional supplement for dietary management of disease-related malnutrition in patients with chronic obstructive pulmonary disease and body-mass index less than 20.	Respifor milkshake style liquid: chocolate, strawberry, vanilla 500 mL = £8.48
Supportan® (Fresenius Kabi Ltd)	Liquid (sip feed) per 100 mL	630 kJ (150 kcal)	10 g cows' milk	12.4 g (sugars 7.5 g)	6.7 g	1.5 g	Gluten-free Residual lactose Contains fish oil	Nutritional supplement in patients with pancreatic cancer or with lung cancer undergoing chemotherapy Not suitable for child under 1 year; use with caution in child 1–4 years	Supportan drink: cappuccino, tropical fruits 800 mL = £10.64

Table 4 Feed supplements
High-energy supplements

High-energy supplements: carbohydrate

Flavoured carbohydrate supplements are not suitable for child under 1 year; liquid supplements should be diluted before use in child under 5 years

Product	Formulation	Energy	Protein	Carbohydrate	Fat	Fibre	Special Characteristics	ACBS Indications	Presentation & Flavour
Caloreen® (Nestle Health Science)	Powder per 100 g	1640 kJ (390 kcal)	Nil	96 g Maltodextrin	Nil	Nil	Gluten-free Lactose-free	Disease-related malnutrition, malabsorption states, or other conditions requiring fortification with a high or readily available carbohydrate supplement. Not suitable for child under 3 years.	Caloreen powder: 500 gram = £3.69
Maxijul® Super Soluble (Nutricia Ltd)	Powder per 100 g	1615 kJ (380 kcal)	Nil	95 g Glucose polymer (sugars 8.6 g)	Nil	Nil	Gluten-free Lactose-free	Disease-related malnutrition, malabsorption states, or other conditions requiring fortification with a high or readily available carbohydrate supplement.	Maxijul Super Soluble powder: 200 gram = £2.60; 528 gram = £6.48; 25000 gram = £155.56
Polycal® (Nutricia Ltd)	Liquid per 100 mL	1050 kJ (247 kcal)	Nil	61.9 g Maltodextrin (sugars 12.2 g)	Nil	Nil	Gluten-free Lactose-free	Disease-related malnutrition, malabsorption states, or other conditions requiring fortification with a high or readily available carbohydrate supplement. Liquid not suitable for child under 3 years.	Polycal liquid: neutral, orange 200 mL = £1.72
	Powder per 100 g	1630 kJ (384 kcal)	Nil	96 g Maltodextrin (sugars 6 g)	Nil	Nil	Gluten-free Lactose-free	Disease-related malnutrition, malabsorption states, or other conditions requiring fortification with a high or readily available carbohydrate supplement.	powder: 400 gram = £4.28

High-energy supplements: carbohydrate (product list continued)

Flavoured carbohydrate supplements are not suitable for child under 1 year; liquid supplements should be diluted before use in child under 5 years

Product	Formulation	Energy	Protein	Carbohydrate	Fat	Fibre	Special Characteristics	ACBS Indications	Presentation & Flavour
S.O.S.® (Vitaflo International Ltd)	Powder per 100 g	1590 kJ (380 kcal)	Nil	95 g (sugars 9 g)	Nil	Nil	S.O.S. products are age-range specific–consult product literature	For use as an emergency regimen in the dietary management of inborn errors of metabolism in adults and children from birth.	S.O.S. 15 oral powder 31g sachets 30 sachet = £10.79; S.O.S. 10 oral powder 21g sachets 30 sachet = £7.31; S.O.S. 20 oral powder 42g sachets 30 sachet = £14.62; S.O.S. 25 oral powder 52g sachets 30 sachet = £18.09

Contents of each sachet should be reconstituted with water to a total volume of 200 mL

Product	Formulation	Energy	Protein	Carbohydrate	Fat	Fibre	Special Characteristics	ACBS Indications	Presentation & Flavour
Vitajoule® (Vitaflo International Ltd)	Powder per 100 g	1590 kJ (380 kcal)	Nil	95 g Dried glucose syrup (sugars 9 g)	Nil	Nil	Gluten-free Lactose-free	Disease-related malnutrition, malabsorption states, or other conditions requiring fortification with a high or readily available carbohydrate supplement.	Vitajoule powder: 500 gram = £4.38

High-energy supplements: fat

Liquid supplements should be diluted before use in child under 5 years

Product	Formulation	Energy	Protein	Carbohydrate	Fat	Fibre	Special Characteristics	ACBS Indications	Presentation & Flavour
Calogen® (Nutricia Ltd)	Liquid (emulsion) per 100 mL	1850 kJ (450 kcal)	Nil	100 mg	50 g (LCT 100 %)	Nil	Gluten-free Lactose-free	Disease-related malnutrition, malabsorption states, or other conditions requiring fortification with a high fat (or fat and carbohydrate) supplement.	Calogen emulsion: banana 500 ml = £10.72 neutral, strawberry 200 ml = £4.36 500 ml = £10.72
Fresubin® 5 kcal Shot (Fresenius Kabi Ltd)	Liquid (emulsion) per 100 mL	2100 kJ (500 kcal)	Nil	4.0 g (sucrose)	53.8 g	400 mg	Gluten-free Lactose-free	Disease-related malnutrition, malabsorption states, or other conditions requiring fortification with a high fat (or fat and carbohydrate) supplement. Not suitable for child under 3 years.	Fresubin 5kcal shot drink neutral: 480 ml = £11.20
Liquigen® (Nutricia Ltd)	Liquid (emulsion) per 100 mL	1850 kJ (450 kcal)	Nil	Nil	50 g (MCT 97 %) Fractionated coconut oil	Nil	Gluten-free Lactose-free	Steatorrhoea associated with cystic fibrosis of the pancreas, intestinal lymphangiectasia, intestinal surgery, chronic liver disease, liver cirrhosis, other proven malabsorption syndromes, ketogenic diet in epilepsy, and in type 1 lipoproteinaemia Not suitable for child under 1 year	Liquigen emulsion: 250 ml = £9.26
Medium-chain Triglyceride (MCT) Oil (Nutricia Ltd)	Liquid per 100 mL	3515 kJ (855 kcal)	Nil	Nil	MCT 100 %	Nil		Nutritional supplement for steatorrhoea associated with cystic fibrosis of the pancreas, intestinal lymphangiectasia, intestinal surgery, chronic liver disease and liver cirrhosis, other proven malabsorption syndromes, ketogenic diet in management of epilepsy, type 1 hyperlipoproteinaemia	MCT oil: 500 ml = £14.68

FAT AND CARBOHYDRATE

Product	Formulation	Energy	Protein	Carbohydrate	Fat	Fibre	Special Characteristics	ACBS Indications	Presentation & Flavour
Duocal® Super Soluble (Nutricia Ltd)	Powder per 100 g	2061 kJ (492 kcal)	Nil	72.7 g (sugars 6.5 g)	22.3 g (MCT 35 %)	Nil	Gluten-free Lactose-free	Disease-related malnutrition, malabsorption states, or other conditions requiring fortification with a high fat (or fat and carbohydrate) supplement.	Duocal Super Soluble powder: 400 gram = £18.09
Energivit® (Nutricia Ltd)	Standard dilution (15%) of powder per 100 mL	309 kJ (74 kcal)	Nil	10 g (sugars 900 mg)	3.75 g	Nil	Lactose-free With vitamins minerals and trace elements	For children requiring additional energy, vitamins, minerals, and trace elements following a protein-restricted diet	Energivit powder: 400 gram = £21.99

Powder provides: carbohydrate 66.7 g, fat 25 g, energy 2059 kJ (492 kcal)/100 g

High-energy supplements: protein

Product	Formulation	Energy	Protein	Carbohydrate	Fat	Fibre	Special Characteristics	ACBS Indications	Presentation & Flavour
ProSource® jelly (Nutrinovo Ltd)	Semi-solid per 100 mL	315 kJ (75 kcal)	16.9 g collagen protein hydrolysate whey protein isolate	Less than 1 g	Nil	Less than 1 g	Gluten-free Lactose-free Contains porcine derivatives	Hypoproteinaemia Not recommended for child under 3 years	ProSource jelly: fruit punch, orange 118 ml = £1.80
Protifar® (Nutricia Ltd)	Powder per 100 g	1580 kJ (373 kcal)	88.5 g cows' milk	less than 1.5 g	1.6 g	Nil	Gluten-free Residual lactose Electrolytes/100 mL: Na⁺ 1.3 mmol K⁺ 1.28 mmol Ca²⁺ 33.75 mmol P⁺ 22.58 mmol	Nutritional supplement for use in biochemically proven hypoproteinaemia.	Protifar powder: 225 gram = £8.69

Powder provides: protein 2.2 g per 2.5 g scoopful

Borderline substances | **Appendix 2**

A2

High-energy supplements: protein (product list continued)

PROTEIN AND CARBOHYDRATE

Product	Formulation	Energy	Protein	Carbohydrate	Fat	Fibre	Special Characteristics	ACBS Indications	Presentation & Flavour
Dialamine® (Nutricia Ltd)	Standard dilution (20%) of powder per 100 mL	264 kJ (62 kcal)	4.3 g protein equivalent (essential and non-essential amino acids)	11.2 g (sugars 10.2 g)	Nil	Nil	Contains vitamin C	Hypoproteinaemia, chronic renal failure, wound fistula leakage with excessive protein loss, conditions requiring a controlled nitrogen intake, and haemodialysis. Not suitable for child under 6 months.	Dialamine powder: 400 gram = £73.46

Powder provides: protein equivalent 25 g, carbohydrate 65 g, vitamin C 125 mg, energy 1530 kJ (360 kcal)/100 g

Product	Formulation	Energy	Protein	Carbohydrate	Fat	Fibre	Special Characteristics	ACBS Indications	Presentation & Flavour
ProSource® Liquid (Nutrinovo Ltd)	Liquid per 30 mL	420 kJ (100 kcal)	10 g collagen protein whey protein isolate	15 g (sugars 8 g)	Nil	Nil	Gluten-free Lactose-free May contain porcine derivatives	Biochemically proven hypoproteinaemia Not recommended for child under 3 years.	ProSource liquid 30ml sachets: citrus berry, lemon, orange creme, original 100 sachet = £97.23
ProSource® Plus (Nutrinovo Ltd)	Liquid per 30 mL	420 kJ (100 kcal)	15 g collagen protein whey protein isolate	11 g (sugars 10 g)	Nil	Nil	Gluten-free Lactose-free May contain porcine derivatives	Hypoproteinaemia Not recommended for child under 3 years	ProSource plus liquid 100 x 30ml sachets: unflavoured: £140.53

PROTEIN, FAT, AND CARBOHYDRATE

Product	Formulation	Energy	Protein	Carbohydrate	Fat	Fibre	Special Characteristics	ACBS Indications	Presentation & Flavour
Calogen® Extra (Nutricia Ltd)	Liquid per 100 mL	1650 kJ (400 kcal)	5 g cows' milk	4.5 g (sugars 3.5 g)	40.3 g	Nil	Gluten-free Residual lactose Contains vitamins and minerals	Disease-related malnutrition, malabsorption states, or other conditions requiring fortification with a high fat or carbohydrate (with protein) supplement. Not suitable for child under 3 years; use with caution in child 3–6 years. May require dilution for child 3–5 years.	Calogen Extra emulsion: neutral, strawberry 200 ml = £4.98
Calogen® Extra Shots (Nutricia Ltd)	Liquid per 100 mL	1650 kJ (400 kcal)	5 g cows' milk	4.5 g (sugars 3.5 g)	40.3 g	Nil	Gluten-free Residual lactose With vitamins and minerals	Disease-related malnutrition, malabsorption states, or other conditions requiring fortification with a high fat or carbohydrate (with protein) supplement. Not suitable for child under 3 years; use with caution in child 3–6 years. May require dilution for child 3–5 years.	Calogen Extra Shots emulsion: neutral, strawberry 240 ml = £5.75

Product	Form	Energy	Protein	Carbohydrate	Fat		Contents	Indications	Price
Calshake® (Fresenius Kabi Ltd)	Powder per 87 g	1841 kJ (439 kcal)	4.1 g cows' milk	56.4 g (sugars 20 g)	22 g	Nil	Contains lactose, Gluten-free	Disease-related malnutrition, malabsorption states, or other conditions requiring fortification with a high fat or carbohydrate (with protein) supplement. Not suitable for child under 1 year.	Calshake powder: chocolate 7 x 90 g sachets = £16.73 banana, neutral, strawberry, vanilla 7 x 87 g sachets = £16.73

Powder: one sachet reconstituted with 240 mL whole milk provides approx. 2 kcal/mL and protein 12 g

Product	Form	Energy	Protein	Carbohydrate	Fat		Contents	Indications	Price
Enshake® (Abbott Laboratories Ltd)	Powder per 100 g	1893 kJ (450 kcal)	8.4 g cows' milk soy protein isolate	69 g (sugars14.5 g)	15.6 g	Nil	Residual lactose, Contains vitamins and minerals	Disease-related malnutrition, malabsorption states, or other conditions requiring fortification with a high fat or carbohydrate (with protein) supplement. Not suitable for child under 1 year; use with caution in child 1-6 years.	Enshake oral powder 96.5g sachets: banana, chocolate, strawberry, vanilla 6 sachet = £12.93

Powder: one sachet reconstituted with 240 mL whole milk provides approx. 2 kcal/mL and protein 16 g

Product	Form	Energy	Protein	Carbohydrate	Fat		Contents	Indications	Price
MCT Procal® (Vitaflo International Ltd)	Powder per 100 g	2742 kJ (657 kcal)	12.5 g cows' milk	20.6 g (sugars 3.1 g)	63.1 g (MCT 99%)	Nil	Contains lactose	Dietary management of disorders of long-chain fatty acid oxidation, fat malabsorption, and other disorders requiring a low LCT, high MCT supplement. Not suitable for child under 1 year.	MCT procal oral powder 16g sachets: 30 sachet = £23.76

Powder 16 g provides: protein 2 g, carbohydrate 3.3 g, fat 10.1 g, energy 439 kJ (105 kcal)

Product	Form	Energy	Protein	Carbohydrate	Fat		Contents	Indications	Price
Pro-Cal® (Vitaflo International Ltd)	Powder per 100 g	2787 kJ (667 kcal)	13.6 g cows' milk	28.2 g (sugars 16 g)	55.5 g	Nil	Contains lactose, Gluten-free	Disease-related malnutrition, malabsorption states, or other conditions requiring fortification with a high fat or carbohydrate (with protein) supplement. Not suitable for child under 1 year; use with caution in child 1-5 years.	Pro-Cal powder: 375 gram = £15.83; 510 gram = £14.67; 1500 gram = £29.88; 3000 gram = £70.54; 12500 gram = £212.37

Powder 15 g provides: protein 2 g, carbohydrate 4.2 g, fat 8.3 g, energy 418 kJ (100 kcal)

Product	Form	Energy	Protein	Carbohydrate	Fat		Contents	Indications	Price
Pro-Cal® Shot (Vitaflo International Ltd)	Liquid per 100 mL	1385 kJ (334 kcal)	6.7 g cows' milk	13.4 g (sugars 13.3 g)	28.2 g	Nil	Contains lactose, Gluten-free, Contains soya	Disease-related malnutrition, malabsorption states, or other conditions requiring fortification with a high fat or carbohydrate (with protein) supplement. Not suitable for child under 3 years.	Pro-Cal: shot starter pack 360 ml = £7.23 neutral, strawberry 720 ml = £14.44 banana 720 ml = £14.44

Product	Form	Energy	Protein	Carbohydrate	Fat		Contents	Indications	Price
Scandishake® Mix (Nutricia Ltd)	Powder per 100 g	2099 kJ (500 kcal)	4.7 g cows' milk	65 g (sugars 14.3 g)	24.7 g	Nil	Gluten-free, Contains lactose	Disease-related malnutrition, malabsorption states, or other conditions requiring fortification with a high fat or carbohydrate (with protein) supplement. Not suitable for child under 3 years.	Scandishake Mix oral powder 85g sachets: banana, caramel, chocolate, strawberry, unflavoured, vanilla 6 sachet = £14.70

Powder: 85 g reconstituted with 240 mL whole milk provides: protein 11.7 g, carbohydrate 66.8 g, fat 30.4 g, energy 2457 kJ (588 kcal)

A2

Borderline substances | **Appendix 2**

Borderline substances | **Appendix 2**

A2

High-energy supplements: protein (product list continued)

PROTEIN, FAT, AND CARBOHYDRATE

Product	Formulation	Energy	Protein	Carbohydrate	Fat	Fibre	Special Characteristics	ACBS Indications	Presentation & Flavour
Vitasavoury® (Vitaflo International Ltd)	Powder per 100 g	2562 kJ (619 kcal)	12 g cows' milk	22.5 g (sugars 1.4 g)	52 g	6.4 g	Contains lactose Contains soya (chicken flavour)	Disease-related malnutrition, malabsorption states, or other conditions requiring fortification with a high fat or carbohydrate (with protein) supplement. Not suitable for child under 3 years.	Vitasavoury powder: chicken, golden vegetable, leek & potato, mushroom 500 g = £18.97 Vitasavoury powder starter pack: 400 g = £15.18

Fibre, vitamin, and mineral supplements

High-fibre supplements

Product	Formulation	Energy	Protein	Carbohydrate	Fat	Fibre	Special Characteristics	ACBS Indications	Presentation & Flavour
Resource® Optifibre® (Nestle Health Science)	Powder per 100 g	323 kJ (76 kcal)	Nil	19 g guar gum partially hydrolysed	Nil	78 g	Gluten-free Lactose-free	Standard, p. 1335 except dysphagia Not suitable for child under 5 years	Resource Optifibre powder: 80 gram = £4.18; 250 gram = £10.28

Vitamin and Mineral supplements

Product	Formulation	Energy	Protein	Carbohydrate	Fat	Fibre	Special Characteristics	ACBS Indications	Presentation & Flavour
FruitiVits® (Vitaflo International Ltd)	Powder per 100 g	133 kJ (33 kcal)	Nil	8.3 g (sugars 400 mg)	less than 100 mg	3.3 g		Vitamin, mineral, and trace element supplement in children 3–10 years with restrictive therapeutic diets	Sachets: 30 × 6 g = £64.23 orange
Paediatric Seravit® (Nutricia Ltd)	Powder per 100 g	1275 kJ (300 kcal)	Nil	75 g (sugars 6.75 g)	Nil	Nil	Pineapple flavour not suitable for child under 6 months	Vitamin, mineral, and trace element supplement in infants and children with restrictive therapeutic diets.	Seravit Paediatric powder: pineapple 200 gram = £19.08 unflavoured 200 gram = £17.91
Renavit® (Stanningley Pharma Ltd)	Tablet per 450 mg	3.15 kJ (0.75 kcal)	Nil	170 mg	Nil	Nil		Dietary management of water-soluble vitamin deficiency in adults with renal failure on dialysis	Renavit tablets: 100 tablet = £12.50

Feed additives

Special additives for conditions of intolerance

Colief®

▸ For the relief of symptoms associated with lactose intolerance in infants, provided that lactose intolerance is confirmed by the presence of reducing substances and/or excessive acid in stools, a low concentration of the corresponding disaccharide enzyme on intestinal biopsy or by breath hydrogen test or lactose intolerance test. For dosage and administration details, consult product literature.
LIQUID, lactase 50 000 units/g

Colief 50,000units/g infant drops (Forum Health Products Ltd)
7 ml (ACBS) · NHS indicative price = £8.40

Fructose

▸ (Laevulose) For proven glucose/galactose intolerance

Glucose

▸ (Dextrose monohydrate) For use as an energy supplement in sucrose-isomaltase deficiency

VSL#3®

▸ Nutritional supplement for use under the supervision of a physician, for the maintenance of remission of ileoanal pouchitis induced by antibacterials in adults. For dosage and administration details, consult product literature.
POWDER, containing 8 strains of live, freeze-dried, lactic acid bacteria. Contains traces of soya, gluten, and lactose.

VSL#3 Probiotic Food Supplement oral powder 4.4g sachets (Ferring Pharmaceuticals Ltd)
10 sachet (ACBS) · NHS indicative price = £14.64 | 30 sachet (ACBS) · NHS indicative price = £33.89

Feed thickeners and pre-thickened drinks

Carobel, Instant®

▸ For thickening feeds in the treatment of vomiting.
POWDER, carob seed flour.

Instant Carobel powder (Cow & Gate Ltd)
135 gram (ACBS) · NHS indicative price = £2.80

Multi-thick®

▸ For thickening of liquids and foods in dysphagia. Not suitable for children under 1 year except in cases of failure to thrive.
POWDER, modified maize starch, gluten- and lactose-free.

Multi-thick powder (Abbott Laboratories Ltd)
250 gram (ACBS) · NHS indicative price = £4.83

Nutilis® Clear

▸ For thickening of liquids or foods in dysphagia. Not suitable for children under 3 years.
POWDER, maltodextrin, xanthan gum, guar gum, gluten- and lactose-free.

Nutilis Clear powder (Nutricia Ltd)
175 gram (ACBS) · NHS indicative price = £8.46

Nutilis® Powder

▸ For thickening of foods in dysphagia. Not suitable for child under 3 years.
POWDER, carbohydrate 86 g, energy 1520 kJ (358 kcal)/100 g, modified maize starch, gluten- and lactose-free.

Nutilis powder (Nutricia Ltd)
240 gram (ACBS) · NHS indicative price = £6.40 | 300 gram (ACBS) · NHS indicative price = £5.01

Resource® ThickenUp Clear

▸ For thickening of liquids or foods in dysphagia. Not suitable for children under 3 years.
POWDER, maltodextrin, xanthum gum, gluten- and lactose-free.

Resource ThickenUp Clear powder (Nestle Health Science)
24 x 1.2 g sachets (ACBS) · NHS indicative price = £5.28 | 125 gram (ACBS) · NHS indicative price = £8.46

Resource® ThickenUp®

▸ For thickening of foods in dysphagia. Not suitable for children under 1 year.
POWDER, modified maize starch. Gluten- and lactose-free.

Resource ThickenUp powder (Nestle Health Science)
227 gram (ACBS) · NHS indicative price = £4.66 | 337.5 gram (ACBS) · NHS indicative price = £17.86

Resource® Thickened Drink

▸ For dysphagia. Not suitable for children under 1 year.
LIQUID, carbohydrate 22 g, energy: orange 382 kJ (90 kcal); apple 376 kJ (89 kcal)/100 mL. Gluten- and lactose-free.

Resource Thickened Drink custard (Nestle Health Science)
apple, orange 114 ml (ACBS) · NHS indicative price = £0.73

Resource Thickened Drink syrup (Nestle Health Science)
apple, orange 114 ml (ACBS) · NHS indicative price = £0.73

SLO Drinks®

▸ Nutritional supplement for patient hydration in the dietary management of dysphagia. Not suitable for children under 3 years.
POWDER, carbohydrate content varies with flavour and chosen consistency (3 consistencies available), see product literature.

SLO Drink 1 oral powder (SLO Drinks Ltd)
lemon, orange, hot chocolate, white coffee, white tea 25 cup (ACBS) · NHS indicative price = £7.50

SLO Drink 2 oral powder (SLO Drinks Ltd)
hot chocolate, lemon, orange, white tea 25 cup (ACBS) · NHS indicative price = £7.50

SLO Drink 3 oral powder orange (SLO Drinks Ltd)
25 cup (ACBS) · NHS indicative price = £7.50

SLO Milkshakes+®

▸ Nutritional supplement in the dietary management of dysphagia. Not suitable for children under 3 years.
POWDER, carbohydrate content varies with flavour and chosen consistency (2 consistencies available), see product literature.

SLO Milkshake+ 1 oral powder chocolate (SLO Drinks Ltd)
7 x 50 gram (ACBS) · NHS indicative price = £5.88

SLO Milkshake+ 1 oral powder strawberry (SLO Drinks Ltd)
7 x 50 gram (ACBS) · NHS indicative price = £5.88

SLO Milkshake+ 2 oral powder chocolate (SLO Drinks Ltd)
7 x 50 gram (ACBS) · NHS indicative price = £5.88

SLO Milkshake+ 2 oral powder strawberry (SLO Drinks Ltd)
7 x 50 gram (ACBS) · NHS indicative price = £5.88

Thick and Easy®

▸ For thickening of foods in dysphagia. Not suitable for children under 1 year except in cases of failure to thrive.
POWDER, modified maize starch

Thick & Easy powder (Fresenius Kabi Ltd)
225 gram (ACBS) · NHS indicative price = £5.12 | 900 gram (ACBS) · NHS indicative price = £31.00 | 4540 gram (ACBS) · NHS indicative price = £85.64

Thicken Aid®

▸ For thickening of foods in dysphagia. Not suitable for children under 1 year.
POWDER, modified maize starch, maltodextrin, gluten- and lactose-free.

Thicken Aid powder (M & A Pharmachem Ltd)
225 gram (ACBS) · NHS indicative price = £3.71 | 900 gram (ACBS) · NHS indicative price = £22.40

Thixo-D®

▸ For thickening of foods in dysphagia. Not suitable for children under 1 year except in cases of failure to thrive.
POWDER, modified maize starch, gluten-free.

Thixo-D (Sutherland Health Ltd)
Cal-Free powder 30 gram · NHS indicative price = £2.85 powder 375 gram (ACBS) · NHS indicative price = £7.15

Vitaquick®

▸ For thickening of foods in dysphagia. Not suitable for children under 1 year except in cases of failure to thrive.
POWDER, modified maize starch.

Vitaquick powder (Vitaflo International Ltd)
300 gram (ACBS) · NHS indicative price = £7.13

Flavouring preparations

Flavour Mix®

POWDER

Nestle Nutrition Flavour (Nestle Health Science)
Mix banana, Mix chocolate 60 gram (ACBS) · NHS indicative price = £7.17

FlavourPac®
▸ For use with Vitaflo's range of unflavoured protein substitutes for metabolic diseases; not suitable for child under 3 years.

POWDER

FlavourPac oral powder 4g sachets (Vitaflo International Ltd)
blackcurrant, lemon, orange, raspberry, tropical 30 sachet (ACBS) · NHS indicative price = £13.79 | 120 sachet (ACBS) · No NHS indicative price available

Foods for special diets

Gluten-free foods

ACBS indications: established gluten-sensitive enteropathies including steatorrhoea due to gluten sensitivity, coeliac disease, and dermatitis herpetiformis.

Bread

LOAVES

Barkat® **Loaf**

GLUTEN-FREE

Barkat gluten free (Gluten Free Foods Ltd)
wholemeal bread sliced 500 gram (ACBS) · NHS indicative price = £3.98
brown rice bread, wheat free multigrain bread, white rice bread 500 gram (ACBS) · NHS indicative price = £5.73
par baked white bread sliced 300 gram (ACBS) · NHS indicative price = £4.13
home fresh country loaf 250 gram (ACBS) · NHS indicative price = £4.35

Ener-G® **Loaves**

GLUTEN-FREE

Ener-G gluten free (General Dietary Ltd)
Seattle brown loaf 454 gram · NHS indicative price = £6.22
rice loaf 612 gram (ACBS) · NHS indicative price = £5.41
white rice bread 456 gram (ACBS) · NHS indicative price = £5.41
tapioca bread 480 gram (ACBS) · NHS indicative price = £5.41
brown rice bread 474 gram (ACBS) · NHS indicative price = £5.41

Genius Gluten Free® **Loaf**

GLUTEN-FREE

Genius gluten free brown bread (Genius Foods Ltd)
unsliced 400 gram (ACBS) · NHS indicative price = £2.73
sliced 400 gram (ACBS) · NHS indicative price = £2.83

Genius gluten free brown sandwich bread sliced (Genius Foods Ltd)
535 gram (ACBS) · NHS indicative price = £3.67

Genius gluten free white bread (Genius Foods Ltd)
unsliced 400 gram (ACBS) · NHS indicative price = £2.73
sliced 400 gram (ACBS) · NHS indicative price = £2.83

Genius gluten free white sandwich bread sliced (Genius Foods Ltd)
535 gram (ACBS) · NHS indicative price = £3.67

Glutafin® **Loaves**

GLUTEN-FREE

Glutafin gluten free (Dr Schar UK Ltd)
fibre loaf sliced, white loaf sliced 400 gram (ACBS) · NHS indicative price = £3.85

Glutafin® **Select Loaves**

GLUTEN-FREE

Glutafin gluten free Select fibre loaf sliced (Dr Schar UK Ltd)
400 gram (ACBS) · NHS indicative price = £3.43

Glutafin gluten free Select fresh (Dr Schar UK Ltd)
brown loaf sliced, white loaf sliced 400 gram (ACBS) · NHS indicative price = £3.43

Glutafin gluten free Select seeded loaf sliced (Dr Schar UK Ltd)
400 gram (ACBS) · NHS indicative price = £3.72

Glutafin gluten free Select white loaf sliced (Dr Schar UK Ltd)
400 gram (ACBS) · NHS indicative price = £3.43

Juvela® **Loaf**

GLUTEN-FREE

Juvela gluten free fibre loaf (Hero UK Ltd)
sliced, unsliced 400 gram (ACBS) · NHS indicative price = £3.54

Juvela gluten free fresh (Hero UK Ltd)
fibre loaf sliced 400 gram (ACBS) · NHS indicative price = £3.39
white loaf sliced 400 gram (ACBS) · NHS indicative price = £3.69

Juvela gluten free loaf unsliced (Hero UK Ltd)
400 gram (ACBS) · NHS indicative price = £3.54

Juvela gluten free part baked (Hero UK Ltd)
fibre loaf 400 gram (ACBS) · NHS indicative price = £3.80
loaf 400 gram (ACBS) · NHS indicative price = £3.95

Lifestyle® **Loaf**

GLUTEN-FREE

Lifestyle gluten free (Ultrapharm Ltd)
high fibre bread sliced 400 gram · NHS indicative price = £2.82
brown bread sliced, white bread sliced 400 gram (ACBS) · NHS indicative price = £2.82

Livwell® **Loaf**

GLUTEN-FREE

Livwell gluten free (Livwell Ltd)
multi grain bread sliced 200 gram · NHS indicative price = £2.25
white bread sliced 200 gram (ACBS) · NHS indicative price = £2.25

Warburtons® **Loaf**

GLUTEN-FREE

Warburtons gluten free (Warburtons Ltd)
brown bread sliced, white bread sliced 400 gram (ACBS) · NHS indicative price = £3.06

Wellfoods® **Loaf**

GLUTEN-FREE

Wellfoods gluten free loaf (Wellfoods Ltd)
unsliced 600 gram (ACBS) · NHS indicative price = £4.85
sliced 600 gram (ACBS) · NHS indicative price = £4.95

BAGUETTES, BUNS AND ROLLS

Barkat® **Baguettes and rolls**

GLUTEN-FREE

Barkat gluten free par baked (Gluten Free Foods Ltd)
baguettes 200 gram (ACBS) · NHS indicative price = £4.35
rolls 200 gram (ACBS) · NHS indicative price = £3.98

Ener-G® **Rolls**

GLUTEN-FREE

Ener-G gluten free (General Dietary Ltd)
white round rolls, white long rolls 220 gram (ACBS) · NHS indicative price = £2.95
dinner rolls 280 gram (ACBS) · NHS indicative price = £3.67

Glutafin® **Baguettes and rolls**

GLUTEN-FREE

Glutafin gluten free (Dr Schar UK Ltd)
4 white rolls, part baked 4 fibre rolls 200 gram (ACBS) · NHS indicative price = £3.68
baguettes 350 gram (ACBS) · NHS indicative price = £3.51

Glutafin® **Select Rolls**

GLUTEN-FREE

Glutafin gluten free part baked (Dr Schar UK Ltd)
2 long white rolls 150 gram (ACBS) · NHS indicative price = £2.81
4 white rolls 200 gram (ACBS) · NHS indicative price = £3.68

Juvela® **Rolls**

GLUTEN-FREE

Juvela gluten free bread rolls (Hero UK Ltd)
425 gram (ACBS) · NHS indicative price = £4.77

Juvela gluten free fibre bread rolls (Hero UK Ltd)
425 gram (ACBS) · NHS indicative price = £4.77

Juvela gluten free fresh (Hero UK Ltd)
fibre rolls, white rolls 425 gram (ACBS) · NHS indicative price = £4.42

Juvela gluten free part baked (Hero UK Ltd)
fibre bread rolls, white bread rolls 375 gram (ACBS) · NHS indicative price = £4.94

Lifestyle® Rolls
GLUTEN-FREE

Lifestyle gluten free (Ultrapharm Ltd)
brown bread rolls, high fibre bread rolls, white bread rolls 400 gram (ACBS) · NHS indicative price = £2.82

Livwell® Baguettes, buns and rolls
GLUTEN-FREE

Livwell gluten free (Livwell Ltd)
toasting bread buns 180 gram (ACBS) · NHS indicative price = £2.40
white baguettes 140 gram (ACBS) · NHS indicative price = £2.15
part baked square dinner rolls 160 gram (ACBS) · NHS indicative price = £2.09

Proceli® Baguettes, buns and rolls
GLUTEN-FREE

Proceli gluten free (Ambe Ltd)
part baked baguettes 250 gram (ACBS) · NHS indicative price = £3.24

Warburtons® Baguettes and rolls
GLUTEN-FREE

Warburtons gluten free (Warburtons Ltd)
brown rolls, white rolls 220 gram (ACBS) · NHS indicative price = £2.55
baguettes 150 gram (ACBS) · NHS indicative price = £2.86

Wellfoods® Buns and rolls
GLUTEN-FREE

Wellfoods gluten free (Wellfoods Ltd)
burger buns 380 gram (ACBS) · NHS indicative price = £3.95
rolls 360 gram (ACBS) · NHS indicative price = £3.65

SPECIALITY BREADS

Livwell® Flat bread
GLUTEN-FREE

Livwell gluten free (Livwell Ltd)
tear drop flat bread 180 gram (ACBS) · NHS indicative price = £3.00
flat bread 220 gram (ACBS) · NHS indicative price = £3.00

Cereals

Juvela® Fibre flakes and oats
GLUTEN-FREE

Juvela gluten free (Hero UK Ltd)
fibre flakes, flakes 300 gram (ACBS) · NHS indicative price = £2.78
pure oats 500 gram (ACBS) · NHS indicative price = £2.78

Nairns® Porridge
GLUTEN-FREE

Nairn's gluten free oat porridge (Nairn's Oatcakes Ltd)
500 gram (ACBS) · NHS indicative price = £3.05

Cookies and biscuits

Barkat® Biscuits
GLUTEN-FREE

Barkat gluten free (Gluten Free Foods Ltd)
digestive biscuits 175 gram (ACBS) · NHS indicative price = £2.61
coffee biscuits 200 gram (ACBS) · NHS indicative price = £3.38

Ener-G® Cookies
GLUTEN-FREE

Ener-G gluten free vanilla cookies (General Dietary Ltd)
435 gram (ACBS) · NHS indicative price = £6.16

Glutafin® Cookies and biscuits
GLUTEN-FREE

Glutafin gluten free (Dr Schar UK Ltd)
digestive biscuits, sweet biscuits 150 gram (ACBS) · NHS indicative price = £2.13
tea biscuits 150 gram (ACBS) · NHS indicative price = £2.09
biscuits 200 gram (ACBS) · NHS indicative price = £4.14
savoury short biscuits 130 gram (ACBS) · NHS indicative price = £2.80
shortbread biscuits 100 gram (ACBS) · NHS indicative price = £1.73

Juvela® Biscuits
GLUTEN-FREE

Juvela gluten free (Hero UK Ltd)
sweet biscuits 150 gram (ACBS) · NHS indicative price = £2.88
digestive biscuits, tea biscuits 150 gram (ACBS) · NHS indicative price = £3.05
savoury biscuits 150 gram (ACBS) · NHS indicative price = £3.82

Crackers, crispbreads, and breadsticks

Barkat® Crackers
GLUTEN-FREE

Barkat gluten free matzo crackers (Gluten Free Foods Ltd)
200 gram (ACBS) · NHS indicative price = £3.52

Glutafin® Crackers
GLUTEN-FREE

Glutafin gluten free (Dr Schar UK Ltd)
mini crackers 175 gram (ACBS) · NHS indicative price = £2.96
crackers 200 gram (ACBS) · NHS indicative price = £3.46
high fibre crackers 200 gram (ACBS) · NHS indicative price = £2.90

Juvela® Crispbread
GLUTEN-FREE

Juvela gluten free crispbread (Hero UK Ltd)
200 gram (ACBS) · NHS indicative price = £4.64

Warburtons® Crackers
GLUTEN-FREE

Warburtons gluten free bran crackers (Warburtons Ltd)
150 gram (ACBS) · NHS indicative price = £2.34

Flour mixes and xanthan gum

FLOUR MIXES

Barkat® Flour mix
GLUTEN-FREE

Barkat gluten free (Gluten Free Foods Ltd)
bread mix 500 gram (ACBS) · NHS indicative price = £6.81
flour mix 500 gram (ACBS) · NHS indicative price = £4.65

Finax® Flour mix
GLUTEN-FREE

Finax gluten free (Drossa Ltd)
coarse flour mix, flour mix 900 gram (ACBS) · NHS indicative price = £8.66
fibre bread mix 1000 gram (ACBS) · NHS indicative price = £9.92

Glutafin® Flour mix
GLUTEN-FREE

Glutafin gluten free multipurpose white mix (Dr Schar UK Ltd)
500 gram (ACBS) · NHS indicative price = £6.66

Glutafin Select® Flour mix
GLUTEN-FREE

Glutafin gluten free Select bread mix (Dr Schar UK Ltd)
500 gram (ACBS) · NHS indicative price = £6.66

Glutafin gluten free Select fibre bread mix (Dr Schar UK Ltd)
500 gram (ACBS) · NHS indicative price = £6.66

Glutafin gluten free Select multipurpose (Dr Schar UK Ltd)
fibre mix, white mix 500 gram (ACBS) · NHS indicative price = £6.66

Heron Foods® Flour mix
GLUTEN-FREE

Heron Hi-Fibre gluten free (Gluten Free Foods Ltd)
organic bread mix, wheat free organic bread mix 500 gram (ACBS) · NHS indicative price = £8.96

Juvela® Flour mix
GLUTEN-FREE

Juvela gluten free (Hero UK Ltd)
fibre mix, harvest mix, mix 500 gram (ACBS) · NHS indicative
price = £7.35

Mrs Crimbles® Flour mixes
GLUTEN-FREE

Mrs Crimble's gluten free (Stiletto Foods (UK) Ltd)
pastry mix 200 gram (ACBS) · NHS indicative price = £1.09
bread mix 275 gram (ACBS) · NHS indicative price = £1.09

Orgran® Flour mix
GLUTEN-FREE

Orgran gluten free (Naturally Good Food Ltd)
pizza & pastry mix 375 gram (ACBS) · NHS indicative price =
£3.80
self-raising flour 500 gram (ACBS) · NHS indicative price =
£3.10
all purpose plain flour 500 gram · NHS indicative price = £3.10

Proceli® Flour mix
GLUTEN-FREE

Proceli gluten free white plain flour (Ambe Ltd)
1000 gram (ACBS) · NHS indicative price = £9.95

Pure® Flour mix
GLUTEN-FREE

Innovative Solutions Pure gluten free blended flour (Innovative
Solutions (UK) Ltd)
1000 gram (ACBS) · NHS indicative price = £4.23

Innovative Solutions Pure gluten free brown rice flour (Innovative
Solutions (UK) Ltd)
500 gram (ACBS) · NHS indicative price = £1.58

Innovative Solutions Pure gluten free white rice flour (Innovative
Solutions (UK) Ltd)
500 gram (ACBS) · NHS indicative price = £1.68

Innovative Solutions Pure gluten free potato flour (Innovative
Solutions (UK) Ltd)
500 gram (ACBS) · NHS indicative price = £1.68

Innovative Solutions Pure gluten free tapioca flour (Innovative
Solutions (UK) Ltd)
500 gram (ACBS) · NHS indicative price = £2.26

Innovative Solutions Pure gluten free brown teff flour (Innovative
Solutions (UK) Ltd)
1000 gram (ACBS) · NHS indicative price = £4.77

Innovative Solutions Pure gluten free white teff flour (Innovative
Solutions (UK) Ltd)
1000 gram (ACBS) · NHS indicative price = £4.77

Tobia® Flour mix
GLUTEN-FREE

Tobia Teff gluten free (Tobia Teff UK Ltd)
brown teff flour, white teff flour 1000 gram (ACBS) · NHS
indicative price = £3.35

Tritamyl® Flour mix
GLUTEN-FREE

Tritamyl gluten free (Gluten Free Foods Ltd)
brown bread mix 1000 gram (ACBS) · NHS indicative price =
£7.10
flour mix, white bread mix 2000 gram (ACBS) · NHS indicative
price = £14.26

Wellfoods® Flour mix
GLUTEN-FREE

Wellfoods gluten free flour alternative (Wellfoods Ltd)
1000 gram (ACBS) · NHS indicative price = £7.65

XANTHAN GUM

Ener-G® Xanthan gum
GLUTEN-FREE

Ener-G xanthan gum (General Dietary Ltd)
170 gram (ACBS) · NHS indicative price = £8.53

Pure® Xanthan gum
GLUTEN-FREE

Innovative Solutions Pure xanthan gum (Innovative Solutions (UK)
Ltd)
100 gram (ACBS) · NHS indicative price = £6.66

Pasta

Barkat® Pasta
GLUTEN-FREE

macaroni (Gluten Free Foods Ltd)
500 gram (ACBS) · NHS indicative price = £5.88

spaghetti (Gluten Free Foods Ltd)
500 gram (ACBS) · NHS indicative price = £5.88

spirals (Gluten Free Foods Ltd)
500 gram (ACBS) · NHS indicative price = £5.88

tagliatelle (Gluten Free Foods Ltd)
500 gram (ACBS) · NHS indicative price = £5.88

Barkat gluten free pasta animal shapes (Gluten Free Foods Ltd)
500 gram (ACBS) · NHS indicative price = £5.88

Barkat gluten free pasta buckwheat (Gluten Free Foods Ltd)
penne, spirals 250 gram (ACBS) · NHS indicative price = £2.93

BiAlimenta® Pasta
GLUTEN-FREE

BiAlimenta gluten free Pasta (Drossa Ltd)
spirals, sagnette 500 gram (ACBS) · NHS indicative price = £5.97

Glutafin® Pasta
GLUTEN-FREE

Glutafin gluten free pasta (Dr Schar UK Ltd)
lasagne, tagliatelle nests 250 gram (ACBS) · NHS indicative price
= £3.53
fibre spaghetti 500 gram (ACBS) · NHS indicative price = £5.74
macaroni penne, shells, spirals, long-cut spaghetti 500 gram
(ACBS) · NHS indicative price = £6.73

Juvela® Pasta
GLUTEN-FREE

Juvela gluten free fibre penne (Hero UK Ltd)
500 gram (ACBS) · NHS indicative price = £6.61

Juvela gluten free pasta (Hero UK Ltd)
tagliatelle 250 gram (ACBS) · NHS indicative price = £3.47
fusilli, macaroni, spaghetti 500 gram (ACBS) · NHS indicative
price = £7.21
lasagne 250 gram (ACBS) · NHS indicative price = £3.68

Orgran® Pasta
GLUTEN-FREE

Orgran gluten free pasta brown rice spirals (Naturally Good Food
Ltd)
250 gram (ACBS) · NHS indicative price = £2.42

Orgran gluten free pasta buckwheat spirals (Naturally Good Food
Ltd)
250 gram (ACBS) · NHS indicative price = £2.42

Orgran gluten free pasta corn spirals (Naturally Good Food Ltd)
250 gram (ACBS) · NHS indicative price = £2.42

Orgran gluten free pasta rice & corn (Naturally Good Food Ltd)
macaroni, spirals 250 gram (ACBS) · NHS indicative price =
£2.42
lasagne 200 gram (ACBS) · NHS indicative price = £3.13

Orgran gluten free pasta rice & millet spirals (Naturally Good Food
Ltd)
250 gram (ACBS) · NHS indicative price = £2.42

Rizopia® Pasta
GLUTEN-FREE

Rizopia gluten free organic brown rice pasta (PGR Health Foods Ltd)
lasagne 375 gram (ACBS) · NHS indicative price = £2.72
fusilli, penne, spaghetti 500 gram (ACBS) · NHS indicative price
= £2.72

Pizza bases

Barkat®, Pizza crust
GLUTEN-FREE

Barkat gluten free (Gluten Free Foods Ltd)
brown rice pizza crust, white rice pizza crust 150 gram (ACBS) ·
NHS indicative price = £5.00

Glutafin® Pizza base
GLUTEN-FREE

Glutafin gluten free pizza base (Dr Schar UK Ltd)
300 gram (ACBS) · NHS indicative price = £6.56

Juvela® Pizza base
GLUTEN-FREE

Juvela gluten free pizza base (Hero UK Ltd)
360 gram (ACBS) · NHS indicative price = £8.78

Proceli® Pizza base
GLUTEN-FREE

Proceli gluten free pizza base (Ambe Ltd)
250 gram (ACBS) · NHS indicative price = £3.90

Wellfoods® Pizza base
GLUTEN-FREE

Wellfoods gluten free pizza base (Wellfoods Ltd)
600 gram (ACBS) · NHS indicative price = £8.95

Gluten- and wheat-free foods

ACBS indications: established gluten-sensitive
enteropathies with coexisting established wheat sensitivity
only.

Ener-G® (General Dietary Ltd)
Gluten-free, wheat-free. Rolls, Seattle brown, round
(hamburger) 4 x 80 gram (ACBS) · NHS indicative price = £4.08
long (hot dog) 4 x 80 gram (ACBS) · NHS indicative price = £4.08
Pizza base 3 x 124 gram (ACBS) · NHS indicative price = £4.74

Glutafin® (Dr Schar UK Ltd)
Gluten-free, wheat-free. Flour mix, bread, fibre 500 gram
(ACBS) · NHS indicative price = £6.66
Crispbread 150 gram (ACBS) · NHS indicative price = £3.25

Heron Foods® (Gluten Free Foods Ltd)
Gluten-free, wheat-free. Flour mix, organic, bread, fibre
500 gram (ACBS) · NHS indicative price = £8.96
Bread and cake mix 500 gram (ACBS) · NHS indicative price =
£8.96

Low-protein foods

ACBS indications: inherited metabolic disorders, renal or
liver failure, requiring a low-protein diet

Bread

Ener-G® Rice bread
LOW PROTEIN

Ener-G low protein rice bread (General Dietary Ltd)
600 gram (ACBS) · NHS indicative price = £5.54

Juvela® Loaf and rolls
LOW PROTEIN

Juvela gluten free loaf sliced (Hero UK Ltd)
400 gram (ACBS) · NHS indicative price = £3.54

Juvela low protein (Hero UK Ltd)
loaf sliced 400 gram (ACBS) · NHS indicative price = £3.64
bread rolls 350 gram (ACBS) · NHS indicative price = £4.52

Loprofin® Bread
LOW-PROTEIN

Loprofin low protein part baked (Nutricia Ltd)
loaf sliced 400 gram (ACBS) · NHS indicative price = £3.98
bread rolls 260 gram (ACBS) · NHS indicative price = £4.20

PK Foods® Loaf
LOW PROTEIN

PK Foods low protein white bread sliced (Gluten Free Foods Ltd)
550 gram (ACBS) · NHS indicative price = £4.75

Cake, biscuits, and snacks

Juvela® Cookies
LOW-PROTEIN

Juvela low protein (Hero UK Ltd)
chocolate chip cookies 110 gram (ACBS) · NHS indicative price =
£7.62
cinnamon cookies, orange cookies 125 gram (ACBS) · NHS
indicative price = £7.62

Loprofin® Wafers
LOW-PROTEIN

Loprofin low protein (Nutricia Ltd)
chocolate cream wafers, vanilla cream wafers 100 gram (ACBS) ·
NHS indicative price = £2.58
crackers, herb crackers 150 gram (ACBS) · NHS indicative price =
£3.62

PK Foods® Biscuits
LOW-PROTEIN

PK Foods Aminex low protein (Gluten Free Foods Ltd)
biscuits, rusks 200 gram (ACBS) · NHS indicative price = £5.04
cookies 150 gram (ACBS) · NHS indicative price = £5.04

PK Foods low protein (Gluten Free Foods Ltd)
crispbread 75 gram (ACBS) · NHS indicative price = £2.42
chocolate chip cookies, cinnamon cookies, orange cookies
150 gram (ACBS) · NHS indicative price = £5.04

Promin® Cooked and flavoured pasta snax
LOW-PROTEIN

Promin low protein (Firstplay Dietary Foods Ltd)
Snax salt & vinegar 25g sachets, Snax ready salted 25g sachets,
Snax cheese & onion 25g sachets 3 sachet · No NHS indicative
price available

Taranis® Cake bars
LOW-PROTEIN

Taranis low protein (Firstplay Dietary Foods Ltd)
apricot cake, lemon cake, pear cake 240 gram (ACBS) · NHS
indicative price = £6.08

Vita Bite®
▶ Not recommended for any child under 1 year.
LOW PROTEIN.Bar, protein 30 mg (less than 2.5 mg
phenylalanine), carbohydrate 15.35 g, fat 8.4 g, energy 572 kJ
(137 kcal)/25 g.

VitaBite bar (Vitaflo International Ltd)
175 gram (ACBS) · NHS indicative price = £8.61

Vitaflo Choices® Mini crackers
LOW-PROTEIN

Vitaflo Choices mini crackers (Vitaflo International Ltd)
40 gram (ACBS) · NHS indicative price = £0.85

Cereals

Loprofin® Breakfast cereal
LOW-PROTEIN

loops (Nutricia Ltd)
375 gram (ACBS) · NHS indicative price = £8.12

Loprofin low protein breakfast cereal flakes (Nutricia Ltd)
apple, chocolate, strawberry 375 gram (ACBS) · NHS indicative
price = £7.98

Promin® Hot breakfast
LOW-PROTEIN

Promin low protein hot breakfast powder sachets (Firstplay Dietary
Foods Ltd)
apple & cinnamon, banana, chocolate 342 gram (ACBS) · NHS
indicative price = £8.09
original 336 gram (ACBS) · NHS indicative price = £8.09

Desserts

Loprofin® Powder
LOW-PROTEIN

Loprofin low protein dessert (Nutricia Ltd)
mix chocolate, mix strawberry, mix vanilla 150 gram (ACBS) ·
NHS indicative price = £4.88

PK Foods® Jelly
LOW-PROTEIN

PK Foods low protein jelly mix dessert (Gluten Free Foods Ltd)
cherry, orange 320 gram (ACBS) · NHS indicative price = £8.03

Promin® Desserts
LOW-PROTEIN

Promin low protein imitation rice pudding (Firstplay Dietary Foods Ltd)
apple, banana, original, strawberry 276 gram (ACBS) · NHS indicative price = £6.33

Flour mixes and egg substitutes

Ener-G® Egg replacer
LOW-PROTEIN

Ener-G low protein egg replacer (General Dietary Ltd)
454 gram (ACBS) · NHS indicative price = £5.11

Fate® Flour mix
LOW PROTEIN

Fate low protein (Fate Special Foods)
all purpose mix, chocolate cake mix, plain cake mix 500 gram (ACBS) · NHS indicative price = £6.97

Juvela® Mix
LOW-PROTEIN

Juvela low protein mix (Hero UK Ltd)
500 gram (ACBS) · NHS indicative price = £7.79

Loprofin® Flour mixes and egg substitutes
LOW-PROTEIN

mix (Nutricia Ltd)
500 gram (ACBS) · NHS indicative price = £8.43

Loprofin low protein cake (Nutricia Ltd)
mix lemon, mix chocolate 500 gram (ACBS) · NHS indicative price = £8.93

Loprofin low protein egg (Nutricia Ltd)
white replacer 100 gram (ACBS) · NHS indicative price = £9.98
replacer 500 gram (ACBS) · NHS indicative price = £15.51

PK Foods® Flour mix and egg substitute
LOW-PROTEIN

PK Foods low protein (Gluten Free Foods Ltd)
egg replacer 200 gram (ACBS) · NHS indicative price = £4.08
flour mix 750 gram (ACBS) · NHS indicative price = £10.71

Pasta

Loprofin® Pasta
LOW-PROTEIN

rice (Nutricia Ltd)
500 gram

Loprofin low protein pasta (Nutricia Ltd)
penne, long cut spaghetti 500 gram (ACBS) · NHS indicative price = £8.82
animal shapes 500 gram (ACBS) · NHS indicative price = £8.49
tagliatelle, macaroni elbows 250 gram (ACBS) · NHS indicative price = £4.24
lasagne 250 gram (ACBS) · NHS indicative price = £4.29

Promin® Pasta
LOW-PROTEIN

Promin Plus low protein pasta (Firstplay Dietary Foods Ltd)
macaroni, flat noodles 500 gram (ACBS) · NHS indicative price = £6.99

Promin low protein imitation rice (Firstplay Dietary Foods Ltd)
500 gram (ACBS) · NHS indicative price = £6.99

Promin low protein lasagne sheets (Firstplay Dietary Foods Ltd)
200 gram (ACBS) · NHS indicative price = £3.03

Promin low protein pasta (Firstplay Dietary Foods Ltd)
alphabets, shells, short cut spaghetti, spirals 500 gram (ACBS) · NHS indicative price = £6.99

Promin low protein tricolour pasta (Firstplay Dietary Foods Ltd)
spirals, alphabets, shells 500 gram (ACBS) · NHS indicative price = £6.99

Pizza bases

Juvela® Pizza base
LOW-PROTEIN

Juvela low protein pizza base (Hero UK Ltd)
360 gram (ACBS) · NHS indicative price = £8.61

Savoury meals and mixes

Promin® Savoury meals and mixes
LOW-PROTEIN

pastameal (Firstplay Dietary Foods Ltd)
500 gram (ACBS) · NHS indicative price = £6.99

elbows (Firstplay Dietary Foods Ltd)
500 gram (ACBS) · NHS indicative price = £6.99

macaroni (Firstplay Dietary Foods Ltd)
500 gram (ACBS) · NHS indicative price = £6.99

Promin Plus low protein pasta spirals (Firstplay Dietary Foods Ltd)
500 gram (ACBS) · NHS indicative price = £6.99

Promin low protein X-Pot (Firstplay Dietary Foods Ltd)
all day scramble, beef & tomato, chip shop curry, rogan style curry 240 gram (ACBS) · NHS indicative price = £20.94

Promin low protein burger mix (Firstplay Dietary Foods Ltd)
124 gram (ACBS) · NHS indicative price = £6.36

Promin low protein cous cous (Firstplay Dietary Foods Ltd)
500 gram (ACBS) · NHS indicative price = £6.99

Promin low protein lamb and mint burger mix (Firstplay Dietary Foods Ltd)
124 gram (ACBS) · NHS indicative price = £6.36

Promin low protein pasta in (Firstplay Dietary Foods Ltd)
cheese and broccoli sauce 264 gram (ACBS) · NHS indicative price = £8.31
tomato, pepper and herb sauce 288 gram (ACBS) · NHS indicative price = £8.31

Promin low protein pasta spirals in Moroccan sauce (Firstplay Dietary Foods Ltd)
288 gram (ACBS) · NHS indicative price = £8.31

Promin low protein potato pot (Firstplay Dietary Foods Ltd)
onion, cabbage & bacon, sausage 200 gram (ACBS) · NHS indicative price = £16.40

Promin low protein sausage (Firstplay Dietary Foods Ltd)
mix apple and sage, mix original, mix tomato and basil 120 gram (ACBS) · NHS indicative price = £7.15

Spreads

Taranis® Spread
LOW-PROTEIN

Taranis low protein hazelnut spread (Firstplay Dietary Foods Ltd)
230 gram (ACBS) · NHS indicative price = £7.87

Nutritional supplements for metabolic diseases

Glutaric aciduria (type 1)

GA1 Anamix® Infant
▸ Nutritional supplement for the dietary management of proven glutaric aciduria (type 1) in children from birth to 3 years.
POWDER, protein equivalent (essential and non-essential amino acids except lysine, and low tryptophan) 13.1 g, carbohydrate 49.5 g, fat 23 g, fibre 5.3 g, energy 1915 kJ (457 kcal)/100 g, with vitamins, minerals, and trace elements; standard dilution (15%) provides protein equivalent 2 g, carbohydrate 7.4 g, fat 3.5 g, fibre 800 mg, energy 287 kJ (69 kcal)/100 mL.

GA Gel®
▸ Nutritional supplement for dietary management of type 1 glutaric aciduria in children 6 months–10 years.
GEL, protein equivalent (essential and non-essential amino acids except lysine, and low tryptophan) 10 g, carbohydrate 10.3 g, fat trace, energy 339 kJ (81 kcal)/24 g, with vitamins, minerals, and trace elements.

GA gel oral powder 24g sachets (Vitaflo International Ltd)
30 sachet (ACBS) · NHS indicative price = £212.44

XLYS, Low TRY, Maxamaid®
▸ Nutritional supplement for the dietary management of type 1 glutaric aciduria.
POWDER, protein equivalent (essential and non-essential amino acids except lysine, and low tryptophan) 25 g, carbohydrate 51 g, fat less than 500 mg, energy 1311 kJ (309 kcal)/100 g, with vitamins, minerals, and trace elements.

XLYS LOW TRY Maxamaid powder (Nutricia Ltd)
500 gram (ACBS) · NHS indicative price = £98.23

XLYS, TRY Glutaridon®
▸ Nutritional supplement for the dietary management of type 1 glutaric aciduria in children and adults; requires additional source of vitamins, minerals, and trace elements.
POWDER, protein equivalent (essential and non-essential amino acids except lysine and tryptophan) 79 g, carbohydrate 4 g, energy 1411 kJ (332 kcal)/100 g.

XLYS TRY Glutaridon powder (Nutricia Ltd)
500 gram (ACBS) · NHS indicative price = £186.08

Glycogen storage disease
Corn flour and corn starch
For glycogen storage disease

Glycosade®
▸ A nutritional supplement for use in the dietary management of glycogen storage disease and other metabolic conditions where a constant supply of glucose is essential. Not suitable for use in children under 2 years.
POWDER, protein 200 mg, carbohydrate (maize starch) 47.6 g, fat 100 mg, fibre less than 600 mg, energy 803 kJ (192 kcal)/60 g.

Glycosade oral powder 60g sachets (Vitaflo International Ltd)
30 sachet (ACBS) · NHS indicative price = £111.65

Homocystinuria or hypermethioninaemia

HCU Anamix® Infant
▸ Nutritional supplement for the dietary management of proven vitamin B6 non-responsive homocystinuria or hypermethioninaemia in children from birth to 3 years.
POWDER, protein equivalent (essential and non-essential amino acids except methionine) 13.1 g, carbohydrate 49.5 g, fat 23 g, fibre 5.3 g, energy 1915 kJ (457 kcal)/100 g, with vitamins, minerals, and trace elements; standard dilution (15%) provides protein equivalent 2 g, carbohydrate 7.4 g, fat 3.5 g, fibre 800 mg, energy 287 kJ (69 kcal)/100 mL.

HCU Anamix Infant powder (Nutricia Ltd)
400 gram (ACBS) · NHS indicative price = £38.91

HCU cooler® 15
▸ A methionine-free protein substitute for use as a nutritional supplement in patients over 3 years with homocystinuria.
LIQUID, protein (essential and non-essential amino acids except methionine) 15 g, carbohydrate 7 g, fat 500 mg, energy 393 kJ (92 kcal)/130 mL, with vitamins, minerals, and trace elements.

HCU orange cooler 15 liquid (Vitaflo International Ltd)
130 ml (ACBS) · NHS indicative price = £11.21

HCU Express® 15
▸ A methionine-free protein substitute for use as a nutritional supplement in children over 8 years with homocystinuria.
POWDER, protein (essential and non-essential amino acids except methionine) 15 g, carbohydrate 3.8 g, fat 30 mg, energy 315 kJ (75.3 kcal)/25 g with vitamins, minerals, and trace elements.

HCU express 15 oral powder 25g sachets (Vitaflo International Ltd)
30 sachet (ACBS) · NHS indicative price = £329.89

HCU Express® 20
▸ A methionine-free protein substitute for use as a nutritional supplement in children over 8 years with homocystinuria.
POWDER, protein (essential and non-essential amino acids except methionine) 20 g, carbohydrate 4.7 g, fat 70 mg, energy 416 kJ (99 kcal)/34 g with vitamins, minerals, and trace elements.

HCU express 20 oral powder 34g sachets (Vitaflo International Ltd)
30 sachet (ACBS) · NHS indicative price = £426.21

HCU gel®
▸ A methionine-free protein substitute for use as a nutritional supplement for the dietary management of children 1–10 years with homocystinuria.
POWDER, protein (essential and non-essential amino acids except methionine) 10 g, carbohydrate 10.3 g, fat 20 mg, energy 339 kJ (81 kcal)/24 g with vitamins, minerals, and trace elements.

HCU gel oral powder 24g sachets (Vitaflo International Ltd)
30 sachet (ACBS) · NHS indicative price = £212.38

HCU Lophlex® LQ 20
▸ Nutritional supplement for the dietary management of homocystinuria in patients over 3 years.
LIQUID, protein equivalent (essential and non-essential amino acids except methionine) 20 g, carbohydrate 8.8 g, fat 440 mg, energy 509 kJ (120 kcal)/125 mL, with vitamins, minerals, and trace elements.

HCU Lophlex LQ 20 liquid (Nutricia Ltd)
125 ml (ACBS) · NHS indicative price = £16.05

HCU LV®
▸ Nutritional supplement for the dietary management of hypermethioninaemia or vitamin B6 non-responsive homocystinuria in children over 8 years.
POWDER, protein (essential and non-essential amino acids except methionine) 20 g, carbohydrate 2.5 g, fat 190 mg, energy 390 kJ (92 kcal)/27.8-g sachet, with vitamins, minerals, and trace elements.

HCU-LV oral powder 27.8g sachets (Nutricia Ltd)
tropical, unflavoured 30 sachet (ACBS) · NHS indicative price = £493.20

XMET Homidon®
▸ Nutritional supplement for the dietary management of hypermethioninaemia or homocystinuria in children and adults.
POWDER, protein equivalent (essential and non-essential amino acids, except methionine) 77 g, carbohydrate 4.5 g, fat nil, energy 1386 kJ (326 kcal)/100 g.

XMET Homidon powder (Nutricia Ltd)
500 gram (ACBS) · NHS indicative price = £186.08

XMET Maxamaid®
▸ Nutritional supplement for the dietary management of hypermethioninaemia or homocystinuria.
POWDER, protein equivalent (essential and non-essential amino acids except methionine) 25 g, carbohydrate 51 g, fat less than 500 mg, energy 1311 kJ (309 kcal)/100 g, with vitamins, minerals, and trace elements.
Maxamaid products are generally intended for use in children 1–8 years.

XMET Maxamaid powder (Nutricia Ltd)
500 gram (ACBS) · NHS indicative price = £98.23

XMET Maxamum®
▸ Nutritional supplement for the dietary management of hypermethioninaemia or homocystinuria.
POWDER, protein equivalent (essential and non-essential amino acids except methionine) 39 g, carbohydrate 34 g, fat less than 500 mg, energy 1260 kJ (297 kcal)/100 g, with vitamins, minerals, and trace elements.
Maxamum products are generally intended for use in children over 8 years.

XMET Maxamum powder (Nutricia Ltd)
500 gram (ACBS) · NHS indicative price = £157.46

Hyperlysinaemia

HYPER LYS Anamix® Infant
▸ Nutritional supplement for the dietary management of proven hyperlysinaemia in children from birth to 3 years.
POWDER, protein equivalent (essential and non-essential amino acids except lysine) 13.1 g, carbohydrate 49.5 g, fat 23 g, fibre

A2

Borderline substances | Appendix 2

5.3 g, energy 1915 kJ (457 kcal)/100 g, with vitamins, minerals, and trace elements; standard dilution (15%) provides protein equivalent 2 g, carbohydrate 7.4 g, fat 3.5 g, fibre 800 mg, energy 287 kJ (69 kcal)/100 mL.

HYPER LYS Anamix Infant powder (Nutricia Ltd)
400 gram (ACBS) · NHS indicative price = £38.91

XLYS Maxamaid®
▸ Nutritional supplement for the dietary management of hyperlysinaemia.
POWDER, protein equivalent (essential and non-essential amino acids except lysine) 25 g, carbohydrate 51 g, fat less than 500 mg, energy 1311 kJ (309 kcal)/100 g with vitamins, minerals, and trace elements.

XLYS Maxamaid powder (Nutricia Ltd)
500 gram (ACBS) · NHS indicative price = £98.23

Isovaleric acidaemia

IVA Anamix® Infant
▸ Nutritional supplement for the dietary management of proven isovaleric acidaemia or other proven disorders of leucine metabolism in children from birth to 3 years.
POWDER, protein equivalent (essential and non-essential amino acids except leucine) 13.1 g, carbohydrate 49.5 g, fat 23 g, fibre 5.3 g, energy 1915 kJ (457 kcal)/100 g, with vitamins, minerals, and trace elements; standard dilution (15%) provides protein equivalent 2 g, carbohydrate 7.4 g, fat 3.5 g, fibre 800 mg, energy 287 kJ (69 kcal)/100 mL.

IVA Anamix Infant powder (Nutricia Ltd)
400 gram (ACBS) · NHS indicative price = £38.91

XLEU Faladon®
▸ Nutritional supplement for the dietary management of isovaleric acidaemia.
POWDER, protein equivalent (essential and non-essential amino acids except leucine) 77 g, carbohydrate 4.5 g, fat nil, energy 1386 kJ (326 kcal)/100 g.

XLEU Maxamaid®
▸ Nutritional supplement for the dietary management of isovaleric acidaemia.
POWDER, protein equivalent (essential and non-essential amino acids except leucine) 25 g, carbohydrate 51 g, fat less than 500 mg, energy 1311 kJ (309 kcal)/100 g with vitamins, minerals, and trace elements.

XLEU Maxamaid powder (Nutricia Ltd)
500 gram (ACBS) · NHS indicative price = £98.23

Maple syrup urine disease

MSUD Aid III®
▸ Nutritional supplement for the dietary management of maple syrup urine disease and related conditions in children and adults where it is necessary to limit the intake of branched chain amino acids.
POWDER, protein equivalent (essential and non-essential amino acids except isoleucine, leucine, and valine) 77 g, carbohydrate 4.5 g, fat nil, energy 1386 kJ (326 kcal)/100 g.

MSUD Aid 111 powder (Nutricia Ltd)
500 gram (ACBS) · NHS indicative price = £186.08

MSUD Anamix® Infant
▸ Nutritional supplement for the dietary management of proven maple syrup urine disease in children from birth to 3 years.
POWDER, protein equivalent (essential and non-essential amino acids except isoleucine, leucine, and valine) 13.1 g, carbohydrate 49.5 g, fat 23 g, fibre 5.3 g, energy 1915 kJ (457 kcal)/100 g, with vitamins, minerals, and trace elements; standard dilution (15%) provides protein equivalent 2 g, carbohydrate 7.4 g, fat 3.5 g, fibre 800 mg, energy 287 kJ (69 kcal)/100 mL.

MSUD Anamix Infant powder (Nutricia Ltd)
400 gram (ACBS) · NHS indicative price = £38.91

MSUD Anamix® Junior
▸ Nutritional supplement for the dietary management of maple syrup urine disease in children 1–10 years.
POWDER, protein equivalent (essential and non-essential amino acids except isoleucine, leucine, and valine) 8.4 g, carbohydrate 11 g, fat 3.9 g, energy 474 kJ (113 kcal)/29-g sachet, with vitamins, minerals, and trace elements.

MSUD Anamix Junior oral powder 36g sachets (Nutricia Ltd)
30 sachet (ACBS) · NHS indicative price = £207.90

MSUD Anamix® Junior LQ
▸ Nutritional supplement for the dietary management of maple syrup urine disease in children 1–10 years.
LIQUID, protein equivalent (essential and non-essential amino acids except isoleucine, leucine, and valine) 10 g, carbohydrate 8.8 g, fat 4.8 g, fibre 310 mg, energy 497 kJ (118 kcal)/125 mL, with vitamins, minerals, and trace elements. Lactose-free.

MSUD Anamix Junior LQ liquid (Nutricia Ltd)
125 ml (ACBS) · NHS indicative price = £9.02

MSUD cooler® 15
▸ Nutritional supplement for the dietary management of maple syrup urine disease in children over 3 years and adults.
LIQUID, protein equivalent (essential and non-essential amino acids except leucine, isoleucine, and valine) 15 g, carbohydrate 7 g, fat 500 mg, energy 393 kJ (92 kcal)/130-mL pouch, with vitamins, minerals, and trace elements.

MSUD (Vitaflo International Ltd)
orange cooler 15 liquid, red cooler 15 liquid 130 ml (ACBS) · NHS indicative price = £11.21

MSUD express® 15
▸ Nutritional supplement for the dietary management of maple syrup urine disease in children over 8 years and adults.
POWDER, protein equivalent (essential and non-essential amino acids except leucine, isoleucine, and valine) 15 g, carbohydrate 3.8 g, fat less than 100 mg, energy 315 kJ (75 kcal)/25 g, with vitamins, minerals, and trace elements.

MSUD express 15 oral powder 25g sachets (Vitaflo International Ltd)
30 sachet (ACBS) · NHS indicative price = £329.89

MSUD express® 20
▸ Nutritional supplement for the dietary management of maple syrup urine disease in children over 8 years and adults.
POWDER, protein equivalent (essential and non-essential amino acids except leucine, isoleucine, and valine) 20 g, carbohydrate 4.7 g, fat less than 100 mg, energy 416 kJ (99 kcal)/34 g, with vitamins, minerals, and trace elements.

MSUD express 20 oral powder 34g sachets (Vitaflo International Ltd)
30 sachet (ACBS) · NHS indicative price = £426.21

MSUD Gel®
▸ Nutritional supplement for the dietary management of maple syrup urine disease in children 1–10 years.
POWDER, protein equivalent (essential and non-essential amino acids except leucine, isoleucine, and valine) 10 g, carbohydrate 10.3 g, fat less than 100 mg, energy 339 kJ (81 kcal)/24 g, with vitamins, minerals, and trace elements.

MSUD gel 24g sachets (Vitaflo International Ltd)
30 sachet (ACBS) · NHS indicative price = £214.88

MSUD Lophlex® LQ 20
▸ Nutritional supplement for the dietary management of maple syrup urine disease in children over 3 years and adults.
LIQUID, protein equivalent (essential and non-essential amino acids except isoleucine, leucine, and valine) 20 g, carbohydrate 8.8 g, fat less than 500 mg, energy 509 kJ (120 kcal)/125 mL, with vitamins, minerals, and trace elements.

MSUD Lophlex LQ 20 liquid (Nutricia Ltd)
125 ml (ACBS) · NHS indicative price = £16.05

MSUD Maxamaid®
▸ Nutritional supplement for the dietary management of maple syrup urine disease.
POWDER, protein equivalent (essential and non-essential amino acids except isoleucine, leucine, and valine) 25 g, carbohydrate 51 g, fat less than 500 mg, energy 1311 kJ (309 kcal)/100 g, with vitamins, minerals, and trace elements.

Maxamaid products are generally intended for use in children 1–8 years.

MSUD Maxamaid powder (Nutricia Ltd)
500 gram (ACBS) · NHS indicative price = £98.23

MSUD Maxamum®
▸ Nutritional supplement for the dietary management of maple syrup urine disease.
POWDER, protein equivalent (essential and non-essential amino acids except isoleucine, leucine, and valine) 39 g, carbohydrate 34 g, fat less than 500 mg, energy 1260 kJ (297 kcal)/100 g, with vitamins, minerals, and trace elements.
Maxamum products are generally intended for use in children over 8 years.

MSUD Maxamum powder (Nutricia Ltd)
orange, unflavoured 500 gram (ACBS) · NHS indicative price = £157.46

Methylmalonic or propionic acidaemia

MMA/PA Anamix® Infant
▸ Nutritional supplement for the dietary management of proven methylmalonic acidaemia or propionic acidaemia in children from birth to 3 years.
POWDER, protein equivalent (essential and non-essential amino acids except methionine, threonine, and valine, and low isoleucine) 13.1 g, carbohydrate 49.5 g, fat 23 g, fibre 5.3 g, energy 1915 kJ (457 kcal)/100 g, with vitamins, minerals, and trace elements; standard dilution (15%) provides protein equivalent 2 g, carbohydrate 7.4 g, fat 3.5 g, fibre 800 mg, energy 287 kJ (69 kcal)/100 mL.

MMA PA Anamix Infant powder (Nutricia Ltd)
400 gram (ACBS) · NHS indicative price = £38.91

XMTVI Asadon®
▸ Nutritional supplement for the dietary management of methylmalonic acidaemia or propionic acidaemia in children and adults.
POWDER, protein equivalent (essential and non-essential amino acids except methionine, threonine, and valine, and low isoleucine) 77 g, carbohydrate 4.5 g, fat nil, energy 1386 kJ (326 kcal)/100 g.

XMTVI Asadon powder (Nutricia Ltd)
200 gram (ACBS) · NHS indicative price = £74.43

XMTVI Maxamaid®
▸ Nutritional supplement for the dietary management of methylmalonic acidaemia or propionic acidaemia.
POWDER, protein equivalent (essential and non-essential amino acids except methionine, threonine, and valine, and low isoleucine) 25 g, carbohydrate 51 g, fat less than 500 mg, energy 1311 kJ (309 kcal)/100 g, with vitamins, minerals, and trace elements.

XMTVI Maxamaid powder (Nutricia Ltd)
500 gram (ACBS) · NHS indicative price = £98.23

XMTVI Maxamum®
▸ Nutritional supplement for the dietary management of methylmalonic acidaemia or propionic acidaemia.
POWDER, protein equivalent (essential and non-essential amino acids except methionine, threonine, and valine, and low isoleucine) 39 g, carbohydrate 34 g, fat less than 500 mg, energy 1260 kJ (297 kcal)/100 g, with vitamins, minerals, and trace elements.

XMTVI Maxamum powder (Nutricia Ltd)
500 gram (ACBS) · NHS indicative price = £157.46

Other inborn errors of metabolism

Cystine500®
▸ Nutritional supplement for the dietary management of inborn errors of amino acid metabolism in adults and children from birth.
POWDER, cystine 500 mg, carbohydrate 3.3 g, fat nil, energy 63 kJ (15 kcal)/4 g

DocOmega®
▸ Nutritional supplement for the dietary management of inborn errors of metabolism for adults and children from birth.
POWDER, protein (cows' milk, soya) 100 mg, carbohydrate 3.2 g, fat 500 mg (of which docosahexaenoic acid 200 mg), fibre nil, energy 74 kJ (18 kcal)/4 g, with minerals

DocOmega oral powder 4g sachets (Vitaflo International Ltd)
30 sachet (ACBS) · NHS indicative price = £39.06

EAA® Supplement
▸ Nutritional supplement for the dietary management of disorders of protein metabolism including urea cycle disorders. Not suitable for children under 3 years.
POWDER, protein equivalent (essential amino acids) 5 g, carbohydrate 4 g, fat nil, energy 151 kJ (36 kcal)/12.5 g, with vitamins, minerals, and trace elements.

EAA Supplement oral powder 12.5g sachets (Vitaflo International Ltd)
50 sachet (ACBS) · NHS indicative price = £203.64

Isoleucine50®
▸ Nutritional supplement for use in the dietary management of inborn errors of amino acid metabolism in adults and children from birth.
POWDER, isoleucine 50 mg, carbohydrate 3.8 g, fat nil, energy 63 kJ (15 kcal)/4 g

Isoleucine50 oral powder 4g sachets (Vitaflo International Ltd)
30 sachet (ACBS) · NHS indicative price = £53.97

KeyOmega®
▸ Nutritional supplement for the dietary management of inborn errors of metabolism.
POWDER, protein (cows' milk, soya) 170 mg, carbohydrate 2.8 g, fat 800 mg (of which arachidonic acid 200 mg, docosahexaenoic acid 100 mg), energy 80 kJ (19 kcal)/4 g.

KeyOmega oral powder 4g sachets (Vitaflo International Ltd)
30 sachet (ACBS) · NHS indicative price = £39.94

Leucine100®
▸ Nutritional supplement for the dietary management of inborn errors of amino acid metabolism in adults and children from birth.
POWDER, leucine 100 mg, carbohydrate 3.7 g, fat nil, energy 63 kJ (15 kcal)/4 g

Leucine100 oral powder sachets (Vitaflo International Ltd)
30 sachet (ACBS) · NHS indicative price = £53.97

Low protein drink
▸ Nutritional supplement for the dietary management of inborn errors of amino acid metabolism in adults and children over 1 year.
POWDER, protein (cows' milk) 4.5 g (phenylalanine 100 mg), carbohydrate 59.5 g, fat 29.9 g, fibre nil, energy 2194 kJ (528 kcal)/100 g, with vitamins, minerals, and trace elements. Contains lactose.

Milupa LP drink (Nutricia Ltd)
400 gram (ACBS) · NHS indicative price = £9.23

Phenylalanine50®
▸ Nutritional supplement for use in the dietary management of inborn errors of metabolism in adults and children from birth.
POWDER, phenylalanine 50 mg, carbohydrate 3.8 g, fat nil, energy 63 kJ (15 kcal)/4 g

Phenylalanine50 oral powder sachets (Vitaflo International Ltd)
30 sachet (ACBS) · NHS indicative price = £52.40

ProZero®
▸ A protein-free nutritional supplement for the dietary management of inborn errors of metabolism in children over 6 months and adults.
LIQUID, carbohydrate 8.1 g (of which sugars 3.5 g), fat 3.8 g, energy 278 kJ (66 kcal)/100 mL. Contains lactose.

ProZero liquid (Vitaflo International Ltd)
250 ml (ACBS) · NHS indicative price = £1.44 | 1000 ml (ACBS) · NHS indicative price = £5.75

A2

Borderline substances | Appendix 2

Tyrosine1000®
▶ Nutritional supplement for the dietary management of inborn errors of amino acid metabolism in adults and children from birth.
POWDER, tyrosine 1 g, carbohydrate 2.9 g, fat nil, energy 63 kJ (15 kcal)/4-g sachet.

Tyrosine1000 oral powder 4g sachets (Vitaflo International Ltd)
30 sachet (ACBS) · NHS indicative price = £4.95

Valine50®
▶ Nutritional supplement for the dietary management of inborn errors of amino acid metabolism in adults and children from birth.
POWDER, valine 50 mg, carbohydrate 3.8 g, fat nil, energy 63 kJ (15 kcal)/4 g

Valine50 oral powder 4g sachets (Vitaflo International Ltd)
30 sachet (ACBS) · NHS indicative price = £53.97

Phenylketonuria

Add-Ins®
▶ Nutritional supplement for the dietary management of proven phenylketonuria. Not suitable for children under 4 years.
POWDER, protein equivalent (containing essential and non-essential amino acids except phenylalanine) 10 g, carbohydrate nil, fat 5.1 g, energy 359 kJ (86 kcal)/18.2-g sachet, with vitamins, minerals, and trace elements.

Add Ins oral powder 18.2g sachets (Nutricia Ltd)
60 sachet (ACBS) · NHS indicative price = £375.60

Easiphen®
▶ Nutritional supplement for the dietary management of proven phenylketonuria. Not suitable for children under 8 years.
LIQUID, protein equivalent (containing essential and non-essential amino acids except phenylalanine) 6.7 g, carbohydrate 5.1 g, fat 2 g, energy 275 kJ (65 kcal)/100 mL with vitamins, minerals, and trace elements.

Easiphen liquid (Nutricia Ltd)
250 ml (ACBS) · NHS indicative price = £9.65

Lophlex®
▶ Nutritional supplement for the dietary management of proven phenylketonuria in children over 8 years and adults including pregnant women.
POWDER, protein equivalent (essential and non-essential amino acids except phenylalanine) 20 g, carbohydrate 2.5 g, fat 60 mg, fibre 220 mg, energy 385 kJ (91 kcal)/27.8-g sachet, with vitamins, minerals, and trace elements.

Lophlex powder 27.8g sachets (Nutricia Ltd)
berry, orange, unflavoured 30 sachet (ACBS) · NHS indicative price = £289.80

Loprofin® PKU Drink
▶ Nutritional supplement for the dietary management of phenylketonuria in children over 1 year and adults.
LIQUID, protein (cows' milk) 400 mg (phenylalanine 10 mg), lactose 9.4 g, fat 2 g, energy 165 kJ (40 kcal)/100 mL.

Loprofin PKU drink (Nutricia Ltd)
200 ml (ACBS) · NHS indicative price = £0.75

Loprofin® Sno-Pro
▶ Nutritional supplement for the dietary management of phenylketonuria, chronic renal failure and other inborn errors of amino acid metabolism.
LIQUID, protein (cows' milk) 220 mg (phenylalanine 12.5 mg), carbohydrate 8 g, fat 3.8 g, energy 273 kJ (65 kcal)/100 mL. Contains lactose.

Loprofin SNO-PRO drink (Nutricia Ltd)
200 ml (ACBS) · NHS indicative price = £1.25

Phlexy-10® Exchange System
▶ Nutritional supplement for the dietary management of phenylketonuria.
CAPSULES, protein equivalent (essential and non-essential amino acids except phenylalanine) 416.5 mg/capsule.

Phlexy-10 500mg capsules (Nutricia Ltd)
200 capsule (ACBS) · NHS indicative price = £42.80

DRINK MIX, powder, protein equivalent (essential and non-essential amino acids except phenylalanine) 8.33 g, carbohydrate 8.8 g/20-g sachet.

Phlexy-10 drink (Nutricia Ltd)
mix apple & blackcurrant, mix citrus burst, mix tropical surprise 600 gram (ACBS) · NHS indicative price = £128.40
TABLETS, protein equivalent (essential and non-essential amino acids except phenylalanine) 833 mg tablet.

tablets (Nutricia Ltd)
75 tablet (ACBS) · NHS indicative price = £27.75

Phlexy-Vits®
▶ For use as a vitamin and mineral component of restricted therapeutic diets in children over 11 years and adults with phenylketonuria and similar amino acid abnormalities.
POWDER, vitamins, minerals, and trace elements

Phlexy-Vits (Nutricia Ltd)
powder 210 gram (ACBS) · NHS indicative price = £71.40

Phlexy-Vits (Nutricia Ltd)
tablets 180 tablet (ACBS) · NHS indicative price = £81.00

PK Aid 4®
▶ Nutritional supplement for the dietary management of phenylketonuria in children and adults.
POWDER, protein equivalent (essential and non-essential amino acids except phenylalanine) 79 g, carbohydrate 4.5 g, fat nil, energy 1420 kJ (334 kcal)/100 g.

PK Aid 4 powder (Nutricia Ltd)
500 gram (ACBS) · NHS indicative price = £143.04

PKU Anamix® Infant
▶ Nutritional supplement for the dietary management of proven phenylketonuria in children from birth to 3 years.
POWDER, protein equivalent (essential and non-essential amino acids except phenylalanine) 13.1 g, carbohydrate 49.5 g, fat 23 g, fibre 5.3 g, energy 1915 kJ (457 kcal)/100 g, with vitamins, minerals, and trace elements; standard dilution (15%) provides protein equivalent 2 g, carbohydrate 7.4 g, fat 3.5 g, fibre 800 mg, energy 287 kJ (69 kcal)/100 mL

PKU Anamix Infant powder (Nutricia Ltd)
400 gram (ACBS) · NHS indicative price = £35.36

PKU Anamix® Junior
▶ Nutritional supplement for the dietary management of phenylketonuria in children 1–10 years.
POWDER, protein equivalent (essential and non-essential amino acids except phenylalanine) 8.4 g, carbohydrate 9.9 g, fat 3.9 g, energy 455 kJ (108 kcal)/29-g sachet, with vitamins, minerals, and trace elements

PKU Anamix Junior powder (Nutricia Ltd)
chocolate, neutral 870 gram (ACBS) · NHS indicative price = £123.90 | 1080 gram (ACBS) · NHS indicative price = £126.30

PKU Anamix® Junior LQ
▶ Nutritional supplement for the dietary supplement of phenylketonuria in children 1–10 years.
LIQUID, protein equivalent (essential and non-essential amino acids except phenylalanine) 10 g, carbohydrate 8.8 g, fat 4.8 g, fibre 310 mg, energy 497 kJ (118 kcal)/125 mL, with vitamins, minerals, and trace elements. Lactose-free.

PKU Anamix Junior LQ liquid (Nutricia Ltd)
berry, orange 125 ml (ACBS) · NHS indicative price = £5.61

PKU cooler10®
▶ Nutritional supplement for the dietary management of phenylketonuria. Not recommended for children under 3 years.
LIQUID, protein equivalent (essential and non-essential amino acids except phenylalanine) 10 g, carbohydrate 5.1 g, energy 258 kJ (62 kcal)/87-mL pouch, with vitamins, minerals, and trace elements.

PKU (Vitaflo International Ltd)
orange cooler 10 liquid, purple cooler 10 liquid, red cooler 10 liquid, white cooler 10 liquid 87 ml (ACBS) · NHS indicative price = £4.56

PKU cooler15®

▸ Nutritional supplement for the dietary management of phenylketonuria. Not recommended for children under 3 years.
LIQUID, protein equivalent (essential and non-essential amino acids except phenylalanine) 15 g, carbohydrate 7.8 g, energy 386 kJ (92 kcal)/130-mL pouch, with vitamins, minerals, and trace elements.

PKU (Vitaflo International Ltd)
orange cooler 15 liquid, purple cooler 15 liquid, red cooler 15 liquid, white cooler 15 liquid 130 ml (ACBS) · NHS indicative price = £6.80

PKU cooler20®

▸ Nutritional supplement for the dietary management of phenylketonuria. Not recommended for children under 3 years.
LIQUID, protein equivalent (essential and non-essential amino acids except phenylalanine) 20 g, carbohydrate 10.2 g, energy 517 kJ (124 kcal)/174-mL pouch, with vitamins, minerals, and trace elements.

PKU (Vitaflo International Ltd)
orange cooler 20 liquid, purple cooler 20 liquid, red cooler 20 liquid, white cooler 20 liquid 174 ml (ACBS) · NHS indicative price = £9.12

PKU express15®

▸ Nutritional supplement for the dietary management of phenylketonuria. Not recommended for children under 3 years.
POWDER, protein equivalent (essential and non-essential amino acids except phenylalanine) 15 g, carbohydrate 2.4 g, energy 293 kJ (70 kcal)/25 g, with vitamins, minerals, and trace elements.

PKU express 15 powder (Vitaflo International Ltd)
lemon, orange, tropical, unflavoured 750 gram (ACBS) · NHS indicative price = £200.00

PKU express20®

▸ Nutritional supplement for the dietary management of phenylketonuria. Not recommended for children under 3 years.
POWDER, protein equivalent (essential and non-essential amino acids except phenylalanine) 20 g, carbohydrate 3.3 g, energy 389 kJ (93 kcal)/34 g, with vitamins, minerals, and trace elements.

PKU express 20 powder (Vitaflo International Ltd)
lemon, orange, tropical, unflavoured 1020 gram (ACBS) · NHS indicative price = £258.39

PKU gel®

▸ For use as part of the low-protein dietary management of phenylketonuria in children 1–10 years
POWDER, protein equivalent (essential and non-essential amino acids except phenylalanine) 10 g, carbohydrate 8.9 g, fat less than 100 mg, energy 318 kJ (76 kcal)/24 g, with vitamins, minerals, and trace elements.

PKU gel powder (Vitaflo International Ltd)
orange, raspberry, unflavoured 720 gram (ACBS) · NHS indicative price = £138.36

PKU Lophlex® LQ 10

▸ Nutritional supplement for the dietary management of phenylketonuria in children over 4 years and adults including pregnant women.
LIQUID, protein equivalent (essential and non-essential amino acids except phenylalanine) 10 g, carbohydrate 4.4 g, fibre 250 mg, energy 245 kJ (58 kcal)/62.5 mL, with vitamins, minerals, and trace elements.

PKU Lophlex LQ 10 liquid juicy (Nutricia Ltd)
berries, orange 62.5 ml (ACBS) · NHS indicative price = £5.18

PKU Lophlex® LQ 20

▸ Nutritional supplement for the dietary management of phenylketonuria in children over 4 years and adults including pregnant women.
LIQUID, protein equivalent (essential and non-essential amino acids except phenylalanine) 20 g, carbohydrate 8.8 g, fibre 340 mg, energy 490 kJ (115 kcal)/125 mL, with vitamins, minerals, and trace elements.

PKU Lophlex LQ 20 liquid (Nutricia Ltd)
berry, juicy berries, orange 125 ml (ACBS) · NHS indicative price = £10.33

PKU Lophlex® Sensation 20

▸ Nutritional supplement for the dietary management of phenylketonuria in children over 4 years and adults including pregnant women.
SEMI-SOLID, protein equivalent (containing essential and non-essential amino acids except phenylalanine) 20 g, carbohydrate 20.2 g, fibre 1 g, energy 706 kJ (166 kcal)/109 g, with vitamins, minerals, and trace elements.

PKU Lophlex Sensation 20 (Nutricia Ltd)
berries, orange 327 gram (ACBS) · NHS indicative price = £33.00

PKU squeezie®

▸ Nutritional supplement for the dietary management of phenylketonuria in children from 6 months to 10 years.
LIQUID, protein equivalent (essential and non-essential amino acids except phenylalanine) 10 g, carbohydrate 22.5 g, fat 500 mg, energy 565 kJ (135 kcal)/85 g, with vitamins, minerals, and trace elements.

PKU squeezie liquid (Vitaflo International Ltd)
2550 gram (ACBS) · NHS indicative price = £132.27

L-Tyrosine

▸ Nutritional supplement for the dietary management of phenylketonuria in pregnant women with low plasma tyrosine concentrations.
POWDER, L-tyrosine 20 g, carbohydrate 76.8 g, fat nil, energy 1612 kJ (379 kcal)/100 g.

L-Tyrosine powder (Nutricia Ltd)
100 gram (ACBS) · NHS indicative price = £21.91

XP Maxamaid®

▸ Nutritional supplement for the dietary management of phenylketonuria in children 1–8 years.
POWDER, protein equivalent (essential and non-essential amino acids except phenylalanine) 25 g, carbohydrate 51 g, fat less than 500 mg, energy 1311 kJ (309 kcal)/100 g, with vitamins, minerals, and trace elements.

XP Maxamaid powder (Nutricia Ltd)
orange, unflavoured 500 gram (ACBS) · NHS indicative price = £58.11

XP Maxamum®

▸ Nutritional supplement for the dietary management of phenylketonuria in children over 8 years and adults.
POWDER, protein equivalent (essential and non-essential amino acids except phenylalanine) 39 g, carbohydrate 34 g, fat less than 500 mg, energy 1260 kJ (297 kcal)/100 g, with vitamins, minerals, and trace elements.

XP Maxamum oral powder 50g sachets (Nutricia Ltd)
orange, unflavoured 30 sachet (ACBS) · NHS indicative price = £269.40

XP Maxamum powder (Nutricia Ltd)
orange, unflavoured 500 gram (ACBS) · NHS indicative price = £89.88

Tyrosinaemia

Methionine-free TYR Anamix® Infant

▸ Nutritional supplement for the dietary management of proven tyrosinaemia type 1 in children from birth to 3 years.
POWDER, protein equivalent (essential and non-essential amino acids except methionine, phenylalanine, and tyrosine) 13.1 g, carbohydrate 49.5 g, fat 23 g, fibre 5.3 g, energy 1915 kJ (457 kcal)/100 g, with vitamins, minerals, and trace elements; standard dilution (15%) provides protein equivalent 2 g, carbohydrate 7.4 g, fat 3.5 g, fibre 800 mg, energy 287 kJ (69 kcal)/100 mL.

TYR Anamix Infant methionine free powder (Nutricia Ltd)
400 gram (ACBS) · NHS indicative price = £38.91

A2

Borderline substances | Appendix 2

TYR Anamix® Infant

▸ Nutritional supplement for the dietary management of proven tyrosinaemia where plasma-methionine concentrations are normal in children from birth to 3 years.

POWDER, protein equivalent (essential and non-essential amino acids except phenylalanine and tyrosine) 13.1 g, carbohydrate 49.5 g, fat 23 g, fibre 5.3 g, energy 1915 kJ (457 kcal)/100 g, with vitamins, minerals, and trace elements; standard dilution (15%) provides protein equivalent 2 g, carbohydrate 7.4 g, fat 3.5 g, fibre 800 mg, energy 287 kJ (69 kcal)/100 mL.

TYR Anamix Infant (Nutricia Ltd)
methionine free powder, powder 400 gram (ACBS) · NHS indicative price = £38.91

TYR Anamix® Junior

▸ Nutritional supplement for the dietary management of proven tyrosinaemia in children 1–10 years.

POWDER, protein equivalent (essential and non-essential amino acids except phenylalanine and tyrosine) 8.4 g, carbohydrate 11 g, fat 3.9 g, energy 475 kJ (113 kcal)/29-g sachet, with vitamins, minerals, and trace elements.

TYR Anamix Junior oral powder 29g sachets (Nutricia Ltd)
30 sachet (ACBS) · NHS indicative price = £206.40

TYR Anamix® Junior LQ

▸ Nutritional supplement for the dietary management of tyrosinaemia type 1 (when nitisinone (NTBC) is used, see), type II, and type III, in children over 1 year.

LIQUID, protein equivalent (essential and non-essential amino acids except phenylalanine and tyrosine) 10 g, carbohydrate 8.8 g, fat 4.8 g, fibre 310 mg, energy 500 kJ (119 kcal)/125 mL, with vitamins, minerals and trace elements.

TYR Anamix Junior LQ liquid (Nutricia Ltd)
125 ml (ACBS) · NHS indicative price = £9.02

TYR cooler® 15

▸ Nutritional supplement for the dietary management of tyrosinaemia in children over 3 years and adults.

LIQUID, protein equivalent (essential and non-essential amino acids except tyrosine and phenylalanine) 15 g, carbohydrate 7 g, fat 500 mg, energy 393 kJ (92 kcal)/130 mL, with vitamins, minerals, and trace elements.

TYR orange cooler 15 liquid (Vitaflo International Ltd)
130 ml (ACBS) · NHS indicative price = £11.21

TYR red cooler (Vitaflo International Ltd)
15 liquid 130 ml (ACBS) · NHS indicative price = £11.21

TYR express15®

▸ Nutritional supplement for the dietary management of tyrosinaemia in children over 8 years and adults.

POWDER, protein equivalent (essential and non-essential amino acids except tyrosine and phenylalanine) 15 g, carbohydrate 3.4 g, fat less than 100 mg, energy 310 kJ (74 kcal)/25 g, with vitamins, minerals, and trace elements.

TYR express 15 oral powder 25g sachets (Vitaflo International Ltd)
30 sachet (ACBS) · NHS indicative price = £329.89

TYR express20®

▸ Nutritional supplement for the dietary management of tyrosinaemia. Not recommended for children under 8 years.

POWDER, protein equivalent (essential and non-essential amino acids except tyrosine and phenylalanine) 20 g, carbohydrate 4.7 g, fat less than 100 mg, energy 416 kJ (99 kcal)/34 g, with vitamins, minerals, and trace elements.

TYR express 20 oral powder 34g sachets (Vitaflo International Ltd)
30 sachet (ACBS) · NHS indicative price = £426.21

TYR Gel®

▸ Nutritional supplement for the dietary management of tyrosinaemia in children 1–10 years.

GEL, protein equivalent (essential and non-essential amino acids except tyrosine and phenylalanine) 10 g, carbohydrate 10.3 g, fat less than 100 mg, energy 339 kJ (81 kcal)/24 g, with vitamins, minerals, and trace elements.

TYR gel oral powder 24g sachets (Vitaflo International Ltd)
30 sachet (ACBS) · NHS indicative price = £212.38

TYR Lophlex® LQ 20

▸ Nutritional supplement for the dietary management of tyrosinaemia in children over 3 years and adults.

LIQUID, protein equivalent (essential and non-essential amino acids except phenylalanine and tyrosine) 20 g, carbohydrate 8.8 g, fat less than 500 mg, fibre 500 mg, energy 509 kJ (120 kcal)/125 mL, with vitamins, minerals, and trace elements.

TYR Lophlex LQ 20 liquid (Nutricia Ltd)
125 ml (ACBS) · NHS indicative price = £16.05

XPHEN TYR Maxamaid®

▸ Nutritional supplement for the dietary management of tyrosinaemia in children 1–8 years.

POWDER, protein equivalent (essential and non-essential amino acids except phenylalanine and tyrosine) 25 g, carbohydrate 51 g, fat less than 500 mg, energy 1311 kJ (309 kcal)/100 g, with vitamins, minerals, and trace elements.

XPHEN TYR Maxamaid powder (Nutricia Ltd)
500 gram (ACBS) · NHS indicative price = £98.23

XPHEN TYR Tyrosidon®

▸ Nutritional supplement for the management of tyrosinaemia in children and adults where plasma-methionine concentrations are normal.

POWDER, protein equivalent (essential and non-essential amino acids except phenylalanine and tyrosine) 77 g, carbohydrate 4.5 g, fat nil, energy 1386 kJ (326 kcal)/100 g.

XPHEN TYR Tyrosidon Free AA Mix powder (Nutricia Ltd)
500 gram (ACBS) · NHS indicative price = £186.08

XPTM Tyrosidon®

▸ Nutritional supplement for the dietary management of tyrosinaemia type I in children and adults where plasma-methionine concentrations are above normal.

POWDER, protein equivalent (essential and non-essential amino acids except methionine, phenylalanine, and tyrosine) 77 g, carbohydrate 4.5 g, fat nil, energy 1386 kJ (326 kcal)/100 g.

XPTM Tyrosidon powder (Nutricia Ltd)
500 gram (ACBS) · NHS indicative price = £91.31

Appendix 3
Cautionary and advisory labels for dispensed medicines

Guidance for cautionary and advisory labels

Medicinal forms within BNF publications include code numbers of the cautionary labels that pharmacists are recommended to add when dispensing. It is also expected that pharmacists will counsel patients and carers when necessary.

Counselling needs to be related to the age, experience, background, and understanding of the individual patient or carer. The pharmacist should ensure understanding of how to take or use the medicine and how to follow the correct dosage schedule. Any effects of the medicine on co-ordination, performance of skilled tasks (e.g. driving or work), any foods or medicines to be avoided, and what to do if a dose is missed should also be explained. Other matters, such as the possibility of staining of the clothes or skin, or discolouration of urine or stools by a medicine should also be mentioned.

For some medicines there is a special need for counselling, such as an unusual method or time of administration or a potential interaction with a common food or domestic remedy, and this should be mentioned where necessary.

Original packs

Most preparations are dispensed in unbroken original packs that include further advice for the patient in the form of patient information leaflets. Label 10 may be of value where appropriate. More general leaflets advising on the administration of preparations such as eye drops, eye ointments, inhalers, and suppositories are also available.

Scope of labels

In general no label recommendations have been made for injections on the assumption that they will be administered by a healthcare professional or a well-instructed patient. The labelling is not exhaustive and pharmacists are recommended to use their professional discretion in labelling new preparations and those for which no labels are shown.

Individual labelling advice is not given on the administration of the large variety of antacids. In the absence of instructions from the prescriber, and if on enquiry the patient has had no verbal instructions, the directions given under 'Dose' should be used on the label.

It is recognised that there may be occasions when pharmacists will use their knowledge and professional discretion and decide to omit one or more of the recommended labels for a particular patient. In this case counselling is of the utmost importance. There may also be an occasion when a prescriber does not wish additional cautionary labels to be used, in which case the prescription should be endorsed 'NCL' (no cautionary labels). The exact wording that is required instead should then be specified on the prescription.

Pharmacists label medicines with various wordings in addition to those directions specified on the prescription. Such labels include 'Shake the bottle', 'For external use only', and 'Store in a cool place', as well as 'Discard.... days after opening' and 'Do not use after....', which apply particularly to antibiotic mixtures, diluted liquid and topical preparations, and to eye-drops. Although not listed in the BNF these labels should continue to be used when appropriate; indeed, 'For external use only' is a legal requirement on external liquid preparations, while 'Keep out of the reach of children' is a legal requirement on all dispensed medicines. Care should be taken not to obscure other relevant information with adhesive labelling.

It is the usual practice for patients to take standard tablets with water or other liquids and for this reason no separate label has been recommended.

The label wordings recommended by the BNF apply to medicines dispensed against a prescription. Patients should be aware that a dispensed medicine should never be taken by, or shared with, anyone other than for whom the prescriber intended it. Therefore, the BNF does not include warnings against the use of a dispensed medicine by persons other than for whom it was specifically prescribed.

The label or labels for each preparation are recommended after careful consideration of the information available. However, it is recognised that in some cases this information may be either incomplete or open to a different interpretation. The BNF will therefore be grateful to receive any constructive comments on the labelling suggested for any preparation.

Recommended label wordings

For BNF 61 (March 2011), a revised set of cautionary and advisory labels were introduced. All of the existing labels were user-tested, and the revised wording selected reflects terminology that is better understood by patients.

Wordings which can be given as separate warnings are labels 1–19, 29–30, and 32. Wordings which can be incorporated in an appropriate position in the directions for dosage or administration are labels 21–28. A label has been omitted for number 20; labels 31 and 33 no longer apply to any medicines in the BNF and have therefore been deleted.

If separate labels are used it is recommended that the wordings be used without modification. If changes are made to suit computer requirements, care should be taken to retain the sense of the original.

Welsh labels

Comprehensive Welsh translations are available for each cautionary and advisory label. These appear directly under the English label.

Labels

1 **Warning: This medicine may make you sleepy**
   Rhybudd: Gall y feddyginiaeth hon eich gwneud yn gysglyd
   To be used on *preparations for children* containing antihistamines, or other preparations given to children where the warnings of label 2 on driving or alcohol would not be appropriate.

2 **Warning: This medicine may make you sleepy. If this happens, do not drive or use tools or machines. Do not drink alcohol**
   Rhybudd: Gall y feddyginiaeth hon eich gwneud yn gysglyd. Peidiwch â gyrru, defnyddio offer llaw neu beiriannau os yw hyn yn digwydd. Peidiwch ag yfed alcohol
   To be used on *preparations for adults that can cause drowsiness*, thereby affecting coordination and the ability to drive and operate hazardous machinery; label 1 is more appropriate for children. *It is an offence to drive while under the influence of drink or drugs.*

   Some of these preparations only cause drowsiness in the first few days of treatment and some only cause drowsiness in higher doses.

   In such cases the patient should be told that the advice applies until the effects have worn off. However many of these preparations can produce a slowing of reaction time and a loss of mental concentration that can have the same effects as drowsiness.

   Avoidance of alcoholic drink is recommended because the effects of CNS depressants are enhanced by alcohol. Strict prohibition however could lead to some patients not taking the medicine. Pharmacists should therefore explain the risk and encourage compliance, particularly in patients who may think they already tolerate the effects of alcohol (see also label 3). Queries from patients with epilepsy regarding fitness to drive should be referred back to the patient's doctor.

Side-effects unrelated to drowsiness that may affect a patient's ability to drive or operate machinery safely include *blurred vision, dizziness, or nausea*. In general, no label has been recommended to cover these cases, but the patient should be suitably counselled.

3 **Warning: This medicine may make you sleepy. If this happens, do not drive or use tools or machines**
Rhybudd: Gall y feddyginiaeth hon eich gwneud yn gysglyd. Peidiwch â gyrru, defnyddio offer llaw neu beiriannau os yw hyn yn digwydd
To be used on *preparations containing monoamine-oxidase inhibitors*; the warning to avoid alcohol and dealcoholised (low alcohol) drink is covered by the patient information leaflet.

Also to be used as for label 2 but where alcohol is not an issue.

4 **Warning: Do not drink alcohol**
Rhybudd: Peidiwch ag yfed alcohol
To be used on *preparations where a reaction such as flushing may occur if alcohol is taken* (e.g. metronidazole). Alcohol may also enhance the hypoglycaemia produced by some oral antidiabetic drugs but routine application of a warning label is not considered necessary.

Patients should be advised not to drink alcohol for as long as they are receiving/using a course of medication, and in some cases for a period of time after the course is finished.

5 **Do not take indigestion remedies 2 hours before or after you take this medicine**
Peidiwch â chymryd meddyginiaethau camdreuliad 2 awr cyn neu ar ôl y feddyginiaeth hon
To be used with label 25 on *preparations coated to resist gastric acid* (e.g. enteric-coated tablets). This is to avoid the possibility of premature dissolution of the coating in the presence of an alkaline pH.

Label 5 also applies to drugs such as gabapentin *where the absorption is significantly affected by antacids*. Pharmacists will be aware (from a knowledge of physiology) that the usual time during which indigestion remedies should be avoided is at least 2 hours before and after the majority of medicines have been taken; when a manufacturer advises a different time period, this can be followed, and should be explained to the patient.

6 **Do not take indigestion remedies, or medicines containing iron or zinc, 2 hours before or after you take this medicine**
Peidiwch â chymryd meddyginiaethau camdreuliad neu feddyginiaethau sy'n cynnwys haearn neu sinc, 2 awr cyn neu ar ôl y feddyginiaeth hon
To be used on *preparations containing ofloxacin and some other quinolones, doxycycline, lymecycline, minocycline, and penicillamine*. These drugs chelate calcium, iron, and zinc and are less well absorbed when taken with calcium-containing antacids or preparations containing iron or zinc. Pharmacists will be aware (from a knowledge of physiology) that these incompatible preparations should be taken at least 2 hours apart for the majority of medicines; when a manufacturer advises a different time period, this can be followed, and should be explained to the patient.

7 **Do not take milk, indigestion remedies, or medicines containing iron or zinc, 2 hours before or after you take this medicine**
Peidiwch â chymryd llaeth, meddyginiaethau camdreuliad, neu feddyginiaethau sy'n cynnwys haearn neu sinc, 2 awr cyn neu ar ôl cymryd y feddyginiaeth hon
To be used on *preparations containing ciprofloxacin, norfloxacin, or tetracyclines that chelate calcium, iron, magnesium, and zinc*, and are thus less available for absorption. Pharmacists will be aware (from a knowledge of physiology) that these incompatible preparations should be

taken at least 2 hours apart for the majority of medicines; when a manufacturer advises a different time period, this can be followed, and should be explained to the patient. Doxycycline, lymecycline, and minocycline are less liable to form chelates and therefore only require label 6 (see above).

8 **Warning: Do not stop taking this medicine unless your doctor tells you to stop**
Rhybudd: Peidiwch â stopio cymryd y feddyginiaeth hon, oni bai fod eich meddyg yn dweud wrthych am stopio
To be used on *preparations that contain a drug which is required to be taken over long periods without the patient necessarily perceiving any benefit* (e.g. antituberculous drugs).

Also to be used on *preparations that contain a drug whose withdrawal is likely to be a particular hazard* (e.g. clonidine for hypertension). Label 10 (see below) is more appropriate for corticosteroids.

9 **Space the doses evenly throughout the day. Keep taking this medicine until the course is finished, unless you are told to stop**
Gadewch yr un faint o amser rhwng pob dôs yn ystod y dydd. Parhewch i gymryd y feddyginiaeth nes bod y cyfan wedi'i orffen, oni bai eich bod yn cael cyngor i stopio
To be used on *preparations where a course of treatment should be completed* to reduce the incidence of relapse or failure of treatment.

The preparations are antimicrobial drugs given by mouth. Very occasionally, some may have severe side-effects (e.g. diarrhoea in patients receiving clindamycin) and in such cases the patient may need to be advised of reasons for stopping treatment quickly and returning to the doctor.

10 **Warning: Read the additional information given with this medicine**
Rhybudd: Darllenwch y wybodaeth ychwanegol gyda'r feddyginiaeth hon
To be used particularly on *preparations containing anticoagulants, lithium, and oral corticosteroids*. The appropriate treatment card should be given to the patient and any necessary explanations given.

This label may also be used on other preparations to remind the patient of the instructions that have been given.

11 **Protect your skin from sunlight—even on a bright but cloudy day. Do not use sunbeds**
Diogelwch eich croen rhag golau'r haul, hyd yn oed ar ddiwrnod braf ond cymylog. Peidiwch â defnyddio gwely haul
To be used on *preparations that may cause phototoxic or photoallergic reactions* if the patient is exposed to ultraviolet radiation. Many drugs other than those listed in Appendix 3 (e.g. phenothiazines and sulfonamides) may, on rare occasions, cause reactions in susceptible patients. Exposure to high intensity ultraviolet radiation from sunray lamps and sunbeds is particularly likely to cause reactions.

12 **Do not take anything containing aspirin while taking this medicine**
Peidiwch â chymryd unrhyw beth sy'n cynnwys aspirin gyda'r feddyginiaeth hon
To be used on *preparations containing sulfinpyrazone* whose activity is reduced by aspirin.

Label 12 should not be used for anticoagulants since label 10 is more appropriate.

13 **Dissolve or mix with water before taking**
Gadewch i doddi mewn dŵr cyn ei gymryd
To be used on *preparations that are intended to be dissolved in water* (e.g. soluble tablets) or *mixed with water* (e.g. powders, granules) before use. In a few cases other liquids such as fruit juice or milk may be used.

14 **This medicine may colour your urine. This is harmless**
Gall y feddyginiaeth hon liwio eich dŵr. Nid yw hyn yn arwydd o ddrwg
To be used on *preparations that may cause the patient's urine to turn an unusual colour*. These include triamterene (blue under some lights), levodopa (dark reddish), and rifampicin (red).

15 Caution: flammable. Keep your body away from fire or flames after you have put on the medicine

Rhybudd: Fflamadwy. Ar ôl rhoi'r feddyginiaeth ymlaen, cadwch yn glir o dân neu fflamau

To be used on *preparations containing sufficient flammable solvent to render them flammable if exposed to a naked flame.*

16 Dissolve the tablet under your tongue—do not swallow. Store the tablets in this bottle with the cap tightly closed. Get a new supply 8 weeks after opening

Rhowch y dabled i doddi dan eich tafod - peidiwch â'i lyncu. Cadwch y tabledi yn y botel yma gyda'r caead wedi'i gau yn dynn. Gofynnwch am dabledi newydd 8 wythnos ar ôl ei hagor

To be used on *glyceryl trinitrate tablets* to remind the patient not to transfer the tablets to plastic or less suitable containers.

17 Do not take more than... in 24 hours

Peidiwch â chymryd mwy na... mewn 24 awr

To be used on *preparations for the treatment of acute migraine* except those containing ergotamine, for which label 18 is used. The dose form should be specified, e.g. tablets or capsules.

It may also be used on preparations for which no dose has been specified by the prescriber.

18 Do not take more than... in 24 hours. Also, do not take more than... in any one week

Peidiwch â chymryd mwy na... mewn 24 awr. Hefyd, peidiwch â chymryd mwy na... mewn wythnos

To be used on preparations containing ergotamine. The dose form should be specified, e.g. tablets or suppositories.

19 Warning: This medicine makes you sleepy. If you still feel sleepy the next day, do not drive or use tools or machines. Do not drink alcohol

Rhybudd: Bydd y feddyginiaeth hon yn eich gwneud yn gysglyd. Os ydych yn dal i deimlo'n gysglyd drannoeth, peidiwch â gyrru, defnyddio offer llaw neu beiriannau. Peidiwch ag yfed alcohol

To be used on *preparations containing hypnotics (or some other drugs with sedative effects) prescribed to be taken at night.* On the rare occasions when hypnotics are prescribed for daytime administration (e.g. nitrazepam in epilepsy), this label would clearly not be appropriate. Also to be used as an *alternative to the label 2 wording* (the choice being at the discretion of the pharmacist) *for anxiolytics prescribed to be taken at night.*

It is hoped that this wording will convey adequately the problem of residual morning sedation after taking 'sleeping tablets'.

21 Take with or just after food, or a meal

Cymerwch gyda neu ar ôl bwyd

To be used on *preparations that are liable to cause gastric irritation, or those that are better absorbed with food.*

Patients should be advised that a *small amount of food is sufficient.*

22 Take 30 to 60 minutes before food

Cymerwch 30 i 60 munud cyn bwyd

To be used on some preparations *whose absorption is thereby improved.*

Most oral antibacterials require label 23 instead (see below).

23 Take this medicine when your stomach is empty. This means an hour before food or 2 hours after food

Cymerwch y feddyginiaeth hon ar stumog wag. Mae hyn yn golygu awr cyn, neu 2 awr ar ôl bwyd

To be used on *oral antibacterials whose absorption may be reduced by the presence of food and acid in the stomach.*

24 Suck or chew this medicine

Bydd angen cnoi neu sugno'r feddyginiaeth hon

To be used on *preparations that should be sucked or chewed.*

The pharmacist should use discretion as to which of these words is appropriate.

25 Swallow this medicine whole. Do not chew or crush

Llyncwch yn gyfan. Peidiwch â chnoi neu falu'n fân

To be used on *preparations that are enteric-coated or designed for modified-release.*

Also to be used on *preparations that taste very unpleasant or may damage the mouth* if not swallowed whole.

Patients should be advised (where relevant) that some modified-release preparations can be broken in half, but that the halved tablet should still be swallowed whole, and not chewed or crushed.

26 Dissolve this medicine under your tongue

Gadewch i'r feddyginiaeth hon doddi o dan y tafod

To be used on *preparations designed for sublingual use.* Patients should be advised to hold under the tongue and avoid swallowing until dissolved. The buccal mucosa between the gum and cheek is occasionally specified by the prescriber.

27 Take with a full glass of water

Cymerwch gyda llond gwydr o ddŵr

To be used on *preparations that should be well diluted* (e.g. chloral hydrate), *where a high fluid intake is required* (e.g. sulfonamides), or *where water is required to aid the action* (e.g. methylcellulose). The patient should be advised that 'a full glass' means at least 150 mL. In most cases fruit juice, tea, or coffee may be used.

28 Spread thinly on the affected skin only

Taenwch yn denau ar y croen sydd wedi'i effeithio yn unig

To be used on *external preparations* that should be applied sparingly (e.g. corticosteroids, dithranol).

29 Do not take more than 2 at any one time. Do not take more than 8 in 24 hours

Peidiwch â chymryd mwy na 2 ar unrhyw un adeg. Peidiwch â chymryd mwy nag 8 mewn 24 awr

To be used on containers of dispensed *solid dose preparations containing paracetamol for adults when the instruction on the label indicates that the dose can be taken on an 'as required' basis.* The dose form should be specified, e.g. tablets or capsules.

This label has been introduced because of the serious consequences of overdosage with paracetamol.

30 Contains paracetamol. Do not take anything else containing paracetamol while taking this medicine. Talk to a doctor at once if you take too much of this medicine, even if you feel well

Yn cynnwys paracetamol. Peidiwch â chymryd unrhyw beth arall sy'n cynnwys paracetamol tra'n cymryd y feddyginiaeth hon. Siaradwch gyda'ch meddyg ar unwaith os ydych yn cymryd gormod, hyd yn oed os ydych yn teimlo'n iawn

To be used on all containers of dispensed *preparations containing paracetamol.*

32 Contains aspirin. Do not take anything else containing aspirin while taking this medicine

Yn cynnwys aspirin. Peidiwch â chymryd unrhyw beth arall sy'n cynnwys aspirin tra'n cymryd y feddyginiaeth hon

To be used on containers of dispensed *preparations containing aspirin when the name on the label does not include the word 'aspirin'.*

A3

Cautionary and advisory labels | **Appendix 3**

Appendix 4
Wound management products and elasticated garments

CONTENTS

The correct dressing for wound management depends not only on the type of wound but also on the stage of the healing process. The principal stages of healing are: cleansing, removal of debris; granulation, vascularisation; epithelialisation. The ideal dressing for moist wound healing needs to ensure that the wound remains: moist with exudate, but not macerated; free of clinical infection and excessive slough; free of toxic chemicals, particles or fibres; at the optimum temperature for healing; undisturbed by the need for frequent changes; at the optimum pH value. As wound healing passes through its different stages, different types of dressings may be required to satisfy better one or other of these requirements. Under normal circumstances, a moist environment is a necessary part of the wound healing process; exudate provides a moist environment and promotes healing, but excessive exudate can cause maceration of the wound and surrounding healthy tissue. The volume and viscosity of exudate changes as the wound heals. There are certain circumstances where moist wound healing is not appropriate (e.g. gangrenous toes associated with vascular disease).

Advanced wound dressings are designed to control the environment for wound healing, for example to donate fluid (hydrogels), maintain hydration (hydrocolloids), or to absorb wound exudate (alginates, foams).

Practices such as the use of irritant cleansers and desloughing agents may be harmful and are largely obsolete; removal of debris and dressing remnants should need minimal irrigation with lukewarm sterile sodium chloride 0.9% solution or water.

Hydrogel, hydrocolloid, and medical grade honey dressings can be used to deslough wounds by promoting autolytic debridement; there is insufficient evidence to support any particular method of debridement for difficult-to-heal surgical wounds. Sterile larvae (maggots) are also available for biosurgical removal of wound debris.

There have been few clinical trials able to establish a clear advantage for any particular product. The choice between different dressings depends not only on the type and stage of the wound, but also on patient preference or tolerance, site of the wound, and cost. For further information, see Buyers' Guide: Advanced wound dressings (October 2008); NHS Purchasing and Supply Agency, Centre for Evidence-based Purchasing.

Prices quoted in Appendix 4 are basic NHS net prices; for further information see *Prices in the BNF* under How to use the BNF.

The table below gives suggestions for choices of primary dressing depending on the type of wound (a secondary dressing may be needed in some cases).

Basic wound contact dressings

Low adherence dressing

Low adherence dressings are used as interface layers under secondary absorbent dressings. Placed directly on the wound bed, non-absorbent, low adherence dressings are suitable for clean, granulating, lightly exuding wounds without necrosis, and protect the wound bed from direct contact with secondary dressings. Care must be taken to avoid granulation tissue growing into the weave of these dressings.

Wound contact material for different types of wounds

Wound PINK (epitheliasing)

Low Exudate	Moderate Exudate	
Low adherence p. 1368	Soft ploymer p. 1374	
Vapour-permeable film p. 1372	Foam, low absorbent p. 1377	
Soft polymer p. 1374	Alginate p. 1378	
Hydrocolloid p. 1375		

Wound RED (granulating)
Symptoms or signs of infection, see Wounds with signs of infection

Low Exudate	Moderate Exudate	Heavy Exudate
Low adherence p. 1368	Hydrocolloid-fibrous p. 1375	Foam with extra absorbency p. 1377
Soft polymer p. 1374	Foam p. 1377	Hydrocolloid-fibrous p. 1375
Hydrocolloid p. 1375	Alginate p. 1378	Alginate p. 1378
Foam, low absorbent p. 1377		

Wound YELLOW (Sloughy) (granulating)
Symptoms or signs of infection, see Wounds with signs of infection

Low Exudate	Moderate Exudate	Heavy Exudate
Hydrogel p. 1371	Hydrocolloid-fibrous p. 1375	Hydrocolloid-fibrous p. 1375
Hydrocolloid p. 1375	Alginate p. 1378	Alginate p. 1378
		Capillary-action p. 1379

Wound BLACK (Necrotic/ Eschar)
Consider mechanical debridement alongside autolytic debridement

Low Exudate	Moderate Exudate	Heavy Exudate
Hydrogel p. 1371	Hydrocolloid p. 1375	Seek advice from wound care specialist
Hydrocolloid p. 1375	Hydrocolloid-fibrous p. 1375	
	Foam p. 1377	

Wounds with signs of infection
Consider systemic antibacterials if appropriate; also consider odour-absorbent dressings. For malodourous wounds with slough or necrotic tissue, consider mechanical or autolytic debridement

Low Exudate	Moderate Exudate	Heavy Exudate
Low adherence with honey p. 1380	Hydrocolloid-fibrous with silver p. 1382	Hydrocolloid-fibrous with silver p. 1382
Low adherence with iodine p. 1380	Foam with silver p. 1381	Foam extra absorbent, with silver p. 1381
Low adherence with silver p. 1381	Alginate with silver p. 1381	Alginate with honey p. 1380
Hydrocolloid with silver p. 1382	Honey-topical p. 1380	Alginate with silver p. 1381
Honey-topical p. 1380	Cadexomer-iodine p. 1380	

Note In each section of this table the dressings are listed in order of increasing absorbency.
Some wound contact (primary) dressings require a secondary dressing

Tulle dressings are manufactured from cotton or viscose fibres which are impregnated with white or yellow soft paraffin to prevent the fibres from sticking, but this is only partly successful and it may be necessary to change the dressings frequently. The paraffin reduces absorbency of the dressing. Dressings with a reduced content (light loading) of soft paraffin are less liable to interfere with absorption; dressings with 'normal loading' (such as Jelonet®) have been used for skin graft transfer. Knitted viscose primary dressing is an alternative to tulle dressings for exuding wounds; it can be used as the initial layer of multi-layer compression bandaging in the treatment of venous leg ulcers.

Knitted polyester primary dressing
Atrauman
Non-adherent knitted polyester primary dressing impregnated with neutral triglycerides
Atrauman dressing (Paul Hartmann Ltd) 10cm × 20cm = £0.63, 20cm × 30cm = £1.74, 5cm × 5cm = £0.27, 7.5cm × 10cm = £0.28

Knitted viscose primary dressing
N-A Dressing
Warp knitted fabric manufactured from a bright viscose monofilament.
N-A dressing (Systagenix Wound Management Ltd) 19cm × 9.5cm = £0.67, 9.5cm × 9.5cm = £0.35
N-A Ultra
Warp knitted fabric manufactured from a bright viscose monofilament.

N-A Ultra dressing (Systagenix Wound Management Ltd) 19cm × 9.5cm = £0.63, 9.5cm × 9.5cm = £0.33
Profore
Warp knitted fabric manufactured from a bright viscose monofilament.
Profore (Smith & Nephew Healthcare Ltd) wound contact layer 14cm × 20cm = £0.32
Tricotex
Warp knitted fabric manufactured from a bright viscose monofilament.
Tricotex dressing (Smith & Nephew Healthcare Ltd) 9.5cm × 9.5cm = £0.34

Paraffin Gauze Dressing
Cuticell
(Tulle Gras). Fabric of leno weave, weft and warp threads of cotton and/or viscose yarn, impregnated with white or yellow soft paraffin; for light or normal loading
Cuticell (BSN medical Ltd) Classic dressing 10cm × 10cm = £0.29
Jelonet
(Tulle Gras). Fabric of leno weave, weft and warp threads of cotton and/or viscose yarn, impregnated with white or yellow soft paraffin; for light or normal loading
Jelonet dressing (Smith & Nephew Healthcare Ltd) 10cm × 10cm = £0.41

A4

Wound management | Appendix 4

Neotulle

(Tulle Gras). Fabric of leno weave, weft and warp threads of cotton and/or viscose yarn, impregnated with white or yellow soft paraffin; for light or normal loading
Neotulle (Neomedic Ltd) dressing 10cm × 10cm = £0.29

Paragauze

(Tulle Gras). Fabric of leno weave, weft and warp threads of cotton and/or viscose yarn, impregnated with white or yellow soft paraffin; for light or normal loading
Paragauze (C D Medical Ltd) dressing 10cm × 10cm = £0.28

Paranet

(Tulle Gras). Fabric of leno weave, weft and warp threads of cotton and/or viscose yarn, impregnated with white or yellow soft paraffin; for light or normal loading
Paranet (Synergy Health Plc) dressing 10cm × 10cm = £0.25

Absorbent dressings

Perforated film absorbent dressings are suitable only for wounds with mild to moderate amounts of exudate; they are not appropriate for leg ulcers or for other lesions that produce large quantities of viscous exudate. Dressings with an absorbent cellulose or polymer wadding layer are suitable for use on moderately to heavily exuding wounds.

Absorbent cellulose dressing
CelluDress

Absorbent Cellulose Dressing with Fluid Repellent Backing
CelluDress dressing (Medicareplus International Ltd) 10cm × 10cm = £0.19, 10cm × 15cm = £0.20, 10cm × 20cm = £0.22, 15cm × 20cm = £0.30, 20cm × 25cm = £0.40, 20cm × 30cm = £0.85

Eclypse

Absorbent Cellulose Dressing with Fluid Repellent Backing
Eclypse (Advancis Medical) Boot dressing 60cm × 70cm = £13.78, dressing 15cm × 15cm = £0.97, 20cm × 30cm = £2.14, 60cm × 40cm = £8.15,

Exu-Dry

Absorbent Cellulose Dressing with Fluid Repellent Backing
Exu-Dry dressing (Smith & Nephew Healthcare Ltd) 10cm × 15cm = £1.13, 15cm × 23cm = £2.30, 23cm × 38cm = £5.34

Mesorb

Cellulose wadding pad with gauze wound contact layer and non-woven repellent backing
Mesorb dressing (Molnlycke Health Care Ltd) 10cm × 10cm = £0.62, 10cm × 15cm = £0.81, 10cm × 20cm = £1.00, 15cm × 20cm = £1.43, 20cm × 25cm = £2.25, 20cm × 30cm = £2.55

Telfa Max

Absorbent Cellulose Dressing with Fluid Repellent Backing

Zetuvit E

Absorbent Cellulose Dressing with Fluid Repellent Backing; sterile or non-sterile
Zetuvit E (Paul Hartmann Ltd) non-sterile dressing 10cm × 10cm = £0.07, 10cm × 20cm = £0.09, 20cm × 20cm = £0.14, 20cm × 40cm = £0.28, sterile dressing 10cm × 10cm = £0.21, 10cm × 20cm = £0.25, 20cm × 20cm = £0.39, 20cm × 40cm = £1.11,

Absorbent perforated dressing
Adpore

Low-adherence primary dressing consisting of viscose and rayon absorbent pad with adhesive border.
Adpore dressing (Medicareplus International Ltd) 10cm × 10cm = £0.10, 10cm × 15cm = £0.16, 10cm × 20cm = £0.30, 10cm × 25cm = £0.34, 10cm × 30cm = £0.42, 10cm × 35cm = £0.50, 7cm × 8cm = £0.08

Cosmopore E

Low-adherence primary dressing consisting of viscose and rayon absorbent pad with adhesive border.
Cosmopor E dressing (Paul Hartmann Ltd) 10cm × 20cm = £0.46, 10cm × 25cm = £0.56, 10cm × 35cm = £0.78, 5cm × 7.2cm = £0.08, 8cm × 15cm = £0.18, 8cm × 15cm = £0.28

Cutiplast Steril

Low-adherence primary dressing consisting of viscose and rayon absorbent pad with adhesive border.

Cutiplast Steril dressing (Smith & Nephew Healthcare Ltd) 10cm × 20cm = £0.31, 10cm × 25cm = £0.32, 10cm × 30cm = £0.42, 8cm × 10cm = £0.11, 8cm × 15cm = £0.24

Leukomed

Low-adherence primary dressing consisting of viscose and rayon absorbent pad with adhesive border.
Leukomed dressing (BSN medical Ltd) 10cm × 20cm = £0.43, 10cm × 25cm = £0.49, 10cm × 30cm = £0.63, 10cm × 35cm = £0.72, 5cm × 7.2cm = £0.09, 8cm × 10cm = £0.18, 8cm × 15cm = £0.32

Medipore + Pad

Low-adherence primary dressing consisting of viscose and rayon absorbent pad with adhesive border.
Medipore + Pads dressing (3M Health Care Ltd) 10cm × 10cm = £0.15, 10cm × 15cm = £0.25, 10cm × 20cm = £0.37, 10cm × 25cm = £0.46, 10cm × 35cm = £0.64, 5cm × 7.2cm = £0.07

Medisafe

Low-adherence primary dressing consisting of viscose and rayon absorbent pad with adhesive border.
Medisafe dressing (Neomedic Ltd) 6cm × 8cm = £0.08, 8cm × 10cm = £0.13, 8cm × 12cm = £0.23, 9cm × 15cm = £0.29, 9cm × 20cm = £0.34, 9cm × 25cm = £0.36

Mepore

Low-adherence primary dressing consisting of viscose and rayon absorbent pad with adhesive border.
Mepore dressing (Molnlycke Health Care Ltd) 10cm × 11cm = £0.22, 11cm × 15cm = £0.36, 7cm × 8cm = £0.11, 9cm × 20cm = £0.44, 9cm × 25cm = £0.61, 9cm × 30cm = £0.70, 9cm × 35cm = £0.76

PremierPore

Low-adherence primary dressing consisting of viscose and rayon absorbent pad with adhesive border.
PremierPore dressing (Shermond) 10cm × 10cm = £0.12, 10cm × 15cm = £0.18, 10cm × 20cm = £0.32, 10cm × 25cm = £0.36, 10cm × 30cm = £0.45, 10cm × 35cm = £0.52, 5cm × 7cm = £0.05

Primapore

Low-adherence primary dressing consisting of viscose and rayon absorbent pad with adhesive border.
Primapore dressing (Smith & Nephew Healthcare Ltd) 10cm × 20cm = £0.43, 10cm × 25cm = £0.50, 10cm × 30cm = £0.63, 10cm × 35cm = £0.96, 6cm × 8.3cm = £0.18, 8cm × 10cm = £0.19, 8cm × 15cm = £0.33

Softpore

Low-adherence primary dressing consisting of viscose and rayon absorbent pad with adhesive border.
Softpore dressing (Richardson Healthcare Ltd) 10cm × 10cm = £0.13, 10cm × 15cm = £0.20, 10cm × 20cm = £0.35, 10cm × 25cm = £0.40, 10cm × 30cm = £0.49, 10cm × 35cm = £0.58, 6cm × 7cm = £0.06

Sterifix

Low-adherence primary dressing consisting of viscose and rayon absorbent pad with adhesive border.

Telfa Island

Low-adherence primary dressing consisting of viscose and rayon absorbent pad with adhesive border.
Telfa Island dressing (Aria Medical Ltd) 10cm × 12.5cm = £0.27, 10cm × 20cm = £0.35, 10cm × 25.5cm = £0.45, 10cm × 35cm = £0.62, 5cm × 10cm = £0.08

Absorbent perforated plastic film faced dressing
Absopad

Low-adherence primary dressing consisting of 3 layers—perforated polyester film wound contact layer, absorbent cotton pad, and hydrophobic backing.
Absopad dressing (Medicareplus International Ltd) 10cm × 10cm = £0.13, 20cm × 10cm = £0.28

Askina Pad

Low-adherence primary dressing consisting of 3 layers—perforated polyester film wound contact layer, absorbent cotton pad, and hydrophobic backing.
Askina (B.Braun Medical Ltd) Pad dressing 10cm × 10cm = £0.21

Cutisorb LA

Low-adherence primary dressing consisting of 3 layers—perforated polyester film wound contact layer, absorbent cotton pad, and hydrophobic backing.

Interpose

Low-adherence primary dressing consisting of 3 layers—perforated polyester film wound contact layer, absorbent cotton pad, and hydrophobic backing.

Melolin

Low-adherence primary dressing consisting of 3 layers—perforated polyester film wound contact layer, absorbent cotton pad, and hydrophobic backing.

Melolin dressing (Smith & Nephew Healthcare Ltd) 10cm × 10cm = £0.27, 20cm × 10cm = £0.54, 5cm × 5cm = £0.17

Skintact

Low-adherence primary dressing consisting of 3 layers—perforated polyester film wound contact layer, absorbent cotton pad, and hydrophobic backing.

Skintact dressing (Robinson Healthcare) 10cm × 10cm = £0.17, 20cm × 10cm = £0.34, 5cm × 5cm = £0.10

Solvaline N

Low-adherence primary dressing consisting of 3 layers—perforated polyester film wound contact layer, absorbent cotton pad, and hydrophobic backing.

Solvaline N dressing (Lohmann & Rauscher (UK) Ltd) 10cm × 10cm = £0.18, 20cm × 10cm = £0.36, 5cm × 5cm = £0.10

Telfa

Low-adherence primary dressing consisting of 3 layers—perforated polyester film wound contact layer, absorbent cotton pad, and hydrophobic backing.

Telfa dressing (Aria Medical Ltd) 10cm × 7.5cm = £0.16, 15cm × 7.5cm = £0.18, 20cm × 7.5cm = £0.29, 7.5cm × 5cm = £0.12

Super absorbent cellulose and polymer primary dressing

Curea P1

Super absorbent cellulose and polymer primary dressing.

Curea P1 dressing (Charles S. Bullen Stomacare Ltd) 10cm × 10cm square = £2.15, 10cm × 20cm rectangular = £3.64, 10cm × 30cm rectangular = £5.20, 12cm × 12cm square = £2.65, 20cm × 20cm square = £6.89, 20cm × 30cm rectangular = £10.03, 7.5cm × 7.5cm square = £1.72

Curea P2

Super absorbent cellulose and polymer primary dressing (non-adherent)

Curea P2 dressing (Charles S. Bullen Stomacare Ltd) 10cm × 20cm rectangular = £4.49, 11cm × 11cm square = £2.47, 20cm × 20cm square = £7.82, 20cm × 30cm rectangular = £10.60

Cutisorb Ultra

Super absorbent cellulose and polymer primary dressing

Cutisorb Ultra dressing (BSN medical Ltd) 10cm × 10cm square = £2.13, 10cm × 20cm rectangular = £3.56, 20cm × 20cm square = £6.68, 20cm × 30cm rectangular = £10.06

DryMax Extra

Super absorbent cellulose and polymer primary dressing

DryMax Extra dressing (Aspen Medical Europe Ltd) 10cm × 10cm square = £0.87, 10cm × 20cm rectangular = £1.04, 20cm × 20cm square = £1.84, 20cm × 30cm rectangular = £2.33

ELECT Superabsorber

Super absorbent cellulose and polymer primary dressing

ELECT Superabsorber dressing (Smith & Nephew Healthcare Ltd) 10cm × 10cm square = £0.96, 10cm × 20cm rectangular = £1.13, 20cm × 20cm square = £2.01, 20cm × 30cm rectangular = £2.54

Zetuvit Plus

Super absorbent cellulose primary dressing

Zetuvit Plus dressing (Paul Hartmann Ltd) 10cm × 10cm = £0.64, 10cm × 20cm = £0.88, 15cm × 20cm = £1.01, 20cm × 25cm = £1.38, 20cm × 40cm = £2.13

Super absorbent hydroconductive dressing

Drawtex

Super absorbent hydroconductive dressing with absorbent, cross-action structures of viscose, polyester and cotton

Drawtex dressing (Martindale Pharmaceuticals Ltd) 10cm × 1.3m = £16.00, 10cm × 10cm = £2.24, 10cm × 1m = £16.00, 15cm × 20cm = £6.00, 20cm × 1m = £25.00, 20cm × 20cm = £6.98, 5cm × 5cm = £0.95, 7.5cm × 1m = £15.50, 7.5cm × 7.5cm = £1.77

Advanced wound dressings

Advanced wound dressings can be used for both acute and chronic wounds. Categories for dressings in this section start with the least absorptive, moisture-donating hydrogel dressings, followed by increasingly more absorptive dressings. These dressings are classified according to their primary component; some dressings are comprised of several components.

Hydrogel dressings

Hydrogel dressings are most commonly supplied as an amorphous, cohesive topical application that can take up the shape of a wound. A secondary, non-absorbent dressing is needed. These dressings are generally used to donate liquid to dry sloughy wounds and facilitate autolytic debridement of necrotic tissue; some also have the ability to absorb very small amounts of exudate. Hydrogel products that do not contain propylene glycol should be used if the wound is to be treated with larval therapy. Hydrogel sheets have a fixed structure and limited fluid-handling capacity; hydrogel sheet dressings are best avoided in the presence of infection, and are unsuitable for heavily exuding wounds.

Hydrogel application (amorphous)

ActivHeal Hydrogel

Hydrogel containing guar gum and propylene glycol

ActivHeal (Advanced Medical Solutions Ltd) Hydrogel dressing = £1.41

Aquaform

Hydrogel containing modified starch copolymer

AquaForm (Aspen Medical Europe Ltd) Hydrogel dressing = £2.02

Askina Gel

Hydrogel containing modified starch and glycerol

Askina (B.Braun Medical Ltd) Gel dressing = £2.01

Cutimed

Hydrogel

Cutimed (BSN medical Ltd) Gel dressing = £3.02

Flexigran

Hydrogel containing modified starch and glycerol

Flexigran (A1 Pharmaceuticals) Gel dressing = £1.90

GranuGel

Hydrogel containing carboxymethylcellulose, pectin and propylene glycol

GranuGEL (ConvaTec Ltd) Hydrocolloid Gel dressing = £2.33

Intrasite Gel

Hydrogel containing modified carmellose polymer and propylene glycol

IntraSite (Smith & Nephew Healthcare Ltd) Gel dressing = £3.59

Nu-Gel

Hydrogel containing alginate and propylene glycol

Nu-Gel (Systagenix Wound Management Ltd) dressing = £2.09

Purilon Gel

Hydrogel containing carboxymethylcellulose and calcium alginate

Purilon (Coloplast Ltd) Gel dressing = £2.27

Hydrogel sheet dressings

ActiFormCool

Hydrogel dressing

ActiFormCool sheet (Activa Healthcare Ltd) 10cm × 10cm square = £2.63, 10cm × 15cm rectangular = £3.79, 20cm × 20cm square = £7.93, 5cm × 6.5cm rectangular = £1.79

Aquaflo

Hydrogel dressing

Aquaflo (Covidien (UK) Commercial Ltd) sheet 7.5cm discs = £2.60

Coolie

Hydrogel dressing (without adhesive border)

Coolie (Zeroderma Ltd) sheet 7cm discs = £1.96

Gel FX
Hydrogel dressing (without adhesive border)
Gel FX sheet (Synergy Health Plc) 10cm × 10cm square = £1.60,
15cm × 15cm square = £3.20

Geliperm
Hydrogel sheets
Geliperm (Geistlich Sons Ltd) sheet 10cm × 10cm square = £2.53

Hydrosorb
Absorbent, transparent, hydrogel sheets containing
polyurethane polymers covered with a semi-permeable film
Hydrosorb sheet (Paul Hartmann Ltd) 10cm × 10cm square = £2.26,
20cm × 20cm square = £6.77, 5cm × 7.5cm rectangular = £1.58

Hydrosorb Comfort
Absorbent, transparent, hydrogel sheets containing
polyurethane polymers covered with a semi-permeable film
(with adhesive border, waterproof)
Hydrosorb Comfort sheet (Paul Hartmann Ltd) 12.5cm × 12.5cm
square = £3.61, 4.5cm × 6.5cm rectangular = £1.87, 7.5cm ×
10cm rectangular = £2.48

Intrasite Conformable
Soft non-woven dressing impregnated with Intrasite gel
IntraSite Conformable dressing (Smith & Nephew Healthcare Ltd) 10cm
× 10cm square = £1.80, 20cm rectangular = £2.44, 40cm
rectangular = £4.35

Novogel
Glycerol-based hydrogel sheets (standard or thin)
Novogel sheet (Ford Medical Associates Ltd) 10cm × 10cm square =
£3.18, 15cm × 20cm rectangular = £6.07, 20cm × 40cm
rectangular = £11.56, 30cm × 30cm (0.15cm thickness) square =
£12.71, (0.30cm thickness) square = £13.47, 5cm × 7.5cm
rectangular = £1.99, 7.5cm diameter circular = £2.89,

SanoSkin NET
Hydrogel sheet (without adhesive border)
SanoSkin (Ideal Medical Solutions Ltd) NET sheet 8.5cm × 12cm
rectangular = £2.28

Vacunet
Non-adherent, hydrogel coated polyester net dressing
Vacunet dressing (Protex Healthcare Ltd) 10cm square = £1.93, 10cm
× 15cm rectangular = £2.86

Sodium hyaluronate dressings
The hydrating properties of sodium hyaluronate promote
wound healing, and dressings can be applied directly to the
wound, or to a primary dressing (a secondary dressing should
also be applied). The iodine and potassium iodide in these
dressings prevent the bacterial decay of sodium hyaluronate
in the wound.
Hyiodine® should be used with caution in thyroid disorders.

Hyiodine
Sodium hyaluronate 1.5%, potassium iodide 0.15%, iodine
0.1%, in a viscous solution
Hyiodine (H & R Healthcare Ltd) dressing = £35.00

Vapour-permeable films and membranes
Vapour-permeable films and membranes allow the passage
of water vapour and oxygen but are impermeable to water
and micro-organisms, and are suitable for lightly exuding
wounds. They are highly conformable, provide protection,
and a moist healing environment; transparent film dressings
permit constant observation of the wound. Water vapour
loss can occur at a slower rate than exudate is generated, so
that fluid accumulates under the dressing, which can lead to
tissue maceration and to wrinkling at the adhesive contact
site (with risk of bacterial entry). Newer versions of these
dressings have increased moisture vapour permeability.
Despite these advances, vapour-permeable films and
membranes are unsuitable for infected, large heavily
exuding wounds, and chronic leg ulcers. Vapour-permeable
films and membranes are suitable for partial-thickness
wounds with minimal exudate, or wounds with eschar. Most
commonly, they are used as a secondary dressing over
alginates or hydrogels; film dressings can also be used to

protect the fragile skin of patients at risk of developing
minor skin damage caused by friction or pressure.

Non-woven fabric dressing with viscose-rayon pad.

Niko Fix
For intravenous and subcutaneous catheter sites
Niko (Unomedical Ltd) Fix dressing 7cm × 8.5cm = £0.19

*Vapour-permeable Adhesive Film Dressing (Semi-permeable
Adhesive Dressing)*
Extensible, waterproof, water vapour-permeable
polyurethane film coated with synthetic adhesive mass;
transparent. Supplied in single-use pieces.

Askina Derm
Extensible, waterproof, water vapour-permeable
polyurethane film coated with synthetic adhesive mass;
transparent. Supplied in single-use pieces
Askina Derm dressing (B.Braun Medical Ltd) 10cm × 12cm = £1.08,
10cm × 20cm = £2.06, 15cm × 20cm = £2.50, 20cm × 30cm =
£4.46, 6cm × 7cm = £0.37

C-View
Extensible, waterproof, water vapour-permeable
polyurethane film coated with synthetic adhesive mass;
transparent. Supplied in single-use pieces
C-View dressing (Aspen Medical Europe Ltd) 10cm × 12cm = £1.02,
12cm × 12cm = £1.09, 15cm × 20cm = £2.36, 6cm × 7cm = £0.38

Dressfilm
Extensible, waterproof, water vapour-permeable
polyurethane film coated with synthetic adhesive mass;
transparent. Supplied in single-use pieces
Dressfilm (St Georges Medical Ltd) dressing 15cm × 20cm = £1.90

Hydrofilm
Extensible, waterproof, water vapour-permeable
polyurethane film coated with synthetic adhesive mass;
transparent. Supplied in single-use pieces
Hydrofilm dressing (Paul Hartmann Ltd) 10cm × 12.5cm = £0.42,
10cm × 15cm = £0.53, 10cm × 25cm = £0.82, 12cm × 25cm =
£0.87, 15cm × 20cm = £0.97, 20cm × 30cm = £1.61, 6cm × 7cm
= £0.23

Hypafix Transparent
Extensible, waterproof, water vapour-permeable
polyurethane film coated with synthetic adhesive mass;
transparent. Supplied in single-use pieces
Hypafix Transparent (BSN medical Ltd) dressing 10cm × 2m = £8.79

Leukomed T
Extensible, waterproof, water vapour-permeable
polyurethane film coated with synthetic adhesive mass;
transparent. Supplied in single-use pieces
Leukomed T dressing (BSN medical Ltd) 10cm × 12.5cm = £1.02,
11cm × 14cm = £1.24, 15cm × 20cm = £2.37, 15cm × 25cm =
£2.53, 7.2cm × 5cm = £0.38, 8cm × 10cm = £0.70

Mepitel Film
Extensible, waterproof, water vapour-permeable
polyurethane film coated with synthetic adhesive mass;
transparent. Supplied in single-use pieces
Mepitel Film dressing (Molnlycke Health Care Ltd) 10.5cm × 12cm =
£1.31, 10.5cm × 25cm = £2.55, 15.5cm × 20cm = £3.24, 6.5cm ×
7cm = £0.49

Mepore Film
Extensible, waterproof, water vapour-permeable
polyurethane film coated with synthetic adhesive mass;
transparent. Supplied in single-use pieces
Mepore Film dressing (Molnlycke Health Care Ltd) 10cm × 12cm =
£1.23, 10cm × 25cm = £2.39, 15cm × 20cm = £3.04, 6cm × 7cm
= £0.46

OpSite Flexifix
Extensible, waterproof, water vapour-permeable
polyurethane film coated with synthetic adhesive mass;
transparent. Supplied in single-use pieces
OpSite Flexifix dressing (Smith & Nephew Healthcare Ltd) 10cm × 1m
= £6.60, 5cm × 1m = £3.91

OpSite Flexigrid

Extensible, waterproof, water vapour-permeable polyurethane film coated with synthetic adhesive mass; transparent. Supplied in single-use pieces

OpSite Flexigrid dressing (Smith & Nephew Healthcare Ltd) 12cm × 12cm = £1.13, 15cm × 20cm = £2.85, 6cm × 7cm = £0.40

Polyskin II

Extensible, waterproof, water vapour-permeable polyurethane film coated with synthetic adhesive mass; transparent. Supplied in single-use pieces

Kendall Film dressing (Aria Medical Ltd) 10cm × 12cm = £1.03, 10cm × 20cm = £2.04, 15cm × 20cm = £2.35, 20cm × 25cm = £4.11, 4cm × 4cm = £0.36, 5cm × 7cm = £0.40

ProtectFilm

Extensible, waterproof, water vapour-permeable polyurethane film coated with synthetic adhesive mass; transparent. Supplied in single-use pieces

ProtectFilm dressing (Wallace, Cameron & Company Ltd) 10cm × 12cm = £0.20, 15cm × 20cm = £0.40, 6cm × 7cm = £0.11

Suprasorb F

Extensible, waterproof, water vapour-permeable polyurethane film coated with synthetic adhesive mass; transparent. Supplied in single-use pieces

Suprasorb F dressing (Lohmann & Rauscher (UK) Ltd) 10cm × 12cm = £0.81, 15cm × 20cm = £2.52, 5cm × 7cm = £0.34

Tegaderm

Extensible, waterproof, water vapour-permeable polyurethane film coated with synthetic adhesive mass; transparent. Supplied in single-use pieces

Tegaderm Film dressing (3M Health Care Ltd) 12cm × 12cm = £1.11, 15cm × 20cm = £2.41, 6cm × 7cm = £0.39

Tegaderm diamond

Extensible, waterproof, water vapour-permeable polyurethane film coated with synthetic adhesive mass; transparent. Supplied in single-use pieces

Tegaderm Diamond dressing (3M Health Care Ltd) 10cm × 12cm = £1.21, 6cm × 7cm = £0.45

Vacuskin

Extensible, waterproof, water vapour-permeable polyurethane film coated with synthetic adhesive mass; transparent. Supplied in single-use pieces

Vellafilm

Extensible, waterproof, water vapour-permeable polyurethane film coated with synthetic adhesive mass; transparent. Supplied in single-use pieces

Vellafilm dressing (Advancis Medical) 12cm × 12cm = £1.10, 12cm × 35cm = £2.75, 15cm × 20cm = £2.10

Vapour-permeable Adhesive Film Dressing with absorbent pad
Adpore Ultra

Film dressing with absorbent pad

Adpore Ultra dressing (Medicareplus International Ltd) 10cm × 10cm = £0.14, 10cm × 15cm = £0.22, 10cm × 20cm = £0.33, 10cm × 25cm = £0.35, 10cm × 30cm = £0.52, 7cm × 8cm = £0.12

Vapour-permeable Adhesive Film Dressing with absorbent pad
Alldress

Film dressing with absorbent pad

Alldress dressing (Molnlycke Health Care Ltd) 10cm × 10cm = £0.96, 15cm × 15cm = £2.08, 15cm × 20cm = £2.57

C-View Post-Op

Film dressing with absorbent pad

C-View Post-Op dressing (Aspen Medical Europe Ltd) 10cm × 12cm = £1.10, 10cm × 25cm = £1.60, 10cm × 35cm = £2.60, 6cm × 7cm = £0.40

Clearpore

Film dressing with absorbent pad

Clearpore dressing (Richardson Healthcare Ltd) 10cm × 10cm = £0.20, 10cm × 15cm = £0.24, 10cm × 20cm = £0.36, 10cm × 25cm = £0.40, 10cm × 30cm = £0.65, 6cm × 10cm = £0.15, 6cm × 7cm = £0.12

Hydrofilm Plus

Film dressing with adsorbent pad

Hydrofilm Plus dressing (Paul Hartmann Ltd) 10cm × 20cm = £0.45, 10cm × 25cm = £0.60, 10cm × 30cm = £0.68, 7.2cm × 5cm = £0.18, 9cm × 10cm = £0.27, 9cm × 15cm = £0.30

Leukomed T Plus

Film dressing with adsorbent pad

Leukomed T plus dressing (BSN medical Ltd) 10cm × 20cm = £1.35, 10cm × 25cm = £1.51, 10cm × 30cm = £2.53, 10cm × 35cm = £3.07, 7.2cm × 5cm = £0.27, 8cm × 10cm = £0.54, 8cm × 15cm = £0.81

Mepore Film & Pad

Film dressing with adsorbent pad

Mepore Film & Pad dressing (Molnlycke Health Care Ltd) 4cm × 5cm = £0.24, 5cm × 7cm = £0.24, 9cm × 10cm = £0.62, 9cm × 15cm = £0.92, 9cm × 20cm = £1.36, 9cm × 25cm = £1.50, 9cm × 30cm = £2.01, 9cm × 35cm = £2.50

Mepore Ultra

Film dressing with adsorbent pad

Mepore Ultra dressing (Molnlycke Health Care Ltd) 10cm × 11cm = £0.79, 11cm × 15cm = £1.17, 7cm × 8cm = £0.40, 9cm × 20cm = £1.51, 9cm × 25cm = £1.67, 9cm × 30cm = £2.75

OpSite Plus

Film dressing with adsorbent pad

OpSite Plus dressing (Smith & Nephew Healthcare Ltd) 10cm × 12cm = £1.20, 10cm × 20cm = £2.02, 10cm × 35cm = £3.34, 6.5cm × 5cm = £0.32, 8.5cm × 9.5cm = £0.88

OpSite Post-op

Film dressing with adsorbent pad

OpSite Post-Op dressing (Smith & Nephew Healthcare Ltd) 10cm × 12cm = £1.18, 10cm × 20cm = £1.98, 10cm × 25cm = £2.49, 10cm × 30cm = £2.95, 10cm × 35cm = £3.28, 8.5cm × 15.5cm = £1.20, 8.5cm × 9.5cm = £0.87

Pharmapore-PU

Film dressing with adsorbent pad

Pharmapore-PU dressing (Wallace, Cameron & Company Ltd) 10cm × 25cm = £0.38, 10cm × 30cm = £0.58, 8.5cm × 15.5cm = £0.20

PremierPore VP

Film dressing with adsorbent pad

PremierPore VP dressing (Shermond) 10cm × 10cm = £0.16, 10cm × 15cm = £0.24, 10cm × 20cm = £0.36, 10cm × 25cm = £0.38, 10cm × 30cm = £0.57, 10cm × 35cm = £0.69, 5cm × 7cm = £0.13

Tegaderm

Film dressing with adsorbent pad

Tegaderm + Pad dressing (3M Health Care Ltd) 5cm × 7cm = £0.26, 9cm × 10cm = £0.65, 9cm × 15cm = £0.95, 9cm × 20cm = £1.40, 9cm × 25cm = £1.57, 9cm × 35cm = £2.60

Tegaderm Absorbent Clear

Film dressing with clear acrylic polymer oval-shaped pad or rectangular-shaped pad

Tegaderm Absorbent Clear Acrylic dressing (3M Health Care Ltd) 11.1cm × 12.7cm oval = £4.11, 14.2cm × 15.8cm oval = £5.78, 14.9cm × 15.2cm rectangular = £8.66, 16.8cm × 19cm sacral = £10.37, 20cm × 20.3cm rectangular = £13.91, 7.6cm × 9.5cm oval = £3.17

Vapour–permeable transparent film dressing with adhesive foam border.
Central Gard

For intravenous and subcutaneous catheter sites

Central Gard dressing (Unomedical Ltd) 16cm × 7cm = £0.95, 8.8cm = £1.04

EasI-V

For intravenous and subcutaneous catheter sites

EasI-V (ConvaTec Ltd) dressing 7cm × 7.5cm = £0.38

Vapour–permeable transparent, adhesive film dressing.
Hydrofilm I.V. Control

For intravenous and subcutaneous catheter sites

Hydrofilm (Paul Hartmann Ltd) I.V. Control dressing 7cm × 9cm = £0.31

Vapour–permeable, transparent, adhesive film dressing.
IV3000
For intravenous and subcutaneous catheter sites
IV3000 dressing (Smith & Nephew Healthcare Ltd) 10cm × 12cm = £1.40, 5cm × 6cm = £0.43, 6cm × 7cm = £0.56, 7cm × 9cm = £0.73, 9cm × 12cm = £1.45

Mepore IV
For intravenous and subcutaneous catheter sites
Mepore IV dressing (Molnlycke Health Care Ltd) 10cm × 11cm = £1.07, 5cm × 5.5cm = £0.31, 8cm × 9cm = £0.40

Pharmapore-PU IV
For intravenous and subcutaneous catheter sites
Pharmapore-PU-I.V dressing (Wallace, Cameron & Company Ltd) 6cm × 7cm = £0.08, 7cm × 8.5cm = £0.07, 7cm × 9cm = £0.17

Tegaderm IV
For intravenous and subcutaneous catheter sites
Tegaderm IV dressing with securing tapes (3M Health Care Ltd) 10cm × 15.5cm = £1.67, 7cm × 8.5cm = £0.59, 8.5cm × 10.5cm = £1.16

Soft polymer dressings
Dressings with soft polymer, often a soft silicone polymer, in a non-adherent or gently adherent layer are suitable for use on lightly to moderately exuding wounds. For moderately to heavily exuding wounds, an absorbent secondary dressing can be added, or a soft polymer dressing with an absorbent pad can be used. Wound contact dressings coated with soft silicone have gentle adhesive properties and can be used on fragile skin areas or where it is beneficial to reduce the frequency of primary dressing changes. Soft polymer dressings should not be used on heavily bleeding wounds; blood clots can cause the dressing to adhere to the wound surface. For silicone keloid dressings see p. 1383.

Cellulose dressings
Sorbion Sachet Border
Absorbent polymers in cellulose matrix, hypoallergenic polypropylene envelope, with adhesive border
Cutimed Sorbion Sachet Border dressing (BSN medical Ltd) 10cm × 10cm square = £2.95, 15cm × 15cm square = £4.49, 25cm × 15cm rectangular = £6.99

Sorbion Sachet EXTRA
Absorbent polymers in cellulose matrix, hypoallergenic polypropylene envelope
Cutimed Sorbion Sachet Extra dressing (BSN medical Ltd) 10cm × 10cm = £2.25, 20cm × 10cm = £3.73, 20cm × 20cm = £7.00, 30cm × 20cm = £9.99, 5cm × 5cm = £1.45, 7.5cm × 7.5cm = £1.78

Sorbion Sachet Multi Star
Absorbent polymers in cellulose matrix, hypoallergenic polypropylene envelope
Cutimed Sorbion Sachet Multi Star dressing (BSN medical Ltd) 14cm × 14cm = £4.89, 8cm × 8cm = £2.99

Sorbion Sachet S Drainage
Absorbent polymers in cellulose matrix, hypoallergenic polypropylene envelope ('v' shaped dressing)
Cutimed (BSN medical Ltd) Sorbion Sachet S drainage dressing 10cm × 10cm = £2.64

Suprasorb X
Biosynthetic cellulose fibre dressing
Suprasorb X dressing (Lohmann & Rauscher (UK) Ltd) 14cm × 20cm rectangular = £8.46, 2cm × 21cm rope = £6.58, 5cm × 5cm square = £2.05, 9cm × 9cm square = £4.27

With absorbant pad
Advazorb Border
Soft silicone wound contact dressing with polyurethane foam film backing and adhesive border
Advazorb Border dressing (Advancis Medical) 10cm × 10cm = £2.10, 10cm × 20cm = £2.90, 10cm × 30cm = £4.25, 12.5cm × 12.5cm = £2.58, 15cm × 15cm = £3.15, 20cm × 20cm = £5.46, 7.5cm × 7.5cm = £1.19

Advazorb Border Lite
Soft silicone wound contact dressing with polyurethane foam film backing and adhesive border

Advazorb Border Lite dressing (Advancis Medical) 10cm × 10cm = £1.89, 10cm × 20cm = £2.61, 10cm × 30cm = £3.83, 12.5cm × 12.5cm = £2.32, 15cm × 15cm = £2.84, 20cm × 20cm = £4.91, 7.5cm × 7.5cm = £1.07

Advazorb Silfix
Soft silicone wound contact dressing with polyurethane foam film backing
Advazorb Silfix dressing (Advancis Medical) 10cm × 10cm = £1.85, 10cm × 20cm = £3.18, 12.5cm × 12.5cm = £2.59, 15cm × 15cm = £3.36, 20cm × 20cm = £4.98, 7.5cm × 7.5cm = £0.99

Advazorb Silfix Lite
Soft silicone wound contact dressing with polyurethane foam film backing
Advazorb Silfix Lite dressing (Advancis Medical) 10cm × 10cm = £1.67, 10cm × 20cm = £2.86, 12.5cm × 12.5cm = £2.33, 15cm × 15cm = £3.02, 20cm × 20cm = £4.48, 7.5cm × 7.5cm = £0.89

Allevyn Gentle
Soft gel wound contact dressing, with polyurethane foam film backing
Allevyn Gentle dressing (Smith & Nephew Healthcare Ltd) 10cm × 10cm = £2.50, 10cm × 20cm = £4.02, 15cm × 15cm = £4.20, 20cm × 20cm = £6.71, 5cm × 5cm = £1.26

Allevyn Gentle Border
Silicone gel wound contact dressing, with polyurethane foam film backing
Allevyn Gentle Border (Smith & Nephew Healthcare Ltd) Heel dressing 23cm × 23.2cm = £9.64, dressing 10cm × 10cm = £2.19, 12.5cm × 12.5cm = £2.68, 17.5cm × 17.5cm = £5.29, 7.5cm × 7.5cm = £1.49,

Allevyn Gentle Border Lite
Silicone gel wound contact dressing, with polyurethane foam film backing
Allevyn Gentle Border Lite dressing (Smith & Nephew Healthcare Ltd) 10cm × 10cm = £2.16, 15cm × 15cm = £3.81, 5.5cm × 12cm = £1.85, 5cm × 5cm = £0.90, 8cm × 15cm = £3.43

Allevyn Life
Soft silicone wound contact dressing, with central mesh screen, polyurethane foam film backing and adhesive border
Allevyn Life dressing (Smith & Nephew Healthcare Ltd) 10.3cm × 10.3cm = £1.69, 12.9cm × 12.9cm = £2.48, 15.4cm × 15.4cm = £3.03, 21cm × 21cm = £5.97

Cutimed Siltec
Soft silicone wound contact dressing, with polyurethane foam film backing
Cutimed Siltec (BSN medical Ltd) Heel dressing 16cm × 24cm = £7.22, Sacrum dressing 17.5cm × 17.5cm = £4.60, 23cm × 23cm = £7.36, dressing 10cm × 10cm = £2.48, 10cm × 20cm = £4.10, 15cm × 15cm = £4.64, 20cm × 20cm = £7.03, 5cm × 6cm = £1.33,

Cutimed Siltec B
Soft silicone wound contact dressing, with polyurethane foam film backing, with adhesive border, for lightly to moderately exuding wounds
Cutimed Siltec B dressing (BSN medical Ltd) 12.5cm × 12.5cm = £3.27, 15cm × 15cm = £5.03, 17.5cm × 17.5cm = £5.29, 22.5cm × 22.5cm = £8.55, 7.5cm × 7.5cm = £1.54

Cutimed Siltec L
Soft silicone wound contact dressing, with polyurethane foam film backing, for lightly to moderately exuding wounds
Cutimed Siltec L dressing (BSN medical Ltd) 10cm × 10cm = £2.14, 15cm × 15cm = £3.52, 5cm × 6cm = £1.06

Eclypse Adherent
Soft silicone wound contact layer with absorbent pad and film backing
Eclypse Adherent dressing (Advancis Medical) 10cm × 10cm = £2.99, 10cm × 20cm = £3.75, 15cm × 15cm = £4.99, 20cm × 30cm = £9.99, 17cm × 19cm sacral = £3.76, 22cm × 23cm sacral = £6.23,

Flivasorb
Absorbent polymer dressing with non-adherent wound contact layer

Flivasorb dressing (Lohmann & Rauscher (UK) Ltd) 10cm × 10cm square = £0.88, 10cm × 20cm rectangular = £1.05, 20cm × 20cm square = £1.86, 20cm × 30cm rectangular = £2.35

Flivasorb Adhesive
Absorbent polymer dressing with non-adherent wound contact layer and adhesive border
Flivasorb Adhesive dressing (Lohmann & Rauscher (UK) Ltd) 12cm × 12cm square = £3.35, 15cm × 15cm square = £4.58

Mepilex
Absorbent soft silicone dressing with polyurethane foam film backing
Mepilex (Molnlycke Health Care Ltd) Heel dressing 13cm × 20cm = £5.41, 15cm × 22cm = £6.22, XT dressing 10cm × 11cm = £2.66, 11cm × 20cm = £4.39, 15cm × 16cm = £4.82, 20cm × 21cm = £7.28, dressing 5cm × 5cm = £1.21,

Mepilex Border
Absorbent soft silicone dressing with polyurethane foam film backing and adhesive border
Mepilex Border (Molnlycke Health Care Ltd) Heel dressing 18.5cm × 24cm = £6.63, Sacrum dressing 18cm × 18cm = £4.85, 23cm × 23cm = £7.91, dressing 10cm × 12.5cm = £2.72, 10cm × 20cm = £3.69, 10cm × 30cm = £5.55, 15cm × 17.5cm = £4.74, 17cm × 20cm = £6.07,

Mepilex Border Lite
Thin absorbent soft silicone dressing with polyurethane foam film backing and adhesive border
Mepilex Border Lite dressing (Molnlycke Health Care Ltd) 10cm × 10cm = £2.53, 15cm × 15cm = £4.13, 4cm × 5cm = £0.92, 5cm × 12.5cm = £2.01, 7.5cm × 7.5cm = £1.39

Mepilex Lite
Thin absorbent soft silicone dressing with polyurethane foam film backing
Mepilex Lite dressing (Molnlycke Health Care Ltd) 10cm × 10cm = £2.17, 15cm × 15cm = £4.22, 20cm × 50cm = £26.66, 6cm × 8.5cm = £1.82

Mepilex Transfer
Soft silicone exudate transfer dressing
Mepilex Transfer dressing (Molnlycke Health Care Ltd) 10cm × 12cm = £3.51, 15cm × 20cm = £10.64, 20cm × 50cm = £27.20, 7.5cm × 8.5cm = £2.23

Sorbion Sana
Non-adherent polyethylene wound contact dressing with absorbent core
Cutimed Sorbion Sana Gentle dressing (BSN medical Ltd) 12cm × 12cm = £2.49, 12cm × 22cm = £4.49, 22cm × 22cm = £7.99, 8.5cm × 8.5cm = £1.99

Urgotul Duo
Non-adherent soft polymer wound contact dressing with absorbent pad
UrgotulDuo dressing (Urgo Ltd) 10cm × 12cm = £3.83, 15cm × 20cm = £8.89, 5cm × 10cm = £2.48

Urgotul Duo Border
Non-adherent soft polymer wound contact dressing with absorbent pad and adhesive polyurethane film backing

Without absorbant pad
Adaptic Touch
Non-adherent soft silicone wound contact dressing
Adaptic Touch dressing (Systagenix Wound Management Ltd) 12.7cm × 15cm = £4.65, 20cm × 32cm = £12.50, 5cm × 7.6cm = £1.13, 7.6cm × 11cm = £2.25

Askina SilNet
Soft silicone-coated wound contact dressing
Askina SilNet dressing (B.Braun Medical Ltd) 10cm × 18cm = £4.98, 20cm × 30cm = £12.20, 5cm × 7.5cm = £1.13, 7.5cm × 10cm = £2.28

Mepitel
Soft silicone, semi-transparent wound contact dressing
Mepitel dressing (Molnlycke Health Care Ltd) 12cm × 15cm = £6.45, 5cm × 7cm = £1.59, 8cm × 10cm = £3.19

Mepitel One
Soft silicone, thin, transparent wound contact dressing
Mepitel One dressing (Molnlycke Health Care Ltd) 13cm × 15cm = £6.45, 24cm × 27.5cm = £17.38, 6cm × 7cm = £1.59, 9cm × 10cm = £3.19

Physiotulle
Non-adherent soft polymer wound contact dressing
Physiotulle dressing (Coloplast Ltd) 10cm × 10cm = £2.26, 5cm × 20cm = £6.89

Silflex
Soft silicone-coated polyester wound contact dressing
Silflex dressing (Advancis Medical) 12cm × 15cm = £4.58, 20cm × 30cm = £11.79, 35cm × 60cm = £39.54, 5cm × 7cm = £1.11, 8cm × 10cm = £2.27

Silon-TSR
Soft silicone polymer wound contact dressing
Silon-TSR dressing (Bio Med Sciences) 13cm × 13cm = £3.52, 13cm × 25cm = £5.47, 28cm × 30cm = £7.37

Sobion Contact
Non-adherent soft polymer wound contact dressing
Cutimed Sorbion Contact dressing (BSN medical Ltd) 10cm × 10cm = £1.99, 10cm × 20cm = £3.99, 20cm × 20cm = £6.99, 20cm × 30cm = £9.99, 7.5cm × 7.5cm = £1.49

Tegaderm Contact
Non-adherent soft polymer wound contact dressing
Tegaderm Contact dressing (3M Health Care Ltd) 20cm × 25cm = £10.86, 7.5cm × 10cm = £2.27

Urgotul
Non-adherent soft polymer wound contact dressing
Urgotul dressing (Urgo Ltd) 10cm × 10cm = £3.07, 10cm × 40cm = £10.33, 15cm × 15cm = £6.53, 15cm × 20cm = £8.70, 20cm × 30cm = £13.99, 5cm × 5cm = £1.54

Hydrocolloid dressings
Hydrocolloid dressings are usually presented as a hydrocolloid layer on a vapour-permeable film or foam pad. Semi-permeable to water vapour and oxygen, these dressings form a gel in the presence of exudate to facilitate rehydration in lightly to moderately exuding wounds and promote autolytic debridement of dry, sloughy, or necrotic wounds; they are also suitable for promoting granulation. Hydrocolloid-fibrous dressings made from modified carmellose fibres resemble alginate dressings; hydrocolloid-fibrous dressings are more absorptive and suitable for moderately to heavily exuding wounds.

Hydrocolloid-fibrous dressings
Aquacel
Soft non-woven pad containing hydrocolloid-fibres
Aquacel (ConvaTec Ltd) Ribbon dressing 1cm × 45cm = £1.84, 2cm × 45cm = £2.45, dressing 10cm × 10cm square = £2.42, 15cm × 15cm square = £4.55, 4cm × 10cm rectangular = £1.30, 4cm × 20cm rectangular = £1.92, 4cm × 30cm rectangular = £2.89, 5cm × 5cm square = £1.02,

Aquacel Foam
Soft non-woven pad containing hydrocolloid-fibres with foam layer; with or without adhesive border
Aquacel Foam dressing (ConvaTec Ltd) (adhesive) 10cm × 10cm = £2.14, 12.5cm × 12.5cm = £2.65, 17.5cm × 17.5cm = £5.30, 19.8cm × 14cm heel = £5.43, 20cm × 16.9cm sacral = £4.87, 21cm × 21cm = £7.76, 25cm × 30cm = £10.05, 8cm × 8cm = £1.39, (non-adhesive) 10cm × 10cm = £2.53, 15cm × 15cm = £4.25, 15cm × 20cm = £5.81, 20cm × 20cm = £6.94,

UrgoClean Pad
Pad, hydrocolloid fibres coated with soft-adherent lipo-colloidal wound contact layer
UrgoClean Pad dressing (Urgo Ltd) 10cm × 10cm square = £2.12, 20cm × 15cm rectangular = £3.98, 6cm × 6cm square = £0.95

UrgoClean Rope
Rope, non-woven rope containing hydrocolloid fibres
UrgoClean rope dressing (Urgo Ltd) 2.5cm × 40cm = £2.38, 5cm × 40cm = £3.15

A4

Wound management | Appendix 4

Polyurethane matrix dressing
Cutinova Hydro
Polyurethane matrix with absorbent particles and waterproof polyurethane film
Cutinova Hydro dressing (Smith & Nephew Healthcare Ltd) 10cm × 10cm square = £2.54, 15cm × 20cm rectangular = £5.38, 5cm × 6cm rectangular = £1.26

With adhesive border
Biatain Super
Semi-permeable hydrocolloid dressing; without adhesive border
Biatain Super dressing (adhesive) (Coloplast Ltd) 10cm × 10cm square = £2.18, 12.5cm × 12.5cm square = £3.60, 12cm × 20cm rectangular = £3.61, 15cm × 15cm square = £4.35, 20cm × 20cm square = £6.78

Granuflex Bordered
Hydrocolloid wound contact layer bonded to plastic foam layer, with outer semi-permeable polyurethane film
Granuflex Bordered dressing (ConvaTec Ltd) 10cm × 10cm square = £3.33, 10cm × 13cm triangular = £3.93, 15cm × 15cm square = £6.36, 15cm × 18cm triangular = £6.13, 6cm × 6cm square = £1.76

Hydrocoll Border
Hydrocolloid dressing with adhesive border and absorbent wound contact pad
Hydrocoll Border (bevelled edge) dressing (Paul Hartmann Ltd) 10cm × 10cm square = £2.43, 12cm × 18cm sacral = £3.64, 15cm × 15cm square = £4.57, 5cm × 5cm square = £1.01, 7.5cm × 7.5cm square = £1.67, 8cm × 12cm concave = £2.14

Tegaderm Hydrocolloid
Hydrocolloid dressing with adhesive border; normal or thin
Tegaderm Hydrocolloid (3M Health Care Ltd) Thin dressing 10cm × 12cm oval = £1.55, 13cm × 15cm oval = £2.89, dressing 10cm × 12cm oval = £2.33, 13cm × 15cm oval = £4.34, 17.1cm × 16.1cm sacral = £4.85,

Ultec Pro
Semi-permeable hydrocolloid dressing with adhesive border
Ultec Pro dressing (adhesive) (Covidien (UK) Commercial Ltd) 15cm × 18cm sacral = £3.30, 19.5cm × 23cm sacral = £4.98, 21cm × 21cm square = £4.67

Without adhesive border
ActivHeal Hydrocolloid
Semi-permeable polyurethane film backing, hydrocolloid wound contact layer, with or without polyurethane foam later
ActivHeal Hydrocolloid (Advanced Medical Solutions Ltd) dressing 10cm × 10cm square = £1.58, 15cm × 15cm square = £3.43, 15cm × 18cm sacral = £3.98, 5cm × 7.5cm rectangular = £0.78, foam backed dressing 10cm × 10cm square = £1.55, 15cm × 15cm square = £2.91, 15cm × 18cm sacral = £3.36, 5cm × 7.5cm rectangular = £0.97,

Askina Biofilm Transparent
Semi-permeable, polyurethane film dressing with hydrocolloid adhesive
Askina Biofilm Transparent dressing (B.Braun Medical Ltd) 10cm × 10cm square = £1.07, 20cm × 20cm square = £3.17

Biatain Super
Semi-permeable, hydrocolloid film dressing without adhesive border
Biatain Super dressing (non-adhesive) (Coloplast Ltd) 10cm × 10cm square = £2.18, 12.5cm × 12.5cm square = £3.60, 12cm × 20cm rectangular = £3.61, 15cm × 15cm square = £4.35, 20cm × 20cm square = £6.78

Comfeel Plus Contour
Hydrocolloid dressings containing carmellose sodium and calcium alginate
Comfeel Plus Contour dressing (Coloplast Ltd) 6cm × 8cm = £2.20, 9cm × 11cm = £3.83

Comfeel Plus Pressure Relieving
Hydrocolloid dressings containing carmellose sodium and calcium alginate

Comfeel Plus Pressure Relieving dressing (Coloplast Ltd) 10cm diameter circular = £4.61, 15cm diameter circular = £6.94, 7cm diameter circular = £3.44

Comfeel Plus Transparent
Hydrocolloid dressings containing carmellose sodium and calcium alginate
Comfeel Plus Transparent dressing (Coloplast Ltd) 10cm × 10cm square = £1.27, 15cm × 15cm square = £3.31, 15cm × 20cm rectangular = £3.36, 20cm × 20cm square = £3.38, 5cm × 15cm rectangular = £1.57, 5cm × 25cm rectangular = £2.56, 5cm × 7cm rectangular = £0.66, 9cm × 14cm rectangular = £2.42, 9cm × 25cm rectangular = £3.43

Comfeel Plus Ulcer
Hydrocolloid dressings containing carmellose sodium and calcium alginate
Comfeel Plus Ulcer (bevelled edge) dressing (Coloplast Ltd) 10cm × 10cm square = £2.43, 18cm × 20cm triangular = £5.67, 20cm × 20cm square = £7.51, 4cm × 6cm rectangular = £0.95

DuoDERM Extra Thin
Semi-permeable hydrocolloid dressing
DuoDERM Extra Thin dressing (ConvaTec Ltd) 10cm × 10cm square = £1.32, 15cm × 15cm square = £2.85, 5cm × 10cm rectangular = £0.76, 7.5cm × 7.5cm square = £0.80, 9cm × 15cm rectangular = £1.77, 9cm × 25cm rectangular = £2.82, 9cm × 35cm rectangular = £3.94

DuoDERM Signal
Semi-permeable hydrocolloid dressing with 'Time to change' indicator
DuoDERM Signal dressing (ConvaTec Ltd) 10cm × 10cm square = £2.12, 11cm × 19cm oval = £3.25, 14cm × 14cm square = £3.71, 18.5cm × 19.5cm heel = £5.19, 20cm × 20cm square = £7.38, 22.5cm × 20cm sacral = £6.07

Flexigran
Semi-permeable hydrocolloid dressing without adhesive border; normal or thin
Flexigran (A1 Pharmaceuticals) Thin dressing 10cm × 10cm square = £1.08, dressing 10cm × 10cm square = £2.19

Granuflex
Hydrocolloid wound contact layer bonded to plastic foam layer, with outer semi-permeable polyurethan film
Granuflex (modified) dressing (ConvaTec Ltd) 10cm × 10cm square = £2.80, 15cm × 15cm square = £5.30, 15cm × 20cm rectangular = £5.75, 20cm × 20cm square = £7.98

Hydrocoll Basic
Hydrocolloid dressing with absorbent wound contact pad
Hydrocoll (Paul Hartmann Ltd) Basic dressing 10cm × 10cm square = £2.47

Hydrocoll Thin Film
Thin hydrocolloid dressing with absorbent wound contact pad
Hydrocoll Thin Film dressing (Paul Hartmann Ltd) 10cm × 10cm square = £1.16, 15cm × 15cm square = £2.61, 7.5cm × 7.5cm square = £0.70

Nu-Derm
Semi-permeable hydrocolloid dressing (normal and thin)
Nu-Derm dressing (Systagenix Wound Management Ltd) 10cm × 10cm square = £1.56, 15cm × 15cm square = £3.18, 15cm × 18cm sacral = £4.45, 20cm × 20cm square = £6.36, 5cm × 5cm square = £0.85, 8cm × 12cm heel/elbow = £3.18, thin 10cm × 10cm square = £1.06

Tegaderm Hydrocolloid
Hydrocolloid dressing without adhesive border; normal and thin
Tegaderm Hydrocolloid (3M Health Care Ltd) Thin dressing 10cm × 10cm square = £1.55, dressing 10cm × 10cm square = £2.37

Ultec Pro
Semi-permeable hydrocolloid dressing; without adhesive border
Ultec Pro dressing (Covidien (UK) Commercial Ltd) 10cm × 10cm square = £2.28, 15cm × 15cm square = £4.44, 20cm × 20cm square = £6.69

Foam dressings

Dressings containing hydrophilic polyurethane foam (adhesive or non-adhesive), with or without plastic film-backing, are suitable for all types of exuding wounds, but not for dry wounds; some foam dressings have a moisture-sensitive film backing with variable permeability dependant on the level of exudate Foam dressings vary in their ability to absorb exudate; some are suitable only for lightly to moderately exuding wounds, others have greater fluid-handing capacity and are suitable for heavily exuding wounds. Saturated foam dressings can cause maceration of healthy skin if left in contact with the wound. Foam dressings can be used in combination with other primary wound contact dressings. If used under compression bandaging or compression garments, the fluid-handling capacity of the foam dressing may be reduced. Foam dressings can also be used to provide a protective cushion for fragile skin. A foam dressing containing ibuprofen is available and may be useful for treating painful exuding wounds.

Cavi-Care
Soft, conforming cavity wound dressing prepared by mixing thoroughly for 15 seconds immediately before use and allowing to expand its volume within the cavity

Polyurethane Foam Dressing
Cutimed Cavity
Cutimed Cavity dressing (BSN medical Ltd) 10cm × 10cm = £3.12, 15cm × 15cm = £4.68, 5cm × 6cm = £1.88

Kendall
Kendall Foam dressing (Aria Medical Ltd) 10cm × 10cm square = £1.06, 10cm × 20cm rectangular = £2.05, 12.5cm × 12.5cm square = £1.80, 15cm × 15cm square = £2.60, 20cm × 20cm square = £3.01, 5cm × 5cm square = £0.71, 7.5cm × 7.5cm square = £1.21, 8.5cm × 7.5cm rectangular (fenestrated) = £0.91

Polyurethane Foam Film Dressing with Adhesive Border
ActivHeal Foam Adhesive
ActivHeal Foam Adhesive dressing (Advanced Medical Solutions Ltd) 10cm × 10cm square = £1.63, 12.5cm × 12.5cm square = £1.68, 15cm × 15cm square = £2.15, 20cm × 20cm square = £4.50, 7.5cm × 7.5cm square = £1.18

Allevyn Adhesive
Allevyn Adhesive dressing (Smith & Nephew Healthcare Ltd) 10cm × 10cm square = £2.18, 12.5cm × 12.5cm square = £2.67, 12.5cm × 22.5cm rectangular = £4.16, 17.5cm × 17.5cm square = £5.27, 17cm × 17cm anatomically shaped sacral = £3.96, 22.5cm × 22.5cm square = £7.67, 22cm × 22cm anatomically shaped sacral = £5.70, 7.5cm × 7.5cm square = £1.49

Allevyn Plus Adhesive
Allevyn Plus Adhesive dressing (Smith & Nephew Healthcare Ltd) 12.5cm × 12.5cm square = £3.35, 12.5cm × 22.5cm rectangular = £5.94, 17.5cm × 17.5cm square = £6.47, 17cm × 17cm anatomically shaped sacral = £4.89, 22cm × 22cm anatomically shaped sacral = £7.07

Biatain Adhesive
Biatain Adhesive dressing (Coloplast Ltd) 10cm × 10cm square = £1.75, 12.5cm × 12.5cm square = £2.55, 17cm diameter contour = £4.96, 18cm × 18cm square = £5.16, 18cm × 28cm rectangular = £7.63, 19cm × 20cm heel = £5.16, 23cm × 23cm sacral = £4.41

Biatain Silicone

Kendall Island
Kendall Foam Island dressing (Aria Medical Ltd) 10cm × 10cm square = £1.54, 15cm × 15cm square = £2.90, 20cm × 20cm square = £5.46

PermaFoam
PermaFoam dressing (adhesive) (Paul Hartmann Ltd) 16.5cm × 18cm concave = £4.06, 18cm × 18cm sacral = £3.34, 22cm × 22cm sacral = £3.84

PermaFoam Comfort
PermaFoam Comfort dressing (Paul Hartmann Ltd) 10cm × 20cm rectangular = £3.38, 11cm × 11cm square = £2.14, 15cm × 15cm

square = £3.50, 20cm × 20cm square = £5.08, 8cm × 8cm square = £1.13

PolyMem
PolyMem dressing (Aspen Medical Europe Ltd) (adhesive) 10cm × 13cm rectangular = £2.18, 15cm × 15cm square = £2.93, 16.5cm × 20.9cm oval = £6.74, 18.4cm × 20cm sacral = £4.53, 5cm × 7.6cm oval = £1.15, 8.8cm × 12.7cm oval = £2.05,

PolyMem
PolyMem (Aspen Medical Europe Ltd) dressing (adhesive) 5cm × 5cm square = £0.52

Tegaderm Foam Adhesive
Tegaderm Foam dressing (adhesive) (3M Health Care Ltd) 10cm × 11cm oval = £2.39, 13.9cm × 13.9cm circular (heel) = £4.22, 14.3cm × 14.3cm square = £3.54, 14.3cm × 15.6cm oval = £4.24, 19cm × 22.2cm oval = £6.96, 6.9cm × 6.9cm soft cloth border = £1.71, 6.9cm × 7.6cm oval = £1.46

Tielle
Tielle (Systagenix Wound Management Ltd) Lite dressing 11cm × 11cm square = £2.28, dressing 15cm × 15cm square = £3.89, 15cm × 20cm rectangular = £4.87, 18cm × 18cm square = £4.95, 7cm × 9cm rectangular = £1.28,

Tielle Lite
Tielle Lite dressing (Systagenix Wound Management Ltd) 11cm × 11cm square = £2.28, 7cm × 9cm rectangular = £1.21, 8cm × 15cm rectangular = £2.81, 8cm × 20cm rectangular = £2.97

Tielle Plus
Tielle Plus dressing (Systagenix Wound Management Ltd) 11cm × 11cm square = £2.63, 15cm × 15cm sacrum = £3.13, square = £4.30, 15cm × 20cm rectangular = £5.39, 20cm × 26.5cm heel = £4.45,

Trufoam
Trufoam Border dressing (Aspen Medical Europe Ltd) 11cm × 11cm square = £1.70, 15cm × 15cm square = £2.23, 15cm × 20cm rectangular = £4.04, 7cm × 9cm rectangular = £1.16

Polyurethane Foam Film Dressing without Adhesive Border
ActivHeal Foam Non-Adhesive
ActivHeal Non-Adhesive Foam polyurethane dressing (Advanced Medical Solutions Ltd) 10cm × 10cm square = £1.13, 10cm × 20cm rectangular = £2.34, 20cm × 20cm square = £3.92, 5cm × 5cm square = £0.75

Advazorb
Advazorb (Advancis Medical) Heel dressing 17cm × 21cm = £4.75, dressing 10cm × 10cm square = £1.08, 10cm × 20cm rectangular = £3.35, 12.5cm × 12.5cm square = £1.59, 15cm × 15cm square = £2.10, 20cm × 20cm square = £3.75, 5cm × 5cm square = £0.65, 7.5cm × 7.5cm square = £0.78,

Advazorb Lite
Advazorb Lite dressing (Advancis Medical) 10cm × 10cm square = £0.97, 10cm × 20cm rectangular = £3.02, 12.5cm × 12.5cm square = £1.43, 15cm × 15cm square = £1.89, 20cm × 20cm square = £3.38, 7.5cm × 7.5cm square = £0.70

Allevyn Cavity, circular
Allevyn Cavity dressing (Smith & Nephew Healthcare Ltd) 10cm diameter circular = £10.04, 12cm × 4cm tubular = £7.19, 5cm diameter circular = £4.21, 9cm × 2.5cm tubular = £4.08

Allevyn Compression
Allevyn Compression dressing (Smith & Nephew Healthcare Ltd) 10cm × 10cm square = £2.58, 15cm × 15cm square = £4.37, 15cm × 20cm rectangular = £4.90, 5cm × 6cm rectangular = £1.25

Allevyn Lite
Allevyn Lite dressing (Smith & Nephew Healthcare Ltd) 10cm × 20cm rectangular = £3.51, 15cm × 20cm rectangular = £4.38, 5cm × 5cm square = £1.13

Allevyn Non-Adhesive
Allevyn dressing (non-adhesive) (Smith & Nephew Healthcare Ltd) 10.5cm × 13.5cm heel (cup shaped) = £5.11, 10cm × 10cm square = £2.49, 10cm × 20cm rectangular = £4.01, 20cm × 20cm square = £6.69, 5cm × 5cm square = £1.26

Allevyn Plus Cavity
Allevyn Plus Cavity dressing (Smith & Nephew Healthcare Ltd) 10cm × 10cm = £3.15, 15cm × 20cm = £6.31, 5cm × 6cm = £1.89

Askina Foam
Askina (B.Braun Medical Ltd) Foam Cavity dressing 2.4cm × 40cm = £2.44, Foam dressing 10cm × 10cm square = £2.19, 10cm × 20cm rectangular = £3.45, 20cm × 20cm square = £5.77, Heel dressing 12cm × 20cm = £4.68,

Biatain -Ibu Non-Adhesive
Biatain-Ibu Non-Adhesive dressing (Coloplast Ltd) 10cm × 12cm rectangular = £3.31, 10cm × 22.5cm rectangular = £5.20, 15cm × 15cm square = £5.20, 20cm × 20cm square = £8.85, 5cm × 7cm rectangular = £1.72

Biatain -Ibu Soft-Hold
Biatain-Ibu Soft-Hold dressing (Coloplast Ltd) 10cm × 12cm rectangular = £3.31, 10cm × 22.5cm rectangular = £5.20, 15cm × 15cm square = £5.20

Biatain Non-Adhesive
Biatain Non-Adhesive dressing (Coloplast Ltd) 10cm × 10cm square = £2.38, 10cm × 20cm rectangular = £3.92, 15cm × 15cm square = £4.38, 20cm × 20cm square = £6.50, 5cm × 7cm rectangular = £1.31

Biatain Soft-Hold
Biatain Soft-Hold dressing (Coloplast Ltd) 10cm × 10cm square = £2.59, 10cm × 20cm rectangular = £3.92, 15cm × 15cm square = £4.29, 5cm × 7cm rectangular = £1.31

Kendall Plus
Kendall Foam Plus dressing (Aria Medical Ltd) 10cm × 10cm square = £1.47, 10cm × 20cm rectangular = £2.69, 15cm × 15cm square = £3.38, 20cm × 20cm square = £4.04, 5cm × 5cm square = £0.82, 7.5cm × 7.5cm square = £1.42, 8.5cm × 7.5cm rectangular (fenestrated) = £1.24

Kerraheel
Kerraheel (Crawford Healthcare Ltd) dressing 12cm × 20cm heel = £4.65

Lyofoam Max
Lyofoam Max dressing (Molnlycke Health Care Ltd) 10cm × 10cm square = £1.14, 10cm × 20cm rectangular = £2.01, 15cm × 15cm square = £2.15, 15cm × 20cm rectangular = £2.71, 20cm × 20cm square = £3.99, 7.5cm × 8.5cm rectangular = £1.09

PermaFoam
PermaFoam (Paul Hartmann Ltd) Cavity dressing 10cm × 10cm = £2.03, dressing (non-adhesive) 10cm × 10cm square = £2.14, 10cm × 20cm rectangular = £3.67, 15cm × 15cm square = £4.06, 20cm × 20cm square = £6.20, 6cm diameter circular = £1.11, 8cm × 8cm square (fenestrated) = £1.26,

PolyMem
PolyMem dressing (Aspen Medical Europe Ltd) 7cm × 7cm tube = £1.72, 9cm × 9cm tube = £2.17, finger/toe size 1 = £2.50, 2 = £2.50, 3 = £2.50,

PolyMem
PolyMem dressing (non-adhesive) (Aspen Medical Europe Ltd) 10cm × 10cm square = £2.47, 10cm × 61cm rectangular = £13.10, 13cm × 13cm square = £4.12, 17cm × 19cm rectangular = £6.08, 20cm × 60cm rectangular = £30.90, 8cm × 8cm square = £1.59

PolyMem Max
PolyMem Max dressing (Aspen Medical Europe Ltd) 11cm × 11cm square = £2.97, 20cm × 20cm square = £11.68

PolyMem WIC
PolyMem (Aspen Medical Europe Ltd) WIC dressing 8cm × 8cm = £3.69

Tegaderm Foam
Tegaderm Foam dressing (3M Health Care Ltd) 10cm × 10cm square = £2.19, 10cm × 20cm rectangular = £3.71, 10cm × 60cm rectangular = £12.54, 20cm × 20cm square = £5.92, 8.8cm × 8.8cm square (fenestrated) = £2.23

Tielle Plus Borderless

Tielle Xtra
Tielle Xtra dressing 1 (Systagenix Wound Management Ltd) 1cm × 11cm square = £2.24, 5cm × 15cm square = £3.37, 5cm × 20cm rectangular = £5.51

Transorbent
Transorbent dressing (adhesive) (B.Braun Medical Ltd) 10cm × 10cm square = £1.98, 15cm × 15cm square = £3.65, 20cm × 20cm square = £5.83, 5cm × 7cm rectangular = £1.05

Trufoam NA
Trufoam Non Adhesive dressing (Aspen Medical Europe Ltd) 10cm × 10cm square = £1.34, 15cm × 15cm square = £2.63, 5cm × 5cm square = £0.71

UrgoCell TLC
UrgoTul Absorb dressing (Urgo Ltd) 10cm × 10cm = £2.68, 15cm × 20cm = £6.09, 6cm × 6cm = £1.85, 12cm × 19cm heel = £4.80,

Alginate dressings

Non-woven or fibrous, non-occlusive, alginate dressings, made from calcium alginate, or calcium sodium alginate, derived from brown seaweed, form a soft gel in contact with wound exudate. Alginate dressings are highly absorbent and suitable for use on exuding wounds, and for the promotion of autolytic debridement of debris in very moist wounds. Alginate dressings also act as a haemostatic, but caution is needed because blood clots can cause the dressing to adhere to the wound surface. Alginate dressings should not be used if bleeding is heavy and extreme caution is needed if used for tumours with friable tissue. Alginate sheets are suitable for use as a wound contact dressing for moderately to heavily exuding wounds and can be layered into deep wounds; alginate rope can be used in sinus and cavity wounds to improve absorption of exudate and prevent maceration. If the dressing does not have an adhesive border or integral adhesive plastic film backing, a secondary dressing will be required.

ActivHeal Alginate
Calcium sodium alginate dressing
ActivHeal Alginate dressing (Advanced Medical Solutions Ltd) 10cm × 10cm = £1.15, 10cm × 20cm = £2.83, 5cm × 5cm = £0.59

ActivHeal Aquafiber
Non-woven, calcium sodium alginate dressing
ActivHeal Aquafiber (Advanced Medical Solutions Ltd) Rope dressing 2cm × 42cm = £1.81, dressing 10cm × 10cm = £1.80, 15cm × 15cm = £3.40, 5cm × 5cm = £0.76,

Algisite M
Calcium alginate fibre, non-woven dressing
Algisite M (Smith & Nephew Healthcare Ltd) Rope dressing 2cm × 30cm = £3.47, dressing 10cm × 10cm = £1.91, 15cm × 20cm = £5.14, 5cm × 5cm = £0.92,

Algosteril
Calcium alginate dressing
Algosteril (Smith & Nephew Healthcare Ltd) Rope dressing 2g = £3.79, dressing 10cm × 10cm = £2.10, 10cm × 20cm = £3.55, 5cm × 5cm = £0.92,

Biatain Alginate
Alginate and carboxymethylcellulose dressing, highly absorbent, gelling dressing
Biatain Alginate dressing (Coloplast Ltd) 10cm × 10cm = £2.31, 15cm × 15cm = £4.38, 44cm = £2.72, 5cm × 5cm = £0.97

Cutimed Alginate
Calcium sodium alginate dressing
Cutimed Alginate dressing (BSN medical Ltd) 10cm × 10cm = £1.56, 10cm × 20cm = £2.94, 5cm × 5cm = £0.75

Kaltostat
Calcium alginate fibre, non-woven
Kaltostat dressing (ConvaTec Ltd) 10cm × 20cm = £4.08, 15cm × 25cm = £7.01, 2g = £3.82, 5cm × 5cm = £0.95, 7.5cm × 12cm = £2.08

Kendall
Calcium alginate dressing
Kendall Calcium Alginate (Aria Medical Ltd) Rope dressing 30cm = £2.89, 61cm = £5.07, 91cm = £5.46, dressing 10cm × 10cm = £1.52, 10cm × 14cm = £2.45, 10cm × 20cm = £2.98, 15cm × 25cm = £5.25, 30cm × 61cm = £27.56, 5cm × 5cm = £0.72,

Kendall Plus
Calcium alginate dressing
Kendall (Aria Medical Ltd) Foam Plus dressing 10cm × 10cm square = £1.47

Melgisorb
Calcium sodium alginate fibre, highly absorbent, gelling dressing, non-woven
Melgisorb (Molnlycke Health Care Ltd) Cavity dressing 2.2cm × 32cm = £3.55, dressing 10cm × 10cm = £1.88, 10cm × 20cm = £3.52, 5cm × 5cm = £0.90,

Sorbalgon
Calcium alginate dressing
Sorbalgon (Paul Hartmann Ltd) T dressing 2g = £3.51, dressing 10cm × 10cm = £1.72, 5cm × 5cm = £0.82,

Sorbsan Flat
Calcium alginate fibre, highly absorbent, flat non-woven pads
Sorbsan Flat dressing (Aspen Medical Europe Ltd) 10cm × 10cm = £1.71, 10cm × 20cm = £3.20, 5cm × 5cm = £0.81

Sorbsan Plus
Alginate dressing bonded to a secondary absorbent viscose pad
Sorbsan Plus dressing (Aspen Medical Europe Ltd) 10cm × 15cm = £3.10, 10cm × 20cm = £3.96, 15cm × 20cm = £5.49, 7.5cm × 10cm = £1.76

Sorbsan Ribbon
Alginate dressing bonded to a secondary absorbent viscose pad
Sorbsan (Aspen Medical Europe Ltd) Ribbon dressing 40cm = £2.04

Sorbsan Surgical Packing
Alginate dressing bonded to a secondary absorbent viscose pad
Sorbsan (Aspen Medical Europe Ltd) Packing dressing 2g = £3.47

Suprasorb A
Calcium alginate dressing
Suprasorb A (Lohmann & Rauscher (UK) Ltd) alginate dressing 10cm × 10cm = £1.23, 5cm × 5cm = £0.63, cavity dressing 2g = £2.28,

Tegaderm Alginate
Calcium alginate dressing
Tegaderm Alginate dressing (3M Health Care Ltd) 10cm × 10cm = £1.72, 2cm × 30.4cm = £2.87, 5cm × 5cm = £0.81

Urgosorb
Alginate and carboxymethylcellulose dressing without adhesive border
Urgosorb (Urgo Ltd) Pad dressing 10cm × 10cm = £2.11, 10cm × 20cm = £3.87, 5cm × 5cm = £0.88, Rope dressing 30cm = £2.76,

Capillary-acting dressings
Advadraw
Non-adherent dressing consisting of a soft viscose and polyester absorbent pad with central wicking layer between two perforated permeable wound contact layers
Advadraw dressing (Advancis Medical) 10cm × 10cm = £0.88, 10cm × 15cm = £1.19, 15cm × 20cm = £1.57, 5cm × 7.5cm = £0.57

Advadraw Spiral
Advadraw (Advancis Medical) Spiral dressing 0.5cm × 40cm = £0.82

Cerdak Aerocloth
Non-adhesive wound contact sachet containing ceramic spheres, with non-woven fabric adhesive backing
Cerdak Aerocloth dressing (Apollo Medical Products Ltd) 5cm × 10cm = £1.94, 5cm × 5cm = £1.37

Cerdak Aerofilm
Non-adhesive wound contact sachet containing ceramic spheres, with waterproof transparent adhesive film backing
Cerdak Aerofilm dressing (Apollo Medical Products Ltd) 5cm × 10cm = £2.07, 5cm × 5cm = £1.51

Cerdak Basic
Non-adhesive wound contact sachet containing ceramic spheres
Cerdak Basic dressing (Apollo Medical Products Ltd) 10cm × 10cm = £1.56, 10cm × 15cm = £2.08, 5cm × 5cm = £0.70

Sumar Lite
Sumar Lite dressing (Lantor (UK) Ltd) 10cm × 10cm = £1.59, 10cm × 15cm = £2.12, 5cm × 5cm = £0.93

Sumar Max
Sumar Max dressing (Lantor (UK) Ltd) 10cm × 10cm = £1.61, 10cm × 15cm = £2.15, 5cm × 5cm = £0.95

Sumar Spiral
Sumar (Lantor (UK) Ltd) Spiral dressing 0.5cm × 40cm = £1.57

Vacutex
Low-adherent dressing consisting of two external polyester wound contact layers with central wicking polyester/cotton mix absorbent layer
Vacutex dressing (Protex Healthcare (UK) Ltd) 10cm × 10cm = £1.66, 10cm × 15cm = £2.23, 10cm × 20cm = £2.68, 5cm × 5cm = £0.94

Odour absorbent dressings
Dressings containing activated charcoal are used to absorb odour from wounds. The underlying cause of wound odour should be identified. Wound odour is most effectively reduced by debridement of slough, reduction in bacterial levels, and frequent dressing changes. Fungating wounds and chronic infected wounds produce high volumes of exudate which can reduce the effectiveness of odour absorbent dressings. Many odour absorbent dressings are intended for use in combination with other dressings; odour absorbent dressings with a suitable wound contact layer can be used as a primary dressing.

Askina Carbosorb
Activated charcoal and non-woven viscose rayon dressing
Askina Carbosorb dressing (B.Braun Medical Ltd) 10cm × 10cm = £2.89, 10cm × 20cm = £5.58

CarboFLEX
Dressing in 5 layers: wound-facing absorbent layer containing alginate and hydrocolloid; water-resistant second layer; third layer containing activated charcoal; non-woven absorbent fourth layer; water-resistant backing layer
CarboFlex dressing (ConvaTec Ltd) 10cm × 10cm = £3.21, 15cm × 20cm = £7.30, 8cm × 15cm oval = £3.85,

Carbopad VC
Activated charcoal non-absorbent dressing
Carbopad VC dressing (Synergy Health Plc) 10cm × 10cm = £1.62, 10cm × 20cm = £2.19

CliniSorb Odour Control Dressings
Activated charcoal cloth enclosed in viscose rayon with outer polyamide coating
CliniSorb dressing (CliniMed Ltd) 10cm × 10cm = £1.89, 10cm × 20cm = £2.51, 15cm × 25cm = £4.05

Sorbsan Plus Carbon
Alginate dressing with activated carbon
Sorbsan Plus Carbon dressing (Aspen Medical Europe Ltd) 10cm × 15cm = £4.96, 10cm × 20cm = £5.94, 15cm × 20cm = £6.84, 7.5cm × 10cm = £2.56

Antimicrobial dressings
Spreading infection at the wound site requires treatment with systemic antibacterials. For local wound infection, a topical antimicrobial dressing can be used to reduce the level of bacteria at the wound surface but will not eliminate a spreading infection. Some dressings are designed to release the antimicrobial into the wound, others act upon the bacteria after absorption from the wound. The amount of exudate present and the level of infection should be taken into account when selecting an antimicrobial dressing. Medical grade honey, has antimicrobial and anti-inflammatory properties. Dressings impregnated with iodine below, can be used to treat clinically infected wounds. Dressings containing silver p. 1381, should be used only when clinical signs or symptoms of infection are present. Dressings containing other antimicrobials p. 1382 such as polihexanide (polyhexamethylene biguanide) or dialkylcarbamoyl chloride are available for use on infected wounds. Although hypersensitivity is unlikely with

chlorhexidine impregnated tulle dressing, the antibacterial efficacy of these dressings has not been established.

Honey

Medical grade honey has antimicrobial and anti-inflammatory properties and can be used for acute or chronic wounds. Medical grade honey has osmotic properties, producing an environment that promotes autolytic debridement; it can help control wound malodour. Honey dressings should not be used on patients with extreme sensitivity to honey, bee stings or bee products. Patients with diabetes should be monitored for changes in blood-glucose concentrations during treatment with topical honey or honey-impregnated dressings.

For *Activon Tulle*®, where no size is stated by the prescriber the 5 cm size is to be supplied.

Medihoney® *Antimicrobial Wound Gel* is not recommended for use in deep wounds or body cavities where removal of waxes may be difficult.

Honey-based topical application

Activon Honey
Medical grade manuka honey

L-Mesitran SOFT ointment dressing
Honey (medical grade) 40%
L-Mesitran (Aspen Medical Europe Ltd) SOFT ointment dressing = £3.59

MANUKApli Honey
Medical grade manuka honey
MANUKApli (Manuka Medical Ltd) dressing = £5.90

Medihoney Antibacterial Medical Honey
Medical grade, Leptospermum sp.
Medihoney (Derma Sciences Europe, Ltd) Antibacterial Medical Honey dressing = £9.90

Medihoney Antibacterial Wound Gel
Medical grade, Leptospermum sp. 80% in natural waxes and oils
Medihoney (Derma Sciences Europe, Ltd) Antibacterial Wound Gel dressing = £4.02

Melladerm Plus Honey
(Medical grade; Bulgarian, mountain flower) 45% in basis containing polyethylene glycol

Mesitran Oinment
Honey (medical grade) 47% Excipients include lanolin
Mesitran (Aspen Medical Europe Ltd) ointment dressing = £9.90

Sheet dressing

Actilite
Knitted viscose impregnated with medical grade manuka honey and manuka oil
Actilite gauze dressing (Advancis Medical) 10cm × 10cm = £0.98, 10cm × 20cm = £1.90, 5cm × 5cm = £0.57

Activon Tulle
Knitted viscose impregnated with medical grade manuka honey
Activon Tulle gauze dressing (Advancis Medical) 10cm × 10cm = £2.97, 5cm × 5cm = £1.80

Algivon
Absorbent, non-adherent calcium alginate dressing impregnated with medical grade manuka honey
Algivon dressing (Advancis Medical) 10cm × 10cm = £3.40, 5cm × 5cm = £1.98

Algivon Plus
Reinforced calcium alginate dressing impregnated with medical grade manuka honey
Algivon Plus (Advancis Medical) Ribbon dressing 2.5cm × 20cm = £3.36, dressing 10cm × 10cm = £3.36, 5cm × 5cm = £1.96,

L-Mesitran Border
Hydrogel, semi-permeable dressing impregnated with medical grade honey, with adhesive border
L-Mesitran (Aspen Medical Europe Ltd) Border sheet 10cm × 10cm square = £2.74

L-Mesitran Hydro
Hydrogel, semi-permeable dressing impregnated with medical grade honey, without adhesive border
L-Mesitran Hydro sheet (Aspen Medical Europe Ltd) 10cm × 10cm square = £2.63, 15cm × 20cm rectangular = £5.48

L-Mesitran Net
Hydrogel, non-adherent wound contact layer, without adhesive border
L-Mesitran (Aspen Medical Europe Ltd) Net sheet 10cm × 10cm square = £2.53

Medihoney Antibacterial Honey Apinate
Non-adherent calcium alginate dressing, impregnated with medical grade honey
Medihoney Antibacterial Honey Apinate (Derma Sciences Europe, Ltd) dressing 10cm × 10cm square = £3.40, 5cm × 5cm square = £2.00, rope dressing 1.9cm × 30cm = £4.20,

Medihoney Antibacterial Honey Tulle
Woven fabric impregnated with medical grade manuka honey
Medihoney (Derma Sciences Europe, Ltd) Tulle dressing 10cm x10cm = £2.98

Medihoney Gel sheet
Sodium alginate dressing impregnated with medical grade honey
Medihoney Gel Sheet dressing (Derma Sciences Europe, Ltd) 10cm × 10cm = £4.20, 5cm × 5cm = £1.75

MelMax
Acetate wound contact layer impregnated with buckwheat honey 75% in ointment basis
MelMax dressing (CliniMed Ltd) 5cm × 6cm rectangular = £4.82, 8cm × 10cm rectangular = £9.90, 8cm × 20cm rectangular = £19.79

Melladerm Plus Tulle
Knitted viscose impregnated with medical grade honey (Bulgarian, mountain flower) 45% in a basis containing polyethylene glycol
Melladerm (SanoMed Manufacturing BV) Plus Tulle dressing 10cm × 10cm = £2.10

Iodine

Cadexomer–iodine, like povidone–iodine, releases free iodine when exposed to wound exudate. The free iodine acts as an antiseptic on the wound surface, the cadexomer absorbs wound exudate and encourages de-sloughing. Two-component hydrogel dressings containing glucose oxidase and iodide ions generate a low level of free iodine in the presence of moisture and oxygen. Povidone–iodine fabric dressing is a knitted viscose dressing with povidone–iodine incorporated in a hydrophilic polyethylene glycol basis; this facilitates diffusion of the iodine into the wound and permits removal of the dressing by irrigation. The iodine has a wide spectrum of antimicrobial activity but it is rapidly deactivated by wound exudate. Systemic absorption of iodine may occur, particularly from large wounds or with prolonged use.

Iodoflex® and *Iodosorb*® are used for the treatment of chronic exuding wounds; max. single application 50 g, max. weekly application 150 g; max. duration up to 3 months in any single course of treatment. They are contra-indicated in patients receiving lithium, in thyroid disorders, in pregnancy and breast feeding, and in children; they should be used with caution in patients with severe renal impairment or history of thyroid disorder.

Iodozyme® is an antimicrobial dressing used for lightly to moderately exuding wounds. It is contra-indicated in thyroid disorders and in patients receiving lithium; it should be used with caution in children and in women who are pregnant or breast-feeding.

Oxyzyme® is used for non-infected, dry to moderately exuding wounds. It is contra-indicated in thyroid disorders and in patients receiving lithium; it should be used with caution in children and in women who are pregnant or breast-feeding.

Povidone-iodine Fabric Dressing is used as a wound contact layer for abrasions and superficial burns. It is contra-indicated in patients with severe renal impairment and in women who are pregnant or breast-feeding; it should be used with caution in patients with thyroid disease and in children under 6 months.

Iodoflex Paste

Iodine 0.9% as cadexomer–iodine in a paste basis with gauze backing

Iodosorb Ointment

Iodine 0.9% as cadexomer–iodine in an ointment basis
Iodosorb (Smith & Nephew Healthcare Ltd) ointment dressing = £9.12

Iodosorb Powder

Iodine 0.9% as cadexomer–iodine microbeads, 3-g sachet
Iodosorb (Smith & Nephew Healthcare Ltd) powder dressing sachets = £1.95

Iodozyme Hydrogel

Hydrogel (two-component dressing containing glucose oxidase and iodide ions)
Iodozyme dressing (Crawford Healthcare Ltd) 10cm × 10cm square = £12.62, 6.5cm × 5cm rectangular = £7.57

Oxyzyme Hydrogel

Hydrogel (two-component dressing containing glucose oxidase and iodide ions)
Oxyzyme dressing (Crawford Healthcare Ltd) 10cm × 10cm square = £10.10, 6.5cm × 5cm rectangular = £6.06

Povidone-iodine fabric dressing
Inadine

(Drug Tariff specification 43). Knitted viscose primary dressing impregnated with povidone–iodine ointment 10%
Inadine dressing (Systagenix Wound Management Ltd) 5cm × 5cm = £0.33, 9.5cm × 9.5cm = £0.49

Silver

Antimicrobial dressings containing silver should be used only when infection is suspected as a result of clinical signs or symptoms (see also notes above). Silver ions exert an antimicrobial effect in the presence of wound exudate; the volume of wound exudate as well as the presence of infection should be considered when selecting a silver-containing dressing. Silver-impregnated dressings should not be used routinely for the management of uncomplicated ulcers. It is recommended that these dressings should not be used on acute wounds as there is some evidence to suggest they delay wound healing. Dressings impregnated with silver sulfadiazine have broad antimicrobial activity; if silver sulfadiazine is applied to large areas, or used for prolonged periods, there is a risk of blood disorders and skin discoloration (see p. 1075). The use of silver sulfadiazine-impregnated dressings is contra-indicated in neonates, in pregnancy, and in patients with significant renal or hepatic impairment, sensitivity to sulfonamides, or G6PD deficiency. Large amounts of silver sulfadiazine applied topically may interact with other drugs—see Appendix 1 (sulfonamides).

Alginate dressings
Algisite Ag

Calcium alginate dressing, with silver
Algisite Ag dressing (Smith & Nephew Healthcare Ltd) 10cm × 10cm = £4.16, 10cm × 20cm = £7.65, 2g = £5.74, 5cm × 5cm = £1.66

Askina Calgitrol Ag

Calcium alginate and silver alginate dressing with polyurethane foam backing
Askina Calgitrol Ag dressing (B.Braun Medical Ltd) 10cm × 10cm square = £3.24, 15cm × 15cm square = £6.27, 20cm × 20cm square = £14.62

Askina Calgitrol Thin

Calcium alginate and silver alginate matrix, for use with absorptive secondary dressings

Askina Calgitrol Thin dressing (B.Braun Medical Ltd) 10cm × 10cm square = £4.08, 15cm × 15cm square = £9.16, 20cm × 20cm square = £16.18, 5cm × 5cm square = £1.97

Melgisorb Ag

Alginate and carboxymethylcellulose dressing, with ionic silver
Melgisorb Ag (Molnlycke Health Care Ltd) Cavity dressing 3cm × 44cm = £4.49, dressing 10cm × 10cm = £3.60, 15cm × 15cm = £7.63, 5cm × 5cm = £1.80,

Silvercel

Alginate and carboxymethylcellulose dressing impregnated with silver
Silvercel dressing (Systagenix Wound Management Ltd) 10cm × 20cm rectangular = £7.68, 11cm × 11cm square = £4.14, 2.5cm × 30.5cm rectangular = £4.45, 5cm × 5cm square = £1.68

Silvercel Non-adherent

Alginate and carboxymethylcellulose dressing with film wound contact layer, impregnated with silver
Silvercel Non-Adherent (Systagenix Wound Management Ltd) cavity dressing 2.5cm × 30.5cm = £3.94, dressing 10cm × 20cm rectangular = £7.25, 11cm × 11cm square = £3.89, 5cm × 5cm square = £1.62,

Sorbsan Silver Flat

Calcium alginate fibre, highly absorbent, flat non-woven pads, with silver
Sorbsan Silver Flat dressing (Aspen Medical Europe Ltd) 10cm × 10cm = £3.97, 10cm × 20cm = £7.26, 5cm × 5cm = £1.57

Sorbsan Silver Plus

Calcium alginate dressing with absorbent backing, with silver
Sorbsan Silver Plus dressing (Aspen Medical Europe Ltd) 10cm × 15cm = £5.56, 10cm × 20cm = £6.77, 15cm × 20cm = £9.08, 7.5cm × 10cm = £3.35

Sorbsan Silver Ribbon

With silver
Sorbsan (Aspen Medical Europe Ltd) Silver Ribbon dressing 1g = £4.15

Sorbsan Silver Surgical Packing

With silver
Sorbsan (Aspen Medical Europe Ltd) Silver Packing dressing 2g = £5.76

Suprasorb A + Ag

Calcium alginate dressing, with silver
Suprasorb A + Ag (Lohmann & Rauscher (UK) Ltd) dressing 10cm × 10cm = £4.11, 10cm × 20cm = £7.59, 5cm × 5cm = £1.63, rope dressing 2g = £6.08,

Tegaderm Alginate Ag

Calcium alginate and carboxymethylcellulose dressing, with silver
Tegaderm Alginate Ag dressing (3M Health Care Ltd) 10cm × 10cm = £3.24, 3cm × 30cm = £3.70, 5cm × 5cm = £1.39

Urgosorb Silver

Alginate and carboxymethylcellulose dressing, impregnated with silver
Urgosorb Silver (Urgo Ltd) Rope dressing 2.5cm × 30cm = £3.67, dressing 10cm × 10cm = £3.65, 10cm × 20cm = £6.88, 5cm × 5cm = £1.53,

Foam dressings
Acticoat Moisture Control

Three layer polyurethane dressing consisting of a silver coated layer, a foam layer, and a waterproof layer
Acticoat Moisture Control dressing (Smith & Nephew Healthcare Ltd) 10cm × 10cm square = £16.78, 10cm × 20cm rectangular = £32.70, 5cm × 5cm square = £7.18

Allevyn Ag

Silver sulfadiazine impregnated polyurethane foam film dressing with or without adhesive border
Allevyn Ag (Smith & Nephew Healthcare Ltd) Adhesive dressing 10cm × 10cm square = £5.50, 12.5cm × 12.5cm square = £7.23, 17.5cm × 17.5cm square = £13.90, 17cm × 17cm sacral = £10.85, 22cm × 22cm sacral = £14.54, 7.5cm × 7.5cm square = £3.49,

Heel Non-Adhesive dressing 10.5cm × 13.5cm = £10.76, Non-Adhesive dressing 10cm × 10cm square = £6.14, 15cm × 15cm square = £11.64, 20cm × 20cm square = £17.04, 5cm × 5cm square = £3.26,

Biatain Ag

Silver impregnated polyurethane foam film dressing, with or without adhesive border

Biatain Ag (Coloplast Ltd) cavity dressing 5cm × 8cm = £4.02, dressing 10cm × 10cm square = £8.08, 10cm × 20cm rectangular = £14.84, 12.5cm × 12.5cm square = £9.24, 15cm × 15cm square = £16.21, 18cm × 18cm square = £18.54, 19cm × 20cm heel = £18.28, 20cm × 20cm square = £22.87, 23cm × 23cm sacral = £19.43, 5cm × 7cm rectangular = £3.32,

PolyMem Silver

Silver impregnated polyurethane foam film dressing, with or without adhesive border

PolyMem Silver (Aspen Medical Europe Ltd) WIC dressing 8cm × 8cm = £7.05, dressing 10.8cm × 10.8cm square = £8.86, 12.7cm × 8.8cm oval = £5.60, 17cm × 19cm rectangular = £17.76, 5cm × 7.6cm oval = £2.27,

UrgoCell Silver

Non-adherent, polyurethane foam film dressing with silver in wound contact layer

UrgoCell Silver dressing (Urgo Ltd) 10cm × 10cm = £5.89, 15cm × 20cm = £10.79, 6cm × 6cm = £4.28

Hydrocolloid dressings
Aquacel Ag

Soft non-woven pad containing hydrocolloid fibres, (silver impregnated),

Aquacel Ag (ConvaTec Ltd) Ribbon dressing 1cm × 45cm = £3.08, 2cm × 45cm = £4.71, dressing 10cm × 10cm square = £4.69, 15cm × 15cm square = £8.82, 20cm × 30cm rectangular = £21.89, 4cm × 10cm rectangular = £2.85, 4cm × 20cm rectangular = £3.72, 4cm × 30cm rectangular = £5.57,

Physiotulle Ag

Non-adherent polyester fabric with hydrocolloid and silver sulfadiazine

Physiotulle (Coloplast Ltd) dressing 10cm × 10cm = £2.26

Low adherence dressing
Acticoat

Three-layer antimicrobial barrier dressing consisting of a polyester core between low adherent silver-coated high density polyethylene mesh (for 3-day wear)

Acticoat dressing (Smith & Nephew Healthcare Ltd) 10cm × 10cm square = £8.56, 10cm × 20cm rectangular = £13.39, 20cm × 40cm rectangular = £45.80, 5cm × 5cm square = £3.51

Acticoat 7

Five-layer antimicrobial barrier dressing consisting of a polyester core between low adherent silver-coated high density polyethylene mesh (for 7-day wear)

Acticoat 7 dressing (Smith & Nephew Healthcare Ltd) 10cm × 12.5cm rectangular = £18.15, 15cm × 15cm square = £32.63, 5cm × 5cm square = £6.09

Acticoat Flex 3

Conformable antimicrobial barrier dressing consisting of a polyester core between low adherent silver-coated high density polyethylene mesh (for 3-day wear)

Acticoat Flex 3 dressing (Smith & Nephew Healthcare Ltd) 10cm × 10cm square = £8.64, 10cm × 20cm rectangular = £13.50, 20cm × 40cm rectangular = £46.21, 5cm × 5cm square = £3.54

Acticoat Flex 7

Conformable antimicrobial barrier dressing consisting of a polyester core between low adherent silver-coated high density polyethylene mesh (for 7-day wear)

Acticoat Flex 7 dressing (Smith & Nephew Healthcare Ltd) 10cm × 12.5cm rectangular = £18.31, 15cm × 15cm square = £32.92, 5cm × 5cm square = £6.15

Atrauman Ag

Non-adherent polyamide fabric impregnated with silver and neutral triglycerides

Atrauman Ag dressing (Paul Hartmann Ltd) 10cm × 10cm = £1.26, 10cm × 20cm = £2.47, 5cm × 5cm = £0.52

Soft polymer dressings
Allevyn Ag Gentle

Soft polymer wound contact dressing, with silver sulfadiazine impregnated polyurethane foam layer, with or without adhesive border

Allevyn Ag Gentle (Smith & Nephew Healthcare Ltd) Border dressing 10cm × 10cm = £6.36, 12.5cm × 12.5cm = £8.18, 17.5cm × 17.5cm = £15.58, 7.5cm × 7.5cm = £4.23, dressing 10cm × 10cm = £6.18, 10cm × 20cm = £10.21, 15cm × 15cm = £11.49, 20cm × 20cm = £17.02, 5cm × 5cm = £3.31,

Mepilex Ag

Soft silicone wound contact dressing with polyurethane foam film backing, with silver, with or without adhesive border

Mepilex (Molnlycke Health Care Ltd) Ag dressing 10cm × 10cm = £6.12, 10cm × 20cm = £10.09, 15cm × 15cm = £11.36, 20cm × 20cm = £16.84, 20cm × 50cm = £63.20, Border Ag dressing 10cm × 12.5cm = £6.16, 10cm × 20cm = £8.97, 10cm × 30cm = £13.46, 15cm × 17.5cm = £11.31, 17cm × 20cm = £14.66, 7cm × 7.5cm = £3.41, Border Sacrum Ag dressing 18cm × 18cm = £11.83, 20cm × 20cm = £12.33, 23cm × 23cm = £18.89, Heel Ag dressing 13cm × 20cm = £12.78, 15cm × 22cm = £14.32,

Urgotul SSD

Non-adherent, soft polymer wound contact dressing, with silver sulfadiazine

Urgotul Silver

Non-adherent soft polymer wound contact dressing, with silver

Urgotul Silver dressing (Urgo Ltd) 10cm × 12cm = £3.54, 15cm × 20cm = £9.65

UrgotulDuo Silver

Non-adherent soft polymer wound contact dressing, with silver

With charcoal
Actisorb Silver 220

Knitted fabric of activated charcoal, with one-way stretch, with silver residues, within spun-bonded nylon sleeve

Actisorb Silver 220 dressing (Systagenix Wound Management Ltd) 10.5cm × 10.5cm = £2.58, 10.5cm × 19cm = £4.70, 6.5cm × 9.5cm = £1.64

Other antimicrobials
Cutimed Siltec Sorbact

Polyurethane foam dressing with acetate fabric coated with dialkylcarbamoyl chloride, with adhesive border

Cutimed Siltec Sorbact dressing (BSN medical Ltd) 12.5cm × 12.5cm = £6.44, 15cm × 15cm = £7.98, 17.5cm × 17.5cm = £11.17, 22.5cm × 22.5cm = £16.99, 7.5cm × 7.5cm = £2.51, 17.5cm × 17.5cm sacral = £8.07, 23cm × 23cm sacral = £12.14,

Cutimed Sorbact

Low adherence acetate tissue impregnated with dialkylcarbamoyl chloride; dressign pad, swabs, round swabs or ribbon gauze, cotton

Cutimed Sorbact (BSN medical Ltd) Ribbon dressing 2cm × 50cm = £4.03, 5cm × 200cm = £7.95, Round swab 3cm = £3.30, dressing pad 10cm × 10cm = £5.50, 10cm × 20cm = £8.58, 7cm × 9cm = £3.52, swab 4cm × 6cm = £1.65, 7cm × 9cm = £2.75,

Cutimed Sorbact Gel

Hydrogel dressing impregnated with dialkylcarbamoyl chloride

Cutimed Sorbact Gel dressing (BSN medical Ltd) 7.5cm × 15cm rectangular = £4.48, 7.5cm × 7.5cm square = £2.65

Cutimed Sorbact Hydroactive

Non-adhesive gel dressing with hydropolymer matrix and acetate fabric coated with dialkylcarbamoyl chloride

Cutimed Sorbact Hydroactive dressing (BSN medical Ltd) 14cm × 14cm = £5.37, 14cm × 24cm = £8.60, 19cm × 19cm = £10.10, 24cm × 24cm = £15.31, 7cm × 8.5cm = £3.68

Cutimed Sorbact Hydroactive B

Gel dressing with hydropolymer matrix and acetate fabric coated with dialkylcarbamoyl chloride, with adhesive border
Cutimed Sorbact Hydroactive B dressing (BSN medical Ltd) 10cm × 10cm = £7.08, 10cm × 20cm = £11.35, 15cm × 15cm = £13.34, 5cm × 6.5cm = £3.97

Flaminal Forte gel

Alginate with glucose oxidase and lactoperoxidase, for moderately to heavily exuding wounds
Flaminal Forte gel dressing (Flen Health UK Ltd) 15g = £7.68, 50g = £25.42

Flaminal Hydro gel

Alginate with glucose oxidase and lactoperoxidase, for lightly to moderately exuding wounds
Flaminal Hydro gel dressing (Flen Health UK Ltd) 15g = £7.68, 50g = £25.42

Kendall AMD

Foam dressing with polihexanide, without adhesive border
Kendall AMD Antimicrobial foam dressing (Aria Medical Ltd) 10cm × 10cm square = £4.71, 10cm × 20cm rectangular = £8.92, 15cm square = £8.92, 20cm × 20cm square = £13.07, 5cm × 5cm square = £2.50, 8.8cm × 7.5cm rectangular (fenestrated) = £4.23

Kendall AMD Plus

Foam dressing with polihexanide, without adhesive border
Kendall AMD Antimicrobial Plus foam dressing (Aria Medical Ltd) 10cm × 10cm square = £4.94, 8.8cm × 7.5cm rectangular (fenestrated) = £4.43

Octenilin Wound gel

Wound gel, hydroxyethylcellulose and propylene glycol, with octenidine hydrochloride
Octenilin Wound Gel dressing (Schulke & Mayr Ltd) 20mL = £4.78

Prontosan Wound Gel

Hydrogel containing betaine surfactant and polihexanide
Prontosan Wound Gel dressing (B.Braun Medical Ltd) 30mL = £6.38

Suprasorb X + PHMB

Biosynthetic cellulose fibre dressing with polihexanide
Suprasorb X + PHMB dressing (Lohmann & Rauscher (UK) Ltd) 14cm × 20cm rectangular = £11.64, 2cm × 21cm rope = £7.25, 5cm × 5cm square = £2.57, 9cm × 9cm square = £5.12

Telfa AMD

Low adherence absorbent perforated plastic film faced dressing with polihexanide
Telfa AMD dressing (Aria Medical Ltd) 10cm × 7.5cm = £0.18, 20cm × 7.5cm = £0.28

Telfa AMD Island

Low adherence dressing with adhesive border and absorbent pad, with polihexanide
Telfa AMD Island dressing (Aria Medical Ltd) 10cm × 12.5cm = £0.59, 10cm × 20cm = £0.86, 10cm × 25.5cm = £0.98, 10cm × 35cm = £1.22

Chlorhexidine gauze dressing
Bactigras

Fabric of leno weave, weft and warp threads of cotton and/or viscose yarn, impregnated with ointment containing chlorhexidine acetate
Bactigras gauze dressing (Smith & Nephew Healthcare Ltd) 10cm × 10cm = no price available, 5cm × 5cm = no price available

Irrigation fluids
Octenilin Wound irrigation solution

Aqueous solution containing glycerol, ethylhexylglycerin and octenidine hydrochloride
Octenilin irrigation solution (Schulke & Mayr Ltd) 350mL bottles = £4.60

Prontosan Wound Irrigation Solution

Aqueous solution containing betaine surfactant and polihexanide
Prontosan irrigation solution (B.Braun Medical Ltd) 350ml bottles = £4.78, 40ml unit dose = £14.18

Specialised dressings

Protease-modulating matrix dressings
Cadesorb Ointment

Cadesorb (Smith & Nephew Healthcare Ltd) ointment = £9.22

Catrix

Catrix dressing (Cranage Healthcare Ltd) sachets = £3.80

Promogran

Collagen and oxidised regenerated cellulose matrix, applied directly to wound and covered with suitable dressing
Promogran dressing (Systagenix Wound Management Ltd) 123 square cm = £15.62, 28 square cm = £5.19

Promogran Prisma Matrix

Collagen, silver and oxidised regenerated cellulose matrix, applied directly to wound and covered with suitable dressing
Promogran Prisma dressing (Systagenix Wound Management Ltd) 123 square cm = £17.98, 28 square cm = £6.31

UrgoStart

Soft adherent polymer matrix containing nano-oligosaccharide factor (NOSF), with polyurethane foam film backing
UrgoStart dressing (Urgo Ltd) 10cm × 10cm = £6.10, 15cm × 20cm = £10.96, 6cm × 6cm = £4.41, 12cm × 19cm heel = £8.40,

UrgoStart Contact

Non-adherent soft polymer wound contact dressing containing nano-oligosaccharide factor (NOSF)
UrgoStart (Urgo Ltd) Contact dressing 5cm × 7cm = £2.97

Silicone keloid dressings

Silicone gel and gel sheets are used to reduce or prevent hypertrophic and keloid scarring. They should not be used on open wounds. Application times should be increased gradually. Silicone sheets can be washed and reused.

Silicone gel
Bapscarcare

Silicone gel
Bapscarcare (BAP Medical UK Ltd) gel = £17.00

Ciltech

Silicone gel
Ciltech (Su-Med International (UK) Ltd) gel = £50.00

Dermatix

Silicone gel
Dermatix gel (Meda Pharmaceuticals Ltd) = £60.53

Kelo-cote UV

Silicone gel with SPF 30 UV protection
Kelo-cote (Sinclair IS Pharma Plc) UV gel = £17.88

Kelo-cote gel

Silicone gel
Kelo-cote (Sinclair IS Pharma Plc) gel = £51.00

Kelo-cote spray

Silicone spray
Kelo-cote (Sinclair IS Pharma Plc) spray = £51.00

NewGel+E

Silicone gel with vitamin E
NewGel+E (Advantech Surgical Ltd) gel = £17.70

ScarSil

Silicone gel
ScarSil (Jobskin Ltd) gel = £15.19

Silgel STC-SE

Silicone gel
Silgel (Nagor Ltd) STC-SE gel = £19.00

Silicone sheets
Advasil Conform

Self-adhesive silicone gel sheet with polyurethane film backing
Advasil Conform sheet (Advancis Medical) 10cm × 10cm square = £5.20, 15cm × 10cm rectangular = £9.17

Bapscarcare T

Self-adhesive silicone gel sheet

A4

Wound management | Appendix 4

Bapscarcare T sheet (BAP Medical UK Ltd) 10cm × 15cm rectangular = £9.00, 5cm × 30cm rectangular = £9.00, 5cm × 7cm rectangular = £3.15

Cica-Care

Soft, self-adhesive, semi-occlusive silicone gel sheet with backing

Cica-Care sheet (Smith & Nephew Healthcare Ltd) 15cm × 12cm rectangular = £28.52, 6cm × 12cm rectangular = £14.63

Ciltech

Silicone gel sheet

Ciltech sheet (Su-Med International (UK) Ltd) 10cm × 10cm square = £7.50, 10cm × 20cm rectangular = £12.50, 15cm × 15cm square = £14.00

Dermatix

Self-adhesive silicone gel sheet (clear- or fabric-backed)

Dermatix (Meda Pharmaceuticals Ltd) Clear sheet 13cm × 13cm square = £15.79, 13cm × 25cm rectangular = £28.53, 20cm × 30cm rectangular = £51.97, 4cm × 13cm rectangular = £6.88, Fabric sheet 13cm × 13cm square = £15.79, 13cm × 25cm rectangular = £28.53, 20cm × 30cm rectangular = £51.97, 4cm × 13cm rectangular = £6.88,

Mepiform

Self-adhesive silicone gel sheet with polyurethane film backing

Mepiform sheet (Molnlycke Health Care Ltd) 4cm × 31cm rectangular = £10.90, 5cm × 7cm rectangular = £3.45, 9cm × 18cm rectangular = £13.49

Scar FX

Self-adhesive, transparent, silicone gel sheet

Scar Fx sheet (Jobskin Ltd) 10cm × 20cm rectangular = £16.00, 22.5cm × 14.5cm shaped = £12.00, 25.5cm × 30.5cm rectangular = £60.00, 3.75cm × 22.5cm rectangular = £12.00, 7.5cm diameter shaped = £8.50

Silgel

Silicone gel sheet

Silgel sheet (Nagor Ltd) 10cm × 10cm square = £13.50, 10cm × 30cm rectangular = £31.50, 10cm × 5cm rectangular = £7.50, 15cm × 10cm rectangular = £19.50, 20cm × 20cm square = £40.00, 25cm × 15cm shaped = £21.12, 30cm × 5cm rectangular = £19.50, 40cm × 40cm square = £144.00, 46cm × 8.5cm shaped = £39.46, 5.5cm diameter shaped = £4.00

Adjunct dressings and appliances

Surgical absorbents

Surgical absorbents applied directly to the wound have many disadvantages—dehydration of and adherence to the wound, shedding of fibres, and the leakage of exudate ('strike through') with an associated risk of infection. Gauze and cotton absorbent dressings can be used as secondary layers in the management of heavily exuding wounds (but see also Capillary-action dressings, p. 1379). Absorbent cotton gauze fabric can be used for swabbing and cleaning skin. Ribbon gauze can be used post-operatively to pack wound cavities, but adherence to the wound bed will cause bleeding and tissue damage on removal of the dressing—an advanced wound dressing (e.g. hydrocolloid-fibrous p. 1375, foam p. 1377, or alginate p. 1378) layered into the cavity is often more suitable.

Cotton

Absorbent Cotton, BP

Carded cotton fibres of not less than 10 mm average staple length, available in rolls and balls

Absorbent (Robert Bailey & Son Plc) cotton BP 1988

Absorbent Cotton, Hospital Quality

As for absorbent cotton but lower quality materials, shorter staple length etc.

Absorbent (Robert Bailey & Son Plc) cotton hospital quality

Gauze and cotton tissue

Gamgee Tissue (blue)

Consists of absorbent cotton enclosed in absorbent cotton gauze type 12 or absorbent cotton and viscose gauze type 2

Gamgee (Robinson Healthcare) tissue blue label

Gamgee Tissue (pink)

Consists of absorbent cotton enclosed in absorbent cotton gauze type 12 or absorbent cotton and viscose gauze type 2

Gamgee (Robinson Healthcare) tissue pink label DT

Gauze and tissue

Absorbent Cotton Gauze, BP 1988

Cotton fabric of plain weave, in rolls and as swabs (see below), usually Type 13 light, sterile

Absorbent (Robert Bailey & Son Plc) cotton BP 1988

Alvita (Alliance Healthcare (Distribution) Ltd) absorbent cotton BP 1988

Clini (CliniSupplies Ltd) absorbent cotton BP 1988

Vernaid (Synergy Health Plc) absorbent cotton BP 1988

Absorbent Cotton and Viscose Ribbon Gauze, BP 1988

Woven fabric in ribbon form with fast selvedge edges, warp threads of cotton, weft threads of viscose or combined cotton and viscose yarn, sterile

Vernaid Fast Edge ribbon gauze sterile (Synergy Health Plc) 1.25cm, 2.5cm

Lint

Absorbent Lint, BPC

Cotton cloth of plain weave with nap raised on one side from warp yarns

Absorbent (Robinson Healthcare) lint

Alvita (Alliance Healthcare (Distribution) Ltd) absorbent lint BPC

Clini (CliniSupplies Ltd) absorbent lint BPC

Pads

Drisorb

Absorbent Dressing Pads, Sterile

Drisorb (Synergy Health Plc) dressing pad 10cm × 20cm = £0.17

PremierPad

Absorbent Dressing Pads, Sterile

PremierPad dressing pad (Shermond) 10cm × 20cm = £0.18, 20cm × 20cm = £0.25

XuPad

Absorbent Dressing Pads, Sterile

Xupad dressing pad (Richardson Healthcare Ltd) 10cm × 20cm = £0.17, 20cm × 20cm = £0.28, 20cm × 40cm = £0.40

Wound drainage pouches

Wound drainage pouches can be used in the management of wounds and fistulas with significant levels of exudate.

Biotrol Draina S

Wound drainage pouch

Biotrol Draina S wound drainage bag (B.Braun Medical Ltd) large (Transparent) = £95.45, medium (Transparent) = £77.61, mini (Transparent) = £77.84

Biotrol Draina S Vision

Wound drainage pouch

Draina S Vision (B.Braun Medical Ltd) 100 wound drainage bag = £123.94, 50 wound drainage bag = £101.11, 75 wound drainage bag = £106.82

Eakin Access window

For use with Eakin pouches

Eakin (Pelican Healthcare Ltd) access window = £37.74

Eakin Wound pouch, bung closure

Wound pouch, bung closure

Eakin wound drainage bag with bung closure (Pelican Healthcare Ltd) large = £102.45, medium = £75.49, small = £53.92, and access window for horizontal wounds, extra large = £102.45, for horizontal wounds, extra large = £91.66, for vertical incision wounds, extra large = £91.66, wounds, extra large = £91.66,

Eakin Wound pouch, fold and tuck closure

Wound pouch, fold and tuck closure

Eakin wound drainage bag with fold and tuck closure, (Pelican Healthcare Ltd) large = £91.66, medium = £70.10, small = £48.53, extra large = £80.88,

Option Wound Manager

Wound drainage bag

Option wound manager bag (Oakmed Ltd) large = £160.22, medium = £134.42, small = £131.50, square = £140.27, extra small = £118.23,

Option Wound Manager with access port
Wound drainage bag, with access port
Option wound manager bag with access port, (Oakmed Ltd) large = £171.27, medium = £140.27, small = £137.34, square = £146.11, extra small = £129.28,

Option Wound Manager, cut to fit
Wound drainage bag, cut to fit
Option wound manager bag (Oakmed Ltd) large = £84.23, medium = £80.42, small = £72.59

Welland Fistula bag
Wound drainage bag, cut-to-fit
Welland (Welland Medical Ltd) Fistula wound drainage bag = £82.07

Physical debridement pads
DebriSoft® is a pad that is used for the debridement of superficial wounds containing loose slough and debris, and for the removal of hyperkeratosis from the skin. DebriSoft® must be fully moistened with a wound cleansing solution before use and is not appropriate for use as a wound dressing.

DebriSoft Pad
Polyester fibres with bound edges and knitted outer surface coated with polyacrylate
DebriSoft (Lohmann & Rauscher (UK) Ltd) pad 10cm × 10cm = £6.45

Complex adjunct therapies

Topical negative pressure therapy
Accessories
Renasys
Soft port and connector
Renasys (Smith & Nephew Healthcare Ltd) Soft Port = £11.21, connector for use with soft port = £3.25

V.A.C.
Drape, gel for canister, Sensa T.R.A.C. Pad
SensaT.R.A.C. (KCI Medical Ltd) pad = £10.95
T.R.A.C. (KCI Medical Ltd) connector = £3.13
V.A.C. (KCI Medical Ltd) drape = £9.39, gel strips = £3.76

Venturi
Gel patches, adhesive, and connector
Venturi (Talley Group Ltd) adhesive gel patch = £15.00, connector = £15.00

WoundASSIST gel strip
WoundASSIST (Huntleigh Healthcare Ltd) TNP gel strip = £3.37

Vacuum assisted closure products
Exsu-Fast kit 1
Dressing Kit
Exsu-Fast (Synergy Health Plc) dressing kit 1 = £28.04

Exsu-Fast kit 2
Dressing Kit
Exsu-Fast (Synergy Health Plc) dressing kit 2 = £35.83

Exsu-Fast kit 3
Dressing Kit
Exsu-Fast (Synergy Health Plc) dressing kit 3 = £35.83

Exsu-Fast kit 4
Dressing Kit
Exsu-Fast (Synergy Health Plc) dressing kit 4 = £28.04

V.A.C GranuFoam
Polyurethane foam dressing (with adhesive drapes and pad connector); with or without silver
V.A.C. GranuFoam (KCI Medical Ltd) Bridge dressing kit = £32.04, Silver with SensaT.R.A.C dressing kit medium = £38.04, small = £32.79, dressing kit large = £31.70, medium = £27.32, small = £22.95,

V.A.C Simplace
Spiral-cut polyurethane foam dressings, vapour-permeable adhesive film dressings (with adhesive drapes and pad connector)

V.A.C. Simplace EX dressing kit (KCI Medical Ltd) medium = £30.58, small = £26.60

V.A.C WhiteFoam
Polyvinyl alcohol foam dressing or dressing kit
V.A.C. WhiteFoam dressing (KCI Medical Ltd) large = £17.04, small = £10.64, kit large = £33.54, small = £25.91,

Venturi
Wound sealing kit, flat drain; with or without channel drain
Venturi wound sealing kit with (Talley Group Ltd) channel drain = £15.00, flat drain, large = £17.50, standard = £15.00,

WoundASSIST
Wound pack and channel drain
WoundASSIST TNP dressing pack (Huntleigh Healthcare Ltd) medium/large = £23.85, small/medium = £20.81, channel drain medium/large = £23.85, small/medium = £20.81, extra large = £34.05,

Wound drainage collection devices
ActiV.A.C.
Canister with gel
ActiV.A.C (KCI Medical Ltd) canister with gel = £28.42

S-Canister
Canister kit
S-Canister (Smith & Nephew Healthcare Ltd) kit = £19.00

V.A.C Freedom
Canister with gel
V.A.C. (KCI Medical Ltd) Freedom Canister with gel = £28.85

Venturi
Canister kit with solidifier
Venturi (Talley Group Ltd) Compact canister kit = £12.50, canister kit = £12.50

WoundASSIST wound pack
Canister
WoundASSIST (Huntleigh Healthcare Ltd) TNP canister = £20.30

Wound care accessories

Dressing packs
The role of dressing packs is very limited. They are used to provide a clean or sterile working surface; some packs shown below include cotton wool balls, which are not recommended for use on wounds.

Multiple Pack Dressing No. 1
Contains absorbent cotton, absorbent cotton gauze type 13 light (sterile), open-wove bandages (banded)
Vernaid (Synergy Health Plc) multiple pack dressing

Non-drug tariff specification sterile dressing packs
Dressit
Vitrex gloves, large apron, disposable bag, paper towel, softswabs, adsorbent pad, sterile field
Dressit sterile dressing pack (Richardson Healthcare Ltd) with medium/large gloves = £0.60, small/medium gloves = £0.60

Nurse It
Contains latex-free, powder-free nitrile gloves, sterile laminated paper sheet, large apron, non-woven swabs, paper towel, disposable bag, compartmented tray, disposable forceps, paper measuring tape
Nurse It sterile dressing pack (Medicareplus International Ltd) with medium/large gloves = £0.55, small/medium gloves = £0.55

Polyfield Nitrile Patient Pack
Contains powder-free nitrile gloves, laminate sheet, non-woven swabs, towel, polythene disposable bag, apron
Polyfield Nitrile Patient Pack (Shermond) with large gloves = £0.52, medium gloves = £0.52, small gloves = £0.52

Sterile Dressing Pack with Non-Woven Pads
Vernaid
(Drug Tariff specification 35). Contains non-woven fabric covered dressing pad, non-woven fabric swabs, absorbent cotton wool balls, absorbent paper towel, water repellent inner wrapper
Vernaid (Synergy Health Plc) sterile dressing pack with non-woven pads

A4

Wound management | Appendix 4

Sterile dressing packs
Vernaid
(Drug Tariff specification 10). Contains gauze and cotton tissue pad, gauze swabs, absorbent cotton wool balls, absorbent paper towel, water repellent inner wrapper
Vernaid (Synergy Health Plc) sterile dressing pack

Woven and fabric swabs
Gauze Swab, PB 1988
Consists of absorbent cotton gauze type 13 light or absorbent cotton and viscose gauze type 1 folded into squares or rectangles of 8-ply with no cut edges exposed, sterile or non-sterile
Alvita gauze swab 8ply (Alliance Healthcare (Distribution) Ltd) non-sterile 10cm × 10cm, sterile 7.5cm × 7.5cm
CS (CliniSupplies Ltd) gauze swab 8ply non-sterile 10cm × 10cm
Clini gauze swab 8ply (CliniSupplies Ltd) non-sterile 10cm × 10cm, sterile 7.5cm × 7.5cm
Gauze (Robert Bailey & Son Plc) swab 8ply non-sterile 10cm × 10cm
MeCoBo gauze swab 8ply (MeCoBo Ltd) non-sterile 10cm × 10cm, sterile 7.5cm × 7.5cm
Propax gauze (BSN medical Ltd) swab 8ply sterile 7.5cm × 7.5cm
Sovereign (Waymade Healthcare Plc) gauze swab 8ply sterile 7.5cm × 7.5cm
Steraid (Robert Bailey & Son Plc) gauze swab 8ply sterile 7.5cm × 7.5cm
Vernaid gauze swab 8ply (Synergy Health Plc) non-sterile 10cm × 10cm, sterile 7.5cm × 7.5cm

Non-woven Fabric Swab
(Drug Tariff specification 28). Consists of non-woven fabric folded 4-ply; alternative to gauze swabs, type 13 light, sterile or non-sterile
CS (CliniSupplies Ltd) non-woven fabric swab 4ply non-sterile 10cm × 10cm
Clini non-woven fabric swab 4ply (CliniSupplies Ltd) non-sterile 10cm × 10cm, sterile 7.5cm × 7.5cm
CliniMed (CliniMed Ltd) non-woven fabric swab 4ply non-sterile 10cm × 10cm
MeCoBo (MeCoBo Ltd) non-woven fabric swab 4ply non-sterile 10cm × 10cm
Multisorb (BSN medical Ltd) non-woven fabric swab 4ply sterile 7.5cm × 7.5cm
Sofsorb non-woven fabric swab 4ply (Synergy Health Plc) non-sterile 10cm × 10cm, sterile 7.5cm × 7.5cm
Softswab non-woven fabric swab 4ply (Richardson Healthcare Ltd) non-sterile 10cm × 10cm, sterile 7.5cm × 7.5cm
Topper 8 non-woven fabric swab 4ply (Systagenix Wound Management Ltd) non-sterile 10cm × 10cm, sterile 7.5cm × 7.5cm

Filmated non-woven Fabric Swab
Regal
(Drug Tariff specification 29). Film of viscose fibres enclosed within non-woven viscose fabric folded 8-ply, non-sterile
Regal (Systagenix Wound Management Ltd) filmated swab 8ply 10cm × 10cm

Surgical adhesive tapes
Adhesive tapes are useful for retaining dressings on joints or awkward body parts. These tapes, particularly those containing rubber, can cause irritant and allergic reactions in susceptible patients; synthetic adhesives have been developed to overcome this problem, but they, too, may sometimes be associated with reactions. Synthetic adhesive, or silicon adhesive, tapes can be used for patients with skin reactions to plasters and strapping containing rubber, or undergoing prolonged treatment.
Adhesive tapes that are occlusive may cause skin maceration. Care is needed not to apply these tapes under tension, to avoid creating a tourniquet effect. If applied over joints they need to be orientated so that the area of maximum extensibility of the fabric is in the direction of movement of the limb.

Occlusive adhesive tapes
Blenderm
(Impermeable Plastic Adhesive Tape, BP 1988). Extensible water-impermeable plastic film spread with a polymericadhesive mass
Blenderm tape (3M Health Care Ltd) 2.5cm = £1.77, 5cm = £3.37

Sleek
(Impermeable Plastic Adhesive Tape, BP 1988). Extensible water-impermeable plastic film spread with an adhesive mass
Leukoplast Sleek tape (BSN medical Ltd) 2.5cm, 5cm, 7.5cm

Permeable adhesive tapes
3m Kind Removal Silicone Tape
Soft silicone, water-resistant, knitted fabric, polyurethane film adhesive tape
3M Kind removal tape (3M Health Care Ltd) 2.5cm = £3.58, 5cm = £6.48

Chemifix
(Permeable, Apertured Non-Woven Synthetic Adhesive Tape, BP 1988). Non-woven fabric with a polyacrylate adhesive
Chemifix tape (Medicareplus International Ltd) 10cm = £2.10, 2.5cm = £0.90, 5cm = £1.40

Chemipore
(Permeable Non-Woven Synthetic Adhesive Tape, BP 1988). Backing of paper-based or non-woven textile material spread with a polymeric adhesive mass
Chemipore tape (Medicareplus International Ltd) 1.25cm = £0.27, 2.5cm = £0.70, 5cm = £0.95

Clinipore
(Permeable Non-Woven Synthetic Adhesive Tape, BP 1988). Backing of paper-based or non-woven textile material spread with a polymeric adhesive mass
Clinipore tape (CliniSupplies Ltd) 1.25cm = £0.35, 2.5cm = £0.73, 5cm = £0.99

Elastoplast
(Elastic Adhesive Tape, BP 1988). Woven fabric, elastic in warp (crepe-twisted cotton threads), weft of cotton and/or viscose threads, spread with adhesive mass containing zinc oxide
Tensoplast (BSN medical Ltd) elastic adhesive tape 2.5cm

Hypafix
(Permeable, Apertured Non-Woven Synthetic Adhesive Tape, BP 1988). Non-woven fabric with a polyacrylate adhesive
Hypafix tape (BSN medical Ltd) 10cm = £4.67, 15cm = £6.92, 2.5cm = £1.69, 20cm = £9.18, 30cm = £13.27, 5cm = £2.68

Insil
Soft silicone, water-resistant, knitted fabric, polyurethane film adhesive tape
Insil tape (Insight Medical Products Ltd) 2cm = £5.77, 4cm = £5.77

Leukofix
(Permeable Non-Woven Synthetic Adhesive Tape, BP 1988). Backing of paper-based or non-woven textile material spread with a polymeric adhesive mass
Leukofix tape (BSN medical Ltd) 1.25cm = £0.55, 2.5cm = £0.90, 5cm = £1.57

Leukopor
(Permeable Non-Woven Synthetic Adhesive Tape, BP 1988). Backing of paper-based or non-woven textile material spread with a polymeric adhesive mass
Leukopor tape (BSN medical Ltd) 1.25cm = £0.49, 2.5cm = £0.77, 5cm = £1.35

Mediplast
(Permeable Non-Woven Synthetic Adhesive Tape, BP 1988). Backing of paper-based or non-woven textile material spread with a polymeric adhesive mass
Mediplast tape (Neomedic Ltd) 1.25cm = £0.30, 2.5cm = £0.50

Mediplast

Fabric, plain weave, warp and weft of cotton and /or viscose, spread with an adhesive containing zinc oxide

Mediplast Zinc Oxide plaster (Neomedic Ltd) 1.25cm = £0.82, 2.5cm = £1.19, 5cm = £1.99, 7.5cm = £2.99

Mefix

(Permeable, Apertured Non-Woven Synthetic Adhesive Tape, BP 1988). Non-woven fabric with a polyacrylate adhesive

Mefix tape (Molnlycke Health Care Ltd) 10cm = £2.90, 15cm = £3.95, 2.5cm = £1.03, 20cm = £5.07, 30cm = £7.27, 5cm = £1.81

Mepitac

Soft silicone, water-resistant, knitted fabric, polyurethane film adhesive tape

Mepitac tape (Molnlycke Health Care Ltd) 2cm = £6.96, 4cm = £6.96

Micropore

(Permeable Non-Woven Synthetic Adhesive Tape, BP 1988). Backing of paper-based or non-woven textile material spread with a polymeric adhesive mass

Micropore tape (3M Health Care Ltd) 1.25cm = £0.62, 2.5cm = £0.92, 5cm = £1.62

Omnifix

(Permeable, Apertured Non-Woven Synthetic Adhesive Tape, BP 1988). Non-woven fabric with a polyacrylate adhesive

Omnifix tape (Paul Hartmann Ltd) 10cm = £4.08, 15cm = £6.02, 5cm = £2.42

OpSite Flexifix Gentle

Soft silicone, water-resistant, knitted fabric, polyurethane film adhesive tape

OpSite Flexifix Gentle tape (Smith & Nephew Healthcare Ltd) 2.5cm = £10.30, 5cm = £19.31

Primafix

(Permeable, Apertured Non-Woven Synthetic Adhesive Tape, BP 1988). Non-woven fabric with a polyacrylate adhesive

Primafix tape (Smith & Nephew Healthcare Ltd) 10cm = £2.33, 15cm = £3.45, 20cm = £4.24, 5cm = £1.59

Scanpor

(Permeable Non-Woven Synthetic Adhesive Tape, BP 1988). Backing of paper-based or non-woven textile material spread with a polymeric adhesive mass

Scanpor tape (Bio-Diagnostics Ltd) 1.25cm = £0.55, 2.5cm = £0.92, 5cm = £1.75, 7.5cm = £2.56

Siltape

Soft silicone, water-resistant, knitted fabric, polyurethane film adhesive tape

Siltape (Advancis Medical) 2cm = £5.60, 4cm = £5.60

Strappal

Fabric, plain weave, warp and weft of cotton and /or viscose, spread with an adhesive containing zinc oxide

Strappal adhesive tape (BSN medical Ltd) 2.5cm = £1.39, 5cm = £2.34, 7.5cm = £3.53

Transpore

(Permeable Non-Woven Synthetic Adhesive Tape, BP 1988). Backing of paper-based or non-woven textile material spread with a polymeric adhesive mass

Transpore tape (3M Health Care Ltd) 2.5cm = £0.84, 5cm = £1.48

Zinc Oxide Adhesive Tape, BP 1988

Fabric, plain weave, warp and weft of cotton and /or viscose, spread with an adhesive containing zinc oxide

Fast Aid zinc oxide adhesive tape (Robinson Healthcare) 1.25cm, 2.5cm, 5cm, 7.5cm

Skin closure dressings

Skin closure strips are used as an alternative to sutures for minor cuts and lacerations. Skin tissue adhesive (section 13.10.5) can be used for closure of minor skin wounds and for additional suture support.

Skin closure strips, sterile

Leukostrip

Drug Tariff specifies that these are specifically for personal administration by the prescriber

Leukostrip (Smith & Nephew Healthcare Ltd) skin closure strips 6.4mm × 76mm = £6.31

Omnistrip

Drug Tariff specifies that these are specifically for personal administration by the prescriber

Omnistrip (Paul Hartmann Ltd) skin closure strips sterile 6mm × 76mm = £24.34

Steri-strip

Drug Tariff specifies that these are specifically for personal administration by the prescriber

Steri-strip (3M Health Care Ltd) skin closure strips 6mm × 75mm = £8.77

Bandages

Non-extensible bandages

Skin closure strips are used as an alternative to sutures for minor cuts and lacerations. Skin tissue adhesive (section 13.10.5) can be used for closure of minor skin wounds and for additional suture support.

Open-wove Bandage, Type 1 BP 1988

Cotton cloth, plain weave, warp of cotton, weft of cotton, viscose, or combination, one continuous length

Clini open wove bandage Type 1 BP 1988 (CliniSupplies Ltd) 10cm × 5m, 2.5cm × 5m, 5cm × 5m, 7.5cm × 5m

Vernaid white open wove bandage (Synergy Health Plc) 10cm × 5m, 2.5cm × 5m, 5cm × 5m, 7.5cm × 5m

White open wove bandage (Robert Bailey & Son Plc) 10cm × 5m, 2.5cm × 5m, 5cm × 5m, 7.5cm × 5m

Triangular Calico Bandage, BP 1980

Unbleached calico right-angled triangle

Clini (CliniSupplies Ltd) triangular calico bandage BP 1980 90cm × 127cm

Triangular (BSN medical Ltd) calico bandage 90cm × 127cm

Light-weight conforming bandages

Lightweight conforming bandages are used for dressing retention, with the aim of keeping the dressing close to the wound without inhibiting movement or restricting blood flow. The elasticity of conforming-stretch bandages (also termed contour bandages) is greater than that of cotton conforming bandages.

Acti-Wrap

Fabric, plain weave, warp of polyamide filament, weft of cotton or viscose, fast edges, one continuous length, 4 m stretched (all)

Acti-Wrap (cohesive/latex free) bandage (Activa Healthcare Ltd) 10cm × 4m = £0.80, 6cm × 4m = £0.46, 8cm × 4m = £0.68

Cotton Conforming Bandage, BP 1988

Cotton fabric, plain weave, treated to impart some elasticity to warp and weft

Easifix Crinx bandage (BSN medical Ltd) 10cm × 3.5m = £1.03, 15cm × 3.5m = £1.41, 5cm × 3.5m = £0.68, 7.5cm × 3.5m = £0.84

Easifix

Fabric, plain weave, warp of polyamide filament, weft of cotton or viscose, fast edges, one continuous length, 4 m stretched (all)

Easifix bandage (BSN medical Ltd) 10cm × 4m = £0.51, 15cm × 4m = £0.86, 5cm × 4m = £0.35, 7.5cm × 4m = £0.43

Easifix K

Fabric, knitted warp of polyamide filament, weft of cotton or viscose, fast edges, one continuous length. 4 m stretched

Easifix K bandage (BSN medical Ltd) 10cm × 4m = £0.18, 15cm × 4m = £0.32, 2.5cm × 4m = £0.10, 5cm × 4m = £0.11, 7.5cm × 4m = £0.16

Hospiform

Fabric, plain weave, warp of polyamide, weft of viscose

Hospiform bandage (Paul Hartmann Ltd) 10cm × 4m = £0.19, 12cm × 4m = £0.24, 6cm × 4m = £0.14, 8cm × 4m = £0.17

K-Band

Fabric, knitted warp of polyamide filament, weft of cotton or viscose, fast edges, one continuous length. 4 m stretched
K-Band bandage (Urgo Ltd) 10cm × 4m = £0.28, 15cm × 4m = £0.50, 5cm × 4m = £0.20, 7cm × 4m = £0.26

Knit Fix

Fabric, knitted warp of polyamide filament, weft of cotton or viscose, fast edges, one continuous length. 4 m stretched
Knit Fix bandage (Robert Bailey & Son Plc) 10cm × 4m = £0.17, 15cm × 4m = £0.33, 5cm × 4m = £0.12, 7cm × 4m = £0.17

Knit-Band

Fabric, knitted warp of polyamide filament, weft of cotton or viscose, fast edges, one continuous length. 4 m stretched
Knit-Band bandage (CliniSupplies Ltd) 10cm × 4m = £0.17, 15cm × 4m = £0.30, 5cm × 4m = £0.10, 7cm × 4m = £0.15

Kontour

Fabric, plain weave, warp of polyamide filament, weft of cotton or viscose, fast edges, one continuous length, 4 m stretched (all)
Kontour bandage (Easigrip Ltd) 10cm × 4m = £0.40, 15cm × 4m = £0.66, 5cm × 4m = £0.28, 7.5cm × 4m = £0.35

Mollelast

Fabric, plain weave, warp of polyamide filament, weft of cotton or viscose, fast edges, one continuous length, 4 m stretched (all)
Mollelast (Lohmann & Rauscher (UK) Ltd) bandage 4cm × 4m = £0.30

Peha-haft

Polyamide and Cellulose Contour Bandage, cohesive, latex-free
Peha-haft bandage (Paul Hartmann Ltd) 10cm × 4m = £0.77, 12cm × 4m = £0.91, 2.5cm × 4m = £0.74, 4cm × 4m = £0.48, 6cm × 4m = £0.56, 8cm × 4m = £0.67

PremierBand

Polyamide and Cellulose Contour Bandage
PremierBand bandage (Shermond) 10cm × 4m = £0.17, 15cm × 4m = £0.25, 5cm × 4m = £0.12, 7.5cm × 4m = £0.14

Slinky

Fabric, plain weave, warp of polyamide filament, weft of cotton or viscose, fast edges, one continuous length, 4 m stretched (all)
Slinky bandage (Molnlycke Health Care Ltd) 10cm × 4m = £0.71, 15cm × 4m = £1.03, 7.5cm × 4m = £0.59

Stayform

Fabric, plain weave, warp of polyamide filament, weft of cotton or viscose, fast edges, one continuous length, 4 m stretched (all)
Stayform bandage (Robinson Healthcare) 10cm × 4m = £0.40, 15cm × 4m = £0.68, 5cm × 4m = £0.29, 7.5cm × 4m = £0.36

Tubular bandages and garments

Tubular bandages are available in different forms, according to the function required of them. Some are used under orthopaedic casts and some are suitable for protecting areas to which creams or ointments (other than those containing potent corticosteroids) have been applied. The conformability of the elasticated versions makes them particularly suitable for retaining dressings on difficult parts of the body or for soft tissue injury, but their use as the only means of applying pressure to an oedematous limb or to a varicose ulcer is not appropriate, since the pressure they exert is inadequate. Compression hosiery reduces the recurrence of venous leg ulcers and should be considered for use after wound healing. Silk clothing is available as an alternative to elasticated viscose stockinette garments, for use in the management of severe eczema and allergic skin conditions.

Elasticated Surgical Tubular Stockinette, Foam padded is used for relief of pressure and elimination of friction in relevant area; porosity of foam lining allows normal water loss from skin surface.

For *Elasticated Tubular Bandage, BP* 1993, where no size stated by the prescriber, the 50 cm length should be supplied and width endorsed.

Non-elasticated Cotton Stockinette, Bleached, BP 1988 1m lengths is used as basis (with wadding) for Plaster of Paris bandages etc.; 6 m length, compression bandage.

For *Non-elasticated Ribbed Cotton and Viscose Surgical Tubular Stockinette, BP* 1988, the Drug Tariff specifies various combinations of sizes to provide sufficient material for part or full body coverage. It is used as protective dressings with tar-based and other steroid ointments.

Elasticated

Acti-Fast

(Drug Tariff specification 46). Lightweight plain-knitted elasticated tubular bandage
Acti-Fast 2-way stretch stockinette (Activa Healthcare Ltd) 10.75cm = £6.04, 17.5cm = £1.83, 20cm = £3.20, 3.5cm = £0.56, 5cm = £0.58, 7.5cm = £0.77

Clinifast

(Drug Tariff specification 46). Lightweight plain-knitted elasticated tubular bandage; various colours and sizes
CliniFast stockinette (CliniSupplies Ltd) 10.75cm = £6.04, 17.5cm = £1.83, 3.5cm = £0.56, 5cm = £0.58, 7.5cm = £0.77, clava 5-14 years = £6.75, 6 months-5 years = £5.85, cycle shorts large adult = £16.25, medium adult = £14.25, small adult = £12.50, gloves large adult = £4.99, child/small adult = £4.99, gloves medium adult = £4.99, child = £4.99, gloves small child = £4.99, leggings (Blue, Pink, White) 11-14 years = £9.50, 5-8 years = £10.69, 8-11 years = £11.88, mittens 2-8 years = £2.97, 8-14 years = £2.97, up to 24 months = £2.97, socks 8-14 years = £2.97, up to 8 years = £2.97, tights (Blue, Pink, White) 6-24 months = £7.13, vest long sleeve (Blue, Pink, White) 11-14 years = £11.88, 2-5 years = £9.50, 5-8 years = £10.69, 6-24 months = £7.13, 8-11 years = £11.88, vest short sleeve large adult = £16.25, medium adult = £14.25, small adult = £12.50,

Comfifast

(Drug Tariff specification 46). Lightweight plain-knitted elasticated tubular bandage; various colours and sizes
Comfifast stockinette (Synergy Health Plc) 10.75cm = £6.04, 17.5cm = £1.83, 3.5cm = £0.56, 5cm = £0.58, 7.5cm = £0.77

Comfifast Easywrap

(Drug Tariff specification 46). Lightweight plain-knitted elasticated tubular bandage; various colours and sizes
Comfifast Easywrap stockinette (Synergy Health Plc) clava 5-14 years = £6.75, 6 months-5 years = £5.85, leggings 11-14 years = £11.88, 2-5 years = £9.50, 5-8 years = £10.69, 8-11 years = £11.88, mittens 2-8 years = £2.97, 8-14 years = £2.97, up to 24 months = £2.97, socks 8-14 years = £2.97, up to 8 years = £2.97, tights 6-24 months = £7.13, vest long sleeve 11-14 years = £11.88, 2-5 years = £9.50, 5-8 years = £10.69, 6-24 months = £7.13, 8-11years = £11.88,

Comfifast Multistretch

(Drug Tariff specification 46). Lightweight plain-knitted elasticated tubular bandage; various colours and sizes
Comfifast MultiStretch stockinette (Synergy Health Plc) 10.75cm = £8.21, 17.5cm = £2.49, 3.5cm = £0.72, 5cm = £0.78, 7.5cm = £5.12

Coverflex

(Drug Tariff specification 46). Lightweight plain-knitted elasticated tubular bandage; various colours and sizes
Coverflex stockinette (Paul Hartmann Ltd) 10.75cm = £9.59, 17.5cm = £2.53, 3.5cm = £0.83, 5cm = £0.86, 7.5cm = £5.68

Easifast

(Drug Tariff specification 46). Lightweight plain-knitted elasticated tubular bandage; various colours and sizes
Easifast stockinette (Easigrip Ltd) 10.75cm = £7.23, 17.5cm = £1.91, 3.5cm = £0.65, 5cm = £0.69, 7.5cm = £0.94

Elasticated Surgical Tubular Stockinette, Foam padded or Tupipad

(Drug Tariff specification 25). Fabric as for Elasticated Tubular Bandage with polyurethane foam lining.

Elasticated Tubular Bandage, BP 1993

(Drug Tariff specification 25). Fabric as for Elasticated Tubular Bandage with polyurethane foam lining; lenghts 50 cm and 1 m

CLINIgrip bandage (CliniSupplies Ltd) 10cm size F = £0.74, 12cm size G = £0.77, 6.25cm size B = £0.61, 6.75cm size C = £0.65, 7.5cm size D = £0.66, 8.75cm size E = £0.74

Comfigrip bandage (Synergy Health Plc) 10cm size F = £0.74, 12cm size G = £0.77, 6.25cm size B = £0.61, 6.75cm size C = £0.65, 7.5cm size D = £0.66, 8.75cm size E = £0.74

Eesiban ESTS bandage (E Sallis Ltd) 10cm size F = £1.80, 12cm size G = £2.09, 6.25cm size B = £0.87, 6.75cm size C = £0.95, 7.5cm size D = £0.95, 8.75cm size E = £1.80

Tubigrip bandage (Molnlycke Health Care Ltd) 10cm size F = £2.04, 12cm size G = £2.35, 6.25cm size B = £0.99, 6.75cm size C = £1.88, 7.5cm size D = £1.88, 8.75cm size E = £2.04

easiGRIP bandage (Easigrip Ltd) 10cm size F = £0.75, 12cm size G = £0.78, 6.25cm size B = £0.62, 6.75cm size C = £0.66, 7.5cm size D = £0.68, 8.75cm size E = £0.75

Skinnies

(Drug Tariff specification 46). Lightweight plain-knitted elasticated tubular bandage; various colours and sizes

Skinnies stockinette (Dermacea Ltd) body suit (Blue, Ecru, Pink) 3-6 months = £16.18, 6-12 months = £18.21, premature = £16.18, up to 3 months = £16.18, clava (Blue, Ecru, Pink) 5-14 years = £7.73, 6 months-5 years = £6.74, gloves large (Beige, Blue, Ecru, Grey, Pink) adult = £5.34, child = £5.34, gloves medium (Beige, Blue, Ecru, Grey, Pink) adult = £5.34, child = £5.34, gloves small (Blue, Ecru, Grey, Pink) adult = £5.29, child = £5.29, knee socks extra (Black, Natural, White) large adult 11+ = £13.94, knee socks large (Black, Natural, White) adult 8-11 = £13.94, child 2-4 = £13.94, knee socks medium (Black, Natural, White) adult 6-8 = £13.94, child 1-2 = £13.94, knee socks small (Black, Natural, White) adult 4-6 = £13.94, child 0-1 = £13.94, leggings (Beige, Blue, Ecru, Grey, Pink) 11-14 years = £17.20, 2-5 years = £13.74, 5-8 years = £15.52, 6-24 months = £10.48, 8-11 years = £17.20, large adult = £25.13, medium adult = £23.20, small adult = £21.27, mittens (Blue, Ecru, Pink) 2-8 years = £3.87, 8-14 years = £3.87, up to 24 months = £3.87, socks (Blue, Ecru, Pink) 6 months-8 years = £4.27, 8-14 years = £4.27, vest long sleeve (Beige, Blue, Ecru, Grey, Pink) 11-14 years = £17.20, 2-5 years = £13.74, 5-8 years = £15.52, 6-24 months = £10.48, 8-11 years = £17.20, large adult = £25.13, medium adult = £23.20, small adult = £21.27, vest short sleeve (White) 11-14 years = £17.09, 2-5 years = £13.63, 5-8 years = £15.36, 6-24 months = £10.38, 8-11 years = £17.09, large adult = £25.03, medium adult = £23.10, small adult = £21.16, vest sleeveless (White) 11-14 years = £17.09, 2-5 years = £13.63, 5-8 years = £15.42, 6-24 months = £10.38, 8-11 years = £17.09, large adult = £25.03, medium adult = £23.10, small adult = £21.16,

Tubifast 2-way stretch

(Drug Tariff specification 46). Lightweight plain-knitted elasticated tubular bandage; various colours and sizes

Tubifast 2-way stretch stockinette (Molnlycke Health Care Ltd) 10.75cm = £6.45, 20cm = £3.42, 3.5cm = £0.61, 5cm = £0.63, 7.5cm = £0.83, gloves extra small child = £5.69, medium/large adult = £5.69, small child = £5.69, small/medium adult, medium/large child = £5.69, leggings 2-5 years = £15.14, 5-8 years = £17.04, 8-11 years = £18.93, socks (one size) = £4.79, tights 6-24 months = £11.36, vest long sleeve 11-14 years = £18.93, 2-5 years = £15.14, 5-8 years = £17.04, 6-24 months = £11.36, 8-11 years = £18.93,

Non-elasticated

Cotton Stockinette, Bleached, BP 1988

Knitted fabric, cotton yarn, tubular length, 1m

Cotton stockinette bleached heavyweight (E Sallis Ltd) 10cm, 2.5cm, 5cm, 7.5cm

Silk Clothing

DermaSilk

Knitted silk fabric, hypoallergenic, sericin-free

DermaSilk (Espere Healthcare Ltd) medium/large = £41.63, medium-large = £30.97, body suit 0-3 months = £38.13, 12-18 months = £40.40, 18-24 months = £41.41, 24-36 months = £41.49, 3-

6 months = £38.21, 6-9 months = £39.31, 9-12 months = £40.32, boxer shorts male adult extra large/XX large = £41.63, small/small = £41.63, briefs female adult extra large-XX large = £30.97, small-small = £30.97, facial mask adult = £20.91, child = £16.40, infant = £16.40, teen = £20.91, gloves extra large adult = £20.68, gloves large adult = £20.72, gloves medium adult = £20.72, child = £14.76, gloves small adult = £20.72, child = £14.76, leggings 0-3 months = £27.22, leggings 12-18 months = £29.47, leggings 18-24 months = £30.51, leggings 3-4 years = £31.65, leggings 3-6 months = £27.28, leggings 6-9 months = £28.37, leggings 9-12 months = £29.41, leggings adult female XX large = £78.31, extra large = £78.31, large = £78.31, medium = £78.31, small = £78.31, leggings adult male XX large = £78.31, extra large = £78.31, large = £78.31, medium = £78.31, small = £78.31, pyjamas 10-12 years = £81.95, 3-4 years = £71.01, 5-6 years = £75.39, 7-8 years = £78.67, roll neck shirt 10-12 years = £54.42, 3-4 years = £47.09, 5-6 years = £50.23, 7-8 years = £52.33, round neck shirt adult female XX large = £77.40, extra large = £77.40, large = £77.40, medium = £77.40, small = £77.40, round neck shirt adult male XX large = £77.40, extra large = £77.40, large = £77.40, medium = £77.40, small = £77.40, tubular sleeves = £33.67, sleeves = £27.28, undersocks adult 11-13 = £18.42, 5 1/2 - 6 1/2 = £18.42, 7 - 8 1/2 = £18.42, 9 - 10 1/2 = £18.42, undersocks child 2-5 = £18.42, 3-8 = £18.42, 9-1 = £18.42, unisex roll neck shirt adult XX large = £77.40, extra large = £77.40, large = £77.40, medium = £77.40, small = £77.40,

DreamSkin

Knitted silk fabric, hypoallergenic, sericin-free, with methyacrylate copolymer and zinc-based antibacterial

DreamSkin (DreamSkin Health Ltd) baby leggings with foldaway feet 0-3 months = £25.19, 12-18 months = £28.07, 18-24 months = £28.59, 3-4 years = £30.15, 3-6 months = £25.69, 6-9 months = £27.03, 9-12 months = £27.55, body suit 0-3 months = £35.48, 12-18 months = £38.49, 18-24 months = £39.01, 3-4 years = £40.57, 3-6 months = £35.99, 6-9 months = £37.44, 9-12 months = £37.99, boxer shorts 11-12 years = £21.39, boxer shorts 3-4 years = £21.39, boxer shorts 5-6 years = £21.39, boxer shorts 7-8 years = £21.39, boxer shorts 9-10 years = £21.39, boxer shorts male adult XX large = £33.65, extra large = £33.65, large = £33.65, medium = £33.65, small = £33.65, briefs 11-12 years = £21.39, briefs 3-4 years = £21.39, briefs 5-6 years = £21.39, briefs 7-8 years = £21.39, briefs 9-10 years = £21.39, briefs female adult XX large = £31.60, extra large = £31.60, large = £31.60, medium = £31.60, small = £31.60, eye mask = £10.16, footless leggings 11-12 years boys = £33.18, girls = £33.18, footless leggings 3-4 years boys = £30.15, girls = £30.15, footless leggings 5-6 years boys = £31.64, girls = £31.64, footless leggings 7-8 years boys = £32.15, girls = £32.15, footless leggings 9-10 years boys = £32.67, girls = £32.67, footless leggings adult female XX large = £76.32, extra large = £76.32, large = £76.32, medium = £76.32, small = £76.32, footless leggings adult male XX large = £76.32, extra large = £76.32, large = £76.32, medium = £76.32, small = £76.32, gloves extra large adult = £20.03, gloves large adult = £20.03, gloves medium adult = £20.03, child = £14.28, gloves small adult = £20.03, child = £14.28, head mask child = £15.62, infant = £15.62, teenager = £20.38, heel-less undersocks = £23.61, liner socks adult female 4 - 5 1/2 = £17.95, 6 - 8 1/2 = £17.95, liner socks adult male 6 - 8 1/2 = £17.95, 9 - 11 = £17.95, liner socks child 12 1/2 - 3 1/2 = £17.95, 3 - 5 1/2 = £17.95, 4 - 5 1/2 = £17.95, 6 - 8 1/2 = £17.95, 9 - 12 = £17.95, polo neck shirt 11-12 years boy = £53.04, girl = £53.04, polo neck shirt 3-4 years boy = £45.89, girl = £45.89, polo neck shirt 5-6 years boy = £48.95, girl = £48.95, polo neck shirt 7-8 years boy = £50.99, girl = £50.99, polo neck shirt 9-10 years boy = £52.02, girl = £52.02, polo neck shirt adult female XX large = £75.43, extra large = £75.43, large = £75.43, medium = £75.43, small = £75.43, polo neck shirt adult male XX large = £75.43, extra large = £75.43, large = £75.43, medium = £75.43, small = £75.43, pyjamas 11-12 years boy = £78.06, girl = £78.06, pyjamas 3-4 years boy = £67.65, girl = £67.65, pyjamas 5-6 years boy = £71.81, girl = £71.81, pyjamas 7-8 years boy = £74.94, girl = £74.94, pyjamas 9-10 years boy = £76.53, girl = £76.53, round neck shirt 3-4 years = £45.90, round neck shirt 5-6 years = £47.94, round neck shirt 7-8 years = £49.98, round neck shirt 9-10 years = £51.00, round neck shirt adult female XX large = £75.43, extra large = £75.43, large = £75.43, medium = £75.43, small =

£75.43, round neck shirt adult male XX large = £75.43, extra large = £75.43, large = £75.43, medium = £75.43, small = £75.43, tubular sleeves = £26.38, sleeves = £32.81,

Support bandages

Light support bandages, which include the various forms of crepe bandage, are used in the prevention of oedema; they are also used to provide support for mild sprains and joints but their effectiveness has not been proven for this purpose. Since they have limited extensibility, they are able to provide light support without exerting undue pressure. For a warning against injudicious compression see p. 1391.

CliniLite

Knitted fabric, viscose and elastomer yarn. Type 2 (light support bandage)

CliniLite bandage (CliniSupplies Ltd) 10cm × 4.5m = £0.80, 15cm × 4.5m = £1.16, 5cm × 4.5m = £0.44, 7.5cm × 4.5m = £0.61

CliniPlus

Knitted fabric, viscose and elastomer yarn. Type 2 (light support bandage)

CliniPlus (CliniSupplies Ltd) bandage 10cm × 8.7m = £1.80

Cotton Crepe Bandage

Light support bandage, 4.5 m stretched (all)

Hospicrepe 239 bandage (Paul Hartmann Ltd) 10cm × 4.5m = £0.81, 15cm × 4.5m = £1.18, 5cm × 4.5m = £0.44, 7.5cm × 4.5m = £0.63

Cotton Crepe Bandage, BP 1988

Fabric, plain weave, warp of crepe-twisted cotton threads, weft of cotton and/or viscose threads; stretch bandage. 4.5 m stretched (both)

Elastocrepe bandage (BSN medical Ltd) 10cm × 4.5m, 7.5cm × 4.5m

Flexocrepe bandage (Robinson Healthcare) 10cm × 4.5m, 7.5cm × 4.5m

Sterocrepe bandage (Steroplast Healthcare Ltd) 10cm × 4.5m, 7.5cm × 4.5m

Cotton Suspensory Bandage

(Drug Tariff). Type 1: cotton net bag with draw tapes and webbing waistband; small, medium, and large (all)

Crepe Bandage, BP 1988

Fabric, plain weave, warp of wool threads and crepe-twisted cotton threads, weft of cotton threads; stretch bandage; 4.5 m stretched

Alvita crepe bandage (Alliance Healthcare (Distribution) Ltd) 10cm × 4.5m, 15cm × 4.5m, 5cm × 4.5m, 7.5cm × 4.5m

Clinicrepe bandage (CliniSupplies Ltd) 10cm × 4.5m, 15cm × 4.5m, 5cm × 4.5m, 7.5cm × 4.5m

Crepe bandage (Robert Bailey & Son Plc) 10cm × 4.5m, 15cm × 4.5m, 5cm × 4.5m, 7.5cm × 4.5m

Propax crepe bandage (BSN medical Ltd) 10cm × 4.5m, 15cm × 4.5m, 5cm × 4.5m, 7.5cm × 4.5m

Vernaid crepe bandage (Synergy Health Plc) 10cm × 4.5m, 15cm × 4.5m, 5cm × 4.5m, 7.5cm × 4.5m

Elset

Knitted fabric, viscose and elastomer yarn. Type 2 (light support bandage)

Elset (Molnlycke Health Care Ltd) S bandage 15cm × 12m = £5.55, bandage 10cm × 6m = £2.58, 10cm × 8m = £3.31, 15cm × 6m = £2.77,

Hospicrepe 233

Fabric, plain weave, warp of crepe-twisted cotton threads, weft of cotton threads; stretch bandage, lighter than cotton crepe, 4.5 m stretched (all)

Hospicrepe 233 bandage (Paul Hartmann Ltd) 10cm × 4.5m = £0.96, 15cm × 4.5m = £1.36, 5cm × 4.5m = £0.52, 7.5cm × 4.5m = £0.72

Hospilite

Fabric, cotton, polyamide, and elastane; light support bandage (Type 2), 4.5 m stretched (all)

Hospilite bandage (Paul Hartmann Ltd) 10cm × 4.5m = £0.62, 15cm × 4.5m = £0.91, 5cm × 4.5m = £0.37, 7.5cm × 4.5m = £0.51

K-Lite

Knitted fabric, viscose and elastomer yarn. Type 2 (light support bandage)

K-Lite (Urgo Ltd) Long bandage 10cm × 5.25m = £1.14, bandage 10cm × 4.5m = £1.00, 15cm × 4.5m = £1.45, 5cm × 4.5m = £0.55, 7cm × 4.5m = £0.76,

K-Plus

Knitted fabric, viscose and elastomer yarn. Type 2 (light support bandage)

K-Plus (Urgo Ltd) Long bandage 10cm × 10.25m = £2.62, bandage 10cm × 8.7m = £2.27

Knit-Firm

Knitted fabric, viscose and elastomer yarn. Type 2 (light support bandage)

Knit-Firm bandage (Millpledge Healthcare) 10cm × 4.5m = £0.66, 15cm × 4.5m = £0.96, 5cm × 4.5m = £0.36, 7cm × 4.5m = £0.51

L3

Knitted fabric, viscose and elastomer yarn. Type 2 (light support bandage)

L3 (Smith & Nephew Healthcare Ltd) bandage 10cm × 8.6m = £2.20

Neosport

Fabric, cotton, polyamide, and elastane; light support bandage (Type 2), 4.5 m stretched (all)

Neosport bandage (Neomedic Ltd) 10cm × 4.5m = £0.91, 15cm × 4.5m = £1.12, 5cm × 4.5m = £0.54, 7.5cm × 4.5m = £0.73

PremierBand

Fabric, plain weave, warp of crepe-twisted cotton threads, weft of cotton threads; stretch bandage, lighter than cotton crepe, 4.5 m stretched (all)

PremierBand bandage (Shermond) 10cm × 4.5m = £0.79, 15cm × 4.5m = £1.18, 5cm × 4.5m = £0.45, 7.5cm × 4.5m = £0.63

Profore #2

Fabric, cotton, polyamide, and elastane; light support bandage (Type 2), 4.5 m stretched (all)

Profore #2 (Smith & Nephew Healthcare Ltd) bandage 10cm × 4.5m = £1.35, latex free bandage 10cm × 4.5m = £1.43

Profore #3

Knitted fabric, viscose and elastomer yarn. Type 2 (light support bandage)

Profore #3 (Smith & Nephew Healthcare Ltd) bandage 10cm × 8.7m = £3.92, latex free bandage 10cm × 8.7m = £4.26

Setocrepe

Fabric, cotton, polyamide, and elastane; light support bandage (Type 2), 4.5 m stretched (all)

Setocrepe (Molnlycke Health Care Ltd) bandage 10cm × 4.5m = £1.19

Soffcrepe

Fabric, cotton, polyamide, and elastane; light support bandage (Type 2), 4.5 m stretched (all)

Soffcrepe bandage (BSN medical Ltd) 10cm × 4.5m = £1.24, 15cm × 4.5m = £1.80, 5cm × 4.5m = £0.69, 7.5cm × 4.5m = £0.98

Adhesive bandages

Elastic adhesive bandages are used to provide compression in the treatment of varicose veins and for the support of injured joints; they should no longer be used for the support of fractured ribs and clavicles. They have also been used with zinc paste bandage in the treatment of venous ulcers, but they can cause skin reactions in susceptible patients and may not produce sufficient pressures for healing (significantly lower than those provided by other compression bandages).

Elastic Adhesive Bandage, BP 1993

Woven fabric, elastic in warp (crepe-twisted cotton threads), weft of cotton and/or viscose threads spread with adhesive mass containing zinc oxide. 4.5 m stretched

Tensoplast bandage (BSN medical Ltd) 10cm × 4.5m, 5cm × 4.5m, 7.5cm × 4.5m

Cohesive bandages

Cohesive bandages adhere to themselves, but not to the skin, and are useful for providing support for sports use where ordinary stretch bandages might become displaced and adhesive bandages are inappropriate. Care is needed in their application, however, since the loss of ability for movement between turns of the bandage to equalise local areas of high tension carries the potential for creating a tourniquet effect. Cohesive bandages can be used to support sprained joints and as an outer layer for multi-layer compression bandaging; they should not be used if arterial disease is suspected.

Cohesive extensible bandages
Coban
Bandage
Coban (3M Health Care Ltd) self-adherent bandage 10cm × 6m = £2.93

K Press
Bandage
K Press bandage (Urgo Ltd) 10cm × 6.5m = £2.90, 10cm × 7.5m = £3.39, 12cm × 7.5m = £4.26, 8cm × 7.5cm = £3.19

Profore #4
Bandage
Profore #4 (Smith & Nephew Healthcare Ltd) bandage 10cm × 2.5m = £3.24, latex free bandage 10cm × 2.5m = £3.53

Ultra Fast
Bandage
Ultra (Robinson Healthcare) Fast cohesive bandage 10cm × 6.3m = £2.59

Compression bandages
High compression products are used to provide the high compression needed for the management of gross varices, post-thrombotic venous insufficiency, venous leg ulcers, and gross oedema in average-sized limbs. Their use calls for an expert knowledge of the elastic properties of the products and experience in the technique of providing careful graduated compression. Incorrect application can lead to uneven and inadequate pressures or to hazardous levels of pressure. In particular, injudicious use of compression in limbs with arterial disease has been reported to cause severe skin and tissue necrosis (in some instances calling for amputation). Doppler testing is required before treatment with compression. Oral pentoxifylline p. 217 can be used as adjunct therapy if a chronic venous leg ulcer does not respond to compression bandaging [unlicensed indication].

High compression bandages
High Compression Bandage
Cotton, viscose, nylon, and Lycra extensible bandage, 3 m (unstretched)
K-ThreeC (Urgo Ltd) bandage 10cm × 3m = £2.82
SurePress (ConvaTec Ltd) bandage 10cm × 3m = £3.61

PEC High Compression Bandages
Polyamide, elastane, and cotton compression (high) extensible bandage, 3.5 m unstretched
Setopress (Molnlycke Health Care Ltd) bandage 10cm × 3.5m = £3.51

VEC High Compression Bandages
Viscose, elastane, and cotton compression (high) extensible bandage, 3 m unstretched (both)
Tensopress bandage (BSN medical Ltd) 10cm × 3m = £3.45, 7.5cm × 3m = £2.68

Short stretch compression bandages
Actico
Bandage
Actico bandage (Activa Healthcare Ltd) 10cm × 6m = £3.34, 12cm × 6m = £4.26, 4cm × 6m = £2.39, 6cm × 6m = £2.80, 8cm × 6m = £3.22

Comprilan
Bandage
Comprilan bandage (BSN medical Ltd) 10cm × 5m = £3.37, 12cm × 5m = £4.11, 6cm × 5m = £2.67, 8cm × 5m = £3.14

Rosidal K
Bandage
Rosidal K bandage (Lohmann & Rauscher (UK) Ltd) 10cm × 10m = £6.02, 10cm × 5m = £3.46, 12cm × 5m = £4.20, 6cm × 5m = £2.65, 8cm × 5m = £3.17

Silkolan
Bandage

Sub-compression wadding bandage
Cellona Undercast Padding
Padding
Cellona Undercast padding bandage (Lohmann & Rauscher (UK) Ltd) 10cm × 2.75m = £0.47, 15cm × 2.75m = £0.60, 5cm × 2.75m = £0.31, 7.5cm × 2.75m = £0.38

Flexi-Ban
Padding
Flexi-Ban (Activa Healthcare Ltd) bandage 10cm × 3.5m = £0.50

K Tech Reduced
Padding
K Tech Reduced bandage (Urgo Ltd) 10cm × 6m = £4.70, 10cm × 7.3m = £5.13

K-Soft
Padding
K-Soft (Urgo Ltd) Long bandage 10cm × 4.5m = £0.57, bandage 10cm × 3.5m = £0.45

K-Tech (K Tech in DMD)
Padding
K Tech (Urgo Ltd) Reduced bandage 10cm × 7.3m = £5.13, bandage 10cm × 5m = £3.92, 10cm × 6m = £4.70, 12cm × 6m = £5.93, 12cm × 7.3m = £6.47, 8cm × 6m = £4.44, 8cm × 7.3m = £4.84,

Ortho-Band Plus
Padding
Ortho-Band (Millpledge Healthcare) Plus bandage 10cm × 3.5m = £0.37

Profore #1
Padding
Profore #1 (Smith & Nephew Healthcare Ltd) bandage 10cm × 3.5m = £0.70, latex free bandage 10cm × 3.5m = £0.76

Softexe
Padding
Softexe (Molnlycke Health Care Ltd) bandage 10cm × 3.5m = £0.62

SurePres
Padding
SurePress (ConvaTec Ltd) bandage 10cm × 3m = £3.61

Ultra Soft
Padding
Ultra (Robinson Healthcare) Soft wadding bandage 10cm × 3.5m = £0.39

Velband
Padding
Velband (BSN medical Ltd) absorbent padding bandage 10cm × 4.5m = £0.73

Multi-layer compression bandaging
Multi-layer compression bandaging systems are an alternative to High Compression Bandages for the treatment of venous leg ulcers. Compression is achieved by the combined effects of two or three extensible bandages applied over a layer of orthopaedic wadding and a wound contact dressing.

Four layer systems
K-Four
Padding

K-Four
Multi-layer compression bandaging kit, four layer system
K-Four (Urgo Ltd) Reduced Compression multi-layer compression bandage kit 18cm+ ankle circumference = £4.47, multi-layer compression bandage kit 18cm-25cm ankle circumference = £6.83, 25cm-30cm ankle circumference = £6.83, greater than 30cm ankle circumference = £9.41, less than 18cm ankle circumference = £7.14,

Profore
Wound contact layer

Profore
Multi-layer compression bandaging kit, four layer system

Profore (Smith & Nephew Healthcare Ltd) Lite latex free multi-layer compression bandage kit = £5.94, multi-layer compression bandage kit = £5.46, latex free multi-layer compression bandage kit 18cm-25cm ankle circumference = £10.11, multi-layer compression bandage kit 18cm-25cm ankle circumference = £9.47, 25cm-30cm ankle circumference = £7.86, above 30cm ankle circumference = £11.77, up to 18cm ankle circumference = £10.16,

Ultra Four
Wound contact layer

Ultra Four
Multi-layer compression bandaging kit, four layer system
Ultra Four (Robinson Healthcare) Reduced Compression multi-layer compression bandage kit = £4.14, multi-layer compression bandage kit 18cm-25cm ankle circumference = £5.67, up to 18cm ankle circumference = £6.41,

Two layer systems
Coban 2
Multi-layer compression bandaging kit, two layer system (latex-free, foam bandage and cohesive compression bandage
Coban 2 (3M Health Care Ltd) Lite multi-layer compression bandage kit = £8.24, multi-layer compression bandage kit = £8.24

K Two
Multi-layer compression bandaging kit, two layer system
UrgoKTwo (Urgo Ltd) Reduced latex free multi-layer compression bandage kit (10cm) 18cm-25cm ankle circumference = £8.59, 25cm-32cm ankle circumference = £9.39, Reduced multi-layer compression bandage kit 18cm-25cm ankle circumference = £8.09, 25cm-32cm ankle circumference = £8.84, latex free multi-layer compression bandage kit (10cm) 18cm-25cm ankle circumference = £8.59, 25cm-32cm ankle circumference = £9.39, multi-layer compression bandage kit (10cm) 18cm-25cm ankle circumference = £8.09, 25cm-32cm ankle circumference = £8.84, multi-layer compression bandage kit (12cm) 18cm-25cm ankle circumference = £10.20, 25cm-32cm ankle circumference = £11.15, multi-layer compression bandage kit (8cm) 18cm-25cm ankle circumference = £7.63, 25cm-32cm ankle circumference = £8.30, multi-layer compression bandage kit size 0 short 18cm-25cm ankle circumference = £6.83, with UrgoStart multi-layer compression bandage kit 18cm-25cm ankle circumference = £10.08, 25cm-32cm ankle circumference = £10.75,

Medicated bandages
Zinc Paste Bandage has been used with compression bandaging for the treatment of venous leg ulcers. However, paste bandages are associated with hypersensitivity reactions and should be used with caution. Zinc paste bandages are also used with coal tar or ichthammol in chronic lichenified skin conditions such as chronic eczema (ichthammol often being preferred since its action is considered to be milder). They are also used with calamine in milder eczematous skin conditions.
Zipzoc® can be used under appropriate compression bandages or hosiery in chronic venous insufficiency.

Zinc Paste Bandage, BP 1993
Cotton fabric, plain weave, impregnated with suitable paste containing zinc oxide; requires additional bandaging Excipients: may include cetostearyl alcohol, hydroxybenzoates
Viscopaste (Smith & Nephew Healthcare Ltd) PB7 bandage 7.5cm × 6m = £3.65

Zinc Paste and Ichthammol Bandage, BP 1993
Cotton fabric, plain weave, impregnated with suitable paste containing zinc oxide and ichthammol; requires additional bandaging Excipients: may include cetostearyl alcohol
Ichthopaste (Smith & Nephew Healthcare Ltd) bandage 7.5cm × 6m = £3.68

Medicated stocking
Zipzoc
Sterile rayon stocking impregnated with ointment containing zinc oxide 20%
Zipzoc (Smith & Nephew Healthcare Ltd) stockings = £31.26

Compression hosiery and garments
Compression (elastic) hosiery is used to treat conditions associated with chronic venous insufficiency, to prevent recurrence of thrombosis, or to reduce the risk of further venous ulceration after treatment with compression bandaging. Doppler testing to confirm arterial sufficiency is required before recommending the use of compression hosiery.
Before elastic hosiery can be dispensed, the quantity (single or pair), article (including accessories), and compression class must be specified by the prescriber. There are different compression values for graduated compression hosiery and lymphoedema garments (see table below). All dispensed elastic hosiery articles must state on the packaging that they conform with Drug Tariff technical specification No. 40, for further details see Drug Tariff.
Graduated Compression hosiery, Class 1 Light Support is used for superficial or early varices, varicosis during pregnancy.
Graduated Compression hosiery, Class 2 Medium Support is used for varices of medium severity, ulcer treatment and prophylaxis, mild oedema, varicosis during pregnancy.
Graduated Compression hosiery, Class 3 Strong Support is used for gross varices, post thrombotic venous insufficiency, gross oedema, ulcer treatment and prophylaxis.

Compression values for hosiery and lymphoedema garments
Class 1: Compression hosiery (British standard) 14–17 mmHg, lymphoedema garments (European classification) 18–21 mmHg; *Class* 2 Compression hosiery (British standard) 18–24 mmHg, lymphoedema garments (European classification) 23–32 mmHg; *Class* 3 Compression hosiery (British standard) 25–35 mmHg, lymphoedema garments (European classification) 34–46 mmHg; *Class* 4 Compression hosiery (British standard)—not available, lymphoedema garments (European classification) 49–70 mmHg; *Class* 4 super Compression hosiery (British standard)—not available, lymphoedema garments (European classification) 60–90 mmHg.

Graduated compression hosiery
Class 1 Light Support
Hosiery, compression at ankle 14–17 mmHg, thigh length or below knee with knitted in heel

Class 2 Light Support
Hosiery, compression at ankle 14–17 mmHg, thigh length or below knee with knitted in heel

Accessories
Suspender
Suspender, for thigh stockings

Anklets
Class 2 Medium Support
Anklets, compression 18–24 mmHg, circular knit (standard and made-to-measure),

Class 3 Strong Support
Anklets, compression 18–24 mmHg, circular knit (standard and made-to-measure),

Knee caps
Class 2 Medium Support
Kneecaps, compression 18–24 mmHg, circular knit (standard and made-to-measure)

Class 3 Strong Support
Kneecaps, compression 18–24 mmHg, circular knit (standard and made-to-measure)

Lymphoedema garments
Lymphoedema compression garments are used to maintain limb shape and prevent additional fluid retention. Either flat-bed or circular knitting methods are used in the manufacture of elasticated compression garments. Seamless, circular-knitted garments (in standard sizes) can be used to prevent swelling if the lymphoedema is well controlled and if the limb is in good shape and without skin folds. Flat-knitted

garments (usually made-to-measure) with a seam, provide greater rigidity and stiffness to maintain reduction of lymphoedema following treatment with compression bandages. A standard range of light, medium, or high compression garments are available, as well as low compression (12–16 mmHg) armsleeves, made-to-measure garments up to compression 90 mmHg, and accessories—see Drug Tariff for details. Note There are different compression values for lymphoedema garments and graduated compression hosiery, see p. 1392.

Dental Practitioners' Formulary

List of Dental Preparations

The following list has been approved by the appropriate Secretaries of State, and the preparations therein may be prescribed by dental practitioners on form FP10D (GP14 in Scotland, WP10D in Wales).

Licensed **sugar-free** versions, where available, are preferred. Licensed **alcohol-free** mouthwashes, where available, are preferred.

Aciclovir Cream, BP
Aciclovir Oral Suspension, BP, 200 mg/5 mL
Aciclovir Tablets, BP, 200 mg
Aciclovir Tablets, BP, 800 mg
Amoxicillin Capsules, BP
Amoxicillin Oral Powder, DPF
Amoxicillin Oral Suspension, BP
Artificial Saliva Gel, DPF
Artificial Saliva Oral Spray, DPF
Artificial Saliva Pastilles, DPF
Artificial Saliva Protective Spray, DPF
Artificial Saliva Substitutes as listed below (to be prescribed only for indications approved by ACBS (patients suffering from dry mouth as a result of having or, having undergone, radiotherapy or sicca syndrome):
  BioXtra® Gel Mouthspray
  BioXtra® Moisturising Gel
  Glandosane®
  Saliveze®
Artificial Saliva Substitute Spray, DPF
Aspirin Tablets, Dispersible, BP
Azithromycin Capsules, 250 mg, DPF
Azithromycin Oral Suspension, 200 mg/5 mL, DPF
Azithromycin Tablets, 250 mg, DPF
Azithromycin Tablets, 500 mg, DPF
Beclometasone Pressurised Inhalation, BP, 50 micrograms/metered inhalation, CFC-free, as:
  Clenil Modulite®
Benzydamine Mouthwash, BP 0.15%
Benzydamine Oromucosal Spray, BP 0.15%
Betamethasone Soluble Tablets, 500 micrograms, DPF
Carbamazepine Tablets, BP
Cefalexin Capsules, BP
Cefalexin Oral Suspension, BP
Cefalexin Tablets, BP
Cefradine Capsules, BP
Cetirizine Oral Solution, BP, 5 mg/5 mL
Cetirizine Tablets, BP, 10 mg
Chlorhexidine Gluconate Gel, BP
Chlorhexidine Mouthwash, BP
Chlorhexidine Oral Spray, DPF
Chlorphenamine Oral Solution, BP
Chlorphenamine Tablets, BP
Choline Salicylate Dental Gel, BP
Clarithromycin Oral Suspension, 125 mg/5 mL, DPF
Clarithromycin Oral Suspension, 250 mg/5 mL, DPF
Clarithromycin Tablets, BP
Clindamycin Capsules, BP
Co-amoxiclav Tablets, BP, 250/125 (amoxicillin 250 mg as trihydrate, clavulanic acid 125 mg as potassium salt)
Co-amoxiclav Oral Suspension, BP, 125/31 (amoxicillin 125 mg as trihydrate, clavulanic acid 31.25 mg as potassium salt)/5 mL
Co-amoxiclav Oral Suspension, BP, 250/62 (amoxicillin 250 mg as trihydrate, clavulanic acid 62.5 mg as potassium salt)/5 mL
Diazepam Oral Solution, BP, 2 mg/5 mL

Diazepam Tablets, BP
Diclofenac Sodium Tablets, Gastro-resistant, BP
Dihydrocodeine Tablets, BP, 30 mg
Doxycycline Tablets, Dispersible, BP
Doxycycline Capsules, BP, 100 mg
Doxycycline Tablets, 20 mg, DPF
Ephedrine Nasal Drops, BP
Erythromycin Ethyl Succinate Oral Suspension, BP
Erythromycin Ethyl Succinate Tablets, BP
Erythromycin Stearate Tablets, BP
Erythromycin Tablets, Gastro-resistant, BP
Fluconazole Capsules, 50 mg, DPF
Fluconazole Oral Suspension, 50 mg/5 mL, DPF
Hydrocortisone Cream, BP, 1%
Hydrocortisone Oromucosal Tablets, BP
Hydrogen Peroxide Mouthwash, BP, 6%
Ibuprofen Oral Suspension, BP, sugar-free
Ibuprofen Tablets, BP
Lansoprazole Capsules, Gastro-resistant, BP
Lidocaine Ointment, BP, 5%
Lidocaine Spray 10%, DPF
Loratadine Syrup, 5 mg/5 mL, DPF
Loratadine Tablets, BP, 10 mg
Menthol and Eucalyptus Inhalation, BP 1980
Metronidazole Oral Suspension, BP
Metronidazole Tablets, BP
Miconazole Cream, BP
Miconazole Oromucosal Gel, BP
Miconazole and Hydrocortisone Cream, BP
Miconazole and Hydrocortisone Ointment, BP
Nystatin Oral Suspension, BP
Omeprazole Capsules, Gastro-resistant, BP
Oxytetracycline Tablets, BP
Paracetamol Oral Suspension, BP
Paracetamol Tablets, BP
Paracetamol Tablets, Soluble, BP
Phenoxymethylpenicillin Oral Solution, BP
Phenoxymethylpenicillin Tablets, BP
Promethazine Hydrochloride Tablets, BP
Promethazine Oral Solution, BP
Saliva Stimulating Tablets, DPF
Sodium Chloride Mouthwash, Compound, BP
Sodium Fluoride Mouthwash, BP
Sodium Fluoride Oral Drops, BP
Sodium Fluoride Tablets, BP
Sodium Fluoride Toothpaste 0.619%, DPF
Sodium Fluoride Toothpaste 1.1%, DPF
Sodium Fusidate Ointment, BP
Temazepam Oral Solution, BP
Temazepam Tablets, BP
Tetracycline Tablets, BP

Preparations in this list which are not included in the BP or BPC are described under Details of DPF preparations. For details of preparations that can be prescribed, see individual entries under the relevant drug monographs throughout the BNF publications.

Details of DPF preparations

Preparations on the List of Dental Preparations which are specified as DPF are described as follows in the DPF. Although brand names have sometimes been included for identification purposes preparations on the list should be prescribed by non-proprietary name.

Amoxicillin Oral Powder
amoxicillin (as trihydrate) 3 g sachet

Artificial Saliva Gel
(proprietary product: *Biotene Oralbalance*), lactoperoxidase, lactoferrin, lysozyme, glucose oxidase, xylitol in a gel basis

Artificial Saliva Oral Spray
(proprietary product: *Xerotin*) consists of water, sorbitol, carmellose (carboxymethylcellulose), potassium chloride, sodium chloride, potassium phosphate, magnesium chloride, calcium chloride and other ingredients, pH neutral

Artificial Saliva Pastilles
(proprietary product: *Salivix*), consists of acacia, malic acid, and other ingredients

Artificial Saliva Protective Spray
(proprietary product: *Aquoral*) consists of oxidised glycerol triesters, silicon dioxide, flavouring agents, aspartame

Artificial Saliva Substitute Spray
(proprietary product: *AS Saliva Orthana Spray*) consists of mucin, methylparaben, benzalkonium chloride, EDTA, xylitol, peppermint oil, spearmint oil, mineral salts

Azithromycin Capsules
azithromycin 250 mg

Azithromycin Oral Suspension 200 mg/5 mL
azithromycin 200 mg/5 mL when reconstituted with water

Azithromycin Tablets
azithromycin 250 mg and 500 mg

Betamethasone Soluble Tablets 500 micrograms
betamethasone (as sodium phosphate) 500 micrograms

Chlorhexidine Oral Spray
(proprietary product: *Corsodyl Oral Spray*), chlorhexidine gluconate 0.2%

Clarithromycin Oral Suspension 125 mg/5 mL
clarithromycin 125 mg/5 mL when reconstituted with water

Clarithromycin Oral Suspension 250 mg/5 mL
clarithromycin 250 mg/5 mL when reconstituted with water

Doxycycline Tablets 20 mg
(proprietary product: *Periostat*), doxycycline (as hyclate) 20 mg

Fluconazole Capsules 50 mg
fluconazole 50 mg

Fluconazole Oral Suspension 50 mg/5 mL
(proprietary product: *Diflucan*), fluconazole 50 mg/5 mL when reconstituted with water

Lidocaine Spray 10%
(proprietary product: *Xylocaine Spray*), lidocaine 10% supplying 10 mg lidocaine/spray

Loratadine Syrup 5 mg/5 mL
loratadine 5 mg/5 mL

Saliva Stimulating Tablets
(proprietary product: *SST*), citric acid, malic acid and other ingredients in a sorbitol base

Sodium Fluoride Toothpaste 0.619%
(proprietary product: *Duraphat* '2800 *ppm*' *Toothpaste*), sodium fluoride 0.619%

Sodium Fluoride Toothpaste 1.1%
(proprietary product: *Duraphat* '5000 *ppm*' *Toothpaste*), sodium fluoride 1.1%

Nurse Prescribers' Formulary

Nurse Prescribers' Formulary for Community Practitioners

List of preparations approved by the Secretary of State which may be prescribed on form FP10P (form HS21(N) in Northern Ireland, form GP10(N) in Scotland, forms WP10CN and WP10PN in Wales) by Nurses for National Health Service patients.

Community practitioners who have completed the necessary training may only prescribe items appearing in the nurse prescribers' list set out below. Community Practitioner Nurse Prescribers are recommended to prescribe generically, except where this would not be clinically appropriate or where there is no approved generic name.

Medicinal Preparations

Preparations on this list which are not included in the BP or BPC are described under Details of NPF preparations, p. 1397.

Almond Oil Ear Drops, BP
Arachis Oil Enema, NPF
Aspirin Tablets, Dispersible, 300 mg, BP (max. 96 tablets; max. pack size 32 tablets)
Bisacodyl Suppositories, BP (includes 5-mg and 10-mg strengths)
Bisacodyl Tablets, BP
Catheter Maintenance Solution, Sodium Chloride, NPF
Catheter Maintenance Solution, 'Solution G', NPF
Catheter Maintenance Solution, 'Solution R', NPF
Chlorhexidine Gluconate Alcoholic Solutions containing at least 0.05%
Chlorhexidine Gluconate Aqueous Solutions containing at least 0.05%
Choline Salicylate Dental Gel, BP
Clotrimazole Cream 1%, BP
Co-danthramer Capsules, NPF
Co-danthramer Capsules, Strong, NPF
Co-danthramer Oral Suspension, NPF
Co-danthramer Oral Suspension, Strong, NPF
Co-danthrusate Capsules, BP
Co-danthrusate Oral Suspension, NPF
Crotamiton Cream, BP
Crotamiton Lotion, BP
Dimeticone barrier creams containing at least 10%
Dimeticone Lotion, NPF
Docusate Capsules, BP
Docusate Enema, NPF
Docusate Oral Solution, BP
Docusate Oral Solution, Paediatric, BP
Econazole Cream 1%, BP
Emollients as listed below:
    Aquadrate® 10% w/w Cream
    Arachis Oil, BP
    Balneum® Plus Cream
    Cetraben® Emollient Cream
    Dermamist®
    Diprobase® Cream
    Diprobase® Ointment
    Doublebase®
    Doublebase® Dayleve Gel
    E45® Cream
    E45® Itch Relief Cream
    Emulsifying Ointment, BP
    Eucerin® Intensive 10% w/w Urea Treatment Cream
    Eucerin® Intensive 10% w/w Urea Treatment Lotion
    Hydromol® Cream

    Hydromol® Intensive
    Hydrous Ointment, BP
    Lipobase®
    Liquid and White Soft Paraffin Ointment, NPF
    Neutrogena® Norwegian Formula Dermatological Cream
    Nutraplus® Cream
    Oilatum® Cream
    Oilatum® Junior Cream
    Paraffin, White Soft, BP
    Paraffin, Yellow Soft, BP
    Ultrabase®
    Unguentum M®
Emollient Bath and Shower Preparations as listed below:
    Aqueous Cream, BP
    Balneum® (except pack sizes that are not to be prescribed under the NHS (see Part XVIIIA of the Drug Tariff, Part XI of the Northern Ireland Drug Tariff))
    Balneum Plus® Bath Oil (except pack sizes that are not to be prescribed under the NHS (see Part XVIIIA of the Drug Tariff, Part XI of the Northern Ireland Drug Tariff))
    Cetraben® Emollient Bath Additive
    Dermalo® Bath Emollient
    Doublebase® Emollient Bath Additive
    Doublebase® Emollient Shower Gel
    Doublebase® Emollient Wash Gel
    Hydromol® Bath and Shower Emollient
    Oilatum® Emollient
    Oilatum® Gel
    Oilatum® Junior Bath Additive
    Zerolatum® Emollient Medicinal Bath Oil
Folic Acid Tablets 400 micrograms, BP
Glycerol Suppositories, BP
Ibuprofen Oral Suspension, BP (except for indications and doses that are prescription-only)
Ibuprofen Tablets, BP (except for indications and doses that are prescription-only)
Ispaghula Husk Granules, BP
Ispaghula Husk Granules, Effervescent, BP
Ispaghula Husk Oral Powder, BP
Lactulose Solution, BP
Lidocaine Ointment, BP
Lidocaine and Chlorhexidine Gel, BP
Macrogol Oral Liquid, Compound, NPF
Macrogol Oral Powder, Compound, NPF
Macrogol Oral Powder, Compound, Half-strength, NPF
Magnesium Hydroxide Mixture, BP
Magnesium Sulfate Paste, BP
Malathion aqueous lotions containing at least 0.5%
Mebendazole Oral Suspension, NPF
Mebendazole Tablets, NPF
Methylcellulose Tablets, BP
Miconazole Cream 2%, BP
Miconazole Oromucosal Gel, BP
Mouthwash Solution-tablets, NPF
Nicotine Inhalation Cartridge for Oromucosal Use, NPF
Nicotine Lozenge, NPF
Nicotine Medicated Chewing Gum, NPF
Nicotine Nasal Spray, NPF
Nicotine Oral Spray, NPF
Nicotine Sublingual Tablets, NPF
Nicotine Transdermal Patches, NPF
Nystatin Oral Suspension, BP
Olive Oil Ear Drops, BP
Paracetamol Oral Suspension, BP (includes 120 mg/5 mL and 250 mg/5 mL strengths—both of which are available as sugar-free formulations)

Paracetamol Tablets, BP (max. 96 tablets; max. pack size 32 tablets)

Paracetamol Tablets, Soluble, BP (includes 120-mg and 500-mg tablets; max. 96 tablets; max. pack size 32 tablets)

Permethrin Cream, NPF

Phosphates Enema, BP

Povidone–Iodine Solution, BP

Senna Oral Solution, NPF

Senna Tablets, BP

Senna and Ispaghula Granules, NPF

Sodium Chloride Solution, Sterile, BP

Sodium Citrate Compound Enema, NPF

Sodium Picosulfate Capsules, NPF

Sodium Picosulfate Elixir, NPF

Spermicidal contraceptives as listed below:
  Gygel® Contraceptive Jelly

Sterculia Granules, NPF

Sterculia and Frangula Granules, NPF

Titanium Ointment, NPF

Water for Injections, BP

Zinc and Castor Oil Ointment, BP

Zinc Oxide and Dimeticone Spray, NPF

Zinc Oxide Impregnated Medicated Bandage, NPF

Zinc Oxide Impregnated Medicated Stocking, NPF

Zinc Paste Bandage, BP 1993

Zinc Paste and Ichthammol Bandage, BP 1993

Appliances and Reagents (including Wound Management Products)

Community Practitioner Nurse Prescribers in England, Wales and Northern Ireland can prescribe any appliance or reagent in the relevant Drug Tariff. In the Scottish Drug Tariff, Appliances and Reagents which may **not** be prescribed by Nurses are annotated **Nx**.

Appliances (including Contraceptive Devices) as listed in Part IXA of the Drug Tariff (Part III of the Northern Ireland Drug Tariff, Part 3 (Appliances) and Part 2 (Dressings) of the Scottish Drug Tariff). (Where it is not appropriate for nurse prescribers in family planning clinics to prescribe contraceptive devices using form FP10(P) (forms WP10CN and WP10PN in Wales), they may prescribe using the same system as doctors in the clinic.)

Incontinence Appliances as listed in Part IXB of the Drug Tariff (Part III of the Northern Ireland Drug Tariff, Part 5 of the Scottish Drug Tariff).

Stoma Appliances and Associated Products as listed in Part IXC of the Drug Tariff (Part III of the Northern Ireland Drug Tariff, Part 6 of the Scottish Drug Tariff).

Chemical Reagents as listed in Part IXR of the Drug Tariff (Part II of the Northern Ireland Drug Tariff, Part 9 of the Scottish Drug Tariff).

The Drug Tariffs can be accessed online at:
National Health Service Drug Tariff for England and Wales:
www.ppa.org.uk/ppa/edt_intro.htm

Health and Social Care, Business Services Organisation, Northern Ireland Drug Tariff:
http://www.hscbusiness.hscni.net/services/2034.htm

Scottish Drug Tariff: www.isdscotland.org/Health-topics/Prescribing-and-Medicines/Scottish-Drug-Tariff/

Details of NPF preparations

Preparations on the Nurse Prescribers' Formulary which are not included in the BP or BPC are described as follows in the Nurse Prescribers' Formulary. Although brand names have sometimes been included for identification purposes, it is recommended that non-proprietary names should be used for prescribing medicinal preparations in the NPF except where a non-proprietary name is not available.

Arachis Oil Enema
arachis oil 100%

Catheter Maintenance Solution, Sodium Chloride
(proprietary products: *OptiFlo S; Uro-Tainer Sodium Chloride; Uriflex-S*), sodium chloride 0.9%

Catheter Maintenance Solution, 'Solution G'
(proprietary products: *OptiFlo G; Uro-Tainer Suby G; Uriflex G*), citric acid 3.23%, magnesium oxide 0.38%, sodium bicarbonate 0.7%, disodium edetate 0.01%

Catheter Maintenance Solution, 'Solution R'
(proprietary products: *OptiFlo R; Uro-Tainer Solution R; Uriflex R*), citric acid 6%, gluconolactone 0.6%, magnesium carbonate 2.8%, disodium edetate 0.01%

Chlorhexidine gluconate alcoholic solutions
(proprietary products: *ChloraPrep; Hydrex Solution; Hydrex spray*), chlorhexidine gluconate in alcoholic solution

Chlorhexidine gluconate aqueous solutions
(proprietary product: *Unisept*), chlorhexidine gluconate in aqueous solution

Co-danthramer Capsules PoM
co-danthramer 25/200 (dantron 25 mg, poloxamer '188' 200 mg)

Co-danthramer Capsules, Strong PoM
co-danthramer 37.5/500 (dantron 37.5 mg, poloxamer '188' 500 mg)

Co-danthramer Oral Suspension PoM
(proprietary product: *Codalax*), co-danthramer 25/200 in 5 mL (dantron 25 mg, poloxamer '188' 200 mg/5 mL)

Co-danthramer Oral Suspension, Strong PoM
(proprietary product: *Codalax Forte*), co-danthramer 75/1000 in 5 mL (dantron 75 mg, poloxamer '188' 1 g/5 mL)

Co-danthrusate Oral Suspension PoM
(proprietary product: *Normax*), co-danthrusate 50/60 (dantron 50 mg, docusate sodium 60 mg/5 mL)

Dimeticone barrier creams
(proprietary products *Conotrane Cream*, dimeticone '350' 22%; *Siopel Barrier Cream*, dimeticone '1000' 10%), dimeticone 10–22%

Dimeticone Lotion
(proprietary product: *Hedrin*), dimeticone 4%

Docusate Enema
(proprietary product: *Norgalax Micro-enema*), docusate sodium 120 mg in 10 g

Liquid and White Soft Paraffin Ointment
liquid paraffin 50%, white soft paraffin 50%

Macrogol Oral Liquid, Compound
(proprietary product: *Movicol Liquid*), macrogol '3350' (polyethylene glycol '3350') 13.125 g, sodium bicarbonate 178.5 mg, sodium chloride 350.7 mg, potassium chloride 46.6 mg/25 mL

Macrogol Oral Powder, Compound
(proprietary products: *Laxido Orange, Molaxole, Movicol*), macrogol '3350' (polyethylene glycol '3350') 13.125 g, sodium bicarbonate 178.5 mg, sodium chloride 350.7 mg, potassium chloride 46.6 mg/sachet; (amount of potassium chloride varies according to flavour of *Movicol®* as follows: plain-flavour (sugar-free) = 50.2 mg/sachet; lime and lemon flavour = 46.6 mg/sachet; chocolate flavour = 31.7 mg/sachet. 1 sachet when reconstituted with 125 mL water provides K^+ 5.4 mmol/litre)

Macrogol Oral Powder, Compound, Half-strength
(proprietary product: *Movicol-Half*), macrogol '3350' (polyethylene glycol '3350') 6.563 g, sodium bicarbonate 89.3 g, sodium chloride 175.4 mg, potassium chloride 23.3 mg/sachet

Malathion aqueous lotions
(proprietary product: *Derbac-M Liquid*), malathion 0.5% in an aqueous basis

Mebendazole Oral Suspension PoM
(proprietary product: *Vermox*), mebendazole 100 mg/5 mL

Nurse Prescribers' Formulary

Mebendazole Tablets PoM
(proprietary products: *Ovex, Vermox*), mebendazole 100 mg
(can be supplied for oral use in the treatment of enterobiasis
in adults and children over 2 years provided its container or
package is labelled to show a max. single dose of 100 mg and
it is supplied in a container or package containing not more
than 800 mg)

Mouthwash Solution-tablets
consist of tablets which may contain antimicrobial,
colouring and flavouring agents in a suitable soluble
effervescent basis to make a mouthwash

Nicotine Inhalation Cartridge for Oromucosal Use
(proprietary products: *NicAssist Inhalator, Nicorette
Inhalator*), nicotine 15 mg (for use with inhalation
mouthpiece; to be prescribed as either a starter pack
(6 cartridges with inhalator device and holder) or refill pack
(42 cartridges with inhalator device))

Nicotine Lozenge
nicotine (as bitartrate) 1 mg or 2 mg (proprietary product:
Nicorette Mint Lozenge, Nicotinell Mint Lozenge), or nicotine
(as resinate) 1.5 mg, 2 mg, or 4 mg (proprietary product:
NiQuitin Lozenges, NiQuitin Minis, NiQuitin Pre-quit)

Nicotine Medicated Chewing Gum
(proprietary products: *NicAssist Gum, Nicorette Gum,
Nicotinell Gum, NiQuitin Gum*), nicotine 2 mg or 4 mg

Nicotine Nasal Spray
(proprietary product: *NicAssist Nasal Spray, Nicorette Nasal
Spray*), nicotine 500 micrograms/metered spray

Nicotine Oral Spray
(proprietary product: *Nicorette Quickmist*), nicotine
1 mg/metered spray

Nicotine Sublingual Tablets
(proprietary product: *NicAssist Microtab, Nicorette Microtab*),
nicotine (as a cyclodextrin complex) 2 mg (to be prescribed
as either a starter pack (2 × 15-tablet discs with dispenser)
or refill pack (7 × 15-tablet discs))

Nicotine Transdermal Patches
releasing in each 16 hours, nicotine approx. 5 mg, 10 mg, or
15 mg (proprietary products: *Boots NicAssist Patch, Nicorette
Patch*), or releasing in each 16 hours approx. 10 mg, 15 mg, or
25 mg (proprietary products: *NicAssist Translucent Patch,
Nicorette Invisi Patch*), or releasing in each 24 hours nicotine
approx. 7 mg, 14 mg, or 21 mg (proprietary products:
Nicopatch, Nicotinell TTS, NiQuitin, NiQuitin Clear)
(prescriber should specify the brand to be dispensed)

Permethrin Cream
(proprietary product: *Lyclear Dermal Cream*), permethrin 5%

Senna Oral Solution
(proprietary product: *Senokot Syrup*), sennosides 7.5 mg/5 mL

Senna and Ispaghula Granules
(proprietary product: *Manevac Granules*), senna fruit 12.4%,
ispaghula 54.2%

Sodium Citrate Compound Enema
(proprietary products: *Micolette Micro-enema; Micralax
Micro-enema; Relaxit Micro-enema*),sodium citrate 450 mg
with glycerol, sorbitol and an anionic surfactant

Sodium Picosulfate Capsules
(proprietary products: *Dulcolax Perles*), sodium picosulfate
2.5 mg

Sodium Picosulfate Elixir
(proprietary product: *Dulcolax Liquid*), sodium picosulfate
5 mg/5 mL

Sterculia Granules
(proprietary product: *Normacol Granules*), sterculia 62%

Sterculia and Frangula Granules
(proprietary product: *Normacol Plus Granules*), sterculia 62%,
frangula (standardised) 8%

Zinc Oxide and Dimeticone Spray
(proprietary product: *Sprilon*), dimeticone 1.04%, zinc oxide
12.5% in a pressurised aerosol unit

Zinc Oxide Impregnated Medicated Bandage
(proprietary product: *Steripaste*), sterile cotton bandage
impregnated with paste containing zinc oxide 15%

Zinc Oxide Impregnated Medicated Stocking
(proprietary product: *Zipzoc*), sterile rayon stocking
impregnated with ointment containing zinc oxide 20%

Non-medical prescribing

Overview

A range of non-medical healthcare professionals can prescribe medicines for patients as either Independent or Supplementary Prescribers.

Independent prescribers are practitioners responsible and accountable for the assessment of patients with previously undiagnosed or diagnosed conditions and for decisions about the clinical management required, including prescribing. They are recommended to prescribe generically, except where this would not be clinically appropriate or where there is no approved non-proprietary name.

Supplementary prescribing is a partnership between an independent prescriber (a doctor or a dentist) and a supplementary prescriber to implement an agreed Clinical Management Plan for an individual patient with that patient's agreement.

Independent and Supplementary Prescribers are identified by an annotation next to their name in the relevant professional register.

Information and guidance on non-medical prescribing is available on the Department of Health website at www.dh.gov.uk/health/2012/04/prescribing-change.

For information on the mixing of medicines by Independent and Supplementary Prescribers, see *Mixing of medicines prior to administration in clinical practice— responding to legislative changes*, National Prescribing Centre, May 2010 (available at www.npc.nhs.uk/improving_safety/ mixing_meds/resources/mixing_of_medicines.pdf).

For information on the supply and administration of medicines to groups of patients using Patient Group Directions see Guidance on prescribing p. 1.

Nurses

Nurse Independent Prescribers (formerly known as Extended Formulary Nurse Prescribers) are able to prescribe any medicine for any medical condition.

Nurse Independent Prescribers are able to prescribe, administer, and give directions for the administration of Schedule 2, 3, 4, and 5 Controlled Drugs. This extends to diamorphine, dipipanone, or cocaine for treating organic disease or injury, but not for treating addiction.

Nurse Independent Prescribers must work within their own level of professional competence and expertise.

The Nurse Prescribers' Formulary for Community Practitioners p. 1396 provides information on prescribing.

Pharmacists

Pharmacist Independent Prescribers can prescribe any medicine for any medical condition.

They are also able to prescribe, administer, and give directions for the administration of Schedule 2, 3, 4, and 5 Controlled Drugs. This extends to diamorphine, dipipanone, or cocaine for treating organic disease or injury, but not for treating addiction.

Pharmacist Independent Prescribers must work within their own level of professional competence and expertise.

Optometrists

Optometrist Independent Prescribers can prescribe any licensed medicine for ocular conditions affecting the eye and the tissues surrounding the eye, except Controlled Drugs or medicines for parenteral administration. Optometrist Independent Prescribers must work within their own level of professional competence and expertise.

Index of proprietary manufacturers

Alphabetical list of manufacturers and other companies

The following is an alphabetical list of manufacturers and other companies referenced in the BNF, with their medicines information or general contact details. For information on 'special-order' manufacturers and specialist importing companies see 'Special-order manufacturers'.

3M Health Care Ltd, Tel: (01509) 611 611

Allen & Hanburys Ltd, Tel: 0800 221 441, customercontactuk@gsk.com

A1 Pharmaceuticals Plc, Tel: (01708) 528 900, sales@a1plc.co.uk

Abbott, Tel: (01628) 773 355

Abbott Healthcare Products Ltd, Tel: (01628) 773 355, medinfo.shl@abbott.com

Abbot Medical Optics, Tel: 0800 376 7950

AbbVie Ltd, Tel: (01628) 561 090, ukmedinfo@abbvie.com

Abraxis BioScience Ltd, Tel: (020) 7081 0850, abraxismedical@idispharma.com

Acorus Therapeutics Ltd, Tel: (01244) 625 152

Actavis UK Ltd, Tel: (01271) 311 257, medinfo@actavis.co.uk

Actelion Pharmaceuticals UK Ltd, Tel: (020) 8987 3333, medinfo_uk@actelion.com

Activa Healthcare, Tel: 0845 060 6707, advice@activahealthcare.co.uk

Adienne Pharma and Biotech, Tel: 0039 (0) 335 873 8731

ADI Medical UK, Tel: (01628) 485159, info@adimedical.co.uk

Advanced Medical Solutions Group Plc, Tel: (01606) 863 500

Advancis Medical Ltd, Tel: (01623) 751 500, info@advancis.co.uk

Advantech Surgical Ltd, Tel: 0845 130 5866, customerservice@newgel.co.uk

Aegerion Pharmaceuticals Ltd, Tel: 00800 2343 7466, medinfo.emea@aegerion.com

AgaMatrix Europe Ltd, Tel: (01235) 838 639, info@wavesense.co.uk

Agepha GmbH, Tel: (020) 3239 6241, uk@agepha.com

Aguettant Ltd, Tel: (01934) 835 694, info@aguettant.co.uk

Air Products plc, Tel: 0800 373 580

Alan Pharmaceuticals, Tel: (020) 7284 2887, info@alanpharmaceuticals.com

Alcon Laboratories (UK) Ltd, Tel: 0345 266 9363, gbmedicaldepartment@alcon.com

Alexion Pharma UK Ltd, Tel: (01932) 359 220, alexion.uk@alxn.com

Alimera Sciences Limited, Tel: 0800 019 1253, medicalinformation@alimerasciences.com

Alissa Healthcare, Tel: (01489) 80 759, enquiries@alissahealthcare.com

ALK-Abelló (UK) Ltd, Tel: (0118) 903 7940, info@uk.alk-abello.com

Alkopharma Sarl, Tel: (0041) 277 206 969, regulatory@alkopharma.com

Allergan Ltd, Tel: (01628) 494 026

Allergy Therapeutics Ltd, Tel: (01903) 844 702

Alliance Pharmaceuticals Ltd, Tel: (01249) 466 966, info@alliancepharma.co.uk

Almirall Ltd, Tel: 0800 008 7399, medinfouk@almirall.com

Altacor Ltd, Tel: (01223) 421 411, info@altacor-pharma.com

Amdipharm Mercury Company Ltd, Tel: 08700 70 30 33, medicalinformation@amcolimited.com

Amgen Ltd, Tel: (01223) 420 305, gbinfoline@amgen.com

Amred Healthcare Ltd, Tel: (0330) 333 0079, info@amredhealthcare.com

Apollo Medical Technologies Ltd, Tel: (01636) 831 201, supercheck2@btinternet.com

Archimed, Tel: 0800 756 9951, enquiries@archimed.co.uk

Archimedes Pharma UK Ltd, Tel: (0118) 931 5094, medicalinformationuk@archimedespharma.com

Arctic Medical Ltd, Tel: (01303) 277 751, sales@arcticmedical.co.uk

Ardana Bioscience Ltd, Tel: (0131) 226 8550

ARIAD Pharma UK Ltd, Tel: 0800 0002 7423, eumedinfo@ariad.com

Ark Therapeutics Group Plc, Tel: (020) 7388 7722, info@arktherapeutics.com

Aspen, Tel: 0800 008 7392, aspenmedinfo@professionalinformation.co.uk

Aspen Medical Europe Ltd, Tel: (01527) 587 728, customers@aspenmedicaleurope.com

AS Pharma Ltd, Tel: 0870 066 4117, info@aspharma.co.uk

Aspire Pharma Ltd, Tel: (01730) 231 148, info@aspirepharma.co.uk

Astellas Pharma Ltd, Tel: (020) 3379 8000, medinfo.gb@astellas.com

AstraZeneca UK Ltd, Tel: 0800 783 0033, medical.information@astrazeneca.com

Auden Mckenzie (Pharma Division) Ltd, Tel: (01895) 627 420

Auxilium, Tel: 0845 017 2315, auxilium@pilglobal.com

Axcan Pharma SA, Tel: (0033) 130 461 900

AYMES International Ltd, Tel: 0845 6805 496, info@aymes.com

Ayrton Saunders Ltd, Tel: (0151) 709 2074, info@ayrtons.com

BAP Medical UK Ltd, Tel: 0844 879 7689

Bard Ltd, Tel: (01293) 527 888

Basilea Pharmaceuticals Ltd, Tel: (01483) 790 023, ukmedinfo@basilea.com

Bausch & Lomb UK Ltd, Tel: (01748) 828 864, medicalinformationuk@bausch.com

Baxter Healthcare Ltd, Tel: (01635) 206 345, surecall@baxter.com

Bayer Healthcare Pharmaceuticals, Tel: (01635) 563 000, medical.information@bayer.co.uk

BBI Healthcare, Tel: (01792) 229 333, info@bbihealthcare.com

B. Braun Medical Ltd, Tel: (0114) 225 9000, info.bbmuk@bbraun.com

Beacon Pharmaceuticals Ltd, Tel: (01892) 600 930, info@beaconpharma.co.uk

Beiersdorf UK Ltd, Tel: (0121) 329 8800

Besins Healthcare (UK) Ltd, Tel: (01748) 828 789, information@besins-healthcare.com

BHR Pharmaceuticals Ltd, Tel: (024) 7637 7210, info@bhr.co.uk

Biogen Idec Ltd, Tel: 0800 008 7401

Biolitec Pharma Ltd, Tel: (00353) 1463 7415

BioMarin Europe Ltd, Tel: (020) 7420 0800, biomarin-europe@bmrn.com

BioMonde, Tel: 0845 230 1810, info@biomonde.com

Biotest (UK) Ltd, Tel: (0121) 733 3393, medicinesinformation@biotestuk.com

Blackwell Supplies Ltd, Tel: (01634) 877 620

BOC Medical, Tel: 0800 111 333

Boehringer Ingelheim Ltd, Tel: (01344) 424 600, medinfo@bra.boehringer-ingelheim.com

The Boots Company PLC, Tel: (0115) 959 5165

BPC 100 Ltd, Tel: 01942 852085

Bio Products Laboratory Ltd, Tel: (020) 8957 2255, medinfo@bpl.co.uk

Bray Healthcare, Tel: (01367) 240 736, info@bray-healthcare.com

Bristol-Myers Squibb Pharmaceuticals Ltd, Tel: (01895) 523 000, medical.information@bms.com

Britannia Pharmaceuticals, Tel: 0870 851 0207, enquiries@medinformation.co.uk

BSN Medical Ltd, Tel: 0845 122 3600

BTG International Ltd, Tel: (0207) 575 0000, medical.services@btgplc.com

Bullen Healthcare, Tel: 0800 269 327

Cambridge Medical Aesthetics Ltd, Tel: (01733) 396171, info@cambridgemedicalaesthetics.com

Cambridge Sensors Ltd, Tel: (01480) 482 920, sales-orders@cs-limited.co.uk

CareFusion UK 244 Ltd, Tel: 0800 043 7546, enquiries@chloraprep.co.uk

Casen-Fleet, Tel: (0034) 913 518 800

C D Medical Ltd, Tel: (01942) 816 184

Celgene Ltd, Tel: 0844 801 0045, medinfo.uk.ire@celgene.com

Chanelle Medical UK Ltd, Tel: (01233) 822 297

Chattem UK Ltd, Tel: (01256) 844 144

Chefaro UK Ltd, Tel: (01748) 828 860, info@omegapharma.co.uk

Chemidex Pharma Ltd, Tel: (01784) 477 167, info@chemidex.co.uk

C. H. Fox Ltd, Tel: (020) 7240 3111

Chiesi Ltd, Tel: (0161) 488 5555, medinfo.uk@chiesi.com

Cambridge Healthcare Supplies Ltd, Tel: (01953) 607 856, customerservices@cambridge-healthcare.co.uk

Chugai Pharma UK Ltd, Tel: (020) 8987 5680

Clement Clarke International Ltd, Tel: (01279) 414 969, resp@clement-clarke.com

Clinigen Group Plc, Tel: (01748) 828 375, clinigeneu@professionalinformation.co.uk

CliniMed Ltd, Tel: (01628) 535 250

Clinisupplies Ltd, Tel: (020) 8863 4168, info@clinisupplies.co.uk

Colgate-Palmolive Ltd, Tel: (01483) 302 222

Coloplast Ltd, Tel: (01733) 392 000

Community Foods Ltd, Tel: (020) 8450 9411, email@communityfoods.co.uk

Complan Foods Ltd, Tel: (020) 7395 7565

Consilient Health UK Ltd, Tel: (020) 8956 2310, drugsafety@consilienthealth.com

ConvaTec Ltd, Tel: (01895) 628 400

Co-Pharma Ltd, Tel: 0870 851 0207

Correvio GmbH, Tel: (020) 3002 8114, info@correvio.com

Covidien UK Commercial Ltd, Tel: (01329) 224 226

Cow & Gate, Tel: 0845 762 3624

Cranage Healthcare Ltd, Tel: (01477) 549 392, db@cranagehealth.com

Crawford Healthcare Ltd, Tel: (01565) 654 920

Crescent Pharma, Tel: (01256) 772 730, info@crescentpharma.com

Crucell (UK) Ltd, Tel: 0844 800 3907, info@crucell.co.uk

CSL Behring UK Ltd, Tel: (01444) 447 400, medinfo@cslbehring.com

CTI Life Sciences Ltd, Tel: (01628) 643 974

Daiichi Sankyo UK Ltd, Tel: (01753) 482 771, medinfo@daiichi-sankyo.co.uk

Danetre Health Products Ltd, Tel: (01327) 310 909, enquiries@danetrehealthproducts.com

DDD Ltd, Tel: (01923) 229 251

Dee Pharmaceuticals Ltd, Tel: (01978) 661993, enquiries@deepharmaceuticalsltd.co.uk

Dental Health Products Ltd, Tel: (01622) 749 222

Dentsply Ltd, Tel: (01932) 837 279

Derma Pharma Ltd, Tel: (01462) 733 500, info@dermauk.co.uk

Derma Sciences Europe Ltd, Tel: (01628) 625 916, cs@dermasciences.com

Derma UK Ltd, Tel: (01462) 733 500, info@dermauk.co.uk

Dermal Laboratories Ltd, Tel: (01462) 458 866

Dermato Logical Ltd, Tel: (0208) 449 2931, enquiries@aqua-max.co.uk

Dermatonics Ltd, Tel: (01480) 462 910, sales@dermatonics.co.uk

Desitin Pharma Ltd, Tel: (01483) 688 240, medinfo@desitin.co.uk

DeVilbiss Healthcare UK Ltd, Tel: (01384) 446 688

Dexcel-Pharma Ltd, Tel: (01327) 312 266, office@dexcelpharma.co.uk

DHP Healthcare Ltd, Tel: (01622) 749 222, sales@dhphealthcare.co.uk

DiME, Tel: (01483) 715 008, info@dime-med.com

Dreamskin Health Ltd, Tel: (01707) 228 688

Dr Falk Pharma UK Ltd, Tel: (01628) 536 600

Drossa Ltd, Tel: (020) 3393 0859, info@drossa.co.uk

Durbin plc, Tel: (020) 8869 6500, info@durbin.co.uk

T G Eakin, Tel: (028) 9187 1000, mail@eakin.co.uk

Easigrip Ltd, Tel: (01926) 497 108, enquiry@easigrip.co.uk

Ecolab UK, Tel: (0113) 232 0066, info.healthcare@ecolab.co.uk

Egis Pharmaceuticals UK Ltd, Tel: (020) 7266 2669, enquiries@medimpexuk.com

Eisai Ltd, Tel: (020) 8600 1400, eumedinfo@eisai.net

Encysive (UK) Ltd, Tel: (01895) 876 168

Entra Health Systems, Tel: (0113) 815 5108

Espere Healthcare Ltd, Tel: (01462) 346 100, info@esperehealth.co.uk

Essential Pharmaceuticals Ltd, Tel: (01784) 477 167, info@essentialpharmaceuticals.com

Ethicon Ltd, Tel: (01506) 594 500

Eumedica S.A., Tel: (020) 8444 3377, enquiries@eumedica.com

European Pharma Group, Tel: 0031 (0) 20 316 0140, info@insujet.com

EUSA Pharma (Europe) Ltd, Tel: (01438) 740 720, medinfo-uk@eusapharma.com

Pierre Fabre Ltd, Tel: (01962) 874 435, medicalinformation@pierre-fabre.co.uk

Fate Special Foods, Tel: (01215) 224 433

Fenton Pharmaceuticals Ltd, Tel: (020) 7224 1388, mail@fent-pharm.co.uk

Ferndale Pharmaceuticals Ltd, Tel: (01937) 541 122, info@ferndalepharma.co.uk

Ferring Pharmaceuticals (UK), Tel: 0844 931 0050, medical@ferring.com

Finox Biotech AG, Tel: 00 800 3466 9246, finoxEY@piglobal.cpm

Firstplay Dietary Foods Ltd, Tel: (0161) 474 7576

Flynn Pharma Ltd, Tel: (01438) 727 822, medinfo@flynnpharma.com

Focus Pharmaceuticals Ltd, Tel: (01283) 495 280, medinfo@focuspharma.co.uk

Foodlink (UK) Ltd, Tel: (01752) 344 544, info@foodlinkltd.co.uk

Ford Medical Associates Ltd, Tel: (01233) 633 224, enquiries@fordmedical.co.uk

Forest Laboratories UK Ltd, Tel: (01322) 421 800, medinfo@forest-labs.co.uk

Forum Health Products Ltd, Tel: (01737) 857 700, enquiries@forumgroup.co.uk

Fresenius Biotech GmbH, Tel: 0049 (0) 893 065 9311, med.info@fresenius-biotech.com

Fresenius Kabi Ltd, Tel: (01928) 533 533, med.info-uk@fresenius-kabi.com

Fresenius Medical Care UK Ltd, Tel: (01623) 445 171, medinfo-uk@fmc-ag.com

Frontier Multigate, Tel: (01495) 233 050, multigate@frontier-group.co.uk

Fyne Dynamics Ltd, Tel: (01279) 423 423, info@fyne-dynamics.com

Galderma (UK) Ltd, Tel: (01923) 208 950, medinfo.uk@galderma.com

Galen Ltd, Tel: (028) 3833 4974, customer.services@galen.co.uk

Gedeon Richter UK Ltd, Tel: (020) 7604 8806, drugsafety.uk@gedeonrichter.eu

GE Healthcare, Tel: (01494) 544 000

Geistlich Pharma, Tel: (01244) 347 534

General Dietary Ltd, Tel: (0203) 044 2933, info@generaldietary.com

Genius Foods Ltd, Tel: 0845 874 4000, info@geniusglutenfree.com

Genus Pharmaceuticals, Tel: (01635) 568 400, info@genuspharma.com

Genzyme Therapeutics, Tel: (01865) 405 200, ukmedinfo@genzyme.com

GF Foods Ltd, Tel: (01757) 289 207, admin@gffdirect.co.uk

Gilead Sciences Ltd, Tel: 0800 011 3700, ukmedinfo@gilead.com

Glenwood GmbH, Tel: (0049) 815 199 8790, info@glenwood.de

GlucoRx Ltd, Tel: (01483) 755 133, info@glucorx.co.uk

Gluten Free Foods Ltd, Tel: (020) 8953 4444, info@glutenfree-foods.co.uk

Grifols UK Ltd, Tel: (01223) 395 700, medinfo.uk@grifols.com

Grünenthal Ltd, Tel: 0870 351 8960, medicalinformationuk@grunenthal.com

GlaxoSmithKline, Tel: 0800 221 441, customercontactuk@gsk.com

GlaxoSmithKline Consumer Healthcare, Tel: (020) 8047 2500, customer.relations@gsk.com

H&R Healthcare Ltd, Tel: (01482) 631 606, info@hrhealthcare.co.uk

Paul Hartmann Ltd, Tel: (01706) 363 200, info@uk.hartmann.info

Henleys Medical Supplies Ltd, Tel: (01707) 333 164

Hennig Arzneimittel GmbH & Co., Tel: 0844 504 0866

HFA Healthcare Ltd, Tel: 0844 335 8270

HK Pharma Ltd, Tel: 0845 519 1609

Hollister Ltd, Tel: (0118) 989 5000

Hospira UK Ltd, Tel: 0800 088 5133, hospirami@pi-arm.co.uk

HRA Pharma UK & Ireland Ltd, Tel: 0800 917 9548, med.info.uk@hra-pharma.com

Huntleigh Healthcare Ltd, Tel: (01582) 413 104

Huxley Europe Ltd, Tel: (0161) 773 0485

Idis Ltd, Tel: (01932) 824 000, mi@idispharma.com

iMed Systems Ltd, Tel: (0203) 397 8020, emerade@imed-systems.com

INCA-Pharm UK, Tel: (01748) 828 812, info@inca-pharm.com

Infai UK Ltd, Tel: (01904) 435 228, info@infai.co.uk

Injex UK Ltd, Tel: 0845 126 8900, enquiries@injexuk.com

Innovative Solutions UK Ltd, Tel: (01706) 746 713, enquiries@innovative-solutions.org.uk

Insight Medical Products Ltd, Tel: (01666) 500 055, info@insightmedical.ne

InterMune, Tel: (03308) 080 960, med-info@intermune.co.uk

Internis Pharmaceuticals Ltd, Tel: (020) 8346 5588, regulatory@jensongroup.com

Intrapharm Laboratories Ltd, Tel: (01628) 771 800, sales@intrapharmlabs.com

Ipsen Ltd, Tel: (01753) 627 777, medical.information.uk@ipsen.com

Warner Chilcott UK Ltd, Tel: (01932) 824 700

Welsh Blood Service, Tel: (01443) 622 000, donor.care@wales.nhs.uk

Wellfoods Ltd, Tel: (01226) 381 712, wellfoods@wellfoods.co.uk

Williams Medical Supplies Ltd, Tel: (01685) 844 739

Wockhardt UK Ltd, Tel: (01978) 661 261

Wyeth Pharmaceuticals, Tel: (01628) 604 377, eumedinfo@pfizer.com

Wynlit Laboratories, Tel: (07903) 370 130

Wyvern Medical Ltd, Tel: (01531) 631 105

Zentiva, Tel: (01483) 554 101, gb-zentivamedicalinformation@sanofi.com

Zeroderma Ltd, Tel: (01858) 525 643

Special-order manufacturers

Unlicensed medicines are available from 'special-order' manufacturers and specialist-importing companies; the MHRA maintains a register of these companies at tinyurl.com/cdslke.

Licensed **hospital manufacturing units** also manufacture 'special-order' products as unlicensed medicines, the principal NHS units are listed below. A database (*Pro-File*; www.pro-file.nhs.uk) provides information on medicines manufactured in the NHS; access is restricted to NHS pharmacy staff.

The Association of Pharmaceutical Specials Manufacturers may also be able to provide further information about commercial companies (www.apsm.com).

The MHRA recommends that an unlicensed medicine should only be used when a patient has special requirements that cannot be met by use of a licensed medicine.

As well as being available direct from the hospital manufacturer(s) concerned, many NHS-manufactured Specials may be bought from the Oxford Pharmacy Store, owned and operated by Oxford Health NHS Foundation Trust.

England

London

Barts and the London NHS Trust
Mr J. A. Rickard, Head of Barts Health Pharmaceuticals
Barts Health NHS Trust
The Royal London Hospital
Pathology and Pharmacy Building
80 Newark St
Whitechapel
London
E1 2ES
(020) 3246 0394 (order/enquiry)
barts.pharmaceuticals@bartshealth.nhs.uk

Guy's and St. Thomas' NHS Foundation Trust
Mr P. Forsey, Associate Chief Pharmacist
Guy's and St. Thomas' NHS Foundation Trust
Guy's Hospital
Pharmacy Department
Great Maze Pond
London
SE1 9RT
(020) 7188 4992 (order)
(020) 7188 5003 (enquiry)
Fax: (020) 7188 5013
paul.forsey@gstt.nhs.uk

Moorfields Pharmaceuticals
Mr. T. Record, Technical Director
Moorfields Pharmaceuticals
25 Provost St
London
N1 7NH
(020) 7684 9090 (order/enquiry)
Fax: (020) 7502 2332

London North West Healthcare NHS Trust
Mr K. Wong,
London North West Healthcare NHS Trust
Northwick Park Hospital
Watford Rd
Harrow
Middlesex
HA1 3UJ
(020) 8869 2295 (order)
(020) 8869 2204/2223 (enquiry)
kwong@nhs.net

Royal Free Hampstead NHS Trust
Ms C. Trehane, Production Manager
Royal Free Hampstead NHS Trust
Pond St
London
NW3 2QG
(020) 7830 2424 (order)
(020) 7830 2282 (enquiry)
Fax: (020) 7794 1875
christine.trehane@nhs.net

St George's Healthcare NHS Trust
Mr V. Kumar, Assistant Chief Pharmacist
St George's Hospital
Technical Services
Blackshaw Rd
Tooting
London
SW17 0QT
(020) 8725 1770/1768
Fax: (020) 8725 3947
vinodh.kumar@stgeorges.nhs.uk

University College Hospital NHS Foundation Trust
Mr T. Murphy, Production Manager
University College Hospital
235 Euston Rd
London
NW1 2BU
(020) 7380 9723 (order)
(020) 7380 9472 (enquiry)
Fax: (020) 7380 9726
tony.murphy@uclh.nhs.uk

Midlands and Eastern

Barking, Havering and Redbridge University Trust
Mr N. Fisher, Senior Principal Pharmacist
Queen's Hospital
Pharmacy Department
Romford
Essex
RM7 0AG
(01708) 435 463 (order)
(01708) 435 042 (enquiry)
neil.fisher@bhrhospitals.nhs.uk

Burton Hospitals NHS Foundation Trust
Mr D. Raynor, Head of Pharmacy Manufacturing Unit
Queens Hospital
Burton Hospitals NHS Foundation Trust
Pharmacy Manufacturing Unit
Belvedere Rd
Burton-on-Trent
DE13 0RB
(01283) 511 511 ext: 5275 (order/enquiry)
Fax: (01283) 593 036
david.raynor@burtonft.nhs.uk

Colchester Hospital University NHS Foundation Trust
Mr S. Pullen, Pharmacy Production Manager
Colchester General Hospital
Main Pharmacy
Turner Rd
Colchester
Essex
CO4 5JL
(01206) 742 007 (order)
(01206) 744 208 (enquiry)
Fax: (01206) 841 249
pharmacy.stores@colchesterhospital.nhs.uk (order)
psu.enquiries@colchesterhospital.nhs.uk (enquiry)

Ipswich Hospital NHS Trust
Dr J. Harwood, Production Manager
Ipswich Hospital NHS Trust
Pharmacy Manufacturing Unit
Heath Rd
Ipswich
IP4 5PD
(01473) 703 440 (order)
(01473) 703 603 (enquiry)
Fax: (01473) 703 609
john.harwood@ipswichhospital.nhs.uk

Nottingham University Hospitals NHS Trust
Mr J. Graham, Senior Pharmacist, Production
Nottingham University Hospitals NHS Trust
Pharmacy Production Units
Queens Medical Centre Campus
Nottingham
NG7 2UH
(0115) 924 9924 ext: 66521 (enquiry/order)
Fax: (0115) 970 9780
jeff.graham@nuh.nhs.uk

University Hospital of North Staffordshire NHS Trust
Ms K. Ferguson, Chief Technician
University Hospital of North Staffordshire NHS Trust
Pharmacy Technical Services
City General Site
Stoke-on-Trent
ST4 6QG
(01782) 674 568 (order)
(01782) 674 568 (enquiry)
Fax: (01782) 674 575
caroline.ferguson@uhns.nhs.uk

North East

The Newcastle upon Tyne Hospitals NHS Foundation Trust
Mr Y. Hunter-Blair, Production Manager
Royal Victoria Infirmary
Newcastle Specials
Pharmacy Production Unit
Queen Victoria Rd
Newcastle-upon-Tyne
NE1 4LP
(0191) 282 0395 (order)
(0191) 282 0389 (enquiry)
Fax: (0191) 282 0469
yan.hunter-blair@nuth.nhs.uk

North West

Preston Pharmaceuticals

Ms A. Bolch, Deputy Chief Pharmacist (PMU)
Preston Pharmaceuticals
Royal Preston Hospital
Fulwood
Preston
PR2 9HT
(01772) 523 617 (order)
(01772) 522 593 (enquiry)
Fax: (01772) 523 645
angela.bolch@lthtr.nhs.uk

Stockport Pharmaceuticals

Mr A. Singleton, Head of Production
Stepping Hill Hospital
Stockport NHS Foundation Trust
Stockport Pharmaceuticals
Stockport
SK2 7JE
(0161) 419 5666 (order)
(0161) 419 5657 (enquiry)
Fax: (0161) 419 5426
andrew.singleton@stockport.nhs.uk

South

Portsmouth Hospitals NHS Trust

Mr R. Lucas, Product Development Manager
Portsmouth Hospitals NHS Trust
Pharmacy Manufacturing Unit
Unit D2, Railway Triangle Industrial Estate
Walton Road
Farlington
Portsmouth
PO6 1TF
(02392) 389 078 (order)
(02392) 316 312 (enquiry)
Fax: (02392) 316 316
robert.lucas@porthosp.nhs.uk

South East

East Sussex Healthcare NHS Trust

Mr P. Keen, Business Manager
Eastbourne District General Hospital
East Sussex Hospitals NHS Trust
Eastbourne Pharmaceuticals
Kings Drive
Eastbourne
BN21 2UD
(01323) 414 906 (order)
(01323) 417 400 ext: 3076 (enquiry)
Fax: (01323) 414 931
paul.keen@esht.nhs.uk

South West

Torbay PMU

Mr P. Bendell, Pharmacy Manufacturing
Services Manager
South Devon Healthcare NHS Foundation Trust
Torbay PMU
Kemmings Close, Long Rd
Paignton
TQ4 7TW
(01803) 664 707
Fax: (01803) 664 354
phil.bendell@nhs.net

Yorkshire

Calderdale and Huddersfield NHS Foundation Trust

Dr B. Grewal, Managing Director
Calderdale and Huddersfield NHS Foundation Trust
Huddersfield Pharmacy Specials
Gate 2 - Acre Mills, School St West
Huddersfield
HD3 3ET
(01484) 355 388 (order/enquiry)
info.hps@cht.nhs.uk

Northern Ireland

Victoria Pharmaceuticals

Mr S. Cameron, Production Manager - Pharmacy
Victoria Pharmaceuticals
Royal Hospitals
Plenum Building
Grosvenor Road
Belfast
BT12 6BA
(028) 9063 0070 (order/enquiry)
Fax: (028) 9063 5282 (order/enquiry)
samuel.cameron@belfasttrust.hscni.net

Scotland

NHS Greater Glasgow and Clyde

Mr G. Conkie, Production Manager
Western Infirmary
Dumbarton Rd
Glasgow
G11 6NT
(0141) 211 2754 (order)
(0141) 211 2882 (enquiry)
Fax: (0141) 211 1967
graham.conkie@ggc.scot.nhs.uk

Tayside Pharmaceuticals

Mr S. Bath, Production Manager
Ninewells Hospital
Tayside Pharmaceuticals
Dundee
DD1 9SY
(01382) 632 052 (order)
(01382) 632 273 (enquiry)
Fax: (01382) 632 060
sbath@nhs.net

Wales

Cardiff and Vale University Health Board

Mr P. Spark, Principal Pharmacist (Production)
Cardiff and Vale University Health Board
20 Fieldway
Cardiff
CF14 4HY
(029) 2074 8120
Fax: (029) 2074 8130
paul.spark@wales.nhs.uk

Index

C

BNF

YellowCard
COMMISSION ON HUMAN MEDICINES (CHM)

It's easy to report online at:
www.mhra.gov.uk/yellowcard

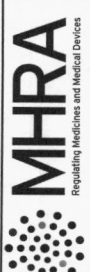

MHRA
Regulating Medicines and Medical Devices

REPORT OF SUSPECTED ADVERSE DRUG REACTIONS

If you suspect an adverse reaction may be related to one or more drugs/vaccines/complementary remedies, please complete this Yellow Card. See 'Adverse reactions to drugs' section in BNF or **www.mhra.gov.uk/yellowcard** for guidance. Do not be put off reporting because some details are not known.

PATIENT DETAILS

Patient Initials:＿＿＿＿   Sex: M / F   Is the patient pregnant? Y / N   Ethnicity:＿＿＿＿

Age (at time of reaction):＿＿＿＿   Weight (kg):＿＿＿＿   Identification number (e.g. Practice or Hospital Ref):＿＿＿＿

SUSPECTED DRUG(S)/VACCINE(S)

Drug/Vaccine (Brand if known)	Batch	Route	Dosage	Date started	Date stopped	Prescribed for

SUSPECTED REACTION(S)
Please describe the reaction(s) and any treatment given. (Please attach additional pages if necessary):

Outcome

☐ Recovered

☐ Recovering

☐ Continuing

☐ Other

Date reaction(s) started:＿＿＿＿   Date reaction(s) stopped:＿＿＿＿

Do you consider the reactions to be serious?   Yes / No

If yes, please indicate why the reaction is considered to be serious (please tick all that apply):

☐ Patient died due to reaction   ☐ Involved or prolonged inpatient hospitalisation

☐ Life threatening   ☐ Involved persistent or significant disability or incapacity

☐ Congenital abnormality   ☐ Medically significant; please give details:＿＿＿＿

If the reactions were not serious according to the categories above, how bad was the suspected reaction?

☐ Mild   ☐ Unpleasant, but did not affect everyday activities   ☐ Bad enough to affect everyday activities

It's easy to report online: www.mhra.gov.uk/yellowcard

OTHER DRUG(S) (including self-medication and complementary remedies)

Did the patient take any other medicines/vaccines/complementary remedies in the last 3 months prior to the reaction? Yes / No

If yes, please give the following information if known:

Drug/Vaccine (Brand if known)	Batch	Route	Dosage	Date started	Date stopped	Prescribed for

Additional relevant information e.g. medical history, test results, known allergies, rechallenge (if performed). For reactions relating to use of a medicine during pregnancy please state all other drugs taken during pregnancy, the last menstrual period, information on previous pregnancies, ultrasound scans, any delivery complications, birth defects or developmental concerns.

Please list any medicines obtained from the internet:

REPORTER DETAILS
Name and Professional Address:

Postcode: _____ Tel No: _____
Email: _____
Speciality: _____
Signature: _____ Date: _____

CLINICAN (if not the reporter)
Name and Professional Address:

Postcode: _____ Tel No: _____
Email: _____
Speciality: _____
Date: _____

Information on adverse drug reactions received by the MHRA can be downloaded at www.mhra.gov.uk/daps
Stay up-to-date on the latest advice for the safe use of medicines with our monthly bulletin *Drug Safety Update* at: www.mhra.gov.uk/drugsafetyupdate

Please attach additional pages if necessary. Send to: FREEPOST YELLOW CARD (no other address details required)

YellowCard

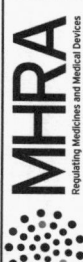

COMMISSION ON HUMAN MEDICINES (CHM)

It's easy to report online at:

www.mhra.gov.uk/yellowcard

MHRA Regulating Medicines and Medical Devices

REPORT OF SUSPECTED ADVERSE DRUG REACTIONS

If you suspect an adverse reaction may be related to one or more drugs/vaccines/complementary remedies, please complete this Yellow Card. See 'Adverse reactions to drugs' section in BNF or **www.mhra.gov.uk/yellowcard** for guidance. Do not be put off reporting because some details are not known.

PATIENT DETAILS

Patient Initials: _____   Sex: M / F   Is the patient pregnant? Y / N   Ethnicity: _____

Age (at time of reaction): _____   Weight (kg): _____   Identification number (e.g. Practice or Hospital Ref): _____

SUSPECTED DRUG(S)/VACCINE(S)

Drug/Vaccine (Brand if known)	Batch	Route	Dosage	Date started	Date stopped	Prescribed for

SUSPECTED REACTION(S)

Please describe the reaction(s) and any treatment given. (Please attach additional pages if necessary):

Outcome

Recovered ☐

Recovering ☐

Continuing ☐

Other ☐

Date reaction(s) started: _____   Date reaction(s) stopped: _____

Do you consider the reactions to be serious?   Yes / No

If yes, please indicate why the reaction is considered to be serious (please tick all that apply):

☐ Patient died due to reaction   ☐ Involved or prolonged inpatient hospitalisation

☐ Life threatening   ☐ Involved persistent or significant disability or incapacity

☐ Congenital abnormality   ☐ Medically significant; please give details: _____

If the reactions were not serious according to the categories above, how bad was the suspected reaction?

☐ Mild   ☐ Unpleasant, but did not affect everyday activities   ☐ Bad enough to affect everyday activities

It's easy to report online: www.mhra.gov.uk/yellowcard

OTHER DRUG(S) (including self-medication and complementary remedies)

Did the patient take any other medicines/vaccines/complementary remedies in the last 3 months prior to the reaction? Yes / No

If yes, please give the following information if known:

Drug/Vaccine (Brand if known)	Batch	Route	Dosage	Date started	Date stopped	Prescribed for

Additional relevant information e.g. medical history, test results, known allergies, rechallenge (if performed). For reactions relating to use of a medicine during pregnancy please state all other drugs taken during pregnancy, the last menstrual period, information on previous pregnancies, ultrasound scans, any delivery complications, birth defects or developmental concerns.

Please list any medicines obtained from the internet:

REPORTER DETAILS
Name and Professional Address:

Postcode: _____ Tel No: _____
Email:
Speciality:
Signature: _____ Date: _____

CLINICIAN (if not the reporter)
Name and Professional Address:

Postcode: _____ Tel No: _____
Email:
Speciality:
Date:

Information on adverse drug reactions received by the MHRA can be downloaded at **www.mhra.gov.uk/daps**

Stay up-to-date on the latest advice for the safe use of medicines with our monthly bulletin *Drug Safety Update* at: **www.mhra.gov.uk/drugsafetyupdate**

Please attach additional pages if necessary. Send to: FREEPOST YELLOW CARD (no other address details required)

Adult Advanced Life Support Algorithm

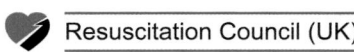 Resuscitation Council (UK)   GUIDELINES 2015   **Adult Advanced Life Support**

Unresponsive and not breathing normally

Call resuscitation team

CPR 30:2
Attach defibrillator/monitor
Minimise interruptions

Assess rhythm

Shockable (VF/Pulseless VT)

Return of spontaneous circulation

Non-shockable (PEA/Asystole)

1 Shock
Minimise interruptions

Immediate post cardiac arrest treatment
- Use ABCDE approach
- Aim for SpO₂ of 94-98%
- Aim for normal PaCO₂
- 12-lead ECG
- Treat precipitating cause
- Targeted temperature management

Immediately resume **CPR for 2 min**
Minimise interruptions

Immediately resume **CPR for 2 min**
Minimise interruptions

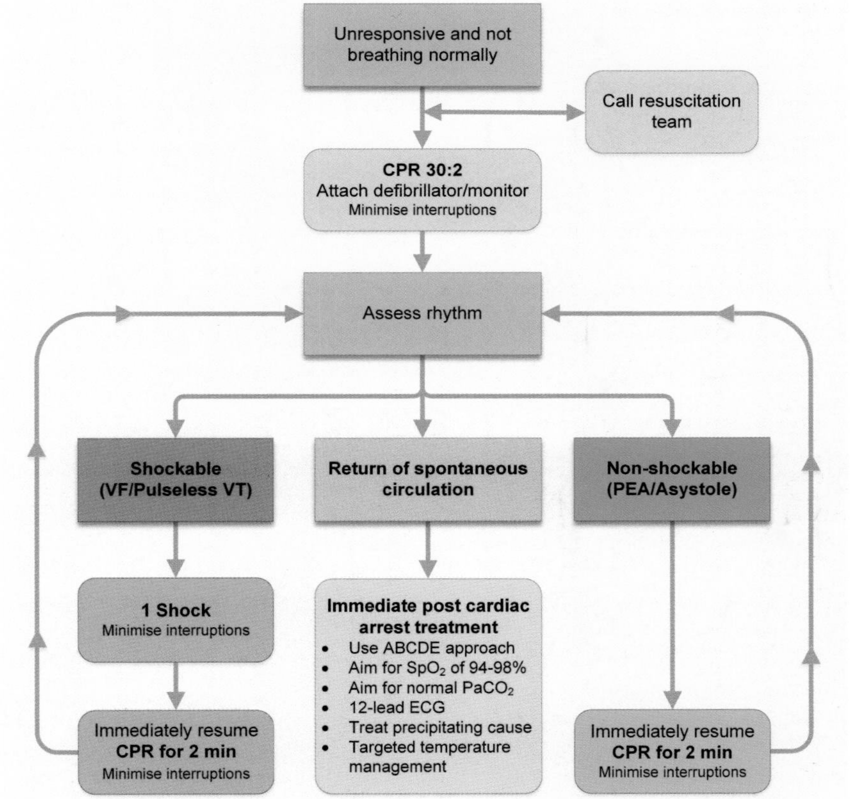

During CPR
- Ensure high quality chest compressions
- Minimise interruptions to compressions
- Give oxygen
- Use waveform capnography
- Continuous compressions when advanced airway in place
- Vascular access (intravenous or intraosseous)
- Give adrenaline every 3-5 min
- Give amiodarone after 3 shocks

Treat Reversible Causes
- Hypoxia
- Hypovolaemia
- Hypo-/hyperkalaemia/metabolic
- Hypothermia

- Thrombosis - coronary or pulmonary
- Tension pneumothorax
- Tamponade – cardiac
- Toxins

Consider
- Ultrasound imaging
- Mechanical chest compressions to facilitate transfer/treatment
- Coronary angiography and percutaneous coronary intervention
- Extracorporeal CPR

Medical emergencies in the community

Overview

Drug treatment outlined below is intended for use by appropriately qualified healthcare professionals. Only drugs that are used for immediate relief are shown; advice on supporting care is not given. Where the patient's condition requires investigation and further treatment, the patient should be transferred to hospital promptly.

Acute coronary syndromes

► **ANGINA: UNSTABLE**
Aspirin dispersible tablets p. 109 (75 mg, 300 mg)
BY MOUTH (DISPERSED IN WATER OR CHEWED)
► Adult: 300 mg

► PLUS

► EITHER **Glyceryl trinitrate aerosol spray p. 201**
(400 micrograms/metered dose)
SUBLINGUALLY
► Adult: 1–2 sprays, repeated as required

► OR **Glyceryl trinitrate tablets p. 201** (300 micrograms, 500 micrograms, 600 micrograms)
SUBLINGUALLY
► Adult: 0.3–1 mg, repeated as required

► **MYOCARDIAL INFARCTION: NON-ST-SEGMENT ELEVATION**
Treat as for Angina: unstable

► **MYOCARDIAL INFARCTION: ST-SEGMENT ELEVATION**
Aspirin dispersible tablets (75 mg, 300 mg)
BY MOUTH (DISPERSED IN WATER OR CHEWED)
► Adult: 300 mg

Glyceryl trinitrate aerosol spray (400 micrograms/metered dose)
SUBLINGUALLY
► Adult: 1–2 sprays, repeated as required

► OR **Glyceryl trinitrate tablets** (300 micrograms, 500 micrograms, 600 micrograms)
SUBLINGUALLY
► Adult: 0.3–1 mg, repeated as required

Metoclopramide hydrochloride injection p. 395 (5 mg/mL)
BY INTRAVENOUS INJECTION
► Adult 18-19 years (body-weight up to 60 kg): 5 mg
► Adult 18-19 years (body-weight 60 kg and above): 10 mg
► Adult over 19 years: 10 mg

Diamorphine hydrochloride injection p. 415 (5 mg powder for reconstitution)
BY SLOW INTRAVENOUS INJECTION (1-2 mg/minute)
► Adult: 5 mg followed by a further 2.5–5 mg if necessary
► Elderly or frail patients: reduce dose by half

► OR **Morphine sulfate injection p. 421** (10 mg/mL)
BY SLOW INTRAVENOUS INJECTION (1-2 mg/minute)
► Adult: 5–10 mg followed by a further 5–10 mg if necessary
► Elderly or frail patients: reduce dose by half

Oxygen, if appropriate

Airways disease, obstructive

► **ASTHMA: ACUTE**
Regard each emergency consultation as being for **severe acute asthma** until shown otherwise; failure to respond adequately **at any time** requires immediate transfer to hospital

► EITHER **Salbutamol aerosol inhaler p. 233**
(100 micrograms/metered inhalation)
BY AEROSOL INHALATION VIA LARGE-VOLUME SPACER
(AND A CLOSE-FITTING FACE MASK IF CHILD UNDER 3 YEARS)
► Adult and Child: 2–10 puffs each inhaled separately, repeated every 10–20 minutes or as necessary

► OR **Salbutamol nebuliser solution** (1 mg/mL, 2 mg/mL)
BY INHALATION OF NEBULISED SOLUTION (VIA OXYGEN-DRIVEN NEBULISER IF AVAILABLE)
► Child 4 years and below: 2.5 mg every 20–30 minutes or as necessary
► Child 5-11 years: 2.5–5 mg every 20–30 minutes or as necessary
► Child 12-17 years: 5 mg every 20–30 minutes or as necessary
► Adult: 5 mg every 20–30 minutes or as necessary

► OR **Terbutaline sulfate nebuliser solution p. 235** (2.5 mg/mL)
BY INHALATION OF NEBULISED SOLUTION (VIA OXYGEN-DRIVEN NEBULISER IF AVAILABLE)
► Child 4 years and below: 5 mg every 20–30 minutes or as necessary
► Child 5-11 years: 5–10 mg every 20–30 minutes or as necessary
► Child 12-17 years: 10 mg every 20–30 minutes or as necessary
► Adult 10: mg every 20–30 minutes or as necessary

► PLUS **(in all cases)**

► EITHER **Prednisolone tablets p. 614 (*or* prednisolone soluble tablets)** (5 mg)
BY MOUTH
► Child 11 years and below: 1–2 mg/kg (max. 40 mg) once daily for up to 3 days or longer if necessary; if child has been taking an oral corticosteroid for more than a few days, give prednisolone 2 mg/kg (max. 60 mg) once daily
► Child 12-17 years: 40–50 mg once daily for at least 5 days
► Adult: 40–50 mg once daily for at least 5 days

► OR **Hydrocortisone p. 612 (preferably as sodium succinate)**
BY INTRAVENOUS INJECTION
► Child 17 years and below: 4 mg/kg (max.100 mg) every 6 hours until conversion to oral prednisolone is possible; alternative dose if weight unavailable:
► Child 1 year and below: 25 mg
► Child 2-4 years: 50 mg
► Child 5-17 years: 100 mg
► Adult: 100 mg every 6 hours until conversion to oral prednisolone is possible

High-flow **oxygen** should be given if available (via face mask in children)

Monitor response 15 to 30 minutes after nebulisation; if any signs of acute asthma persist, arrange hospital admission. While awaiting ambulance, repeat **nebulised beta$_2$ agonist** (as above) and give with

Ipratropium bromide nebuliser solution p. 228
(250 micrograms/mL)
BY INHALATION OF NEBULISED SOLUTION (VIA OXYGEN-DRIVEN
NEBULISER IF AVAILABLE)
- Child 11 years and below: 250 micrograms, repeated every 20–30 minutes for the first 2 hours, then every 4–6 hours as necessary
- Child 12-17 years: 500 micrograms every 4–6 hours as necessary
- Adult: 500 micrograms every 4–6 hours as necessary

▶ CROUP
Dexamethasone oral solution p. 610 (2 mg/5 mL)
BY MOUTH
- Child 1 month-2 years: 150 micrograms/kg as a single dose

Anaphylaxis

▶ ANAPHYLAXIS
Adrenaline/epinephrine injection p. 205 (1 mg/mL (1 in 1000))
BY INTRAMUSCULAR INJECTION
- Child 5 years and below: 150 micrograms (0.15 mL), repeated every 5 minutes if necessary
- Child 6-11 years: 300 micrograms (0.3 mL), repeated every 5 minutes if necessary
- Child 12-17 years: 500 micrograms (0.5 mL), repeated every 5 minutes if necessary; 300 micrograms (0.3 mL) should be given if child is small or prepubertal
- Adult: 500 micrograms (0.5 mL), repeated every 5 minutes if necessary

High-flow **oxygen** and **intravenous fluids** should be given as soon as available.

Chlorphenamine maleate injection p. 260
BY INTRAMUSCULAR OR INTRAVENOUS INJECTION
May help counter histamine-mediated vasodilation and bronchoconstriction.

Hydrocortisone (preferably as sodium succinate)
BY INTRAVENOUS INJECTION
Has delayed action but should be given to severely affected patients to prevent further deterioration.

Bacterial infection

▶ MENINGOCOCCAL DISEASE
Benzylpenicillin sodium injection p. 496 (600 mg, 1.2 g)
BY INTRAVENOUS INJECTION (OR BY INTRAMUSCULAR INJECTION IF VENOUS ACCESS NOT AVAILABLE)
- Neonate: 300 mg
- Child 1 month-11 months: 300 mg
- Child 1-9 years: 600 mg
- Child 10-17 years: 1.2 g
- Adult: 1.2 g
NOTE A single dose should be given before urgent transfer to hospital, so long as this does not delay the transfer.

▶ OR **if history of allergy to penicillin**
Cefotaxime injection p. 479 (1 g)
BY INTRAVENOUS INJECTION (OR BY INTRAMUSCULAR INJECTION IF VENOUS ACCESS NOT AVAILABLE)
- Neonate: 50 mg/kg
- Child 1 month-11 years: 50 mg/kg (max. 1 g)
- Child 12-17 years: 1 g
- Adult 18 years and over: 1 g
NOTE A single dose can be given before urgent transfer to hospital, so long as this does not delay the transfer.

▶ OR **if history of immediate hypersensitivity reaction (including anaphylaxis, angioedema, urticaria, or rash immediately after administration) to penicillin or to cephalosporins**
Chloramphenicol injection p. 517 (1 g)
BY INTRAVENOUS INJECTION
- Child: 12.5–25 mg/kg
- Adult: 12.5–25 mg/kg
NOTE A single dose can be given before urgent transfer to hospital, so long as this does not delay the transfer.
See also Central nervous system infections, bacterial p. 465.

Hypoglycaemia

▶ DIABETIC HYPOGLYCAEMIA
Glucose or sucrose
BY MOUTH
- Adult and Child over 2 years: approx. 10–20 g (55–110 mL *Lucozade*® *Energy Original* or 100–200 mL *Coca-Cola*®—both non-diet versions *or* 2–4 teaspoonfuls of sugar *or* 3–6 sugar lumps) repeated after 10–15 minutes if necessary

▶ OR **if hypoglycaemia unresponsive *or* if oral route cannot be used**

Glucagon injection p. 652 (1 mg/mL)
BY SUBCUTANEOUS OR INTRAMUSCULAR INJECTION
- Child body-weight up to 25 kg: 500 micrograms (0.5 mL)
- Child body-weight 25 kg and above: 1 mg (1 mL)
- Adult: 1 mg (1 mL)

▶ OR **if hypoglycaemia prolonged *or* unresponsive to glucagon after 10 minutes**

Glucose intravenous infusion p. 903 (10%)
BY INTRAVENOUS INJECTION INTO LARGE VEIN
- Child: 5 mL/kg (glucose 500 mg/kg)

Glucose intravenous infusion p. 903 (20%)
BY INTRAVENOUS INJECTION INTO LARGE VEIN
- Adult: 50 mL

Seizures

▶ CONVULSIVE (INCLUDING FEBRILE) SEIZURES LASTING LONGER THAN 5 MINUTES
▶ EITHER **Diazepam rectal solution p. 313** (2 mg/mL, 4 mg/mL)
BY RECTUM
- Neonate: 1.25–2.5 mg, repeated once after 10–15 minutes if necessary
- Child 1 month-1 year: 5 mg, repeated once after 10–15 minutes if necessary
- Child 2-11 years: 5–10 mg, repeated once after 10–15 minutes if necessary
- Child 12-17 years: 10–20 mg, repeated once after 10–15 minutes if necessary
- Adult: 10–20 mg, repeated once after 10–15 minutes if necessary
- Elderly: 10 mg, repeated once after 10–15 minutes if necessary

▶ OR **Midazolam oromucosal solution p. 310**
BY BUCCAL ADMINISTRATION, REPEATED ONCE AFTER 10 MINUTES IF NECESSARY
- Neonate: 300 micrograms/kg [unlicensed]
- Child 1-2 months: 300 micrograms/kg (max. 2.5 mg) [unlicensed]
- Child 3 months-11 months: 2.5 mg
- Child 1-4 years: 5 mg
- Child 5-9 years: 7.5 mg
- Child 10-17 years: 10 mg
- Adult: 10 mg [unlicensed]

Approximate Conversions and Units

Conversion of pounds to kilograms

lb	kg
1	0.45
2	0.91
3	1.36
4	1.81
5	2.27
6	2.72
7	3.18
8	3.63
9	4.08
10	4.54
11	4.99
12	5.44
13	5.90
14	6.35

Conversion of stones to kilograms

stones	kg
1	6.35
2	12.70
3	19.05
4	25.40
5	31.75
6	38.10
7	44.45
8	50.80
9	57.15
10	63.50
11	69.85
12	76.20
13	82.55
14	88.90
15	95.25

Conversion from millilitres to fluid ounces

mL	fl oz
50	1.8
100	3.5
150	5.3
200	7.0
500	17.6
1000	35.2

Length

1 metre (m) = 1000 millimetres (mm)
1 centimetre (cm) = 10 mm
1 inch (in) = 25.4 mm
1 foot (ft) = 12 inches
12 inches = 304.8 mm

Mass

1 kilogram (kg) = 1000 grams (g)
1 gram (g) = 1000 milligrams (mg)
1 milligram (mg) = 1000 micrograms
1 microgram = 1000 nanograms
1 nanogram = 1000 picograms

Volume

1 litre = 1000 millilitres (mL)
1 millilitre (1 mL) = 1000 microlitres
1 pint ≈ 568 mL

Other units

1 kilocalorie (kcal) = 4186.8 joules (J)
1000 kilocalories (kcal) = 4.1868 megajoules (MJ)
1 megajoule (MJ) = 238.8 kilocalories (kcal)
1 millimetre of mercury (mmHg) = 133.3 pascals (Pa)
1 kilopascal (kPa) = 7.5 mmHg (pressure)

Plasma-drug concentrations

Plasma-drug concentrations in BNF publications are expressed in mass units per litre (e.g. mg/litre). The approximate equivalent in terms of amount of substance units (e.g. micromol/litre) is given in brackets.

Prescribing for children: weight, height, and gender

The table below shows the **mean values** for weight, height, and gender by age; these values have been derived from the UK-WHO growth charts 2009 and UK1990 standard centile charts, by extrapolating the 50th centile, and may be used to calculate doses in the absence of measurements. However, an individual's weight and height might vary considerably from the values in the table and it is important to ensure that the value chosen is appropriate. In most cases the actual measurement should be obtained as soon as possible and the dose re-calculated.

Age	Weight (kg)	Height (cm)
Full-term neonate	3.5	51
1 month	4.3	55
2 months	5.4	58
3 months	6.1	61
4 months	6.7	63
6 months	7.6	67
1 year	9	75
3 years	14	96
5 years	18	109
7 years	23	122
10 years	32	138
12 years	39	149
14 year old boy	49	163
14 year old girl	50	159
Adult male	68	176
Adult female	58	164

Recommended wording of cautionary and advisory labels

For details including Welsh Language translation see p. 1365

1   Warning: This medicine may make you sleepy

2   Warning: This medicine may make you sleepy. If this happens, do not drive or use tools or machines. Do not drink alcohol

3   Warning: This medicine may make you sleepy. If this happens, do not drive or use tools or machines

4   Warning: Do not drink alcohol

5   Do not take indigestion remedies 2 hours before or after you take this medicine

6   Do not take indigestion remedies, or medicines containing iron or zinc, 2 hours before or after you take this medicine

7   Do not take milk, indigestion remedies, or medicines containing iron or zinc, 2 hours before or after you take this medicine

8   Warning: Do not stop taking this medicine unless your doctor tells you to stop

9   Space the doses evenly throughout the day. Keep taking this medicine until the course is finished, unless you are told to stop

10 Warning: Read the additional information given with this medicine

11 Protect your skin from sunlight—even on a bright but cloudy day. Do not use sunbeds

12 Do not take anything containing aspirin while taking this medicine

13 Dissolve or mix with water before taking

14 This medicine may colour your urine. This is harmless

15 Caution: flammable. Keep your body away from fire or flames after you have put on the medicine

16 Dissolve the tablet under your tongue—do not swallow. Store the tablets in this bottle with the cap tightly closed. Get a new supply 8 weeks after opening

17 Do not take more than... in 24 hours

18 Do not take more than... in 24 hours. Also, do not take more than... in any one week

19 Warning: This medicine makes you sleepy. If you still feel sleepy the next day, do not drive or use tools or machines. Do not drink alcohol

21 Take with or just after food, or a meal

22 Take 30 to 60 minutes before food

23 Take this medicine when your stomach is empty. This means an hour before food or 2 hours after food

24 Suck or chew this medicine

25 Swallow this medicine whole. Do not chew or crush

26 Dissolve this medicine under your tongue

27 Take with a full glass of water

28 Spread thinly on the affected skin only

29 Do not take more than 2 at any one time. Do not take more than 8 in 24 hours

30 Contains paracetamol. Do not take anything else containing paracetamol while taking this medicine. Talk to a doctor at once if you take too much of this medicine, even if you feel well

32 Contains aspirin. Do not take anything else containing aspirin while taking this medicine